Adams and Victor's

Principles of NEUROLOGY

NOTICE

Adams and Victor's

Principles of NEUROLOGY

SEVENTH EDITION

Maurice Victor, M.D.

Professor of Medicine and Neurology, Dartmouth Medical School
Hanover, New Hampshire
Distinguished Physician of the Veterans Administration
White River Junction, Vermont

Allan H. Ropper, M.D.

Professor and Chairman of Neurology, Tufts University School of Medicine
Chief, Neurology Service
St. Elizabeth's Medical Center
Boston, Massachusetts

McGraw-Hill
MEDICAL PUBLISHING DIVISION

New York St. Louis San Francisco Auckland Bogotá Caracas Lisbon London Madrid
Mexico City Milan Montreal New Delhi San Juan Singapore Sydney Tokyo Toronto

McGraw-Hill 

A Division of The **McGraw-Hill** *Companies*

ADAMS AND VICTOR'S
PRINCIPLES OF NEUROLOGY

1234567890 DOCDOC 09876543210

ISBN 0-07-067497-3 (domestic)
ISBN 0-07-116333-6 (international)

This book was set in Times Roman by Better Graphics, Inc.
The editors were Martin J. Wonsiewicz, Michael P. Medina, and Muza Navrozov.
The production supervisor was Catherine H. Saggese.
The index was prepared by Alexandra Nickerson.
R. R. Donnelley & Sons Company was printer and binder.

This book is printed on acid-free paper.

Library of Congress Cataloging in Publication Data

Victor, Maurice
Adams and Victor's principles of neurology / Maurice Victor, Allan H. Ropper—7th ed.
p. cm
Includes bibliographical references and index.
ISBN 0-07-067497-3 (alk. paper)
1. Nervous system—Diseases. 2. Neuropsychiatry. I. Title: Principles of neurology
II. Ropper, Allan H.
[DNLM: 1. Nervous System Diseases. 2. Mental Disorders. WL 100 V644a2001]
RC346.A3 2001
616.8—dc21

Shaila Bokkala-Pinninti

CONTENTS

PREFACE

In the first edition of the *Principles of Neurology*, we remarked that the preface to a textbook is often an unnecessary appendage, doing little more than adding to the book's weight or distracting critics from its contents. The value of the book should be judged by its substance and composition. In his foreword to *Cromwell*, Victor Hugo expressed this sentiment more figuratively: one seldom inspects the cellar of a house after visiting its salons or examines the roots of a tree after eating its fruit.

Yet there has to be a place where authors can state the purpose of their work, the manner in which it was conceived, and the reasons for foisting yet another book on a medical public already overburdened with an immense literature. To sustain our analogy, although one seldom derives pleasure from inspecting the cellar of a house, one is not sorry to have done so, especially if one is to purchase it.

In writing the *Principles of Neurology*, we adopted a method that had for long been espoused on the Neurology Service of the Massachusetts General Hospital. Instead of the customary recitation of many diseases of the nervous system, we chose to introduce the subject with a consideration of the phenomenology, or cardinal manifestations, of neurologic disease. Thus the first part of this book consists of a detailed exposition of the symptoms and signs of disordered nervous function, their analysis in terms of anatomy and physiology, and their clinical implications. This is followed by an account of the natural clusterings of these phenomena, or syndromes, which are the lore of clinical neurology, and this, in turn, by a description of all the main categories and types of disease that express themselves by each syndrome. We believe this approach to neurologic disease to be a logical one, for in practice the patient presents with symptoms of disordered nervous function, from which the clinician reasons to a diagnosis. This sequence of symptom to syndrome to disease recapitulates the rational process by which this is achieved. In teaching students and residents, we have found this clinical method to be eminently successful.

The compass of our book differs in several other ways from most contemporary textbooks of neurology. We have included discussions of a number of subjects that form the core of pediatric neurology, which is heavily weighted with developmental anomalies and hereditary metabolic diseases. These are presented in the context of normal development and maturation of the nervous system. And the effects of aging and age-linked diseases (geriatric neurology) have been accorded a separate chapter. No distinction is drawn between neurosurgical neurology and medical neurology, since they differ only with reference to mode of therapy. A significant portion of the book has been allotted to psychiatric syndromes and the major psychiatric diseases. This has been done in the belief that these diseases are neurologic in the strict sense. Further, it is our belief that all physicians, including neurologists, should be knowledgeable about the diagnosis of depressive states, neuroses, and eccentricities of personality which are commonly associated with all manner of medical illnesses. The neuropsychiatric effects of alcoholism and drug abuse are also included. Finally, we have consigned a section of the book to a description of muscle diseases, which increasingly are coming under the purview of neurologists. Thus our book provides information that is essential not only to the practice of neurology and neurosurgery, but also to the practice of internal medicine, pediatrics, and psychiatry. To aid readers from these various specialties in finding relevant material, we suggest they turn their attention to the following chapters: internists: 8, 10, 11, 16, 18, 32, 33, 34; pediatricians: 16, 28, 37, 38; emergency and intensive care physicians: 16, 17, 18, 34, 35; orthopedists: 8, 11, 44, 45; psychiatrists: 20, 21, 22, 24, 25, 56, 57, 58.

Throughout this text the emphasis is on the clinical aspects of disease. Of course, pertinent neurobiologic data are not disregarded, but always they are presented with the view of how they bear upon and explain neurologic phenomena and disease. One of our primary aims, in conformity with Oslerian tradition, is to present the clinical phenomena that we ourselves have observed. We persist in our belief that there are advantages to limited authorship. It enables the authors to select what they believe to be essential knowledge about common diseases and to view them from a particular perspective. Also it assures an evenness and uniformity of style that is more likely to please the reader.

The warm reception accorded the first six editions of *Principles of Neurology* has led us to believe that our plan of exposition has filled a need and has emboldened us to carry this work forward. During the editing of the seventh edition, each of us has undertaken a deliberate and critical review of new ideas and developments in clinical neurology and has endeavored to incorporate them. Every chapter has thus been thoroughly revised. The newest discoveries of molecular genetics have been added where relevant. The clarification of physiologic function obtained by PET and SPECT scanning and functional MRI has been expanded. Considerably greater use has been made of tables and MRI illustrations as refinements of biopathology of disease. A special effort has been made to provide the most detailed and current information about the treatment of neurologic diseases.

It is hardly possible to enumerate and adequately thank our many colleagues who in one way or another have been instrumental in the development and growth of this textbook. Foremost is our indebtedness to colleagues and teachers who had an abiding influence in shaping our ideas—Derek Denny-Brown, C. M. Fisher, Paul Yakovlev, E. P. Richardson, and Mandel Cohen. A special debt is owed to Betty Banker for her assistance in revising the chapters on muscle disease and for her help on all matters, large and small, pertaining to this book, since its inception. We are grateful also to the many colleagues with whom we have repeatedly discussed the substantive material of previous editions—Robert Young, Jay Mohr, Hugo Moser, Edwin Kolodny, and Shirley Wray.

Individual chapters or parts of chapters for the current edition were graciously reviewed by Michael Worthington (Chap 32), David Weinberg (Chap 45), and Richard Blair (neuroimaging) of St. Elizabeth's Medical Center; and by Peter Williamson and Vijay Thadani (Chap 16) and James Filiano (Chap 39) of Dartmouth-Hitchcock Medical Center. Expert advice on particularly difficult topics was provided by Harvey Levy (inherited metabolic disorders), John Leigh (the anatomy of vertical eye movements), Pauline Filipek (autism), and Paul Chapman (arteriovenous malformations). Other colleagues too numerous to mention have been sources of constant reference and constructive criticism in this and previous editions.

Finally, we wish to express our gratitude to Richard Haver, librarian at Vermont Veterans Administration Medical Center, and to Sandra Ropper, both of whom were assiduous in searching out innumerable references; to Dolores Altavilla and Dorothy Sweet for their help in preparation of the manuscript; to Winifred Quick for her generous support of the Department of Neurology at St. Elizabeth's Medical Center; to Muza Navrozov of McGraw-Hill, whose dedication and editing skills have ensured repeated editions of readable text; and to Catherine Saggese for her successful efforts in achieving the timely production of the book.

With the publication of the seventh edition of the *Principles*, readers will recognize a change in the book's format. Raymond D. Adams, who conceived the book and was its senior author through six editions, is relinquishing his role of active authorship and will henceforth have his name incorporated in the title of the book. Although no longer burdened with the day-to-day demands of editors and publishers, Dr. Adams has retained a keen interest in the book. He has read virtually the entire seventh edition, throughout which time we have had both the pleasure and the benefit of his guiding hand and his many suggestions and contributions.

Maurice Victor
Allan H. Ropper

Part 1

APPROACH TO THE PATIENT WITH NEUROLOGIC DISEASE

Chapter 1

THE CLINICAL METHOD OF NEUROLOGY

Neurology is regarded by many as the most difficult and exacting medical specialty. Students and residents coming to the neurology ward or clinic for the first time are easily discouraged by what they see. Having had brief contact with neuroanatomy, neurophysiology, and neuropathology, they are already somewhat intimidated by the complexity of the nervous system. The ritual they then witness of putting the patient through a series of maneuvers designed to evoke certain mysterious signs, the names of which are difficult to pronounce, is hardly reassuring; in fact, the procedure often appears to conceal the very intellectual processes by which neurologic diagnosis is attained. Moreover, the students have had little or no experience with the many special tests used in neurologic diagnosis—such as lumbar puncture and electroencephalographic, angiographic, and imaging procedures—nor do they know how to interpret the results of such tests. Neurology textbooks only confirm their fears as they read the detailed accounts of the many rare diseases of the nervous system.

The authors believe that many of the difficulties in comprehending neurology can be overcome by adhering to the basic principles of clinical medicine. First and foremost, it is necessary to learn and acquire facility in the use of the *clinical method*. Without a full appreciation of this method, the student is virtually as helpless with a new clinical problem as a botanist or chemist who would undertake a research problem without understanding the steps in the scientific method.

The importance of the clinical method stands out more clearly in the study of neurologic disease than in certain other fields of medicine. In most cases, the clinical method will prove to consist of an orderly series of steps, as follows:

1. The symptoms and signs are secured by history and physical examination, respectively.

2. The symptoms and physical signs considered relevant to the problem at hand are interpreted in terms of physiology and anatomy—that is, one identifies the disorder(s) of function and the anatomic structure(s) implicated by such a disorder. Often one recognizes a characteristic clustering of symptoms and signs, constituting a *syndrome*. The formulation of symptoms and signs in syndromic terms is particularly helpful in ascertaining the locus and nature of the disease. This step may be called *syndromic diagnosis*.

3. These correlations permit the physician to localize the disease process, i.e., to name the part or parts of the nervous system involved. This step is called the *anatomic*, or *topographic, diagnosis*.

4. From the anatomic diagnosis and other medical data—particularly the mode of onset, evolution, and course of the illness, the involvement of nonneurologic organ systems, the relevant past and family histories, and the laboratory findings—one deduces the *pathologic diagnosis* and, when the mechanism and causation of the disease can be determined, the *etiologic diagnosis*.

5. Finally, the physician should assess the degree of disability and determine whether it is temporary or permanent (*functional diagnosis*). This is important in managing the patient's illness and judging the potential for restoration of function, i.e., prognosis.

The foregoing approach to the diagnosis of neurologic disease is summarized in Fig. 1-1, a procedural diagram by which the clinical problem is solved in a series of sequential finite steps. This systematic approach, allowing the confident localization and often precise diagnosis of disease, is one of the intellectual attractions of neurology.

Of course, the solution to a clinical problem need not always be schematized in this way. The clinical

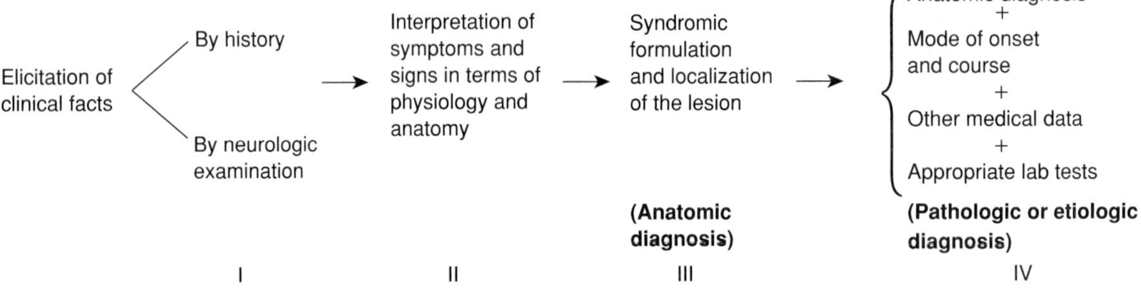

Figure 1-1

Steps in the diagnosis of neurologic disease.

method offers a much wider choice in the order and manner by which information is collected and interpreted. In fact, in some cases, adherence to a formal sequence is not necessary at all. The clinical picture of Parkinson disease, for example, is usually so characteristic that the nature of the illness is at once apparent. In other cases it is not necessary to carry the clinical analysis beyond the stage of the anatomic diagnosis, which in itself may suggest the cause of a disease. For example, when a unilateral Horner syndrome, cerebellar ataxia, paralysis of a vocal cord, and analgesia of the face of acute onset are combined with loss of pain and temperature sensation in the opposite arm, trunk, and leg, the most likely cause is an occlusion of the vertebral artery, because all the involved structures can be localized to the lateral medulla, within the territory of this artery. Thus, the anatomic diagnosis determines and limits the disease possibilities. If the signs point to disease of the peripheral nerves, it is usually not necessary to consider the causes of disease of the spinal cord. Some signs themselves are almost specific, e.g., opsoclonus for paraneoplastic cerebellar degeneration, and Argyll Robertson pupils for neurosyphilitic or diabetic oculomotor neuropathy.

Irrespective of the intellectual process that one utilizes in solving a particular clinical problem, the fundamental steps in diagnosis always involve the accurate elicitation of symptoms and signs and their correct interpretation in terms of disordered function of the nervous system. Most often, when there is uncertainty or disagreement as to diagnosis, it will be found later that the symptoms of disordered function were incorrectly interpreted in the first place. Thus, if a complaint of dizziness is identified as vertigo instead of light-headedness or if partial continuous epilepsy is mistaken for an extrapyramidal movement disorder such as choreoathetosis, then the clinical method is derailed from the beginning. Repeated examinations may be necessary to establish the fundamental clinical findings beyond doubt and to ascertain the course of the illness. Hence the aphorism that a second examination is the most helpful diagnostic test in a difficult neurologic case.

Different disease processes may cause identical symptoms, which is understandable in view of the fact that the same parts of the nervous system may be affected by any one of several diseases. For example, a spastic paraplegia may result from spinal cord tumor, a genetic defect, or multiple sclerosis. Conversely, one disease may present with different groups of symptoms and signs. However, despite the many possible combinations of symptoms and signs in a particular disease, a few combinations occur with greater frequency than others and can be recognized as highly characteristic of that disease. The experienced clinician acquires the habit of attempting to categorize every case in terms of a characteristic symptom complex, or *syndrome*. One must always keep in mind that syndromes are not disease entities but rather abstractions set up by clinicians in order to facilitate the diagnosis of disease. For example, the symptom complex of right-left confusion and inability to write, calculate, and identify individual fingers constitutes the so-called Gerstmann syndrome, recognition of which determines the anatomic locus of the disease (region of the left angular gyrus) and at the same time narrows the range of possible etiologic factors.

In the initial analysis of a neurologic disorder, anatomic diagnosis takes precedence over etiologic diagnosis. To seek the cause of a disease of the nervous system without first ascertaining the parts or structures that are affected would be analogous in internal medicine to attempting an etiologic diagnosis without knowing whether the disease involved the lungs, stomach, or kidneys. Discerning the cause of a clinical syndrome (etiologic diagnosis) requires knowledge of an entirely different order. Here one must be conversant with the clinical details, including the mode of onset, course, and natural history of a multiplicity of disease entities. Many of these facts are well known and not difficult to master; they form the substance of later chapters.

TAKING THE HISTORY

In neurology more than any other specialty, the physician is dependent upon the cooperation of the patient for a reliable history, especially for a description of symptoms that are unaccompanied by observable signs of disease. And if the symptoms are in the sensory sphere, only the patient can tell what he* sees, hears, or feels. The first step in the clinical encounter is to enlist the patient's trust and cooperation and make him realize the importance of the examination procedure. The following points about taking the neurologic history deserve further comment:

1. Special care must be taken to avoid suggesting to the patient the symptoms that one seeks. The clinical interview is a bipersonal engagement, and the conduct of the examiner has a great influence on the patient. Repetition of this truism may seem tedious, but it is evident that conflicting histories can often be traced to leading questions that either suggested symptoms to the patient or led to a distortion of the patient's story. Errors and inconsistencies in the recorded history are as often the fault of the physician as of the patient. As a corollary, the patient should be discouraged from framing his symptom(s) in terms of a diagnosis that he may have heard, but should be urged to give as accurate a description of the symptom as possible—being asked, for example, to choose a single word that best describes the quality of his pain.

2. The practice of making notes at the bedside or in the office is particularly recommended. The patient who is given to highly circumstantial and rambling accounts can be kept on the subject of his illness by discrete questions that draw out essential points. Immediate recording of the history assures maximal reliability. Of course, no matter how reliable the history appears to be, verification of the patient's account by a knowledgeable and objective informant is always desirable.

3. The setting in which the illness occurred, its mode of onset and evolution, and its course are of paramount importance. One must attempt to learn precisely how each symptom began and progressed. Often the nature of the disease process can be decided from these data alone. If such information cannot be supplied by the patient or his family, it may be necessary to judge the course of the illness by what the patient was able to do at different times (e.g., how far he could walk, when he could no longer negotiate stairs or carry on his usual work) or by changes in the clinical findings between successive examinations, provided that the physician had recorded the findings accurately and quantitated them in some way.

4. Since neurologic diseases often impair mental function, it is necessary, in every patient who might have cerebral disease, for the physician to decide, by an initial assessment of the mental status and the circumstances under which symptoms occurred, whether or not the patient is competent to give a history of the illness. If the patient's power of attention, memory, and coherence of thinking are inadequate, the history must be obtained from a relative, friend, or employer. Also, illnesses that are characterized by seizures or other forms of episodic confusion abolish or impair the patient's memory of events occurring during these episodes. In general, students (and some physicians as well) tend to be careless in estimating the mental capacities of their patients. Attempts are sometimes made to take histories from patients who are feebleminded or so confused that they have no idea why they are in a doctor's office or a hospital, or from patients who for other reasons could not possibly have been aware of the details of their illnesses.

THE NEUROLOGIC EXAMINATION

The neurologic examination begins with observation of the patient while the history is being obtained. The manner in which the patient tells the story of his illness may betray confusion or incoherence in thinking, impairment of memory or judgment, or difficulty in comprehending or expressing ideas. Observation of such matters is an integral part of the examination and provides information as to the adequacy of cerebral function. The physician should learn to obtain this type of information without embarrassment to the patient. A common error is to pass lightly over inconsistencies in history and inaccuracies about dates and symptoms, only to discover later that these flaws in memory were the essential features of the illness. Asking the patient to give his own interpretation

*Throughout this text we follow the traditional English practice of using the pronoun *he, his,* or *him* in the generic sense whenever it is not intended to designate the gender of a specific individual.

of the possible meaning of symptoms may sometimes expose unnatural concern, anxiety, suspiciousness, or even delusional thinking.

The remainder of the neurologic examination should be performed as the last part of the general physical examination, proceeding from an examination of the cranial nerves, neck, and trunk to the testing of motor, reflex, and sensory functions of the upper and lower limbs. This is followed by an assessment of the function of sphincters and the autonomic nervous system and suppleness of the neck and spine (meningeal irritation). Gait and station (standing position) should be observed before or after the rest of the examination. The neurologic examination is always performed and recorded in a sequential and uniform manner in order to avoid omissions and to facilitate the subsequent analysis of case records. In addition, it is often instructive to observe the patient in the course of his natural activities, such as walking or dressing; this may disclose subtle abnormalities of gait and movement that might not be evident in formal testing.

The thoroughness of the neurologic examination must of necessity be governed by the type of clinical problem presented by the patient. To spend a half hour or more testing cerebral, cerebellar, cranial nerve, and sensorimotor function in a patient seeking treatment for a simple compression palsy of an ulnar nerve is pointless and uneconomical. The examination must also be modified according to the condition of the patient. Obviously many parts of the examination cannot be carried out in a comatose patient; also, infants and small children as well as patients with psychiatric disease need to be examined in special ways. The following comments apply to the examination procedure in these and other particular clinical circumstances.

PATIENTS WHO PRESENT SYMPTOMS OF NERVOUS SYSTEM DISEASE

Numerous guides to the examination of the nervous system are available. For a full account of the methods, the reader is referred to the monographs of DeMyer, Ross, Mancall, Bickerstaff and Spillane, Glick, and the staff members of the Mayo Clinic, each of which approaches the subject from a somewhat different point of view. The monograph of DeMyer is particularly recommended to students. An inordinately large number of tests of neurologic function have been devised, and it is not proposed to review all of them here. Some are described in subsequent chapters dealing with disorders of mentation, cranial nerves, and motor, sensory, and autonomic functions. Many tests are of doubtful value and should not be taught to students of neurology. Merely to perform all of them on one patient would require several hours and probably, in most instances, would not make the examiner any the wiser. The danger with all clinical tests is to regard them as indisputable indicators of disease rather than as ways of uncovering disordered functioning of the nervous system. The following tests are relatively simple and provide the most useful information.

Testing of Higher Cortical Functions

These functions are tested in detail if the patient's history or behavior during the general examination has provided reason to suspect some cognitive defect. Questions should then be directed toward determining the patient's orientation in time (day and date) and place and insight into his current medical problem. Attention, speed of response, ability to give relevant answers to simple questions, and the capacity for sustained mental effort all lend themselves to straight-forward observation. Useful bedside tests of attention, concentration, memory, and clarity of thinking include the repetition of a series of seven digits in forward and five in reverse order, serial subtraction of 3s and 7s from 100, recall of three items of information or a short story after an interval of 3 min, and naming the last five presidents or prime ministers. The patient's account of his recent illness, medical consultations, dates of hospitalization, and the day-to-day recollection of medical procedures, meals, and other incidents in the hospital are excellent tests of memory; the narration of how the tests were done and the patient's choice of words (vocabulary) provide information about his intelligence and coherence of thinking. Many other tests can be devised for the same purpose. Often the examiner can obtain a better idea of the clarity of the patient's sensorium and soundness of intellect by using these few tests and noting the manner in which he deals with them than by relying on the score of a formal intelligence test.

If there is any suggestion of a speech or language disorder, the nature of the patient's spontaneous speech should be noted. In addition, his ability to read, write, and spell; execute spoken commands; repeat words and phrases spoken by the examiner; name objects and parts of objects; and solve simple arithmetical problems should be assessed. Bisecting a line, drawing a clock or the floor plan of one's home or a map of one's country, and copying figures are useful tests of visuospatial perception in cases of suspected cerebral disease. The testing of language, cognition, and other aspects of higher cerebral function are considered in Chaps. 21, 22, and 23.

Testing of Cranial Nerves

The function of the cranial nerves must be investigated more fully in patients who have neurologic symptoms than in those who do not. If one suspects a lesion in the anterior fossa, the sense of smell should be tested in each nostril, and then it should be determined whether odors can be discriminated. Visual fields should be outlined by confrontation testing, in some cases by testing each eye separately; if any abnormality is suspected, it should be checked on a perimeter and scotomas sought on the tangent screen or, more accurately, by computed perimetry. Pupil size and reactivity to light and accommodation (during convergence), the range and rate of ocular movements, and the presence or absence of nystagmus should next be observed. Details of these test procedures and their interpretation are described in Chaps. 12, 13, and 14.

Sensation over the face is tested with a pin and wisp of cotton; also, the presence or absence of the corneal reflexes should be determined. Facial movements should be observed as the patient speaks and smiles, for a slight weakness may be more evident in these circumstances than on movements to command. The auditory meati and tympanic membranes should be inspected with an otoscope. A 256 double-vibration tuning fork held next to the ear and on the mastoid discloses hearing loss and distinguishes middle ear (conductive) from neural deafness. The vocal cords need to be inspected with special instruments in cases of suspected medullary or vagus nerve disease, especially when there is hoarseness. Pharyngeal reflexes are meaningful if there is a difference on the two sides; bilateral absence of these reflexes is seldom significant. Inspection of the tongue, when protruded and at rest, is helpful; atrophy and fasciculations may be seen and weakness detected. Slight deviation of the protruded tongue as a solitary finding can usually be disregarded. Any abnormality in pronunciation should be noted. The jaw jerk and the snout, buccal, and sucking reflexes should be sought, particularly if there is a question of dysphagia, dysarthria, or dysphonia.

Tests of Motor Function

In the assessment of motor function, it should be kept in mind that observations of the speed and strength of movements and of muscle bulk, tone, and coordination are usually more informative than the tendon reflexes. It is essential to have the limbs fully exposed and to inspect them for atrophy and fasciculations as well as to watch the patient maintain the arms outstretched in the prone and supine positions; perform simple tasks, such as alternately touching his nose and the examiner's finger; make rapid alternating movements, particularly such movements that necessitate sudden acceleration and deceleration and changes in direction; rapidly touch the thumb to each fingertip and supinate and pronate the forearm; and accomplish simple tasks such as buttoning clothes, opening a safety pin, or handling common tools. Estimates of the strength of leg muscles with the patient in bed are often unreliable; there may seem to be little or no weakness even though the patient cannot step up on a footstool without help or arise from a kneeling position. Running the heel down the front of the shin and rhythmically tapping the heel on the shin are the only tests of coordination that need be carried out in bed. The maintenance of the outstretched and supinated arms against gravity is a useful test; the weak one, tiring first, soon begins to sag, or, in the case of a corticospinal lesion, to resume the more natural pronated position. The strength of the legs can be similarly tested, either with the patient supine and the legs flexed at hips and knees, or with the patient prone and the knees bent. Also, abnormalities of movement and posture and tremors may be exposed (see Chaps. 4 and 6).

Tests of Reflex Function

Testing of the biceps, triceps, supinator (radial-periosteal), patellar, Achilles, and cutaneous abdominal and plantar reflexes permits an adequate sampling of reflex activity of the spinal cord. Elicitation of tendon reflexes requires that the involved muscles be relaxed. Underactive or barely elicitable reflexes can be facilitated by voluntary contraction of other muscles (Jendrassik maneuver). The interpretation of the plantar response offers special difficulty because several different reflex responses can be evoked by stimulating the sole of the foot along its outer border from heel to toes. These are (1) the quick, high-level withdrawal-avoidance response; (2) the slower, spinal flexor noci-fensor reflex (flexion of knee and hip and dorsiflexion of toes and foot); dorsiflexion of the large toe as part of this reflex is the well-known Babinski sign; and (3) the plantar grasp reflex. Avoidance and withdrawal responses interfere with the interpretation of the Babinski sign and can sometimes be overcome by utilizing the several alternative stimuli that are known to elicit the Babinski response (squeezing the calf or Achilles tendon, flicking the fourth toe, downward scraping of the shin, lifting the straight leg, etc.). An absence of the superficial cutaneous reflexes of the abdominal, cremasteric, and other muscles is a useful ancillary test for detecting corticospinal lesions.

Testing of Sensory Function

This is undoubtedly the most difficult part of the neurologic examination. Usually sensory testing is reserved for the end of the examination and, if the findings are to be reliable, it should not be prolonged for more than a few minutes. Each test should be explained briefly; too much discussion of these tests with a meticulous, introspective patient may encourage the reporting of useless minor variations of stimulus intensity.

It is not necessary to examine all areas of the skin surface. A quick survey of the face, neck, hands, trunk, and feet with a pin takes only a few seconds. Usually one is seeking differences between the two sides of the body (it is preferable to ask whether stimuli on opposite sides of the body feel the same rather than to ask if they feel different), a level below which sensation is lost, or a zone of relative or absolute anesthesia. Regions of sensory deficit can then be tested more carefully and mapped out. Moving the stimulus from an area of diminished sensation into a normal area enhances the perception of a difference.

The finding of a zone of heightened sensation ("hyperesthesia") calls attention to a disturbance of superficial sensation. Variations in sensory findings from one examination to another most often reflect differences in technique of examination as well as inconsistencies in the responses of the patient.

Sensory testing is considered in greater detail in Chap. 9.

Testing of Stance and Gait

No examination is complete without watching the patient stand and walk. An abnormality of stance and gait may be the most prominent or the only neurologic abnormality, as in certain cases of cerebellar or frontal lobe disorder. Also, an impairment of posture and highly automatic adaptive movements in walking may provide the most definite diagnostic clues in the early stages of Parkinson disease and progressive supranuclear palsy (Chap. 7). Walking is the most effective way to bring out dystonic postures in the hands, feet, and trunk. And having the patient walk tandem or on the sides of the soles may disclose a lack of balance. Hopping or standing on one foot may also betray a lack of balance or weakness, and standing with feet together and eyes closed will bring out a disequilibrium that is due to impairment of labyrinthine-vestibular function or deep sensory loss (Romberg test).

THE MEDICAL OR SURGICAL PATIENT WITHOUT NEUROLOGIC SYMPTOMS

In this situation, brevity is desirable, but any test that is undertaken should be done carefully and recorded accurately and legibly. The patient's orientation, insight, and judgment and the integrity of speech and language functions are readily assessed in the course of taking the history. With respect to the cranial nerves, the size of the pupils and their reaction to light, ocular movements, visual and auditory acuity (by questioning), and movements of the face, palate, and tongue should be tested. Observing the bare outstretched arms for atrophy, weakness (pronating drift), tremor, or abnormal movements; checking the strength of hand grip and dorsiflexion at the wrist; inquiring about sensory disturbances; and eliciting the supinator, biceps, and triceps reflexes are usually sufficient for the upper limbs. Inspection of the legs as the feet, toes, and knees are actively flexed and extended; elicitation of the patellar, Achilles, and plantar reflexes; testing of vibration and position sense in the fingers and toes; and assessment of coordination by having the patient alternately touch his nose and the examiner's finger and run his heel up and down the front of the opposite leg complete the essential parts of the neurologic examination. This entire procedure does not add more than 3 or 4 min to the physical examination. The routine performance of these few simple tests may provide clues to the presence of disease of which the patient is not aware. For example, the finding of absent Achilles reflexes and diminished vibratory sense in the feet and legs alerts the physician to the possibility of diabetic or alcoholic-nutritional neuropathy even when the patient has no symptoms referable to these disorders.

Accurate recording of negative data may be useful in relation to some future illness that requires examination.

THE COMATOSE PATIENT

Although subject to obvious limitations, careful examination of the stuporous or comatose patient yields considerable information concerning the function of the nervous system. The demonstration of signs of focal cerebral or brainstem disease or of meningeal irritation is particularly useful in the differential diagnosis of diseases that cause stupor and coma. The adaptation of the neurologic examination to the comatose patient is described in Chap. 17.

THE PSYCHIATRIC PATIENT

One is compelled in the examination of psychiatric patients to rely less on the cooperation of the patient and to be unusually critical of his statements and opinions. The depressed patient, for example, may claim to have impaired memory or weakness when actually there is neither amnesia nor diminution in muscular power, or the sociopath or hysteric may feign paralysis. The opposite is sometimes true—a psychotic patient may make accurate observations of his own symptoms, only to have them ignored because of his mental state.

If the patient will speak and cooperate even to a slight degree, much may be learned about the functional integrity of different parts of the nervous system. Aphasia can, in nearly every instance, be recognized by the manner in which the patient expresses ideas, reads and writes, and responds to spoken or written requests. Often it is possible to determine whether there are hallucinations or delusions, defective memory, or other recognizable symptoms of brain disease merely by watching and listening to the patient. Ocular movements and visual fields can be tested with fair accuracy by observing the patient's response to a moving stimulus or threat in all four quadrants of the fields. Cranial nerve, motor, and reflex functions are tested in the usual manner, but it must be remembered that the neurologic examination is never complete unless the patient will speak and cooperate in testing. On occasion, mute and resistive patients judged to be schizophrenic prove to have some widespread cerebral disease such as hypoxic or hypoglycemic encephalopathy, a brain tumor, a vascular lesion, or extensive demyelinative lesions.

INFANTS AND SMALL CHILDREN

The reader is referred to the methods of examination described by Gesell and Amatruda, Dubowitz et al, and textbooks of pediatric neurology (e. g., Berg), which are listed in the references and described in Chap. 28.

THE GENERAL MEDICAL EXAMINATION

Never to be overlooked in the assessment of a neurologic problem are the findings on general medical examination. Often they disclose evidence of an underlying systemic disease that has secondarily affected the nervous system. In fact, many of the most serious neurologic problems are of this type. A few common examples will suffice: the finding of adenopathy or a lung infiltrate implicates neoplasia or sarcoidosis as the cause of multiple cranial nerve palsies; the presence of low-grade fever, anemia, a heart murmur, and splenomegaly in a case of unexplained stroke points to a diagnosis of subacute bacterial endocarditis with embolic occlusion of brain arteries. Certainly no examination of a patient with stroke is complete without a search for hypertension, carotid bruits, heart murmurs, or irregular pulse.

IMPORTANCE OF A WORKING KNOWLEDGE OF NEUROANATOMY, NEUROPHYSIOLOGY, AND NEUROPATHOLOGY

Once the technique of obtaining reliable clinical data is mastered, students and residents may find themselves handicapped in the interpretation of the findings by a lack of knowledge of neuroanatomy and neurophysiology. For this reason, each of the later chapters dealing with the motor system, sensation, special senses, consciousness, language, etc., is introduced by a review of the anatomic and physiologic facts that are necessary for an understanding of their clinical disorders.

At a minimum, physicians should know the anatomy of the corticospinal tract; the motor unit (anterior horn cell, nerve, and muscle); the basal ganglionic and cerebellar motor connections; the sensory pathways; the cranial nerves; the hypothalamus and pituitary; the reticular formation of brainstem and thalamus; the limbic system; the functional areas of the cerebral cortex and their major connections; the visual, auditory, and autonomic systems; and the cerebrospinal fluid pathways. A working knowledge of neurophysiology should include an understanding of the nerve impulse, neuromuscular transmission, and the contractile process of muscle; spinal reflex activity; central neurotransmission; the processes of neuronal excitation, inhibition, and release; and cortical activation and seizure production.

From a practical diagnostic and therapeutic point of view, the neurologist is helped most by a knowledge of neuropathology—i.e., the changes that are produced by disease processes such as infarction, hemorrhage, demyelination, physical trauma, compression, inflammation, neoplasm, and infection, to name the more common ones. Experience with the gross and microscopic appearances of these disease processes greatly enhances one's ability to explain their clinical behavior. The ability to visualize the effects of disease on nerve and muscle, brain and spinal cord, meninges, and blood vessels gives one a strong sense of the clinical features that one might expect of a particular disease and which features are untenable or inconsistent with a particular diagnosis. An additional advantage of being exposed to neuropathology, of course, is that the clinician is better able to evaluate pathologic changes and reports of material obtained by biopsy.

LABORATORY DIAGNOSIS

From the foregoing description of the clinical method and its application, it is evident that the use of laboratory aids in the diagnosis of diseases of the nervous system is always preceded by rigorous clinical examination. Laboratory study can be planned intelligently only on the basis of clinical information. To reverse this process is wasteful of medical resources. However, in neurology, the ultimate goal is the prevention of disease, because the brain changes induced by many neurologic diseases are irreversible. In the prevention of neurologic disease, the clinical method in itself is inadequate, and of necessity one resorts to two other methods, namely, the use of genetic information and laboratory screening tests. Genetic information enables the neurologist to identify patients at risk of developing certain diseases and prompts the search for biologic markers before the advent of symptoms or signs. Biochemical screening tests are applicable to an entire population and permit the identification of neurologic disease in individuals who have yet to show their first symptom; in some such diseases, treatment can be instituted before the nervous system has suffered damage. In preventive neurology, therefore, laboratory methodology may take precedence over clinical methodology.

The laboratory methods that are available for neurologic diagnosis are discussed in the next chapter and in Chap. 45, on clinical electrophysiology. The relevant principles of genetic and laboratory screening methods that are presently available for the prediction of disease are presented in the discussion of the disease(s) to which they are applicable.

SHORTCOMINGS OF THE CLINICAL METHOD

If one adheres faithfully to the clinical method outlined here, neurologic diagnosis is greatly simplified. In most cases, one can reach an anatomic diagnosis. The cause of the disease may prove more elusive and usually entails the intelligent and selective employment of a number of the laboratory procedures described in the next chapter.

However, even after the most assiduous application of the clinical method and laboratory procedures, there are numerous patients whose diseases elude diagnosis. In such circumstances we have often been aided by the following *rules of thumb*: (1) Focus the clinical analysis on the principal symptoms and signs and avoid being distracted by minor signs and uncertain clinical data. As mentioned earlier, when the main sign has been mistakenly interpreted—say a tremor has been taken for ataxia, or fatigue for weakness—the clinical method is derailed from the start. (2) Avoid early closure of diagnosis. Often this is the result of premature fixation on some item in the history or examination, closing the mind to alternative diagnostic considerations. The first diagnostic formulation should be regarded as only a testable hypothesis, subject to modification when new items of information are secured. Should the disease be in a stage of transition, time will allow the full picture to emerge and the diagnosis to be clarified. (3) When several of the main features of a disease under consideration are lacking, an alternative diagnosis should always be entertained. In general, however, one is more likely to encounter rare manifestations of common diseases than the typical manifestations of rare diseases (a paraphrasing of Bayes' theorem). (4) It is preferable to base diagnosis on one's experience with the dominant symptoms and signs and not on statistical analyses of the frequency of clinical phenomena. For the most part, the methods of probability-based decision analysis have proved to be disappointing in relation to neurologic disease because of the impossibility of weighing the importance of each clinical datum. (5) Whenever reasonable and safe, obtain tissue for examination, for this adds the dimension of histopathology to the clinical study.

As pointed out by Chimowitz, students tend to err in failing to recognize a disease they have not seen, and experienced clinicians may fail to recognize a rare variant of a common disease. There is no doubt that some clinicians are more adept than others at solving difficult clinical problems. Their talent is not intuitive, as sometimes is presumed, but is attributable to having paid close attention to the details of their experience with many diseases and having catalogued them for future reference. The unusual case is recorded in memory and can be resurrected when another one like it is encountered. Long experience also teaches one not to immediately accept the obvious explanation.

THE PURPOSE OF THE CLINICAL METHOD OF NEUROLOGY

Accurate diagnosis serves four main purposes: (1) it enables the physician to determine the proper treatment of the patient; (2) it is helpful in prognosis, i.e., in predicting the outcome of the illness; (3) if the disease is hereditary, it allows for genetic counseling; and (4) it is the essential initial step in the scientific study of clinical phenomena and disease. The medical profession is primarily concerned with the prevention and cure of illness, and all our knowledge is applied to this well-defined end. A major aim of the neurologist, therefore, is not to overlook a disease for which there is an effective treatment. Each of the treatable causes of a given syndrome must be carefully considered and excluded by clinical and laboratory methods. For example, in the study of a patient with disease of the spinal cord, one must take special care to exclude the presence of a tumor, subacute combined degeneration (vitamin B_{12} deficiency), spinal syphilis, epidural abscess or hematoma, herniated disc, and cervical spondylosis, for these are all treatable. In this respect, failure to recognize amyotrophic lateral sclerosis is a less serious error.

THERAPEUTICS IN NEUROLOGY

Among medical specialties, neurology has traditionally occupied a somewhat anomalous position, being thought of by many as little more than an intellectual exercise concerned with making diagnoses of untreatable diseases. This disdainful view of our profession is no longer valid. There are a growing number of diseases, some medical and others surgical, for which specific therapy is now available, and—through advances in neuroscience—their number is steadily increasing. Matters pertaining to these therapies and to the dosages, timing, and manner of administration of particular drugs are considered in later chapters, in relation to the description of individual diseases.

There are, in addition, many diseases in which neurologic function can be restored to a varying degree by appropriate rehabilitation measures or by the judicious use of therapeutic agents that have not been fully validated. Claims for the effectiveness of a particular therapy, based on statistical analysis of large-scale clinical studies, must be treated circumspectly. Was the study well conceived, was there rigid adherence to the criteria for randomization and admission of cases into the study, were the statistical methods standardized, were the controls truly comparable? And most importantly, were the patients in a particular study strictly comparable to the clinical problem at hand? Also, it has been our experience, based on participation in a number of such multicenter trials, that the original claims must be accepted with caution. Since newly proposed therapeutic agents are often risky and expensive, it is often prudent to wait until further studies confirm the benefits that have been claimed for them or expose flaws in the design or fundamental assumptions of the original study.

Even when no treatment is possible, neurologic diagnosis is far more than an intellectual pastime. The first step in the scientific study of a disease process is its identification in the living patient. Until this is achieved, it is impossible to apply adequately the "master method of controlled experiment." The clinical method of neurology thus serves both the physician in the practical matters of diagnosis, prognosis, and treatment and the clinical scientist in the search for the mechanism and cause of the disease.

REFERENCES

BERG BO (ed): *Principles of Child Neurology*. New York, McGraw-Hill, 1996, pp 5–22.

BICKERSTAFF ER, SPILLANE JA: *Neurological Examination in Clinical Practice*, 5th ed. Oxford, Blackwell Scientific, 1989.

CHIMOWITZ MI, LOGIGIAN EL, CAPLAN LP: The accuracy of bedside neurological diagnoses. *Ann Neurol* 28:78, 1990.

DEMYER WE: *Technique of the Neurologic Examination: A Programmed Text*, 4th ed. New York, McGraw-Hill, 1994.

DUBOWITZ LM, DUBOWITZ V, MERCURI E: *The Neurological Assessment of the Preterm and Full-term Newborn Infant*, 2nd ed. Clinics in Developmental Medicine 148. Mac Keith Press, 1999.

GESELL A, AMATRUDA CS: in Knoblock H, Pasamanick B (eds): *Gesell and Amatruda's Developmental Diagnosis*, 3rd ed. Hagerstown, MD, Harper & Row, 1974.

GLICK T: *Neurologic Skills: Examination and Diagnosis*. Boston, Blackwell, 1993.

HOLMES G: *Introduction to Clinical Neurology*, 3rd ed. Revised by Bryan Matthews. Baltimore, Williams & Wilkins, 1968.

MANCALL EL: *Alpers and Mancall's Essentials of the Neurologic Examination*, 2nd ed. Philadelphia, Davis, 1981.

MAYO CLINIC: *Examinations in Neurology*, 7th ed. St. Louis, Mosby, 1998.

ROSS RT: *How to Examine the Nervous System*, 3rd ed. Stamford, CT, Appleton Lange, 1999.

Chapter 2

SPECIAL TECHNIQUES FOR NEUROLOGIC DIAGNOSIS

The analysis and interpretation of data elicited by a careful history and examination may prove to be adequate for diagnosis. Special laboratory examinations then do no more than corroborate the clinical impression. However, it happens more often that the nature of the disease is not discerned by "case study" alone; the diagnostic possibilities may be reduced to two or three, but the correct one is uncertain. Under these circumstances, one resorts to the ancillary examinations outlined below. The aim of the neurologist is to arrive at a final diagnosis by artful analysis of the clinical data aided by the least number of laboratory procedures. Moreover, the strategy of laboratory study of disease should be based purely on therapeutic and prognostic considerations, not on the physician's curiosity or presumed medicolegal exigencies.

A few decades ago the only laboratory procedures available to the neurologist were lumbar puncture and examination of a sample of cerebrospinal fluid, radiology of the skull and spinal column, contrast myelography, pneumoencephalography, and electroencephalography. Now, through formidable advances in scientific technology, the physician's armamentarium has been expanded to include a multitude of neuroimaging, biochemical, and genetic methods. Some of these new methods are so impressive that there is a temptation to substitute them for a careful, detailed history and physical examination. Use of the laboratory in this way should be avoided; it certainly does not guarantee a diagnosis. In fact, in a carefully examined series of 86 consecutively hospitalized neurologic patients, laboratory findings [including magnetic resonance imaging (MRI)] clarified the clinical diagnosis in 40 patients but failed to do so in the remaining 46 patients (Chimowitz et al). The physician should always keep in mind the primacy of the clinical method and judge the relevance and significance of each laboratory datum only in the context of clinical findings. Hence the neurologist must be familiar with all laboratory procedures relevant to neurologic disease, their reliability, and their hazards.

Below is a description of laboratory procedures that have application to a diversity of neurologic diseases. Procedures that are pertinent to a particular symptom complex or category of disease—e.g., audiogram (deafness); electronystagmogram, or ENG (vertigo); electromyogram (EMG) and nerve conduction studies (neuromuscular disease)—are presented in the chapters devoted to these disorders.

LUMBAR PUNCTURE AND EXAMINATION OF CEREBROSPINAL FLUID

The information yielded by examination of the cerebrospinal fluid (CSF) is often crucial in the diagnosis of neurologic disease.

Indications for Lumbar Puncture (LP)

1. To obtain pressure measurements and procure a sample of the CSF for cellular, cytologic, chemical, and bacteriologic examination.

2. To aid in therapy by the administration of spinal anesthetics and occasionally antibiotics or antitumor agents, or by reduction of CSF pressure.

3. To inject a radiopaque substance, as in myelography, or a radioactive agent, as in scintigraphic cisternography.

LP carries a certain risk if the CSF pressure is very high (evidenced by headache and papilledema), for it increases the possibility of a fatal cerebellar or transtentorial herniation. The risk is considerable when papilledema is due to an intracranial mass, but it is much lower in patients with subarachnoid hemorrhage or pseudotumor cerebri, conditions in which repeated lumbar punctures have actually been employed as a therapeutic measure. In patients with purulent meningitis, there is also a small risk of herniation, but this is far outweighed by the need for a definitive diagnosis and the institution of appropriate treatment at the earliest moment. With this exception, therefore, lumbar puncture should be preceded by computed tomography (CT) or magnetic resonance imaging (MRI) whenever an elevation of intracranial pressure is suspected. If the latter procedures do not disclose a mass lesion that causes displacement of tissue toward the tentorial opening or into the foramen magnum (the presence of a mass alone is of less concern) and it is considered essential to have the information yielded by CSF examination, the LP should be performed—with certain precautions. A fine-bore (no. 22 or 24) needle should be used, and if the pressure proves to be very high—over 400 mmH_2O—one should obtain the necessary sample of fluid and then, according to the suspected disease and patient's condition, administer urea or mannitol and watch the manometer until the pressure falls. Dexamethasone or an equivalent corticosteroid should then be given in an initial intravenous dose of 10 mg, followed by doses of 4 to 6 mg every 6 h in order to produce a sustained reduction in intracranial pressure.

Cisternal puncture and *cervical subarachnoid puncture*, although safe in the hands of an expert, are too hazardous to entrust to those without experience. Lumbar puncture is preferred except in obvious instances of spinal block requiring a sample of cisternal fluid or myelography above the lesion.

Technique of Lumbar Puncture Experience teaches the importance of meticulous technique. LP should always be done under sterile conditions. Local anesthetic is injected in and beneath the skin, which should render the procedure painless. Warming of the analgesic by rolling the vial between the palms seems to diminish the burning sensation that accompanies cutaneous infiltration. The patient is positioned on his side, preferably on the left side for right-handed physicians, with hips and knees flexed and his head as close to his knees as comfort permits. The patient's back should be aligned near the edge of the bed and a small pillow placed under the ear. The trochar should be removed slowly from the needle in order to avoid sucking a nerve rootlet into the lumen and causing radicular pain. Otherwise, sciatic pain during the procedure indicates that the needle is placed too far laterally. If the flow of CSF slows, the head can be elevated slowly. When drops of CSF contact the edge of a collecting tube, capillary action can also be utilized to speed up flow. Occasionally, one resorts to gentle aspiration with a small-bore syringe to overcome the resistance of proteinaceous and viscous CSF. The puncture is easiest to perform at the L3-L4 interspace, which corresponds to the axial plane of the iliac crests, or in the space above or below. In infants and young children, in whom the spinal cord may extend to the level of the L3-L4 interspace, lower spaces should be used. Failure to enter the lumbar subarachnoid space after two or three trials can usually be overcome by doing the puncture with the patient in the sitting position and then assisting him to lie on one side for pressure measurements and fluid removal. The "dry tap" is more often due to an improperly placed needle than to obliteration of the subarachnoid space by a compressive lesion of the cauda equina or chronic adhesive arachnoiditis.

There are few serious complications of lumbar puncture beyond the risk of inducing brain herniation. The most common is headache, the result of a reduction of CSF pressure and the tugging of cerebral and dural vessels as the patient assumes the erect posture. The syndrome of low CSF pressure and other complications of lumbar puncture are considered further in Chap. 30. Bleeding into the spinal meningeal spaces can occur in patients who are taking anticoagulants [prothrombin time >13.5 or an International Normalized Ratio (INR) >1.3], have low platelet counts ($<30,000$ to 50,000/mm^3), or have impaired platelet function (alcoholism, uremia). Purulent meningitis and disc space infections have been known to complicate lumbar puncture, the result of imperfect sterile technique; and the introduction of particulate matter (e.g., talc) can produce a sterile meningitis. Diplopia, facial paresis, and tinnitus or deafness have reportedly complicated lumbar puncture on very rare occasions.

Examination Procedures

Once the subarachnoid space has been entered, the pressure and—in special cases—"dynamics" of the CSF are determined (see below) and samples of fluid obtained. The gross appearance of the fluid is noted, after which the CSF, in separate tubes, can be examined for (1) number and type of cells and presence of micro-organisms; (2) protein and glucose content; (3) tumor cells, using a Millipore filter or similar technique; (4) content of gamma globulin and other protein fractions and presence of oligoclonal bands; (5) pigments, lactate, NH_3, pH, CO_2, enzymes, and substances elaborated by tumors; and (6) bacteria and fungus (by culture), cryptococcal antigen, mycobacteria, herpesvirus and cytomegalovirus DNA (by polymerase chain reaction), and viral isolation.

Pressure and Dynamics With the patient in the lateral decubitus position, the CSF pressure is measured by a manometer attached to the needle in the subarachnoid space. In the normal adult, the opening pressure varies from 100 to 180 mmH_2O, or 8 to 14 mmHg. In children, the pressure is in the range of 30 to 60 mmH_2O. A pressure above 200 mmH_2O with the patient relaxed and legs straightened reflects the presence of increased intracranial pressure. In an adult, a pressure of 50 mmH_2O or below indicates intracranial hypotension, generally due to leakage of spinal fluid or systemic dehydration. When measured with the needle in the lumbar sac and the patient in a sitting position, the fluid in the manometer rises to the level of the cisterna magna (pressure is approximately double that obtained in the recumbent position). It fails to reach the level of the ventricles because the latter are in a closed system under slight negative pressure, whereas the fluid in the manometer is influenced by atmospheric pressure. Normally, with the needle properly placed in the subarachnoid space, the fluid in the manometer oscillates through a few millimeters in response to the pulse and respiration and rises promptly with coughing, straining, or abdominal compression.

The presence of a spinal subarachnoid block can be confirmed by jugular compression. First one side of the neck is compressed, then the other, and then both sides simultaneously, with enough pressure to compress the veins but not the carotid arteries (Queckenstedt test). In the absence of subarachnoid block, there is a rapid rise in pressure of 100 to 200 mmH_2O and a return to its original level within 10 s after release. Failure of the pressure to rise with this maneuver usually means that the needle is improperly placed. A rise in pressure in response to abdominal compression (or coughing or straining) but not to jugular compression indicates a spinal subarachnoid block. Failure of the pressure to rise with compression of one jugular vein but not the other (Tobey-Ayer test) may indicate lateral sinus thrombosis. These tests are now rarely used, having been replaced by more precise and less hazardous imaging techniques, but they remain useful in appropriate circumstances. Jugular compression should never be performed when an intracranial tumor or other mass lesion is present or suspected.

Gross Appearance and Pigments Normally the CSF is clear and colorless, like water. Minor degrees of color change are best detected by comparing tubes of CSF and water against a white background (by daylight rather than fluorescent illumination) or by looking down into the tubes from above. The presence of red blood cells imparts a hazy or ground-glass appearance; at least 200 red blood cells (RBC) per cubic millimeter (mm^3) must be present to detect this change. The presence of 1000 to 6000 RBC per cubic millimeter imparts a hazy pink to red color, depending on the amount of blood; centrifugation of the fluid or allowing it to stand causes sedimentation of the RBC. Several hundred or more white blood cells in the fluid (pleocytosis) may cause a slight opaque haziness.

A traumatic tap (in which blood from the epidural venous plexus has been introduced into the spinal fluid) may seriously confuse the diagnosis if it is incorrectly interpreted to indicate a pre-existent subarachnoid hemorrhage. To distinguish between these two types of "bloody tap," two or three serial samples of fluid should be taken at the time of the LP. With a traumatic tap, there is usually a decreasing number of RBC in the second and third tubes. Also with a traumatic tap, the CSF pressure is usually normal, and if a large amount of blood is mixed with the fluid, it will clot or form fibrinous webs. These are not seen with pre-existent hemorrhage because the blood has been greatly diluted with CSF and defibrinated. With subarachnoid hemorrhage, the RBC begin to hemolyze within a few hours, imparting a pink-red discoloration (erythrochromia) to the supernatant fluid; allowed to stand for a day or more, the fluid becomes yellow-brown (xanthocromia). Prompt centrifugation of bloody fluid from a traumatic tap will yield a colorless supernatant; only with large amounts of blood (RBC over 100,000/mm^3) will the supernatant fluid be faintly xanthochromic due to contamination with serum bilirubin and lipochromes.

The fluid from a traumatic tap should contain one or two white blood cells (WBC) per 1000 RBC assuming that the hematocrit is normal, but in reality this ratio varies widely. With subarachnoid hemorrhage, the proportion of WBC rises as RBC hemolyze, sometimes reaching a level of several hundred per cubic millimeter; but the vagaries of this reaction are such that it, too, cannot be relied upon to distinguish traumatic from pre-existent bleeding. The same can be said for crenation of RBC, which occurs in both types of bleeding.

The reason that red corpuscles undergo rapid hemolysis in the CSF is not clear. It is surely not due to osmotic differences, insofar as the osmolarity of plasma and CSF is essentially the same. Fishman suggests that the low protein content of CSF disequilibrates the red cell membrane in some way. The explanation for the rapid phagocytosis of RBC in the CSF, which begins within 48 h, is also obscure.

The pigments that discolor the CSF following subarachnoid hemorrhage are oxyhemoglobin, bilirubin, and methemoglobin; in pure form, these pigments are colored

red (orange to orange-yellow with dilution), canary yellow, and brown, respectively. Mixtures of these pigments produce combinations of these colors. Oxyhemoglobin appears first, within several hours of the hemorrhage, becomes maximal in about 36 h, and if no further bleeding occurs, diminishes over a 7- to 9-day period. Bilirubin begins to appear in 2 to 3 days and increases in amount as the oxyhemoglobin decreases. Following a single brisk bleed, bilirubin persists in the CSF for 2 to 3 weeks, the duration varying with the number of RBC that were present originally. Methemoglobin appears when blood is loculated or encysted and isolated from the flow of CSF. Spectrophotometric techniques can be used to distinguish the various hemoglobin breakdown products and thus determine the approximate time of bleeding.

Not all xanthochromia of the CSF is due to hemolysis of RBC. With severe jaundice, bilirubin of both the direct- and indirect-reacting types will diffuse into the CSF. The quantity of bilirubin is from one-tenth to one-hundredth that in the serum. Elevation of CSF protein from whatever cause results in a faint opacity and xanthochromia, more or less in proportion to the albumin-bound fraction of bilirubin. Only at levels of more than 150 mg/100 mL does the coloration due to protein become visible to the naked eye. Hypercarotenemia and hemoglobinemia (through hemoglobin breakdown products, particularly oxyhemoglobin) also impart a yellow tint to the CSF, as do blood clots in the subdural or epidural space of the cranium or spinal column. Myoglobin does not enter the CSF, probably because a low renal threshold for this pigment permits rapid clearing of the blood.

Cellularity During the first month of life, the CSF may contain a small number of mononuclear cells. Beyond this period, the CSF normally contains no cells or at most up to five lymphocytes or other mononuclear cells per cubic millimeter. An elevation of WBC in the CSF always signifies a reactive process to bacteria or other infectious agents, blood, chemical substances, or a neoplasm or vasculitis. The WBC can be counted in an ordinary counting chamber, but their identification requires centrifugation of the fluid and a Wright stain of the sediment or the use of a Millipore filter, cell fixation, and staining. One can then recognize and count differentially neutrophilic and eosinophilic leukocytes (the latter being prominent in Hodgkin disease, parasitic infection, cholesterol emboli), lymphocytes, plasma cells, mononuclear cells, arachnoidal lining cells, macrophages, and tumor cells. Bacteria, fungi, and fragments of echinococci and cysticerci can also be seen in cell-stained or Gram-stained preparations. An India-ink preparation is useful in distinguishing between lymphocytes and cryptococci or *Candida*. On occasion, acid-fast bacilli will be found in appropriately stained samples. The monographs of Dufresne and of den Hartog-Jager and the article of Bigner are excellent references on CSF cytology. Special immunostaining techniques applied to cells of the CSF permit the recognition of lymphoma cell markers, glial fibrillary protein, and carcinoembryonic and other antigens. Electron microscopy permits more certain identification of tumor cells and may demonstrate such substances as phagocytosed fragments of myelin (e.g., in multiple sclerosis). These and other special methods for the examination of cells in the CSF are mentioned in the appropriate chapters.

Proteins In contrast to the high protein content of blood (5500 to 8000 mg/dL), that of the lumbar spinal fluid is 45 mg/dL or less in the adult. The protein content of CSF from the basal cisterns is 10 to 25 mg/dL and that from the ventricles is 5 to 15 mg/dL, reflecting a ventricular-lumbar gradient in the permeability of capillary endothelial cells to protein (blood-CSF barrier) and a lesser degree of circulation in the lumbosacral region. In children, the protein concentration is somewhat lower at each level (less than 20 mg/dL in the lumbar subarachnoid space). Levels higher than normal indicate a pathologic process in or near the ependyma or meninges—in either the brain, spinal cord, or nerve roots—though the cause of modest elevations of the CSF protein frequently remains obscure.

As one would expect, bleeding into the ventricles or subarachnoid space results in spillage not only of RBC but of serum proteins. If the serum protein concentrations are normal, the CSF protein should increase by about 1 mg per 1000 RBC provided that the same tube of CSF is used in determining the cell count and protein content. Because of the irritating effect of hemolyzed RBC upon the leptomeninges, the CSF protein may be increased by many times this ratio.

The protein content of the CSF in bacterial meningitis, in which choroidal and meningeal perfusion are increased, often reaches 500 mg/dL or more. Viral infections induce a less intense and mainly lymphocytic reaction and a lesser elevation of protein—usually 50 to 100 mg but sometimes up to 200 mg/dL; in some instances the protein content is normal. Paraventricular tumors, by reducing the blood-CSF barrier, often raise the total protein to over 100 mg/dL. Protein values as high as 500 mg/dL or even higher are found in exceptional cases of the Guillain-Barré syndrome and chronic inflammatory demyelinating polyneuropathy. Values of 1000 mg/dL or more usually indicate loculation of the lumbar CSF (CSF block); the fluid is then deeply yellow and clots readily because of the presence of fibrinogen. This combination of CSF abnormalities is called the *Froin syndrome*. Partial CSF blocks by ruptured discs or tumor may elevate the protein to 100 to 200 mg/dL. Low CSF protein values are sometimes found in meningismus (a febrile illness with signs of meningeal irritation but normal CSF), in the condition known as meningeal hydrops (Chap. 30), in hyperthyroidism, or after a recent lumbar puncture.

The quantitative partition of CSF proteins by electrophoretic and immunochemical methods demonstrates the presence of most of the serum proteins with a molecular weight of less than 150,000 to 200,000. The protein fractions that have been identified electrophoretically are prealbumin and albumin as well as alpha$_1$, alpha$_2$, beta$_1$, beta$_2$, and gamma globulin fraction, the last of these being accounted for mainly by immunoglobulins (the major immunoglobulin in normal CSF is IgG). Quantitative values of the different fractions are given in Table 2-1. Immunoelectrophoretic methods have also demonstrated the presence of glycoproteins, haptoproteins, ceruloplasmin, transferrin, and hemopexin. Large molecules—such as fibrinogen, IgM, and lipoproteins—are mostly excluded from the CSF.

There are other notable differences between the protein fractions of CSF and plasma. The CSF always contains a prealbumin fraction and the plasma does not. Although derived from plasma, this fraction, for an unknown reason, concentrates in the CSF, and the level is greater in ventricular than in lumbar CSF (perhaps because of its concentration by choroidal cells). Also, the CSF beta$_2$ or tau fraction (transferrin) is proportionally larger than that in the plasma and again higher in the ventricular than in the spinal fluid. The gamma globulin fraction in CSF is about 70 percent of that in serum.

At present only a few of these proteins are known to be associated with specific diseases of the nervous system. The most important is IgG, which may exceed 12 percent of the total CSF protein in diseases such as multiple sclerosis, neurosyphilis, subacute sclerosing panencephalitis, and other chronic viral meningoencephalitides. The serum IgG is not correspondingly increased, which means that this immune globulin originates in the nervous system. However, an elevation of serum gamma globulin—as occurs in cirrhosis, sarcoidosis, myxedema, and multiple myeloma—will be accompanied by a rise in the CSF globulin. Therefore, in patients with an elevated CSF gamma globulin, it is necessary to determine the electrophoretic pattern of the serum proteins as well. Certain qualitative changes in the CSF immunoglobulin pattern, particularly the demonstration of several discrete (oligoclonal) bands, are of special diagnostic importance in multiple sclerosis.

The albumin fraction of the CSF increases in a wide variety of central nervous system (CNS) and craniospinal nerve root diseases that increase the perme-

Table 2-1
Average values of constituents of normal CSF and serum

	Cerebrospinal fluid	*Serum*
Osmolarity	295 mosmol/L	295 mosmol/L
Sodium	138.0 meq/L	138.0 meq/L
Potassium	2.8 meq/L	4.1 meq/L
Calcium	2.1 meq/L	4.8 meq/L
Magnesium	2.3 meq/L	1.9 meq/L
Chloride	119 meq/L	101.0 meq/L
Bicarbonate	23.0 meq/L	23.0 meq/L
Carbon dioxide tension	48 mmHg	38 mmHg (arterial)
pH	7.33	7.41 (arterial)
Nonprotein nitrogen	19.0 mg/dL	27.0 mg/dL
Ammonia	30.0 g/dL	70.0 g/dL
Uric acid	0.24 mg/dL	5.5 mg/dL
Urea	4.7 mmol/L	5.4 mmol/L
Creatinine	1.1 mg/dL	1.8 mg/dL
Phosphorus	1.6 mg/dL	4.0 mg/dL
Total lipid	1.5 mg/dL	750.0 mg/dL
Total cholesterol	0.4 mg/dL	180.0 mg/dL
Cholesterol esters	0.3 mg/dL	126.0 mg/dL
Glucose	60 mg/dL	90.0 mg/dL
Lactate	1.6 meq/L	1.0 meq/L
Total protein	15–50 mg/dL	6.5–8.4 g/100 dL
Prealbumin	1–7%	Trace
Albumin	49–73%	56%
Alpha$_1$ globulin	3–7%	4%
Alpha$_2$ globulin	6–13%	10%
Beta globulin (beta$_1$ plus tau)	9–19%	12%
Gamma globulin	3–12%	14%

Source: Reproduced by permission from Fishman.

ability of the blood-CSF barrier, but no specific clinical correlations can be drawn. Certain enzymes that originate in the brain, especially the brain-derived fraction of creatine kinase (CK-BB) but also enolase and neopterin, are found in the CSF after stroke or trauma and have been used as markers of damage in experimental work.

Glucose Normally the CSF glucose concentration is in the range of 45 to 80 mg/dL, i.e., about two-thirds of that in the blood (0.6 to 0.7 of serum concentrations). Higher levels parallel the blood glucose; but with marked hyperglycemia, the ratio of CSF to blood glucose is reduced (0.5 to 0.6). With extremely low serum glucose, the ratio becomes higher, approximating 0.85. In general, CSF values below 40 mg/dL are abnormal. After the intravenous injection of glucose, 2 to 4 h is required to reach equilibrium with the CSF; a similar delay follows the lowering of blood glucose. For these reasons, samples of CSF and blood for glucose determinations should ideally be drawn simultaneously in the fasting state. Low values of CSF glucose in the presence of pleocytosis usually indicate pyogenic, tuberculous, or fungal meningitis, although low values are observed in some patients with widespread neoplastic infiltration of the meninges and occasionally with sarcoidosis and subarachnoid hemorrhage (usually in the first week).

The almost invariable rise of CSF lactate in purulent meningitis probably means that some of the glucose is undergoing anaerobic glycolysis by polymorphonuclear leukocytes and cells of the meninges and adjacent brain tissue. For a long time it was assumed that in meningitis the bacteria lowered the CSF glucose by their active metabolism, but the fact that the glucose remains at a subnormal level for 1 to 2 weeks after effective treatment of the meningitis suggests that another mechanism may be operative in the production of this hypoglycorrhachia. Theoretically at least, an inhibition of the entry of glucose into the CSF, due to an impairment of the membrane transfer system, can be implicated. As a rule, viral infections of the meninges and brain do not lower the CSF glucose or raise the lactate levels, although low glucose values have been reported in a small number of patients with mumps meningoencephalitis and rarely with herpes simplex and zoster infections.

Serologic and Virologic Tests It has become routine practice to test the CSF for cryptococcal surface antigen as a rapid method of detecting this fungal infection. On occasion, a false-positive reaction is obtained in the presence of high titers of rheumatoid factor or antitreponemal antibodies, but otherwise the test is diagnostically more dependable than the conventional India-ink preparation (page 772). The nontreponemal antibody tests of the blood—Venereal Disease Research Laboratories (VDRL) slide flocculation test and rapid plasma reagin (RPR) agglutination test—can also be performed on the CSF. When positive, these tests are diagnostic of neurosyphilis, but false-positive reactions may occur with collagen diseases, malaria, and yaws or with contamination of the CSF by seropositive blood. Tests that depend on the use of treponemal antigens, including the *Treponema pallidum* immobilization test and the fluorescent treponemal antibody test, are more specific and assist in the interpretation of false-positive reactions. The value of CSF examinations in the diagnosis and treatment of neurosyphilis is discussed in Chap. 32, but routine testing of CSF for treponemal antibodies is no longer practiced.

The utility of serum serologic tests for viruses is limited by the time required to obtain results, but they are useful in determining retrospectively the source of meningitis or encephalitis. More rapid tests that utilize the polymerase chain reaction (PCR) in CSF, which amplifies viral DNA fragments, are now widely available for diagnosis, particularly for herpesviruses and cytomegalovirus. These tests are most useful in the first week of infection, when the virus is being reproduced and its genomic material is most prevalent; afterwards, serologic techniques for viral infection are more sensitive. Amplification of DNA by PCR is particularly useful in the more rapid detection of tubercle bacilli in the CSF, the conventional culture of which takes several weeks at best. New tests for the detection of prion proteins in the spinal fluid are available and may aid in the diagnosis of the spongiform encephalopathies.

Changes in Solutes and Other Components The average osmolality of the CSF (295 mosmol/L) is identical to that of plasma. As the osmolality of the plasma is increased by the intravenous injection of hypertonic solutions such as mannitol or urea, there is a delay of several hours in the rise of osmolality of the CSF. It is during this period that the hyperosmolality of the blood dehydrates the brain and decreases the volume of CSF.

The CSF and serum levels of sodium, potassium, calcium, and magnesium are listed in Table 2-1. Neurologic disease does not alter the CSF concentrations of these constituents in any characteristic way. The low CSF concentration of chloride that occurs in bacterial meningitis is not specific but a reflection of hypochloremia and, to a slight degree, of a greatly elevated CSF protein.

Acid-base balance in the CSF is of considerable interest in relation to metabolic acidosis and alkalosis. Normally the pH of the CSF is about 7.31—i.e., somewhat lower than that of arterial blood, which is 7.41. The P_{CO_2} in the CSF is in the range of 45 to 49 mmHg—i.e., higher than in arterial blood (about 40 mmHg). The bicarbonate levels of the two fluids are about the same, 23 meq/L. The pH of the CSF is precisely regulated, and it tends to remain relatively unchanged even in the face of severe systemic acidosis and alkalosis. Measurements of acid-base balance in the CSF, while of interest, have only limited clinical value. Acid-base changes in the lumbar CSF do not necessarily reflect the presence of similar changes in the brain, nor are the CSF data as accurate an index of the systemic changes as direct measurements of arterial blood gases.

The *ammonia content* of the CSF is one-third to one-half that of the arterial blood; it is increased in hepatic encephalopathy, the inherited hyperammonemias and in Reye syndrome; the concentration corresponds roughly with the severity of the encephalopathy. The uric acid content of CSF is about 5 percent of that in serum and varies with changes in the serum level (high in gout, uremia, and meningitis and low in Wilson disease). The urea concentration in the CSF is slightly less than in the serum (see Table 2-1), and in uremia it rises in parallel with that in the blood. An intravenous injection of urea raises the blood level immediately and the CSF level more slowly, exerting an osmotic dehydrating effect on the central nervous tissues and CSF. All 24 of the amino acids have been isolated from the CSF. The concentration of the total amino acids is about one-third that of plasma. Elevations of glutamine are found in hepatic coma and the Reye syndrome and of phenylalanine, histidine, valine, leucine, isoleucine, tyrosine, and homocystine in the corresponding aminoacidurias.

Many of the *enzymes* found in serum are known to rise in CSF under conditions of disease, usually in relation to a rise in the CSF protein. None of the enzyme changes has proved to be a specific indicator of neurologic disease, with the possible exception of *lactic dehydrogenase*, especially isoenzymes 4 and 5, which are derived from granulocytes and are elevated in bacterial meningitis but not in aseptic or viral meningitis. Lactic dehydrogenase is also elevated in cases of carcinomatous meningitis, as is carcinoembryonic antigen; the latter, however, is not elevated in bacterial, viral, or fungal meningitis. As to *lipids*, the quantities in CSF are small and their measurement is difficult.

The catabolites of the *catecholamines* can now be measured in the CSF. Homovanillic acid (HVA), the major catabolite of dopamine, and 5-hydroxyindoleacetic acid (5-HIAA), the major catabolite of serotonin, are normally present in the spinal fluid; both are five or six times higher in the ventricular than in the lumbar CSF. The levels of both catabolites are reduced in patients with idiopathic and drug-induced parkinsonism.

Finally, it may be said that with continued development of microchemical techniques for the analysis of the CSF, we can look forward to a better understanding of the metabolic mechanisms of the brain, particularly in the hereditary metabolic diseases. Ultrarefined methods such as gas-liquid chromatography will probably reveal many new catabolic products, the measurement of which will be of value in diagnosis and therapy. Thompson has reviewed the biochemical analysis of CSF and its use for diagnostic purposes.

RADIOGRAPHIC EXAMINATION OF SKULL AND SPINE

For a long time, plain films of the cranium constituted a "routine" part of the study of the neurologic patient, but it is now evident that the yield of useful information from this procedure is relatively small. Even in patients with head injury, where radiography of the skull would seem to be an optimal method of examination, a fracture is found in only 1 out of 16 cases, at a cost of thousands of dollars per fracture and a small risk from radiation exposure. Nevertheless plain skull films are eminently useful in demonstrating fractures, changes in contour of the skull, bony erosions and hyperostoses, infection in paranasal sinuses and mastoids, and changes in the basal foramina. Plain films of the spine are able to demonstrate destructive lesions of vertebrae, fracture-dislocations, and Paget disease.

Sequential refinements of technique—such as pneumoencephalography, carotid and vertebral arteriography, and tomography—have greatly increased the yield of valuable information in special cases, but without question the most important recent advances in neuroradiology, and indeed in neurology, have come about with the development of computed tomography (CT) and magnetic resonance imaging (MRI). They represent a quantum leap in our ability to visualize pathology in the living person. A new field of bioneuropathology has been created.

Computed Tomography

In this procedure, conventional x-radiation is attenuated as it passes successively through the skull, CSF, cerebral gray and white matter, and blood vessels. The intensity of the exiting radiation relative to the incident radiation is measured, the data are integrated, and images are reconstructed by computer. This major achievement in mathematical methodology, attributed to Hounsfield and others, permitted the astonishing technologic advance from plain radiographs of the skull to reconstructed images of the cranium and its contents in any plane. More than thirty thousand 2- to 4-mm x-ray beams are directed successively at several horizontal levels of the cranium. The differing densities of bone, CSF, blood, and gray and white matter are distinguishable in the resulting picture. One can see hemorrhage, softened and edematous brain, abscess, and tumor tissue and also the precise size and position of the ventricles and midline structures. The radiation exposure is not significantly greater than that from plain skull films.

The latest generation of CT scanners afford pictures of brain, spine, and orbit of great clarity. As illustrated in Fig. 2-1, in transverse section of the brain one actually sees displayed the caudate and lenticular nuclei and the internal capsules and thalami. The position and width of all the main sulci can be measured, and the optic nerve and medial and lateral rectus muscles stand out clearly in the posterior parts of the orbit. The brainstem, cerebellum, and spinal cord are easily visible in the scan at appropriate levels. The scans are also useful in imaging parts of the body that surround peripheral nerves and plexuses, thereby demonstrating tumors, inflammatory lesions, and hematomas that involve these nerves. In imaging of the head, CT has a number of advantages over MRI, the most important being safety when metal is present in the body and the clarity of imaging of blood from the moment it is shed. Other advantages are its lower cost, easy availability, shorter examination time, and superior visualization of calcium, fat, and bone, particularly of the skull base and vertebrae. Also, if constant monitoring and use of life-support equipment is required during the imaging procedure, it is accomplished more readily in the CT than in the MRI machine. Recent advances in CT technology (spiral or helical CT) have greatly increased the speed of the scanning procedure and have made possible the visualization, with great clarity, of the cerebral vasculature (CT angiography, see further on).

Magnetic Resonance Imaging

Magnetic resonance imaging, formerly referred to as nuclear magnetic resonance, also provides "slice" images of the brain in any plane, but it has the great advantages over CT of using nonionizing energy and providing better resolution of different structures within the brain and other organs. For the visualization of most neurologic diseases, MRI is the procedure of choice.

MRI is accomplished by placing the patient within a powerful magnetic field, causing certain endogenous isotopes (atoms) of the tissues and CSF to align themselves in the longitudinal orientation of the magnetic field. Application of a brief (few milliseconds) radiofrequency (RF) pulse into the field changes the axis of alignment of the atoms from the longitudinal to the transverse plane. When the RF pulse is turned off, the atoms return to their original alignment. The RF energy that was absorbed and then emitted results in a magnetic signal that is detected by electromagnetic receiver coils. To create contrasting tissue images from these signals, the RF pulse must be repeated many times (a pulse sequence), the signals being measured after the application of each pulse. The scanner stores the signals as a matrix of data, which is subjected to computer analysis and from which an image is constructed.

Nuclear magnetic resonance can be accomplished with several isotopes, but current technology uses signals derived from hydrogen atoms (^{1}H), because hydrogen is the most abundant isotope and yields the strongest magnetic signal. The image is essentially a map of the hydrogen content of tissue, influenced also by the physical and chemical environment of the hydrogen atoms. Different tissues have different rates of proton relaxation, yielding different signal intensities and hence tissue contrast. The terms *T1* and *T2* refer to the time constants for proton relaxation; these may be altered to highlight certain features of tissue structure. In the T1-weighted image, the CSF appears dark and the cortical border and cortical–white matter junction are well defined, as in CT images, whereas T2-weighted images show the CSF as white. T2-weighted images highlight alterations in white matter such as infarction, demyelination, and edema. So-called FLAIR (fluid-attenuated inversion recovery) imaging is a technique that gives a high signal for parenchymal lesions and a low signal for CSF. It is sensitive to calcium and iron within brain tissue, shows the earliest stages of infarction, and accentuates inflammatory demyelinating lesions.

The images generated by the latest MRI machines are truly remarkable (Fig. 2-2*A* to *C*). Because of the high degree of contrast between white and gray matter, one can identify all discrete nuclear structures and lesions within them. Deep lesions in the temporal lobe and structures in the posterior fossa and at the cervicomedullary junction are seen much better than with CT;

Figure 2-1

Normal axial CT scans of the brain, orbits, and lumbar spine from a young healthy man. A. *Image through the cerebral hemispheres at the level of the corona radiata. The dense bone of the calvarium is white. Gray matter appears denser than white matter. The triangular shape of the sagittal sinus in axial section is seen posteriorly.* B. *Image at the level of the lenticular nuclei. The caudate and lenticular nuclei are more dense than the internal capsule. CSF within the frontal and occipital horns of the lateral ventricle as well as surrounding the pineal body appears dark.* C. *Image at the level of the posterior fossa. Again, the CSF within the fourth ventricle and prepontine cisterns appears dark. The basilar artery is seen as a small, round, dense focus anterior to the pons. Typical artifact generated by temporal bones creates streaking across the inferior temporal lobes. The mastoid and sphenoid sinuses are black due to their aeration.* D. *Thin-section axial image through the midorbits. The sclera appears as a dense band surrounding the globe. Medial and lateral rectus muscles have a fusiform shape. Orbital fat appears dark due to its low attenuation value. Air contained within the sphenoid sinus and ethmoid air cells appears black.*

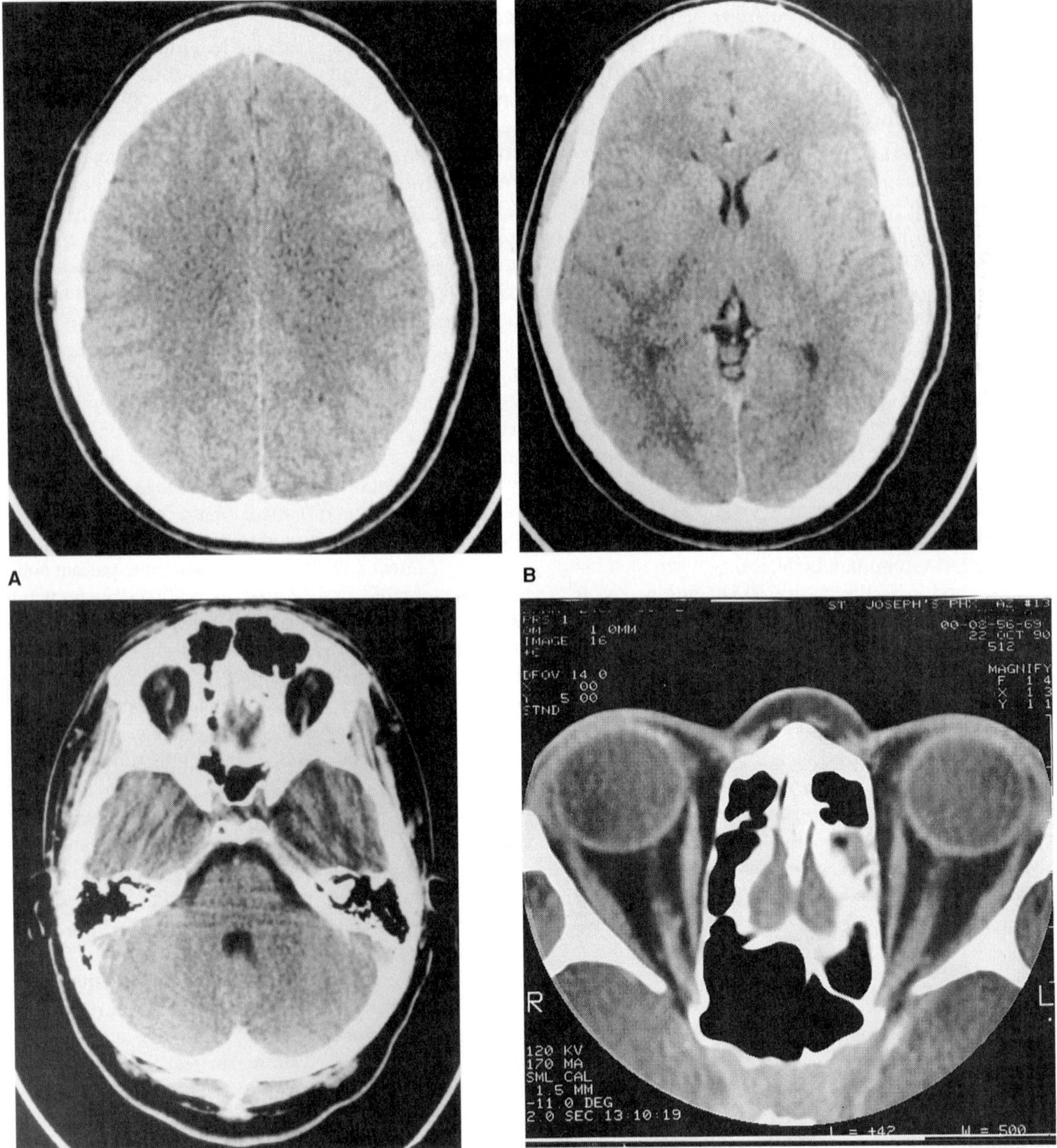

Figure 2-1 *(Continued)*

E. and F. *Axial images of the lumbar spine following myelography. Contrast contained within the thecal sac appears white. The filling defects are caused by nerve roots at the L3-4 and L5-S1 levels. Bony structures appear dense, and the facet joints are well seen. There is no evidence of disc herniation or canal stenosis. (Illustrations courtesy of Dr. Burton Drayer and Dr. Andrew Mancall.)*

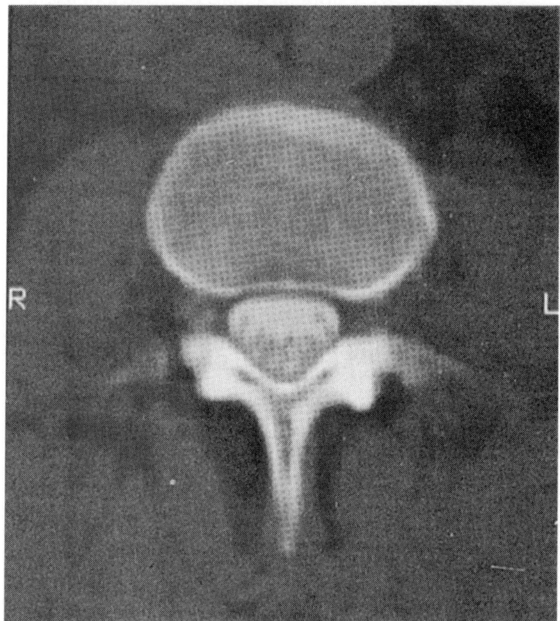

E

F

the structures can be displayed in three planes and are unmarred by signals from adjacent skeletal structures (bony artifact). Demyelinative lesions stand out with greater clarity and infarcts can be seen at an earlier stage than with CT. Each of the products of disintegrated RBC—methemoglobin, hemosiderin, and ferritin—can be recognized, enabling one to date the age of hemorrhages and to follow their resolution. Similarly, CSF, fat, calcium, and iron have their own signal characteristics in different imaging sequences.

MRI imaging of the spine provides clear images of the vertebral bodies, intervertebral discs, spinal cord, and cauda equina (Fig. 2-2*D* to *F*), and of syringomyelia and other lesions (herniated discs, tumors, epidural or subdural hemorrhages and abscesses). It has practically replaced contrast myelography except in certain circumstances where very high resolution images of nerve roots and spinal cord are required.

The administration of gadolinium, a so-called paramagnetic agent that enhances the process of proton relaxation during the T1 sequence of MRI, permits even sharper definition and highlights regions surrounding many types of lesions where the blood-brain barrier has been disrupted.

The degree of cooperation that is required to perform MRI limits its use in young children and in the mentally confused or retarded. Studying a patient who requires a ventilator is difficult but manageable by using either hand ventilation or nonferromagnetic ventilators (Barnett et al). The main dangers in the use of MRI are torque or dislodgement of metal clips on blood vessels, of dental devices and other ferromagnetic objects, and of small metal fragments in the orbit, often acquired unnoticed by operators of machine tools. For this reason it is wise, in appropriate patients, to obtain plain radiographs of the skull so as to detect metal in these regions. The presence of a cardiac pacemaker is an absolute contraindication to the use of MRI, since the magnetic field induces unwanted currents in the device and the wires exiting from it.

Because of the development of cataracts in fetuses of animals exposed to MRI, there has been hesitation in performing MRI in pregnant patients, especially in the first trimester. However, current data indicate that it may be performed in such patients provided that the study is medically indicated. In a study of 1000 pregnant MRI technicians who entered the magnetic field frequently (the magnet remains on between procedures), no adverse

Figure 2-2

Normal MRI of the brain and the cervical and lumbar spine. A. *T2-weighted (SE 2500/90) axial image at the level of the lenticular nuclei. Note that gray matter appears brighter than white matter. The CSF within the lateral ventricles is very bright. The caudate nuclei, putamen, and thalamus appear brighter than the internal capsule, while the globus pallidus is darker.* B. *T2-weighted (SE 2500/90) axial image at the level of the midbrain. The red nucleus and the substantia nigra are dark due to normal iron accumulation. The CSF within the lateral ventricles and subarachnoid spaces appears bright, as does the vitreous. Signal is absent ("flow void") from the rapidly flowing anterior, middle, and posterior cerebral arteries.* C. *T1-weighted (SE 700/17) midline sagittal image of the brain. Note that white matter appears brighter than gray matter and the corpus callosum is well defined. Subcutaneous fat and calvarial marrow appear very bright. The pons, medulla, and cervicomedullary junction are well delineated, and the region of the pituitary gland is normally demonstrated.* D. *Gradient echo sagittal image of the cervical spine. Note the bright signal intensity of the CSF, which provides a "myelographic" effect. Intervertebral discs also demonstrate high signal intensity. The spinal cord and brain demonstrate intermediate signal intensity, and the craniocervical junction is clearly defined.*

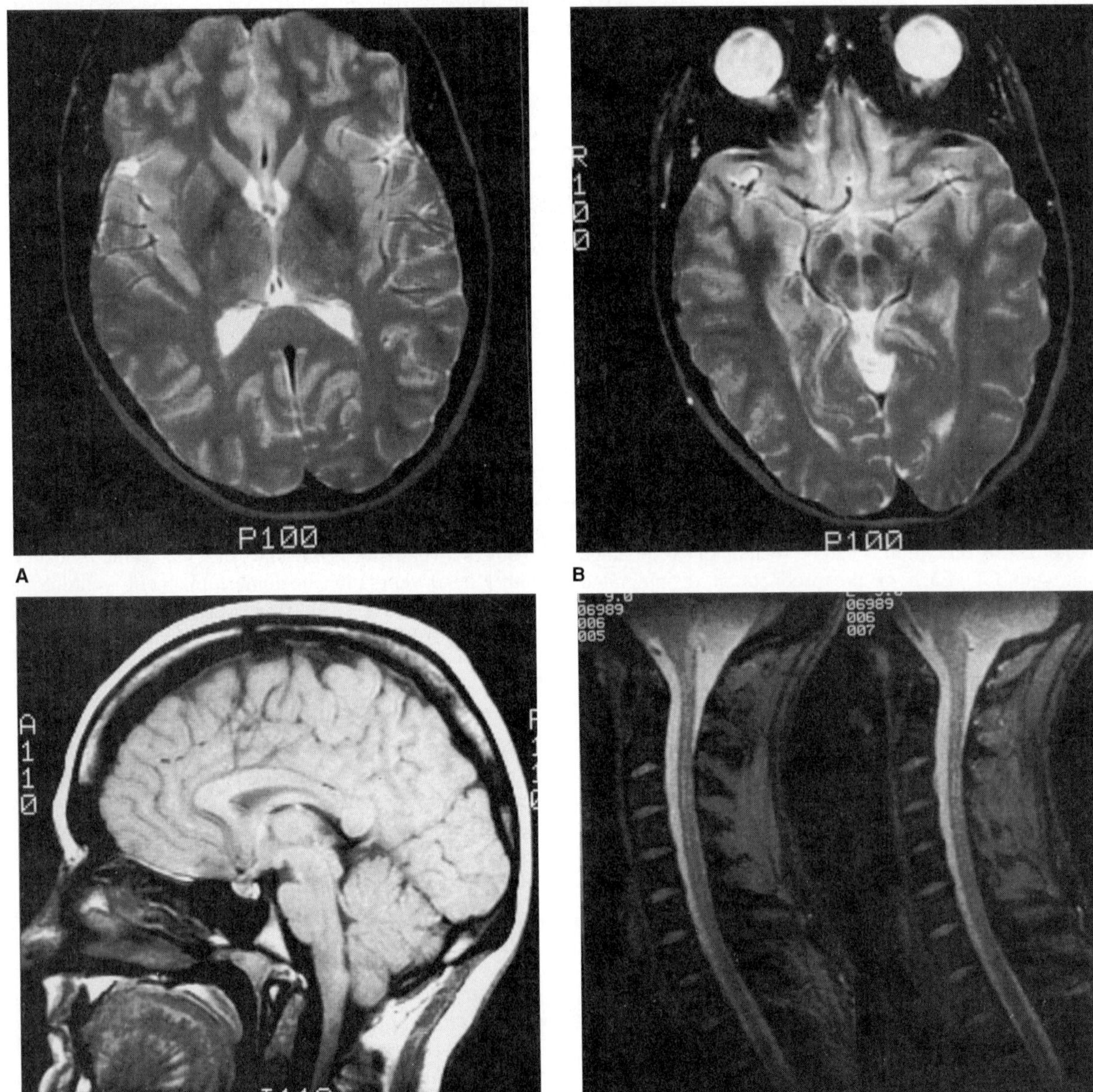

C

D

Figure 2-2 *(Continued)*

E. *T1-weighted (SE 600/20) axial image of the lumbar spine at the L3-4 level. Note that bone marrow appears brighter than disc material. The neural foramina are filled with fat, which demonstrates high signal intensity, and a small amount of fat is present within the spinal canal posterior to the thecal sac. The CSF within the thecal sac is dark, and nerve roots of intermediate signal intensity are demonstrated posteriorly. The facet joints are well seen.* F. *Gradient-echo sagittal image of the lumbar spine. Again, note the bright signal intensity of the CSF, creating a "myelographic" effect. The conus medullaris is well demonstrated, and individual nerve roots can be seen streaming inferiorly.*

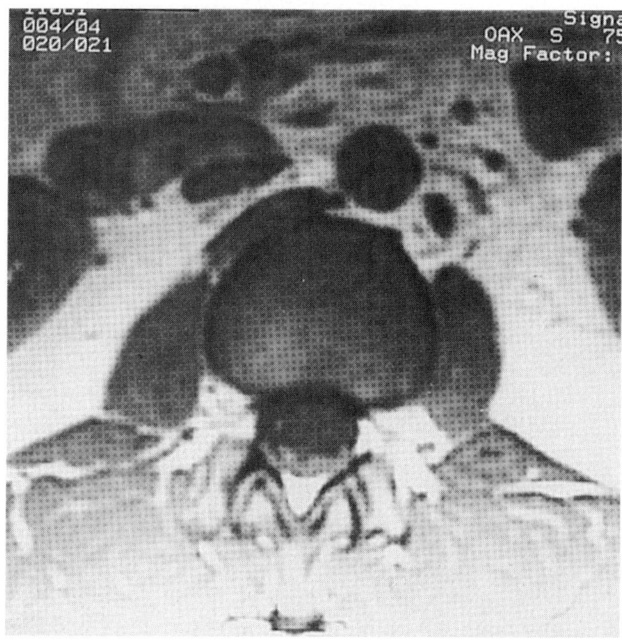

E

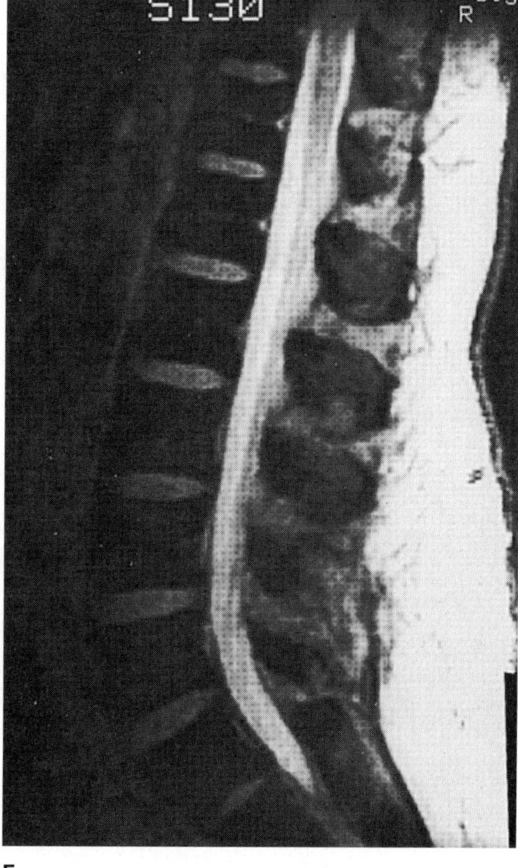

F

effects upon the fetus could be discerned (Kanal et al). It is also considered safe to perform cranial MRI in patients with hip prostheses, wire sutures, and some types of heart valves as well as special cerebral aneurysm clips composed of titanium (Shellock et al). The procedure is not safe if conventional stainless-steel aneurysm clips were used. MRI entails some risk in these situations unless there is direct knowledge of the type of material that had been used. There have been several instances over the years in which physicians have rushed into the MRI room to assist an acutely ill patient, only to have their metal instruments drawn from their pockets and forcibly strike the patient or magnet.

Many types of MRI artifacts are known, most having to do with malfunctioning of the electronics of the magnetic field or of the mechanics involved in the imaging procedure (for details, see the monograph of Huk et al). Among the most common and problematic are CSF flow artifacts in the thoracic spinal cord, giving the impression of an intradural mass; distortions of the appearance of structures at the base of the brain from ferromagnetic dental appliances; and lines across the entire image, induced by blood flow and patient movement.

The MRI device is costly and requires special housing and cooling to contain its powerful magnetic field. Nevertheless, as with CT earlier, MRI machines have proliferated and the technique has become indispensable for neurologic diagnosis. In most clinical circumstances, as noted above, it is advantageous to proceed directly to MRI after the clinical analysis.

The technology of MRI is evolving constantly. The visualization of blood vessels in the brain (MR angiography, see further on), of tumors, compressive lesions, traumatic discontinuities of peripheral nerves (Filler et al), and of developmental defects of the CNS are among the more refined and promising applications of MRI. Diffusion-weighted imaging (DWI) is a new imaging procedure that takes only a minute to accomplish and can detect evidence of infarction within 2 h of the onset of a stroke; it is also particularly useful in distinguishing between cerebral metastases and abscesses. Every few months there appears some refinement in the interpretation of signal characteristics and morphologic changes as well as new ways of using this technology in the study of brain metabolism and blood flow ("functional" MRI or fMRI). These functional images taken in normal patients during the performance of cognitive and motor tasks and in those with neurologic and psychiatric disease are exposing novel patterns of cerebral activation and altering some of the traditional concepts of cortical function and localization. The capacity of MRI to quantitate the volume of anatomic structures offers the prospect of demonstrating neuronal atrophies. Physiologists and experimental psychologists are adapting MRI techniques to study changes in blood flow during nervous and mental activity.

The uses of CT scanning and MRI in the diagnosis of particular neurologic disorders are considered in their appropriate chapters (see also Gilman).

Angiography

This technique has evolved over the last 50 years to the point where it is relatively safe and an extremely valuable method for the diagnosis of aneurysms, vascular malformations, narrowed or occluded arteries and veins, arterial dissections, and angiitis. Since the advent of CT and MRI, the use of angiography has practically been limited to the diagnosis of these disorders, and refinements in the former two techniques (MR angiography and spiral and helical CT scanning, described further on) threaten to eliminate even these applications of conventional x-ray angiography.

Following local anesthesia, a needle is placed in the femoral or brachial artery; a cannula is then threaded through the needle and along the aorta and the arterial branches to be visualized. In this way, a contrast medium can be injected to visualize the arch of the aorta, the origins of the carotid and vertebral systems, and the extent of these systems through the neck and into the cranial cavity. Highly experienced arteriographers can visualize the cerebral and spinal cord arteries down to about 0.1 mm in lumen diameter (under optimal conditions) and small veins of comparable size.

Angiography is not altogether without risk. High concentrations of the injected medium may induce vascular spasm and occlusion, and clots may form on the catheter tip and embolize the artery. Overall morbidity from the procedure is about 2.5 percent, mainly in the form of worsening of a pre-existent vascular lesion or from complications at the site of artery puncture. Occasionally a frank ischemic lesion is produced, leaving the patient hemiplegic, quadriplegic, or blind; for these reasons the procedure should not be undertaken unless it is absolutely necessary. A cervical myelopathy is an infrequent but disastrous complication of vertebral artery dye injection; the problem is heralded by pain in the back of the neck immediately after injection. Progressive cord ischemia from an ill-defined vascular pathology ensues over the following hours. This same complication may occur at other levels of the cord with visceral angiography.

A refinement of radiologic technique—digital subtraction angiography—uses digital computer processing of radiologic data to produce images of the major cervical and intracranial arteries. The great advantages of this procedure are that the vessels can be visualized with relatively small amounts of dye and that this can be accomplished with smaller catheters than those used in standard angiography. The arterial route is now used exclusively for dye injection in preference to the venous route.

Magnetic Resonance and Computed Tomographic (Spiral, Helical) Angiography

These are the newest noninvasive techniques for visualizing the main intracranial arteries and can reliably detect intracranial vascular lesions and extracranial carotid artery stenosis. These techniques approach but have not yet reached the radiographic resolution of invasive angiography for distal vessels and for the fine detail of occlusive lesions, but they are very useful in gauging the patency of the large cervical and basal vessels (Fig. 2-2*G* to *I*). Unlike MR angiography, the CT technique requires the injection of intravenous dye but has the great advantage of showing blood vessels and their anomalies in relation to adjacent brain and bone. The use of these and

Figure 2-2 *(Continued)*

G. *Magnetic resonance angiogram (MRA) of the intracranial vessels (anterior-posterior projection). Visualized are the large carotid arteries ascending on either side of the smaller vertebral arteries, which join to form the basilar artery in the midline. This technique allows resolution of the middle and anterior cerebral arteries beyond their first branchings.* H. *Lateral views of the MRA showing the two large carotid arteries superimposed on each other anteriorly, giving rise to the middle and anterior cerebral arteries, and the vertebral and basilar arteries posteriorly, giving rise to the posterior cerebral arteries.* I. *Normal MRA of the cervical portions of the common, internal and external carotid arteries, and the lone, smaller vertebral artery.*

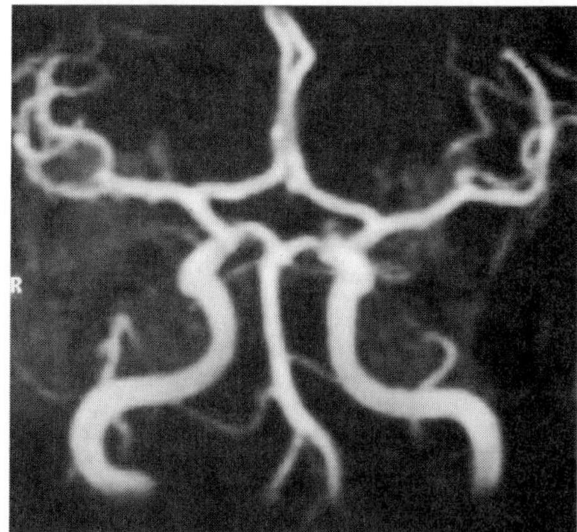

G

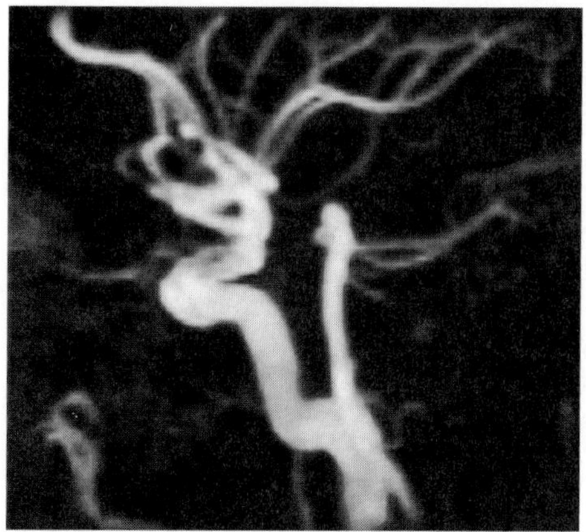

H

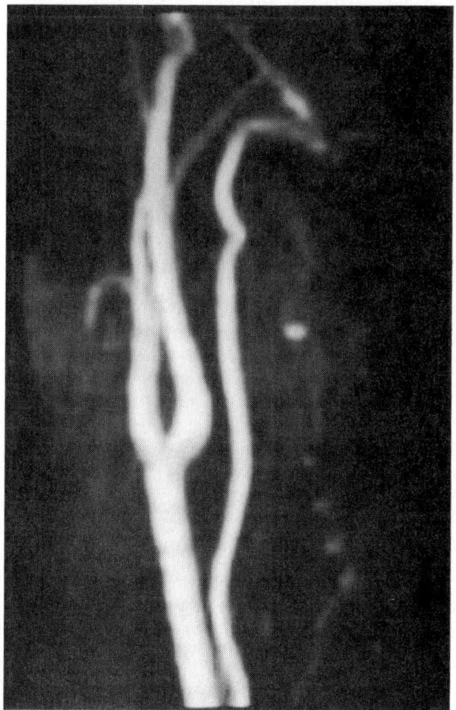

I

other methods for the investigation of carotid artery disease (ultrasound Doppler flow and imaging techniques) are discussed further in Chap. 34, on cerebral vascular disease.

Positron Emission Tomography

This technique, commonly known as PET, measures the cerebral concentration of systemically administered radioactive tracers. Positron-emitting isotopes (usually ^{11}C, ^{18}F, ^{13}N, and ^{15}O) are produced in a cyclotron or linear accelerator and incorporated into biologically active compounds in the body. The concentration of the tracers in various parts of the brain is determined noninvasively, by detectors outside the body, and tomographic images are constructed by techniques similar to those used in CT and MRI.

Local patterns of cerebral blood flow, oxygen uptake, and glucose utilization can be measured by PET scanning, and the procedure has proved to be of value in grading primary brain tumors, distinguishing tumor tissue from radiation necrosis, localizing epileptic foci, and differentiating types of dementing diseases. The ability of the technique to quantitate neurotransmitters and their receptors promises to be of importance in the study of Parkinson disease and other degenerative diseases. This technology is found in relatively few medical centers and requires costly facilities and support staff, for which reasons it is not available for routine diagnosis.

Single Photon Emission Computed Tomography (SPECT)

This technique, which has evolved from PET, utilizes isotopes that do not require a cyclotron for their production. Here also radioligands (usually containing iodine) are incorporated into biologically active compounds which, on decay, emit only a single photon. This procedure allows the study of regional cerebral blood flow under conditions of cerebral ischemia or during intense tissue metabolism. The restricted anatomic resolution provided by SPECT has limited its clinical usefulness, but its wider availability makes it appealing for clinical use. This has proved particularly true in helping to distinguish between Alzheimer dementia and a number of focal cerebral (lobar) atrophies and in the localization of epileptic foci in patients who are candidates for cortical resection. Once injected, the isotope localizes rapidly in the brain, with regional absorption proportional to blood flow, and is then stable for an hour or more. It is thus possible to inject the isotope at the time of the seizure onset, while the patient is undergoing video and EEG monitoring, and to scan the patient later. As with PET, the clinical potential of this technique has yet to be fully realized.

Ultrasound Scanning

In recent years this technique has been refined to the point where it has become the principal methodology for clinical study of the fetal and neonatal brain. The instrument for this application consists of a transducer capable of converting electrical energy to ultrasound waves of a frequency ranging from 5 to 20 kHz. These are transmitted through the intact skull into the brain. The different tissues have a variable acoustic impedance and send echoes back to the transducer, which displays them as waves of variable height or as points of light of varying intensity. In this way one can obtain images of choroid plexuses, ventricles, and central nuclear masses. Usually several coronal and parasagittal views are obtained. Intracerebral and subdural hemorrhages, mass lesions, and congenital defects can readily be visualized.

Similar instruments are used to insonate the basal vessels of the circle of Willis, the cervical carotid and vertebral arteries, and the temporal arteries for the study of cerebrovascular disease. Their greatest use is in estimating the degree of stenosis of the origin of the internal carotid artery.

This methodology has several advantages, notably that it is noninvasive, harmless (hence can be used repeatedly), convenient because of the portability of the instrument, and inexpensive. More specific applications of this technique are discussed in Chap. 38, on developmental disorders of the nervous system, and in Chap. 34, on stroke.

Contrast Myelography

By injecting 5 to 25 mL of a radiopaque dye—e.g., iopamidol (Isovue)—through a lumbar puncture needle and then tipping the patient on a tilt table, the entire spinal subarachnoid space can be visualized. The procedure is almost as harmless as the lumbar puncture except for cases of complete spinal block, in which high concentrations of dye near the block can cause pain and regional myoclonus. Ruptured lumbar and cervical discs, cervical spondylotic bars and bony spurs encroaching on the spinal cord or roots, and spinal cord tumors can be diagnosed accurately. Iophendylate (Pantopaque), a formerly used fat-soluble dye, is still approved by the FDA but is now employed only in special circumstances (e.g., visualizing the upper level of a spinal canal lesion that completely obstructs the flow of dye from below). If iophendylate is left in the subarachnoid space, particularly in the presence of blood or inflammatory exudate, it may incite a severe arachnoiditis of the spinal cord and brain.

The CT body scan also provides excellent images of the spinal canal and intervertebral foramina in three planes, making the combination of water-soluble dye and CT scanning a useful means of visualizing spinal and posterior fossa lesions (Fig. 2-1*E* and *F*). Contrast myelography is particularly useful in visualizing small areas within the spinal canal, such as the lateral recesses and spinal nerve root sleeves. MRI provides even sharper visualization of the spinal canal and its contents as well as the vertebrae and intervertebral discs. It has largely replaced contrast myelography because it does not require lumbar puncture and it images lesions (in three planes) within the spinal cord with greater clarity.

ELECTROENCEPHALOGRAPHY

The electroencephalographic examination, for many years a standard laboratory procedure in the study of all forms of cerebral disease, has to a large extent been supplanted by CT and MRI. Nevertheless, it continues to be an essential part of the study of patients with seizures and those suspected of having seizures. It is also used in evaluating the cerebral effects of many systemic metabolic diseases, in the study of sleep, and in the operating room to monitor cerebral activity in anesthetized patients. For a few diseases, such as subacute spongiform encephalopathy (page 815), it can be the defining laboratory test. It is described here in some detail, since it cannot suitably be assigned to any other single chapter.

The electroencephalograph records spontaneous electrical activity generated in the cerebral cortex. This activity reflects the electrical currents that flow in the extracellular spaces of the brain, and these, in turn, reflect the summated effects of innumerable excitatory and inhibitory synaptic potentials upon the cortical neurons. This spontaneous activity of cortical neurons is much influenced by subcortical structures, particularly the thalamus and high brainstem reticular formation. Afferent impulses from these deep structures are probably responsible for entraining cortical neurons to produce characteristic rhythmic brain-wave patterns, such as alpha rhythm and sleep spindles (see further on).

Electrodes, which are solder or silver-silver chloride discs 0.5 cm in diameter, are attached to the scalp by means of adhesive material such as collodion and conductive paste (or conductive paste alone). The electroen-cephalograph has 8 to 24 or more amplifying units capable of recording from many areas of the scalp at the same time. The amplified brain rhythms are strong enough to move an ink-writing pen, which produces waveforms of brain activity in the frequency range of 0.5 to 30 Hz (cycles per second) on paper moving at a standard speed of 3 cm/s. The resulting electroencephalogram (EEG), essentially a *voltage-versus-time graph*, is recorded as a number of parallel wavy lines, or "channels." Each channel represents the electrical potential between two electrodes (a common or ground electrode may be used as one recording site, but the channel still represents a bipolar recording). The channels are arranged for viewing into standard montages that generally compare the activity from one region of the cerebral cortex to that from the corresponding region of the opposite side. Conventional ink-written EEGs are gradually being replaced by a digital format, in which the digitized waveforms are viewed on the computer screen. The latter does not always provide the clarity of the conventional EEG but has the great advantage of providing many more channels and requiring practically no storage space.

Patients are usually examined with their eyes closed and while relaxed in a comfortable chair or bed. The ordinary EEG, therefore, represents the electrocerebral activity that is recorded under restricted circumstances, usually during the waking state, from several parts of the cerebral convexities during an almost infinitesimal segment of the person's life.

In addition to the resting record, a number of so-called activating procedures are usually carried out.

1. The patient is asked to breathe deeply 20 times a minute for 3 min. Hyperventilation, through a mechanism yet to be determined, may activate characteristic seizure patterns or other abnormalities.

2. A powerful strobe light is placed about 15 in. from the patient's eyes and flashed at frequencies of 1 to 20 per second with the patient's eyes open and closed. The occipital EEG leads may then show waves corresponding to each flash of light (photic driving, Fig. 2-3*B*) or abnormal discharges (Fig. 2-3*C*).

3. The EEG is recorded after the patient is allowed to fall asleep naturally or following sedative drugs given by mouth or by vein. Sleep is extremely helpful in bringing out abnormalities, especially where

Figure 2-3

A. *Normal alpha (9- to 10-per-second) activity is present posteriorly (bottom channel). The top channel contains a large blink artifact. Note the striking reduction of the alpha rhythm with eye opening.* B. *Photic driving. During stroboscopic stimulation of a normal subject, a visually evoked response is seen posteriorly after each flash of light (signaled on the bottom channel).* C. *Stroboscopic stimulation at 14 flashes per second (bottom channel) has produced a photoparoxysmal response in this epileptic patient, evidenced by the abnormal spike and slow-wave activity toward the end of the period of stimulation.*

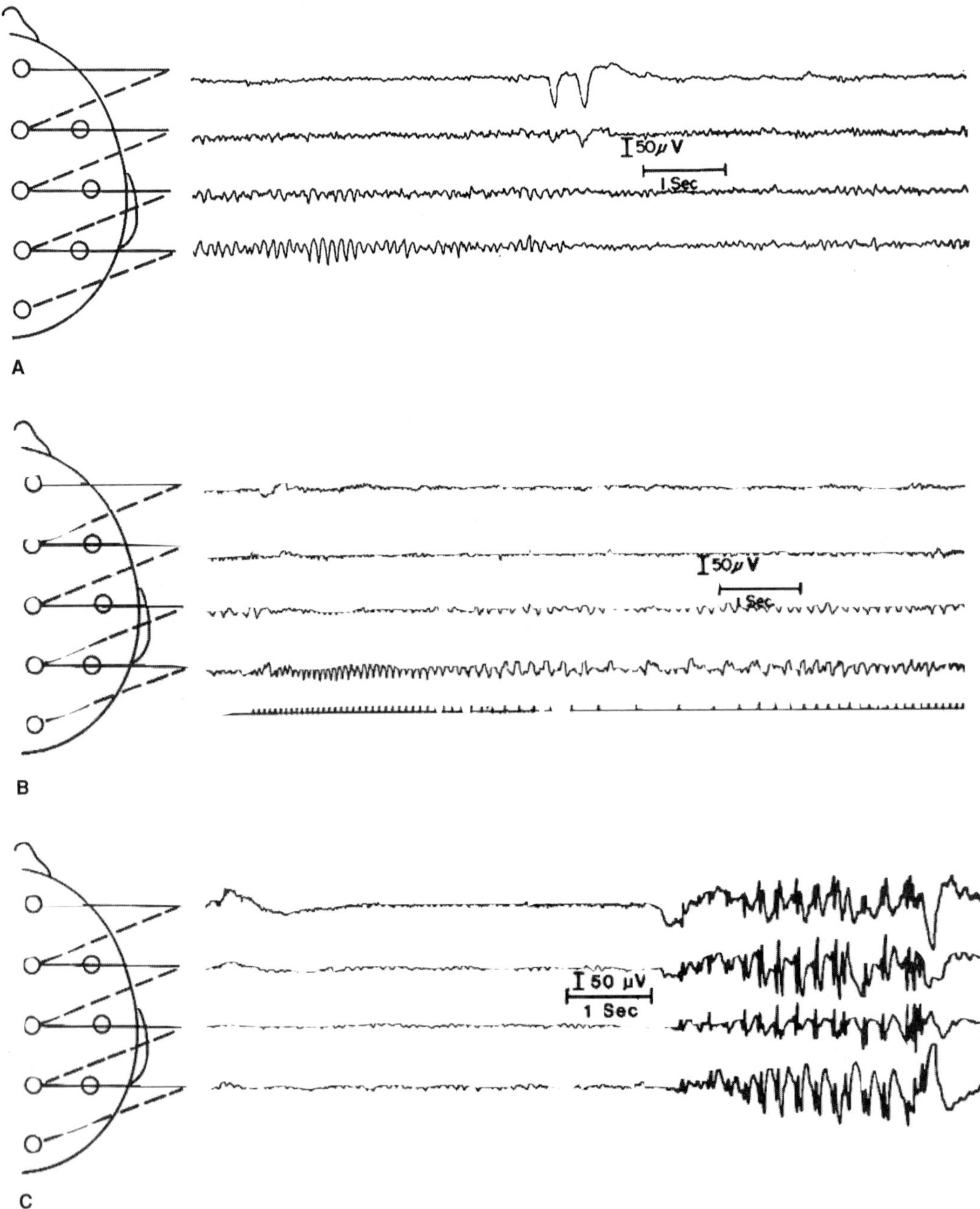

Figure 2-3 *(Continued)*

D. *An EEG from a patient with focal motor seizures of the left side. Note focal spike and wave discharge in right frontal region (channels 1 to 3). The activity from the left hemisphere (not shown here) was relatively normal.* E. *Absence seizures, showing generalized 3-per-second spike-and-wave discharge. The abnormal activity ends abruptly and normal background activity appears.* F. *Large, slow, irregular delta waves are seen in the right frontal region (channels 1 and 2). In this case a glioblastoma was found in the right cerebral hemisphere, but the EEG picture does not differ basically from that produced by a stroke, abscess, or contusion.*

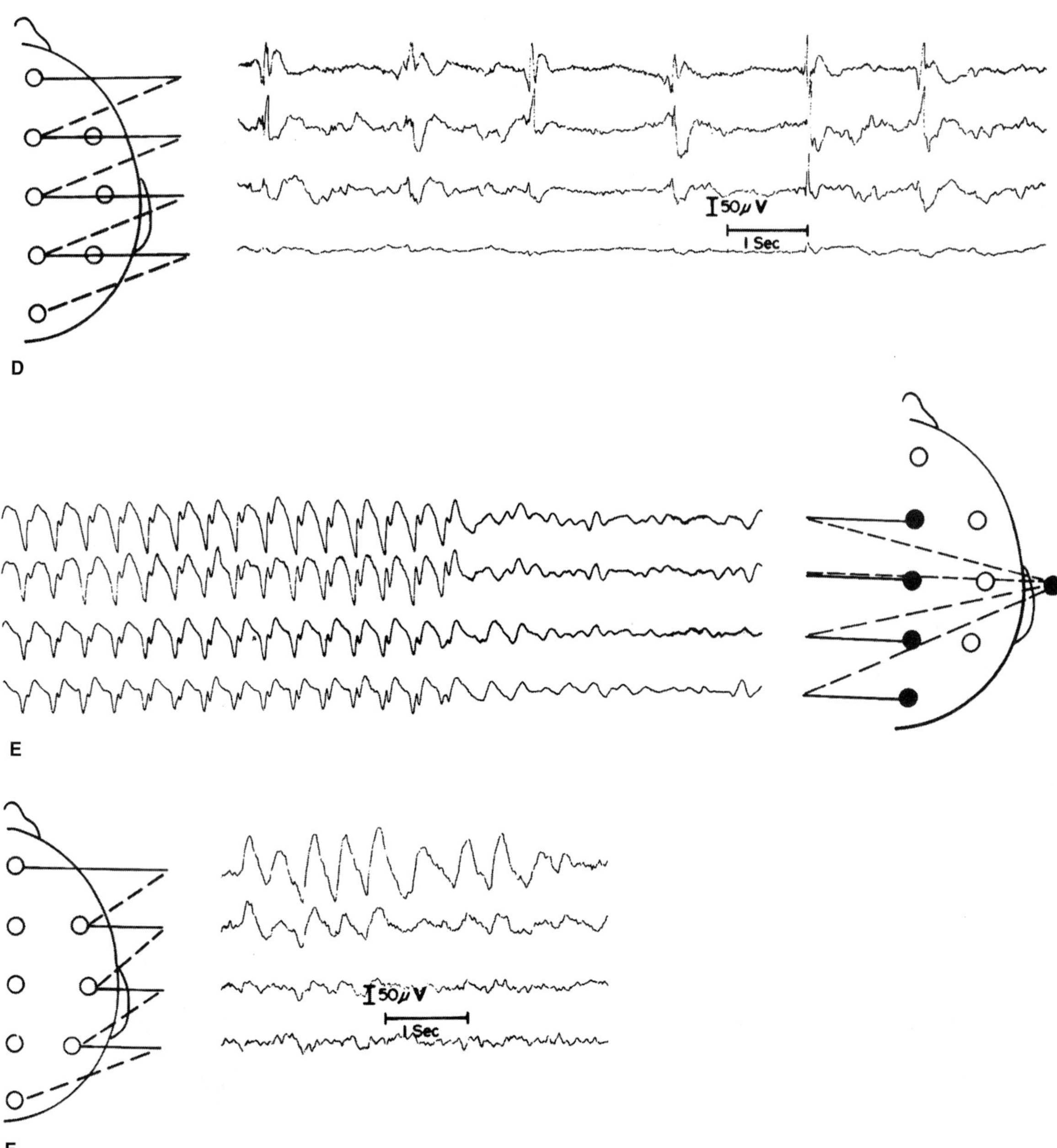

Figure 2-3 *(Continued)*

G. *Grossly disorganized background activity interrupted by repetitive "pseudoperiodic" discharges consisting of large, sharp waves from all leads about once per second. This pattern is characteristic of Creutzfeldt-Jakob disease.* H. *Advanced hepatic coma. Slow (about 2-per-second) waves have replaced the normal activity in all leads. This record demonstrates the triphasic waves sometimes seen in this disorder (channel 1).* I. *Deep coma following cardiac arrest, showing electrocerebral silence. With the highest amplification, ECG and other artifacts may be seen, so that the record is not truly "flat" or isoelectric. However, no cerebral rhythms are visible. Note the ECG (channel 5). (Illustrations courtesy of Dr. Susan Chester.)*

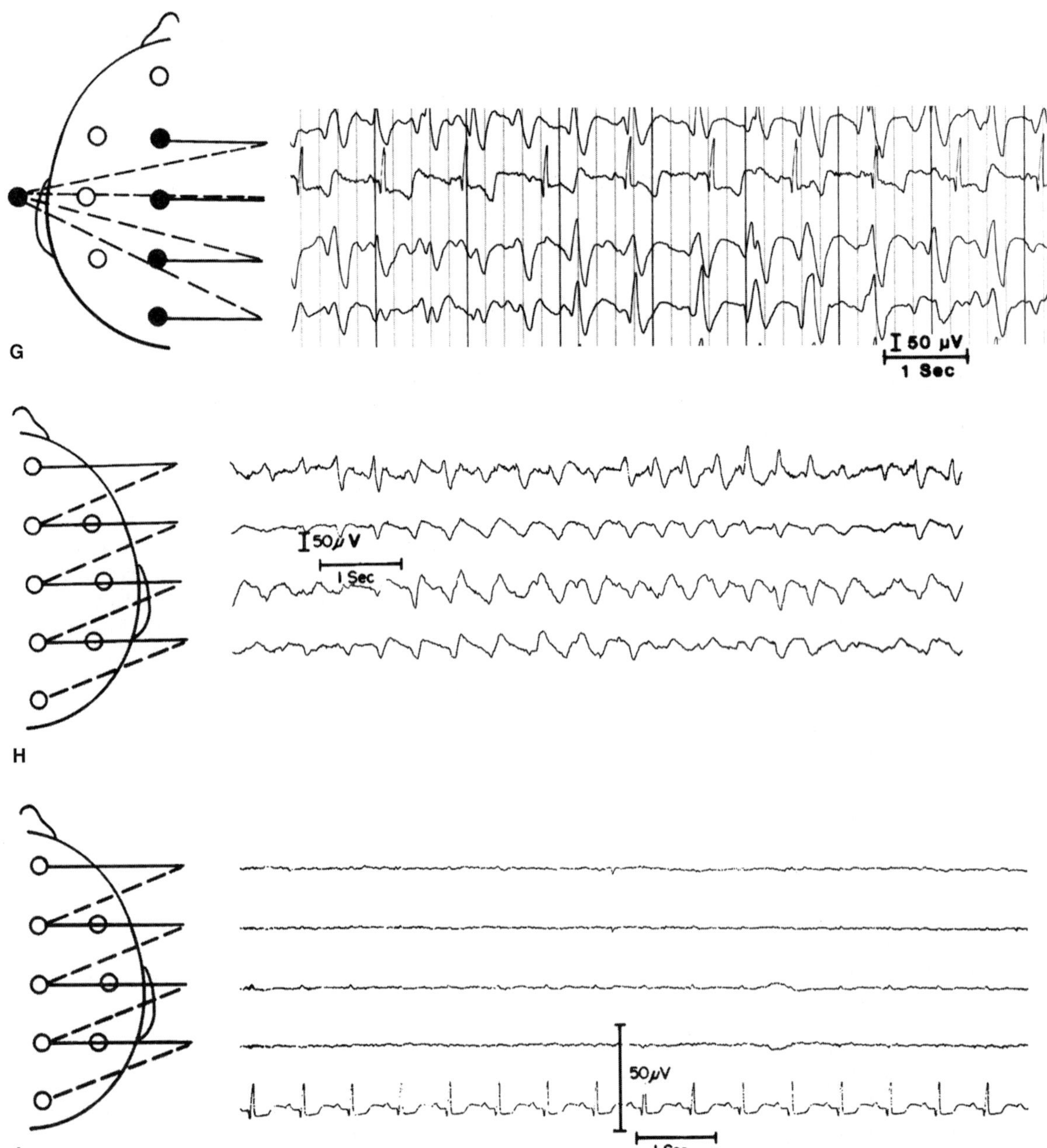

temporal lobe epilepsy and certain other seizures are suspected.

Through the medium of lengthy EEG recordings, many abnormalities associated with sleep can be demonstrated and EEG activity can be synchronized with videographically recorded seizure activity. Also important clinically are EEGs recorded by small tape recorders or telemetry from freely moving ambulatory patients with suspected seizure disorders. These techniques are discussed more fully in Chap. 16.

The EEG consists of 150 to 300 or more pages, each representing 10 s in time. It is obtained by a technician who is primarily responsible for the entire procedure, including notation of movements or other events responsible for artifacts and successive modifications of technique based upon what the record shows. Certain precautions are necessary if electroencephalography is to be most useful. The patient should not be sedated (except as noted above) and should not have been without food for a long time, for both sedative drugs and relative hypoglycemia modify the normal EEG pattern. The same may be said of mental concentration and extreme nervousness or drowsiness, all of which tend to suppress the normal alpha rhythm and increase muscle and other artifacts. When dealing with patients who are suspected of having epilepsy and are already being treated for it, most physicians prefer to record the EEG while the patient continues to receive anticonvulsant drugs. Under special circumstances these drugs may be omitted for a day or two in order to increase the chance of recording a seizure discharge.

The proper interpretation of EEGs involves the recognition of the characteristic normal and abnormal patterns and background rhythms (in accordance with the age of the patient), the detection of asymmetries and periodic changes in rhythm, and, importantly, the differentiation of artifacts from genuine abnormalities.

Types of Normal Recordings

The normal record in adults shows somewhat asymmetrical 8- to 12-per-second 50-μV sinusoidal *alpha* waves in both occipital and parietal regions. These waves wax and wane spontaneously and are attenuated or suppressed completely with eye opening or mental activity (see Fig. 2-3*A*). The frequency of the alpha rhythm is invariant for an individual patient, although the rate may slow during aging. Also, waves faster than 12 Hz and of lower amplitude (10 to 20 μV), called *beta* waves, are recorded from the frontal regions symmetrically. When the normal subject falls asleep, the alpha rhythm slows symmetrically and characteristic waveforms (vertex sharp waves and sleep spindles) appear; if sleep is induced by barbiturate or benzodiazepine drugs, an increase in the fast frequencies occurs and is considered to be normal. A small amount of theta (4- to 7-Hz) activity may normally be present over the temporal regions, somewhat more so in persons over 60 years of age. Delta (1- to 3-Hz) activity is not present in the normal waking adult.

During stroboscopic stimulation, an occipital response to each flash of light may normally be seen (*photic* or *occipital driving*). The visual response arrives in the calcarine cortex 20 to 30 ms after the flash of light. The presence of such a response indicates that the patient can at least perceive light, and if there is a claim to the contrary, the patient is either hysterical or malingering. The evoked visual responses (see further on) are an even more sensitive means of detecting hysterical blindness than occipital driving, since the latter may be absent in normal persons. Spread of the occipital response to photic stimulation, with the production of abnormal waves, provides evidence of abnormal excitability (Fig. 2-3*B* and *C*). Seizure patterns may be produced during this type of EEG testing, accompanied by gross myoclonic jerks of the face, neck, and limbs (photomyogenic or photomyoclonic response) or by major convulsions (photoparoxysmal or photoconvulsive response). Such effects occur with some frequency during periods of withdrawal from alcohol and other sedative drugs. These responses are to be differentiated from purely myoclonic ones that are produced normally by contracting scalp muscles and are often visible in the routine EEG.

Children and adolescents are more sensitive than adults to all the activating procedures mentioned. It is customary for children to develop slow activity (3 to 4 Hz) during the middle and latter parts of a period of overbreathing. This activity, referred to as "breakdown," disappears soon after hyperventilation has stopped. The frequency of the dominant rhythms in infants is normally about 3 Hz, and they are very irregular. With maturation, there is a gradual increase in frequency and regularity of these occipital rhythms; by the age of 12 to 14 years, normal alpha waves are the dominant pattern (see Chap. 28 for further discussion of maturation of the brain as expressed in the EEG). The records of infants and children are difficult to interpret because the wide range of normal patterns at each age period makes rigid classification using frequency criteria impossible (see Hahn and Tharp). Nevertheless, asymmetrical records or records with seizure patterns are clearly abnormal in children of any age. Also, normal patterns in the fetus, from the seventh month onward, have been established. Certain changes in these patterns, as described by Stockard-Pope et al and by deWeerd, are clearly indicative of a developmental disorder or disease.

Types of Abnormal Recordings

The most pathologic finding of all is the replacement of the normal EEG pattern by "electrocerebral silence," meaning that the electrical activity of the cortical mantle, recorded from the scalp, is absent. Artifacts of various types should be seen as the amplifier gains are increased; if not, there is a risk that the leads are not connected to the machine. Acute intoxication with high levels of drugs such as barbiturates can produce this sort of isoelectric EEG (Fig. 2-3*I*). However, in the absence of nervous system depressants or extreme degrees of hypothermia, a record that is "flat" (less than 2 μV except for artifacts) over all parts of the head is almost always a result of profound cerebral hypoxia or ischemia or of trauma and raised intracranial pressure. Such a patient—without EEG activity, brainstem reflexes, and spontaneous respiratory or muscular activity of any kind for 6 h or more—is said to be "brain dead." The brain of such a patient is largely necrotic, and there is no chance of neurologic recovery. The topic of brain death is discussed further in Chap. 17.

Localized regions of absent brain waves may rarely be seen when there is a particularly large area of infarction, traumatic necrosis, or tumor or when an extensive clot lies between the cerebral cortex and the electrodes. With such a finding, the EEG localization of the abnormality is reasonably precise—but, of course, the nature of the lesion is not disclosed. However, most such lesions are not large enough, relative to the recording arrangement, to abolish the brain waves, and the EEG may then record abnormal waves arising from functioning though damaged brain at the borders of the lesion.

Two types of abnormal waves, already mentioned, are of lower frequency and higher amplitude than normal. Waves of fewer than 4 Hz with amplitudes from 50 to 350 μV are called *delta* waves (Fig. 2-3*G* and *H*); those with a frequency of 4 to 7 Hz are called *theta* waves. Fast (*beta*) activity tends to be prominent frontally and usually reflects the effects of sedative drugs or, if focal, an immediately underlying skull defect (bone filters the normally abundant fast activity of the cortex). *Spikes* or *sharp waves* are transient high-voltage waveforms that have a pointed peak at conventional paper speeds and a duration of 20 to 70 ms (Fig. 2-3*D*). Spikes or sharp waves that occur interictally in epileptics or in individuals with a genetic disposition to seizures are referred to as *epileptiform discharges*.

These abnormal fast and slow waves may be combined, and when a series of them interrupts relatively normal EEG patterns in a paroxysmal fashion, they are highly suggestive of epilepsy. The ones associated with *absence seizures* are 3-per-second spike-and-wave complexes that characteristically appear in all leads of the EEG simultaneously and disappear almost as suddenly at the end of the seizure (Fig. 2-3*E*). This finding led to the theoretic localization of a pacemaker for primary generalized seizure discharges in the thalamus or other deep gray structures ("centrencephalic seizures"), but such a center has not been verified anatomically or physiologically.

Neurologic Conditions with Abnormal Electroencephalograms

Epilepsy All types of generalized epileptic seizures (grand mal and typical and atypical absence—see Chap. 16) are associated with some abnormality in the EEG provided that it is being recorded at the time of the seizure. Also, the EEG is usually abnormal during more restricted types of seizure activity. Exceptions are seizure states that originate in deep temporal, mesial, or orbital frontal foci, from which the discharge fails to reach the scalp in sufficient amplitude to be seen against the normal background activity of the EEG, particularly if there is well-developed alpha rhythm. In these cases, extra scalp leads in the anterior frontal and temporal regions (which are the most free of alpha frequencies) may pick up the discharge, especially during sleep. In some such cases, the only way in which this deep activity can be sampled is by inserting an electrode into the substance of the brain or placing a grid of electrodes in the subdural space, but this procedure is applicable only to the relatively few patients who are undergoing craniotomy. Occasionally one may fail to record an EEG abnormality in the course of one of the types of focal seizure (sensory, jacksonian, partial complex, epilepsia partialis continua) or in polymyoclonus. Presumably this means that the neuronal discharge is too deep, discrete, fast, or asynchronous to be transmitted by volume conduction through the skull and recorded via the EEG electrode, which is some 2 cm from the cortex. More often, a completely normal EEG during a seizure indicates a "pseudoseizure".

Some of the different types of seizure patterns are shown in Fig. 2-3*C*, *D*, and *E*. The absence, myoclonic, and grand mal patterns correlate closely with the clinical seizure type and may be present in milder form in the interictal EEG.

A fact of importance is that between seizures a single EEG recording will show a normal pattern in as many as 20 percent of patients with absence seizures and 40 percent of those with grand mal epilepsy (this percentage is less with repeated recordings). Anticonvulsant therapy also tends to diminish the interictal EEG abnormalities. The records of another 30 to 40 percent of epileptics, though abnormal between seizures, are nonspecifically so; therefore the diagnosis of epilepsy can be made only by the correct interpretation of clinical data in relation to the EEG abnormality.

Brain Tumor, Abscess, Subdural Hematoma, and Encephalitis Intracranial mass lesions are associated with characteristic abnormalities in the EEG, depending on their type and location, in some 90 percent of patients. In addition to diffuse changes, the classic abnormalities are focal or localized slow-wave activity (usually delta, as in Fig. 2-3*F*) or, occasionally, seizure activity and decreased amplitude and synchronization of normal rhythms. Although the EEG may be diagnostically helpful in cases of brain tumor or abscess, particularly when integrated with the other laboratory and clinical findings, reliance is now placed almost exclusively on CT and MRI.

However, EEG may be of considerable value in the diagnosis of herpes simplex encephalitis; periodic high-voltage sharp waves and slow-wave complexes at intervals of 2 to 3 per second in the temporal regions are characteristic. The other infectious encephalitides are often associated with sharp or spike activity, particularly if there have been seizures. The highly characteristic pattern of Creutzfeldt-Jakob disease is shown in Fig. 2-3*G*.

Cerebrovascular Disease The EEG is now little used in the differential diagnosis of vascular hemiplegia. The main practical value of the EEG lies in its ability to distinguish an acute lesion in the distribution of the internal carotid or other major cerebral artery, which produces an area of slowing in the appropriate region. By contrast, with a lacunar infarction deep in the cerebrum or brainstem, the surface EEG is usually normal despite prominent clinical abnormalities. After 3 to 6 months, roughly 50 percent of patients with infarction in the territory of the middle cerebral artery have a normal EEG. Perhaps half these patients will have had normal EEGs even in the week or two following the stroke. A persistent abnormality is associated with a poor prognosis for further recovery. Large lesions of the diencephalon or midbrain produce bilaterally synchronous slow waves, but those of the pons and medulla (i.e., below the mesencephalon) are usually associated with a normal or near-normal EEG pattern despite catastrophic clinical changes.

Cerebral Trauma A brief episode of cerebral concussion in animals is accompanied by a transitory disturbance in the EEG, but in humans this is usually no longer evident by the time a recording can be made. Large cerebral contusions produce EEG changes similar to those described for cerebral infarction. Diffuse changes often give way to focal ones, especially if the lesions are on the superolateral surfaces of the brain, and these, in turn, usually disappear over a period of weeks or months. Sharp waves or spikes sometimes emerge as the focal slow-wave abnormality resolves and may precede the occurrence of posttraumatic epilepsy; serial EEGs may be of prognostic value in this regard. They may also aid in evaluating patients for subdural hematoma.

Diseases That Cause Coma and States of Impaired Consciousness The EEG is abnormal in almost all conditions in which there is impairment of consciousness. There is a fairly close correspondence between the severity of acute anoxic damage from cardiac arrest and the degree of EEG slowing. The mildest forms are associated with generalized theta activity, intermediate forms with widespread delta waves and the loss of normal background activity, and the most severe forms with "burst suppression," in which the recording is almost isoelectric for several seconds, followed by high-voltage sharp and irregular delta activity.

The term *alpha coma* refers to a unique EEG pattern in which an apparent alpha activity in the 8- to 12-Hz range is distributed widely over the hemispheres rather than posteriorly. When analyzed carefully, this apparent alpha, unlike the normal rhythm, is found not to be monorhythmic; instead, it varies in frequency in a narrow band. This is usually a transitional pattern after global anoxia; less often, alpha coma may be seen with acute large pontine lesions. Both burst suppression and alpha coma are usually transitional patterns leading to severe generalized slowing and voltage reduction or to electrocerebral silence. With severe *hypothyroidism*, the brain waves are normal in configuration but usually of decreased frequency.

In altered states of consciousness, the more profound the depression of consciousness, in general, the more abnormal the EEG recording. In states of deep stupor or coma, the slow (delta) waves are bilateral and of high amplitude and tend to be more conspicuous over the frontal regions (Fig. 2-3*H*). This pertains in such differing conditions as acute meningitis or encephalitis and disorders that severely derange blood gases, glucose, electrolytes, and water balance; uremia; diabetic coma; and impairment of consciousness accompanying the large cerebral lesions discussed above. In *hepatic coma*, the degree of abnormality in the EEG corresponds closely with the degree of confusion, stupor, or coma. Characteristic of hepatic coma are paroxysms of bilaterally synchronous large, sharp "triphasic waves" (Fig. 2-3*H*), although such waveforms may also be seen with encephalopathies related to renal or pulmonary failure and with acute hydrocephalus.

An EEG may also be of help in the diagnosis of coma when the pertinent history is unavailable. Perhaps its greatest value in this situation is the disclosure of status epilepticus in the absence of obvious convulsions ("spike-wave stupor," epileptic fugue state). It may also point to an otherwise unexpected cause, such as hepatic encephalopathy, intoxication with barbiturates or other sedative-hypnotic drugs, the effects of diffuse anoxia-ischemia, or hysteria (in which case the EEG is normal).

Diffuse Degenerative Diseases Alzheimer disease and other degenerative diseases that cause serious impairment of cerebrocortical function are accompanied by relatively slight degrees of diffuse slow-wave abnormality in the theta (4- to 7-Hz) range. More rapidly progressive disorders—such as subacute sclerosing panencephalitis (SSPE), Creutzfeldt-Jakob disease, and to a lesser extent the cerebral lipidoses—often have, in addition, very characteristic and almost pathognomonic EEG changes consisting of periodic bursts of high-amplitude sharp waves, usually bisynchronous and symmetrical (Fig. 2-3*G*). In a negative sense, a normal EEG in a patient who is profoundly apathetic is a point in favor of the diagnosis of catatonia, an affective disorder, or schizophrenia (see below).

Other Diseases of the Cerebrum Many disorders of the brain cause little or no alteration in the EEG. Multiple sclerosis and other demyelinating diseases are examples, though as many as 50 percent of advanced cases will have an abnormal record of nonspecific type (focal or diffuse slowing). Delirium tremens and Wernicke-Korsakoff disease, despite the dramatic nature of the clinical picture, cause little or no change in the EEG. Some degree of slowing usually accompanies confusional states that have been designated by some clinicians as hypokinetic delirium (Chap. 20). Interestingly, the neuroses, psychoses (such as manic-depressive disorders or schizophrenia), intoxication with hallucinogenic drugs such as LSD, and the majority of cases of mental retardation are associated either with no modification of the normal record or with only minor nonspecific abnormalities unless seizures are present.

Clinical Significance of Minor EEG Abnormalities

The gross EEG abnormalities discussed above are by themselves clearly abnormal, and any formulation of the patient's clinical state should attempt to account for them. These abnormalities include seizure discharges, generalized and extreme slowing, definite slowing with a clear-cut asymmetry or a focus, and absence of normal rhythms. Lesser degrees of these abnormalities form a continuum between the undoubtedly abnormal and the completely normal and are of correspondingly minor significance. Findings such as 14- and 6-per-second positive spikes, small sharp waves, scattered 5- or 6-per-second slowing, voltage asymmetries, and persistence of "breakdown" for a few minutes after hyperventilation are interpreted as *borderline*. The latter abnormalities may be meaningful, but only if correlated with particular clinical phenomena. Whereas borderline deviations in an otherwise entirely normal person have no clinical significance, the same EEG findings associated with particular clinical signs and symptoms—even if they, too, are of minimal severity—become important. The significance of a normal or "negative" EEG in certain patients suspected of having a cerebral lesion has been discussed above.

In summary, the results of the EEG, like those of the EMG and electrocardiogram, are meaningful only in relation to the clinical state of the patient at the time the recordings were made.

Evoked Potentials

The stimulation of sense organs or peripheral nerves evokes a response in the appropriate cortical receptive areas and a number of subcortical relay stations as well. However, one cannot place a recording electrode near the relay stations, nor can one detect tiny potentials of only a few microvolts among the much larger background activity in the EEG or EMG. The use of averaging methods, introduced by Dawson in 1954, and the subsequent development of computer techniques have provided the means of overcoming these problems. Initially, emphasis was on the study of late waves (over 75 ms after the stimulus) because they are of high amplitude and easy to obtain. However, there is more clinical utility in recording the much smaller, so-called short-latency waveforms, which are modified at each nuclear relay station and recorded by distant electrodes ("far-field recording"). These waveforms are maximized by the computer to a point where their latency and voltage can easily be measured. One of the most remarkable properties of evoked potentials is their resistance to anesthesia, sedative drugs, and—in comparison with EEG activity—even damage of the cerebral hemispheres. This permits their use for monitoring the integrity of cerebral pathways in situations that render the EEG useless. The details of these techniques are reviewed in the monograph edited by Chiappa. The interpretation of afferent evoked potentials (visual, auditory, and somatosensory) is based on the prolongation of the latencies of the waveforms after the stimulus, the interwave latencies, and asymmetries in timing. Norms have been established, but it is still advisable to confirm these in each laboratory. Typically 2.5 or 3 standard deviations above the mean latency for any measurement is taken as the definition of abnormality (Table 2-2). The amplitudes of the waves are less informative.

Table 2-2
Main sensory evoked potential latencies from stimulus, milliseconds[a]

Type of evoked potential	*Mean*	*Upper limit (mean + 2.5 S.D.)*
PSVER (*70-min check size*)		
P100 absolute latency	104	118
Intereye difference	2	8
BAER (*60 dBSL, 10/s monoaural stimuli*)		
Interwave latency		
I–III	2.1	2.6
III–V	1.9	2.4
I–V	4.0	4.7
Interside difference for most latencies	0.1	0.4
SSEP—median nerve (*wrist stimulation*)		
Absolute latency		
Erb's point	9.7	12.0
P/N 13 (cervicomedullary)	13.5	16.3
N 19/P 21 (cortical)	19.0	22.1
Interwave latency		
Erb's-P/N 13	3.8	5.2
P/N 13–N 19	5.5	4.7
Interside difference		
P/N 13–N 19	0.3	1.1
SSEP—tibial nerve (*ankle stimulation; Fz-Cz recording; 165-cm height; absolute latencies are shorter for stimulation at the knee*)		
Absolute latency		
Lumbar point (cauda equina)	20	25
N/P 37 (cortex)	36	42.5
Interwave latency		
Lumbar–N/P 37	16.4	21.6
Interside difference		
Lumbar–N/P 37	0.7	1.9

[a]Norms must be verified in each laboratory; in most instances they are sensitive to the technique and stimulus used and to height in the cases of limb stimulation. PSVER, pattern shift visual evoked response; BAER, brainstem auditory evoked response; SSEP, somatosensory evoked response.

Visual Evoked Potentials For many years it had been known that a light stimulus flashing on the retina often initiates a discernible waveform over the occipital lobes. In the EEG, such responses to fast rates of stimulation are referred to as the occipital driving response (Fig. 2-3*B* and *C*). In 1969, Regan and Heron observed that a visual evoked response could be produced by the sudden change of a viewed checkerboard pattern. The responses produced in this way, by rapidly repeating the pattern reversal, were easier to detect and measure than flash responses and more consistent in waveform from one individual to another. It became apparent that this type of stimulus, applied first to one eye and then to the other, could demonstrate conduction delays in the visual pathways of patients who had formerly suffered a disease of the optic nerve—even though in some instances there were no residual signs of reduced visual acuity, visual field abnormalities, alterations of the optic nerve head, or changes in pupillary reflexes.

This procedure, called pattern-shift visual evoked responses (PSVER) or pattern-reversal visual evoked potentials, has been widely adopted as one of the most delicate tests of lesions in the visual system. Figure 2-4 illustrates the normal PSVER and two types of delayed responses. Usually, abnormalities in the amplitude and duration of PSVER accompany the abnormally prolonged latencies, but they are difficult to quantify. The expected latency for the positive polarity PSVER is near 100 ms (thus the term "P 100"); an absolute latency over approximately 118 ms or a difference in latencies of greater than 9 ms between the two eyes signifies involvement of one optic nerve (Table 2-2). Bilateral prolongation of latencies, demonstrated by separate stimulation of each eye, can be due to lesions in both optic nerves, in the optic chiasm, or in the visual pathways posterior to the chiasm.

As indicated above, PSVER is especially valuable in proving the existence of active or residual disease of an optic nerve. Examinations of large numbers of patients who were known to have had retrobulbar (optic) neuritis showed that among 51 such patients, only 4 had normal latencies (Shahrokhi and coworkers). These authors found similar abnormalities of PSVER in about one-third of multiple sclerosis patients who had no history or clinical evidence of optic nerve involvement. The finding of abnormal PSVER in a patient with a clinically apparent lesion elsewhere in the CNS may usually be taken as evidence of multiple sclerosis.

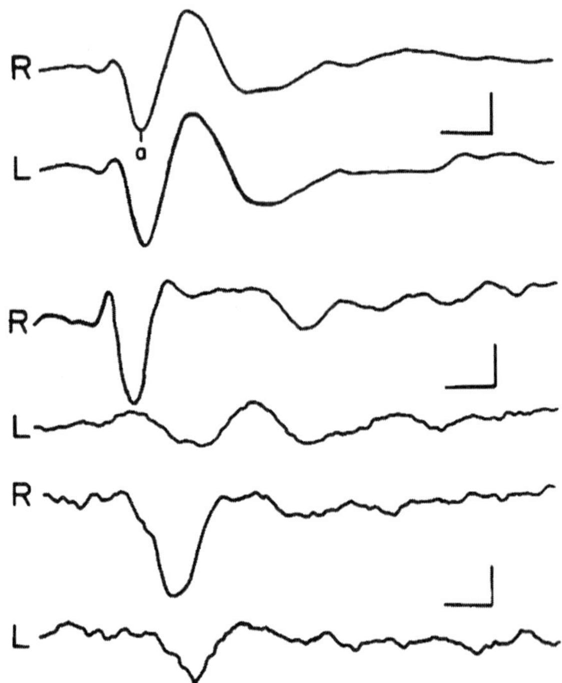

Figure 2-4

Pattern-shift visual evoked responses (PSVER). Latency measured to first major positive peak (a). *Upper two tracings: These, from the right and left eyes, are normal. Middle tracings: PSVER from the right eye is normal but the latency of the response from the left eye is prolonged and its duration is increased. Lower tracings: PSVER from both eyes show abnormally prolonged latencies, somewhat greater on the left than on the right. Calibration: 50 ms, 2.5 μV. (Adapted by permission from Shahrokhi et al.)*

A compressive lesion of an optic nerve will have the same effect as a demyelinative one. Many other diseases of the optic nerves—including toxic and nutritional amblyopias, ischemic optic neuropathy, and the Leber type of hereditary optic neuropathy—show abnormalities of the PSVER. Glaucoma and other diseases involving structures anterior to the retinal ganglion cells may also produce increased latencies. Impaired visual acuity has little effect on the latency but does correlate well with the amplitude of the PSVER. By presenting the pattern-shift stimulus to one hemifield, it is sometimes possible to isolate a lesion to an optic tract or radiation, or one occipital lobe, but with less precision than that provided by the usual monocular test.

Brainstem Auditory Evoked Potentials The effects of auditory stimuli can be studied in the same way as visual ones by a procedure called *brainstem auditory evoked responses* or *potentials* (BAERs or BAEPs). Between 1000 and 2000 clicks, delivered first to one ear and then to the other, are recorded through scalp electrodes and maximized by computer. A series of seven waves appears at the scalp within 10 ms after each stimulus. On the basis of depth recordings and the study of lesions produced in cats as well as pathologic studies of the brainstem in humans, it has been determined that each of the first five waves is generated by the brainstem structures indicated in Fig. 2-5. The generators of waves VI and VII are uncertain. Clinical interpretations of BAERs are based mainly on latency measurements of waves I, III, and V. The most important are the interwave latencies between I and III and III and V (see Table 2-2). The presence of wave I and its absolute latency are of particular value in testing the integrity of the auditory nerve.

Figure 2-5

Short-latency brainstem auditory evoked responses (BAERs). Diagram of the proposed electrophysiologic-anatomic correlations in human subjects. Waves I through V are the ones measured in clinical practice.

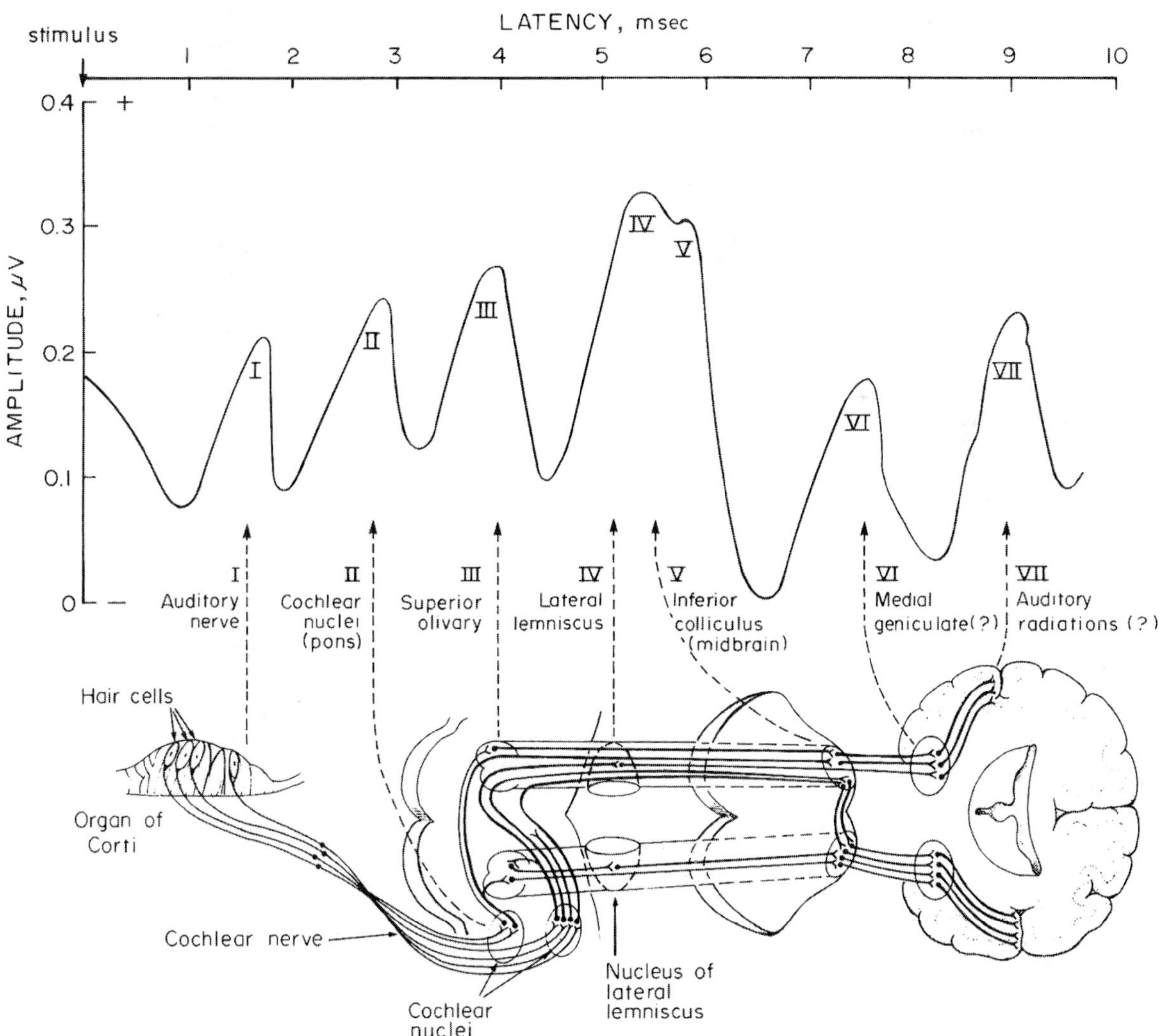

A lesion that affects one of the relay stations or its immediate connections manifests itself by a delay in its appearance and an absence or reduction in amplitude of subsequent waves. These effects are more pronounced on the side of the stimulated ear than contralaterally. This is difficult to understand, since a majority of the cochlear-superior olivary-lateral lemniscal-medial geniculate fibers cross to the opposite side. It is also surprising that a severe lesion of one relay station would allow impulses, even though delayed, to continue their ascent and be recordable in the cerebral cortex.

As indicated above, BAEPs are a particularly sensitive means of detecting lesions of the eighth cranial nerve (acoustic neuroma and other tumors of the cerebellopontine angle) and of the auditory pathways of the brainstem. Almost one-half of patients with definite multiple sclerosis and a lesser number with a possible or probable diagnosis of this disease will show abnormalities of the BAEPs (usually a prolongation of interwave latencies I-III or III-V), even in the absence of clinical symptoms and signs of brainstem disease. The BAEPs are also useful in assessing hearing in infants who have been exposed to ototoxic drugs, in young children, and in hysterical patients who feign deafness.

Somatosensory Evoked Potentials *Somatosensory evoked potentials* (SEPs) are used in most clinical neurophysiology laboratories to confirm lesions in the somatic sensory systems. The technique consists of applying 5-per-second painless transcutaneous electrical stimuli to the median, peroneal, and tibial nerves and recording the evoked potentials (for the upper limb) over Erb's point above the clavicle, over the C-2 spine and over the opposite parietal cortex, and (for the lower limb) over the lumbar and cervical spines and the opposite parietal cortex. The impulses generated in large touch fibers by 500 or more stimuli and averaged by computer can be traced through the peripheral nerves, spinal roots, and posterior columns to the nuclei of Burdach and Goll in the lower medulla, through the medial lemniscus to the contralateral thalamus, and thence to the sensory cortex of the parietal lobe. Delay between the stimulus site and Erb's point or lumbar spine indicates peripheral nerve disease; delay from Erb's point (or lumbar spine) to C-2 implies an abnormality in the appropriate nerve roots or more frequently in the posterior columns; the presence of lesions in the medial lemniscus and thalamoparietal pathway can be inferred from delays of subsequent waves recorded from the parietal cortex (Fig. 2-6). The normal waveforms are designated by the symbol P (positive) or N (negative), with a number indicating the interval of time in milliseconds from stimulus to recording (e.g., N 11, N 13, P 13, P 22, etc.). As shorthand for the polarity and approximate latency, the summated wave that is recorded at the cervicomedullary junction is termed "N/P 13," and the cortical potential from median nerve stimulation is seen in two contiguous waves of opposite polarity, called "N 19–P 22." The corresponding cortical wave after tibial or peroneal nerve stimulation is called "N/P 37."

For purposes of clinical interpretation, the SEPs are assumed to be linked in series, so that interwave abnormalities in latency indicate a conduction defect between the generators of the two peaks involved (Chiappa and Ropper). Normal values are shown in Table 2-2. Recordings with pathologically verified lesions at these levels are to be found in the monograph by Chiappa. This test has been most helpful in establishing the existence of lesions in spinal roots, posterior columns, and brainstem in disorders such as the Guillain-Barré syndrome, ruptured lumbar and cervical discs, multiple sclerosis, and lumbar and cervical spondylosis even when the clinical data are uncertain. The counterpart also pertains—namely, that obliteration of the cortical waves (assuming that all preceding waves are unaltered) reflects profound damage to the somatosensory pathways in the hemisphere or to the cortex itself. As a corollary, the bilateral absence of cortical somatosensory waves after cardiac arrest is a powerful predictor of a poor clinical outcome. Likewise, the persistent absence of a cortical potential after stroke usually indicates such profound damage that only a limited clinical recovery is to be expected.

Evoked potential techniques have also been used in the experimental study of olfactory sensation (see Chap. 12).

Transcranial Motor Cortex Stimulation

It is now possible, by using single-pulse high-voltage magnetic stimulation, to directly activate the motor cortex and cervical spine segments and to detect delays or lack of conduction in descending motor pathways. This technique, introduced by Marsden and associates, painlessly stimulates only the largest motor neurons (presumably Betz cells) and the fastest-conducting axons. Cervical cord stimulation is believed to activate the anterior roots. The difference in time between the motor cortical and cervical activation of hand or forearm muscles represents the conduction velocity of the cortical–cervical cord motor neurons. Berardelli and colleagues, who have applied the technique to 20 hemi-

Figure 2-6

*Short-latency SSEPs produced by stimulation of the **median nerve** at the wrist. The set of responses shown at left is from a normal subject; the set at right is from a patient with multiple sclerosis who had no sensory symptoms or signs. In the patient, note the preservation of the brachial-plexus component (EP), the absence of the cervical-cord (N 11) and lower-medullary components (N/P 13), and the latency of the thalamocortical components (N 19 and P 22), prolonged markedly above the normal mean +3 SD for the separation from the brachial plexus. Unilateral stimulation occurred at a frequency of 5 per second. Each trace is the averaged response to 1024 stimuli; the superimposed trace represents a repetition to demonstrate waveform consistency. Recording-electrode locations are as follows: FZ denotes midfrontal; EP, Erb's point (the shoulder); C2, the middle back of the neck over the C2 cervical vertebra; and Cc, the scalp overlying the sensoriparietal cortex contralateral to the stimulated limb.*

Relative negativity at the second electrode caused an upward trace deflection. Amplitude calibration marks denote 2 μV. (Reproduced by permission from Chiappa and Ropper.)

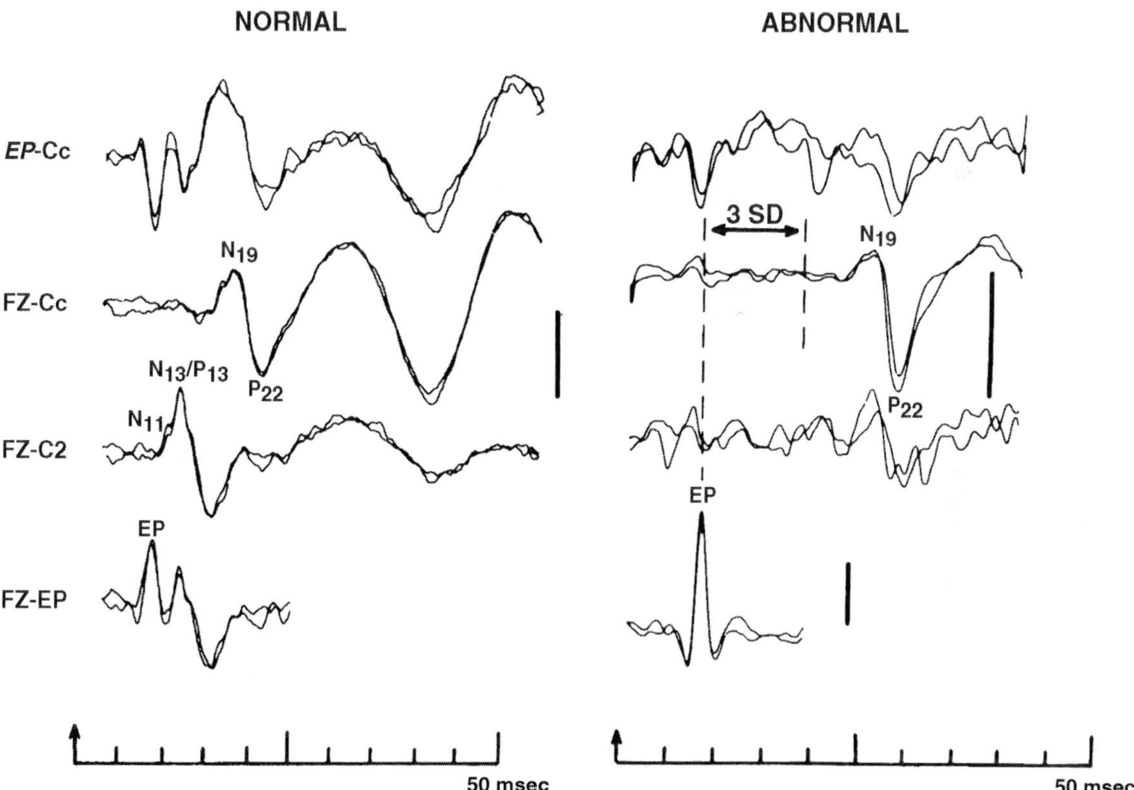

plegic patients with cerebrovascular lesions, found that in 15 there was no descending influence in comparison with the normal side. Although the degree of functional deficit does not correlate with the degree of electrophysiologic change, one expects that refinements of this technique will be useful in evaluating the status of the corticospinal motor system as well as other cortically based functions.

Endogenous Event-Related Evoked Potentials

Among the very late brain electrical potentials (>100-ms latency), which can be extracted from background activity by computer methods, are a group that cannot be classified as sensory or motor but rather as psychophysical responses to environmental stimuli. These responses are of very low voltage, often fleeting and inconsistent, and of unknown anatomic origin. The most studied types occur approximately 300 ms (P 300) after an attentive subject identifies an unexpected or novel stimulus that has been inserted into a regular train of stimuli. Almost any modality can be used and the potential occurs even when a stimulus has been omitted from a regular pattern. The amplitude of the response depends on the difficulty of the task and has an inverse relationship to the frequency of the unexpected or "odd" event; the latency depends on the task difficulty and other features of testing. There is therefore no single P 300; instead, there are numerous components, depending on the experimental paradigm. A prolongation of the latency is found with aging and in dementia as well as with degenerative diseases such as Parkinson disease, progressive supranuclear palsy, and Huntington chorea, and the amplitude is depressed in schizophrenia and depression. The potential has been interpreted by some as a reflection of the subject's orienting behavior or attention, and by others, including Donchin, who discovered the phenomenon, as related to updating the brain's representation of the environment. The P 300 remains a curiosity for the clinical neurologist because abnormalities are detected only when large groups are compared to normals, and the technique is hardly as standardized as the conventional evoked potentials. A review of the subject can be found in sections by Altenmüller and Gerloff and by Polich in the Niedermeyer and Lopes DaSilva text on electroencephalography.

Electromyography and Nerve Conduction Studies

These are discussed in Chap. 45.

Psychometry, Perimetry, Audiometry, and Tests of Labyrinthine Function

These methods are used in quantitating and defining the nature of the psychologic or sensory deficits produced by disease of the nervous system. The indications for doing these tests are (1) to obtain confirmation of a disorder of function in particular parts of the nervous system and to ascertain its nature or (2) to quantitate the disorder and to determine, by subsequent examinations, the course of the underlying illness. A description of these methods and their clinical use will be found in the chapters dealing with developmental disorders of the cerebrum (Chap. 28), dementia (Chap. 21), and disorders of vision (Chap. 13) and of hearing and equilibrium (Chap. 15).

Biopsy of Muscle, Nerve, Skin, Temporal Artery, Brain, and Other Tissue

The application of light, phase, and electron microscopy to the study of these tissues may be highly informative. The findings are discussed in Chaps. 45 (muscle), 46 (nerve), and 37 (skin and conjunctivum in the diagnosis of storage diseases). Temporal artery biopsy is indicated when giant cell arteritis is suspected. Brain biopsy, aside from the direct sampling of a suspected neoplasm, is often diagnostic in cases of granulomatous angiitis, some forms of encephalitis, subacute spongiform encephalopathy (biopsy performed infrequently because of the risk of transmitting the infectious agent), and a number of other rare diseases. An important advance in recent years has been the use of CT-guided stereotactic biopsy, which is particularly valuable in tumor diagnosis and exposes the patient to less risk than does a craniotomy and open biopsy. In choosing to perform a biopsy in any of these clinical situations, the paramount issue is the likelihood of establishing a definitive diagnosis—one that would permit successful treatment or otherwise enhance the management of the disease.

REFERENCES

Altenmüller EO, Gerloff C: Psychophysiology and the EEG, in Niedermeyer E, Lopes DaSilva F (eds): *Electroencephalography: Basic Principles, Clinical Applications, and Related Fields*, 4th ed. Baltimore, Williams & Wilkins, 1999, pp 637–665.

American Electroencephalographic Society: Guidelines in electroencephalography, evoked potentials, and polysomnography. *J Clin Neurophysiol* 11:1–147, 1994.

Barnett GH, Ropper AH, Johnson KA: Physiological support and monitoring of critically ill patients during magnetic resonance imaging. *J Neurosurg* 68:246, 1988.

Barrows LJ, Hunter FT, Banker BQ: The nature and clinical significance of pigments in the cerebrospinal fluid. *Brain* 78:59, 1955.

Berardelli A, Inghilleri M, Manfredi M, et al: Cortical and cervical stimulation after hemispheric infarctions. *J Neurol Neurosurg Psychiatry* 50:861, 1987.

Bigner SH: Cerebrospinal fluid (CSF) cytology: Current status and diagnostic applications. *J Neuropathol Exp Neurol* 51:235, 1992.

Blume WT: *Atlas of Pediatric Electroencephalography*. New York, Raven Press, 1982.

Chiappa KH (ed): *Evoked Potentials in Clinical Medicine*, 3rd ed. Philadelphia, Lippincott-Raven, 1997.

Chiappa KH, Ropper AH: Evoked potentials in clinical medicine. *N Engl J Med* 306:1140, 1205, 1982.

Chimowitz MI, Logigian EL, Caplan LR: The accuracy of bedside neurological diagnoses. *Ann Neurol* 28:78, 1990.

Daly DD, Pedley TA (eds): *Current Practice of Clinical EEG*, 2nd ed. New York, Raven Press, 1990.

Dawson GD: A summation technique for the detection of small evoked potentials. *Electroencephalogr Clin Neurophysiol* 6:65, 1954.

deWeerd AW: *Atlas of EEG in the First Months of Life*. New York, Elsevier, 1995.

den Hartog-Jager WA: *Color Atlas of CSF Cytopathology*. New York, Elsevier-North Holland, 1980.

Dufresne JJ: *Cytopathologie de CSF*. Basel, Ciba Foundation, 1973.

Filler AG, Kliot M, Howe FA, et al: Application of magnetic resonance in the evaluation of patients with peripheral nerve pathology. *J Neurosurg* 85:299, 1996.

Fishman RA: *Cerebrospinal Fluid in Diseases of the Nervous System*, 2nd ed. Philadelphia, Saunders, 1992.

Gilman S: Imaging of the brain. *N Engl J Med* 338:812, 889, 1998.

Goldenshohn ES, Wolf S, Koszer S, Legatt A (eds): *EEG Interpretation*, 2nd ed. New York, Futura, 1998.

Greenberg JO (ed): *Neuroimaging: A Companion to Adams and Victor's Principles of Neurology*, 2nd ed. New York, McGraw-Hill, 1999.

Hahn JS, Tharp BR: Neonatal and pediatric electroencephalography, in Aminoff MJ (ed): *Electrodiagnosis in Clinical Neurology*, 4th ed. New York, Churchill Livingstone, 1999, pp 81–128.

Horowitz AL: *MRI Physics for Radiologists*, 2nd ed. New York, Springer, 1992.

Hughes JR: *EEG in Clinical Practice*, 2nd ed. Woburn, MA, Butterworth, 1994.

Huk WN, Gademann G, Friedman G: *MRI of Central Nervous System Diseases*. Berlin, Springer Verlag, 1990.

Kanal E, Gillen J, Evans JA, et al: Survey of reproductive health among female MR workers. *Radiology* 187:395, 1993.

Latchaw RE (ed): *MRI and CT Imaging of the Head, Neck, and Spine*, 2nd ed. St. Louis, Mosby–Year Book, 1991.

Marsden CD, Merton PA, Morton HB: Direct electrical stimulation of corticospinal pathways through the intact scalp and in human subjects. *Adv Neurol* 39:387, 1983.

Modic MT, Masaryk TJ, Ross JS, et al: *Magnetic Resonance Imaging of the Spine*, 2nd ed. St. Louis, Mosby–Year Book, 1994.

Newton TH, Hasso AN, Dillon WP (eds): *Modern Neuroradiology*: Vol 3. *Computed Tomography of the Head and Neck*. San Anselmo, CA, Clavadel Press, 1988.

Polich J: P300 in clinical applications, in Niedermeyer E, Lopes DaSilva F (eds): *Electroencephalography: Basic Principles, Clinical Applications, and Related Fields*, 4th ed. Baltimore, Williams & Wilkins, 1999, pp 1073–1091.

Regan D, Heron JR: Clinical investigation of lesions of the visual pathway: A new objective technique. *J Neurol Neurosurg Psychiatry* 32:479, 1969.

Scher MS, Painter MJ: Electroencephalographic diagnosis of neonatal seizures, in Wasterlain CG, Vert P (eds): *Neonatal Seizures*. New York, Raven Press, 1990.

Shahrokhi F, Chiappa KH, Young RR: Pattern shift visual evoked responses. *Arch Neurol* 35:65, 1978.

Shellock FG, Morisoli S, Kanal E: MR procedures and biomedical implants, materials, and devices: 1993 update. *Radiology* 189:587, 1993.

Stockard-Pope JE, Werner SS, Bickford RG: *Atlas of Neonatal Electroencephalography*, 2nd ed. New York, Raven Press, 1992.

Thompson EJ: Cerebrospinal fluid. *J Neurol Neurosurg Psychiatry* 59:349, 1995.

Part 2

CARDINAL MANIFESTATIONS OF NEUROLOGIC DISEASE

Section 1

DISORDERS OF MOTILITY

The control of motor function, to which much of the human nervous system is committed, is accomplished through the integrated action of a vast array of segmental and suprasegmental motor neurons. As originally conceived by Hughlings Jackson in 1858, purely on the basis of clinical observations, the motor system is organized hierarchically in three levels, each higher level controlling the one below. It was Jackson's concept that the spinal and brainstem neurons represent the lowest, simplest, and most closely organized motor centers; that the motor neurons of the posterior frontal region represent a more complex and less closely organized second motor center; and that the prefrontal parts of the cerebrum are the third and highest motor center. This scheme is still regarded as being essentially correct, though Jackson failed to recognize the importance of the parietal lobe and basal ganglia in motor control.

Since Jackson's time, physiologists have repeatedly analyzed these three levels of motor organization and have found their relationships to be remarkably complex. Motor and sensory systems, although separated for practical clinical purposes, are not independent entities but are closely integrated. Without sensory feedback, motor control is ineffective. And at the higher cortical levels of motor control, motivation, planning, and other frontal lobe activities that subserve volitional movement are always preceded and modulated by activity in the parietal sensory cortex.

Motor activities include not only those that alter the position of a limb or other part of the body (isotonic contraction) but also those that stabilize posture (isometric contraction). Movements that are performed slowly are called *ramp movements*. Very rapid movements, too fast for sensory control, are called *ballistic*. Another way of classifying movements, stressed by Hughlings Jackson, is in terms of their automaticity: reflex movements are the most automatic, willed movements the least. Physiologic studies, cast in their simplest terms, indicate that the following parts of the nervous system are engaged primarily in the control of movement and, in the course of disease, yield a number of characteristic derangements.

1. *The large motor neurons in the anterior horns of the spinal cord and the motor nuclei of the brainstem.* The axons of these nerve cells comprise the anterior spinal roots, the spinal nerves, and the cranial nerves, and they innervate the skeletal muscles. These nerve cells and their axons constitute the primary, or lower, motor neurons, complete lesions of which result in a loss of all movement—voluntary, automatic, postural, and reflex. The lower motor neurons are the *final common path* by which all neural impulses are transmitted to muscle.

2. *The motor neurons in the frontal cortex adjacent to the rolandic fissure* connect with the spinal motor neurons by a system of fibers known, because of their collective shape in transverse sections through the medulla, as the *pyramidal tract.* Since the motor fibers that extend from the cerebral cortex to the spinal cord are not confined to the pyramidal tract, they are more accurately designated as *the corticospinal tract*, or, alternatively, as *the upper motor neurons*, to distinguish them from the lower motor neurons.

3. *Several brainstem nuclei that project to the spinal cord, notably the pontine and medullary reticular nuclei, vestibular nuclei, and red nuclei.* These nuclei and

their descending fibers subserve the neural mechanisms of posture and movement, particularly when movement is highly automatic and repetitive. Certain of these brainstem nuclei are influenced by the motor or premotor regions of the cortex, e.g., via corticoreticulospinal relays.

4. *Two subcortical systems, the basal ganglia (striatum, pallidum, and related structures, including the substantia nigra and subthalamic nucleus)* and the *cerebellum.* Each system plays an important role in the control of muscle tone, posture, and coordination of movement by virtue of its connections, via thalamocortical fibers, with the corticospinal system and other descending cortical pathways.

5. *Several other parts of the cerebral cortex, particularly the premotor and supplementary motor cortices.* These structures are involved in the programming (i.e., the sequencing and modulation) of voluntary movement.

6. *The prefrontal cortex, which is involved in the planning and initiation of willed movement.* Fibers from the prefrontal cortex project to the supplementary and premotor cortex and provide the motor signals to these more strictly motor areas. Similarly, certain *parietal cortical areas (superior parietal lobule)* supply the somatic sensory information that activates the premotor and supplementary motor cortices and leads to directed movement. In addition, other parts of the nervous system concerned with tactile, visual, and auditory sensation are connected by fiber tracts with the motor cortex. These association pathways provide their own sensory regulation of motor function.

The impairments of motor function that result from lesions in these various parts of the nervous system may be subdivided into (1) paralysis (or paresis) due to affection of lower motor neurons, (2) paralysis due to affection of upper motor (corticospinal) neurons, (3) apraxic or nonparalytic disturbances of purposive movement due to involvement of association pathways in the cerebrum, (4) involuntary movements and abnormalities of posture due to disease of the basal ganglia, and (5) abnormalities of coordination (ataxia) due to lesions in the cerebellum. The first two types of motor disorder and the apraxic disorders of movement are discussed in Chap. 3; "extrapyramidal" motor abnormalities are discussed in Chap. 4; and disorders of coordination in Chap. 5. A miscellaneous group of movement disorders—tremor, myoclonus, spasms, and tics—and disorders of stance and gait are considered in Chaps. 6 and 7. Impairment or loss of motor function due to primary disease of peripheral nerves and striated muscle or to a failure of neuromuscular transmission forms the subject matter of Chaps. 46 to 55.

Chapter 3

MOTOR PARALYSIS

Definitions

The term *paralysis* is derived from the Greek words *para*, "beside, off, amiss," and *lysis*, a "loosening" or "breaking up." In medicine it has come to refer to an abolition of function, either sensory or motor. When applied to motor function, *paralysis* means loss of voluntary movement due to interruption of one of the motor pathways at any point from the cerebrum to the muscle fiber. A lesser degree of paralysis is spoken of as *paresis*, but in everyday medical parlance *paralysis* may stand for either partial or complete loss of function. The word *plegia* comes from a Greek word meaning "to strike," and the word *palsy* from an old French word that has the same meaning as *paralysis*. All these words are used interchangeably, though generally one uses *paralysis* or *plegia* for severe or complete loss of motor function and *paresis* for partial loss.

THE LOWER MOTOR NEURON

Anatomic and Physiologic Considerations

Each spinal and cranial motor nerve cell, through the extensive arborization of the terminal part of its efferent fiber, comes into contact with only a few or up to 100 or more muscle fibers; together, they constitute *the motor unit*. All variations in the force, range, rate, and type of movement are determined by the number and size of motor units called into action and the frequency and sequence of firing of each motor unit. Feeble movements involve relatively few small motor units; powerful movements recruit many more units of increasing size. When a motor neuron becomes diseased, as in progressive spinal muscular atrophy, it may manifest increased irritability, i.e., the axon is unstable and capable of ectopic impulse generation, and all the muscle fibers that it controls may discharge sporadically, in isolation from other units. The result of contraction of one or several such units is a visible twitch, or *fasciculation*, which can be recognized in the electromyogram (EMG) as a large spontaneous muscle action potential. Simultaneous or sequential spontaneous contractions of multiple motor units cause a rippling of muscle, a condition known as *myokymia*. If the motor neuron is destroyed, all the muscle fibers that it innervates undergo profound atrophy—namely, *denervation atrophy*. Within a few days after interruption of a motor nerve, the individual denervated muscle fibers begin to contract spontaneously. This isolated activity of individual muscle fibers is called *fibrillation*. Inability of the isolated fiber to maintain a stable membrane potential is a more likely explanation. Fibrillation is so fine that it cannot be seen through the intact skin, but it can be recorded as a small, repetitive, short-duration potential in the EMG (Chap. 45).

The motor nerve fibers of each ventral root intermingle with those of neighboring roots to form plexuses, and although the muscles are innervated roughly according to segments of the spinal cord, each large muscle comes to be supplied by two or more roots. In contrast, a single peripheral nerve usually provides the complete motor innervation of a muscle or group of muscles. For this reason, paralysis due to disease of the anterior horn cells or anterior roots usually has a different pattern than paralysis following interruption of a peripheral nerve.

All motor activity, even the most elementary reflex type, requires the synchronous activity of many muscles. Analysis of a relatively simple movement, such as clenching the fist, conveys some idea of the complexity of the underlying neuromuscular arrangements. In this act the primary movement is a contraction of the flexor muscles of the fingers, the flexor digitorum sublimis and profundus, the flexor pollicis longus and brevis, and the abductor pollicis brevis. In the terminology of Beevor, these muscles act as *agonists*, or *prime movers*. In order for flexion to be smooth and forceful, the extensor muscles (*antagonists*) must relax at the same rate as the flexors contract (reciprocal innervation, or Sherrington's law). The muscles that flex the fingers also flex the wrist; since it is desired that only the fingers flex, the extensors of the wrist must be brought into play to prevent its flexion. In this particular act, the wrist extensors function as *synergists*. Last, during this action of the hand, appropriate flexor and extensor muscles stabilize the wrist, elbow, and shoulder; muscles that accomplish this serve as *fixators*. The coordination of agonists, antagonists, synergists, and fixators is effected mainly by segmental spinal reflexes under the guidance of proprioceptive sensory stimuli. In general, the more delicate the movement, the more precise must be the coordination between agonist and antagonist muscles.

All movements are effected by the activation of motor neurons, large ones supplying large motor units and small ones, small motor units. The latter are more efficiently activated by sensory afferents from muscle spindles, more tonically active, and more readily recruited in reflex activities, postural maintenance, walking, and running. The large motor units participate mainly in phasic movements, which are characterized by an initial burst of activity in the agonist muscles, then a burst in the antagonists, followed by a third burst in the agonists. The strength of the initial agonist burst determines the speed and distance of the movement, but there is always the same triphasic pattern of agonist, antagonist, and agonist activity (Hallett et al). The basal ganglia and cerebellum set the pattern and timing of the muscle action in any projected motor performance. These points are discussed further in Chaps. 4 and 5.

Unlike phasic movements, certain basic motor activities do not involve reciprocal innervation. In support of the body in an upright posture, when the legs must act as rigid pillars, and in shivering, agonists and antagonists contract simultaneously. Locomotion requires that the extensor pattern of reflex standing be inhibited and that the coordinated pattern of alternating stepping movements be substituted; the latter is accomplished by multisegmental spinal and brainstem reflexes, the so-called locomotor centers. Suprasegmental control of the axial and proximal limb musculature (antigravity postural mechanisms) is mediated primarily by the reticulospinal and vestibulospinal tracts and manipulatory movements of the distal extremity muscles, by the rubrospinal and corticospinal tracts. These aspects of motor function are also elaborated further on.

Tendon reflex activity and muscle tone depend on the status of the large motor neurons of the anterior horn (the *alpha motor neurons*), the muscle spindles and their afferent fibers, and the small anterior horn cells (*gamma neurons*) whose axons terminate on the small intrafusal muscle fibers within the spindles. Each anterior horn cell has on its surface membrane approximately 10,000 synaptic terminals (boutons). Some of these terminals are excitatory, others inhibitory; in combination, they determine the activity of the neuron. The largest neurons, in Rexed layer IX (see Fig. 8-1*B*), innervate large muscles with large motor units. Smaller anterior horn cells innervate small muscles and control more delicate movements, particularly those in the fingers and hand. *Beta motor neurons* effect cocontraction of both spindle and nonspindle fibers, but the physiologic significance of this phenomenon is not fully understood. Some of the gamma neurons are tonically active at rest, keeping the intrafusal (nuclear chain) muscle fibers taut and sensitive to active and passive changes in muscle length. A tap on a tendon stretches or perhaps causes a vibration of the spindle and activates its nuclear bag fibers. Afferent projections from these fibers synapse with alpha motor neurons in the same and adjacent spinal segments; these neurons, in turn, send impulses to the skeletal muscle fibers, resulting in the familiar monosynaptic muscle contraction or monophasic (myotatic) stretch reflex (Fig. 3-1). All this occurs within 25 ms of sudden stretch. The alpha neurons of antagonist muscles are simultaneously inhibited, but through disynaptic rather than monosynaptic connections. Mainly this is accomplished through the Renshaw cells, which are stimulated by recurrent collateral branches from alpha motor neurons. Renshaw cell axons end on inhibitory synapses of alpha motor neurons (recurrent inhibition).

Thus the setting of the spindle fibers and the state of excitability of the alpha and gamma neurons (influenced greatly by descending fiber systems) determine the level of activity of the tendon reflexes and muscle tone (the responsiveness of muscle to stretch.) Other mechanisms, of an inhibitory nature, involve the Golgi tendon organs, for which the stimulus is tension produced by active contraction of muscle. These encapsulated receptors, which lie in the tendinous and aponeurotic insertions of muscle, activate afferent fibers that end on internuncial cells, which, in turn, project to alpha motor neurons, thus forming a disynaptic reflex arc. Golgi tendon receptors are silent in relaxed muscle and during passive stretch; they serve, together with muscle spindles, to monitor or calibrate the length and force of muscle contraction under different conditions. They also play a role in naturally occurring limb movements, particularly in locomotion.

Figure 3-1

Patellar tendon reflex. Sensory fibers of the femoral nerve (spinal segments L2 and L3) mediate this myotatic reflex. The principal receptors are the muscle spindles, which respond to brisk stretching of the muscle effected by tapping the patellar tendon. Afferent fibers from muscle spindles are shown entering only the L3 spinal segment, while afferent fibers from the Golgi tendon organ are shown entering only the L2 spinal segment. In this monosynaptic reflex, afferent fibers entering spinal segments L2 and L3 and efferent fibers issuing from the anterior horn cells of these and lower levels complete the reflex arc. Motor fibers shown leaving the S2 spinal segment and passing to the hamstring muscles demonstrate the disynaptic pathway by which inhibitory influences are exerted upon an antagonistic muscle group during the reflex.

The small diagram below illustrates the gamma loop. Gamma efferent fibers pass to the polar portions of the muscle spindle. Contractions of the intrafusal fibers in the polar parts of the spindle stretch the nuclear bag region and thus cause an afferent impulse to be conducted centrally. The afferent fibers from the spindle synapse with many alpha motor neurons, the peripheral processes of which pass to extrafusal muscle fibers, thus completing the loop. Both alpha and gamma motor neurons are influenced by descending fiber systems from supraspinal levels. (Adapted by permission from Carpenter MB, Sutin J: Human Neuroanatomy, 8th ed. Baltimore, Williams & Wilkins, 1983.)

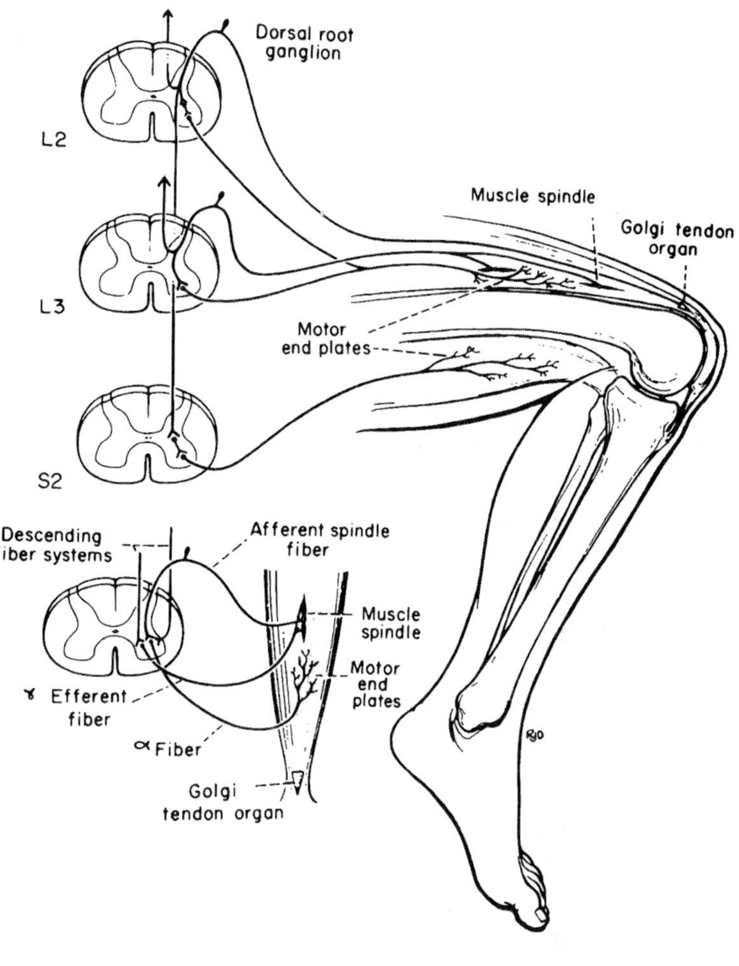

The alpha neurons of the medial parts of the anterior horn supply trunk or axial muscles, and neurons of the lateral parts supply the appendicular muscles. Both groups of alpha neurons receive projections from neurons in the intermediate Rexed layers (V to VIII) and from propriospinal neurons in the fasciculi proprii of adjacent spinal segments (see Fig. 8-1*B*). All the facilitatory and inhibitory influences supplied by cutaneous and proprioceptive afferent and descending suprasegmental neurons are coordinated at segmental interneuronal levels in such activities as phasic and tonic reflexes, flexor withdrawal and crossed extensor reflexes, postural support, tonic neck and lumbar reflexes, and more complex synergies such as rhythmic stepping (e.g., the reflex stepping of neonates). For details, see Burke and Lance and also Davidoff (1992).

There is also considerable information concerning the pharmacology of motor neurons. The large neurons of the anterior horns of the spinal cord contain high concentrations of choline acetyltransferase and utilize acetylcholine as their transmitter. Glycine is the neurotransmitter released by Renshaw cells, which are responsible for recurrent inhibition, and by interneurons that mediate reciprocal inhibition during reflex action. Gamma-aminobutyric acid (GABA) serves as the inhibitory neurotransmitter of interneurons in the posterior horn. L-glutamate and L-aspartate are released by primary afferent terminals and interneurons and act specifically on excitatory amino acid receptors. There are also descending cholinergic, adrenergic, and dopaminergic axons, which play a less well defined role in reflex functions.

Paralysis Due to Lesions of the Lower Motor Neurons

If all or practically all peripheral motor fibers supplying a muscle are interrupted, all voluntary, postural, and reflex movements of that muscle are abolished. The muscle becomes lax and soft and does not resist passive stretching, a condition known as *flaccidity*. Muscle tone—the slight resistance that normal relaxed muscle offers to passive movement—is reduced (*hypotonia* or *atonia*). The denervated muscle undergoes extreme atrophy, being reduced to 20 or 30 percent of its original bulk within 3 to 4 months. The reaction of the muscle to sudden stretch, as by tapping its tendon, is lost (*areflexia*). Affection of only a portion of the motor fibers supplying the muscle results in partial paralysis, or paresis, and a proportionate diminution in the speed of contraction. The atrophy will be less and the tendon reflex will be reduced instead of lost. The electrodiagnosis of denervation depends upon finding fibrillations, fasciculations, and other abnormalities on needle electrode examination. These abnormalities appear several days or a week or two after nerve injury (see Chap. 45).

Lower motor neuron paralysis is the direct result of loss of function or destruction of anterior horn cells or their axons in anterior roots and nerves. The signs and symptoms vary according to the location of the lesion. In any individual case, the most important clinical question is whether sensory changes coexist. The combination of a flaccid, areflexic paralysis and sensory changes usually indicates involvement of mixed motor and sensory nerves or of both anterior and posterior roots. If sensory changes are absent, the lesion must be situated in the anterior gray matter of the spinal cord, in the anterior roots, in a purely motor branch of a peripheral nerve, or in motor axons alone. At times it may be impossible to distinguish between nuclear (spinal) and anterior root (radicular) lesions.

Acute and profound spinal cord lesions and, to a lesser extent, corticospinal lesions in the brainstem and cerebrum temporarily abolish spinal myotatic reflexes ("spinal shock"). This is due to the interruption of descending tonic excitatory impulses, which normally maintain a sufficient level of excitation in spinal motor neurons to permit the peripheral activation of segmental reflexes. Preserved and often heightened tendon reflexes and spasticity in muscles weakened by lesions of the corticospinal systems attest to the integrity of the spinal segments below the level of the lesion.

THE UPPER MOTOR NEURONS

Anatomic and Physiologic Considerations

The terms *pyramidal, corticospinal*, and *upper motor neuron* are often used interchangeably, although they are not altogether synonymous. The pyramidal tract, strictly speaking, designates only those fibers that course longitudinally in the pyramid of the medulla oblongata. Of all the fiber bundles in the brain, the pyramidal tract has been known for the longest time, the first accurate description having been given by Turck in 1851. It descends from the cerebral cortex; traverses the subcortical white matter (corona radiata), internal capsule, cerebral peduncle, basis pontis, and pyramid of the upper medulla; decussates in the lower medulla; and continues its caudal course in the lateral funiculus of the spinal cord—hence the alternative name *corticospinal tract*. This is the only *direct* long-fiber connection between the cerebral cortex and the spinal cord (Fig. 3-2). The *indirect* pathways through which the cortex influences spinal motor neurons are the corticorubrospinal, corticoreticulospinal, corticovestibulospinal, and corticotectospinal; these tracts do not run in the pyramid. All of these pathways, direct and indirect, are embraced by the term *upper motor neuron*.

A major source of confusion about the pyramidal tract stems from the traditional view, formulated at the turn of the century, that it originates entirely from the large motor cells of Betz in the fifth layer of the precentral convolution, or area 4 of Brodmann (Figs. 3-3 and 22-1). However, there are only some 25,000 to 35,000 Betz cells, whereas the medullary pyramid contains about 1 million axons (Lassek). The pyramidal tract, therefore, contains many fibers that arise from cortical neurons other than Betz cells, particularly those in Brodmann areas 4 and 6 (the frontal cortex immediately rostral to area 4, including the posterior portion of the superior frontal gyrus, i.e., the supplementary motor area); in the primary somatosensory cortex (Brodmann's areas 3, 1, and 2); and in the superior parietal lobule (areas 5 and 7). Data concerning the origin of the pyramidal tract in humans are scanty, but in the monkey, by counting the pyramidal axons that remained after cortical excisions and long survival periods, Russell and DeMyer found that 40 percent of the descending axons arose in the parietal lobe, 31 percent in area 4, and the remaining 29 percent in area 6. Studies of retrograde transport of tracer substance in the monkey have confirmed these findings.

Fibers from the motor and premotor cortices (Brodmann areas 4 and 6, Fig. 22-1), supplementary motor cortex, and portions of parietal cortex (areas 1, 3,

Figure 3-2

Corticospinal and corticobulbar tracts. Variable lines indicate the trajectories of these pathways, from their origin in particular parts of the cerebral cortex to their nuclei of termination.

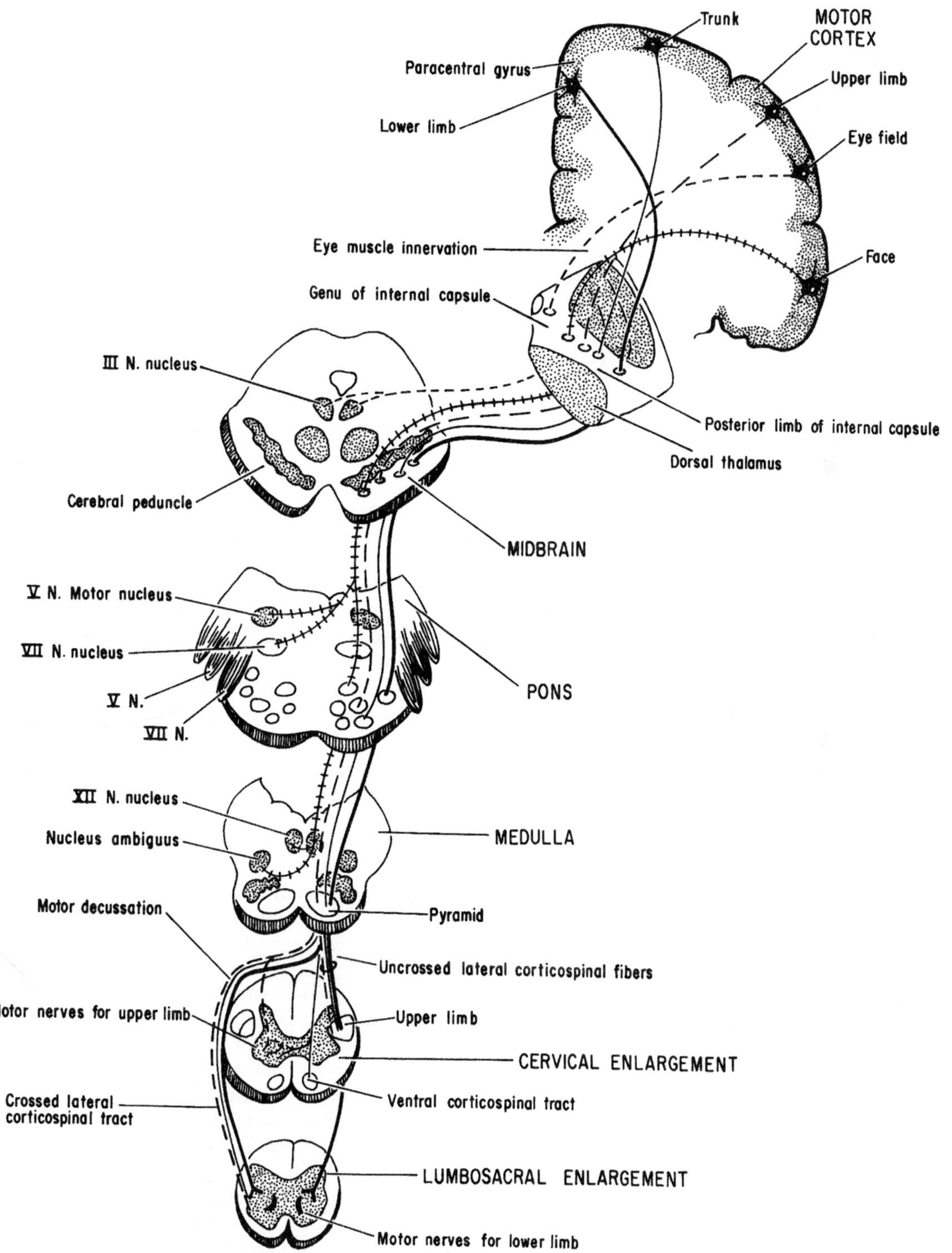

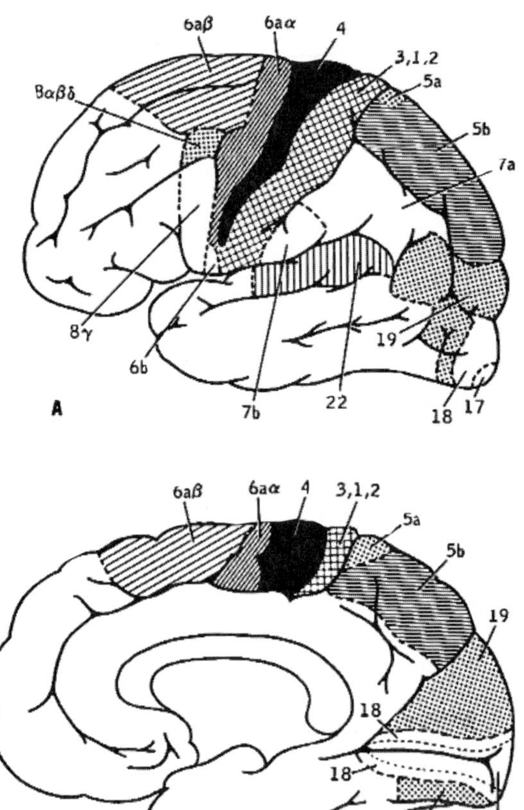

Figure 3-3

Lateral (A) and medial (B) surfaces of the human cerebral hemispheres, showing the areas of excitable cortex, i.e., areas, numbered according to the scheme of Brodmann, from which movement can be elicited by electrical stimulation. (Reprinted with permission from House EL, Pansky B: A Functional Approach to Neuroanatomy, *2nd ed. New York, McGraw-Hill, 1967.)*

5, and 7) converge in the corona radiata and descend through the posterior limb of the internal capsule, basis pedunculi, basis pontis, and medulla. As the corticospinal tracts descend in the cerebrum and brainstem, they send collaterals to the striatum, thalamus, red nucleus, cerebellum, and reticular formations. Accompanying the corticospinal tracts in the brainstem are the corticobulbar tracts, which are distributed to motor nuclei of the cranial nerves, ipsilaterally and contralaterally (Fig. 3-2). Iwatsubo and colleagues, using histologic techniques, have traced the direct projection of axons of cortical neurons to the trigeminal, facial, ambiguus, and hypoglossal nuclei. No axons were seen to terminate directly in the oculomotor, trochlear, abducens, or vagal nuclei. Insofar as the corticobulbar and corticospinal fibers have a similar origin and the motor nuclei of the brainstem are the homologues of the motor neurons of the spinal cord, the term *upper motor neurons* may suitably be applied to both these systems of fibers.

The corticospinal tracts *decussate* at the lower end of the medulla, although some of their fibers may cross above this level. The proportion of crossed and uncrossed fibers varies to some extent from one person to another. Most textbooks state that 75 to 80 percent of the fibers cross and that the remainder descend ipsilaterally, mostly in the uncrossed ventral corticospinal tract. In exceptional cases, these tracts cross completely; equally rarely, they remain uncrossed. These variations are probably of functional significance in determining the amount of neurologic deficit that results from a unilateral lesion such as capsular infarction.

Beyond their decussation, the corticospinal pathways descend as well-defined bundles in the anterior and posterolateral columns of white matter (funiculi) of the spinal cord (Fig. 3-2). The course of the noncorticospinal motor pathways (vestibulospinal, reticulospinal, and descending propriospinal) have been traced in man by Nathan and his colleagues. The lateral vestibulospinal tract lies at the periphery of the cord, where it occupies the most anterolateral portion of the anterior funiculus. The medial vestibulospinal fibers mingle with those of the medial longitudinal fasciculus. Reticulospinal fibers are less compact; they descend bilaterally, and most of them come to lie just anterior to the lateral corticospinal tract. The descending propriospinal pathway consists of a series of short fibers (one or two segments long) lying next to the gray matter.

The *somatotopic organization* of the corticospinal system is of importance in clinical work, especially in relation to certain stroke syndromes. As the descending axons subserving limb and facial movements emerge from the cortical motor strip, they maintain the anatomic specificity of the overlying cortex; therefore, a discrete cortical-subcortical lesion will result in a restricted weakness of the hand and arm or the foot and leg. More caudally the descending motor fibers converge and are collected in the posterior limb of the internal capsule, so that even a small lesion there may cause a "pure motor hemiplegia," in which the face, arm, hand, leg and foot are affected to more or less the same degree (page 851). The axons subserving facial movement are situated rostrally in the posterior limb of the capsule, those for hand and arm in the central port and those for foot and leg, caudally (see Brodal).

This topographic distribution is more or less maintained in the cerebral peduncle, where the corticospinal fibers occupy approximately the middle of the peduncle, the fibers destined to innervate the facial nuclei lying most medially. More caudally, in the basis pontis, the descending motor tracts separate into bundles that are interspersed with masses of pontocerebellar neurons and their cerebellopetal fibers. A somatotopic organization can be recognized here as well, exemplified by selective weakness of the face and hand with dysarthria, or of the leg, which may occur with pontine lacunar infarctions. Anatomic studies in nonhuman primates indicate that arm-leg distribution of fibers in the rostral pons is much the same as in the basis pedunculi; in the caudal pons this distinction is less well defined. In man, a lack of systematic study leaves the precise somatotopic organization of corticospinal fibers in the pons uncertain.

The descending pontine bundles, now devoid of their corticopontine fibers, reunite to form the medullary pyramid. The brachial-crural pattern may persist in the pyramids and is certainly reconstituted in the lateral columns of the spinal cord (Fig. 8-3), but it should be emphasized that the topographic separation of motor fibers at cervical, thoracic, lumbar, and sacral levels is not as discrete as usually shown in schematic diagrams of the spinal cord.

The corticospinal tracts and other upper motor neurons terminate mainly in relation to nerve cells in the intermediate zone of spinal gray matter (internuncial neurons), from which motor impulses are then transmitted to the anterior horn cells. Only 10 to 20 percent of corticospinal fibers (presumably the thick, rapidly conducting axons derived from Betz cells) establish direct synaptic connections with the large motor neurons of the anterior horns.

The Motor, Premotor, and Supplementary Motor Cortex and the Control of Movement

The *motor area of the cerebral cortex* is defined physiologically as the region of electrically excitable cortex from which isolated movements can be evoked by stimuli of minimal intensity (Fig. 3-3). The muscle groups of the contralateral face, arm, trunk, and leg are represented in the primary motor cortex (area 4), those of the face being in the most inferior part of the precentral gyrus on the lateral surface of the cerebral hemisphere and those of the leg in the paracentral lobule on the medial surface of the cerebral hemisphere. The parts of the body capable of the most delicate movements have, in general, the largest cortical representation.

Area 6, the premotor area, is also electrically excitable but requires more intense stimuli than area 4 to evoke movements. Stimulation of its caudal aspect (area 6aα) produces responses that are similar to those elicited from area 4. These responses are probably effected by transmission of impulses from area 6a to area 4 (since they cannot be obtained after ablation of area 4) and discharge via the corticospinal tract. Stimulation of the rostral premotor area (area 6aβ) elicits more general movement patterns, predominantly of proximal limb musculature. The latter movements are effected via pathways other than those derived from area 4 (hence, "extrapyramidal"). Very strong stimuli elicit movements from a wide area of premotor frontal and parietal cortex, and the same movements may be obtained from several widely separated points. From this it may be assumed, as Alexander and DeLong point out, that the premotor cortex includes several anatomically distinct subregions with different afferent and efferent connections. In general, it may be said that the motor-premotor cortex is capable of synthesizing agonist actions into an infinite variety of finely graded, highly differentiated patterns. These are directed by visual (area 7) and tactile (area 5) sensory information and supported by appropriate postural mechanisms.

The *supplementary motor area* is the most anterior portion of area 6 on the medial surface of the cerebral hemisphere. Stimulation of this area may induce relatively gross homolateral or contralateral movements, bilateral tonic contractions of the limbs, contraversive movements of the head and eyes with tonic contraction of the contralateral arm, and sometimes inhibition of voluntary motor activity and vocal arrest.

How the motor cortex controls movements is still a controversial matter. The traditional view, based on the interpretations of Hughlings Jackson and of Sherrington, is that the motor cortex is organized not in terms of individual muscles but of movements, i.e., the coordinated contraction of groups of muscles. Jackson visualized a widely overlapping representation of muscle groups in the cerebral cortex, based on his observation that a patient could recover the use of a limb following destruction of the limb area as defined by cortical stimulation. This view was supported by Sherrington's observations that stimulation of the cortical surface activated not solitary muscles but a combination of muscles, and always in a reciprocal fashion—i.e., in a manner that maintained the expected relationship between agonists and antagonists. He also noted the inconstancy of stimulatory effects; the stimulation of a given cortical point that initiated flexion of a part on one occasion might initiate extension on another.

These interpretations must be viewed with circumspection, as must all observations based on the electrical stimulation of the surface of the cortex. It has been shown that to stimulate motor cells from the surface, the electric current has to penetrate the cortex to layer V, where these neurons are located, inevitably activating a large number of other cortical neurons. The elegant experiments of Asanuma and of Evarts and his colleagues, who stimulated the depths of the cortex with microelectrodes, demonstrated the existence of discrete zones of efferent neurons that control the contraction of individual muscles; moreover, the continued stimulation of a given efferent zone often facilitated rather than inhibited the contraction of the antagonists. These investigators have also shown that cells in the efferent zone receive afferent impulses from the particular muscle to which the efferent neurons project. When the effects of many stimulations at various depths were correlated with the exact sites of each penetration, cells that projected to a particular pool of spinal motor neurons were found to be arranged in radially aligned columns about 1 mm in diameter. The columnar arrangement of cells in the sensorimotor cortex had been appreciated for many years; the wealth of radial interconnections between the cells in these columns led Lorente de Nó to suggest that these "vertical chains" of cells were the elementary functional units of the cortex. On the sensory side, this notion received strong support from Mountcastle's observations that all the neurons in a somatosensory column receive impulses of the same sensory modality, from the same part of the body. In regard to the functional organization of the columns of motor neurons, it is still not entirely clear whether they contribute to a movement as units or whether individual cells within many columns are selectively activated to produce a movement. The evidence for these disparate views has been summarized by Henneman and by Asanuma (see References).

The role of cerebrocortical motor neurons in sensory evoked or planned movement has also been elucidated by Evarts and his colleagues. Using single cell recording techniques, they showed that pyramidal cells fire about 60 ms prior to the onset of a movement in a sequence determined by the required pattern and force of the movement. But other, more complex properties of the pyramidal cells were also noted. Some of them received a somatosensory input transcortically from the parietal lobe (areas 3, 1, and 2), which could be turned on or off or gated according to whether the movement was to be controlled, i.e., guided, by sensory input. Many neurons of the supplementary and premotor parts of the motor cortical area were activated in a "set discharge" that preceded (anticipated) a planned movement. Thus, pyramidal (area 4) motor neurons were prepared for the oncoming activation; i.e., they were triggered by a number of transcortical impulses from the parietal, prefrontal, premotor, and auditory and visual areas of the cortex. This set signal could occur in the absence of any segmental activity in the spinal cord and muscles. The source of this set signal was found to be mainly in the supplementary motor cortex, which appears to be under the direct influence of the readiness stimuli (Bereitschaft) reaching it from the prefrontal areas (for planned movements) and the posterior parietal cortex (for motor activities initiated by visual, tactile, and auditory perceptions). Also, there are fibers that reach the motor area from the limbic system, presumably subserving motivation and attention. The blood flow to each of the cortical motor zones increases with an increase in their synaptic activity, and the measurement of blood flow has been used to follow these neural events (Roland).

Thus the prefrontal cortex, supplementary motor cortex, premotor cortex, and motor cortex are all responsive to various afferent stimuli and are involved in set discharges prior to and in coordinated fashion with a complex movement. And, as will be remarked later on, the striatopallidum and cerebellum, which project to these cortical areas, are also activated prior to or concurrently with the discharge of corticospinal neurons (see Thach and Montgomery for a critical review of the physiologic data).

Termination of the Corticospinal and Other Descending Motor Tracts

This has been studied in the monkey by interrupting the descending motor pathways in the medulla and more rostral parts of the brainstem and tracing the distribution of the degenerating elements in the spinal gray matter. On the basis of such experiments and other physiologic data, Lawrence and Kuypers proposed that the functional organization of the descending cortical and subcortical pathways is determined more by their patterns of termination and the motor capacities of the internuncial neurons upon which they terminate than by the location of their cells of origin. Three groups of motor fibers were distinguished according to their differential terminal distribution: (1) A *ventromedial pathway*, which arises in the tectum, vestibular nuclei, and pontine and medullary reticular cells and terminates principally on the internuncial cells of the ventromedial part of the spinal gray matter. This system is mainly concerned with axial movements—the maintenance of posture, integrated movements of body and limbs, and total-limb movements. (2) A *lateral pathway*, which is derived mainly from the magnocellular part of the red nucleus and terminates in the dorsal and lateral parts of the internuncial zone. This pathway adds the capacity for independent use of the extremities, especially of the hands. (3) A major portion of the *corticospinal pathway*, which terminates diffusely throughout the nucleus proprius of the dorsal horn and the intermediate zone and greatly amplifies the control of hand movements. This portion of the corticospinal projection arises from the sensory cortex and appears to function in the control of afferent projection neurons. Finally, there is a portion of the corticospinal tract that synapses directly with the large motor neurons that innervate the muscles of the fingers, face, and tongue; this system provides the capacity for a high degree of fractionation of movements, as exemplified by independent finger movements.

Other Descending Cerebrospinal Motor Systems

Reference has already been made to the corticomesencephalic, corticopontine, and corticomedullary fiber systems which project onto the reticulospinal, vestibulospinal, rubrospinal, and tectospinal nuclei. These control stability of the head (via labyrinthine reflexes) and of the neck and body in relation to the head (tonic neck reflexes) as well as postures of the body in relation to limb movements. Lesions in these systems are less well understood than those of the corticospinal system. They cause no paralysis of muscles but result in the liberation of unusual postures (e.g., hemiplegic dystonia), heightened tonic neck and labyrinthine reflexes, and decerebrate rigidity. In a strict sense these are all "extrapyramidal." They are discussed further in the following chapter.

Paralysis due to Lesions of the Upper Motor Neurons

The corticospinal pathway may be interrupted by a lesion at any point along its course—at the level of the cerebral cortex, subcortical white matter, internal capsule, brainstem, or spinal cord. Usually, when hemiplegia is severe and permanent as a consequence of disease, much more than the long, direct corticospinal pathway is involved. In the cerebral white matter (corona radiata) and internal capsule, the corticospinal fibers are intermingled with corticostriate, corticothalamic, corticorubral, corticopontine, cortico-olivary, and corticoreticular fibers. It is noteworthy that thalamocortical fibers, which are a vital link in an ascending fiber system from the basal ganglia and cerebellum, also pass through the internal capsule and cerebral white matter. Thus lesions in these parts simultaneously affect both corticospinal and extrapyramidal systems. Attribution of a capsular hemiplegia to a lesion of the corticospinal or pyramidal pathway is therefore not entirely correct. The term *upper motor neuron paralysis*, which recognizes the involvement of several descending fiber systems that influence and modify the lower motor neuron, is more suitable.

In primates, lesions limited to area 4 of Brodmann, the motor cortex, cause only hypotonia and weakness of the distal limb muscles. Lesions of the premotor cortex (area 6) result in weakness, spasticity, and increased stretch reflexes (Fulton). Lesions of the supplementary motor cortex lead to involuntary grasping. These clinical effects have not been as clearly defined in humans as in monkeys. Resection of cortical areas 4 and 6 and subcortical white matter causes complete and permanent paralysis and spasticity (Laplane et al).

The one place where corticospinal fibers are entirely isolated as the pyramidal tract is in the medullary pyramids. In humans there are a few documented cases of a lesion more or less confined to this location (Ropper et al). The result of such lesions has been an initial flaccid hemiplegia (with sparing of the face), from which there is considerable recovery. Similarly in monkeys—as shown by Tower in 1940 and subsequently by Lawrence and Kuypers and by Gilman and Marco—interruption of both pyramidal tracts results in a hypotonic paralysis; ultimately, these animals regain a wide range of movements, though slowness of all movements and loss of individual finger movements remain as permanent deficits. Also, the cerebral peduncle has been sectioned in patients in an effort to abolish involuntary movements (Bucy et al); in some of these patients, a slight degree of weakness or only a Babinski sign was produced but no spasticity developed. These observations and those in monkeys indicate that a pure pyramidal tract lesion does not result in spasticity and that control over a wide range of voluntary movements depends at least in part on nonpyramidal motor pathways. Animal experiments suggest that the corticoreticulospinal pathways are particularly important in this respect, since their fibers are arranged somatotopically and are able to influence stretch reflexes. Further studies in humans are necessary to settle problems related to volitional movement and spasticity. The motor organization of the cat and even of the monkey is so different from that of humans, and the range of volitional activity and motor skills is so much less in animals, that direct comparisons are not justified.

The distribution of the paralysis due to upper motor neuron lesions varies with the locale of the lesion, but certain features are characteristic of all of them. A group of muscles is always involved, never individual muscles, and if any movement is possible, the proper relationships between agonists, antagonists, synergists, and fixators are preserved. The paralysis never involves all the muscles on one side of the body, even in the severest forms of hemiplegia. Movements that are invariably bilateral—such as those of the eyes, jaw, pharynx, larynx, neck, thorax, diaphragm, and abdomen—are little or not at all affected. This comes about because the muscles involved in bilateral movements are bilaterally innervated; i.e., stimulation of either the right or left motor cortex results in contraction of these muscles on both sides of the body. Upper motor neuron paralysis is rarely complete for any long period of time; in this respect it differs from the absolute paralysis due to destruction of anterior horn cells or interruption of their axons.

Upper motor neuron lesions are characterized further by certain peculiarities of residual movement. There is decreased voluntary drive on spinal motor neurons (fewer motor units are recruitable and their firing rates are slower). There is an increased degree of cocontraction of antagonistic muscles, reflected in a decreased rate of rapid alternating movements. These abnormalities probably account for the greater sense of effort and the manifest fatigability in effecting voluntary movement of the weakened muscles. Another phenomenon is the activation of paralyzed muscles as parts of certain automatisms (synkinesias). The paralyzed arm may move suddenly during yawning and stretching. Attempts by the patient to move the hemiplegic limbs may result in a variety of associated movements. Thus, flexion of the arm may result in involuntary pronation and flexion of the leg, in dorsiflexion and eversion of the foot. Also, volitional movements of the paretic limb may evoke imitative (mirror) movements in the normal one or vice versa. In some patients, as they recover from hemiplegia, a variety of movement abnormalities emerge, such as tremor, ataxia, athetosis, and chorea on the affected side. These are expressions of damage to basal ganglionic and thalamic structures and are discussed in Chap. 4.

If the upper motor neurons are interrupted above the level of the facial nucleus in the pons, hand and arm muscles are affected most severely and the leg muscles to a lesser extent; of the cranial musculature, only muscles of the tongue and lower part of the face are involved to any significant degree. Since Broadbent was the first to call attention to this distribution of paralysis, it is sometimes referred to as "Broadbent's law." At lower levels, such as the cervical cord, complete acute lesions of the upper motor neurons not only cause a paralysis of voluntary movement but also abolish temporarily the spinal reflexes subserved by segments below the lesion. This is the condition referred to above as *spinal shock*, a state of acute flaccid paralysis that is replaced later by *spasticity*. A comparable state of shock may occur with acute cerebral lesions but is less sharply defined than the spinal state. With some acute cerebral lesions, spasticity and paralysis develop together; in others, especially with parietal lesions, the limbs remain flaccid but reflexes are retained.

Spasticity A predilection for involvement of certain muscle groups, a specific pattern of response of muscles to passive stretch (where resistance increases linearly in relation to velocity of stretch), and a manifest exaggeration of tendon reflexes are the identifying characteristics of *spasticity*. The antigravity muscles—the flexors of the arms and the extensors of the legs—are predominantly affected. The arm tends to assume a flexed and pronated position and the leg an extended and adducted one, indicating that certain spinal neurons are reflexly more active than others. At rest, with the muscles shortened to midposition, they are flaccid to palpation and electromyographically silent. If the arm is extended or the leg flexed very slowly, there may be little or no change in muscle tone. By contrast, if the muscles are briskly stretched, the limb moves freely for a very short distance (free interval), beyond which there is an abrupt catch and then a rapidly increasing muscular resistance up to a point; then, as passive extension of the arm or flexion of the leg continues, the resistance melts away. This sequence constitutes the classic "clasp-knife" phenomenon. With the limb in the extended or flexed position, a new passive movement may not encounter the same sequence; this entire pattern of response constitutes the lengthening and shortening reaction. Thus the essential feature of spasticity is a velocity-dependent increase in the resistance of muscles to a passive stretch stimulus.

Although a clasp-knife relaxation following peak resistance is highly characteristic of cerebral hemiplegia, it is by no means found consistently. In some cases, the arm flexors and leg extensors are spastic, while the antagonist muscles show an even resistance throughout the range of passive movement—i.e., rigidity (Chap. 4); or rigidity may be more prominent than spasticity in all muscles. This plastic resistance, in Denny-Brown's view, is the mild form or precursor of an altered posture or attitude that he called *dystonic* and considered to be a characteristic feature of hemiplegic spasticity. Nor is there a constant relationship between spasticity and weakness. In some cases, severe weakness may be associated with only the mildest signs of spasticity, detectable as a "catch" in the pronators on passive supination of the forearm and in the flexors of the hand on extension of the wrist. Contrariwise, the most extreme degrees of spasticity, observed in certain patients with cervical spinal cord disease, may so vastly exceed paresis of voluntary movement as to indicate that these two states depend on separate mechanisms. Indeed, the selective blocking of small gamma neurons is said to abolish spasticity as well as hyperactive segmental tendon reflexes but to leave motor performance unchanged.

Until recently, it was taught that the heightened myotatic or stretch reflexes ("tendon jerks") of the spastic state are "release" phenomena—the result of interruption of descending inhibitory pathways. This appears to be only a partial explanation. Animal experiments have demonstrated that this aspect of the spastic state is also mediated through spindle afferents (increased tonic activity of gamma motor neurons) and, centrally, through reticulospinal and vestibulospinal pathways that act on alpha motor neurons. The clasp-knife phenomenon appears to derive at least partly from a lesion (or presumably a change in central control) of a specific portion of the reticulospinal system.

Brown, in a discussion of the pathophysiology of spasticity, has emphasized the importance of two systems of fibers: (1) the dorsal reticulospinal tract, which has inhibitory effects on stretch reflexes, and (2) the medial reticulospinal and vestibulospinal tracts, which together facilitate extensor tone. He postulates that in cerebral and capsular lesions, cortical inhibition is weakened, resulting in spastic hemiplegia. In spinal cord lesions that involve the corticospinal tract, the dorsal reticulospinal tract is usually involved as well. If the latter tract is spared, only paresis, loss of support reflexes, and possibly release of flexor reflexes (Babinski phenomenon) occur. Pantano and colleagues have suggested that primary involvement of the lentiform nucleus and thalamus is the feature that determines the persistence of flaccidity after stroke, but the anatomic and physiologic evidence for this view is insecure.

The hyperreflexic state that characterizes spasticity often takes the form of *clonus*, a series of rhythmic involuntary muscular contractions occurring at a frequency of 5 to 7 Hz in response to an abruptly applied and sustained stretch stimulus. It is usually designated in terms of the part of the limb to which the stimulus is applied (e.g., patella, ankle). The frequency is constant within 1 Hz and is not appreciably modified by altering peripheral or central nervous system activities. Clonus depends for its elicitation on an appropriate degree of muscle relaxation, integrity of the spinal stretch reflex mechanisms, sustained hyperexcitability of alpha and gamma motor neurons (suprasegmental effects), and synchronization of the contraction-relaxation cycle of muscle spindles. The cutaneomuscular abdominal and cremasteric reflexes are usually abolished in these circumstances, and a Babinski sign is usually but not invariably present.

Irradiation, or *spread of reflexes*, is regularly associated with spasticity, although the former phenomenon may be observed in normal persons with brisk tendon reflexes. Tapping of the radial periosteum, for example, may elicit a reflex contraction not only of the brachioradialis but also of the biceps, triceps, or finger flexors. This spread of reflex activity is probably due not to an irradiation of impulses in the spinal cord, as is often taught, but to the propagation of a vibration wave from bone to muscle, stimulating the excitable muscle spindles in its path (Lance). The same mechanism is probably operative in other manifestations of the hyperreflexic state, such as the Hoffmann sign and the crossed adductor reflex of the thigh muscles. Also, reflexes may be "inverted," as in the case of a lesion of the fifth or sixth cervical segment; here the biceps and brachioradialis reflexes are abolished and only the triceps and finger flexors, whose reflex arcs are intact, respond to a tap over the distal radius.

There have been many investigations of the biochemical changes that underlie spasticity and the mechanisms of action of antispasticity drugs. These have been reviewed by Davidoff. Since glutamic acid is the neurotransmitter of the corticospinal tracts, one would expect its action on inhibitory interneurons to be lost. As mentioned earlier, gamma-aminobutyric acid (GABA) and glycine are the major inhibitory transmitters in the spinal cord; GABA functions as a presynaptic inhibitor, suppressing sensory signals from muscle and cutaneous receptors. Baclofen, a derivative of GABA, as well as diazepam and progabide, are thought to act by reducing the release of excitatory transmitter from the presynaptic terminals of primary afferent terminals. Actually, none of these agents is particularly effective in the treatment of spasticity when administered orally; the administration of baclofen intrathecally may have a beneficial effect. Glycine is the transmitter released by inhibitory interneurons and is measurably reduced in quantity, uptake, and turnover in the spastic animal. There is some evidence that the oral administration of glycine reduces experimentally induced spasticity, but its value in patients is uncertain. Interruption of descending noradrenergic, dopaminergic, and serotoninergic fibers is undoubtedly involved in the genesis of spasticity, although the exact mode of action of these neurotransmitters on the various components of spinal reflex arcs remains to be defined.

In addition to hyperactive *phasic myotatic reflexes* ("tendon jerks"), certain lesions, particularly of the cervical segments of the spinal cord, may result in great enhancement of *tonic myotatic reflexes*. These are stretch reflexes in which a stimulus produces a prolonged asynchronous discharge of motor neurons, causing sustained muscle contraction. As the patient stands or attempts voluntary movement, the entire limb may become involved in intense muscular spasm, sometimes lasting for several minutes. During this period the limb is quite useless. Presumably there is both an interruption of lateral reticulospinal inhibitory influences on the anterior horn cells and a release of the medial reticulospinal facilitatory effects needed in antigravity support (Henneman).

The *nociceptive spinal flexion reflexes*, of which the Babinski sign is a part, are not essential components of spasticity. They, too, are exaggerated because of disinhibition or release in cases of paraparesis or paraplegia of spinal origin. Important characteristics of these responses are their capacity to be induced by weak superficial stimuli (such as a series of pinpricks) and their tendency to persist after the stimulation ceases. In their most complete form, a nocifensive flexor synergy occurs, involving flexion of the knee and hip and dorsiflexion of the foot and big toe (*triple flexion response*). With incomplete suprasegmental lesions, the response may be fractionated; for example, the hip and knee may flex but the foot may not dorsiflex, or vice versa. In the more chronic stages of hemiplegia the upper limb is characteristically held stiffly in partial flexion.

With bilateral cerebral lesions, exaggerated stretch reflexes can be elicited in cranial as well as limb and trunk muscles because of interruption of the corticobulbar pathways. These are seen as easily triggered masseter contractions in response to a brisk downward tap on the chin (jaw jerk) and brisk contractions of the orbicularis oris muscles in response to tapping the philtrum or corners of the mouth. In advanced cases, weakness or paralysis of voluntary movements of the face, tongue, larynx, and pharynx are added (bulbar spastic or "pseudobulbar" palsy; see pages 517 and 541).

Table 3-1 summarizes the main attributes of upper motor neuron lesions and contrasts them with those of the lower motor neuron.

Table 3-1
Differences between upper and lower motor neuron paralysis

Upper motor neuron or supranuclear paralysis	*Lower motor neuron or nuclear-infranuclear paralysis*
Muscles affected in groups, never individual muscles	Individual muscles may be affected
Atrophy slight and due to disuse	Atrophy pronounced, up to 70% of total bulk
Spasticity with hyperactivity of the tendon reflexes and extensor plantar reflex (Babinski sign)	Flaccidity and hypotonia of affected muscles with loss of tendon reflexes Plantar reflex, if present, is of normal flexor type
Fascicular twitches absent	Fasciculations may be present
Normal nerve conduction studies; no denervation potentials in EMG	Abnormal nerve conduction studies; denervation potentials (fibrillations, fasciculations, positive sharp waves) in EMG

Motor Disturbances due to Lesions of the Parietal Lobe

As indicated earlier in this section, a significant portion of the pyramidal tract originates in neurons of the parietal cortex. Also, the parietal lobes are important sources of visual and tactile information necessary for the control of movement. Pause and colleagues have described the motor disturbances due to lesions of the parietal cortex. The patient is unable to maintain stable postures of the outstretched hand when his eyes are closed and cannot exert a steady contraction. Exploratory movements and manipulation of small objects are impaired, and the speed of tapping is diminished. Posterior parietal lesions (involving areas 5 and 7) are more detrimental in this respect than anterior ones (areas 1, 3, and 5), but in patients with the most severe deficits both regions are affected.

APRAXIA AND OTHER NONPARALYTIC DISORDERS OF MOTOR FUNCTION

All that has been said about the cortical and spinal control of the motor system gives one only a limited idea of human motility. Viewed objectively, the conscious and sentient human organism is continuously active—fidgeting, adjusting posture and position, sitting, standing, walking, running, speaking, manipulating tools, or performing the intricate sequences of movements involved in athletic or musical skills. Some of these activities are relatively simple, automatic, and stereotyped. Others have been learned and mastered through intense conscious effort and with long practice have become habitual—i.e., reduced to an automatic level—a process not at all understood physiologically. Still others are complex and voluntary, parts of a carefully formulated plan, and demand continuous attention and thought. What is more remarkable, one can be occupied in several of these variably conscious and habitual activities simultaneously, such as driving through heavy traffic while lighting a cigarette and engaging in animated conversation. Moreover, when an obstacle prevents a particular sequence of movements from accomplishing its goal, a new sequence can be undertaken automatically for the same purpose. As stated above, these activities, in the scheme of Hughlings Jackson, represent the third and highest level of motor function.

How is all this made possible? Neuropsychologists, on the basis of studies of large numbers of patients with lesions of different parts of the cerebrum, believe that the planning of complex activities, conceptualizing their final purpose, and continuously modifying the individual components of a motor sequence until the goal is achieved are initiated and directed by the frontal lobes. Lesions of the frontal lobes have the effect of reducing the impulse to think, speak, and act (i.e., abulia or reduced "cortical tone," to use Luria's expression), and a complex activity will not be initiated or sustained long enough to permit its completion.

The term *apraxia* is applied to a state in which a clear-minded patient with no weakness, ataxia, or other extrapyramidal derangement and no defect of the primary modes of sensation loses the ability to execute highly complex and previously learned skills and gestures. This was the meaning given to *apraxia* by Liepmann, who introduced the term in 1900. It was his view, on the basis of subsequent case studies, that apraxia could be subdivided into three types—ideational, ideomotor, and kinetic. His anatomic data indicated that planned or commanded action is normally developed not in the frontal lobe but in the parietal lobe of the dominant hemisphere, where visual, auditory, and somasthetic information is integrated. Presumably the formation of engrams of skilled movements depends on the integrity of this part of the brain; if it is damaged, the engrams cannot be activated at all or the movements are faltering and inappropriate. The failure to conceive or formulate an action, either spontaneously or to command, was referred to by Liepmann as *ideational apraxia*. From sensory areas 5 and 7 in the dominant parietal lobe there are connections with the supplementary and premotor cortices of both cerebral hemispheres, wherein reside the innervatory mechanisms for patterned movement. The patient may know and remember the planned action, but because these connections are interrupted, he cannot execute it with either hand. This was Liepmann's concept of *ideomotor apraxia*. *Kinetic limb apraxia* refers to clumsiness and maladroitness of a limb in the performance of a skilled act that cannot be accounted for by paresis, ataxia, or sensory loss (see also Chap. 22).

These high-order abnormalities of learned movement patterns have several unique features. Seldom are they evident to the patient himself, and therefore they are not sources of complaint; or, if they are appreciated by the patient, he has difficulty describing the problem except in narrow terms of the activity that is impaired, such as using a phone or dressing. For this reason they are often overlooked by the examining physician. Their evocation requires special types of testing that may be difficult because of the presence of other neurologic deficits. Obviously, if the patient is confused or aphasic, spoken or written requests to perform an act will not be understood and one must find ways of persuading him to imitate the movements of the examiner. Moreover, the patient must be able to recognize and name the articles that he attempts to manipulate; i.e., there must not be an agnosia.

In a practical sense, the lesions responsible for *ideomotor apraxia of both arms* usually reside in the left parietal region. Kertesz and colleagues have provided evidence that separate lesions are responsible for aphasia and apraxia, though the two conditions are frequently associated. Surprisingly, there are but a few cases of ideomotor apraxia with proven premotor lesions. The exact location of the parietal lesion, whether in the supramarginal gyrus or in the superior parietal lobe (areas 5 and 7) and whether subcortical or cortical, is still uncertain. Geschwind accepted Liepmann's proposition that a lesion of a subcortical tract (presumably the arcuate fasciculus) disconnects the parietal from the left frontal cortex, accounting for the ideomotor apraxia of the right limbs, and that the left limb apraxia is due to a callosal disconnection of the left and right premotor association cortices. In a right-handed person, the lesion that gives rise to a *left limb apraxia* is usually in the left frontal lobe and includes Broca's area, the left motor cortex, and the deep underlying white matter. Clinically there is a motor speech disorder, a right hemiparesis, and apraxia of the nonparalyzed hand—i.e., "sympathetic apraxia." If the lesion in the deep white matter separates the language areas from the right motor cortex but not from the left, the patient can write with the right hand but not with the left, or he may write correctly with the right hand and aphasically with the left. That such a syndrome is attributable to interruption of a pathway that traverses the genu of the corpus callosum, as depicted by Geschwind, is questionable, insofar as sympathetic apraxia has not been observed in patients with lesions (or surgical sections) confined to the anterior third of the corpus callosum (see page 494). The disconnection syndromes are discussed further in Chaps. 22 and 23.

Facial-oral apraxia is probably the most common of all apraxias. It may occur with lesions that undercut the left supramarginal gyrus or the left motor association cortex and may be associated with apraxia of the limbs. Such patients are unable to carry out facial movements to command (lick the lips, blow out a match, etc.), although they may do better when asked to imitate the examiner or when holding a lighted match. With lesions that are restricted to the facial area of the left motor cortex, the apraxia will be limited to the facial musculature and may be associated with a verbal apraxia or cortical dysarthria (page 505). So-called apraxia of gait is considered in Chap. 7. The terms *dressing apraxia* and *constructional apraxia* are sometimes used to describe certain manifestations of parietal lobe disease. These abnormalities are not apraxias in the strict sense as defined above but are symptoms of contralateral extinction or neglect of the body and extrapersonal space (anosognosia, page 484).

Testing for apraxia is carried out in several ways. First, one observes the actions of the patient as he engages in such tasks as dressing, washing, shaving, and using eating utensils. Second, the patient is asked to carry out familiar symbolic acts—wave good-bye, shake his fist as though angry, salute, or blow a kiss. Third, if he fails, he is asked to imitate such acts made by the examiner. Finally, he is asked to show how he would hammer a nail, brush his teeth, comb his hair, cross himself, and so forth, or to execute a more complex act, such as lighting and smoking a cigarette or opening a bottle of soda, pouring some into a glass, and drinking it. These last actions, involving more complex sequences, are said to be tests of ideational apraxia, and the simpler acts, tests of ideomotor apraxia. To perform these tasks in the absence of the tool or utensil is always more demanding because the patient must mentally formulate a plan of action rather than engage in a habitual motor sequence. The patient may fail to carry out a commanded or suggested activity (e.g., to take a pipe out of his pocket), yet a few minutes later he may perform the same motor sequence automatically. One may think of such an ideomotor deficit, if it can be singled out (no confusion or defect in comprehension), as a kind of amnesia for certain learned patterns of movement, analogous to the amnesia for words in aphasia.

Children with cerebral diseases that retard mental development are often unable to learn the sequences of movement required in hopping, jumping over a barrier, hitting or kicking a ball, or dancing. They suffer a developmental motor apraxia. Certain tests quantitate failure in these age-linked motor skills (see Chap. 28).

In the authors' opinion, the time-honored division of apraxia into ideational, ideomotor (idiokinetic), and kinetic types is unsatisfactory. It is more helpful to think of the apraxias in an anatomic sense, as disorders of association between different parts of the cerebral cortex, as described above. We have been unable to confidently separate ideomotor from ideational apraxia. The patient with a severe ideomotor apraxia nearly always has difficulty at the ideational level. Furthermore, in view of the complexity of the motor system, we are frequently uncertain whether a clumsiness or ineptitude of a hand in performing a motor skill represents a kinetic apraxia or some other fault in the intrinsic organization of hand control.

A related but poorly understood disorder of movement has been termed the *alien hand*. In the absence of volition, the hand and arm undertake complex and seemingly purposeful movements such as reaching into a pocket or handbag, placing the hand behind the head, and tugging on the opposite hand or other body part, and these activities may occur even during sleep. The patient has the sense that the actions are beyond his control, and there is often an impression that the hand is estranged as if controlled by an external agent (although the limb is recognized as one's own—there is no anosognosia); a grasp reflex and a tendency to grope are usually added. Most instances arise as a result of infarction in the territory of the opposite anterior cerebral artery including the corpus callosum; when the latter structure is involved, Feinberg and colleagues find that frequently there appears to be a conflict between the actions of the hands, the normal one restraining the alien one. Damage in the left supplementary motor area as well as the disease corticobasal ganglionic degeneration (page 140) is associated with a similar syndrome. A form that results from sensory loss has also been suggested.

Finally, it should be remarked once again that the complexity of motor activity is almost beyond imagination. Reference was made earlier to the reciprocal innervation involved in "making a fist." But what must be involved in playing a piano concerto? Over a century ago Hughlings Jackson commented that "There are, we shall say, over thirty muscles in the hand; these are represented in the nervous centers in thousands of different combinations, that is, as very many movements; it is just as many chords, musical expressions and tunes can be made out of a few notes." The execution of these complex movements, many of them learned and habitual, is made possible by the cooperative activities of the basal ganglia, cerebellum, reticular formation of the brainstem, and sensory and motor spinal neurons. All are continuously integrated and controlled by feedback mechanisms. Even the spinal stretch reflex has connections with the motor cortex. These points, already touched upon in this chapter, are elaborated in the following three chapters.

PATTERNS OF PARALYSIS AND THEIR DIAGNOSIS

The diagnostic considerations in cases of paralysis can be simplified by utilizing the following subdivision, based on the location and distribution of the muscle weakness.

1. *Monoplegia* refers to weakness or paralysis of all the muscles of one leg or arm. This term should not be applied to paralysis of isolated muscles or groups of muscles supplied by a single nerve or motor root.

2. *Hemiplegia*, the commonest form of paralysis, involves the arm, the leg, and sometimes the face on one side of the body. With rare exceptions, mentioned further on, hemiplegia is attributable to a lesion of the corticospinal system on the side opposite to the paralysis.

3. *Paraplegia* indicates weakness or paralysis of both legs. It is most often the result of spinal cord disease, rarely of the medial frontal motor cortices, cauda equina, or peripheral nerves.

4. *Quadriplegia (tetraplegia)* denotes weakness or paralysis of all four extremities. It may result from disease of the peripheral nerves, muscles, or myoneural junctions; gray matter of the spinal cord; or the upper motor neurons bilaterally in the cervical cord, brainstem, or cerebrum. *Diplegia* is a special form of quadriplegia in which the legs are affected more than the arms. *Triplegia* occurs most often as a transitional condition in the development of or partial recovery from tetraplegia.

5. Isolated paralysis of one or more muscle groups.

6. Nonparalytic disorders of movement (apraxia, ataxia, etc.).

7. Muscular paralysis without visible changes in motor neurons, roots, or nerves.

8. Hysterical paralysis.

Monoplegia

The examination of patients who complain of weakness of one limb often discloses an asymptomatic weakness of another, and the condition is actually a hemiparesis or paraparesis. Or, instead of weakness of all the muscles in a limb, only isolated groups are found to be affected. Ataxia, sensory disturbances, or reluctance to move the limb because of pain must not be misinterpreted as weakness. The presence of parkinsonism may give rise to the same error, as can rigidity or bradykinesia of other causation, or a mechanical limitation due to arthritis and bursitis. The presence or absence of atrophy of muscles in a monoplegic limb is of particular diagnostic help, as indicated below.

Monoplegia without Muscular Atrophy This is most often due to a lesion of the cerebral cortex. Only infrequently does it result from a subcortical lesion that interrupts the motor pathways. A cerebral vascular lesion (thrombotic or embolic infarction) is the commonest cause; a circumscribed tumor or abscess may have the same effect. Multiple sclerosis and spinal cord tumor, early in their course, may cause weakness of one limb, usually the leg. Monoplegia due to a lesion of the upper motor neuron is usually accompanied by spasticity, increased reflexes, and an extensor plantar reflex (Babinski sign); exceptionally, a small lesion of the motor cortex will not result in spasticity. In either event, nerve conduction studies are normal. In acute diseases of the lower motor neurons, the tendon reflexes are reduced or abolished, but atrophy may not appear for several weeks. Hence, before reaching an anatomic diagnosis, one must take into account the mode of onset and duration of the disease.

Monoplegia with Muscular Atrophy This is more frequent than monoplegia without muscular atrophy. Long-continued disuse of one limb may lead to atrophy, but it is usually of lesser degree than atrophy due to lower motor neuron disease (denervation atrophy). In disuse atrophy, the tendon reflexes are retained and nerve conduction studies are normal. With denervation of muscles, there may be visible fasciculations and reduced or abolished tendon reflexes in addition to paralysis. If the limb is partially denervated, the electromyogram shows reduced numbers of motor unit potentials (often of large size) as well as fasciculations and fibrillations. The location of the lesion (in nerves, spinal roots, or spinal cord) can usually be determined by the pattern of weakness, by the associated neurologic symptoms and signs, and by special tests—magnetic resonance imaging (MRI) of the spine, examination of the cerebrospinal fluid (CSF), and electrical studies of nerve and muscle.

A *complete atrophic brachial monoplegia* is uncommon; more often, only parts of a limb are affected. When present in an infant, it should suggest brachial plexus trauma from birth; in a child, poliomyelitis or other viral infection of the spinal cord; and in an adult, poliomyelitis, syringomyelia, amyotrophic lateral sclerosis, or a brachial plexus lesion. *Crural (leg) monoplegia* is more frequent than brachial monoplegia and may be caused by any lesion of the thoracic or lumbar cord—i.e., trauma, tumor, myelitis, multiple sclerosis, progressive muscular atrophy, late radiation effect, etc. These disorders rarely cause severe atrophy; neither does infarction in the territory of the anterior cerebral artery. A prolapsed intervertebral disc and the several varieties of mononeuropathy almost never paralyze all or most of the muscles of a limb. The effects of a centrally prolapsed disc or other compressive lesion of the cauda equina are rarely confined to one leg. However, a unilateral retroperitoneal tumor or hematoma may paralyze the leg by compressing the lumbosacral plexus. The mode of onset and temporal course differentiate these diseases.

Hemiplegia

This is the most frequent form of paralysis. With rare exceptions (a few unusual cases of poliomyelitis or motor system disease), this pattern of paralysis is due to involvement of the corticospinal pathways.

Location of Lesion Producing Hemiplegia The site or level of the lesion—i.e., cerebral cortex, corona radiata, capsule, brainstem, or spinal cord—can usually be deduced from the associated neurologic findings. Diseases localized to the cerebral cortex, cerebral white matter (corona radiata), and internal capsule usually manifest themselves by weakness or paralysis of the leg, arm, and lower face on the opposite side. The occurrence of seizures or the presence of a language disorder (aphasia), a loss of discriminative sensation (astereognosis, impairment of tactile localization, etc.), anosognosia, or a homonymous visual field defect suggests a contralateral cortical or subcortical location.

Damage to the corticospinal and corticobulbar tracts in the upper portion of the brainstem also causes paralysis of the face, arm, and leg of the opposite side (see Fig. 3-2). The lesion in such cases may in some patients be localized by the presence of a third-nerve palsy (Weber syndrome) or other segmental abnormality on the same side as the lesion. With low pontine lesions, an ipsilateral abducens or facial palsy is combined with a contralateral weakness or paralysis of the arm and leg (Millard-Gubler syndrome). Lesions in the medulla affect the tongue and sometimes the pharynx and larynx on one side and the arm and leg on the other. These "crossed paralyses," so characteristic of brainstem lesions, are described further in Chap. 47.

Even lower in the medulla, a unilateral infarct in the pyramid causes a flaccid paralysis followed by slight spasticity of the contralateral arm and leg, with sparing of the face and tongue. Some motor function may be retained, as in the case described by Ropper and coworkers; interestingly, in this case and in three others previously reported, there was considerable recovery of voluntary power even though the pyramid was almost completely destroyed.

Rarely, an ipsilateral hemiplegia may be caused by a lesion in the lateral column of the cervical spinal cord. In this location, however, the pathologic process more often induces bilateral signs, with resulting quadriparesis or quadriplegia. A homolateral paralysis that spares the face, if combined with a loss of vibratory and position sense on the same side and a contralateral loss of pain and temperature, signifies disease of one side of the spinal cord (*Brown-Séquard syndrome*).

As indicated above, muscle atrophy that follows upper motor neuron lesions never reaches the proportions seen in diseases of the lower motor neuron. The atrophy in the former cases is due to disuse. When the motor cortex and adjacent parts of the parietal lobe are damaged in infancy or childhood, normal development of the muscles as well as the skeletal system in the affected limbs is retarded. The limbs and even the trunk are smaller on one side than on the other. This does not happen if the paralysis occurs after puberty, by which time the greater part of skeletal growth has been attained. In hemiplegia due to spinal cord lesions, muscles at the level of the lesion may atrophy as a result of damage to anterior horn cells or ventral roots.

In the causation of hemiplegia, hemorrhagic and ischemic vascular diseases of the cerebrum and brainstem exceed all others in frequency. Trauma (brain contusion, epidural and subdural hemorrhage) ranks second. Other important causes, less acute in onset, are, in order of frequency, brain tumor, brain abscess, demyelinative diseases, and the vascular complications of meningitis and encephalitis. Most of these diseases can be recognized by their mode of evolution and characteristic clinical and laboratory findings, which are presented in the chapters on neurologic diseases. Alternating transitory hemiparesis may be due to a special type of migraine (see discussion in Chap. 10).

Paraplegia

Paralysis of both lower extremities may occur with diseases of the spinal cord, nerve roots, or, less often, the peripheral nerves. If the onset is acute, it may be difficult to distinguish spinal from neuropathic paralysis because of the element of spinal shock, which results in abolition of reflexes and flaccidity. In acute spinal cord diseases with involvement of corticospinal tracts, the paralysis or weakness affects all muscles below a given level; usually, if the white matter is extensively damaged, sensory loss below a particular level is conjoined (loss of pain and temperature sense due to spinothalamic tract damage, and loss of vibratory and position sense due to posterior column involvement). Also, in bilateral disease of the spinal cord, the bladder and bowel and their sphincters are usually affected. These abnormalities may be due to an intrinsic lesion of the cord or to an extrinsic mass that narrows the spinal canal, both types of lesion being evident on MRI.

In peripheral nerve diseases, motor loss tends to involve the distal muscles of the legs more than the proximal ones (exceptions are certain varieties of the Guillain-Barré syndrome and diabetic neuropathy); sphincteric function is usually spared or impaired only transiently. Sensory loss, if present, is also more prominent in the distal segments of the limbs and the degree of loss is often more for one modality than for another.

For clinical purposes it is helpful to separate the acute paraplegias from the chronic ones and to divide the latter into two groups: those beginning in adult life and those occurring in infancy.

The most common cause of *acute paraplegia* (or *quadriplegia*, if the cervical cord is involved) is spinal cord trauma, usually associated with fracture-dislocation of the spine. Less common causes are hematomyelia due to a vascular malformation, an arteriovenous malformation of the cord that causes ischemia by an obscure mechanism, or infarction of the cord due to occlusion of the anterior spinal artery or, more often, to occlusion of segmental branches of the aorta (due to dissecting aneurysm or atheroma, vasculitis, and nucleus pulposus embolism).

Paraplegia or quadriplegia due to postinfectious myelitis, demyelinative or necrotizing myelopathy, or epidural abscess or tumor with spinal cord compression tends to develop somewhat more slowly, over a period of hours or days or longer. Epidural or subdural hemorrhage from bleeding diseases or warfarin therapy causes an acute or subacute paraplegia; in a few instances the bleeding has followed a lumbar puncture. Paralytic poliomyelitis and acute polyneuritis (Guillain-Barré)—the former, a purely motor disorder with mild meningitis (now rare), the latter predominantly motor but often with sensory disturbances—must be distinguished from the acute and subacute myelopathies and from each other.

In adult life, multiple sclerosis and tumor account for most cases of *subacute and chronic spinal paraplegia*, but a wide variety of extrinsic and intrinsic processes may produce the same effect: protruded cervical disc and cervical spondylosis (often with a congenitally narrow canal), epidural abscess and other infections (tuberculous, fungal, and other granulomatous diseases), syphilitic meningomyelitis, motor system disease, subacute combined degeneration (vitamin B_{12} deficiency), syringomyelia, and degenerative disease of the lateral and posterior columns of unknown cause. (See Chap. 44 for discussion of these spinal cord diseases.) Several varieties of polyneuropathy and polymyositis must also be considered in the differential diagnosis of paraplegia or paraparesis.

In pediatric practice, delay in starting to walk and difficulty in walking are common problems. These conditions may indicate a systemic disease (such as rickets), mental deficiency, or, more commonly, some muscular or neurologic disease. Congenital cerebral disease from periventricular leukomalacia accounts for a majority of cases of infantile diplegia (weakness predominantly of the legs, with minimal affection of the arms). Present at birth, it becomes manifest in the first months of life and may appear to progress, but actually the disease is stationary and the progression is only apparent, being exposed as the motor system develops; later there may seem to be slow improvement as a result of the normal maturation processes of childhood. Congenital malformation or birth injury of the spinal cord are other possibilities. Friedreich ataxia and familial paraplegia, muscular dystrophy, tumor, and the chronic varieties of polyneuropathy tend to appear later, during childhood and adolescence, and are slowly progressive. Acute transverse (demyelinative) myelitis is a rare condition of childhood.

Quadriplegia (Tetraplegia)

All that has been said about the spinal causes of paraplegia applies to quadriplegia, the lesion being in the cervical rather than the thoracic or lumbar segments of the spinal cord. If the lesion is situated in the low cervical segments and involves the anterior half of the spinal cord, as typified by the anterior spinal artery syndrome (but occurring also in some cases of myelitis and fracture-dislocations of the cervical spine), the paralysis of the arms may be flaccid and areflexic in type and that of the legs, spastic. There is usually pain in the neck and shoulders and numbness of the hands; elements of ataxia from posterior column lesions accompany the paraparesis. Dislocation of the odontoid process with compression of the C1 and C2 spinal cord segments may occur with rheumatoid arthritis and Morquio disease; in the latter there may also be pronounced dural thickening.

A progressive syndrome of monoparesis, biparesis, and then triparesis is caused by tumors and a variety of other compressive lesions in the region of the foramen magnum and high cervical cord. Bilateral infarction of the medullary pyramids from occlusion of the vertebral arteries or their anterior spinal branches is a very rare cause of quadriplegia. Repeated cerebrovascular accidents may lead to bilateral hemiplegia, usually accompanied by pseudobulbar palsy. In infants and young children, aside from developmental abnormalities and anoxia of birth, certain metabolic cerebral diseases (metachromatic and other forms of leukoencephalopathy, lipid storage disease) may be responsible for a quadriparesis or quadriplegia, but always with severe psychomotor retardation. Congenital forms of muscular dystrophy and muscular atrophy (Werdnig-Hoffmann disease) may be recognized soon after birth or later and progress slowly.

Triplegia Paralysis that remains confined to three limbs is observed only rarely; more often the fourth limb is weak or hyperreflexic, and the syndrome is really an incomplete tetraplegia. Also, as indicated earlier, this pattern of involvement is important, because it may signify an evolving lesion of the upper cervical cord or cervicomedullary junction. A meningioma of the foramen magnum, for example, may begin with spastic weakness of one limb, followed by sequential involvement of the other limbs in an "around the clock" pattern. There are usually bilateral Babinski signs early in the process, but there may be few sensory findings. We have also seen this pattern in patients with multiple sclerosis and other intrinsic inflammatory and neoplastic lesions. These same diseases may produce triplegia (or triparesis) by a combination of paraplegia from a thoracic spinal cord lesion and a separate unilateral lesion in the cervical cord or higher that results in a hemiparesis.

Paralysis of Isolated Muscle Groups

This condition usually indicates a lesion of one or more peripheral nerves or of several adjacent spinal roots. The diagnosis of an individual peripheral nerve lesion is made on the basis of weakness or paralysis of a particular muscle or group of muscles and impairment or loss of sensation in the distribution of the nerve. Complete or extensive interruption of a peripheral nerve is followed by atrophy of the muscles it innervates and by loss of tendon reflexes of the involved muscles; abnormalities of vasomotor and sudomotor functions and trophic changes in the skin, nails, and subcutaneous tissue may also occur.

Knowledge of the motor and sensory innervation of the peripheral nerve in question is needed for a satisfactory diagnosis. It is not practical to memorize the precise sensorimotor distribution of each peripheral nerve, and special manuals, such as *Aids to the Examination of the Peripheral Nervous System*, should be consulted (see also Chap. 46). In addition, it is important to decide whether the lesion is a temporary one of conduction alone or whether there has been a structural interruption of nerve fibers, requiring nerve regeneration or corrective surgery for recovery. Electromyography and nerve conduction studies are of great value here.

If there is no evidence of upper or lower motor neuron disease but certain movements are nonetheless imperfectly performed, one should look for a disorder of position sense or cerebellar coordination, or for rigidity with abnormalities of posture and movement due to disease of the basal ganglia (Chap. 4). In the absence of these disorders, the possibility of an apraxic disorder should be investigated by the methods outlined earlier.

Hysterical Paralysis

Hysterical paralysis may involve one arm or leg, both legs, or all of one side of the body. Tendon reflexes are retained and severe atrophy is lacking in hysterical paralysis, features that distinguish it from chronic lower motor neuron disease. Diagnostic difficulty arises only in certain acute cases of upper motor neuron disease that lack the usual changes in reflexes and muscle tone. The hysterical gait is often diagnostic (page 131). Sometimes there is loss of sensation in the paralyzed parts and loss of sight, hearing, and smell on the paralyzed side—a pattern of sensory changes that is never seen in organic brain disease. When the hysterical patient is asked to move the affected limbs, the movements tend to be slow, hesitant, and jerky, often with contraction of agonist and antagonist muscles simultaneously and intermittently. Lack of effort is usually obvious, despite facial and other expressions to the contrary. Power of contraction improves with encouragement. The weakness is inconsistent; some movements are performed tentatively and moments later another movement involving the same muscles is performed naturally. Hoover's sign and the trunk-thigh sign of Babinski are helpful in distinguishing hysterical from organic hemiplegia. To elicit Hoover's sign, the examiner places both hands under the heels of the recumbent patient, who is asked to press the heels down forcefully. With organic hemiplegia, pressure will be felt entirely or almost entirely from the nonparalyzed leg. The examiner then removes his hand from under the nonparalyzed leg, places it on top of the nonparalyzed foot, and asks the patient to raise that leg. In true hemiplegia, no added pressure will be felt by the hand that remained beneath the heel of the paralyzed leg. In hysteria, the heel of the supposedly paralyzed leg will press down on the examiner's hand. To carry out Babinski's trunk-thigh test, the examiner asks the recumbent patient to sit up while keeping his arms crossed in front of his chest. In the patient with organic hemiplegia, there is an involuntary flexion of the paretic lower limb; in paraplegia, both limbs are flexed as the trunk is flexed; in hysterical hemiplegia, only the normal leg may be flexed; and in hysterical paraplegia, neither leg is flexed.

Muscular Paralysis and Spasm Unattended by Visible Changes in Nerve or Muscle

A discussion of motor paralysis would not be complete without some reference to a group of diseases in which muscle weakness may be profound but there are no overt structural changes in motor nerve cells or nerve fibers. This group comprises myasthenia gravis; myotonia congenita (Thomsen disease); familial periodic paralysis; disorders of potassium, sodium, calcium, and magnesium metabolism; tetany; tetanus; poisoning by *Clostridium botulinum*; black widow spider bite; and the thyroid and other endocrine myopathies. In these diseases, each with a fairly distinctive clinical picture, the abnormality is essentially biochemical, and their investigation requires special biochemical and histochemical tests and electron microscopic study. These subjects are discussed in the section on muscle disease.

REFERENCES

Aids to the Examination of the Peripheral Nervous System. London, Baillière Tindall/Saunders, 1986.

Alexander GE, DeLong MR: Mechanisms of the initiation and control of movement, in Asbury AK, McKhann GM, McDonald WI (eds): *Diseases of the Nervous System: Clinical Neurobiology*, 2nd ed. Philadelphia, Saunders, 1992, chap 21, pp 285–308.

Asanuma H: Cerebral cortical control of movement. *Physiologist* 16:143, 1973.

Asanuma H: The pyramidal tract, in Brooks VB (ed): *Handbook of Physiology*. Sec 1: *The Nervous System*. Vol 2: *Motor Control*, Part 2. Bethesda, MD, American Physiological Society, 1981, pp 702–733.

Brodal P: *The Central Nervous System: Structure and Function*, 5th ed. New York, Oxford University Press, 1992.

Brown P: Pathophysiology of spasticity. *J Neurol Neurosurg Psychiatry* 57:773, 1994.

Bucy PC, Keplinger JE, Siqueira EB: Destruction of the pyramidal tract in man. *J Neurosurg* 21:385, 1964.

Burke D, Lance JW: Myotatic unit and its disorders, in Asbury AK, McKhann GM, McDonald WI (eds): *Diseases of the Nervous System: Clinical Neurobiology*, 2nd ed. Philadelphia, Saunders, chap 20, pp 270–284.

Davidoff RA: Antispasticity drugs: Mechanisms of action. *Ann Neurol* 17:107, 1985.

Davidoff RA: Skeletal muscle tone and the misunderstood stretch reflex. *Neurology* 42:951, 1992.

Denny-Brown D: *The Cerebral Control of Movement*. Springfield, IL, Charles C Thomas, 1966.

Denny-Brown D: The nature of apraxia. *J Nerv Ment Dis* 12:9, 1958.

DiRenzi E, Faglioni PR, Sorgato P: Modality-specific and supramodal mechanisms of apraxia. *Brain* 105:301, 1982.

Evarts EV, Shinoda Y, Wise SP: *Neurophysiological Approaches to Higher Brain Functions*. New York, Wiley, 1984.

Faglioni PR, Basso A: Historical perspectives on neuroanatomical correlates of limb apraxia, in Roy EA (ed): *Neuropsychological Studies of Apraxia and Related Disorders*. Amsterdam, North Holland, 1985, pp 3–44.

Feinberg TE, Schindler RJ, Flanagan NG, Haber LD: Two alien hand syndromes. *Neurology* 42:19, 1992.

Fulton JF: *Physiology of the Nervous System*. New York, Oxford University Press, 1938, chap 20.

Geschwind N: The apraxias: Neural mechanisms of disorders of learned movement. *Am Sci* 63:188, 1975.

Gilman S, Marco LA: Effects of medullary pyramidotomy in the monkey. *Brain* 94:495, 515, 1971.

Hallett M, Shahani BT, Young RR: EMG analysis of stereotyped voluntary movements in man. *J Neurol Neurosurg Psychiatry* 38:1154, 1975.

Henneman E: Organization of the spinal cord and its reflexes, in Mountcastle VB (ed): *Medical Physiology*, 14th ed. Vol 1. St Louis, Mosby, 1980, pp 762–786.

Iwatsubo T, Kuzuhara S, Kanemitsu A, et al: Corticofugal projections to the motor nuclei of the brain stem and spinal cord in humans. *Neurology* 40:309, 1990.

Kertesz A, Ferro JM, Shewan CM: Apraxia and aphasia: The functional anatomical basis for their dissociation. *Neurology* 34:40, 1984.

Lance JW: The control of muscle tone, reflexes and movement: Robert Wartenburg Lecture. *Neurology* 30:1303, 1980.

Laplane D, Talairach J, Meininger V, et al: Motor consequences of motor area ablations in man. *J Neurol Sci* 31:29, 1977.

Lassek AM: *The Pyramidal Tract*. Springfield, IL, Charles C Thomas, 1954.

Lawrence DG, Kuypers HGJM: The functional organization of the motor system in the monkey. *Brain* 91:1, 15, 1968.

Liepmann H: Das Krankheitsbild der Apraxie (motorische Asymbolie auf Grund eines Falles von einseitiger Apraxie). *Monatsschr Psychiatry Neurol* 8:15, 102, 182, 1900.

Lorente de Nó R: Cerebral cortex: Architecture, intracortical connections, motor projections, in Fulton JF (ed): *Physiology of the Nervous System*, 3rd ed. New York, Oxford University Press, 1949, pp 288–330.

Luria AR: *The Working Brain: An Introduction to Neuropsychology*. New York, Basic Books, 1973.

Mountcastle VB: Central nervous mechanisms in sensation, in Mountcastle VB (ed): *Medical Physiology*, 14th ed. Vol 1: Part 5. St Louis, Mosby, 1980, chaps 11–19, pp 327–605.

Nathan PW, Smith M, Deacon P: Vestibulospinal, reticulospinal and descending propriospinal nerve fibers in man. *Brain* 119:1809, 1996.

Nyberg-Hansen R, Rinvik E: Some comments on the pyramidal tract with special reference to its individual variations in man. *Acta Neurol Scand* 39:1, 1963.

Pantano P, Formisano R, Ricci M, et al: Prolonged muscular flaccidity after stroke. Morphological and functional brain alterations. *Brain* 118:1329, 1995.

Pause M, Kunesch F, Binkofski F, Freund H-J: Sensorimotor disturbances in patients with lesions of the parietal cortex. *Brain* 112:1599, 1989.

Roland PE: Organization of motor control by the normal human brain. *Hum Neurobiol* 2:205, 1984.

Ropper AH, Fisher CM, Kleinman GM: Pyramidal infarction in the medulla: A cause of pure motor hemiplegia sparing the face. *Neurology* 29:91, 1979.

Russell JR, DeMyer W: The quantitative cortical origin of pyramidal axons of Macaca rhesus, with some remarks on the slow rate of axolysis. *Neurology* 11:96, 1961.

Thach WT Jr, Montgomery EB Jr: Motor system, in Pearlman AL, Collins RC (eds): *Neurobiology of Disease*. New York, Oxford University Press, 1990, pp 168–196.

Tower SS: Pyramidal lesion in the monkey. *Brain* 63:36, 1940.

Chapter 4

ABNORMALITIES OF MOVEMENT AND POSTURE DUE TO DISEASE OF THE BASAL GANGLIA

In this chapter, the disorders of the automatic, static, postural, and other less modifiable motor activities of the nervous system are discussed. They are believed, on good evidence, to be an expression of the *extrapyramidal* motor system, meaning—according to S. A. K. Wilson, who introduced this term—the motor structures of the basal ganglia and certain related thalamic and brainstem nuclei.

In health, the activities of the basal ganglia and the cerebellum are blended with and modulate the corticospinal and cortical-brainstem-spinal systems. The static postural activities of the former are indispensable to the voluntary movements of the latter. The close association of these two systems also becomes evident in the course of neurologic disease. Cerebral lesions that involve the corticospinal tracts predominantly result not only in a contralateral paralysis of volitional movements but also in a fixed posture or attitude in which the arm is flexed and the leg extended (predilection type of Wernicke-Mann or hemiplegic dystonia of Denny-Brown). As noted in Chap. 3, interruption of the motor projection pathways by a lesion in the upper pons or midbrain may release another posture in which all four limbs or the arm and leg on one side are extended and the cervical and thoracolumbar portions of the spine are hyperextended (*decerebrate rigidity*). In these released motor patterns, one has evidence of labyrinthine, tonic neck, and other postural reflexes that are mediated through descending nonpyramidal bulbospinal and other brainstem motor systems. Observations such as these and the anatomic data presented in Chap. 3 have blurred the classic distinctions between pyramidal and extrapyramidal motor systems. Nevertheless, this division remains a useful if not an essential concept in clinical work, since it compels us to distinguish several motor syndromes from one another—one that is characterized by a loss of volitional movement and spasticity; a second by akinesia, rigidity, and tremor without loss of voluntary movement; a third by involuntary movements (choreoathetosis and dystonia); and yet another by incoordination (ataxia). The clinical differences between corticospinal and extrapyramidal syndromes are summarized in Table 4-1.

Much of the criticism of the pyramidal-extrapyramidal concept derives from the terms themselves. The ambiguity related to the term *pyramidal* was discussed in Chap. 3, in which it was pointed out that pure pyramidal lesions do not cause total paralysis; when the latter exists, there is always involvement of other descending pathways as well. The term *extrapyramidal* is equally imprecise. Strictly interpreted, it refers to all the motor pathways except the pyramidal one, making this term so all-embracing as to be practically meaningless. The concept of an extrapyramidal motor system becomes more meaningful if it is subdivided into two parts: (1) the striatopallidonigral system (basal ganglia) and (2) the cerebellum. These parts function very differently in the control of movement and posture, and disease in each of them results in particular disturbances of movement and posture without paralysis. The basal ganglia and the symptoms that result when they are diseased are described in the pages that follow. The disorders of movement and posture due to cerebellar disease are described in Chap. 5.

Table 4-1
Clinical differences between corticospinal and extrapyramidal syndromes

	Corticospinal	*Extrapyramidal*
Character of the alteration of muscle tone	Clasp-knife effect (spasticity); ± rigidity	Plastic, equal throughout passive movement (rigidity), or intermittent (cogwheel rigidity)
Distribution of hypertonus	Flexors of arms, extensors of legs	Generalized but predominates in flexors of limbs and of trunk
Shortening and lengthening reaction	Present	Absent
Involuntary movements	Absent	Presence of tremor, chorea, athetosis, dystonia
Tendon reflexes	Increased	Normal or slightly increased
Babinski sign	Present	Absent
Paralysis of voluntary movement	Present	Absent or slight

THE STRIATOPALLIDONIGRAL SYSTEM (BASAL GANGLIA)

Anatomic and Physiologic Considerations

As an anatomic entity, the basal ganglia have no precise definition. Principally they include the caudate nucleus and the lentiform nucleus with its two subdivisions, the putamen and globus pallidus. Insofar as the caudate nucleus and putamen are really a continuous structure (separated only incompletely by fibers of the internal capsule) and are cytologically and functionally distinct from the pallidum, it is more meaningful to divide these nuclear masses into the striatum (or neostriatum), comprising the caudate nucleus and putamen, and the paleostriatum or pallidum, which has a medial (internal) and a lateral (external) segment. The putamen and pallidum lie on the lateral aspect of the internal capsule, which separates them from the caudate nucleus, thalamus, subthalamic nucleus, and substantia nigra on its medial side (Figs. 4-1 and 4-2). By virtue of their close connections with the caudate and lenticular nuclei, the subthalamic nucleus (nucleus of Luys) and the substantia nigra are usually considered as parts of the basal ganglia. The claustrum and amygdaloid nuclear complex, because of their largely different connections and functions, are usually excluded.

For reasons indicated further on, some physiologists have expanded the list of basal ganglionic structures to include the red nucleus, the intralaminar thalamic nuclei, and the reticular formations of the upper brainstem. These structures receive direct cortical projections and give rise to rubrospinal and reticulospinal tracts which run parallel to the corticospinal (pyramidal) ones; hence they were referred to as *extrapyramidal*. However, these nonpyramidal linkages are structurally independent of the major nonpyramidal circuit that includes the striatum, pallidum, thalamus, and premotor and supplementary motor cortices. Insofar as the final links in this circuit—the premotor and supplementary motor cortices—ultimately project onto the motor cortex, this circuit is more aptly referred to as *prepyramidal* (Thach and Montgomery).

Earlier views of basal ganglionic organization emphasized the serial connectivity of the basal ganglionic structures and the funneling of efferent projections to the ventrolateral thalamus and thence to the motor cortex (Fig. 4-3). This concept was based largely on the seminal experimental work of Whittier and Mettler and of Carpenter, in the late 1940s. These investigators demonstrated, in monkeys, that a characteristic movement disorder, which they termed *choreoid dyskinesia*, could be produced consistently in the limbs of one side of the body by a lesion localized to the opposite subthalamic nucleus. They also showed that for such a lesion to provoke dyskinesia, the adjacent pallidum and pallidofugal fibers had to be preserved; furthermore, a secondary lesion—placed in the medial segment of the pallidum, in the fasciculus lenticularis, or in the ventrolateral thalamic nuclear group—could abolish the dyskinesia. This experimental hyperkinesia could be abolished permanently by interruption of the lateral corticospinal tract but not by interruption of the other motor or sensory pathways in the spinal cord. These observations were interpreted to mean that the subthalamic nucleus normally exerts an inhibitory or regulating influence on the globus pallidus and ventral thalamus. Removal of this influence by selective destruction of the subthalamic nucleus is expressed physiologically by bursts of irregular choreoid activity, presumably arising from the intact pallidum and conveyed by pallidofugal fibers to the ventrolateral thalamic nuclei, thence by thalamocortical fibers to the ipsilateral premotor cortex, and

Figure 4-1

Diagram of the striatal afferent pathways. Corticostriate fibers from broad cortical areas project to the putamen; fibers from the cortex on the medial surface project largely to the caudate nucleus. Nigrostriatal fibers arise from the pars compacta of the substantia nigra. Thalamostriate fibers arise from the centromedian-parafascicular complex of the thalamus. CM, centromedian nucleus; DM, dorsomedial nucleus; GP, globus pallidus; IC, internal capsule; PUT, putamen; RN, red nucleus; SN, substantia nigra; VPL, ventral posterolateral nucleus; VPM, ventral posterior medial nucleus. (Redrawn by permission from Carpenter MB, Sutin J: Human Neuroanatomy, 8th ed. Baltimore, Williams & Wilkins, 1983.)

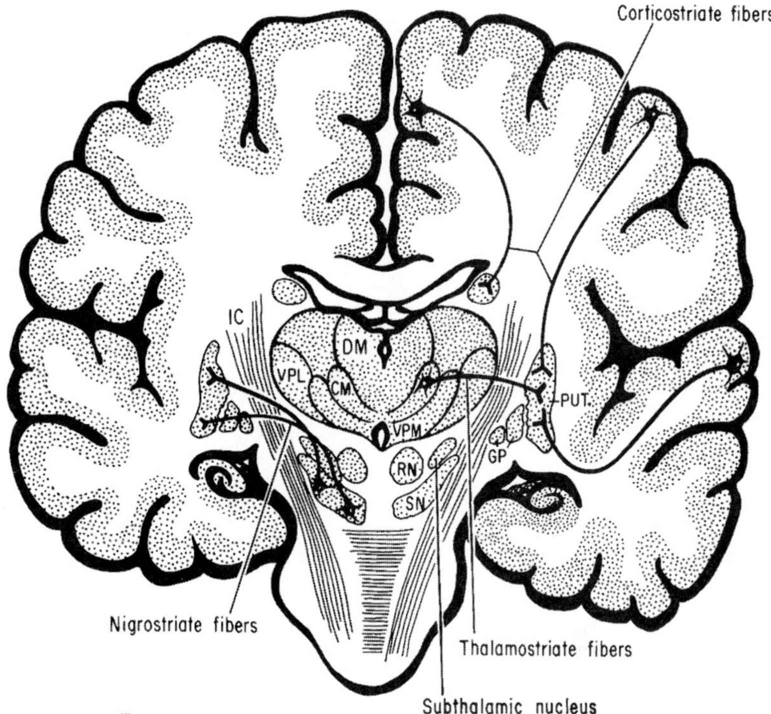

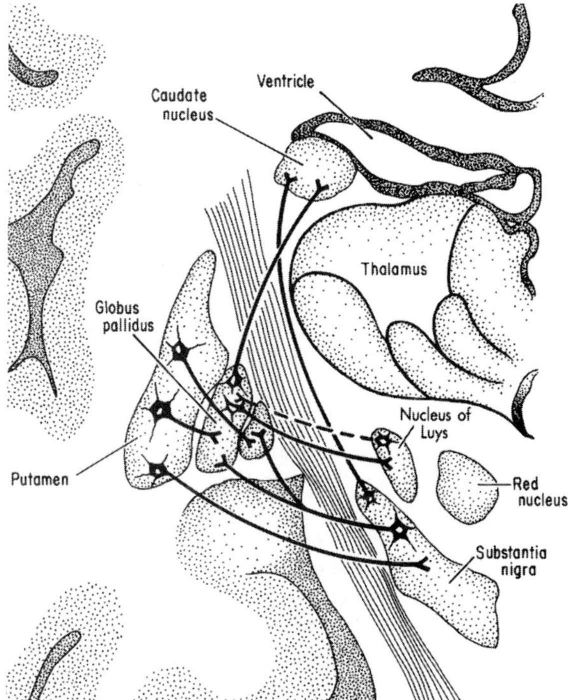

Figure 4-2

Diagram of the basal ganglia in the coronal plane, illustrating the main striatal efferent pathways (details in text). The pallidothalamic connections are illustrated in Fig. 4-3.

from there by short association fibers to the motor cortex. Ultimately the abnormal movement is expressed via the lateral corticospinal tract, which in this instance functions as the final executive pathway.

A general principle that emerged from these observations was the central role of the ventrolateral and ventroanterior nuclei of the thalamus. Together, they form a vital link in an ascending fiber system, not only from the basal ganglia but also from the cerebellum, to the motor and premotor cortex. Thus both basal ganglionic and cerebellar influences are brought to bear, via thalamocortical fibers, on the corticospinal system and on other descending pathways from the cortex. Direct descending pathways from the basal ganglia to the spinal cord are relatively insignificant.

The foregoing view of basal ganglionic organization has been broadened considerably, the result of new anatomic, physiologic, and pharmacologic data (see in particular the reviews of Alexander and Crutcher, of DeLong, and of Penney and Young). Whereas earlier concepts emphasized the serial connectivity of the basal ganglionic structures and the funneling of efferent projections to the ventrolateral thalamus and then to the motor cortex, current evidence indicates an organization into several parallel basal ganglionic–cortical circuits. Although these circuits run parallel to the premotor or prepyramidal pathway, they remain separate from it,

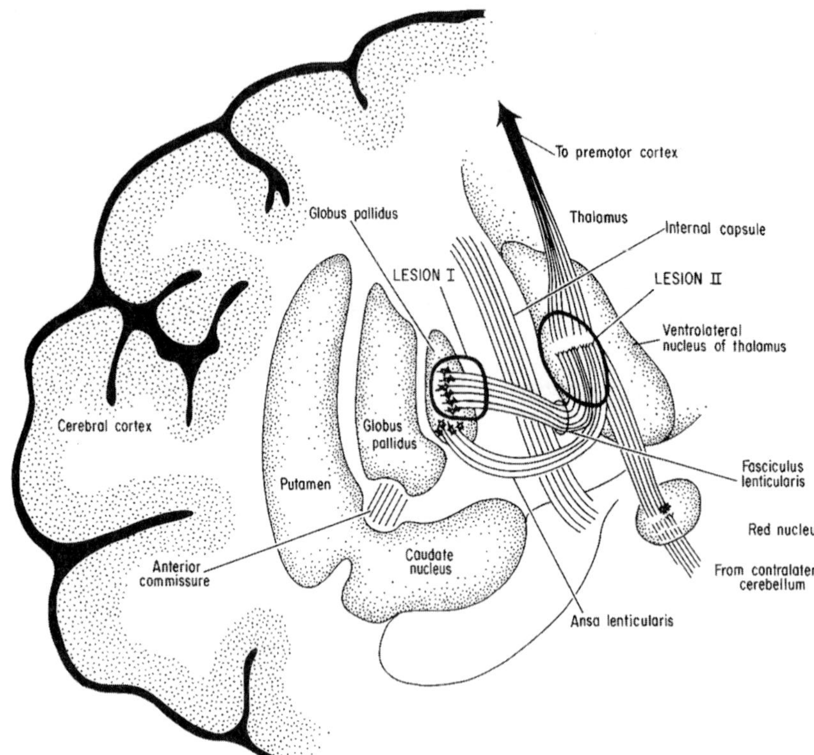

Figure 4-3

Basal ganglia in the horizontal plane, illustrating the main efferent projections from the medial segment of the pallidum to the ventral nuclei of the thalamus (details in text).

anatomically and physiologically. At least five such circuits have been described, each focused on a different portion of the frontal lobe: the prototypical motor circuit, converging on the premotor cortex; the oculomotor circuit, on the frontal eye fields; two prefrontal circuits, on the dorsolateral prefrontal and lateral orbitofrontal cortex, respectively; and a limbic circuit, on the anterior cingulate and medial orbitofrontal cortex.

An additional and most important feature of basal ganglionic structure and function, also relatively recently appreciated, is the nonequivalence of all parts of the striatum. Particular cell types and zones of cells within this structure appear to mediate different aspects of motor control and utilize specific neurochemical transmitters (Albin et al, DeLong).

The most important basal ganglionic connections and circuitry are indicated in Figs. 4-1, 4-2, and 4-3. Conventionally it has been taught that the striatum, mainly the putamen, is the *receptive part* of the basal ganglia, receiving topographically organized fibers from all parts of the cerebral cortex and from the pars compacta (pigmented neurons) of the substantia nigra; and that the *output* nuclei of the basal ganglia consist of the medial (internal) pallidum and the nonpigmented portion of the substantia nigra (pars reticulata).

It has been proposed—on the basis of physiologic, lesional, and pharmacologic studies—that there are two main efferent projections from the putamen, but these models, being quite incomplete, should be viewed as provisional. Nonetheless, there are reasons to conceptualize a *direct* efferent system from the putamen onto the medial (internal) pallidum and then onto the substantia nigra, particularly the nonpigmented (pars reticulata) cells, and an *indirect* system that traverses the lateral (external) pallidum and continues on to the subthalamic nucleus, with which it has strong to-and-fro connections. In some ways the subthalamic nucleus and lateral pallidum operate as a single functional unit (at least in terms of the effects of lesions in those locations on parkinsonian symptoms and the neurotransmitters involved; see further on). The medial pallidum and reticular part of the nigra can be viewed in a similar unitary way, sharing the same input and output patterns. Within the indirect pathway, an internal loop is created by projections from the subthalamic nucleus to the medial segment of the pallidum and pars reticulata. A second offshoot of the indirect pathway, recently uncovered, consists of projections from the lateral pallidum to the medial pallidonigral output nuclei.

From the internal pallidum, two bundles of fibers reach the *thalamus*—the ansa and the fasciculus lenticularis (Fig. 4-3). The ansa sweeps around the internal capsule; the fasciculus traverses the internal capsule in a number of small fascicles and then continues medially and caudally to join the ansa in the prerubral field. Both these fiber bundles join the thalamic fasciculus, which then contains not only the pallidothalamic projections but also mesothalamic, rubrothalamic, and dentatothalamic ones. These projections are directed to separate targets in the ventrolateral nucleus of the thalamus and to a lesser extent in the ventral anterior and intralaminar thalamic nuclei. The centromedian nucleus of the intralaminar group projects back to the putamen and, via the parafascicular nucleus, to the caudate. A major projection from the ventral thalamic nuclei to the ipsilateral premotor cortex completes the large *cortical-striatal-pallidal-thalamic-cortical* motor loop—(the prepyramidal circuit, mentioned above)—with conservation of the somatotopic arrangement of motor fibers.

There is pharmacologic and physiologic evidence that a balanced functional architecture, one excitatory and the other inhibitory, is operative within individual circuits. The *direct* striato-medial pallidal-nigral pathway is activated by *glutaminergic* projections from the sensorimotor cortex and by *dopaminergic* nigral (pars compacta)-striatal projections. Stimulation of this direct pathway inhibits the medial pallidum, which, in turn, disinhibits the ventrolateral and ventroanterior nuclei of the thalamus. As a consequence, thalamocortical drive is enhanced and cortically initiated movements are facilitated. The *indirect* circuit arises from putaminal neurons that contain *gamma-aminobutyric acid* (GABA) and smaller amounts of enkephalin. These striatal projections have an inhibitory effect on the lateral pallidum, which, in turn, disinhibits the subthalamic nucleus through GABA release, providing excessive subthalamic drive to the medial pallidum and substantia nigra pars reticulata. The net effect is thalamic inhibition and reduced thalamocortical input to the precentral motor fields. These complex anatomic and physiologic relationships have been summarized in numerous schematic figures, such as Fig. 4-4 (see also the review by Lang and Lozano).

It has been suggested that enhanced conduction through the indirect pathway leads to hypokinesia (by increasing pallidothalamic inhibition), whereas enhanced conduction through the direct pathway results in hyperkinesia (by reducing pallidothalamic inhibition). The direct pathway is perceived by Marsden and Obeso as

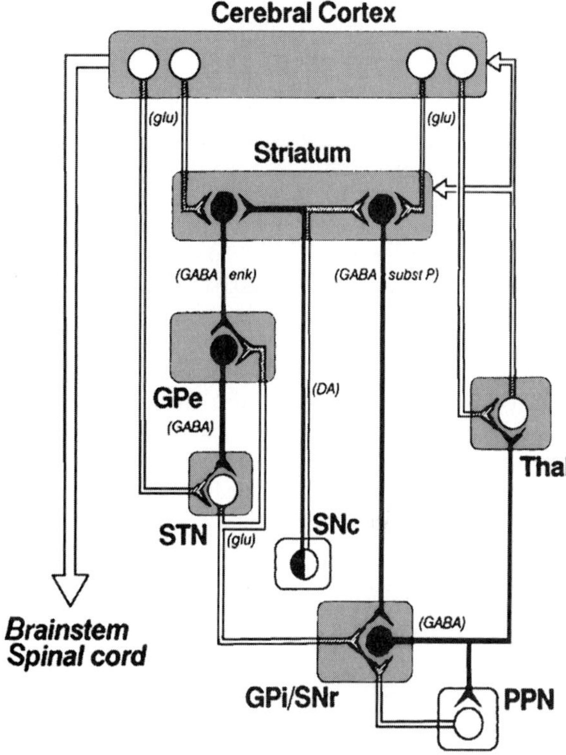

Figure 4-4

Schematic diagram of the main putative neurotransmitter pathways and their effects in the cortical-basal ganglia-thalamic circuits. The solid circles and lines indicate neurons with excitatory effects, and the white circles and lines indicate inhibitory influences. The internal (medial) segment of the globus pallidus (GPi) and the zona reticulata of the substantia nigra (SNr) are believed to act as one entity that projects via GABA-containing neurons to the thalamus (ventrolateral and ventroanterior nuclei) and to the pedunculopontine nuclei (PPN). Dopaminergic neurons arising in the pars compacta of the substantia nigra (SNc) have an excitatory influence on one portion of the striatum and an inhibitory effect on the portion of the striatum that projects to the external (lateral) pallidum (GPe) and subthalamic nucleus (STN). This scheme is inferred from the effects of pharmacologic agents on the motor and electrophysiologic activities of each structure, but the results of surgical lesions are not always concordant with these principles. Substance P and enkephalin act as modulating neurotransmitters for GABA in pathways that project from the striatum. (glu = glutamine; DA = dopamine.) (Reprinted by permission from Alexander GE, Crutcher MD: Functional architecture of basal ganglia circuits: neural substrates of parallel processing. Trends Neurosci 13:266, 1990.)

facilitating cortically initiated movements, and the indirect pathway as suppressing potentially conflicting and unwanted motor patterns. This view is supported by studies of motor organization in acquired hemidystonia (Ceballos-Baumann and colleagues) and lesioning studies in Parkinson disease.

In more conventional physiologic terms, Denny-Brown and Yanagisawa, who studied the effects of ablation of individual extrapyramidal structures in monkeys, concluded that the basal ganglia function as a kind of clearinghouse where, during an intended or projected movement, one set of activities is facilitated and all other unnecessary ones are suppressed. Another theory, stated somewhat differently, suggests that the basal ganglia function as a brake or switch. The tonic inhibitory ("brake") action of the basal ganglia prevents their target structures from generating unwanted motor activity. The "switch" function refers to the capacity of the basal ganglia to select which of many available motor programs will be active at any given time. Still other theories focus on the role of the basal ganglia in the initiation, sequencing, and modulation of motor activity ("motor programming"). Also, it appears that the basal ganglia participate in the constant priming of the motor system, enabling the rapid execution of motor acts without premeditation—e.g., hitting a baseball. In most ways, these conceptualizations restate the same notions of balance and selectivity imparted to all motor actions by the basal ganglia. Despite the recent impressive expansion of knowledge, the precise mechanisms by which the basal ganglia control motor function remains elusive. The manner in which excessive or depleted activity of various components of the basal ganglia gives rise to hypokinetic and hyperkinetic movement disorders is discussed further on under "Symptoms of Basal Ganglia Disease."

Pharmacologic Considerations

During the past three decades, a series of pharmacologic observations—some abstracted above—has considerably enhanced our understanding of basal ganglionic function and led to the discovery of a rational treatment of Parkinson disease and other extrapyramidal syndromes. Whereas physiologists had for years failed to discover the functions of the basal ganglia by stimulation and crude ablation experiments, clinicians became aware that the use of certain drugs, such as reserpine and the phenothiazines, regularly produced extrapyramidal syndromes (parkinsonism, choreoathetosis, dystonia, etc.). These observations greatly stimulated the study of central nervous system transmitter substances in general. The current view is that the integrated basal ganglionic control of movement can be best understood by considering, in the context of the anatomy described above, the physiologic effects of neurotransmitters that convey the signals between cortex, striatum, globus pallidus, subthalamic nucleus, substantia nigra, and thalamus.

The most important neurotransmitter substances from the point of view of basal ganglionic function are glutamate, GABA, dopamine, acetylcholine, and serotonin, as already alluded to. They are summarized in Fig. 4-4, and a more complete account of this subject than is possible here may be found in the recent reviews of Penney and Young and of Ciliax and colleagues referenced at the end of this chapter.

Glutamate is the neurotransmitter of the corticostriatal excitatory projections and of the excitatory neurons of the subthalamic nucleus. GABA is the inhibitory neurotransmitter of striatal, pallidal, and substantia nigra (pars reticulata) projection neurons. Acetylcholine (ACh), long established as the neurotransmitter at the neuromuscular junction as well as in the autonomic ganglia, is also physiologically active in the basal ganglia. The highest concentration of ACh as well as of choline acetylase and acetylcholinesterase (the enzymes necessary for the synthesis and degradation, respectively, of ACh) is in the striatum. Acetylcholine is synthesized and released by the large but sparse (Golgi type 2) nonspiny neurons. It has a mixed but mainly excitatory effect upon the more numerous spiny neurons within the putamen that constitute the main origin of the direct and indirect pathways. Dopamine, by contrast, has an inhibitory effect on these neurons (see below). It is likely that the effectiveness of the belladonna alkaloids and other atropinic agents—which have been used empirically for many years in the treatment of Parkinson disease and dystonia—depends on their capacity to antagonize ACh at sites within the basal ganglia and in projections from the pedunculopontine nuclei. Acetylcholine appears also to act on the presynaptic membrane of striatal cells and to influence their release of neurotransmitters, as discussed below.

In addition, the basal ganglia contain other biologically active substances—substance P, enkephalin, cholecystokinin, somatostatin, and neuropeptide Y—which may enhance or diminish the effects of other neurotransmitters, i.e., they act as *neuromodulators*. The neurons utilizing these substances are just now being identified.

Of the catecholamines, dopamine has the most pervasive role in the functioning of the basal ganglia.

The areas richest in dopamine are the substantia nigra, where it is synthesized in the nerve cell bodies of the pars compacta, and the termination of these fibers in the striatum. In the most simplified models, stimulation of the dopaminergic neurons of the substantia nigra induces a specific response in the striatum—namely, an inhibitory effect on the already low firing rate of neostriatal neurons. However, the effects of dopamine have proved more difficult to unravel, in large part because there are now four known types of postsynaptic receptors (D_1 to D_4), each with its particular anatomic distribution and pharmacologic action. This heterogeneity is reflected in the excitatory effect of dopamine on the small spiny neurons of the putamen and an inhibitory effect on others.

Certain drugs—namely reserpine, the phenothiazines, and the butyrophenones, notably haloperidol—may induce parkinsonian syndromes in humans. Reserpine acts by depleting the striatum and other parts of the brain of dopamine; haloperidol and the phenothiazines produce parkinsonism by a different mechanism, probably by causing a blockade of dopamine receptors within the striatum.

New insight into Parkinson disease has come from the discovery that it can be faithfully reproduced in humans and primates by the toxin1-methyl-4-phenyl-1,2,3,6-tetrahydropyridine (MPTP). This toxin was discovered accidentally in drug addicts who self-administered an analogue of meperidine. The toxin binds with high affinity to monoamine oxidase (MAO), an extraneural enzyme that transforms it to a toxic metabolite—pyridinium. The latter is bound by melanin in the dopaminergic nigral neurons in sufficient quantities to destroy the cells. In monkeys made parkinsonian by the administration of MPTP, electrophysiologic studies have shown increased activity in the medial globus pallidus and decreased activity in the lateral globus pallidus, as predicted from the previously described models. This comes about because of the differential loss of activity of dopaminergic striatal neurons that project to each of these parts of the pallidum. The end result is increased inhibition of thalamocortical neurons. As pointed out by Bhatia and Marsden, it is difficult to explain why medial pallidal lesions do not regularly cause parkinsonism. Perhaps it is because the subtle imbalance between the medial and lateral pallidal circuits that exists in Parkinson disease is not reproduced. This may also explain why crude lesions such as infarcts, hemorrhages, and tumors rarely produce the complete parkinsonian syndrome of tremor, bradykinesia, and rigidity without paralysis or reflex changes. Indeed, striking improvements in parkinsonian symptoms are obtained by placing lesions in the medial pallidum (pallidotomy), as discussed on page 1136.

In order to correct the basic nigral dopamine deficiency, attempts were at first made to administer dopamine to Parkinson patients. However, dopamine as such cannot pass the blood-brain barrier and has no therapeutic effect. But the immediate dopamine precursor, L-dopa, does cross the barrier and is effective in decreasing the akinesia, rigidity, and tremor of Parkinson disease as well as of MPTP-induced parkinsonism. This effect is greatly enhanced by the inhibition of dopadecarboxylase, an important enzyme in the catabolism of dopamine. The addition of this enzyme inhibitor (carbidopa or benserazide) to L-dopa results in a marked increase of dopamine concentration in the brain, while sparing other organs from exposure to high levels of the drug. Similarly, drugs that inhibit catechol O-methyltransferase (COMT), another enzyme that breaks down dopamine, can prolong the effects of administered L-dopa.

Because of the pharmacologic activities of ACh and dopamine, it was originally postulated by Hornykiewicz that a functional equilibrium exists in the striatum between the excitatory activity of ACh and the inhibitory activity of dopamine. In Parkinson disease, the decreased release of dopamine by the substantia nigra onto the striatum disinhibits neurons that synthesize ACh, resulting in a predominance of cholinergic activity—a notion supported by the observation that parkinsonian symptoms are aggravated by centrally acting cholinergic drugs and improved by anticholinergic drugs. According to this theory, administration of anticholinergic drugs restores the ratio between dopamine and acetylcholine, with the new equilibrium being set at a lower-than-normal level because the striatal levels of dopamine are low to begin with. The use of drugs that enhance dopamine synthesis or dopamine release or that directly stimulate dopaminergic receptors in the striatum (e.g., bromocriptine) represents a more physiologic method of treating Parkinson disease.

The Pathology of Basal Ganglionic Disease

The extrapyramidal motor syndrome as we know it today was first delineated on clinical grounds and so named by S. A. K. Wilson in 1912. In the disease that now bears his name and that he called *hepatolenticular degeneration*, the most striking abnormality in the nervous system was a bilaterally symmetrical degeneration of the putamens, sometimes to the point of cavitation. To these lesions Wilson attributed the characteristic symptoms of rigidity and tremor. Shortly thereafter, van Woerkom described a similar clinical syndrome in a patient with acquired liver disease (Wilson's cases were familial); in the acquired form also, the most prominent lesions consisted of foci of neuronal degeneration in the striatum. Clinicopathologic studies of Huntington chorea—beginning with those of Meynert (1871) and followed by those of Jelgersma (1908) and Alzheimer (1911)—related the movement disorder as well as the rigidity to a loss of nerve cells in the striatum. In 1920, Oskar and Cecile Vogt gave a detailed account of the neuropathologic changes in several patients who had been afflicted with choreoathetosis since early infancy; the changes, which they described as a status fibrosis or status dysmyelinatus, were said to be confined to the caudate and lenticular nuclei. Tretiakoff (1919) was the first to demonstrate the consistent pathology of the substantia nigra in cases of paralysis agitans. A series of observations, culminating with those of J. Purdon Martin and later of Mitchell and colleagues, related hemiballismus to lesions in the subthalamic nucleus of Luys and its immediate connections.

More recently, Bhatia and Marsden, relying on published imaging studies, reviewed some 240 cases in which there were lesions in the caudate, putamen, and globus pallidus associated with movement and behavioral abnormalities. Dystonia had occurred in 36 percent, chorea in 8 percent, parkinsonism in only 6 percent, and dystonia-parkinsonism in 3 percent. Bilateral lesions of the subthalamic nuclei resulted in parkinsonism in 19 percent and dystonia-parkinsonism in 6 percent. The commonest persisting behavioral abnormality was abulia (apathy and loss of initiative, spontaneous thought, and emotional responsivity), occurring in 28 percent of those with caudate lesions. The deficiencies of this type of case analysis, conceded by the authors, included the crudity of the anatomy (judged by early computed tomography studies) and the lack of precise information regarding the temporal aspects of the functional disorder—time of onset, duration, and changes during the course of the illness. We find it surprising that choreoathetosis was not more frequent. Needed, of course, are detailed anatomic (postmortem) studies of cases in which the disturbances of function were stable for many months or years. Such an example is the case of generalized dystonia with pallidoluysian atrophy reported by Wooten and coworkers.

Table 4-2 summarizes the clinicopathologic correlations accepted by most neurologists, but it must be emphasized that there is still much uncertainty as to the finer details.

Table 4-2
Clinicopathologic correlations of extrapyramidal motor disorders

Symptoms	*Principal location of morbid anatomy*
Unilateral plastic rigidity with static tremor (Parkinson disease)	Contralateral substantia nigra plus (?) other mesencephalic structures
Unilateral hemiballismus and hemichorea	Contralateral subthalamic nucleus of Luys or luysial pallidal connections
Chronic chorea of Huntington type	Caudate nucleus and putamen
Athetosis and dystonia	Contralateral striatum. Pathology of dystonia musculorum deformans (Oppenheim) unknown
Cerebellar incoordination, intention tremor, and hypotonia	Ipsilateral cerebellar hemisphere; ipsilateral middle or inferior cerebellar peduncle; brachium conjunctivum (ipsilateral if below decussation, contralateral if above)
Decerebrate rigidity, i.e., extension of arms and legs, opisthotonos	Usually bilateral in tegmentum of upper brainstem, at level of red nucleus or between red and vestibular nuclei
Palatal and facial myoclonus (rhythmic)	Ipsilateral central tegmental tract, with denervation of inferior olivary nucleus and nucleus ambiguus
Diffuse myoclonus	Neuronal degeneration, usually diffuse or predominating in cerebral or cerebellar cortex and dentate nuclei

SYMPTOMS OF BASAL GANGLIA DISEASE

In broad terms, all motor disorders may be considered to consist of primary functional deficits (or *negative* symptoms) and secondary effects (*positive* symptoms), the latter being ascribed to the release or disinhibition of the activity of undamaged parts of the motor nervous system. When diseases of the basal ganglia are analyzed along these classic lines, bradykinesia, hypo- or akinesia, and loss of normal postural reflexes stand out as the primary negative symptoms, and tremor, rigidity, and involuntary movements (chorea, athetosis, ballismus, and dystonia) as the positive ones. Disorders of phonation, articulation, and locomotion are more difficult to classify. In some instances they are clearly a consequence of rigidity and postural disorders, while in others, where rigidity is slight or negligible, they seem to represent primary deficiencies. In some cases that present as slowness of movement alone, examination may reveal only a slight delay in the initiation of movement and slight irregularity and clumsiness of movement (e.g., maladroitness in children) that is sometimes misinterpreted as apraxia. Stress and nervous tension characteristically worsen both the motor deficiency and the abnormal movements in all extrapyramidal syndromes, just as relaxation improves them. The particular symptoms of basal ganglia disease are elaborated below.

Hypokinesia and Bradykinesia

The terms *hypokinesia* and *akinesia* refer to a disinclination on the part of the patient to use an affected part and to engage it freely in all the natural actions of the body. There may, in addition, be slowness in the initiation and execution of a movement. In contrast to what occurs in paralysis (the primary symptom of corticospinal tract lesions), strength is not significantly diminished. Also, hypokinesia is unlike apraxia, in which a lesion erases the memory of the pattern of movements necessary for an intended act, leaving other actions intact. Clinically, the phenomenon of hypokinesia or akinesia is expressed most clearly in the parkinsonian patient and takes the form of an extreme underactivity (poverty of movement). The frequent automatic, habitual movements observed in the normal individual—such as putting the hand to the face, folding the arms, or crossing the legs—are absent or greatly reduced. In looking to one side, the eyes move, not the head. In arising from a chair, there is a failure to make the usual small preliminary adjustments, such as pulling the feet back, putting the hands on the arms of the chair, and so forth. Blinking is infrequent. Saliva is not swallowed as quickly as it is produced, and drooling results. The face lacks expressive mobility ("masked facies," hypomimia). Speech is rapid and monotonic and the voice is soft.

Bradykinesia, which connotes slowness rather than lack of movement, is probably another aspect of the same physiologic difficulty. Not only is the parkinsonian patient slightly "slow off the mark" (displaying a longer-than-normal interval between a command and the first contraction of muscle—i.e., increased reaction time), but the velocity of movement, or the time from onset to completion of movement, is slower than normal. Hallett distinguishes between akinesia and bradykinesia, equating akinesia with a prolonged reaction time and bradykinesia with a prolonged time of execution. But he concedes that if bradykinesia is severe, it may result in akinesia. There is no slowness in formulating the plan of movement; that is to say, there is no bradyphrenia. For a time, bradykinesia was attributed to the frequently associated rigidity, which could reasonably hamper all movements, but the incorrectness of this explanation became apparent when it was discovered that an appropriately placed stereotactic lesion in a patient with Parkinson disease may abolish rigidity while leaving the akinesia unaltered. Thus it appears that apart from their contribution to the maintenance of posture, the basal ganglia provide an essential element for the performance of the large variety of voluntary and semiautomatic actions required for the full repertoire of natural human motility. Hallett and Khoshbin, in an analysis of ballistic (rapid) movements in the parkinsonian patient, found that the normal triphasic sequence of agonist-antagonist-agonist is intact but lacks the energy (number of activated motor units) to complete the movement. Several triphasic sequences are then needed, which slows the movement. That cells in the basal ganglia participate in the initiation of movement is also evident from the fact that the firing rates in these cells increase before movement is detected clinically.

In terms of pathologic anatomy and physiology, bradykinesia may be caused by any process or drug that interrupts some component of the cortico-striato-pallido-thalamic circuit. Rigidity (discussed further on) is frequently combined. Clinical examples include reduced dopaminergic input from the substantia nigra to the striatum, as in Parkinson disease; dopamine receptor blockade by neuroleptic drugs; extensive degeneration of striatal neurons, as in striatonigral degeneration and the rigid form of Huntington chorea; and destruction of the medial pallidum, as in Wilson and Hallervorden-Spatz disease.

A number of other disorders of voluntary movement may also be observed in patients with diseases of the basal ganglia. A persistent voluntary contraction of hand muscles, as in holding a pencil, may fail to be inhibited, so that there is interference with the next willed movement. This has been termed "tonic innervation" and may be brought out by asking the patient to repetitively open and close a fist. Attempts to perform an alternating sequence of movements may be blocked at one point with a tendency for the voluntary movement to adopt the frequency of the coexistent tremor. Muscles fatigue more readily on repeated activity. In still other cases, performance of a simple movement (e.g., touching finger to nose, forcefully striking an object with the fisted hand) is rendered impossible by the simultaneous contraction of agonist and antagonist muscles not only of the arm and hand but also of the neck, trunk, and even the legs ("intention spasm").

Disorders of Postural Fixation, Equilibrium, and Righting

These deficits are also demonstrated most clearly in the parkinsonian patient. The prevailing posture is one of involuntary flexion of the trunk and limbs and of the neck. The inability of the patient to make appropriate postural adjustments to tilting or falling and the inability to move from the reclining to the standing position are closely related phenomena. A gentle push on the patient's sternum or back may start a series of small corrective steps that the patient cannot control (festination). These postural abnormalities are not the result of weakness or of defects in proprioceptive, labyrinthine, or visual function, the principal forces that control the normal posture of the head and trunk. Anticipatory and compensatory righting reflexes are also manifestly impaired—early in progressive supranuclear palsy and later in Parkinson disease. These postural abnormalities have been compared to the flexed postures of the head and neck and disorders of equilibrium and righting that have been produced in monkeys by the ablation of the globus pallidus bilaterally (Richter).

A point of interest is whether akinesia and disorders of postural fixation are invariable negative manifestations of all extrapyramidal diseases and whether, without them, there could be any secondary release effects such as dystonia, choreoathetosis, and rigidity. The question has no clear answer. Akinesia and abnormalities of posture are invariable features of both Parkinson and Wilson diseases; they seem to be present also in Huntington chorea and in the double athetosis of cerebral palsy, but one cannot be sure of their existence in hemiballismus.

Rigidity

In the form of altered muscle tone known as *rigidity*, the muscles are continuously or intermittently firm and tense. Although brief periods of electromyographic silence can be obtained in selected muscles by persistent attempts to relax the limb, there is obviously a low threshold for involuntary sustained muscle contraction, and this is present during most of the waking state, even when the patient appears quiet and relaxed. In contrast to spasticity, the increased resistance on passive movement that characterizes rigidity is not preceded by an initial "free interval" and has an even or uniform quality through-out the range of movement of the limb, like that experienced in bending a lead pipe or pulling a strand of toffee. When released, the limb does not resume its original position, as happens in spasticity.

Rigidity usually involves all muscle groups, both flexor and extensor, but it tends to be more prominent in muscles that maintain a flexed posture, i.e., in the flexor muscles of trunk and limbs. It appears to be somewhat greater in the large muscle groups, but this may be merely a matter of muscle mass. Certainly the small muscles of the face and tongue and even those of the larynx are often affected. The tendon reflexes are not enhanced. Nevertheless, like spasticity, rigidity represents a lower threshold for synaptic excitation of spinal and cranial motor neurons. It can be abolished by the extradural or subarachnoid injection of local anesthesia, and, as claimed by Foerster many years ago, by posterior root section, presumably by interrupting the afferent fibers of the gamma loop. Recording from muscle spindles has not confirmed this spindle overdrive, and although the phasic myotatic (tendon) reflexes are not increased, the tonic stretch reflexes are. In the electromyographic tracing, motor-unit activity is more continuous in rigidity than in spasticity, persisting even after apparent relaxation.

A special type of rigidity, first noted by Negro in 1901, is the *cogwheel phenomenon*. When the hypertonic muscle is passively stretched, e.g., when the hand is dorsiflexed, one encounters a rhythmically interrupted, ratchet-like resistance. Most likely this phenomenon represents an associated static or action tremor that is masked by rigidity but emerges faintly during manipulation.

Rigidity is a prominent feature of many basal ganglionic diseases such as Parkinson disease (late stages), Wilson disease, striatonigral degeneration (multiple system atrophy), progressive supranuclear palsy, dystonia musculorum deformans (all discussed in Chap. 39), intoxication with neuroleptic drugs, and calcinosis of the basal ganglia. The rigidity is characteristically variable in degree, and in some patients with involuntary movements, particularly in those with chorea or dystonia, the limbs may be intermittently or persistently hypotonic.

A distinctive type of variable resistance to passive movement is that in which the patient seems unable to relax a group of muscles on request. When the limb muscles are passively stretched, the patient appears to actively resist the movement (*gegenhalten, paratonia,* or oppositional resistance). Natural relaxation requires concentration on the part of the patient. If there is inattentiveness—as happens with diseases of the frontal lobes, dementia, or other confusional states—this type of oppositional resistance may raise a question of parkinsonian rigidity. Actually this is not a manifestation of basal ganglia disorder per se but may indicate that the connections of the basal ganglia to the frontal lobes are impaired. A similar difficulty in relaxation is observed normally in children.

As to pathophysiology, it is generally agreed that rigidity and bradykinesia result from lesions of the nigrostriatal system and that such lesions produce their effects through a series of sequential inhibitory and excitatory events involving the components and circuitry of the basal ganglia. The normal activating effects of dopamine on both the direct and indirect striatal-pallidal systems and their effects on thalamocortical drive have been described earlier. Degeneration of the pigmented cells of the substantia nigra deprives striatal neurons of their dopaminergic innervation, with the ultimate result that the normal thalamocortical drive is inhibited. Impulses that do reach the cortex are translated through successive stations in the cerebral cortex and spinal cord and culminate in rigidity, hypo- or akinesia, and bradykinesia.

Involuntary Movements (Chorea, Athetosis, Ballismus, Dystonia)

In deference to usual practice, these symptoms are described separately, as though each represented a discrete clinical phenomenon readily distinguishable from the others. In reality, they usually occur together and have many points of clinical similarity, and there are reasons to believe that they have a common anatomic and physiologic basis. One must be mindful that chorea, athetosis, and dystonia are symptoms and are not to be equated with disease entities that happen to incorporate one of these terms in their names (e.g., Huntington chorea, dystonia musculorum deformans). Here the discussion is limited to the symptoms. The diseases of which these symptoms are a part are considered elsewhere, mainly in Chap. 39.

Chorea Derived from the Greek word meaning "dance," *chorea* refers to involuntary arrhythmic movements of a forcible, rapid, jerky type. These movements may be simple or quite elaborate and of variable distribution. Although the movements are purposeless, the patient may incorporate them into a deliberate act, as if to make them less noticeable. When superimposed on voluntary actions, they may assume an exaggerated and bizarre character. Grimacing and peculiar respiratory sounds may be other expressions of the movement disorder. Usually the movements are discrete, but if they are very numerous, they become confluent and then resemble athetosis, as described below. In moments when the involuntary movements are absent or briefly held in abeyance, volitional movements of normal strength are possible, since there is no paralysis; but these movements tend also to be excessively quick and poorly sustained. The limbs are often slack or hypotonic and, because of this, the knee jerks tend to be pendular; with the patient sitting on the edge of the examining table and the foot free of the floor, the leg swings back and forth four or five times in response to a tap on the patellar tendon, rather than once or twice, as it does normally. A choreic movement may be superimposed on the reflex movement, checking it in flight, so to speak, and giving rise to the "hung-up" reflex.

The hypotonia in chorea as well as the pendular reflexes may suggest a disturbance of cerebellar function. Lacking, however, are "intention" tremor and true incoordination or ataxia. In patients with hypernatremia and other metabolic disorders, it may be necessary to distinguish chorea from myoclonus. Chorea differs from myoclonus mainly with respect to the speed of the movements; the myoclonic jerk is much faster and may involve single muscles or part of a muscle as well as groups of muscles.

Diseases that are characterized by chorea are listed in Table 4-3. Chorea is a major feature of Huntington disease (hereditary or chronic chorea), in which the movements tend more typically to be choreoathetotic. Also, there is an inherited form of chorea without dementia. Not infrequently, chorea has its onset in late life without the other identifying features of Huntington disease. It is referred to as *senile chorea,* a term that is hardly helpful in understanding the process. Its relation to Huntington chorea is unsettled. It may be a delayed form of the disease, and a few such patients we have seen have had atypical depressions or mild psychosis; but others remain for a decade with only chorea. A number of

Table 4-3
Diseases characterized by chorea

Inherited disorders
Huntington disease
Benign hereditary chorea
Neuroacanthocytosis
Rheumatic chorea (Sydenham, chorea gravidarum)
Drug-induced chorea
Neuroleptics (phenothiazines, haloperidol, and others)
Oral contraceptives
Phenytoin (occasionally other anticonvulsants)
Chorea symptomatic of systemic disease
Lupus erythematosus
Thyrotoxicosis
Polycythemia vera
Hyperosmolar, nonketotic hyperglycemia
AIDS
Hemichorea, rarely associated with
Stroke
Tumor
Vascular malformation
Other rare causes (Wilson disease, Hallervorden-Spatz disease, dentatorubropallidoluysian atrophy, paraneoplastic)

far less common degenerative conditions are associated with chorea, among them dentatorubropallidoluysian atrophy. These are discussed in Chap. 39.

Typical choreic movements are the dominant feature of Sydenham chorea and of the variety of that disease associated with pregnancy (chorea gravidarum), disorders that are related in some way to streptococcal infection. Striatal abnormalities have been demonstrated by MRI in some cases, usually transient but rarely persistent (Emery and Vieco). Also, in recent years it has been suggested that the spectrum of poststreptococcal disorders be extended to tic and obsessive-compulsive behavior in children. In these cases the neurologic problems arise suddenly, subside, and return with future streptococcal infections, as discussed in Chap. 6.

The use of phenothiazine drugs or haloperidol (or an idiosyncratic reaction to these drugs) is a common cause of extrapyramidal movement disorders of all types, including chorea. Rarely chorea complicates hyperthyroidism, polycythemia vera, lupus erythematosus or other forms of cerebral arteritis, and the use of phenytoin or other anticonvulsant drugs. A transitory chorea may occur in the course of an acute metabolic derangement such as hyperosmolar hyperglycemia or hyponatremia. AIDS has emerged as a cause of a number of subacutely progressive movement disorders, initially asymmetrical in our experience, and chorea has been one manifestation. The usual associations have been with toxoplasmosis, progressive multifocal leukoencephalopathy, and lymphoma, but some instances are apparently the result of encephalitis due to the AIDS virus. Chorea may be limited to one side of the body (*hemichorea*). When the involuntary movements involve proximal limb muscles and are of wide range and flinging in nature, the condition is called *hemiballismus* (see further on).

A number of rare *paroxysmal kinesigenic* disorders that are discussed later in this chapter may have a choreic component.

To put these various causes into perspective Piccolo et al reviewed 7829 consecutive neurologic admissions to two general hospitals. They identified 23 cases of chorea, of which 5 were drug-induced, 5 were AIDS-related, and 6 were due to stroke. Sydenham chorea and arteritis were each found in 1 case. In 4 cases no cause could be determined, and 1 case proved to have Huntington disease. In only 3 cases were basal ganglionic lesions considered to be causative.

The anatomic basis of chorea is uncertain. In Huntington chorea, there are obvious lesions in the caudate nucleus and putamen. Yet one often observes vascular lesions in these parts without chorea. The localization of lesions in Sydenham chorea and other choreic diseases has not been completely determined. It is of interest that in instances of chorea related to acute metabolic disturbances, there are sometimes small infarctions in the basal ganglia or metabolic changes in the lenticular nucleus, as shown by imaging studies. One suspects that chorea and hemiballismus relate to disorders of the same system of neurons; however, the subthalamic nucleus is affected only slightly in Huntington chorea.

Athetosis This term stems from a Greek word meaning "unfixed" or "changeable." The condition is characterized by inability to sustain the fingers and toes, tongue, or any other part of the body in one position. The maintained posture is interrupted by relatively slow, sinuous, purposeless movements that have a tendency to flow into one another. As a rule, the abnormal movements are most pronounced in the digits and hands, face, tongue, and throat, but no group of muscles is spared. One can detect as basic patterns of movement an alternation between extension-pronation and flexion-supination of the arm and between flexion and extension of the fingers, the flexed and adducted thumb being trapped by the flexed fingers as the hand closes. Other characteristic movements are eversion-inversion of the foot, retraction and pursing of the lips, twisting of the neck and torso, and alternate wrinkling and relaxation of the forehead or forceful opening and closing of the eyelids. The movements appear to be slower than those of chorea, but all gradations between the two are seen; in some cases, it is impossible to distinguish between them, hence the term *choreoathetosis*. Discrete voluntary movements of the hand are executed more slowly than normal, and attempts to perform them may result in a cocontraction of antagonistic muscles and a spread (overflow) of contraction to muscles not normally required in the movement ("intention spasm"). The overflow appears related to a failure of the striatum to suppress the activity of unwanted muscle groups. Like polymyoclonus, some forms of athetosis occur only during the performance of projected movement (*intention* or *action athetosis*). In other forms, the spasms appear to occur spontaneously, i.e., they are involuntary and, if persistent, give rise to more or less fixed dystonic postures (Yanagisawa and Goto).

Athetosis may affect all four limbs or may be unilateral, especially in children who have suffered a hemiplegia at some previous date (*posthemiplegic athetosis*). Many athetotic patients exhibit variable degrees of rigidity and motor deficit due to associated corticospinal tract disease, and these may account for the slower quality of athetosis compared to chorea. In other patients with generalized choreoathetosis, as pointed out above, the limbs may be intermittently hypotonic.

The combination of athetosis and chorea of all four limbs is a cardinal feature of Huntington disease and of a state known as *double athetosis*, which begins in childhood. Athetosis appearing in the first years of life is usually the result of a congenital or postnatal condition such as hypoxia or rarely kernicterus. Postmortem examinations in some of the cases have disclosed a peculiar pathologic change of probable hypoxic etiology, a *status marmoratus*, in the striatum (Chap. 38); in other cases, of probable kernicteric etiology, there has been a loss of nerve cells and medullated fibers—a *status dysmyelinatus*—in the same regions. In adults, athetosis may occur as an episodic or persistent disorder in hepatic encephalopathy, as a manifestation of chronic intoxication with phenothiazines or haloperidol, and as a feature of certain degenerative diseases, most notably Huntington chorea but also Wilson disease, Hallervorden-Spatz disease, Leigh disease, and other mitochondrial disease variants; less frequently, athetosis may be seen with Niemann-Pick (type C) disease, Kufs disease, neuroacanthocytosis, and ataxia telangiectasia. It may also occur as an effect of excessive L-dopa in the treatment of Parkinson disease, in which case it appears to be due to a decrease in the activity of the subthalamic nucleus and the medial segment of the globus pallidus (Mitchell et al). Athetosis, usually in combination with chorea, may occur rarely in patients with AIDS and in those taking anticonvulsants. Localized forms of athetosis may occasionally follow vascular lesions of the lenticular nucleus or thalamus (Dooling and Adams).

Ballismus The term *ballismus* designates an uncontrollable, poorly patterned flinging movement of an entire limb. As remarked earlier, it is closely related to chorea and athetosis, indicated by the frequent coexistence of these movement abnormalities and the tendency for ballismus to devolve into a less obtrusive choreoathetosis of the distal parts of the affected limb. Ballistic movements are usually unilateral (*hemiballismus*) and the result of an acute lesion of the contralateral subthalamic nucleus or immediately surrounding structures (infarction or hemorrhage, rarely a demyelinative or other lesion). Rarely, a transitory form is linked to a subdural hematoma or thalamic or parietal lesion. The flinging movements may be almost continuous or intermittent, occurring several times a minute, and of such dramatic appearance that it is not unusual for an untutored physician to regard them as hysterical in nature.

Bilateral ballismus is very infrequent and usually asymmetrical; here a metabolic disturbance, particularly nonketotic hyperosmolar coma, is the usual cause.

When ballismus persists for weeks on end, as it often did before effective treatment became available, the continuous forceful movements can result in exhaustion and even death. In most cases, medication with haloperidol or phenothiazine suppresses the violent movements. In extreme cases stereotactic lesions placed in the ventrolateral thalamus and zona incerta have proved effective (Krauss and Mundinger).

Dystonia (Torsion Spasm) (See also Chap. 6 on focal dystonias.) Dystonia is a persistent attitude or posture in one or the other of the extremes of athetoid movement, produced by cocontraction of agonist and antagonist muscles in one region of the body. It may take the form of an overextension or overflexion of the hand, inversion of the foot, lateral flexion or retroflexion of the head, torsion of the spine with arching and twisting of the back, forceful closure of the eyes, or a fixed grimace (Fig. 4-5). Defined in this way, dystonia is closely allied to athetosis, differing only in the persistence or fixity of the postural abnormality and the disproportionate involvement of the large axial muscles (those of the

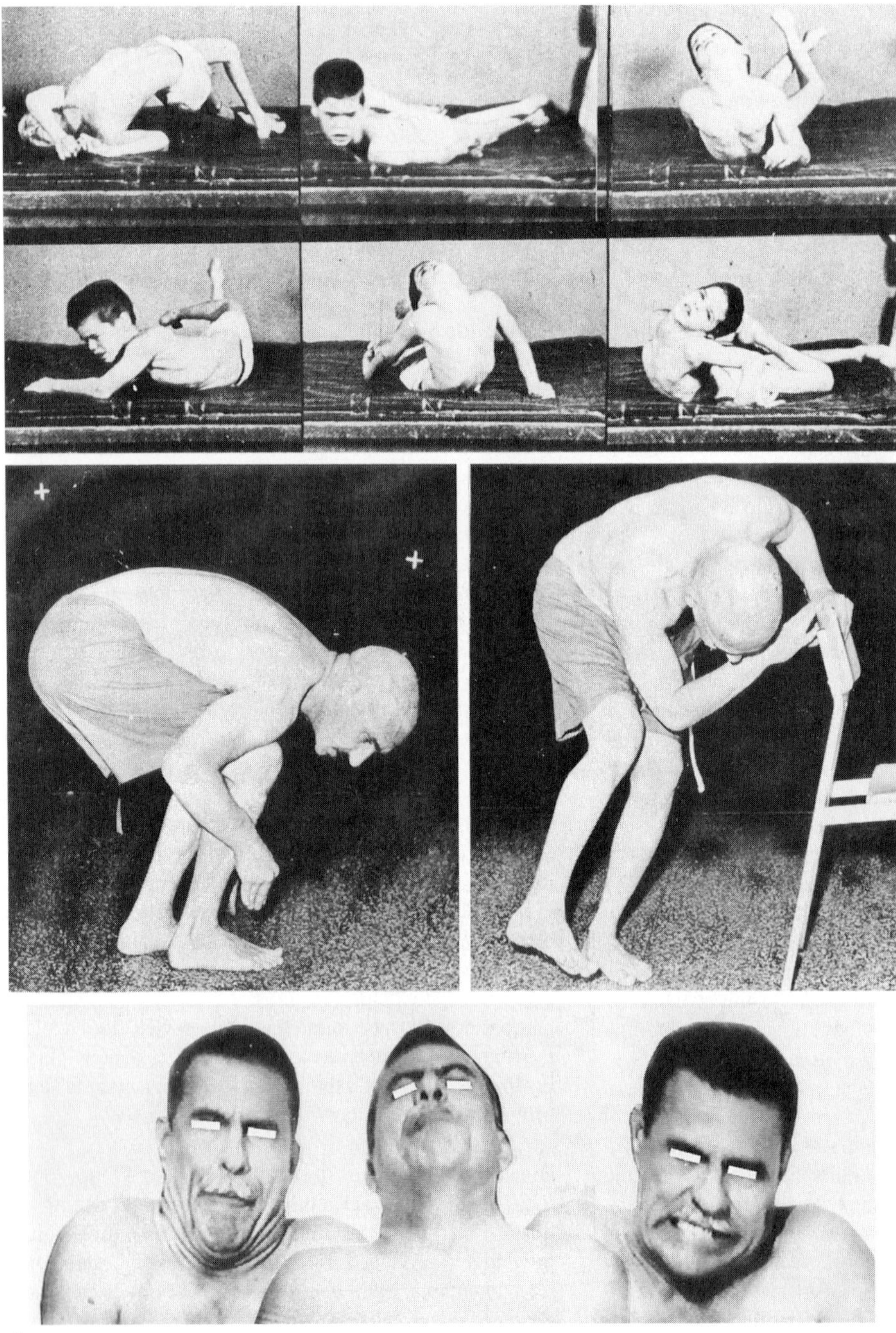

A

Figure 4-5

A. (Top) *Characteristic dystonic deformities in a young boy with dystonia musculorum deformans.* (Middle) *Sporadic instance of dystonia with onset in adult life.* (Bottom) *Patient with Meige syndrome, showing spasms of platysma and facial muscles and grimacing combined with retrocollic spasms. (Top and middle photos courtesy of the late Dr. I.S. Cooper. Bottom photos, courtesy of Dr. Joseph M. Waltz.)*

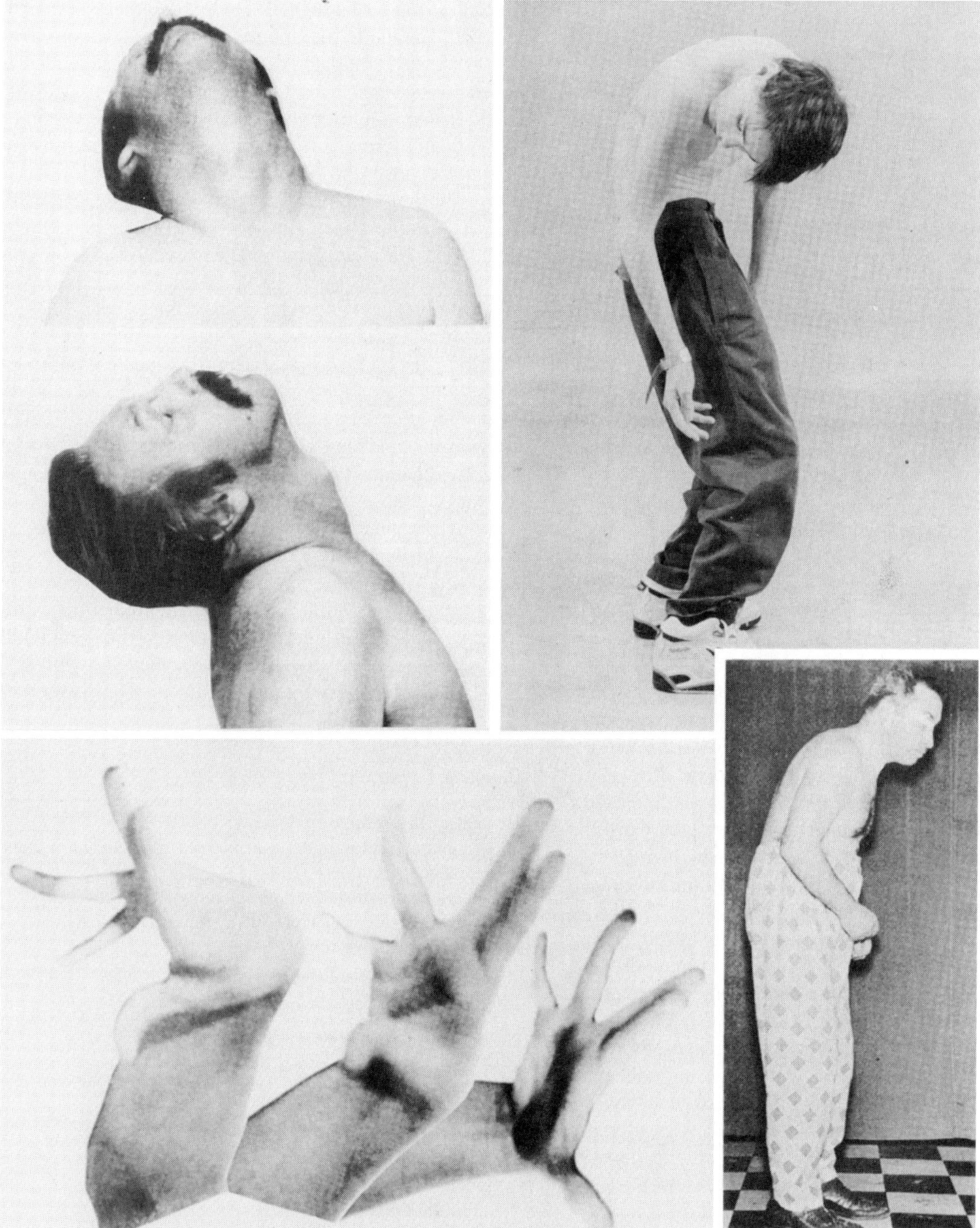

B

Figure 4-5 *(Continued)*

B. (Upper left) *Young adult with severe spasmodic retrocollis. Note hypertrophy of sternocleidomastoid muscles.* (Upper right) *Incapacitating postural deformity in a young man with dystonia.* (Lower left) *Characteristic athetoid-dystonic deformities of the hand in a patient with tardive dyskinesia.* (Lower right) *Typical postural abnormality in Parkinson disease. (Photos courtesy of Dr. Joseph M. Waltz.)*

trunk and limb girdles). The term *dystonia* is now generally used in this way, but it has been given other meanings as well. Wilson referred to any variability in muscle tone as dystonia. This term has also been applied to fixed abnormalities of posture that may be the end result of certain diseases of the motor system; thus Denny-Brown speaks of "hemiplegic dystonia" and the "flexion dystonia of parkinsonism." If the term is to be used in the latter sense, it would be better to speak of the persistent but reversible athetotic movements of the limbs and trunk as "torsion spasms" or "phasic dystonia," in contrast to "fixed dystonia."

Dystonia, like athetosis, may vary considerably in severity and may show striking fluctuations in individual patients. In its early stages it may be interpreted as an annoying mannerism or hysteria, and only later—in the face of persisting postural abnormality, lack of the usual psychologic features of hysteria, and the emerging character of the illness—is the correct diagnosis made. Dystonia may be limited to the facial, cervical, or trunk muscles or to those of one limb and may cease when the body is in repose. Severe instances result in grotesque movements and distorted positions of the body; sometimes the whole musculature seems to be thrown into spasm by an effort to move an arm or to speak.

Generalized dystonia is seen in its most pronounced form as an uncommon heritable disease, dystonia musculorum deformans, in which case it is associated with a specific mutation on chromosome 9, termed DYT1 (page 1141). It was in relation to this disease that Oppenheim and Vogt, in 1911, introduced the term *dystonia*. Widespread torsion spasm may also be a prominent feature of certain other heredodegenerative disorders, such as familial striatal necrosis with affection of the optic nerves and other parts of the nervous system (Marsden et al, Novotny et al). Nygaard and colleagues have described yet another familial form in which one of several types of dystonia is coupled with elements of parkinsonism and is responsive to minute doses of L-dopa, as described below (Segawa disease).

Restricted or fragmentary forms of dystonia (*dyskinesias*) are the types most commonly encountered in clinical practice. Characteristically the spasms involve only the orbicularis oculi and face or mandibular muscles (blepharospasm-oromandibular dystonia), tongue, cervical muscles (spasmodic torticollis), hand (writer's cramp), or foot. These are described more fully in Chap. 6 as well as in Chap. 39. Dystonia also occurs as a manifestation of many other diseases ("symptomatic dystonias"). The latter include double athetosis due to hypoxic damage to the brain, kernicterus, Hallervorden-Spatz disease, Huntington disease, Wilson hepatolenticular degeneration, Parkinson disease, lysosomal storage diseases, striatopallidodentatal calcification (due sometimes to hypoparathyroidism), thyroid disease, and chronic or previous exposure to phenothiazines.

The most frequent cause of *acute dystonic reactions* is drug intoxication—with phenothiazines, butyrophenones, or metoclopramide and even with the newer neuroleptic agents such as olanzipine, which have the relative advantage of producing these side effects far less frequently than the other drugs mentioned above. These reactions respond to some extent to diphenhydramine or benztropine given two or three times in 24 to 48 h. Also, L-dopa, calcium channel blockers, and a number of anticonvulsants and anxiolytics are among a long list of other medications that may on occasion induce dystonia, the various causes of which are listed in Table 4-4.

All manner of drugs have been used in the treatment of chronic dystonia, with a notable lack of success. However, Fahn has reported beneficial effects (more so in children than in adults) with the anticholinergic agents trihexyphenidyl (Artane) and ethopropazine (Parsidol) given in massive doses—which are achieved by increasing the dosage very gradually. A distinct subset of

Table 4-4
Causes of dystonia

Hereditary dystonias
- Dystonia musculorum deformans (recessive and autosomal dominant forms)
- Dystonia with other heredodegenerative disorders (neural deafness; striatal necrosis with optic nerve affection; paraplegic amyotrophy)
- Juvenile dystonia—Parkinson syndrome (L-dopa responsive)

Idiopathic (primary) dystonias

Symptomatic (secondary) dystonias
- Double athetosis due to cerebral hypoxia
- Kernicterus
- Hallervorden-Spatz disease
- Huntington chorea
- Wilson disease
- Acquired hepatocerebral degeneration
- Parkinson disease
- Lysosomal storage diseases
- Striatopallidodentatal calcification
- Acute and chronic phenothiazine and haloperidol intoxication

Focal dystonias
- Spasmodic torticollis, blepharospasm, hemifacial spasm, oromandibular dystonia, spasmodic dysphonia, writer's cramp and other craft spasms, etc.

dystonic patients (described by Nygaard et al) have responded to extremely small doses of L-dopa. The disease is familial, usually autosomal dominant, and the dystonia-athetosis may be combined with elements of parkinsonism. Marked diurnal fluctuation of symptoms is characteristic. In one autopsied case there was hypopigmentation of the substantia nigra. It is discussed in greater detail in Chap. 39.

Another rare hereditary dystonia that has its onset in adolescence or early adulthood is of interest because of the rapid evolution, at times within an hour but more often over days, of severe dystonic spasms, dysarthria, dysphagia, and postural instability with bradykinesia, which may follow (Dobyns et al). A few cases have followed a febrile episode. The disorder is termed *rapid-onset dystonia-parkinsonism*. It is our understanding from the authors that the latter features are mild and not responsive to L-dopa.

In the focal dystonias, the most effective treatment has proved to be the periodic injection of botulinum toxin into the affected muscles. Stereotactic surgery on the pallidum and ventrolateral thalamus has given rather unpredictable results, but in recent years there has been a renewed interest in this form of treatment (see page 1136).

Paroxysmal Choreoathetosis and Dystonia Under the names *paroxysmal kinesigenic dyskinesia, familial paroxysmal choreoathetosis*, and *periodic dystonia*, among others, there has been described an uncommon sporadic or familial disorder characterized by paroxysmal attacks of choreoathetotic movements or dystonic spasms of the limbs and trunk. Both children and young adults are affected.

There are two main forms of familial paroxysmal choreoathetosis. One, which has an autosomal dominant or recessive pattern of inheritance, is characterized by numerous brief (less than 2 s) attacks of choreoathetosis provoked by startle or sudden movement—hence the title *paroxysmal kinesigenic choreoathetosis*. This disorder responds well to anticonvulsant medication, notably to phenytoin or carbamazepine.

In other families, such as those originally described by Mount and Reback and subsequently by Lance and by Plant et al, the attacks take the form of persistent (5 min to 4 h) dystonic spasms and have reportedly been precipitated by the ingestion of alcohol or coffee, by fatigue, and rarely by prolonged exercise (nonkinesigenic type). The attacks may be predominantly one-sided or bilateral. This form of the disease is inherited as an autosomal dominant trait. A favorable response to benzodiazepines (clonazepam) has been reported, even when the drug is given on alternate days (Kurlan and Shoulson).

Because of their paroxysmal nature and the response (of the kinesigenic type) to anticonvulsant drugs these familial disorders have been thought to represent seizures originating in the basal ganglia. However, consciousness is not lost and the electroencephalogram is normal, even when recorded during an attack of choreoathetosis, arguing against an epileptic discharge.

More common than these familial dyskinesias are sporadic cases and those secondary to focal brain lesions, such as the ones reported by Demirkirian and Jankovic. They classify these dyskinesias according to the duration of each attack and the event or activity that precipitates the abnormal movements (kinesigenic, non-kinesigenic, exertional, or hypnagogic). As with the familial cases, kinesigenic-induced movements improve with anticonvulsants, and the others respond better to clonazepam.

Some cases can be an expression of a serious neurologic or metabolic disease, or may follow injuries such as stroke, trauma, encephalitis, perinatal anoxia, multiple sclerosis, hypoparathyroidism, or thyrotoxicosis. The most severe instances in our experience have been of the kinesigenic variety due to demyelinating disease and, in a few recent cases, to HIV, as a result of either toxoplasmosis, lymphoma, or a presumed encephalitis due to the retrovirus. These patients were relatively unresponsive to medications. Also, it should be recalled that oculogyric crises and other nonepileptic spasms have occurred episodically in patients with postencephalitic parkinsonism; now these phenomena are seen with acute and chronic phenothiazine intoxication and with Niemann-Pick disease (type C).

The Identity of Chorea, Athetosis, and Dystonia It must be evident from the foregoing descriptions that the distinctions between chorea and athetosis are probably not fundamental. Even their most prominent differences—the discreteness and rapidity of choreic movements and the slowness and confluence of athetotic ones—may be more apparent than real. As pointed out by Kinnier Wilson, involuntary movements may follow one another in such rapid succession that they become confluent and therefore appear to be slow. In practice, one finds that the patient with relatively slow, confluent movements also shows discrete, rapid ones, and vice versa, and that many patients with chorea and athetosis also exhibit the persistent disorder of movement and posture that is generally designated as dystonia.

In a similar vein, no meaningful distinction except one of degree can be made between choreoathetosis and ballismus. Particularly forceful movements of large amplitude (ballismus) are observed in certain patients with Sydenham and Huntington chorea, who, according to traditional teaching, exemplify pure forms of chorea and athetosis, respectively. The close relationship between these involuntary movements is illustrated by the patient with hemiballismus, who, at the onset of the illness, exhibits wild flinging movements of the arm and, after a period of partial recovery, shows only choreoathetotic flexion-extension movements that are limited to the fingers and hand. For this reason, the terms *hemiballismus* and *hemichorea* have sometimes been used interchangeably.

Finally, it should be pointed out that all disorders of movement due to lesions of the extrapyramidal system have certain other attributes in common. The abnormalities of movement are superimposed on relatively intact praxic and voluntary movements, implying integrity of the cerebral control of the corticospinal systems. The persistence of the abnormal movements indicates that they are veritable release phenomena; they are abolished by sleep and enhanced by anxiety and excitement; they are caused by a variety of diseases, some of which evoke one type of movement disorder more than another; and they can be altered by certain pharmacologic agents and by stereotactic lesions in certain parts of the motor systems. To the clinician, the most difficult examples are those in which all types of involuntary movement and tremors are combined—a gestalt of dyskinesias.

REFERENCES

ALBIN RL, YOUNG AB, PENNEY JB: The functional anatomy of basal ganglia disorders. *Trends Neurosci* 12:366, 1989.

ALEXANDER GE: Anatomy of the basal ganglia and related motor structures, in Watts RL, Koller WC (eds): *Movement Disorders*. New York, McGraw-Hill, 1997, pp 73–85.

ALEXANDER GE, CRUTCHER MD: Functional architecture of basal ganglia circuits: Neural substrates of parallel processing. *Trends Neurosci* 13:266, 1990.

ALEXANDER GE, DELONG MR: Macrostimulation of the primate neostriatum. *J Neurophysiol* 53:1417, 1433, 1985.

BERGMAN H, WICHMANN T, DELONG MR: Reversal of experimental parkinsonism by lesions of the subthalamic nucleus. *Science* 249:1436, 1990.

BHATIA KP, MARSDEN CD: The behavioral and motor consequence of focal lesions of the basal ganglia in man. *Brain* 117:859, 1994.

BROOKS VB: *The Neural Basis of Motor Control*. New York, Oxford University Press, 1986.

CARPENTER MB: Brainstem and infratentorial neuraxis in experimental dyskinesia. *Arch Neurol* 5:504, 1961.

CARPENTER MB: Anatomy of the corpus striatum and brainstem integrating systems, in Brooks VB (ed): *Handbook of Physiology*. Sec 1: *The Nervous System*. Vol 2: *Motor Control*, part 2. Bethesda, MD, American Physiological Society, 1981, pp 947–995.

CARPENTER MB, WHITTIER JR, METTLER FA: Analysis of choreoid hyperkinesia in the rhesus monkey: Surgical and pharmacological analysis of hyperkinesia resulting from lesions of the subthalamic nucleus of Luys. *J Comp Neurol* 92:293, 1950.

CEBALLOS-BAUMANN AO, PASSINGHAM RE, et al: Motor reorganization in acquired hemidystonia. *Ann Neurol* 37:746, 1995.

CILIAX BJ, GREENAMYRE T, LEVEY, AI: Functional biochemistry and molecular neuropharmacology of the basal ganglia and motor systems, in Watts RL, Koller WC: *Movement Disorders*. New York, McGraw-Hill, 1997, pp 99–116.

COOPER IS: *Involuntary Movement Disorders*. New York, Hoeber-Harper, 1969.

DELONG MR: Primate models of movement disorders of basal ganglia origin. *Trends Neurosci* 13:281, 1990.

DEMIRKIRIAN M, JANKOVIC J: Paroxysmal dyskinesias: Clinical features and classification. *Ann Neurol* 38:571, 1995.

DENNY-BROWN D, YANAGISAWA N: The role of the basal ganglia in the initiation of movement, in Yahr MD (ed): *The Basal Ganglia*. New York, Raven Press, 1976, pp 115–148.

DOBYNS WB, OZELIUS LJ, KRAMER PL, et al: Rapid-onset dystonia-parkinsonism. *Neurology* 43:2596, 1993.

DOOLING EC, ADAMS RD: The pathological anatomy of posthemiplegic athetosis. *Brain* 98:29, 1975.

EMERY SE, VIECO PT: Sydenham chorea: Magnetic resonance imaging reveals permanent basal ganglia injury. *Neurology* 48:531, 1997.

FAHN S: High-dosage anticholinergic therapy in dystonia. *Neurology* 33:1255, 1985.

HALLETT M: Clinical neurophysiology of akinesia. *Rev Neurol* 146:585, 1990.

HALLETT M, KHOSHBIN S: A physiological mechanism of bradykinesia. *Brain* 103:301, 1980.

HUDGINS RL, CORBIN KB: An uncommon seizure disorder: Familial paroxysmal choreoathetosis. *Brain* 91:199, 1968.

JANKOVIC J, TOLOSA ES (eds): *Parkinson's Disease and Movement Disorders*, 3rd ed. Baltimore, Lippincott, Williams & Wilkins, 1998.

KRAUSS JK, MUNDINGER F: Functional stereotactic surgery for hemiballism. *J Neurosurg* 58:278, 1996.

KURLAN R, SHOULSON I: Familial paroxysmal dystonic choreoathetosis and response to alternate-day oxazepam therapy. *Ann Neurol* 13:456, 1983.

LANCE JW: Familial paroxysmal dystonic choreoathetosis and its differentiation from related syndromes. *Ann Neurol* 2:285, 1977.

LANG EA, LOZANO AM: Parkinson's disease: Second of two parts. *N Engl J Med* 339:1130, 1998.

MARSDEN CD, OBESO JA: The functions of the basal ganglia and the paradox of stereotaxic surgery in Parkinson's disease. *Brain* 117:877, 1994.

Marsden CD, Lang AE, Quinn NP, et al: Familial dystonia and visual failure with striatal CT lucencies. *J Neurol Neurosurg Psychiatry* 49:500, 1986.

Martin JP: *Papers on Hemiballismus and the Basal Ganglia.* London, National Hospital Centenary, 1960.

Martin JP: *The Basal Ganglia and Posture.* Philadelphia, Lippincott, 1967.

Mitchell IJ, Boyce S, Sambrook MA, et al: A 2-deoxyglucose study of the effects of dopamine agonists on the parkinsonian primate brain. *Brain* 115:809, 1992.

Mount LA, Reback S: Familial paroxysmal choreoathetosis: Preliminary report on a hitherto undescribed clinical syndrome. *Arch Neurol Psychiatry* 44:841, 1940.

Novotny EJ Jr, Dorfman LN, Louis A, et al: A neurodegenerative disorder with generalized dystonia: A new mitochondriopathy? *Neurology* 35(suppl 1):273, 1985.

Nygaard TG, Trugman JM, Yebenes JG: Dopa-responsive dystonia: The spectrum of clinical manifestations in a large North American family. *Neurology* 40:66, 1990.

Penney JB, Young AB: Biochemical and functional organization of the basal ganglia, in Jankovic J, Tolosa ES (eds): *Parkinson's Disease and Movement Disorders*, 3rd ed. Baltimore, Lippincott, Williams & Wilkins, 1998, pp 1–13.

Piccolo I, Sterzi R, Thiella G, et al: Sporadic choreas: Analysis of a general hospital series. *Eur Neurol* 41:143, 1999.

Plant GT, Williams AC, Earl CJ, Marsden CD: Familial paroxysmal dystonia induced by exercise. *J Neurol Neurosurg Psychiatry* 47:275, 1984.

Richter R: Degeneration of the basal ganglia in monkeys from chronic carbon disulfide poisoning. *J Neuropathol Exp Neurol* 4:324, 1945.

Segawa M, Hosaka A, Miyagawa F, et al: Hereditary progressive dystonia with marked diurnal fluctuation. *Adv Neurol* 14:215, 1976.

Thach WT Jr, Montgomery EB Jr: Motor system, in Pearlman AL, Collins RC (eds): *Neurobiology of Disease.* New York, Oxford University Press, 1992, pp 168–196.

van Woerkom W: La cirrhose hepatique avec alterations dans les centres nerveux evoluant chez des sujets d'age moyen. *Nouv Iconogr Saltpétrière* 7:41, 1914.

Watts RL, Koller WC (eds): *Movement Disorders: Neurologic Principles and Practice.* New York, McGraw-Hill, 1997.

Wichmann T, DeLong M: Physiology of the basal ganglia and pathophysiology of movement disorders of basal ganglia origin, in Watts RL, Koller WC (eds): *Movement Disorders: Neurologic Principles and Practice.* New York, McGraw-Hill, 1997, pp 87–97.

Whittier JR, Mettler FA: Studies on the subthalamus of the rhesus monkey. *J Comp Neurol* 90:281, 319, 1949.

Wilson SAK: Disorders of motility and of muscle tone, with special reference to corpus striatum: The Croonian Lectures. *Lancet* 2:1, 53, 169, 215, 1925.

Wooten GF, Lopes MBS, Harris WO, et al: Pallidoluysian atrophy: Dystonia and basal ganglia functional anatomy. *Neurology* 43:1764, 1993.

Yanagisawa N, Goto A: Dystonia musculorum deformans: Analysis with electromyography. *J Neurol Sci* 13:39, 1971.

Young AB, Penney JB: Biochemical and functional organization of the basal ganglia, in Jankovic J, Tolosa ES: *Parkinson's Disease and Movement Disorders*, 3rd ed. Baltimore, Lippincott, Williams & Wilkins, 1998, pp 1–11.

Zeman W: Pathology of the torsion dystonias (dystonia musculorum deformans). *Neurology* 20:79, 1970.

Chapter 5

INCOORDINATION AND OTHER DISORDERS OF CEREBELLAR FUNCTION

The cerebellum, principally a motor organ, is responsible for the *regulation of muscular tone; the coordination of movements, especially skilled voluntary ones; and the control of posture and gait*. The mechanisms by which these functions are accomplished have been the subject of intense investigation by anatomists and physiologists. Their studies have yielded a mass of data, testimony to the complexity of the organization of the cerebellum and its afferent and efferent connections. A coherent picture of cerebellar function is now emerging, although it is not yet possible, with a few notable exceptions, to relate each of the symptoms of cerebellar disease to a derangement of a discrete anatomic or functional unit of the cerebellum.

Knowledge of cerebellar function has been derived mainly from the study of natural and experimental ablative lesions and to a lesser extent from stimulation of the cerebellum, which produces little in the way of movement or alterations of induced movement. Notably, none of the motor activities of the cerebellum reach conscious kinesthetic perception; its main role is to assist in the initiation and modulation of willed movements that are generated in the cerebral hemispheres. The following outline of cerebellar structure and function has of necessity been simplified; a full account can be found in the writings of Jansen and Brodal, Gilman, Ito, and Thach and colleagues, listed at the end of this chapter.

ANATOMIC AND PHYSIOLOGIC CONSIDERATIONS

The classic studies of the comparative anatomy and fiber connections of the cerebellum have led to its subdivision into three parts (Fig. 5-1): (1) The *flocculonodular lobe*, located inferiorly, which is phylogenetically the oldest portion of the cerebellum and is much the same in all animals (hence *archicerebellum*). It is separated from the main mass of the cerebellum, or corpus cerebelli, by the posterolateral fissure. (2) The *anterior lobe*, or *paleocerebellum*, which is the portion of the corpus cerebelli rostral to the primary fissure. In lower animals, the anterior lobe constitutes most of the cerebellum, but in humans it is relatively small, consisting of the anterosuperior vermis and the contiguous paravermian cortex. (3) The *posterior lobe*, or *neocerebellum*, consisting of the middle divisions of the vermis and their large lateral extensions. The major portions of the human cerebellar hemispheres fall into this subdivision.

This anatomic subdivision corresponds roughly with the distribution of cerebellar function, based on the arrangement of its afferent fiber connections. The flocculonodular lobe receives special proprioceptive impulses from the vestibular nuclei and is therefore also referred to as the *vestibulocerebellum*; it is concerned essentially with equilibrium. The anterior vermis and part of the posterior vermis are referred to as the *spinocerebellum*, since projections to these parts derive to a large extent from the proprioceptors of muscles and tendons in the limbs and are conveyed to the cerebellum in the dorsal spinocerebellar tract (from the lower limbs) and the ventral spinocerebellar tract (upper limbs). The main influence of the spinocerebellum appears to be on posture and muscle tone. The neocerebellum derives its afferent fibers from the cerebral cortex via the pontine nuclei and brachium pontis, hence the designation *pontocerebellum*; this portion of the cerebellum is concerned primarily with the coordination of skilled movements that are initiated at a cerebral cortical level. These divisions are necessarily incomplete because it is now appreciated that certain portions of the cerebellar hemispheres are involved to some extent in tactual, visual, auditory, and even visceral functions.

On the basis of ablation experiments in animals, three characteristic clinical syndromes, corresponding to these major divisions of the cerebellum, have been delineated. Lesions of the nodulus and flocculus have been associated with a disturbance of equilibrium and fre-

Figure 5-1

Diagram of the cerebellum, illustrating the major fissures, lobes, and lobules and the major phylogenetic divisions (left).

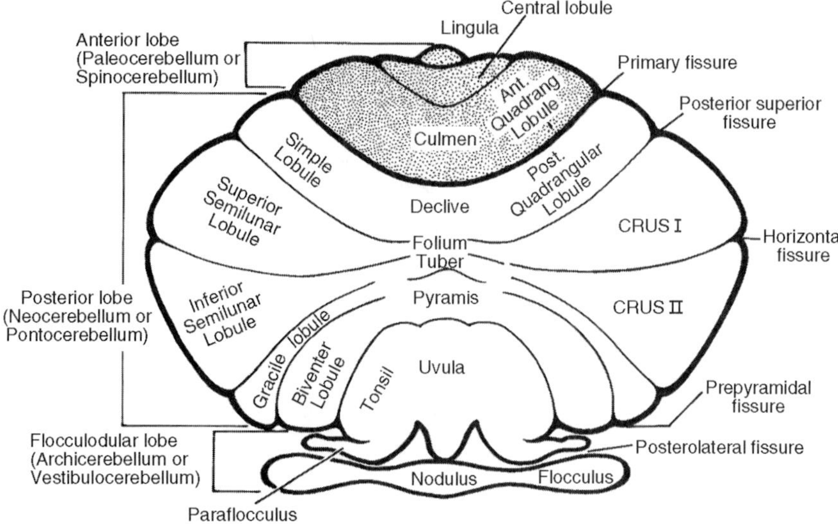

quently with a positional nystagmus; individual movements of the limbs are not affected. Anterior lobe ablation in primates results in increased shortening and lengthening reactions, somewhat increased tendon reflexes, and an exaggeration of the postural reflexes, particularly the "positive supporting reflex," which consists of an extension of the limb in response to light pressure on the foot pad. Ablation of a cerebellar hemisphere in cats and dogs yields inconsistent results, but in monkeys it causes hypotonia and clumsiness of the ipsilateral limbs; if the dentate nucleus is included in the hemispheric ablation, these abnormalities are more enduring and the limbs also show an ataxic or "intention" tremor.

As one might expect, cerebellar function and structure are hardly as simple or precise as the preceding outline might suggest. The seminal studies of Chambers and Sprague and of Jansen and Brodal indicate that in respect to both its afferent and efferent projections, the cerebellum is organized into longitudinal (sagittal) rather than transverse zones. There are three longitudinal zones—the vermian, paravermian or intermediate, and lateral—and there seems to be considerable overlapping from one to another. Chambers and Sprague, on the basis of their investigations in cats, concluded that the vermian zone coordinates movements of the eyes and body with respect to gravity and movement of the head in space. Interruption of vestibulocerebellar connections disturbs the posture, tone, locomotion, and equilibrium of the entire body and results in instability of ocular fixation and nystagmus. The intermediate zone, which receives both peripheral and central projections (from motor cortex), influences postural tone and also individual movements of the ipsilateral limbs. The lateral zone is concerned mainly with coordination of movements of the ipsilateral limbs but is involved in other functions as well.

The efferent fibers of the cerebellar cortex, which consist essentially of the axons of Purkinje cells, project onto the deep cerebellar nuclei. The projections from Purkinje cells are inhibitory, and those from the nuclei are excitatory. According to the scheme of Jansen and Brodal, cells of the vermis project mainly to the fastigial nucleus; those of the intermediate zone, to the globose and emboliform nuclei (represented by the interpositus nucleus in animals); and those of the lateral zone, to the dentate nucleus. The deep cerebellar nuclei, in turn, project to the cerebral cortex and certain brainstem nuclei via two main pathways: fibers from the dentate, emboliform, and globose nuclei form the superior cerebellar peduncle, enter the upper pontine tegmentum as the brachium conjunctivum, decussate completely at the level of the inferior colliculus, and ascend to the ventrolateral nucleus of the thalamus and, to a lesser extent, to the intralaminar thalamic nuclei (Fig. 5-2). Some of the ascending fibers, soon after their decussation, synapse in the red nucleus, but most of them traverse this nucleus without synapsing. Ventral thalamic nuclear groups that receive these ascending efferent fibers project to the supplementary motor cortex of that side. Since the pathway from the cerebellar nuclei to the thalamus and then on to the motor cortex is crossed and the connection from the motor cortex through the corticospinal is again crossed, *the effects of a lesion in one cerebellar hemisphere*

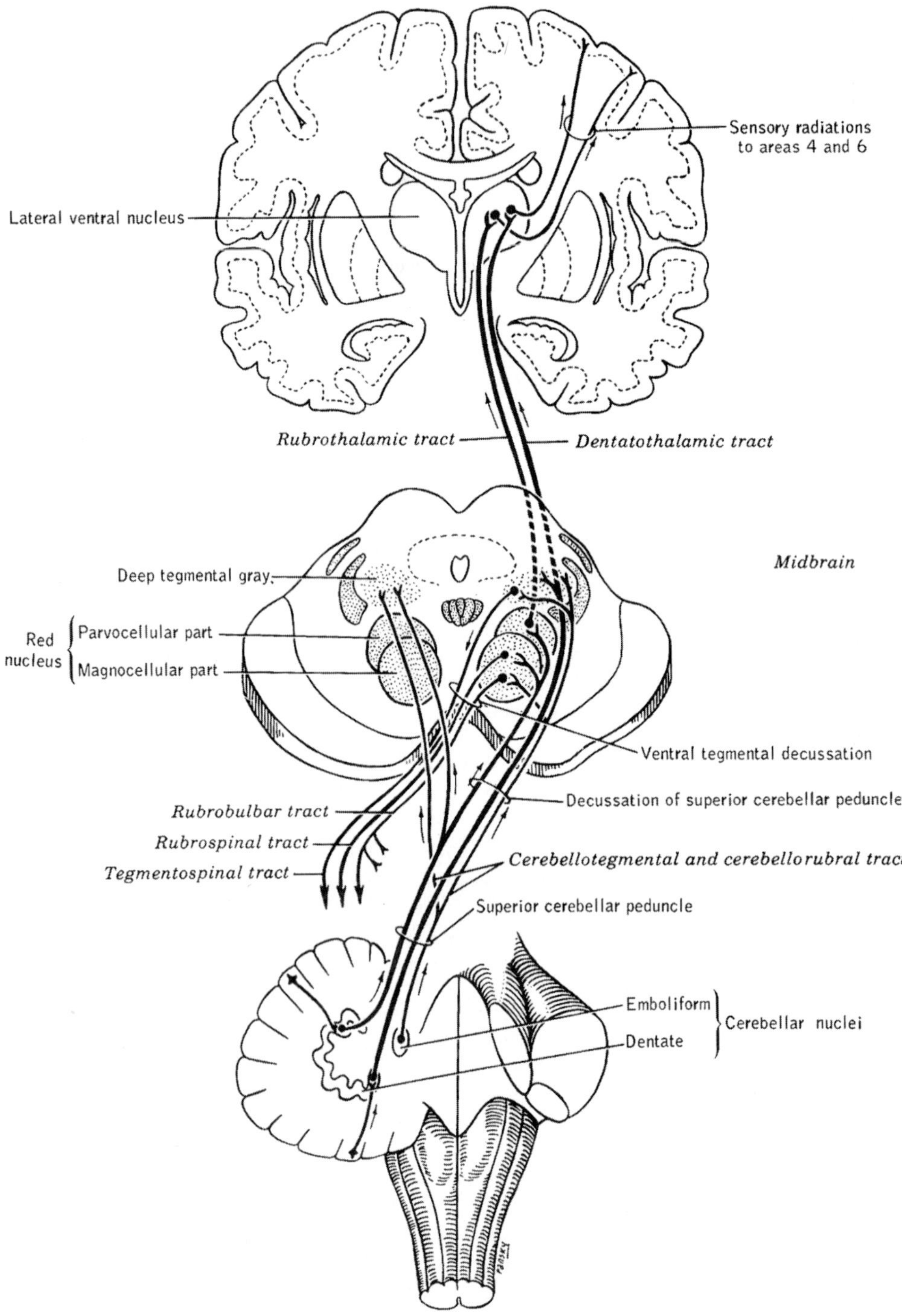

Figure 5-2

Cerebellar projections to the red nucleus, thalamus, and cerebral cortex. (Adapted from House EL et al: A Systematic Approach to Neuroscience, 3rd ed. New York, McGraw-Hill, 1979.)

are manifest on the ipsilateral side of the body (see also page 69).

A small group of fibers of the superior cerebellar peduncle, following their decussation, descend in the ventromedial tegmentum of the brainstem and terminate in the reticulotegmental and paramedian reticular nuclei of the pons and inferior olivary nuclei of the medulla. These nuclei, in turn, project via the inferior cerebellar peduncle to the cerebellum, mainly the anterior lobe, thus completing a cerebellar-reticular-cerebellar feedback system (Mollaret triangle, page 106) (Fig. 5-3). The fastigial nucleus sends fibers to the vestibular nuclei of both sides and, to a lesser extent, to other nuclei of the reticular formation of the pons and medulla. There are also direct fiber connections with the alpha and gamma motor neurons of the spinal cord. The inferior olivary nuclei project via the restiform body (inferior cerebellar peduncle) to the contralateral cerebellar cortex and

Figure 5-3

Dentatothalamic and dentatorubrothalamic projections via the superior cerebellar peduncle. The "feedback" circuit via the reticular nuclei and reticulocerebellar fibers is also shown.

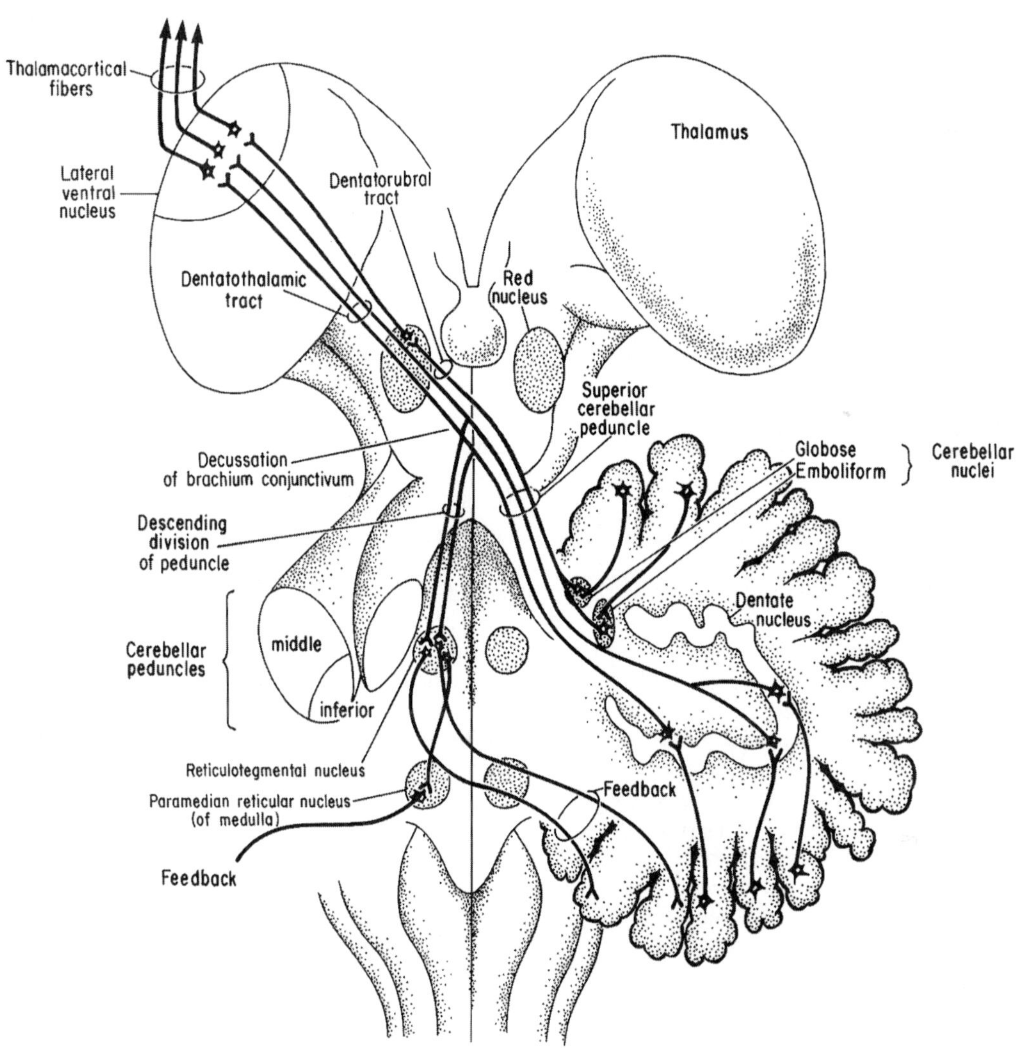

corresponding parts of the deep cerebellar nuclei. Thus the cerebellum influences motor activity through its connections with the motor cortex and brainstem nuclei and their descending motor pathways. The integration at the thalamic level of basal ganglionic influences with those of the cerebellum is detailed in Chap. 4.

The disturbances of movement and posture that result from lesions of the human cerebellum were first cogently analyzed by two eminent neurologists, Joseph Babinski and Gordon Holmes. For Babinski, the essential function of the cerebellum was the orchestration of muscle synergies in the performance of voluntary movement. A loss or impairment of this function—i.e., *asynergia* or *dyssynergia*—resulted in irregularity or fragmentation of the normal motor sequences involved in any given act. This deficit, most apparent in the execution of rapidly alternating movements, was referred to by Babinski as *dys-* or *adiadochokinesis*. He also pointed out that this was accompanied by certain maladjustments of stance and by catalepsy (perseveration of a posture), features that are not as widely appreciated nowadays.

The abnormalities observed by Holmes were in the acceleration and deceleration of movement and, in general, in the rate, range, and force of movement, resulting in an undershooting or overshooting of the target. He used the term *decomposition of movements* to describe the fragmentation of a smooth movement into a series of irregular, jerky components. In Holmes's view, these abnormalities were largely attributable to an underlying hypotonia. The terminal ("intention") tremor, for example, and the inability to check the displacement of an outstretched limb were attributed to this defect (see further on).

The hypotheses of both Babinski and Holmes have been sustained by modern physiologic studies. In their analysis of rapid (ballistic) projected movements, Hallett and colleagues have demonstrated that the cerebellum is essential for the proper timing of agonist and antagonist muscle action in the course of a coordinated act. With cerebellar lesions, there is a prolongation of the interval between the commanded act and the onset of movement. Also, there is a derangement of the triphasic agonist-antagonist-agonist motor sequence, referred to in Chaps. 3 and 4; the agonist burst may be too long or too short, or it may continue into the antagonist burst, resulting in excessive agonist-antagonist cocontraction at the onset of movement. These findings could explain what has variously been described as asynergia, decomposition of movement, and dysmetria, as alluded to above. Diener and Dichgans confirmed these fundamental abnormalities in the timing and amplitude of reciprocal inhibition and of cocontraction of agonist-antagonist muscles and remarked that these were particularly evident in pluriarticular movements. The observations of Ugawa and coworkers are pertinent in this regard; they found that contraction of hand muscles evoked by stimulation of the motor cortex was reduced when preceded (by 5 to 7 ms) by magnetic stimulation over the cerebellum.

Role of the Deep Cerebellar Nuclei The physiologic studies of Allen and Tsukahara and those of Thach and his colleagues have greatly increased our knowledge of the role of the deep cerebellar nuclei. These investigators studied the effects of cooling the deep nuclei during a projected movement in the awake macaque monkey. Their observations, coupled with established anatomic data, permit the following conclusions. The *dentate nucleus* receives information from the premotor and supplementary motor cortices via the pontocerebellar system and helps to initiate volitional movements. The latter are accomplished via efferent projections from the dentate nucleus to the ventrolateral thalamus and motor cortex. The dentatal neurons were shown to fire just before the onset of volitional movements, and inactivation of the dentatal neurons delayed the initiation of such movements. The *interpositus nucleus* also receives cerebrocortical projections via the pontocerebellar system; in addition, it receives spinocerebellar projections via the intermediate zone of the cerebellar cortex. The latter projections convey information from Golgi tendon organs, muscle spindles, cutaneous afferents, and spinal cord interneurons involved in movement. The interpositus nucleus fires in relation to a movement once it has started. Also, the prepositus nucleus appears to be responsible for making volitional oscillations (alternating movements). Its cells fire in tandem with these actions and their regularity and amplitude are impaired when these cells are inactivated. In addition, Thach has pointed out that the nucleus interpositus normally damps physiologic tremor and has suggested that this may play a part in the genesis of so-called intention tremor. The *fastigial nucleus* controls antigravity and other muscle synergies in standing and walking; ablation of this nucleus greatly impairs these motor activities.

Neuronal Organization of the Cerebellum Coordinated and fluid movements result from a neuronal organization in the cerebellum, which permits a computational comparison between desired and actual movements while the latter are being carried out. An enormous number of neurons are committed to these tasks as attested by the fact that the cerebellum contributes only 10 percent to the total weight and volume of the brain, but contains half of the brain's neurons. Also, it has been estimated that there are forty times more afferent axons than efferent axons in the various cerebellar pathways, a reflection of the enormous amount of information that is required for the control of motor function.

The cerebellar cortex is a stereotyped three-layered structure containing five types of neurons (Figs. 5-4 and 5-5). In its relatively regular geometry it is similar to

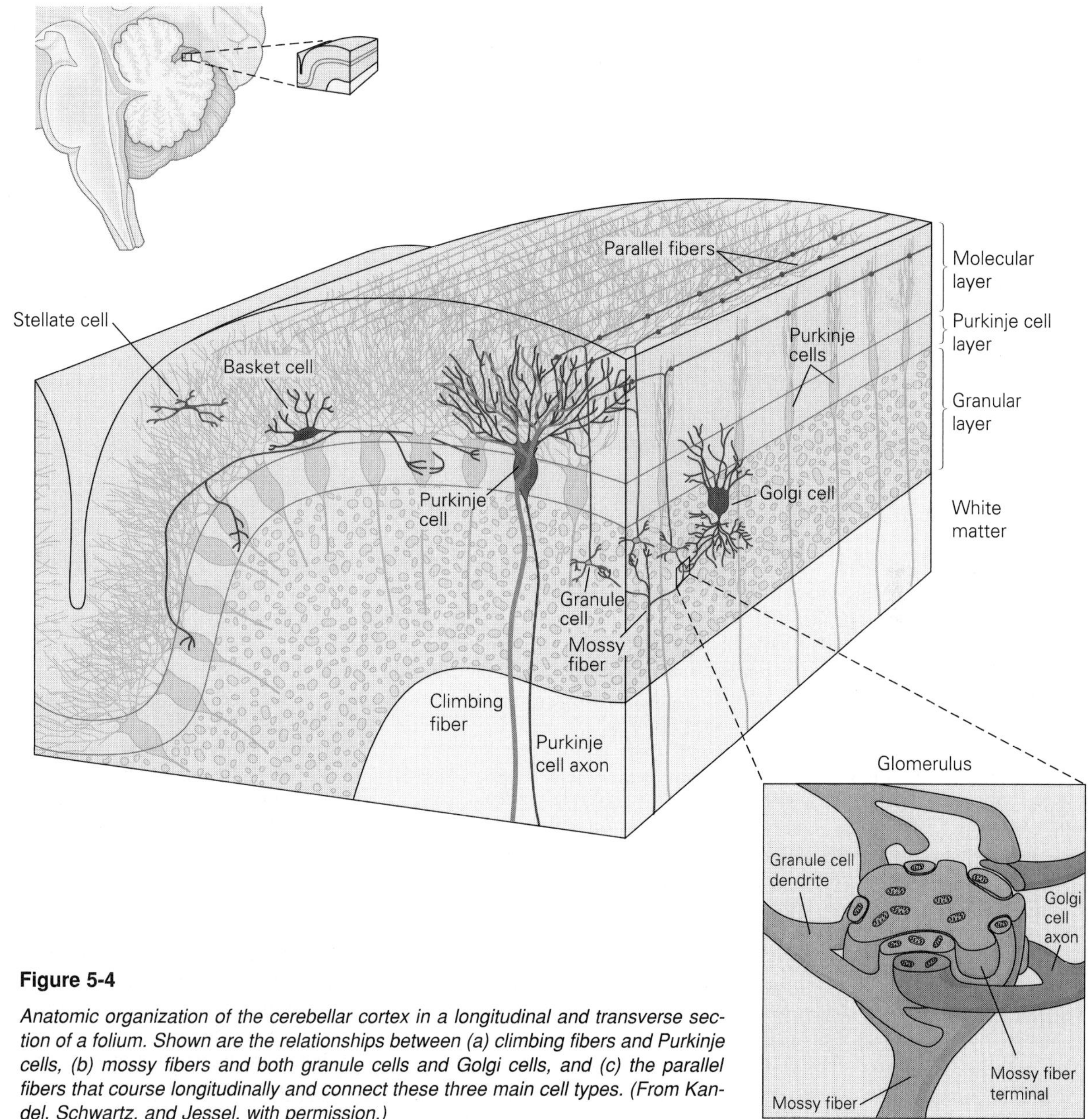

Figure 5-4

Anatomic organization of the cerebellar cortex in a longitudinal and transverse section of a folium. Shown are the relationships between (a) climbing fibers and Purkinje cells, (b) mossy fibers and both granule cells and Golgi cells, and (c) the parallel fibers that course longitudinally and connect these three main cell types. (From Kandel, Schwartz, and Jessel, with permission.)

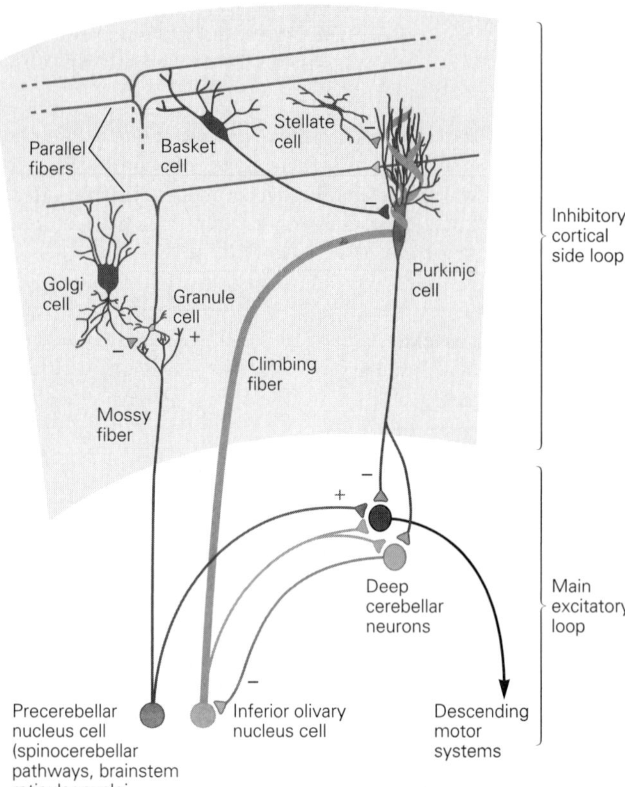

Figure 5-5

The physiologic organization of cerebellar circuitry. The main output of the deep cerebellar nuclei is excitatory and is transmitted through mossy and climbing fibers. This "main loop" is modulated by an inhibitory cortical loop, which is effected by Purkinje cell output but indirectly includes the other main cell types through their connections with Purkinje cells. Recurrent pathways between the deep nuclei and cortical cells via mossy and climbing fibers complete the cerebellar servo-mechanism for motor control. (From Kandel, Schwartz, and Jessel, with permission.)

the columnar architecture of the cerebral cortex (page 467), but it differs in the greater degree of intracortical feedback between neurons and the convergent nature of input fibers. The outermost "molecular" layer of the cerebellum contains two types of inhibitory neurons, the *stellate* and the *basket cells*. They are interspersed among the dendrites of the *Purkinje cells*, the somites of which lie in the underlying layer. The Purkinje cell axons constitute the main output of the cerebellum, which is directed at the deep cerebellar and the vestibular nuclei. Purkinje cells are likewise entirely inhibitory and utilize the neurotransmitter GABA. The innermost "granular" layer contains an enormous number of densely packed *granule cells* and a few larger *Golgi interneurons*. Axons of granule cells travel long distances as "parallel fibers," which are oriented along the long axis of the folia and form excitatory synapses with Purkinje cells. Each Purkinje cell is influenced by as many as a million granule cells to produce a single "simple spike."

The predominant afferent input to the cerebellum is via the mossy fibers, which excite Golgi and granule neurons through special synapses termed *cerebellar glomeruli*. The other main afferent input is via the *climbing fibers,* which originate in the inferior olives and communicate somatosensory, visual, and cerebral cortical signals (Figs. 5-4 and 5-5). The climbing fibers, so named because of their vine-like configuration around Purkinje cells and their axons, preserve a topographic arrangement from olivary neuronal groups; a similar topographic arrangement is maintained in the Purkinje cell projections. The climbing fibers have specific excitatory effects on Purkinje cells that result in prolonged "complex spike" depolarizations. The firing of stellate and basket cells is facilitated by the same parallel fibers that excite Purkinje cells, and these smaller cells in turn inhibit the Purkinje cells. These reciprocal relationships form the feedback loops that permit the exquisitely delicate inhibitory smoothing of limb movements that are lost when the organ is damaged.

Pharmacologic Considerations A number of pharmacologic and biochemical considerations are of interest in this context. Four of the five cell types of the cerebellar cortex (Purkinje, stellate, basket, Golgi) are inhibitory; the granule cells are an exception and are excitatory. Afferent fibers to the cerebellum are of three types, two of which have been mentioned above: (1) *Mossy fibers*, which are the axons of the spinocerebellar tracts and of the pontine, vestibular, and reticular nuclei; they enter through all three cerebellar peduncles and project to the granule cell layer. (2) *Climbing fibers*, which are the axons of cells in the inferior olivary nucleus and project to the Purkinje cells of the opposite cerebellar hemisphere. The mossy fibers utilize aspartate, but the neurotransmitter of the climbing fibers is unknown. Noradrenalin is the transmitter of the afferent fibers from the locus ceruleus. (3) *Aminergic fibers*, which project through the superior cerebellar peduncle and terminate on the Purkinje and granule cells in all parts of the cerebellar cortex. They are of two types: *dopaminergic fibers,* which arise in the ventral mesencephalic tegmentum and project to the interpositus and dentate nuclei and to the granule and Purkinje cells throughout the cortex, and *serotoninergic neurons*, which are located in the raphe nuclei of the brainstem and project diffusely to the granule cell and molecular layer. The granule cell axons elaborate the excitatory transmitter glutamate. All the inhibitory cerebellar cortical neurons appear to utilize gamma-aminobutyric acid (GABA). The neurotransmitters of the deep nuclei have not been fully elucidated.

CLINICAL FEATURES OF CEREBELLAR DISEASE

The symptoms produced in animals by ablation of discrete anatomic or functional zones of the cerebellum bear only an imperfect relationship to the symptoms of cerebellar disease in humans. This is understandable for several reasons. Most of the lesions that occur in humans do not respect the boundaries established by experimental anatomists. Even with lesions that are more or less confined to discrete functional zones (e.g., flocculonodular lobe, anterior lobe), it is difficult to identify the resultant clinical syndromes with those produced by ablation of analogous zones in cats, dogs, and even monkeys, indicating that the functional organization of these parts varies from species to species.

Our own observations affirm what was stated above—that lesions of the cerebellum in humans give rise to the following abnormalities: (1) incoordination (ataxia) of volitional movement; (2) a characteristic tremor ("intention" or ataxic tremor), described in detail in Chap. 6; (3) disorders of equilibrium and gait; and (4) diminished muscle tone, particularly with acute lesions.

In general, extensive lesions of one cerebellar hemisphere, especially of the anterior lobe, cause hypotonia, postural abnormalities, ataxia, and perhaps mild weakness of the ipsilateral arm and leg. Lesions of the deep nuclei and cerebellar peduncles have the same effects as extensive hemispheral lesions. If the lesion involves a limited portion of the cerebellar cortex and subcortical white matter, there may be surprisingly little disturbance of function, or the abnormality may be greatly attenuated with the passage of time. For example, a congenital developmental defect or an early life sclerotic cortical atrophy of half of the cerebellum may produce no clinical abnormalities. Lesions involving the superior cerebellar peduncle or the dentate nucleus cause the most severe and enduring cerebellar symptoms, manifest mostly in the ipsilateral limbs. Disorders of stance and gait depend more upon vermian than upon hemispheral or peduncular involvement.

Incoordination The most prominent manifestations of cerebellar disease, namely, the abnormalities of intended (volitional) movement, are classified under the general heading of *cerebellar incoordination* or *ataxia*. Following Babinski, the terms *dyssynergia*, *dysmetria*, and *dysdiadochokinesis* came into common usage to describe cerebellar abnormalities of movement. Holmes's characterization of these disturbances as abnormalities in the *rate*, *range*, and *force* of movement is at once less confusing and more accurate, as becomes apparent from an analysis of even simple movements—e.g., those elicited by finger-to-nose or by toe-to-finger testing, running the heel down the opposite shin, or tracing a square in the air with a hand or foot. In performing these tests, the patient should be asked to move the limb to the target or trace a figure accurately and rapidly.

The *speed of initiating movement* is slowed somewhat in cerebellar disease. In a detailed electrophysiologic analysis of this defect, Hallett and colleagues noted, in both slow and fast movements, that the initial agonist burst was prolonged and the peak force of the agonist contraction was reduced. Also, there is irregularity and slowing of the movement itself, in both acceleration and deceleration. These abnormalities are particularly prominent as the finger or toe approaches its target. Normally, deceleration of movement is smooth and accurate, even if sharp changes in direction are demanded by a moving target. With cerebellar disease, the velocity and force of the movement are not checked in the normal manner. The excursion of the limb may be arrested prematurely, and the target is then reached by a series of jerky movements. Or the limb overshoots the mark (*hypermetria*), due to delayed activation and diminished contraction of antagonist muscles; then the error is corrected by a series of secondary movements in which the finger or toe sways around the target before coming to rest, or moves from side to side a few times on the target itself. This side-to-side movement of the finger as it approaches its mark tends to assume a rhythmic quality; it has traditionally been referred to as *intention tremor* but in reality reflects defective fixation at the shoulder (see Chap. 6). Gilman and coworkers have provided evidence that more than hypotonia is involved in the tremor of cerebellar incoordination. They found that deafferentation of the forelimb of a monkey resulted in dysmetria and kinetic tremor; subsequent cerebellar ablation significantly increased both the dysmetria and tremor, indicating the presence of a mechanism as yet unidentified in addition to depression of the fusimotor efferent–spindle afferent circuit.

In addition to intention tremor, there may be a coarse, irregular, wide-range tremor that appears whenever the patient activates limb muscles, either to sustain a posture or to effect a movement (*wing-beating tremor*). Its anatomy is not fully known. The cerebellar cortex, the interpositus nucleus (globose and fastigial nuclei), and their connections with the brainstem are probably involved. Holmes called it *rubral tremor*, and although the lower part of the red nucleus may be the site of the lesion, the nucleus itself is probably not involved in this type of tremor. Probably the tremor is due to interruption of the fibers of the superior cerebellar peduncle, which traverse the lesion. Also, with certain sustained postures (e.g., with arms extended and hands on knees) the patient with cerebellar disease may develop a rhythmic oscillation of the fingers, having much the same tempo as a parkinsonian tremor. A rhythmic tremor of the head or upper trunk (3 to 4 per second), mainly in the anteroposterior plane, often accompanies midline cerebellar disease. This is called *titubation*.

All of the foregoing defects in volitional movement are more noticeable in acts that require alternation or rapid change in direction of movement, such as pronation-supination of the forearm or successive touching of each fingertip to the thumb. The normal rhythm of these movements is interrupted by irregularities of force and speed. This is the abnormality that Babinski called *adiadochokinesis*. Even a simple movement may be fragmented ("decomposition" of movement), each component being effected with greater or lesser force than is required. These movement abnormalities together impart a highly characteristic clumsiness to the cerebellar syndromes, an appearance that is not simulated by the weakness of upper or lower motor neuron disorders or by diseases of the basal ganglia. As pointed out by Babinski, extension of the neck in the upright posture is not compensated for by flexion of the knees—another mark of asynergia.

Cerebellar lesions commonly give rise to a disorder of speech, which may take one of two forms, either a slow, *slurring dysarthria*, like that following interruption of the corticobulbar tracts, or a *scanning dysarthria* with variable intonation, so called because words are broken up into syllables, as when a line of poetry is scanned for meter. The latter disorder is uniquely cerebellar; in addition to its scanning quality, speech is slow, and each syllable, after an involuntary interruption, may be uttered with less force or more force ("explosive speech") than is natural.

Myoclonic movements—i.e., brief (50- to 100-ms), random contractions of muscles or groups of muscles—are frequently combined with cerebellar ataxia. When multiple jerks mar a volitional movement, it may be mistaken for an ataxic tremor. (The same error may be caused by asterixis.) Ramsey Hunt described this symptom in connection with a rare heredodegenerative disease (see page 1150), but it has also been observed in neuronal storage diseases of various kinds. *Action myoclonus* may be the principal residual sign of hypoxic encephalopathy, as described on page 110, and it has been proposed that these conditions have a cerebellar orign. Myoclonus is described more fully in Chap. 6.

Ocular movement may be altered as a result of cerebellar disease, specifically if vestibular connections are involved. Patients with cerebellar lesions are unable to hold eccentric positions of gaze, resulting in the need to make rapid repetitive saccades to look eccentrically—i.e., *gaze-paretic nystagmus*. Conjugate voluntary gaze is then accomplished by a series of jerky movements (*saccadic dysmetria*). Smooth pursuit movements are slower than normal and require that the patient make catch-up saccades in an attempt to keep the moving target near the fovea. On attempted refixation, the eyes may overshoot the target and then oscillate through several corrective cycles until precise fixation is attained. It will be recognized that these abnormalities, as well as those of speech, resemble the abnormalities of volitional movements of the limbs. Currently it is believed that nystagmus due to cerebellar disease depends upon lesions of the vestibulocerebellum (Thach and Montgomery). Skew deviation (vertical displacement of one eye), ocular flutter, and ocular myoclonus (opsoclonus) may also be related to cerebellar disease; these abnormalities and other effects of cerebellar lesions on ocular movement are discussed in Chap. 14.

Disorders of Equilibrium and Gait The patient with cerebellar disease has variable degrees of difficulty in standing and walking, as described more fully in Chap. 7. Standing with feet together may be impossible or maintained only briefly before pitching to one side or backward. Closing the eyes worsens this difficulty slightly, though the Romberg sign is absent. In walking, the steps are uneven and placement of the foot is misaligned, resulting in unexpected lurching.

The evidence that flocculonodular lesions in humans cause a disturbance of equilibrium is not conclusive. It rests on the observation that with certain tumors of childhood, namely, medulloblastomas, there may be an unsteadiness of stance and gait but no tremor or incoordination of the limbs. Insofar as these tumors are thought to originate from cell rests in the posterior medullary velum, at the base of the nodulus, it has been inferred that the disturbance of equilibrium results from involvement of this portion of the cerebellum. However, the validity of this deduction remains to be proved. By the time such tumors are inspected at operation or autopsy, they have spread beyond the confines of the nodulus, and strict clinicopathologic correlations are not possible.

Data from patients in whom accurate clinicoanatomic correlations can be made indicate that the disequilibrium syndrome, with normality of movements of the limbs, corresponds more closely with lesions of the anterior vermis than with lesions of the flocculus and nodulus. This conclusion is based on the study of a highly stereotyped form of cerebellar degeneration in alcoholics (Chap. 42). In such patients the cerebellar disturbance is often limited to one of stance and gait, in which case the pathologic changes are restricted to the anterior parts of the superior vermis. In more severely affected patients, in whom there is also incoordination of individual movements of the limbs, the changes are found to extend laterally from the vermis, involving the anterior portions of the anterior lobes (in patients with ataxia of the legs) and the more posterior portions of the anterior lobes (in patients whose arms are affected). In other diseases, involvement of the posterior vermis and its connections with the pontine and mesencephalic reticular formations have caused abnormalities of ocular movement (see Chap. 14). Similar clinicopathologic relationships pertain in patients with familial cerebellar cortical degeneration of the "Holmes type" (page 1148). In both the alcoholic and familial degenerative cases, despite a serious disturbance of stance and gait, the flocculonodular lobe may be spared completely.

These clinicopathologic observations indicate that the cerebellar cortex, and the anterior lobe in particular, is organized somatotopically, as described earlier. This view has been amply confirmed experimentally by the mapping of evoked potentials from the cerebellar cortex, elicited by a variety of sensory stimuli, and an analysis of the motor effects produced by stimulation of specific parts of the cerebellar cortex. The topographic representation of body parts based on these experimental observations is illustrated in Fig. 5-6. The similarities between this scheme and the one derived from the study of human disease are at once apparent.

Hypotonia The term *hypotonia* refers to a decrease in the normal resistance that is offered by muscles to palpation or to passive manipulation (e.g., flexion and extension of a limb). It appears to be related to a depression of gamma and alpha motor neuron activity, as discussed in Chap 3. Experimentally, in cats and monkeys, acute cerebellar lesions and hypotonia are associated with a depression of fusimotor efferent and spindle afferent activity; both static and dynamic afferents are depressed, but not the secondary afferents. With the passage of time, fusimotor activity is restored as hypotonia disappears (Gilman et al). As indicated earlier, Holmes believed that hypotonia was a fundamental defect in cerebellar disease, accounting not only for the defects in postural fixation (see below) but also for certain elements of ataxia and so-called intention tremor.

Hypotonia is much more apparent with acute than with chronic lesions and may be demonstrated in a number of ways. There may be mild flabbiness of the muscles on the affected side. Segments of the limbs may be displaced by the examiner through a wider range than normal. With recent, severe cerebellar lesions, there may be gross asymmetries of posture, so that the shoulder slumps or the body tilts to the ipsilateral side. A conventional test for hypotonia is to tap the wrists of the outstretched arms, in which case the affected limb (or both limbs in diffuse cerebellar disease) will be displaced through a wider range than normal and may oscillate;

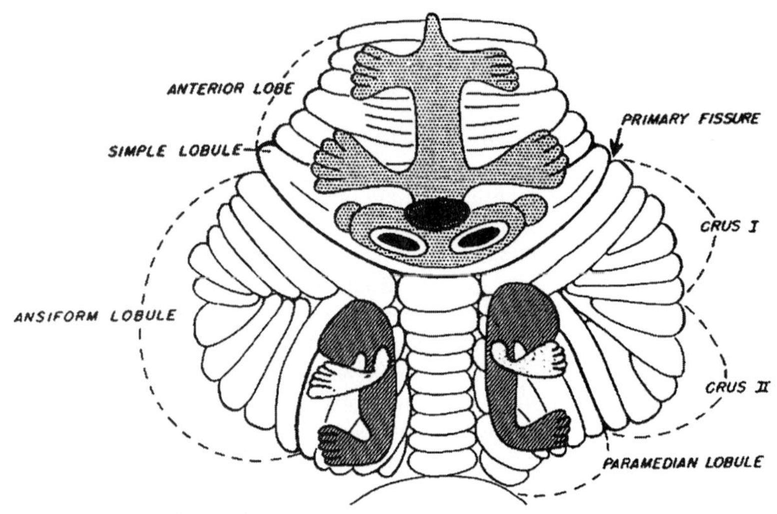

Figure 5-6

Somatotopic localization of motor and sensory function in the cerebellum. See text for explanation. (From Victor M et al: Arch Neurol 1:579, 1959.)

this is due to a failure of the hypotonic muscles to fixate the arm at the shoulder. When an affected limb is shaken, the flapping movements of the hand are of wider excursion than normal. If the patient places his elbows on the table with the arms flexed and the hands are allowed to hang limply, the hand of the hypotonic limb will sag more than that of the normal one. Forced flexion of a hypotonic arm at the elbow may obliterate the space between the volar aspect of the wrist and the deltoid. Babinski also was impressed with gross alterations of posture, apparently related to hypotonia. These alterations take the form of a passive extension of the neck and an involuntary bending of the knees, apparent when the patient is lifted from a bed or chair or upon first standing.

Failure to check a movement is a closely related phenomenon. Thus, after strongly flexing one arm against a resistance that is suddenly released, the patient may be unable to check the flexion movement, to the point where the arm may strike the face. This is due to a delay in contraction of the triceps muscle, which ordinarily would arrest overflexion of the arm. This abnormality, incorrectly referred to as *Holmes's rebound phenomenon,* is more appropriately designated as an *impairment of the check reflex.* Stewart and Holmes, who first described this test, made the point that when resistance to flexion is suddenly removed, the normal limb moves only a short distance in flexion and then recoils or rebounds in the opposite direction. In this sense, rebound of the limb is actually deficient in cerebellar disease but is exaggerated in spastic states.

Patients with these various abnormalities of tone may show little or no impairment of motor power, indicating that the maintenance of posture involves more than the voluntary contraction of muscles. Also, it is noteworthy that most of the signs of cerebellar hypotonia are absent in the flaccid muscles of peripheral nerve disease—indicating that the cerebellum exerts a unique modulating effect at spinal segmental levels.

Other Symptoms of Cerebellar Disease A slight loss of muscular power and excessive fatigability of muscle may occur with acute cerebellar lesions. Also, in unilateral cerebellar disease, the ipsilateral arm may not swing normally in walking. Insofar as these symptoms cannot be explained by other disturbances of motor function, they must be regarded as primary manifestations of cerebellar disease, but they are never severe or persistent and are of little clinical importance; anything approaching a hemiparesis in distribution or severity should not be attributed to cerebellar disease.

More abstruse than the role of the cerebellum in motor control is the alleged participation of this structure in all manner of cognitive function and behavior (see reviews of Leiner et al and of Schmahmann and Sherman). These authors and others have described a wide range of deficits of memory and cognition, language function, and behavior in patients with disease apparently limited to the cerebellum (as determined by computed tomography and magnetic resonance imaging). It is true that cerebellar lesions interfere with the establishment of conditioned reflexes. To date, however, a uniform clinical pathologic syndrome in which a distinctive cognitive-behavioral deficit or group of deficits is related to a particular cerebellar lesion has not emerged, and the proposed mechanisms by which discrete cerebellar lesions might influence cognitive function remain somewhat speculative.

Differential Diagnosis of Ataxia

The ataxia of severe sensory neuropathy may simulate cerebellar ataxia; presumably this is due to involvement of the large peripheral spinocerebellar afferent fibers. However, seldom should there be difficulty in separating the two if one takes note of the loss of distal joint position sense, absence of associated cerebellar signs such as dysarthria or nystagmus, loss of tendon reflexes, and the corrective effects of vision on sensory ataxia. In the Miller Fisher syndrome, which is considered to be a variant of Guillain-Barré neuropathy, sensation is intact or affected only slightly and the ataxia is presumably due to a selective peripheral disorder of spinocerebellar nerve fibers. Affection of these fibers in the cervical cord may produce the same effects. *Vertiginous ataxia* is primarily an ataxia of gait and is distinguished by the obvious complaint of vertigo and listing to one side, past-pointing, and rotary nystagmus. The *nonvertiginous ataxia* of gait due to vestibular paresis (e.g., streptomycin toxicity) has special qualities that are described in Chap. 7. Vertigo and cerebellar ataxia may be concurrent, as in some patients with a paraneoplastic disease and in those with infarction of the lateral medulla and inferior cerebellum, but the two conditions are usually separable. An unusual and transient ataxia of the contralateral limbs occurs acutely after infarction or hemorrhage in the anterior thalamus (*thalamic ataxia*); in addition to neighborhood signs, there is often an accompanying unilateral asterixis. Also, a lesion of the superior parietal lobule (areas 5 and 7 of Brodmann) may result in a similar ataxia of the contralateral limbs.

In the diagnosis of disorders characterized by generalized cerebellar ataxia, the mode of onset (rate of development) and degree of permanence of the ataxia are of particular importance, as summarized in Table 5-1. Unilateral ataxia is most often caused by infarction or tumor in the cerebellar hemisphere or by demyelinating disease affecting cerebellar connections, while the causes of generalized ataxia and of pure gait ataxia are many.

Table 5-1
Diagnosis of generalized cerebellar ataxia

Mode of development	*Causes*
Acute-transitory	Intoxication with alcohol, lithium, barbiturate, phenytoin or other anticonvulsants (associated with dysarthria, nystagmus, and sometimes confusion; Chaps. 42, 43). Diamox responsive episodic ataxia (Chap. 37). Childhood hyperammonemias (Chap. 37).
Acute but usually reversible	Postinfectious, with mild inflammatory changes in CSF (Chap. 36). Viral cerebellar encephalitis (Chap. 33).
Acute-enduring	Hyperthermia with coma at onset (Chap. 17). Intoxication with mercury compounds or toluene (glue sniffing; spray painting; Chap. 43).
Subacute (over weeks)	Brain tumors such as medulloblastoma, astrocytoma, hemangioblastoma (usually with headache and papilledema; Chap. 31). Alcoholic-nutritional (Chaps. 41 and 42). Paraneoplastic, often with opsoclonus and specific anticerebellar antibodies (particularly with breast and ovarian carcinoma; Chap. 31.) Creutzfeldt–Jakob disease (Chap. 33). Abscess (Chap. 32). Idiopathic
Chronic (months to years)	Friedreich ataxia and other spinocerebellar degenerations; other hereditary cerebellar degenerations [olivopontocerebellar degenerations; cerebellar cortical degenerations (Chap. 39)]. Hereditary metabolic diseases, often with myoclonus (Chap. 37). Childhood ataxias, including ataxia telangiectasia, cerebellar agenesis, and dyssynergia cerebellaris myoclonica of Ramsay Hunt (Chap. 39).

REFERENCES

Allen GI, Tsukahara N: Cerebrocerebellar communication systems. *Physiol Rev* 54:957, 1974.

Babinski J: De l'asynergie cerebelleuse. *Rev Neurol* 7:806, 1899.

Chambers WW, Sprague JM: Functional localization in the cerebellum: I. Organization in longitudinal cortico-nuclear zones and their contribution to the control of posture, both extrapyramidal and pyramidal. *J Comp Neurol* 103:104, 1955.

Chambers WW, Sprague JM: Functional localization in the cerebellum: II. Somatotopic organization in cortex and nuclei. *Arch Neurol Psychiatry* 74:653, 1955.

Diener HC, Dichgans J: Pathophysiology of cerebellar ataxia. *Mov Disord* 7:95, 1992.

Evarts EV, Thach WT: Motor mechanism of the CNS: Cerebrocerebellar interrelations. *Annu Rev Physiol* 31:451, 1969.

Gilman S: Cerebellar control of movement. *Ann Neurol* 35:3, 1994.

Gilman S, Bloedel J, Lechtenberg R: *Disorders of the Cerebellum.* Philadelphia, Davis, 1980, pp 159–177.

Hallett M, Berardelli A, Matheson J, et al: Physiological analysis of simple rapid movement in patients with cerebellar deficits. *J Neurol Neurosurg Psychiatry* 53:124, 1991.

Hallett M, Shahani BT, Young RR: EMG analysis of patients with cerebellar deficits. *J Neurol Neurosurg Psychiatry* 38:1163, 1975.

Holmes G: The cerebellum of man: Hughlings Jackson Lecture. *Brain* 62:1, 1939.

Ito M: *The Cerebellum and Neural Control.* New York, Raven Press, 1984.

Jansen J, Brodal A: *Aspects of Cerebellar Anatomy.* Oslo, Johan Grundt Tanum Forlag, 1954.

Kandel ER, Schwartz JH, Jessel TM (eds): *Principles of Neural Science*, 4th ed. New York, McGraw-Hill, 2000.

Leiner HC, Leiner AL, Dow RS: Does the cerebellum contribute to mental skills? *Behav Neurosci* 100:443, 1986.

Schmahmann JD. Sherman JC: The cerebellar cognitive affective syndrome. *Brain* 121:561, 1998.

Sprague JM, Chambers WW: Control of posture by reticular formation and cerebellum in the intact, anesthetized and unanesthetized and in the decerebrated cat. *Am J Physiol* 176:52, 1954.

Stewart TG, Holmes G: Symptomatology of cerebellar tumors: A study of forty cases. *Brain* 27:522, 1904.

Thach WT Jr, Goodkin HP, Keating JG: The cerebellum and the adaptive coordination of movement. *Annu Rev Neurosci* 150:403, 1992.

Thach WT Jr, Montgomery EB Jr: Motor system, in Pearlman AL, Collins RC (eds): *Neurobiology of Disease.* New York, Oxford University Press, 1992, pp 168–196.

Ugawa Y, Uesaka Y, Terao Y, et al: Magnetic stimulation over the cerebellum in humans. *Ann Neurol* 37:703, 1995.

Chapter 6

TREMOR, MYOCLONUS, FOCAL DYSTONIAS, AND TICS

The subject of tremor may suitably be considered at this point because of its association with diseases of the basal ganglia and cerebellum. In addition, a group of miscellaneous movement disorders—myoclonus, facial and cervical dyskinesias, occupational spasms (dystonias), and tics—are described in this chapter. These disorders are largely involuntary in nature and can be quite disabling, but they have an uncertain pathologic basis and an indefinite relationship to the extrapyramidal motor disorders or to other standard categories of neurologic disease. They are brought together here mainly for convenience of exposition.

TREMOR

Tremor may be defined as a more or less involuntary and rhythmic oscillatory movement produced by alternating or irregularly synchronous contractions of reciprocally innervated muscles. The rhythmic quality distinguishes tremor from other involuntary movements, and the involvement of agonist and antagonistic muscles distinguishes it from clonus. Two general categories are recognized: normal (or physiologic) and abnormal (or pathologic). The former, as the name indicates, is a normal phenomenon; it is present in all contracting muscle groups and persists throughout the waking state and even in certain phases of sleep. The movement is so fine that it can barely be seen by the naked eye, and then only if the fingers are firmly outstretched; in most instances special instruments are required for its detection. It ranges in frequency between 8 and 13 Hz, the dominant rate being 10 Hz in adulthood and somewhat less in childhood and old age. Several hypotheses have been proposed to explain physiologic tremor, a traditional one being that it reflects the passive vibration of body tissues produced by mechanical activity of cardiac origin (ballistocardiogram). Assuredly this is not the whole explanation of physiologic tremor. As Marsden has pointed out, several additional factors—such as spindle input, the unfused grouped firing rates of motor neurons, and the natural resonating frequencies and inertia of the muscles and other structures—are probably of greater significance. Certain abnormal tremors, namely, the metabolic varieties of postural or action tremor and at least one type of familial tremor, are believed by some workers to be variants or exaggerations of physiologic tremor—i.e., "enhanced physiologic tremor" (see further on).

Abnormal or pathologic tremor, which is what one means when the term *tremor* is used clinically, preferentially affects certain muscle groups—the distal parts of the limbs (especially the fingers and hands); less often, the proximal parts; the head, tongue, jaw, or vocal cords; and rarely the trunk—and is present only in the waking state. The rate in most forms is from 4 to 7 Hz, or about half that of physiologic tremor. In any one individual, the rate is fairly constant in all affected parts. With the advent of electromyography (EMG) and mechanical recording devices, abnormal tremors were subdivided according to their rate, their relationship to posture of the limbs and volitional movement, their pattern of EMG activity (synchronous or alternating) in opposing muscle groups, and their response to certain drugs. The following types of tremor, the features of which are summarized in Table 6-1, are the ones encountered most frequently in clinical practice.

Postural and Action Tremors

These terms, which are used interchangeably, refer to a tremor that is present when the limbs and trunk are actively maintained in certain positions (such as holding the arms outstretched) and that may persist throughout active movement. More particularly, the tremor is absent when the limbs are relaxed but becomes evident when the muscles are activated. It is accentuated as greater

Table 6-1
Main types of tremor

Type of tremor	*Frequency Hz*	*Predominant location(s)*	*Enhancing agents*	*Attenuating agents*
Physiologic (enhanced)	8–13	Hands	Epinephrine, β-adrenergics	Alcohol, β-adrenergic antagonists
Parkinson (rest)	3–5	Hands and forearms, fingers, feet, lips, tongue	Emotional stress	L-dopa, anticholinergics
Cerebellar (intention, ataxic, "rubral")	2–4	Limbs, trunk, head	Emotional stress	Alcohol
Postural, or action	5–8	Hands	Anxiety, fright, β-adrenergics, alcohol withdrawal, xanthines, lithium, exercise, fatigue	β-adrenergic antagonists in some cases
Essential (familial, senile)	4–8	Hands, head, vocal cords	Same as above	Alcohol, propranolol, primidone
Alternate beat	3.5–6	Hands, head	Same as above	Clonazepam, alcohol, β-adrenergic antagonists
Orthostatic	4–8, irregular	Legs	Quiet standing	Repose, walking, clonazepam, valproate
Tremor of neuropathy	4–7	Hands	—	
"Palatal-myoclonus"	60–100/min 1–2	Palate, sometimes facial, pharyngeal, proximal limb muscles	—	Clonazepam, valproate

precision of movement is demanded, but it does not approach the degree of augmentation seen with so-called intention tremor, which is associated with cerebellar disease. In contrast to rest or static (parkinsonian) tremor, which is characterized electromyographically by alternating activity in agonist and antagonist muscles, most cases of action tremor are characterized by relatively rhythmic bursts of grouped alpha motor neuron discharges that occur not quite synchronously and simultaneously in opposing muscle groups. Slight inequalities in the strength and timing of contraction of opposing muscle groups account for the tremor.

Action tremors are of several different types, a feature that makes them more difficult to interpret than other tremors.

Enhanced Physiologic Tremor One type of action tremor seems merely to be an exaggeration of normal or physiologic tremor; it has the same frequency as physiologic tremor but a greater amplitude. Such a tremor, best elicited by holding the arms outstretched with fingers spread apart, is characteristic of intense fright and anxiety, certain metabolic disturbances (hyperthyroidism, hypercorticolism, hypoglycemia), pheochromocytoma, intense physical exertion, withdrawal from alcohol and other sedative drugs, and the toxic effects of several drugs—lithium, nicotinic acid, xanthines (coffee, tea, aminophylline, colas), and corticosteroids. It is noteworthy that a transient action tremor of this type can be reproduced by the intravenous injection of epinephrine or beta-adrenergic drugs such as isoproterenol. Young and colleagues have adduced evidence that the enhancement of physiologic tremor that occurs in these various metabolic and toxic states is due to stimulation of muscular tremorogenic beta-adrenergic receptors by increased levels of circulating catecholamines. Thus it appears that synchronization of motor units in physiologic tremor, though not primarily of neural origin, is nevertheless influenced by central and peripheral nervous activity.

Alcohol Withdrawal Tremor This, the most prominent feature of the alcohol withdrawal syndrome, is a special type of action tremor, closely related to enhanced physiologic tremor. Withdrawal of other sedative drugs (benzodiazepines, barbiturates) following a sustained period of use may produce much the same effect. Using surface electrodes on agonist and antagonist muscles of the outstretched limb, Lefebvre-D'Amour and colleagues have described two somewhat different types of tremor in the alcohol withdrawal period: In the first, with frequency greater than 8 Hz, EMG recordings show continuous activity in antagonistic muscles. Thus it resembles physiologic tremor but is of greater amplitude (enhanced physiologic tremor) and is responsive to propranolol (Koller et al). The second, of less than 8 Hz, is characterized by discrete bursts of EMG activity occurring synchronously in antagonistic muscles, like that observed in one type of familial tremor (see below). Either of these types may occur after a relatively short period of intoxication ("morning shakes"). A number of alcoholics, upon recovery from the withdrawal state, exhibit a persistent tremor of essential-familial type, described below. In such patients, the additive effects of an enhanced physiologic tremor probably account for the severity of tremor during alcohol withdrawal. The mechanisms involved in alcohol withdrawal symptoms are discussed in Chap. 42.

Essential Tremor This, the commonest type of *action tremor*, is of lower frequency (4 to 8 Hz) than physiologic tremor. Tremor of this relatively slow type may occur as the only neurologic abnormality in several members of a family, in which case it is called *familial* or *hereditary tremor*. Such a tremor is inherited as an autosomal dominant trait with virtually complete penetrance. If the inherited nature of the tremor is not evident, it is referred to as *essential tremor*—and, if it becomes evident only in late adult life, as *senile tremor*. Sometimes referred to as "benign," it is hardly so in many patients, in whom it worsens with age and interferes with normal activities. These tremors cannot be distinguished on the basis of their physiologic and pharmacologic properties and probably should not, therefore, be considered as separate entitities.

Clinically, it may be difficult to distinguish essential and hereditary forms of tremor from enhanced physiologic tremor. One type of essential tremor is of the same frequency (6 to 8 Hz) as enhanced physiologic tremor, which has led several clinicians to declare their identity. However, there are certain clinical and physiologic differences, as indicated below.

Familial or *essential tremor* most often makes its appearance in the second decade, but it may begin in childhood and then persist. A second peak of increased incidence occurs in adults over 35 years of age. Both sexes are affected. It is a relatively common disorder, with an estimated prevalence of 415 per 100,000 persons over the age of 40 years (Haerer et al). The tremor frequency is 4 to 8 Hz, usually at the lower end of this range, and it is of variable amplitude. *The identifying feature is its appearance or marked enhancement with attempts to maintain a static limb posture.* Like most tremors, essential tremor is worsened by emotion, exercise, and fatigue. The tremor practically always begins in the arms and is usually symmetrical, but in approximately 15 percent of patients it may appear first in the dominant hand. A severe isolated arm or leg tremor should suggest another disease (Parkinson disease or focal dystonia, as described further on). The tremor may be limited to the upper limbs or a side-to-side or nodding movement of the head may be added or occur independently. Infrequently, the tremor of the head precedes that of the hands. The head tremor is also postural in nature and disappears when the head is supported. In advanced cases, there is involvement of the jaw, lips, tongue, and larynx, the latter imparting a quaver to the voice. In the large series of familial case studies by Bain and colleagues, solitary jaw or head tremor was not found. Nor was there an association with Parkinson disease, cerebellar ataxia, or dystonia. Many patients with essential tremor will have identified the amplifying effects of anxiety and the ameliorating effects of alcohol on their tremor.

The lower limbs are usually spared or only minimally affected. Rare cases, in which the legs are affected disproportionately, have been described under the title of *orthostatic tremor* (Heilman, Thompson et al, Wee et al). This tremor is most prominent or may occur only during quiet standing; it diminishes with walking and disappears when the patient is seated or reclining. In the latter positions, the tremor can be evoked by strong contraction of the leg muscles against resistance. In such patients, the arms are affected little or not at all. Some of these cases have reportedly responded to the administration of clonazepam and sodium valproate.

Electromyographic studies of familial essential tremors reveal that the tremor is generated by more or less rhythmic and almost simultaneous bursts of activity in pairs of agonist and antagonist muscles (Fig. 6-1*B*). Less often, especially in the lower-frequency tremors, the activity in agonist and antagonist muscles alternates, a feature more characteristic of parkinsonism (see below). Tremor of either pattern may be disabling, but the slower, alternating-beat tremor is more of a handicap. Both types occur not only during volitional movement (kinetic tremor) but also during the maintenance of certain postures (postural tremor).

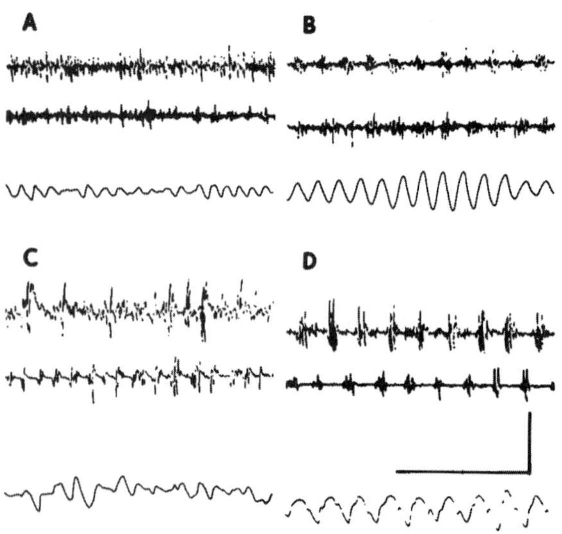

Figure 6-1

Types of tremor. In each, the lowest trace is an accelerometric recording from the outstretched hand; the upper two traces are surface electromyographs from the wrist extensor (upper) *and flexor* (middle) *muscle groups.* A. *A physiologic tremor; there is no evidence of synchronization of electromyographic (EMG) activity.* B. *Essential-familial tremor; the movements are very regular and EMG bursts occur simultaneously in antagonistic muscle groups.* C. *Neuropathic tremor; movements are irregular and EMG bursts vary in timing between the two groups.* D. *Parkinsonian ("rest") tremor; EMG bursts alternate between antagonistic muscle groups. Calibration is 1 s. (Courtesy of Dr. Robert R. Young.)*

This type of tremor may increase in severity to a point where handwriting becomes illegible and the patient cannot bring a spoon or glass to his lips without spilling its contents. Eventually all tasks that require manual dexterity become difficult or impossible. Treatment of these tremors is discussed further on.

Other Forms of Action Tremor Action tremors are seen in a number of clinical settings in addition to those already mentioned. A coarse action tremor, sometimes combined with myoclonus, accompanies various types of meningoencephalitis (e.g., general paresis) and certain intoxications (methyl bromide and bismuth). Its anatomy and mechanism are obscure. Also, it is important to repeat that an action tremor of either the high-frequency or slower (essential) variety may occur in certain diseases of the basal ganglia, including Parkinson disease, in which case both the action and the more typical static tremor are superimposed, with either one predominating. Adams and coworkers have also described a disabling action tremor in patients with chronic demyelinating and paraproteinemic polyneuropathies. It is also a prominent feature of the neuropathy caused by IgM antibodies to myelin-associated glycoprotein (MAG). It simulates a coarse essential tremor and typically worsens if the patient is asked to hold his finger near a target. The EMG pattern in this neuropathic tremor is more irregular than that in the essential-familial tremor; it is hypothesized that there is a disturbance of muscle spindle afferents. Occasionally an inflammatory large-fiber neuropathy, acute or chronic in type, is marked by a prominent ataxic (intention) tremor and a faster action tremor. Also, peroneal muscular atrophy may be associated with tremor of the essential-familial type; this combination of symptoms was the basis upon which Roussy and Levy incorrectly set it apart as a distinct disease.

Management of Essential Tremor A curious fact about the familial and essential tremors of the non-alternate-beat type is that they can be suppressed by a few drinks of alcohol in more than 75 percent of patients; but once the effects of the alcohol have worn off, the tremor returns and may even be worse. Also, this type of tremor can often be inhibited by the beta-adrenergic antagonist propranolol (between 120 and 300 mg per day in divided doses or as a sustained-release preparation) taken orally over a long period of time. However, the benefit is variable and often incomplete; most studies indicate that 50 to 70 percent of patients have some symptomatic relief. Several but not all of the other beta-blocking drugs are similarly effective; metoprolol and nadolol, which may be better tolerated than propranolol (bronchospasm, sleepiness, impotence, etc.), are the ones most extensively studied. Young and associates have shown that neither propranolol nor ethanol, when injected intra-arterially into a limb, decreases the amplitude of essential tremor. These findings suggest that the therapeutic effects of these agents are due less to blockade of the peripheral beta-adrenergic tremorogenic receptors than to the action of these agents on structures within the central nervous system.

The anticonvulsant primidone (Mysoline, in low doses of 25 to 50 mg initially, and raised slowly) has also been found to be effective in controlling essential tremor and should be tried in patients who do not respond to or cannot tolerate beta-blocking medications. Amantadine has a modest effect on tremor and may be used as an adjunct.

The alternate-beat, kinetic-predominant type of essential tremor is said to respond well to clonazepam (Biary and Koller). Alcohol and primidone have been less effective in our experience. Injections of botulinum toxin, as for focal dystonia, can reduce the severity of essential tremor, but the accompanying weakness of arm and hand muscles often proves unacceptable to the patient. The apparent benefit of valproate and clonazepam for the lower limb (orthostatic) form of essential tremor has already been mentioned.

Parkinsonian (Rest) Tremor

This is a coarse, rhythmic tremor with a frequency of 3 to 5 Hz. Electromyographically, it is characterized by bursts of activity that alternate between opposing muscle groups. The tremor is most often localized in one or both hands and forearms and less frequently in the feet, jaw, lips, or tongue (Fig. 6-1*D*). It occurs when the limb is in an *attitude of repose* and is suppressed or diminished by willed movement, at least momentarily, only to reassert itself once the limb assumes a new position. For this reason the parkinsonian tremor is often referred to as a *resting tremor* or *tremor at rest*, but these terms need to be qualified. Maintaining the arm in an attitude of repose or keeping it still in other positions requires a certain degree of muscular contraction, albeit slight. If the tremulous hand is completely relaxed, as it is when the arm is fully supported at the wrist and elbow, the tremor usually disappears; however, the patient rarely achieves this state. Usually he maintains a state of slight tonic contraction of the trunk and proximal muscles of the limbs. Under conditions of complete rest, i.e., in all except the lightest phases of sleep, the tremor disappears, as do most abnormal tremors except palatal and ocular myoclonus.

Parkinsonian tremor takes the form of flexion-extension or abduction-adduction of the fingers or the hand; pronation-supination of the hand and forearm is also a common presentation. Flexion-extension of the fingers in combination with adduction-abduction of the thumb yields the classic "pill-rolling" tremor. It continues while the patient walks, unlike essential tremor; indeed, it may first become apparent or be exaggerated during walking. When the legs are affected, the tremor takes the form of a flexion-extension movement of the foot, sometimes the knee; in the jaw and lips, it is seen as an up-and-down and a pursing movement, respectively. The eyelids, if they are closed lightly, tend to flutter rhythmically (blepharoclonus), and the tongue, when protruded, may move in and out of the mouth at about the same tempo as the tremor elsewhere. The so-called cogwheel effect, which is perceived by the examiner on passive movement of the extremities (Negro's sign), is probably no more than a palpable tremor superimposed on rigidity and as such is not specific for Parkinson disease. The tremor frequency is surprisingly constant over long periods, but the amplitude is variable. Emotional stress augments the amplitude and may add the effects of an enhanced physiologic tremor; increasing rigidity of the limbs, with advance of the disease, reduces it. The tremor interferes surprisingly little with voluntary movement; for example, it is possible for a tremulous patient to raise a full glass of water to his lips and drain its contents without spilling a drop.

Resting tremor is most often a manifestation of the Parkinson syndrome, whether the idiopathic variety described by James Parkinson (paralysis agitans) or the drug-induced type. In the former, the tremor is relatively gentle and more or less limited to the distal muscles; often it is asymmetrical and, at the outset, it may be unilateral. The tremor of postencephalitic parkinsonism (which is now extinct) often had a greater amplitude and involved proximal muscles. In neither disease is there a close correspondence between the degree of tremor and the degree of rigidity or akinesia. A parkinsonian type of tremor may also be seen in elderly persons without akinesia, rigidity, or mask-like facies. In some of these patients, the tremor is followed years later by the other manifestations of paralysis agitans, but in the majority it is not, the tremor remaining stationary for many years or progressing very slowly, unaffected by anti-Parkinson drugs. Patients with the familial (wilsonian) or the acquired form of hepatocerebral degeneration may also show a tremor of parkinsonian type, usually mixed with ataxic tremor and other extrapyramidal motor abnormalities.

Parkinsonian tremor is suppressed to some extent by the phenothiazine derivative ethopropazine (Parsidol), by trihexyphenidyl (Artane) and other anticholinergic drugs, and somewhat less consistently but sometimes quite impressively by L-dopa and dopaminergic agonist drugs that are the mainstay of treatment for the other features of parkinsonism. Stereotactic lesions in the basal ventrolateral nucleus of the thalamus diminish or abolish tremor contralaterally. A parkinsonian tremor is sometimes associated with an additional tremor of faster frequency (see above and page 1129); the latter is of action or postural type and responds better to beta-blocking drugs and primidone than to anti-Parkinson medications. Treatment is discussed in greater detail in Chap. 39.

Intention (Ataxic) Tremor

The word *intention* is ambiguous in this context because the tremor itself is not intentional and occurs not when the patient intends to make a movement but only during the most demanding phases of active performance. In this sense it is a *kinetic*, or *action, tremor*, but the latter term has other connotations to neurologists, as described above. The term *ataxic* is a suitable substitute for *intention* because this tremor is always combined with and adds to cerebellar ataxia. Its salient feature is that it requires for its full expression the performance of an exacting, precise, projected movement. The tremor is absent when the limbs are inactive and during the first part of a voluntary movement, but as the action continues and fine adjustments of the movement are demanded (e.g., in touching the tip of the nose or the examiner's finger), an irregular, more or less rhythmic (2- to 4-Hz) interruption of forward progression with side-to-side oscillation appears and may continue for several beats after the target has been reached. Unlike familial tremor, the oscillations occur in more than one plane (Young). The tremor and ataxia may seriously interfere with the patient's performance of skilled acts. In some patients there is a rhythmic oscillation of the head on the trunk (titubation), or of the trunk itself, at approximately the same rate. As indicated above, this type of tremor invariably indicates disease of the cerebellum or its connections, particularly via the superior cerebellar peduncle.

As remarked on page 94, there is another, more violent type of tremor associated with cerebellar ataxia, in which every movement, even lifting the arm slightly or the maintenance of static postures with the arms held out to the side, results in a wide-ranging, rhythmic 2- to 5-Hz "wing beating" movement, sometimes of sufficient force to throw the patient off balance. In such cases, the lesion is usually in the midbrain, involving the upward projections of the dentatorubrothalamic fibers and the medial part of the ventral tegmental reticular nucleus. Because of the location of the lesion in the region of the red nucleus, Holmes originally called this a *rubral* tremor. However, experimental evidence in monkeys indicates that the tremor is produced not by a lesion of the red nucleus per se but by interruption of dentatothalamic fibers that traverse this nucleus—i.e., the cerebellar efferent fibers that form the superior cerebellar peduncle and brachium conjunctivum (Carpenter). This type of tremor is seen in some patients with multiple sclerosis and Wilson disease, occasionally with vascular and other lesions of the tegmentum of the midbrain and subthalamus, and rarely as an effect of antipsychotic medications. It is abolished by a lesion in the opposite ventrolateral nucleus of the thalamus. Beta-adrenergic blocking agents, anticholinergic drugs, isoniazid, and L-dopa have little therapeutic effect.

The mechanisms involved in the production of intention or ataxic tremor have been discussed in Chap. 5.

Hysterical Tremor

Tremor is a relatively rare manifestation of hysteria, but it may simulate some types of organic tremor, thereby causing difficulty in diagnosis. Hysterical tremors are usually restricted to a single limb; they are gross in nature, are less regular than the common static or action tremors, and diminish in amplitude or disappear if the patient is distracted, as, for example, when asked to make a complex movement with the opposite hand. If the affected hand and arm are restrained by the examiner, the tremor may move to a more proximal part of the limb or to another part of the body ("chasing the tremor"). Hysterical tremor persists in repose and during movement and is less subject than nonhysterical tremors to the modifying influences of posture and willed movement.

Tremors of Mixed Type

Not all tremors correspond exactly with the ones described above. There is frequently a variation in one or more particulars from the classic pattern, or one type of tremor may show a feature ordinarily considered characteristic of another. In some parkinsonian patients, for example, the tremor is accentuated rather than dampened by active movement; in others, the tremor may be very mild or absent "at rest" and become obvious only with movement of the limbs. As mentioned above, a patient with classic parkinsonian tremor may, in addition, show a fine tremor of the outstretched hands, i.e., a postural or action tremor, and occasionally an element of ataxic tremor as well. In a similar vein, essential or familial tremor may, in its advanced stages, assume the aspects of a cerebellar, or intention, tremor. Gordon Holmes was careful to note that patients with acute cerebellar lesions sometimes show a parkinsonian tremor in addition to the usual signs of ataxia and ataxic tremor.

The features of one type of tremor may be so mixed with those of another that satisfactory classification is not possible. For example, in certain patients with essential or familial tremor or with cerebellar degeneration, one may observe a rhythmic tremor, characteristically parkinsonian in tempo, which is not apparent in repose but appears with certain sustained postures. It may take the form of an abduction-adduction or flexion-extension of the fingers when the patient's weight is partially supported by the hands, as in the writing position, or it may appear as a tremor of the outstretched fingers or of the thigh when the patient is seated.

Also difficult to classify are tremors that are intermixed with dystonia. These are discussed further on, in the section on cervical dystonia.

The Pathophysiology of Tremor

The exact anatomic basis of *parkinsonian tremor* is not known. In Parkinson disease, the visible lesions predominate in the substantia nigra and this was true also of the postencephalitic form of the disease. In animals, however, experimental lesions confined to the substantia nigra do not result in tremor; neither do lesions in the striatopallidal parts of the basal ganglia. Moreover, not all patients with lesions of the substantia nigra have tremor; in some there are only bradykinesia and rigidity. In a group of eight patients poisoned with the meperidine analogue MPTP, which destroys the neurons of the pars compacta of the substantia nigra (page 1133), four developed a tremor, and it had more the characteristics of a proximal action or postural tremor than of a rest tremor (Burns et al).

Ward and others have produced a Parkinson-like tremor in monkeys by placing a lesion in the ventromedial tegmentum of the midbrain, just caudal to the red nucleus and dorsal to the substantia nigra. Ward postulated that interruption of the descending fibers at this site liberates an oscillating mechanism in the lower brainstem; the latter presumably involves the limb innervation via the reticulospinal pathway. Alternative possibilities are that the lesion in the ventromedial tegmentum interrupts the brachium conjunctivum, or a tegmental-thalamic projection, or the descending limb of the superior cerebellar peduncle, which functions as a link in a dentate-reticular-cerebellar feedback mechanism (Fig. 5-3).

Ataxic tremor has been consistently produced in monkeys by inactivating the deep cerebellar nuclei or sectioning the superior cerebellar peduncle or the brachium conjunctivum below its decussation. A lesion of the nucleus interpositus or dentate nucleus causes an ipsilateral tremor of ataxic type, as one might expect, associated with other manifestations of cerebellar ataxia. In addition, such a lesion gives rise to a "simple tremor," which is the term that Carpenter applied to a "resting," or parkinsonian, tremor. He found that the latter tremor was most prominent during the early postoperative period and was less enduring than ataxic tremor. Nevertheless, the concurrence of the two types of tremor and the fact that both can be abolished by ablation of the contralateral ventrolateral thalamic nucleus suggest that they have closely related neural mechanisms. The conflicting observations regarding the role of the inferior olives and olivocerebellar system in the genesis of essential tremor have been mentioned earlier.

To date, only a few cases of *essential tremor* have been examined postmortem, and these have disclosed no consistent lesion to which the tremor could indisputably be attributed (Herskovits and Blackwood; Koller and Busenbark). Essential tremors of sporadic and familial type, like parkinsonian and ataxic (intention) tremors, can be abolished or diminished by small stereotactic lesions of the basal ventrolateral nucleus of the thalamus and are abolished by strokes that cause corticospinal or gross unilateral cerebellar lesions; in these respects also they differ from enhanced physiologic tremor. Colebatch and coworkers, who studied cerebral and cerebellar blood flow in patients with essential tremor, found that the cerebellum was selectively activated; they postulated a release of an oscillatory mechanism of the cerebello-olivary pathway. Dubinsky and Hallett have demonstrated that the inferior olives become hypermetabolic in patients with essential tremor when their tremor is activated. However, the inferior olivary localization has been questioned by Wills and colleagues, who recorded an increased blood flow in the cerebellum and red nuclei but not in the olive. The fact that the tremor can be ablated by lesions in the cerebellum as well as in the ventrolateral thalamus suggests that the oscillatory activity is conducted to the motor cortex via the dentatothalamic system. These mechanisms have been reviewed by Elble.

In patients with tremor of either the parkinsonian, postural, or intention type, Narabayashi has recorded rhythmic burst discharges of unitary cellular activity in the nucleus intermedius ventralis of the thalamus (as well as in the medial pallidum and subthalamic nucleus), synchronous with the beat of the tremor. Neurons that exhibit the synchronous bursts are arranged somatotopically and respond to kinesthetic impulses from the muscles and joints involved in the tremor. A stereotaxic lesion in any of these sites abolishes the tremor. The effectiveness of the thalamic lesion may be due to interruption of pallidothalamic and dentatotha-lamic projections or, more likely, to interruption of projections from the ventrolateral thalamus to the premotor cortex, since the impulses responsible for cerebellar tremor, like those for choreoathetosis, are ultimately mediated by the lateral corticospinal tract. This concept would explain why a lesion of the subthalamic nucleus causes *contralateral* dyskinesia, whereas a lesion of the dentate nucleus or of the brachium conjunctivum, before its decussation, gives rise to *ipsilateral* ataxia and tremor.

In the clinical analysis of tremor in humans, the aforementioned types are usually distinguishable on the basis of rhythmicity, amplitude, frequency, relation to movement, postural set, and relaxation. Such analysis also differentiates tremors from a large array of nontremorous states, such as fasciculations, sensory ataxia, myoclonus, asterixis, epilepsia partialis continua, clonus, and shivering.

Palatal Tremor

This is a rare and unique disorder consisting of rapid, rhythmic, involuntary movements of the soft palate. For many years it was considered to be a form of uniphasic myoclonus (hence the terms *palatal myoclonus* or *palatal nystagmus*). Because of the ongoing rhythmic movement, it is now classified as a tremor. There are two forms of this movement, according to Deuschl and colleagues. One is called *essential palatal tremor* and reflects the rhythmic activation of the tensor veli palatini muscles; it has no known pathologic basis. The palatal movement imparts a repetitive audible click, which ceases during sleep. The second, more common form is a *symptomatic palatal tremor;* it involves the levator veli palatini muscles and is due to a diverse group of brainstem lesions that interrupt the central tegmental tract(s), which contain descending fibers from midbrain nuclei to the inferior olivary complex. In patients with this tremor, the frequency of the tremor is 26 to 420 cycles per minute in the essential form and 107 to 164 cycles per minute in the symptomatic form.

Symptomatic palatal tremor, in contrast to the essential type and all other tremors, persists during sleep and is often associated with oscillopsia and unilateral or bilateral cerebellar signs. In some cases of the symptomatic type, the pharynx as well as the facial and extraocular muscles (pendular or convergence nystagmus), diaphragm, vocal cords, and even the muscles of the neck and shoulders partake of the persistent rhythmic movements. A similar phenomenon, in which contraction of the masseters occurs concurrently with pendular ocular convergence, has been observed in Whipple disease (*oculomasticatory myorhythmia*).

Magnetic resonance imaging reveals no lesions to account for essential palatal tremor, but in the symptomatic form one can see the tegmental brainstem lesions and conspicuous enlargement of the inferior olivary nucleus, unilaterally or bilaterally. With unilateral palatal tremor, it is the contralateral olive that becomes enlarged. It has been proposed that the lesions in the symptomatic form interrupt the circuit (dentate nucleus–brachium conjunctivum–central tegmental tract–olivary nucleus–dentate nucleus) that Lapresle and Ben Hamida call the *triangle of Guillain and Mollaret*, after the persons who first carefully studied the condition (page 89). Our own pathologic material confirms the central tegmental-olivary lesions but contains no examples of the production of palatal myclonus by lesions of the cerebellum or of the dentate and red nuclei. The lesions have been vascular, neoplastic, demyelinating (multiple sclerosis), or traumatic and have been found in the midbrain or pontine tegmentum. There are no reports on the pathologic anatomy of essential palatal tremor.

The physiologic basis of palatal tremor remains conjectural. Matsuo and Ajax postulated a denervation hypersensitivity of the inferior olivary nucleus and its dentate connections; Kane and Thach have adduced evidence that the critical event in the genesis of palatal tremor is denervation not of the olive but of the nucleus ambiguus and the dorsolateral reticular formation adjacent to it. More recently, Hallett and Dubinsky have suggested that palatal tremor may be based on the same mechanism as postural tremor—i.e., presumably a disinhibition of the olive and a rhythmic coupling of neurons in the olive induced by a lesion of the dentato-olivary pathway. We are uncertain whether to designate these rhythmic disorders as uniphasic myoclonus or as tremors.

The use of drugs in treating this movement disorder has met with variable success. Clonazepam (0.25 to 0.5 mg/day, increasing gradually to 3.0 to 6.0 mg/day) and sodium valproate (250 mg/day, increasing to 1000 mg/day) have suppressed the movement in some cases. Also, tetrabenazine and haloperidol have been helpful on occasion. Selective injection of the palatal muscles with botulinum toxin affords modest relief.

ASTERIXIS

The movement disorder known as *asterixis* was described by Adams and Foley in 1953. It consists essentially of arrhythmic lapses of sustained posture. These sudden interruptions in sustained muscular contraction allow gravity or the inherent elasticity of muscles to produce a movement, which the patient then corrects, sometimes with overshoot. Later Adams and Schwab demonstrated that the initial movement or lapse in posture is associated with EMG silence for a period of 35 to 200 ms. By interlocking EMG and electroencephalographic (EEG) recordings, Ugawa et al found that a sharp wave, probably generated in the motor cortex, immediately precedes the period of EMG silence. This confirmed that asterixis differs physiologically from both tremor and myoclonus, with which it was formerly confused; it has incorrectly been referred to as a "negative tremor."

Asterixis is most readily evoked by asking the patient to hold his arms outstretched with hands dorsiflexed or to dorsiflex the hands and extend the fingers while resting the forearms on the bed or the arms of a chair. Flexion movements of the hands may then occur once or several times a minute. The lapses in sustained muscle contraction and the corresponding lapses in EMG activity are usually generalized and can be provoked by the persistent contraction of any muscle group—including, for example, the protruded tongue, the closed eyelids, or the trunk muscles. If small finger muscles are affected, an EMG may be required to separate asterixis from tremor and myoclonus.

This sign was first observed in patients with hepatic encephalopathy but was later noted in those with hypercapnia, uremia, and other metabolic and toxic encephalopathies. However, lapses of this type may sometimes appear in the neck and arms of a normal person during a period of drowsiness. They may be evoked by phenytoin and other anticonvulsants, suggesting that these drugs are present in excessive concentrations.

Unilateral asterixis has been noted in an arm and leg on the side opposite an infarction in the territory of the anterior cerebral artery, contralateral to a stereotaxic thalamotomy, thalamic infarction or hemorrhage, and with an upper midbrain lesion, usually as a transient phenomenon after stroke. Montalban and colleagues observed unilateral asterixis in 45 patients without metabolic or toxic abnormalities and in more than half the patients, there were lesions in the contralateral thalamus; in the remainder, there was an abnormality in the pons or a cerebral hemisphere.

CLONUS, MYOCLONUS, AND POLYMYOCLONUS

The terms *clonus* (or *clonic*), *myoclonus* (or *myoclonic*), and *polymyoclonus* have been used indiscriminately to designate any rhythmic or arrhythmic series of brief, shock-like muscular contractions attendant upon disease of the central nervous system. In this text, the terms are used as follows: *Clonus* refers to a series of *rhythmic, uniphasic* or *monophasic* (i.e., *unidirectional*) *contractions and relaxations* of a group of muscles, differing in this way from tremors, which are always diphasic or bidirectional. *Myoclonus* specifies the shock-like contraction(s) of a group of muscles, irregular in rhythm and amplitude, and, with few exceptions, asynchronous and asymmetrical in distribution; if such contractions occur singly or are repeated in a restricted group of muscles, such as those of an arm or leg, we designate the phenomenon as *segmental myoclonus* or *myoclonus simplex*. Widespread, lightning-like, arrhythmic con-tractions are referred to as *myoclonus multiplex* or *polymyoclonus*. In the discussion that follows, it will become evident that this is not a matter of mere pedantry but that each of the three phenomena has a distinctive pathophysiology and particular clinical implications.

Clonus

Reference has already been made to the type of clonus that appears in relation to spasticity and heightened tendon reflexes in diseases affecting the corticospinal tract (page 56). *Epilepsia partialis continua* is a special type of rhythmic clonus in which one group of muscles, usually of the face, arm, or leg, is continuously (day and night) involved in a series of rhythmic monophasic contractions. These may continue for weeks, months, or years. In most cases there is a corresponding EEG abnormality. The disorder appears to be cerebral in origin, but its precise anatomic and physiologic basis cannot be determined in most cases (see Chap. 16 for further discussion).

Myoclonus Simplex

Patients with idiopathic epilepsy may complain of a localized myoclonic jerk or a short burst of myoclonic jerks, occurring particularly on awakening and on the day or two preceding a major generalized seizure, after which these movements cease. Very few patients with this type of myoclonus show progressive mental and physical deterioration. One-sided myoclonic jerks are the dominant feature of a particular form of childhood epilepsy—so-called benign epilepsy with rolandic spikes (page 342). Diffuse myoclonic jerks are the main or only manifestation of a fairly common seizure disorder with distinctive EEG features called juvenile myoclonic epilepsy; this diagnosis is suggested by an onset during adolescence and symptoms that become prominent with sleep deprivation and alcohol consumption (page 335). Myoclonus may be associated with atypical petit mal and akinetic seizures in the Lennox-Gastaut syndrome (page 335); the patient often falls during the brief lapse of postural mechanisms that follows a single myoclonic contraction. Similarly, in the West syndrome of infantile spasms, the arms and trunk are suddenly flexed or extended in a single massive myoclonic jerk ("jackknife" or "salaam" seizures); mental regression occurs in fully 80 to 90 percent of cases, even when the seizures are successfully treated with adrenocorticotropic hormone (ACTH).

Diffuse Myoclonus (Myoclonus Multiplex, or Polymyoclonus)

Under the title *paramyoclonus multiplex*, Friedreich in 1881 described a sporadic instance of widespread muscle jerking in an adult. It was probably in the course of this description that the term *myoclonus* was used for the first time. Muscles were involved diffusely, particularly those of the lower face and proximal segments of the limbs, and the myoclonus persisted for many years, being absent only during sleep. No other neurologic abnormalities accompanied the movement abnormality. The nature and pathologic basis of this disorder were never determined, and its status as a clinical entity has never been secure. Over the years, the term *paramyoclonus multiplex* has been applied to all varieties of myoclonic disorder (and other motor phenomena as well), to the point where it has nearly lost its specific clinical connotation. Myoclonus multiplex of the type described by Friedreich may occur in pure or "essential" form as a benign, often familial, nonprogressive disease or as part of a more complex progressive syndrome that may prove disabling and fatal. Some have specified the first as primary and the latter as secondary forms, but these designations have little fundamental value, serving only to indicate differences in severity and clinical course.

Essential Myoclonus So-called essential myoclonus may begin at any period of life but usually appears first in childhood and is of unknown etiology. An autosomal dominant mode of inheritance is evident in some families. The myoclonus takes the form of irregular twitches of one or another part of the body, involving groups of muscles, single muscles, or even a portion of a muscle. As a result, an arm may suddenly flex, the head may jerk backward or forward, or the trunk may curve or straighten. The face, neck, jaw, tongue, and ocular muscles may twitch; also the diaphragm. Some muscle contractions cause no visible displacement of a limb. Even fascicles of the platysma may twitch, according to Wilson. In this and other forms of myclonus, the muscle contraction is brief (20 to 50 ms), i.e., faster than that of chorea, with which it may be confused. The speed of the myoclonic contraction is the same, whether it involves a part of a muscle, a whole muscle, or a group of muscles. Many of the patients register little complaint, accepting the constant intrusions of motor activity with stoicism, and lead relatively normal, active lives. Seizures, dementia, and other neurologic deficits are notably absent. Occasionally there is hint of a mild cerebellar ataxia and, in one family studied by R. D. Adams, essential tremor was present as well, both in family members with polymyoclonia and in those without. Both the tremor and myoclonus were dramatically suppressed by the ingestion of alcohol. Similar families have been observed by others (Marsden et al). In a Mayo Clinic series, 19 of 94 patients with polymyoclonus were of this "essential" type (Aigner and Mulder).

Several of the sleep-related syndromes that involve repetitive leg movements include an element of myoclonus. In a few patients, mainly older ones with severe "restless legs syndrome", the myoclonus and dyskinesias are troublesome in the daytime as well. Marching in place and body rocking have been observed in some patients with the restless legs syndrome (Walters et al). Opiates may be helpful in suppressing the movements. These disorders are discussed in Chap. 19.

Myoclonic Epilepsy (see also page 335) Myoclonic epilepsy, or myoclonus epilepsy, constitutes another important syndrome of multiple etiologies. A relatively benign idiopathic form, juvenile myoclonic epilepsy, has been mentioned and is discussed further on page 335. A more serious type of myoclonus epilepsy, which in the beginning may be an isolated phenomenon, is eventually associated with dementia and other signs of progressive neurologic disease (familial variety of Unverricht and Lundborg, page 349). An outstanding feature of the latter is a remarkable sensitivity of the myoclonus to stimuli of all sorts. If a limb is passively or actively displaced, the resulting myoclonic jerk may lead, through a series of progressively larger and more or less synchronous jerks, to a generalized convulsive seizure. In late childhood this type of stimulus-sensitive myoclonus is usually a manifestation of the juvenile form of lipid storage disease, which, in addition to myoclonus, is characterized by seizures, retinal degeneration, dementia, rigidity, pseudobulbar paralysis, and, in the late stages, by quadriplegia in flexion. Another form of stimulus-sensitive (reflex) myoclonus, inherited as an autosomal recessive trait, begins in late childhood or adolescence and is associated with neuronal inclusions (Lafora bodies) in the cerebral and cerebellar cortex and in brainstem nuclei (page 349). In yet another familial form (described under the title of *Baltic myoclonus* by Eldridge and associates, necropsy has disclosed a loss of Purkinje cells but no inclusion bodies. Unlike Lafora disease, the Baltic variety of myoclonic epilepsy has a favorable prognosis, particularly if the seizures are treated with valproic acid.

Under the title of *cherry-red-spot myoclonus syndrome*, Rapin and associates have drawn attention to a familial (autosomal recessive) form of diffuse, incapacitating intention myoclonus associated with visual loss and ataxia. This disorder develops insidiously in adolescence. The earliest sign is a cherry-red spot in the macula that may fade in the chronic stages of the illness. The intellect is relatively unimpaired. The specific enzyme defect appears to be a deficiency of lysosomal α-neuroaminidase (sialidase), resulting in the excretion of large amounts of sialylated oligosaccharides in the urine. Lowden and O'Brien refer to this disorder as *type 1 sialidosis* and distinguish it from a second type, in which patients are of short stature (due to chondrodystrophy) and often have a deficiency of β-galactosidase in tissues and body fluids. In patients with sialidosis, a mucopolysaccharide-like material is stored in liver cells, but neurons show only a nonspecific accumulation of lipofuscin. A similar clinical syndrome of myoclonic epilepsy is seen in a variant form of neuroaxonal dystrophy and in the late childhood–early adult neuronopathic form of Gaucher disease, in which it is associated with supranuclear gaze palsies and cerebellar ataxia (page 997).

Diffuse Myoclonus with Neurologic Disease of Diverse Type (Table 6-2) The clinical settings in which one observes widespread random myoclonic jerks as a transient or persistent phenomenon are viral encephalitis, Creutzfeldt-Jakob disease, general paresis, advanced Alzheimer and Lewy-body disease, occasionally in Wilson disease, and most often with acquired metabolic disorders (prototypically uremic and anoxic encephalopathy) and certain drug intoxications, notably with haloperidol and amphetamines. An acute onset of polymyoclonus with confusion may occur with lithium intoxication; once ingestion is discontinued, there is improvement (slowly over days to weeks) and the myoclonus is replaced by diffuse action tremors, which later subside. Diffuse, severe myoclonus may be a prominent feature of early tetanus and strychnine poisoning. A polymyoclonus that occurs in acute anoxic encephalopathy should be distinguished from postanoxic action, or intention, myoclonus that emerges with recovery (see below). Encephalopathy with diffuse myoclonus may occur in Hashimoto thyroiditis and in Whipple disease with central nervous system involvement (both are discussed in Chap. 40). The factor common to all these disorders is the presence of diffuse neuronal disease and, as a group, they account for most of the instances of polymyoclonus observed by the neurologist.

Myoclonus in association with signs of cerebellar incoordination, including *opsoclonus* (rapid, irregular, but predominantly conjugate movements of the eyes in all planes), is another syndrome that has been described in both children and adults under a variety of names. Most cases run a chronic course, waxing and waning in severity. Many of the childhood cases have been associated with occult *neuroblastoma*, and some have responded to the administration of corticosteroids. In adults, a similar syndrome has been described as a remote effect of carcinoma (mainly of lung, breast, and ovary), but it also occurs at all ages as a relatively benign manifestation of a benign postinfectious (possibly viral) illness (Baringer et al). In some cases, myoclonus is associated only with cerebellar ataxia and tremor, opsoclonus being absent; in others, myoclonus, seizures, retinal degeneration, cerebellar tremor, and ataxia have been combined

Table 6-2
Causes of generalized and regional myoclonus

Epileptic forms (myoclonic epilepsies)
- *Unverricht-Lundborg disease*
- *Lafora body disease*
- *Baltic myoclonus*
- *Benign epilepsy with rolandic spikes*
- *Juvenile myoclonic epilepsy*
- *Infantile spasms (West syndrome)*
- *Cherry-red spot–myoclonus*
- *Mitochondrial myoclonic epilepsy (MERRF)*
- *Ceroid lipofuscinosis (Kuf disease)*
- *Tay-Sachs disease*

Essential and heredofamilial forms

Myoclonic dementias
- *Creutzfeldt-Jakob disease*
- *Subacute sclerosing panencephalitis*
- *Familial progressive poliodystrophy*
- *Alzheimer, Lewy-body, and Wilson diseases (occasional in late stages)*
- *Whipple disease of the central nervous system*
- *Corticobasal degeneration*
- *Dentoatorubropallidoluysian atrophy*
- *AIDS dementia*

Myoclonus with cerebellar disease (myoclonic ataxia)
- *Opsoclonus-myoclonus syndrome [Paraneoplastic (anti-Ri), neuroblastoma, post- and parainfectious]*
- *Postanoxic myoclonus (Lance Adams)*
- *Ramsay-Hunt dyssynergia cerebellaris myoclonica*

Metabolic and toxic disorders
- *Cerebral hypoxia (acute variety)*
- *Uremia*
- *Hashimoto thyroiditis*
- *Lithium intoxication*
- *Haloperidol and sometimes phenothiazine intoxication*
- *Hepatic encephalopathy (rare)*
- *Cyclosporine toxicity*
- *Nicotinic acid deficiency encephalopathy*
- *Tetanus*
- *Other drug toxicities*

Focal and spinal forms of myoclonus
- *Herpes zoster myelitis*
- *Other unspecified viral myelitis*
- *Multiple sclerosis*
- *Traumatic spinal cord injury*
- *Arteriovenous malformation of spinal cord*
- *Subacute myoclonic spinal neuronitis*

(dyssynergia cerebellaris myoclonica of Ramsay Hunt; see page 1150).

As mentioned above, diffuse myoclonus is a prominent feature of a unique transmissible subacute illness in adults, commonly referred to as *Creutzfeldt-Jakob* disease and characterized by dementia, disturbances of gait and coordination, and all manner of mental and visual aberrations. Originally the jerks are random in character, but late in the disease they may attain a certain rhythmicity and symmetry. In addition, there is an exaggerated startle response and violent myoclonus may be elicited by tactile, auditory, or visual stimuli in advanced stages of the disease. In this condition, too, there is a progressive destruction of nerve cells, mainly but not exclusively of the cerebral and cerebellar cortices, and a striking degree of gliosis. In addition to parenchymal destruction, the cortical tissue shows a fine-meshed vacuolation; hence the preferable designation *subacute spongiform encephalopathy*. Both the sporadic and rare familial forms of this disease are due to an unconventional transmissible agent, or prion (see also page 914).

In yet another group of "myoclonic dementias," the most prominent associated abnormality is a progressive deterioration of intellect. Like the myoclonic epilepsies, the myoclonic dementias may be sporadic or familial and may affect both children and adults. A rare childhood type is subacute sclerosing panencephalitis (SSPE), which is an acquired subacute or chronic (occasionally remitting) disease, related in some way to infection with the measles virus (page 810). Another type, familial in nature and affecting infants and young children, has been described by Ford, who called it *progressive poliodystrophy*. On a background of normal birth and development over the first few months or years of life, there occurs a progressive psychomotor deterioration, with spastic quadriplegia, seizures, myoclonus, and blindness. The fundamental pathologic alteration is a destruction of nerve cells in the cerebral and cerebellar cortices with replacement gliosis.

Intention, or Action, Myoclonus (Postanoxic) This type of myoclonus was described by Lance and Adams in 1963 in a group of patients who were recovering from hypoxic encephalopathy. When the patient is relaxed, the limb and other skeletal muscles are quiet (except in the most severe cases), and only seldom does the myoclonus appear during slow, smooth (ramp) movements. Fast (ballistic) movements, however, especially when directed to a target, as in touching the examiner's finger, elicit a series of irregular myoclonic jerks that differ in speed and rhythmicity from intention tremor. For this reason it was called *intention*, or *action*, *myoclonus*. Only the limb that is moving is involved; hence it is a localized, stimulus-evoked myoclonus. Speech may be affected; it is fragmented by the myoclonic jerks, and a syllable or word may be almost compulsively repeated, as in palilalia.

Action myoclonus is always associated with cerebellar ataxia. The pathologic anatomy has not been ascertained. Lance and Adams found the irregular discharges to be transmitted via the corticospinal tracts, preceded in some cases by a discharge from the motor cortex. Chadwick and coworkers postulated a reticular loop reflex mechanism. Hallett and colleagues found that a cortical reflex mechanism was operative in some cases and a reticular reflex mechanism in others. Whether these are two aspects of one mechanism could not be decided. Barbiturates and valproic acid have been helpful in some cases. Clonazepam is our preference in combination with valproate. Several clinical trials have suggested that the experimental drug piracetam may be useful.

Spinal, or Segmental, Myoclonus

The notion that monophasic restricted myoclonus emanates from the cerebellum or brainstem cannot be sustained, for there are forms that are traceable to a purely spinal lesion. A form that has been termed "propriospinal" involves repetitive flexion or extension myoclonus of the torso that is aggravated by stretching or action; it has been attributed, on the grounds of its electrophysiologic features, to a spinal origin.

A sharply demarcated segmental myoclonus has been induced in spinal animals by the Newcastle disease virus, and examples of myelitis with irregular segmental myoclonic jerks (either rhythmic or arrhythmic) have been reported in humans. In our experience, the phenomenon has usually occurred with zoster myelitis and rarely with multiple sclerosis or after spinal traumatic injury. A subacute spinal myoclonus of obscure origin was described many years ago by Campbell and Garland and similar cases continue to be cited in the literature. When highly ionic contrast media were used for myelography, painful spasms and myoclonus sometimes occurred in segments where the dye was concentrated by a block.

Pathophysiology of Myoclonus Multiplex

It seems logical to assume that myoclonus is caused by abnormal discharges of aggregates of motor neurons or interneurons because of the directly enhanced excitability of these cells or the removal of some inhibitory mechanism.

Sensory relationships are a prominent feature of myoclonus multiplex, particularly those related to metabolic disorders, and will eventually shed some light on the mechanism. Flickering light, a loud sound, or an unexpected tactile stimulus to some part of the body initiates a jerk so quickly and consistently that it must utilize a direct sensorimotor pathway or the mechanism involved in the startle reaction. Repeated stimuli may recruit a series of incremental myoclonic jerks that culminate in a generalized convulsion, as often happens in the familial myoclonic syndrome of Unverricht-Lundborg. Another type of sensory myoclonus is the audiogenic form, characteristic of Tay-Sachs disease. Each auditory stimulus results in blinking, abrupt elevation of the arms, and other movements. This generalized myoclonic jerk does not fatigue with successive stimuli and is modality-specific.

Evidence implicating cortical hyperexcitability in myoclonus is indirect, being based mainly on the finding that the cortical components of the somatosensory evoked potential are exceedingly large. In some such instances, the myoclonic jerks also have a strict time relationship ("time-locked") to preceding spikes in the contralateral rolandic area, indicating that the cerebral cortex may play an active and perhaps primary role in the elaboration of myoclonus (Marsden et al; Brown et al); however, it is just as likely that the cortical potentials are projected from subcortical structures. In humans, the indication is that postanoxic action myoclonus has its basis in reflex hyperactivity of the reticular formation and that the only consistent damage is in the cerebellum rather than in the cerebral cortex (see above, under "Intention, or Action, Myoclonus").

Pathologic examinations have been of little help in determining the essential sites of this unstable neuronal discharge because, in most cases, the neuronal disease is so diffuse. The most restricted lesions associated with myoclonus are seemingly located in the cerebellar cortex, dentate nuclei, and pretectal region. A lack of modulating influence of the cerebellum on the thalamocortical system of neurons has been postulated as a likely mechanism, but it is uncertain whether the disinhibited motor activity is then expressed through corticospinal or reticulospinal pathways. Pentylenetetrazol injections evoke myoclonus in the limbs of animals, and the myoclonus persists after transection of corticospinal and other descending tracts until the lower brainstem (medullary reticular) structures are destroyed.

PATHOLOGIC STARTLE SYNDROMES

To some degree, everyone startles or jumps in reaction to a totally unanticipated, potentially frightening stimulus. This is the normal startle reflex. It is probably a protective reaction, being seen also in animals, and its purpose seemingly is to prepare the organism for escape. By *pathologic startle* we refer to a greatly exaggerated startle reflex and to a group of other stimulus-induced disorders of which startle is a predominant part. In most ways, startle cannot be separated from myoclonus (simplex) except for its generalized nature and a striking evocation by various stimuli.

Aside from exaggerated forms of the normal startle reflex, the commonest startle syndrome is so-called startle disease, also referred to as *hyperexplexia* or *hyperekplexia* (Gastaut and Villeneuve). There is a familial proclivity to this disease (e.g., the "jumping Frenchmen of Maine," and others as described further on). The subject has been reviewed by Wilkins and colleagues and by Ryan et al; the latter authors, by linkage analysis, have localized the gene to chromosome 5q. The resulting biochemical change is now known to be in the α_1-subunit of the inhibitory glycine receptor (Shiang et al).

With the description of an increasing number of cases of startle disease, the special attributes of the condition have become more familiar. Any stimulus—most often an auditory one but also a flash of light, a tap on the neck, back, or nose, or even the presence of someone behind the patient—normally evinces a sudden contraction of the orbicularis, neck, and spinal musculature and even the legs on occasion. In the abnormal startle response, the contraction is more severe and widespread, with less tendency to habituate. There may be a jump and occasionally an involuntary shout and fall to the ground. As pointed out by Suhren and associates and by Kurczynski, the condition is transmitted in some families as an autosomal dominant trait. In the proband described by the latter author, affected infants were persistently hypertonic and hyperreflexic (up to 2 to 4 years of age) and had nocturnal and sometimes diurnal generalized myoclonic jerks, all of which subsided with maturation of the nervous system. Later in life, excessive startle must be distinguished from epileptic seizures, which may begin with a startle or massive myoclonic jerk (startle epilepsy) and from Gilles de la Tourette syndrome, of which startle may be a prominent manifestation. With startle disease, even with a fall, there is no loss of consciousness, and the manifestations of tic and other neurologic abnormalities are absent.

The auditory startle response may be a manifestation of other neurologic diseases. It is a prominent feature of Tay-Sachs disease (page 996) and of some cases of the "stiff-man syndrome" (page 1569). Auditory, visual, and somatic startle reactions are conspicuous features of some of the lipid storage diseases and Creutzfeldt-Jakob disease. During the startle, the EEG may show a vertex or frontal spike–slow wave complex, followed by a general desynchronization of the cortical rhythms; between startles the EEG is normal.

The mechanism of the startle disorder has been a matter of speculation. In animals, the anatomic substrate has been localized in the pontine reticular nuclei, with transmission to the lower brainstem and spinal motor neurons via the reticulospinal tracts. Some authors have postulated a disinhibition of certain brainstem centers. Others, on the basis of testing by somatosensory evoked potentials, have suggested that hyperactive long-loop reflexes constitute the physiologic basis of startle disease (Markand et al). Wilkins and coworkers consider hyperexplexia to be an independent phenomenon (different from the normal startle reflex) and to fall within the spectrum of stimulus-sensitive myoclonic disorders. Clonazepam controls the startle disorder to a varying degree. Sedative drugs relieve the rigidity in infants and the startle reaction to a lesser extent.

The relationship of hyperexplexia to the phenomenon displayed by the "jumping Frenchmen of Maine" is not altogether clear. The latter was described originally by James Beard, in 1868, among small pockets of socially backward, French-speaking lumberjacks in northern Maine. The subjects displayed a greatly excessive response to minimal stimuli, to which no adaptation was possible. The reaction consisted of jumping, raising the arms, screaming, and flailing of limbs, sometimes with echolalia, echopraxia, and a forced obedience to commands, even if this entailed a risk of serious injury. A similar syndrome in Malaysia and Indonesia is known as *latah* and in Siberia as *myriachit*. This syndrome has been explained in psychologic terms as operant-conditioned behavior (Saint-Hilaire et al) or as culturally determined behavior (Simons). Possibly the complex secondary phenomena can be explained in this way, but the stereotyped onset with an uncontrollable startle and the familial occurrence described earlier attest to a biologic basis akin to that of hyperexplexia.

SPASMODIC TORTICOLLIS AND OTHER FOCAL DYSTONIAS

These focal or segmental dystonias, in contrast to the generalized dystonic disorders described in Chap. 4, are intermittent, arrhythmic, brief or prolonged spasms or contractions of a muscle or adjacent group of muscles that places the body part in a forced and unnatural position. When limited to the neck muscles, the spasms may be more pronounced on one side, with rotation and partial extension of the head (*idiopathic cervical dystonia* or *torticollis*), or the posterior or anterior neck muscles may be involved predominantly and the head hyperextended (retrocollic spasm, *retrocollis*) or inclined forward (antero- or procollic spasm, *anterocollis*). Other dystonias restricted to craniocervical muscle groups are spasms of the orbicularis oculi, causing forced closure of the eyelids (*blepharospasm*); contraction of the muscles of the mouth and jaw, which may cause forceful opening or closure of the jaw and retraction or pursing of the lips (*oromandibular dystonia*). With the latter condition, the tongue may undergo forceful involuntary protrusion; the throat and neck muscles may be thrown into violent spasm when the patient attempts to speak or the facial muscles may contract in a grimace; and the laryngeal muscles may be involved, imparting a high-pitched, strained quality to the voice (*spasmodic dysphonia*). More often, spasmodic dysphonia occurs as an isolated phenomenon. Of the large number of focal dystonias seen in the movement disorder clinic of Columbia Presbyterian Hospital, 44 percent were classified as torticollis, 26 percent as spasmodic dysphonia, 14 percent as blepharospasm, 10 percent as focal dystonia of the right hand and arm (writer's cramp), and 3 percent as oromandibular dystonia.

These movement disorders are involuntary and cannot be inhibited, thereby differing from habit spasms or tics. For many years torticollis was thought to be a type of neurosis, but all neurologists now agree that it is a localized form of dystonia. As discussed in Chap. 4, it is characteristic of these spasms and similar focal dystonias that occur in the hands or feet to display a simultaneous activation of agonist and antagonist muscles (cocontraction), a tendency for the spasm to spread to adjacent muscle groups that are not normally activated in the movement (overflow), and an arrhythmic intermixed tremor; but these features tend not to be as prominent in focal dystonias as in the generalized varieties (described in Chap. 4).

Any of the typical forms of restricted dystonia may represent a tardive dyskinesia; i.e., they complicate treatment with neuroleptic drugs (see pages 1264 and 1637). The most common of these is combined with a more or less constant movement of the tongue and lips, which may include lip smacking, tongue protrusion, and similar unnatural movements. Also, restricted dystonias of the hand or foot often emerge as components of a number of degenerative diseases—Parkinson disease, corticobasal ganglionic degeneration, and progressive supranuclear palsy (all described in Chap. 39). These dystonias may also occur in metabolic diseases such as Wilson disease and nonwilsonian hepatolenticular degeneration. Rarely, a dystonia emerges transiently after a stroke that involves the striatopallidal system or the thalamus, but the varied locations of these infarctions makes it difficult to draw conclusions about the mechanism of dystonia. Several such cases are described by Krystkowiak and colleagues and all fall into the category of *symptomatic or secondary dystonias*. The ones due to acquired systemic disorders are summarized by Janavs and Aminoff.

The pathogenesis of the idiopathic (primary) focal dystonias is uncertain, although there is evidence that a large proportion are genetically determined. Authoritative commentators including Marsden have classed the adult-onset focal dystonias with the broader category of idiopathic torsion dystonia. This view is based on the recognition of each of the focal dystonias as an early component of the idiopathic syndrome in children, the occurrence of focal and segmental dystonias in family members of these children, as well as a tendency of the dystonia in some adult patients to spread to other body parts. There are families in which the only manifestation of the DYT1 mutation (the gene abnormality associated with dystonia musculorum deformans) is a late-onset writer's cramp, described further on. The genetics of torsion dystonia has been reviewed by Korf.

It is noteworthy that no consistent pathologic changes have been demonstrated in any of the idiopathic and genetically determined dystonias. Most physiologists cast the disorder in terms of reduced cortical inhibition of unwanted muscle contractions, as summarized in the review by Berardelli and colleagues. Specific changes in the cortical areas that are pertinent to the dystonias associated with overuse of certain body parts (craft and occupational dystonias) are described below.

Spasmodic Torticollis (Idiopathic Cervical Dystonia)

This is the most frequent form of restricted dystonia, localized to the neck muscles (see also page 1144). It usually begins in early to middle adult life (peak incidence in the fifth decade) and tends to worsen slowly. A condition of unknown cause, almost always sporadic, it is somewhat more common in women. The quality of the neck and head movements varies; they may be deliberate and smooth or jerky or cause a persistent deviation of the head to one side. Sometimes brief bursts of myoclonic twitching or a slightly irregular, high-frequency kinetic tremor accompanies deviation of the head, possibly representing an effort to overcome the contraction of the neck muscles. The tremor tends to beat in the direction of the dystonic movement, which has been termed a directional "vector." The spasms are worse when the patient stands or walks and are characteristically reduced or abolished by a contactual stimulus, such as placing a hand on the chin or neck or exerting mild but steady counterpressure on the side of the deviation or sometimes on the opposite side, or bringing the occiput in contact with the back of a high chair. These maneuvers become less effective as the disease progresses. In the majority of cases, the spasms cease when the patient lies down. In chronic cases, the affected muscles may undergo hypertrophy. Pain in the contracting muscles is a common complaint, especially if there is associated cervical arthropathy. Although the most prominently affected muscles are the sternomastoid and trapezius, EMG studies also show sustained or intermittent activity in the posterior cervical muscles on both sides of the neck. In most patients the spasms remain confined to the neck muscles and persist in unmodified form, but in some the muscle spasms spread beyond the neck, involving muscles of the shoulder girdle and back or the face and limbs. The distinction between these two forms is not fundamental. About 15 percent of patients with torticollis also have oral, mandibular, or hand dystonia, 10 percent have blepharospasm, and a similarly small number have a family history of dystonia or tremor (Chan et al). No neuropathologic changes were found in the single case studies reported by Tarlov and by Zweig and colleagues.

Spasmodic torticollis is resistant to treatment with L-dopa and other antiparkinsonian agents, although occasionally they give slight relief. In a few of our patients (four or five of several hundred), the condition disappeared without therapy, an occurrence observed in 10 to 20 percent in the series of Dauer et al. In their experience, remissions usually occurred during the first few years after onset in patients whose disease began relatively early in life; however, nearly all these patients relapsed within 5 years.

The periodic (every 3 to 4 months) injection of minute amounts of botulinum toxin type A directly into several sites in the affected muscles is by far the most effective form of treatment. The injections are best guided by clinical and EMG analysis to determine which tonically contracted muscles are most responsible for the aberrant postures. All but 10 percent of patients with torticollis have had some degree of relief from symptoms with this treatment. Adverse effects (excessive weakness of injected muscles, local pain and dysphagia—the latter from a systemic effect of the toxin) are usually mild and transitory. Five to 10 percent of patients become resistant to repeated injections because of the development of neutralizing antibodies to the toxin (see Brin; Dauer et al).

In the most severe cases and those refractory to treatment with botulinum toxin, a combined sectioning of the spinal accessory nerve (of the more affected sternomastoid) and of the first three cervical motor roots bilaterally has been successful in reducing spasm of the muscles without totally paralyzing them. Considerable relief has been achieved for as long as 6 years in one-third to one-half of cases treated in this way (Krauss et al, Ford et al). Bilateral thalamotomy has also been tried, but since it is less effective and carries a considerable risk, particularly to speech and swallowing, it should be reserved for the most severely affected patients with more widespread dystonia. These surgical procedures are rarely necessary now that botulinum toxin treatment has been refined.

Blepharospasm

From time to time, patients in late adult life, predominantly women, present with the complaint of inability to keep their eyes open. Any attempt to look at a person or object is associated with a persistent tonic spasm of the eyelids. During conversation, the patient struggles to overcome the spasms and is distracted by them. All customary activities are hampered to a varying extent. Reading and watching television are impossible at some times but surprisingly easy at other. Jankovic and Orman, in a survey of 250 such patients, found that the condition of 75 percent progressed in severity over the years to the point, in about 15 percent of cases, where the patients were, in effect, legally blind.

One's first inclination is to think of this disorder as photophobia, and indeed the patient may state that bright light is annoying (ocular inflammation, especially of the iris, may produce severe blepharospasm). However, the spasms persist in dim light and even after anesthesia of the corneas. Extraocular movements are quite normal. Blepharospasm may occur as an isolated phenomenon, but just as often it is combined with oromandibular spasms (see below) and sometimes with spasmodic dysphonia, torticollis, and other dystonic fragments. Again, it has been postulated that these various focal dystonias have a psychiatric basis, but with the exception of a depressive reaction in some patients, psychiatric symptoms are lacking and the use of psychotherapy, acupuncture, behavioral modification therapy, hypnosis, etc., has generally failed to cure the spasms. Again, no neuropathologic lesion or uniform pharmacologic profile has been established in any of these disorders (Marsden et al; see also Hallett).

In the treatment of blepharospasm, a variety of antiparkinsonian, anticholinergic, and tranquilizing medications may be tried, but one should not be sanguine about the chances of success. A very few of our patients have had temporary and partial relief from L-dopa. Sometimes the blepharospasm disappears spontaneously (in 13 percent of the cases in the series of Jancovic and Orman). The most effective treatment consists of the injection of botulinum toxin into several sites in the orbicularis oculi and adjacent facial muscles. The benefit lasts for 3 to 5 months and several cycles of treatment are usually required. There appear to be no adverse systemic effects. Thermolytic destruction of part of the fibers in the branches of the facial nerves that innervate the orbicularis oculi muscles is reserved for the most resistant and disabling cases.

Other Causes of Blepharospasm There are several clinical settings other than the one described above in which blepharospasm may be observed. In the days following cerebral infarction or hemorrhage, the stimulus of lifting the patient's eyelids may lead to strong involuntary closure of the lids. *Reflex blepharospasm*, as Fisher has called this phenomenon, is more commonly associated with a left than a right hemiplegia and is more prominent on the nonparalyzed side. A homolateral blepharospasm has also been observed with a small thalamomesencephalic infarct. In patients with Parkinson disease, progressive supranuclear palsy, or Wilson disease, and with other lesions in the rostral brainstem, light closure of the eyelids may induce blepharospasm and an inability to open the eyelids voluntarily.

We have seen an instance of blepharospasm as part of a paraneoplastic midbrain encephalitis, and there have been several reports of it with autoimmune disease such as systemic lupus and myasthenia gravis, but the mechanism in these cases is as obscure as for the ideopathic variety.

Lingual, Facial, and Oromandibular Spasms

These special varieties of involuntary movements also appear in later adult life, with a peak age of onset in the sixth decade. Women are affected more frequently than men. The most common type is characterized by forceful opening of the jaw, retraction of the lips, spasm of the platysma, and protrusion of the tongue; or the jaw may be clamped shut and the lips may purse. Other patterns include lateral jaw deviation and bruxism. Common terms for this condition are the *Meige syndrome*, after the French neurologist who gave an early description of it, and the *Brueghel syndrome*, because of the similarity of the grotesque grimace to that of a subject in a Brueghel painting called *De Gaper*. Difficulty in speaking and swallowing (spastic or spasmodic dysphonia) and blepharospasm are frequently conjoined, and occasionally patients with these disorders develop torticollis or dystonia of the trunk and limbs. A number have tremor of affected muscles or of the hands as well. All these prolonged, forceful spasms of facial, tongue, and neck muscles have resulted from the administration of phenothiazine and butyrophenone drugs. More often, however, the disorder induced by neuroleptics is different, consisting of choreoathetotic chewing, lip smacking, and licking movements (tardive orofacial dyskinesia; see pages 1264 and 1637).

Very few cases of the Meige syndrome have been studied neuropathologically. In some of them no lesions were found. In one case there were foci of neuronal loss in the striatum (Altrocchi and Forno); another case showed a loss of nerve cells and the presence of Lewy bodies in the substantia nigra and related nuclei (Kulisevsky et al).

Many drugs have been used in the treatment of these craniocervical spasms, but none has effected a cure. Much greater success has been obtained with injections of botulinum toxin into the masseter, temporal, and internal pterygoid muscles. This is true also for spasmodic dysphonia (page 519), which responds favorably to injections of the toxin into the thyroaretynoid vocalis muscles.

A form of focal dystonia that affects only the jaw muscles has been described (*masticatory spasm* of Romberg); a similar dystonia may be a component of orofacial and generalized dystonias. In the cases described by Thompson and colleagues, the problem began with brief periods of spasm of the pterygoid or masseter muscle on one side. Early on, the differential diagnosis includes bruxism, hemifacial spasm, and tetanus. As the illness progresses, forced opening of the mouth and lateral deviation of the jaw may last for days and adventitious lingual movements may be added. A form that occurs with hemifacial atrophy has been described by Kaufman. High doses of benztropine may be helpful, but local botulinum toxin injection is probably the best alternative. A spasm that is confined to one side of the face (hemifacial spasm) is not, strictly speaking, a dystonia and is considered with disorders of the facial nerve on page 1455.

Writer's Cramp, Musician's Spasm, and Other Craft (Occupational) Dystonias

The so-called craft or occupational cramps or spasms should be mentioned here, since the prevailing opinion is that they are restricted or focal "task-specific" dystonias. Men and women are equally affected, most often between the ages of 20 and 50 years. In the commonest form, *writer's cramp*, the patient observes, upon attempting to write, that all the muscles of thumb and fingers either go into spasm or are inhibited by a feeling of stiffness and pain or hampered in some other inexplicable way. The spasm may be painful and spread into the forearm or even the upper arm and shoulder. Sometimes the spasm fragments into a tremor that interferes with the execution of fluid, cursive movements. Immediately upon cessation of writing, the spasm disappears. Although the disturbance in writer's cramp is usually limited to the specific act of writing, it may involve other equally demanding manual tasks. At all other times and in the execution of grosser movements, the hand is normal, and there are no other neurologic abnormalities. Many patients learn to write in new ways or to use the other hand, though that, too, may become involved. A few of our younger patients have developed spasmodic torticollis at a later date.

The performance of other highly skilled motor acts, such as playing the piano or fingering the violin, may be similarly affected. The "loss of lip" in trombonists and other instrumentalists may represent an analogous phenomenon, seen only in experienced musicians. In each case a delicate motor skill, perfected by years of practice and performed almost automatically, suddenly comes to require a conscious and labored effort for its execution. Discrete movements are impaired by a spreading innervation of unneeded muscles (intention spasm), a feature common to athetotic states.

The nature of these disorders is quite obscure. They have been classed traditionally as "occupational neuroses," and a psychiatric causation has been suggested repeatedly, but careful clinical analysis has not borne this out. Once developed, the disability persists in varying degrees of severity, even after long periods of inactivity of the affected part.

In monkeys, Byl and colleagues found that sustained, rapid, and repetitive highly stereotypical movements greatly expanded and degraded the cortical representation of sensory information from the hand. These authors hypothesized that degradation of sensory feedback to the motor cortex was responsible for excessive and persistent motor activity, including dystonia. Such a change in cortical responses to magnetic stimulation has also been found by a number of investigators in patients with writer's cramp. Other theories pertaining to the physiology of the focal dystonias have been reviewed by Berardelli et al.

A high degree of therapeutic success has reportedly been obtained by injections of botulinum toxin into specifically involved muscles of the hand and forearm (Cohen et al, Rivest et al) and this is now the most widely used form of therapy. It has been claimed that the patient can be helped by a deconditioning procedure that delivers an electric shock whenever the spasm occurs or by biofeedback, but these forms of treatment have not been rigorously tested.

TICS AND HABIT SPASMS

Many persons throughout their lives are given to habitual movements. They range from simple, highly personalized, idiosyncratic mannerisms (e.g., of the lips and tongue) to repetitive actions such as sniffing, clearing the throat, protruding the chin, or blinking whenever these individuals become tense. Stereotypy and irresistibility are the main identifying features of these phenomena. The patient admits to making the movements and feels compelled to do so in order to relieve perceived tension. Such movements can be suppressed for a short time by an effort of will, but they reappear as soon as the subject's attention is diverted. In certain cases the tics become so ingrained that the person is unaware of them and seems unable to control them. An interesting feature of many tics is that they correspond to purposive, coordinated acts that normally serve the organism. It is only their incessant repetition when uncalled for that marks them as habit spasms or tics. The condition varies widely in its expression from a single isolated movement (e.g., blinking, sniffing, throat clearing, or stretching the neck) to a complex of movements.

Children between 5 and 10 years of age are especially likely to develop habit spasms. These consist of blinking, hitching up one shoulder, sniffing, throat clearing, jerking the head or eyes to one side, grimacing, etc. If ignored, such spasms seldom persist for longer than a few weeks; providing more rest and a calmer environment may be helpful. In adults, relief of nervous tension by sedative or tranquilizing drugs and psychotherapy may be helpful, but the disposition to tics persists. A putative relationship to streptococcal infection is mentioned below.

When idle, adults often display a wide variety of fidgeting types of movement, gestures, and mannerisms that vary in degree from one person to another. Lay persons refer to them as "bad habits." Special types of rocking, head bobbing, and other movements, particularly self-stimulating movements, are disorders of motility unique to the mentally retarded. These "rhythmias" have no known pathologic anatomy in the basal ganglia or elsewhere in the brain. Apparently they represent a persistence of some of the rhythmic, repetitive movements (head banging, etc.) of normal infants. In some cases of impaired vision and photic epilepsy, eye rubbing or moving the fingers rhythmically across the field of vision is observed, especially in mentally retarded children.

Gilles de la Tourette Syndrome

Multiple tics—associated with sniffing, snorting, involuntary vocalization, and troublesome compulsive and aggressive impulses—constitute the rarest and most severe tic syndrome. The Tourette syndrome begins in childhood, usually as a simple tic; as the condition progresses, new tics are added to the repertoire. It is the multiplicity of tics and the combination of motor and vocal tics that distinguish the Tourette syndrome from the more benign, restricted tic disorders.

Vocal tics, usually loud and irritating in pitch, are characteristic. Some patients display repetitive and annoying motor behavior, such as jumping, squatting, or turning in a circle. Other common types of repetitive behavior include the touching of other persons and repeating one's own words (palilalia) and the words or movements of others. Explosive and involuntary cursing and the compulsive utterance of obscenities (coprolalia) are the most dramatic manifestations. Interestingly, the latter phenomena are uncommon in Japanese patients, whose decorous culture and language contain few obscenities. The full repertoire of tics and compulsions comprised by the Tourette syndrome has been described by Tolosa and Jankovic.

Stone and Jankovic have noted the occurrence of persistent blepharospasm, torticollis, and other dystonic fragments in a small number of patients with Tourette syndrome. Feinberg and associates have described four patients with arrhythmic myoclonus and vocalization, but it is not clear whether these symptoms represent an unusual variant of Tourette disease or a new syndrome. So-called soft neurologic signs are noted in half of the patients, and hyperactivity and disorders of attention and perception are frequent. Evidence of "organic" impairment by psychologic tests was found in 40 to 60 percent of Shapiro's series; however, intelligence does not deteriorate. Nonspecific abnormalities of the EEG occur in more than half of the patients.

In one-third of the cases reported by Shapiro and colleagues, tics were observed in other members of the family. Several other studies have reported a familial clustering of cases in which the pattern of transmission appears to be autosomal dominant with incomplete penetrance (Pauls and Leckman). Support for the primary genetic nature of Tourette syndrome derives also from twin studies, which have revealed higher concordance rates in monozygotic twin pairs than in dizygotic pairs. An ethnic bias (Ashkenzai Jews) has been reported, ranging from 19 to 62 percent in several series, but this has not been borne out in equally large series outside of New York (Lees et al).

As to causation, little is known. The disease, if it is such, is unrelated to social class or to psychiatric illness; there is no consistent association with infection, trauma, or other disease. Hyperactive children who have been treated with stimulants appear to be at increased risk of developing or exacerbating tics (Price et al), but a causal relationship has not been established beyond doubt. Reports of a relationship to obsessive-compulsive neurosis have also been inconsistent. MRI and CT and positron emission tomography (PET) have shown no uniform abnormalities, and histopathologic changes have not been discerned in the few brains examined by the usual methods. However, Singer and coworkers, who analyzed pre- and postsynaptic dopamine markers in postmortem striatal tissue, found a significant alteration of dopamine uptake mechanisms; more recently, Wolf et al have found that differences in D_2 dopamine receptor binding in the head of the caudate nucleus predicted differences in the phenotypic severity of Tourette syndrome. These observations, coupled with the facts that L-dopa exacerbates the symptoms of Tourette syndrome and that the highly effective therapeutic agent haloperidol blocks dopamine (particularly D_2) receptors, support the notion of a dopaminergic abnormality in the basal ganglia, more specifically in the caudate nucleus. In this latter respect, reported instances of compulsive behavior in relation to lesions in the head of the caudate nucleus and its projections from orbitofrontal and cingulate cortices may be pertinent.

Using the model of Sydenham chorea, a recent line of investigation has implicated streptococcal infection in the genesis of abruptly appearing Tourette syndrome and of less generalized tics in children. This association has also been adopted by some authors to explain obsessive-compulsive behavior of sudden and unexplained onset. These putative disorders have been summarized by Swedo and colleagues under the acronym PANDAS (pediatric autoimmune neuropsychiatric disorders with streptococcal infection). In a few cases there has been a relapsing course that is similar to some Sydenham cases. This information is intriguing but not confirmed.

The course of the illness is unpredictable. In some adolescents it subsides spontaneously and permanently or undergoes long remissions, but in other patients it persists throughout life. This variability emphasizes the difficulty in separating transient habit spasms from the Tourette chronic multiple tic syndrome. Haloperidol has proved to be an effective therapeutic agent, but it should be used only in severely affected patients and in small doses (0.25 mg initially, increasing the dosage gradually to 2 to 10 mg daily). The addition of benztropine mesylate (0.5 mg daily) at the outset of treatment may help to prevent the adverse effects of haloperidol. Patients who do not respond to haloperidol may respond to the neuroleptic pimozide, which has a more specific antidopaminergic action than haloperidol. Pimozide should be given in small amounts (0.5 mg daily) to begin with and increased gradually to 8 to 9 mg daily. The antispasticity agent tetrabenazine may also be useful if high doses can be tolerated. Kurlan and associates have noted a lessening of tics after treatment with naltrexone, 50 mg daily.

Akathisia

The term *akathisia* was coined by Haskovec in 1904 to describe an inner feeling of restlessness, an inability to sit still, and a compulsion to move about. When sitting, the patient constantly shifts his body and legs, crosses and uncrosses his legs, and swings the free leg. Running in place and persistent pacing are also characteristic. This abnormality of movement is most prominent in the lower extremities and may not be accompanied, at least in mild forms of akathisia, by perceptible rigidity or other neurologic abnormalities. In its advanced form, patients complain of difficulty in concentration, distracted no doubt by the constant movement.

First noted in patients with Parkinson disease and senile dementia, akathisia is now observed most often in patients receiving neuroleptic drugs (page 1132). However, this disorder may be observed in psychiatric patients who are receiving no medication and in some patients with Parkinson disease; it can also be induced in normal individuals by the administration of neuroleptic drugs or L-dopa.

The main diagnostic considerations are an agitated depression, particularly in patients already on neuroleptic medications, and the "restless legs" syndrome of Ekbom (page 412). Patients with the latter affliction describe a crawling sensation in the legs rather than an inner restlessness, although both disorders create an irresistible desire for movement. At times these distinctions are blurred and treatment must be empiric. Many of the medications utilized for the restless legs syndrome, such as propoxyphene or clonazepam, may be tried, or treatment can be directed to the akathisia by selecting a less potent neuroleptic (if it is the suspected cause), or by using an anticholinergic medication, amantadine, or—perhaps the most effective and best tolerated—beta-adrenergic blocking drugs.

REFERENCES

Adams RD, Foley JM: The neurological disorder associated with liver disease. *Res Publ Assoc Nerv Ment Dis* 32:198, 1953.

Adams RD, Shahani B, Young RR: Tremor in association with polyneuropathy. *Trans Am Neurol Assoc* 97:44,1972.

Aigner BR, Mulder DW: Myoclonus: Clinical significance and an approach to classification. *Arch Neurol* 2:600, 1960.

Altrocchi PH, Forno LS: Spontaneous oral-facial dyskinesia: Neuropathology of a case. *Neurology* 33:802, 1983.

Bain PG, Findley LJ, Thompson PD, et al: A study of hereditary essential tremor. *Brain* 117:805, 1994.

Baringer JR, Sweeney VP, Winkler GF: An acute syndrome of ocular oscillations and truncal myoclonus. *Brain* 91:473, 1968.

Berardelli A, Rothwell JC, Hallett M, et al: The pathophysiology of primary dystonia. *Brain* 121:1195, 1998.

Biary N, Koller W: Kinetic-predominant essential tremor: Successful treatment with clonazepam. *Neurology* 37:471, 1987.

Brin MF: Botulinum toxin. *Neurosci Forum* 4:1, 1994.

Brown P, Ridding MC, Werhaus KJ, et al. Abnormalities of the balance between inhibition and excitation in the motor cortex of patients with cortical myoclonus. *Brain* 119:309, 1996.

Burns RS, LeWitt PA, Ebert MH, et al: The classical syndrome of striatal dopamine deficiency: Parkinsonism induced by MPTP. *N Engl J Med* 312:1418, 1985.

Byl NN, Merzenich MM, Jenkins WM: A primate genesis model of focal dystonia and repetitive strain injury: I. Learning-induced differentiation of the representation of the hand in the primary somatosensory cortex in adult monkey. *Neurology* 47:508, 1996.

Campbell AMG, Garland H: Subacute myoclonic spinal neuronitis. *J Neurol Neurosurg Psychiatry* 19:268, 1956.

Carpenter MB: Functional relationships between the red nucleus and the brachium conjunctivum: Physiologic study of lesions of the red nucleus in monkeys with degenerated superior cerebellar brachia. *Neurology* 7:427, 1957.

Chadwick D, Hallett M, Harris R, et al: Clinical, biochemical, and physiological features distinguishing myoclonus responsive to 5-hydroxy-tryptophan, tryptophan with a monoamine oxidase inhibitor, and clonazepam. *Brain* 100:455, 1977.

Chan J, Brin MF, Fahn S: Idiopathic cervical dystonia: Clinical characteristics. *Mov Disord* 6:119, 1991.

Cohen LG, Hallett M, Geller BD, Hochberg F: Treatment of focal dystonias of the hand with botulinum toxin injections. *J Neurol Neurosurg Psychiatry* 52:355, 1989.

Colebatch JG, Findley LJ, Frakowiak RSJ, et al: Preliminary report: Activation of the cerebellum in essential tremor. *Lancet* 336:1028, 1990.

Dauer WT, Burke RE, Greene P, Fahn S: Current concepts on the clinical features, aetiology, and management of idiopathic cervical dystonia. *Brain* 121:547, 1998.

Dubinsky R, Hallett M: Glucose hypermetabolism of the inferior olive in patients with essential tremor. *Ann Neurol* 22:118, 1987.

Elble RJ: Origins of tremor. *Lancet* 355:1113, 2000.

Eldridge R, Iivanainen M, Stern R, et al: "Baltic" myoclonus epilepsy: Hereditary disorders of childhood made worse by phenytoin. *Lancet* 2:838, 1983.

Feinberg TE, Shapiro AK, Shapiro E: Paroxysmal myoclonic dystonia with vocalisations: New entity or variant of pre-existing syndromes? *J Neurol Neurosurg Psychiatry* 49:52, 1986.

Fisher CM: Reflex blepharospasm. *Neurology* 13:77, 1963.

Ford FR: Degeneration of the cerebral gray matter, in *Diseases of the Nervous System in Infancy, Childhood and Adolescence*, 6th ed. Springfield, IL, Charles C Thomas, 1973, p 305.

Ford B, Louis ED, Greene P, Fahn S: Outcome of selective ramisectomy for botulinum toxin resistant torticollis. *J Neurol Neurosurg Psychiatry* 65:472, 1998.

Gastaut R, Villeneuve A: A startle disease or hyperekplexia. *J Neurol Sci* 5:523, 1967.

Haerer AF, Anderson DW, Schoenberg BS: Prevalence of essential tremor. *Arch Neurol* 39:750, 1982.

Hallett M: Blepharospasm: Report of a workshop. *Neurology* 46:1213, 1996.

Hallett M, Chadwick P, Marsden CD: Ballistic movement overflow myoclonus: A form of essential myoclonus. *Brain* 100:299, 1977.

Hallett M, Chadwick D, Marsden CD: Cortical reflex myoclonus. *Neurology* 29:1107, 1979.

Hallett M, Chadwick D, Adams J, et al: Reticular reflex myoclonus: A physiological type of human post-hypoxic myoclonus. *J Neurol Neurosurg Psychiatry* 40:253, 1977.

Hallett M, Dubinsky RM: Glucose metabolism in the brain of patients with essential tremor. *J Neurol Sci* 113:45, 1993.

Heilman KH: Orthostatic tremor. *Arch Neurol* 41:880, 1984.

Herskovits E, Blackwood W: Essential (familial, hereditary) tremor: A case report. *J Neurol Neurosurg Psychiatry* 32:509, 1969.

Hunt JR: Dyssynergia cerebellaris myoclonica—Primary atrophy of the dentate system: A contribution to the pathology and symptomatology of the cerebellum. *Brain* 44:490, 1921.

Janavs JL, Aminoff MJ: Dystonia and chorea in acquired systemic disorders. *J Neurol Neurosurg Psychiatry* 65:436, 1998.

Jankovic J, Brin MF: Therapeutic uses of botulinum toxin. *N Engl J Med* 324:1186, 1991.

Jankovic J, Orman J: Blepharospasm: Demographic and clinical survey of 250 patients. *Ann Ophthalmol* 16:371, 1984.

Kane SA, Thach WT Jr: Palatal myoclonus and function of the inferior olive: Are they related? in Strata P (ed): *Olivocerebellar System in Motor Control*. Published by *Exp Brain Res*, suppl 11, Berlin, Springer-Verlag, 1988.

Kaufman MD: Masticatory spasm in hemifacial atrophy. *Ann Neurol* 7:585, 1980.

Koller WC, Busenbark KL: Essential tremor, in Watts RL, Koller WC (eds): *Movement Disorders*. New York, McGraw-Hill, 1997, pp 365–385.

Koller W, O'Hara R, Dorus W, Bauer J: Tremor in chronic alcoholism. *Neurology* 35:1660, 1985.

Korf BR: The hereditary dystonias: An emerging story with a twist. *Ann Neurol* 44:4, 1998.

Krauss JK, Toups EG, Jankovic J, Grossman RG: Symptomatic and functional outcome of surgical treatment of cervical dystonia. *J Neurol Neurosurg Psychiatry* 63:642, 1997.

Krystkowiak P, Martinat P, Defebvre L, et al: Dystonia after striatopallidal and thalamic stroke: Clinicoradiological correlations and pathophysiological mechanisms. *J Neurol Neurosurg Psychiatry* 665:703, 1998.

Kulisevsky J, Marti MJ, Ferrer I, Tolosa E: Meige syndrome: Neuropathology of a case. *Mov Disord* 3:170, 1988.

Kurczynski TW: Hyperexplexia. *Arch Neurol* 40:246, 1983.

Kurlan R, Majumdar L, Deeley C, et al: A controlled trial of propoxyphene and naltrexone in patients with Tourette's syndrome. *Ann Neurol* 30:19, 1991.

Lance JW, Adams RD: The syndrome of intention or action myoclonus as a sequel to hypoxic encephalopathy. *Brain* 87:111, 1963.

Lapresle J, Ben Hamida M: The dentato-olivary pathway. *Arch Neurol* 22:135, 1970.

Lees AS, Robertson M, Trimble MR, Murray HMF: A clinical study of Gilles de la Tourette syndrome in the United Kingdom. *J Neurol Neurosurg Psychiatry* 47:1, 1984.

LeFebvre-D'Amour M, Shahani BT, Young RR: Tremor in alcoholic patients, in Desmedt JE (ed): *Physiological Tremor and Clonus*. Basel, Karger, 1978, pp 160–164.

Markand ON, Garg BP, Weaver DD: Familial startle disease (hyperexplexia). *Arch Neurol* 41:71, 1984.

Marsden CD: Blepharospasm-oromandibular dystonia syndrome (Brueghel's syndrome). *J Neurol Neurosurg Psychiatry* 39:1204, 1976.

Marsden CD: The problem of adult-onset idiopathic torsion dystonia and other isolated dyskinesias in adult life (including blepharospasm, oromandibular dystonia, dystonic writers cramp, and torticollis, or axial dystonia). *Adv Neurol* 14:259, 1976.

Marsden CD, Hallett M, Fahn S: The nosology and pathophysiology of myoclonus, in Marsden CD, Fahn S (eds): *Movement Disorders*. London, Butterworth, 1982, pp 196–248.

MATSUO F, AJAX ET: Palatal myoclonus and denervation super-sensitivity in the central nervous system. *Ann Neurol* 5:72, 1979.

MOE PG, NELLHAUS G: Infantile polymyoclonia—opsoclonus syndrome and neural crest tumors. *Neurology* 20:756, 1970.

MONTALBAN RJ, PUJEDAS F, ALVAREZ-SABIB J, et al: Asterixis associated with anatomic cerebral lesions: A study of 45 cases. *Acta Neurol Scand* 91:377, 1995.

NARABAYASHI H: Surgical approach to tremor, in Marsden CD, Fahn S (eds): *Movement Disorders*. London, Butterworth, 1982, pp 292–299.

PAULS DL, LECKMAN JF: The inheritance of Gilles de la Tourette's syndrome and associated behaviors: Evidence for autosomal dominant transmission. *N Engl J Med* 315:993, 1986.

PRICE RA, LECKMAN JF, PAULS DL, et al: Gilles de la Tourette's syndrome: Tics and central nervous stimulants in twins and nontwins. *Neurology* 36:232, 1986.

RAPIN I, GOLDFISCHER S, KATZMAN R, et al: The cherry-red spot–myoclonus syndrome. *Ann Neurol* 3:234, 1978.

RIVEST J, LEES AJ, MARSDEN CD: Writer's cramp: Treatment with botulinum toxin injections. *Mov Disord* 6:55, 1990.

RYAN SG, SHERMAN SL, TERRY JC, et al: Startle disease, or hyperekplexia: Response to clonazepam and assignment of the gene (STHE) to chromosome 5q by linkage analysis. *Ann Neurol* 31:663, 1992.

SAINT-HILAIRE M-H, SAINT-HILAIRE J-M, GRANGER L: Jumping Frenchmen of Maine. *Neurology* 36:1269, 1986.

SHAPIRO AK, SHAPIRO ES, BRUUN RD, et al: Gilles de la Tourette's syndrome: Summary of clinical experience with 250 patients and suggested nomenclature for tic syndromes, in Eldridge R, Fahn S (eds): *Advances in Neurology*. Vol 14: *Dystonia*. New York, Raven Press, 1976, pp 277–283.

SHEEHY MP, MARSDEN CD: Writer's cramp—A focal dystonia. *Brain* 105:461, 1982.

SHIANG R, RYAN SG, ZHU Z, et al: Mutations in the α_1-subunit of the inhibitory glycine receptor causes the dominant neurologic disorder, hyperexplexia. *Nature Genet* 5:351, 1993.

SIMONS RC: The resolution of the Latah paradox. *J Nerv Ment Dis* 168:195, 1980.

SINGER HS, HAHN I-H, MORAN TH: Abnormal dopamine uptake sites in postmortem striatum from patients with Tourette's syndrome. *Ann Neurol* 30:558, 1991.

STONE LA, JANKOVIC J: The coexistence of tics and dystonia. *Arch Neurol* 48:862, 1991.

SUHREN D, BRUYN GW, TUYMAN JA: Hyperexplexia, a hereditary startle syndrome. *J Neurol Sci* 3:577, 1966.

SUTTON GG, MAYER RF: Focal reflex myoclonus. *J Neurol Neurosurg Psychiatry* 37:207, 1974.

SWANSON PD, LUTTRELL CN, MAGLADERY JW: Myoclonus: A report of 67 cases and review of the literature. *Medicine* 41:339, 1962.

SWEDO SE, RAPPAPORT JL, CHESLOW DL, et al: High prevalence of obsessive-compulsive symptoms in patients with Sydenham chorea. *Am J Psychiatry* 146:246, 1989.

TARLOV E: On the problem of spasmodic torticollis in man. *J Neurol Neurosurg Psychiatry* 33:457, 1970.

THOMPSON PD, OBESO JA, DELGADO G, et al: Focal dystonia of the jaw and the differential diagnosis of unilateral jaw and masticatory spasm. *J Neurol Neurosurg Psychiatry* 49:651, 1986.

THOMPSON PD, ROTHWELL JC, DAY BL, et al: The physiology of orthostatic tremor. *Arch Neurol* 43:584, 1986.

TOLOSA ES, JANKOVIC J: Tics and Tourette's syndrome, in Jankovic J, Tolosa ES (eds): *Parkinson's Disease and Movement Disorders*, 3rd ed. Baltimore, Lippincott Williams & Wilkins, 1998, pp 491–512.

UGAWA Y, GENBA K, SHIMPO T, MANNEN T: Onset and offset of electromyographic (EMG) silence in asterixis. *J Neurol Neurosurg Psychiatry* 53:260, 1990.

WALTERS AS, HENING WA, CHOKROVERTY S: Frequent occurrence of myoclonus while awake and at rest, body rocking and marching in place in a subpopulation of patients with restless legs syndrome. *Acta Neurol Scand* 77:418, 1988.

WARD AAR: The function of the basal ganglia, in Vinken PJ, Bruyn GW (eds): *Handbook of Clinical Neurology*. Vol 6: *Basal Ganglia*. Amsterdam, North-Holland, 1968, chap 3, pp 90–115.

WATSON CW, DENNY-BROWN DE: Myoclonus epilepsy as a symptom of diffuse neuronal disease. *Arch Neurol Psychiatry* 70:151, 1953.

WEE AS, SUBRAMONY SH, CURRIER RD: "Orthostatic tremor" in familial-essential tremor. *Neurology* 36:1241, 1986.

WILKINS DE, HALLETT M, WESS MM: Audiogenic startle reflex of man and its relationship to startle syndromes. *Brain* 109:561, 1986.

WILLS AJ, JENKINS IH, THOMPSON PD: Red nuclear and cerebellar but no olivary activation associated with essential tremor: A positron emission tomographic study. *Ann Neurol* 36:636, 1994.

WILSON SAK: *Neurology*. London, Edward Arnold, 1940.

WOLF SS, JONES DW, KNABLE MB, et al: Tourette syndrome: Prediction of phenotypic variation in monozygotic twins by caudate nucleus D_2 receptor binding. *Science* 273:1225, 1996.

YOUNG RR: Tremor, in Asbury AK, McKhann GM, McDonald WI (eds): *Diseases of the Nervous System*, 2nd ed. Philadelphia, Saunders, 1992, chap 25, pp 353–367.

YOUNG RR, GROWDON JH, SHAHANI BT: Beta-adrenergic mechanisms in action tremor. *N Engl J Med* 293:950, 1975.

ZWEIG RM, JANKEL WR, WHITEHOUSE PJ, et al: Brainstem pathology in dystonia. *Neurology* 36(suppl 1):74, 1986.

Chapter 7

DISORDERS OF STANCE AND GAIT

Certain disorders of motor function manifest themselves most clearly as impairments of upright stance and locomotion, and their evaluation depends on a knowledge of the neural mechanisms underlying these peculiarly human functions. Analysis of stance, carriage, and gait is a particularly rewarding medical exercise; with some experience, the examiner can sometimes reach a neurologic diagnosis merely by noting the manner in which the patient enters the office. Considering the frequency of falls that result from gait disorders and their consequences, such as hip fractures, and the resultant need for hospital and nursing home care, this is an important subject for all physicians (Tinetti and Williams).

NORMAL GAIT

The normal gait seldom attracts attention, but it should be observed with care if slight deviations from normal are to be appreciated. The body is erect, the head is straight, and the arms hang loosely and gracefully at the sides, each moving rhythmically forward with the opposite leg. The feet are slightly everted, the steps are approximately equal, and the internal malleoli almost touch as each foot passes the other. The medial edges of the heels, as they strike the ground with each step, form a straight line. As each leg moves forward, there is coordinated flexion of the hip and knee, dorsiflexion of the foot, and a barely perceptible elevation of the hip so that the foot clears the ground. Also, with each step, the thorax advances slightly on the side opposite the swinging lower limb. The heel strikes the ground first, and inspection of the shoes will show that this part is most subject to wear. The muscles of greatest importance in maintaining the erect posture are the erector spinae and the extensors of the hips and knees.

The normal *gait cycle*, defined as the period between successive points at which the heel of the same foot strikes the ground, is illustrated in Fig. 7-1; it is based on the studies of Murray and coworkers and of Olsson. In this figure, the cycle is initiated by the heel strike of the right foot. The *stance phase*, during which the foot is in contact with the ground, occupies 60 to 65 percent of the cycle. The *swing phase* begins when the right toes leave the ground. Noteworthy is the fact that for 20 to 25 percent of the walking cycle, both feet are in contact with the ground (*double limb support*). In later life, when the steps shorten and cadence (the rhythm and number of steps per minute) decreases, the proportion of double limb support increases (see further on). Surface electromyograms show an alternating pattern of activity in the legs, predominating in the flexors during the swing phase and in the extensors during the stance phase.

When analyzed in greater detail, the requirements for locomotion in an upright, bipedal position may be reduced to the following elements: (1) antigravity support of the body, (2) stepping, (3) the maintenance of equilibrium, and (4) a means of propulsion. Locomotion is impaired in the course of neurologic disease when one or more of these mechanical principles are prevented from operating normally.

The upright support of the body is provided by *righting* and *antigravity reflexes*, which allow a person to arise from a lying or sitting position to an upright bipedal stance and to maintain firm extension of the knees, hips, and back, modifiable by the position of the head and neck. These postural reflexes depend on the afferent vestibular, somatosensory (proprioceptive and tactile), and visual impulses, which are integrated in the spinal cord, brainstem, and basal ganglia. (Transection of the neuraxis between the red and vestibular nuclei leads to exaggeration of these antigravity reflexes—decerebrate rigidity.)

Stepping, the second element, is a basic movement pattern present at birth and integrated at the spinal-midbrain-diencephalic level. Its appropriate stimuli are contact of the sole with a flat surface and a shifting of the

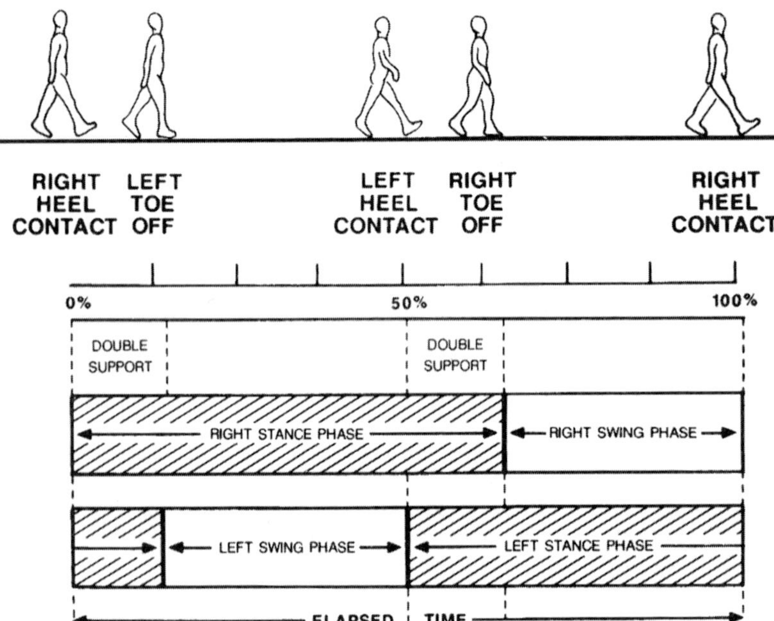

Figure 7-1

The normal gait cycle, based on the studies of Olsson and of Murray et al. See text for details.

center of gravity—first laterally onto one foot, allowing the other to be raised, and then forward, allowing the body to move onto the advancing foot. Rhythmic stepping movements can be initiated and sustained in decerebrate or "spinal" cats and dogs. This is accomplished through the activity of interneurons that are organized as rhythmic "locomotor generators," akin to the pattern generators that permit the rhythmic movement of wings or fins. There is no evidence for a similar system of locomotor control in monkeys or humans, in whom the spinal mechanisms for walking cannot function independently but depend upon higher command centers. The latter are located in the posterior subthalamic region, caudal midbrain tegmentum, and pontine reticular formation; they control the spinal gait mechanisms through the reticulospinal, vestibulospinal, and tectospinal pathways in the ventral cord (Eidelberg et al; Lawrence and Kuypers). Probably, in the human, the brainstem locomotor regions are activated by cerebral cortical centers.

Equilibrium involves the maintenance of balance at right angles to the direction of movement. The center of gravity during the continuously unstable equilibrium that prevails in walking must shift within narrow limits from side to side and forward as the weight is borne first on one foot, then on the other. This is accomplished through the activity of highly sensitive postural and righting reflexes, both peripheral (stretch reflexes) and central (vestibulocerebellar reflexes). These reflexes are activated within 100 ms of each shift in the support surface and require reliable afferent information from the visual, vestibular, and proprioceptive systems.

Propulsion is provided by leaning forward and slightly to one side and permitting the body to fall a certain distance before being checked by the support of the leg. Here, both forward and alternating lateral movements must occur. But in running, where at one moment both feet are off the ground, a forward drive or thrust by the hind leg is also needed.

Obviously gait varies considerably from one person to another, and it is a commonplace observation that a person may be identified by the sound of his footsteps, notably the pace and the lightness or heaviness of tread. The manner of walking and the carriage of the body may even provide clues to an individual's personality and occupation; Sherlock Holmes was proud of his talent for reading such clues. Furthermore, the gaits of men and women differ, a woman's steps being quicker and shorter and movement of the trunk and hips more graceful and delicate. Certain female characteristics of gait, if observed in the male, immediately impart an impression of femininity; or male characteristics, observed in the female, suggest masculinity. The changes in stance and gait that accompany aging—the slightly stooped posture and slow, stiff tread—are so familiar that they are not perceived as abnormalities.

ABNORMAL GAITS

Since normal body posture and locomotion require intact vestibular function, proprioception, and vision (we see where we are going and pick our steps), the effects on normal function of deficits in these senses are worth noting.

A blind person—or a normal one who is blindfolded or walks in the dark—moves cautiously, with arms slightly forward to avoid collisions, and shortens his step slightly on a smooth surface; with shortening of the step, there is less rocking of the body and the gait is unnaturally stiff.

Disorders of vestibular function are most often the result of prolonged administration of aminoglycoside antibiotics or other toxic medications, which destroy the hair cells of the vestibular labyrinth. This also occurs in some patients in the late stages of Ménière disease and, infrequently, for no definable reason. Patients with vestibulopathy show unsteadiness in standing and walking, often without widening their base, and an inability to descend stairs without holding onto the banister. They complain of a sense of imbalance, usually with movement but at times when standing still—a sensation that may be likened to being on the deck of a rolling ship. Running and turning quickly are even more impaired, with lurching in all directions. The patient has great difficulty in focusing his vision on a fixed target when he is moving or on a moving target when he is either stationary or moving. When the body is in motion or the head is moved suddenly, objects in the environment appear blurred or actually jiggle up and down or from side to side (oscillopsia). Driving a car or reading on a train is difficult or impossible; even when walking, the patient may need to stop in order to read a sign. These abnormalities indicate a loss of stabilization of ocular fixation by the vestibular system during body movements. An elderly person, unlike a child or young adult, has difficulty compensating for these abnormalities. Proof that the gait of such persons is dependent on visual clues comes from their performance blindfolded or in the dark, when their unsteadiness and staggering increase to the point of falling. The diagnosis is confirmed by testing labyrinthine function (caloric and rotational testing, electronystagmography, and posture platform testing).

A loss of proprioception—as occurs in patients with severe large-fiber polyneuropathy, posterior root lesions (e.g., tabes dorsalis, lumbosacral compression), or complete interruption of the posterior columns in the cervical spinal cord (multiple sclerosis, vitamin B_{12} deficiency, spondylotic or neoplastic compression)—abolishes or seriously impairs the capacity for independent locomotion. After years of training, such patients still have difficulty in initiating gait and in forward propulsion. As Purdon Martin has illustrated, they hold their hands in front of the body, bend the body and head forward, walk with a wide base and irregular, uneven steps, but still rock the body. If they are tilted to one side, they fail to compensate for their abnormal posture. If they fall, they cannot arise without help; they are unable to crawl or to get into an "all fours" posture. They have difficulty in getting up from a chair. When standing, if instructed to close their eyes, they sway markedly and may fall (*Romberg sign*). This informs us that static postural reactions are primarily dependent on proprioceptive rather than on visual or labyrinthine information.

With lesions of the basal ganglia, both in monkeys and in humans, the posture of the body and the postural responses to disturbed equilibrium are faulty. There is difficulty in taking the first step; once it is taken, the body pitches forward and a fall can be prevented only by catch-up stepping (propulsion). Similarly, a step backward may induce a series of quickening steps in that direction (retropulsion). Corrective righting reflexes are clearly in abeyance when the patient is pushed off balance (Denny-Brown). These abnormalities are elaborated further on, under "Festinating Gait."

Examination of the Patient with Abnormal Gait

When confronted with a disorder of gait, the examiner must observe the patient's stance and the attitude and dominant positions of the legs, trunk, and arms. It is good practice to watch patients as they walk into the examining room, when they are apt to walk more naturally than during the performance of special tests. They should be asked to stand with feet together and head erect, with eyes open and then closed. A normal person can stand with feet together and eyes closed while moving the head from side to side, a test that eliminates both visual and vestibular cues and induces certain compensatory trunk and leg movements that depend on proprioceptive afferent mechanisms (Ropper). A Romberg sign—marked swaying or falling with the eyes closed but not with the eyes open—usually indicates a loss of postural sense, not of cerebellar function, although with vestibular or cerebellar dysfunction there may be a less pronounced exaggeration of swaying with eyes closed and feet together. Swaying due to nervousness may be overcome by asking the patient to touch the tip of his nose alternately with the forefinger of one hand and then the other.

Next, the patient should be asked to walk, noting in particular any hesitation in starting and negotiating turns, width of base, length of stride, foot clearance, arm swing, and cadence. A tendency to veer to one side, as with unilateral cerebellar disease, can be brought out by having the patient walk around a chair. When the affected side is toward the chair, the patient tends to walk into it; when it is away from the chair, there is a veering outward in ever-widening circles. More delicate tests of gait are walking a straight line heel to toe and having the patient arise quickly from a chair, walk briskly, stop and turn suddenly, and then sit down again.

It is instructive to observe the patient's postural reaction to a sudden push backward and forward or to the side. With postural instability there is a delay or inadequacy of corrective actions. Finally, the patient should be asked to hop on one leg and to jog. If all these tests are successfully executed, it may be assumed that any difficulty in locomotion is not due to impairment of a proprioceptive, labyrinthine-vestibular, basal ganglionic, or cerebellar mechanism. Detailed musculoskeletal and neurologic examination is then necessary to determine which of several other disturbances of function is responsible for the patient's disorder of gait.

The following types of abnormal gait are so distinctive that, with a little practice, they can be recognized at a glance.

Cerebellar Gait

The main features of this gait are a wide base (separation of legs), unsteadiness, irregularity of steps, and lateral veering. Steps are uncertain, some are shorter and others longer than intended, and the patient may compensate for these abnormalities by shortening his steps and shuffling, i.e., keeping both feet on the ground simultaneously. Cerebellar gait is often referred to as "reeling" or "drunken," but these adjectives are not entirely apt, as explained further on.

With cerebellar ataxia, the unsteadiness and irregular swaying of the trunk are more prominent when the patient arises from a chair or turns suddenly while walking and may be most evident when he has to stop walking abruptly and sit down; it may be necessary for him to grasp the chair for support. It is noteworthy that patients with purely cerebellar gait abnormalities may not complain of imbalance or vertigo. Cerebellar ataxia may be so severe that the patient cannot stand without assistance. If it is less severe, standing with feet together and head erect is difficult. In its mildest form, the ataxia is best demonstrated by having the patient walk a line heel to toe; after a step or two, he loses his balance and finds it necessary to place one foot to the side to avoid falling.

The patient with cerebellar ataxia who sways perceptibly when standing with feet together and eyes open will sway somewhat more with eyes closed. By contrast, removal of visual clues from a patient with proprioceptive loss causes a marked increase in swaying or falling (Romberg test). Thus, the defect in cerebellar gait is not primarily in antigravity support, steppage, or propulsion but in the coordination of proprioceptive, labyrinthine, and visual information in reflex movements, particularly those that are required to make rapid adjustments to changes in posture and position.

Cerebellar abnormalities of stance and gait are usually accompanied by signs of cerebellar incoordination of the arms and legs, but they need not be. The presence of the latter signs depends on involvement of the cerebellar hemispheres as distinct from the anterosuperior (vermian) midline structures. With thalamic and midbrain lesions (beyond the decussation of the brachium conjunctivum), the ataxic signs are on the opposite side. If the lesions are bilateral, there is often titubation (tremor) of the head and trunk.

Cerebellar gait is seen most commonly in patients with multiple sclerosis, cerebellar tumors (particularly those affecting the vermis disproportionately—e.g., medulloblastoma), stroke, and the cerebellar degenerations. In certain forms of cerebellar degeneration in which the disease process remains stable for many years, e.g., the type associated with chronic alcoholism, the gait disorder becomes altered as compensations are acquired. The base is wide and the steps are still short but more regular, the trunk is inclined slightly forward, the arms are held somewhat away from the body, and the gait assumes a more mechanical, rhythmic quality. In this way the patient can walk for long distances, but he still lacks the capacity to make the necessary postural adjustments in response to sudden changes in position, such as occur in walking on uneven ground.

Many patients with cerebellar disease, particularly of acute type, also show pendularity of the patellar reflexes and other signs of hypotonia of the limbs when they are examined in the sitting or recumbent position, as discussed in Chap. 5. Paradoxically, walking without the support of a cane or the arm of a companion brings out a certain stiffness of the legs and firmness of the muscles. The latter abnormality may be analogous to positive supporting reactions observed in cats and dogs following ablation of the anterior vermis; such animals react to pressure on the foot pad with an extensor thrust of the leg.

Drunken, or Reeling, Gait

This is characteristic of intoxication with alcohol and other sedative drugs. The drunken patient totters, reels, tips forward and then backward, appearing each moment to be on the verge of losing his balance and falling. Control over the trunk and legs is greatly impaired. The steps are irregular and uncertain. Such patients appear stupefied and indifferent to the quality of their performance, but under certain circumstances they can momentarily correct the defect. As indicated above, the adjectives *drunken* and *reeling* are used frequently to describe the gait of cerebellar disease, but the similarities between them are only superficial. The severely intoxicated patient reels or sways in many different directions and seemingly makes little or no effort to correct the staggering by watching his legs or the ground, as in cerebellar or sensory ataxia. Also, the variability of the drunken gait is noteworthy. Despite wide excursions of the body and deviation from the line of march, the drunken patient may, for short distances, be able to walk on a narrow base and maintain his balance. In contrast, the patient with cerebellar gait has great difficulty in correcting his balance if he sways or lurches too far to one side. Milder degrees of the drunken gait more closely resemble the gait disorder that follows loss of labyrinthine function (see earlier discussion).

Gait of Sensory Ataxia

This disorder of gait is due to an impairment of joint-position or muscular kinesthetic sense resulting from interruption of afferent nerve fibers in the peripheral nerves, posterior roots, posterior columns of the spinal cords, or medial lemnisci and occasionally from a lesion of both parietal lobes. Whatever the location of the lesion, its effect is to deprive the patient of knowledge of the position of his limbs and, more relevant to gait, to interfere with afferent kinesthetic information that does not attain conscious perception. A sense of imbalance is usually present. These patients are aware that the trouble is in the legs and not in the head, that foot placement is awkward, and that the ability to recover quickly from a misstep is impaired. The resulting disorder is characterized by varying degrees of difficulty in standing and walking; in advanced cases, there is a complete failure of locomotion, although muscular power is retained.

The principal features of the gait disorder are the brusqueness of movement of the legs and stamp of the feet. The feet are placed far apart to correct the instability, and patients carefully watch the ground and their legs. As they step out, the legs are flung abruptly forward and outward, in irregular steps of variable length and height. Many steps are attended by an audible stamp as the foot is forcibly brought down onto the floor (possibly to enhance joint-position sense). The body is held in a slightly flexed position, and some of the weight is supported on the cane that the severely ataxic patient usually carries. To use Ramsay Hunt's characterization, the patient with this gait disorder is recognized by his "stamp and stick." The ataxia is markedly exaggerated when the patient is deprived of his visual cues, as in walking in the dark. Such patients, when asked to stand with feet together and eyes closed, show greatly increased swaying or falling (the latter being the actual sign described by Romberg). It is said that in cases of sensory ataxia, the shoes do not show wear in any one place because the entire sole strikes the ground at once. Examination invariably discloses a loss of position sense in the feet and legs and usually of vibratory sense as well.

Formerly, a disordered gait of this type was observed most frequently with tabes dorsalis, hence the term *tabetic gait*; but it is also seen in Friedreich ataxia and related forms of spinocerebellar degeneration, subacute combined degeneration of the cord (vitamin B_{12} deficiency), syphilitic meningomyelitis, chronic sensory polyneuropathy, and those cases of multiple sclerosis or compression of the spinal cord (spondylosis and meningioma are the common causes) in which the posterior columns are predominantly involved.

Steppage, or Equine, Gait

This is caused by paralysis of the pretibial and peroneal muscles, with resultant inability to dorsiflex and evert the foot (foot drop). The steps are regular and even, but the advancing foot hangs with the toes pointing toward the ground. Walking is accomplished by excessive flexion at the hip, the leg being lifted abnormally high in order for the foot to clear the ground. There is a slapping noise as the foot strikes the floor. Thus there is a superficial similarity to the tabetic gait, especially in severe polyneuropathy, where the features of steppage and sensory ataxia may be combined. However, patients with steppage gait alone are not troubled by a perception of imbalance; they fall mostly from tripping on carpet edges and curbstones.

Foot drop may be unilateral or bilateral and occurs in diseases that affect the peripheral nerves of the legs or motor neurons in the spinal cord, such as chronic acquired axonal neuropathies, Charcot-Marie-Tooth disease (peroneal muscular atrophy), progressive spinal muscular atrophy, and poliomyelitis. It may also be observed in certain types of muscular dystrophy in which the distal musculature of the limbs is involved.

A particular disorder of gait, also of peripheral origin and resembling steppage gait, may be observed in patients with painful dysesthesias of the soles of the feet. Because of the exquisite pain evoked by tactile stimulation of the feet, the patient treads gingerly, as though walking barefoot on hot sand or pavement, with the feet rotated in such a way as to limit contact with their most painful portions. Peripheral neuropathy (most often of the alcoholic-nutritional type), causalgia, and erythromelalgia are the usual causes.

Hemiplegic and Paraplegic (Spastic) Gaits

The patient with hemiplegia or hemiparesis holds the affected leg stiffly and does not flex it freely at the hip, knee, and ankle. The leg tends to rotate outward to describe a semicircle, first away from and then toward the trunk (circumduction). The foot scrapes the floor, and the toe and outer sole of the shoe are worn. One can recognize a spastic gait by the sound of slow, rhythmic scuffing of the foot and wearing of the medial toe of the shoe. The arm on the affected side is weak and stiff to a variable degree; it is carried in a flexed position and does not swing naturally. In the hemiparetic child, the arm tends to abduct as he steps forward. This type of gait disorder is most often a sequela of stroke or trauma but may result from a number of other cerebral conditions that damage the corticospinal pathway on one side.

The spastic paraplegic or paraparetic gait is, in effect, a bilateral hemiplegic gait affecting only the lower limbs. Each leg is advanced slowly and stiffly, with restricted motion at the hips and knees. The legs are extended or slightly bent at the knees and the thighs may be strongly adducted, causing the legs almost to cross as the patient walks (scissors gait). The steps are regular and short, and the patient advances only with great effort, as though wading waist-deep in water. An easy way to remember the main features of the hemiplegic and paraplegic gaits is through the letter S, for *slow, stiff,* and *scraping*. The defect is in the stepping mechanism and in propulsion, not in support or equilibrium.

A spastic paraparetic gait is the major manifestation of cerebral diplegia (cerebral palsy), the result of anoxic or other damage to the brain in the perinatal period. Also, this disorder of gait is seen in a variety of chronic spinal cord diseases involving the dorsolateral and ventral funiculi, including multiple sclerosis, syringomyelia, any type of chronic meningomyelitis, combined system disease of both the pernicious anemia (PA) and non-PA types, chronic spinal cord compression, and familial forms of spastic paraplegia. Frequently, the effects of posterior column disease are added, giving rise to a mixed gait disturbance—a spinal spastic ataxia.

Festinating and Parkinsonian Gait

The term "festination" derives from the Latin *festinare*, "to hasten," and appropriately describes the involuntary acceleration or hastening that characterizes the gait of Parkinson disease (page 1130). Diminished or absent arm swing, turning en bloc, hesitation in starting to walk, shuffling, or "freezing" briefly when encountering doorways or other obstacles are the other stigmata of the parkinsonian gait. When they are joined to the typical tremor, unblinking and mask-like facial expression, general attitude of flexion, immobility, and poverty of movement, there can be little doubt as to the diagnosis. The arms are carried slightly flexed and ahead of the body and do not swing. The legs are stiff and bent at the knees and hips. The steps are short, and the feet barely clear the ground as the patient shuffles along. Once walking has started, the upper part of the body advances ahead of the lower part, and the patient is impelled to take increasingly short and rapid steps as though trying to catch up to his center of gravity. The steps become more and more rapid, and the patient could easily break into a trot and collide with an obstacle or fall if not assisted. Festination may be apparent when the patient is walking forward or backward. The defects are in rocking the body from side to side, so that the feet may clear the floor, and in moving the legs quickly enough to overtake the center of gravity. The problem is compounded by the inadequacy of postural support reflexes, demonstrable, in the standing patient, by a push against the sternum or a tug backward on the shoulder. A normal person readily retains his stability or adjusts to modest displacement of the trunk with a single step backward, but the parkinsonian patient may stagger or fall unless someone stands by to prevent it.

Other unusual gaits are sometimes observed in Parkinson disease and were particularly prominent in the postencephalitic form, now practically extinct. For example, such a patient may be unable to take a step forward or does so only after he takes a few hops or one or two steps backward. Or walking may be initiated by a series of short steps or a series of steps of increasing size. Occasionally such a patient may run better than he walks or walk backward better than forward. Often, walking so preoccupies the patient that talking simultaneously is impossible and he must stop to answer a question.

Choreoathetotic and Dystonic Gaits

Diseases characterized by involuntary movements and dystonic postures seriously affect gait. In fact, a disturbance of gait may be the initial and dominant manifestation of such diseases, and the testing of gait often brings out abnormalities of movement of the limbs and posture that are otherwise not conspicuous.

As the patient with congenital athetosis or Huntington chorea stands or walks, there is a continuous play of irregular movements affecting the face, neck, hands, and, in the advanced stages, the large proximal joints and trunk. The position of the arms and upper parts of the body varies with each step, at times giving the impression of a puppet. There are jerks of the head, grimacing, squirming and twisting movements of the trunk and limbs, and peculiar respiratory noises. One arm may be thrust aloft and the other held behind the body, with wrist and fingers undergoing alternate flexion and extension, supination and pronation. The head may incline in one direction or the other, the lips alternately retract and purse, and the tongue intermittently protrudes from the mouth. The legs advance slowly and awkwardly, the result of superimposed involuntary movements and postures. Sometimes the foot is plantarflexed at the ankle, and the weight is carried on the toes; or it may be dorsiflexed or inverted. An involuntary movement may cause the leg to be suspended in the air momentarily, imparting a lilting or waltzing character to the gait, or it may twist the trunk so violently that the patient may fall.

In dystonia musculorum deformans and in focal axial dystonias, the first symptom may be a limp due to inversion or plantar flexion of the foot or a distortion of the pelvis. One leg may be rigidly extended or one shoulder elevated, and the trunk may assume a position of exaggerated flexion, lordosis, or scoliosis. Because of the muscle spasms that deform the body in this manner, the patient may have to walk with knees flexed. The gait may seem normal as the first steps are taken, the abnormal postures asserting themselves as the patient continues to walk. Prominence of the buttocks, owing to a lumbar lordosis, combined with flexion of one leg or both legs at the hip, give rise to the so-called dromedary gait of Oppenheim. In the more advanced stages, walking becomes impossible owing to torsion of the trunk or the continuous flexion of the legs.

The general features of choreoathetosis and dystonia are described more fully in Chap. 4.

Waddling (Gluteal or Trendelenburg) Gait

This gait is characteristic of progressive muscular dystrophy, but it occurs as well in chronic forms of spinal muscular atrophy, in certain inflammatory myopathies, and with congenital dislocation of the hips.

In normal walking, as weight is placed alternately on each leg, the hip is fixated by the gluteal muscles, particularly the gluteus medius, allowing for a slight rise of the opposite hip and tilt of the trunk to the weight-bearing side. With weakness of the glutei, there is a failure to stabilize the weight-bearing hip, causing it to bulge outward and the opposite side of the pelvis to drop, with inclination of the trunk to that side. The alternation in lateral trunk movements results in the roll or waddle.

In progressive muscular dystrophy, an accentuation of the lumbar lordosis is often associated. Also, childhood cases may be complicated by muscular contractures leading to an equinovarus position of the foot, so that the waddle is combined with circumduction of the legs and "walking on the toes."

With unilateral gluteal weakness, often the result of damage to the first sacral nerve root, tilting and drooping of the pelvis is apparent on only one side as the patient overlifts the leg when walking.

Toppling Gait

Toppling, meaning tottering and falling, may occur with brainstem and cerebellar lesions, especially in the older person following a stroke. It is a frequent feature of the lateral medullary syndrome, in which falling occurs to the side of the infarction. In patients with vestibular neuronitis, falling also occurs to the same side as the lesion. With the Tullio phenomenon (vertigo induced by loud high-pitched sounds, or yawning following a fenestration operation on the vestibule), the toppling is contraversive; with midbrain strokes, the falls tend to be backward. In patients with *progressive supranuclear palsy* (see page 1139), where dystonia of the neck is combined with paralysis of vertical gaze and pseudobulbar features, unexplained falling is often an early and prominent feature. In addition, the gait is uncertain and hesitant—features that are enhanced, no doubt, by the hazard of falling unpredictably. The cause of the toppling phenomenon is unclear; it does not have its basis in weakness, ataxia, or loss of deep sensation. It appears to be a disorder of balance that is occasioned by precipitant action or the wrong placement of a foot and by a failure of the righting reflexes. Slowness of motor response is another factor. When the defect is due to a central vestibular disorder, the patient may describe a sense of being pushed (pulsion) rather than of imbalance. In midbrain disease, including progressive supranuclear palsy, a remarkable feature is the lack of appreciation of a sense of imbalance. In the advanced stages of Parkinson disease, falling of a similar type may be a serious problem.

Gait Disorder in Normal-Pressure Hydrocephalus

Progressive difficulty in walking is usually the initial and most prominent symptom of normal-pressure hydrocephalus (NPH), a disorder of cerebrospinal fluid (CSF) circulation described on page 663. The gait disturbance in NPH has few specific features. Certainly it cannot be categorized as an ataxic or spastic gait or what has been described as an "apraxic" gait; nor does it have more than a superficial resemblance to the parkinsonian gait. Its main features—diminished cadence, widened base, short steps, and shuffling—are the natural compensations observed in patients with all manner of gait disorders. Patients with the gait disorder of NPH often complain of a sense of imbalance or even of dizziness, but most of them have difficulty in articulating the exact problem. Like patients with other disorders of frontal lobe function, they can carry out the motions of stepping while supine or sitting but have difficulty in taking steps when upright or attempting to walk. There appears to be a dyscontrol of the entire axial musculature as the patient awkwardly assumes the erect posture—with hips and knees only slightly flexed and stiff and a delay in swinging the legs over the side of the bed.

Sudarsky and Simon have quantified these defects by means of high-speed cameras and computer analysis. They have also demonstrated a reduction in height of step, an increase in sway, and a decrease in rotation of the pelvis and counterrotation of the torso. Tone in the leg muscles of the NPH patient is increased, with a tendency to cocontraction of flexor and extensor muscle groups. Walking is perceptibly slower than normal, the body is held stiffly and moves en bloc, arm swing is diminished, and there is a tendency to fall backwards—features that are reminiscent of the gait in Parkinson disease. In general, the lack of arm swing and the stooped posture are more prominent in Parkinson disease than in NPH, and, of course, most of the other features of Parkinson disease are lacking. There is no hint of ataxia of arm and leg movements. As with the related "frontal gait," described below, patients who have difficulty initiating gait or whose steps are so short as to be ineffective are helped by marching to a cadence or in step with the examiner. In patients with untreated NPH, one observes a progressive deterioration of stance and gait—from an inability to walk to an inability to stand, sit, and rise from or turn over in bed.

Frontal Lobe Disorder of Gait

Standing and walking may be severely disturbed by diseases that affect the frontal lobes, particularly their medial parts and their connections with the basal ganglia. This disorder is sometimes spoken of as a frontal lobe ataxia or as an apraxia of gait, since the difficulty in walking cannot be accounted for by weakness, loss of sensation, cerebellar incoordination, or basal ganglionic abnormality. Whether the gait disorder should be designated as an apraxia, in the sense of Liepmann's concept of arm and hand apraxia, is questionable, since walking is instinctual and not learned. Patients with so-called apraxia of gait do not have apraxia of individual limbs, particularly of the lower limbs; conversely, patients with apraxia of the limbs usually walk normally. More likely, the disorder represents a loss of integration, at the cortical and basal ganglionic levels, of the essential instinctual elements of stance and locomotion that are acquired in infancy and often lost in old age.

Patients assume a posture of slight flexion, with the feet placed farther apart than normal. They advance slowly, with small, shuffling, hesitant steps. At times they halt, unable to advance without great effort, although they do much better with a little assistance or with exhortation to walk in step with the examiner or to a marching cadence. Turning is accomplished by a series of tiny, uncertain steps that are made with one foot, the other foot being planted on the floor as a pivot. There is a need to seek support from a companion's arm or nearby furniture. The initiation of walking becomes progressively more difficult; in advanced cases, the patient makes only feeble, abortive stepping movements in place, unable to move his feet and legs forward; in even more advanced cases, the patient can make no stepping movements whatsoever, as though his feet were glued to the floor. These late phenomena have been referred to colloquially as "magnetic feet" or the "slipping clutch" syndrome (Denny-Brown) and as "gait ignition failure" (Atchison et al). In some patients, difficulty in the initiation of gait may be an early and apparently isolated phenomenon, but invariably, with the passage of time, sometimes of years, the other features of the frontal lobe gait disorder become evident. Finally, as in untreated

NPH, these patients become unable to stand or even to sit; without support, they fall helplessly backward or to one side.

Most patients, while seated or supine, are able to make complex movements with their legs, such as drawing imaginary figures or pedaling a bicycle, at a time when their gait is seriously impaired. Eventually, however, all movements of the legs become slow and awkward, and the limbs, when passively moved, offer variable resistance (*gegenhalten*). Difficulty in turning over in bed is highly characteristic and may eventually become complete. These advanced motor disabilities are usually associated with dementia, but the two disorders need not evolve in parallel. Thus, some patients with Alzheimer disease may show a serious degree of dementia for several years before a gait disorder becomes apparent; in other conditions, such as NPH and Binswanger disease, the opposite pertains. Or both the dementia and gait disorder may evolve more or less together. Grasping, groping, hyperactive tendon reflexes, and Babinski signs may or may not be present. The end result in some cases is a "cerebral paraplegia in flexion" (Yakovlev), in which the patient lies curled up in bed, immobile and mute, with the limbs fixed by contractures in an attitude of flexion (Fig. 7-2).

In addition to NPH and Alzheimer disease, the causes of frontal lobe gait disorder include widespread neoplasm (meningioma, infiltrating glioma), subcortical arteriosclerotic encephalopathy (Binswanger disease; see Thompson and Marsden) Pick disease, and frontal lobe damage from trauma, stroke, or a ruptured anterior communicating aneurysm.

Gait of the Aged

An alteration of gait unrelated to overt cerebral disease is an almost universal accompaniment of aging (Fig. 7-3). Lost with aging are the speed, balance, and many of the quick and graceful adaptive movements that characterize the gait of younger individuals. A slightly stooped posture, varying degrees of slowness and stiffness of walking, shortening of the stride, slight widening of the base, and a tendency to turn en bloc are the main objective characteristics. The shortening of stride and widening of the base provide the support that enables the elderly individual to more confidently maintain his balance but result in a somewhat guarded gait, like that of a person walking on a slippery surface or in the dark.

Lacking to a varying degree in the elderly is the ability to make the rapid compensatory postural changes ("rescue responses") that are necessary to cushion or prevent a fall. A slight misstep, a failure to elevate the foot sufficiently, or tipping of the center of gravity to one side often cannot be corrected—features, no doubt, that account for the frequency of falls and fear of falling. Most persons with this type of gait disturbance are aware of impaired balance and their need for caution to avoid falls (the "cautious gait"; see Nutt et al). As such, this gait disorder lacks specificity, being a general adaptive or defensive reaction to all forms of defective locomotion.

The nature of this gait disorder is not fully understood. It may simply represent a mild degree of neuronal

Figure 7-2

The evolution of erect stance and gait and paraplegia in flexion of cerebral origin according to Yakovlev. The ripening forebrain of the fetus drives the head and body up and moves the individual onward. When the "driving brain" (frontal lobe, striatum, and pallidum) degenerates, the individual "curls up" again. (Adapted by permission from Yakovlev.) Lesser degrees of this sequence, indicated by the upper line, may account for the changes in gait and posture that accompany normal aging (see Fig. 7-3).

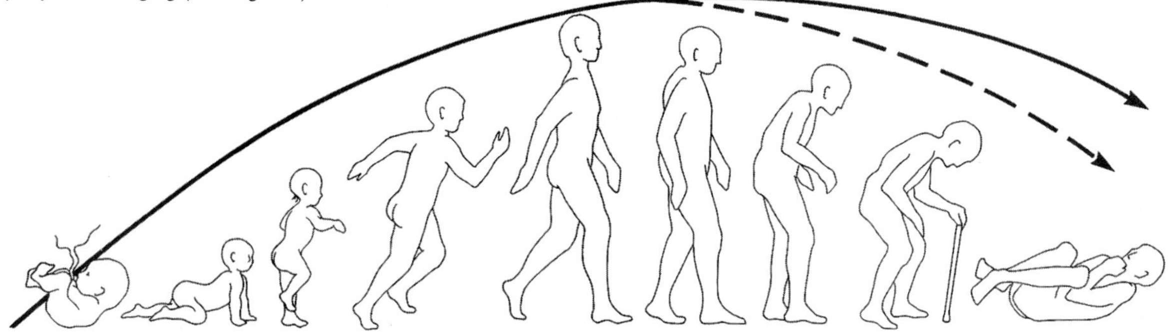

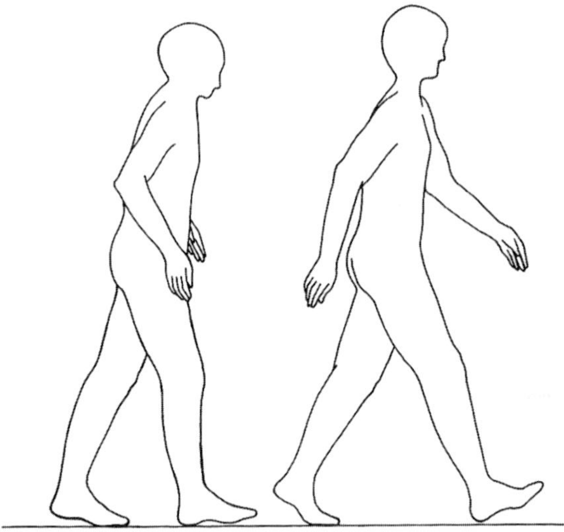

Figure 7-3

Diagram illustrating the changes in posture and gait that accompany aging ("senile gait"). With aging (figure on left) *there occurs a decrease in the length of stride, excursion of the hip, elevation of the toes of the forward foot and the heel of the rear foot, shoulder flexion on forward arm swing, and elbow extension on backward swing. (Redrawn permission from Murray et al.)*

loss, attributable to aging itself, which in a severe (pathologic) form is referred to as a "frontal lobe disorder of gait" (as discussed above). Inadequate proprioception, slowness in making corrective postural responses, diminished vestibular function of varying degree, and weakness of pelvic and thigh muscles are probably contributing factors, as are degenerative joint changes of the spine, hips, and knees. Fisher has remarked upon the similarity of the senile gait to that of NPH and suggests that this form of hydrocephalus underlies the gait disorder of many elderly but mentally competent persons. The changes in gait due to aging are discussed further in Chap. 29.

Gaits of the Mentally Retarded

There are, in addition to the disorders described above, peculiarities of gait that defy analysis. One has only to observe the assortment of gait abnormalities among the institutionalized mentally handicapped to appreciate this fact. An ungainly stance with the head too far forward or the neck extended and arms held in odd positions, a wide-based gait with awkward lurches or feet stomping the floor—each patient with his own ungraceful style—these are but a few of the peculiarities that meet the eye. One tries in vain to relate them to a disorder of proprioception, cerebellar deficit, or pyramidal or extrapyramidal disease.

The only plausible explanation that comes to mind is that these pathologic variants of gait are based on a retardation of the natural developmental sequence of the cerebral and spinal mechanisms involved in bipedal locomotion, posture, and righting. The acquisition of the refinements of locomotion—such as running, hopping, jumping, dancing, balancing on one foot, kicking a ball, etc.—are age-linked; i.e., each has its average age of acquisition. There are wide individual variations, but the most striking extremes are found in the mentally handicapped, who may be retarded in these ways as well as in cognitive development. The rhythmic rocking movements and hand clapping, odd mannerisms, waving of the arms, tremors, and other stereotyped patterns mentioned in Chap. 28 make their performances even more eccentric. The Lincoln-Oseretsky scale is an attempt to quantitate maturational delays in the locomotor sphere (Chap. 28).

Hysterical Gait

This may take one of several forms. There may be a hysterical monoplegia, hemiplegia, or paraplegia. In walking, the patient may hesitate and advance the leg in a grossly ataxic or tremulous manner. Typically, patients with a hysterical paralysis of the leg do not lift the foot from the floor while walking; instead, they tend to drag the leg as a useless member or push it ahead of them as though it were on a skate. In hysterical hemiparesis, the characteristic circumduction of the leg is absent, as are the usual hemiparetic postures, hyperactive tendon reflexes, and Babinski sign. The hysterical paraplegic cannot very well drag both legs and usually depends on canes or crutches or remains helpless in bed or in a wheelchair; the muscles may be flaccid or rigid, with development of contractures. The hysterical gait may take other dramatic forms. Some patients look as though they were walking on stilts, others assume extreme dystonic postures, and still others lurch wildly in all directions without falling, actually demonstrating by their gyrations a normal ability to make rapid and appropriate postural adjustments. The gait disorder may be accompanied by similarly exaggerated movements of the arms, as though to impress the observer with the great effort required to walk and maintain balance. The many forms of hysterical gait have been well described by

Keane. Leg movements in bed may be unimpaired or the patient may display a Hoover sign (page 65). Many of the patients exhibit abnormalities of the voice and visual fields, tremors, and weakness of muscle contraction.

Astasia-abasia—in which patients, though unable to either stand or walk, display more or less normal use of their legs while in bed and have an otherwise normal neurologic examination and body carriage—is nearly always a hysterical condition. When such patients are placed on their feet, they may take a few steps and then become unable to advance their legs; they lurch in all directions and crumple to the floor if not assisted. On the other hand, one should not assume that a patient who manifests a disorder of gait but no other neurologic abnormality is necessarily suffering from hysteria. Lesions that are restricted to the anterosuperior cerebellar vermis may cause an ataxia that becomes manifest only when the patient attempts to stand and walk; this is true of normal-pressure hydrocephlaus and frontal lobe disease as well (see above).

Rehabilitative Measures

Once the gait abnormality is stable, i.e., neither progressive nor regressive, one should explore the possibility of rehabilitation by a combination of medical therapy and other corrective measures. The antispasticity agents baclofen and tizanidine are somewhat helpful when stiffness of the limbs exceeds weakness. They may reduce spasticity of the legs, but sometimes at the expense of exposing, to a greater degree than before, a loss of muscle power—the net effect being to the patient's disadvantage. Hypofunction of the labyrinths, as in drug-induced or idiopathic vestibulopathy, has greatly challenged physiatrists. Balance training and the more effective use of postural correction and vision have helped some of these patients to be more steady and better able to function in the activities of daily living and at work (Baloh and Honrubia). Exercises to strengthen leg muscles can be beneficial, as can weight loss. Likewise, gait ataxia from proprioceptive defects can probably be corrected to some extent by careful attention to visual control and proper placement of the feet. Some success has been reported by Heitmann and colleagues in training elderly who fall frequently. Ventricular shunting in idiopathic hydrocephalus has restored locomotion in patients with this syndrome. Once dementia becomes conjoined with any of the gait disorders that occur in older age, rehabilitation stands little chance of success, since the ability to attend to small changes in terrain and posture are lost. Progression from the use of a cane, to a pronged cane, and finally to a four-posted walker allows patients with all types of gait disorders to maintain some mobility. The optimal use of these orthoses is best directed by an experienced physical therapist.

REFERENCES

Atchison PR, Thompson PD, Frackowiak RS, Marsden CD: The syndrome of gait ignition failure: A report of six cases. *Mov Disord* 8:285, 1993.

Baloh RW, Honrubia V: *Clinical Neurophysiology of the Vestibular System*, 2nd ed. Philadelphia, Davis, 1990, pp 137–143.

Baloh RW, Yue Q, Socotch TM, Jacobson KM. White matter lesions and disequilibrium in older people: I. Case control comparison. *Arch Neurol* 52:970,1995.

Denny-Brown D: *The Basal Ganglia and Their Relation to Disorders of Movement*. London, Oxford University Press, 1962.

Eidelberg E, Walden JG, Nguyen LH: Locomotor control in macaque monkeys. *Brain* 104:647, 1981.

Fife TD, Baloh RW: Disequilibrium of unknown cause in older people. *Ann Neurol* 34:694, 1993.

Fisher CM: Hydrocephalus as a cause of disturbances of gait in the elderly. *Neurology* 32:1358, 1982.

Heitmann DK, Gossman MR, Shaddeau SA, Jackson JR: Balance performance and step width in noninstitutionalized, elderly, female fallers and nonfallers. *Phys Ther* 69:923, 1989.

Keane JR: Hysterical gait disorders. *Neurology* 39:586, 1989.

Lawrence DG, Kuypers HGSM: The functional organization of the motor system in the monkey: II. The effects of lesions of the descending brainstem pathways. *Brain* 91:15, 1968.

Martin JP: The basal ganglia and locomotion. *Ann R Coll Surg Engl* 32:219, 1963.

Masdeu JP, Sudarsky L, Wolfson L (eds): *Gait Disorders of Aging*. Philadelphia, Lippincott-Raven, 1997.

Meyer JS, Barron D: Apraxia of gait: A clinico-physiologic study. *Brain* 83:261, 1960.

Murray MP, Kory RC, Clarkson BH: Walking patterns in healthy old men. *J Gerontol* 24:169, 1969.

Nutt JG, Marsden CD, Thompson PD: Human walking and higher-level gait disorders, particularly in the elderly. *Neurology* 43:268, 1993.

Olsson E: Gait analysis in hip and knee surgery. *Scand J Rehabil Med Suppl* 15:1, 1986.

Ropper AH: Refined Romberg test. *Can J Neurol Sci* 12:282, 1985.

Sudarsky L: Geriatrics: Gait disorders in the elderly. *N Engl J Med* 322:1441, 1990.

Sudarsky L, Simon S: Gait disorder in late-life hydrocephalus. *Arch Neurol* 44:263, 1987.

Thompson PD, Marsden CD: Gait disorder of subcortical arteriosclerotic encephalopathy: Binswanger's disease. *Mov Disord* 2:1, 1987.

Tinetti ME, Williams CS: Falls, injuries due to falls, and the risk of admission to a nursing home. *N Engl J Med* 337:1279, 1997.

Yakovlev PI: Paraplegia in flexion of cerebral origin. *J Neuropathol Exp Neurol* 13:267, 1954.

Section 2

PAIN AND OTHER DISORDERS OF SOMATIC SENSATION, HEADACHE, AND BACKACHE

Chapter 8

PAIN

Pain, it has been said, is one of "nature's earliest signs of morbidity," and it stands pre-eminent among all the sensory experiences by which humans judge the existence of disease within themselves. Indeed, pain is the most common symptom of disease. Relatively few diseases do not have a painful phase, and in many pain is a characteristic without which diagnosis must be in doubt.

The painful experiences of the sick pose manifold problems in virtually every field of medicine, and physicians must learn something of these problems and their management if they are to practice their profession effectively. They must be prepared to recognize disease in patients who have felt only the first rumblings of discomfort, before other symptoms and signs have appeared. Even more problematic are patients who seek treatment for pain that appears to have little or no structural basis; further inquiry may disclose that fear of serious disease, worry, or depression has aggravated some relatively minor ache or that the complaint of pain has become the means of seeking drugs or monetary compensation. They must also cope with the "difficult" pain cases in which no amount of investigation brings to light either medical or psychiatric illness. Finally, the physician must be prepared to manage patients who demand relief from intractable pain caused by established and incurable disease. To deal intelligently with such pain problems requires familiarity with the anatomy of sensory pathways and the sensory supply of body segments as well as insight into the psychologic factors that influence the perception of and reaction to pain.

The dual nature of pain is responsible for some of our difficulty in understanding it. One aspect, the easier to comprehend, is its evocation by particular stimuli and the transmission of pain impulses along certain pathways, i.e., the sensation of pain. Far more abstruse is its quality as a mental state intimately linked to emotion, i.e., the quality of anguish or suffering—"a passion of the soul," in the words of Aristotle—which defies definition and quantification. This duality is of practical importance, for certain drugs or surgical procedures, such as cingulotomy, may reduce the patient's reaction to painful stimuli, leaving his awareness of the sensation largely intact. Alternatively, interruption of certain neural pathways may abolish all sensation in an affected part, but the symptom of pain may persist (i.e., denervation dysesthesia or anesthesia dolorosa), even in an amputated limb ("phantom pain"). Unlike most sensory modalities—which are aroused by a specific stimulus such as touch-pressure, heat, or cold—pain can be evoked by any one of these stimuli if it is intense enough.

It is apparent to the authors that in highly specialized medical centers, and often even in "pain centers", few physicians are capable of handling difficult and unusual pain problems in any comprehensive way. In fact, it is to the neurologist that other physicians regularly turn for help with these matters. Although much has been learned about the anatomy of pain pathways, their physiologic mechanisms, and which structures to ablate in order to produce analgesia, relatively little is known about which patients should be subjected to these destructive operations or how to manage their pain by medical means. Here is a subspecialty that should challenge every thoughtful physician, for it demands the highest skill in medicine, neurology, and psychiatry.

ANATOMY AND PHYSIOLOGY OF PAIN

Historical Perspective

For more than a century, views on the nature of pain sensation have been dominated by two major theories. One, known as the *specificity theory*, was from the beginning associated with the name of von Frey. He asserted that the skin consisted of a mosaic of discrete sensory spots and that each spot, when stimulated, gave rise to one sensation—either pain, pressure, warmth, or cold; in his view, each of these sensations had a distinctive end organ in the skin and each stimulus-specific end organ was connected by its own private pathway to the brain. A second theory was that of Goldscheider, who abandoned his own earlier discovery of pain spots to argue that they simply represented pressure spots, a sufficiently intense stimulation of which could produce pain. According to the latter theory, there were no distinctive pain receptors, and the sensation of pain was the result of the summation of impulses excited by pressure or thermal stimuli applied to the skin. Originally called the intensivity theory, it later became known as the *pattern* or *summation theory*.

In an effort to conciliate the pattern and specificity theories, Head and his colleagues, in 1905, formulated a novel concept of pain sensation, based on observations that followed division of the cutaneous branch of the radial nerve in Head's own forearm. The zone of impaired sensation contained an innermost area in which superficial sensation was completely abolished. This was surrounded by a narrower ("intermediate") zone, in which pain sensation was preserved but poorly localized; extreme degrees of temperature were recognized in the intermediate zone, but perception of touch, lesser differences of temperature, and two-point discrimination were abolished. To explain these findings, Head postulated the existence of two systems of cutaneous receptors and conducting fibers: (1) an ancient *protopathic* system, subserving pain and extreme differences in temperature and yielding ungraded, diffuse impressions of an all-or-none type, and (2) a more recently evolved *epicritic* system, which mediated touch, two-point discrimination, and lesser differences in temperature as well as localized pain. The pain and hyperesthesia that follow damage to a peripheral nerve were attributed to a loss of inhibition that was normally exerted by the epicritic upon the protopathic system. This theory was used for many years to explain the sensory alterations that occur with both peripheral and central (thalamic) lesions. It lost credibility for several reasons, but mainly because Head's original observations (and deductions upon which they were based) could not be corroborated (see Trotter and Davies; also Walshe). Nevertheless, both a fast and a slow form of pain conduction were later corroborated (see below).

A much later refinement of the pattern and specificity concepts of pain was made in 1965, when Melzack and Wall propounded their "gate-control" theory. They observed, in decerebrate and spinal cats, that peripheral stimulation of large myelinated fibers produced a negative dorsal root potential and that stimulation of small C (pain) fibers caused a positive dorsal root potential. They postulated that these potentials, which were a reflection of presynaptic inhibition or excitation, modulated the activity of secondary transmitting neurons (T cells) in the dorsal horn, and that this modulation was mediated through inhibitory (I) cells. The essence of this theory is that the large-diameter fibers excite the I cells, which, in turn, cause a presynaptic inhibition of the T cells; conversely, the small pain afferents inhibit the I cells, leaving the T cells in an excitatory state. Melzack and Wall emphasized that pain impulses from the dorsal horn must also be under the control of a descending system of fibers from the brainstem, thalamus, and limbic lobes.

At first the gate-control mechanisms seemed to offer an explanation of the pain of ruptured disc and of certain chronic neuropathies (large fiber outfall), and attempts were made to relieve pain by subjecting the peripheral nerves and dorsal columns (presumably their large myelinated fibers) to sustained, transcutaneous electrical stimulation. Such selective stimulation would theoretically "close" the gate. In some clinical situations, these procedures have indeed given relief from pain, but not necessarily due to stimulation of large myelinated fibers alone (see Taub and Campbell). And in a number of other instances relating to pain in large- and small-fiber neuropathies, the clinical behavior has been quite out of keeping with what one would expect on the basis of the gate-control mechanism. As with preceding pain theories, flaws have been exposed in the physiologic observations on which the theory is based. These and other aspects of the gate-control theory of pain have been critically reviewed by P. W. Nathan.

During the last few decades there has been a significant accrual of information on cutaneous sensibility, demanding a modification of earlier anatomic-physiologic and clinical concepts. Interestingly, much of this information is still best described and rationalized in the general framework of specificity, as will be evident from the ensuing discussion on pain and that on other forms of cutaneous sensibility in the chapter that follows.

Pain Receptors and Peripheral Afferent Pathways

In terms of peripheral pain mechanisms, as already implied, there is indeed a high degree of specificity, though not an absolute specificity in the von Frey sense. It is now well established that two types of afferent fibers in the distal axons of primary sensory neurons respond maximally to nociceptive (i.e., potentially tissue-damaging) stimuli. One type is the very fine, unmyelinated, slowly conducting C fiber (0.4 to 1.1 mm in diameter), and the other is the thinly myelinated, more rapidly conducting A-delta (A-δ) fiber (1.0 to 5.0 mm in diameter). The peripheral terminations of both these primary pain afferents, or receptors, are the free, profusely branched nerve endings in the skin and other organs; these are covered by Schwann cells and contain little or no myelin.

There is considerable evidence, based on their response characteristics, that a degree of subspecialization exists within these freely branching, nonencapsulated endings and their small fiber afferents. Three broad categories of free endings, or receptors, are recognized: mechanoreceptors, thermoreceptors, and polymodal nociceptors. Each ending transduces stimulus energy into an action potential in nerve membranes. The first two types of receptors are activated by innocuous mechanical and thermal stimulation, respectively; the mechanoeffects are transmitted by both A-δ and C fibers and the thermal effects only by C fibers. The polymodal afferents are most effectively excited by noxious or tissue-damaging stimuli, but they can respond as well to both mechanical and thermal stimuli and to chemical mediators such as those associated with inflammation. Moreover, certain A-δ fibers respond to light touch, temperature, and pressure as well as to pain stimuli and are capable of discharging in proportion to the intensity of the stimulus. The stimulation of single fibers by intraneural electrodes indicates that they can also convey information concerning the nature and location of the stimulus (local sign). These observations on the polymodal functions of A-δ and C fibers would explain the earlier observations of Lele and Weddell that modes of sensation other than pain can be evoked from structures such as the cornea, which is innervated solely by free nerve endings.

The peripheral afferent pain fibers of both A-δ and C types have their cell bodies in the dorsal root ganglia; central extensions of these nerve cells project, via the dorsal root, to the dorsal horn of the spinal cord (or, in the case of cranial pain afferents, to the nucleus of the trigeminal nerve, the medullary analogue of the dorsal horn). The pain afferents occupy mainly the lateral part of the root entry zone. Within the spinal cord, many of the thinnest fibers (C fibers) form a discrete bundle, the tract of Lissauer (Fig. 8-1*A*). That Lissauer's tract is predominantly a pain pathway is shown (in animals) by the ipsilateral segmental analgesia that results from its transection, but it contains deep sensory, or propriospinal, fibers as well. Although it is customary to speak of a lateral and medial division of the posterior root (the former contains small pain fibers and the latter, large myelinated fibers), the separation into discrete functional bundles is not complete, and in humans the two groups of fibers cannot be differentially interrupted by selective rhizotomy.

Dermatomic Distribution of Pain Fibers

Each sensory unit (the sensory nerve cell in the dorsal root ganglion, its central and peripheral extensions, and cutaneous and visceral endings) has a unique topography that is maintained throughout the sensory system from the periphery to the sensory cortex. The discrete segmental distribution of the sensory units permits the construction of sensory maps, so useful to clinicians. This aspect of sensory anatomy is elaborated in the next chapter, which includes maps of the sensory dermatomes and cutaneous nerves. However, as a means of quick orientation to the topography of peripheral pain pathways, it is useful to remember that the facial structures and anterior cranium lie in the fields of the trigeminal nerves; the back of the head, second cervical; the neck, third cervical; the epaulet area, fourth cervical; the deltoid area, fifth cervical; the radial forearm and thumb, sixth cervical; the index and middle fingers, seventh cervical; the little finger and ulnar border of hand and forearm, eighth cervical–first thoracic; the nipple, fifth thoracic; the umbilicus, tenth thoracic; the groin, first lumbar; the medial side of the knee, third lumbar; the great toe, fifth lumbar; the little toe, first sacral; the back of the thigh, second sacral; and the genitoanal zones, the third, fourth, and fifth sacrals. The distribution of pain fibers from deep structures, though not fully corresponding to those from the skin, also follows a segmental pattern. The first to fourth thoracic nerve roots are the important sensory pathways for the heart and lungs; the sixth to eighth thoracic, for the upper abdominal organs; and the lower thoracic and upper lumbar, for the lower abdominal viscera.

The Dorsal Horn

The afferent pain fibers, after traversing Lissauer's tract, terminate in the posterior gray matter or dorsal horn, predominantly in the marginal zone. Most of the fibers terminate within the segment of their entry into the cord; some extend ipsilaterally to one or two adjacent rostral and caudal segments; and some project, via the anterior commissure, to the contralateral dorsal horn. The cytoarchitectonic studies of Rexed in the cat (the same organization pertains in primates and probably in humans) have shown that second-order neurons, the sites of synapse of afferent sensory fibers in the dorsal horn, are arranged in a series of six layers or laminae (Fig. 8-1*B*). Fine, myelinated (A-δ) fibers terminate principally in lamina I of Rexed (marginal cell layer of Waldeyer) and also in the outermost part of lamina II; some A-δ pain fibers penetrate the dorsal gray matter and terminate in the lateral part of lamina V. Unmyelinated (C) fibers terminate in lamina II (substantia gelatinosa). Yet other

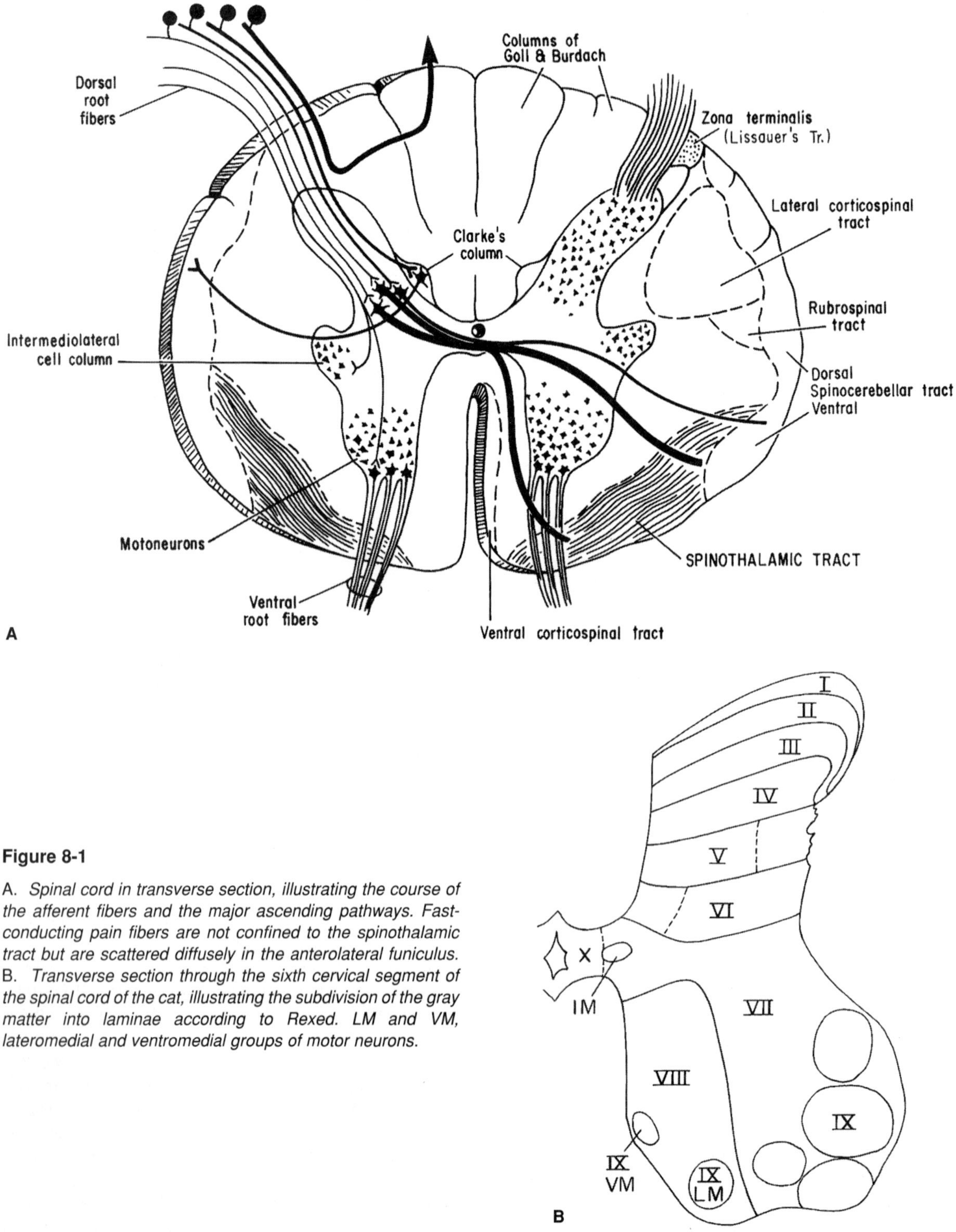

Dorsal root fibers
Columns of Goll & Burdach
Zona terminalis (Lissauer's Tr.)
Lateral corticospinal tract
Clarke's column
Rubrospinal tract
Intermediolateral cell column
Dorsal Spinocerebellar tract Ventral
Motoneurons
SPINOTHALAMIC TRACT
Ventral root fibers
Ventral corticospinal tract

A

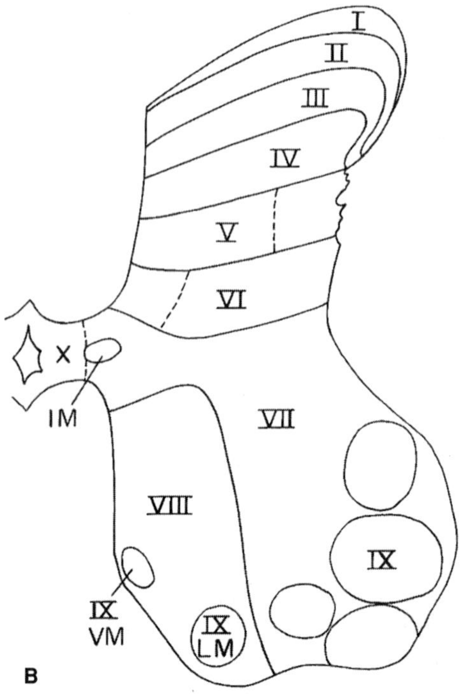

B

Figure 8-1

A. *Spinal cord in transverse section, illustrating the course of the afferent fibers and the major ascending pathways. Fast-conducting pain fibers are not confined to the spinothalamic tract but are scattered diffusely in the anterolateral funiculus.* B. *Transverse section through the sixth cervical segment of the spinal cord of the cat, illustrating the subdivision of the gray matter into laminae according to Rexed. LM and VM, lateromedial and ventromedial groups of motor neurons.*

cells that respond to painful cutaneous stimulation are located in ventral horn laminae VII and VIII. The latter neurons are responsive to descending impulses from brainstem nuclei as well as segmental sensory impulses. From these cells of termination, second-order axons connect with ventral and lateral horn cells in the same and adjacent spinal segments and subserve both somatic and autonomic reflexes. The main bundle of secondary neurons subserving pain sensation projects contralaterally (and to a lesser extent ipsilaterally) to higher levels.

In recent years, a number of important observations have been made concerning the mode of transmission and modulation of pain impulses in the dorsal horn and brainstem. Excitatory amino acids (glutamate, aspartate) and nucleotides such as adenosine triphosphate (ATP) are the putative transmitters at terminals of primary A-δ sensory afferents. Also, A-δ pain afferents, when stimulated, release several neuromodulators that play a role in the transmission of pain sensation. Slower neurotransmission by C neurons involves other substances, of which the most important is the 11–amino acid peptide known as substance P. In animals, substance P has been shown to excite nociceptive dorsal root ganglion and dorsal horn neurons; furthermore, destruction of substance P fibers produces analgesia. In patients with the rare condition of congenital neuropathy and insensitivity to pain, there is a marked depletion of dorsal horn substance P.

A large body of evidence indicates that opiates are important modulators of pain impulses that are relayed through the dorsal horn and centers in the medulla and pons. Thus, opiates have been noted to decrease substance P; at the same time, flexor spinal reflexes, which are evoked by segmental pain, are reduced. Opiate receptors of three types are found on both presynaptic primary afferent terminals and postsynaptic dendrites of small neurons in lamina II. Moreover, lamina II neurons, when activated, release enkephalins, endorphins, and dynorphins—all of which are endogenous, morphine-like peptides that bind specifically to opiate receptors and inhibit pain transmission at the dorsal horn level. The subject of pain modulation by opiates and endogenous morphine-like substances is elaborated further on.

Spinal Afferent Tracts for Pain

Lateral Spinothalamic Tract As indicated above, axons of secondary neurons that subserve pain sensation originate in laminae I, II, V, VII, and VIII of the spinal gray matter. The principal bundle of these axons decussates in the anterior spinal commissure and ascends in the anterolateral fasciculus to terminate in several brainstem and thalamic structures (Fig. 8-2). It is of clinical consequence that the axons from each dermatome decussate one to three segments above the level of root entry; in this way a discrete lesion of the lateral spinal cord creates a loss of pain and thermal sensation of the contralateral trunk, the dermatomal level of which is *two to three segments below that of the spinal cord lesion*. As the ascending fibers cross the cord, they are added to the inner side of the *spinothalamic tract* (the principal afferent pathway of the anterolateral fasciculus), so that the longest fibers from the sacral segments come to lie most superficially and fibers from successively more rostral levels occupy progressively deeper positions (Fig. 8-3). This somatotopic arrangement is of importance to the neurosurgeon insofar as the depth to which the funiculus is cut will govern the level of analgesia that is achieved; for the neurologist, it provides an explanation of the "sacral sparing" of sensation created by centrally placed lesions of the spinal cord.

Other Spinocerebral Afferent Tracts In addition to the lateral spinothalamic tract—the fast-conducting pathway that projects directly to the thalamus—the anterolateral fasciculus of the cord contains several more slowly conducting, medially placed systems of fibers. One such group of fibers projects directly to the reticular core of the medulla and midbrain and then to the medial and intralaminar nuclei of the thalamus; this group of fibers is referred to as the *spinoreticulothalamic* or *paleospinothalamic* pathway (Fig. 8-4). At the level of the medulla, these fibers synapse in the nucleus gigantocellularis; more rostrally, they connect with nuclei of the parabrachial region, midbrain reticular formation, periaqueductal gray matter, and hypothalamus. A second, more medially placed pathway ascends to the brainstem reticular core via a series of short interneuronal links. It is not clear whether these spinoreticular fibers are collaterals of the spinothalamic tracts, as Cajal originally stated, or whether they represent an independent system, as more recent data seem to indicate. Probably both statements are correct. There is also a third, direct spinohypothalamic pathway. All three spinoreticular fiber systems lie in the posteromedial part of the lateral column. The conduction of diffuse, poorly localized pain arising from deep and visceral structures (gut, periosteum) has been ascribed to these pathways. Melzack and Casey have proposed that this fiber system (which they refer to as *paramedian*), with its diffuse projection via brainstem and thalamus to the limbic and frontal lobes,

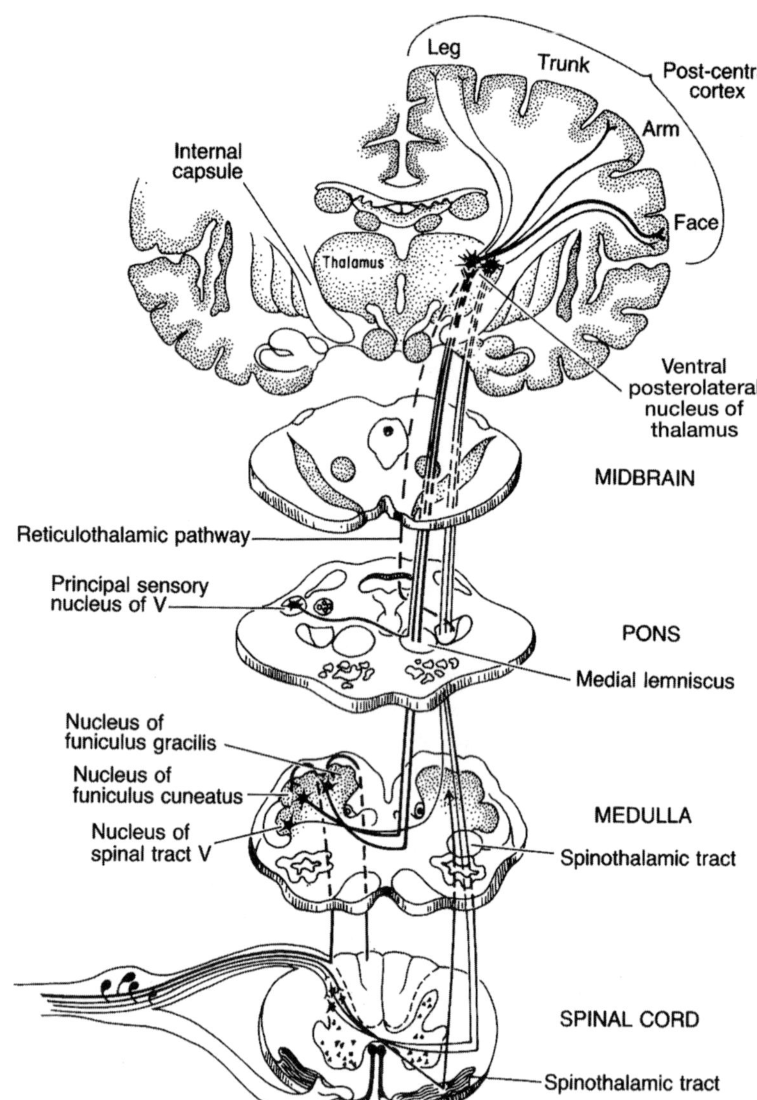

Figure 8-2

The main somatosensory pathways. Offsets from the ascending anterolateral fasciculus (spinothalamic tract) to nuclei in the medulla, pons, and mesencephalon and nuclear terminations of the tract are indicated in Fig. 8-4.

subserves the affective aspects of pain, i.e., the unpleasant feelings engendered by pain. It is evident that these spinoreticulothalamic pathways continue to evoke the psychic experience of pain even when the direct (anterolateral) spinothalamic pathways have been interrupted. However, it is the lateral pathway, which projects to the ventroposterolateral (VPL) nucleus of the thalamus and thence to discrete areas of the sensory cortex, that subserves the *sensory-discriminative* aspects of pain, i.e., the processes that underlie the localization, quality, and possibly the intensity of the noxious stimulus. Also, the pathways for *visceral pain* from the esophagus, stomach, small bowel, and proximal colon are carried largely in the vagus nerve and terminate in the nucleus of the solitary tract (NTS) before projecting to the thalamus, as described below. Other abdominal viscera still activate the NTS when the vagus is severed in animals, probably passing through the splanchnic plexus.

It should be emphasized that the foregoing data concerning the cells of termination of cutaneous nociceptive stimuli and the cells of origin of ascending spinal afferent pathways have all been obtained from studies in animals (including monkeys). In humans, the cells of origin of the long (direct) spinothalamic tract fibers have

Figure 8-3

Spinal cord showing the segmental arrangement of nerve fibers within major tracts. On the left side are indicated the "sensory modalities" that appear to be mediated by the two main ascending pathways. Note the broad zone close to the gray matter occupied by propriospinal fibers. C, cervical; L, lumbar; S, sacral; Th, thoracic. (Adapted by permission from Brodal A: Neurological Anatomy, *3rd ed. New York, Oxford University Press, 1981.)*

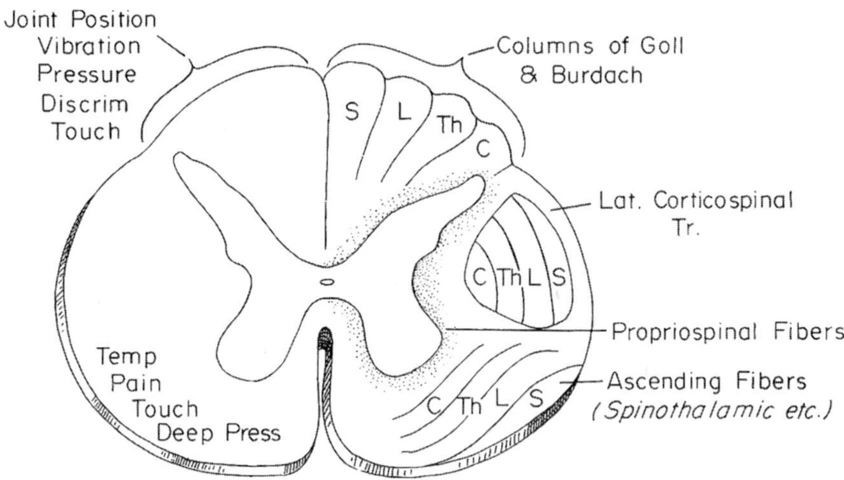

not been fully identified. Information about this pathway in humans has been derived from the study of postmortem material and from the examination of patients subjected to anterolateral cordotomy for intractable pain. As mentioned above, unilateral section of the anterolateral funiculus produces a relatively complete loss of pain and thermal sense on the opposite side of the body, extending to a level two or three segments below the lesion. After a variable period of time, pain sensation usually returns, probably being conducted by pathways that lie outside the anterolateral quadrants of the spinal cord and which gradually increase their capacity to conduct pain impulses. One of these is a longitudinal polysynaptic bundle of small myelinated fibers in the

Figure 8-4

The paleospinothalamic tract is illustrated on the right. This is a slow-conducting multineuron system that mediates poorly localized pain from deep somatic and visceral structures. On the left is the major descending inhibitory pathway, derived mainly from the periaqueductal gray matter and brainstem raphe nuclei. It modulates pain input at the dorsal horn level.

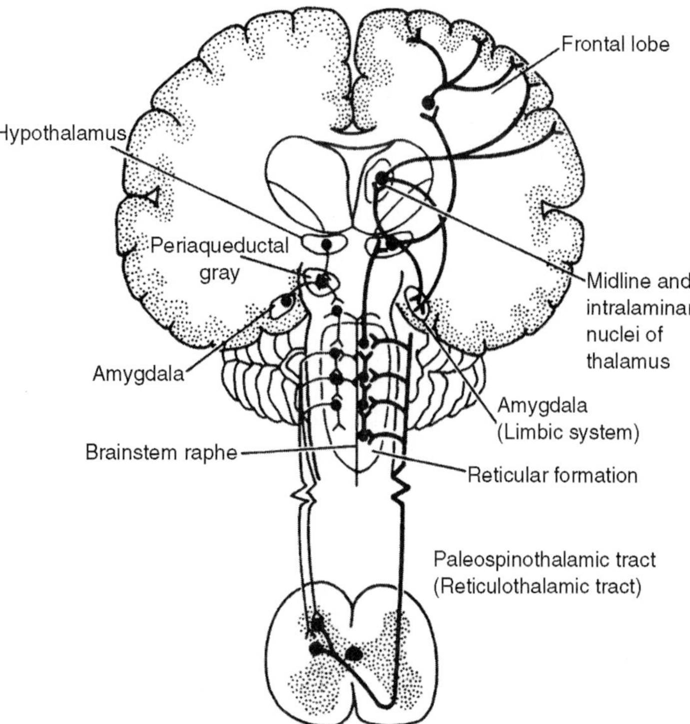

center of the dorsal horn (the dorsal intracornual tract); another consists of axons of lamina I cells that travel in the dorsal part of the lateral funiculus.

Thalamic Terminus of Pain Fibers

The direct spinothalamic fibers separate into two bundles as they approach the thalamus. The lateral division terminates in the ventrobasal and posterior groups of nuclei. The medial contingent terminates mainly in the intralaminar complex of nuclei and in the nucleus submedius. Spinoreticulothalamic (paleospinothalamic) fibers project onto the medial intralaminar (primarily parafascicular and centrolateral) thalamic nuclei; i.e., they overlap with the terminations of the medially projecting direct spinothalamic pathway. Projections from the dorsal column nuclei, which have a modulating influence on pain transmission, are mainly to the ventrobasal and ventroposterior group of nuclei. Each of the four thalamic nuclear groups that receives nociceptive projections from the spinal cord has a distinct cortical projection, and each is thought to play a different role in pain sensation (see below).

One practical conclusion to be reached from these anatomic and physiologic studies is that at thalamic levels, fibers and cell stations transmitting the nociceptive impulses are not organized into discrete loci. In general, neurophysiologic evidence indicates that as one ascends from peripheral nerve to spinal, medullary, mesencephalic, thalamic, and limbic levels, the predictability of neuron responsivity to noxious stimuli diminishes. Thus it comes as no surprise that neurosurgical procedures for interrupting afferent pathways become less and less successful at progressively higher levels of the brainstem and thalamus.

Thalamocortical Projections

The ventrobasal thalamic complex and the ventroposterior group of nuclei project to two main cortical areas: the primary sensory (postcentral) cortex (a small number terminate in the precentral cortex) and the upper bank of the sylvian fissure. These cortical areas are described more fully in Chap. 9, but it can be stated here that they are concerned mainly with the reception of tactile and proprioceptive stimuli and with all discriminative sensory functions, including pain. The extent to which either cortical area is activated by thermal and painful stimuli is uncertain. Certainly, stimulation of these (or any other) cortical areas in a normal, alert human being does not produce pain. The intralaminar nuclei, which also project to the hypothalamus, amygdaloid nuclei, and limbic cortex, probably mediate the arousal and affective aspects of pain and the autonomic responses.

Thalamic and cerebral cortical localization of visceral sensation is not well known. However, cerebral evoked potentials and increased cerebral blood flow (by PET studies) have been demonstrated in the thalamus and pre- and postcentral gyri of patients undergoing rectal balloon distention (Silverman et al; Rothstein et al).

Descending Pain-Modulating Systems

Of great importance was the discovery of a system of descending fibers and way stations that modulate activity in nociceptive pathways. The one system that has been studied most extensively emanates from the frontal cor-

Figure 8-5

Pain-modulating pathways in the CNS. Impulses originating in the frontal cortex and hypothalamus project to cells in the periaqueductal gray matter of the midbrain, which control dorsal horn pain transmission cells via cells in the rostroventral medulla. Details in text. (Adapted, by permission from Fields 1987.)

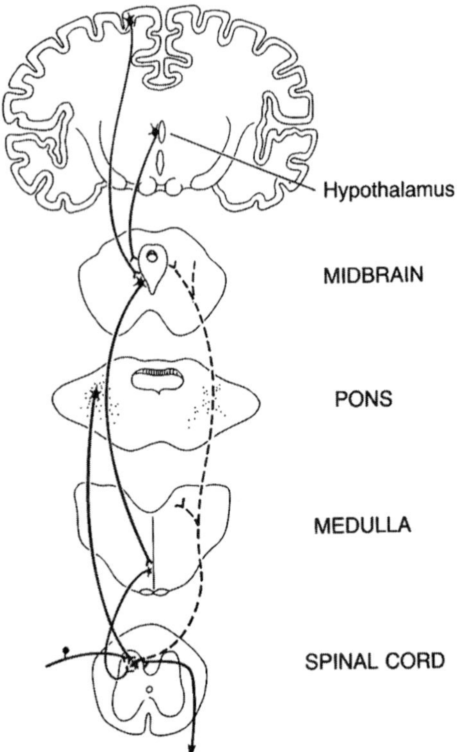

tex and hypothalamus and projects to cells in the periaqueductal region of the midbrain and then passes to the ventromedial medulla. From there it descends in the dorsal part of the lateral fasciculus of the spinal cord to the posterior horns (laminae I, II, and V; see further discussion under "Endogenous Pain-Control Mechanisms" and Fig. 8-5). Several other descending pathways, noradrenergic and serotoninergic, arise in the locus ceruleus, dorsal raphe nucleus, and nucleus reticularis gigantocellularis and are also important modifiers of the nociceptive response. The significance of these pain-modulating pathways is discussed further on.

PHYSIOLOGIC ASPECTS OF PAIN

The stimuli that activate pain receptors vary from one tissue to another. As pointed out above, the adequate stimulus for skin is one that has the potential to injure tissue, i.e., pricking, cutting, crushing, burning, and freezing. These stimuli are ineffective when applied to the stomach and intestine, where pain is produced by an engorged or inflamed mucosa, distention or spasm of smooth muscle, and traction on the mesenteric attachment. In skeletal muscle, pain is caused by ischemia (the basis of intermittent claudication), necrosis, hemorrhage, and injection of irritating solutions, as well as by injuries of connective tissue sheaths. Prolonged contraction of skeletal muscle evokes an aching type of pain. Ischemia is also the most important cause of pain in cardiac muscle. Joints are insensitive to pricking, cutting, and cautery, but pain can be produced in the synovial membrane by inflammation and by exposure to hypertonic saline. The stretching and tearing of ligaments around a joint can evoke severe pain. Injuries to the periosteum give rise to pain but probably not to other sensations. Arteries are a source of pain when pierced by a needle or involved in an inflammatory process. Distention of arteries, as occurs with thrombotic or embolic occlusion, and excessive arterial pulsation, as in migraine, may be sources of pain; other mechanisms of headache relate to traction on arteries and the meningeal structures by which they are supported (see Chap. 10). Pain due to intraneural lesions probably arises from the sheaths of the nerves. Nerve root(s) and sensory ganglia, when compressed (e.g., by a ruptured disc), give rise to pain.

With damage to tissue, there is a release of proteolytic enzymes, which act locally on tissue proteins to liberate substances that excite peripheral nociceptors. These pain-producing substances—which include histamine, prostaglandins, serotonin, and similar polypeptides as well as potassium ions—elicit pain when they are injected intra-arterially or applied to the base of a blister. Other pain-producing substances such as kinins are released from sensory nerve endings or are carried there by the circulation. Also, vascular permeability may be increased by these substances.

In addition, direct stimulation of nociceptors releases polypeptide mediators that enhance pain perception. The best-studied of these is substance P, which is released from the nerve endings of C fibers in the skin during peripheral nerve stimulation. It causes erythema by dilating cutaneous vessels and edema by releasing histamine from mast cells; it also acts as a chemoattractant for leukocytes. This reaction, called *neurogenic inflammation* by White and Helme, is mediated by antidromic action potentials from the small nerve cells in the spinal ganglia and is the basis of the axon reflex of Lewis. This reaction is abolished in certain peripheral nerve diseases and can be studied electrophysiologically as an aid to clinical localization.

Perception of Pain

The *threshold for perception of pain*, i.e., the lowest intensity of a stimulus recognized as pain, is approximately the same in all persons. It is lowered by inflammation, a process that is called *sensitization* and is clinically important because in sensitized tissues ordinarily innocuous stimuli can produce pain. The pain threshold is, of course, raised by local anesthetics and by certain lesions of the nervous system as well as by centrally acting analgesic drugs. Mechanisms other than lowering or raising the pain threshold are important as well. Placebos reduce pain in about one-third of the groups of patients in which such effects have been recorded. Acupuncture at sites anatomically remote from painful operative fields apparently reduces the pain in some individuals. Distraction and suggestion, by turning attention away from the painful part, reduce the awareness of and response to pain. Strong emotion (fear or rage) suppresses pain, presumably by activation of the above-described descending adrenergic system. The experience of pain appears to be lessened in manic states and enhanced in depression. Neurotic patients in general have the same pain threshold as normal subjects, but their reaction may be excessive or abnormal. The pain thresholds of frontal lobotomized subjects are also unchanged, but they react to painful stimuli only briefly or casually if at all. The degrees of emotional reaction and verbalization (complaint) also vary with the personality and character of the patient.

The conscious awareness or perception of pain occurs only when pain impulses reach the thalamocortical level. The precise roles of the thalamus and cortical sensory areas in this mental process are not fully understood, however. For many years it was taught that the recognition of a noxious stimulus as such is a function of the thalamus and that the parietal cortex is necessary for appreciation of the intensity, localization, and other discriminatory aspects of sensation. This traditional separation of sensation (in this instance awareness of pain) and perception (awareness of the nature of the painful stimulus) has been abandoned in favor of the view that sensation, perception, and the various conscious and unconscious responses to a pain stimulus comprise an indivisible process. That the cerebral cortex governs the patient's reaction to pain cannot be doubted, however. It is also likely that the cortex can suppress or otherwise modify the perception of pain in the same way that corticofugal projections from the sensory cortex modify the rostral transmission of other sensory impulses from thalamic and dorsal column nuclei. It has been shown that central transmission in the spinothalamic tract can be inhibited by stimulation of the sensorimotor areas of the cerebral cortex, and, as indicated above, a number of descending fiber systems have been traced to the dorsal horn laminae from which this tract originates.

Endogenous Pain-Control Mechanisms

In recent years, the most important contribution to our understanding of pain has been the discovery of a neuronal analgesia system, which can be activated by the administration of opiates or by naturally occurring brain substances with the pharmacologic properties of opiates. This endogenous system was first demonstrated by Reynolds, who found that stimulation of the ventrolateral periaqueductal gray matter in the rat produced a profound analgesia without altering behavior or motor activity. Subsequently, stimulation of other discrete sites in the medial and caudal regions of the diencephalon and rostral bulbar nuclei (notably raphe magnus and paragigantocellularis) were shown to have the same effect. Under the influence of such electrical stimulation, the animal could be operated upon without anesthesia and move around in an undisturbed manner despite the administration of noxious stimuli. Investigation disclosed that the effect of stimulation-produced analgesia (SPA) is to inhibit the neurons of laminae I, II, and V of the dorsal horn, i.e., the neurons that are activated by noxious stimuli. In human subjects, stimulation of the midbrain periaqueductal gray matter through stereotactically implanted electrodes has also produced a state of analgesia, though not consistently. Other sites in which electrical stimulation is effective in suppressing nociceptive responses are the rostroventral medulla (nucleus raphe magnus and adjacent reticular formation) and the dorsolateral pontine tegmentum. These effects are relayed to the dorsal horn gray matter via a pathway in the dorsolateral funiculus of the spinal cord. Ascending pathways from the dorsal horn, conveying noxious somatic impulses, are also important in activating the modulatory network. These connections are illustrated in Fig. 8-5.

As indicated earlier, opiates also act pre- and postsynaptically on the neurons of laminae I and V of the dorsal horn, suppressing afferent pain impulses from both the A-δ and C fibers. Furthermore, these effects can be reversed by the narcotic antagonist naloxone. Interestingly, naloxone can reduce some forms of stimulation-produced analgesia. Levine and colleagues have demonstrated that not only does naloxone enhance clinical pain but it also interferes with the pain relief produced by placebos. These observations suggest that the heretofore mysterious beneficial effects of placebos (and perhaps of acupuncture) may be due to activation of an endogenous system that shuts off pain through the release of pain-relieving endogenous opioids, or *endorphins* (see below). Prolonged pain and fear are the most powerful activators of this endogenous opioid-mediated modulating system. The same system is probably operative under a variety of other stressful conditions; for example, some soldiers, wounded in battle, require little or no analgesic medication ("stress-induced analgesia"). The opiates also act at several loci in the brainstem, at sites corresponding with those producing analgesia when stimulated electrically and generally conforming to areas in which neurons with endorphin receptors are localized.

Soon after the discovery of specific opiate receptors in the central nervous system (CNS), several naturally occurring peptides, which proved to have a potent analgesic effect and to bind specifically to opiate receptors, were identified (Hughes et al). These endogenous, morphine-like compounds are generically referred to as *endorphins*, meaning "the morphines within." The most widely studied of these compounds are β-endorphin, a peptide sequence of the pituitary hormone β-lipotropin, and two other peptides, *enkephalin* and *dynorphin*. They are found in greatest concentration in relation to opiate receptors in the midbrain. At the level of the spinal cord, opiate receptors are essentially enkephalin receptors. A theoretical construct of the roles

Figure 8-6

Theoretical mechanism of action of enkephalin (endorphin) and morphine on the transmission of pain impulses from the periphery to the CNS. Spinal interneurons containing enkephalin synapse with the terminals of pain fibers and inhibit the release of the presumptive transmitter, substance P. As a result, the receptor neuron in the dorsal horn receives less excitatory (pain) impulses and transmits fewer pain impulses to the brain. Morphine binds to unoccupied enkephalin receptors, mimicking the pain-suppressing effects of the endogenous opiate enkephalin.

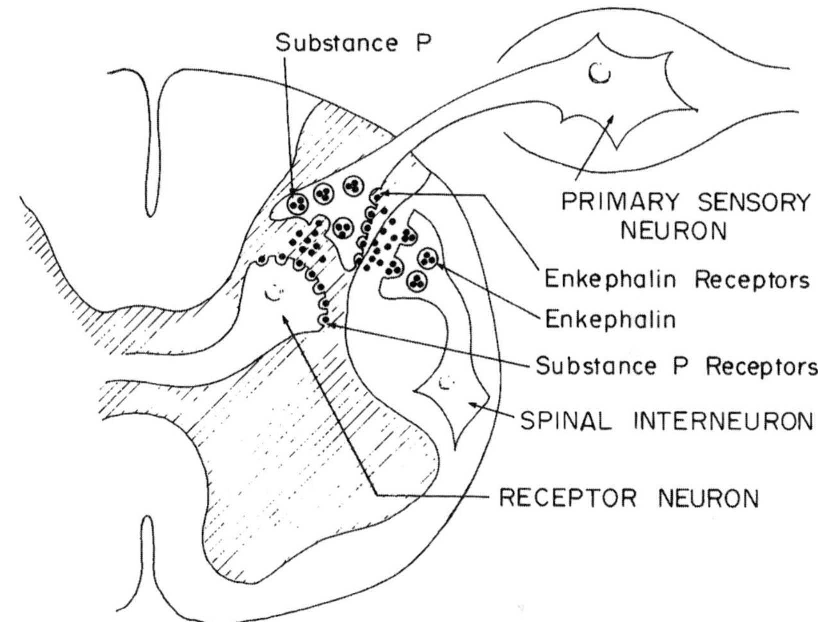

of enkephalin (and substance P) at the point of entry of pain fibers into the spinal cord is illustrated in Fig. 8-6. A subgroup of dorsal horn interneurons also contain enkephalin; they are in contact with spinothalamic tract neurons.

Thus it would appear that the central effects of a painful condition are determined by many ascending and descending systems utilizing a variety of transmitters. A deficiency in a particular region would explain persistent or excessive pain. Opiate addiction might conceivably be accounted for in this way, and also the discomfort that follows withdrawal of the drug. Indeed, it is known that some of these peptides not only relieve pain but suppress withdrawal symptoms. It has been speculated that in the limbic regions, disturbances in the formation of neurotransmitters could be the basis of unpleasant and distressing emotional states (e.g., depression).

Finally it should be noted that the descending pain-control systems probably contain noradrenergic and serotoninergic as well as opiate links. A descending norepinephrine-containing pathway, as mentioned, has been traced from the dorsolateral pons to the spinal cord, and its activation blocks spinal nociceptive neurons. The rostroventral medulla contains a large number of serotoninergic neurons. Descending fibers from the latter site inhibit dorsal horn cells concerned with pain transmission, perhaps providing a rationale for the use of certain serotonin agonists in patients with chronic pain.

CLINICAL AND PSYCHOLOGIC ASPECTS OF PAIN

Terminology Several terms related to the experience of altered sensations and pain are often used interchangeably, but each has specific meaning. *Hyperesthesia* is a general term for heightened cutaneous sensitivity. The term *hyperalgesia* refers to an increased sensitivity and a lowered threshold to painful stimuli. Inflammation and burns of the skin are common causes of hyperalgesia. The term *hypalgesia*, or *hypoalgesia*, refers to the opposite state—i.e., a decreased sensitivity and a raised threshold to painful stimuli. A demonstrable defect in pain perception (i.e., an elevated threshold) in the affected part, associated with an increased reaction to the stimulus once it is perceived, is sometimes referred to as *hyperpathia* (subtly different from hyperalgesia). In this circumstance there is an excessive reaction to all stimuli, even those (such as light touch) that normally do not evoke pain, a symptom termed *allodynia*. The elicited allodynic pain may have unusual features, being diffuse, modifiable by fatigue, emotion, etc., and often mixed with other sensations. The mechanism of these abnormalities is not clear, but both hyperpathia and allodynia are common features of neuropathic or neurogenic pain, i.e., pain generated by peripheral neuropathy. These features are exemplified by causalgia, a special type of burning pain that results from interruption of a peripheral nerve (see page 1438).

Skin Pain and Deep Sensibility As indicated earlier, the nerve endings in each tissue are activated by different mechanisms, and the pain that results is characterized by its quality, locale, and temporal attributes. *Skin pain* is of two types: a pricking pain, evoked immediately on penetration of the skin by a needle point, and a stinging or burning pain, which follows in a second or two. Together they constitute the "double response" of Lewis. Both types of dermal pain can be localized with precision. Ischemia of nerve by the application of a tourniquet to a limb abolishes pricking pain before burning pain. The first (fast) pain is thought to be transmitted by the larger (A-δ) fibers and the second (slow) pain, which is somewhat more diffuse and longer-lasting, by the thinner, unmyelinated C fibers.

Deep pain from visceral and skeletomuscular structures is basically aching in quality; if intense, it may be sharp and penetrating (knife-like). Occasionally there is a burning type of pain, as in the "heartburn" of esophageal irritation and rarely in angina pectoris. The pain is felt as being deep to the body surface. The pain is diffuse and poorly localized, and the margins of the painful zone are not well delineated, presumably because of the relative paucity of nerve endings in viscera.

Referred Pain The localization of deep pain raises a number of problems. Although deep pain has indefinite boundaries, its location always bears a fixed relationship to the skeletal or visceral structure that is involved. It tends to be referred not to the skin overlying the viscera of origin but to other areas of skin innervated by the same spinal segment (or segments). This pain, projected to some fixed site at a distance from the source, is called *referred pain*. Small-caliber pain afferents from deep structures project to a wide range of lamina V neurons in the dorsal horn, as do cutaneous afferents. The convergence of deep and cutaneous afferents on the same dorsal horn cells, coupled with the fact that cutaneous afferents are far more numerous than visceral afferents and have direct connections with the thalamus, probably explains the phenomenon of referred pain.

Since the nociceptive receptors and nerves of any given visceral or skeletal structure may project upon the dorsal horns of several adjacent spinal or brainstem segments, the pain may be fairly widely distributed. For example, afferent pain fibers from cardiac structures, distributed through segments T1 to T4, may be projected superficially to the inner side of the arm and the ulnar border of the hand and arm (T1 and T2) as well as the precordium (T3 and T4). Once this pool of sensory neurons in the dorsal horns of the spinal cord is activated, additional noxious stimuli may heighten the activity in the whole sensory field ipsilaterally and, to a lesser extent, contralaterally.

Another peculiarity of localization is aberrant reference, explained by an alteration of the physiologic status of the pools of neurons in adjacent segments of the spinal cord. For example, cervical arthritis or gallbladder disease, causing low-grade discomfort by constantly activating their particular segmental neurons, may induce a shift of cardiac pain cephalad or caudad from its usual locale. Any pain, once it becomes chronic, may spread quite widely in a vertical direction on one side of the body. On the other hand, painful stimuli arising from a distant site exert an inhibitory effect upon segmental nociceptive flexion reflexes in the leg (DeBroucker et al). Yet another clinical peculiarity of segmental pain is the reduction in power of muscle contraction that it may cause (reflex paralysis, or algesic weakness).

In an injured nerve, the unmyelinated sprouts of A-δ and C fibers become capable of spontaneous ectopic excitation and afterdischarge and susceptible to ephaptic activation (Rasminsky). They are also sensitive to locally applied or intravenous catecholamines because there are adrenergic receptors on the regenerating fibers. Either this mechanism or ephapsis (nerve-to-nerve cross-activation) is thought to be the basis of causalgia and other forms of reflex sympathetic dystrophy; either mechanism would explain the relief afforded by sympathetic block. This subject is discussed in greater detail in relation to peripheral nerve injuries (see page 1438).

Central sensory structures, e.g., sensory neurons in the dorsal horns of the spinal cord or thalamus, if chronically bombarded with pain impulses, may become autonomously overactive (being maintained in this state perhaps by excitatory amino acids) and may remain so after the peripheral pathways have been interrupted. Peripheral nerve lesions have been shown to induce enduring derangements of central (spinal cord) processing (Fruhstorfer and Lindblom). Avulsion of nerves or nerve roots may cause chronic pain even in analgesic zones (anesthesia dolorosa or "deafferentation pain"). In experimentally deafferented animals, neurons of lamina V begin to discharge irregularly in the absence of stimulation. Later the abnormal discharge subsides in the spinal cord but can still be recorded in the thalamus. Hence, painful states such as causalgia, spinal cord pain, and phantom pain are not abolished simply by cutting spinal nerves or spinal tracts.

Pain has several other singular attributes. It does not appear to be subject to negative adaptation—i.e., pain may persist as long as the stimulus is operative—

whereas other somatic stimuli, if applied continuously, soon cease to be effective. Furthermore, prolonged stimulation of pain receptors sensitizes them, so that they become responsive to even low grades of stimulation, such as touch (allodynia). Another remarkable characteristic of pain is the strong feeling or affect with which it is endowed, nearly always unpleasant. Since pain has this affective element, psychologic conditions assume great importance in all persistent painful states. It is of interest that despite this strong affective aspect of pain, it is difficult to recall precisely, or to re-experience from memory, a previously experienced acute pain. Also, the patient's tolerance of pain and capacity to experience it without verbalization are influenced by race, culture, and religion. Some individuals—by virtue of training, habit, and phlegmatic temperament—remain stoic in the face of pain, and others react in an opposite fashion. Pain may be the presenting or predominant symptom in a depressive illness (Chap. 57).

Finally, a comment should be made about the devastating behavioral effects of chronic pain. To quote from Ambroise Paré, a sixteenth-century French surgeon, "There is nothing that abateth so much the strength as paine." Continuous pain increases irritability and fatigue, disturbs sleep, and impairs appetite. Ordinarily strong persons can be reduced to a whimpering, pitiable state that may arouse the scorn of healthy observers. Patients in pain may seem irrational about their illness and make unreasonable demands on family and physician. Characteristic also is an unwillingness to engage in or continue any activity that might enhance their pain. They withdraw from the main current of daily affairs. Their thoughts and speech come to be dominated by the pain. Once a person is subjected to the tyranny of chronic pain, depressive symptoms are practically always added. The demand for and dependence on narcotics often complicate the clinical problem.

APPROACH TO THE PATIENT WITH PAIN AS THE PREDOMINANT SYMPTOM

One learns quickly in dealing with such patients that not all pain is the consequence of serious disease. Every day, healthy persons of all ages have pains that must be taken as part of normal sensory experience. To mention a few, there are the "growing pains" of children; the momentary hard pain over an eye or in the temporal or occipital regions, which strikes with such suddenness as to raise the suspicion of a ruptured intracranial aneurysm; the more persistent ache in the fleshy part of the shoulder, hip, or extremity that subsides spontaneously or in response to a change in position; the fluctuant precordial discomfort of gastrointestinal origin, which conjures up fear of cardiac disease; the breathtaking "stitch in the side," due to intercostal or diaphragmatic cramp. These normal pains, as they should be called, tend to be brief and to depart as obscurely as they came. Such pains come to notice only when elicited by an inquiring physician or when experienced by a patient given to worry and introspection. They must always be distinguished from the pain of disease.

Whenever pain—by its intensity, duration, and the circumstances of its occurrence—appears to be abnormal or when it constitutes the chief complaint or one of the principal symptoms, the physician must attempt to reach a tentative decision as to its mechanism and cause. This is accomplished by a thorough interrogation of the patient, with the physician carefully seeking out the main characteristics of the pain in terms of

1. Location
2. Mode of onset
3. Provoking and relieving factors
4. Quality and time-intensity attributes
5. Duration
6. Severity

Knowledge of these factors in every common disease is the lore of medicine. The severity of pain is often difficult to assess. Extreme degrees of pain are betrayed by the patient's demeanor, but lesser degrees can be roughly estimated by the extent to which the pain has interfered with the patient's sleep, work, and other activities or by the patient's need for bed rest. Some physicians find it helpful, particularly in gauging the effects of analgesic agents, to use a "pain scale," i.e., to have the patient rate the intensity of his pain on a scale of zero (no pain) to ten (worst pain) or to mark it on a line. Needless to say, this general approach is put to use every day in the practice of internal medicine. Together with the physical examination, including tests designed to reproduce and relieve the pain, and ancillary diagnostic procedures, it enables the physician to identify the source of most pains and the diseases of which they are a part.

Once the pains due to the more common and readily recognized diseases of each organ system are eliminated, there remain a significant number of chronic pains that fall into one of four categories: (1) pain from an obscure medical disease, the nature of which has not yet been disclosed by diagnostic procedures; (2) pain associated with disease of the central or peripheral nervous system (i.e., neurogenic or neuropathic pain); (3) pain associated with psychiatric disease; and (4) pain of unknown cause.

Pain due to Undiagnosed Medical Disease

Here the source of the pain is usually peripheral and caused by a lesion that irritates and destroys nerve endings. Hence the term *nociceptive pain* is often used, but it is ambiguous. It usually means an involvement of structures bearing the termination of pain fibers. Carcinomatosis is the most frequent example. Osseous metastases, peritoneal implants, invasion of retroperitoneal tissues or the hilum of the lung, and implication of nerves of the brachial or lumbosacral plexuses can be extremely painful, and the origin of the pain may remain obscure for a long time. Sometimes it is necessary to repeat all diagnostic procedures after an interval of a few months, even though at first they were negative. From experience one learns to be cautious about reaching a diagnosis from insufficient data. Treatment is directed to the relief of pain, at the same time instilling in the patient a need to cooperate with a program of expectant observation.

Neurogenic, or Neuropathic, Pain

These terms are generally used interchangeably to designate pain that arises from direct stimulation of nervous tissue itself, central or peripheral, exclusive of pain due to stimulation of sensitized C fibers (i.e., the nociceptive pain described above). This category comprises a variety of disorders involving single and multiple nerves, notably trigeminal neuralgia and those due to herpes zoster, diabetes, and trauma (including causalgia); a number of polyneuropathies of diverse type; root irritation, e.g., from a prolapsed disc; spinal arachnoiditis and spinal cord injuries; the thalamic pain syndrome of Déjerine-Roussy; and rarely parietal lobe infarction (Schmahmann and Leifer). The clinical features that characterize central pain have been reviewed by Schott. As a rule, lesions of the cerebral cortex and white matter are associated not with pain but with hypalgesia. Particular diseases giving rise to neuropathic pain are considered in their appropriate chapters. The following remarks are of a general nature, applicable to all of the painful states that compose this group.

The features that characterize neurogenic and neuropathic pain are their persistence and generally poor response to analgesic medication; their burning, gnawing, aching, and often shooting or lancinating quality; their frequent association with hyperesthesia, hyperalgesia, allodynia, and hyperpathia (see above); the presence in many cases of a sensory deficit and some autonomic dysfunction; and the variable temporal relationship of the pain to the disease of which it is an expression.

Peripheral Nerve Pain Painful states that fall into this category are in most cases related to disease of the peripheral nerves, and it is to pain from this source that the term *neuropathic* is more strictly applicable. Pain states of peripheral nerve origin far outnumber those due to spinal cord, brainstem, thalamic, and cerebral disease. Although the pain is localized to a sensory territory supplied by a nerve plexus or nerve root, it often radiates to adjacent areas. Sometimes the onset of pain is immediate on receipt of injury; more often it appears at some point during the evolution or recession of the disorder. The disease of the nerve may be obvious, expressed by the usual sensory, motor, reflex, and autonomic changes, or these changes may be undetectable by standard tests. In the latter case, the term *neuralgia* is the preferred term.

The postulated mechanisms of peripheral nerve pain are diverse and probably differ from those of central diseases. In peripheral nerve, one mechanism is denervation hypersensitivity, first described by Walter Cannon. He noted that when a group of neurons is deprived of its natural innervation, they become hyperactive. Some neurologists point to a reduced density of certain types of fibers in nerves supplying a causalgic zone as the basis of the burning pain, but the comparison of nerves from painful and nonpainful neuropathies has not proved to be consistently different. Dyck and colleagues, in a study of painful versus nonpainful axonal neuropathies, concluded that there was no difference between them in terms of the type of fiber degeneration. The occurrence of ectopic impulse generation all along the surface of injured axons and the possibility of ephaptic activation of unsheathed axons seems applicable particularly to causalgic states in which nerve pain appears to be abolished by sympathetic denervation. Stimulation of the nervi nervorum of larger nerves by an expanding intraneural lesion or a vascular change was postulated by Asbury and Fields as the mechanism of nerve trunk pain. Regenerating axonal sprouts, as in a neuroma, are also hypersensitive to mechanical stimuli. On a molecular level, it has been shown that sodium channels accumulate at the site of a neuroma and all along the axon after nerve injury, and this gives rise to ectopic and spontaneous activity of the sensory nerve cell and nerve fiber.

Such firing has been demonstrated in humans after nerve injury. This mechanism is concordant with the relief of neurogenic pain by sodium channel–blocking anticonvulsants. Spontaneous activity in nociceptive C fibers is thought to give rise to burning pain; firing of large myelinated A fibers is believed to produce dysesthetic pain induced by tactile stimuli. The abnormal response to stimulation is also influenced by sensitization of central pain pathways. Hyperalgesia is proposed to result from such a mechanism (see Woolf and Mannion). Possibly more than one of these mechanisms is operative in a given peripheral nerve disease.

Central Pain In central lesions, deafferentation of secondary neurons in the posterior horns or of sensory ganglion cells that terminate on them may cause the deafferented cells to become continuously active and, if stimulated by a microelectrode, to reproduce pain. In the patient whose spinal cord has been transected, there may be intolerable pain in regions below the level of the lesion. It may be exacerbated or provoked by movement, fatigue, or emotion and projected to areas disconnected from suprasegmental structures (akin to the phantom pain in the missing part of an amputated limb). Here, and in the rare cases of intractable pain with lateral medullary or pontine lesions, loss of the descending inhibitory systems seems a likely explanation. This may also explain the pain of the Déjerine-Roussy thalamic syndrome described on page 172. Altered sensitivity and hyperactivity of central neurons is an alternative possibility.

Further details concerning the subject of neuropathic pain can be found in the writings of Scadding and of Woolf and Mannion (see References).

Pain in Association with Psychiatric Diseases

It is not unusual for patients with endogenous depression to have pain as the predominant symptom. And most patients with chronic pain of all types are depressed. Wells and colleagues, in a survey of a large number of depressed and chronic pain patients, have convincingly corroborated this clinical impression. Fields has elaborated a theoretical explanation of the overlap of pain and depression. In such cases one is faced with an extremely difficult clinical problem—that of determining whether a depressive state is primary or secondary. In some instances the diagnostic criteria cited in Chap. 57 provide the answer, but in others it is impossible to make this distinction. Empiric treatment with antidepressant medication or, failing this, with electroconvulsive therapy is one way out of the dilemma.

Intractable pain may be the leading symptom of both hysteria and compensation neurosis. Every experienced physician is familiar with the "battle-scarred abdomen" of the woman with hysteria (so-called Briquet disease) who has demanded and yielded to one surgical procedure after another, losing appendix, ovaries, fallopian tubes, uterus, gallbladder, etc., in the process ("diagnosis by evisceration"). The recognition and management of hysteria are discussed in Chap. 56.

Compensation neurosis is often colored by persistent complaints of headaches, neck pain (whiplash injuries), low-back pain, etc. The question of ruptured disc is often raised, and laminectomy and spinal fusion may be performed (sometimes more than once) on the basis of dubious radiologic findings. Complaints of weakness and fatigue, depression, anxiety, insomnia, nervousness, irritability, palpitations, etc., are woven into the clinical syndrome, attesting to the prominence of psychiatric disorder. Long delay in settlement of litigation, allegedly to determine the seriousness of the injury, only enhances the symptoms and prolongs the disability. The medical and legal professions have no certain approach to such problems and often work at cross-purposes. We have found that a frank, objective appraisal of the injury, an assessment of the psychiatric problem, and encouragement to settle the legal claims as quickly as possible work in the best interests of all concerned. While hypersuggestibility and relief of pain by placebos, etc., may reinforce the physician's belief that there is a prominent factor of hysteria or malingering (see Chap. 56), such data are difficult to interpret and are not acceptable in court.

Chronic Pain of Indeterminate Cause

This is the most difficult group of all—pain in the thorax, abdomen, flank, back, face, or other part that cannot be traced to any visceral abnormality. Supposedly all neurologic sources, such as a spinal cord tumor, have been excluded by repeated examinations and imaging procedures. A psychiatric disorder to which the patient's symptoms and behavior might be attributed cannot be discerned. Yet the patient complains continuously of pain, is disabled, and spends a great deal of effort and money seeking medical aid.

In such a circumstance, some physicians and surgeons, rather than concede their helplessness, may resort to extreme measures such as exploratory thoracotomy, laparotomy, or laminectomy. Or they may injudiciously attempt to alleviate the pain and avoid drug addiction by severing roots and spinal tracts, often with the result that the pain moves to an adjacent segment or to the other side of the body.

This type of patient should be seen frequently by the physician. All the medical facts should be reviewed and the clinical and laboratory examinations repeated if some time has elapsed since they were last done. Tumors in the hilum of the lung or mediastinum, in the retropharyngeal, retroperitoneal, and paravertebral spaces, or in the uterus, testicle, kidney, and prostate offer special difficulty in diagnosis, often being undetected for many months. Neurofibroma causing pain in an unusual site, such as one side of the rectum or vagina, is another type of tumor that may defy diagnosis for a long time. Neurologic pain is almost invariably accompanied by alterations in cutaneous sensation and other neurologic signs, the finding of which facilitates diagnosis; the appearance of the neurologic signs may be long delayed, however. The possibility of drug addiction as a motivation should be eliminated. It is impossible to assess pain in the addicted individual, for the patient's complaints are woven into his need for medication. Temperament and mood should be evaluated carefully from day to day; the physician must remember that the depressed patient often denies being depressed and may occasionally smile. When no medical, neurologic, or psychiatric disease can be established, one must be resigned to managing the painful state by the use of nonnarcotic medications and frequent clinical re-evaluations. Such a course, though not altogether satisfactory, is preferable to prescribing excessive opioids or subjecting the patient to ablative surgery.

Because of the complexity and difficulty in diagnosis and treatment of chronic pain, most medical centers have found it advisable to establish *pain clinics*. Here a staff of internists, anesthesiologists, neurologists, neurosurgeons, and psychiatrists are able to review each patient in terms of drug dependence, neurologic disease, and psychiatric problems. Success is achieved by treating each aspect of chronic pain, with emphasis on increasing the patient's tolerance of pain by means of biofeedback, meditation and related techniques, by using special invasive anesthetic special procedures (discussed later in the chapter), by establishing a regimen of pain medication, and by controlling depressive illness.

Rare and Unusual Disturbances of Pain Perception

Lesions of the parieto-occipital regions of one cerebral hemisphere sometimes have peculiar effects on the patient's capacity to feel and react to pain. Under the title of *pain hemiagnosia*, Hecaen and Ajuriaguerra described several cases of left-sided paralysis from a right parietal lesion which, at the same time, rendered the patient hypersensitive to noxious stimuli. When pinched on the affected side, the patient, after a delay, became agitated, moaned, and seemed distressed but made no effort to fend off the painful stimulus with the other hand or to withdraw from it. In contrast, if the good side was pinched, the patient reacted normally and moved the normal hand at once to the site of the stimulus to remove it. The motor responses seem no longer to be guided by sensory information from one side of the body.

There are also two varieties of rare individuals who from birth are totally indifferent to pain ("congenital insensitivity to pain") or are incapable of feeling pain ("universal analgesia"). The former have an uncertain congenital deficiency of a neurotransmitter or an equally obscure peculiarity of the central receptive apparatus (see Chap. 9), and the second group suffers from either a congenital lack of pain neurons in dorsal root ganglia, a polyneuropathy, or a lack of pain receptors in the primary afferent neuron.

The phenomenon of *asymbolia for pain* is another rare and unusual condition, wherein the patient, although capable of distinguishing the different types of pain stimuli from one another and from touch, is said to make none of the usual emotional, motor, or verbal responses to pain. This patient seems totally unaware of the painful or hurtful nature of stimuli delivered to any part of the body, whether on one side or the other. The current interpretation of asymbolia for pain is that it represents a particular type of agnosia (analgagnosia) or apractagnosia (cf. Chap. 22), in which the organism loses its ability to adapt its emotional, motor, and verbal actions to the consciousness of a nociceptive impression. "*Le sujet a perdu la compréhension de la signification de la douleur*." We have been unable to corroborate the existence of this syndrome from our own clinical experience.

Treatment of Intractable Pain

Once the nature of the patient's pain and underlying disease have been determined, therapy must include some type of pain control. Initially, of course, attention is directed to the underlying disease, with the idea of eliminating the source of the pain by appropriate medical, surgical, or radiotherapeutic measures.

If the patient is ridden with disease and will not live more than a few weeks or months, is opposed to surgery, or has widespread pain, surgical measures are out of the question. However, pain from widespread osseous metastases, even in patients with hormone-insensitive tumors, may be relieved by radiation therapy or by hypophysectomy. Pain confined to a restricted area of the jaw or face may be relieved by nerve root blocks; by radiofrequency destruction of the trigeminal nerve, roots, or ganglion; or in some cases by decompressive surgery of an aberrant vascular loop that abuts a root in the posterior fossa. Usually, nerve section is not a satisfactory way of relieving restricted pain of the trunk and limbs because the overlap of adjacent nerves prevents complete denervation. Another procedure to be considered before undertaking the section of several contiguous sensory roots is the regional delivery of narcotic analogues, such as fentanyl or ketamine, by means of an external pump and a catheter that is implanted percutaneously in the epidural space in proximity to the dorsal nerve roots in the affected region; this device can be used safely at home.

If radiation therapy and other medical and surgical measures are not feasible or fail to relieve the pain, a program utilizing analgesic medication must be undertaken. Central to such a program is the use of opioids, which to this day represent the most effective analgesic agents for the management of severe chronic pain due to medical disease.

A useful way in which to undertake the management of chronic pain that affects several parts of the body, as in the patient with metastases, is with codeine, oxycodone, or propoxyphene taken together with aspirin, acetaminophen, or another nonsteroidal anti-inflammatory agent. The analgesic effects of these two types of drugs are additive, which is not the case when narcotics are combined with diazepam or phenothiazine. Antidepressants may have a beneficial effect on pain, even in the absence of overt depression. This is true particularly in cases of neuropathic pain (painful polyneuropathy and some types of radicular pain). Sometimes these nonnarcotic agents may in themselves or in combination with other treatment modalities be sufficient to control the patient's pain, and the use of narcotics can be kept in reserve.

Use of Opioids and Opiates Should the foregoing measures prove to be ineffective, one must turn to more potent narcotic agents. Methadone and levorphanol are the most useful drugs with which to begin, because of their effectiveness by mouth and the relatively slow development of tolerance. The oral route should be utilized whenever possible, since it is more comfortable for the patient than the parenteral route. Also, the oral route is associated with less side effects, except for nausea and vomiting, which tend to be worse than with parenteral administration. Should the latter become necessary, one must be aware of the ratios of oral to parenteral dosages required to produce equivalent analgesia. These are indicated in Table 8-1.

If oral medication fails to control the pain, the parenteral administration of codeine or more potent opioids becomes necessary. Again, one may begin with methadone, dihydromorphone (Dilaudid), or levorphanol, given at intervals of 4 to 6 h, because of their relatively long duration of action (particularly in comparison to meperidine). Alternatively, one may first resort to the use of transdermal patches of drugs such as fentanyl, which provide relief for 24 to 72 h and which we have found particularly useful in the treatment of pain from brachial or lumbosacral plexus invasion by tumor. Long-acting morphine preparations are useful alternatives. Should long-continued injections of opiates become necessary, the optimal dose for the relief of pain should be established and the drug then given at regular intervals around the clock, rather than "as needed." The administration of morphine (and other narcotics) in this way represents a laudable shift in attitude among physicians. For many years it was taught that the drug should be given in the smallest possible doses, spaced as far apart as possible, and repeated only when severe pain reasserted itself. It has become clear that such usage of the drug results in unnecessary discomfort and, in the end, the need to use larger doses. The fear of creating narcotic dependence and the expected phenomenon of increasing tolerance must be balanced against the overriding need to relieve pain. The most pernicious aspect of addiction, that of compulsive drug-seeking behavior and self-administration of the drug, occurs only rarely in this setting and usually in patients with a previous history of addiction or alcoholism, with depression as the primary problem, or with certain character defects that have been loosely referred to as "addiction proneness." Even in patients with severe acute or postoperative pain, the best results are obtained by allowing the patient to determine the dose and frequency of intravenous medication, so-called patient-controlled analgesia, or PCA. Again, the danger of producing addiction is minimal.

Excellent guidelines for the use of orally and parenterally administered opioids for cancer-related pain

Table 8-1
Common drugs for the management of chronic pain

Nonopioid analgesics			
Generic name	*Oral dose, mg*	*Interval*	*Comments*
Acetylsalicylic acid	650	q4h	Enteric-coated preparations available
Acetaminophen	650	q4h	Side effects uncommon
Ibuprofen	400	q4–6h	
Naproxen	250–500	q12h	Delayed effects may be due to long half-life
Ketorolac	10–20	q4–6h	Useful postoperatively and for weaning from narcotics. Can be used IM
Trisalicylate	1000–1500	q12h	Fewer gastrointestinal or platelet effects
Indomethacin	25–50	q8h	Gastrointestinal side effects common
Tramadol	50	q6h	Potent nonnarcotic with similar side effects but less respiratory depression

Narcotic analgesics			
Generic name	*Oral dose, mg*	*Interval*	*Comments*
Codeine	30–60	q4h	Nausea common
Oxycodone	—	5–10 q4–6h	Usually available only combined with acetaminophen or aspirin
Morphine	10 q4h	60 q4h	
Morphine, sustained release	—	90 q12h	Oral slow-release preparation
Hydromorphone	1–2 q4h	2–4 q4h	Shorter-acting than morphine sulfate
Levorphanol	2 q6–8h	4 q6–8h	Longer-acting than morphine sulfate; absorbed well orally
Methadone	10 q6–8h	20 q6–8h	Delayed sedation due to long half-life
Meperidine	75–100 q3–4h	300 q4h	Poorly absorbed orally; normeperidine is a toxic metabolite
Fentanyl	—	—	Parenteral and transcutaneous ("patch") use

Anticonvulsants and related drugs		
Generic name	*Oral dose, mg*	*Interval*
Phenytoin	100	q6–8h
Carbamazepine	200–300	q6h
Clonazepam	1	q6h
Mexiletine	150–200	q4–6h
Gabapentin	300–2700	q8h

Tricyclic antidepressants

Generic name	*Sedative potency*	*Anticholinergic potency*	*Orthostatic hypotension*	*Cardiac arrhythmia*	*Dose, mg/day*	*Range, ng/l00 mL*
Doxepin	High	Mod	Mod	Less	200	75–400
Amitriptyline	High	Highest	Mod	Yes	150	75–300
Imipramine	Mod	Mod	High	Yes	200	75–400
Nortriptyline	Mod	Mod	Low	Yes	100	40–150
Desipramine	Low	Low	Low	Yes	150	75–300

are contained in the article of Cherny and Foley and in the publication of the U.S. Department of Health and Human Services (see References).

The regimen outlined above conforms with current information about pain-control mechanisms. Aspirin and other nonsteroidal anti-inflammatory analgesics are believed to prevent the activation of nociceptors by inhibiting the synthesis of prostaglandins in skin, joints, viscera, etc. Morphine and meperidine given orally, parenterally, or intrathecally presumably produce analgesia by acting as "false" neurotransmitters at receptor sites in the posterior horns of the spinal cord—sites that are normally activated by endogenous opioid peptides (see Fig. 8-5). The separate sites of action of nonsteroidal analgesics and opioids provide an explanation for the therapeutic usefulness of combining these drugs. Yet another mechanism, described earlier in this chapter, consists of the physiologic activation of the intrinsic analgesic system (descending pathways from brain to spinal cord) by electrical stimulation, administration of placebo, and possibly acupuncture; short bursts of transcutaneous electrical stimulation may also suppress pain in this way. Not only do opioids act directly on the central pain-conducting sensory systems but they also exert a powerful action on the affective component of pain. Serotoninergic neurons are also thought to play a role in pain modulation.

Other Supplemental Medications Tricyclic antidepressants, especially the methylated forms (imipramine, amitriptyline, and doxepin), block serotonin reuptake and thus enhance the action of this neurotransmitter at synapses and putatively facilitate the action of the intrinsic opiate analgesic system. As a general rule, relief is afforded with tricyclic antidepressants in the equivalent dose range of 75 to 125 mg daily of amitriptyline, but little benefit accrues with higher doses. The newer serotoninergic antidepressants seem not to be as effective for the treatment of chronic neuropathic pain (see review by McQuay and colleagues), but these agents have not yet been extensively investigated in this clinical condition.

Anticonvulsants have a beneficial effect on many central and peripheral neuropathic pain syndromes but are generally less effective for causalgic pain due to partial injury of a peripheral nerve. The mode of action of phenytoin, carbamazepine, neurontin, and other anticonvulsants in suppressing the lancinating pains of tic douloureux and certain polyneuropathies as well as pain after spinal cord injury and myelitis is not understood. The biphosphate compound pamidronate, known to relieve several painful bone disorders, is being adopted increasingly for the treatment of causalgic pain, but the precise indications for its use remain to be defined.

The use of analgesic (nonnarcotic and narcotic), anticonvulsant, and antidepressant drugs in the management of chronic pain are summarized in Table 8-1.

Treatment of Neuropathic Pain

The treatment of pain induced by nerve root compression or intrinsic peripheral nerve disease utilizes several special techniques, some of which fall in the province of the anesthesiologist. If the pain is regional and has a predominantly burning quality, capsaicin cream can be applied locally, care being taken to avoid contact with the eyes and mouth. The irritative effect of this chemical seems in some cases to mute the pain. Concoctions of "eutectic" mixtures of local anesthetic creams (EMLA) and the simpler lidocaine gel preparation may provide relief in postherpetic neuralgia and painful peripheral neuropathies.

Injections of epidural corticosteroids or mixtures of analgesic and steroids are helpful in selected cases of lumbar or thoracic nerve root pain and occasionally in painful peripheral neuropathy, but precise criteria for the use of this measure are not well established. Root blocks with lidocaine or with longer-acting local anesthetics are helpful at times in establishing the precise source of radicular pain. Their main therapeutic use in our experience has been for thoracic radiculitis from shingles, chest wall pain after thoracotomy, and diabetic radiculopathy. Similar local injections are used in the treatment of occipital neuralgia.

The infusion of lidocaine has a brief beneficial effect on many types of pain, including neuropathic varieties, localized headaches, and facial pain, and it is said to be useful in predicting the response to longer-acting agents such as its oral analogue, mexiletine, although this relationship has been erratic in our experience (see Table 8-1). Mexiletine is given in an initial dose of 150 mg per day and slowly increased to a maximum of 300 mg three times daily; it should be used very cautiously in patients with heart block.

Finally, reducing sympathetic activity within somatic nerves by direct injection of the sympathetic ganglia in affected regions of the body (stellate ganglion for arm pain and lumbar ganglia for leg pain) has met with mixed success in neuropathic pain, including that of causalgia and reflex sympathetic dystrophy. A variant of this technique utilizes regional intravenous infusion of a sympathetic blocking drug (bretylium, guanethidine, reserpine) into a limb that is isolated from the systemic circulation by the use of a tourniquet. It is known as a "Bier block," after the developer of regional anesthesia for single-limb surgery. The use of these techniques, and the intravenous infusion of the adrenergic blocker phentolamine, is predicated on the concept of "sympathetically sustained pain," meaning pain that is mediated by the interaction of sympathetic and pain nerve fibers ("false synapse" or "ephapsis") or by the sprouting of adrenergic axons in partially damaged nerves. This form of treatment is still under study, but the most consistent responses to sympathetic blockade are obtained in cases of true causalgia that results from partial nerve injury and in reflex sympathetic dystrophy. These pain syndromes have been referred to by a number of different names, most recently as the "complex regional pain syndrome," but all refer to the same constellation of burning and other regional pains that may or may not conform to a nerve or root distribution (see page 1438). A number of other treatments have proven successful in some patients with reflex sympathetic dystrophy, but the clinician should not be sanguine about their chances of success over the long run. Perhaps the most novel and promising of these has been the use of bisphosphonates (pamidronate, alendronate), which have been beneficial in painful disorders of bone, e.g., Paget disease and metastatic bone lesions. Another treatment of last resort is the epidural infusion of drugs such as ketamine; sometimes this has a lasting effect on causalgic pain.

The therapeutic approaches enumerated here are usually undertaken in sequence. They reflect the general ineffectiveness of currently available treatments and our uncertainty as to the mechanisms of neuropathic pain. There are occasional successes, most of them temporary. Further references can be found in the article by Katz.

Use of Ablative Surgery in the Control of Pain

It is the authors' considered opinion that a program of medical therapy should always precede ablative surgical measures. Only when a variety of analgesic medications (including opioids) combined with phenothiazines and anticonvulsants, and only when certain practical measures, such as regional analgesia or anesthesia, have completely failed should one turn to neurosurgical procedures. Also, one should be very cautious in suggesting a procedure of last resort for pain that has no established cause, as, for example, limb pain that has been incorrectly identified as causalgic because of a burning component of the pain but in which there has been no nerve injury.

The least destructive procedure consists of implantation of an electrical stimulator, usually adjacent to the posterior columns. This procedure, which enjoyed a brief period of popularity, affords only incomplete relief and is difficult to maintain in place; it is now little used. The use of nerve section and dorsal rhizotomy as definitive measures for the relief of regional pain has already been discussed, under "Treatment of Intractable Pain," above.

Spinothalamic tractotomy, in which the anterior half of the spinal cord on one side is sectioned at an upper thoracic level, effectively relieves pain in the opposite leg and lower trunk. This may be done as an open operation or as a transcutaneous procedure in which a radiofrequency lesion is produced by an electrode. The analgesia and thermoanesthesia may last a year or longer, after which the level of analgesia tends to descend and the pain to return. Bilateral cordotomy is also feasible, but with greater risk of loss of sphincteric control and, at higher levels, of respiratory paralysis. Motor power is nearly always spared because of the position of the corticospinal tract in the posterior part of the lateral funiculus.

Pain in the arm, shoulder, and neck is more difficult to relieve surgically. High cervical transcutaneous cordotomy has been used successfully, with achievement of analgesia up to the chin. Commissural myelotomy by longitudinal incision of the anterior or posterior commissure of the spinal cord over many segments has also been performed, with variable success. Lateral medullary tractotomy is another possibility but must be carried almost to the midline to relieve cervical pain. The risks of this latter procedure and also of lateral mesencephalic tractotomy (which may actually produce pain) are so great that neurosurgeons have to all intents abandoned these operations.

Stereotactic surgery on the thalamus for one-sided chronic pain is still used in a few clinics, and the results have been instructive. Lesions placed in the ventroposterior nucleus are said to diminish pain and thermal sensation over the contralateral side of the body while leaving the patient with all the misery or affect of pain; lesions in the intralaminar or parafascicular-centromedian nuclei relieve the painful state without altering sensation (Mark). Since these procedures have not yielded predictable benefits to the patient, they are now seldom practiced. The same unpredictability pertains to cortical ablations. Patients in whom a severe depression of mood is associated with a chronic pain syndrome have been subjected to bilateral stereotactic cingulotomy or the equivalent, subcaudate tractotomy. A considerable degree of success has been claimed for these operations, but the results are difficult to evaluate. Orbitofrontal leukotomy has been virtually discarded because of the personality change that it produces (see Chap. 22).

Unconventional Methods for the Treatment of Pain

Included under this heading are certain techniques such as biofeedback, meditation, imagery, acupuncture, some forms of spinal manipulation, as well as transcutaneous electrical stimulation. Each of these may be of value in the context of a comprehensive pain management program, conducted usually in a pain clinic, as a means of providing relief from pain and suffering, reducing anxiety, and diverting the patient's attention, even if only temporarily, from the painful body part. Attempts to quantify the benefits of these techniques—judged usually by a reduction of drug dosage in response to a particular form of treatment—have given mixed results. Nevertheless, it is unwise for physicians to dismiss these methods out of hand, since well-motivated and apparently well-balanced persons have reported subjective improvement with one or another of these methods and, in the final analysis, this is what really matters. Conventional psychotherapy in combination with the use of medication and, at times, of electroconvulsive therapy can be of great benefit in the treatment of associated depressive symptoms, as discussed above (under "Pain in Association with Psychiatric Disease").

REFERENCES

Amit Z, Galina ZH: Stress-induced analgesia: Adaptive pain suppression. *Physiol Rev* 66:1091, 1986.

Asbury AK, Fields HL: Pain due to peripheral nerve damage: An hypothesis. *Neurology* 34:1587, 1984.

Cherny NI, Foley KM: Nonopioid and opioid analgesic pharmacotherapy of cancer pain. *Hematol Oncol Clin North Am* 10:79, 1996.

Cline MA, Ochoa J, Torebjork HE: Chronic hyperalgesia and skin warming caused by sensitized C nociceptors. *Brain* 112:621, 1989.

DeBroucker TH, Cesaro P, Willer JC, LeBars D: Diffuse noxious inhibitory controls in man: Involvement of the spinoreticular tract. *Brain* 113:1223, 1990.

Dyck PJ, Lambert EH, O'Brien PC: Pain in peripheral neuropathy related to rate and kind of fiber degeneration. *Neurology* 26:466, 1976.

Fields HL (ed): *Pain Syndromes in Neurology*. London, Butterworth, 1990.

Fields NL: Depression and pain: A neurobiological model. *Neuropsychiatry Neuropsychol Behav Neurol* 4:83, 1991.

Fields HL: *Pain*. New York, McGraw-Hill, 1987.

Fields HL, Heinricher MM, Mason P: Neurotransmitters in nociceptive modulatory circuits. *Annu Rev Neurosci* 14:219, 1991.

Fields HL, Levine JD: Placebo analgesia—A role for endorphins? *Trends Neurosci* 7:271, 1984.

Friehs GM, Schröttner O, Pendl G: Evidence for segregated pain and temperature conduction within the spinothalamic tract. *J Neurosurg* 83:8, 1995.

Fruhstorfer H, Lindblom U: Sensibility abnormalities in neuralgic patients studied by thermal and tactile pulse stimulation, in von Euler C et al (eds): *Somatosensory Mechanisms*. New York, Plenum Press, 1984, pp 353–361.

Goldscheider A: *Ueber den Schmerz in Physiologischer und Klinischer Hinsicht*. Berlin, Hirschwald, 1884.

Head H, Rivers WHR, Sherren J: The afferent nervous system from a new aspect. *Brain* 28:99, 1905.

Hecaen H, Ajuriaguerra J: Asymbolie à la douleur, étude anatomoclinique. *Rev Neurol* 83:300, 1950.

Hughes J (ed): Opioid peptides. *Br Med Bull* 39:1, 1983.

Hughes J, Smith TW, Kosterlitz HW, et al: Identification of two related pentapeptides from the brain with potent opiate agonist activity. *Nature* 258:577, 1975.

Katz N: Role of invasive procedures in chronic pain management. *Semin Neurol* 14:225, 1994.

Lele PP, Weddell G: The relationship between neurohistology and corneal sensibility. *Brain* 79:119, 1956.

Levine JD, Gordon NC, Fields HL: The mechanism of placebo analgesia. *Lancet* 2:654, 1978.

Light AR, Perl ER: Peripheral sensory systems, in Dyck PJ, Thomas PK, et al (eds): *Peripheral Neuropathy*, 3rd ed. Philadelphia, Saunders, 1993, pp 149–165.

Mark VH: Stereotactic surgery for the relief of pain, in White JC, Sweet WH (eds): *Pain and the Neurosurgeon*. Springfield, IL, Charles C Thomas, 1969, chap 18, pp 843–887.

McQuay HJ, Tramer M, Nye BA, et al: A systematic review of antidepressants in neuropathic pain. *Pain* 68:217, 1996.

Melzack R, Casey KL: Localized temperature changes evoked in the brain by somatic stimulation. *Exp Neurol* 17:276, 1967.

Melzack R, Wall PD: Pain mechanism: A new theory. *Science* 150:971, 1965.

Mountcastle VB: Central nervous mechanisms in sensation, in Mountcastle VB (ed): *Medical Physiology*, 14th ed. Vol 1, Part 5. St Louis, Mosby, 1980, chaps 11–19, pp 327–605.

Nathan PW: The gate-control theory of pain: A critical review. *Brain* 99:123, 1976.

Rasminsky M: Ectopic impulse generation in pathologic nerve fibers, in Dyck PJ et al (eds): *Peripheral Neuropathy*, 2nd ed. Vol 1. Philadelphia, Saunders, 1984, chap 40, pp 911–918.

Rexed B: A cytotectonic atlas of the spinal cord in the cat. *J Comp Neurol* 100:297, 1954.

Reynolds DV: Surgery in the rat during electrical analgesia induced by focal brain stimulation. *Science* 164:444, 1969.

Rothstein RD, Stecker M, Reivich M, et al: Use of positron emission tomography and evoked potentials in the detection of cortical afferents from the gastrointestinal tract. *Am J Gastroenterol* 91:2372, 1996.

SCADDING JW: Neuropathic pain, in Asbury AK, McKhann GM, McDonald WI (eds): *Diseases of the Nervous System: Clinical Neurobiology*, 2nd ed. Philadelphia, Saunders, 1992, pp 858–872.

SCHMAHMANN JD, LEIFER D: Parietal pseudothalamic pain syndrome: Clinical features and anatomic correlates. *Arch Neurol* 49:1032, 1992.

SCHOTT GD: From thalamic syndrome to central poststroke pain. *J Neurol Neurosurg Psychiatry* 61:560, 1995.

SILVERMAN DH, MUNAKATA JA, ENNES H, et al: Regional cerebral activity in normal and pathological perception of visceral pain. *Gastroenterology* 112:64, 1997.

SINCLAIR D: *Mechanisms of Cutaneous Sensation*. Oxford, England, Oxford University Press, 1981.

SNYDER SH: Opiate receptors in the brain. *N Engl J Med* 296:266, 1977.

TAUB A, CAMPBELL JN: Percutaneous local electrical analgesia: Peripheral mechanisms, in *Advances in Neurology*. Vol 4: *Pain*. New York, Raven Press, 1974, pp 727–732.

TROTTER W, DAVIES HM: Experimental studies in the innervation of the skin. *J Physiol* 38:134, 1909.

U.S. DEPARTMENT OF HEALTH AND HUMAN SERVICES: *Management of Cancer Pain: Clinical Practice Guideline Number 9*. AHCPR Publications No. 94-0592 and 94-0593. March 1994. (Available by calling 1-800-4-CANCER.)

VON FREY M: Untersuchungen über die Sinnesfunctionen der menschlichen Haut: I. Druckempfindung und Schmerz. *Königl Sächs Ges Wiss Math-Phys Kl* 23:175, 1896.

WALL PD, MELZACK R (eds): *Textbook of Pain*, 4th ed. New York, Churchill-Livingstone, 1999.

WALSHE FMR: The anatomy and physiology of cutaneous sensibility. A critical review. *Brain* 65:48, 1942.

WEDDELL G: The anatomy of cutaneous sensibility. *Br Med Bull* 3:167, 1945.

WELLS KB, STEWART A, HAYS RD, et al: The functioning and well-being of depressed patients. *JAMA* 262:914, 1989.

WHITE D, HELME RD: Release of substance P from peripheral nerve terminals following electrical stimulation of sciatic nerve. *Brain Res* 336:27, 1985.

WOOLF CJ, MANNION RJ: Neuropathic pain: Aetiology, symptoms, mechanisms, and management. *Lancet* 353:1959, 1999.

YAKSH TL, HAMMOND DL: Peripheral and central substrates involved in the rostrad transmission of nociceptive information. *Pain* 13:1, 1982.

Chapter 9
OTHER SOMATIC SENSATION

Under normal conditions, sensory and motor functions are interdependent, as was dramatically illustrated by the early animal experiments of Claude Bernard and Sherrington, in which practically all effective movement of a limb was abolished by eliminating only its sensory innervation (sectioning of posterior roots). Interruption of other sensory pathways and destruction of the parietal cortex also have a profound effect upon motility. Sensory and motor neurons are intimately connected at all levels of the nervous system, from the spinal cord to the cerebrum. To a large extent, human motor activity depends upon a constant influx of sensory impulses (most of them not consciously perceived). Truly, in a physiologic sense, "movement is sensation."

However, under conditions of disease, motor or sensory function may be affected independently. There may be loss or impairment of sensory function, and this may represent the principal manifestation of neurologic disease. The logic of this is clear enough, since the major anatomic pathways of the sensory system are distinct from those of the motor system and can be selectively disturbed by disease. The analysis of sensory symptoms involves the use of special tests, designed to elicit the nature of the sensory alteration and its location, and it is from this point of view that disorders of sensory function are considered here.

This chapter deals with general somatic sensation, i.e., afferent impulses that arise in the skin, muscles, or joints. One form of somatic sensation—pain—has already been discussed (Chap. 8). Because of its overriding clinical importance, pain has been accorded a chapter of its own, but the two chapters are of one piece and should be read together. The special senses—vision, hearing, taste, and smell—are considered in the next section (Chaps. 12 to 15), and visceral (interoceptive) sensation, most of which does not reach consciousness, is considered with the disorders of the autonomic nervous system (Chap. 26).

ANATOMIC AND PHYSIOLOGIC CONSIDERATIONS

An understanding of sensory disorders depends upon a knowledge of functional anatomy. It is necessary to be familiar with the sensory receptors in the skin and deeper structures, the distribution of the peripheral nerves and roots, and the pathways by which sensory impulses are conveyed from the periphery and through the spinal cord and brainstem to the thalamus and cerebral cortex. These aspects of sensory anatomy and physiology have already been touched upon in Chap. 8, in relation to the perception of pain, and are elaborated here to include all forms of somatic sensation. Charts showing the cutaneous distribution of the peripheral nerves are included (Fig. 9-1).

All sensation depends on impulses that are excited by adequate stimulation of receptors and conveyed to the central nervous system by afferent, or sensory, fibers. Sensory receptors are of two general types: those in the skin, mediating superficial sensation (*exteroceptors*), and those in the deeper somatic structures (*proprioceptors*). The skin receptors are particularly numerous and transduce four types of sensory experience: warmth, cold, touch, and pain; these are conventionally referred to as *sensations* or *senses*, e.g., tactile sensation or sense of touch. The proprioceptors inform us of the position of our body or parts of our body; of the force, direction, and range of movement of the joints (kinesthetic sense); and of a sense of pressure, both painful and painless. Histologically, a wide variety of sensory receptors has been described, varying from simple, free axon terminals to highly branched and encapsulated structures, the latter bearing the names of the anatomists who first described them (see below).

Mechanisms of Cutaneous Sensation

As indicated in the preceding chapter, it was common teaching for many years that each of the primary modalities

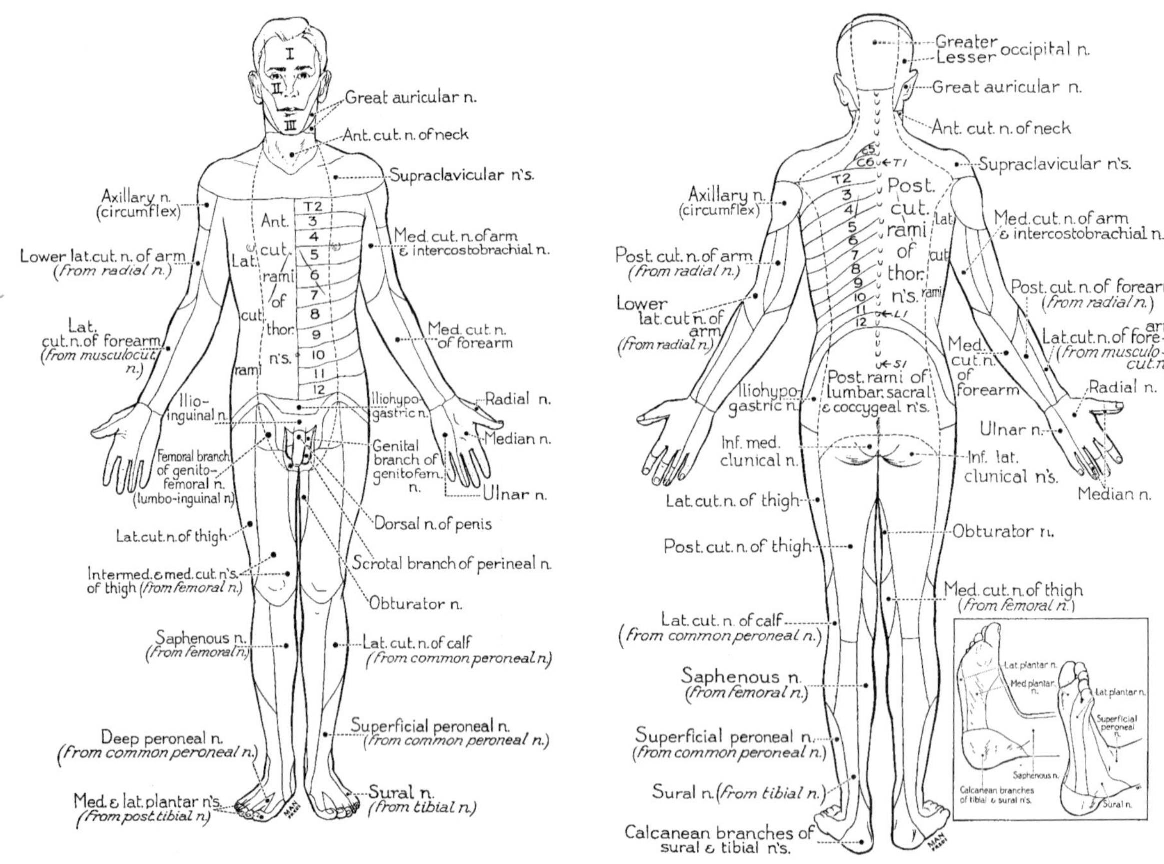

Figure 9-1

The cutaneous fields of peripheral nerves. (From Haymaker W, Woodhall B: Peripheral Nerve Injuries, 2nd ed. Philadelphia, Saunders, 1953, by permission.)

of cutaneous sensation is subserved by a morphologically distinct end organ, each with its separate peripheral nerve fibers. According to this formulation, traditionally associated with the name of von Frey, each type of end organ was thought to respond only to a particular type of stimulus and to subserve a specific modality of sensation: Meissner corpuscles, touch; Merkel discs, pressure; Ruffini plumes, heat; Krause end bulbs, cold; pacinian corpuscles, vibration and tickle; and freely branching endings, pain.

This *specificity theory*, as it came to be called, has held up best in respect to the peripheral mechanisms for pain, insofar as certain primary afferent fibers, namely the C and A-δ fibers and their free nerve-ending type of receptors, respond maximally to noxious stimuli. But even these freely branching receptor endings and their so-called pain fibers convey considerable nonnoxious information; that is, their specificity as pain fibers is not absolute (Chap. 8). Nor has it been possible to ascribe a specific function to each of the many other types of receptors. Thus, Merkel discs, Meissner corpuscles, nerve plexuses around the hair follicles, and free nerve endings can all be activated by moving or stationary tactile stimuli. Conversely, a single type of receptor seems capable of generating more than one sensory modality. Lele and Weddell found that with appropriate stimulation of the cornea, each of the four primary modalities of somatic sensibility (touch, warmth, cold, pain) could be recognized, even though the cornea contains only fine, freely ending nerve filaments. In the outer ear, which is also sensitive to these four modalities, only two types of receptors—freely ending and perifollicular—are present. The lack of organized receptors—e.g., the end bulbs of Krause and Ruffini—in the cornea and ear makes it evident that these types of receptors are not essential for the recognition of cold and warmth, as von Frey and other early anatomists had postulated.

Particularly instructive in this regard are the observations of Kibler and Nathan, who studied the responses of warm and cold spots to different stimuli. (Warm and cold spots are those small areas of skin that respond most consistently to thermal stimuli with a sensation of warmth or cold.) They found that a cold stimulus applied to a warm spot gave rise to a sensation of cold and that a noxious stimulus applied to a warm or cold spot gave rise only to a painful sensation; they also noted that mechanical stimulation of these spots gave rise to a sensation of touch or pressure. These observations indicate that cutaneous receptors, some not easily distinguishable from one another on morphologic grounds, are probably endowed with a degree of specificity, in the sense that each responds *preferentially* (i.e., has a lower threshold) to one particular form of stimulation. Even among the freely branching nociceptors there is some degree of specialization, as discussed in Chap. 8 (page 136). Such end organs can then be classed as mechanoreceptors, thermoreceptors, or nociceptors, depending on their selective sensitivity to mechanical, thermal, or noxious stimuli, respectively (Sinclair; Light and Perl).

Recent physiologic studies have shown that the *quality* of sensation depends on the type of nerve fiber that is activated. Different diseases therefore evoke a variety of sensory deficits. Microstimulation of single sensory fibers in a peripheral nerve of an awake human subject arouses different sensations, depending on which fibers are stimulated and not on the frequency of stimulation. On the other hand, the frequency of stimulation does govern the *intensity* of sensation, as does the number of sensory units that are stimulated. Stated somewhat differently, afferent impulse frequency (*temporal summation*) is encoded by the brain in terms of magnitude or intensity of sensation. In addition, as the intensity of stimulation increases, more sensory units are activated (*spatial summation*).

Localization of a stimulus was formerly thought to depend on the simultaneous activation of overlapping sensory units. Tower defined a peripheral sensory unit as a monopolar dorsal root ganglion cell, its central and distal axon extensions, and all the sensory endings in the territory supplied by the distal extension (receptive field). In the very sensitive pulp of the finger, where the error of localization is less than 1.0 mm, there are 240 overlapping, low-threshold mechanoreceptors per square centimeter. Highly refined physiologic techniques have demonstrated that activation of even a single sensory unit is sufficient to localize the point stimulated and that the body map in the parietal lobe is capable, by its modular columnar organization, of encoding such information. Noteworthy also is the fact that each point in the skin that is stimulated may involve more than one type of receptor. It is possible, therefore, that a stimulus of increased intensity, e.g., a mechanical one, will activate a related pain ending.

A stimulus, in order to gain access to its receptor, must pass through the skin and possess sufficient energy to transduce, i.e., depolarize, the nerve ending. Not only does the threshold of stimulation vary but the nerve impulse that is generated is a graded one, not an all-or-none phenomenon like an action potential in nerve. This poorly understood peripheral generator potential determines the frequency of impulse in the nerve and to what degree it is sustained or fades out (i.e., adapts to the stimulus or fatigues). The mechanism by which a stimulus is translated into a sensory experience, i.e., is encoded, is obscure. It is probably fair to say that each type of specialized ending has a membrane structure that facilitates the transducive process for a particular type of stimulus. In general, the encapsulated endings are more deeply situated, are of low-threshold type, are variably adaptable to continued stimulation (the Meissner and pacinian corpuscles are rapidly adapting; the Merkel disc and Ruffini endings are slowly adapting) and are connected to large sensory fibers (see Lindblom and Ochoa). Pain receptors lie deeper in the skin than those for touch.

Sensory Pathways

Sensory Nerves Fibers that mediate superficial sensation are located in cutaneous sensory or mixed sensorimotor nerves. In cutaneous nerves, unmyelinated pain and autonomic fibers exceed myelinated fibers by a ratio of 3 or 4:1. The myelinated fibers are of two types, small, lightly myelinated, A-δ fibers for pain and cold, as already mentioned, and larger, faster-conducting A-α fibers for touch and pressure. The nonmyelinated autonomic fibers are efferent (postganglionic) and innervate piloerector muscles, sweat glands, and blood vessels. Proprioceptive fibers are located in deeper, predominantly motor nerves. In addition, these nerves contain afferent and efferent spindle and Golgi tendon organ fibers and thinner pain afferents. The differing conduction velocities of these fibers are discussed in Chap. 45.

A single cutaneous (touch, pain, and temperature) axon connects to several receptors, all of one type, which are irregularly distributed in the skin and account for sensory spots. Stimuli from a given spot are conveyed by two or more fibers. The proprioceptive fibers subserve pressure sense and, with endings in articular structures, the sense of position and movement; they enable one to discriminate the form, size, texture, and weight of objects. Sensations of tickle, itch, and wetness are believed to arise from combinations of several types of receptors. The pathophysiology of itching has been discussed by Greaves and Wall.

Spinal Roots All the sensory neurons have their cell bodies in the dorsal root ganglia. The peripheral extensions of these cells constitute the sensory nerves; the central projections of these same cells form the posterior (dorsal) roots and enter the spinal cord. Each dorsal root contains all the fibers from skin, muscles, connective tissue, ligaments, tendons, joints, bones, and viscera that lie within the distribution of a single body segment, or somite. This segmental innervation has been amply demonstrated in humans and animals by observing the effects of lesions that involve one or two spinal nerves, such as (1) herpes zoster, which also causes visible vesicles in the corresponding area of skin; (2) the effects of a prolapsed intervertebral disc, which causes hypalgesia in a single root zone; and (3) surgical section of several roots on each side of an intact root (method of remaining sensibility). Maps of the dermatomes derived from these several types of data are shown in Fig. 9-2. It should be noted that there is considerable overlap from one dermatomal segment to the other, more so for touch than for pain. By contrast, there is little overlap between branches of the trigeminal nerve. Also, the maps differ somewhat according to the methods used in constructing them. In contrast to most dermatomal charts, those of Keegan and Garrett (based on the injection of local anesthetic into single dorsal root ganglia) show bands of hypalgesia to be continuous longitudinally from the periphery to the spine (Fig. 9-3). The distribution of pain fibers from deep structures, though not exactly corresponding to that of pain fibers from the skin, also follows a segmental pattern.

In the dorsal roots, the sensory fibers are first rearranged according to function. Large and heavily myelinated fibers enter the cord just medial to the dorsal horn and divide into ascending and descending branches. The descending fibers and some of the ascending ones enter the gray matter of the dorsal horn within a few segments of their entrance and synapse with nerve cells in the posterior horns as well as with large ventral horn cells that subserve segmental reflexes. Some of the ascending fibers run uninterruptedly in the dorsal columns of the *same side of the spinal cord*, terminating in the gracile and cuneate nuclei. The central axons of the primary sensory neurons are joined in the posterior columns by other secondary neurons whose cell bodies lie in the posterior horns of the spinal cord (see below). The fibers in the posterior columns are displaced medially as new fibers

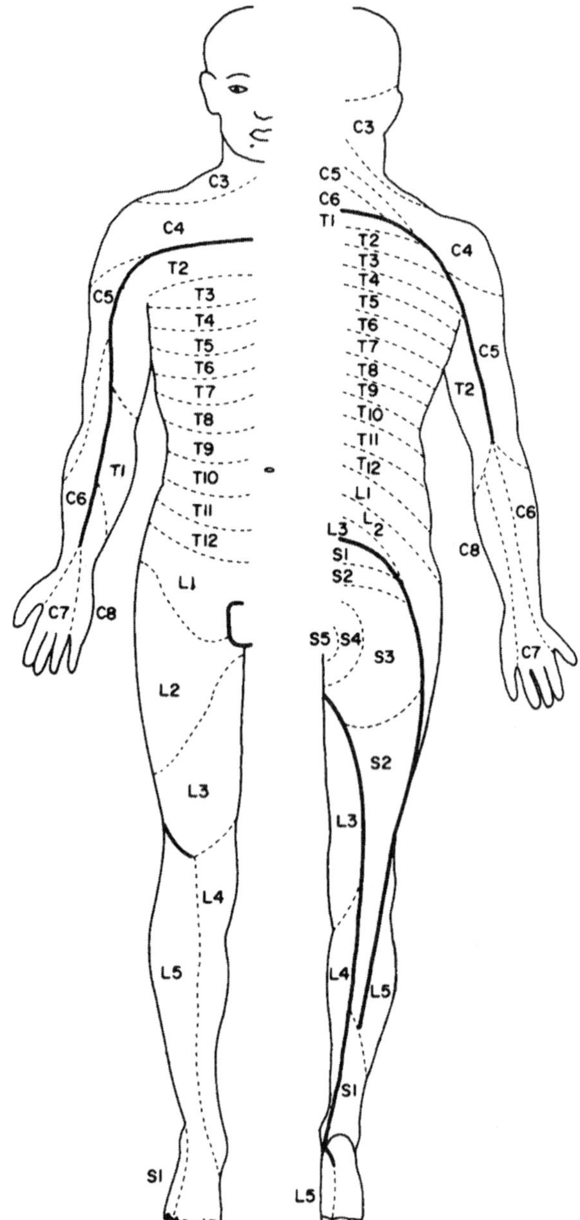

Figure 9-2

Distribution of the sensory spinal roots on the surface of the body. (Reproduced by permission from Sinclair.)

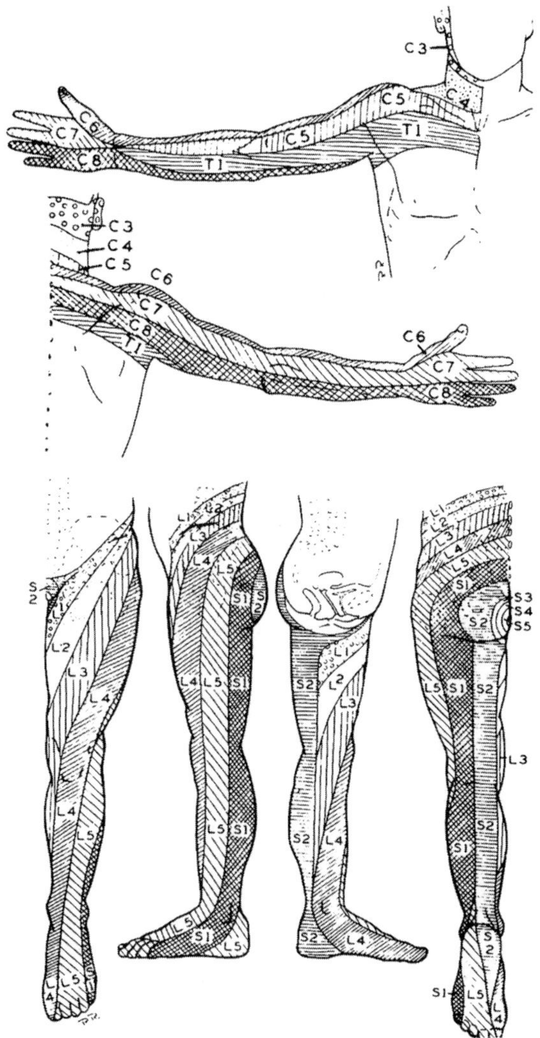

Figure 9-3

Dermatomes of the upper and lower extremities, outlined by the pattern of sensory loss following lesions of single nerve roots. (Reproduced by permission from Keegan and Garrett.)

from each successively higher root are added (Figs. 8-1 and 8-3).

Posterior Columns Of the long ascending posterior column fibers, which are activated by mechanical stimuli of skin and subcutaneous tissues and by movement of joints, only about 25 percent (from the lumbar region) reach the gracile nuclei. The rest give off collaterals to or terminate in the dorsal horns of the spinal cord, at least in the cat (Davidoff). An estimated 20 percent of ascending fibers originate from cells in Rexed layers IV and V of the posterior horns and convey impulses from low-threshold mechanoreceptors that are sensitive to hair movement, to skin pressure, or to noxious stimuli. There are also descending fibers in the posterior columns, including fibers from cells in the dorsal column nuclei.

The posterior columns contain a portion of the fibers for the sense of touch as well as the fibers mediating the senses of touch-pressure, vibration, direction of movement and position of joints, stereoesthesia—recognition of surface texture, shape, numbers and figures written on the skin, and two-point discrimination—all of which depend on patterns of touch-pressure (Fig. 8-3). However, the fiber pathways in the posterior columns are not the sole mediators of proprioception in the spinal cord (see "Posterior Column Syndrome," further on). The nerve cells of the nuclei gracilis and cuneatus and accessory cuneate nuclei give rise to a secondary afferent path, which crosses the midline in the medulla and ascends as the medial lemniscus to the posterior thalamus (see further on).

In addition to these well-defined posterior column pathways, there are cells in the "reticular" part of the dorsal column nuclei that receive secondary ascending fibers from the dorsal horns of the spinal cord and from ascending fibers in the posterolateral columns. These dorsal column fibers project to brainstem nuclei, cerebellum, and thalamic nuclei. Many other cells of the dorsal column nuclei are interneurons, with both excitatory and inhibitory effects on local reflexes or on the primary ascending neurons. They are under the influence of the sensorimotor cortex. Some act on descending corticospinal motor neurons. The functions of many of the extrathalamic projections of dorsal column cells are unknown (Davidoff).

Thinly myelinated or unmyelinated fibers enter the cord on the lateral aspect of the dorsal horn and synapse with dorsal horn cells, mainly within a segment or two of their point of entry into the cord. The dorsal horn cells, in turn, give rise to secondary sensory fibers, some of which may ascend ipsilaterally but most of which decussate and ascend in the spinothalamic tracts, as described in Chap. 8 (Figs. 8-1 and 8-2). Observations based on surgical interruption of the anterolateral funiculus indicate that fibers mediating pain and temperature occupy the dorsolateral part of the funiculus (lateral spinothalamic tract), and those for touch and deep pressure occupy the ventromedial part (anterior spinothalamic tract). Also, as remarked in Chap. 8, an ascending tract of secondary sensory axons lies in or medial to the descending corticospinal system.

Trigeminal Connections The pathways mediating cutaneous sensation from the face and head, especially touch, pain, and temperature, are conveyed to the brainstem by the trigeminal nerve. After entering the pons, the pain and temperature fibers turn caudally and run through the medulla as the descending trigeminal tract, terminating in a long, vertically oriented nucleus that lies beside it and extends to the second or third cervical segment of the cord, where it becomes continuous with the posterior horn of the spinal gray matter. Axons from the neurons of this nucleus cross the midline and ascend as the trigeminal lemniscus along the medial side of the spinothalamic tract (Fig. 8-2).

Ascending fibers from the reticular nuclei, medial lemniscus, trigeminal lemniscus, and spinothalamic pathways merge in the midbrain and terminate in the posterior complex of thalamic nuclei, particularly in the ventral posterolateral nucleus (VPL).

Thalamocortical Connections The posterior thalamic complex projects mainly to two somatosensory cortical areas. The first area (S1) corresponds to the postcentral cortex or Brodmann's areas 3, 1, and 2. S1 afferents are derived primarily from VPL and VPM (ventral posteromedial nucleus—the terminus of trigeminal fibers) and are distributed somatotopically, with the leg represented uppermost and the face lowermost (face and hand are juxtaposed). Electrical stimulation of this area yields sensations of tingling, numbness, and warmth in specific regions on the *opposite* side of the body. The information transmitted to S1 is tactile and proprioceptive, derived mainly from the dorsal column–medial lemniscus system and concerned mainly with sensory discrimination. The second somatosensory area (S2) lies on the upper bank of the sylvian fissure, adjacent to the insula. Localization of function is less discrete in S2 than in S1, but S2 is also organized somatotopically, with the face rostrally and the leg caudally. The sensations evoked by electrical stimulation of S2 are much the same as those of S1 but, in distinction to the latter, may be felt bilaterally. Of note is the failure of cortical stimulation to evoke pain sensation.

Undoubtedly, the perception of sensory stimuli involves more of the cerebral cortex than the two discrete areas described above. Some sensory fibers probably project to the precentral gyrus and others to the superior parietal lobule. Moreover, S1 and S2 are not purely sensory in function; motor effects can be obtained by stimulating them electrically. It has been shown that sensory neurons in VPL, cuneate and gracile nuclei, and sensory neurons in the dorsal horns of the spinal cord all receive descending cortical projections as well as ascending ones. This reciprocal arrangement probably influences movement and the transmission and interpretation of pain, as discussed in Chap. 8.

Provided that the subcortical structures, especially the thalamus, are intact, certain sensations such as pain, touch, pressure, and extremes of temperature can reach consciousness. Their accurate localization, however, as well as the patient's ability to make other fine sensory discriminations, depends to a large extent on the integrity of the sensory cortex. This clinical distinction is elaborated in the discussion of the sensory syndromes, further on.

From this brief account of the various channels of sensory information, the conclusion is inevitable that at every level there is the possibility of feedback control from higher levels. Most external and some internal stimuli are highly complex and induce activity in more than one sensory system. In every system, there is sufficient redundancy to allow lesser used systems to compensate for the deficits incurred by disease.

EXAMINATION OF SENSATION

Most neurologists would agree that sensory testing is the most difficult part of the neurologic examination. For one thing, test procedures are relatively crude and inadequate and are unlike natural modes of stimulation with which the patient is familiar. It is also fair to say that few diagnoses are made solely on the basis of the sensory examination; more often it serves to complement the motor examination. Embarrassingly often, no objective sensory loss can be demonstrated despite symptoms that suggest the presence of such an abnormality. Rarely, the opposite pertains, i.e., one sometimes discovers a sensory deficit when there has been no complaint of sensory symptoms. In the former instance, sensory symptoms in the nature of paresthesias or dysesthesias may be generated along axons of nerves not sufficiently diseased to impair or reduce sensory function; in the latter instance, loss of function may have been so mild and gradual as to pass unnoticed. Always there is some difficulty in evaluating the response to sensory stimuli, since it depends on the patient's interpretation of sensory experiences. This, in turn, will depend on his general awareness and responsiveness and ability to cooperate as well as his intelligence, education, and suggestibility. At times, children and relatively uneducated persons, by virtue of their simple and direct responses, are better witnesses than more sophisticated individuals, who are likely to analyze their feelings minutely and report small and insignificant differences in stimulus intensity.

General Considerations

Before proceeding to sensory testing, the physician should question patients about their symptoms, and this too poses special problems. Patients are confronted with derangements of sensation that may be unlike anything they have previously experienced, and they have few words to describe what they feel. They may say that a limb feels "numb" and "dead" when in fact they mean that it is weak. Occasionally a loss of sensation is discovered almost accidentally, e.g., by a lack of pain on touching an object hot enough to blister the skin, or unawareness of articles of clothing and other objects in contact with the skin. But more often disease induces new and unnatural sensory experiences.

If nerves, sensory roots, or spinal tracts are damaged or partially interrupted, the patient may complain of tingling or prickling feelings ("like Novocain" or like the feelings in a limb that has "fallen asleep," the common colloquialism for nerve compression), cramp-like sensations, or burning or cutting pain occurring either spontaneously or in response to stimulation.

Experimental data support the view that partially damaged touch, pressure, thermal, and pain fibers become hyperexcitable and generate ectopic impulses along their course, either spontaneously or in response to a natural volley of stimulus-evoked impulses (Ochoa and Torebjork). These abnormal sensations are called *paresthesias*, or *dysesthesias* if they are severe and distressing. Another positive sensory symptom is *allodynia*, referring to a phenomenon in which one type of stimulus evokes another type of sensation—e.g., touch may induce pain.

The clinical characteristics of a sensation may divulge the particular sensory fibers that are involved. It has been shown that stimulation of touch fibers gives rise to a sensation of tingling and buzzing; of muscle proprioceptors, to pseudocramp; of thermal fibers, to hotness and coldness; and of A-δ fibers, to prickling and pain. Paresthesias arising from ectopic discharges in large sensory fibers can be induced by compression, by hypocalcemia, and by diverse diseases of nerves.

The presence of persistent paresthesias should always raise the suspicion of a lesion involving sensory pathways in nerves, spinal cord, or higher structures. Evanescent paresthesias, of course, may be of no significance. Every person has had the experience of resting a limb on the ulnar, sciatic, or peroneal nerve and having the extremity "fall asleep." This is due to compressive interruption of axonal transport and not to ischemia of the nerve or other components of the limb, as is commonly assumed. The hyperventilation of anxiety may cause paresthesias of the lips and hands (sometimes unilateral) from diminution of CO_2 and thereby of ionized calcium; tetany may also occur, with carpopedal spasms. Severe acral and peripheral paresthesias with perversion of hot and cold sensations are characteristic of certain neurotoxic shellfish poisonings (*ciguatera*).

Effect of Age on Sensory Function A matter of importance in the testing of sensation is the progressive impairment of sensory perception that occurs with advancing age. This requires that sensory thresholds, particularly in the feet and legs, always be assessed in relation to age standards. The effect of aging is most evident in relation to vibratory sense, but proprioception, touch, and fast pain are also diminished with age. Sweating and vasomotor reflexes are reduced as well. These changes, which are discussed further in Chap. 29, are probably due to neuronal loss in dorsal root ganglia and are reflected in a progressive depletion of fibers in the posterior columns. Receptors in the skin and special sense organs (taste, smell) also wither with age.

Terminology A few additional terms require definition, since they may be encountered in discussions of sensation. Some of these, relating to pain sensation, were alluded to in Chap. 8. *Anesthesia* refers to a complete loss and *hypesthesia* to a partial loss of all forms of sensation. Loss or impairment of specific cutaneous sensations may be indicated by an appropriate prefix or suffix, e.g., *thermoanesthesia* or *thermohypesthesia*, *analgesia* (loss of pain sense), *hypalgesia* (reduction in pain sensibility), *tactile anesthesia*, and *pallanesthesia* (loss of vibratory sense). The term *hyperesthesia*, as explained in Chap. 8, refers to an increased sensitivity to various stimuli and is usually used with respect to cutaneous sensation. It implies a heightened activity of the sensory apparatus. Under certain conditions (e.g., sunburn), there does appear to be an enhanced sensitivity of cutaneous receptors, but usually the presence of hyperesthesia betrays an underlying sensory defect. Careful testing will demonstrate an elevated threshold to tactile, painful, or thermal stimuli, but once the stimulus is perceived, it may have a severely painful or unpleasant quality (*hyperpathia*). Some clinicians use the latter term to denote an exaggerated response to a painful stimulus (hyperalgesia). In *alloesthesia*, or *allesthesia*, a tactile or painful stimulus delivered on the side of hemisensory loss is experienced in a corresponding area of the opposite side. The latter phenomenon is observed most frequently with right-sided putaminal lesions (usually hemorrhage) and with anterolateral lesions of the cervical spinal cord; it presumably depends on the existence of an uncrossed ipsilateral spinothalamic pathway (Ray and Wolff).

The Bedside Testing of Sensory Function

The detail with which sensation is tested is determined by the clinical situation. If the patient has no sensory complaints, it is sufficient to test vibration and position sense in the fingers and toes and the perception of pinprick over the face, trunk, and extremities, and to determine whether the findings are the same in symmetrical parts of the body. A rough survey of this sort occasionally detects sensory defects of which the patient was unaware. On the other hand, more thorough testing is in order if the patient has complaints referable to the sensory system or if one finds localized atrophy or weakness, ataxia, trophic changes of joints, or painless ulcers.

A few other general rules should be mentioned. One should not press the sensory examination in the presence of fatigue, for an inattentive patient is a poor witness. Also, the examiner must avoid suggesting symptoms to the patient. After explaining in the simplest terms what is required, the examiner interposes as few questions and remarks as possible. Consequently, patients should not be asked, "Do you feel that?" each time they are touched; they are simply told to say "yes" or "sharp" every time they are touched or feel pain. Repetitive pinpricks within a small area of skin should be avoided, since this will make inapparent a subtle hypalgesia. In patients who may be overinterpreting subtle changes in pinprick, differentiating between warm and cold is often more informative than differentiating between "sharp" and "dull." The patient should not see the part under examination. However, a cooperative patient may, if asked to use a pin or his fingertips, outline an analgesic or anesthetic area or determine if there is a graduated loss of sensation in the distal parts of a leg or arm. Finally, the findings of the sensory examination should be accurately recorded on a chart by shading affected regions on a preprinted figure of the body or a sketch of a hand, foot, face, or limb.

Described below are the usual bedside methods of testing sensory function. With attention to certain details of procedure, these tests are quite sufficient for most clinical purposes. For clinical investigation and research into the physiology of pain, which require the detection of threshold values and quantification of sensory impairment, a wide range of instruments are available. Their use has been described by Dyck et al (see also Lindblom and Ochoa, and Bertelsmann et al).

Testing of Tactile Sensation This is usually done with a wisp of cotton. Patients are first acquainted with the nature of the stimulus by applying it to a normal part of the body. Then, with eyes closed, they are asked to say "yes" each time various other parts are touched. A patient who is simulating sensory loss may say "no" in response to a tactile stimulus. Cornified areas of skin, such as the soles and palms, will require a heavier stimulus than other areas and the hair-clad parts a lighter one because of the numerous nerve endings around the follicles. The patient is more sensitive to a moving contactual stimulus of any kind than to a stationary one. The deft application of the examiner's or preferably the patient's roving fingertips is a useful refinement and aids in demarcating an area of tactile loss, as Trotter and Davies originally showed.

More precise testing is possible by using a von Frey hair. By this method, a stimulus of constant strength can be applied and the threshold for tactile sensation determined by measuring the force required to bend a hair of known length. Special difficulties arise in the testing of tactile perception, when a series of contactual stimuli lead to a decrement of sensation, either through adaptation of the end organ or because the initial sensation outlasts the stimulus and seems to spread. The patient may then fail to report tactile stimuli in an area where they were previously present, or he may report contact without being touched.

Testing of Pain Perception This is most efficiently assessed by pinprick, although it may be evoked by a great diversity of noxious stimuli. Patients must understand that they are to report the feeling of sharpness, not simply the feeling of contact or pressure of the pin point. If pinpricks are applied rapidly in one area, their effect may be summated and a heightened perception of pain may result; therefore, they should be delivered about one per second, and not over the same spot.

It is almost impossible, using an ordinary pin, to apply each stimulus with equal intensity. A pinwheel is sometimes more effective because it allows the application of a more constant pressure. This difficulty can be overcome to some extent by the use of an algesimeter, which enables one to deliver stimuli of constant intensity and also to grade the intensity and determine threshold values. Even with this instrument, an isolated stimulus may be reported as being excessively sharp, apparently because of direct contact with a pain spot.

If an area of diminished or absent touch or pain sensation is encountered, its boundaries should be demarcated to determine whether it has a segmental or peripheral nerve distribution or is lost below a certain level on the trunk. Such areas are best delineated by proceeding from the region of impaired sensation toward the normal. The changes may be confirmed by dragging a pin lightly over the parts in question.

Testing of Deep Pressure-Pain One can estimate this modality simply by lightly pinching or pressing deeply on the tendons, muscles, or bony prominences. Pain can often be elicited by heavy pressure even when superficial sensation is diminished; conversely, in some diseases, such as tabetic neurosyphilis, loss of deep pressure-pain may be more striking than loss of superficial pain.

Testing of Thermal Sense A rough but quick way to assess thermal loss (or to corroborate a previously found zone of hypalgesia) is to apply alternate sides of a tuning fork to the skin, one side of which has been warmed by rubbing it briskly against the palm. Usually more careful examination is required, in which case the areas of skin to be tested should be exposed to room air for a brief time before the examination. The test objects should be large, preferably two stoppered test tubes containing hot (45°C) and cold (20°C) tap water. Thermometers, which extend into the water through the flask stoppers, indicate the temperature of the water at the moment of testing. At first, extreme degrees of heat and cold (e.g., 10 and 45°C) are employed to delineate roughly an area of thermal sensory impairment. The side of each tube is applied successively to the skin for a few seconds and the patient is asked to report whether the flask feels "less hot" or "less cold" over an area of suspected impairment in comparison to a normal part. The qualitative change should then be quantitated as far as possible by estimating the differences in temperature that the patient is able to recognize. The difference in temperature between the two tubes is gradually reduced. A normal person can detect a difference of 1°C or even less when the temperature of the tubes is in the range of 28 to 32°C; in the warm range, differences between 35 and 40°C can be recognized, and in the cold range, between 10 and 20°C. If the temperature of the test object is below 10°C or above 50°C, sensations of cold or heat become confused with pain.

Testing of Proprioceptive Sense Awareness of the position and movements of our limbs, fingers, and toes is derived from receptors in the muscles, tendons (Golgi tendon organs, according to Roland et al), and joints and is probably facilitated by activation of skin receptors (Moberg). The two modalities comprised by proprioception, i.e., sense of movement and of position, are usually lost together, although clinical situations do arise in which perception of the position of a limb or digits is lost while that of passive and active movement (kinesthesia) of these parts is retained. The opposite has also been said to occur but must be very rare.

Abnormalities of position sense may be disclosed in several ways. When the patient has his arms outstretched and eyes closed, the affected arm will wander from its original position; if the fingers are spread apart, they may undergo a series of changing postures ("piano-playing" movements, or pseudoathetosis); in attempting to touch the tip of his nose with his index finger, the patient may miss the target repeatedly, but he corrects his performance with the eyes open.

The lack of position sense in the legs is demonstrated by displacing the limb from its original position and having the patient, with eyes closed, place the other leg in the same position or point to the great toe. If position sense is defective in both legs, the patient will be unable to maintain his balance with feet together and eyes closed (*Romberg sign*). The latter term is often used imprecisely. In the Romberg position, even a normal person whose eyes are closed will sway slightly, and the patient who lacks balance due to cerebellar ataxia or vestibulopathy or to some other motor disorder will sway considerably more if his visual cues are removed. In performing this test, the patient should optimally be barefoot. Only a marked discrepancy in balance with eyes open and with eyes closed qualifies as a Romberg sign. The best indication of abnormality is the need to step to the side in order to avoid falling. Mild degrees of unsteadiness in nervous or suggestible patients may be overcome by diverting their attention, e.g., by having them touch the index finger of each hand alternately to the nose while they are standing with eyes closed or by following the examiner's finger with their eyes.

Perception of passive movement is first tested in the fingers and toes, since the defect, when present, is reflected maximally in these parts. It is important to grasp the digit firmly at the sides perpendicular to the plane of movement; otherwise the pressure applied by the examiner in displacing the digit may allow the patient to identify the direction of movement. This applies as well to testing of the more proximal segments of the limb. Also, the patient should be instructed to report each movement as being "up" or "down" from the previous position (directional kinesthesia). It is useful to demonstrate the test with a large and easily identified movement, but once the idea is clear to the patient, the smallest detectable changes should be determined. The sensitivity of testing is enhanced by using the third and fourth fingers and toes. The part being tested should be moved rapidly. Normally, a very slight degree of movement is appreciated in the digits (as little as 1 degree of an arc). The test should be repeated enough times to eliminate chance (50 percent of responses). Defective perception of passive movement is judged by comparison with a normal limb or, if perception is bilaterally defective, on the basis of what the examiner has learned through experience to be normal. Slight impairment may be disclosed by a slowness of response or, if the digit is displaced very slowly, by an unawareness or uncertainty that movement has occurred; or, after the digit has been displaced in the same direction several times, the patient may misjudge the first movement in the opposite direction; or, after the examiner has moved the toe, the patient may make a number of small voluntary movements of the toe in an apparent attempt to determine its position or the direction of the movement. Inattentiveness will also cause some of these errors.

Testing of Vibratory Sense This is a composite sensation comprising touch and rapid alterations of deep-pressure sense. The only cutaneous structure capable of registering such rapid stimuli is the rapidly adapting pacinian corpuscle. The conduction of vibratory sense depends on both cutaneous and deep afferent fibers that ascend mainly in the dorsal columns of the cord. It is therefore rarely affected by lesions of single nerves but will be disturbed in patients with disease of multiple peripheral nerves, dorsal columns, medial lemniscus, and thalamus. Vibration and position sense are usually lost together, although one of them (most often vibration sense) may be affected disproportionately. With advancing age, vibration is the sensation most commonly diminished, at the toes and ankles.

Vibration sense is tested by placing a tuning fork with a low rate and long duration of vibration (128 Hz) over the bony prominences, making sure that the patient responds to the vibration, not simply to the pressure of the fork, and that he is not trying to listen to it. There are mechanical devices to quantitate vibration sense, but it is sufficient for clinical purposes to compare the point tested with a normal part of the patient or the examiner. The examiner may detect the vibration after it ceases for the patient by holding a finger under the distal interphalangeal joint, the handle of the tuning fork being placed on the dorsal aspect of the joint. Or, the vibrating fork is allowed to run down until the moment that vibration is no longer perceived, at which point the fork is transferred quickly to the corresponding part of the examiner and the time to extinction is noted. There is a small degree of accommodation to the vibration stimulus, so that slight asymmetries detected by rapidly shifting from a body part on one side to the other should be interpreted with caution. The perception of vibration at the tibial tuberosity after it has disappeared at the ankle or at the anterior iliac spine after it has disappeared at the tibial tuberosity is indicative of a peripheral neuropathy. The approximate level of a spinal cord lesion can be corroborated by testing vibratory sensation over the iliac crests and successive vertebral spines.

Testing of Discriminative Sensation Damage to the sensory cortex or to the thalamocortical projections results in a special type of disturbance—namely, an inability to make sensory discriminations. Lesions in these structures usually disturb position sense but leave the so-called primary modalities (touch, pain, temperature, and vibration sense) relatively little affected. In such a situation, or if a cerebral lesion is suspected on other grounds, discriminative function should be tested further by the following tests:

Two-Point Discrimination The ability to distinguish two points from one is tested by using a compass, the points of which should be blunt and applied simultaneously and painlessly. The distance at which such stimuli can be recognized as double varies but is roughly 1 mm at the tip of the tongue, 2 to 3 mm on the lips, 3 to 5 mm at the fingertips, 8 to 15 mm on the palm, 20 to 30 mm on the dorsa of the hands and feet, and 4 to 7 cm on the body surface. It is characteristic of the patient with a lesion of the sensory cortex to mistake two points for one, although occasionally the opposite occurs.

Cutaneous Localization and Figure Writing (Graphesthesia) Localization of cutaneous tactile or painful stimuli is tested by touching various points on the body and asking the patient to place the tip of his index finger on the point stimulated or on the corresponding point of the examiner's limb. Recognition of numbers or letters (these should be larger than 4 cm on the palm) or the direction of lines drawn on the skin also depends on localization of tactile stimuli. Normally, traced numbers as small as 1 cm can be detected on the pulp of the fingers if drawn with a sharp pencil. According to Wall and Noordenbos, these are also the most useful and simplest tests of posterior column function.

Appreciation of Texture, Size, and Shape Appreciation of texture depends mainly on cutaneous impressions, but the recognition of the shape and size of objects is based on impressions from deeper receptors as well. The lack of recognition of shape and form is frequently a manifestation of cortical disease, but a similar clinical defect will occur if tracts that transmit proprioceptive and tactile sensation are interrupted by lesions of the spinal cord and brainstem (and, of course, of the peripheral nerves). The latter type of sensory defect is called *stereoanesthesia* and must be distinguished from *astereognosis*, which connotes an inability to identify an object by palpation, even though the primary sense data (touch, pain, temperature, and vibration) are intact. In practice, a pure astereognosis is rarely encountered, and the term is employed when the impairment of superficial and vibratory sensation in the hands seems to be of insufficient severity to account for the defect in tactile object identification. Defined in this way, astereognosis is either right- or left-sided and, with the qualifications mentioned below, is the product of a lesion in the opposite hemisphere, involving the sensory cortex, particularly S2, or the thalamoparietal projections.

The classic doctrine that somatic sensation is represented only in the contralateral parietal lobe is not absolute. Beginning with Oppenheim in 1906, there have been sporadic reports of patients who showed bilateral astereognosis or loss of tactile sensation as a result of an apparently unilateral cerebral lesion. The correctness of these observations was corroborated by Semmes and colleagues, who tested a large series of patients with traumatic lesions involving either the right or left cerebral hemisphere. They found that the impairment of sensation (particularly discriminative sensation) following right- and left-sided lesions was not strictly comparable; the left hand as well as the right tended to be impaired by injury to the left sensorimotor region, whereas only the left hand tended to be affected by injury to the right sensorimotor region. These observations, with minor qualifications, were also confirmed by Carmon and by Corkin and associates, who investigated the sensory effects of cortical excisions in patients with focal epilepsy. Caselli has described six patients with extensive right-sided cerebral infarctions, associated in each case with bilateral impairment of tactile object recognition but without impairment of the primary sense modalities in the right hand. In each of these patients, there was also a profound hemineglect, which confounded the interpretation of left-sided sensory signs. Thus it appears that certain somatosensory functions are mediated not only by the contralateral hemisphere but also by the ipsilateral one, although the contribution of the former is undoubtedly the more significant.

Finally, there is a distinction to be made between astereognosis and tactile agnosia. Some authors (e.g., Caselli) have defined tactile agnosia as a strictly unilateral disorder, right or left, in which the impairment of tactile object recognition is unencumbered by a disturbance of the primary sensory modalities. Such a disorder would be designated by others as a pure form of astereognosis (see above). In our view, *tactile agnosia* is a disturbance in which a one-sided lesion lying posterior to the postcentral gyrus of the *dominant* parietal lobe results in an inability to recognize an object by touch in *both* hands. According to this view, tactile agnosia is a disorder of apperception of stimuli and of translating them into symbols, akin to the defect in naming parts of the body, visualizing a plan or a route, or understanding the meaning of the printed or spoken word (visual or auditory verbal agnosia). These and other agnosias are discussed in Chap. 22.

The traditional concept of left hemispheric dominance in respect to tactile perception has been questioned by Carmon and Benton, who found that the right hemisphere is particularly important in perceiving the direction of tactile stimuli. Also, Corkin observed that patients with right-hemisphere lesions show a consistently greater failure of tactile-maze learning than those with left-sided lesions, pointing to a relative dominance of the right hemisphere in the mediation of tactile performance involving a spatial component. Certainly the phenomenon of sensory inattention or extinction is more prominent with right than with left parietal lobe lesions and is most informative if the primary and secondary sensory cortical areas are spared. These matters are considered further on in this chapter and in Chap. 22.

SENSORY SYNDROMES

Sensory Changes due to Interruption of a Single Peripheral Nerve

These changes will vary, depending on whether the nerve involved is predominantly muscular, cutaneous, or mixed. Following division of a *cutaneous nerve*, the area of sensory loss is always less than its anatomic distribution because of overlap from adjacent nerves. That the area of tactile loss is greater than the one for pain relates both to a lack of collateralization (regeneration) from adjacent tactile fibers (in contrast to rapid collateral regeneration of pain fibers) and to a greater overlap of pain sensory units. If a large area of skin is involved, the sensory defect characteristically consists of a central portion, in which all forms of cutaneous sensation are lost, surrounded by a zone of partial loss, which becomes less marked as one proceeds from the center to the periphery. Perceptions of deep pressure and passive movement are intact because these modalities are mediated by nerve fibers from subcutaneous structures and joints. Along the margin of the hypesthetic zone, the skin becomes excessively sensitive (dysesthetic); light contact may be felt as smarting and mildly painful, more so as one proceeds from the periphery of the area to its center. According to Weddell, the dysesthesias are attributable to the greater sensitivity of collateral regenerating fibers that have made their way from surrounding healthy pain fibers into the denervated region.

Particular types of lesions have differing effects upon sensory nerve fibers but are nearly always multimodal. *Compression* may ablate the function of large touch and pressure fibers and leave the function of small pain, thermal, and autonomic fibers intact; procaine and ischemia have the opposite effect. The tourniquet test is instructive in this respect. A sphygmomanometer cuff is applied above the elbow, inflated to a point well above the systolic pressure, and maintained there for as long as 30 min. (This is not particularly painful if the patient does not contract the forearm and hand muscles.) Paresthesias appear within a few minutes, followed by sensory loss—first of touch and vibration, then of cold, fast pain, heat, and slow pain, in that order and spreading centripetally. Physiologic studies have confirmed the theory of Lewis and colleagues that compression blocks the function of nerve fibers in order of their size. Release of the cuff results in postcompression paresthesias, which have been shown to arise spontaneously along the myelinated nerve fibers, from ectopic sites at a distance from the compression. Within seconds, postischemic changes appear—the cold, blanched hand becomes red and hot and there is an array of tingling, stinging, cramp-like sensations that reach maximum intensity in 90 to 120 s and slowly fade (Lewis). Function is recovered in an order inverse to that in which it was lost. Similar spontaneous and ectopic discharges explain the predominance of paresthetic symptoms early in the acute demyelinating neuropathies, even before the appearance of sensory loss or numbness.

Certain classic maneuvers for the provocation of positive sensory phenomena—the *Tinel sign* of tingling upon percussion of a regenerating peripheral nerve and the *Phalen sign* of paresthesias in the territory of the median nerve on wrist flexion—are examples of the susceptibility of a damaged nerve to pressure. In the case of a severed nerve, regeneration from the proximal end begins within days. The thin, regenerating sprouts are unusually sensitive to substance P as well as to pressure and to tapping, which produces tingling, or Tinel's sign.

Sensory Changes Due to Involvement of Multiple Nerves (Polyneuropathy)

In most instances of polyneuropathy, the sensory changes are accompanied by varying degrees of motor and reflex loss. Usually the sensory impairment is bilaterally symmetrical, with the notable exception of some instances of diabetic, inflammatory, and vasculitic neuropathy. Since in most types of polyneuropathy the longest and largest fibers are the most affected, sensory loss is most severe over the feet and legs and, if the upper limbs are affected, over the hands. The abdomen, thorax, and face are spared except in the most severe cases, in which sensory changes may be found over the escutcheon and around the mouth. When the neuropathy is primarily demyelinative rather than axonal, paresthesias are an early feature, and they are reported in the distal territories of nerves; when short nerves (e.g., the trigeminal) are involved, the paresthesias appear in proximal body parts, such as the perioral region. The sensory loss usually involves all modalities of sensation, and—although it is difficult to equate the degrees of impairment of pain, touch, temperature, vibration, and position senses—one modality may seemingly be impaired out of proportion to the others. This clinical feature can probably be explained by the fact that disease of the peripheral nerves may selectively damage sensory fibers of different size. For example, axonal degeneration or demyelination of the large kinesthetic fibers causes a loss of vibratory and position sense and relative sparing of pain, temperature, and to some degree tactile perception; it may result in sensory ataxia. Involuntary movements of digits may also be based on a loss of sense of position and movement coupled with coarse myokymic motor nerve discharges (dancing toes, pseudoathetosis of fingers). By contrast, involvement of small caliber myelinated and unmyelinated axons affects pain, temperature, and autonomic sensation, with preservation of proprioceptive, vibration, and tactile sense—producing a pseudosyringomyelic syndrome. Prolonged analgesia may lead to trophic ulcers and Charcot joints. These special patterns of loss as well as those produced by plexopathies and mononeuritis multiplex are discussed further in Chap. 46. One cannot accurately predict from the patient's symptoms which mode of sensation will be disproportionately affected. The term *glove-and-stocking anesthesia*, frequently employed to describe the sensory loss of polyneuropathy, draws attention to the predominantly distal pattern of involvement but fails to indicate that the change from normal to impaired sensation is characteristically gradual. In hysteria, by contrast, the border between normal and absent sensation is usually sharply defined.

Sensory Changes due to Involvement of Nerve Roots (Radiculopathy)

Because of considerable overlap from adjacent roots, division of a single sensory root does not produce complete loss of sensation in any area of skin. However, compression of a single sensory cervical or lumbar root (e.g., by a herniated intervertebral disc) can cause a segmental impairment of cutaneous sensation. When two or more contiguous roots have been completely divided, a zone of sensory loss can be demonstrated, surrounded by a narrow zone of partial loss, in which a raised threshold accompanied by excessive sensitivity (dysesthesia) may or may not be evident. For reasons not altogether clear, partial sensory loss from root lesions is easier to demonstrate by the use of a painful stimulus than by a tactile or pressure stimulus. Tendon and cutaneomuscular (abdominal, cremasteric) reflexes may be lost. If pain is present, it may be intensified by movement of the spine and radiates in a proximal-distal direction.

Disease of the nerve roots frequently gives rise to "shooting pains" and burning sensations that project down the course of their sensory nerves. The common examples are sciatica, from lower lumbar or upper sacral root compression, and sharp pain radiating from the shoulder and down the upper arm, from cervical disc protrusion.

When multiple roots are affected (polyradiculopathy) by an infiltrative, inflammatory, or compressive process, the syndrome is more complex and needs to be differentiated from polyneuropathy. Its distinguishing features are an asymmetrical muscle weakness, the differential involvement of proximal and distal limb parts, and pain and sensory loss consistent with affection of several roots, not necessarily contiguous ones. Details will be found in Chap. 46.

Sensory Changes due to Involvement of Sensory Ganglia (Sensory Neuronopathy)

Widespread disease of the dorsal root ganglia (paraneoplastic, toxic, and inflammatory, as in Sjögren syndrome and other connective tissue diseases) produces many of the same sensory defects as disease of the roots but is unique in that proximal areas of the body show pronounced sensory loss; the face, oral mucosa, scalp, trunk, and genitalia may be sites of hypesthesia and hypalgesia. Proprioception is diminished or lost in distal and, to some extent, proximal body parts, giving rise also to ataxia, sometimes prominent, and pseudoathetosis. Tendon reflexes are lost. Often there are features of dysautonomia, but strength is entirely spared. Recognition of this unusual pattern of pansensory loss is of considerable diagnostic importance, since it raises for consideration a number of underlying diseases that might otherwise be missed; these are discussed in Chap. 46. The tabetic syndrome, described below, may also be considered a special type of polyradiculopathy or ganglionopathy.

Sensory Spinal Cord Syndromes (Fig. 9-4; see also Chap. 44)

Tabetic Syndrome This results from damage to the large proprioceptive and other fibers of the posterior lumbosacral (and sometimes cervical) roots. It is typically caused by neurosyphilis but also by diabetes mellitus and other diseases that involve the posterior roots and/or dorsal root ganglia. Numbness or paresthesias and lightning or lancinating pains are frequent complaints; areflexia, abnormalities of gait (page 125), and hypotonia without significant muscle weakness are found on examination. The sensory loss may involve only vibration and position senses in the lower extremities, but in severe cases, loss or impairment of superficial or deep pain sense or of touch may be added. Romberg's sign is prominent. The feet and legs are most affected, much less often the arms and trunk. Frequently, atonicity of the bladder with retention of urine and trophic joint changes (Charcot joints) are associated.

Complete Spinal Sensory Syndrome With a complete transverse lesion of the spinal cord, all forms of sensation are abolished below a level that corresponds to the lesion. There may be a narrow zone of hyperesthesia at the upper margin of the anesthetic zone. Loss of pain,

Figure 9-4

Some of the sites of lesions that produce characteristic spinal cord syndromes (shaded areas indicate lesions).

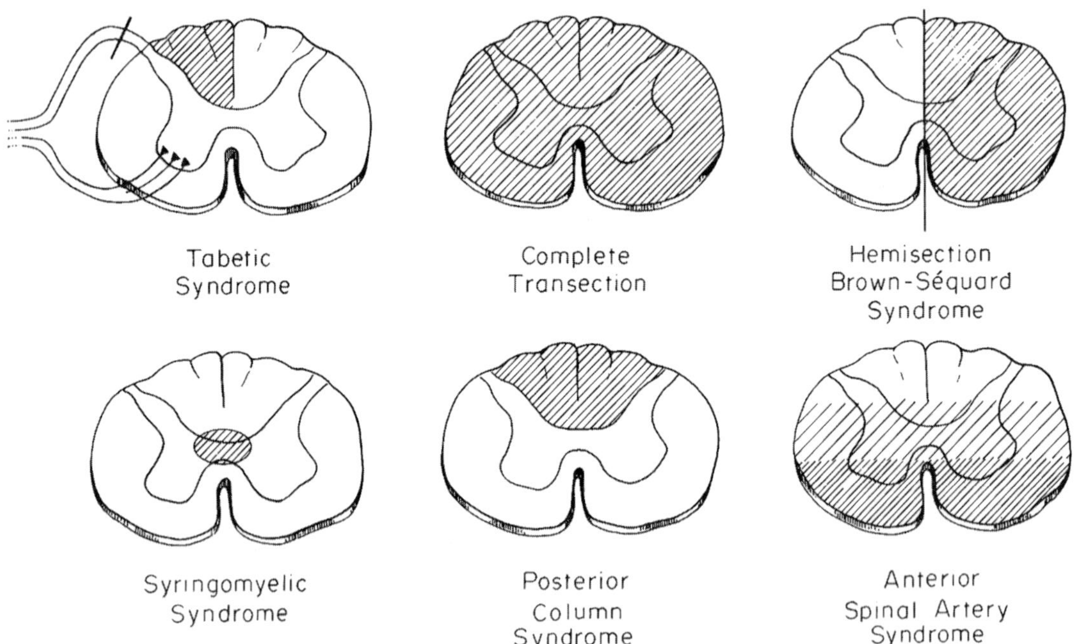

temperature, and touch sensation begins one or two segments below the level of the lesion; vibratory and position senses have less discrete levels. The sensory (and motor) loss in spinal cord lesions that involve both gray and white matter is expressed in patterns corresponding to bodily segments or dermatomes. These are shown in Figs. 9-2 and 9-3 and are most obvious on the trunk, where each intercostal nerve has a transverse distribution.

Also, it is important to remember that during the subacute and chronic evolution of a transverse spinal cord lesion, there may be a greater discrepancy between the level of the lesion and that of the sensory loss, the latter ascending as the lesion progresses. This can be understood if one conceives of a lesion evolving from the periphery to the center of the cord, affecting first the outermost fibers carrying pain and temperature sensation from the legs. Conversely, a lesion advancing from the center of the cord will affect these modalities in the reverse order, with so-called sacral sparing.

Hemisection of the Spinal Cord (Brown-Séquard Syndrome) In rare instances, disease is confined to or predominates on one side of the spinal cord; pain and thermal sensation are affected on the opposite side of the body, and proprioceptive sensation is affected on the same side as the lesion. The loss of pain and temperature sensation begins one or two segments below the lesion. An associated spastic motor paralysis on the side of the lesion completes the syndrome (Fig. 9-4). Tactile sensation is not affected, since the fibers from one side of the body are distributed in tracts (posterior columns, anterior and lateral spinothalamic) on both sides of the cord.

Syringomyelic Syndrome (Lesion of the Central Gray Matter) Since fibers conducting pain and temperature sensation cross the cord in the anterior commissure, a lesion of considerable vertical extent in this location will characteristically abolish these modalities on one or both sides over several segments (dermatomes) but will spare tactile sensation (Fig. 9-4). The most common cause of such a lesion in the cervical region is developmental syringomyelia; less common causes are intramedullary tumor, trauma, and hemorrhage. This type of *dissociated sensory loss* usually occurs in a segmental distribution, and since the lesion frequently involves other parts of the gray matter, varying degrees of segmental amyotrophy and reflex loss are usually present as well. If the lesion has spread to the white matter, corticospinal, spinothalamic, and posterior column signs will be conjoined. A *pseudosyringomyelic* syndrome has been alluded to above (see also page 1376).

Posterior Column Syndrome Loss of vibratory and position sense occurs below the lesion, but the perception of pain and temperature is affected relatively little or not at all. Since posterior column lesions are due to the interruption of central projections of the dorsal root ganglia cells, they may be difficult to distinguish from an affection of large fibers in sensory roots (tabetic syndrome). In some diseases that involve the dorsal columns, vibratory sensation may be involved predominantly, whereas in others position sense is more affected. With complete posterior column lesions, only a few of which have been verified by postmortem examinations (see Nathan et al for a review of the literature), not only is the patient deprived of knowledge of movement and position of parts of the body below the lesion, but all types of sensory discrimination are impaired as well. If the lesion is in the high cervical region, there is clumsiness in the palpation of objects and an inability to recognize the qualities of objects by touch, even though touch-pressure sensation is relatively intact. The stereoanesthesia is expressed also by impaired graphesthesia, tactile localization, and ability to detect the direction of lines drawn on the skin. There may be unusual disturbances of touch and pressure, manifest as lability of threshold, persistence of sensation after removal of the stimulus, and sometimes tactile and postural hallucinations. Nathan and colleagues have confirmed older observations that lesions of the posterior columns cause only slight defects in touch and pressure sensation and that lesions of the anterolateral spinothalamic tracts cause minimal or no defects in these modalities. However, a combined lesion in both pathways causes a total loss of tactile and pressure sensibility below the lesion.

The loss of sensory functions that follows a posterior column lesion—such as impaired two-point discrimination; figure writing; detection of size, shape, weight, and texture of objects; and ability to detect the direction and speed of a moving stimulus on the skin—may simulate a parietal "cortical" lesion but differs in that vibratory sense is also lost in the spinal cord lesion. Paresthesias in the form of tingling and pins-and-needles sensations or girdle- and band-like sensations are common complaints with posterior column disease, and in some cases pinprick may produce a diffuse, burning, unpleasant sensation.

In several cases on record, interruption of the posterior columns by surgical incision or other type of injury did not cause a permanent loss of the sensory modalities thought to be subserved by these pathways (Cook and Browder, Wall and Noordenbos). Since postmortem studies of these cases were not carried out, it is possible that some of the posterior column fibers had been spared. Also, it should be realized that not all proprioceptive fibers ascend to the gracile and cuneate nuclei; some proprioceptive fibers leave the posterior columns in the lumbar region and synapse with secondary neurons in the spinal gray matter and ascend in the ipsilateral posterolateral funiculus. Only cutaneous fibers continue to the gracile and cuneate nuclei. The proposition of Wall and Noordenbos, which is debatable, is that such patients lose not the modalities conventionally attributed to the posterior columns but the ability to perform tasks that demand simultaneous analysis of spatial and temporal characteristics of the stimulus.

Anterior Myelopathy (Anterior Spinal Artery Syndrome) With infarction of the spinal cord in the territory of supply of the anterior spinal artery or with other destructive lesions that affect the ventral portion of the cord predominantly, as in some cases of myelitis, one finds a loss of pain and temperature sensation below the level of the lesion and a relative or absolute sparing of proprioceptive sensation (see also page 1317). Since the corticospinal tracts and the ventral gray matter also lie within the area of distribution of the anterior spinal artery, spastic paralysis is a prominent part of this syndrome (Fig. 9-4).

Disturbances of Sensation due to Lesions of the Brainstem

A characteristic feature of medullary lesions is the occurrence, in many instances, of a crossed sensory disturbance, i.e., a loss of pain and temperature sensation on one side of the face and on the opposite side of the body. This is accounted for by involvement of the descending trigeminal tract or its nucleus and the crossed lateral spinothalamic tract on one side of the brainstem and is nearly always caused by a lateral medullary infarction (Wallenberg syndrome). In the upper medulla, pons, and midbrain, the crossed trigeminothalamic and lateral spinothalamic tracts run together, and a lesion at these levels causes loss of pain and temperature sense on the opposite half of the face and body. There are no tactile paresthesias, only thermal or painful dysesthesias. In the upper brainstem, the spinothalamic tract and the medial lemniscus become confluent, so that an appropriately placed lesion causes a contralateral loss of all superficial and deep sensation.

Cranial nerve palsies, cerebellar ataxia, or motor paralysis are often associated, as indicated in the discussion of strokes in this region (Chap. 34).

Sensory Loss due to a Lesion of the Thalamus (Syndrome of Déjerine-Roussy)

Involvement of the ventral posterolateral (VPL) and posteromedial (VPM) nuclei of the thalamus, usually due to a vascular lesion, less often to a tumor, causes loss or diminution of all forms of sensation on the opposite side of the body. Position sense is affected more frequently than any other sensory function and is usually but not always more profound than loss of touch and pinprick. With partial recovery of sensation, spontaneous pain or discomfort (thalamic pain), sometimes of the most distressing type, may appear on the affected side of the body, and any stimulus may then have a diffuse, unpleasant, lingering quality (page 840). Thermal, especially cold, stimuli, emotional disturbance, loud sounds, and even certain types of music may aggravate the painful state. In spite of this overresponse to pinprick, or to thermal or other stimuli, the patient usually shows an elevated pain threshold, i.e., a stronger stimulus than normal is necessary to produce a sensation of pain (hypalgesia with hyperpathia). The same type of pain syndrome may occasionally accompany lesions of the white matter of the parietal lobe or the medial lemniscus or even the posterior columns of the spinal cord.

Sensory Loss due to Lesions of the Parietal Lobe

In the best-known anterior parietal lobe syndrome, that of Verger-Déjerine, there are disturbances mainly of discriminative sensory functions of the opposite leg, arm, and side of face without impairment of the primary modalities of sensation (unless the lesion is deep). Loss of position sense and sense of movement, impaired ability to localize touch and pain stimuli (topagnosia), widening of two-point threshold, and astereognosis are the most prominent findings, as described earlier in this chapter and on page 483.

Another characteristic manifestation of parietal lobe lesions is *sensory inattention*, *extinction*, or *neglect*. In response to bilateral simultaneous testing of symmetrical parts, using either tactile or painful stimuli, the patient may acknowledge only the stimulus on the sound side; or, if the face and hand or foot on the affected side is touched or pricked, only the stimulus to the face may be noticed. Apparently, cranial structures command more attention than other less richly innervated parts. A similar phenomenon occurs when visual stimuli are simultaneously delivered to both right and left peripheral fields. Yet each stimulus, when applied separately to each side or to each part of the affected side, is properly perceived and localized. In sensory neglect, the patient ignores one side of the body and extrapersonal space, contralateral to the parietal lesion, which is usually in the nondominant hemisphere. Left parietal lesions may also cause (right) sensory neglect, but less frequently. This type of sensory neglect, or extinction, which may also occur occasionally with posterior column and medial lemniscus lesions, may be detected in persons who disclaim any sensory symptoms. These phenomena and other features of parietal lobe lesions are considered further in Chap. 22.

Yet another parietal lobe syndrome (Déjerine-Mouzon) is featured by a severe impairment of the primary modalities of sensation (pain, thermal, tactile, and vibratory sense) over half of the body. Motor paralysis is variable and, with partial recovery, there may be a clumsiness that resembles cerebellar ataxia. Since the sensory disorder simulates that due to a thalamic lesion, it was called *pseudothalamic* by Foix and coworkers. Hyperpathia, much like that of the Déjerine-Roussy syndrome (see above), has also been observed in patients with cortical-subcortical parietal lesions. The pseudothalamic syndrome was related by Foix and colleagues to a sylvian infarct; Bogousslavsky and associates traced it to a parietal infarct due to occlusion of the ascending parietal branch of the middle cerebral artery. In each of the aforementioned parietal lobe syndromes, if the dominant hemisphere is involved, there may be an aphasia, a bimanual tactile agnosia, or a Gerstmann syndrome; with nondominant lesions, there may be anosognosia (page 485).

Often with parietal lesions, the patient's responses to sensory stimuli are variable. A common mistake is to attribute this abnormality to hysteria. A lesion confined to only a part of the parietal cortex (the best examples have been due to glancing bullet or shrapnel wounds of the skull) may result in a circumscribed loss of superficial sensation in an opposite limb, mimicking a root or peripheral nerve lesion.

Sensory Loss due to Suggestion and Hysteria

The possibility of suggesting sensory loss to a patient is a very real one, as has already been indicated. Hysterical patients rarely complain spontaneously of cutaneous sensory loss, although they may use the term *numbness* to indicate paralysis of a limb. Examination, on the other hand, may disclose a complete hemianesthesia—often with reduced hearing, sight, smell, and taste—as well as impaired vibration sense over only half the skull, most being anatomic impossibilities. Anesthesia of an entire limb or a sharply defined sensory loss over part of a limb, not conforming to the distribution of a root or cutaneous nerve, may also be observed. The diagnosis of hysterical hemianesthesia is best made by eliciting the other relevant symptoms of hysteria or, if this is not possible, by noting the discrepancies between this type of sensory loss and that which occurs as part of the known, anatomically verified sensory syndromes. Sometimes, in a patient with no other neurologic abnormality or in one with a definite neurologic syndrome, one is dismayed by sensory findings that are completely inexplicable and discordant. In such cases one must try to reason through to the diagnosis by disregarding the sensory findings.

Diagnosis of Somatosensory Syndromes

Affirmation of the clinical sensory syndromes is often possible by the application of *electrophysiologic testing*. Slowing and reduced amplitude of sensory nerve conduction is found with lesions of nerve, but only if the lesion lies distal to the sensory ganglion. Severe sensory loss in a neuropathic pattern with preserved sensory nerve action potentials therefore points to a radiculopathy. Loss of or slowing of H and F responses corroborates the presence of lesions in proximal parts of nerves, plexuses, and roots. By the use of somatosensory evoked potentials, it is possible to demonstrate slowing of conduction in the peripheral nerve, in the spinal cord to a point in the lower medulla, in the medial lemniscus to the thalamus, and in the pathway from the thalamus to the cerebral cortex. These tests require little cooperation on the part of the patient and can be employed in the analysis of sensory systems even in patients who are comatose. (See Chap. 2 for further discussion.)

In practice, it is seldom necessary to examine all modalities of sensation and perception. With single peripheral nerve lesions, touch and pinprick testing are the most informative. With spinal cord disease, pinprick and thermal stimuli are most revealing of lateral column lesions; testing the senses of vibration, position, and movement, and particularly the sense of direction of a dermal stimulus, reliably indicates posterior column lesions. Touch is the least useful. In brainstem lesions, all modes of sensation including touch are regularly affected, and this applies in general to thalamic lesions. Thus, one is guided in the selection of tests by the locale of the disease.

REFERENCES

Bertelsmann FW, Heimans JJ, Weber EJM, et al: Thermal discrimination thresholds in normal subjects and in patients with diabetic neuropathy. *J Neurol Neurosurg Psychiatry* 48:686, 1985.

Bogousslavsky J, Assal G, Regli F: Aphasie afferente motrice et hemisyndrome sensitif droite. *Rev Neurol* 138:649, 1982.

Brodal A: The somatic afferent pathways, in *Neurological Anatomy*, 3rd ed. New York, Oxford University Press, 1981, pp 46–147.

Carmon A: Disturbances of tactile sensitivity in patients with unilateral cerebral lesions. *Cortex* 7:83, 1971.

Carmon A, Benton AL: Tactile perception of direction and number in patients with unilateral cerebral disease. *Neurology* 19:525, 1969.

Caselli RJ: Rediscovering tactile agnosia. *Mayo Clin Proc* 66:129, 1991.

Cook AW, Browder EJ: Function of the posterior column. *Trans Amer Neurol Assoc* 89:193, 1964.

Corkin S, Milner B, Rasmussen T: Tactually guided maze learning in man: Effects of unilateral cortical excision and bilateral hippocampal lesions. *Neuropsychologia* 3:339, 1965.

Corkin S, Milner B, Rasmussen T: Effects of different cortical excisions on sensory thresholds in man. *Trans Am Neurol Assoc* 89:112, 1964.

Davidoff RA: The dorsal columns. *Neurology* 39:1377, 1989.

Dyck PJ, Karnes J, O'Brien PC, Zimmerman IR: Detection thresholds of cutaneous sensation in humans, in Dyck PJ, Thomas PK, et al (eds): *Peripheral Neuropathy*, 3rd ed. Philadelphia, Saunders, 1993, pp 706–728.

Foix C, Chavany JA, Levy M: Syndrome pseudothalamique d'origine parietale. *Rev Neurol* 35:68, 1965.

Greaves MS, Wall PD: Pathophysiology of itching. *Lancet* 348:938, 1996.

Holmes GM: *Introduction to Clinical Neurology*, 2nd ed. Baltimore, Williams & Wilkins, 1952, chaps 8 and 9, pp 67–97.

Keegan JJ, Garrett FD: The segmental distribution of the cutaneous nerves in the limbs of man. *Anat Rec* 102:409, 1948.

Kibler RF, Nathan PW: A note on warm and cold spots. *Neurology* 10:874, 1960.

Lele PP, Weddell G: The relationship between neurohistology and corneal sensibility. *Brain* 79:119, 1956.

Lewis T, Pickering GW, Rothschild P: Centrifugal paralysis arising out of arrested blood flow to the limb, including notes on a form of tingling. *Heart* 16:1, 1931.

Light AR, Perl ER: Peripheral sensory systems, in Dyck PJ, Thomas PK, et al (eds): *Peripheral Neuropathy*, 3rd ed. Philadelphia, Saunders, 1993, chap 8, pp 149–165.

Lindblom U, Ochoa J: Somatosensory function and dysfunction, in Asbury AK, McKhann GM, McDonald IW (eds): *Diseases of the Nervous System*, 2nd ed. Philadelphia, Saunders, 1992, chap 16, pp 213–228.

Loh L, Nathan PW: Painful peripheral states and sympathetic blocks. *J Neurol Neurosurg Psychiatry* 41:664, 1978.

Markel R: Human cutaneous mechanoreceptors during regeneration: Physiology and interpretation. *Ann Neurol* 18:165, 1985.

Mayo Clinic: *Examinations in Neurology*, 7th ed. St Louis, Mosby, 1998.

Moberg E: The role of cutaneous afferents in position sense, kinaesthesia and motor function of the hand. *Brain* 106:1, 1983.

Mountcastle VG: Central nervous mechanisms in sensation, in Mountcastle VB (ed): *Medical Physiology*, 14th ed. Vol 1. Part 5. St Louis, Mosby, 1980, chaps 11–19, pp 327–605.

Nathan PW, Smith MC, Cook AW: Sensory effects in man of lesions in the posterior columns and of some other afferent pathways. *Brain* 109:1003, 1986.

Ochoa JL, Torebjork HE: Paraesthesiae from ectopic impulse generation in human sensory nerves. *Brain* 103:835, 1980.

Ray BS, Wolff HG: Studies on pain: Spread of pain: Evidence on site of spread within the neuraxis of effects of painful stimulation. *Arch Neurol Psychiatry* 53:257, 1945.

Roland PE, Ladegaard-Pederson H: A quantitative analysis of sensations of tension and of kinaesthesia in man. *Brain* 100:671, 1977.

Semmes J, Weinstein S, Ghent L, Teuber H-L: *Somatosensory Changes after Penetrating Brain Wounds in Man*. Cambridge, MA, Harvard University Press, 1960.

Sinclair D: *Mechanisms of Cutaneous Sensation*. Oxford, England, Oxford University Press, 1981.

Torebjork HE, Vallbo AB, Ochoa JL: Intraneural microstimulation in man: Its relation to specificity of tactile sensations. *Brain* 110:1509, 1987.

Tower SS: Unit for sensory reception in the cornea. *J Neurophysiol* 3:486, 1940.

Trotter W, Davies HM: Experimental studies in the innervation of the skin. *J Physiol* 38:134, 1909.

Wall PD, Noordenbos W: Sensory functions which remain in man after complete transection of dorsal columns. *Brain* 100: 641, 1977.

Weddell G: The multiple innervation of sensory spots in the skin. *J Anat* 75:441, 1941.

Chapter 10

HEADACHE AND OTHER CRANIOFACIAL PAINS

Of all the painful states that afflict humans, headache is undoubtedly the most frequent and rivals backache as the most common reason for seeking medical help. In fact, there are so many cases of headache that special headache clinics have been established in many medical centers. Insofar as many headaches are due to medical rather than neurologic diseases, the subject is the legitimate concern of the general physician. Yet always there is the question of intracranial disease, so that it is difficult to approach the subject without a knowledge of neurologic medicine.

Why so many pains are centered in the head is a question of some interest. Several explanations come to mind. For one thing, the face and scalp are more richly supplied with pain receptors than many other parts of the body, perhaps in order to protect the precious contents of the skull. Also, the nasal and oral passages, the eye, and the ear, all delicate and highly sensitive structures, reside here and must be protected; when afflicted by disease, each is capable of inducing pain in its own way. Finally, for the intelligent person, there is greater concern about what happens to the head than to other parts of the body, since the former houses the brain, and headache frequently raises the specter of brain tumor or other cerebral disease.

Semantically, the term *headache* should encompass all aches and pains located in the head, but in practice its application is restricted to discomfort in the region of the cranial vault. Facial, lingual, and pharyngeal pains are put aside as something different and are discussed separately in the latter part of this chapter.

GENERAL CONSIDERATIONS

In the introductory chapter on pain, reference was made to the necessity, when dealing with any painful state, of determining its quality, severity, location, duration, and time course as well as the conditions that produce, exacerbate, or relieve it. When headache is considered in these terms, a certain amount of useful information is obtained, but often less than one might expect. Auscultation of the skull may disclose a bruit (with large arteriovenous malformations) and palpation may disclose the tender, hardened arteries of temporal arteritis, sensitive areas overlying a cranial metastasis, an inflamed sinus, or a tender occipital nerve. However, apart from such special instances, examination of the head itself, though always necessary, is seldom revealing.

As to the *quality* of cephalic pain, the patient's description may or may not be helpful. Persistent questioning on this point may even occasion surprise, for the patient often assumes that the word *headache* should have conveyed enough information to the examiner about the nature of the discomfort. Most headaches, regardless of type, tend to be dull, aching, and not sharply localized, as is usually the case with disease of structures deep to the skin. Seldom does the patient describe the pricking or stinging type of pain that arises from the skin. When asked to compare the pain to some other sensory experience, the patient may allude to tightness, pressure, bursting, sharpness, or stabbing. The most important information to be obtained is whether the headache throbs, indicating a vascular sensitivity. But one must keep in mind that patients often use the word *throbbing* to refer to a waxing and waning of the headache, without any relation to the pulse, whereas authentic pulsatile throbbing, especially if hemicranial, is highly characteristic of migraine.

Similarly, statements about *the intensity of the pain* must be accepted with caution, since they reflect as much the patient's attitudes and customary ways of experiencing and reacting to pain as its true severity. By temperament, some persons tend to minimize discomfort and others to dramatize it. A better index of severity is the degree to which the pain has incapacitated the patient, especially if he is not prone to illness. A severe migraine attack seldom allows performance of the day's work. Another rough index of the severity of headache is its propensity to awaken the patient from sleep or to prevent sleep. The most intense cranial pains are those associated with meningitis and subarachnoid hemorrhage, which have grave implications, and with migraine, cluster headache, or tic douloureux, which do not.

Data regarding the *location* of a headache are apt to be more informative. Inflammation of an extracranial artery causes pain localized to the site of the vessel. Lesions of paranasal sinuses, teeth, eyes, and upper cervical vertebrae induce a less sharply localized pain, but still one that is referred to a certain region, usually to the forehead or maxilla, or around the eyes. Intracranial lesions in the posterior fossa usually cause pain in the occipitonuchal region and usually are homolateral if the lesion is one-sided. Supratentorial lesions induce frontotemporal pain, again approximating the site of the lesion. Localization, however, may also be deceiving. Pain in the frontal regions may be due to such diverse lesions and mechanisms as glaucoma, sinusitis, thrombosis of the vertebral or basilar artery, pressure on the tentorium, or increased intracranial pressure. Similarly, ear pain may signify disease of the ear itself, but more often it is referred from other regions, such as the throat, cervical muscles, spine, or structures in the posterior fossa. Periorbital and supraorbital pain, while sometimes indicative of local disease, may reflect dissection of the cervical portion of the internal carotid artery. Headaches localized to the vertex or biparietal regions are infrequent and should raise the suspicion of sphenoid or ethmoid sinus disease or thrombosis of the superior sagittal sinus.

The *mode of onset*, *time-intensity curve*, and *duration* of the headache, with respect both to a single attack and to the temporal profile of the headache over a period of years, are also useful data. The headache of subarachnoid hemorrhage (due to a ruptured aneurysm) occurs as an abrupt attack that attains its maximal severity in a matter of seconds or minutes; or, in the case of meningitis, it may come on more gradually, over several hours or days. Brief sharp pain, lasting a few seconds, in the eyeball (ophthalmodynia) or cranium ("icepick") pains; "ice-cream headache," due to pharyngeal cooling, are more common in migraineurs, with or without the characteristic headache, but otherwise are uninterpretable and are significant only for reason of their benignity. Migraine of the classic type has its onset in the early morning hours or daytime, reaches its peak of severity rapidly or gradually, and lasts, unless treated, for 4 to 24 h, occasionally for as long as 72 h. Often it is terminated by sleep. More than a single attack of migraine every few weeks is exceptional. A migrainous patient having several attacks per week usually proves to have a combination of migraine and tension headaches, an analgesic "rebound headache" or, rarely, some new, unexpected intracranial lesion. By contrast, the occurrence of unbearably severe unilateral orbitotemporal pain coming on within an hour or two after falling asleep or at predictable times during the day and recurring nightly or daily for a period of several weeks to months is typical of cluster headache; usually an individual attack dissipates in 30 to 45 min. The headaches of intracranial tumor may appear at any time of the day or night, interrupt sleep, vary in intensity, and last a few minutes to hours; as the tumor raises intracranial pressure, or with posterior fossa masses, the headache tends to be worse in the morning on awakening. Tension headaches, described further on, may persist with varying intensity for weeks to months or even longer. In general, headaches that have recurred regularly for many years prove to be vascular or tension in type.

The more or less constant *relationship of headache to certain biologic events and also to certain precipitating or aggravating (or relieving) factors* must always be noted. Headaches that occur regularly in the premenstrual period are usually generalized and mild in degree ("premenstrual tension"), but attacks of migraine may also occur at this time. Headaches that have their origin in cervical spine disease are most typically intense after a period of inactivity, such as a night's sleep, and the first movements of the neck are stiff and painful. Headache from infection of the nasal sinuses may appear, with clocklike regularity, upon awakening or in midmorning; it is characteristically worsened by stooping and changes in atmospheric pressure. Eyestrain headaches, of course, follow prolonged use of the eyes, as after long-sustained periods of reading, peering into glaring headlights, or exposure to the glare of video displays. In certain individuals, alcohol, intense exercise (such as weightlifting), stooping, straining, coughing, and sexual intercourse are known to initiate a special type of bursting headache, lasting a few seconds to minutes. If the headache is made worse by sudden movement or by coughing or straining, an intracranial source is suggested. Anger, excitement, or worry may initiate migraine in certain disposed persons. In other patients, migraine occurs several hours or a day following a period of intense activity and stress ("weekend migraine"). Some patients have discovered that their migraine is relieved momentarily by gentle compression of the carotid or superficial temporal artery on the painful side, and others have noted that the carotid itself is tender during the headache.

Pain-Sensitive Cranial Structures

Understanding of headache has been greatly augmented by observations made during operations on the brain (Ray and Wolff). These observations inform us that only certain cranial structures are sensitive to pain: (1) skin, subcutaneous tissue, muscles, extracranial arteries, and periosteum of the skull; (2) delicate structures of the eye, ear, nasal cavities, and sinuses; (3) intracranial venous sinuses and their large tributaries, especially pericavernous structures; (4) parts of the dura at the base of the brain and the arteries within the dura and pia-arachnoid, particularly the proximal parts of the anterior and middle cerebral arteries and the intracranial segment of the internal carotid artery; (5) the middle meningeal and superficial temporal arteries; and (6) the optic, oculomotor, trigeminal, glossopharyngeal, vagus, and first three cervical nerves. Interestingly, pain is practically the only sensation produced by stimulation of these structures; the pain arises in the walls of small blood vessels containing pain fibers (the nature of vascular pain is discussed further on).

Of importance also are the reference sites of pain from the aforementioned structures. Pain impulses that arise from distention of the middle meningeal artery are projected to the back of the eye and temporal area. Pain from the intracranial segment of the internal carotid artery and proximal parts of the middle and anterior cerebral arteries is felt in the eye and orbitotemporal regions. The bony skull, much of the pia-arachnoid and dura over the convexity of the brain, the parenchyma of the brain, and the ependyma and choroid plexuses lack sensitivity.

The pathways whereby sensory stimuli, whatever their nature, are transmitted to the central nervous system (CNS) are the trigeminal nerves, particularly their first and, to some extent, second divisions, which convey impulses from the forehead, orbit, anterior and middle fossae of the skull, and the upper surface of the tentorium. The sphenopalatine branches of the facial nerve convey impulses from the naso-orbital region. The ninth and tenth cranial nerves and the first three cervical nerves transmit impulses from the inferior surface of the tentorium and all of the posterior fossa. Sympathetic fibers from the three cervical ganglia and parasympathetic fibers from the sphenopalatine ganglia are mixed with the trigeminal and other sensory fibers. The tentorium roughly demarcates the trigeminal and cervical innervation zones. The central sensory connections, which ascend through the cervical spinal cord and brainstem to the thalamus, have been described in the preceding chapter.

To summarize, pain from supratentorial structures is referred to the anterior two-thirds of the head, i.e., to the territory of sensory supply of the first and second divisions of the trigeminal nerve; pain from infratentorial structures is referred to the vertex and back of the head and neck by the upper cervical roots. The seventh, ninth, and tenth cranial nerves refer pain to the naso-orbital region, ear, and throat. There may be local tenderness of the scalp at the site of the referred pain. Dental or temporomandibular joint pain may also have cranial reference. With the exception of the cervical portion of the internal carotid artery, from which pain is referred to the eyebrow and supraorbital region, and the upper cervical spine, from which pain may be referred to the occiput, pain due to disease in extracranial parts of the body is not referred to the head.

Mechanisms of Cranial Pain

The studies of Ray and Wolff have also demonstrated that relatively few mechanisms are operative in the genesis of cranial pain. More specifically, *intracranial mass lesions* cause headache only if in a position to deform, displace, or exert traction on vessels and dural structures at the base of the brain, and this may happen long before intracranial pressure rises. In fact, artificially raising the intraspinal and intracranial pressure by the subarachnoid or intraventricular injection of sterile saline solution does not consistently result in headache. This has been interpreted to mean that raised intracranial pressure does not cause headache—a questionable conclusion when one considers the relief of headache that follows lumbar puncture and lowering of the cerebrospinal fluid (CSF) pressure in some patients. Actually, most patients with high intracranial pressure complain of bioccipital and bifrontal headaches that fluctuate in severity, probably because of traction on vessels or dura.

Dilatation of intracranial or extracranial arteries (and possibly sensitization of these vessels), of whatever cause, is likely to produce headache. The headaches that follow seizures, infusion of histamine, and ingestion of alcohol are probably all due to cerebral vasodilatation. Nitroglycerin, nitrites in cured meats ("hot-dog headache"), and monosodium glutamate in Chinese food may cause headache by the same mechanism. It seems probable that the throbbing or steady headache that accompanies febrile illnesses has a vascular origin as well; it is likely that the increased pulsation of meningeal vessels activates pain-sensitive structures around the base of the brain. Certain infectious agents, enumerated further on, seem to have a proclivity to cause severe headache. The febrile headache may be generalized or predominate in the frontal or occipital regions and is much like histamine headache in being relieved on one side by carotid or superficial temporal artery compression and on both sides by jugular vein compression. It, like migraine, is increased by shaking the head.

A similar mechanism may be operative in the severe, bilateral, throbbing headaches associated with extreme rises in blood pressure, as occurs with pheochromocytoma, malignant hypertension, sexual activity, and in patients being treated with monoamine oxidase inhibitors. Patents should be informed that mild to moderate degrees of hypertension do not cause headaches. So-called cough and exertional headaches may also have their basis in distention of intracranial vessels.

For many years, following the investigations of Harold Wolff, the headache of migraine was attributed to dilatation of the extracranial arteries. Now it appears that this is not a constant relationship and that the headache is of intracranial as much as extracranial origin, perhaps related to the sensitization of blood vessels and their surrounding structures. Activation of the trigeminovascular system (the trigeminal nerves and the blood vessels they supply), leading to "sterile inflammation," has also been assigned a role in the genesis of migraine headache. These and other theories of causation are discussed further on in this chapter.

Extracranial temporal and occipital arteries, when involved in giant-cell arteritis (cranial or "temporal" arteritis), give rise to severe, persistent headache, at first localized and then more diffuse. With occlusion or dissection of the vertebral artery, the pain is postauricular or in the low occipital region; basilar artery thrombosis causes pain to be projected to the occiput and sometimes to the forehead. The ipsilateral eye and brow and the forehead above it are the most common sites of projected pain from dissection of the carotid and the stem of the middle cerebral arteries. Expanding or ruptured intracranial aneurysms may cause pain projected from the posterior communicating artery to the eye.

Infection or blockage of paranasal sinuses is accompanied by pain over the affected maxillary or frontal sinuses. Usually it is associated with tenderness of the skin in the same distribution. Pain from the ethmoid and sphenoid sinuses is localized deep in the midline behind the root of the nose or occasionally at the vertex (especially with disease of the sphenoid sinus) or other part of the cranium. The mechanism in these cases involves changes in pressure and irritation of pain-sensitive sinus walls. Sinus pain recurs and subsides periodically, depending on drainage from the sinus. With frontal and ethmoidal sinusitis, the pain tends to be worse on awakening and gradually subsides when the patient is upright; the opposite pertains with maxillary and sphenoidal sinusitis. These relationships are believed to disclose their mechanism; pain is ascribed to filling of the sinuses and its relief to their emptying, induced by the dependent position of the ostia. Bending over intensifies the pain by causing changes in pressure, as does blowing the nose if the ostium of the infected sinus is patent; during air travel, both earache and sinus headache tend to occur on descent, when the relative pressure in the blocked viscus rises. Sympathomimetic drugs such as phenylephrine hydrochloride, which reduce swelling and congestion, tend to relieve the pain. However, the pain may persist after all purulent secretions have disappeared, probably because of blockage of the orifice by boggy membranes and absorption of air from the blocked sinus (*vacuum sinus headaches*). The condition is relieved when aeration is restored.

Headache of ocular origin, located as a rule in the orbit, forehead, or temple, is of the steady, aching type and tends to follow prolonged use of the eyes in close work. The main faults are hypermetropia and astigmatism (rarely myopia), which result in sustained contraction of extraocular as well as frontal, temporal, and even occipital muscles. Correction of the refractive error abolishes the headache. Traction on the extraocular muscles or the iris during eye surgery will evoke pain. Patients who develop diplopia from neurologic causes or are forced to use one eye because the other has been occluded by a patch often complain of frontal headache. Another mechanism is involved in *iridocyclitis* and in *acute glaucoma*, in which raised intraocular pressure causes steady, aching pain in the region of the eye, radiating to the forehead. As for headache in general, it is important that the eyes be refracted, but eyestrain is probably not as frequent a cause as one would expect from the wholesale dispensing of eyeglasses for its relief.

Headaches that accompany disease of ligaments, muscles, and apophyseal joints in the upper part of the spine are referred to the occiput and nape of the neck on the same side and sometimes to the temple and forehead. These headaches have been reproduced in part by the injection of hypertonic saline solution into the affected ligaments, muscles, and zygoapophyseal joints. Such pains are especially frequent in late life because of the prevalence of degenerative changes in the cervical spine and tend also to occur after whiplash injuries or other forms of sudden flexion, extension, or torsion of the head on the neck. If the pain is arthritic in origin, the first movements after being still for some hours are stiff and painful. The pain of fibromyalgia, evidenced by tender areas near the cranial insertion of cervical and other muscles, is a controversial entity. There are no pathologic data as to the nature of these vaguely palpable lesions, and it is uncertain whether the pain actually arises in them. They may represent only the deep tenderness felt in the region of referred pain or the involuntary secondary protective spasm of muscles. Sleep disturbance is often associated, as is depression. Massage of muscles, heat, and injection of the tender spots with local anesthetic have unpredictable effects but relieve the pain in some cases. Unilateral occipital headache is often misinterpreted as occipital neuralgia (see further on).

The headache of meningeal irritation (infection or hemorrhage) is acute in onset, usually severe, generalized, deep-seated, constant, and associated with stiffness of the neck, particularly on forward bending. It has been ascribed to increased intracranial pressure; indeed, the withdrawal of CSF may afford some relief. However, dilatation and inflammation of meningeal vessels and the chemical irritation of pain receptors in the large vessels and meninges by chemical agents, particularly serotonin and plasma kinins, are probably more important factors in the production of pain and spasm of the neck extensors. In the chemically induced meningitis from rupture of an epidermoid cyst, for example, the spinal fluid pressure is usually normal but the headache is severe.

Lumbar puncture (LP) headache is characterized by a steady occipitonuchal and frontal pain coming on within a few minutes after arising from a recumbent position and relieved within a minute or two by lying down. Its cause is a persistent leakage of CSF into the lumbar tissues through the needle track. The CSF pressure is low (often zero in the lateral decubitus position), and the injection of sterile isotonic saline solution intrathecally or the placing of an epidural "blood patch" relieves the headache. Usually this type of headache is increased by compression of the jugular veins but is unaffected by digital obliteration of one carotid artery. It seems probable that, in the upright position, a low intraspinal and negative intracranial pressure permits caudal displacement of the brain, with traction on dural attachments and dural sinuses. Pannullo and colleagues, with magnetic resonance imaging, have demonstrated this downward displacement of the cranial contents. Understandably, then, headache following cisternal puncture is less frequent. As soon as the leakage of CSF stops and CSF pressure is restored (usually within hours or a few days), the headache disappears. "Spontaneous" low-pressure headache may follow a sneeze, strain, or athletic injury, presumably because of rupture of the arachnoid sleeve along a nerve root (page 671). Less frequently, lumbar puncture is complicated by severe stiffness of the neck and pain over the back of the neck and occiput (page 670); a second spinal tap in some instances discloses slight pleocytosis but no decrease in glucose—a sterile or chemical meningitis. This benign reaction must be distinguished from the rare occurrence of bacterial meningitis due to introduction of bacteria by the LP needle.

Headaches that are aggravated by lying down occur with chronic subdural hematoma and some tumors, especially with those in the posterior fossa. The headaches of pseudotumor cerebri are also generally worse in the supine position.

Exertional headaches are usually benign but are sometimes related to pheochromocytoma, arteriovenous malformation, or other intracranial lesions. The same applies to headaches induced by stooping (see further on).

The identification of a number of neurotransmitters has helped in the understanding of headache mechanisms. These are considered below in the section on migraine, since they have been best studied in this form of headache.

PRINCIPAL VARIETIES OF HEADACHE

There should be little difficulty in recognizing the acute headaches of glaucoma, purulent sinusitis, subarachnoid hemorrhage, and bacterial or viral meningitis and the subacute or more chronic headache of brain tumor provided that these sources of headache are kept in mind. A fuller account of these types of headache may be found in later chapters of this book, where the underlying diseases are described. When the headache is chronic, recurrent, and unattended by other symptoms and signs of neurologic disease, the physician faces a more difficult diagnostic problem.

The following types of headaches should then be considered (see Table 10-1). In general, the classification of these headaches and other types of craniofacial pain follow those of the International Headache Society (see Olesen). One area of controversy in classification concerns the status (and indeed the existence) of tension headache. A currently held view, with which the authors do not entirely agree, is that there is a continuum between migraine and tension headache. This relationship is considered further on.

Table 10-1
Common types of headache

Type	*Site*	*Age and sex*	*Clinical characteristics*	*Diurnal pattern*	*Life profile*	*Provoking factors*	*Associated features*	*Treatment*
Migraine without aura (common migraine)	Frontotemporal Uni- or bilateral	Adolescents, young to middle-aged adults, sometimes children, more common in women	Throbbing (pulsatile); worse behind one eye or ear Becomes dull ache and generalized Scalp sensitive	Upon awakening or later in day Duration: 4–24 h in most cases, sometimes longer	Irregular intervals, weeks to months Tends to decrease in middle age and during pregnancy	Bright light, noise, tension, alcohol Relieved by darkness and sleep	Nausea and vomiting in some cases	Ergotamine sumatriptan, nonsteroidal anti-inflammatory agents Propranolol or amitriptyline for prevention
Migraine with aura (neurologic migraine)	Same as above	Same as above	Same as above Family history frequent	Same as above	Same as above	Same as above	Scintillating lights, visual loss, and scotomas Unilateral paresthesias, weakness, dysphasia, vertigo, rarely confusion	Same as above
Cluster (histamine headache, migrainous neuralgia)	Orbito-temporal Unilateral	Adolescent and adult males (90%)	Intense, nonthrobbing	Usually nocturnal, 1–2 h after falling asleep Occasionally diurnal	Nightly or daily for several weeks to months Recurrence after many months or years	Alcohol in some	Lacrimation Stuffed nostril Rhinorrhea Injected conjunctivum Ptosis	Ergotamine before anticipated attack O_2, sumatriptan Methysergide, corticosteroids, Verampil, Valproate, and lithium in recalcitrant cases

Tension headaches	Generalized	Mainly adults, both sexes, more in women	Pressure (nonthrobbing), tightness, aching	Continuous, variable intensity, for days, weeks, or months	One or more periods of months to years	Fatigue and nervous strain	Depression, worry, anxiety	Antianxiety and antidepressant drugs
Meningeal irritation (meningitis, subarachnoid hemorrhage)	Generalized, or bioccipital or bifrontal	Any age, both sexes	Intense, steady deep pain, may be worse in neck	Rapid evolution—minutes to hours	Single episode	None	Neck stiff on forward bending Kernig and Brudzinski signs	For meningitis or bleeding (see text)
Brain tumor	Unilateral or generalized	Any age, both sexes	Variable intensity May awaken patient Steady pain	Lasts minutes to hours; worse in early A.M., increasing severity	Once in a lifetime: weeks to months	None Sometimes position	Papilledema Vomiting Impaired mentation Seizures Focal signs	Corticosteroids Mannitol Treatment of tumor
Temporal arteritis	Unilateral or bilateral, usually temporal	Over 50 years, either sex	Throbbing, then persistent aching and burning, arteries thickened and tender	Intermittent, then continuous	Persists for weeks to months	None	Loss of vision Polymyalgia rheumatica Fever, weight loss, increased sedimentation rate	Corticosteroids

MIGRAINE

Migraine is a ubiquitous familial disorder characterized by periodic, commonly unilateral, often pulsatile headaches which begin in childhood, adolescence, or early adult life and recur with diminishing frequency during advancing years.

Two closely related clinical syndromes have been identified. The first is called *migraine with aura* and the second, *migraine without aura* (terminology of the International Headache Society). For many years the first syndrome was referred to as *classic* or *neurologic* migraine, and the second, as *common* migraine. The ratio of classic to common migraine is 1:5. Either type may be preceded by vague premonitory changes in mood and appetite (a prodrome). Migraine with aura, the term now used to denote classic migraine, is ushered in by an evident disturbance of nervous function, most often visual, followed in a few minutes by hemicranial or, in about one-third of cases, by bilateral headache, nausea, and sometimes vomiting, all of which last for hours or as long as a day or two. Migraine without aura is characterized by an unheralded onset of hemicranial headache or, less often, by generalized headache with or without nausea and vomiting, which then follows the same temporal pattern as the migraine with aura. Sensitivity to light and noise attends both types and intensification with movement of the head is common. If the pain is severe, the patient prefers to lie down in a quiet, darkened room and tries to sleep. Both headache syndromes usually respond to ergotamine, sumatriptan, and related drugs.

The genetic nature of classic migraine (with an aura) is apparent from its occurrence in several members of the family of the same and successive generations in 60 to 80 percent of cases. Twin and sibling studies have not revealed a consistent mendelian pattern in either the classic or common form, and the inheritance in all likelihood is polygenic. Certain rare forms of migraine, such as familial hemiplegic migraine, appear to be monogenic disorders, but the role of these genes, one of which codes for a calcium channel (see below), in classic and common migraine is speculative.

Migraine, with or without aura, is a remarkably common condition; its prevalence among Caucasians is in the range of 4 to 6 percent among men and 13 to 18 percent among women (see Stewart et al). The numbers are lower in Asians. Migraine may have its onset in childhood but usually begins in adolescence; in more than 80 percent of patients, the onset is before 30 years of age. Both the prevalence and gender ratio vary with age, increasing to about 40 years of age and declining thereafter. The headaches tend to occur during the premenstrual period; in about 15 percent of women migraineurs, the attacks are exclusively perimenstrual ("true menstrual migraine"), although estrogen and progesterone levels throughout the menstrual cycle are the same in normal and migrainous women. Menstrual migraine, discussed further on, is thought to be related to the withdrawal of estradiol rather than progesterone (Somerville). The attacks cease during pregnancy in 75 to 80 percent of women, and in others they continue at a reduced frequency; less often, attacks of migraine or the associated neurologic symptoms first appear during pregnancy, usually in the first trimester. Although migraine usually diminishes in severity and frequency with age, it may actually worsen in some postmenopausal women, and estrogen therapy may either increase, or, paradoxically, diminish the incidence of headaches. The use of birth control pills has been associated with an increased frequency and severity of migraine and in rare instances has resulted in a permanent neurologic deficit. Some patients link their attacks to certain dietary items—particularly chocolate, cheese, fatty foods, oranges, tomatoes, and onions—but these connections seem to us to be overrated. Some of these foods are rich in tyramine, which has been incriminated as a provocative factor in migraine. Alcohol, particularly red wine or port, regularly provokes an attack in some persons; in others, headaches are consistently induced by exposure to glare or other strong sensory stimuli, sudden jarring of the head ("footballer's migraine"), or by rapid changes in barometric pressure.

Migraine with aura frequently has its onset soon after awakening, but it may occur at any time of day. During the preceding day or so, there may have been mild changes in mood (sometimes a surge of energy or a feeling of well-being), hunger or anorexia, drowsiness, and frequent yawning. Then, abruptly, there is a disturbance of vision consisting usually of unformed flashes of white or, rarely, of multicolored lights (photopsia), an enlarging blind spot with a shimmering edge (*scintillating scotoma*), or formations of dazzling zigzag lines (arranged like the battlements of a castle, hence the term *fortification spectra* or *teichopsia*). Some patients complain of blurred or shimmering or cloudy vision, as though they were looking through thick or smoked glass or the wavy distortions produced by heat rising from asphalt. These luminous hallucinations move slowly across the visual field for several minutes and may leave an island of visual loss in their wake (scotomatous defects); the latter are usually bilateral and often homonymous (involving corresponding parts of the field of vision of each eye), pointing to their origin in the visual cortex. Visual abnormalities of retinal and optic nerve origin have also been described (see further on).

Other focal neurologic symptoms, much less common than visual ones, include numbness and tingling of the lips, face, and hand (on one or both sides); slight confusion of thinking; weakness of an arm or leg; mild aphasia or dysarthria, dizziness, and uncertainty of gait; or drowsiness. Only one or a few of these neurologic phenomena are present in any given patient, and they tend to occur in more or less the same combination in each attack. If weakness or paresthetic numbness spreads from one part of the body to another or if one neurologic symptom follows another, this occurs relatively slowly over a period of minutes (not over seconds, as in a seizure). These neurologic symptoms last for 1 to 15 min, sometimes longer; as they begin to recede, they are followed by a unilateral dull pain that progresses to a throbbing headache (usually but not always on the side of the cerebral disturbance), which slowly increases in intensity. At its peak, within minutes to an hour, the patient is forced to lie down and to shun light and noise. Light is irritating and may be painful to the globes, or it is perceived as overly bright (dazzle) and strong odors are very disagreeable. Nausea and, less often, vomiting may occur. The headache lasts for hours and sometimes for a day or even longer and is always the most unpleasant feature of the illness. The temporal vessels may be tender and the headache may be worsened by strain or jarring of the body or rapid movement of the head. Pressure on the scalp vessels or carotid artery may momentarily reduce the pain.

Between attacks, the migrainous patient is normal. For a time, when psychosomatic medicine was much in vogue, there was insistence on a migrainous personality, characterized by tenseness, rigidity of attitudes and thinking, meticulousness, and perfectionism. Further analyses, however, have not established a particular personality type in the migraineur. Moreover, the fact that the headaches may begin in early childhood, when the personality is relatively amorphous, would argue against this idea. There is no clear relationship, despite many statements to the contrary, between migraine and neurosis. Some patients have noted that their attacks of migraine tend to occur during the "let-down period," after many days of hard work or nervous tension, but the temporal relations between headache and the day's or week's activities have not proved to be consistent. The relationship to epilepsy is also tenuous; the incidence of seizures is slightly higher in migrainous patients and their relatives than in the general population. Lance and Anthony find no mechanism common to migraine and epilepsy. There does seem to be in migraineurs an overrepresentation of motion sickness and of fainting.

Migraine Variants Much variation occurs. The headache may be exceptionally severe and abrupt in onset ("crash migraine"), raising the specter of subarachnoid hemorrhage. Careful questioning reveals that the headache did not attain its peak of severity instantaneously but evolved over several minutes. The headache may accompany rather than follow the neurologic abnormalities. Though typically hemicranial (the French word migraine is said to be derived from *megrim*, which in turn was derived from the Latin *hemicrania* and its corrupted forms *hemigranea* and *migranea*), the pain may be frontal, temporal, or generalized.

Milder forms of migraine, especially if partially controlled by medication, may not force withdrawal from accustomed activities. Any one of the three principal components—neurologic abnormality, headache, and nausea and vomiting—may be absent. With advancing age, there is a tendency for the headache and nausea to become less severe, finally leaving only the neurologic abnormality ("aura without migraine"), which itself recurs with decreasing frequency. The latter is also subject to variation. Visual disturbances, by far the most common, differ in detail from patient to patient; numbness and tingling of the lips and the fingers of one hand are probably next in frequency, followed by transient aphasia or a thickness of speech and hemiparesis. Rarely, there is sudden blindness or a hemianopia at the onset accompanied by only a mild headache.

Basilar Migraine A less common form of the migraine syndrome, with prominent brain symptoms, was described by Bickerstaff. The patients, usually young women with a family history of migraine, first develop visual phenomena like those of typical migraine except that they occupy the whole of both visual fields (temporary cortical blindness may occur). There may be associated vertigo, staggering, incoordination of the limbs, dysarthria, and tingling in both hands and feet and sometimes around both sides of the mouth. Exceptionally there is an alarming period of coma or quadriplegia. These symptoms last 10 to 30 min and are followed by headache, which is usually occipital. Some patients, at the stage when the headache is likely to begin, may faint, and others become confused or stuporous, a state that may persist for several hours or longer. The symptoms closely resemble those due to ischemia in the territory of the basilar-posterior cerebral arteries—hence the name *basilar artery* or *vertebrobasilar migraine*. Subsequent studies have indicated that basilar migraine, though more common in children and adolescents, affects men and women more or less equally over a wide age range, and that the condition is not always benign and transient (see further on, under "Complicated Migraine").

Ophthalmoplegic and Retinal Migraine The former are recurrent unilateral headaches associated with weakness of extraocular muscles. A transient third-nerve palsy with ptosis, with or without involvement of the pupil, is the usual picture; rarely, the sixth nerve is affected. This disorder is more common in children. The paresis often outlasts the headache by days or weeks; after many attacks, a slight mydriasis and, rarely, ophthalmoparesis may remain as permanent defects.

Retinal and anterior optic nerve ischemia have also been documented. In some cases, the retinal arterioles are attenuated and sometimes there are retinal hemorrhages; in other cases, narrowing of retinal venules has been observed during an attack. In still other cases, monocular blindness is associated with disc edema and peripapillary hemorrhages, and vision recovers only partially after several months (Hupp et al). Such events, referred to as *retinal migraine*, are more accurately termed *ocular migraine*, since either the retinal or the ciliary circulation may be involved. It is well to remember that in adults the syndrome of headache, unilateral ophthalmoparesis, and loss of vision may have more serious causes, including temporal (cranial) arteritis.

Migraine Following Head Injury A particularly troublesome migraine variant occurs in a child or adolescent who, after a trivial head injury, may lose sight, suffer severe headache, or be plunged into a state of confusion, with belligerent and irrational behavior that lasts for hours or several days before clearing. In yet another variant there is an abrupt onset of either one-sided paralysis or aphasia after virtually every minor head injury (we have seen this condition several times in college athletes), but without visual symptoms and little or no headache. Although a family history of migraine is frequent in such cases, there has been no hemiplegia in other family members.

Young Children Migraine may present particular difficulties in diagnosis in a young child, whose capacity for accurate description is limited. Instead of complaining of headache, the child appears limp and pale and complains of abdominal pain; vomiting is more frequent than in the adult and there may be fever. Recurrent attacks are referred to by pediatricians as the "periodic syndrome." Another variant in the child is episodic vertigo and staggering (paroxysmal disequilibrium) followed by headache (Watson and Steele). Also, there are the puzzling patients with bouts of fever or transient disturbances in mood (psychic equivalents) and abdominal pain (*abdominal migraine*), dubious entities at best. We have also seen several infants and young children who have had attacks of hemiplegia (without headache), first on one side then the other, every few weeks. Recovery was complete, and arteriography in one child, after more than 70 attacks, was normal. The relationship of this condition to neurologic migraine remains uncertain. The only advantage of considering such attacks as migrainous is that it may protect some patients from unnecessary diagnostic procedures and surgical intervention; but, by the same token, it may delay appropriate investigation and treatment.

Hemiplegic Migraine In a related disorder known as *hemiplegic migraine*, an infant, child, or adult has episodes of unilateral paralysis that may long outlast the headache. Several families have been described in which this condition was inherited as an autosomal dominant trait (*familial hemiplegic migraine*). In the latter disorder, linkage-analysis studies have localized the responsible gene to chromosome 19 in one-third of families (Joutel et al); in other families, the gene has localized to chromosome 1; and in yet others, no linkage has been found. The gene on chromosome 19 codes for a voltage-gated calcium channel protein, which raises the provocative possibility that other forms of migraine are also due to an ion channel disorder. Instances of hemiplegic migraine may account for some of the inexplicable strokes in young women and older adults of both sexes. The mode of onset, lack of seizures, and an apparent relationship to anticardiolipin and antiphospholipid antibodies in some instances stamp the illness as vascular.

Stroke and Transient Ischemic Attacks (TIA) with Migraine Attacks of migraine, instead of beginning in childhood (see pages 880 and 913) and recurring in stereotyped fashion every few weeks or months with diminishing frequency in middle and late adult years, may have their onset in the latter periods or suddenly increase in frequency during menopause or in association with hypertension and vascular disease. Some of the transient hemianesthetic or hemiplegic strokes of later life may be of migrainous origin ("migrainous accompaniments"); Fisher has provided support for this hypothesis.

Rarely, neurologic symptoms, instead of being transitory, may leave a permanent deficit (e.g., a homonymous visual field defect), like an ischemic stroke. This is called *complicated migraine* or *migrainous infarction*. Platelet aggregation, edema of the arterial wall, increased coagulability of the blood, and intense, prolonged spasm of vessels have all been implicated in the pathogenesis of arterial occlusion and strokes that complicate migraine (Rascol et al). The reported incidence of this complication has varied. At the Mayo Clinic, in a group of 4874 patients aged 50 years or younger with a diagnosis of migraine, migraine equivalent, or vascular headache, 20 patients had migraine-associated infarctions (Broderick and Swanson). The reports of Dorfman and coworkers, in which cerebral infarction was revealed by computed tomography (CT) in four young adults (16 to 32 years of age) with migraine, and of Caplan, who described seven patients in whom attacks of migraine were complicated by strokes in the vertebrobasilar territory, matches our experience and suggests that these complications may be more prevalent than is generally appreciated. There is a paucity of useful pathology by which to interpret the mechanism of migraine-associated stroke. In children with the mitochondrial disease MELAS (page 1044) and in adults with the rare vasculopathy CADASIL (page 879) migraine may be a prominent feature. These issues are addressed further in Chap. 34.

Other Variations In some individuals, the migraine, for unaccountable reasons, may increase in frequency for several months. As many as three or four attacks may occur each week, leaving the scalp continuously tender. An even more difficult clinical problem is posed by migraine patients who lapse into a condition of daily or virtually continuous migraine (*status migrainosus*); the pain is unilateral, throbbing, and disabling. In such instances the illness has sometimes followed immediately upon a head injury or viral infection. Relief is sought by increasing the intake of ergot preparations or even opiate medications, often to an alarming degree, with only temporary relief. The mechanism of migraine being obscure, one can only surmise that the basic process has been greatly intensified. However, always to be considered in the diagnosis of such cases is the possibility that migraine has been combined with tension headache (migraine-tension or mixed-pattern headache) or transformed to so-called analgesia-rebound headache or ergotamine-dependency headache. Ergot intoxication or narcotic addiction are other diagnostic considerations. It has been our practice to admit such patients to the hospital, discontinue all ergot and narcotic medication, and administer corticosteroids intravenously or ergots intravenously in selected patients (see further on for details of treatment).

The relationships between migraine, menses, and pregnancy have already been addressed. In general, headaches can be expected to abate during pregnancy, but—in our experience—a few women have an intensification or the appearance of auras in the third trimester.

Under the title "Pseudomigraine with Temporary Neurological Symptoms and Lymphocytic Pleocytosis," Gomez-Aranda and colleagues have described what is possibly yet another migraine variant. Their series comprised 50 adolescents and young adults, predominantly males, who developed several episodes of transient (hours) neurologic deficits, accompanied by migraine-like headaches and sometimes fever. One-quarter of this group had a history of migraine and a similar number had a viral-like illness within 3 weeks before the onset of the syndrome. The CSF contained from 10 to 760 lymphocytes per cubic millimeter and the total protein was elevated. Neurologic deficits were mainly sensorimotor and aphasic; only six patients had visual symptoms. The patients were asymptomatic between attacks and in none did the entire illness persist beyond 7 weeks. The causation and pathophysiology of this syndrome and its relation to migraine are entirely obscure, although an aseptic inflammation of the leptomeningeal vasculative has been proposed. We have observed several similar cases, presumably parainfectious, and have tentatively found corticosteroids to be useful.

Cause and Pathogenesis So far, it has not been possible to determine, from the many clinical observations and investigations, a unifying theory as to the cause and pathogenesis of migraine. Tension and other emotional states, which are claimed by some migraineurs to precede their attacks, are so inconsistent as to be no more than aggravating factors. Clearly, an underlying genetic factor is implicated, although it is expressed in a recognizable mendelian pattern (autosomal dominant) in a relatively small number of families (see above). The puzzle is how this genetic fault is translated periodically into a regional neurologic deficit, unilateral headache, or both. For many years, our thinking about the pathogenesis of migraine was dominated by the views of Harold Wolff and others—that the headache was due to the distention and excessive pulsation of branches of the external carotid artery. Certainly the throbbing, pulsating quality of the headache and its relief by compression of the common carotid artery supported this view, as did the early observation of Graham and Wolff that the headache and amplitude of pulsation of the extracranial arteries diminished after the intravenous administration of ergotamine tartrate.

The importance of vascular factors continues to be emphasized by more recent findings. In a group of 11 patients with classic migraine, Olsen and colleagues, using the xenon inhalation method, noted a regional reduction in cerebral circulation during the period when neurologic symptoms appear. They concluded that the reduction in blood flow was sufficient to cause both ischemia and the neurologic deficits and that the latter had a vascular origin. In a subsequent study, Woods and colleagues described a patient who, during positron emission tomography (PET), fortuitously had an attack of common migraine. Highly sophisticated measurements showed a reduction in blood flow that started in the occipital cortex and spread slowly forward on both sides, in a manner much like that of the spreading depression of Leão (see below). Cutter et al, using perfusion-weighted MRI, corroborated the finding of diminished occipital cerebral blood flow during the aura in four patients. However, a study using single photon emission computed tomography (SPECT) in 20 patients during and after attacks of migraine without aura, disclosed no detectable focal changes of cerebral blood flow; also, no changes occurred after treatment of the attacks with 6 mg of subcutaneous sumatriptan (Ferrari et al). This matter must be regarded as unresolved, but clearly there is an alteration in blood flow during auras and a vascular element is likely in both types of migraine. Iversen and associates, by means of ultrasound measurements, documented a dilatation of the superior temporal artery on the side of the migraine during the headache period. The same dilatation has been inferred to occur in the middle cerebral arteries from observations with transcranial Doppler imaging. The well-established complication of cerebral infarction is also in keeping with a vascular hypothesis, but it involves only a tiny proportion of migraineurs.

Several other relationships between the vascular changes and evolving neurologic symptoms of migraine are noteworthy. Lashley, who plotted his own visual aura, calculated that the cortical impairment progressed at a rate of 2 to 3 mm/min. Also, during the aura, there occurs a regional reduction in blood flow, as noted above. It begins in one occipital lobe and extends forward slowly (2.2 mm/min) as a wave of "spreading oligemia" that does not respect arterial boundaries (Lauritzen and Olesen). Both of these events are intriguingly similar to the phenomenon of "spreading cortical depression," first observed by Leão in experimental animals. He demonstrated that a noxious stimulus applied to the rat cortex was followed by vasoconstriction and slowly spreading waves of inhibition of the electrical activity of cortical neurons, moving at a rate of approximately 3 mm/min. Lauritzen and Olesen attribute both the aura and the spreading oligemia to the spreading cortical depression of Leão, and considerable work since then has corroborated this idea. These observations, however, apply only to migraine with aura; the blood flow during common migraine has generally remained normal.

Another hypothesis linking the aura and the painful phase of migraine has been proposed by Moskowitz. The linkage is based on the fact that the involved vessels, both extracranial and intracranial, are innervated by small unmyelinated fibers, which are derived from the trigeminal nerve and subserve both pain and autonomic functions (trigeminovascular complex). Moskowitz found that activation of these fibers releases substance P and other peptides into the vessel wall. He has postulated that the released peptides serve to dilate the cerebral vessels and increase their permeability, culminating in a throbbing unilateral headache. More recently, nitric oxide that is generated by endothelial cells has been implicated as the cause of the pain of migraine headache, but the reason for its release and the relationship to blood flow changes is unclear.

The foregoing observations leave a number of questions unanswered. Is one to conclude that migraine with and without aura are different diseases, involving extracranial arteries in one instance and intracranial ones in another? Is the circulatory change the primary cause of headache, or is it a secondary or coincidental phenomenon? Is diminished neuronal activity (spreading depression) the primary cause of neurologic symptoms (it seems so) and headache (unclear), and is the diminished regional blood flow secondary to reduced metabolic demand? Why are the posterior portions of the brain so often implicated? Blau and Dexter and also Drummond and Lance are confident that the presence or absence of headache does not depend on extracranial vascular factors. These authors point to their findings that occlusion of blood flow through the scalp or common carotid circulation fails to alleviate the pain of migraine in one-third to one-half the patients. Alternatively, Lance has suggested that the trigeminal pathways are in a state of persistent hyperexcitability in the migraine patient and that they discharge periodically, perhaps in response to a hypothalamic stimulus. This is in keeping with current theories of central sensitization to pain from repeated noxious stimulation from one region. Also, there is a considerable body of circumstantial evidence that serotonin acts as a neurotransmitter and humoral mediator in the neural and vascular components of the migraine headache. This evidence and the role of other factors in the pathogenesis of migraine have been reviewed in detail by Lance and Goadsby. The potential role of nitric oxide has been mentioned, and its importance in migraine is bolstered by the observation that drugs blocking the production of nitric acid ameliorate the headache.

No final reconciliation of all these conflicting data is possible at this time and the mechanism of migraine remains incompletely explained. Several aspects seem clear, however. The authors continue to favor the unique mechanism of spreading depression as the best explanation of the neurologic deficit, as well as the view that a trigeminal vascular reflex, which releases vasogenic substances into the vessel walls, is the most plausible explanation of the headache. The neural mechanisms that underlie these changes and precisely what is altered by the genetic predisposition to migraine are unresolved. There are consistent vascular changes during the aura (reduced regional flow, mainly in posterior regions of the cerebrum) and, at the same time, dilation of both basal brain and scalp vessels; but the connection of this change in caliber to pain, the traditional explanation for headache, is not certain. Perhaps emotion, fatigue, fasting, mild head injury, and so forth serve, in vulnerable individuals, to activate the neural mechanisms intermittently.

Diagnosis Neurologic migraine should occasion no difficulty in diagnosis if the above facts are kept in mind and a good history is obtained. The difficulties come from a lack of awareness that (1) a progressively unfolding neurologic syndrome may be migrainous in origin, (2) the neurologic disorder may occur without headache, and (3) recurrent headaches, which may be an isolated phenomenon, may take many forms, some of which may prove difficult to distinguish from the other common types of headache. Some of these problems merit elaboration because of their practical importance.

The neurologic part of the migraine syndrome may resemble focal epilepsy, the clinical effects of a slowly evolving hemorrhage from an arteriovenous malformation or aneurysm, a transient ischemic attack, or a thrombotic or embolic stroke. It is the pace of the neurologic symptoms of migraine, more than their character, that reliably distinguishes the condition from epilepsy.

Ophthalmoplegic migraine will always suggest a carotid aneurysm, but in normotensive children saccular aneurysm is a great rarity, and in very few adult cases has carotid arteriography revealed such an abnormality. There have been many claims that the habitual occurrence of migraine on the same side of the head increases the likelihood of an underlying arteriovenous malformation (AVM). R. D. Adams, who studied more than 1200 patients with AVMs, found that the headaches, which occurred in over 30 percent of cases, usually did not have the other features of either migraine or cluster headache. However, in about 5 percent the headaches were associated with visual aura, indistinguishable from neurologic migraine. Stated somewhat differently, the incidence of classic migraine is more than five times greater in patients with AVMs than in the general population. In most of the patients, the AVM was in the occipital region, on the side of the headache; and in most, there was an initial visual aura. Approximately half of the patients with AVM and migraine had a family history of migraine. Thus, AVM must be regarded as an acknowledged cause of recurrent headache, and the latter may be frequent and troublesome for years before the malformation is revealed by a hemorrhage or discovered by other manifestations.

A special problem relates to paroxysms of throbbing headache that is not hemicranial in distribution, not preceded by a neurologic aura, and not accounted for by other known cause. Are these cases examples of common (nonneurologic) migraine or of some other type of cephalalgia? Unfortunately, since diagnosis depends on the interpretation of the patient's symptoms and since there is as yet no valid confirmatory laboratory test, the controversy as to where migraine begins and ends is of the armchair type. Favoring the diagnosis of migraine are onset in childhood or adolescence, lifelong history, positive family history, and response of the headache to ergotamine or sumatriptan. The observation that pattern and flash visual stimulation induces fast waves of high amplitude in children with migraine may, if corroborated, prove to be helpful (Mortimer et al).

Treatment of Migraine This topic may logically be subdivided into two parts—control of the individual attack and prevention. The time to initiate treatment of an attack is during the neurologic (visual) prodrome at the very onset of the headache (see below). If the headaches are mild, the patient may already have learned that acetylsalicylic acid, acetaminophen, or a nonsteroidal anti-inflammatory drug (the most effective drugs for mild and moderate cases in our experience) will suffice to control the pain. Insofar as a good response may be obtained from one type of nonsteroidal anti-inflammatory drug and not from another, it is advisable to try two or three preparations in several successive attacks of headache. Reliable patients can be given small amounts of codeine or oxycodone, usually combined with aspirin or acetaminophen, for limited periods. The combination of aspirin or acetaminophen, caffeine, and butalbital, though popular with some patients, is usually incompletely effective if the headache is severe, and is capable of causing dependence. Numerous other agents have proved to be effective and each has had a period of popularity among neurologists (Schulman and Silberstein).

Overall, for severe attacks, the ergot alkaloids, ergotamine tartrate, and particularly dihydroergotamine (DHE) and sumatriptan or one of the newer "triptans" (e.g., zolimtriptan, rizatriptan) are probably the most effective forms of treatment and are best administered early in the attack. Ergotamine is an alpha-adrenergic agonist with strong serotonin (5HT) receptor affinity and vasoconstrictor action. The drug is taken as an uncoated 1- to 2-mg tablet of ergotamine tartrate, held under the tongue until dissolved (or swallowed), and repeated every half hour until the headache is relieved or until a total of 8 mg is taken. A single oral dose of promethazine (Phenergan), 50 mg, or of metoclopramide (Reglan), 20 mg, given with the ergotamine, relaxes the patient and allays nausea and vomiting. Patients in whom vomiting prevents oral administration may be given ergotamine by rectal suppository or DHE by nasal spray or inhaler (one puff at onset and another at 30 min) or learn to give themselves a subcutaneous injection of DHE (usual dosage 1 mg). Caffeine, 100 mg, is thought, on slim evidence, to potentiate the effects of ergotamine and other medications for migraine. When ergotamine is administered early in the attack, the headache will be abolished or reduced in severity and duration in some 70 to 75 percent of patients.

A single 6-mg dose of sumatriptan (a selective agonist of 5HT receptors), given subcutaneously, is an equally effective and well-tolerated treatment for migraine attacks. An advantage of this drug is the ease of self-administration using prepackaged injection kits, thus avoiding frequent and inconvenient visits to the emergency department. Sumatriptan can also be given orally in a 50-or 100-mg tablet, zolmitriptan in a 2.5 or 5 mg tablet, and rizatriptan in a 10 mg dose repeated if needed in 2 h, but their latencies are considerably longer than that of the subcutaneous injection. Sumatriptan is available as an intranasal spray, which is particularly useful in patients with nausea and vomiting. The response rate after 2 h is similar to that of the orally administered drug, although the nasal spray acts more rapidly.

For severe cases that arrive in the emergency department or physician's office having failed to obtain relief with the above medications, Raskin has found metoclopramide 10 mg IV, followed by dihydroergotamine 0.5 to 1 mg PO every 8 h for 2 days, to be effective. Intravenous and oral corticosteroids have also been useful in some refractory cases and in terminating migraine status, but they should not be given continuously. If a depressive illness emerges as an important problem, as it frequently does, it is treated along the lines described in Chap. 57.

The sympathomimetic drug isometheptene combined with a sedative and acetaminophen (Midrin) has been useful for some patients and probably acts in a similar way to ergotamine and sumatriptan. A wide array of other drugs have been recommended as therapeutic adjuncts, e.g., metoclopramide, prochlorperazine, chlorpromazine, ketorolac, and intranasal lidocaine. Each of these drugs, given alone, is effective in alleviating the headache in about half of patients. This fact emphasizes the need for blinded placebo trials for any new drug that is introduced for the treatment of headache.

Because of the danger of prolonged arterial spasm in patients who have vascular (particularly coronary) disease or are pregnant, they should not be given ergotamine and DHE. Elderly patients should have electrocardiographic and blood pressure monitoring during and after administration of the drugs. Even in healthy individuals, more than 10 to 15 mg of ergotamine or 6 mg of DHE per week is not advised. Similarly, sumatriptan should not be given to patients with coronary artery disease or uncontrolled hypertension or to patients taking serotoninergic and tricyclic antidepressants. Contraceptive agents taken orally or implanted subcutaneously have had a propensity to induce migraine, but this risk has been reduced greatly with the introduction of low-estrogen agents.

If, in an individual attack, all of the foregoing measures fail, it is best to resort to narcotics, which usually give the patient a restful, pain-free sleep. Halfway measures at this point are usually futile. However, the use of narcotics as the mainstay of acute or prophylactic therapy is to be avoided.

Prophylactic Treatment In individuals with frequent migrainous attacks, efforts at prevention are worthwhile. The most effective agents have been beta blockers, anticonvulsants, and antidepressants. Considerable success has been obtained with propranolol (Inderal), beginning with 20 mg three times daily and increasing the dosage gradually to as much as 240 mg daily, probably best given as a long-acting preparation in the higher dosage ranges. Underdosing is a major reason for ineffectiveness. If propranolol is unsuccessful, one of the other beta blockers—atenolol (40 to 160 mg/day), timolol (20 to 40 mg/day), or metoprolol (100 to 200 mg/day)—may prove to be effective. In patients who do not respond to these drugs over a period of 4 to 6 weeks, valproic acid 250 mg taken three to four times daily or one of the antidepressants (amitriptyline, 75 to 125 mg nightly) may be tried. Calcium channel blockers (verapamil, 320 to 480 mg/day; nifedipine, 90 to 360 mg/day) are also effective in decreasing the frequency and severity of migraine attacks in some patients, but there is typically a lag of several weeks before benefit is attained. Methysergide (Sansert), an ergot-like preparation, in doses of 2 to 6 mg daily for several weeks or months, has proven to be a useful agent in the prevention of migraine. Retroperitoneal and pulmonary fibrosis are rare but serious complications that can be avoided by discontinuing the medication for 3 to 4 weeks after every 5-month course of treatment. Clonidine, 0.05 mg three times daily; Midrin; indomethacin, 150 to 200 mg/day; and cyproheptadine (Periactin), 4 to 16 mg/ day are found to be helpful in some patients and may be particularly useful in preventing predictable attacks of perimenstrual migraine. A typical experience is for one of these medications to reduce the number and severity of headaches for several months and then to become less effective, whereupon an increase in the dosage, if tolerated, may help; or one of the many alternatives can be tried. The newest putative treatment for headaches, both migraine and tension, is the injection of botulinum toxin (Botox) into sensitive temporalis and other cranial muscles. Elimination of headaches for 2 to 4 months has been reported—a claim that justifies further study.

A group of relatively uncommon headaches respond very well to indomethacin, so much so that some authors have defined a category of *indomethacin-responsive headaches*. These include orgasmic migraine, chronic paroxysmal hemicrania (see further on), and hemicrania continua, exertional headache, and some instances of premenstrual migraine.

Some patients know or allege to know that certain items of food induce attacks (chocolate, hot dogs, smoked meats, oranges, and red wine are the ones most commonly mentioned), and it is obvious enough that they should avoid these foods if possible. Limiting caffeinated beverages may be helpful. In certain cases the correction of a refractive error, an elimination diet, or behavioral modification is said to have reduced the frequency and severity of migraine and of tension headaches. However, the methods of study and the results are so poorly controlled that it is difficult to evaluate them. All experienced physicians appreciate the importance of helping patients rearrange their schedules with a view to controlling tensions and hard-driving ways of living. There is no one way of accomplishing this. Psychotherapy has not been helpful, or at least one can say that there is no critical evidence of its value. The claims for sustained improvement of migraine with chiropractic manipulation are similarly unsubstantiated and do not accord with our experience. Meditation, acupuncture, and biofeedback techniques all have their advocates, but again the results, while not to be discounted, are uninterpretable.

Cluster Headache

This type of headache has been described under a variety of names, including paroxysmal nocturnal cephalalgia (Adams), migrainous neuralgia (Harris), histamine cephalalgia (Horton), red migraine, erythromelalgia of the head, and others. Kunkle and colleagues, who were impressed with the characteristic "cluster pattern" of the attacks, coined the term in current use—"*cluster headache*." This type of headache occurs predominantly in young adult men (range 20 to 50 years; male-to-female ratio about 5:1) and is characterized by a consistent unilateral orbital localization. The pain is felt deep in and around the eye. It is intense and nonthrobbing as a rule and often radiates into the forehead, temple, and cheek—less often to the ear, occiput, and neck. The headache tends to occur nightly, between 1 and 2 h after the onset of sleep, or several times during the night and day, unattended by aura or vomiting. The headache recurs with remarkable regularity each day for periods that last over 6 to 12 weeks, followed then by complete freedom for many months or even years (hence the term *cluster*). However, in approximately 10 percent of our patients, the headache has become chronic, persisting over years. The associated phenomena, by which cluster headache can be identified, are a blocked nostril, rhinorrhea, injected conjunctivum, lacrimation, miosis, and a flush and edema of the cheek, all lasting on average for 45 min (range 15 to 180 min). Some of our patients, when alerted to the sign, report a slight ptosis on the side of the orbital pain; in a few, the ptosis becomes permanent after repeated attacks. The homolateral temporal artery may become prominent and tender during an attack, and the skin over the scalp and face may be hyperalgesic. Most patients arise from bed during an attack and sit in a chair and rock or pace the floor, holding a hand to the side of the head. The pain of a given attack may leave as rapidly as it began or fade away gradually. Almost always the same orbit is involved during a cluster of headaches as well as in recurring bouts. A similar type of head pain may occasionally be confined to the lower facial, postauricular, or occipital areas. Ekbom distinguished yet another "lower cluster headache" syndrome with infraorbital radiation of the pain, an ipsilateral partial Horner syndrome, and ipsilateral hyperhydrosis. During the period of freedom from pain, alcohol, which commonly precipitates headaches during a cluster, no longer has the capacity to do so.

The picture of cluster headache is usually so characteristic that it cannot be confused with any other disease, though those unfamiliar with it may entertain a diagnosis of migraine, trigeminal neuralgia, carotid aneurysm, temporal arteritis, or pheochromocytoma. To be distinguished also are the *Tolosa-Hunt syndrome* of ocular pain and ocular motor paralyses (see further on) and the *paratrigeminal syndrome of Raeder*, which consists of paroxysms of pain somewhat like that of tic douloureux in the distribution of the ophthalmic and maxillary divisions of the fifth nerve, in association with ocular sympathetic paralysis (ptosis and miosis but with preservation of sweating); loss of sensation in a trigeminal nerve distribution and weakness of muscles innervated by the fifth nerve are often added. We have seen instances of head pain, particularly in women, in which the features of both cluster headache and Raeder syndrome could be recognized; no lesion in or near the trigeminal ganglion was found. Many of the cases of paroxysmal pain behind the eye or nose or in the upper jaw or temple—associated with blocking of the nostril or lacrimation and described under the titles of *sphenopalatine* (Sluder), *petrosal*, *vidian*, and *ciliary neuralgia* (Charlin or Harris, "lower half" headache)—probably represent instances of cluster headache or its variants. There is no evidence to support the separation of these neuralgias as distinct entities.

Chronic paroxysmal hemicrania is the name given by Sjaastad and Dale to a unilateral form of headache that resembles cluster headache in some respects but has several distinctive features. Like cluster headaches, these are of short duration (2 to 45 min), and usually affect the temporo-orbital region of one side, accompanied by conjunctival hyperemia, rhinorrhea, and in some cases a partial Horner syndrome. Unlike cluster headache, however, the paroxysms occur many times each day, recur daily for long periods (the patient of Price and Posner had an average of 16 attacks daily for more than 40 years) and, most importantly, respond dramatically to the administration of indomethacin, 25 to 50 mg tid. Also unlike the usual form of cluster headache, chronic paroxysmal hemicrania is more common in women than in men, in a ratio of 3:1.

The relationship of the cluster headache to migraine remains conjectural. No doubt the headaches in some persons have some of the characteristics of both, hence the terms *migrainous neuralgia* and *cluster migraine* (Kudrow). Lance and others, however, have pointed out differences that seem important to the authors: flushing of the face on the side of a cluster headache and pallor in migraine; increased intraocular pressure in cluster headache, normal pressure in migraine; increased skin temperature over the forehead, temple, and cheek in cluster headache, decreased temperature in migraine; and notable distinctions in sex distribution, age of onset, rhythmicity, and other clinical features, as described above. Cluster has been observed to be triggered in sensitive patients by the use of nitroglycerin; the same occurs rarely in migraine.

The cause and mechanism of the cluster headache syndrome are unknown. Gardner and coworkers originally postulated a paroxysmal parasympathetic discharge mediated through the greater superficial petrosal nerve and sphenopalatine ganglion. These authors obtained inconsistent results by cutting the nerve, but others (Kittrelle et al) have reported that application of cocaine or lidocaine to the region of the sphenopalatine fossa (via the nostril) consistently aborts attacks of cluster headache. Capsaicin, applied over the affected region of the forehead and scalp, may have the same effect. Stimulation of the ganglion is said to reproduce the syndrome. Kunkle, on the basis of a large personal experience, concluded that the pain arises from the internal carotid artery, in the canal through which it ascends in the petrous portion of the temporal bone. In the course of an arteriogram, during which a patient with cluster headaches fortuitously developed an attack, Ekbom and Greitz noted a narrowing of the ipsilateral internal carotid artery. This was interpreted as being due to swelling of the arterial wall, which in turn compromised the pericarotid sympathetic plexus and caused the Horner syndrome. On rather speculative grounds, the cyclic nature of the attacks has been linked to the hypothalamic mechanism that governs the circadian rhythm. At the onset of the headache, the region of the suprachiasmatic nucleus appears to be active on PET scanning (May et al). The fact that cluster headaches could be reproduced by the intravenous injection of 0.1 mg histamine (an early experimental technique for studying the mechanism of headache) led to the notion, popular for many years, that this form of headache was caused by the spontaneous release of histamine and to a form of treatment that consisted of "desensitizing" the patient by slow intravenous injections of this drug given daily for several weeks. Experience has shown that this form of treatment accomplishes nothing more than temporization. It should be pointed out that the intravenous injection of histamine induces or worsens many forms of focal or generalized headache (due to fever, trauma, brain tumor) that are dependent upon activation of pain-sensitive tissue around the vessels derived from the internal carotid artery.

Treatment of Cluster Headache The usual nocturnal attacks of cluster headache can be treated with a single anticipatory dose of ergotamine at bedtime (2 mg orally). Inhalation of 100% oxygen for 10 to 15 min at the onset of headache may also abort the attack, but is not always practical. Intranasal lidocaine, or "triptan" drugs (as for migraine, see above) can be used to abort an attack. In other patients, ergotamine has to be given once or twice during the day at times when an attack of pain is expected. If ergotamine and triptans are not effective or become ineffective in subsequent bouts, methysergide (2 to 8 mg daily) has been successful as a prophylactic measure in some cases. We prefer a course of prednisone, beginning with 75 mg daily for 3 days and then reducing the dose at 3-day intervals. Usually it can be decided within a week if any of these medications is effective. If not, verapamil up to 480 mg per day should be tried. Ekbom introduced lithium therapy for cluster headache (600 mg up to 900 mg daily) and Kudrow has confirmed its efficacy in chronic cases. Lithium and veramapil may be given together. The blood level of lithium must be kept between 0.7 and 1.2 meq/L; toxicity is a frequent problem (manifest by nausea, vomiting, tremor, blurred vision, fasciculations, and choreoathetosis). Indomethacin (Indocin, 75 to 200 mg/day) has reportedly been efficacious in the chronic form of cluster headache but was ineffective in several of our own cases. In brief, no method is effective in all cases.

Tension Headache

This, the most common variety of headache, is usually bilateral, with occipitonuchal, temporal, or frontal predominance or diffuse extension over the top of the cranium. The pain is usually described as dull and aching, but questioning often uncovers other sensations, such as fullness, tightness, or pressure (as though the head were surrounded by a band or clamped in a vise) or a feeling that the head is swollen and may burst. On these sensations, waves of aching pain are superimposed. The latter may be interpreted as paroxysmal or throbbing and, if the pain is more on one side, the headache may suggest a migraine without aura. However, it lacks the persistent throbbing quality, nausea, photophobia, and phonophobia of the latter. Nor do most tension headaches seriously interfere with daily activities. The onset is more gradual than that of migraine, and the headache, once established, may persist with only mild fluctuations for days, weeks, months, or even years. In fact, this is the only type of headache that exhibits the peculiarity of being present throughout the day, day after day, for long periods of time. The term *chronic tension-type headache* is used to signify this type of chronic daily headache. Although sleep is usually undisturbed, the headache is present when the patient awakens or develops soon afterward, and the common analgesic remedies have little or no beneficial effect if the pain is of more than mild to moderate severity.

The incidence of tension headache is certainly greater than that of migraine. However, many patients treat tension headaches themselves and do not seek medical advice. Like migraine, tension headaches are more common in women than in men. Unlike migraine, they infrequently begin in childhood or adolescence but are more likely to occur in middle age and to coincide with anxiety, fatigue, and depression in the trying times of life. In the large series of Lance and Curran, about one-third of patients with tension headaches had readily recognized symptoms of depression. In our experience, chronic anxiety or depression of varying degrees of severity is present in the majority of cases with protracted headaches. Migraine and traumatic headaches may be complicated by tension headache, which, because of its persistence, often arouses fears of a brain tumor or other intracranial disease. However, as Patten points out, not more than one or two patients out of every thousand with tension headaches will be found to harbor an intracranial tumor.

In a substantial group of patients, the headache, when severe, develops a pulsating quality, to which the term *tension-vascular* headache has been applied (Lance and Curran). This is particularly the case in patients with protracted and chronic daily headaches. Observations such as these have tended to blur the sharp distinctions between migrainous and tension headaches.

For many years it was taught that tension headaches were due to excessive contraction of craniocervical muscles and an associated constriction of the scalp arteries. However, it is not clear that either of these mechanisms contributes to the genesis of tension headache, at least in its chronic form. Until recently it has been felt that in most patients with tension headache, the craniocervical muscles are quite relaxed (by palpation) and show no evidence of persistent contraction when measured by surface electromyographic (EMG) recordings. Anderson and Frank found no difference in the degree of muscle contraction between migraine and tension headache. However, using an ingenious laser device, Sakai et al have reported that the pericranial and trapezius muscles are hardened in patients with tension headaches. Recently, nitric oxide has been implicated in the genesis of tension-type headaches, specifically by creating a central sensitization to sensory stimulation from cranial structures. The strongest support of this concept comes from several reports that an inhibitor of nitric oxide reduces muscle hardness and pain in patients with chronic tension headache (Ashina et al). At present, this is an interesting but speculative idea.

Treatment of Tension Headache Simple analgesics, such as aspirin or acetaminophen or other nonsteroidal anti-inflammatory drugs, may be helpful but only for brief periods. Tension headaches respond best to the cautious use of one of several drugs that relieve anxiety or depression, when the latter symptoms are present. Some patients respond to ancillary measures such as massage, meditation, and biofeedback techniques. Stronger analgesic medication should be avoided. Raskin reports success with calcium channel blockers, phenelzine, or cyproheptadine. Ergotamine and propranolol are not effective unless there are symptoms of both migraine and tension headache. Relaxation techniques may be helpful in teaching patients how to deal with underlying anxiety and stress (Lance).

Headaches in the Elderly

In several surveys of an elderly population, headache with onset in this age period was found to be a prominent symptom in as many as one of six persons and more often to have serious import than headache in a younger population. In one series of such patients reported by Pascual and Berciano, more than 40 percent had tension headaches (women more than men) and there was a wide variety of diseases in the others (posttraumatic headaches, cerebrovascular disease, intracranial tumors, cranial arteritis, severe hypertension). Cough headache and cluster headache were present in some of the men. New-onset migraine in this age group is a rarity.

Raskin has described a headache syndrome in older patients that shares with cluster headache a nocturnal occurrence (hypnic headache). It may occur with daytime naps as well. However, it differs in being bilateral and unaccompanied by lacrimation and rhinorrhea. Also, it differs from migraine. Raskin has successfully treated a number of his patients with 300 mg of lithium carbonate at bedtime. The nosologic position of this hypnic headache syndrome is undetermined.

Despite these considerations, the most treacherous and neglected cause of headache in the elderly is temporal (cranial) arteritis with or without polymyalgia rheumatica, as discussed further on.

Headache and Other Craniofacial Pain with Psychiatric Disease

In our outpatient clinics the most common cause of generalized persistent headache, both in adolescents and adults, is depression or anxiety in one of its several forms. The authors have noted that many seriously ill psychiatric patients complain of frequent headaches that are not typically of the tension type. These patients report unilateral or generalized throbbing cephalic pain lasting for hours every day or two. The nature of these headaches, which in some instances resemble common migraine, is unsettled. Others have delusional symptoms involving physical distortion of cranial structures. As the psychiatric symptoms subside, the headaches usually disappear.

Odd cephalic pains, e.g., a sensation of having a nail driven into the head (*clavus hystericus*), may occur in hysteria and raise perplexing problems in diagnosis. The bizarre character of these pains, their persistence in the face of every known therapy, the absence of other signs of disease, and the presence of other manifestations of hysteria provide the basis for correct diagnosis. Older children and adolescents sometimes have peculiar behavioral reactions to headache: screaming, looking dazed, clutching the head with an agonized look. Usually, migraine is the underlying disorder, the additional manifestations responding to therapeutic support and suggestion.

Posttraumatic Headache

Severe, chronic, continuous, or intermittent headaches appear as the cardinal symptom of several posttraumatic syndromes, separable in each instance from the headache that immediately follows head injury (i.e., scalp laceration and cerebral contusion with blood in the CSF and increased intracranial pressure) and which may last several days or a week or two.

The *headache of chronic subdural hematoma* is deep-seated, steady, unilateral or generalized, and usually accompanied or followed by drowsiness, confusion, stupor, and hemiparesis. The head injury may have been minor and forgotten by the patient and family and mild degrees of confusion may be attributed to inattention and distractability. Typically the headache and other symptoms increase in frequency and severity over several weeks or months. Diagnosis is usually established by CT and MRI.

Headache is a prominent feature of a complex syndrome comprising giddiness, fatigability, insomnia, nervousness, trembling, irritability, inability to concentrate, and tearfulness—a syndrome that we have called *posttraumatic nervous instability*. This type of headache and associated symptoms, which resemble the tension headache syndrome, are described fully in Chap. 35, "Craniocerebral Trauma." The patient with posttraumatic nervous instability requires supportive therapy in the form of repeated reassurance and explanations of the benign nature of the symptoms, a program of increasing physical activity, and the use of drugs that allay anxiety and depression. The early settlement of litigation, which is often an issue, works to the patient's advantage.

Tenderness and aching pain sharply localized to the scar of a scalp laceration represent in all probability a different problem and raise the question of a traumatic neuralgia. Tender scars from scalp lacerations may be treated by repeated subcutaneous injections of local anesthetics such as 5 mL of 1% procaine.

With *whiplash injuries* of the neck, there may be unilateral or bilateral retroauricular or occipital pain, due probably to stretching or tearing of ligaments and muscles at the occipitonuchal junction or to a worsening of a preexistent cervical arthropathy. Much less frequently, cervical intervertebral discs and nerve roots are involved.

Under the heading of *posttraumatic dysautonomic cephalalgia*, Vijayan and Dreyfus have described a syndrome comprising severe, episodic, throbbing, unilateral headaches sometimes accompanied by ipsilateral mydriasis and excessive sweating of the face, thus simulating migraine or cluster headache. Between bouts of headache, a few of the patients showed partial ptosis and miosis as well as pharmacologic evidence of partial sympathetic denervation. The condition followed injury to the soft tissues of the neck in the region of the carotid artery sheath. The headaches did not respond to treatment with ergotamine, but prompt relief was obtained in each case with the beta-adrenergic blocking agent propranolol.

Headaches of Brain Tumor

Headache is said to be a significant symptom in about two-thirds of all patients with brain tumor (Rooke), but it is considerably less frequent in our experience, particularly as the heralding symptom in an adult. The pain has no specific features; it tends to be deep-seated, usually nonthrobbing (occasionally throbbing), and is described as aching or bursting. Attacks of pain last a few minutes to an hour or more and occur once or many times during the day. Physical activity and changes in position of the head may provoke pain, whereas rest diminishes its frequency. Nocturnal awakening because of pain occurs in only a small proportion of patients and is by no means diagnostic. Unexpected forceful (projectile) vomiting may punctuate the illness in its later stages. If unilateral, the headache is nearly always on the same side as the tumor. Pain from supratentorial tumors is felt anterior to the interauricular circumference of the skull; from posterior fossa tumors, it is felt behind this line. Bifrontal and bioccipital headaches, coming on after unilateral headaches, signify the development of increased intracranial pressure.

Harris described headaches of paroxysmal type with intra- and periventricular brain tumors, and many others have commented on the same type of headache with parenchymal tumors. These are severe headaches that reach their peak intensity in a few seconds, last for several minutes or as long as an hour, and then subside quickly. When they are associated with vomiting, transient blindness, leg weakness with "drop attacks," and loss of consciousness, there is a high likelihood of brain tumor. With respect to its onset, this headache resembles that of subarachnoid hemorrhage, but the latter is far more long-lasting. In its entirety, this paroxysmal headache is most typical of a colloid cyst of the third ventricle, but it can occur with other tumors as well, including craniopharyngiomas, pinealomas, and cerebellar masses. One cannot help but be impressed with the frequency of headache as a manifestation of colloid cysts, and we have several times stumbled on the correct diagnosis when an odd, unexplained headache led to brain imaging. The mechanism of headache in cases of colloid cyst is not simply one of blocking the flow of CSF at the foramina of Monro and is not predicated on the development of hydrocephalus.

Temporal Arteritis (Giant-Cell Arteritis, Cranial Arteritis)

This particular type of inflammatory disease of cranial arteries is an important cause of headache in elderly persons. All of our patients have been more than 50 years of age, most of them more than age 65. From a state of normal health, the patient develops an increasingly intense throbbing or nonthrobbing headache, often with superimposed sharp, stabbing pains. In a few patients the headache has had an almost explosive onset. The headache is usually unilateral, sometimes bilateral, and often localized to the site of the affected arteries. The pain persists to some degree throughout the day and is particularly severe at night. It lasts for many months if untreated (average duration, 1 year). The superficial temporal and other scalp arteries are frequently thickened and tender and without pulsation. Jaw claudication and ischemic nodules on the scalp, with ulceration of the overlying skin, have been described in severe cases. Many of the patients feel generally unwell and have lost weight; some have a low-grade fever and anemia. Usually the sedimentation rate is greatly elevated (>50 mm/h) and a few patients have a neutrophilic leukocytosis. As many as 50 percent of patients have generalized aching of proximal limb muscles, reflecting the presence of polymyalgia rheumatica (see page 230).

The importance of early diagnosis relates to the threat of blindness from thrombosis of the ophthalmic and, less often, of the posterior ciliary arteries. This may be preceded by several episodes of amaurosis fugax (page 263). Ophthalmoplegia may also occur but is less frequent, and its cause, whether neural or muscular, is not settled. The large intracranial vessels are occasionally affected. Once vision is lost, it is seldom recoverable. For this reason *the earliest suspicion* of cranial arteritis should lead to biopsy of the appropriate scalp artery *and the immediate administration of corticosteroids.* Microscopic examination discloses an intense granulomatous or "giant-cell" arteritis. If biopsy on one side fails to clarify the situation and there are sound clinical reasons for suspecting the diagnosis, the other side should be sampled. Arteriography of the external carotid artery branches is probably the most sensitive test but is seldom used; ultrasound examination has recently been introduced to display the irregularly thickened vessel wall of the temporal arteries. This technique, which shows promise, requires further study.

Treatment consists of the administration of prednisone, 45 to 60 mg/day in single or divided doses over a period of several weeks, with gradual reduction to 10 to 20 mg/day and maintenance at this dosage for several months or years if necessary to prevent relapse. The headache can be expected to improve within a day or two of beginning treatment and failure to do so brings the diagnosis into question. When the sedimentation rate or C-reactive protein are elevated, their return to normal is a reliable index of therapeutic response.

Pseudotumor Cerebri (Benign or Idiopathic Intracranial Hypertension)

The headache of pseudotumor cerebri assumes a variety of forms. Typical is a feeling of occipital pressure that is greatly worsened by lying down, but many patients have—in addition or only—headaches of migraine or tension type. Indeed, some of them respond to medications such as propranolol or ergot compounds. None of the proposed mechanisms for pain in pseudotumor cerebri seems to be adequate as an explanation, particularly the idea that cerebral vessels are displaced or compressed, since neither has been demonstrated. It is worth noting that facial pain may also be a feature of the illness, albeit rare. A more complete description can be found on page 667.

SPECIAL VARIETIES OF HEADACHE

Low-Pressure and Spinal Puncture Headache These are commonly known to neurologists and the latter type is an unavoidable part of lumbar punctures. The headache is associated with the greatly reduced pressure of the CSF compartment and probably caused by traction or cranial blood vessels. Assuming the supine position almost immediately relieves the cranial pain and eliminates vomiting, but a blood-patch procedure may be required in persistent cases. In a limited number of cases we have had success in aborting the headache by the use of intravenous caffeine injections. The condition and its treatment are discussed on pages 670–671.

Menstrual Migraine and Other Headaches Linked to the Hormonal Cycle The relation of headache to a drop in estradiol levels has been mentioned on page 182. Premenstrual headache, taking the form of migraine or a combined tension-migraine headache, usually responds to the administration of a nonsteroidal anti-inflammatory drug begun 3 days before the anticipated onset of the menstrual period; oral sumatriptan (25 to 50 mg q.i.d.) and zolmitriptan (2.5 to 5 mg bid.) are equally effective. Manipulation of the hormonal cycle with danazol (a testosterone derivative) or estradiol has also been effective but is rarely necessary.

Cough and Exertional Headache A patient may complain of very severe, transient cranial pain on coughing, sneezing, laughing heartily, lifting heavy objects, stooping, and straining at stool. Pain is usually felt in the front of the head, sometimes occipitally, and may be unilateral or bilateral. As a rule, it follows the initiating action within a second or two and lasts a few seconds to a few minutes. The pain is often described as having a bursting quality and may be of such severity as to cause the patient to cradle his head in his hands, simulating the headache of acute subarachnoid hemorrhage.

Most often this syndrome takes the form of a benign idiopathic state that recurs over a period of several months to a year or two and then disappear. In a report of 103 patients followed for 3 years or longer, Rooke found that additional symptoms of neurologic disease developed in only 10; Symonds also has attested to the usual benignity of the condition. Its cause and mechanism have not been determined. During the attack, the CSF pressure is normal. Bilateral jugular compression may induce an attack, possibly because of traction on the walls of large veins and dural sinuses. In a few instances, we have observed this type of headache after lumbar puncture or after a hemorrhage from an arteriovenous malformation.

Aside from a rare instance of subarachnoid hemorrhage, patients with cough or strain headache may occasionally be found to have serious intracranial disease, most often of the posterior fossa and foramen magnum: arteriovenous malformation, Chiari malformation, platybasia, basilar impression, or tumor. It may be necessary, therefore, to supplement the neurologic examination by appropriate skull films, CT, and MRI. Far more common, of course, are the temporal and maxillary pains that are due to dental or sinus disease and are induced by coughing.

A special variant of exertional headache is "weight-lifter's headache." It occurs either as a single event or repeatedly over a period of several months, but each episode of headache may last many hours or days, again raising the suspicion of subarachnoid hemorrhage. If the pain resolves in an hour or less and there is no meningismus or sign of bleeding on the CT, we have foregone lumbar puncture and angiography but have suggested that weight-lifting not be resumed for several weeks. Athletes and runners in general seem to suffer exertional headaches quite often in our experience, and the episodes usually have migrainous features.

Indomethacin may be quite effective in controlling exertional headaches, and this has been confirmed in controlled trials. Useful alternatives are nonsteroidal anti-inflammatory agents, ergot preparations, and phenelzine. In a few of our cases, lumbar puncture appeared to resolve the problem in some inexplicable way.

Headaches Related to Sexual Activity Lance has described 21 cases of this type of headache, 16 in males and 5 in females. The headache took one of two forms: one in which headache of the tension type developed as sexual excitement increased and another in which a severe, throbbing, "explosive" headache occurred at the time of orgasm and persisted for several minutes or hours. The latter headaches were of such abruptness and severity as to suggest a ruptured aneurysm, but the neurologic examination was negative in every instance, as was arteriography in seven patients who were subjected to this procedure. In 18 patients who were followed for a period of 2 to 7 years, no other neurologic symptoms developed. Characteristically, the headache occurred on several consecutive occasions and then inexplicably disappeared. In cases of repeated coital headache, indomethacin is effective. Of course, so-called orgasmic headache is not always benign; a hypertensive hemorrhage, rupture of an aneurysm or vascular malformation, or myocardial infarction may occur during the exertion of sexual intercourse.

Erythrocyanotic Headache On rare occasions, an intense, generalized, throbbing headache may occur in conjunction with flushing of the face and hands and numbness of the fingers (erythromelalgia). Episodes tend to be present on awakening from sound sleep. This condition has been reported in a number of unusual settings: (1) in mastocytosis (infiltration of tissues by mast cells, which elaborate histamine, heparin, and serotonin); (2) with carcinoid tumors; (3) with serotonin-secreting tumors; (4) with some tumors of the pancreatic islets; and (5) with pheochromocytoma. Seventy-five percent of patients with pheochromocytoma reportedly have vascular-type headaches coincident with paroxysms of hypertension and elaboration of catecholamines (Lance and Hinterberger).

Headache Related to Medical Diseases

Severe headache may occur with a number of infectious illnesses caused by banal viral upper respiratory infections, by organisms such as *Mycoplasma*, or *Coxiella* (Q fever), and particularly by influenza. The suspicion of meningitis is raised, even subarachnoid hemorrhage, but almost invariably there is no reaction in the CSF.

About 50 percent of patients with hypertension complain of headache, but the relationship of one to the other is not clear. Minor elevations of blood pressure may be a result rather than the cause of tension headaches. Severe (malignant) hypertension, with diastolic pressures of more than 120 mmHg, is regularly associated with headache, and measures that reduce the blood pressure relieve it. Abrupt elevations of blood pressure, as occur in patients taking monoamine oxidase inhibitors and then ingest tyramine-containing food, can cause headaches that are abrupt and severe enough to simulate subarachnoid hemorrhage. However, it is the individual with moderately severe hypertension and frequent severe headaches who causes the most concern. In some of these patients the headache is of the common migrainous or tension type, but in others they defy classification. According to Wolff, the mechanism of the hypertensive headache is similar to that of migraine, i.e., increased vascular pulsations. The headaches, however, bear no clear relation to modest peaks in blood pressure. Curiously, headaches that occur toward the end of renal dialysis or soon after its completion are associated with a fall in blood pressure (as well as a decrease in blood sodium levels and osmolality). The latter type of headache is bifrontal and throbbing, and is accompanied sometimes by nausea and vomiting. The mechanism of occipital pain that may awaken the hypertensive patient and wear off during the day is not understood.

Headaches frequently follow a seizure, having been recorded in half of one large series of epileptic patients analyzed in Great Britain. In migraineurs, the postictal headache may reproduce a typical migraine attack. Rarely, in patients with a vascular malformation, a migraine-like attack precedes a seizure.

Experienced physicians are aware of many other conditions in which headache may be a dominant symptom. These include fevers of any cause, carbon monoxide exposure, chronic lung disease with hypercapnia (headaches often nocturnal), hypothyroidism, Cushing disease, withdrawal from corticosteroid medication, hypoglycemia, mountain sickness, chronic exposure to nitrates, occasionally adrenal insufficiency, aldosterone-producing adrenal tumors, use of "the pill," and development of acute anemia with hemoglobin below 10 g.

No attempt is made here to discuss the symptomatic treatment of headache that may accompany these many medical conditions. Obviously the guiding principle in management is to uncover and remove the underlying disease or functional disturbance.

Headache Related to Diseases of the Cervical Spine

Headaches that accompany diseases of the upper cervical spine are well recognized, but their mechanism is obscure. Recent writings have focused on a wide range of causative lesions, such as zygoapophyseal arthropathy, C2 dorsal root entrapment, calcified ligamentum flavum, hypertrophied posterior longitudinal ligament, and rheumatoid arthritis of the atlantoaxial region. CT and MRI have divulged a number of these abnormalities. They are discussed below, under the heading of "Third Occipital Nerve Headache," below, and in Chap. 11.

OTHER CRANIOFACIAL PAINS

(See Table 10-2)

Trigeminal Neuralgia (Tic Douloureux)

This is a common disorder of middle age and later life and consists of paroxysms of intense, stabbing pain in the distribution of the mandibular and maxillary divisions (rarely the ophthalmic division) of the fifth cranial nerve. The pain seldom lasts more than a few seconds or a minute or two but may be so intense that the patient involuntarily winces; hence the term *tic*. It is uncertain whether the tic is reflexive or quasi-voluntary. The paroxysms recur frequently, both day and night, for several weeks at a time. Another characteristic feature of trigeminal neuralgia is the initiation of pain by stimulation of certain areas of the face, lips, or gums, as in shaving or brushing the teeth, or by movement of these parts in chewing, talking, or yawning—the so-called trigger zones. Sensory or motor loss in the distribution of the fifth nerve cannot be demonstrated in these cases, though there are minor exceptions to this rule. In addition to the paroxysmal pain, some of the patients complain of a more or less continuous discomfort, itching, and sensitivity of the face, features always regarded as atypical even though not infrequent.

In studying the relationship between stimuli applied to the trigger zones and the paroxysms of pain, the latter are found to be induced by touch and possibly tickle rather than by a painful or thermal stimulus. Usually a spatial and temporal summation of impulses is necessary to trigger a paroxysm of pain, which is followed by a refractory period of up to 2 or 3 min. This suggests that the mechanism of the paroxysmal pain is in the nature of allodynia, a feature of other neuropathic pains (see page 145).

The *diagnosis* of tic douloureux must rest upon the strict clinical criteria enumerated above, and the condition must be distinguished from other forms of facial and cephalic neuralgia and pain arising from diseases of the jaw, teeth, or sinuses. Most cases of trigeminal neuralgia are without assignable cause (idiopathic), in contrast to

Table 10-2
Types of facial pain

Type	*Site*	*Clinical characteristics*	*Aggravating-relieving factors*	*Associated diseases*	*Treatment*
Trigeminal neuralgia (tic douloureux)	Second and third divisions of trigeminal nerve, unilateral	Men/women = 1:3 Over 50 years Paroxysms (10–30 s) of stabbing, burning pain; persistent for weeks or longer Trigger points No sensory or motor paralysis	Touching trigger points, chewing, smiling, talking, blowing nose, yawning	Idiopathic If in young adults, multiple sclerosis Vascular anomaly Tumor of fifth cranial nerve	Carbamazepine, phenytoin, gabapentin, Alcohol injection, coagulation, or surgical (vascular) decompression of root
Postzoster neuralgia	Unilateral Usually ophthalmic division of fifth nerve	History of zoster Aching, burning pain; jabs of pain Paresthesiae, slight sensory loss Dermal scars	Contact, movement	Herpes zoster	Carbamazepine, antidepressants, and sedatives
Costen syndrome	Unilateral, behind or front of ear, temple, face	Severe aching pain, intensified by chewing Tenderness over temporo-mandibular joints Malocclusion, missing molars	Chewing, pressure over temporo-mandibular joints	Loss of teeth, rheumatoid arthritis	Correction of bite Surgery in some
Tolosa-Hunt syndrome	Unilateral, mainly retro-orbital	Intense sharp, aching pain, associated with ophthalmoplegias and sensory loss over forehead; pupil usually spared	None	Granulomatous lesion of cavernous sinus or superior orbital fissure	Corticosteroids
Raeder paratrigeminal syndrome	Unilateral, frontotemporal and maxilla	Intense sharp or aching pain, ptosis, miosis, preserved sweating	None	Parasellar tumors, granulomatous lesions, trauma, idiopathic	Depends on type of lesion
"Migrainous neuralgia"	Orbitofrontal, temple, upper jaw, angle of nose and cheek	See cluster headache, Table 10-1	Alcohol in some		Ergotamine before anticipated attack
Carotidynia, lower-half headache, sphenopalatine neuralgia, etc.	Unilateral face, ear, jaws, teeth, upper neck	Both sexes, constant dull ache 2–4 h	Compression of common carotid at or below bifurcation reproduces pain in some	Occasionally with cranial arteritis, carotid tumor, migraine and cluster headache	Ergotamine acutely; methysergide for prevention Lithium Ca blockers
Atypical facial neuralgia (facial pain of indeterminate cause)	Unilateral or bilateral; cheek or angle of cheek and nose; deep in nose	Predominantly female 30 –50 years Continuous intolerable pain Mainly maxillary areas	None	Depressive and anxiety states Hysteria Idiopathic	Antidepressant and antianxiety medication

symptomatic trigeminal neuralgia, in which paroxysmal facial pain is due to involvement of the fifth nerve by some other disease: multiple sclerosis (may be bilateral), aneurysm of the basilar artery, or tumor (acoustic or trigeminal neuroma, meningioma, epidermoid) in the cerebellopontine angle. Sometimes it is due to compression of the trigeminal roots by a tortuous blood vessel, as originally pointed out by Dandy. Currently there is some disagreement as to the importance of the vascular lesion and its management. Jannetta has observed it in most of his patients and has relieved their pain by surgical decompression of the trigeminal root. Others declare a vascular compressive causation to be less frequent (Adams et al). Each of the forms of symptomatic trigeminal neuralgia may give rise only to pain in the distribution of the fifth nerve, or it may produce a loss of sensation as well. This and other disorders of the fifth nerve, some of which give rise to facial pain, are discussed in Chap. 47, "Diseases of the Cranial Nerves."

Treatment Anticonvulsant drugs such as phenytoin (300 to 400 mg/day), valproic acid (800 to 1200 mg/day), clonazepam (2 to 6 mg/day), gabapentin (300 to 900 mg/day), and particularly carbamazepine (600 to 1200 mg/day), alone or in combination, suppress or shorten the duration and severity of the attacks. Carbamazepine is effective in 70 to 80 percent of patients, but half of them become tolerant over a period of several years. Baclofen may be useful in patients who cannot tolerate carbamazepine or gabapentin, but it is most effective as an adjunct to one of the anticonvulsant drugs. Capsaicin applied locally to the trigger zones or the topical instillation in the eye of an anesthetic (proparacaine 0.5%) has been helpful in some patients. By temporizing and using these drugs, one may permit a spontaneous remission to occur.

Most of the patients with intractable pain come to surgery. The commonly used procedures are stereotactically controlled thermocoagulation of the trigeminal roots using a radio-frequency generator (Sweet and Wepsic) and the procedure of vascular decompression, popularized by Jannetta, which requires a posterior fossa craniotomy but leaves no sensory loss. Barker and colleagues have reported that 70 percent of 1185 patients were relieved of pain by repositioning a small branch of the basilar artery that was found to compress the fifth nerve, and this effect persisted, with an annual recurrence rate of less than 1 percent per year for 10 years. The therapeutic efficacy of these two surgical approaches is roughly equivalent; in recent years there has been a preference for microvascular decompression, especially late in the course of the illness (Fields).

Glossopharyngeal Neuralgia

This syndrome is much less common than trigeminal neuralgia but resembles the latter in many respects. The pain is intense and paroxysmal; it originates in the throat, approximately in the tonsillar fossa, and is provoked most commonly by swallowing but also by talking, chewing, yawning, laughing, etc. The pain may be localized in the ear or radiate from the throat to the ear, implicating the auricular branch of the vagus nerve. For this reason, White and Sweet suggested the term *vagoglossopharyngeal neuralgia*. This is the only craniofacial neuralgia that may be accompanied by bradycardia and even by syncope, presumably because of the triggering of cardioinhibitory reflexes by afferent pain impulses. There is no demonstrable sensory or motor deficit. Rarely, carcinoma or epithelioma of the oropharyngeal-infracranial region or peritonsillar abscess may give rise to pain clinically indistinguishable from glossopharyngeal neuralgia. For idiopathic glossopharyngeal neuralgia, a trial of carbamazepine, gabapentin, or baclofen may be useful. If these are unsuccessful, the conventional surgical procedure has been to interrupt the glossopharyngeal nerve and upper rootlets of the vagus nerve near the medulla. Recent observations suggest that a vascular decompression procedure similar to the one used for tic but directed to a small vascular loop under the ninth nerve relieves the pain in a proportion of patients.

Acute Zoster and Postherpetic Neuralgia

Neuralgia associated with a vesicular eruption due to the herpes zoster virus may affect cranial as well as peripheral nerves. In the region of the cranial nerves, two syndromes are frequent: herpes zoster auricularis and herpes zoster ophthalmicus. Both may be exceedingly painful in the acute phase of the infection. In the former, herpes of the external auditory meatus and pinna and sometimes of the palate and occipital region—with or without deafness, tinnitus, and vertigo—is combined with facial paralysis. This syndrome, since its original description by Ramsay Hunt, has been known as geniculate herpes, despite the lack, to this day, of pathologic proof that it depends solely upon a herpetic infection of the geniculate ganglion (see Chap. 47). Pain and herpetic eruption due to herpes zoster infection of the gasserian ganglion and the peripheral and central pathways of the trigeminal nerve are practically always limited to the first division (herpes zoster ophthalmicus). Ordinarily, the eruption will appear within 4 to 5 days after the onset of the pain and, if it does not, some cause other than herpes zoster will almost invariably declare itself. Nevertheless, a few cases have been reported in which the characteristic localization of pain to a dermatome, with serologic evidence of herpes zoster infection, was not accompanied by skin lesions.

The acute discomfort associated with the herpetic eruption usually subsides after several weeks, or it may linger for several months. Treatment with acyclovir, along the lines indicated in Chap. 33, will shorten the period of eruption and pain, but the drug does not prevent the occurrence of chronic pain. In the elderly the pain often becomes chronic and intractable. It is described as a constant burning, with superimposed waves of stabbing pain, and the skin in the territory of the preceding eruption is exquisitely sensitive to the slightest tactile stimuli, while the threshold of pain and thermal perception is elevated. Allodynia is frequent. This unremitting *postherpetic neuralgia* of long duration represents one of the most difficult pain problems with which the physician has to deal. Some relief may be provided by application of capsaicin cream, use of a mechanical vibrator, or administration of phenytoin, gabapentin, or carbamazepine. Antidepressants such as amitriptyline and fluoxetine, are helpful in some patients, and Bowsher has suggested, on the basis of a small placebo-controlled trial, that treatment with amitriptyline during the acute phase may prevent persistent pain. The addition of a phenothiazine to an antidepressant (e.g., amitriptyline 75 mg at bedtime and fluphenazine 1 mg tid) has proved to be a useful measure, but the long-term use of phenothiazines carries with it all the well-known risks, including that of inducing a movement disorder. Probably equivalent results are obtained by a combination of valproic acid and an antidepressant, as reported by Raftery. King has reported that two (5-grain) aspirin tablets crushed and mixed with cold cream or chloroform (15 mL) and spread over the painful zone on the the face or trunk relieved the pain for several hours in most patients with postzoster neuralgia. The authors have limited personal experience with this treatment. Extensive trigeminal rhizotomy or other destructive procedures should be avoided, since these surgical measures are not universally successful and may superimpose a diffuse refractory dysesthetic component upon the neuralgia.

Otalgia

Pain localized in and around one ear is occasionally a primary complaint. This can have a number of different causes and mechanisms. During neurosurgical operations in awake patients, stimulation of cranial nerves V, VII, IX, and X causes ear pain, yet interruption of these nerves usually causes no demonstrable loss of sensation in the ear canal or ear itself (superficial sensation in this region is supplied by the great auricular nerve, which is derived from the C2 and C3 roots). The neurosurgical literature cites examples of otalgia that were relieved by section of the nervus intermedius (sensory part of VII) or nerves IX and X. One is prompted to search for a nasopharyngeal tumor or vertebral artery aneurysm in such cases. Formerly, lateral sinus thrombosis was a common cause in children. But when this possibility is eliminated by appropriate studies, there will always remain examples of primary idiopathic otalgia, lower cluster headache, and glossopharyngeal neuralgia. Some patients with common migraine have pain centered in the ear region and occiput, but we have never observed a trigeminal neuralgia in which the ear was the predominant site of pain.

Occipital Neuralgia

Paroxysmal pain may occasionally occur in the distribution of the greater or lesser occipital nerves (suboccipital, occipital, and posterior parietal areas). There may be tenderness where these nerves cross the superior nuchal line, but there is only questionable evidence of an occipital nerve lesion in such cases. Carbamazepine may provide some relief. Blocking the nerves with lidocaine may abolish the pain and encourage attempts to section one or more occipital nerves or the second or third cervical dorsal root, but the results have rarely been successful, and several such patients who had these procedures were later referred to us with disabling anesthesia dolorosa. We have advised repeated injections of local anesthetic agents and the use of steroids, traction, local heat, and analgesic and anti-inflammatory drugs. The pain at times may be difficult to distinguish from that arising in the upper three cervical apophyseal joints, one type of which is discussed below.

Third Occipital Nerve Headache This condition, a unilateral occipital and suboccipital ache, is a prominent symptom in patients with neck pain, particularly after whiplash injuries (a prevalence of 27 percent, according to Lord et al). Bogduk and Marsland attribute this type of headache to a degenerative or traumatic arthropathy involving the C2 and C3 apophyseal joints with impingement on the third occipital nerve (a branch of the C3 dorsal ramus that crosses the lateral and dorsal aspects of the apophyseal joint). Ablation of the neck pain and headache by percutaneous blocking of the third occipital nerve under fluoroscopic control is diagnostic. More sustained relief (weeks to months) may be obtained by radio frequency coagulation of the nerve or steroid injections of the zygapophyseal joint. Nonsteroidal anti-inflammatory medications may provide some relief.

Carotidynia

This term was coined by Temple Fay in 1927 to designate a special type of cervicofacial pain that could be elicited by pressure on the common carotid arteries of patients with *atypical facial neuralgia*, or the so-called lower-half headache of Sluder. Compression of the artery in these patients, or mild electrical stimulation at or near the bifurcation, produced a dull ache that was referred to the ipsilateral face, ear, jaws, and teeth or down the neck. This type of carotid sensitivity occurs rarely as part of cranial (giant-cell) arteritis and during attacks of migraine or cluster headache; it has also been described with displacement of the carotid artery by tumor and dissecting aneurysm of its wall.

A variant of carotidynia, with a predilection for young adults, has been described by Roseman. This syndrome takes the form of recurrent, self-limited attacks of pain in the aforementioned distribution lasting a week or two. During the attack, aggravation of the pain by head movement, chewing, and swallowing is characteristic. This condition is treated with simple analgesics. Yet another variety of carotidynia appears at any stage of adult life and recurs in attacks lasting minutes to hours in association with throbbing headaches indistinguishable from common migraine (Raskin and Prusiner). This form responds favorably to the administration of ergotamine, methysergide, and other drugs that are effective in the treatment of migraine.

Costen Syndrome (Temporomandibular Joint Pain)

This is a form of craniofacial pain consequent upon dysfunction of one temporomandibular joint. Malocclusion due to ill-fitting dentures or loss of molar teeth on one side, with alteration of the normal bite, may lead to distortion of and ultimately degenerative changes in the joint and to pain in front of the ear, with radiation to the temple and over the face. The diagnosis is supported by the findings of tenderness over the joint, crepitus on opening the mouth, and limitation of jaw opening. The favored diagnostic maneuver involves palpating the joint from its posterior aspect by placing a finger in the external auditory meatus and pressing forward. The diagnosis can be made with some confidence if this reproduces the patient's pain. CT and plain films are rarely helpful, but effusions have been shown in the joints by MRI. Management consists of careful adjustment of the bite by a dental specialist and should be undertaken only when the patient meets the strict diagnostic criteria for this condition. In our experience, most of the diagnoses of Costen syndrome that reach the neurologist have been erroneous and the number of headaches and facial pains that are attributed to "temporomandibular joint dysfunction" is excessive, especially if judged by the response to treatment. The temporomandibular joint may also be the source of pain when involved by rheumatoid arthritis.

Facial Pain of Dental or Sinus Origin

Maxillary and mandibular discomfort are common effects of nerve irritation from deep caries, dental pulp degeneration, or periodontal abscess. The pain of dental nerve origin is most severe at night, slightly pulsating, and often associated with local tenderness at the root of the tooth in response to heat, cold, or pressure. It usually responds to denervation of the tooth.

Trigeminal neuritis following dental extractions or oral surgery is another vexing problem. There may be sensory loss in the tongue or lower lip and weakness of the masseter or pterygoid muscle.

Sometimes the onset of "atypical facial pain" (see below) can be dated to a dental procedure such as tooth extraction, and, as usually happens, neither the dentist nor the neurologist is able to find a source for the pain or any malfunction of the trigeminal nerve. Roberts and coworkers as well as Ratner and associates have pointed out that residual microabscesses and subacute bone infection account for some of these cases. They isolated the affected region by local anesthetic blocks, curetted the bone, and administered antibiotics, following which the pain resolved. The removed bone fragments showed vascular and inflammatory changes and infection with oral bacterial flora.

Facial Pain of Uncertain Origin ("Atypical" Facial Pain)

There remains—after all the aforementioned pain syndromes and all the possible intracranial and local sources of pain from throat, mouth, sinuses, orbit, and carotid vessels have been excluded—a small number of patients with pain in the face for which no cause can be found.

These patients are most often young women who describe the pain as constant and unbearably severe, deep in the face, or at the angle of cheek and nose and unresponsive to all varieties of analgesic medication. Because of the failure to identify an organic basis for the pain, one is tempted to attribute it to psychologic or emotional factors or to abnormal personality traits. Only a small proportion of the patients satisfy the diagnostic criteria for hysteria, but depression of varying severity is found in nearly half of them. Many such patients, with or without depression, respond to tricyclic antidepressants and monoamine oxidase inhibitors. Always to be differentiated from this group is the condition of trigeminal neuropathy, described in Chap. 47. Facial pain of the "atypical type," like other chronic pain of indeterminate cause, requires close observation of the patient, looking for lesions such as nasopharyngeal carcinoma to declare themselves. The pain should be managed by the conservative methods outlined in the preceding chapter and not by destructive cerebral surgery.

Other Rare Types of Facial Pain These include ciliary, nasociliary, supraorbital, and Sluder neuralgia. These are vague entities at best, and some merely represent different descriptive terms given to pains localized around the eye and nose (see "Cluster Headache" above; also Table 10-2). The Tolosa-Hunt syndrome of pain behind the eye and granulomatous involvement of some combination of cranial nerves III, IV, VI, and ophthalmic V, responsive to steroids, are discussed in Chap. 47.

A kind of *reflex sympathetic dystrophy of the face* is postulated as another rare form of persistent facial pain that may follow dental surgery or penetrating injuries to the face. It is characterized by severe burning pain and hyperpathia in response to all types of stimuli. Sudomotor, vasomotor, and trophic changes are lacking, unlike causalgia that affects the limbs. Nevertheless, this form of facial pain responds to repeated blockade or resection of the stellate ganglion.

Under the title of *neck-tongue syndrome*, Lance and Anthony have described the occurrence of a sharp pain and tingling in the upper neck or occiput on sudden rotation of the neck, associated with numbness of the ipsilateral half of the tongue. They attribute the syndrome to stretching of the C2 ventral ramus, which contains proprioceptive fibers from the tongue; these fibers run from the lingual nerve to the hypoglossal nerve and thence to the second cervical root.

The vexing problem that has gone by the self-evident name *burning mouth syndrome* occurs mainly in middle-aged and older women. The oral mucosa is normal and no one treatment has been consistently effective but gabapentin combined with antidepressants may be tried. One of our patients with a limited form of this condition, which affected only the upper palate and gums, benefitted from dental nerve blocks with lidocaine.

REFERENCES

Adams CBT, Kaye AH, Teddy PJ: The treatment of trigeminal neuralgia by posterior fossa microsurgery. *J Neurol Neurosurg Psychiatry* 45:1020, 1982.

Anderson CD, Frank RD: Migraine and tension headache: Is there a physiological difference? *Headache* 21:63, 1981.

Anthony M, Lance JM: Plasma serotonin in patients with chronic tension headaches. *J Neurol Neurosurg Psychiatry* 52:182, 1989.

Ashina M, Lassin LH, Bendsten L, et al: Effect of inhibition of nitric oxide synthetase on chronic tension type headache: a randomised crossover trial. *Lancet* 353:287, 1999.

Barker FG, Jannetta PJ, Bissonette DJ, et al: The long-term outcome of microvascular decompression for trigeminal neuralgia. *N Engl J Med* 334:1077, 1996.

Bickerstaff ER: Basilar artery migraine. *Lancet* 1:15, 1961.

Blau JN, Dexter SL: The site of pain origin during migraine attacks. *Cephalalgia* 1:143, 1981.

Bogduk N, Marsland A: On the concept of third occipital headache. *J Neurol Neurosurg Psychiatry* 49:775, 1986.

Bowsher D: The effects of pre-emptive treatment of postherpetic neuralgia with amitriptyline: A randomized, double-blind, placebo-controlled trial. *J Pain Symptom Mgt* 13:327, 1997.

Broderick JP, Swanson JW: Migraine-related strokes. *Arch Neurol* 44:868, 1987.

Caplan LR: Migraine and vertebrobasilar ischemia. *Neurology* 41:55, 1991.

Cole AJ, Aube M: Migraine with vasospasm and delayed intracerebral hemorrhage. *Arch Neurol* 47:53, 1990.

Cutter FM, Sorensen AG, Weisskoff RM, et al: Perfusion-weighted imaging defects during spontaneous migraine aura. *Ann Neurol* 43:25, 1998.

Dalessio DJ (ed): *Wolff's Headache and Other Head Pain*, 5th ed. New York, Oxford University Press, 1987.

Dandy WE: Concerning the cause of trigeminal neuralgia. *Am J Surg* 24:447, 1934.

Dorfman LS, Marshall WH, Enzmann DR: Cerebral infarction and migraine: Clinical and radiologic correlations. *Neurology* 29:317, 1979.

Drummond PD, Lance JW: Contribution of the extracranial circulation to the pathophysiology of headache, in Olesen J, Edvinsson L (eds): *Basic Mechanisms of Headache*. Amsterdam, Elsevier, 1988, pp 321–330.

Ekbom K: cited by Kudrow L (see below).

Ekbom K, Greitz T: Carotid angiography in cluster headache. *Acta Radiol (Diagn)* 10:177, 1970.

Feinmann C: Pain relief by antidepressants: Possible modes of action. *Pain* 23:1, 1985.

Ferrari MD, Haan J, Blokland JAK, et al: Cerebral blood flow during migraine attacks without aura and effect of sumatriptan. *Arch Neurol* 52:135, 1995.

Fields HL: Treatment of trigeminal neuralgia. *N Engl J Med* 334:1125, 1996.

Fisher CM: Late-life migraine accompaniments—Further experience. *Stroke* 17:1033, 1986.

Gardner WJ, Stowell A, Dutlinger R: Resection of the greater superficial petrosal nerve in the treatment of unilateral headache. *J Neurosurg* 4:105, 1947.

Gomez-Aranda F, Cañadillas F, Marti-Masso JF, et al: Pseudomigraine with temporary neurological symptoms and lymphocytic pleocytosis: A report of 50 cases. *Brain* 120:1105, 1997.

Graham JR, Wolff HG: Mechanism of migraine headache and action of ergotamine tartrate. *Arch Neurol Psychiatry* 39:737, 1938.

Guralnick W, Kaban LB, Merrill RG: Temporomandibular-joint afflictions. *N Engl J Med* 299:123, 1978.

Harris N: Paroxysmal and postural headaches from intraventricular cysts and tumours. *Lancet* 2:654, 1944.

Herold S, Gibbs JM, Jones AKP, et al: Oxygen metabolism in classical migraine. *J Cereb Blood Flow Metab* 5(suppl 5):5445, 1985.

Hupp SL, Kline LB, Corbett JJ: Visual disturbances of migraine. *Surv Ophthalmol* 33:221, 1989.

Iversen HK, Nielsen TH, Olesen J: Arterial responses during migraine headache. *Lancet* 336:837, 1990.

Jannetta PJ: Structural mechanisms of trigeminal neuralgia: Arterial compression of the trigeminal nerve at the pons in patients with trigeminal neuralgia. *J Neurosurg* 26:159, 1967.

Joutel A, Bousser MG, Brousse V, et al: Migraine hémiplégique familiale: Localisation d'un gène responsable sur le chromosome 19. *Rev Neurol* 150:340, 1994.

King RB: Topical aspirin in chloroform and the relief of pain due to herpes zoster and postherpetic neuralgia. *Arch Neurol* 50:1046, 1993.

Kittrelle JP, Grouse DS, Seybold ME: Cluster headache. *Arch Neurol* 42:496, 1985.

Kudrow L: *Cluster Headache: Mechanisms and Management.* Oxford, England, Oxford University Press, 1980.

Kunkle EC: Clues in the tempos of cluster headache. *Headache* 22:158, 1982.

Kunkle EC, Pfeiffer JB, Wilhoit WM, Lamrick LW: Recurrent brief headaches in "cluster" pattern. *NC Med J* 15:510, 1954.

Lance JW: Headaches related to sexual activity. *J Neurol Neurosurg Psychiatry* 39:1226, 1976.

Lance JW: *Migraine and Other Headaches.* Simon & Schuster, Australia, 1998.

Lance JW, Anthony M: Neck-tongue syndrome on sudden turning of the head. *J Neurol Neurosurg Psychiatry* 43:97, 1980.

Lance JW, Curran DA: Treatment of chronic tension headache. *Lancet* 1:1236, 1964.

Lance JW, Goadsby PJ: *The Mechanism and Management of Headache*, 6th ed. London, Butterworth-Heinemann, 1998.

Lance JW, Hinterberger H: Symptoms of pheochromocytoma, with particular reference to headache, correlated with catecholamine production. *Arch Neurol* 33:281, 1976.

Lashley KS: Pattern of cerebral integration indicated by the scotomas of migraine. *Arch Neurol Psychiatry* 46:331, 1941.

Lauritzen M, Olesen J: Regional cerebral blood flow during migraine attacks by xenon 133 inhalation and emission tomography. *Brain* 107:447, 1984.

Leão AAP: Spreading depression of activity in cerebral cortex. *J Neurophysiol* 7:359, 1944.

Lord SM, Barnsley L, Wallis BJ, Bogduk N: Third occipital nerve headache: A prevalence study. *J Neurol Neurosurg Psychiatry* 57:1187, 1994.

May A, Bahra A, Büchel C, et al: Hypothalamic activation in cluster headache attacks. *Lancet* 352:275, 1998.

Mortimer MJ, Good PA, Marsters JB, Addy DP: Visual evoked responses in children with migraine: A diagnostic test. *Lancet* 335:75, 1990.

Moskowitz MA: Neurogenic inflammation in the pathophysiology and treatment of migraine. *Neurology* 43(suppl 3):S16, 1993.

Olesen J: Headache Classification Committee of the International Headache Society: Classification and diagnostic criteria for headache disorders, cranial neuralgia, and facial pain. *Cephalalgia* 8 (suppl 7):1, 1988.

Olesen J: The ischemic hypothesis of migraine. *Arch Neurol* 44:321, 1987.

Olsen TS, Friberg L, Lassen NA: Ischemia may be the primary cause of the neurologic defects in classic migraine. *Arch Neurol* 44:156, 1987.

Pannullo SC, Reich JB, Krol G, et al: MRI changes in intracranial hypotension. *Neurology* 43:919, 1993.

Pascual J, Berciano J: Experience with headaches that start in elderly people. *J Neurol Neurosurg Psychiatry* 57:1255, 1994.

Patten J: *Neurological Differential Diagnosis.* London, Harold Starke, 1977.

Price RW, Posner JB: Chronic paroxysmal hemicrania: A disabling headache syndrome responding to indomethacin. *Ann Neurol* 3:183, 1978.

Raftery H: The management of postherpetic pain using sodium valproate and amitriptyline. *Irish Med J* 72:399, 1979.

Rascol A, Cambier J, Guiraud B, et al: Accidents ischemiques cerebraux au cours de crises migraineuses. *Rev Neurol* 135:867, 1979.

Raskin NH: Repetitive intravenous dihydroergotamine as therapy for intractable migraine. *Neurology* 36:995, 1986.

Raskin NH: Serotonin receptors and headache. *N Engl J Med* 325:353, 1991.

Raskin NH: The hypnic headache syndrome. *Headache* 28:534, 1988.

Raskin NH, Prusiner S: Carotidynia. *Neurology* 27:43, 1977.

Ratner EJ, Person P, Kleinman JD, et al: Jawbone cavities and trigeminal and atypical facial neuralgias. *Oral Surg* 48:3, 1979.

Ray BS, Wolff HG: Experimental studies on headache: Pain sensitive structures of the head and their significance in headache. *Arch Surg* 41:813, 1940.

Roberts AM, Person P, Chandra NB, Hori JM: Further observations on dental parameters of trigeminal and atypical facial pain. *Oral Surg* 58:121, 1984.

ROOKE ED: Benign exertional headache. *Med Clin North Am* 52:801, 1968.

ROSEMAN DM: Carotidynia. *Arch Otolaryngol* 85:103, 1967.

SAKAI F, EBIHARA S, AKIYAMA M, HORIKAWA M: Pericranial muscle hardness in tension-type headache: A non-invasive measurement method and its clinical application. *Brain* 118:523, 1995.

SCHULMAN EA, SILBERSTEIN SD: Symptomatic and prophylactic treatment treatment of migraine and tension-type headache. *Neurology* 42(suppl 2): 16, 1992.

SJAASTAD O, DALE I: A new (?) clinical headache entity "chronic paroxysmal hemicrania." *Acta Neurol Scand* 54:140, 1976.

SOMERVILLE BW: The role of estradiol withdrawal in the etiology of menstrual migraine. *Neurology* 22:355, 1972.

STEWART WF, SHECHTER A, RASMUSSEN BK: Migraine prevalence: A review of population-based studies. *Neurology* 44(suppl 4): S17, 1994.

Subcutaneous Sumatriptan International Study Group: Treatment of migraine attacks with sumatriptan. *N Engl J Med* 325:316, 1991.

SWEET WH: The treatment of trigeminal neuralgia (tic douloureux). *N Engl J Med* 315:174, 1986.

SWEET WH, WEPSIC JG: Controlled thermocoagulation of trigeminal ganglion and rootlets for differential destruction of pain fibers. *J Neurosurg* 40:143, 1974.

SYMONDS CP: Cough headache. *Brain* 79:557, 1956.

VIJAYAN N, DREYFUS PM: Posttraumatic dysautonomic cephalalgia. *Arch Neurol* 32:649, 1975.

WATSON P, STEELE JC: Paroxysmal dysequilibrium in the migraine syndrome of childhood. *Arch Otolaryngol* 99:177, 1974.

WELCH KMA: Migraine: A behavioral disorder. *Arch Neurol* 44:323, 1987.

WHITE JC, SWEET WH: *Pain and the Neurosurgeon*. Springfield, IL, Charles C Thomas, 1969, p 265.

WOLFF HG: *Headache and Other Head Pain*, 2nd ed. New York, Oxford University Press, 1963.

WOODS RP, IACOBONI M, MAZZIOTTA JC: Bilateral spreading cerebral hypoperfusion during spontaneous migraine headache. *N Engl J Med* 331:1690, 1994.

ZIEGLER DK, HURWITZ A, HASSANEIN RS, et al: Migraine prophylaxis: A comparison of propranolol and amitriptyline. *Arch Neurol* 44:486, 1987.

Chapter 11

PAIN IN THE BACK, NECK, AND EXTREMITIES

The diagnosis of pain in these parts of the body often requires the assistance of a neurologist. His task is to determine whether a disease of the spine has implicated the spinal cord or the spinal roots and nerves. To do this effectively, some knowledge of orthopedics and rheumatology is requisite. We include a chapter on this subject in recognition of the fact that back pain is among the most frequent of medical complaints. Up to 80 percent of adults have low-back pain at some time in their lives, and an even larger percentage of adults will be found at autopsy to have degenerative disc disease, according to Kelsey and White. Similar changes are disclosed by imaging studies of the lower spine. Our purpose in this chapter is to focus on the neurologic implications of back and neck pain and to assist the clinician in developing a systematic approach to patients with such complaints.

Since pains in the lower part of the spine and legs are caused by rather different types of disease than those in the neck, shoulder, and arms, they are considered separately.

PAIN IN THE LOWER BACK AND LIMBS

The lower parts of the spine and pelvis, with their massive muscular attachments, are relatively inaccessible to palpation and inspection. Although some physical signs and radiographs are helpful, diagnosis often depends on the patient's description of the pain and his or her behavior during the execution of certain maneuvers. Seasoned clinicians, for these reasons, have come to appreciate the need for a systematic inquiry and method of examination, the descriptions of which are preceded here by a brief consideration of the anatomy and physiology of the spine.

Anatomy and Physiology of the Lower Part of the Back

The bony spine is a complex structure, roughly divisible into an anterior and a posterior part. The former consists of a series of cylindric vertebral bodies, articulated by the intervertebral discs and held together by the anterior and posterior longitudinal ligaments. The posterior elements are more delicate and extend from the bodies as pedicles and laminae that form, with the posterior aspects of the bodies and ligaments, the vertebral canal. Stout transverse and spinous processes project laterally and posteriorly, respectively, and serve as the origins and insertions of the muscles that support and protect the spinal column. The bony processes are also held together by sturdy ligaments, the most important being the ligamentum flavum. The posterior parts of the vertebrae articulate with one another at the diarthrodal apophyseal (facet) joints, each of which is composed of the inferior facet of the vertebra above and the superior facet of the one below. These anatomic features are illustrated in Figs. 11-1 and 11-2. The facet and sacroiliac joints, covered by synovia, the compressible intervertebral discs, and the collagenous and elastic ligaments permit a limited degree of flexion, extension, rotation, and lateral motion of the spine.

The stability of the spine depends on the integrity of the vertebral bodies and intervertebral discs and on two types of supporting structures, ligamentous (passive) and muscular (active). Although the ligamentous structures are quite strong, neither they nor the vertebral body–disc complexes have sufficient integral strength to resist the enormous forces that may act on the spinal column; the stability of the lower back is therefore largely dependent on the voluntary and reflex activity of

Figure 11-1

The fifth lumbar vertebra viewed from above (A) *and from the side* (B).

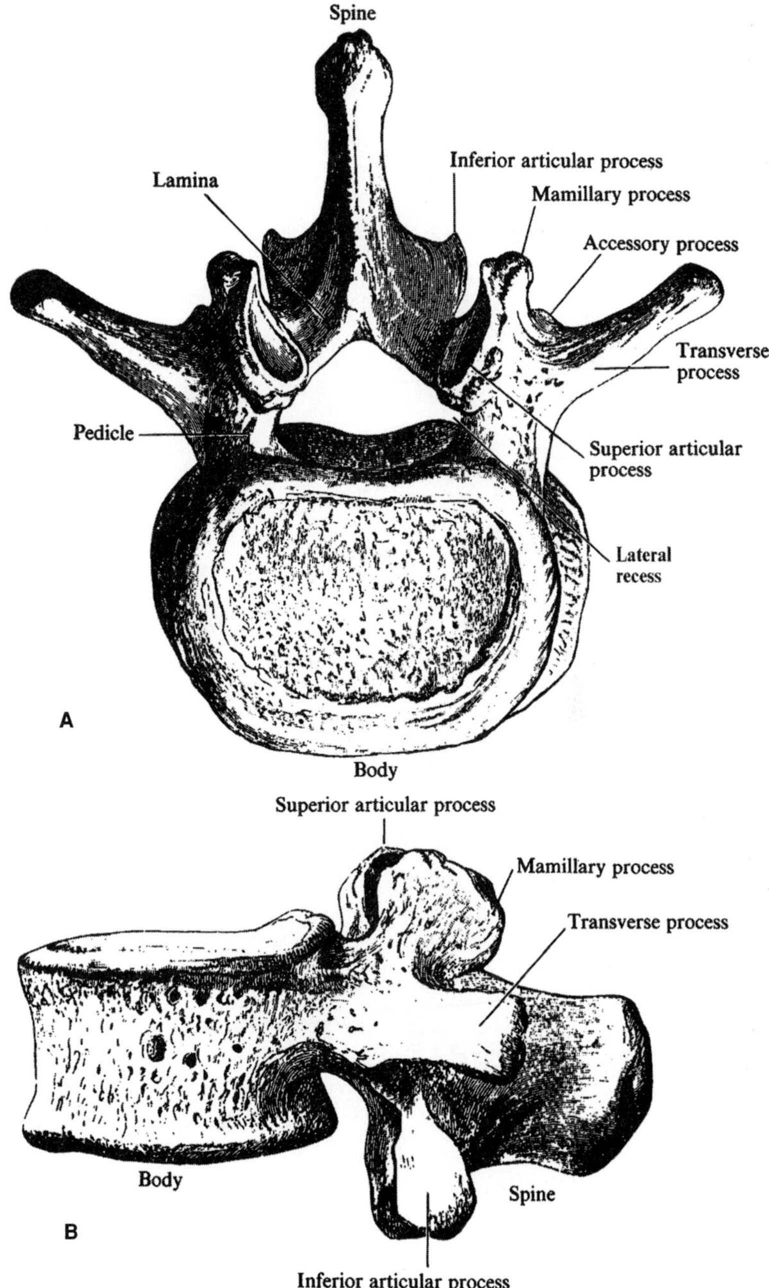

the sacrospinalis, abdominal, gluteus maximus, and hamstring muscles.

The vertebral and paravertebral structures derive their innervation from the meningeal branches of the spinal nerves (also known as recurrent meningeal or sinuvertebral nerves). These meningeal branches spring from the posterior divisions of the spinal nerves just distal to the dorsal root ganglia, re-enter the spinal canal through the intervertebral foramina, and supply pain fibers to the intraspinal ligaments, periosteum of bone, outer layers of the annulus fibrosus (that enclose the disc), and capsule of the articular facets. Coppes and associates have found A-δ and C pain fibers extending into the inner layers of the annulus and even the nucleus

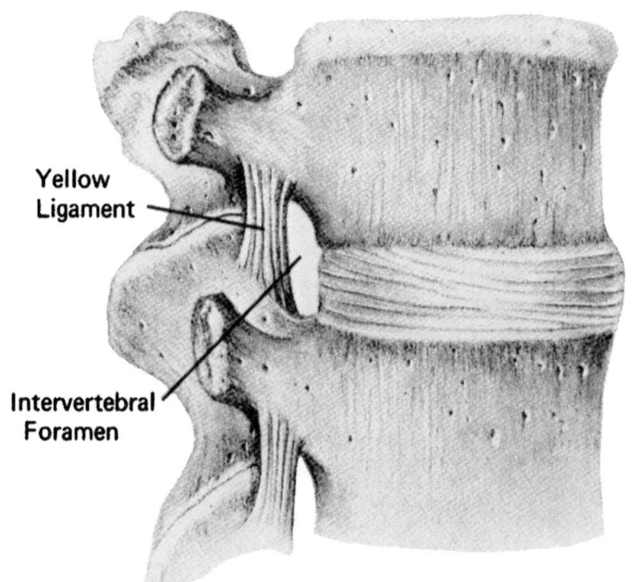

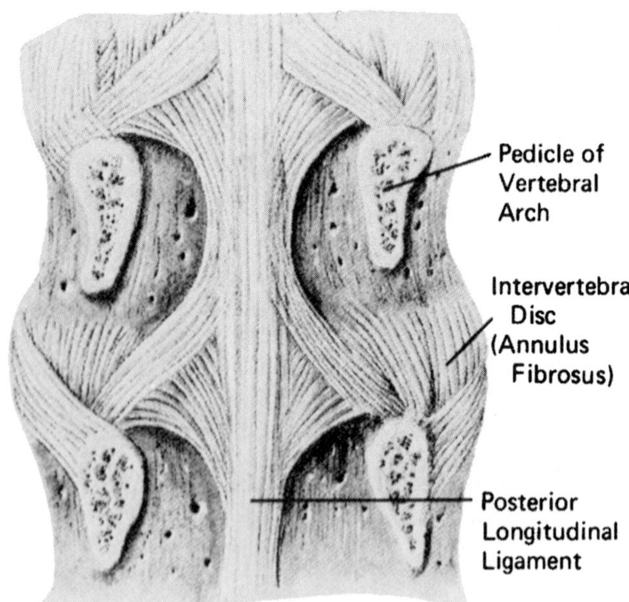

Figure 11-2

The main ligamentous structures of the spine. A. *Buckling of the yellow ligament (ligamentum flavum) may compress the nerve root or the spinal nerve at its origin in the intervertebral foramen, particularly if the foramen is narrowed by osteophytic overgrowth.* B. *Posterior aspect of the vertebral bodies. Fibers of the posterior longitudinal ligament merge with the posteromedial portion of the annulus fibrosus, leaving the posterolateral portion of the annulus relatively unsupported. (Reprinted by permission from Finneson.)*

pulposus. Although the spinal cord itself is insensitive, many of the conditions that affect it produce pain by involving these adjacent structures. The sensory fibers from these structures and the lumbosacral and sacroiliac joints enter the spinal cord via the fifth lumbar and first sacral roots. Motor fibers exit through the corresponding anterior roots and form the efferent limb of segmental reflexes. The sympathetic nerves contribute only to the innervation of blood vessels. The spinal roots in the lumbar region, after exiting from the spinal cord, course downward in the spinal canal and are gradually displaced laterally until they angulate and exit at the intervertebral foramina. Prior to entering the short foraminal canal, the spinal root lies in a shallow furrow along the inner surface of the pedicle termed the *lateral recess*. This is a common site of root entrapment by disc fragments and bony overgrowth.

The parts of the back that possess the greatest freedom of movement and hence are most frequently subject to injury are the lumbar, lumbosacral, and cervical. In addition to bending, twisting, and other voluntary movements, many actions of the spine are reflexive in nature and are the basis of posture.

Aging Changes in Spinal Structures Changes in the intervertebral discs and ligaments as a consequence of aging and perhaps a succession of minor traumas begin to occur as early as the first part of the third decade. Deposition of collagen and elastin and alterations of glycosaminoglycans combine to decrease the water content of the nucleus pulposus; concomitantly, the cartilagenous end plate becomes less vascular (Hassler). The dehydrated disc thins out and becomes more fragile. Similar changes occur in the annulus of the disc, which frays to an increasing degree with the passage of time, permitting the nucleus pulposus to bulge and, sometimes with injury, to extrude. This process can be observed by magnetic resonance imaging (MRI), which shows a gradual reduction in the high signal of the nucleus pulposus with the passage of time. In women who had MRI for gynecologic reasons, Powell and coworkers found an increasing frequency of lumbar disc degeneration and bulging, approaching 70 percent by the fiftieth year of life. Similar abnormalities in asymptomatic men and women have been recorded by Jensen and colleagues. The shrinkage of the disc alters the alignment of the articular facets and vertebral bodies, leading sometimes to facet arthropathy and spur formation. The latter changes may contribute to stenosis of the spinal canal and compromise the lateral recesses of the canal and the intervertebral foramina, where they may impinge on nerve roots. Osteoporosis, especially in older women, is an important cause of vertebral flattening or collapse, additionally narrowing the spinal canal.

General Clinical Features of Low-Back Pain

Types of Low-Back Pain Of the several symptoms of spinal disease (pain, stiffness, limitation of movement, and deformity), pain is of foremost importance. Four types of pain may be distinguished: local, referred, radicular, and that arising from secondary (protective) muscular spasm. These several types of pain can often be discerned from the patient's description; reliance is placed mainly on the character of the pain, its location, and conditions that modify it.

Local pain is caused by any pathologic process that impinges upon structures containing sensory endings. Involvement of the periosteum, capsule of apophyseal joints, muscles, annulus fibrosus, and ligaments is often exquisitely painful, whereas destruction of the vertebral body or nucleus pulposus alone produces little or no pain. Local pain is most often described as steady and aching, but it may be intermittent and sharp and, though not well circumscribed, is always felt in or near the affected part of the spine. Usually there is involuntary protective splinting of the corresponding spinal segments by reflex activity in paravertebral muscles, and certain movements or postures that counteract the spasm and alter the position of the injured tissues tend to aggravate the pain. Also, the superficial structures in the involved region are tender and direct pressure on them evokes pain. Muscles that are continually in reflex spasm may also become tender and sensitive to deep pressure.

Referred pain is of two types, one that is projected from the spine to viscera and other structures lying within the territory of the lumbar and upper sacral dermatomes and another that is projected from pelvic and abdominal viscera to the spine. Pain due to disease of the upper part of the lumbar spine is often referred to the flank, lateral hip, groin, and anterior thigh. This has been attributed to irritation of the superior cluneal nerves, which are derived from the posterior divisions of the first three lumbar spinal nerves and innervate the superior portions of the buttocks. Pain from the lower part of the lumbar spine is usually referred to the lower buttocks and posterior thighs and is due to irritation of lower spinal nerves, which activate the same pool of intraspinal neurons as the nerves that innervate the posterior thighs. Pain of this type is usually rather diffuse and has a deep, aching quality, but it tends at times to be more superficially projected. McCall and colleagues and Kellgren have verified these areas of reference by the injection of hypertonic saline into the apophyseal joints. But, as Sinclair and coworkers have pointed out, the sites of reference are inexact and cannot be relied upon for the precise anatomic localization of lesions. In general, the intensity of the referred pain parallels that of the local pain. In other words, maneuvers that alter local pain have a similar effect on referred pain, though lacking the precision and immediacy of so-called root pain.

Pain from visceral diseases is usually felt within the abdomen, flanks, or lumbar region and may be modified by the state of activity of the viscera and sometimes by assuming an upright or supine posture. Its character and temporal relationships have little relationship to movement of the back.

Radicular, or "root," pain has some of the characteristics of referred pain but differs in its greater intensity, distal radiation, circumscription to the territory of a root, and factors that excite it. The mechanism is stretching, irritation, or compression of a spinal root, within or central to the intervertebral foramen. The pain is sharp, often intense, and usually superimposed on the dull ache of referred pain; it nearly always radiates from a paracentral position near the spine to some part of the lower limb. Coughing, sneezing, and straining characteristically evoke this sharp radiating pain, although each of these actions may also jar or move the spine and enhance local pain; jugular vein compression, which raises intraspinal pressure and may cause a shift in position of the root, has a similar effect. In fact, any maneuver that stretches the nerve root—e.g., "straight-leg raising" in cases of sciatica—evokes radicular pain. The patterns of radicular pain due to involvement of particular roots are described in the sections on prolapsed discs (pages 214 and 225–226). The most common pattern is *sciatica, pain that originates in the buttock and is projected along the posterior or posterolateral thigh.* It results from irritation of the L5 or S1 nerve root. Paresthesias or superficial sensory loss, soreness of the skin, and tenderness in certain circumscribed regions along the nerve usually accompany radicular pain. If the anterior roots are involved as well, there may be reflex loss, weakness, atrophy, and fascicular twitching.

In patients with severe circumferential constriction of the cauda equina due to spondylosis (*lumbar stenosis*), sensorimotor impairment and sometimes referred pain are elicited by standing and walking. The neurologic symptoms involve the calves and the back of the thighs, simulating the exercise-induced symptoms due to vascular insufficiency—hence the term *spinal claudication* (see page 218).

Of importance is the observation that referred pain from the lower back (sometimes called *pseudoradicular*) does not, as a rule, project below the knees and is not accompanied by neurologic changes other than a vague numbness without demonstrable sensory impairment. The subcutaneous tissues within the area of referred pain may be tender. Of course, local, referred, and radicular pain may occur together.

Pain resulting from muscular spasm usually occurs in relation to local pain. The spasm may be thought of as a nocifensive reflex for the protection of the diseased parts against injurious motion. Muscle spasm is associated with many disorders of the low back and can distort normal posture. Chronic muscular contraction may give rise to a dull, sometimes cramping ache. One can feel the tautness of the sacrospinalis and gluteal muscles and demonstrate by palpation that the pain is localized to them. However, except for the most severe degrees of spasm in acute injury of the back, the contribution of this component to back pain is relatively small.

Other pains, often of undetermined origin, are sometimes described by patients with chronic disease of the lower part of the back: drawing and pulling in the legs, cramping sensation (without involuntary muscle spasm), tearing, throbbing, or jabbing pains, and feelings of burning or coldness. These sensations, like paresthesias and numbness, should always suggest the possibility of nerve or root disease.

In addition to assessing the character and location of the pain, one should determine the factors that aggravate and relieve it, its constancy, and its relationship to activity and rest, posture, forward bending, and cough, sneeze, and strain. Frequently the most important lead comes from knowledge of the mode of onset and the circumstances that initiated the pain. Inasmuch as many painful affections of the back are the result of injuries incurred during work or in automobile accidents, the possibility of exaggeration or prolongation of pain for purposes of compensation must always be kept in mind.

Examination of the Lower Back

Some information may be gained by inspection of the back, buttocks, and lower limbs in various positions. The normal spine shows a thoracic kyphosis and lumbar lordosis in the sagittal plane, which in some individuals may be exaggerated (swayback). In the coronal plane, the spine is normally straight or shows a slight curvature, particularly in women. One should observe the spine closely for excessive curvature, a list, flattening of the normal lumbar lordosis, presence of a gibbus (a sharp, kyphotic angulation usually indicative of a fracture), pelvic tilt or obliquity (Trendelenburg sign), and asymmetry of the paravertebral or gluteal musculature. A sagging gluteal fold suggests involvement of the S1 root. In sciatica one may observe a flexed posture of the affected leg, presumably to reduce tension on the irritated nerve. Patients in whom a free fragment of lumbar disc material has migrated posterolaterally may be unable to lie down and extend the spine.

The next step in the examination is *observation of the spine, hips, and legs during certain motions*. It is well to remember that no advantage accrues from determining how much pain the patient can tolerate. More important is to determine when and under what conditions the pain begins or worsens. Observation of the patient's gait when he is unaware of being watched may disclose a subtle limp, a pelvic tilt, a shortening of step, or a stiffness of bearing—indicative of a disinclination to bear weight on a painful leg. One looks for limitation of motion while the patient is standing, sitting, and reclining. When standing, the motion of forward bending normally produces flattening and reversal of the lumbar lordotic curve and exaggeration of the thoracic curve. With lesions of the lumbosacral region that involve the posterior ligaments, articular facets, or sacrospinalis muscles and with ruptured lumbar discs, protective reflexes prevent flexion, which stretches these structures. As a consequence, the sacrospinalis muscles remain taut and prevent motion in the lumbar part of the spine. Forward bending then occurs at the hips and at the thoracolumbar junction; also, the patient bends in such a way as to avoid tensing the hamstring muscles and putting undue leverage on the pelvis. In the presence of degenerative disc disease, straightening up from a flexed position is performed with difficulty and is aided to some extent by flexing the knees.

Lateral bending is usually less instructive than forward bending. In unilateral ligamentous or muscular strain, bending to the opposite side aggravates the pain by stretching the damaged tissues. With unilateral sciatica, the patient lists to one side and strongly resists bending to the opposite side, and his preferred posture in standing is with the leg slightly flexed at the hip and knee. When the herniated disc lies lateral to the nerve root and displaces it medially, tension on the root is reduced by bending the trunk to the side opposite the lesion; with herniation medial to the root, tension is reduced by inclining the trunk to the side of the lesion.

In the sitting position, flexion of the spine can be performed more easily, even to the point of bringing the knees in contact with the chest. The reason for this is that knee flexion relaxes tightened hamstring muscles and relieves the stretch on the sciatic nerve. Asking the seated patient to extend the leg so that the sole of the foot can be inspected is a way of checking for a feigned Lasègue sign (see below).

Examination in the reclining position yields much the same information as in the standing and sitting positions. With lumbosacral disc lesions and sciatica, passive lumbar flexion causes little pain and is not limited as long as the hamstrings are relaxed and there is no stretching of the sciatic nerve. Thus, with the knees flexed to 90 degrees, sitting up from the reclining position is unimpeded and not painful; with knees extended, there is pain and limited motion (Kraus-Weber test). With vertebral disease (e.g., arthritis), passive flexion of the hips is free, whereas flexion of the lumbar spine may be impeded and painful.

Passive *straight-leg raising* (possible up to 90 degrees in normal individuals), like forward bending in the standing posture with the legs straight, places the sciatic nerve and its roots under tension, thereby producing radicular radiating pain. It may also cause an anterior rotation of the pelvis around a transverse axis, increasing stress on the lumbosacral joint and causing pain if this joint is arthritic or otherwise diseased. Consequently, in diseases of the lumbosacral joints and roots, passive straight-leg raising evokes pain and is limited on the affected side and, to a lesser extent, on the opposite side (Lasègue sign). *Straight raising of the opposite leg* may also cause pain on the affected side and is believed by some to be an even more reliable sign of prolapsed disc than a Lasègue sign. It is important to remember that the evoked pain is always referred to the diseased side, no matter which leg is elevated. While in the supine position, leg length (anterosuperior iliac spine to medial malleolus) and the circumference of the thigh and calf should be measured.

Hyperextension may be performed with the patient standing or lying prone. If the condition causing back pain is acute, it may be difficult to extend the spine in the standing position. A patient with lumbosacral strain or disc disease (except in the acute phase or if the disc fragment has migrated laterally) can usually extend or hyperextend the spine with little or no aggravation of pain. If there is an active inflammatory process or fracture of the vertebral body or posterior elements, hyperextension may be markedly limited. In disease of the upper lumbar roots, hyperextension is the motion that is limited and reproduces pain; however, in some cases of lower lumbar disc disease with thickening of the ligamentum flavum, this movement is also painful. In patients with narrowing of the spinal canal (spondylosis, spondylolisthesis), upright stance and extension may produce neurologic symptoms (see further on).

Maneuvers in the *lateral decubitus position* yield less information as a rule. In cases of sacroiliac joint disease, abduction of the upside leg against resistance reproduces pain in the sacroiliac region, with radiation of the pain to the buttock, posterior thigh, and symphysis pubis. Hyperextension of the upside leg with the downside leg flexed is another test for sacroiliac disease. Rotation and abduction of the leg evoke pain in a diseased hip joint and with trochanteric bursitis. Another helpful indicator of hip pain is the Patrick test: with the patient supine, the heel of the offending leg is placed on the opposite knee and pain is evoked by depressing the flexed leg and externally rotating the hip.

Gentle palpation and percussion of the spine are the last steps in the examination. It is preferable to first palpate the regions that are the least likely to evoke pain. At all times the examiner should know what structures are being palpated (see Fig. 11-3). Localized tenderness is seldom pronounced in disease of the spine because the involved structures are so deep. Nevertheless, tenderness over a spinous process or jarring by gentle percussion may indicate the presence of inflammation (as in disc space infection), pathologic fracture, a spinal metastasis, or a disc lesion at the site deep to it.

Tenderness over the costovertebral angle often indicates genitourinary disease, adrenal disease, or an injury to the transverse process of the first or second lumbar vertebra [Fig. 11-3, (1)]. Tenderness on palpation of the paraspinal muscles may signify a strain of muscle attachments or injury to the underlying transverse processes of the lumbar vertebrae. Focal pain in the same sagittal line along the thoracic spine points to inflammation of the costotransverse articulation between spine and rib (*costotransversitis*).

Figure 11-3

(1) *Costovertebral angle.* (2) *Spinous process and interspinous ligament.* (3) *Region of articular facet (fifth lumbar to first sacral).* (4) *Dorsum of sacrum.* (5) *Region of iliac crest.* (6) *Iliolumbar angle.* (7) *Spinous processes of fifth lumbar and first sacral vertebrae (tenderness = faulty posture or occasionally spina bifida occulta).* (8) *Region between posterior superior and posterior inferior spines. Sacroiliac ligaments (tenderness = sacroiliac sprain, often tender with fifth lumbar or first sacral disc).* (9) *Sacrococcygeal junction (tenderness = sacrococcygeal injury, i.e., sprain or fracture).* (10) *Region of sacrosciatic notch (tenderness = fourth or fifth lumbar disc rupture and sacroiliac sprain).* (11) *Sciatic nerve trunk (tenderness = ruptured lumbar disc or sciatic nerve lesion).*

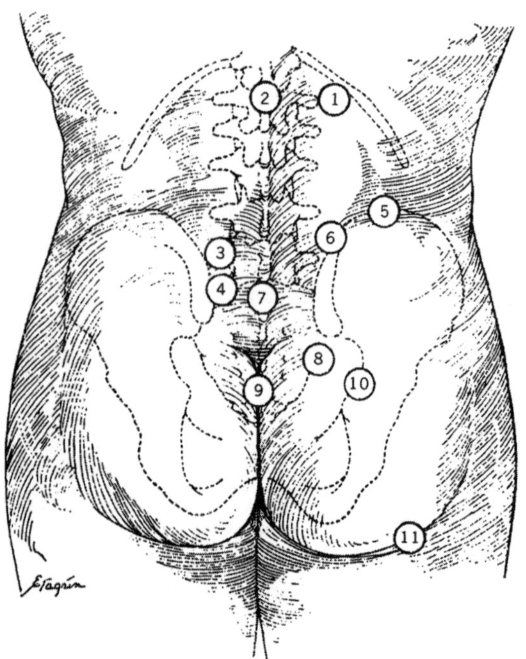

In palpating the spinous processes, it is important to note any deviation in the lateral plane (this may be indicative of fracture or arthritis) or in the anteroposterior plane. A "step-off" forward displacement of the spinous process and exaggerated lordosis are important clues to the presence of *spondylolisthesis* (see further on). Tenderness over the interspinous ligaments is indicative of disc lesions [Fig. 11-3, (2)]. Tenderness over the region of the articular facets between the fifth lumbar and first sacral vertebrae is consistent with lumbosacral disc disease [Fig. 11-3, (3)]. Tenderness in this region and in the sacroiliac joints is also a frequent manifestation of ankylosing spondylitis.

Abdominal, rectal, and pelvic examinations are essential elements in the study of the patient with low back symptoms that fail to be clarified by the aforementioned spinal maneuvers. Neoplastic, inflammatory, or degenerative disorders may produce symptoms referred to the lower part of the spine.

Upon completion of the examination of the back and legs, one turns to a search for motor, reflex, and sensory changes in the lower extremities (see "Protrusion of Lumbar Intervertebral Discs," further on in this chapter).

Ancillary Diagnostic Procedures

Depending on the circumstances, these may include a blood count and erythrocyte sedimentation rate (especially helpful in screening for infection or myeloma); calcium, phosphorus, uric acid, alkaline phosphatase, acid phosphatase, and prostate-specific antigen (if one suspects metastatic carcinoma of the prostate); a serum protein electrophoresis (myeloma proteins); in special cases, a tuberculin test or serologic test for *Brucella*; a test for rheumatoid factor; and HLA typing (for ankylosing spondylitis). Radiographs of the lumbar spine (preferably with the patient standing) in the anteroposterior, lateral, and oblique planes are still useful in the routine evaluation of low back pain and sciatica. Readily demonstrable in plain films are narrowing of the intervertebral disc spaces, bony facetal or vertebral overgrowth, displacement of vertebral bodies (spondylolisthesis), and an unsuspected infiltration of bone by cancer. In cases of suspected disc herniation or tumor infiltration of the spinal canal, one proceeds directly to MRI. Although these imaging procedures have largely replaced conventional myelography, the latter examination, when combined with computed tomography (CT), provides detailed information about the dural sleeves that surround the spinal roots, at times disclosing subtle truncations caused by laterally situated disc herniations and at times revealing surface abnormalities of the spinal cord, such as arteriovenous malformations. Administration of gadolinium at the time of MRI enhances regions of inflammation and tumor.

Injection of contrast medium directly into the intervertebral disc (discogram) is still practiced in a few institutions but is more difficult to interpret than CT-myelography and MRI and carries the risk of damage to nerve roots or the introduction of infection. Discography is indicated only in special circumstances and should be undertaken only by those who are specialized in its performance. Isotope bone scans are useful in demonstrating tumors and inflammatory processes such as osteomyelitis.

Nerve conduction studies and electromyography (EMG) are particularly helpful in suspected root and nerve diseases, as indicated further on in the discussion of protruded lumbar discs. However, as for all the aforementioned tests, they are useful only in the context of the history and clinical examination; otherwise they are subject to overuse and overinterpretation.

Principal Conditions Giving Rise to Pain in the Lower Back

Congenital Anomalies of the Lumbar Spine

Anatomic variations of the spine are frequent, and though rarely of themselves the source of pain and functional derangement, they may predispose an individual to discogenic and spondylotic complications by virtue of altering the mechanics and alignment of the vertebrae or size of the spinal canal.

The commonest anomaly is a lack of fusion of the laminae of one or several of the lumbar vertebrae or of the sacrum (spina bifida). Occasionally, a subcutaneous mass, hypertrichosis, or hyperpigmentation in the sacral area betrays the condition, but in most patients it remains occult until it is disclosed radiologically. The anomaly may be accompanied by malformation of vertebral joints and usually induces pain only when aggravated by injury. The neurologic aspects of defective fusion of the spine (dysraphism) are discussed in Chap. 38.

Many other congenital anomalies affect the lower lumbar vertebrae: asymmetrical facetal joints, abnormalities of the transverse processes, "sacralization" of the fifth lumbar vertebra (in which L5 appears to be fixed to the sacrum), or "lumbarization" of the first sacral vertebra (in which S1 looks like a sixth lumbar vertebra) are seen occasionally in patients with low back symptoms, but apparently with no greater frequency than in asymptomatic individuals. The role of these anomalies in the genesis of low back derangement is unclear, but in the authors' opinion they are rarely the cause of specific symptoms.

Spondylolysis consists of a bony defect in the pars interarticularis (the segment at the junction of pedicle and lamina) of the lower lumbar vertebrae. The defect is remarkably common; it affects approximately 5 percent of the North American population, is probably genetic, and predisposes to fracture at this location. Radiographically, the pars interarticularis defect is best visualized on oblique projections. In some persons it is unilateral and may cause unilateral aching back pain that is accentuated by hyperextension and twisting. It is not uncommon in athletes. In the usual bilateral form, small fractures at the pars interarticularis allow the vertebral body, pedicles, and superior articular facets to move anteriorly, leaving the posterior elements behind. This latter deformity, known as *spondylolisthesis*, is mainly a disease of children (peak incidence between 5 and 7 years of age). It may cause little difficulty at first but eventually becomes symptomatic. The patient complains of limitation of motion and pain in the low back, radiating into the thighs. Examination discloses tenderness near the segment that has "slipped" (most often L5, occasionally L4), a palpable "step" of the spinous process forward from the segment below, hamstring spasm, and, in severe cases (*spondyloptosis*), shortening of the trunk and protrusion of the lower abdomen (both of which result from the abnormal forward shift of L5 on S1) as well as signs of involvement of spinal roots—paresthesias and sensory loss, muscle weakness, and reflex impairment. These neurologic symptoms and signs tend not to be severe.

Sometimes, the fourth lumbar vertebra may slip forward on the fifth, narrowing the spinal canal, without the presence of a defect in the pars interarticularis. This is termed *intact arch spondylolisthesis* and occurs most often in middle-aged or elderly women. This form of spondylolisthesis is probably due to degenerative disease of the inferior and superior facets. It causes severe low back pain, made worse by standing or walking and relieved by bed rest. Symptoms of root compression are common (Alexander et al).

Patients with progressive vertebral displacement and neurologic deficits require surgery, usually posterolateral fusion and excision of the posterior elements. Reduction of displaced vertebral bodies before fusion and direct repair of pars defects are possible in special cases.

Traumatic Disorders of the Low Back Traumatic disorders constitute the most frequent cause of low back pain. In severe acute injuries, the examiner must be careful to avoid further damage. All movements must be kept to a minimum until an approximate diagnosis has been made and adequate measures have been instituted for the proper care of the patient. If the patient complains of pain in the back and cannot move his legs, the spine may have been fractured and the cord or cauda equina compressed or crushed. The neck should not be manipulated, and the patient should not be allowed to sit up. (See Chap. 44 for further discussion of spinal cord injury.)

Sprains and Strains The terms *lumbosacral strain*, *sprain*, and *derangement* are used loosely by most physicians, and it is probably not possible to differentiate them. What was formerly referred to as "sacroiliac strain" or "sprain" is now known to be due, in many instances, to disc disease. The authors prefer the term *acute low back* or *myofascial strain* for minor, self-limited injuries that are usually associated with lifting heavy loads in a mechanically disadvantaged position, a fall, stiffness that arises from prolonged uncomfortable postures such as air travel or car rides, or sudden unexpected motion, as may occur in an auto accident.

The discomfort of acute low-back strain is often severe, and the patient may assume unusual postures related to spasm of the lower lumbar and sacrospinalis muscles. The pain is usually confined to the lower part of the back, in the midline or just to one side or other of the spine. The diagnosis of lumbosacral strain depends upon the description of the injury or activity that precipitated the pain, the localization of the pain, the finding of localized tenderness, the augmentation of pain by postural changes, e.g., bending forward, twisting, or standing up from a sitting position, and the absence of signs of radicular involvement. In more than 80 percent of cases of acute low-back strain of this type, the pain resolves in a matter of several days or a week even with no specific treatment.

Sacroiliac strain is the most likely diagnosis when there is tenderness over the sacroiliac joint and pain radiating to the buttock and posterior thigh, but this always needs to be distinguished from a ruptured intervertebral disc (see further on). Strain is characteristically worsened by abduction of the thigh against resistance and is also felt in the symphysis pubis or groin. It, too, responds within days or a week or two to conservative management.

Treatment of Acute Low-Back Strains The pain of muscular and ligamentous strains is usually self-limited, responding to simple measures in a relatively short period of time. The basic principle of therapy in both disorders is rest, in a recumbent position, for several days. Lying on the side with knees and hips flexed or supine with a pillow under the knees are the favored positions. With strains of the sacrospinalis muscles and sacroiliac ligaments, the optimal position is hyperextension. This position is best maintained by having the patient lie with a small pillow or folded blanket under the lumbar portion of the spine or by lying face down. Physical measures—such as application of ice in the acute phase (30 min on, 60 min off) and heat after the third or fourth day, diathermy, and massage—can be tried but are of limited value. Nonsteroidal anti-inflammatory medication should be given liberally during the first few days. Muscle relaxants are of little use, serving mainly to make bed rest more tolerable. When weight bearing is resumed, discomfort may be diminished by a light lumbosacral support, but many orthopedists refrain from prescribing this aid. Thereafter, corrective exercises are prescribed, designed to stretch and strengthen trunk (especially abdominal) muscles, overcome faulty posture, and increase the mobility of the spinal joints.

The use of spinal manipulation—practiced by chiropractors, osteopaths, and others—has always been a contentious matter in the United States, partly because of unrealistic therapeutic claims made in diseases other than low back derangements. By contrast, in certain parts of Europe, orthopedists often incorporate manipulative procedures into conventional practice. A type of slow muscle stretching and joint distraction (axial traction on a joint) administered by physiatrists is quite similar. It must be recognized that many patients seek chiropractic manipulation on their own, often before seeing a physician, and may not disclose this information to the physician. When the supporting elements of the spine (pedicles, facets, and ligaments) are not disrupted, chiropractic manipulation of the lumbar spine has provided relief to a considerable number of patients with low-back strain or facet pain. A randomized British trial has shown manipulation to be superior to analgesics and bed rest in returning patients to work after minor back injury (Meade et al). Some trials have corroborated this finding (Hadler et al), while others have not or the results have been ambiguous. In the study by Cherkin and colleagues comparing chiropractic, physical therapy (McKenzie method), and simple instruction to the patient from a booklet, manipulation yielded a slightly better outcome at the end of a month. Despite several hypotheses that have been offered by practitioners of spinal manipulation, the mechanism of pain relief is not known. The sound created by rapid and forceful distraction of the facet joints, similar to cracking the knuckles, seems not to be necessary for pain relief. Whether all forms of low-back pain represent minor subluxations, as claimed by chiropractors, is undocumented and seems unlikely. Chronic low back pain has, in the authors' experience, been even less successfully treated by manipulative procedures, but there are patients who testify to improvement in their clinical state, and admittedly the medical profession has little to offer many of these patients. The commitment of patients to a regime of anti-inflammatory agents for many months or to narcotic analgesics is a hazard always to be avoided.

The Degenerative Low-Back Syndrome Often the symptoms of low-back strain are recurrent and more chronic in nature, being regularly exacerbated by bending or lifting, suggesting that postural, muscular, and arthritic factors play a role. This is the most common syndrome seen in orthopedic clinics, more in men than in women.

After some unusual activity, raising the question of trauma, especially if it happens in the workplace, the patient develops deep aching pain in the low back, increased by certain movements and attended by stiffness. The pain often has a restricted radiation into the buttocks and posterior thigh. There are no motor, sensory, or reflex abnormalities. Plain films and imaging procedures reveal some combination of osteoarthropathy, changes in vertebral discs, osteoarthritic changes in apophyseal joints, and sometimes osteoporosis or slight spondylosis. Treatment with short-duration bed rest, analgesics, and physiotherapy, as outlined for acute strains, help to relieve the symptoms and the majority of patients recover within a month. Chiropractic manipulation has the same uncertain effect as for acute low-back symptoms. Usually the origin of the pain cannot be determined and special diagnostic procedures are not helpful. Only if the pain persists for longer than a month is MRI indicated. Recurrent attacks are typical of degenerative spine disease. Workers' compensation problems add to the disability, especially in older workers.

Vertebral Fractures Fractures of a lumbar vertebral body are usually the result of flexion injuries. Such trauma may occur in a fall or jump from a height (if the patient lands on his feet, the calcanei may also be fractured) or as a result of an auto accident or other violent injury. If the injury is severe, it may cause a fracture dislocation, a "burst" fracture of one or more vertebral bodies, or an asymmetrical fracture of a pedicle, lamina, or spinous process, but most often there is asymmetrical loss of height of a vertebral body (*compression fracture*), which may be extremely painful at the onset. When compression or other fractures occur with minimal trauma (or spontaneously), the bone has presumably been weakened by some pathologic process. Most of the time, particularly in older individuals, osteoporosis is the cause of such an event, but there are many other causes, including osteomalacia, hyperparathyroidism, prolonged use of corticosteroids, ankylosing spondylitis, myeloma, metastatic carcinoma, and a number of local conditions. Spasm of the lower lumbar muscles, limitation of all movements of the lumbar section of the spine, and the radiographic appearance of the damaged lumbar portion (with or without neurologic abnormalities) are the basis of clinical diagnosis. The pain is usually immediate, though occasionally it may be delayed for days.

A fractured transverse process, which is almost always associated with tearing of the paravertebral muscles and a local hematoma, causes deep tenderness at the site of the injury, local muscle spasm, and limitation of all movements that stretch the lumbar muscles. The radiologic findings, particularly MRI, confirm the diagnosis. In some circumstances, tears of the paravertebral musculature may be associated with extensive bleeding into the retroperitoneal space and proximal leg weakness.

Herniation of Lumbar Intervertebral Discs This condition is a major cause of severe and chronic or recurrent low back and leg pain. It occurs mainly during the third and fourth decades of life, when the nucleus pulposus is still gelatinous. The disc between the fifth lumbar and first sacral vertebrae (L5-S1) is the one most often involved, and, with decreasing frequency, that between the fourth and fifth (L4-5), third and fourth (L3-4), second and third (L2-3), and quite infrequently, the first and second (L1-2) lumbar vertebrae. Relatively rare but well described in the thoracic portion of the spine, disc disease is again frequent at the fifth and sixth and the sixth and seventh cervical vertebrae (see further on).

The cause of a herniated lumbar disc is usually a flexion injury, but a considerable proportion of patients do not recall a traumatic episode. Degeneration of the nucleus pulposus, the posterior longitudinal ligaments, and the annulus fibrosus may have taken place silently or have been manifest by mild, recurrent lumbar ache. A sneeze, lurch, or other trivial movement may then cause the nucleus pulposus to prolapse, pushing the frayed and weakened annulus posteriorly. Fragments of the nucleus pulposus protrude through rents in the annulus, usually to one side or the other (sometimes in the midline), where they impinge upon a root or roots. In more severe cases of disc disease, the nucleus may protrude through the annulus or be extruded and lie epidurally, as a free fragment. A large protrusion may compress the root(s) against the articular apophysis or lamina. The protruded material may be resorbed to some extent and become reduced in size, but often it does not, causing chronic irritation of the root or a discarthrosis with posterior osteophyte formation.

The Clinical Syndrome The fully developed syndrome of prolapsed intervertebral lumbar disc consists of: (1) pain in the sacroiliac region, radiating into the buttock, thigh, calf, and foot and broadly termed *sciatica*; (2) a stiff or unnatural spinal posture; and (3) some combination of paresthesias, weakness, and reflex impairment.

The pain of herniated intervertebral disc varies in severity from a mild discomfort to the most severe knife-like stabs that radiate the length of the leg and are superimposed on a constant intense ache. Abortive forms of sciatica may produce aching discomfort only in the lower buttock and thigh and occasionally only in the lower hamstring or upper calf. With the most severe pain, the patient is forced to stay in bed, avoiding the slightest movement; a cough, sneeze, or strain is intolerable. The patient is usually most comfortable lying on his back with legs flexed at the knees and hips (dorsal decubitus position) and with the shoulders raised on pillows to obliterate the lumbar lordosis. For some patients, a particular lateral decubitus position is more comfortable. As mentioned earlier, free fragments of disc that find their way to a lateral and posterior position in the spinal canal may produce the opposite situation, one of being unable to extend the spine and lie supine. When the condition is less severe, walking is possible, though fatigue sets in quickly, with a feeling of heaviness and drawing pain. Sitting and standing up from a sitting position are particularly painful. The pain is usually located deep in the buttock, just lateral to and below the sacroiliac joint, and in the posterolateral region of the thigh, with radiation to the calf and infrequently to the heel and other parts of the foot. Radiation of pain into the foot should at least raise the suspicion of an alternative cause of nerve damage. It is noteworthy and surprising to patients that a lumbar disc protrusion sometimes causes little back pain, although in these circumstances there is often, in our experience, deep tenderness over the lateral process or facet joint adjacent to the protrusion. Pain is also characteristically provoked by pressure over the course of the sciatic nerve at the classic points of Valleix (sciatic notch, retrotrochanteric gutter, posterior surface of thigh, head of fibula). Pressure at one point may cause radiation of pain and tingling down the leg.

Elongation of the nerve root by straight-leg raising or by flexing the leg at the hip and extending it at the knee (Lasègue maneuver) is the most consistent of all pain-provoking signs. When sciatica is severe, straight-leg raising is restricted to 20 to 30 degrees of elevation; when the condition is less severe or with improvement, the angle formed by the leg and bed widens, finally to almost 90 degrees, in patients with flexible backs and limbs. During straight-leg raising, the patient can distinguish between the discomfort of ordinary tautness of the hamstring and the sharper, less familiar root pain, particularly when asked to compare the experience with that on the normal side. Many variations of the Lasègue maneuver have been described (all with eponyms), the most useful of which is accentuation of the pain by dorsiflexion of the foot (Bragard sign) or of the great toe (Sicard sign). The Lasègue maneuver with the healthy leg may evoke pain, but usually of lesser degree and always on the side of the spontaneous pain (Fajerstagn sign). The presence of a crossed straight-leg-raising sign is strongly indicative of a ruptured disc as the cause of sciatica (in 56 of 58 cases in the series of Hudgkins). With the patient standing, forward bending of the trunk will cause flexion of the knee on the affected side (Neri sign); the degree of limitation of forward bending approximates that of straight-leg raising. Sciatica may be provoked by forced flexion of the head and neck, coughing, or pressure on both jugular veins, all of which increase the intraspinal pressure (Naffziger sign). Marked inconsistencies in response to these tests raise the suspicion of psychologic factors.

In the upright position, the posture of the body is altered by the pain. The patient stands with the affected leg slightly flexed at the knee and hip, so that only the ball of the foot rests on the floor. The trunk tends to tilt forward and to one side or the other, depending on the relationship of the protruded disc material to the root (see above). This antalgic posture is referred to as *sciatic scoliosis* and is maintained by reflex contraction of the paraspinal muscles, which can be both seen and palpated. In walking, the knee is slightly flexed, and weight bearing on the painful leg is brief and cautious, giving a limp. It is particularly painful for the patient to go up and down stairs.

The signs of severe spinal root compression are impairment of sensation, loss or diminution of tendon reflexes, and muscle weakness. The hypotonia is evident on inspection and palpation of the buttock and calf, and the Achilles tendon tends to be less salient. Paresthesias (rarely hyperesthesia or hypoesthesia) are reported by one-third of patients; usually they are felt in the foot, sometimes in the leg. Often there is a diminution of pain perception over the appropriate dermatome. Muscle weakness occurs, but less frequently. The ankle or knee jerk is usually diminished or lost on the side of the lesion. The reflex changes have little relationship to the severity of the pain or sensory loss. Furthermore, compression of the fourth or fifth lumbar root may occur without any change in the tendon reflexes. Bilaterality of symptoms and signs is rare, as is sphincteric paralysis, but they may occur with large central protrusions. The cerebrospinal fluid (CSF) protein is then predictably elevated, usually in the range of 55 to 85 mg/dL, sometimes higher.

As indicated above, herniations of the intervertebral lumbar discs occur most often between the fifth lumbar and first sacral vertebrae (compressing the S1 root; see Fig 11-4) and between the fourth and fifth lumbar vertebrae (compressing the L5 root). It is important, therefore, to recognize the clinical characteristics of root compression at these two sites. *Lesions of the fifth lumbar root* produce pain in the region of the hip, posterolateral thigh, lateral calf (to the external malleolus), dorsal surface of the foot, and the first or second and third toes. Paresthesias may be felt in the entire territory or only in its distal parts. The tenderness is in the lateral gluteal region and near the head of the femur. Weakness, if present, involves the extensors of the big toe and of the foot. The ankle jerk may be diminished (more often it is normal), but the knee jerk is hardly ever altered. Walking on the heels may be more difficult and uncomfortable than walking on the toes because of weakness of dorsiflexion.

With *lesions of the first sacral root*, the pain is felt in the midgluteal region, posterior part of the thigh, posterior region of the calf to the heel, outer plantar surface of the foot, and fourth and fifth toes. Tenderness is most pronounced over the midgluteal region (in the region of the sacroiliac joint), posterior thigh areas, and calf. Paresthesias and sensory loss are mainly in the lower part of the leg and outer toes, and weakness, if present, involves the flexor muscles of the foot and toes, abductors of the toes, and hamstring muscles. The Achilles reflex is diminished or absent in the majority of cases. In fact, loss of the Achilles reflex is often the first and only objective sign. Walking on the toes is more difficult and uncomfortable than walking on the heels because of weakness of the plantar flexors.

The rarer lesions of the *third and fourth lumbar roots* give rise to pain in the anterior part of the thigh and knee and anteromedial part of the leg (fourth lumbar), with corresponding sensory impairment. The knee jerk is diminished or abolished. L3 motor root lesions may weaken the quadriceps, thigh adductor, and iliopsoas; L4 root lesions weaken the anterior tibial innervated muscles. L1 root pain is projected to the groin and L2 to the lateral hip. Motion of the spine and certain positions are most evocative of root pain; if the pain is constant in all positions, root irritation is seldom the cause.

Much has been made of a distinctive syndrome associated with extreme lateral disc protrusions, particularly those lying within the proximal portion of the intervertebral spinal foramina. Unremitting radicular pain without back pain and a tendency to worsen with extension of the back and torsion toward the side of the herniation are said to be characteristic. Similarly, in rare instances of lumbar intradural disc rupture, there may not be sciatic pain because the free fragment does not impinge on the roots of the cauda equina. Both of these configurations may confound radiologic diagnosis and make surgery more difficult.

Rarer still are protrusions of *thoracic intervertebral discs* (0.5 percent of all surgically verified disc protrusions, according to Love and Schorn). The four lowermost thoracic interspaces are the most frequently involved. Trauma, particularly hard falls on the heels or buttocks, is an important causative factor. Deep boring spine pain, root pain circling the body or projected to the abdomen or thorax (sometimes simulating visceral disease), paresthesias below the level of the lesion, loss of sensation, both deep and superficial, and paraparesis or paraplegia are the usual clinical manifestations.

Frequently, a herniated disc at one interspace compresses more than one root (Fig. 11-4), and it follows that the symptoms will then reflect this involvement. Anomalies of the lumbosacral roots may lead to errors in localization (see descriptions by Postaccini et al). The combined rupture of two or more discs occurs occasionally and further complicates the clinical picture. When both the L5 and S1 roots are compressed by a large herniated disc, the signs of the S1 lesion usually predominate.

Low-back pain may also be caused by degeneration of the intervertebral disc, without frank extrusion of disc tissue, or by degenerative arthritic changes of the spine, described further on, under lumbar spondylosis. Or the herniation may occur into the adjacent vertebral body, giving rise to a so-called Schmorl nodule. In such cases there are no signs of nerve root involvement, although back pain may be present, sometimes recurrent and referred to the thigh. And not to be forgotten as a cause of low-back pain is the implication of a root or nerve by an intrinsic tumor.

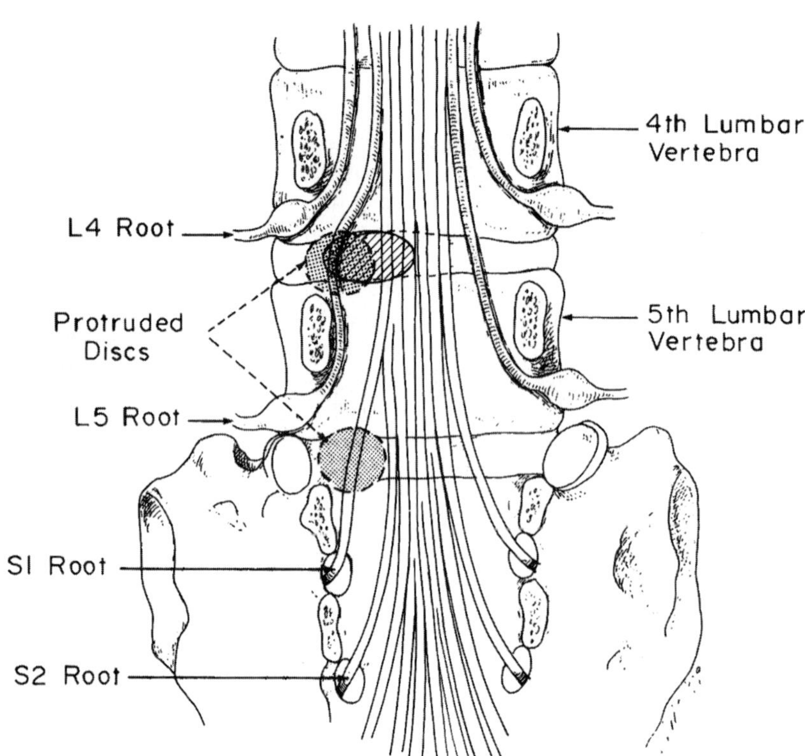

Figure 11-4

Mechanisms of compression of the fifth lumbar and first sacral roots. A lateral disc protrusion at the L4-5 level usually involves the fifth lumbar root and spares the fourth; a protrusion at L5-S1 involves the first sacral root and spares the fifth lumbar root. Note that a more medially placed disc protrusion at the L4-5 level (cross-hatched) may involve the fifth lumbar root as well as the first (or second and third) sacral root.

Diagnosis When all components of the syndrome are present, diagnosis is easy; but most neurologists prefer to corroborate their clinical impression by CT, with or without contrast myelography, or by MRI of the L3-S1 spine. Most neurologists favor MRI, in part because of the advantages of the sagittal image; however, the differences are slight except when the extruded fragment is molded into the adjacent bone (as it is prone to be with laterally extruded fragments) and becomes inevident on CT (see Forristall et al). As indicated earlier, we turn to CT-myelography for refined definition of the root sleeves and use the EMG to corroborate subtle findings. Usually MRI will demonstrate the extruded disc at the suspected site and will also exclude herniations at other sites or an unsuspected tumor (Fig. 11-5). At the lumbosacral junction there is a wide gap between the posterior margins of the vertebrae and the dural sac, so that a lateral or central protrusion of the L5-S1 disc may fail to distort the dural margin as seen on myelography. In this situation (and in others where the disc is not evident), nerve conduction studies and electromyography are useful. We find, as do Leyshon and coworkers, that the needle study in particular is abnormal showing fibrillation potentials in denervated muscles after one or two weeks in over 90 percent of cases. Loss or marked asymmetry of the H reflex is a particularly useful sign of S1 radiculopathy. The finding of denervation potentials in the paraspinal muscles (indicating root rather than peripheral nerve lesions) and in other muscles in a root distribution is also helpful, provided that at least 2 or 3 weeks have elapsed from the onset of root pain.

It is most important to keep in mind that a number of disc abnormalities, frequently observed on MRI and loosely referred to as "herniation," may be incidental findings, unrelated to the patient's symptoms. Jensen and colleagues, in an MRI study of the lumbar spine in 98 asymptomatic adults, found that in more than half of them there was a symmetrical extension of a disc (or discs) beyond the margins of the interspace (*bulging*). In 27 percent, there was a focal or asymmetrical extension of the disc beyond the interspace (*protrusion*), and in only 1 percent was there more extreme extension of the disc (*extrusion*). These findings emphasize the importance of using precise morphologic terms in describing the MRI abnormalities and always evaluating these abnormalities in the light of the patient's symptoms.

Management of Ruptured Lumbar Disc In the treatment of an *acute or chronic rupture of a lumbar disc*, complete bed rest is usually advised and appears to be

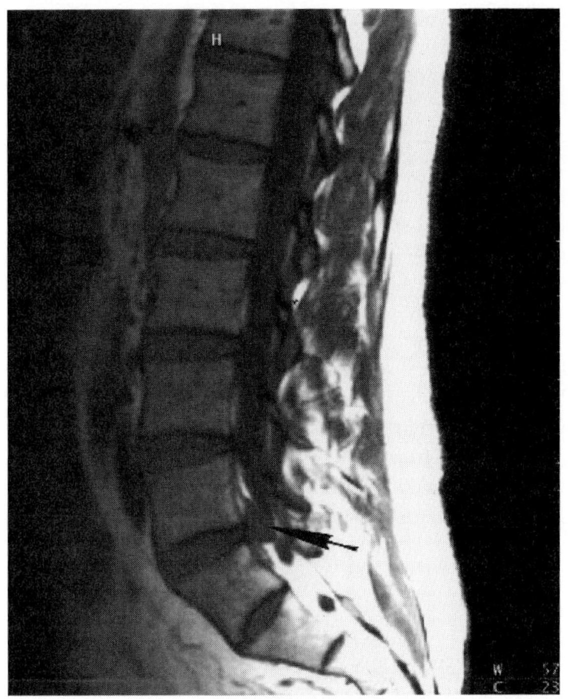

A

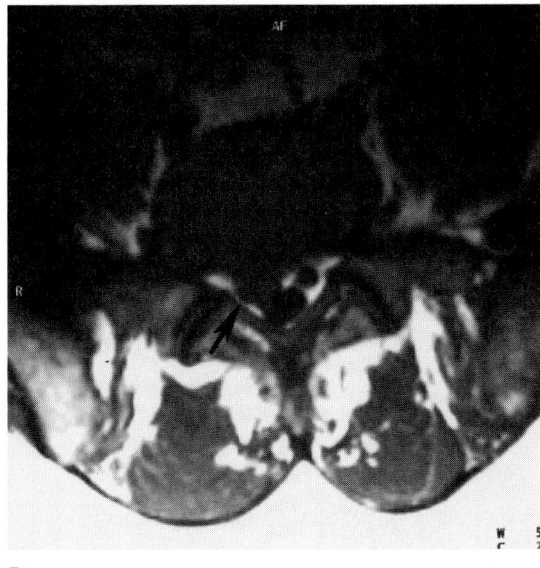

B

Figure 11-5

Lumbar disc herniation on T-1 weighted MRI. A. *Sagittal view of large L5-S1 herniated nucleus pulposis* (arrow). *The extruded material has the same signal characteristics as the normal adjacent disc.* B. *Axial view of same disc* (arrow) *showing the paracentral mass that obliterates the epidural fat signal and compresses the S1 root.*

helpful, although even this time-honored tenet has been questioned by the results of a randomized study (Vroomen et al). Nonetheless we adhere to this form of treatment and it results in marked improvement in over 80 percent of patients. Analgesic medication, either nonsteroidal anti-inflammatory agents or narcotics, may be required for a few days. In some patients with severe sciatica, we have been impressed with the relief afforded by administration of oral dexamethasone for several days, 4 mg every 8 h, although this has not been studied systematically. The only indication for emergency surgery is an acute compression of the cauda equina by massive disc extrusion, causing bilateral sensorimotor loss and sphincteric paralysis or severe unilateral motor loss. Although not the recommended course for most patients, it should be pointed out that there are instances where even a dramatic syndrome of cauda equina compression has cleared up after several weeks of bed rest. Traction is of little value in lumbar disc disease, and it is best to permit the patient to find the most comfortable position. After 1 or 2 weeks at rest, the patient can be allowed to resume activities gradually, sometimes with the protection of a brace or light spinal support. The patient may suffer minor recurrence of the pain but should be able to continue his usual activities and eventually will recover.

If the pain and neurologic findings do not subside in response to this type of conservative management or the patient suffers frequent disabling acute episodes, surgical treatment must be considered. This should be preceded by CT-myeolography or MRI to localize the lesion (and exclude intra- or extradural tumors). The surgical procedure most often indicated for lumbar disc disease is a hemilaminectomy, with excision of the disc involved. In cases with sciatic pain due to L4-5 or L5-S1 disc ruptures, 85 to 90 percent are relieved by operation. Rerupture occurs in approximately 5 percent (Shannon and Paul). Arthrodesis (spinal fusion) of the involved segments is indicated only in cases in which there is extraordinary instability, usually related to an anatomic abnormality (such as spondylolysis). The treatment of nerve root compression with repeated epidural injections of methylprednisolone enjoyed a period of popularity, but controlled studies of this procedure have failed to confirm its sustained efficacy (White et al; Cuckler et al) and the procedure is not without complications. Carette et al have found only short-term improvement with facet injection, but the ultimate need for surgery was not altered (see further on). Nevertheless, many neurologists have not discarded this form of treatment in view of notable success in selected patients.

Chemonucleolysis has been used for the management of lumbar disc lesions; however, as experience with this procedure increased, so did the number of failures and adverse effects, and the procedure has been abandoned. The same is true for the intradural injection of methylprednisolone.

Other Causes of Sciatica and Low-Back Pain

An increasing experience with lumbar back pain, gluteal neuralgia, and sciatica has impressed the authors with the large number of such cases that are unsolvable. At one time all these cases were classified as sciatic neuritis or "sacroiliac strain." After Mixter and Barr popularized the concept of prolapsed disc, all sciatica and lumbar pains were ascribed to this condition. Operations became widely practiced, not only for frank disc protrusion but also for "hard discs" (unruptured) and related pathologies of the spine. The surgical results became less and less satisfactory until recently, in large referral centers, as many patients were being seen with unrelieved postlaminectomy pain as with unoperated ruptured discs. To explain these chronic pain cases, a number of new pathologic entities, some of uncertain status, have been described. Entrapment of lumbar roots appears to be the consequence not only of disc rupture but also of spondylotic spurs with *stenosis of the lateral recess*, hypertrophy of apophyseal facets, compression of the nerve by the pyriformis muscle, and arachnoiditis. Lateral recess stenosis in particular may be a cause of sciatica not relieved by disc surgery. Another surprising finding in the course of imaging the spinal canal is a cystlike dilatation of the perineurial sheath (Tarlov cysts). One or more sacral roots may be involved at points where they penetrate the dura and be associated with radicular symptoms. There are reports of relief from opening the cysts and freeing the roots. Sciatica that is temporally linked to the premenstrual period is not uncommon and is almost always due to endometriosis that involves the nerve at the sciatic notch. We have also observed cases of sciatica that occurred with each pregnancy.

These are but a few of the large number of spinal abnormalities disclosed by newer radiologic techniques. An atlas of these abnormalities—congenital and developmental stenoses, Paget disease, apophyseal joint abnormalities including synovial cysts arising from the joint, unilateral spondylolisthesis, trochanteric and ischiogluteal bursitis—are admirably presented in the symposium on CT of the lumbar spine (see References, under "Symposium").

Compression of the cauda equina by epidural tumor, as described further on, most often begins with back pain or sciatica, most often as a result of deposits of prostatic or breast cancer or myeloma. The sciatic nerve or the plexus from which it originates may be implicated in tumor growths (lymphoma, neurofibrosarcoma). Several inflammatory diseases of the cauda equina produce back pain and bilateral sciatica and may be mistaken for the more usual types of cauda equina compression—cytomegalovirus infection in AIDS patients, Lyme disease, herpetic infection, and neoplastic meningitis at times behave in this fashion. In all of these, the CSF shows an intense pleocytosis. The Guillain-Barré syndrome may also produce misleading back and radicular pain before weakness is apparent. The caudal roots in these diseases enhance with gadolinium on MRI.

Finally one must not overlook the possible occurrence of a *lumbosacral plexus neuritis*, a unilateral (occasionally bilateral) disorder akin to brachial neuritis, and acute or subacute sciatic or femoral neuropathy due to diabetes, herpes zoster, or a retroperitoneal mass, any of which may produce a syndrome similar to that of ruptured disc (see Chap. 46).

Lumbar Stenosis and Spondylotic Caudal Radiculopathy In the lumbar region, osteoarthritic or spondylotic changes may lead to compression of one or more caudal roots. The problem is exaggerated if there is a congenitally narrow lumbar canal. The roots are caught between the posterior surface of the vertebral body and the ligamentum flavum posterolaterally. Lateral recess stenosis, alluded to above, may also contribute to root compression. Upon standing or walking (downhill walking is especially difficult), there is in many cases a gradual onset of numbness and weakness of the legs, which forces the patient to sit down. When this condition is more severe, the patient gains relief by squatting or lying down with the legs flexed at the hips and knees. Usually the numbness begins in one leg, spreads to the other, and ascends as standing or walking continues. Tendon reflexes may disappear, only to return on flexing the spine. Pain in the low back and gluteii is variable. Disturbances of micturition and impotence are rare. In some patients with lumbar stenosis, neurologic symptoms persist without relation to body position. The clinical picture, with its intermittency, corresponds to the so-called intermittent claudication of the cauda equina described by van Gelderen in 1948. Soon thereafter, it was shown by Verbiest to be due not to ischemia but to encroachment on the cauda by hypertrophied apophyseal joints, thickened ligaments, and small protrusions of disc material engrafted upon a canal that is developmentally shallow in the anteroposterior diameter. Sometimes a slight subluxation at L3-4 or at L4-5 is also present. Later it became evident that the canal in these cases is also narrow from side to side (reduced interpedicular distance radiographically). Decompression of the spinal canal relieves the symptoms in a considerable proportion of the cases.

Spondylotic caudal radiculopathy is the lumbar equivalent of spondylotic cervical myelopathy and radiculopathy. Insofar as the former is a cauda equina syndrome, its differential diagnosis is also discussed in Chap. 44, "Diseases of the Spinal Cord."

Osteoarthritis or Osteoarthropathy This, the most frequent type of arthritic disease, usually occurs in later life and may involve all or any part of the spine. However, it is most prevalent in the cervical and lumbar regions, where it is sometimes confused with discogenic syndromes. The pain is centered in the affected part of the spine, is increased by movement, and is associated with stiffness and limitation of motion. There is a notable absence of systemic symptoms such as fatigue, malaise, and fever, and the pain can usually be relieved by rest. A slightly flexed posture is preferred. The sitting position is usually comfortable, although stiffness and discomfort are accentuated when the erect posture is resumed. There are no neurologic signs except in association with disc disease. The severity of the symptoms often bears little relation to the radiologic findings; pain may be present despite minimal radiographic findings; conversely, marked osteophytic overgrowth with spur formation, ridging, bridging of vertebrae, narrowing of disc spaces, subluxation of posterior joints on flexion, and air in the disc spaces can be seen in both symptomatic and asymptomatic persons.

The Facet Syndrome This syndrome has been clarified in recent years, but its definition is still somewhat imprecise. It appears that two distinct painful states can be related to disease of the facet joint and adjacent lateral recess. In one type, facet hypertrophy gives rise to a lumbar monoradiculopathy, indistinguishable from that due to a ruptured disc. Reynolds et al have documented 22 such cases. Of these patients, 16 had an L5 radiculopathy, 3 an S1 radiculopathy, and 3 an L4 radiculopathy; in 15 of the patients there was coexisting back pain. At operation, the spinal root was compressed against the floor of the intervertebral canal by overgrowth of an inferior or superior facet. Foraminotomy and facetectomy, after exploration of the root from the dural sac to the pedicle, relieved the pain in 12 of the 15 operated cases.

In a second type, facet hypertrophy gives rise to lumbar back pain, often parasagittal, sometimes in the midline, with variable tenderness over the joint but without signs of root compression; it is relieved for a variable period by injection of the joint with lidocaine or its derivatives. Often one is uncertain whether it was the analgesic effect on the joint or the infiltration of the region around the nerve root that relieved the pain. Two controlled studies have provided evidence of the inefficacy of another popular treatment for this type of low-back pain, namely, corticosteroid injections into the facet joints (Carette et al; Lilius et al). Notwithstanding these studies, we have found the injection of analgesics and steroids in and around the facet to be a useful temporizing measure in some patients. In any case, this group of patients does not require operation.

Lumbar Adhesive Arachnoiditis This also is a somewhat vague entity, in which the arachnoid membrane is thickened and opaque in the vicinity of the cauda equina. The term is also applied to thickening of the arachnoidal sheaths around roots (roots have essentially no epineurium). It can be seen in lumbar myelograms in which the contrast material fails to outline the roots and flow freely in the subarachnoid space. According to a British review, lumbar arachnoiditis is rare, having been seen in only 80 of 7600 myelograms. Judging by American writings, it is much more frequent (see "Symposium," in the References). The usual clinical features are intractable low-back and leg pain and paresthesias, all positional, in combination with neurologic abnormalities referable to lumbar spinal roots. In our patients, multiple myelograms, disc rupture, operative procedures, infections, and subarachnoid bleeding have been causally involved. Some cases have followed spinal anesthesia and even epidural anesthesia by a period of months or years. The presumption is that the dura had been breached and often there were clinical signs of an aseptic meningitis soon after the procedure. The MRI may show eccentrically thickened meninges in the spinal canal with arachnoid adhesions and collections of CSF that displace nerve roots (Fig. 11-6). Treatment is unsatisfactory. Lysis of adhesions and administration of intrathecal steroids have been of no value. Epidural injection of steroids is occasionally helpful, according to some orthopedists.

Ankylosing Spondylitis This disorder, referred to in the past as *rheumatoid spondylitis* and as *von Bechterew* or *Marie-Strumpell arthritis*, affects young adult males predominantly. Its prevalence in the general population has been variously estimated at 1 to 3 per 1000. Approximately 95 percent of patients with ankylosing spondylitis are marked by the histocompatibility antigen HLA-B27 (which is present in only 7 percent of nonaffected persons). Pain, usually centered in the low back, is the main complaint, at least in the initial stages of the disease. Often it radiates to the back of the thighs and groin. At first the symptoms are vague (tired back, "catches" up and down the back, sore back), and the diagnosis may be overlooked for many years. Although the pain is recurrent, limitation of movement is constant and progressive; over time, it dominates the clinical picture. Early in the course, this is experienced as "morning stiffness" or an increase in stiffness after periods of inactivity; these findings may be present long before radiologic changes are manifest. Rarely, a cauda equina syndrome may complicate ankylosing spondylitis, the result apparently of an inflammatory reaction and later a proliferation of connective tissue in the caudal canal (Matthews). Limitation of chest expansion, tenderness over the sternum, decreased motion and tendency to progressive flexion of the hips, and the characteristic immobility and flexion deformity of the spine ("poker spine") may be present early in the course of the disease. The radiologic hallmarks are, at first, destruction and subsequently obliteration of the sacroiliac joints, followed by bony bridging of the vertebral bodies to produce the characteristic "bamboo spine." When this occurs, the pain usually subsides, but the patient has by then little motion of the back and neck. Ankylosing spondylitis may also be accompanied by the Reiter syndrome, psoriasis, and inflammatory diseases of the intestine (see also Chap. 44). The great risk in this disease is fracture dislocation of the spine from relatively minor trauma, particularly flexion-extension injuries.

Occasionally ankylosing spondylitis is complicated by destructive vertebral lesions. This complication should be suspected whenever the pain returns after a period of quiescence or becomes localized. The cause of these lesions is not known, but they may represent a response to nonunion of fractures, taking the form of an excessive production of fibrous inflammatory tissue. Ankylosing spondylitis, when severe, may involve both hips, greatly accentuating the back deformity and disability.

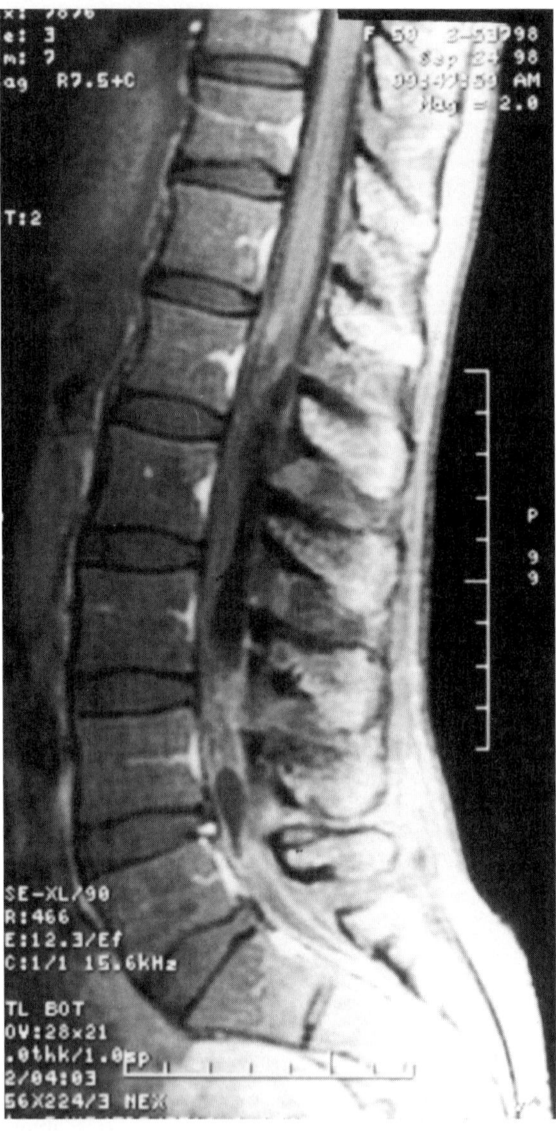

Figure 11-6

Severe lumbar arachnoiditis causing back pain, sciatica, and paresthesias years after spinal analgesia. Lumbar MRI performed with infusion of gadolinium showing thickened arachnoid and displacement of cauda equine roots by acquired arachnoid cysts.

Rheumatoid arthritis, when it affects the spine, may be confined to the cervical region and is considered further on in this chapter.

Neoplastic and Infectious Diseases of the Spine *Metastatic carcinoma* (breast, bronchus, prostate, thyroid, kidney, stomach, uterus), multiple myeloma, and lymphoma are the common malignant tumors that involve the spine. The primary lesion may be small and asymptomatic and the first manifestation of the tumor may be pain in the back due to metastatic deposits. The pain is described as constant and dull; it is often unrelieved by rest and may be worse at night. Radicular pain may be added, as described earlier in the chapter. At the time of onset of the back pain, there may be no radiographic changes; when such changes do appear, they usually take the form of destructive lesions in one or several vertebral bodies with little or no involvement of the disc space, even in the face of a compression fracture. Before such destructive changes become evident, a CT or radioactive isotope scan may be helpful in detecting areas of osteoblastic activity due to neoplastic or inflammatory disease and characteristic changes are also evident on MRI.

Infection of the vertebral column, *osteomyelitis*, is usually caused by staphylococci and less often by coliform and tubercule bacilli. The patient complains of pain in the back, of subacute or chronic nature, which is exacerbated by movement but not materially relieved by rest. Motion becomes limited, and there is percussion-induced tenderness over the spine in the involved segments and pain with jarring of the spine, as occurs when the heels strike the floor. Often these patients are afebrile and do not have a leukocytosis. The erythrocyte sedimentation rate is elevated as a rule. CT scanning and MRI will usually demonstrate the involved vertebra(e) and intervertebral disc—*the finding of a breached disc space is one of the features that differentiates infectious from neoplastic diseases of the spine*. A paravertebral mass is often found, indicating an abscess, which may, in the case of tuberculosis, drain spontaneously at sites quite remote from the vertebral column. We have also encountered a number of patients with subacute bacterial endocarditis who complained of severe midline thoracic and lumbar back pain but had no evident infection of the spine.

Special mention should be made of *spinal epidural abscess*, which necessitates urgent surgical treatment. Most often this is due to staphylococcal infection, which is carried in the bloodstream from a septic focus (e.g., furuncle) or is introduced into the epidural space from an osteomyelitic lesion. Another important avenue of infection is the intravenous self-administration of adulterated drugs and use of contaminated needles. Rarely the infection is introduced in the course of a lumbar puncture, epidural injection, or laminectomy for disc excision. In some instances the source of the epidural infection cannot be ascertained. The main symptoms are fever, leukocytosis, and persistent and severe localized pain, intensified by percussion and pressure over the vertebral spines; additionally the pain may acquire a radicular radiation. These symptoms mandate immediate investigation by MRI or CT-myelography and surgical intervention, preferably before the signs of paraplegia, sphincter dysfunction, and sensory loss become manifest. Exceptionally small abscesses can be treated successfully with antibiotics alone. A noninflammatory form of acute epidural compression may be due to hemorrhage (anticoagulant therapy, vascular malformation) and, in the cervical region, to rheumatoid arthritis (see further on).

Intraspinal Hemorrhage Sudden, excruciating midline back pain (*le coup de poignard* or "the strike of the dagger")—often with rapidly evolving paraparesis, urinary retention, and numbness of the legs—may announce the occurrence of subarachnoid, subdural, or epidural bleeding. The commonest cause of such an event is a spinal arteriovenous malformation (AVM), as discussed on page 1318. Spinal arterial aneurysms are much less common. It should be mentioned that back pain of comparable intensity may mark the onset of acute myelitis, spinal cord infarction, compression fracture, and occasionally Guillain-Barré syndrome.

Pain from Visceral Disease Peptic ulcer disease and carcinoma of the stomach most typically induce pain in the epigastrium. However, if the posterior stomach wall is involved, particularly if there is retroperitoneal extension, the pain may be felt in the thoracic spine, centrally or to one side, or in both locations. If intense, it may seem to encircle the body. The back pain tends to reflect the characteristics of the pain from the affected organ; e.g., if due to peptic ulceration, it appears about 2 h after a meal and is relieved by food and antacids.

Diseases of the pancreas are apt to cause pain in the back, being more to the right of the spine if the head of the pancreas is involved and to the left if the body and tail are implicated. Retroperitoneal neoplasms—e.g., lymphomas, hypernephromas, sarcomas, and carcinomas—may evoke pain in the thoracic or lumbar spine with a tendency to radiate to the lower part of the abdomen, groins, anterior thighs, or flank. A tumor in the iliopsoas region often produces a unilateral lumbar ache with radiation toward the groin and labia or testicle; there may also be signs of involvement of the upper lumbar spinal roots. An aneurysm of the abdominal aorta may induce pain that is localized to an analogous region of the spine. The sudden appearance of lumbar pain in a patient receiving anticoagulants should arouse suspicion of retroperitoneal bleeding. This pain may also be referred to the groin.

Inflammatory diseases and neoplasms of the colon cause pain that may be felt in the lower abdomen, the midlumbar region, or both. As with intense pain higher in the spine, it may have a belt-like distribution. Pain from a lesion in the transverse colon or first part of the descending colon may be central or left-sided; its level of reference is to the second and third lumbar vertebrae. If the sigmoid colon is implicated, the pain is lower, in the upper sacral spine and anteriorly in the suprapubic region or left lower quadrant of the abdomen. Retroperitoneal appendicitis may have an odd referral of pain to the low flank and back.

Gynecologic disorders often manifest themselves by back pain, but their diagnosis is seldom difficult. Thorough abdominal palpation as well as vaginal and rectal examination, supplemented by ultrasound and CT scanning or MRI, usually discloses the source of pain. The uterosacral ligaments are the most important pelvic source of chronic back pain. Endometriosis or carcinoma of the uterus (body or cervix) may invade these structures, causing pain that is localized to the sacrum either centrally or more to one side. In endometriosis, the pain begins premenstrually and often merges with menstrual pain, which also may be felt in the sacral region. Rarely, cyclic engorgement of ectopic endometrial tissue may give rise to sciatica and other radicular pain. Malposition of the uterus (retroversion, uterus descensus, and prolapse) characteristically gives rise to sacral pain, especially after the patient has been standing for several hours. Changes in posture may also evoke pain here when a fibroma of the uterus pulls on the uterosacral ligaments. Low-back pain with radiation into one or both thighs is a common phenomenon during the last weeks of pregnancy.

Pain due to carcinomatous infiltration of pelvic nerve plexuses is continuous and becomes progressively more severe; it tends to be more intense at night and may have a burning quality. The primary lesion can be inconspicuous and may be overlooked on pelvic examination.

Coccydynia This is the name applied to pain that is localized to the "tail piece," the three or four small vestigial bones at the lowermost part of the sacrum. The trauma of childbirth, a fall on the buttocks, avascular necrosis, a glomus tumor, or one of a variety of other rare tumors and anal disorders can sometimes be established as the cause of pain in this region. Far more often, the source remains obscure. In the past, patients in this latter group were indiscriminately subjected to coccygectomy, but more recent studies have demonstrated that most cases respond favorably to injections of local anesthetic and methylprednisolone or to manipulation of the coccyx under anesthesia (Wray et al).

Obscure Types of Low-Back Pain and the Question of Psychiatric Disease It is a safe clinical rule that all patients who complain of low-back pain have some type of primary or secondary disease of the spine and its supporting structures or of the abdominal or pelvic viscera. However, even after careful examination, there remains a sizable group of patients in whom no pathologic basis can be found for the back pain. Two categories can be recognized: one with postural back pain and another with aggravating psychiatric illness, but there are always cases where the diagnosis remains obscure.

Postural Back Pain Many slender, asthenic individuals and some fat, middle-aged ones have chronic discomfort in the back, and the pain interferes with effective work. The physical examination is unrevealing except for slack musculature and poor posture. The pain is diffuse in the middle or lower region of the back; characteristically, it is relieved by bed rest and induced by the maintenance of a particular posture over a period of time. Spinal manipulation is said to have helped a number of these patients. Pain in the neck and between the shoulder blades is a common complaint among thin, tense, active women and seems to be related to taut trapezius muscles.

Adolescent girls and boys are subject to an obscure form of epiphyseal disease of the spinal vertebrae (Scheuermann disease), which, over a period of 2 to 3 years, may cause low-back pain upon exercise.

Psychiatric Illness Low-back pain may be a major symptom in patients with hysteria, malingering, anxiety neurosis, depression, and hypochondriasis as well as in many nervous persons whose symptoms do not conform to any of these psychiatric illnesses. Again, it is good practice to assume that pain in the back in such patients may signify disease of the spine or adjacent structures, and this should always be carefully sought. However, even when some organic factors are found, the pain may be exaggerated, prolonged, or woven into a pattern of invalidism because of coexistent primary or secondary psychologic factors. This is especially true when there is the possibility of secondary gain (notably workers' compensation or settlement of personal injury claims). Patients seeking compensation for protracted low-back pain without obvious structural disease tend, after a time, to become suspicious, uncooperative, and hostile toward their physicians or anyone who might question the authenticity of their illness. One notes in them a tendency to describe their pain vaguely and a preference to discuss the degree of their disability and their mistreatment at the hands of the medical profession. The description of the pain may vary considerably from one examination to another. Often also, the region(s) in which pain is experienced and its radiation are nonphysiologic, and the condition fails to respond to rest and inactivity. These features and a negative examination of the back should lead one to suspect a psychologic factor. A few patients, usually frank malingerers, adopt the most bizarre gaits and attitudes, such as walking with the trunk flexed at almost a right angle (camptocormia), and are unable to straighten up. Or the patient may be unable to bend forward even a few degrees, despite the absence of muscle spasm, and may wince at the slightest pressure, even over the sacrum, which is seldom a site of tenderness unless there is pelvic disease.

The depressed and anxious patient with back pain represents a troublesome problem. A common error is to minimize the importance of anxiety and depression or to ascribe them to worry over the illness and its social effects. In these circumstances, common and minor back ailments, e.g., those due to osteoarthritis and postural ache, etc., are enhanced and rendered intolerable. Such patients are often subjected to unnecessary surgical procedures. The disability seems excessive for the degree of spinal malfunction, and misery, irritability, and despair are the prevailing features of the syndrome. One of the most reliable diagnostic features is the response to drugs or other measures that alleviate the depression (see Chap. 57).

Failed Back Syndrome

Surely the most difficult patients to manage are those with chronic low-back pain who have already had one or more laminectomies and sometimes a fusion without substantial relief. In one large series of patients operated on for proven disc prolapse, 25 percent were left with troublesome symptoms and 10 percent required further surgery (Weir and Jacobs). In such patients our practice has been to repeat the MRI and CT-myelography. In a small number of the patients, it will be found that the disc has reruptured, or that there is a lateral recess stenosis, or that a disc has ruptured at another level. It may happen that the surgeon did not remove all the disc tissue, in which case another operation to remove the remainder will be successful. Electromyography and nerve conduction studies, searching for evidence of a radiculopathy, are helpful. If there is evidence of a radiculopathy but no disc material, or only scar tissue is seen, one does not know whether the pain is due to injury from the initial rupture or was the aftermath of surgery. Various explanations are then invoked—radiculitis, lateral recess syndrome, facet syndrome, unstable spine, and lumbar arachnoiditis described earlier in the chapter (see reviews by Quiles et al and by Long as well as the "Symposium" listed in the References).

One would suppose that these chronic pain cases could be subdivided into a group with continued radicular pain and another with referred pain from disease of the spine. However, once the pain becomes chronic, the separation is not easy. Pressure over the spine, buttock, or thigh may cause pain to be projected into the leg. Lidocaine blocks of nerve roots have yielded inconsistent results. Occupational injuries, in which workers' compensation or litigation is a factor, make the patient's report of therapeutic effects almost worthless. Transcutaneous stimulators, posterior column stimulators, intrathecal injections of analgesics, and epidural steroid injections have seldom helped for long in our experience. At present the best that can be offered the patient is weight reduction (if he is obese), stretching and progressive exercise to strengthen abdominal and back muscles, as well as nonsteroidal anti-inflammatory and antidepressant drugs. A trial of massage therapy or a limited course of spinal manipulation is reasonable.

Preventive Aspects of Lower Back Pain

Without doubt these are important. There would be many fewer back problems if adults kept their trunk muscles in optimal condition by *regular slow stretching* and exercise such as swimming, walking briskly, running, and calisthenic programs of the Canadian Air Force type. Morning is the ideal time for exercising, since the back of the older adult tends to be stiffest following a night of inactivity. This happens regardless of whether a bed board or stiff mattress is used. Sleeping with the back hyperextended and sitting for long periods in an overstuffed chair or a badly designed car seat are particularly likely to aggravate backache. It is estimated that intradiscal pressures are increased 200 percent by changing from a recumbent to a standing position and 400 percent when slumped in an easy chair. Correct sitting posture lessens this pressure. Long trips in a car or plane without change in position put maximal strain on discal and ligamentous structures in the spine. Lifting from a position in which the back is flexed, as in removing a heavy suitcase from the trunk of a car, is risky (always lift with the object close to the body). Also, sudden strenuous activity without conditioning and warmup is likely to injure discs and their ligamentous envelopes. Certain families seem disposed to injury of these structures.

PAIN IN THE NECK, SHOULDER, AND ARM

General Considerations

In this connection, it is useful to distinguish *three major categories of painful disease*—that originating in the *spine*, in the *brachial plexus*, and in the *shoulder*. Although the distribution of pain from each of these sources may overlap, the patient can usually indicate its site of origin.

Pain arising from the *cervical part of the spine* is felt in the neck and back of the head and may be projected to the shoulder and upper arm; it is evoked or enhanced by certain movements or positions of the neck and is accompanied by limitation of motion of the neck and by tenderness to palpation over the cervical spine.

Pain of brachial plexus origin is experienced in the supraclavicular region, or in the axilla and around the shoulder; it is induced by certain maneuvers and positions of the arm, and is sometimes associated with tenderness of structures above the clavicle. There may be a palpable abnormality above the clavicle (aneurysm of the subclavian artery, tumor, cervical rib). The combination of circulatory abnormalities and signs referable to the medial cord of the brachial plexus is characteristic of the *thoracic outlet syndrome*, which is described further on.

Pain localized to the shoulder region, worsened by motion, and associated with tenderness and limitation of movement, especially internal and external rotation and abduction, points to a tendonitis, subacromial bursitis, or tear of the rotator cuff, which is made up of the tendons of the muscles surrounding the shoulder joint. The term *bursitis* is often used loosely to designate these disorders. Shoulder pain, like spine and plexus pain, may radiate into the arm and rarely into the hand, but sensorimotor and reflex changes—which always indicate disease of nerve roots, plexus, or nerves—are absent. Shoulder pain of this type is very common in middle and late adult life. It may arise spontaneously or after unusual or vigorous use of the arm. Local tenderness over the greater tuberosity of the humerus is characteristic. Plain x-rays of the shoulder may be normal or show a calcium deposit in the supraspinatus tendon or subacromial bursa; MRI is able to demonstrate more subtle abnormalities such as muscle and tendon tears of the rotator cuff. In most patients the pain subsides gradually with immobilization and analgesics, followed by a program of increasing shoulder mobilization. If it does not, the injection of small amounts of corticosteroids into the bursa, or the site of major pain indicated by passive shoulder movement in the case of rotator cuff injuries, is often temporarily effective and allows the patient to mobilize the shoulder.

Osteoarthritis and osteophytic spur formation of the cervical spine may cause pain that radiates into the back of the head, shoulders, and arm on one or both sides. Coincident compression of nerve roots is manifest by paresthesias, sensory loss, weakness and atrophy, and tendon reflex changes in the arms and hands. Should bony ridges form in the spinal canal, as described in detail in Chap. 44, the spinal cord may be compressed, with resulting spastic weakness, ataxia, and loss of vibratory and position sense in the legs (*cervical spondylosis*). The bony changes are evident on plain films but are better seen by CT. There may be difficulty in distinguishing cervical spondylosis with root and spinal cord compression from a primary neurologic disease (syringomyelia, amyotrophic lateral sclerosis, or tumor) with an unrelated cervical osteoarthritis, particularly at the C5-6 and C6-7 levels. Here the CT-myelogram and MRI are of particular diagnostic importance in revealing compression of the spinal cord, generally with narrowing of the spinal canal to less than 10 to 11 mm in the anteroposterior diameter (see also pages 1322–1326).

A combination of osteoarthritis of the cervical spine with injury to ligaments and muscles when the neck has been forcibly extended and flexed (e.g., the acceleration or "whiplash injury" in rear-end automobile collisions) can create a number of difficult clinical problems. The injury ranges from a minor sprain of muscles and ligaments to severe tearing of these structures, to avulsion of muscle and tendon from vertebral body, and even to vertebral and intervertebral disc damage. The latter lesions can be seen with MRI and, if severe, can result in root or spinal cord compression or, occasionally, in cartilagenous embolization of the spinal cord (see page

1321). Milder degrees of whiplash injury are often complicated by psychologic and compensation factors (see LaRocca for a review of this subject).

Spinal rheumatoid arthritis may be restricted to the cervical apophyseal (facet) joints and the atlantoaxial articulation. The usual manifestations are pain, stiffness, and limitation of motion in the neck and pain in the back of the head. In contrast to ankylosing spondylitis, rheumatoid arthritis is rarely confined to the spine. Because of major affection of other joints, the diagnosis is relatively easy to make, but significant involvement of the cervical spine may be overlooked in patients with diffuse disease. In the advanced stages of the disease, one or several of the vertebrae may become displaced anteriorly, or a synovitis of the atlantoaxial joint may damage the transverse ligament of the atlas, resulting in forward displacement of the atlas on the axis, i.e., atlantoaxial subluxation. Pain in the neck may project into and cause numbness or burning of one half the tongue (the "neck-tongue syndrome"; see page 201). In either instance, serious and even life-threatening compression of the spinal cord may occur gradually or suddenly. Cautiously performed lateral radiographs in flexion and extension are useful in visualizing atlantoaxial dislocation or subluxation of the lower segments. Occipital headache and neck pain related to degenerative changes in the upper cervical facets is discussed with other cranial pains on page 199 (so-called third occipital nerve pain).

Cervical Disc Protrusion

A common cause of neck, shoulder, and arm pain is disc herniation in the lower cervical region (Fig. 11-7*A* and *B*). It may develop after trauma, which may be major or minor (from sudden hyperextension of the neck, falls, diving accidents, forceful chiropractic manipulations, etc.). The roots most commonly involved in cervical disc protrusion are the seventh (in 70 percent of cases) and the sixth (20 percent); fifth- and eighth-root involvement make up the remaining 10 percent (Yoss et al).

When the protruded disc lies between the sixth and seventh vertebrae, there is involvement of the *seventh cervical root*. The pain is in the region of the shoulder blade, pectoral region and medial axilla, posterolateral upper arm, elbow and dorsal forearm, index and middle fingers, or all the fingers. Tenderness is most pronounced

Figure 11-7

Cervical disc herniation. A. *Schematic of the mechanism of root and cord compression from central and paracentral herniation.* B. *T-1 weighted MRI of a disc extrusion at C5-6 (arrow) that caused a myelopathy and radicular pain.*

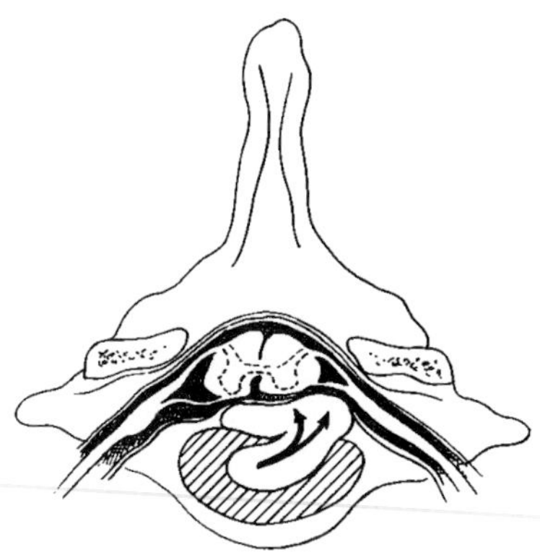

A

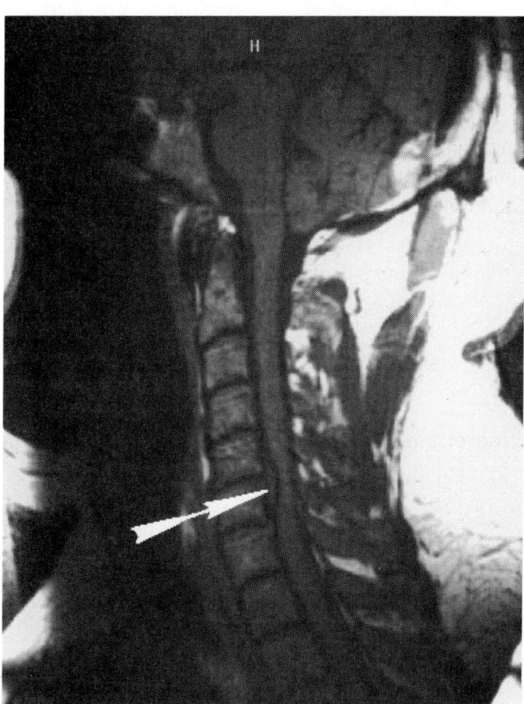

B

over the medial aspect of the shoulder blade opposite the third to fourth thoracic spinous processes and in the supraclavicular area and triceps region. Paresthesias and sensory loss are most evident in the second and third fingers or may be experienced in the tips of all the fingers. Weakness involves the extensors of the forearm and sometimes of the wrist; occasionally the hand grip is weak as well; the triceps reflex is diminished or absent; and the biceps and supinator reflexes are preserved.

With a laterally situated disc protrusion between the fifth and sixth cervical vertebrae, the symptoms and signs are referred to the *sixth cervical root*. The full syndrome is characterized by pain at the trapezius ridge and tip of the shoulder, with radiation into the anterior-upper part of the arm, radial forearm, often the thumb, and sometimes the lateral aspect of the index finger as well; paresthesias and sensory impairment in the same regions; tenderness in the area above the spine of the scapula and in the supraclavicular and biceps regions; weakness in flexion of the forearm; and diminished to absent biceps and supinator reflexes (triceps reflex retained or exaggerated).

The *fifth cervical root* syndrome, produced by disc herniation between the fourth and fifth vertebral bodies, is characterized by pain in the shoulder and trapezius region and by supra- and infraspinatus weakness, manifest by an inability to abduct the arm and rotate it externally with the shoulder adducted.

Compression of the *eighth cervical root* at C7-T1 may mimic an ulnar palsy. The pain is along the medial side of the forearm and the sensory loss is in the distribution of the medial cutaneous nerve of the forearm and of the ulnar nerve in the hand. The weakness involves the muscles supplied by the ulnar nerve (page 1434).

These syndromes are usually incomplete in that only one or several of the typical findings are present. Particularly noteworthy is the occurrence, in laterally placed cervical disc rupture, of isolated weakness without pain, especially with discs at the fifth and sixth levels. Friis and coworkers have described the distribution of pain in 250 cases of herniated disc or spondylotic nerve root compression in the cervical region. Virtually every patient, irrespective of the particular root(s) involved, showed a *limitation in the range of motion of the neck and aggravation of pain with movement (particularly hyperextension)*. Coughing, sneezing, and downward pressure on the head in the hyperextended position usually exacerbated the pain, and traction (even manual) tended to relieve it. Nerve conduction studies, F responses, and EMG are extremely helpful in confirming the level of root compression and distinguishing pain of radicular origin from that originating in the brachial plexus (see page 1357).

In many of the cervical radicular syndromes, the onset is acute and no traumatic incident can be documented. It is difficult to relate the syndrome to osseous changes that must have been present for years. Even more difficult to explain is the tendency to recovery within a few weeks when movement of the neck is limited by traction or a collar. Conservative measures should always be tried before turning to laminectomy and foraminotomy unless there are additional signs of a myelopathy, such as weakness, gait ataxia, or sphincteric dysfunction.

Unlike herniated lumbar discs, cervical ones, if large and centrally situated, may result in compression of the spinal cord (central disc, all of the cord; paracentral disc, asymmetrical but bilateral parts of the cord; Fig. 11-7*B*). The centrally situated disc may be painless, and the cord syndrome may simulate a degenerative disease (amyotrophic lateral sclerosis, combined system disease). Failure to think of a protruded cervical disc in patients with obscure symptoms in the legs, including stiffness and falling, is a common error. A vague sensory change can often be detected several dermatomes below the level of compression. The diagnosis and the level of disc protrusion should be confirmed by CT myelography or by MRI (Fig. 11-7B).

Management of Herniated Cervical Disc In some cases of herniated cervical disc, a sustained period of inactivity and immobilization of the head and neck by use of a close-fitting soft cervical collar may be all that is necessary for treatment. In the case of a ruptured cervical disc, in distinction to lumbar disc, traction with a halter may be of considerable benefit. Traction can be administered with the patient recumbent, or it can be performed intermittently in the sitting position, using special equipment, the simplest of which applies 2 to 10 lb of upward traction while the patient is seated with his back to a door and the weight attached to a rope over the top of the door. This should be performed two or three times daily. After 1 or 2 weeks of rest and traction, the patient can be allowed to resume activities gradually, usually with the protection of a soft collar. The patient may suffer minor recurrence but should be able to continue his usual activities and eventually will recover.

If the pain and neurologic findings do not subside in response to this type of conservative management or the patient suffers frequent disabling acute episodes, surgical treatment must be considered. This should always be preceded by a CT-myelogram or MRI to localize the lesion (and to exclude intra- or extradural tumors). The surgical procedure most often indicated is a hemilaminectomy, with excision of the disc involved. Arthrodesis (spinal fusion) of the involved segments is indicated only in cases in which there is extraordinary instability, usually related to an extensive laminectomy that has rendered the spine unstable. Large, centrally placed cervical disc protrusions may require an anterior approach, which is accomplished by displacing the trachea and esophagus and drilling through the disc from its ventral aspect.

Cervical Spondylosis

This is basically a chronic degenerative disease of the lower cervical spine that narrows the spinal canal and intervertebral foramina, causing compressive injury of the spinal cord. Since the main effects of cervical spondylosis are on the cord, it is discussed in detail in Chap. 44. Cervical spondylosis is also a common cause of neck and arm pain as described earlier, symptoms that are helped by bed rest and traction; if signs of spinal cord and root involvement are present, a collar to limit movement of the head and neck may halt the progression and even lead to improvement. Decompressive laminectomy or anterior excision of single spondylotic spurs and fusion is reserved for instances of the disease with advancing neurologic symptoms or intractable pain (see Chap. 44).

Thoracic Outlet Syndromes

A number of anatomic anomalies occur in the lateral cervical region; these may, under certain circumstances, compress the brachial plexus, the subclavian artery, and the subclavian vein, causing muscle weakness and wasting, pain, and vascular abnormalities in the hand and arm. The most frequent of these abnormalities are an incomplete cervical rib, with a sharp fascial band passing from its tip to the first rib; a taut fibrous band passing from an elongated, down-curving transverse process of C7 to the first rib; less often, a complete cervical rib, which articulates with the first rib; and anomalies of the position and insertion of the anterior and medial scalene muscles. Thus, the sites of potential neurovascular compression extend all the way from the intervertebral foramina and superior mediastinum to the axilla. Depending on the postulated abnormality and mechanism of symptom production, the terms *cervical rib*, *anterior scalene*, *costoclavicular*, and *neurovascular compression* have been applied to this syndrome. The international anatomic term is *superior thoracic aperture syndrome*.

Variations in regional anatomy could theoretically explain these several postulated mechanisms, but to this day there is not full agreement about the anterior scalene and costoclavicular syndromes. An anomalous cervical rib, which arises from the seventh cervical vertebra and extends laterally between the anterior and medial scalene muscles and then under the brachial plexus and subclavian artery to attach to the first rib, obviously disturbs the anatomic relationships of these structures and may compress them (Fig. 11-8). However, since an estimated 1.0 percent of the population has cervical ribs, usually on both sides, and only about 10 percent of these persons have neurologic or vascular symptoms (almost always one-sided), other factors must be operative in most instances. A majority of the patients are women in early or mid-adult life (female-to-male ratio 5:1) in whom sagging of the shoulders, large breasts, and poor muscular tone may be of importance. Clavicular abnormalities, both congenital and traumatic, and certain occupational activities may also play a part.

The anterior and middle scalene muscles, which flex and rotate the neck, are both inserted into the first rib; the subclavian artery and vein and the brachial plexus must pass between them. Hence abnormalities of insertion and hypertrophy of these muscles were once thought to be causes of the syndrome. However, section of these muscles (scalenectomy) so rarely altered the symptoms that this mechanism is no longer given credence.

Three neurovascular syndromes have been associated with a rudimentary cervical rib (rarely with a complete cervical rib) and related abnormalities at the thoracic outlet. These syndromes sometimes coexist, but more often each occurs independently.

1. *Compression of the subclavian vein*, causing a dusky discoloration, venous distention, and edema of the arm. The vein may become thrombosed after prolonged exercise, the so-called effort-thrombotic syndrome of Paget and Schroetter.

2. *Compression of the subclavian artery*, which results in ischemia of the limb, may be complicated by digital gangrene and retrograde embolization. A unilateral Raynaud phenomenon, brittle nails, and ulceration of the fingertips are important diagnostic findings. A supraclavicular bruit is suggestive but not in itself diagnostic of subclavian artery compression. The conven-

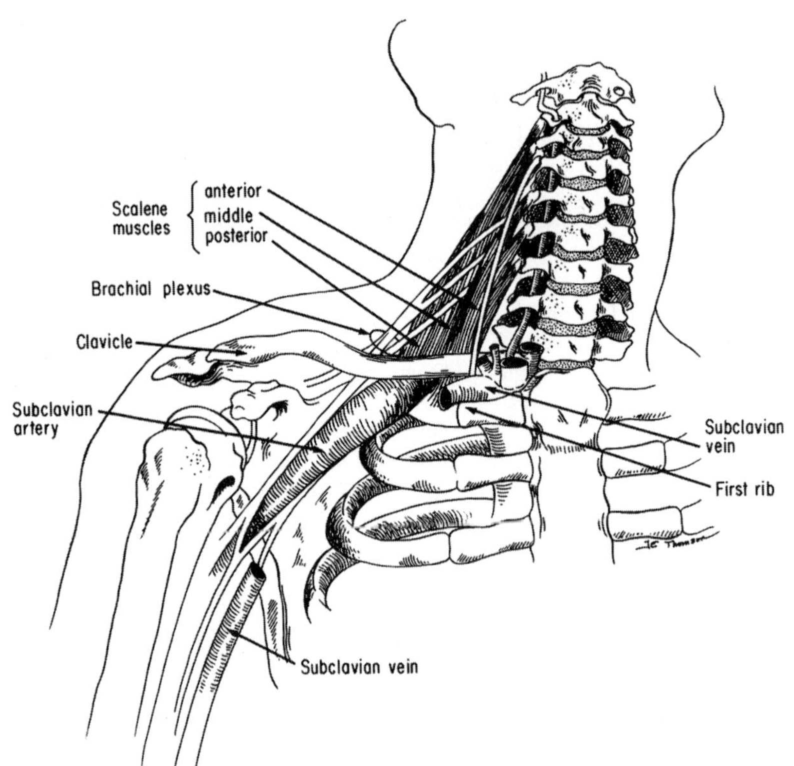

Figure 11-8

Course of the brachial plexus and subclavian artery between the anterior scalene and middle scalene muscles. Dilatation of the subclavian artery just distal to the anterior scalene muscle is illustrated. Immediately distal to the anterior and middle scalene muscles is another potential area of constriction, between the clavicle and the first rib. With extension of the neck and turning of the chin to the affected side (Adson maneuver), the tension on the anterior scalene muscle is increased and the subclavian artery compressed, resulting in a supraclavicular bruit and obliteration of the radial pulse.

tional tests for vascular compression—diminution or obliteration of the pulse when the patient, seated and with the arm dependent, takes and holds a full breath, tilts the head back, and turns it to the affected side (Adson test) or abducts and externally rotates the arm and braces the shoulders (Wright maneuver)—are not entirely reliable. Sometimes these maneuvers fail to obliterate the radial pulse in cases of proved compression; contrariwise, these tests may be positive in normal persons. Nevertheless, a positive test on the symptomatic side (with reproduction of the patient's symptoms) but not on the other side should always suggest a local lesion. The addition of plethysmographic recording of the radial pulse and ultrasound of the vessel adds greatly to the accuracy of these positional tests.

3. *A primarily neurologic syndrome*, characterized by slight wasting and weakness of the hypothenar, interosseous, adductor pollicis, and deep flexor muscles of the fourth and fifth fingers (i.e., the muscles innervated by the lower trunk of the brachial plexus and ulnar nerve). Weakness of the flexor muscles of the forearm may be present in advanced cases. Tendon reflexes are usually preserved. In addition, most patients with this form of the syndrome complain of an intermittent aching of the arm, particularly of the ulnar side, and about half of them complain also of numbness and tingling along the ulnar border of the forearm and hand. A loss of superficial sensation in these areas is a variable finding. It may be possible to reproduce the sensory symptoms by firm pressure just above the clavicle or by simple traction on the arm. Vascular features are often absent or minimal in patients with the neurologic form of the syndrome.

In all three forms of the syndrome, shoulder and arm pain is a prominent complaint. The discomfort is of the aching type and is felt in the posterior hemithorax, pectoral region, and upper arm.

Diagnostic measures should include the Adson test or preferably the Wright maneuver, described earlier, with digital plethysmography to quantitate the degree of positional vascular compromise; also films of the cervical spine should be obtained, looking for a cervical rib or an elongated C7 transverse process (the fibrous bands are not visualized). Typically, nerve conduction studies disclose a reduced amplitude of the ulnar sensory potentials. There may be a decreased amplitude of the median motor evoked potentials, a mild but *uniform* slowing of the median motor conduction velocity, and a prolongation of the F-wave latency. Concentric needle examination of affected hand muscles reveals large-amplitude motor units, suggesting collateral reinnervation. The application of somatosensory evoked potentials may prove to be a useful adjunct to the conventional nerve conduction and EMG studies (Yiannikas and Walsh). Brachial artery angiography is usually reserved for patients with a suspected arterial occlusion, an aneurysm, or an obvious cervical rib. The place of venography in the diagnostic workup is uncertain, for a number of otherwise normal individuals can occlude the subclavian vein by fully abducting the arm.

In the authors' experience, unambiguous instances of thoracic outlet syndrome are not common. This has also been the experience of Wilbourn, whose review of this subject is recommended. Neck and arm pain in slender, neurotic women presents particularly difficult problems in diagnosis; often the physician assumes the presence of a thoracic outlet syndrome, only to discover that operation affords little or no lasting relief. One should be skeptical of the diagnosis unless the rigid clinical and EMG criteria enumerated above have been met. Common mistakes are to confuse the thoracic outlet syndrome with carpal tunnel syndrome, ulnar neuropathy or entrapment at the elbow, or cervical radiculopathy due to arthritis or disc disease. Imaging studies and careful nerve conduction and EMG studies may be necessary to exclude latter disorders.

Treatment of the Thoracic Outlet Syndrome In the management of this syndrome, a conservative approach is advisable. If the main symptoms are pain and paresthesias, Leffert advises the use of local heat, analgesics, muscle relaxants, and an assiduous program of special exercises to strengthen the shoulder muscles. Twice a day, holding a 1- or 2-lb weight in each hand, the patient intermittently shrugs and relaxes the shoulders forward and upward, then backward and upward, and then upward, each performed 10 times. In a second exercise, with the weights held at the side, the extended arms are lifted over the head until the backs of the hands meet; again this done 10 times. In a third exercise, the patient faces a corner of a room and places one hand on each wall; with elbows bent, he leans into the wall and at the same time inhales, then exhales as he pushes away. A full range of neck motions is then practiced. On such a regimen some patients experience a relief of symptoms after 2 to 3 weeks.

If pain is severe and persistent and is clearly associated with the vascular and/or neurogenic features of the syndrome, surgery is indicated. The usual approach is through the supraclavicular space, with cutting of fibrous bands and excision of the rudimentary rib. In cases of venous or minor arterial forms of the syndrome, some thoracic surgeons favor the excision of a segment of the first rib through the axilla. Pain is often dramatically relieved but the sensorimotor defects improve only slightly. Atherosclerosis with thrombosis and embolism of the subclavian artery and thrombosis of the vein require decompression and arterioplasty and venous thrombectomy, respectively. Brachial sympathectomy may be necessary in exceptional patients with a persistent Raynaud phenomenon.

As mentioned earlier, vasomotor, sudomotor, and trophic changes in the skin, with atrophy of the soft tissues and decalcification of bone, may follow the prolonged immobilization and disuse of an arm or leg for whatever reason. The patient may be reluctant to move the limb because of pain or a lack of motivation to get well or for reasons of monetary gain. Surgery in this group of patients is ill advised, and the physician's efforts should be directed to mobilization of the affected part through an intensive physical therapy program and settlement of litigation if this is a factor.

Other Painful Conditions Originating in the Neck, Brachial Plexus, and Shoulder

The brachial plexus is an important source of shoulder and arm pain. The main disorders are brachial neuritis and metastatic infiltration and radiation damage to the plexus. These disorders are discussed in detail in Chap. 46.

Metastases to the cervical region of the spine are less common than to other parts of the vertebral column. They are frequently painful and may cause root compression. Posterior extension of the tumor from the vertebral bodies or compression fractures may lead to the rapid development of quadriplegia.

The Pancoast tumor, usually a squamous cell carcinoma in the superior sulcus of the lung, may implicate the lower cervical and upper thoracic (T1 and T2) spinal nerves as they exit from the spine. In these cases, a Horner syndrome, numbness of the inner side of the arm and hand, and weakness of all muscles of the hand and of the triceps muscle are combined with pain beneath the upper scapula and in the arm. The neurologic abnormalities may occur long before the tumor becomes visible radiographically.

Shoulder injuries (rotator cuff), subacromial or subdeltoid bursitis, periarthritis or capsulitis ("frozen shoulder"), tendonitis, and arthritis may develop in patients who are otherwise well, but these conditions also occur occasionally as complications of hemiplegia. The pain tends to be severe and extends toward the neck and down the arm into the hand. The dorsum of the hand may tingle without other signs of nerve involvement. Immobility of an arm following myocardial infarction may be associated with pain in the shoulder and arm and with vasomotor changes and secondary arthropathy of the hand joints (shoulder-hand syndrome); after a time, osteoporosis and atrophy of cutaneous and subcutaneous structures occur (Sudeck atrophy or Sudeck-Leriche syndrome). Similar changes may occur in the foot and leg or all articular structures on the side of a hemiplegia or in association with the painful lesions described in the first part of this chapter. These conditions fall within the province of the orthopedist and are not discussed in detail. The neurologist, however, should know that they can be prevented by proper exercises and relieved by cooling of the affected limb, exercises, and physiotherapy (see further on).

Medial and lateral epicondylitis (tennis elbow) are readily diagnosed by demonstrating tenderness over the affected parts and an aggravation of pain on certain movements of the wrist. We have observed entrapment of the ulnar nerve in some cases of medial epicondylitis.

The pain of the carpal tunnel syndrome (page 1433) often extends into the forearm and sometimes higher and may be mistaken for disease of the shoulder or neck. Similarly, involvement of the ulnar, radial, or median nerves may be mistaken for brachial plexus or root lesions. Electromyography and nerve conduction studies are helpful in these circumstances.

PAIN CONFINED TO THE EXTREMITIES

Arthritis of the Extremities The principal symptom of *osteoarthritis* is pain that is brought on by activity and relieved by rest. Stiffness after sitting and immediately upon arising in the morning is common but seldom persists for more than a few minutes. The more common locations are the terminal phalanges, carpal-metacarpal joint of the thumb, knees, hips, and spine. *Rheumatoid arthritis* most commonly involves the proximal interphalangeal and metacarpophalangeal joints, toes, wrists, ankle, knee, elbow, hip, and shoulder.

Polymyalgia Rheumatica This syndrome is observed in middle-aged and elderly persons and is characterized by severe pain, aching, and stiffness in the proximal muscles of the limbs and a markedly elevated erythrocyte sedimentation rate. Constitutional symptoms (loss of weight, fever, and anemia) and articular swelling are less consistent manifestations. Activity of the disease correlates with elevation of the sedimentation rate; unlike the case in polymyositis, with which it is confused by the uninitiated, creatine kinase levels are normal. In many patients, polymyalgia rheumatica is associated with giant-cell (temporal, or cranial) arteritis, which may be the only symptomatic expression of the disease (pages 193, 263 and 907). The arteritis may affect one or both optic nerve heads, and blindness is the main risk of the disease. This disorder is self-limited, lasting 6 months to 2 years, and responds dramatically to corticosteroid therapy, although the latter may need to be continued in low dosage for several months or a year or longer, using the sedimentation rate or C-reactive protein and hip and shoulder pain as guides.

Arteriosclerosis Obliterans Atherosclerosis of large and medium-sized arteries, the most common vascular disease of humans, often leads to symptoms that are induced by exercise (intermittent claudication) but may also occur at rest (ischemic rest pain). The diabetic patient is especially susceptible. The muscle pain that is brought on by exercise and promptly relieved by rest most frequently involves the calf and thigh muscles. If the atherosclerotic narrowing or occlusion implicates the aorta and iliac arteries, it may also cause hip and buttock claudication and impotence in the male (Leriche syndrome). Ischemic rest pain—and sometimes attendant ulceration and gangrene, usually localized to the foot and toes—is the consequence of multiple sites of vascular occlusion. Pain at rest is characteristically worse at night and totally or partially relieved by dependency.

The examination of such patients will reveal a loss of one or more peripheral pulses, trophic changes in the skin and nails (in advanced cases), and the presence of bruits over or distal to sites of narrowing. The ankle reflexes are often diminished.

Raynaud Phenomenon Painful blanching of the fingers with emotional stress or exposure to cold is the main feature. In many cases, no cause can be discerned. Other so-called secondary cases are due to partial obstruction of the brachial circulation, as occurs with some of the forms of the thoracic outlet syndrome, with repeated trauma to the hands, as in sculling or with use of a jackhammer, or with cryoglobulinemia, osteosclerotic myeloma, and autoimmune diseases. The Raynaud phenomenon is discussed further on page 569.

Reflex Sympathetic Dystrophy and Causalgia This is an excessive or abnormal response to injury of the shoulder, arm, or leg, particularly if an incomplete nerve injury is associated. It consists of protracted pain, characteristically described as "burning," together with cyanosis or pallor, swelling, coldness, pain on passive motion, osteoporosis, and marked sensitivity of the effected part to tactile stimulation. The condition is variously described under such terms as *Sudeck atrophy*, *posttraumatic osteoporosis* (in which case the bone scan may show increased local uptake of radioactive nuclide), and the related *shoulder-hand syndrome*. The unique pain syndrome is referred to as *causalgia*. Pharmacologic or surgical sympathectomy appears to relieve the symptoms in some patients. In others, with a hypersensitivity of both C-fiber receptors and postganglionic sympathetic fibers, it is not helpful (Lindblom and Ochoa). This subject is discussed further on pages 148 and 1438.

Neuroma Formation after Nerve Injury Persistent and often incapacitating pain and dysesthesias may follow any type of injury that leads to partial or complete interruption of a nerve with subsequent *neuroma formation or intraneural scarring*—fracture, contusion of the limbs, compression from lying on the arm in a drunken stupor, severing of sensory nerves in the course of surgical operations or biopsy of nerve, or incomplete regeneration after nerve suture. It is stated that the nerves in these cases contain a preponderance of unmyelinated C fibers and a reduced number of A-δ fibers; this imbalance is presumably related to the genesis of painful dysesthesias. These cases are best managed by complete excision of the neuromas with end-to-end suture of healthy nerve, but not all cases lend themselves to this procedure.

Another special type of neuroma is the one that forms at the end of a nerve severed at amputation (stump neuroma). Pain from this source is occasionally abolished by relatively simple procedures such as resection of the distal neuroma, proximal neurotomy, or resection of the regional sympathetic ganglia. Anterolateral cordotomy with attainment of complete analgesia may abolish pain from a stump neuroma (as well as pain from a phantom limb), but it is of limited value since there is usually a return of sensation and of pain after several months (6 months in the case of the lower extremities and earlier in the arms).

Erythromelalgia This rare disorder of the microvasculature produces a burning pain and bright red color change, usually in the toes and forefoot and sometimes in the hands, usually in association with changes in ambient temperature. Since it was first described by Weir Mitchell in 1878, many articles have been written about it, but the cause of the primary form is still obscure. Each patient has a temperature threshold above which symptoms appear and the feet become bright red and warm. The afflicted patient rarely wears stockings or regular shoes, since these tend to bring out the symptoms. The pain is relieved by walking on a cold surface or soaking the feet in ice water and by rest and elevation of the legs. The peripheral pulses are intact, and there are no motor, sensory, or reflex changes. There are rare secondary forms of the disease associated with myeloproliferative disorders, particularly polycythemia vera, thrombocythemia, and occlusive vascular diseases; in some instances it is a manifestation of a painful neuropathy (Chap. 46). The ergot-based dopamine agonists that are used in the treatment of Parkinson disease sometime cause this syndrome. Aspirin and methysergide have been recommended in the treatment of this disease but we have not had the opportunity of confirming their efficacy.

Myofascial Pain Syndrome (Fibromyalgia) A confusing problem in the differential diagnosis of neck and limb pain is posed by the patient with pains that are clearly musculoskeletal in origin but are not attributable to any of the aforementioned diseases of the spine, articular structures, or nerves. The pain is localized to certain points in skeletal muscles, particularly the large muscles of the neck and shoulder girdle, arms, and thighs. Ill-defined, tender nodules or cords can be felt in the muscle tissue (page 1572). Excision of such nodules reveals no sign of inflammation or other disease process. The currently fashionable terms *myofascial pain syndrome*, *fibromyalgia*, and *fibrositis* have been attached to the syndrome, depending on the particular interest or personal bias of the physician. Many of the patients are tense, sedentary women and there is a strong association with the equally vague chronic fatigue syndrome (page 528). Some relief is afforded by procaine injections, administration of local vapocoolants, stretching of underlying muscles ("spray and stretch"), massage, etc., but the results in any given individual are unpredictable.

REFERENCES

Alexander E Jr, Kelly DL, Davis CH Jr, et al: Intact arch spondylolisthesis: A review of 50 cases and description of surgical treatment. *J Neurosurg* 63:840, 1985.

Carette S, Leclaire R, Marcoux S, et al: Epidural corticosteroid injections for sciatica due to herniated nucleus pulposus. *N Engl J Med* 336:1634, 1997.

Carette S, Marcoux S, Truchon R, et al: A controlled trial of corticosteroid injections into facet joints for chronic low back pain. *N Engl J Med* 325:1002, 1991.

Cherkin DC, Devo RA, Battié M: A comparison of physical therapy, chiropractic manipulation, and provision of an educational booklet for the treatment of patients with low back pain. *N Engl J Med* 339:1021, 1998.

Collier B: Treatment for lumbar sciatic pain in posterior articular lumbar joint syndrome. *Anesthesia* 34:202, 1979.

Coppes MH, Marani E, Thomeer RTWM: Innervation of annulus fibrosus in low back pain. *Lancet* 1:189, 1990.

Cuckler JM, Bernini PA, Wiesel SW, et al: The use of epidural steroids in the treatment of lumbar radicular pain. *J Bone Joint Surg* 67:63, 1985.

Epstein NE, Epstein JA, Carras R, Hyman RA: Far lateral lumbar disc herniations and associated structural abnormalities: An evaluation in 60 patients of the comparative value of CT, MRI and myelo-CT in diagnosis and management. *Spine* 15:534, 1990.

Evans BA, Stevens JC, Dyck PJ: Lumbosacral plexus neuropathy. *Neurology* 31:1327, 1981.

Finneson BE: *Low Back Pain*, 2nd ed. Philadelphia, Lippincott, 1981.

Forristall RM, Marsh HO, Pay NT: Magnetic resonance imaging and contrast CT of the lumbar spine: Comparison of diagnostic methods and correlation with surgical findings. *Spine* 13:1049, 1988.

Friis ML, Bulliksen GC, Rasmussen P: Distribution of pain with nerve root compression. *Acta Neurosurg* 39:241, 1977.

Hadler NM, Curtis P, Gillings DB: A benefit of spinal manipulation as adjunctive therapy for acute low-back pain: A stratified controlled trial. *Spine* 12:703, 1987.

Hassler O: The human intervertebral disc: A micro-angiographical study on its vascular supply at various ages. *Acta Orthop Scand* 40:765, 1970.

Hudgkins WR: The crossed straight leg raising sign (of Fajerstagn). *N Engl J Med* 297:1127, 1977.

Jensen MC, Brant-Zawadzki MN, Obuchowski N, et al: Magnetic resonance imaging of the lumbar spine in people without back pain. *N Engl J Med* 331:69, 1994.

Kellgren JH: On the distribution of pain arising from deep somatic structures with charts of segmental pain areas. *Clin Sci* 4:35, 1939.

Kelsey JL, White AA: Epidemiology and impact of low back pain. *Spine* 5:133, 1980.

Kristoff FV, Odom GL: Ruptured intervertebral disc in the cervical region. *Arch Surg* 54:287, 1947.

LaRocca H: Acceleration injuries of the neck. *Clin Neurosurg* 25:209, 1978.

Leffert RD: Thoracic outlet syndrome, in Omer G, Springer M (eds): *Management of Peripheral Nerve Injuries*. Philadelphia, Saunders, 1980.

Leyshon A, Kirwan E O'G, Parry CB: Electrical studies in the diagnosis of compression of the lumbar root. *J Bone Joint Surg* 63B:71, 1981.

Lilius G, Laasonen EM, Myllynen P, et al: Lumbar facet joint syndrome: A randomized clinical trial. *J Bone Joint Surg (Br)* 71:681, 1989.

Lindblom U, Ochoa J: Somatosensory function and dysfunction, in Asbury AK, McKhann, GM, McDonald WI (eds): *Diseases of the Nervous System*, 2nd ed. Philadelphia, Saunders, 1992, pp 213–228.

Long DM: Low-back pain, in Johnson RT, Griffin JW (eds): *Current Therapy in Neurologic Disease 5*. St. Louis, Mosby, 1997, pp 71–76.

Lord SM, Barnsley L, Wallis BJ, et al: Percutaneous radiofrequency neurotomy for chronic cervical zygoapophyseal joint pain. *N Engl J Med* 335:1721, 1996.

Love JG, Schorn VG: Thoracic-disc protrusions. *JAMA* 191:627, 1965.

Matthews WB: The neurological complications of ankylosing spondylitis. *J Neurol Sci* 6:561, 1968.

McCall IW, Park WM, O'Brian JP: Induced pain referral from posterior lumbar elements in normal subjects. *Spine* 4:441, 1979.

Meade TW, Dyer S, Browne W, et al: Low back pain of mechanical origin: Randomised comparison of chiropractic and hospital outpatient treatment. *BMJ* 300:1431, 1990.

Michiels JJ, van Joost TH, Vuzevski VD: Idiopathic erythermalgia: A congenital disorder. *J Am Acad Dermatol* 21:1128, 1989.

Mikhael MA, Ciric I, Tarkington JA, et al: Neurologic evaluation of lateral recess syndrome. *Radiology* 140:97, 1981.

Mixter WJ, Barr JS: Rupture of the intervertebral disc with involvement of the spinal canal. *N Engl J Med* 211:210, 1934.

Postaccini F, Urso S, Ferro L: Lumbosacral nerve root anomalies. *J Bone Joint Surg* 64A:721, 1982.

Powell MC, Szypryt P, Wilson M, et al: Prevalence of lumbar disc degeneration observed by magnetic resonance in symptomless women. *Lancet* 2:1366, 1986.

Quiles M, Marchisello PJ, Tsairis R: Lumbar adhesive arachnoiditis: Etiologic and pathologic aspects. *Spine* 3:45, 1978.

Reynolds AF, Weinstein PR, Wachter RD: Lumbar monoradiculopathy due to unilateral facet hypertrophy. *Neurosurgery* 10:480, 1982.

Shannon N, Paul EA: L4/5, L5/S1 disc protrusions: Analysis of 323 cases operated on over 12 years. *J Neurol Neurosurg Psychiatry* 42:804, 1979.

Sinclair DC, Feindel WH, Weddell G, et al: The intervertebral ligaments as a source of segmental pain. *J Bone Joint Surg* 30B:515, 1948.

Symposium: Computerized tomography of the lumbar spine. *Spine* 4:281, 1979.

Tarlov IM: Perineurial cysts of the spinal nerve roots. *Arch Neurol Psychiatry* 40:1067, 1938.

van Gelderen C: Ein orthotisches (lordotisches) Kaudasyndrom. *Acta Psychiatr Neurol Scand* 23:57, 1948.

Verbiest H: Further experiences on the pathological influence of a developmental narrowness of the bony lumbar vertebral canal. *J Bone Joint Surg* 37B:576, 1955.

VROOMEN P, DEKROM M, WILMINK JT, et al: Lack of effectiveness of bed rest for sciatica. *N Engl J Med* 340:418, 1999.

WEIR BKA, JACOBS GA: Reoperation rate following lumbar discectomy. *Spine* 5:366, 1980.

WILBOURN AJ: The thoracic outlet syndrome is overdiagnosed. *Arch Neurol* 47:328, 1990.

WILBOURN AJ: Thoracic outlet syndromes: Plea for conservatism. *Neurosurg Clin North Am* 2:235, 1991.

WHITE AH, DERBY R, WYNNE G: Epidural injections for the diagnosis and treatment of low-back pain. *Spine* 5:78, 1980.

WRAY CC, EASOM S, HOSKINSON J: Coccydynia: Aetiology and treatment. *J Bone Joint Surg* 73B:335, 1991.

YIANNIKAS C, WALSH JC: Somatosensory evoked responses in the diagnosis of the thoracic outlet syndrome. *J Neurol Neurosurg Psychiatry* 46:234, 1983.

YOSS RE, CORBIN KB, MACCARTY CS, LOVE JG: Significance of symptoms and signs in localization of involved root in cervical disc protrusion. *Neurology* 7:673, 1957.

Section 3

DISORDERS OF THE SPECIAL SENSES

The four chapters in this section are concerned with the clinical aspects of the highly specialized functions of taste and smell, vision, hearing, and the sense of balance. These special senses and the cranial nerves that subserve them represent the most finely developed parts of the sensory nervous system. The sensory dysfunctions of the eye and ear are, of course, the domain of the ophthalmologist and otologist, but they are of interest to the neurologist as well. Some of them reflect the presence of serious systemic disease, and others represent the initial or leading manifestation of neurologic disease. It is from both these points of view that they are considered here. In keeping with the general scheme of this text, the disorders of the special senses (and of ocular movement) are considered in a particular sequence: first, the presentation of certain facts of anatomic and physiologic importance, followed by their cardinal clinical manifestations and then by a consideration of the syndromes of which these manifestations are a part. Because of their specialized nature, some of the diseases that produce these syndromes are discussed here rather than in later chapters of the book.

Chapter 12

DISORDERS OF SMELL AND TASTE

The sensations of smell (olfaction) and taste (gustation) are suitably considered together. Physiologically, these modalities share the singular attribute of responding primarily to chemical stimuli; i.e., the end organs that mediate olfaction and gustation are chemoreceptors. Also, taste and smell are interdependent clinically; appreciation of the flavor of food and drink depends to a large extent on their aroma, and an abnormality of one of these senses is frequently misinterpreted as an abnormality of the other. In comparison to sight and hearing, taste and smell play a relatively unimportant role in the life of the individual. However, the role of chemical stimuli in communication between humans has not been fully explored. Pheromones (*pherein*, "to carry"; *hormon*, "exciting"), that is, odorants exuded from the body and perfumes, play a part in sexual attraction (Agosta); noxious body odors repel. In certain vertebrates the olfactory system is remarkably well developed, rivaling the sensitivity of the visual system, but it has been stated that even humans, in whom the sense of smell is relatively weak, have the capacity to discriminate between as many as 10,000 different odorants (Reed).

Clinically, disorders of taste and smell can be persistently unpleasant, but only rarely is the loss of either of these modalities a serious handicap. Nevertheless, since all foods and inhalants pass through the mouth and nose, these two senses serve to detect noxious odors (e.g., smoke) and to avoid tainted food and potential poisons; loss of these senses could then have serious consequences. Also, a loss of taste and smell may signify a number of intracranial and systemic disorders, and assume clinical importance from this point of view.

OLFACTORY SENSE

Anatomic and Physiologic Considerations

Nerve fibers subserving the sense of smell have their cells of origin in the mucous membrane of the upper and posterior parts of the nasal cavity (superior turbinates and nasal septum). The entire olfactory mucosa covers an area of about 2.5 cm^2 and contains three cell types—the olfactory or receptor cells (which number between 6 and 10 million in each nasal cavity); sustentacular or supporting cells; which maintain the electrolyte (particularly K) levels in the extracellular milieu; and basal cells, which are stem cells and the source of both the olfactory and sustentacular cells during regeneration. The olfactory cells are actually bipolar neurons. Each of these cells has a peripheral process (the olfactory rod), from which project 10 to 30 fine hairs, or cilia. These hair-like processes, which lack motility, are the sites of olfactory receptors. The central processes of these cells, or *olfactory fila*, are very fine (0.2 mm in diameter), unmyelinated fibers that converge to form small fascicles enwrapped by Schwann cells that pass through openings in the cribriform plate of the ethmoid bone into the olfactory bulb (Fig. 12-1). Collectively, the central processes of the olfactory receptor cells constitute the *first cranial, or olfactory, nerve*. Notably, this is the only site in the organism where neurons are in direct contact with the external environment. The epithelial surface is covered by a layer of mucus, which is secreted by tubuloalveolar cells (Bowman's glands) and within which there are immunoglobulins A and M, lactoferrin, and lysoenzyme as well as odorant-binding proteins. These molecules are

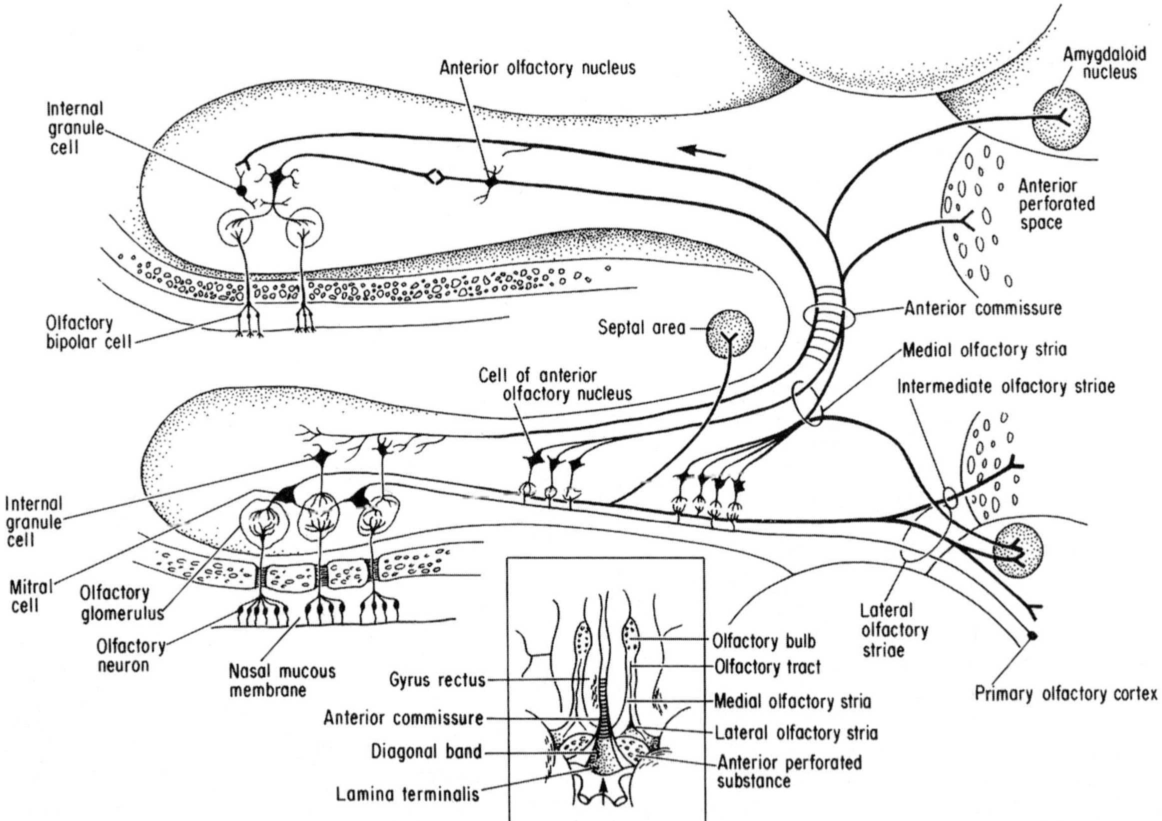

Figure 12-1

Diagram illustrating the relationships between the olfactory receptors in the nasal mucosa and neurons in the olfactory bulb and tract. Cells of the anterior olfactory nucleus are found in scattered groups caudal to the olfactory bulb. Cells of the anterior olfactory nucleus make immediate connections with the olfactory tract. They project centrally via the medial olfactory stria and to contralateral olfactory structures via the anterior commissure. Inset: diagram of the olfactory structures on the inferior surface of the brain (see text for details).

thought to prevent the intracranial entry of pathogens via the olfactory pathway (Kimmelman).

In the olfactory bulb, the receptor-cell axons synapse with granule cells and mitral cells (triangular, like a bishop's miter), the dendrites of which form brush-like terminals or olfactory glomeruli (Fig. 12-1). Smaller, so-called tufted cells in the olfactory bulb also contribute dendrites to the glomerulus. Approximately fifteen thousand olfactory-cell axons converge on a single glomerulus. This high degree of convergence is thought to account for an integration of afferent information. The mitral and tufted cells are excitatory; the granule cells—along with centrifugal fibers from the olfactory nuclei, locus ceruleus, and piriform cortex—inhibit mitral cell activity. Presumably, interaction between these excitatory and inhibitory neurons provides the basis for the special physiologic aspects of olfaction.

The axons of the mitral and tufted cells form the olfactory tract, which courses along the olfactory groove of the cribriform plate to the cerebrum. Lying caudal to the olfactory bulbs are groups of cells that constitute the anterior olfactory nucleus (Fig. 12-1). Dendrites of these cells synapse with fibers of the olfactory tract, while their axons project to the olfactory nucleus and bulb of the opposite side; these neurons are thought to function as a reinforcing mechanism for olfactory impulses.

Posteriorly, the olfactory tract divides into medial and lateral olfactory striae. The medial stria contains fibers from the anterior olfactory nucleus, which pass to the opposite side via the anterior commissure. Fibers in the lateral stria originate in the olfactory bulb, give off collaterals to the anterior perforated substance, and terminate in the medial and cortical nuclei of the amygdaloid complex and the prepiriform area (also referred to as the lateral olfactory gyrus). The latter represents the *primary olfactory cortex*, which in humans occupies a restricted area on the anterior end of the parahippocampal gyrus and uncus (area 34 of Brodmann; see Figs. 22-1 and 22-2). Thus olfactory impulses reach the cerebral cortex without relay through the thalamus; in this respect also, olfaction is unique among sensory systems. From the prepiriform cortex, fibers project to the neighboring entorhinal cortex (area 28 of Brodmann) and the medial dorsal nucleus of the thalamus; the amygdaloid nuclei connect with the hypothalamus and septal nuclei. The role of these latter structures in olfaction is not well understood, but presumably they subserve reflexes related to eating and sexual function. As with all sensory systems, feedback regulation occurs at every point in the afferent olfactory pathway.

In quiet breathing, little of the air entering the nostril reaches the olfactory mucosa; sniffing carries the air into the olfactory crypt. To be perceived as an odor, an inhaled substance must be volatile—i.e., spread in the air as very small particles—and soluble in water. Molecules provoking the same odor seem to be related more by their shape than by their chemical quality. When a jet of scented vapor is directed to the sensory epithelium, as by sniffing, a slow negative potential shift called the *electro-olfactogram* (EOG) can be recorded from an electrode placed on the mucosa. The conductance changes that underlie the receptor potential are induced by molecules of odorous material dissolved in the mucus overlying the receptor. The transduction of odorant stimuli to electrical signals appears to be mediated in part by a GTP-dependent adenylyl cyclase ("G protein"); like other cyclic AMP pathways, it utilizes an intracellular second messenger, but in the case of olfaction, the responsible molecule has not been definitely identified. There follow conformational changes in transmembrane receptor proteins and a series of intracellular biochemical events that generate axon potentials. Intensity of olfactory sensation is determined by the frequency of firing of afferent neurons. The quality of the odor is thought to be provided by "cross-fiber" activation, since the individual receptor cells are responsive to a wide variety of odorants and exhibit different types of responses to stimulants—excitatory, inhibitory, and on-off responses have been obtained. The olfactory potential can be eliminated by destroying the olfactory receptor surface or the olfactory filaments. The loss of EOG occurs 8 to 16 days after severance of the nerve; the receptor cells disappear, but the sustentacular cells are not altered. Most significant is the fact that, as a result of division of the basal cells of the olfactory epithelium, the olfactory receptor cells are constantly dying and being replaced by new ones. In this respect the chemoreceptors, both for smell and for taste, are unique, constituting the only examples of neuronal regeneration in humans.

The trigeminal system also participates in chemesthesia through undifferentiated receptors in the nasal mucosa. These receptors have little discriminatory ability but a great sensitivity to all irritant stimuli. The trigeminal afferents also release neuropeptides that result in hypersecretion of mucus, local edema, and sneezing. Finally, it should be noted that stimulation of the olfactory pathway at sites other than the receptor cells may also induce olfactory experiences.

The olfactory system adapts quickly to the sensory stimulus, and for sensation to be sustained, there must be repeated stimulation. The olfactory sense differs from other senses in yet another way. It is common experience that an aroma can restore long-forgotten memories of complex experiences. That olfactory and emotional stimuli are strongly linked is not surprising in view of their common roots in the limbic system. Yet the ability to recall an odor is negligible in comparison with the ability to recall sounds and sights. As Vladimir Nabokov has remarked: "Memory can restore to life everything except smells."

Clinical Manifestations

Disturbances of olfaction may be subdivided into four groups, as follows:

1. Quantitative abnormalities: loss or reduction of the sense of smell (anosmia, hyposmia) or, rarely, increased olfactory acuity (hyperosmia)

2. Qualitative abnormalities: distortions or illusions of smell (dysosmia or parosmia)

3. Olfactory hallucinations and delusions caused by temporal lobe disorders or psychiatric disease

4. Higher-order loss of olfactory discrimination (olfactory agnosia)

Anosmia (Loss of Sense of Smell) This is the most frequent clinical abnormality, and, if unilateral, will usually not be recognized by the patient. Unilateral anosmia can sometimes be demonstrated in the hysterical patient on the side of anesthesia, blindness, or deafness. Bilateral anosmia, on the other hand, is a not uncommon complaint, and the patient is usually convinced that the sense of taste has been lost as well (*ageusia*). This calls attention to the fact that taste depends largely on the volatile particles in foods and beverages, which reach the olfactory receptors through the nasopharynx, and that the perception of flavor is a combination of smell, taste, and tactile sensation. This can be proved by demonstrating that such patients are able to distinguish the elementary taste sensations (sweet, sour, bitter, and salty). The olfactory defect can be verified readily enough by presenting a series of nonirritating olfactory stimuli (vanilla, peanut butter, coffee, tobacco, etc.), first in one nostril, then in the other, and asking the patient to sniff and identify them. If the odors can be detected and described, even if they cannot be named, it may be assumed that the olfactory nerves are relatively intact (humans can distinguish many more odors than they can identify by name). Ammonia and similar pungent substances are unsuitable stimuli because they do not test the sense of smell but have a primary irritating effect upon the free nerve endings of the trigeminal nerves.

A more elaborate scratch and sniff test has been developed and standardized by Doty and colleagues (University of Pennsylvania Smell Identification Test). In this test the patient attempts to identify 40 microencapsulated odorants and his olfactory performance is compared with that of age- and sex-matched normal individuals. Unique features of this test are a means for detecting malingering and amenability to self-administration. Air-dilution olfactory detection is a more refined way of determining thresholds of sensation and of demonstrating normal olfactory perception in the absence of identification. Olfactory evoked potentials are being used in some electrophysiology laboratories, but their reliability is uncertain. These refined techniques are essentially research tools and are not used in neurologic practice.

The loss of smell usually falls into one of three categories: *nasal* (in which odorants do not reach the olfactory receptors), *olfactory neuroepithelial* (due to destruction of receptors or their axon filaments), and *central* (olfactory pathway lesions). In an analysis of 4000 cases of anosmia from specialized clinics, Hendriks found that three categories of pathology—nasal or paranasal sinus disease, viral infection of the upper respiratory tracts (the largest group), and head injury—accounted for most of the cases. Regarding the nasal diseases responsible for bilateral hyposmia or anosmia, the most frequent are those in which hypertrophy and hyperemia of the nasal mucosa prevent olfactory stimuli from reaching the receptor cells. Heavy smoking is said to be the most frequent cause of hyposmia. Chronic atrophic rhinitis; sinusitis of allergic, vasomotor, or infective types; nasal polyposis; and overuse of topical vasocontrictors are other common causes. Biopsies of the olfactory mucosa in cases of allergic rhinitis have shown that the sensory epithelial cells are still present, but their cilia are deformed and shortened and are buried under other mucosal cells. Influenza, herpes simplex, and hepatitis virus infections may be followed by hyposmia or anosmia due to destruction of receptor cells, and, if the basal cells are also destroyed, this may be permanent. These cells may also be affected as a result of atrophic rhinitis and local radiation therapy or by a very rare type of tumor (*esthesioneuroblastoma*) that originates in the olfactory epithelium. There is also a group of rare diseases in which the primary receptor neurons are congenitally absent or hypoplastic and lack cilia. One of these is the Kallman syndrome of congenital anosmia and hypogonadotropic hypogonadism. A similar disorder occurs in the Turner syndrome and in albinos, because of the absence of "olfactory pigment" or some other congenital structural defect.

Anosmia that follows head injury is most often due to tearing of the delicate filaments of the receptor cells as they pass through the cribriform plate, especially if the injury is severe enough to cause fracture. The damage may be unilateral or bilateral. With closed head injury, anosmia is relatively infrequent (6 percent of Sumner's series of 584 cases). Some recovery of olfaction occurs in about one-third of all head trauma cases over a period of several days to months. Beyond 6 to 12 months, recovery is negligible. Cranial surgery, subarachnoid hemorrhage, and chronic meningeal inflammation may have a similar effect. Strangely, in some of the cases of traumatic anosmia, there is also a loss of taste (ageusia). Ferrier, who first described traumatic ageusia in 1876, noted that there was always anosmia as well—an observation subsequently corroborated by Sumner. Often the ageusia clears within a few weeks. A bilateral lesion near the frontal operculum and paralimbic region, where olfactory and gustatory receptive zones are in close proximity, would best explain this concurrence. Obviously the interruption of olfactory filaments alone would not explain ageusia.

In women, olfactory acuity varies throughout the menstrual cycle and may be disordered during pregnancy. Nutritional and metabolic diseases such as thiamine deficiency, vitamin A deficiency, adrenal and perhaps thyroid insufficiency, cirrhosis, and chronic renal failure may give rise to transient anosmia, all as a result of sensorineural dysfunction. A large number of toxic agents—the more common ones being organic solvents (benzene), metals, dusts, cocaine, corticosteroids, methotrexate, aminoglycoside antibiotics, tetracyclines, opiates, and L-dopa—can damage the olfactory epithelium (Doty et al).

It has been reported that a large proportion of patients with degenerative disease of the brain show anosmia or hyposmia, for reasons that are quite unclear. Included in this group are Alzheimer, Parkinson, Huntington, and Pick disease and the Parkinson-dementia syndrome of Guam. The studies relating to this subject have been reviewed in detail by Doty. A number of theories have been proposed to explain these findings, but they are conjectural. It has been known for some time that alcoholics with Korsakoff psychosis have a defect in odor discrimination (Mair et al). In the latter disorder, anosmia is presumably due to degeneration of neurons in the higher-order olfactory systems involving the medial thalamic nuclei. Hyman and colleagues have remarked on the early neuronal degeneration in the region of the hippocampus in cases of Alzheimer disease, but we know of no studies of the central olfactory connections in this or any other degenerative disorder. Anosmia has been found in some patients with temporal lobe epilepsy and in some such patients who had been subjected to anterior temporal lobectomy. In these conditions, Andy and coworkers have found an impairment in discriminating the quality of odors and in matching odors with test objects seen or felt.

As with other sensory modalities, olfaction (and taste) are diminished with aging. The receptor cell population is depleted, and if the loss is regional, neuroepithelium is slowly replaced with respiratory epithelium (which is normally present in the nasal cavity and serves to filter, humidify, and warm incoming air). Neurons of the olfactory bulb may also be reduced as part of the aging process.

Bilateral anosmia is an increasingly common manifestation of *malingering*, now that it has been recognized as a compensable disability by insurance companies. The fact that true anosmics will complain inordinately of a loss of taste (but show normal taste sensation) may help to separate them from malingerers. Testing of olfactory evoked potentials, if perfected, would be of use here.

The nasal epithelium or the olfactory nerves themselves may be affected in Wegener granulomatosis and by craniopharyngioma. A meningioma of the olfactory groove may implicate the olfactory bulb and tract and may extend posteriorly to involve the optic nerve, sometimes with optic atrophy; these abnormalities, if combined with papilledema on the opposite side, are known as The Foster Kennedy syndrome (page 260). A large aneurysm of the anterior cerebral or anterior communicating artery may produce a similar syndrome. With tumors confined to one side, the anosmia may be strictly unilateral, in which case it will not be reported by the patient but will be found on examination. Children with anterior meningoencephaloceles are usually anosmic and, in addition, may exhibit cerebrospinal fluid (CSF) rhinorrhea when the head is held in certain positions. Injury of the cribriform plate and hydrocephalus are other causes of CSF rhinorrhea. These defects in the sense of smell are attributable to lesions of either the receptor cells and their axons or the olfactory bulbs, and current test methods do not distinguish between lesions in these two localities. It is not known whether olfactory symptoms may be produced by lesions of the anterior perforated space or of the medial and lateral olfactory striae. In some cases of increased intracranial pressure, olfactory sense has been impaired without evidence of lesions in the olfactory bulbs.

The term *specific anosmia* has been applied to an unusual olfactory phenomenon, in which a person with normal olfactory acuity for most substances encounters a particular compound or class of compounds that is odorless to him, although obvious to others. In a sense, this is a condition of "smell blindness," analogous to color blindness. The basis of this disorder is unclear, although there is evidence that specific anosmia for musky and urinous odors is inherited as an autosomal recessive trait (see Amoore).

Whether a true *hyperosmia* exists is a matter of conjecture. Neurotic individuals may complain of being unduly sensitive to odors, but there is no proof of an actual change in their threshold of perception of odors. During migraine attacks and in some cases of aseptic meningitis, the patient may be unusually sensitive not only to light and sound but sometimes to odors as well.

Dysosmia or Parosmia These terms refer to distortions of odor perception, where an odor is present. Parosmia may occur with local nasopharyngeal conditions such as empyema of the nasal sinuses and ozena. In some instances the abnormal tissue itself may be the source of unpleasant odors; in others, where partial injuries of the olfactory bulbs have occurred, parosmia is in the nature of an olfactory illusion. Parosmia may also be a troublesome symptom in middle-aged and elderly persons with a depressive illness, who may report that every article of food has an extremely unpleasant odor (cacosmia). Sensations of disagreeable taste are often associated (cacogeusia). Nothing is known of the basis of this state; there is usually no loss of discriminative sensation.

The treatment of parosmia is difficult. The use of antipsychotic drugs has given unpredictable results. Claims for the efficacy of zinc and vitamins have not been verified. Some reports indicate that repeated anesthetization of the nasal mucosa reduces or abolishes the parosmic disturbance. In many cases the disorder subsides spontaneously. Minor degrees of parosmia are not necessarily abnormal, for unpleasant odors have a way of lingering for several hours and of being reawakened by other olfactory stimuli (phantosmia), as every pathologist knows.

Olfactory Hallucinations These are always of central origin. The patient claims to smell an odor that no one else can detect (phantosmia). Most often this is due to temporal lobe seizures ("uncinate fits"), in which circumstances the olfactory hallucinations are brief and accompanied by an alteration of consciousness and other manifestations of epilepsy (page 339).

If the patient is convinced of the presence of a hallucination and also gives it personal reference, the symptom assumes the status of a delusion. The combination of olfactory hallucinations and delusions of this type signifies a psychiatric illness. Zilstorff has written informatively on this subject. There is often a complaint of a large array of odors, most of them foul. In most cases, the smells seem to emanate from the patient (intrinsic hallucinations); in others, they seem to come from an external source (extrinsic hallucinations). Both types vary in intensity and are remarkable with respect to their persistence. They may be combined with gustatory hallucinations. According to Pryse-Phillips, who took note of the psychiatric illness in a series of 137 patients with olfactory hallucinations, most were associated with endogenous depression and schizophrenia. In schizophrenia, the olfactory stimulus is usually interpreted as arising externally and as being induced by someone for the purpose of upsetting the patient. In depression, the stimulus is usually intrinsic and is more overwhelming. The patient uses all manner of ways to get rid of the perceived stench, the usual ones being excessive washing and use of deodorants; the condition may lead to social withdrawal. There is some reason to believe that the amygdaloid group of nuclei is the source of the hallucinations, since stereotactic lesions here have reportedly abolished both the olfactory hallucinations and the psychiatric disorder (Chitanondh).

Olfactory hallucinations and delusions may occur in conjunction with senile dementia, but when this happens one should also consider the possibility of an associated late-life depression. Occasionally olfactory hallucinations are part of an alcohol withdrawal syndrome. Peculiar reactions to smell characterize certain sexual psychopathies. Usually the stimuli appear to be extrinsic, but in this regard it should be noted that odors imagined by normal individuals are also perceived as coming from outside the person through inspired air, and unpleasant ones are more clearly represented than pleasant ones.

In lower vertebrates, these functions and similar ones (modulation of menstrual and reproductive behavior) have been attributed to the activities of a subset of olfactory receptors in the rostral end of the nasal mucosa. The axons of these cells penetrate the cribriform plate and synapse with secondary neurons in a discrete portion of the olfactory bulb (accessory olfactory bulb). This functionally and anatomically distinct olfactory tissue is referred to as the *vomeronasal system or organ of Jacobson* (see review of Wysocki and Meredith).

Loss of Olfactory Discrimination (Olfactory Agnosia) Finally, one must consider a disorder in which the primary perceptual aspects of olfaction (detection of odors, adaptation to odors, and recognition of different intensities of the same odor) are intact but the capacity to distinguish between odors and their recognition by quality is impaired or lost. In the writings on this subject, this deficit is usually referred to as a disorder of olfactory discrimination. In dealing with other sense modalities, however, the inability to identify and name a perceived sensation would be called an *agnosia*. To recognize this deficit requires special testing, such as matching to sample, the identification and naming of a variety of scents, and determining whether two odors are identical or different. Such an alteration of olfactory function has been shown to characterize patients with the alcoholic form of Korsakoff psychosis; this impairment is not attributable to impaired olfactory acuity or to failure of learning and memory (Mair et al). As indicated above, the olfactory disorder in the alcoholic Korsakoff patient is most likely due to lesions in the medial dorsal nucleus of the thalamus; several observations in animals indicate that this nucleus and its connections with the orbitofrontal cortex give rise to deficits in odor discrimination (Mair et al; Slotnick and Kaneko). Eichenbaum and associates demonstrated a similar impairment of olfactory capacities in a patient who had undergone extensive bilateral medial temporal lobe resections. The operation was believed to have eliminated a substantial portion of the olfactory afferents to the frontal cortex and thalamus, though there was no anatomic verification of this. In patients with stereotactic or surgical amygdalotomies, Andy and coworkers noted a similar reduction in odor discrimination. Thus it appears that both portions of the higher olfactory pathways (medial temporal lobes and medial dorsal nuclei) are necessary for the discrimination and identification of odors.

GUSTATORY SENSE

Anatomic and Physiologic Considerations

The sensory receptors for taste (taste buds) are distributed over the surface of the tongue and, in smaller numbers, over the soft palate, pharynx, larynx, and esophagus. Mainly they are located in the epithelium along the lateral surfaces of the circumvallate and foliate papillae and to a lesser extent on the surface of the fungiform papillae (Fig. 12-2). The taste buds are round or oval structures, each composed of up to two hundred vertically oriented receptor cells arranged like the staves of a barrel. The superficial portion of the bud is marked by a small opening, the taste pore or pit, which opens onto the mucosal surface. The tips of the sensory cells project through the pore as a number of filiform microvilli ("taste hairs"). Fine, unmyelinated sensory fibers penetrate the base of the taste bud and synapse directly with the sensory taste cells, which have no axons.

The taste receptors are activated by chemical substances in solution and transmit their activity along the sensory nerves to the brainstem. As stated earlier, there are four primary and readily tested taste sensations—salty, sweet, bitter, and sour; the full range of taste sensations is much broader, consisting of combinations of these elementary gustatory sensations. Any one taste bud is capable of responding to a number of sapid substances, but always it is preferentially sensitive to one type of stimulus (Fig. 12-2). In other words, the receptors are only relatively specific. The sensitivity of these receptors is remarkable: as little as 0.05 mg/dL of quinine sulfate will arouse a bitter taste when applied to the base of the tongue.

If the gustatory impairment is unilateral, taste is tested by withdrawing the tongue with a gauze sponge and using a moistened applicator to place a few crystals of salt or sugar on discrete parts of the tongue; the tongue is then wiped clean and the subject is asked to report what he had sensed. A useful stimulus for sour sensation is a low-voltage direct current, the electrodes of which can be accurately placed on the tongue surface. If the taste loss is bilateral, mouthwashes with a dilute solution of sucrose, sodium chloride, citric acid, and caffeine may be used. After swishing, the test fluid is spat out and the mouth rinsed with water. The patient indicates whether he had tasted a substance and is asked to identify it. Special types of apparatus (electrogustometers) have been devised for the measurement of taste intensity and for determining the detection and recognition thresholds of taste and olfactory stimuli (Krarup;

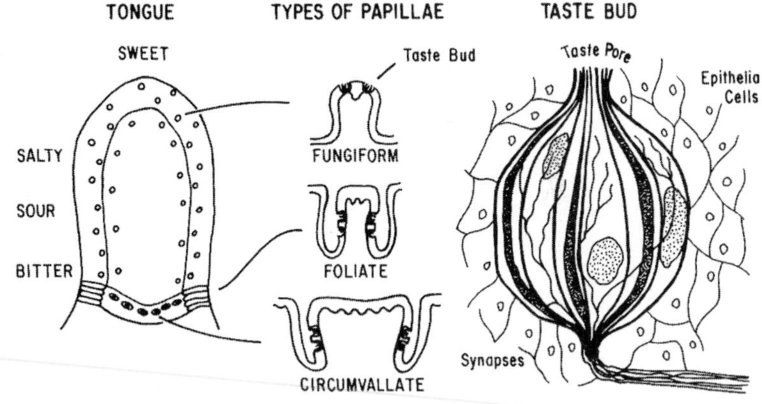

Figure 12-2

The distribution and structure of taste buds on the human tongue. Each taste bud can respond to all four primary taste sensations, but certain ones are preferentially sensitive to one modality, as indicated in the diagram on the left. Taste buds of the fungiform and foliate papillae are innervated by the chorda tympani (cranial nerve VII), and those of the circumvallate papillae by cranial nerve IX. Note that sensory fibers penetrate the base of the taste bud and synapse directly with the sensory taste cells. The darker segments of the taste bud represent taste cells in stages of degeneration and regeneration. (Adapted by permission, from Shepherd GM, Neurobiology, New York, Oxford University Press, 1983.)

Henkin et al), but these are beyond the scope of the usual clinical examination.

The receptor cells of the taste buds have a brief life cycle (about 10 days), being replaced constantly by mitotic division of adjacent basal epithelial cells. The number of taste buds, not large to begin with, is gradually reduced with age; also, changes occur in the taste cell membranes, with impaired function of ion channels and receptors (Mistretta). Both gustatory (and olfactory) acuity diminish (everything begins to taste and smell the same). According to Schiffman, taste thresholds for salt, sweeteners, and amino acids are 2 to 2½ times higher in the elderly than in the young. The reduction in the acuity of taste and smell with aging may lead to a distortion of food habits (e.g., excessive use of salt and other condiments) and contribute to the anorexia and weight loss of elderly persons.

Sensory impulses for taste arise from several sites in the oropharynx and are transmitted to the medulla via several cranial nerves (V, VII, IX, and X). The main pathway arises on the anterior two-thirds of the tongue; the taste fibers first run in the lingual nerve (a major branch of the mandibular-trigeminal nerve). After coursing within the lingual nerve for a short distance, the taste fibers diverge to enter the chorda tympani (a branch of the seventh nerve); thence they pass through the pars intermedia and geniculate ganglion of the seventh nerve to the rostral part of the nucleus of the tractus solitarius in the medulla, where all taste afferents converge (see below). Fibers from the palatal taste buds pass through the pterygopalatine ganglion and greater superficial petrosal nerve, join the facial nerve at the level of the geniculate ganglion, and proceed to the nucleus of the solitary tract (see Fig. 47-2). Possibly, taste fibers from the tongue may also reach the brainstem via the mandibular division of the trigeminal nerve. The presence of this alternative pathway probably accounts for reported instances of unilateral taste loss that have followed section of the root of the trigeminal nerve and instances in which no loss of taste has occurred with section of the chorda tympani. From the posterior third of the tongue, soft palate, and palatal arches, the sensory taste fibers are conveyed via the glossopharyngeal nerve and ganglion nodosum to the nucleus of the tractus solitarius. Taste fibers from the extreme dorsal part of the tongue and the few that arise from taste buds on the pharynx and larynx run in the vagus nerve. Rostral and lateral parts of the *nucleus tractus solitarius*, which receive the special afferent (taste) fibers from the facial and glossopharyngeal nerves, constitute the *gustatory nucleus*. Probably both sides of the tongue are represented in this nucleus.

The second sensory neuron for taste has been difficult to track. Neurons of the nucleus solitarius project to adjacent nuclei (e.g., dorsal motor nucleus of the vagus, ambiguus, salivatorius superior and inferior, trigeminal, and facial nerves), which serve viscerovisceral and viscerosomatic reflex functions, but those concerned with the conscious recognition of taste are believed to form an ascending pathway to a pontine parabrachial nucleus. From the latter, two ascending pathways have been traced (in animals). One is the solitariothalamic lemniscus to the ventroposteromedial nucleus. A second passes to the ventral parts of the forebrain, to parts of the hypothalamus (which probably influences autonomic function), and to other basal forebrain limbic areas in or near the uncus of the temporal lobe. Other ascending fibers lie near the medial lemniscus and are both crossed and uncrossed. Experiments in animals indicate that taste impulses from the thalamus project to the tongue-face area of the postrolandic sensory cortex. This is probably the end station of gustatory projections in humans as well, insofar as gustatory hallucinations have been produced by electrical stimulation of the parietal and/or rolandic opercula (Hausser-Hauw and Bancaud). Penfield and Faulk evoked distinct taste sensations by stimulating the anterior insula.

Richter has explored the biologic role of taste in normal nutrition. Animals made deficient in sodium, calcium, certain vitamins, proteins, etc., will automatically select the correct foods, on the basis of their taste, to compensate for their deficiency.

Clinical Manifestations

Apart from the loss of taste sensation that accompanies normal aging (see above), heavy smoking, particularly pipe smoking, is probably the commonest cause of impairment of taste sensation. Extreme drying of the tongue from any cause may lead to temporary loss or reduction of the sense of taste (*ageusia* or *hypogeusia*), since saliva is essential for normal taste function. Saliva acts as a solvent for chemical substances in food and for conveying them to taste receptors. Dryness of the mouth (xerostomia) from inadequate saliva, as occurs in the Sjögren syndrome; hyperviscosity of saliva, as in cystic fibrosis; irradiation of head and neck; and pandysautonomia all interfere with taste. Also, in familial dysautonomia (Riley-Day syndrome), the number of circumvallate and fungiform papillae are reduced, accounting for a diminished ability to taste sweet and salty foods. If unilateral, ageusia is seldom the source of complaint. Taste is frequently lost over one-half of the tongue (except posteriorly) in cases of Bell's palsy (as indicated on page 1452).

A permanent decrease in acuity of taste and smell (hypogeusia and hyposmia), sometimes associated with perversions of these sensory functions (dysgeusia and dysosmia), may follow influenza-like illnesses. These abnormalities have been associated with pathologic changes in the taste buds as well as in the nasal mucous membranes. In a group of 143 patients who presented with hypogeusia and hyposmia, 87 were of this postinfluenzal type (Henkin et al); the remainder developed their symptoms in association with scleroderma, acute hepatitis, viral encephalitis, myxedema, adrenal insufficiency, malignancy, deficiency of vitamins B and A, and the administration of a wide variety of drugs (see further on).

Distortions of taste and loss of taste are sources of complaint in patients with a variety of malignant tumors. Oropharyngeal tumors may, of course, abolish taste by invading the chorda tympani or lingual nerves. Malnutrition due to neoplasm or radiation therapy may also cause ageusia, as pointed out by Settle and colleagues. Some patients with certain carcinomas remark on an increase in their threshold for bitter foods, and some who have been radiated for breast cancer or sublingual or oropharyngeal tumors find sour foods intolerable. The loss of taste from radiation of the oropharynx is usually recovered within a few weeks or months; the reduced turnover of taste buds caused by radiation therapy is only temporary.

Persistent misinterpretations and distortions of taste (and smell) have been reported with a wide variety of drugs. According to Schiffman, more than 250 drugs have been implicated in the alteration of taste sensation. Lipid lowering drugs, antihistamines, antimicrobials, antineoplastics, bronchodilators, antidepressants, and anticonvulsants are the main offenders. Little is known about the mechanisms by which drugs induce these effects.

An interesting syndrome, called *idiopathic hypogeusia*, in which a decreased taste acuity is associated with dysgeusia, hyposmia, and dysosmia has been described by Henkin and coworkers. Food has an unpleasant taste and aroma, to the point of being revolting (cacogenusia and cacosmia); the persistence of these symptoms may lead to a loss of weight, anxiety, and depression. Patients with this disorder were said to have a decreased concentration of zinc in their parotid saliva and to respond to small oral doses of zinc sulfate. The authors have had no opportunity to confirm these observations.

Another poorly defined disorder is the so-called *burning mouth syndrome*, which occurs mainly in postmenopausal women and is characterized by persistent, severe intra-oral pain (particularly of the tongue). We have seen what we believe to be fragmentary forms of the syndrome in which pain and burning are isolated to the alveolar ridge or gingival mucosa. The oral mucosa appears normal and some patients may report a diminution of taste sensation. A small number of such patients prove to have diabetes or vitamin B_{12} deficiency, but in most no systemic illness or local abnormality can be found. The few such cases that we have encountered appeared to have a depressive illness and responded variably to administration of tricyclic antidepressants.

Unilateral lesions of the medulla oblongata have not been reported to cause ageusia, perhaps because the nucleus of the tractus solitarius is usually outside the zone of infarction. Unilateral thalamic and parietal lobe lesions have both been associated with contralateral impairment of taste sensation. As indicated above, a gustatory aura occasionally marks the beginning of a seizure originating in the frontoparietal (suprasylvian) cortex or in the uncal region. This implies that taste fibers terminate in the amygdala, in close association with olfactory fibers. Gustatory hallucinations are much less frequent than olfactory ones. Nevertheless, the former were found in 30 of 718 cases of intractable epilepsy (Hausser-Hauw and Bancaud). During surgery, these investigators produced an aura of disagreeable taste by electrical stimulation of the parietal and frontal opercula and also by stimulation of the hippocampus and amygdala (uncinate seizures). In their view, the low-threshold seizure focus for taste in the temporal lobe is secondary to functional disorganization of the opercular gustatory cortex by the seizure. Gustatory hallucinations were more frequent with right-hemisphere lesions, and in half of the cases, the gustatory aura was followed by a convulsion.

REFERENCES

Agosta WC: *Chemical Communication: The Language of Pheromones*. New York, Scientific American Library, Freeman, 1992.

Amoore JE: Specific anosmias, in Getchell TV, Bartoshuk LM, Doty RL, Snow JB (eds): *Smell and Taste in Health and Disease*. New York, Raven Press, 1991, pp 655–664.

Andy OJ, Jurko MF, Hughes JR: The amygdala in relation to olfaction. *Confin Neurol* 37:215, 1975.

Buck LB: Smell and taste: The chemical senses, in Kandel ER, Schwartz JH, Jessel TM (eds): *Principles of Neural Science*, 4th ed., New York, McGraw-Hill, 2000, pp 625–647.

CHITANONDH H: Stereotaxic amygdalotomy in the treatment of olfactory seizures and psychiatric disorders with olfactory hallucinations. *Confin Neurol* 27:181, 1966.

DOTY RL: Olfactory dysfunction in neurodegenerative disorders, in Getchell TV et al (eds): *Smell and Taste in Health and Disease*. New York, Raven Press, 1991, pp 735–751.

DOTY RL, SHAMAN P, APPLEBAUM SL: Smell identification ability: Changes with age. *Science* 226:1441, 1984.

DOTY RL, SHAMAN P, DANN M: Development of University of Pennsylvania Smell Identification Test. *Physiol Behav* 32:489, 1984.

EICHENBAUM H, MORTON TH, POTTER H, CORKIN S: Selective olfactory deficits in case H.M. *Brain* 106:459, 1983.

GETCHELL TV, DOTY RL, BARTOSHUK LM, SNOW JB JR (eds): *Smell and Taste in Health and Disease*. New York, Raven Press, 1991.

HAUSSER-HAUW C, BANCAUD J: Gustatory hallucinations in epileptic seizures. *Brain* 110:339, 1987.

HENDRIKS AP: Olfactory dysfunction. *Rhinology* 4:229, 1988.

HENKIN RI, GILL JR JR, BARTTER FC: Studies on taste thresholds in normal man and in patients with adrenal cortical insufficiency: The effect of adrenocorticosteroids. *J Clin Invest* 42:727, 1963.

HENKIN RI, LARSON AL, POWELL RD: Hypogeusia, dysgeusia, hyposmia and dysosmia following influenza-like infection. *Ann Otol* 84:672, 1975.

HENKIN RI, SCHECHTER PJ, HOYE R, MATTERN CFT: Idiopathic hypogeusia with dysgeusia, hyposmia, and dysosmia: A new syndrome. *JAMA* 217:434, 1971.

HYMAN BT, VAN HOESEN GW, DAMASIO AR: Alzheimer disease: Cell specific pathology isolates the hippocampal formation. *Science* 225:1168, 1984.

KIMMELMAN CP: Clinical review of olfaction. *Am J Otolaryngol* 14:227, 1993.

KRARUP B: Electrogustometry: A method for clinical taste examinations. *Acta Otolaryngol* 69:294, 1958.

MAIR R, CAPRA C, MCENTEE WJ, ENGEN T: Odor discrimination and memory in Korsakoff's psychosis. *J Exp Psychol [Hum Percept]* 6:445, 1980.

MISTRETTA CM: Aging effects on anatomy and neurophysiology of taste and smell. *Gerontology* 3:131, 1984.

PENFIELD W, FAULK ME: The insula: Further observations on its function. *Brain* 78:445, 1955.

PRYSE-PHILLIPS W: Disturbances in the sense of smell in psychiatric patients. *Proc R Soc Med* 68:26, 1975.

QUINN NP, ROSSOR MN, MARSDEN CD: Olfactory threshold in Parkinson's disease. *J Neurol Neurosurg Psychiatry* 50:88, 1987.

REED RR: The molecular basis of sensitivity and specificity in olfaction. *Cell Biol* 5:33, 1994.

RICHTER CP: Total self-regulatory functions in animals and human beings. *Harvey Lect* 38:63, 1942–1943.

SCHIFFMAN SS: Drugs influencing taste and smell perception, in Getchell TV et al (eds): *Smell and Taste in Health and Disease*. New York, Raven Press, 1991, pp 845–850.

SCHIFFMAN SS: Taste and smell losses in normal aging and disease. *JAMA* 276: 1357, 1997.

SETTLE RG, QUINN MR, BREND JG: Gustatory evaluation of cancer patients, in Von Eys J, Nichols BL, Seeling MS (eds): *Nutrition and Cancer*. New York, Spectrum, 1979.

SLOTNICK BM, KANEKO N: Role of mediodorsal thalamic nucleus in olfactory discrimination learning in rats. *Science* 214:91, 1981.

SUMNER D: Disturbances of the senses of smell and taste after head injuries, in Vinken PJ, Bruyn GW (eds): *Handbook of Clinical Neurology*. Vol 24. Amsterdam, North-Holland, 1975, pp 1–25.

SUMNER D: Post-traumatic ageusia. *Brain* 90:187, 1967.

WYSOCKI CJ, MEREDITH H: The vomeronasal system, in Finger TE, Silver WL (eds): *Neurobiology of Taste and Smell*. New York, Wiley, 1987, pp 125–150.

ZILSTORFF W: Parosmia. *J Laryngol Otol* 80:1102, 1966.

Chapter 13

COMMON DISTURBANCES OF VISION

The faculty of vision is our most important source of information about the world. Attesting to the importance of visual function is the magnitude of its representation in the central nervous system. The largest part of the cerebrum is involved in vision: the visual control of movement as well as the perception of printed words and the form and color of objects. The optic nerve, which is a central nervous system (CNS) structure, contains over a million fibers (compared to 50,000 in the auditory nerve). The visual system has special significance in several other respects, and study of this system has greatly advanced our knowledge of the nervous system. Indeed, we know more about vision than about any other sensory system. Because of its diverse composition of epithelial, vascular, collagenous, neural, and pigmentary tissues, the eye is virtually a medical microcosm, susceptible to many diseases. Moreover, the eye's transparent media permit direct inspection of these tissues and afford an opportunity to observe, during life, many lesions of neurologic and systemic medical disease.

Since the eye is the sole organ of vision, impairment of visual function (defect in acuity and visual fields) obviously stands as the most frequent and important symptom of eye disease. A number of terms are commonly used to describe visual loss. *Amaurosis* refers to blindness, especially blindness that is not due to an error of refraction or to intrinsic disease of the eye itself. *Amblyopia* has much the same meaning—dimness of vision from any cause, ocular or nonocular. *Nyctalopia* is the term for poor twilight or night vision and is associated with vitamin A deficiency, retinitis pigmentosa, and, often, color blindness. There are also positive symptoms (phosphenes, visual illusions, and hallucinations), but they are less significant than symptoms of visual loss. Irritation, redness, photophobia, pain, diplopia and strabismus, changes in pupillary size, and drooping or closure of the eyelids are the other major symptoms and signs. The impairment of vision may be unilateral or bilateral, sudden or gradual, episodic or enduring. The common causes of failing eyesight vary with age. In infancy, congenital defects, severe myopia, hypoplasia of the optic nerve, optic pits, and coloboma are the main causes. In late childhood and adolescence, nearsightedness, or myopia, is the usual cause, though a pigmentary retinopathy or a retinal, optic nerve, or suprasellar tumor must not be overlooked. In middle age, beginning usually in the fifth decade, farsightedness (presbyopia) is almost invariable. Still later in life, cataracts, glaucoma, retinal hemorrhages and detachments, macular degeneration, and tumor, unilateral or bilateral, are the most frequent causes of visual impairment.

As a rule, episodic visual loss in early adult life, often hemianopic, is due to migraine. One or more attacks of retrobulbar neuritis, often a harbinger of multiple sclerosis, is the other important cause of transient (weeks) monocular visual loss in this age period. Later in life, transient monocular blindness, or *amaurosis fugax*, is more common; it is related to stenosis of the ipsilateral carotid artery or less often to embolism of retinal arterioles. Rarely, amaurosis occurs in the child or young adult, in which case systemic lupus erythematosus or the antiphospholipid syndrome may be responsible. Or there may be no discernible cause. Cerebrovascular disease deranges vision with increasing frequency in later life.

APPROACH TO THE PROBLEM OF VISUAL LOSS

In the investigation of a disturbance of vision, one must always inquire as to what the patient means when he claims not to see properly, for the disturbance in question may vary from near- or farsightedness to excessive tearing, diplopia, partial syncope, or even giddiness or dizziness. Fortunately the patient's statement can be checked by the measurement of visual acuity, which is the single most important part of the ocular examination. Inspection of the refractive media and the optic fundi—

especially the macular region, the testing of pupillary reflexes, and the plotting of visual fields complete the examination.

In the measurement of visual acuity the *Snellen Chart*, which contains rows of letters of diminishing size, is utilized. The letter at the top of the chart subtends 5 min of an arc at a distance of 200 ft (or roughly 60 m). The patient follows rows of letters that can normally be read at lesser distances. Thus, if the patient can read only the top letter at 20 rather than 200 ft, the acuity is expressed as 20/200 (*V* + 20/200, or 6/60 if distances are measured in meters rather than feet). If the patient's eyesight is normal, the visual acuity will equal 20/20, or 6/6 using the metric scale. Many persons, especially during youth, can read at 20 ft the line that can normally be read at 15 ft from the chart (*V* + 20/15). Patients with a corrected refractive error should wear their glasses for the test. For bedside testing, a "near card" or newsprint held 14 in. from the eyes can be used. In young children, acuity can be estimated by having them mimic the examiner's finger movements at varying distances or recognize and pick up objects of different sizes from varying distances.

If the visual acuity (with glasses) is less than 20/20, either the refractive error has not been properly corrected or there is some other reason for the diminished acuity. The possibility of a refractive error can be ruled out if the patient can read the 20/20 line at a distance (not on a near card) through a pinhole in a cardboard held in front of the eye; the pinhole permits a narrow shaft of light to fall on the macular fovea (the area of greatest visual acuity) without distortion by the curvature of the lens. Minor degrees of visual impairment may be disclosed by alternately stimulating each eye with a bright white or colored object, enabling the patient to compare the intensity of vision in the two eyes. Objects look less bright and colors less saturated when viewed by the faulty eye.

Light entering the eye is focused by the biconvex lens onto the outer layer of the retina. Consequently the cornea, the fluid of the anterior chamber, the lens, the vitreous, and the retina itself must be transparent. The clarity of these media can be determined ophthalmoscopically, and a complete examination requires that the pupil be dilated to at least 6 mm in diameter. This is best accomplished by instilling two drops of 2.5 to 10% phenylephrine (Neosynephrine) or 0.5 to 1.0% tropicamide (Mydriacyl) in each eye after the visual acuity has been measured, the pupillary responses recorded, and the intraocular pressure estimated. In elderly persons, the lower concentrations of these mydriatics should be used. The mydriatic action of phenylephrine lasts for 3 to 6 h. Very rarely, an *attack of angle-closure glaucoma* (manifesting itself by diminished vision, ocular pain, nausea, and vomiting) may be precipitated by pupillary dilation; this requires the immediate attention of an ophthalmologist.

By looking through a high-plus lens of the ophthalmoscope from a distance of 6 to 12 in., the examiner can visualize opacities in the refractive media; by adjusting the lenses from a high-plus to a zero or minus setting, it is possible to "depth-focus" from the cornea to the retina. Depending upon the refractive error of the examiner, lenticular opacities are best seen within the +20 to +12 range. The retina comes into focus with +1 to −1 lenses. The pupil appears as a red circular structure (red reflex), the color being provided by blood in the capillaries of the choroid layer. If all the refractile media are clear, reduced vision that is uncorrectable by glasses is due to a defect in the macula, the optic nerve, or parts of the brain with which they are connected.

NONNEUROLOGIC CAUSES OF REDUCED VISION

It is hardly possible, within the confines of this chapter, to describe all the causes of opacification of the refractive media. Those with the most important medical or neurologic implications are briefly commented upon. Although changes in the refractive media do not involve neural tissue primarily, certain ones are often associated with neurologic disease and provide clues to its presence.

In the *cornea*, the most common abnormality is scarring due to trauma and infection. Ulceration and subsequent fibrosis may occur with recurrent herpes simplex, herpes zoster, and trachomatous infections or with certain mucocutaneous-ocular syndromes (Stevens-Johnson, Reiter). Hypercalcemia secondary to sarcoid, hyperparathyroidism, and vitamin D intoxication or milk-alkali syndrome may give rise to precipitates of calcium phosphate and carbonate beneath the corneal epithelium, primarily in a plane corresponding to the interpalpebral fissure—so-called band keratopathy. Polysaccharides are deposited in the corneas in some of the mucopolysaccharidoses (page1015), and copper in hepatolenticular degeneration (Kayser-Fleischer ring, page 1026). Crystal deposits may be observed in multiple myeloma and cryoglobulinemia. The corneas are also diffusely clouded in certain lysosomal storage diseases (Chap. 37). Arcus senilis occurring at an early age (due to hypercholesterolemia), sometimes combined with yellow lipid deposits in the eyelids and periorbital skin (xanthelasma), serve as markers of atheromatous vascular disease.

In relation to the *anterior chamber* of the eye, the common problem is one of impediment to the outflow of aqueous fluid, leading to excavation of the optic disc and visual loss, i.e., *glaucoma*. In more than 90 percent of cases (of the open-angle type), the cause of this syndrome is unknown; a genetic factor is suspected. The drainage channels in this type appear normal. In about 5 percent, the angle between pupil and lateral cornea is narrow and blocked when the pupil is dilated (angle-closure glaucoma). In the remaining cases, the condition is secondary to some disease process that blocks outflow channels—inflammatory debris of uveitis, red blood cells from hemorrhage in the anterior chamber (hyphema), or new formation of vessels and connective tissue on the surface of the iris (rubeosis iridis), a rare complication of ocular ischemia secondary to diabetes mellitus or carotid artery occlusion. The visual loss is gradual in open-angle glaucoma and the eye looks normal, unlike the red, painful eye of angle-closure glaucoma. However, some cases of open-angle glaucoma may progress to rapid loss of vision. Intraocular pressures that are persistently above 20 mmHg may damage the optic nerve. This may be manifest first as an arcuate defect in the upper or lower nasal field or as an enlargement of the blind spot (Bjerrum field defect), which, if untreated, may go on to blindness. Other characteristic field patterns are winged extensions from the blind spot (Seidel scotoma) and a narrowing of the superior nasal quadrant that may progress to a horizontal edge, corresponding to the horizontal raphe of the retina (nasal step). The damage is at the optic nerve head; with the ophthalmoscope, the optic disc appears excavated and any pallor that is present extends only to the rim of the disc and not beyond, thus distinguishing it from optic neuropathy.

In the *lens*, cataract formation is the common abnormality. The cause of the common type in the elderly is unknown. The "sugar cataract" of diabetes mellitus is the result of sustained high levels of blood glucose, which is changed in the lens to sorbitol, the accumulation of which leads to a high osmotic gradient with swelling and disruption of the lens fibers. Galactosemia is a much rarer cause, but the mechanism of cataract formation is similar, i.e., the accumulation of dulcitol in the lens. In hypoparathyroidism, lowering of the concentration of calcium in the aqueous humor is in some way responsible for the opacification of newly forming superficial lens fibers. Prolonged high doses of chlorpromazine and corticosteroids as well as radiation therapy are believed to induce lenticular opacities as well. Down syndrome and oculocerebrorenal syndrome (Chap. 38), spinocerebellar ataxia with oligophrenia (Chap. 39), and certain dermatologic syndromes (atopic dermatitis, congenital ichthyosis, incontinentia pigmenti) are also accompanied by lenticular opacities. Myotonic dystrophy (Chap. 48) and, rarely, Wilson disease (Chap. 37) are associated with special types of cataract. Subluxation of the lens, the result of weakening of its zonular ligaments, occurs in syphilis, Marfan syndrome, and homocystinuria.

In the *vitreous humor*, hemorrhage may occur from rupture of a ciliary or retinal vessel. On ophthalmoscopic examination, the hemorrhage appears as a diffuse haziness of part or all of the vitreous or, if the blood is between the retina and the vitreous and displaces the latter rather than mixing with it, takes the form of a sharply defined mass. The common causes are orbital or cranial trauma, rupture of an intracranial aneurysm or arteriovenous malformation with high intracranial pressure, rupture of newly formed vessels of proliferative retinopathy in patients with diabetes mellitus, and retinal tears, in which the hemorrhage breaks through the internal limiting membrane of the retina. The commonest vitreous opacities are the benign "floaters" or "spots before the eyes," which appear as gray flecks or threads with changes in the position of the eyes; they may be annoying or even alarming until the person stops looking for them. A sudden burst of flashing lights associated with an increase in floaters may mark the onset of retinal detachment. Another common occurrence, with advancing age, is shrinkage of the vitreous humor and retraction from the retina, causing persistent streaks of light (phosphenes), usually in the periphery of the visual field. The phosphenes, known as "*Moore's lightning streaks*," are quite benign. They are most prominent on movement of the globe, on closure of the eyelids, at the moment of accommodation, with saccadic eye movements, and with sudden exposure to dark. The vitreous may be infiltrated by lymphoma that originates in the brain; biopsy by planar vitrectomy has been used to establish the diagnosis.

The term *uveitis* refers to an infective or noninfective inflammatory disease that affects any of the uveal structures (iris, ciliary body, and choroid.). According to Bienfang and colleagues, uveitis accounts for 10 percent of all cases of legal blindness in the United States. Infective causes are toxoplasma and cytomegalic inclusion disease. Noninfective autoimmune types are more frequent in the adult. The inflammation may be in the anterior part of the eye or in the posterior part, behind the iris and extending to the retina and choroid. Anterior uveitis is sometimes linked to ankylosing spondylitis, and the posterior forms are associated with sarcoidosis, Behçet disease, multiple sclerosis, and lymphoma.

NEUROLOGIC CAUSES OF REDUCED VISION

Certain anatomic and physiologic facts are requisite for an interpretation of the neurologic lesions that affect vision. Visual stimuli entering the eye traverse the inner layers of the retina to reach its outer (posterior) layer, which contains two classes of photoreceptor cells—the flask-shaped cones and the slender rods. The photoreceptors rest on a single layer of pigmented epithelial cells, which form the outermost surface of the retina. The rods and cones and pigmentary epithelium receive their blood supply from the capillaries of the choroid, not from the retinal arterioles. The rod cells contain rhodopsin, a conjugated protein in which the chromophore group is a carotenoid akin to vitamin A. The rods function in the perception of visual stimuli in subdued light (twilight or scotopic vision), and the cones are responsible for color discrimination and the perception of stimuli in bright light (photopic vision). Most of the cones are concentrated in the macular region, particularly in its central part, the *fovea*, and are responsible for the highest level of visual acuity. Specialized pigments in the rods and cones absorb light energy and transform it into electrical signals, which are transmitted to the bipolar cells of the retina and then, in turn, to the superficially (anteriorly) placed neurons, or ganglion cells (Fig. 13-1). There are no ganglion cells in the fovea.

Three types of retinal ganglion cells, referred to as X, Y, and W, have been identified in nonhuman primates on the basis of their retinal topography and terminations. The X cells are centered in the maculae and project to the striate cortex. The Y cells are distributed throughout the retina and project to both the striate cortex and the superior colliculi. The W cells terminate only in the superior colliculi. Presumably the same neuronal types exist in humans, but in different proportions.

The axons of the retinal ganglion cells, as they stream across the inner surface of the retina, pursue an arcuate course. Being unmyelinated, they are not visible, although fluorescein retinography shows a tracery of their outlines and an experienced examiner, using a bright light and deep green filter, can visualize the fibers through direct ophthalmoscopy. The ganglion cell axons are collected in the optic discs and then run uninterruptedly through the *optic nerves*, *optic chiasm*, and *optic tracts* to reach the lateral geniculate nuclei and superior colliculi (Figs. 13-3 and 13-4). The fibers derived from macular cells form a discrete bundle that first occupies the temporal side of the disc and optic nerve and then assumes a more central position within the nerve (papillomacular bundle). These fibers are of smaller caliber than the peripheral optic nerve fibers. It is important to keep in mind the retinal ganglion cells and their axonic extensions are, properly speaking, an exteriorized part of the brain and that the pathologic reactions in this part reflect their CNS origin.

In the optic chiasm, the fibers derived from the nasal half of each retina decussate and continue in the optic tract with uncrossed temporal fibers of the other eye (Figs. 13-2 and 13-3). Thus, interruption of the left optic tract causes a right hemianopic defect in each eye, i.e., a homonymous (left nasal and right temporal) field defect (Fig. 13-3*D*). In partial tract lesions, the visual defects in the two eyes are not exactly congruent, since the tract fibers are not evenly admixed. A variable bundle of fibers from the inferior-nasal part of the optic nerve turns anteriorly into the opposite optic nerve as it crosses in the chiasm (Wilbrand's knee). Lesions at this "junctional" point of the optic nerve and the chiasm are therefore able to cause a contralateral quadrantic defect in addition to the central scotoma that is due to the ipsilateral optic nerve lesion, as shown in Fig. 13-2*B*. The optic chiasm lies just above the pituitary body and also forms part of the anterior wall of the third ventricle; hence the crossing fibers may be compressed from below by a pituitary tumor, a meningioma of the tuberculum sellae, or an aneurysm, and from above by a dilated third ventricle or craniopharyngioma. The resulting field defect is bitemporal (Fig. 13-2*C*); if one optic nerve is also implicated, there will be a loss of full-field vision in that eye. Optic tract lesions, in comparison with chiasmatic and nerve lesions, are relatively rare. Surprisingly, in albinism, there is an abnormality of chiasmatic decussation, in which a majority of the fibers, including many that would not normally cross to the other side, decussate. How this relates to the defect in the pigment epithelium is not known.

The optic tract terminates mainly in the lateral geniculate body and synapses with the six laminae of neurons. Three of these laminae (1, 4, 6), which constitute the large dorsal nucleus receive crossed (nasal) fibers from the contralateral eye, and three laminae (2, 3, 5) receive uncrossed (temporal) fibers from the ipsilateral eye. The geniculate cells project to the visual

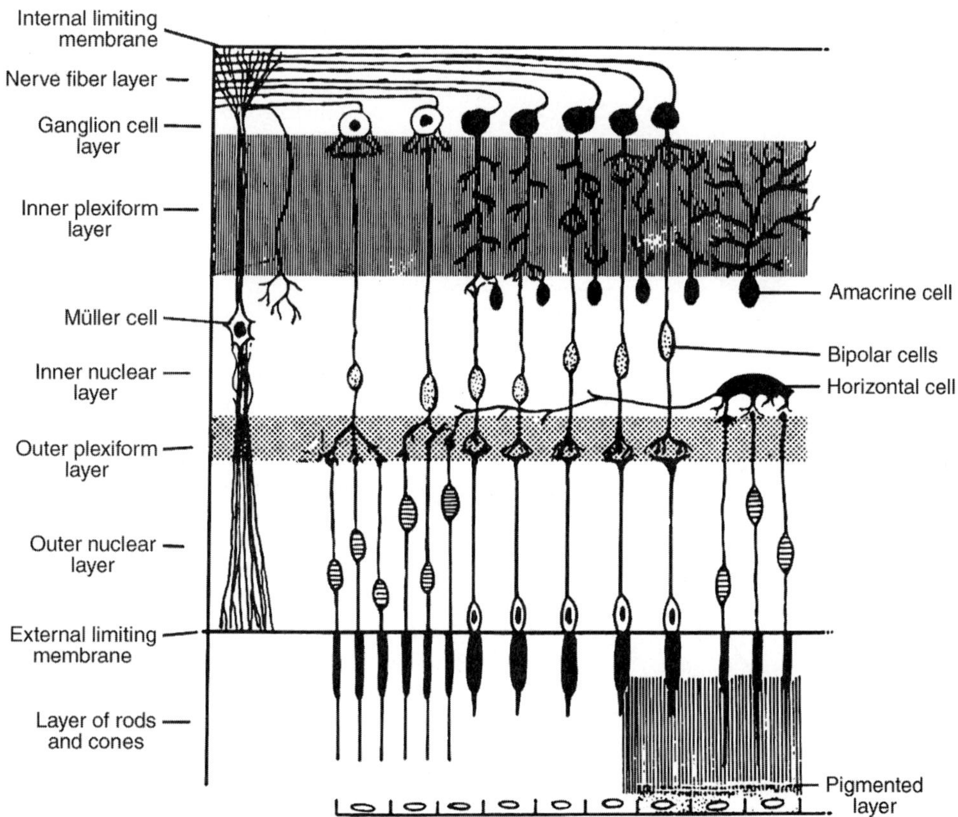

Figure 13-1

Diagram of the cellular elements of the retina. Light entering the eye passes through the full thickness of the retina to reach the rods and cones (first system of retinal neurons). Impulses arising in these cells are transmitted by the bipolar cells (second system of retinal neurons) to the ganglion cell layer. The third system of visual neurons consists of the ganglion cells and their axons, which run uninterruptedly through the optic nerve, chiasm, and optic tracts, synapsing with cells in the lateral geniculate body. (Courtesy of Dr. E. M. Chester.)

(striate) cortex, also called area 17 or V_1. Other optic tract fibers terminate in the pretectum and innervate both Edinger-Westphal nuclei, which subserve pupillary constriction (see Fig. 14-7). If there is a lesion in one optic nerve, a light stimulus to the ipsilateral eye will have no effect on the pupil of either eye, although the ipsilateral pupil will still constrict consensually, i.e., in response to a light stimulus from the normal eye. This is called the *afferent pupillary defect*. Other tract fibers terminate in the pretectal and suprachiasmatic hypothalamic nuclei. The lateral geniculate body is supplied by the posterior and anterior choroidal and thalamogeniculate arteries and is rarely infarcted or exclusively involved in any disease process other than one affecting these vessels.

In their course through the temporal lobes, the fibers from the lower and upper quadrants of each retina diverge. The lower ones arch around the anterior pole of the temporal horn of the lateral ventricle before turning posteriorly; the upper ones follow a more direct path through the white matter of the uppermost part of the temporal lobe (Fig. 13-3) and possibly of the adjacent parietal lobe. Both groups of fibers merge posteriorly at the internal sagittal stratum. For these reasons, incomplete lesions of the geniculocalcarine pathways cause visual field defects that are partial and often not fully congruent (Fig. 13-2*E* and *F*).

It is in Brodmann area 17, embedded in the medial lip of the occipital pole, that cortical processing of the

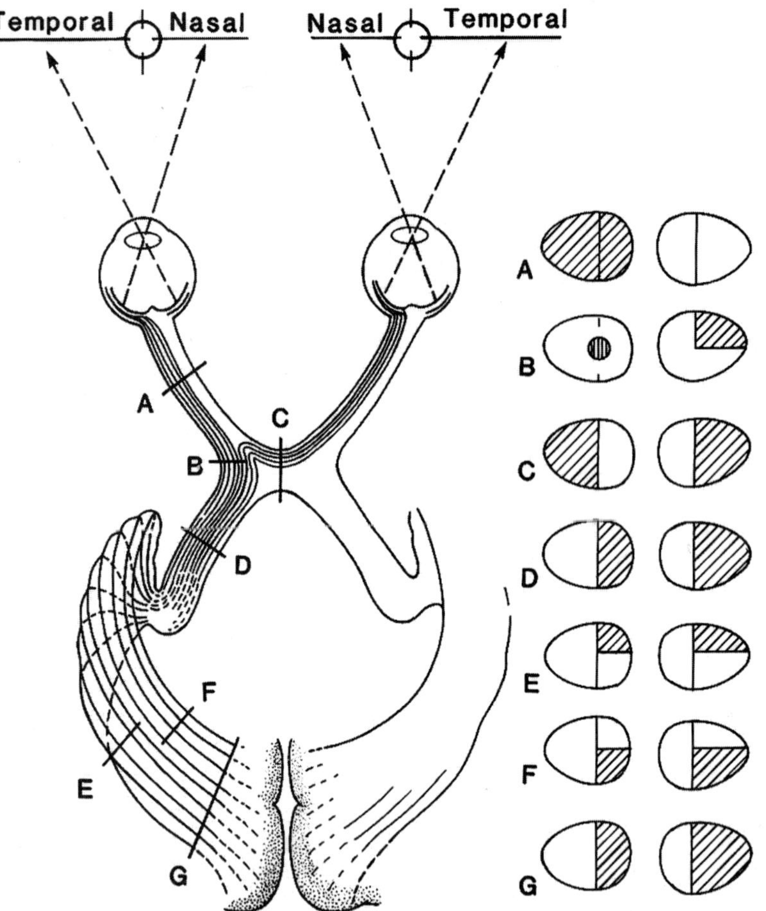

Figure 13-2

Diagram showing the effects on the fields of vision produced by lesions at various points along the optic pathway: A. *Complete blindness in left eye from an optic nerve lesion.* B. *The usual effect is a left-junction scotoma in association with a right upper quadrantanopia. The latter results from interruption of right retinal nasal fibers that project into the base of the left optic nerve (Wilbrand's knee). A left nasal hemianopia could occur from a lesion at this point but is exceedingly rare.* C. *Chiasmatic lesion causing bitemporal hemianopia.* D. *Right homonymous hemianopia from optic tract lesion.* E *and* F. *Right superior and inferior quadrant hemianopia from interruption of visual radiations.* G. *Right homonymous hemianopia due to lesion of striate cortex.*

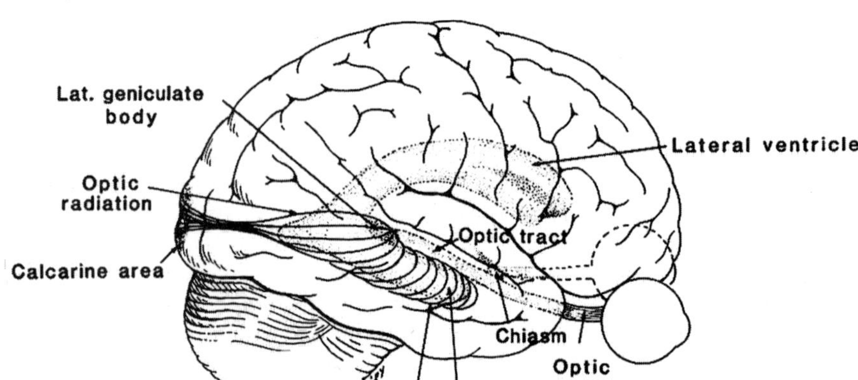

Figure 13-3

The geniculocalcarine projection, showing the detour of lower fibers around the temporal horn. Note that practically none of the pathway traverses the parietal lobe.

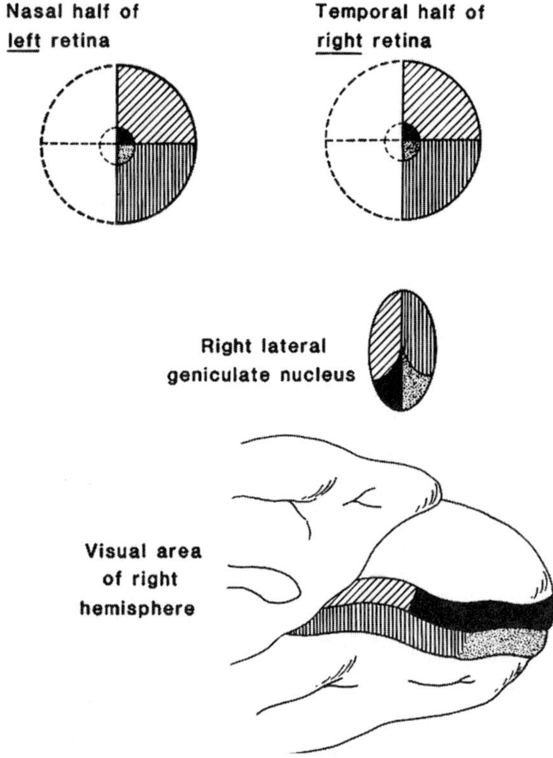

Figure 13-4

Diagrammatic depiction of the retinal projections, showing the disproportionately large representation of the macula in the lateral geniculate nucleus and visual (striate) cortex. (Redrawn by permission from Barr ML, Kiernan J: The Human Nervous System, 4th ed. Philadelphia, Lippincott, 1983.)

retinogeniculate projections occurs. The receptive neurons are arranged in columns, some of which are activated by form and others by moving stimuli or by color. Some of the afferent fibers terminate in the fourth cortical layer and others just above or below it. The neurons for each eye are grouped together and have concentric center-surround receptive fields.

The deep neurons of area 17 project to the secondary and tertiary visual areas of the occipitotemporal cortex of the same and opposite cerebral hemispheres and also to other multisensory parietal and temporal cortices. Several of these extrastriate connections are just now being identified. Separate visual systems are utilized in the perception of motion, color, stereopsis, contour, and depth. The classic studies of Hubel and Wiesel have elucidated much of this visual cortical physiology.

The *normal development* of the connections described above requires that the visual system be activated at each of several critical periods of development. The early deprivation of vision in one eye causes a failure of development of the geniculate and cortical receptive fields of that eye. Moreover, the cortical receptive fields of the seeing eye become abnormally large and usurp the monocular dominance columns of the blind eye (Hubel and Wiesel). In children with congenital cataracts, the eye will remain amblyopic if the opacity is removed later, after this critical period of development. A severe strabismus in early life, especially an esotropia, will have the same effect.

In regard to the *vascular supply* of the eye, the *ophthalmic branch of the internal carotid artery* supplies the retina, posterior coats of the eye, and optic nerve head. This artery gives origin to the posterior ciliary arteries; the latter form a rich circumferential plexus of vessels (arterial circle of Zinn-Haller) located deep to the lamina cribrosa. This arterial circle supplies the optic disc and adjacent part of the optic nerve, the choroid, and the ciliary body; it anastamoses with the pial arterial plexus that surrounds the optic nerve. The other major branch of the ophthalmic artery is the *central retinal artery*. It supplies the inner retinal layers and issues from the optic disc, where it divides into four branches, each of which supplies a quadrant of the retina; it is these vessels and their branches that are visible by ophthalmoscopy. A short distance from the disc, these vessels lose their internal elastic lamina and the media (muscularis) becomes thin; they are properly classed as arterioles. The inner layers of the retina, including the ganglion and bipolar cells, receive their blood supply from these arterioles and their capillaries, whereas the deeper photoreceptor elements and the fovea are nourished by the underlying choroidal vascular bed, by diffusion through the retinal pigmented cells and the semipermeable Bruch's membrane upon which they rest.

Abnormalities of the Retina

As indicated above, this thin (100- to 350-μm) sheet of transparent tissue, and the optic nerve head, into which all visual information flows are an exteriorized part of the CNS and the only part of the nervous system that can be inspected directly by ophthalmoscopic examination. Common mistakes in funduscopic examination are a failure to carefully inspect the macular zone (which is located 3 to 4 mm lateral to the optic disc and provides for 95 percent of visual acuity) and to search the periphery of the retina through a dilated pupil. There are variations in the appearance of the normal macula and optic disc, and these may prove troublesome. A normal macula may be called abnormal because of a slight aberration of the retinal pigment epithelium or a few drusen (see further on). With experience, the unmyelinated nerve fiber layer of the retina can be visualized by using bright-green (red-free) illumination. This is most often helpful in detecting demyelinative lesions of the optic nerve, which produce a loss of discrete bundles of the radially arranged and arching retinal fibers as they converge onto the disc.

The normal optic disc varies in color, being paler in infants and in blond individuals; and the prominence of the lamina cribrosa (a sieve-like structure in the central and nasal part of the disc through which run the fascicles of unmyelinated axons of the retinal ganglion cells) differs from one individual to another. The absence of receptive elements in the optic disc, or papilla, accounts for the normal blind spot. The ganglion-cell axons normally acquire their myelin sheaths after penetration of the lamina cribrosa, but they sometimes do so in their intraretinal course, as they approach the disc. The myelinated fibers adjacent to the disc appear as white patches with fine-feathered edges and are a normal variant, not to be confused with exudates.

In evaluating changes *in the retinal vessels*, one must remember that these are arterioles and not arteries. Since the walls of retinal arterioles are transparent, what is seen with the ophthalmoscope is the column of blood within them. The central light streak of many normal arterioles is thought to represent the reflection of light from the ophthalmoscope as it strikes the interface of the column of blood and the concave vascular wall. In *arteriolosclerosis* (usually coexistent with hypertension), the lumina of the vessels are segmentally narrowed because of fibrous tissue replacement of the media and thickening of the basement membrane. Straightening of the arterioles and arteriolar-venular compression are other signs of hypertension and arteriolosclerosis. It is generally believed that the vein is compressed by the thickened arteriole within the adventitial envelope shared by both vessels at the site of crossing; this compression may lead to occlusion of branches of the retinal veins. Progressive arteriolar disease, to the point of occlusion of the lumen, results in a narrow, white ("silver-wire") vessel with no visible blood column. This change is associated most often with severe hypertension but may follow other types of occlusion of the central retinal artery or its branches (see descriptions and retinal illustrations further on). Sheathing of the venules, probably representing focal leakage of cells from the vessels, is observed in approximately 25 percent of patients with multiple sclerosis. Similar alterations are also seen in leukemia, malignant hypertension, sarcoid, Behçet disease, and other forms of vasculitis.

In *malignant hypertension* there are, in addition to the retinal arteriolar changes noted above, a number of extravascular lesions: the so-called soft exudates or cotton-wool patches, sharply marginated and glistening "hard" exudates, retinal hemorrhages, and edema of the disc. In many patients who show these retinal changes, analogous lesions are to be found in the brain (necrotizing arteriolitis and microinfarcts). These are the changes that underlie hypertensive encephalopathy.

The ophthalmoscopic appearance of *retinal hemorrhages* is determined by the structural arrangements of the particular tissue in which they occur. In the superficial layer of the retina, they are linear or flame-shaped ("splinter" hemorrhages) because of their confinement by the horizontally coursing nerve fibers in that layer. These hemorrhages usually overlie and obscure the retinal vessels. Round or oval ("dot-and-blot") hemorrhages lie behind the vessels, in the outer plexiform layer of the retina (synaptic layer between bipolar cells and nuclei of rods and cones—Fig. 13-1); in this layer, blood accumulates in the form of a cylinder between vertically oriented nerve fibers and appears round or oval when viewed end-on with the ophthalmoscope. Rupture of arterioles on the inner surface of the retina—as occurs with ruptured intracranial saccular aneurysms, arteriovenous malformations, and other conditions causing sudden severe elevation of intracranial pressure—permits the accumulation of a sharply outlined lake of blood between the internal limiting membrane of the retina and the coalescing vitreous or hyaloid membrane (the condensed gel at the periphery of the vitreous body); this is the subhyaloid or preretinal hemorrhage. Either the small superficial or deep retinal hemorrhage may show a central or eccentric pale (Roth) spot, which is caused by an accumulation of white blood cells, fibrin, histiocytes, or amorphous material between the vessel and the hemorrhage. This lesion is said to be characteristic of bacterial endocarditis, but is also seen in leukemia and in embolic retinopathy due to carotid disease.

Cotton-wool patches or soft exudates, like splinter hemorrhages, overlie and tend to obscure the retinal blood vessels. These patches, even large ones, rarely cause serious disturbances of vision unless they involve the macula. Soft exudates are in reality infarcts of the nerve fiber layer, due to occlusion of arterioles and capillaries; they are composed of clusters of ovoid structures called *cytoid bodies*, representing the terminal swellings of interrupted axons. *Hard exudates* appear as punctate white or yellow bodies; they lie in the outer plexiform layer, behind the retinal vessels, like the punctate hemorrhages. If present in the macular region, they are arranged in lines radiating toward the fovea (*macular star*). Hard exudates consist of fibrin strands, neutral fat, and fatty acids; their pathogenesis is not understood. They are observed most often in cases of diabetes mellitus and accelerated hypertension. *Drusen (colloid bodies)* appear ophthalmoscopically as pale yellow spots and are difficult to distinguish from hard exudates except when they occur alone; as a rule, hard exudates are accompanied by other funduscopic abnormalities. The source of retinal drusen is uncertain; probably they represent benign accumulations of lipofuscin and other cellular debris derived from the retinal pigment epithelium (D'Amico). *Hyaline bodies*, located on or near the optic disc, are also referred to as drusen but must be distinguished from those occurring peripherally. Drusen of the optic discs are probably mineralized residues of dead axons and can be seen on computed tomography (CT) in some cases. Their main significance for neurologists is that they are often associated with anomalous elevation of the disc and can be mistaken for papilledema (Table 13-1).

Aneurysms of retinal vessels appear as small, discrete red dots and are located in largest number in the paracentral region. They are most often a sign of diabetes mellitus, sometimes appearing before the usual clinical manifestations of that disease have become obvious. The use of the red-free (green) light on the ophthalmoscope helps to pick out microaneurysms from the background. Microscopically, the aneurysms take the form of small (20- to 90-mm) saccular outpouchings from the walls of capillaries, venules, or arterioles. The vessels of origin of the aneurysms are invariably abnormal, being either acellular branches of occluded vessels or themselves occluded by fat or fibrin.

Finally, the periphery of the retina may harbor a hemangioblastoma, which may appear during adolescence, before the more characteristic cerebellar lesion. A large retinal artery may be seen leading to it and a large vein draining it. Occasionally, retinal examination discloses the presence of a vascular malformation that may be coextensive with a much larger malformation of the optic nerve and basilar portions of the brain.

Ischemic Lesions of the Retina Occlusion of the internal carotid artery may cause no disturbance of vision whatsoever provided that there are adequate anastomotic branches from the external carotid artery in the orbit. Rarely, carotid occlusion with inadequate collateralization is associated with a chronic ischemic oculopathy, which may predominantly affect the anterior or posterior segment or both. Insufficient circulation to the anterior segment is manifest by episcleral vascular congestion, cloudiness of the cornea, anterior chamber flare, rubeosis and iris atrophy (rubeosis iridis) and an abnormally low or high intraocular pressure. Ischemia of the posterior segment is manifest by circulatory changes in the retina and optic nerve and venous stasis. Other neurologic signs of carotid disease may be present (pages 829–834).

More often, ischemia of the retina can be traced to the central retinal artery or its branches, which may be occluded by thrombi or emboli. Occlusion of the main artery is attended by sudden blindness. The retina becomes opaque and has a gray-yellow appearance; the arterioles are narrowed, with segmentation of columns of blood and a cherry-red appearance of the fovea (Fig. 13-5)*. With branch occlusions by emboli, one may be able to see the occluding material. Most frequently observed are so-called Hollenhorst plaques—glistening, white-yellow atheromatous particles (Fig. 13-6) seen in 40 of 70 cases of retinal embolism in the series of Arruga and Sanders. The remainder are white calcium particles, from calcified aortic or mitral valves or atheroma of the great vessels, and red or white fibrin-platelet emboli. The latter may be asymptomatic or associated with transient blindness and may be difficult to see without fluorescein retinography; these emboli

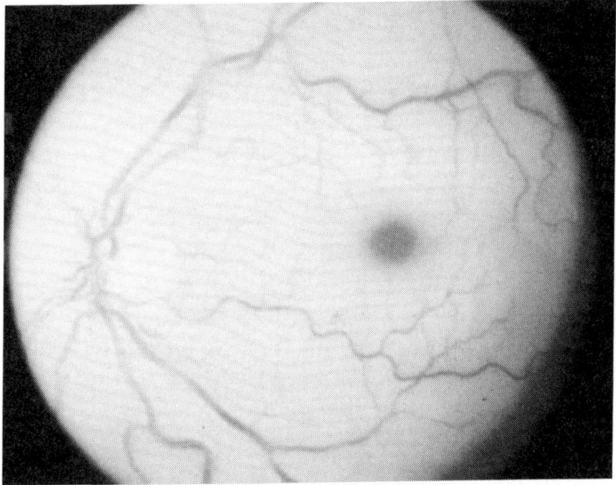

Figure 13-5

Appearance of the fundus in central retinal artery occlusion. In addition to the paucity of blood flow in retinal vessels, the retina has a creamy gray appearance and there is a "cherry red spot" at the fovea.

*Figure 13-5 and subsequent fundoscopic illustrations courtesy of Dr. Shirley Wray.

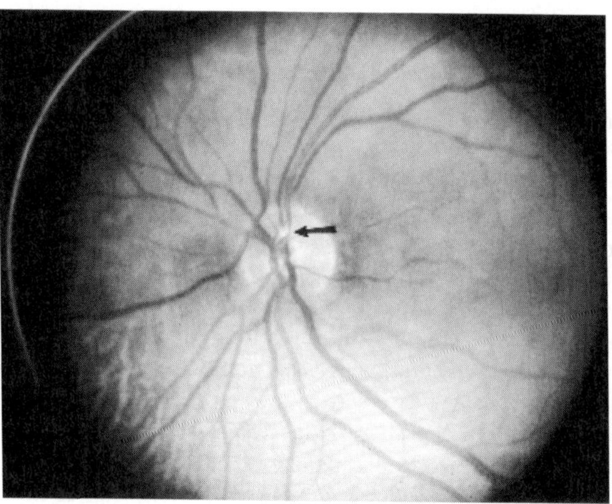

Figure 13-6

Glistening "Hollenhorst plaque" occlusion of a superior retinal artery branch (arrow). These occlusions represent atheromatous particles or platelet-fibrin emboli. Some are asymptomatic and others are associated with segmental visual loss or are seen after central retinal artery occlusion.

soon disappear. Transient ischemic attacks of visual loss, involving all or part of the field of vision of one eye, are referred to as *amaurosis fugax* or *transient monocular blindness (TMB)* and are common manifestations of atherosclerotic carotid stenosis or ulceration. Inspection of the retina during an attack shows stagnation of arterial blood flow, which returns within seconds or minutes as vision is restored (Fisher). One or a hundred attacks may precede infarction of a cerebral hemisphere in the territory of the anterior or middle cerebral artery. In one series of 80 such patients followed by Marshall and Meadows for 4 years, 16 percent developed permanent unilateral blindness, a completed hemispheral stroke, or both. If one eye is affected in this way, there is one chance in four that the other will be involved, usually within the first year (Sawle et al). This subject is discussed further in Chap. 34, on cerebrovascular diseases.

Since the central retinal artery and vein share a common adventitial sheath, atheromatous plaques in the artery are said to be associated in some instances with thrombosis of the retinal vein. There is then a spectacular display of retinal lesions that differs from the picture of central retinal artery occlusion. The veins are engorged and tortuous, and there are diffuse "dot-and-blot" and streaky linear retinal hemorrhages (Fig. 13-7).

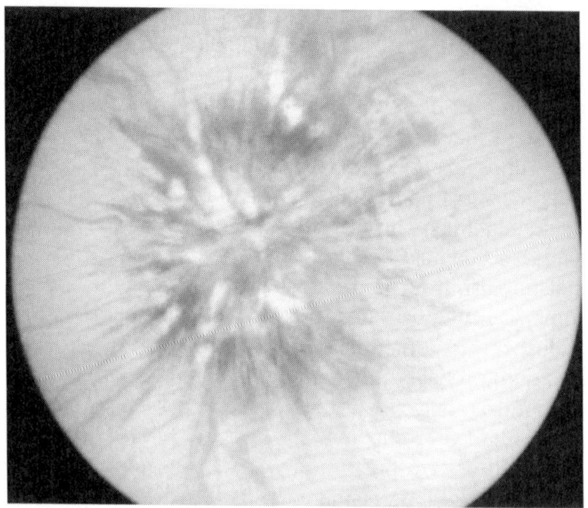

Figure 13-7

Occlusion of the central retinal vein with suffusion of the veins, swelling of the disc, and florid retinal hemorrhages.

This lesion is observed most frequently with diabetes mellitus, hypertension, and leukemia; less frequently with sickle cell disease; and rarely with multiple myeloma and macroglobulinemia, in relation to the hyperviscosity they cause. Sometimes no associated systemic disease can be identified, in which case the possibility of an orbital mass (e.g., optic nerve glioma) should always be considered. In retinal vein thrombosis, visual loss is variable and there may be recovery of useful vision.

A transitory retinal ischemia is observed occasionally as a manifestation of migraine; it has also been observed in polycythemia, hyperglobulinemia, and sickle cell anemia. Massive blood loss or intraoperative hypotension, particularly in association with the use of a heart bypass pump, may also produce visual loss and ischemic infarction of the retina and optic nerve. In younger persons, transient monocular blindness is relatively uncommon and the cause is often not immediately apparent, although ischemia related to the antiphospholipid antibody or migraine is presumed to be responsible for many cases.

More common than retinal ischemia as a cause of sudden monocular blindness, especially in elderly persons, is *ischemic optic neuropathy*. It is due to infarction of the optic disc and sometimes of the retrobulbar portion of the optic nerve, for which reason it is considered further on with diseases of the optic nerve.

In summary, sudden painless monocular loss of vision should always raise the question of ischemia of the retina, due either to occlusive disease of the central retinal artery or vein or to ischemic optic neuropathy.

Detachment of the retina, macular or vitreous hemorrhage, and acute glaucoma are less common but obvious causes.

Other Diseases of the Retina Aside from vascular lesions, other alterations of the retina, namely tears and detachments, may impair vision acutely. One form of retinal detachment is really an intraretinal detachment due to a collection of blood or fluid separating the photoreceptive layer from the pigment epithelium. In so-called traction detachment—observed in cases of premature birth or proliferative retinopathy secondary to diabetes or other vascular disease—contracting fibrous tissue may forcibly elevate the entire retina from the choroid.

Serous retinopathy and chorioretinitis represent another category of retinal disease. In serous retinitis, a condition that occurs most often in young or middle-aged males, the entire perimacular zone is elevated by edema fluid. Vision is usually distorted but acuity is not much impaired. The optic disc remains normal. The retinal change is best revealed by fluorescein angiography. In chorioretinitis, there may also be difficulty in diagnosis and, in a few of our cases, the initial diagnosis had been retrobulbar neuritis. One cannot depend upon the appearance of a macular star (see above) for diagnosis.

A majority of patients with acquired immunodeficiency syndrome (AIDS) develop retinal lesions. Infarcts of the nerve-fiber layer (cotton-wool patches), hemorrhages, and perivascular sheathing are the usual findings. Toxoplasmosis is the most common infective lesion, followed by cytomegalovirus (CMV), but histoplasmosis, syphilis, and tuberculosis have also been implicated. Both the retina and choroid may be involved by these diseases, in which case the ophthalmoscopic picture is characteristic. Destruction of the retina and the pigment epithelium of the choroid produces punched-out lesions, exposing the whitish sclera and deposits of black pigment in various forms. The choroid may be the site of viral and noninfective inflammatory reactions, often in association with recurrent iridocyclitis and lacrimal inflammation.

Degenerations of the retina are an important cause of chronic visual loss. They assume several forms and may be associated with other neurologic abnormalities. The most frequent in youth and middle age is *retinitis pigmentosa*, a hereditary disease of the outer photoreceptor layer and subjacent pigment epithelium. The retina is thin, and there are fine deposits of black pigment in the shape of bone corpuscles, more in the periphery; later the optic discs become pale. Clinically this disorder is marked by constriction of the fields with relative sparing of central vision ("gun-barrel" vision), metamorphopsia (distorted vision), delayed recovery from glare, and nyctalopia (reduced twilight vision). It may be associated with the Laurence-Moon-Biedl syndrome, with certain mitochondrial diseases (Kearns-Sayre syndrome), and with certain degenerative and metabolic diseases (e.g., Refsum disease) of the nervous system. In one form of retinitis pigmentosa, which follows an autosomal dominant pattern of inheritance and is linked to chromosome 3, the gene for rhodopsin (a combination of vitamin A and the rod-cell protein opsin) produces a defective opsin. This results in a diminution of rhodopsin in rod cells, a diminished response to light, and eventual degeneration of the rod cells (Dryja et al).

Another early-life hereditary retinal degeneration, characterized by massive central retinal lesions, is the autosomal recessive Stargardt form of juvenile tapetoretinal degeneration. Like retinitis pigmentosa, Stargardt disease may be accompanied by progressive spastic paraparesis or ataxia. *Nonpigmentary retinal degeneration* is a familiar feature of a number of other rare syndromes and diseases, such as neuronal ceroid lipofuscinosis (pages 1014 and 1024), Bassen-Kornzweig disease (pages 1021 and 1421), Refsum disease (page 1421), Batten-Mayou disease (page 1014), and others (see Chap. 37).

Macular degeneration is the most important cause of visual loss in the elderly. Examination discloses central scotomata and an alteration of the retina around the maculae. Central vision gradually diminishes, preventing reading, but these patients can still get about because of retained peripheral vision.

Phenothiazine derivatives may conjugate with the melanin of the pigment layer, resulting in degeneration of the outer layers of the retina and a characteristic "bull's eye retinopathy," demonstrated by fluorescein angiography. These drugs should be administered in their lowest effective dosage and the patient tested frequently for defects in visual fields and color vision.

Retinal degeneration may also occur in patients with an oat cell carcinoma of the lung. Antiretinal ganglion cell antibodies, presumably produced by the tumor cells, have been demonstrated in the serum of such patients by several authors (Grunwald; Kornguth et al; Jacobson et al).

Certain lysosomal diseases of infancy and early childhood are characterized by an abnormal accumulation of undegraded proteins, polysaccharides, and lipids in cerebral neurons as well as in the macula and other parts of the retina (hence the terms *storage diseases* and *cerebromacular degenerations*). Corneal clouding, cherry-red spot and graying of the retina, and later optic atrophy are the observed ocular abnormalities. These diseases are discussed in Chap. 37.

In some of these retinal diseases, minimal changes in the pigment epithelium or other layers of the retina, enough to reduce visual acuity, may not be readily detected by ophthalmoscopy. In these circumstances, it is helpful to estimate the time required for recovery of visual acuity following light stimulation (macular photostress test). This test consists of shining a strong light through the pupil of an affected eye for 10 s and measuring the time necessary for the acuity to return to the pretest level (normally 50 s or less). With macular lesions, recovery time is prolonged, but with lesions of the optic nerve, it is not affected. Retinal diseases reduce or abolish the electrical activity generated by the outer layers of the retina, and this can be measured in the electroretinogram. Fluorescein retinography may also be helpful.

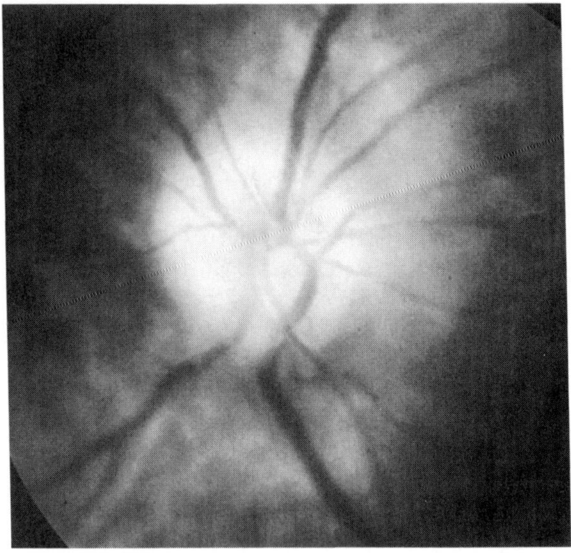

Figure 13-8

Mild papilledema with hyperemia of the disc and slight blurring of the disc margins.

Papilledema and Raised Intracranial Pressure

Of the various abnormalities of the optic disc, *papilledema*, or *optic disc swelling*, has the greatest neurologic implication, for it signifies the presence of increased intracranial pressure. It must be made clear, however, that an ophthalmoscopic appearance identical to that of papilledema can be produced by infarction of the optic nerve head (anterior ischemic optic neuropathy) and by inflammatory changes in the intraorbital portion of the optic nerve (papillitis," or optic neuritis). Certain additional clinical and funduscopic findings, listed in Table 13-1 and described below, assist in distinguishing these processes, although all share the basic feature of conspicuous disc swelling.

In its mildest form, the papilledema may take the form of only slight elevation of the disc and blurring of the disc margins, especially of the superior and inferior aspects and a mild fullness of the veins in the disc. Since many normal individuals, especially those with hypermetropia, have ill-defined disc margins, this early stage of papilledema may be difficult to detect (Fig. 13-8). Pulsations of the retinal veins, best seen where the veins turn to enter the disc, will have disappeared by the time intracranial pressure is raised, but this criterion is not absolute, since venous pulsations cannot be seen in 10 to 15 percent of normal individuals. On the other hand, the presence of spontaneous venous pulsations is a reliable indicator of an intracranial pressure below 180 to 190 mmH_2O and thus usually excludes the presence of early papilledema. Fluorescein angiography, red-free fundus photos (which highlight the retinal nerve fibers), and stereoscopic fundus photography may be helpful in detecting early edema of the optic discs.

More pronounced degrees of papilledema appear as a "mushrooming" of the entire disc and surrounding retina, with edema and obscuration of vessels at the disc margins and in some instances, peripapillary hemorrhages (Fig. 13-9). When advanced, papilledema is almost always bilateral, although it may be more pronounced on the side of an intracranial tumor. A purely unilateral edema of the optic disc is usually associated with perioptic meningioma or other tumor involving the optic nerve, but it can occur at an early stage of increased intracranial pressure. As the papilledema becomes chronic, elevation of the disc margin becomes less prominent and pallor of the optic nerve head more evident (Fig. 13-10). Varying degrees of secondary optic atrophy follow, leaving the disc pale and shrunken. Unlike the case in primary optic atrophy, the disc margins are irregular, often with peripapillary pigment deposits.

It is important to emphasize that *acute papilledema* from raised intracranial pressure does not affect visual acuity except transiently during spontaneous waves of greatly increased pressure. Therefore optic disc

Table 13-1
Main causes of swelling of the optic disc

Ophthalmic abnormality	*Underlying cause*	*Visual loss*	*Associated symptoms*	*Pupils*
Papilledema	Increased intracranial pressure	None or transient blurring; constriction of visual fields and enlargement of blind spot; findings almost always binocular	Headache; signs of intracranial mass	Normal unless succeeded by optic atrophy
Anterior ischemic optic neuropathy (AION)	Infarction of disc and intraorbital optic nerve due to atherosclerosis or temporal arteritis	Acute visual loss, monocular (usually); may be an altitudinal defect	Headache with temporal arteritis	Afferent pupillary defect
Optic neuritis[a] ("papillitis")	Inflammatory changes in disc and intraorbital part of optic nerve—usually due to MS, sometimes to ADEM	Rapidly progressive visual loss; usually monocular	Tender globe, pain on ocular movement	Afferent pupillary defect
Hyaline bodies[b] (drusen)	Congenital, familial	Usually none; may be slowly progressive enlargement of blindspot or arcuate inferior nasal defect	Usually none; rarely transient visual obscurations	Afferent pupillary defect Normal

Key: MS, multiple sclerosis; ADEM, acute disseminated encephalomyelopathy.
[a]Optic neuritis affecting the retrobulbar portion of the nerve shows no funduscopic changes.
[b]May be mistaken for papilledema (pseudopapilledema).

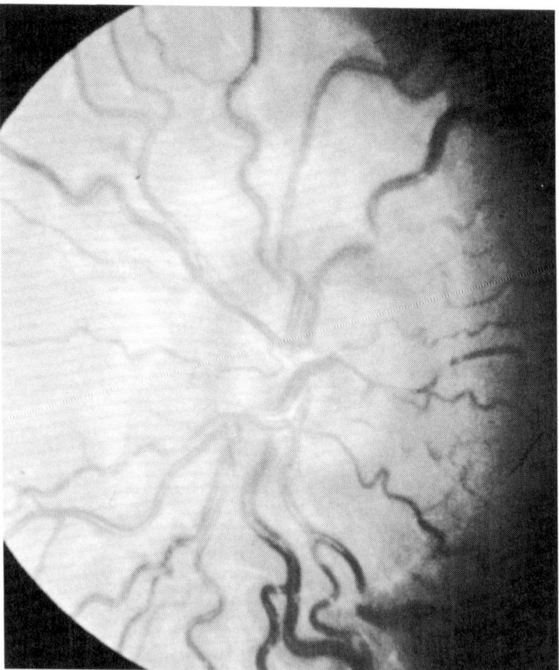

Figure 13-9

Fully developed papilledema. The main characteristics are marked swelling and enlargement of the disc, vascular engorgement, obscuration of small vessels at the disc margin as a result of nerve fiber edema, and white "cotton-wool spots" that represent superficial infarcts of the nerve fiber layer.

swelling in a patient with severely reduced vision is usually due not to papilledema but to intraorbital optic neuritis (papillitis) or to infarction of the nerve head (ischemic optic neuropathy), both of which are described further on. The examiner is aided by the fact that papilledema is generally bilateral, although the degree of disc swelling tends not to be symmetrical; in contrast, papillitis and infarction of the nerve head usually affect one eye, but there are exceptions to both of these statements. Also, the pupillary reaction to light is muted only with the latter disorders, not with papilledema. The occurrence of papilledema on one side and optic atrophy on the other is referred to as the Foster Kennedy syndrome and is attributable to a frontal lobe tumor or an olfactory meningioma on the side of the atrophic disc. In its complete form, which is seen only rarely, there is also anosmia on the side of the optic atrophy.

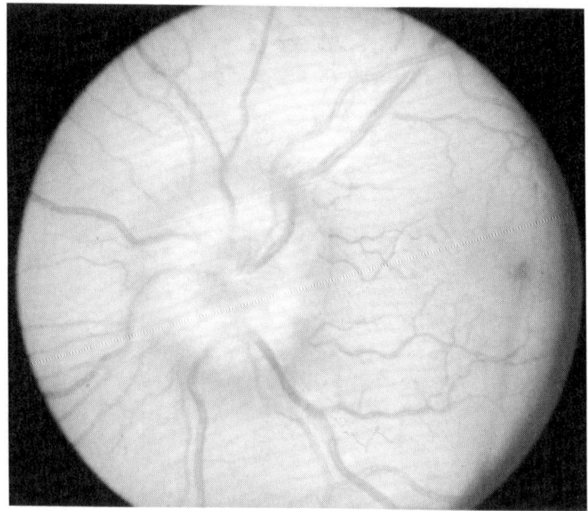

Figure 13-10

Chronic papilledema with beginning optic atrophy, in which the disc stands out like a champagne cork. The hemorrhages and exudates have been absorbed, leaving a glistening residue around the disc.

Papilledema due to increased intracranial pressure must be distinguished from combined edema of the optic nerve and retina, which typifies both malignant hypertension and posterior uveitis with retinitis as well as infarction of the disc, described further on. Papilledema due to infarction of the nerve head is characterized by extension of the swelling beyond the nerve head, as described below, whereas the papilledema of increased pressure is associated with peripapillary hemorrhages. Often this distinction cannot be made on the basis of the funduscopic appearance alone, in which case the most reliable distinguishing feature is the presence or absence of visual loss (Table 13-1).

The essential element in the pathogenesis of papilledema is an increase in pressure in the sheaths of the optic nerve, which communicate directly with the subarachnoid space of the brain. This was demonstrated convincingly by Hayreh (1964), who produced bilateral chronic papilledema in monkeys by inflating balloons in the temporal subarachnoid space and then opening the sheath of one optic nerve; the papilledema promptly subsided on the operated side but not on the opposite side. Many years ago, Paton and Holmes hypothesized that the increased pressure in the perioptic subarachnoid spaces blocks the central retinal vein, leading to congestion in the capillary circulation of the optic nerve head. However, the picture of central retinal vein obstruction—consisting of rapidly evolving retinal edema, marked venous dilatation, and florid retinal hemorrhages—is quite different from that of papilledema.

Furthermore, the capillaries that become congested in papilledema are derived not from the central retinal vein but from the short ciliary arteries (Hayreh). More recently, the pathogenesis of papilledema has been restudied in terms of axoplasmic flow in the optic nerve fibers (Minckler et al; Tso and Hayreh). These investigators found that compression of the optic nerve fibers by the elevated cerebrospinal fluid (CSF) pressure resulted in swelling of axons behind the optic nerve head and leakage of their contents into the extracellular spaces of the disc; these changes were thought to be responsible for the swelling of the optic disc and blurring of the disc margins. The vascular changes (hyperemia of the disc, capillary dilatation, and hemorrhages) appeared later and were considered to be secondary to edema of the optic disc. In our opinion, the block in axonic flow alone could not account for the marked congestion of vessels and hemorrhages.

The mechanism of papilledema that rarely accompanies spinal tumors, particularly oligodendrogliomas, and the Guillain-Barré syndrome is not entirely clear. Usually the CSF protein is more than 1000 mg/100 mL, but this cannot be the entire explanation, since cases occur in which the protein concentration is only slightly elevated. (See Chap. 30.) In other diseases that at times give rise to papilledema—e.g., chronic lung disease with hypercarbia, leukemia with meningeal infiltration, or dural arteriovenous malformation—the mechanism is most often one of generalized increase of intracranial pressure. Puzzling, however, are cases of papilledema without raised intracranial pressure, as may occur in children with cyanotic congenital heart disease and other forms of polycythemia.

Abnormalities of the Optic Nerves

These structures, which constitute the axonic projections of the retinal ganglion cells to the lateral geniculate bodies and superior colliculi (the third visual neurons), can be inspected only in the optic nerve head. Observable changes in the optic disc are, therefore, of particular importance. They may reflect the presence of raised intracranial pressure (papilledema or "choked disc"), as already described, optic neuritis ("papillitis"), infarction of the optic nerve head, congenital defects of the optic nerves (optic pits and colobomas), hypoplasia and atrophy of the optic nerves, and glaucoma. Illustrations of these and other abnormalities of the disc and ocular fundus can be found in the atlas by E. M. Chester and in the text by Glaser, listed in the References.

The main causes of visual loss from optic neuropathy are listed in Table 13-2 and are discussed in subsequent portions of this chapter.

Table 13-2
Main Causes of Unilateral and Bilateral Optic Neuropathy

I. Demyelinative (optic neuritis)
- Multiple sclerosis
- Postinfectious and viral neuroretinitis

II. Ischemic
- Arteriosclerotic (usually in-situ occlusion; rarely carotid artery disease)
- Granulomatous (giant cell) arteritis
- Syphilitic arteritis

III. Parainfectious
- Cavernous sinus thrombosis
- Paranasal sinus infection

IV. Toxins and drugs
- Methanol
- Ethambutol
- Chloroquine
- Streptomycin
- Chlorpropamide
- Chloramphenicol
- Ergot compounds, etc.

V. Deficiency states
- Vitamin B_{12}
- Thiamine or possibly several B vitamins ("tobacco-alcohol" amblyopia)
- Epidemic nutritional types (Cuban, Jamaican)

VI. Heredofamilial and developmental
- Dominant juvenile optic atrophy
- Leber optic atrophy (see page 1164)
- Developmental failure of disc or papillomacular bundle
- Progressive hyaline body encroachment

VII. Compressive and infiltrative
- Meningioma of sphenoid wing or olfactory groove
- Metastasis to optic nerve or chiasm
- Glioma of optic nerve (neurofibromatosis type I)
- Optic atrophy following long-standing papilledema
- Pituitary tumor and apoplexy (page 717)
- Thyroid ophthalmopathy
- Sarcoid
- Lymphoma
- Wegener granulomatosis

Optic Neuritis (Papillitis; Retrobulbar Neuritis; See page 963**)** Acute impairment of vision in one eye or both eyes (in the latter case the eyes may be affected either simultaneously or successively) develops in a number of clinical settings. The most frequent is one in which an adolescent or young adult (rarely a child) notes a rapid diminution of vision in one eye (as though a veil had covered the eye), sometimes progressing within hours or days to complete blindness. The optic disc and retina may appear normal (retrobulbar neuritis), but if the lesion of the optic nerve is near the nerve head, there may be swelling of the disc, i.e., papillitis (Fig. 13-11); the disc margins are then seen to be elevated, blurred, and rarely surrounded by hemorrhages. As indicated above, papillitis is associated with marked impairment of vision and a scotoma, thus distinguishing it from the papilledema of increased intracranial pressure. Pain on movement and tenderness on pressure of the globe and a difference between the two eyes in the perception of brightness of light are other consistent findings (Table 13-1). The patient may report an increase in blurring of vision with exertion or following a hot bath (Uthoff phenomenon). In addition to papillitis, examination may disclose an impairment of color vision and variable haziness of the vitreous that causes difficulty in visualizing the retina. Inflammatory sheathing of the retinal veins, as described by Rucker, has been an uncommon finding in our cases of optic neuritis and papillitis. Edema may suffuse from the disc to cause a rippling in the adjacent retina. In about 10 percent of cases, both eyes are involved, either simultaneously or in rapid succession.

In a large proportion of such patients, at least initially, no cause of the retrobulbar neuropathy can be found. After several weeks there is spontaneous recovery; vision returns to normal in more than two-thirds of instances. Regression of symptoms may occur spontaneously or may be hastened by the intravenous administration of high doses of corticosteroids, but the oral administration of the same drugs appears to increase the frequency of a relapse of optic neuritis (page 973). Occasionally, diminution of brightness, dyschromatopsia, or a scotoma is left; much more rarely, the patient is left blind. The optic disc later becomes slightly pale, especially on the temporal side, and the pallor extends beyond the margins of the disc into the peripapillary retinal nerve fiber layer. The CSF may be normal or may contain from 10 to 100 lymphocytes, an elevated total protein and gamma globulin, and oligoclonal bands.

As time progresses, approximately half of such patients will develop other symptoms and signs of multiple sclerosis within 5 years, and probably even more do so when they are observed for longer periods. Conversely, in approximately 15 percent of patients with multiple sclerosis, the history discloses that retrobulbar neuritis was the first symptom. Multiple sclerosis is the most common cause of a unilateral retrobulbar neuritis, but post-infectious demyelinative disease is a probable cause of the minority that do not progress to multiple sclerosis. Less is known about children with retrobulbar neuropathy, in whom the disorder is more often bilateral and frequently related to a preceding viral infection ("neuroretinitis," see below). Their prognosis is better than that of adults. Formerly, the syndrome was often blamed on sinus disease, but this rarely affects vision and should be considered only in the face of other evidence of infection, such as fever, purulent nasal discharge, leukocytosis, etc. Treatment of optic neuritis is discussed in the context of multiple sclerosis on page 973. Occasionally, a sphenoidal or ethmoidal mucocele can compress the optic nerve. *Leber hereditary optic atrophy* may simulate retrobulbar neuropathy even in causing a relatively abrupt onset of visual loss and some degree of recovery (page 1164).

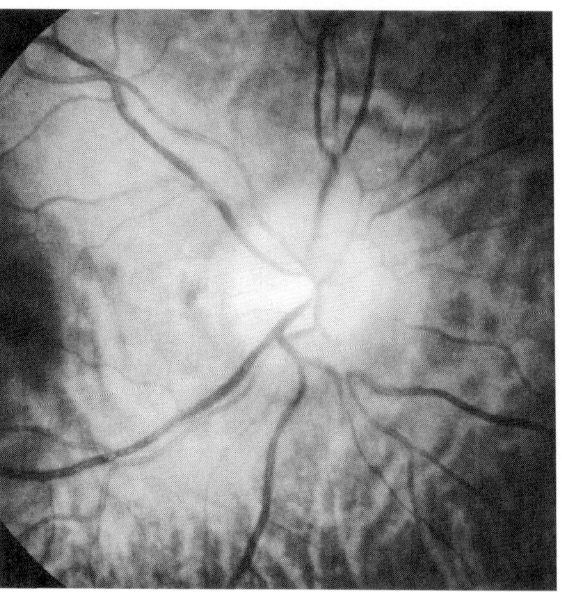

Figure 13-11

Acute optic neuritis in a patient with multiple sclerosis. The disc is swollen from an inflammatory process near the nerve head (papillitis) and the patient is virtually blind.

In a condition that is related to optic neuritis known as *neuroretinitis*, papillitis is accompanied by macular edema and exudates, a "macular star" appearance. This is a rare parainfectious process seen mostly in children and young adults.

Anterior Ischemic Optic Neuropathy (ION: Anterior ION) In persons over 50 years of age, *ischemic infarction of the optic nerve head* is the most common cause of a persistent monocular loss of vision (Fig. 13-12). The onset is abrupt and painless, and the visual loss may be progressive for several days. The field defect is often altitudinal and involves the area of central fixation, accounting for the severe loss of acuity. Swelling of the optic disc, extending for a short distance beyond the disc margin and associated small, flamed-shaped hemorrhages, is typical, or the disc may appear entirely normal. As the disc edema subsides, optic atrophy becomes evident. The second eye is similarly affected at a later date in approximately one-third of patients, particularly those with hypertension and diabetes mellitus. Usually there are no premonitory symptoms or episodes of transient visual loss.

As to the pathogenesis of ION, the usual (anterior) form has been attributed by Hayreh to ischemia in the posterior ciliary artery circulation and more specifically to occlusion of the branches of the peripapillary choroidal arterial system. Infarction of the more posterior portions of the optic nerve(s) is uncommon. Most cases occur on a background of hypertensive vascular disease and diabetes, but not necessarily in relation to carotid artery stenosis, which in our experience has accounted for very few cases. The retina is not affected, as it is in cases of embolic occlusion of the central retinal artery. ION may also complicate intraocular surgery or follow an episode of severe blood loss or other causes of ischemia and hypotension.

Cranial, or giant-cell, arteritis (pages 193 and 907) is the other important cause of ION. In some of the arteritic cases, fleeting premonitory symptoms of visual loss (amaurosis fugax) may precede infarction of the nerve. Unlike the common atherosclerotic type of ION, infarction due to cranial arteritis may affect both optic nerves in close succession and, less often, ocular motor function as well. Also, the arteritis may present with the picture of central retinal artery occlusion. Systemic lupus erythematosus, diabetes, Lyme disease, neurosyphilis, and AIDS rarely give rise to the syndrome of retrobulbar neuropathy but should be considered only after optic nerve compression has been excluded.

Figure 13-12

Anterior ischemic optic neuropathy (AION) related to hypertension and diabetes. There is diffuse disc swelling from infarction that extends into the retina as a milky edema. The veins are engorged. "Cotton-wood" infarcts can be seen to the left of the disc and a "flame" hemorrhage extends from the right disc margin.

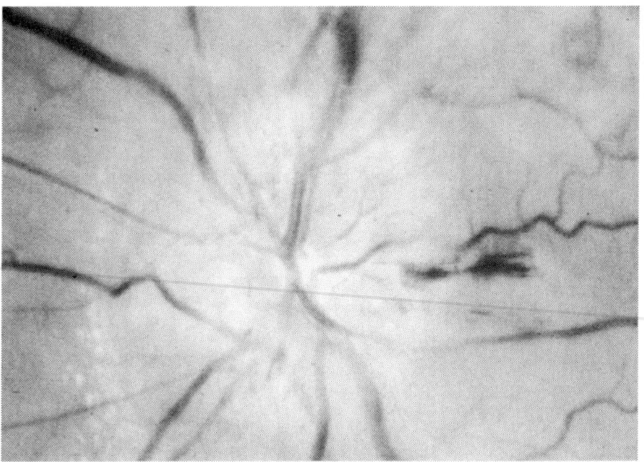

Optic Neuropathy due to Acute Cavernous and Paranasal Sinus Disease A number of disease processes adjacent to the orbit and optic nerve can cause blindness, usually with signs of compression or infarction of the optic and ocular motor nerves. They are seen far less frequently than ischemic optic neuropathy and optic neuritis. Septic cavernous sinus thrombosis (see page 750) may be accompanied by blindness of one eye or both eyes in succession and asymmetrically. In our experience, the visual loss has appeared days after the chemosis and ocular motor palsies. The mechanism of visual loss in this setting, sometimes without swelling of the optic nerve head, is unclear but most likely relates to a retrobulbar ischemia of the nerve. Similarly, optic and ocular motor disorders may complicate ethmoid or sphenoid sinus infections. Severe diabetes with mucormycosis or other invasive fungal or bacterial infection is the usual setting for these complications. Although the formerly held notion that uncomplicated sinus disease is a common cause of optic neuropathy is no longer tenable, there are still a few instances in which such an association occurs and the nature of the visual loss is unclear. Slavin and Glaser described loss of vision from a sphenoethmoidal sinusitis with cellulitis at the orbital apex. Visual symptoms in these circumstances can occur prior to overt signs of local inflammation.

Toxic and Nutritional Optic Neuropathies Simultaneous impairment of vision in the two eyes, with central or centrocecal scotomas, is usually caused not by a demyelinative process but by a toxic or nutritional one. The latter condition is observed most often in the chronically alcoholic patient. Impairment of visual acuity evolves over several days or a week or two, and examination discloses bilateral, roughly symmetrical central or centrocecal scotomas, the peripheral fields being intact. With appropriate treatment (nutritious diet and

B vitamins) instituted soon after the onset of amblyopia, complete recovery is possible; if treatment is delayed, patients are left with varying degrees of permanent defect in central vision and pallor of the temporal portions of the optic discs. This disorder has commonly been referred to as "tobacco-alcohol amblyopia," the implication being that it is due to the toxic effects of tobacco or alcohol, or both. In fact, the disorder is one of nutritional deficiency and is more properly designated as *deficiency amblyopia* or *nutritional optic neuropathy* (Chap. 41). The same disorder may be seen under conditions of severe dietary deprivation and in patients with vitamin B_{12} deficiency. Another cause is Leber hereditary optic atrophy, which is discussed in Chap. 37.

A subacute optic neuropathy has been described in Jamaican natives. It is characterized by a bilaterally symmetrical central visual loss and is occasionally accompanied by nerve deafness, ataxia, and spasticity. A similar condition has been described in other Caribbean countries, most recently in Cuba, where an optic neuropathy of epidemic proportions was associated with a sensory polyneuropathy. A nutritional etiology, rather than an increased risk from tobacco use (especially cigars in the Cuban epidemic), is likely but has not been proved conclusively (see Sadun et al and The Cuba Neuropathy Field Investigation report).

Impairment of vision due to *methyl alcohol intoxication* is abrupt in onset and characterized by large symmetrical central scotomas as well as by symptoms of systemic disease and acidosis. Treatment is directed mainly to correction of the acidosis. The subacute development of central field defects has also been attributed to several other toxins and the chronic administration of certain therapeutic agents: halogenated hydroxyquinolines (clioquinol), chloramphenicol, ethambutol, isoniazid, streptomycin, chlorpropamide (Diabinese), and various ergot preparations. Grant has catalogued the many drugs reported to have a toxic effect on the optic nerves.

Developmental Abnormalities Congenital cavitary defects due to defective closure of the optic fissure may be a cause of impaired vision because of failure of development of the papillomacular bundle. Usually the optic pit or a larger coloboma is unilateral and unassociated with developmental abnormalities of the brain (optic disc dysplasia and dysplastic coloboma). A hereditary form is known (Brown and Tasman). Vision may be impaired as a result of developmental anomalies of the optic nerves; the discs are of small diameter (hypoplasia of the optic disc or micropapilla).

Other Optic Neuropathies

Optic nerve and chiasmal involvement by gliomas, meningiomas, craniopharyngiomas, and metastatic tumors (most often from lung or breast) may cause scotomas and optic atrophy (Chap. 31). Pituitary tumors characteristically cause bitemporal hemianopia, but very large adenomas, as in pituitary apoplexy, can cause blindness in one or both eyes (see page 717). Infiltration of an optic nerve may occur in sarcoidosis, Wegener granulomatosis, and with certain neoplasms, notably leukemia and lymphoma. Of particular importance is the optic nerve glioma that occurs in 15 percent of patients with type I von Recklinghausen neurofibromatosis. Usually it develops in children, often before the fourth year, causing a mass within the orbit and progressive loss of vision. If the eye is blind, the recommended therapy is surgical removal, to prevent extension into the optic chiasm and hypothalamus. If vision is retained, radiation and chemotherapy are the recommended forms of treatment.

Thyroid ophthalmopathy with orbital edema, exophthalmos, and usually a swelling of extraocular muscles is an occasional cause of optic nerve compression.

Radiation-induced damage of the optic nerves and chiasm has been well documented. In a series of 219 patients at the M. D. Anderson Cancer Center who received radiotherapy for carcinomas of the nasal or paranasal region, retinopathy occurred in 7, optic neuropathy with blindness in 8, and chiasmatic damage with bilateral visual impairment in 1. These complications followed the use of more than 50 Gy (5000 rad) of radiation (Jiang et al).

Finally, it should be mentioned again that long-standing papilledema from any cause may eventually lead to optic atrophy and blindness. In the case of pseudotumor cerebri, the visual loss may be unexpectedly abrupt, appearing in a day or less and even sequentially in both eyes. This seems to happen most often in patients with constitutionally small optic nerves, no optic cup of the nerve head, and, presumably, a small aperture of the lamina cribosa.

NEUROLOGY OF THE CENTRAL VISUAL PATHWAYS

From the retina there is a point-to-point projection to the lateral geniculate ganglion and from the latter to the calcarine cortex of the occipital lobe. Thus the visual cortex receives a spatial pattern of stimulation that corresponds with the retinal image of the visual field. Visual impairments due to lesions of the central pathways usually involve only a part of the visual fields, and a plotting of the latter provides information as to the site of the lesion.

For purposes of description of the visual fields, each retina and macula are divided into a temporal and nasal half by a vertical line passing through the fovea centralis. A horizontal line represented roughly by the junction of the superior and inferior retinal vascular arcades also passes through the fovea and divides each half of the retina and macula into upper and lower quadrants. Visual field defects are always described in terms of the field defect from the patient's view rather than the retinal defect. The retinal image of an object in the visual field is inverted and reversed from right to left, like the image on the film of a camera. Thus the left visual field of each eye is represented in the opposite half of each retina, with the upper part of the field represented in the lower part of the retina (see Fig. 13-2). The retinal projections to the geniculate nuclei and occipital cortex are illustrated in Fig. 13-4.

Testing for Abnormalities of the Visual Fields

Visual field defects caused by lesions of the retina, optic nerve and tract, lateral geniculate body, geniculocalcarine pathway, and striate cortex of the occipital lobe are illustrated in Fig. 13-3. In the alert, cooperative patient, the visual fields can be plotted accurately at the bedside. With one of the patient's eyes covered and the other aligned with the corresponding eye of the examiner (patient's right with examiner's left), a target—such as a moving finger, a cotton pledget, or a white disc mounted on a stick—is brought from the periphery toward the center of the visual field (confrontational testing). With the target at an equal distance between the eye of the examiner and that of the patient, the fields of the patient and examiner are then compared. Similarly, the patient's blind spot can be aligned with the examiner's and its size determined by moving the target outward from the blind spot until it is seen. Central and paracentral defects in the field can be outlined the same way. For reasons not known, red-green test objects are more sensitive than white ones in detecting defects of the visual pathways.

It should be emphasized that movement of the visual target provides the coarsest stimulus to the retina, so that a perception of its motion may be preserved while a stationary target of the same size may not be seen. In other words, moving targets are less useful than static ones in confrontational testing of visual fields. Rapid finger counting and comparison of color intensity of a red object or the examiner's hand from quadrant to quadrant are simple confrontation tests that will disclose even subtle field defects. Glaser uses a simple and effective method for the detection of hemianopic defects. The examiner's hands are presented simultaneously, one on each side of the vertical meridian separating the temporal from the nasal hemifield; the hand in the hemianopic field appears blurred or darker than the other. Similarly, a scotoma may be defined by asking the patient to report changes in color or brightness of a red test object as it is moved toward or away from the point of fixation.

A central scotoma may be identified by having the patient fixate with one eye on the examiner's nose, on which the examiner places the index finger of one hand or a white-headed pin and has the patient compare it for brightness, clarity, and color with a finger or pin held in the periphery. Alternatively, two test objects can be used, one placed centrally and the other eccentrically, and the patient is asked to describe differences in color intensity. Finally, if any defect is found or suspected by confrontation testing, the fields should be charted and scotomas outlined on a tangent screen or perimeter. Highly accurate computer-assisted perimetry is now available in most ophthalmology clinics.

The method of testing by double simultaneous stimulation may elicit defects in the central processing of vision that are undetected by conventional perimetry. Movement of one finger in all parts of each temporal field may disclose no abnormality, but if movement is simultaneous in analogous parts of both temporal fields, the patient with a parietal lobe lesion, especially on the right, may see only the one in the normal right hemifield. In young children or uncooperative patients, the integrity of the fields may be roughly estimated by observing whether the patient is attracted to objects in the peripheral field or blinks in response to sudden threatening gestures in half of the visual field.

A common abnormality disclosed by visual field examination is *concentric constriction*. This may be due to papilledema, in which case it is usually accompanied by an enlargement of the blind spot. A progressive constriction of the visual fields, at first unilateral and later bilateral, associated with pallor of the optic discs (optic atrophy), should suggest a chronic meningeal process involving the optic nerves (syphilis, cryptococcosis, sarcoid, lymphoma). Long-standing, untreated glaucoma and retinitis pigmentosa are other causes of concentric constriction. Marked constriction of the visual fields of unvarying degree, regardless of the distance of the visual stimulus from the eye, ("gun-barrel" or "tunnel" vision), is a sign of hypersuggestibility or hysteria. With organic disease, the constricted visual field naturally enlarges as the distance between the patient and the test object increases.

Prechiasmal Lesions

Lesions of the macula, retina, or optic nerve cause either a *scotoma* (an island of impaired vision surrounded by normal vision) or a defect that extends to the periphery of one visual field. Scotomas are named according to their position (central, cecocentral) or their shape (ring, arcuate). A small scotoma in the macular part of the visual field may seriously impair visual acuity. Demyelinative disease (retrobulbar neuritis), Leber hereditary optic atrophy, toxins (methyl alcohol, quinine, chloroquine, and certain phenothiazine drugs), nutritional deficiency (so-called tobacco-alcohol amblyopia), and vascular disease (ischemic optic neuropathy or occlusion of a branch of the retinal artery) are the usual causes of scotomas. Orbital or retro-orbital tumors and infectious or granulomatous processes (e.g., sarcoid, retinal toxoplasmosis in AIDS) are other common causes. Certain toxic states are characterized by symmetrical bilateral scotomas and the nutritional disorders by more or less bilaterally symmetrical central scotomas (involving the fixation point) or cecocentral ones (involving both the fixation point and the blind spot). The cecocentral scotoma, which tends to have an arcuate border, represents a lesion that is predominantly in the distribution of the papillomacular bundle. However, finding this visual field abnormality does not establish whether the primary defect is in the cells of the origin of the bundle, i.e., the retinal ganglion cells, or in their fibers. Demyelinative disease is characterized by unilateral or asymmetrical bilateral scotomas. Vascular lesions that take the form of retinal hemorrhages or infarctions of the nerve-fiber layer (cotton- wool patches) give rise to unilateral scotomas; occlusion of the central retinal artery or its branches causes infarction of the retina and, as a rule, a loss of central vision. As pointed out earlier, anterior ischemic optic neuropathy causes sudden monocular blindness or an altitudinal field defect. Since the optic nerve also contains the afferent fibers for the pupillary light reflex, lesions of the nerve will cause a so-called afferent pupillary defect, which has been alluded to on page 252 and is considered further in Chap. 14.

With most diseases of the optic nerve, the optic disc will eventually become pale. This usually requires 4 to 6 weeks to develop. If the optic nerve degenerates (e.g., in multiple sclerosis, Leber hereditary optic atrophy, traumatic transection, tumor of nerve, or syphilitic optic atrophy), the disc becomes chalk white, with sharp, clean margins. If the atrophy is secondary (consecutive) to papillitis or papilledema, the disc margins are indistinct and irregular; the disc has a pallid, yellow-gray appearance, like candle tallow; the vessels are partially obscured and may be sheathed; and the adjacent retina is altered.

Visual evoked potentials from the stimulation of one eye may be slowed even if the optic disc appears normal and there is no perimetric abnormality. This may be the only sign of a previously unrecorded optic neuritis or of a compressive optic neuropathy even though sight has been fully restored.

Lesions of the Chiasm, Optic Tract, and Geniculocalcarine Pathway

Hemianopia (hemianopsia) means blindness in half of the visual field. *Bitemporal hemianopia* indicates a lesion of the decussating fibers of the optic chiasm and is usually caused by the extrasellar extension of a tumor of the pituitary gland including pituitary apoplexy. It may also be caused by a craniopharyngioma, a saccular aneurysm of the circle of Willis, and a meningioma of the tuberculum sellae; less often, it may be due to sarcoidosis, metastatic carcinoma, ectopic pinealoma or dysgerminoma, Hand-Schüller-Christian disease, or hydrocephalus with dilation and downward herniation of the posterior part of the third ventricle (Corbett). The lesion is usually at the chiasm, involving the decussating nasal fibers from each retina (Fig. 13-2*C*), although in some instances a tumor pushing upward presses the medial parts of the optic nerves, just anterior to the chiasm, against the anterior cerebral arteries. Heteronymous field defects, i.e., scotomas or field defects that differ in the two eyes, are also a sign of involvement of the optic chiasm or the adjoining optic nerves or tracts; they are caused by craniopharyngiomas or other suprasellar tumors and rarely by mucoceles, angiomas, giant carotid aneurysm, and opticochiasmic arachnoiditis.

The pattern created by a lesion in the optic nerve as it joins the chiasm typically includes a scotomatous defect on the affected side coupled with a contralateral quadrantanopia. As noted previously, the latter is caused by interruption of nasal retinal fibers which, after crossing in the chiasm, project into the base of the affected optic nerve (Wilbrand's knee, see Fig. 13-2*B*). A sharply defined pattern of this type is relatively uncommon. Variations in the pattern of visual loss in the case of these "junctional" lesions are frequent, in part accounted for by the location of the chiasm—a prefixed chiasm making unilateral eye findings more common.

Homonymous hemianopia (a loss of vision in corresponding halves of the visual fields) signifies a lesion of the visual pathway behind the chiasm and, if complete, gives no more information than that. *Incomplete homonymous hemianopia* has more localizing value. As a general rule, if the field defects in the two eyes are identical (congruous), the lesion is likely to be in the calcarine cortex and subcortical white matter of the occipital lobe; if they are *incongruous*, the visual fibers in the optic tract or in the parietal or temporal lobe are more likely to be implicated. Lesions of the optic tract give the most incongruous defects; only when the lesion is complete is the defect congruous. Actually, absolute congruity of field defects is rare, even with occipital lesions.

The lower fibers of the geniculocalcarine pathway (from the inferior retinas) swing in a wide arc over the temporal horn of the lateral ventricle and then proceed posteriorly to join the upper fibers of the pathway on their way to the calcarine cortex (Fig. 13-3). This arc of fibers is known variously as the Flechsig, Meyer, or Archambault loop, and a lesion that interrupts these fibers will produce a *superior homonymous quadrantanopia* (contralateral upper temporal and ipsilateral upper nasal quadrants; Fig. 13-2*E*). This clinical effect was first described by Harvey Cushing, so that his name also has been applied to the loop of temporal visual fibers. Parietal lobe lesions are said to affect the inferior quadrants of the visual fields more than the superior ones, but this is difficult to document; with a lesion of the right parietal lobe, the patient ignores the left half of space; with a left parietal lesion, the patient is often aphasic. As to the localizing value of *quadrantic defects*, the report of Jacobson is of interest; he found, in reviewing the imaging studies of 41 patients with inferior quadrantanopia and 30 with superior quadrantanopia, that in 76 percent of the former and 83 percent of the latter the lesions were confined to the occipital lobe.

If the entire optic tract or calcarine cortex on one side is destroyed, the homonymous hemianopia is complete. But often that part of the field subserved by the macula is spared, i.e., there is a 5- to 10-degree island of vision around the fixation point on the side of the hemianopia (sparing of fixation or *macular sparing*). With infarction of the occipital lobe due to occlusion of the posterior cerebral artery, the macular region, represented in the most posterior port of the striate cortex, may be spared by virtue of collateral circulation from the middle cerebral artery. Incomplete lesions of the optic tract and radiation usually spare central (macular) vision. We have nevertheless observed a lesion of the tip of one occipital lobe that produced central homonymous hemianopic scotomata, bisecting the maculae. Lesions of both occipital poles (as in embolization of the posterior cerebral arteries) result in bilateral central scotomas; if all the calcarine cortex or all the subcortical geniculocalcarine fibers on both sides are completely destroyed, there is cerebral, or *"cortical," blindness*.

An *altitudinal defect* is one that is confined to the upper or lower half of the visual field but crosses the vertical meridian. *Homonymous altitudinal hemianopia* is usually due to lesions of both occipital lobes below or above the calcarine sulcus and rarely to a lesion of the optic chiasm or nerves. The most common cause of a homonymous altitudinal hemianopia is infarction due to occlusion of the posterior cerebral arteries. However, the most common cause of a monocular altitudinal hemianopia is ischemic optic neuropathy.

In certain instances of homonymous hemianopia, the patient is capable of some visual perception in the hemianopic fields, a circumstance that permits the study of the vulnerability of different visual functions. Colored targets may be detected in the hemianopic fields, whereas achromatic ones cannot. But even in seemingly complete hemianopic defects, in which the patient admits to being blind, it has been shown that he may still react to visual stimuli when forced-choice techniques are used. This type of residual visual function has been called "blindsight" by Weiskrantz and colleagues. Blythe and coworkers found that 20 percent of their patients with no pattern discrimination in the hemianopic field could still reach accurately and look at a moving light in the "blind" field. These residual visual functions are generally attributed to the preserved function of retinocollicular or geniculoprestriate cortical connections, but they may as likely be due to sparing of small islands of calcarine neurons.

In yet other instances of an occipital lesion and a dense homonymous hemianopia, the patient may be little disabled by his visual field loss (Benton et al; Meienberg). This is due to preservation of vision in a small monocular part of the visual field known as the "*temporal crescent*." The latter is a peripheral unpaired portion of the visual field, between 60 and 100 degrees from the fixation point, and is represented in the most anterior part of the visual striate cortex. In particular, the temporal crescent is sensitive to moving stimuli, allowing the patient to avoid collisions with people and objects.

Blindness in the Hysterical or Malingering Patient

Hysterical blindness is described on page 1596, but a few

comments are in order here. Feigned or hysterical visual loss is usually detected by attending to the patient's activities when he thinks he is unobserved and can be confirmed by a number of simple tests. Complete feigned blindness is exposed directly by observing the normal ocular jerk movements in response to a rotating optokinetic drum or strip or by noting that the patient's eyes follow their own image in a moving mirror. The simplest way to establish the hysterical nature of monocular blindness is to note the presence of a normal pupillary response to light. An optokinetic response in the nonseeing eye (with the good eye covered) is an even more convincing test; also, the visual evoked potential from the allegedly blind eye is normal. *Hysterical homonymous hemianopia* is exceedingly rare and is only displayed by practiced malingerers and psychopaths. Lateral hemianopias of every variety are common (Keane). The uniformly constricted, tubular field defect of hysteria has already been mentioned.

Visual Agnosias In distinction to blindness, there is another, far less common category of visual impairment in which the patient cannot understand the meaning of what he sees, i.e., *visual agnosia*. Primary visual perception is more or less intact, and the patient may describe accurately the shape, color, and size of objects and draw copies of them. Despite this, he cannot identify the objects unless he hears, smells, tastes, or palpates them. The failure of visual recognition of words alone is called *visual verbal agnosia*, or *alexia*. The ability to recognize visually presented objects and words depends upon the integrity not only of the visual pathways and primary visual area of the cerebral cortex (area 17 of Brodmann) but also of those cortical areas that lie just anterior to area 17 (areas 18 and 19 of the occipital lobe and area 39—the angular gyrus of the dominant hemisphere). Visual-object agnosia rarely occurs as an isolated finding: as a rule, it is combined with visual verbal agnosia, homonymous hemianopia, or both. These abnormalities arise from lesions of the dominant occipital cortex and adjacent temporal and parietal (angular gyrus) cortex or from a lesion of the left calcarine cortex combined with one that interrupts the fibers crossing from the right occipital lobe (see Fig. 22-7). Failure to understand the meaning of an entire picture even though some of its parts are recognized is referred to as *simultanagnosia*, and a failure to recognize familiar faces is called *prosopagnosia*. These and other variants of visual agnosia (including visual neglect) and their pathologic bases are dealt with more fully in Chap. 22.

Other Cerebral Disturbances of Vision These include various types of distortion in which images seem to recede into the distance (teleopsia), appear too small (micropsia), or, less frequently, seem too large (macropsia). If such distortions are perceived with only one eye, a local retinal lesion should be suspected. If perceived with both eyes, they usually signify disease of the temporal lobes, in which case the visual disturbances tend to occur in attacks and are accompanied by other manifestations of temporal lobe seizures (Chap. 16). With parietal lobe lesions, objects may appear to be askew or even turned upside down. More often lesions of the vestibular nucleus or its immediate connections produce the illusion that objects are tilted (tortopia; page 290) or that straight lines are curved. Presumably this is due to a mismatch between the visual image and the otolithic or vestibular input to the visual system.

Abnormalities of Color Vision

Normal color vision depends on the integrity of cone cells, which are most numerous in the macular region. When activated, they convey information to special columns of cells in the striate cortex. Three different cone pigments with optimal sensitivities to blue, green, and orange-yellow wavelengths are said to characterize these cells; presumably each cone possesses only one of these pigments. Transmission to higher centers for the perception of color is believed to be effected by neurons and axons that encode at least two pairs of complementary colors: red-green in one system and yellow-blue in the other. In the optic nerves and tracts, the fibers for color are of small caliber and seem to be preferentially sensitive to certain noxious agents and to pressure. The geniculostriate fibers for color are separate from fibers that convey information about form and brightness but course along with them; hence there may be a homonymous color hemianopia (hemiachromatopsia). The visual fields for blue-yellow are smaller than those for white light, and the red and green fields are smaller than those for blue-yellow.

Diseases may affect color vision by abolishing it completely (*achromatopsia*) or partially by quantitatively reducing one or more of the three attributes of color—brightness, hue, and saturation. Or, only one of the complementary pairs of colors may be lost, usually red-green. The disorder may be congenital and hereditary or acquired. The commonest form, and the one to which the term *color blindness* is usually applied, is a male sex-linked inability to see red and green while normal visual acuity is retained. A genetic abnormality of cone pigments is postulated, but the defect cannot be seen by inspecting the retina. A failure of the cones to develop or a degeneration of cones may cause a loss of color vision, but in these conditions visual acuity is often diminished, a central scotoma may be present, and, although the macula appears to be normal ophthalmoscopically, fluorescein angiography shows the pigment epithelium to be defective. Congenital color vision defects are usually protan (red) or detan (green), leaving yellow-blue color vision intact; acquired lesions may affect all colors. Lesions of the optic nerves usually affect red-green more than blue-yellow; the opposite is true of retinal lesions. An exception is a rare dominantly inherited optic atrophy, in which the scotoma mapped by a large blue target is larger than that for red.

Damasio has drawn attention to a group of acquired deficits of color perception with preservation of form vision, the result of focal damage (usually infarction) of the visual association cortex and subjacent white matter. Color vision may be lost in a quadrant, half of the visual field, or the entire field. The latter, or full-field achromatopsia, is the result of bilateral occipitotemporal lesions involving the fusiform and lingual gyri, a localization that accounts for its frequent association with visual agnosia (especially prosopagnosia; see page 491) and some degree of visual field defect. A lesion restricted to the inferior part of the right occipitotemporal region, sparing both the optic radiations and striate cortex, causes the purest form of achromatopsia (left hemiachromatopsia). With a similar left-sided lesion, alexia may be associated with the right hemiachromatopsia.

Other Visual Disorders Finally, in addition to the losses of perception of form, movement, and color, lesions of the visual system may also give rise to a variety of positive sensory visual experiences. The simplest of these are called phosphenes, i.e., flashes of light and colored spots in the absence of luminous stimuli. Mechanical pressure on the normal eyeball may induce them at the retinal level, as every child discovers. Or they may occur with disease of the visual system at many different sites. As mentioned earlier, elderly patients commonly complain of flashes of light in the peripheral field of one eye, most evident in the dark (*Moore's lightning streaks*); these are related to vitreous tags that rest on the retinal equator and are quite benign. In patients with migraine, ischemia of nerve cells in the occipital lobe gives rise to the bright zigzag lines of a fortification spectrum. Stimulation of the cortical terminations of the visual pathways accounts for the simple or unformed visual hallucinations in epilepsy. Formed or complex visual hallucinations (of people, animals, landscapes, etc.) are observed in a variety of conditions, notably in old age when vision fails (Bonnet syndrome), in the withdrawal state following chronic intoxication with alcohol and other sedative-hypnotic drugs (Chaps. 42 and 43), in Alzheimer disease, and in infarcts of the occipitoparietal or occipitotemporal regions (release hullucinations) or the diencephalon ("peduncular hallucinosis").

Occasionally, patients in whom a hemianopia is only evident when tested by double simultaneous stimulation ("attention hemianopia") may displace an image to the nonaffected half of the field of vision (*visual allesthesia*), or a visual image may persist for minutes to hours or reappear episodically, after the exciting stimulus has been removed (*palinopsia* or *paliopsia*); the latter disorder also occurs in defective but not blind homonymous fields of vision. *Polyopia*, the perception of multiple images when a single stimulus is presented, is said to be associated predominantly with right occipital lesions and can occur with either eye. Usually there is one primary and a number of secondary images, and their relationships may be constant or changing. Bender and Krieger, who described several such patients, attributed the polyopia to unstable fixation. *Oscillopsia*, or illusory movement of the environment, occurs mainly with lesions of the labyrinthine-vestibular apparatus and is described with disorders of ocular movement (see page 292). A rare idiopathic myoclonus of one superior oblique muscle may produce a monocular oscillopsia.

Clinical effects and syndromes that result from occipital lobe lesions are discussed further in Chap. 22.

REFERENCES*

ARRUGA J. SANDERS M: Ophthalmologic findings in 70 patients with evidence of retinal embolism. *Ophthalmology* 89:1336, 1982.

BENDER MB, KRIEGER HP: Visual function in perimetric blind fields. *Arch Neurol Psychiatry* 65:72, 1951.

BENTON S, LEVY I, SWASH M: Vision in the temporal crescent in occipital infarction. *Brain* 103:83, 1980.

BIENFANG DC, KELLY LD, NICHOLSON DH, et al: Ophthalmology. *N Engl J Med* 323:956, 1990.

BLYTHE IM, KENNARD C, RUDDOCK KH: Residual vision in patients with retrogeniculate lesions of the visual pathways. *Brain* 110:887, 1987.

*See also References in Chap. 14.

Brown GC, Tasman WS: *Congenital Anomalies of the Optic Disc*. New York, Grune & Stratton, 1983.

Chester EM: *The Ocular Fundus in Systemic Disease*. Chicago, Year Book, 1973.

Corbett JJ: Neuro-ophthalmologic complications of hydrocephalus and shunting procedures. *Semin Neurol* 6:111, 1986.

Damasio AR: Disorder of complex visual processing: Agnosia, achromatopsia, Balint's syndrome and related difficulties of orientation and construction, in Mesulam M-M (ed): *Principles of Behavioral Neurology*. Philadelphia, Davis, 1985, pp 259–288.

D'Amico DJ: Disease of the retina. *N Engl J Med* 331:95, 1994.

Digre KB, Kurcan FJ, Branch DW, et al: Amaurosis fugax associated with antiphospholipid antibodies. *Ann Neurol* 25:228, 1989.

Dryja TP, McGee TL, Reichel E, et al: A point mutation of the rhodopsin gene in one form of retinitis pigmentosa. *Nature* 343:364, 1990.

Fisher CM: Observations on the fundus in transient monocular blindness. *Neurology* 9:333, 1959.

Glaser JS (ed.): *Neuro-ophthalmology*, 3rd ed. Philadelphia, Lippincott Williams and Wilkins, 1999.

Grant WM: *Toxicology of the Eye*. Springfield, IL, Charles C Thomas, 1986.

Grunwald GB, Klein R, Simmonds MA, Kornguth SE: Autoimmune basis for visual paraneoplastic syndrome in patients with small cell lung carcinoma. *Lancet* 1:658, 1985.

Hayreh SS: Anterior ischemic optic neuropathy. *Arch Neurol* 38:675, 1981.

Hayreh SS: Blood supply of the optic nerve head and its role in optic atrophy, glaucoma, and oedema of the optic disc. *Br J Ophthalmol* 53:721, 1969.

Hayreh SS: Pathogenesis of oedema of the optic disc (papilloedema). *Br J Ophthalmol* 48:522, 1964.

Hubel DH, Wiesel TN: Functional architecture of macaque monkey visual cortex. *Proc R Soc Lond [Biol]* 198:1, 1977.

Jacobson DM: The localizing value of a quadrantanopia. *Arch Neurol* 54:401, 1997.

Jacobson DM, Thurkill CE, Tipping SJ: A clinical triad to diagnose paraneoplastic retinopathy. *Ann Neurol* 28:162, 1990.

Jiang GL, Tucker SL, Guttenberger R, et al: Radiation-induced injury to the visual pathway. *Radiother Oncol* 30:17, 1994.

Keane JR: Patterns of hysterical hemianopia. *Neurology* 51:1230, 1998.

Kornguth SE, Klein R, Appen R, Choate J: The occurrence of anti-retinal ganglion cell antibodies in patients with small cell carcinoma of the lung. *Cancer* 50:1289, 1982.

Leibold JE: Drugs having a toxic effect on the optic nerve. *Int Ophthalmol Clin* 11:137, 1971.

Levin BE: The clinical significance of spontaneous pulsations of the retinal vein. *Arch Neurol* 35:37, 1978.

Marshall J, Meadows S: The natural history of amaurosis fugax. *Brain* 91:419, 1968.

McDonald WI, Barnes D: Diseases of the optic nerve, in Asbury AK, McKhann GM, McDonald WI (eds): *Diseases of the Nervous System*, 2nd ed. Philadelphia, Saunders, 1992, chap 29, pp 421–433.

Meienberg O: Sparing of the temporal crescent in homonymous hemianopia and its significance for visual orientation. *Neuroophthalmology* 2:129, 1981.

Minckler DS, Tso MOM, Zimmerman LE: A light microscopic autoradiographic study of axoplasmic transport in the optic nerve head during ocular hypotony, increased intraocular pressure, and papilledema. *Am J Ophthalmol* 82:741, 1976.

Newman NJ: Optic neuropathy. *Neurology* 46:315, 1996.

Paton L, Holmes G: The pathology of papilloedema: A histological study of 60 eyes. *Brain* 33:389, 1911.

Pearlman AJ: Visual system, in Pearlman AL, Collins RC (eds): *Neurobiology of Disease*. New York, Oxford University Press, 1990, chap 7, pp 124–148.

Rucker CW: Sheathing of retinal venus in multiple sclerosis. *Mayo Clin Proc* 47:335, 1972.

Sadun RA, Martone JF, Muci-Mendoza R, et al: Epidemic optic neuropathy in Cuba:. Eye findings. *Arch Ophthalmol* 112:691, 1994.

Savino PJ, Paris M, Schatz NJ, et al: Optic tract syndrome. *Arch Ophthalmol* 96:656, 1978.

Sawle GV, James CB, Ross M, Russell RW: The natural history of non-arteritic anterior ischemic optic neuropathy. *J Neurol Neurosurg Psychiatry* 53:830, 1990.

Slavin M, Glaser JS: Acute severe irreversible visual loss with sphenoethmoiditis-posterior orbital cellulitis. *Arch Ophthalmol* 105:345, 1987.

Smith JL, Hoyt WP, Susac JO: Optic fundus in acute Leber's optic atrophy. *Arch Ophthalmol* 90:349, 1973.

The Cuba Neuropathy Field Investigation Team: Epidemic optic neuropathy in Cuba—Clinical characteristics and risk factors. *N Engl J Med* 333:1176, 1995.

Tso MOM, Hayreh SS: Optic disc edema in raised intracranial pressure: III. A pathologic study of experimental papilledema. *Arch Ophthalmol* 95:1448, 1977; IV: Axoplasmic transport in experimental papilledema, *Arch Ophthalmol* 95:1458, 1977.

Weiskrantz L, Warrington EK, Sanders MD, Marshall J: Visual capacity in the hemianopic field following a restricted occipital ablation. *Brain* 97:709, 1974.

Wray SH: Neuro-ophthalmologic diseases, in Rosenberg RN (ed): *Comprehensive Neurology*. New York, Raven Press, 1991, chap 20.

Wray SH: Visual aspects of extracranial carotid artery disease, in Bernstein EF (ed): *Amaurosis Fugax*. New York, Springer-Verlag, 1988, pp 72–80.

Young LHY, Appen RE: Ischemic oculopathy. *Arch Neurol* 38:358, 1981.

Chapter 14

DISORDERS OF OCULAR MOVEMENT AND PUPILLARY FUNCTION

Ocular movement and vision are virtually inseparable. A moving object evokes ocular movement and almost simultaneously arouses attention and initiates the perceptive process. To look searchingly, i.e., to peer, requires stable fixation of the visual image on the center of the two retinas. One might say that the ocular muscles are at the beck and call of our visual sense. This is the logic of juxtaposing Chaps. 13 and 14 and suggesting that they be read together.

Abnormalities of ocular movement are of four basic types. One disorder of motility can be traced to a lesion of the extraocular muscles themselves, the neuromuscular junction, or to the cranial nerves that supply them (*nuclear* or *infranuclear palsy*). The second type, of particular neurologic interest, is a derangement in the highly specialized neural mechanisms that enable the eyes to move together (*supranuclear or internuclear palsies*). Such a distinction, in keeping with the general concept of upper and lower motor neuron paralysis, hardly portrays the complexity of the neural mechanisms governing ocular motility; nevertheless, it constitutes an essential step in the approach to the patient with defective eye movements. In the third type, there is a mechanical restriction of the globe because of a mass or infiltrating lesion within the orbit. In all three types, a knowledge of the anatomic basis of normal movement is essential to an understanding of abnormal movement. Perhaps more common but not primarily neurologic is the fourth type, concomitant strabismus, in which there is a congenital imbalance of the yoked muscles of extraocular movement.

SUPRANUCLEAR CONTROL OF EYE MOVEMENT

Anatomic and Physiologic Considerations

In no aspect of human anatomy and physiology is the sensory guidance of muscle activity more instructively revealed than in the neural control of coordinated ocular movement. To focus the eyes voluntarily in searching the environment, to stabilize objects for scrutiny when one is moving, to maintain clear images of moving objects, to bring into sharp focus near and far objects—all require the perfect coordination of six sets of extraocular muscles and three sets of intrinsic muscles (ciliary muscles and sphincters and dilators of the iris). The neural mechanisms that govern these functions reside in the medulla, pons, midbrain, cerebellum, basal ganglia, and the frontal, parietal, and occipital lobes of the brain. Most of the nuclear structures and pathways concerned with fixation and stable ocular movements are now known, and much has been learned of their physiology both from clinical-pathologic correlations in humans and from experiments in monkeys. Different diseases may give rise to particular defects in ocular movement and pupillary function, and these are of diagnostic importance.

Accurate binocular vision is achieved by the associated action of the ocular muscles, which allows a visual stimulus to fall on exactly corresponding parts of the two retinas. The symmetrical and synchronous movement of the eyes is termed *conjugate movement* or *gaze* (*conjugate* = yoked or joined together). The simultaneous movement of the eyes in opposite directions, as in convergence, is termed *disconjugate* or *disjunctive*. These two forms of normal ocular movement—conjugate and disconjugate—are also referred to as *versional* and *vergence*, respectively. *Vergence movements* are of two types—fusional and accommodative. *Fusional movements* are the convergence and divergence movements that maintain binocular single vision and depth perception (stereopsis); they are necessary at all times to prevent visual images from falling on noncorresponding parts of the retinas. *Accommodative vergence movements* are brought into action when one looks at a near object. The eyes turn inward (off their parallel axes) and at the same time the pupils constrict and the ciliary muscles relax to thicken the lens (*accommodation*). This synkinesis is called the *near reflex* or *accommodative triad.*

Voluntary conjugate movements of the eyes to the opposite side are probably initiated in area 8 of the frontal lobe and relayed to the pons. These movements are characteristically rapid or *saccadic* (peak velocity may exceed 700 degrees per second). Their purpose is to quickly change ocular fixation in order to bring images of new objects of interest onto the foveas. They can be elicited by instructing the individual to look to the right or left (commanded saccades) or to move the eyes to fixate on a target (refixation saccades). Saccadic movements, or saccades, may also be elicited reflexly, as when a sudden sound or the appearance of an object in the peripheral field of vision attracts attention and triggers an automatic movement of the eyes in the direction of the stimulus. Saccadic latency, the interval between the appearance of a target and the initiation of a saccade, is approximately 200 ms.

The neuronal firing pattern of pontine neurons that produces a saccade has been characterized as "pulse-step" in type. This refers to the sudden increase in neuronal firing (the pulse) that is necessary to overcome the inertia and viscous drag of the eyes and to move them into their new position; this is followed by a return to a new baseline firing level (the step), which maintains the eyes in their new position by constant tonic contraction of the extraocular muscles (*gaze holding*). Saccades are so rapid that there is no subjective awareness of any movement and objectively only one swift unbroken conjugate movement is observed.

Saccades are distinguished from the slower and smoother, largely involuntary *pursuit*, or *following, movements*, for which the major stimulus is a moving target upon which the eyes are fixated. The function of pursuit movements is to stabilize the image of a moving object on the foveas as the fixated object is tracked by the eyes ("smooth tracking") and thus to maintain a continuous clear image of the object as it moves in the environment. Pursuit movements to each side appear to be generated in the ipsilateral parieto-occipital cortex, but the ipsilateral cerebellum, especially the vestibulocerebellum (flocculus and nodulus), is also involved. Another portion of the cerebellum, the posterior vermis, modulates saccadic movements (see further on).

If, when following a moving target, the visual image slips off the foveas, the firing rate of the governing motor neurons increases in proportion to the speed of the moving target, so that normally eye velocity matches target velocity. If, during pursuit, the eyes fall behind the target, supplementary catch-up saccades are required for refixation. The pursuit movement is then not smooth but jerky ("cogwheel" or "saccadic" pursuit). A lesion of one cerebral hemisphere may cause pursuit movements to that side to break up into saccades. This is often associated with but not dependent upon a homonymous hemianopia. Diseases of the basal ganglia are a common cause of saccadic pursuit in all directions.

If a series of visual targets enters the visual field, as when one is watching trees from a moving car or the stripes on a rotating drum, repeated quick saccades refocus the eyes centrally; the resulting repeated cycles of pursuit and refixation are termed *optokinetic nystagmus.* This phenomenon is described more fully further on, in the section on nystaginus.

Vestibular influences are of particular importance in stabilizing images on the retina. By means of the *vestibulo-ocular reflex (VOR)*, a movement of the eyes is produced that is equal and opposite to movement of the head. The VOR generates a prompt (short latency) response to rapid transient head movements. During sustained rotation of the head, the VOR is supplemented by the optokinetic system, which enables one to maintain compensatory eye movements for a more prolonged period. If the VOR is lost, as occurs with disease of the vestibular apparatus or eighth nerve, the slightest movements of the head, especially those occurring during locomotion, cause a movement of images across the retina large enough to impair vision. When objects are tracked using both eye and head movements, the vestibulo-ocular movements induced by head turning must be suppressed, otherwise the eyes would remain stabilized in space; it appears likely that the smooth pursuit signals cancel the unwanted vestibular ones (Leigh and Zee).

Horizontal Gaze

Saccades As already mentioned, the signals for volitional horizontal gaze saccades originate in the eye field of the opposite frontal lobe (area 8 of Brodmann) and are modulated by the adjacent supplementary motor eye field and the posterior visual cortical areas. The corticofugal pathways for saccadic horizontal gaze have been traced in the monkey by Leichnetz. He found that these fibers traverse the internal capsule and separate at the level of the rostral diencephalon into two bundles: a primary but indirect ventral "capsular-peduncular" bundle, which descends through the internal capsule and most medial part of the basis pedunculi. This more ventral pathway undergoes a partial decussation in the low midbrain, at the level of the trochlear nucleus, and terminates mainly in the paramedian pontine reticular formation (PPRF), which in turn projects to the sixth nerve nucleus (Fig. 14-1). A second, more dorsal "transthalamic" bundle is predominantly uncrossed and courses through the internal medullary lamina and paralaminar parts of the thalamus to terminate diffusely in the pretectum, superior colliculus, and periaqueductal gray matter. An offshoot of these fibers (the prefrontal oculomotor bundle) projects to the rostral part of the oculomotor nucleus and to the ipsilateral rostral interstitial nucleus of the medial longitudinal fasciculus (ri MLF) and to the interstitial nucleus of Cajal (INC), which are involved in vertical eye movements, as discussed in the next section.

Pursuit The cortical pathways for smooth pursuit movements are less well known. One pathway probably originates in the posterior parietal cortex and the adjacent temporal and anterior occipital cortex (area MT of the monkey), and descends to the ipsilateral dorsolateral pontine nuclei. Also contributing to smooth pursuit

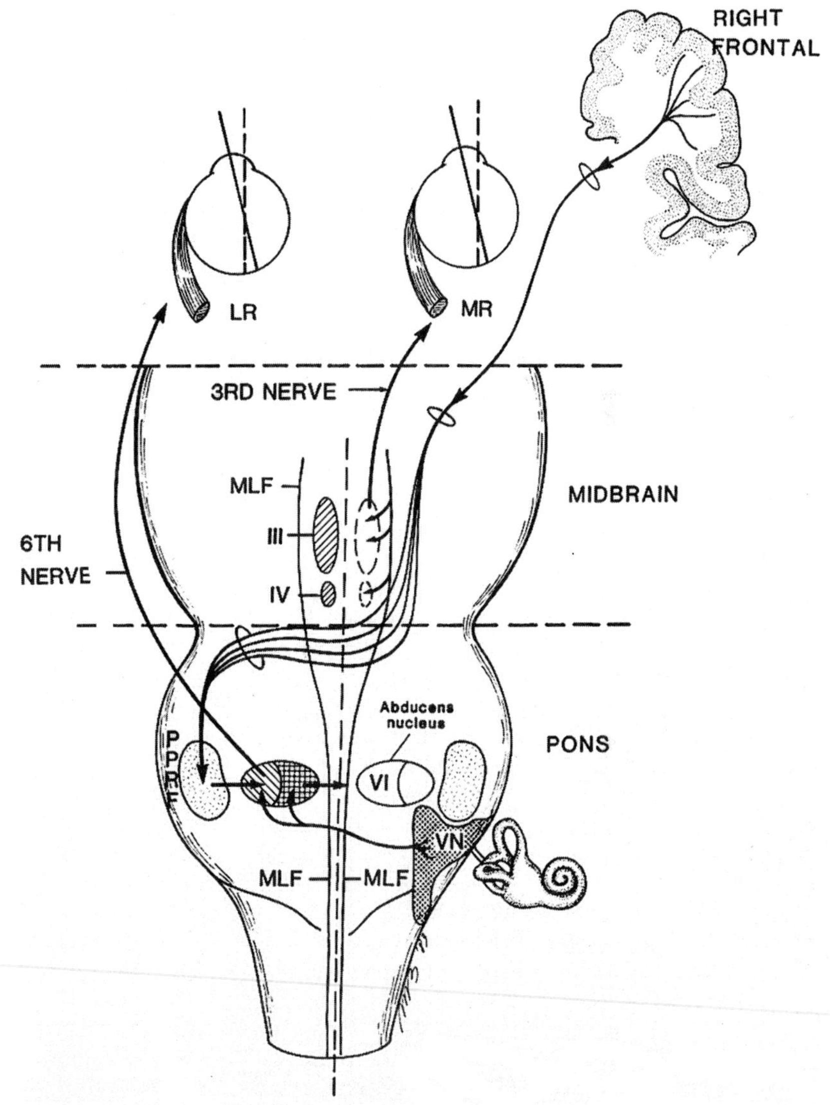

Figure 14-1

The supranuclear pathways subserving saccadic horizontal gaze to the left. The pathway originates in the right frontal cortex, descends in the internal capsule, decussates at the level of the rostral pons, and descends to synapse in the left pontine paramedian reticular formation (PPRF). Further connections with the ipsilateral sixth nerve nucleus and contralateral medial longitudinal fasciculus are also indicated. Cranial nerve nuclei III and IV are labeled on left; nucleus of VI and vestibular nuclei (VN) are labeled on right. LR, lateral rectus; MR, medial rectus; MLF, medial longitudinal fasciculus.

movements are projections from the frontal eye fields to the ipsilateral dorsolateral pontine nuclei. The latter, in turn, project to the flocculus and dorsal vermis of the cerebellum.

Brainstem Pathways Ultimately, all the pathways mediating saccadic and pursuit movements in the horizontal plane as well as vestibular and optokinetic movements converge upon the pontine centers for horizontal gaze. These comprise the PPRF, the nuclei prepositus hypoglossi and commissure, the abducens and medial vestibular nuclei, and pathways in the pontine and mesencephalic tegmentum that interconnect the ocular motor nuclei (Fig. 14-1). (Conventionally, the term *ocular motor nuclei* refers to the nuclei of the third, fourth, and sixth cranial nerves; the term *oculomotor nucleus* refers to the third nerve nucleus alone.) The pathway connecting the third and sixth nerve nuclei, and connecting both these nuclei with the vestibular nuclei, lies in the medial tegmentum of the brainstem; this pathway is termed the *medial longitudinal fasciculus* (MLF).

The PPRF and the prepositus and medial vestibular nuclei function as a neural integrator and relay station for horizontal saccade pathways. However, the neural signals that encode smooth pursuit and vestibular and optokinetic movements bypass the PPRF and project independently to the abducens nuclei (Hanson et al).

The abducens nucleus contains two groups of neurons, each with distinctive morphologic and pharmacologic properties: (1) abducens motor neurons, which project to the ipsilateral lateral rectus muscle, and (2) abducens internuclear neurons, which project via the contralateral MLF to the medial (internal) rectus neurons of the oculomotor nucleus. Conjugate lateral gaze is accomplished by the simultaneous innervation of the ipsilateral external rectus and the contralateral medial rectus, the latter through fibers that run in the medial portion of the MLF. Interruption of the MLF accounts for the discrete impairment or loss of adduction of the eye ipsilateral to the MLF lesion, while the medial rectus still contracts and the eye adducts on convergence, a phenomenon referred to as *internuclear ophthalmoplegia*, the details of which are discussed further on (Fig. 14-1). Two other ascending pathways between the pontine centers and the mesencephalic reticular formation have been traced: one traverses the central tegmental tract and terminates in the pretectum, in the nucleus of the posterior commissure; the other is a bundle separate from the MLF that passes around the nuclei of Cajal and Darkschewitz to the rostral interstitial nucleus of the MLF (ri MLF). These nuclei are involved more in vertical gaze and are described below. In addition, each vestibular nucleus projects onto the abducens nucleus and the MLF of the opposite side; the functional significance of the latter pathways is not entirely clear.

Although projections from the frontal eye fields to the ocular motor nuclei, as described above, undoubtedly exist, indirect projections are probably more important in the voluntary control of conjugate eye movements. According to Leigh and Zee, a more accurate conceptualization of these voluntary influences is one of a hierarchy of cell stations and parallel pathways that do not project directly to ocular motor nuclei but to adjacent *premotor* or *burst neurons*, which discharge at high frequencies immediately preceding the saccade. The premotor or burst neurons for horizontal saccades lie within the PPRF and those for vertical saccades in the ri MLF (see below). Yet a third class of neurons (pause cells), lying in the midline of the pons, is involved in the inhibition of unwanted saccadic discharges.

Vertical Gaze In contrast to horizontal gaze, which is generated by unilateral aggregates of cerebral and pontine neurons, vertical eye movements, with few exceptions, are under bilateral control of the cerebral cortex and upper brainstem. The groups of nerve cells and fibers that govern upward and downward gaze as well as torsional saccades are situated in the pretectal areas of the midbrain and involve three integral structures—the rostral interstitial nucleus of the medial longitudinal fasciculus (ri MLF), the interstitial nucleus of Cajal (INC), and the nucleus and fibers of the posterior commissure (Fig. 14-2).

The ri MLF lies at the junction of the midbrain and thalamus, at the rostral end of the medial longitudinal fasciculus, just dorsomedial to the rostral pole of the red nucleus. The ri MLF functions as the "premotor" nucleus or "burst cells" for the production of fast (saccadic) versional and torsional movements. Input to the ri MLF arises both from the PPRF and the vestibular nuclei. Each ri MLF projects mainly ipsilaterally to the oculomotor and trochlear nuclei, but each ri MLF is connected to its counterpart by fibers that traverse the posterior commissure. Bilateral lesions of the ri MLF or of their interconnections in the posterior commisure (see below) are more common than unilateral ones and cause a loss either of downward saccades or of all vertical saccades.

The *interstitial nucleus of Cajal (INC)* is a small collection of cells that lies just caudal to the ri MLF on each side. Each nucleus projects to the motor neurons of the elevator muscles (superior rectus and inferior oblique) by fibers that cross through the posterior com-

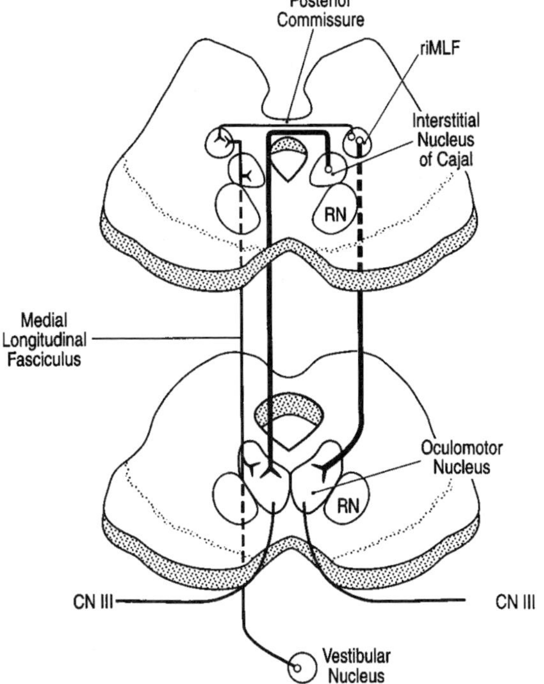

Figure 14-2

Pathways for the control of vertical eye movements. The main structures are the interstitial nucleus of Cajal (INC), the rostral interstitial nucleus of the medial longitudinal fasciculus (riMLF), and the subnuclei of the third nerve, all located in the dorsal midbrain. Voluntary vertical movements are initiated by the simultaneous activity of both frontal cortical eye fields. The riMLF serves as the generator of vertical saccades and the INC acts tonically to hold eccentric vertical gaze. The INC and riMLF connect with their contralateral nuclei via the posterior commissure where fibers are subject to damage. Projections for upgaze cross through the commissure before descending to innervate the third nerve nucleus, while those for downgaze may travel directly to the third nerve thus accounting for the frequency of selective upgaze palsies (see text). The MLF carries signals from the vertibular nuclei, mainly ipsilaterally, to stabilize the eyes in the vertical plane (VOR) and maintain tonic vertical position.

missure and project ipsilaterally to the depressor muscles (inferior rectus and superior oblique). The functional role of the INC appears to be in holding eccentric vertical gaze, especially after a saccade; it is also integral to the vestibulo-ocular reflex. Lesions of the INC produce a vertical gaze-evoked and torsional nystagmus and an ocular tilt reaction (page 278) and probably impair all conjugate eye movements, mainly vertical ones, to some extent.

Lesions of the *posterior commissure* interrupt signals crossing from the INC and the ri MLF and characteristically produce a paralysis of upward gaze and of convergence, often associated with mydriasis and lid retraction (Collier's "tucked lid" sign) and less commonly with ptosis. This is the *Parinaud syndrome*, also referred to as the pretectal, dorsal midbrain, or Sylvian aqueduct syndrome (see page 277). The same syndrome may be produced by unilateral lesions of the posterior commissure, presumably by interrupting its afferent and efferent connections. With acute lesions of the commissure, there may be a tonic downward deviation of the eyes and lid retraction ("setting-sun sign").

The MLF is the main conduit of vertical gaze signals from the vestibular nuclei in the medulla to the midbrain centers. For this reason, vertical pursuit and VOR are impaired with internuclear ophthalmoplegia (INO), particularly when the lesion is bilateral, and a vertical deviation of the ipsilateral globe (*skew*; see further on) may be seen in cases of unilateral INO, as discussed in a later section

Vestibulocerebellar Influences on Eye Movements

There are important vestibulocerebellar influences on both smooth pursuit and saccadic movements (see also Chap. 5). The flocculus and posterior vermis of the cerebellum receive abundant sensory projections from proprioceptors of the cervical musculature (responsive to head velocity), the retinas (sensitive to target velocity), proprioceptors of eye muscles (eye position and eye velocity), auditory and tactile receptors, and the superior colliculi and PPRF. Cerebellar efferents concerned with ocular movement project onto the vestibular nuclei, and the latter, in turn, influence gaze mechanisms through several projection systems: one, for horizontal movements, consists of direct projections from the vestibular nuclei to the contralateral sixth nerve nucleus; another, for vertical movements, projects, via the contralateral MLF, to third and fourth nerve nuclei (Figs. 14-1 and 14-2).

Lesions of the flocculus and posterior vermis (lobules VI and VII) are consistently associated with deficits in smooth pursuit movements and an inability to suppress the vestibulo-ocular reflex by fixation (Baloh et al). Floccular lesions are also an important cause of downbeat nystagmus. Also, as indicated in Chap. 5, patients with cerebellar (floccular) lesions are unable to hold eccentric positions of gaze and must make repeated saccades to look at a target that is away from the neutral position (*gaze-paretic nystagmus*). This phenomenon is explained by the fact that with acute, one-sided lesions of the vestibulocerebellum, the inhibitory discharges of the Purkinje cells onto the ipsilateral medial vestibular nucleus are removed and the eyes deviate away from the lesion. When gaze to the side of the lesion is attempted, the eyes drift back to the midline and can be corrected only by a saccadic jerk. The head and neck may also turn away from the lesion (the occiput toward the lesion and the face away). In addition, the vestibular ocular reflexes, which coordinate eye movements with head movements, are improperly adjusted (Thach and Montgomery). The interested reader will find further details concerning cerebellar influences on ocular movements in the monograph by Leigh and Zee and the review by Lewis and Zee.

Testing of Conjugate Gaze

It is apparent from the foregoing remarks that there is considerable clinical information to be obtained about ocular movements and their central control mechanisms by the simple expedients of asking the patient to look quickly to each side as well as up and down and to follow a moving target (a light, the examiner's or the patient's finger, or an optokinetic drum) or, in patients with stupor and coma, by passively turning the head and irrigating the external auditory canals—the last two being vestibular stimuli.

Most individuals make accurate saccades to a target. Persistent alterations of saccadic movements, particularly overshooting of the eyes (*hypermetria*), is characteristic of a cerebellar lesion. *Slowness of saccadic movements* are sometimes extreme in degree. Slow saccades may be seen in Huntington disease and also in Wilson disease, ataxia-telangiectasia, progressive supranuclear palsy, olivopontocerebellar degeneration, and certain lipid storage diseases. Lesions involving the PPRF may be accompanied by slow saccadic movements to the affected side. Hypometric, slow saccades, occurring only in the adducting eye on quick lateral gaze, indicate an internuclear ophthalmoparesis due to a lesion of the ipsilateral MLF. When slow saccades are first observed in the vertical plane early in an extrapyramidal disease, the likeliest diagnosis is progressive supranuclear palsy; if upward gaze saccades are lost late in an extrapyramidal process, advanced Parkinson disease may be the explanation or any of a number of diseases that affect vertical gaze (Table 14-1). Slow up-and-down saccades are also a consistent finding in Niemann-Pick disease type C (page1014).

Yet another saccadic disorder takes the form of an *inability to initiate voluntary movements*, either vertically or horizontally. This abnormality may be congenital in nature, as in the ocular "apraxia" of childhood (Cogan syndrome, see below) and ataxia-telangiectasia; difficulty in the initiation of saccadic movements as an acquired abnormality may be seen in patients with Huntington disease or with a lesion of the contralateral frontal lobe or ipsilateral pontine tegmentum.

In addition to abnormalities of the saccades themselves, saccadic latency or reaction time (the interval between the impulse to move and movement) is prolonged in Huntington chorea and Parkinson disease. Saccade latency is also increased in cerebral-basal ganglionic degeneration, in which case it seems to correlate with the degree of apraxia.

Fragmentation of smooth pursuit movement is a frequent neuro-ophthalmic finding. Drug intoxication—with phenytoin, barbiturates, diazepam, and other sedative drugs—is probably the most common cause. As a manifestation of structural disease, it points to a lesion of the vestibulocerebellum. Smooth pursuit movements are found to be impaired in all basal ganglionic degenerations, according to Vidailhet and colleagues. Also, in certain extrapyramidal diseases, such as Parkinson disease, Huntington disease, and progressive supranuclear palsy—there is often an impairment of smooth pursuit movements in association with slow, hypometric saccades ("saccadic pursuit"). Asymmetrical impairment of smooth pursuit movements is indicative of a parietal lobe lesion; a right

Table 14-1
Diseases exhibiting upgaze or vertical gaze palsy

Midbrain infarction and hemorrhage
Midbrain region tumor (e.g., pinealoma)
Advanced hydrocephalus with third ventricular enlargement
Progressive supranuclear palsy
Parkinson disease
Lewy body disease
Cortical basal ganglionic degeneration
Whipple disease
Metabolic diseases of childhood (Niemann-Pick C, Gaucher, Tay-Sachs, etc.)
Any cause of bilateral internuclear palsy (e.g., multiple sclerosis)

parietal lesion causes an impairment of smooth tracking to the patient's right and a consequent decrease in the corrective nystagmus on rotating the optokinetic drum in that direction.

Zee has described a simple means of *evaluating the VOR*. In a dimly lit room, the patient is instructed to fixate on a distant target with one eye while the examiner observes the optic nerve head of the other eye with an ophthalmoscope. The subject is then instructed to rotate his head back and forth at a rate of one to two cycles per second. In a normal subject, the optic nerve head remains stationary; if the VOR is impaired, the optic nerve head appears to oscillate. Normally, movement of the head at this rate does not cause blurring of vision, because of the rapidity with which the VOR accomplishes compensatory eye movements. By contrast with the head in a fixed position, to-and-fro movement of the environment will cause blurring of vision because normal tracking movements are too slow to fixate the object in space. As a rule, the patient with impairment of smooth pursuit movements will have a commensurate inability to suppress the VOR.

Combined fusional-accommodative movements (tested by asking the patient to look at his thumbnail as it is brought toward the eyes) are frequently impaired in the elderly and in confused or inattentive patients. In others, the absence or impairment of these movements should suggest the presence of basal ganglionic disease, more particularly progressive supranuclear palsy, Parkinson disease, or some other lesion in the rostral midbrain. *Convergence spasms* and *retraction nystagmus* may accompany paralysis of vertical gaze. Such spasms, occurring alone, are characteristic of hysteria. In such patients, full movement can usually be obtained if each eye is tested separately. A cycloplegic (homatropine eyedrops) will abolish the accommodation and pupillary miosis, but its effect on the convergence spasm is less predictable.

Paralysis of Conjugate Gaze

Horizontal Gaze Palsy An *acute lesion of one frontal lobe*, such as an infarct, usually causes impersistence or paresis of contralateral gaze, and the eyes will turn involuntarily toward the side of the cerebral lesion. Occasionally a deep cerebral lesion, particularly a thalamic hemorrhage extending into the midbrain, will cause the eyes to deviate conjugately to the side opposite the lesion ("wrong-way" gaze). In most cases of cerebral infarction, the gaze palsy is incomplete and temporary, lasting for a day or two or for as long as a week. Almost invariably, it is accompanied by hemiparesis. In this circumstance, forced closure of the eyelids may cause the eyes to move paradoxically to the side of the hemiparesis rather than upward. During sleep, the eyes deviate conjugately from the side of the lesion to the side of the hemiplegia. Also, as indicated above, pursuit movements to the side of the lesion tend to fragment. With bilateral frontal lesions, the patient may be unable to turn his eyes voluntarily in any direction but retains fixation and following movements, probably because pursuit movements are initiated in the parieto-occipital cortex. Gaze paralysis of central origin is not attended by strabismus or diplopia. The usual causes are vascular occlusion with infarction, hemorrhage, and abscess or tumor of the frontal lobe.

A *unilateral lesion in the rostral midbrain tegmentum*, by interrupting the cerebral pathways for horizontal conjugate gaze before their decussation, will cause a gaze palsy to the opposite side. A lesion in the pontine horizontal gaze complex (PPRF) involving the abducens nucleus causes ipsilateral gaze palsy and deviation of the eyes to the opposite side. As a rule, the horizontal gaze palsies of cerebral and pontine origin are readily distinguished. The former are usually accompanied by hemiparesis, and the paralysis of gaze is on the same side as the hemiparesis. Palsies of pontine origin are associated with other signs of pontine disease, particularly peripheral facial and external rectus palsies and internuclear ophthalmoplegia on the same side as the paralysis of gaze; hemiparesis, if present, is on the side opposite to the gaze palsy. Gaze palsies due to cerebral lesions tend not to be as long-lasting as those due to pontine lesions. Also, in the case of a cerebral lesion (but not a pontine lesion), the eyes can be turned to the paralyzed side if they are fixated on the target and the head is rotated passively to the opposite side (i.e., by utilizing the VOR).

Vertical Gaze Palsy Midbrain lesions affecting the pretectum on both sides of the midline (or at times a lesion confined to one side) and lesions in the region of the posterior commissure interfere with conjugate movements in the vertical plane. Restated, paralysis of vertical gaze is a prominent feature of the *Parinaud, or dorsal midbrain, syndrome* (see above). Upward gaze is affected far more frequently than downward gaze because, as already explained, some of the fibers subserving upgaze cross rostrally and posteriorly between the ri MLF and INC nuclei and are subject to interruption before descending to the oculomotor nuclei, whereas the pathways for downgaze apparently project directly downward from the two controlling nuclei. Optokinetic nystagmus in the vertical plane is usually lost in association with these abnormalities.

The range of upward gaze is frequently restricted by a number of extraneous factors, such as drowsiness, increased intracranial pressure, and particularly by aging. In patients who cannot elevate their eyes voluntarily, the presence of reflex upward deviation of the eyes in response to forced flexion of the head ("doll's-head maneuver") or to forced closure of the eyelids (*Bell's phenomenon*) usually indicates that the nuclear and infranuclear mechanisms for upward gaze are intact and that the defect is supranuclear. However useful this rule may be, in some instances of Guillain-Barré syndrome and myasthenia gravis, in which voluntary upgaze is limited, the strong stimulus of eye closure may also cause upward deviation, whereas voluntary attempts at upgaze are unsuccessful. About 15 percent of normal adults do not show a Bell's phenomenon, and in others deviation of the eyes is paradoxically downward.

In several patients who during life had shown an isolated palsy of downward gaze, autopsy has disclosed bilateral lesions (infarction) of the rostral midbrain tegmentum, just medial and dorsal to the red nuclei. In monkeys, a defect in downward gaze has been produced of bilateral circumscribed lesions centered in these regions (Kompf et al). A unique case, described by Bogousslavsky and colleagues, suggests that a paralysis of vertical gaze may follow a strictly unilateral infarction involving the posterior commissure, ri MLF, and INC. Hommel and Bogousslavsky have summarized the location of infarctions that cause monocular and binocular vertical gaze palsies.

Several *degenerative and related processes* exhibit selective upgaze or vertical gaze palsies (Table 14-1). In progressive supranuclear palsy, a characteristic feature is a selective paralysis of upward and then downward gaze, initially evident as difficulty with saccades (page 1139). Parkinson and Lewy body diseases (Chap. 39), corticobasalganglionic degeneration (Chap. 39), and Whipple disease of the brain (Chap. 40) may produce vertical gaze palsies as the diseases progress.

Other Gaze Palsies *Skew deviation* is a poorly understood disorder in which there is vertical deviation of one eye above the other. The deviation may be the same (comitant) in all fields of gaze or it may vary with different directions of gaze. The patient complains of vertical diplopia. Skew deviation does not have precise localizing value but occurs with a variety of lesions of the cerebellum and the brainstem, particularly those involving the MLF. With skew deviation due to cerebellar disease, the eye on the side of the lesion is usually lower but sometimes higher than the other eye (in a ratio of 2:1 in Keane's series), in distinction to unilateral internuclear ophthalmoplegia, in which the eye is typically higher on the side of the lesion. (Recall that the image from the affected eye is always projected in the opposite direction to eye deviation.) Skew deviation has been known to alternate from one side to the other and has been seen with the condition known as periodic alternating nystagmus. Ford and coworkers have described a rare form of skew deviation due to monocular elevation palsy from a lesion immediately rostral to the ipsilateral oculomotor nucleus; a lesion of upgaze efferents from the ipsilateral ri MLF was postulated, but an abnormality of the vertical gaze holding mechanism related to the INC is an alternative explanation.

The *ocular tilt reaction*, in which skew deviation is combined with ocular torsion and head tilt, is usually attributed to an imbalance in otolith-ocular and otolith-collic reflexes. In unilateral lesions involving the vestibular nuclei, as in lateral medullary infarction, the eye is lower on the side of the lesion. With lesions of the MLF or INC, which can also cause an ocular tilt reaction, the eye is higher on the side of the lesion.

Another unusual and now almost vanished disturbance of gaze is the *oculogyric crisis*, or *spasm*, which consists of a tonic spasm of conjugate deviation of the eyes, usually upward and less frequently laterally or downward. Recurrent attacks, sometimes associated with spasms of the neck, mouth, and tongue muscles and lasting from a few seconds to an hour or two, were pathognomonic of postencephalitic parkinsonism. Now this phenomenon is observed rarely as an acute reaction in patients being given phenothiazine drugs (page 1264) and in Niemann-Pick disease. The pathogenesis of these ocular spasms is not known.

Congenital ocular motor "apraxia" (Cogan syndrome) is a disorder characterized by abnormal eye and head movements during attempts to change the position of the eyes. The patient is unable to make normal voluntary *horizontal* saccades when the head is stationary. If the head is free to move and the patient is asked to look at an object to either side, the head is thrust to one side and the eyes turn in the opposite direction; the head overshoots the target, and the eyes, as they return to the central position, fixate on the target. Both voluntary saccades and the quick phase of vestibular nystagmus are defective. The pathologic anatomy has never been studied. This phenomenon is also seen in ataxia-telangiectasia (page 1011) and in association with agenesis of the corpus callosum, in which both horizontal and vertical saccades may be affected.

NUCLEAR AND INFRANUCLEAR DISORDERS OF EYE MOVEMENT

Anatomic Considerations

The third (oculomotor), fourth (trochlear), and sixth (abducens) cranial nerves innervate the extrinsic muscles of the eye. Since their actions are closely integrated and many diseases involve all of them at once, they are suitably considered together.

The *oculomotor (third-nerve)* nuclei consist of several paired groups of nerve cells, adjacent to the midline and ventral to the aqueduct of Sylvius, at the level of the superior colliculi. A centrally located group of nerve cells that innervate the pupillary sphincters and ciliary bodies (muscles of accommodation) is situated dorsally in the Edinger-Westphal nucleus; this is the parasympathetic portion of the oculomotor nucleus. Ventral to this nuclear group are cells that mediate the actions of the levator of the lid, superior and inferior recti, inferior oblique, and medial rectus in this dorsal-ventral order. This functional arrangement has been determined in cats and monkeys by extirpating individual extrinsic ocular muscles and observing the retrograde cellular changes (Warwick). Subsequent studies, utilizing radioactive tracer techniques, have shown that the medial rectus neurons occupy three disparate locations within the oculomotor nucleus rather than being confined to its ventral tip (Büttner-Ennever and Akert). These experiments also indicate that the medial and inferior recti and the inferior oblique have a strictly homolateral representation in the oculomotor nuclei; the superior rectus receives only crossed fibers; and the levator palpebrae superioris has a bilateral innervation. Vergence movements are under the control of medial rectus neurons and not an unpaired medial group of cells ("nucleus of Perlia"), as was once supposed.

It is important to note that the efferent fibers of the oculomotor and abducens nuclei have a considerable intramedullary extent (Fig. 14-3*A* and *B*). The fibers of the third-nerve nucleus course ventrally in the brainstem, crossing the medial longitudinal fasciculus, red nucleus, substantia nigra, and medial part of the cerebral peduncle; lesions involving these structures may therefore interrupt oculomotor fibers in their intramedullary course. The *sixth nerve (abducens)* arises at the level of the lower pons, from a paired group of cells in the floor of the fourth ventricle, adjacent to the midline. The intrapontine portion of the facial nerve loops around

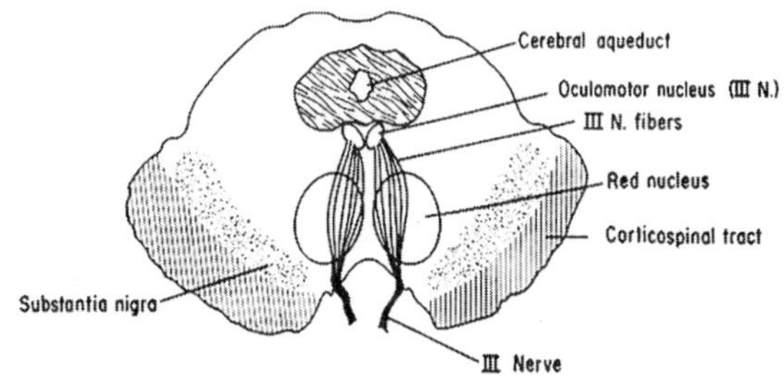

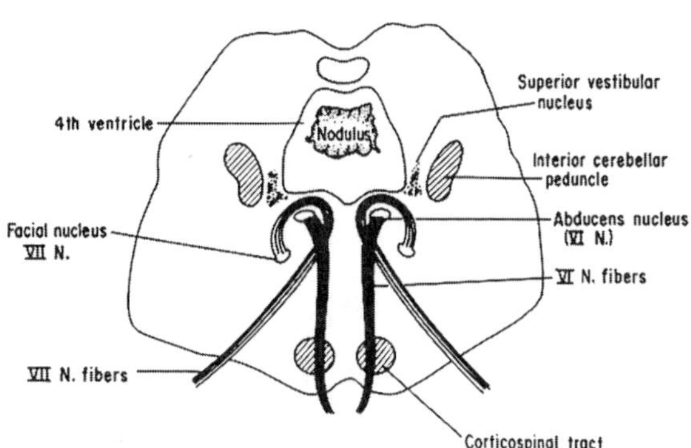

Figure 14-3

A. *Midbrain in horizontal section, indicating the effects of lesions at different points along the intramedullary course of the third nerve fibers. Lesion at level of oculomotor nucleus results in homolateral third nerve paralysis and homolateral anesthesia of the cornea. Lesion at level of red nucleus results in homolateral third nerve paralysis and contralateral ataxic tremor (Benedikt and Claude syndromes). Lesion near point of exit of third nerve fibers results in homolateral third nerve paralysis and crossed corticospinal tract signs (Weber syndrome; see Table 47-2).* B. *Brainstem at the level of the sixth nerve nuclei, indicating effects of lesions at different loci. Lesion at level of the nucleus results in homolateral sixth and seventh nerve paralyses with varying degrees of nystagmus and weakness of conjugate gaze to the homolateral side. Lesion at level of corticospinal tract results in homolateral sixth nerve paralysis and crossed hemiplegia (Millard-Gubler syndrome).*

the sixth-nerve nucleus before it turns anterolaterally to make its exit; a lesion in this locality therefore causes a homolateral paralysis of the lateral rectus and facial muscles.

The cells of origin of the *trochlear nerves* are just caudal to those of the oculomotor nerves. Unlike the third and sixth nerves, the fourth nerve courses posteriorly and decussates a short distance from its origin before emerging from the dorsal surface of the brainstem, just caudal to the inferior colliculi. It therefore innervates the *contralateral* superior oblique muscle.

The oculomotor nerve, soon after it emerges from the brainstem, passes between the superior cerebellar and posterior cerebral arteries. The nerve (and posterior cerebral artery) may be compressed at this point by herniation of the uncus through the tentorium (see Chap. 17). The sixth nerve, after leaving the brainstem, sweeps upward and runs alongside the third and fourth cranial nerves; together they course anteriorly, pierce the dura just lateral to the posterior clinoid process, and run in the lateral wall of the cavernous sinus, where they are closely applied to the cavernous portion of the internal carotid artery and first and second divisions of the fifth nerve (Fig. 14-4).

Retrocavernous compressive lesions, notably infraclinoid aneurysms and tumors, tend to involve all three sensory divisions of the trigeminal nerve, together with the ocular motor nerves. In the posterior portion of the cavernous sinus, the first and second trigeminal divisions tend to be involved along with the ocular motor nerves; in the anterior portion, only the ophthalmic division is affected. Just posterior and superior to the cavernous sinus, the oculomotor nerve crosses the terminal portion of the internal carotid artery at its junction with the posterior communicating artery. An aneurysm at the latter site frequently damages the third nerve, and this serves to localize the site of compression or bleeding.

Together with the first division of the fifth nerve, the third, fourth, and sixth nerves enter the orbit through the superior orbital fissure. The oculomotor nerve, as it

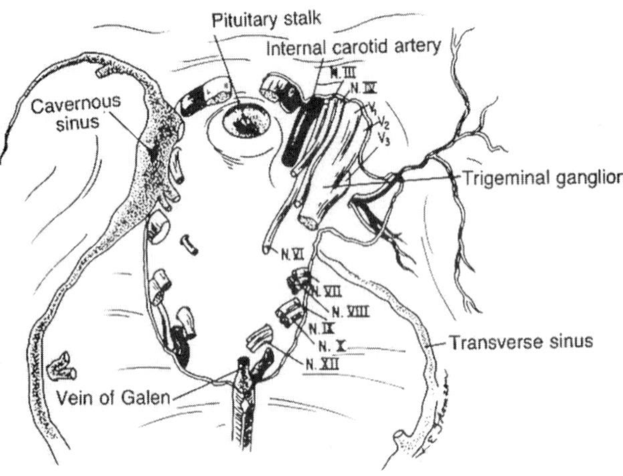

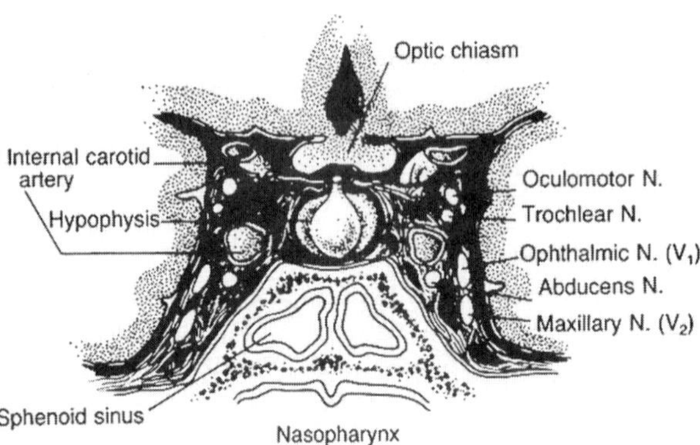

Figure 14-4

The cavernous sinus and its relation to the cranial nerves. A. *Base of the skull; the cavernous sinus has been removed on the right.* B. *The cavernous sinus and its contents viewed in the coronal plane.*

enters the orbit, divides into superior and inferior branches, although a functional division occurs well before the anatomic bifurcation. The superior branch supplies the superior rectus and the voluntary (striated) part of the levator palpebrae (the involuntary part is under the control of sympathetic fibers); the inferior branch supplies the pupillary and ciliary muscles and all the other extrinsic ocular muscles except two—the superior oblique and the external rectus—which are innervated by the trochlear and abducens nerves, respectively. Superior branch lesions caused by an aneurysm or associated with diabetes or a viral infection cause ptosis and uniocular upgaze paresis.

Under normal conditions, all the extraocular muscles probably participate in every movement of the eyes; for proper movement, the contraction of any muscle requires relaxation of its antagonist. Clinically, however, an eye movement should be thought of in terms of the one muscle that is predominantly responsible for an agonist movement in that direction: e.g., outward rotation of the eye requires the action of the lateral rectus; inward rotation, action of the medial rectus. The action of the superior and inferior recti and the oblique muscles varies according to the position of the eye. When the eye is turned outward, the elevator is the superior rectus and the depressor is the inferior rectus. When the eye is turned inward, the elevator and depressor are the inferior and superior oblique muscles, respectively. The actions of the ocular muscles in different positions of gaze are illustrated in Fig. 14-5 and Table 14-2. The clinical implications of flaws in these muscle actions are discussed below.

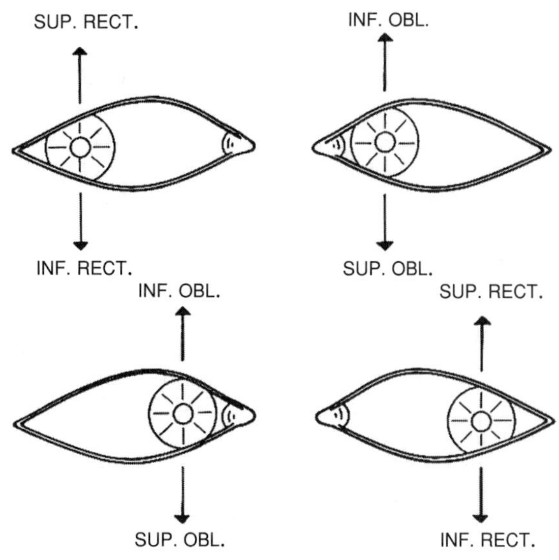

Figure 14-5

Muscles chiefly responsible for vertical movements of the eyes in different positions of gaze. (Adapted by permission from Cogan DG: Neurology of the Ocular Muscles, 2nd ed, Springfield, IL, Charles C Thomas, 1956.)

Strabismus (Squint)

This refers to a muscle imbalance that results in a misalignment of the visual axes of the two eyes. It may be caused by weakness of an individual eye muscle (*paralytic strabismus*) or by an imbalance of muscular tone, presumably due to a faulty "central" mechanism that normally maintains a proper angle between the two visual axes (*nonparalytic strabismus*). It is in the latter sense that the term is generally used. Almost everyone has a slight tendency to strabismus, i.e., to misalign the visual axes when a target is viewed with one eye. This tendency is referred to as a *phoria* and is normally overcome by the fusion mechanisms. A misalignment that is manifest during binocular viewing of a target and cannot be overcome, even when the patient is forced to fixate with the deviant eye, is called a *tropia*. The prefixes *eso-* and *exo-* indicate that the phoria or tropia is directed inward or outward, respectively, and the prefixes *hyper-* and *hypo-*, that the deviation is upward or downward. Paralytic strabismus is primarily a neurologic problem; nonparalytic strabismus (referred to as *comitant strabismus* if the angle between the visual axes is the same in all fields of gaze) is more strictly an ophthalmologic problem.

Once binocular fusion is established, usually by 6 months of age, any type of ocular muscle imbalance will cause diplopia, since images then fall on disparate or noncorresponding parts of the two functionally active retinas. After a time, however, the child eliminates the diplopia by suppressing the image in one eye. After a variable period, the suppression becomes permanent, and

Table 14-2
Actions of the extraocular muscles (see also Fig. 14-5)

Muscle	*Primary action*	*Secondary action*
Medial rectus	Adduction	—
Lateral rectus	Abduction	—
Superior rectus	Elevation	Intorsion
Inferior rectus	Depression	Extorsion
Superior oblique	Intorsion	Depression
Inferior oblique	Extorsion	Elevation

the individual grows up with a diminished visual acuity in that eye, the result of prolonged disuse (*amblyopia ex anopsia*). With proper early treatment, the amblyopia can be reversed; but if it persists beyond the age of 5 or 6 years, recovery of vision rarely occurs. Occasionally, when the eyes are used alternately for fixation (*alternating strabismus*), visual acuity remains good in each eye.

Nonparalytic strabismus may pose a problem for neurologists. It has a way of appearing in early childhood for unclear reasons and conjures up possibilities of serious neurologic disease. Sometimes it is first noticed after a head injury or an infection, or it may be exposed by some other neurologic disorder or drug intoxication that impairs fusional mechanisms (vergence). In a cooperative patient, nonparalytic strabismus may be demonstrated by showing that each eye can be moved fully when the other eye is covered. Tropias and phorias can readily be detected by means of the simple "cover" and "cover-uncover" tests. In the case of a tropia, in which one eye is not aligned with the target (for example when viewing the large E at 20 ft), covering the fixating eye will force the uncovered (deviating) eye to change its position abruptly and focus on the target (movement of redress). Similarly, the cover-uncover test can detect latent phorias that are suppressed by the fusion mechanism as long as both eyes are used. When fusion is disrupted by covering one eye, the covered eye will deviate as just noted; uncovering the eye results in a quick corrective movement designed to re-establish the fusion mechanism.

Clinical Effects of Lesions of Individual Ocular Nerves

Characteristic clinical disturbances result from lesions of the third, fourth, and sixth cranial nerves. A complete *third-nerve lesion* causes ptosis or drooping of the upper eyelid (since the levator palpebrae is supplied mainly by the third nerve) and an inability to rotate the eye upward, downward, or inward. When the lid is passively elevated, *the eye is found to be deviated outward and slightly downward* because of the unopposed actions of the intact lateral rectus and superior oblique muscles. In addition, one finds a dilated nonreactive pupil (iridoplegia) and paralysis of accommodation (cycloplegia) due to interruption of the parasympathetic fibers in the third nerve. However, the extrinsic and intrinsic eye muscles may be affected separately. Infarction of the central portion of the oculomotor nerve, as occurs in diabetic ophthalmoplegia, typically spares the pupil, since the parasympathetic preganglionic pupilloconstrictor fibers lie near the surface. Conversely, compressive lesions of the nerve usually dilate the pupil. After injury, regeneration of the third nerve fibers may be aberrant. For example, some of the fibers that originally moved the eye in a particular direction now reach another muscle or the iris; in the latter instance the pupil, which is unreactive to light, may constrict when the eye turns up and in.

A *fourth nerve* lesion is the commonest cause of symptomatic vertical diplopia. Paralysis of the superior oblique muscle results in extorsion and weakness of downward movement of the affected eye, most marked when the eye is turned inward, so that the patient complains of special difficulty in reading or going down stairs. The affected eye tends *to deviate upward and inward*. This defect may be overlooked in the presence of a third nerve palsy if the examiner fails to note the absence of intorsion as the patient tries to move the paretic eye downward. Head tilting to the opposite shoulder (Bielschowsky sign) is especially characteristic of fourth nerve lesions; this maneuver causes a compensatory intorsion of the unaffected eye and ameliorates the double vision. Bilateral trochlear palsies, as occur after head trauma, give a characteristic alternating hyperdeviation depending on the direction of gaze.

Lesions of the *sixth nerve* result in a paralysis of lateral or outward movement and a crossing of the visual axes. The affected eye *deviates medially*, i.e., in the direction of the opposing muscle. With incomplete sixth nerve palsies, turning the head toward the side of the paretic muscle may overcome the diplopia. The main causes of individual oculomotor palsies and of combined palsies are listed in Table 14-3 and are analyzed in Fig. 14-6 and below.

The Analysis of Diplopia Almost all instances of diplopia (i.e., seeing a single object as double) are the result of an acquired paralysis or paresis of one or more extraocular muscles. The signs of the oculomotor palsies, as described above, are manifest in various degrees of completeness. Noting the relative positions of the corneal light reflections and having the patient perform common versional movements will usually *disclose the faulty muscle(s) as the eyes are turned into the field of action of the paretic muscle*. The muscle weakness may be so slight, however, that no squint or defect in ocular movement is obvious, yet the patient experiences diplopia. It is then necessary to study the relative positions of the images of the two eyes as a means of determining which muscle might be involved. Several tests are useful for this purpose.

Table 14-3
Main causes of individual and combined oculomotor palsies

Lesions of the third (oculomotor) nerve

Nuclear and intramedullary (fasciular)
- Infarction
- Demyelination
- Tumor
- Trauma
- Wernicke disease

Radicular (subarachnoid space and tentorial edge)
- Aneurysm (posterior communicating or basilar)
- Meningitis (infectious, neoplastic, granulomatous)
- Diabetic infarction
- Tumor
- Raised intracranial pressure (horizontal shift and herniation of medial temporal lobe, hydrocephalus)

Cavernous sinus and superior orbital fissure
- Diabetic infarction of nerve
- Aneurysm of internal carotid artery
- Carotid-cavernous fistula
- Cavernous thrombosis (septic and bland)
- Tumor (pituitary, meningioma, nasopharyngeal carcinoma, metastasis)
- Pituitary apoplexy
- Sphenoid sinusitis and mucocele
- Herpes zoster
- Tolosa-Hunt syndrome
- Macroglobulinemia-hyperviscosity

Orbit
- Trauma
- Fungal infection (mucormycosis, etc.)
- Tumor and granuloma

Uncertain localization
- Migraine
- Postinfectious

Lesions of the fourth (trochlear) nerve

Nuclear and intramedullary (fascicular)
- Midbrain hemorrhage and infarction
- Tumor
- Arteriovenous malformation
- Demyelination

Radicular (subarachnoid space)
- Tumor (pineal, meningioma, metastasis, etc.)
- Hydrocephalus
- Pseudotumor cerebri and increased intracranial pressure
- Mastoiditis
- Meningitis (Infectious, neoplastic, granulomatous)
- Raised intracranial pressure

Cavernous sinus and superior orbital fissure
- Tumor
- Tolosa-Hunt syndrome
- Internal carotid aneurysm
- Herpes zoster
- Diabetic infarction

Orbit
- Trauma
- Tumor and granuloma

Lesions of the sixth (abducens) nerve

Nuclear (characterized by gaze palsy) and intramedullary (fascicular)
- Möbius syndrome
- Wernicke syndrome
- Infarction
- Demyelination
- Tumor
- Lupus

Radicular (subarachnoid)
- Aneurysm
- Trauma
- Meningitis
- Tumor (clivus, fifth- and eighth-nerve schwannoma, meningioma)

Petrous
- Infection of mastoid and petrous bone
- Thrombosis of inferior petrosal vein
- Trauma

Cavernous sinus and superior orbital fissure
- Carotid aneurysm
- Cavernous sinus thrombosis
- Tumor (pituitary, nasopharyngeal, meningioma)
- Tolosa-Hunt syndrome
- Diabetic infarction
- Herpes zoster

Orbit
- Tumor and granulomas

Uncertain localization
- Migraine
- Viral and postviral
- Transient in newborns

Source: Adapted by permission from Leigh and Zee.

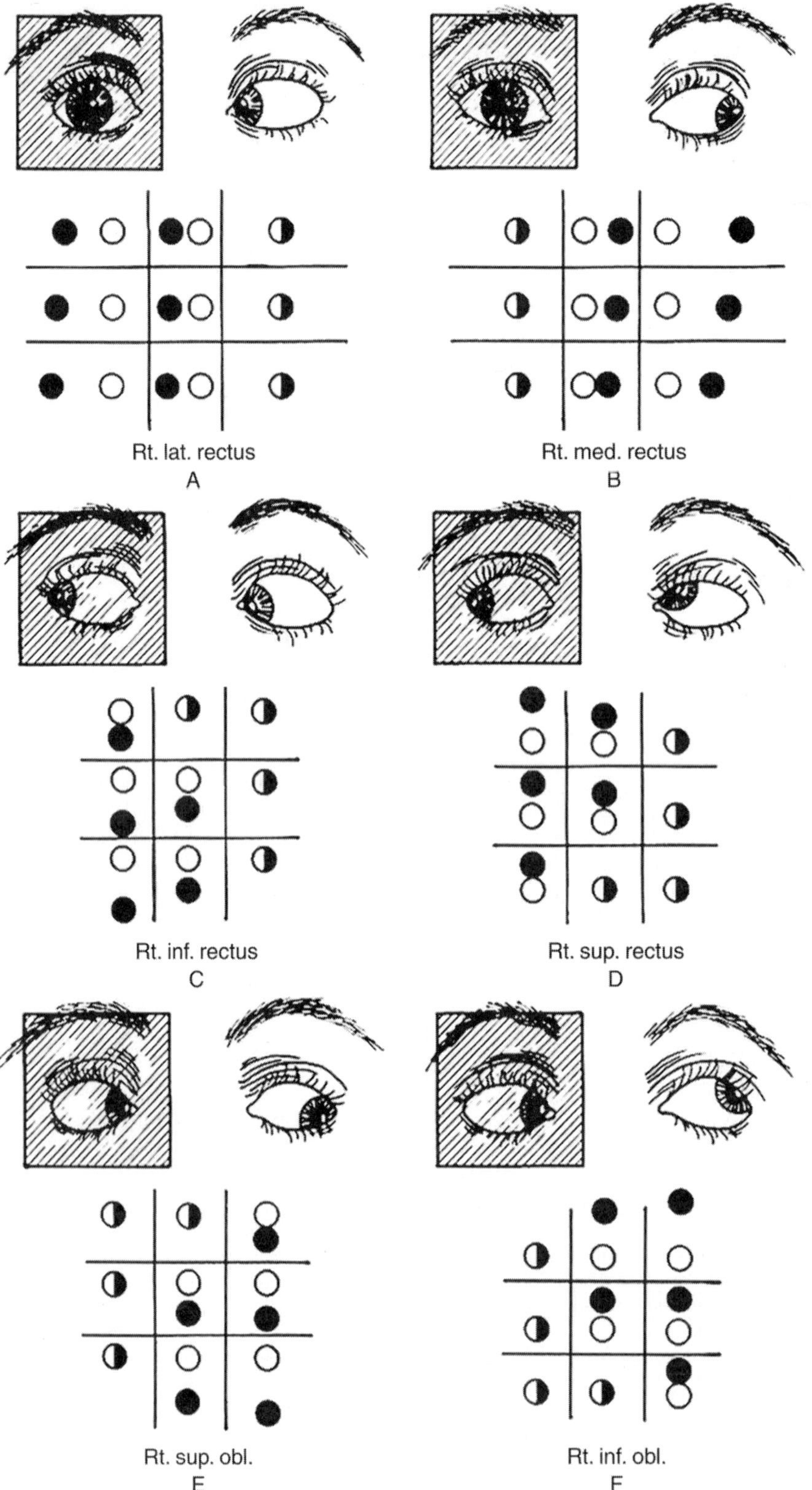
Rt. lat. rectus
A
Rt. med. rectus
B
Rt. inf. rectus
C
Rt. sup. rectus
D
Rt. sup. obl.
E
Rt. inf. obl.
F

Perhaps the simplest maneuver consists of asking the patient to follow an object or penlight into the six cardinal positions of gaze. When the position of maximal separation of images is identified, one eye is covered and the patient is asked to identify which image disappears. A more reliable way of distinguishing the weak muscle is by the *red-glass test*. The essential strategy of this test is also to determine the position of gaze that produces maximum diplopia. A red glass is placed in front of the patient's right eye (the choice of the right eye is arbitrary, but if the test is always done in the same way, interpretation is simplified). The patient is then asked to look at a flashlight (held at a distance of 1 m), to turn both eyes to the six cardinal points in the visual fields, and to state or indicate with his index fingers the position of the red and white images and the relative distances between them. The positions of the two images are plotted as the patient indicates them to the examiner (Fig. 14-6).

Three rules aid in the analysis of ocular movements by the red-glass test or simply from the reported separation of the images as viewed with both eyes:

1. The direction in which the images are maximally separated is the direction of action of a pair of muscles, one of which is paretic. For example, if the greatest horizontal separation is in looking to the right, either the right abductor (lateral rectus) or the left adductor (medial rectus) muscle is weak; when looking to the left, the left lateral rectus and right medial rectus are implicated (Fig. 14-6*A* and *B*).

2. If the separation is mainly horizontal, the paresis will be found in one of the horizontally acting recti (a small vertical disparity should be disregarded); if the separation is mainly vertical, the paresis will be found in the vertically acting muscles, and a small horizontal deviation should be disregarded.

3. The image projected farther from the center belongs to the paretic eye. With a red glass over the right eye, if the patient looks to the right and the red image is farther to the right, then the right lateral rectus muscle is weak.

It must be remembered that the red-glass test distinguishes *one* of *two* muscles responsible for the movement in the direction of maximal separation of images. If the white image on right lateral gaze is to the right of the red (i.e, the image from the left eye is projected outward), then the left medial rectus muscle is weak. In testing vertical movements, again, the image seen with the eye with the paretic muscle is the one projected most peripherally in the visual field. For example, if the maximum vertical separation of images occurs on looking downward and to the *left* and the white image is projected farther down than the red, the paretic muscle is the left inferior rectus; if the red image is lower than the white, the paretic muscle is the right superior oblique. As already mentioned for a supplementary test, correction of vertical diplopia by a tilting of the head implicates the superior oblique muscle of the opposite side. Separation of images on looking up and to the right or left will similarly distinguish paresis of the inferior oblique and superior rectus muscles. The examiner is aided by committing to memory the cardinal actions of the ocular muscles shown in Fig. 14-5 and Table 14-2.

The red-glass test and other similar tests are most useful when a single muscle is responsible for the diplopia. If more than one muscle seems to be involved, one must be certain not to overlook myasthenia gravis and thyroid ophthalmopathy.

There are several alternative methods for studying the relative positions of the images of the two eyes. One, a refinement of the red-glass test, is the *Maddox rod*, in

Figure 14-6

Diplopia fields with individual muscle paralysis. The dark glass is in front of the right eye, and the fields are projected as the patient sees the images. A. *Paralysis of right lateral rectus. Characteristic: right eye does not move to the right. Field: horizontal homonymous diplopia increasing on looking to the right.* B. *Paralysis of right medial rectus. Characteristic: right eye does not move to the left. Field: horizontal crossed diplopia increasing on looking to the left.* C. *Paralysis of right inferior rectus. Characteristic: right eye does not move downward when eyes are turned to the right. Field: vertical diplopia (image of right eye lowermost) increasing on looking to the right and down.* D. *Paralysis of right superior rectus. Characteristic: right eye does not move upward when eyes are turned to the right. Field: vertical diplopia (image of right eye uppermost) increasing on looking to the right and up.* E. *Paralysis of right superior oblique. Characteristic: right eye does not move downward when eyes are turned to the left. Field: vertical diplopia (image of right eye lowermost) increasing on looking to left and down.* F. *Paralysis of right inferior oblique. Characteristic: right eye does not move upward when eyes are turned to the left. Field: vertical diplopia (image of right eye uppermost) increasing on looking to left and up. (Adapted by permission from Cogan DG: Neurology of the Ocular Muscles, 2nd ed. Springfield, IL, Charles C. Thomas, 1956.)*

which the occluder consists of a transparent red lens with series of parallel cylindrical bars that transform a point source of light into a red perpendicular to the cylinder axes; the position of the red line is compared with the position of a white point source of light seen with the other eye. Another, the *alternate cover test*, requires less cooperation than the red-glass test and is, therefore, more useful in the examination of young and inattentive patients. It does, however, require sufficient visual function to permit central fixation with each eye. The test consists of rapidly alternating an occluder from one eye to another and observing the deviations from and return to the point of fixation, as described above in the discussion of tropias and phorias. Detailed descriptions of the Maddox rod and alternate cover test, which are the ones favored by neuro-ophthalmologists, can be found in the monographs of Leigh and Zee and of Glaser, listed with the references.

Monocular diplopia occurs most commonly in relation to diseases of the cornea and lens rather than the retina; usually the images are overlapping or superimposed rather than discrete. In most cases, monocular diplopia can be traced to a lenticular distortion or displacement, but in some no abnormality can be found. Monocular diplopia has been reported in association with cerebral disease (Safran et al), but this must be a very rare occurrence. Occasionally patients with homonymous scotomas due to a lesion of the occipital lobe will see multiple images (polyopia) in the defective field of vision, particularly when the target is moving.

Rarely, the acute onset of convergence paralysis may give rise to diplopia and blurred vision at all near points; most cases are due to head injury, some to encephalitis or multiple sclerosis. Many cases of convergence paralysis do not have a demonstrable neurologic basis. The acute onset of divergence paralysis causes diplopia at a distance because of crossing of the visual axes; in patients with divergent paralysis, images fuse only at a near position. This disorder, the pathologic basis of which is unknown, is difficult to distinguish from mild bilateral sixth nerve palsies and from convergence spasm, which is common in malingerers and hysterics.

Causes of Third, Fourth, and Sixth Nerve Palsies (Table 14-3) Ocular palsies may be central—i.e., due to a lesion of the nucleus or the intramedullary (fascicular) portion of the cranial nerve—or they may be peripheral. Weakness of ocular muscles due to a lesion in the brainstem is usually accompanied by involvement of other cranial nerves or long tracts. Peripheral lesions, which may or may not be solitary, have a great variety of causes. Rucker (1958, 1966), who analyzed 2000 cases of paralysis of the oculomotor nerves, found that the most common causes were tumors at the base of the brain (primary, metastatic, meningeal carcinomatosis), head trauma, ischemic infarction of a nerve (generally associated with diabetes), and aneurysms of the circle of Willis, in that order. In Rucker's series, the sixth nerve was affected in about half of the cases; third nerve palsies were about half as common as those of the sixth nerve; and the fourth nerve was involved in less than 10 percent of cases. In a series of 1000 unselected cases reported subsequently by Rush and Younge, trauma was a more frequent cause than neoplasm and the frequency of aneurysm-related cases had declined somewhat; otherwise the findings were little changed from those of the earlier studies. Less common causes of paralysis of the oculomotor nerves include variants of Guillain-Barré syndrome, herpes zoster, giant-cell arteritis, ophthalmoplegic migraine, carcinomatous or lymphomatous meningitis, and sarcoidosis as well as fungal, tuberculous, syphilitic, and other chronic forms of meningitis. *Myasthenia gravis* must always be considered in cases of ocular muscle palsy, particularly if several muscles are involved with ptosis as a prominent feature. Thyroid ophthalmopathy, discussed further on, presents in the same way but without ptosis and is less common than myasthenia. Actually, in the single largest group (20 to 30 percent) in each of the aforementioned series of cases, no cause could be assigned, although more cases are now being resolved with MRI, and newly available serological tests of CSF. Fortunately, in many cases of undetermined cause, the palsy disappears in a few weeks to months.

Sixth Nerve Palsy An isolated sixth nerve palsy frequently proves to be caused by neoplasm. In children, the most common tumor involving the sixth nerve is a pontine glioma; in adults, it is a metastatic tumor arising from the nasopharynx. Thus it is essential that the nasopharynx be examined carefully in every case of unexplained sixth nerve palsy, particularly if it is accompanied by sensory symptoms on the side of the face. As the abducens nerve passes near the apex of the petrous bone, it is in close relation to the trigeminal nerve. Both may be implicated by petrositis, manifest by facial pain and diplopia (Gradenigo syndrome). Fractures at the base of the skull and petrous clivus tumors may have a similar effect. Infarction of the nerve is a common cause of sixth nerve palsy in diabetics, in which case there is usually pain near the inner canthus of the eye. An idiopathic form that occurs in the absence of diabetes, possibly arteritic or phlebitic, is also well known.

Unilateral or bilateral abductor weakness may be a nonspecific sign of increased intracranial pressure from any source—including brain tumor, meningitis, and pseudotumor cerebri; rarely, it may appear after lumbar puncture, epidural injections, or insertion of a ventricular shunt. Occasionally the nerve is compressed by a congenitally persistent trigeminal artery.

Fourth Nerve Palsy The fourth nerve is particularly vulnerable to head trauma (this was the cause in 43 percent of 323 cases of trochlear nerve lesions collected by Wray from the literature). A fair number of cases remain idiopathic even after careful investigation. The fourth and sixth nerves are practically never involved by aneurysm. This reflects the relative infrequency of carotid artery aneurysms in the infraclinoid portion of the cavernous sinus, where they could impinge on the sixth nerve. (In contrast, supraclinoid aneurysms commonly involve the third nerve.) Herpes zoster ophthalmicus may affect any of the ocular motor nerves but particularly the trochlear, which shares a common sheath with the ophthalmic division of the trigeminal nerve. Diabetic infarction of the fourth nerve occurs, but far less frequently than infarction of the third or sixth nerves. Trochlear nerve palsy may also be a false localizing sign in cases of increased intracranial pressure, but again not nearly as often as abducens palsy. Entrapment of the superior oblique tendon is a rare cause (Brown syndrome). In addition to the appropriate diplopia, there is focal pain at the corner of the orbit; hence it may be mistaken for the Tolosa-Hunt syndrome, discussed further on. Most cases are idiopathic. There have been instances of trochlear nerve palsy in patients with lupus erythematosus and with Sjögren syndrome, but their fundamental nature is not known.

Superior oblique myokymia is another unusual condition, characterized by recurrent episodes of diplopia, monocular blurring of vision, and a tremulous sensation in the affected eye. It is usually benign and responds to carbamazepine, but rare instances presage pontine glioma or demyelinating disease. Compression of the fourth nerve by a small looped branch of the basilar artery has been suggested as the cause of the idiopathic variety, analogous to several other better documented cranial nerve vascular compression syndromes.

Third Nerve Palsy The third nerve is commonly compressed by aneurysm, tumor, or temporal lobe herniation. In a series of 206 cases of third nerve palsy collected by Wray and Taylor, neoplastic diseases accounted for 25 percent and aneurysms for 18 percent. Of the neoplasms, 25 percent were parasellar meningiomas and 4 percent pituitary adenomas. The palsy is usually chronic, progressive, and painless. As mentioned earlier, enlargement of the pupil is a sign of extramedullary third nerve compression because of the peripheral location in the nerve of the pupilloconstrictor fibers. By contrast, as indicated above, infarction of the nerve, as occurs in diabetics, usually spares the pupil, since the lesion characteristically involves the central portion of the nerve. The oculomotor palsy that complicates diabetes (this was the cause in 11 percent of the Wray and Taylor series) develops over a few hours and is accompanied by pain, usually severe, in the forehead and around the eye. The prognosis for recovery (as in other nonprogressive lesions of the ocular motor nerves) is usually good because of the potential of the nerve to regenerate. Infarction of the third nerve may occur in nondiabetics as well.

In chronic compressive lesions of the third nerve (distal carotid, basilar, or, most commonly, posterior communicating artery aneurysm; pituitary tumor, meningioma, cholesteatoma, etc.), the chronicity of the lesion may permit aberrant nerve regeneration. This is manifest by pupillary constriction on adduction of the eye or by retraction of the upper lid on downward gaze or adduction.

Rarely, children or young adults may have one or more attacks of ocular palsy in conjunction with an otherwise typical migraine (ophthalmoplegic migraine). The muscles (both extrinsic and intrinsic) innervated by the oculomotor or, very rarely, by the abducens nerve are affected. Presumably, intense spasm of the vessels supplying these nerves or compression by edematous arteries causes a transitory ischemic paralysis. Arteriograms done after the onset of the palsy usually disclose no abnormality. The oculomotor palsy of migraine tends to recover; after repeated attacks, however, there may be permanent paresis.

Painful Ophthalmoplegia The slow development of a *painful unilateral ophthalmoplegia* is most often traceable to an aneurysm, a tumor, or an inflammatory or granulomatous process in the anterior portion of the cavernous sinus or at the superior orbital fissure—*Tolosa-Hunt syndrome*, or an extension of the process known as *orbital pseudotumor*. Although there is little pathology on which to base an understanding of the latter two processes, they are both idiopathic orbital inflammations—Tolosa-Hunt syndrome involving the superior orbital fissure or the anterior cavernous sinus, and orbital pseudotumor causing inflammatory infiltration and enlargement of the extraocular muscles but sometimes including the globe and other orbital contents.

Orbital pseudotumor is accompanied by injection of the conjunctiva and lid and slight proptosis; the Tolosa-Hunt syndrome lacks these features but causes intra- and retro-orbital pain that may simulate migraine or cluster headache. In pseudotumor, a single muscle or several may be involved and there is a tendency to relapse and later to involve the opposite globe. Visual loss from compression of the optic nerve is a rare complication. Associations with connective tissue disease have been reported, but most cases in our experience have occurred in isolation. Ultrasound examination or CT scans of the orbit shows enlargement of the orbital contents in pseudotumor, mainly the muscles, similar to the findings in thyroid ophthalmopathy. The inflammatory changes of Tolosa-Hunt syndrome are limited to the superior orbital fissure and can sometimes be detected by MRI. Both the Tolosa-Hunt syndrome and orbital pseudotumor should be treated with corticosteroids for several weeks or longer.

In the *cavernous sinus syndrome*, involvement of the oculomotor nerve on one or both sides is accompanied by periorbital pain and chemosis (Fig. 14-4*B*). In a series of 151 such cases reported by Keane, the third nerve (usually with pupillary abnormalities) and sixth nerve were affected in almost all and the fourth nerve in one-third of them; complete ophthalmoplegia, usually unilateral, was present in 28 percent. Sensory loss in the distribution of the ophthalmic division of the trigeminal nerve was often added, a finding that is helpful in the diagnosis of orbital edema and obscure ocular muscle infiltration. Trauma and neoplastic invasion were the most frequent inciting causes, whereas conditions that in the past were commonly responsible (thrombophlebitis, intracavernous carotid aneurysm or fistula, fungal infection, meningioma) accounted for only 6 percent (see pages 722 and 911). A dural arteriovenous fistula is a rare cause. The diagnosis is confirmed and the disorder is distinguished from orbital pseudotumor by the finding of thrombosis in the sinus by imaging studies such as MRI, MRV, or MRA.

The other main differential diagnostic considerations in older patients with painful ophthalmoplegia are *temporal arteritis* (pages 193 and 907) and *thyroid ophthalmopathy* (although pain tends not to be so prominent in the latter), which are discussed further on. When only the superior oblique muscle is involved, the Brown syndrome, alluded to earlier, must be considered. The various intramedullary and extramedullary syndromes involving the oculomotor and other cranial nerves are summarized in Tables 47-1 and 47-2.

Acute Bilateral Ophthalmoplegia When this syndrome evolves within a day or days, it raises a number of diagnostic considerations. Keane, who analyzed 60 such cases, found the responsible lesion to lie within the brainstem in 18 (usually infarction and less often Wernicke disease), in the cranial nerves in 26 (Guillain-Barré syndrome or tuberculous meningitis), within the cavernous sinus in 8 (tumors or infection), and at the myoneural junction in 8 (myasthenia gravis and botulism). The Guillain-Barré ophthalmoplegic form is almost always associated with circulating antibodies to GQ1b ganglioside. The *chronic development of bilateral ophthalmoplegia* is most often due to an ocular myopathy [the mitochondrial disorder known as progressive external ophthalmoplegia (page 1503), a restricted muscular dystrophy (page 1503), or thyroid ophthalmopathy (see page 1520)].

Several causes of *pseudoparalysis of ocular muscles* must be distinguished. In *thyroid disease*, a swollen and tight inferior or superior rectus muscle may limit upward and downward gaze; less frequently, involvement of the medial rectus limits abduction. In most instances of thyroid ophthalmopathy, diagnosis is not difficult. This disorder is discussed further, on page 1520. In a significant number of cases, however (10 percent, according to Bahn and Heufelder), there are no signs of hyperthyroidism. However, most of these patients have laboratory evidence of thyroid autoimmune disease. The extraocular muscle enlargement can be demonstrated by CT scans and ultrasonography, and their inelasticity by *forced duction tests* (the insertions of the extraocular muscles are anesthetized and grasped by toothed forceps and attempts to move the globe are restricted).

The *Duane retraction syndrome* (so called because of the retraction of the globe and narrowing of the palpebral fissure that are elicited by attempted adduction) is due to a congenital absence or hypoplasia of the abducens nucleus and nerve and aberrant innervation of the lateral rectus by branches of the third nerve. Cocontraction of the medial and lateral recti results in retraction of the globe in all directions of ocular movement. The isolated occurrence of *convergence spasm*, in which both eyes converge on attempted fixation straight ahead or to the side, is usually hysterical, as already alluded to. An old squint or tropia with secondary fibrosis of an ocular muscle should also be considered.

Mixed Gaze and Ocular Muscle Paralysis

We have already considered two types of paralysis of the extraocular muscles: paralysis of conjugate movements (gaze) and neural paralysis of individual ocular muscles. Here we discuss a third more complex one—namely, mixed gaze and ocular muscle paralysis. The mixed type is always a sign of an intrapontine or mesencephalic lesion due to a wide variety of pathologic changes.

Internuclear Ophthalmoplegia (INO) and Other Pontine Gaze Palsies This abnormality has been alluded to sever times earlier as it is involved in numerous brainstem syndromes affecting both horizontal and vertical gaze. A lesion of the lower pons in or near the sixth nerve nucleus causes a homolateral paralysis of the lateral rectus muscle and a failure of adduction of the opposite eye—i.e., a combined paralysis of the sixth nerve and of conjugate lateral gaze. As already indicated, the pontine center accomplishes horizontal conjugate gaze by simultaneously innervating the ipsilateral lateral rectus (via the abducens neurons) and the contralateral medial rectus via fibers that originate in the internuclear neurons of the abducens nucleus and cross at the level of the nucleus to run in the medial longitudinal fasciculus (MLF) of the opposite side (Fig. 14-1). With a lesion of the left MLF, the left eye fails to adduct when the patient looks to the right; this condition is referred to as *left internuclear ophthalmoplegia*. With a lesion of the right MLF, the right eye fails to adduct when the patient looks to the left (*right internuclear ophthalmoplegia*). The limitation of ocular adduction is most evident with saccadic movements, brought out by large side-to-side refixation between two targets or by observing the deficient and slanted corrective saccades induced by optokinetic stimulation. The two medial longitudinal fasciculi lie close together, each being situated adjacent to the midline, so that they are frequently affected together, yielding a bilateral internuclear ophthalmoplegia; this condition should always be suspected when adduction of both eyes is affected. Quite often, rather than a complete paralysis of adduction, there are greatly slowed adducting saccades in the affected eye while its opposite quickly arrives at its fully abducted position upon commanded gaze or refixation.

A second component of the INO is nystagmus that is limited to or more prominent in the abducting eye. Several explanations have been offered to account for this dissociated nystagmus, all of them hypothetical. The most favored explanation invokes Hering's law—that activated yoke muscles receive equal and simultaneous innervation; because of an adaptive increase in innervation of the weak adductor, a commensurate increase in innervation to the strong abductor occurs (manifest as nystagmus). Whatever the afferent stimulus for this overdrive, it is probably proprioceptive, since occluding the affected eye does not suppress the nystagmus. Since the MLF contains axons that originate in the vestibular nuclei and govern vertical eye movements, a lesion of the MLF may also cause vertical nystagmus and impairment of vertical fixation and pursuit.

Lesions involving the MLF in the high midbrain may be associated with a loss of convergence ("anterior" internuclear ophthalmoplegia); if the MLF is involved by a lesion in the pons, convergence is spared, but some degree of horizontal gaze or sixth nerve palsy is often associated ("posterior" internuclear ophthalmoplegia).

The main cause of *unilateral INO* is a small paramedian pontine infarction. Other common causes are lateral medullary infarction (where skew deviation is often added), multiple sclerosis (more common as a cause of bilateral INO), lupus erythematosus, and infiltrative brainstem and fourth ventricular tumors. Occasionally INO is an unexplained finding after mild head injury or with subdural hematoma or hydrocephalus.

Bilateral INO is most often the result of a demyelinating lesion (multiple sclerosis) in the posterior part of the midpontine tegmentum. Pontine myelinolysis, infarction, Wernicke disease, or infiltrating tumors are other causes bilateral INO.

Another pontine disorder of ocular movement combines an internuclear ophthalmoplegia in one direction and a horizontal gaze palsy in the other. One eye lies fixed in the midline for all horizontal movements; the other eye can make only abducting movements and may be engaged in horizontal nystagmus in the direction of abduction ("*one-and-a-half syndrome*" of Fisher; see Wall and Wray). The lesion in such cases involves the pontine center for gaze plus the ipsilateral MLF; it is usually due to vascular or demyelinative disease. Caplan has summarized the features of other mixed oculomotor defects that occur with thrombotic occlusion of the upper part of the basilar artery ("top of the basilar" syndromes). These include upgaze or complete vertical gaze palsy and so-called pseudoabducens palsy. The latter is characterized by bilateral incomplete esotropia that simulates bilateral sixth nerve paresis but appears to be a type of sustained convergence or a paresis of divergence; it can be overcome by vestibular stimulation.

Among the most unusual of the complex ocular disturbances is a subjective tilting of the entire visual field that may produce any angle of divergence but most often creates an illusion of tilting of 45 to 90 degrees (*tortopia*) or of 180-degree vision (*upside-down vision*). Objects normally on the floor, such as chairs and tables, are perceived to be on the wall or ceiling. Although this symptom may arise as a result of a lesion of the parietal lobe or in the otolithic apparatus, it is most often associated with an internuclear ophthalmoplegia and presumably with impaired function of the vestibular-otolithic nucleus or its central connections. Lateral medullary infarction has been the most common cause in our experience (Ropper).

Nystagmus

Nystagmus refers to involuntary rhythmic movements of the eyes and is of two general types. In the more common *jerk nystagmus*, the movements alternate between a slow component and a fast corrective component, or jerk, in the opposite direction. In *pendular nystagmus*, the oscillations are roughly equal in rate in both directions, although on lateral gaze the pendular type may be converted to the jerk type, with the fast component to the side of gaze.

Jerk nystagmus is the more common type. It may be horizontal or vertical, particularly on ocular movement in these planes, or it may be rotatory and rarely retractory or vergent. By custom in the English-speaking world, the direction of the nystagmus is named according to the direction of the fast component. There are several varieties of jerk nystagmus. Some occur spontaneously; others are readily induced in normal persons by drugs or by labyrinthine or visual stimulation. Deviations from the patterns of normally induced nystagmus may provide important clues to the locus of disease.

In testing for nystagmus, the eyes should be examined first in the central position and then during upward, downward, and lateral movements. Nystagmus of labyrinthine origin is best thought out by eliminating visual fixation, facilitated by the use of Frenzel lenses. On the other hand, nystagmus of brainstem and cerebellar origin is brought out best by having the patient fixate upon and follow a moving target. Characteristically, labyrinthine nystagmus varies with position of the head. In particular, the benign positional vertigo of Barany (described more fully on page 321) is evoked by hyperextension and rotation of the neck, with the head being placed below the horizontal plane of the bed and turned to the side. Nystagmus of the vertical torsional type and vertigo develop in 10 to 15 s and persist for another 10 to 15 s. When the patient sits up quickly, the nystagmus reappears in the opposite direction.

In some normal individuals, a few irregular jerks are observed as they turn their eyes far to one side ("nystagmoid" jerks), but no sustained rhythmic movements occur once fixation is attained. A fine rhythmic nystagmus may occur in extreme lateral gaze, beyond the range of binocular vision; but if it is bilateral and disappears as the eyes move a few degrees toward the midline, it usually has no clinical significance. These movements are probably analogous to the tremulousness of skeletal muscles that are maximally contracted.

Pendular nystagmus is found in a variety of conditions in which central vision is lost early in life, such as albinism and various other diseases of the retina and refractive media (congenital ocular nystagmus). Occasionally it is observed as a congenital abnormality, even without poor vision. The defect is postulated to be an instability of smooth pursuit or gaze-holding mechanisms. Examples are occasionally seen in multiple sclerosis. The nystagmus is always binocular and in one plane; i.e., it will remain horizontal even during vertical movement. It is purely pendular (sinusoidal) except in extremes of gaze, when it comes to resemble jerk nystagmus. Head oscillation may accompany the nystagmus and is probably compensatory. The formerly common syndrome of "miner's nystagmus" occurs in patients who have worked for many years in comparative darkness. The oscillations of the eyes are usually very rapid, increase on upward gaze, and may be associated with compensatory oscillations of the head and intolerance of light. *Spasmus nutans*, a specific type of pendular nystagmus of infancy, is accompanied by head nodding and occasionally by wry positions of the neck. Most cases begin between the fourth and twelfth months of life, never after the third year. The nystagmus may be horizontal, vertical, or rotatory; it is usually more pronounced in one eye than the other (or limited to one eye) and can be intensified by immobilizing or straightening the head. Most infants recover within a few months or years. Rarely, symptoms like those of spasmus nutans betray the presence of a chiasmal or third ventricular tumor.

Apart from the pendular variety, *nystagmus occurring spontaneously* may signify the presence of labyrinthine-vestibular, brainstem, or cerebellar disease. Labyrinthine-vestibular nystagmus may be horizontal, vertical, or oblique, and that of purely labyrinthine origin characteristically has a torsional component. Tinnitus and hearing loss are often associated with disease of the peripheral labyrinthine mechanism; vertigo, nausea, vomiting, and staggering may accompany disease of any part of the labyrinthine-vestibular apparatus or its central connections. These points are elaborated in Chap. 15.

Nystagmus due to Brainstem-Cerebellar Disease Brainstem lesions often cause a coarse, unidirectional, *gaze-dependent nystagmus*, which may be horizontal or vertical, meaning that the nystagmus is exaggerated when the eyes sustain a position of gaze; vertical nystagmus is brought out usually on upward gaze, less often on downward gaze. The presence of bidirectional *vertical nystagmus* usually indicates disease in the pontomedullary or pontomesencephalic tegmentum. Vertigo is uncommon, but signs of disease of other nuclear structures and tracts in the brainstem are frequent. *Upbeat nystagmus* is observed frequently in patients with demyelinative or vascular disease, tumors, and Wernicke disease. There is still uncertainty about the precise anatomy of coarse upbeat nystagmus. According to some authors, it has been associated with lesions of the anterior vermis, but we have not observed such an association. Kato and associates cite cases with a lesion at the pontomedullary junction, involving the nucleus prepositus hypoglossi, which receives vestibular connections and projects to all brainstem and cerebellar regions concerned with oculomotor functions.

Downbeat nystagmus, which is always of central origin, may be observed in Wernicke disease and is characteristic of syringobulbia, Chiari malformation, basilar invagination, and floccular and other lesions in the medullary-cervical region. Halmagyi and coworkers, who studied 62 patients with downbeat nystagmus, found that in half of them this abnormality was associated with the Chiari malformation and various forms of cerebellar degeneration; in most of the remainder, the cause could not be determined. Downbeat nystagmus, in association with oscillopsia, has also been observed in patients with lithium intoxication or with profound magnesium depletion (Saul and Selhorst). The paraneoplastic opsoclonic disorder can begin with downbeat nystagmus.

Cerebellopontine-angle tumors may cause a coarse bilateral horizontal nystagmus, coarser to the side of the lesion. Nystagmus of several types—including gaze-evoked nystagmus, downbeat nystagmus, and "rebound nystagmus" (gaze-evoked nystagmus that changes direction with fatigue or refixation to the primary position)—occurs with cerebellar disease (more specifically with lesions of the vestibulocerebellum) or with brainstem lesions that involve the nucleus prepositus hypoglossi and medial vestibular nucleus (see above, in relation to upbeat nystagmus). Characteristic also of cerebellar disease are several closely related disorders of saccadic movement (opsoclonus, flutter, dysmetria) described below.

Nystagmus that occurs only in the abducting eye is referred to as *dissociated nystagmus* and is a common sign of multiple sclerosis. Probably it represents an incompletely developed form of internuclear ophthalmoplegia; on attempted lateral gaze, the adducting eye (which does not show nystagmus) lags behind the abducting one.

Drug intoxication is the most frequent cause of induced nystagmus. Alcohol, barbiturates, other sedative-hypnotic drugs, and phenytoin are the common offenders. This form of nystagmus is most prominent on deviation of the eyes in the horizontal plane, but occasionally it may appear in the vertical plane as well. It rarely appears in the vertical plane alone, suggesting then a tegmental brainstem disorder. It may be asymmetrical in the two eyes, for no known reason.

Optokinetic Nystagmus When one is watching a moving object (e.g., the passing landscape from a train window or a rotating drum with vertical stripes or a strip of cloth with similar stripes), a rhythmic jerk nystagmus, *optokinetic nystagmus (OKN)*, normally appears. The usual explanation of this phenomenon is that the slow component of the nystagmus represents an involuntary pursuit movement to the limit of comfortable conjugate gaze; the eyes then make a quick saccadic movement in the opposite direction in order to fixate a new target that is entering the visual field. With unilateral lesions of the parietal region (and transiently with acute frontal lobe lesions), OKN may be lost or diminished when a moving stimulus, e.g., the striped OKN drum, is rotated *toward* the side of the lesion, whereas rotation of the drum to the opposite side elicits a normal response. It should be again noted that patients with hemianopia may show a normal optokinetic response; patients with a parietal lobe lesion, with or without hemianopia, frequently have an abnormal optokinetic response with the stripes moving in the direction of the affected hemisphere. These observations indicate that an abnormal response does not depend upon a lesion of the geniculocalcarine tract. Presumably it is due to interruption of efferent pathways from the parietal cortex to the brainstem centers for conjugate gaze. Frontal lobe lesions allow the eyes to deviate tonically in the direction of the target, with little or no fast-phase correction. An important fact about OKN is that its demonstration proves that the patient is not blind. Each eye can be tested separately to exclude monocular blindness. Thus it is of particular value in the examination of hysterical patients and malingerers who claim that they cannot see and of neonates and infants (a nascent OKN is established in within hours after birth and becomes more easily elicitable over the first few months of life).

Labyrinthine stimulation—e.g., irrigation of the external auditory canal with warm or cold water—produces nystagmus; cold water induces a slow tonic deviation of the eyes in a direction opposite to that of the nystagmus; warm water does the reverse. The slow component reflects the effect of impulses originating in the semicircular canals, and the fast component is a corrective movement. Smooth pursuit movements remain intact, indicating that labyrinthine vestibular nystagmus is suppressed during fixation. The production of nystagmus by labyrinthine stimulation and other features of vestibular nystagmus are discussed further in Chap. 15.

Other Types of Nystagmus *Convergence nystagmus* refers to a rhythmic oscillation in which a slow abduction of the eyes in respect to each other is followed by a quick movement of adduction. It is usually accompanied by quick rhythmic retraction movements of the eyes (*nystagmus retractorius*) and by one or more features of the Parinaud syndrome. There may also be rhythmic movements of the eyelids or a maintained spasm of convergence, best brought out on attempted elevation of the eyes to command or downward rotation of an OKN drum. These unusual phenomena all point to a lesion of the upper midbrain tegmentum and are usually manifestations of vascular disease, traumatic disease, or tumor, notably pinealoma. *Seesaw nystagmus* is a torsional-vertical oscillation in which the intorting eye moves up and the opposite (extorting) eye moves down, then both move in the reverse direction. It is occasionally observed in conjunction with bitemporal hemianopia due to sellar or parasellar masses. So-called *palatal nystagmus*, which is really a tremor, is due to a lesion of the central tegmental tract and may be accompanied by a convergence-retraction nystagmus that has the same beat as the palatal and pharyngeal muscles as discussed on page 106.

Other Spontaneous Ocular Movements

Oscillopsia is the illusory movement of the environment in which stationary objects seem to move back and forth, up and down, or from side to side. It may be associated with ocular flutter or with coarse nystagmus of any type due to brainstem lesions that involve the vestibular nuclei on one or both sides. With lesions of the labyrinths (as in aminoglycoside toxicity), oscillopsia is characteristically provoked by motion, e.g., walking or riding in an automobile, and indicates an impaired ability of the vestibular system to stabilize ocular fixation during body movement (i.e., impaired VOR function). In these circumstances cursory examination of the eyes may disclose no abnormalities; however, if the patient's head oscillates while attempting to fixate a target, impairment of smooth eye movements and their replacement by saccadic movements are evoked. If briefly episodic and involving only one eye, oscillopsia may be due to myokymia of an ocular muscle (usually the superior oblique).

Roving conjugate eye movements are characteristic of light coma. Slow horizontal ocular deviations that shift every few seconds from side to side ("ping-pong gaze") is a variant of roving eye movements that occurs with bihemispheric infarctions or sometimes with posterior fossa lesions, Fisher has noted a similar slow, side-to-side pendular oscillation of the eyes ("windshield-wiper eyes"). This phenomenon has been associated with bilateral hemispheric lesions that have presumably released a brainstem pacemaker. *Ocular bobbing* is a term coined by Fisher to describe a distinctive spontaneous fast downward jerk of the eyes followed by a slow upward drift to the midposition. It is usually observed in comatose patients in whom horizontal eye movements are absent and has been associated most often with large destructive lesions of the pons, less often of the cerebellum. The eye movements may be disconjugate in the vertical plane, especially if there is an associated third nerve palsy on one side.

Other spontaneous vertical eye movements, many identical to each other, have been given a variety of confusing names: *atypical bobbing*, *inverse bobbing*, *reverse bobbing*, and *ocular dipping*. For the most part, they are observed in coma of metabolic or anoxic origin and in the context of preserved horizontal eye movements (in distinction to ocular bobbing). *Ocular dipping* is a term we have used to describe an arrhythmic slow conjugate downward movement followed in several seconds by a more rapid upward movement; it occurs spontaneously but may at times be elicited by moving the limbs or neck. Anoxic encephalopathy has been the most common cause.

Opsoclonus is the term applied to rapid, conjugate oscillations of the eyes in horizontal, rotatory, and vertical directions, made worse by voluntary movement or the need to fixate the eyes. These movements are continuous and chaotic, without an intersaccadic pause (saccadomania), and persist in sleep. Often, as indicated in Chap. 6, they are part of a widespread myoclonus (associated with parainfectious disease, occasionally with AIDS and rickettsial infections, but most characteristically they occur as a paraneoplastic manifestation (page 725). Opsoclonus may also be observed in patients intoxicated with antidepressants, anticonvulsants, organophosphates, cocaine, lithium, thallium, and haloperidol; in the nonketotic hyperosmolar state; and in cerebral Whipple disease, where it is coupled with rhythmic jaw movements (page 748). A childhood form associated with limb ataxia and myoclonus that is responsive to adrenocorticotropic hormone (ACTH) may persist for years without explanation, as in the "dancing eyes" of children (Kinsbourne syndrome), although neuroblastoma remains the main consideration. There is also a self-limited benign form in neonates. Similar movements have been produced in monkeys by creating bilateral lesions in the pretectum.

Ocular dysmetria consists of an overshoot of the eyes on attempted fixation followed by several cycles of oscillation of diminishing amplitude until fixation is attained. The overshoot may occur on eccentric fixation or on refixation to the primary position of gaze. This abnormality probably reflects dysfunction of the anterosuperior vermis and underlying deep cerebellar nuclei. *Ocular flutter* refers to occasional bursts of very rapid horizontal oscillations around the point of fixation; this abnormality is also associated with cerebellar disease. Flutter at the end of a saccade, called *flutter dysmetria* ("*fish-tail nystagmus*)," has the appearance of dysmetria, but careful analysis indicates that it is probably a different phenomenon. Whereas the inaccurate saccades of ataxia are separated by normal intersaccadic intervals, flutter dysmetria consists of consecutive saccades without an intersaccadic interval (Zee and Robinson).

Opsoclonus, ocular dysmetria, and flutter-like oscillations may occur together, or a patient may show only one or two of these ocular abnormalities, either simultaneously or in sequence. One hypothesis relates opsoclonus and ocular flutter to a disorder of the saccadic "pause neurons" (see above), but their exact anatomic basis has not been elucidated.

Disorders of the Eyelids and Blinking

A consideration of oculomotor disorders would be incomplete without some reference to the eyelids and blinking. In the normal individual, the eyelids on both sides are at the same level with respect to the limbus of the cornea and there is a variable prominence of the eyes, depending on the width of the palpebral fissure. The function of the eyelids is to protect the delicate corneal surfaces against injury and the retinae against glare; this is done by blinking and lacrimation. Eyelid movement is normally coordinated with ocular movement—the upper lids elevate when looking up and descend when looking down. Turning the eyes quickly to the side is usually attended by a single blink, which is necessarily brief so as not to interfere with vision.

Closure and opening of the eyelids is accomplished through the reciprocal action of the levator palpebrae and orbicularis oculi muscles. Relaxation of the levator and contraction of the orbicularis effect closure; the reverse action of these muscles effects opening of the closed eyelids. Opening of the lids is aided by the tonic sympathetic innervation of Müller's muscles. The levator is innervated by the oculomotor nerve, and the orbicularis, by the facial nerve. The trigeminal nerves provide sensation to the eyelids and are also the afferent limbs of corneal and palpebral reflexes. Central mechanisms for the control of blinking, in addition to the reflexive brainstem connections between the third, fifth, and seventh nerve nuclei, include the cerebrum, basal ganglia, and hypothalamus. Voluntary closure is initiated through frontobasal ganglionic connections.

The eyelids are kept open by the tonic contraction of the levator muscles, which overcomes the elastic properties of the periorbital muscles. The eyelids close during sleep and certain altered states of consciousness due to relaxation of the levator muscles. Facial paralysis causes the closure to be incomplete.

Blinking occurs irregularly at a rate of 12 to 20 times a minute, the frequency varying with the state of concentration and with emotion. The natural stimuli for the blink reflex (blinking is always bilateral) are corneal contact (corneal reflex), a tap on the brow or around the eye, visual threat, an unexpected loud sound, and, as indicated above, turning of the eyes to one side. There is normally a rapid adaptation of blink to visual and auditory stimuli but not to corneal stimulation.

Electromyography of the orbicularis oculi reveals two components of the blink response, an early and late one, a feature that is readily corroborated by clinical observation. The early response consists of only a slight movement of the upper lids; the later response is more forceful and approximates the upper and lower lids. Whereas the early part of the blink reflex is beyond volitional control, the second part can be inhibited voluntarily.

Blepharospasm, an excessive and forceful closure of the lids, which is described on page 114, is a common disorder that occurs in isolation or as part of a number of dyskinesias and drug-induced movement disorders (pages 1264 and 1637). Increased blink frequency occurs with corneal irritation, with sensitization of trigeminal nerve endings, and in oculofacial dyskinetic syndromes, such as blepharospasm. A reduced frequency of blinking (<10 per minute) is characteristic of progressive supra–nuclear palsy and Parkinson disease. In the latter, adaptation to repeated supraorbital tapping at a rate of about 1 per second is impaired; therefore the patient continues to blink with each tap on the forehead or glabella. The failure to inhibit this response is referred to as the glabellar, or *Myerson sign*.

A lesion of the oculomotor nerve, by paralyzing the levator muscle, causes *ptosis*, i.e., drooping of the upper eyelid. A lesion of the facial nerve, as in Bell's palsy, results in an inability to close the eyelids due to weakness of orbicularis oculi, a slight retraction of the upper lid (due to the unopposed action of the levator), and loss of the blink reflex. In some instances of Bell's palsy, even after nearly full recovery of facial movements, the blink frequency may be reduced on the affected side. Of neurologic importance is the fact that a trigeminal nerve lesion on one side, by reducing corneal sensation, interferes with the blink reflex on both sides, while a Bell's palsy does not abolish the contralateral blink. Aberrant regeneration of the third nerve may result in a condition wherein the upper lid retracts on lateral or downward gaze (pseudo–von Graefe sign). Aberrant regeneration of the facial nerve after Bell's palsy has an opposite effect—closure of the lid with jaw movements or speaking. A useful clinical rule is that a combined paralysis of the levator and orbicularis oculi muscles (i.e., the muscles that open and close the lids) nearly always indicates a myopathic disease, such as myasthenia gravis or myotonic dystrophy. This is because the third and seventh cranial nerves are rarely affected together in peripheral nerve or brainstem disease.

Bilateral ptosis is a characteristic feature of muscular dystrophies and myasthenia gravis; congenital ptosis and progressive sagging of the upper lids in the elderly are other common forms. Unilateral ptosis is a notable feature of third nerve lesions (see above) and of sympathetic paralysis, as in the Horner syndrome. It may be accompanied by an overaction (compensation) of the frontalis and the contralateral levator palpebrae muscles. This combination of abnormalities may be observed with myasthenia gravis and with compensatory ptosis in diplopic states. In patients with myasthenia, Cogan has described a "lid twitch" phenomenon, in which there is a transient retraction of the upper lid when the patient moves visual fixation from the down position to straight ahead. Brief fluttering of the lid margins is also characteristic of myasthenia.

The opposite of ptosis, i.e., *retraction of the upper lids*, often with a staring expression, is observed with orbital tumors and thyroid disease, the most common causes of unilateral and bilateral proptosis. A staring appearance alone is observed in Parkinson disease, progressive supranuclear palsy, and hydrocephalus, in which there is downturning of the eyes ("sunset sign") and paralysis of upward gaze. Retraction of the eyelids (Collier sign), when part of a dorsal midbrain syndrome, is accompanied by a light-near pupillary dissociation; it is not accompanied by a lid lag (von Graefe sign) on downward gaze, in distinction to what is observed in thyroid ophthalmopathy. Lid retraction has been observed in patients with hepatic cirrhosis, Cushing disease, chronic steroid myopathy, and hyperkalemic periodic paralysis; in these conditions, lid lag is also absent. Lid retraction can be a reaction to ptosis on the other side; this is clarified by lifting the ptotic lid manually and observing the disappearance of contralateral retraction.

In myotonic dystrophy and other less common myotonic disorders, forceful closure of the eyelids may induce a strong aftercontraction. In certain extrapyramidal diseases, particularly progressive supranuclear palsy and Parkinson disease, even gentle closure may elicit blepharoclonus and blepharospasm on attempted opening of the lids; or there may be a delay in the opening of the tightly closed eyelids. An acute right parietal lesion or bifrontal lesions often produce a peculiar disinclination to open the eyelids, even to the point of offering active resistance upon attempts at forced opening.

THE PUPILS

The testing of pupillary size and reactivity, which can be accomplished by the use of a flashlight and simple pupillometer (we have used the circular laminated card known as the *Iowa pupil gauge*), yields important, often vital clinical information. Essential, of course, is the proper interpretation of the pupillary reactions, and this requires some knowledge of their underlying neural mechanisms.

The diameter of the pupil is determined by the balance of innervation between the autonomically innervated sphincter and radially arranged dilator muscles of the iris, the sphincter muscle playing the major role. The *pupilloconstrictor (parasympathetic)* fibers arise in the Edinger-Westphal nucleus in the high midbrain, join the third cranial (oculomotor) nerve, and synapse in the ciliary ganglion, which lies in the posterior part of the orbit. The postganglionic fibers then enter the globe via the short ciliary nerves; approximately 3 percent of the fibers innervate the sphincter pupillae and 97 percent, the ciliary body. The sphincter of the pupil comprises 50 motor units, according to Corbett and Thompson. The *pupillodilator (sympathetic)* fibers arise in the posterolateral part of the hypothalamus and descend, uncrossed, in the lateral tegmentum of the midbrain, pons, medulla, and cervical spinal cord to the eighth cervical and first and second thoracic segments, where they synapse with the lateral horn cells. The latter cells give rise to preganglionic fibers, most of which leave the cord by the second ventral thoracic root and proceed through the stellate ganglion to synapse in the superior cervical ganglion; the postganglionic fibers course along the internal carotid artery and traverse the cavernous sinus, where they join the first division of the trigeminal nerve, finally reaching the eye as the long ciliary nerve. Some of the postganglionic fibers also innervate the sweat glands and arterioles of the face and Müller's muscle in the eyelid.

The Pupillary Light Reflex

The commonest stimulus for pupillary constriction is exposure of the retina to light. Reflex pupillary constriction is also part of the act of convergence and accommodation for near objects (near-synkinesis).

The pathway for the pupillary light reflex consists of three parts (Fig. 14-7):

1. *An afferent limb*,whose fibers originate in the retinal receptor cells, pass through the bipolar cells, and synapse with the retinal ganglion cells; axons of these cells run in the optic nerve and tract. The light reflex fibers leave the optic tract just rostral to the lateral geniculate body and enter the high midbrain, where they synapse in the pretectal nucleus.

2. *Intercalated neurons* that give rise to the pupillomotor fibers, which pass ventrally to the ipsilateral

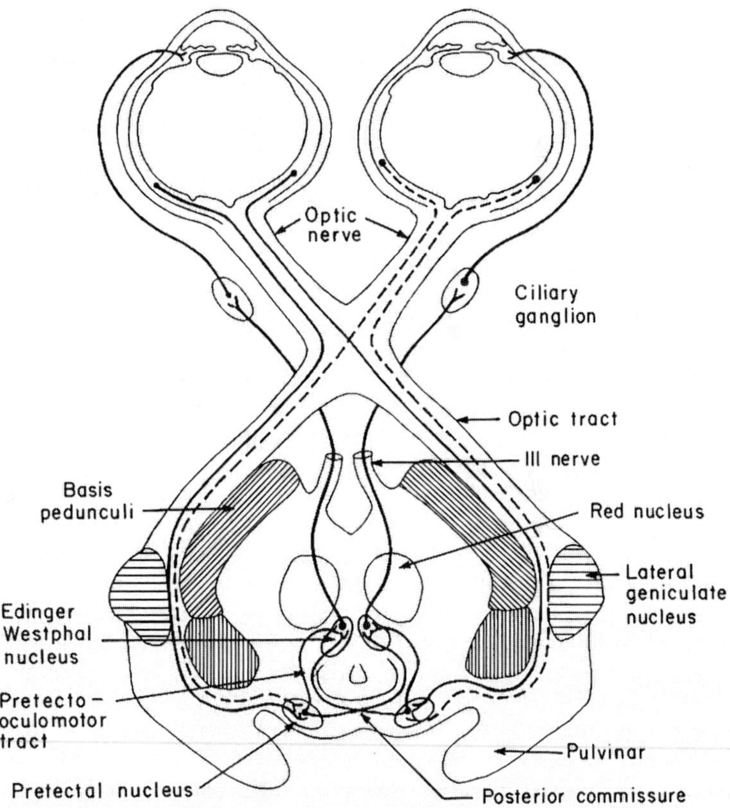

Figure 14-7

Diagram of the pupillary light reflex. (Redrawn, with permission from Walsh FB, Hoyt WF. Clinical Neuro-Ophthalmology, 3rd ed. Baltimore, Williams & Wilkins, 1969.)

Edinger-Westphal nucleus and, via fibers that cross in the posterior commissure, to the contralateral Edinger-Westphal nucleus (labeled "pretecto-oculomotor" tract in Fig. 14-7).

3. *An efferent two-neuron pathway from the Edinger-Westphal nucleus,* synapsing in the ciliary ganglion, by which all motor impulses reach the pupillary sphincter, as described above.

Alterations of the Pupils

The pupils tend to be large in children and small in the aged, sometimes markedly miotic but still reactive (senile miosis). An asymmetry of the pupils of 0.3 to 0.5 mm is found in 20 percent or more of normal individuals. A lesion that destroys only a small number of nerve cells in the Edinger-Westphal nucleus or ciliary ganglion will cause paralysis of a sector or sectors of the iris and deform the pupil.

Normally the pupil constricts under a bright light (direct reflex), and the other unexposed pupil also constricts (consensual reflex). With complete or nearly complete interruption of the optic nerve, the pupil will fail to react to direct light stimulation; however, the pupil of the blind eye will still show a consensual reflex, i.e., it will constrict when light is shone in the healthy eye. The lack of a direct reflex in the blind eye together with lack of a consensual reflex in the sound one means that the afferent limb of the reflex arc (optic nerve) is the site of the lesion. A lack of direct and consensual light reflex with retention of the consensual reflex in the opposite eye places the lesion in the efferent limb of the reflex arc, i.e., in the homolateral oculomotor nerve or its nucleus. A lesion of the afferent limb of the light reflex pathway will not affect the near responses of the pupil and lesions of the visual pathway caudal to the point where the light reflex fibers leave the optic tract will not alter the pupillary light reflex (Fig. 14-7).

Following initial constriction, the pupil may dilate slightly in spite of a light shining steadily in one or both eyes. Slowness of response along with failure to sustain pupillary constriction, or "pupillary escape," is sometimes referred to as the *Gunn pupillary sign*; a mild degree of it may be observed in normal persons, but it is far more prominent in cases of damage to the retina or optic nerve. A variant of this pupillary response may be used to expose mild degrees of retrobulbar neuropathy (relative afferent pupillary defect). This is best tested in a dimly lighted room with the patient fixating on a distant target. If a light is shifted quickly from the normal to the impaired eye, the direct light stimulus is no longer sufficient to maintain the previously evoked consensual pupillary constriction and both pupils dilate. These abnormal pupillary responses form the basis of "the swinging-flashlight test," in which each pupil is alternately exposed to light at 3-s intervals.

The Gunn pupillary sign is not to be confused with the Gunn "jaw-winking" phenomenon, a congenital and sometimes hereditary anomaly, in which a ptotic eyelid retracts momentarily when the mouth is opened or the jaw is moved to one side. In other cases, inhibition of the levator muscle and ptosis occurs with opening of the mouth ("inverse Marcus Gunn phenomenon," or Marin Amat syndrome). *Hippus*, a rapid alternation in pupillary size, is common in metabolic encephalopathy but has no particular significance.

Interruption of the sympathetic fibers—either centrally, between the hypothalamus and their points of exit from the spinal cord (C8 to T3, mainly T2), or peripherally (cervical sympathetic chain, superior cervical ganglion, or along the carotid artery)—results in miosis and ptosis (because of paralysis of the pupillary dilator muscle and of Müller's muscle, respectively), loss of sweating on the same side of the face, and redness of the conjunctiva. The entire complex is called the *Horner syndrome, Bernard-Horner syndrome,* or oculosympathetic palsy (page 566). It may be due to ipsilateral lesions of the medulla or cervical cord or to peripheral lesions. The pattern of sweating may be helpful in localizing the lesion (Morris et al). With lesions of the common carotid artery, loss of sweating involves the entire side of the face. With lesions distal to the bifurcation, loss of sweating is confined to the medial aspect of the forehead and side of the nose. Retraction of the eyeball (enophthalmos) is probably an illusion created by narrowing of the palpebral fissure. A hereditary form (autosomal dominant) of the Horner syndrome is known, associated with a congenital absence of pigment in the affected iris (heterochromia iridis). *Bilateral Horner syndrome* is a rare occurrence; usually it is found in autonomic neuropathies and in high cervical cord transection. Although difficult to appreciate, it may be detected (using pupillometry) by noting a lag in the redilation of the initially small pupils when light is withdrawn (Smith and Smith).

Stimulation or irritation of the sympathetic fibers has the opposite effect, i.e., lid retraction, dilatation of the pupil, and apparent proptosis. The *ciliospinal pupillary reflex*, evoked by pinching the neck (afferent, C2, C3), is effected through the efferent sympathetic fibers, but we have not found it to be a reliable test.

Extreme constriction of the pupils (miosis) is commonly observed with pontine lesions, presumably because of bilateral interruption of the pupillodilator fibers. Narcotic ingestion is the commonest cause. Interruption of the parasympathetic fibers causes an abnormal dilatation of the pupils (mydriasis), often with loss of pupillary light reflexes; this is frequently the result of midbrain lesions and is a common finding in cases of deep coma (the "blown pupil," or Hutchinson pupil, described in Chap. 17) and with direct compression of the oculomotor nerve, as by cerebral aneurysm, tumor, or temporal lobe herniation. Other signs of oculomotor palsy are usually conjoined.

The functional integrity of the sympathetic and parasympathetic nerve endings in the iris may also be determined by the use of certain drugs. Atropinics dilate the pupils by paralyzing the parasympathetic nerve endings; physostigmine and pilocarpine constrict the pupils, the former by inhibiting cholinesterase activity at the neuromuscular junction and the latter by direct stimulation of the sphincter muscle of the iris. Epinephrine and phenylephrine dilate the pupils by direct stimulation of the dilator muscle. Cocaine dilates the pupils by preventing the reabsorption of norepinephrine into the nerve endings. Morphine and other narcotics act centrally to constrict the pupils.

In *diabetes mellitus*, where spinal and cranial nerves are often involved, the pupils are affected in the majority of cases. They are smaller than would be expected for age due to involvement of pupillodilator sympathetic fibers, and mydriasis is excessive upon instillation of sympathomimetic drugs. The light reflex, mediated by parasympathetic fibers (which are also damaged), is reduced, usually to a greater degree than constriction on accommodation (Smith and Smith). Some of these abnormalities require special methods of pupillometry for their demonstration.

In the forms of late syphilis, particularly tabes dorsalis, the pupils are usually small, irregular, and unequal; they fail to react to light, although they do constrict on accommodation (light-near dissociation) and do not dilate properly in response to mydriatic drugs. Atrophy of the iris is associated in some cases. This is known as the *Argyll Robertson pupil*. The exact locality of the lesion is not certain; it is generally believed to be in the tectum of the midbrain proximal to the oculomotor nuclei, where the descending pupillodilator fibers are in close proximity to the light reflex fibers (Fig. 14-7). The possibility of a partial third nerve lesion extending to the ciliary ganglion seems more plausible to us. A similar pupillary abnormality has also been observed in the meningoradiculitis of Lyme disease. A dissociation of the light reflex from the accommodation-convergence reaction is also sometimes observed with a variety of midbrain lesions—e.g., pinealoma, multiple sclerosis—and occasionally in patients with diabetes mellitus; in these diseases, miosis, irregularity of pupils, and failure to respond to a mydriatic are usually not present. S. A. K. Wilson referred to this condition as the *Argyll Robertson pupillary phenomenon*, in contrast to the Argyll Robertson pupil.

Another interesting pupillary abnormality is the tonic reaction, also referred to as the *Adie pupil*. This syndrome is due to a degeneration of the ciliary ganglia and the postganglionic parasympathetic fibers that normally constrict the pupil and effect accommodation. The patient may complain of unilateral blurring of vision or may have noticed that one pupil is larger than the other. The affected pupil is slightly enlarged in ambient light and the reaction to light is absent or greatly reduced if tested in the customary manner, although the size of the pupil will change slowly with prolonged maximal stimulation. Characteristically, there is a light-near dissociation, i.e., the Adie pupil responds better to near than it does to light. Once the pupil has constricted, it tends to remain tonically constricted and redilates very slowly. Once dilated, the pupil remains in this state for many seconds, up to a minute or longer. Light and near paralysis of a segment or segments of the pupillary sphincter is also characteristic of the syndrome; this segmental irregularity can be seen with the high plus lenses of an ophthalmoscope. The affected pupil constricts promptly in response to the common miotic drugs and is unusually sensitive to a 0.1% solution of pilocarpine, a concentration that has only minimal effect on a normal pupil (denervation supersensitivity). The tonic pupil usually appears during the third or fourth decade of life and is much more common in women than in men; it may be associated with absence of knee or ankle jerks (*Holmes-Adie syndrome*) and hence be mistaken for tabes dorsalis. From all available data, it represents a mild polyneuropathy, often familial.

Finally, mention should be made of a rare pupillary phenomenon characterized by transient episodes of unilateral mydriasis for which no cause can be found (the "*springing pupil*"). These episodes of mydriasis, which are more common in women, last for minutes to days and may recur at random intervals. Ocular motor palsies and ptosis are notably lacking, but sometimes the pupil is distorted during the attack. Some patients complain of blurred vision and head pain on the side of the mydriasis, suggesting an atypical form of ophthalmoplegic migraine. In children, following a minor or major seizure, one pupil may remain dilated for a protracted period of time. The main consideration in an awake patient is that the cornea has inadvertently (or purposefully) been exposed to mydriatic solutions, among them vasopressor agents used in cardiac resuscitation.

Differential Diagnosis of Anisocoria

In regard to pupillary disorders, there are two main issues with which the neurologist has to contend. One is the problem of the relative afferent pupillary defect and how to recognize it; this is discussed above. The second problem is one of unequal pupils (anisocoria) and determining whether this abnormality depends upon sympathetic or parasympathetic denervation.

As stated above, in dealing with anisocoria, it is important to remember that at any given examination, 20 percent of normal persons show an inequality of 0.3 to 0.5 mm or more. This is "simple" or physiologic anisocoria, and it may be a source of confusion in patients with small pupils. It is characteristically variable from day to day and even from hour to hour and often will have disappeared at the time of the second examination (Loewenfeld; Lam et al). Also, in first dealing with the problem of pupillary asymmetry, one has to determine which of the pupils is abnormal. If it is the larger one, the light reaction will be muted on that side; if it is the smaller pupil, it will fail to enlarge in response to shading both eyes. More simply stated, *light exaggerates the anisocoria due to a third-nerve lesion, and darkness accentuates the anisocoria in the case of a Horner syndrome.*

A *persistently small pupil* always raises the question of a Horner syndrome, a diagnosis that may be difficult if the ptosis is slight and facial anhidrosis undetectable. In darkness, the Horner pupil dilates more slowly and to a lesser degree than the normal one because it lacks the pull of the dilator muscle (dilation lag). The diagnosis can be confirmed by placing 1 or 2 drops of 2 to 10% cocaine in each eye; the Horner pupil dilates not at all or much less than the normal one—a response that can be documented by photos taken after 5 and 15 s of darkness. Such a response to cocaine will occur with a defect at any point along the sympathetic pathway (page 562) because lesions of the first- or second-order sympathetic neurons deplete norepinephrine at the synapses with third-order neurons. The reduction of neurotransmitter at the nerve endings in the ciliary dilator muscle greatly reduces the reuptake blocking effects of cocaine. If the subsequent (24 h after cocaine) application of the adrenergic mydriatic hydroxyamphetamine (1%) has no effect, the lesion can be localized to the postganglionic portion of the pathway since this drug releases any norepinephrine that may remain in the third order neuron. Localization of the lesion to the central or preganglionic parts of the sympathetic pathway depends upon the associated symptoms and signs (Chap. 26).

A variety of lesions, some of them purely ocular, such as uveitis, may give rise to a *dilated pupil*. Neurologically, there are three main diagnostic considerations:

1. An interruption of the parasympathetic preganglionic pupilloconstrictor fibers in the third nerve. It is a safe clinical rule that the interruption of these fibers is practically always associated with ptosis, palsy of the extraocular muscles, or signs of other brainstem or cerebral disease. The importance of unilateral pupillary enlargements in the diagnosis of coma is discussed in Chap. 17. Often in this circumstance the pupil goes through an early phase of miosis followed by irregularly shaped enlargement.

2. The presence of a tonic, or *Adie*, pupil. Here one requires that the pupillary abnormalities conform to the diagnostic criteria for this disorder, enumerated above.

3. Drug-induced iridoplegia. Not infrequently, particularly among nurses and pharmacists, a mydriatic fixed pupil is the result of accidental or deliberate application of an atropinic or sympathomimetic drug. Failure of 1% pilocarpine drops to contract the pupil provides proof that the iris sphincter has been blocked by atropine or some other anticholinergic agent.

As a rule, bilateral smallness of pupils does not pose a difficult diagnostic problem. The clinical associations, acute and chronic, have already been discussed. Long-standing bilateral Adie pupils tend to be small and show tonic near responses. They can be readily distinguished from Argyll Robertson pupils, which constrict quickly to near and redilate quickly on release from the near stimulus.

Figure 14-8 is a useful schematic, devised by Thompson and Pilley, for sorting out the various types of anisocoria.

Orbital Mass Lesions

Ocular movement, pupillary reaction, and visual acuity may be affected by diseases that alter the contents of the orbit. The most frequent of these is thyroid disease, causing bilateral or unilateral exophthalmos. Orbital tumors (dermoids, hemangiomas, adenoma of lacrimal gland,

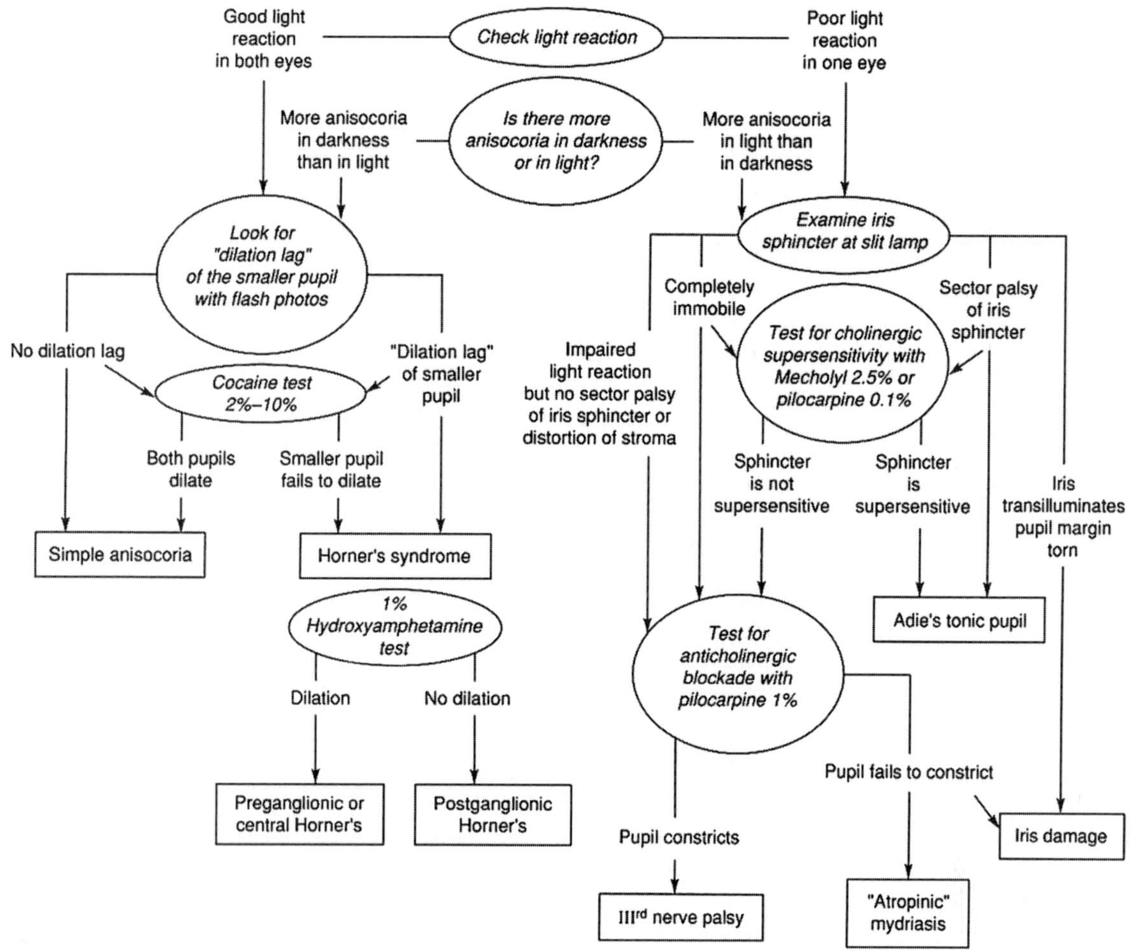

Figure 14-8

A schematic for sorting out the nature of anisocoria. (From Thompson and Pilley, reprinted by permission.)

optic nerve glioma, neurofibroma, metastatic carcinoma, meningioma), granuloma (including sarcoid and orbital pseudotumor), orbital cellulitis or abscess, or cavernous sinus thrombosis are other causes of unilateral exophthalmos.

REFERENCES

Aramideh M, Ongerboer de Visser BW, Devriese PP, et al: Electromyographic features of levator palpebrae superioris and orbicularis oculi muscles in blepharospasm. *Brain* 117:27, 1994.

Bahn RS, Heufelder AE: Pathogenesis of Graves' ophthalmopathy. *N Engl J Med* 329:1468, 1993.

Baloh RW, Yee RD, Honrubia V: Late cortical cerebellar atrophy: Clinical and oculographic features. *Brain* 109:159, 1986.

Bogousslavsky J, Miklossy J, Deruaz JP, et al: Unilateral left paramedian infarction of thalamus and midbrain: A clinicopathological study. *J Neurol Neurosurg Psychiatry* 49:686, 1986.

Büttner-Ennever JA, Akert K: Medial rectus subgroups of the oculomotor nucleus and their abducens internuclear input in the monkey. *J Comp Neurol* 197:17, 1981.

Caplan LR: "Top of the basilar" syndrome. *Neurology* 30:72, 1980.

Cogan DG: A type of congenital ocular motor apraxia presenting jerky head movements. *Am J Ophthalmol* 36:433, 1953.

Cogan DG: *Neurology of the Ocular Muscles*, 2nd ed. Springfield, IL, Charles C Thomas, 1956.

Cogan DG: *Neurology of the Visual System*. Springfield, IL Charles C Thomas, 1966.

Corbett JJ, Thompson HS: Pupillary function and dysfunction, in Asbury AK, McKhann GM, McDonald WI (eds): *Diseases of the Nervous System*, 2nd ed. Philadelphia, Saunders, 1992, chap 34, pp 490–500.

Daroff RB: Ocular oscillations. *Ann Otol Rhinol Laryngol* 86:102, 1977.

Fisher CM: Some neuro-ophthalmological observations. *J Neurol Neurosurg Psychiatry* 30:383, 1967.

Ford CS, Schwartze GM, Weaver RG, Troost BT:Monocular elevation paresis caused by an ipsilateral lesion. *Neurology* 34: 1264, 1984.

Glaser JS (ed): *Neuro-ophthalmology*, 3rd ed. Philadelphia, Lippincott, Williams and Wilkins, 1999.

Goldberg ME, Bushnell MC: Behavioral enhancement of visual responses in monkey cerebral cortex: II. Modulation in frontal eye fields specifically related to saccades. *J Neurophysiol* 46: 773, 1981.

Halmagyi GM, Rudge P, Griesty M, Sanders MD: Downbeating nystagmus. *Arch Neurol* 40:777, 1983.

Hanson MR, Hamid MA, Tomsak RL, et al: Selective saccadic palsy caused by pontine lesions: Clinical, physiological and pathological correlations. *Ann Neurol* 20:209, 1986.

Hommel M, Bogousslavsky J: The spectrum of vertical gaze palsy following unilateral brainstem stroke. *Neurology* 41:1229, 1991.

Hotson R: Cerebellar control of fixation eye movements. *Neurology* 32:31, 1982.

Jacobs L, Anderson PJ, Bender MG: The lesions producing paralysis of downward but not upward gaze. *Arch Neurol* 28:319, 1973.

Kato I, Nakamura T, Watanabe J, et al: Primary posterior upbeat nystagmus: Localizing value. *Arch Neurol* 42:819, 1985.

Keane JR: Acute bilateral ophthalmoplegia: 60 cases. *Neurology* 36:279, 1986.

Keane JR: Cavernous sinus syndrome: Analysis of 151 cases. *Arch Neurol* 53:967, 1996.

Keane JR: Ocular skew deviation. *Arch Neurol* 32:185, 1975.

Kompf D, Pasik T, Pasik P, Bender MB: Downward gaze in monkeys: Stimulation and lesion studies. *Brain* 102:527, 1979.

Lam BL, Thompson HS, Corbett JJ: The prevalence of simple anisocoria. *Am J Ophthalmol* 104:69, 1987.

Leichnetz GR: The prefrontal cortico-oculomotor trajectories in the monkey. *J Neurol Sci* 49:387, 1981.

Leigh RJ, Zee DS: *The Neurology of Eye Movements*, 2nd ed. Philadelphia, Davis, 1991.

Lewis RF, Zee DS: Ocular motor disorders associated with cerebellar lesions: Pathophysiology and topical localization. *Rev Neurol* 149:665, 1993.

Loewenfeld IE: "Simple, central" anisocoria: A common condition seldom recognized. *Trans Am Acad Ophthalmol Otolaryngol* 83: 832, 1977.

Morris JGL, Lee J, Lim CL: Facial sweating in Horner's syndrome. *Brain* 107:751, 1984.

Ranalli PJ, Sharpe JA, Fletcher WA: Palsy of upward and downward saccadic, pursuit, and vestibular movements with a unilateral midbrain lesion: Pathophysiologic correlations. *Neurology* 38:114, 1988.

Ropper AH: Ocular dipping in anoxic coma. *Arch Neurol* 38:297, 1981.

Ropper AH: Illusion of tilting of the visual environment. *J Clin Neuroophthalmol* 3:147, 1983.

Rucker CW: Paralysis of the third, fourth, and sixth cranial nerves. *Am J Ophthalmol* 46:787, 1958.

Rucker CW: The causes of paralysis of the third, fourth and sixth cranial nerves. *Am J Ophthalmol* 61:1293, 1966.

Rush JA, Younge BR: Paralysis of cranial nerves III, IV, and VI: Cause and prognosis in 1000 cases. *Arch Ophthalmol* 99:76, 1981.

Safran AB, Kline LB, Glaser JS, Daroff RB: Television-induced formed visual hallucinations and cerebral diplopia. *Br J Ophthalmol* 65:707, 1981.

Saul RF, Selhorst JB: Downbeat nystagmus with magnesium depletion. *Arch Neurol* 38:650, 1981.

Smith SA, Smith SE: Bilateral Horner's syndrome: Detection and occurrence. *J Neurol Neurosurg Psychiatry* 66:48, 1999.

Smith AS, Smith SC: Assessment of pupillary function in diabetic neuropathy, in Dyck PJ, Thomas PK, Asbury AK, et al (eds): *Diabetic Neuropathy*. Philadelphia, Saunders, 1987, chap 13, pp 134–139.

Thach WT, Montgomery EB: Motor system, in Pearlman AL, Collins RC (eds): *Neurobiology of Disease*. New York, Oxford University Press, 1990, pp 168–196.

Thompson HS: Diagnosing Horner's syndrome. *Trans Am Acad Ophthalmol Otolaryngol* 83:OP840, 1977.

Thompson HS, Pilley SFJ: Unequal pupils: A flow chart for sorting out the anisocorias. *Surv Ophthalmol* 21:45, 1976.

Vidailhet M, Rivaud S, Gouider-Khouja N, et al: Eye movements in parkinsonian syndromes. *Ann Neurol* 35:420, 1994.

Von Noorden GK: *Van Noorden-Maumenee's Atlas of Strabismus*, 3rd ed. St Louis, Mosby, 1977.

Wall M, Wray SH: The one and a half syndrome—A unilateral disorder of the pontine tegmentum: A study of 20 cases and review of the literature. *Neurology* 33:971, 1983.

Warwick R: Representation of the extraocular muscles in the oculomotor nuclei of the monkey. *J Comp Neurol* 98:449, 1953.

Warwick R: The so-called nucleus of convergence. *Brain* 78:92, 1955.

White OB, St Cyr JA, Sharpe JA: Ocular motor deficits in Parkinson's disease. *Brain* 106:555, 571, 1983.

Wray SH: Neuro-ophthalmologic diseases, in Rosenberg RN (ed): *Comprehensive Neurology*. New York, Raven Press, 1991, chap 20, pp 659–697.

Wray SH, Taylor J: Third nerve palsy: A review of 206 cases. Unpublished data, quoted in Wray SH (above).

Zee DS: Ophthalmoscopy in examination of patients with vestibular disorders. *Ann Neurol* 3:373, 1978.

Zee DS, Robinson DA: A hypothetical explanation of saccadic oscillations. *Ann Neurol* 5:405, 1979.

Zee DS, Yee RD, Cogan DG, et al: Ocular motor abnormalities in hereditary cerebellar ataxia. *Brain* 99:207, 1976.

Chapter 15

DEAFNESS, DIZZINESS, AND DISORDERS OF EQUILIBRIUM

Hearing is one of our most precious possessions. Sounds alert us to danger; spoken words are the universal means of communication; music is one of our most exalted esthetic pleasures. The loss of this sense excludes the individual from much of what is going on around him, and adjustment to this deprivation imposes a profound reorientation. Prevention of deafness is a goal toward which medicine strives. Likewise, our vestibular function assures our ability to stand steadily and erect and to move about gracefully. Hence an understanding of the functions of the eighth cranial nerves and their derangements by disease is the legitimate concern of the neurologist.

ANATOMIC AND PHYSIOLOGIC CONSIDERATIONS

The vestibulocochlear or eighth cranial nerve has two separate components: the cochlear nerve, which subserves hearing, or acoustic function, and the vestibular nerve, which is concerned with equilibrium, or balance, and orientation of the body to the surrounding world.

The acoustic division has its cell bodies in the spiral ganglion of the cochlea. This ganglion is composed of bipolar cells, the peripheral processes of which convey auditory impulses from the specialized neuroepithelium of the inner ear, the spiral organ of Corti. This is the end organ of hearing, wherein sound is transduced into nerve impulses. It consists of approximately 15,000 neuroepithelial (hair) cells, resting on the basilar membrane, which extends along the entire 2½ turns of the cochlea. Projecting from the inner surface of each hair cell are approximately 60 very fine filaments, or stereocilia, which are embedded in the tectorial membrane, a gelatinous structure overlying the organ of Corti (Fig. 15-1). Sound causes the basilar membrane to vibrate; upward displacement of the basilar membrane bends the relatively fixed stereocilia and provides the adequate stimulus for activating the hair cells. The stimulus is then transmitted to the sensory fibers of the cochlear nerve, which end synaptically at the base of each hair cell. Each afferent auditory fiber and the hair cell with which it is connected has a minimum threshold at one frequency ("characteristic" or "best" frequency). The basilar membrane vibrates at different frequencies throughout its length, according to the frequency of the sound stimulus. In this way the fibers of the cochlear nerve respond to the full range of audible sound and can differentiate and resolve complexes of sounds.

The so-called inner hair cells, numbering about 3500, are of particular importance, since they synapse with about 90 percent of the 30,000 afferent cochlear neurons. The central processes of the primary auditory neurons constitute the cochlear division of the eighth cranial nerve. In addition, the nerve contains approximately 500 efferent fibers, which arise from the superior olivary nuclei (80 percent from the contralateral nucleus and 20 percent from the ipsilateral one) and synapse with the afferent neurons from the hair cells (Rasmussen). The function of this efferent pathway is not clear. It is thought to play some part in the auditory activity that is generated in the ear itself, possibly to enhance the sharpness of sound perception by some feedback mechanism (Kemp). The eighth nerve also contains adrenergic postganglionic fibers that are derived from the cervical autonomic chain and innervate the cochlea and labyrinth.

The vestibular division arises from cells in the vestibular, or Scarpa's, ganglion, which is situated in the internal auditory meatus. This ganglion is also composed of bipolar cells, the peripheral processes of which terminate in hair cells of the specialized sensory epithelium of the labyrinth (semicircular canals, saccule, and utricle). The sensory epithelium is located on hillocks (cristae) in the dilated openings or ampullae of the semicircular canals, where they are called the *cristae ampullaris*, and

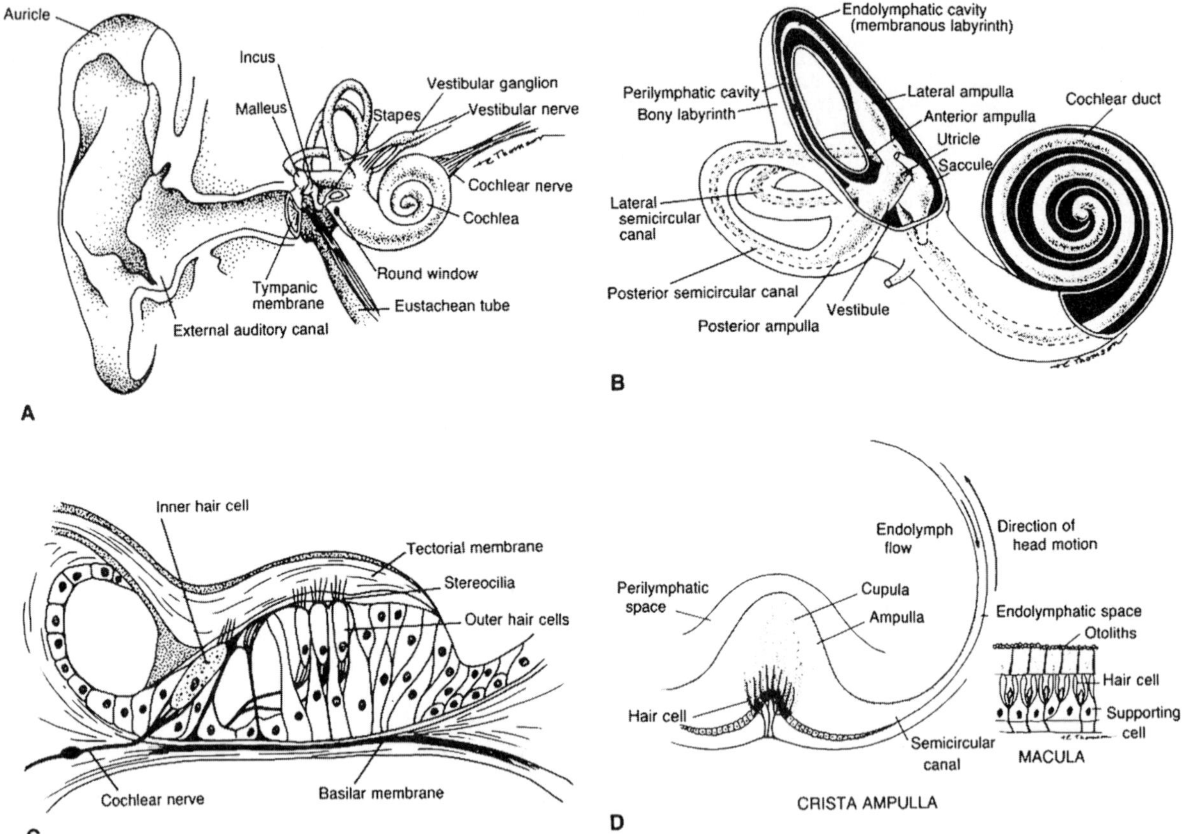

Figure 15-1

The auditory and vestibular systems. A. *The right ear, viewed from the front, showing the external ear and auditory canal, the middle ear and its ossicles, and the inner ear.* B. *The main parts of the right inner ear, viewed from the front. The* perilymph *is located between the wall of the bony labyrinth and the membranous labyrinth. In the cochlea, the perilymphatic space takes the form of two coiled tubes—the* scala vestibuli *and* scala tympani. *The* endolymph *is located within the membranous labyrinth, which includes the three semicircular canals, utricle, and saccule.* C. *The* organ of Corti. *This is the end organ of hearing; it consists of a single row of inner hair cells and three rows of outer hair cells. The stereocilia of the hair cells are embedded in the tectorial membrane.* D. *Diagram of a crista ampulla, the specialized sensory epithelium of a semicircular canal. The crista senses the displacement of endolymph during head rotation. The direction of head rotation is indicated by the large arrow, and endolymph flow by the small arrow. The* macula *is the locus of the sensory epithelium in the utricle and saccule. Note that the tips of the hair cells are in contact with the otoliths (calcareous material), which are embedded in a gelatinous mass called the* cupula.

in the utricle and saccule, where they are called *maculae acusticae*. The hair cells of the maculae are covered by the *otolithic membrane*, or *otolith*, which is composed of calcium carbonate crystals embedded in a gelatinous matrix. The sensory cells of the cristae are covered by a sail-shaped gelatinous mass called a *cupula* (Fig. 15-1). The labyrinthine semicircular canals transduce angular movements of the head, and the otoliths transduce linear movement.

The central fibers from the cells of the spiral and vestibular ganglia are united in a common trunk, which enters the cranial cavity through the internal auditory meatus (accompanied by the facial and intermediate nerves), traverses the cerebellopontine angle, and enters the brainstem at the junction of the pons and medulla. Here the cochlear and vestibular fibers become separated. The cochlear fibers bifurcate and terminate almost at once in the dorsal and ventral cochlear nuclei. The fibers from each cochlear nucleus pursue separate crossing and ascending pathways; they are transmitted to both inferior colliculi (mainly to the opposite side) via the lateral lemnisci. Secondary acoustic fibers project via the trapezoid body and lateral lemniscus to the medial geniculate bodies (Fig. 15-2). Some fibers terminate in the trapezoid body and superior olivary complex and subserve such reflex functions as auditory attention, sound localization, auditory startle, and oculo-postural orientation to sound. Both excitatory and inhibitory neurons are located at every level of these pathways. From the medial geniculate bodies fibers project to the cortex via the auditory radiations—relatively compact bundles that course ventrolaterally to the posterior parts of the putamens before dispersing and ending in the transverse gyri of Heschl and other auditory cortical areas (Tanaka et al).

The auditory cortical field comprises the superior temporal gyrus and the upper bank of the sylvian fissure (area 41), or primary auditory cortex, and the surrounding secondary and tertiary cortices in the adjacent temporal lobe. The latter are of particular importance in the interpretation of sound (Celesia). Bilateral temporal lobe lesions involving the geniculocortical fasciculi result in cortical deafness although such lesions are rare; unilateral cortical lesions do not affect hearing. At every

Figure 15-2

The ascending auditory pathways. The lower part of the diagram is a horizontal section through the upper medulla. (Reproduced with permission from Noback CR: The Human Nervous System, *3rd ed. New York, McGraw-Hill, 1981.*

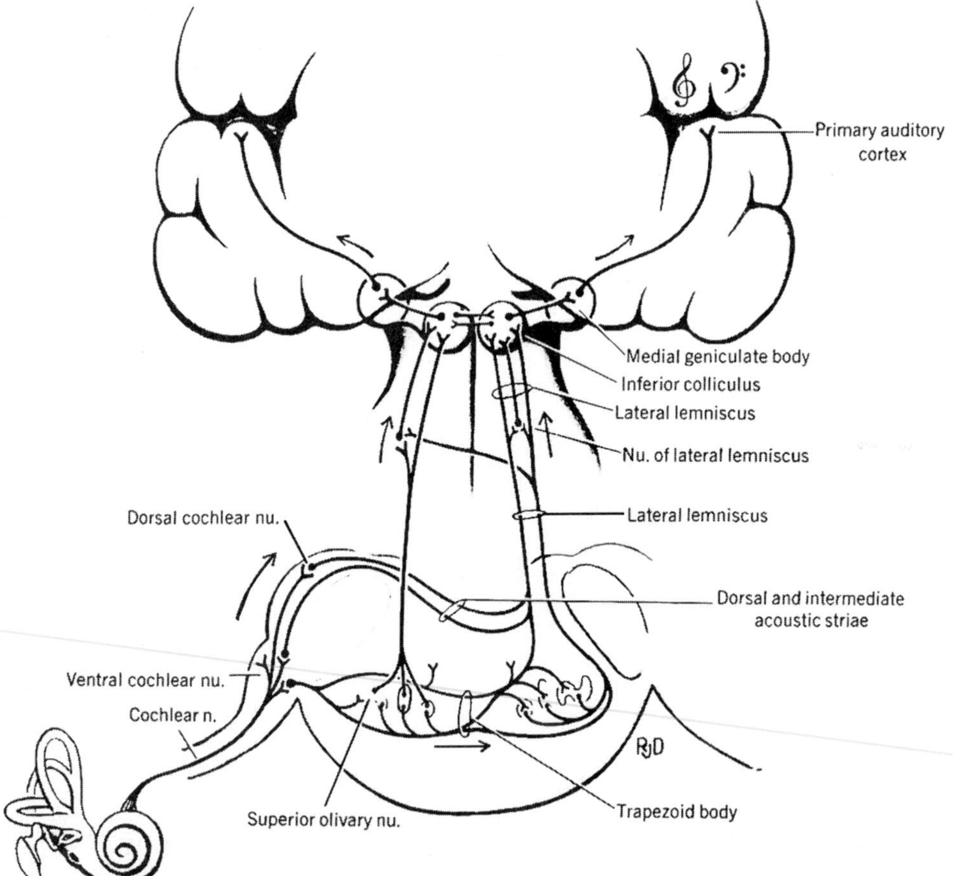

level of these ascending fiber systems there is feedback to lower structures.

The vestibular fibers of the eighth nerve terminate in the four vestibular nuclei: superior (Bechterew), lateral (Deiters), medial (triangular, or Schwalbe), and inferior (spinal, or descending). In addition, some of the fibers from the semicircular canals project directly to the cerebellum via the juxtarestiform body and terminate in the flocculonodular lobe and adjacent vermian cortex ("vestibulocerebellum"). Efferent fibers from this portion of the cerebellar cortex project ipsilaterally to the vestibular nuclei and to the fastigial nucleus; in turn, fibers from the fastigial nucleus project to the contralateral vestibular nuclei, again via the juxtarestiform body. Thus each side of the cerebellum exerts an influence on the vestibular nuclei of both sides (Fig. 15-3; see also Chap. 5).

The lateral and medial vestibular nuclei also have important connections with the spinal cord, mainly via the uncrossed lateral vestibulospinal tract and the crossed and uncrossed medial vestibulospinal tracts (Fig. 15-4). Presumably, vestibular effects on posture are mediated via these pathways—the axial muscles being acted upon predominantly by the medial vestibulospinal tract and

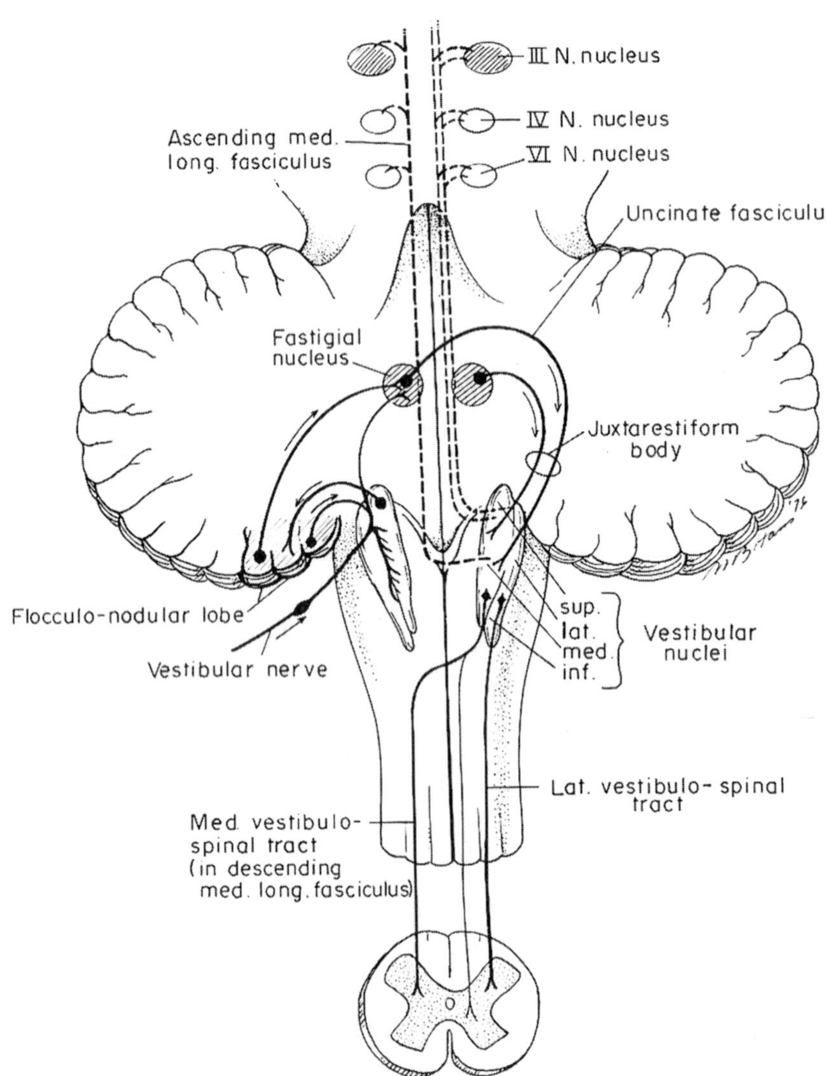

Figure 15-3

A simplified diagram of the vestibulocerebellar and vestibulospinal pathways and connections between vestibular and ocular motor nuclei. The medial longitudinal fasciculi (dotted vertical lines) are the main pathways for ascending vestibular impulses. (See text and also Fig. 14-1.)

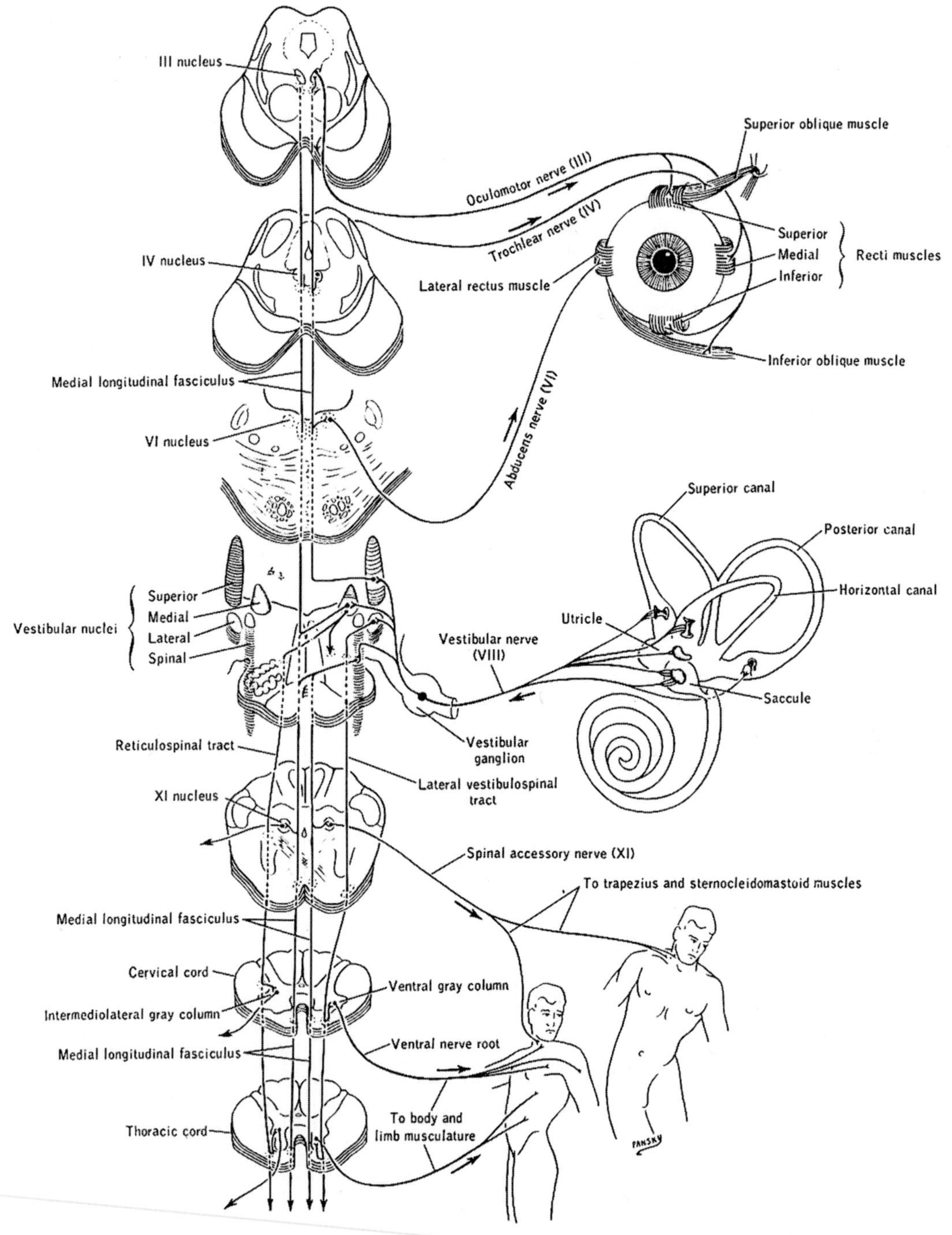

Figure 15-4

The vestibular reflex pathways. (Reproduced by permission from House EL, et al: A Systematic Approach to Neuroscience. *New York, McGraw-Hill, 1979.)*

the limb muscles, by the lateral tract. The nuclei of the third, fourth, and sixth cranial nerves come under the influence of the vestibular nuclei, mainly the superior and medial nuclei, through the projection pathways, mainly the medial longitudinal fasciculus described in Chap. 14. In addition, all the vestibular nuclei have afferent and efferent connections with the pontine reticular formation (Fig. 15-4). The latter connections subserve vestibulo-ocular and vestibulospinal reflexes that are essential for clear vision and stable posture. Finally, there are projections from the vestibular nuclei to the cerebral cortex, specifically to the regions of the intraparietal sulcus and superior sylvian gyrus. In the monkey, these projections are almost exclusively contralateral, terminating near the "face area" of the first somatosensory cortex (area 2 of Brodmann). Lesions in the posterior insula impair the sense of verticality, body orientation, and movement.

These brief remarks convey some notion of the complexity of the anatomic and functional organization of the vestibular system (for a full discussion, see the monographs of Brodal and of Baloh and Honrubia). In view of the proximity of cochlear and vestibular elements, it is understandable that acoustic and vestibular function are often affected together in the course of disease; each may be affected separately, however.

DEAFNESS, TINNITUS, AND OTHER DISORDERS OF AUDITORY PERCEPTION

Deafness

This is a problem of immense proportions. In 1969, Konigsmark estimated that there were in the United States at least 6 million persons with hearing loss of sufficient severity to impair the understanding of speech; there were probably three times this many with some impairment of hearing. Konigsmark also estimated that in about half of the affected children and about one-third of the affected adults, the deafness was on a hereditary basis. Figures from a more recent (1989) National Health Survey indicated that approximately 28 million Americans of all ages had a significant degree of deafness and that 2 million of this group were profoundly deaf. More than one-third of persons over the age of 75 were handicapped to some extent by hearing loss.

Deafness is of three general types: (1) *Conductive deafness*, due to a defect in the mechanism by which sound is transformed (amplified) and conducted to the cochlea. Disorders of the external or middle ear—obstruction of the external auditory canal by atresia or cerumen, thickening of the tympanic membrane from infection or trauma, chronic otitis media, otosclerosis (the main cause of deafness in early adult life), and obstruction of the eustachian tube—are the main causes. (2) *Sensorineural deafness* (also called *nerve deafness*), which is due to disease of the cochlea or of the cochlear division of the eighth cranial nerve. Although cochlear and eighth nerve causes of deafness have conventionally been combined in one (sensorineural) category, the neurologist recognizes that the symptoms and causes of the two are quite different and that it is more practical to think of them separately. (3) *Central deafness*, due to lesions of the cochlear nuclei and their connections with the primary auditory receptive areas in the temporal lobes. Complete tone deafness, which is probably inherited as an autosomal dominant trait, is another central disorder.

The two peripheral forms of deafness, conductive and nerve deafness, must be distinguished, since important remedial measures are available for the former. In differentiating conductive from nerve deafness, the tuning-fork tests are often of value. When a vibrating fork, preferably of 512-Hz frequency, is held about 2.5 cm from the ear (the test for air conduction), sound waves can be appreciated only as they are transmitted through the middle ear; they will be reduced with disease in this location. When the vibrating fork is applied to the skull (test for bone conduction), the sound waves are conveyed directly to the cochlea, without intervention of the sound-transmission apparatus of the middle ear, and will therefore not be reduced or lost. Normally air conduction is better than bone conduction. These principles form the basis for several simple tests of auditory function.

In the *Weber test*, the vibrating fork is applied to the forehead in the midline. A normal person hears the bone-conducted sound equally in both ears. In nerve deafness, the sound is localized in the normal ear; in conductive deafness, the sound is localized in the affected ear. In the *Rinne test*, the fork is applied to the mastoid process. At the moment the sound ceases, the fork is held at the auditory meatus. In middle ear deafness, the sound cannot be heard by air conduction after bone conduction has ceased (abnormal or negative Rinne test). In nerve deafness, the reverse is true (normal or positive Rinne test), although both air and bone conduction may be quantitatively decreased. The *Schwabach test* consists of comparing the patient's bone conduction with that of a normal examiner.

In general, early sensorineural deafness is characterized by a partial loss of perception of high-pitched sounds and conductive deafness by a partial loss of low-pitched sounds. This can be ascertained by the use of tuning forks of different frequencies but most accurately by the use of an audiometer and the construction of an audiogram, which reveals the entire range of hearing at a glance. The audiogram is the one essential test in the evaluation of hearing loss and the point of departure for subsequent diagnostic evaluation.

A cochlear type of hearing loss can be recognized by eliciting the symptoms of recruitment and diplacusis. There is a heightened perception of loudness, or *recruitment*, once the threshold for hearing has been exceeded; thus the common retort "You don't have to shout" when the examiner raises his voice. *Diplacusis* refers to a defect in frequency discrimination that is manifest by a lack of clarity of spoken syllables or by the perception that music is out of tune and unpleasant.

Since each cochlear nucleus is connected with the cortex of both temporal lobes, hearing is unaffected by unilateral cerebral lesions. Deafness due to brainstem lesions is observed only rarely, since a massive lesion is required to interrupt both the crossed and uncrossed projections from the cochlear nuclei—so massive, as a rule, that other neurologic abnormalities make the testing of hearing impossible.

The main causes of sensorineural and conductive hearing loss are discussed further on.

Special Audiologic Procedures

A number of special tests have proved to be helpful in distinguishing cochlear from retrocochlear (nerve) lesions. Although an absolute distinction cannot be made on the basis of any one test, the results of the tests when taken together (particularly loudness recruitment and threshold tone decay) make it possible to predict the site of the lesion with considerable accuracy. These tests, usually carried out by an otologist or audiologist, include the following:

1. *Loudness recruitment.* This phenomenon, alluded to above, is thought to depend upon the selective destruction of low-intensity elements subserved by the external hair cells of the organ of Corti. The high-intensity elements are preserved, so that loudness is appreciated only at high intensities. In testing for loudness recruitment, the difference in hearing between the two ears is estimated and the loudness of the pure tone stimulus of a given frequency delivered to each ear is then increased by regular increments. In *nonrecruiting deafness* (characteristic of a nerve lesion), the original difference in hearing persists in all comparisons of loudness above threshold, since both high- and low-intensity fibers are affected. In *recruiting deafness* (which occurs with a lesion in the organ of Corti—e.g., Ménière disease), the more affected ear gains in loudness and may finally be equal to the better one. In bilateral disease, recruitment is assessed by the intensity of the stimulus that causes discomfort. In the normal person, the threshold of discomfort is about 100 dB (decibels).

2. *Threshold "tone decay" (abnormal auditory adaptation).* This test requires only a conventional pure-tone audiometer. With lesions of the nerve, e.g., acoustic neuroma, a continuous tone presented at or above threshold intensity gradually seems to decrease in loudness, in contrast to what happens with cochlear lesions.

3. *Short-increment sensitivity index (SiSi).* The patient is asked to respond to a series of twenty 1-dB increments in amplitude superimposed on a steady tone of the same frequency presented at a sensation level of 20 dB. In normal persons and in those with retrocochlear (nerve) lesions, most of these small 1-dB pips of sound are not heard; with cochlear lesions, most of them are heard.

4. *Speech discrimination.* This consists of presenting the patient with a list of 50 phonetically balanced monosyllabic words (e.g., *thin, sin*) at suprathreshold levels. The speech-discrimination score is the percentage of the 50 words correctly repeated by the patient. Marked reduction (less than 30 percent) in the speech-discrimination test scores is characteristic of eighth nerve lesions.

5. *Békésy audiometry.* Continuous and interrupted tones are presented at various frequencies. Tracings are made, measuring the increments by which the patient must increase the volume in order to continue to hear the continuous and interrupted tones just above threshold. Analysis of many tracings has shown that there are four basic configurations, referred to as types I to IV Békésy audiograms. Types III or IV usually indicate the presence of a retrocochlear lesion, the type II response points to a lesion of the cochlea itself, and type I is considered normal.

6. The *acoustic-stapedial reflex* can be used as a measure of conduction in the auditory (and the facial) nerve. This reflex normally protects the cochleas from excessively loud sound. When sound of greater intensity than 70 to 90 dB above threshold hearing reaches the inner ear, the stapedius muscles on both sides contract reflexly, relaxing the tympanum and offering impedance to further sound. It may be tested by insufflating the external auditory canal with pressured air and measuring

the change in pressure that follows immediately after a loud sound is introduced to either ear. The response is muted in patients with conductive hearing loss because of the mechanical restriction of ossicular movement, but otherwise the test is sensitive to cochlear and acoustic nerve lesions and also can be used to test recruitment.

7. *Brainstem auditory evoked potentials* (BAER; page 36). This method provides information as to the integrity of primary and secondary auditory pathways from the cochlea to the temporal lobe cortex. This method can be used in uncooperative and even comatose patients. It is of particular value in detecting small acoustic neuromas; in localizing brainstem lesions such as areas of demyelination; in corroborating the state of brain death, where all waves except occasionally the eighth nerve (wave I) responses are abolished; and in assessing sensorineural damage in neonates who have had meningitis or been exposed to ototoxic medications.

Tinnitus

This is the other major manifestation of cochlear and auditory disease. *Tinnitus aurium* literally means "ringing of the ears" (Latin *tinnire*, "to ring or jingle") and refers to sounds originating in the ear, although they need not be ringing in character. Buzzing, humming, whistling, roaring, hissing, clicking, chirping, or pulse-like sounds are also reported. Some otologists use the term *tinnitus cerebri* to distinguish other head noises from those that arise in the ear, but the term *tinnitus* when used without qualification refers to tinnitus aurium.

Tinnitus is a remarkably common symptom, affecting more than 37 million Americans, according to Marion and Cevette. It may be defined as any sensation of sound for which there is no source outside the individual. Two basic types are recognized, *tonal* and *nontonal* (nonvibratory and vibratory, in the terminology of Fowler). The tonal type is by far the more common and is also called *subjective tinnitus*, because it can be heard only by the patient. The nontonal form is sometimes *objective*, in the sense that under certain conditions the tinnitus can be heard by the examiner as well as by the patient. In either case, whether tinnitus is produced in the inner ear or in some other part of the head and neck, sensory auditory neurons must be stimulated, for only the auditory neural pathways can transmit an impulse that will be perceived as sound.

Nontonal and Pulsatile Tinnitus These head noises are mechanical in origin and are conducted to the inner ear through the various hard or soft structures or the fluid or gaseous media of the body. They are not due to a primary dysfunction of the auditory neural mechanism but have their origin in the contraction of muscles of the eustachian tube, middle ear (stapedius, tensor tympani), palate (palatal myoclonus) or pharynx (muscles of deglutition), or in vascular structures near the ear. One of the most common forms of subjective tinnitus is a self-audible bruit, the source of which is the turbulent flow of blood in the large vessels of the neck or in an arteriovenous malformation or glomus jugulare tumor. The sound is pulsatile and asymmetrically appreciated by the patient but is rarely detectable by the examiner. Normal variations in the size and location of the jugular bulb may explain the symptom in some patients (Adler and Ropper). Other noteworthy causes of pulsatile tinnitus are pseudotumor cerebri or raised intracranial pressure of any type, in which the pulsatile quality is attributed to a pressure gradient between the cranial and cervical venous structures, thyroid enlargement with increased venous blood flow, intracranial aneurysm, aortic stenosis, and vascular tumors of the skull, such as histiocytosis X. In the case of a vascular tumor or a large arteriovenous malformation, the examiner may hear the bruit over the mastoid process. Obliteration of the sound by gentle compression of the jugular vein on the symptomatic side is a useful indicator of a venous origin. Carotid artery disease is a relatively uncommon cause of a self-audible bruit. A flow-related bruit originating from fibromuscular dysplasia, atherosclerotic stenosis, dissection, and enhanced blood flow in a vessel contralateral to a carotid occlusion have all been incriminated. In 100 consecutive cases of pulsatile tinnitus, intracranial hypertension, glomus tumors, and carotid disease were found to be the most common causes (Sismanis and Smoker). One must always be cautious in interpreting this symptom, because normal persons can hear their pulse when lying with one ear on a pillow, and introspective individuals may worry about it.

Tonal Tinnitus This form of tinnitus arises in the middle or inner ear. Under ideal acoustic circumstances (in a soundproof room having an ambient noise level of 18 dB or less), it is present in 80 to 90 percent of adults ("physiologic tinnitus"). The ambient noise level in ordinary living conditions usually exceeds 35 dB and is of sufficient intensity to mask physiologic tinnitus, which remains inaudible. Tinnitus due to disease of the middle ear and auditory neural mechanisms may also be masked by environmental noise and hence becomes troublesome only in quiet surroundings—at night, in the country, etc.

Most often, tinnitus signifies a disorder of the tympanic membrane, ossicles of the middle ear, inner ear, or eighth nerve. A majority of patients who complain of persistent tinnitus have some degree of deafness as well. Tinnitus that is localized to one ear and is described as having a tonal character (such as a ringing, bell-like, or high steady musical tone) is usually associated with an impairment of cochlear or neural function. Tinnitus associated with sensorineural hearing loss of high frequency is often described as "chirping" and that of low frequency as "whooshing" or blowing (Marion and Cevette). Tinnitus due to middle ear disease (e.g., otosclerosis) tends to be more constant than the tinnitus of sensorineural disorders, is of variable intensity and lower pitch, and is characterized by clicks, pops, and rushing sounds. The more common of these are the rhythmic clicking of palatal myoclonus and intermittent clicking from contraction of the tensor tympani or stapedius muscles, termed "middle ear myoclonus." The latter has been treated with a variety of medications, including diazepam, or, in extremely annoying cases, by section of the offending muscles (Badia et al). Ear-clicking noises due to palatal myoclonus have been successfully treated by botulinum toxin injections of the soft palatal tissues (Jamieson et al).

As was remarked, the pitch of tinnitus associated with a conductive hearing loss is of low frequency (median frequency of 490 Hz, with a range of 90 to 1450 Hz). That which accompanies sensorineural loss is higher (median frequency of 3900 Hz, with a range of 545 to 7500 Hz). This rule does not apply to Ménière disease, in which the tinnitus is usually described as a low-pitched whoosh, buzz, or roar (median frequency of 320 Hz, with a range of 90 to 900 Hz), thus resembling the tinnitus that accompanies a conductive rather than a sensorineural hearing loss (Nodar and Graham). The tinnitus of Ménière disease often fluctuates in intensity, like the hearing loss.

The mechanism of tonal tinnitus has not been established, although a number of theories have been postulated. One supposition attributes tinnitus to an overactivity or disinhibition of hair cells adjacent to a part of the cochlea that has been injured. Another postulates a decoupling of hair cells from the tectorial membrane. Yet another theory is based on the finding of an abnormal discharge pattern of afferent neurons, attributed to ephaptic transmission between nerve fibers that have been damaged by vascular compression (Møller). Relief of tinnitus in special cases has reportedly been achieved by vascular decompression of the eighth nerve (Jannetta).

For most forms of tinnitus, there is little effective treatment. Most patients become reconciled to its presence once the nature of the disorder is explained to them. It is possible to fit some patients with a special audiologic instrument, like a hearing aid, which masks the tinnitus by delivering a sound of like pitch and intensity. Also, a hearing aid that improves audition may suppress or diminish tinnitus. Drugs such as anticonvulsants and tocainide hydrochloride have not been helpful in our experience. If tinnitus is the basis of persistent complaints, one often discovers that the patient is anxious or depressed, in which case a careful medical history will reveal the other symptoms of the psychiatric illness. Treatment then must be directed to the psychiatric symptoms.

Tinnitus that is unilateral, pulsatile, or fluctuating and associated with vertigo must be investigated by appropriate neurologic and audiologic studies.

Other Disorders of Auditory Perception

On occasion, pontine lesions may be accompanied by complex auditory illusions, sometimes with the qualities of true hallucinations (*pontine auditory hallucinosis*). These consist of alternating musical tones, like an organ; a jumble of sound, like a symphony orchestra tuning up; or siren-like or buzzing sounds, like a swarm of bees. These auditory sense disturbances are more complex than neurosensory tinnitus but less formed than temporal lobe hallucinations. They are usually associated with impairment of hearing in one or both ears and other neurologic signs related to the pontine lesion. An unpleasant degree of hyperacusis in the contralateral ear has also been reported with upper pontine tegmental lesions. Brainstem evoked potentials reveal intact cochlear, auditory nerve, and cochlear nuclear responses. As in the case of peduncular visual hallucinosis, patients realize that the sounds are unreal, i.e., they have insight into their illusory nature (Cascino and Adams).

Another well-recognized but inexplicable type of auditory hallucinosis occurs in aged patients with long-standing neurosensory deafness. All day long, they hear songs, symphonies, choral music, or familiar or unfamiliar melodies interrupted only by other ambient noise, sleep, or when they are engaged in conversation. Our cases, like those reported by Hammeke and colleagues, have been neither depressed nor demented, and anticonvulsant and antipsychotic drugs have had no effect. Activation of the right auditory cortex on single photon emission tomography (SPECT) and magnetoencephalography has been reported in such a case by Kasai et al.

Complex auditory hallucinations may occur as part of temporal-lobe seizures, arising from a variety of temporal-lobe lesions. Conversely, seizures may be induced by musical sounds as well as by other auditory stimuli. These topics are discussed in Chaps. 16 and 22. Paracusis, a condition in which a sound, tune, or voice is repeated for several seconds, is also a cerebral auditory phenomenon similar in a sense to the visual phenomenon of palinopsia. The precise anatomy is unknown.

Causes of Middle Ear Deafness

The common causes are otosclerosis, otitis media, and trauma. Of the various types of progressive conductive deafness, otosclerosis is the most frequent, being the cause of about half the cases of bilateral (but not necessarily symmetrical) deafness that have their onset in early adult life (usually in the second or third decade). Otosclerosis is transmitted as an autosomal dominant trait with variable penetrance; pathologically, it is characterized by an overgrowth of labyrinthine capsular bone around the oval window, leading to progressive fixation of the stapes. The remarkable advances in micro-otologic surgery, designed to mobilize or replace the stapes and to reconstruct the ossicular chain, have greatly altered the prognosis in this disease; significant improvement in hearing can now be achieved in the majority of such patients.

The use of antibiotic drugs has markedly reduced the incidence of suppurative otitis media, both the acute and chronic forms, which in former years were common causes of conductive hearing loss. Repeated attacks of serous otitis media are still an important cause of this type of deafness.

Fractures of the temporal bone, particularly those in the long axis of the petrous pyramid, may damage middle ear structures; frequently there is bleeding into the middle ear as well, and a ruptured tympanic membrane. Transverse fractures through the petrous pyramid are more likely to damage both the cochlear-labyrinthine structures and the facial nerve. Other diseases of the temporal bone such as Paget disease, fibrous dysplasia, and osteopetrosis may impair hearing by compression of the cochlear nerve.

Causes of Sensorineural Deafness

This has many causes. Explosions or intense, sustained noise in certain industrial settings or from gun blasts or even rock music may result in a high-tone sensorineural hearing loss. Certain antimicrobial drugs (namely, the aminoglycoside group and vancomycin) damage cochlear hair cells and, after prolonged use, can result in severe hearing loss. If these drugs have been used to treat bacterial meningitis, it may be difficult to determine if the antibiotic or the infection is the cause. A variety of other commonly used drugs have been reported to be ototoxic (see Nadol). Quinine and acetylsalicylic acid may impair sensorineural function transiently. The common high-frequency sensorineural type of hearing loss in the aged (presbycusis) is probably due to neuronal degeneration, i.e., progressive loss of spiral ganglion neurons (Suga and Lindsay).

The cochlea may be damaged by rubella in the pregnant mother. Mumps, acute purulent meningitis (particularly from pneumococcus and Haemophilus), or chronic infection spreading from the middle to the inner ear may cause nerve deafness in childhood. The meningeal infection may spread along the cochlear aqueduct, a structure that connects the cerebrospinal fluid (CSF) space with the perilymph of the cochlea. The inner ear contains melanocytes, and their involvement in Vogt-Koyanagi-Harada disease adds dysacusis, tinnitus, and sensorineural deafness to the usual manifestations of vitiligo of the eyebrows, iridocyclitis, retinal depigmentation, and recurrent meningitis. Measles vaccination, *Mycoplasma pneumoniae* infection, and scarlet fever are sometimes associated with acute deafness with or without vestibular symptoms. It is uncertain whether the deafness in these cases is due to direct infection or represents an autoimmune reaction directed to the inner ear. Meningeal hemosiderosis, a rare process that results from repeated bouts of subarachnoid hemorrhage, also causes eighth nerve damage and deafness, presumably as a toxic effect of iron deposition in the meninges.

Of most concern to neurologists is the onset, in an adult, of sudden unilateral hearing loss without vertigo. Many patients can date the onset by noting that they have changed from their customary ear when using the telephone or that they need to turn their head in order to carry on a conversation. Little is known about the pathogenesis of this syndrome. A vascular causation (occlusion of the auditory artery or its cochlear branch or presumed arterial spasm in the course of migraine) has been postulated, on uncertain grounds. A few cases have complicated herpes zoster and mumps parotitis, but aside from these there is no proven relationship to the usual viral respiratory infections. *Episodic deafness in one ear without vertigo* proves in most instances to be *Ménière disease* (see further on). In a prospective study of 88 cases of acute sensorineural hearing loss, two-thirds recovered their hearing completely within a few days or a week or two (Mattox and Simmons). In the remaining patients, recovery was much slower and often incomplete; in this latter group, the hearing loss was predominantly for high tones and in some cases was associated with varying degrees of vertigo and hypoactive caloric responses.

The *sudden onset of bilateral sensorineural hearing loss* has been reported to follow cardiopulmonary bypass surgery and has been ascribed to microemboli. Less often such an event follows general anesthesia for nonotologic surgery (Evan et al); the pathogenesis is quite obscure. None of the currently popular therapeutic agents—such as histamine, calcium channel blockers, anticoagulants, carbogen inhalation, and steroids—seem to affect the outcome of sudden unilateral or bilateral deafness without vertigo.

Otologists have described a progressive sensorineural type of hearing loss as a late manifestation of congenital syphilis, allegedly occurring despite prior treatment with adequate doses of penicillin. It has been claimed that the long-term administration of steroids may be useful in such cases. The pathologic basis of the hearing loss has not been determined and the causal relationship to congenital syphilis remains to be established.

The *auditory* nerve may be involved by tumors of the cerebellopontine angle or by mycotic, lymphomatous, carcinomatous, tuberculous, or other types of chronic meningitis. Lymphomatous meningitis appears particularly liable to cause unilateral hearing loss, and we have seen several such cases in which no other cranial nerves were infiltrated. Of the solid tumors, the ones that involve the auditory nerve most frequently are neurofibromas (schwannomas), meningiomas, dermoids, and metastatic carcinoma. In central neurofibromatosis (type II) the involvement by acoustic neuromas is often bilateral. Unilateral deafness may also result from demyelinative plaques, infarction, or tumor involving the cochlear nerve fibers or nuclei in the brainstem. Rarely, deafness is the result of bilateral lesions of the temporal lobes (Chap. 22). The condition called pure word deafness is also due to temporal lobe disease; despite normal pure-tone perception and audiometry and normal brainstem auditory evoked potentials, spoken words cannot be understood. This condition is discussed in Chap. 23.

A large number of *genetically determined syndromes* that feature a neural or conductive type of deafness—some congenital and others having their onset in childhood or early adult life—have come to light (see articles by Konigsmark and by Proctor and Proctor). About 70 percent of cases of congenital deafness are inherited as an autosomal recessive trait. In most of the remainder, inheritance is autosomal dominant in type and in 2 percent it is sex-linked (Sank and Kallman). The most important advance in this field has been the identification in recessive nonsyndromic deafness of a mutation of the connexin-26 gene on chromosome 13. This mutation is found in half of recessive familial cases and, what is more striking, the same gene abnormality occurs in 37 percent of cases of apparently sporadic congenital deafness (Estivill et al, and Morell et al). The connexin protein is a component of gap junctions and the mutation is theorized to interfere with the recycling of potassium from the cochlear hair cells to the endolymph. There are few complete histopathologic studies of congenital and hereditary deafness. From available data, two groups can be recognized—aplasias and degenerations. Four types of inner ear aplasia have been described: (1) *Michel defect*, a complete absence of the otic capsule and eighth nerve; (2) *Mondini defect*, an incomplete development of the bony and membranous labyrinths and the spiral ganglion; (3) *Scheibe defect*, a membranous cochleosaccular dysplasia with atrophy of the vestibular and cochlear nerves; and (4) rare chromosomal aberrations (trisomies) characterized by abnormality of the end organ and absence of the spiral ganglion.

In addition to these more or less pure aplasias of the peripheral auditory system, cochleovestibular atrophies and degenerations occur as part of many other developmental and heredodegenerative syndromes. Konigsmark has classified these hereditary forms of deafness on the basis of associated defects caused by the same gene: malformations of the external ear; integumentary abnormalities such as hyperkeratosis, hyperplasia or scantiness of eyebrows, albinism, large hyperpigmented or hypopigmented areas, brittle twisted hair, and coniform and missing teeth; ocular abnormalities such as hypertelorism, severe myopia, optic atrophy, congenital and juvenile cataracts, and retinitis pigmentosa; neurologic abnormalities such as polyneuropathy and sensory ataxia (Refsum disease), progressive ophthalmoplegia and cerebellar ataxia, bilateral acoustic neuromas, photomyoclonic seizures, and mental deficiency; skeletal abnormalities; and renal, thyroid, or cardiac abnormalities. Deafness is also a feature of several mitochondrial disorders, particularly the Kearns-Sayre syndrome and occasionally the MELAS syndrome (page 1042). The Wolfram syndrome can have either a nuclear or mitochondrial genetic origin. This and other hereditary syndromes are summarized in Table 15-1, and the mitochondrial causes of deafness have recently been summarized by Chinnery et al. The

Table 15-1
Hereditary cochlear and cochleovestibular atrophies
Type I: Progressive hearing loss with involvement of kidneys, skin, or bones

Mode of inheritance	*Age of onset*	*Type of hearing loss*	*Associated abnormalities*	*Eponymic disease or syndrome*
Autosomal dominant	Childhood	Onset with loss of low, mid, or high frequencies, variably progressive	None	
Autosomal recessive	Congenital	Neural, rapidly progressive with failure of speech development	None	
Sex-linked recessive	Early childhood	Neural, rapidly progressive with speech impairment	None	
Autosomal dominant or recessive	Early adulthood	Neural, with tinnitus; progressive with unilateral or bilateral vestibular paresis	Episodic paroxysmal vertigo ("hereditary Ménière")	
Autosomal dominant	Congenital or first decade	Sensorineural; variable severity and progression	Progressive nephritis with uremia	Alport
Autosomal recessive	Childhood	Neural; progressive	Renal tubular acidosis	
Autosomal dominant	Childhood or adolescence	Sensorineural; slowly progressive	Nephrotic syndrome with amyloidosis; recurrent urticaria and fever	Muckle-Wells
Autosomal dominant (probable)	Childhood	Neural; progressive	Ichthyosis of extremities; prolinuria; glomerulosclerosis and uremia in some cases	Goyer
Autosomal dominant	Early adulthood	Neural; progressive	Congenital anhidrosis with absence of sweat and sebaceous glands	Helweg-Larsen
Autosomal dominant	Middle age	Conductive loss at onset, then sensorineural; progressive	Osteitis deformans	Paget
Autosomal dominant	Childhood	Conductive or neural or mixed; usually progressive	Craniometaphyseal dysplasia with sclerosis of base of skull and narrowing of foramina; sometimes optic atrophy and facial palsy	Pyle
Autosomal recessive	Childhood or adolescence	Neural or mixed; progressive	Osteosclerosis of skull and mandible with narrowing of foramina; facial paresis	Van Buchem
Autosomal dominant	Second or third decade	Conductive; sometimes neural or mixed	Osteogenesis imperfecta tarda	Ekman-Lobstein or Van der Hoeve

Table 15-1 *(Continued)*
Hereditary cochlear and cochleovestibular atrophies
Type II: Hereditary hearing loss with retinal disease

Mode of inheritance	*Age of onset*	*Type of hearing loss*	*Associated abnormalities*	*Eponymic disease or syndrome*
Autosomal recessive	Congenital	Sensorineural, with vestibular hypofunction	Progressive retinitis pigmentosa and ataxia beginning in late childhood or adolescence. Sometimes mental defect, cataracts, and glaucoma	Usher
Autosomal recessive	Early in second decade	Sensorineural; progressive	Retinitis pigmentosa, polyneuropathy, ataxia, mental deterioration	Refsum
Autosomal recessive	Infancy	Sensorineural; progressive	Retinal pigmentary degeneration, cataracts, diabetes mellitus	Alström
Autosomal recessive	Childhood	Sensorineural; variable progression	Dwarfism, senile appearance, variable mental retardation	Cockayne
Autosomal dominant	Childhood	Neural; variably progressive	Optic atrophy, ataxia, wasting of shoulder girdle and hand muscles, mental dullness, degeneration of optic nerves, posterior columns, spinocerebellar and corticospinal tracts	Sylvester
Autosomal recessive	Infancy	Neural; progressive with failure of speech development	Optic atrophy, polyneuropathy	Rosenberg-Chutorian
Autosomal recessive	First decade	Neural; progressive	Optic atrophy, juvenile diabetes mellitus	Turnbridge-Paley
Autosomal recessive	Infancy	Neural; progressive	Opticocochleodentate degeneration, progressive quadriparesis and mental deterioration	Nyssen-Van Bogaert
Sex-linked recessive	Congenital (ocular signs)	Onset of neural deafness in second and third decades; progressive	Retinal vascular and glial proliferation, progressive microphthalmia and mental retardation	Norrie
Autosomal recessive	Congenital	Neural	Tortuosity of retinal vessels and exudative retinitis, muscle wasting, immobile facies	Small

(continued)

Table 15-1 *(Continued)*
Hereditary cochlear and cochleovestibular atrophies
Type II: Hereditary hearing loss with retinal disease

Mode of inheritance	*Age of onset*	*Type of hearing loss*	*Associated abnormalities*	*Eponymic disease or syndrome*
Autosomal dominant	Third decade	Neural, progressive	Nephropathy, photomyoclonic seizures, mental deterioration, diabetes mellitus. Diffuse cerebral and cerebellar cortical neuronal loss	Hermann
Autosomal dominant	Childhood	Neural, slowly progressive	Myoclonus, progressive ataxia and dysarthria	May-White
Autosomal recessive	Congenital	Neural, with failure of speech development	Mild chronic myoclonic epilepsy	Latham-Munro
Autosomal dominant	Congenital	Neural, varying severity	Piebald trait and variable absence of pigmentation of skin; ataxia and mental retardation frequent	Telfer
Autosomal dominant	Second or third decade	Sensorineural	Hyperuricemia, decreased renal function, progressive ataxia and dysarthria, proximal muscle weakness and wasting	Rosenberg-Bergstrom
Autosomal recessive	Childhood	Progressive, severe	Progressive ataxia, hypotonia and dysarthria, mild mental retardation	Lichtenstein-Knorr
Autosomal recessive	Infancy or early childhood	Neural, slowly progressive	Progressive ataxia of gait, hypogonadism, mental deficiency, wasting and weakness of distal limb muscles	Richards-Rundle
Autosomal recessive	Childhood	Neural, rapidly progressive	Progressive cerebellar ataxia, mental deficiency, extensor plantar signs, pigmented spots on face and limbs; heart block	Jeune-Tommasi
Autosomal dominant	Second or third decade	Neural; progressive with tinnitus and loss of vestibular function	Bilateral acoustic neuromas	Gardner
Autosomal dominant	Childhood	Neural deafness, not in all cases	Progressive sensory radicular neuropathy	Denny-Brown
Autosomal dominant	First or second decade	Neural; progressive	Myopia, cataracts and retinitis pigmentosa; sensorimotor peripheral neuropathy; skin atrophy with ulceration; dental caries; kyphoscoliosis, cystic bone changes	Flynn-Aird

Table 15-1 *(Continued)*
Hereditary cochlear and cochleovestibular atrophies
Type II: Hereditary hearing loss with retinal disease

Mode of inheritance	*Age of onset*	*Type of hearing loss*	*Associated abnormalities*	*Eponymic disease or syndrome*
Autosomal recessive	Childhood	Neural, progressive	Proteinuria, progressive distal muscle wasting and weakness with claw hand and foot	Lemieux-Neemeh
? Dominant with incomplete penetrance	Congenital	Auditory imperception with failure of speech development	Indifference to pain	Osuntokun
Autosomal recessive	Childhood or adolescence	Progressive; neural with loss of vestibular function	Slowly progressive bulbar palsy	
Autosomal recessive	Childhood	Neurosensory	Optic atrophy Diabetes mellitus Diabetes insipidus	Wolfram
Mitochondrial (point mutations and deletions), maternal	Childhood	Neurosensory	Diabetes mellitus; progressive external ophthalmoplegia; myopathy	Kearns-Sayre, MELAS

Source: Adapted from Konigsmark (1975), with permission.

association of neurosensory deafness with degenerative neurologic disease is discussed further in Chaps 37 and 39.

Hysterical Deafness

It is possible to distinguish hysterical and feigned deafness from that due to structural disease in several ways. In the case of bilateral deafness, the distinction can be made by observing a blink (cochleo-orbicular reflex) or an alteration in skin sweating (psychogalvanic skin reflex) in response to loud sound. Unilateral hysterical deafness may be detected by an audiometer, with both ears connected, or by whispering into the bell of a stethoscope attached to the patient's ears, closing first one and then the other tube without the patient's knowledge. The elicitation of the first several waves of the brainstem auditory evoked potentials provides indisputable evidence that sounds are reaching the receptive auditory structures. It should be kept in mind that a brief episode of deafness with fully preserved consciousness may be caused by seizure activity in one temporal lobe (epileptic suppression of hearing).

DIZZINESS AND VERTIGO

Dizziness and other sensations of imbalance are, along with headache, back pain, and fatigue, the most frequent complaints among medical out-patients (Kroenke and Mangelsdorff). The significance of these complaints varies greatly. For the most part they are benign, but always there is the possibility that they signal the presence of an important neurologic disorder. Diagnosis of the underlying disease demands that the complaint of dizziness be analyzed correctly—the nature of the disturbance of function being determined first and then its anatomic localization. This classic approach to neurologic diagnosis is nowhere more valuable than in the patient whose main complaint is dizziness.

The term *dizziness* is applied by the patient to a number of different sensory experiences—a feeling of rotation or whirling as well as nonrotatory swaying, weakness, faintness, light-headedness, or unsteadiness. Blurring of vision, feelings of unreality, syncope, and even petit mal or other seizure phenomena may be called "dizzy spells." Hence a close questioning of the patient as to how he is using the term becomes a necessary first step in clinical study. Essentially, the physician must determine whether the symptoms have the specific qualities of vertigo—which in this chapter refers to all subjective and objective illusions of motion or position—or whether they are more properly categorized as nonrotatory giddiness or pseudovertigo. The distinction between these two groups of symptoms is elaborated after a brief discussion of the factors involved in the maintenance of equilibrium.

Physiologic Considerations

Several mechanisms are responsible for the maintenance of a balanced posture and for awareness of the position of the body in relation to its surroundings. Continuous afferent impulses from the eyes, labyrinths, muscles, and joints inform us of the position of different parts of the body. In response to these impulses, the adaptive movements necessary to maintain equilibrium are carried out. Normally we are unaware of these adjustments, since they operate largely at a reflex level. The most important of the afferent impulses are the following:

1. Visual impulses from the retinae and possibly proprioceptive ones from the ocular muscles, which enable us to judge the distance of objects from the body. This information is coordinated with sensory information from the labyrinths and neck (see below) to stabilize gaze during movements of the head and body.

2. Impulses from the labyrinths, which function as highly specialized spatial proprioceptors and register changes in the velocity of motion (either acceleration or deceleration) and position of the body. The cristae of the three semicircular canals sense angular acceleration of the head (side-to-side or rotary), and the maculae of the saccule and utricle sense linear acceleration and gravity. In each of these structures displacement of the sensory hair cells is the effective stimulus. In the semicircular canals, this is accomplished by movement of the endolymphatic fluid, which, in turn, is induced by rotation of the head and results in an illusion of rotation. In the utricle and saccule, the hairs are displaced in response to the force of gravity on the otoliths, giving rise to a sensation of linear displacement or tilt. In either case, the movement generates an electrical charge in the hair cells, causing depolarization of the nerve terminals and initiating impulses in the vestibular nerve, with the production of two main reflex responses: the vestibulo-ocular, which stabilizes the eyes, and the vestibulospinal, which stabilizes the position of the head and body.

3. Impulses from the proprioceptors of the joints and muscles, which are essential to all reflex, postural, and volitional movements. Those from the neck are of special importance in relating the position of the head to the rest of the body. The sense organs listed above are connected with the cerebellum and with certain ganglionic centers and pathways in the brainstem, particularly the vestibular nuclei, and, via the medial longitudinal fasciculi, with the ocular motor nuclei. These cerebellar and brainstem structures are the important coordinators of the sensory data and provide for postural adjustments and the maintenance of equilibrium. They are the basis of what is called the "space constancy mechanisms," whereby the perceptions of one's self (the body schema) and one's surroundings (the environmental schema) are matched. Conversely, any disease that disrupts these neural mechanisms may give rise to vertigo and disequilibrium. The interdependence of the two schemata (self and environment) is ascribed to the fact that the various sense organs—retinal, labyrinthive, and proprioceptive—are usually activated simultaneously by any body movement. Through a process of learning, we come to see objects as stationary while we are moving and moving objects as having motion when we are either moving or stationary. At times, especially when our own sensory information is incomplete, we mistake movement of our surroundings for movements of our own body. A well-known example is the feeling of movement that one experiences in a stationary train when a neighboring train is moving. In this frame of reference, the orientation of the body to its surroundings depends on the maintenance of an orderly relationship between the bodily schema and the schema of the surround; as a corollary, disorientation in space, or disequilibrium, occurs when this relationship is upset.

Yet another factor that influences equilibrium is the effect of aging (page 643). Old people may lose their balance on extending the neck, and their peripheral sensory afferents are often impaired, as are the protective postural mechanisms, making falls more frequent. A destructive lesion of one or both labyrinths may leave an elderly person permanently unbalanced, while a younger person compensates for the loss.

Clinical Characteristics of Vertigo and Giddiness (Pseudovertigo)

Vertigo A careful history and physical examination usually afford the basis for separating true vertigo from the dizziness of the anxious patient and from the other types of pseudovertigo. The recognition of vertigo is not difficult when the patient states that objects in the environment spun around or moved rhythmically in one direction or that he had a sensation of whirling of the head and body. (A distinction is sometimes drawn between subjective vertigo, meaning a sense of turning of one's body, and objective vertigo, an illusion of movement of the environment, but its significance is doubtful.) Often, however, the patient is not so explicit.

The feeling may be described as a to-and-fro or up-and-down movement of the body, usually of the head, or the patient may compare the feeling to that imparted by the pitch and roll of a ship. Or the floor or walls may seem to tilt or to sink or rise up. In walking, the patient may have felt unsteady and veered to one side. Or he may have had a sensation of leaning or being pulled to the ground or to one side or another (a static tilt), as though being drawn by a strong magnet. This feeling of impulsion, or pulsion, is particularly characteristic of vertigo. Oscillopsia, an illusory movement of the environment, is another effect of vestibular disorder, especially if induced by movement of the head. Some observant patients may actually note a rhythmic movement of the environment due to nystagmus.

Some patients may be able to identify their symptoms only when asked to compare them with the feeling of movement they experience when they come to a halt after rapid rotation. If the patient is unobservant or imprecise in his descriptions, a helpful tactic is to provoke a number of dissimilar sensations by rotating him rapidly, irrigating his ears with warm and cold water, and then asking him to stoop for a minute and straighten up; having him stand relaxed for 3 min and checking his blood pressure for orthostatic effect; and having him hyperventilate for 3 min. Should the patient be unable to distinguish among these several types of induced dizziness or to ascertain the similarity of one of the types to his own condition, the history is probably too inaccurate for purposes of diagnosis.

When the patient's symptoms are mild or poorly described, small items of the history—a disinclination to stoop or walk during an attack; a tendency to list to one side; an aggravation of symptoms by turning over in bed or closing his eyes; a sense of imbalance when making a quick turn on foot or in a car; and a preference for one position of the body or head—help to identify them as vertigo. At the other end of the scale are attacks of such abruptness and severity as to virtually throw the patient to the ground. Independently occurring vertiginous attacks of the usual variety mark these falling episodes as part of Ménière disease (see further on).

All but the mildest forms of vertigo are accompanied by some degree of nausea, vomiting, pallor, perspiration, and some difficulty with walking. The patient may simply be disinclined to walk or walk unsteadily and veer to one side, or he may be unable to walk at all if the vertigo is intense. Forced to lie down, the patient realizes that one position, usually on one side with his eyes closed, reduces the vertigo and nausea, and that the slightest motion of the head aggravates them. One form of vertigo, the benign positional vertigo of Bárány (see further on), occurs only with the repositioning that accompanies lying down, sitting up, or turning. The source of the gait ataxia associated with vertigo (vertiginous ataxia) is recognized as being "in the head," not in the control of the legs and trunk. It is noteworthy that the coordination of individual movements of the limbs is not impaired in these circumstances—a point of difference from most instances of cerebellar disease. There may be headache, generalized or in the region of the offending ear. Loss of consciousness as part of a vertiginous attack nearly always signifies another type of disorder (seizure or faint).

Pseudovertigo To be distinguished from true vertigo are symptoms of *giddiness and other types of pseudovertigo*. The patient, who may complain only of dizziness, will, on closer questioning, describe his symptoms as a feeling of swaying, light-headednes, a swimming sensation, or, less often, a feeling of uncertainty or imbalance, "walking on air," faintness, or some other unnatural sensation in the head. These sensory experiences are particularly common in states characterized by anxiety or panic attacks—namely, anxiety neurosis, hysteria, and depression. They are in part reproduced by hyperventilation, and then it may be appreciated that varying degrees of apprehension, palpitation, breathlessness, trembling, and sweating are concurrent.

This constellation of nonvertiginous symptoms has been loosely referred to as "functional," "psychic," psychogenic," and "psychiatric dizziness." We agree with Furman and Jacobs that the term *psychiatric dizziness*, if used at all, should be restricted to dizziness that occurs as part of a recognized psychiatric syndrome, notably anxiety disorder. There seems to be little point in dignifying the nonvertiginous symptoms with separate designations based on the settings in which they commonly occur ("supermarket syndrome," "motorist disorientation syndrome," "phobic postural vertigo," "street neurosis," etc.). Furman and Jacobs have related psychiatric dizziness to minor degrees of vestibular dysfunction, but we have not found it possible to determine if there is a genuine labyrinthine disorder in these patients.

Oculomotor disorders, such as ophthalmoplegia with diplopia of abrupt onset, may be a source of spatial disorientation and brief sensations of vertigo, mild nausea, and staggering. These symptoms are maximal when the patient looks in the direction of action of the paralyzed muscle; it is attributable to the receipt of two conflicting visual images. Some normal persons may experience such symptoms for brief periods when first adjusting to bifocal glasses. In a peculiar symptom called the *Tullio phenomenon*, a loud sound or, rarely, yawning produces a brief sensation of vertigo. Some patients with this symptom are found to have an absence or thinning of the bony roof of the superior semicircular canal. Occasionally, this symptom is reported by patients with Ménière disease.

Other pseudovertiginous symptoms are less definite. In severe anemic states, particularly pernicious anemia, and in aortic stenosis, easy fatigability and languor may be attended by light-headedness, related particularly to postural change and exertion. In the emphysematous patient, physical effort may be associated with weakness and peculiar cephalic sensations, and violent paroxysms of coughing may lead to giddiness and even fainting (tussive syncope) because of impaired venous return to the heart. The dizziness that often accompanies hypertension is difficult to evaluate; sometimes it is an expression of anxiety, or it may conceivably be due to an unstable adjustment of cerebral blood flow. Postural dizziness is another state in which unstable vasomotor reflexes prevent a constant cerebral circulation; it is frequent in persons with primary orthostatic hypotension and in those taking antihypertensive drugs, and in patients with a polyneuropathy that has an autonomic component. Such persons, on rising abruptly from a recumbent or sitting position, experience a swaying type of dizziness, dimming of vision, and spots before the eyes that last for several seconds. The patient is forced to stand still and steady himself by holding onto a nearby object. Occasionally, a syncopal attack may occur at this time (see Chap. 18). Hypoglycemia gives rise to another form of pseudovertigo, marked by a sense of hunger and attended by trembling, sweating, and other autonomic symptoms. Drug intoxication—particularly with alcohol, sedatives, and anticonvulsants—may induce a nonspecific dizziness and, at advanced stages of intoxication, true vertigo.

In practice, it is usually not difficult to separate these types of pseudovertigo from true vertigo, for there is none of the feeling of rotation, impulsion, up-and-down movement, oscillopsia, or other disturbance of motion so characteristic of the latter. Lacking also are the ancillary symptoms of true vertigo—namely, nausea, vomiting, tinnitus and deafness, staggering, and the relief obtained by sitting or lying still.

The Neurologic and Otologic Causes of Vertigo

The fact that vertigo may constitute the aura of an epileptic seizure supports the view that this symptom may have a cerebrocortical origin. Indeed, electrical stimulation of the cerebral cortex in an unanesthetized patient, either of the posterolateral aspects of the temporal lobe or the inferior parietal lobule adjacent to the sylvian fissure, may evoke intense vertigo (page 338). The occurrence of vertigo as the initial symptom of a seizure is infrequent, however. In such cases, a sensation of movement—either of the body away from the side of the lesion or of the environment in the opposite direction—lasts for a few seconds before being submerged in other seizure activity. *Vertiginous epilepsy* of this type should be differentiated from *vestibulogenic seizures*, in which an excessive vestibular discharge serves as the stimulus for a seizure. The latter is a rare form of reflex epilepsy, in which tests that induce vertigo may provoke the seizure.

Whether lesions of the cerebellum produce vertigo seems to depend on which part of this structure is involved. Large, destructive processes in the cerebellar hemispheres and vermis may cause no vertigo. However, strokes in the territory of the medial branch of the posterior inferior cerebellar artery (which arises distal to the branches to the medulla and therefore does not involve the lateral medulla) may cause intense vertigo that is *indistinguishable from that due to labyrinthine disorder*. In two such pathologically studied cases, a large zone of infarction extended to the midline and involved the flocculonodular lobe (Duncan et al). Falling, in these cases, was toward the side of the lesion; nystagmus was present on gaze to each side but was more prominent on gaze to the side of the infarct. These findings have been confirmed by CT scanning and MRI (Amarenco et al). Labyrinthine disease, on the other hand, causes predominantly unidirectional nystagmus to the side opposite the impaired labyrinth and swaying or falling toward the involved side—i,e., the direction of the nystagmus is opposite to that of the falling and past pointing (the latter referring to overshooting a target with eyes closed, as originally described by Bárány). Early in the course of an acute attack of vertigo, when it may be difficult to assess the gait and the quality of nystagmus, it is necessary to exclude a cerebellar infarct or hemorrhage by use of imaging procedures.

Biemond and DeJong have described a kind of nystagmus and vertigo originating in the upper cervical roots and the muscles and ligaments that they innervate (so-called cervical vertigo). Spasm of the cervical muscles, trauma to the neck, and irritation of the upper cervical sensory roots are said to produce asymmetrical spinovestibular stimulation and thus to evoke nystagmus, prolonged vertigo, and disequilibrium. Downbeat nystagmus, vertigo, and postural instability have been observed with paramedian lesions at the craniocervical junction, and upbeat nystagmus with oscillopsia and vertigo has been traced to two separate brainstem lesions—one in the perihypoglossal nuclei and the other in the pontomesencephalic tegmentum (Brandt). Cervical vertigo has also been attributed to circulatory insufficiency in the vertebrobasilar territory. Toole and Tucker demonstrated a reduced flow through these vessels (in cadavers) when the head was rotated or hyperextended. In our view, the existence of "cervical vertigo" and nystagmus, or at least these interpretations of it, are still open to question. Occasionally, vertigo lasting a few minutes occurs as a prelude to a basilar migraine headache (Grad and Baloh).

In summary, although lesions of the cerebral cortex, eyes, cerebellum, and perhaps the cervical muscles may give rise to vertigo, they are not common sources of vertigo, and vertigo is rarely the dominant manifestation of disease in these parts. For all practical purposes, vertigo indicates a disorder of the vestibular end organs, the vestibular division of the eighth nerve, or the vestibular nuclei in the brainstem and their immediate connections. The clinical problem resolves itself into deciding which portion of the labyrinthine-vestibular apparatus is primarily involved. Usually this decision can be made on the basis of the form of the vertiginous attack, on the nature of the ancillary symptoms and signs, and tests of labyrinthine function. The latter are described below, followed by a description of the common labyrinthine-vestibular syndromes.

Tests of Labyrinthine Function

Irrigation of the ear canal alternately with cold and warm water (caloric, or oculovestibular, testing) may be used to disclose an impairment or loss of thermally induced nystagmus on the involved side. In caloric testing, the patient's head is tilted forward 30° from the horizontal; this brings the horizontal semicircular canal into a vertical plane, the position of maximal sensitivity of this canal to thermal stimuli. Each external auditory canal is irrigated for 30 s, first with water at 30°C and then at 44°C (7°C below and above body temperature), with a pause of at least 5 min between each irrigation. In normal persons, cold water induces a slight tonic deviation of the eyes to the side being irrigated, followed, after a latent period of about 20 s, by nystagmus to the opposite side (direction of the fast phase). Warm water induces nystagmus to the irrigated side. In normal subjects, the nystagmus usually persists for 90 to 120 s, although the range is considerably larger. Nausea and symptoms of excessive reflex vagal activity may occur in sensitive individuals.

Simultaneous irrigation of both canals with cold water causes a tonic downward deviation of the eyes, with nystagmus (quick component) upward. Bilateral irrigation with warm water yields a tonic upward movement and nystagmus in the opposite direction.

Caloric testing, as described above, will reliably answer whether the vestibular end organs react, and comparison of the responses from the two ears will indicate which one is paretic. The presence of "directional preponderance" can be determined (if the two stimuli that induce nystagmus to one side provoke a stronger reaction than the two stimuli that induce nystagmus to the other side) and is a means of quantifying the caloric responses. Galvanic stimulation of the labyrinths offers no particular advantage over caloric stimulation.

Vestibular (labyrinthine) stimulation can also be produced by rotating the patient in a Bárány chair or any type of swivel chair. The patient's eyes are kept closed or blindfolded or defocused with Frenzel lenses during rotation to avoid the effects of optokinetic nystagmus. Electronystagmography provides a more refined method of detecting disordered labyrinthine function.

Ménière Disease and Other Forms of Labyrinthine Vertigo

Labyrinthine disease is the most common cause of true vertigo. The classic variety, Ménière disease, is characterized by recurrent attacks of vertigo associated with fluctuating tinnitus and deafness. One or the other of the latter symptoms—rarely both—may be absent during the initial attacks of vertigo, but invariably they assert themselves as the disease progresses and increase in severity during an acute attack. Ménière disease affects the sexes about equally and has its onset most frequently in the fifth decade of life, although it may begin earlier or later. Cases of Ménière disease are usually sporadic, but hereditary forms, both autosomal dominant and recessive, have been described (see reviews by Konigsmark). The main pathologic changes consist of an increase in the volume of endolymph and distention of the endolymphatic system (endolymphatic hydrops). It has been speculated that the paroxysmal attacks of vertigo are related to ruptures of the membranous labyrinth and a dumping of potassium-containing endolymph into the perilymph, changes that have a paralyzing effect on vestibular nerve fibers and lead to degeneration of the delicate cochlear hair cells (Friedmann).

In typical *Ménière disease* the attacks of vertigo are characteristically abrupt and last for several minutes to an hour or longer. The vertigo is unmistakably whirling or rotational in type and usually so severe that the patient cannot stand or walk. Varying degrees of nausea and vomiting, low-pitched tinnitus, a feeling of fullness in the ear, and a diminution in hearing are practically always associated. Nystagmus is present during the acute attack; it is horizontal in type, usually with a rotary component and with the slow phase to the side of the affected ear. On attempting to touch a target with the eyes closed, there is past pointing as well as a tendency to fall toward the affected ear. The patient prefers to lie with the faulty ear uppermost and is disinclined to look toward the normal side, which exaggerates the nystagmus and dizziness. As the attack subsides, hearing improves, as does the sensation of fullness in the ear; with further attacks, however, there is a progressive increase of deafness.

The attacks vary considerably in frequency and severity. They may recur several times weekly for many weeks on end, or there may be remissions of several years' duration. Frequently recurring attacks may give rise to a mild chronic state of disequilibrium and a reluctance to move the head or to turn quickly. With milder forms of the disease, the patient may complain more of head discomfort and of difficulty in concentrating than of vertigo and may be considered neurotic. Symptoms of anxiety are common in patients with Ménière disease, particularly in those who suffer frequent severe attacks.

As indicated earlier a small proportion of patients with Ménière disease experience sudden, violent falling attacks. These episodes have been referred to by the quaint name of "otolithic catastrophe of Tumarkin", who attributed them, with little evidence, to deformation of the otolithic membrane of the utricle and saccule. Patients characteristically describe a sensation of being pushed or knocked to the ground without warning, or there may be a sudden movement or tilt of the environment just before the fall. Consciousness is not lost, and vertigo of the usual type and its accompaniments are not part of the falling attack, although some patients become aware of these symptoms after falling. The attacks may occur early or late in the course of the disease. Typically, several attacks occur over a period of a year or less and remit spontaneously (Baloh et al). An initial attack must be distinguished from other types of drop attacks (see page 399), but the occurrence of the more typical vertiginous attacks of Ménière disease, with deafness and tinnitus, clarifies the diagnosis.

The hearing loss in Ménière disease usually precedes the first attack of vertigo, but it may appear later. Episodic deafness without vertigo has been called *cochlear Ménière syndrome*. As already mentioned, with recurrent attacks, there is a saltatory progressive unilateral hearing loss (in most series only 10 percent of cases involve both ears, but Baloh places the figure closer to 30 percent). Early in the disease, deafness affects mainly the low tones and fluctuates in severity. Without the fluctuations in pure-tone audiometric thresholds, the diagnosis is uncertain. Later the fluctuations cease and high tones are affected. Speech discrimination is relatively preserved. The attacks of vertigo usually cease when the hearing loss is complete. Audiometry reveals a sensorineural type of deafness, with air and bone conduction equally depressed. Provided that deafness is not complete, loudness recruitment can be demonstrated in the involved ear (see above). In general, the association of vertigo and deafness signifies a disease process of the end organ or eighth nerve. The precise locus of the disease is determined by tests of labyrinthine and auditory function described above and by findings, on neurologic examination and imaging studies, that implicate structures adjacent to the eighth cranial nerve.

During an acute attack of Ménière disease, rest in bed is the most effective treatment, since the patient can usually find a position in which vertigo is minimal. The antihistaminic agents cyclizine (Marezine), meclizine (Bonine, Antivert), or transdermal scopolamine are useful in the more protracted cases. Promethazine (Phenergan) helps to suppress the nausea and vomiting, as does trimethobenzamide (Tigan), given in 200-mg suppositories. For many years a low-salt diet in combination with ammonium chloride, and diuretics had been used in the treatment of Ménière disease, but the value of this regimen has never been established. The same is true for dehydrating agents such as oral glycerol and the more recently popular calcium channel blockers. Mild sedative drugs may help the anxious patient between attacks. If the attacks are very frequent and disabling, permanent relief can be obtained by surgical means. Destruction of the labyrinth should be considered only in patients with strictly unilateral disease and complete or nearly complete loss of hearing. In patients with bilateral disease or significant retention of hearing, the vestibular portion of the eighth nerve can be sectioned. An endolymphatic-subarachnoid shunt is the operation favored by some surgeons, and selective destruction of the vestibule by a cryogenic probe or transtympanic injection of streptomycin is favored by others. Decompression of the eighth cranial nerve, by separating it from an adjacent vessel, as suggested by Janetta, is still a controversial measure and probably better suited to the treatment of sustained and disabling but unexplained vertigo, as discussed further on, than to the treatment of classic Ménierè disease. The decision to undertake any surgical procedure must be tempered by the fact that a majority of the patients, who are middle-aged, stabilize spontaneously in a few years.

Benign Positional Vertigo (of Bárány)

This disorder of labyrinthine function is more frequent than Ménière disease. It is characterized by *paroxysmal vertigo* and nystagmus that occur *only with the assumption of certain critical positions of the head*, particularly lying down or rolling over in bed, bending over and straightening up, and tilting the head backward. Brandt prefers the descriptive adjective positioning to positional, insofar as this type of vertigo is induced not by a particular head position relative to the gravitational vector, but only by rapid changes in head position. This disorder was first described by Bárány; Dix and Hallpike were responsible for its further characterization and emphasized its benign nature. Individual episodes last for less than a minute, but these may recur periodically for several days or for many months—rarely for years. As a rule, examination discloses no abnormalities of hearing or other identifiable lesions in the ear or elsewhere. However, if patients are subjected to careful bithermal caloric testing, a considerable number will show mild abnormalities of vestibular function (Baloh et al).

The *diagnosis* of this disorder is settled at the bedside by quickly moving the patient from the sitting position to recumbency, with the head tilted 30 to 40 degrees over the end of the table and 30 to 45 degrees to one side, as originally described by Dix and Hallpike. After a latency of a few seconds, this maneuver provokes a paroxysm of vertigo; the patient may become frightened and grasp the examiner or the table or struggle to sit up. The vertigo is accompanied by oscillopsia and nystagmus, predominantly torsional in type, with the upper pole of the eye beating toward the floor. Electronystagmography discloses both a vertical and horizontal nystagmus, with the rapid components in the direction of the forehead and away from the floor, respectively (Baloh et al). The vertigo and nystagmus last no more than 30 to 40 s and usually less than 15 s. *Changing from a recumbent to a sitting position often reverses the direction of vertigo and nystagmus* (position changing nystagmus). With repetition of the maneuver, vertigo and nystagmus become less apparent, and after three or four trials, they can no longer be elicited (referred to as "fatigue"); they can be reproduced in their original severity only after a protracted period of rest. The head-hanging maneuver does not always evoke vertigo and nystagmus in patients whose histories are otherwise consistent with the diagnosis of benign paroxysmal vertigo—for which reason Froehling and co-workers do not insist upon it for diagnosis.

A common variant of benign positional vertigo is one in which sudden turning induces vertigo for a few seconds. Such attacks of vertigo may come and go for years, particularly in the elderly, and require no treatment. At the other end of the scale is the rare patient with positional vertigo of such persistence and severity as to require surgical intervention.

Baloh and colleagues, in their study of 240 cases of benign positional vertigo, found that 17 percent had their onset within several days or weeks after cerebral trauma and 15 percent after presumed viral neurolabyrinthitis. The significance of these preceding events is unclear, insofar as they did not appear to influence the clinical symptoms or course of the otologic disorder. It should be pointed out that sudden changes in position, particularly of the head, may induce vertigo and nystagmus or cause a worsening of these symptoms in patients with all types of vestibular-labyrinthine disease, including Ménière disease and the types associated with vertebral-basilar stroke, trauma, and posterior fossa tumors. However, only if the paroxysm has the special characteristics noted above—namely, latency of onset, brevity, reversal of direction of nystagmus on sitting up, fatigability with repetition of the test, and the presence of distressing subjective symptoms of vertigo or its recurrence for months or years without other symptoms—can it be regarded as "benign paroxysmal" in type.

Shuknecht originally proposed that benign positional vertigo was due to cupulolithiasis, in which otolithic crystals become detached and attach themselves to the cupula of the posterior semicircular canal. It is now generally believed that the debris, probably detached from the otolith, forms a free-floating clot in the endolymph of the canal (canalolithiasis), and as such gravitates to the most dependent part of the canal during changes in the position of the head (see Brandt et al). The clot is thought to act as a plunger, inducing push-and-pull forces on the cupula and triggering an attack of vertigo. Based on this presumed mechanism, a canalith repositioning maneuver has been devised (Semont et al; Epley), allowing the clot to gravitate out of the semicircular canal into the utricle where it will not induce a current during angular acceleration.

The first part of the canalith repositioning maneuver (Fig. 15-5) is identical to the diagnostic Hallpike maneuver, outlined above. With the patient in the head-hanging position that causes symptoms, the head is turned in a series of three steps, each separated by about 20 s: first the head is turned 45 to 60 degrees toward the opposite ear; the patient is then turned onto his side and the head turned an additional 45 degrees, until the head is parallel to the ground; then the head is turned once more until it nearly faces the floor. After 20 s, the patient is returned to the upright position, and must remain at least 45 degrees upright for the next 24 h. Often a single sequence suffices to terminate a period of positional vertigo.

It is important to reiterate that in some patients with positional vertigo, the disorder is neither benign nor paroxysmal. Jannetta and colleagues have described a group of patients in whom symptoms of vertigo and disequilibrium were almost constant (even in the upright position) and disabling and unresponsive to habituation and other medical therapy (*disabling positional vertigo*). They attributed this disorder to cross-compression of the root entry zone of the eighth cranial nerve by an adjacent blood vessel and have reported that decompression of the nerve provides lasting relief of symptoms.

Toxic and Idiopathic Bilateral Vestibulopathy

The common and serious ototoxic effects of the aminoglycoside antibiotics have already been mentioned—both upon the cochlear hair cells, with loss of hearing (page 310), and, often independently, upon the vestibular labyrinth. Prolonged exposure to these agents can produce a bilateral vestibulopathy without vertigo. Instead, there tends to be a disequilibrium associated with oscillopsia (page 292). The symptoms are especially troublesome when the patient moves. Often the disequilibrium is not discovered until a bedfast patient tries to walk.

Less well appreciated is the occurrence of a slowly progressive vestibulopathy for which no cause can be discerned. The latter disorder affects men and women alike, with onset in middle or late adult life. The main abnormalities are unsteadiness of gait, which is worse in the dark or with eyes closed, and oscillopsia, which occurs with head movements and is particularly noticeable when walking. Vertigo and hearing loss are notably absent, as are other neurologic abnormalities. The bilateral vestibular loss can be documented with caloric and rotational testing. Baloh and colleagues, in a report of 22 patients with bilateral idiopathic vestibulopathy, found that a significant proportion (9 of 22 cases) had a prior history of prolonged episodes of vertigo consistent with the diagnosis of bilateral sequential vestibular neuronitis.

Vestibular Neuronitis (Labyrinthitis)

This is the term applied originally by Dix and Hallpike to a distinctive disturbance of vestibular function, characterized clinically by a paroxysmal and usually a single attack of vertigo and by a conspicuous absence of tinnitus and deafness.

This disorder occurs mainly in young to middle-aged adults (children and older individuals may be affected), without preference for either sex. The patient frequently gives a history of an antecedent upper respiratory infection of nonspecific type. Usually the onset of vertigo is abrupt, although some patients describe a prodromal period of several hours or days in which they felt "top-heavy" or "off balance." The vertigo is severe as a rule and is associated with nausea, vomiting, and the need to remain immobile. Examination discloses vestibular paresis on one side, i.e., an absent or diminished response to caloric stimulation of the horizontal semicircular canal. Halmagyi and Cremer, whose review of the assessment of dizziness is recommended, favor the *rapid head impulse test* as the best means of demonstrating absent function of one lateral semicircular canal. This test is essentially a method of comparing the vestibulo-ocular reflex (VOR) between the two sides. It consists of performing a quick 10 degree rotation of the patient's head while he is fixating a distant target. The patient with vestibular neuronitis is unable to maintain fixation when the head is turned toward the affected side and must make a saccade to stay on target. The test does not elicit a corrective eye movement in cases of cerebellar infarction. Nystagmus (quick component) and sense of body motion are to the opposite side, whereas falling and past pointing are to the side of the lesion. In some patients the caloric responses are abnormal bilaterally, and in some the vertigo may recur, affecting the same or the other ear. Auditory function is normal.

Vestibular neuronitis is a benign disorder. The severe vertigo and associated symptoms subside in a matter of several days, but lesser degrees of these symptoms, made worse by rapid movements of the head, may persist for several weeks or months. The caloric responses are gradually restored to normal as well. In

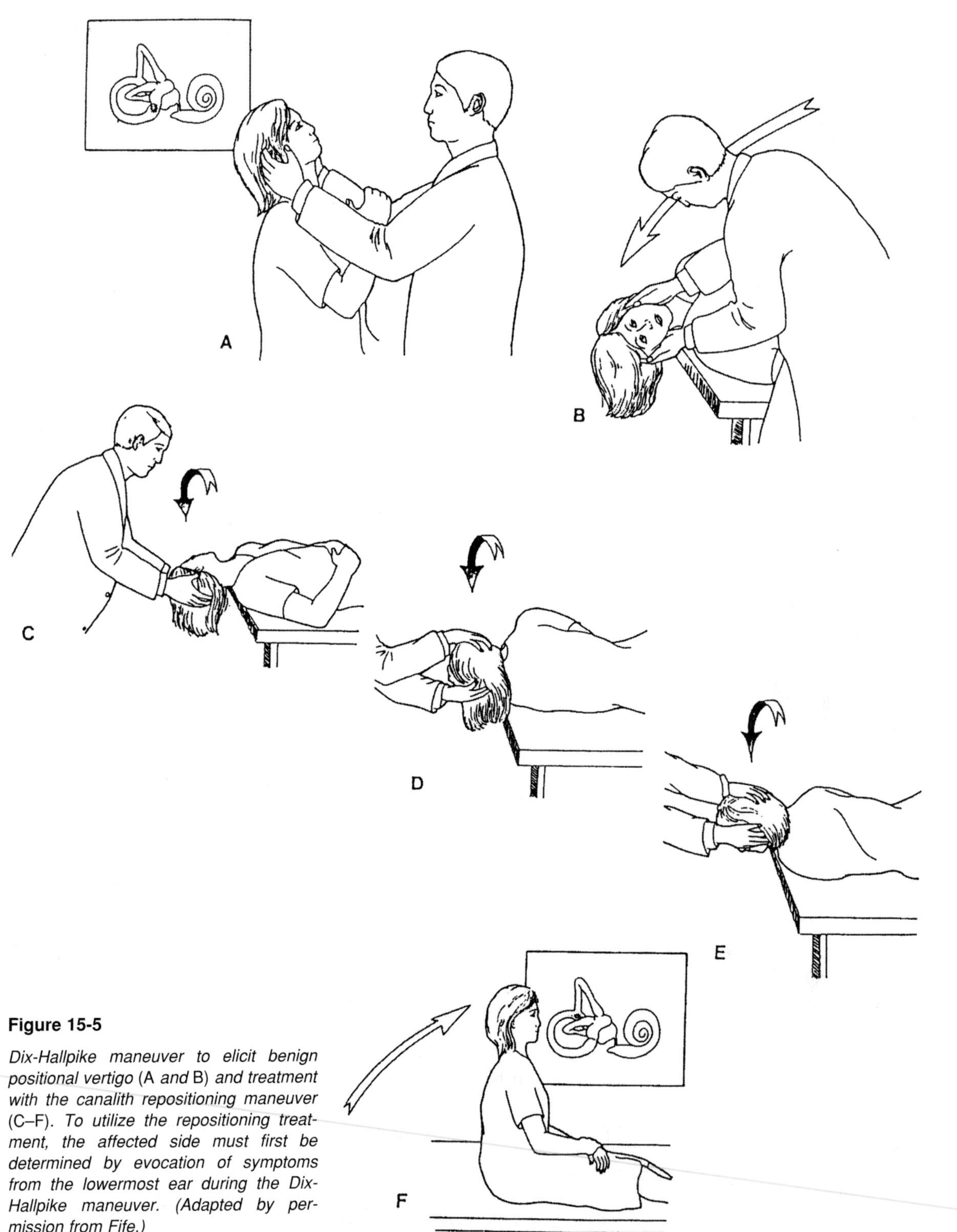

Figure 15-5

Dix-Hallpike maneuver to elicit benign positional vertigo (A *and* B) *and treatment with the canalith repositioning maneuver* (C–F). *To utilize the repositioning treatment, the affected side must first be determined by evocation of symptoms from the lowermost ear during the Dix-Hallpike maneuver. (Adapted by permission from Fife.)*

some patients there has been a recurrence months or years later.

The portion of the vestibular pathway that is primarily affected in this disease is thought to be the superior part of the vestibular nerve trunk, which was observed to show degenerative changes by Shuknecht and Kitamura. Earlier, Dix and Hallpike had reasoned that the lesion was located central to the labyrinth, since hearing is spared and vestibular function usually returns to normal. They used the term vestibular neuronitis because of the uncertainty of more precise localization within the peripheral vestibular pathway. The cause is uncertain. It may be a viral infection, analogous to Bell's palsy, and from time to time enhancement of the eighth nerve or the membranous labyrinth is seen after gadolinium administration on MRI. For want of more specific etiologic or pathologic data, many neurologists prefer the term *vestibular neuropathy* or *neuritis*, or *acute unilateral peripheral vestibulopathy*. It is likely that many of the conditions described under the terms *epidemic vertigo, epidemic labyrinthitis,* and *acute labyrinthitis* or *neurolabyrinthitis*. These many names attest to the fact that the distinction between vestibular neuronitis and labyrinthitis has never been clarified; some otolaryngologists consider labyrinthitis to be a vestibular neuronitis with mild hearing loss. Certainly herpes zoster oticus causes this syndrome (as well as affecting the seventh nerve (Ramsay Hunt syndrome; page 799).

During the acute stage, antihistamine drugs, phenergan, and scopolamine may be helpful in reducing the symptoms.

Other Causes of Vertigo of Vestibular Nerve Origin

This may occur with diseases that involve the nerve in the petrous bone or the cerebellopontine angle. Aside from vestibular neuronitis, discussed above, the most common cause of vertigo of eighth nerve origin is probably an acoustic neuroma. Vertigo is rarely the initial symptom; the usual sequence is deafness affecting the high-frequency tones initially, followed some months or years later by chronic vertigo and impaired caloric responses, and then by additional cranial nerve palsies (involving the seventh, fifth, and tenth nerves), ipsilateral ataxia of limbs, and headache (see page 709). Variations in the sequence of development of symptoms are frequent, however. In the diagnosis of acoustic neuroma, MRI and BAER are the most important ancillary examinations. Others include the special audiologic tests that have been described on page 307 and serve to separate lesions of the eighth nerve from those of the cochlea (absence of loudness recruitment, low SiSi scores, poor speech discrimination, pronounced tone decay, and type III or IV Békésy audiograms).

As mentioned earlier, a disabling positional vertigo may be due to compression of the eighth nerve by an abnormal vessel (Jannetta et al).

A clinical syndrome of unknown nature consists of a single abrupt attack of severe vertigo, nausea, and vomiting without tinnitus or hearing loss but with permanent ablation of labyrinthine function on one side. It has been suggested that this syndrome is due to occlusion of the labyrinthine division of the internal auditory artery, but so far anatomic confirmation of this idea has not been obtained. Labyrinthine hemorrhage has been demonstrated by MRI in some of these patients.

A particular form of paroxysmal vertigo occurs in childhood. The attacks occur in a setting of good health and are of sudden onset and brief duration. Pallor, sweating, and immobility are prominent manifestations; occasionally vomiting and nystagmus occur. No relation to posture or movement has been observed. The attacks are recurrent but tend to cease spontaneously after a period of several months or years. The outstanding abnormality is demonstrated by caloric testing, which shows impairment or loss of vestibular function, bilateral or unilateral, frequently persisting after the attacks have ceased. Cochlear function is unimpaired. The pathologic basis of this disorder has not been determined and a suggested connection with migraine is tenuous. The special case of basilar artery migraine is discussed below.

Cogan has described a not infrequent syndrome in young adults in which a *nonsyphilitic interstitial keratitis* is associated with vertigo, tinnitus, nystagmus, and rapidly progressive deafness. The prognosis for vision is good, but the deafness and loss of vestibular function are usually permanent. The cause and pathogenesis of this syndrome are unknown, although approximately half of the patients later develop aortic insufficiency or a systemic vasculitis that resembles polyarteritis nodosa. These vascular complications proved fatal in 7 of 78 cases reviewed by Vollertsen and colleagues.

There are many other causes of aural vertigo, such as purulent labyrinthitis complicating mastoiditis or meningitis; serous labyrinthitis due to infection of the middle ear; "toxic labyrinthitis" due to intoxication with alcohol, quinine, or salicylates; motion sickness; and hemorrhage into the inner ear. Bárány was the first to draw attention to the nystagmus and positional vertigo, worse on closing the eyes, that occurs at a certain level of intoxication with alcohol and lasts only a few hours. Such an episode of alcohol-induced vertigo tends to last longer than a vertiginous attack of Ménière disease, but in other respects the symptoms are similar.

Vertigo with varying degrees of spontaneous or positional nystagmus and reduced vestibular responses is a frequent complication of *head trauma*. Vertigo, often of the nonrotatory, to-and-fro type, may follow cerebral concussion or whiplash injury, in which the head has not been impacted. Brandt has attributed this vertigo to a loosening or dislodgement of the otoconia in the otoliths. The vertigo in these circumstances usually improves in a few days or weeks and is rarely accompanied by impairment of hearing—in distinction to the vertigo that follows fractures of the temporal bones (as described earlier in this chapter in the discussion of deafness). Dizziness is also a common complaint as part of the syndrome of posttraumatic nervous instability (page 945); usually this proves to be giddiness rather than true vertigo.

Vertigo of Brainstem Origin

Reference was made above to the occurrence of vertigo and nystagmus with lower and upper brainstem lesions. In these cases, vestibular nuclei and their connections are implicated. Auditory function is nearly always spared, since the vestibular and cochlear fibers diverge upon entering the brainstem, at the junction of the medulla and pons. The vertigo of brainstem origin as well as the accompanying nausea, vomiting, nystagmus, and dis-equilibrium are generally more protracted than with labyrinthine lesions, but one can think of exceptions to this statement. Nevertheless, with brainstem lesions, one often observes marked nystagmus without the slightest degree of vertigo—which does not happen with labyrinthine disease. The nystagmus of brainstem origin may be uni- or bidirectional, purely horizontal, vertical or rotary, and is characteristically worsened by attempted visual fixation. In contrast, nystagmus of labyrinthine origin is unidirectional, and past pointing and falling are in the direction of the slow phase; a purely vertical nystagmus does not occur, and a purely horizontal nystagmus without a rotary component is unusual. Furthermore, labyrinthine nystagmus is inhibited by visual fixation.

The central localization of vertigo is confirmed by finding signs of involvement of other structures within the brainstem (cranial nerves, sensory and motor tracts, etc.). Mode of onset, duration, and other features of the clinical picture depend upon the nature of the causative disease, which may be vascular, demyelinative, or neoplastic.

Vertigo is a prominent symptom of ischemic attacks and brainstem infarction occurring in the territory of the vertebrobasilar arteries, particularly the Wallenberg syndrome of lateral medullary infarction (page 844). On the other hand, vertigo as the *sole* manifestation of brainstem disease is rare. Unless other symptoms and signs of brainstem disorder appear within several days, one can postulate that the vertigo has an aural origin and nearly always exclude vascular disease of the brainstem. The same is true of multiple sclerosis, which may be the explanation of a persistent vertigo in an adolescent or young adult. Vertigo of cerebellar origin is exceptional in this respect in that it may be the sole manifestation of cerebellar infarction or hemorrhage, as described on pages 846 and 885. One explanation attributes the vertigo to small concomitant infarctions or compression of the lateral medulla, but this does not appear to be necessary. The nystagmus and ataxia of gait that accompany the cerebellar lesions do not differentiate them from acute vestibulopathies, but limb ataxia and dysarthria are reliable indicators of a cerebellar origin.

Attacks of vertigo followed by an intense unilateral and often suboccipital headache and vomiting are the characteristic features of *basilar artery migraine* (see page 183). The prodromal visual symptoms take the form of blindness or of photopsia that occupies all of the visual fields. Between headaches, tests of cochlear and vestibular function in these patients are normal. The relationship of this form of migraine to disease of the vertebral and basilar arteries is obscure.

Finally, mention should be made of a *familial vestibulocerebellar syndrome*, beginning in childhood or early adult life and characterized by recurrent episodes of vertigo and imbalance. Diplopia and dysarthria complicate some attacks, which seem to be precipitated by extreme exertion and emotion. Repeated attacks are followed by a mild, persistent ataxia, mainly of the trunk. This disorder was first described by Farmer and Mustian and more recently by Baloh and Winder, who have pointed out that both the episodic vertigo and ataxia are markedly reduced or abolished by the administration of acetazolamide.

The features of the various vertiginous syndromes are summarized in Table 15-2.

Table 15-2
Vertiginous syndromes with lesions of different parts of the vestibular system

	Findings on ear exam	*Other neurologic findings*	*Disorders of equilibrium*	*Type of nystagmus*[a]	*Hearing*	*Laboratory exam*
Labyrinths (postural vertigo, trauma, Ménière disease, aminoglycoside toxicity, labyrinthitis)	Usually negative	None	Ipsilateral past pointing and lateral propulsion to side of lesion	Horizontal or rotary to side opposite lesion, positional and position changing, fatigable	Normal or conduction or neurosensory deafness with recruitment	Vestibular paresis by caloric testing, directional preponderance
Vestibular nerve and ganglia (vestibular neuronitis, herpes zoster)	Vesicles in external auditory canal and palate in herpes zoster	Auditory eighth and seventh cranial nerve abnormalities; abnormal head impulse test to affected side	Ipsilateral past pointing and lateral propulsion to side of lesion	Unidirectional positional	Sometimes sensorineural deafness, without recruitment (vestibulo-labyrinthitis)	Radiography and CT may be normal or abnormal Vestibular paresis on caloric testing Directional preponderance
Cerebellopontine angle (acoustic neuroma, glomus and other tumors)	Negative	Ipsilateral fifth, seventh, ninth, tenth cranial nerves, cerebellar ataxia Increased intracranial pressure (late)	Ataxia and falling ipsilaterally	Gaze-paretic, positional, coarser to side of lesion	Sensorineural deafness without recruitment	CT and MRI abnormal Vestibular paresis on caloric testing BAERs abnormal Increased CSF protein
Brainstem and cerebellum (infarcts, tumors, viral infections)	Negative	Multiple cranial nerves, brainstem tract signs, cerebellar ataxia	Ataxia present with eyes open	Coarse horizontal and vertical, gaze-paretic	Usually normal	Hyperactive labyrinths or directional preponderance on caloric testing CT, MRI, and BAERs abnormal in most cases
Higher (cerebral) connections	Negative	Aphasia, visual field, hemimotor, hemisensory, and other cerebral abnormalities, seizures	No change	Usually absent	Normal	No change in caloric responses CT and EEG may be abnormal

[a]See text and Chap. 14 for description of types of nystagmus.

REFERENCES

ADLER JR, ROPPER AH: Self-audible venous bruits and high jugular bulb. *Arch Neurol* 43:257, 1986.

AMARENCO P, ROULLET E, HOMMEL M, et al: Infarction in the territory of the medial branch of the posterior inferior cerebellar artery. *J Neurol Neurosurg Psychiatry* 53:731, 1990.

BADIA L, PARIKH A, BOOKES GB: Management of middle ear myoclonus. *J Laryngol Otol* 108:380, 1994.

BALOH RW: *Clinical Neurotology*. London, Bailliére Tindall, 1994.

BALOH RW: Vertigo. *Lancet* 352, 1841, 1998.

BALOH RW, HONRUBIA V: *Clinical Neurophysiology of the Vestibular System*, 2nd ed. Philadelphia, Davis, 1990.

BALOH RW, HONRUBIA V, JACOBSON K: Benign positional vertigo: Clinical and oculographic features in 240 cases. *Neurology* 37:371, 1987.

BALOH RW, JACOBSON K, HONRUBIA V: Idiopathic bilateral vestibulopathy. *Neurology* 39:272, 1989.

BALOH RW, JACOBSON K, WILSON T: Drop attacks with Ménière's syndrome. *Ann Neurol* 28:384, 1990.

BALOH RW, WINDER A: Acetazolamide responsive vestibulo-cerebellar syndrome. Clinical and oculographic features. *Neurology* 41:429, 1991.

BÁRÁNY R: Experimentelle Alkohol-intoxication. *Monatsschr Ohrenheilk* 45:959, 1911.

BÁRÁNY R: Diagnose von Krankheitserscheinungen im Bereiche des Otolithenapparatus. *Acta Otolaryngol* 2:234, 1921.

BIEMOND A, DEJONG JMBV: On cervical nystagmus and related disorders. *Brain* 92:437, 1969.

BRANDT TH: Man in motion: Historical and clinical aspects of vestibular function—A review. *Brain* 114:2159, 1991.

BRANDT TH, STEDDIN S, DAROFF RB: Therapy for benign paroxysmal positioning vertigo, revisited. *Neurology* 44:796, 1994.

BRODAL A: The cranial nerves, in *Neurological Anatomy*, 3rd ed. New York, Oxford University Press, 1981, pp 448–577.

CASCINO G, ADAMS RD: Brainstem auditory hallucinosis. *Neurology* 36:1042, 1986.

CELESIA GG: Organization of auditory cortical areas in man. *Brain* 99:403, 1976.

CHINNERY PF, ELLIOTT C, GREEN GR, et al: The spectrum of treating loss due to mitochondrial DNA defects. *Brain* 123:82, 2000.

COGAN DG: Syndrome of nonsyphilitic interstitial keratitis and vestibuloauditory symptoms. *Arch Ophthalmol* 34:144, 1945.

DIX M, HALLPIKE C: Pathology, symptomatology and diagnosis of certain disorders of the vestibular system. *Proc R Soc Lond* 1952.

DUNCAN GW, PARKER SW, FISHER CM: Acute cerebellar infarction in the PICA territory. *Arch Neurol* 32:364, 1975.

EPLEY JM: The canalith repositioning procedure for treatment of benign paroxysmal positional vertigo. *Otolaryngol Head Neck Surg* 107:399, 1992.

ESTIVILL X, FORTINA P, SURREY S, et al: Connexin-26 mutations in sporadic and inherited sensorineural deafness. *Lancet* 351:394, 1998.

EVAN KE, TAVILL MA, GOLDBERG AN, SIVERSTEIN H: Sudden sensorineural hearing loss after general anesthesia for nonotologic surgery. *Laryngoscope* 107:747, 1997.

FARMER TW, MUSTIAN VM: Vestibulocerebellar ataxia. *Arch Neurol* 8:471, 1963.

FETTERMAN BL, LUXFORD WM, SAUNDERS JE: Sudden bilateral sensorineural hearing loss. *Lanryngoscope* 106:1347, 1996.

FIFE TD: Bedside cure for benign positional vertigo. *Barrows Neurological Inst Q* 10:2, 1994.

FOWLER EP: Head noises in normal and in disordered ears. *Arch Otolaryngol* 39:498, 1944.

FRIEDMANN I: Ultrastructure of ear in normal and diseased states, in Hinchcliffe R, Harrison D (eds): *Scientific Foundations of Otolaryngology*. London, Heinemann, 1976, pp 202–211.

FROEHLING DA, SILVERSTEIN MD, MOHR DN, et al: Benign positional vertigo: Incidence and prognosis in a population-based study in Olmsted County, Minnesota. *Mayo Clinic Proc* 16:596, 1991.

FURMAN JM, JACOB RG: Psychiatric dizziness. *Neurology* 48:1161, 1997.

GRAD A, BALOH RW: Vertigo of vascular origin. *Arch Neurol* 46:281, 1989.

GRAHAM JT, NEWBY HA: Acoustical characteristics of tinnitus. *Arch Otolaryngol* 75:162, 1962.

HALMAGYI GM, CREMER PD: Assessment and treatment of dizziness. *J Neurol Neurosurg Psychiatry* 68:129, 2000.

HAMMEKE TA, MCQUILLEN MP, COHEN BA: Musical hallucinations associated with acquired deafness. *J Neurol Neurosurg Psychiatry* 46:570, 1983.

HOTSON JR, BALOH RW: Acute vestibular syndrome. *N Engl J Med* 339:680, 1998.

JAMIESON DRS, MANN C, O'REILLY B, THOMAS AM: Ear click in palatal tremor caused by activity of the levator veli palatini. *Neurology* 46:1168, 1996.

JANNETTA PJ: Neurovascular decompression in cranial nerve and systemic disease. *Am J Surg* 192:518, 1980.

JANNETTA PJ, MOLLER MB, MOLLER AR: Disabling positional vertigo. *N Engl J Med* 310:1700, 1984.

KASAI K, ASADA T, YUMOTO M, et al: Evidence for functional abnormality in the right auditory cortex during musical hallucinosis. *Lancet* 354:1703, 1999.

KONIGSMARK BW: Hereditary deafness in man. *N Engl J Med* 281:713, 774, 827, 1969.

KONIGSMARK BW: Hereditary diseases of the nervous system with hearing loss, in Vinken PJ, Bruyn GW (eds): *Handbook of Clinical Neurology*. Vol 22. Amsterdam, North-Holland, 1975, chap 23, pp 499–526.

KONIGSMARK BW: Hereditary progressive cochleovestibular atrophies, in Vinken PJ, Bruyn GW (eds): *Handbook of Clinical Neurology*. Vol 22. Amsterdam, North-Holland, 1975, chap 22, pp 481–497.

KROENKE K, MANGELSDORFF AD: Common symptoms in ambulatory care: Incidence, evaluation, therapy, and outcome. *Am J Med* 86:262, 1989.

LEIGH RJ, ZEE DS: *The Neurology of Eye Movements*, 2nd ed. Philadelphia, Davis, 1991.

MARION MS, CEVETTE MJ: Tinnitus. *Mayo Clin Proc* 66:614, 1991.

MATTOX DE, SIMMONS FB: Natural history of sudden sensorineural hearing loss. *Ann Otol* 86:463, 1977.

MØLLER AR: Pathophysiology of tinnitus. *Ann Otol Rhinol Laryngol* 93:39, 1984.

Morell RJ, Kim HJ, Hood LJ, et al: Mutations in the connexin 26 gene (GJB2) among Ashkenazi Jews with nonsyndromic recessive deafness. *N Engl J Med* 339:1500, 1998.

Nadol JB Jr: Hearing loss. *N Engl J Med* 329:1092, 1993.

National Institute on Deafness and Other Communication Disorders: *A Report of the Task Force on the National Strategic Research Plan.* Bethesda, MD, National Institutes of Health, 1989.

Nodar RH, Graham JT: An investigation of frequency characteristics of tinnitus associated with Ménière's disease. *Arch Otolaryngol* 82:28, 1965.

Page J: Audiologic tests in the differential diagnosis of vertigo. *Otolaryngol Clin North Am* 6:53, 1973.

Proctor CA, Proctor B: Understanding hereditary nerve deafness. *Arch Otolaryngol* 85:23, 1967.

Rasmussen GI: An efferent cochlear bundle. *Anat Rec* 82:441, 1942.

Rudge P: *Clinical Neuro-otology.* Edinburgh, Churchill-Livingstone, 1983.

Sank D, Kallman FJ: The role of heredity in early total deafness. *Volta Rev* 65:461, 1963.

Schuknecht HF: Cupulolithiasis. *Arch Otolaryngol Head Neck Surg* 90:765, 1969.

Schuknecht HF, Kitamura K: Vestibular neuronitis. *Ann Otol Rhinol Laryngol* 90:1, 1981.

Semont A, Freyss G, Vitte E: Curing the BPPV with a liberatory maneuver. *Adv Otorhinolaryngol* 42:290, 1988.

Sismanis A, Smoker WR: Pulsatile tinnitus: Recent advances in diagnosis. *Laryngoscope* 104:681, 1994.

Suga S, Lindsay JR: Histopathological observations of presbyacusis. *Ann Otol Rhinol Laryngol* 85:169, 1976.

Tanaka Y, Kamo T, Yoshida M, Yamadori A: So-called cortical deafness. *Brain* 114:2385, 1991.

Tillman TW: Special hearing tests in otoneurologic diagnosis. *Arch Otolaryngol* 89:51, 1968.

Toole JF, Tucker H: Influence of head position upon cerebral circulation. *Arch Neurol* 2:616, 1960.

Tumarkin A: The otolithic catastrophe: A new syndrome. *BMJ* 1:175, 1936.

Vollertsen RS, McDonald TJ, Younge BR et al: Cogan's syndrome: 18 cases and a review of the literature. *Mayo Clin Proc* 61:344, 1986.

Section 4

EPILEPSY AND DISORDERS OF CONSCIOUSNESS

Chapter 16

EPILEPSY AND OTHER SEIZURE DISORDERS

In contemporary society, the frequency and importance of epilepsy can hardly be overstated. From the epidemiologic studies of Hauser and colleagues, it can be extrapolated that, at the time of the last census, approximately 1.77 million individuals in the United States were subject to epilepsy (i.e., chronically recurrent cerebral cortical seizures) and that about 44 new cases per 100,000 population occur each year. These figures are exclusive of patients in whom convulsions complicate febrile and other intercurrent illnesses or injuries. It has also been estimated that approximately 1 percent of persons in the United States will have epilepsy by the age of 20 years (Hauser and Annegers). Over two-thirds of all epileptic seizures begin in childhood (most in the first year of life), and this is the age period when seizures assume the widest array of forms. The incidence increases again slightly after age 60. In the practice of pediatric neurology, epilepsy is one of the most common disorders. The chronicity of childhood forms and their persistence in patients of all ages adds to their importance. For all these reasons, every physician should know something of the nature of seizure disorders and their treatment.

Epilepsy may be defined as an intermittent derangement of the nervous system due to "an excessive and disorderly discharge of cerebral nervous tissue on muscles." This was the postulate, in 1870, of Hughlings Jackson, the eminent British neurologist, and modern electrophysiology offers no evidence to the contrary. The discharge may result in an almost instantaneous loss of consciousness, alteration of perception or impairment of psychic function, convulsive movements, disturbance of sensation, or some combination thereof. A terminologic difficulty arises from the diversity of the clinical manifestations. The term *convulsion*, referring as it does to an intense paroxysm of involuntary repetitive muscular contractions, is inappropriate for a disorder that may consist only of an alteration of sensation or consciousness. *Seizure* is preferable as a generic term, since it embraces a diversity of paroxysmal events and also for the reason that it lends itself to qualification. The term *motor* or *convulsive seizure* is therefore not tautologic, and one may likewise speak of a *sensory seizure* or *psychic seizure*. The word *epilepsy* is derived from Greek words meaning "to seize upon" or a "taking hold of." Our predecessors referred to it as the "falling sickness" or the "falling evil." Although it is a useful medical term to denote recurrent seizures, the words *epilepsy* and *epileptic* still have unpleasant connotations to the laity and should be used advisedly in dealing with patients.

Viewed in its many clinical contexts, the first solitary seizure or brief outburst of seizures may occur during the course of many medical illnesses. It always indicates that the cerebral cortex has been affected by disease, either primarily or secondarily. By their nature, if repeated every few minutes, as in status epilepticus, convulsive seizures may threaten life. Equally important, a seizure or a series of seizures may be the manifestation of an ongoing neurologic disease that demands the employment of special diagnostic and therapeutic measures, as in the case of a brain tumor.

A more common and less grave circumstance is for a seizure to be but one in an extensive series occurring over a long period of time, with most of the attacks being more or less similar in type. In this instance they may be the result of a burned-out lesion that originated in the past and remains as a scar. The original disease may have passed unnoticed; or perhaps it occurred in utero, at birth, or in infancy, in parts of the brain too immature to manifest signs. It may have affected a very small or "silent" area in a mature brain. The increasingly refined techniques of magnetic resonance imaging (MRI) are revealing small zones of cortical dysplasia and hippocampal sclerosis, both of which tend to be epileptogenic. Patients with such long-standing lesions probably make up the majority of those with recurrent seizures but are necessarily classified as having "idiopathic" or "cryptogenic epilepsy," because it is impossible to ascertain the nature of the original disease and the seizures may be the only sign of brain abnormality.

There are other types of epilepsy for which no pathologic basis has been established and for which there is no apparent underlying cause except perhaps a genetic one. These epilepsies have been referred to as *primary*. Included in this category are hereditary forms, such as certain generalized tonic-clonic (grand mal) and absence seizure states. Some authors (Lennox and Lennox; Forster) have reserved the term *idiopathic* for recurrent seizures of the latter types.

CLASSIFICATION OF SEIZURES

Seizures have been classified in several ways: according to their supposed etiology, i.e, idiopathic (primary) or symptomatic (secondary); their site of origin; or on the basis of their clinical form (generalized or focal), their frequency (isolated, cyclic, prolonged, or repetitive), or their electrophysiologic correlates. A distinction needs to be drawn between the classification of *seizures*, considered below, and the classification of the *epilepsies*, or *epileptic syndromes*, which will be commented upon later in the chapter.

The classification to be followed here was first proposed by Gastaut in 1970 and was then refined repeatedly by the Commission on Classification and Terminology of the International League Against Epilepsy (1981). This classification, based mainly on the clinical form of the seizure and its electroencephalographic (EEG) features, has been adopted worldwide and is generally referred to as the International Classification of Epileptic Seizures. A modified version of it is reproduced in Table 16-1.

The strength of the International Classification lies in its easy applicability to patients with epilepsy and its clinical usefulness. The main value of classifying a seizure by its clinical and EEG features is the reasonable predictability of response to specific medications and to some extent its prognosis. Basically, this classification divides seizures into two types—*partial*, in which a focal or localized onset can be discerned, and *generalized*, in which the seizures appear to begin bilaterally. Seizures that begin locally may evolve into generalized tonic-clonic seizures, in which case they are called *secondarily generalized seizures*.

Table 16-1
International Classification of Epileptic Seizures

I. Generalized seizures (bilaterally symmetrical and without local onset)
   A. Tonic, clonic, or tonic-clonic (grand mal)
   B. Absence (petit mal)
      1. With loss of consciousness only
      2. Complex—with brief tonic, clonic, or automatic movements
   C. Lennox-Gastaut syndrome
   D. Juvenile myoclonic epilepsy
   E. Infantile spasms (West syndrome)
   F. Atonic (astatic, akinetic) seizures (sometimes with myoclonic jerks)

II. Partial, or focal, seizures (seizures beginning locally)
   A. Simple (*without* loss of consciousness or alteration in psychic function)
      1. Motor–frontal lobe origin (tonic, clonic, tonic-clonic; jacksonian; benign childhood epilepsy; epilepsia partialis continua)
      2. Somatosensory or special sensory (visual, auditory, olfactory, gustatory, vertiginous)
      3. Autonomic
      4. Pure psychic
   B. Complex (*with* impaired consciousness)
      1. Beginning as simple partial seizures and progressing to impairment of consciousness
      2. With impairment of consciousness at onset

III. Special epileptic syndromes
   A. Myoclonus and myoclonic seizures
   B. Reflex epilepsy
   C. Acquired aphasia with convulsive disorder
   D. Febrile and other seizures of infancy and childhood
   E. Hysterical seizures

Partial or *focal seizures* are classified as *simple* when consciousness is undisturbed and *complex* when consciousness is altered or impaired. Simple partial seizures are further classified according to their main clinical manifestations—motor, sensory, autonomic, or psychic. When one of these subjective manifestations precedes the progression of the attack to a loss of consciousness, it is referred to as an *aura* and has commonly been regarded as a premonitory sign or warning of the impending seizure. In reality, the aura represents the initial phase of a focal or partial seizure; and in some instances it may constitute the entire epileptic attack.

Generalized seizures are of two types—*convulsive* and *nonconvulsive*. The common convulsive type is the *tonic-clonic (grand mal) seizure*. Less common is a purely tonic, purely clonic, or clonic-tonic-clonic generalized seizure. The classic nonconvulsive generalized seizure is the brief lapse of consciousness or absence (*petit mal*); included also under this heading are minor motor phenomena such as brief myoclonic, atonic, or tonic seizures.

The classification of seizures and of the epilepsies is constantly being modified. In the latest version, the so-called syndromic classification (*Epilepsia* 30:389, 1989), an attempt has been made to incorporate all of the seizure types, epilepsies, and epileptic syndromes and to categorize them not only as partial and generalized but also according to their age of onset, their primary or secondary nature, the cortical loci of the epileptogenic lesions, and the many clinical settings in which they occur. This classification is semantically difficult and, in our view, too complicated as yet for general clinical application. Since many epileptic syndromes share overlapping features, it is often not possible to fit a newly diagnosed case of epilepsy into a specific category of this new classification (Manford et al). Currently the commission is engaged in an extensive revision of terminology and classification in the field of epilepsy. Until this revision is agreed upon, we propose to begin our discussion with the 1981 classification of seizures, with certain modifications and additions, to be followed by a consideration of a number of well-defined epilepsies and epileptic syndromes.

GENERALIZED SEIZURES

The Generalized Tonic-Clonic Seizure (Grand Mal)

As has already been intimated, it is always important to distinguish between a primary (generalized) type of seizure, with widespread EEG abnormalities at the onset, and a secondarily generalized type, which begins as a focal, or partial, seizure and then becomes generalized.

The patient sometimes senses the approach of a seizures by one of several subjective phenomena (a *prodrome*). For some hours, the patient may feel apathetic, depressed, irritable, or, very rarely, the opposite—ecstatic. One or more myoclonic jerks of the trunk or limbs on awakening may herald a seizure later in the day. In more than half the cases, there is some type of movement for a few seconds before consciousness is lost (turning of the head and eyes or whole body or intermittent jerking of a limb). Abdominal pains or cramps, a sinking, rising, or gripping feeling in the epigastrium, pallor or redness of the face, throbbing headache, constipation, or diarrhea have also been given prodromal status, but we have not found them consistently enough to be helpful.

Most often, the seizure strikes "out of the blue," i.e., without warning, beginning with a sudden loss of consciousness and fall to the ground. The initial motor signs are a brief flexion of the trunk, an opening of the mouth and eyelids, and upward deviation of the eyes. The arms are elevated and abducted, the elbows semiflexed, and the hands pronated. These are followed by a more protracted extension (*tonic*) phase, involving first the back and neck, then the arms and legs. There may be a piercing cry as the whole musculature is seized in a spasm and air is forcibly emitted through the closed vocal cords. Since the respiratory muscles are caught up in the tonic spasm, breathing is suspended, and after some seconds the skin and mucous membranes become cyanotic. The pupils are dilated and unreactive to light. The bladder may empty at this stage or later, during the postictal coma. This is the tonic phase of the seizure and lasts for 10 to 20 s.

There then occurs a transition from the tonic to the *clonic phase* of the convulsion. At first there is a mild generalized tremor, which is, in effect, a repetitive relaxation of the tonic contraction. It begins at a rate of 8 per second and coarsens to 4 per second and then rapidly gives way to brief violent flexor spasms that come in rhythmic salvos and agitate the entire body. The face becomes violaceous and contorted by a series of grimaces, and often the tongue is bitten. Autonomic signs are prominent: the pulse is rapid, blood pressure is elevated, pupils are dilated, and salivation and sweating are abundant; bladder pressure may increase sixfold during this phase. The clonic jerks decrease in amplitude and frequency over a period of about 30 s. The patient remains apneic until the end of the clonic phase, which is marked by a deep inspiration.

In the terminal phase of the seizure, all movements have ended and the patient lies still and limp, in a deep coma. The pupils, equal or unequal, now begin to contract to light. Breathing may be quiet or stertorous. This state persists for several minutes, after which the patient opens his eyes, begins to look about, and is obviously bewildered and confused. The patient may speak and later not remember anything that was said. Often, undisturbed, he becomes drowsy and falls asleep for several hours, then awakens with a pulsatile headache. When fully recovered, such a patient has no memory of any part of the spell but knows that something has happened because of the strange surroundings (in ambulance or hospital), the obvious concern of those around him, and a sore, bitten tongue and aching muscles from the violent contractions. The contractions may even have crushed a vertebral body, or a serious injury (fracture, periorbital hemorrhages, subdural hematoma, or burn) may have been sustained in the fall.

Each of these phases of the generalized tonic-clonic seizure has its characteristic electroencephalographic (EEG) accompaniment. Initially, the EEG changes are obscured by movement artifacts; sometimes there are repetitive spikes or spike-wave discharges lasting a few seconds, followed by an approximately 10-s period of 10-Hz spikes. As the clonic phase asserts itself, the spikes become mixed with slow waves and then the EEG slowly assumes a polyspike-and-wave pattern. When all movements have ceased, the EEG tracing is nearly flat for a variable time, and then the brain waves resume their preseizure pattern.

Convulsions of this type ordinarily come singly or in groups of two or three and may occur when the patient is awake and active or during sleep or frequently when he is falling asleep or awakening. Some 5 to 8 percent of such patients will at some time have a prolonged series of such seizures without completely regaining consciousness between them; this is called *convulsive status epilepticus* and demands urgent treatment. Sometimes the first outburst of seizures takes the form of convulsive status. Instead of the whole dramatic sequence described above, the seizures may be abbreviated or limited in scope by anticonvulsive medications.

Few clinical states closely simulate a grand mal convulsion, but several are worthy of mention. One is a clonic jerking of the extended limbs (usually less severe than those of a grand mal seizure) that occurs with vasodepressor syncope or a Stokes-Adams attack. In contrast to an epileptic type of EEG, the brain waves are slow and flat during the jerking movements. A rarer phenomenon that may be indistinguishable from a generalized convulsion occurs as part of basilar artery occlusion (Ropper). This presumably has its basis in ischemia of the corticospinal tracts in the pons; a similar mechanism has been invoked for "limb-shaking TIAs" (transient ischemic attacks), in which there are clonic movements of one limb or one side of the body during an episode of cerebral ischemia. Hysterical (nonepileptogenic, "psychogenic") seizures, as discussed further on, are often difficult to distinguish from the true variety. Rarely, in adults, an attack of panic (page 531) or the rare entity of rapid-eye-movement (REM) sleep behavior disorder may resemble a seizure. In infants, a breath-holding spell may resemble the tonic phase of a generalized seizure.

Idiopathic Nonconvulsive Seizures (Absence, Petit Mal)

In contrast to major generalized seizures, absence seizures (formerly referred to as *petit mal* or *pyknoepilepsy*) are notable for their brevity and the paucity of motor activity. Indeed, they may be so brief that the patients themselves are sometimes not aware of them; to an onlooker, they resemble a moment of absentmindedness or daydreaming.

The attack, coming without warning, consists of a sudden interruption of consciousness, for which the French word *absence* ("not present," "not in attendance") has been retained. The patient stares and briefly stops talking or ceases to respond. Only about 10 percent of such patients are completely motionless during the attack; in the remainder, one observes a brief burst of fine clonic movements of the eyelids, facial muscles, or fingers or synchronous movements of both arms at a rate of 3 per second, i.e., a rate that corresponds to that of the EEG abnormality, which takes the form of a generalized 3 per second spike-and-wave pattern (Fig. 2-3*E*). Minor automatisms—in the form of lip-smacking, chewing, and fumbling movements of the fingers—are common during an attack but do not assume prominence. Postural tone may be slightly decreased or increased, and occasionally there is a mild vasomotor disorder. As a rule, such patients do not fall; they may even continue such complex acts as walking or riding a bicycle. After 2 to 10 s, occasionally longer, the patient reestablishes full contact with the environment and resumes his preseizure activity. Only a loss of the thread of conversation or the place in reading betrays the occurrence of a momentary "blank" period (the absence). In many such patients, voluntary hyperventilation for 2 to 3 min is an effective way of inducing absence attacks.

Typical absence seizures constitute the most characteristic epilepsy of childhood; rarely do the seizures begin before 4 years of age or after puberty. Another attribute is their great frequency (hence the old term *pykno*, meaning "compact" or "dense"). As many as several hundred may occur in a single day, sometimes in bursts at certain times of the day. Most often they relate to periods of inattention and may appear in the classroom when the child is sitting quietly rather than participating actively in his lessons. If frequent, they may disturb attention and thinking to the point that the child does poorly in school. Such attacks may last for hours with no interval of normal mental activity between them—so-called *absence* or *petit mal status*. Small, subtle 3-per-second myoclonic movements are the only motor display (myoclonic petit mal), and are accompanied by a continuous 3-per-second spike-wave abnormality in the

EEG. Most cases of absence status have been described in adults with frontal lobe epilepsy (see below). Such attacks begin or end with a generalized tonic-clonic seizure or a burst of seizures and may be provoked by the abrupt withdrawal of anticonvulsant drugs.

Absence may be the only type of seizure during childhood. The attacks tend to diminish in frequency in adolescence and often disappear, only to be replaced in many instances by major generalized seizures. Absence epilepsy responds well to treatment with ethosuximide or valproate.

Absence or Petit Mal Variants To be distinguished from typical absence seizures are varieties in which the loss of consciousness is less complete or in which myoclonus is prominent, and others in which the EEG abnormalities are less regularly of a 3-per-second spike-and-wave type (they may occur at the rate of 2 to 2.5 per second or take the form of 4- to 6-Hz polyspike-and-wave complexes). *Atypical petit mal* is a term that was coined to describe long runs of slow spike-and-wave activity, usually with no apparent loss of consciousness. External stimuli such as asking the patient to answer a question or to count will interrupt the run of abnormal EEG activity.

About 30 percent of children with absence attacks will, in addition, display symmetrical or asymmetrical myoclonic jerks without loss of consciousness, and about 50 percent will also at some time have major generalized (tonic-clonic) convulsions. As described further on, a common variety of myoclonic seizures occurs in late childhood and adolescence (*juvenile myoclonic epilepsy*).

In sharp contrast to the aforementioned epilepsies is a form that has its onset between 2 and 6 years of age and is characterized by atonic, or astatic, seizures (i.e., falling attacks), often succeeded by various combinations of minor motor, tonic-clonic, and partial seizures and by intellectual impairment, in association with a distinctive, slow (1- to 2-Hz) spike-and-wave EEG pattern. This is the *Lennox-Gastaut syndrome*. Often it is preceded in earlier life by infantile spasms, a characteristic EEG picture ("hypsarrhythmia"), and an arrest in mental development, a triad sometimes referred to as the *West syndrome* (see further on). The early onset of atonic seizures with abrupt falls, injuries, and associated abnormalities nearly always has a grave implication—namely, the presence of serious neurologic disease. Prematurity, perinatal injury, and metabolic diseases of infancy are the most common underlying conditions. This is essentially a symptomatic generalized epilepsy, in contrast to the foregoing idiopathic types. The Lennox-Gastaut syndrome may persist into adult life and is one of the most difficult forms of epilepsy to treat.

The notion that absence, myoclonic, and akinetic seizures constitute a petit mal triad, as originally proposed by Lennox, has been generally abandoned. Akinesia (motionlessness) is not unique to any seizure type. The typical absence, with or without myoclonic jerks, rarely causes the patient to fall and should be considered a separate entity because of its relative benignity.

Myoclonus and Myoclonic Seizures

The phenomenon of myoclonus has already been discussed in Chap. 6, where the relationship to seizures was indicated. Characterized by a brusque, brief, muscular contraction, some myoclonic jerks are so small as to involve only one muscle or part of a muscle; others are so large as to implicate a limb on one or both sides of the body or the entire trunk musculature. Many are brief, lasting 50 to 100 ms. They may occur intermittently and unpredictably or present as a single jerk or a brief salvo.

As mentioned earlier, several small, rhythmic myoclonic jerks occur with varying frequency as part of absence seizures and as isolated events in patients with generalized clonic-tonic-clonic or tonic-clonic seizures. As a rule, these types of myoclonus are quite benign and respond well to medication. In contrast, *disseminated myoclonus (polymyoclonus)*, having its onset in childhood, raises the suspicion of acute viral encephalitis, the myoclonus-opsoclonus-ataxia syndrome of Kinsbourne, lithium or other drug toxicity, or, if lasting a few weeks, subacute sclerosing panencephalitis. Chronic progressive polymyoclonus with dementia characterizes the group of juvenile lipidosis, Lafora-type familial myoclonic epilepsy, certain mitochondrial disorders, or other chronic familial degenerative diseases of undefined type (paramyoclonus multiplex of Friedreich, dyssynergia cerebellaris myoclonica of Ramsay Hunt). In middle and late adult years, disseminated myoclonus joined with dementia usually indicates the presence of so-called Creutzfeldt-Jakob disease (page 814) and sometimes of Alzheimer disease. Myoclonus may be the main manifestation of juvenile myoclonic epilepsy, as discussed below. Uremia, at any age, gives rise to myoclonus, twitching, and sometimes to seizures. The large number of diseases causative of seizure disorders are discussed in Chaps. 33, 37, and 39.

Juvenile Myoclonic Epilepsy This is probably the most common form of idiopathic generalized epilepsy. It begins in adolescence, typically about age 15. The patient comes to attention because of a generalized seizure, often upon awakening; less often, for morning myoclonic jerks that involve the entire body; or for absence seizures. The family reports that the patient has occasional myoclonic jerks of the arm and upper trunk that become prominent with fatigue, during early stages of sleep, or after alcohol ingestion. A few patients in our experience have had only the myoclonic phenomena and rare absence seizures that went unnoticed for years. The EEG characteristically shows bursts of 4- to 6-Hz irregular polyspike- and-wave activity. A linkage has been established to chromosome 6 in some cases of this illness and in some other forms of juvenile-onset epilepsy, but no mendelian pattern of inheritance has been established. The disorder does not impair intelligence and tends not to be progressive, but a proclivity to infrequent seizures usually persists throughout life. Valproic acid and other drugs are very effective in eliminating the seizures and myoclonus.

PARTIAL, OR FOCAL, SEIZURES

As indicated earlier, the International Classification divides all seizures into two types—generalized (described above), in which the clinical and EEG manifestations indicate bilateral and diffuse cerebral cortical involvement from the onset, and focal of partial (more recently termed *localization-related*) in which the seizure is the product of a demonstrable focal lesion or EEG abnormality in some part of the cerebral cortex (or perhaps in a deep nuclear structure). As noted, partial seizures vary with the locale of the lesion and are conventionally divided into two groups, *simple* and *complex*, depending on whether consciousness is retained or impaired. Simple partial seizures most often arise from foci in the sensorimotor cortex. Complex partial seizures most often have their focus in the temporal lobe on one side or the other. Localization of the offending lesions and the types of seizures to which they give rise are listed in Table 16-2. These relationships are so helpful in diagnosis that they should be known to all neurologists.

Table 16-2
Common seizure patterns

Clinical type	*Localization*
Somatic motor	
Jacksonian (focal motor)	Prerolandic gyrus
Masticatory, salivation, speech arrest	Amygdaloid nuclei, opercular
Simple contraversive	Frontal
Head and eye turning associated with arm movement or athetoid-dystonic postures	Supplementary motor cortex
Somatic and special sensory (auras)	
Somatosensory	Contralateral postrolandic
Unformed images, lights, patterns	Occipital
Auditory	Heschl's gyri
Vertiginous	Superior temporal
Olfactory	Mesial temporal
Gustatory	Insula
Visceral: autonomic	Insular-orbital-frontal cortex
Complex partial seizures	
Formed hallucinations	Temporal neocortex or amygdaloid-hippocampal complex
Illusions	
Dyscognitive experiences (déjà vu, dreamy states, depersonalization)	
Affective states (fear, depression, or elation)	Temporal
Automatism (ictal and postictal)	Temporal and frontal
Absence	Frontal cortex, amygdaloid-hippocampal complex, reticular-cortical system
Bilateral epileptic myoclonus	Reticulocortical, frontocentral

Source: Modified from Penfield and Jasper.

Frontal Lobe Partial Seizures (Focal Motor and Jacksonian Seizures)

Focal or partial motor seizures are attributable to a discharging lesion of the opposite frontal lobe. The most common type, attributable to a focus in the supplementary motor area, takes the form of a turning movement of the head and eyes to the side opposite the irritative focus, often associated with a tonic contraction of the trunk and limbs on that side. This may constitute the entire seizure, or it may be followed by focal and then generalized clonic movements; generalization of the seizure may occur just before or simultaneously with loss of consciousness. On the other hand, a lesion in one frontal lobe may give rise to a major generalized convulsion without an initial turning of the head and eyes. It has been postulated that in both types of seizure, the one with and the one without turning movements, there is an immediate spread of the discharge from the frontal lobe to integrating centers in the thalamic or high midbrain reticular formation, accounting for the loss of consciousness.

Seizures that begin with forceful, sustained deviation of the head and eyes, and sometimes of the entire body, are referred to as *versive* or *adversive*. Since the turning movements are usually to the side opposite the irritative focus (sometimes to the same side), *contraversive* and *ipsiversive* respectively would be preferable terms. Nonforceful, unsustained, or seemingly random lateral head movements during the ictus do not have localizing value. The same is true for the head and eye turning that occurs at the end of the generalized tonic-clonic phase of versive seizures (Wylie et al). Contraversive deviation of only the head and eyes can be induced most consistently by electrical stimulation of the superolateral frontal region (area 8), just anterior to area 6 (see Fig. 22-1). Less consistently, the same movements can be obtained by stimulating the more anterior portions of the frontal cortex, the posterior part of the superior frontal gyrus (the supplementary motor area), and the temporal or occipital cortex—presumably through propagation of the ictal discharge to the frontal contraversive area. In seizures of temporal lobe origin, early in the seizure, there may be head turning ipsilaterally followed by forceful, contraversive head (and body) turning. These head and body movements, if they occur, are preceded by quiet staring and automatisms.

The *jacksonian motor seizure* begins with a tonic contraction of the fingers of one hand, the face on one side, or the muscles of one foot. This transforms into clonic movements in these parts in a fashion analogous to that in a generalized clonic-tonic-clonic convulsion. Sometimes a series of clonic movements of increasing frequency build up to a tonic contraction. The movements may remain localized or spread ("march") from the part first affected to other muscles on the same side of the body. In the latter, or "classic," jacksonian form, which is relatively uncommon, the seizure spreads from the hand, up the arm, to the face, and down the leg; or, if the first movement is in the foot, the seizure marches up the leg, down the arm, and to the face, usually in a matter of 20 to 30 s. Interestingly, spontaneously occurring focal motor seizures, e.g., those beginning in the toes or fingers, may sometimes be arrested (inhibited) by applying a ligature above the affected part or, in the case of focal sensory seizures, by applying a vigorous sensory stimulus ahead of the advancing sensory aura. Rarely, the first muscular contraction is in the abdomen, thorax, or neck. In some cases, the one-sided seizure activity is followed by turning of the head and eyes to the convulsing side, occasionally to the opposite side, and then by a generalized seizure with loss of consciousness. Consciousness is not lost if the sensorimotor symptoms remain confined to one side.

The high incidence of onset of focal motor epilepsy in the face, hands, and toes is probably related to the disproportionately large cortical representation of these parts. The disease process or focus of excitation is usually in or near the rolandic cortex, i.e., area 4 of Brodmann (Figs. 3-3 and 22-1); in some cases, and especially if there is a sensory accompaniment, it has been found in the postrolandic convolution. Lesions confined to the motor cortex are reported to assume the form of clonic contractions, and those confined to the premotor cortex (area 6), tonic contractions of the contralateral arm, face, neck, or all of one side of the body. Tonic elevation and extension of the contralateral arm ("fencer's posture") and choreoathetotic and dystonic postures have been associated with high medial frontal lesions (area 8 and supplementary motor cortex), as have complex, bizarre, and flailing movements of a contralateral limb. Perspiration and piloerection occur occasionally in parts of the body involved in a focal motor seizure, suggesting that these autonomic functions have a cortical representation in or adjacent to the rolandic area. Focal motor and jacksonian seizures have essentially the same localizing significance.

Seizure discharges arising from the cortical language areas may give rise to a brief aphasic disturbance (*ictal aphasia*) or, more frequently, to vocal arrest. Ictal aphasia is usually succeeded by other focal or generalized seizure activity but may occur in isolation, without loss of consciousness, in which case it can later be described by the patient. Postictal aphasia is more common and has much the same localizing value. Vocalization at the onset of a seizure has no such significance. These disturbances should be distinguished from the stereotyped repetition of words or phrases or the garbled speech that characterizes some cases of complex partial seizures or the postictal confusional state.

As pointed out by Manford and colleagues, relatively few focal seizures can be localized precisely from clinical data alone. However, when combined with scalp and intracranial EEG recording and MRI, the data are reasonably accurate.

Somatosensory, Visual, and Other Types of Sensory Seizures

Somatosensory seizures, either focal or "marching" to other parts of the body on one side, are nearly always indicative of a focus in or near the postrolandic convolution of the opposite cerebral hemisphere. Penfield and Kristiansen found the seizure focus in the postcentral or precentral convolution in 49 of 55 such cases. The sensory disorder is usually described as numbness, tingling, or a "pins-and-needles" feeling and occasionally as a sensation of crawling (formication), electricity, or movement of the part. Pain and thermal sensations may occur but are exceedingly rare. In the majority of cases, the onset of the sensory seizure is in the lips, fingers, or toes, and the spread to adjacent parts of the body follows a pattern determined by sensory arrangements in the postcentral (postrolandic) convolution of the parietal lobe. If the sensory symptoms are localized to the head, the focus is in or adjacent to the lowest part of the convolution, near the sylvian fissure; if the symptoms are in the leg or foot, the upper part of the convolution, near the superior sagittal sinus or on the medial surface of the hemisphere, is involved.

Visual seizures are relatively rare but also have localizing significance. Lesions in or near the striate cortex of the occipital lobe usually produce elemental visual sensations of darkness or sparks and flashes of light, which may be stationary or moving and colorless or colored. According to Gowers, red is the most frequently reported color, followed by blue, green, and yellow. These images may be referred to the visual field on the side opposite the lesion or may appear straight ahead. If they occur on one side of the visual field, patients usually report that only one eye is affected (the one opposite the lesion), probably because most persons are aware of only the temporal half of a homonymous field defect. Curiously, a seizure arising in one occipital lobe may cause momentary blindness in both fields. It has been noted that lesions on the lateral surface of the occipital lobe (Brodmann areas 18 and 19) are likely to cause a sensation of twinkling or pulsating lights. More complex or formed visual hallucinations are usually due to a focus in the posterior part of the temporal lobe, near its junction with the occipital lobe, and may be associated with auditory hallucinations. The localizing value of visual auras has been confirmed recently by Bien and colleagues in a group of 20 surgically treated patients with intractable seizures. They found that elementary visual hallucinations and visual loss were typical of occipital lobe epilepsy but could also occur with seizures foci in the anteromedial temporal and occipitotemporal regions.

Auditory hallucinations are infrequent as an initial manifestation of a seizure. Occasionally a patient with a focus in one superior temporal convolution will report a buzzing or roaring in the ears. A human voice, sometimes repeating unrecognizable words, has been noted a few times with lesions in the more posterior part of one temporal lobe.

Vertiginous sensations of a type suggesting a vestibular origin may be the first symptom of a seizure. The lesion is usually localized to the superoposterior temporal region or the junction between parietal and temporal lobes. In one of the cases reported by Penfield and Jasper, a sensation of vertigo was evoked by stimulating the cortex at the junction of the parietal and occipital lobes. Occasionally, with a temporal focus, the vertigo is followed by an auditory sensation. Giddiness, or light-headedness, is a frequent prelude to a seizure, but this symptom has so many different connotations that it is of little diagnostic value.

Olfactory hallucinations are often associated with disease of the inferior and medial parts of the temporal lobe, usually in the region of the parahippocampal convolution or the uncus (hence Jackson's term *uncinate seizures*, pages 242 and 481). Usually the perceived odor is exteriorized, i.e., projected to someplace in the environment, and is described as disagreeable or foul, though otherwise unidentifiable. *Gustatory hallucinations* have also been recorded in proven cases of temporal lobe disease (see page 245) and with lesions of the insula and parietal operculum; salivation and a sensation of thirst may be associated. Electrical stimulation in the depths of the sylvian fissure, extending into the insular region, has produced peculiar sensations of taste.

Vague and often indefinable visceral sensations arising in the thorax, epigastrium, and abdomen are among the most frequent of auras, as already indicated. Most often they have a temporal lobe origin although in several such cases the seizure discharge has been localized to the upper bank of the sylvian fissure; in a few others, the focus was located in the upper or middle frontal gyrus or in the medial frontal area near the cingulate gyrus. Palpitation and acceleration of the pulse at the beginning of the attack have also been related to a temporal lobe focus.

Complex Partial Seizures (Psychomotor Seizures, Temporal Lobe Seizures)

These differ from the major generalized and absence seizures discussed above in that (1) the aura (i.e., the initial event in the seizure) may be either a focal seizure of simple type or a hallucination or perceptual illusion, indicating (usually) a temporal lobe origin, and (2) instead of a complete loss of control of thought and action, there is a period of altered behavior and consciousness, for which the patient is later found to be amnesic.

Although it is difficult to enumerate all the psychic experiences that may occur during complex partial seizures, they may be categorized into a somewhat arbitrary hierarchy of illusions, hallucinations, dyscognitive states, and affective experiences. Sensory illusions, or distortions of ongoing perceptions, are the most common. Objects or persons in the environment may shrink or recede into the distance, or, less frequently, they may enlarge (micropsia and macropsia). Tilting of the visual environment has been reported. Hallucinations are most often visual or auditory, consisting of formed or unformed visual images, sounds, and voices; less frequently, they may be olfactory (usually unpleasant, unidentifiable sensations of smell), gustatory, or vertiginous. The term *dyscognitive* state refers to feelings of increased reality or familiarity (déjà vu) or of strangeness or unfamiliarity (jamais vu) or a stated depersonalization. Fragments of certain old memories or scenes may insert themselves into the patient's mind and recur with striking clarity, or there may be an abrupt interruption of memory. (See Gloor for a more detailed description of the experiential phenomena of temporal lobe epilepsy.) Epigastric and abdominal sensations have been alluded to above.

Emotional experiences, while less common, may be dramatic—sadness, loneliness, anger, happiness, and sexual excitement have all been recorded. Fear and anxiety are the most common affective experiences, while occasionally the patient describes a feeling of rage or intense anger as part of a complex partial seizure. Ictal fear may have no apparent connection to objective experience and is generally not related to the situation in which the patient finds himself during the seizure.

Each of these subjective psychic experiences may constitute the entire seizure (simple partial seizure), or some combination may occur and proceed to a period of unresponsiveness. The motor components of the seizure occur during the latter phase and take the form of automatisms such as lip smacking, chewing or swallowing movements, salivation, fumbling of the hands, or shuffling of the feet. The patient may walk around in a daze or act inappropriately (undressing in public, speaking incoherently, etc.). Certain complex acts that were initiated before the loss of consciousness—such as walking, chewing food, turning the pages of a book, or even driving—may continue. However, when asked a specific question or given a command, the patient is obviously out of contact with his surroundings. There may be no response at all, or the patient may look toward the examiner in a perplexed way or utter a few stereotyped phrases. In a very small number of patients with temporal lobe seizures (7 of 123 patients studied by Ebner et al), some degree of responsiveness (to simple questions and motor commands) was preserved in the presence of prominent automatisms such as lip smacking and swallowing. Interestingly, in this small group of partially responsive patients, the seizures lateralized to the right temporal lobe.

The patient, in his confused and irritable state, may resist or strike out at the examiner. The *violence and aggression* that are said to characterize patients with temporal lobe seizures usually take this form of nondirected oppositional resistance in response to restraint during the period of automatic behavior (so called because the patient presumably acts like an automaton) or, more often, in the postictal period. Unprovoked assault or outbursts of intense rage or blind fury are very unusual; Currie and associates found such outbursts in only 16 of 666 patients (2.4 percent) with temporal lobe epilepsy. Penfield once commented that he had never observed a rage state as a result of temporal lobe stimulation. It is exceedingly unlikely that an organized violent act requiring several sequential steps in its performance, such as obtaining a gun and using it, could represent a temporal lobe seizure.

Rarely, laughter (*gelastic epilepsy*) may be the most striking feature of an automatism. (A particular combination of gelastic seizures and precocious puberty is due to a hamartoma of the hypothalamus.) Or the patient may walk repetitively in small circles (*volvular epilepsy*), run (*epilepsia procursiva*), or simply wander aimlessly, either as an ictal or postictal phenomenon (*poriomania*). These forms of seizure are actually more common with frontal lobe than with temporal lobe foci.

Dystonic posturing of the arm and leg contralateral to the seizure focus is found to be a frequent accompaniment if sought—again, the origin is more often in the frontal than the temporal lobes localizing particularly to the supplementary motor area. After the attack, the patient usually has no memory or only fragments of recall for what was said or done. Any type of complex partial seizures may proceed to other forms of secondary generalized seizures. The tendency to generalization holds true for all types of partial or focal epilepsy.

The patient with temporal lobe seizures may exhibit only one of the foregoing manifestations of seizure activity or various combinations of them. In a series of 414 patients studied by Lennox, 43 percent displayed some of the motor changes; 32 percent, automatic behavior; and 25 percent, alterations in psychic function. Because of the frequent concurrence of these symptom complexes, he referred to them as the *psychomotor triad*. Probably the clinical pattern varies with the precise locality of the lesion and the direction and extent of spread of the electrical discharge. Because of their focal origin and complex symptomatology, all these types of seizures are subsumed under the title of *complex partial seizures*. This term is preferable to *temporal lobe seizures*, since typical complex partial seizures sometimes arise from a focus in the medial-orbital part of the frontal lobe, and the seizure discharge in such cases can be limited to the frontal lobe. Also, seizures originating in the parietal or occipital lobes may be manifested as complex partial seizures because of seizure spread into the temporal lobes. Often the brief ictal aura is not reflected in cortical epileptic activity and therefore may be missed by routine EEG recordings.

Complex partial seizures are not peculiar to any period of life but show an increased incidence in adolescence and the adult years. In the series of Ounsted and coworkers, about one-third of such cases could be traced to the occurrence of severe febrile convulsions in early life (see further on). As a corollary, about 5 percent of all their patients with febrile seizures continued to have seizures during adolescence and adult life; in the latter group there were many in whom the seizures were of the temporal lobe type. Also, in Falconer's series of temporal lobectomies for intractable epilepsy, there were many patients who had previously had this complicated type of febrile seizure. Neonatal convulsions, head trauma, and various other nonprogressive perinatal neurologic disorders are other factors that place a child at risk of developing complex partial seizures (Rocca et al). Two-thirds of patients with complex partial seizures also have generalized tonic-clonic seizures or have had them at some earlier time, and the generalized seizures may have led to secondary ischemic damage to the hippocampal portions of the temporal lobes. In the latter cases, carefully performed and quantitated MRI in the coronal plane may disclose a loss of volume in the hippocampi and adjacent gyri on one or both sides—*medial temporal sclerosis* (Fig. 16-1).

Complex partial seizures are notably variable in duration. Behavioral automatisms rarely last longer than a minute or two, although postictal confusion and amnesia may persist for a considerably longer time. Some complex partial seizures consist only of a momentary change in facial expression and a blank spell, resembling an absence. Almost always, however, the former are characterized by distinct ictal and postictal phases, whereas patients with absence attacks usually have an instantaneous return of full consciousness following the ictus.

Postictal behavior after partial complex seizures is often accompanied by widespread slowing in the EEG. With seizures of left-sided origin there is likely to be global and nonfluent aphasia. Prolonged disorientation for time and place suggests a right-sided source. Automatisms in the postictal period have no lateralizing connotation (Devinsky et al). However, postictal posturing and paresis of an arm (*Todd's paralysis*) or an aphasic difficulty are helpful in determining the side of the lesion (Cascino). Also, postictal nose wiping, is carried out by the hand ipsilateral to the seizure focus in 97 percent of patients, according to Leutzmezer and colleagues, but the authors are in no position to confirm this.

Amnesic Seizures Rarely, brief, recurrent attacks of transient amnesia are the only manifestations of temporal lobe epilepsy, although it is unclear whether the amnesia in such patients represents an ictal or postictal phenomenon. These attacks of pure amnesia have been referred to as *transient epileptic amnesia*, or TEA (Palmini et al; Zeman et al). If the patient functions at a fairly high level during the attack, as may happen, there is some resemblance to transient global amnesia (page 457). However, the brevity and frequency of the TEA spells, their tendency to occur on awakening, the impaired performance on complex cognitive tasks, and, of course, a history of epilepsy and associated seizure discharges in the EEG help to make the distinction.

Behavioral and Psychiatric Disorders Some comments are in order concerning the issues of *personality*, *behavioral*, and *psychiatric disorders* in patients with complex partial seizures. Data as to prevalence of these

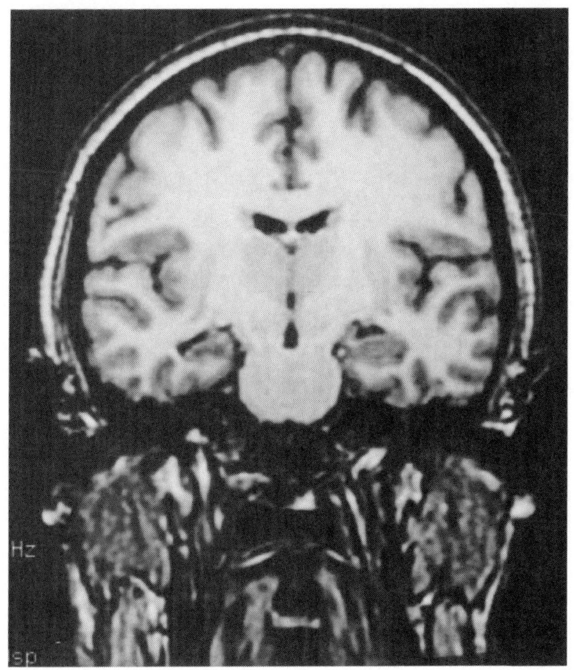

A

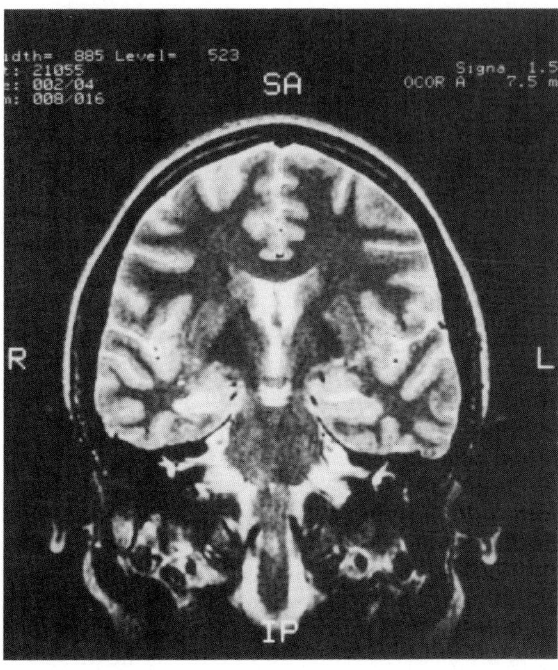

B

Figure 16-1

Medial temporal sclerosis. A. *Thin slice volumetric MR image in the coronal plane, showing shrinkage of the right hippocampus and secondary enlargement of the temporal horn of the lateral ventricle.* B. *T2-weighted image showing signal change in the hippocampi. (Courtesy of Dr. Peter Williamson)*

disorders are limited and have been derived mainly from studies of selected groups of patients attending university hospital and other specialty clinics that tend to treat the most difficult and complicated cases. In one such study (Victoroff), about one-third of the patients had a history of major depressive illness and an equal number had symptoms of anxiety disorder; psychotic symptoms were found in 10 percent. Similar figures, also from a university-based epilepsy center, have been reported by Blumer et al. It must be emphasized that these remarkable rates of psychiatric morbidity do not reflect the prevalence in the entire population of epileptics.

The postictal state in patients with temporal lobe epilepsy sometimes takes the form of a protracted *paranoid-delusional state*. Indeed, some patients lapse into a paranoid-delusional or amnesic psychosis lasting for days or weeks. The EEG during this period may show no seizure discharge, though this does not exclude repeated or sustained seizure activity in the amygdala and other deep temporal lobe structures. This disorder, virtually indistinguishable from schizophrenia, may also present in the interictal period. Again, the frequency of this association is uncertain. An excess of psychosis has been reported only in studies emanating from specialized centers; epidemiologic studies provide only limited evidence of an excess of psychosis in the overall population of epileptics (see Trimble and Schmitz and the review by Trimble for a critical discussion of this subject).

Epileptic Personality Disorder It has long been observed that some patients with temporal lobe seizures also exhibit a number of *abnormalities of behavior and personality* during the interictal period. Often they are slow and rigid in their thinking, verbose, circumstantial and tedious in conversation, inclined to mysticism, and preoccupied with rather naive religious and philosophical ideas. Also they are often subject to outbursts of bad temper and aggressiveness. Obsessionalism, humorless sobriety, emotionality (mood swings, sadness and anger) and a tendency to paranoia are other frequently described traits. Diminished sexual interest and potency in men and menstrual problems in women, not readily attributable to anticonvulsant drugs, are common among patients with complex partial seizures of temporal lobe origin.

Geschwind proposed that a triad of behavioral abnormalities—hyposexuality, hypergraphia and hyperreligiosity—constitute a characteristic syndrome in such patients.

Bear and Fedio have suggested that certain of these traits (obsessionalism, elation, sadness, and emotionality) are more common with *right* temporal lesions and that anger, paranoia, and cosmologic or religious conceptualizing are more characteristic of *left* temporal lesions. However, Rodin and Schmaltz, who administered the Bear-Fedio inventory to patients with both primary generalized and temporal lobe epilepsy, found no features that would distinguish patients with right-sided temporal foci from those with left-sided foci. Moreoever, they found no behavioral changes that would distinguish patients with temporal lobe epilepsy from other groups of epileptics. The problem of personality disturbances in epilepsy remains to be clarified (see review by Trimble).

SPECIAL EPILEPTIC SYNDROMES

There remain to be considered several epileptic syndromes and other seizure states that cannot be readily classified with the usual types of generalized or partial seizures. These special types are described below.

Benign Childhood Epilepsy with Centrotemporal Spikes (Rolandic Epilepsy, Sylvian Epilepsy) or with Occipital Spikes

This type of focal motor epilepsy is unique among the partial epilepsies of childhood in that it tends to be a self-limited disorder, transmitted in families as an autosomal dominant trait. The convulsive disorder begins between 5 and 9 years of age and usually announces itself by a nocturnal tonic-clonic seizure with focal onset. Thereafter, the seizures take the form of clonic contractions of one side of the face, less often of one arm or leg, and the interictal EEG shows high-voltage spikes in the contralateral lower rolandic or centrotemporal area. The seizures are readily controlled by a single anticonvulsant drug and gradually disappear during adolescence. The relation of this syndrome to acquired aphasia with convulsive disorder in children, described by Landau and Kleffner, is unsettled.

A similar type of epilepsy, usually benign in the sense that there is no intellectual deterioration and a cessation of seizures in adolescence, has been associated with spike activity over the occipital lobes. In both of these types of childhood epilepsy, the observation that spikes are greatly accentuated by sleep is a useful diagnostic aid.

Infantile Spasms (West Syndrome)

This is the term applied to a particular form of epilepsy of infancy and early childhood. West, in the mid-nineteenth century, described the condition in his son in exquisite detail. This seizure disorder, which in most cases appears during the first year of life, is characterized by recurrent, gross flexion movements of the trunk and limbs and, less frequently, by extension movements (hence the alternative terms *infantile spasms or salaam or jackknife seizures*). Most but not all patients with this disorder show severe EEG abnormalities, consisting of continuous multifocal spikes and slow waves of large amplitude. However, this pattern, referred to originally by Gibbs and Gibbs as *hypsarrhythmia* ("mountainous" dysrhythmia), is not specific for infantile spasms, being frequently associated with other developmental or acquired abnormalities of the brain. As the child matures, the seizures diminish and usually disappear by the fourth to fifth year. If MRI and CT scans are more or less normal, the usual pathologic findings according to Jellinger are cortical dysgeneses. Both the seizures and the EEG abnormalities may respond dramatically to treatment with adrenocorticotropic hormone (ACTH), corticosteroids, or the benzodiazepine drugs, of which clonazepam is probably the most widely used. However, most patients, even those who were apparently normal when the seizures appeared, are left mentally impaired. Infantile spasms may also be part of the Lennox-Gastaut syndrome, a seizure disorder of early childhood of grave prognosis (see page 335).

Febrile Seizures

The well-known *febrile seizure*, peculiar to infants and children between 6 months and 5 years of age (peak incidence 9 to 20 months) and with a strong tendency to be inherited, is generally regarded as a benign condition. Usually it takes the form of a single, generalized motor seizure occurring as the temperature rises or reaches its peak. Seldom does the seizure last longer than a few minutes; by the time an EEG can be obtained, there is usually no abnormality. Recovery is complete. Except for a presumed genetic relationship with benign epilepsy of childhood (Luders et al), which in itself is transient in nature, these patients' risk of developing epilepsy in later life is only slightly greater than that of the general population.

This benign type of febrile seizure should not be confused with a second and more serious type of illness in which an acute encephalitic or encephalopathic state presents as a febrile illness with focal or prolonged seizures, generalized or focal EEG abnormalities, and repeated episodes of febrile convulsions with the same or different illnesses (*complicated febrile seizures*). These seizures may recur not only with infections but also at other times. When patients with both types are lumped together under the rubric of *febrile convulsions*, it is not surprising that a high percentage are complicated by atypical petit mal, atonic, and astatic spells followed by tonic seizures, mental retardation, and partial complex epilepsy. Falconer, who studied psychomotor seizures in adults, noted retrospectively a high incidence of "febrile seizures" during the infancy and childhood of his subjects. The present authors believe that he was referring to complicated febrile seizures, i.e., fever and convulsions with structural brain disease, which should be kept separate from the common benign febrile seizures. In a later study of 67 patients with proven medial temporal lobe epilepsy (French et al), 70 percent had a history of complicated febrile seizures during the first 5 years of life, although many did not develop temporal lobe epilepsy until their teens. Bacterial meningitis was another important risk factor; head and birth trauma were less common factors. All of the patients had complex partial seizures and half of them, in addition, had secondarily generalized tonic-clonic seizures.

Epidemiologic studies have substantiated this clinical point of view. Annegers and colleagues observed a cohort of 687 children for an average of 18 years after their initial febrile convulsion. Overall, these children had a fivefold excess of unprovoked seizures in later life. Among the children with simple febrile convulsions, the risk was only 2.4 percent. By contrast, children with what Annegers et al called complex febrile convulsions (focal, prolonged, or repeated episodes of febrile seizures) had a greatly increased risk—8, 17, or 49 percent, depending on the association of one, two, or three of the complex features.

Reflex Epilepsy

For a long time it has been known that seizures could be evoked in certain epileptic individuals by a discrete physiologic or psychologic stimulus. The term *reflex epilepsy* is reserved for this small subgroup. Forster has classified these seizures in accordance with their evocative stimuli into five types: (1) *visual*—flickering light, visual patterns, and specific colors (especially red), leading to rapid blinking or eye closure; (2) *auditory*—sudden unexpected noise (startle), specific sounds, musical themes, and voices; (3) *somatosensory*—either a brisk unexpected tap or sudden movement after sitting or lying still, or a prolonged tactile or thermal stimulus to a certain part of the body; (4) *writing* or *reading* of words or numbers; and (5) *eating*.

Visually induced seizures are by far the commonest type of reflex epilepsy. The seizures are generalized and are most often triggered by the photic stimulation of television or an EEG examination or by the photic or pattern stimulation of video games. In other types of reflex epilepsy, the evoked seizure may be focal (beginning often in the part of the body that was stimulated) or generalized and may take the form of one or a series of myoclonic jerks or of an absence or tonic-clonic seizure. Seizures induced by reading, voices, or eating are most often of the complex partial type; seizures induced by music are usually myoclonic. A few such instances of reflex epilepsy have been due to focal cerebral disease, particularly occipital lesions.

Clonazepam, valproate, carbamazepine, and phenytoin are all effective in controlling individual instances of reflex epilepsy. Some patients learn to avert the seizure by undertaking a mental task, e.g., thinking about some distracting subject, counting, etc., or by initiating some type of physical activity. Forster has demonstrated that in certain types of reflex epilepsy, the repeated presentation of the noxious stimulus may eventually render the stimulus innocuous. This technique requires a great deal of time and assiduous reinforcement, which limits its therapeutic value.

Epilepsia Partialis Continua

This is another special type of focal motor epilepsy characterized by persistent rhythmic clonic movements of one muscle group—usually of the face, arm, or leg—which are repeated at fairly regular intervals every few seconds and continue for hours, days, weeks, or months without spreading to other parts of the body. Thus epilepsia partialis continua is, in effect, a highly restricted focal motor status epilepticus. The distal muscles of the leg and arm, especially the flexors of the hand and fingers, are affected more frequently than the proximal ones. In the face, the recurrent contractions involve either the corner of the mouth, or one or both eyelids. Occasionally, isolated muscles of the neck or trunk are affected on one side. The clonic spasms may be accentuated by active or passive movement of the involved muscles and may be reduced in severity but not abolished during sleep.

First described by Kozhevnikov in patients with Russian spring-summer encephalitis, these partial seizures may be induced by a variety of acute or chronic cerebral lesions. In some cases the underlying disease is not apparent and the clonic movements are mistaken for some type of slow tremor or extrapyramidal movement disorder. Most patients with epilepsia partialis continua show focal EEG abnormalities, either repetitive slow-wave abnormalities or sharp waves or spikes over the central areas of the contralateral hemisphere. In some cases, the spike activity can be related precisely in location and time to the clonic movements (Thomas et al). In the series of cases collected by Obeso and colleagues, there were various combinations of epilepsia partialis continua and cutaneous reflex myoclonus (cortical mycolonus occurring only in response to a variety of afferent stimuli); these investigators view epilepsia partialis continua as part of a spectrum of motor disorders that also includes stimulus-sensitive myoclonus, focal motor seizures, and grand mal seizures. As would be expected, a wide range of causative lesions has been implicated—developmental anomalies, encephalitis, demyelinative diseases, brain tumors, and degenerative diseases. In our experience, epilepsia partialis continua has been particularly common in patients with Rassmussen's encephalitis (page 352). As a rule, this type of seizure activity responds poorly or not at all to anticonvulsant medications.

Whether cortical mechanisms or subcortical ones are responsible for epilepsia partialis continua is an unresolved question. The electrophysiologic evidence adduced by Thomas and colleagues favors a cortical origin. The pathologic evidence is less definite. In each of eight cases in which the brain was examined postmortem, they found some degree of involvement of the motor cortex or adjacent cortical area contralateral to the affected limbs. However, all but one of these patients also had some involvement of deeper structures on the same side as the cortical lesion, on the opposite side, or on both sides.

Hysterical Seizures

These seizures, also referred to as "psychogenic" seizures, are nonepileptic in nature—i.e., they are not caused by an abnormal neuronal discharge. They are mentioned here because they are frequently mistaken for epileptic seizures and treated with anticonvulsant drugs, to which they are characteristically unresponsive. Such seizures are most often a symptom of hysteria in the female ("Briquet disease") or of compensation neurosis and malingering in males and females, in which case the terms "sham seizures" and "pseudoseizures" are appropriate. Of course, patients with true epileptic seizures sometimes exhibit hysterical seizures as well, and distinguishing the two may be difficult. Usually, however, the motor display in the course of a nonepileptic seizure is sufficient to identify it as such: completely asynchronous thrashing of the limbs and repeated side-to-side movements of the head; striking out at a person restraining the patient; hand-biting, kicking, trembling, and quivering; pelvic thrusting and opisthotonic arching postures; and screaming or talking during the ictus. In general, pseudoseizures tend to occur in the presence of other people, to be precipitated by emotional factors, and to be prolonged for many minutes or hours; with few exceptions, tongue-biting, incontinence, hurtful falls, or postictal confusion are lacking. No single one of these features is determinative, however.

Prolonged *fugue states* usually have proved to be manifestations of hysteria or a psychopathy even in a known epileptic. The serum creatine kinase and prolactin levels are normal after hysterical seizures; this may be helpful in distinguishing them from genuine convulsions. Where doubt remains, a recording of the ictal or postictal EEG or the combined video and EEG recording of an attack will settle the issue. This subject is discussed further in Chap. 56.

THE NATURE OF THE DISCHARGING LESION

Physiologically, the epileptic seizure has been defined as a sudden alteration of central nervous system (CNS) function resulting from a paroxysmal high-frequency or synchronous low-frequency, high-voltage electrical discharge. This discharge arises from an assemblage of excitable neurons in any part of the cerebral cortex and possibly in secondarily involved subcortical structures as well. Of course, there need not be a visible lesion. Under the proper circumstances, a seizure discharge can be initiated in an entirely normal cerebral cortex, as when the cortex is activated by ingestion or injection of drugs, by withdrawal from alcohol or other sedative drugs, or by repeated stimulation with subconvulsive electrical pulses ("kindling phenomenon").

Just why the neurons in or near a focal cortical lesion discharge abnormally is not fully understood. Some of the electrical properties of a cortical epileptogenic focus suggest that its neurons have been deafferented. Such neurons are known to be hyperexcitable, and they may remain so chronically, in a state of partial depolarization, able to fire irregularly at rates of 700 to 1000 per second. The cytoplasmic membranes of such cells appear to have an increased ionic permeability, which renders them susceptible to activation by hyperthermia, hypoxia, hypoglycemia, hypocalcemia, and hyponatremia, as well as by repeated sensory (e.g., photic) stimulation and during certain phases of sleep (where *hypersynchrony* of neurons is known to occur).

Epileptic foci induced in the animal cortex by the application of penicillin are characterized by spontaneous interictal discharges, during which the neurons of the discharging focus exhibit large, presumably Ca-mediated paroxysmal depolarizing shifts (PDSs), followed by prolonged after-hyperpolarizations (AHPs). The latter also are due in part to Ca-dependent K currents but are better explained by enhanced synaptic inhibition. The PDSs occur synchronously in the penicillin focus and summate to produce surface-recorded interictal EEG spikes; the AHPs correspond to the slow wave of the EEG spike-and-wave complex (Engel).

The neurons surrounding the epileptogenic focus are hyperpolarized from the beginning and are mainly GABAergic, thereby inhibiting the neurons within the focus. Seizure spread probably depends on any factor or agent that activates neurons in the focus or inhibits those surrounding it. The precise mechanisms that govern the transition from a circumscribed interictal discharge to a widespread seizure state are not understood.

Biochemical studies of neurons from a seizure focus have not clarified the problem. Levels of extracellular K are found to be elevated in glial scars near epileptic foci, and a defect in voltage-sensitive Ca channels has also been postulated. Epileptic foci are known to be sensitive to acetylcholine and to be slower in binding and removing it than is normal cerebral cortex. A deficiency of the inhibitory neurotransmitter GABA, increased glycine, decreased taurine, and either decreased or increased glutamic acid have been variously reported in excised human epileptogenic tissue, but whether these changes are the cause or result of seizure activity has not been determined. The interpretation of reported abnormalities of GABA, biogenic amines, and acetylcholine in the cerebrospinal fluid (CSF) of epileptic patients poses similar difficulties.

Concurrent EEG recordings from an epileptogenic cortical focus and subcortical, thalamic, and brainstem centers in the animal model have enabled investigators to construct a sequence of electrical and clinical events that characterize an evolving focal seizure. Firing of the involved neurons in the cortical focus is reflected in the EEG as a series of periodic spike discharges, which increase progressively in amplitude and frequency. Once the intensity of the seizure discharge exceeds a certain point, it overcomes the inhibitory influence of surrounding neurons and spreads to neighboring cortical regions via short corticocortical synaptic connections. If the abnormal discharge remains confined to the cortical focus and the immediate surrounding cortex, there are probably no clinical symptoms or signs of seizure, and the EEG abnormality that persists during the interseizure period reflects this restricted type of abnormal cortical activity.

If unchecked, cortical excitation spreads to the adjacent cortex and to the contralateral cortex via interhemispheric pathways and also to anatomically and functionally related pathways in subcortical nuclei (particularly the basal ganglionic, thalamic, and brainstem reticular nuclei). It is then that the first clinical manifestations of the seizure begin, the initial signs and symptoms depending upon the portion of the brain from which the seizure originates. The excitatory activity from the subcortical nuclei is fed back to the original focus and to the other parts of the forebrain, a mechanism that serves to amplify their excitatory activity and to give rise to the characteristic high-voltage polyspike discharge in the EEG. There is propagation downward to spinal neurons as well, via corticospinal and reticulospinal pathways, yielding a generalized tonic-clonic convulsion.

The spread of excitation to the subcortical, thalamic, and brainstem centers are thought to correspond to the tonic phase of the seizure and loss of consciousness, as well as to the signs of autonomic nervous system overactivity (salivation, mydriasis, tachycardia, increase in blood pressure). Vital functions may be arrested, but usually for only a few seconds. In rare instances, however, death may occur owing to a sustained cessation of respiration, a derangement of cardiac action, or some unknown cause. The development of unconsciousness and the generalized tonic contraction of muscles is reflected in the EEG by a diffuse high-voltage discharge pattern appearing simultaneously over the entire cortex.

Soon after the spread of excitation, a diencephalo-cortical inhibition begins and intermittently interrupts the seizure discharge, changing it from the persistent discharge of the tonic phase to the intermittent bursts of the clonic phase. Electrically, a transition occurs from a continuous polyspike to a spike-and-wave pattern. The intermittent clonic bursts become less and less frequent and finally cease altogether, leaving in their wake an "exhaustion" of the neurons of the epileptogenic focus and a regional increase in permeability of the blood-brain barrier. An overshoot of these inhibitory mechanisms is thought to be the basis of *Todd's postepileptic paralysis* (and of postictal stupor, sensory loss, aphasia, hemianopia, headache, diffuse slow waves in the EEG) and regional edema in T2-weighted MR images. Plum and associates have observed a two- to threefold increase in glucose utilization during seizure discharges, and the paralysis that follows might be due to neuronal depletion of glucose and increase in lactic acid. However, inhibition of epileptogenic neurons may occur in the absence of neuronal exhaustion. The exact roles played by each of these factors in postictal paralysis of function is not settled.

Bilaterally synchronous 3-per-second high-voltage spike-and-wave discharges and seizures resembling absence attacks have been produced in animals by a number of experimental procedures. The spike-and-wave complex, which represents brief excitation followed by slow-wave inhibition, is the type of EEG pattern that characterizes the clonic (inhibitory) phase of the focal motor or grand mal seizure. By contrast, this strong element of inhibition is present diffusely throughout an "absence" attack, a feature that perhaps accounts for the failure of excitation to spread to lower brainstem and spinal structures (tonic-clonic movements do not occur). However, the absence seizure can also at times activate the mechanism for rhythmic myoclonus, probably at an upper brainstem level.

Current physiologic data indicate that the characteristic EEG patterns of both generalized forms of epilepsy (i.e., tonic or tonic-clonic and absence) are generated in the neocortex and are enhanced by the synchronizing influences of subcortical structures. In both instances, the generalization of the clinical and electrical manifestations depends upon activation of a deep, centrally located physiologic mechanism which, for reasons outlined in Chap. 17, includes the midbrain reticular formation and its diencephalic extension, the intralaminar and nonspecific thalamic projection systems (originally referred to by Penfield as the "centrencephalon"). There is no evidence, however, that seizure activity originates in these deep activating structures, for which reason the term *centrencephalic epilepsy* has been replaced by *corticoreticular epilepsy*.

Complex partial seizures are almost always of temporal lobe origin, arising in foci in the medial temporal lobe, amygdaloid nuclei, and hippocampus. Only rarely do they originate in the convexity of the temporal lobe and propagate to the amygdaloid nuclei, hippocampus, and posteroinferior parts of the frontal lobe. Electrical stimulation in these areas reproduces feelings of depersonalization, emotionality, and automatic behavior, the characteristic features of psychomotor epilepsy. The automatic behavior appears to be a direct effect of the temporal lobe discharge in some instances and a postexcitatory or inhibitory effect in others. Loss of memory for the events of the episode may be due to the paralytic effect of the discharge on neurons of the hippocampus.

Of theoretical importance is the observation that a seizure focus, if active for a time, may sometimes establish, via commissural connections, a persistent secondary focus in the corresponding cortical area of the opposite hemisphere (*mirror focus*). The nature of this phenomenon is obscure; it may be similar to the "kindling" phenomenon mentioned earlier in animals, where a repeated nonconvulsive stimulation induces a permanent epileptic focus. No morphologic change is visible in the mirror focus, at least by light microscopy. The mirror focus may be a source of confusion in trying to identify the side of the primary lesion by EEG, but there is little evidence that it can produce chronic seizures in humans. Similarly, there are no firm data supporting a role for kindling in the diagnosis and management of patients with epilepsy (Goldensohn).

Severe seizures may be accompanied by a systemic lactic acidosis with a fall in arterial pH, reduction in arterial oxygen saturation, and rise in P_{CO_2}. These effects are secondary to the respiratory arrest and excessive muscular activity. If prolonged, they may cause hypoxic-ischemic damage to remote areas in the cerebrum, basal ganglia, and cerebellum. In paralyzed and artificially ventilated subjects receiving electroconvulsive therapy, these changes are less marked and the oxygen tension in cerebral venous blood may actually rise. Heart rate, blood pressure, and particularly CSF pressure rise briskly during the seizure. According to Plum and colleagues, the rise in blood pressure evoked by the seizure usually causes a sufficient increase in cerebral blood flow to meet the increased metabolic needs of the brain.

The Electroencephalogram in Epilepsy

The EEG provides confirmation of Hughlings Jackson's concept of epilepsy—that it represents a recurrent, sudden, excessive discharge of cortical neurons. The EEG is undoubtedly the most sensitive, indeed indispensable, tool for the diagnosis of epilepsy, but, like other laboratory tests, it must be used in conjunction with clinical data. In patients with idiopathic generalized seizures and in a high proportion of their relatives, interictal spike-and-wave abnormalities, without any clinical seizure activity are common, especially if the EEG is repeated several times. Contrariwise, a proportion of epileptic patients have a perfectly normal interictal EEG; occasionally, using standard methods of scalp recording, the EEG may even be normal during a simple or complex partial seizure. Furthermore, a small number of healthy persons (approximately 2 to 3 percent) show paroxysmal EEG abnormalities; some of them have a family history of epilepsy (particularly of absence seizures) and may themselves later develop seizures.

EEG abnormalities that characterize a spreading epileptogenic focus and generalization of seizure activity, both the grand mal and absence types, have been described in the preceding section and are illustrated in Chap. 2. At first there was thought to be a characteristic EEG picture for seizures, but further studies have not confirmed this, many patterns being possible. One consistent observation, however, has been that the region of earliest spike activity corresponds best to the epileptogenic focus. This rule guides epilepsy surgery. The postseizure, or postictal, state following generalized seizures also has its EEG correlate, taking the form of random generalized slow waves. Following partial, or focal, seizures, the EEG shows focal slowing. With clinical recovery, the EEG returns to normal or to the preseizure state. A single EEG tracing obtained during the interictal state is abnormal to some degree in 30 to 50 percent of epileptic patients; this figure rises to 60 to 70 percent if patients are subjected to three or more studies utilizing standard activating measures (hyperventilation, photic stimulation, and sleep; see Chap. 2). With structural lesions, focal slow and sharp activity, which is not clearly epileptiform, may be the only clue to a seizure focus.

A higher yield of abnormalities and a more precise definition of seizure types can be obtained by the use of several special EEG procedures. Overnight EEG recording are particularly helpful because focal abnormalities, particularly in the temporal lobes, are most prominent in stage II sleep. Sphenoidal leads have been used to detect inferomedial temporal seizure activity, but they are uncomfortable and probably add no more information than can be obtained by the placement of additional subtemporal scalp electrodes. In our experience, nasopharyngeal electrode recordings are too contaminated by artifact to be clinically useful. Activating procedures such as hyperventilation, photic stroboscopic stimulation, and sleep increase the yield of EEG recordings, as detailed in Chap. 2.

Several *long-term monitoring procedures* are now in common use and are of particular value in the investigation of patients with surgically removable epileptogenic foci. The most common of these makes use of telemetry systems, in which the patient is attached to the EEG machine by cable or radio transmitter without unduly limiting his freedom of movement. The telemetry system is joined to an audiovisual recording system, making it possible to record seizure phenomena (even at night, under dim infrared light) and to synchronize them with the EEG abnormalities. An alternative is the use of a small cassette recorder that is attached to a miniature EEG machine worn by the patient at home and at work. The patient is instructed to push a button if he experiences an "event," which can later be correlated with EEG activity. The role of intensive neurodiagnostic monitoring in the investigation and treatment of seizures is described in detail in the monographs of Engel and of Niedermeyer.

The EEG changes in epilepsy are discussed further in Chap. 2.

Other Laboratory Abnormalities Associated with Seizures

MRI is the most important diagnostic tool for the detection of structural abnormalities underlying epilepsy. Medial temporal sclerosis, glial scars, porenecephaly, heterotopias, and other disorders of neuronal migration can be clearly visualized. After a seizure, particularly one with a focal component, MRI sometimes discloses subtle focal cortical swelling, or, if a contrast agent is administered, an ill-defined cortical blush may be visible on CT or MRI. There is a rough relationship between the duration of seizure activity and the intensity and size of these cortical changes. Likewise, angiography performed soon after a seizure may show a focal area of enhanced flow. This phenomenon was often a source of confusion when radionuclide scans were routinely performed for the evaluation of new seizures—focal increased uptake being mistaken for a tumor or stroke. All of these imaging abnormalities are thought to reflect transient disruption of the blood-brain barrier, and they rarely persist for more than a day or two. Less well understood is the occasional finding on MRI of increased T-2 signal (probably due to hypoxia) in the hippocampi after a prolonged seizure or status epilepticus.

The CSF is known to contain a small number of white blood cells (rarely up to 50/mm^3, but more often in the range of 10/mm^3) in about 15 percent of patients after a seizure. A slight increase in protein is also possible. Like the imaging abnormalities just mentioned, these findings may lead to spurious conclusions about the presence of an intracranial infection, particularly if polymorphonuclear leukocytes predominate. Nonetheless, a significant pleocytosis after a seizure should always be construed as a sign of inflammatory or infectious disease.

Systemic acidosis is a common result of convulsive seizures, and it is not unusual for the serum pH to reach levels near 7 if taken immediately after a seizure. Almost all convulsions produce a rise in serum creatine kinase activity, a finding that could be used more frequently in emergency departments to assist in distinguishing seizures from fainting. Of course, extensive muscle injury from a fall or prolonged compression during a period of unconsciousness can produce the same abnormality.

Concentrations of serum prolactin, like those of other hypothalamic hormones, rise after all types of generalized seizures, including complex partial seizures, but not in absence or myoclonic types. An elevation may help differentiate a hysterical seizure from a genuine one; however, serum prolactin may also be slightly elevated after a syncopal episode. Elevations persist for 10 to 20 min after the seizure. Detection is facilitated by collecting capillary blood from the finger on filter paper for analysis (Fisher et al). There is also a postictal rise in ACTH and serum cortisol, but these changes have a longer latency and briefer duration. If changes in these hormonal levels are used as diagnostic tests, one must have information about normal baseline levels, diurnal variations, and the effects of concurrent medications. Changes in body temperature, sometimes even preceding a seizure, may reflect hypothalamic changes but are far less consistent and therefore difficult to use in clinical work.

Pathology of Epilepsy

In most autopsied cases of primary generalized epilepsy of the grand mal and absence types, the brains have been said to be grossly and microscopically normal. However, it is unlikely that the brains in these cases were examined completely—at least there is not a single case that has been subjected to whole-brain serial sectioning in a search for disorders of neural migration and old scars. Not surprisingly, there are also no visible lesions in the seizure states complicating drug intoxication and withdrawal, and transient hyper- and hyponatremia, and hyper- and hypoglycemia, which presumably represent derangements at the cellular level.

In contrast, most of the so-called secondary epilepsies have definable lesions. These include zones of neuronal loss and gliosis (scars) or other signs of tissue loss such as a porencephaly, dysgenetic cortex, heterotopias, hamartomas, vascular malformations, and tumors. The frequency of these lesions is not fully known. Certainly the focal epilepsies have the highest incidence of structural abnormalities, although in certain cases no morphologic change is visible. In several series of cases of temporal lobe excisions, such as that of Falconer, a specific pattern of neuronal loss with gliosis (sclerosis) in the hippocampal and amygdaloid region was found in the majority, and this abnormality is being increasingly recognized with MRI, as noted below. Vascular malformations, hamartomas, and low-grade astrocytomas were less frequent; in a small number, no abnormalities could be found.

The widespread use of CT and MRI has offered an important surrogate approach to the pathologic study of epilepsy. More than 20 years ago, Gastaut and Gastaut reported that in primary grand mal and absence epilepsies, a CT abnormality was found in approximately 10 percent of cases, whereas in the Lennox-Gastaut syndrome, the West syndrome, and partial complex epilepsies it was found in 52, 77, and 63 percent, respectively. Atrophy, calcification, and malformations were the most frequent changes. MRI and particularly the FLAIR images have proved to be a particularly sensitive means of detecting epileptogenic lesions of the medial-basal portion of the temporal lobes (mesial temporal sclerosis; Fig. 16-1) and cortical heterotopias and other developmental abnormalities that give rise to seizures. Repeatedly, patients are observed in whom MRI disclosed a cortical or subcortical developmental malformation or another surgically treatable lesion of the temporal lobe, even after CT scanning had failed to do so. More subtle epileptogenic foci (areas of hypometabolism or hypoperfusion) may be demonstrated by positron emission tomography (PET) or interictal single photon emission computed tomography (SPECT). Ictal SPECT, which shows hyperperfusion of the seizure focus, is a more demanding but also more sensitive and specific procedure.

With reference to the focal epilepsies, it has not been possible to determine which component of the lesion is responsible for the seizures. Gliosis, fibrosis, vascularization, and meningocerebral cicatrix have all been incriminated, but they are found in nonepileptic foci as well. The Scheibels' Golgi studies of neurons from epileptic foci in the temporal lobe showed distortions of dendrites, loss of dendritic spines, and disorientation of neurons near the scars, but these findings have dubious status since they were not usually compared with similar nonepileptic lesions. Moreover, changes such as these have proved to be nonspecific and artifactual. Once a gliotic focus of whatever cause, bordered by groups of discharging neurons, becomes epileptogenic, it may remain so throughout the patient's lifetime. Nevertheless, with the passage of years, seizures cease in as many as half of childhood epilepsies.

The most common histologic finding in the brains of epileptics is a bilateral loss of neurons in the CA1 segment (Sommer sector) of the pyramidal cell layer of the hippocampus, extending into contiguous segments of the pyramidal layer and the underlying dentate gyrus. It is still undecided whether this neuronal loss is primary or secondary and, if the latter, whether it was incurred at birth (as alluded to above) or happened later as the consequence of seizures. The cessation of seizures in many patients following surgical resection of the medial temporal lobe favors the first interpretation.

Role of Heredity

Most primary epilepsies are thought to have a genetic basis and—as in many other idiopathic diseases, such as diabetes and atherosclerosis—a complex or polygenic inheritance is common. That a genetic factor is operative in primary generalized tonic-clonic seizures is suggested by the finding of a familial incidence in 5 to 10 percent of such patients and, in particular families, the inheritance of a generalized seizure disorder through specific chromosomal regions (Berkovic). The importance of genetic factors in the primary (idiopathic) epilepsies is also underscored by evidence from twin studies; in six major studies, the overall concordance rate was 60 percent for monozygotic twins and 13 percent for dizygotic pairs.

In only a few of the idiopathic seizure disorders is a simple (mendelian) pattern of inheritance recognized. The idiopathic epileptic syndromes of proven inherited type are benign neonatal familial convulsions, inherited as an autosomal dominant trait (Leppert et al), a similar disorder of infantile onset, and the benign myoclonic epilepsy of childhood (autosomal recessive). Another group displays mendelian inheritance, but these are symptomatic epilepsies in which the primary condition is a generalized myoclonic disorder (Lafora disease, Unverricht-Lundborg disease, neuronal ceroid lipofuscinosis and so-called Northern epilepsy syndrome, see page 109). Inherited diseases such as tuberous sclerosis could be added to this group.

A more complex genetic element is clearly discerned in several classic childhood types—absence epilepsy with 3-per-second spike-and-wave discharges and benign epilepsy of childhood with centrotemporal spikes—both of which are transmitted as incompletely penetrant autosomal dominant traits or perhaps in a more complicated manner. Interest has been aroused by the finding that the aberrant genes in the first of these conditions code for abnormal neuronal potassium channels that interfere with cellular repolarization. Certain other primary generalized epilepsies that begin in later childhood are inherited as well; the gene predisposing to juvenile myoclonic epilepsy has been mapped to chromosome 6p and in some cases to 15q (Delgado-Escueta et al). Undoubtedly inherited is the tendency to develop simple febrile convulsions, although it is not clear whether the mode of inheritance is polygenic or autosomal dominant with incomplete penetrance; perhaps either type may explain the occurrence in individual families.

In the partial, or focal, epilepsies (which is the form that seizures take in two-thirds of adults and almost half of the children with epilepsy), the role of heredity is not nearly so clear. However, numerous studies have shown a greater-than-expected incidence of seizures, EEG abnormalities, or both among first-degree relatives of patients with partial epilepsy. Among the familial cortical epilepsies, both a temporal and frontal lobe type has been identified. Both are inherited in a polygenic fashion or as autosomal dominant traits. In the frontal lobe type, not only the chromosome but the gene defect (a mutant neuronal acetylcholine receptor) has been identified. An autosomal dominant familial partial epilepsy with frontal or temporal foci has also been described. The genetics of epilepsy has been reviewed in detail by Anderson and Hauser and by Andermann and by Berkovic.

CLINICAL APPROACH TO THE EPILEPSIES

A physician faced with a patient who seeks advice about an episodic disorder of nervous function must determine, first, whether the episode in question is indeed a seizure; if so, he must determine its pattern and other characteristics; and, finally, he must undertake a search for its cause.

In the diagnosis of epilepsy, history is the key; in most cases the physical examination is relatively unrevealing. A number of laboratory studies should routinely be included in the initial diagnostic workup—CBC, blood chemistries, liver and thyroid function tests, EEG, and most importantly an imaging study of the brain, preferably MRI. CT scanning may be the only feasible study in an emergency or for very young children. Some patients may later need protracted video/EEG monitoring, either in the hospital or with portable equipment at home. Other forms of testing—e.g., cardiac stress tests, Holter monitors, tilt-table testing, long-term patient activated cardiac monitors, and sleep studies—are sometimes indicated in order to exclude some of the disorders listed below.

The conditions most likely to simulate a seizure are syncope and transient ischemic attacks, but also to be considered are migraine, unexplained falls (drop attacks), sleepwalking and rapid-eye-movement (REM) sleep behavior disorder, panic attacks, hypoglycemia, cataplexy, paroxysmal ataxia and choreoathetosis, recurrent transient global amnesia, and the hysterical pseudoseizures discussed above. Often, in emergency departments, it is difficult to differentiate the postictal effects of an unwitnessed seizure from mild confusion following cerebral concussion or a brief loss of consciousness with subarachnoid hemorrhage.

The clinical differences between a seizure and a *syncopal attack* are considered in Chap. 18. It must be emphasized that no single criterion stands inviolate. The authors have erred in mistaking akinetic seizures for simple faints and vasovagal and cardiac faints for seizures. If blood is obtained soon after an episode, elevations in creatine kinase and prolactin may be helpful in the diagnosis of a convulsive seizure. Postictal confusion, incontinence, and a bitten tongue bespeak seizure rather than syncope. Absence attacks may be difficult to identify because of their brevity. Helpful maneuvers are to have the patient hyperventilate in order to elicit an attack or to count aloud for 5 min. Those with frequent absence attacks will pause or skip one or two numbers. The diagnosis of complex partial seizures is the most difficult. These attacks are so variable and so often induce disturbances of behavior and psychic function—rather than obvious interruptions of consciousness—that they may be mistaken for temper tantrums, hysteria, sociopathic behavior, or acute psychosis. The careful questioning of witnesses of an attack is essential. Verbalizations that cannot be remembered, walking aimlessly, or inappropriate actions and social behavior are characteristic. As stated above, we have placed emphasis on amnesia for the events of at least part of the seizure as a crucial criterion for the diagnosis of temporal lobe epilepsy. In all obscure forms of epilepsy, prolonged EEG and video monitoring may prove diagnostic. A mild complex partial seizure, consisting of a brief loss of consciousness and lip smacking, may be mistaken for an absence unless it is kept in mind that the former (but not the latter) is commonly followed by a period of confusion and dysphasia when the language areas are involved.

Epilepsy complicated by states of constitutional mental dullness and confusion poses special problems in diagnosis. Most epileptic patients seen in a general hospital or in office practice show no evidence of mental retardation, regardless of the type of seizure. Undoubtedly, seizures are more common in the mentally retarded, but recurrent seizures in themselves seldom cause intellectual deterioration (Ellenberg et al); when this does happen, one should suspect an underlying degenerative or hereditary metabolic disease. An exception to this statement is the patient with frequent and uncontrolled subclinical seizures (nonconvulsive status) who is drugged or in a postseizure psychotic state. Hospital admission and a systematic study of the seizure state and drug levels is necessary in the analysis of this problem.

Migraine should not be mistaken for a seizure, for reasons discussed on page 187. One feature of the focal neurologic disorder of classic migraine is particularly helpful—namely, the pace of the sequence of cerebral malfunction, over a period of minutes rather than seconds, as in partial epilepsy. Even this criterion may fail occasionally, especially if both migraine and partial seizures are joined, e.g., as expressions of a vacular malformation of the brain.

Useful in the identification of a *transient ischemic attack* (TIA) and its separation from partial epilepsy are the patient's age, evidence of disease of the heart or carotid arteries, and the lack of disorder of consciousness or amnesia. Again, if the ischemic attack is marked by an evolution of symptoms, they tend to develop more slowly than those of a seizure, and by their nature TIAs tend to produce a focal loss of function, while seizures generally cause limb movements and positive sensory phenomena. However, a type of "limb-shaking" TIA and seizures during basilar artery occlusion may be nearly impossible to distinguish from epilepsy.

Drop attacks (falling to the ground without loss of consciousness) remain an enigma (page 399). In most cases, we have failed to substantiate their association with circulatory disturbances of the vertebrobasilar system, and seldom have we observed them to be an expression of atonic or myoclonic epilepsy, but such an occurrence has been reported with the Lennox-Gastaut syndrome. In some instances they represent unexpected falls, especially in stout older women who are sedentary.

Regarding the distinction of narcolepsy, paroxysmal ataxia or choreoathetosis, transient global amnesia, hysterical fugues, panic attacks, and REM sleep behavior disorder from seizures, it is sufficient to be aware of the diagnostic criteria for each of these conditions.

The Probable Causes of Seizure(s) at Different Age Periods (See Table 16-3)

Having concluded that the neurologic disturbance under consideration is one of seizure, the next question is whether it should be subjected to treatment with anti-seizure drugs. This will depend on the seizure type, age of onset, and the clinical setting in which it occurs. Since there are so many seizure types, especially in childhood and adolescence, each one tending to predominate in a certain age period, a clinical advantage accrues to considering seizure problems from just this point of view, i.e., the problem of epilepsy as it presents in each period of life, along with the neurologic and EEG findings, response to drugs, etiology, and prognosis.

Neonatal Seizures The neonatologist is often confronted by a baby who begins to convulse in the first days of postnatal life. In most instances, the seizures are fragmentary—an abrupt movement or posturing of a limb, stiffening of the body, rolling up of the eyes, a pause in respirations, lip smacking, chewing, or bicycling movements of the legs. Even the experienced observer may have difficulty at times in distinguishing seizure activity from the normal movements of the neonate. If manifest seizures are frequent, respiratory support may be needed. The seizures correlate with focal or multifocal cortical discharges. Presumably, the immaturity of the cerebrum prevents the development of a fully organized seizure pattern. The EEG is helpful in diagnosis. Periods of EEG suppression may alternate with sharp or slow waves, or there may be discontinuous theta activity. However, electrical seizure activity may be unattended by clinical manifestations. Aicardi finds an early onset of myoclonic jerks, either fragmentary or massive, with an EEG showing alternation of suppression and complex bursts of activity to be particularly ominous. An extremely malignant form of neonatal seizure evolving later into infantile spasms and Lennox-Gastaut syndrome and leaving in its wake severe brain damage was described by Ohtahara. Most of the reported patients later were mentally retarded (Brett).

Neonatal seizures occurring within 24 to 48 h of a difficult birth are usually indicative of severe cerebral damage, usually anoxic either antenatal or parturitional. Such infants often succumb, and about half of the survivors are seriously handicapped. *Seizures having their onset several days or weeks after birth* are more often an expression of acquired or hereditary metabolic disease. Hypoglycemia is the most frequent cause; hypocalcemia with tetany has become infrequent. A hereditary form of pyridoxine deficiency is a rare cause, sometimes also inducing seizures in utero and characteristically responding promptly to massive doses (100 mg) of vitamin B_6 given intravenously. Biotinidase deficiency is another rare but correctable cause. Nonketotic hyperglycemia, maple syrup urine disease, and other metabolic disorders

Table 16-3
Causes of recurrent seizures in different age groups

Age of onset	*Probable cause*[a]
Neonatal	Congenital maldevelopment, birth injury, anoxia, metabolic disorders (hypocalcemia, hypoglycemia, vitamin B_6 deficiency, biotinidase deficiency, phenylketonuria, and others)
Infancy (1–6 months)	As above Infantile spasms
Early childhood (6 months–3 years)	Infantile spasms, febrile convulsions, birth injury and anoxia, infections, trauma, metabolic disorders, cortical dysgenesis, accidental drug poisoning
Childhood (3–10 years)	Perinatal anoxia, injury at birth or later, infections, thrombosis of cerebral arteries or veins, metabolic disorders, or cortical malformations, "idiopathic," probably inherited, epilepsy (Rolandic epilepsy, etc.)
Adolescence (10–18 years)	Idiopathic epilepsy, including genetically transmitted types, juvenile myoclonic epilepsy, trauma, drugs
Early adulthood (18–25 years)	Idiopathic epilepsy, trauma, neoplasm, withdrawal from alcohol or other sedative drugs
Middle age (35–60 years)	Trauma, neoplasm, vascular disease, alcohol or other drug withdrawal
Late life (over 60 years)	Vascular disease (usually post-infarction), tumor, abscess degenerative disease, trauma (cortical-subcortical encephalomalacia)

[a] *Meningitis* or encephalitis and their complications may be a cause of seizures at any age. This is true also of severe metabolic disturbances. In tropical and subtropical countries, parasitic infection of the CNS is a common cause.

may lead to seizures in the first week or two of life and are expressive of a more diffuse encephalopathy.

Benign forms of neonatal seizures have also been identified. Plouin has described a form of benign neonatal clonic convulsions beginning on days 2 and 3, up to day 7, without specific EEG changes. They then remit. The inheritance is autosomal dominant. In nonfamilial cases with onset on days 4 to 6, the partial seizures may increase to status epilepticus. The EEG consists of discontinuous theta activity. In both these groups, the outlook for normal development is good and seizures seldom recur later in life. There are also benign forms of polymyoclonus without seizures or EEG abnormality in this age period. Some occur only with slow-wave sleep or feeding. They disappear after a few months and require no treatment. A form of benign nocturnal myoclonus in the neonate has also been documented.

Infantile Seizures (Occurring in the First Months, Up to 2 Years) Neonatal seizures may continue into the infantile period, or seizures may begin in an infant who seemed to be normal up to the time of the first convulsive attack. The most characteristic pattern at this age is the massive myoclonic jerk of head and arms leading to flexion or, less often, to extension of the body (infantile spasms, salaam spasms). The latter form, known as the West syndrome and described earlier, is the most threatening. We have observed the same seizure pattern in infants with tuberous sclerosis (diagnosed in infancy by dermal white spots), phenylketonuria, Sturge-Weber angiomatosis, and other diseases beginning in this age period. West syndrome is probably a metabolic encephalopathy of unknown type or, in some cases, a cortical dysgenesis (Jellinger) and is identified by an EEG picture of large bilateral slow waves and multifocal spikes (*hypsarrhythmia*). Again, there is a benign form of infantile myoclonic epilepsy in which repetitive myoclonic jerking occurs in otherwise normal infants and whose EEG shows only spike waves in early sleep.

However, when the myoclonus begins in infancy with fever and unilateral or bilateral clonic seizures or with partial seizures that are followed by focal neurologic abnormalities, there is a likelihood of developmental delay. The latter types are sometimes referred to as febrile seizures, but, as indicated above, they must be distinguished from the benign familial febrile seizure syndrome. Infantile spasms cease by the fifth year and are replaced by partial and generalized grand mal seizures.

Seizures Presenting in Early Childhood (Onset during the First 5 to 6 Years) At this age, the first burst of seizures may take the form of status epilepticus and, if not successfully controlled, may end fatally. Or the convulsive state may present around the age of 4 years as a focal myoclonus with or without astatic seizures, atypical absence, or generalized tonic-clonic seizures. The EEG, repeated if initially normal, is most helpful in diagnosis; it reveals a paroxysmal 2- to 2.5-per-second spike-and-wave pattern on a background of predominant 4- to 7-Hz slow waves. This syndrome is difficult to separate from the Lennox-Gastaut syndrome. It proves difficult to treat and is likely to be associated with developmental retardation. The MRI may be helpful in identifying a birth injury or cortical dysgenesis.

In contrast, the more typical absence, with its regularly recurring 3-per-second spike-and-wave EEG abnormality, also begins in this age period (rarely before 4 years) and carries a good prognosis. This seizure disorder responds well to medications, as indicated further on. Its features are fully described on page 334.

A number of partial epilepsies may appear for the first time during this age period and carry a good prognosis, i.e., the neurologic and intellectual capacities remain relatively unimpaired and seizures may cease in adolescence. These disorders begin between 3 and 13 years of age, and there is often a familial predisposition. Most are marked by distinctive focal spike activity that is greatly accentuated by sleep (see above, in reference to benign childhood epilepsy with centrotemporal or occipital spikes). In one form, unilateral tonic or clonic contractions of the face and limbs recur repeatedly with or without paresthesias; anarthria follows the seizure. There are central and temporal spikes in the EEG interictally. The focus may involve an occipital lobe with EEG spiking on eye closure, according to Gastaut. An acquired aphasia was noted by Landau and Kleffner to mark the beginning of an illness in which there are partial or generalized motor seizures and multifocal spike or spike-and-wave discharges in the EEG. Tumor and arteriovenous malformation are rare causes in this age group.

Rasmussen encephalitis In other rare cases, a lesion, usually identified at operation, takes the form of a chronic focal encephalitis. In 1958, Rasmussen described three children in each of whom the clinical problem consisted of intractable focal epilepsy in association with a progressive hemiparesis. Biopsies of the cerebral cortex disclosed a mild meningeal infiltration of inflammatory cells and an encephalitic process marked by neuronal destruction, neuronophagia, some degree of tissue necrosis, and perivascular cuffing. Many additional cases were soon uncovered, and by 1991, in a publication devoted to this subject (edited by Andermann), Rasmussen was able to report on the natural history of 48 personally observed patients.

The expanded view of the syndrome has added several interesting features. All the patients were children aged 3 to 15 years, more girls than boys. Half of them had epilepsia partialis continua. The progression of the disease led to hemiplegia or other deficits and brain atrophy in most cases. The CSF has shown pleocytosis and sometimes oligoclonal bands. Focal cortical and subcortical lesions have been well visualized by MRI and are bilateral in some cases. The neuropathology of five fully autopsied cases revealed extensive destruction of the cortex and white matter with intense gliosis but with lingering inflammatory reactions. The recent finding of antibodies to glutamate receptors in a proportion of patients has raised interest in an immune causation (see review by Antel and Rasmussen). Also an autoimmune hypothesis has been proposed based on the findings of Twyman and colleagues that these antibodies cause seizures in rabbits and lead to the release of the neurotoxin kainate in cell cultures.

The unrelenting course of the disease has defied medical therapy. In some patients the process has eventually burned out, but in those with continuous focal epilepsy the seizures continued despite all antiepileptic drugs. The use of full doses of corticosteroids, if started within the first year of the disease, proved beneficial in 5 of the 8 patients treated by Chinchilla and colleagues. Repeated plasma exchanges or immune globulin have been tried, but the results are difficult to interpret. When the disease is extensive and unilateral, neurosurgeons have in the past resorted to hemispherectomy. The authors have cared for a number of such patients with the same discouraging results.

Seizures in Later Childhood and Adolescence

These represent the most common epileptic problem in general practice. Here, we face two different issues: one relates to the nature and management of the first seizure in an otherwise normal person and the other to the management of a patient who has had one or more seizures at some time in the past. With respect to the first, a search for a cause by CT, MRI, CSF examination, and EEG rarely discloses a tumor or a vascular malformation and the epilepsy is classed as idiopathic. The type of seizure that first brings the child or adolescent to medical attention is most likely to be a generalized tonic-clonic convulsion and often marks the beginning of a juvenile myoclonic epilepsy, as described on page 335. In the second type of case, in which there had been some type of seizure at an earlier period, one should suspect a developmental disorder, parturitional hypoxic-ischemic encephalopathy (birth injury), or one of the hereditary metabolic diseases.

Several groups of patients fall between these two distinct types. Development may have been slightly delayed, but reportedly no seizures had occurred earlier in life. Closer investigation may disclose absence seizures, not always recognized as such by parents or teachers, and a typical absence EEG which points more directly to a genetic factor and to a more favorable prognosis.

When the seizures are an expression of a longstanding epileptic focus or foci that had been associated with mental backwardness, scholastic failure, and inadequacy of social adjustment, the problem is much more difficult and demanding. Poor compliance with therapy, muddled thinking, and bizarre ideation on the part of the patient and unintelligent parents may pose problems as difficult as the seizures themselves. Some patients of this latter group will eventually fall into the category of epilepsy with complex partial seizures. In adulthood, the seizures may continue to interfere with work, marriage, and family relationships. In the interictal periods, the patients may exhibit bursts of bad temper, and they commonly have wide mood swings of sadness and anger or elation. As indicated earlier, paranoid ideation or a frank hallucinatory-delusional psychosis sometimes appears and lasts for weeks after a single seizure, without any specific EEG changes.

In the large group with *intractable seizures in early life*, many of which are indiscriminately called febrile seizures, nearly half end up in the group identified as temporal lobe epilepsies. Huttenlocher and Hapke, in a follow-up study of 145 infants and children with intractable epilepsy, found that the majority had borderline or subnormal intelligence. This group stands in contrast to the group of otherwise normal adolescents with a first seizure, whose scholastic progress and social and emotional adjustment are little affected.

Finally, a first generalized seizure may bring to attention an adolescent who is abusing alcohol or another drug. Usually it is difficult from the clinical information alone to determine the type and quantity of the drug(s) and the setting in which the seizure occurred—whether in relation to overdose or withdrawal. While steps must be taken to exclude an infection of the nervous system, vascular occlusion, or trauma, the more important issue is generally not the seizure but the addiction and its control.

Regarding treatment, opinion is divided on whether treatment is required for the older child or adolescent who comes to medical attention because of a first seizure. When a large number of such cases have been left untreated, such as in the series reported by Hesdorfer and colleagues, the risk of another seizure over 10 years was 13 percent unless the first episode was status epilepticus, in which case the risk was 41 percent. Age, sex, and the circumstances of the seizure (withdrawal from drugs or alcohol, myoclonic episodes, family history, etc.) all figured into the risk.

Seizures with Onset in Adult Life, Secondary to Medical Disease Several primary diseases of the brain often announce themselves by an acute convulsive state, particularly *primary and metastatic brain tumors*; these are discussed further on in the section on seizures of late adult life. Here we focus on generalized medical disorders as causes of single and repeated seizures.

Withdrawal Seizures The possibility of abstinence seizures in patients who had chronically abused alcohol, barbiturates, or benzodiazepine sedative drugs must always be considered when seizures occur for the first time in adult life (or even in adolescence) Suspicion of this mechanism is raised by the stigmata of alcohol abuse or a history of prolonged nervousness and depression requiring sedation. Also, sleep disturbance, tremulousness, disorientation, illusions, and hallucinations are often associated with the convulsive phase of the illness. Seizures in this setting may occur singly, but more often they occur in a brief flurry, the entire convulsive period lasting for several hours and rarely for a day or longer, during which time the patient may be unduly sensitive to photic stimulation. Alcohol and other drug-related seizures are discussed in more detail on pages 1241 and 1261.

Infections An outburst of seizures is also a prominent feature of all varieties of *bacterial meningitis*, more so in children than in adults. Fever, headache, and stiff neck usually provide the clues to diagnosis, and lumbar puncture yields the salient data. Myoclonic jerking and seizures appear early in acute *herpes simplex encephalitis* and other forms of viral, treponemal, and parasitic encephalitis including those derived from HIV infection, both directly and indirectly, through toxoplasmosis and brain lymphoma, in subacute sclerosing panencephalitis, and in lipid storage diseases. In tropical countries, cysticercosis and tuberculous granulomas of the brain are common causes of epilepsy. Seizure(s) without fever or stiff neck may be the initial manifestation of syphilitic meningitis.

Endogenous Metabolic Encephalopathies *Uremia* is a condition with a strong convulsive tendency. Of interest is the relation of seizures to the development of anuric renal failure, generally from acute tubular necrosis but occasionally due to glomerular disease. Uremia may be tolerated for several days, without the appearance of neurologic signs, and then there is an abrupt onset of twitching, trembling, myoclonic jerks, and generalized motor seizures. Tetany may be added. The motor display, one of the most dramatic in medicine, lasts several days until the patient sinks into terminal coma or recovers, depending on the outcome of the renal disease and its treatment by dialysis. When this twitch-convulsive syndrome accompanies lupus erythematosus, seizures of undetermined cause, or generalized neoplasia, one can nearly always be sure that it has its basis in renal failure.

Other *acute metabolic illnesses and electrolytic disorders* complicated by generalized and multifocal motor seizures are hyponatremia and its opposite, a hypernatremic hyperosmolar state, thyrotoxic storm, porphyria, hypoglycemia, hyperglycemia, hypomagnesemia, and hypocalcemia. In all these cases *rapidly evolving electrolyte abnormalities are more likely to cause seizures than those occurring gradually*. For this reason it is not possible to assign absolute levels of electrolyte, BUN, or glucose concentrations above or below which seizures are likely to occur. Lead (in children) and mercury (in children and adults) are the most frequent of the metallic poisons that cause convulsions.

In most cases of seizures due to metabolic and withdrawal states, treatment with anticonvulsants is not necessary as long as the underlying disturbance is rectified. Indeed, anticonvulsants are often ineffective if the metabolic disorder persists.

Generalized seizures, with or without twitching, may occur in the advanced stages of many other illnesses, such as *hypertensive encephalopathy*, sepsis—especially gram-negative septicemia with shock—hepatic stupor, and intractable congestive heart failure. Usually, seizures in these circumstances can be traced to an associated metabolic abnormality and are revealed by appropriate studies of the blood.

Medications A large number of medications can cause seizures, usually when toxic blood levels are attained. The antibiotic imipenem and excessive doses of other penicillin congeners will on occasion cause seizures, particularly if renal failure leads to their accumulation. Cefapime, a fourth generation cephalosporin, widely used for the treatment of gram negative sepsis, can result in status epilepticus, especially if given in excessive dosage (Dixit et al). The tricyclic antidepressants, bupropion (Wellbutrin), and lithium may cause seizures, particularly in the presence of a structural brain lesion. Lidocaine and aminophylline are known to induce a single convulsion if administered too quickly or in excessive doses. The list of medications that at one time or another have been associated with a convulsion is long, and if no other explanation for a single seizure is evident, the physician is advised to look up in standard references the side effects of the drugs being given to the patient. In a few of our otherwise healthy adult patients, extreme *sleep deprivation* coupled with ingestion of large doses of antibiotics or adrenergic medications or other remedies that are used indiscriminately for the symptomatic relief of colds has been the only plausible explanation after extensive search for the cause of a single or doublet seizure.

Global Arrest of Circulation and Cerebrovascular Diseases Cardiac arrest, suffocation or respiratory failure, CO poisoning, or other causes of *hypoxic encephalopathy* tend to induce diffuse myoclonic jerking and generalized seizures as cardiac function is resumed. The myoclonic-convulsive phase of this condition may last only a few hours or days, in association with coma, stupor, and confusion; or it may persist indefinitely as an intention myoclonus-convulsive state.

Convulsive seizures are relatively uncommon occurrences in the evolving phases of an arterial stroke. Only exceptionally will acute embolic infarction of the brain cause a focal fit at its onset, though embolic infarcts involving the cortex later become epileptogenic in almost 25 percent of cases. Similarly, thrombotic infarcts are almost never convulsive at their onset. On the other hand, *cortical venous thrombosis* with ischemia and infarction is highly epileptogenic, but fortunately rare. The same is true for hypertensive encephalopathy. The rupture of a saccular aneurysm is sometimes marked by one or two generalized convulsions. Subcortical cerebral hemorrhages occasionally become sources of recurrent focal seizures.

Seizures in Pregnancy Here one contends with two types of problem: one, the woman with epilepsy who becomes pregnant; the other, the woman who has her first seizure during pregnancy. In respect to the first group, about half of the epileptic women who become pregnant have no change in seizure frequency or severity; in about 25 percent, the frequency increases; and in an equal number, it lessens. In a large cohort of such women, there was a slight increase in the number of stillbirths and a doubling in the expected incidence of mental retardation and nonfebrile seizures in their offspring. Parturition itself was unaffected except that in those taking phenytoin, bleeding was slightly increased (but easily controlled with vitamin K). Plasma levels of most anticonvulsant drugs, both free and protein-bound fractions, fall slightly in pregnancy, since the drugs are cleared more rapidly from the blood. The conventional drugs (phenytoin, carbamazepine, phenobarbital, valproate) are all appropriate in pregnancy. The main practical issue is the potential teratogenicity of anticonvulsant drugs. The most common recorded teratogenic effects have been cleft lip and cleft palate, but a subtle facial dysmorphism ("fetal anticonvulsant syndrome"), similar to the fetal alcohol syndrome, has also been described. In general the risk of congenital defects is low—2 to 3 percent in the overall population of pregnant women—which increases to 4 to 5 percent in women taking anticonvulsant drugs during pregnancy. This risk is shared more or less equally by all the major anticonvulsants (lamotrigine and several other new drugs may not carry the risk).

The newer anticonvulsants should probably be avoided until greater experience has been obtained. The risk of neural tube defects (possibly increased by anticonvulsants and greatest with valproate) can be reduced by giving folate before pregnancy has begun. Also, these risks are greater in women taking more than one anticonvulsant, so that monotherapy is a desirable goal. And since it is essential to prevent convulsions in the pregnant epileptic, anticonvulsant medication should not be discontinued or arbitrarily reduced, particularly if there have been convulsions in the recent past.

The conventional anticonvulsants also seem to be safe for the baby during breast-feeding in that only small amounts are excreted in lactated milk. For example, carbamazepine in human milk is found to be 40 percent of the mother's serum concentration, and this results in a neonatal blood level that is below the conventionally detectable amount. Phenytoin is excreted at 15 percent of maternal serum concentration, and valproate, being highly protein-bound, is virtually absent in breast milk. No adverse effects have been attributed to these small amounts of drug.

Eclampsia during the last trimester of pregnancy may announce itself by hypertension and convulsions; the latter are generalized and occur in a cluster. The standard practice is to induce labor or perform cesarean section and manage the seizures as one would manage those of hypertensive encephalopathy (of which this is one type). The administration of magnesium sulfate continues to be the favored treatment for the prevention of eclamptic seizures; two randomized trials have re-established its value in preventing seizures in pre-eclamptic women (Lucas et al) and in avoiding a second convulsion once one had occurred (Eclampsia Trial Collaborative Group). Magnesium sulfate, 10 g intramuscularly, followed by 5 g every 4 h, proved comparable to standard doses of phenytoin as prophylaxis for seizures. Our colleagues use a regimen of 4 g intravenously over 5 to 10 min followed by a maintenance dose of 5 g every 4 h intramuscularly or 1 to 2 g per hour intravenously. Whether magnesium is as effective in the management of active convulsions of toxemia remains uncertain. In nontoxic gestational epilepsy, about 25 percent of patients are found to have some disease (neoplastic, vascular, or traumatic) that will persist after the pregnancy is terminated.

Focal or Generalized Seizures in Late Adult Life

Hauser and Kurland have reported a marked increase in the incidence of seizures as the population ages—from 11.9 per 100,000 in the 40- to 60-year age group to 82 per 100,000 in those 60 years of age or older. A person in the latter age group who begins to have seizures of either partial or generalized type is always to be suspected of harboring a primary or secondary tumor or an infarct that had not declared itself clinically. This is a matter usually settled by the neurologic examination and by CT scans or MRI. Tumor, either primary or secondary, will be found to account for about half the cases of seizures occurring for the first time in late adult life. In our clinical material, almost 25 percent of patients with infarction involving the cerebral cortex later developed recurrent partial or generalized seizures. According to Sung and Chu, previous infarcts are by far the most common lesions underlying status epilepticus in late adult life. Cortical and subcortical encephalomalacia, the result of previous traumatic contusions, are another important cause of seizures, particularly among alcoholics; the lesions are revealed by brain imaging and are typically located in the anterior frontal and temporal lobes. Brain abscess and other inflammatory and infectious illnesses are less common except in tropical regions. Seizures as a result of Alzheimer and other degenerative diseases are decidedly rare.

In the not infrequent cases of an adult with a first seizure that remains unexplained after thorough evaluation, it has been our practice to administer an anticonvulsant and to reevaluate the situation in a matter of 6 to 12 months, with the goal of eventually discontinuing medication. Sometimes, a second MRI and EEG are performed to exclude focal abnormalities that were not appreciated during the initial evaluation, but usually these studies are again unrevealing. This approach has been prompted by data such as those of Hauser and colleagues, who found that about one-third of patients with a single unprovoked seizure will have another seizure within 5 years; the risk is even greater if there is a history of seizures in a sibling, a complex febrile convulsion in childhood, or a spike-and-wave abnormality in the EEG. Moreover, the risk of recurrence is greatest in the first 24 months. In patients with two or three unexplained seizures, three-quarters have further seizures in the subsequent 4 years.

TREATMENT

The treatment of epilepsy of all types can be divided into four parts: the use of antiepileptic drugs, the surgical excision of epileptic foci and other surgical measures, the removal of causative and precipitating factors, and the regulation of physical and mental activity.

The Use of Antiepileptic Drugs—General Principles

The use of antiepileptic drugs is the most important facet of treatment. In approximately 70 percent of all patients with epilepsy, the seizures are controlled completely or almost completely by the use of antiepileptic drugs; in an additional 20 to 25 percent, the attacks are significantly reduced in frequency and severity. The most commonly used drugs are listed in Table 16-4, along with their dosages, effective blood levels, and serum half-lives. Because of the long half-lives of phenytoin, phenobarbital, and ethosuximide, these drugs need be taken only once daily, preferably at bedtime. Valproate and carbamazepine have shorter half-lives, and their administration should be spaced during the day. It is also useful to be familiar with the serum protein-binding characteristics of antiepileptic drugs and the interactions among these drugs, and between antiepileptic and other drugs.

Certain drugs are more effective in one type of seizure than in another, and it is necessary to use the proper drugs in optimum dosages for the different types of seizures. Initially, only one drug should be used and the dosage increased until sustained therapeutic levels have been assured. If seizures are not controlled by the first drug, a different drug should be tried, but frequent

Table 16-4
Common antiepileptic drugs

Generic name	Trade name	Usual dosage: Children, mg/kg	Usual dosage: Adults, mg/day	Principal therapeutic indications	Serum half-life, hours	Effective blood level,[a] μg/mL
Major anticonvulsants used as monotherapy						
Valproate	Depakote	30–60	1000–3000	Generalized tonic-clonic, complex partial, absence, myoclonic	6–15	50–100
Phenytoin	Dilantin	4–7	300–400	Generalized tonic-clonic, complex partial, absence, myoclonic	12–36	10–20
Carbamazepine	Tegretol	20–30	600–1200[b]	Tonic-clonic, complex partial	14–25	4–12
Phenobarbital	Luminal	3–5 (8 for infants)	90–200	Tonic-clonic, simple and complex	40–120	15–40
Lamotrigine	Lamicatal	0.5	3–500	Generalized	15–60	
Adjuvant and special use anticonvulsants						
Topiramate	Topimax		400	Partial	20–30	
Vigabatrin			4000	Partial and secondary generalizing	20–40	
Tiagabine			30–60	Partial	7–9	
Gabapentin	Neurontin	30–60	900–1800[b]	Partial	5–7	
Primidone	Mysoline	10–25	750–1500[b]	Tonic-clonic, simple and complex partial	6–18	5–12
Ethosuximide	Zarontin	20–40	750–1500	Absence	20–60	50–100
Methosuximide	Celontin	10–20	500–1000	Absence	28–50	40–100
ACTH		40–60 Units daily		Infantile spasms		
Clonazepam	Klonipin	0.01–0.2	2–10	Absence, myoclonus	18–50	0.01–0.07
Anticonvulsants for status epilepticus (initial loading or continuous infusion doses shown)[c]- phenytoin and phenobarbital used in doses higher than shown above						
Diazepam	Valium	0.15–2	2–20	Status epilepticus		
Lorazepam	Ativan	0.03–0.22	2–20	Status epilepticus		
Midazolam	Versed		0.1–0.4 mg/kg/h	Status epilepticus		
Propofol	Diprivan	2.5–3.5	2-8 mg/kg/h	Status epilepticus		
Fosphenytoin	Cerebyx	30–50 mg	1000–1500	Status epileptics		10–20

[a] Average trough values.
[b] May require slow dose escalation.
[c] Administered intravenously.

shifting of drugs is not advisable; each should be given an adequate trial before another is substituted. In changing medication, the dosage of the new drug should be increased gradually to an optimum level while the dosage of the old drug is gradually decreased; the sudden withdrawal of a drug may lead to an increase in seizure frequency or status epilepticus, even though a new drug is substituted. If seizures are still not controlled, a second drug can then be added. Seldom if ever are more than two drugs necessary; the physician should make an effort to succeed with one drug and with no more than two, given in adequate dosage. Once an anticonvulsant or a combination of anticonvulsants is found to be effective, their use in most cases should be maintained for a period of years.

The therapeutic dose for any given patient must be determined, to some extent, by trial and error and by measurement of serum levels, as described below. Not uncommonly a drug is discarded as being ineffective, when a slight increase in dosage would have led to disappearance of the attacks. It is, however, also an error to administer a drug to the point where the patient is so dull and stupefied that the toxic effects are more incapacitating than the seizures. It is highly doubtful that prolonged administration of anticonvulsant medication is a factor in the development of the mental deterioration that occurs in a small percentage of patients with convulsive seizures. In fact, improvement in mentation sometimes occurs following control of the seizures by the proper dosage of appropriate antiepileptic drugs.

The management of seizures with drugs is greatly facilitated by having the patient chart his daily medication and the number, time, and circumstances of seizures. Some patients find it helpful to use a dispenser that is filled on Sunday, for example, with sufficient medication to last the week. This indicates to the patient whether a dose had been missed and whether the supply of medications is running low.

The proper use of anticonvulsant drugs is considerably enhanced by the measurement of their *serum levels*. The concentrations of almost all the commonly used drugs can be measured on a single specimen by immunoassay or by the older gas-liquid chromatography method. These measurements are helpful in regulating dosage, detecting irregular drug intake, identifying the toxic agent in patients taking more than one drug, and assuring patient compliance. Blood for serum levels is ideally drawn in the morning before breakfast and the first ingestion of anticonvulsants ("trough levels"), a practice that introduces consistency in the measurement of drug concentrations.

The effective serum levels for each of the commonly used anticonvulsant drugs are indicated in Table 16-4. The upper and lower levels of the "therapeutic range" are not to be regarded as immutable limits within which the serum values must fit. In some patients, seizures are controlled at serum levels below the therapeutic range; in others, the seizures continue despite serum values within this range. In the latter patients, seizures are sometimes controlled by raising levels above the therapeutic range but not to the point of producing clinical toxicity. In general, higher serum concentrations of drugs are necessary for the control of simple or complex partial seizures than for the control of tonic-clonic seizures alone (Schmidt et al). It is to be noted that the blood level is not a precise measure of the amount of drug entering the brain, because—in the case of the most widely used anticonvulsants—the larger proportion of drug is bound to albumin and does not penetrate nervous tissue. Laboratory measurements of the serum concentration, however, detect only the protein-bound fraction. In patients who are malnourished or chronically ill or who have a constitutional reduction in proteins, this may lead to intoxication at low total serum levels. Certain anticonvulsants also have active metabolites that may produce toxicity but are not measured by methods ordinarily used to determine serum concentrations of antiepileptic drugs. This is particularly true for the epoxide of carbamazepine. The situation may be further complicated by interactions between one anticonvulsant and the metabolites of another, as, for example, the inhibition of epoxide hydrolase by valproic acid, leading to toxicity through the buildup of carbamazepine epoxide. In circumstances of unexplained toxicity in the face of conventionally obtained serum levels that are normal, it is therefore important to measure the levels of free drug and the concentration of active metabolites by chromatographic techniques.

Finally, the pharmacokinetics of each drug play a role in toxicity and the serum level that is achieved with each alteration in the dose. This is particularly true of phenytoin, which has nonlinear kinetics once serum concentrations reach 10 μg/mL, as the result of saturation of liver enzymatic capacity. For this reason, the typical increase in dose from 300 to 400 mg daily often results in a disproportionate elevation of the serum level and toxic side effects. These elevations are also accompanied by a prolongation of the serum half-life, which increases the time to reach a steady-state phenytoin concentration after dosage adjustments. Similarly, carbamazepine is known to induce its own metabolism, so that doses adequate to control seizures at the outset of therapy are no longer effective several weeks later.

Always to be considered in the use of an antiepileptic drug, as already mentioned, is its possible interactions with other drugs. Many such interactions have been demonstrated, but only a few are of clinical significance, requiring adjustment of drug dosages (Kutt). Important drugs in this respect are chloramphenicol, which causes the accumulation of phenytoin and phenobarbital, and erythromycin, which causes the accumulation of carbamazepine. Antacids reduce the blood phenytoin concentration, whereas cimetidine does the opposite. Salicylates may reduce the plasma levels of anticonvulsant drugs. Among anticonvulsant drugs, valproate often leads to accumulation of phenytoin and of phenobarbital by displacing them from serum proteins; equally important, warfarin levels are decreased by the addition of phenobarbital or carbamazepine and may be increased by phenytoin. Enzyme-inducing drugs such as phenytoin, carbamazepine, and barbiturates can greatly increase the chance of breakthrough menstrual bleeding in women taking oral contraceptives, and adjustments in the amount of estradiol must be made.

Hepatic failure can seriously affect antiepileptic anticonvulsant drug concentrations, since most of these drugs are metabolized in the liver. Serum levels must be checked frequently, and if there is hypoalbuminemia, it is advisable to obtain free drug levels for reasons just mentioned. Renal failure has only an indirect effect on the concentrations of the commonly used anticonvulsants, but some newer agents, such as vigabatrin and gabapentin, are renally excreted. The main renal effects have to do with alterations in protein binding that are induced by uremia. In end-stage renal failure, serum levels are not an accurate guide to therapy, and the goal should be to attain free phenytoin concentrations of 1 to 2 μg/mL. In addition, uremia causes the accumulation of phenytoin metabolites, which are measured with the parent drug by enzyme-multiplied immunoassay techniques. In patients who are being dialyzed, total blood levels of phenytoin tend to be low because of decreaed protein binding; in this situation it is also necessary to track free (unbound) phenytoin levels. Dialysis does remove phenobarbital and ethosuximide, and dosage may need to be increased. Decreased phenytoin levels are also known to occur during viral illnesses, and supplementary doses are occasionally necessary.

Once an effective anticonvulsant regimen has been established, it must usually be continued for many years. Because of the long-term toxic effects of such a regimen, many neurologists choose not to institute anticonvulsant therapy after the occurrence of a single generalized seizure in an otherwise normal child or adult (normal EEG and MRI; no family history of seizures). Our more conservative approach of administering an anticonvulsant for 6 to 12 months and then re-evaluating the patient has already been mentioned.

Discontinuing Anticonvulsants Withdrawal of anticonvulsant drugs may be undertaken in patients who have been free of seizures for a prolonged period. There are few firm rules to guide the physician in this decision. A safe plan, applicable to most forms of epilepsy, is to obtain an EEG whenever withdrawal of medication is contemplated; if the EEG is abnormal, it is generally better to continue treatment. A prospective study by Callaghan and colleagues has shown that in patients who had been seizure-free during 2 years of treatment with a single drug, one-third relapsed after discontinuation of the drug, and this relapse rate was much the same in adults and children and whether the drug was reduced over a period of weeks or months. The relapse rate was less in patients with absence and generalized-onset seizures than in those with complex partial seizures and secondary generalization. Other authors have suggested that a longer seizure-free period is associated with a lesser rate of relapse (see reviews of Todt and of Pedley and comments above, under "Focal or Generalized Seizures in Late Adult Life"). Patients with juvenile myoclonic epilepsy, even those with long seizure-free periods, should probably continue with medication lifelong. The appropriate duration of treatment for postinfarction epilepsy has not been studied and most neurologists continue to use one drug indefinitely. Interestingly, epilepsy caused by military brain wounds tends to be reduced in frequency or to disappear in 20 to 30 years, no longer requiring treatment.

The Use of Specific Drugs in Treatment of Seizures

Phenytoin, *carbamazepine*, and *valproate* are more or less equally effective in the treatment of both generalized and partial seizures (see Table 16-4 for typical initial dosages). Valproate is probably less effective in the treatment of complex partial seizures. The first two of these drugs putatively act by blocking sodium channels, thus preventing abnormal neuronal firing and seizure spread.

Since carbamazepine has somewhat fewer side effects it is preferred as the initial drug by many neurologists, but phenytoin and valproate have very similar therapeutic and side-effect profiles. Carbamazepine and valproate are probably preferable to phenytoin for epileptic children because they do not coarsen facial features and do not produce gum hypertrophy or breast enlargment. In many cases, phenytoin or carbamazepine alone will control the seizures. If not, the use of valproate (which facilitates GABA activity) alone or the combined use of phenytoin and carbamazepine is sometimes effective. In others, the addition of valproate to carbamazepine may prove effective.

Rash, fever, lymphadenopathy, eosinophilia and other blood dyscrasias, and polyarteritis are manifestations of an idiosyncratic *phenytoin hypersensitivity*; their occurrence calls for discontinuation of the medication. *Overdose with phenytoin* causes ataxia, diplopia, and stupor. The prolonged use of phenytoin often leads to hirsutism (mainly in young girls), hypertrophy of gums, and coarsening of facial features in children. Chronic phenytoin intoxication may rarely be associated with peripheral neuropathy and probably with a form of cerebellar degeneration (Lindvall and Nilsson). An antifolate effect on blood and interference with vitamin K metabolism have also been reported. The pregnant woman taking phenytoin should be given vitamin K before delivery and the newborn infant should receive vitamin K as well, to prevent bleeding. Phenytoin should not be used together with disulfiram (Antabuse), chloramphenicol, sulfamethizole, phenylbutazone, or cyclophosphamide, and the use of either phenobarbital or phenytoin is not advisable in patients receiving warfarin (Coumadin) because of the undesirable interactions already described.

Carbamazepine causes many of the same side effects as phenytoin, but to a slightly lesser degree. Leukopenia is common and rare instances of pancytopenia, hyponatremia, and diabetes insipidus have been reported as idiosyncratic reactions. It is essential, therefore, that a complete blood count be done before treatment is instituted, and that the white cell count be checked regularly. A newly introduced analogue of carbamazepine *oxcarbazepine* is said to have even fewer side effects than the parent drug, but its long-term therapeutic effects still have to be established.

Valproate is occasionally hepatotoxic, an adverse effect that is usually (but not invariably) limited to children 2 years of age and younger. The use of valproate with hepatic enzyme–inducing drugs increases the risk of liver toxicity. However, mild elevations of serum ammonia and mild impairments of liver function tests in an adult do not require discontinuation of the drug.

Phenobarbital, which was introduced as an antileptic drug in 1912, is still highly effective, but because of its toxic effects—drowsiness and mental dullness, nystagmus, and staggering—is seldom used as a first-line drug. The adverse effects of *primidone* are much the same. Both drugs may provoke behavioral problems in retarded children. It is still used to advantage as an adjunctive anticonvulsant.

A newer drug, the folate antagonist *lamotrigine*, closely resembles phenytoin in its antiseizure activity and toxicity and is thought to have less risk of teratogenic effects. It is effective as a first-line drug for generalized and focal seizures. *Felbamate*, a drug similar to meprobamate, has shown promise as an adjunctive form of treatment of generalized seizures, complex partial seizures, and Lennox-Gastaut syndrome, but its use has been limited because of the rare occurrence of bone marrow suppression and liver failure. Two other new drugs, *gabapentin* and *vigabatrin*, were synthesized specifically to enhance the intrinsic inhibitory system of GABA in the brain. Gabapentin is chemically similar to GABA, but actually its anticonvulsant mechanism is not known. It is moderately effective in partial and secondary generalized seizures and has the advantage of not being metabolized by the liver. Vigabatrin and the related drugs *progabide* and *tiagabine* are inhibitors of GABA transaminase and are effective in the treatment of partial seizures and, to a lesser extent, primary generalized seizures. Neither is bound to plasma protein, and they have few toxic effects and no known adverse drug interactions. *Topiramate*, another new antiepileptic agent, has much the same mode of action and degree of effectiveness as tiagabine. It may cause serious dermatologic side effects, especially if used with valproate and appears to induce renal stones in 1.5 percent of patients.

Ethosuximide (Zarontin) and valproate are equally effective for the treatment of absence seizures, the latter one being used mainly in children more than 4 years of age. It is good practice, in order to avoid excessive sleepiness, to begin with a single dose of 250 mg of ethosuximide per day and to increase it every week until the optimum therapeutic effect is achieved. *Methsuximide* (Celontin) is useful in individual cases where ethosuximide and valpraote have failed. In patients with benign absence attacks that are associated with photosensitivity, myoclonus, and clonic-tonic-clonic seizures (including juvenile myoclonic epilepsy), valproate is the drug of choice. Valproate is particularly useful in children who have both absence and grand mal attacks, since the use of this drug alone often permits the control of both types of seizure. The concurrent use of valproate and clonazepam has been known to produce absence status.

Treatment of the *special types of convulsions in the neonatal period* and in infancy and childhood is discussed by Fenichel and by Volpe. In general, phenobarbital is preferred for seizure control in infancy.

Probably the form of epilepsy that is most difficult to treat is the *Lennox-Gastaut* syndrome. Some of these patients have as many as 50 or more seizures per day, and every combination of anticonvulsant medications may have no effect. Valproic acid (900 to 2400 mg/day) will reduce the frequency of spells in approximately half the cases. The newer drugs—lamotrigine, topiramate, vigabatrine—are each beneficial in about 25 percent of cases. Clonazepam also has had limited success.

Seizure states in which myoclonus is a major element (absence, juvenile myoclonic, and certain cases of tonic-clonic epilepsy) respond particularly well to valproate. Even the myoclonus of certain progressive diseases, such as the Unverricht-Lundborg syndrome, may be suppressed by this drug. Methsuximide is preferred by some physicians. In the treatment of infantile spasms, ACTH or adrenal corticosteroids have been the most effective. Postanoxic intention myoclonus (page 110) can be suppressed to some extent by clonazepam and by Valproate, combined with other drugs.

Restricted forms of myoclonus or polymyoclonus, discussed in Chap. 6, may respond to special drugs in combination.

Status Epilepticus

Recurrent generalized convulsions at a frequency that prevents the regaining of consciousness in the interval between seizures (grand mal status) constitute the most serious therapeutic problem (an overall mortality of 20 to 30 percent, according to Towne and colleagues, but probably lower in recent years). Most patients who die of epilepsy do so because of uncontrolled seizures of this type, complicated by the effects of the underlying illness or an injury sustained as a result of a seizure. Rising temperature, acidosis, hypotension, and renal failure from myoglobinuria is a sequence of life-threatening events that may be encountered in cases of status epilepticus. Prolonged convulsive status (for longer than 30 min) also carries a risk of serious neurologic sequelae ("epileptic encephalopathy"). The MRI frequently shows signal abnormalities in the hippocampi, most often reversible, but we have had several such patients who awakened and were left in a permanent amnesic state. From time to time a case of neurogenic pulmonary edema is encountered during or just after the convulsions.

The many regimens that have been proposed for the treatment of status attest to the fact that no one of them is altogether satisfactory and none is clearly superior (Treiman et al). The present authors have had the most success with the following program: when the patient is first seen, an initial assessment of cardiorespiratory function is made and an oral airway is established. A large-bore intravenous line is inserted; blood is drawn for glucose, blood urea nitrogen, electrolytes, and a metabolic and drug screen; and a normal saline infusion is begun. Diazepam is given intravenously at a rate of about 2 mg/min until the seizures stop or a total of 20 mg has been given. Or lorazepam may be administered, being marginally more effective than diazepam because of its putative longer duration of action in the central nervous system. Lorazepam 0.1 mg/kg is given by intravenous push at a rate not to exceed 2 mg/min.

Immediately thereafter a loading dose (15 to 18 mg/kg) of phenytoin is administered by vein at a rate of less than 50 mg/min. Faster administration risks hypotension and heart block; it is therefore recommended that the blood pressure and electrocardiogram be monitored during the infusion. Phenytoin must be given through a freely running line with normal saline (it precipitates in other fluids) and should not be injected intramuscularly. A large study by Treiman and colleagues has demonstrated the superiority of using lorazepam instead of phenytoin as the first drug to control status, but this is not surprising considering the longer latency of action of phenytoin. Nonetheless, a long-acting anticonvulsant such as phenytoin must be administered immediately after diazepam has controlled the initial seizures. An alternative is the water-soluble drug *fosphenytoin*, which is administered in the same doses as phenytoin but can be given at twice the maximum rate. Moreover, it can be given intramuscularly in cases where venous access is difficult. Because of the delay in the hepatic conversion of fosphenytoin to active phenytoin, the latency of clinical effect is the same for both drugs.

In an epileptic patient known to be taking anticonvulsants chronically, but in whom the serum level of drug is unknown, it is probably best to administer the full recommended dose of phenytoin or fosphenytoin. If the serum phenytoin can be established at a level above 10 μg/mL, a lower loading dose can be given. If seizures continue, an additional 5 mg/kg is indicated. If this fails to suppress the seizures and status has persisted for 20 to 30 min, an endotracheal tube should be inserted and O_2 administered.

Several regimens have been suggested if status persists after these efforts. The conventional and still dependable one is infusion of phenobarbital at a rate of 100 mg/min until the seizures stop or to a total dose of 20 mg/kg. In our experience, a long subsequent period of stupor must be anticipated, but some epileptologists still prefer this as the initial treatment. Alternatively, at this stage, we prefer the approach of Kumar and Bleck, using high doses of *midazolam* (0.2 mg/kg loading dose followed by an infusion of 0.1 to 0.4 mg/kg/h as determined by clinical and EEG monitoring). If status continues, the dose can be raised as blood pressure permits. We have had occasion to use in excess of 20 mg/h because of a diminishing effect over days. This regimen of midazolam and phenytoin may be maintained for days without major ill effect in previously healthy patients. Propofol given in a bolus of 2 mg/kg and then as an intravenous drip of 2 to 8 mg/kg/h is an alternative to midazolam, but after 24 h the drug behaves like a high dose of barbiturate and there may be difficulty due to hypotension.

If none of these measures controls the seizures, all medication except phenytoin should be discontinued and a more aggressive approach taken to subdue all brain electrical activity. The preferred medications for this purpose have been pentobarbital and propofol, which, despite their poor record as anticonvulsants, are easier to use than the alternative inhalational anesthetic agents. An initial intravenous dose of 5 mg/kg pentobarbital or 2 mg/kg propofol is given slowly to induce an EEG burst-suppression pattern, which is then maintained by the administration of 0.5 to 2 mg/kg/h pentobarbital or 10 mg/kg/h of propofol. Every 12 to 24 h, the rate of infusion is slowed to determine whether the seizures have stopped. The experience of Lowenstein and colleagues, like our own, is that the majority of instances of status epilepticus that cannot be controlled with the standard anticonvulsants and midazolam will respond to high doses of barbiturates (or propofol) but that the infusions cause hypotension and cannot be carried out for long periods.

Should the seizures continue either clinically or electrographically despite all these medications, one is justified in the assumption that the convulsive tendency is so strong that it cannot be checked by reasonable quantities of anticonvulsants. A few patients in this predicament have survived and awakened, even at times with minimal neurologic damage. Isoflurane (Forane) has been used in these circumstances with good effect, but continuous administration of such inhalational agents is impractical in most critical care units. Halothane has been ineffective as an anticonvulsant, but ether, also impractical, had in the past been effective in some cases. In these patients with intractable status, one usually depends entirely on phenytoin, 0.5 g, and phenobarbital, 0.4 g/day (smaller doses in infants and children, as shown in Table 16-4), and on measures that safeguard the patient's vital functions.

A word must be added concerning neuromuscular paralysis and continuous EEG monitoring in status epilepticus. With failure of aggressive anticonvulsant and anesthetic treatment, there may be a temptation to paralyze all muscular activity, something easily accomplished with drugs such as pancuronium, while neglecting the underlying seizures. The use of neuromuscular blocking drugs without a concomitant attempt to suppress seizure activity is a mistake. If such measures are undertaken and the paralysis continued for more than several hours, continuous or frequent intermittent EEG monitoring is virtually obligatory, and it is also helpful in the early stages of status epilepticus in adjusting the doses of anticonvulsants that are required to suppress the seizures.

In the related but less serious condition of *acute repetitive seizures*, a diazepam gel, which is well absorbed if given rectally, is available and has been found useful in institutional and home care of epileptics patients, although it is quite expensive. A similar effect has been attained by the nasal or buccal (transmucosal) administration of midazolam, which is quickly absorbed from these sites (5 mg/mL, 0.2 mg/kg nasally; 2 ml to 10 mg buccally). These approaches have found their main use in children with frequent seizures who live in supervised environments where a nurse or parent can administer the medication.

Petit mal status should be managed by intravenous lorazepam, valproic acid, or both, followed by ethosuximide. Nonconvulsive status is treated along the lines of grand mal status, usually stopping short of using anesthetic agents.

Surgical Treatment of Epilepsy

The surgical excision of epileptic foci in simple and complex partial epilepsies that have not responded to intensive and prolonged medical therapy is being used with increasing effectiveness in a large number of specialized epilepsy centers. At these centers, it has been estimated that approximately 25 percent of all patients with epilepsy are candidates for surgical therapy and more than half of these may benefit from surgery. To locate the discharging focus requires a careful analysis of clinical and EEG findings, often including those obtained by long-term video/EEG monitoring and sometimes intracranial EEG recording by means of intraparenchymal depth electrodes, subdural strip electrodes, and subdural grids. The most favorable candidates for surgery are those with complex partial seizures and a unilateral temporal lobe focus, in whom rates of cure and significant improvement approach 90 percent. Outside of the temporal lobe, complete seizure-free states are attained in about 50 percent. Only about 10 percent of patients obtain no improvement at all and less than 5 percent are worse.

Other surgical procedures of value in selected cases are section of the corpus callosum and hemispherectomy. The most encouraging results with callosotomy have been obtained in the control of partial and secondarily generalized seizures, particularly when atonic drop attacks are the most disabling seizure type. Removal of all of the cortex of one hemisphere, in addition to the amygdala and hippocampus, may be of value in young children and also in some adults with severe cerebral disease of that hemisphere and intractable unilateral motor seizures and hemiplegia. Rasmussen encephalitis, Sturge-Weber disease, and large porencephalic cysts at times fall into this category. Surgical or endovascular reduction of arteriovenous malformations generally reduce the frequency of associated seizures, but the results in this regard are somewhat unpredictable (see Chap. 34).

Regulation of Physical and Mental Activity

The most important factors in seizure breakthrough, next to the abandonment of medication, are loss of sleep and abuse of alcohol or other drugs. The need for moderation in the use of alcohol must be stressed, as well as the need to maintain regular hours of sleep.

A moderate amount of physical exercise is desirable. With proper safeguards, even potentially more dangerous sports, such as swimming, may be permitted. However, a person with incompletely controlled epilepsy should not be allowed to drive an automobile, operate unguarded machinery, climb ladders, or take tub baths behind locked doors; such a person should swim only in the company of a good swimmer and wear a life preserver when boating.

Psychosocial difficulties must be identified and addressed early. Simple advice and reassurance will frequently help to prevent or overcome the feelings of inferiority and self-consciousness of many epileptic patients. Patients and their families may benefit from more extensive counseling and proper family attitudes should be cultivated. Oversolicitude and overprotection should be discouraged. It is important that the patient be allowed to live as normal a life as possible Every effort should be made to keep children in school, and adults should be encouraged to work. Once seizures have ceased under medical control for a period varying from 6 months to a year, driving an automobile is allowed in most western countries. Many communities have vocational rehabilitation centers and special social agencies for epileptics, and advantage should be taken of such facilities.

Other Therapeutic Measures

Ketogenic Diet Since the 1920s interest in this form of seizure control has vacillated, being revived periodically in centers caring for many children with intractable epilepsy. Despite the absence of controlled studies showing its efficacy or a reasonable hypothesis for its mechanism, several trials in the first half of the century and again more recently have demonstrated a reduction in seizures in half of the patients, including handicapped children with severe and sometimes intractable fits. The regimen is initiated by starvation for a day or so to induce ketosis followed by a diet in which 80 to 90 percent of the calories are derived from fat (Vining). The difficulties in making such a diet palatable leads to its abandonment by about one-third of children and their families.

Vagal Nerve Stimulation This experimental technique has found favor in cases of intractable partial and secondarily generalizing seizures. A pacemaker-like device is implanted in the anterior chest wall and stimulating electrodes are connected to the vagus at the left carotid bifurcation. The procedure is well tolerated except for hoarseness in some cases. Several trials have demonstrated an average of one-quarter or greater reduction in seizure frequency among patients who were resistant to all manner of anticonvulsant drugs (Wilder). The mechanism by which vagal stimulation produces its effects is unclear, and its role in the management of seizures is still being defined. Cerebellar stimulation has also been used in the control of seizures, with no clear evidence of success.

REFERENCES

AICARDI J: Early myoclonic encephalopathy, in Roger J, Drevet C, Bureau M, et al (eds): *Epileptic Syndromes in Infancy, Childhood, and Adolescence*. London, John Libbey Eurotext, 1985, pp 12–21.

ANDERSON VE, HAUSER WA: Genetics of epilepsy, in Laidlaw JP, Richens A, Chadwick D (ed): *Textbook of Epilepsy*, 4th ed. New York, Churchill Livingstone, 1992, pp 47–75.

ANDERMANN F (ed): *Chronic Encephalitis and Epilepsy: Rasmussen Syndrome*. Boston, Butterworth-Heineman, 1991.

ANNEGERS JF, HAUSER WA, SHIRTS SB, KURLAND LT: Factors prognostic of unprovoked seizures after febrile convulsions. *N Engl J Med* 316:493, 1987.

ANTEL JP, RASMUSSEN T: Rasmussen's encephalitis and the new hat. *Neurology* 46:9, 1996.

BEAR DM, FEDIO P: Quantitative analysis of interictal behavior in temporal lobe epilepsy. *Arch Neurol* 34:454, 1977.

BERKOVIC SF: Genetics of epilepsy, in *Epilepsy: A Comprehensive Textbook*. Philadelphia, Lippincott-Raven, 1997, pp 217–224.

BIEN CG, BENNINGER FD, URBACH H, et al: Localizing value of epileptic visual auras. *Brain* 123:244, 2000.

BLECK TP: Refractory status epilepticus. *Neurol Chronicle* 2:1, 1992.

BLUMER D, MONTOURIS G, HERMANN B: Psychiatric morbidity in seizure patients on a neurodiagnostic monitoring unit. *J Neuropsychiatry Clin Neurosci* 7:445, 1995.

BRETT EM: Epilepsy. In Brett EM (ed): *Pediatric Neurology*, 2nd ed. London, Churchill Livingstone, 1991.

CALLAGHAN N, GARRETT A, GOGGIN T: Withdrawal of anticonvulsant drugs in patients free of seizures for two years. *N Engl J Med* 318:942, 1988.

CASCINO GD: Intractable partial epilepsy: Evaluation and treatment. *Mayo Clin Proc* 65:1578, 1990.

CHINCHILLA D, DULAC O, ROBAN O, et al: Reappraisal of Rasmussen syndrome with special emphasis on treatment with high dose steroids. *J Neurol Neurosurg Psychiatry* 57:1325, 1994.

COLE AJ, ANDERMANN F, TAYLOR L, et al: The Landau-Kleffner syndrome of acquired epileptic aphasia: Unusual clinical outcome, surgical experiences, and absence of encephalitis. *Neurology* 38:31, 1988.

Commission on Classification and Terminology of the International League Against Epilepsy: Proposal for revised clinical and electroencephalographic classification of epileptic seizures. *Epilepsia* 22:489, 1981.

Commission on Classification and Terminology of the International League Against Epilepsy: Classification of Epilepsy and Epileptic Syndromes. *Epilepsia* 30:389, 1989.

CURRIE S, HEATHFIELD KWG, HENSON RA, SCOTT DF: Clinical course and prognosis of temporal lobe epilepsy. *Brain* 94:173, 1970.

DALY DD, PEDLEY TA: *Current Practice of Clinical Electroencephalography*, 2nd ed. New York, Raven Press, 1990.

DELGADO-ESCUETA AV, GREENBERG DA, TREIMAN L, et al: Mapping the gene for juvenile myoclonic epilepsy. *Epilepsia* 30:S8, 1989.

DEVINSKY O, KELLEY K, YACUBIAN EM, et al: Postictal behavior: A clinical and subdural electroencephalographic study. *Arch Neurol* 51:254, 1994.

DIXIT S, KURLE P, BUYAN-DENT L, SHETH RD: Status epilepticus associated with cefepime. *Neurology* 54:2153, 2000.

EADIE MJ, TYRER JH: *Anticonvulsant Therapy: Pharmacological Basis and Practice*, 3rd ed. New York, Churchill Livingstone, 1989.

EBNER A, DINNER DS, NOACHTAR S, LUDERS H: Automatisms with preserved responsiveness: A lateralizing sign in psychomotor seizures. *Neurology* 45:61, 1995.

ECLAMPSIA TRIAL COLLABORATIVE GROUP: Which anticonvulsant for women with eclampsia? Evidence from the Collaborative Eclampsia Trial. *Lancet* 345:1455, 1995.

ELLENBERG JG, HIRTZ DG, NELSON KB: Do seizures in children cause intellectual deterioration? *N Engl J Med* 314:1085, 1986.

ENGEL J JR: Surgery for epilepsy. *N Eng J Med* 334:647, 1996.

ENGEL J JR, PEDLEY TA: *Epilepsy: A Comprehensive Textbook*. Philadelphia, Davis, 1998.

FALCONER MA: Genetic and related aetiological factors in temporal lobe epilepsy: A review. *Epilepsia* 12:13, 1971–1972.

FISHER RS, CHAN DW, BARE M, LESSER RP: Capillary prolactin measurements for diagnosis of seizures. *Ann Neurol* 29:187, 1991.

FORSTER FM: *Reflex Epilepsy, Behavioral Therapy, and Conditional Reflexes*. Springfield, IL, Charles C Thomas, 1977.

FRENCH JA, WILLIAMSON PD, THADANI VM, et al: Characteristics of medial temporal lobe epilepsy: I. Results of history and physical examination. *Ann Neurol* 34:774,1993.

GASTAUT H, AGUGLIA U, TINUPER P: Benign versive or circling epilepsy with bilateral 3-cps spike and wave discharges in late childhood. *Ann Neurol* 9:301, 1986.

GASTAUT H, GASTAUT JL: Computerized transverse axial tomography in epilepsy. *Epilepsia* 47:325, 1978.

GESCHWIND N: Interictal behavioral changes in epilepsy. *Epilepsia* 24(suppl):523, 1983.

GLOOR P: Experiential phenomena of temporal lobe epilepsy: Facts and hypothesis. *Brain* 113:1673, 1990.

GOLDENSOHN E: The relevance of secondary epileptogenesis to the treatment of epilepsy: Kindling and the mirror focus. *Epilepsia* 25(suppl 2):156, 1984.

GOWERS WR: *Epilepsy and Other Chronic Convulsive Diseases: Their Causes, Symptoms and Treatment*. New York, Dover, 1964 (originally published in 1885; reprinted as Vol 1 in The Amer Acad of Neurol Reprint Series).

HAUSER WA, ANNEGERS JF: Epidemiology of epilepsy, in Laidlaw JP, Richens A, Chadwick D (eds): *Textbook of Epilepsy*, 4th ed. New York, Churchill Livingstone, 1992, pp 23–45.

HAUSER WA, ANNEGERS JF: Incidence of epilepsy and unprovoked seizures in Rochester, Minnesota, 1935–1984. *Epilepsia* 34:453, 1993.

HAUSER WA, KURLAND LT: The epidemiology of epilepsy in Rochester, Minnesota, 1935–1967. *Epilepsia* 16:1, 1975.

HAUSER WA, RICH SS, LEE JR, et al: Risk of recurrent seizures after two unprovoked seizures. *N Engl J Med* 338:429, 1998.

HESDORFER DC, LOGROSCINA G, CASCINO G, et al: Risk of unprovoked seizure after acute symptomatic seizure: effect of sttatus epilepticus. *Ann Neurol* 44:908, 1998.

HUTTENLOCHER PR, HAPKE RJ: A follow-up study of intractable seizures in childhood. *Ann Neurol* 28:699, 1990.

JELLINGER K: Neuropathologic aspects of infantile spasms. *Brain Dev* 9:349, 1987.

KUMAR A, BLECK TP: Intravenous midazolam for the treatment of status epilepticus. *Crit Care Med* 20:438, 1992.

KUTT H: Interactions between anticonvulsants and other commonly prescribed drugs. *Epilepsia* 25(suppl 2):188, 1984.

LANDAU WM, KLEFFNER FR: Syndrome of acquired aphasia with convulsive disorder in children. *Neurology* 7:523, 1957.

LENNOX MA: Febrile convulsions in childhood. *Am J Dis Child* 78:868, 1949.

LENNOX W, LENNOX MA: *Epilepsy and Related Disorders*. Boston, Little, Brown, 1960.

LEPPERT M, ANDERSON VE, QUATTELBAUM T, et al: Benign familial neonatal convulsions linked to genetic markers on chromosome 20. *Nature* 337:647, 1989.

LEUTZMEZER F, SERLES W, LEHNER J, et al: Postical nose wiping: A lateralizing sign in temporal lobe complex partial seizures. *Neurology* 51: 1175, 1998.

LINDVALL O, NILSSON B: Cerebellar atrophy following phenytoin intoxication. *Ann Neurol* 16:258, 1984.

LOWENSTEIN DH, ALDREDGE BK: Status epilepticus. *N Engl J Med* 338:970, 1998.

LUCAS MJ, LEVENO KJ, CUNNINGHAM FG: A comparison of magnesium sulfate with phenytoin for the prevention of eclampsia. *N Engl J Med* 333:201, 1995.

LUDERS H, LESSER RP, DIMMER DS, MORRIS HH III: Benign focal epilepsy of childhood, in Luders H, Lesser RP (eds): *Epilepsy: Electroclinical Syndromes*. London, Springer-Verlag, 1987, pp 303–346.

MANFORD M, HART YM, SANDER JW, SHORVON SD: The national general practice study of epilepsy: The syndromic classification of the International League Against Epilepsy, applied to epilepsy in a general population. *Arch Neurol* 49:801, 1992.

MANFORD M, FISH DR, SHORVON SD: An analysis of clinical seizure patterns and their localizing value in frontal and temporal lobe epilepsies. *Brain* 119:17, 1996.

MATTSON RH, CRAMER JA, COLLINS JF, et al: Comparison of carbamazepine, phenobarbital, phenytoin, and primidone in partial and secondarily generalized tonic-clonic seizures. *N Engl J Med* 313:145, 1985.

NIEDERMEYER E: *The Epilepsies: Diagnosis and Management.* Baltimore, Urban and Schwarzenberg, 1990.

OBESO JA, ROTHWELL JC, MARSDEN CD: The spectrum of cortical myoclonus. *Brain* 108:193, 1985.

OHTAHARA S: Seizure disorders in infancy and childhood. *Brain Dev* 6:509, 1984.

OUNSTED C, LINDSAY J, NORMAN RA: *Biological Factors in Temporal Lobe Epilepsy: Clinics in Developmental Medicine,* Vol 22. London, Heineman/Spastics Society, 1986.

PALMINI AL, GLOOR P, JONES-GOTMAN M: Pure amnestic seizures in temporal lobe epilepsy. *Brain* 115:749, 1992.

PEDLEY TA: Discontinuing antiepileptic drugs. *N Engl J Med* 318:982, 1988.

PENFIELD W, JASPER HH: *Epilepsy and Functional Anatomy of the Human Brain.* Boston, Little, Brown, 1954.

PENFIELD W, KRISTIANSEN K: *Epileptic Seizure Patterns.* Springfield, Ill, Charles C Thomas, 1951.

PENRY JK, PORTER RV, DREIFUSS FE: Simultaneous recording of absence seizures with video tape and electroencephalography. *Brain* 98:427, 1975.

PLOUIN P: Benign neonatal convulsions (familial and nonfamilial), in Roger J, Drevet C, Bureau M, et al (eds): *Epileptic Syndromes in Infancy, Childhood, and Adolescence.* London, John Libbey Eurotext, 1985, pp 2–9.

PLUM F, HOWSE DC, DUFFY TE: Metabolic effects of seizures. *Res Publ Assoc Res Nerv Ment Dis* 53:141, 1974.

PORTER RJ: *Epilepsy: 100 Elementary Principles,* 2nd ed. Philadelphia, Saunders, 1989.

RASMUSSEN T, OLSZEWSKI J, LLOYD-SMITH D: Focal seizures due to chronic localized encephalitis. *Neurology* 8:435, 1958.

RASMUSSEN T: Further observations on the syndrome of chronic encephalitis and epilepsy. *Appl Neurophysiol* 41:1, 1978.

RIVERA R, SEGNINI M. BALTODANO A, et al: Midazolam in the treatment of status epilepticus in children. *Crit Care Med* 21:991, 1993.

ROCCA WA, SHARBROUGH FW, HAUSER A, et al: Risk factors for complex partial seizures: A population-based case-control study. *Ann Neurol* 21:22, 1987.

RODIN E, SCHMALTZ S: The Bear-Fedio personality inventory and temporal lobe epilepsy. *Neurology* 34:591, 1984.

ROPPER AH: "Convulsions" in basilar artery disease. *Neurology* 38:1500, 1988.

SALANOVA V, ANDERMANN F, RASMUSSEN T, et al: Parietal lobe epilepsy. Clinical manifestations and outcome in 82 patients treated surgically between 1929 and 1988. *Brain* 118:607, 1995.

SCHEIBEL ME, SCHEIBEL AB: Hippocampal pathology in temporal lobe epilepsy: A Golgi survey, in Brazier MAB (ed): *Epilepsy: Its Phenomena in Man.* New York, Academic Press, 1973, pp 315–357.

SCHOMER DL: Partial epilepsy. *N Engl J Med* 309:536, 1983.

SUNG C, CHU N: Status epilepticus in the elderly: Aetiology, seizure type and outcome. *Acta Neurol Scand* 80:51, 1989.

THOMAS JE, REGAN TJ, KLASS DW: Epilepsia partialis continua: A review of 32 cases. *Arch Neurol* 34:266, 1977.

TODT H: The late prognosis of epilepsy in childhood: Results of a prospective follow-up study. *Epilepsia* 25:137, 1984.

TOWNE AR, MCGEE FE, MERCER EL, et al: Mortality in a community-based status epilepticus study. *Neurology* 40(suppl 1):229, 1990.

TREIMAN DM, MEYERS PD, WALTON NY, et al: A comparison of four treatments for generalized status epilepticus. *N Engl J Med* 339:792, 1998.

TRIMBLE MR: Personality disturbance in epilepsy. *Neurology* 33:1332, 1983.

TRIMBLE MR, SCHMITZ B: The psychosis of epilepsy/schizophrenia, in Engel J Jr, Pedley TA (eds): *Epilepsy: A Comprehensive Textbook.* Philadelphia, Lippincott-Raven, 1998, pp 2071–2081.

TWYMAN RE, GAHRING LC, SPIESS J, ROGERS SW: Glutamate receptor antibodies activate a subset of receptors and reveal an agonist binding site. *Neuron* 14:755, 1995.

VICTOROFF J: DSM-III-R psychiatric diagnoses in candidates for epilepsy surgery: lifetime prevalence. *Neuropsychiatry Neuropsychol Behav Neurol* 7:87, 1994.

VOLPE JJ: *Neurology of the Newborn,* 3rd ed. Philadelphia, Saunders, 1995.

WILDER BJ: Vagal nerve stimulation, in Engel J Jr, Pedley TA: *Epilepsy: A Comprehensive Textbook.* Philadelphia, Davis, 1998, chap. 125.

WYLIE E, LUDERS H, MORRIS HH, et al: The lateralizing significance of versive head and eye movements during epileptic seizures. *Neurology* 36:606, 1212, 1986.

ZEMAN AZ, BONIFACE SJ, HODGES JR: Transient epileptic amnesia: A description of the clinical and neuropsychological features in 10 cases and a review of the literature. *J Neurol Neurosurg Psychiatry* 64:435, 1998.

Chapter 17

COMA AND RELATED DISORDERS OF CONSCIOUSNESS

In hospital neurology, the clinical analysis of unresponsive and comatose patients becomes a practical necessity. There is always an urgency about such medical problems—a need to determine the underlying disease process and the direction in which it is evolving and to protect the brain against more serious or irreversible damage. When called upon, the physician must therefore be prepared to implement a rapid, systematic investigation of the comatose patient; the need for prompt therapeutic and diagnostic action allows no time for deliberate, leisurely investigation.

Some idea of the dimensions of this category of neurologic disease can be obtained from published statistics. Many years ago, in two large municipal hospitals, it was estimated that 3 percent of all admissions to the emergency wards were for diseases that had caused coma. Alcoholism, cerebral trauma, and cerebrovascular diseases were the most common causes, accounting for 82 percent of the comatose patients admitted to the Boston City Hospital in past years (Solomon and Aring). Epilepsy, drug intoxication, diabetes, and severe infections were the other major causes for admission. Recent figures from municipal hospitals are much the same, emphasizing that the common conditions underlying coma are relatively invariant in general medical practice. In university hospitals, which tend to attract more obscure cases, the statistics may be somewhat different. For example, in the series of Plum and Posner (Table 17-1), only one-quarter proved to have cerebrovascular disease, and only in 6 percent was coma the consequence of trauma. Indeed, all "mass lesions,"—such as tumors, abscesses, hemorrhages, and infarcts—made up less than one-third of the coma-producing diseases. A majority were the result of exogenous (drug overdose) and endogenous (metabolic) intoxications and hypoxia. Subarachnoid hemorrhage, meningitis, and encephalitis made up another 5 percent of the total. Thus the order is reversed, but still intoxication, stroke, and cranial trauma stand as the "big three" of coma-producing conditions. Equally common in some series, albeit obvious

Table 17-1
Final diagnosis in 500 patients admitted to hospital with "coma of unknown etiology"

Supratentorial mass lesions	101
Intracerebral hematoma	44
Subdural hematoma	26
Epidural hematoma	4
Cerebral infarct	9
Thalamic infarct	2
Brain tumor	7
Pituitary apoplexy	2
Brain abscess	6
Closed-head injury	1
Subtentorial lesions	65
Brainstem infarct	40
Pontine hemorrhage	11
Brainstem demyelination	1
Cerebellar hemorrhage	5
Cerebellar tumor	3
Cerebellar infarct	2
Cerebellar abscess	1
Posterior fossa subdural hemorrhage	1
Basilar migraine	1
Metabolic and other diffuse disorders	326
Anoxia or ischemia	87
Hepatic encephalopathy	17
Uremic encephalopathy	8
Pulmonary disease	3
Endocrine disorders (including diabetes)	12
Acid-base disorders	12
Temperature regulation	9
Nutritional	1
Nonspecific metabolic coma	1
Encephalomyelitis and encephalitis	14
Subarachnoid hemorrhage	13
Drug poisoning	149
Psychiatric disorders	8

Note: Listed here are only those patients in whom the initial diagnosis was uncertain and a final diagnosis was established. Thus, obvious poisonings and closed-head injuries are underrepresented.
Source: Plum and Posner, by permission.

and usually transient, is coma that follows seizures and resuscitation from cardiac arrest.

The terms *consciousness*, *confusion*, *stupor*, *unconsciousness*, and *coma* have been endowed with so many different meanings that it is almost impossible to avoid ambiguity in their usage. They are not strictly medical terms but literary, philosophic, and psychologic ones as well. The word *consciousness* is the most difficult of all. William James once remarked that everyone knows what consciousness is until he attempts to define it. To the psychologist, consciousness denotes a state of continuous awareness of one's self and environment. Knowledge of self includes all "feelings, attitudes and emotions, impulses, volitions, and the active or striving aspects of conduct," in short, an awareness of all one's own mental functioning, particularly of the cognitive processes, and their relation to past memories and experience. These can be judged only by the patient's verbal account of his introspections and, indirectly, by his actions. Physicians, being more practical and objective for the most part, give greater credence to the patient's behavior and reactions to overt stimuli than to what the patient says. For this reason they usually give the term *consciousness* its commonest and simplest operational meaning—namely, the state of the patient's awareness of *self and environment* and his responsiveness to external stimulation and inner need. This narrow definition has another advantage in that *unconsciousness* has the opposite meaning—a state of unawareness of self and environment or a suspension of those mental activities by which people are made aware of themselves and their environment, coupled with a diminished responsiveness to environmental stimuli. Some authors make a distinction between the *level of consciousness*—meaning the state of arousal or the degree of variation from normal alertness as judged by the appearance of facial muscles, fixity of gaze, and body posture—and the *content of consciousness*, i.e., the quality and coherence of thought and behavior. For medical purposes, the loss of normal arousal is by far the more important and dramatic aspect of disordered consciousness and the one identified by laypersons and physicians as being the central issue in coma. To add to the ambiguity, psychoanalysts have given the word *unconscious* a still different meaning; for them it is a repository of impulses and memories of previous experiences that cannot immediately be recalled to the conscious mind.

Much more could be said about the history of our ideas concerning consciousness and the theoretic problems with regard to its definition, but this would serve no practical purpose. The interested reader is referred to the discussions of consciousness by Young and by Plum and Posner listed in the references.

Description of States of Normal and Impaired Consciousness

The following definitions, though probably not acceptable to all psychologists, are of service to clinicians and will provide the student and practitioner with a convenient terminology for describing the states of awareness and responsiveness of their patients.

Normal Consciousness This is the condition of the normal person when awake. In this state the individual is fully responsive to stimuli and indicates by his behavior and speech the same awareness of self and environment as that of the examiner. This normal state may fluctuate during the day from one of keen alertness or deep concentration with a marked constriction of the field of attention to one of mild general inattentiveness. From this state, the normal individual can be brought immediately to a state of full alertness and function.

Confusion In this condition the patient does not take into account all elements of his immediate environment. This state always implies a degree of imperceptiveness and distractibility, referred to traditionally as "clouding of the sensorium." The term *confusion* lacks precision, but in general it denotes an inability to think with customary speed and clarity, usually marked by some degree of *inattentiveness* and *disorientation*. Here the difficulty is to define *thinking*, a term that refers variably to problem solving or to coherence of ideas and formation of memories. Confusion results most often from a process that influences the brain globally, such as a toxic or metabolic disturbance or a dementia. Any condition that causes drowsiness or stupor, including the natural state that comes from sleep deprivation, results in some degradation of mental performance and inattentiveness. A confusional state can also accompany focal cerebral disease in various locations, particularly in the right hemisphere, or result from disorders that also disturb language, memory, or visuospatial orientation, but these are readily distinguished from the global confusional state.

The mildest degree of confusion may be so slight that it can be overlooked unless the examiner searches for deviations from the patient's normal behavior and liveliness of conversation. The patient may even be roughly oriented as to time and place, with only occasional irrelevant remarks betraying an incoherence of thinking. *Moderately confused* persons can carry on a simple conversation for short periods of time, but their thinking is slow and incoherent, their responses are inconsistent, and they are unable to stay on one topic and to inhibit inappropriate responses. Usually they are disoriented in time and place. They are distractible and at the mercy of every stimulus. Periods of irritability and excitability may alternate with drowsiness and diminished vigilance. Movements are often tremulous, jerky, and ineffectual. Sequences of movement also reveal impersistence. *Severely confused* and inattentive persons are usually unable to do more than carry out the simplest commands, and these only inconsistently and in brief sequence. Few if any thought processes are in operation. Their speech is usually limited to a few words or phrases; infrequently these individuals are voluble. They are unaware of much that goes on around them, are often disoriented in time and place, do not grasp their immediate situation, and may misidentify people or objects. Illusions may lead to fear or agitation. Occasionally, hallucinatory or delusional experiences impart a psychotic cast to the clinical picture, obscuring the deficit in attention.

The degree of confusion often varies from one time of day to another. It tends to be least pronounced in the morning but increases as the day wears on ("sundowning"), when the patient is fatigued and environmental cues are less clear-cut. Many events that involve the confused patient leave no trace in memory; in fact, the capacity to recall events of the past hours or days is one of the most delicate tests of mental clarity. So is the use of so-called working memory, which requires the temporary storage of the solution of one task for use in the next. This deficit, which is such a common feature of the confusional states, can be demonstrated by tests of serial subtraction and the spelling of words (or repeating a phone number) forward and then backward. Careful analysis will show these defects to be tied to inattention and impaired perception, or registration of information, rather than a fault in retentive memory.

In some medical writings, the terms *delirium* and *confusion* are used interchangeably, the former connoting nothing more than a nondescript confusional state in which hyperactivity may be prominent. However, in the syndrome of delirium tremens (observed most often but not exclusively in alcoholics), the vivid hallucinations, inaccessibility of the patient to events other than those to which he is reacting at any one moment, extreme agitation, tendency to tremble as well as to startle easily and to convulse, and the signs of overactivity of the autonomic nervous system suggest that the term *delirium* should be reserved for a highly distinctive confusional syndrome (elaborated in Chap. 20). The clearest evidence of the relationship of inattention, confusion, stupor, and coma is that patients may pass through each of these states as they become comatose or emerge from coma. The authors have not observed such a relationship between coma and delirium except possibly in patients suffering from bacterial meningitis or hepatic stupor and coma, which in some few instances may be *preceded* by a brief period of delirium. In certain acute mental syndromes, it can no doubt be difficult to distinguish between delirium and other confusional states, since some of the attributes of delirium may be lacking.

Drowsiness and Stupor In these states, mental, speech, and physical activity are reduced. *Drowsiness* denotes an inability to sustain a wakeful state without the application of external stimuli. Inattentiveness and mild confusion are the rule, both improving with arousal. The lids droop without closing completely; there may be snoring, the jaw and limb muscles are slack, and the limbs are relaxed. This state is indistinguishable from light sleep, with slow arousal elicited by speaking to the patient or applying a tactile stimulus.

Stupor describes a patient who can be roused only by vigorous and repeated stimuli, at which time he opens his eyes, looks at the examiner, and does not appear to be unconscious; response to spoken commands is either absent or slow and inadequate. Restless or stereotyped motor activity is common in stuporous patients and they do not shift position as frequently as patients who are only drowsy. When left unstimulated, they quickly drift back into a sleep-like state. The eyes move outward and upward, a feature that is shared with sleep (see further on). Tendon and plantar reflexes and breathing pattern may or may not be altered, depending on how the underlying disease has affected the nervous system. In psychiatry, the term *stupor* has been used in a second sense—to denote an uncommon condition in which the perception of sensory stimuli is presumably normal but activity is suspended or marked by negativism (catatonic stupor).

Coma The patient who appears to be asleep and is at the same time incapable of being aroused by external stimuli or inner need is in a state of coma. There are variations in the degree of coma; in its deepest stages, no reaction of any kind is obtainable: corneal, pupillary, pharyngeal, tendon, and plantar reflexes are in abeyance, and tone in the limb muscles is diminished. With lesser degrees of coma, pupillary reactions, reflex ocular movements, and corneal and other brainstem reflexes are preserved in varying degree, and muscle tone in the limbs may be increased. Respiration may be slow or rapid, periodic, or deranged in other ways (see further on). In still lighter stages, sometimes referred to by the ambiguous term *semicoma*, most of the above reflexes can be elicited, and the plantar reflexes may be either flexor or extensor (Babinski sign). Moreover, vigorous stimulation of the patient or distention of the bladder may cause a stirring or moaning and a quickening of respiration. These physical signs vary somewhat depending on the cause of coma. For example, patients with alcoholic coma may be areflexic and unresponsive to noxious stimuli, even when respiration and other vital functions are not threatened. The depth of coma and stupor, when compared in serial examinations, is most useful in assessing the direction in which the disease is evolving.

Relationship of Sleep to Coma Persons in sleep give little evidence of being aware of themselves or their environment; in this respect they are unconscious. Sleep shares a number of other features with the pathologic states of drowsiness, stupor, and coma. These include yawning, closure of the eyelids, cessation of blinking and swallowing, upward deviation or divergence or roving movements of the eyes, loss of muscular tone, decrease or loss of tendon reflexes, and even the presence of Babinski signs and irregular respirations, sometimes Cheyne-Stokes in type. Upon being awakened from deep sleep, a normal person may be confused for a few moments, as every physician knows. Nevertheless, sleeping persons may still respond to unaccustomed stimuli and at times are capable of some mental activity in the form of dreams that leave traces of memory, thus differing from persons in stupor or coma. The most important difference, of course, is that persons in sleep, when stimulated, can be roused to normal consciousness. There are important physiologic differences as well. Cerebral oxygen uptake does not decrease during sleep, as it usually does in coma. Recordable electrical activity—electroencephalographic (EEG) and cerebral evoked responses—and spontaneous motor activity differ in the two states, as indicated later in this chapter and in Chap. 19. The anatomic basis for these differences is not clear.

The Persistent Vegetative State, Locked-in Syndrome, and Akinetic Mutism

With increasing refinements in the treatment of severe systemic diseases and cerebral injury, more and more patients who formerly would have died have survived for indefinite periods without regaining any meaningful mental function. For the first week or two after the cerebral injury, these patients are in a state of deep coma. Then they begin to open their eyes, at first in response to painful stimuli and later spontaneously and for increasingly prolonged periods. The patient may blink in response to threat or to light and intermittently the eyes move from side to side, seemingly following objects or fixating momentarily on the physician or a family member and giving the erroneous impression of recognition. Respiration may quicken in response to stimulation and certain automatisms—such as swallowing, bruxism, grimacing, grunting, and moaning—may be observed (Zeman). However, the patient remains totally inattentive, does not speak, and shows no signs of awareness of the environment or inner need; responsiveness is limited to primitive postural and reflex movements of the limbs. In brief, there is arousal or wakefulness and alternating arousal-nonarousal cycles may be established, but the patient regains neither awareness nor purposeful behavior of any kind. This state is characterized by a number of EEG abnormalities. After global anoxic injury, the EEG tends to display the most profound abnormalities, even to the point of being isoelectric. However, predominantly low-amplitude delta-frequency background activity, burst suppression, widespread alpha and theta activity, an alpha coma pattern, and sleep spindles have all been described in this syndrome, as summarized by Hansotia (see Chap. 2). Moreover, the transition from coma to a state of partial awakening is generally not marked by a change in the EEG pattern.

If lasting, the above described syndrome is most appropriately referred to as the *persistent vegetative state* or PVS (Jennett and Plum). This term has gained wide acceptance and applies to the clinical situation whatever the underlying cause. The most common pathologic bases of this state are diffuse cerebral injury due to closed head trauma, widespread laminar necrosis of the cortex after cardiac arrest, and thalamic necrosis from a number of causes. Occasionally, the most prominent changes are in the thalamic and subthalamic nuclei, as in the celebrated Quinlan case (Kinney et al). It is noteworthy that a persistent vegetative state may also be the terminal phase of progressive degenerative processes such as Alzheimer disease and of Creutzfeldt-Jakob disease. The profound and widespread dysfunction of the cerebrum is reflected by extreme reductions in cerebral blood flow and metabolism, measured with positron emission tomography (PET) and other techniques. On the basis of PET studies in a patient with carbon monoxide poinsoning, Laureys and colleagues observed that the main difference between the PVS and the recovered state was the presence of hypometabolism in the parietal lobe association areas in the former. However, it is quite clear that the neuroanatomic basis of the vegetative state is far more complex.

Additional terms that have been used to describe this syndrome of preserved autonomic and respiratory function without cognition include *apallic syndrome* and *neocortical death*. A recent position paper has codified the features of the persistent vegetative state and suggests dropping a number of related ambiguous terms, although some, such as *akinetic mutism*, discussed further on, have a more specific neurologic meaning and still find use (see Multi-Society Task Force on PVS).

It is difficult to predict which patients will fall permanently into the PVS category (see pages 1178 to 1179). Plum and Posner have reported that of 45 patients with signs of the vegetative state at 1 week, 13 awakened and 5 had satisfactory outcomes; after being vegetative for close to 2 weeks, only one recovered to a level of moderate disability. And after 2 weeks, the prognosis was uniformly poor. Larger studies by Higashi and colleagues have given similar results. As a rough guide to prognosis in head injury, Braakman and colleagues found that among a large group of comatose patients, 59 percent regained consciousness within 6 hours; of those in a vegetative state at 3 months, none became independent. At no time after the onset of coma was it possible to distinguish patients who would remain in a vegetative state from those who would die. If one allows the term *vegetative state* to be applied soon after the onset of coma, rather than requiring coma to persist for several months, then fewer cases would be "persistent." For this reason and because of the anxiety created for families by such a final diagnosis, it has been suggested that the term be abandoned (Kennard and Illingworth); a more meaningful goal would be to insist on strict adherence to the clinical diagnostic criteria.

It is useful to maintain a critical view of news reports of remarkable recuperation from prolonged coma or the vegetative state. When the details of such cases become known, it is evident that recovery might reasonably have been expected. There are, however, numerous reported instances of partial recovery in patients—particularly children—who display vegetative features for several weeks or, as Andrews describes, even several months after injury. Such observations cast doubt on unqualified claims of success with various therapies such as sensory stimulation. Nevertheless, the occurrence of rare instances of very late recovery in adults must be acknowledged [see Andrews; Higashi et al; and Rosenberg et al (1977)].

The states of coma described above and the PVS must be clearly distinguished from a clinical state in which there is little or no disturbance of awareness (consciousness) but only an inability of the patient to respond adequately. The latter is referred to as the *locked-in*, syndrome or the *de-efferented* state. The term *pseudocoma* as a synonym for this state is best avoided, since it is used by some physicians to connote the feigned unconsciousness of the hysteric or malingerer. The locked-in syndrome is due most often to a lesion of the ventral pons (basis pontis) as a result of basilar artery occlusion. Such an infarction may spare both the somatosensory pathways and the ascending neuronal systems that are responsible for arousal and wakefulness as well as certain midbrain elements that allow the eyelids to be raised and give the appearance of wakefulness; the lesion interrupts the corticobulbar and corticospinal pathways, depriving the patient of speech and the capacity to respond in any way except by vertical gaze and blinking. Severe motor neuropathy (e.g., Guillain-Barré syndrome), pontine myelinolysis, or periodic paralysis may have a similar effect. One could logically refer to this state as *akinetic mutism* insofar as the patient is akinetic (motionless) and mute, but this is not the sense in which the term was originally used by Cairns and colleagues. They described a patient who appeared to be awake but was unresponsive (actually their patient was able to answer in whispered monosyllables). Following each of several evacuations of a third ventricular cyst, the patient would become aware and responsive but would have no memory for any of the events that had taken place when she was in the akinetic-mute state. This rare state of apparent vigilance in an imperceptive and unresponsive patient has been referred to by French authors as *coma vigile*.

The term *akinetic mutism* has been applied to yet another group of patients who are silent and inert as a result of bilateral lesions of the anterior parts of the frontal lobes, leaving intact the motor and sensory pathways; the patient is profoundly apathetic, lacking to an extreme degree the psychic drive or impulse to action (*abulia*) (page 544). The abulic patient, unlike Cairns's patient, registers most of what is happening about him and forms memories.

The psychiatric patient with *catatonia* appears unresponsive, simulating stupor, light coma, or the akinetic mute state. There are no signs of structural brain disease such as pupillary or reflex abnormalities. Oculocephalic responses are preserved as in the awake state, i.e. the eyes move concurrently as the head is turned. There is usually resistance to eye opening, and some patients display a waxy flexibility of passive limb movement that gives the examiner a feeling of bending a wax rod (flexibilitas cerea); there is also the retention for a long period of seemingly uncomfortable limb postures (catalepsy). Peculiar motor mannerisms or repetitive motions, seen in a number of these patients, may give the impression of seizures; choreiform jerking has been reported. The EEG shows normal posterior alpha activity that is attenuated by stimulation. Catatonia is discussed further on pages 435 and 1628.

Since there is considerable imprecision in the use of terms by which these states are designated, the student would be better advised to supplement designations such as *coma* and *akinetic mutism* by simple descriptions indicating whether the patient appears awake or asleep, drowsy or alert, aware or unaware of his surroundings, and responsive or unresponsive to a variety of stimuli.

Brain Death

In the late 1950s European neurologists called attention to a state of coma in which the brain was irreversibly damaged and had ceased to function but pulmonary and cardiac function could still be maintained by artificial means. Mollaret and Goulon referred to this condition as *coma dépassé* (a state beyond coma). A Harvard Medical School committee, in 1968, called it *brain death* and established a set of clinical criteria by which it could be recognized (Beecher et al). The concept that a person is dead if the brain is dead and that death of the brain may precede the cessation of cardiac function has posed a number of important ethical, legal, and social problems as well as medical ones. The various aspects of brain death have been the subject of close study by several professional committees, which have for the most part confirmed the 1968 guidelines for determining that the brain is dead.

The central considerations in the diagnosis of brain death are (1) absence of cerebral functions (unreceptivity and unresponsivity); (2) absence of brainstem functions, including spontaneous respiration; and (3) irreversibility of the state. To these is usually added evidence of catastrophic brain damage (trauma, cardiac arrest, cerebral hemorrhage, etc.).

The *absence of cerebral function* is judged by the presence of deep coma and total lack of spontaneous movement and of motor and vocal responses to all visual, auditory, and cutaneous stimulation. Spinal reflexes may persist in some cases, and the toes often flex slowly in response to plantar stimulation; but a well-developed Babinski sign is unusual. Extensor or flexor posturing is seen from time to time as a transitional phenomenon just after brain death becomes evident. The *absence of brainstem function* is judged by absence of spontaneous eye movements, midposition of the eyes, and lack of response to oculocephalic and caloric (oculovestibular) testing; presence of dilated or midposition fixed pupils (not smaller than 3 mm); paralysis of bulbar musculature (no facial movement or gag, cough, corneal, or sucking reflexes); absence of decerebrate responses to noxious stimuli; and absence of respiratory movements. As a final test of *complete apnea*, the patient, after preoxygenation for several minutes, can be disconnected from the respirator for a few minutes (during which time 100% O_2 is being delivered by cannula), allowing the P_{CO_2} to rise to 50 to 60 mmHg as a stimulus to the medullary respiratory centers. If no breaths are observed and examination of the blood gases shows that an adequate level of P_{CO_2} has been attained, the presence of brain death is corroborated. Most but not all patients have the signs of diabetes insipidus when the other criteria for brain death are fulfilled, reflecting the imprecision of clinical features in detecting the total loss of brain function.

The authors have observed a number of dramatic spontaneous movements when severely hypoxic levels are attained by apnea testing or disconnection from the ventilator for several minutes. These include opisthotonos with chest expansion that simulates a breath, raising the arms and crossing them in front of the chest or neck (Lazarus sign), head turning, shoulder shrugging, and variants of these movements (Ropper 1984). For this reason it is advisable that the family not be in attendance immediately after mechanical ventilation has been discontinued.

The EEG provides confirmation of cerebral death, and most institutions still prefer corroboration of the clinical features by the demonstration of electrocerebral silence (flat or isoelectric EEG), which is considered to be present if there is no electrical potential of more than 2 μV (except for artifacts created by the ventilator, ECG, or surrounding electrical devices) during a 30-min recording.

It must be emphasized that cerebral unresponsivity and a flat EEG do not always signify brain death but that both may occur and may be reversible in states of profound hypothermia or intoxication with sedative-hypnotic drugs and immediately following cardiac arrest. For this reason, it has been recommended that the diagnosis of brain death not be entertained until several hours have passed from the time of initial observation. If the examination is performed at least 6 h after the ictus and there is prima facie evidence of overwhelming brain injury from trauma, anoxia, or massive cerebral hemorrhage (the most common conditions causing brain death), there is no need for serial testing. If cardiac arrest was the antecedent event, or the cause of neurologic damage is unclear, or drug or alcohol intoxication could reasonably have played a role in suppressing the brainstem's reflexes, it is advisable to wait about 24 h before pronouncing the patient dead. Toxicologic screening of the serum or urine is requisite in the latter circumstances. Evoked potentials show interesting and variable abnormalities in brain-dead patients but are not of primary value in the diagnosis. Some centers utilize nuclide brain scanning or cerebral angiography to demonstrate an absence of blood flow to the brain, equating this with brain death, but there are technical pitfalls in the use of these methods and it is preferable to keep the diagnosis of death primarily clinical. The same can be said for transcranial Doppler sonography, which in brain death shows a to-and-fro "pendelfluss" blood-flow pattern in the basal vessels.

In our experience the main difficulties that arise in relation to brain death are not the technical issues but those involving the sensitive relationship with the family and other medical professionals. The task of dealing with these matters most often falls to the neurologist. It is best not to embark on clinical or EEG testing for brain death unless there is a clear intention on the part of the physician to remove the ventilator or request organ donation at the end of the process. The process and its intended outcome should be explained to the family and no intimation given that they have a role in deciding whether to remove the ventilator. The family's desires regarding organ transplantation should be sought after adequate time has passed for them to absorb the shock of the circumstances. Neurologists must, of course, resist pressures from diverse sources that might lead them to the premature designation of a state of brain death. The clinical findings should show complete absence of brain function, not an approximation that might be reflected, for example, by small or poorly reactive pupils, slight eye deviation with oculovestibular stimulation, flexor posturing of the limbs, and the like. At the same time, it should be clarified that while brain death is an operational state that allows transplantation to proceed and mandates withdrawal of ventilation and blood pressure support, patients with overwhelming brain injuries need not fulfill these absolute criteria in order for medical support to be withdrawn.

A task force for the determination of brain death in children has recommended the adoption of essentially the same criteria as for adults. Because of the great difficulty in evaluating the status of nervous function in relation to perinatal insults, they have suggested that a diagnosis of brain death not be made before the seventh postnatal day and that the period of observation be extended to 48 h. As with adults, the possibility of reversible brain dysfunction from toxins, drugs, hypothermia, and hypotension must always be considered.

The Electroencephalogram and Disturbances of Consciousness

One of the most delicate confirmations of the fact that the states of impaired consciousness are expressions of neurophysiologic changes in the cerebrum is the altered EEG. Some alteration of brain waves occurs in all disturbances of consciousness except the milder degrees of confusion and in catatonia. These alterations usually consist of a disorganization of the EEG pattern, including disappearance of alpha rhythm and replacement by random slow waves of low to moderate voltage in the initial stages of confusion; a more regular pattern of slow, 2- to 3-per-second waves of high voltage in stupor; slow low-voltage waves or intermittent suppression of organized electrical activity in the deep coma of hypoxia and ischemia; and ultimately a complete absence of electrical activity in brain death.

In some deeply comatose patients, the EEG may transiently show diffuse and variable (8- to 12-Hz) activity, which may be mistaken for physiologic alpha rhythm. However, the former pattern (so-called *alpha coma*) is not limited to the posterior cerebral regions, is not monorhythmic like normal alpha activity, and displays no reactivity to sensory stimuli. This alpha-like activity pattern may be associated with pontine or diffuse cortical lesions and has a poor prognosis (Iragui and McCutchen; page 33). A rarer EEG abnormality is "*spindle coma,*" in which sleep spindles dominate the record (page 415).

The EEG accurately reflects the depth of certain metabolic comas, particularly those due to hepatic or renal failure. In these conditions the slow waves become higher in amplitude as coma deepens, ultimately assuming a high-voltage rhythmic delta pattern and a triphasic configuration. There is also a general correspondence between the intensity of stimuli required to elicit motor activity and the degree of slowing of the background rhythm. Not all cerebral disorders that cause confusion, stupor, and coma have the same effects on the EEG. In cases of intoxication with sedatives, exemplified by barbiturates, fast activity initially replaces normal rhythms. Coma in which myoclonus or twitching is a major clinical feature may show frequent sharp waves or a sharpness to the background slowing of the EEG. The differences in EEG changes among metabolic derangements probably represent important biologic distinctions at the neuronal level that have not yet been elucidated (see also Chap. 2).

The Anatomy and Neurophysiology of Coma

Our current understanding of the anatomy and physiology of alertness comes largely from the elegant experiments of F. G. Bremer and of Magoun and Moruzzi in the 1930s and 1940s. Observing cats in whom he had sectioned the brainstem between the pons and midbrain and at the level of the lower medulla, Bremer found that the rostral section caused a sleep-like state and "synchronized" EEG rhythms that were characteristic of sleep; animals with the lower section remained awake, with appropriate "desynchronized" EEG rhythms. He interpreted this to mean that a constant stream of sensory stimuli, provided by trigeminal and other cranial sources, was required to maintain the awake state. Several years later, Morrison and Dempsey demonstrated a system of "nonspecific" projections from the thalamus to all cortical regions, independent of any specific sensory nucleus. A critical refinement of this concept resulted from the observation, by Moruzzi and Magoun, that electrical stimulation of the medial midbrain tegmentum and adjacent areas just above this level caused a lightly anesthetized animal to become suddenly alert and its EEG to change correspondingly, i.e., to become "desynchronized," in a manner identical to normal arousal by sensory stimuli. The sites at which stimulation led to arousal consisted of a series of points extending from the non-specific medial thalamic nuclei down through the caudal midbrain. These points were situated along the loosely organized core of neurons that anatomists had referred to as the *reticular system* or *formation*. The anatomic studies of the Scheibels described widespread innervation of the reticular formation by multiple bifurcating and collateral axons of the ascending sensory systems, implying that the this area was maintained in a tonically active state by ascending sensory stimulation. Because this region, especially the medial thalamus, projected widely to the cerebral hemispheres, there arose the concept of a *reticular activating system* (RAS) that maintained the alert state and the inactivation of which led to an unarousable state. In this way, despite a number of experimental inconsistencies (see Steriade) the paramedian upper brainstem tegmentum and lower diencephalon came to be conceived as the locus of the alerting system of the brain.

The anatomic boundaries of the high brainstem reticular activating system are somewhat indistinct. This system is interspersed throughout the paramedian regions of the upper (rostral) pontine and midbrain tegmentum; at the thalamic level, it includes the functionally related posterior paramedian, parafascicular, and medial portions of the centromedian and adjacent intralaminar nuclei. In the brainstem, nuclei of the reticular formation receive collaterals from the direct spinothalamic pathways and project not just to the sensory cortex of the parietal lobe, as do the thalamic relay nuclei for somatic sensation, but to the whole of the cerebral cortex. Thus, it would seem that sensory stimulation has a double effect—it conveys information to the brain from somatic structures and the environment and also activates those parts of the nervous system on which the maintenance of consciousness depends. The cerebral cortex not only receives impulses from the ascending reticular activating system but also modulates this incoming information via corticofugal projections to the reticular formation. Although the physiology of the reticular activating system is far more complicated than this simple formulation would suggest, it nevertheless, as a working idea, retains a great deal of clinical credibility and makes some of the neuropathologic observations noted further on, under "Pathologic Anatomy of Coma," more comprehensible.

Metabolic Mechanisms That Disturb Consciousness

In a number of disease processes that disturb consciousness there is direct interference with the metabolic activities of the nerve cells in the cerebral cortex and the central nuclei of the brain. Hypoxia, global ischemia, hypoglycemia, hyper- and hypo-osmolar states, acidosis, alkalosis, hypokalemia, hyperammonemia, hypercalcemia, hypercarbia, drug intoxication, and severe vitamin deficiencies are well-known examples (see Chap. 40 and Table 40-1). In general, the loss of consciousness in these conditions parallels the reduction in cerebral metabolism or blood flow. For example, in the case of global ischemia, an acute drop in cerebral blood flow (CBF) to 25 mL/min/100 g brain tissue from its normal 55 mL/min/l00 g causes slowing of the EEG and syncope or impaired consciousness; a drop in CBF below 12 to 15 mL/min/100 g causes electrocerebral silence, coma, and cessation of most neuronal metabolic and synaptic functions. Lower levels are tolerated if arrived at more slowly, but neurons cannot survive when flow is reduced below 8 to 10 mL/min/100 g. There is a corresponding reduction in the cerebral metabolic rate. In other cases of metabolic encephalopathy or widespread anatomic damage to the hemispheres, blood flow stays near normal levels while metabolism is greatly reduced. Oxygen consumption of 2 mg/min/100 g (approximately half of normal) is incompatible with an alert state. The exception is coma from seizures, in which metabolism and blood flow are greatly increased during the seizure. Extremes of body temperature (above 41°C or below 30°C) also induce coma through a nonspecific effect on the metabolic activity of neurons. These metabolic changes are probably epiphenomena reflecting, in each particular type of encephalopathy, a specific dysfunction in neurons and their supporting cells.

The endogenous metabolic toxin(s) that are responsible for coma cannot always be identified. In diabetes, acetone bodies (acetoacetic acid, β-hydroxybutyric acid, and acetone) are present in high concentration; in uremia, there is probably an accumulation of dialyzable small molecular toxins, notably phenolic derivatives of the aromatic amino acids. In hepatic coma, elevation of blood NH_3 to five to six times normal levels has been found. Lactic acidosis may affect the brain by lowering arterial blood pH to less than 7.0. The impairment of consciousness that accompanies pulmonary insufficiency is related mainly to hypercapnia (see page 1181). In hyponatremia (Na<120 meq/L) from whatever cause, neuronal dysfunction is due to the intracellular movement of water, leading to neuronal swelling and loss of potassium chloride from the cells. The mode of action of bacterial toxins is not fully understood.

Drugs such as general anesthetics, alcohol, opiates, barbiturates, phenytoin, antidepressants, and diazepines induce coma by their direct effects on neuronal membranes in the cerebrum and diencephalon or on neurotransmitters and their receptors. Others, such as methyl alcohol and ethylene glycol, act by producing a metabolic acidosis. Although the coma of toxic and metabolic diseases usually evolves through stages of drowsiness, confusion, and stupor (and the reverse sequence occurs during emergence from coma), each disease imparts its own characteristic clinical features. Probably this means that each disease has a distinctive mechanism and that the locus of the metabolic effect is somewhat different from one disease to another.

The sudden and excessive neuronal discharge that characterizes an epileptic seizure is a common coma-producing mechanism. Usually focal seizure activity has little effect on consciousness until it spreads from one side of the brain (and body if there is a convulsion) to the other. Coma then ensues, presumably because the spread of the seizure discharge to deep central neuronal structures paralyzes their function. In other types of seizure, in which consciousness is interrupted from the very beginning, a diencephalic origin has been postulated (centrencephalic seizures of Penfield).

Concussion exemplifies another special pathophysiologic mechanism of coma. In "blunt" or closed head injury, it has been shown that at the moment of the concussive injury there is an enormous increase in intracranial pressure, on the order of 200 to 700 lb/in^2, lasting a few thousandths of a second. The vibration set up in the skull and transmitted to the brain was for many years thought to be the basis of the abrupt paralysis of nervous function that characterizes concussive head injury. Instead it is more likely that the sudden swirling motion of the brain induced by the blow to the head, producing a rotation (torque) of the cerebral hemispheres around the axis of the upper brainstem, is the proximate cause of loss of consciousness. These same physical forces, when extreme, cause multiple shearing lesions or hemorrhages in the diencephalon and upper brainstem. The subject of concussion is discussed fully in Chap. 35.

Yet another unique form of coma is that produced by inhalation anesthetics. Current theories attribute the effects of general anesthesia to changes in the physical chemistry of neuronal membranes and perhaps to consequent alterations in neurotransmitter function. Inhalation anesthetics are unusual among coma-producing drugs in respect to the sequence of inhibitory and excitatory effects that they produce at different concentrations. During anesthesia, sufficient inhibition of brainstem activity can be attained to eliminate the pupillary responses and the corneal reflex. Both return to normal by the time the patient is able to speak. Sustained clonus, exaggerated tendon reflexes, and Babinski signs are common during the process of arousal. These findings have been studied systematically by Rosenberg et al and reviewed by Ropper and Kennedy. Pre-existing focal deficits from strokes often worsen transiently with the administration of anesthetics, as is true for other sedatives, metabolic encephalopathies, and hyperthermia.

Recurring Stupor and Coma Aside from repeated drug overdose, recurring episodes of stupor are usually due to the decompensation of an encephalopathy from an underlying biochemical derangement, hepatic failure being the most common. A similar condition of periodic hyperammonemic coma in children and adults can come about from urea cycle enzyme defects, such as ornithine transcarbamylase deficiency. These are discussed in Chap. 37 in the section on inherited hyperammonemias.

Under the title of *idiopathic recurring stupor*, a rare condition has been described in adult men who displayed a prolonged state of deep sleepiness lasting from hours to days intermittently over a period of many years. Despite the impression of a sleep disorder related to narcolepsy, the electroencephalogram (EEG) showed widespread fast (beta) activity, and both the stupor and EEG changes were promptly reversed by flumazenil, a benzodiazepine receptor antagonist. During the bouts, a hundredfold increase of circulating endozepine-4, a naturally occurring diazepine agonist, was found in the serum and spinal fluid. Subsequently, the authors of the original reports (Lugaresi et al) found, by the use of more advanced techniques, that intoxication with lorazepam may have accounted for at least some of the cases; the status of this entity is therefore unclear.

It is uncertain to us whether migraine can cause a similar syndrome, as suggested in the study of familial hemiplegic migraine by Fitzsimmons and Wolfenden. Basilar migraine may exceptionally cause transient stupor and coma. Catatonic stupor and Kleine–Levin syndrome also need to be considered.

Pathologic Anatomy of Coma

Coma-producing alterations in the brain are divided into two broad groups: The first is clearly morphologic, consisting either of discrete lesions in the upper brainstem and lower diencephalon (which may be primary or secondary to compression), or of more widespread changes throughout the hemispheres. The second is metabolic or submicroscopic, resulting in suppression of neuronal activity. The clinical examination in coma is designed to separate these various mechanisms and to gauge the depth of brain dysfunction.

The study of a large number of human cases in which coma preceded death by several days has disclosed three main types of lesion, each of which ultimately deranges the function of the reticular activating system directly or indirectly. In the *first type*, a readily discernible mass lesion—chiefly a tumor, abscess, meningitis, massive edematous infarct, or intracerebral, subarachnoid, subdural, or epidural hemorrhage—is demonstrable. Usually the lesion involves only a portion of the cortex and white matter, leaving much of the cerebrum intact but nonetheless it distorts deeper structures. In most instances, these mass lesions in or surrounding the hemispheres cause coma by a lateral displacement of deep central structures, sometimes, but not always, with herniation of the temporal lobe into the tentorial opening, resulting in compression, ischemia, and secondary hemorrhages in the midbrain and subthalamic region including the reticular activating system (see below and also Chap. 31). Likewise, a cerebellar lesion may secondarily compress the adjacent upper brainstem reticular region by displacing it forward and perhaps upward. A detailed clinical record will show the coma to have coincided with these displacements and herniations. The anatomical displacements caused by herniations are discussed in more detail below.

In *a second type*, less frequent than the first, the lesion is located in the thalamus or midbrain, in which case the reticular activating neurons are involved directly. This pathoanatomic pattern characterizes brainstem stroke from basilar artery occlusion, and thalamic–upper brainstem hemorrhage.

In *a third type*, widespread bilateral damage to the cortex and white matter is found—the result of traumatic damage (contusions, diffuse axonal injury), bilateral infarcts or hemorrhages, viral encephalitis, meningitis, hypoxia, or ischemia, as occurs after cardiac arrest. The coma in these cases results either from interruption of corticopetal impulses or from generalized destruction of cortical neurons, which prevents their activation by the upper reticular formation. Only if the cerebral lesions are bilateral and extensive is consciousness markedly impaired. Thus, pathologic changes are compatible with physiologic deductions—that the state of prolonged coma correlates with lesions of all parts of the cortical-diencephalic system of neurons; but it is only in the upper brainstem that the coma-producing lesions may be small and discrete.

In yet another, larger group of cases, no lesion is visible to the naked eye. Sometimes no abnormality is divulged by any technique of pathology; the lesion, caused by a metabolic or toxic abnormality or a generalized electrical discharge (seizure), is presumably subcellular or molecular, or the visible microscopic lesions are too diffuse for clinicoanatomic correlation, as discussed below.

Pathoanatomy of Brain Displacement and Herniations

As was pointed out earlier, large, destructive, and space-consuming lesions of the cerebrum—such as hemorrhage, tumor, abscess, or infarction—impair consciousness in one of two ways. One is by direct extension of the lesion into the diencephalon and midbrain. The other, far more frequent, is by lateral and downward displacement of the subthalamic–upper brainstem structures with or without herniation of the medial part of the temporal lobe (uncus, hippocampus) through and below the opening in the tentorium. One consequence of lateral displacement is that the upper midbrain, particularly the cerebral peduncle, is crushed against the opposite free edge of the tentorium (the resulting creasing of the lateral edge of the peduncle is called Kernohan's notch or, more properly, the Kernohan-Woltman phenomenon), causing a Babinski sign ipsilateral to the hemispheral lesion. The posterior cerebral artery is also compressed at the edge of the tentorium, leading to hemorrhagic infarction of the ipsilateral occipital lobe (see also page 682).

It follows from the foregoing discussion that unilateral destructive lesions of the hemispheres, such as infarcts or hemorrhages, do not cause coma unless they create some degree of mass effect, usually delayed in onset, which secondarily compresses the upper brainstem. There are exceptions in which patients with massive strokes affecting the territory of the internal carotid artery are drowsy from the onset, even before brain swelling occurs, but more often they are simply apathetic with a tendency to keep their eyes closed, a state that may be misinterpreted as stupor.

Plum and Posner, following upon earlier observations of McNealy and Plum, subdivided the brainstem displacements by supratentorial masses into two groups: one a central syndrome with downward displacement and bilateral compression of the upper brainstem and the other a unilateral displacement with medial temporal lobe and particularly uncal gyrus herniation into the tentorial opening. Both are types of *transtentorial herniation*. According to these authors, the *central syndrome* takes the form of a rostral-caudal deterioration of function: there is first confusion, apathy, and drowsiness and often Cheyne-Stokes respiration (CSR); then the pupils become small and react very little to light; "doll's-head" (oculocephalic) eye movements are elicitable, as are deviations of the eyes in response to cold-water caloric testing (the compensatory fast component of the response is impaired or absent, however). Bilateral Babinski signs can be detected early; later, grasp reflexes and decorticate postures appear. These signs give way to a downward gradient of brainstem signs—coma, central hyperventilation, medium-sized fixed pupils, bilateral decerebrate postures, loss of oculovestibular (caloric) responses, slow, irregular breathing, and death.

The *uncal syndrome*, thought traditionally to be the result of herniation of the medial temporal lobe downward through the tentorial opening, differs mainly in that drowsiness in the early stages is accompanied or preceded by unilateral pupillary dilatation, most often on the side of a mass. These herniations between dural compartments are illustrated in Fig. 17-1 and Table 31-2, page 683.

Our own experience does not fully substantiate this distinction between the two syndromes, and seldom have we been able to follow such an orderly sequence of neural dysfunction from the diencephalic to the medullary level. With lateral shift and uncal herniation, one sometimes observes smallness of the pupils, rather than ipsilateral pupillary dilatation, as drowsiness develops. Or, infrequently, the contralateral pupil may dilate

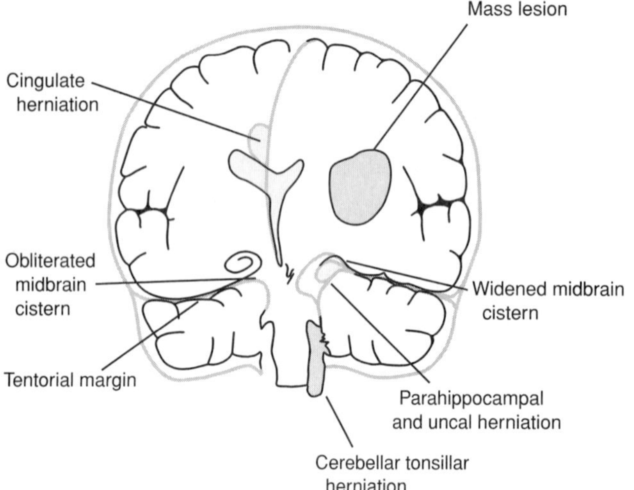

Figure 17-1

Brain herniations between dural compartments. Transfalcial, uncal-parahippocampal, and cerebellar herniations are shown.

before the ipsilateral one. Nor is it clear that the dilatation of one pupil is always due to trapping or compression of the oculomotor nerve by the herniated uncus, as traditionally taught. More often the third nerve is stretched and angulated over the clivus or compressed under the descended posterior cerebral artery. Involvement of the third nerve nucleus or its fibers of exit may be responsible for the dilatation of the opposite pupil, the usual occurrence after the pupil on the side of the mass has become fixed. In a serial study of 12 patients with brain edema and lateral diencephalic-mesencephalic shifts due to hemispheral infarcts, 4 patients initially had no ipsilateral pupillary enlargement; in 1 patient, the pupillary enlargement was contralateral; in 3 patients, the pupils were symmetrical when drowsiness gave way to stupor or coma (Ropper and Shafran). Cyclic Cheyne-Stokes breathing was an early sign of deterioration. In one patient, the first motor sign was an ipsilateral decerebrate rigidity rather than decorticate posturing; most of the patients had bilateral Babinski signs by the time they became stuporous. Indeed, the appearance of a Babinski sign on the nonhemiparetic side has been one of the best sentinels of secondary brain tissue shift. These signs often progressed to deep coma and decerebration within hours and they fluctuated widely, worsening with waves of high intracranial pressure.

As the primary explanation for coma from a large mass in one hemisphere, we favor a mechanism of predominantly lateral displacement that causes compression of subthalamic and mesencephalic structures. This is often but not invariably associated with temporal lobe herniation. The resulting neural dysfunction of deep structures is probably due to ischemia. This view is supported by findings on CT scans and MRI, which have been used to study the earliest structural displacements in patients with acute hemispheral mass lesions. In our experience, the early disturbances of consciousness (drowsiness and stupor) are related to the degree of lateral displacement of high brainstem and subthalamic structures (judged by shifts in the position of the pineal body and, with less accuracy, the septum pellucidum), all occurring in the absence of transtentorial herniation which arises later. With acute masses, a 3- to 5-mm horizontal displacement of the pineal calcification is associated with drowsiness; 5 to 8 mm, with stupor; and greater than 8 or 9 mm, with coma (Ropper, 1986).

The location as well as the size of a mass determines the degree of brain distortion and displacement of crucial structures in the lower diencephalon and upper midbrain. Andrews and colleagues have pointed out that frontal and occipital hemorrhages are less likely to displace deep structures and to cause coma than are clots of equivalent size in the parietal or temporal lobes. Nor is it surprising that slowly enlarging masses such as brain tumors may sometimes cause massive shifts of brain tissue yet result in few clinical changes.

Downward movement of the upper brainstem occurs, but its role in the production of coma in comparison to horizontal shift is not entirely settled. In our view, the importance of direct downward displacement may be overestimated as the main pathoanatomic cause of coma. Although in some cases the predominant shift is downward and in others it is horizontal, horizontal displacement on MRI is usually disproportionate to vertical displacement, and the clinical state corresponds better with the degree of lateral shift. Others, notably Reich and colleagues, disagree with these observations and find the argument for vertical shift to be more compelling. It is noteworthy that the brainstem can usually tolerate, without inducing a change in consciousness, a large downward movement that occurs as part of the syndrome of low cerebrospinal fluid (CSF) pressure following lumbar puncture. This is not always the case, however, as in the patient reported by Pleasure and colleagues who became stuporous with low CSF pressure from a spinal leak and aroused when the pressure was normalized.

CLINICAL APPROACH TO THE COMATOSE PATIENT

It must be repeated that coma is always a symptomatic expression of an underlying disease. Sometimes the primary disorder is perfectly obvious, as with severe cranial trauma. All too often, however, the patient is brought to the hospital in a state of coma and little pertinent medical information is immediately available. The need for efficiency in reaching a diagnosis and providing appropriate acute care demands that the physician have a methodical approach that leaves none of the common and treatable causes of coma unexplored.

When the comatose patient is first seen, one must quickly make sure that the patient's airway is clear and the patient is not in shock; if trauma has occurred, one must check for bleeding from a wound or ruptured organ (e.g., spleen or liver). If hypotension is present, certain therapeutic measures—placement of a central venous line and administration of fluids and pressor agents, oxygen, blood, or glucose solutions (*after* blood is drawn for glucose determinations and thiamine is administered)—take precedence over diagnostic procedures. If respirations are shallow or labored or if there is emesis with a threat of aspiration, tracheal intubation and mechanical ventilation are required. An oropharyngeal airway is usually adequate in a comatose patient who is breathing normally. Deeply comatose patients with shallow respirations require endotracheal intubation. The patient with a head injury may also have suffered a fracture of the cervical vertebrae, in which case caution must be exercised in moving the head and neck, and in intubation, lest the spinal cord be inadvertently damaged.

There must then be an inquiry as to the previous health of the patient—whether there was a history of diabetes, a head injury, a convulsion, alcohol or drug use, or a prior episode of coma or attempted suicide—and the circumstances in which the person was found. Persons who accompany the comatose patient to the hospital should be encouraged not to leave until they have been questioned.

From an initial survey, many of the common causes of coma—such as severe head injury, alcoholic or other forms of drug intoxication, and hypertensive brain hemorrhage—are readily recognized.

General Examination Alterations in vital signs—temperature, pulse, respiratory rate, and blood pressure—are important aids in diagnosis. Fever is most often due to a systemic infection such as pneumonia or to bacterial meningitis or viral encephalitis. An excessively high body temperature (42 or 43°C) associated with dry skin should arouse suspicion of heat stroke or intoxication by a drug with anticholinergic activity. Fever should not be ascribed to a brain lesion that has disturbed the temperature-regulating center—so-called central fever, which is a very rare occurrence. *Hypothermia* is observed in patients with alcoholic or barbiturate intoxication, drowning, exposure to cold, peripheral circulatory failure, and myxedema.

Slow breathing points to opiate or barbiturate intoxication and occasionally to hypothyroidism, whereas deep, rapid breathing (Kussmaul respiration) should suggest the presence of pneumonia, diabetic or uremic acidosis, pulmonary edema, or the less common occurrence of an intracranial disease that causes central neurogenic hyperventilation. Diseases that elevate intracranial pressure or damage the brain often cause slow, irregular, or cyclic Cheyne-Stokes respiration (see further on). The various disordered patterns of breathing and their clinical significance are described further on and on page 579. *Vomiting* at the outset of sudden coma, particularly if combined with pronounced hypertension, is highly characteristic of cerebral hemorrhage within the hemispheres, brainstem, cerebellum, or subarachnoid space. When occurring with coma of more gradual onset, it may signify drug or alcohol intoxication.

The *pulse rate*, if exceptionally slow, should suggest heart block from medications such as tricyclic antidepressants or anticonvulsants, or—if combined with periodic breathing and hypertension—an increase in intracranial pressure. Marked hypertension is observed in patients with cerebral hemorrhage and hypertensive encephalopathy and, at times, in those with greatly increased intracranial pressure. Hypotension is the usual finding in states of depressed consciousness due to diabetes, alcohol or barbiturate intoxication, internal hemorrhage, myocardial infarction, dissecting aortic aneurysm, septicemia, Addison disease, or massive brain trauma.

Inspection of the skin may yield valuable information. Cyanosis of the lips and nail beds signifies inadequate oxygenation. Cherry-red coloration is typical of carbon monoxide poisoning. Multiple bruises (particularly a bruise or boggy area in the scalp), bleeding, CSF leakage from an ear or the nose, or periorbital hemorrhage greatly raises the likelihood of cranial fracture and intracranial trauma. Telangiectases and hyperemia of the face and conjunctivae are the common stigmata of alcoholism; myxedema imparts a characteristic puffiness of the face, and hypopituitarism, an equally characteristic sallow complexion. Marked pallor suggests internal hemorrhage. A maculohemorrhagic rash indicates the possibility of meningococcal infection, staphylococcal endocarditis, typhus, or Rocky Mountain spotted fever. Excessive sweating suggests hypoglycemia or shock, and excessively dry skin, diabetic acidosis or uremia. Skin turgor is reduced in dehydration. Large blisters, sometimes bloody, may form over pressure points if the patient has been motionless for a time; they are particularly characteristic of acute barbiturate, alcohol, or opiate intoxication. Thrombotic thrombocytopenic purpura, disseminated intravascular coagulation, and fat embolism may cause diffuse petechiae.

The *odor of the breath* may provide a clue to the etiology of coma. The odor of alcohol is easily recognized (except for vodka, which is odorless). The spoiled-fruit odor of diabetic coma, the uriniferous odor of uremia, the musty fetor of hepatic coma, and the burnt almond odor of cyanide poisoning are distinctive enough to be identified by physicians who possess a keen sense of smell.

Neurologic Examination of the Stuporous or Comatose Patient Although limited in many ways, the neurologic examination is of crucial importance.

Simply watching the patient for a few moments often yields considerable information. The predominant postures of the limbs and body; the presence or absence of spontaneous movements on one side; the position of the head and eyes; and the rate, depth, and rhythm of respiration should be noted. The state of responsiveness is then estimated by noting the patient's reaction to calling his name, to simple commands, or to noxious stimuli such as supraorbital or sternal pressure, pinching the side of the neck or inner parts of the arms or thighs, or applying pressure to the knuckles. By gradually increasing the strength of these stimuli, one can roughly estimate both the degree of unresponsiveness and changes from hour to hour. Vocalization may persist in stupor and is the first response to be lost as coma appears. Grimacing and deft avoidance movements of the stimulated parts are preserved in light coma; their presence substantiates the integrity of corticobul-bar and corticospinal tracts. Yawning and spontaneous shifting of body positions indicate a minimal degree of unresponsiveness. The Glasgow Coma Scale, constructed originally as a quick and simple means of quantitating the responsiveness of patients with severe cerebral trauma, can be used in the grading of other acute coma-producing diseases (see Chap. 35).

It is usually possible to determine whether coma is associated with *meningeal irritation* or with focal cerebral or brainstem disease. In all but the deepest stages of coma, meningeal irritation—from either bacterial meningitis or subarachnoid hemorrhage—will cause resistance to passive flexion of the neck but not to extension, turning, or tilting of the head. It should be noted that in some patients the signs of meningeal irritation do not develop for 12 to 24 h after the onset of subarachnoid hemorrhage, during which time CT scanning and lumbar puncture are the most reliable diagnostic measures. Resistance to movement of the neck in all directions may be part of generalized muscular rigidity (as in phenothiazine intoxication) or indicate disease of the cervical spine. In the infant, bulging of the anterior fontanel is at times a more reliable sign of meningitis than stiff neck. A temporal lobe or cerebellar herniation or decerebrate rigidity may also limit passive flexion of the neck and be confused with meningeal irritation.

A lesion in a cerebral hemisphere can usually be detected, even though the patient is comatose, by careful observation of the patient's spontaneous movements, responses to stimulation, prevailing postures, respiratory rate and rhythm, and by examination of the cranial nerves. A hemiplegia is revealed by a lack of restless movements of the limbs and of aversive or protective movements in response to painful stimuli. The paralyzed limbs are usually slack; they tend to remain in passive positions and, if lifted from the bed, "fall flail." The hemiplegic leg lies in a position of external rotation (this may also be due to a fractured femur), and the thigh may appear wider and flatter than the nonhemiplegic one. In expiration, the cheek and lips puff out on the paralyzed side. With hemispheric lesions, the eyes are often turned away from the paralyzed side (toward the lesion, as described below); the opposite may occur with brainstem lesions. In most cases, a hemiplegia and an accompanying Babinski sign are indicative of a contralateral hemispheral lesion; but with lateral mass effect and compression of the opposite cerebral peduncle against the tentorium, extensor rigidity, a Babinski sign, and weakness of arm and leg may also occur ipsilateral to the lesion (Kernohan-Woltman sign). A moan or grimace may be provoked by painful stimuli on one side but not on the other, reflecting the presence of a hemianesthesia; also during grimacing, facial weakness may be noted.

Of the various indicators of brainstem function, the most useful are pupillary size and reactivity, ocular movements, oculovestibular reflexes, and, to a lesser extent, the pattern of breathing. These functions, like consciousness itself, are to a large extent dependent on the integrity of structures in the midbrain and rostral pons.

The Pupillary Reactions These are of great diagnostic importance in the comatose patient. A unilaterally enlarged pupil (>5.5 mm diameter) is an early indicator of stretching or compression of the third nerve as a secondary effect of an ipsilateral hemispheral mass. First there is usually a loss of light reaction alone. With continued compression of the nerve, the pupil may, as a transitional phenomenon, become oval or pear-shaped and appear to be off center (corectopia) due to a differential loss of innervation of a portion of the pupillary sphincter. The light-unreactive pupil continues to enlarge to a size of 6 to 9 mm diameter, associated with slight outward deviation of the globe, as noted below. In unusual instances, for an unknown reason, the pupil contralateral to the mass may enlarge first; this has been reported in 10 percent of cases of unilateral subdural hematomas but has been far less frequent in our experience with other mass lesions. As midbrain displacement continues, both pupils dilate and become unreactive to light (Ropper, 1990). The last step in the evolution of brainstem compression tends to be a slight reduction in pupillary size, to 5 to 7 mm; contrariwise, normal pupillary size, shape, and light reflexes indicate integrity of midbrain structures and a cause of coma other than a mass lesion.

Pontine tegmental lesions cause extremely miotic pupils (<1 mm in diameter) with only a slight reaction to strong light; this is characteristic of the early phase of pontine hemorrhage. The ipsilateral pupillary dilatation from pinching the side of the neck (the ciliospinal reflex, page 296) is also lost in brainstem lesions. A Horner syndrome (miosis, ptosis, apparent enophthalmos, and reduced sweating) may be observed homolateral to a lesion of the brainstem or hypothalamus or as a sign of dissection of the internal carotid artery.

With coma due to drug intoxications and metabolic disorders, pupillary reactions are usually spared, but there are notable exceptions. Opiates cause pinpoint pupils with so slight a constriction to light that it can be seen only with a magnifying glass. High-dose barbiturates may act similarly, but the pupillary diameter tends to be 1 mm or more. Poisoning with atropine or atropinic drugs, especially tricyclic antidepressants, is characterized by wide dilation and fixity of pupils, which cannot be reversed by physostigmine. Hippus, or fluctuating pupillary size, is said by some observers to be characteristic of the metabolic encephalopathies.

Movements of Eyes and Eyelids and Corneal Responses
These may be altered in a variety of ways. In light coma of metabolic origin, the eyes rove conjugately from side to side in random fashion, sometimes resting briefly in an eccentric position. These movements disappear as coma deepens and the eyes then remain motionless in slightly exotropic positions.

A lateral and slight downward deviation of one eye suggests the presence of a third nerve palsy, and a medial deviation, a sixth nerve palsy. There may be a persistent conjugate deviation of the eyes to one side—away from the side of the paralysis with a large cerebral lesion (looking toward the lesion) and toward the side of the paralysis with a unilateral pontine lesion (looking away from the lesion). "Wrong-way" conjugate deviation may sometimes occur with thalamic and upper brainstem lesions (page 277). During a one-sided seizure, the eyes turn or jerk toward the convulsing side (opposite to the irritative focus). The eyes may be turned down and inward (looking at the nose) with hematomas or ischemic lesions of the thalamus and upper midbrain (a variant of Parinaud syndrome; see page 277). Retraction and convergence nystagmus and "ocular bobbing," described on page 293, occur with lesions in the tegmentum of the midbrain and pons, respectively. "Ocular dipping," in which the eyes move down slowly and return rapidly to the meridian, may be observed with coma due to anoxia and drug intoxications; horizontal eye movements are preserved (page 293). The coma-producing structural lesions of the brainstem abolish most if not all conjugate ocular movements, whereas metabolic disorders generally do not (except for rare instances of hepatic coma and anticonvulsant drug overdose).

Oculocephalic reflexes (doll's-eye movements), are elicited by briskly turning or tilting the head. The response in coma consists of conjugate movement of the eyes in the opposite direction and is not present in the normal alert person. Elicitation of these reflexes in a comatose patient provides two pieces of information: (1) evidence of unimpeded function of the oculomotor nerves and of the midbrain and pontine tegmental structures that integrate ocular movements, and (2) loss of the cortical inhibition that normally holds these movements in check. The presence of unimpaired reflex eye movements implies that coma is not due to a mass lesion causing secondary compression or one that directly destroys the upper midbrain. Instead, it must be the result of widespread cortical dysfunction such as occurs with cerebral anoxia or metabolic-toxic suppression of cortical activity. It must be conceded, however, that although the failure to elicit eye movements implies brainstem dysfunction, *sedative or anticonvulsant intoxication serious enough to cause coma may obliterate the brainstem mechanisms for oculocephalic reactions and, in extreme cases, even the oculovestibular responses*, described below. Asymmetry in elicited eye movements remains a dependable sign of focal brainstem disease. In instances of coma due to a large mass in one cerebral hemisphere that secondarily compresses the upper brainstem, the oculocephalic reflexes are usually present but the movement of the eye on the side of the mass is often impeded in adduction, as a result of a third nerve paresis.

Irrigation of each ear with 10 mL of cold water (or room-temperature water if the patient is not comatose) normally causes slow conjugate deviation of the eyes toward the irrigated ear, followed in a few seconds by compensatory nystagmus (fast component away from the stimulated side). This is the *oculovestibular* or *caloric* response (page 319). The ears are irrigated separately several minutes apart. In comatose patients, the fast "corrective" phase of nystagmus is lost and the eyes are tonically deflected to the side irrigated with cold water or away from the side irrigated with warm water; this position may be held for 2 to 3 min. With brainstem lesions, these vestibulo-ocular reflexes are lost or disrupted.

If, on attempted lateral gaze, only one eye abducts and the other fails to adduct, one can conclude that the medial longitudinal fasciculus has been interrupted (on the side of adductor paralysis). The opposite, an abducens palsy, is indicated by an esotropic resting position and a lack of outward deviation of one eye with the reflex maneuvers.

Reduction in frequency and eventual loss of spontaneous blinking, then loss of blink in response to touching the eyelashes, and finally a lack of response to corneal touch (afferent limb–trigeminal nerve; efferent limb–both facial nerves) are among the most dependable signs of deepening coma. A marked asymmetry in corneal responses indicates either an acute lesion of the opposite hemisphere or, less often, an ipsilateral lesion in the brainstem.

Spontaneous Limb Movements Restless movements of both arms and both legs and grasping and picking movements signify that the corticospinal tracts are more or less intact. Variable oppositional resistance to passive movement (paratonic rigidity), complex avoidance movements, and discrete protective movements have the same meaning; if these movements are bilateral, the coma is usually not profound. The occurrence of focal motor epilepsy usually indicates that the corresponding corticospinal pathway is intact. With massive destruction of a cerebral hemisphere, as occurs in hypertensive hemorrhage or internal carotid–middle cerebral artery occlusion, focal seizures are seldom seen on the paralyzed side; seizure activity may be manifest solely in the ipsilateral limbs, the contralateral limbs being prevented from participating by the hemiplegia. Often, elaborate forms of semivoluntary movement are present on the "good side" in patients with extensive disease in one hemisphere; they probably represent some type of disequilibrium or disinhibition of cortical and subcortical movement patterns. Definite choreic, athetotic, or hemiballistic movements indicate a disorder of the basal ganglionic and subthalamic structures, just as they do in the alert patient.

Postural Changes in the Comatose Patient One of these abnormal postures is *decerebrate rigidity*, which in its fully developed form consists of opisthotonos, clenching of the jaws, and stiff extension of the limbs, with internal rotation of the arms and plantar flexion of the feet. This postural pattern was first described by Sherrington, who produced it in cats and monkeys by transecting the brainstem at the intercollicular level. The decerebrate pattern was noted to be ipsilateral to a one-sided lesion, hence not due to involvement of the corticospinal tracts. Such a precise correlation is rarely possible in patients who develop this stereotyped extensor posturing in a variety of clinical settings—with midbrain compression due to a hemispheral mass; with cerebellar or other posterior fossa lesions; with certain metabolic disorders, such as anoxia and hypoglycemia; and rarely with hepatic coma and profound intoxication. Patients with an acute lesion of one cerebral hemisphere may show a similar type of extensor posturing of the contralateral and sometimes ipsilateral limbs, and this may coexist with the ability to make purposeful movements of the same limbs. The extensor postures, unilateral or bilateral, may seemingly occur spontaneously, but more often they occur in response to manipulation of the limbs and all varieties of noxious stimuli. Also characteristic is the extensor posturing of arm and leg on one side and flexion and abduction of the opposite arm. These reactions are analogous to the tonic reflexes described by Magnus in decerebrate animals.

In some patients with the foregoing postural changes the lesions are clearly in the cerebral white matter or basal ganglia, which is difficult to reconcile with the classic physiologic explanation of decerebrate posturing; presumably there is a functional derangement of structures in the midbrain in these cases due to brain swelling and distortion. Decerebrate posturing, either in experimental preparations or in humans, is usually not a persistent steady state but an intermittent and transient one. Hence the term *decerebrate state* is preferable to *decerebrate rigidity*, which implies a fixed, tonic extensor attitude (Feldman).

Decorticate rigidity, with arm or arms in flexion and adduction and leg(s) extended, signifies lesions at a higher level—in the cerebral white matter or internal capsule and thalamus. Bilateral decorticate rigidity is essentially a bilateral spastic hemiplegia. *Diagonal postures*, e.g., flexion of one arm and extension of the opposite arm and leg, usually indicate a supratentorial lesion. Forceful extensor postures of the arms and weak flexor responses of the legs are probably due to lesions at about the level of the vestibular nuclei. Lesions below this level lead to flaccidity and abolition of all postures and movements. The coma is then usually profound and often progresses to brain death.

Only in the most advanced forms of intoxication and metabolic coma, as might occur with anoxic necrosis of neurons throughout the entire brain, are coughing, swallowing, hiccoughing, and spontaneous respiration all abolished. Further, the tendon and plantar reflexes may give little indication of what is happening. Tendon reflexes are usually preserved until the late stages of coma due to metabolic disturbances and intoxications. In coma due to a large cerebral infarct or hemorrhage, the tendon reflexes may be normal or only slightly reduced on the hemiplegic side and the plantar reflexes may be absent or extensor. Plantar flexor responses, succeeding extensor responses, signify ether a return to normalcy or, in the context of deepening coma, a transition to brain death.

Patterns of Breathing** **(see pages 579–580) A massive supratentorial lesion, bilateral deep-seated cerebral lesions, or metabolic disturbances of the brain give rise to a characteristic pattern of breathing, in which a period of waxing and waning hyperpnea regularly alternates with a shorter period of apnea (*Cheyne-Stokes* respiration, or CSR). This phenomenon has been attributed to isolation of the brainstem respiratory centers from the cerebrum, rendering them more sensitive than usual to CO_2 (hyperventilation drive). As a result of overbreathing, the blood CO_2 drops below the concentration required to stimulate the centers, and breathing gradually stops. Carbon dioxide then reaccumulates until it exceeds the respiratory threshold, and the cycle then repeats itself. Alternatively, CSR has been attributed to the stimulating effect of a low arterial P_{O_2} on a depressed respiratory center. In either case, the presence of CSR signifies bilateral dysfunction of cerebral structures, usually those deep in the hemispheres or diencephalon, and is seen with states of drowsiness or stupor. Coma with CSR is usually due to intoxication or a severe metabolic derangement and occasionally to bilateral lesions, such as subdural hematomas. In itself, CSR is not a grave sign. It may occur during sleep in elderly individuals and can be a manifestation of cardiopulmonary disorders in awake patients. Only when it gives way to other abnormal respiratory patterns that implicate the brainstem more directly is the patient in imminent danger.

A number of other aberrant breathing rhythms occur with brainstem lesions (reviewed in Chap. 26), but few are as specifically localizing as are abnormalities of the pupils and eye movements. The more conspicuous respiratory arrhythmias are associated with brainstem lesions below the level of the reticular activating system and are therefore found in the late stages of brainstem compression or with large brainstem lesions such as infarction, primary hemorrhage, or infiltrating tumor.

Lesions of the lower midbrain–upper pontine tegmentum, either primary or secondary to a tentorial herniation, may give rise to *central neurogenic hyperventilation* (CNH). This disorder is characterized by an increase in the rate and depth of respiration to the extent that respiratory alkalosis results. CNH is thought to represent a release of the reflex mechanisms for respiratory control in the lower brainstem. It must be distinguished from hyperventilation caused by medical illnesses, particularly pneumonia and acidosis. Mild degrees of hyperventilation are common after a number of acute neurologic events, notably head injury. The neurologic basis of CNH is uncertain. It has been observed with tumors of the medulla, lower pons, and midbrain. However, North and Jennett, in a study of respiratory abnormalities in neurosurgical patients, found no consistent correlation between tachypnea and the site of the lesion. It is noteworthy that primary brain lymphoma *without* brainstem involvement has emerged as a common cause of CNH (Pauzner et al).

Low pontine lesions, usually due to basilar artery occlusion, sometimes cause *apneustic breathing* (a pause of 2 to 3 s in full inspiration) or so-called *short-cycle CSR*, in which a few rapid deep breaths alternate with apneic cycles. With lesions of the dorsomedial part of the medulla, the rhythm of breathing is chaotic, being irregularly interrupted and each breath varying in rate and depth (Biot breathing). This has also been called "ataxia of breathing"—not an appropriate term. The latter progresses to intermittent prolonged inspiratory gasps and finally to apnea; in fact, respiratory arrest is the mode of death of most patients with serious central nervous system (CNS) disease.

Probably all of these erratic patterns are related in some manner; Webber and Speck have shown that apnea, Biot breathing, and gasping could be produced in the same animal with lesions in the dorsolateral pontine tegmentum by altering the depth of anesthesia. As has been pointed out by Fisher and by Plum and Posner, when certain supratentorial lesions progress to the point of temporal lobe and cerebellar herniation, one may observe a succession of respiratory patterns (CSR-CNH-Biot breathing), indicating an extension of the functional disorder from upper to lower brainstem; but, again, such a sequence is seldom observed in clinical practice. Rapidly evolving lesions of the posterior fossa may cause acute apnea without any of the aforementioned abnormalities of breathing.

Signs of Increased Intracranial Pressure A history of headache before the onset of coma, recurrent vomiting, severe hypertension beyond the patient's static level, and subhyaloid retinal hemorrhages are immediate clues to the presence of increased intracranial pressure, usually from one of the types of cerebral hemorrhage. Papilledema develops within 12 to 24 h in cases of brain trauma and hemorrhage, but if it is pronounced, it usually signifies brain tumor or abscess—i.e., a lesion of longer duration. Increased intracranial pressure produces coma by impeding global cerebral blood flow; however, this occurs only at extremely high levels of pressure. High pressure within one compartment, produce shifts of central structures and a series of "false localizing" signs, due to lateral displacements and herniations, as previously discussed.

The syndrome of *acute hydrocephalus*, most often from subarachnoid hemorrhage or from rapid obstruction of the ventricular system by a tumor in the posterior fossa, induces a state of abulia (page 633), followed by stupor and then coma with bilateral Babinski signs, small pupils and increased tone in the legs, as well as the systemic features of raised intracranial pressure, noted above. This subject is discussed further in Chap. 30.

Laboratory Procedures

Unless the diagnosis is established at once by history and physical examination, it is necessary to carry out a number of laboratory procedures. In patients with evidence of a cerebral mass or acute hydrocephalus, as evidenced by signs of raised intracranial pressure or indications of brain displacements (asymmetry of limb movements, pupillary enlargement), a CT scan or MRI should be obtained as a primary procedure. As discussed in Chap. 2, lumbar puncture, although carrying a certain small risk of promoting further herniation, is nevertheless necessary in some instances to exclude bacterial meningitis or encephalitis. If poisoning is suspected, aspiration and analysis of the gastric contents is sometimes helpful, but greater reliance should be placed on chromatographic analysis of the blood and urine. Accurate means are available for measuring the blood concentrations of phenytoin and other anticonvulsants, opiates, diazepines, barbiturates, alcohol, and a wide range of other toxic substances. A specimen of urine is obtained by catheter for determination of specific gravity and for glucose, acetone, and protein content. Proteinuria may also be found for 2 or 3 days after a subarachnoid hemorrhage or with fever. Urine of high specific gravity, glycosuria, and acetonuria occur almost invariably in diabetic coma; but transient glycosuria and hyperglycemia may result from a massive cerebral lesion. Blood counts should be obtained, and in malarial districts a blood smear is examined for parasites. Neutrophilic leukocytosis occurs in bacterial infections and also with brain hemorrhage and infarction, although the elevation of leukocytes in the latter conditions rarely exceeds 12,000/mm^3. Venous blood should be examined for glucose, urea, carbon dioxide, bicarbonate, ammonium, sodium, potassium, chloride, calcium, and SGOT (serum glutamic oxaloacetic transaminase) and analysis of blood gases should be obtained in appropriate cases.

It should be kept in mind that disorders of water and sodium balance, reflected in hyper- or hyponatremia, may be the result of cerebral disease (excess ADH secretion, diabetes insipidus, atrial natriuretic factor release), as well as the cause of coma.

Classification of Coma and Differential Diagnosis (Table 17-2)

The demonstration of focal brain disease or of meningeal irritation with abnormalities of the CSF is of particular help in the differential diagnosis of coma and serves to divide the diseases that cause coma into three classes, as follows:

I. Diseases that cause *no focal or lateralizing neurologic signs*, usually with normal brainstem functions. CT scan and cellular content of the CSF are normal.
   A. *Intoxications*: alcohol, barbiturates and other sedative drugs, opiates, etc. (Chaps. 42 and 43).
   B. *Metabolic disturbances*: anoxia, diabetic acidosis, uremia, hepatic failure, nonketotic hyperosmolar hyperglycemia, hypo- and hypernatremia, hypoglycemia, addisonian crisis, profound nutritional deficiency, thyroid states (Chaps. 40 and 41).
   C. *Severe systemic infections*: pneumonia, peritonitis, typhoid fever, malaria, septicemia, Waterhouse-Friderichsen syndrome.
   D. Circulatory collapse (shock) from any cause.
   E. Postseizure states and convulsive and non-convulsive status epilepticus (Chap. 16).
   F. Hypertensive encephalopathy and eclampsia (Chap. 34).
   G. Hyperthermia and hypothermia.
   H. Concussion (Chap. 35).
   I. Acute hydrocephalus (Chap 30).
   J. Late stages of certain degenerative diseases and Creutzfeldt-Jakob disease.

II. Diseases that cause *meningeal irritation* with or without fever, and with an excess of WBCs or RBCs in the CSF, usually without focal or lateralizing cerebral or brainstem signs. CT scanning or MRI, (which preferably should precede lumbar puncture) may be normal or abnormal.

A. Subarachnoid hemorrhage from ruptured aneurysm, arteriovenous malformation, occasionally trauma (Chaps. 34 and 35).
B. Acute bacterial meningitis (Chap. 32).
C. Some forms of viral encephalitis (Chap. 33).
D. Neoplastic and parasitic meningitides.

III. Diseases that cause *focal brainstem or lateralizing cerebral signs*, with or without changes in the CSF. CT scanning and MRI are usually abnormal.
A. Hemispheral hemorrhage or massive infarction (Chap. 34).
B. Brainstem infarction due to basilar artery thrombosis or embolism (Chap. 34).
C. Brain abscess, subdural empyema (Chap. 32).
D. Epidural and subdural hemorrhage and brain contusion (Chap. 35).
E. Brain tumor (Chap. 31).
F. Cerebellar and pontine hemorrhage.
G. Miscellaneous: cortical vein thrombosis, some forms of viral encephalitis (herpes), focal embolic infarction due to bacterial endocarditis, acute hemorrhagic leukoencephalitis, disseminated (postinfectious) encephalomyelitis, intravascular lymphoma, thrombotic thrombocytopenic purpura, diffuse fat embolism, and others.

Using the clinical criteria outlined above, one can usually ascertain whether a given case of coma falls into one of these three categories. Concerning the group without focal or lateralizing or meningeal signs (which includes most of the metabolic encephalopathies, intoxications, concussion, and postseizure states), it must be kept in mind that residua from previous neurologic disease may confuse the clinical picture. Thus, an earlier hemiparesis from vascular disease or trauma may reassert itself in the course of uremic or hepatic coma with hypotension, hypoglycemia, diabetic acidosis, or following a seizure. In hypertensive encephalopathy, focal signs may also be present. Occasionally, for no understandable reason, one leg may seem to move less, one plantar reflex may be extensor, or seizures may be predominantly or entirely unilateral in a metabolic coma, particularly in the hyperglycemic–hyperosmolar state. Babinski signs and extensor rigidity, conventionally considered to be indicators of structural disease, do occur in profound intoxications with a number of agents.

The diagnosis of concussion or of postictal coma depends on observation of the precipitating event or indirect evidence thereof. Often a convulsive seizure is marked by a bitten tongue, urinary incontinence, and an elevated CK-skeletal muscle fraction and may be followed by another seizure or burst of seizures. The presence of small convulsive movements of a hand or foot or fluttering of the eyelids requires that an EEG be performed to determine whether status epilepticus is the cause of coma. This state, called *nonconvulsive status* or *spike-wave stupor* and described in Chap. 16, must always be considered in the diagnosis of unexplained coma, especially in known epileptics (Table 17-2).

With respect to the second group in the above classification, the signs of meningeal irritation (head retraction, stiffness of neck on forward bending, Kernig and Brudzinski signs) can usually be elicited in both bacterial meningitis and subarachnoid hemorrhage. However, in infants and in adults, if the coma is profound, stiff neck may be absent. In such cases the spinal fluid has to be examined in order to establish the diagnosis. In most cases of bacterial meningitis, the CSF pressure is not exceptionally high (usually less than 400 mmH_2O). However, in cases associated with brain swelling, the CSF pressure is greatly elevated; the pupils become fixed and dilated, and there may be signs of compression of the brainstem with arrest of respiration. Patients in coma from ruptured aneurysms also have high CSF pressure; the CSF is overtly bloody and the blood is invariably visible in the CT scan throughout the basal cisterns and ventricles if the bleeding has been severe enough to cause coma.

In the third group of patients, it is the focality of sensorimotor signs and the abnormal pupillary and ocular reflexes, postural states, and breathing patterns that provide the clues to serious structural lesions in the cerebral hemispheres and their effects upon segmental brainstem functions. As the brainstem effects become prominent, they may obscure earlier signs of cerebral disease.

It is worth emphasizing once more that hepatic, hypoglycemic, hyperglycemic, and hypoxic coma sometimes resemble coma due to brainstem lesions by causing asymmetrical motor signs, focal seizures, and decerebrate postures and that deep coma from drug intoxication may obliterate reflex eye movements. Also, certain structural lesions of the cerebral hemispheres are so diffuse as to produce a picture that simulates a metabolic disturbance; thrombotic thrombocytopenic purpura (TTP), fat embolism, and the late effects of global ischemia-anoxia are examples of such states. At other times they cause a diffuse encephalopathy with superimposed focal signs. Unilateral infarction due to anterior, middle, or posterior cerebral artery occlusion produces no more than drowsiness, as a rule; however, with massive unilateral infarction due to carotid artery occlusion, coma can occur if extensive brain edema and secondary tissue shift are associated. Edema of this degree seldom develops before 12 or 24 h. Rapidly evolving hydrocephalus causes smallness of the pupils, rapid respiration, extensor rigidity of the legs, Babinski signs, and sometimes a loss of eye movements.

Finally, it should be restated that diagnosis has as its prime purpose the direction of therapy. The treatable causes of coma are: drug and alcohol intoxications, shock due to infection, cardiac failure, or systemic bleeding, epidural and subdural hematomas, brain abscess, bacterial and fungal meningitis, diabetic acidosis or hyperosmolar state, hypoglycemia, hypo- or hypernatremia, hepatic coma, uremia, status epilepticus, and hypertensive encephalopathy. Also treatable to a varying degree are uremia; putaminal and cerebellar hemorrhages, which can sometimes be evacuated successfully; edema from massive stroke, which may be ameliorated by hemicraniectomy; and hydrocephalus from any cause, which may respond to ventricular drainage.

Management of the Acutely Comatose Patient

Seriously impaired states of consciousness, regardless of their cause, are often fatal not only because they represent an advanced stage of many diseases but also because they add their own particular burdens to the primary disease. The physician's main objective, of course, is to find the cause of the coma and to treat it appropriately. It often happens, however, that the disease process is one for which there is no specific therapy; or, as in hypoxia or hypoglycemia, the acute, irreversible effects already have occurred before the patient comes to the attention of the physician. Again, the problem may be highly complex, for the disturbance may be attributable not to a single cause but to several factors acting in unison, no one of which could account for the total clinical picture. In lieu of specific therapy, supportive measures must be used; indeed, the patient's chances of surviving the original disease often depend on the effectiveness of these measures.

The successful management of the insensate patient requires the services of a well-coordinated team of nurses under the close guidance of a physician. Necessary treatment must be instituted immediately, even before all the diagnostic steps have been completed; diagnosis and treatment may have to proceed concurrently. The following is a brief outline of the principles involved in the treatment of such patients. The details of management of shock, fluid and electrolyte imbalance, and other complications that threaten the comatose patient (pneumonia, urinary tract infections, deep venous thrombosis, etc.) are found in *Harrison's Principles of Internal Medicine.*

1. The management of shock, if present, takes precedence over all other diagnostic and therapeutic measures.

2. Shallow and irregular respirations, stertorous breathing (indicating obstruction to inspiration), and cyanosis require the establishment of a clear airway and delivery of oxygen. The patient should initially be placed in a lateral position so that secretions and vomitus do not enter the tracheobronchial tree. Secretions should be removed by suctioning as soon as they accumulate; otherwise they will lead to atelectasis and bronchopneumonia. Arterial blood gases should be measured and further observed by monitoring of oxygen saturation. A patient's inability to protect against aspiration and the presence of either hypoxia or hypoventilation dictates the use of endotracheal intubation and a positive-pressure respirator.

3. Concomitantly, an intravenous line is established and blood samples are drawn for determination of glucose, drugs, and electrolytes and for tests of liver and kidney function. Naloxone, 0.5 mg, should be given intravenously if a narcotic overdose is a possibility. Hypoglycemia that has produced stupor or coma demands the infusion of glucose, usually 25 to 50 mL of a 50% solution followed by a 5% infusion; this must be supplemented with thiamine. A urine sample is obtained for drug and glucose testing.

4. With the development of elevated intracranial pressure from a mass lesion, mannitol, 25 to 50 g in a 20% solution, should be given intravenously over 10 to 20 min and hyperventilation instituted if deterioration occurs, as judged by pupillary enlargement or deepening coma. Repeated CT scanning allows the physician to follow the size of the lesion and degree of localized edema and to detect displacements of cerebral tissue. With massive cerebral lesions, it may be appropriate to place a pressure-measuring device in the cranium of selected patients (see Chap. 35 for details of intracranial pressure monitoring and treatment).

5. A lumbar puncture should be performed if meningitis or subarachnoid hemorrhage is suspected, keeping in mind the risks of this procedure and the means of dealing with them. A CT scan may have disclosed a primary subarachnoid hemorrhage, in which case lumbar puncture is not necessary.

TABLE 17-2
Important Points in the Differential Diagnosis of the Common Causes of Coma

General group	*Specific disorder*	*Important clinical findings*	*Important laboratory findings*	*Remarks*
Coma *with* focal or lateralizing signs	Cerebral hemorrhage	Hemiplegia, hypertension, cyclic breathing, specific ocular signs (See Chaps. 14 and 33)	CT scan +	Sudden onset, often with headache, vomiting; history of chronic hypertension; late pupillary enlargement
	Basilar artery occlusion (thrombotic or embolic)	Extensor posturing and bilateral Babinski signs; early loss of oculocephalic responses; ocular bobbing	Normal early CT; MRI shows cerebellar and brainstem or thalamic infarction, normal CSF	Onset subacute (thrombosis), or sudden (rostral basilar embolism)
	Massive infarction and edema in carotid territory	Hemiplegia, unilateral unresponsive or enlarged pupil	CT and MRI show massive edema of hemisphere	Coma preceded by drowsiness for several days after stroke
	Subdural hematoma	Slow or cyclic respiration, rising blood pressure, hemiparesis, unilateral enlarged pupil	CT scan +; CSF xanthochromic with relatively low protein	Signs or history of trauma, headache, confusion, progressive drowsiness
	Trauma	Signs of cranial and facial injury	CT and MRI show brain contusions and other injuries (see Chap. 34)	Unstable blood pressure, associated systemic injuries
	Brain abscess	Neurologic signs depending on location	CT scan and MRI +	Systemic infection or neurosurgical procedure, fever
	Hypertensive encephalopathy; eclampsia	Blood pressure > 210/110 (lower in eclampsia and in children), headache, seizures, hypertensive retinal changes	CT ±; CSF pressure elevated	Acute or subacute evolution, use of aminophylline or catecholamine medications
	Thrombotic thrombocytopenic purpura (TTP)	Petechiae, seizures shifting focal signs	Multiple small cortical infarctions; thrombocytopenia	Similar to fat embolism
Coma *without* focal or lateralizing signs, *with* signs of meningeal irritation	Meningitis and encephalitis	Stiff neck, Kernig sign, fever, headache	CT scan ±; pleocytosis, increased protein, low glucose in CSF	Subacute or acute onset
	Subarachnoid hemorrhage	Stertorous breathing, hypertension, stiff neck, Kernig sign	CT scan may show blood and aneurysm; bloody or xanthochromic CSF under increased pressure	Sudden onset with severe headache
Coma *without* focal neurologic signs or meningeal irritation; CT scan and CSF normal	Alcohol intoxication	Hypothermia, hypotension, flushed skin, alcohol breath	Elevated blood alcohol	May be combined with head injury, infection, or hepatic failure

TABLE 17-2 ***(Continued)***
Important Points in the Differential Diagnosis of the Common Causes of Coma

General group	*Specific disorder*	*Important clinical findings*	*Important laboratory findings*	*Remarks*
	Sedative intoxication	Hypothermia, hypotension	Drug in urine and blood; EEG often shows fast activity	History of intake of drug; suicide attempt
	Opioid intoxication	Slow respiration, cyanosis, constricted pupils		Administration of naloxone causes awakening and withdrawal signs
	Carbon monoxide intoxication	Cherry-red skin	Carboxyhemoglobin	
	Global ischemia–anoxia	Rigidity, decerebrate postures, fever, seizures, myoclonus	CSF normal; EEG may be isoelectric or show high-voltage delta	Abrupt onset following cardiopulmonary arrest; damage permanent if anoxia exceeds 3–5 min
	Hypoglycemia	Same as in anoxia	Low blood and CSF glucose	Characteristic slow evolution through stages of nervousness, hunger, sweating, flushed face; then pallor, shallow respirations and seizures
	Diabetic coma	Signs of extracellular fluid deficit, hyperventilation with Kussmaul respiration, "fruity" breath	Glycosuria, hyperglycemia, acidosis; reduced serum bicarbonate; ketonemia and ketonuria, or hyperosmolarity	History of polyuria, polydipsia, weight loss, or diabetes
	Uremia	Hypertension; sallow, dry skin, uriniferous breath, twitch-convulsive syndrome	Protein and casts in urine; elevated BUN and serum creatinine; anemia, acidosis, hypocalcemia	Progressive apathy, confusion, and asterixis precede coma
	Hepatic coma	Jaundice, ascites, and other signs of portal hypertension; asterixis	Elevated blood NH_3 levels; CSF yellow (bilirubin) with normal or slightly elevated protein	Onset over a few days or after paracentesis or hemorrhage from varices; confusion, stupor, asterixis, and characteristic EEG changes precede coma
	Hypercapnia	Papilledema, diffuse myoclonus, asterixis	Increased CSF pressure; P_{CO_2} may exceed 75 mmHg; EEG theta and delta activity	Advanced pulmonary disease; profound coma and brain damage uncommon
	Severe infections (septic shock); heat stroke	Extreme hyperthermia, rapid respiration	Vary according to cause	Evidence of a specific infection or exposure to extreme heat
	Seizures	Episodic disturbance of behavior or convulsive movements	Characteristic EEG changes	History of previous attacks

6. Convulsions should be controlled by measures outlined in Chap. 16.

7. As indicated above, gastric aspiration and lavage with normal saline may be diagnostically and therapeutically useful in some instances of coma due to drug ingestion. Salicylates, opiates, and anticholinergic drugs (tricyclic antidepressants, phenothiazines, scopolamine), all of which induce gastric atony, may be recovered many hours after ingestion. Caustic materials should not be lavaged because of the danger of gastrointestinal perforation. The administration of activated charcoal is indicated in certain drug poisonings. Measures to prevent gastric hemorrhage and excessive gastric acid secretion are usually advisable.

8. The temperature-regulating mechanisms may be disturbed, and extreme hypothermia, hyperthermia, or poikilothermia should be corrected. In severe hyperthermia, evaporative-cooling measures are indicated in addition to antipyretics.

9. The bladder should not be permitted to become distended; if the patient does not void, decompression should be carried out with an indwelling catheter. Needless to say, the patient should not be permitted to lie in a wet or soiled bed.

10. Diseases of the CNS may disrupt the control of water, glucose, and sodium. The unconscious patient can no longer adjust the intake of food and fluids by hunger and thirst. Both salt-losing and salt-retaining syndromes have been described with brain disease (see Chap. 27). Water intoxication and severe hyponatremia may of themselves prove damaging. If coma is prolonged, the insertion of a nasogastric tube will ease the problems of feeding the patient and maintaining fluid and electrolyte balance. It is quite acceptable to leave the tube in place for long periods. Otherwise, approximately 35 mL/kg of isotonic fluid should be administered per 24 h (5% dextrose in 0.45% saline with potassium supplementation unless there is brain edema, in which case the use of isotonic normal saline is indicated).

11. Aspiration pneumonia is avoided by prevention of vomiting (gastric tube and endotracheal intubation), proper positioning of the patient, and restriction of oral fluids. Should aspiration pneumonia occur, it requires treatment with appropriate antibiotics, and aggressive pulmonary physical therapy.

12. Leg vein thrombosis—a common occurrence in comatose and hemiplegic patients—often does not manifest itself by obvious clinical signs. An attempt may be made to prevent it by the subcutaneous administration of heparin, 5000 units q 12 h, and by the use of intermittent pneumatic compression boots.

13. If the patient is capable of moving, suitable restraints should be used to prevent falling out of bed and self-injury from convulsions.

14. Regular conjunctival lubrication and oral cleansing should be instituted.

Prognosis of Coma (See also page 1179)

As a general rule, recovery from coma of metabolic and toxic causes is far better than from anoxic coma, with head injury occupying an intermediate prognostic position. Most comatose stroke patients die. If there are no pupillary, corneal, or oculovestibular responses within several hours of the onset of coma, the chances of regaining independent function are practically nil (see Levy et al). Other signs that predict a poor outcome are absence of corneal reflexes and eye-opening responses and atonia of the limbs at 1 and 3 days after the onset of coma and absence of the cortical component of the somatosensory evoked responses on both sides. It is the unfortunate survivor from this latter group who may remain in a vegetative state for months or years, breathing without aid and with preserved hypothalamopituitary functions. The frequency of this persistent vegetative state after head injury and the negligible chances of improvement if the condition persists for several weeks have already been discussed (page 370).

REFERENCES

Andrews K: Recovery of patients after four months or more in the persistent vegetative state. *BMJ* 306:1597, 1993.

Andrews BT, Chiles BW, Olsen WL, et al: The effects of intracerebral hematoma location on the risk of brainstem compression and outcome. *J Neurosurg* 69:518, 1988.

Beecher HK, Adams RD, Sweet WH: A definition of irreversible coma: Report of the Committee of Harvard Medical School to examine the definition of brain death. *JAMA* 205:85, 1968.

Braakman R, Jennett WB, Minderhound JM: Prognosis of the posttraumatic vegetative state. *Acta Neurochir* 95:49, 1988.

Bremer F: L'activité cerebralé au cours du sommeil et de la narcose. *Bull Acad R Soc Belg* 2:68, 1937.

Cairns H, Oldfield RC, Pennybacker JB, et al: Akinetic mutism with an epidermoid cyst of the third ventricle. *Brain* 64:273, 1941.

Feldman MH: The decerebrate state in the primate: I. Studies in monkeys. *Arch Neurol* 25:501, 1971.

Feldman MH, Sahrmann S: The decerebrate state in the primate: II. Studies in man. *Arch Neurol* 25:517, 1971.

Fisher CM: The neurological examination of the comatose patient. *Acta Neurol Scand* Suppl 36: 1969.

Fitzsimmons RB, Wolfenden WH: Migraine coma: Meningitic migraine with cerebral oedema associated with a new form of autosomal dominant cerebellar ataxia. *Brain* 108:555, 1985.

Frederiks JAM: Consciousness, in Vinken PJ, Bruyn GW (eds): *Disorders of Higher Nervous Function: Handbook of Clinical Neurology*. Vol 4. Amsterdam, North-Holland, 1969, chap 4, p 48.

Guidelines for the detection of brain death in children. *Ann Neurol* 21:616, 1987.

Hansotia PL: Persistent vegetative state: Review and report of electrodiagnostic studies in eight cases. *Arch Neurol* 42:1048, 1985.

Higashi K, Sakata Y, Hatano M, et al: Epidemiologic studies on patients with a persistent vegetative state. *J Neurol Neurosurg Psychiatry* 40:876, 1977.

Iragui VJ, McCutchen CB: Physiologic and prognostic significance of "alpha coma." *J Neurol Neurosurg Psychiatry* 46:632, 1983.

Jennett B, Plum F: Persistent vegetative state after brain damage. *Lancet* 1:734, 1972.

Kennard C, Illingworth R: Persistent vegetative state. *J Neurol Neurosurg Psychiatry* 59:347, 1995.

Kernohan JW, Woltman HW: Incisura of the crus due to contralateral brain tumor. *Arch Neurol Psychiatry* 21:274, 1929.

Kinney HC, Korein J, Panigraphy A, et al: Neuropathological findings in the brain of Karen Ann Quinlan—The role of thalamus in the persistent vegetative state. *N Engl J Med* 330:1469, 1994.

Laureys S, Lemaire C, Maquet P, et al: Cerebral metabolism during vegetative state and after recovery of consciousness. *J Neurol Neurosurg Psychiatry* 67:121, 1999.

Levy DE, Bates D, Caronna JJ: Prognosis in nontraumatic coma. *Ann Intern Med* 94: 293, 1981.

Lugaresi E, Montagna P, Tinuper P, et al: Suspected covert loiazepam administration misdiagnosed as recurrent endozepine stupor. *Brain* 121:2201, 1998.

Magnus R: Some results of studies in the physiology of posture. *Lancet* 2:531, 585, 1926.

Moruzzi G, Magoun H: Brain stem reticular formation and activation of EEG. *Electroencephalogr Clin Neurophysiol* 1:455, 1949.

McNealy DE, Plum FP: Brainstem dysfunction with supratentorial mass lesions. *Arch Neurol* 7:10, 1962.

Mollaret P, Goulon M: Le coma dépassé. *Rev Neurol* 101:3, 1959.

Multi-Society Task Force on PVS. Medical aspects of the persistent vegetative state: Parts I and II. *N Engl J Med* 330:1499, 1572, 1994.

North JB, Jennett B: Abnormal breathing patterns associated with acute brain damage. *Arch Neurol* 32:338, 1974.

Pleasure SJ, Abosch A, Friedman J, et al: Spontaneous intracranial hypotension resulting in stupor caused by diencephalic compression. *Neurology* 50:1854, 1998.

Pauzner R, Mouallem M, Sadeh M, et al: High incidence of primary cerebral lymphoma in tumor-induced central neurogenic hyperventilation. *Arch Neurol* 46:510, 1989.

Plum F: Coma and related global disturbances of the human conscious state, in Peters A (ed): *Cerebral Cortex*. Vol 9. New York, Plenum Press, 1991, pp 359–425.

Plum F, Posner JB: *Diagnosis of Stupor and Coma*, 3rd ed. Philadelphia, Davis, 1980.

Reich JB, Sierra J, Camp W, et al: Magnetic resonance imaging measurement and clinical changes accompanying transtentorial and foramen magnum brain herniation. *Ann Neurol* 33:159, 1993.

Ropper AH: Lateral displacement of the brain and level of consciousness in patients with an acute hemispheral mass. *N Engl J Med* 314:953, 1986.

Ropper AH: Unusual spontaneous movements in brain-dead patients. *Neurology* 34:1089, 1984.

Ropper AH: The opposite pupil in herniation. *Neurology* 40:1707, 1990.

Ropper AH, Kennedy SK: Postoperative neurosurgical care, in Ropper AH (ed): *Neurological and Neurosurgical Intensive Care*, 3rd ed. New York, Raven Press, 1993, pp 185–196.

Ropper AH, Shafran B: Brain edema after stroke: Clinical syndrome and intracranial pressure. *Arch Neurol* 41:26, 1984.

Rosenberg GA, Johnson SF, Brenner RP: Recovery of cognition after prolonged vegetative state. *Ann Neurol* 2:167, 1977.

Rosenberg H, Clofine R, Bialik O: Neurologic changes during awakening from anesthesia. *Anesthesiology* 45:898, 1981.

Scheibel AB: On detailed connections of the medullary and pontine reticular formation. *Anat Rec* 109:345, 1951.

Sherrington CS: Decerebrate rigidity and reflex coordination of movements. *J Physiol* 22:319, 1898.

Solomon P, Aring CD: Causes of coma in patients entering a general hospital. *Amer J Med Sci* 188:805, 1934.

Steriade M: Arousal: Revisiting the reticular activating system. *Science* 272:225, 1996.

Webber CL, Jr., Speck DF: Experimental Biot periodic breathing in cats: Effects of changes in PiO_2 and $PiCO_2$. *Respir Physiol* 46:327, 1981.

Young BG: Consciousness, in Young GB, Ropper AH, Bolton CG: *Coma and Impaired Consciousness: A Clinical Perspective*, McGraw Hill, New York, 1998.

Zeman A: Persistent vegetative state. *Lancet* 350:795, 1997.

Chapter 18

FAINTNESS AND SYNCOPE

The term *syncope* (Greek, *synkope*) literally means a "cessation," a "cutting short" or "pause." Medically, it refers to an episodic loss of consciousness and postural tone and an inability to stand, due to a diminished flow of blood to the brain. It is synonymous in everyday language with *fainting*. *Feeling faint* and a *feeling of faintness* are also commonly used terms to describe the sudden loss of strength and other symptoms that characterize the impending or incomplete fainting spell. This latter state is referred to as *presyncope*. Relatively abrupt onset, brief duration, and spontaneous and complete recovery not requiring specific resuscitative measures are other distinguishing features.

Faintness and syncope are among the most common of all medical phenomena. Practically every adult has experienced some presyncopal symptoms if not a fully developed syncopal attack or has observed such attacks in others. Description of these symptoms, as with other predominantly subjective states, is often ambiguous. The patient may refer to the experience as light-headedness, giddiness, dizziness, a "drunk feeling," a weak spell, or, if consciousness was lost, a "blackout." Careful questioning may be necessary to ascertain the exact meaning of these words. In many instances the nature of the symptoms is clarified by the fact that they include a sensation of faintness and then a momentary loss of consciousness, which is easily recognized as a faint, or syncope. This sequence also informs us that under certain conditions any difference between faintness and syncope is only one of degree. These symptoms must be clearly set apart from certain types of epilepsy, the other major cause of episodic unconsciousness, and disorders such as cataplexy, transient ischemic attacks, "drop attacks," and vertigo, which are also characterized by episodic attacks of generalized weakness or inability to stand upright but not by a loss of consciousness.

CLINICAL FEATURES OF SYNCOPE

The clinical manifestations of fainting attacks vary to some extent, depending on their mechanisms and the settings in which they occur.

The commonest type of faint—namely, *vasodepressor* or *vasovagal syncope*, defined more precisely further on—conforms more or less to the following pattern. The patient is usually in the upright position at the beginning of the attack, either sitting or standing. Certain subjective symptoms, the prodrome, mark the onset of the faint. The person feels queasy, is assailed by a sense of giddiness and apprehension, may sway, and sometimes develops a headache. What is most noticeable at the beginning of the attack is pallor or an ashen-gray color of the face; often the face and body become bathed in cold perspiration. Salivation, epigastric distress, nausea, and sometimes vomiting accompany these symptoms, and the patient tries to suppress them by yawning, sighing, or breathing deeply. Vision may dim or close in concentrically, the ears may ring, and it may be impossible to think clearly ("gray-out").

The duration of the prodromal symptoms is variable, from a few minutes to only a few seconds, but it is doubtful that consciousness is ever abolished as abruptly as with a seizure. If, during the prodromal period, the person is able to lie down promptly, the attack can be averted before complete loss of consciousness occurs; otherwise, consciousness is lost and the patient falls to the ground. The more or less deliberate onset of this type of syncope enables patients to lie down or at least to protect themselves as they slump. A hurtful fall is exceptional in the young, though an elderly person may be injured.

The depth and duration of unconsciousness vary. Sometimes the person is not completely oblivious to his surroundings; he may still hear voices or see the blurred outlines of people. More often there is a complete lack of awareness and responsiveness. The patient lies motionless, with skeletal muscles fully relaxed. Sphincteric control is maintained in nearly all cases. The pupils are dilated. The pulse is thin and slow or cannot be felt; the systolic blood pressure is reduced (to 60 mmHg or less, as a rule), and breathing is almost imperceptible. The depressed vital functions, striking facial pallor, and unconsciousness simulate death.

Once the patient is horizontal, the flow of blood to the brain is no longer hindered. The strength of the pulse soon improves and color begins to return to the face. Breathing becomes quicker and deeper. Then the eyelids flutter and consciousness is quickly regained. However, should unconsciousness persist for 15 to 20 s, convulsive movements may occur (*convulsive syncope*). These movements, which are often mistaken for a seizure, usually take the form of brief, mild, clonic jerks of the limbs and trunk and twitchings of the face or a tonic extension of the trunk and clenching of the jaw. Occasionally the extensor rigidity and jerking flexor movements are more severe, but very rarely is there urinary incontinence or biting of the tongue, features that characterize a generalized tonic-clonic convulsion.

From the moment that consciousness is regained, there is a correct perception of the environment. Confusion, headache, and drowsiness, the common sequelae of a convulsive seizure, do not follow a syncopal attack. Nevertheless, the patient often feels weak and groggy after a vasodepressor faint and, by arising too soon, may precipitate another faint.

The clinical features of *cardiac* and *carotid sinus syncope* are much the same as those described above except that the onset of these forms of syncope may be absolutely abrupt, without any warning symptoms, and is much less dependent upon the patient being in an upright posture. The clinical particularities of these and other forms of syncope are described further on.

CAUSES OF EPISODIC FAINTNESS AND SYNCOPE

From a clinical and pathophysiologic perspective, syncope is essentially of three main types, each of which may lead to a temporary reduction in the flow of blood to the brain:

1. Sudden loss of vascular sympathetic tone (vasodepressor effect), often associated with excessive vagal effect and bradycardia (vasovagal effect) triggered by the centrally mediated inhibition of the normal tonic sympathetic influences. These are referred to as the *neurogenic* or *neurocardiogenic syncopes*.

2. A failure of sympathetic innervation of blood vessels and of autonomically activated compensatory responses (reflex tachycardia and vasoconstriction), which occurs with assumption of the upright body position and leads to pooling of blood in the lower parts of the body—causing *orthostatic hypotension* and syncope. Typically, in individuals with these first two forms of syncope, there is no evidence of underlying cardiac disease.

3. A diminished cardiac output due to disease of the heart itself (as in the Stokes-Adams attack); or to greatly reduced blood volume from dehydration or blood loss.

The three main types of syncope and several other types that cannot readily be included within these categories can be further subdivided as follows:

- I. Neurogenic vasodepressor reactions
  - A. Elicited by *extrinsic signals* to the medulla from baroreceptors
    1. Vasodepressor (vasovagal)
    2. Neurocardiogenic
    3. Carotid sinus hypersensitivity
    4. Vagoglossopharyngeal
  - B. Coupled with diminished venous return to the heart
    1. Micturitional
    2. Tussive
    3. Valsalva, straining, breath holding, weight lifting
    4. Postprandial
  - C. Intrinsic psychic stimuli
    1. Fear, anxiety (presyncope more common)
    2. Sight of blood
    3. Hysterical
- II. Failure of sympathetic nervous system innervation (postural-orthostatic hypotension)
  - A. Peripheral nervous system autonomic failure
    1. Diabetes
    2. Pandysautonomia
    3. Guillain-Barré syndrome
    4. Amyloid neuropathy
    5. Surgical sympathectomy
    6. Antihypertensive medications and other blockers of vascular innervation
  - B. Central nervous system autonomic failure

1. Primary autonomic failure (idiopathic orthostatic hypotension)
2. Multiple system atrophy (parkinsonism, ataxia, orthostatic hypotension)
3. Spinal cord trauma, infarction, and necrosis
4. Centrally acting antihypertensive and other medications

III. Reduced cardiac output or inadequate intravascular volume (hypovolemia)
   A. Reduced cardiac output
      1. Cardiac arrhythmias
         i. Bradyarrhythmias
            a. Atrioventricular (AV) block (second and third degree) with Stokes-Adams attacks
            b. Ventricular asystole
            c. Sinus bradycardia, sinoatrial block, sinus arrest, sick-sinus syndrome
         ii. Tachyarrhythmias
            a. Episodic ventricular tachycardia
            b. Supraventricular tachycardia (infrequently causes syncope)
      2. Myocardial: infarction or severe congestive heart failure
      3. Obstruction to left ventricular outflow: aortic stenosis; hypertrophic subaortic stenosis
      4. Obstruction to pulmonary flow: pulmonic stenosis, tetralogy of Fallot, primary pulmonary hypertension, pulmonary embolism
      5. Pericardial tamponade
   B. Inadequate intravascular volume (hemorrhage); dehydration

IV. Other causes of episodic faintness and syncope
   A. Hypoxia
   B. Anemia
   C. Diminished CO_2 due to hyperventilation (faintness common, syncope rare)
   D. Hypoglycemia (faintness frequent, syncope rare)
   E. Anxiety (panic) attacks
   F. Environmental overheating

This list of conditions causing faintness and syncope is deceptively long and involved. It will be recognized that the usual types are reducible to a few well-established mechanisms, all resulting in a temporary reduction of blood flow to the brain. In order not to obscure these mechanisms by too many details, only the varieties of fainting commonly encountered in clinical practice or those of particular neurologic interest are discussed below.

Neurogenic Syncope

This term refers to all forms of syncope that result directly from the vascular effects of neural signals coming from the central nervous system, primarily the nucleus tractus solitarius. A number of stimuli, mostly from the viscera but some of psychologic origin, are capable of eliciting this response, which consists of a reduction or loss of sympathetic vascular tone coupled with a heightened vagal activity. The nucleus tractus solitarius (NTS) in the medulla integrates these afferent stimuli and normal baroreceptor signals with the efferent sympathetic mechanisms that maintain vascular tone (see further on and Chap. 26). By the use of microneurography, Wallin and Sundlof have demonstrated that sympathetic outflow in peripheral nerves is greatly increased just prior to syncope, but at the onset of fainting sympathetic activity ceases. This signifies that *there is an initial attempt to compensate for falling blood pressure by enhanced sympathetic tone, following which there is a centrally mediated withdrawal of sympathetic activity that results in fainting*.

It has been suggested, on the basis of reasonable but not conclusive physiologic evidence, that the early sympathotonic attempt to maintain blood pressure leads to overly vigorous contractions of the cardiac chambers, and this, in turn, acts as the afferent stimulus for withdrawal of sympathetic tone (see "Neurocardiogenic Syncope," below). It is also possible that the initial adrenergic discharge that precedes syncope causes a vasodilation in muscular blood vessels and initiates hypotension. The vasodilating effects of nitric oxide on vascular endothelium and the greatly augmented levels of circulating acetylcholine in syncope have also been invoked as factors in the vasodepressor phenomenon.

In essence all the following types of syncope are "vasovagal," meaning a combination of vasodepressor and vagal effects in varying proportions; the only differences are in the stimuli that elicit the response from the medulla.

Vasodepressor Syncope This is the common faint, fully described above and seen mainly in young individuals. A familial proclivity is known (Mathias et al). The evocative factors are usually strong emotion, physical injury—particularly to viscera (testicles, gut)—or other factors (see below). As described above, the vasodilatation of adrenergically innervated "resistance vessels" leads to a reduction in peripheral vascular resistance, but cardiac output fails to exhibit the compensatory rise that normally occurs in hypotension. Some physiologic studies suggest that the dilatation of intramuscular vessels, innervated by beta-adrenergic fibers, may be more important than dilatation of the splanchnic ones. Skin vessels are constricted. Vagal stimulation may then occur (hence the term *vasovagal*), causing bradycardia and leading possibly to a slight further drop in blood pressure. Other vagal effects are perspiration, increased peristaltic activity, nausea, and salivation.

As already mentioned, bradycardia probably contributes little to the hypotension and syncope. The term *vasovagal*, used originally by Thomas Lewis to designate this type of faint, is therefore not entirely apt and should be avoided as a synonym for vasodepressor syncope. As Lewis himself pointed out, atropine, "while raising the pulse rate up to and beyond normal levels during the attack, leaves the blood pressure below normal and the patient still pale and not fully conscious."

In summary, the vasodepressor faint occurs (1) in normal health under the influence of strong emotion, particularly in some susceptible individuals (sight of blood or an accident) or in conditions that favor peripheral vasodilatation, e.g., hot, crowded rooms ("heat syncope"), especially if the person is hungry or tired or has had a few alcoholic drinks, or (2) during a painful illness or after bodily injury (especially of the abdomen or genitalia), as a consequence of fright, pain, and other factors (where pain is involved, the vagal element tends to be more prominent in the genesis of the faint), and (3) during exercise in some sensitive persons (see further on).

Neurocardiogenic Syncope This entity, a component or perhaps a subtype of vasodepressor syncope, has received attention as a cause of otherwise unexplained fainting in children and young adults. As alluded to above, it may be the final precipitant in the common vasodepressor faint, and the term is used synonymously with vasovagal or vasodepressor syncope by some authors (Kosinski et al).

Oberg and Thoren were the first to observe that the left ventricle itself can be the source of neurally mediated syncope in much the same way as the carotid sinus, when stimulated, produces vasodilation and bradycardia. During acute blood loss in cats, they noted a paradoxical bradycardia that was preceded by increased afferent activity in autonomic fibers arising from the ventricles of the heart, a reaction that could be eliminated by sectioning these nerves. This concept of the heart as a source of vasodepressor reflexes had been suggested earlier by Bezold as well as by Jarisch and Zoterman and came to be known as the "Bezold-Jarisch reflex." The inferoposterior wall of the left ventricle is the site of most of the subendocardial mechanoreceptors that are responsible for the afferent impulses.

In order for this mechanism to become active, very vigorous cardiac contractions must occur in the presence of deficient filling of the cardiac chambers (hence "neurocardiogenic"). In the simple faint, an initial burst of sympathetic activity is thought to precipitate these physiologic circumstances of excessive cardiac activity. Echocardiographic findings of a greatly diminished ventricular chamber size and vigorous contractions just prior to syncope support this notion (the "empty heart syndrome"). However, the ability to induce a similar neurally mediated syncope in cardiac transplantation patients, whose hearts are denervated, leads one to question this concept. Perhaps the remaining baroreceptors in the aorta are responsible in this instance.

According to Kaufmann, patients with a proclivity to primary neurocardiogenic syncope can be identified by the finding of delayed fainting when the patient is placed at a 60-degree upright position on a tilt table. After approximately 10 min of upright posture, the blood pressure drops below 100 mmHg; soon thereafter patients complain of dizziness and sweating, and subsequently faint. In contrast, patients with primary sympathetic failure will faint soon after upward tilting. Half of patients with unexplained syncope display this delayed tilt-table reaction, but it is seen also in 5 percent of controls (see page 401). The value of isoproteronol as a cardiac stimulant and peripheral vasodilator to enhance the effect of upright posture and expose neurocardiogenic syncope during the tilt-table test is controversial (see further on).

Exercise-Induced Syncope Aerobic exercise, particularly running, is known to induce fainting in some persons, a trait that may become apparent in late childhood or later and may be familial. There is nausea as well as other presyncopal symptoms, and the faint can be avoided by discontinuing exercise or not exceeding a threshold of effort set by the patient himself. Such persons do not seem unduly sensitive to nonaerobic exercise and have no recognizable electrocardiographic (ECG) or structural heart problems. They have a predilection to faint with prolonged tilt-table testing and with isoproterenol infusion, suggesting an excessive muscular vasodilatory response, as described above with neurocardiogenic syncope. These patients may benefit from beta-adrenergic blocking drugs if given under careful supervision. As discussed further on, exercise can also precipitate syncope in patients with a number of underlying cardiac conditions (myocardial ischemia, prolonged–QT interval syndrome, aortic outflow obstruction, cardiomyopathy, structural chamber anomalies, exercise-induced ventricular tachycardia, and, less often, supraventricular tachycardias).

Athletes who faint unpredictably during exercise pose a particularly difficult problem. Obviously those found to have serious heart disease should give up competitive sports, but the majority have no demonstrable cardiac abnormality. Subjecting these patients to intense exercise and other testing sometimes fails to elicit the faints, but many of them have varying degrees of hypotension when subjected to prolonged head-up tilt, again suggesting "neurocardiogenic" syncope (see above). Standard pacemakers are not curative in these vasodepressor faints, since the main deficiency is in vascular resistance. Unless the results of tilt testing are unequivocal and reproducible, it is best to consider the more serious causes of exercise-induced syncope and to treat the patient appropriately.

Carotid Sinus Syncope The carotid sinus is normally sensitive to stretch and gives rise to sensory impulses carried via the nerve of Hering, a branch of the glossopharyngeal nerve, to the medulla. Massage of one of the carotid sinuses or of both of them alternately, particularly in elderly persons, causes (1) a reflex cardiac slowing (sinus bradycardia, sinus arrest, or even atrioventricular block)—the *vagal type* of response, or (2) a fall of arterial pressure without cardiac slowing—the *vasodepressor type* of response. Another ("central") type of carotid sinus syncope was in the past ascribed to cerebral arteriolar constriction, but such an entity has never been validated.

Faintness or syncope due to carotid sinus sensitivity has reportedly been initiated by turning of the head to one side while wearing a tight collar or even by shaving over the region of the sinus. However, the absence of a history of such an association does not exclude the diagnosis. The attack nearly always occurs when the patient is upright, usually standing. The onset is sudden, often with falling. Small convulsive movements occur quite frequently in both the vagal and vasodepressor types of carotid sinus syncope. The period of unconsciousness in carotid sinus syncope seldom lasts longer than 30 s, and the sensorium is immediately clear when consciousness is regained. The majority of the reported cases have involved men.

As intimated above, in a patient displaying faintness on massage of one carotid sinus, it is important to distinguish between the benign disorder (hypersensitivity of the carotid sinus) and a more serious condition—atheromatous narrowing of the basilar or opposite carotid artery (see Chap. 34). In testing for carotid sinus sensitivity in the latter circumstance, it is important to avoid compression of the carotid artery, which may represent the major vascular supply to both hemispheres; testing should be avoided altogether if a carotid bruit is heard in either vessel.

A number of other types of purely reflexive cardiac slowing can be traced to direct irritation of the vagus nerves (from esophageal diverticula, mediastinal tumors, gallbladder stones, carotid sinus disease, bronchoscopy, and needling of body cavities). Here, the reflex bradycardia is more often of sinoatrial than atrioventricular type. Weiss and Ferris called such faints *vagovagal.*

Gastaut and Fischer-Williams used the oculocardiac inhibitory reflex to study this form of syncope. They found that the heightened vagal discharge produced by compression of the eyeballs (oculovagal reflex, a cause of syncope in acute glaucoma) could produce brief periods of cardiac arrest and syncope. This effect was produced in 20 of 100 patients who had a history of syncopal attacks, mainly of the vasodepressor type. These investigators found that after a 7- to 13-s period of cardiac arrest, there was a loss of consciousness, pallor, and muscle relaxation. Toward the end of this period, runs of bilaterally synchronous theta and delta waves appeared in the EEG, predominantly in the frontal lobes; in some patients there were one or more myoclonic jerks, synchronous with the slow waves. If the cardiac arrest persisted beyond 14 or 15 s, the EEG became flat. This period of electrical silence lasted for 10 to 20 s and was sometimes accompanied by a generalized tonic spasm with incontinence. Following the spasm, heartbeats and large-amplitude delta waves reappeared, and after another 20 to 30 s, the EEG reverted to normal. It is noteworthy that rhythmic clonic seizures or epileptiform EEG activity were not observed at any time during the periods of cardiac arrest, syncope, and tonic spasm.

Tumors or lymph node enlargements at the base of the skull or in the neck which impinge on the carotid artery, as well as post radiation fibrosis are capable of causing dramatic syncopal attacks, sometimes preceded by unilateral head or neck pain. Often the episodes are unpredictable, but some patients find that turning the head stimulates an attack. The mechanism in our experience has been primarily a vasodepressor response; patients with prominent bradycardia have generally had tumors that impinged directly on the glossopharyngeal and vagus nerves (Frank et al; Macdonald et al). If the tumor can be safely removed from the carotid region, the syncope often abates; in many cases, however, intracranial section of the ninth and upper rootlets of the vagus nerves on the side of the mass is necessary.

Syncope in Association with Glossopharyngeal Neuralgia *Glossopharyngeal neuralgia* (also referred to as *vagoglossopharyngeal neuralgia*) (page 1456) typically begins in the sixth decade with paroxysms of pain localized to the base of the tongue, pharynx or larynx, tonsillar area, or an ear. In only a small proportion of cases (estimated at 2 percent) are the paroxysms of pain complicated by syncope. Always, the sequence is pain, then bradycardia, and finally syncope. Presumably the pain gives rise to a massive volley of afferent impulses along the ninth cranial nerve, activating the medullary vasomotor centers via collateral fibers from the nucleus of the tractus solitarius. An increase in parasympathetic (vagal) activity slows the heart. Wallin and colleagues have demonstrated that, in addition to bradycardia, there is an element of hypotension, due to inhibition of peripheral sympathetic activity. The effects of the bradycardia greatly exceed those of the vasodepressor hypotension, sometimes to the point of asystole, thus differing from the related condition of carotid sinus syncope and from most other types of syncope.

The medical treatment of this type of syncope parallels that of trigeminal neuralgia (which is associated in approximately 10 percent of cases, usually on the same side). Anticonvulsants and baclofen are helpful in some patients. Vascular decompression procedures involving small branches of the basilar artery that impinge on the ninth nerve are said to be useful, but such patients but have not been extensively studied. Conventional surgical treatment, which consists of sectioning the ninth cranial nerve and upper rootlets of the tenth, has proved to be effective.

The same mechanism is probably operative in so-called *deglutitional syncope*, in which consciousness is lost during or immediately after a forceful swallow. The administration of anticholinergic drugs (propantheline 15 mg tid) has abolished these attacks (Levin and Posner).

Micturition Syncope This condition is usually seen in men, sometimes in young adults but more often in the elderly, who arise from bed at night to urinate. The syncope occurs at the end of micturition or soon thereafter, and the loss of consciousness is abrupt, with rapid and complete recovery. Several factors are probably operative. A full bladder causes reflex vasoconstriction; as the bladder empties, this gives way to vasodilatation, which, combined with an element of postural hypotension, might be sufficient to cause fainting in some individuals. Vagus-mediated bradycardia and, in some cases, a mild Valsalva effect may also be factors, and alcohol ingestion, hunger, fatigue, and upper respiratory infection are common predisposing factors. In some instances, especially in the elderly, the nocturnal collapse has caused serious head injury.

Tussive and Valsalva Syncope Syncope as a result of a severe paroxysm of coughing was first described by Charcot in 1876. Patients with this type of syncope are usually heavy-set males who smoke and have chronic bronchitis. Occasionally it occurs in children, particularly following the paroxysmal coughing spells of pertussis and laryngitis. After sustained hard coughing, the patient suddenly becomes weak and may lose consciousness momentarily. This is mainly attributable to the greatly elevated intrathoracic pressure, which interferes with venous return to the heart. Increased cerebrospinal fluid (CSF) pressure and diminished P_{CO_2}, with resultant cerebral vasoconstriction, are probably contributing factors.

Powerful efforts to exhale against a closed glottis (as occurs in tussive syncope) is referred to as the *Valsalva maneuver*. The unconsciousness that results from *breath-holding spells* in infants is probably based on this mechanism as well; the so-called pallid attacks in infants probably represent reflex vasodepression. Also, the loss of consciousness that occurs during competitive weight lifting ("weight lifters' blackout") is mainly the effect of a Valsalva maneuver, added to which are the effects of vascular dilatation produced by squatting and hyperventilation. Lesser degrees of this phenomenon (faintness and light-headedness) not infrequently follow other kinds of strenuous activity, such as unrestrained laughing, straining at stool, heavy lifting, underwater diving, or effortful trumpet playing. Rarely, a brief faint may occur in each of these circumstances.

Syncope may occur occasionally in the course of prostatic or rectal examination, but only if the patient is standing (prostatic syncope). A Valsalva effect and reflex vagal stimulation appear to be contributing factors. *Postprandial hypotension* may occasionally lead to syncope in elderly persons, in whom impaired baroreflex function cannot compensate for pooling of blood in splanchnic vessels.

Primary Failure of the Sympathetic Nervous System

Postural (Orthostatic) Hypotension This type of syncope affects persons whose peripheral vasomotor reflexes are defective. Although the character of the faint differs little from that of vasodepressor syncope, the effect of posture in its initiation is its most typical attribute. Standing still for prolonged periods or arising quickly from a recumbent position are the two circumstances under which it is most likely to happen. The patient, on assuming an upright position, shows a steady decline in blood pressure to a level at which the cerebral circulation cannot be supported. *It should be emphasized that the bedside testing of orthostatic blood pressure is best performed by having the patient stand quickly, and taking readings immediately, at 1 and at 3 min, rather than using the lying-sitting-standing sequence.* With few exceptions (see Chap. 26), peripheral autonomic failure precludes a compensatory tachycardia, and contrary to what happens in vasodepressor syncope, there are no autonomic responses such as pallor, sweating, nausea, or release of norepinephrine. Mild mental clouding with staggering or falling may precede unconsciousness or be the only evidence of cerebral disorder.

The maintenance of blood pressure during various levels of activity and with postural changes depends on pressure-sensitive receptors (baroreceptors) in the aortic arch and carotid sinus and mechanoreceptors in the walls of the heart. These receptors, which are the sensory nerve endings of the glossopharyngeal and vagus nerves, send afferent impulses to the vasomotor centers in the medulla, more specifically the nucleus of the tractus solitarius (NTS). Axons from the NTS project to the reticular formation of the ventrolateral medulla, which, in turn, sends fibers to the intermediolateral cell column of the spinal cord, thereby controlling vasomotor tone in skeletal muscles, skin, and the splanchnic bed. A diminution of sensory impulses from baroreceptors increases the flow of excitatory signals, which raise the blood pressure and cardiac output, thus restoring cerebral perfusion. This subject is discussed further in relation to the regulation of blood pressure, in Chap. 26.

Postural syncope occurs under a wide variety of clinical conditions: (1) in otherwise normal individuals who, in certain circumstances, experience a failure of pressor-receptor reflex function, as described earlier; (2) as part of a chronic syndrome known as idiopathic orthostatic hypotension or primary autonomic insufficiency (see further on); (3) after a period of prolonged illness with recumbency, especially in elderly individuals with poor muscle tone; (4) in association with diseases of the peripheral nerves that involve autonomic nerve fibers—diabetes, tabes dorsalis, amyloidosis, Guillain-Barré syndrome, a primary idiopathic autonomic neuropathy, pandysutonomia, and several other polyneuropathies, all of which interrupt vasomotor reflexes; (5) after sympathectomy or high vagotomy; (6) in patients receiving L-dopa, antihypertensive agents and certain sedative and antidepressant drugs; (7) in spinal cord transection above the T6 level, particularly in the acute stage; and (8) in patients with hypovolemia.

These conditions are easily understood if one keeps in mind that, on assuming the erect posture, the pooling of blood in the lower parts of the body is normally prevented by (1) reflex arteriolar and arterial constriction, through alpha- and beta-adrenergic effector mechanisms; (2) reflex acceleration of the heart by means of aortic and carotid reflexes, as described above; and (3) muscular activity, which improves venous return. Unmyelinated (postganglionic sympathetic) fibers cease firing during vasovagal fainting at a point when the blood pressure falls below 80/40 mmHg and the pulse below 60. Lipsitz has pointed out that aging is associated with a progressive impairment of these compensatory mechanisms, thus rendering the older person especially vulnerable to syncope. However, even in some younger persons, after the blood pressure has fallen slightly and stabilized at a lower level, the compensatory reflexes may fail suddenly, with a precipitant drop in blood pressure.

Postural Orthostatic Tachycardia Syndrome ("POTS") The authors have limited experience with this process and are uncertain about its validity as an entity apart from an aversion of the patient to assume an upright posture and the tendency to become weak and tremulous. As described by Low et al, it consists of intolerance of the standing position accompanied by tachycardia up to 120 beats per minute or more, but *without* orthostatic hypotension. Dyspnea, fatigue, and tremulousness and a complaint of "dizziness" accompany the assumption of an upright posture, and the same constellation of symptoms may be brought out by upright tilting. There is a frequent association with fatigue and with exercise intolerance. The situation is comparable to orthostatic intolerance in the chronic fatigue syndrome (page 528), with which POTS shares many features. An impairment of cerebral autoregulation has been hypothesized; others consider it to be a limited form of dysautonomia.

Primary Autonomic Insufficiency (Idiopathic Orthostatic Hypotension) This presents in two forms. In one form (Bradbury-Eggleston) there is probably a selective degeneration of neurons in the sympathetic ganglia with denervation of smooth muscle vasculature and adrenal glands. The pathology has not been fully delineated but lesions in other parts of the nervous system are not evident. In the second type (Shy-Drager) there is a degeneration of preganglionic neurons in the lateral columns of gray matter in the spinal cord, leaving postganglionic neurons isolated from spinal control. The latter lesion is often associated with degeneration of other systems of neurons in the central nervous system. Three such system degenerations have been identified, occurring singly or in combination: (1) degeneration of the substantia nigra and locus ceruleus (Parkinson disease), (2) striatonigral degeneration, and (3) olivopontocerebellar degeneration. In the first two syndromes, orthostatic hypotension is combined with a parkinsonian syndrome; in the third, it is associated with cerebellar ataxia. These forms of degenerative disease have their onset in adult life, and the associated hypotension and syncope are usually part of a more widespread autonomic dysfunction that includes a fixed cardiac rate, vocal cord paralysis, a loss of sweating in the lower parts of the body, atonicity of the bladder, constipation, and impotence in the male. As indicated on page 1137, the symptoms of Parkinson disease, autonomic failure, and cerebellar atrophy are often associated—a distinctive combination that has been subsumed under the term *multiple system atrophy*.

Syncope of Cardiac Origin

This is due to a sudden reduction in cardiac output, usually because of an arrhythmia, predominantly a bradyarrhythmia. Normally, a pulse as low as 35 to 40 beats per minute or as high as 150 beats per minute is well tolerated, especially if the patient is recumbent. Changes in pulse rate beyond these extremes impair cardiac output and may lead to syncope. Upright posture, anemia, and coronary, myocardial, and valvular disease all render the individual more susceptible to these alterations. Detailed discussions of the various valvular and myocardial abnormalities and arrhythmias that may compromise cardiac output and lead to syncope are to be found in the articles by Lipsitz, by Manolis, and by Kapoor and colleagues, listed in the references.

Syncope of cardiac origin occurs most frequently in patients with *complete atrioventricular block* and a pulse rate of 40 or less per minute (Adams-Stokes-Morgagni syndrome). The block may be persistent or intermittent; it is often preceded by fascicular or second-degree heart block. Ventricular arrest of 4 to 8 s, if the patient is upright, is enough to cause syncope; if the patient is supine, the asystole must last 12 to 15 s. After asystole of 12 s, according to Engel, the patient turns pale and becomes momentarily weak or may lose consciousness without warning; this may occur regardless of the position of the body. If the duration of cerebral ischemia exceeds 15 to 20 s, there are a few clonic jerks. With still longer asystole, the clonic jerks merge with tonic spasms and stertorous respirations and the ashen-gray pallor gives way to cyanosis, incontinence, fixed pupils, and bilateral Babinski signs. As heart action resumes, the face and neck become flushed. The report of this sequence of signs by a dependable observer helps to distinguish syncope from epilepsy. In cases of even more prolonged asystole (4 to 5 min), there may be cerebral injury, caused by a combination of hypoxia and ischemia. Coma may persist or may be replaced by confusion and other neurologic signs. Focal ischemic changes, often irreversible, may then be traced to the fields of occluded atherosclerotic cerebral arteries or the border zones between the areas of supply of major arteries. Cardiac faints of the Stokes-Adams type may recur several times a day. The heart block is usually intermittent at first, and between attacks the ECG may show only evidence of myocardial disease. A continuous ECG using a Holter monitor or telemetry is then needed to demonstrate the arrhythmia (see further on).

Less easily recognized are faintness and syncope due to *dysfunction of the sinus node*, manifest by marked sinus bradycardia, sinoatrial block, or sinus arrest ("sick-sinus syndrome"). The nodal block results in prolonged atrial asystole (>3 s). Supraventricular tachycardia or atrial fibrillation may occur, alternating with sinus bradycardia (bradycardia-tachycardia syndrome).

Tachyarrhythmias alone are less likely to produce syncope. Certainly intermittent ventricular fibrillation can cause fainting, and supraventricular tachycardias with rapid ventricular responses (usually over 180 beats per minute) cause syncope when sustained, predominantly in patients who are upright at the time. *The long–QT interval syndrome* is a rare familial condition in which syncope and ventricular arrhythmias are prone to occur. Another inherited syndrome with right bundle branch block and ST segment elevation in the right precordial leads is known to cause syncope and even sudden death (Brugada syndrome). Some patients with mitral valve prolapse seem disposed to syncope and presyncope and an inordinate number also have panic attacks.

Aortic stenosis or *subaortic stenosis* from cardiomyopathy often sets the stage for exertional syncope, because cardiac output cannot keep pace with the demands of exercise. Primary pulmonary hypertension and obstruction of right ventricular outflow (pulmonic valvular or infundibular stenosis) or intracardiac tumors may also be associated with exertional syncope. Vagal overactivity may be the factor responsible for the syncope in these conditions and possibly for the syncope that accompanies pulmonary embolism and aortic outflow obstruction. Tetralogy of Fallot is the congenital cardiac malformation that most often leads to syncope. Other cardiac causes are listed in the classification given at the opening of this chapter.

Syncope Associated with Cerebrovascular Disease

Syncope is an uncommon manifestation of cerebrovascular disease; cases that do occur are usually associated with occlusion of the large arteries in the neck. The best examples are found in patients with the aortic-arch syndrome (Takayasu pulseless disease, page 908), in which the brachiocephalic, common carotid, and vertebral arteries have become narrowed. Physical activity may then critically reduce blood flow to the upper part of the brainstem, causing abrupt loss of consciousness. Stenosis or occlusion of vertebral arteries and the "subclavian steal syndrome" are other examples (page 843). Fainting is said also to occur occasionally in patients with congenital anomalies of the upper cervical spine (Klippel-Feil syndrome) or cervical spondylosis, in which the vertebral circulation is compromised. Head turning may then cause vertigo, nausea and vomiting, visual scotomas, and finally unconsciousness. Syncope does not occur with ischemic attacks that are confined to the territory of the internal carotid artery. Nor, in the authors' experience, do pure syncopal attacks occur with vertebrobasilar ischemia (see further on).

Cerebral Hemorrhage and Syncope The onset of a subarachnoid hemorrhage may be signaled by a syncopal episode, often with transient apnea. Because the bleeding is arterial, there is a momentary cessation of cerebral circulation as intracranial pressure and blood pressure approach one another. Unless there has been vomiting, a complaint of headache immediately preceding the syncope, or the discovery of hypertension or stiff neck when the patient awakens, the diagnosis may not be suspected until a CT scan or lumbar puncture is performed.

An associated problem, with which we have had numerous unsatisfactory encounters, is posed by the patient who is seen to fall suddenly forward without apparent cause, awakens with headache, and is found to have bifrontal hematomas and subarachnoid blood on CT. These cases highlight the difficulty of distinguishing a primary aneurysmal subarachnoid hemorrhage from an accidental fall or syncope with secondary frontal brain contusions; in almost every case, we have felt obliged to perform cerebral angiography to exclude an anterior communicating artery aneurysm but we have rarely found one.

Fainting in Hysteria

Hysterical fainting is rather frequent and usually occurs under dramatic circumstances (Chap. 56). The evident lack of change in pulse, blood pressure, or color of the skin or any outward display of anxiety distinguishes it from the vasodepressor faint. Irregular jerking movements and generalized spasms without loss of consciousness or change in the EEG are typical features. The diagnosis is based on these negative findings in a person who exhibits the general personality and behavioral characteristics of hysteria. Several interesting instances of mass faintness and syncope of hysterical type have been described in school marching bands (Levine RJ).

Syncope of Unknown Cause

Finally, it should be pointed out that after careful evaluation of patients with syncope and the exclusion of the many forms of the condition described above, there remains a significant proportion of patients (one-third to one-half, according to Kapoor) in which a cause for the syncope cannot be ascertained. The question of whether a single positive tilt table test signifies that a prior episode of syncope was neurocardiogenic is not resolved; this obviously has a bearing on the proportion of cases that remain without a diagnosis. If the episodes are repetitive and erratically spaced, a cardiac arrhythmia or intraventricular conduction defect should be sought by use of special monitoring devices and conduction studies.

DIFFERENTIAL DIAGNOSIS

Conditions Associated with Episodic Weakness and Faintness but Rarely with Syncope

Anxiety Attacks and the Hyperventilation Syndrome These are probably the most important diagnostic considerations in unexplained faintness without syncope. The light-headedness of anxiety and hyperventilation are frequently described as a feeling of faintness, but a loss of consciousness does not follow (see Linzer et al). Such symptoms are not accompanied by facial pallor or relieved by recumbency. The diagnosis is made on the basis of the associated symptoms, the absence of laboratory and tilt-table abnormalities, and the finding that part of the attack can be reproduced by having the patient hyperventilate. The symptoms produced in this way mimic the persistent or episodic dizziness that accompanies anxiety and panic states (Chap. 15). When anxiety attacks are combined with a Valsalva effect or prolonged standing, fainting may occur. The relationship of anxiety-panic to the previously described postural orthostatic tachycardia syndrome is uncertain.

Hypoglycemia In nondiabetics, hypoglycemia may be an obscure cause of episodic weakness and very rarely of syncope. With progressive lowering of blood glucose, the clinical picture is one of hunger, trembling, flushed facies, sweating, confusion, and finally, after many minutes, seizures and coma. The diagnosis depends largely upon the history, the documentation of reduced blood glucose during an attack, and reproduction of the patient's spontaneous attacks by an injection of insulin or an oral dose of tolbutamide (or ingestion of a high-carbohydrate meal in the case of reactive hypoglycemia).

Acute Blood Loss Acute hemorrhage, usually within the gastrointestinal tract, is a cause of weakness, faintness, or even unconsciousness when the patient stands suddenly. The cause (gastric or duodenal ulcer is the most common) may remain obscure until the passage of black stools.

Transient Cerebral Ischemic Attacks The many symptoms comprised by these attacks in the carotid system are fully described on page 859, but syncope is not one of the clinical presentations. In the case of attacks in the vertebrobasilar territory, an impairment of consciousness is a rare manifestation, but almost always in the context of additional signs of upper brainstem dysfunction.

Drop Attacks This term is generally applied to falling spells that occur without warning and *without* loss of consciousness or postictal symptoms. The patient, usually elderly and more often female, suddenly falls down while walking or standing, rarely while stooping. The knees inexplicably buckle. There is no dizziness or impairment of consciousness, and the fall is usually forward, with scuffing of the knees and sometimes the nose. The patient, unless obese, is able to right herself and to rise immediately and go her way, quite embarrassed. There may be several attacks during a period of a few weeks and none thereafter. The interval EEGs are normal. One potential mechanism is a lapse of tone in leg muscles during the silent phase of an unnoticed myoclonic jerk. Drop attacks also occur in hydrocephalics, and these patients, though conscious, may not be able to arise for several hours. Drop attacks as defined above are usually without an identifiable mechanism, requiring no treatment if cardiologic studies are normal. On uncertain grounds, they are often attributed to brainstem ischemia. In only about one-quarter such cases, according to Meissner and coworkers, can an association be made with cardiovascular or cerebrovascular disease, to which treatment should be directed. Rare instances of Meniere disease, in which the patient is suddenly thrown to the ground ("otolithic catastrophe of Tumarkin", page 320) may be mistaken for a syncopal attack, but only briefly, until vertigo becomes prominent.

Seizures and Syncope In the final analysis, the loss of consciousness in the different types of syncope must be caused by impaired function of the neural elements in those parts of the brain subserving consciousness, i.e., in the high brainstem reticular activating system. In this respect syncope and primary generalized (so-called centrencephalic) epilepsy have a common ground; yet there is a fundamental difference. In epilepsy, whether major or minor, the arrest in consciousness is almost instantaneous, and, as revealed by the EEG, is accompanied by a paroxysm of electrical activity occurring simultaneously in all of the cerebral cortex and thalamus. The EEG changes (delta waves) in syncope appear later in the course of the attack. The difference relates to the essential pathophysiology—the rapid spread of an electrical discharge in epilepsy and a more gradual failure of cerebral circulation in syncope.

There are also a number of important clinical distinctions between epileptic and syncopal attacks. The epileptic attack may occur day or night, regardless of the position of the patient; syncope rarely appears when the patient is recumbent, the only common exception being the Stokes-Adams attack. The patient's color usually does not change at the onset of an epileptic attack; pallor is an early and invariable finding in all types of syncope except those due to chronic orthostatic hypotension or hysteria, and it precedes unconsciousness. An epileptic attack, as indicated above, is more sudden in onset; if an aura is present, it rarely lasts longer than a few seconds before consciousness is abolished. The onset of syncope is usually more gradual, and the prodromal symptoms are quite distinctive and different from those of seizures. In general, injury from falling is more frequent in epilepsy than in syncope, because protective reflexes are instantaneously abolished in the former. Nevertheless, cardiogenic syncope is an important cause of hurtful falls, especially in the elderly. Tonic spasm of muscles with upturning of the eyes is a prominent and often initial feature of epilepsy, but this occurs only rarely and late in the course of a faint; however, twitching and a few clonic contractions of the limbs may occur several seconds after the patient has fainted (see above). Urinary incontinence is a frequent occurrence in epilepsy, but it need not occur during an epileptic attack and may occur with syncope, so that it cannot be used as a means of excluding the latter disorder. The return of consciousness is slow in epilepsy, prompt in syncope; mental confusion, headache, and drowsiness are common sequelae of seizures, and physical weakness with clear sensorium of syncope (a brief period of grogginess may follow vasodepressor syncope). Repeated spells of unconsciousness in a young person at a rate of several per day or month are much more suggestive of epilepsy than of syncope.

The EEG may be helpful in differentiating syncope from epilepsy. In the interval between epileptic seizures, the EEG, particularly if repeated once or twice, shows some degree of abnormality in 50 to 75 percent of cases, whereas it should be normal between syncopal attacks. Sometimes one must resort to continuous EEG monitoring by tape recording or telemetry to clarify the situation (this can be combined with continuous ECG recording.) Cases in which vertebrobasilar ischemia is the suspected cause of syncope may be clarified by Doppler flow studies, magnetic resonance angiography, or, if necessary, by angiography (Chap. 34). Another useful laboratory marker of a seizure, especially if unwitnessed, is an elevation of the serum creatine kinase (CK) concentration; such a finding could conceivably occur only in the very rare case of syncope associated with extensive muscle trauma. Prolactin levels have not proved discriminating enough for routine use in separating seizure from syncope but remain useful in distinguishing both of these from other causes of loss of consciousness, particularly hysteria (see page 344).

No single one of these criteria will absolutely differentiate epilepsy from syncope, but taken as a group and supplemented by the EEG, they usually enable one to distinguish the two conditions.

SPECIAL METHODS OF EXAMINATION

In patients who complain of recurrent faintness or syncope but do not have a spontaneous attack while under observation of the physician, an attempt to reproduce attacks may prove to be of great assistance in diagnosis. Here it is important to recall that normal persons can faint if made to squat and overbreathe and then to stand erect and hold their breath (Valsalva maneuver). Prolonged standing at attention in the heat often causes even well-conditioned soldiers to faint, as does compression of the chest and abdomen while holding one's breath, as in the parlor trick of adolescents ("fainting lark").

When an anxiety state is accompanied by faintness, the pattern of symptoms can often be reproduced by having the subject hyperventilate—that is, breathe rapidly and deeply for 2 to 3 min. This test may also be of therapeutic value, because the underlying anxiety tends to be lessened when the patient learns that the symptoms can be produced and alleviated at will simply by controlling breathing.

Most patients with tussive syncope cannot reproduce an attack by the Valsalva maneuver but can sometimes do so by voluntary coughing if severe enough. Another useful procedure is to have the patient perform the Valsalva maneuver for more than 10 s (thus trapping blood behind closed valves in the veins) while the pulse and blood pressure are measured (see "Tests for Abnormalities of the Autonomic Nervous System," Chap. 26).

In each of the aforementioned instances, the crucial point is not whether symptoms are produced but whether they reproduce the exact pattern of symptoms that occurs in the spontaneous attacks.

Other conditions in which the diagnosis is clarified by reproducing the attacks are carotid sinus hypersensitivity (massage of one or the other carotid sinus) and orthostatic hypotension (observations of pulse rate, blood pressure, and symptoms in the recumbent and standing positions or, even better, with the patient on a tilt table). The latter is now a regularly used procedure when the diagnosis of syncope is not evident from physical examination and routine studies such as ECG, blood count, and bedside sphygmomanometry. There is a distinct difference in the cardiovascular challenge imposed by a tilt table and that created by the simple act of standing up from a sitting or recumbent position. It is re-emphasized that, from the perspective of uncovering autonomic failure, having the patient stand abruptly from a lying position and then recording the blood pressure at intervals is more informative than interposing a period of sitting between the lying and standing positions.

The measurement of beat-to-beat variation in heart rate is a simple but sensitive means of detecting vagal dysfunction, as described in Chap. 26.

Careful, continuous monitoring of the ECG in the hospital or by using a portable recorder may determine whether an arrhythmia is responsible for the syncopal episode. A continuous cardiac loop ECG recorder (which continually records and erases cardiac rhythm) permits prolonged (a month or longer) ambulatory monitoring at reasonable cost. The diagnostic yield from loop recording is much greater than that from Holter monitoring (Linzer et al). The signal-averaged ECG is reportedly a useful means of identifying individuals at risk for ventricular tachycardia as a cause of syncope (Manolis).

Tilt Table Testing There are two types of abnormal response to upright tilting: early hypotension (occurring within moments of tilting), which signifies inadequate sympathetic tone and baroreceptor function; and a delayed (several minutes) hypotension and syncope, which indicates a neurocardiogenic mechanism or an idiopathic type. The normal response to an 60- to 80-degree head-up tilt for 10 min is a transient drop in systolic blood pressure (5 to 15 mmHg), a rise in diastolic pressure (5 to 10 mmHg), and a rise in heart rate (10 to 15 beats per minute). Abrupt and persistent declines in blood pressure of greater than 20 to 30 mmHg systolic and 10 mmHg diastolic and a drop (or failure to rise) of the heart rate are considered abnormal; often these findings are associated with faintness and sometimes with syncope. Although controversial, in some circumstances the infusion of the catecholamine isoproterenol (1 to 5 mg/min for 30 min during head-up tilt) may be a more effective means of producing hypotension (and syncope) than the standard tilt test alone (Almquist et al; Waxman et al).

It should be repeated that the presence of a delayed faint with tilting only demonstrates a proclivity to neurocardiogenic fainting since it occurs in a proportion of individuals who have never fainted; it is not to be taken as incontrovertible evidence that a recent spell is explained by this mechanism.

TREATMENT

Patients seen during the preliminary stages of fainting or after they have lost consciousness should be placed in a position that permits maximal cerebral blood flow, i.e., with head lowered between the knees if sitting or preferably in the supine position with legs elevated. All tight clothing and other constrictions should be loosened and the head and body positioned so that the tongue does not fall back into the throat and the possible aspiration of vomitus is avoided. Nothing should be given by mouth until the patient has regained consciousness. The patient should not be permitted to rise until the sense of physical weakness has passed and he should be watched carefully for a few minutes after arising.

As a rule, the physician sees the patient after recovery from the faint and is asked to explain why it happened and how it can be prevented in the future. One should think first of those causes of fainting that constitute a therapeutic emergency. Among them are massive internal hemorrhage and myocardial infarction, which may be painless, and cardiac arrhythmias. In an elderly person, a sudden faint without obvious cause must always arouse the suspicion of a complete heart block or other cardiac arrhythmia, even though all findings are negative when the physician sees the patient.

The prevention of fainting depends on the mechanisms involved. In the usual vasodepressor faint of adolescents—which tends to occur in circumstances favoring vasodilatation (warm environment, hunger, fatigue, alcohol intoxication) and periods of emotional excitement—it is enough to advise the patient to avoid such circumstances. In postural hypotension, patients should be cautioned against arising suddenly from bed. Instead, they should first exercise the legs for a few seconds, then sit on the edge of the bed and make sure they are not light-headed or dizzy before starting to walk. Standing for prolonged periods can sometimes be tolerated without fainting by crossing the legs forcefully. Sleeping with the headposts of the bed elevated on wooden blocks 8 to 12 in. high and wearing a snug elastic abdominal binder and elastic stockings are measures that often prove helpful. Alternatives should be found for medications that are conceivable causes of orthostasis. Beta-adrenergic blocking agents, diuretics, antidepressants, and sympatholytic antihypertensive drugs are the common culprits.

In the syndrome of chronic orthostatic hypotension, special corticosteroid preparations—such as fludrocortisone acetate (Florinef) 0.05 to 0.4 mg/day in divided doses—and increased salt intake to expand blood volume are helpful. Recently the alpha$_1$ agonist, midodrine, beginning with 2.5 mg every 4 h and slowly increasing the dose to 5 mg every 4 to 6 hours, has been successful in small studies, but this medication has the potential to worsen the situation, and must be used with care. Binding of the legs and sleeping with the head and shoulders elevated are other useful measures. Tyramine and monoamine oxidase inhibitors have given limited relief in some cases of Shy-Drager syndrome, and beta blockers (propranolol or pindolol) and indomethacin (25 to 50 mg tid) in others. The approaches that have proved useful in treating orthostatic hypotension are reviewed by Mathias and Kimber.

Neurally mediated syncope (neurocardiogenic, or vasodepressor syncope), identified by upright tilt-table testing, may be prevented by the use of beta-adrenergic blocking agents (we have used acebutolol) or the anticholinergic agent disopyramide (Milstein et al). Several other drugs (e.g., ephedrine, metoclopramide, dihydroergotamine) have been variably successful in individiual patients, but their utility as standard medications remains to be established; the beta-blocking agents are generally preferred.

The treatment of carotid sinus syncope involves, first of all, instructing the patient in measures that minimize the hazards of a fall (see below). Loose collars should be worn, and the patient should learn to turn the whole body, rather than the head alone, when looking to one side. Atropine or one of the ephedrine group of drugs should be used, respectively, in patients with pronounced bradycardia or hypotension during attacks. If atropine is not successful and the syncopal attacks are incapacitating, the insertion of a dual-chamber pacemaker should be considered. Radiation or surgical denervation of the carotid sinus has apparently yielded favorable results in some patients, but it is rarely necessary. Vagovagal attacks usually respond well to an anticholinergic agent (propantheline, 15 mg tid).

Treatment of the hyperventilation syndrome and of hysteria are considered in Chap. 56. For a discussion of the treatment of hypoglycemia and the various cardiac arrhythmias that may induce syncope, the reader is referred to *Harrison's Principles of Internal Medicine*.

In the elderly person, a faint carries the additional hazard of a fracture or other trauma due to the fall. Therefore, the patient subject to recurrent syncope should cover the bathroom floor and bathtub with mats and have as much of his home carpeted as is feasible. Especially important is the floor space between the bed and the bathroom, because this is the route along which faints in elderly persons most commonly occur. Outdoor walking should be on soft ground rather than hard surfaces, and the patient should avoid standing still for prolonged periods, which is more likely than walking to induce an attack.

REFERENCES

ABBOUD FM: Neurocardiogenic syncope. *N Engl J Med* 328:1117, 1993.

ALMQUIST A, GOLDENBERG IF, MILSTEIN S, et al: Provocation of bradycardia and hypotension by isoproterenol and upright posture in patients with unexplained syncope. *N Engl J Med* 320:346, 1989.

BANNISTER R, MATHIAS W (eds): *Autonomic Failure: A Textbook of Clinical Disorders of the Autonomic Nervous System*, 4th ed. New York, Oxford University Press, 1999.

COMPTON D, HILL PM, SINCLAIR JD: Weight-lifters' blackout. *Lancet* 2:1234, 1973.

ENGEL GL: *Fainting*, 2nd ed. Springfield, IL, Charles C Thomas, 1962.

FRANK JI, ROPPER AH, ZUNIGA G: Vasodepressor carotid sinus syncope associated with a neck mass. *Neurology* 42:1194, 1992.

GASTAUT H, FISCHER-WILLIAMS M: Electro-encephalographic study of syncope: Its differentiation from epilepsy. *Lancet* 2:1018, 1957.

JARISCH A, ZOTERMAN Y: Depressor reflexes from the heart. *Acta Physiol Scand* 16:31, 1948.

KAPOOR WN: Evaluation and management of the patient with syncope. *JAMA* 268:2553, 1992.

KAPOOR WN, KARPF M, MAHER Y, et al: Syncope of unknown origin. *JAMA* 247:2687, 1982.

KAUFMANN H: Neurally mediated syncope: Pathogenesis, diagnosis, and treatment. *Neurology* 45(suppl 5):s12, 1995.

KONTOS HA, RICHARDSON DW, NORVELL JE: Norepinephrine depletion in idiopathic orthostatic hypotension. *Ann Intern Med* 82:336, 1975.

KOSINSKI D, GRUBB BP, TEMESY-ARMOS P: Pathophysiologic aspects of neurocardiogenic syncope: Current concepts and new perspectives. *PACE* 18:716, 1995.

LEVINE B, POSNER JB: Swallow syncope: Report of a case and review of the literature. *Neurology* 22:1086, 1972.

LEVINE RJ: Epidemic faintness and syncope in a school marching band. *JAMA* 238:2373, 1977.

LEWIS T: A lecture on vasovagal syncope and the carotid sinus mechanism. *BMJ* 1:873, 1932.

LINZER M, PRITCHETT ELC, PONTINEN M, et al: Incremental diagnostic yield of loop electrocardiographic recorders in unexplained syncope. *Am J Cardiol* 66:214, 1990.

LINZER M, VARIA I, PONTINEN M, et al: Medically unexplained syncope: Relationship to psychiatric illness. *Am J Med* 92:185, 1992.

LIPSITZ LA: Orthostatic hypotension in the elderly. *N Engl J Med* 321:952, 1989.

LIPSITZ LA: Syncope in the elderly. *Ann Intern Med* 99:92, 1983.

LOW PA, OPFER-GEHRKING TL, TEXTOR SC, BENARROCH EE, et al: Postural tachycardia syndrome (POTS). *Neurology* 45(suppl 5):19, 1995.

MACDONALD DR, STRONG E, NIELSEN S, POSNER JB: Syncope from head and neck cancer. *J Neurooncol* 1:257, 1983.

MANOLIS AS: The clinical spectrum and diagnosis of syncope. *Herz* 18:143, 1993.

MARK AL: The Bezold-Jarisch reflex revisited: Clinical implications of inhibitory reflexes originating in the heart. *J Am Coll Cardiol* 1:90, 1983.

Mathias CJ, Keguchi K, Bleasdale-Barr K, Kimber JR: Frequency of family history in vasovagal syncope. *Lancet* 352:33, 1998.

Mathias CJ, Kimber JR: Treatment of postural hypotension. *J Neurol Neurosurg Psychiatry* 65:285, 1998.

Meissner L, Wiebers DO, Swanson JW, O'Fallon WM: The natural history of drop attacks. *Neurology* 36:1029, 1986.

Milstein S, Buetikofer J, Dunnigan A, et al: Usefulness of disopyramide for prevention of upright tilt-induced hypotension-bradycardia. *Am J Cardiol* 65:1339, 1990.

Oberg B, Thoren P: Increased activity in left ventricular receptors during hemorrhage or occlusion of caval veins in the cat: A possible cause of the vasovagal reaction. *Acta Physiol Scand* 85:164, 1972.

Ross RT: *Syncope*. Philadelphia, Saunders, 1988.

Schoenberg BS, Kuglitsch JF, Karnes WE: Micturition syncope—Not a single entity. *JAMA* 229:1631, 1974.

Shy GM, Drager GA: A neurological syndrome associated with orthostatic hypotension: A clinical-pathologic study. *Arch Neurol* 2:511, 1960.

Wallin BG: New aspects of sympathetic function in man, in Stalberg E, Young RR (eds): *Clinical Neurophysiology*. London, Butterworth, 1981, pp 145–167.

Wallin BG, Sundlof G: Sympathetic outflow to muscles during vasovagal syncope. *J Auton Nerv Syst* 6:287, 1982.

Wallin BG, Westerberg CE, Sundlof G: Syncope induced by glossopharyngeal neuralgia: Sympathetic outflow to muscle. *Neurology* 34:522, 1984.

Waxman MB, Yao L, Cameron DA, et al: Isoproterenol induction of vasodepressor-type reaction in vasodepressor-prone persons. *Am J Cardiol* 63:58, 1989.

Weiss S, Capps RB, Ferris EB Jr, Munro D: Syncope and convulsions due to a hyperactive carotid sinus reflex: Diagnosis and treatment. *Arch Intern Med* 58:407, 1936.

Weiss S, Ferris EB Jr: Adams-Stokes syndrome with transient complete heart block of vagovagal reflex origin: Mechanism and treatment. *Arch Intern Med* 54:931, 1934.

Chapter 19

SLEEP AND ITS ABNORMALITIES

Sleep, that familiar yet inexplicable condition of repose in which consciousness is in abeyance, is obviously not abnormal, yet it is not illogical to consider it in connection with abnormal phenomena. There are a number of interesting irregularities of sleep, some of which approach serious extremes, just as there are unnatural forms of waking consciousness.

Everyone has had a great deal of personal experience with sleep, or lack of it, and has observed people in sleep, so it requires no special knowledge to know something about this condition or to appreciate its importance to health and well-being. The psychologic and physiologic benefits of sleep have seldom been so eloquently expressed as in the words of Tristram Shandy:

> *"Tis the refuge of the unfortunate—the enfranchisement of the prisoner, the downy lap of the hopeless, the weary, the broken-hearted; of all the soft delicious functions of nature this is the chiefest; what a happiness it is to man, when the anxieties and passions of the day are over."*

Physicians are often consulted by patients who suffer some derangement of sleep. Most often the problem is one of sleeplessness, but sometimes it concerns excessive sleep or some other peculiar phenomenon occurring in connection with sleep. Certain points concerning normal sleep and the sleep-wake mechanisms are worth reviewing, since familiarity with them is necessary for an understanding of disorders of sleep. A great deal of information about sleep and sleep abnormalities is now available as a result of the development, in relatively recent years, of the subspecialty of sleep medicine and the creation of a large number of centers for the diagnosis and treatment of sleep disorders.

Most disorders of sleep can be readily recognized and managed if one attends closely to the patient's description of his sleep disturbance. Only complex or odd cases or those requiring the documentation of apneic episodes or seizures and other motor disorders during sleep need study in special sleep laboratories.

Physiology of Sleep and Sleep-Wake Mechanisms

Sleep, as everyone knows, is an elemental phenomenon of life and an indispensable phase of human existence. It represents one of the basic 24-h (circadian) rhythms, traceable through all mammalian, avian, and reptilian species. The neural control of circadian rhythms is thought to reside in the ventral-anterior region of the hypothalamus—more specifically, in the suprachiasmatic nuclei. Lesions in these nuclei result in a disorganization of the sleep-wake cycles as well as of the rest-activity, temperature, and feeding rhythms. The ancillary role of melatonin and the pineal body in modulating this cyclic activity is described in Chap. 27.

Effects of Age Observations of the human sleep-wake cycle show it to be age-linked. The newborn baby sleeps from 16 to 20 h a day and the child, 10 to 12 h. Total sleep time drops to 9 to 10 h at age 10 and to about 7 to 7.5 h during adolescence. A gradual decline to about 6.5 h develops in late adult life. However, there are wide individual differences in the length and depth of sleep, due apparently to genetic factors, early-life conditioning, the amount of physical activity, and particular psychologic states.

The pattern of sleeping, which in terrestrial life is adjusted to the 24-h day, also varies in the different epochs of life. The circadian rhythm, with predominance of daytime wakefulness and nighttime sleep, begins to appear only after the first few weeks of postnatal life of the full-term infant; as the child matures, the morning nap is omitted, then the afternoon nap; by the fourth or fifth year, sleep becomes consolidated into a single long nocturnal period. (Actually, a large part of the world's population continues to have an afternoon nap, or siesta, as a lifelong sleep-wake pattern.) This alternating pattern of sleeping and waking persists throughout the adolescent and adult years unless it is altered by emotional or physical disease; fragmentation of the sleep pattern begins in late adult life. Over ensuing years, night awakenings tend to increase in frequency and the daytime waking period tends to be interrupted by episodic sleep lasting seconds to minutes (microsleep) as well as by longer naps. From about 35 years of age onward, women tend to sleep slightly more than men.

Stages of Sleep Seminal contributions to our understanding of the physiology of sleep were made by Loomis and associates and by Aserinsky, Dement, and Kleitman through EEG and polygraphic analysis. As a result of their studies, five stages of sleep, representative of two alternating physiologic mechanisms, were defined. In each stage, the electrical activity of the brain occurs in organized and recurring cycles, referred to as the *architecture of sleep*. These findings put to rest the antiquated ideas that sleep is a purely passive state and simply reflects fatigue and reduction in environmental stimuli, and that sleep and coma have fundamentally the same anatomic-physiologic basis. As the electrophysiologic stages of sleep progress, sleep becomes deeper, meaning that arousal requires a more intense stimulus.

Relaxed wakefulness with the eyes closed is accompanied in the electroencephalogram (EEG) by sinusoidal alpha waves of 9 to 11 Hz (cycles per second) and low-voltage fast activity of mixed frequency (as well as a 30- to 40-Hz gamma rhythm that is not evident on the routine EEG). The electromyogram (EMG) is silent when the patient is sitting or lying quietly except for the facial (mimetic) muscles. With drowsiness, as the first stage of sleep sets in, the eyelids begin to droop, the eyes may rove slowly from side to side, and the pupils become smaller. As the early stage of sleep evolves, the muscles relax, and the EEG pattern changes to one of progressively lower voltage and mixed frequency, with a loss of alpha waves; this is associated with slow, rolling eye movements and is called *stage 1 sleep*. As this changes into *stage 2 sleep*, 1/2- to 2-s bursts of biparietal 12- to 14-Hz waves (sleep spindles) and high-amplitude, sharp slow-wave (K) complexes appear (Fig. 19-1). The deep sleep of *stages 3 and 4*, also called *slow-wave sleep*, is composed of an increasing proportion of high-amplitude (>75-mV), delta (1- to 2-Hz) waves in the EEG. If the eyelids are raised gently, the globes are usually seen to be exotropic and the pupils are even smaller than before, but with retained responses to light. The last, or fifth, stage of the sleep cycle is associated with further reduction in muscle tone, except in the extraocular muscles, and with bursts of rapid eye movements (REMs) behind the closed lids. Concomitantly, the EEG becomes desynchronized, i.e., it has a low-voltage and high-frequency discharge pattern. The first four stages of sleep are called *non–rapid eye movement (NREM) sleep or quiet or synchronized sleep*; the last stage is variously designated as *rapid-eye-movement (REM), fast-wave, nonsynchronized, or desynchronized sleep* (these features are illustrated in Fig. 19-2).

In the first portion of a typical night's sleep, the normal young and middle-aged adult passes successively through stages 1, 2, 3, and 4 of NREM sleep. After about 70 to 100 min, a large proportion of which consists of stages 3 and 4 sleep, the first REM period occurs, usually heralded by a transient increase in body movements and a shift in the EEG pattern from that of stage 4 to stage 2. This NREM-REM cycle is repeated at about the same interval four to six times during the night, depending on the total duration of sleep. The first REM period may be brief; the later cycles have less stage 4 sleep or none at all. In the latter portion of a night's sleep, the cycles consist essentially of two alternating stages—REM sleep and stage 2 (spindle-K-complex) sleep.

Newborn full-term infants spend about 50 percent of their sleep in the REM stage (although they have different EEG and eye movement characteristics than adults). The newborn sleep cycle lasts about 60 min (50 percent REM, 50 percent NREM, generally alternating through a 3- to 4-h interfeeding period); with age, the sleep cycle lengthens to 90 to 100 min. About 20 to 25 percent of total sleep time in young adults is spent in REM sleep, 3 to 5 percent in stage 1, 50 to 60 percent in stage 2, and 10 to 20 percent in stages 3 and 4 combined. The amount of sleep in stages 3 and 4 decreases with age, and persons more than 70 years of age have virtually no stage 4 sleep and only small amounts of stage 3 sleep (Fig. 19-3). The 90- to 100-min cycle is fairly stable in any one person and is believed to continue to operate to a less perceptible degree during wakefulness in relation to cyclic gastric motility, hunger, degrees of alertness, and capacity for cognitive activity.

Physiologic Changes and Dreaming in NREM and REM Sleep A comparison of the physiologic changes in NREM and REM sleep is instructive. The change in the EEG pattern has already been indicated. Cortical neurons tend to discharge in synchronized bursts during NREM sleep and in nonsynchronized bursts in the wake-

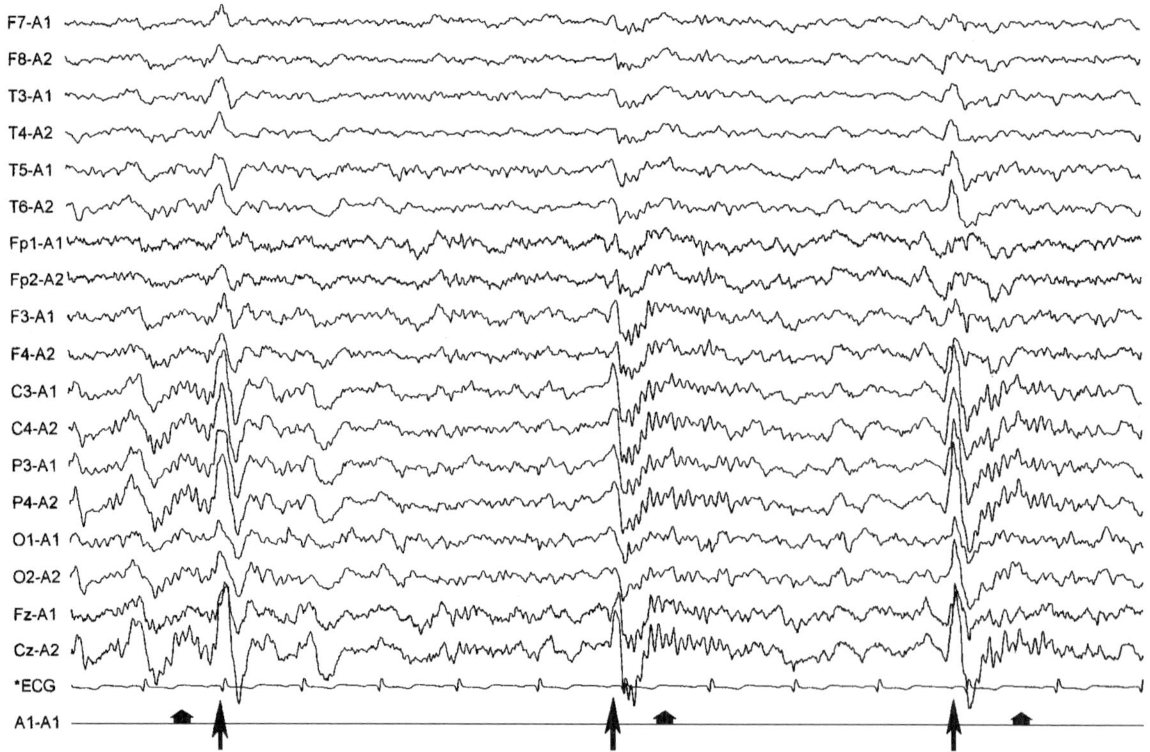

Figure 19-1

Conventional EEG (30 mm/s) of a young healthy woman in stage 2 sleep showing vertex waves (large arrows) *and sleep spindles* (small arrows) *best seen in the central regions.*

ful states; in REM sleep, the EEG pattern is generally asynchronous as well. Most complex visual dreaming has been thought to occur in the REM period and is recalled most consistently if the subject is awakened at this time. Similar mental activity may be reported by subjects awakened from NREM sleep, though to a lesser extent. Since the time spent in NREM is so much greater than that in REM, a substantial portion of dreaming occurs outside of REM periods. Subjects are easily aroused from REM sleep, but arousing a person during stage 3 or stage 4 of NREM sleep is more difficult; full arousal may take 5 min or more, during which time the subject may be disoriented and confused (physicians called at night should, if possible, avoid making medical decisions during this brief period).

As mentioned above, tonic muscle activity is minimal during REM sleep, although small twitches in facial and digital muscles (hand and foot) can still be detected. Eye movements of REM sleep are conjugate and occur in all directions (horizontal more than vertical). Gross body movements occur every 15 min or so in all stages of sleep but are maximal in the transition between REM and NREM sleep, at which time the sleeping person changes position, usually from side to side (most people sleep on their sides). On closer study, REM sleep has been found to have phasic and tonic components. In addition to the rapid eye movements, phasic phenomena include alternate dilatation and constriction of the pupils and an increase in the blood pressure as well as fluctuation of the blood pressure, pulse, and respiration. The phasic activities are related to bursts of neuronal activity in the vestibular nuclei and are mediated through the medial longitudinal fasciculi and ocular motor nuclei, the median raphe nuclei, and the corticobulbar and corticospinal tracts. In the nonphasic periods of REM sleep, alpha and gamma spinal neurons are inhibited, the H responses diminish, and the tendon (phasic myotatic) and postural and flexor reflexes diminish or are abolished. This flaccidity or atonia—which is prominent in the abdominal, upper airway, and intercostal muscles—may compromise breathing during REM sleep and pose a threat in infants with excessive respiratory difficulty and in patients with obesity, kyphoscoliosis, muscular dystrophy, and other neuromuscular paralyses (Guilleminault and Dement).

It has long been known that body temperature falls slightly during sleep; however, if sleep does not occur, there is still a drop in body temperature as part of the circadian (24-h) temperature curve. This drop in temperature is also independent of the 24-h recumbency-ambulatory cycle. During sleep, the decline in temperature occurs mainly during the NREM period, and the same is true of the heartbeat and respiration, both of which become slow and more regular in this period. Cerebral blood flow and oxygen consumption in muscle diminish during NREM sleep and increase during REM sleep. Also, cerebral blood flow and metabolism are markedly reduced across the entire brain during deep NREM sleep; during REM sleep, metabolism and blood flow are restored to that of the waking state (Madsen and Vorstrup). Braun and colleagues, who used positron emission tomography (PET) to study REM sleep, observed selective activation of the extrastriate visual cortices and limbic–paralimbic regions, with concomitant attenuation of activity in the primary visual cortex and frontal association areas. These authors have speculated that dreaming activates the visual association areas and their paralimbic connections and that these regions operate independently of frontal lobe modulation, perhaps explaining the uncritical acceptance of the bizarre content of dreams and the disordered temporal relationships and heightened emotionality that characterize dreams.

Urine excretion decreases during sleep, and the absolute quantity of sodium and potassium that is eliminated also decreases; however, urine specific gravity and osmolality increase, presumably because of increased antidiuretic hormone excretion and reabsorption of water. Parasympathetic outflow is activated periodically in REM sleep; sympathetic activity is suppressed. Breathing is more irregular and heart rate and blood pressure fluctuate. Penile erections appear periodically, usually during REM periods.

A number of hormonal changes have a regular relationship to the sleep-wake cycle. The secretion of cortisol and particularly of thyroid-stimulating hormone is diminished at the onset of sleep. High concentrations of cortisol are characteristically found on awakening. Melatonin, elaborated by the pineal gland, is produced at night and ceases upon retinal stimulation by sunlight (see Chap. 27). During the first 2 h of sleep there is a surge of growth hormone secretion, mainly during sleep stages 3 and 4. This feature persists through middle and late adult life and then disappears. Prolactin secretion increases during the night in both men and women, the highest plasma concentrations being found soon after the onset of sleep. Also, an increased sleep-associated secretion of luteinizing hormone occurs in pubertal boys and girls.

Neurophysiology of Sleep Evidence from animal studies suggest that the physiologic mechanisms governing NREM and REM sleep lie in the pontine reticular formation and are influenced by acetylcholine and by the two biogenic amines 5-hydroxytryptamine (serotonin) and norepinephrine. *Serotoninergic neurons* are located in and near the midline or raphe regions of the pons; the lower groups of raphe cells project to the medulla and spinal cord; the more rostral groups project to the medial temporal (limbic) cortex, and the dorsal raphe nuclei project to the neostriatum, cerebral and cerebellar cortices, and thalamus. *Norepinephrine-rich neurons* are concentrated in the locus ceruleus and related nuclei in the central tegmentum of the caudal mesencephalon as well as in other lateral-ventral tegmental regions. These neurons project downward to the lateral horn cells of the spinal cord and upward via centrally located tegmental tracts to specific thalamic and hypothalamic nuclei and all of the cerebral cortex, and, via the superior cerebellar peduncle, to the cerebellar cortex. *Cholinergic neurons* are found in two major loci in the parabrachial region of the dorsolateral pontine tegmentum—in the pedunculopontine group of nuclei and the lateral dorsal tegmental group. The cholinergic cell groups project rostrally, but the precise anatomy of this projection system has not been defined. Cells from these groups make up parts of the ascending reticular activating system.

Hobson originally proposed that the basic oscillation of the sleep cycle is the result of reciprocal interaction of excitatory and inhibitory neurotransmitters. Single-cell recordings from the pontine reticular formation have suggested that there are two interconnected neuronal populations whose levels of activity fluctuate periodically and reciprocally. During wakefulness, according to this theory, the activity of aminergic (inhibitory) neurons is high, and, because of this inhibition, the activity of the cholinergic neurons is low. During NREM sleep, aminergic inhibition gradually declines and cholinergic excitation increases; REM sleep occurs when the shift is complete.

Despite the undoubted heuristic value of Hobson's reciprocal-interaction hypothesis, some of its features remain controversial. Although it is generally agreed that cholinergic mechanisms selectively promote REM sleep and its components—rapid eye movements, absence of

Figure 19-2

Representative polysomnographic recordings from adults in the awake state and various stages of sleep. Upper tracings: *Awake state (with eyes closed). Alpha rhythms are prominent in EEG. Normally active chin EMG.* Middle tracings: *Stage 1 sleep. Onset of sleep is defined by the diminished amplitude of alpha waves in the occipital EEG channel ("flat" appearance).* Lower tracings: *Stage 2 sleep, characterized by appearance of high amplitude, single-complex (K) waves and bursts of 13- to 16-Hz waves (sleep spindles) on a background of low frequency.*

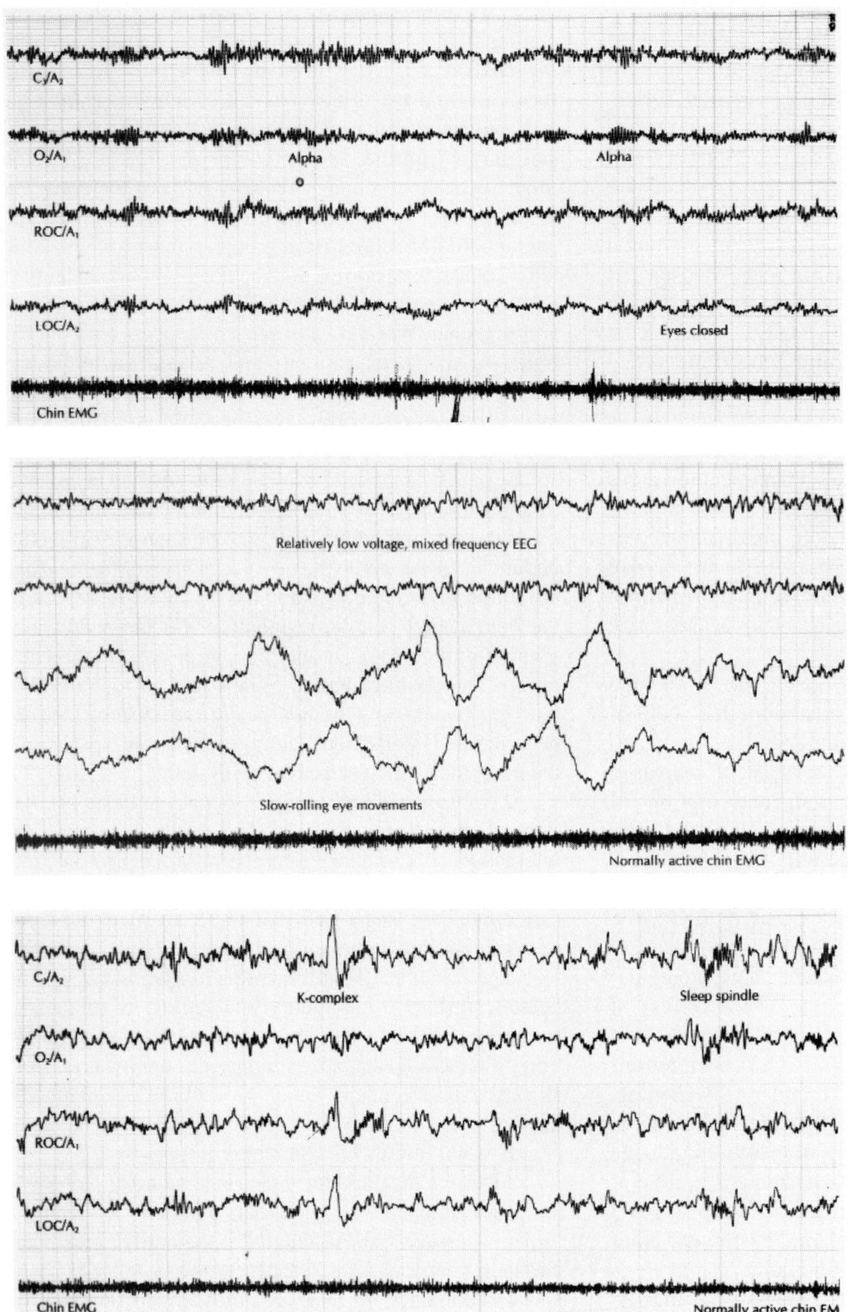

Figure 19-2 (Continued)

Upper tracings: *Stage 3 sleep. Appearance of high-voltage, slow (delta) waves.* Middle tracings: *Stage 4—deepest stage of sleep, with predominant delta wave activity occupying > 50 percent of a 30 s tracing.* Lower tracings: *REM sleep, characterized by episodes of rapid eye movement and occasional muscle twitches in an otherwise flat chin EMG.*

Technical Note: *Four sites from the same montage are illustrated in each recording: C_3/A_2, left central to right mastoid; O_2/A_1, right occipital to left mastoid; ROC/A_1, right outer canthus to left mastoid. LOC/A_2, left outer canthus to right mastoid. A chin EMG tracing is added to each recording. Recordings were made at conventional sleep laboratory speed of 10 mm/s (i.e., at the paper speed of one-third standard clinical EEG recordings). (Adapted, with permission, from Nic Butkov,* Atlas of Clinical Polysomnography, *vol. 1, Synapse Media, Inc., 1996.)*

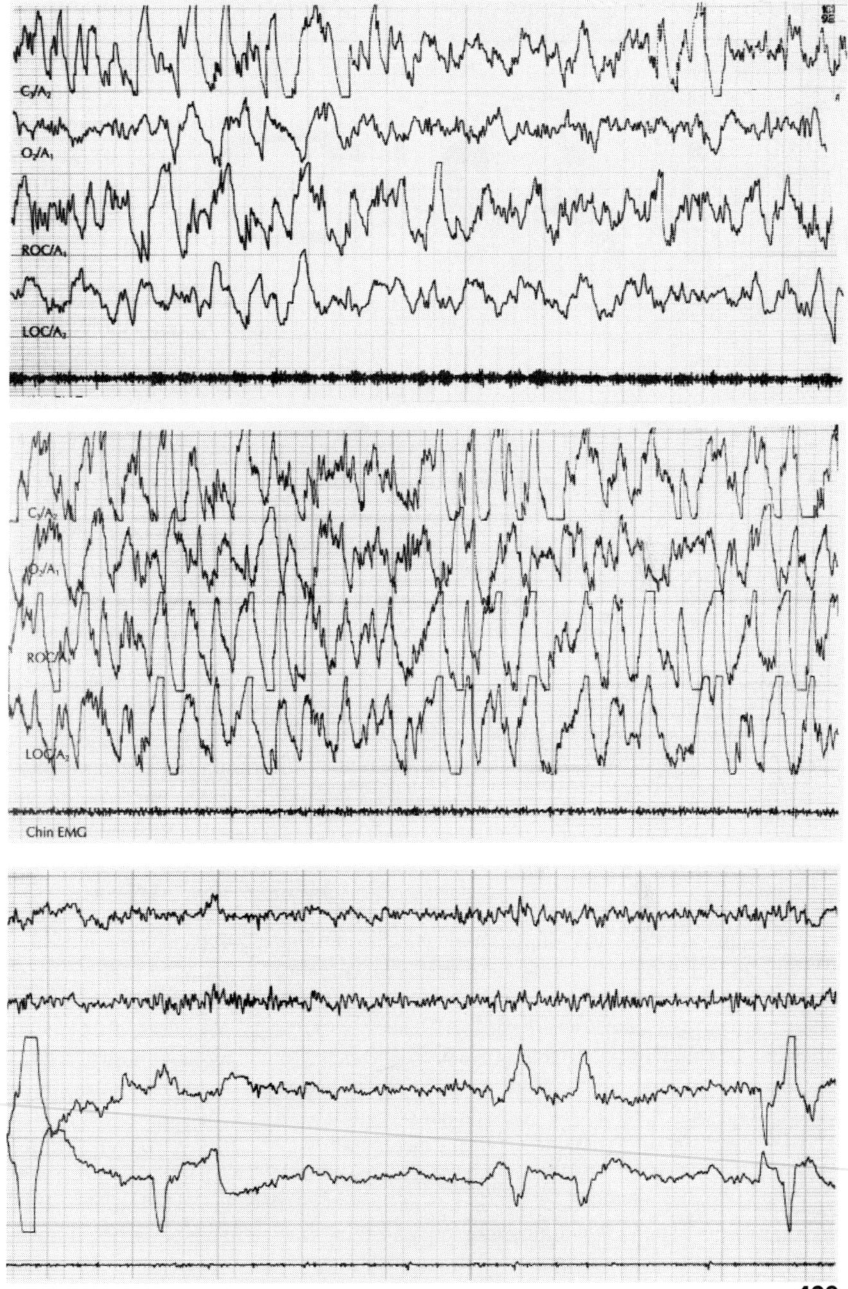

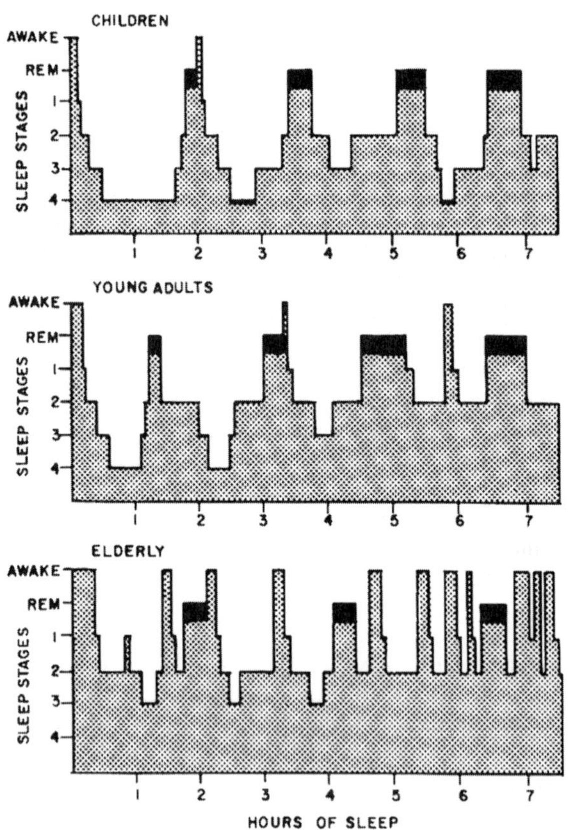

Figure 19-3

Normal sleep cycles. REM sleep (darkened areas) occurs cyclically throughout the night at intervals of approximately 90 min in all age groups. REM sleep shows little variation in the different age groups, whereas stage 4 sleep decreases with age. (Redrawn from Kales and Kales et al. by permission.)

activity in the antigravity muscles (i.e., atonia), and desynchronized EEG—the role of amines has been more difficult to establish. Thus, lesions of the locus ceruleus and raphe nuclei, which contain neurons rich in norepinephrine, do not alter REM sleep. Nevertheless, a considerable body of pharmacologic data suggests that a decrease in monoamines causes an increase in REM activity and vice versa. Insofar as the bulk of cholinergic and aminergic neurons are found in the pedunculopontine group of nuclei, Shiromani and colleagues have suggested that interaction between these neurons occurs in the region of the pedunculopontine nuclei rather than in the medial pontine reticular formation, as suggested by Hobson and associates.

The traditional view that dreaming and REM sleep are obligately or even closely connected has been further questioned by Solms. Among patients with lesions that eliminate or disrupt REM sleep he cites several cases in which dreaming was retained. Conversely, in nine of his patients with basal forebrain (frontal) lesions, dreaming was lost, at least for a time, while REM periods remained undisturbed through the night. This same observation had been made many years ago in patients who had prefrontal leukotomies. Solms has proposed that the dopaminergic systems in the basal forebrain areas elicit or modulate dreaming. This view is supported by the reports of diminished breathing in patients being treated with dopminergic blockers and the enhancement of dreaming reported by patients taking L-dopa (major intracortical dopaminergic pathways originate in the frontal lobes).

Braun and colleagues, who used positron emission tomography (PET) to study REM sleep, observed selective activation of the extrastriate visual cortices and limbic-paralimbic regions, with concomitant attenuation of activity in the primary visual cortex and frontal association areas. The relation of these findings to the nature of dreams is discussed below.

It is evident from the comprehensive review of Culebras and other authors that there is as yet no agreement concerning the integration of all these brainstem mechanisms in the production of sleep and dreams.

The Function of Sleep and Dreams

This has been pondered by physiologists and psychiatrists. Parkes has reviewed the main theories—body restitution, facilitation of motor function, consolidation of learning and memory—and tends to agree with the ungrammatical but unambiguous conclusion of Popper and Eccles that "Sleep is a natural repeated unconsciousness that we do not even know the reason for." There is no convincing proof that we stabilize learned material while asleep, nor can one logically entertain the notion that the function of sleep is to produce dreams, at least until the utility and meaning of dreams becomes known. On the basis of plausibility and logic, we favor the simple notion that sleep restores strength and physical and mental energy.

Based on the PET studies mentioned above, several authors have speculated that the suppression of frontal activity during dreaming at a time when visual association areas and their paralimbic connections are activated might explain the uncritical acceptance of the bizarre visual content, the disordered temporal relationships, and the heightened emotionality characterizing dreams. This would be in keeping with Hobson's most recently expressed view of dreams as a form of delirium. This is an interesting idea but explains little, since the nature of delirium is obscure. In contrast, Solms has suggested that activation of frontal dopaminergic systems, the same pathways that participate in biologic drives, implies that dreams may express latent wishes and drives—a psychoanalytical interpretation expressed by Freud in his book *The Interpretation of Dreams*. The authors remain skeptical of these views.

The Effects of Total and Partial Sleep Deprivation

Deprived of sleep, experimental animals will die within a few weeks, no matter how well they are fed, watered, and housed (Rechtschaffen et al); but whether a similar degree of sleep deprivation leads to death in humans is unknown. Nevertheless, humans being deprived of sleep do suffer a variety of unpleasant symptoms quite distinct from the effects of the usual types of insomnia.

Despite many studies of the deleterious emotional and cognitive effects of sleeplessness, we still know little about them. If deprived of sleep (NREM and REM) for periods of 60 to 200 h, human beings experience increasing sleepiness, fatigue, irritability, and difficulty in concentration. Performance of skilled motor activities also deteriorates: if the tasks are of short duration and slow pace, the subject can manage them; but if speed and perseverance are demanded, he cannot. Self-care is neglected, incentive to work wanes, sustained thought and action are interrupted by lapses of attention, judgment is impaired, and the subject becomes less and less inclined to communicate. With sustained deprivation, sleepiness becomes increasingly more intense, momentary periods of sleep ("microsleep") become more intrusive, and the tendency to all types of errors and accidents becomes more marked. Eventually, subjects fail to perceive accurately and to maintain their orientation. Illusions and hallucinations, mainly visual and tactile ones, intrude into consciousness and become more persistent as the period of sleeplessness is prolonged.

Neurologic signs to be noted include a mild and inconstant nystagmus, impairment of saccadic eye movements, loss of accommodation, exophoria, a slight tremor of the hands, ptosis of the eyelids, expressionless face, and thickness of speech, with mispronunciations and incorrect choice of words. The EEG shows a decrement of alpha waves, and closing of the eyes no longer generates alpha activity. The seizure threshold is reduced and seizure foci in the EEG may be activated. The concentration of 17-hydroxycorticosteroids increases in the blood, and catecholamine output rises.

Rarely, and probably only in predisposed persons, loss of sleep provokes a psychotic episode (2 to 3 percent of 350 sleep-deprived patients studied by Tyler). The subject may go berserk, screaming, sobbing, and muttering incoherently about seeing things and frequently expressing fragmentary delusions and paranoid thoughts.

During recovery from prolonged sleep deprivation, the amount of sleep obtained is never equal to the amount lost. This is probably due to the intrusion of brief sleep periods during the waking state and represents a sizable amount of time if summated (it is virtually impossible to deprive a human being or animal totally of sleep). When falling asleep after a long period of deprivation, the subject rapidly enters stage 4 of NREM sleep, which continues for several hours at the expense of stage 2 and REM sleep. But by the second recovery night, REM sleep rebounds and exceeds that of the predeprivation period. Stage 4 NREM sleep seems to be the most important sleep stage in restoring the altered functions that result from prolonged sleep deprivation.

The effects of differential sleep deprivation are more difficult to interpret than the effects of total or near total deprivation. Some subjects in whom REM sleep is prevented night after night show an increasing tendency to hyperactivity, emotional lability, and impulsivity—a state that has been compared to the heightened activity, excessive appetite, and hypersexuality of animals deprived of REM sleep. It is noteworthy, however, that in humans, monoamine inhibitors—e.g., phenelzine—will completely suppress REM sleep for months to years without obvious harm. Differential deprivation of NREM sleep (stages 3 and 4) leads, instead, to hyporesponsiveness and excessive sleepiness.

Since the need for sleep varies considerably from person to person, it is difficult to decide what is partial sleep deprivation. Certain rare individuals apparently function well on 4 h or even less of sleep per 24-h period, and others, who sleep long hours, claim not to obtain maximum benefit from this.

SLEEP DISORDERS

Insomnia

The word *insomnia* signifies a chronic inability to sleep despite adequate opportunity to do so; it is used popularly to indicate any impairment in the duration, depth, or restorative properties of sleep. There may be difficulty in falling asleep or remaining asleep, awakening may come too early, or a combination of these complaints may be made. Precision as to what constitutes insomnia is impossible at the present time because of our uncertainty as to the exact amounts of sleep required and the role of sleep in the economy of the human body. All that can be said is that some form of sleeplessness is a frequent complaint (20 to 40 percent of the population) and is more prominent in the elderly and in women. Only a small proportion of persons who perceive their sleep to be inadequate seek professional help or use sleeping pills (Mellinger et al).

Two general classes of insomnia can be recognized—one in which there appears to be a primary abnormality of the normal sleep mechanism and another in which the sleep disturbance is secondary to a medical or psychologic disorder. Polygraphic studies have defined yet another subgroup—"pseudoinsomniacs"—who actually sleep enough but who perceive their sleep time to be shortened.

Primary Insomnia This term should be reserved for the condition in which nocturnal sleep is disturbed for prolonged periods and none of the symptoms of neurosis, depression, or other psychiatric or medical diseases can be invoked to explain the sleep disturbance. In some of the patients, like those described by Hauri and Olmstead, the disorder is lifelong. Unlike the rare individuals who seem to be satisfied with 4 h or even less of sleep a night, insomniacs suffer the effects of partial sleep deprivation and resort to all manner of drugs and various techniques to induce or maintain sleep. Their lives come to revolve around sleep to such an extent that they have been called "sleep pedants" or "sleep hypochondriacs." Although statements of insomniacs are often not to be trusted, Rechtschaffen and Monroe have confirmed that most of them do indeed sleep for shorter periods, move and awaken more often, spend less time in stage 4 sleep than normal persons, and show a heightened physiologic arousal. Personality inventories have disclosed a high incidence of psychologic disturbances in this group, but whether these are cause or effect is not clear. Although victims of insomnia, regardless of the cause, tend to exaggerate the amount of sleep lost, primary insomnia should be recognized as an entity and not passed off as a neurotic quirk.

Secondary or Situational Insomnia This type of insomnia, which is usually transitory, can often be ascribed to pain or some other recognizable bodily disorder, such as drug or alcohol abuse or, most commonly, to anxiety, worry, or depression. Of the medical disorders conducive to abnormal wakefulness, certain ones stand out—pain in the joints or in the spine, abdominal discomfort from peptic ulcer and carcinoma, pulmonary and cardiovascular insufficiency, prostatism, and the "restless legs" syndrome and periodic leg movements of sleep.

"Restless Legs" and Periodic Leg Movements of Sleep The disorder known as the *restless legs syndrome* (anxietas tibiarum) may regularly delay the onset of sleep or occur in its early stages. The patient complains of unpleasant aching and drawing sensations in the calves and thighs, often associated with creeping or crawling feelings—symptoms that are temporarily relieved by moving the legs. A compulsion to move the legs can be suppressed voluntarily for a brief period but is ultimately irresistible. The syndrome is usually benign but is occasionally a prelude to a peripheral neuropathy, particularly uremic polyneuropathy. Excessive fatigue may give rise to abnormal ("drawing") muscular sensations, but careful questioning will distinguish the latter disorder as well as benign nocturnal cramping of leg muscles from the restless legs syndrome.

A closely related disturbance and one resulting in sleep deprivation and daytime somnolence is *periodic leg movements during sleep*. Originally described as "nocturnal myoclonus," periodic leg movements are slower than myoclonic jerks.

Gross jerks that occur in normal persons on falling asleep (sleep starts, described further on under "Parasomnic Disturbances") and nocturnal muscle cramps are also to be distinguished from periodic leg movements. The latter consist of a series of repetitive movements of the feet and legs occurring every 20 to 90 s for several minutes to an hour; mainly the anterior tibialis is involved, with dorsiflexion of the foot and big toe, sometimes followed by flexion of the hip and knee. The movements are similar to the triple flexion (Babinski) response, which can be elicited in normal sleeping persons. These movements produce frequent microarousals or, if severe and periodic, full arousals. The patient, usually unaware of these sleep-related movements at the time they occur, is told of them by a bedmate or suspects their occurrence from the disarray of the bedclothes. This type of periodic leg movement may be associated with "restless legs"—as well as with narcolepsy, sleep apnea, the use of tricyclic antidepressants and L-dopa, and withdrawal from anticonvulsants and hypnotic-sedative drugs.

There are, in addition, a few patients who have true *myoclonic jerks* in the legs or trunk muscles, often associated with *dyskinesias* that are difficult to characterize but may include walking-like movements and arrhythmic abduction-adduction of one or both legs or of an arm as discussed in a later section. In a few patients, mainly older ones with a severe form of the nighttime disorder, these movements and the myoclonus spill over into wakefulness and are accompanied by foot stamping, body rocking, and marching in place that are only partly under voluntary control. These phenomena may be responsive to opiates in some cases.

Several medications have proved helpful in the treatment of both the restless-legs syndrome and periodic leg movements. Long-acting combinations of L-dopa/carbidopa (12.5/50 or 25/100 dose) taken at bedtime have been the most successful. L-dopa causes some patients to develop the movements earlier, i.e., in the daytime, or to have an exaggeration of the movements later in the night as the effect of the drug wears off. Bromocriptine (1.25 or 2.5 mg) and pergolide (0.15 to 1 mg in divided doses during the day) may be equally effective and do not appear to augment the problem, as L-dopa may. Clonazepam (0.5 to 2.0 mg), temazepam (30 mg), propoxyphene, (65 mg), or imipramine (25 mg) taken l/2 h before retiring are also useful in diminishing the number of movements, but their main benefit is to reduce the fragmentation of sleep.

Other Causes of Secondary Insomnia *Acroparesthesias*, a predominantly nocturnal tingling and numbness of the fingers and palms due to tight carpal ligaments (carpal-tunnel syndrome), may awaken the patient at night (see further on, under "Sleep Palsies"). *Cluster headaches* characteristically awaken the patient within 1 to 2 h after falling asleep (page 189). In a few patients the headaches were found to occur during or immediately after the REM period.

Among the secondary insomnias, those due to some type of *psychologic disturbance* are particularly common. Domestic or business worries may keep the patient's mind in a turmoil (situational insomnia). A strange bed or unfamiliar surroundings may prevent drowsiness and sleep. Under these circumstances the main difficulty is in falling asleep, with a tendency to sleep late in the morning. These facts emphasize that, to a certain degree, conditioning and environmental factors (social and learned) are normally involved in readying the mind and body for sleep.

Illnesses in which anxiety and fear are prominent symptoms also result in difficulty in falling asleep and in light, fitful, or intermittent sleep. Disturbing dreams are frequent in these situations and may awaken the patient. Exceptionally, a patient may even try to stay awake in order to avoid them. In contrast, the *depressive illnesses* characteristically produce early-morning waking and inability to return to sleep; the quantity of sleep is reduced, and nocturnal motility is increased; REM sleep, although not always reduced, comes earlier in the night. If anxiety is combined with depression, there is a tendency for both the above patterns to be observed. Yet another pattern of disturbed sleep can be discerned in individuals who are under great tension and worry or are overworked and tired out. These people sink into bed and sleep through sheer exhaustion, but they awaken early with their worries and are unable to get back to sleep.

In states of mania and acute agitation, sleep diminishes and REM sleep may be abolished. Chronic and even short-term use of alcohol, barbiturates, and certain nonbarbiturate sedative-hypnotic drugs markedly reduces REM sleep as well as stages 3 and 4 of NREM sleep. Following withdrawal of these drugs, there is a rapid and marked increase of REM sleep, sometimes with vivid dreams and nightmares. "Rebound insomnia," a worsening of sleep compared with pretreatment levels, has also been reported upon discontinuation of short-half-life benzodiazepine hypnotics, notably triazolam (Gillin et al). Furthermore, a form of drug-withdrawal or rebound insomnia may actually occur during the night in which the drug is administered. The drug produces its hypnotic effect in the first half of the night and a worsening of sleep during the latter half of the night, as the effects of the drug wear off; the patient and the physician may be misled into thinking that these latter symptoms require more of the hypnotic drug or a different one. Alcohol taken in the evening acts in the same way.

A wide variety of other pharmacologic agents may give rise to sporadic or persistent disturbances of sleep. Caffeine-containing beverages, steroids, bronchodilators, central adrenergic blocking agents, amphetamines, certain "activating" antidepressants such as fluoxetine, and cigarettes are the most common offenders. Others are listed in the extensive review of Kupfer and Reynolds.

The sleep rhythm may be totally deranged in acute confusional states and especially in delirium, and the patient may doze for only short periods, both day and night, the total amount and depth of sleep in a 24-h period being reduced. Frightening hallucinations may prevent sleep. The senile patient tends to catnap during the day and to remain alert for progressively longer periods during the night, until sleep is obtained in a series of short naps throughout the 24 h; the total amount of sleep may be increased or decreased.

Treatment of Insomnia In general, a sedative-hypnotic drug for the management of insomnia should be prescribed only as a short-term adjuvant during an illness or some unusual circumstance. For patients who have difficulty falling asleep, staying asleep, or both, a quick-acting, fairly rapidly metabolized hypnotic is useful. The ones most commonly used are flurazepam (Dalmane), 15 to 30 mg, triazolam (Halcion) 0.25 to 0.5 mg and the non-bezodiazepine hypnotic zolpidem (Ambien) 10 mg. Barbiturates are no longer used because they so often produce dependence and, after a few consecutive nights, unpleasant aftereffects. Chloral hydrate occupies a position between these two groups. All of these drugs are more or less equally effective in inducing and maintaining sleep, although they affect sleep stages somewhat differently. Flurazepam reduces stage 4 but not REM sleep, whereas the barbiturates reduce both stage 4 and REM sleep. If flurazepam or triazolam are given for longer than a week or two, they may have a cumulative effect and lead to daytime drowsiness and even dependence. Melatonin (300 to 900 mg) is sometimes as effective as the sedative-hypnotics and may have fewer short-term side effects and withdrawal symptoms. Amitriptyline (25 to 50 mg at bedtime) appears to be a sleep-enhancing drug even in those who are not anxious or depressed. When pain is a factor in insomnia, the sedative may be combined with a suitable analgesic. Nonprescription drugs, such as Nytol and Sleepeze, contain diphenhydramine (Benadryl) or doxylamine, which are minimally effective in inducing sleep but may impair the quality of sleep and lead to drowsiness the following morning.

The chronic insomniac who has no other symptoms should not be permitted to use sedative drugs as a crutch on which to limp through life. The solution of this problem is rarely to be found in medication. One should search out and correct, if possible, any underlying situational or psychologic difficulty, using medication only as a temporary measure. Patients should be encouraged to regularize their daily schedules, including their bedtimes, and to be physically active during the day but to avoid strenuous physical and mental activity before bedtime. It has been suggested that illumination from broad-spectrum light (television) in the late evening is detrimental. Dietary excesses must be corrected and all nonessential medications interdicted. A number of simple behavioral modifications may be useful, such as using the bedroom only for sleeping, arising at the same time each morning regardless of the duration of sleep, avoiding daytime naps, and limiting the time spent in bed strictly to the duration of sleep. A helpful approach is to lessen the patient's concern about sleeplessness by pointing out that the human organism will always get as much sleep as needed and that there is pleasure to be derived from staying awake and reading a good book.

Disorders of Sleep due to Neurologic Disease

Many neurologic diseases seriously derange the total amount and patterns of sleep (see Culebras). Lesions in the upper pons, near the locus ceruleus, are particularly prone to do so. Markand and Dyken have described cases of pontine infarction with involvement of the tegmental raphe nuclei; the clinical abnormality took the form of diminished NREM sleep and near abolition of REM sleep lasting for weeks or months. Bilateral lacunar infarctions in the pontine tegmentum, demonstrable by MRI, also appear to be the basis of some instances of the so-called REM sleep behavior disorder (Culebras and Moore), described further on, with the other parasomnias. Bilateral paramedian thalamic infarctions are a potent cause of hypersomnia, the result of disruption of both arousal mechanisms and NREM sleep (Bassetti et al).

Medullary lesions may affect sleep by altering automatic ventilation; the most extreme examples occur with bilateral tegmental lesions that may completely abolish breathing during sleep ("Ondine's curse," as described in Chap. 26). Lesser degrees of tegmental damage—as might occur with Chiari malformations, unilateral medullary infarction, syringobulbia, or poliomyelitis—may cause sleep apnea and daytime drowsiness. Patients with large hemispheric strokes may also be left with daytime lethargy on the basis of inversion of sleep-wake rhythm. Certain instances of mesencephalic infarction that are characterized by vivid visual hallucinations (peduncular hallucinosis) may be associated with disruption of sleep.

Von Economo encephalitis, now extinct, was usually associated with a hypersomnolent state, but caused persistent insomnia in some instances. The latter was related to a predominance of lesions in the anterior hypothalamus and basal frontal lobes, in distinction to hypersomnia, which was related to lesions mainly in the dorsal hypothalamus and subthalamus. This subject and other forms of hypersomnia are elaborated further on, under "Excessive Sleep." A remarkable form of *fatal familial insomnia* has been described by Lugaresi and colleagues. This disorder, with onset in middle age and a clinical course of 7 to 36 months, is characterized by a virtual incapacity to sleep and to generate EEG sleep patterns. The cerebral changes consist mainly of profound neuronal loss in the anterior or anteroventral and medial-dorsal thalamic nuclei. These cases are thought to represent a familial form of prion disease similar to those that cause subacute spongiform encephalopathy and Gerstmann-Sträussler- Scheinker disease (see Chap. 33). Interestingly, the alcoholic form of the Korsakoff amnesic state, associated with less severe lesions in the same thalamic nuclei, is also characterized by a sleep disturbance, taking the form of an increased frequency of intermittent periods of wakefulness (Martin et al).

Major *head injury* is an important cause of sleep disturbance. The abnormalities, which may persist for months or years, consist mainly of a decrease in stages 1 and 2 of NREM sleep and less than the expected amounts of REM sleep and dreaming. Some patients in the persistent vegetative state show a cycle of changes in the EEG, progressing from a picture of abortive spindles and K complexes with cyclic alterations in respiration and pupil size to the acquisition of a more normally structured sleep activity. This sequence usually presages the change from a state of coma to one of wakefulness. Organized sleep activity is absent in virtually all types of coma that are the result of anatomic damage to the brain. A possible exception occurs in the unusual condition known as "spindle coma," in which persistent coma and the electrographic features of sleep coexist. This particular combination of events has been described after head trauma and rarely in association with profound metabolic encephalopathies. Despite what appears to be a genuine comatose state (not simply hypersomnolence) from a lesion of the reticular activating system, the EEG displays frequent spindle activity and vertex waves, attesting to the integrity of thalamocortical pathways for sleep activity (see Nogueira de Melo et al).

Disturbed sleep patterns have been described in patients with Alzheimer disease, Huntington chorea, olivopontocerebellar degeneration, and progressive supranuclear palsy (Parkes). Dreaming is absent in some of these conditions. The peculiarities of sleep in *Parkinson disease* have been extensively studied; many patients in early stages of the disease complain of fragmented and unrestful sleep, particularly in the early morning hours. The loss of natural body movements and the alerting effects of L-dopa contribute to the insomnia. In striatonigral degeneration (multiple system atrophy), Lewy-body disease, and other parkinsonian syndromes, REM sleep is particularly affected, although some of the effects may be the result of abnormal respiratory patterns and obstructive sleep apnea.

Migraine, cluster headaches, and paroxysmal hemicrania all have been linked to certain sleep stages. Additionally, patients with epilepsy and myasthenia gravis and motor neuron disease may have sleep-related complaints; in the latter two the cause can be traced to mild respiratory failure or to pharyngeal weakness leading to apneic periods or aspiration.

Disorders of Sleep Associated with Changes in Circadian Rhythm

Sleep is also disturbed and diminished when the normal circadian rhythm of the sleep-wake cycle is exogenously altered. This is observed most often in shift workers, who periodically change their work schedule from day to night, and as a result of transmeridional air travel i.e., jet lag (Baker and Lee). Eastbound travelers fall asleep late and face an early sunrise. The consequent fatigue is a product of both sleep deprivation and a phase change required by changing time zones. One antidote is to reset one's watch on the plane and conform to the routine of the destination—i.e., to stay awake all day until the usual evening hour for sleep—and to take a short-acting sedative (e.g., triazolam) at bedtime. Melatonin is also used for this purpose, but its effects have not been studied extensively. These measures facilitate the resetting of the circadian rhythm. Westbound travelers face a late sunset and a long night's sleep and adjust more readily to resetting of the circadian rhythm. Exposure to light during the extended day is helpful in entraining the sleep cycle; this adjustment is accomplished more easily when traveling west than east. Shifting of the circadian rhythm in animals suggests that brief exposure to light at crucial times effectively resets the sleep-wake cycle; apparently the period just before 4 A.M. is a nodal time for susceptibility to this phase shift. The sleep problems caused by shift work are more complicated (see Monk).

The *delayed-sleep-phase syndrome* is a chronic inability to fall asleep and to arise at conventional clock times. Sleep onset is delayed until 3 to 6 A.M., and the subject then sleeps normally until 11 A.M. to 2 P.M. An imposed sleep period from 11 P.M. to 7 A.M.. leads to a prolonged sleep latency and daytime sleepiness. The *advanced-sleep-phase syndrome* is characterized by an early-evening sleep onset (8 to 9 P.M.) and early-morning awakening (3 to 5 A.M.). Delaying the onset of sleep usually fails to prevent early-morning awakening. This pattern is not uncommon among healthy elderly persons, in whom it should probably not be dignified as an insomnia syndrome. Still other persons show a completely *irregular sleep-wake pattern*; sleep consists of persistent but variable short or long naps throughout the night and day, with a nearly normal 24-h accumulation of sleep.

Parasomnic Disturbances

Included under this title are several diverse disorders, the distinctive feature of which is their occurrence only during sleep—somnolescent starts, sensory paroxysms, nocturnal paroxysmal dystonia, sleep paralysis, night terrors and nightmares, somnambulism, and REM sleep behavior disorder.

Somnolescent (Sleep, Hypnic) Starts As sleep comes on, certain motor centers may be excited to a burst of insubordinate activity. The result is a sudden "start" or bodily jerk of large amplitude, which rouses the incipient sleeper. It may involve one or both legs or the trunk (less often, the arms) and may be associated with a frightening dream or sensory experience. If the start occurs repeatedly during the process of falling asleep and is a nightly event, it may become a matter of great concern to the patient. The starts are more apt to occur in individuals in whom the sleep process develops slowly; they are especially frequent under conditions of tension and anxiety. Polygraphic recordings have shown that these bodily jerks occur at the moment of falling asleep or during the early stages of sleep. Sometimes they appear as part of an arousal response to a faint external stimulus and are then associated with a frontal K complex in the EEG. It is probable that some relationship exists between these brusque nocturnal jerks and the sudden isolated jerk of a leg, or arm and leg, that occurs occasionally in a healthy, fully conscious person. These bodily jerks are not variants of epilepsy. Nor should these "somnolescent starts" be referred to as nocturnal myoclonus, a term that has also been used incorrectly to designate the relatively mild, repetitive leg movements that occur *during* sleep, mainly in stages 3 and 4 (see above, under "Insomnia").

A small proportion of otherwise healthy infants exhibit rhythmic jerking of the hands, arms, and legs or abdomen, both at the onset and in the later stages of sleep (*benign neonatal myoclonus*). The movements begin in the first days of life and disappear within months. There may be a familial proclivity to these movements. Coulter and Allen differentiate this state from myoclonic epilepsy and neonatal seizures by the absence of EEG changes and its occurrence only during sleep.

Sensory Paroxysms Sensory centers may be disturbed in a similar way, either as an isolated phenomenon or in association with motor phenomena. The patient, dropping off to sleep, may be roused by a sensation that darts through the body, a sudden flash of light, or a sudden crashing sound or thunderclap sensation—"the exploding head syndrome" (Pearce). Sometimes there is a sensation of being turned or lifted and dashed to the ground; conceivably these are sensory paroxysms involving the labyrinthine-vestibular mechanism. A paroxysm of head pain (cephalalgia fugax) is yet another example. Though causes for concern, these sensory paroxysms are benign.

Nocturnal Paroxysmal Dystonia This is yet another parasomnic disorder, characterized by paroxysmal bursts of generalized choreoathetotic, ballistic, and dystonic movements occurring during NREM sleep (Lugaresi et al). Sometimes the patient appears awake and has a fearful or astonished expression, or there are repetitive utterances and an appearance of distress, similar to what is seen in night terrors, discussed further on. The attacks may begin at any age, affect both sexes alike, and are usually nonfamilial. Two forms of this disorder have been recognized: in one, the attacks last 60 s or less; they may be diurnal as well as nocturnal; some patients in addition have epileptic seizures of the more usual type; and all respond to treatment with carbamazepine. The studies of Tinuper and co-workers, utilizing prolonged video-EEG monitoring, indicate that these brief attacks of nocturnal paroxysmal dystonia may actually be epileptic seizures of frontal lobe origin. In a second and much rarer type, the attacks are longer lasting (2 to 40 min). Again, ictal and interictal EEGs during wakefulness and sleep are normal, but these attacks do not respond to anticonvulsants of any type. Except for the lack of familial incidence, the disorder is very much the same as the "familial paroxysmal dystonic choreoathetosis" decribed by Lance (see page 83).

Sleep Paralysis Curious paralytic phenomena, referred to as *pre- and postdormital paralyses*, may occur in the transition from the sleeping to the waking state. Sometimes in the morning and less frequently when falling asleep, otherwise healthy persons—though awake, conscious, and fully oriented—are seemingly unable to activate their muscles. Respiratory and diaphragmatic function and eye movements are usually not affected, although a few patients have reported a sensation of being unable to breathe. They lie as though still asleep, with eyes closed, and may become quite frightened while engaged in a struggle for movement. They have the impression that if they could move one muscle, the paralysis would be dispelled instantly and they would regain full power. It has been stated that the slightest stimulus, such as the touch of a hand or calling the patient's name, will abolish the paralysis. Such attacks are observed in patients with narcolepsy (discussed later in this chapter) and with the hypersomnia of the pickwickian syndrome and other forms of sleep apnea. Some cases are familial. The weakness or paralysis is thought to be a dissociated form of the atonia of REM sleep. Usually the attacks are brief (minutes) and transient; if they occur in isolation and only on rare occasions, they are of no special significance. If frequent, as in narcolepsy, they can be prevented by the use of tricyclic antidepressants or clomipramine.

Night Terrors and Nightmares The night terror (*pavor nocturnus*) is mainly a problem of childhood. It usually occurs soon after falling asleep, during stage 3 or 4 sleep. The child awakens abruptly in a state of intense fright, screaming or moaning, with marked tachycardia (150 to 170 beats per minute) and deep, rapid respirations. Children with night terrors are often sleepwalkers as well, and both kinds of attack may occur simultaneously. The entire episode lasts only a minute or two, and in the morning the child recalls nothing of it or only a vague unpleasant dream. It has been suggested that night terrors and somnambulism represent impaired or partial arousal from deep sleep, since EEGs taken during such episodes show a waking type of mixed frequency and alpha pattern. Children with night terrors and somnambulism do not show an increased incidence of psychologic abnormalities and tend to outgrow these disorders. The persistence of such problems into adult life, however, is said to be associated with significant psychopathology (Kales et al). It has been said that diazepam, which reduces the duration of stages 3 and 4 sleep, will prevent night terrors. Selective serotonin reuptake inhibitors have also been used successfully, especially when night terrors are associated with sleepwalking. Frequent night terrors have reportedly been eliminated by having parents awaken the child for several successive nights, just prior to the usual time of the attack or at the first sign of restlessness and autonomic arousal (Lask).

Frightening dreams or nightmares are far more frequent than night terrors and affect children and adults alike. They occur during periods of normal REM sleep and are particularly prominent during periods of increased REM sleep (REM rebound), following the withdrawal of alcohol or other sedative-hypnotic drugs that had suppressed REM sleep chronically. Autonomic changes are slight or absent, and the content of the dreams can usually be recalled in considerable detail. Some of these dreams (e.g., the ones occurring in the alcohol-withdrawal period) are so vivid that the patient may later have difficulty in separating them from reality; they may merge with the hallucinations of delirium tremens. Nightmares are of little significance as isolated events. Fevers dispose to them, as do conditions such as indigestion and the reading of bloodcurdling stories or exposure to terrifying movies or television programs before bedtime. Some patients report nightmares when first taking certain medications such as beta blockers or L-dopa. We have also seen a few patients who complain of almost nightly nightmares and concurrent severe headaches, but without apparent depression or other psychiatric illness. Persistent nightmares may be a pressing medical complaint and are said to be accompanied frequently by other behavioral disturbances or neuroses.

Somnambulism and Sleep Automatism This condition occurs far more often in children (average age, 4 to 6 years) than in adults and is often associated with nocturnal enuresis and night terrors, as indicated above. It is estimated that 15 percent of children have at least one episode of sleepwalking, and that 1 in 5 sleepwalkers has a family history of this disorder. Motor performance and responsiveness during the sleepwalking incident vary considerably. The most common behavioral abnormality is for a patient to sit up in bed or on the edge of the bed without actually walking. When walking about the house, he may turn on a light or perform some other familiar act. There may be no outward show of emotion, or the patient may be frightened (night terror), but in the child, the frenzied, aggressive behavior of the adult sleepwalker, described below, is rare. Usually the eyes are open, and such sleepwalkers are guided by vision, thus avoiding familiar objects; the sight of an unfamiliar object may awaken them. Sometimes they make no attempt to avoid obstacles and may injure themselves. If spoken to, they make no response; if told to return to bed, they may do so, but more often they must be led back. Sometimes they repeatedly mutter strange phrases or perform certain repetitive acts, such as pushing against a wall or turning a doorknob back and forth. The episode lasts for only a few minutes, and the following morning they usually have no memory of it or only a fragmentary recollection.

A popular belief is that the sleepwalker is acting out a dream. The observations of sleep laboratories are at variance with this view, since somnambulism has been found to occur almost exclusively during stage 4 of NREM sleep and during the first third of the night, when stage 4 sleep is most prominent and dreaming is least likely to occur. In fact, the entire nocturnal sleep pattern of such individuals does not differ from normal. Also, there is no evidence that somnambulism is a form of epilepsy. It is probably allied to talking in one's sleep, although the two conditions seldom occur together. Sleepwalking must be distinguished from fugue states and ambulatory automatisms of complex partial seizures (pages 339–340).

The major consideration in the treatment of childhood somnambulism is to guard patients against injury by locking doors and windows, removing dangerous objects from the patients' usual routes of march, having them sleep on the ground floor, etc. Children usually outgrow this disorder; parents should be reassured on this score and disabused of the notion that somnambulism is a sign of psychiatric disease.

Somnabulism in Adults The onset of sleepwalking or night terrors in adult life is most unusual and suggests the presence of psychiatric disease or drug intoxication. Almost always, the adult sleepwalker has a history of sleepwalking as a child, although there may have been a period of freedom between the childhood episodes and their reemergence in the third and fourth decades. Adult somnambulism also occurs during stages 3 and 4 of NREM sleep but, unlike the childhood type, need not be confined to the earlier part of the night. Somnambulism in the adult, as in the child, can be a purely passive event unaccompanied by fear or other signs of emotion. More frequently, however, the attack is characterized by frenzied or violent behavior associated with fear and tachycardia, like that of a night terror and often with self-injury. Very rarely, crimes have been committed during sleepwalking; there is some anecdotal evidence that large bedtime doses of psychotropic or sedative drugs may have induced this phenomenon (Luchins et al). Polysomnography distinguishes these attacks from complex partial seizures. These attacks can be eliminated or greatly reduced by the administration of clonazepam (0.5 to 1.0 mg) at bedtime. Some patients respond better to a combination of clonazepam and phenytoin or to flurazepam (Kavey et al).

Half-waking somnambulism, or sleep automatism, is a closely related disorder in which an adult, half-roused from sleep, goes through a fairly complex series of purposeful but inappropriate acts, such as going to a window, opening it, and looking out, but afterward recalling the episode only vaguely and partially.

REM Sleep Behavior Disorder This is a more recently recognized parasomnic disorder, occurring in adult life, most commonly in older men without a history of childhood sleepwalking. It is characterized by attacks of vigorous and often dangerous motor activity that accompanies vivid dreams (Mahowald and Schenck). The episodes are of varying frequency, occurring once every week or two or several times nightly. The characteristic features are angry speech with shouting, violent activity with injury to self and bedmate, a very high arousal threshold, and the detailed recall of a nightmare of being attacked and fighting back or attempting to flee. The violent episodes, which occur *exclusively during REM sleep*, are out of keeping with the patient's waking personality. Polysomnographic recordings during these episodes have disclosed augmented muscle tone (i.e., absence of intermittent atonia) but no seizure activity. The rare appearance of this disorder with pontine infarctions has already been mentioned (page 414). In a series of 93 such cases reported by Olson et al, more than one-half were associated with some other neurologic disorder, such as Parkinson disease, multiple system atrophy, and dementia.

These episodes can be successfully suppressed by the administration of clonazepam in doses of 0.5 to 1.0 mg at bedtime. Discontinuation of medication, even after years of effective control, has resulted in relapse.

Nocturnal Epilepsy

It has long been known that convulsive seizures often occur during sleep, especially in children. This is such a frequent occurrence that the practice of inducing sleep has been adopted as an activating EEG procedure to obtain confirmation of epilepsy. Seizures may occur soon after the onset of sleep or at any time during the night, but mainly in stage 4 of NREM sleep or in REM sleep. They are also common during the first hour after awakening. On the other hand, deprivation of sleep may be conducive to a seizure.

Sleeping epileptic patients attract attention to their seizures by a cry, violent motor activity, unusual but stereotyped actions, such as sitting up and crossing the arms over the chest, or labored breathing. As in diurnal seizures, after the tonic-clonic phase, patients become quiet and fall into a state resembling sleep, but they cannot be roused from it. The appearance of such a seizure depends on the phase of the seizure in which the patient happens to be when first observed. If the nocturnal seizure is unobserved, the only indication of it may be disheveled bedclothes, a few drops of blood on the pillow from a bitten tongue, wet bed linen from urinary incontinence, or sore muscles. Or the occurrence of a seizure may be betrayed only by confusion or headache, the common aftermaths of a major generalized seizure.

Rarely, a patient may die in an epileptic seizure during sleep, sometimes from smothering in the bedclothes or aspirating vomitus or for some obscure reason (possibly respiratory or cardiac dysrhythmia). These accidents and similar ones in awake epileptics account for the higher mortality rate in epileptics than in nonepileptics.

Rarely, epilepsy occurs in conjunction with night terrors and somnambulism; the question then arises whether the latter disorders represent postepileptic automatisms. Usually no such relationship is established. Electroencephalographic (EEG) studies during a nocturnal period of sleep are most helpful in such cases.

Excessive Sleep (Hypersomnia) and Reversal of Sleep-Wake Rhythm

Encephalitis lethargica, or von Economo "epidemic encephalitis," the remarkable illness that appeared on the medical horizon as a pandemic following World War I, provided some of the most dramatic instances of pathologic somnolence. In fact, protracted sleep lasting for days to weeks was such a prominent symptom of this disease that it was called *sleeping sickness*. The patient appeared to be in a state of continuous sleep, or *somnosis*, and could be kept awake only by constant stimulation. Although the infective agent was never isolated, the pathologic anatomy was fully divulged by many excellent studies, all of which demonstrated a destruction of neurons in the midbrain, subthalamus, and hypothalamus. Patients who survived the acute phase of the illness often had difficulty in reestablishing their normal sleep-wake rhythm. As the somnolence disappeared, some patients exhibited a reversal of the normal pattern, tending to sleep by day and stay awake at night; many of them also developed a parkinsonian syndrome months or years later. Possibly the hypersomnia was related to destruction or functional paralysis of dopamine-rich neurons in the substantia nigra, resulting in overactivity of the raphe (serotoninergic) neurons.

Hypersomnia is also a manifestation of *trypanosomiasis*, the common cause of "*sleeping sickness*" in Africa, and of other diseases localized to the mesencephalon and the floor and walls of the third ventricle, as indicated earlier in this chapter. Small tumors in this area have been associated with arterial hypotension, diabetes insipidus, hypo- or hyperthermia, and protracted somnolence lasting many weeks. Such patients can be aroused; but, if left alone, they immediately fall asleep. Traumatic and vascular lesions and other diseases affecting the mesencephalon may have a similar effect.

"*Sleep drunkenness*" is the name given to a special form of hypersomnia, characterized by a failure of the patient to attain full alertness for a protracted period after awakening. Unsteadiness, drowsiness, disorientation, and automatic behavior are the main features. This disorder is usually associated with sleep apnea or other forms of sleep deprivation, but sometimes no such connection can be discerned, in which case a motivational factor should be suspected.

Kleine-Levin Syndrome This form of hypersomnia occurs three or four times a year, for periods lasting a few days to several weeks. These patients (most often adolescent boys), after a brief prodromal period of inertia and drowsiness, have daily attacks of prolonged diurnal sleep lasting many hours, or the duration of nocturnal sleep may be greatly prolonged, or they may sleep for days on end. Nevertheless, the organization of components of the sleep cycle is normal. Food intake during and around the period of hypersomnia may exceed three times the normal (bulimia), and to a variable extent there are other behavioral changes such as social withdrawal, negativism, slowness of thinking, incoherence, inattentiveness, and disturbances of memory. The basis of this condition has never been elucidated. A psychogenic mechanism has been proposed, but without foundation. The condition usually disappears during adulthood, and there is limited pathologic material (see page 598).

Finally, it should be mentioned that sleep laboratories now recognize a form of *idiopathic hypersomnia* in which there are repeated episodes of drowsiness throughout the day. This condition is discussed further on, in relation to the diagnosis of narcolepsy, with which it is most often confused.

Sleep Apnea and Excessive Daytime Sleepiness

Excessive daytime sleepiness is a common complaint in general medical practice (see Table 19-1). Certainly the most frequent cause is the use of any one of the large variety of medications that are not prescribed for their sedative effect. Abuse of alcohol and illicit drugs should also be included in this category. Most conditions associated with severe fatigue produce daytime sleepiness and a desire to nap. One notable medical cause is infectious mononucleosis, but many other viral infections have the same effect. Certain chronic neurologic conditions produce fatigue and sleepiness, multiple sclerosis being the outstanding example. Among general medical conditions, hypothyroidism and hypercapnia must always be considered when daytime sleepiness is a prominent

Table 19-1
Causes of daytime sleepiness

1. Medications (including many types of sedatives, tranquilizers, anticonvulsants, antihistaminics, antidepressants, beta adrenergic blockers, and atropinic drugs), abuse of alcohol and illicit drugs
2. Acute medical illness of the mononucleosis type, including mundane respiratory and gastrointestinal infections
3. Postsurgical and postanesthetic states
4. Chronic neurologic diseases: multiple sclerosis, dementias
5. Depression
6. Metabolic derangements: hypothyroidism, Addison disease
7. Encephalitic diseases
   A. Following viral encephalitis
   B. Trypanosomiasis
   C. Encephalitis lethargica (historical)
8. Lesions of the hypothalamus
   A. Kleine-Levin syndrome
   B. Hypothalamic tumor or granuloma
9. Sleep apnea syndromes
10. Narcolepsy-cataplexy
11. Idiopathic hypersomnia

feature. Also, one must not overlook the possibility that excessive daytime drowsiness is the result of repeated episodes of sleep apnea and the disruption of nocturnal sleep by disorders such as the restless legs syndrome.

As mentioned above, REM sleep is characterized by irregular breathing, and this may include several brief periods of apnea up to 10 s in duration. Such apneas and those occurring at the onset of sleep are not in themselves considered to be pathologic. In some individuals, however, sleep-induced apneic periods are particularly frequent and prolonged (greater than 10 s), and such a condition may be responsible for a variety of clinical disturbances in children and adults. This pathologic form of sleep apnea may be due to a cessation of respiratory drive (so-called central apnea), an obstruction of the upper airway, or a combination of these two mechanisms.

Central sleep apnea has been observed in patients with a variety of severe and life-threatening lower brainstem lesions—bulbar poliomyelitis, lateral medullary infarction, spinal (high cervical) surgery, syringobulbia, brainstem encephalitis, striatonigral degeneration, Creutzfeldt-Jakob disease, anoxic encephalopathy, olivopontocerebellar degeneration—and with a disorder referred to as the *primary*, or *idiopathic, hypoventilation syndrome* ("Ondine's curse," as described in Chap. 26). This last term is now applied to many forms of total loss of automatic breathing, especially during sleep. When a unilateral lesion (e.g., infarction) of the medulla is the cause, there is almost always involvement of crossing fibers between respiratory nuclei (page 578). In the few autopsied cases of congenital central hypoventilation, Liu and colleagues found the external arcuate nuclei of the medulla to be absent and the neuron population in the medullary respiratory areas to be depleted. Patients with *primary hypoventilation syndromes* are usually of normal body habitus. Awakenings during the night are frequent, usually after an apneic period, and insomnia is a common complaint. Snoring is mild and intermittent.

Apnea of the *obstructive type* is more common than the purely central variety. Obstructive apnea is often associated with obesity and less frequently with acromegaly, myxedema, micrognathia, and myotonic dystrophy. In children, far more than in adults, adenotonsillar hypertrophy may be a factor. Other instances occur in neuromuscular diseases that weaken the posterior pharyngeal musculature; motor neuron disease is the most common example of this group. Obstructive sleep apnea is characterized by noisy snoring of a special type. After a period of regular albeit noisy breathing, there occurs a waning of breathing efforts; then, despite repeated inspiratory efforts, airflow ceases. After a prolonged period of apnea (10 to 30 s or even longer), the patient makes a series of progressively greater breathing efforts until breathing resumes, accompanied by very loud snorting sounds and a brief arousal.

Obstructive sleep apnea occurs during both REM and NREM sleep. The upper respiratory muscles (genioglossus, geniohyoid, tensor veli palatini, and medial pterygoid) normally contract just before the diaphragm contracts, resisting the collapse of the oropharynx. If the airway is obstructed or the muscles are weakened and then go slack, the negative intrathoracic pressure causes narrowing of this passage. Sedative medications, excessive tiredness, a recent stroke, head trauma or other acute neurologic disease, and primary pulmonary disease may all exaggerate obstructive sleep apnea, particularly in the obese patient with a tendency to snore.

The occurrence of a prolonged period of apnea, from whatever cause, is accompanied by progressive hemoglobin desaturation, hypercapnia and hypoxia, a transient increase in systemic and pulmonary arterial pressures, and sinus bradycardia or other arrhythmias. The blood gas changes or perhaps other stimuli induce an arousal response, either a lightening of sleep or a very brief awakening, which is followed by an immediate resumption of breathing. The patient quickly falls asleep again and the sequence is repeated, several hundred times a night in severe cases, greatly disrupting the sleep pattern and reducing the total sleep time. Paradoxically, these patients are very difficult to rouse at all times during the night.

Sleep apnea syndromes occur in persons of all ages. In adults, obstructive sleep apnea is predominantly a disorder of overweight, middle-aged men and usually presents as *excessive daytime sleepiness*, a complaint that is often mistaken for narcolepsy (see below). Other patients, usually those with the much less common central form of apnea, complain mainly of a disturbance of sleep at night, or insomnia, which may be incorrectly attributed to anxiety or depression. Morning headache, inattentiveness, and decline in school or work performance are other symptoms attributable to sleep apnea. Ultimately, systemic and pulmonary arterial hypertension, cor pulmonale, polycythemia, and heart failure may develop, particularly in patients with obstructive apnea. These symptoms, if combined with obesity, are frequently referred to as the pickwickian syndrome, so named by Burwell and coworkers (1956), who identified this clinical syndrome with that of the extraordinarily sleepy, red-faced fat boy described by Dickens in *The Pickwick Papers*. The term is no longer apt, since it fails to take note of the facilitatory role of reduced respiratory drive of central type in the genesis of obstructive apnea. Furthermore, obesity need not be present in patients with sleep apnea; conversely, sleep apnea occurs in only a small proportion of obese persons.

In infants with delayed maturation of the respiratory centers, sleep apnea is not infrequent and not without danger, accounting for a certain number of crib deaths. In approximately half of the observed infants with this condition, the apnea represents a respiratory arrest during a seizure. This can be demonstrated by EEG.

The full-blown syndrome of sleep apnea is readily recognized. In patients who complain only of excessive daytime sleepiness or insomnia, the diagnosis may be elusive and require special tests of respiratory function in addition to all-night polygraphic sleep monitoring. Treatment is governed by the severity of symptoms and the predominant type of apnea, central or obstructive. In *central apnea*, any underlying abnormality, such as congestive heart failure or nasal obstruction, should, of course, be treated insofar as possible. Trazodone (50 mg at bedtime) has reportedly been successful in reducing sleep apnea associated with olivopontocerebellar degeneration (Salazar-Grueso et al). Where no underlying cause can be found, one of several medications—acetazolamide, medroxyprogesterone, protriptyline, and particularly clomipramine—may be helpful in the short run (Brownell et al). Low-flow oxygen may also be useful in reducing central sleep apnea.

In the treatment of *obstructive apnea*, continuous positive airway pressure (CPAP, or BIPAP) is the most useful measure. This is delivered by a tight-fitting nasal mask that is worn at night and connected to a pressure-cycled ventilator circuit triggered by the patient's breath. Patients also benefit from losing weight, lateral positioning during sleep, avoidance of alcohol and other sedative drugs, and the use of the medications mentioned above. Surgical correction of an upper airway defect may be helpful, but it is difficult to predict which patients will benefit and there are no clear guidelines for procedures such as uvulectomy or tonsillectomy. Patients with severe hypersomnia and cardiopulmonary failure may require tracheostomy and nocturnal respirator care. (See Parkes for a full account of therapeutic measures.) Some patients with nonobstructive apnea may also benefit from nighttime treatment with CPAP, but the results are far less consistent than with the obstructive type.

Narcolepsy and Cataplexy

This clinical entity has long been known to the medical profession. Gelineau gave it the name *narcolepsy* in 1880, although several authors had described the recurring attacks of irresistible sleep even before that time. Gelineau had also mentioned that the sleep attacks were sometimes accompanied by falls ("astasias"), but it was probably Loewenfeld (1902) who first recognized the common association between the sleep attacks and the temporary paralysis of the somatic musculature during bouts of laughter, anger, and other emotional states; this was referred to as cataplectic inhibition by Henneberg (1916) and later as cataplexy by Adie (1926). The term *sleep paralysis*—used to designate the brief, episodic loss of voluntary movement that occurs during the period of falling asleep (hypnagogic or predormital) or less often when awakening (hypnopompic or postdormital)—was introduced by Kinnier Wilson in 1928. Actually, Weir Mitchell had described this latter disorder in 1876, under the title of *night palsy*. Sometimes sleep paralysis is accompanied or just preceded by vivid and terrifying hallucinations (*hypnagogic hallucinations*), which may be visual, auditory, vestibular (a sense of motion), or somatic (a feeling that a limb or finger or other part of the body is enlarged or otherwise transformed). The association of hypnagogic hallucinations with narcolepsy was first noted by Lhermitte and Tournay in 1927. These four conditions—narcolepsy, cataplexy, hypnagogic paralysis, and hallucinations—constitute a clinical tetrad. The historical aspects and early accounts of this subject have been reviewed by Wilson.

Clinical Features This syndrome is not infrequent, as shown by the fact that Daly and Yoss recorded the occurrence of about 100 new cases a year at the Mayo Clinic. Dement and his colleagues have estimated the prevalence at 50 to 70 per 100,000 in the San Francisco and Los Angeles areas. Men and women are affected about equally. Family studies have disclosed an increased incidence of excessive sleep disturbances among the parents, siblings, and children of probands with narcolepsy, but a recessive or dominant pattern of transmission has not been identified (Kessler et al). Nevertheless, tissue typing of narcoleptics defined by strict clinical and laboratory criteria has disclosed an almost universal association with specific alleles of the HLA-DQ histocompatibility antigens, suggesting a genetically determined susceptibility to the disease (Neely et al; Kramer et al).

As a rule, narcolepsy has a gradual onset between the ages of 15 and 35 years; in fully 90 percent of narcoleptics, the condition is established by the 25th year. Narcolepsy is usually the first symptom, less often cataplexy, and rarely sleep paralysis. The essential disorder is one of frequent attacks of sleepiness, which are irresistible. Several times a day, usually after meals or while sitting in class or in other boring or sedentary situations, the affected person is assailed by an uncontrollable desire to sleep. The eyes close, the muscles relax, breathing deepens slightly, and by all appearances the individual is dozing. A noise, a touch, or even the cessation of the lecturer's voice is enough to awaken the patient. The periods of sleep rarely last longer than 15 min unless the patient is reclining, when he may continue to sleep for an hour or longer. At the conclusion of a nap, the patient feels somewhat refreshed. There are, however, some narcoleptics who tend to be pervasively drowsy throughout the day. What distinguishes the typical narcoleptic sleep attacks from commonplace postprandial drowsiness is the frequent occurrence of the former (two to six times every day, as a rule), their irresistibility, and their occurrence in unusual situations, as while standing, eating, or carrying on a conversation. Blurring of vision, diplopia, and ptosis may attend the drowsiness and may bring the patient first to an ophthalmologist.

It is not generally appreciated that, in addition to episodes of outright sleep, narcoleptics, like other very drowsy persons, may experience episodes of automatic behavior and amnesia. These episodes may last for a few seconds or as long as an hour or more and occur more often in the afternoon and evening than in the morning, usually when the patient is alone and performing some monotonous task, such as driving. Initially the patient feels drowsy and may recall attempts to fight off the drowsiness, but gradually he loses track of what is going on. The patient may continue to perform routine tasks automatically but does not respond appropriately to a new demand or answer complex questions. Often there is a sudden burst of words, without meaning or relevance to what was just said. Such an outburst may terminate the attack, for which there is complete or nearly complete amnesia. In many respects the attacks resemble episodes of nocturnal sleepwalking. Such attacks of automatic behavior and amnesia are common, occurring in more than half of a large series of patients with narcolepsy-cataplexy (Guilleminault and Dement). Such patients are frequently involved in driving accidents, even more frequently than epileptics.

Nocturnal sleep is often disrupted and reduced in amount. The number of hours in a 24-h day spent in sleep by the narcoleptic is no greater than that of a normal individual. Narcoleptics have an increased incidence of sleep apnea and periodic leg and body movements, but not of somnambulism.

Approximately 70 percent of narcoleptics first seeking professional help will report having some form of cataplexy, and about half of the remainder will develop cataplexy later in life. *Cataplexy* refers to a sudden loss of muscle tone brought on by strong emotion—that is, circumstances in which hearty laughter or, more rarely, excitement, surprise, anger, or intense athletic activity cause the patient's head to fall forward, the jaw to drop, the knees to buckle, even with sinking to the ground—all with perfect preservation of consciousness. Cataplectic attacks occur without provocation in perhaps 5 percent of cases. The attacks last only a few seconds or a minute or two and are of variable frequency. In most of our cases they have appeared at intervals of a few days or weeks. Exceptionally there are many attacks daily and even status cataplexicus, in which the atonia lasts for hours. This is more likely to happen at the beginning of the illness or upon discontinuing tricyclic medication.

Most attacks of cataplexy are partial (e.g., only a dropping of the jaw). Wilson found that the tendon reflexes were abolished during the attack. Pupillary reflexes are absent in some cases and preserved in others.

Rarely, cataplexy precedes the advent of sleep attacks, but usually it follows them, sometimes by many years. Sleep paralysis and hypnagogic hallucinations together are stated to occur in about half the patients, but the incidence has been far less in our personally observed cases. It should also be noted that hypnagogic paralysis and hallucinations occur occasionally in otherwise normal persons and that normal children, especially when tickled, may laugh to the point of cataplexy. About 10 percent of persons with sleep attacks like those of narcolepsy have none of the associated phenomena ("independent narcolepsy"), and in these cases REM periods are not found consistently at the onset of sleep (see further on).

Once established, narcolepsy and cataplexy usually continue for the remainder of the patient's life. The degree of sleepiness, once it has stabilized, rarely lessens, although cataplexy, sleep paralysis, and hallucinations improve or disappear with age in about one-third of patients (Billiard and Cadilhac). No other condition is consistently associated with narcolepsy-cataplexy and none develops later.

Cause and Pathogenesis Narcolepsy bears no relation to epilepsy or migraine. Narcolepsy and cataplexy, as well as unambiguous sleep-onset REM periods, have been described in several breeds of dogs—discrediting the notion that this condition might be psychogenic. Neuronal defects have been found in the septal nuclei, diagonal band of Broca, and amygdaloid nuclei of these animals. One of the most promising insights into the disease has been the identification by Lin and colleagues of a canine narcolepsy gene that encodes the receptor for a little understood neuropeptide, orexin (also called hypocretin). This peptide appears to regulate feeding behavior and energy metabolism in the lateral and posterior hypothalamus, but precisely how this affects sleep is unclear.

Rarely, the narcolepsy-cataplexy syndrome follows cerebral trauma or accompanies multiple sclerosis, craniopharyngioma or other tumors of the third ventricle or brainstem, or a sarcoid granuloma in the hypothalamus (Servan et al) (*secondary or symptomatic narcolepsy*).

Our understanding of narcolepsy was greatly advanced by the demonstration, by Dement and his group, that this disorder is associated with a reversal in the order of the two states of sleep, with REM rather than NREM sleep occurring at the onset of the sleep attacks. Not all the diurnal sleep episodes of the narcoleptic begin with REM sleep, but almost always a number of sleep attacks with such an onset can be identified in narcoleptic-cataplectic patients in the course of a polygraphic sleep study. The hypnagogic hallucinations (which in this formulation are viewed as dream phenomena), cataplexy, and sleep-onset paralysis (inhibition of anterior horn cells) all coincide with the REM period. These investigators have also shown that the night sleep pattern of patients with narcolepsy-cataplexy may begin with a REM period. This, too, almost never occurs in normal subjects. Furthermore, the nocturnal sleep pattern is altered in narcoleptics, who have frequent body movements and transient awakenings and a decrease in sleep stages 3 and 4 as well as in total sleep. Another important finding in narcoleptics is that *sleep latency* (the interval between the point when an individual tries to sleep and the point of onset of EEG sleep patterns), measured repeatedly in diurnal nap situations, is greatly reduced. Thus narcolepsy is not simply a matter of excessive diurnal sleepiness (essential daytime drowsiness) or even a disorder of REM sleep but a generalized disorganization of sleep-wake function.

Diagnosis The greatest difficulty in diagnosis relates to the problem of separating narcolepsy from the daytime sleepiness of certain sedentary, obese adults who, if unoccupied, doze readily after meals, while watching television, or in the theater. (Many of these patients prove to have obstructive sleep apnea.) A more serious form of recurrent daytime sleepiness, referred to as *independent narcolepsy* or *essential narcolepsy*, is described further on. However, both of these forms of daytime drowsiness are isolated disturbances, lacking the other sleep and motor disturbances that characterize the narcolepsy syndrome. The distinguishing features of narcolepsy are the imperative need for sleep, even under unusual circumstances, and the tendency of the sleep attacks to recur, sometimes abruptly, several times each day. When cataplexy is conjoined, diagnosis becomes certain. The brief attacks of automatic behavior and amnesia of the narcoleptic must be distinguished from hysterical fugues and complex partial seizures. Excessive daytime somnolence, easily mistaken for idiopathic narcolepsy, may attend sleep apnea syndromes (the most frequent cause), obesity, heart failure, hypothyroidism, excessive use of barbiturates and other anticonvulsants, abuse of alcohol, cerebral trauma, and certain brain tumors (e.g., craniopharyngioma; see Table 19-1). Interestingly, excessive daytime sleepiness is not a frequent part of the chronic fatigue syndrome, although there may be prolonged periods of sleepiness if the latter illness begins with a mononucleosis-like syndrome.

Cataplexy must also be distinguished from syncope, drop attacks (page 399), and atonic seizures; in the latter, consciousness is temporarily abolished. The careful documentation of narcolepsy by laboratory techniques is imperative when the diagnosis is in doubt, in part because of the potential for abuse of stimulant drugs used for treatment. Overnight polysomnography followed by a standardized multiple sleep latency test in which the patient is afforded opportunities for napping at 2-h intervals permit the quantification of drowsiness and increase the probability of detecting short-latency REM activity (within 5 min from the onset of each sleep period). We would comment, however, that we rarely resort to these studies in clinically typical cases.

Treatment No single therapy will control all the symptoms. The narcolepsy responds best to (1) strategically placed 15- to 20-min naps (during lunch hour, before or after dinner, etc.); (2) the use of stimulant drugs—modafinil, dextroamphetamine sulfate (Dexedrine), methylphenidate hydrochloride (Ritalin), or pemoline (Cylert)—to heighten alertness; and (3) a tricyclic antidepressant (protryptiline, imipramine, or clomipramine) for control of cataplexy. All these drugs are potent suppressants of REM sleep.

The timing and frequency of the scheduled naps has to be individualized, depending on the pattern of hypersomnolence and the work and social demands for full wakefulness. Similarly, the medication schedule should be adjusted to the study or work habits of the patient. Until now the drug of choice has been methylphenidate, because of its prompt action and relative lack of side effects. It is usually, given in doses of 10 to 20 mg three times daily, on an empty stomach. Alternatively amphetamine 5 to 10 mg may be given three to five times a day; this is ordinarily well tolerated and does not cause wakefulness at night. Pemoline (50 to 75 mg daily) and mazindol (1 mg tid) may also be useful in reducing daytime sleep episodes. These drugs have rather little effect on cataplexy but are partially effective in the Kleine-Levin syndrome. A recently introduced drug, modafinil (200 mg once daily) may prove to be the safest of the stimulants (Fry), but experience with this agent is still being acquired. Protryptiline (Vivactil) 5 to 15 mg in the morning, imipramine (Tofranil), in doses of 25 mg three to four times a day, and clomipramine (10 mg daily) are effective in preventing cataplexy.

The combined use of these stimulant and tricyclic antidepressant drugs is often indicated. A problem with the stimulant drugs is the development of tolerance over a 6- to 12-month period, which requires the switching and periodic discontinuation of drugs. Excessive amounts of amphetamines may induce a schizophreniform psychosis (page 1268). The stimulant drugs and the tricyclic antidepressants increase catecholamine levels; their chronic administration may produce hypertension.

Narcoleptics must be warned of the dangers of falling asleep and lapses of consciousness while driving or during engagement in other activities that require constant alertness. The earliest feeling of drowsiness should prompt the patient to pull off the road and take a nap. Long-distance driving should probably be avoided completely.

Idiopathic Hypersomnia (Essential Hypersomnolence; Independent Narcolepsy)

As has been indicated, recurrent daytime sleepiness may be the presenting symptom in a varied number of disorders other than narcolepsy and cataplexy. When chronic daytime sleepiness occurs repeatedly and persistently without known cause, it is classified as essential or idiopathic hypersomnolence. Roth distinguishes this state from narcolepsy on the basis of longer and unrefreshing daytime sleep periods, deep and undisturbed night sleep, difficulty in awakening in the morning or after a nap ("sleep drunkenness"), all of these occurring in the absence of REM-onset sleep and cataplexy. Admittedly this condition proves difficult to distinguish from narcolepsy unless laboratory studies exclude the latter, and even then there is in some cases overlap between the two syndromes (Bassetti and Aldrich). Treatment, however, is the same as that for narcolepsy. Idiopathic hypersomnia, as defined in this manner, proves to be a rare syndrome, once narcolepsy and all other causes of daytime sleepiness have been excluded.

Pathologic Wakefulness

This state, as remarked earlier, has been induced in animals by lesions in the tegmentum (median raphe nuclei) of the pons. Comparable states are known to occur in humans but are very rare (Lugaresi et al; see page 414). The commonest causes of asomnia in hospital practice are delirium tremens and certain other drug-withdrawal psychoses. Drug-induced psychoses and mania (bipolar disease) may induce a similar state. We have seen a number of patients with a delirious hyperalertness lasting a few days to a week or more after temporofrontal trauma or in association with a hypothalamic tumor (lymphoma). None of the various treatments we have tried has been successful in suppressing this state. Fortunately, it was transitory in the traumatic cases.

Sleep Palsies and Acroparesthesias

Several types of paresthetic disturbances, sometimes distressing in nature, may arise during sleep. Everyone is familiar with the phenomenon of an arm or leg "falling asleep." Immobility of the limbs and maintenance of uncomfortable postures, without any awareness of them, permit undue pressure to be applied on peripheral nerves (especially the ulnar, radial, and peroneal). Pressure of the nerve against the underlying bone may interfere with intraneural function in the compressed segment of nerve. Sustained pressure may result in a sensory and motor paralysis—sometimes referred to as *sleep or pressure palsy*. Usually, this condition lasts only a few hours or days, but if compression is prolonged, the nerve may be severely damaged, so that recovery of function awaits remyelination or regeneration. Deep sleep or stupor, as in alcohol intoxication or anesthesia, renders patients especially liable to pressure palsies merely because they do not heed the discomfort of a sustained unnatural posture. A form of familial pressure palsies in which there is a disposition to involvement of one nerve after another under conditions not usually conducive to the condition is also known (page 1417).

Acroparesthesias are frequent in adult women and are not unknown to men. The patient, after being asleep for a few hours, is awakened by a numbness, tingling, prickling, "pins-and-needles" feeling in the fingers and hands. There are also aching, burning pains or tightness and other unpleasant sensations. With vigorous rubbing or shaking of the hands or extension of the wrists, the paresthesias subside within a few minutes, only to return later, or upon first awakening in the morning. At first, there is a suspicion of having slept on an arm, but the frequent bilaterality of the symptoms and their occurrence regardless of the position of the arms dispels this notion. Usually the paresthesias are in the distribution of the median nerves, and almost invariably the symptoms prove to be due to carpal tunnel syndrome (see page 1433).

Bruxism

Nocturnal grinding of the teeth, sometimes diurnal as well, occurs at all ages and may be as distressing to the bystander as it is to the patient. It may also cause serious dental problems unless the teeth are protected in some way. There are many hypothetical explanations, all without proof. Stress is most often blamed, and claimants point to EMG studies that show the masseter and temporalis muscles to be excessively contracted in states of nervous tension. We are more inclined to regard it as a tic or automatism. When present in the daytime, it may also represent a fragment of segmental dystonia or tardive dyskinesia.

Nocturnal Enuresis

Nocturnal bedwetting with daytime continence is a frequent disorder during childhood, and it may persist into adult life. Approximately 1 of 10 children 4 to 14 years of age is affected, boys more frequently than girls (in a ratio of 4:3); even among adults (military recruits), the incidence is 1 to 3 percent. The incidence is much higher if one or both parents were enuretic. Though the condition was formerly thought to be functional, i.e., psychogenic, the studies of Gastaut and Broughton revealed a peculiarity of bladder physiology. The intravesicular pressure periodically rises to much higher levels in the enuretic than in normal persons, and the functional bladder capacity of the enuretic is smaller than normal. This suggests a maturational failure of certain modulating nervous influences.

An enuretic episode is most likely to occur 3 to 4 h after sleep onset and usually but not necessarily in stages 3 and 4 sleep. It is preceded by a burst of rhythmic delta waves associated with a general body movement. If the patient is awakened at this point, he does not report any dreams. Imipramine (10 to 75 mg at bedtime) has proved to be an effective agent in reducing the frequency of enuresis. A series of training exercises designed to increase the functional bladder capacity and sphincter tone may also be helpful. Sometimes all that is required is to proscribe fluid intake for several hours prior to sleep and to awaken the patient and have him empty his bladder about 3 h after going to sleep. One interesting patient, an elderly physician with lifelong enuresis, reported that he had finally obtained relief (after all other measures had failed) by using a nasal spray of an analogue of antidiuretic hormone (desmopressin) at bedtime. This has now been adopted for the treatment of intractable cases. Diseases of the urinary tract, diabetes mellitus or diabetes insipidus, epilepsy, sleep apnea syndrome, sickle cell anemia, and spinal cord or cauda equina disease must be excluded as causes of symptomatic enuresis.

Relation of Sleep to Other Medical Illnesses

The high incidence of thrombotic stroke that is apparent upon awakening, a phenomenon long known to neurologists, has been studied epidemiologically by Palomaki and colleagues. These authors have summarized the evidence for an association between snoring, sleep apnea, and an increased risk for stroke. As already mentioned, cluster headache and migraine have an intricate relationship to sleep, the former almost always occurring during or soon after the first REM period, and the latter often curtailed by a sound sleep.

Patients with duodenal ulcer secrete more HCl during sleep (peaks coincide with REM sleep) than normal subjects. Patients with coronary arteriosclerosis may show ECG changes during REM sleep, and nocturnal angina has been recorded at this time. Snoring is strongly associated with hypertension. Asthmatics frequently have their attacks at night, but not concomitantly with any specific stage of sleep; they do have a decreased amount of stage 4 NREM sleep and frequent awakenings, however. Patients with hypothyroidism have shown a decrease of stages 3 and 4 NREM sleep and a return to a normal pattern when they become euthyroid. Demented patients exhibit reduced amounts of REM sleep and stage 4 NREM sleep, as do children with Down syndrome, phenylketonuria, and other forms of brain damage. A correlation has been demonstrated between the level of intelligence and the amount of REM sleep in all these conditions and in normal persons as well. Alcohol, barbiturates, and other sedative-hypnotic drugs, which suppress REM sleep, permit extraordinary excesses of it to appear during withdrawal periods, which may in part account for the hyperactivity and confusion and perhaps the hallucinosis seen in these states.

REFERENCES

ALDRICH MS: Diagnostic aspects of narcolepsy. *Neurology* 50 (suppl):S2, 1998.

ASERINSKY E, KLEITMAN N: A motility cycle in sleeping infants as manifested by ocular and gross bodily activity. *J Appl Physiol* 8:11, 1955.

BAKER SK, ZEE PC: Circadian disorders of the sleep-wake cycle, in Keyger MH, Roth T, Dement WC (eds): *Principles and Practice of Sleep Medicine*, 3rd ed. Philadelphia, Saunders, 2000, pp 606–614.

BASSETTI C, ALDRICH MS: Idiopathic hypersomnia: A series of 42 patients. *Brain* 120:1423, 1997.

BASSETTI C, MATHIS J, GUGGER M, et al: Hypersomnia following paramedian thalamic stroke: A report of 12 patients. *Ann Neurol* 39:471, 1996.

BILLIARD M, CADILHAC J: Narcolepsy. *Rev Neurol (Paris)* 141:515, 1985.

BRAUN AR, BALKIN TJ, WESENTEN NJ, et al: Dissociated pattern of activity in visual cortices and their projections during human rapid eye movement sleep. *Science* 279:91, 1998.

BROWNELL LG, WEST PR, SWEATMAN P, et al: Protriptyline in obstructive sleep apnea. *N Engl J Med* 307:1037, 1982.

BURWELL CS, ROBIN ED, WHALEY RD, BICKELMANN AG: Extreme obesity associated with alveolar hypoventilation: A pickwickian syndrome. *Am J Med* 21:811, 1956.

COULTER DL, ALLEN RJ: Benign neonatal sleep myoclonus. *Arch Neurol* 39:192, 1982.

CULEBRAS A (ed): The neurology of sleep. *Neurology* 42(suppl 6): 1–94, 1992.

CULEBRAS A, MOORE JT: Magnetic resonance findings in REM sleep behavior disorder. *Neurology* 39:1519, 1989.

DALY D, YOSS R: Narcolepsy, in Vinken PJ, Bruyn GW (eds): *Handbook of Clinical Neurology*. Vol 15: *The Epilepsies*. Amsterdam, North-Holland, 1974, chap 43, pp 836–852.

DEMENT WC, CARSKADON MA, LEY R: The prevalence of narcolepsy. *Sleep Res* 2:147, 1973.

DEMENT WC, KLEITMAN N: Cyclic variations in EEG during sleep and their relation to eye movements, bodily motility and dreaming. *EEG Clin Neurophysiol* 9:673, 1957.

FORD DE, KAMEROW DB: Epidemiologic study of sleep disturbances and psychiatric disorders. *JAMA* 262:1479, 1989.

FRY JM: Treatment modalities for narcolepsy. *Neurology* 50(suppl):S43, 1998.

GASTAUT H, BROUGHTON R: A clinical and polygraphic study of episodic phenomena during sleep. *Recent Adv Biol Psychiatry* 7:197, 1965.

GILLIN JC, SPINWEBER CL, JOHNSON LC: Rebound insomnia: A critical review. *J Clin Psychopharmacol* 9:161, 1989.

GUILLEMINAULT C, DEMENT WC: 235 cases of excessive daytime sleepiness: Diagnosis and tentative classification. *J Neurol Sci* 31:13, 1977.

GUILLEMINAULT C, DEMENT WC: *Sleep Apnea Syndromes*. New York, Liss, 1978.

GUILLEMINAULT C, FLAGG W: Effect of baclofen on sleep-related periodic leg movements. *Ann Neurol* 15:234, 1984.

HAURI P, OLMSTEAD E: Childhood onset insomnia. *Sleep* 3:59, 1980.

HOBSON JA: Dreaming as delirium: A mental status analysis of our nightly madness. *Semin Neurol* 17:121, 1997.

HOBSON JA, LYDIC R, BAGHDOYAN H: Evolving concepts of sleep cycle generation: From brain centers to neuronal populations. *Behav Brain Sci* 9:371, 1986.

KALES A: Chronic hypnotic use: Ineffectiveness, drug withdrawal insomnia and hypnotic drug dependence. *JAMA* 27:513, 1974.

KALES A, CADIEUX RJ, SOLDATOS CR, et al: Narcolepsy-cataplexy: 1. Clinical and electrophysiologic characteristics. *Arch Neurol* 39:164, 1982.

KALES AL, KALES JD, SOLDATOS CR: Insomnia and other sleep disorders. *Med Clin North Am* 66:971, 1982.

KAVEY NB, WHYTE J, RESOR SR JR, GIDRO-FRANK S: Somnambulism in adults. *Neurology* 40:749, 1990.

KESSLER S, GUILLEMINAULT C, DEMENT W: A family study of 50 REM narcoleptics. *Acta Neurol Scand* 50:503, 1974.

KRAMER RE, DINNER DS, BRAUN WE, et al: HLA-DR2 and narcolepsy. *Arch Neurol* 44:853, 1987.

KRUEGER BR: Restless legs syndrome and periodic movements of sleep. *Mayo Clinic Proc* 65:999, 1990.

KRYGER MH, ROTH T, DEMENT WC (eds): *Principles and Practice of Sleep Medicine*, 3rd ed. Philadelphia, Saunders, 2000.

KUPFER DL, REYNOLDS CF: Management of insomnia. *N Engl J Med* 336:341, 1998.

LASK B: Novel and non-toxic treatment for night terrors. *BMJ* 297:592, 1988.

LIN L, FARACO J, LI R, KADOTANI H, et al: The sleep disorder canine narcolepsy is caused by a mutation in the hypocretin (orexin) receptor 2 gene. *Cell* 98:365, 1999.

LIU HM, LOEW JM, HUNT CE: Congenital central hypoventilation syndrome: A pathologic study of the neuromuscular system. *Neurology* 28:1013, 1978.

LOOMIS AL, HARVEY EN, HOBART G: Cerebral states during sleep as studied by human brain potentials. *J Exp Psychol* 21:127, 1937.

LUCHINS DJ, SHERWOOD PM, GILLIN JC, et al: Filicide during psychotic-induced somnambulism: A case report. *Am J Psychiatry* 135:1404, 1978.

LUGARESI E, CIRIGNORRA F, MONTAGNA P: Nocturnal paroxysmal dystonia. *J Neurol Neurosurg Psychiatry* 49:375, 1986.

LUGARESI E, MEDORI R, MONTAGNA P, et al: Fatal familial insomnia and dysautonomia with selective degeneration of thalamic nuclei. *N Engl J Med* 315:997, 1986.

MADSEN PL, VORSTRUP S: Cerebral blood flow and metabolism during sleep. *Cerebrovasc Brain Metab Rev* 3:281, 1991.

MAHOWALD MW, SCHENCK CH: REM sleep parasomnias, in Kryger MH, Roth T, Dement WC (eds): *Principles and Practice of Sleep Medicine*, 3rd ed. Philadelphia, Saunders, 2000, pp 724–741.

MARKAND OHN, DYKEN ML: Sleep abnormalities in patients with brainstem lesions. *Neurology* 26:769, 1976.

MARTIN PR, LOEWENSTEIN RJ, KAYE WJ, et al: Sleep EEG in Korsakoff's psychosis and Alzheimer's disease. *Neurology* 36:411, 1986.

MELLINGER GD, BALTER MB, UHLENHOTH EH: Insomnia and its treatment: Prevalence and correlates. *Arch Gen Psychiatry* 42:225, 1985.

MITLER MM: Toward an animal model of narcolepsy-cataplexy, in Guilleminault C, Dement WC, Passouant P (eds): *Narcolepsy*. New York, Spectrum, 1976, pp 387–409.

MONK TH: Shift work, in Kryger MH, Roth T, Dement WC (eds): *Principles and Practice of Sleep Medicine*, 3rd ed. Philadelphia, Saunders, 2000, pp. 600–605.

NEELY SE, ROSENBERG RS, SPIRE JP, et al: HLA antigens in narcolepsy. *Neurology* 137:1858, 1987.

NOGUEIRA DE MELO A, KRAUS GL, NIEDERMEYER E: Spindle coma: Observations and thoughts. *Clin Electroencephalogr* 21(suppl 3):151, 1990.

OLSON EJ, BOEVE BF, SILBER MH: Rapid eye movement sleep behavior disorder: Demographic, clinical, and laboratory findings in 93 cases. *Brain* 123:331, 2000.

PALOMAKI H, PARTINEN M, ERKINJUNTTI T, et al: Snoring, sleep apnea syndrome, and stroke. *Neurology* 42(suppl 6):75, 1992.

PARKES JD: *Sleep and Its Disorders*. Philadelphia, Saunders, 1985.

PEARCE JMS: Clinical features of the exploding head syndrome. *J Neurol Neurosurg Psychiatry* 52:907, 1989.

POPPER KR, ECCLES JC: *The Self and the Brain*. Berlin, Springer-Verlag, 1977.

RECHTSCHAFFEN A, GILLILAND MA, BERGMAN BM, et al: Physiological correlates of prolonged sleep deprivation in rats. *Science* 221:182, 1983.

RECHTSCHAFFEN A, MONROE LJ: Laboratory studies of insomnia, in Kales A (ed): *Sleep: Physiology and Pathology—A Symposium*. Philadelphia, Lippincott, 1969, p 158.

ROTH B: *Narcolepsy and Hypersomnia*. Basel, Springer-Verlag, 1980.

SALAZAR-GRUESO EF, ROSENBERG RS, ROOS RP: Sleep apnea in olivopontocerebellar degeneration: Treatment with trazodone. *Ann Neurol* 23:399, 1988.

SERVAN J, MARCHAND F, GARMA L, et al: Narcolepsie revelatrice d'une neurosarcoidose. *Rev Neurol* 151:281, 1995.

SHIROMANI PJ, ARMSTRONG DM, BERKOWITZ A, et al: Distribution of choline acetyltransferase immunoreactive somata in the feline brainstem: Implications for REM sleep generation. *Sleep* 11:1, 1988.

SOLMS M: *The Neuropshycology of Dreams: A Clinico-Anatomical Study*. London, Lawrence Erlbaum Associates, 1996.

SOLMS M: New findings on the neurological organization of dreaming: implications for psychoanalysis. *Psychoanal Q* 64:43, 1995.

TINUPER P, CERULLO A, CIRIGNOTTA F, et al: Nocturnal paroxysmal dystonia with short lasting attacks: three cases with evidence for an epileptic frontal lobe origin for seizures. *Epilepsia* 31:549, 1990.

TYLER DB: Psychological change during experimental sleep deprivation. *Dis Nerv Syst* 16:239, 1955.

WEITZMAN ED, BOYAR RM, KAPEN S, HELLMAN L: The relationship of sleep and sleep stages to neuroendocrine secretion and biological rhythms in man. *Recent Prog Horm Res* 31:399, 1975.

WILSON SAK: *Neurology*. London, Edward Arnold, 1940, pp 1545–1560.

Section 5

INCOORDINATION AND OTHER DISORDERS OF CEREBELLAR FUNCTION

Physicians sooner or later discover, through clinical experience, the need for special competence in assessing the mental faculties of their patients. They must be able to observe with detachment and complete objectivity the patient's intelligence, memory, judgment, mood, character, and other attributes of personality in much the same fashion as they observe the patient's nutritional state and the color of the mucous membranes. The systematic examination of these intellectual and affective functions permits the physician to reach certain conclusions regarding the patient's mental status and its relationship to his illness. Without such data, one cannot judge the reliability of the history, and errors will be made in the diagnosis and treatment of the patient's neurologic or psychiatric disease.

Perhaps the content of this section will be more clearly understood if we anticipate a few of the introductory remarks to the section on psychiatric diseases. The main thesis of the neurologist is that mental and physical functions of the nervous system are simply two aspects of the same neural process. Mind and behavior both have their roots in the self-regulating, goal-seeking activities of the organism, the same ones that provide impulse to all forms of mammalian life. The prodigious complexity of the human brain permits, to an extraordinary degree, the solving of difficult problems, the capacity for remembering past experiences and casting them in a symbolic language that can be written and read, and the planning of events that have yet to take place. Somehow there emerges in the course of these complex cerebral functions a more complete and continuous awareness of one's self and the operation of one's psychic processes than is found in any other species. It is this continuous inner consciousness of one's self and one's past experiences and ongoing cognitive activities that is called mind. Any separation of the mental from the observable behavioral aspects of cerebral function is illusory. Biologists and psychologists have reached this view by placing all protoplasmic activities of the nervous system (growth, development, behavior, and mental function) on a continuum and noting the inherent purposiveness and creativity common to all of them. The physician is persuaded of the truth of this view through daily clinical experience, in which every known aberration of behavior and intellect appears at some time or other as an expression of cerebral disease. Further, in many brain diseases one witnesses parallel disorders of the patient's behavior and the introspective awareness of his own psychic capacities.

The reader will find that in this section of the book, Chapters 20 and 21 are concerned with common disturbances of the sensorium and of cognition, which stand as cardinal manifestations of certain cerebral diseases. The most frequent of these are delirium and other acute confusional states as well as disorders of learning, memory, and other intellectual functions. A consideration of these abnormalities—indicative, as a rule, of a diffuse disturbance of cerebral function—leads naturally to an examination of the symptoms consequent upon focal cerebral lesions (Chap. 22), and of derangements of language (Chap. 23), which fall between the readily localizable functions of the cerebrum and those that cannot be localized.

Chapter 20

DELIRIUM AND OTHER ACUTE CONFUSIONAL STATES

The singular event in which a patient with previously intact mentality becomes acutely confused is observed almost daily on the medical and surgical wards of a general hospital. Occurring, as it often does, during an infection with fever or in the course of a toxic or metabolic disorder (such as renal or hepatic failure) or as an effect of medication or alcohol, it never fails to create grave problems for the physician, nursing personnel, and family. The physician has to cope with the problem of diagnosis, often without the advantage of a lucid history, and any program of therapy to be initiated is constantly threatened by the patient's agitation, sleeplessness, and inability to cooperate. The nursing personnel are burdened with the need of providing satisfactory care for the patient and, at the same time, maintaining a tranquil atmosphere for other patients. The family must be supported as it faces the appalling specter of a deranged mind and all it signifies.

These difficulties are greatly magnified when the patient arrives in the emergency ward, having behaved in some irrational way, and the physician must begin the clinical analysis without knowledge of the patient's background and underlying medical illnesses. Such patients should be admitted to a general medical or neurologic ward and not to a purely psychiatric unit, which often lacks the wherewithal to properly investigate and manage the great variety of medical diseases with which the confusional state may be associated. Transfer of the patient to a psychiatric service is undertaken only if the behavioral disorder proves impossible to manage in a general hospital, or, if warranted, when the underlying medical problems have been identified and a program of treatment has been started.

DEFINITION OF TERMS

The definition of normal and abnormal states of mind is difficult, because the terms used to describe these states have been given so many different meanings in both medical and nonmedical writings. Compounding the difficulty is the fact that the pathophysiology of the confusional states and delirium is not fully understood, and the definitions depend on their clinical relationships, with all the imprecision that this entails. The following nomenclature, though tentative, has proved useful to us and is employed in this and subsequent chapters throughout this textbook.

Confusion is a general term denoting the patient's incapacity to think with customary speed, clarity, and coherence. Its most conspicuous attributes are impaired attention and concentration, manifest disorientation, an inability to properly register immediate events and to recall them later, an appearance of bewilderment, and a diminution of all mental activity, including the normally constant inner ideation. Thinking, speech, and the performance of goal-directed actions may be impersistent or abruptly arrested by the intrusion of irrelevant thoughts. Reduced perceptiveness with visual and auditory illusions and even hallucinations and paranoid delusions (a veritable psychosis) are variable features.

These psychologic disturbances may appear in many contexts. Confusion, as defined above, is an essential ingredient of *delirium* (discussed further on), in which case the disorder of attention and perception is associated with agitation, hallucinations, convulsions, and tremor. As pointed out in Chap. 17, a confusional state may appear at any stage in the evolution and devolution of a number of diseases that lead to drowsiness, stupor, and coma—typically in the metabolic encephalopathies but also in diseases affecting the anatomic regions that maintain normal arousal; in the latter instances the confusional state is closely aligned with diminished levels of consciousness. Confusion is also a characteristic feature of the chronic syndrome of *dementia*, where it is the product of a progressive failure of language, memory, and other intellectual functions. Intense emotional disturbances, of either *manic or depressive* type, may interfere with attentiveness and coherence of thinking and thereby produce an apparent confusional state. Finally, an element of confusion may appear in association with focal cerebral lesions, particularly of the frontoparietal and sometimes the temporal lobe association areas. Then, instead of tremor, asterixis, and myoclonus—the generalized motor abnormalities that characterize confusional states of toxic-metabolic origin—there may be unilateral neglect of self and environment and unilateral motor-sensory defects.

The many mental and behavioral aberrations that are seen in confused patients, and their occurrence in various combinations and clinical contexts, make it unlikely that they all derive from a single psychologic abnormality such as a disturbance of attention. Phenomena as diverse as drowsiness and stupor, hallucinations and delusions, disorders of perception and registration, impersistence and perseveration, and so forth cannot logically be reduced to a disorder of one psychologic or physiologic mechanism. More likely, a number of separable disorders of function are involved, all acute and usually reversible. All of them are included under the rubric of the confusional states, for want of a better term.

We use the term *delirium* to denote a special type of confusional state. In addition to many of the negative elements mentioned above, delirium is marked by a prominent disorder of perception, terrifying hallucinations and vivid dreams, a kaleidoscopic array of strange and absurd fantasies and delusions, inability to sleep, a tendency to twitch and convulse, and intense fear or other emotional reactions. Delirium is distinguished not only by extreme inattentiveness but also by a state of heightened alertness, i.e., an increased readiness to respond to stimuli, and by overactivity of psychomotor and autonomic nervous system functions, sometimes striking in degree. Implicit in the term *delirium* are its nonmedical connotations as well—intense agitation, frenzied excitement, and trembling. All these positive aspects of disordered consciousness, after the classic studies of French authors, are designated by the term *oneirism* or *oneiric consciousness* (from the Greek *oneiros*, "dream"). The *twilight states* are closely related disorders, but the clinical descriptions have been so diverse that the term now has little useful meaning.

It should be noted that this distinction between delirium and other acute confusional states is not universally accepted. Some authors attach no particular significance to the autonomic and psychomotor overactivity and the dreamlike features of delirium, or to the underactivity and somnolence that characterize certain other confusional states. All such states are lumped together under headings such as *organic brain syndrome, acute organic reaction, toxic-infective psychosis, febrile delirium, exogenous reaction type of psychosis, acute organic reaction*, and *symptomatic psychosis*, with the implication that they are induced by toxic or metabolic disturbances of the brain. (The term *organic* is unfortunate, for it implies the existence of other nonorganic states.) We believe that delirium should be set apart from other confusional states because the two conditions are descriptively different and tend to occur in different clinical contexts, as indicated further on. Nevertheless, implicit in both designations is the idea of an acute, transient, completely reversible disorder—modified, of course, by the underlying cause, clinical setting, and age of the patient.

An impairment of memory is often included among the symptoms of delirium and other confusional states. More precisely, the term *amnesia* should refer to a loss of past memories as well as to an inability to form new ones, despite an alert state of mind and normal attentiveness; the definition further presupposes an ability of the patient to grasp the meaning of what is going on around him, to use language normally, and to maintain adequate motivation to learn and to recall. Only if defined this way does the term *amnesia* have any clinical usefulness. The failure in the amnesic state is mainly one of retention, recall, and reproduction and must be distinguished from states of drowsiness, acute confusion, and delirium, in which information and events seem never to have been adequately perceived and registered in the first place. In the latter circumstances the patient will, of course, be left with a permanent gap in memory for his acute illness.

In a similar way, the term *dementia* (literally, an undoing of the mind) denotes a deterioration of all intellectual or cognitive functions with little or no disturbance of consciousness or perception. Implied by the word is the idea of a gradual enfeeblement of mental powers in a person who formerly possessed a normal mind. *Amentia*, by contrast, indicates a congenital feeblemindedness more commonly referred to as *mental retardation*. Dementia and amnesia are defined more explicitly in Chap. 21.

OBSERVABLE ASPECTS OF BEHAVIOR AND INTELLECTION IN STATES OF CONFUSION, DELIRIUM, AMNESIA, AND DEMENTIA

The intellectual, emotional, and behavioral activities of the human organism are so complex and varied that one may question the feasibility of using derangements of these activities as reliable indicators of cerebral disease. Certainly they do not have the same reliability and ease of anatomic and physiologic interpretation as sensory and motor paralysis or aphasia. Yet one observes particular patterns of disturbed higher cerebrocortical function recurring with such regularity as to be clinically useful in identifying certain diseases. And some of these disturbances gain in specificity because they are often combined in certain ways to form syndromes, which are essentially what states of confusion, delirium, amnesia, and dementia are.

The components of mentation and behavior that lend themselves to bedside examination are (1) the processes of attention, sensation, and perception; (2) the capacity to memorize and to recall events of the recent and distant past; (3) the ability to think and reason; (4) temperament, mood, and emotion; (5) initiative, impulse, and drive; (6) social behavior; and (7) insight. Of these, the first is *sensorial*, the second and third are *cognitive*, the fourth is *affective*, the fifth is *conative* or volitional, the sixth refers to the patient's relationships with those around him, and the seventh refers to the patient's capacity to assess his own normal or disordered functioning. Each component of behavior and intellect has its objective side, expressed in the behavioral responses produced by certain stimuli, and its subjective side, expressed in the thinking and feeling described by the patient in relation to the stimuli. Less accessible to the examiner but nevertheless possible to study by repeated questioning of the patient is the constant stream of inner thought, memories, planning, and other psychic activities that continuously occupy the mind of an alert person. They, too, are deranged or quantitatively diminished by cerebral disease.

Disturbances of Perception

Perception—i.e., the process of acquiring through the senses a knowledge of the "world about" or of one's self (apperception, in classic psychology)—involves much more than the simple sensory process of being aware of the attributes of a stimulus. New visual stimuli, for example, activate the striate cortex and visual association areas wherein are stored the coded past representations of these stimuli. Recognition involves the reactivation of this system by the same or similar stimuli at a later time. *Essential elements in the perceptual process are the maintenance of attention, the selective focusing on a stimulus, elimination of all extraneous stimuli, and identification of the stimulus by recognizing its relationship to personal remembered experience.*

The perception of stimuli undergoes predictable types of derangement in disease. Most often there is a reduction in the number of perceptions in a given unit of time and a failure to synthesize them properly and relate them to the ongoing activities of the mind. Or there may be apparent inattentiveness or fluctuations of attention, distractibility (pertinent and irrelevant stimuli now having equal value), and inability to concentrate and persist in an assigned task. This often leads to disorientation in time and place. Qualitative changes also appear, mainly in the form of sensory distortions, causing misinterpretations of environmental stimuli (illusions) and misidentifications of persons; these, at least in part, form the basis of hallucinatory experience in which the patient reports and reacts to environmental stimuli that are not evident to the examiner. There is an inability to perceive simultaneously all elements of a large complex of stimuli, a defect that is sometimes explained as a "failure of subjective organization." These major disturbances in the perceptual sphere, traditionally referred to as "clouding of the sensorium," are characteristic of delirium and other acute confusional states, but a quantitative deficiency may also become evident in the advanced stages of mental retardation and dementia.

More specific partial losses of perception are manifest in the "neglect syndromes" (amorphosynthesis). The most dramatic examples are observed with right parietal lesions, which render a patient unaware of the left half of his body and the environment on the left side. There are numerous other examples of focal cerebral lesions that disturb or distort sensory perceptions, each subject to neurologic testing; these are discussed in Chap. 22.

Disturbances of Memory

Memory, i.e., the retention of learned information and experiences, is involved in all mental activities. It may be arbitrarily subdivided into several parts: (1) registration, which includes all that was mentioned under perception; (2) fixation, mnemonic integration, and retention; (3) recognition and recall; and (4) reproduction. As stated above, there may be a failure of learning and memory in patients with impaired perception and attention because the material to be learned was never registered and assimilated in the first place. In the Korsakoff amnesic syndrome, newly presented material appears to be correctly registered but cannot be retained for more than a few minutes (*anterograde amnesia* or failure of learning). There is always an associated defect in the recall and reproduction of memories that had been formed several days, weeks, or even years before the onset of the illness (*retrograde amnesia*). The fabrication of stories, called *confabulation*, constitutes a third feature of the syndrome, but is neither specific nor invariably present. Intact retention with failure of recall (retrograde amnesia without anterograde amnesia) is at times a normal state; when it is severe and extends to all events of past life and even personal identity, it is usually a manifestation of hysteria or malingering. Proof that the processes of registration and recall are indeed intact under these circumstances comes from hypnosis and suggestion, by means of which the lost items are fully recalled. Since memory is involved to some extent in all mental processes, it becomes the most testable component of mentation and behavior.

Disturbances of Thinking

Thinking, the highest order of intellectual activity, remains one of the most elusive of all mental operations. If by thinking one means the selective ordering of symbols for learning and organizing information and for problem solving as well as the capacity to reason and form sound judgments, then the working units of this type of mental activity are words and numbers. The substitution of words and numbers for the objects for which they stand (symbolization) is a fundamental part of the process. These symbols are formed into ideas or concepts, and the arrangement of new and remembered ideas into certain orders or relationships, according to the rules of logic, constitutes another intricate part of thought, presently beyond the scope of analysis. On page 474, reference is made to Luria's analysis of the steps involved in problem solving in connection with frontal lobe function; but actually, as he himself points out, the whole cerebrum is implicated. In a general way one may examine thinking in terms of speed and efficiency, ideational content, coherence and logical relationships of ideas, quantity and quality of associations to a given idea, and the propriety of the feeling and behavior engendered by an idea.

Information concerning the thought processes and associative functions is best obtained by analyzing the patient's spontaneous verbal productions and by engaging him in conversation. If the patient is taciturn or mute, one may have to depend on responses to direct questions or upon written material, i.e., letters, etc. One notes the prevailing trends of the patient's thoughts; whether the ideas are reasonable, precise, and coherent or vague, circumstantial, tangential, and irrelevant, indicating that the thought processes are shallow and fragmented.

Disorders of thinking are prominent in delirium and other confusional states, in mania, in dementia, and in schizophrenia. In confusional states of all types, the organization of thought processes is disrupted, with fragmentation, repetition, and perseveration; this is spoken of as an "incoherence of thinking." The patient may be excessively critical, rationalizing, and hairsplitting; this disturbance of thinking is often seen in depressive psychoses. Derangements of thinking may also take the form of a flight of ideas; patients move nimbly from one idea to another, and their associations are numerous and loosely linked. This is a common feature of hypomanic and manic states. The opposite condition, poverty of ideas, is characteristic both of depressive illnesses, in which it is combined with gloomy thoughts, and of dementing diseases, in which it is part of a reduction of all inner psychic intellectual activity. Thinking may be distorted in such a way that ideas are not checked against reality. When a false belief is maintained in spite of convincing evidence to the contrary, the patient is said to have a *delusion*. This abnormality is common to several illnesses, particularly manic-depressive, schizophrenic, and paranoid states as well as the early stages of dementia. Some patients believe that ideas have been implanted in their minds by some outside agency, such as radio, television, or atomic energy; these "passivity feelings" are highly characteristic of schizophrenia and sometimes of manic disease. Also diagnostic of schizophrenia are distortions of logical thought, such as gaps in sequential thinking, intrusion of irrelevant ideas, and condensation of associations.

Disturbances of Emotion, Mood, and Affect

The emotional life of the patient is expressed in a variety of ways. In the first place, rather marked individual differences in basic temperament are observed in the normal population; some persons are throughout their lives cheerful, gregarious, optimistic, and free from worry, whereas others are just the opposite. The usually volatile, cyclothymic person is said to be liable to manic-depressive disease, and the suspicious, withdrawn, introverted person to schizophrenia and paranoia, but there are frequent exceptions to this statement. Strong, persistent emotional states, such as fear and anxiety, may occur as reactions to life situations and may be accompanied by derangements of visceral function. If excessive and disproportionate to the stimulus, they are usually manifestations of an anxiety neurosis or depression. In the latter state, all stimuli tend to enhance the somber mood of unhappiness. Emotional responses that are excessively labile and poorly controlled or uninhibited are a common manifestation of many cerebral diseases, particularly those involving the corticopontine and corticobulbar pathways. This disorder constitutes part of the syndrome of spastic bulbar (pseudobulbar) palsy (pages 517 and 541). Conversely, all emotional feeling and expression may be lacking, as in states of profound apathy or severe depression. Or excessive cheerfulness may be maintained in the face of serious, potentially fatal disease or other adversity; this is called *euphoria*. Finally, the emotional response may be inappropriate to the stimulus, e.g., a depressing or morbid thought may seem amusing and be attended by a smile, as in schizophrenia.

Temperament, mood, and other emotional experiences described above are evaluated by observing the patient's behavior and appearance and questioning him about his feelings. For these purposes it is convenient to divide emotionality into *mood* and *affect*. By mood is meant the prevailing emotional state of an individual without reference to the stimuli immediately impinging upon him. It may be cheerful and optimistic or gloomy and melancholic. The patient's language (e.g., the adjectives used), facial expression, attitude, posture, and speed of movement most reliably reflect his prevailing mood. By contrast, *affect* (or *feeling*) refers to the emotional reactions evoked by a thought or an environmental stimulus. As such, it is the observable aspect of emotion. According to some psychiatrists, feeling is the subjective component and affect is the overt manifestation. Others use either term to describe the subjective emotional reaction. These distinctions may seem rather tenuous, but they are considered valuable by psychiatrists.

The emotional disturbances are discussed more fully in Chap. 25.

Disturbances of Impulse (Conation) and Activity

Reference was made, in Chaps. 3 and 4, to motor weakness, akinesia, and bradykinesia as cardinal manifestations of corticospinal and extrapyramidal disease. Disorders of these parts of the motor system interfere with voluntary or automatic movements, much to the distress of the patient. But motility and activity can be impaired for other reasons, one of which is a lack of *conation*, or *impulse*. These terms designate that basic biologic urge, driving force, or purpose by which every organism is motivated to achieve an endless series of objectives. Indeed, motor activity is a necessary and satisfying objective in itself, for few individuals can remain still for long (fidgets, doodling), and even the severely retarded obtain gratification from certain rhythmic movements, such as rocking, head-banging, etc.

It is the authors' impression that a quantitative reduction in spontaneous activity, i.e., in the amount of activity per unit of time, is one of the most important manifestations of cerebral disease. And an important aspect of this state, called *abulia*, is the concomitant reduction in speech, ideation, and emotional reaction (apathy). It is well known that individuals vary greatly in strength of impulse, drive, and energy. Some are born low in impulse, with a lifelong tendency to inactivity, a constitutional inadequacy that Kahn called *asthenic psychopathy*; others are excessively active from early life. But with certain cerebral diseases the disinclination to move and act may reach an extreme degree, to a point where a wide-awake person, perceptive of the environment, does not speak or move for weeks on end (akinetic mutism, see page 371). Such patients seem indifferent to what is happening around them and unconcerned about the consequences of their inactivity.

Abulia must be distinguished from two allied states, *catatonia* and the *psychomotor retardation* of depression. Kahlbaum, who first used the term catatonia in 1874, described it as a condition in which the patient sits or lies silent and motionless, with a staring countenance, completely without volition and without reaction to sensory impressions. Sometimes there is resistance to the examiner's efforts to move the patient (negativism), which is separable from an inability to relax (paratonia or gegenhalten); or there are certain movements or phrases that are repeated hour after hour. If the limbs are moved passively, they may retain their new position for a prolonged period (*flexibilitas cerea*), but usually there is no rigidity except that of voluntary resistance. The psychomotor retardation of depression may be so profound that the patient makes no attempt to help himself in any way and ultimately starves unless fed with a nasogastric tube. The speech and demeanor of such patients express their sadness and desire to die.

In both catatonia and depression, the mind is usually sufficiently alert to record events and later to remember them, in which respect these states differ from stupor. But this distinction is not always valid, for we have seen catatonic schizophrenic and retarded depressive patients who occasionally could not recall what had happened during the period of catatonia or depression. Moreover, Stauder has described a form of "lethal catatonia" in which the completely inert patient develops a high fever, collapses, and dies. In some respects this state resembles the neuroleptic malignant syndrome, the consequence of intoxication with neuroleptic drugs (page 1265). Also, there is a close relationship if not identity between catatonia and some forms of akinetic mutism.

Pathologic degrees of restlessness and hyperactivity represent the opposite extreme to abulia. *Akathisia* refers to the constant restless movements and inability to sit still consequent upon the prolonged use of phenothiazines, butyrophenones, and L-dopa (pages 1264 and 1637). On page 629 is described the hyperactivity-inattention syndrome of children, mostly boys. In the manic form of manic-depressive disease (and to a lesser extent in hypomania), continuous activity and insomnia are added to the flight of ideas and the euphoric though somewhat irritable mood. Following certain cerebral diseases, notably some forms of encephalitis, the patient may remain in a state of constant activity, destroying uncontrollably whatever he can reach. Kahn referred to this state as "organic drivenness."

Disorders of Social Behavior

Behavioral disturbances of this type are common manifestations of all delirious-confusional states, particularly those of toxic-metabolic origin but also those due to more obvious structural disease of the brain. The patient may be completely indifferent to all persons around him. Close relatives may not be recognized or the physician may be mistaken for a relative. Any person approaching the patient may excite anger and aggressive action. Family members may be treated with disrespect, regarded with suspicion, or falsely accused of harming the patient, stealing his possessions, or trying to poison him. The embarrassment of urinating in public or soiling the bed may be lost and, particularly in men, there may be lewd behavior towards the opposite sex. In its most extreme form, usually seen in the later stages of dementing diseases, irascible behavior degenerates to kicking, screaming, biting, spitting, and an aversion to being touched, producing a complete inability to approach the patient. These aspects of disordered mental function are the most alarming to the family and difficult to manage in the hospital.

In contrast, docility and amiable social behavior characterize the Down and Williams syndromes (pages 1066 and 1098), and social indifference is a major feature of autism (page 1098).

Loss of Insight

Insight, the state of being aware of the nature and degree of one's deficits and their consequences, becomes manifestly impaired or abolished in relation to all types of cerebral disease that cause complex disorders of behavior. Lack of insight is a far more complex phenomenon than this operational definition suggests. There are many restricted forms of unawareness of particular neurologic deficits. These are inseparable from the agnosias, which are discussed in several other parts of this book (see Chap. 22). Patients with these diseases rarely seek advice or help for their illness; instead, the family usually brings the patient to the physician. And, after the diagnosis has been made, the loss of insight may be reflected in a lack of compliance with planned therapy.

Thus, diseases that produce the aforementioned abnormalities of mentation not only evoke observable changes in behavior but also alter or reduce the capacity of the patient to make accurate introspections concerning his psychic function. This fact stands as proof that the brain is the organ both of behavior and of all inner psychic activity (thoughts, imaginations, and plans); i.e., mind and behavior are two inseparable aspects of the function of the nervous system (psycho-physical monism).

COMMON SYNDROMES

To summarize, the entire group of acute confusional and delirious states is characterized principally by an alteration of consciousness and prominent disorders of attention and perception, which interfere with the speed, clarity, and coherence of thinking, the formation of memories, and the capacity for performance of self-directed and commanded activities. Three major clinical syndromes can be recognized. One is an *acute confusional state* in which there is manifest reduction in alertness and psychomotor activity. A second syndrome, here called *delirium*, is marked by overactivity, sleeplessness, tremulousness, and prominence of vivid hallucinations, with convulsions often preceding or associated with the delirium. These two illnesses tend to develop acutely, to have multiple causes, and, except for certain cerebral diseases, to terminate within a relatively short period of time (days to weeks), leaving the patient without residual damage or with whatever defects were present before their onset. The third syndrome is one in which a confusional state occurs in persons with some underlying, more chronic medical or cerebral disease. The cerebral disease may be focal or diffuse and, in the latter case, may dispose the patient to an acute psychosis, which we have chosen to designate as a *beclouded dementia*. From the neurologic perspective, the generic term *psychosis* applies to states of confusion in which elements of hallucinations, delusions, and disordered thinking make up prominent elements.

Acute Confusional States Associated with Reduced Alertness and Psychomotor Activity

Clinical Features Some features of this syndrome have already been described in Chap. 17, "Coma and Related Disorders of Consciousness." In the most typical examples, all mental functions are reduced to some degree; but alertness, attentiveness, orientation, and the ability to concentrate and to grasp all elements of the immediate situation suffer most. Characteristically, these abnormalities *fluctuate in severity*, typically being worse at night ("sundowning"). In the mildest form of the syndrome, the patient appears alert and may even pass for normal; only the failure to recollect and accurately reproduce happenings of the past few hours or days reveals the subtle inadequacy of mental function. The more obviously confused patients spend much of their time in idleness, and what they do may be inappropriate and annoying to others. Only the more automatic acts and verbal responses are performed properly, but these may permit the examiner to obtain from the patient a number of relevant and accurate replies to questions about age, occupation, and residence. Answers tend to be slow and indecisive. Orientation to the date, day, and place is frequently imprecise, often with the exact date being off by several days, the year being given as several years or one decade previous, or with the last two numbers transposed, i.e., 2002 given as 2020 (see page 441 for techniques of testing for confusion). Such patients may, before answering, repeat every question that is put to them, and their responses tend to be brief and mechanical. It is difficult or impossible for them to sustain a conversation. Their attention wanders and they constantly have to be brought back to the subject at hand. They may even fall asleep during the interview, and, if left alone, are observed to sleep more hours each day than is natural or to sleep at irregular intervals.

Frequently there are perceptual disturbances in which voices, common objects, and the actions of other persons are misinterpreted. Frank hallucinations may occur, but often one cannot discern whether these patients hear voices and see things that do not exist, i.e., whether they are hallucinating or are merely misinterpreting stimuli in the environment (illusions). Some patients are irritable and others are suspicious; in fact, a paranoid trend may be a pronounced and troublesome feature of the illness. There may also be mild degrees of anomia and dysphasia and a labile affect.

As the confusion deepens, conversation becomes more difficult, and at a certain stage these patients no longer notice or respond to much of what is happening around them. Questions may be answered with a single word or a short phrase, spoken in a soft tremulous voice or whisper, or the patient may be mute. Asterixis is a common accompaniment if a metabolic or toxic encephalopathy is responsible for the confusional state. In the most advanced stages of the illness, confusion gives way to stupor and finally to coma (see Chap. 17). As these patients improve, they may pass again through the stages of stupor and confusion in the reverse order. All this informs us that at least one category of confusion is but a manifestation of the same disease processes that in their severest form cause coma.

Typical confusional states, in which impairments of alertness and attention dominate, are readily distinguished from delirium; in others, with more than the usual degree of irritability and restlessness, and perhaps a fleeting hallucination, one cannot fail to notice their resemblance to one another. Further, when a delirium is complicated by an illness that superimposes stupor (e.g., delirium tremens with pneumonia, meningitis, or hepatic encephalopathy), it may be difficult to differentiate from other acute confusional states. This explains why some psychiatrists (Engel and Romano, Lipowski) insist that there is only one disorder, which they call delirium.

Etiology The many causes of this type of confusional state are listed in Table 20-1. The most frequent are drug intoxications and metabolic encephalopathies: electrolyte imbalance, disorders of water metabolism (hypo- and hypernatremia, hyperosmolarity), hypercalcemia, etc., disorders of acid-base balance, renal and hepatic failure, hyper- and hypoglycemia, septic states, and chronic cardiac and pulmonary insufficiency as well as

Table 20-1
Classification of delirium and acute confusional states

- **I. Acute confusional states associated with psychomotor underactivity**
  - A. Associated with a medical or surgical disease (no focal or lateralizing neurologic signs; CSF clear)
    1. Metabolic disorders; hepatic stupor, uremia, hypo- and hypernatremia, hypercalcemia, hypo- and hyperglycemia, hypoxia, hypercapnia, porphyria, and some endocrinopathies
    2. Infectious illnesses (pneumonia, endocarditis, urosepsis, peritonitis, and other illnesses causing bacteremia and septicemia—septic encephalopathy
    3. Congestive heart failure
    4. Postoperative and posttraumatic states
  - B. Associated with drug intoxication (no focal or lateralizing signs; CSF clear): opiates, barbiturates and other sedatives, trihexyphenidyl, etc.
  - C. Associated with diseases of the nervous system (with focal or lateralizing neurologic signs and/or CSF changes)
    1. Cerebrovascular disease, tumor, abscess (especially of the right parietal, left temporal and occipital, and inferofrontal lobes)
    2. Subdural hematoma
    3. Meningitis
    4. Encephalitis
    5. Cerebral vasculitis (e.g., granulomatous, lupus)
    6. Hypertensive encephalopathy
- **II. Delirium**
  - A. In a medical or surgical illness [no focal or lateralizing neurologic signs; cerebrospinal fluid (CSF) usually clear]
    1. Pneumonia
    2. Septicemia and bacteremia (septic encephalopathy)
    3. Postoperative and postconcussive states
    4. Thyrotoxicosis and corticosteroid excess (exogenous or endogenous)
    5. Typhoid and other infectious fevers
  - B. In neurologic disease that causes focal or lateralizing signs or changes in the CSF
    1. Vascular, neoplastic, or other diseases, particularly those involving the temporal lobes and upper part of the brainstem
    2. Concussion and contusion (traumatic delirium)
    3. Meningitis of acute purulent, fungal, tuberculous and neoplastic types (Chap. 32)
    4. Encephalitis due to viral (e.g., herpes simplex, infectious mononucleosis) bacterial (mycoplasma, etc.), and other causes (Chap. 33)
    5. Subarachnoid hemorrhage
  - C. Abstinence states, exogenous intoxications, and postconvulsive states (signs of other medical, surgical, and neurologic illnesses absent or coincidental)
    1. Withdrawal of alcohol (delirium tremens), barbiturates, and nonbarbiturate sedative drugs, following chronic intoxication (Chaps. 42 and 43)
    2. Drug intoxications: scopolamine, atropine, amphetamine, cocaine, and other illicit drugs
    3. Postconvulsive delirium
- **III. Confusional states due to focal cerebral lesions**
- **IV. Beclouded dementia**, i.e., dementing or other brain disease in combination with infective fevers, drug reactions, trauma, heart failure, or other medical or surgical diseases

hypertensive encephalopathy. Concussion and seizures, especially petit mal or psychomotor status, and certain focal (e.g., right parietal and temporal) cerebral lesions may also be followed by a period of confusion.

Pathophysiology of Confusional States All that has been said on this subject in Chap. 17, "Coma and Related Disorders of Consciousness," is applicable to at least one subgroup of the confusional states. In most cases no consistent pathologic change has been found because the abnormalities are metabolic and subcellular. As discussed in Chap. 2, the electroencephalogram (EEG) is almost invariably abnormal in even mild forms of this syndrome, in contrast to delirium, where the changes may be relatively minor. Bilateral high-voltage slow waves in the 2- to 4-per-second (delta) range or the 5- to 7-per-second (theta) range are the usual findings. These changes surely reflect one aspect of the central problem—the diffuse impairment of the cerebral mechanisms governing alertness and attention.

Delirium

Clinical Features These are most perfectly depicted in the patient undergoing withdrawal from alcohol after a sustained period of intoxication. The symptoms usually develop over a period of 2 or 3 days. The first indications of the approaching attack are difficulty in concentration, restless irritability, increasing tremulousness, insomnia, and poor appetite. The patient's sleep is troubled by unpleasant or terrifying dreams. There may be momentary disorientation, an occasional inappropriate remark, or transient illusions or hallucinations. One or several generalized convulsions often precede or initiate the delirium.

These initial symptoms rapidly give way to a clinical picture that, in severe cases, is one of the most colorful in medicine. There is "clouding of the sensorium," that is, the patient is inattentive and unable to perceive all elements of his situation. He may talk incessantly and incoherently and look distressed and perplexed; his expression is in keeping with his vague notions of being annoyed or threatened by someone who seeks to harm him. From his manner and the content of his speech, it is evident that he misinterprets the meaning of ordinary objects and sounds, misidentifies the people around him, and is experiencing vivid visual, auditory, and tactile hallucinations, often of a most unpleasant type. At first the patient can be brought into touch with reality and may, in fact, identify the examiner and answer other questions correctly; but almost at once he relapses into a preoccupied, confused state, giving wrong answers and being unable to think coherently. As the process evolves the patient cannot shake off his hallucinations even for a second and does not recognize his physician or even his family. He is unable to make meaningful responses to the simplest questions and is, as a rule, profoundly disoriented.

Tremor of fast frequency and jerky restless movements are practically always present and may be violent. Sleep is impossible or occurs only in brief naps. Speech is reduced to an unintelligible muttering. The face is flushed, the pupils are dilated, and the conjunctivae are injected; the pulse is rapid and soft, and the temperature may be raised. There is much sweating. The signs of overactivity of the autonomic nervous system, more than any others, distinguish delirium from all other confusional states.

After 2 or 3 days, the symptoms abate, either suddenly or gradually, although in exceptional cases they may persist for several weeks. The most certain indication of the subsidence of the attack is the occurrence of lucid intervals of increasing length and sound sleep. Recovery is usually complete. In retrospect, the patient has only a few vague memories of his illness or none at all.

Delirium is subject to all degrees of variability, not only from patient to patient but in the same patient from day to day and even hour to hour. The entire syndrome may be observed in one patient and only a few fragments in another. In its mildest form, as so often occurs in febrile diseases, the delirium consists of an occasional wandering of the mind and incoherence of verbal expression. This form, lacking motor and autonomic overactivity, is sometimes referred to as a quiet or hypokinetic delirium and can hardly be distinguished from the confusional states described above.

Pathology and Pathophysiology of Delirium The brains of patients who have died in delirium tremens, without associated disease or injury usually show no pathologic changes of significance. Delirium may also occur in association with a number of recognizable pathologic states, such as viral encephalitis or meningoencephalitis, Wernicke disease, trauma, or multiple focal embolic strokes due to subacute bacterial endocarditis, cholesterol or fat embolism, or cardiac surgery. The topography of the lesions in these conditions is of particular interest. They tend to be localized in the midbrain and hypothalamus and in the temporal lobes, where they involve the reticular activating and limbic systems. Involvement of the hypothalamus probably accounts for the autonomic hyperactivity that characterizes delirium.

Electrical stimulation studies of the human cerebral cortex during surgical exploration and studies by positron emission tomography (PET) have indicated the importance of the temporal lobe in the genesis of complex visual, auditory, and olfactory hallucinations. Subthalamic and midbrain lesions may give rise to visual hallucinations that are not unpleasant and are accompanied by good insight ("peduncular hallucinosis" of Lhermitte). With pontine-midbrain lesions, there may be unformed auditory hallucinations (page 309).

The EEG may show symmetrical, generalized slow activity in the 5- to 7-per-second range, a state that rapidly returns to normal as the delirium clears. In other cases, only activity in the fast beta frequency range is seen; in milder degrees of delirium, there is usually no abnormality at all.

Analysis of the several conditions conducive to delirium suggests at least three physiologic mechanisms. The withdrawal of alcohol or other sedative-hypnotic drugs, following a period of chronic intoxication, is the most common (see Chap. 43). These drugs are known to have a strong depressant effect on certain regions of the central nervous system; presumably, the disinhibition and overactivity of these parts after withdrawal of the drug are the basis of delirium. In this respect it is of interest that the symptoms of delirium tremens are the antithesis of those of alcoholic intoxication. Another mechanism is operative in the case of bacterial infections and poisoning by certain drugs, such as atropine and scopolamine, in which visual hallucinations are a prominent feature. Here the delirious state probably results from the direct action of the toxin or chemical agent on the same parts of the brain. Third, destructive lesions of the undersurfaces of the temporal lobes, as occur in herpes simplex encephalitis or severe concussive injury, may cause delirium.

Psychophysiologic mechanisms have also been postulated in the genesis of delirium. It has long been suggested that some persons are much more liable to delirium than others, but there is reason to doubt this hypothesis. Many years ago, Wolff and Curran showed that all of a group of randomly selected persons developed delirium if the causative mechanisms were strongly operative. This is not surprising, for any normal person may, under certain circumstances, experience phenomena akin to those of delirium. After a sustained period of auditory or visual stimulation, the same impressions may continue to be perceived even though the stimuli are no longer present. The whine of artillery shells may continue to be heard long after the bombardment has ceased. Also, a healthy person can be induced to hallucinate by being isolated for several days in an environment free of sensory stimulation (sensory deprivation). A relationship of delirium to dream states has been postulated; both are characterized by a loss of appreciation of time, a richness of visual imagery, indifference to inconsistencies, and "defective reality testing." Patients may refer to delirious symptoms as a "bad dream," and normal persons may experience so-called hypnagogic hallucinations in the period between waking and sleeping. Formulations in the field of dynamic psychiatry seem more reasonably to explain the topical content of delirium than its occurrence. Wolff and Curran, having observed the same content in repeated attacks of delirium due to different causes, concluded that the content depends more on the age, sex, intellectual endowment, occupation, personality traits, and past experiences of the patient than on the cause or mechanism of the delirium.

The main difficulty in understanding delirium derives from the fact that it has not been possible to ascertain which of the many symptoms have physiologic significance. What is the basis of the altered consciousness, the sensorial disturbance, and the lack of congruence between actual sensory impressions of the present and memory of those in the past? Obviously, something has been removed from the perceptive process, something that leaves the patient at the mercy of certain sensory stimuli and unable to attend to others and at the same time incapable of discriminating between sense impression and fantasy. The lack of inhibition of sensory stimuli may also be the basis of the sleeplessness that characterizes delirium.

Confusional States Complicating Focal and Diffuse Cerebral Disease

Confusional States due to Focal Cerebral Lesions

A variety of cerebral diseases may be associated with confusional states. Among these are meningitis, encephalitis, disseminated intravascular coagulation, tumors, and trauma. As remarked above, focal lesions (most often infarcts) of the right cerebral hemisphere may evoke an acute confusional state. Such states have been described with strokes in the territory of the right middle cerebral artery (Mesulam et al; Caplan et al; Mori and Yamadori); mainly the infarcts have involved the posterior parietal lobe or inferior frontostriatal regions, but they have also occurred with strokes in the territory of one posterior cerebral artery. An acute agitated delirium has been noted at one time or another with lesions involving the fusiform and lingual gyri and calcarine cortex (Horenstein et al); the hippocampal, and lingual gyri (Medina et al); or the middle temporal gyrus (Mori and Yamadori). Of course, there may be elements of confusion with stroke in almost any cerebral territory, but with the aforementioned lesions the confusional state has occasionally been unattended by other paralytic motor and sensory disorders.

Confusional States Complicating Diffuse Cerebral Disease: Beclouded Dementia Apart from the aforementioned types of focal cerebral disease, there are many elderly patients who enter the hospital with a medical or surgical illness and a newly acquired state of mental confusion. Presumably the liability to this state is determined by preexisting brain disease, most often Alzheimer disease, which may or may not have been obvious to the family before the onset of the complicating illness. The effects of other cerebral diseases (vascular, neoplastic, demyelinative) may also have been too subtle to be appreciated by the patient or the family. All the clinical features that one observes in the acute confusional states may be present. The severity varies greatly. The confusion may be reflected only in the patient's inability to relate the history of the illness sequentially, or it may be so severe that the patient is virtually non compos mentis.

Although almost any complicating illness may bring out a confusional state in an elderly person, the most common are febrile infectious diseases, especially cases that resist the effects of antibiotics; trauma, notably concussive brain injuries; surgical operations, particularly those requiring general anesthesia and pre- and postoperative medication; even small amounts of pain or sedative medications used for any cause; and congestive heart failure, chronic respiratory disease, and severe anemia, especially pernicious anemia. Often it is difficult to determine which of several possible factors is responsible for the patient's confusion, and there may be more than one. In a cardiac patient, for example, there may be fever, a marginally reduced cerebral blood flow, intoxication with one or more drugs, and electrolyte imbalance. The same may be true of a patient in a *postoperative confusional state*, in which a number of factors such as fever, infection, dehydration, and drug effects may be incriminated. In a study of 1218 postoperative patients by Moller and colleagues, increasing age was by far the most important association with confusion that persisted for weeks and months after an operation; but a number of factors—including the duration of anesthesia, need for a second operation soon after the first, postoperative infection, and respiratory complications—were each predictive of cognitive difficulty in the days after the procedure. Alcoholism and withdrawal effects may further complicate the problem. A more extensive review of this subject has been written by Kaplan and Ropper (see also page 881).

When such patients recover from the medical or surgical illness, they usually return to their premorbid state, though their shortcomings, now drawn to the attention of the family and physician, may be more obvious than before. In this case, families will date the onset of a dementia to the time of the medical illness and minimize the previous decline in cognition.

Development of Schizophrenic or Manic-Depressive Psychosis during a Medical or Surgical Illness

A small proportion of psychoses of schizophrenic or manic-depressive type first become manifest during an acute medical illness or following an operation or parturition and need to be distinguished from an acute confusional state. Rarely, a catatonic state will make its first appearance in these circumstances. A causal relationship between the psychosis and medical illness is sought but cannot be established. The psychosis may have preceded the medical illness but was not recognized, or it may have emerged during the convalescent period. The diagnostic study of the psychiatric illness must proceed along the lines suggested in Chaps. 57 and 58. Close observation will usually disclose a clear sensorium and relatively intact memory, features that permit differentiation from an acute confusional or delirious state or dementia.

Classification and Diagnosis of Acute Confusional States

The syndromes themselves and their main clinical relationships are the only satisfactory basis for classification until such time as their actual causes and pathophysiology are discovered (Table 20-1). The practice of classifying the syndromes according to their most prominent symptom or degree of severity—e.g., "picking delirium," "microptic delirium," "acute delirious mania," "muttering delirium"—has no fundamental value.

The first step in diagnosis is to recognize that the patient is confused. This is obvious in most cases, but, as pointed out above, the mildest forms of confusion, particularly when some other alteration of personality is prominent, may be overlooked. In these mild forms, a careful analysis of the patient's thought processes, as details of the history of the illness and the patient's personal life are obtained, will usually reveal an incoherence. A subtle disorder of orientation may be betrayed by an incorrect response regarding dates (off by more than one day of the month or day of the week), or in misnaming the hospital. Digit span forward (normally 7) and backward (normally 5), spelling the word *world* backward, reciting the months of the year in their reverse order, and serial subtraction of 3s from 30 or 7s from 100 are useful bedside tests of the patient's capacity for attentiveness and sustained mental activity. Another is his efficiency in performing dual tasks such as tapping alternately with each hand while reading aloud. Memory of recent events is one of the most delicate tests of adequate mental function and is readily accomplished by having the patient relate the details of entry to the hospital; ancillary examinations; naming the president, vice president, and mayor; and summarizing major current events, etc., as outlined in Chap. 21.

Once it is established that the patient is confused, the differential diagnosis must be made between delirium, an acute confusional state associated with psychomotor underactivity, a beclouded dementia, and a confusional state that complicates focal cerebral disease.

This is done by taking into account the degree of the patient's alertness, wakefulness, psychomotor and hallucinatory activity, and disturbances of memory and impulse as well as the presence or absence of asterixis or myoclonus or signs of overactivity of the autonomic nervous system and of generalized or focal cerebral disease.

At times, a left hemispheral lesion causing a mild Wernicke aphasia resembles a confusional state in that the stream of thought, as judged by verbal output, is incoherent. The prominence of paraphasias and neologisms in spontaneous speech, difficulties in auditory comprehension, and normal nonverbal behavior mark the disorder as aphasic in nature.

The distinction between an acute confusional state and dementia may be difficult at times, particularly if the mode of onset and the course of the mental decline are not known. The patient with an acute confusional state is said to have a "clouded sensorium" (a somewhat ambiguous term referring to a symptom complex of inattention, disorientation, perhaps drowsiness, and an inclination to inaccurate perceptions and sometimes to hallucinations and delusions), whereas the patient with dementia usually has a clear sensorium. In the demented patient, there are usually a number of "frontal-release" signs such as grasping, groping, sucking, and paratonic rigidity of the limbs. However, some demented patients are as beclouded and bewildered as those with confusional psychosis, and the two conditions are distinguishable only by differences in their mode of onset and clinical course. This suggests that the affected parts of the nervous system may be the same in both conditions. As indicated earlier, schizophrenia and manic-depressive psychosis can usually be separated from the confusional states by the presence of a clear sensorium and relatively intact memory function.

Once a case has been appropriately classified, it is important to determine its clinical associations (Table 20-1). A thorough medical and neurologic examination, computed tomography or magnetic resonance imaging, and—in cases with fever or with no other apparent cause—lumbar puncture should be performed. The medical, neurologic, and laboratory findings (including measurements of Na, Ca, CO_2, BUN, NH_3, calcium, glucose, "toxic screen," etc.) determine the underlying disease and its treatment, and they also give information concerning prognosis. In the neurologic examination particular attention should be given to the presence or absence of focal neurologic signs and to asterixis, myoclonus, and seizures.

Care of the Delirious and Confused Patient

The primary therapeutic effort is directed to the control of the underlying medical disease. Other important objectives are to quiet the patient and protect him from injury. A nurse, attendant, or member of the family should be with such a patient at all times if this can be arranged. Depending on the degree of restlessness and hyperactivity, a locked room, screened windows that cannot be opened by the patient, and a low bed are desirable. It is often better to let such a patient walk about the room than to tie him in bed, which may increase his fright or excitement and cause him to struggle to the point of exhaustion and collapse. The less active patient can usually be kept in bed by side rails, wrist restraints, or a restraining sheet or vest. The patient should be permitted to sit up or walk about the room part of the day unless this is contraindicated by the primary disease.

All drugs that could possibly be responsible for the acute confusional state or delirium should be discontinued if this can be done safely. In particular, these include sedating, antianxiety, narcotic, anticholinergic, antispasticity, and corticosteroid medications, L-dopa, metoclopramide (Reglan), and cimetidine (Tagamet) as well as antidepressants, antiarrhythmics, anticonvulsants, and antibiotics. Despite the need to be sparing with medications in these circumstances, haloperidol, quetiapine, and risperidone are helpful in calming the agitated and hallucinating patient, but they too should be used in the lowest effective doses. Another exception is alcohol or sedative withdrawal, in which chlordiazepoxide (Librium) is the drug favored by most physicians, but chloral hydrate, lorazepam, and diazepam are trustworthy and equally effective sedatives if given in full doses (see Chap. 42). In delirious patients, the purpose of sedation is to assure rest and sleep, avoid exhaustion, and facilitate nursing care, but one must be cautious in attempting to suppress delirium completely. Warm baths are also effective in quieting the delirious patient, but few hospitals have facilities for this valuable method of treatment.

It would seem obvious that attempts should be made to preempt the onset of confusion (beclouded dementia) in the hospitalized elderly patient. Inouyue and colleagues have devised an intervention program that includes frequent reorientation to the surroundings, mentally stimulating activities, ambulation at least three times a day or similar exercises when possible, and attention to the need for visual and hearing aids in patients with these impairments. They recorded a 40-percent reduction in the frequency of a confusional illness in comparison to patients who did not receive this type or attention. Preventive strategies of the type they outline are most important in the elderly, even those without overt dementia, and they must be assiduously applied by nurses and ancillary staff.

Finally, the physician should be aware of the benefit of many small therapeutic measures that allay fear and suspicion and reduce the tendency to hallucinations. The room should be kept dimly lighted at night and, if possible, the patient should not be moved from one room to another. Every procedure should be explained to the patient, even such simple ones as the taking of blood pressure or temperature. The presence of a member of the family may help the patient to maintain contact with reality.

It may be some consolation and also a source of professional satisfaction to remember that most confused and delirious patients recover if they receive competent medical and nursing care. The family should be reassured on this point but forewarned that improvement may take several days or more. They must also understand that the patient's abnormal behavior is not willful but rather symptomatic of a brain disease. (See also Chaps. 42 and 43 for specific aspects of management of delirium due to withdrawal of alcohol and other sedative-hypnotic drugs.)

REFERENCES

Caplan LR, Kelly M, Kase CS, et al: Mirror image of Wernicke's aphasia. *Neurology* 36:1015, 1986.

Engel GL, Romano J: Delirium: A syndrome of cerebral insufficiency. *J Chronic Dis* 9:260, 1959.

Ey H: Disorders of consciousness in psychiatry, in Vinken PJ, Bruyn GW (eds): *Handbook of Clinical Neurology*, Vol 3: *Disorders of Higher Nervous Activity*. Amsterdam, North-Holland, 1969, chap 7, pp 112–136.

Horenstein S, Chamberlin W, Conomy T: Infarction of the fusiform and calcarine regions: Agitated delirium and hemianopia. *Trans Am Neurol Assoc* 92:85, 1967.

Inouye SK, Bogardus ST, Charpentier PA, et al: A multicomponent intervention to prevent delirium in hospitalized older patients. *N Engl J Med* 340:669, 1999.

Kahn E: *Psychopathic Personalities*. New Haven, CT, Yale University Press, 1931.

Kaplan J, Ropper AH: Postoperative confusion, in Grenvik A, Ayers SM, Holbrook WC, Shoemakder WC (eds): *Textbook of Critical Care,* 4th ed. Philadelphia, Saunders, 2000, pp 1825–1830.

Lipowski ZJ: *Delirium: Acute Confusional States*. New York, Oxford University Press, 1990.

Medina JL, Rubino FA, Ross A: Agitated delirium caused by infarction of the hippocampal formation, fusiform and lingual gyri. *Neurology* 24:1181, 1974.

Mesulam MM: Attention, confusional states, and neglect, in Mesulam MM (ed), *Principles of Behavioral Neurology*. Philadelphia, Davis, 1985, pp 125–168.

Mesulam MM, Waxman SG, Geschwind N, et al: Acute confusional states with right middle cerebral infarctions. *J Neurol Neurosurg Psychiatry* 39:84, 1976.

Moller JT, Cluitmans P, Rasmussen LS: Long-term postoperative cognitive dysfunction in the elderly: ISPOCD1 study. *Lancet* 351:857, 1998.

Mori E, Yamadori A: Acute confusional state and acute agitated delirium. *Arch Neurol* 44:1139, 1987.

Stauder HK: Die todliche Katatonie. *Arch Psychiatr Nervenkr* 102:614, 1934.

Wolff HG, Curran D: Nature of delirium and allied states. *Arch Neurol Psychiatry* 33:1175, 1935.

Chapter 21

DEMENTIA AND THE AMNESIC (KORSAKOFF) SYNDROME: With Comments on the Neurology of Intelligence and Memory

Increasingly, as the number of elderly in our population rises, the neurologist is consulted because an otherwise healthy person begins to fail mentally and lose his capacity to function effectively at work or in his household. This may indicate the development of a degenerative brain disease, a brain tumor, multiple strokes, a chronic subdural hematoma, chronic drug intoxication, chronic meningoencephalitis (such as caused by acquired immunodeficiency syndrome or syphilis), normal-pressure hydrocephalus, or a depressive illness. Formerly, when there was little that could be done about these clinical states, no great premium was attached to diagnosis. But modern medicine offers the means of treating several of these conditions and in some instances of restoring the patient to normal mental competence. Moreover, a number of modern diagnostic technologies now allow earlier recognition of the underlying pathologic process, improving the chances of recovery or preventing its progression.

DEFINITIONS

The definitions of normal and abnormal states of mind have already been considered in Chap. 20. There it was pointed out that the term *dementia* denotes a deterioration of intellectual, or cognitive, function, with little or no disturbance of consciousness or perception. In current neurologic parlance the term is commonly used to designate a syndrome of failing memory and impairment of other intellectual functions due to chronic progressive degenerative disease of the brain. Such a definition is too narrow. The term more accurately includes a number of closely related syndromes characterized not only by intellectual deterioration but also by certain behavioral abnormalities and changes in personality. Moreover, it is not entirely logical to set apart any one constellation of cerebral symptoms on the basis of their speed of onset, rate of evolution, severity, or duration. Alternatively, we would propose that there are several states of dementia of differing causes and mechanisms and that a degeneration of widely distributed systems of cerebral neurons, albeit common, is only one of the many causes. Therefore it is more correct to speak of the *dementias* or the *dementing diseases*.

To understand the phenomenon of intellectual deterioration, it is helpful to have some idea of how intellectual functions, in particular intelligence and memory, are normally organized and sustained and the manner in which deficits in these functions relate to diffuse and focal cerebral lesions. The neurology of intelligence is considered first, as a prelude to a discussion of the dementias, and the neurology of memory further on, in relation to the clinical amnesic syndromes.

THE NEUROLOGY OF INTELLIGENCE

Intelligence, or *intelligent behavior*, has been variously defined as a "general mental efficiency," as an "innate cognitive ability," or as "the aggregate or global capacity of an individual to act purposefully, to think rationally, and to deal effectively with his environment" (Wechsler). It is global because it characterizes an individual's behavior as a whole; it is an aggregate in the sense that it is composed of a number of independent and qualitatively distinguishable cognitive abilities.

As every educated person knows, intelligence has something to do with normal cerebral function. It is also apparent that the level of intelligence differs widely from one person to another, and members of certain families are exceptionally bright and intellectually accomplished while members of other families are just the opposite. If properly motivated, intelligent children excel in school and score high on intelligence tests. Indeed, the first intelligence tests, devised by Binet and Simon in 1905, were for the purpose of predicting scholastic success. The term *intelligence quotient*, or *IQ*, was introduced by Terman in 1916; it denotes the figure that is obtained by dividing the subject's mental age (as determined by the Binet-Simon scale) by his chronologic age (up to the fourteenth year) and multiplying the result by 100. The IQ correlates with achievement in school and eventual success in professional work. IQ increases with age up to the fourteenth to sixteenth year and then remains stable, at least until late adult life. At any given age a large sample of normal children attain test scores that range in conformity with the normal, or Gaussian, distribution.

The original studies of pedigrees of highly intelligent and mentally inferior families, which revealed a striking concordance between parent and child, lent support to the idea that intelligence is to a large extent inherited. However, it became evident that the tests being used depended also on skill with words and verbal relationships and on specific cultural experiences provided to children by educated parents, and that the tests were less reliable in identifying children who were talented but never had similar educational opportunities. This led to the widespread belief that intelligence tests are only achievement tests and that environmental factors fostering high performance are the important factors determining intelligence. Neither of these views is entirely correct. Studies of monozygotic and dizygotic twins raised in the same or different families have put the matter in a clearer light. Identical twins reared together or apart are more alike in intelligence than nonidentical twins brought up in the same home (see reviews of Willerman, of Shields, and of Slater and Cowie). A more recent study of elderly twins, by McLean and colleagues, has shed further light on the issue; even in twins who were above 80 years of age, a substantial part (an estimated 62 percent) of cognitive performance could be accounted for by genetic traits. These findings suggest that life experience alters intelligence in only a limited way. There can be no doubt, therefore, that genetic endowment is the more important factor, a view that has long been championed by Piercy and more recently by Herrnstein and Murray (*The Bell Curve*). However, there is also convincing evidence that early learning can modify the level of ability that is finally attained. The latter should be looked upon not as the sum of genetic and environmental factors but as the product of the two. Moreover, it is generally appreciated that nonscholastic achievement or success is governed by a number of factors other than intellectual ones, such as a readiness to learn, interest, persistence, and ambition or motivation—factors that vary considerably from person to person and are not measured by tests of intelligence. Not surprisingly, severe malnutrition in utero or early-life exposure to lead and other toxins have a detrimental effect on brain weight and IQ.

As to the genetic mechanisms involved in the inheritance of intelligence, very little is known. Based on the excess of males with mental retardation, the common inheritance of mental retardation in an X-linked pattern, and the somewhat different patterns of subtest performance between males and females (males perform better on subtests of spatial ability and certain mathematical tasks), Lehrke has proposed that genes coding for intelligence reside on the X chromosome. This view has received support from Turner and his associates on the basis of their extended study of families in which the sole manifestation of an X-linked disorder was a nonspecific mental retardation. Turner has suggested that the male is more likely to be affected by advantageous or aberrant genes on a single X chromosome, while the female benefits from the mosaic provided by two X chromosomes. Turner also alludes to pedigrees in which high intelligence segregates to certain individuals through an X-linked pattern. Further study will determine the validity of this view and its contribution to our understanding of what will certainly prove to be a polygenic inheritance of intellectual traits.

One would think that neurologic structure and function would correlate in some way with intelligence; but except in the pathologically retarded (Chap. 38), such an association has been difficult to document. Brain weight has a weak correlation with IQ. Only laboratory measures of vigilance and facility of sensory registration (speed of motor responses and rapid recognition of differences between lines, shapes, or pictures) have definite but modest correlations with IQ.

As to psychologic theories of intelligence, two have traditionally held sway. One is the two-factor theory of Spearman, who noted that all the separate tests of cognitive abilities correlated with each other, suggesting that a general factor (*"g" factor*) enters into all performance. Since none of the correlations between subtests approached unity, he postulated that each test measures not only this general ability (commonly identified with intelligence) but also a subsidiary factor or factors specific to the individual tests. The latter he designated the *"s" factors*. A second theory, the multifactorial theory of Thurstone, proposed that intelligence consists of a number of primary mental abilities such as memory, verbal facility, numerical ability, visuospatial perception, and capacity for problem solving, all of them more or less equivalent. These primary abilities, although correlated, are not subordinate to a more general ability. Another theory, that of Alexander, supported Spearman's notion of a g factor. For Eysenck, intelligence exists in three forms: biologic (the genetic component), social (development of the genetic component in relation to personal relationships), and a number of specific abilities subject to measurement by psychometric tests.

The most recent elaboration of Thurstone's multifactorial theory of intelligence is that of Gardner. He recognizes six categories of high-order cerebral function: the linguistic (encompassing all language functions); the musical (including composition and performance); the logical-mathematical (the ideas and works of mathematicians); the spatial (including artistic talent and the creation of visual impressions); the bodily-kinesthetic (including dance and athletic performance); and the personal (consciousness of self and others in social interactions). He refers to each of these as an *intelligence*, defined as the ability to solve problems or resolve difficulties within the particular field, and to be creative. The following lines of evidence are marshaled in support of this parceling of what are really separable skills and abilities: (1) each of these abilities may be developed to an exceptionally high level in certain individuals, constituting virtuosity or genius; (2) each can be destroyed or spared in isolation as a consequence of a lesion in a certain part of the nervous system; (3) in certain individuals, i.e., in prodigies, special competence in one of these abilities is evident at an unusually early age; (4) in the autistic mentally retarded, one of these abilities may be spared (idiot savant). Each of these abstracted entities is genetic but the full development of each is influenced by environmental factors.

There are only limited data regarding the highest levels of intelligence identified as genius. Terman and Ogden's longitudinal study of 1500 California school children, who were initially tested in 1921, supported the idea that an extremely high IQ predicted future scholastic accomplishments (though not necessarily occupational success). On the other hand, most individuals recognized as geniuses have been especially skilled in one domain—such as painting, linguistics, music, chess, or mathematics—and such "domain genius" is not necessarily predicated on IQ, although certain individuals display cross-modal superiorities, for example, in mathematics and music.

Concerning the way in which intelligence develops, the most widely known theory is that of Piaget, who proposed that this is accomplished in discrete stages related to age: sensorimotor, from 0 to 2 years; preconceptual thought, from 2 to 4 years; intuitive thought, from 4 to 7 years; concrete operations (conceptualization), from 7 to 11 years; and finally the period of "formal operations" (logical or abstract thought), from 11 years on. This scheme implies that the capacity for logical thought, developing as it does according to an orderly timetable, is coded in the genes. Surely one can recognize these states of intellectual development in the child, but Piaget's theory has been criticized as being too anecdotal and lacking the quantitative validation that could be derived only from studies of a large normal population. Further, it does not take into account the individual's special abilities, which do not develop and reach their maximum at the same time as the more general intellectual capacities.

One would suppose that in neurology, where one is exposed to so many diseases affecting the cerebrum, it might be possible to verify one of these several theories of intelligence and to determine its anatomy. Presumably the g factor of intelligence would be maximally impaired by diffuse lesions, in proportion to the mass of brain involved (mass-action principle of Lashley). Indeed, according to Chapman and Wolff, there is a correlation between the volume of tissue lost and a general deficit of cerebral function. Others have disagreed, claiming that no universal psychologic deficit can be recognized with lesions affecting particular parts of the brain. Probably the truth lies between these two divergent points of view. According to Tomlinson and colleagues, who studied the effects of vascular lesions in the aging brain, lesions that involve more than 50 mL of tissue cause some general reduction in performance, especially in speed and capacity to solve problems. Piercy, on the other hand, found positive correlations only between specific intellectual deficits and lesions of particular parts of the left and right hemispheres. (These are discussed in Chap. 22.) It is surprising that lesions of the frontal lobes, and particularly the prefrontal regions, which so profoundly disorder planning and "executive" functions, do not measurably affect IQ except in subtests specific to these skills.

The authors conclude from personal experience and from evidence provided by neurologic studies that intelligence is a gestalt of multiple primary abilities, each of which seems to be inherited and each of which has a separate but as yet poorly delineated anatomy. We would disagree with Thurstone and with Gardner that these special abilities are of equivalent rank with regard to what is generally considered as "intelligence" and would attach a disproportionate importance to some of them (linguistic and mathematical and perhaps spatial-dimensional abilities). These last abilities are integral to ideation and problem solving and are accomplished by forming associations with a previously established informational skill, which is largely absent in the mentally retarded and is lost early in dementing diseases. Also, we would insist that retentive memory and capacity to learn constitute a cognitive entity with its own neuroanatomic localization. The relationships of some of these special abilities have been thoughtfully analyzed by Luria (see the section on frontal lobes in Chap. 22). Neurologic data do not exclude the possibility of a g factor—one that is unavoidably measured in many different tests of cerebral function. It is expressed in thinking and abstract reasoning and is operative only if the connections between the frontal lobes and other parts of the brain are intact. Attention, drive, and motivation are non-cognitive psychologic attributes of fundamental importance, the precise anatomy and physiology of which remain to be identified. A current account of the subject of IQ and intelligence can be found in the monograph by Mackintosh.

THE NEUROLOGY OF DEMENTIA

Dementia is a syndrome, consisting of a loss of several separable but overlapping intellectual abilities and presenting in a number of different combinations. These varied constellations of intellectual deficits constitute the preeminent clinical abnormalities in several cerebral diseases and are sometimes (e.g., in Alzheimer disease) virtually the only abnormalities, in which case the syndrome is virtually equivalent to the disease. The most common types of dementing diseases and their relative frequency are listed in Table 21-1.

What is noteworthy about the figures in this table is the apparently high level of accuracy of diagnosis. Rather consistently, postmortem examination confirms the diagnosis in about 80 percent of cases or a larger percentage when research criteria are used for the clinical diagnosis of Alzheimer disease (Table 21-2). In many cases, the degenerative diseases can be differentiated by one or two characteristic clinical features, but these distinctions may be difficult to discern early in the disease process. In particular, a small proportion of patients thought to have Alzheimer disease are found to have multi-infarct dementia or a combination of the two disorders. Less often, they are found to have other types of cerebral atrophy, such as progressive supranuclear palsy, Pick, Huntington, Parkinson, or Lewy-body disease; or a variety of other processes. Of special importance is the fact that approximately 10 percent of patients who are referred to a neurologic center with a question of dementia prove to have a potentially reversible psychiatric or metabolic disorder simulating degenerative brain disease.

Table 21-1
The common types of dementing diseases and their approximate frequencies

Dementing disease	*Relative frequency, %*
Cerebral atrophy, mainly Alzheimer but including Lewy-body, Parkinson, frontotemporal, and Pick disease	50
Multi-infarct dementia	10
Alcoholic dementia	7
Intracranial tumors	5
Normal-pressure hydrocephalus	5
Huntington chorea	2
Chronic drug intoxications	3
Miscellaneous diseases (hepatic failure; pernicious anemia; hypo- or hyperthyroidism; dementias with Parkinson disease, amyotrophic lateral sclerosis, cerebellar atrophy; neurosyphilis; Cushing syndrome, Lewy-body disease, Creutzfeldt-Jakob disease; multiple sclerosis; epilepsy)	6
Cerebral trauma	2
AIDS dementia complex	2
Pseudodementias (depression, hypomania, schizophrenia, hysteria, undiagnosed)	8

Sources: Van Horn; Mayeux et al; Cummings and Benson (see References).

In the following pages we consider the prototype syndromes. They are observed most frequently with degenerative diseases of the brain (Chap. 39) and less often as part of other categories of disease (vascular, traumatic, infectious, demyelinative, etc.), which are considered in their appropriate chapters.

Dementia due to Degenerative Diseases

The earliest signs of dementia due to degenerative disease may be so subtle as to escape the notice of the most discerning physician. An observant relative of the patient or an employer may become aware of a certain lack of initiative or lack of interest in work, a neglect of routine tasks, or an abandonment of pleasurable pursuits. Initially, these changes may be attributed to fatigue or boredom. More often, gradual development of forgetfulness is the

Table 21-2
Neuropathologic diagnoses for 261 cases with a clinical diagnosis of Alzheimer disease: Data from the Massachusetts ADRC Brain Registry, 1984–1993[a]

Neuropathologic diagnosis	*Number of cases*	*Percent*
Alzheimer disease	218	83.5
Parkinson and Alzheimer disease	16	6.1
Lewy-body disease	8	3.1
Pick disease	6	2.3
Multiple infarcts	5	1.9
Binswanger disease	1	0.4
Corticobasal ganglionic degeneration	1	0.4
Mixed dementia	1	0.4
Other	5	1.9
Total	261	100

[a]Courtesy of Dr. John Growdon.

most prominent early symptom. Proper names are no longer remembered, to a far greater extent than can be attributed to so-called benign senescent forgetfulness (see page 641). Difficulty in balancing a checkbook and making change becomes evident. The purpose of an errand is forgotten, appointments are not kept, a recent conversation or social event has been forgotten. The patient may ask the same question repeatedly, having failed to retain the answers that were previously given.

Later it becomes evident that the patient is easily distracted by every passing incident. No longer is it possible to think about or discuss a problem with customary clarity or to comprehend all aspects of complex situations. The patient's judgement and ability to make proper deductions and inferences from given premises are greatly reduced. One feature of a situation or some relatively unimportant event may become a source of unreasonable concern or worry. Tasks that require several steps cannot be accomplished, and all but the simplest directions cannot be followed. The patient may get lost, even along habitual routes of travel. Day-to-day events are not recalled, and perseveration or impersistence in speech, action, and thought becomes evident.

In yet other instances, an early abnormality may be in the nature of emotional instability, taking the form of unreasonable outbursts of anger, easy tearfulness, or aggressiveness. Frequently a change in mood becomes apparent, deviating more toward depression than elation. Apathy is common. Some patients are grumpy and irascible; a few are cheerful and facetious. The direction of the mood change is said to depend on the previous personality of the patient rather than on the character of the disease, but one can think of glaring exceptions to this dictum. Excessive lability of mood may also be observed—for example, easy fluctuation from laughter to tears on slight provocation.

A few patients come to the physician with physical complaints, the most common being dizziness, a vague mental "fogginess," and nondescript headaches. The patient's inability to give a coherent account of his symptoms bears witness to the presence of a dementia. Sometimes the mental failure is brought to light more dramatically by a severe confusional state attending a febrile illness, a concussive head injury, an operative procedure, or the administration of some new medicine, as discussed in Chap. 20. As noted there, the family may mistakenly date an abrupt onset of dementia to the time of the intercurrent illness.

Loss of social graces and indifference to social customs occur, but usually later in the course of illness. Judgment becomes impaired, early in some, late in others. At certain phases of the illness, suspiciousness or frank paranoia may develop. Visual and auditory hallucinations, sometimes quite vivid in nature, may be added. Wandering, pacing, and other aimless activities are common in the intermediate stage of the illness, while other patients sit placidly for hours. As a rule, these patients have little or no realization of such changes within themselves; i.e., they lack insight.

As the condition progresses, all intellectual faculties are impaired; but in the commonest degenerative diseases, memory is most affected. Up to a certain point in the illness, memories of the distant past are relatively well retained at a time when more recently acquired information has been lost (Ribot's law). Eventually patients also fail to retain remote memories, to recognize their relatives, or even to recall the names of their children. Apraxias and agnosias may be prominent, and these defects may alter the performance of the simplest tasks, such as preparing a meal, setting the table, or even using the telephone or a knife and fork, dressing, or walking.

Language functions tend to be impaired almost from the beginning of certain forms of dementia. Lost is the capacity to understand nuances of the spoken and written word, as are the suppleness and spontaneity of verbal expression. Vocabulary becomes restricted and conversation is rambling and repetitious. The patient gropes for proper names and common nouns and no longer formulates ideas with well-constructed phrases or sentences. Instead, there is a tendency to resort to cliches, stereotyped phrases, and exclamations, which may hide the underlying defect during conversation. Paraphasias and difficulty in comprehending complex conversations are almost universal abnormalities. Subsequently, more severe degrees of aphasia, dysarthria, palilalia, and echolalia may be added to the clinical picture.

As pointed out by Chapman and Wolff, there is loss also of the capacity to express feelings, to suppress impulses, and to tolerate frustration and restrictions. If the patient is restrained, disagreeable behavior, petulance, agitation, shouting, and whining may occur. Nighttime confusion and inversion of the normal sleep pattern as well as increased confusion and restlessness in the early evening ("sundowning") are common.

It would be an error to think that the abnormalities in the atrophic-degenerative dementing diseases are confined to the intellectual sphere. The appearance of the patient and the physical examination yield highly informative data. The first impression is often revealing; the patient may be unkempt and unbathed. He may look bewildered, as though lost, or his expression may be vacant, and he does not maintain a lively interest or participate in the interview. There is a kind of psychic inertia. Deference to a spouse or child when the patient is unable to answer the examiner's questions is characteristic. All movements are slightly slow, sometimes suggesting an oncoming Parkinson syndrome.

Sooner or later gait is characteristically altered (Chap. 7). Passive movements of the limbs encounter a fluctuating resistance, or paratonia (gegenhalten). Mouthing movements and a number of abnormal reflexes—grasping and sucking (in response to visual as well as tactile stimuli), inability to inhibit blink on tapping the glabella, snout reflex (protrusion of the lips in response to perioral tapping), biting or jaw clamping (bulldog) reflex, corneomandibular reflex (jaw clenching when the cornea is touched), and palmomental reflex (retraction of one side of the mouth and chin caused by contraction of the mentalis muscle when the thenar eminence of the palm is stroked)—all occur with increasing frequency in the advanced stages of the dementia. Many of these abnormalities are considered to be motor disinhibitions that appear when the premotor areas of the brain are involved.

In the later stages, physical deterioration is inexorable. Food intake, which may be increased at the onset of the illness, sometimes to the point of gluttony, is in the end reduced, with resulting emaciation. Any febrile illness, drug intoxication, or metabolic upset is poorly tolerated, leading to severe confusion, stupor, or coma—an indication of the precarious state of cerebral compensation (see "Beclouded Dementia," page 441). Finally, these patients remain in bed most of the time, oblivious of their surroundings, and succumb to pneumonia or to some other intercurrent infection. Some patients, should they not succumb in this way, become virtually decorticate—totally unaware of their environment, unresponsive, mute, incontinent, and, in the end, adopting a posture of paraplegia in flexion. They lie with their eyes open but do not look about. Food and drink are no longer requested but are swallowed if placed in the mouth. The term *persistent vegetative state* is appropriately applied to these patients, although it was originally devised to describe patients in this same state after cardiac arrest or head injury. Occasionally diffuse choreoathetotic movements or random myoclonic jerking can be observed, and seizures occur in a few advanced cases. Pain or an uncomfortable posture goes unheeded. The course of Alzheimer disease extends for 5 to 10 years or more from the time that the memory defect becomes evident.

Naturally, every case does not follow the exact sequence outlined above. Not infrequently a patient is brought to the physician because of an impaired facility with language. In other patients, impairment of retentive memory with relatively intact reasoning power may be the dominant clinical feature in the first months or even years of the disease; or low impulsivity (apathy and abulia) may be the most conspicuous feature, resulting in obscuration of all the more specialized higher cerebral functions. Gait disorder, though usually a late development, may occur early, particularly in patients in whom the dementia is associated with or superimposed on Parkinson disease, normal pressure hydrocephalus, cerebellar ataxia, or progressive supranuclear palsy. Insofar as the several types of degenerative disease do not affect certain parts of the brain equally, it is not surprising that their symptomatology varies. Moreover, frank psychosis with delusions and hallucinations may be woven into the dementia. These variations and others are discussed more fully in Chap. 39.

The aforementioned alterations of intellect and behavior are the direct consequence of neuronal loss in certain parts of the cerebrum. In other words, the symptoms are the primary manifestations of neurologic disease. However, some symptoms are secondary; i.e., they may represent the patient's reactions to his mental incapacity. For example, a demented person may seek solitude to hide his affliction and thus may appear to be asocial or apathetic. Again, excessive orderliness may be an attempt to compensate for failing memory; apprehension, gloom, and irritability may reflect a general dissatisfaction with a necessarily restricted life. According to Goldstein, who has written about these "catastrophic reactions," as he called them, even patients in a state of fairly advanced deterioration are still capable of reacting to their illness and to persons who care for them.

In the early and intermediate stages of the illness, special psychologic tests aid in the quantitation of some of these abnormalities, as indicated in the latter part of this chapter.

Frontotemporal Dementia As indicated above, not all degenerative dementias have a uniform mode of onset and clinical course. Several clinical variants have long been recognized and in recent years; three of them—frontotemporal dementia, primary progressive aphasia, and semantic dementia—have been subsumed under a newly minted term, *frontotemporal dementia.* Two consensus statements on the clinical diagnostic criteria for these syndromes were published relatively recently, although not all writings on this subject are in agreement (see Morris).

The most common clinical syndrome is characterized by features that would be expected of diffuse cortical degeneration of the frontal lobes (see also Chap. 22): early personality changes, particularly apathy or disinhibition, euphoria, perseveration in motor and cognitive tasks, ritualistic and repetitive behaviors, laconic speech leading to mutism—all with relative preservation of memory and orientation. With anterior temporal lobe involvement, hyperorality, excessive smoking or overeating occur and there may be added anxiety, depression, and anomia. Diminished capacity for abstraction, attention, planning, and problem solving may be observed as the degenerative process continues.

Primary progressive (nonfluent) aphasia is a highly circumscribed syndrome, characterized by effortful speech, agrammatism, and impairment of reading and writing, with relative preservation of the understanding of the meaning of words. Such aphasic syndromes may persist in isolation for several years before other features of cognitive decline become evident. *Semantic dementia* is the least common and most poorly defined of the three syndromes. It is said to be characterized by a fluent aphasia in which impaired semantic memory causes severe anomia and impaired word comprehension.

Certainly frontotemporal dementia, however it is defined, does not have a unique pathology; the same degenerative diseases that cause primary dementia (prototype Alzheimer but also Pick and Lewy-body disease) also underlie so-called frontotemporal dementia. Furthermore, dementias, in which language problems are early and preeminent, have long been known to result from Pick or Alzheimer disease and at other times to have an ambiguous pathology, i.e., an ill-defined neuronal loss and gliosis. It is specifically to this latter type of nondescript pathologic change that the term *frontotemporal dementia* is now being applied by some authors, and this at least has the advantage of separating one category of cerebral degeneration on clinical and pathologic grounds from Alzheimer disease. Current opinion supports the separation of one subgroup of cases on the basis of a heritable frontotemporal dementia; these and the sporadic cases share the pathologic features of cell loss, microvacuolation of the frontal and temporal cortex, gliosis, and the ubiquitous deposition of tau protein. A separate group is similar in clinical presentation but displays Pick bodies as well as deposition of tau (Neary et al; Morris).

It is evident that a wide variety of pathologic entities underlie the clinical conditions subsumed under the rubric of fronto-temporal dementia; moreover, a full clinical classification of this presumed entity remains to be completed. (See also Chap. 39.)

Subcortical Dementia McHugh, who introduced the concept of subcortical dementia, pointed out that the dementias of certain predominantly basal ganglionic diseases such as progressive supranuclear palsy, Huntington chorea, and Parkinson disease, though similar to one another, are different in several respects from the cortical dementia of Alzheimer disease. The former diseases, in addition to the obvious disorders of motility and involuntary movements, are characterized by lesser degrees of forgetfulness, slowed thought processes, lack of initiative, and depression of mood. Relatively spared are vocabulary, naming, and praxis. By contrast, the "cortical dementias" (exemplified by Alzheimer disease) are distinguished by more severe disturbances of memory, language, and calculation, prominent signs of apraxia and agnosia, and impaired capacity for abstract thought.

The pathologic changes underlying the subcortical dementias predominate in the basal ganglia, thalamus, rostral brainstem nuclei, and the ill-defined projections from these regions to the cortex, particularly of the frontal lobes.

Certain authors, notably Mayeux and Stern and their colleagues as well as Tierney and coworkers, have been critical of the concept of subcortical dementia. They have argued that the distinctions between cortical and subcortical dementias are not fundamental and that any differences between them are probably attributable to differences in the relative severity of the dementing processes. Nonetheless, a number of recent studies do indeed indicate that the constellations of cognitive impairments in the two groups of dementias differ along the lines indicated above (Brandt et al; Pillon et al).

One of the problems with the concept of subcortical dementia is the name itself, implying as it does that symptoms of dementia are attributable to lesions confined to subcortical structures. Anatomically, none of the neurodegenerative dementias is strictly cortical or subcortical. The attribution of dementia to subcortical gliosis, for example, has always proved to be incorrect; invariably there are cortical neuronal changes as well. In a similar way, the changes of Alzheimer disease may extend well beyond the cerebral cortex, involving the striatum, thalamus, and even cerebellum. Also, functionally, it is unlikely that the symptoms of dementia are due to the basal ganglionic lesions themselves. More likely these lesions produce their effects by interrupting neural links to the frontal and other parts of the cerebral cortex. McHugh has suggested, and we would concur, that *dementia without aphasia or apraxia* is a more apt term than *subcortical dementia* for the dementia associated with basal ganglionic-thalamic disease.

Pathology and Pathogenesis of Dementia

Attempts to relate the impairment of particular intellectual functions to lesions in certain parts of the brain have been, with a few notable exceptions, unsuccessful. Two types of difficulty have obstructed progress in this field. First, there is the problem of defining and analyzing the nature of the so-called intellectual functions. Second, the pathologic anatomy of the dementing diseases is often so diffuse and complex that it cannot be fully localized and quantitated. Memory impairment, which is a constant feature of most dementias, may occur with extensive disease in several different parts of the cerebrum. Yet it is important to note that the integrity of certain discrete parts of the diencephalon and inferomedial parts of the temporal lobes is more fundamental to retentive memory than is the rest of the brain. Impairment of language function is closely associated with disease of the dominant cerebral hemisphere, particularly the perisylvian parts of the frontal, temporal, and parietal lobes. Loss of capacity for reading and calculation is related to lesions in the posterior part of the left (dominant) cerebral hemisphere; loss of use of tools and imitation of gestures (apraxias) is related to loss of tissue in the dominant parietal region. Impairment in drawing or constructing simple and complex figures with blocks, sticks, picture arrangements, etc., is observed with parietal lobe lesions, more often with right-sided (nondominant) than with left-sided ones. And problems with modulation of behavior and stability of personality are generally related to frontal lobe degeneration. Thus, the *clinical picture resulting from cerebral disease depends in part on the extent of the lesion, i.e., the amount of cerebral tissue destroyed, and in part on the region of the brain that bears the brunt of the pathologic change*.

Dementia of the degenerative type is usually related to obvious structural diseases mainly of the cerebral cortex, but also of the diencephalon and possibly the basal ganglia. In some pathologic entities, such as Alzheimer disease, the main process is a degeneration and loss of nerve cells in the cortical association areas and medial temporal lobes. In Pick disease and the primary frontotemporal dementia group, the atrophy is mainly frontal or temporal or both and sometimes quite asymmetrical. In other diseases, such as Huntington chorea, the neuronal degeneration predominates in the caudate nuclei, putamens, and other parts of the basal ganglia. In general, dementia associated with basal ganglia degenerations is of "subcortical" type, described earlier. Rarely, purely thalamic degenerations may be the basis of a dementia because of the integral relationship of the thalamus to the cerebral cortex.

Arteriosclerotic cerebrovascular disease, which pursues a different course than the neurodegenerative diseases, results in multiple foci of infarction throughout the thalami, basal ganglia, brainstem, and cerebrum and, in the latter, in the motor, sensory, or visual projection areas as well as in the association areas. There is no evidence, however, that arteriosclerosis per se, without thrombotic occlusion and infarction or globally diminished blood flow, is a cause of progressive dementia. Undoubtedly, the cumulative effects of recurrent strokes impair the intellect; usually, but not always, the stroke-by-stroke advance of the disease is apparent in such patients (multi-infarct dementia). Far more uncertain is the notion that a characteristic decline in mental function can be attributed to periventricular white matter changes (leukoaraiosis), which are observed in CT scans and MR images of many elderly patients and are presumed to be ischemic and hypertensive in nature (see review of Van Gijn). Also, the notion that small strokes exaggerate or in some way produce an Alzheimer neuropathologic process has been uncritically accepted in some quarters. The special problem of arteriosclerotic or multi-infarct dementia is discussed further in Chap. 34 and addressed in relation to Alzheimer disease on page 1109.

The lesions of severe *trauma*, if they result in dementia, are to be found in the cerebral convolutions (mainly frontal and temporal poles), corpus callosum, and mesencephalon; rarely, there is widespread degeneration of the white matter and hydrocephalus. Most traumatic lesions that produce dementia are quite extensive.

Mechanisms other than the overt destruction of brain tissue may operate in some cases. *Chronic hydrocephalus*, regardless of cause, is often associated with a general impairment of mental function. Compression of the cerebral white matter is probably the main factor. The compression of one or both of the cerebral hemispheres by *chronic subdural hematomas* may have the same effect. A *diffuse inflammatory process* is at least in part the basis of dementia in syphilis, cryptococcosis, other chronic meningitides, and viral infections such as AIDS, herpes simplex encephalitis, and subacute sclerosing panencephalitis; presumably there is a loss of some neurons and an inflammatory derangement of function in the neurons that remain. The prior diseases (Creutzfeldt-Jakob disease) cause a diffuse loss of cortical neurons, replacement gliosis, and spongiform change and produce special patterns of cognitive dysfunction.

The adult forms of *leukodystrophy* (Chap. 37) also give rise to a dementing syndrome, generally with a "subcortical" syndrome and prominent frontal lobe features. Or extensive lesions in the white matter may be due to advanced cerebral multiple sclerosis, progressive multifocal leukoencephalitis, or some of the vascular dementias already alluded to (Binswanger disease). Last, several of the metabolic and toxic disorders discussed in Chaps. 37, 40, and 43 may interfere with nervous function over a period of time and create a clinical picture similar if not identical to that of one of the dementias. One must suppose that the altered biochemical environment has affected neuronal function.

Bedside Classification of the Dementing Diseases

Conventionally, the dementing diseases have been classified according to cause, if known, to the pathologic changes, or more recently, to a genetic mutation. Another, more practical approach, which follows logically from the method by which much of the subject matter is presented in this book, is to subdivide the diseases into three categories on the basis of the neurologic signs and associated clinical and laboratory signs of medical disease (see Table 21-3). Once it has been determined that the patient suffers from a dementing illness, it must then be decided from the medical, neurologic, and ancillary data into which category the case fits. This classification may at first seem somewhat cumbersome. However, it is likely to be more useful to the student or physician not conversant with the many diseases that cause dementia than a classification based on pathology or genetics.

Differential Diagnosis

Although confusion or dementia per se does not indicate a particular disease, certain combinations of symptoms and neurologic signs are more or less characteristic and may aid in diagnosis. The age of the patient, the mode of onset of the dementia, its clinical course and time span, the associated neurologic signs, and the accessory laboratory data constitute the basis of differential diagnosis. It must be admitted, however, that some of the rarer types of degenerative brain disease are at present recognized only by pathologic examination. The correct diagnosis of treatable forms of dementia—subdural hematoma, certain brain tumors, chronic drug intoxication, normal-pressure hydrocephalus, AIDS (treatable to some extent), neurosyphilis, cryptococcosis, pellagra, vitamin B_{12} and thiamine deficiency states, hypothyroidism, and other metabolic and endocrine disorders—is, of course, of greater practical importance than the diagnosis of the untreatable ones. Important also is the detection of a *depressive illness*, which may masquerade as a dementia and is treatable.

The first task in dealing with this class of patients is to verify the presence of intellectual deterioration and personality change. *It may be necessary to examine the patient serially before one is confident of the clinical findings.*

There is always a tendency to assume that mental function is normal if a patient complains only of nervousness, fatigue, insomnia, or vague somatic symptoms and to label the patient as neurotic. This will be avoided if one keeps in mind that a neurosis rarely has its onset in middle or late adult life. A practical rule is to assume that all mental illnesses beginning during this period are due either to structural disease of the brain or to depression.

A mild aphasia must not be mistaken for dementia. Aphasic patients appear uncertain of themselves, and their speech may be incoherent. Furthermore, they may be anxious and depressed over their ineptitude. Careful attention to the patient's language performance will lead to the correct diagnosis in most instances. Further observation will disclose that the patient's behavior, except that which is related to the language disorder or to an

Table 21-3
Bedside classification of the dementias

I. Diseases in which dementia is associated with clinical and laboratory signs of other medical diseases
  A. AIDS
  B. Endocrine disorders: hypothyroidism, Cushing syndrome, rarely hypopituitarism
  C. Nutritional deficiency states: Wernicke-Korsakoff syndrome, subacute combined degeneration (vitamin B_{12} deficiency), pellagra
  D. Chronic meningoencephalitis: general paresis, meningovascular syphilis, cryptococcosis
  E. Hepatolenticular degeneration—familial (Wilson disease) and acquired
  F. Chronic drug intoxications (including CO poisoning)
  G. Prolonged hypoglycemia or hypoxia
  H. Paraneoplastic "limbic" encephalitis
  I. Heavy metal exposure: arsenic, bismuth, gold, manganese, mercury
  J. Dialysis dementia (now rare)

II. Diseases in which dementia is associated with other neurologic signs but not with other obvious medical diseases
  A. Invariably associated with other neurologic signs
    1. Huntington chorea (choreoathetosis)
    2. Multiple sclerosis, Schilder disease, adrenal leukodystrophy, and related demyelinative diseases (spastic weakness, pseudobulbar palsy, blindness)
    3. Lipid-storage diseases (myoclonic seizures, blindness, spasticity, cerebellar ataxia)
    4. Myoclonic epilepsy (diffuse myoclonus, generalized seizures, cerebellar ataxia)
    5. Subacute spongiform encephalopathy; Creutzfeldt-Jakob disease; Gerstmann-Strausler-Scheinker disease (prion, myoclonic dementias)
    6. Cerebrocerebellar degeneration (cerebellar ataxia)
    7. Cerebral-basal ganglionic degenerations (apraxia-rigidity)
    8. Dementia with spastic paraplegia
    9. Progressive supranuclear palsy
    10. Parkinson disease
    11. Amyotrophic lateral sclerosis (ALS) and ALS-Parkinson-dementia complex
    12. Other rare hereditary metabolic diseases
  B. Often associated with other neurologic signs
    1. Multiple thrombotic or embolic cerebral infarctions and Binswanger disease
    2. Brain tumor (primary or metastatic) or abscess
    3. Brain trauma, such as cerebral contusions, midbrain hemorrhages, chronic subdural hematoma
    4. Lewy-body disease (parkinsonian features)
    5. Communicating, normal-pressure, or obstructive hydrocephalus (usually with ataxia of gait)
    6. Progressive multifocal leukoencephalitis
    7. Marchiafava-Bignami disease (often with apraxia and other frontal lobe signs)
    8. Granulomatous and other vasculitides of the brain
    9. Viral encephalitis (herpes simplex)

III. Diseases in which dementia is usually the only evidence of neurologic or medical diseases
  A. Alzheimer disease
  B. Pick disease
  C. Some cases of AIDS
  D. Progressive aphasia syndromes
  E. Frontotemporal and "frontal lobe" dementias associated with tau deposition, Alzheimer change, or with no specific pathologic alteration
  F. Degenerative disease of unspecified type

Note: The special clinical features and morbid anatomy of these many dementing diseases are discussed in appropriate chapters throughout this book, particularly Chap. 39 on degenerative disorders, Chaps. 37 and 41 on metabolic and nutritional disturbances, and Chap. 33 on chronic infections.

associated apraxia, is not abnormal. Also, progressive deafness or loss of sight in an elderly person may sometimes be misinterpreted as dementia.

Clues to the diagnosis of depression are the presence of sighing, crying, loss of energy, psychomotor underactivity or its opposite, agitation with pacing, persecutory delusions, persistent hypochondriasis, and a history of depression in the past and in the family. Although depressed patients may complain of memory failure, scrutiny of their complaints will show that they can usually remember the details of their illness and that no qualitative change in other intellectual functions has taken place. Their difficulty is either a lack of energy and interest or preoccupation with personal worries and anxiety, which prevent the focusing of attention on anything except their own problems. Even during mental tests, their performance may be impaired by emotional blocking, in much the same way as the worried student blocks during an examinations ("experiential confusion"). When such patients are calmed by reassurance and encouraged to try harder, their mental function improves, indicating that intellectual deterioration has not occurred. Conversely, it is helpful to remember that demented patients rarely have sufficient insight to complain of mental deterioration; if they admit to poor memory, they do so without conviction or full appreciation of the degree of their disability. The physician must never rely on the patient's statements alone in gauging the efficiency of mental function. Yet another problem is that of the impulsive, cantankerous, and quarrelsome patient who is a constant source of distress to employer and family. Such changes in personality and behavior (as, for example, in Huntington disease) may precede or mask early intellectual deterioration.

It is a clinical truism that the abrupt onset of mental symptoms points to a delirium or other type of acute confusional state and occasionally to a stroke; inattention, perceptual disturbances, and often drowsiness are conjoined (Chap. 20). Inasmuch as these latter conditions are practically always reversible, it is important that they be distinguished from dementia. The neuropsychiatric symptoms associated with metabolic, endocrine, or toxic disorders may present difficulties in diagnosis because of the wide variety of clinical pictures by which they manifest themselves. Whenever any such disorder is suspected, a thorough review of the patient's medications is crucial. Medications with atropinic activity, for example, can produce an apparent dementia or worsen a structurally based dementia. Occupational exposure to toxins and heavy metals should also be explored.

Once it is decided that the patient suffers from a dementing condition, the next step is to determine by careful physical examination whether there are other neurologic signs or indications of a particular medical disease. This enables the physician to place the case in one of the three categories in the bedside classification (see above and Table 21-3). Ancillary examinations—such as CT, MRI, EEG, lumbar puncture, measurement of blood urea nitrogen and serum concentrations of calcium and electrolytes, and liver function tests—should be carried out in most cases. The MRI and CT are or major importance in objectifying hydrocephalus, lobar atrophy, leukoencephalopathy, cerebrovascular disease, tumor, and subdural hematoma. Testing for syphilis, vitamin B_{12} deficiency, and thyroid function is also done almost as a matter of routine because the tests are simple and the dementias they cause are reversible. These are supplemented in individual circumstances by serologic testing for human immunodeficiency virus (HIV) infection, measurement of copper and ceruloplasmin levels, (Wilson disease), heavy metal concentrations in urine or tissues, serum cortisol levels, and drug toxicology screening. The final step is to determine, from the total clinical picture, the particular disease within any one category.

THE AMNESIC SYNDROME (KORSAKOFF SYNDROME; AMNESIC OR AMNESIC-CONFABULATORY SYNDROME); See also Chap. 41

Definition The terms listed above are used interchangeably to designate a unique but common disorder of cognitive function in which memory and learning are deranged out of proportion to all other components of mentation and behavior. The amnesic state, as originally defined by Ribot, possesses two salient features that may vary in severity but are always conjoined: (1) an impaired ability to recall events and other information that had been firmly established before the onset of the illness (*retrograde amnesia*) and (2) an impaired ability to acquire certain types of new information, i.e., to learn or to form new memories (*anterograde amnesia*). This dual aspect inspired one of Lewis Carroll's characters to say that one's memory works both ways, past and future. In other words, memory and learning are inseparable. A third invariable feature of the Korsakoff syndrome, contingent upon the retrograde amnesia, is an impaired temporal localization of past experience (see below, under "Confabulation"). Other cognitive functions (particularly the capacity for concentration, spatial organization, as well as visual and verbal abstraction), which depend little or not at all on memory, are usually impaired as well, but to a lesser degree than memory function. The patient is usually lacking in initiative, spontaneity, and insight.

Equally important in the definition of the *Korsakoff syndrome* or *amnesic state* (these terms are preferable to *Korsakoff psychosis*) is the integrity of certain aspects of behavior and mental function. The patient must be awake, attentive, and responsive—capable of perceiving and understanding the written and spoken word, of making appropriate deductions from given premises, and of solving such problems as can be included within his forward memory span. These "negative" features are of particular diagnostic importance because they help to distinguish the Korsakoff amnesic state from a number of other disorders in which the basic defect is not in retentive memory but in some other psychologic abnormality—e.g., an impairment in attention and perception (as in the delirious, confused, or stuporous patient), in recall (as in the hysterical patient), or in volition, i.e., the will to learn (as in the apathetic or abulic patient with frontal lobe disease or depression).

So-called short-term or working memory, as demonstrated by the ability to repeat a string of digits, is intact, but this is more a measure of attention and registration than of retentive memory. Remote memory is relatively less affected than recent memory (Ribot's rule, as discussed below).

Confabulation The creative falsification of memory in an alert, responsive individual is often included in the definition of the Korsakoff amnesic state but is not a requisite for diagnosis. It can be provoked by questions as to the patient's recent activities. The replies may be recognized as partially remembered events and personal experiences that are inaccurately localized in the past and related with no regard to their proper temporal sequence. Whether one calls this a memory defect or confabulation is an academic matter. Far less frequent but more dramatic is a spontaneous recital of personal experiences, many of which are fantasies. These two forms of confabulation have been referred to as "momentary" and "fantastic," respectively, and it has been claimed, on uncertain grounds, that the latter form reflects an associated lesion in the frontal lobes (Berlyne). In our patients with the alcoholic Korsakoff syndrome, so-called fantastic confabulation was observed mainly in the initial phase of the illness, in which it could be related to a state of profound general confusion; "momentary confabulation" came later, in the convalescent stage. In the chronic, stable stage of the illness, confabulation was rarely elicitable irrespective of how broadly this symptom was defined.

Neuropsychology of Memory Loss It is noteworthy that memory function obeys certain neurologic laws. As memory fails, it first loses its hold on recent events. The degree of retrograde amnesia is proportionate to the magnitude of the underlying neurologic disorder. Early life memories are better preserved and integrated into habitual responses; nevertheless, with natural aging, there is also a gradual loss of early life memories. In transitory amnesias (e.g., concussive head injury), memories are recovered in reverse order, i.e., first the remote and then the more recent. All these principles were enunciated by Ribot in the latter half of the nineteenth century. The enduring aspect of early life memories in contrast to more recently experienced and learned material, a restatement of Ribot's rule, is apparent in both normal adults and in demented patients.

In the further analysis of the Korsakoff amnesic syndrome, it is necessary to consider the proposition that memory is not a unitary function but takes several forms. Thus, a patient with virtually no capacity to learn any newly presented information can still acquire some simple manual and pattern-analyzing skills (e.g., mirror reading). Moreover, having acquired these skills, the patient may have no memory of the circumstances in which they were acquired (implicit memory). The learning of simple mechanical skills has been referred to as *procedural memory*, in distinction to learning new data-based information, referred to as nonprocedural or *declarative memory*. Cohen and Squire have described this dichotomy as "knowing how" as opposed to "knowing that."

Much has also been written in the psychologic literature about two systems of memory referred to as *episodic* and *semantic*. A pervasive problem with these terms is the lack of uniformity in defining them. To Tulving, whose writings on this subject are recommended, the term "episodic" denotes a memory system for dating personal experiences and their temporal relationships; semantic memory is one's repository of perceptual and factual knowledge, which make it possible to comprehend language and make inferences. The latter hardly constitutes a novel concept; Korsakoff himself clearly recognized that certain aspects of mental function (among them the ones now being defined as semantic memory) remain intact, despite the profound impairment of retentive (episodic) memory. Gadian and colleagues have described a group of five young patients who showed severe impairments of episodic memory with relative preservation of semantic memory, attributable to hypoxic-ischemic injury (bilateral hippocampal atrophy) sustained early in life.

Damasio has introduced yet another set of terms—*generic*, in place of semantic and *contextual*, for episodic. To Damasio, generic memory denotes the basic properties of acquired information, such as its class membership and function; he makes the point that in the amnesic syndrome, this component of declarative memory remains intact and only the contextual component is impaired.

The full significance of these categorizations is still being explored. The categorical purity of semantic memory is open to question, as is the notion of a strict dichotomy between semantic and episodic memory. Most importantly, a separate anatomic basis for these systems of memory has not be established (see below).

Anatomic Basis of the Amnesic Syndrome

The anatomic structures of particular importance in memory function are the diencephalon (specifically the medial portions of the dorsomedial and adjacent midline nuclei of the thalamus) and the hippocampal formations (dentate gyrus, hippocampus, parahippocampal gyrus, subiculum, and entorhinal cortex). Discrete bilateral lesions in these regions derange memory and learning out of all proportion to other cognitive functions, and a unilateral lesion of these structures, especially of the dominant hemisphere, can produce a lesser degree of the same effect. A severe but less enduring defect in retentive memory has also been observed with infarction of the septal gray matter, a cluster of midline nuclei at the base of the frontal lobes, just below the interventricular septum and including the septal nucleus, nucleus accumbens, diagonal band of Broca, and paraventricular hypothalamic gray matter (Phillips et al). These septal nuclei have connections with the hippocampus through the precommissural fornix and with the amygdala through the diagonal band. The amnesic syndrome that follows ruptured anterior communicating aneurysm is due to a lesion involving these nuclei. The clinical-anatomic relationships that bear on this subject are discussed in detail by Aggleton and Saunders and by Victor, Adams, and Collins.

Experimental studies in monkeys have confirmed the importance of the diencephalic-hippocampal structures in memory function. (The reviews of these studies by Zola-Morgan et al are recommended.) The difficulty of evaluating memory function in monkeys has been largely overcome by use of the delayed nonmatching-to-sample task, which is essentially a refined test of recognition memory and is impaired both in patients with the amnesic syndrome and in monkeys with lesions of the mediodorsal nuclei of the thalamus and inferomedial temporal cortical regions (Mishkin and Delacour). Using this method of testing and several others that are sensitive to human amnesia, Zola-Morgan and colleagues have shown that bilateral lesions of the hippocampal formation cause an enduring impairment of memory function. Lesions confined to the fornices or mammillary bodies and stereotaxic lesions of the amygdala that spared the adjacent cortical regions (entorhinal and perirhinal cortices) failed to produce a memory defect. However, lesions that were confined to the perirhinal and entorhinal cortex (Brodmann areas 35 and 36) and the closely associated parahippocampal cortex did cause a persistent memory defect, presumably by interrupting major afferent pathways conveying cortical information to the hippocampus. Lesions of the anteromedial parts of the diencephalon, which receive and send fibers to the amygdala and hippocampus, similarly abolished memory function.

These observations indicate that integrity of the hippocampal formations and the mediodorsal nuclei of the thalamus are essential for normal memory and learning. Interestingly, there are only sparse direct anatomic connections between these two regions. The importance assigned to the hippocampal formations and medial thalamic nuclei in memory function does not mean that the mechanisms governing this function are confined to these structures or that these parts of the brain form a "memory center." It means only that these are the sites where the smallest lesions have the most devastating effects on memory and learning. Normal memory function involves many parts of the brain in addition to diencephalic-hippocampal structures. It is also clear that extensive lesions of the neocortex may cause impairment of retentive memory and learning and that this effect is probably more dependent upon the size of the lesion than upon its locus. Of particular importance are the circumscribed areas of the cerebral cortex that are related to special forms of learning and memory (so-called modality-based memory), a subject that is considered in detail in the next chapter. Thus, a lesion of the dominant temporal lobe impairs the ability to remember words (loss of explicit semantic memory), and a lesion of the inferior parietal lobule undermines the recognition of written or printed words as well as the ability to relearn them. The dominant parietal lobe is related to recollection of geometric figures and numbers; the nondominant parietal lobe, to visuospatial relations; the inferoposterior temporal lobes, to the recognition of faces; and the dominant posterofrontal region, to acquiring and remembering motor skills and their affective associations.

Any hypothesis concerning the anatomic substratum of learning and retentive memory must therefore include not only the diencephalic-hippocampal structures but also special parts of the neocortex and midbrain reticular formation (for maintaining alertness). We would suggest that the diencephalic-hippocampal structures are involved in all active phases of learning and integration of new information, regardless of the sense avenue through which this information reaches the organism in order to be assimilated or of the final pathway of its expression, and it seems to make little difference whether the newly acquired information involves functions classed as purely cognitive or as emotional. This general aspect of memory function may suitably be designated as the "universal" or "U" factor of memory. Restricted regions of the temporal, parietal, and occipital cortex have particular relationships to the several special (modality-specific) memories, which may be designated as the "S" factors of memory.

It is a remarkable feature of the Korsakoff amnesic state that no matter how severe the defect in retentive memory may be, it is never complete. Certain past memories can be recalled, but imperfectly and with no regard for their normal temporal relationships, giving them a fictional quality and explaining many instances of confabulation. Another noteworthy fact is that long-standing social habits, automatic motor skills, and memory for words (language) and visual impressions (visual or pictorial attributes of persons, objects, and places) are unimpaired. Long periods of repetition and usage have made these implicit or procedural memories virtually automatic; they no longer require the participation of the diencephalic-hippocampal structures that were necessary to learn them originally. All of this suggests that these special memories, or coded forms of them, through a process of relearning and habituation, come to be stored or filed in other regions of the brain; i.e., they acquire a separate and autonomous anatomy.

Several fundamental questions concerning the amnesic syndrome remain unanswered. Not known is how a disease process, acting over a brief period of time, not only impairs all future learning but also wipes out a vast reservoir of past memories that had been firmly established for many years before the onset of the illness. Also unknown are the anatomic and physiologic mechanisms that govern immediate registration, which remains intact in even the most severely damaged patients with the Korsakoff amnesic syndrome. Equally obscure are the anatomic arrangements that enable the patient with virtually no capacity to retain any newly presented factual information to still learn some simple perceptual-motor and cognitive skills, even though there may be no memory of having been taught these skills in the first place. Other psychologic features of human memory that must be accounted for by any model purporting to explain this function are the importance of cueing in eliciting learned material and the imprecision of past memories, allowing for unwitting embellishment and false recollection, to the point of fabrication. The latter aspect has been a topic of considerable importance in children who have (or have not) been subjected to sexual abuse and in adults and children whose memories of past abuse have been suggested by the examiners (see Schacter).

The cellular mechanisms that are involved in learning and the formation of memories are only beginning to be understood. Kandel has provided a detailed review of current information on this subject (see references).

Classification of Diseases Characterized by an Amnesic Syndrome

The amnesic (Korsakoff) syndrome, as defined above, may be a manifestation of several neurologic disorders, identified by their mode of onset and clinical course, the associated neurologic signs, and ancillary findings (see Table 21-4). Each of the amnesic states listed in this table is considered at an appropriate point in subsequent chapters of this book. The only exception is so-called *transient global amnesia*, the nature of which is not entirely certain. It cannot with assurance be included with the epilepsies or the cerebrovascular diseases or any other category of disease and is therefore considered here.

Transient Global Amnesia

This is the name applied by Fisher and Adams to a particular type of memory disorder that occurs not infrequently in middle-aged and elderly persons and is characterized by an episode of amnesia and bewilderment lasting for several hours. The symptoms have their basis in an amnesia for events of the present and the recent past coupled with an ongoing anterograde amnesia. During the attack, there is no impairment in the state of consciousness and no overt sign of seizure activity; personal identification is intact, as are motor, sensory, and reflex functions. The patient's behavior is normal except for incessant, repetitive questioning about his immediate circumstances (e.g., "What am I doing here?"; "How did we get here?"). Unlike those with psychomotor epilepsy, the patient is alert, in contact with his surroundings, and capable of high-level intellectual activity and language function during the attack. As soon as the attack has ended, no abnormality of mental function is apparent except for a permanent gap in memory for the period of the attack itself and for a brief period (hours or days) preceding the attack. The patient may be left with a mild headache.

Table 21-4
Classification of the amnesic states

I. Amnesic syndrome of sudden onset—usually with gradual but incomplete recovery
   A. Bilateral or left (dominant) hippocampal infarction due to atherosclerotic-thrombotic or embolic occlusion of the posterior cerebral arteries or their inferior temporal branches
   B. Bilateral or left (dominant) infarction of anteromedial thalamic nuclei
   C. Infarction of the basal forebrain due to occlusion of anterior cerebral-anterior communicating arteries
   D. Subarachnoid hemorrhade (usually rupture of anterior communicating artery aneurysm)
   E. Trauma to the diencephalic, inferomedial temporal, or orbitofrontal regions
   F. Cardiac arrest, carbon monoxide poisoning, and other hypoxic states (hippocampal damage)
   G. Following prolonged status epilepticus
   H. Following delirium tremens

II. Amnesia of sudden onset and short duration
   A. Temporal lobe seizures
   B. Postconcussive states
   C. Transient global amnesia
   D. Hysteria

III. Amnesic syndrome of subacute onset with varying degrees of recovery, usually leaving permanent residua
   A. Wernicke-Korsakoff syndrome
   B. Herpes simplex encephalitis
   C. Tuberculous and other forms of meningitis characterized by a granulomatous exudate at the base of the brain

IV. Slowly progressive amnesic states
   A. Tumors involving the floor and walls of the third ventricle and limbic cortical structures
   B. Alzheimer disease (early stage) and other degenerative disorders with disproportionate affection of the temporal lobes
   C. Paraneoplastic "limbic" encephalitis

Hodges and Ward have made detailed psychologic observations in five patients during an attack. The psychologic deficit, except for its transience, was much the same as that in the permanent amnesia syndrome. Personality, cognition involving high-level functioning, semantic language, and visuospatial discrimination were all preserved. So-called immediate memory, i.e., registration (see above), was intact, but retentive memory was severely deranged. The extent of retrograde amnesia was highly variable, but characteristically it shrank after the attack, leaving a permanent retrograde gap of about 1 h. Some impairment of new learning persisted for up to a week after the acute attack.

In the Rochester, Minnesota, area, transient global amnesia (TGA) occurred at an annual rate of 5.2 cases per 100,000 population. The recurrence of such attacks is not uncommon, having been noted in 66 of 277 patients who were observed for an average period of 80 months (Miller et al) and in 16 of 74 patients followed for 7 to 210 months (Hinge et al). The latter authors estimate the mean annual recurrence rate to be so low (4.7 percent) that most elderly patients are likely to experience only one attack. One of our patients had more than 50 attacks, but among all the rest (more than 100 cases), 5 was the maximum. It seems children are not susceptible to the condition; however, a 13-year-old and 16-year-old with migraine were reported to have had similar attacks during participation in sports (Tosi and Righetti).

No consistent antecedent events have been identified, but certain ones—such as a highly emotional experience, pain, exposure to cold water, sexual intercourse, and mild head trauma—have been reported in some cases (Haas and Ross; Fisher). We have also seen several patients in whom the attacks appeared after minor diagnostic procedures such as colonoscopy, but the residual effects of sedation are suspect in some of these instances. Several cases have been reported in high-altitude climbers and created difficulty in distinguishing TGA from altitude sickness. One of the difficulties in judging the accuracy of the many published reports of TGA is whether, during the attack, the patient was or was not in contact with the environment and capable of high-level mental performance and whether a retrograde amnesia was present—important features in differentiating the attack from a partial complex seizure.

The pathogenesis of TGA has not been settled. It has been suggested that it represents an unusual form of temporal lobe epilepsy, but this seems unlikely. A large number of patient's have been studied with EEGs during an attack or shortly thereafter and have not shown seizure activity (Miller et al). Moreover, amnesic episodes due to seizures are usually much briefer than those of TGA, and most or all temporal lobe seizures are associated with impairment of consciousness and an inability to interact fully with the social and physical environment. Using EEG and nasopharyngeal leads, Rowan and Protass found mesiotemporal spike discharges in 5 of 7 patients. They attributed the discharges to ischemic lesions during drug-induced sleep. Palmini and coworkers cite exceptional cases of pure amnesic seizures in temporal lobe epilepsy, but even in their best examples, ictal and postictal function was not normal. More likely, transient global amnesia is ischemic in nature, though not athero-sclerotic-thrombotic. Rarely do the attacks progress to stroke. In the series of Hinge and associates, the observed rates of death and stroke were similar to the expected rates in the Danish population matched for age and sex. Hodges and Warlow, in a case-control study of 114 patients with transient global amnesia, also found no evidence of an association with cerebrovascular disease; there was, however, a significantly increased history of migraine in this group of patients, as there was in the series of Miller and coworkers (14 percent) and of Caplan and colleagues. The most compelling case for an ischemic basis, perhaps related in some way to migraine, comes from Stillhard and colleagues, who demonstrated bitemporal hypoperfusion during an attack of TGA, and from Strupp et al, who demonstrated left mediotemporal changes (interpreted as cellular edema) with diffusion-weighted MRI in 7 of 10 patients. The precipitation of identical attacks by vertebrobasilar and coronary angiography is also suggestive of an ischemic causation.

The benignity of episodic global amnesia in most patients is noteworthy. Once the history and examination have excluded vertebrobasilar ischemia and temporal lobe epilepsy, no treatment is required other than an explanation of the nature of the attack and reassurance, although we often hospitalize such patients briefly to be certain that the episode clears without further incident.

APPROACH TO THE PATIENT WITH DEMENTIA AND THE AMNESIC STATE

The physician presented with a patient suffering from dementia and amnesia must adopt an examination technique designed to expose the intellectual defect fully. Abnormalities of posture, movement, sensation, and reflexes cannot be relied upon to disclose the disease process, since the association areas of the brain may be severely damaged without demonstrable neurologic signs of these types. Suspicion of a dementing disease is aroused when the patient presents multiple complaints that seem totally unrelated to one another and to any known syndrome; when symptoms of irritability, nervousness, and anxiety are vaguely described and do not fit exactly into one of the major psychiatric syndromes; and when the patient is incoherent in describing the illness and the reasons for consulting a physician.

Three categories of data are required for the recognition and differential diagnosis of dementing brain disease:

1. A reliable history of the illness

2. Findings on mental examination, i.e., the mental status, as well as on the rest of the neurologic examination

3. Ancillary examinations: CT, MRI, sometimes lumbar puncture, EEG, and appropriate laboratory procedures, as described in Chap. 2

The history should generally be supplemented by information obtained from a person other than the patient, because, through lack of insight, the patient will have no grasp of his illness or its gravity; indeed, he may be ignorant even of his chief complaint. Special inquiry should be made about the patient's general behavior, capacity for work, personality changes, language, mood, special preoccupations and concerns, delusional ideas, hallucinatory experiences, personal habits, and such faculties as memory and judgment.

The examination of the mental status must be systematic and should include most of the following categories:

1. *Insight* (patient's replies to questions about the chief symptoms): What is your difficulty? Are you ill? When did your illness begin?
2. *Orientation* (knowledge of personal identity and present situation): What is your name, address, telephone number? What is your occupation? Are you married?
   a. *Place*: What is the name of the place where you are now (building, city, state)? How did you get here? What floor is it on? Where is the bathroom?
   b. *Time*: What is the date today (day of week and of month, month, year)? What time of the day is it? What meals have you had? When was the last holiday?
3. *Memory*.
   a. *Remote*: Tell me the names of your children and their birth dates. When were you married? What was your mother's maiden name? What was the name of your first schoolteacher? What jobs have you held? We find it useful to quiz the patient about cultural icons of the past that are appropriate to his age. Most patients should be able to name the presidents in reverse order dating to their twenties.
   b. *Recent past*: Tell me about your recent illness (compare with previous statements). What is my name (or the nurse's name)? When did you see

me for the first time? What tests were done yesterday? What were the headlines of the newspaper today?

   c. *Immediate recall—("short-term memory")*: Repeat these numbers after me (give series of 3, 4, 5, 6, 7, 8 digits at a speed of one per second). Now when I give a series of numbers, repeat them in reverse order.
   d. *Memorization (learning)*: The patient is given four simple data (examiner's name, date, time of day, and a fruit, structure, or trait, such as honesty) or a brief story containing several facts and is asked to repeat them. The capacity to reproduce them at intervals after committing them to memory is a test of *retentive memory span*.
   e. Another test of memory and verbal fluency we have found useful is to ask the patient to give the names of animals, vegetables, or makes of cars, as many as come to mind; most individuals can list at least 12 items in each category.
   f. *Visual span*: Show the patient a picture of several objects; then ask him to name the objects.

4. *Capacity for sustained mental activity and working memory*: Crossing out all the a's on a printed page; counting forward and backward; saying the months of the year forward and backward; spelling *world* forward and then backward.
   a. *Calculation*: Test ability to add, subtract, multiply, and divide. Subtraction of serial 3's and 7's from 100 is a good test of calculation as well as of concentration.
   b. *Constructions*: Ask the patient to draw a clock and place the hands at 7:45, a map of the United States, a floor plan of his house; ask him to copy a cube and other figures.
   c. *Abstract thinking*: See if the patient can describe the similarities and differences between classes of objects (orange and apple, horse and dog, desk and bookcase, newspaper and radio) or explain a proverb or fable.
5. *General behavior*: Attitudes, general bearing, evidence of hallucinosis, stream of coherent thought and attentiveness (ability to maintain a sequence of mental operations), mood, manner of dress, etc.
6. *Special tests of localized cerebral functions*: Grasping, sucking, aphasia battery, praxis with both hands, and cortical sensory function.

In order to enlist the full cooperation of the patient, the physician must prepare him for questions of this type. Otherwise, the patient's first reaction will be one of embarrassment or anger because of the implication that his mind is unsound. It should be pointed out to the patient that some individuals are rather forgetful or have difficulty in concentrating, or that it is necessary to ask specific questions in order to form some impression about his degree of nervousness when being examined. Reassurance that these are not tests of intelligence or of sanity is helpful. If the patient is extremely agitated, suspicious, or belligerent, intellectual functions must be inferred from his remarks and from information supplied by the family.

This type of mental status survey can be accomplished in about 10 min. In our experience, a high level of performance on all tests eliminates the possibility of dementia in 95 percent of cases. It may fail to identify a dementing disease in an uncooperative patient and in a highly intelligent individual in the earliest stages of disease.

The question of whether to resort to formal psychologic tests is certain to arise. Such tests yield quantitative data of comparative value but cannot of themselves be used for diagnostic purposes. A number of tests that measure the degree of dementia (Roth, Pfeiffer, Blessed, Mattis) rely essentially on the points mentioned above and a brief assessment of the patient's ability to accomplish the activities of daily living, which is lost in the later stages of disease. Probably the Wechsler Adult Intelligence Scale (WAIS) is the most useful. In this test, an index of deterioration is provided by the discrepancy between the vocabulary, picture-completion, and object-assembly tests as a group (these correlate well with premorbid intelligence and are relatively insensitive to dementing brain disease) and other measures of general performance, namely arithmetic, block-design, digit-span, and digit-symbol tests. The Wechsler Memory Scale estimates the degree of memory failure and can be used to distinguish the amnesic state from a more general dementia (discrepancy of more than 25 points between the WAIS and the memory scale). The Mini-Mental Status examination of Folstein and coworkers and the Short Test of Mental Status of Kokmen and colleagues are useful bedside methods of scoring cognitive impairment and following its progress. Questions that measure spatial and temporal orientation and retentive memory are the key items in most of these abbreviated scales of dementia. All of the aforementioned clinical and psychologic tests, and others as well, measure the same aspects of behavior and intellectual function. The WAIS and the

Mini-Mental Status examination of Folstein and associates are the most widely used clinically.

Management of the Demented Patient

Dementia is a clinical state of the most serious nature; though now sometimes impractical, it is usually worthwhile to admit patients to the hospital for a period of observation. Alternatively, the physician can see the patient serially over a period of weeks, during which time the appropriate laboratory tests (blood, cerebrospinal fluid analysis, and CT or MRI) can be carried out. The management of demented patients in the hospital may be relatively simple if they are quiet and cooperative. If the disorder of mental function is severe, it is helpful if a nurse, attendant, or member of the family can stay with the patient at all times.

The primary responsibility of the physician is to diagnose the treatable forms of dementia and to institute appropriate methods of therapy. Once it is established that the patient has an untreatable dementing brain disease and the diagnosis is sufficiently certain, a responsible member of the family should be informed of the medical facts and prognosis and assisted in the initiation of social and support services. Patients themselves need be told only that they have a nervous condition for which they are to be given rest and treatment. Little is accomplished by telling them more. If the dementia is slight and circumstances are suitable, patients should remain at home, continuing the activities of which they are capable. They should be spared responsibility and guarded against injury that might result from imprudent action. If they are still at work, plans for occupational retirement should be carried out. In more advanced stages of the disease, when mental and physical enfeeblement become pronounced, nursing home or institutional care should be arranged. So-called nerve tonics, vitamins, vasodilators, and hormones are of no value in checking the course of the illness or in regenerating atrophic tissue. The value of newer, centrally acting cholinergic agents in the treatment of Alzheimer disease is questionable and should be weighed against the need for repeated blood testing. They may, however, offer some psychologic support to the patient and family. Undesirable restlessness, nocturnal wandering, and belligerency may be reduced by administration of one of the antipsychotic or benzodiazepine drugs (see Chaps. 20, 43 and 48). Emotional lability and paranoid tendencies may be managed by the judicious use of olanzapine, risperidone, or haloperidol. Some patients are helped by short-acting sedatives such as lorazepam without worsening the mental condition, but all these drugs must be given with caution.

Questions asked by the patient's family must be answered patiently and sensitively by the physician. Common questions are: "Should I correct or argue with the patient?" (No.) "Can the patient be left alone?" "Must I be there constantly?" (Depends on specific circumstances and the severity of dementia.) "Should the patient manage his own money?" (Generally not.) "Will a change of environment or a trip help?" (Generally not—often the disruption in daily routine worsens behavior and orientation.) "Can he drive?" (Best to advise against driving in most instances.) "What shall we do about the patient's fears at night and his hallucinations?" (Medication under supervision may help.) "When is a nursing home appropriate?" "How will the condition worsen? What should the family expect, and when?" (Uncertain, but guided by one's understanding of the natural history of the disease.)

Visiting nurses, social agencies, live-in health care aides, day care settings, and respite care to relieve families from the constant burden of caring for the patient should all be used to advantage. Some of the inevitable practical problems accompanying the dissolution of personal life caused by dementia can be ameliorated by judicious use of powers of attorney, guardianship, and similar legal vehicles.

REFERENCES

AGGLETON JP, SAUNDERS RC: The relationships between temporal lobe and diencephalic structures implicated in anterograde amnesia. *Memory* 5:49, 1997.

ALEXANDER WP: Intelligence, concrete and abstract. *Br J Psychol* 1:1, 1935.

BERLYNE N: Confabulation. *Br J Psychiatry* 120:31, 1972.

BOLLER F, LOPEZ OL, MOOSY J: Diagnosis of dementia: Clinicopathologic correlations. *Arch Neurol* 39:1559, 1989.

BRANDT J, FOLSTEIN SE, FOLSTEIN MF: Differential cognitive impairment in Alzheimer's disease and Huntington's disease. *Ann Neurol* 23:555, 1988.

CAPLAN L, CHEDRU F, LHERMITTE F, MAYMAN G: Transient global amnesia and migraine. *Neurology* 31:1167, 1981.

CHAPMAN LF, WOLFF HF: The cerebral hemispheres and the highest integrative functions. *Arch Neurol* 1:357, 1959.

CUMMINGS JL, BENSON DF: *Dementia: A Clinical Approach*, 2nd ed. Boston, Butterworth, 1992.

EYSENCK HJ: Revolution in the theory and measurement of intelligence. *Eval Psicol* 1:99, 1985.

FISHER CM: Transient global amnesia: Precipitating activities and other observations. *Arch Neurol* 39:605, 1982.

FISHER CM, ADAMS RD: Transient global amnesia. *Acta Neurol Scand* 40(suppl 9):1, 1964.

FOLSTEIN MF, FOLSTEIN SE, MCHUGH PR: "Mini-mental status": A practical method for grading the cognitive state of patients for the clinician. *J Psychiatr Res* 12:189, 1975.

GADIAN DG, AICARDI J, WATKINS KE, et al: Developmental amnesia associated with early hypoxic–ischaemic injury. *Brain* 123:499, 2000.

GARDNER H: *Mutiple Intelligences: The Theory in Practice*. New York, Basic Books, 1993.

GOLDSTEIN K: *The Organism: A Holistic Approach to Biology*. New York, American Book Company, 1939, pp 35–61.

GROWDON JH, ROSSOR MN: *The Dementias*. Boston, Butterworth-Heinemann, 1998.

HAAS DC, ROSS GS: Transient global amnesia triggered by mild head trauma. *Brain* 109:251, 1986.

HERRNSTEIN RJ, MURRAY C: *The Bell Curve: Intelligence and Class Structure in American Life*. New York, Free Press, 1994.

HINGE HH, JENSEN TS, KJAER M, et al: The prognosis of transient global amnesia. *Arch Neurol* 43:673, 1986.

HODGES JR, WARD CD: Observations during transient global amnesia: A behavioral and neuropsychological study of five cases. *Brain* 112:595, 1989.

HODGES JR, WARLOW CP: The aetiology of transient global amnesia: A case-control study of 114 cases with prospective follow-up. *Brain* 113:639, 1990.

KANDEL ER: Cellular mechanisms of learning and the biological basis of individuality, in Kandel ER, Schwartz JH, Jessel TM (eds): *Principles of Neural Science,* 4th ed, New York, McGraw-Hill, 2000, pp 1247–1279.

KOKMEN E, SMITH GE, PETERSEN RC, et al: The short test of mental status: Correlations with standardized psychometric testing. *Arch Neurol* 48:725, 1991.

LASHLEY KS: *Brain Mechanisms and Intelligence*. Chicago, University of Chicago Press, 1929.

LEHRKE R: A theory of X-linkage of major intellectual traits. *Am J Ment Defic* 76:611, 1972.

MAYEUX R, FOSTER NL, ROSSOR MN, WHITEHOUSE PJ: The clinical evaluation of patients with dementia, in Whitehouse PJ (ed): *Dementia*. Philadelphia, Davis, 1993, pp 92–129.

MAYEUX R, STERN Y: Subcortical dementia. *Arch Neurol* 44:129, 1987.

MACKINTOSH NJ: *IQ and Human Intelligence*. Oxford, Oxford University Press, 1998.

MCHUGH PR: The basal ganglia: The region, the integration of its symptoms and implications for psychiatry and neurology, in Franks AJ, Ironside JW, Mindham RHS, et al (eds): *Function and Dysfunction in the Basal Ganglia*. New York, Manchester Press, 1990, pp 259–268.

MCHUGH PR, FOLSTEIN MF: Psychiatric syndromes of Huntington's chorea: A clinical and phenomenologic study, in Benson DF, Blumer D (eds): *Psychiatric Aspects of Neurologic Disease*. New York, Grune & Stratton, 1975, pp 267–286.

MCLEAN GE, JOHANSSON B, BERG S, et al: Substantial genetic influence on cognitive abilities in twins 80 or more years old. *Science* 276:1560, 1997.

MILLER JW, PETERSON RC, METTER EJ, et al: Transient global amnesia: Clinical characteristics and prognosis. *Neurology* 37:733, 1987.

MILLER JW, YANAGIHARA T, PETERSON RC, KLASS DW: Transient global amnesia and epilepsy. *Arch Neurol* 44:629, 1987.

MISHKIN M: A memory system in the monkey. *Phil Trans R Soc Lond B* 298:85, 1982.

MISHKIN M, DELACOUR J: An analysis of short term visual memory in the monkey. *J Exp Psychol Anim Behav Proc* 1:326, 1975.

MORRIS JC: Frontotemporal dementias, in Clark, CM, Trojanowski, JQ: *Neurodegenerative Dementias*. New York, McGraw-Hill, 2000, pp 279–290.

NEARY D, SNOWDEN JS, GUSTAFSON L, et al: Frontotemporal lobar degeneration:. A consensus on clinical diagnostic criteria. *Neurology* 51:1546, 1998.

PALMINI AL, GLOOR P, JONES-GOTMAN M: Pure amnestic seizures in temporal lobe epilepsy. *Brain* 115:749, 1992.

PHILLIPS S, SANGELANG V, STERNS G: Basal forebrain infarction. *Arch Neurol* 44:1134, 1987.

PIAGET J: *The Psychology of Intelligence*. London, Routledge & Kegan Paul, 1950.

PIERCY M: Neurological aspects of intelligence, in Vinken PJ, Bruyn GW (eds): *Handbook of Clinical Neurology*. Vol 3: *Disorders of Higher Nervous Activity*. Amsterdam, North-Holland, 1969, chap 18, pp 296–315.

PILLON B, DUBOIS B, PLOSKA A, AGID Y: Severity and specificity of cognitive impairment in Alzheimer's, Huntington's, and Parkinson's diseases and progressive supranuclear palsy. *Neurology* 41:634, 1991.

RIBOT TH: *Diseases of Memory: An Essay in Positive Psychology*. New York, Appleton, 1882.

ROWAN AJ, PROTASS LM: Transient global amnesia: Clinical and electroencephalographic findings in 10 cases. *Neurology* 29:869, 1979.

SCHACTER DL: *Searching for Memory*. New York, Basic Books, 1996.

SHIELDS J: *Monozygotic Twins Brought Up Apart and Brought Up Together: An Investigation into the Genetic and Environmental Causes of Variation in Personality*. London, Oxford University Press, 1962.

SHIELDS J: Heredity and psychological abnormality, in Eysenck HJ (ed): *Handbook of Abnormal Psychology*, 2nd ed. London, Pitman, 1973.

SLATER E, COWIE V: *The Genetics of Mental Disorders*. London, Oxford University Press, 1971, pp 196–200.

SPEARMAN CE: *The Abilities of Man*. London, Macmillan, 1927.

Stillhard G, Landis T, Schiess R, et al: Bitemporal hypoperfusion in transient global amnesia: 99m-Tc-HM-PAO SPECT and neuropsychological findings during and after an attack. *J Neurol Neurosurg Psychiatry* 53:339, 1990.

Strupp M, Br¸ning R, Hua R, et al: Diffusion-weighted MRI in transient global amnesia: Elevated signal intensity in the left mesial temporal lobe in 7 of 10 patients. *Ann Neurol* 43:164, 1998.

Terman LM, Ogden MH: *The Gifted Group at Mid-life: Genetic Studies of Genius*. Vol IV. Stanford, CA, Stanford University Press, 1959.

The Lund and Manchester Groups: Consensus statement: Clinical and neuropathological criteria for fronto-temporal dementia. *J Neurol Neurosurg Psychiatry* 57:416, 1994.

Tierney MC, Snow WG, Reid DW, et al: Psychometric differentiation of dementia. *Arch Neurol* 44:720, 1987.

Thurstone LL: *The Vectors of the Mind*. Chicago, University of Chicago Press, 1953.

Tomlinson BE, Blessed G, Roth M: Observations on the brains of demented old people. *J Neurol Sci* 11:205, 1970.

Tosi L, Righetti CA: Transient global amnesia and migraine in young people. *Clin Neurol Neurosurg* 99:63, 1997.

Turner G: Intelligence and the X chromosome. *Lancet* 347:1814, 1996.

Van Gijn J: Leukoaraiosis and vascular dementia. *Neurology* 51(suppl 3):83, 1998.

Van Horn G: Dementia. *Am J Med* 83:101, 1987.

Victor M, Agamanolis D: Amnesia due to lesions confined to the hippocampus: A clinical-pathologic study. *J Cog Neurosci* 2:246, 1990.

Victor M, Adams RD, Collins GH: *The Wernicke-Korsakoff Syndrome*, 2nd ed. Philadelphia, Davis, 1989.

Wade JPH, Mirsen TR, Hachinski VC, et al: The clinical diagnosis of Alzheimer's disease. *Arch Neurol* 44:24, 1987.

Wechsler D: *The Measurement of Adult Intelligence*, 3rd ed. Baltimore, Williams & Wilkins, 1944.

Willerman L: *The Psychology of Individual and Group Differences*. San Francisco, Freeman, 1978, pp 106–129.

Zola-Morgan S, Squire LR, Amaral DG: Lesions of the amygdala that spare adjacent cortical regions do not impair memory or exacerbate the impairment following lesions of the hippocampal formation. *J Neurosci* 9:1922, 1989.

Zola-Morgan S, Squire LR, Amaral DG: Lesions of the hippocampal formation but not lesions of the fornix or the mammillary nuclei produce long-lasting memory impairment in monkeys. *J Neurosci* 9:898, 1989.

Zola-Morgan S, Squire LR, Amaral DG: Lesions of perirhinal and parahippocampal cortex that spare the amygdala and hippocampal formation produce severe memory impairment. *J Neurosci* 9:4355, 1989.

Chapter 22

NEUROLOGIC DISORDERS CAUSED BY LESIONS IN PARTICULAR PARTS OF THE CEREBRUM

The age-old controversy about cerebral functions—whether they are diffusely represented in the cerebrum, with all parts roughly equivalent, or localized to certain lobes or regions—was resolved long ago. Clinicians and physiologists have demonstrated beyond doubt that particular cortical regions are related to certain functions. For example, the pre- and postrolandic zones are motor and sensory, the striate-parastriate occipital zones are visual, the superior temporal and transverse gyri of Heschl are auditory. Beyond these broad correlations, however, there is a notable lack of precision in the cortical localization of many of the behavioral and mental operations described in Chaps. 20 and 21. As to the higher-order physiologic and psychologic functions—such as attention, vigilance, apperception, thinking, etc.—virtually none has been assigned a precise and predictable anatomy; or, more accurately, the neural systems on which they depend are widely distributed.

One may suitably pause and inquire into what precisely is meant by *cerebral localization*. Does it refer to the physiologic function of a circumscribed aggregate of neurons in the cerebral cortex, indicated clinically by a loss of that function (negative symptom) when the neurons in question are paralyzed or destroyed? From what we know of the rich connectivity of all parts of the so-called cortical centers, one must assume that this is not the case, but only that a lesion in a particular part or in the fiber systems with which it is connected is most consistently associated with certain impairments of function. It is therefore appropriate for the clinician to operate on the principle of correlation between certain neurologic signs or syndromes and damage (lesion) in particular regions of the brain. Nevertheless, it must be readily apparent, but is worth repeating, that certain positive symptoms resulting from the lesion—e.g., the grasping and sucking responses—cannot arise from destroyed neurons but are attributable to the now deranged or disinhibited functions of closely related intact parts of the cerebrum. And how is one to interpret the seeming inconsistencies from one case report to another, in which several different functions have been assigned to the same region of the brain and any one region appears to be the anatomic substratum of multiple functions? Most modern theorists who deal with this subject believe that the organization of cerebral function is based on discrete networks of closely interconnected afferent and efferent neurons in each region of the brain. These networks must be linked by both regional and more widespread systems of fibers.

Pertinent to this topic are a number of morphologic and physiologic data. Along strictly histologic lines, Brodmann distinguished 47 different areas of cerebral cortex (Figs. 22-1 and 22-2), and von Economo identified more than twice this number. Although this parceling was criticized by Bailey and von Bonin, it is still used by physiologists and clinicians, who find that Brodmann's areas do indeed approximate certain functional zones of the cerebral cortex (Fig. 22-3). Also, the cortex has been shown to differ in its various parts by virtue of its particular connections with other areas of the cortex and with the thalamic nuclei and other lower centers. Hence, one must regard the cortex as a heterogeneous array of many anatomic systems, each with highly organized intercortical and central (thalamic) connections.

Some general aspects of cerebrocortical anatomy are noteworthy. The sheer size of the cortex is remarkable. Unfolded, it has a surface extent of about 4000 cm^2—about the size of a full sheet of newsprint (right and left pages). Contained in the cortex are many

Figure 22-1

Cytoarchitectural zones of the human cerebral cortex, according to Brodmann. A. Lateral surface. B. Medial surface. The functional zones of the cortex are illustrated in Fig. 22-3.

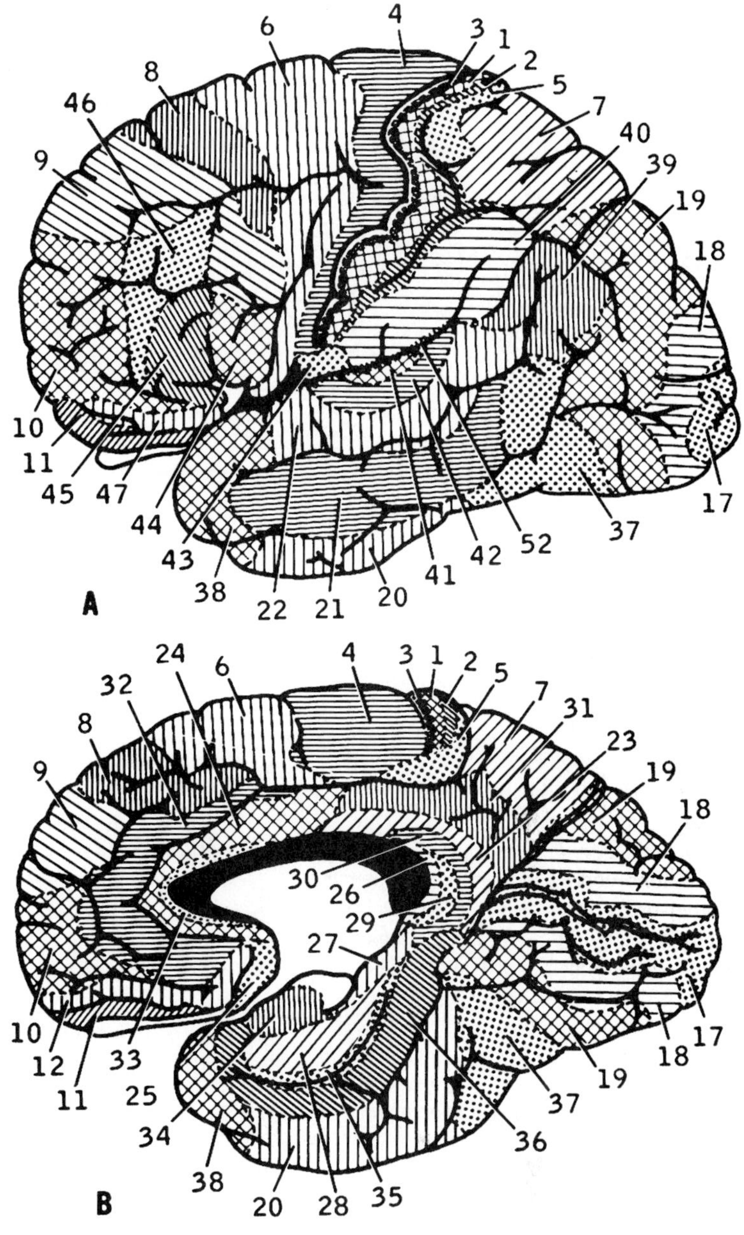

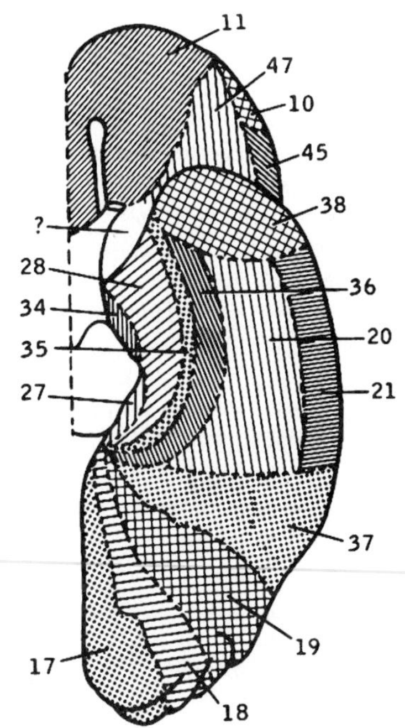

Figure 22-2

Cytoarchitectural zones of the cerebral cortex, basal inferior surface, according to Brodmann.

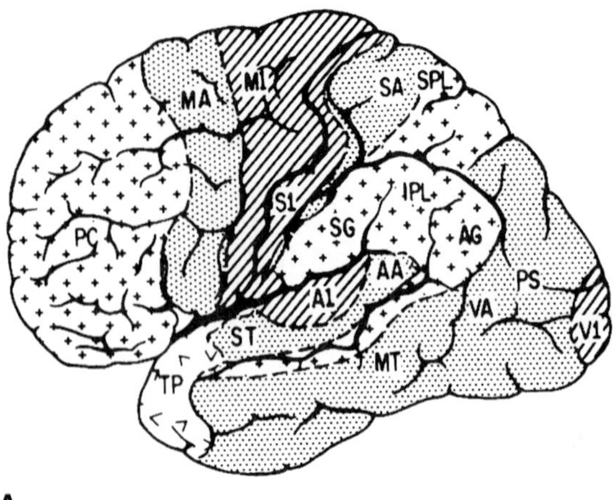

A

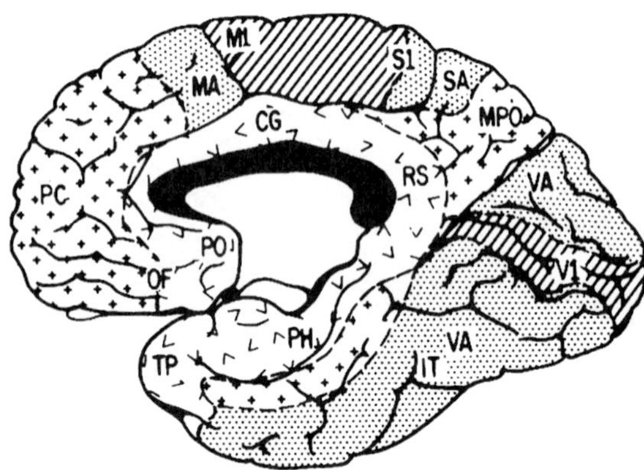

B

Figure 22-3

A *and* B. *Approximate distribution of functional zones on lateral (above) and medial (below) aspects of the cerebral cortex. Abbreviations: AA, auditory association cortex; AG, angular gyrus; A1, primary auditory cortex; CG, cingulate cortex; INS, insula; IPL, inferior parietal lobule; IT, inferior temporal gyrus; MA, motor association cortex; MPO, medial parieto-occipital area; MT, middle temporal gyrus; M1, primary motor area; OF, orbitofrontal region; PC, prefrontal cortex; PH, parahippocampal region; PO, parolfactory area; PS, peristriate cortex; RS, retrosplenial area; SA, somatosensory association cortex; SG, supramarginal gyrus; SPL, superior parietal lobule; ST, superior temporal gyrus; S1, primary somatosensory area; TP, temporopolar cortex; VA, visual association cortex; V1, primary visual cortex. (Redrawn from Mesulam M-M, by permission.)*

billions of neurons (estimated at 10 to 30 billion) and five times this number of glial cells. The intercellular synaptic connections number in the trillions. Since nerve cells look alike and presumably function alike, the remarkable diversity in human intelligence, store of knowledge, and behavior must depend on infinite variations in neuronal interconnectivity.

Most of the human cerebral cortex is phylogenetically recent, hence the term *neocortex*. It has also been referred to as *isocortex* (Vogt) because of its uniform embryogenesis and morphology. These latter features distinguish the neocortex from the older and less uniform cortex, which comprises mainly the hippocampus and olfactory cortex and is referred to as the *allocortex* ("other cortex").

Concerning the detailed histology of the neocortex, six layers (laminae) can be distinguished, from the pial surface to the underlying white matter: molecular (or plexiform) external granular, external pyramidal, internal granular, ganglionic (or internal pyramidal), and multiform (or fusiform). These are illustrated in Fig. 22-4. Two cell types—relatively large pyramidal cells and smaller, more numerous rounded (granular) cells—predominate, and variations in the lamination of the neocortex are largely determined by variations in the size and density of these neuronal types. Many variations in lamination have been described by the cortical mapmakers, but two main types of neocortex are recognized: (1) the *homotypical cortex*, in which the six-layered arrangement is readily discerned, and (2) the *heterotypical cortex*, in which the layers are less distinct. The association cortex—the large areas (75 percent of the surface) that are not obviously committed to primary motor or sensory functions—is generally of this latter type. The homotypical cortex is characterized by either granular or agranular nerve cells. The precentral cortex (Brodmann's areas 4 and 6, mainly motor region) is dominated by pyramidal rather than granular cells, especially in layer V; hence the term *agranular* (Fig. 22-5). In contrast, primary sensory cortex—postcentral gyrus (areas 3, 1, 2), banks of the calcarine sulcus (area 17), and the transverse gyri of Heschl (areas 41 and 42)—where layers II and IV are strongly developed for the receipt of afferent impulses, has been termed *granular cortex* (koniocortex in older nomeclature) because of the marked predominance of granular cells (Fig. 22-5).

The intrinsic organization of the neocortex follows the pattern elucidated by Lorente de Nó. He described vertical chains of neurons that are arranged in cylindrical modules or columns, each containing 100 to 300 neurons and heavily interconnected up and down between cortical layers and to a lesser extent horizontally. Figure 22-6

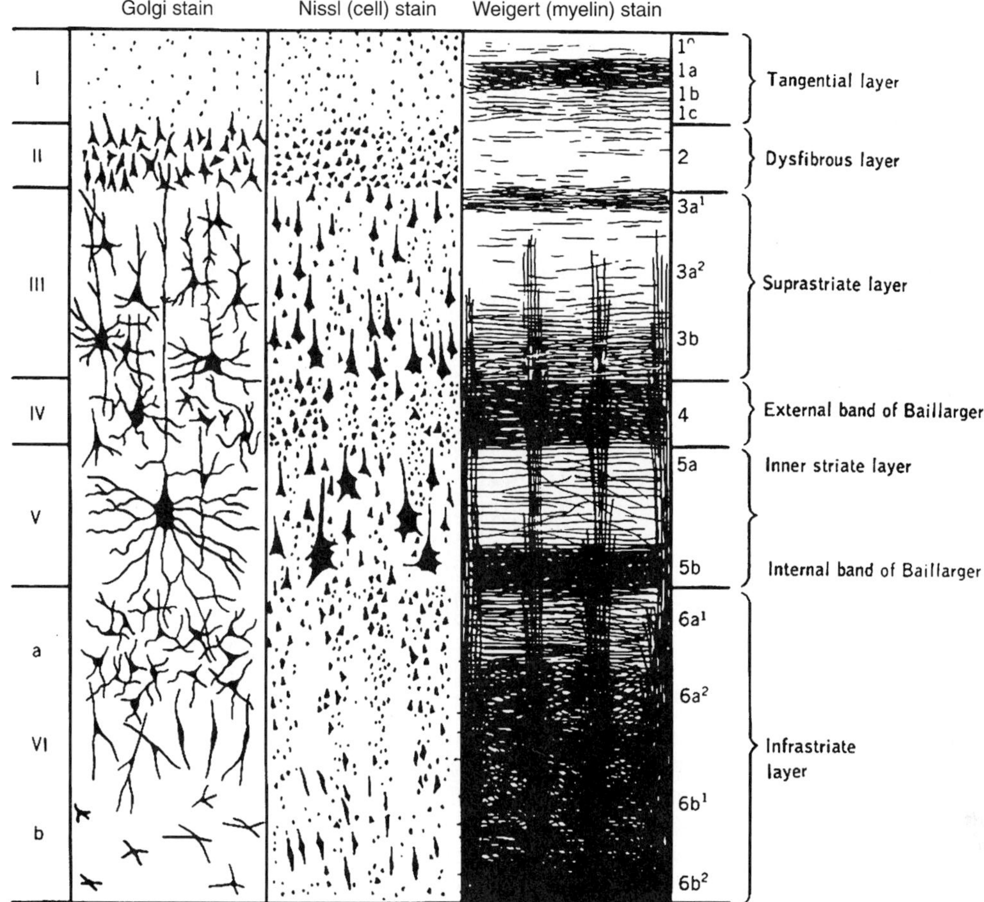

Figure 22-4

The basic cytoarchitecture of the cerebral cortex, adapted from Brodmann. The six basic cell layers are indicated on the left, and the fiber layers on the right.

illustrates the fundamental vertical (columnar) organization of these neuronal systems. Afferent fibers activated by various sensory stimuli terminate in layers IV and II. These impulses are then transmitted by internuncial neurons (interneurons) to adjacent superficial and deep layers and then to appropriate efferent neurons in layer V. Neurons of lamina III send axons to other parts of the association cortex in the same and opposite hemisphere. Neurons of layer VI project mainly to the thalamus. In the macaque brain, each pyramidal neuron in layer V has about 60,000 synapses, and one afferent axon may synapse with dendrites of as many as 5000 neurons; these figures convey some idea of the wealth and complexity of cortical connections. These columnar ensembles of neurons, on both the sensory and motor sides, function as the elementary working units of the cortex, in a manner indicated in Chaps. 3, 8, and 9.

Whereas certain regions of the cerebrum are committed to special perceptual, motor, sensory, mnemonic, and linguistic activities, the intricacy of the anatomy and psychophysical mechanisms in each region are just beginning to be envisioned. The lateral geniculate-occipital organization in relation to color vision and recognition of form, stemming from the work of Hubel and Wiesel, may be taken as an example. In area 17, the polar region of the occipital lobe, there are discrete, highly specialized groups of neurons, each of which is activated in a small area of lamina 4 by spots of light or lines and transmitted via particular cells in the lateral geniculate bodies; other groups of adjacent cortical

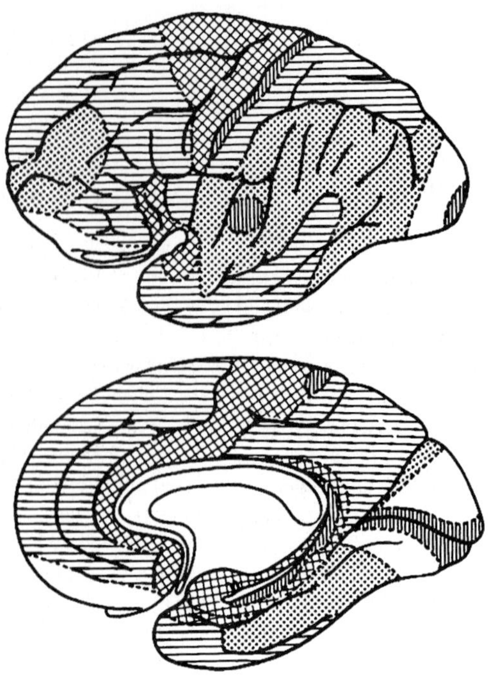

Figure 22-5

The five fundamental types of cerebral cortex, according to von Economo: 1, agranular; 2, frontal; 3, parietal; 4, polar; and 5, granular.

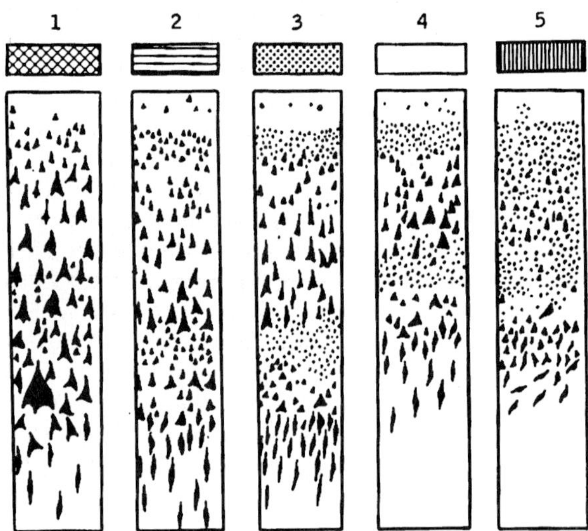

neurons are essential for the perception of color (see also page 487). Preparedness for all types of visual stimulation and recognition of objects, faces, and verbal and mathematical symbols also involves these areas but is integrated with other cortical regions. Lying between the main unimodal receptive areas for vision, audition, and somesthetic perception are zones of integration called *heteromodal* cortices. In the latter regions, neurons respond to more than one sensory modality or neurons responsive to one sense are interspersed with neurons responsive to another sense.

Cortical-subcortical integrations are reflected in volitional or commanded movements. A simple movement of the hand, for example, requires activation of the premotor cortex (also called *accessory motor cortex*), which projects to the striatum and cerebellum and back to the motor cortex via a complex thalamic circuitry before the direct and indirect corticospinal pathways can activate certain combinations of spinal motor neurons (see Chaps. 3 and 4).

Interregional connections of the cerebrum are required for all natural sensorimotor functions; moreover, as indicated above, their destruction disinhibits or releases other areas. Denny-Brown has referred to these as cortical tropisms. Thus, destruction of the premotor areas, leaving precentral and parietal lobes intact, results in release of the sensorimotor automatisms of groping, grasping, and sucking. Parietal lesions result in complex avoidance movements to contactual stimuli. Temporal lesions lead to a visually activated reaction to every observed object and its oral exploration, and limbic sexual mechanisms are rendered hyperactive.

Some of the aforementioned disorders and others known simplistically as *disconnection syndromes* depend not merely on involvement of certain cortical regions but also on the interruption of inter- and intrahemispheral fiber tracts. Some of these disconnections are indicated in Fig. 22-7; the involved fiber systems include the corpus callosum, anterior commissure, uncinate temporofrontal fasciculus, occipito- and temporoparietal tracts, etc. Extensive white matter lesions may virtually isolate certain cortical zones. Another example is the isolation of the perisylvian language areas from the rest of the cortex, as occurs with anoxic-ischemic infarction of border zones between major cerebral arteries.

These aspects of cerebral localization—brought out so clearly in the writings of Wernicke, Déjerine, and Liepmann and resurrected more recently by Geschwind—have been elaborated by the Russian school of physiologists and psychologists. They view function not as the direct property of a particular, highly specialized group of cells in one region of the cerebrum but as the product of complex, diffusely distributed activity by which sensory stimuli are analyzed and integrated at various levels of the nervous system and are united, through a system of temporarily acquired (experientially derived)

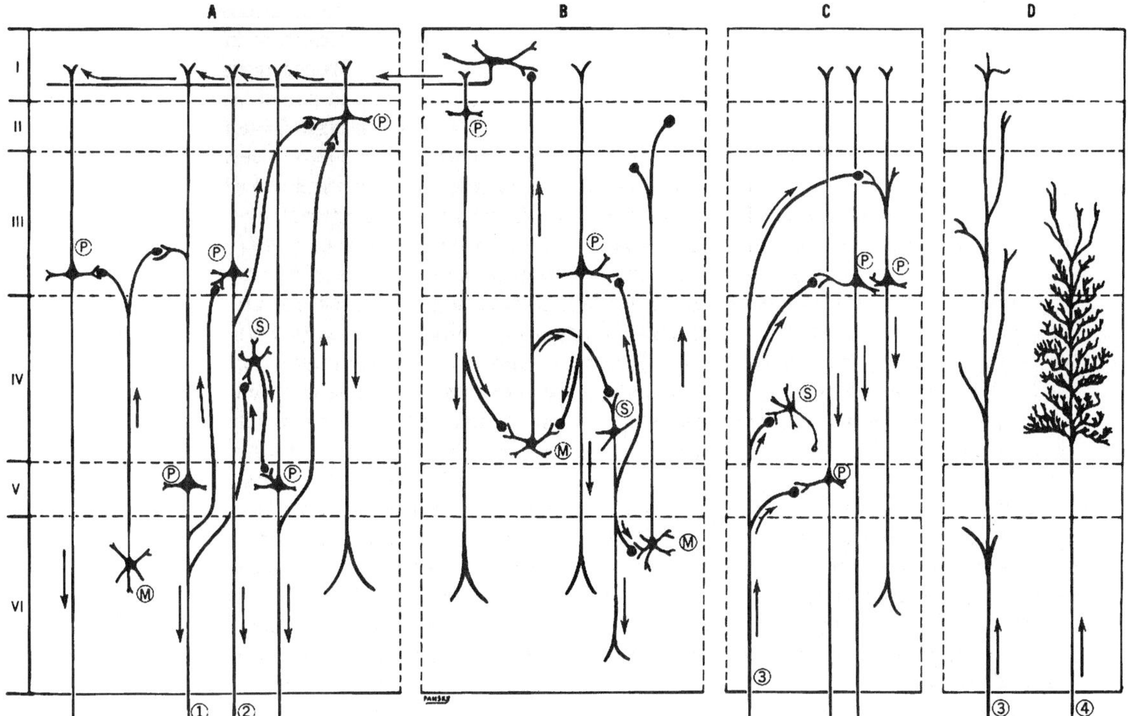

Figure 22-6

The organization of neuronal systems in the granular cortex, following the plan of Lorente de Nó. The black spheres represent points of synapse. A. *Connections of efferent cortical neurons.* B. *Connections of intracortical neurons.* C. *Connections of afferent (thalamocortical) neurons.* D. *Mode of termination of afferent cortical fibers. P, pyramidal cell; M, Martinotti cell; S, spindle cell; 1, projection efferent; 2, association efferent; 3, specific afferent; 4, association afferent.*

connections, into a working mosaic adapted to accomplish a particular task. To some extent, this model has been corroborated by functional imaging studies [positron emission tomography (PET) and functional magnetic resonance imaging (fMRI)], which show increased metabolic activity in several cortical regions during any human behavior, including willed motor acts, language tasks, and perceptive and apperceptive sensory experiences. Within such a functional system, the initial and final links (the task and the effect) remain unchanged, but the intermediate links (the means of performance of a given task) may be modified within wide limits and will never be exactly the same on two consecutive occasions. Thus, when a certain act is called for by a spoken command, the dominant temporal lobe must receive the message and transmit it to the premotor areas. Or it may be initiated by the intention of the individual, in which case the first measurable cerebral activity (a negative readiness potential) occurs anterior to the premotor cortex. The motor cortex is always under the dynamic control of the proprioceptive, visual, and vestibular systems. These are some of the recognizable elements in motor performance; loss of a skilled act may be caused by a lesion that affects any one of several elements in the act, either the motor centers themselves or their connections with the other elements.

This concept of cerebral function and localization, which applies to all mental activities, contradicts both the concept that postulates the functional equivalence of all cerebral regions and also the one that assumes strict localization of any given activity within one part of the brain. It is open to neuropsychologic analysis, which has been the approach of A. R. Luria and others of the Russian school and of behavioral psychologists of the Skinner school.

Another theoretical scheme of cerebral anatomy and function systematizes cortices of similar overall structure and divides the cerebral mantle into three

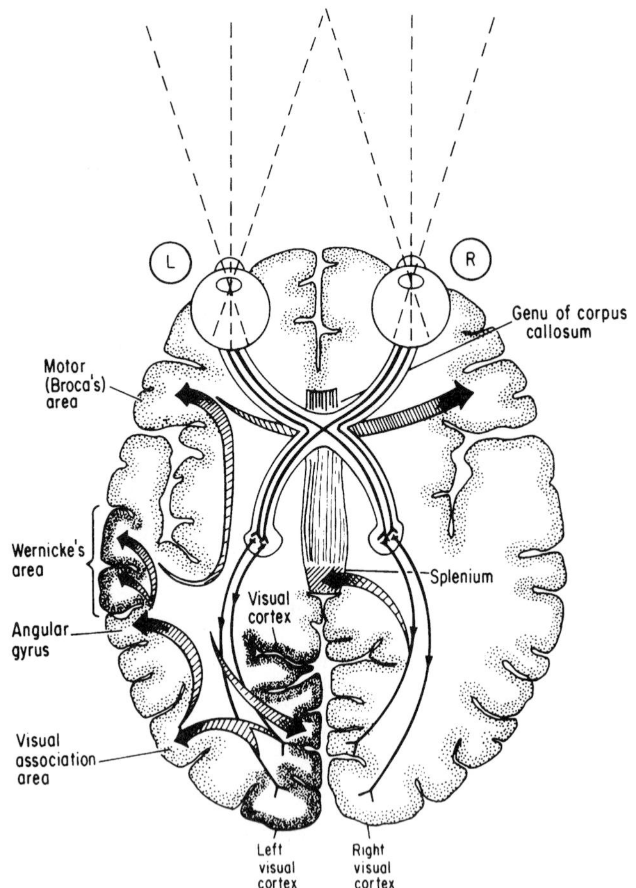

Figure 22-7

Connections involved in naming a seen object and in reading. The visual pattern is transferred from the visual cortex and association areas to the angular gyrus, which arouses the auditory pattern in the Wernicke area. The auditory pattern is transmitted to the Broca area, where the articulatory form is aroused and transferred to the contiguous face area of the motor cortex. With destruction of the left visual cortex and splenium (or intervening white matter), words perceived in the right visual cortex cannot cross over to the language areas and the patient cannot read.

longitudinally oriented zones. The central vegetative neuronal system (allocortex and hypothalamus) provides the mechanisms for all internal functions—the *milieu interieur* of Bernard and Cannon. The outer zone, comprising the sensorimotor and association cortices and their projections, provides the mechanisms for perceiving the external world and interacting with it. The region between (limbic-paralimbic cortices) provides the bridges that permit the adaptation of organismal needs to the external environment. This concept of central nervous system function, first proposed by Broca, was elaborated by Yakovlev and has been adopted more recently by Mesulam and by Benson. Such a model retains to a large degree the cytoarchitectural similarities among areas that serve similar functions (i.e., the scheme of Brodmann) and also respects the sequence of maturation (myelination) of connecting pathways proposed by Flechsig (Fig. 28-3), which corresponds to the functional development of the primary, secondary, and tertiary associative cortical regions. In this way, localization may be viewed as the product of genetic patterns of structure, which mature during development, and their synaptic formations, which permit the development of complex circuits during lifelong learning and experience.

From these remarks it follows that subdivision of the cerebrum into frontal, temporal, parietal, and occipital lobes is somewhat of an anachronism and has a limited functional validity (although, in clinical work, it still serves a practical purpose as a shorthand way of localizing a lesion). These delineations were made long before our first glimmer of knowledge about the function of the cerebrum. Even when the neurohistologists began parceling the neocortex, they found that their areas did not fall within zones bounded by sulci and fissures. Therefore, when the terms *frontal*, *parietal*, *temporal*, and *occipital* are used in the text below, it is mainly to provide the reader with familiar anatomic landmarks.

SYNDROMES CAUSED BY LESIONS OF THE FRONTAL LOBES

Anatomic and Physiologic Considerations

The frontal lobes lie anterior to the central, or rolandic, sulcus and superior to the sylvian fissure (Fig. 22-8). They are larger in humans (30 percent of the cerebrum) than in any other primate (9 percent in the macaque). Several different systems of neurons are located here, and they subserve different functions. Brodmann's areas 4, 6, 8, and 44 relate specifically to motor activities. The *primary motor cortex*, i.e., area 4, is directly connected with somatosensory neurons of the anterior part of the postcentral gyrus as well as with other parietal areas, thalamic and red nuclei, and the reticular formation of the brainstem. The supplementary motor cortex, a portion of area 6, shares most of these connections. As pointed out in earlier chapters, all motor activity needs sensory guidance, and this comes from the somesthetic, visual, and auditory cortices and from the cerebellum via the ventral tier of thalamic nuclei.

Area 8 is concerned with turning the eyes and head contralaterally. Area 44 of the dominant hemisphere (Broca's area) and the contiguous part of area 4 are "centers" of motor speech and related functions of the lips, tongue, larynx, and pharynx; bilateral lesions in these areas cause paralysis of articulation, phonation, and deglutition. The medial-orbital gyri and anterior parts of the cingulate gyri, which are the frontal components of the limbic system, take part in the control of respiration, blood pressure, peristalsis, and other autonomic functions. The most anterior parts of the frontal lobes (areas 9 to 12 and 45 to 47), sometimes referred to as the

Figure 22-8

Photograph of lateral surface of the human brain. (From Carpenter MB, Sutin J: Human Neuroanatomy, 8th ed. Baltimore, Williams & Wilkins, 1982, by permission.)

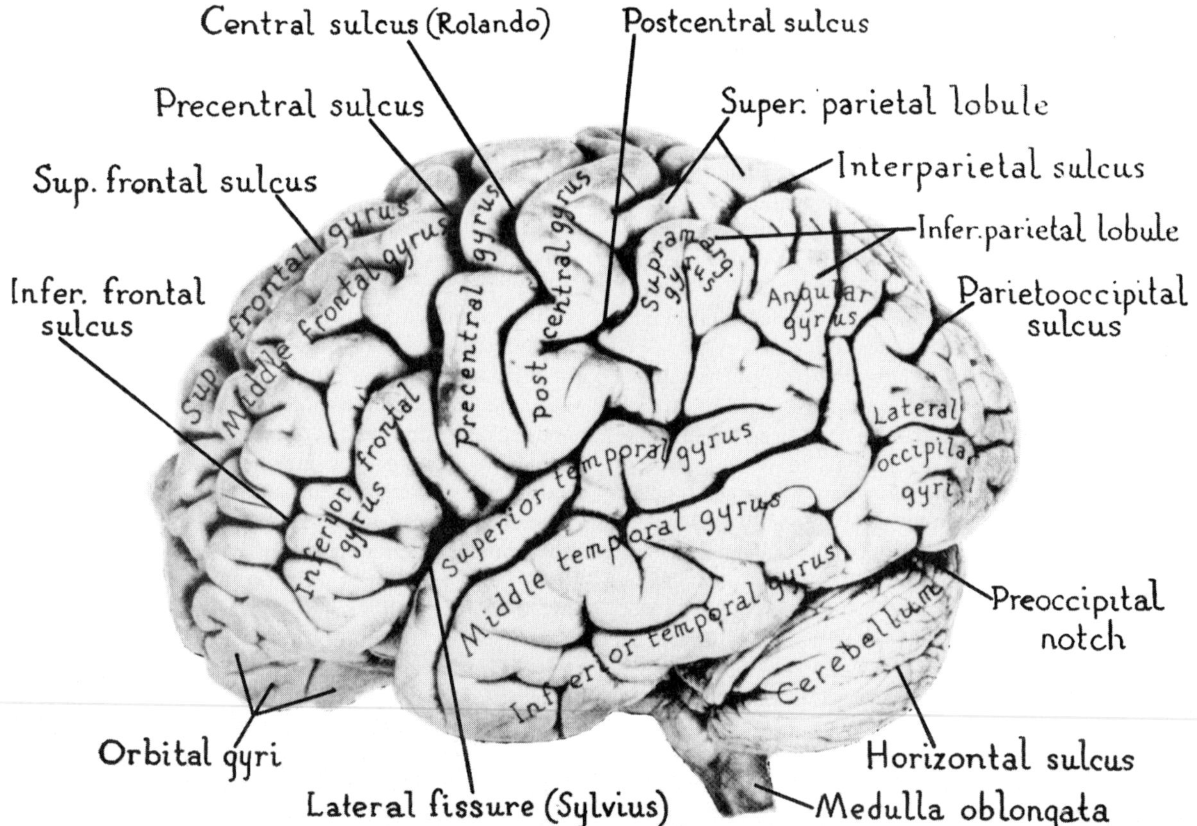

prefrontal areas, are particularly well developed in human beings but have imprecisely determined functions. They are not, strictly speaking, parts of the motor cortex, in the sense that electrical stimulation evokes no direct movement; the prefrontal cortex is said to be inexcitable. Yet these areas are involved in the initiation of planned action and executive control of all mental operations, including emotional expression.

The frontal agranular cortex (areas 4 and 6) and, more specifically, pyramidal cells of layer V of the pre- and postcentral convolutions provide most of the cerebral efferent motor system known as the pyramidal, or corticospinal, tract (see Figs. 3-2 and 3-3). Another massive projection from these regions is the frontopontocerebellar tract. In addition, there are other fiber systems that pass from frontal cortex to the caudate and putamen, subthalamic and red nuclei, brainstem reticular formation, substantia nigra, and inferior olive as well as to the ventrolateral, mediodorsal, and dorsolateral nuclei of the thalamus. Areas 8 and 6 are connected with the ocular and other brainstem motor nuclei and with identical areas of the other cerebral hemisphere through the corpus callosum. A massive bundle connects the frontal with the occipital lobe, and an uncinate bundle connects the orbital part of the frontal lobe with the temporal lobe.

The granular frontal cortex has a rich system of connections both with lower levels of the brain (medial and ventral nuclei and pulvinar of the thalamus) and with virtually all other parts of the cerebral cortex, including its limbic and paralimbic parts. As to its limbic connections, the frontal lobe is unique among cerebrocortical areas. Electrical stimulation of the orbitofrontal cortex and cingulate gyrus has manifest effects on respiratory, circulatory, and other vegetative functions. These parts of the frontal cortex also receive major afferent projections from other parts of the limbic system, presumably to mediate the emotional responses to sensory experiences, and they project to other parts of the limbic and paralimbic cortices (hippocampus, parahippocampus, anterior pole of the temporal lobe), amygdala, and midbrain reticular formation. The frontal-limbic connections are described in greater detail in Chap. 25.

Blood is supplied to the medial parts of the frontal lobes by the anterior cerebral artery and to the convexity and deep regions by the superior (rolandic) division of the middle cerebral artery.

With respect to the physiology of the frontal lobes, the literature is replete with unsubstantiated claims. Here are presumed to reside the mechanisms that govern personality, character, motivation, and our unique capacities for abstract thinking, introspection, and planning. These qualities and traits do not lend themselves to easy definition and study or to discrete localization. Most of them are too subtle to isolate and measure. Except for the more posterior frontal mechanisms subserving motor speech and motility and certain behaviors relating to impulse, neurologists have had great difficulty in delineating a group of symptoms indicative of frontal lobe disease, as will be evident in further discussion.

Clinical Effects of Frontal Lobe Lesions

In a general sense, the anterior half of the brain is committed to the monitoring and execution of all cerebral activity. This means that all activities—be they motor, cognitive, or emotional—are planned and initiated here. Of necessity in such a scheme, there must also be inhibitory mechanisms that control or modulate behavior. Thus, aside from the overt abnormalities of motor, speech, and voluntary movement, lesions of the frontal lobes give rise to a loss of drive, impairment of consecutive planning, inability to maintain serial relationships of events and to shift easily from one mental activity to another—at times in combination with the release (disinhibition) of sucking, grasping, and groping reflexes and other so-called utilization behaviors. Furthermore, in the emotional sphere, frontal lobe lesions may cause anhedonia, apathy, loss of self-control, disinhibited social behavior, and euphoria.

For descriptive purposes, the clinical effects of frontal lobe lesions can be grouped under the following categories: (1) motor abnormalities related to the prerolandic motor cortex; (2) speech and language disorders related to the dominant hemisphere; (3) impairment of certain cognitive functions, especially attention, concentration, capacity for sustained mental activity, and ability to shift from one line of thought or action to another—i.e., both impersistence and perseveration; (4) akinesia and lack of initiative and spontaneity (apathy and abulia); (5) other changes in personality, particularly in mood and self-control (disinhibition of behavior); (6) incontinence of bladder and bowel; and (7) a distinctive abnormality of gait (page 128).

Motor Abnormalities Of the various effects of frontal lobe lesions, most is known about the motor abnormalities. Electrical stimulation of the motor cortex elicits contraction of corresponding muscle groups, and focal seizure activity has a similar effect. Stimulation of Brodmann area 4 produces movement of discrete muscle groups or, if sufficiently refined, of individual muscles. Repertoires of larger coordinated movements are evoked by stimulation of area 6, the premotor cortex. Voluntary movement involves the motor cortex in its entirety. Lesions in the posterior part of the frontal lobe cause spastic paralysis of the contralateral face, arm, and leg. Involved are the direct corticospinal tract and other indirect tracts that descend from the motor, premotor, supplementary motor, and anterior parietal cortex to the spinal cord, either directly or via the red and pontomedullary reticular nuclei in the brainstem. Lesions of the more anterior and medial parts of the motor cortex (area 6 and supplementary motor area of 8—the *premotor cortex*) result in less paralysis and more spasticity as well as a release of sucking, groping, and grasping reflexes, the mechanisms of which reside in the parietal lobe and which, according to Denny-Brown, are tropisms, or automatisms, that are normally inhibited by the frontal cortex.

Mutism, contralateral motor neglect, and impairment of bibrachial coordination were found by Laplane and his colleagues to follow ablation of the right or left supplementary motor area. On the basis of radioactive blood flow studies, Roland and colleagues and Fuster have suggested that an important function of the supplementary motor area is the ordering of motor tasks or the recall of memorized motor sequences—further evidence of the executive functions of the frontal lobes. Temporary paralysis of contralateral eye turning and sometimes head turning follows a destructive lesion in area 8, on the dorsolateral aspect (convexity) of the cerebral cortex, often referred to as the frontal eye field (see Fig. 22-1). Seizure activity in this area causes a tonic deviation of the head and eyes to the opposite side. Destruction of Broca's convolution (areas 44 and 45) and adjacent insular and motor cortex results in a reduction or loss of motor speech, agraphia, and apraxia of the face, lips, and tongue (see Chap. 23).

When the lesions of the motor parts of the frontal lobe are bilateral, there is a quadriplegia or quadriparesis in which the weakness is not only more severe but also more extensive, affecting cranial muscles (pseudobulbar palsy) as well as spinal ones.

Damage to the cortices anterior to areas 6 and 8—i.e., to areas 9, 10, 45, and 46—the *prefrontal cortex*, and also the anterior cingulate gyri—has less easily defined effects on motor behavior. The prefrontal cortex is heteromodal and has strong reciprocal connections with the visual, auditory, and somatosensory cortices. Of these, the visuomotor mechanisms are the most powerful. These frontal areas as well as the supplementary motor areas are involved in the planning and initiation of sequences of movement, as indicated in Chap. 4. In the monkey, for example, when a visual signal evokes movement, some of the prefrontal neurons become active immediately preceding the motor response; other prefrontal neurons are activated if the response is to be delayed. With prefrontal lesions on one side or the other, a series of motor abnormalities occur, ranging through slight grasping and groping responses ("instinctive grasping" of Denny-Brown), a tendency to imitate the examiner's gestures and to compulsively manipulate objects that are in front of the patient (imitation and utilization behavior of Lhermitte), reduced and delayed motor and mental activity (abulia), motor perseveration or impersistence (with left and right hemispheric lesions, respectively), and paratonic rigidity on passive manipulation of the limbs (oppositional resistance, or gegenhalten).

An ataxia of the contralateral limbs has been attributed to prefrontal lesions, but careful anatomic verification is lacking. Instead, in our experience, a unilateral ataxia from a cerebral lesion has been related to a lesion of the opposite parietal lobe. The condition described by Bruns due to a frontal lobe lesion was designated by him as an *ataxia of gait*; he made no reference to an ataxia of limb movements. This disorder is often referred to as an apraxia of gait, inappropriately in our opinion, because the term *apraxia* is best used to describe the inability to perform a commanded or learned motor task, not an ingrained one (page 59). Also, with bilateral frontal lobe degeneration, there may be a characteristic disturbance of stance and gait (probably the basal ganglia and their conections to the frontal lobes are involved in these cases as well). Here the steps are shortened to a shuffle and balance is precarious; with further deterioration, the patient can no longer walk or even stand (*astasia-abasia*). *Cerebral paraplegia in flexion* is the end stage; the affected individual lies curled up in bed, unable even to turn over (see Chap. 7).

Less is known about the extreme degrees of hyperactivity ("organic drivenness") induced in the macaque by bilateral lateral-orbital lesions and occasionally observed in humans after encephalitis or trauma, as noted below. Possibly, compulsive behavior (and tic) is related in some manner to caudatal-frontal lesions.

Incontinence is another manifestation of frontal lobe disease. Right- or left-sided lesions involving the posterior part of the superior frontal gyrus, the anterior cingulate gyrus, and the intervening white matter result in a loss of control of micturition and defecation (Andrew and Nathan). There is no warning of fullness of the bladder and imminence of urination or bowel evacuation, and the patient is surprised and embarrassed at suddenly being wet or soiled. Less complete forms of the syndrome are associated with frequency and urgency of urination during waking hours. An element of indifference to being incontinent is added when the more anterior (nonmotor) parts of the frontal lobes are the sites of disease.

In the spheres of *speech and language*, a number of abnormalities other than Broca's aphasia appear in conjunction with disease of the frontal lobes—laconic speech, lack of spontaneity of speech, telegraphic speech (agrammatism), loss of fluency, perseveration of speech, tendency to whisper instead of speaking aloud, and dysarthria. These are more prominent with left-sided lesions and are fully described in Chap. 23.

In sum, one can say that all parts of the frontal lobes are involved in all spheres of motor activity, from the planning stages to ultimate execution. This applies not only to willed movement but to all postural reactions and habitual activity as well.

Cognitive and Intellectual Changes In general, when one speaks of cognitive and behavioral aspects of frontal lobe function, reference is made to the more anterior (prefrontal) parts rather than the motor and linguistic parts. Here one faces a paradox. These most recently developed parts of the human brain, sometimes called the "organ of civilization," have the most elusive functions.

The effects of lesions of the frontal lobes were first divulged by the famous case of Harlow, published in 1868. His patient, Phineas Gage, was a capable, God-fearing foreman of a railroad gang who became irreverent, dissipated, irresponsible, and vacillating (he also confabulated freely) following an injury in which an explosion drove a large iron tamping bar into his frontal lobes. In Harlow's words, "he was no longer Gage." Another similarly dramatic example was Dandy's patient (the subject of a monograph by Brickner), who underwent a bilateral frontal lobotomy during the removal of a meningioma. Feuchtwanger, in a clinical study of 200 cases of frontal lobe injury, was impressed with the lack of initiative, vacillation, changes in mood (euphoria), and inattentiveness, without intellectual and memory deficits; and Rylander, in a classic monograph, described similar changes in patients with unilateral and bilateral frontal lobectomies (see below). Kleist, under the caption of "alogia," stressed the importance of loss of capacity for abstract thought, as shown in tests of analogies, proverbs, definitions, etc. In chimpanzees, Jacobsen observed that the removal of the premotor parts of the frontal lobes led to social indifference, tameness, placidity, forgetfulness, and difficulty in problem solving—findings that led Egas Moniz, in 1936, to perform prefrontal lobotomies on psychotic patients (see Damasio). This operation and its successor, prefrontal leukotomy (undercutting of the prefrontal white matter), reached their height of popularity in the 1940s and provided the opportunity to study the effects of a wide range of frontal lobe lesions in a large number of patients.

The findings in patients subjected to frontal leukotomy have been the subject of endless controversy. Some workers claimed that there were few or no discernible effects of the operation, even with bilateral lesions. Others insisted that if the proper tests were used, a series of predictable and diagnostic changes in cognition and behavior could be demonstrated. The arguments pro and con and the inadequacies of many of the studies, both in methods of testing and in anatomic verification of the lesions (the extent and location of the lesions varied considerably, and this influenced the clinical effects), have been well summarized by Walsh. Admittedly, in patients who underwent bilateral frontal lobotomy, there was little if any impairment of memory function or of cognitive function as measured by intelligence tests and certainly no loss of alertness and orientation. And some patients who had been disabled by schizophrenia, anxious depression, obsessive-compulsive neurosis, or a chronic pain syndrome did improve in respect to their psychiatric and pain symptoms. However, many patients were left with changes in personality, much to the distress of their families. These patients were indifferent to the problems of others; gave no thought to the effects of their conduct; were tactless, distractible, and socially inept; and were given to euphoria and emotional outbursts.

Luria had an interesting conception of the role of the frontal lobes in intellectual activity. He postulated that problem solving of whatever type (perceptual, constructive, arithmetical, psycholinguistic, or logical—definable also as goal-related behavior) proceeds in four steps: (1) the specification of a problem and the conditions in which it has arisen (in other words, a goal is perceived and the conditions associated with it are set); (2) formulation of a plan of action or strategy for the solution of the problem, requiring that certain linguistic activities be simultaneously initiated in orderly sequence; (3) execution, including implementation and control of the plan; and (4) checking or comparison of the results against the original plan to see if it was adequate. Obviously such complex psychologic activity must implicate many parts of the cerebrum and will suffer as a result of a lesion in any of the parts that contribute to the functional system. Luria found that when the frontal lobes are injured by disease, there was not only a general psychomotor slowing and easy distractibility but also an erroneous analysis of the above-listed conditions of the problem. "The plan of action that is selected quickly loses its regulating influence on behavior as a whole and is replaced by a perseveration of one particular link of the motor act or by the influence of some connection established during the patient's past experience." Furthermore, there was a failure to distinguish the essential sequences in the analysis and to compare the final solution with the original conception of the problem.

Plausible as this scheme appears, like Goldstein's "loss of the abstract attitude" (the patient thinks concretely, i.e., he thinks and reacts directly to the stimulus situation), such psychophysiologic analyses of the mental processes are highly theoretical, and the factors to which they refer are not easily measured.

Other Alterations of Behavior and Personality A lack of initiative and spontaneity is the most common effect of frontal lobe disease, and it is much easier to observe than to quantitate. With relatively mild forms of this disorder, patients exhibit an idleness of thought, speech, and action and they lapse into this state without complaint. They are tolerant of most conditions in which they are placed, though they may act unreasonably for brief periods if irritated, seemingly unable to think through the consequences of their remonstrances. They let members of the family answer questions and "do the talking," interjecting a remark only rarely and unpredictably. Questions directed to such patients may evoke only brief, unqualified answers. Once started on a task, they may persist in it ("stimulus bound"); i.e., they tend to perseverate. Fuster, in his studies of the prefrontal cortex, emphasizes the failure over time to maintain events in serial order (impairment of temporal grading) and to integrate new events and information with previously learned data. Placidity is a notable feature of the behavior. Worry, anxiety, self-concern, hypochondriasis, complaints of chronic pain, and depression are all reduced by frontal lobe disease, as they are by frontal lobotomy.

Extensive bilateral disease is accompanied by a quantitative reduction in all psychomotor activity. The number of movements, spoken words, and thoughts per unit of time diminish. Relatively mild degrees of this state, associated with a delay in responses, are called *abulia*; the most severe degrees take the form of *akinetic mutism* (page 371), wherein a nonparalyzed patient, alert and capable of movement and speech, lies or sits motionless and silent for days or weeks on end. The localization of this condition is quite imprecise. It has been attributed to bilateral lesions in the ventromedial frontal regions or frontal-diencephalic connections. Laplane finds the lack of motivation of the patient with bifrontal lesions and bipallidal lesions to be the same, though one would expect the latter to be manifest more as a bradykinesia than as a bradyphrenia (slowness of thinking). Benson (and Kleist and others before him) related the syndrome of apathy and lack of initiative to lesions in the sagittal or mediodorsal convexities, and the facetious, unguarded, and socially inappropriate state (see below) to orbital and dorsolateral frontal lesions.

The opposite state, in a sense, is the hyperactivity syndrome or "organic drivenness" described by von Economo in children who had survived an attack of encephalitis lethargica. In our patients, the latter syndrome has been associated with combined frontal and temporal lobe lesions, usually traumatic but also encephalitic, although exact clinicopathologic correlations could not be made. Such patients may also exhibit brief but intense involvement with some meaningless activity, such as sorting papers in an attic or hoarding objects or food. Combativeness and extreme insomnia or an otherwise disrupted sleep cycle are often part of the syndrome. The hyperactivity of young boys and the mania or hypomania of manic-depressive disease, despite similar symptoms, also lack a known anatomic basis.

In addition to the disorders of initiative and spontaneity, frontal lobe lesions result in a number of other changes in personality and behavior. These, too, are easier to observe in the patient's natural environment, by his family, than to measure by psychologic tests. It has been difficult to find a term for all these personality changes. Analytical psychiatrists have referred to them as a loss of ego strength—a lessening of the integrative and constructive forces within the personality. Some patients, particularly those with inferofrontal lesions, feel compelled to make silly jokes that are inappropriate to the situation—so-called Witzelsucht or moria; they are socially uninhibited and lack awareness of their abnormal behavior. The patient is no longer the sensitive, compassionate, effective human being that he once was, having lost his usual ways of reacting with affection to family and friends. In more advanced instances, there is a reduced regard for social conventions and an interest only in immediate personal gratification. These changes, observed characteristically in lobotomized patients, came to be recognized as too great a price to pay for the loss of neurotic traits, pain, depression, and "tortured self-concern," for which reasons lobotomies were done; hence the procedure became obsolete.

The effect of unilateral prefrontal lesions is a question that continues to vex clinicians. If the lesions are small, their effects are undetectable; even a large lesion, such as a tumor, may long escape detection. Rylander, by careful psychologic testing, has shown that patients with lesions of either frontal lobe manifest a slight elevation of mood, with increased talkativeness and a tendency to joke, lack of tact, inability to adapt to a new situation, instability of mood, and loss of initiative—changes that are more readily recognized if the frontal lobe lesions are bilateral.

Our experience with frontal lobe lesions, derived mainly from patients with trauma or ruptured anterior communicating aneurysms, affirms most of the statements above. Most apparent is the abulic-hypokinetic disorder that seems to slow the mental processes involved in all forms of cerebral performance. Inattentiveness, impersistence in all assigned tasks, and sometimes perseveration are the major features of this disorder. Such a state cannot be specifically ascribed to prefrontal lesions, since it may be a reflection of a more general impairment of the thalamolimbic or reticular activating thalamocortical system. Indeed, bilateral medial thalamic lesions may give rise to the same syndrome, and Degos and colleagues have described a severe "frontal lobe syndrome" in association with bilateral lesions of the anterior cingulate gyrus. It is noteworthy that these structures have close connections with the prefrontal cortices.

In general, we agree that the greatest cognitive-intellectual deficits relate to lesions in the dorsolateral parts of the prefrontal lobes and the personality, mood, and behavioral changes to lesions of the medial-orbital parts, although the two types of disorder often merge with one another. The diagnosis of lesions in the orbital regions is facilitated by the finding of unilateral anosmia or optic atrophy, as occurs with a meningioma of the olfactory groove.

Although frontal lobe function is the subject of a vast literature and endless speculation (see reviews of Stuss and Benson and of Damasio), a unified concept of this function has not emerged—probably because the frontal lobes are so large and include several heterogeneous systems. There is no doubt that the mind is changed by disease of the prefrontal parts of the frontal lobes, but often it is difficult to say exactly how it is changed. Perhaps at present it is best to regard the frontal lobes as the part of the brain that quickly and effectively orients and drives the individual, with all the percepts and concepts formed from past life experiences, toward action that is projected into the future.

Psychologic tests of particular value are the card-sorting test, proverb interpretation, sequencing of pictures, and the three-step hand posture test of Luria. The last test is a popular part of the bedside neurologic evaluation of patients with suspected frontal lobe lesions. The patient is asked to imitate, then reproduce on his own, a sequence of three hand gestures, typically performed by slapping the opposite outstretched palm, followed by hitting the palm with a closed fist, and then by striking it with the side of the open hand. Patients with frontal lesions on either or both sides have difficulty performing the test in correct sequence, often perseverating, balking, or making unwanted gestures, but it should be kept in mind that similar impairments of performance may occur with all manner of confusional and inattentive states and apraxias.

Effects of frontal lobe disease may be summarized as follows:

I. Effects of unilateral frontal disease, either left or right
   - *A.* Contralateral spastic hemiplegia
   - *B.* Slight elevation of mood, increased talkativeness, tendency to joke (Witzelsucht), lack of tact, difficulty in adaptation, loss of initiative
   - *C.* If entirely prefrontal, no hemiplegia; grasp and suck reflexes or instinctive grasping may be released
   - *D.* Anosmia with involvement of orbital parts

II. Effects of right frontal disease
   - *A.* Left hemiplegia
   - *B.* Changes as in I.*B*, *C*, and *D*

III. Effects of left frontal disease
   - *A.* Right hemiplegia
   - *B.* Motor speech disorder with agraphia, with or without apraxia of the lips and tongue (see Chap. 23)
   - *C.* Sympathetic apraxia of left hand (see page 60)
   - *D.* Loss of verbal associative fluency; perseveration
   - *E.* Changes as in I.*B*, *C*, and *D*

IV. Effects of bifrontal disease
   - *A.* Bilateral hemiplegia
   - *B.* Spastic bulbar (pseudobulbar) palsy
   - *C.* If prefrontal, abulia or akinetic mutism, lack of ability to sustain attention and solve complex problems, rigidity of thinking, bland affect, social ineptitude, behavioral disinhibition, in-

ability to anticipate, labile mood, and varying combinations of grasping, sucking, decomposition of gait, and sphincteric incontinence

SYNDROMES CAUSED BY LESIONS OF THE TEMPORAL LOBES

Anatomic and Physiologic Considerations

The boundaries of the temporal lobes are indicated in Fig. 22-8. The sylvian fissure separates the superior surface of each temporal lobe from the frontal lobe and anterior parts of the parietal lobe. There is no definite anatomic boundary between the temporal lobe and the occipital or posterior part of the parietal lobe, but the angular gyrus serves as a landmark for the latter.

The inferior branch of the middle cerebral artery supplies the convexity of the lobe, and the temporal branch of the posterior cerebral artery supplies the medial and inferior aspects, including the hippocampus.

The temporal lobe includes the superior, middle, and inferior temporal, lateral occipitotemporal, fusiform, lingual, parahippocampal, and hippocampal convolutions and the transverse gyri of Heschl; the last of these constitute the primary auditory receptive area and are located within the sylvian fissure. This area has a tonotopic arrangement: fibers carrying high tones terminate in the medial portion of the gyrus and those carrying low tones, in the lateral and more rostral portions (Merzenich and Brugge). The planum temporale (area 22), an integral part of the auditory cortex, lies immediately posterior to Heschl's convolutions, on the superior surface of the temporal lobe. The left planum is larger in right-handed individuals. There are rich reciprocal connections between the medial geniculate bodies and Heschl's gyri. The latter project to the unimodal association cortex of the superior temporal gyrus, which, in turn, projects to the paralimbic and limbic regions of the temporal lobe and to temporal and frontal heteromodal association cortices and the inferior parietal lobe. There is also a system of fibers that projects back to the medial geniculate body and to lower auditory centers. The cortical receptive zone for labyrinthine impulses is less well demarcated than the one for hearing but is probably situated on the inferior bank of the sylvian fissure, just posterior to the auditory area. Least well delimited is the role of the medial parts of the temporal lobe in olfaction and gustatory perception, although seizure foci in the region of the uncus (uncinate seizure) will excite hallucinations of olfaction and occasionally of taste.

The middle and inferior temporal gyri (areas 21 and 37) receive a massive contingent of fibers from the striate cortex (area 17) and the parastriate visual association areas (areas 18 and 19). These temporal visual areas make abundant connections with the medial limbic, rhinencephalic (olfactory brain), orbitofrontal, parietal, and occipital cortices. Here the cortices subserving vision and hearing are intimately interconnected.

The superior part of the dominant temporal lobe is concerned with the acoustic or receptive aspects of language (page 500) and the middle and inferior convolutions, with visual discriminations. The latter convolutions receive fiber systems from the striate and parastriate visual cortices and, in turn, project to the contralateral visual association cortex, to the prefrontal heteromodal cortex, to the superior temporal cortex, and to the limbic and paralimbic cortex. Presumably these systems subserve visual discriminative functions such as spatial orientation, estimation of depth and distance, stereoscopic vision, and hue perception. Similarly, the unimodal auditory cortex is closely connected with a series of auditory association areas in the superior temporal convolution, and the latter are connected with prefrontal and temporal-parietal heteromodal areas and the limbic areas (Mesulam). Most of these auditory systems have been worked out in the macaque, but they are probably involved in complex verbal and nonverbal auditory discriminations in humans.

The hippocampus was formerly thought to be related to the olfactory system, but now it is known that lesions here do not alter the sense of smell. Most important is the role of the hippocampus and other structures of the hippocampal formation (dentate gyrus, subiculum, entorhinal cortex, and parahippocampal gyrus) in learning and memory functions, already discussed in Chap. 21. There is an abundance of connections between the medial temporal lobe and the entire limbic system. For this reason MacLean referred to these parts as the "visceral brain," and Williams, as the "emotional brain." Included in this anatomic concept are the hippocampus, the amygdaloid nuclei, the fornices and limbic portions of the inferior and medial frontal regions, the cingulate cortices, and the septal and associated subcortical nuclei (see Chap. 25).

Most of the temporal lobe cortex, including Heschl's gyri, has fairly equally developed pyramidal and granular layers. In this respect, it resembles more the granular cortex of the frontal and prefrontal regions and inferior parts of the parietal lobes (see Fig. 22-5). Unlike the six-layered neocortex, the hippocampus and dentate gyrus are typical of the phylogenetically older three-layered allocortex.

A massive fiber system projects from the striate and parastriate zones of the occipital lobes to the inferior and medial parts of the temporal lobes. The temporal lobes are connected to one another through the anterior commissure and middle part of the corpus callosum; the inferior, or uncinate, fasciculus connects the anterior temporal and orbital frontal regions. The arcuate fasciculus connects the posterosuperior temporal lobe to the motor cortex and Broca's area (see page 501). The medial parts of the temporal lobe are supplied by the posterior cerebral artery and the superior and lateral parts by the temporal branches of the middle cerebral artery.

Physiologically, two ideas stand out—that the temporal lobe is the great integrator of "sensations, emotions, and behavior" (Williams) and that it is continuously active throughout life. The temporal lobe seems to be the site where sensory modalities are integrated into ultimate self-awareness (the cartesian view of consciousness of one's self as a person with a mind). Similar suprasensory integrative mechanisms are operative in the parietal lobe, but only in the temporal lobe are they brought into close relationship to one's instinctive and emotional life. Probably self-awareness also requires a coherent and sequential stream of thought. Where precisely the inner stream of consciousness is perceived is still an open question, but given the requirement that it be close to other integrated sensory experiences, the main locus is likely to be in the temporal lobes. Also, the stream of thinking (the internal conversation that is constant in the waking state—James's "stream of consciousness") requires both language and memory function (inner language comprises thought and memories); both these functions involve the temporal lobe.

During the middle years of the twentieth century, the temporal lobe was the principal focus of studies of cerebral function. Some hint of its role in our personal and emotional life had been suggested by Hughlings Jackson, in the nineteenth century, derived from his insightful analysis of the psychic states accompanying temporal lobe seizures. Later, the observations of Penfield and his collaborators on the effects of stimulating the temporal lobes in the conscious epileptic patient revealed something of its complex functions. There followed a large volume of writings on its anatomy, the neuronal networks and circuits by which it was connected to other cortical and subcortical structures, and the effects of ablation on emotion, behavior, and sensory perception. The classic writings on this subject include Williams's chapter on temporal lobe syndromes in the *Handbook of Clinical Neurology* and the monographs by Penfield and Rasmussen (*The Cerebral Cortex of Man*) and by Alajouanine and colleagues (*Les Grandes Activités du Lobe Temporale*).

Clinical Effects of Temporal Lobe Lesions

The symptoms consequent to disease of the temporal lobes may, for convenience of exposition, be divided into disorders of the special senses (visual, auditory, olfactory, and gustatory), time perception, language, memory, emotion, and behavior. Of central importance are the roles of the superior part of the dominant lobe and its hippocampal and limbic parts in language, memory and learning functions, and the emotional life of the individual. Several of these functions and their derangements are of such scope and importance that they have been accorded separate chapters. Language is discussed in Chap. 23, memory in Chap. 21, and the neurology of emotion and behavior in Chap. 25; these subjects are omitted from further discussion here.

Visual Disorders Already in Chap. 13 (on vision) it was pointed out that lesions of the white matter of the central and posterior parts of the temporal lobe characteristically involve the lower arching fibers of the geniculocalcarine pathway (Meyer's loop). This results in an upper homonymous quadrantanopia, usually not perfectly congruent. There is considerable variability in the arrangement of visual fibers as they pass around the temporal horn of the lateral ventricle; this accounts for the smallness of the field defect in some patients after temporal lobectomy or stroke and extension into the inferior field in others. Quadrantanopia from a dominant lesion is often combined with aphasia.

Bilateral lesions of the temporal lobes render a monkey psychically blind. He can see and pick up objects but does not recognize them until they are explored orally. Natural emotional reactions such as fear are lost. This syndrome, named for Klüver and Bucy, has been identified in partial form in humans (page 545). Lesser degrees of visual imperception have been uncovered by Milner and by McFie and colleagues, using special tests.

Visual hallucinations of complex form, including ones of the patient himself (autoscopy), appear during temporal lobe seizures. In stimulation studies, Penfield was able to induce what he called "interpretive illusions" (altered impressions of the present) and to reactivate past experiences quite completely and vividly in association with their original emotions. Temporal lobe abnormalities may also distort visual perception; seen objects may appear too large (macropsia) or small (micropsia), too close or far away, or unreal. Some visual hallucinations have an auditory component: an imaginary figure may speak and move and, at the same time, arouse intense emotion in the patient. The entire experience may seem unnatural and unreal but is unlike the visuospatial disorders of the body schema, which are considered with disorders of the parietal lobe, further on.

Cortical Deafness Bilateral lesions of the transverse gyri of Heschl are known to cause deafness. Henschen, in his famous review of 1337 cases of aphasia that had been reported up to 1922, found 9 in which these parts were destroyed by restricted vascular lesions, with resulting deafness. There are now many more cases of this type in the medical literature; lesions in other parts of the temporal lobes have no effect on hearing. These observations are the basis for the localization of the primary auditory receptive area in the cortex of the transverse gyri (chiefly the first), on the posterior-superior surface of the temporal lobe, deep within the sylvian fissure (areas 41 and 42). Subcortical lesions, which interrupt the fibers from both medial geniculate bodies to the transverse gyri, as in the two cases of Tanaka and colleagues, have the same effect. With left-sided superotemporal lesions, there is usually an aphasia as well, because of the proximity of the transverse gyri to the superotemporal association cortex. Hécaen has remarked that cortically deaf persons may seem to be unaware of their deafness, a state similar to that of blind persons who act as though they could see (Anton syndrome, see further on).

Unlike the marked visual and somatic sensory defects with unilateral cerebral lesions, unilateral lesions of Heschl's gyri were for a long time believed to have no effect on hearing; it has been found, however, that if very brief auditory stimuli are delivered, the threshold of sensation is elevated in the ear opposite the lesion. Also, while unilateral lesions do not diminish the perception of pure tones or clearly spoken words, the ear contralateral to a temporal lesion is less efficient if the conditions of hearing are rendered more difficult (binaural test). For example, if words are slightly distorted (electronically filtered to alter consonants), they are heard less well in the ear contralateral to the lesion. In addition, the patient has more difficulty in equalizing the volume of sounds that are presented to both ears and in perceiving rapidly spoken numbers or different words presented to the two ears (dichotic listening).

Auditory Agnosias Lesions of the secondary (unimodal association) zones of the auditory cortex—area 22 and part of area 21—have no effect on the perception of sounds and pure tones. However, the perception of complex combinations of sounds is severely impaired. This impairment, or auditory agnosia, takes several forms—inability to recognize sounds, different musical notes (amusia), or words—and presumably each has a slightly different anatomic basis.

In *agnosia for sounds*, auditory sensations cannot be distinguished from one another. Such varied sounds as the tinkling of a bell, the rustling of paper, running water, and a siren all sound alike. The condition is usually associated with word deafness (page 510 and below) or with amusia. Hécaen observed an agnosia for sounds alone in only two cases; one patient could identify only half of 26 familiar sounds, and the other could recognize no sound other than the ticking of a watch. Yet in both patients the audiogram was normal, and neither had trouble understanding spoken words. In both, the lesion involved the right temporal lobe and the corpus callosum was intact.

Amusia proves to be more complicated, for the appreciation of music has several aspects: the recognition of a familiar melody and the ability to name it; the perception of pitch and timbre; and the ability to produce, read, and write music. There are many reports of musicians who became word-deaf with lesions of the dominant temporal lobe but retained their recognition of music and their skill in producing it. Others became agnosic for music but not for words, and still others were agnosic for both words and music. According to Segarra and Quadfasel, impaired recognition of music results from lesions in the middle temporal gyrus and not from lesions at the pole of the temporal lobe, as had been postulated by Henschen.

That the appreciation of music is impaired by lesions of the nondominant temporal lobe finds support in Milner's studies of patients who had undergone temporal lobectomy. She found a statistically significant lowering of the patient's appreciation of the duration of notes, timbre, intensity of sounds, and memory of melodies following right temporal lobectomy; these abilities were preserved in patients with left temporal lobectomies, regardless of whether Heschl's gyri were included. Similar observations had been made by Shankweiler, but in addition he found that patients had difficulty in denominating a note or naming a melody following left temporal lobectomies.

More recent observations permit somewhat different interpretations. Tramo and Bharucha examined the mechanisms mediating the recognition and discrimination of timbre (the distinctive tonal quality produced by a particular musical instrument) in patients whose right and left hemispheres had been separated by callosotomy. They found that timbre could be recognized by *each* hemisphere—somewhat better by the left hemisphere than by the right. Also, it was observed that lesions of the right auditory cortex impair the recognition of melody (the temporal sequence of pitches) and of harmony (the sounding of simultaneous pitches). However, if words are added to the melody, then either a left- or right-sided lesion impairs its recognition (Samson and Zatorre). From functional imaging studies, it appears that the left inferior frontal region is activated by tasks that involve the identification of familiar music (Platel et al), as if this were a semantic test, but passively listening to melodies activates the right superior temporal and occipital regions (Zatorre et al).

Taken together, these data suggest that the nondominant hemisphere is important for the recognition of harmony and melody (in the absence of words), but that the naming of musical scores and all the semantic (writing and reading) aspects of music require integrity of the dominant temporal and probably the frontal lobes as well.

Word Deafness (Auditory Verbal Agnosia) In essence, word deafness is a failure of the left temporal lobe function in decoding the acoustic signals of speech and converting them into understandable words. This is the essential element in Wernicke's aphasia and is discussed in Chap. 23. However, word deafness can occur by itself, without other features of Wernicke's aphasia. Also, verbal agnosia may be combined with agnosia for sounds and music, or the two may occur separately.

Auditory Illusions Temporal lobe lesions that leave hearing intact may cause a hearing disorder in which sounds are perceived as being louder or less loud than normal. Sounds or words may seem strange or disagreeable, or they may seem to be repeated, a kind of sensory perseveration. If auditory hallucinations are also present, they may undergo similar alterations. Such paracusias may last indefinitely and, by changing timbre or tonality, alter musical appreciation as well.

Auditory Hallucinations These may be elementary (murmurs, blowing, sound of running water or motors, whistles, clangs, sirens, etc.), or they may be complex (musical themes, choruses, voices). Usually sounds and musical themes are heard more clearly than voices. Patients may recognize the illusions and hallucinations for what they are, or they may be convinced that the voices are real and respond to them with intense emotion. Hearing may fade before or during the hallucination.

In temporal lobe epilepsy, the auditory hallucinations may occur alone or in combination with visual or gustatory hallucinations, visual distortions, dizziness, and aphasia. There may be hallucinations based on remembered experiences (experiential hallucinations, in the terminology of Penfield and Rasmussen).

The anatomy of lesions underlying auditory illusions and hallucinations has been incompletely studied. In some instances these sensory phenomena have been combined with auditory verbal (or nonverbal) agnosia; the superior and posterior parts of the dominant or both temporal lobes were then involved. Clinicoanatomic correlation is difficult in cases of tumors that distort the brain without completely destroying it and also cause edema of the surrounding tissue. Moreover, it is often uncertain whether symptoms have been produced by destruction of tissue or by excitation, i.e., by way of seizure discharges, which act in a fashion similar to electrical stimulation of the auditory cortical areas. Elementary hallucinations and dreamy states have been reported with lesions of either temporal lobe, whereas the more complex auditory hallucinations and particularly polymodal ones (visual plus auditory) occur more often with left-sided lesions. Also, it should be noted that elementary or unformed auditory hallucinations (e.g., the sound of an orchestra tuning up) as well as entire strains of music and singing, occur with lesions that appear to be restricted to the pons ("pontine auditory hallucinosis").

It is tempting to relate complex auditory hallucinations to disorders in the auditory association areas surrounding Heschl's gyri, but the data do not fully justify such an assumption. In schizophrenic patients, the areas activated during a period of active auditory hallucinosis include not only Heschl's gyri but also the hippocampus and other widely distributed structures in the dominant hemisphere (see Chap. 58)

Vestibular Disturbances In the superior and posterior part of the temporal lobe (posterior to the primary auditory cortex), there is an area that responds to vestibular stimulation by altering one's sense of verticality in relation to the environment. If this area is destroyed on one side, the only clinical effect may be a subtle change in eye movements on optokinetic stimulation (more often a result of parietal damage). Epileptic activation of this area may occur, inducing vertigo or a sense of disequilibrium. As pointed out on page 338, pure vertiginous epilepsy does occur but is a rarity, and if vertigo does precede a seizure, it is usually momentary and is quickly submerged in other components of the seizure.

Disturbances of Time Perception These may occur with lesions of either temporal lobe. In a temporal lobe seizure, time may seem to stand still or to pass with great speed. On recovery from such a seizure, the patient, having lost all sense of time, may repeatedly look at the clock. Amentias (mental retardation) and dementias prevent or abolish the capacity to reckon personal events in terms of a subjective time scale. The patient with a Korsakoff amnesic state is unable to place events in their proper time relationships, presumably because of failure of retentive memory. Assal and Bindschaedler have reported an extraordinary abnormality of time sense in which the patient invariably placed the day and date 3 days ahead of the actual ones. There had been aphasia from a left hemispheral stroke years before, but the impairment of time sense occurred after a left temporal stroke that also produced cortical deafness.

Certainly the commonest disruptions of the sense of time occur as part of confusional states of any type. The usual tendency is for the patient to report the current date as an earlier one, much less often as a later one. Characteristically, in this situation the responses vary from one examination to the next.

Smell and Taste The central anatomy and physiology of these two senses have been elusive. Brodal concluded that the hippocampus was not involved. However, seizure foci in the medial part of the temporal lobe (in the region of the uncus) may evoke olfactory hallucinations. This "uncinate fit," as originally pointed out by Jackson and Stewart, was often accompanied by a dreamy state, or, in the words of Penfield, an "intellectual aura." The central areas identified physiologically with olfaction are the posterior orbitofrontal, subcallosal, anterior temporal, and insular cortices, i.e., the areas that mediate visceral functions.

In comparison, hallucinations of taste are rare. Stimulation of the posterior insular area elicited a sensation of taste along with disturbances of alimentary function (Penfield and Faulk). There are cases in which a lesion in the medial temporal lobe caused both gustatory and olfactory hallucinations. Sometimes the patient cannot decide whether he experienced an abnormal odor, taste, or both. The anatomy and physiology of smell and taste are discussed further in Chap. 12.

Other (Nonauditory) Syndromes Between the hippocampal formation (on the inferomedial surface of the temporal lobe) and the primary and secondary auditory areas (Heschl's transverse gyri and superior temporal convolution, respectively), there is a large inferolateral expanse of temporal lobe that has only vaguely assignable integrative functions. With lesions in these parts of the dominant temporal lobe, a defect in the retrieval of words (*amnesic dysnomia*) has been a frequently observed abnormality. Stimulation of the posterior parts of the first and second temporal convolutions of fully conscious epileptic patients can arouse complex memories and visual and auditory images, some with strong emotional content (Penfield and Roberts).

Careful psychologic studies have disclosed a difference between the effects of dominant and nondominant partial temporal lobectomy (Milner). With the former, there was dysnomia and impairment in the learning of material presented through the auditory sense; with the latter, there was impairment in the learning of visually presented material. In addition, about 20 percent of patients who had undergone temporal lobectomy, left or right, showed a syndrome similar to that which results from lesions of the prefrontal regions. Perhaps more significant is the observation that the remainder of the cases showed little or no defect in personality or behavior.

Disorders of Memory, Emotion, and Behavior Finally, attention must be drawn to the central role of the temporal lobe, notably its hippocampal and limbic parts, in memory and learning and in the emotional life of the individual. As indicated earlier, these functions and their derangements have been accorded separate chapters. Memory is discussed in Chap. 21 and the neurology of emotion and behavior in Chap. 25.

To summarize, human temporal lobe syndromes include the following:

I. Effects of unilateral disease of the dominant temporal lobe
   A. Homonymous upper quadrantanopia
   B. Wernicke's aphasia (word deafness—auditory verbal agnosia)
   C. Amusia (some types)
   D. Impairment in tests of verbal material presented through the auditory sense
   E. Dysnomia or amnesic aphasia
   F. Visual agnosia
   G. Occasionally amnesic (Korsakoff) syndrome
II. Effects of unilateral disease of the nondominant temporal lobe
   A. Homonymous upper quadrantanopia
   B. Inability to judge spatial relationships in some cases

    C. Impairment in tests of visually presented nonverbal material
    D. Agnosia for sounds and some qualities of music
III. Effects of disease of either temporal lobe
    A. Auditory, visual, olfactory, and gustatory hallucinations
    B. Dreamy states with uncinate seizures
    C. Emotional and behavioral changes
    D. Delirium (usually nondominant)
    E. Disturbances of time perception
IV. Effects of bilateral disease
    A. Korsakoff amnesic defect (hippocampal formations)
    B. Apathy and placidity
    C. Hypermetamorphopsia (compulsion to attend to all visual stimuli), hyperorality, hypersexuality, blunted emotional reactivity (Klüver-Bucy syndrome; the full syndrome is rarely seen in man)

SYNDROMES CAUSED BY LESIONS OF THE PARIETAL LOBES

Anatomic and Physiologic Considerations

This part of the cerebrum, lying behind the central sulcus and above the sylvian fissure, is the least well demarcated (Fig. 22-8). Its posterior boundary, where it merges with the occipital lobe, is obscure, as is part of the inferior boundary, where it merges with the temporal lobe. On its medial side, the parieto-occipital sulcus marks the posterior border, which is completed by extending the line of the sulcus downward to the preoccipital notch on the inferior border of the hemisphere. Within the parietal lobe, there are two important sulci: the postcentral sulcus, which forms the posterior boundary of the somesthetic cortex, and the interparietal sulcus, which runs anteroposteriorly from the middle of the posterior central sulcus and separates the mass of the parietal lobe into superior and inferior lobules (Figs. 22-3 and 22-8). The inferior parietal lobule (Ecker's lobule in older terminology) is composed of the supramarginal gyrus (Brodmann's area 40) and the angular gyrus (area 39). These two gyri and the posterior third of the first temporal gyrus make up what has been called *Wernicke's language area*.

The architecture of the postcentral convolution is typical of all primary receptive areas (homotypical granular cortex). The rest of the parietal lobe resembles the association cortex, both unimodal and heteromodal, of the frontal and temporal lobes. The superior and inferior parietal lobules and adjacent parts of the temporal and occipital lobes are relatively much larger in humans than in any of the other primates and are relatively slow in attaining their fully functional state (beyond the seventh year of age). This area of heteromodal cortex has large fiber connections with the frontal, occipital, and temporal lobes of the same hemisphere and, through the middle part of the corpus callosum, with corresponding parts of the opposite hemisphere.

The postcentral gyrus or primary somatosensory cortex receives most of its afferent projections from the ventroposterior thalamic nucleus, which is the terminus of the ascending somatosensory pathways. The contralateral half of the body is represented somatotopically on the posterior bank of the rolandic sulcus. It has been shown in the macaque that spindle afferents project to area 3a, cutaneous afferents to areas 3b and 1, and joint afferents to area 2 (Kaas). Stimulation of the posterior bank of the rolandic sulcus elicits a numb, tingling sensation and sense of movement. Penfield remarked that rarely are these tactile illusions accompanied by pain, warmth, or cold. Stimulation of the motor cortex may produce similar sensations, as do discharging seizure foci from these regions. The primary sensory cortex projects to the superior parietal lobule (area 5), which is the somatosensory association cortex. Some parts of areas 1, 3, and 5 (except the hand and foot representations) probably connect, via the corpus callosum, with the opposite somatosensory cortex. There is some uncertainty as to whether area 7 (which lies posterior to area 5) is unimodal somatosensory or heteromodal visual and somatosensory; certainly it receives a large contingent of fibers from the occipital lobe.

In humans, electrical stimulation of the cortex of the superior and inferior parietal lobules evokes no specific motor or sensory effects. Overlapping here, however, are the tertiary zones for vision, hearing, and somatic sensation, the supramodal integration of which is essential to our awareness of space and person and certain aspects of language and calculation, as mentioned below.

The parietal lobe is supplied by the middle cerebral artery, the inferior and superior divisions supplying the inferior and superior lobules, respectively, although the vascular distribution in this area is variable.

Despite Critchley's pessimistic prediction that to establish a formula of normal parietal function will prove to be a "vain and meaningless pursuit," our concepts of the activities of this part of the brain are now assuming some degree of order. There is little reason to doubt that the anterior parietal cortex contains the mechanisms for tactile percepts. Discriminative tactile functions, listed below, are organized in the more posterior, secondary sensory areas. But the greater part of the parietal lobe functions as a center for integrating somatosensory with visual and auditory information in order to construct an awareness of one's own body (body schema) and its relation to extrapersonal space. Connections with the frontal and occipital lobes provide the necessary proprioceptive and visual information for movement of the body and manipulation of objects and for certain constructional activities. Impairment of these functions implicates the parietal lobes, more clearly the one on the right. The understanding of spoken and written words is a function of the supramarginal and angular gyri of the dominant parietal lobe, as elaborated in Chap. 23. The recognition and utilization of numbers, arithmetic principles, and calculation, which have important spatial attributes, are other functions integrated principally through these structures.

Clinical Effects of Parietal Lobe Lesions

Within the brain, no other territory surpasses the parietal lobes in the rich variety of clinical phenomena that are exposed under conditions of disease. Our current understanding of the effects of parietal lobe disease contrasts sharply with that of the late nineteenth century, when these lobes, in the classic textbooks of Oppenheim and Gowers, were considered to be "silent areas." However, the clinical manifestations of parietal lobe disease may be subtle, requiring special techniques for their elicitation; even more difficult is the interpretation of these abnormalities of function in terms of a coherent and plausible physiology.

Cortical Sensory Syndromes The effects of a parietal lobe lesion on somatic sensation were first described by Verger and then more completely by Déjerine, in his monograph *L'agnosie corticale*, and by Head and Holmes. The latter, in their important paper of 1911, noted the close interrelationships between the thalamus and the sensory cortex. As pointed out on page 172, the defect is essentially one of *sensory discrimination*, i.e., an impairment or loss of the sense of position and passive movement and the ability to localize tactile, thermal, and noxious stimuli applied to the body surface; to distinguish objects by their size, shape, and texture (astereognosis); to recognize figures written on the skin; to distinguish between single and double contacts (two-point discrimination); and to detect the direction of movement of a tactile stimulus. In contrast, the perception of pain, touch, pressure, vibratory stimuli, and thermal stimuli is *relatively intact*. This type of sensory defect is sometimes referred to as "cortical," although it can be produced just as well by lesions of the subcortical connections. Clinicoanatomic studies indicate that parietocortical lesions that spare the postcentral gyrus produce only transient somatosensory changes or none at all (Corkin et al; Carmon and Benton).

The question of bilateral sensory deficits with lesions in only one postcentral convolution was raised by the studies of Semmes and of Corkin and their associates. In tests of pressure sensitivity, two-point discrimination, point localization, position sense, and tactile object recognition, they found bilateral disturbances in nearly half of their patients with unilateral lesions, but the deficits were always more severe contralaterally and mainly in the hand. These disturbances of discriminative sensation and the subject of tactile agnosia are discussed more fully in Chap. 9.

Déjerine and Mouzon described another parietal sensory syndrome in which touch, pressure, pain, thermal, vibratory, and position sense are all lost on one side of the body or in a limb. This syndrome, usually associated with a thalamic lesion, may also occur with large, acute lesions (infarcts, hemorrhages) in the central and subcortical white matter of the contralateral parietal lobe; in the latter case these symptoms recede in time, leaving more subtle defects in sensory discrimination. As indicated in Chap. 9, smaller lesions, particularly ones that result from a glancing blow to the skull or a small infarct or hemorrhage, may cause a defect in cutaneous-kinesthetic perception in a discrete part of a limb, e.g., the ulnar or radial half of the hand and forearm; these cerebral lesions may mimic a peripheral nerve or root lesion (Dodge and Meirowsky). Also, a *pseudothalamic pain syndrome* on the side deprived of sensation has been described (Biemond). In a series of 12 such patients described by Michel and colleagues, burning or constrictive pain, identical to the thalamic pain syndrome (page 172), resulted from vascular lesions restricted to the cortex. The discomfort involved the entire half of the body or matched the region of cortical hypesthesia; in a few cases it was paroxysmal.

Head and Holmes drew attention to a number of interesting points about patients with parietal sensory defects—the easy fatigability of their sensory perceptions; the inconsistency of responses to painful and tactile stimuli; the difficulty in distinguishing more than one contact at a time; the disregard of stimuli on the affected side when the healthy side is stimulated simultaneously (tactile inattention or extinction); the tendency of superficial pain sensations to outlast the stimulus and to be hyperpathic; and the occurrence of hallucinations of touch. An interesting observation, for which there is no cogent explanation, is the temporary elimination of hemineglect in patients with right parietal infarcts by caloric or electrical stimulation of the ipsilateral vestibular apparatus.

With anterior parietal lobe lesions there is often an associated hemiparesis, since this portion of the parietal lobe contributes a considerable number of fibers to the corticospinal tract. Or there is only a poverty of movement or a weak effort of the opposite side in the absence of somatic neglect. The affected limbs, if involved with this apparent weakness solely from a parietal lesion, tend to remain hypotonic and the musculature may undergo atrophy of a degree not explained by inactivity alone. In some cases, as noted below, there is clumsiness in reaching for and grasping an object under visual guidance (optic ataxia), and exceptionally, at some phase in recovery from the hemisensory deficit, there is incoordination of movement and intention tremor of the contralateral arm and leg, simulating a cerebellar deficit (pseudocerebellar syndrome). While relatively rare, it is authenticated by our own case studies. With parietal lesions, the arm and hand may sometimes be held in a fixed dystonic posture.

The Asomatognosias This term denotes the inability to recognize part of one's body. The idea that visual and tactile sensory information is synthesized during development into a body schema or image (perception of one's body and the relations of bodily parts to one another) was first clearly formulated by Pick and extensively elaborated by Brain. Long before their time, however, it was suggested that such information was the basis of our emerging awareness of ourselves as persons, and philosophers had assumed that this comes about by the constant interplay between percepts of ourselves and of the surrounding world.

The formation of the body schema is thought to be based on the constant influx and storage of sensations from our bodies as we move about; hence, motor activity is important in its development. Always, however, a sense of extrapersonal space is involved as well, and this depends upon visual and labyrinthine stimulation. The mechanisms upon which these perceptions depend are best appreciated by studying their derangements in the course of neurologic disease.

Anosognosia (Unilateral Asomatognosia; Anton-Babinski Syndrome) The observation that a patient with a dense hemiplegia, usually of the left side, may be indifferent to, or unaware of, the paralysis was first made by Anton; later, Babinski named this disorder *anosognosia*. It may express itself in several ways: The patient may act as if nothing were the matter. If asked to raise the paralyzed arm, he may raise the intact one or do nothing at all. If asked whether the paralyzed arm has been moved, the patient may say yes. If the failure to do so is pointed out, the patient may admit that the arm is slightly weak. If told it is paralyzed, the patient may deny that this is so or offer an excuse: "My shoulder hurts." If asked why the paralysis went unnoticed, the response may be, "I'm not a doctor." Some patients report that they feel as though their left side had disappeared, and when shown the paralyzed arm, they may deny it is theirs and assert that it belongs to someone else or even take hold of it and fling it aside. This mental derangement, which Hughlings Jackson referred to as "a kind of imbecility," obviously includes a somatosensory defect and loss of the stored engrams of the body schema as well as a conceptual negation of paralysis and even a disturbed visual perception and neglect of half of the body.

The lesion responsible for the various forms of unilateral asomatognosia lies in the cortex and white matter of the superior parietal lobule but may extend variably into the postcentral gyrus, frontal motor areas, and temporal and occipital lobes, accounting for some of the associated abnormalities described below. Rarely, a deep lesion of the ventrolateral thalamus and juxtaposed white matter of the parietal lobe will produce contralateral neglect. Unilateral asomatognosia is seven times as frequent with right (nondominant) parietal lesions as with left-sided ones, according to Hécaen's statistics. The apparent infrequency of right-sided symptoms is attributable only in part to their obscuration by an associated aphasia.

Anosognosia is usually associated with a number of additional abnormalities. Often, in this state, there is a blunted emotionality. The patient looks dull, is inattentive and apathetic, and shows varying degrees of general confusion. There may be an indifference to failure, a feeling that something is missing, visual and tactile illusions when sensing the paralyzed part, hallucinations of movement, and allocheiria (one-sided stimuli are felt on the other side).

A particularly common group of parietal symptoms, easily tested at the bedside, consists of neglect of one side of the body in dressing and grooming ("dressing apraxia"), recognition only on the intact side of bilaterally and simultaneously presented stimuli ("sensory extinction"), deviation of head and eyes to the side of the lesion and torsion of the body in the same direction (failure of directed attention to the body and to extrapersonal space on the side opposite the lesion). The patient may fail to shave one side of the face, apply lipstick or comb the hair only on one side, or find it impossible to put on eyeglasses, insert dentures, or put on a dressing gown when one sleeve has been turned inside out. Unilateral spatial neglect is brought out by having the patient bisect a line, draw a daisy or a clock, or name all the objects in the room. Homonymous hemianopia and varying degrees of hemiparesis may or may not be present. Unilateral spatial neglect is further reflected in the patient's inability to reproduce geometric figures ("constructional apraxia"). A number of tests have been designed to elicit these disturbances, such as indicating the time by placement of the hands on a clock, drawing a map, copying a complex figure, reproducing stick-pattern constructions and block designs, making three-dimensional constructions, and reconstructing puzzles.

According to Denny-Brown and coworkers, the basic disturbance in such cases is an inability to summate a series of "spatial impressions"—tactile, kinesthetic, visual, or auditory—a defect they refer to as *amorphosynthesis*. In their view, imperception or neglect of one side of the body and of extrapersonal space represents the full extent of the disturbance, which in lesser degree consists only of tactile and visual extinction. They make the additional points that the disorder of spatial summation is strictly contralateral to the damaged parietal lobe, right or left, and must be distinguished from a true agnosia, which is a conceptual disorder and involves *both* sides of the body and extrapersonal space as a result of damage to one (the dominant) hemisphere. More recent observations indicate that patients with right parietal lesions show variable but lesser elements of ipsilateral neglect in addition to the striking degree of contralateral neglect, suggesting that, *in respect to spatial attention, the right parietal lobe is truly dominant* (Weintraub and Mesulam).

An interesting observation of Bisiach and Luzzatti suggests that the loss of attention to one side of the environment extends to the mental representation of space. Their patient with a right parietal lesion was asked to describe from memory the buildings lining the Piazza del Duomo, first as if seen from one corner of the piazza and then from the opposite corner. In each instance the description omitted the left side of the piazza. We have been unable to elicit this effect in our patients.

Perhaps another aspect of parietal lobe physiology, revealed by human disease, is the loss of exploratory and orienting behavior with the contralateral arm and even a tendency to avoid tactile stimuli. Mori and Yamadori call this "rejection behavior." Denny-Brown and Chambers attribute the released grasping and exploring that follow frontal lobe lesions to a disinhibition of parietal lobe automatisms. It is of interest that demented patients with prominent grasp reflexes tend not to grasp parts of their own bodies unless there has been a parietal lesion, in which case there may be "self-grasping" of the forearm opposite the lesion (Ropper).

Bilateral Asomatognosia (Gerstmann Syndrome) This syndrome provides the most striking example of bilateral asomatognosia and is due to a left, or dominant, parietal lesion. The characteristic features are inability to designate or name the different fingers of the two hands (finger agnosia), confusion of the right and left sides of the body, and inability to calculate (dyscalculia) and to write (dysgraphia). One or more of these manifestations may be associated with word blindness (alexia) and homonymous hemianopia or a lower quadrantanopia, of which the patient is usually unaware. The lesion can then be placed in the angular gyrus or subjacent white matter of the left hemisphere ("angular gyrus syndrome").

There has been a dispute as to whether the four main elements of the Gerstmann syndrome have a common basis or only a chance association. Benton states that they occur together in a parietal lesion no more often than do constructional apraxia, alexia, and loss of visual memory and that every combination of these symptoms and those of the Gerstmann syndrome occurs with equal frequency in parietal lobe disease. Others, including the authors, tend to disagree and believe that right-left confusion, digital agnosia, agraphia, and acalculia have special significance, being linked through a unitary defect in spatial orientation of fingers, body sides, and numbers.

Lesions of the superior parietal lobule may interfere with voluntary movement of the opposite limbs, particularly the arm, as pointed out by Holmes. In reaching for a visually presented target in the contralateral visual field and to a lesser extent in the ipsilateral field, the movement is misdirected and dysmetric (the distance to the target is misjudged). This disorder of movement, alluded to above in the general discussion of parietal signs and sometimes referred to as optic ataxia, resembles cerebellar ataxia and is explained by the fact that cortical areas 7 and 5 receive visual projections from the parastriate areas and proprioceptive ones from the cerebellum, both of which are integrated in the multimodal parietal cortex. Areas 5 and 7, in turn, project to frontal areas 6, 8, and 9, where ocular scanning and reaching are coordinated.

Dyscalculia has attracted little critical attention, perhaps because it occurs most often as a byproduct of aphasia and an inability of the patient to appreciate numerical language. The latter difficulty is usually associated with other elements of the Gerstmann syndrome. Computational difficulty may also be part of the more complex visuospatial abnormality of the nondominant parietal lobe; there is then difficulty in the placing of numbers in specific spatial relationships while calculating. In such cases, there is no difficulty in reading or writing the numbers and the rules governing the calculation can be described, but the computation cannot be accomplished correctly with pencil and paper. Hécaen has made a distinction between dyscalculia and anarithmetria; in the former, the process of calculation alone has been disturbed; in the latter, there is an inability to manipulate numbers. Recognition and reproduction of numbers are intact in both. An analysis of how the computation goes awry in each individual case is therefore required.

Ideomotor and Ideational Apraxia As discussed in Chap. 3, patients with *dominant* parietal lesions who exhibit no defects in motor or sensory function lose the ability to perform learned motor skills on command or by imitation. Common implements and tools can no longer be used, either in relation to the patient's body (e.g., comb or brush) or in relation to objects in the environment. It is as though the patient had forgotten the sequences of learned movements. The effects are bilateral. It is of interest that, in both agraphia and acalculia, the motor defect appears to be intertwined with agnosic defects; hence the term *apractognosia* seems appropriate.

From the above descriptions it is evident that the left and right parietal lobes function differently. The most obvious difference, of course, is that language and arithmetical functions are centered in the left hemisphere. It is hardly surprising, therefore, that verbally mediated or verbally associated spatial functions are more affected with left-sided than with right-sided lesions. It must also be realized that language function involves cross-modal connections and is central to all cognitive functions. Hence cross-modal matching tasks (auditory-visual, visual-auditory, visual-tactile, tactile-visual, auditory-tactile, etc.) are most clearly impaired with lesions of the dominant hemisphere. Such patients can read and understand spoken words but cannot grasp the meaning of a sentence if it contains elements of relationship (e.g., "the mother's daughter" versus "the daughter's mother," "the father's brother's son," "Jane's complexion is lighter than Marjorie's but darker than her sister's"). There are similar difficulties with calculation, as just described. The recognition and naming of parts of the body and the distinction of right from left and up from down are other learned, verbally mediated spatial concepts that are disturbed by lesions in the dominant parietal lobe.

Visual Disorders with Parietal Lesions A lesion deep to the inferior part of the parietal lobe, at its junction with the temporal lobe, may involve the geniculocalcarine radiations and result in an incongruous homonymous hemianopia; but just as often, in practice, the defect is complete or almost complete and congruous. If the lesion is incomplete, the lower quadrants of the visual fields are affected predominantly (quadrantanopia). An alexia or components of the Gerstmann syndrome may be associated. If the lesion is predominantly cortical, optokinetic nystagmus is usually retained; with deep lesions, it is abolished, with the target moving ipsilaterally (Chap. 14). With posterior parietal lesions, as noted by Holmes and Horrax, there are deficits in localization of visual stimuli, inability to compare the sizes of objects, failure to avoid objects when walking, inability to count objects, disturbances in smooth pursuit eye movements, and loss of stereoscopic vision. Cogan observed that the eyes may deviate away from the lesion on forced lid closure, a "spasticity of conjugate gaze."

Visual Disorientation and Disorders of Spatial (Topographic) Localization Spatial orientation depends upon visual, tactile, and kinesthetic perceptions, but there are instances in which the defect in visual perception predominates. Patients with this disorder are unable to orient themselves in an abstract spatial setting (*topographagnosia*). Such patients cannot draw the floor plan of their house or a map of their town or the United States and cannot describe a familiar route—from their home to their place of work, for example—or find their way in familiar surroundings. In brief, they have lost topographic memory. This disorder is almost invariably caused by lesions in the dorsal convexity of the right parietal lobe.

A common and striking disorder of motor behavior of the eyelids is seen in most patients with large acute lesions of the right parietal lobe. Its mildest form is a disinclination to open the lids when spoken to. This gives the erroneous impression that a patient is drowsy or stuporous, but it will be found that a quick reply can be given to whispered questions. In more severe cases, the lids are held shut and opening is strongly resisted, to the point of making an examination of the globes impossible.

The effects of disease of the parietal lobes may be summarized as follows:

I. Effects of unilateral disease of the parietal lobe, right or left
   A. Corticosensory syndrome and sensory extinction (or total hemianesthesia with large acute lesions of white matter)
   B. Mild hemiparesis, unilateral muscular atrophy in children, hypotonia, poverty of movement, hemiataxia
   C. Homonymous hemianopia or inferior quadrantanopia (incongruent or congruent) or visual inattention, and sometimes anosognosia, neglect of one-half of the body and of extrapersonal space (amorphosynthesis, observed more frequently with right than with left parietal lesions)
   D. Abolition of optokinetic nystagmus with target moving toward side of the lesion
II. Effects of unilateral disease of the dominant parietal lobe (left hemisphere in right-handed patients)—additional phenomena include
   A. Disorders of language (especially alexia)
   B. Gerstmann syndrome (dysgraphia, dyscalculia, finger agnosia, right-left confusion)
   C. Tactile agnosia (bimanual astereognosis)
   D. Bilateral ideomotor and ideational apraxia
III. Effects of unilateral disease of the nondominant (right) parietal lobe
   A. Visuospatial disorders
   B. Topographic memory loss
   C. Anosognosia, dressing and constructional apraxias. (These disorders may occur with lesions of either hemisphere but have been observed more frequently with lesions of the nondominant one.)
   D. Confusion
   E. Tendency to keep the eyes closed, resist opening, and blepharospasm
IV. Effects of bilateral disease of the parietal lobes
   A. Visual spatial imperception, spatial disorientation, and complete or partial Balint syndrome

In all these lesions, if the disease is sufficiently extensive, there may be a reduction in the capacity to think clearly, as well as inattentiveness and impaired memory.

It is still not possible to present an all-embracing formula of parietal lobe function. It does seem reasonably certain that, in addition to the perception of somatosensory impulses (postcentral gyrus), the parietal lobe participates in the integration of all sensory data, especially those that provide an awareness of one's body as well as a percept of one's surroundings and of the relation of one's body to extrapersonal space and of objects in the environment to one another. In this respect, the parietal lobe may be regarded as a special, high-order sensory organ—the locus of transmodal (intersensory) integrations, particularly tactile and visual ones, which are the basis of our concepts of spatial relations.

Useful references on parietal function include Critchley's monograph on the parietal lobes and the chapter by Botez et al in the *Handbook of Clinical Neurology*.

SYNDROMES CAUSED BY LESIONS OF THE OCCIPITAL LOBES

Anatomic and Physiologic Considerations

The occipital lobes are the terminus of the geniculocalcarine pathways and are essential for visual perception and recognition. This part of the brain has a large medial surface and somewhat smaller lateral and inferior surfaces (Fig. 22-8). The parieto-occipital fissure is its obvious medial boundary with the parietal lobe, but laterally it merges with the parietal and temporal lobes. The large calcarine fissure courses in an anteroposterior direction from the pole of the occipital lobe to the splenium of the corpus callosum; area 17, the primary idiotypic visual receptive cortex, lies on its banks (Fig. 22-3). It is typical homotypical cortex but is unique in that its fourth receptive layer is divided into two granular cell laminae by a greatly thickened band of myelinated fibers, the external band of Baillarger. This stripe in area 17, also called the *line* or *band of Gennari*, is grossly visible and has given this area its name—*striate cortex*. The largest part of area 17 is the terminus of the retinal macular fibers (see Fig. 13-2). The parastriate cortex (areas 18 and 19) lacks the line of Gennari and resembles the granular unimodal association cortex of the rest of the cerebrum. Area 17 contains cells that are activated by the homolateral geniculocalcarine pathway; these cells are interconnected and project also to cells in areas 18 and 19. The latter are connected with one another and with the angular gyri, lateral and medial temporal gyri, frontal motor areas, limbic and paralimbic areas, and corresponding areas of the opposite hemisphere through the posterior third (splenium) of the corpus callosum.

The occipital lobes are supplied by the posterior cerebral arteries and their branches, either directly in most individuals or through an embryologically persistent branch of the internal carotid arteries in a few ("fetal" posterior cerebral artery).

The connections among these several areas in the occipital lobe are complicated, and the old idea that area 17 is activated by the lateral geniculate neurons and that this activity is then transferred and elaborated in areas 18 and 19 is surely not the complete story. Actually four or five occipital receptive fields are activated by the lateral geniculate neurons, and fibers from area 17 project to approximately 20 other visual areas, of which 5 are identified most clearly. These extrastriate visual areas lie in the lingula and posterior regions. Monkeys with bilateral lesions in the temporal visual zones lose the ability to identify objects; with posterior parietal lesions, there is loss of ability to locate objects. And, as Hubel and Wiesel have shown, the response patterns of neurons in both occipital lobes to edges and moving visual stimuli, to on-and-off effects of light, and to colors are much different from what was originally supposed. Hence, form, location, color, and movement each have separate localizable mechanisms. The monographs of Polyak and of Miller contain detailed information about the anatomy and physiology of this part of the brain.

Clinical Effects of Occipital Lobe Lesions

Visual Field Defects The most familiar clinical abnormality resulting from a lesion of one occipital lobe, *homonymous hemianopia*, has already been discussed in Chap. 13. Extensive destruction abolishes all vision in the corresponding half of each visual field. With a neoplastic lesion that eventually involves the entire striate region, the field defect may extend from the periphery toward the center, and loss of color vision (hemiachromatopsia) precedes loss of black and white. Lesions that destroy only part of the striate cortex on one side yield characteristic field defects that accurately indicate the loci of the lesions. A lesion confined to the pole of the occipital lobe results in a central hemianopic defect that splits the macula and leaves the peripheral fields intact. This observation indicates that half of each macula is unilaterally represented and that the maculae may be involved (split) in hemianopia. Bilateral lesions of the occipital poles, as in embolism of the posterior cerebral arteries, result in bilateral central hemianopias. Quadrant defects and altitudinal field defects due to striate lesions indicate that the cortex on one side, above or below the calcarine fissure, is damaged. The cortex below the fissure is the terminus of fibers from the lower half of the retina; the resulting field defect is in the upper quadrant, and vice versa. Most bilateral altitudinal defects are traceable to incomplete bilateral occipital lesions (cortex or terminal parts of geniculocalcarine pathways). Head and Holmes described several such cases due to gunshot wounds; embolic or thrombotic infarction is now the common cause.

As indicated in Chap. 13, the homonymous hemianopia that results from ablation of one occipital lobe is not absolute. In monkeys, visuospatial orientation and the capacity to reach for moving objects in the defective field are preserved (Denny-Brown and Chambers). In humans also, flashing light and moving objects can sometimes be seen in the blind field even without the patient's full awareness. Weiskrantz and colleagues have referred to these preserved functions as "blindisms" or "blindsight."

Cortical Blindness With bilateral lesions of the occipital lobes (destruction of area 17 of both hemispheres), there is a loss of sight and a loss of reflex closure of the eyelids to a bright light or threat. The degree of blindness may be equivalent to that which follows enucleation of the eyes or severing of the optic nerves. The pupillary light reflexes are preserved, since they depend upon visual fibers that terminate in the midbrain, short of the geniculate bodies (see Fig. 14-6). Usually no changes are detectable in the retinas, though van Buren has described slight optic atrophy in monkeys long after occipital ablations. The eyes are still able to move through a full range, but optokinetic nystagmus cannot be elicited. Visual imagination and visual imagery in dreams are preserved. With very rare exceptions, no cortical potentials can be evoked in the occipital lobes by light flashes or pattern changes (visual evoked response), and the alpha rhythm is lost in the electroencephalogram (EEG) (see Chap. 2).

Less complete lesions leave the patient with varying degrees of visual perception. There may also be visual hallucinations of either elementary or complex types. The mode of recovery from cortical blindness has been studied carefully by Gloning and colleagues, who describe a regular progression from cortical blindness through visual agnosia and partially impaired perceptual function to recovery. Even with recovery, the patient may complain of visual fatigue (asthenopia) and difficulties in fixation and fusion.

The usual cause of cortical blindness is occlusion of the posterior cerebral arteries (embolic or thrombotic) or the equivalent, occlusion of the distal basilar artery. The infarct may also involve the medial temporal regions or thalami with a resulting Korsakoff amnesic defect and a variety of other neurologic deficits referable to the high midbrain and diencephalon (see pages 838–842). Hypertensive, eclamptic, and hypoxic-ischemic encephalopathy, Schilder disease and other leukodystrophies, CreutzfeldtJakob disease, progressive multifocal leukoenalopathy, cerebral infarctions following cardiac arrest, and bilateral gliomas are other causes of cortical blindness. A transitory form of cortical blindness may occur with head injury, migraine, or the antiphospholipid antibody syndrome of lupus erythematosus, and as a consequence of intravascular dye injection and administration of a number of drugs such as interferon-alpha or cyclosporine. In the case of the latter drugs, imaging studies have disclosed a reversible posterior leukoencephalopathy, similar in appearance to what occurs in hypertensive encephalopathy.

Visual Anosognosia (Anton Syndrome) The main characteristic is denial of blindness by a patient who obviously cannot see. The patient acts as though he can see, and when attempting to walk, collides with objects, even to the point of injury. He may offer excuses for his difficulties: "I lost my glasses," "The light is dim," etc., or there may be only an indifference to the loss of sight. The lesions in cases of negation of blindness extend beyond the striate cortex to involve the visual association areas.

Rarely, the opposite condition may arise: a patient can see small objects but claims to be blind. This individual walks about avoiding obstacles, picks up crumbs or pills from the table, and catches a small ball thrown from a distance. Damasio suggests that this might be a type of visual disorientation but with sufficient residual visual information to guide the hand, and that the lesion will be in the visual association areas superior to the calcarine cortex.

Visual Illusions (Metamorphopsias) These may present as distortions of form, size, movement, or color. In a group of 83 patients with visual perceptual abnormalities, Hécaen found that 71 fell under one of four headings: deformation of the image, change in size, illusion of movement, or a combination of all three. Illusions of these types have been reported with lesions confined to the occipital lobes but are more frequently due to shared occipitoparietal or occipitotemporal lesions, for which reason they are also considered in earlier sections of this chapter as well as in Chaps. 13 and 16. The right hemisphere appears to be involved more often than the left. Illusions of movement occur more frequently with posterior temporal lesions, polyopia (one object appearing as two or more objects) more frequently with occipital lesions (although it may occur in hysteria), and palinopsia (perseveration of visual images) with both parietal and occipital lesions. Visual field defects are present in many of the cases. In all these conditions the anatomic correlates are imprecise.

It is likely that an element of vestibular disorder underlies the metamorphopsias of parieto-occipital lesions (the vestibular and proprioceptive systems are represented in the parietal lobes of each side and the lesions there are responsible for misperceptions of movement and spatial relations). The illusion of tilting of the environment or upside-down vision has been known to occur as a result of parieto-occipital lesions but occurs more often with abnormalities of the vestibular nuclei.

Pharmacologic agents may also alter visual experience, and one may surmise that occipital or temporo-occipital regions are involved. Atropine, lysergic acid, and mescaline, but also other anticholinergic and dopaminergic drugs used for therapeutic purposes cause many of the aforementioned illusory and hallucinatory phenomena.

Visual Hallucinations These phenomena may be elementary or complex, and both types have sensory as well as cognitive aspects. Elementary (or unformed) hallucinations include flashes of light, colors, luminous points, stars, multiple lights (like candles), and geometric forms (circles, squares, and hexagons). They may be stationary or moving (zigzag, oscillations, vibrations, or pulsations). They are much the same as the effects that Foerster and Penfield obtained by stimulating the calcarine cortex in a conscious patient. Complex (formed) hallucinations include objects, persons, or animals. They are indicative of lesions in the visual association areas or their connections with the temporal lobes. They may be of natural size, lilliputian, or grossly enlarged. With hemianopia, they may appear in the defective field or move from the intact field toward the hemianopic one. The patient may realize that the hallucinations are false experiences or may be convinced of their reality. Since the patient's response is usually in accord with the nature of the hallucination, he may react with fear to a threatening vision or casually if its content is benign.

The clinical setting for the occurrence of visual hallucinations varies. The simplest black-and-white moving scintillations are part of migraine. Others, some colored, can occur as a seizure aura. Often they are associated with a homonymous hemianopia, as indicated earlier. Frequently they occur as part of a confusional state or delirium (Chap. 20). In the "peduncular hallucinosis" of Lhermitte, the hallucinations are purely visual, appear natural in form and color—sometimes in pastels, move about as in an animated cartoon, and are usually considered by the patient to be unreal, abnormal phenomena (preserved insight). Similar phenomena may occur as part of hypnagogic hallucinations in the narcolepsy-cataplexy syndrome. In our material, hallucinosis of this type (erroneously called "peduncular") has been associated mainly with high mesencephalic lesions. As indicated above, the hallucinations in this disorder are purely visual; if hallucinations are polymodal, the lesion is always in the occipitotemporal parts of the cerebrum.

A special syndrome of ophthalmopathic hallucinations occurs in the blind person. The visual images may be of elementary or complex type, usually of people or animals, and are polychromic (vivid colors). The hallucinations may occupy all of the visual field (in the totally blind person), the field of one eye, or corresponding blind fields in the patient with homonymous hemianopia. Moving the eyes or closing the affected eye has variable effects, sometimes abolishing the hallucinations.

A similar phenomenon in elderly patients with partially impaired vision has been called the *syndrome of Charles Bonnet*, following the report by this author of visual hallucinations occurring in a "sane" person. The topic of senile hallucinosis has been reviewed by Gold and Rabin and 60 such patients were reported in detail by Teunisse and colleagues. The latter authors found that 11 percent of older persons with reduced vision experienced these phenomena at one time or another. In the majority of their cases the hallucinations lacked any personal meaning and were usually not distressing, but the patients were greatly relieved to hear that they did not have mental disease.

Traditionally it has been taught that the lesions responsible for visual hallucinations, if identifiable, are situated in the occipital lobe or posterior part of the temporal lobe, and that elementary hallucinations have their origin in the occipital cortex and complex ones, in the temporal cortex. However, the opposite may pertain; in some cases, formed hallucinations are related to lesions of the occipital lobe and unformed ones to lesions of the temporal lobe (Weinberger and Grant). Also, as emphasized by these authors, lesions that give rise to visual hallucinations, simple or elaborate, need not be confined to central nervous structures but may be caused by lesions at every level of the neuro-optic apparatus (retina, optic nerve, chiasm, etc.).

The hallucinatory phenomena of delirium are nonlocalizable, as pointed out in Chap. 20, but sometimes the evidence points to an origin in the temporal lobe.

The Visual Agnosias ***Visual Object Agnosia*** This rare condition, first described by Lissauer in 1890, consists of a failure to name and indicate the use of a seen object by spoken or written word or by gesture. The patient cannot even tell the generic class of the seen object. Visual acuity is intact, the mind is clear, and the patient is not aphasic—conditions requisite for the diagnosis of agnosia. If the object is palpated, it is recognized at once, and it can also be identified by smell or sound if it has an odor or makes a noise. Moving the object or placing it in its customary surroundings facilitates recognition. In most reported instances of object agnosia, the patient retains normal visual acuity but cannot identify, match, or name objects presented in any part of the visual fields; if misnamed, the object is used in a fashion that reflects the incorrect perception. Amazingly, one encounters patients who have lost the capacity to recognize only one class of objects, e.g., animals or vegetables, suggesting that, in the human, stored information is grouped and classified in a way that is necessary for visual perception. Lissauer conceived of visual object recognition as consisting of two distinct processes—the construction of a perceptual representation from vision (apperception) and the mapping of this perceptual representation onto stored percepts or engrams of the object's functions and associations. Lissauer proposed that impairment of either of these processes could give rise to a defect in visual object recognition.

As indicated in Chap. 13, visual object agnosia is usually associated with *visual verbal agnosia* (*alexia*) and homonymous hemianopia. *Prosopagnosia* (the inability to identify faces; see further on) is also present in most cases. The underlying lesions are usually bilateral, although McCarthy and Warrington have related an instance of visual object agnosia to a restricted lesion of the left occipitotemporal region (by MRI). Several of our patients with visual object agnosia had an incomplete amnesic syndrome and a left-sided inferior occipital and medial temporal infarction, reflecting a proximal occlusion of the posterior cerebral artery.

Simultanagnosia Wolpert originally described a patient who demonstrated a "spelling dyslexia" (an inability to read all but the shortest words, spelled out letter by letter) and a failure to perceive simultaneously all the elements of a scene and to properly interpret the scene. In the framework of gestalt psychology, the patient could recognize the parts but not the whole. A cognitive defect of synthesis of the visual impressions was thought to be the basis of this condition, which Wolpert called *simultanagnosia*. Some patients with this disorder have a right homonymous hemianopia; in others, the visual fields are full but there is one-sided extinction when tested with double simultaneous stimulation. This is part of the Balint syndrome (see below), the other components of which are faulty visual scanning (ocular apraxia) and visual reaching (optic ataxia), suggesting that a fault in ocular scanning might underlie all the defects. Through tachistoscopic testing, Kinsbourne and Warrington have noted that reducing the time of stimulus exposure permits single objects to be perceived in an instant, but not two objects. Rizzo and Robin have proposed that the primary defect is in sustained attention to incoming visuospatial information. Nielsen has attributed this disorder to a lesion of the inferolateral part of the dominant occipital lobe (area 18). In a patient who presented with an isolated "spelling dyslexia" and simultanagnosia, Kinsbourne and Warrington found a lesion localized within the inferior part of the left occipital lobe. In other instances the lesions have been bilateral in the superior parts of the occipital association cortices.

Balint Syndrome This not uncommon syndrome consists of (1) an inability to project gaze voluntarily into the peripheral field and to scan it despite the fact that eye movements are full (psychic paralysis of fixation of gaze); (2) a failure to precisely grasp or touch an object under visual guidance, as though hand and eye were not coordinated (inappropriately called *optic ataxia*); and (3) visual inattention mainly to the periphery of the visual field, attention to other sensory stimuli being intact. Balint, a Hungarian neurologist, was the first to recognize this constellation of findings.

The psychic paralysis of gaze is apparent when the patient attempts to turn his eyes to fixate an object in the right or left visual field and to follow a moving object into all four quadrants of the field once the eyes are fixated on it. So-called optic ataxia is detected when the patient reaches for an object, either spontaneously or in response to verbal command. To reach the object, the patient engages in a tactile search with the palm and fingers, presumably using somatosensory cues to compensate for a lack of visual information. This may give the erroneous impression that the patient is blind. In contrast, movements that do not require visual guidance, such as those directed to the body or movements of the body itself, are performed naturally. This disorder may involve one or both hands. The presence of visual inattention is tested by asking the patient to carry out tasks such as looking at a series of objects or connecting a series of dots by lines; often only one of a series of objects can be found, even though the visual fields seem to be full.

The essential feature of the Balint syndrome appears to be a failure to properly direct oculomotor function in the exploration of space. Thus it is closely related, to simultanagnosia and to a disorder of spatial summation (amorphosynthesis). In all reported cases of the Balint syndrome, the lesions have been bilateral, often in the vascular border zones (areas 19 and 7) of the parieto-occipital regions, although instances of optic ataxia alone have been described within a single visual field, contralateral to a right or left parieto-occipital lesion.

Prosopagnosia (Greek *prosopon*, "face," and *gnosis*, "knowledge.") This term was introduced by Bodamer for a type of visual defect in which the patient cannot identify a familiar face, by looking at either the person or a picture, even though he knows that a face is a face and can point out the features. Such patients cannot learn to recognize new faces. They may also be unable to interpret the meaning of facial expressions or to judge the ages or distinguish the genders of faces. In identifying persons, the patient depends on other data, such as the presence and type of spectacles or moustache, the type of gait, or sound of the voice. Similarly, species of animals and birds and specific models or types of cars cannot be distinguished from one another, but the patient can still recognize an animal, bird, or car as such. As a rule, other agnosias are present in such cases (color agnosia, simultanagnosia), and there may be topographic disorientation, disturbances of body schema, and constructional or dressing apraxia. Visual field defects are nearly always present, a left upper quadrantanopia being the most frequent. Some neurologists have interpreted this condition as a simultanagnosia involving facial features. Another interpretation is that the face, though satisfactorily perceived, cannot be matched to a memory store of faces. Levine has found a deficit in perception, characterized by insufficient feature analysis of visual stimuli. The small number of cases that have been studied anatomically and by computed tomography scanning and MRI indicate that prosopagnosia is associated with bilateral lesions of the ventromesial occipitotemporal regions (Damasio et al).

A variant of this disorder is characterized by a specific difficulty with facial matching or discrimination from partial cues, such as portions of the face or a profile. The distinction between this deficit and the usual type of prosopagnosia rests on the use of tests that do not require memory of a specific face. This difficulty with facial matching and discrimination is more likely to be seen with lesions of the right than of the left posterior hemisphere.

Closely allied and often associated with prosopagnosia is the syndrome of loss of environmental familiarity, in which the patient is unable to recognize familiar places. The patient may be able to describe a familiar environment from memory and locate it on a map, but he experiences no sense of familiarity and gets lost when faced with the actual landscape. In essence, this is an *environmental agnosia*. This syndrome is associated with right-sided, medial temporo-occipital lesions, although in some patients, as in those with prosopagnosia, the lesions are bilateral (Landis et al).

To be distinguished from environmental agnosia is the visual disorientation and disorder of spatial (topographic) localization, already discussed under "Parietal Lobes" (page 486). Patients with the latter disorder, in distinction to those with environmental agnosia, are unable to orient themselves in an abstract spatial setting (*topographagnosia* or loss of topographic memory). Such patients cannot draw the floor plan of their house or a map of their town or the United States and cannot describe a familiar route, from their home to their place of work or find their way in familiar surroundings. This disorder is of interest insofar as it suggests that there are two separate processes for spatial orientation—one for the actual space, i.e. environmental (temporo-occipital), and one for the abstract topography of space (parietal).

Visual Agnosia for Words (Alexia without Agraphia) See Chap. 23 and further on in the present chapter, under the "Disconnection Syndromes."

Color Agnosia Here one must distinguish several different aspects of identification of colors, such as the correct perception of color (the loss of which is called *color blindness*) or the naming of a color. The common form of retinal color blindness is congenital and is readily tested by the use of Ishihara plates. Acquired color blindness with retention of form vision, due to a cerebral lesion, is referred to as *central achromatopsia*. Here the disturbance is one of hue discrimination; the patient cannot sort a series of colored wools according to hue (Holmgren test) and may complain that colors have lost their brightness or that everything looks gray. Achromatopsia is frequently associated with visual field defects and with prosopagnosia. Most often the field defects are bilateral and tend to affect the upper quadrants. However, full-field achromatopsia may exist with retention of visual acuity and form vision. There may also be a hemi- or quadrantachromatopsia without other abnormalities. These features, together with the associated prosopagnosia, point to involvement of the inferomesial occipital and temporal lobe(s) and the lower part of the striate cortex or optic radiation (Meadows; Damasio et al). These clinical findings are not surprising in view of the animal studies of Hubel, which identified sets of cells in areas 17 and 18 that are activated only by color stimuli.

A second group of patients with color agnosia have no difficulty with color perception (i.e., they can match seen colors), but they cannot reliably name them or point out colors in response to their names. They have a *color anomia*, of which there are at least two varieties. One is typically associated with pure word blindness, i.e., alexia without agraphia, and is best explained by a disconnection of the primary visual areas from the language areas (see further on). In the second variety, the patient fails not only in tasks that require the matching of a seen color with its spoken name but also in purely verbal tasks pertaining to color naming, such as naming the colors of common objects (e.g., grass, banana). This latter disorder is probably best regarded as a form of anomic aphasia, in which the aphasia is more or less restricted to the naming of colors (Meadows). According to Damasio and associates, the lesion has invariably involved the mesial part of the left hemisphere at the junction of the occipital and temporal lobes, just below the splenium of the corpus callosum. All their patients also had a right homonymous hemianopia because of destruction of the left lateral geniculate body, optic radiation, or calcarine cortex.

The Theoretical Problem of Visual and Other Agnosias From the foregoing discussion, it is apparent that the term *visual agnosia* applies to a series of visual perceptive disorders that include, in varying combinations, faults of discrimination, identification, and recognition of faces, objects, pictures, colors, spatial arrangements, and words. The diagnosis of these states is predicated on the assumption that the failure in perception occurs in spite of intact visual acuity and adequate language and mental function. When examined carefully, agnosic patients usually do not satisfy all these criteria and instead have a number of other derangements that may at least in part explain their perceptual incompetence. Often there is a unisensory or polysensory disturbance, an inadequacy of memory or of naming, or an impairment of visual oculomotor or visuomanual control. Anatomic studies have established that disturbances of recognition of complex forms, human faces, and spatial arrangements accompany right (nondominant) parieto-occipital lesions more often than left-sided ones. Disturbances of perception of graphic symbols of objects, of color discrimination and naming—in short, all of the lexical aspects of recognition—are virtually always associated with left parieto-occipital lesions. Variations in the clinical effects of such lesions are dependent not only on their location and size but also on the particular tests used to elicit these effects and whether they involve learning, recognition, and recall.

There have been many critics of the concept of agnosia as a higher-order perceptual disturbance that can be clearly separated from loss of elementary sensation. Such a division is said to perpetuate an archaic view of sensory reception in the brain as consisting of two separable functional attributes: elementary sensation and perception. Bay, for example, claimed that careful testing of patients with visual agnosia always brings to light some degree of diminished vision in combination with general defects such as confusion and mental deterioration. Others (Geschwind; Sperry and colleagues) have emphasized that the visual agnosias depend upon disconnections of the visual receptive zones of the brain from the language areas of the left hemisphere, the learning and memory zones of the temporal lobes, the suprasensory zones of the parietal lobes, and the motor regions. Hécaen, Gassel, and McCarthy and Warrington have presented the evidence for and against these points of view, the first of which argues for a diminution of sensory function and the second, for a disconnection.

The reported cases of visual agnosia emphasize the complexity of the perceptive process and the inadequacy of our knowledge of the physiology of the several receptive zones of the occipital lobes. The fact that in some cases there are impairments of primary sensation that can be elicited by careful testing of visual function—using tachistoscopic stimuli, visual adaptation, perception of pattern, flicker-fusion, etc.—cannot be disputed. However, even when present, such abnormalities would not fully explain the loss of discrimination and the inability to visualize or imagine the form and color of objects, their spatial arrangements, and their names. Failure of a sensation to activate these visual memories must involve a higher-order disturbance of cerebral function in the heteromodal association areas. Here sensory and motor functions are always integrated, the latter being essential for proper scanning and exploring by the sense organs. To reduce the agnosias to a series of disconnections between the striate and parastriate cortex and other parts of the brain, although an interesting approach, leads to an overly simplified mechanistic view of cerebral activity, which probably will not be sustained as more knowledge of cerebral physiology is acquired. There is still a great need of cases in which sensation and perception have been tested in detail and the anatomy of the lesion, in its stable end stage, has been carefully studied.

The effects of disease of the occipital lobes may be summarized as follows:

I. Effects of unilateral disease, either right or left
   A. Contralateral (congruent) homonymous hemianopia, which may be central (splitting the macula) or peripheral; also homonymous hemiachromatopsia
   B. Elementary (unformed) hallucinations—usually due to irritative lesions
II. Effects of left occipital disease
   A. Right homonymous hemianopia
   B. If deep white matter or splenium of corpus callosum is involved, alexia and color-naming defect
   C. Visual object agnosia
III. Effects of right occipital disease
   A. Left homonymous hemianopia
   B. With more extensive lesions, visual illusions (metamorphopsias) and hallucinations (more frequent with right-sided than left-sided lesions)
   C. Loss of topographic memory and visual orientation
IV. Bilateral occipital disease
   A. Cortical blindness (pupils reactive)
   B. Anton syndrome (denial of cortical blindness)
   C. Loss of perception of color
   D. Prosopagnosia, simultanagnosia
   E. Balint syndrome

Disturbances of the Nondominant Cerebral Hemisphere

A line of disagreement, as old as neurology itself, pertains to the relationship between the two cerebral hemispheres. Fechner, in 1860, speculated that since the two cerebral hemispheres, joined by the corpus callosum, were virtual mirror images of one another and functioned in totality in conscious life, separating them would result in two minds. William McDougall rejected this idea and is said to have offered to have his own brain divided by Charles Sherrington should he have an incurable disease. He died of cancer and the callosotomy was considered unnecessary, for already there were indications that, when separated, the two hemispheres had different functions (Sperry and colleagues), as indicated in the next section, on "Disconnection Syndromes."

The practice of surgical sectioning of the corpus callosum for the control of epilepsy had greatly stimulated interest in the functions of the right cerebral hemisphere when isolated from the left. It is in the sphere of visuospatial perception that right hemispheral dominance is most convincing. Lesions of the right posterior cerebral region result in an inability to utilize information about spatial relationships in making perceptual judgments and in responding to objects in a spatial framework. This is manifest in constructing figures (constructional apraxia), in the spatial orientation of the patient (topographic agnosia), in identifying faces (prosopagnosia), and in relating to one another a scattering of visual stimuli (simultanagnosia). Also, there are claims that the right hemisphere is more important than the left in visual imagery, attention, emotion (both in feeling and in the perception of emotion in others), and manual drawing (but not writing); in respect to these functions, however, the evidence is less firm. The idea that attention is a function of the right hemisphere derives from the neglect of left visual space and of somatic sensation in the anosognosic syndrome and also from the apathy that characterizes such patients. Certainly the popular notion of the right hemisphere as "emotional" in contrast to the left one as "logical" has no basis in fact and represents a gross oversimplification of brain function and localization.

DISCONNECTION SYNDROMES

Following the insightful clinical observations and anatomic studies of Wernicke, Déjerine, and Liepmann, the concept of disconnection of parts of one or both cerebral hemispheres as a cause of neurologic syndromes was introduced to neurologic thinking. In more recent years, these ideas were resurrected and modernized by Geschwind. He called attention to several clinical syndromes resulting from interruption of the connections between the two cerebral hemispheres in the corpus callosum or adjacent white matter (commissural syndromes) or between different parts of one hemisphere (intrahemispheral disconnection syndromes). Some of these are illustrated in Fig. 22-7.

When the entire corpus callosum has been destroyed by tumor or surgical section, the language and perception areas of the left hemisphere are isolated from the right hemisphere. Patients with such lesions, if blindfolded, are unable to match an object held in one hand with that in the other. Objects placed in the right hand are named correctly, but not those in the left. Furthermore, if rapid presentation is used to avoid bilateral visual scanning, such patients cannot match an object seen in the right half of the visual field with one in the left half, and they cannot read words projected to the left visual field. They are alexic in the left visual fields, since the verbal symbols that are seen there have no access to the language areas of the left hemisphere. If given a verbal command, they execute it correctly with the right hand but not with the left. For example, if asked to write from dictation with the left hand, they produce only an illegible scrawl.

In most lesions confined to the posterior portion of the corpus callosum (splenium), only the visual part of the disconnection syndrome occurs. Occlusion of the left posterior cerebral artery provides the best examples. Since infarction of the left occipital lobe causes a right homonymous hemianopia, all visual information needed for activating the speech areas of the left hemisphere must thereafter come from the right occipital lobe. The patient with a lesion of the splenium of the corpus callosum or the adjacent white matter cannot read or name colors because the visual information cannot reach the left language areas. There is no difficulty in copying words; presumably the visual information for activating the left motor area crosses the corpus callosum more anteriorly. Spontaneous writing and writing to dictation are also intact because the language areas, including the angular gyrus, Wernicke's and Broca's areas, and the left motor cortex, are intact and connected. After a delay, the patient is unable to read what he has previously written unless it was memorized. This is the syndrome of *alexia without agraphia* alluded to earlier and is discussed further on page 511.

A lesion that is limited to the anterior third of the corpus callosum (or a surgical section of this part, as in patients with intractable epilepsy) does not result in an apraxia of the left hand, i.e., a failure of only the left hand to obey spoken commands, the right one performing normally. A section of the entire corpus callosum does result in such an apraxia, indicating that the fiber systems that connect the left to the right motor areas cross in the corpus callosum posterior to the genu (but anterior to the splenium). Object naming and matching of colors without naming them are done without error. Blinded, the patient cannot name a finger touched on the left hand or use it to touch a designated part of the body.

Of interest to the authors is the fact that one sometimes encounters patients with a lesion in all or some part of the corpus callosum without being able to demonstrate the aforementioned disconnection syndromes. Is the lesion incomplete? Probably not in every case. Notable is the observation that in some patients with a congenital agenesis of the corpus callosum (a not uncommon developmental abnormality), none of the interhemispheral disconnection syndromes can be found. One can only suppose that in such patients information is transferred by another route—perhaps the anterior or posterior commissure—or that dual dominance for language was established during early development. (See review of this subject by Lassonde and Jeeves.)

In addition to alexia without agraphia, the following intrahemispheral disconnections have received the most attention. They are mentioned here only briefly and are considered in detail in the following chapter.

1. *Conduction* (also called "central") *aphasia*. The patient has fluent but paraphasic speech and writing, impaired repetition, but relatively intact comprehension of spoken and written language. Wernicke's area in the temporal lobe is separated from Broca's area, presumably by a lesion in the arcuate fasciculus or external capsule or subcortical white matter.

2. *Ideomotor ("sympathetic") apraxia in Broca's aphasia*. By destroying the origin of the fibers that connect the left and right motor association cortices, a lesion in the more anterior parts of the corpus callosum or the subcortical white matter underlying Broca's area and contiguous frontal cortex causes an apraxia of commanded movements of the left hand (see above).

3. *Pure word deafness*. Although the patient is able to hear and to identify nonverbal sounds, there is loss of ability to discriminate speech sounds, i.e., to comprehend spoken language. The patient's speech may be paraphasic, presumably because of the inability to monitor his own speech. This defect has been attributed to a subcortical lesion of the left temporal lobe, spanning Wernicke's area and interrupting also those auditory fibers that cross in the corpus callosum from the opposite side. Thus there is a failure to activate the left auditory language area (Wernicke's area). Bilateral lesions of the auditory cortex have the same effect.

Special Neuropsychologic Tests

In the study of focal cerebral disease, there are two approaches—the clinical-neurologic and the neuropsychologic. The first consists of the observation and recording of qualitative changes in behavior and performance and the identification of syndromes from which one may deduce the locus and nature of certain diseases. The second consists of recording a patient's performance on a variety of psychologic tests that have been standardized in a large population of age-matched normal individuals. These tests provide data that can be graded and treated statistically. An example is the *deterioration index*, deduced from the difference in performance on subtest items of the Wechsler Adult Intelligence Scale that hold up well in cerebral diseases (vocabulary, information, picture completion, and object assembly) and those that undergo impairment (digit span, similarities, digit symbol, and block design). A criticism of this index and others is the implicit assumption that cerebral cortical activity is a unitary function. However, it cannot be denied that certain psychometric scales reveal disease in certain parts of the cerebrum more than in others. These tests allow comparison of the patient's deficits from one point in the course of an illness to another. Walsh has listed the ones that he finds most valuable. In addition to the Wechsler Adult Intelligence Scale, Wechsler Memory Scale, and an aphasia screening test, he recommends the following for quantifying particular psychologic abilities and skills:

I. *Frontal lobe disorders*
   A. Milan Sorting Test, Halstead Category Test, and Wisconsin Card-Sorting Test, as tests of ability to abstract
   B. The Porteus Maze Test, Reitan Trail Making Test, and the recognition of figures in the Figure of Rey as tests of planning, regulating, and checking programs of action
   C. Benton's Verbal Fluency Test for estimating verbal skill and verbal regulation of behavior
II. *Temporal lobe disorders*
   A. Figure of Rey, Benton Visual Retention Test, Illinois Nonverbal Sequential Memory Test, Recurring Nonsense Figures of Kimura, and Facial Recognition Test as modality-specific memory tests
   B. Milner's Maze Learning Task and Lhermitte-Signoret amnesic syndrome tests for general retentive memory
   C. Seashore Rhythm Test, Speech-Sound Perception Test from the Halstead-Reitan battery, Environmental Sounds Test, and Austin Meaningless Sounds Test as measures of auditory perception
III. *Parietal lobe disorders*
   A. Figure of Rey, Wechsler Block Design and Object Assembly, Benton Figure Copying Test, Halstead-Reitan Tactual Performance Test, and Fairfield Block Substitution Test as tests of constructional praxis
   B. Several mathematical and logicogrammatical tests as tests of spatial synthesis

C. Cross-modal association tests as tests of suprasensory integration

D. Benson-Barton Stick Test, Cattell's Pool Reflection Test, and Money's Road Map Test, as tests of spatial perception and memory

IV. *Occipital lobe disorders*

A. Color naming, color form association, and visual irreminiscence, as tests of visual perception; recognition of faces of prominent people, map drawing

It is the authors' opinion that the data obtained from the above tests should supplement clinical observations. Taken alone, they cannot be depended upon for the localization of cerebral lesions.

REFERENCES

ALAJOUANINE T, AUBREY M, PIALOUX P: *Les Grandes Activités du Lobe Temporale*. Paris, Masson, 1955.

ANDREW J, NATHAN PW: Lesions of the anterior frontal lobes and disturbances of micturition and defaecation. *Brain* 87:233, 1964.

ASSAL G, BINDSCHAEDLER C: Délire temporal systèmatise et trouble auditif d'origine corticale. *Rev Neurol* 146:249, 1990.

BAILEY P, VON BONIN G: *The Isocortex in Man*. Urbana, IL, University of Illinois Press, 1951.

BALINT R: Seelenlahmung des "Schauens" optische Ataxie, raumliche Storung der Aufmerksamkeit. *Monatsschr Psychiatr Neurol* 25:51, 1909.

BAY E: Disturbances of visual perception and their examination. *Brain* 76:515, 1953.

BENSON DF: *The Neurology of Thinking*. New York, Oxford University Press, 1994.

BENSON DF, GESCHWIND N: Psychiatric conditions associated with focal lesions of the central nervous system, in Arieti S, Reiser MF (eds): *American Handbook of Psychiatry*. Vol 4. New York, Basic Books, 1975, pp 208–243.

BENTON AL: The fiction of Gerstmann's syndrome. *J Neurol Neurosurg Psychiatry* 24:176, 1961.

BIEMOND A: The conduction of pain above the level of the thalamus opticus. *Arch Neurol Psychiatry* 75:231, 1956.

BISIACH E, LUZZATTI C: Unilateral neglect of representational space. *Cortex* 14:129, 1978.

BLUMER D, BENSON DF: Personality changes with frontal and temporal lobe lesions, in Blumer D, Benson DF (eds): *Psychiatric Aspects of Neurologic Disease*. Philadelphia, Grune & Stratton, 1975, pp 151–170.

BODAMER J: Die Prosopagnosie. *Arch Psychiatr Nervenkr* 179:6, 1947.

BOTEZ TH, OLIVIER M: Parietal lobe syndrome, in Vinken PJ, Bruyn GW, Klawans HL (eds): Vol. 45. *Handbook of Clinical Neurology*. Amsterdam, Elsevier, 1985, pp. 63–85.

BRAIN R: Visual disorientation with special reference to lesions of the right hemisphere. *Brain* 64:244, 1941.

BRICKNER RM: *The Intellectual Functions of the Frontal Lobes*. New York, Macmillan, 1936.

BRODAL A: The hippocampus and the sense of smell. *Brain* 70:179, 1947.

BROWN JW: Frontal lobe syndromes, in Vinken PJ, Bruyn GW, Klawans HL (eds): Vol 45: *Handbook of Clinical Neurology*. Amsterdam, Elsevier, 1985, pp 23–43.

CARMON A: Sequenced motor performance in patients with unilateral cerebral lesions. *Neuropsychologia* 9:445, 1971.

CARMON A, BENTON AL: Tactile perception of direction and number in patients with unilateral cerebral disease. *Neurology* 19:525, 1969.

CHAPMAN LF, WOLFF HF: The cerebral hemispheres and the highest integrative functions of man. *Arch Neurol* 1:357, 1959.

COGAN DG: Brain lesions and eye movements in man, in Bender MB (ed): *The Oculomotor System*. New York, Harper & Row, 1964.

CORKIN S, MILNER B, RASMUSSEN T: Effects of different cortical excisions on sensory thresholds in man. *Trans Am Neurol Assoc* 89:112, 1964.

CRITCHLEY M: *The Parietal Lobes*. London, Arnold, 1953.

DAMASIO AR: Egas Moniz, pioneer of angiography and leucotomy. *Mt Sinai J Med* 42:502, 1975.

DAMASIO AR: The frontal lobes, in Heilman KM, Valenstein E (eds): *Clinical Neuropsychology*, 3rd ed. New York, Oxford University Press, 1993, pp 409–459.

DAMASIO AR, BENTON AL: Impairment of hand movements under visual guidance. *Neurology* 29:170, 1979.

DAMASIO AR, DAMASIO H, VAN HOESEN GW: Prosopagnosia: Anatomic basis and behavioral mechanisms. *Neurology* 32:331, 1982.

DAMASIO AR, VAN HOESEN GW: Emotional disturbances associated with focal lesions of the limbic frontal lobe, in Heilman KM, Satz P (eds): *Neuropsychology of Human Emotion*. New York, Guilford Press, 1983, pp 85–110.

DAMASIO A, YAMADA T, DAMASIO H, et al: Central achromatopsia: Behavioral, anatomic, and physiologic aspects. *Neurology* 30:1064, 1980.

DEGOS J-D, DAFONSECA N, GRAY F, CESARO P: Severe frontal syndrome associated with infacts of the left anterior cingulate gyrus and the head of the right caudate nucleus. *Brain* 116:1541, 1993.

DÉJERINE J, MOUZON J: Un nouveau type de syndrome sensitif corticale observé dans un cas de monoplégie corticale dissociée. *Rev Neurol* 28:1265, 1914–1915.

DENNY-BROWN D: The frontal lobes and their functions, in Feiling A (ed): *Modern Trends in Neurology*. New York, Hoeber-Harper, 1951, pp 13–89.

DENNY-BROWN D, BANKER B: Amorphosynthesis from left parietal lesion. *Arch Neurol Psychiatry* 71:302, 1954.

DENNY-BROWN D, CHAMBERS RA: Physiologic aspects of visual perception: 1. Functional aspects of visual cortex. *Arch Neurol* 33:219, 1976.

DENNY-BROWN D, MEYER JS, HORENSTEIN S: Significance of perceptual rivalry resulting from parietal lesions. *Brain* 75:433, 1952.

DODGE PR, MEIROWSKY AM: Tangential wounds of skull and scalp. *J Neurosurg* 9:472, 1952.

FEUCHTWANGER E: Die Functionen des Stirnhirns. *Monogr Neurol Psychiatr* 38:194, 1923.

FLECHSIG P: *Anatomie der menschlichen Gehirns und Ruckenmarks auf myelogenetischer Grundlage*. Leipzig, Thieme, 1920.

FUSTER JM: *The Prefrontal Cortex*, 2nd ed. New York, Raven Press, 1989.

GASSEL MM: Occipital lobe syndromes (excluding hemianopia), in Vinken PJ, Bruyn GW (eds): *Handbook of Clinical Neurology*. Vol 2. New York, American Elsevier, 1969, chap 19, pp 640–679.

GESCHWIND N: Disconnexion syndromes in animals and man. *Brain* 88:237, 585, 1965.

GESCHWIND N, QUADFASEL FA, SEGARRA J: Isolation of the speech area. *Neuropsychologia* 6:327, 1968.

GLONING I, GLONING K, HAFF H: *Neuropsychological Symptoms and Syndromes in Lesions of the Occipital Lobes and Adjacent Areas*. Paris, Gauthier-Villars, 1968.

GOLD K, RABIN PV: Isolated visual hallucinations and the Charles Bonnet syndrome: A review of the literature and presentation of six cases. *Comp Psychiatry* 30:90, 1989.

GOLDSTEIN K: The significance of the frontal lobes for mental performance. *J Neurol Psychopathol* 17:27, 1936.

HALSTEAD WC: *Brain and Intelligence*. Chicago, University of Chicago Press, 1947.

HARLOW JM: Quoted in Denny-Brown D: The frontal lobes and their functions, in Feiling A (ed): *Modern Trends in Neurology*. New York, Hoeber–Harper, 1951, p 65.

HEAD H, HOLMES G: Sensory disturbances from cerebral lesions. *Brain* 34:102, 1911.

HÉCAEN H: Clinical symptomatology in right and left hemispheric lesions, in Mountcastle VB (ed): *Interhemispheric Relations and Cerebral Dominance*. Baltimore, Johns Hopkins University Press, 1962, chap 10, pp 215–263.

HEILMAN KA, VALENSTEIN E: *Clinical Neuropsychology*, 3rd ed. New York, Oxford University Press, 1993.

HENSCHEN SE: *Klinische und anatomische Beitrage zur Pathologie des Gehirns*. Vols 5–7. Stockholm, Nordiska Bokhandeln, 1920–1922.

HOLMES G: Disturbances of visual orientation. *Br J Ophthalmol* 2: 449, 506, 1918.

HOLMES G, HORRAX G: Disturbances of spatial orientation and visual attention with loss of stereoscopic vision. *Arch Neurol Psychiatry* 1:385, 1919.

HUBEL D: Exploration of the primary visual cortex. *Nature* 299:515, 1982.

HUBEL DH, WIESEL TN: Receptive fields, binocular interaction and functional architecture in the cat's visual cortex. *J Physiol* 160:106, 1962.

JACKSON JH, STEWART P: Epileptic attacks with a warning of crude sensation. *Brain* 22:534, 1899.

JACOBSEN CF: Functions of frontal association in primates. *Arch Neurol Psychiatry* 33:558, 1935.

KAAS JH: What if anything is S1? Organization of the first somatosensory area of cortex. *Physiol Rev* 63:206, 1983.

KINSBOURNE M, WARRINGTON EK: A disorder of simultaneous form perception. *Brain* 85:461, 1962.

KINSBOURNE M, WARRINGTON EK: The localizing significance of limited simultaneous visual form perception. *Brain* 86:697, 1963.

KLEIST K: *Sensory Aphasia and Amusia: The Myeloarchitectonic Basis*. Tr. by Fish FJ, Stanton JB. Oxford, England, Pergamon Press, 1962.

KLEIST K: *Gehirnpathologie*. Leipzig, Barth, 1934.

KLÜVER H, BUCY PC: An analysis of certain effects of bilateral temporal lobectomy in the rhesus monkey with special reference to psychic blindness. *J Psychol* 5:33, 1938.

LANDIS T, CUMMINGS JL, BENSON F, PALMER EP: Loss of topographic familiarity: An environmental agnosia. *Arch Neurol* 43:132, 1986.

LAPLANE D: La perte d'auto-activation psychique. *Rev Neurol* 146:397, 1990.

LAPLANE D, TALAIRACH J, MEININGER V, et al: Motor consequences of motor area ablations in man. *J Neurol Sci* 31:29, 1977a.

LAPLANE D, TALAIRACH J, MEININGER V, et al: Clinical consequences of corticectomies involving supplementary motor area in man. *J Neurol Sci* 34:301, 1977b.

LASSONDE M, JEEVES MA (eds): *Callosal Agenesis: A Natural Split Brain*? New York, Plenum Press, 1994.

LEVINE DN: Prosopagnosia and visual object agnosia. *Brain Lang* 5:341, 1978.

LEVINE DN, CALVANIO R: A study of the visual defect in verbal alexia-simultanagnosia. *Brain* 101:65, 1978.

LHERMITTE F: Human autonomy and the frontal lobes: II. Patient behavior in complex and social situations—The "environmental dependency syndrome." *Ann Neurol* 19:335, 1986.

LHERMITTE F: Utilization behavior and its relation to lesions of the frontal lobes. *Brain* 106:237, 1983.

LILLY R, CUMMINGS SL, BENSON F, FRANKEL M: The human Klüver-Bucy syndrome. *Neurology* 33:1141, 1983.

LURIA AR: *Higher Cortical Functions in Man*. New York, Basic Books, 1966.

LURIA AR: Frontal lobe syndromes, in Vinken PJ, Bruyn GW (eds): *Handbook of Clinical Neurology*. Vol 2. Amsterdam, North-Holland, 1969, chap 23, pp 725–759.

LURIA AR: *The Working Brain*. London, Allen Lane, 1973.

MACLEAN PD: Chemical and electrical stimulation of hippocampus in unrestrained animals: II. Behavioral findings. *Arch Neurol Psychiatry* 78:128, 1957.

MARLOWE WB, MANCALL EL, THOMAS JJ: Complete Klüver-Bucy syndrome in man. *Cortex* 11:53, 1975.

MCCARTHY RA, WARRINGTON EK: Visual associative agnosia: A clinico-anatomical study of a single case. *J Neurol Neurosurg Psychiatry* 49:1233, 1986.

MCFIE J, PIERCY MF, ZANGWILL OL: Visual-spatial agnosia associated with lesions of the right cerebral hemisphere. *Brain* 73:167, 1950.

MEADOWS JC: The anatomical basis of prosopagnosia. *J Neurol Neurosurg Psychiatry* 37:489, 1974.

MEADOWS JC: Disturbed perception of colors associated with localized cerebral lesions. *Brain* 97:615, 1974.

MERZENICH MM, BRUGGE JF: Representation of the cochlear partition on the superior temporal plane of the macaque monkey. *Brain Res* 50:275, 1973.

MESULAM M-M (ed): *Principles of Behavioral Neurology*. Philadelphia, Davis, 1985.

MESULAM M-M: From sensation to cognition. *Brain* 121:1013, 1998.

MICHEL D, LAURENT B, CONVERS P, et al: Douleurs corticales: Etude clinique, electrophysiologique, et topographique de 12 cas. *Rev Neurol* 146:405, 1990.

MILLER NR: *Walsh and Hoyt's Clinical Neuro-ophthalmology*, 4th ed. Vol 1. Baltimore, Williams & Wilkins, 1982, pp 83–103.

MILNER B: Psychological defects produced by temporal lobe excision. *Res Publ Assoc Res Nerv Ment Dis* 36:1956, pp. 244–257.

MILNER B: Interhemispheric differences in the localization of psychological processes in man. *Br Med Bull* 27:272, 1971.

MORI E, YAMADORI A: Rejection behavior: A human analogue of the abnormal behavior of Denny-Brown and Chambers' monkey with bilateral parietal ablation. *J Neurol Neurosurg Psychiatry* 52:1260, 1989.

NEILSEN JM: *Agnosia, Apraxia, Aphasia: Their Value in Cerebral Localization*, 2nd ed. New York, Hoeber, 1946.

OBRADOR S: Temporal lobotomy. *J Neuropathol Exp Neurol* 6:185, 1947.

PAPEZ JW: A proposed mechanism of emotion. *Arch Neurol Psychiatry* 38:725, 1937.

PENFIELD W, ERICKSON TC: *Epilepsy and Cerebral Localization*. Springfield, IL, Charles C Thomas, 1941.

PENFIELD W, FAULK ME: The insula: Further observations of its function. *Brain* 78:445, 1953.

PENFIELD W, RASMUSSEN P: *The Cerebral Cortex of Man*. New York, Macmillan, 1950.

PENFIELD W, ROBERTS L: *Speech and Brain Mechanisms*. Princeton, NJ, Princeton University Press, 1956.

PHILLIPS S, SANGALANG V, STERNS G: Basal forebrain infarction: A clinicopathologic correlation. *Arch Neurol* 44:1134, 1987.

PLATEL H, PRICE C, BARON JC, et al: The structural components of music perception. A functional anatomical study. *Brain* 120:229, 1997.

POLYAK SL: *The Vertebrate Visual System*. Chicago, University of Chicago Press, 1957.

PORTER R, LEMON R: *Corticospinal Function and Voluntary Movement*. London, Oxford University Press, 1994.

REITAN RW: Psychological deficits resulting from cerebral deficits in man, in Warren JM, Akert K (eds): *The Frontal Granular Cortex and Behavior*. New York, McGraw-Hill, 1964, chap 14.

RIZZO M, ROBIN DA: Simultanagnosia: A defect of sustained attention yields insights on visual information processing. *Neurology* 40:447, 1990.

ROLAND PE, LARSEN B, LASSEN NA, SKINHOJ E: Supplementary motor area and other cortical areas in organization of voluntary movements in man. *J Neurophysiol* 43:118, 1980.

ROPPER AH: Self-grasping: A focal neurological sign. *Ann Neurol* 12:575, 1982.

RYLANDER G: Personality changes after operations on the frontal lobes. *Acta Psychiatr Scand Suppl* 20: 1939.

SAMSON S, ZATORRE RJ: Recognition memory for text and melody of songs after unilateral temporal lobe lesion: Evidence for dual encoding. *J Exp Psychol Learn Mem Cogn* 17:793, 1991.

SEGARRA JM, QUADFASEL FA: Destroyed temporal lobe tips: Preserved ability to sing. *Proc VII Internat Congr Neurol* 2:377, 1961.

SEMMES J, WEINSTEIN S, GHENT L, TEUBER HL: *Somatosensory Changes after Penetrating Brain Wounds in Man*. Cambridge, MA, Harvard University Press, 1960.

SEYFFARTH H, DENNY-BROWN D: The grasp reflex and instinctive grasp reaction. *Brain* 71:109, 1948.

SHANKWEILER DP: Performance of brain-damaged patients on two tests of sound localization. *J Comp Physiol Psychol* 54:375, 1961.

SPERRY RW, GAZZANIGA MS, BOGEN JE: The neocortical commissures: Syndrome of hemisphere disconnection, in Vinken PJ, Bruyn GW (eds): *Handbook of Clinical Neurology*. Vol 4. Amsterdam, North-Holland, 1969, chap 14, pp 273–290.

STUSS DT, BENSON DF: *The Frontal Lobes*. New York, Raven Press, 1986.

TANAKA Y, KAMO T, YOSHIDA M, YAMADORI A: So-called cortical deafness, clinical, neurophysiological, and radiological observations. *Brain* 114:2385, 1991.

TEUNISSE RJ, CRUYSBERG JR, HOEFNAGELS WH, et al: Visual hallucinations in psychologically normal people: Charles Bonnet syndrome. *Lancet* 347:794, 1996.

TRAMO MJ, BHARUCHA JJ: Musical priming by the right hemisphere post-callosotomy. *Neuropsychologia* 29:313, 1991.

VAN BUREN JM: Trans-synaptic retrograde degeneration in the visual system of primates. *J Neurol Neurosurg Psychiatry* 26:402, 1963.

VON ECONOMO: *Encephalitis Lethargica: Its Sequelae and Treatment*. London, Oxford University Press, 1931.

WALSH KW: *Neuropsychology: A Clinical Approach*, 3rd ed. New York, Churchill Livingstone, 1994.

WEINBERGER LM, GRANT FC: Visual hallucinations and their neuro-optical correlates. *Arch Ophthalmol* 23:166, 1941.

WEINTRAUB S, MESULAM M-M: Right cerebral dominance in spatial attention. *Arch Neurol* 44:621, 1987.

WEISKRANTZ L, WARRINGTON EK, SAUNDERS MD, et al: Visual capacity in the blind field following a restricted occipital ablation. *Brain* 97:709, 1974.

WILLIAMS W: Temporal lobe syndromes, in Vinken PJ, Bruyn GW (eds): *Handbook of Clinical Neurology*. Vol. 2. Amsterdam, North-Holland, 1969, chap 22, pp 700–724.

WOLPERT I: Die Simultanagnosie-Storung der Gesamtauffassung. *Z Gesamte Neurol Psychiatr* 93:397, 1924.

YAKOVLEV PI: Motility, behavior; and the brain: Stereodynamic organization and neural co-ordinates of behavior. *J Nerv Ment Dis* 107:313, 1948.

ZATORRE RJ, EVANS AC, MEYER E: Neural mechanisms underlying melodic perception and memory for pitch. *J Neuroscience* 14:1908, 1994.

Chapter 23

DISORDERS OF SPEECH AND LANGUAGE

Speech and language functions are of fundamental human significance, both in social interaction and in private intellectual life. When they are disturbed as a consequence of brain disease, the resultant functional loss exceeds all others in gravity—even blindness, deafness, and paralysis.

The neurologist is concerned with all derangements of speech and language, including those of reading and writing, because they are the source of great disability and are almost invariably manifestations of disease of the brain. Broadly viewed, language is the mirror of all higher mental activity. In a narrower context, language is the means whereby patients communicate their complaints and problems to the physician and at the same time the medium for all delicate interpersonal transactions. Therefore any disease process that interferes with speech or the understanding of spoken words touches the very core of the physician-patient relationship. Finally, the study of language disorders serves to illuminate the abstruse relationship between psychologic functions and the anatomy and physiology of the brain. Language mechanisms fall somewhere between the well-localized sensorimotor functions and the more widely distributed complex mental operations such as imagination and thinking, which cannot be localized.

General Considerations

It has been remarked that as human beings, we owe our commanding position in the animal world to two faculties: (1) the ability to develop and employ verbal symbols as a background for our own ideation and as a means of transmitting thoughts, by spoken and written word, to others of our kind and (2) the remarkable facility in the use of our hands. One curious and provocative fact is that both language and manual dexterity have evolved in relation to particular aggregates of neurons and pathways in one (the dominant) cerebral hemisphere. This is a departure from most other localized neurophysiologic activities, which are organized according to a contralateral or bilateral and symmetrical plan. The dominance of one hemisphere, usually the left, emerges together with speech and the preference for the right hand, especially for writing. A lack of development or loss of cerebral dominance as a result of disease deranges both these traits causing aphasia and apraxia.

There is abundant evidence that higher animals are able to communicate with one another by vocalization and gesture. However, the content of their communication is their feeling or reaction of the moment. This emotional language, as it is called, was studied by Charles Darwin, who noted that it undergoes increasing differentiation in the animal kingdom. Only in the chimpanzee do the first semblances of propositional language become recognizable.

Similar instinctive patterns of emotional expression are observed in human beings. They are the earliest modes of expression to appear (in infancy) and may have been the original forms of speech in primitive human beings. Moreover, the utterances we use to express joy, anger, and fear are retained even after destruction of all the language areas in the dominant cerebral hemisphere. The neural arrangement for this paralinguistic form of communication (intonation, exclamations, facial expressions, eye movements, body gestures), which subserves emotional expression, is bilateral and symmetrical and does not depend solely on the cerebrum. The experiments of Cannon and Bard demonstrated that emotional expression is possible in animals after removal of both cerebral hemispheres provided that the diencephalon, particularly its hypothalamic part, remains intact. In the human infant, emotional expression is well developed at a time when much of the cerebrum is still immature.

Propositional, or symbolic, language differs from emotional language in several ways. Instead of communicating feelings, it is the means of transferring ideas from one person to another, and it requires the substitution of a series of sounds or marks for objects, persons, and concepts. This is the essence of language. It is not instinctive but learned and is therefore subject to all the modifying social and cultural influences of the environment. However, the learning process becomes possible only after the nervous system has attained a certain degree of maturation. Facility in symbolic language, which is acquired over a period of 15 to 20 years, depends then on maturation of the nervous system and on education.

Although speech and language are closely interwoven functions, they are not synonymous. A derangement of language function is always a reflection of an abnormality of the brain and, more specifically, of the dominant cerebral hemisphere. A disorder of speech may have a similar origin, but not necessarily; it may be due to abnormalities in different parts of the brain or to extracerebral mechanisms. Language function involves the comprehension, formulation, and transmission of ideas and feelings by the use of conventionalized verbal symbols, sounds, and gestures and their sequential ordering according to accepted rules of grammar. Speech, on the other hand, refers more to the articulatory and phonetic aspects of verbal expression.

The profound importance of language may not be fully appreciated unless one reflects on the proportion of our time devoted to purely verbal pursuits. *External speech*, or exophasy, by which is meant the expression of thought by spoken or written words and the comprehension of the spoken or written words of others, is an almost continuous activity when human beings gather together; *inner speech*, or endophasy, i.e., the silent processes of thought and the formulation in our minds of unuttered words on which thought depends, is "the coin of mental commerce." The latter is almost incessant during our preoccupations, since we think always with words. Thought and language are inseparable. In learning to think, the child talks aloud to himself and only later learns to suppress the vocalization. Even adults may mutter subconsciously when pondering a difficult proposition. As Gardiner remarks, any abstract thought can only be held in mind by the word or mathematic symbol denoting it. It is entirely impossible to comprehend what is meant by "religion," for example, without the controlling and limiting consciousness of the word itself. Words have thus become an integral part of the mechanism of our thinking and remain for ourselves and for others the guardians of our thoughts (quoted from Brain). This is the reasoning that persuaded Head, Wilson, Goldstein, and others that any comprehensive theory of language must include explanations in terms not only of cerebral anatomy and physiology but also of the psycholinguistic processes that are involved.

Anatomy of the Language Functions

The conventional teaching, based on correlations between various disorders of language and damage to particular areas of the brain, postulates four main language areas, situated, in most persons, in the left cerebral hemisphere (Fig. 23-1). The entire language zone that encompasses these areas is perisylvian, i.e., it borders the sylvian fissure. Two language areas are receptive and two are executive, i.e., concerned with the production (output) of language. The two receptive areas are closely related and embrace what has been referred to as the *central language zone*. One, subserving the perception of spoken language, occupies the posterior-posterosuperior temporal area (the posterior portion of area 22) and Heschl's gyri (areas 41 and 42); the posterior part of area 22 in the planum temporale is referred to as *Wernicke's area*. A second area, subserving the perception of written language, occupies the angular gyrus (area 39) in the inferior parietal lobule, anterior to the visual receptive areas. The supramarginal gyrus, which lies between

Figure 23-1

Diagram of the brain showing the classic language areas, numbered according to the scheme of Brodmann. The elaboration of speech and language probably depends on a much larger area of cerebrum, indicated roughly by the entire shaded zone (see text). Note that areas 41 and 42, the primary auditory receptive areas, are shown on the lateral surface of the temporal lobe but extend to its superior surface, deep within the sylvian fissure.

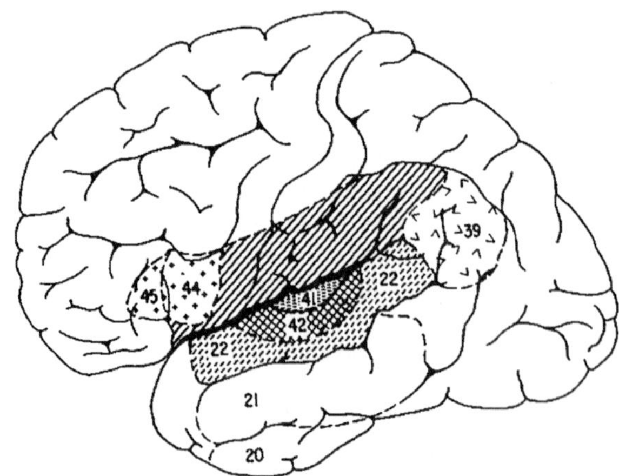

these auditory and visual language "centers," and the inferior temporal region, just anterior to the visual association cortex, are probably part of this central language zone as well. Here are located the integrative centers for cross-modal visual and auditory language functions.

The main executive region, situated at the posterior end of the inferior frontal convolution (Brodmann areas 44 and 45), is referred to as *Broca's area* and is concerned with motor aspects of speech. Visually perceived words are given expression in writing through a fourth language area, the so-called Exner writing area in the posterior part of the second frontal convolution, a concept that is still controversial in view of the fact that widely separated parts of the language zone may cause a disproportionate disorder of writing. Thus there are two parallel systems for understanding the spoken word and producing speech and for the understanding of the written word and producing writing. They develop separately but are the integral components of the semantic system.

These sensory and motor areas are intricately connected with one another by a rich network of nerve fibers, one large bundle of which, the arcuate fasciculus, passes through the isthmus of the temporal lobe and around the posterior end of the sylvian fissure; other connections may traverse the external capsule of the lenticular nucleus (subcortical white matter of the insula). Many additional corticocortical connections and other fiber systems lead into the perisylvian zones and project from them to other parts of the brain. The visual receptive and somatosensory zones are integrated in the parietal lobe, and the auditory receptive zones, in the temporal lobe. Of special importance are the short association fibers that join Broca's area with the lower rolandic cortex, which, in turn, innervates the speech apparatus, i.e., the muscles of the lips, tongue, pharynx, and larynx. The Exner writing area is similarly integrated with the motor apparatus for the muscles of the hand. The perisylvian language areas are also connected with the striatum and thalamus and with corresponding areas in the minor (nondominant) cerebral hemisphere through the corpus callosum and anterior commissure (Fig. 22-7).

There has been much difference of opinion concerning the cortical language areas, and objection has been made to calling them "centers," for they do not represent histologically circumscribed structures of constant function. Moreover, a competent neuroanatomist would not be able to distinguish the cortical language areas microscopically from the cerebral cortex that surrounds them. Some of the perceptive areas are polymodal, i.e., they are activated by auditory, visual, and tactile stimuli. Presumably, their function is integrative. Electrical stimulation of the anterior cortical language areas while the patient is alert and talking (during craniotomy under local anesthesia) may induce a simple vocalization, usually a single-vowel monotone, but otherwise causes only an arrest of speech. Electrical stimulation of Wernicke's area causes errors of speech, such as stumbling over a word or saying the wrong word.

As indicated earlier, knowledge of the anatomy of language has come almost exclusively from the postmortem study of humans with focal brain diseases. Two major theories emerged from these studies. One subdivided the language zone into separate afferent (auditory and visual) receptive parts, connected by identifiable tracts to the executive (efferent-expressive) centers. Depending on the exact anatomy of the lesions, a number of special syndromes are elicited. The other theory, advanced originally by Marie (he later changed his mind) and supported by Head, Wilson, Brain, and Goldstein, favored a single language mechanism, roughly localized in the opercular, or perisylvian, region of the dominant cerebral hemisphere. The aphasia in any particular case was presumably due to the summation of damage to input or output modalities consequent upon damage to this central language process. Undeniably, there is, within the language area, a recognizable afferent and efferent localization, as discussed above, but there is also an undifferentiated central integrative mass action, in which the degree of deficit is to a considerable extent influenced by the size of the lesion. Thus a strict division of aphasias into executive and receptive is not fully borne out by clinical observation.

Carl Wernicke, of Breslau, more than any other person, must be credited with the anatomic-psychologic scheme upon which many contemporary ideas of aphasia rest. Earlier, Paul Broca (1865), and, even before him, Dax (1836), had made the fundamental observations that a lesion of the insula and the overlying operculum deprived a person of speech and that such lesions were always in the left hemisphere. Wernicke's thesis was that there were two major anatomic loci for language: (1) an anterior locus, in the posterior part of the inferior frontal lobe (Broca's area), in which were contained the "memory images" of speech movements, and (2) the insular region and adjoining parts of the posterior perisylvian cortex, in which were contained the images of sounds (Meynert had already shown that aphasia could occur with lesions in the temporal lobe, Broca's area being intact). Wernicke believed that the fibers between these regions ran in the insula and mediated the psychic reflex arc between the heard and spoken word. Later, Wernicke came to accept von Monakow's view that the connecting fibers ran around the posterior end of the sylvian fissure, in the arcuate fasciculus.

Wernicke gave a comprehensive description of the receptive or sensory aphasia that now bears his name. The four main features, he pointed out, were (1) a disturbance of comprehension of spoken language and (2) of written language (alexia), (3) agraphia, and (4) fluent paraphasic speech. In Broca's aphasia, by contrast, comprehension was intact, but the patient was mute or employed only a few simple words. Wernicke theorized that a lesion interrupting the connecting fibers between the two cortical speech areas would leave the patient's comprehension undisturbed but would prevent the intact sound images from exerting an influence on the choice of words. Wernicke proposed that this variety of aphasia be called Leitungsaphasie, or *conduction aphasia* (later called *central aphasia* by Kurt Goldstein and *deep aphasia* by Martin and Saffran).

Careful case analyses since the time of Broca and Wernicke have repeatedly borne out these associations between a receptive (Wernicke) type of aphasia and lesions in the posterior perisylvian region and between a predominantly (Broca) motor aphasia and lesions in the posterior part of the inferior frontal lobe and the adjacent, insular, and opercular regions of the cortex. The concept of a conduction aphasia, based upon an interruption of pathways between Wernicke's and Broca's zones, has been the most difficult to accept, because it presupposes a neat separation of sensory and motor functions, which is not in line with contemporary views of sensorimotor physiology of the rest of the nervous system or with the recent analyses of language by cognitive neuropsychologists (Margolin). Nevertheless, there are in the medical literature a number of descriptions and we have certainly encountered a few cases that conform to the Wernicke model of conduction aphasia; the lesion in these cases most often lies in the parietal operculum, involving the white matter deep to the supramarginal gyrus, where it presumably interrupts the arcuate fasciculus and posterior insular subcortex.

How these regions of the brain are organized into separable but interactive information processing modules and how they can be activated (controlled) by a variety of visual and auditory stimuli and bifrontal motivational mechanisms, resulting in the complex behavior of which we make casual daily use in interpersonal communication, is just beginning to be studied by linguists and cognitive neuropsychologists. They are dissecting language into its most basic elements—phonemes (the smallest units of sound recognizable as language), morphemes (the smallest meaningful units of a word), graphemes, lexical and semantic elements (words and their meanings), and syntax (sentence structure). In general, as a restatement of the Wernicke-Broca scheme, *phonologic difficulties correlate with left frontal lesions; semantic-comprehension difficulties, with left temporal lesions; and alexia and agraphia, with inferior parietal lesions.* These elements, or modules, have been diagrammed as a series of boxes and are connected to one another by arrows, to indicate the flow of information and the manner in which it influences the spoken output of language. These "boxologies," as they are called, are not inconsistent with current psychologic theory that views language functions as the result of synchronized activity in vast neuronal networks made up of many cerebrocortical regions and their interconnecting pathways (Damasio and Damasio, 1989).

Despite this level of theoretical sophistication, attempts to delineate the anatomy of speech and language disorders by means of brain imaging techniques have been disappointing. Using computed tomography (CT) scanning, Roch-LeCours and Lhermitte were unable to establish a correspondence between the type of aphasia and the demonstrable lesion. Also, Willmes and Poeck, in a retrospective study of 221 aphasic patients, failed to demonstrate an unequivocal association between the type of aphasia and the CT localization of the lesion. This poor correlation may be related to the timing of the CT scan; images of infarcts may not be evident for several days and, when they do appear, the functional disorder at first extends beyond the margins of the visible anatomic lesion. Functional magnetic resonance imaging may prove to be superior to conventional scanning for understanding the language process, but so far only the broadest rules of localization can be confirmed. Studies of blood flow and topographic physiology during the acts of reading and speaking have shown widespread activation of Wernicke's and Broca's areas as well as the supplementary motor area and even the opposite hemisphere.

Although localization of the lesion that produces aphasia is in most instances roughly predictable from the clinical deficit, there are wide variations in the degree of deficit that follows focal brain disease. Inconsistency of anatomic findings in certain types of aphasia has several explanations, the most popular being that the net effect of any lesion depends not only on its locus and extent but also on the degree of cerebral dominance, i.e., on the degree to which the minor hemisphere assumes language function after damage to the major one. According to this view, a left-sided lesion has less effect on language function if cerebral dominance is poorly established than if dominance is strong. Another explanation invokes the poorly understood concept that individuals differ in the ways in which they acquire language as children. This is believed to play a role in making available alternative means for accomplishing language tasks when the method initially learned has been impaired through brain disease. The extent to which improvement of aphasia represents "recovery" of function or generation of new response methods has not been settled to the present day.

Cerebral Dominance and Its Relation to Language and Handedness

The functional supremacy of one cerebral hemisphere is fundamental to language function. There are many ways of determining that the left side of the brain is dominant: (1) by the loss of speech that occurs with disease in certain parts of the left hemisphere and its preservation with lesions involving corresponding parts of the right hemisphere; (2) by preference for and greater facility in the use of the right hand, foot, and eye; (3) by the arrest of speech with magnetic cortical stimulation or a focal seizure or with electrical stimulation of the anterior language area during a surgical procedure; (4) by the injection of sodium amytal into the left internal carotid artery (Wada test—a procedure that produces mutism for a minute or two, followed by misnaming, including perseveration and substitution; misreading; and paraphasic speech—effects lasting 8 to 9 min in all); (5) by the dichotic listening test, in which different words or phonemes are presented simultaneously to the two ears (yielding a right ear–left hemisphere advantage); (6) by observing increases in cerebral blood flow during language processing; and (7) by lateralization of speech and language functions following commissurotomy.

Approximately 90 to 95 percent of the general population is right-handed; i.e., they choose the right hand for intricate, complex acts and are more skillful with it. The preference is more complete in some persons than in others. Most individuals are neither completely right-handed nor completely left-handed but favor one hand for more complicated tasks.

The reason for hand preference is not fully understood. There is strong evidence of a hereditary factor, but the mode of inheritance is uncertain. Yakovlev and Rakic, in a study of infant brains, observed that the corticospinal tract coming from the left cerebral hemisphere contains more fibers and decussates higher than the tract from the right hemisphere. Learning is also a factor; many children are shifted at an early age from left to right (shifted sinistrals) because it is a handicap to be left-handed in a right-handed world. Most right-handed persons sight with the right eye, and it has been said that eye preference determines hand preference. Even if true, this still does not account for eye dominance. It is noteworthy that handedness develops simultaneously with language, and the most that can be said at present is that localization of language; preference for one eye, hand, and foot; and praxis of the right hand are all manifestations of some fundamental, inherited tendency not yet defined.

There are slight but definite anatomic differences between the dominant and the nondominant cerebral hemispheres. The *planum temporale*, the region on the superior surface of the temporal lobe, posterior to Heschl's gyri and extending to the posterior end of the sylvian fissure, has been found to be slightly larger on the left in 65 percent of brains and larger on the right in only 11 percent (Geschwind and Levitsky). LeMay and Culebras noted in cerebral angiograms that the left sylvian fissure is longer and more horizontal than the right and that there is a greater mass of cerebral tissue in the area of the left temporoparietal junction. CT scanning has shown the right occipital horn to be smaller than the left, indicative perhaps of a greater right-sided development of visuospatial connections. Also, subtle cytoarchitectonic asymmetries of the auditory cortex and posterior thalamus have been described; these and other biologic aspects of cerebral dominance have been reviewed by Geschwind and Galaburda.

Left-handedness may result from disease of the left cerebral hemisphere in early life; this probably accounts for its higher incidence among the mentally retarded and brain-injured. Presumably the neural mechanisms for language then come to be represented in the right cerebral hemisphere. Handedness and cerebral dominance may fail to develop in some individuals, and this is particularly true in certain families. In these individuals, defects in reading, stuttering, mirror writing, and general clumsiness are much more frequent and persistent during development.

In right-handed individuals, aphasia is almost invariably related to a left cerebral lesion; aphasia in such individuals as a result of purely right cerebral lesions ("crossed aphasia") is very rare, occurring in only 1 percent of cases (Joanette et al). Cerebral dominance in ambidextrous and left-handed persons is not nearly so uniform. In a large series of left-handed patients with aphasia, 60 percent had lesions confined to the left cerebral hemisphere (Goodglass and Quadfasel). In the relatively rare case of an aphasia due to a right cerebral lesion, the patient is nearly always left-handed; moreover, the language disorder in some such patients is less severe and enduring than in right-handed patients with comparable lesions in the left hemisphere (Gloning, Subirana). The latter findings suggest a bilateral albeit unequal representation of language functions in non-right-handed patients. Using the Wada test, Milner and colleagues found evidence of bilateral speech representation in about 15 percent of 212 consecutively studied left-handed patients.

The language capacities of the nondominant hemisphere have not been documented by careful anatomic studies. As mentioned above, there is always some uncertainty as to whether residual function after lesions of the dominant hemisphere can be traced to recovery of parts of its language zones or to activity of the minor hemisphere. The observations of Levine and Mohr suggest that the nondominant hemisphere has only a limited capacity to produce oral speech after extensive damage to the dominant hemisphere; their patient recovered the ability to sing, recite, curse, and utter one- or two-word phrases, all of which were abolished by a subsequent minor hemisphere infarction. The fact that varying amounts of language function may remain after dominant hemispherectomy in adults with glioma also suggests a definite though limited capacity of the minor hemisphere for language production. Kinsbourne's observations of the effect of amytal injections into the right-hemispheral arteries of patients aphasic from left-sided lesions make the same point. However, congenital absence (or surgical section) of the corpus callosum, permitting the testing of each hemisphere, has shown virtually no language functions of the right hemisphere. Some of these differences are attributable to variations in the clinical state of the subjects being tested and in the methods of language testing.

Despite its minimal contribution to the purely linguistic or propositional aspects of language, the right hemisphere does have an important role in the communication of feelings and emotion. It has long been known that globally aphasic patients, when angered, can shout or curse. These aspects of language are subsumed under the term prosody, by which is meant the melody of speech—its intonation, inflection, and pauses—all of which have emotional overtones. These prosodic components of speech and the gestures that accompany them enhance the meaning of the spoken word and endow language with its richness and vitality.

Many diseases and focal cerebral lesions mute the prosody of speech, the most dramatic examples being the hypophonic monotone of Parkinson disease and the effortful utterances of Broca's aphasia. But in recent years, largely through the work of Ross, it has been shown that this deficit in prosody is also present in patients with strokes involving the territory of the right middle cerebral artery, i.e., in portions of the nondominant hemisphere that mirror the language areas of the left hemisphere. There is an impairment both of comprehending and of producing the emotional content of speech and its accompanying gestures. A prospective study of middle cerebral artery infarctions by Darby has corroborated this view; *aprosodia* was present only in those patients with lesions in the territory of the inferior division of the right middle cerebral artery. The deficit was most prominent soon after the stroke and was not found with lacunar lesions.

Interest has been expressed in a possible role for the cerebellum in language function, based partly on observations in the Williams syndrome, in which mental retardation is associated with preservation of language skills that is sometimes striking in degree. In this disease, the cerebellum is spared in the face of greatly diminished volume of the cerebral hemispheres (see also Leiner et al). Based on our clinical experience, we would judge any language (though not speech) deficits from cerebellar disease to be subtle or nonexistent.

DISORDERS OF SPEECH AND LANGUAGE DUE TO DISEASE

These may be divided into four categories:

1. A loss or impairment of the production and/or the comprehension of spoken or written language due to an acquired lesion of the brain. This condition is called *aphasia* or *dysphasia*.

2. Disturbances of speech and language with diseases that globally affect higher-order mental function, i.e., in confusion, delirium, mental retardation, and dementia. Speech and language functions are seldom lost in these conditions but are deranged as part of a general impairment of perceptual and intellectual functions. In Alzheimer disease, for example, a gradual impairment of all elements of language without the emergence of any of the classic aphasic syndromes constitutes an important part of the clinical picture (Chap. 21). Common to this category are certain special disorders of speech such as extreme perseveration (*palilalia*) and *echolalia*, in which the patient repeats, parrot-like, words and phrases that he hears (see further on). The odd constructs of language and other disorders of verbal communication of schizophrenics and some autistic individuals—extending to the

production of meaningless phrases, neologisms or jargon—probably belong in this category as well.

3. A defect in articulation with intact mental functions and comprehension of spoken and written language and normal syntax (grammatical construction of sentences). This is a pure motor disorder of the muscles of articulation and may be due to flaccid or spastic paralysis, rigidity, repetitive spasms (stuttering), or ataxia. The terms *dysarthria* and *anarthria* are applied to this category of speech disorder.

4. An alteration or loss of voice due to a disorder of the larynx or its innervation—*aphonia* or *dysphonia*. Articulation and language are unaffected.

The important category of *developmental disorders of speech and language* is considered fully in Chap. 28.

Clinical Varieties of Aphasia

Systematic examination will usually enable one to decide whether a patient has a predominantly *motor*, or *Broca's, aphasia*, sometimes called "expressive," "anterior," or "nonfluent" aphasia; a *sensory*, or *Wernicke's, aphasia*, referred to also as "receptive," "posterior," or "fluent" aphasia; a *total*, or *global, aphasia*, with loss of all or nearly all speech and language functions; or one of the *dissociative language syndromes*, such as conduction aphasia, word deafness (auditory verbal agnosia), word blindness (visual verbal agnosia or alexia), and several types of mutism. The last of these, *mutism*, does not permit one to predict the exact locus of the lesion. Anomia (also called nominal or amnesic aphasia) and the impaired ability to communicate by writing (agraphia) are found to some degree in practically all types of aphasia. Only rarely does agraphia exist alone. The main aphasic syndromes are summarized in Table 23-1.

Broca's Aphasia

Although the precise nature of Broca's aphasia remains somewhat in doubt, we have chosen to apply the term, as have others, to a primary deficit in language output or speech production, with relative preservation of comprehension. There is a wide range of variation in the motor speech deficit, from the mildest types of poverty of speech and so-called cortical dysarthria with intact comprehension and ability to write (Broca's area aphasia; "mini-Broca"), to a complete loss of all means of lingual, phonetic, and gestural communication. Since the muscles that can no longer be used in speaking may still function in other learned acts, i.e., they are not paralyzed, the term *apraxia* seems applicable to certain elements of the deficit.

In the most advanced form of the syndrome, patients will have lost all power of speaking aloud. Not a word can be uttered in conversation, in attempting to read aloud, or in trying to repeat words that are heard. One might suspect that the lingual and phonatory apparatus is paralyzed, until patients are observed to have no difficulty chewing, swallowing, clearing the throat, crying or shouting, and even vocalizing without words. Occasionally, the words *yes* and *no* can be uttered, usually in the correct context. Or patients may repeat a few stereotyped utterances over and over again, as if compelled to do so—a disorder referred to as *monophasia* (Critchley), *recurring utterance* (Hughlings Jackson), *verbal stereotypy*, or verbal automatism. If speech is possible at all, certain habitual expressions, such as "hi," "fine, thank you," or "good morning," seem to be the easiest to elicit, and the words of well-known songs may be sung or counting by consecutive numbers may remain facile. When angered or excited, the patient may utter an expletive, thus emphasizing the fundamental distinction between propositional and emotional speech (see above). The patient recognizes his ineptitude and mistakes. Repeated failures in speech may cause exasperation or despair.

Often the arm and lower part of the face are weak on the right side, and occasionally the leg as well. The tongue may deviate away from the lesion, i.e., to the right, and be slow and awkward in rapid movements. For a time, despite the relative preservation of auditory comprehension and ability to read, commands to purse, smack, or lick the lips or to blow and whistle and make other purposeful movements are poorly executed, which means that an apraxia has extended to certain other learned acts involving the lips, tongue, and pharynx. In these circumstances, imitation of the examiner's actions is performed better than execution of acts on command. Self-initiated actions, by contrast, may be normal. By implication from CT and MRI findings in patients with apractic speech, the coordination of orobuccolingual movements, which are responsible for articulation, takes place in the left insular cortex (Dronkers). Scanning by positron emission tomography (PET) shows activation of the same insular region as well as of the lateral premotor cortex and the anterior pallidum during repetition of single words (Wise et al). It would be incorrect, however, to conclude from these studies that Broca's area itself does not participate in the composition of articulatory movements during natural speech.

In the milder form of Broca's aphasia and in the recovery phase of the severe form, patients are able to

Table 23-1
The aphasic syndromes

Type of aphasia	*Speech*	*Comprehension*	*Repetition*	*Associated signs*	*Localization*[a]
Broca	Nonfluent, effortful, agrammatical, paucity of output but transmits ideas	Relatively preserved	Impaired	Right arm and face weakness	Frontal suprasylvian
Wernicke	Fluent, voluble, well articulated but lacking meaning	Greatly impaired	None	Hemi- or quadrantanopia, no paresis	Temporal, infrasylvian including angular and supramarginal gyri
Conduction	Fluent	Relatively preserved	None	Usually none	Supramarginal gyrus or insula
Global	Scant, nonfluent	Very impaired	None	Hemiplegia usual	Large perisylvian or separate frontal and temporal
Transcortical motor	Nonfluent	Good	Largely preserved	Variable	Anterior or superior to Broca's area
Transcortical sensory	Fluent	Impaired as Wernicke	Largely preserved	Variable	Surrounding Wernicke's area
Pure word deafness	Mildly paraphasic or normal	Impaired	Impaired	None or quadrantanopia	Bilateral (or left) middle of superior temporal gyrus
Pure word blindness (and alexia without agraphia)	Normal but unable to read aloud	Normal	Normal	Right hemianopia; unable to read own writing	Calcarine and white matter or callosum (or angular gyrus)
Pure word mutism (aphemia)	Mute, but able to write	Normal	None	None	Region of Broca's area
Anomic aphasia	Isolated word finding difficulty	Normal	Normal	Variable	Deep temporal lobe, various sites

[a] Lesion in dominant (left) hemisphere unless noted.

Source: Adapted from Damasio AR: Aphasia. *N Engl J Med* 326:531, 1992.

speak aloud to some degree, but the normal melody of speech is entirely lacking. Words are uttered slowly and laboriously and are enunciated poorly. Lacking is the normal inflection, intonation, phrasing of words in a series, and the pacing of word utterances. This labored, uninflected speech stands in contrast to the fluent speech of Wernicke's aphasia. Speech in Broca's aphasia is sparse (10 to 15 words per minute as compared with the normal 100 to 115 words per minute) and consists mainly of nouns, transitive verbs, or important adjectives; phrase length is abbreviated and many of the small words (articles, prepositions, conjunctions) are omitted, giving the speech a telegraphic character (so-called agrammatism). The substantive content of the patient's language permits the crude communication of ideas, despite the gross expressive difficulties. Repetition of the examiner's spoken language is as abnormal as the patient's own speech. If a patient with nonfluent aphasia has no difficulty in repetition, the condition is termed *transcortical motor aphasia* (see further on).

Most patients with Broca's aphasia have a correspondingly severe impairment in writing. Should the right hand be paralyzed, the patient cannot print with the left one, and if the right hand is spared, the patient fails as miserably in writing to request and replying to questions as in speaking them. Letters are malformed and words misspelled. While writing to dictation is impossible, letters and words can still be copied.

The comprehension of spoken and written language, though seemingly normal under many conditions of testing, is usually defective in Broca's aphasia and will break down under stringent testing, especially when novel or complicated material is introduced. The naming of objects and particularly parts of objects is usually faulty. These are the most variable and controversial aspects of Broca's aphasia. In some patients with a loss of motor speech and agraphia as a result of cerebral infarction, the understanding of spoken and written language may be virtually normal. Mohr has pointed out that in such patients an initial mutism is usually replaced by a rapidly improving dyspraxic and effortful articulation, leading to complete recovery (the above noted "mini-Broca's aphasia"); the lesion in such cases is restricted to a zone in and immediately around the posterior part of the inferior frontal convolution (Broca's area). Mohr has stressed the distinction between this relatively mild and restricted type of motor speech disorder and the more complex syndrome that is traditionally referred to as *Broca's aphasia*. The lesion in the major form of Broca's aphasia is much larger than originally described, involving not only the inferior frontal gyrus but also the subjacent white matter and even the head of the caudate nucleus and putamen (Fig. 23-2), the anterior insula, frontoparietal operculum, and adjacent cerebrum. In other words, the lesion in the usual form of Broca's aphasia extends well beyond the so-called Broca's area (Brodmann areas 44 and 45). The persistence of Broca's aphasia is associated with the type of extensive lesion illustrated in Fig. 23-2).

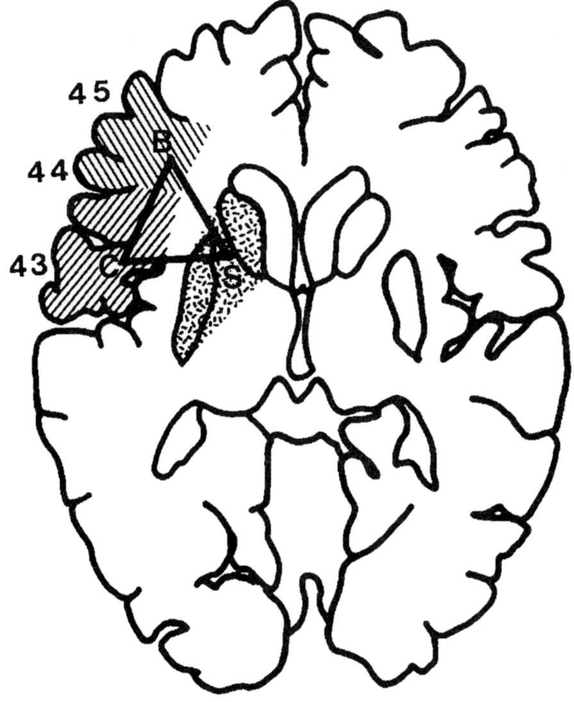

Figure 23-2

Cerebral structures concerned with language output and articulation. B = *Broca's area;* C = *pre- and postcentral gyri;* S = *striatum. Areas 43, 44, and 45 are Brodmann's cytoarchitectonic areas. A lesion in any one of the components of this output network* (B, C, *or* S) *can produce a mild and transient Broca's aphasia. Large lesions, damaging all three components, produce severe, persistent Broca's aphasia with sparse, labored, agrammatic speech but well-preserved comprehension. (Illustration courtesy of Dr. Andrew Kertesz.)*

It is noteworthy that in one of Broca's original patients, whose expressive language had been limited to a few verbal stereotypes for 10 years before his death, inspection of the surface of the brain (the brain was never cut, although CT scans have since been made) disclosed an extensive lesion encompassing the left insula; the frontal, central, and parietal operculum; and even part of the inferior parietal lobe posterior to the sylvian fissure. The Wernicke area was spared, refuting the prediction of Marie. Inexplicably, Broca attributed the aphasic disorder to the lesion of the frontal operculum alone. (The term *operculum* refers to the cortex that borders the sylvian fissure and covers or forms a lid over the insula, or island of Reil.) Broca ignored the rest of the lesion, which he considered to be a later spreading effect of the stroke. Perhaps Broca was influenced by the prevailing opinion of the time (1861) that articulation was a function of the inferior parts of the frontal lobes. The fact that Broca's name later became attached to a discrete part of the inferior frontal cortex helped to entrench the idea that Broca's aphasia equated with a lesion in the Broca's area. However, as pointed out above, a lesion confined to the Broca's area gives rise to a relatively modest and transient motor speech disorder (Mohr et al) or to no disorder of speech at all (Goldstein).

Motor speech disorders, both severe Broca's aphasia and the more restricted and transient types, are most often due to a vascular lesion. Embolic infarction in the territory of the upper main (rolandic) division of the middle cerebral artery is probably the most frequent type of vascular lesion and results in the most abrupt onset and sometimes the most rapid regression (hours or days), depending on whether the ischemia proceeds to tissue necrosis. Even with the latter, however, transient ischemia around the zone of infarction causes a more extensive syndrome than one might expect from the infarct itself, i.e., the physiologic impairment exceeds the pathologic. Because of the distribution of the upper, or superior, branch of the middle cerebral artery, there are a frequently associated *right*-sided faciobrachial paresis and a *left*-sided brachial apraxia (so-called sympathetic apraxia), due probably to interruption of the fibers that connect the left and right motor cortices. Atherosclerotic thrombosis, tumor, subcortical hypertensive hemorrhage, traumatic hemorrhage, seizure, etc., should they involve the appropriate parts of the motor cortex, may also declare themselves by a Broca's aphasia.

A closely related syndrome, *pure word mutism*, also causes the patient to be wordless but leaves inner speech intact and writing undisturbed. Anatomically, this is believed to be in the nature of a disconnection of the motor cortex for speech from lower centers and is described with the dissociative speech syndromes discussed further on in this chapter.

Wernicke's Aphasia

This syndrome comprises two main elements: (1) an impairment in the comprehension of speech—basically an inability to differentiate word elements or phonemes, both spoken and written—which reflects involvement of auditory association areas or their separation from the primary auditory cortex (transverse gyri of Heschl) and (2) a relatively fluent but paraphasic speech, which reveals the major role of the auditory region in the regulation of language. The defect in language is manifest further by a varying inability to repeat spoken and written words. The involvement of visual association areas or their separation from the primary visual cortices is reflected in an inability to read (alexia).

In contrast to Broca's aphasia, the patient with Wernicke's aphasia talks volubly, gestures freely, and appears strangely unaware of his deficit. Speech is produced without effort; the phrases and sentences appear to be of normal length and are properly intoned and articulated. These attributes, in the context of aphasic disturbances, are referred to as "fluency" of speech. Despite the fluency and normal prosody, the patient's speech is remarkably devoid of meaning. The patient with Wernicke's aphasia produces many nonsubstantive words, and the words themselves are often malformed or inappropriate, a disorder referred to as *paraphasia*. A phoneme (the minimum unit of sound recognizable as language) or a syllable may be substituted within a word (e.g., "The grass is greel"); this is called *literal paraphasia*. The substitution of one word for another ("The grass is blue") is called *verbal paraphasia*, or *semantic substitution*. Neologisms—i.e., phonemes, syllables, or words that are not part of the language—may also appear ("The grass is grumps"). Fluent paraphasic speech may be entirely incomprehensible (gibberish or *jargon aphasia*). Fluency is not an invariable feature of Wernicke's aphasia. Speech may be hesitant, in which case the block tends to occur in part of the phrase that contains the central communicative (predicative) item, such as a key noun, verb, or descriptive phrase. The patient with such a disorder conveys the impression of constantly searching for the correct word and of having difficulty in finding it.

Although the motor apparatus required for the expression of language may be intact, patients with Wernicke's aphasia have great difficulty in functioning as social organisms because they are deprived of the main means of communication. They cannot understand fully what is said to them; a few simple commands may still be executed, but there is failure to carry out complex ones. They cannot read aloud or silently with comprehension, tell others what they want or think, or write spontaneously. Written letters are often combined into meaningless words, but there may be a scattering of correct words. In trying to designate an object that they see or feel, they cannot find the name, even though they can sometimes repeat it from dictation; nor can they write from dictation the very words that they can copy. The copying performance is notably slow and laborious and conforms to the contours of the model, including the examiner's handwriting style. All these defects, of course, may be present in varying degrees of severity. In general, the disturbances in reading, writing, naming, and repetition parallel in severity the impairment in comprehension. There are, however, exceptions in which either reading or the understanding of spoken language is disproportionately affected. Some aphasiologists thus speak of two Wernicke syndromes.

In terms of the Wernicke schema, the motor language areas are no longer under control of the auditory and visual areas. The disconnection of the motor speech areas from the auditory and visual ones accounts for the impairment of repetition and the inability to read aloud. Reading may remain fluent, but with the same paraphasic errors that mar conversational language. The occurrence of dyslexia (impaired visual perception of letters and words) with lesions in the temporal lobe is explained by the fact that most individuals learn to read by transforming the printed word into the auditory form before it can gain access to the integrative centers in the posterior perisylvian region. Only in the congenitally deaf is there thought to be a direct pathway between the visual and central integrative language centers.

Wernicke's aphasia that is due to stroke usually improves in time, sometimes to the point where the deficits can be detected only by asking the patient to repeat unfamiliar words, to name unusual objects or parts of objects, to spell difficult words, or to write complex self-generated sentences. A more favorable prognosis attends those forms of Wernicke's aphasia in which some of the elements, e.g., reading, are only slightly impaired.

As a rule, the lesion lies in the posterior perisylvian region (comprising posterosuperior temporal, opercular supramarginal, angular, and posterior insular gyri) and is usually due to embolic (less often thrombotic) occlusion of the lower (inferior) division of the left middle cerebral artery. A hemorrhage confined to the subcortex of the temporoparietal region or involvement of this area by tumor, abscess, or extension of a small putaminal or thalamic hemorrhage may have similar effects but a different prognosis. A lesion that involves structures deep to the posterior temporal cortex will cause an associated homonymous quadrant- or hemianopia. Often there is no associated weakness of limbs or face and the aphasic patient may be misdiagnosed as psychotic, especially if there is jargon aphasia. According to Kertesz and Benson, persistence of Wernicke's aphasia is related to a lesion that involves both the supramarginal and angular gyri.

The posterior perisylvian region appears to encompass a variety of language functions, and seemingly minor changes in the size and locale of the lesion are associated with important variations in the elements of Wernicke's aphasia or lead to *conduction aphasia* or to *pure word deafness* (see below). The interesting theoretical problem is whether all the deficits observed are indicative of a unitary language function that resides in the posterior perisylvian region or, instead, of a series of separate sensorimotor activities whose anatomic pathways happen to be crowded together in a small region of the brain. In view of the multiple ways in which language is learned and deteriorates in disease, the latter hypothesis seems more likely.

Total, or Global, Aphasia

This syndrome is due to destruction of a large part of the language zone, embracing both Broca's and Wernicke's areas and much of the territory between them. The lesion is usually due to occlusion of the left internal carotid artery or middle cerebral artery, but it may be caused by hemorrhage, tumor, or other lesions, and it may occur briefly as a postictal effect. The middle cerebral artery perfuses all of the language area, and nearly all the aphasic disorders due to vascular occlusion are caused by involvement of this artery or its branches.

All aspects of speech and language are affected. At most, the patients can say only a few words, usually some cliché or habitual phrase, and they can imitate single sounds. Or they can only emit a syllable, such as "ah," or cry, shout, or moan. In other words, they are not mute. They may understand a few words and phrases, but—because of rapid fatigue and verbal and motor perseveration (the obligate repetitive evocation of a word or motor act just after it has been employed)—they characteristically fail to carry out a series of simple commands or to name a series of objects. They cannot read or write or repeat what is said to them. The patient may participate in common gestures of greeting, show modesty and avoidance reactions, and engage in self-help activities. With the passage of time, some degree of comprehension of language may return, and the clinical picture that is then most likely to emerge is closest to that of a severe Broca's aphasia.

Varying degrees of right hemiplegia, hemianesthesia, and homonymous hemianopia almost invariably accompany global aphasia of vascular origin. In such patients, language function rarely recovers to a significant degree. On the other hand, improvement frequently occurs when the main cause is cerebral trauma, compression from edema, postconvulsive paralysis, or a transient metabolic derangement such as hypoglycemia, hyponatremia, etc., which may worsen an old lesion that had involved language areas.

Disconnection (Dissociative) Syndromes

This term refers to certain disorders of language that result not from lesions of the cortical language areas themselves but from an apparent interruption of association pathways joining the primary receptive (sensory) areas to the language areas. Included also in this category are aphasias due to lesions that separate the more strictly receptive parts of the language mechanism itself from the purely motor ones (conduction aphasia—see below) and to lesions that isolate the perisylvian language areas, separating them from the other parts of the cerebral cortex ("transcortical aphasias").

The anatomic basis for most of these so-called disconnection syndromes is poorly defined. The concept, however, is an interesting one and emphasizes the importance of afferent, intercortical, and efferent connections of the language mechanisms. The weakness of the concept is that it may lead to premature acceptance of anatomic and physiologic mechanisms that are overly simplistic. The locale of the lesion that causes loss of a language function does not localize the language function itself, a warning enunciated long ago by Hughlings Jackson. Nevertheless, the language disorders described below occur with sufficient regularity and clinical uniformity to be as useful as the more common types of aphasia in revealing the complexity of language functions.

Conduction Aphasia As indicated earlier, Wernicke theorized that certain clinical symptoms would follow a lesion that effectively separated the auditory and motor language areas without directly damaging either of them. Since then, a number of well-studied cases have been described that conform to Wernicke's proposed model of *Leitungsaphasie* (conduction aphasia), which is the name he gave to it. Characteristically, *repetition is severely affected both for single words and for nonwords in the face of relatively preserved comprehension.* This dichotomy is said to be the essential feature of conduction aphasia.

In other respects, the features of conduction aphasia resemble those of Wernicke's aphasia. There is a similar fluency and paraphasia in self-initiated speech, in repeating what is heard, and in reading aloud; writing is invariably impaired. Dysarthria and dysprosody are usually lacking. Speech output is normal or somewhat reduced. But, compared with the one who has Wernicke's aphasia, the patient with conduction aphasia has relatively little difficulty in understanding words that are heard or seen and is aware of his deficit.

The lesion in autopsied cases has been located in the cortex and subcortical white matter in the upper bank of the left sylvian fissure, sometimes involving the supramarginal gyrus and occasionally the most posterior part of the superior temporal region. According to Damasio and Geschwind, Wernicke's and Broca's areas are spared, and the critical structure involved is the arcuate fasciculus. This fiber tract streams out of the temporal lobe, proceeding somewhat posteriorly, around the posterior end of the sylvian fissure; there it joins the superior longitudinal fasciculus, deep in the anteroinferior parietal region, and proceeds forward, deep to the suprasylvian operculum, to the motor association cortex, including the Broca and Exner areas (Fig. 22-7). However, in most of the reported cases, such as those of the Damasios, the left auditory complex, insula, and supramarginal gyrus were also involved. The usual cause of conduction aphasia is an embolic occlusion of the ascending parietal or posterior temporal branch of the middle cerebral artery, but other forms of vascular disease, neoplasm, or trauma in this region may produce the same syndrome.

The concept of conduction aphasia, as outlined above, remains a useful theoretic construct, although not all authors are in agreement as to its purity as an aphasic syndrome. Mohr, in his analysis of the writings on this subject, found that the distinction between conduction aphasia and Wernicke's aphasia, mainly one of degree of auditory comprehension, was ambiguous clinically and that the lesions in the two syndromes were much the same.

"Pure" Word Deafness This uncommon disorder, originally described by Lichtheim in 1885, is characterized by an impairment of auditory comprehension and repetition and an inability to write to dictation. Self-initiated utterances are usually correctly phrased but sometimes paraphasic; spontaneous writing and ability to comprehend written language are preserved, thus distinguishing this disorder from classic Wernicke's aphasia. Patients with pure word deafness may declare that they cannot hear, but shouting does not help, sometimes to their surprise. Audiometric testing and auditory evoked potentials disclose no hearing defect, and nonverbal sounds, such as a doorbell, can be heard without difficulty. The patient is forced to depend heavily on visual cues and frequently uses them well enough to understand most of what is said. However, tests that prevent the use of visual cues readily uncover the deficit. If able to describe the auditory experience, the patient says that words sound like a jumble of noises. As in the case of visual verbal agnosia (see below), the syndrome of pure auditory verbal agnosia is not pure, particularly at its onset, and paraphasic and other elements of Wernicke's aphasia may be detected (Buchman et al). At times this syndrome is the result of resolution of a more typical Wernicke's aphasia, and it will be recognized that word deafness is an integral feature of all instances of Wernicke's aphasia. Conceptually it has been thought of as an exclusive injury of the auditory processing system.

In most recorded autopsy studies, the lesions have been bilateral, in the middle third of the superior temporal gyri, in a position to interrupt the connections between the primary auditory cortex in the transverse gyri of Heschl and the association areas of the superoposterior cortex of the temporal lobe. In a few cases unilateral lesions have been localized in this part of the dominant temporal lobe (see page 495). Requirements of small size and superficiality of the lesion in the cortex and subcortical white matter are best fulfilled by an embolic occlusion of a small branch of the lower division of the middle cerebral artery.

"Pure" Word Blindness (Alexia without Agraphia, Visual Verbal Agnosia) This is a not uncommon syndrome, in which a literate person loses the ability to read aloud, to understand written script, and, often, to name colors—i.e., to match a seen color to its spoken name—*visual verbal color anomia*. Such a person can no longer name or point on command to words, although he is sometimes able to read letters or numbers. Understanding spoken language, repetition of what is heard, writing spontaneously and to dictation, and conversation are all intact. The ability to copy words is impaired but is better preserved than reading, and the patient may even be able to spell a word or to identify a word by having it spelled to him or by reading one letter at a time (letter-by-letter reading). In some cases, the patient manages to read single letters but not to join them together (*asyllabia*). The most striking feature of this syndrome is the retained capacity to write fluently, after which the patient cannot read what has been written (*alexia without agraphia*). And when the patient with alexia or dyslexia also has difficulty in auditory comprehension and in repeating spoken words, the syndrome corresponds to Wernicke's aphasia.

Autopsies of such cases have usually demonstrated a lesion that destroys the left visual cortex and underlying white matter, particularly the geniculocalcarine tract, as well as the connections of the right visual cortex with the intact language areas of the dominant hemisphere. In the case originally described by Déjerine (1892), the disconnection occurred in the posterior part (splenium) of the corpus callosum, wherein lie the connections between the visual association areas of the two hemispheres (Fig. 22-7). More often the callosal pathways are interrupted in the forceps major or in the paraventricular region (Damasio and Damasio). In either event, the patient is blind in the right half of each visual field by virtue of the left occipital lesion, and visual information reaches only the right occipital lobe; however, this information cannot be transferred, via the callosal pathways, to the angular gyrus of the left (dominant) hemisphere.

A rare variant of this syndrome takes the form of *alexia without agraphia and without hemianopia*. A lesion deep in the white matter of the left occipital lobe, at its junction with the parietal lobe, interrupts the projections from the intact (right) visual cortex to the language areas but spares the geniculocalcarine pathway (Greenblatt). This lesion, coupled with one in the splenium, prevents all visual information from reaching the language areas, including the angular gyrus and Wernicke's area.

In yet other cases, the lesion is confined to the angular gyrus or the subjacent white matter. In such cases also, a right homonymous hemianopia will be absent, but the *alexia may be combined with agraphia* and other elements of the Gerstmann syndrome—i.e., right-left confusion, acalculia, and finger agnosia (page 485). This constellation of symptoms is sometimes referred to as the *syndrome of the angular gyrus*. Anomic aphasia may be added (see below).

"Pure" Word Mutism (Aphemia, Pure Motor Aphasia of Déjerine) Occasionally, as a result of a vascular lesion or other type of localized injury of the dominant frontal lobe, the patient loses all capacity to speak while retaining perfectly the ability to write, to understand spoken words, to read silently with comprehension, and to repeat spoken words. Facial and brachial paresis may be associated. From the time speech becomes audible, language may be syntactically complete, showing neither loss of vocabulary nor agrammatism; or there may be varying degrees of dysarthria (hence "cortical dysarthria"), anomia, and paraphasic substitutions, especially for consonants. The most notable feature of this type of speech disorder is its transience; within a few weeks or months, language is restored to normal. Bastian and more recently other authors have called this syndrome *aphemia*, a term that was used originally by Broca in another context—to describe the severe motor aphasia that now carries his name. Probably the syndrome is closely allied to the "mini-Broca's aphasia" described on page 505.

The anatomic basis of pure word mutism has not been determined precisely. In a few postmortem cases, reference is made to a lesion in Broca's area. Damasio and Geschwind state that the lesion is anterior and superior to this area. A particularly well-studied case has been reported by Roch-LeCours and Lhermitte. Their patient uttered only a few sounds for 4 weeks, after which he recovered rapidly and completely. From the onset of the stroke, the patient showed no disturbance of comprehension of language or of writing. Autopsy, 10 years later, disclosed an infarct that was confined to the cortex and subjacent white matter of the lowermost part of the precentral gyrus; Broca's area, one gyrus forward, was completely spared.

Anomic (Amnesic, Nominal) Aphasia Some degree of word-finding difficulty is probably part of every type of language disorder, including that which occurs with the confusional states and dementia. In fact, without an element of anomia, a diagnosis of aphasia is usually incorrect. Only when this feature is the most notable aspect of language difficulty is the term *anomic aphasia* employed. In this latter condition, a relatively uncommon form of aphasia, the patient loses only the ability to name people and objects. There are typical pauses in speech, groping for words, circumlocution, and substitution of another word or phrase that is intended to convey the meaning. Or the patient may simply fail to name a shown object, in contrast to the usual aphasic patient, who produces a paraphasic error. Less frequently used words give more trouble. When shown a series of common objects, the patient may tell of their use instead of giving their names. The difficulty applies not only to objects seen but to the names of things heard or felt (Geschwind), but this is more difficult to demonstrate.

Beauvois and coworkers have described a form of bilateral tactile aphasia in which objects seen and verbally mentioned could be named, but not those felt with either hand. Recall of the names of letters, digits, and other printed verbal material is almost invariably preserved, and immediate repetition of a spoken name is intact. That the deficit is principally one of naming is shown by the patient's correct use of the object and, usually, by an ability to point to the correct object on hearing or seeing the name and to choose the correct name from a list. The patient's understanding of what is heard or read is normal. There is a tendency for patients to attribute their failure to forgetfulness or to give some other lame excuse for the disability, suggesting that they are not completely aware of the nature of their difficulty.

Of course, there are patients who fail not only to name objects but also to recognize the correct word when it is given to them. In such patients, the understanding of what is heard or read is not normal, i.e., the naming difficulty is but one symptom of another type of aphasic disorder.

Anomic aphasia has been associated with lesions in different parts of the language area, classically in the temporal lobe. In these cases the lesion has been deep in the basal portion of the posterior temporal lobe or in the middle temporal convolution, in position to interrupt connections between sensory language areas and the hippocampal regions concerned with learning and memory. Mass lesions—such as a tumor, herpes encephalitis, or an abscess—are the most frequent causes; as these lesions enlarge, a contralateral upper quadrantic visual field defect or a Wernicke's aphasia is added. Occasionally, anomia appears with lesions due to occlusion of the temporal branches of the posterior cerebral artery. Anomia may be a prominent manifestation of transcortical motor aphasia (see below) and may be associated with the Gerstmann syndrome, in which case the lesions are found in the frontal lobe and angular gyrus, respectively. An anomic type of aphasia is often an early sign of Alzheimer and Pick disease, and minor degrees of it are common in old age. Finally, anomic aphasia may be the only residual abnormality after partial recovery from Wernicke's, conduction, transcortical sensory, or (rarely) Broca's aphasia (Benson).

Isolation of the Language Areas (Transcortical Aphasias) Destruction of the border zones between anterior, middle, and posterior cerebral arteries—usually as a result of prolonged hypotension, carbon monoxide poisoning, or other forms of anoxic-ischemic injury—may effectively isolate the intact motor and sensory language areas, all or in part, from the rest of the cortex of the same hemisphere. In the case of Assal and colleagues, for example, multiple infarcts had isolated all of the language area.

In *transcortical sensory aphasia*, so named by Lichtheim and later defined by Goldstein, the patient suffers a deficit of auditory and visual word comprehension, and writing and reading are impossible. Speech remains fluent, with marked paraphasia, anomia, and empty circumlocutions. However, the central feature of transcortical aphasia is that *repetition is remarkably preserved*, unlike the deficit in Wernicke's and conduction aphasia, in which ability to repeat the spoken word is lost or severely impaired. Facility in repetition, in extreme degree, takes the form of echoing, parrot-like, word phrases and songs that are heard (echolalia). In a series of 15 such patients, CT and isotope scans have uniformly disclosed a lesion in the posterior parieto-occipital region (Kertesz et al). This locale explains the frequent concurrence of transient visual agnosia and hemianopia. In general, this disorder has a good prognosis.

Presumably, in transcortical aphasia, information from the nonlanguage areas of the cerebrum cannot be transferred to Wernicke's area for conversion into verbal form. The paraphasia is thought to result from the weakened control of the motor language areas by the auditory and visual areas, though the direct connection between them, presumably the arcuate fasciculus, is preserved. Preservation of this direct connection is said to account for the ability to repeat. Reading and auditory comprehension suffer because the sensory information does not reach the central integrative centers.

In *transcortical motor aphasia* ("anterior isolation syndrome," "dynamic aphasia" of Luria) the patient is unable to initiate conversational speech, producing only a few grunts or syllables. Comprehension is relatively preserved, but *repetition is strikingly intact*, distinguishing this syndrome from pure word mutism (see above). Transcortical motor aphasia occurs in two clinical contexts: (1) in a mild or partially recovered Broca's aphasia in which repetition remains superior to conversational speech (repeating and reading aloud are generally easier than self-generated speech) and (2) in states of abulia and akinetic mutism with frontal lobe damage, for the same reason. Several of our cases have resulted from infarctions in the watershed zone between the anterior and middle cerebral arteries, after cardiac arrest or shock.

These transcortical syndromes are of great theoretical interest and are probably more common than is currently appreciated.

The Agraphias

Writing is, of course, an integral part of language function but a less essential and universal component, for a considerable segment of the world's population speaks but does not read or write. It might be supposed that all the rules of language derived from the study of motor aphasia would be applicable to agraphia. In part this is true. One must be able to formulate ideas in words and phrases in order to have something to write as well as to say; hence disorders of writing, like disorders of speaking, reflect all the basic defects of language. But there is an obvious difference between these two expressive modes. In speech, only one final motor pathway coordinating the movements of lips, tongue, larynx, and respiratory muscles is available, whereas if the right hand is paralyzed, one can still write with the left one, or with a foot, and even with the mouth by holding a pencil between the teeth.

The writing of a word can be accomplished either by the direct lexical method of recalling its spelling or by sounding out its phonemes and transforming them into learned graphemes (motor images)—i.e., the phonologic method. Some authors state that in agraphia there is a specific difficulty in transforming phonologic information, acquired through the auditory sense, into orthographic forms; others see it as a block between the visual form of phonemes and the cursive movements of the hand (Basso et al). In support of the latter idea is the fact that reading and writing usually develop together and are long preceded by the development and elaboration of auditory-articular mechanisms.

Pure agraphia as the initial and sole disturbance of language function is a great rarity, but such cases have been described (see the review of Rosati and de Bastiani). Pathologically verified cases are virtually nonexistent, but CT examination of the case of Rosati and de Bastiani disclosed a lesion of the posterior perisylvian area. This is in keeping with the observation that a lesion in or near the angular gyrus will occasionally cause a disproportionate disorder of writing as part of the Gerstmann syndrome. As mentioned earlier, the notion of a specific center for writing in the posterior part of the second frontal convolution ("Exner's writing area") has been questioned by some aphasiologists (see Leischner). However, Croisile and associates do cite cases of pure dysgraphia in which a lesion (in their case, a hematoma) was located in the centrum semiovale beneath the motor parts of the frontal cortex.

Quite apart from these *aphasic agraphias*, in which spelling and grammatical errors abound, there are special forms of agraphia caused by abnormalities of spatial perception and praxis. Disturbances in the perception of spatial relationships appear to underlie *constructional agraphia*. In this circumstance, letters and words are formed clearly enough but are wrongly arranged on the page. Words may be superimposed, reversed, written diagonally or in haphazard arrangement, or from right to left; with right parietal lesions, only the right half of the page is used. Usually one finds other constructional difficulties as well, such as inability to copy geometric figures or to make drawings of clocks, flowers, and maps, etc.

A third group may be called the *apraxic agraphias*. Here language formulation is correct and the spatial arrangements of words are respected, but the hand has lost its skill in forming letters and words. Handwriting becomes a scrawl, losing all personal character. There may be an uncertainty as to how the pen should be held and applied to paper; apraxias (ideomotor and ideational) are present in the right-hander. As a rule, other learned manual skills are simultaneously disordered. Speculations as to the basic fault here are discussed in Chap. 3, under "Apraxia and Other Nonparalytic Disorders of Motor Functions," and in Chap. 22, in relation to functions of the frontal and parietal lobes.

In addition to the neurologic forms of agraphia, described above, psychologists have defined a group of "*linguistic*" *agraphias*, subdivided into phonologic, lexical, and semantic types (Roeltgen). These linguistic models are based on loss of the ability to write (and to spell) particular classes of words. For example, the patient may be unable to spell pronounceable nonsense words, with preserved ability to spell real words (phonologic agraphia); or there may be preserved ability to write nonsense words but not irregular words, such as *island* (lexical agraphia); patients with semantic agraphia have difficulty incorporating meaning into the written word, e.g., "the moon comes out at knight." For the most part these linguistic agraphias have no well-established cerebral localization and only tenuous associations with the classic aphasias, for which reason this subject is of greater interest to linguists and psychologists than to neurologists.

Subcortical Aphasia (Thalamic and Striatocapsular Aphasias)

A lesion of the dominant thalamus, usually vascular and involving the posterior nuclei, may cause an aphasia, the clinical features of which are not entirely uniform. Usually there is mutism initially and comprehension is impaired. With beginning recovery, spontaneous speech is reduced in amount; less often, speech is fluent and paraphasic to the point of jargon. Reading and writing may or may not be affected. Anomia has been described with a ventrolateral lesion (Ojemann). Characteristically the patient's ability to repeat dictated words and phrases is unimpaired, as in transcortical sensory aphasia. Complete recovery, in a matter of weeks, is the rule, often with persistence of the thalamic lesion.

Aphasia has also been described with dominant striatocapsular lesions, particularly if they extend laterally into the subcortical white matter of the temporal lobe and insula. The head of the caudate, anterior limb of the internal capsule, and the anterosuperior aspect of the putamen appear to be the critically involved structures. The aphasia is characterized by nonfluent, dysarthric, paraphasic speech and varying degrees of difficulty with comprehension of language, naming, and repetition. The lesion is vascular as a rule, and a right hemiparesis is usually associated. In general, striatocapsular aphasia recovers more slowly and less completely than thalamic aphasia.

These two subcortical aphasias—thalamic and striatocapsular—resemble but are not identical to the Wernicke and Broca types of aphasia. For further discussion of the subcortical aphasias, the reader is directed to the articles of Naeser and of Alexander and their colleagues.

Other Cerebral Disorders of Language

It would be incorrect to conclude that the syndromes described above, all of which are related to perisylvian lesions of the dominant cerebral hemisphere, represent all the ways in which cerebral disease disturbs language. The effects on speech and language of diffuse cerebral disorders, such as delirium tremens and Alzheimer disease, have already been mentioned (see pages 505 and 512). Pathologic changes in parts of the cerebrum other than the perisylvian regions may secondarily affect language function. The lesions that occur in the border zones between major cerebral arteries and effectively isolate perisylvian areas from other parts of the cerebrum fall into this category (transcortical aphasias, see above). Other examples are the lesions in the medio-orbital or superior and lateral parts of the frontal lobes, which impair all motor activity, to the point of abulia or akinetic mutism (pages 369–370). The mute patient, in contrast to the aphasic one, emits no sounds. If the patient is less severely hypokinetic, his speech tends to be laconic, with long pauses and an inability to sustain a monologue. Extensive occipital lesions will, of course, impair reading, but they also reduce the utilization of all visual and lexical stimuli. Deep cerebral lesions, by causing fluctuating states of inattention and disorientation, induce fragmentation of words and phrases and sometimes protracted, uncontrollable talking (logorrhea). Strong stimulation, which momentarily stabilizes behavior and speech, proves the essential integrity of language mechanisms.

Severe mental retardation often results in failure to acquire even spoken language, as pointed out in Chaps. 28 and 38. If there is any language skill, it consists only of the understanding of a few simple spoken commands. The subject of developmental dyslexia is discussed on page 628.

Approach to the Patient with Language Disorders

In the investigation of aphasia, it is first necessary to inquire into the patient's native language, handedness, and previous level of literacy and education. For many years it has been taught that following the onset of aphasia, individuals who had been fluent in more than one language (polyglots) improved more quickly in their native language than in a subsequently acquired one (a derivative of Ribot's law of retained distant memory). This rule seems to hold if the patient is not truly fluent in the more recently acquired language, or has not used it for a long time. More often, the language most used before the onset of the aphasia will recover first (Pitres' law). Usually, if adequate testing is possible, more or less the same aphasic abnormalities are found in both the first and the more recently acquired language.

Many naturally left-handed children are trained to use the right hand for writing; therefore, in determining handedness, one must ask which hand is preferred for throwing a ball, threading a needle, sewing, or using a tennis racket or hammer, and which eye is used for sighting a target with a rifle or other instrument. It is important, before beginning the examination, to determine whether the patient is alert and can participate reliably in testing, since accurate assessment of language depends on these factors.

One should quickly ascertain whether the patient has other gross signs of a cerebral lesion such as hemiplegia, facial weakness, homonymous hemianopia, or corticosensory loss. When such a constellation of major neurologic signs is present, the aphasic disorder is usually of the total (global) type. Dyspraxia of limbs and speech musculature in response to spoken commands or to visual mimicry is generally associated with Broca's aphasia and sometimes with Wernicke's aphasia. Bilateral or unilateral homonymous hemianopia without motor weakness tends often to be linked to pure word blindness, to alexia with or without agraphia, and to anomic aphasia.

The bedside analysis of aphasic disorders entails the systematic testing of six aspects of language function: *conversational speech (fluency), comprehension, repetition, reading, writing, and naming*. Simply engaging the patient in conversation permits quick assessment of the motor aspects of speech (praxis and prosody), fluency, language formulation, and auditory comprehension. If the disability consists mainly of sparse, laborious speech, it suggests, of course, Broca's aphasia, and this possibility can be pursued further by tests of repeating from dictation and by special tests of praxis of the oropharyngeal muscles. Fluent but empty paraphasic speech with impaired comprehension is indicative of Wernicke's aphasia. Impaired comprehension but perfectly normal formulated speech and intact ability to read suggest the rare syndrome of pure word deafness.

When conversation discloses virtually no abnormalities, other tests may still be revealing. The most important of these are reading, writing, repetition, and naming. Reading aloud single letters, words, and text may disclose the dissociative syndrome of pure word blindness. Except for this syndrome and pure word mutism (see above), writing is disturbed in all forms of aphasia. Literal and verbal paraphasic errors may appear in milder cases of Wernicke's aphasia as the patient reads aloud from a text or from words in the examiner's handwriting. Similar errors appear even more frequently when the patient is asked to explain the text, read aloud, or give an explanation in writing.

Testing the patient's ability to repeat spoken language is a simple and important maneuver in the evaluation of aphasic disorders. As with other tests of aphasia, it may be necessary to increase the complexity of the test—from digits and simple words to complex words, phrases, and sentences—in order to disclose the full disability. Defective repetition occurs in all forms of aphasia (Broca's, Wernicke's, and global) due to lesions in the perisylvian language areas. The patient may be unable to repeat what is said to him, despite relatively adequate comprehension—the hallmark of conduction aphasia. Contrariwise, normal repetition in an aphasic patient indicates that the perisylvian area is intact (so-called transcortical aphasia). In fact, the tendency to repeat may be excessive (echolalia). Preserved repetition is also characteristic of anomic aphasia and occurs occasionally with subcortical lesions. Disorders confined to naming, other language functions (reading, writing, spelling, etc.) being adequate, are diagnostic of amnesic, or anomic, aphasia and referable usually to lower temporal lobe lesions.

These deficits can be quantitated by the use of any one of several examination procedures. Those of Goodglass and Kaplan (Boston Diagnostic Aphasia Examination, or BDAE) and of Kertesz (Western Aphasia Battery, or WAB) are the most widely used in the United States. The use of these procedures will enable one to predict the type and localization of the lesion in approximately two-thirds of the patients, which is not much better than detailed bedside examination. Aphasia of the Broca, Wernicke, conduction, global, and anomic types accounted for 392 of 444 unselected cases studied by Benson and his group.

Treatment The sudden onset of aphasia would be expected to cause great apprehension, but except for cases of pure or almost pure motor disorders of speech, most patients show remarkably little concern. It appears that the very lesion that deprives them of speech also causes at least a partial loss of insight into their own disability. This reaches almost a ludicrous extreme in some cases of Wernicke's aphasia, in which the patient becomes indignant when others cannot understand his jargon. Nonetheless, as improvement occurs, many patients do become discouraged. Reassurance and a program of speech rehabilitation are the best ways of helping the patient at this stage.

Whether contemporary methods of speech therapy accomplish more than can be accounted for by spontaneous recovery is still uncertain. Most aphasic disorders are due to vascular disease and trauma, and they are nearly always accompanied by some degree of spontaneous improvement in the days, weeks, and months that follow the stroke or accident. A Veterans Administration Cooperative Study (Wertz et al) has suggested that intensive therapy by a speech pathologist does hasten improvement. Also, Howard and colleagues have shown increased efficacy of word retrieval in a group of chronic stable aphasics treated by two different techniques. More studies of this type, which control for the effects of the patient's motivation and the interest of family and therapist, are needed. In an interesting personal experiment by Wender, a classicist who had become aphasic, practice of Greek vocabulary and grammar led to recovery in that language, but there was little recovery of her facility with Latin, which was not similarly exercised.

One must decide for each patient when speech training should be started. As a rule, therapy is not advisable in the first few days of an aphasic illness, because one does not know how lasting it will be. Also, if the patient suffers a severe global aphasia and can neither speak nor understand spoken and written words, the speech therapist is virtually helpless. Under such circumstances, one does well to wait a few weeks until one of the language functions has begun to return. Then the physician and therapist can begin to help the patient to use that function to a maximum degree. In milder aphasic disorders, the patient may be sent to the speech therapist as soon as the illness has stabilized.

The methods of speech rehabilitation are specialized, and it is advisable to call in a person who has been trained in this field. However, inasmuch as the benefit is also largely psychologic, an interested family member or schoolteacher can be of help if a speech therapist is not available in the community.

Frustration, depression, and paranoia, which complicate some aphasias, may require psychiatric evaluation and treatment. The developmental language disorders of children pose special problems and are considered in Chap. 28.

Prognosis and Recovery Patterns Some aspects of prognosis have been discussed above. In general, recovery from aphasia due to cerebral trauma is usually faster and more complete than that from aphasia due to stroke. The type of aphasia and particularly its initial severity (extent of the lesion) clearly influence recovery: global aphasia usually improves very little, and the same is true of severe Broca's and Wernicke's aphasias (Kertesz and McCabe). The various dissociative speech syndromes and pure word mutism tend to improve rapidly and often completely. Also, in general, the outlook for recovery of any particular aphasia is more favorable in a left-handed person than in a right-handed one. Characteristically, in the course of recovery, one type of aphasia may evolve into another type (global into severe Broca's; Wernicke's, transcortical, and conduction into anomic)—patterns of recovery that may mistakenly be attributed to the effects of therapy. It is because so many factors may influence the mode of recovery from aphasia that the effectiveness of formal speech therapy has never been fully evaluated.

DISORDERS OF ARTICULATION AND PHONATION

The act of speaking involves a highly coordinated sequence of actions of the respiratory musculature, larynx, pharynx, palate, tongue, and lips. These structures are innervated by the vagal, hypoglossal, facial, and phrenic nerves, the nuclei of which are controlled by both motor cortices through the corticobulbar tracts. As with all movements, those involved in speaking are subject to extrapyramidal influences from the cerebellum and basal ganglia. The act of speaking requires that air be expired in regulated bursts, and each expiration must be maintained long enough (by pressure mainly from the intercostal muscles) to permit the utterance of phrases and sentences. The current of expired air is then finely regulated by the activity of the various muscles engaged in speech.

Phonation, or the production of vocal sounds, is a function of the larynx, more particularly the vocal cords. The pitch of the speaking or singing voice depends upon the length and mass of the membranous parts of the vocal cords and can be varied by changing their tension; this is accomplished by means of the intrinsic laryngeal muscles, before any audible sound emerges. The controlled intratracheal pressure forces air past the glottis and separates the margins of the cords, setting up a series of vibrations and recoils. Sounds thus formed are modulated as they pass through the nasopharynx and mouth, which act as resonators. *Articulation* consists of contractions of the pharynx, palate, tongue, and lips, which interrupt or alter the vocal sounds. Vowels are of laryngeal origin, as are some consonants, but the latter are formed for the most part during articulation; the consonants *m*, *b*, and *p* are labial, *l* and *t* are lingual, and *nk* and *ng* are guttural (throat and soft palate).

Defective articulation and phonation are recognized at once by listening to the patient speak during ordinary conversation or read aloud from a newspaper. Test phrases or attempts at rapid repetition of lingual, labial, and guttural consonants (e.g., *la-la-la-la*, *me-me-me-me*, or *k-k-k-k*) bring out the particular abnormality. Disorders of phonation call for a precise analysis of the voice and its apparatus during speech and singing. The movements of the vocal cords should be inspected with a laryngoscope and those of the tongue, palate, and pharynx by direct observation.

Dysarthria and Anarthria

In pure dysarthria or anarthria, there is no abnormality of the cortical language mechanisms. The dysarthric patient is able to understand perfectly what is heard and, if literate, has no difficulty in reading and writing, although he may be unable to utter a single intelligible word. This is the strict meaning of being inarticulate. Defects in articulation (dysarthria, anarthria) may be subdivided into several types: lower motor neuron (neuromuscular); spastic (pseudobulbar); rigid (extrapyramidal); cerebellar-ataxic; and hypo- and hyperkinetic dysarthrias.

Lower Motor Neuron (Neuromuscular) Dysarthria, Atrophic Bulbar Paralysis This is due to weakness or paralysis of the articulatory muscles, the result of disease of the motor nuclei of the medulla and lower pons or their intramedullary or peripheral extensions (*lower motor neuron paralysis*). In advanced forms of this disorder, the shriveled tongue lies inert and fasciculating on the floor of the mouth, and the lips are lax and tremulous. Saliva constantly collects in the mouth because of dysphagia, and drooling is troublesome. Dysphonia—alteration of the voice to a rasping monotone due to vocal cord paralysis—is often added. As this condition evolves, speech becomes slurred and progressively less distinct. There is special difficulty in the enunciation of vibratives, such as *r*, and as the paralysis becomes more complete, lingual and labial consonants are finally not pronounced at all. In the past, bilateral paralysis of the palate, causing nasality of speech, often occurred with diphtheria and poliomyelitis, but now it occurs most often with progressive bulbar palsy, a form of motor neuron disease (page 1154), and with certain neuromuscular disorders. Bilateral paralysis of the lips—as in the facial diplegia of the Guillain-Barré syndrome or of Lyme disease—interferes with enunciation of labial consonants; *p* and *b* are slurred and sound more like *f* and *v*. Degrees of these abnormalities are also observed in myasthenia gravis.

Spastic (Pseudobulbar) Dysarthria Diseases that involve the corticobulbar tracts, usually due to vascular, demyelinative, or motor system disease (amyotrophic lateral sclerosis), result in the syndrome of spastic bulbar (pseudobulbar) palsy. The patient may have had a clinically inevident vascular lesion at some time in the past, affecting the corticobulbar fibers on one side; however, since the bulbar muscles on each side are innervated by both motor cortices, there may be little or no impairment in speech or swallowing from a unilateral corticobulbar lesion. Should another stroke then occur, involving the other corticobulbar tract at the pontine, midbrain, or capsular level, the patient immediately becomes dysphagic, dysphonic, and anarthric or dysarthric, often with paresis of the tongue and facial muscles. This condition, unlike bulbar paralysis due to lower motor neuron involvement, entails no atrophy or fasciculations of the paralyzed muscles; the jaw jerk and other facial reflexes become exaggerated, the palatal reflexes are retained or increased, emotional control is impaired (spasmodic crying and laughing—the pseudobulbar affective state described on page 541), and sometimes breathing becomes periodic (Cheyne-Stokes). Amyotrophic lateral sclerosis is the main condition in which the signs of spastic and atrophic bulbar palsy are combined.

When the dominant frontal operculum alone is involved, speech may be dysarthric, usually without impairment in emotional control. In the beginning, with vascular lesions, the patient may be mute; but with recovery or in mild degrees of the same condition, speech is notably slow, thick, and indistinct, much like that of partial bulbar paralysis. Magnetic stimulation of the cortex in these cases may reveal a delay in corticobulbar conduction. The terms *cortical dysarthria* and *anarthria*, among many others, have been applied to this disorder, which is more closely related to mild forms of Broca's aphasia than to the dysarthrias being considered in this section (see "Pure Word Mutism," page 511). Also, in many cases of partially recovered Broca's aphasia and in the "mini-Broca" syndrome, the patient is left with a dysarthria that may be difficult to distinguish from a pure articulatory defect. Careful testing of other language functions, especially writing, will in this instance reveal the aphasic aspect of the defect.

A severe dysarthria that is difficult to classify but resembles that of cerebellar disease may occur with a left hemiplegia, the result of capsular or right opercular infarction. It tends to improve over several weeks but initially may be so severe as to make speech incomprehensible (Ropper).

Rigid (Extrapyramidal) Dysarthria In Parkinson and other extrapyramidal diseases associated with rigidity of muscles, one observes a rather different disturbance of articulation, characterized by rapid utterance and slurring of words and syllables and trailing off in volume at the ends of sentences. The voice is low-pitched and monotonous, lacking both inflection and volume (hypophonia). The words are spoken hastily and run together in a pattern different from that of spastic dysarthria. In advanced cases, speech is almost unintelligible; only whispering is possible. It may happen that the patient finds it impossible to talk while walking but can speak better if standing still, sitting, or lying down. The terms *hypokinetic* and *festinating* are aptly applied to these aspects of parkinsonian speech. Curiously, in the extrapyramidal disorder of progressive supranuclear palsy, the dysarthria and dysphonia tend to be spastic in nature.

With chorea and myoclonus, speech may also be affected in a highly characteristic way. The speech is loud, harsh, improperly stressed, and poorly coordinated with breathing (*hyperkinetic dysarthria*). Unlike the defect of pseudobulbar palsy or Parkinson disease, chorea and myoclonus cause abrupt interruptions of the words by superimposition of involuntary movements of bulbar muscles. The latter abnormality is best described as "hiccup speech," in that the breaks are unexpected, as in singultation. Grimacing and other characteristic movement abnormalities must be depended upon for diagnosis. The Tourette syndrome of multiple motor and vocal tics is characterized both by startling vocalizations (barking noises, squeals, shrieks, grunting, sniffing, snorting) and by speech disturbances, notably stuttering and the involuntary utterance of obscenities (coprolalia).

Elements of both corticobulbar (spastic) and extrapyramidal speech disturbances may be combined in Wilson disease, in Hallervorden-Spatz disease, and in the form of cerebral palsy called *double athetosis*. The speech is loud, slow, and labored; it is poorly coordinated with breathing and accompanied by facial contortions and athetotic accesses of tone in other muscles. In diffuse cerebral diseases such as general paresis, slurred, tremulous speech is one of the cardinal signs.

Ataxic Dysarthria This is characteristic of acute and chronic cerebellar lesions. It may be observed in multiple sclerosis and various degenerative disorders involving the cerebellum or its peduncles, or as a sequel of anoxic encephalopathy and rarely of heat stroke. The principal abnormalities are slowness of speech, slurring, monotony, and unnatural separation of the syllables of words (scanning). Again, the coordination of speech and respiration is disordered. There may not be enough breath to utter certain words or syllables, and others are expressed with greater force than intended (explosive speech). *Scanning dysarthria* (see page 94) is distinctive and is due most often to mesencephalic lesions involving the brachium conjunctivum. However, in some cases of cerebellar disease, especially if there is an element of spastic weakness of the tongue from corticobulbar tract involvement, there may be only a slurring dysarthria, and it is not possible to predict the anatomy of the lesions from analysis of speech alone. Myoclonic jerks involving the speech musculature may be superimposed on cerebellar ataxia in a number of diseases.

Acquired Stuttering This abnormality, characterized by interruptions of the normal rhythm of speech by involuntary repetition and prolongation or arrest of uttered letters or syllables, is a common developmental disorder, discussed in Chap. 38. But as pointed out by Rosenbek et al and by Helm and colleagues, it may appear in patients who are recovering from aphasic disorders and who had never stuttered in childhood. This acquired stuttering in adults resembles the developmental type in that the repetitions, prolongations, and blocks are restricted to the initial syllables of words, and there is no adaptation. However, it involves grammatical as well as substantive words and is generally unaccompanied by grimacing and associated movements. In many instances, acquired stuttering is transitory; if it is permanent, according to Helm and associates, bilateral cerebral lesions are present. Nevertheless we have observed some cases in which only a left-sided, predominantly motor aphasia provided the background for stuttering and others in which stuttering was an early sign of cerebral glioma originating in the parietal region. Benson also cites patients in whom stuttering accompanied fluent aphasia. Noteworthy is the fact that stuttering differs from palilalia, in which there is repetition of a word or phrase with increasing rapidity, and from echolalia, in which there is an obligate repetition of words or phrases. The treatment of Parkinson disease with L-dopa and occasionally an acquired cerebral lesion may reactivate developmental stuttering.

Aphonia and Dysphonia

Finally, a few points should be made concerning the fourth group of speech disorders, i.e., those due to disturbances of phonation. In adolescence there may be a persistence of the unstable "change of voice" normally seen in boys during puberty. As though by habit, the patient speaks part of the time in falsetto, and the condition may persist into adult life. Its basis is unknown. Probably the larynx is not masculinized, i.e., there is a failure in the spurt of growth (length) of the vocal cords that ordinarily occurs in pubertal boys. Voice training has been helpful in the majority of patients.

Paresis of respiratory movements, as in myasthenia gravis, Guillain-Barré syndrome, and severe pulmonary disease, may affect the voice because insufficient air is provided for phonation. Also, disturbances in the rhythm of respiration may interfere with the fluency of speech. This is particularly noticeable in extrapyramidal diseases, where one may observe that the patient tries to talk during part of inspiration. Another common feature of the latter diseases is the reduction in volume of the voice (hypophonia) due to limited excursion of the breathing muscles; the patient is unable to shout or to speak above a whisper. Whispering speech is also a feature of advanced Parkinson disease, stupor, and occasionally concussive brain injury and frontal lobe lesions, but strong stimulation may make the voice audible.

With paresis of both vocal cords, the patient can speak only in whispers. Since the vocal cords normally separate during inspiration, their failure to do so when paralyzed may result in an inspiratory stridor. If one vocal cord is paralyzed—as a result of involvement of the tenth cranial nerve by tumor, for example—the voice becomes hoarse, low-pitched, rasping, and somewhat nasal in quality, like cleft palate speech, because the posterior nares do not close during phonation. The pronunciation of certain consonants such as *b*, *p*, *n*, and *k* is followed by an escape of air into the nasal passages. The abnormality is sometimes less pronounced in recumbency and increased when the head is thrown forward.

Spasmodic (Spastic) Dysphonia This is a relatively common condition about which little is known. *Spasmodic dysphonia* is a better term than spastic dysphonia, since the adjective *spastic* suggests corticospinal involvement, whereas the disorder is probably of extrapyramidal origin. The authors have seen many patients, middle-aged or elderly men and women, otherwise healthy, who lose the ability to speak quietly and fluently. Any attempt to speak results in contraction of all the speech musculature, so that the patient's voice is strained and speaking is a great effort. The patient sounds as though he were trying to speak while being strangled. Shouting is easier than quiet speech, and whispering is unaltered. Other actions utilizing approximately the same muscles (swallowing and singing) are usually unimpeded.

Spasmodic dysphonia is usually nonprogressive and occurs as an isolated phenomenon, but we have observed exceptions in which it occurs in various combinations with blepharospasm, spasmodic torticollis, writer's cramp, or some other type of segmental dystonia. The nature of spasmodic dysphonia is unclear. As a neurologic disorder, it is akin to writer's cramp, i.e., a restricted dystonia (see Chap. 6). Speech therapists, observing such a patient strain to achieve vocalization, often assume that relief can be obtained by making the patient relax, and psychotherapists believed at first that a search of the patient's personal life around the time when the dysphonia began would enable the patient to understand the problem and regain a normal mode of speaking. But both these methods have failed without exception. Drugs useful in the treatment of Parkinson disease and other extrapyramidal diseases are practically never effective. Crushing of one recurrent laryngeal nerve can be beneficial, but recurrence is to be expected. The most effective treatment consists of the injection of 5 to 20 units of botulinum toxin, under laryngoscopic guidance, into each thyroarytenoid or cricothyroid muscle. Relief lasts for several months. An anatomic abnormality has not been demonstrated, but careful neuropathologic studies have not been made.

Glottis spasm, as in tetanus, tetany, and certain hereditary metabolic diseases, results in crowing, stridulous phonation. Hoarseness and raspiness of the voice may also be due to structural changes in the vocal cords, the result of cigarette smoking, acute or chronic laryngitis, polyps, edema after extubation, etc.

REFERENCES

ALEXANDER MP, BENSON DF: The aphasias and related disturbances, in Joynt RJ (ed): *Clinical Neurology*. Vol 1. New York, Lippincott, 1991, chap 10.

ALEXANDER MP, NAESER MA, PALUMBO CL: Correlation of subcortical CT lesion sites and aphasia profiles. *Brain* 110:961, 1987.

ASSAL G, REGLI F, THUILLARD A, et al: Syndrome de l'isolement de la zone du language. *Rev Neurol* 139:417, 1983.

BASSO A, TABORELLI A, VIGNOLO LA: Dissociated disorders of reading and writing in aphasia. *J Neurol Neurosurg Psychiatry* 41:556, 1978.

BEAUVOIS MF, SAILLANT B, MEININGER V, LHERMITTE F: Bilateral tactile aphasia: A tacto-verbal dysfunction. *Brain* 101:381, 1978.

BENSON DF: *Aphasia, Alexia, and Agraphia*. New York, Churchill Livingstone, 1979.

BRAIN R: *Speech Disorders. Aphasia, Apraxia and Agnosia*. Washington, DC, Butterworth, 1961.

BROCA P: Portée de la parole: Ramollisement chronique et destruction partielle du lobe anterieur gauche du cerveau. *Paris Bull Soc Anthropol* 2:219, 1861.

BUCHMAN AS, GARRON DC, TROST-CARDOMONE JE, et al: Word deafness: One hundred years later. *J Neurol Neurosurg Psychiatry* 49:489, 1986.

CRITCHLEY M: Aphasiological nomenclature and definitions. *Cortex* 3:3, 1967.

CROISILE B, LAURENT B, MICHEL D, et al: Pure agraphia after a deep hemisphere haematoma. *J Neurol Neurosurg Psychiatry* 53:263, 1990.

DAMASIO AR: Aphasia. *N Engl J Med* 326:531, 1992.

DAMASIO AR, DAMASIO H: The anatomic basis of pure alexia. *Neurology* 33:1573, 1983.

DAMASIO AR, GESCHWIND N: Anatomical localization in clinical neuropsychology, in Vinken PJ, Bruyn GW, Klawans HL (eds): *Handbook of Clinical Neurology*. Vol 45. Amsterdam, Elsevier, 1985, chap 2, pp 7–22.

DAMASIO H, DAMASIO AR: The anatomical basis of conduction aphasia. *Brain* 103:337, 1980.

DAMASIO H, DAMASIO AR: *Lesion Analysis in Neuropsychology*. New York, Oxford University Press, 1989.

DARBY DG: Sensory aprosodia: A clinical clue to lesions of the inferior division of the right middle cerebral artery? *Neurology* 43:567, 1993.

DÉJERINE J: Contribution a l'étude anatomo-pathologique et clinique des differentes varietés de cécité verbale. *Mem Soc Biol* 4:61, 1892.

DRONKERS NF: A new brain region for coordinating speech articulation. *Nature* 384:159, 1996.

GARDINER AH: *The Theory of Speech and Language*. Westport, CT, Greenwood Press, 1979.

GESCHWIND N: Disconnection syndromes in animals and man. *Brain* 88:237, 585, 1965.

GESCHWIND N: Wernicke's contribution to the study of aphasia. *Cortex* 3:449, 1967.

GESCHWIND N: The varieties of naming errors. *Cortex* 3:97, 1967.

GESCHWIND N, GALABURDA AM: *Cerebral Dominance: Biological Foundations*. Cambridge, MA, Harvard University Press, 1984.

GESCHWIND N, LEVITSKY W: Human brain: Left-right asymmetries in temporal speech region. *Science* 161:186, 1968.

GLONING K: Handedness and aphasia. *Neuropsychologia* 15:355, 1977.

GOLDSTEIN K: *Language and Language Disturbances*. New York, Grune & Stratton, 1948, pp 190–216.

GOODGLASS H, KAPLAN E: *The Assessment of Aphasia and Related Disorders*. Philadelphia, Lea & Febiger, 1972.

GOODGLASS H, QUADFASEL FA: Language laterality in left-handed aphasics. *Brain* 77:521, 1954.

GREENBLATT SH: Alexia without agraphia or hemianopsia. *Brain* 96:307, 1973.

HEAD H: *Aphasias and Kindred Disorders*. London, Cambridge University Press, 1926.

HELM NA, BUTLER RB, BENSON DF: Acquired stuttering. *Neurology* 28:1159, 1978.

HOWARD D, PATTERSON K, FRANKLIN S: Treatment of word retrieval deficits in aphasia: A comparison of two therapy methods. *Brain* 108:817, 1985.

JOANETTE Y, PUEL JL, NESPOULOSIS A, et al: Aphasie croisee chez les droities. *Rev Neurol* 138:375, 1982.

KERTESZ A: *Aphasia and Associated Disorders*. Needham Heights, MA, Allyn and Bacon, 1989.

KERTESZ A: *The Western Aphasia Battery*. New York, Grune & Stratton, 1982.

KERTESZ A: Clinical forms of aphasia. *Acta Neurochir* 56(Suppl):52, 1993.

KERTESZ A, BENSON F: Neologistic jargon: A clinicopathologic study. *Cortex* 6:362, 1970.

KERTESZ A, MCCABE P: Recovery patterns and prognosis in aphasia. *Brain* 100:1, 1977.

KERTESZ A, SHEPPARD A, MACKENZIE R: Localization in transcortical sensory aphasia. *Arch Neurol* 39:475, 1982.

KINSBOURNE M: *Hemispheric Disconnection and Cerebral Function*. Springfield, IL, Charles C Thomas, 1974.

LEINER HC, LEINER SL, DOW RS: Cognitive and language functions of the human cerebellum. *Trends Neurosci* 16:444, 1993.

LEISCHNER A: The agraphias, in Vinken PJ, Bruyn GW (eds): *Handbook of Clinical Neurology*. Vol 4: *Disorders of Speech, Perception and Symbolic Behavior*. Amsterdam, North-Holland, 1969, pp 141–180.

LeMay M, Culebras A: Human brain morphologic differences in the hemispheres demonstrable by carotid angiography. *N Engl J Med* 287:168, 1972.

Lesser RP, Lueders H, Dinner DS, et al: The location of speech and writing functions in the frontal language area. *Brain* 107:275, 1984.

Levine DN, Mohr JP: Language after bilateral cerebral infarctions: Role of the minor hemisphere in speech. *Neurology* 29:927, 1979.

Margolin DI: Cognitive neuropsychology: Resolving enigmas about Wernicke's aphasia and other higher cortical disorders. *Arch Neurol* 48:751, 1991.

Martin N, Saffran EM: A computational account of deep dysphasia: Evidence from a single case study. *Brain Lang* 43:240, 1992.

Milner B, Branch C, Rasmussen T: Evidence for bilateral speech representation in some non-right-handers. *Trans Am Neurol Assoc* 91:306, 1966.

Mohr JP: Broca's area and Broca's aphasia, in Whitaker H, Whitaker H (eds): *Studies in Neurolinguistics*. Vol 1. New York, Academic Press, 1976, pp 201–235.

Mohr JP: The vascular basis of Wernicke aphasia. *Trans Am Neurol Assoc* 105:133, 1980.

Mohr JP, Pessin MS, Finkelstein S, et al: Broca aphasia: Pathologic and clinical. *Neurology* 28:311, 1978.

Naeser MA, Alexander MP, Helm-Estabrook N, et al: Aphasia with predominantly subcortical lesion sites. *Arch Neurol* 39:2, 1982.

Ojemann G: Cortical organization of language. *J Neurosci* 11:2281, 1991.

Roch-LeCours H, Lhermitte F: The pure form of the phonetic disintegration syndrome (pure anarthria). *Brain Lang* 3:88, 1976.

Roch-LeCours H, Lhermitte F: *Aphasiology*. Eastbourne, England, Ballière-Tindall, 1989.

Roeltgen DP: Agraphia, in Feinberg TE, Farah MJ (eds): *Behavioral Neurology and Neuropsychology*. New York, McGraw-Hill, 1997, pp 219–226.

Ropper AH: Severe dysarthria with right hemisphere stroke. *Neurology* 37:1061, 1987.

Rosati G, de Bastiani P: Pure agraphia: A discrete form of aphasia. *J Neurol Neurosurg Psychiatry* 42:266, 1979.

Rosenbek J, Messert B, Collins M, et al: Stuttering following brain damage. *Brain Lang* 6:82, 1975.

Ross ED: The Aprosodias, in Feinberg TE, Farah MJ (eds): *Behavioral Neurology and Neuropsychology*. New York, McGraw-Hill, 1997, pp 699–717.

Subirana A: Handedness and cerebral dominance, in Vinken PJ, Bruyn GW (eds): *Handbook of Clinical Neurology*. Vol 4: *Disorders of Speech, Perception and Symbolic Behavior*. Amsterdam, North-Holland, 1969, pp 284–292.

Symonds C: Aphasia. *J Neurol Neurosurg Psychiatry* 16:1, 1953.

Wender D: Aphasic victim as investigatior. *Arch Neurol* 46:91, 1989.

Wernicke C: *Der Aphasische Symptomkomplex*. Breslau, Germany, Kohn & Weigert, 1874. English translation by Eggert GH: *Wernicke Works on Aphasia: A Source Book and Review*. The Hague, Mouton, 1977.

Wertz RT, Weiss DG, Aten JL, et al: Comparison of clinic, home, and deferred language treatment for aphasia: A Veterans Administration Cooperative study. *Arch Neurol* 43:653, 1986.

Willmes K, Poeck K: To what extent can aphasic syndromes be localized? *Brain* 116:1527, 1993.

Wilson SAK: *Aphasia*. London, Kegan Paul, 1926.

Wise RJ, Greene J, Büchel C, Scott SK: Brain regions involved in articulation. *Lancet* 353:1057, 1999.

Yakovlev PI, Rakic P: Patterns of decussation of bulbar pyramids and distribution of pyramidal tracts on the two sides of the spinal cord. *Trans Am Neurol Assoc* 91:366, 1966.

Section 6

ANXIETY AND DISORDERS OF ENERGY, MOOD, EMOTION, AND AUTONOMIC AND ENDOCRINE FUNCTIONS

Chapter 24

FATIGUE, ASTHENIA, ANXIETY, AND DEPRESSIVE REACTIONS

In this chapter, we consider the clinical phenomena of lassitude, fatigue, nervousness, irritability, anxiety, and depression. These phenomena, though more abstruse than paralysis, sensory loss, seizures, or aphasia, are no less important, if for no other reason than their frequency in neurologic and general practice. In an audit of one neurologic outpatient department, anxiety-depression was the main preliminary diagnosis in 20 percent of the patients—second only to the complaint of headache (Digon et al). And in two primary care clinics, in Boston and Houston, fatigue was the chief complaint in 21 and 24 percent, respectively. Some of these symptoms, acting through the autonomic nervous system, represent only slight aberrations of function or only a heightening or exaggeration of normal reactions to all manner of medical and neurologic diseases; others are integral features of the diseases themselves; and still others represent subtle and inchoate disturbances of psychiatric function, which are not yet sufficiently advanced to be readily identified as one of the diseases described in the section on psychiatry. It is because of their frequency and clinical significance that we have accorded them a chapter of their own among the cardinal manifestations of neurologic disease.

FATIGUE AND ASTHENIA

Of all the symptoms to be considered in this chapter, lassitude and fatigue are the most frequent and often the most vague. *Fatigue* refers to the universally familiar state of weariness or exhaustion resulting from physical or mental exertion. *Lassitude* has much the same meaning, although more strictly it connotes an inability or disinclination to be active, physically or mentally. More than half of all patients entering a general hospital register a complaint of fatigability or admit to it when questioned. During World War II, fatigue was such a prominent symptom in combat personnel as to be given a separate place in medical nosology, namely *combat fatigue*, a term that came to be applied to practically all acute psychiatric disorders occurring on the battlefield. In subsequent wars it was a key element in the posttraumatic stress and Gulf War syndromes. In civilian life, fatigue is, of course, the central feature of the chronic fatigue syndrome. The common clinical antecedents and accompaniments of fatigue, its significance, and its physiologic and psychologic bases should, therefore, be matters of interest to all physicians. These aspects of the subject will be better understood if we first consider the effects of fatigue on the normal individual.

Effects of Fatigue on the Normal Person

Fatigue has both explicit and implicit effects, grouped under (1) a series of biochemical and physiologic changes in muscles and a reduced capacity to generate force—manifest as weakness, or asthenia; (2) an overt disorder in behavior, taking the form of a reduced output of work (*work decrement*) or a lack of endurance; and (3) a subjective feeling of tiredness and discomfort.

As to the *biochemical and physiologic changes*, continuous muscular work leads to depletion of muscle adenosine triphosphate (ATP), the supply of which is derived from creatine phosphate via phosphorylation of adenosine diphosphate (ADP). With continued and more intense exercise, a further supply of ATP becomes available as a result of anaerobic breakdown of glycogen. When all the muscle glycogen has been consumed, exercise at a maximal level cannot be continued. However, mild to moderate exercise is still possible, since fatty acids provide an increasing share of muscle fuel. Gradually there is an accumulation of lactic acid and other metabolites, which in themselves reduce the power of muscular contraction and delay the recovery of muscle strength. Even in normal persons, extreme degrees of muscular effort, in which activity exceeds the provision of substrates, may result in necrosis of fibers and a rise in serum concentrations of creatine kinase (CK) and aldolase (this effect is much more evident in individuals with one of the hereditary metabolic diseases of muscle described in Chap. 51).

The *decreased productivity and capacity for work*, which is a direct consequence of fatigue, has been investigated by industrial psychologists. Their findings clearly demonstrate the importance of motivational factors on work output, whether the work be of physical or mental type. Also, individual differences in energy potential appear to be important, just as there are differences in physique, intelligence, and temperament. It should be emphasized that *in the majority of persons complaining of fatigue, one does not find true muscle weakness*. This may be difficult to prove, for many such individuals are disinclined to exert full effort in tests of peak power of muscle contraction or endurance of muscular activity.

Aside from feeling weary and tired, the fatigued person is unable to deal effectively with complex problems and may behave unreasonably, often over trivialities. The number and quality of his associations in psychologic tests are reduced. The ability to deliberate and to make sound judgments is impaired. The worker, after a long, hard day, is unable to perform adequately the demanding duties of head of household; the tired business executive who becomes the tyrant of the family is proverbial. A disinclination to make an effort is another characteristics of the fatigued mind.

The Clinical Significance of Lassitude and Fatigue

Patients experiencing lassitude and fatigue have a more or less characteristic way of expressing their symptoms. They say that they are "all done in," "tired all the time," "weary," "exhausted," "turned off," "fed up," or "pooped out"—or that they have "no pep," "no ambition," or "no interest." They manifest their condition by showing an indifference to the tasks at hand, by talking much about how hard they are working and how stressed they are by circumstances; they are inclined to sit around or lie down or to occupy themselves with trivial tasks. On closer analysis, one observes that they have difficulty in initiating activity and also in sustaining it—i.e., endurance is diminished. This condition, of course, is the familiar aftermath of sleeplessness or prolonged mental or physical effort, and under such circumstances it is accepted as a normal physiologic reaction. When, however, similar symptoms appear without relation to such antecedents, they should be suspected of being the manifestations of disease.

The physician's task begins, then, with an attempt to determine whether the patient is merely suffering from the physical and mental effects of overwork without realizing it. Overworked, overwrought people are observable everywhere in our society. Their actions are both instructive and pitiful. Some constitutional inadequacy seems to prevent them from deriving pleasure from any activity except their work, in which they indulge themselves as a kind of defense mechanism. Their behavior is said to be irrational in that they will not listen to reason; they seem to be impelled by certain notions of duty and refuse to think of themselves. They work with great intensity and persistence, which reveals a high degree of emotional involvement. In addition to fatigue, such persons frequently show other symptoms, such as irritability, restlessness, sleeplessness, and anxiety, sometimes to the point of panic attacks and a variety of somatic symptoms, particularly abdominal, thoracic, and cranial discomforts. Formerly, society accepted this state in responsible individuals and prescribed the obvious cure—a vacation. Even Charcot made time for regular "cures" during the year, in which he retired to a spa without family, colleagues, or the drain of work. Nowadays, the need to contain this type of stress, to which some individuals are more prone than others, has spawned a small industry of meditation, yoga, and similar "therapies." Individuals with strong hobbies and athletic interests seem to be less subject to this problem.

Instances of fatigue and lassitude resulting from overwork are not difficult to recognize. A description of the patient's daily routine and a talk with family members and associates will usually suffice. A common error in diagnosis, however, is to ascribe fatigue to overwork when actually it is a manifestation of a neurosis or depression.

Lassitude and Fatigue as Symptoms of Psychiatric Illness

The great majority of patients who seek medical help for unexplained chronic fatigue and lassitude are found to have some type of psychiatric illness. Formerly this state was called "neurasthenia," but since lassitude and fatigue rarely exist as isolated phenomena, the current practice is to label such cases according to the total clinical picture. The usual associated symptoms are nervousness, irritability, anxiety, depression, insomnia, headaches, dizziness, difficulty in concentrating, reduced sexual impulse, and loss of appetite. In one series, 85 percent of persons admitted to a general hospital and seen in consultation by a psychiatrist for the chief complaint of chronic fatigue were diagnosed, finally, as having anxious depression or anxiety neurosis. In a subsequent study, Wessely and Powell found similarly that 72 percent of patients who presented to a neurologic center with unexplained chronic fatigue proved to have a psychiatric disorder, most often a depressive illness.

Several features are common to the psychiatric group. Tests of peak muscle power on command, with the patient exerting full effort, reveal no weakness. The muscles retain their normal bulk and tendon reflex activity. The fatigue may be worse in the morning. There is an inclination to lie down and rest, but sleep does not follow. The fatigue is worsened by mild exertion and relates more to some activities than to others. Inquiry may disclose that the fatigue was first experienced in temporal relation to a grief reaction, a surgical operation, physical trauma such as an automobile accident, or a medical illness such as myocardial infarction. The feeling of fatigue interferes with mental as well as physical activities; the patient is easily worried, is mentally inactive, is "full of complaints," and finds it difficult to concentrate in attempting to solve a problem or to read a book, or in carrying on a complicated conversation. Also, sleep is disturbed, with a tendency to early-morning waking, so that such persons are at their worst in the morning, both in spirit and in energy output. Their tendency is to improve as the day wears on, and they may even feel fairly normal by evening. It may be difficult to decide whether the fatigue is a primary manifestation of the disease or secondary to a lack of interest.

Among chronically fatigued individuals without medical disease, not all deviate enough from normal to justify the diagnosis of neurosis or depression. Many persons, because of circumstances beyond their control, have little or no purpose in life and much idle time. They are bored with the monotony of their routine. Such circumstances are conducive to fatigue, just as the opposite, a strong emotion or a new enterprise that excites optimism and enthusiasm, will dispel fatigue. Also, as mentioned, one must be aware of striking individual differences in energy potential. Some persons are born low in impulse and energy and become more so at times of stress; they have a lifelong inability to play games vigorously, to compete successfully, to work hard without exhaustion, to withstand or recover quickly from illness, or to assume a dominant role in a social group—a constitutional asthenia (Kahn).

Lassitude and Fatigue with Medical Disease

Myopathic Fatigue Not unexpectedly, fatigue and intolerance of exercise (i.e., fatigue with mild exertion) are prominent manifestations of myopathic disease, in which muscles are weak to begin with. Even in a disease such as myasthenia gravis, the muscles exhibiting fatigue are usually weak even in the resting state. The classes of myopathic disease in which weakness, inability to sustain effort, and excessive fatigue are notable features include the following: the muscular dystrophies, congenital myopathies, disorders of neuromuscular transmission (myasthenia gravis, Lambert-Eaton syndrome), some of the glycogen storage myopathies, and mitochondrial myopathies. One type of glycogen storage disease—McArdle phosphorylase deficiency—is exceptional in that fatigue and weakness are accompanied by pain and sometimes by cramps and contracture. The first contractions after rest are of near normal strength, but after 20 to 30 contractions, there occurs a deep ache and an increasing firmness and shortening of the contracting muscles. The characteristics of these diseases are presented in the chapters on muscle disease.

Neurologic Diseases Fatigue of varying degree is a regular feature of all diseases that are marked by denervation of muscle and loss of muscle fiber. Fatigue in these cases is due to the excessive work imposed on the intact muscle fibers (overwork fatigue). This is most characteristic of amyotrophic lateral sclerosis and the postpolio syndrome, but it also occurs in patients who are recovering from Guillain-Barré syndrome and in those with chronic polyneuropathy.

Not surprisingly, many neurologic diseases that are characterized by incessant muscular activity (Parkinson disease, double athetosis, Huntington disease, hemiballismus) induce fatigue. In particular, muscles partially paralyzed by a stroke often feel tired (Brodal). Fatigue is often a major complaint of patients with multiple sclerosis; its cause is unknown, although the effect of CSF interleukins has been postulated. Also, the depression that follows stroke or myocardial infarction frequently presents with the complaint of fatigue rather than other signs of mood disorder. Inordinate fatigue is a common complaint among patients with posttraumatic nervous instability (page 945). Severe degrees of fatigue that cause the patient consistently to go to bed after dinner and make all mental activity effortful should suggest an associated depression.

Systemic Diseases A wide variety of *medications* and other therapeutic agents, particularly when first administered, commonly induce fatigue. The main offenders in this respect are antihypertensive drugs, especially beta-adrenergic blocking agents, anticonvulsants, antispasticity drugs, anxiolytics, chemotherapy and radiation therapy, and, paradoxically, many antidepressant and antipsychotic drugs. Introduction of these medications in gradually escalating doses may obviate the problem, but, just as often, an alternative medicine must be chosen. The administration of beta-interferon for the treatment of multiple sclerosis (and alpha-interferon for other diseases) induces fatigue of varying degree. Plasma exchange for the treatment of immune neuropathies and myasthenia gravis may be followed by fatigue for a day or so; this state should not be mistaken for a worsening of the underlying disease. Surgeons and nurses can testify to fatigue that comes with exposure to anesthetics in inadequately ventilated operating rooms. Similarly, fatigue and headache may result from exposure to carbon monoxide or natural gas in homes with furnaces in disrepair or from leaking gas pipes.

The sleep apnea syndrome is an important cause of fatigue and daytime drowsiness. In overweight men who snore loudly and need to nap frequently, testing for sleep apnea is indicated (page 419).

Acute or chronic infection is an important cause of fatigue. Everyone, of course, has at some time or other sensed the abrupt onset of exhaustion, a tired ache in the muscles, or an inexplicable listlessness, only to discover later that he was "coming down with the flu." Chronic infections such as hepatitis, tuberculosis, brucellosis, infectious mononucleosis [Epstein-Barr virus (EBV) infection], subacute bacterial endocarditis, and Lyme disease may not be evident immediately but should always be suspected when fatigue is a new symptom and disproportionate to other symptoms such as mood change, nervousness, and anxiety. More often, the fatigue begins with an obvious infection (such as influenza, hepatitis, or infectious mononucleosis) but persists for several weeks after the overt manifestations of infection have subsided; it may then be difficult to decide whether the fatigue represents the lingering effects of the infection or the infection has been complicated by psychologic symptoms during convalescence. This difficult problem is discussed below. Patients with systemic lupus, Sjögren syndrome, or polymyalgia rheumatica may complain of severe fatigue; in the latter, fatigue may be the initial symptom.

Metabolic and endocrine diseases of various types may cause inordinate degrees of lassitude and fatigue. Sometimes there is, in addition, a true muscular weakness. In Addison disease and Simmonds disease, fatigue may dominate the clinical picture. Aldosterone deficiency is another established cause of chronic fatigue. In persons with hypothyroidism with or without frank myxedema, lassitude and fatigue are frequent complaints, as are muscle aches and joint pains. Fatigue may also be present in patients with hyperthyroidism, but it is usually less troublesome than nervousness. Uncontrolled diabetes mellitus is accompanied by excessive fatigability, as are hyperparathyroidism, hypogonadism, and Cushing disease.

Reduced cardiac output and diminished pulmonary reserve are important causes of breathlessness and fatigue that are brought out by mild exertion. Anemia, when severe, is another cause, probably predicated on a similar inadequacy of oxygen supply to tissues. Mild grades of anemia are usually asymptomatic; lassitude is far too often ascribed to it. An occult malignant tumor—e.g., pancreatic carcinoma—may announce itself by inordinate fatigue. In patients with metastatic carcinoma, leukemia, and multiple myeloma, fatigue is a prominent symptom. Uremia is accompanied by fatigue; the accompanying anemia may play a role.

Any type of *nutritional deficiency* may, when severe, cause lassitude, and in its early stages this may be the chief complaint. Weight loss and a history of alcoholism and dietary inadequacy provide the clues to the nature of the illness.

For several weeks or months following *myocardial infarction*, most patients complain of fatigue out of all proportion to effort. In many of these patients, there is accompanying anxiety or depression. Much more difficult to understand is the complaint of fatigue that sometimes precedes myocardial infarction.

Pregnancy causes fatigue, which may be profound in the later months. To some extent the underlying causes, including the work of carrying excess weight and an anemia, are obvious; but if weight gain and hypertension are associated, pre-eclampsia should be suspected.

Postviral and Chronic Fatigue Syndromes A particularly difficult problem is that of the patient who complains of severe fatigue for many months or even years after a bout of infectious mononucleosis or some other viral illness. This has been called the *postviral fatigue syndrome*. The majority of patients are women between 20 and 40 years old. A few such patients were found to have unusually high titers of antibody to EBV, which suggested a causal relationship and gave rise to terms such as the *chronic infectious mononucleosis* or *chronic EBV syndrome* (Strauss et al). However, subsequent studies made it clear that a vast majority of patients with complaints of chronic fatigue have neither a clear-cut history of infectious mononucleosis nor serologic evidence of such an infection (Strauss; Holmes et al). In some of these patients the fatigue state has allegedly been associated with obscure immunologic abnormalities such as those attributed (spuriously) to silicone breast implants or minor trauma. The currently fashionable designation for these and other abstruse states of persistent fatigue is the *chronic fatigue syndrome*, although a malady of this nature, under many different names, has long pervaded postindustrial Western society (Shorter). Its attribution to viral infection and ill-defined immune dysfunction are only the latest in a long line of putative explanations. At various times, colitis and other forms of bowel dysfunction, spinal irritation, hypoglycemia, brucellosis, and chronic mononucleosis, among others, have been proposed as causes.

The proposed criteria for the diagnosis of chronic fatigue syndrome are the presence of persistent and disabling fatigue for at least 6 months, coupled with an arbitrary number (6 or 8) of persistent or recurrent somatic and neuropsychologic symptoms—including low-grade fever, cervical or axillary lymphadenopathy, myalgias, migrating arthralgias, sore throat, forgetfulness, headaches, difficulties in concentration and thinking, irritability, and sleep disturbances (Holmes et al). A number of such patients, in our experience, have also complained of *paresthesias* in the feet or hands, and an association is well recognized with a painful *fibromyalgia* state, consisting of neck, shoulder, and paraspinal pain and point tenderness (pages 231 and 1572). Despite these complaints, the patient may look surprisingly rested and robust and the neurologic examination is normal. Complaints of muscle weakness are frequent among such patients, but Lloyd and coworkers, who studied their neuromuscular performance and compared them with control subjects, found no difference in maximal isometric strength or endurance in repetitive submaximal exercise and no change in intramuscular acidosis or serum CK levels, or depletion of energy substrates. These individuals share with depressed patients a subnormal response to cortical magnetic motor stimulation after exercise (Samii et al), which can be said to match their symptoms of reduced endurance but otherwise is difficult to interpret. In a small number of persons, a chronic mild hypotension, elicited mainly with tilt-table testing, has been proposed as a cause of chronic fatigue (Rowe et al). Electromyography and nerve conduction studies are invariably normal, as is the spinal fluid, but the electroencephalogram (EEG) may be mildly and nonspecifically slowed. Batteries of psychologic tests have disclosed variable impairments of cognitive function, misinterpreted by advocates of the "organic" nature of the syndrome as proof of some type of encephalopathy.

In a large group of patients who were studied 6 months after viral infections, Cope and colleagues found that none of the features of the original illness was predictive of the development of chronic fatigue; however, a previous history of fatigue or psychiatric morbidity and an indefinite diagnosis often were associated with persistent disability. One thing is clear to the authors: that applying the label of *chronic fatigue syndrome* in susceptible individuals almost always perpetuates this state.

At the present time, the nature of the chronic fatigue syndrome is undecided. The possibility of some obscure metabolic or immunologic derangement secondary to a viral infection cannot be dismissed (Swartz), but it seems unlikely to us in the majority of cases that lack such a history. In one study of more than 1000 patients who were observed for 6 months following an infective illness, the chronic fatigue syndrome was no more frequent than in the general population (Wessely et al). It is our impression that most such patients are depressed; they are best treated with exercises and antidepressant medication, although this regimen is not always successful. There are anecdotal reports of success in treating these patients with mineralocorticoids (predicated on the above-mentioned orthostatic intolerance), estradiol patches, hypnosis, and a variety of other medical and nonmedical treatments. Only a very few exhibit the special psychologic disorder related to litigation (compensation neurosis). Noteworthy is the frequency with which the syndrome has become the basis of court action against employers, as in the "sick-building syndrome" or claims against the government.

Differential Diagnosis of Fatigue

If one looks critically at patients who seek medical help because of incapacitating exhaustion, lassitude, and fatigability (sometimes incorrectly called "weakness"), it is evident that the most commonly overlooked diagnoses are anxiety and depression. The correct conclusion can usually be reached by keeping these illnesses in mind as one elicits the history from patient and family. Difficulty arises when symptoms of the psychiatric illness are so inconspicuous as not to be appreciated; one comes then to suspect the diagnosis only by having eliminated the common medical causes. Repeated observation may bear out the existence of an anxiety state or gloomy mood, as the patient resists rehabilitation. Strong reassurance in combination with a therapeutic trial of antianxiety or antidepressant drugs may suppress symptoms of which the patient was barely aware, thus clarifying the diagnosis. The constitutionally asthenic individual, described earlier, is recognized by the characteristic lifelong behavioral pattern disclosed by his biography. The best that can be done is to assist the patient in adjusting to the adverse circumstances that have brought him under medical surveillance.

Tuberculosis, brucellosis, Lyme disease, hepatitis, subacute bacterial endocarditis, mycoplasmal pneumonia, EBV, CMV, coxsackie B and other viral infections, and malaria, hookworm, giardiasis, and other parasitic infections need to be included in the differential diagnosis and a search made for their characteristic symptoms, signs, and, when appropriate, laboratory findings. There should also be a search for anemia, azotemia, chronic inflammatory disease such as temporal arteritis–polymyalgia rheumatica (sedimentation rate), and occult tumor; an endocrine survey (thyroid, calcium, and cortisol levels) and an evaluation for sleep apnea are also in order in obscure cases. It must be remembered that chronic intoxication with alcohol, barbiturates, or other sedative drugs, some of which are given to suppress nervousness or insomnia, may contribute to fatigability. The rapid and recent onset of fatigue should always suggest the presence of an infection, a disturbance in fluid balance, gastrointestinal bleeding, or rapidly developing circulatory failure of either peripheral or cardiac origin. The features that suggest sleep apnea have been mentioned above and are discussed further on page 419.

Finally, it bears repeating that lassitude and fatigue must always be distinguished from genuine weakness of muscle. The demonstration of reduced muscular power, reflex changes, fasciculations, and atrophy sets the case analysis along different lines, bringing up for particular consideration diseases of the peripheral nervous system or of the musculature. It must also be kept in mind that weakness may be so slight as to be detectable only by tests of endurance (sustained exercise). Rare, difficult-to-diagnose diseases that cause inexplicable muscle weakness and exercise intolerance are masked hyperthyroidism, hyperparathyroidism, ossifying hemangiomas with hypophosphatemia, some of the kalemic periodic paralyses, hyperinsulinism, disorders of carbohydrate and lipid metabolism, the mitochondrial myopathies, and possibly adenylate deaminase deficiency.

NERVOUSNESS, ANXIETY, STRESS, AND IRRITABILITY

The world is full of nervous, tense, apprehensive, and worried people. The stresses of contemporary society are often blamed for their plight. The poet W. H. Auden referred to our time as "the age of anxiety." But history informs us that our own age is not unique in this respect. Medical historians have identified comparable periods of pervasive anxiety dating back to the time of Marcus Aurelius and Constantine, when societies were undergoing rapid and profound changes and individuals were assailed by an overwhelming sense of insecurity, personal insignificance, and fear of the future (Rosen).

Like lassitude and fatigue, nervousness, irritability, and anxiety are among the most frequent symptoms encountered in office and hospital practice. A British survey found that more than 40 percent of the population, at one time or another, experienced symptoms of anxiety, and about 5 percent suffered from lifelong anxiety states (Lader). The vast amounts of antianxiety drugs and alcohol that are consumed in our society would tend to corroborate these figures. Of course, some degree of nervousness and anxiety is experienced by any person facing a challenging or threatening task for which he may feel unprepared and inadequate. In such cases, anxiety is not abnormal, and the alertness and attentiveness that accompany it may actually improve performance up to a point. In a similar vein, if worry or depression stands in clear relation to serious economic reverses or loss of a loved one, the symptom is usually accepted as normal. Only when it is excessively intense or prolonged or when accompanying visceral derangements are prominent do anxiety and depression become matters of medical concern. Admittedly, the line that separates normal emotional reactions and pathologic (neurotic) ones is not sharp. These matters are dealt with more fully in Chap. 56.

In this chapter we are concerned with *nervousness, irritability, stress, anxiety, and depression as symptoms*, together with currently accepted views of their origins and biologic significance. The *diseases* of which these symptoms may be a part are discussed in Chaps. 56 and 57.

Anxiety Reactions and Panic Attacks

There is no unanimity among psychiatrists as to whether symptoms of nervousness, irritability, anxiety, and fear comprise a single emotional reaction, varying only in its severity or duration, or a group of discrete reactions, each with distinctive clinical features. In some writings, anxiety is classified as a form of subacute or chronic fear. However, there is reason to question this assumption. Anxious patients, when frightened under experimental conditions, state that the fear reaction differs in being more overwhelming. The exceedingly frightened person is "frozen," unable to act or to think clearly, and his responses are automatic and sometimes irrational. The fear reaction is characterized by overactivity of both the sympathetic and parasympathetic nervous systems, and the parasympathetic effects (bradycardia, sphincteric relaxation) may predominate, unlike anxiety, in which sympathetic effects are the more prominent. Long ago, Cicero distinguished between an acute and transient attack of fear provoked by a specific stimulus (*angor*) and a protracted state of fearfulness (*anxietas*). This distinction was elaborated by Freud, who regarded fear as an appropriate response to a sudden, unexpected external threat and anxiety as a neurotic maladjustment (see below).

Less readily distinguishable from anxiety is the complaint of *nervousness*. By this vague term the lay person usually refers to a state of restlessness, tension, uneasiness, apprehension, irritability, or hyperexcitability. Unfortunately, the term may have a wide range of other connotations as well, such as thoughts of suicide, fear of killing one's child or spouse, a distressing hallucination or paranoid idea, a frankly hysterical outburst, or even tics or tremulousness. Obviously, a careful inquiry as to what the patient means in complaining of nervousness is always a necessary first step in the analysis of this complaint.

Most often nervousness represents no more than a transient psychic and behavioral state in which the person is maximally challenged or threatened by difficult personal problems. Some persons claim to have been nervous throughout life or to be nervous periodically for no apparent reason. In these instances the symptoms blend imperceptibly with those of anxiety or depression, described below.

We use the term *anxiety* to denote an *intermittent or sustained emotional state characterized by subjective feelings of nervousness, irritability, uneasy anticipation, and apprehension,* often but by no means always with a definite topical content and the physiologic accompaniments of strong emotion, i.e., one or more of the symptoms of breathlessness, tightness in the chest, choking sensation, palpitation, increased muscular tension, giddiness, trembling, sweating, and flushing. By *topical content* is meant the idea, person, or object about which the person is anxious. The vasomotor and visceral accompaniments are mediated through the autonomic nervous system, particularly its sympathetic part, and involve also the thyroid and adrenal glands.

Panic Attacks The symptoms of anxiety may be manifest either in acute episodes, each lasting several minutes or up to an hour, or as a protracted state that may last for weeks, months, or years. In the *panic attack*, or *panics*, as they are called, the patient is suddenly overwhelmed by feelings of apprehension, or a fear that he may lose consciousness and die, have a heart attack or stroke, lose his reason or self-control, become insane, or commit some horrible crime. These experiences are accompanied by a series of physiologic reactions, mainly sympathoadrenal hyperactivity, resembling the "fight-or-flight" reaction. Breathlessness, a feeling of suffocation, dizziness, sweating, trembling, palpitation, and precordial or gastric distress are typical but not invariable physical accompaniments. As a persistent and less severe state, the patient experiences fluctuating degrees of nervousness, apprehension, palpitation or excessive cardiac impulse, shortness of breath, light-headedness, faintness, easy fatigue, and intolerance of physical exertion. Attacks tend to occur during periods of relative calm and in nonthreatening circumstances. Usually, the apprehension and physical symptoms escalate over a period of minutes to an hour and then abate over 20 to 30 min, leaving the patient tired and asthenic. The dramatic effects of the panic attack have usually abated by the time the patient reaches a doctor's office or an emergency department, but the blood pressure may still be elevated and there may be tachycardia. Otherwise the patient looks remarkably collected. Often, discrete anxiety attacks and persistent states of anxiety merge with one another. The fear of further attacks leads many patients, particularly women, to become agoraphobic and homebound, fearing public places, especially if alone.

Because panic is a common disorder, affecting 1 to 2 percent of the population at some time in their lives, and the symptoms mimic neurologic disease, the neurologist is often called upon to distinguish panic attacks from temporal lobe seizures or from vertiginous diseases. Except for the occasional inability of the patient to think or articulate clearly during a panic, the manifestations of epilepsy are quite different. Practically never is consciousness lost during a panic attack. If dizziness predominates in the attacks, there may be concern about vertebrobasilar ischemia or labyrinthine dysfunction (see Chap. 15). Vertigo from any cause is accompanied by many of the autonomic symptoms displayed during a panic attack, but careful questioning in the latter will elicit the characteristic apprehension, breathlessness, and palpitations, and the absence of ataxia or other neurologic signs. It should be recognized that recurrent panic attacks and chronic anxiety have a familial aspect, with one-fifth of first-degree relatives affected and a high degree of concordance in monozygotic twins. The symptoms tend to be periodic, beginning in the patient's twenties; a later onset is usually coupled with a depression. Treatment of the depression with any number of medications and the sparing use of anxiolytics are relatively successful in controlling panic disorders.

Anxiety Neurosis and Anxious Depression Episodic or sustained anxiety without a disorder of mood (i.e., without depression) is properly classified as *anxiety neurosis*. The term *neurocirculatory asthenia* (among many others) has been applied to the chronic form with prominent exercise intolerance (see Chap. 56). The symptoms of anxiety may, however, be part of several other psychiatric disorders. Anxiety may be combined with other somatic symptoms in hysteria and is the most prominent feature of *phobic neurosis*. Symptoms of persistent anxiety with insomnia, lassitude, and fatigue should always raise the suspicion of a *depressive* illness, especially when they begin in middle adult life or beyond. Also, panic attacks may sometimes herald the onset of a schizophrenic illness. As with fatigue, the symptoms of both anxiety and depression are prominent features of the syndrome *of posttraumatic nervous instability*, also called *posttraumatic stress syndrome* (see page 945). Also, when visceral symptoms predominate or the psychic counterparts of fear and apprehension are absent, the presence of thyrotoxicosis, Cushing disease, pheochromocytoma, hypoglycemia, and menopausal symptoms should be suspected.

Cause, Mechanism, and Biologic Significance of Nervousness and Anxiety

These have been the subjects of much speculation, and completely satisfactory explanations are not available. As noted above, some individuals go through life in a chronic state of low-grade anxiety, the impetus for which may or may not be apparent. They are by nature, or constitutionally, nervous and subject to this character trait. Spontaneous episodes of anxiety demand another explanation. Some psychologists regard anxiety as anticipatory behavior, i.e., a state of uneasiness about something that may happen in the future. William McDougall spoke of it as "an emotional state arising when a continuing strong desire seems likely to miss its goal." The primary emotion, somewhat muted perhaps, may be one of fear, and its arousal under conditions that are not overtly threatening may be explained as a conditioned response to some recondite component of a formerly threatening stimulus.

In psychoanalytic theory, anxiety is regarded as the individual's response to some undefinable threat from within, i.e., it lies in the "subconscious." A primitive drive has been aroused that is not compatible with current social practices and can be satisfied only at the risk of harming the person.

Physicians have searched for evidence of visceral impairment, without success. The patient with anxiety neurosis is often in poor physical condition and has an increased blood lactate concentration in both the resting state and after exercise; infusions of lactic acid are said to make the symptoms of anxiety worse and, in susceptible individuals, to elicit a panic attack. The patient seems not to tolerate the work or exercise needed to build up his stamina. The urinary excretion of epinephrine has been found elevated in some patients; in others, there is an increased urinary excretion of norepinephrine and its metabolites. During periods of intense anxiety, aldosterone excretion is increased to two or three times normal.

There is also suggestive evidence that corticosteroids and corticotropin releasing hormone (CRH) have a role in the genesis of anxiety. A systemic release of corticosteroid accompanies all states of stress, and the administration of corticosteroids may give rise to anxiety and panic in some patients and to depression in others—suggesting a linkage between steroid stimulation of the brain and the limbic system activities that generate these states. In animal models, stress elicited by predators or electric shock as well as by withdrawal of alcohol and other drugs precipitates activity in CRH pathways (amygdala to hypothalamus, raphe nuclei, nucleus ceruleus, and other regions of the brainstem); blocking such activity by drugs or by destruction of the amygdala eliminates anxiety and fear-like behavior. Admittedly the concepts of fear, stress, and anxiety are used interchangeably in these models, but repeated stimuli that produce fear and stress eventually induce a state akin to anxiety, and the amygdala appears to be involved in the perpetuation of this anxiety state. The meaning of these effects, i.e., whether they are primary or secondary, is not certain, but it is evident that prolonged and diffuse anxiety is associated with certain biochemical abnormalities of the blood and probably of the brain.

In addition to the role of the amygdala, animal studies have related acute anxiety to a disturbance of function of the locus ceruleus and the septal and hippocampal areas—the principal norepinephrine-containing nuclei. It is noteworthy that the locus ceruleus is involved in rapid-eye-movement (REM) sleep and that drugs such as the tricyclic antidepressants and monoamine oxidase inhibitors, which suppress REM sleep, also decrease anxiety. Certain of the serotonin receptors in the brain, different from those implicated in depression, have been related to anxiety. Other parts of the brain must also be involved; bifrontal orbital leukotomy also diminishes anxiety, possibly by interrupting the medial forebrain connections with the limbic parts of the brain. Positron emission tomography (PET) studies in subjects who anticipate an electric shock show enhanced activity in the temporal lobes and insula, implicating these regions in the experience of acute anxiety (see also page 547).

Several alterations in neurotransmitter function have been implicated in the anxious state. The finding that a small proportion of the inherited personality trait of anxiety can be accounted for by one polymorphism of the serotonin transporter gene is provocative (Lesch et al) but requires further study.

Anxiety, being so ubiquitous, is probably not without biologic significance. It strengthens social bonds at certain moments in life, among men in combat, for example, or when there is a threat of separation of child and mother (separation anxiety); in the adult period, anxiety can help to stabilize marriage, companionship, and work. Also, intense intellectual activity can be facilitated by controlled amounts of anxiety. Barratt and White found that mildly anxious medical students performed better on examinations than those lacking in anxiety. As anxiety increases, so does the standard of performance, but only to a point, after which increasing anxiety causes a rapid decline in performance (Yerkes-Dodson law).

Stress and Stress Syndromes

The psychologic phenomenon of *stress* is closely allied to nervousness and anxiety, and all of them are pervasive features of modern life. In general terms, stress has been defined as a feeling of self-doubt about being able to cope with some situation over a period of time. The term *stress syndrome* refers to perturbations of behavior and accompanying physiologic changes that are ascribable to environmental challenges of such intensity and duration as to overwhelm the individual's adaptive capacity. The biologic effects of this phenomenon can be recognized in many species—chickens laying fewer eggs when moved to a new coop and cows giving less milk when put in a new barn, or monkeys going berserk when repeatedly frustrated by threats that they cannot control. Human beings forced to work under confined conditions and constant danger and cultural groups removed from their home and traditional way of life lose their coping skills and suffer anxiety. Presumably they have an increased output of "stress hormones" (cortisol and adrenalin). Such psychologic disorders, bearing a direct relationship to environmental stressors, are among the most common occupational health problems. One such stress syndrome, in which an individual develops delayed or recurrent symptoms of anxiety after exposure to extreme psychologic trauma, has been given its own name—*posttraumatic stress disorder*. Stress syndromes are distinguished from anxiety neurosis, in which the psychologic disturbance arises from within the individual and has no definite relationship to environmental stimuli. Whether certain individuals are by nature hyperresponsive to such stimuli is not known. The only therapeutic approach is to attempt to alter the patient's perception of stress—for example, with psychotherapy and meditation exercises—and to remove him, if possible, from recognizable environmental stressors. (See "Editorial" in References.)

Irritability, Irritable Mood, and Aggressive Behavior

The phenomenon of irritability, or an irritable mood, must be familiar to almost everyone, exposed as we are to all of the noise, niggling inconveniences, and annoyances of daily life. It is, nevertheless, a difficult symptom to interpret in the context of psychopathology. Freud used the term *Reisbarkeit* in a restricted sense—to denote an undue sensitivity to noise—and considered it a manifestation of anxiety, but obviously this symptom has a much broader connotation and significance. For one thing, some people are by nature irritable throughout life. Also, irritability is an almost expected reaction in overworked, overwrought individuals, who become irritable by force of circumstances. An irritable mood or feeling may be present without observed manifestations (inward irritability), or there may be an overt loss of control of temper, with irascible verbal and behavioral outbursts, provoked by trivial but frustrating events.

Irritability in the foregoing circumstances can hardly be considered a departure from normal. However, when it becomes a recurrent event in a person of normally placid temperament, it assumes significance, for it may then signify an ongoing anxiety state or depression. Irritability is also a common symptom of obsessional neurosis. Here the irritability tends to be directed inward, indicating perhaps a sense of frustration with personal disability (Snaith and Taylor). Depressed patients are frequently irritable; as a corollary, this symptom should always be sought in patients suspected of being depressed, since it is so readily recognized by both patients and their families. The days preceding menses and the mother's common postnatal mood disorder are characterized by high levels of outwardly directed irritability. Short-temperedness and irritability are also common features of the manic state. The most extreme degrees of irritability, exemplified by repeated quarrelsome and assaultive behavior (irritable aggression), are rarely observed in anxiety neurosis and endogenous depression but are usually the mark of sociopathy and brain disease. Such irritable aggression is also observed in some patients with Alzheimer disease and other types of dementia and following traumatic contusions of the temporal and frontal lobes.

DEPRESSIVE REACTIONS

There are few persons who do not experience periods of discouragement and despair. As with nervousness, irritability, and anxiety, depression of mood that is appropriate to a given situation in life (e.g., grief reaction) is seldom the basis of medical concern. Persons in these situations tend to seek help only when their grief or unhappiness is persistent and beyond control. However, there are numerous instances in which the symptoms of depression assert themselves for reasons that are not apparent. Often the symptoms are interpreted as a medical illness, bringing the patient first to the internist or neurologist. Sometimes another disease is found (such as chronic hepatitis or other infection or postinfectious asthenia) in which chronic fatigue is confused with depression; more often the opposite pertains, i.e., an endogenous depression is the essential problem even when there has been evidence earlier of a viral or bacterial infection. Since the risk of suicide is not inconsiderable in the depressed patient, an error in diagnosis may be life-threatening.

From the patient and the family it is learned that the patient has been "feeling unwell," "low in spirits," "blue," "glum," "unhappy," or "morbid." There has been a change in his emotional reactions of which the patient may not be fully aware. Activities that he formerly found pleasurable are no longer so. Often, however, change in mood is less conspicuous than reduction in psychic and physical energy, and it is this type of case that is so often misdiagnosed by internists and neurologists. A complaint of fatigue is almost invariable; not uncommonly, it is worse in the morning after a night of restless sleep. The patient complains of a "loss of pep," "weakness," "tiredness," "having no energy," and/or that his job has become more difficult. His outlook is pessimistic. The patient is irritable and preoccupied with uncontrollable worry over trivialities. With excessive worry, the ability to think with accustomed efficiency is reduced; the patient complains that his mind is not functioning properly and he is forgetful and unable to concentrate. If the patient is naturally of suspicious nature, paranoid tendencies may assert themselves.

Particularly troublesome is the patient's tendency to *hypochondriasis*. Indeed, most cases formerly diagnosed as hypochondriasis are now regarded as depression. Pain from whatever cause—a stiff joint, a toothache, fleeting chest or abdominal pains, muscle cramps, or other disturbances such as constipation, frequency of urination, insomnia, pruritus, burning tongue, weight loss—may lead to obsessive complaints. The patient passes from doctor to doctor seeking relief from symptoms that would not trouble the normal person, and no amount of reassurance relieves his state of mind. The anxiety and depressed mood of these persons may be obscured by their preoccupation with visceral functions.

When the patient is examined, his facial expression is often plaintive, troubled, pained, or anguished. The patient's attitude and manner betray a prevailing mood of depression, hopelessness, and despondency. Sighing is a frequent sign. In other words, the affect, which is the outward expression of feeling, is consistent with the depressed mood. During the interview the patient may sigh frequently or be tearful and may cry openly. In some, there is a kind of immobility of the face that mimics parkinsonism, though others are restless and agitated (pacing, wringing their hands, etc.). Occasionally the patient will smile, but the smile impresses one as more a social gesture than a genuine expression of feeling.

The stream of speech is slow. There may be long pauses between questions and answers. The latter are brief and may be monosyllabic. There is a paucity of ideas. The retardation extends to all topics of conversation and affects movement of the limbs as well (anergic depression). The most extreme forms of decreased motor activity, rarely seen in the office or clinic, border on muteness and stupor. Conversation is replete with pessimistic thoughts, fears, and expressions of unworthiness, inadequacy, inferiority, hopelessness, and sometimes guilt. In severe depressions, bizarre ideas and bodily delusions ("blood drying up," "bowels are blocked with cement," "I am half dead") may be expressed.

Three theories have emerged concerning the cause of the pathologic depressive state: (1) that the endogenous form is hereditary, (2) that a biochemical abnormality results in a periodic depletion in the brain of serotonin and norepinephrine, and (3) that a basic fault in character development exists. These theories are elaborated in Chap. 57.

It is the authors' belief that depressive states are among the most commonly overlooked diagnoses in clinical medicine. Part of the trouble is with the word itself, which implies being unhappy about something. *Endogenous depression should be suspected in all states of chronic ill health, hypochondriasis, disability that exceeds manifest signs of a medical disease, neurasthenia and ongoing fatigue, chronic pain syndromes—all of which may be termed "masked depressions."* Inasmuch as recovery is the rule, suicide is a tragedy for which the medical profession must often share responsibility.

Depressive illnesses and theories of their causation and management are considered further in Chap. 57.

REFERENCES

BARRATT ES, WHITE R: Impulsiveness and anxiety related to medical students' performance and attitudes. *J Med Ed* 44:604, 1969.

BRODAL A: Self-observations and neuro-anatomical considerations after a stroke. *Brain* 96:675, 1973.

CASSIDY WL, FLANAGAN NB, SPELLMAN M, COHEN ME: Clinical observations in manic depressive disease. *JAMA* 164:1535, 1953.

COPE H, DAVID A, PELOSI A, et al: Predictors of chronic "postviral" fatigue. *Lancet* 344:864, 1994.

DAWSON DM, SABIN TD: *Chronic Fatigue Syndrome*. Boston, Little, Brown, 1993.

DIGON A, GOICOECHEA A, MORAZA MJ: A neurological audit in Vitoria, Spain. *J Neurol Neurosurg Psychiatry* 55:507, 1992.

Editorial: The essence of stress. *Lancet* 344:1713, 1994.

FREUD S: On the grounds for detaching a particular syndrome from neurasthenia under the description "anxiety neurosis," in *The Complete Psychological Works of Sigmund Freud*, standard edition. Vol 3. London, Hogarth Press, 1962, p 90.

HOLMES GP, KAPLAN JE, GLANTZ NM, et al: Chronic fatigue syndrome: A working case definition. *Ann Intern Med* 108:387, 1988.

KAHN E: *Psychopathic Personalities*. New Haven, CT, Yale University Press, 1931.

LADER M: The nature of clinical anxiety in modern society, in Spielberger CD, Sarason IG (eds): *Stress and Anxiety*. Vol 1. New York, Halsted, 1975, pp 3–26.

LESCH KP, BENGEL D, JEILS A, et al: Association of anxiety related traits with a polymorphism in the serotonin transporter gene regulatory system. *Science* 274:1527, 1996.

LLOYD AR, GANDEVIA SC, HALES JP: Muscle performance: Voluntary activation, twitch properties, and perceived effort in normal subjects and patients with chronic fatigue syndrome. *Brain* 114:85, 1991.

MCDOUGALL W: *Outlines of Abnormal Psychology*. New York, Scribner's, 1926.

ROSEN G: Emotions and sensibility in ages of anxiety: A comparative historical review. *Am J Psychiatry* 124:771, 1967.

ROWE PC, BOU-HOLAIGAH I, KAN JS, et al: Is neurally mediated hypotension an unrecognized cause of chronic fatigue? *Lancet* 345:623, 1995.

ROWLAND LP, LAYZER RB, DIMAURO S: Pathophysiology of metabolic myopathies, in Asbury AK, McKhann GM, McDonald WI (eds): *Diseases of the Nervous System*, 2nd ed. Philadelphia, Saunders, 1992, chap 12, pp 135–145.

SAMII A, WASSERMANN EM, IKOMA K, et al: Decreased postexercise facilitation of motor evoked potentials in patients with chronic fatigue or depression. *Neurology* 47:1410, 1996.

SHORTER E: *From Paralysis to Fatigue: A History of Psychosomatic Illness in the Modern Era*. New York, Free Press, 1992.

SNAITH RP, TAYLOR CM: Irritability: Definition, assessment, and associated factors. *Br J Psychiatry* 147:127, 1985.

STRAUSS SE: The chronic mononucleosis syndrome. *J Infect Dis* 157:405, 1988.

STRAUSS SE, DALE JK, TOBI M, et al: Acyclovir treatment of the chronic fatigue syndrome. *N Engl J Med* 319:1692, 1988.

SWARTZ MN: The chronic fatigue syndrome—One entity or many? *N Engl J Med* 319:1726, 1988.

WESSELY S, POWELL R: Fatigue syndromes: A comparison of chronic "postviral" fatigue with neuromuscular and affective disorders. *J Neurol Neurosurg Psychiatry* 52:940, 1989.

WESSELY S, CHALDER T, HIRSCH S, et al: Post infectious fatigue: Prospective cohort study in primary care. *Lancet* 345:1333, 1995.

WHEELER EO, WHITE PD, REED EW, COHEN ME: Neurocirculatory asthenia (anxiety neurosis, effort syndrome, neuroasthenia). *JAMA* 142:878, 1950.

Chapter 25

THE LIMBIC LOBES AND THE NEUROLOGY OF EMOTION

The medical literature is replete with references to illnesses thought to be based on emotional disorders. Careful examination of clinical records discloses that a diversity of phenomena are being so classified: anxiety states, cycles of depression and mania, reactions to distressing life situations, so-called psychosomatic diseases, and illnesses of obscure nature. Obviously great license is being taken with the term *emotional*, the result no doubt of its indiscriminate nonmedical usage. Such ambiguity discourages neurologic analysis. Nevertheless, in certain clinical states, patients appear to be excessively apathetic or elated under conditions that are not normally conducive to such displays of emotion. It is to these disturbances that the following remarks pertain. First, however, one must be clear as to what is meant by "emotion."

Emotion may be defined as any strong feeling state—e.g., fear, anger, excitement, love, or hate—associated with certain types of bodily changes (mainly visceral and under control of the autonomic nervous system) and leading usually to an impulse to action or to a certain type of behavior. If the emotion is intense, there may ensue a disturbance of intellectual functions—that is, a disorganization of rational thought and a tendency toward a more automatic behavior of unmodulated, stereotyped character.

In its most easily recognized human form, emotion is initiated by a stimulus (real or imagined), the perception of which involves recognition, memory, and specific associations. The emotional state that is engendered is mirrored in a psychic experience, i.e., a feeling, or affect, which is purely subjective and known to others only through the patient's verbal expressions or by judging his behavioral reactions. The behavioral aspect, which is in part autonomous (hormonal-visceral) and in part somatic, shows itself in the patient's facial expression, bodily attitude, vocalizations, or directed voluntary activity. Subdivided, the components of emotion appear to consist of (1) the perception of a stimulus, which may be internal (an idea) or external, (2) the affect or feeling, (3) the autonomic-visceral changes, and (4) the impulse to a certain type of activity. In many cases of neurologic disease, however, it is not possible to separate these components from one another, and to emphasize one of them does no more than indicate the particular bias of the examiner. Obviously neural networks of both affective response and cognition are involved.

Anatomic Relationships

The occurrence of deviant emotional reactions in the course of disease is associated with lesions that preferentially involve certain parts of the nervous system. These structures have been grouped under the term *limbic* and are among the most complex and least understood parts of the nervous system. The Latin word *limbus* means "border" or "margin." Credit for introducing the term *limbic* to neurology is usually given to Broca, who used it to describe the ring of gray matter (formed primarily by the cingulate and parahippocampal gyri) that encircles the corpus callosum and underlying upper brainstem. Actually, Thomas Willis had pictured this region of the brain and referred to it as the *limbus* in 1664. Broca preferred his term, *le grand lobe limbique*, to *rhinencephalon*, which was the term then in vogue and referred more specifically to structures having an olfactory function. Neuroanatomists who followed Broca affirmed his position and have extended the boundaries of the *limbic lobe* to include not only the cingulate and parahippocampal gyri but also the underlying hippocampal formation, the subcallosal gyrus, and the paraolfactory area. The terms *visceral brain* and *limbic system*, introduced by MacLean, have an even wider designation; in addition to all parts of the limbic lobe, they include a number of associated subcortical nuclei such as those of the amygdaloid complex, septal region, preoptic area, hypothalamus, anterior thalamus, habenula, and central midbrain tegmentum, including the raphe nuclei and interpeduncular nucleus. The major structures comprised by the limbic system and their relationships are illustrated in Figs. 25-1 and 25-2.

The cytoarchitectonic arrangements of the limbic cortex clearly distinguish it from the surrounding neocortex (isocortex). The latter, as stated in Chap. 22, differentiates into a characteristic six-layered structure. In contrast, the inner part of the limbic cortex (hippocampus) is composed of irregularly arranged aggregates of nerve cells that tend to be trilaminate (archi- or allocortex). The cortex of the cingulate gyrus, which forms the outer ring of the limbic lobe, is transitional between neocortex and allocortex—hence it is known as the mesocortex, or juxtallocortex. Information from a wide array of cortical neurons is funneled into the dentate gyrus and then to the CA (cornu ammonis) pyramidal cells of the hippocampus; output from the hippocampal formation is mainly from the pyramidal cells of the CA1 segment and subiculum. The amygdaloid complex, a subcortical nuclear component of the limbic lobe, also has a unique composition, consisting of several separable nuclei, each with special connections to other limbic structures.

The connections between the orbitofrontal neocortex and limbic lobes, between the individual components of the limbic lobes, and between the limbic lobes and the hypothalamus and midbrain reflect their many functional relationships. At the core of this system lies the medial forebrain bundle, a complex set of ascending and descending fibers that connect the orbitomesiofrontal cortex, septal nuclei, amygdala, and hippocampus rostrally and certain nuclei in the midbrain and pons

Figure 25-1

Sagittal schematic of the limbic system. The location of the major limbic structures and their relation to the thalamus, hypothalamus, and midbrain tegmentum are shown. (From Angevine and Cotman by permission.)

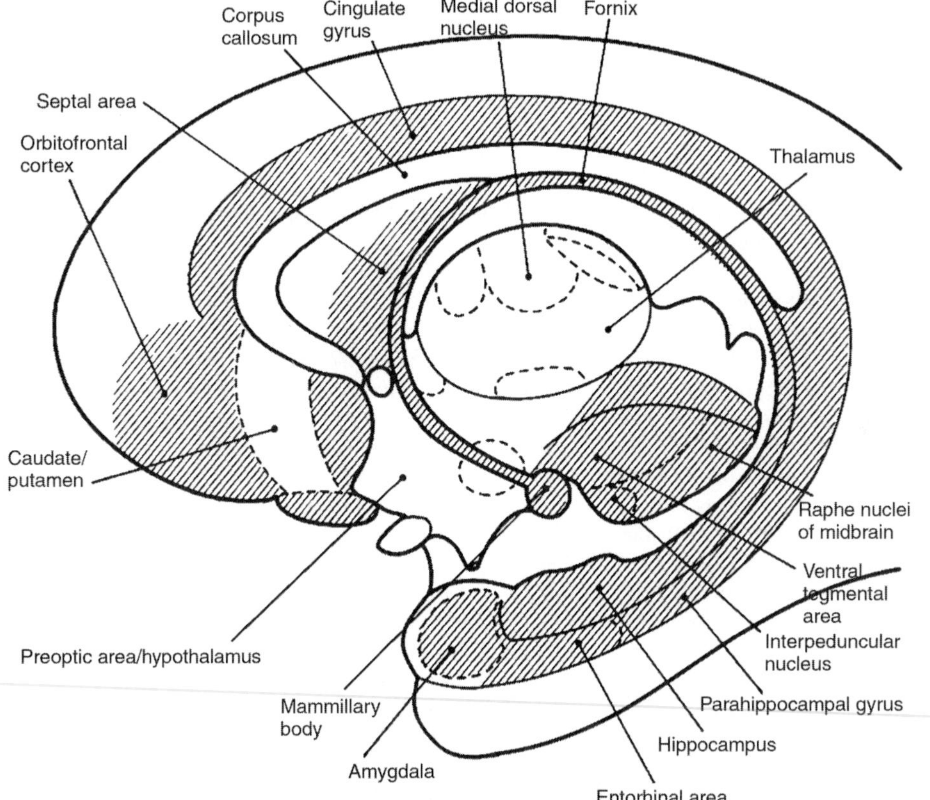

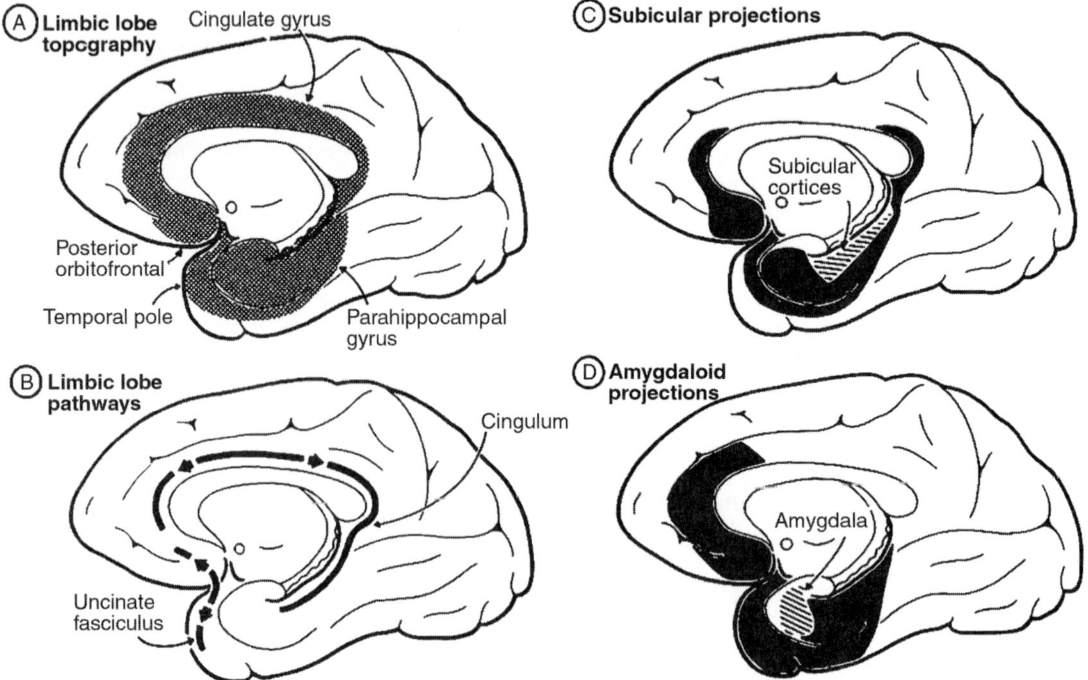

Figure 25-2

Diagrams of the medial surface of the brain, illustrating the topography of the mesocortex and allocortex, which constitute the cortical parts of the limbic system, or limbic lobe (A)*; two major pathways that interconnect various parts of the limbic lobe* (B)*; the topography of allocortical subicular projections to the limbic lobe* (C)*; and the topography of amygdaloid projections to the limbic lobe* (D). *(Reproduced from Damasio and Van Hoesen by permission.)*

caudally. This system, of which the hypothalamus is the central part, was designated by Nauta as the *septohypothalamomesencephalic continuum.*

There are many other interrelationships between various parts of the limbic system, only a few of which can be indicated here. The best-known of these is the so-called *Papez circuit*. It leads from the hippocampus, via the fornix, to the mammillary body and septal and preoptic regions. The bundle of Vicq d'Azyr (mammillothalamic tract) connects the mammillary nuclei with the anterior nuclei of the thalamus, which, in turn, project to the cingulate gyrus and then, via the cingulum, to the hippocampus. The cingulum runs concentric to the curvature of the corpus callosum; it connects various parts of the limbic lobe to one another and projects to the striatum and to certain brainstem nuclei as well. Also, the cingulum receives fibers from the inferior parietal lobule and temporal lobe, which are multimodal suprasensory centers for the integration of visual, auditory, and tactile perceptions. It is connected to the opposite cingulum through the corpus callosum.

Physiology of the Limbic System

The functional properties of the limbic structures first became known during the third and fourth decades of the twentieth century. From ablation and stimulation studies, Cannon, Bard, and others established the fact that the hypothalamus contains the suprasegmental integrations of the autonomic nervous system, both the sympathetic and parasympathetic parts. Soon after, anatomists found efferent pathways from the hypothalamus to the neural structures subserving parasympathetic and sympathetic reflexes. One such segmental reflex, involving the sympathetic innervation of the adrenal gland, served as the basis of Cannon's emergency theory of sympathoadrenal action, which for many years dominated thinking about the neurophysiology of acute emotion (see pages 558–559).

Following Cannon, Bard localized the central regulatory apparatus for respiration, wakefulness, and sexual activity in the hypothalamus. Later, the hypothalamus was also found to contain neurosecretory cells, which control the secretion of the pituitary hormones; within it also are special sensory receptors for the regulation of hunger, thirst, body temperature, and levels of circulating electrolytes. Gradually the idea emerged of a hypothalamic-pituitary-autonomic system that is essential to both the basic homeostatic and emergency reactions of the organism. The functional anatomy of the autonomic and neuroendocrine systems is discussed in Chaps. 26 and 27.

The impressions of the great psychologists of the nineteenth century—that autonomic reactions were the essential motor component of instinctual feeling—have been corroborated. In fact, for a time, it was proposed that emotional experience was merely the self-awareness of these visceral activities (the James-Lange theory of emotion). The fallacy of this theory became evident when it was demonstrated by Cannon that the capacity to manifest emotional changes remained after all visceral afferent fibers had been interrupted.

Although the natural stimuli for emotion involve the same neocortical perceptive-cognitive mechanisms as does any nonemotional sensory experience, there are important differences, which relate to the prominent visceral effects and particular behavioral reactions evoked by emotion. Clearly, specific parts of the nervous system must be utilized. Bard, in 1928, first produced "sham rage" in cats by removing the cerebral hemispheres and leaving the hypothalamus and brainstem intact. This is a state in which the animal reacts to all stimuli with expressions of intense anger and signs of autonomic overactivity. In subsequent studies, Bard and Mountcastle found that only if the ablations included the amygdaloid nuclei on both sides would sham rage be produced; removal of all the neocortex but sparing the limbic structures resulted in placidity. Interestingly, in the macaque monkey, a normally aggressive and recalcitrant animal, removal of the amygdaloid nuclei bilaterally greatly reduced the reactions of fear and anger. Papez, on the basis of these and his own anatomic observations, postulated that the limbic parts of the brain elaborate the functions of central emotion and participate as well in emotional expression. The intermediate position of the limbic structures enables them to transmit neocortical effects from their outer side to the hypothalamus and midbrain on their inner side.

The role of the *cingulate gyrus* in the behavior of animals and humans has been the subject of much discussion. Stimulation is said to produce autonomic effects similar to the vegetative correlates of emotion (increase in heart rate and blood pressure, dilatation of pupils, piloerection, respiratory arrest, breath-holding). More complex responses such as fear, anxiety, or pleasure have been reported during neurosurgical stimulative and ablative procedures, although these results are inconstant. Bilateral cingulectomies have been performed in psychotic and neurotic patients and result in a diminution of emotional reactions (Ballantine et al; Brown). Some investigators believe that the cingulate gyri are involved in memory processing (functioning presumably in connection with the mediodorsal thalamic nuclei and medial temporal lobes) and in exploratory behavior and visually focused attention. In humans, this system appears to be more efficient in the nondominant hemisphere, according to Bear. Baleydier and Mauguiere emphasize the dual function of the cingulate gyrus—in cognition and in emotional reactions.

Another aspect of limbic function has come to light as information is being acquired about neurotransmitters. The concentration of norepinephrine is highest in the hypothalamus and next highest in the medial parts of the limbic system; at least 70 percent of it is concentrated in terminals of axons that arise in the medulla and in the locus ceruleus of the rostral pons. Axons of other ascending fibers, especially those arising in the reticular formation of the midbrain and terminating in the amygdala and septal nuclei as well as in lateral parts of the limbic lobe, are rich in serotonin. The axons of neurons in the ventral tegmental parts of the midbrain, which ascend in the medial forebrain bundle and the nigrostriatal pathway, contain a high content of dopamine. Of unknown significance is the fact that the zinc content of the limbic system is the highest of any part of the nervous system.

All of this having been said, it would be a mistake to assume that the many structures listed above and their connections constitute a unified functional system. The term *limbic system* is a misnomer. The various parts differ in respect to their connections with the neocortex and central nuclei, their transmitters, and their effects when damaged.

EMOTIONAL DISTURBANCES DUE TO DISEASES INVOLVING LIMBIC STRUCTURES

Many of the foregoing ideas about the role of the limbic lobes have come from experimentation in laboratory animals. Only in relatively recent years have neurologists, primed with the knowledge of these studies, begun to relate emotional disturbances in patients with disease of limbic structures. These clinical observations, summarized in the following pages, are beginning to form an interesting chapter in neurology. The most readily recognized derangements of emotion are listed in Table 25-1. The list is tentative, since our understanding of many of these states, particularly their pathologic basis, is incomplete. Only a small number of these derangements can be used as pathognomonic indicators of lesions and diseases in particular parts of the human brain. Panksepp thinks of emotional disturbances and their expression as reflective only of "spheres of influence" of certain brain mechanisms. The authors believe that, taken in context, these disturbances are useful diagnostically. And, as knowledge of emotional disorders increases, it will undoubtedly bring together large segments of psychiatry and neurology.

Emotional Disturbances in Hallucinating and Deluded Patients

These are best portrayed by the patient with a florid delirium. Threatened by imaginary figures and voices that seem real and inescapable, the patient trembles, struggles to escape, and displays the full picture of terror. The patient's affect, emotional reaction, and visceral and somatic motor responses are altogether appropriate to the content of the hallucinations. We have seen a patient slash his wrists and another try to drown himself in response to hallucinatory voices that admonished them for their worthlessness and the shame they had brought upon their families. But the abnormality in these circumstances is one of disordered perception and thinking, and we have no reason to believe that there is a derangement of the mechanisms for emotional expression.

Table 25-1
Neurology of emotional disturbances

I. Disturbances of emotionality due to:
   A. Perceptual abnormalities (illusions and hallucinations)
   B. Cognitive derangements (delusions)
II. Disinhibition of emotional expression
   A. Emotional lability
   B. Pathologic laughing and crying
III. Rage reactions and aggressivity
IV. Apathy and placidity
   A. Klüver-Bucy syndrome
   B. Other syndromes (frontal and thalamic)
V. Altered sexuality
VI. Endogenous fear, anxiety, depression, and euphoria

An excessive or inappropriate emotional outburst is a common occurrence in a manic, hypomanic, or schizophrenic patient. Here the patient's emotional experience and impulse to action are a response to a delusion. Believing that somebody is a threat to himself or to society, the deluded patient may injure or kill his imagined tormentor. Again the emotional state becomes comprehensible once the content of the delusion has been divulged. In other words, the abnormality under these circumstances is primarily in the sphere of cognition and thinking rather than in the mechanisms for emotional expression.

However, many psychotic patients whose hallucinations and delusions persist for months or years appear to become inured to them. No longer do the appropriate emotional reactions and impulses follow. The patient either denies having hallucinations or appears to disregard them. Perhaps we observe here the emergence of the bland affect and inappropriate emotional reaction of the schizophrenic. We have had occasion, in patients with alcoholic auditory hallucinosis, to trace this state from the early terrifying hallucinosis with appropriate emotional response to a chronic hallucinatory state with inappropriate reaction indistinguishable from paranoid schizophrenia (see Chap. 42).

There also occurs a state—difficult to classify—of overwhelming emotionality in patients who are in severe acute pain. The patient's attention can be captured only briefly, but within moments there is a return to an extreme state of angst, groaning, and anger. We have encountered this with spinal subdural hemorrhage, subarachnoid hemorrhage, explosive migraine, trauma with multiple fractures, and intense pelvic, renal, or abdominal pain.

Disinhibition of Emotional Expression

Emotional Lability It is commonplace clinical experience that cerebral diseases of many types, seemingly without respect to location, weaken the mechanism of control of emotional expression—a mechanism that has been acquired over years of maturation. To be grown up implies an ability to inhibit one's emotions—not that one has less feeling with maturation, but rather that it can be hidden from others. The degree to which this pertains varies with gender and ethnicity and has more to do with social norms than with biology. In certain cultures, women are permitted to cry in public, but men are not. Men and women of Mediterranean races exhibit their feelings more openly than do Anglo-Saxons.

A patient whose cerebrum has been damaged by one or more vascular lesions may suffer the humiliation of crying in public upon meeting an old friend or hearing the national anthem. Less often, a mildly amusing remark or an attempt to tell a funny story may cause excessively loud and prolonged laughter. There may also be easy vacillation from one state to another; this is called *emotional lability* and has for more than a century been accepted as a sign of "organic brain disease." In this type of emotional disturbance, the response is excessive but appropriate to the stimulus and the affect is congruent with the visceral and motor components of the expression. The anatomic substrate is obscure. Perhaps lesions of the frontal lobes more than those of other parts of the brain are conducive to this state, but the authors are unaware of a critical clinicoanatomic study that substantiates this impression. Emotional lability is certainly a frequent accompaniment of diffuse cerebral diseases such as Alzheimer disease, but these diseases, of course, also involve the limbic cortex.

Pathologic (Pseudobulbar, Forced, Spasmodic) Laughing and Crying This form of disordered emotional expression, characterized by outbursts of involuntary, uncontrollable laughing or crying, has been well recognized since the late nineteenth century. Numerous references to these conditions (the *Zwangslachen* and *Zwangsweinen* of German neurologists and the *rire et pleurer spasmodiques* of the French) can be found in the writings of Oppenheim, von Monakow, and Wilson (see Wilson for historical references). Not included under this heading are the tearfulness and facile mood that so often accompany chronic diseases of the nervous system, or the shallow facetiousness (*Witzelsucht*) of the patient with frontal lobe disease. Forced laughing and crying always have a pathologic basis in the brain, either diffuse or focal; hence this stands as a syndrome of multiple causes. It may occur with degenerative and vascular diseases of the brain and no doubt is the direct result of them, but often the diffuse nature of the underlying disease precludes useful topographic analysis and clinicoanatomic correlation. More instructive in this regard are cases of forced laughing or crying in which a vascular or demyelinative process is discretely localized; unfortunately, few well-documented clinical cases of these types have been studied by proper anatomic methods.

The best examples of pathologic laughing and crying are provided by lacunar vascular disease and less often by amyotrophic lateral sclerosis, multiple sclerosis, and progressive supranuclear palsy. They may also be part of the residue of the more widespread lesions of hypoxic-hypotensive encephalopathy, Binswanger ischemic encephalopathy, cerebral trauma, or encephalitis. Most often by far, a sudden hemiplegia, engrafted upon a pre-existent (and often clinically silent) lesion in the opposite hemisphere, sets the stage for the pathologic emotionality that emerges as part of the syndrome of *pseudobulbar palsy* (page 517). In the latter state there is a striking incongruity between the loss of voluntary movements of muscles innervated by the motor nuclei of the lower pons and medulla (inability to forcefully close the eyes, elevate and retract the corners of the mouth, open and close the mouth, chew, swallow, phonate, articulate, and move the tongue) and the preservation of movement of the same muscles in yawning, coughing, throat clearing, and spasmodic laughing or crying (i.e., in reflexive pontomedullary activities). In some such cases, on the slightest provocation and sometimes for no apparent reason, the patient is thrown into a stereotyped spasm of laughter that may last for many minutes, to the point of exhaustion. Or, far more often, the opposite happens—the mere mention of the patient's family or the sight of the doctor provokes an uncontrollable spasm of crying or, more accurately stated, a caricature of crying. The severity of the emotional incontinence or the ease with which it is provoked does not always correspond with the severity of the faciobulbar paralysis or with an exaggeration of the facial and masseter ("jaw jerk") tendon reflexes. In some patients with forced crying and laughing, there is little or no detectable weakness of facial and bulbar muscles; in others, forced laughing and crying are lacking despite a severe upper motor neuron weakness of these muscles. In certain diseases, such as progressive supranuclear palsy and central pontine myelinolysis, of which pseudobulbar palsy is a frequent manifestation, forced laughing and crying are less dramatic or, in many cases, absent. Therefore the pathologic emotional state cannot be equated with pseudobulbar palsy even though the two usually occur together.

Is this pathologic state, whether one of involuntary laughing or of crying, activated by an appropriate stimulus? Does the emotional response accurately reflect the patient's affect or feeling? There are no simple answers to these questions. One problem, of course, is to determine what constitutes an appropriate stimulus for the patient in question. Virtually always, the emotional response is set off by some stimulus or thought; but in most cases it is trifling, or at least it appears so to the physician. Merely addressing the patient or making some casual remark in his presence may suffice. Certainly in such cases the emotional response is out of all proportion to the stimulus. As to the affect, Oppenheim and others stated that these patients need not feel sad when crying or mirthful when laughing, and at least in some cases this is in agreement with our experience. Other patients, however, do report a congruence of affect and emotional expression.

Noteworthy also are the invariability of the initial motor response and the relatively undifferentiated nature of the emotional reaction. Laughter or crying, as each proceeds, may merge, one with the other. Poeck puts great emphasis on the latter point, but it does not seem surprising when one considers the closeness of these two forms of emotional expression—a feature that is particularly evident in young children. Normal persons often cry when overjoyed and smile when sad. More impressive to us is the fact that in some patients with pseudobulbar palsy, laughing and crying, or caricatures thereof, are the only available forms of emotional expression; intermediate phenomena, such as smiling and frowning, are lost. In other patients with pseudobulbar palsy, it seems to us, there are lesser degrees of forced laughing and crying, bridging the gap between this phenomenon and emotional lability.

Wilson, in his discussion of the anatomic basis and mechanism of forced laughing and crying, pointed out that both involve the same facial, vocal, and respiratory musculature and have similar visceral accompaniments (dilatation of facial vessels, secretion of tears, etc.). Two major supranuclear pathways control the pontomedullary mechanisms of facial and other movements required in laughing and crying. One is the familiar corticobulbar pathway that runs from the motor cortex through the posterior limb of the internal capsule and controls volitional movements; the other is a more anterior pathway which descends just rostral to the knee of the internal capsule and contains facilitatory and inhibitory fibers. Unilateral involvement of the anterior pathway leaves the opposite side of the face under volitional control but paretic during laughing, smiling, and crying (emotional facial paralysis); the opposite is observed with a unilateral lesion of the posterior pathway. Wilson's argument, based to some extent on clinicopathologic evidence, was that in pseudobulbar palsy the descending motor pathways, which naturally inhibit the expression of the emotions, are interrupted, although he was uncertain of the exact level. Almost 40 years later, Poeck, after reviewing all the published pathologic anatomy in 30 verified cases, was able to do no more than conclude that supranuclear motor pathways are always involved, with loss of a control mechanism somewhere in the brainstem between thalamus and medulla. However, this clinical state is observed in amyotrophic lateral sclerosis, where the corticobulbar tracts may be involved at a cortical and subcortical level. The lesions are bilateral in practically all instances (see Poeck in the References). There are reports of spasmodic laughter that follows unilateral striatocapsular infarction and lasts for a month or two (Ceccaldi et al), but these cases have not been verified pathologically.

Of interest is the effect of drugs such as imipramine and fluoxetine. In a number of personally observed cases, both the emotional lability and pathologic laughter and crying were partially suppressed by these drugs; in others there was no effect.

A rare but probably related syndrome is *le fou rire prodromique* (prodromal laughing madness) of Féré, in which uncontrollable laughter begins abruptly and is followed after several hours by hemiplegia. Martin cites examples where patients laughed themselves to death. Again, the pathologic anatomy is unsettled. Protracted laughing and (less often) crying may occur also as a manifestation of epileptic seizures, usually of psychomotor type. Ictal laughter is usually without affect. Daly and Mulder have referred to these as "gelastic" seizures. The concurrence of gelastic seizures and precocious puberty should suggest an underlying hamartoma (or other lesion) of the hypothalamus (see Chaps. 16 and 27).

Aggressiveness, Anger, Rage, and Violence

Aggressiveness is an integral part of social behavior. The emergence of this trait early in life enables the individual to secure a position in the family and later in an ever-widening social circle. Individual differences, probably inherited, are noteworthy. Timidity, for example, is a persistent trait, recognized in infancy (Kagan). Males tend to be more aggressive than females. The degree to which excessively aggressive behavior is tolerated varies in different cultures. In most civilized societies, tantrums, rage reactions, and outbursts of violence and destructiveness are not condoned, and one of the principal objectives of training and education is the suppression and sublimation of such behavior. The rate at which this developmental process proceeds varies from one individual to another. In some, especially males and the mentally backward, it is not complete until 25 to 30 years of age; until that time, the deviant behavior is called *sociopathy* (see Chap. 28).

That seemingly groundless outbreaks of unbridled rage may represent the initial or main manifestation of disease is not fully appreciated by the medical profession. A patient with these symptoms may, with little provocation, change from a reasonable state to one of the wildest rage, with a blindly furious impulse to violence and destruction. He charges at those around him, strikes, kicks, bites, and throttles whomever he can reach; he smashes every object that he can lay hands on, tears his clothes, shouts, and curses; his face is suffused with blood and his heart beats violently. Every incoming sensation excites him to further frenzy. On attempting to subdue the patient, one finds that he has the strength of five men. In such states the patient appears out of contact with reality and is impervious to all argument or pleading. As far as one can tell, this pattern of behavior is associated with a feeling of anger. What is so obviously abnormal is the provocation of the attack by some trifling event and a degree of violence that is out of all proportion to the stimulus. There are examples also of a dissociation of affect and behavior in which the patient may spit, cry out, attack, or bite without seeming to be angry. This is especially true of the mentally retarded.

Although the functional anatomy of these states of anger, rage, and aggressiveness has not been fully established, all the human and animal data point to an origin in the temporal lobes. *In humans*, stimulation of the corticomedial amygdaloid nuclei, through depth electrodes, evokes a display of anger, whereas stimulation of the basilateral nuclei does not; destruction of the amygdaloid complex bilaterally reportedly reduces aggressiveness (Kiloh; Narabayashi et al). Lesions in the mediodorsal thalamic nuclei, which receive projections from the amygdaloid nuclei, render humans more placid and docile. Sex hormones influence the activity of these temporal lobe circuits; testosterone promotes aggressiveness and estradiol suppresses it, suggesting an explanation for sex differences in the disposition to anger. Surprisingly, propranolol and lithium have benefited such patients much more than haloperidol, the phenothiazine drugs, or sedatives.

Observations *in experimental animals* have corroborated the observations in humans. As mentioned earlier, bilateral removal of the amygdaloid nuclei in the macaque greatly reduces the reactions of fear and anger. Electrical stimulation in or near the amygdala of the unanesthetized cat yields a variety of motor and vegetative responses. One of these has been referred to as the *fear*, or *flight*, response, in which the animal appears frightened and runs away and hides; another is the *anger*, or *defense*, reaction, characterized by growling, hissing, and piloerection. However, structures other than the amygdaloid nuclei are also involved in these reactions. Lesions in the ventromedial nuclei of the hypothalamus (which receive an abundant projection of fibers from the amygdaloid nuclei via the stria medullaris and possibly the ventral amygdala–fugal pathway) have been shown to cause aggressive behavior, and bilateral ablation of neocortical area 24 (rostral cingulate gyrus) has produced the opposite state—tameness and reduced aggressiveness, at least in some species.

Rage reactions of the intensity described above may be encountered in the following medical settings: (1) rarely as part of a temporal lobe seizure; (2) as an episodic reaction without recognizable seizures or other neurologic abnormality, as in certain sociopaths; (3) in the course of a recognizable acute neurologic disease; or (4) with the clouding of consciousness that accompanies a metabolic or toxic encephalopathy. Each of these circumstances is considered below.

Rage in Temporal Lobe Seizures (See also page 339.) According to Gastaut and colleagues, a directed attack of uncontrollable rage may occur either as part of a seizure or as an interictal phenomenon. Some patients describe a gradual heightening of excitability for 2 to 3 days, either before or after a seizure, before bursting into a rage. Certainly such attacks have been observed, but they are very rare. However, a lesser degree of aggressive behavior as part of a temporal lobe seizure is not uncommon; it is usually part of the ictal or postictal behavioral automatism and tends to be brief in duration and poorly directed. Usually the lesion is in the temporal lobe of the dominant hemisphere. Similarly, a feeling of rage or severe anger is relatively rare as an ictal emotion—much less common than feelings of fear, sadness, or pleasure (Williams reported only 17 cases of anger among 165 patients with ictal emotion). Geschwind has emphasized the frequency of a profound deepening of the patient's emotional experiences in temporal lobe epilepsy.

Rage Attacks without Apparent Seizure Activity In some instances of this type, the patient had from early life been hot-headed, intolerant of frustration, and impulsive, exhibiting behavior that would be classed as sociopathic (Chap. 56). There are others, however, who, at certain periods of life, usually adolescence or early adulthood, begin to have episodes of wild, aggressive behavior. Alcohol or some other drug may set them off. One suspects epilepsy, but there is no history of a recognizable seizure and no interruption of consciousness, which is so typical of complex partial epilepsy. The electroencephalogram (EEG) is either normal or nonspecifically abnormal. In a few such cases, in which aggression has resulted in serious injury to others (or homicide), depth electrodes placed in the amygdaloid nuclear complex have recorded seizure discharges.

Attacks of excitement and various autonomic accompaniments have been aroused by stimulation of the same region, and the abnormal behavior has in some instances been relieved by ablation of the abnormally discharging structures. Mark and Ervin have documented a number of examples of this "dyscontrol syndrome."

Violent Behavior in Acute or Chronic Neurologic Disease From time to time one encounters patients in whom intense excitement, rage, and aggressiveness begin abruptly in association with an acute neurologic disease or in a phase of partial recovery. In most cases the medial and anterior temporal lobes are implicated. Cranial trauma is the most frequent cause of what has been called "organic personality disorder of the explosive type." Serious head injury with protracted coma may be followed by personality changes consisting of aggressive outbursts, suspiciousness, poor judgment, indifference to the feelings of family, and variable degrees of cognitive impairment. Hemorrhagic leukoencephalitis, lobar hemorrhage, infarction, and herpes simplex encephalitis affecting the medial-orbital portions of the frontal lobes and inferomedial portions of the temporal lobes may have the same effect. Fisher has noted the occurrence of intense rage reactions as an aftermath of a dominant temporal lobe lesion that had caused a Wernicke type aphasia. Cases of this type have also been reported with ruptured aneurysm of the circle of Willis and extension of a pituitary adenoma; references to these reports can be found in the articles of Poeck (1969) and of Pillieri.

Also of interest in this connection are the effects of slow-growing tumors of the temporal lobe. Malamud described outbursts of rage in association with temporal lobe gliomas. Other patients harboring such tumors had no rage reactions but exhibited a clinical picture resembling schizophrenia. It is noteworthy that 8 of the 9 patients with temporal lobe glioma described by Malamud also had seizures. Many similar examples have been reported (see Poeck for references). The anteromedial part of the left temporal lobe has been the site of the tumor in the majority of cases. Falconer and Serafetinides have described patients with rage reactions in whom there was a hamartoma or sclerotic focus in this region. However, the precise anatomy has not been demarcated.

Aggressive Behavior in Acute Toxic-Metabolic Encephalopathies Here the patient is not in a clear-headed state and rage or aggression is superimposed on an encephalopathy of toxic or metabolic origin. The most dramatic examples in our experience have been associated with hypoglycemic reactions. When the patient is left alone, the aggressive behavior is undirected and disorganized, but anyone in the immediate neighborhood may be struck by flailing limbs. In medical writings, this type of activity is described as "bizarre behavior" but is rarely characterized further. Such patients are clearly out of contact. Their attention cannot be gained for a moment, and attempts at physical restraint provoke an even more violent reaction.

A similar state may occur with phencyclidine and cocaine intoxication and at times with other hallucinogens, always with agitation and usually hallucinosis. Outbursts of rage and violence with alcohol intoxication are somewhat different in nature: some instances represent a rare paradoxical or idiosyncratic reaction to alcohol ("pathologic intoxication," see page 1237); in other cases, alcohol appears to disinhibit an underlying sociopathic behavior pattern.

Placidity and Apathy

The animal organism normally indulges in and displays highly energized, exploratory activity of its environment. Some of this activity is motivated by the drive for sexual satisfaction and procurement of food; in humans, it may be a matter of curiosity. According to Panksepp, these activities are governed by "expectancy circuits," involving nuclear groups in mesolimbic and mesocortical dopaminergic circuits connected with the diencephalon and mesencephalon via the medial forebrain bundles; lesions that interrupt these connections are said to abolish the expectancy reactions. Positron emission tomography (PET) studies correlate functional difficulty in the initiation of movements with impaired activation of the anterior cingulum, putamen, prefrontal cortex, and supplementary motor area (Playford et al).

In our experience, a quantitative reduction in all activity is the most frequent of all psychobehavioral alterations in patients with cerebral disease, particularly in those with involvement of the anterior parts of the frontal lobes. There are fewer thoughts, fewer words uttered, and fewer movements per unit of time. That this is not a purely motor phenomenon is disclosed in conversation with the patient, who seems to perceive and think more slowly, to make fewer associations with a given idea, to initiate speech less frequently, and to exhibit less inquisitiveness and interest. This reduction in psychomotor activity is recognized as a personality change by the family.

Depending upon how this state is viewed, it may be interpreted as a heightened threshold to stimulation, inattentiveness or inability to maintain an attentive attitude, impaired thinking, apathy, or lack of impulse (*abulia*). In a sense, all are correct, for each represents a different aspect of the reduced mental activity. Clinicoanatomic correlates are inexact, but bilateral lesions deep in the septal region (as sometimes occur with bleeding from an anterior communicating aneurysm) have resulted in the most striking lack of impulse, spontaneity, and conation, i.e., akinetic mutism. An impairment of learning and memory functions may be added. Typically the patient is fully conscious, is wide awake, and looks around, i.e., is visually attentive. Upon recovery, memory is retained for all that happened. In this respect abulia differs from stupor and hypersomnolence. Insofar as there is no paralysis, this condition differs from the *locked-in syndrome*. In abulia, we assume the apathy and placidity to be secondary to reduced impulse.

Patients who exhibit abulia are difficult to test because they respond slowly or not at all to every type of test. Yet on rare occasions, when intensely stimulated, they may speak and act normally. It is as though some energizing mechanism (possibly striatocortical), different from the reticular activating system of the upper brainstem, were impaired.

Quite apart from this abulic syndrome, which has already been discussed in relation to coma and to extensive lesions of the frontal lobes (Chaps. 17 and 22), there are lesser degrees of it, in which a lively, sometimes volatile person has been rendered placid (hypobulic) by a disease of the nervous system. The most consistent changes of this type were observed formerly to follow bilateral prefrontal leukotomy, the effects of which have also been discussed in relation to the frontal lobes. Barris and Schuman and many others have documented states of extreme placidity with lesions of the anterior cingulate gyri. Unlike the case in retarded depression, the mood is neutral; the patient is apathetic rather than depressed.

The alteration in emotional behavior described above differs from that observed in the *Klüver-Bucy syndrome*, which results from total bilateral temporal lobectomy in adult rhesus monkeys (see also page 478). While these animals were rather placid and lacked the ability to recognize objects visually (they could not distinguish edible from inedible objects), they had a striking tendency to examine everything orally, were unusually alert and responsive to visual stimuli (they touched or mouthed every object in their visual fields), became hypersexual, and increased their food intake. This constellation of behavioral changes has been sought in human beings, but the complete syndrome has been described only infrequently (Marlowe et al; Terzian and Dalle). Pillieri and Poeck have collected cases that have come closest to reproducing the syndrome (Fig. 25-3*A* and *B*). Unfortunately, many human examples have occurred in conjunction with diffuse diseases (Alzheimer and Pick cerebral atrophies, meningoencephalitis due to toxoplasmosis, herpes simplex, or AIDS) and hence are of little use for anatomic analysis. With bitemporal surgical ablations, placidity and enhanced oral behavior were the most frequent consequences; altered sexual behavior and visual agnosia were less frequent. In all patients who showed placidity and an amnesic state, the hippocampi and medial parts of the temporal lobe had been destroyed, but not the amygdaloid nuclei.

Perhaps the most consistent type of reduced emotionality in humans is that associated with acute lesions (usually infarcts or hemorrhages) in the right or nondominant parietal lobe. Not only is the patient indifferent to the paralysis but, as Bear points out, he is unconcerned about his other diseases as well as personal and family problems, is less able to interpret the emotional facial expressions of others, and is inattentive in general. Dimond and coworkers interpret this to mean that the right hemisphere is more involved in affective-emotional experience than the left, which is committed to language. Observations derived from the study of split-brain patients and from selective anesthetizations of the cerebral hemispheres by intracarotid injection of amobarbital (Wada test) lend some support to this oversimplified view. Rarely, lesions of the left (dominant) hemisphere appear to induce the opposite effect—a frenzied excitement lasting for days or weeks.

The full range of placidity reactions in neurology has not been catalogued. Unfortunately, neurologists and psychiatrists have tended to neglect this aspect of behavior.

Altered Sexuality

The normal pattern of sexual behavior in both males and females may be altered by cerebral disease quite apart from impairment due to obvious physical disability or to diseases that destroy or isolate the segmental reflex mechanisms (see Chap. 26).

Hypersexuality in men or women is a rare but well-documented complication of neurologic disease. It has long been believed that lesions of the orbital frontal lobes may remove moral-ethical restraints and lead to indiscriminate sexual behavior, and that superior frontal lesions may be associated with a general loss of initiative that reduces all impulsivity, including sexual. In rare

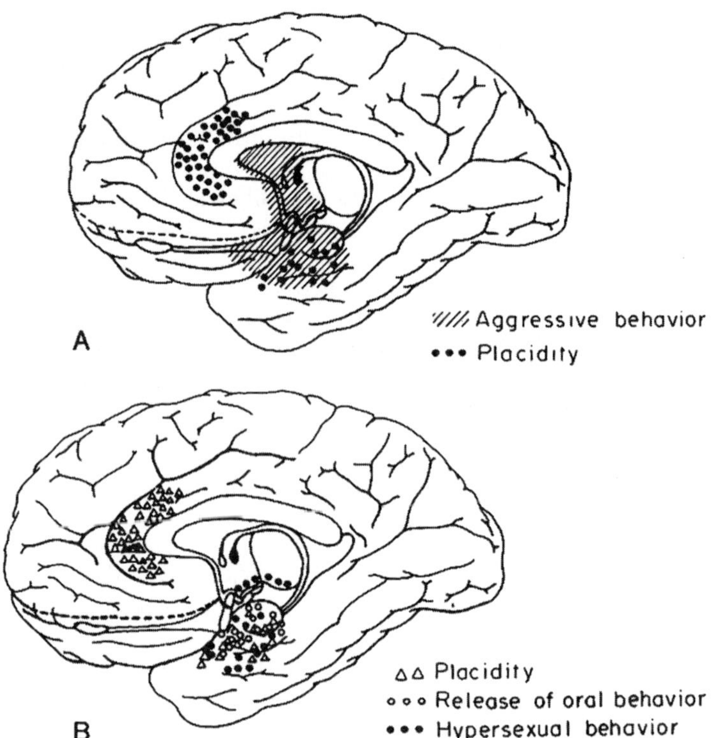

Figure 25-3

A. Localization of lesions which, in humans, can lead to aggressive behavior and placidity. B. Localization of lesions which, in humans, can lead to placidity, release of oral behavior, and hypersexuality. (From Poeck by permission.)

cases, extreme hypersexuality marks the onset of encephalitis or develops gradually with tumors of the temporal region. Persistence of this behavior suggests disinhibition as the mechanism. Possibly the limbic parts of the brain are affected, the ones from which MacLean and Ploog could evoke penile erection and orgasm by electrical stimulation (medial dorsal thalamus, medial forebrain bundle, and septal preoptic region). In humans, Heath has observed that stimulation of the ventroseptal area (through depth electrodes) evokes feelings of pleasure and lust. Also, Gorman and Cummings have described two patients who became sexually disinhibited after a shunt catheter had perforated the dorsal septal region. This is in keeping with the experience of Heath and Fitzjarrell, who found that infusion of acetylcholine into the septal region (an experimental treatment for Parkinson disease) produced euphoria and orgasm, and with Heath's recordings from the septum of patients during sexual intercourse, showing greatly increased activity with spikes and slow waves. However, we know of no case in which a stable lesion that caused abnormal sexual behavior has been studied carefully by serial sections of the critical parts of the brain. In clinical practice the commonest cause of disinhibited sexual behavior, next to the aftermaths of head injury and cerebral hemorrhage, is the use of dopaminergic drugs in Parkinson disease.

Hyposexuality, meaning loss of libido, is most often due to a depressive illness. Certain chemical agents—notably antihypertensive, anticonvulsant, serotoninergic antidepressant, and neuroleptic drugs—may be responsible in individual patients. A variety of cerebral diseases may also have this effect.

Lesions that involve the tuberoinfundibular region of the hypothalamus are known to cause disturbances in sexual function. If such lesions are acquired early in life, pubertal changes are prevented from occurring; hamartomas of the hypothalamus, as in von Recklinghausen neurofibromatosis and tuberous sclerosis, may cause sexual precocity. Autonomic neuropathies and lesions involving the sacral parts of the parasympathetic system, the commonest being prostatectomy, abolish normal sexual performance but do not alter libido or orgasm.

Blumer and Walker have reviewed the literature on the association of epilepsy and abnormal sexual behavior. They note that sexual arousal, as an ictal phenomenon, is apt to occur in relation to temporal lobe seizures, particularly when the discharging focus is in the mediotemporal region. These authors also cite the high incidence of global hyposexuality in patients with temporal lobe epilepsy. Temporal lobectomy in such patients has sometimes been followed by a period of hypersexuality.

Acute Fear, Anxiety, Elation, and Euphoria

The phenomenon of acute fear and anxiety occurring as a prelude to or part of a seizure is familiar to every physician. Williams's study, already alluded to, is of particular interest; from a series of about 2000 epileptics, he was able to cull 100 patients in whom an emotional experience was part of the seizure. Of the latter, 61 experienced feelings of fear and anxiety and 21 experienced depression. Daly has made similar observations. These clinical data call to mind the effects that had been noted by Penfield and Jasper when they stimulated the upper, anterior, and inferior parts of the temporal lobe and cingulate gyrus during surgical procedures; frequently the patient described feelings of strangeness, uneasiness, and fear. In most instances, consciousness was variably impaired at the same time, and some patients had hallucinatory experiences as well.

In these cortical stimulations, neuronal circuits subserving fear are coextensive with those of anger; both are thought to lie in the medial part of the temporal lobe and amygdala, as discussed earlier. Both in animals and in humans, electrical stimulation in this region can arouse each emotion, but the circuitry subserving fear appears to be located lateral to that of anger and rage. Destruction of the central part of the amygdaloid nuclear complex abolishes fear reactions. These nuclei are connected to the lateral hypothalamus and midbrain tegmentum, regions from which Monroe and Heath as well as Nashold and associates have been able to evoke feelings of fear and anxiety by electrical stimulation.

Depression is less frequent as an ictal emotion, although it occurs often enough as an interictal phenomenon (Benson et al). Of interest is the observation that lesions of the dominant hemisphere are more likely than nondominant ones to be attended by an immediate pervasive depression of mood, disproportionate to the degree of severity of physical disability (Robinson et al). We are inclined to the view that the onset of depression after a stroke is a reaction to disability, i.e., a reactive depression, akin to that which follows myocardial infarction (Chap. 57).

Odd mixtures of depression and anxiety are often associated with temporal lobe tumors and less often with tumors of the hypothalamus and third ventricle (see review by Alpers), and they sometimes occur at the onset of a degenerative disease, such as multiple system atrophy.

Elation and *euphoria* are less well documented as limbic phenomena, nor has this elevation in mood in some patients with multiple sclerosis ever been adequately explained. Feelings of pleasure and satisfaction as well as "stirring sensations" are unusual but well-described emotional experiences in patients with temporal lobe seizures, and this type of affective response, like that of fear, has been elicited by stimulating several different parts of the temporal lobe (Penfield and Jasper). In states of hypomania and mania, every experience may be colored by feelings of delight and pleasure and a sense of power, and the patient may remember these experiences after he has recovered.

Differential Diagnosis of Perturbations in Emotion and Affect

Aside from clinical observation, there are no reliable means of evaluating the emotional disorders described above. While neurologic medicine has done little more than describe and classify some of the clinical states dominated by emotional derangements, an activity considered by some to be the lowest level of science, knowledge of this type is nonetheless of both theoretical and practical importance. In theory, it prepares one for the next step, of passing from a superficial to a deeper order of inquiry, where questions of pathogenesis and etiology can be broached. Practically, it provides certain clues that are useful in differential diagnosis. A number of particular neurologic possibilities must always be considered when one is confronted with one of the following clinical states.

Uninhibited Laughter and Crying and Emotional Lability As indicated earlier, one may confidently assume that the syndrome of forced or spasmodic laughing and crying signifies cerebral disease and more specifically bilateral disease of the corticobulbar tracts. Usually the motor and reflex changes of spastic bulbar (pseudobulbar) palsy are associated, especially heightened facial and mandibular reflexes and often corticospinal tract signs as well. Extreme emotional lability also indicates bilateral cerebral disease, although only the signs of unilateral disease may be apparent clinically. The most common pathologic bases for these clinical states are lacunar infarction or other cerebrovascular lesions, diffuse hypoxic-hypotensive encephalopathy, amyotrophic lateral sclerosis, and multiple sclerosis. Abrupt onset, of course, points to vascular disease.

Placidity and Apathy These may be the earliest and most important signs of cerebral disease. Clinically, placidity and apathy must be distinguished from the akinesia or bradykinesia of Parkinson disease and the reduced mental activity of depressive illness. Alzheimer disease, normal-pressure hydrocephalus, and frontal–corpus callosum tumors are the most common pathologic states underlying apathy and placidity, but these disturbances may complicate a variety of other frontal and temporal lesions such as occur with demyelinative disease or as an aftermath of ruptured anterior communicating aneurysm.

An Outburst of Rage and Violence Most often such an outburst is but another episode in a lifelong sequence of sociopathic behavior (see Chap. 56). More significance attaches to its abrupt appearance as a sudden departure from an individual's normal personality. If an outburst of rage accompanies a seizure, the rage should be viewed as the consequence of the disruptive effect of seizure activity on temporal lobe function; however, as indicated earlier, an outburst of uncontrolled rage and violence is a very rare manifestation of psychomotor epilepsy. Lesser degrees of poorly directed combative behavior, as part of ictal or postictal automatism, are more common. Rarely, rage and aggressivity are expressive of an acute neurologic disease that involves the medial temporal and orbitofrontal regions. We have several times observed such states in the course of a dementing disease and in a stable individual as a transient expression of an obscure encephalopathy.

Rage reactions with continuous violent activity must be distinguished from *mania*, in which there is flight of ideation to the point of incoherence, euphoric or irritable mood, and incessant psychomotor activity; from *organic drivenness*, in which continuous motor activity, accompanied by no clear ideation occurs, usually in a child, as an aftermath of encephalitis; and from extreme instances of *akathisia*, where incessant restless movements and pacing may occur in conjunction with extrapyramidal symptoms.

Extreme Fright and Agitation Here the central problem must be clarified by determining whether the patient is delirious (clouding of consciousness, psychomotor overactivity, and hallucinations), deluded (schizophrenia), manic (overactive, flight of ideas), or experiencing an isolated panic attack (palpitation, trembling, feeling of suffocation, etc.). Rarely does panic prove to be an expression of temporal lobe epilepsy. In an adult without a characterologic trait of anxiety, an acute panic attack may signify the onset of a depressive illness or schizophrenia.

Bizarre Ideation Developing over Weeks or Months While these symptoms are usually due to a psychosis (schizophrenia or manic-depressive disease), one should consider a tumor or other lesion of the temporal lobe, particularly when accompanied by psychomotor seizures, aphasic symptoms, rotatory vertigo (rare), and quadrantic visual field defects. Such states have also been described in hypothalamic disease, suggested by somnolence, diabetes insipidus, visual field defects, and hydrocephalus (see Chap. 27).

REFERENCES

ALPERS BJ: Personality and emotional disorders associated with hypothalamic lesions. *Res Publ Assoc Nerv Ment Dis* 20:725, 1939.

ANGEVINE JB JR, COTMAN CW: *Principles of Neuroanatomy.* New York, Oxford University Press, 1981, pp 253–283.

BALEYDIER C, MAUGUIERE F: The duality of the cingulate gyrus in monkey. *Brain* 103:525, 1980.

BALLANTINE HT, CASSIDY WL, FLANAGAN NB, et al: Stereotaxic anterior cingulotomy for neuropsychiatric illness and chronic pain. *J Neurosurg* 26:488, 1967.

BARD P: A diencephalic mechanism for the expression of rage with special reference to the sympathetic nervous system. *Am J Physiol* 84:490, 1928.

BARD P, MOUNTCASTLE VB: Some forebrain mechanisms involved in the expression of rage with special reference to suppression of angry behavior. *Assoc Res Nerv Ment Dis Proc* 27:362, 1947.

BARRIS RW, SCHUMAN HR: Bilateral anterior cingulate gyrus lesions: Syndrome of the anterior cingulate gyri. *Neurology* 3:44, 1953.

BEAR DM: Hemispheric specialization and the neurology of emotion. *Arch Neurol* 40:195, 1983.

BENSON DF, MENDEZ MF, ENGEL J, et al: Affective symptomatology in epilepsy. *Int J Neurol* 19–20:30, 1985–1986.

BLUMER D, WALKER AE: The neural basis of sexual behavior, in Benson F, Blumer D (eds): *Psychiatric Aspects of Neurologic Disease*. New York, Grune & Stratton, 1975, chap 11, pp 199–217.

BROWN JW: Frontal lobe syndromes, in Vinken PJ, Bruyn GW, Klawans HL (eds): Vol 45: *Handbook of Clinical Neurology.* Amsterdam, Elsevier Science Publications, 1984, pp 23–42.

CANNON WB: *Bodily Changes in Pain, Hunger and Fear*, 2nd ed. New York, D. Appleton, 1929.

CECCALDI M, PONCET M, MILANDRE L, ROUYER C: Temporary forced laughter after unilateral strokes. *Eur Neurol* 34:36, 1994.

DALY DD: Ictal affect. *Am J Psychiatry* 115:97, 1958.

DALY DD, MULDER DW: Gelastic epilepsy. *Neurology* 7:189, 1957.

Damasio AR, Van Hoesen GW: The limbic system and the localization of herpes simplex encephalitis. *J Neurol Neurosurg Psychiatry* 48:297, 1985.

Dimond SJ, Farrington L, Johnson P: Differing emotional responses from right and left hemisphere. *Nature* 261:690, 1976.

Engel J Jr, Bandler R, Caldecott-Hazard S: Modification of emotional expression induced by clinical and experimental epileptic disturbances. *Int J Neurol* 19–20:21, 1985–1986.

Falconer MA, Serafetinides EA: A follow-up study of surgery in temporal lobe epilepsy. *J Neurol Neurosurg Psychiatry* 26:154, 1963.

Féré MC: Le fou rire prodromique. *Rev Neurol* 11:353, 1903.

Fisher CM: Anger associated with dysphasia. *Trans Am Neurol Assoc* 95:240, 1970.

Gastaut H, Morin G, Lefevre N: Etude de comportement des épileptiques psychomoteurs dans l'intervalle de leurs crises. *Ann Med Psychol* 1:1, 1955.

Geschwind N: The clinical setting of aggression in temporal lobe epilepsy, in Field WS, Sweet WH (eds): *The Neurobiology of Violence*. St Louis, Warren H Green, 1975.

Gorman DG, Cummings JL: Hypersexuality following septal injury. *Arch Neurol* 49:308, 1992.

Heath RG: Pleasure and brain activity in man. *J Nerv Ment Dis* 154:3, 1972.

Heath RG, Fitzjarrell AT: Chemical stimulation to deep forebrain nuclei in parkinsonism and epilepsy. *Int J Neurol* 18:163, 1984.

Kagan J: *The Nature of the Child*. New York, Basic Books, 1984.

Kiloh LG: The treatment of anger and aggression and the modification of sex deviation, in Smith JS, Kiloh LG (eds): *Psychosurgery and Psychiatry*. Oxford, Pergamon Press, 1977, pp 37–54.

Klüver H, Bucy PC: An analysis of certain effects of bilateral temporal lobectomy in the rhesus monkey with special reference to psychic blindness. *J Psychol* 5:33, 1938.

MacLean PD: Contrasting functions of limbic and neocortical systems of the brain and their relevance to psychophysiological aspects of medicine. *Am J Med* 25:611, 1958.

MacLean PD, Ploog DW: Cerebral representation of penile erection. *J Neurophysiol* 25:29, 1962.

Malamud N: Psychiatric disorder with intracranial tumors of limbic system. *Arch Neurol* 17:113, 1967.

Mark VH, Ervin FR: *Violence and the Brain*. New York, Harper & Row, 1970.

Marlowe WB, Mancall EL, Thomas JJ: Complete Klüver-Bucy syndrome in man. *Cortex* 11:53, 1975.

Martin JP: Fits of laughter (sham mirth) in organic cerebral disease. *Brain* 70:453, 1950.

Monroe RR, Heath RC: Psychiatric observations on the patient group, in Heath RC (ed): *Studies in Schizophrenia*. Cambridge, MA, Harvard University Press, 1983, pp 345–383.

Narabayashi H, Nacao Y, Yoshida M, Nagahata M: Stereotaxic amygdalectomy for behavior disorders. *Arch Neurol* 9:1, 1963.

Nashold BS, Wilson WP, Slaughter DE: Sensations evoked by stimulation in the midbrain of man. *J Neurosurg* 30:14, 1969.

Nauta WJH: The central visceromotor system: A general survey, in Hockman CH (ed): *Limbic System Mechanisms and Autonomic Function*. Springfield, IL, Charles C Thomas, 1972, chap 2, pp 21–33.

Panksepp J: Mood changes, in Vinken PJ, Bruyn GW, Klawans HL (eds): *Handbook of Clinical Neurology*. Vol 45. Amsterdam, North-Holland, 1985, chap 21, pp 271–285.

Papez JW: A proposed mechanism of emotion. *Arch Neurol Psychiatry* 38:725, 1937.

Penfield W, Jasper H: *Epilepsy and the Functional Anatomy of the Human Brain*. Boston, Little, Brown, 1954, pp 413–416.

Pillieri G: The Klüver-Bucy syndrome in man. *Psychiatr Neurol* 152:65, 1967.

Playford ED, Jenkins LH, Passingham RE, et al: Impaired mesial frontal and putamen activation in Parkinson's disease: A positron emission tomography study. *Ann Neurol* 32:151, 1992.

Poeck K: Pathophysiology of emotional disorders associated with brain damage, in Vinken PJ, Bruyn GW (eds): *Handbook of Clinical Neurology*. Vol 3: *Disorders of Higher Nervous Activity*. Amsterdam, North-Holland, 1969, chap 20, pp 343–367.

Poeck K: Pathological laughter and crying, in Vinken PJ, Bruyn GW, Klawans HV (eds): *Handbook of Clinical Neurology*. Vol 45. Amsterdam, North-Holland, 1985, chap 16, pp 219–225.

Robinson RG, Kubos KL, Starr LB, et al: Mood disorders in stroke patients: Importance of location of lesion. *Brain* 107:81, 1984.

Terzian H, Dalle G: Syndrome of Klüver-Bucy reproduced in man by bilateral removal of the temporal lobes. *Neurology* 5:373, 1955.

Williams D: The structure of emotions reflected in epileptic experiences. *Brain* 79:29, 1956.

Wilson SAK: Some problems in neurology. II: Pathological laughing and crying. *J Neurol Psychopathol* 16:299, 1924.

Chapter 26

DISORDERS OF THE AUTONOMIC NERVOUS SYSTEM, RESPIRATION, AND SWALLOWING

The human internal environment is regulated in large measure by the integrated activity of the autonomic nervous system and endocrine glands. Their visceral and homeostatic functions, essential to life and survival, are involuntary. Why nature has divorced them from volition is an interesting question. One would like to think that the mind, being preoccupied with discriminative, moral, and esthetic matters, should not have to be troubled with such mundane functions as breathing, regulation of heart rate, lactation, swallowing, and sleeping. Claude Bernard expressed this idea in more sardonic terms when he wrote that "nature thought it prudent to remove these important phenomena from the caprice of an ignorant will."

While relatively few neurologic diseases exert their effects primarily or exclusively on the autonomic-neuroendocrine axis, there are numerous medical diseases that implicate this system in some way—hypertension, asthma, and certain dramatic disorders of cardiac conduction, such as ventricular tachycardia, to name some of the important ones. And many neurologic diseases involve the autonomic nervous system to a varying extent, giving rise to symptoms such as syncope, sphincteric dysfunction, pupillary abnormalities, diaphoresis, and disorders of thermoregulation. Also, a wide variety of pharmacologic agents influence autonomic functions, making them the concern of every physician. Finally, in addition to their central role in visceral innervation, autonomic parts of the neuraxis and parts of the endocrine system are utilized in all emotional experience and its display.

Breathing is unique among autonomic nervous system functions. While continuous throughout life, it is not altogether automatic and it is partly under volitional control. Current views of the central control of breathing, and the ways in which diseases cause it to break down, should be known to neurologists. Respiratory failure is a major feature of numerous neurologic conditions such as coma, high spinal cord injury, and any number of neuromuscular diseases—the Guillain-Barré syndrome, myasthenia gravis, and poliomyelitis (formerly) being the main ones. Treatment of the respiratory and other aspects of autonomic failure constitutes a most important part of the specialty of neurologic intensive care, for which reason these conditions are brought together here.

The autonomic and endocrine systems, though closely related, give rise to disparate clinical syndromes, so that each is accorded a separate chapter—this chapter dealing with the autonomic nervous system and the next one with the hypothalamus and neuroendocrine disorders. The following discussion of anatomy and physiology serves as an introduction to both chapters.

Anatomic Considerations

The most remarkable feature of the autonomic nervous system (also called the visceral, vegetative, or involuntary nervous system) is that a major part of it is located outside the cerebrospinal system, in proximity to the visceral structures that it innervates. This position alone seems to symbolize its relative independence from the cerebrospinal system. Also, in distinction to the somatic neuromuscular system, where a single motor neuron bridges the gap between the central nervous system and the effector organ, in the autonomic nervous system there are always two efferent neurons serving this function—one (preganglionic) arising from its nucleus in the brainstem or spinal cord and the other (postganglionic) arising from specialized peripheral ganglia. This fundamental anatomic feature is illustrated in Fig. 26-1.

From a strictly anatomic point of view, the autonomic nervous system is divided into two parts: the

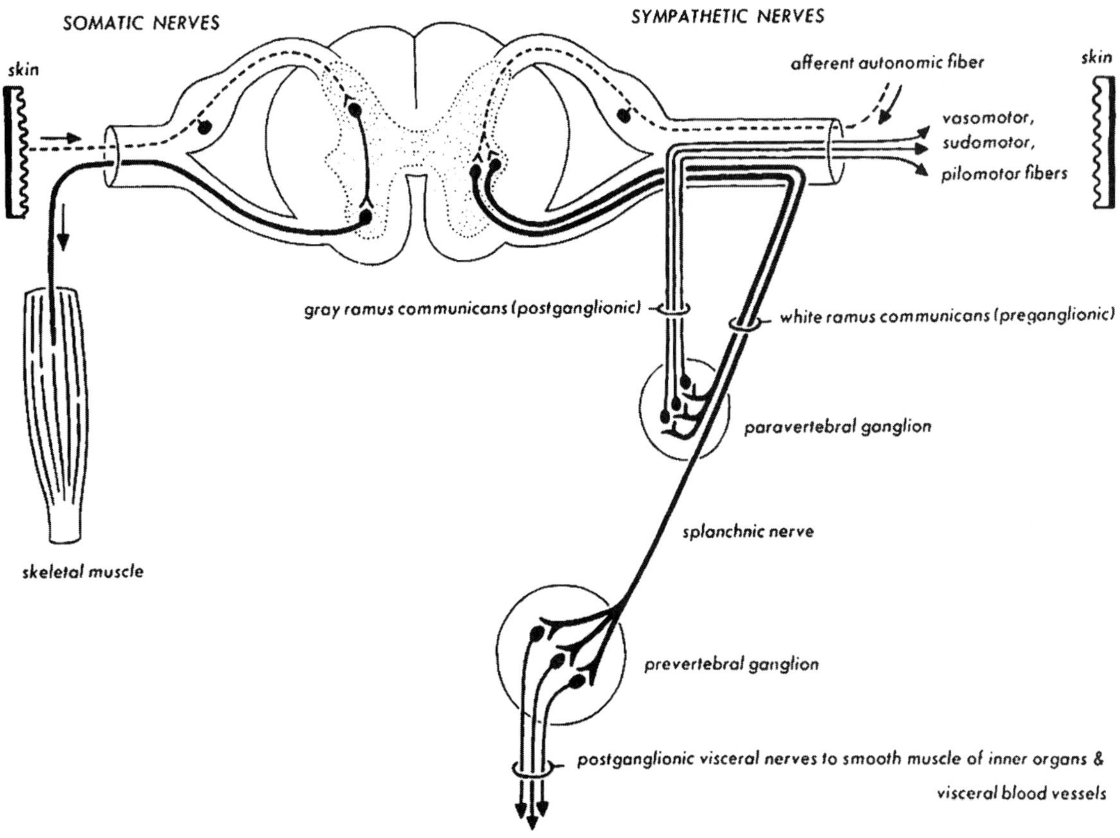

Figure 26-1

Sympathetic outflow from the spinal cord and the course and distribution of sympathetic fibers. The preganglionic fibers are in heavy lines; postganglionic fibers are in thin lines. (From Pick by permission.)

craniosacral, or parasympathetic, and the thoracolumbar, or sympathetic (Figs. 26-2, 26-3, and 26-4). Functionally, the two parts are complementary in maintaining a balance in the tonic activities of many visceral structures and organs. This rigid separation into sympathetic and parasympathetic parts, while useful for purposes of exposition, is not altogether sustainable physiologically. Blessing points out that the scheme does not provide a thorough explanation for each of the homeostatic functions that are under control of complex systems of central and peripheral neurons. From a neurologist's perspective, the two components are often affected together. Nonetheless, the notion of a balanced autonomic system has stood the test of time and remains a primary neuroanatomic and neurophysiologic concept.

The Parasympathetic Nervous System (Fig. 26-2)

There are two divisions of the parasympathetic nervous system—cranial and sacral. The *cranial division* originates in the visceral nuclei of the midbrain, pons, and medulla. These nuclei lie in close proximity to the somatic afferent nuclei and include the Edinger-Westphal nucleus, superior and inferior salivatory nuclei, dorsal motor nucleus of the vagus, and adjacent reticular nuclei.

Axons (preganglionic fibers) of the visceral nuclei course through the oculomotor, facial, glossopharyngeal, and vagus nerves. The preganglionic fibers from the Edinger-Westphal nucleus run in the oculomotor nerve and synapse in the ciliary ganglion in the orbit; axons of the ciliary ganglion cells innervate the ciliary muscle and sphincter pupillae (Fig. 14-7). The preganglionic fibers of the superior salivatory nucleus enter the facial nerve and, at a point near the geniculate ganglion, form the greater superficial petrosal nerve, through which they reach the sphenopalatine ganglion; postganglionic fibers

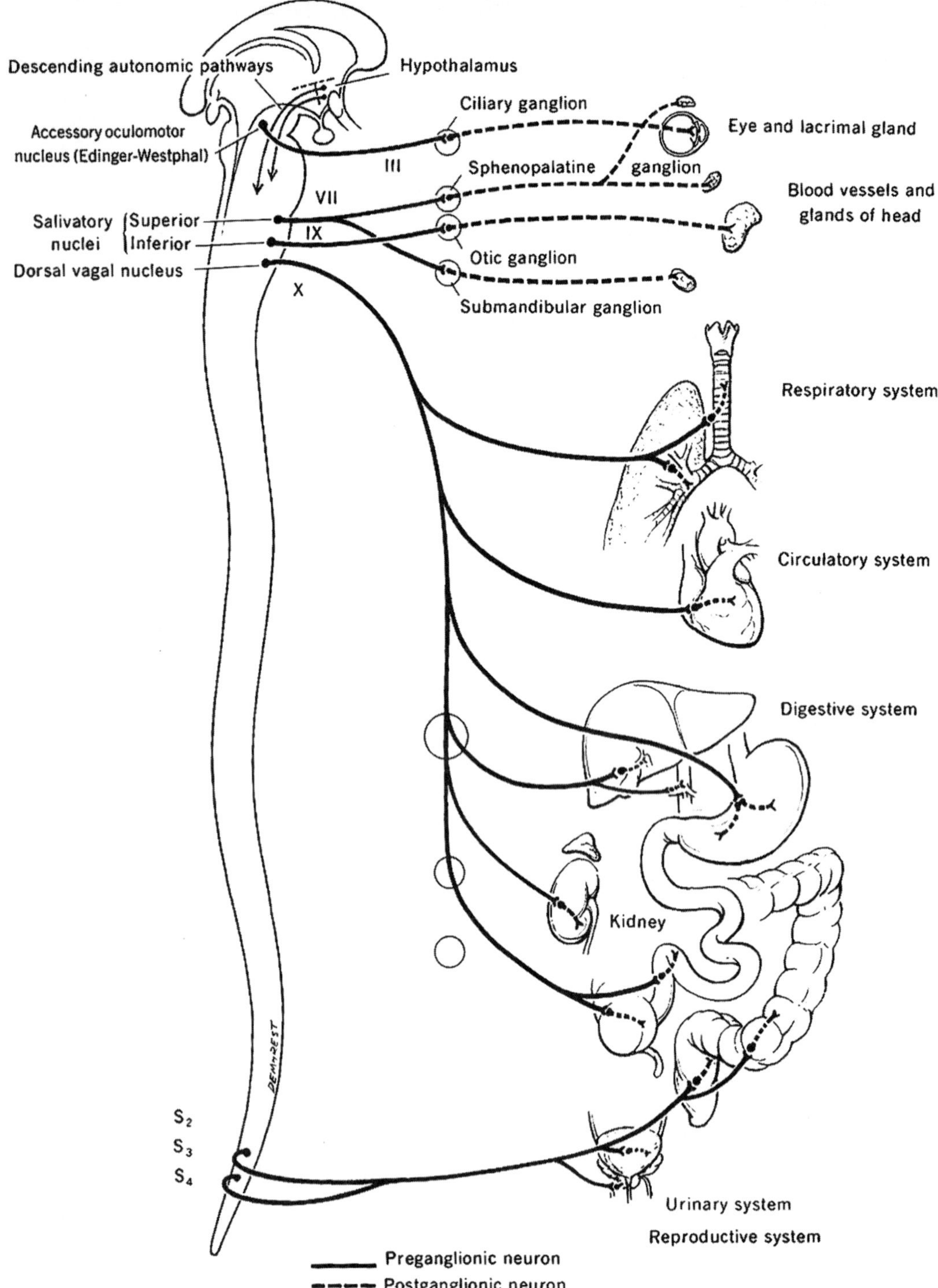

Figure 26-2

The parasympathetic (craniosacral) division of the autonomic nervous system. Preganglionic fibers extend from nuclei of the brainstem and sacral segments of the spinal cord to peripheral ganglia. Short postganglionic fibers extend from the ganglia to the effector organs. The lateral-posterior hypothalamus is part of the supranuclear mechanism for the regulation of parasympathetic activities. The frontal and limbic parts of the supranuclear regulatory apparatus are not indicated in the diagram (see text). (From Noback CL, Demarest R: The Human Nervous System, 3rd ed., New York, McGraw-Hill, 1981, by permission.)

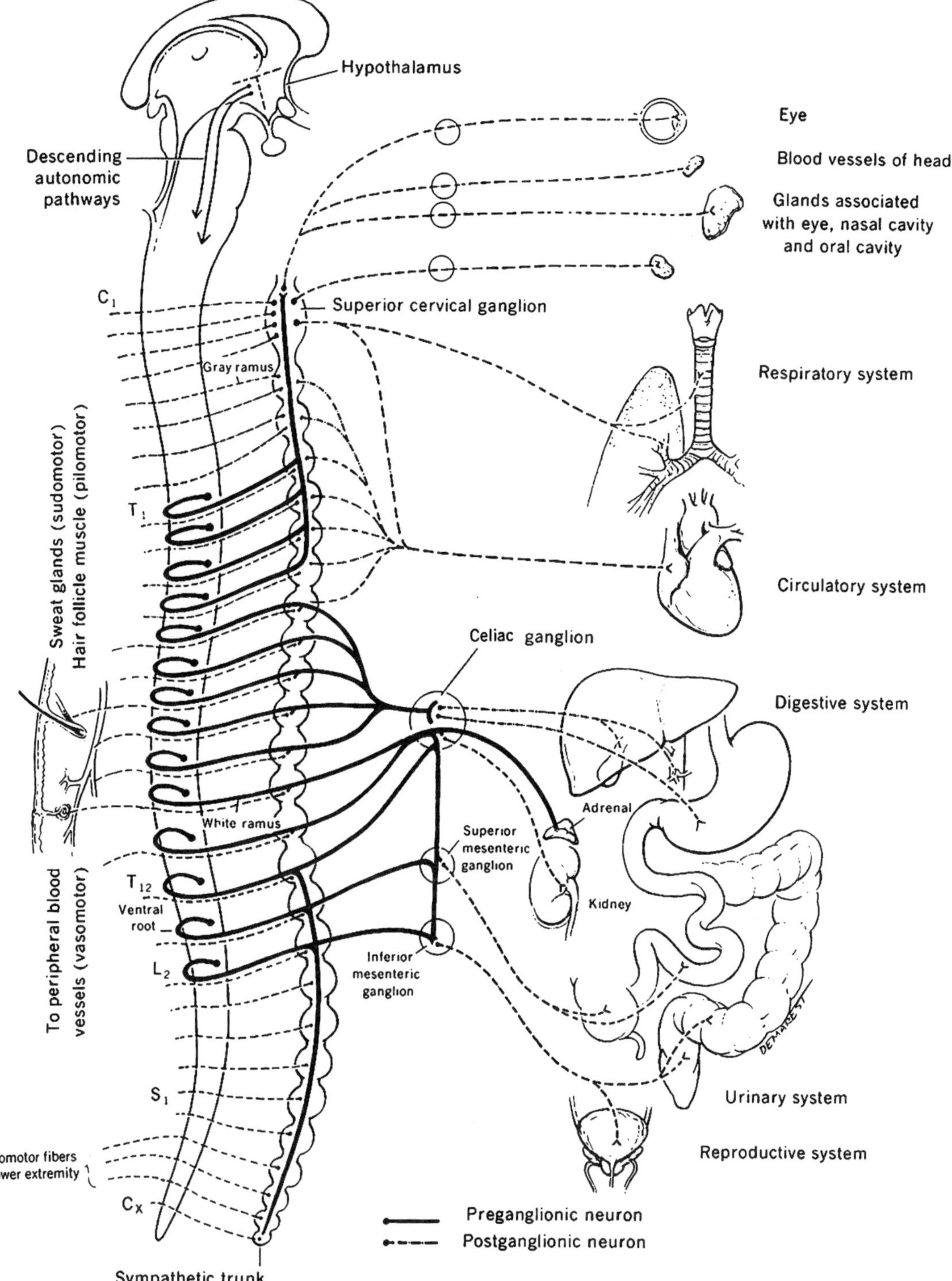

Figure 26-3

The sympathetic (thoracolumbar) division of the autonomic nervous system. Preganglionic fibers extend from the intermediolateral nucleus of the spinal cord to the peripheral autonomic ganglia, and postganglionic fibers extend from the peripheral ganglia to the effector organs, according to the scheme in Fig. 26-1. (From Noback CL, Demarest R: The Human Nervous System, 3rd ed. New York, McGraw-Hill, 1981, by permission.)

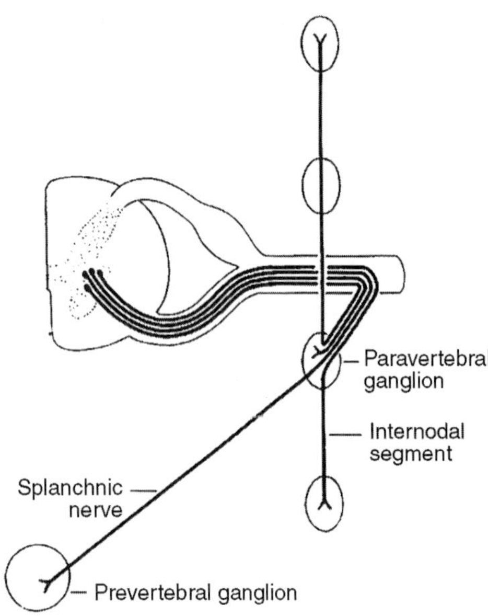

Figure 26-4

The principle of the preganglionic innervation of paravertebral ganglia that are placed beyond the limits of the preganglionic sympathetic outflow from the spinal cord. Preganglionic fibers (heavy lines) *emerging from a spinal segment do not synapse exclusively in the corresponding paravertebral ganglion. Some pass as splanchnic nerves to prevertebral ganglia; some fibers enter the sympathetic trunk, in which they pass up or down for a variable number of segments. (From Pick by permission.)*

from the cells of this ganglion innervate the lacrimal gland (see also Fig. 47-2). Other fibers of the facial nerve traverse the tympanic cavity as the chorda tympani and eventually join the submandibular ganglion; cells of this ganglion innervate the submandibular and sublingual glands. Axons of the inferior salivatory nerve cells enter the glossopharyngeal nerve and reach the otic ganglion through the tympanic plexus and lesser superficial petrosal nerve; cells of the otic ganglion send fibers to the parotid gland. Preganglionic fibers, derived from the dorsal motor nucleus of the vagus and adjacent visceral nuclei in the lateral reticular formation, enter the vagus nerve and terminate in ganglia situated in the walls of many thoracic and abdominal viscera; the ganglionic cells give rise to short postganglionic fibers that activate smooth muscle and glands of the pharynx, esophagus, and gastrointestinal tract (up to the descending colon) and of the heart, pancreas, liver, gallbladder, kidney, and ureter.

The *sacral part of the parasympathetic system* originates in the lateral horn cells of the second, third, and fourth sacral segments. Axons of these sacral neurons, constituting the preganglionic fibers, traverse the sacral nerves and synapse in ganglia that lie within the walls of the distal colon, bladder, and other pelvic organs. Thus, the sacral autonomic neurons, like the cranial ones, have long preganglionic and short postganglionic fibers, a feature that permits a circumscribed influence upon the target organ.

Probably the neurons that activate striated muscle differ from those that innervate glands and smooth muscle. In the sacral segments, for example, the neurons that activate the external sphincters (voluntary muscle) differ from others that supply the smooth muscle of bladder and rectocolon. In 1900, Onufrowicz (calling himself Onuf) described a discrete, compact group of relatively small cells in the anterior horns of sacral segments 2 to 4. These neurons were originally thought to be autonomic in function, mainly because of their histologic features. There is now more compelling evidence that they are somatomotor, innervating the skeletal muscle of the external urethral and anal sphincters (Holstege and Tan). Neurons in the intermediolateral cell column of sacral cord segments innervate the detrusor of the bladder wall. In passing, it is worth noting that in motor system disease, in which bladder and bowel functions are usually preserved until late in the disease, the neurons in Onuf's nucleus (in contrast to other somatomotor neurons in the sacral cord) tend not to be involved in the degenerative process (Mannen et al).

The Sympathetic Nervous System (Fig. 26-3) The *preganglionic neurons of the sympathetic division originate* in the intermediolateral cell column of the spinal gray matter, from the eighth cervical to the second lumbar segments. Low and Dyck have estimated that each segment of the cord contains about 5000 lateral horn cells and that in late adult life there is an attrition of 5 to 7 percent per decade. Axons of the nerve fibers originating in the intermediolateral column are of small caliber and are myelinated; when grouped, they form the *white communicating rami*. These preganglionic fibers synapse with the cell bodies of the postganglionic neurons, which are collected into two large ganglionated chains or cords, one on each side of the vertebral column (paravertebral ganglia), and several single prevertebral ganglia.

Axons of the sympathetic ganglion cells are also of small caliber but are unmyelinated. Most of the postganglionic fibers pass via *gray communicating rami* to spinal nerves of T5 to L2; they supply blood vessels, sweat glands, and hair follicles and also form plexuses that supply the heart, bronchi, kidneys, intestines, pancreas, bladder, and sex organs. The postganglionic fibers of the prevertebral ganglia form the hypogastric, splanchnic, and mesenteric plexuses, which innervate the glands, smooth muscle, and blood vessels of the abdominal and pelvic viscera (Figs. 26-1 and 26-4).

The sympathetic innervation of the adrenal medulla is unique in that its secretory cells receive preganglionic fibers directly, via the splanchnic nerves. This is an exception to the rule that organs innervated by the autonomic nervous system receive only postganglionic fibers. This special arrangement can be explained by the fact that cells of the adrenal medulla are the morphologic homologues of the postganglionic sympathetic neurons and secrete epinephrine and norepinephrine (the postganglionic transmitters) directly into the bloodstream. In this way, the sympathetic nervous system and the adrenal medulla act in unison to produce diffuse effects—as one would expect from their role in emergency reactions. By contrast, the parasympathetic effects, as in the pupil and urinary bladder, are more discrete (see above).

There are three cervical (superior, middle, and inferior, or stellate), eleven thoracic, and four to six lumbar sympathetic ganglia. The head receives its sympathetic innervation from the eighth cervical and first two thoracic cord segments, the fibers of which pass through the inferior to the middle and superior cervical ganglia. Postganglionic fibers from cells of the superior cervical ganglion follow the internal and external carotid arteries and innervate the blood vessels and smooth muscle as well as the sweat, lacrimal, and salivary glands of the head. Included among these postganglionic fibers, issuing mainly from T1, are the pupillodilator fibers and those innervating Müller's muscle of the upper eyelid. The arm receives its postganglionic innervation from the inferior cervical ganglion and uppermost thoracic ganglia (the two are fused to form the stellate ganglion). The cardiac plexus and other thoracic sympathetic nerves are derived from the upper thoracic ganglion and the abdominal visceral plexuses, from the fifth to the ninth or tenth thoracic ganglia. The lowermost thoracic ganglia have no abdominal visceral connections; the upper lumbar ganglia supply the descending colon, pelvic organs, and legs.

The terminals of autonomic nerves and their junctions with smooth muscle and glands have been more difficult to visualize and study than the motor end plates of striated muscle. As the postganglionic axons enter an organ, usually via the vasculature, they ramify into many smaller branches and disperse, without a Schwann cell covering, to innervate the smooth muscle fibers, the glands, and, in largest number, the small arteries, arterioles, and precapillary sphincters (Burnstock). Some of these terminals penetrate the smooth muscle of the arterioles; others remain in the adventitia. At the ends of the postganglionic fibers and in part along their course there are swellings that lie in close proximity to the sarcolemma or gland cell membrane; often the muscle fiber is grooved to accommodate these swellings. The axonal swellings contain synaptic vesicles, some clear and others with a dense granular core. The clear vesicles contain acetylcholine, and those with a dense core contain catecholamines, particularly norepinephrine (Falck). This is well illustrated in the iris, where nerves to the dilator muscle (sympathetic) contain dense-core vesicles and those to the constrictor (parasympathetic), clear vesicles. A single nerve fiber innervates multiple smooth muscle and gland cells.

Visceral Afferents Somewhat arbitrarily, anatomists have declared the autonomic nervous system to be purely efferent motor and secretory in function. However, most autonomic nerves are mixed, also containing afferent fibers that convey sensory impulses from the viscera and blood vessels. The cell bodies of these sensory neurons lie in the posterior root ganglia; some central axons of the ganglionic cells synapse with lateral horn cells of the spinal cord and subserve visceral reflexes; others synapse in the dorsal horn and convey or modulate impulses for conscious sensation. Secondary afferents carry sensory impulses to certain brainstem nuclei, particularly the nucleus tractus solitarius, as described below, and the thalamus via the lateral spinothalamic and polysynaptic pathways.

The Central Regulation of Visceral Function Integration of autonomic function takes place at two levels, the brainstem and the cerebrum. In the brainstem, the main visceral afferent nucleus in the brainstem is the nucleus tractus solitarius (NTS). Cardiovascular, respiratory, and gastrointestinal afferents, carried in cranial nerves X and IX via the nodose and petrose ganglia, terminate on specific subnuclei of the NTS. The caudal subnuclei are the primary receiving site for viscerosensory fibers; other less well defined areas receive baroreceptor and chemoreceptor information. The caudal NTS is thought to integrate these signals and to project to a number of critical areas in the hypothalamus, amygdala, and insular cortex, involved primarily in cardiovascular control, as well as to the pontine and medullary nuclei controlling respiratory rhythms. The NTS therefore serves a critical integratory function for both circulation and respiration, as described further on.

An important advance in our understanding of the autonomic nervous system occurred with the discovery of autonomic regulating mechanisms in the hypothalamus. Small, insignificant-appearing nuclei in the walls of the third ventricle and in buried parts of the limbic cortex, formerly judged to have purely olfactory functions, are now known to have rich bidirectional connections. In fact, the hypothalamus serves as the integrating mechanism of the autonomic nervous system and limbic system, as indicated in Chap. 25. The regulatory activity of the hypothalamus is accomplished in two ways—through direct pathways that descend to particular groups of cells in the brainstem and spinal cord and through the pituitary and thence to other endocrine glands. The supranuclear regulatory apparatus of the autonomic nervous system includes three main cerebral structures: the frontal lobe cortex, the insular cortex, and the amygdaloid and adjacent nuclei.

The ventromedial prefrontal and cingulate cortices function as the highest levels of autonomic integration. Stimulation of one frontal lobe may evoke changes in temperature and sweating in the contralateral arm and leg; massive lesions here, which usually cause a hemiplegia, may modify the autonomic functions in the direction of either inhibition or facilitation. Lesions involving the posterior part of the superior frontal and anterior part of the cingulate gyri (usually bilateral, occasionally unilateral) result in loss of voluntary control of the bladder and bowel (see page 473). Most likely a large contingent of these fibers terminates in the hypothalamus, which, in turn, sends fibers to the brainstem and spinal cord. The descending spinal pathways are believed to lie ventromedial to the corticospinal fibers.

The insular cortex receives projections from the NTS, the parabrachial nucleus of the pons, and the lateral hypothalamic nuclei. Direct stimulation of the insula produces cardiac arrhythmias and a number of other alterations in visceral function.

The cingulate and hippocampal gyri and their associated subcortical structures (substantia innominata and the amygdaloid, septal, piriform, habenular, and midbrain tegmental nuclei) have been identified as important cerebral autonomic regulatory centers. Together they have been called the *visceral brain* (see Chap. 25). Of particular importance in autonomic regulation is the amygdala, the central nucleus of which is a major site of origin of projections to the hypothalamus and brainstem. The anatomy and the effects of stimulation and ablation of the amygdala have been discussed in Chap. 25, on the neurology of emotion.

In addition to the aforementioned central relationships, it should be noted that important interactions between the autonomic nervous system and the endocrine glands occur at a peripheral level. The best-known example is in the adrenal medulla, as already indicated. A similar relationship pertains to the pineal gland; norepinephrine (NE) released from postganglionic fibers that end on pineal cells stimulates several enzymes involved in the biosynthesis of melatonin. Similarly, the juxtaglomerular apparatus of the kidney and the islets of Langerhans of the pancreas may function as neuroendocrine transducers insofar as they convert a neural stimulus (in these cases adrenergic) to an endocrine secretion (renin and glucagon and insulin, respectively). The autonomic–endocrine interactions are elaborated in the next chapter.

Finally, there is the central role of the hypothalamus in the initiation and regulation of autonomic activity, both sympathetic and parasympathetic. Sympathetic responses are most readily obtained by stimulation of the posterior and lateral regions of the hypothalamus, and parasympathetic responses, from the anterior regions. The descending sympathetic fibers are largely or totally uncrossed, although their pathway or pathways have not been sharply defined. According to Carmel, fibers from the caudal hypothalamus at first run in the prerubral field, dorsal and slightly rostral to the red nucleus, and then ventral to the ventrolateral thalamic nuclei; then they descend in the lateral tegmentum of the midbrain, pons, and medulla to the intermediolateral cell column of the spinal cord. Luhan and Pollack demonstrated that a small infarct in the territory of supply of the superior cerebellar artery, involving an area just posterior to the medial lemniscus and extending laterally to the periphery of the rostral pons, causes an ipsilateral ptosis, miosis, and anhidrosis (Horner syndrome). In the medulla, the descending sympathetic pathway is located in the posterolateral retro-olivary area, where it is frequently involved in lateral medullary infarctions; in the cervical cord, the fibers run in the posterior angle of the anterior horn (Nathan and Smith). According to the latter authors, some of the fibers supplying sudomotor neurons run outside this area but also remain ipsilateral. Jansen and colleagues, by the use of viral vectors in rodents, were able to label certain neurons of the hypothalamus and the ventral medulla that stimulated sympathetic activity in both the stellate ganglion and the adrenal gland. They hypothesized that this dual control underlies the fight-or-flight response, as described in Chapter 25.

By contrast, the pathways of descending parasympathetic fibers are not known.

Afferent projections from the spinal cord to the hypothalamus have been demonstrated in animals and provide a potential route by which sensation from somatic and possibly visceral structures may influence autonomic responses.

Physiologic and Pharmacologic Considerations

The function of the autonomic nervous system, in its regulation of the activities of organs, mainly visceral ones, is to a high degree independent. When the autonomic nerves are interrupted, these organs continue to function (the organism survives), but no longer are they as effective in maintaining homeostasis and adapting to the demands of changing internal conditions and external stresses.

It was learned long ago that most viscera have a double nerve supply, sympathetic and parasympathetic, and that in general these two parts of the autonomic nervous system exert opposite effects. For example, the effects of the sympathetic nervous system on the heart are excitatory and those of the parasympathetic, inhibitory. However, some structures—sweat glands, somatic blood vessels, and hair follicles—receive only sympathetic postganglionic fibers, and the adrenal gland, as indicated above, has only a preganglionic sympathetic innervation. Also, some parasympathetic neurons have been identified in sympathetic ganglia.

Neurohumoral Transmission All autonomic functions are mediated through the release of chemical transmitters. The modern concept of neurohumoral transmission had its beginnings in the early decades of the twentieth century. In 1921, Loewi discovered that stimulation of the vagus nerve released a chemical substance ("*Vagustoff*") that slowed the heart. Later this substance was shown by Dale to be acetylcholine (ACh). Also in 1921, Cannon reported that stimulation of the sympathetic trunk released an epinephrine-like substance, which increased the heart rate and blood pressure. He named this substance "sympathin," subsequently shown to be noradrenaline, or norepinephrine (NE). Dale found that ACh had pharmacologic effects similar to those obtained by stimulation of parasympathetic nerves; he designated these effects as "parasympathomimetic." These observations placed neurochemical transmission on solid ground and laid the basis for the distinction between cholinergic and adrenergic transmission in the autonomic nervous system.

The most important of the neurotransmitters are ACh and NE. ACh is synthesized at the terminals of axons and stored in presynaptic vesicles until it is released by the arrival of nerve impulses. ACh is released at the terminals of all preganglionic fibers (in both the sympathetic and parasympathetic ganglia) as well as at the terminals of all postganglionic parasympathetic and a few postganglionic sympathetic fibers. (Of course, ACh is also the chemical transmitter of nerve impulses to the skeletal muscle fibers.) The arrival of nerve impulses releases ACh, which traverses the synaptic cleft and attaches to receptor sites on the next neuron, smooth or striated muscle cell, or glandular cell. There are two distinct types of ACh receptors—*nicotinic* and *muscarinic*, so named by Dale because the choline-induced responses were similar either to those of nicotine or to those of the alkaloid muscarine. The postganglionic parasympathetic receptors are muscarinic, i.e., they are antagonized by atropinic drugs. The receptors in ganglia, like those of skeletal muscle, are not blocked by atropine (i.e., the nicotinic effect) but are blocked by other agents (e.g., tubocurarine).

It is likely that more than ACh is involved in nerve transmission at a ganglionic level. Many peptides—substance P, enkephalins, somatostatin, vasoactive intestinal peptide, adenosine triphosphate (ATP), and most recently nitric oxide—have been identified in the autonomic ganglia, localizing in some cases to the same cell as ACh. Particular neuronal firing rates appear to cause the preferential release of one or another of these substances. Most of the neuropeptides exert their postsynaptic effects through the G-protein transduction system which utilizes adenylcyclase or phospholipase C as intermediaries. The neuropeptides probably act as modulators at transmitter sites, although their exact function in many cases remains to be determined.

As a general rule, postganglionic sympathetic fibers release NE at their terminals, but there are exceptions. The sweat glands and some blood vessels in muscle are innervated by postganglionic sympathetic fibers, but their terminals release ACh. The NE that is discharged into the synaptic space activates specific *adrenergic receptors* on the postsynaptic membrane of target cells.

Adrenergic receptors are of two types, classified originally by Ahlquist as alpha and beta. In general, the alpha receptors mediate vasoconstriction, relaxation of the gut, and dilatation of the pupil; beta receptors mediate vasodilatation, especially in muscles, relaxation of the bronchi, and an increased rate and contractility of the heart. Each of these receptors is subdivided further into two types. $Alpha_1$ receptors are postsynaptic; $alpha_2$ receptors are presynaptic and, when stimulated, diminish the release of the transmitter. $Beta_1$ receptors are, for all practical purposes, limited to the heart; their activation increases the heart rate and contractility. $Beta_2$ receptors, when stimulated, relax the smooth muscle of the bronchi and of most other sites. A comprehensive account of neurohumoral transmission and receptor function can be found in the review by Hoffman and colleagues and in the monograph by Cooper, Bloom, and Roth.

Discussed in the following pages are the ways in which the two divisions of the autonomic nervous system, acting in conjunction with the endocrine glands, maintain the homeostasis of the organism. As stated above, the integration of these two systems is achieved primarily in the hypothalamus. In addition, the endocrine glands are influenced by circulating catecholamines, and some of them are innervated by adrenergic fibers, which terminate not only on blood vessels but also, in some cases, directly on secretory cells. These autonomic-endocrine relations are elaborated in Chap. 27.

Regulation of Blood Pressure

As was indicated briefly in Chap.18, blood pressure depends on the adequacy of intravascular blood volume, on systemic vascular resistance, and on the cardiac output. Both the autonomic and endocrine systems influence the muscular, cutaneous, and mesenteric (splanchnic) vascular beds, pulse rate, and stroke volume of the heart. Together, these serve to maintain normal blood pressure and allow reflex maintenance of blood pressure with changes in body position. Two types of baroreceptors function as the afferent component of this reflex arc by sensing pressure gradients across the walls of large blood vessels. Those in the carotid sinus and aortic arch are sensitive to reductions in pulse pressure (the difference between systolic and diastolic blood pressure), while those in the right heart chambers and pulmonary vessels respond more to alterations in blood volume. The carotid sinus baroreceptors are rapidly responsive and capable of detecting beat-to-beat changes, in contrast to the aortic arch nerves, which have a longer response time and discriminate only the larger and more prolonged alterations in pressure.

The nerves arising from these receptors are small-caliber, thinly myelinated fibers that course in cranial nerves IX and X and terminate in the NTS, as noted earlier. In response to increased stimulation of these receptors, vagal efferent activity is reduced, resulting in cardioacceleration. This is accomplished through polysynaptic connections between the NTS and the dorsal motor nucleus of the vagus, where vagal neurons that project to the sinoatrial node originate. Increased systemic vascular resistance occurs concomitantly in most circumstances through parallel connections between the NTS and medullary pressor areas that project to the intermedolateral cells of the mid-thoracic cord segments. The opposite response, bradycardia and hypotension, results when vagal tone is enhanced and sympathetic tone is reduced. The main sympathetic outflow from these segments is via the greater splanchnic nerve to the celiac ganglion, the postganglionic nerves of which project to the capacitance vessels of the gut. The splanchnic capacitance veins act as a reservoir for as much as 20 percent of the total blood volume, and interruption of the splanchnic nerves results in severe postural hypotension. After a high-carbohydrate meal, there is a marked hyperemia of the gut and compensatory peripheral vasoconstriction in the muscles and skin. It has also been noted that the mesenteric vascular bed is responsive to the orthostatic redistribution of blood volume but not to mental stress.

Two slower-acting humoral mechanisms regulate blood volume and complement the alterations in systemic vascular resistance. Pressure-sensitive renal juxtaglomerular cells release renin, which stimulates production of angiotensin and influences aldosterone production, both of which effect an increase of blood volume. Of lesser influence in the control of blood pressure is antidiuretic hormone, discussed in the next chapter, but the effects of this peptide become more important when autonomic failure forces a dependence on secondary mechanisms for the maintenance of blood pressure.

Emergency and Alarm Reactions Inasmuch as the autonomic nervous system and the adrenal glands were accepted for many years as the neural and humoral basis of all instinctive and emotional behavior, it is remarkable how little sound information has been acquired about their roles in disease. In states of chronic anxiety and acute panic reactions, depressive psychosis, mania, and schizophrenia, all of which are characterized by an altered emotionality, no consistent autonomic or endocrine dysfunction has been demonstrated except perhaps for diminished responses of growth hormone in panic disorders. This has been disappointing, since Cannon, with his emergency theory of sympathoadrenal action, had provided such a promising concept of the neurophysiology of acute emotion and Selye had extended this theory so plausibly to explain all the reactions to stress in animals and humans. According to these theories, strong emotion, such as anger or fear, excites the sympathetic nervous system and the adrenal glands [via corticotropin releasing factor (CRF) and adrenocorticotropic hormone (ACTH)], which are under direct neural as well as endocrine control. These sympathoadrenal reactions are brief and sustain the animal in "flight or fight" (pages 532 and 543). Prolonged stress and production of ACTH activates all the adrenal hormones, referred to collectively as *steroids* (glucocorticoids, mineralocorticoids, and adrenocorticoids).

Animals deprived of adrenal cortex or human beings with Addison disease cannot tolerate stress because they are incapable of mobilizing both the adrenal medulla and adrenal cortex. In animals, exercise, cold, oxygen lack, and surgical injury are all said to evoke the same sympathoadrenal reactions as anger or fear. Selye's extension of Cannon's theory, although attractive, has received little support. Critics have pointed out that the conditions to which his experimental animals had been subjected are so different from human disease that conclusions as to the unity of the two cannot be drawn. More critical studies of the anatomy and physiology of the hypothalamus, hypophysis, adrenal glands, and autonomic nervous system are still needed to fully test these hypotheses.

Tests for Abnormalities of the Autonomic Nervous System

With few exceptions, such as testing pupillary reactions and examination of the skin for abnormalities of color and sweating, the neurologist tends to be casual in evaluating the function of the autonomic nervous system. Nonetheless, several simple but informative tests can be used to confirm one's clinical impressions and to elicit abnormalities of autonomic function that may aid in diagnosis. A combination of tests is usually necessary, because certain ones are particularly sensitive to abnormalities of sympathetic function and others to parasympathetic or baroreceptor afferent function. These are described below and are summarized in Table 26-1. A scheme for the examination of pupillary abnormalities has been presented in Fig. 14-8.

Responses of Blood Pressure and Heart Rate to Changes in Posture and Breathing These are among the simplest and most important tests of autonomic function and are currently automated in most laboratories. McLeod and Tuck state that in changing from the recumbent to the standing position, a fall of more than 30 mmHg systolic and 15 mmHg diastolic is abnormal; others give figures of 20 and 10 mmHg. They caution that the arm on which the cuff is placed must be held horizontally when standing, so that the decline in arm pressure will not be obscured by the added hydrostatic pressure.

The main cause of an orthostatic drop in blood pressure is hypovolemia. In the context of recurrent fainting, however, an excessive drop reflects inadequate sympathetic vasoconstrictor activity. The use of a tilt table, as described in Chap. 18, is the most sensitive means of inducing orthostatic changes and also elicits these changes in patients prone to syncope from an oversensitive cardiac reflex, i.e., one that produces vasodilation (so-called neurocardiogenic syncope), as discussed in Chap. 18. In response to the induced drop in blood pressure, the pulse rate (under vagal control) normally increases. *The failure of the heart rate to rise in response to the slight drop in blood pressure with standing is the simplest bedside indicator of vagal nerve dysfunction.* In addition, the pulse, after rising initially, slows after about 15 beats to reach a stable rate by the 30th beat. The ratio of R–R intervals in the electrocardiogram (ECG), corresponding to the 30th and 15th beats (the 30:15 ratio), is an even more sensitive measure of the integrity of vagal inhibition of the sinus node. A ratio in young adults of less than 1.05 is usually abnormal.

Another simple procedure for quantitating vagal function consists of measuring the *variation in heart rate during deep breathing* (respiratory sinus arrhythmia). The ECG is recorded while the patient first breathes at a regular rate of 6 to 12 per minute. Normally, the heart rate varies by as many as 15 beats per minute or even more; differences of less than 10 beats per minute may be abnormal. A more reliable test of vagal function is the measurement of the ratio of the longest R–R interval during forceful slow expiration to the shortest R–R interval during inspiration, which allows the derivation of an expiration-inspiration (E:I) ratio. This is the best-validated of all the pulse-rate measurements, particularly since computerized methods can be used to display the spectrum of beat-to-beat ECG intervals during breathing. Always, the results of these tests must be compared with those obtained in normal individuals of the same age. Up to age 40, E:I ratios of less than 1.2 are abnormal. The ratio normally decreases with age, and markedly so beyond age 60 (at which time it approaches 1.04 or less), as it does also in the presence of even mild diabetic neuropathy. Thus the test results must be interpreted cautiously in the elderly. Computerized methods of *power spectral analysis* of heart rate are used to express

Table 26-1
Clinical tests of autonomic function

Test	*Normal response*	*Part of reflex arc tested*
	Noninvasive bedside tests	
Blood-pressure response to standing or vertical tilt	Fall in BP ≤ 30/15 mmHg	Afferent and sympathetic efferent limbs
Heart rate response to standing	Increase 11–90 beats/min; 30:15 ratio ≥1.04	Vagal afferent and efferent limbs
Isometric exercise	Increase in diastolic BP, 15 mmHg	Sympathetic efferent limb
Heart rate variation with respiration	Maximum-minimum heart rate ≥15 beats/min; E:I ratio 1.2[a]	Vagal afferent and efferent limbs
Valsalva ratio (see text)	≥1.4[a]	Afferent and efferent limbs
Sweat tests	Sweating over all body and limbs	Sympathetic efferent limb
Axon reflex	Local piloerection, sweating	Postganglionic sympathetic efferent fibers
Plasma noradrenaline level to vertical	Rises on tilting from horizontal to vertical	Sympathetic efferent limb
Plasma vasopressin level	Rise with induced hypotension	Afferent limb
	Invasive tests	
Valsalva maneuver (BP response with indwelling arterial catheter or continuous noninvasive BP measurement)	Phase I: Rise in BP Phase II: Gradual reduction of BP to plateau; tachycardia Phase III: Fall in BP Phase IV: Overshoot of BP, bradycardia[a]	Afferent and sympathetic efferent limbs
Baroreflex sensitivity	(1) Slowing of heart rate with induced rise of BP[a] (2) Steady-state responses to induced rise and fall of BP	(1) Parasympathetic afferent and efferent limbs (2) Afferent and efferent limbs
Infusion of pressor drugs	(1) Rise in BP (2) Slowing of heart rate	(1) Adrenergic receptors (2) Afferent and efferent parasympathetic limbs
	Other tests of vasomotor control	
Radiant heating of trunk	Increased hand blood flow	Sympathetic efferent limb
Immersion of hand in hot water	Increased blood flow of opposite hand	Sympathetic efferent limb
Cold pressor test	Reduced blood flow	Sympathetic efferent limb
Emotional stress	Increased BP	Sympathetic efferent limb
	Tests of pupillary innervation	
4% cocaine	Pupil dilates	Sympathetic innervation
0.1% adrenaline	No response	Postganglionic sympathetic innervation
1% hydroxyamphetamine hydrobromide	Pupil dilates	Postganglionic sympathetic innervation
2.5% methacholine 0.125% pilocarpine	No response	Parasympathetic innervation

[a]Age-dependent response. BP = blood pressure; E:I = expiration: inspiration. *Source*: McLeod and Tuck by permission.

the variance in heart rate as a function of the beat-to-beat interval. Several power peaks are appreciated: one related to the respiratory sinus arrhythmia and others that reflect baroreceptor and cardiac sympathetic activity. All of these tests of heart rate variation are usually combined with the Valsalva maneuver, as described below, and with the prolonged tilt table test, as described in Chap 18.

Tests of Vasomotor Reactions Measurement of the skin temperature is a useful index of vasomotor function. Vasomotor paralysis results in vasodilatation of skin vessels and a rise in skin temperature; vasoconstriction lowers the temperature. With a skin thermometer, one may compare affected and normal areas under standard conditions. The normal skin temperature is 31 to 33°C when the room temperature is 26 to 27°C. Vasoconstrictor tone may also be tested by measuring the skin temperature of the area in question before and after immersing one or both hands in cold water.

The integrity of the sympathetic reflex arc—which includes baroreceptors in the aorta and carotid sinus, their afferent pathways, the vasomotor centers, and the sympathetic and parasympathetic outflow—can be tested in a general way by combining the cold pressor test, grip test, mental arithmetic test, and Valsalva maneuver, as described below.

Vasoconstriction induces an elevation of the blood pressure. This is the basis of the *cold pressor test*. In normal persons, immersing one hand in ice water for 1 to 5 min raises the systolic pressure by 15 to 20 mmHg and the diastolic pressure by 10 to 15 mmHg. Similarly, the *sustained isometric contraction* of a group of muscles (e.g., those of the forearm in handgrip) for 5 min normally increases the heart rate and the systolic and diastolic pressures by 15 mmHg or more. The response in both of these tests is reduced or absent with lesions of the sympathetic reflex arc, particularly of the efferent limb, but neither of these tests has been well validated. The stress involved in doing *mental arithmetic* in noisy and distracting surroundings will normally stimulate a mild but measurable increase in pulse rate and blood pressure. Obviously, this response does not depend upon the afferent limb of the sympathetic reflex arc and must be mediated by cortical-hypothalamic mechanisms.

In the *Valsalva maneuver*, the subject exhales into a manometer or against a closed glottis for 10 to 15 s, creating a markedly positive intrathoracic pressure. Normally, this causes a sharp reduction in venous return and cardiac output, so that the blood pressure falls; the effect on the baroreceptors is to cause a reflex tachycardia and, to a lesser extent, peripheral vasoconstriction. With release of intrathoracic pressure, the venous return, stroke volume, and blood pressure rise to higher than normal levels; parasympathetic influence then predominates and results in bradycardia.

Failure of the heart rate to increase during the positive intrathoracic pressure phase of the Valsalva maneuver points to sympathetic dysfunction, and failure of the rate to slow during the period of blood pressure overshoot points to a parasympathetic disturbance. If the response to the Valsalva maneuver is abnormal and the response to the cold pressor test is normal, the lesion is probably in the baroreceptors or their afferent nerves; such a defect has been found in diabetic and tabetic patients and is common in many neuropathies. A failure of the pulse rate and blood pressure to rise during mental arithmetic, coupled with an abnormal Valsalva maneuver, suggests a defect in the central or peripheral efferent sympathetic pathways. In patients with autonomic failure, the fall in blood pressure is not aborted during the last few seconds of increased intrathoracic pressure, and there is no overshoot of blood pressure when the breath is released.

Tests of Sudomotor Function The integrity of sympathetic efferent pathways can be assessed further by tests of sudomotor activity. There are several of these, all somewhat cumbersome and used mainly in autonomic testing laboratories; furthermore, most of them cannot differentiate central from peripheral causes of anhidrosis. Sweat can be weighed after it is absorbed by small squares of filter paper. Powdered charcoal dusted on the skin will cling to moist areas and not to dry ones.

In the *sympathetic or galvanic skin-resistance* test, a set of electrodes placed on the skin measures the resistance to the passage of a weak current through the skin; in all likelihood, the electrical potential is the result of a change in the ionic current within the sweat glands, not simply an increase in sweating that lowers skin resistance. This method can be used to outline an area of reduced sweating due to a peripheral nerve lesion, since the response depends on sympathetic activation of sweat glands (Gutrecht). The starch-iodine test or use of a color indicator such as quinizarin (gray when dry, purple when wet) and the more recently introduced plastic or silicone method are other acceptable procedures.

A more quantitative and reproducible examination of postganglionic sudomotor function, QSART, has been developed by Low. It is essentially a test of distal sympathetic axonal integrity, utilizing the local axon reflex. A 10% solution of acetylcholine is iontophoresed onto the skin using 2 mA for 5 min. Sweat output is recorded in the adjacent skin by sophisticated circular cells that detect the sweat water. The forearm, proximal leg, distal leg, and foot have been chosen as standardized recording sites. By this test, Low has been able to define patterns of absent or delayed sweating that signify postganglionic sympathetic failure in small-fiber neuropathies and excessive sweating or reduced latency in response, as is seen in reflex sympathetic dystrophy. This is by far the preferred method of studying sweating and the function of distal sympathetic fibers, but its technical complexity makes it available only in specially equipped laboratories.

Lacrimal Function *Tearing* can be estimated roughly by inserting one end of a 5-mm-wide and 25-mm-long strip of thin filter paper into the lower conjunctival sac while the other end hangs over the edge of the lower lid (the Schirmer test). The tears wet the strip of filter paper, producing a moisture front. After 5 min, the moistened area extends for a length of approximately 15 mm in normal persons. An extent of less than 10 mm is suggestive of hypolacrimia. Mainly this test is used to detect the dry eyes (keratoconjunctivitis sicca) of the Sjögren syndrome.

Tests of Bladder, Gastrointestinal, and Penile Erectile Function *Bladder function* is best assessed by the cystometrogram, which measures intravesicular pressure as a function of the volume of saline solution permitted to flow by gravity into the bladder. The rise of pressure as 500 mL of fluid is allowed to flow gradually into the bladder, the emptying contractions of the detrusor, and the volume at which the patient reports a sensation of bladder fullness can be recorded by a manometer. (A detailed account of cystometric techniques can be found in the monograph of Krane and Siroky.) A quick and simple way of determining bladder atony (prostatic obstruction and overdistention having been excluded) is to measure the residual urine (by catheterization of the bladder) immediately after voluntary voiding, or to estimate its volume by intravenous myelography or ultrasound imaging.

Disorders of gastrointestinal motility are readily demonstrated radiologically. In dysautonomic states, a barium swallow may disclose a number of abnormalities, including atonic dilatation of the esophagus, gastric atony and distention, delayed gastric emptying time, and a characteristic small bowel pattern consisting of an increase in frequency and amplitude of peristaltic waves and rapid intestinal transit. A barium enema may demonstrate colonic distention and a decrease in propulsive activity. Sophisticated manometric techniques are now available for the measurement of gastrointestinal motility (see Low et al).

Nocturnal penile tumescence is recorded in many sleep laboratories and may be used as an ancillary test of sacral autonomic (parasympathetic) innervation.

Pharmacologic Tests of Autonomic Function The topical application of pharmacologic agents is particularly useful in evaluating *pupillary denervation*. Part of the rationale behind these special tests is "Cannon's law," or the phenomenon of denervation hypersensitivity, in which an effector organ, 2 to 3 weeks after denervation, becomes hypersensitive to its particular neurotransmitter substance and related drugs.

The instillation of a 1:1000 solution of epinephrine into the conjunctival sac has no effect on the normal pupil but will cause the sympathetically denervated pupil to dilate (3 drops instilled three times at 1-min intervals). The pupillary size is checked after 15, 30, and 45 min. As a rule, hypersensitivity to epinephrine is greater with lesions of postganglionic fibers than of preganglionic fibers. If denervation is incomplete, the hypersensitivity phenomenon may not be demonstrable. Also, in lesions that involve central sympathetic pathways, the pupil rarely reacts to this test.

More reliable as a test of sympathetic denervation is the topical application into the conjunctival sac of a 4 to 10% cocaine solution that potentiates the effects of NE by preventing its uptake. The test should be carried out as described above. A normal response to cocaine consists of pupillary dilatation. In sympathetic denervation caused by lesions of the post- or preganglionic fibers, no change in pupillary size occurs, since no transmitter substance is available. In cases of central sympathetic lesions, slight mydriasis occurs.

These and other pharmacologic methods of evaluating pupillary disturbances are considered more fully in Chap. 14 and are outlined in Fig. 14-8.

Cutaneous Flare Response The intracutaneous injection of 0.05 mL of 1:1000 histamine phosphate normally causes a 1-cm wheal after 5 to 10 min. This is surrounded by a narrow red areola, and it, in turn, by an erythematous flare that extends 1 to 3 cm beyond the border of the wheal. A similar triple response follows the release of histamine into the skin as the result of a scratch. The wheal and the deeply colored red areola are caused by the direct action of histamine on blood vessels, while the flare depends upon the integrity of the axon reflex mediated along sensory fibers by antidromic transmission. In familial dysautonomia, the flare response to histamine and to scratch is absent. It may also be absent in peripheral neuropathies that involve sympathetic nerves (e.g., diabetes, alcoholic-nutritional disease, Guillain-Barré disease, amyloidosis, porphyria, etc.). The quantitative sudomotor response to topical acetylcholine, described above, is preferred for its sensitivity and accuracy but requires special equipment.

Pressor Infusion and Other Direct Cardiovascular Tests The infusion of NE causes a rise in blood pressure, which is usually more pronounced for a given infusion rate in dysautonomic states than with normal subjects. In many instances, e.g., the Guillain-Barré syndrome, the excessive rise in blood pressure is thought to be more a result of inadequate muting of the hypertension by baroreceptors than it is a reflection of true denervation hypersensitivity, i.e., it reflects dysfunction of the afferent limb of the reflex arc. In patients with familial dysautonomia, the infusion of NE also produces erythematous blotching of the skin, like that which may occur under emotional stress, probably representing an exaggerated response to endogenous NE.

The infusion of angiotensin II into patients with idiopathic orthostatic hypotension also causes an exaggerated blood pressure response. A similar response to methacholine and NE has been interpreted as a denervation hypersensitivity to neurotransmitter or related substances. A different mechanism must be invoked for the blood pressure response induced by angiotensin; perhaps it is due to defective baroreceptor function.

The integrity of autonomic innervation of the heart can be evaluated by the intramuscular injection of atropine, ephedrine, and neostigmine while the heart rate is monitored. Normally, the intramuscular injection of 0.8 mg of atropine causes a parasympathetic block and a withdrawal of vagal tone. No such change occurs in cases of parasympathetic denervation of the heart, the most common such conditions being diabetes and the Guillain-Barré syndrome and the most dramatic being the brain death state, in which there is no longer any tonic vagal activity to be ablated by atropine.

Microchemical methods are available for the measurement of norepinephrine (NE) and dopamine β-hydroxylase in the serum. Normally, when a person changes from a recumbent to a standing position. The serum NE levels rise two-or threefold. In patients with central and peripheral autonomic failure, there is little or no elevation upon standing or with exercise. The dopamine β-hydroxylase enzyme is deficient in patients with a rare form of sympathetic dysautonomia.

In summary, the noninvasive tests listed in Table 26-1 and described above are quite adequate for the clinical testing of autonomic function. Low has emphasized that the most informative tests are those that are quantitative and have been standardized and validated in patients with both mild and severe autonomic disturbances. At the bedside, the most convenient ones are measurement of orthostatic pulse and blood pressure changes, blood pressure response to the Valsalva maneuver, estimation of pulse changes with deep breathing, pupillary responses to light and dark, and a rough estimate of sweating of the palms and soles. The results of these tests and the clinical situation will determine whether further testing is needed.

CLINICAL DISORDERS OF THE AUTONOMIC NERVOUS SYSTEM

Acute Autonomic Paralysis (Dysautonomic Polyneuropathy; Pure Pandysautonomia)

Since this condition was first reported by Young and colleagues in 1975, many more cases in both adults and children have been placed on record. Over a period of a week or a few weeks, the patient develops some combination of anhidrosis, orthostatic hypotension, paralysis of pupillary reflexes, loss of lacrimation and salivation, impotence, impaired bladder and bowel function (urinary retention, postprandial bloating, and ileus or constipation), and loss of certain pilomotor and vasomotor responses in the skin (flushing and heat intolerance). Severe fatigue is a prominent complaint in most patients, and abdominal pain and vomiting in others. A few have developed sleep apnea or the syndrome of excessive antidiuretic hormone secretion (leading to hyponatremia). The cerebrospinal fluid (CSF) protein is normal or slightly increased. Clinical and laboratory findings indicate that both the sympathetic and parasympathetic parts of the autonomic nervous system are affected, mainly at the postganglionic level. Somatic sensory and motor nerve fibers appear to be spared or are affected to only a slight extent, although many patients complain of paresthesias and tendon reflexes are frequently lost. In one of the patients described by Low and colleagues, there was physiologic and morphologic (sural biopsy) evidence of loss of small myelinated and unmyelinated somatic fibers and foci of epineurial mononuclear cells; in other cases, sural nerve fiber counts have been normal; and in an autopsied case, in which there had also been sensory loss, there was lymphocytic infiltration in sensory and autonomic nerves (Fagius et al). The original patient described by Young and colleagues and most of the other patients with pure dysautonomia are said to have recovered completely or almost so within several months, but some of our patients have been left with disordered gastrointestinal and sexual functions. In addition to this idiopathic form of autonomic paralysis, some cases are postinfectious, and there is a similar but rare paraneoplastic form. Antibodies against ganglionic acetylcholine receptors have been found in half of idiopathic cases and one-quarter of paraneoplastic cases (Vernino et al).

Some of the children with this disease and a few adults have had a predominantly cholinergic dysautonomia with pain and dysesthesias (Kirby et al). There is little or no postural hypotension in this form of the disease, and the course has been more chronic than that of complete dysautonomia. In view of the occurrence of identical autonomic disturbances in some cases of the Guillain-Barré syndrome and the high incidence of minor degrees of weakness, reflex loss, CSF protein elevation, and especially paresthesias in dysautonomic polyneuropathy, it is likely that the latter disorder is also an immune polyneuropathy affecting the autonomic fibers within peripheral nerves. The autopsy findings reported by Fagius and coworkers support such a relationship. In animals, autonomic paralysis has been produced by injection of extracts of sympathetic ganglia and Freund's adjuvant (Appenzeller et al) similar to the experimental immune neuritis that is used as an animal model of the Guillain-Barré syndrome.

An acquired form of orthostatic intolerance, referred to as *sympathotonic orthostatic hypotension* (Polinsky et al), may represent another variant or partial form of autonomic paralysis. In this syndrome, unlike the common forms of orthostatic hypotension (see below), the fall in blood pressure is accompanied by tachycardia. Hoeldtke and colleagues, who described four such patients, found that the vasomotor reflexes and NE production were normal; these investigators were inclined to attribute the disorder to an affection of lower thoracic and lumbar sympathetic neurons. Its relationship to the similarly indistinct entity of *primary orthostatic tachycardia syndrome* and to the orthostatic intolerance associated with the chronic fatigue syndrome is uncertain, but asthenia is a feature common to all of them. Indeed, similar syndromes in the past have been called neurocirculatory asthenia ("soldiers heart," Da Costa syndrome; see Chap. 24). We are inclined to view those so-called orthostatic intolerance syndromes as part of the asthenia-anxiety disorders. The autonomic changes may represent sympathetic overactivity in susceptible individuals.

Lambert-Eaton Myasthenic Syndrome One of the characteristic features of the fully developed Lambert-Eaton myasthenic syndrome, which is discussed more fully on page 1547, is a *dysautonomia*, characterized by dryness of the mouth, impotence, difficulty in starting the urinary stream, and constipation. Presumably, circulating antibodies interfere with ACh release at both muscarinic and nicotinic sites.

Primary Autonomic Failure (Idiopathic Orthostatic Hypotension, PAF, IOH)

This clinical state is now known to be caused by at least two conditions. One is a degenerative disease of middle and late adult life, first described by Bradbury and Eggleston in 1925 and designated by them as "idiopathic orthostatic hypotension." This term is not entirely apt, since it emphasizes only one feature of the autonomic failure and neglects the disturbances of sweating and of bladder and sexual functions, which are usually associated. In this disorder, the lesions are said to involve mainly the postganglionic sympathetic neurons (Petito and Black); the parasympathetic system is relatively spared and the central nervous system is uninvolved. In the second disorder, described by Shy and Drager, the preganglionic lateral horn neurons of the thoracic spinal segments degenerate; these changes are responsible for the orthostatic hypotension. Later, signs of cerebellar or basal ganglionic disease or both are added, in which case the disorder is called *multiple system atrophy* (page 1137). In the central type of orthostatic hypotension, as in the peripheral type, anhidrosis, impotence, and atonicity of the bladder may be conjoined, but orthostatic fainting is the main problem in both types.

The clinical differentiation of these two types of orthostatic hypotension depends largely on the appearance, with time, of associated central nervous system (CNS) signs. The distinction between the postganglionic and the central preganglionic types of disease is also based on pharmacologic and neurophysiologic evidence, but it must be emphasized that the criteria stated here do not always conform to clinical experience. In the postganglionic type, plasma levels of NE are subnormal while the patient is recumbent because of failure of the damaged nerve terminals to synthesize or release catecholamines. When the patient stands up, the NE levels do not rise, as they do in a normal person. Also, in this type, there is denervation hypersensitivity to infused norepinephrine. In the central preganglionic type, the resting NE levels in the plasma are normal, but again, on standing, there is no rise. However, the response to exogenously administered NE is normal. Cohen and associates, who studied the postganglionic sudomotor and vasomotor functions of 62 patients with idiopathic orthostatic hypotension, found that the signs of postganglionic denervation were uncommon in patients with the central type, a finding that assists in distinguishing the two types. In both, the plasma levels of dopamine β-hydroxylase, the enzyme that converts dopamine to NE, are subnormal (Ziegler et al). The use of these neurochemical tests in clinical practice is difficult and the data in the literature are inconsistent. Low's monograph should be consulted for the procedural details.

Pathologic studies have disclosed the central type of autonomic failure to be somewhat heterogeneous. Oppenheimer, who collected all the reported central cases with complete autopsies, found that they fell into two groups—one in which autonomic failure was associated with a parkinsonian syndrome and often with the presence of cytoplasmic inclusions in sympathetic neurons, the other with involvement of the striatum, cerebellum, pons, and medulla but without inclusions (there are now believed to be glial and neuronal cytoplasmic inclusions in all these cases). Both conditions are now loosely referred to as *multiple system atrophy*, as discussed in Chap. 39. In both groups, the autonomic failure appears to be related to degeneration of lateral horn cells. There is also a degeneration of nerve cells in the vagal nuclei as well as nuclei of the tractus solitarius, locus ceruleus, and sacral autonomic nuclei, accounting for laryngeal abductor weakness (laryngeal paralysis and stridor are features in some cases), incontinence, and impotence. Norepinephrine and dopamine are depleted in the hypothalamus (Spokes et al). The sympathetic ganglia have been normal, an exception being the case of Rajput and Rozdilsky, in which most of the ganglion cells had degenerated. In Parkinson disease, where fainting is sometimes a problem, there are Lewy bodies in sympathetic ganglion cells.

Treatment of orthostatic hypotension consists of having the patient sleep with the head of the bed elevated, administering mineralocorticoid medications such as fludrocortisone acetate (Florinef) 0.1 mg twice daily, or midodrine beginning with 2.5 mg q 4 h, slowly raising the dose to 5 mg q 4 h, and using elastic stockings that compress the veins of the legs and lower abdomen.

Peripheral Neuropathy with Secondary Orthostatic Hypotension

Impairment of autonomic function, of which orthostatic hypotension is the most serious feature, may occur as part of the more common acute or chronic peripheral neuropathies (e.g., Guillain-Barré, diabetic, alcoholic-nutritional, amyloid, heavy metal-toxic, and porphyric). Disease of the peripheral nervous system may affect the circulation in two ways: baroreceptors may be affected, interrupting normal homeostatic reflexes on the afferent side, or postganglionic efferent sympathetic fibers may be involved in the spinal nerves. The severity of the autonomic failure need not parallel the degree of motor weakness. An additional feature of the acute dysautonomias is a tendency to develop hyponatremia, presumably as a result of dysfunction of afferent fibers from aortic arch volume receptors, which elicits a release of vasopressin. The volume receptors are also implicated in the hypertension that sometimes complicates these neuropathies.

Of particular importance is the autonomic disorder that accompanies diabetic neuropathy. It presents as impotence, constipation, or diarrhea (especially at night), hypotonia of the bladder, gastroparesis, and orthostatic hypotension in some combination. There are invariably signs of a sensory polyneuropathy, consisting of a distal loss of vibratory and thermal-pain sensation and reduced or lost ankle reflexes; but again the severity of affection of the two systems of nerve fibers may not be parallel. The pupils are often small and the amplitude of constriction to light is reduced (Argyll-Robertson pupils); this has been attributed to involvement of the ciliary ganglia. The pathologic basis of the other features has been difficult to assess because of the frequency of artifact in the sympathetic ganglia in autopsy material. Duchen and coworkers attributed the autonomic disorder to vacuolization of sympathetic ganglionic neurons, cell necrosis and inflammation, loss of myelinated fibers in the vagi and white rami communicantes, and loss of lateral horn cells in the spinal cord. They believe the latter changes to be secondary.

Another polyneuropathy with an unusually prominent dysautonomia is that due to amyloidosis. Extensive loss of pain and thermal sensation is usually present; other forms of sensation may also be reduced to a lesser degree. Motor function is much less altered. Sympathetic function is more affected than parasympathetic. Iridoplegia (pupillary paralysis) and disturbances of other smooth muscle and glandular functions are variable.

Both the primary and secondary types of orthostatic hypotension are also discussed in connection with syncope in Chap. 18.

Autonomic Neuropathy in Infants and Children (Riley-Day Syndrome) and Other Dysautonomias

This is a familial disease inherited as an autosomal recessive trait. The main symptoms are postural hypotension and lability of blood pressure, faulty regulation of temperature, diminished hearing, hyperhidrosis, blotchiness of the skin, insensitivity to pain, emotional lability, and cyclic vomiting. The tendon reflexes are hypoactive and mild slowing of motor nerve conduction velocities is common. There is denervation sensitivity of the pupils and other structures. A deficiency of neurons in the superior cervical ganglia and in the lateral horns of the spinal cord has been found. Also, a decreased number of unmyelinated nerve fibers in the sural nerve has been reported by Aguayo and by Dyck and their colleagues (see also page 1423). It is likely that this disease represents a failure of embryologic migration or formation of first- and second-order sympathetic neurons.

Autonomic symptoms may also be a prominent feature of the small-fiber neuropathy of Fabry disease (α-galactosidase deficiency) as a result of the accumulation of ceramide in hypothalamic and intermediolateral column neurons (see pages 1037 and 1422).

Another inherited form of peripheral dysautonomia, characterized by severe pain in the feet on exercise and an autosomal dominant pattern of inheritance, has been described by Robinson and colleagues. Stabbing pains in the feet were increased by bending, crouching, and kneeling. There was no sweat response to intradermal injection of 1% ACh and no autonomic fibers were found in punch biopsies of the skin. Fabry disease was excluded.

Autonomic Failure in the Elderly

Orthostatic hypotension is prevalent in the elderly, so much so that norms of blood pressure and pulse changes have been difficult to establish. Caird and coworkers reported that among individuals who were more than 65 years of age and living at home, 24 percent had a fall of systolic blood pressure on standing of 20 mmHg; 9 percent had a fall of 30 mmHg; and 5 percent, a fall of 40 mmHg. An increased frequency of thermoregulatory impairment has been documented as well. The elderly are also more liable to develop hypothermia and, when exposed to high ambient temperature, to hyperthermia. Loss of sweating of the lower parts of the body and increased sweating of the head and arms probably reflect a senile neuropathy or neuronopathy. The number of sensory ganglion cells decreases with age (Castro). Impotence and incontinence also increase with age, but these, of course, may be due to a number of processes besides autonomic failure.

It is of interest that the idiopathic type of small fiber neuropathy that occurs predominantly in elderly women ("burning hands and feet" syndrome) has no associated autonomic features. (See Chap. 46.)

Horner (Oculosympathetic) and Stellate Ganglion Syndromes

Interruption of postganglionic sympathetic fibers at any point along the internal carotid arteries or a lesion of the superior cervical ganglion results in miosis, drooping of the eyelid, and abolition of sweating over one side of the face (see also page 296). The same syndrome in less obvious form may be caused by interruption of the preganglionic fibers at any point between their origin in the intermediolateral cell column of the C8–T2 spinal segments and the superior cervical ganglion or by interruption of the descending, uncrossed hypothalamospinal pathway in the tegmentum of the brainstem or cervical cord. The common causes are neoplastic or inflammatory involvement of the cervical lymph nodes or proximal part of the brachial plexus, surgical and other types of trauma to cervical structures (e.g., jugular venous catheters), carotid artery dissection, syringomyelic or traumatic lesions of the first and second thoracic spinal segments, and infarcts or other lesions of the lateral part of the medulla (Wallenberg syndrome). There is also an idiopathic variety that may sometimes be hereditary. If a Horner syndrome develops early in life, the iris on the affected side fails to become pigmented and remains blue or mottled gray-brown (heterochromia iridis). A lesion of the stellate ganglion, e.g., compression by a tumor arising from the superior sulcus of the lung, produces the interesting combination of a Horner syndrome and paralysis of sympathetic reflexes in the limb (the hand and arm are dry and warm). With preganglionic lesions, facial flushing may develop on the side of the sympathetic disorder; this is brought on in some instances by exercise (harlequin effect).

Keane has provided data as to the relative frequency of the lesions causing oculosympathetic paralysis. In 100 successive cases, 63 were of central type due to brainstem strokes, 21 were preganglionic due to trauma or tumors of the neck, 13 were postganglionic due to miscellaneous causes, and in 3 cases the localization was indeterminate (see Chap. 14 for further discussion).

The pupillary disturbances associated with oculomotor nerve lesions, the Adie pupil, and other parasympathetic and sympathetic abnormalities of pupillary function are considered fully in Chap. 14. The combination of segmental anhidrosis and an Adie pupil is sometimes referred to as the *Ross syndrome*; it may be abrupt in onset and idiopathic or may follow a viral infection.

Sympathetic and Parasympathetic Paralysis in Tetraplegia and Paraplegia

Lesions of the C4 or C5 segments of the spinal cord, if complete, will interrupt suprasegmental control of both the sympathetic and sacral parasympathetic nervous systems. Much the same effects are observed with lesions of the upper thoracic cord (above T6). Lower thoracic lesions leave much of the descending sympathetic outflow intact, only the descending sacral parasympathetic control being interrupted. Traumatic necrosis of the spinal cord is the usual cause of these states, but they may be due as well to infarction, certain forms of myelitis, and tumors.

The initial effect of an acute cervical cord transection is abolition of all sensorimotor and autonomic functions of the isolated spinal cord. The autonomic changes include hypotension, loss of sweating and piloerection, paralytic ileus and gastric atony, and paralysis of the bladder. Plasma epinephrine and NE are reduced. This state, known as spinal shock, lasts for several weeks. The basic mechanisms are not known, but changes in neurotransmitters (catecholamines, endorphins, substance P, and 5-hydroxytryptamine) are under investigation.

After spinal shock dissipates, sympathetic and parasympathetic functions return, since the afferent and efferent autonomic connections within the isolated segments of the spinal cord are intact, although no longer under the control of higher centers. With *cervical cord lesions*, there is a loss of the sympathetically mediated cardiovascular changes in response to stimuli reaching the medulla. However, cutaneous stimuli (pinprick or cold) in segments of the body below the transection will raise the blood pressure. A fall in blood pressure is not compensated by sympathetic vasoconstriction. Hence tetraplegics are prone to orthostatic hypotension. Pinching the skin below the lesion causes gooseflesh in adjacent segments. Heating the body results in flushing and sweating over the face and neck but not the trunk and legs. Bladder and bowel, including their sphincters, which are at first flaccid, become automatic as spinal reflex control returns. There may be reflex penile erection or priapism and even ejaculation, and the female may become pregnant even though voluntary control of sexual activity has been abolished.

After a time the tetraplegic may develop a "*mass reflex*" (page 1297), in which flexor spasms of the legs and involuntary emptying of the bladder are associated with a rise in blood pressure, bradycardia, and sweating and pilomotor reactions in parts below the cervical segments ("autonomic dysreflexia"). These reactions may also be evoked by pinprick, passive movement, contactual stimuli of the limbs and abdomen, and pressure on the bladder. An exaggerated vasopressor reaction also occurs in response to injected NE. In such attacks, the patient experiences paresthesias of the neck, shoulders, and arms; tightness in the chest and dyspnea; pupillary dilatation; pallor followed by flushing of the face; fullness in the head and ears; and a throbbing headache. Plasma NE and dopamine rise slowly during the autonomic discharge. When such an attack is severe and prolonged, myocardial infarction, seizures, and visual defects have been observed. Clonidine, up to 0.2 mg three times daily, has been useful in preventing the hypertensive crises.

Acute Autonomic Crises (Sympathetic Storm and the Cushing Response)

Several toxic and pharmacologic agents such as cocaine and phenylpropanolamine are capable of producing abrupt overactivity of the sympathetic and parasympathetic nervous systems—severe hypertension and mydriasis coupled with signs of central nervous system excitation, including seizures. Tricyclic antidepressants in excessive doses are also known to produce autonomic effects, but in this case there is cholinergic blockade, leading to dryness of the mouth, flushing, absent sweating, and mydriasis. The main concern with tricyclic antidepressant overdose is the development of a ventricular arrhythmia, also on an autonomic basis, presaged by prolongation of the Q-T interval on the ECG. Poisoning with organophosphate insecticides (e.g., Parathion), which are anticholinesterase drugs, causes a combination of *parasympathetic overactivity* and motor paralysis (see page 1281). A severe degree of autonomic disturbance, involving both postganglionic sympathetic and parasympathetic function, is produced by ingestion of the rodenticide *N*-3-pyridylmethyl-*N*'-*p*-nitrophenylurea (PNU, Vacor). The exaggerated sympathetic state that accompanies tetanus, manifest by diaphoresis, mydriasis, and labile or sustained hypertension, has been attributed to circulating catecholamines.

The most dramatic syndromes of unopposed sympathetic-adrenal medullary hyperactivity occur with severe head injury and cerebral hemorrhage. Three mechanisms are observed at different times: an outpouring of adrenal catecholamines at the time of the ictus with acute hypertension and tachycardia; a brainstem-mediated vasopressor reaction (Cushing response); and a later phenomenon, consisting of extreme hypertension, profuse diaphoresis, and pupillary dilation, and coming in episodes of several minutes or more during periods of rigid extensor posturing (the "diencephalic autonomic seizures" of Penfield, described below and in Chap. 35 in relation to head injury).

Experimental evidence suggests that nuclei in the caudal medullary reticular formation (reticularis gigantocelluraris and parvicellularis) can precipitate severe hypertensive reactions. These are tonically inhibited by the nucleus of the tractus solitarius (NTS), which receives afferent input from arterial baroreceptors and chemoreceptors. Bilateral lesions of the NTS therefore produce extreme elevations in blood pressure and probably also play a role in the genesis of "neurogenic" pulmonary edema (see page 597). These effects are eliminated by sectioning of the cervical spinal cord and by alpha-adrenergic blockade.

The *Cushing response*, reflex, or "reaction," as Cushing described it, occurs as a result of an abrupt increase in intracranial pressure. It consists of a triad of hypertension, bradycardia, and slow, irregular breathing elicited by the stimulation of mechanically sensitive regions in the paramedian caudal medulla (Hoff and Reis). Similar pressure-sensitive areas in the upper cervical spinal cord can produce the Cushing response when intraspinal pressure is raised abruptly; a ventral medullary vasodepressor area that acts in the opposite manner has been found in animals. The Cushing response is predicated on mechanical distortion of the lower brainstem, either from a mass in the posterior fossa or, more often, from a large hemorrhage or tumor in one of the hemispheres or a subarachnoid hemorrhage that elevates the pressure within the fourth ventricle. Often, only the hypertensive component of the reaction occurs, with the systolic blood pressure reaching levels of 200 mmHg, suggesting the presence of a pheochromocytoma or renal artery stenosis. In our experience, the most severe instances of this type of centrally provoked hypertensive syndrome have occurred in children with cerebellar tumors who presented with headache and extreme systolic hypertension. Difficulty may arise in differentiating this response from hypertensive encephalopathy, especially from cases that derive from renovascular hypertension, which may likewise be accompanied by headache and papilledema. It is useful to know that hypertensive encephalopathy is associated with a tachycardia or normal heart rate and that systolic blood pressure levels above 210 mmHg are attained only rarely in the Cushing response.

Penfield described paroxysms of hypertension, intense diaphoresis, flushed skin, and mydriasis in comatose patients and attributed them to epilepsy (*diencephalic seizures*), although his original patient had a tumor obstructing the foramen of Munro. Many similar attacks have been described, additional features being a rise in temperature just prior to the paroxysm, cyclic respirations, and shivering. Often the bedsheets are soaked and the patient's forehead is covered by beads of sweat. Most patients who exhibit such paroxysms are decorticate from traumatic lesions of the deep cerebral white matter or from acute hydrocephalus, which was the likely explanation of Penfield's cases; they are clearly not epileptic. These attacks are thought to result from the removal of inhibitory influences on the hypothalamus, creating, in effect, a hypersensitive decorticated autonomic nervous system. The condition is thought to be analogous to overactivity of the extensor and opisthotonic posturing mechanisms that appear with little provocation in the same clinical settings. Morphine and bromocriptine have been helpful in suppressing the syndrome, and beta-adrenergic blockers reduce the hypertension and tachycardia.

During episodes of intense sympathetic discharge, there are *alterations in the ECG*, mainly in the ST segments, and T waves; in extreme cases, evidence of myocardial damage can be observed. The role of direct sympathetic innervation of the heart in producing these myocardial abnormalities is unclear, but the surge in circulating norepinephrine and cortisol consequent to subarachnoid hemorrhage and trauma is postulated as the cause. A similar hyperadrenergic mechanism has been proposed to explain sudden death from fright, asthma, status epilepticus, and cocaine overdose. Recent investigations by Schobel et al have suggested that sustained sympathetic overactivity is responsible for the hypertension of *pre-eclampsia, which* may be considered in some ways as a dysautonomic state. Further information on these topics is contained in the reviews by Samuels and by Ropper.

A role has also been inferred for the ventrolateral medullary pressor centers in the maintenance of *essential hypertension*. Geiger and colleagues removed looped posteroinferior cerebellar artery branches from the ventral surface of the medulla in 8 patients with intractable essential hypertension and found that 7 improved. Vascular decompression of cranial nerves has proved to be a credible therapeutic measure for hemifacial spasm and some cases of vertigo and trigeminal neuralgia, but the notion that vascular compression of the ventral medulla is a valid mechanism of essential hypertension and that decompression is a useful therapeutic measure requires confirmation.

The Effects of Thoracolumbar Sympathectomy Surgical resection of the thoracolumbar sympathetic trunk, widely used in the 1940s in the treatment of hypertension, has provided the clinician with the clearest examples of extensive injury to the peripheral sympathetic nervous system, though a similar defect had long been suspected in primary orthostatic hypotension (see above). In general, bilateral thoracolumbar sympathectomy results in surprisingly few disturbances of function. Aside from loss of sweating over the denervated areas of the body, the most pronounced abnormality is an impairment of vasomotor reflexes. In the upright posture, faintness and syncope are frequent because of pooling of blood in the splanchnic bed and lower extremities; although the blood pressure may fall steadily to shock levels, there is little or no pallor, nausea, vomiting, or sweating—the usual accompaniments of syncope. Bladder, bowel, and sexual function are preserved, though semen is sometimes ejaculated into the posterior urethra and bladder. No consistent abnormalities of renal or hepatic function have been found.

Disorders of Sweating

Hyperhidrosis results from overactivity of sudomotor nerve fibers under a variety of conditions. It may occur as an initial excitatory phase of certain peripheral neuropathies (e.g., due to arsenic or thallium) and be followed by anhidrosis and is one aspect of sympathetic reflex dystrophy. Affections of small nerve fibers, which enhance adrenergic responses, are associated with excessive sweating. This is also observed as a localized effect in painful mononeuropathies (causalgia) and diffusely in certain painful polyneuropathies ("burning foot" syndrome). A type of nonthermoregulatory hyperhidrosis may occur in spinal paraplegics (page 1297). Loss of sweating in one part of the body may require a compensatory increase in normal parts—for example, the excessive facial and upper truncal sweating that occurs in patients with transection of the high thoracic cord.

Localized hyperhidrosis may be a troublesome complaint in some patients. One variety, presumably of congenital origin, affects the palms. The social embarrassment of a "succulent hand" or a "dripping paw" is often intolerable. It is taken to be a sign of nervousness, though many persons with this condition disclaim all other neurotic symptoms. Cold, clammy hands are common in individuals with anxiety, and indeed this has been a useful sign in distinguishing an anxiety state from hyperthyroidism, in which the hands are also moist but warm. Extirpation of T2 and T3 sympathetic ganglia relieves the more severe cases of palmar sweating; a Horner syndrome does not develop if the T1 ganglion is left intact. In other cases, the hyperhidrosis affects mainly the feet.

Anhidrosis in restricted skin areas is a frequent and useful finding in peripheral nerve disease. It is due to the interruption of the postganglionic sympathetic fibers, and its boundaries can be mapped by means of the sweat tests described earlier in the chapter. The loss of sweating corresponds to the area of sensory loss. In contrast, sweating is not affected in spinal root disease because there is much intersegmental mixing of the preganglionic axons once they enter the sympathetic chain.

A postinfectious anhidrosis syndrome is known, sometimes accompanied by mild orthostatic hypotension. The process is thought to be a limited form of the pandysautonomia described earlier. Corticosteroids are said to be beneficial.

Raynaud Syndrome This disorder, characterized by episodic, painful blanching of the fingers and presumably caused by digital artery spasm, was first described by Raynaud in 1862. It occurs in a number of clinical settings. In the most common type, the episodes are brought on by cold or emotional stress and are usually followed by redness on rewarming. In more than half such cases there is an associated connective tissue disease, scleroderma being the main one (Porter et al). In these patients, mainly women, the Raynaud syndrome may antedate systemic symptoms by many years. In a second group, predominantly men, the syndrome is induced by local trauma, such as prolonged sculling on a cold day, and particularly by vibratory injury incurred by the sustained use of a pneumatic drill or hammer and chisel (the syndrome is well known to quarry workers). Obstructive arterial disease, as might occur with the thoracic outlet syndrome, vasospasm due to drugs (ergot, cytotoxic agents), previous cold injury (frostbite), and circulating cryoglobulins are less common causes. In 64 of 219 patients studied by Porter and coworkers, the Raynaud syndrome was classified as idiopathic. Formerly, the idiopathic form was called *Raynaud disease*, and the type with associated disease, *Raynaud phenomenon*.

Irrespective of the associated disease, one of two mechanisms seems to be operative in the pathogenesis of Raynaud syndrome—either an increase in arterial constriction or a decrease in the intraluminal pressure. The former, in purest form, is observed in young women on exposure to cold and aggravated by emotional stress; a decrease in intraluminal pressure is associated with arterial obstruction. Treatment is directed to the associated conditions and prevention of precipitating factors. Cervicothoracic sympathectomy has not proved to be an effective measure.

Lafferty and colleagues have pointed out that, in contrast to many areas of the body, the cutaneous nerves of the hands and feet can induce solely vasoconstrictive effects when stimulated, and dilatation is accomplished by chemical mediators. In the pure vasospastic form of the disease, there is a defect locally in the histaminergic vasodilating system. Cold or emotional activation of the sympathetic vasoconstrictive mechanism is intact, but the neural release of histamine from mast cells in the hands is defective. Mast cells may be injured locally or destroyed by an autoimmune reaction in connective tissue diseases. It is because active vasodilatation is under control of the histaminergic system that sympathectomy is usually ineffective. The vasodilating properties of the various prostaglandins have been exploited to good effect in some cases.

Erythromelalgia, first described by Weir Mitchell, is a condition of unknown cause and mechanism in which the feet and lower extremities become red and painful on exposure to warm temperatures for prolonged periods (see page 231).

Disturbances of Bladder Function

The familiar functions of the bladder and lower urinary tract—the storage and intermittent evacuation of urine—are served by three structural components: the bladder itself, the main component of which is the large detrusor (smooth) muscle; a functional internal sphincter composed of smooth muscle; and the striated external sphincter or urogenital diaphragm. The sphincters assure continence; in the male, the internal sphincter also prevents the reflux of semen from the urethra during ejaculation. For micturition to occur, the sphincters must relax, allowing the detrusor to expel urine from the bladder into the urethra. This is accomplished by a complex mechanism involving mainly the parasympathetic nervous system (the sacral peripheral nerves derived from the second, third, and fourth sacral segments of the spinal cord and their somatic sensorimotor fibers) and to a lesser extent, sympathetic fibers derived from the thorax. The brainstem "micturition centers," with their spinal and suprasegmental connections may contribute (Fig. 26-5).

The detrusor muscle receives motor innervation from nerve cells in the intermediolateral columns of gray matter, mainly from the third and also from the second and fourth sacral segments of the spinal cord (the "detrusor center"). These neurons give rise to preganglionic fibers that synapse in parasympathetic ganglia within the bladder wall. Short postganglionic fibers end on muscarinic acetylcholine receptors of the muscle fibers. There are also beta-adrenergic receptors in the dome of the bladder, which are activated by sympathetic fibers that arise in the intermediolateral nerve cells of T10, T11, and T12 segments. These *preganglionic fibers* pass via inferior splanchnic nerves to the inferior mesenteric ganglia (Figs. 26-1 and 26-4); pre- and postganglionic sympathetic axons are conveyed by the hypogastric nerve to the pelvic plexus and the bladder dome. The internal sphincter and base of the bladder (trigone), consisting of smooth muscle, are also innervated to some extent by the sympathetic fibers of the hypogastric nerves; their receptors are mainly of alpha-adrenergic type.

The external urethral and anal sphincters are composed of striated muscle fibers. Their innervation, via the pudendal nerves, is derived from a densely packed group of somatomotor neurons (nucleus of Onuf) in the anterolateral horns of sacral segments 2, 3, and 4. Cells in the ventrolateral part of Onuf's nucleus innervate the external urethral sphincter, and cells of the mediodorsal part innervate the anal sphincter. The muscle fibers of the sphincters respond to the nicotinic effects of ACh.

The pudendal nerves also contain afferent fibers coursing from the urethra and the external sphincter to the sacral segments of the spinal cord. These fibers convey impulses for reflex activities and, through connections with higher centers, for sensation. Some of these fibers probably course through the hypogastric plexus, as indicated by the fact that patients with complete transverse lesions of the cord as high as T12 may report vague sensations of urethral discomfort. The blad-

Figure 26-5

Innervation of the urinary bladder and its sphincters.

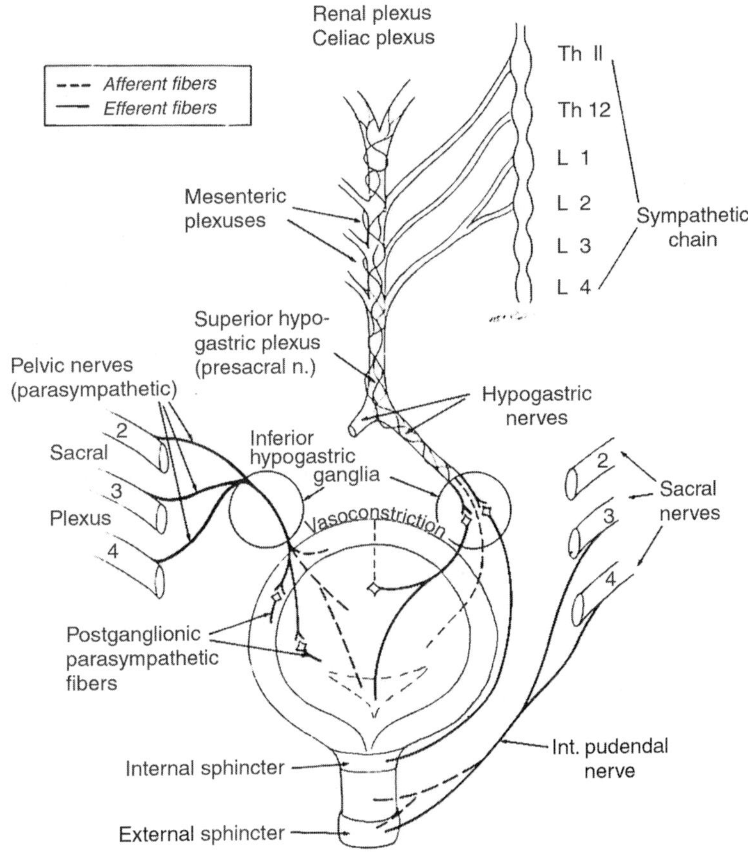

der is sensitive to pain and pressure; these senses are transmitted to higher centers along the sensory pathways described in Chaps. 8 and 9.

Unlike skeletal striated muscle, the detrusor, because of its postganglionic system, is capable of some contractions, imperfect at best, after complete destruction of the sacral segments of the spinal cord. Isolation of the sacral cord centers (transverse lesions of the cord above the sacral levels) and their peripheral nerves permits contractions of the detrusor muscle, but they do not empty the bladder completely; patients with such lesions usually develop dyssynergia of the detrusor and external sphincter muscles (see below), indicating that coordination of these muscles must occur at supraspinal levels (Blaivas). With acute transverse lesions of the upper cord, the function of sacral segments is abolished for several weeks in the same way as the motor neurons of skeletal muscles (the state of spinal shock).

The storage of urine and the efficient emptying of the bladder is possible only when the spinal segments, together with their afferent and efferent nerve fibers, are connected with the so-called micturition centers in the pontomesencephalic tegmentum. In experimental animals, this center (or centers) lies within or adjacent to the locus ceruleus. A medial region apparently triggers micturition, while a lateral area seems more important for continence. These centers receive afferent impulses from the sacral cord segments; their efferent fibers course downward via the reticulospinal tracts in the lateral funiculi of the spinal cord and activate cells in the nucleus of Onuf as well as in the intermediolateral cell groups of the sacral segments (Holstege and Tan). In cats, the pontomesencephalic centers receive descending fibers from anteromedial parts of the frontal cortex, thalamus, hypothalamus, and cerebellum, but the pathways involved have not been precisely defined in humans. Other fibers, from the motor cortex, descend with the corticospinal fibers to the anterior horn cells of the sacral cord and innervate the external sphincter. According to Ruch, the descending pathways from the midbrain tegmentum are inhibitory and those from the pontine tegmentum and posterior hypothalamus are facilitatory. The pathway that descends with the corticospinal tract from the motor cortex is inhibitory. Thus the net effect of lesions in the brain and spinal cord on the micturition reflex, at least in animals, may be either inhibitory or facilitatory (DeGroat).

Almost all of this information has been inferred from animal experiments; there is little human pathologic material to corroborate the role of central nuclei and cortex in bladder control. What information is available is reviewed extensively by Fowler, whose article is recommended. Of interest also is the study of Blok and colleagues, who performed positron emission tomography (PET) in volunteer subjects during micturition. Increased blood flow was detected in the right pontine tegmentum, periaqueductal region, hypothalamus, and right inferior frontal cortex. When the bladder was full but the subjects were prevented from voiding, increased activity was seen in the right ventral pontine tegmentum. The meaning of these lateralized findings is unclear, but the study supports the presumption that pontine centers are involved in the coordination of voiding.

The act of micturition is both reflex and voluntary. When the normal person desires to void, there is first a voluntary relaxation of the perineum, followed sequentially by an increased tension of the abdominal wall, a slow contraction of the detrusor, and an associated opening of the internal sphincter; finally, there is a relaxation of the external sphincter (Denny-Brown and Robertson). It is useful to think of the detrusor contraction as a spinal stretch reflex, subject to facilitation and inhibition from higher centers. Voluntary closure of the external sphincter and contraction of the perineal muscles cause the detrusor contraction to subside. The abdominal muscles have no power to initiate micturition except when the detrusor muscle is not functioning normally. The voluntary restraint of micturition is a cerebral affair and is mediated by fibers that arise in the frontal lobes (paracentral motor region), descend in the spinal cord just anterior and medial to the corticospinal tracts, and terminate on the cells of the anterior horns and intermediolateral cell columns of the sacral segments, as described above. The integration of detrusor and external sphincteric function depends mainly on the descending pathway from the dorsolateral pontine tegmentum.

With regard to the neurologic diseases that cause bladder dysfunction, multiple sclerosis, usually with urinary urgency, is by far the most common. In Fowler's clinic, other spinal cord disorders accounted for 12 percent of cases, degenerative diseases (Parkinson disease and multiple system atrophy) for 14 percent, and frontal lobe lesions for 9 percent.

These data and the physiologic principles elaborated above enable one to understand the effects of the following lesions on bladder function:

1. *Complete destruction of the cord below T12*, as from trauma, myelodysplasias, tumor, venous angioma, and necrotizing myelitis. The bladder is paralyzed and there is no awareness of the state of fullness; voluntary initiation of micturition is impossible; the tonus of the detrusor muscle is abolished and the bladder distends as urine accumulates until there is overflow incontinence; voiding is possible only by the Credé maneuver, i.e., lower abdominal compression and abdominal straining. Usually the anal sphincter and colon are similarly affected, and there is "saddle" anesthesia and abolition of the bulbocavernosus and anal reflexes. The cystometrogram shows low pressure and no emptying contractions.

2. *Disease of the sacral motor neurons in the spinal gray matter, the anterior roots, or peripheral nerves*, as in lumbosacral meningomyelocele and the tethered cord syndrome. This is, in effect, a lower motor neuron paralysis of the bladder. The disturbance of bladder function is the same as in (1) above except that sacral and bladder sensation are intact. Various causes pertain in cauda equina disease, the most frequent being compression by epidural tumor or disc, neoplastic meningitis, and radiculitis from herpes or cytomegalovirus. It is noteworthy that a hysterical patient can suppress motor function and suffer a similar distention of the bladder (see below).

3. *Interruption of sensory afferent fibers* from the bladder, as in diabetes and tabes dorsalis, leaving motor nerve fibers unaltered. This is a primary sensory bladder paralysis. Again, the disturbance in function is the same as in (1) and (2) above. Although a flaccid (atonic) paralysis of the bladder may be purely motor or sensory, as described above, in most clinical situations there is *interruption of both afferent and efferent innervation*, as in cauda equina compression or severe polyneuropathy. Neuropathies affecting mainly the small fibers are the ones usually implicated (diabetes, amyloid, etc.), but urinary retention occurs in Guillain-Barré syndrome as well.

4. *Upper spinal cord lesions*. These result in a *reflex neurogenic (spastic) bladder*. In addition to multiple sclerosis and traumatic myelopathy, which are the commonest causes, myelitis, spondylosis, arteriovenous malformation (AVM), syringomyelia, and tropical spastic paraparesis may cause a bladder disturbance of this type. As stated above, if the cord lesion is of sudden

onset, the detrusor muscle suffers the effects of spinal shock. At this stage, urine accumulates and distends the bladder to the point of overflow. As the effects of spinal shock subside, the detrusor usually becomes overactive, and since the patient is unable to inhibit the detrusor and control the external sphincter, urgency, precipitant micturition, and incontinence result. In addition, initiation of voluntary micturition is impaired and bladder capacity reduced. Bladder sensation depends on the extent of involvement of sensory tracts. Bulbocavernosus and anal reflexes are preserved. The cystometrogram shows uninhibited contractions of the detrusor muscle in response to small volumes of fluid. If the upper motor neuron lesion evolves slowly, spasticity of the bladder will not be preceded by a flaccid stage and the symptoms of urgency and incontinence worsen with time. Most puzzling to the authors have been cases of cervical cord injury in which reflex activity of the sacral mechanism does not return; the bladder remains hypotonic.

5. *Mixed type of neurogenic bladder*. In diseases such as multiple sclerosis, subacute combined degeneration, tethered cord, and syphilitic meningomyelitis, bladder function may be deranged from lesions at multiple levels, i.e., spinal roots, sacral neurons or their fibers of exit, and higher spinal segments. The resultant picture is a combination of sensory, motor, and spastic types of bladder paralysis.

6. *Stretch injury of the bladder wall*, as occurs with anatomic obstruction at the bladder neck and occasionally with repeated voluntary retention of urine, as in hysteria. Repeated overdistention of the bladder wall often results in varying degrees of decompensation of the detrusor muscle and permanent atonia or hypotonia, although the evidence for this mechanism is uncertain. The bladder wall becomes fibrotic and bladder capacity is greatly increased. Emptying contractions are inadequate, and there is a large residual volume even after the Credé maneuver and strong contraction of the abdominal muscles. As with motor and sensory paralyses, the patient is subject to cystitis, ureteral reflux, hydronephrosis and pyelonephritis, and calculus formation.

Urinary retention has been observed in women with polycystic ovaries. In one study of 62 such women, it was found that myotonic-like discharges activated the urethral sphincter, interfering with its relaxation during micturition. There were increasing amounts of residual urine, followed, finally, by complete retention. This obscure mechanism has been offered as an explanation of some cases of *hysterical urinary retention*. Fowler describes unusual patterns of electromyographic (EMG) activity in the bladder and sphincter of patients we would have classified as hysterical urine retainers.

7. *Frontal lobe incontinence*. Often the patient, because of his torpid or confused mental state, ignores the desire to void and the subsequent incontinence. There is also a supranuclear type of hyperactivity of the detrusor and precipitant evacuation. These types of frontal lobe incontinence are considered on page 473.

8. *Nocturnal enuresis, or urinary incontinence during sleep*, due presumably to a delay in acquiring inhibition of micturition, is discussed in Chap. 19.

As alluded to earlier, a role for pontine centers in human micturition is implied from animal experiments, but there are few clinical data except perhaps the PET studies mentioned. Sakakibara and colleagues have reported that half of their patients with brainstem strokes had urinary symptoms, for which lesions in the pons were most often responsible; but the precision of anatomic localization of the strokes was limited and the symptoms varied.

Despite an apparent integratory micturition center in the pons, to our knowledge there are no well-studied examples of human bladder dysfunction due solely to a brainstem lesion.

Therapy of Disordered Micturition Several drugs are useful in the management of flaccid and spastic disturbances of bladder function. In the case of a flaccid paralysis, bethanechol (Urecholine) produces contraction of the detrusor by direct stimulation of its muscarinic cholinergic receptors. In spastic paralysis, the detrusor can be relaxed by propantheline (Pro-Banthine, 15 to 30 mg three times daily) which acts as a muscarinic antagonist, and by oxybutynin (Ditropan, 5 mg two to three times daily), which acts directly on the smooth muscle and also has a muscarinic antagonist action. Atropine, which is mainly a muscarinic antagonist, only partially inhibits detrusor contraction.

Several other drugs may be useful in the treatment of neurogenic bladder but can be utilized rationally only on the basis of sophisticated urodynamic investigations (Krane and Siroky).

Often the patient must resort to intermittent self-catheterization, which can be safely carried out with scrupulous attention to sterile technique (washing hands, disposable catheter, etc.). Some forms of chronic antibiotic therapy and acidification of urine with vitamin C (1000 g/day) are practical aids. In selected paraplegic patients, the implantation of a sacral anterior root stimulator may prove to be helpful in emptying the bladder and achieving continence (Brindley et al).

Disturbances of Bowel Function

The colon and anal sphincters are obedient to the same principles that govern bladder function. Ileus from spinal shock, reflex neurogenic colon, and sensory and motor paralysis with megacolon are all recognized clinical entities. The colon, stomach, and small intestine may be hypotonic and distended and the anal sphincters lax, either from deafferentation, de-efferentation, or both. The anal and, in the male, the bulbocavernosus reflex may be abolished. Defecation may be urgent and precipitant with higher spinal and cerebral lesions. Since the same spinal segments and nearly the same spinal tracts subserve bladder and bowel function, meningomyeloceles, and other cauda equina and spinal cord diseases often cause so-called double incontinence. However, since the bowel is less often filled and its content is usually solid, fecal incontinence is less frequent than urinary incontinence.

In recent years there has been considerable interest in weakness of the muscles of the pelvic floor as a cause of double incontinence, more so in the female. Also, it has been suggested that paradoxical contraction of the puborectus and external anal sphincter may be a cause of severe constipation (anismus). Extreme degrees of descent of the pelvic floor are believed to injure the pudendal nerves, as reflected in prolonged terminal latencies in nerve conduction studies.

Systemic diseases may affect the colonic sphincters; examples are myotonic dystrophy and scleroderma, which may weaken the internal sphincter, and polymyositis and myasthenia gravis, which may impair the function of the external sphincter (Schuster). The inability to control flatulence may be an early sign of sphincteric weakness in myasthenia. Also, sphincteric damage may complicate hemorrhoidectomy.

The serotonin receptor agonist cisapride has been useful in partially restoring gastrointestinal motility in some cases of neurogenic ileus as, for example, the early stages of the Guillain-Barré syndrome. When given orally or by nasogastric tube in doses of 10 to 20 mg every 4 to 6 h, it may restore bowel motility enough to allow parenteral feeding. The drug should not be used if there is any question of bowel obstruction or gastrointestinal hemorrhage.

Many cases of ileus, even to the extent of megacolon, have a pharmacologic basis, and are the effect of drugs that paralyze the parasympathetic system or of narcotics that have a direct effect on the motility of gastrointestinal smooth muscle.

Congenital Megacolon (Hirschsprung Disease)

This is a rare disease affecting mainly male infants and children. It is due to a congenital absence of ganglion cells in the myenteric plexus. The internal anal sphincter and rectosigmoid are involved most often and are the parts affected in restricted forms of Hirschsprung disease (75 percent of cases), but the aganglionosis is sometimes more extensive. The aganglionic segment of the bowel is constricted and cannot relax, thus preventing propagation of peristaltic waves, which, in turn, produces retention of feces and massive distention of the colon above the aganglionic segment. Enterocolitis is the most serious complication and is associated with a high mortality. Some cases of megaloureter are attributed to a similar defect. Hirschsprung disease has been traced to a mutation of either the RET oncogene or the endothelin β receptor.

Disturbances of Sexual Function

Sexual function in the male, which is not infrequently affected in neurologic disease, may be divided into several parts: (1) sexual impulse, drive, or desire, often referred to as *libido*, discussed in Chap. 25; (2) penile erection, enabling the act of sexual intercourse (potency); and (3) ejaculation of semen by the prostate through the urethra.

The arousal of libido in men and women may result from a variety of stimuli, some purely imaginary. Such neocortical influences involve the limbic system and are transmitted to the hypothalamus and spinal centers. The suprasegmental pathways traverse the lateral funiculi of the spinal cord near the corticospinal tracts to reach sympathetic and parasympathetic segmental centers. Penile erection is effected through sacral parasympathetic motor neurons (S3 and S4), the nervi erigentes, and pudendal nerves. There is some evidence also that a sympathetic outflow from thoracolumbar segments (originating in T12–L1) via the inferior mesenteric and hypogastric plexuses can mediate psychogenic erections in patients with complete sacral cord destruction. Activation from these segmental centers opens vascular channels between arteriolar branches of the pudendal arteries and the vascular spaces of the corpora cavernosa and corpus spongiosum (erectile tissues), resulting in tumescence. Deturgescence occurs when venous channels open widely. Copulation consists of a complex series of rhythmic thrusting movements of pelvic musculature, and ejaculation involves rhythmic contractions of the prostate, compressor (sphincter) urethrae, and bulbocavernosus and ischiocavernosus muscles, which are under the control of both the sympathetic and parasympathetic centers. Afferent segmental influences arise in the glans penis and reach parasympathetic centers at S3 and S4 (reflexogenic erections). The organization of this neural system and the locations of lesions that can abolish normal potency are shown in Fig. 26-6. Similar neural arrangements exist in females.

The different aspects of sexual function may be affected separately. Loss of libido may depend upon both psychic and somatic factors. It may be complete, as in old age or in medical and endocrine diseases, or it may occur only in certain circumstances or in relation to a certain situation or individual. In the latter case, which is usually due to psychologic factors, reflex penile erection during REM sleep and even emission of semen may occur, and effective sexual intercourse in other circumstances is possible. Sexual desire can on occasion be altered in the opposite direction, i.e., it may be excessive. This too may be psychologic or psychiatric in origin, as in manic states, but sometimes it occurs with neurologic disease, such as encephalitis and tumors that affect the diencephalon, septal region, and temporal lobes; with the dementias; and as a result of certain medications such as L-dopa, as discussed in Chap. 25. In the instances of neurologic diseases, there are usually other signs of disinhibited behavior as well.

On the other hand, sexual desire may be present but penile erection impossible to attain or sustain, a condition called *impotence*, in which nocturnal erections are usually preserved. The commonest cause of impotence is a depressive state. Prostatectomy is another, the result of

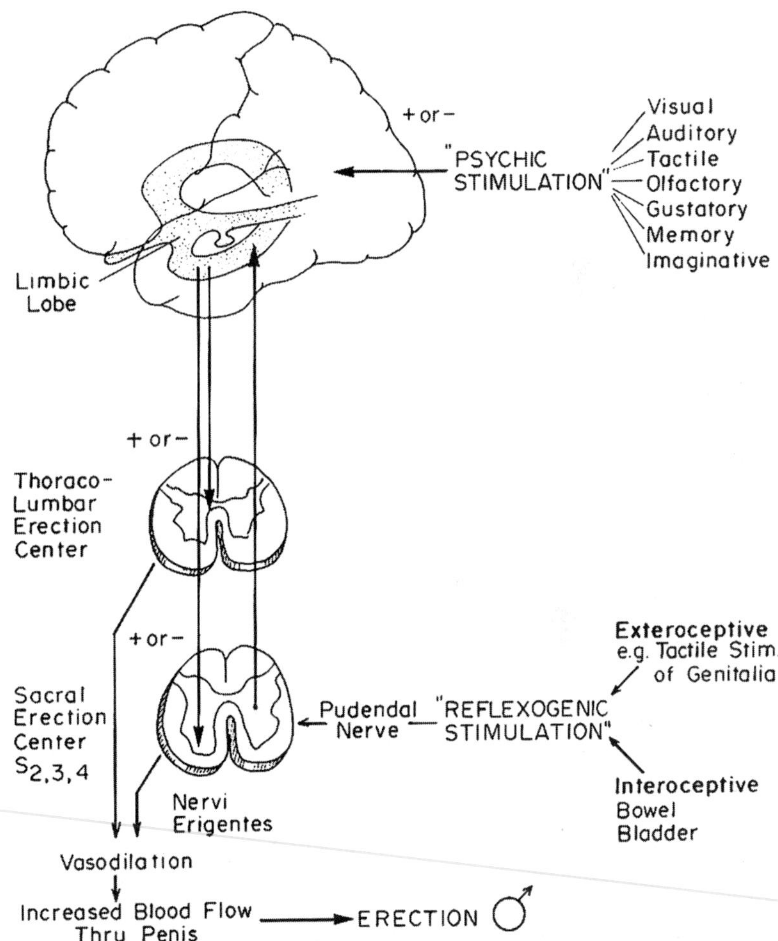

Figure 26-6

The pathways involved in human penile erection. (From Weiss by permission.)

damage to the parasympathetic nerves embedded in the capsule of the gland. It occurs also in patients who suffer disease of the sacral cord segments and their afferent and efferent connections (e.g., cord tumor, myelitis, tabes, and diabetic and many other polyneuropathies), in which case nocturnal erections are absent. The parasympathetic nerves cannot then be activated to cause tumescence of the corpora cavernosa and corpus spongiosum. The phosphodiesterase inhibitor sildenafil (Viagra) has proved to be useful in the treatment of impotence in some patients with sexual dysfunction of neurologic cause. During sexual stimulation, it enhances the effect of local nitrous oxide on the smooth muscle of the corpus cavernosum; this results in relaxation of the smooth muscle and inflow of blood. The high rate of success of this drug in patients with spinal cord injury indicates that segmental innervation is all that is required for reflexive erection.

Diseases of the spinal cord may abolish psychogenic erections, leaving reflexogenic ones intact. In fact, the latter may become overactive, giving rise to sustained painful erections (*priapism*). This indicates that the segmental mechanism for penile erection is relatively intact.

Other sexual difficulties include the premature ejaculation of semen. After lumbar sympathectomy, the semen may be ejected back into the bladder because of paralysis of the periurethral muscle within the prostate, at the verumontanum (colliculus seminalis). Prostatism may have a similar effect.

There are also aberrations of sexual function that occur in the female, but they are more difficult to analyze. Lack of sexual desire or failure to attain orgasm (frigidity) is much more frequent in the female than in the male, occurring in a significant percentage of neurotic women and in others who exhibit no signs of psychic disorder. The activation of the pelvic reflexes involved in female orgasm is highly variable. Often the pelvic reflexes are congenitally deficient and the woman is anorgasmic but still sexually active and fertile. States of excessive sexual excitability are known in sociopathic individuals and, rarely, in those who suffer disease of the brain. Fecundity and sterility are usually unrelated to the other aspects of sexuality.

The genesis of sexual perversions is discussed in Chap. 56. Their origin remains obscure. Endocrine, biochemical, and psychologic studies have failed to clarify the cause and mechanism. Cerebral disorders of sexual function are discussed further in Chap. 25 (page 545) and the development of sexual function in Chap. 28.

NERVOUS SYSTEM CONTROL OF RESPIRATION

Considering the fact that the act of breathing is entirely neurologic, it is surprising how little attention it has received other than from physiologists. Every component of breathing—the lifelong automatic cycling of inspiration, the transmission of coordinated nerve impulses to and from the respiratory muscles, the translation of systemic influences such as acidosis to the neuromuscular apparatus of the diaphragm—is under neural control. Moreover, respiratory failure is one of the most noteworthy disturbances of neurologic function in comatose states and in neuromuscular diseases such as myasthenia gravis, Guillain-Barré syndrome, and poliomyelitis. The major part of the treatment of these disorders consists of measures that assist respiration (mechanical ventilators). Finally, death—or brain death—is now virtually defined in terms of the ability of the nervous system to sustain respiration. A full understanding of respiration requires knowledge of the mechanical and physiologic workings of the lungs as organs of gas exchange; but here we shall limit our remarks to the nervous system control of breathing. Neurologists should be familiar with the alterations of respiration caused by diseases in different parts of the nervous system, the effects of respiratory failure on the brain, and the rationale that underlies modern methods of treatment.

The Central Respiratory Motor Mechanisms

It has been known for more than a century that breathing is controlled mainly by the lower brainstem, and that each half of the brainstem is capable of producing an independent respiratory rhythm. In patients with poliomyelitis, for example, the occurrence of respiratory failure was associated with lesions in the ventrolateral tegmentum of the medulla (Feldman, Cohen). Until recently, thinking on this subject was dominated by Lumsden's scheme of the breathing patterns that resulted from sectioning the brainstem of cats at various levels. He postulated the existence of several centers in the pontine tegmentum, each corresponding to an abnormal breathing pattern—a pneumotaxic center, an apneustic center, and a medullary gasping center. This scheme proves to be oversimplified when viewed in the light of modern physiologic experiments. It appears that neurons in several discrete regions discharge with each breath and generate the respiratory rhythm. However, these sites do not function in isolation, as individual oscillators, but interact with one another to generate the perpetual respiratory cycle; they contain both inspiratory and expiratory components.

Three paired groups of respiratory nuclei are oriented more or less in columns in the pontine and medullary tegmentum (see Fig. 26-7). They comprise (1) a ventral respiratory group (referred to as VRG) extending from the lower to the upper ventral medulla, in the region of the nucleus retroambiguus, (2) a dorsal medullary respiratory group (DRG) located dorsal to the obex and immediately ventromedial to the nucleus of the tractus solitaries (NTS), and (3) two clusters of cells in the dorsolateral pons in the region of the parabrachial nucleus.

From electrical stimulation experiments, it appears that these paired neurons in the dorsal pons may act as "on-off" switches in the transition between inspiration and expiration. Inspiratory neurons are concentrated in the dorsal respiratory group and in the rostral portions of the ventral group, some of which have monosynaptic connections to the motor neurons of the phrenic nerves and the nerves to the intercostal muscles. Normal breathing is actively inspiratory and only passively expiratory; however, under some circumstances of increased respiratory drive, the internal intercostal muscles and abdominal muscles actively expel air. The expiratory neurons that mediate this activity are concentrated in the caudal portions of the ventral respiratory group and in the most rostral parts of the dorsal group. On the basis of both neuroanatomic tracer and physiologic studies, it has been determined that these expiratory neurons project to spinal motor neurons and have an inhibitory influence on inspiratory neurons.

The pathway of descending fibers that arises in the inspiratory neurons and terminates on phrenic nerve motor neurons lies just lateral to the anterior horns of the upper three cervical cord segments. When this region is damaged, automatic but not voluntary diaphragmatic movement on that side is lost. As noted below, the fibers carrying voluntary volleys of motor impulses to the diaphragm course more dorsally in the cord. The phrenic

Figure 26-7

The location of the main centers of respiratory control in the brainstem as currently envisioned from animal experiments and limited human pathology. There are three paired groups of nuclei: A. *The dorsal respiratory group (DRG), containing mainly inspiratory neurons, located in the ventrolateral subnucleus of the nucleus of the tractus solitarius;* B. *A ventral respiratory group (VRG) situated near the nucleus ambiguus and containing, in its caudal part, neurons that fire predominantly during expiration and, in its rostral part, neurons that are synchronous with inspiration—the latter structure merges rostrally with the Botzinger complex, which is located just behind the facial nucleus and contains neurons that are active mostly during expiration;* C. *A pontine pair of nuclei (PRG), one of which fires in the transition between inspiration and expiration and the other between expiration and inspiration. The intrinsic rhythmicity of the entire system probably depends on interactions between all these regions, but the "pre-Botzinger" area in the rostral ventromedial medulla may play a special role in generating the respiratory rhythm. (Adapted from Duffin et al. by permission.)*

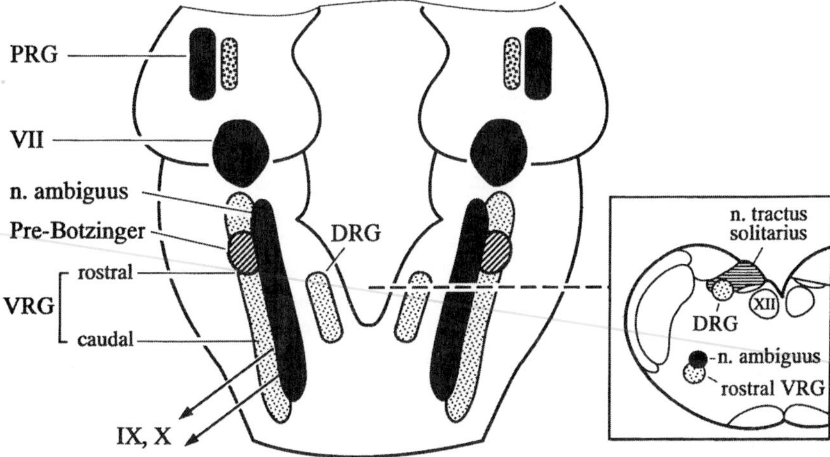

motor neurons form a thin column in the medial parts of the ventral horns, extending from the third through fifth cervical cord segments. Damage to these neurons precludes both voluntary and automatic breathing.

The exact locus in which the breathing rhythm is generated is not known. The conventional teaching has been that the dorsal respiratory group (DRG) was the dominant generator of the respiratory rhythm, but the situation is certainly more complex. Animal experiments have focused attention on the rostral ventrolateral medulla (VRG). This region contains a group of neurons in the vicinity of the "Botzinger complex" (which itself contains neurons that fire mainly during expiration). Cooling of this area or injecting it with neurotoxins that do not affect traversing axons causes the respiratory rhythm to be lost (see the review by Duffin et al). It has been shown that the paired respiratory nuclei in the pons that are thought to act as switches between inspiration and expiration also possess an autonomous rhythmicity, but their role in engendering cyclic breathing has not been clarified. Some workers are of the opinion that two or more sets of neurons in the VRG create a rhythm by their reciprocal activity or that oscillations arise within even larger networks (see Blessing for details). There are also centers in the pons that do not generate respiratory rhythms but may, under extreme circumstances, greatly influence them. One pontine group of respiratory neurons, the "pneumotaxic center," modulates the response to hypoxia, hyopcapnia, and lung inflation. In general, expiratory neurons are located laterally and inspiratory neurons medially in this center, but there is an additional group that lies between them and remains active during the transition between respiratory phases. Also found in the lower pons is a group of neurons that prevent unrestrained activity of the medullary inspiratory neurons ("apneustic center"). In addition to these ambiguities regarding a "center" for the generation of respiratory rhythm, there is the difficulty that the nuclei described above are not well defined in humans.

As to the effects of a unilateral brainstem lesion on ventilation, numerous cases of hypoventilation or total loss of automatic ventilation ("Ondine's curse"—see further on) have been recorded (Bogousslavsky et al). We have observed several such cases as well, due in most instances to a large lateral medullary infarction. If the neural oscillators on each side were totally independent, such a syndrome should not be possible. The explanation may be that a unilateral lesion interrupts the connections between each of the paired groups of nuclei, which normally synchronize the two sides in the generation of rhythmic bursts of excitatory impulses to spinal motor neurons.

Voluntary Control of Breathing During speech, swallowing, breath-holding, or voluntary hyperventilation, the automaticity of the brainstem mechanisms of respiration is arrested in favor of reflexive or of conscious control of diaphragmatic contraction. The observations of Colebatch and coworkers, utilizing PET scanning, indicate that voluntary control of breathing is associated with activity in the motor and premotor cortex. The experiments of Maskill and associates demonstrated that magnetic cortical stimulation of a region near the cranial vertex activates the diaphragm. Although automatic and voluntary breathing utilize the same pools of cervical motor neurons that give rise to the phrenic nerves, the descending cortical pathways for voluntary breathing are distinct from those utilized by automatic brainstem mechanisms. It is not known if the voluntary signal bypasses the brainstem mechanisms or is possibly integrated there. When both dorsal descending tracts subserving voluntary control are interrupted, as in the "locked-in syndrome," the independent, automatic respiratory system in the medulla is capable of maintaining perfectly regular breathing at 16 per minute with uniform tidal volumes.

These essential facts do not fully depict the rich interactions between the neuronal groups that govern respiration and the neurons for laryngeal and glottic activity that come into play during such coordinated acts as swallowing, sneezing, and coughing, and speaking.

Afferent Respiratory Influences A number of signals that modulate respiratory drive originate in chemoreceptors located in the carotid body and throughout the ascending aorta. The former are influenced mainly by changes in pH and the latter more by hypoxia. Chemoreceptor afferents pass along the carotid sinus nerves, which join the glossopharyngeal nerves and terminate in the NTS. Aortic body receptors send afferent volleys to the medulla through the aortic nerves, which join the vagus nerves. There are also chemoreceptors in the brainstem, but their precise location is uncertain. Their main locus is thought to be in the ventral medulla, but other areas that are responsive to changes in pH have been demonstrated in animals. What is clear is that these regions are sensitive not to the pH of CSF, as had been thought, but to the hydrogen content of the extracellular fluid of the medulla.

Numerous stretch receptors within smooth muscle cells of the airways also project via the vagus nerves to the NTS and influence the depth and duration of breathing. Afferent signals from these specialized nerve endings mediate the Hering-Breuer reflex, described in 1868—a shortened inspiration and increased tidal volume triggered by excessive lung expansion. The Hering-Breuer mechanism seems not to be important at rest, since bilateral vagal section has no effect on the rate or depth of respiration. These aspects of afferent pulmonary modulation of breathing have been reviewed by Berger and colleagues. It is interesting, however, that patients with high spinal transections and inability to breathe can still sense changes in lung volume, attesting to a nonspinal afferent route to the brainstem from lung receptors, probably through the vagus nerves. In addition, there are receptors located between pulmonary epithelial cells that respond to irritants such as histamine and smoke. They have been implicated in the genesis of asthma. Also there are "J-type" receptors that are activated by substances in the interstitial fluid of the lungs. These are capable of inducing hyperpnea and probably play a role in driving ventilation under conditions of pulmonary edema. Both the diaphragm and the accessory muscles of respiration contain conventional spindle receptors, but their role is not clear; all that can be said is that the diaphragm has a paucity of these receptors compared with other skeletal muscles and is therefore not subject to spasticity with corticospinal lesions or to the loss of tone in states such as rapid-eye-movement (REM) sleep, in which gamma motor neuron activity is greatly diminished.

Dyspnea The common respiratory sensations of breathlessness, air hunger, chest tightness, or shortness of breath, all subsumed under the term *dyspnea*, have defied neurophysiologic interpretation. In animals, Chen and colleagues have demonstrated that neurons in the thalamus and central midbrain tegmentum fire in a graduated manner as respiratory drive is increased. These neurons are influenced greatly by afferent information from the chest wall, lung, and chemoreceptors and are postulated to be the thalamic representation of sensation from the thorax that is perceived at a cortical level as dyspnea.

Aberrant Respiratory Patterns Many of the most interesting respiratory patterns observed in neurologic disease are found in comatose patients, and several of these patterns have been assigned localizing value of uncertain validity: *central neurogenic hyperventilation, apneusis, and ataxic breathing*. These are discussed in relation to the clinical signs of coma (Chap. 17) and sleep apnea (Chap. 19). Some of the most bizarre cadences of breathing—those in which unwanted breaths intrude on speech or those characterized by incoordination of laryngeal closure, diaphragmatic movement, or swallowing, or by respiratory tics—have been described in paraneoplastic brainstem encephalitis. Similar incoordinated patterns occur in certain extrapyramidal diseases. Patterns such as episodic tachypnea up to 100 breaths per minute and loss of voluntary control of breathing were noteworthy features in patients with postencephalitic parkinsonism. In *Leeuwenhoek disease*, named for the discoverer of the microscope, Leeuwenhoek, who described and suffered from the disease, there is a continuous epigastric pulsation and dyspnea in association with rhythmic bursts of activity in the inspiratory muscles—a respiratory myoclonus akin to palatal myoclonus.

Cheyne-Stokes breathing, the common and well-known waxing and waning type of cyclic ventilation reported by Cheyne in 1818 and elaborated by Stokes, has been ascribed to a prolongation of circulation time, as in congestive heart failure;, but there are data that support a primary neural origin of the disorder, particularly the observation that it occurs most often in patients with deep bilateral hemispheral lesions.

Another striking aberration of ventilation is a loss of automatic respiration during sleep, with preserved voluntary breathing ("*Ondine's curse*"). The term stems from the German myth in which Ondine, a sea nymph, condemns her unfaithful lover to a loss of all movements and functions that do not require conscious will. Patients with this condition are compelled to remain awake lest they stop breathing, and they must have nighttime mechanical ventilation to survive. Presumably the underlying pathology is one that selectively interrupts the ventrolateral descending medullocervical pathways that subserve automatic breathing. The syndrome has been documented in cases of unilateral and bilateral brainstem infarctions, hemorrhage, encephalitis (neoplastic or infectious—for example, due to *Listeria*), Leigh syndrome, and recovery from traumatic Duret hemorrhages. The issue of a loss of automatic ventilation as a result of a unilateral lesion has been addressed above. The converse of this state, in which there is complete loss of voluntary control of ventilation but preserved automatic monorhythmic breathing, has also been described (Munschauer et al). Incomplete variants of this latter phenomenon have been observed in cases of infarction or severe demyelinating disease and may be a component of the "locked-in state."

The *congenital central hypoventilation syndrome* is thought to be an idiopathic version of the loss of automatic ventilation (see Shannon et al). This rare condition begins in infancy with apneas and sleep disturbances of varying severity or later in childhood with signs of chronic hypoxia leading to pulmonary hypertension. As mentioned in Chap. 19, several subtle changes in the arcuate nucleus of the medulla and a depletion of neurons in regions of the respiratory centers have been found in this condition, but further study is necessary.

Neurologic lesions that cause *hyperventilation* are diverse and widely located throughout the brain, not just in the brainstem. In clinical practice, episodes of hyperventilation are most often seen in anxiety and panic states. The traditional view of "central neurogenic hyperventilation" as a manifestation of a pontine lesion has been brought into question by the observation that it may occur as a sign of cerebral lymphoma, in which postmortem examination has failed to show involvement of the brainstem regions controlling respiration (Plum).

Hiccup (singultus) is a poorly understood phenomenon. It does not seem to serve any useful physiologic purpose, existing only as a nuisance, and is not associated with any particular disease. It may occur as a component of the lateral medullary syndrome (page 844), with masses in the posterior fossa or medulla, and occasionally with generalized elevation of intracranial pressure or with metabolic encephalopathies such as uremia. Rarely, singultation may be provoked by medication, one possible offender in our experience being dexamethasone. Since the triggers of hiccup often seem to arise in epigastric organs adjacent to the diaphragm, it is considered to be a gastrointestinal reflex, more than a respiratory one. A physiologic study by Newsom Davis has demonstrated that hiccup is the result of powerful contraction of the diaphragm and intercostal muscles, followed immediately by laryngeal closure. This results in little or no net movement of air. He concluded that the projections from the brainstem responsible for hiccup are independent of the pathways that mediate rhythmic breathing. Within a single burst or run of hiccups, the frequency remains relatively constant, but at any one time it may range anywhere from 15 to 45 per minute. The contractions are most liable to occur during inspiration. They are inhibited by therapeutic elevation of arterial CO_2 tension. We cannot vouch for the numerous other methods that are said to suppress hiccups, but where the neurologist is asked to help in an intractable case, phenothiazines are sometimes effective.

Disorders of Ventilation Due to Neuromuscular Disease

Failure of ventilation in the neuromuscular diseases presents as one of two symptom complexes: one occurs in patients with acute generalized weakness, such as Guillain-Barré syndrome and myasthenia gravis, and the other in patients with subacute or chronic diseases, such as motor neuron disease, certain myopathies (acid maltase), and muscular dystrophy. The review by Polkey and colleagues provides a more extensive list. Patients in whom respiratory failure evolves rapidly, in a matter of hours, become anxious, tachycardic, and diaphoretic; they exhibit the characteristic signs of diaphragmatic paralysis. That is, they experience *paradoxical respiration*, in which the abdominal wall retracts during inspiration, owing to the failure of the diaphragm to contract, while the intercostal and accessory muscles create a negative intrathoracic pressure. Or these patients may have *respiratory alternans*, a pattern of diaphragmatic descent only on alternate breaths (this is more typical of airway obstruction). These signs appear in the acutely ill patient when the vital capacity has been reduced to approximately 25 percent of normal, or approximately 1 L.

In patients with chronic but stable weakness of the respiratory muscles, there occur signs of carbon dioxide (CO_2) retention, such as daytime somnolence, headache upon awakening, nightmares, and, in extreme cases, papilledema. The accessory muscles of respiration attempt to maximize tidal volume, and there is a tendency for the patient to gulp or assume a rounded "fish mouth" appearance in an effort to inhale additional air. In general, patients with chronic respiratory difficulty tolerate lower tidal volumes without dyspnea than do patients with acute disease, and symptoms in the former may occur only at night, when respiratory drive is diminished and compensatory mechanisms for obtaining additional air are in abeyance.

Also, treatment of the two conditions differs. Patients with the chronic type of respiratory failure may need only nighttime support, which can be provided by negative pressure devices such as a cuirass or preferably by intermittent positive pressure applied by a tight-fitting mask over the nose. These measures may also be used temporarily in acute situations, but invariably there will be need of a positive-pressure ventilator that provides a constant volume with each breath. This can be effected only through an endotracheal tube.

Typical ventilator settings in cases of acute mechanical respiratory failure, if there is no pneumonia, are for tidal volumes of 12 to 15 mL/kg, depending on the compliance of the lungs and the patient's comfort, at a ventilator rate between 4 and 12 breaths per minute, adjusted to the degree of respiratory failure. The tidal volume is kept relatively constant in order to prevent atelectasis, and only the rate is changed as the diaphragm becomes weaker or stronger. Decisions regarding the need for these mechanical devices are frequently difficult, since patients with chronic illnesses often become dependent on a ventilator. The presence of oropharyngeal weakness as a result of the underlying neuromuscular disease may leave the patient's airway unprotected and require endotracheal intubation before mechanical ventilation is necessary. It is also difficult to decide when to remove the endotracheal tube in cases of oropharyngeal weakness. Because the safety of the swallowing mechanism cannot be assessed with the tube in place, one must be prepared to reintubate the patient or to have a surgeon prepared to perform a tracheostomy after extubation, in the event that aspiration occurs.

From time to time a patient is encountered in whom the earliest feature of neuromuscular disease is *subacute respiratory failure*, manifest as dyspnea and exercise intolerance but *without other overt signs of neuromuscular disease*. Most such cases turn out to have motor neuron disease, but rare instances of myasthenia gravis, acid maltase deficiency, polymyositis, Lambert-Eaton syndrome, or chronic inflammatory demyelinating polyneuropathy may present in this way. The neurologist may be consulted in these cases after other physicians have found no evidence of intrinsic pulmonary disease. The spirometric flow-volume loop examination in mechanical-neuromuscular forms of respiratory failure shows low airflow rates with diminished lung volumes that together simulate a restrictive lung disease. Among such patients we have also found instances of an apparently isolated unilateral or *bilateral phrenic nerve paresis*, which had followed surgery or an infectious illness. The problem is probably akin to brachial neuritis (Parsonage-Turner syndrome, page 1427), in which the phrenic nerve can be implicated.

Neuromuscular Causes of Respiratory Failure in Critically Ill Patients Neurologists are increasingly being called upon to address the question of an underlying neuromuscular cause for respiratory failure in a *critically ill patient*. Aside from the diseases listed above, Bolton and colleagues have delineated a "critical illness polyneuropathy," which accounts for an inability to wean the patient from a ventilator when alternative causes for diaphragmatic weakness—such as malnutrition and hypokalemia—have been eliminated. Such a polyneuropathy has been identified by EMG in as many as 40 percent of patients in medical intensive care units. Most of the patients have been septic or have had multiorgan failure (see Chap 46). Less often, a "critical illness myopathy" that occurs in relation to administration of high-dose corticosteroids (Chap. 51) has been found as the cause of generalized weakness and respiratory failure. This unique polymyopathy occurs mainly in patients who are receiving postsynaptic blocking drugs such as pancuronium and high-dose steroids (page 1521). Severe hypophosphatemia is another cause of persistent weakness (page 1352).

The Neurology of Swallowing

The act of swallowing, like breathing, continues periodically through waking and sleep largely without conscious will or awareness. Swallowing occurs at a natural frequency of about five to six times per minute while an individual is idle; it is suppressed during concentration and emotional excitement.

The fundamental role of swallowing is to move food from the mouth to the esophagus and thereby to begin the process of digestion, but it also serves to empty the oral cavity of saliva and prevent its entry into the respiratory tract. Since the oropharynx is a shared conduit for breathing and swallowing, obligatory reflexes exist to assure that breathing is held in abeyance during swallowing. Because of this relationship and the frequency with which dysphagia and aspiration complicate neurologic disease, the neural mechanisms that underlie swallowing are of considerable importance to the neurologist and are described here. The reader is also referred to other parts of this book for a discussion of derangements of swallowing consequent upon diseases of the lower cranial nerves (Chap. 47), of muscle (Chap. 48), and of the neuromuscular junction (Chap. 53).

Anatomic and Physiologic Considerations A highly coordinated sequence of muscle contractions is required to move a bolus of food smoothly and safely through the oropharynx. This programmed activity may be elicited voluntarily or by reflex movements that are triggered by sensory impulses from the posterior pharynx. Swallowing normally begins as the tongue, innervated by cranial nerve XII, sweeps food to the posterior oral cavity, and brings the bolus into contact with the posterior wall of the oropharynx. As the food passes the pillars of the fauces, tactile sensation, carried through nerves IX and X, triggers (1) the contraction of levator and tensor veli palatini muscles, which close the nasopharynx and prevent nasal regurgitation, followed by (2) the upward and forward movement of the arytenoid cartilages toward the epiglottis (observed as an upward displacement of the hyoid and thyroid cartilages), which closes the airway. With these movements the epiglottis guides the food into the valleculae and into channels formed by the epiglottic folds and the pharyngeal walls. The airway is closed by sequential contractions of the arytenoid-epiglottic folds, and below them, the false cords, and then the true vocal cords, which seal the trachea. All of these contractions are effected largely by cranial nerve X (vagus). The contractions of the palatopharyngeal muscles pull the pharynx up over the bolus and the stylopharyngeal muscles draw the sides of the pharynx outward (nerve IX). At the same time, the upward movement of the larynx opens the cricopharyngeal sphincter. A wave of peristalsis then begins in the pharynx, pushing the bolus through the sphincter into the esophagus. These muscles relax as soon as the bolus reaches the esophagus.

Reflex swallowing requires only medullary functioning and is known to occur in the vegetative and locked-in states as well as in normal and anencephalic neonates. The sequence of muscle activity for swallowing is organized in a region of brainstem that roughly comprises a swallowing center, located in the region of the NTS and the adjacent reticular formation, close to the respiratory centers. This juxtaposition ostensibly allows the refined coordination of swallowing with the cycle of breathing. Besides a programmed period of apnea, there is a slight forced exhalation after each swallow that further prevents aspiration. The entire swallowing ensemble can be elicited by stimulation of the superior laryngeal nerve; this route is used in experimental studies. The studies of Jean, Kessler, and others (cited by Blessing), using microinjection of excitatory neurotransmitters, have localized the swallowing center in animals to a region adjacent to the termination of the superior laryngeal nerve. Unlike the generators of respiratory rhythm, the entire reflex apparatus for swallowing may be located in the NTS. There is, however, no direct connection between the NTS and the cranial nerve motor nuclei. Therefore it is presumed that control must be exerted through premotor neurons located in lateral brainstem regions. There have been few comparable anatomic studies of the structures responsible for swallowing in humans. As to the cortical regions that are involved in swallowing, it appears from PET studies that the inferior precentral gyrus and the posterior inferior frontal gyrus are activated, and lesions in these parts of the brain give rise to the most profound dysphagia.

Dysphagia and Aspiration Weakness or incoordination of the swallowing apparatus is manifest as dysphagia and, at times, aspiration. The patient himself is often able to discriminate one of several types of defect: (1) difficulty initiating swallowing, which leaves solids stuck in the oropharynx; (2) nasal regurgitation of liquids; (3) frequent coughing and choking immediately after swallowing and a hoarse, "wet cough" following the ingestion of fluids; and (4) some combination of these. It is surprising how often the tongue and the muscles that cause palatal elevation appear on direct examination to act normally despite an obvious failure of coordinated swallowing. In this regard, the utility of the gag reflex as a neurologic sign has been controversial. In our experience, palatal elevation in response to touching the posterior pharynx only assures that cranial nerves IX and X and the local musculature are not entirely dysfunctional; however, the presence of the reflex does not assure the smooth coordination of the swallowing mechanism and does not obviate the risk of aspiration. It should also be mentioned that difficulties with swallowing may begin subtly and express themselves as weight loss or as a noticeable increase in the time required to swallow and to eat a meal. Nodding or sideways head movements to assist the propulsion of the bolus, or the need to repeatedly wash food down with water, are other clues to the presence of dysphagia.

The first type of defect in the initiation of swallowing is usually attributable to weakness of the tongue and may be a manifestation of myasthenia gravis, motor neuron disease, or rarely inflammatory muscle diseases; it may be due to palsies of the twelfth cranial nerve (metastases at the base of the skull or meningoradiculitis) or to a number of other causes. There is usually an associated dysarthria with difficulty pronouncing lingual sounds. The second type of dysphagia, associated with nasal regurgitation of liquids indicates a failure of velopalatine closure and is characteristic of myasthenia gravis, tenth nerve palsy of any cause, or incoordination of swallowing due to bulbar or pseudobulbar palsy. A nasal pattern of speech with air escaping from the nose is a usual accompaniment.

The symptoms of aspiration, such as choking and others mentioned above, or of recurrent unexplained pneumonias ("silent aspiration"), have myriad causes that fall into four main categories: (1) weakness of the responsible musculature, due to lesions of the vagus on one or both sides; (2) a myopathy (myotonic and oculopharyngeal dystrophies) or neuromuscular disease (amyotrophic lateral sclerosis and myasthenia gravis); (3) a medullary lesion that affects the NTS or the cranial motor nuclei (lateral medullary infarction is the prototype) but syringomyelia-syringobulbia and rarely multiple sclerosis, polio, and brainstem tumors may have the same effects; or (4) a less well defined mechanism of slowed or discoordinated swallowing that arises either from corticospinal disease (pseudobulbar palsy, hemispheral stroke) or from diseases of the basal ganglia (mainly Parkinson disease) that alter the timing of breathing and swallowing and permitting the airway to remain open as food passes through the posterior pharynx. In the latter cases a decreased frequency of swallowing also causes saliva to pool in the mouth (leading to drooling) and adds to the risk of aspiration.

Aspiration and swallowing difficulty after severe stroke occur in a surprisingly large number of cases. This tends to happen during the first few days after a hemispheral stroke on either side of the brain (Meadows). These effects last 1 or 2 weeks and render the patient subject to pneumonia and fever even if only saliva is aspirated.

Pain on swallowing occurs under a different set of circumstances, the one of most neurologic interest being glossopharyngeal neuralgia (page 1456).

Videoflouoroscopy has become a very useful tool in determining the presence of aspiration during swallowing and in differentiating the several clinical types of dysphagia. The movement of the bolus by the tongue, the timing of reflex swallowing, and the closure of the pharyngeal and palatal openings are judged directly by observation of a bolus of food mixed with barium or of liquid barium alone. However, authorities in the field, such as Wiles, whose reviews are recommended (also Hughes and Wiles), warn that unqualified dependence on videofluoroscopy is unwise. They remark that observation of the patient swallowing water and repeated observation of the patient while eating can be equally informative. Having the patient swallow water is a particularly effective test of laryngeal closure; the presence of coughing, wet hoarseness or breathlessness, and/or the need to swallow small volumes slowly are indicative of a high risk of aspiration.

Based on bedside observations and videofluoroscopy, an experienced therapist can make recommendations regarding the safety of oral feeding, changes in the consistency and texture of the diet, postural adjustments, and the need to insert a tracheostomy or feeding tube.

REFERENCES

Aguayo AJ, Nair CPV, Bray GM: Peripheral nerve abnormalities in Riley-Day syndrome. *Arch Neurol* 24:106, 1971.

Ahlquist RP: A study of adrenotropic receptors. *Am J Physiol* 153:586, 1948.

Appenzeller O, Arnason BG, Adams RD: Experimental autonomic neuropathy: An immunologically induced disorder of reflex vasomotor function. *J Neurol Neurosurg Psychiatry* 28: 510, 1965.

Berger AJ, Mitchell JH, Severinghaus JW: Regulation of respiration. *N Engl J Med* 297:92, 1977.

Blaivas JG: The neurophysiology of micturition: A clinical study of 550 patients. *J Urol* 127:958, 1982.

Blessing WW: *The Lower Brainstem and Bodily Homeostasis.* New York, Oxford, 1997.

Blok BFM, Willemsen ATM, Holstege G: A PET study on brain control of micturition in humans. *Brain* 120:111, 1997.

Bogousslavsky J, Khurana R, Deruaz JP, et al: Respiratory failure and unilateral caudal brainstem infarction. *Ann Neurol* 28:668, 1990.

Bolton CF, Laverty DA, Brown JD, et al: Critically ill polyneuropathy: Electrophysiological studies and differentiation from Guillain-Barré syndrome. *J Neurol Neurosurg Psychiatry* 49:563, 1986.

Bradbury S, Eggleston C: Postural hypotension: A report of three cases. *Am Heart J* 1:73, 1925.

Brindley GS, Polkey CE, Rushton DN, Cardozo L: Sacral anterior root stimulation for bladder control in paraplegia: The first 50 cases. *J Neurol Neurosurg Psychiatry* 49:104, 1986.

Burnstock G: Innervation of vascular smooth muscle: Histochemistry and electron microscopy. *Clin Exp Pharmacol Physiol* 2(suppl):2, 1975.

Caird FI, Andrews GR, Kennedy RD: Effect of posture on blood pressure in the elderly. *Br Heart J* 35:527, 1973.

Cannon WB: *Bodily Changes in Pain, Hunger, Fear and Rage*, 2nd ed. New York, Appleton, 1920.

Carmel PW: Sympathetic deficits following thalamotomy. *Arch Neurol* 18:378, 1968.

Castro F de: Sensory ganglia of the cranial and spinal nerves: Normal and pathological, in Penfield W (ed): *Cytology of Cellular Pathology of the Nervous System.* New York, Hafner, 1965, pp 93–143.

Chen Z, Eldridge FL, Wagner PG: Respiratory-associated thalamic activity is related to level of respiratory drive. *Respir Physiol* 90:99, 1992.

Cohen J, Low P, Fealey R, et al: Somatic and autonomic function in progressive autonomic failure and multiple system atrophy. *Ann Neurol* 22:692, 1987.

Cohen MI: Neurogenesis of respiratory rhythm in the mammal. *Physiol Rev* 59:1105, 1979.

Colebatch JG, Adams L, Murphy K, et al: Regional cerebral blood flow during volitional breathing in man. *J Physiol (Lond)* 443:91, 1991.

Cooper JR, Bloom FE, Roth RH: *The Biochemical Basis of Neuropharmacology*, 7th ed., New York, Oxford University Press, 1996.

DeGroat WC: Nervous control of urinary bladder of the cat. *Brain Res* 87:201, 1975.

Denny-Brown D, Robertson EG: On the physiology of micturition. *Brain* 56:149, 1933.

Denny-Brown D, Robertson EG: The state of the bladder and its sphincters in complete transverse lesions of the spinal cord and cauda equina. *Brain* 56:397, 1933.

Duchen LW, Anjorin A, Watkins PJ, Mackay JD: Pathology of autonomic neuropathy in diabetes mellitus. *Ann Intern Med* 92:301, 1980.

Duffin J, Kazuhisa E, Lipski J: Breathing rhythm generation: focus on the rostral ventrolateral medulla. *News Physiol Sci* 10:133, 1995.

Dyck PJ, Kawamer Y, Low PA, et al: The number and sizes of reconstituted peripheral, autonomic, sensory, and motor neurons in a case of dysautonomia. *J Neuropathol Exp Neurol* 37:741, 1978.

Fagius J, Westerber CE, Olson Y: Acute pandysautonomia and severe sensory deficit with poor recovery: A clinical, neurophysiological, and pathological case study. *J Neurol Neurosurg Psychiatry* 46:725, 1983.

Falck B: Observations on the possibilities of the cellular localization of monoamines by a fluorescence method. *Acta Physiol Scand* 56(suppl 197), 1962.

Feldman JL: Neurophysiology of breathing in mammals, in FE Bloom (ed): *Handbook of Physiology*. Vol IV: *The Nervous System*. Bethesda, MD, American Physiological Society, chap 9, 1986, pp 463–524.

Fowler CJ: Neurological disorders of micturition and their treatment. *Brain* 122:1213, 1999.

Geiger H, Naraghi R, Schobel HP, et al: Decrease of blood pressure by ventrolateral medullary decompression in essential hypertension. *Lancet* 352:446, 1998.

Gutrecht JA: Sympathetic skin response. *J Clin Neurophysiol* 11:519, 1994.

Hoeldtke RD, Dworkin GE, Gaspar SR, Israel BC: Sympathotonic orthostatic hypotension: A report of 4 cases. *Neurology* 39:34, 1989.

Hoff JT, Reis DJ: Localization of regions mediating the Cushing response in CNS of cat. *Arch Neurol* 23:228, 1970.

Hoffman BB, Lefkowitz RJ, Taylor P: Neurotransmission: The autonomic and somatic motor nervous systems, in Hardman JG, Limbird LE (eds): *Goodman and Gilman's The Pharmacological Basis of Therapeutics*, 9th ed. New York, McGraw-Hill, 1996, pp 105–139.

Holstege G, Tan J: Supraspinal control of motorneurons innervating the striated muscles of the pelvic floor, including urethral and anal sphincters in the cat. *Brain* 110:1323, 1987.

Hughes TA, Wiles CM: Neurogenic dysphagia: the role of the neurologist. *J Neurol Neurosurg Psychiatry*. 64:569, 1998.

Jansen SP, Sguyen XV, Karpitsky V, et al: Central command neurons of the sympathetic nervous system: Basis of the fight-or-flight response. *Science* 270:644, 1995.

Keane JR: Oculosympathetic paresis: Analysis of 100 hospitalized patients. *Arch Neurol* 36:13, 1979.

Kirby R, Fowler CV, Gosling JA, et al: Bladder dysfunction in distal autonomic neuropathy of acute onset. *J Neurol Neurosurg Psychiatry* 48:762, 1985.

Krane RJ, Siroky MD (eds): *Clinical Neurourology*, 2nd ed. Boston, Little, Brown, 1991.

Lafferty K, Roberts VC, deTrafford JC, et al: On the nature of Raynaud's phenomenon: The role of histamine. *Lancet* 2:313, 1983.

Lewis P: Familial orthostatic hypotension. *Brain* 87:719, 1964.

Low PA: *Clinical Autonomic Disorders*, 2nd ed. Philadelphia, Lippincott-Raven, 1997.

Low PA, Dyck PJ: Splanchnic preganglionic neurons in man: II. Morphometry of myelinated fibers of T7 ventral spinal root. *Acta Neuropathol* 40:219, 1977.

Low PA, Dyck PJ, Lambert EH: Acute panautonomic neuropathy. *Ann Neurol* 13:412, 1983.

Luhan JA, Pollack SL: Occlusion of the superior cerebellar artery. *Neurology* 3:77, 1953.

Lumsden T: Observations on the respiratory centers. *J Physiol (Lond)* 57:354, 1923.

Mannen T, Iwata M, Toyokura Y, Nagashima K: Preservation of a certain motoneuron group of the sacral cord in amyotrophic lateral sclerosis: Its clinical significance. *J Neurol Neurosurg Psychiatry* 40:464, 1977.

Maskill D, Murphy K, Mier A, et al: Motor cortical representation of the diaphragm in man. *J Physiol (Lond)* 443:105, 1991.

McLeod JG, Tuck RR: Disorders of the autonomic nervous system. Part I: Pathophysiology and clinical features. Part II: Investigation and treatment. *Ann Neurol* 21:419, 519, 1987.

Meadows JC: Dysphagia in unilateral cerebral lesions. *J Neurol Neurosurg Psychiatry* 36:853, 1973.

Munschauer FE, Mador MJ, Ahuja A, Jacobs L: Selective paralysis of voluntary but not limbically influenced automatic respiration. *Arch Neurol* 48:1190, 1991.

Nathan PW, Smith MC: The location of descending fibers to sympathetic neurons supplying the eye and sudomotor neurons supplying the head and neck. *J Neurol Neurosurg Psychiatry* 49:187, 1986.

Newsom Davis J: An experimental study of hiccup. *Brain* 39:851, 1970.

Onufrowicz B: On the arrangement and function of cell groups of the sacral region of the spinal cord of man. *Arch Neurol Psychopathol* 3:387, 1900.

Oppenheimer D: Neuropathology of autonomic failure, in Bannister R (ed): *Autonomic Failure*, 2nd ed. New York, Oxford University Press, 1988, chap 25, pp 451–463.

Pasztor A, Pasztor E: Spinal vasomotor reflex and Cushing response. *Acta Neurochir* 52:85, 1980.

Penfield W, Jasper H: *Epilepsy and the Functional Anatomy of the Human Brain*. Boston, Little, Brown, 1954, p 414.

Petito CK, Black IB: Ultrastructure and biochemistry of sympathetic ganglia in idiopathic orthostatic hypotension. *Ann Neurol* 4:6, 1978.

Pick J: *The Autonomic Nervous System*. Philadelphia, Lippincott, 1970.

Plum F: Cerebral lymphoma and central hyperventilation. *Arch Neurol* 47:10, 1990.

Polinsky RJ: Neuropharmacological investigation of autonomic failure, in Mathias CJ, Bannister R (eds): *Autonomic Failure: A Textbook of Clinical Disorders of the Autonomic Nervous System*, 4th ed. New York, Oxford University Press, 1999, pp 334–358.

Polinsky RJ, Kopin IJ, Ebert MH, Weise V: Pharmacologic distinction of different orthostatic hypotension syndromes. *Neurology* 31:1, 1981.

Polkey MI, Lyall RA, Moxham J, Leigh PN: Respiratory aspects of neurological disease. *J Neurol Neurosurg Psychiatry* 66:5, 1999.

Porter JM, Rivers SP, Anderson CS, Baur GM: Evaluation and management of patients with Raynaud's syndrome. *Am J Surg* 142:183, 1981.

Rajput AH, Rozdilsky B: Dysautonomia in parkinsonism: A clinico-pathologic study. *J Neurol Neurosurg Psychiatry* 39:1092, 1976.

Robinson B, Johnson R, Abernethy D, Holloway L: Familial distal dysautonomia. *J Neurol Neurosurg Psychiatry* 52:1281, 1989.

Ropper AH: Acute autonomic emergencies and autonomic storm, in Low PA (ed), *Clinical Autonomic Disorders*, 2nd ed. Boston, Little Brown, 1997, chap. 5, pp 791–801.

Ropper AH, Wijdicks WFM, Truax BT: *Guillain-Barré Syndrome*. Philadelphia, Davis, 1991, pp 109–112.

Ruch T: The urinary bladder, in Ruch TC, Patton HD (eds): *Physiology and Biophysics*. Vol 2: *Circulation, Respiration, and Fluid Balance*. Philadelphia, Saunders, 1974, pp 525–546.

Sakakibara R, Hattori T, Yasuda K, et al: Micturitional disturbance and the pontine tegmental lesion: urodynamic and MRI analyses of vascular cases. *J Neurol Sci* 141:105, 1996.

Samuels MA: Cardiopulmonary aspects of acute neurologic disease, in Ropper AH (ed): *Neurological and Neurosurgical Intensive Care*, 3rd ed. New York, Raven Press, 1993, pp 103–120.

Schobel HP, Fischer T, Heuszer K, et al: Preeclampsia—A state of sympathetic overactivity. *N Engl J Med* 335:1480, 1996.

Schuster MM: Clinical significance of motor disturbances of the enterocolonic segment. *Am J Dig Dis* 11:320, 1966.

Selye H: The general adaptation syndrome and the diseases of adaptation. *J Clin Endocrinol Metab* 6:117, 1946.

Shannon DC, Marsland DW, Gould JB, et al: Central hypoventilation during quiet sleep in two infants. *Pediatrics* 57:342, 1976.

Shy GM, Drager GA: A neurological syndrome associated with orthostatic hypotension: A clinical-pathologic study. *Arch Neurol* 2:511, 1960.

Spokes EGS, Bannister R, Oppenheimer DR: Multiple system atrophy with autonomic failure. *J Neurol Sci* 43:59, 1979.

Tansey EM: Chemical neurotransmission in the autonomic nervous system: Sir Henry Dale and acetylcholine. *Clin Auton Res* 1:63, 1991.

Thompson PD, Melmon KL: Clinical assessment of autonomic function. *Anesthesiology* 29:724, 1968.

Vernino S, Low PA, Fealey RD, et al: Autoantibodies to ganglionic acetylcholine receptors in autoimmune autonomic neuropathies. *New Engl J Med* 343:847, 2000.

Weiss HD: The physiology of human penile erection. *Ann Intern Med* 76:792, 1972.

Wiles CM: Neurogenic dysphagia. *J Neurol Neurosurg Psychiatry* 54:1037, 1991.

Young RR, Asbury AK, Corbett JL, Adams RD: Pure pan-dysautonomia with recovery: Description and discussion of diagnostic criteria. *Brain* 98:613, 1975.

Ziegler MG, Lake R, Kopin IJ: The sympathetic nervous system defect in primary orthostatic hypotension. *N Engl J Med* 296:293, 1977.

Chapter 27

THE HYPOTHALAMUS AND NEUROENDOCRINE DISORDERS

The hypothalamus plays a triple role in the actions of the nervous system. The first, as the "head ganglion" of the autonomic nervous system, was described in the preceding chapter; the second, as the circadian and seasonal clock for behavioral and sleep-wake functions, was considered in Chap. 19, on sleep; its third role, as the neural control center of the endocrine system, is the subject of this chapter. In the hypothalamus, these systems are integrated with one another as well as with neocortical, limbic, and spinal influences. Together, they maintain homeostasis and provide the substructure of emotion and affective behavior.

The expansion of knowledge of neuroendocrinology during the past few decades stands as one of the most significant achievements in neurobiology. It has been learned that neurons, in addition to transmitting electrical impulses, can synthesize and discharge complex molecules into the systemic circulation, and that these molecules are capable of activating or inhibiting endocrine, renal, and vascular cells at distant sites.

The concept of neurosecretion probably had its origins in the observations of Speidel, in 1919 (and later, of the Scharrers in 1929), who noted that some of the hypothalamic neurons had the morphologic characteristics of glandular cells. Their suggestion that such cells might secrete hormones into the bloodstream was so novel, however, that it was rejected by most biologists at the time. This seems surprising now that neurosecretion is viewed as a fundamental part of the science of endocrinology.

Following these early observations, it was found that certain peptides secreted by neurons in the central and peripheral nervous systems were also contained in glandular cells of the pancreas, intestines, and heart. This seminal observation was made in 1931 by Euler and Gaddum, who isolated a substance from the intestines that was capable of acting on smooth muscle. But it was not until some 35 years later that Leeman and her associates purified the substance and identified it as substance P (see Aronin et al). Then followed the discovery of somatostatin by Brazeau and colleagues in 1973 and the endogenous opioids (enkephalin) by Hughes and coworkers in 1975; subsequently a series of hypothalamic releasing factors that act on the pituitary gland have been isolated.

THE HYPOTHALAMUS

Anatomic Features

The hypothalamus lies on each side of the third ventricle and is continuous across its floor. It is bounded posteriorly by the mammillary bodies, anteriorly by the optic chiasm and lamina terminalis, superiorly by the hypothalamic sulci, laterally by the optic tracts, and inferiorly by the hypophysis. It comprises three main nuclear groups, the standard nomenclature for which was proposed in 1939 by Rioch and colleagues: (1) the anterior group, which includes the preoptic, supraoptic, and paraventricular nuclei; (2) the middle group, which includes the tuberal, arcuate, ventromedial, and dorsomedial nuclei; and (3) the posterior group, comprising the mammillary and posterior hypothalamic nuclei.

Nauta and Haymaker have subdivided the hypothalamus sagitally. The *lateral part* lies lateral to the fornix; it is sparsely cellular and its cell groups are traversed by the medial forebrain bundle, which carries finely myelinated and unmyelinated ascending and descending fibers to and from the rostrally placed septal nuclei, substantia innominata, nucleus accumbens, amygdala, and piriform cortex, and the caudally placed tegmental reticular formation. The *medial hypothalamus* is rich in cells, some of which are the neurosecretory cells for pituitary regulation and visceral control. It contains two main efferent fiber systems—the mammillothalamic tract of Vicq d'Azyr, which connects the mammillary nuclei with the anterior thalamic nucleus (which, in turn, projects to the cingulate gyrus), and the mammillotegmental tract. Additional structures of importance are the stria terminalis, which runs from the amygdala to the ventromedial hypothalamic nucleus, and the fornix, which connects the hippocampus to the mammillary body, septal nuclei, and periventricular parts of the hypothalamus. The lateral and medial parts of the hypothalamus are interconnected and their functions are integrated.

The inferior surface of the hypothalamus, just posterior to the pituitary stalk, bulges downward slightly; this region is known as the tuber cinerium. From the center of the tuber arises the *median eminence or infundibulum*; the latter stands out because of its vascularity (the hypophysial-portal system of veins courses over the surface). The infundibulum extends into the pituitary stalk, which, in turn, enters the pars nervosa of the hypophysis (Fig. 27-1). The median eminence assumes special importance because of the intimate relation of its cell groups to the anterior lobe of the pituitary gland. It represents the interface between converging pathways from the brain and the master gland of the endocrine system. The supraopticohypophysial fibers terminate on capillaries of the outer zone of the median eminence (Martin and Reichlin). The tuberoinfundibular neurons of the arcuate nucleus and anterior periventricular nuclei synthesize most of the releasing factors described below (Fig. 27-1).

The abundant blood supply of the hypothalamus (from several feeding arteries) is of importance to neurosurgeons who attempt to obliterate aneurysms that derive from adjacent vessels. Many small radicles, arising from the posterior and anterior communicating arteries as well as from the most proximal portions of the anterior and posterior cerebral arteries, form a network of such redundancy that infarction of the hypothalamus is infrequent.

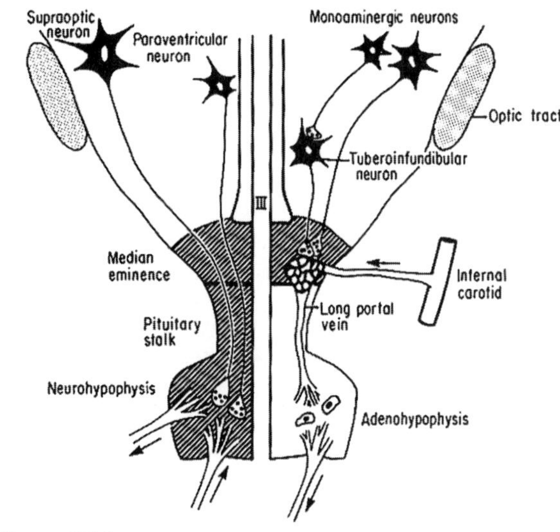

Figure 27-1

Diagram of the hypothalamic-pituitary axis. Indicated on the left is the hypothalamic-neurohypophysial system, consisting of supraoptic and paraventricular neurons, axons of which terminate on blood vessels in the posterior pituitary (neurohypophysis). The hypothalamic-adenohypophysial system is illustrated on the right. Tuberoinfundibular neurons, the source of the hypothalamic regulatory hormones, terminate on the capillary plexus in the median eminence. (Courtesy of Dr. J. B. Martin.)

The Hypothalamic Releasing Hormones

Thyrotropin-Releasing Hormone (TRH) This was the first of the releasing hormones to be identified; its tripeptide structure was determined in 1968. The hormone is elaborated by the anterior periventricular, paraventricular, arcuate, ventromedial, and dorsomedial neurons but not by those of the posterior hypothalamic or thalamic nuclei. Mainly, it stimulates the release of thyroid-stimulating hormone (TSH) from the pituitary gland, and the latter, in turn, effects the release of T_4 (thyroxine) and T_3 (triiodothyronine). Pituitary cells that release dopamine and somatostatin are also stimulated; the latter has an inhibitory effect on TSH. There is also an inhibitory feedback of T_3 on TSH and TRH. Actually, more than half of brain TRH is found outside the hypothalamus—in brainstem raphe nuclei, tractus solitarius, and the anterior and lateral horn cells of spinal cord—suggesting that TRH may function as a central regulator of the autonomic nervous system.

Growth Hormone–Releasing Hormone (GHRH) This hormone and somatostatin (also known as GH-release inhibiting hormone, or SRIH) are both secreted by specialized tuberoinfundibular neurons and released into the hypophysial-portal circulation, by which they are carried to specific GH-secreting cells of the anterior pituitary gland (somatotropes). Immunohistochemical staining has shown the sources of GHRH and somatostatin to be neurons of the posterior part of the arcuate and ventromedian nuclei and other neurons of the median eminence and premammillary area. Somatostatin, a 14–amino acid peptide, is produced more anteriorly by neurons in the periventricular area and small-cell part of the paraventricular nucleus. The amygdala, hippocampus, and other limbic structures project to the arcuate nuclei via the medial corticohypothalamic tract (in the stria terminalis) and are believed to account for the sleep- and stress-induced fluctuations of GH and somatostatin. Also, it has been demonstrated that all four biogenic amines (dopamine, norepinephrine, epinephrine, and serotonin) influence GH regulation, as does acetylcholine, either by direct action on pituitary somatotropic cells or on hypothalamic regulatory neurons. Thyrotropin-releasing hormone also increases GH from somatotropes. Many of the latter pituitary cells contain large eosinophilic granules, but others, previously identified incorrectly as chromophobe cells, also contain GH. Somatomedin C, a basic peptide that is synthesized in the liver, exerts feedback control of GH by inhibiting the pituitary somatotropes and stimulating the release of somatostatin. Growth hormone enhances skeletal growth by stimulating the proliferation of cartilage and growth of muscle. It also regulates lipolysis, stimulates the uptake of amino acids in cells, and has anti-insulin effects. The blood concentrations of GH fluctuate from 1 or 2 to over 60 ng/mL, being highest within the first hour or two after the onset of sleep.

Corticotropin-Releasing Hormone (CRH) This hormone, a 14–amino acid peptide, acts synergistically with vasopressin to release adrenocorticotropic hormone (ACTH) from basophilic cells in the pituitary. ACTH stimulates the synthesis and release of the hormones of the adrenal cortex, mainly glucocorticoids (cortisol or hydrocortisone) but also mineralocorticoids (aldosterone) and androcorticoids (converted in the tissues to testosterone). The neurons of origin of CRH lie in a particular part of the paraventricular nucleus, other cells of which form the paraventricular-supraopticohypophysial tract (neurohypophysis) and elaborate vasopressin and oxytocin and several other substances (neurotensin, dynorphin, vasoactive intestinal peptide). These hypothalamic cells receive an extensive input from other regions of the nervous system, particularly via the noradrenergic pathways (from reticular neurons in the medulla, and those of the locus ceruleus and tractus solitarius) and from many of the limbic structures. Presumably, these extrahypothalamic connections provide the mechanism by which stress and pain activate the secretion of ACTH and cortisol. Corticotropin-releasing hormone itself is widely distributed in the brain. There is feedback control of CRH and ACTH via glucocorticoid receptors in the hypothalamus and anterior lobe of the pituitary. Serotonin and acetylcholine enhance ACTH secretion, whereas the catecholamines are inhibitory.

Gonadotropin-Releasing Hormone (GnRH) This 10–amino acid peptide originates in the arcuate nucleus and is present in highest concentration near the median eminence. It effects the release of the two gonadotropic hormones—luteinizing hormone (LH) and follicle-stimulating hormone (FSH). The ovary and testis, by secreting a peptide called *inhibin*, are able to suppress FSH, as do gonadal steroids, i.e., estrogens. GnRH is under the influence of other neuronal systems, which are modulated by catecholamines, serotonin, acetylcholine, and dopamine. Puberty, menstruation, ovulation, lactation, and menopause are all related to the effects of GnRH, FSH, and LH on the ovaries, uterus, breasts, and testes. Normal levels of blood FSH are 2.5 to 4.9 ng/mL in prepuberty and 7.5 to 11 ng/mL in the adult; levels of blood LH are 2.8 to 9.6 ng/mL in prepuberty and 10 to 18 ng/mL in the adult.

Prolactin-Releasing Hormone (PRH) This hormone is released by neurons in the region of the arcuate nucleus and activates lactotropic cells of the anterior pituitary. However, a number of other peptides—thyroid-releasing factor, vasoactive intestinal peptide, peptide-histidine-isoleucine, and oxytocin—also have the capacity to raise the levels of prolactin in the blood. The hypothalamopituitary axis is responsive to sensory stimuli from the nipples, via pathways in the spinal cord and brainstem, accounting for the effect of suckling on milk production. The normal blood levels of prolactin are 5 to 25 ng/mL. The release of prolactin is also influenced by an inhibitory dopaminergic innervation of pituitary lactotrophic cells. This mechanism accounts for galactorrhea and reproductive disorders, which occur with tumors that compress the pituitary stalk and interrupt the venous portal transport of dopamine from the hypothalamus.

The Neurohypophysis: Vasopressin and Oxytocin

The oliogopeptides *vasopressin* and *oxytocin* are elaborated by cells of the supraoptic and paraventricular nuclei and are transported, via their axons, through the stalk of the pituitary to its posterior lobe, where the substances are stored. Together, these elements constitute the neurohypophysis (posterior pituitary), which develops as an evagination of the floor of the third ventricle. Some of the vasopressin-containing nerve endings also terminate on cells of origin of the autonomic nervous system and on the capillary plexus of the hypophysial portal circulation, through which they influence the secretion of CRH and GH. The peptide parts of vasopressin and oxytocin, whose chemical nature was determined by duVigneaud, are almost identical, differing from one another by only two amino acids.

Vasopressin, acting upon the kidney tubules, serves as the antidiuretic hormone (ADH) and, complemented by thirst mechanisms, maintains the osmolality of the blood. Plasma osmolality modifies vasopressin secretion by acting directly on the supraoptic and paraventricular neurons or on separate osmoreceptors in the hypothalamus. The sensitivity of the vasopressin-ADH mechanism is demonstrated by the absence of antidiuretic effect when vasopressin is below 1 pg/mL and by maximal antidiuresis when plasma ADH reaches 5 pg/mL. If serum osmolality falls below 280 mosm/L, the release of ADH is completely inhibited. This system is most effective in maintaining homeostasis when serum osmolality is relatively close to the normal range, between 280 and 295 mosm/L.

Alterations in blood volume and pressure also affect vasopressin release through neural mechanisms that have their origin in baro- and mechanoreceptors of the aortic arch, carotid sinus, and right atrium. Afferent signals from these regions are conveyed in the vagus and glossopharyngeal nerves, which synapse in the nucleus of the tractus solitarius; the precise pathways to the hypothalamus have not been delineated, however. With severe hypotension, ADH release will continue despite a low serum osmolality. Vasopressin secretion is also influenced by nonosmotic factors. Nausea, for example, is a potent stimulus, raising levels of the hormone 100-fold. Hypoglycemia has a less profound effect. Drugs such as morphine, nicotine, alcohol, and certain chemotherapeutic agents (cyclophosphamide) also cause release of the stored peptide. Pain, emotional stress, and exercise have long been thought to cause release of vasopressin, but it is unclear whether this is a direct effect or is mediated through hypotension or nausea.

Oxytocin initiates uterine contraction and has milk-ejecting effects. Its release is stimulated by distention of the cervix, labor, breast feeding, and estrogen. The effects of oxytocin are inhibited by alcohol.

In summary, it is apparent that the regulatory system of hypothalamic releasing hormones is extremely complex. The releasing factors have overlapping functions, and the hypothalamic nuclei act on many parts of the brain in addition to the pituitary. Conversely, many parts of the brain influence the hypothalamus through neural connections, or modulate its activity and that of the pituitary gland through the action of neurotransmitters and modulators (catecholamines, acetylcholine, serotonin, and dopamine). There is feedback control between every part of the hypothalamus and the endocrine structures on which it acts. The factors that influence hypothalamic neurons have been reviewed in detail by Reichlin. Some of these relationships have been mentioned and others will emerge further on in this chapter and in later chapters, particularly as they relate to behavioral and psychiatric disorders.

Of particular significance is the role of the hypothalamus in the integration of the endocrine and autonomic nervous systems at both the peripheral and central levels. The best-known example of this interaction is in the adrenal medulla, as indicated in Chap. 26. Similarly, the juxtaglomerular apparatus of the kidney and the islets of Langerhans of the pancreas function as neuroendocrine transducers, in that they convert a neural stimulus (in these cases adrenergic) to an endocrine secretion (renin from the kidney and glucagon and insulin from the islet cells).

Role of the Hypothalamus in Sexual Development

The hypothalamus also plays a critical role in the development of human sexuality and its expression, a theme elaborated in the next chapter. The suprachiasmatic nucleus and the number of neurons it contains is considerably larger in men than in women, a dimorphism that becomes evident during postnatal development. The interstitial nucleus of the hypothalamus is reportedly smaller in the homosexual male, evidence perhaps that homosexuality has a recognizable morphologic basis (Levay). This biological evidence has been sharply challenged (Byne). In our opinion, Levay's observations have not been confirmed. The intimate relationship of the hypothalamus with the development of sexual characteristics at all stages of life is shown by the appearance, in the infundibular area, of hypertrophic neurons that are rich in estrogen receptors; it has been proposed that some of the symptoms of menarche are timed and mediated by these hypothalamic neurons. With aging, and even more so with Alzheimer disease, the neuronal population in this region decreases markedly; the sleep disturbances of senescence and some aspects of the "sundowning" syndrome have been attributed to this cell loss.

Regulation of Sympathetic and Parasympathetic Activity

Finally, the central role of the hypothalamus in the regulation of both sympathetic and parasympathetic activities needs to be emphasized. This aspect of hypothalamic function is discussed fully in the preceding chapter (pages 556 and 569).

The Pineal Gland and Melatonin

The pineal gland, or pineal body, is a small glandular structure (about 9 mm in diameter) that projects from the dorsal diencephalon and lies just posterior to the third ventricle. In the past the pineal body figured prominently in philosophic and religious writings; for Descartes it was the seat of the soul. When this idea was discredited, the pineal gland was relegated to the status of a vestigial organ. The identification of the pineal hormone, melatonin—followed by recognition of its role in maintaining biologic rhythms and the modulating effects on its secretion by the circadian light-dark cycle—revived scientific interest in the structure. Even though the hormone was found to have an indirect effect on several other neuroendocrine systems, neurologists took little interest in pineal function because ablation of the gland in humans, with attendant loss of most of the circulating melatonin, led to few if any clinical changes.

It is the cyclic secretion of melatonin that appears to be the most important activity of the pineal gland. However, melatonin secretion is more accurately regarded as a linked manifestation of the circadian rhythm than its controlling mechanism. The main cellular element of the gland, the pinealocyte, is thought to be derived from neural photoreceptors in lower vertebrates. The latter cells, structurally analogous to retinal cones, transduce light directly into neural impulses and are one of the mechanisms for circadian entrainment of hormonal rhythms. In humans, the pineal no longer possesses the ability to transduce light directly. However, it does retain an input from photic stimuli and influences the circadian light-dark cycle through a pathway that originates in the retina, synapses in the suprachiasmatic nucleus, passes through descending sympathetic tracts to the intermediolateral cell columns and superior cervical ganglia, and then ascends to innervate noradrenergic terminals on the pinealocytes. Darkness elicits a release of norepinephrine from the photoreceptors, stimulating the synthesis and release of melatonin. During daylight the retinal photoreceptor cells are hyperpolarized, norepinephrine release is inhibited, and there is little melatonin production. The concentration of the hormone peaks between 2 and 4 A.M. and gradually falls thereafter. An approximate circadian rhythmicity to melatonin release is preserved in continuous darkness, and the blind maintain a light suppression of secretion. It is readily appreciated that, in humans, it is difficult to separate the changes that occur in the suprachiasmatic nucleus from those of the pineal.

Like other neuroendocrine cells, pinealocytes release peptides that are produced in the Golgi apparatus and packaged in secretory granules. Whether secretion is the main mechanism for melatonin release is unclear because these cells can utilize an alternative ependymal type of vacuolar secretion. The entire gland is invested by a rich vasculature to receive the released peptide (in some mammals the blood flow per gram of pineal tissue is surpassed only by that of the kidney). The biochemistry and physiology of melatonin have been extensively reviewed by Brzezinski.

In humans a regular feature of pineal pathology is the accumulation of calcareous deposits, commonly thought to be calcium but actually composed of carbonate-containing hydroxyapatite. These concretions, are formed within vacuoles of pinealocytes and released into the extracellular space. This mineralization of the pineal body provides a convenient marker for its position in plain films and on various imaging studies.

It is of significance that pineal tumors do not secrete melatonin, but the loss of melatonin may be used as a marker for the completeness of surgical pinealectomy. Most interest in the past several years has centered around melatonin as a soporific agent and its potential to reset sleep rhythms. Its concentration in depressive illnesses, especially in the elderly, is also decreased.

HYPOTHALAMIC SYNDROMES

Hypothalamic syndromes are of two distinct types (Martin and Reichlin). In one, all or many hypothalamic functions are disordered, often in combination with signs of disease in contiguous structures ("global hypothalamic syndromes," as described below). The second type is characterized by a selective loss of hypothalamic-hypophysial function, attributable to a discrete lesion of the hypothalamus and often resulting in a deficiency or overproduction of a single hormone—*a partial hypothalamic syndrome.*

Global Hypothalamic Syndromes

A variety of lesions can invade and destroy all or a large part of the hypothalamus. These include sarcoid and other granulomatous diseases (histiocytosis X), an idiopathic inflammatory disease, and germ-cell and other tumors.

The hypothalamus is involved in approximately 5 percent of cases of sarcoidosis, sometimes as the primary manifestation of the disease, more often in combination with facial palsy and hilar lymphadenopathy. An elevation of angiotensin-converting factor, particularly in the cerebrospinal fluid (CSF), confirms the diagnosis. The lesions are visible by MRI (see Fig. 32-2).

Tumors that involve the hypothalamo-pituitary axis include metastatic carcinoma, lymphoma, craniopharyngioma, and a variety of germ-cell tumors. The latter (reviewed by Jennings et al) include germinomas, teratomas, embryonal carcinoma, and choriocarcinoma. They develop during childhood, tend to invade the posterior hypothalamus, and are accompanied in some instances by an increase in serum alpha fetoprotein or the beta subunit of chorionic gonadotropin.

Among the inflammatory conditions, infundibuloneurohypophysitis, or *infundibulitis*, is a cryptogenic inflammation of the neurohypophysis and pituitary stalk, with thickening of these parts by infiltrates of lymphocytes (mainly T cells) and plasma cells (Imura et al). It is thought to be an autoimmune disorder. Histiocytosis X, a group of diseases comprised of (Letterer-Siwe disease, Hand-Schüller-Christian disease, and eosinophilic granuloma) implicates multiple organs, including the hypothalamus and neighboring structures and leptomeninges (often causing cells in CSF). These conditions pursue an indolent course in children. The cell type is a proliferating histiocyte.

Partial Hypothalamic Syndromes

Diabetes Insipidus (DI) As long ago as 1913, Farini of Venice and von den Velden of Dusseldorf (quoted by Martin and Reichlin) independently discovered that diabetes insipidus (DI) was associated with destructive lesions of the hypothalamus. They showed, moreover, that in patients with this disorder, the polyuria could be corrected by injections of extracts of the posterior pituitary. Ranson elucidated the anatomy of the neurohypophysis and the Scharrers traced the posterior pituitary secretion to granules in the cells of the supraoptic and paraventricular nuclei and followed their passage to axon terminals in the posterior lobe of the pituitary. DuVigneaud and colleagues determined the chemical structure of the two neurohypophysial peptides, vasopressin and oxytocin, of which these granules were composed. These observations opened up the entire field of neuroendocrinology.

The usual cause of DI is a lack of vasopressin (antidiuretic hormone, ADH) as a result of a lesion of the neurohypophysis. This leads to a reduction in its action in the kidneys, where it normally promotes the absorption of water. As a consequence there is diuresis of low-osmolar urine (polyuria), reduction in blood volume, and increased thirst and drinking of water (polydipsia) in an attempt to maintain osmolality. A congenital abnormality of renal tubular epithelium or destruction of the epithelium has a similar effect—nephrogenic DI. The latter is of interest to the neurologist because of its association with lithium toxicity.

Among the established *causes of acquired DI*, the most important are brain tumors, infiltrative granulomatous diseases, head injury, and intracranial surgical trauma (which has become less frequent with the transphenoidal approach to pituitary tumors). In one series of 135 cases of persistent DI reported by Moses and Streeten, 25 percent were idiopathic, 15 percent complicated primary brain tumors, 24 percent were postoperative (mostly after hypophysectomy or surgery for craniopharyngioma), 18 percent were due to head trauma, and fewer than 10 percent were associated with intracranial histiocytosis, metastatic cancer, sarcoidosis, and ruptured aneurysm. We have been impressed by hypothalamic disorders that become manifest years after whole-brain radiation for tumor. Such patients exhibit disruption of sleep patterns, diminished libido, and abnormalities of thirst and appetite. Hyperprolactinemia is a regular feature of this condition, as detailed by Mechanick and colleagues. Granulomatous infiltration of the base of the brain by sarcoid, eosinophilic granuloma, Letterer-Siwe disease, or Hand-Schüller-Christian disease is a more frequent cause of DI in young patients. Of the primary tumors, glioma, hamartoma and craniopharyngioma, granular cell tumor (choristoma), large chromophobe adenomas, and pinealoma are notable causes of DI. The primary tumors can present with DI alone, whereas the granulomatous infiltrating processes generally exhibit other systemic manifestations before polydipsia and polyuria appear. Metastatic tumors originating in the lung or breast or leukemic infiltration may cause DI, sometimes in conjunction with pituitary disturbances and impairment of vision. The most extreme cases of hypothalamic destruction occur in brain death, in which DI is a regular component, although not always evident at the time brainstem reflexes are lost.

Pituitary tumors are infrequently associated with DI unless they become massive and invade the stalk of the pituitary and the infundibulum. This has been substantiated by surgical sections of the stalk for metastatic carcinoma and retinitis proliferans, which result in DI only if the section is high enough to produce retrograde degeneration of supraoptic neurons.

Among the idiopathic forms of DI, there also exists a *congenital type of hypothalamic DI* of which only a small number of familial cases has been described. The disorder exists throughout life, owing to a developmental defect of the supraoptic and paraventricular nuclei and smallness of the posterior lobe of the pituitary. This defect has been related in some cases to a point mutation in the vasopressin-neurophysin-glycopeptide gene. It may be combined with other genetic disorders such as diabetes mellitus, optic atrophy, and deafness (Wolfram syndrome), and Friedreich ataxia.

Acquired idiopathic DI may occur at any age, most often in childhood or early adult life and more often in males, and it may not have an apparent cause. Other signs of hypothalamic or pituitary disease are lacking in 80 percent of such patients, but steps must be taken to exclude other disease processes by repeating the endocrine and radiologic studies periodically. In some cases of idiopathic DI, there are serum antibodies that react with the supraoptic neurons, raising the question of an autoimmune disorder. In a few such instances, postmortem examination has disclosed a decreased number of neurons in the supraoptic and paraventricular nuclei. Also, anorexia nervosa is often associated with mild DI.

In all these conditions, the severity and permanence of the DI are determined by the nature of the lesion. In cases of acute onset, three phases have been delineated: first, a severe DI lasting days; then, as the neurohypophysis degenerates, a reduction in severity of DI due to release of stored ADH; and finally a persistent pattern, usually lifelong. The neurohypophysial axons can regenerate, allowing for some degree of recovery, even after years.

Diagnosis of DI This is always suggested by the passage of large quantities of dilute urine accompanied by polydipsia and polyuria lasting throughout the night. The last two signs are, of course, obviated in an unresponsive patient, in which case careful measurement of fluid output and input are needed to expose the disorder. The thirst mechanism and drinking usually prevent dehydration and hypovolemia, but if the patient is stuporous or the thirst mechanism is inoperative, severe dehydration and hypernatremia can occur, leading to stupor, coma, seizures, and death. A 6- to 8-h dehydration test increases urinary osmolality in a person with normal kidneys and neurohypophysis; it is this change in urine concentration that is most useful in the differential diagnosis of polyuria, particularly in distinguishing compulsive water drinkers from those with DI. In DI a low urine osmolality and specific gravity are found, in conjunction with high serum osmolality and sodium values. Proof that the patient has a central cause of DI and not nephrogenic unresponsiveness to vasopressin is obtained by injecting 5 units of vasopressin (Pitressin) subcutaneously; this will diminish urine output and increase osmolality. A radioimmunoassay for plasma ADH is available; ADH is usually reduced to less than 1.0 pg/mL in patients with DI (normal, 1.4 to 2.7 pg/mL). Osmotic dehydration as a cause of the polydipsia-polyuria syndrome, such as glycosuria of diabetes mellitus, must, of course, be excluded.

Treatment of DI Vasopressin tannate in oil, synthetic lysin vasopressin nasal spray, and a long-acting analogue of arginine vasopressin (DDAVP) administered by nasal insufflation (10 to 20 mg or 0.1 to 0.2 mL) are used to control chronic DI. The latter drug is generally preferred because of its long antidiuretic action and few side effects. In unconscious patients, aqueous vasopressin, 5 to 10 units given subcutaneously, is effective for 3 to 6 h; DDAVP, 1 to 4 mg subcutaneously, is effective for 12 to 24 h. These drugs must be given repeatedly, depending on urine output and osmolality (we have also given these drugs intravenously in critical situations). The brief duration of action of the medication is advantageous in postoperative states and after head injury, for it allows the recognition of recovery of neurohypophyseal function and the avoidance of water intoxication. If a longer duration of treatment is anticipated, one uses vasopressin tannate in oil (2.5 units), the action of which persists for 24 to 72 h. In the unconscious patient, great care must be taken in the acute stages to replace the fluid lost in the urine, but not to the point of water intoxication. These problems can be avoided by matching the amount of intravenous fluids to urinary volume and by evaluating serum and urine osmolalities every 8 to 12 h. For patients with partial preservation of ADH function, chlorpropamide, clofibrate, or carbamazepine can be used to stimulate release of the hormone.

Syndrome of Inappropriate Antidiuretic Hormone (SIADH) Secretion As mentioned, blood volume and osmolality are normally maintained within narrow limits by the secretion of ADH and the thirst mechanism. A reduction in osmolality of even 1 percent stimulates osmoreceptors in the hypothalamus to decrease ADH and to suppress thirst and drinking; increased osmolality and reduced blood volume do the opposite. Normally, blood osmolality is about 282 mmol/kg and is maintained within a very narrow range. Release of ADH begins when it reaches 287 mmol/kg (osmotic threshold). At this point, plasma ADH levels are 2 pg/mL and increase rapidly as the osmolality rises. The response of ADH secretion to hyperosmolality is not the same for all plasma solutes; in contrast to hypernatremia, for example, hyperosmolality induced by elevations in urea nitrogen or endogenous glucose produce minimal or no elevations in ADH.

Derangement of this delicately regulated mechanism, taking the form of dilutional hyponatremia and water retention without edema, is observed under a variety of clinical circumstances. Instead of suppression of ADH secretion by water retention, the plasma ADH is above normal or inappropriately normal despite plasma hypo-osmolality. The term *inappropriate secretion of antidiuretic hormone* (SIADH) was applied to this syndrome by Schwartz and Bartter because of its similarity to that produced in animals by the chronic administration of ADH. The same syndrome can arise from ectopic production of the hormone by tumor tissue. In such cases, the thirst mechanism is not inhibited by decreased osmolality, and continued drinking further increases blood volume and reduces its solute concentration. The physiologic hallmarks of this condition are a concentrated urine, usually with an osmolality above 300 mosm/L, and low serum osmolality and sodium concentrations. Because of the dilutional effects, urea nitrogen and uric acid are reduced in the blood and serve as markers for excessive total body water. Tissue edema is not seen because sodium excretion in the urine is maintained by suppression of the renin-angiotensin system and by an increase in atrial natriuretic peptide secretion (see below).

SIADH is observed frequently with a variety of cerebral lesions (infarct, tumor, hemorrhage, meningitis, encephalitis) that do not involve the hypothalamus directly and with many types of local hypothalamic disease (trauma, surgery, vascular lesions). In most cases it tends to be a transient feature of the underlying illness. The acute dysautonomia of Guillain-Barré syndrome is a common cause of SIADH, and hyponatremia is particularly likely to occur in patients being ventilated mechanically. The increased thoracic pressure induced by positive pressure ventilation promotes SIADH in susceptible patients. Acute porphyric episodes have the same effect. Neoplasms, particularly oat-cell tumors and sometimes inflammatory lesions of the lung, may elaborate an ADH-like substance, and certain drugs—such as chlorpromazine, carbamazepine, chlorothiazide, chlorpropamide, clofibrate, nonsteroidal anti-inflammatory agents, and vincristine—also stimulate ADH release. In some cases, no cause or associated disease is apparent.

A fall in serum sodium to 120 to 125 meq/L usually has no apparent clinical effects, although symptoms from an associated neurologic disease, such as a previous stroke or a subdural hematoma, may worsen. Sodium levels of less than 120 meq/L are attended by nausea and vomiting, inattentiveness, drowsiness, stupor, and generalized seizures. As is characteristic of most metabolic encephalopathies, the more rapid the decline of the serum sodium, the more likely it is that there will be accompanying neurologic symptoms.

Treatment of SIADH The rapid restitution of serum sodium to normal or above-normal levels carries a risk of producing central pontine myelinolysis. Our usual procedure in patients with serum sodium concentrations of 117 to 126 meq/L is to slowly correct the sodium concentration by restricting water to 400 to 800 mL/day and to verify the desired urinary loss of water by checking the patient's weight and serum sodium until it reaches the lower 130 meq/L range. If there is drowsiness, confusion, or seizures that cannot be confidently attributed to the underlying neurologic illness or if the serum sodium is in the range of 100 to 115 meq/L, isotonic or 3% NaCl should be infused over 3 to 4 h and furosemide 20 to 40 mg administered to prevent fluid overload. A safe clinical rule is to raise the serum sodium by no more than 12 meq/L in the first 24 h and by no more than 20 meq/L in 48 h (see also page 1193).

Neurogenic (Cerebral) Salt Wasting Moderate lowering of the serum sodium is a common finding in patients with acute intracranial diseases and postoperatively in neurosurgical patients. Originally it was described as a "cerebral salt-wasting" syndrome by Peters and colleagues and later was erroneously identified with the then newly described Schwartz-Bartter syndrome of SIADH. In recent years it has again come to be recognized as being due to natriuresis and not to water retention caused by ADH secretion. As Nelson and colleagues had demonstrated, neurosurgical patients with hyponatremia and ostensibly with SIADH showed, instead, a reduction in blood volume, suggesting sodium loss rather than water retention. This distinction has important clinical implications, because the use of fluid restriction to treat SIADH can have disastrous results if a state of volume contraction exists from salt wasting. A leading hypothesis concerning the mechanism of hyponatremia in these cases is secretion of another oligopeptide, atrial natriuretic factor (ANF), found mainly in the walls of the cardiac atria but also in neurons surrounding the third ventricle in the anteroventral hypothalamic region. Physiologically, ANF activity opposes that of ADH in the kidney tubules and also has a potent inhibitory effect on ADH release from the hypothalamus. (See review by Samson). ANF, like some other neural peptides, may be secreted in bursts, and the natriuresis is evident only if total urinary sodium content is measured over many hours or a day.

The role of ANF in the hyponatremia that follows subarachnoid hemorrhage remains controversial (see Wijdicks et al and Diringer et al for opposing views), but it is our experience that the hyponatremia in this condition comes mainly from salt loss, not from water retention. Often, cerebral salt wasting and SIADH are combined. Because fluid restriction in this setting may lead to cerebral ischemia from vasospasm, the proper approach is to maintain intravascular volume with intravenous fluids and to correct hyponatremia by normal saline infusions. Salt wasting has also been reported with cerebral tumors, after pituitary surgery, and in the dysautonomia that occurs in some cases of Guillain-Barré syndrome, circumstances that have also been associated with SIADH. In each of these disorders, should the patient be hyponatremic, it is desirable to determine the intravascular volume and the urine sodium output before instituting treatment.

Other Disturbances of ADH and Thirst Conditions have been described in which the osmoreceptor control of ADH and of thirst appear to be dissociated. One of our patients, reported by Hayes and coworkers, repeatedly developed severe hypernatremia (levels as high as 180 to 190 meq/L), at which time he became confused and stuporous. Although the patient was able to initiate a release of ADH, his thirst mechanism was nonfunctional. Only when the patient was compelled to drink water at regular intervals did his serum sodium fall. Robertson and others have described similar cases with abnormalities of thirst. These have been reported under the title of "central" or "essential" hypernatremia.

Pituitary Insufficiency

Loss of function of the anterior pituitary gland may result from disease of the pituitary itself or from hypothalamic disease. In either event, it leads to a number of clinical abnormalities, each predicated on the deficiency of one or more hormones that depend on the pituitary trophic factors described earlier. The condition of *panhypopituitarism* represents the more serious illness in that it requires supplementation with multiple hormones. Hypopituitarism may have its onset in childhood, either as an inherited process that affects individual or multiple hormones or as a secondary process due to a destructive lesion of the pituitary or the hypothalamus from tumor, e.g., craniopharyngioma. Later in life the causes vary, but the most common are pituitary surgery, infarct of the gland from a rapidly growing adenoma (*pituitary apoplexy*, page 717), involutional changes that occur at the end of pregnancy (Sheehan syndrome), cranial irradiation for cerebral tumors other than those in the pituitary fossa, lymphocytic hypophysitis, and granulomatous and neoplastic invasion. The clinical features of pituitary failure vary, but impairments of thyroid function tend to be more prominent than those of adrenal failure. The neurologic accompaniments of pituitary failure depend on the underlying cause; Lamberts and colleagues have reviewed the endocrinologic aspects.

Other Hypothalamic Syndromes

Apart from diabetes insipidus and SIADH, there are a variety of other special clinical phenomena attendant upon disease of the hypothalamus. These usually occur not in isolation but in various combinations, comprising a number of rare but widely known syndromes.

Precocious Puberty This term refers to the abnormally early onset of androgen secretion and spermatogenesis in boys and of estrogen secretion and cyclic ovarian secretion in girls. It is associated with the premature development of secondary sexual characteristics. The occurrence of precocious puberty always calls for a neurologic as well as an endocrine investigation. In the male, one searches for evidence of a teratoma of the pineal gland or mediastinum or an androgenic tumor of the testes or adrenals. In the female with early development of secondary sexual characteristics and menstruation, one seeks other evidence of hypothalamic disease as well as an estrogen-secreting ovarian tumor. A hamartoma of the hypothalamus (part of von Recklinghausen disease or of polyostotic fibrous dysplasia) is a leading cause of precocious puberty in both boys and girls; in a number of such cases, so-called *gelastic seizures* have been conjoined (Breningstall). Neurologic study entails CT and MRI imaging of the hypothalamus, ovaries, and adrenals.

Adiposogenital Dystrophy (Froehlich Syndrome) Under this title, in 1901, Froehlich first described the association of obesity and gonadal underdevelopment. He related the disorder to a pituitary tumor. But a few years later, Erdheim recognized that the same syndrome could be a manifestation of a lesion (a suprasellar cyst in his case) involving or restricted to the hypothalamus. Later it was determined that obesity and hypogonadism could occur together or separately and were often combined with a loss of vision and unprovoked rage, aggression, or antisocial behavior. Diabetes insipidus may be conjoined. In some patients, the clinical state is characterized by abulia, apathy, and reduced verbal output. The usual causes of the Froehlich syndrome are craniopharyngioma, adamantinoma, and glioma, but many other tumors have been reported (pituitary adenoma, cholesteatoma, lipoma, meningioma, glioma, angiosarcoma, and chordoma). The condition bears clinical similarities to the Prader-Willi syndrome, in which hypothalamic abnormalities are not found (page 1068).

Hypothalamic Disorders Associated with Alterations in Weight Precise neuroanatomic studies have localized a satiety center in the ventromedial nucleus of the hypothalamus and an appetite center in the ventrolateral nucleus. Lesions in the lateral hypothalamus may result in a failure to eat and, in the neonate, to thrive; lesions in the medial hypothalamus, in overeating and obesity. Bray and Gallagher, who analyzed eight cases of the latter type, concluded that the critical lesion was a bilateral destruction of the ventromedial regions of the hypothalamus. Most of the reported cases of this type have been due to tumors, particularly craniopharyngioma, and some to trauma, inflammatory disease, and hydrocephalus (Suzuki et al). In a case that lent itself to clinicopathologic correlation, Reeves and Plum found that a hamartoma had destroyed the medial eminence and the ventromedial nuclei bilaterally but had spared the lateral hypothalamus. Hyperphagia and rage reactions were the main clinical features; the associated polydipsia and polyuria were due to extension of the tumor to the anterior hypothalamus.

It is evident that in only a tiny fraction of obese persons can the problem be traced to a hypothalamic lesion. Of overriding importance are genetic factors, such as the number of lipocytes that one inherits and their ability to store fat. Stunkard and associates have shown that the body mass (weight in kilograms divided by height in meters) of babies that grow to adulthood in adopted families reflects the weight class of their biologic parents and not that of their adopted ones. This applies to thin adults as well. Swedish twin studies have yielded similar results. This, of course, does not eliminate environmental influences; sedentary life in a food-laden society encourages obesity. Interest in recent years has been centered on the possible role of an obesity (ob) gene and its hormonal product, leptin. Animals with mutations in the ob gene are obese and lose weight when given leptin, and the evidence to date indicates that most obese persons are insensitive to leptin, perhaps explaining their tendency to store fat (Considine et al).

Since obesity is known to have adverse effects on health, preventive efforts should be directed to children at risk of becoming fat. There are no safe, effective antiobesity medications (or surgical measures); reliance must be placed on dieting and educating patients as to the need to change their eating habits. The problem also comes into play in women with pseudotumor cerebri (page 667), in whom marked weight loss is often the most effective treatment. Gastric plication is a popular surgical measure in some institutions for the treatment of morbid obesity, and has been tried in pseudotumor, but it is a hazardous procedure and often proves to be unsuccessful in the long term.

A rare disorder of infants has been described under the title of *diencephalic syndrome*. Progressive and ultimately fatal emaciation (failure to thrive), despite normal or near-normal food intake, in an otherwise alert and cheerful infant is the main clinical feature. The lesion has usually proved to be a low-grade astrocytoma of the anterior hypothalamus or optic nerve (Burr et al).

Extrahypothalamic parts of the brain, if diseased, may also be associated with increased food-seeking behavior, food ingestion, and weight gain. Examples are involvement of limbic structures, as in the Klüver-Bucy syndrome (page 545) and basal frontal lobe lesions leading to gluttony.

Anorexia Nervosa and Bulimia The special syndromes called *anorexia nervosa* and *bulimia* have been difficult to classify and are mentioned in this chapter only because they are associated with alterations in several hypothalamic functions, including appetite, temperature control, and menstruation. In all likelihood, these alterations are not the result of a primary dysfunction of hypothalamic nuclei but are secondary to the extreme weight loss, which is the primary feature of the disease. However, a causal link between these idiopathic diseases and hypothalamic dysfunction has been tentatively suggested by the rare patients with anorexia nervosa who were later found to have hypothalamic tumors (Bhanji and Mattingly, Berek et al, and Lewin et al).

Anorexia nervosa (and bulimia) are probably best regarded as disorders of behavior, in this case an obsession with thinness, for which reason they are discussed with the psychiatric disorders (see page 1604). But the developmental nature of the disease (arising in early adolescence), its virtual absence in men, and the hypothalamic alterations mentioned above do not allow the dismissal of a primary disorder of the brain's appetite centers.

Abnormalities of Growth Presumably, in most instances of growth retardation, there is a deficiency of GHRH or of GH per se. In the Prader-Willi syndrome (obesity, hypogonadism, hypotonia, mental retardation, and short stature) Bray and Gallagher found the deficiency to be one of GHRH. In certain congenital and developmental diseases, the hypothalamus appears to be incapable of releasing GH. This appears to be the case, in the de Morsier septo-optic defect of the brain (median facial cleft, cavum septum pellucidum, optic defect), Stewart and colleagues found an isolated deficiency of GH. In children with idiopathic hypopituitarism in whom stunting of growth is associated with other endocrine abnormalities, the deficiency is probably in the synthesis or release of GHRH. In some dwarfs (Laron dwarf, Seckel bird-headed dwarf), there are extremely high levels of circulating GH, suggesting either a defect in the GH molecule or an unresponsiveness of target organs. Many patients with the more severe forms of mental retardation are subnormal in height and weight, but the explanation for this has not been ascertained. It has not been reducible to changes in the level of GHRH or GH.

Of course, the vast majority of unusually short children who are otherwise healthy do not have a recognizable defect in GH or GHRH. Often their parents are short. The therapeutic use of GH in such children is a controversial matter. The hormone effects a spurt in growth during the first year of its administration, but whether it significantly influences growth in the long term is still under investigation. There is concern about the risk of transmitting prion or viral diseases through administration of the biologically derived hormone; this problem is obviated if genetically produced hormone is used.

In *gigantism*, most of the reported cases have been due to pituitary adenomas that secrete an excess of GH. This must occur prior to closure of the epiphyses. Hypersecretion of GH after closure of the epiphyses results in *acromegaly*. The notion of a purely hypothalamic form of gigantism or acromegaly (hypothalamic acromegaly) has been affirmed by Asa and associates, who described six patients with hypothalamic gangliocytomas that produced GHRH. The possibility of an ectopic source of GH must also be considered.

The mentally retarded individuals with gigantism described by Sotos and coworkers were found to have no abnormalities of GHRH, GH, or somatomedin.

Disturbances of Temperature Regulation Bilateral lesions in the anterior parts of the hypothalamus, specifically of temperature-sensitive neurons in the preoptic area, may result in *hyperthermia*. The heat-dissipating mechanisms of the body, notably vasodilation and sweating, are impaired. This effect has followed operations or other trauma in the region of the floor of the third ventricle but is seen most often after massive rupture of an anterior communicating artery aneurysm. The temperature rises to 41°C (106°F) or higher and remains at that level until death some hours or days later, or it drops abruptly with recovery. Acetylsalicylic acid has little effect on central hyperthermia; the only way to control it is by active evaporative cooling of the body while administering sedation. A less dramatic example of the loss of natural circadian temperature patterns is seen in patients with postoperative damage in the suprachiasmatic area (Cohen and Albers) and suprachiasmatic metastasis (Schwartz et al). These types of lesions are invariably associated with other disorders of intrinsic rhythmicity, including sleep and behavior. It should be emphasized, however, that instances of "central fever" are rare, and unexplained fever of moderate degree should not be attributed to a putative brain lesion.

Hyperthermia is also part of the *malignant hyperthermia* syndrome, in which there is an inherited (autosomal dominant) susceptibility to develop hyperthermia and muscle rigidity in response to inhalation anesthetics and skeletal muscle relaxants (page 1563); it is due to a defective ryanodine receptor on the calcium channel. Closely related is the *neuroleptic malignant syndrome*, which is the result of an idiosyncratic reaction to neuroleptic drugs (page 1265). Wolff and colleagues have described a syndrome of *periodic hyperthermia*, associated with vomiting, hypertension, and weight loss and accompanied by an excessive excretion of glucocorticoids; the symptoms had no apparent explanation, although there was a symptomatic response to chlorpromazine.

Lesions in the posterior part of the hypothalamus have had a different effect; i.e., they often produce *hypothermia* (a persistent temperature of 35°C or less) or *poikilothermia* (equilibration of body and environmental temperatures). The latter may pass unnoticed unless the patient's temperature is taken after lowering and raising the room temperature. Somnolence, confusion, and hypotension may be associated. *Spontaneous periodic hypothermia*, probably first described by Gowers, has been found in association with a cholesteatoma of the third ventricle (Penfield) and with agenesis of the corpus callosum (Noel et al). Episodically, there are symptoms of autonomic disturbance—salivation, nausea and vomiting, vasodilation, sweating, lacrimation, and bradycardia; the rectal temperature may fall to 30°C and seizures may occur. Penfield referred to these attacks incorrectly as "diencephalic epilepsy" (page 567). Between attacks, which last a few minutes to an hour or two, neurologic abnormalities are usually not discernible and temperature regulation is normal.

Chronic hypothermia is a more familiar state than hyperthermia, being recorded in cases of hypothyroidism, hypoglycemia, and uremia; after prolonged immersion or exposure to cold; and in cases of intoxication with barbiturates, phenothiazines, or alcohol. It tends to be more frequent among elderly patients, who are often found to have an inadequate thermoregulatory mechanism.

Cardiovascular Disorders with Hypothalamic Lesions Ranson (1939) demonstrated a number of autonomic effects upon stimulation of the hypothalamus; these effects as well as hypertension were recorded in Penfield's case of "diencephalic epilepsy", mentioned above. Since Byer and colleagues' description of large, upright T waves and prolonged Q-T intervals in patients with stroke, it has been appreciated that acute lesions of the brain—particularly subarachnoid hemorrhage and head trauma—may be accompanied by changes in the electrocardiogram (ECG) as well as by supraventricular tachycardia, ectopic ventricular beats, and ventricular fibrillation. Most of the same effects can be induced by very high levels of circulating norepinephrine and corticosteroids. Considering the numerous catastrophic lesions of the brain as well as extreme emotional states that can provoke arrhythmias and other changes in the ECG, the hypothalamus, with its limbic connections and ability to mount a massive sympathoadrenal discharge, is the likely source of these autonomic changes. Cropp and Manning found that the changes seen in the ECG, particularly "cerebral T waves" and other reversible repolarization abnormalities, could occur almost instantaneously (too quickly for attribution to circulating factors) during surgery for a cerebral aneurysm. Again, the hypothalamus is implicated, but as yet no direct evidence links this structure to direct cardiac control.

Gastric Hemorrhage In experimental animals, lesions placed in or near the tuberal nuclei induce superficial erosions or ulcerations of the gastric mucosa in the absence of hyperacidity (Cushing ulcers). Gastric lesions of similar type are seen in patients with several types of acute intracranial disease (particularly subdural hematoma and other effects of head injury, cerebral hemorrhages, and tumors). In seeking causative lesions, as in patients dying with cardiac changes, one searches in vain for a lesion in the various hypothalamic nuclei. A functional disorder in this region is nonetheless suspected.

"Neurogenic" Pulmonary Edema Following the original observations by Maire and Patton in humans, numerous cases of massive and often fatal pulmonary edema have been described in relation to catastrophic intracranial lesions—head injury, subarachnoid and intracerebral hemorrhage, bacterial meningitis and status epilepticus being the usual ones. A sudden elevation in intracranial pressure occurs in most cases, usually accompanied by a brief bout of extreme systemic hypertension but without left ventricular failure—which is the reason the pulmonary edema has been attributed to a "neurogenic" rather than a cardiogenic cause. It has also been shown that experimental lesions in the caudal hypothalamus are capable of producing this type of pulmonary edema, but almost always in the context of brief and extreme systemic hypertension. The caudal sympathetic part of the hypothalamus is tonically inhibited by adjacent neurons in the lateral preoptic region, and both the pulmonary edema and hypertensive response can be prevented by sympathetic blockade. The rapid rise in vascular resistance and systemic pressure is similar to the pressor reaction obtained by destruction of the nucleus of the tractus solitarius, as described in Chap. 26, and a few instances of neurogenic edema have followed damage to the medullary tegmentum (Brown et al).

The question remains, however, whether the hypothalamus exerts a direct sympathetic influence upon the pulmonary vasculature, allowing a leakage of protein-rich edema fluid, or if the edema is the result of sudden and massive overloading of the pulmonary circulation by a shift of fluid from the systemic vasculature. The latter theory is currently favored. Likewise, the role of circulating catecholamines and adrenal steroids has not been fully elucidated. These issues have been summarized by Samuels.

Disorders of Consciousness and Personality Since Ranson's original experimental work in monkeys (1939), it has been appreciated that acute lesions in the posterior and lateral parts of the hypothalamus are associated in some way with stupor or coma, although it has always been difficult to determine the precise structures that were involved. One can be certain that permanent coma from small lesions in the diencephalon may occur in the absence of any changes in the hypothalamus, and, conversely, that chronic hypothalamic lesions may be accompanied by no more than drowsiness or confusion or no mental change at all. In one of our cases, involving an infundibuloma entirely confined to the hypothalamus, the patient lay for weeks in a state of torpor, drowsy and confused. His blood pressure was low, his body temperature was 34 to 35°C, and he had diabetes insipidus. When aroused, he was aggressive, like the patient of Reeves and Plum (see above). Among the cases of acquired changes in personality and sleep patterns from ventral hypothalamic disease that we have seen, a few have been impressive because of a tendency to a hypomanic, hypervigilant state with insomnia, lasting days on end, and an impulsiveness and disinhibition suggestive of involvement of the frontal connections to the hypothalamus. These and other cognitive disorders with hypothalamic lesions are difficult to interpret and are usually transient. Often the lesions are acute and involve adjacent areas, making it impossible to attribute them to the hypothalamus alone.

Periodic Somnolence and Bulimia (Kleine-Levin Syndrome) Kleine in 1925 and Levin in 1936 described an episodic disorder characterized by somnolence and overeating. For days or weeks, the patients, mostly adolescent boys, sleep 18 or more hours a day, awakening only long enough to eat and attend to toilet needs. They appeared dull, often confused, and restless and were sometimes troubled by hallucinations. In the series of 18 cases collected by Critchley, the age range was from puberty to 45 years. The episodes varied in duration from 2 days to 12 weeks and in frequency from 2 to 12 yearly. The condition has also been seen in females. The somnolence has been well studied by modern laboratory methods and, except for the total duration of sleep, the individual components of the non-rapid-eye-movement (NREM) and rapid-eye-movement (REM) cycles are normal. Between episodes these patients are behaviorally and cognitively normal.

The cause of the condition is disputed. The hyperphagia has suggested a hypothalamic disorder, but anatomic verification is lacking. The case reported by Carpenter and coworkers, in which an acute and chronic inflammation in the medial thalamus but not the hypothalamus was found, must be questioned as representative of the idiopathic adolescent condition. Their patient was a man of 39 years of age who had episodes of diurnal drowsiness, hyperphagia (intermittently relieved by methylphenidate), and hypersexuality over a period of months. In some patients with this disorder, schizophrenic and sociopathic symptoms have been recorded between attacks, raising doubt as to whether all the reported cases are of the same type. In most instances, the disease is self-limited and disappears by early adult life. We have seen variants of this syndrome manifesting themselves by drowsiness and extreme inactivity and lasting for a few weeks, with complete return to normalcy. In two of our patients, the use of serotoninergic antidepressants lengthened the interval between episodes.

Neuroendocrine Syndromes Related to the Adrenal Glands

Cushing Disease and Cushing Syndrome The clinical features of Cushing disease, first described in his classic monograph in 1932, are now familiar to everyone in medicine: truncal obesity with reddish purple cutaneous striae over the abdomen and other parts, dryness and pigmentation of the skin and fragility of skin vessels, excessive facial hair and baldness, cyanosis and mottling of the skin of the extremities, osteoporosis and thoracic kyphosis, generalized muscular weakness, hypertension, glycosuria, and a number of psychologic disturbances. Adrenal hyperplasia secondary to a basophil adenoma of the pituitary (*pituitary basophilia* was Cushing's term) was the established pathology in Cushing's cases. But the same combination of abnormalities may be associated with chronically increased production of cortisol from a primary adrenal tumor, ectopic production of ACTH by carcinoma of the lung or less common carcinomas, and most commonly with the prolonged administration of glucocorticoids (prednisone, methylprednisolone, or ACTH). For these latter conditions, all but the last being associated with secondary adrenal hyperplasia, the term *Cushing syndrome* is appropriate. Some components of the syndrome may be lacking or less conspicuous than in florid Cushing disease; diagnosis is then facilitated by measurements of ACTH and cortisol in the blood and urine.

In Orth's review of 630 cases of Cushing syndrome of endogenous cause, 65 percent were due to hyperpituitarism (Cushing disease), 12 percent to an ectopic production of ACTH, 10 percent to an adrenal adenoma, and 8 percent to adrenal carcinoma.

In *Cushing disease*, as postulated initially, a basophil adenoma produces a hormone, now known to be ACTH or corticotropin, that stimulates the adrenals. Unlike the usual pituitary tumors, the corticotroph (basophil) type are usually microadenomas (<1 cm) and enlarge the sella in only 20 percent of cases. However, by MRI or high-resolution CT through the sella, either micro- or macroadenomas can be visualized in about 85 percent of cases.

The possibility that excess ACTH production by the pituitary might be due to a disorder of the hypothalamus was conceptualized in 1944, and the isolation of a corticotropin-releasing hormone (CRH) was accomplished by Guillemin and Rosenberg in 1955. However, the proof that Cushing syndrome could be due to an excess of CRH or a lack of hypothalamic inhibitor remains unconvincing. There are only a few cases in which a hypothalamic tumor such as a gangliocytoma has caused Cushing syndrome. More firmly established is the *ectopic production of ACTH* by a variety of tumors: oat-cell and squamous-cell carcinoma of the lung, carcinoma of the pancreas, thymoma, and several others in rare instances (pheochromocytoma, medullary carcinoma of the thyroid, islet cell tumors). Cushing syndrome of ectopic type tends to differ clinically from primary pituitary Cushing disease with respect to its more rapid development and greater degrees of skin pigmentation, hypokalemia, hypertension, and glycosuria. Plasma concentrations of ACTH exceed 50 mg/dL in the ectopic type and are not suppressed by dexamethasone administration.

For *diagnostic purposes*, measurement of the excretion of cortisol over 24 h in the urine is the most expeditious test and superior to serum sampling because of fluctuations in the latter. If a 24-h urine collection is not feasible, it is advisable to obtain two or three daily determinations, since the values may vary from day to day in Cushing syndrome and patients are frequently unable to save all their urine. The normal value for urinary excretion of cortisol is approximately 12 to 40 mg in 24 h, but some assays that measure additional metabolites of the hormone may allow normal values up to 100 mg. This should be followed by low- or high-dose dexamethasone suppression testing, as described by Orth. A test using high doses of dexamethasone (2 mg every 6 h orally for 2 days, or a single dose of 8 mg at midnight) is the most dependable screening method for distinguishing Cushing disease from ectopic secretion of ACTH. As mentioned, in the latter, the urinary excretion of cortisol is not suppressed by the administration of dexamethasone, whereas there is a reduction of 90 percent in urinary excretion in 60 to 70 percent of patients with Cushing disease.

Treatment is governed by the cause of the syndrome. A corticotroph adenoma, if not extending out of the sella and encroaching on the optic chiasm, is ideally treated by transsphenoidal pituitary microsurgery. The alternative is focused proton beam or gamma radiation, but the long latency of response to these forms of treatment, 6 months or more, makes them less desirable. If such indirect methods of treatment are used, hypercortisolism may be suppressed in the interim by adrenal enzyme inhibitors such as ketoconazole, metapyrone, or aminoglutethimide. The rate of cure for pituitary microadenoma by transsphenoidal surgery approaches 80 percent, although operative complications—CSF leakage, transient diabetes insipidus, visual abnormalities, meningitis—occur in as many as 10 percent of patients. In about 20 percent of patients, removal of the tumor is incomplete and symptoms persist or recur. In such circumstances reoperation is often undertaken, with total excision of the gland and a consequent requirement for extensive hormone replacement in many cases. As an alternative, radiotherapy may be used. If there is an urgent need to suppress the effects of hypercortisolism, bilateral adrenalectomy is effective but has obvious limitations.

Depending on the functional status of the pituitary after any mode of successful treatment, replacement therapy may be needed for a variable period.

Adrenocortical Insufficiency (Addison Disease)

The classic form of adrenal insufficiency, described by Addison in the nineteenth century, is due to primary disease of the adrenals. It is characterized by pigmentation of the skin and mucous membranes, nausea, vomiting, and weight loss as well as muscle weakness, languor, and a tendency to faint. Since Addison's time, hypotension, hyperkalemia, hyponatremia, and low serum cortisol concentrations have come to be recognized as important laboratory features.

In former times, the most common cause of primary adrenal disease was tuberculosis. Now, most cases are designated as idiopathic and thought to represent an autoimmune disorder, often associated with Hashimoto thyroiditis and diabetes mellitus and rarely with other polyglandular autoimmune endocrine disorders. A less frequent cause is a hereditary metabolic disease of the adrenals—in combination with a demyelinating disease of brain, spinal cord, and nerves and occurring predominantly in males (adrenoleukodystrophy; see page 1035). In primary adrenal disease, plasma concentrations of cortisol are low, in response to which the concentrations of ACTH rise. Adrenal insufficiency of whatever cause is a life-threatening condition; there is always a danger of collapse and even death, particularly during periods of infection, surgery, injury, and the like. Lifelong replacement therapy is usually required, with a glucocorticoid (cortisone, 25 to 50 mg, or prednisone, 7.5 to 15 mg daily) and a mineralocorticoid such as fludrocortisone acetate (Florinef), 0.05 to 0.2 mg daily.

When adrenal insufficiency is secondary to disease of the pituitary, ACTH is low or absent and cortisol secretion is markedly reduced, but aldosterone levels are sustained. Hyperpigmentation is notably absent; it is the elevation of ACTH that causes melanoderma, such as occurs, for example, in patients subjected to bilateral adrenalectomy. Hypothalamic lesions, principally involving the paraventricular nuclei, may also cause adrenal insufficiency, but less frequently than do pituitary lesions.

REFERENCES

Anderson AE: *Practical Comprehensive Treatment of Anorexia Nervosa and Bulimia*. Baltimore, Johns Hopkins University Press, 1985.

Aronin N, diFiglea M, Leeman SE: Substance P, in Krieger DT, Brownstein NJ, Martin JB (eds): *Brain Peptides*. New York, Wiley, 1983, pp 783–804.

Asa SL, Scheithauer BW, Bilbau J, et al: A case of hypothalamic acromegaly: A clinico-pathologic study of 6 patients with hypothalamus gangliocytomas producing growth hormone releasing factor. *J Clin Endocrinol Metab* 58:796, 1984.

Berek K, Aichner F, Schmutzhard E, et al: Intracranial germ cell tumour mimicking anorexia nervosa. *Klin Wochenschr* 69:440, 1991.

Bhanji S, Mattingly D: *Medical Aspects of Anorexia Nervosa*. London, Wright, 1988.

Bray GA, Gallagher TF Jr: Manifestations of hypothalamic obesity in man: A comprehensive investigation of eight patients and a review of the literature. *Medicine* 54:301, 1975.

Brazeau P, Vale W, Bargus R, et al: Hypothalamic polypeptide that inhibits the secretion of immunoreactive pituitary growth hormone. *Science* 179:77, 1973.

Breningstall GN: Gelastic seizures, precocious puberty and hypothalamic hamartoma. *Neurology* 35:1180, 1985.

Brown RH, Beyerl BD, Iseke R, Lavyne MH: Medulla oblongata edema associated with neurogenic pulmonary edema. *J Neurosurg* 64:494, 1986.

Brzezinski A: Melatonin in humans. *N Engl J Med* 336:186, 1997.

Burr IM, Slonim AE, Danish RK: Diencephalic syndrome revisited. *J Pediatr* 88:429, 1976.

Byer E, Ashman R, Toth LA: Electrocardiogram with large upright T-wave and long Q-T intervals. *Am Heart J* 33:796, 1947.

Byne W: The biological evidence challenged, in *The Scientific American Book of the Brain*. New York, Lyons Press, 1999, pp 181–194.

Carmel PW: Sympathetic deficits following thalamotomy. *Arch Neurol* 18:378, 1968.

Carpenter S, Yassa R, Ochs R: A pathologic basis for Kleine-Levin syndrome. *Arch Neurol* 39:25, 1982.

Cavallo A: The pineal gland in human beings:. Relevance to pediatrics. *J Pediatr* 123:843, 1993.

Cohen RA, Albers HE: Disruption of human circadian and cognitive regulation following a discrete hypothalmic lesion: A case study. *Neurology* 41:726, 1991.

Considine RV, Sinha MK, Heiman ML, et al: Serum immunoreactive-leptin concentrations in normal-weight and obese humans. *N Engl J Med* 354:292, 1996.

Critchley M: Periodic hypersomnia and megaphagia in adolescent males. *Brain* 85:627, 1962.

Cropp CF, Manning GW: Electrocardiographic change simulating myocardial ischemia and infarction associated with spontaneous intracranial hemorrhage. *Circulation* 22:24, 1960.

Cushing H: Basophil adenomas of the pituitary body and their clinical manifestations (pituitary basophilia). *Bull Johns Hopkins Hosp* 50:137, 1932.

Diringer M, Ladenson PW, Stern BJ, et al: Plasma atrial natriuretic factor and subarachnoid hemorrhage. *Stroke* 19:1119, 1988.

DuVigneaud V: Hormones of the posterior pituitary gland: Oxytocin and vasopressin. *Harvey Lect* 50:1, 1954–1955.

Erdheim J: Über Hypophysengangs Geschwülste und Hirn Cholesteatome. Sitzungs DK Akad d Wissensch. *Math Natur WC Wien* 113:537, 1904.

Froehlich A: Ein Fall von Tumor der Hypophysis cerebri ohne Akromegalie. *Wien Klin Wochenschr* 15:883, 1901.

Guillemin R, Rosenberg B: Humoral hypothalamic control of anterior pituitary: A study with combined tissue cultures. *Endocrinology* 57:599, 1955.

Hayes R, McHugh PR, Williams H: Absence of thirst in hydrocephalus. *N Engl J Med* 269:277, 1963.

Hughes IT, Smith W, Kosterlitz HW, et al: Identification of two related pentapeptides from the brain with potent opiate agonist activity. *Nature* 258:577, 1975.

Imura H, Nakoa K, Shimatsu A, et al: Lymphocytic infundibuloneurohypophysitis as a cause of central diabetes insipidus. *N Engl J Med* 329:683, 1993.

Jennings MT, Gelman R, Hochberg FH: Intracranial germ-cell tumors: Natural history and pathogenesis. *J Neurosurg* 63:155, 1985.

Kleine W: Periodische Schlafsucht. *Monatsschr Psychiatr Neurol* 57:285, 1925.

LAMBERTS SWJ, DEHERDER WW, VAN DER LELY AJ: Pituitary insufficiency. *Lancet* 352:127, 1998.

LEEMAN SE, MROZ EA: Substance P. *Life Sci* 15:2003, 1975.

LEVAY S: A difference in the hypothalamic structure between heterosexual and homosexual men. *Science* 253:1034, 1991.

LEVIN M: Periodic somnolence and morbid hunger. *Brain* 62:494, 1936.

LEWIN K, MATTINGLY D, MILLS RR: Anorexia nervosa associated with hypothalamic tumour. *BMJ* 2:629, 1972.

MARTIN JB, REICHLIN S: *Clinical Neuroendocrinology*, 2nd ed. Philadelphia, Davis, 1987.

MECHANICK JI, HOCHBERG FH, LAROCQUE A: Hypothalamic dysfunction following whole-brain radiation. *J Neurosurg* 65:490, 1986.

MOSES AM, STRETTEN DHP: Disorders of the neurohypophysis, in Wilson JD, Braunwald E, Isselbacher KJ, et al (eds): *Harrison's Principles of Internal Medicine*, 13th ed. New York, McGraw-Hill, 1994, p 1924.

NAUTA WJH, HAYMAKER W: Hypothalamic nuclei and fiber connections, in Haymaker W, Anderson E, Nauta WJH (eds): *The Hypothalamus*. Springfield, IL, Charles C Thomas, 1969, pp 136–209.

NELSON PB, SEIF SM, MAROON JC, ROBINSON AG: Hyponatremia in intracranial disease: Perhaps not the syndrome of inappropriate secretion of antidiuretic hormone (SIADH). *J Neurosurg* 55:938, 1981.

NOEL P, HUBERT JP, ECTORS M, et al: Agenesis of the corpus callosum associated with relapsing hypothermia. *Brain* 96:359, 1973.

ORTH DN: Cushing's syndrome. *N Engl J Med* 332:791, 1995.

PENFIELD W: Diencephalic autonomic epilepsy. *Arch Neurol Psychiatry* 22:358, 1929.

PETERS JP, WELT LG, SIMS EAH, et al: A salt wasting syndrome associated with cerebral disease. *Trans Assoc Am Physiol* 63:57, 1950.

RANSON SW: Somnolence caused by hypothalamic lesions in the monkey. *Arch Neurol Psychiatry* 41:1, 1939.

REEVES AG, PLUM F: Hyperphagia, rage and dementia accompanying a ventromedial hypothalamic neoplasm. *Arch Neurol* 20:616, 1969.

REICHLIN S: Neuroendocrinology, in Wilson JD, Foster DW (eds): *Williams Textbook of Endocrinology*, 8th ed. Philadelphia, Saunders, 1992, pp 135–219.

RIOCH D MCK, WISLOCKI GB, O'LEARY JL: A precis of preoptic hypothalamic and hypophysial terminology with atlas, in *The Hypothalamus*. Baltimore, Williams & Wilkins, 1940.

ROBERTSON GL: Posterior pituitary, in Selig P, Baxter JD, Broadus AE, Frohman LA (eds): *Endocrinology and Metabolism*, 2nd ed. New York, McGraw-Hill, 1987, pp 338–385.

SAMSON WK: Atrial natriuretic factor and the central nervous system. *Endocrinol Metab Clin North Am* 16:145, 1987.

SAMUELS MA: Cardiopulmonary aspects of acute neurological disease, in *Neurological and Neurosurgical Intensive Care*, 3rd ed. New York, Raven Press, 1993, pp 103–120.

SCHARRER E, SCHARRER B: Secretory cells within the hypothalamus, in *The Hypothalamus*. Baltimore, Williams & Wilkins, 1940, pp 170–194.

SCHEITHAUER BW, KOVACS KT, JARIWALA LK, et al: Anorexia nervosa: An immunohistochemical study of the pituitary gland. *Mayo Clin Proc* 63:23, 1988.

SCHWARTZ WB, BARTTER FC: The syndrome of inappropriate secretion of antidiuretic hormone. *Am J Med* 42:790, 1967.

SCHWARTZ WJ, BUSIS NA, HEDLEY-WHYTE T: A discrete lesion of the ventral hypothalamus and optic chiasm that disrupted the daily temperature rhythm. *J Neurol* 233:1, 1986.

SOTOS JF, DODGE PR, MUIRHEAD D et al: Cerebral gigantism in childhood. *N Engl J Med* 271:109, 1964.

SPEIDEL CG: *Carnegie Inst Wash Publ* 13:1, 1919.

STEWART C, CASTRO-MAGANA M, SHERMAN J, et al: Septo-optic dysplasia and median cleft face syndrome in a patient with isolated growth hormone deficiency and hyperprolactinemia. *Am J Dis Child* 137:484, 1983.

STUNKARD AJ, SORENSEN TIA, HANIS C, et al: An adoption study of human obesity. *N Engl J Med* 314:193, 1986.

SUZUKI N, SHINONAGA M, HIRATA K, et al: Hypothalamic obesity due to hydrocephalus caused by aqueductal stenosis. *J Neurol Neurosurg Psychiatry* 53:1102, 1990.

VON ECONOMO CJ: *Encephalitis Lethargica*. New York, Oxford University Press, 1930.

WIJDICKS EF, ROPPER AH, HUNNICUTT EJ, et al: Atrial natriuretic factor and salt wasting after aneurysmal subarachnoid hemorrhage. *Stroke* 22:1519, 1991.

WOLFF SM, ADLER RC, BUSKIRK ER, et al: A syndrome of periodic hypothalamic discharge. *Am J Med* 36:956, 1964.

Part 3

GROWTH AND DEVELOPMENT OF THE NERVOUS SYSTEM AND THE NEUROLOGY OF AGING

Chapter 28

NORMAL DEVELOPMENT AND DEVIATIONS IN DEVELOPMENT OF THE NERVOUS SYSTEM

In this chapter and the next we consider the effects of growth, maturation, and aging on the nervous system. These are elaborated in some detail because certain aspects of neurologic diseases are meaningful only when viewed against the background of these natural age-linked changes. Developmental diseases of the nervous system, i.e., malformations and diseases that are acquired in the intrauterine period of life, are considered in Chap. 38.

TIME-LINKED SEQUENCES OF NORMAL DEVELOPMENT

The establishment of a biologic time scale of human development requires observation, under standardized conditions, of a large number of normal individuals of known ages and the testing of them for measurable items of behavior. Because of individual variations in the tempo of development, it is equally important to study the growth and development of any one individual for a prolonged period. If these observations are to be correlated with stages of neuroanatomic development, the clinical and morphologic data must be expressed in units that are comparable. Early in life, age periods are difficult to ascertain because of the special difficulty in fixing the time of conception. The average human gestational period is 40 weeks (280 days), but birth may occur with survival as early as 28 or as late as 49 weeks (a time span of almost 5 months), and the extent of nervous system development will vary accordingly.

After birth, any given item of behavior or structural differentiation must always have two reference points: (1) to a particular item of behavior that has already been achieved and (2) to units of chronologic time or duration of life of the organism. The chronologic, or biologic, scale assumes special significance in early prenatal life. Then development proceeds at such a rapid pace that small units of time weigh heavily and the organism appears to change literally day by day. In infancy, the tempo of development slows somewhat but is still very rapid in comparison with later childhood.

The neurologist will find it advantageous to organize his knowledge of normal development and disease around the timetables for human growth and development listed in Tables 28-1 and 28-2. In addition, the last decade has brought startling advances in the understanding of the genetic and molecular control of neural development. The latter topic is quite beyond the scope of this chapter, although some of the mutations that are relevant to the developmental diseases of the nervous system are considered in Chap. 38.

Neuroanatomic Bases of Normal Development

A large body of knowledge has accumulated concerning the functional and structural status of the nervous system during each successive period of life. This information is reviewed briefly in the following paragraphs and is summarized in Table 28-2. It must be kept in mind that development of the nervous system does not proceed stepwise, from one period to the next, but is continuous from conception to maturity. The sequences of development are much the same in all infants, although the rate may vary. Any given function, in order to be expressed, must await the development of its neural substrate. At any given moment in development, several measurable functions appear in parallel, and it is often their dissociation that acquires clinical significance.

Embryonal and Fetal Periods What we know of the nervous system in the germinal and embryonal periods has been derived from the study of a relatively small number of abortuses that have come into the hands of anatomists. Neuroblastic differentiation, migration, and neuronal multiplication are already well under way in the first 3 weeks of embryonic life. The chemical control of each of these phases (and, later, of connectivity of neurons) is determined by the genome of the organism. Primitive cells destined to become neurons originate in or close to the neuroepithelium of the neural tube. These cells proliferate at an astonishingly rapid rate (250,000 per minute, according to Cowan) for a circumscribed period (several days to weeks). They become transformed into bipolar neuroblasts, which migrate in a series of waves toward the marginal layer of what is to become the cortex of the cerebral hemispheres. The first glial cells also appear very early and provide the scaffolding along which the neuroblasts move. Each step in the differentiation and migration of the neuroblasts proceeds in an orderly fashion, and one stage progresses to the next with remarkable precision. The process of migration is largely completed by the end of the fifth fetal month but continues at a much slower rate up to 40 weeks of gestation, according to the classic studies of Conel and of Rabinowicz. Since the migration of most neurons involves postmitotic cells, the cerebral cortex by this time has presumably acquired its full complement of nerve cells, numbered in the many billions. Actually, we have little idea of the number of nerve cells in the cerebral and cerebellar cortices at different ages. More are formed than survive, since programmed cell death (apoptosis) constitutes an important phase of development.

Within a few months of midfetal life, the cerebrum, which begins as a small bihemispheric organ with hardly a trace of surface indentation, evolves into a deeply sulcated structure. Every step in the folding of the surface to form fissures and sulci follows a temporal pattern of such precision as to permit a reasonably accurate estimation of fetal age by this criterion alone. The major sylvian, rolandic, and calcarine fissures take on the adult configuration during the fifth month of fetal life, the secondary sulci in the sixth and seventh months, and the tertiary sulci—which vary from one individual to another—in the eighth and ninth months (see Fig. 28-1 and Table 28-2).

Concomitantly, subtle changes in neuronal organization are occurring in the cerebral cortex and central ganglionic masses. Involved here are the processes of

Table 28-1
Time scale of stages in human growth and development

Growth period	*Approximate age*
Prenatal	From 0 to 280 days
Ovum	From 0 to 14 days
Embryo	From 14 days to 9 weeks
Fetus	From 9 weeks to birth
Premature infant	From 27 to 37 weeks
Birth	Average 280 days
Neonate	First 4 weeks after birth
Infancy	First year
Early childhood (preschool)	From 1 to 6 years
Later childhood (prepubertal)	From 6 to 10 years
Adolescence	Girls, 8 or 10 to 18 years Boys, 10 or 12 to 20 years
Puberty (average)	Girls, 13 years Boys, 15 years

Source: Lowrey GH, *Growth and Development of Children*, 8th ed. Chicago, Year Book, 1986, by permission.

Table 28-2
Timetable of growth and nervous system development in the normal embryo and fetus

Age, days	*Size (crown–rump length), mm*	*Nervous system development*
18	1.5	Neural groove and tube
21	3.0	Optic vesicles
26	3.0	Closure of anterior neuropore
27	3.3	Closure of posterior neuropore; ventral horn cells appear
31	4.3	Anterior and posterior roots
35	5	Five cerebral vesicles
42	13	Primordium of cerebellum
56	25	Differentiation of cerebral cortex and meninges
150	225	Primary cerebral fissures appear
180	230	Secondary cerebral sulci and first myelination appear in brain
8–9 months	240	Further myelination and growth of brain (see text)

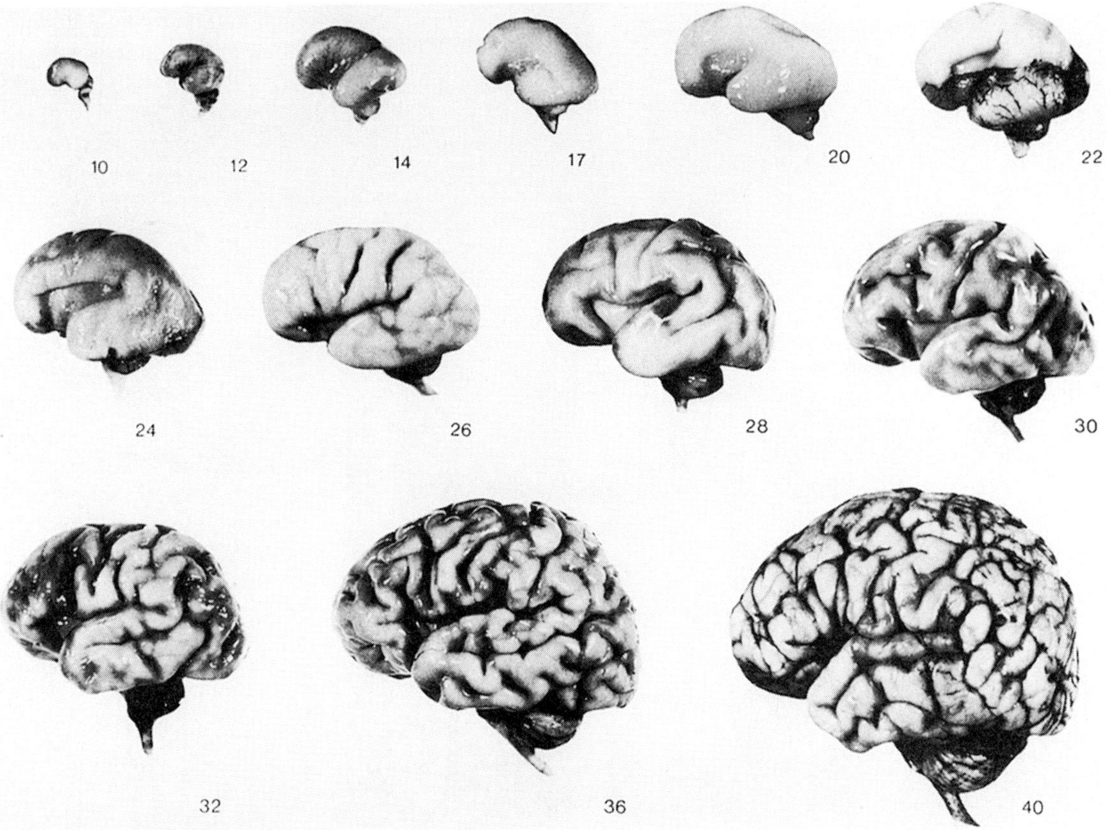

Figure 28-1

Lateral views of the fetal brain, from 10 to 40 weeks of gestational age. (Reproduced from Feess-Higgins and Larroche, with permission.)

synaptogenesis and axonal pathfinding. Neurons become more widely separated as differentiation proceeds, owing to an increase in the size and complexity of dendrites and axons and enlargement of synaptic surfaces (Fig. 28-2). The cytoarchitectural patterns that demarcate one part of the cerebral cortex from another are already in evidence by the thirtieth week of fetal life and become definitive at 40 weeks and in succeeding months. As the maturational process of cortical neurons proceeds, the patterns of neuronal organization in different regions of the brain (motor, premotor, sensory and striate cortices, Broca and Wernicke areas) continue to change.

Myelination provides another index of the development and maturation of the nervous system and is believed to be related to the functional activity of the fiber systems. The acquisition of myelin sheaths by the spinal nerves and roots by the 10th week of fetal life is associated with the beginning of reflex motor activities. Segmental and intersegmental fiber systems in the spinal cord myelinate soon afterward, followed by ascending and descending fibers to and from the brainstem (reticulospinal, vestibulospinal). The acoustic and labyrinthine systems stand out with singular clarity in myelin-stained preparations by the 28th to 30th weeks, and the spinocerebellar and dentatorubral systems by the 37th week (Fig. 28-3).

Neonatal Period and Infancy After birth, the brain continues to grow dramatically. From an average weight of 375 to 400 g at birth (40 weeks), it reaches about 1000 g by the end of the first postnatal year. Glial cells (oligodendrocytes and astrocytes) derived from the matrix zones continue to divide and multiply during the first 6 months of postnatal life. The visual system begins to myelinate about the 40th gestational week; its myelination cycle proceeds rapidly, being nearly complete a

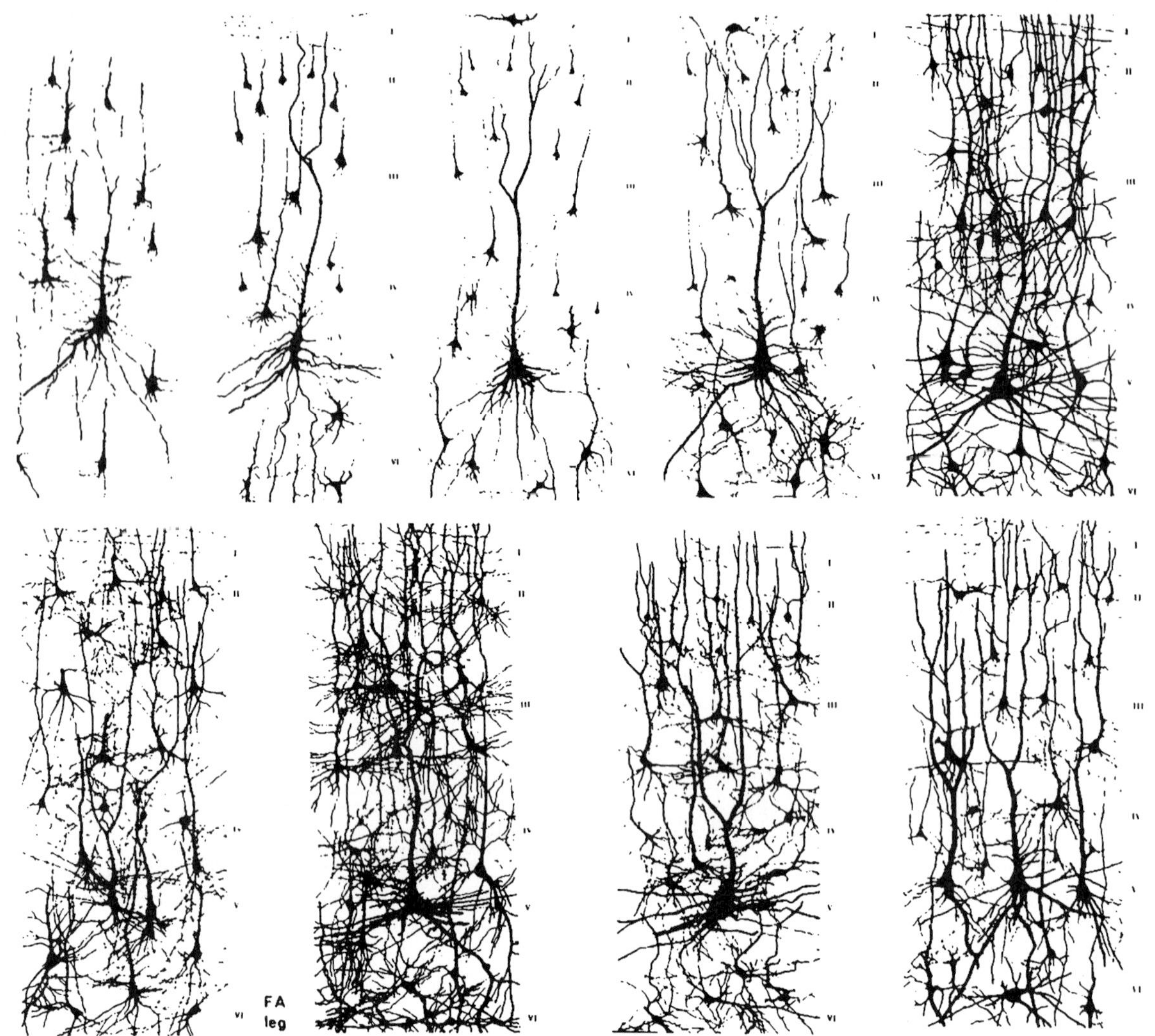

Figure 28-2

Cox-Golgi preparations of the leg area of the motor cortex (area 4). Upper row, left to right: 8 months premature; newborn at term; 1 month; 3 months; and 6 months. Lower row, left to right: 15 months; 2 years; 4 years; 6 years. Magnification, 100×; apical dendrites of Betz cells have been shortened, all to the same degree. (Courtesy of T Rabinowicz, University of Lausanne.)

few months after birth. The corticospinal tracts are not fully myelinated until halfway through the second postnatal year. Most of the principal tracts are myelinated by the end of this period. In the cerebrum, the first myelin is seen at 40 weeks in the posterior frontal and parietal lobes, and the occipital lobes (geniculocalcarine tracts) myelinate soon thereafter. Myelination of the anterior frontal and temporal lobes occurs later, during the first year of postnatal life. By the end of the second year, myelination of the cerebrum is largely complete (Fig. 28-3). These steps in myelination can be followed by MRI. Despite these careful anatomic observations, their correlation with developmental clinical and electroencephalographic (EEG) data has not been successful.

Childhood, Puberty, and Adolescence Growth of the brain continues, at a much slower rate than before, until 12 to 15 years, when the average adult weight of 1230 to 1275 g in females and 1350 to 1410 g in males is attained. Myelination also continues slowly during this

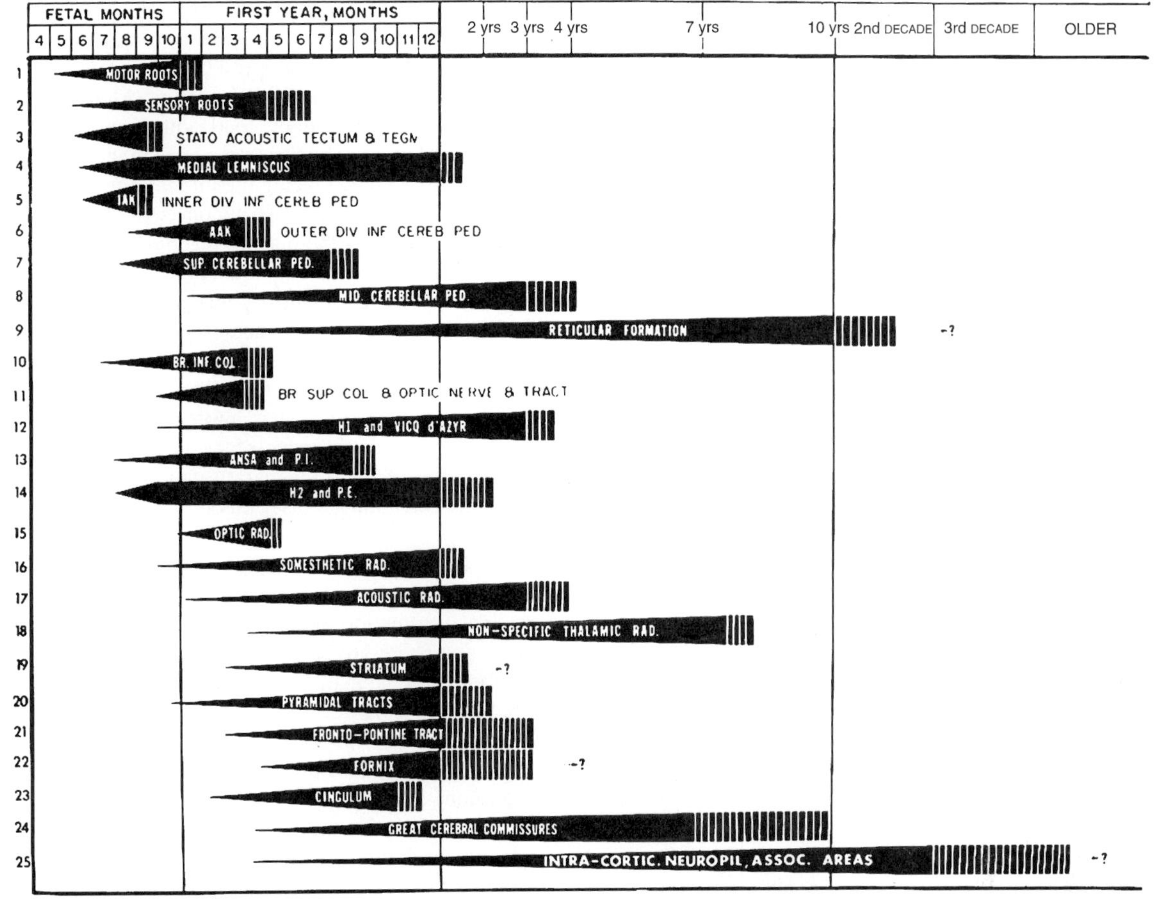

Figure 28-3

The myelogenetic chronology. (From Yakovlev and Lecours, with permission.)

period. Yakovlev and Lecours, who re-examined Flechsig's findings on the ontogeny of myelination, traced the progressive myelination of the middle cerebellar peduncle, acoustic radiation, and bundle of Vicq d'Azyr (mammillothalamic tract) beyond the third postnatal year; the nonspecific thalamic radiations continued to myelinate beyond the seventh year and fibers of the reticular formation, great cerebral commissures, and intracortical association neurons to at least the tenth year and beyond (Fig. 28-3). The investigators noted that there was an increasing complexity of fiber systems through late childhood and adolescence and perhaps even into middle adult life. Similarly, in the classic studies of Conel and Rabinowicz, depicting the cortical architecture at each year from mid–fetal life to the 20th year, the dendritic arborizations and cortical interneuronal connections were observed to increase progressively in complexity, thus reducing the "packing density" of neurons, i.e., the number of neurons in any given volume of tissue (Fig. 28-2).

Interesting questions are (1) whether neurons begin to function only when their axons have acquired a myelin sheath; (2) whether myelination is under the control of the cell body, the axon, or both; and (3) whether the classic myelin stains yield sufficient information as to the time of onset and degree of the myelination process. At best these correlations can be only approximate. It seems likely that systems of neurons begin to function before the first appearance of myelin as shown in conventional myelin stains. These correlations need to be restudied, using more delicate measures of function and finer staining techniques, as well as the techniques of quantitative biochemistry and phase and electron microscopy.

Physiologic and Psychologic Development

Neural Development in the Fetus The human fetus is capable of a complex series of reflex activities, some of which appear as early as 5 weeks of postconceptional age. Cutaneous and proprioceptive stimuli evoke slow, generalized, patterned movements of the head, trunk, and extremities. More discrete movements appear to differentiate from these generalized activities. Reflexes subserving blinking, sucking, grasping, and visceral functions, as well as tendon and plantar reflexes, are all elicitable in late fetal life. They seem to develop along with the myelination of peripheral nerves, spinal roots, spinal cord, and brainstem. By the 24th week of gestation, the neural apparatus is functioning sufficiently well to give the fetus some chance of survival should birth occur at this time. However, most infants fail to survive birth at this age, usually owing to an inadequacy of pulmonary function. Thereafter, the basic neural equipment matures so rapidly that, by the 30th week, postnatal viability is relatively common. It seems that nature prepares the fetus for the contingency of premature birth by hastening the establishment of vital functions necessary for extrauterine existence.

It is in the last trimester of pregnancy that a complete timetable of fetal movements, posture, and reflexes would be of the greatest value, for only during this period does the need for a full clinical evaluation arise. That there are recognizable differences between infants born in the sixth, seventh, eighth, and ninth months of fetal life has been documented by Saint-Anne Dargassies, who applied the neurologic tests earlier devised by André-Thomas and herself. Her observations are in reference to prevailing postures; control and attitude of head, neck, and limbs; muscle tonus; and grasp and sucking reflexes. These findings are of interest and may well prove to be a means of determining exact age, but many more observations are needed with follow-up data on later development before they can be fully accepted as having predictive value. Part of the difficulty here is the extreme variability of the premature infant's neurologic functions, which may change literally from hour to hour. Even at term there is variability in neurologic functions from one day to the next. This variability reflects the traumatic effects of parturition and the effects of drugs and anesthesia given to the mother as well as the inaccurate dating of conception and rapid developmental changes in the brain.

Development During the Neonatal Period, Infancy, and Early Childhood *At term*, effective sucking, rooting, and grasping reactions are present. The infant is able to swallow and cry, and the startle reaction (Moro reflex, page 621) can be evoked by loud sound and sudden extension of the neck. Support and steppage movements can be demonstrated by placing the infant on its feet, and incurvation of the trunk, by stroking one side of the back. Also present at birth is the placing reaction, wherein the foot or hand, brought passively into contact with the edge of a table, is lifted automatically and placed on the flat surface. These neonatal automatisms depend essentially on the functioning of the spinal cord, brainstem, and possibly diencephalon and pallidum. The *Apgar score*, a universally used but somewhat imprecise index of the well-being of the newly born infant, is in reality a numerical rating of the adequacy of brainstem-spinal mechanisms (breathing, pulse, color of skin, tone, and responsivity).

Studies of local cerebral glucose metabolism by positron emission tomography (PET) have provided interesting information about the functional maturation of the brain. There are remarkable differences between the newborn and the mature individual. Neonatal values, adjusted for brain weight, are only one-third those of the adult; except for the primary sensorimotor cortex, they are confined to brainstem, cerebellum, and thalamus. During infancy there occurs a progressive glucose metabolic maturation in the parietal, temporal, striate, dorsolateral occipital, and frontal cortices, in this order. Only by the end of the first year do the glucose metabolic patterns qualitatively resemble those of the normal young adult (Chugani).

Behavior during *infancy and early childhood* is also the subject of a substantial literature, contributed more by psychologists than neurologists. In particular they have explored sensorimotor performance in the first year and language and social development in early childhood. In the first 6 years of life, the infant and young child traverse far more ground developmentally than they ever will again in a similar period. From the newborn state, when the infant is little more than an amorphous mass of protoplasm with a few feeding and postural reflexes, there are acquired, within a few months, smiling and head and hand-eye control; by 6 months, the ability to sit; by 10 months, the strength to stand; by 12 months, the muscle coordination required to walk; by 2 years, the ability to run; and by 6 years, mastery of the rudiments of a game of baseball or a musical skill. On the perceptual side, the neonate progresses, in less than 3 months, from a state in which ocular control is tentative and tonic deviation of the eyes occurs only in response to labyrinthine stimulation to one in which he or she is able to fixate and follow an object. (The latter corresponds to the development of the macula.) Much later the child is able to make fine discriminations of color, form, and size. Gesell has provided a graphic summarization of the variety and developmental sweep of a child's behavior. He writes:

> *At birth the child reflexly grasps the examiner's finger, with eyes crudely wandering or vacantly transfixed . . . and by the sixth year the child adaptively scans the perimeter of a square or triangle, reproducing each form with directed crayon. The birth cry, scant in modulation and social meaning, marks the low level of language, which in two years passes from babbling to word formation that soon is integrated into sentence structure, and in six years to elaborated syntactic speech with questions and even primitive ideas of causality. In personality makeup . . . the school beginner is already so highly organized, both socially and biologically, that he foreshadows the sort of individual he will be in later years.*

The studies of Gesell and Amatruda and of others represent attempts to establish age-linked standards of behavioral development, but the difficulties of using such rating scales are considerable. The components of behavior that have been chosen as a frame of reference are not likely to be of uniform physiologic value or of comparable complexity, and they have seldom been standardized on large populations drawn from different cultures. Also, the examinations at specified ages are cross-sectional assessments, which give little idea of the dynamics of behavioral development. As already stated, temporal patterns of behavior reveal an extraordinary degree of variation in their emergence, increment, and decrement as well as marked variation from one individual to another.

The predictive value of developmental assessment has been the subject of a lively dispute. Gesell took the position that careful observation of a large number of infants, with accurate recording of the age at which various skills are acquired, permits the establishment of norms or averages. From such a framework one can determine the level of developmental attainment, expressed as the development quotient (DQ = developmental age/chronological age), and thus ascertain whether any given child is superior, average, or inferior. After examining 10,000 infants over a period of 40 years, Gesell concluded that "attained growth is an indicator of past growth processes and a foreteller of growth yet to be achieved." In other words, the DQ predicts potential attainment.

The other position—taken by Anderson and others—is that developmental attainments are of no real value in predicting the level of intelligence but are measures of completely different functions. Illingworth and most clinicians, including the authors, have taken an intermediate position, that the developmental scale in early life is a useful source of information, but it must always be combined with a full clinical assessment. When this is done, the clinician has a reasonably certain means of detecting mental retardation and other forms of neurologic impairment.

The trajectory of rapid growth and maturation continues in late childhood and adolescence, though at a slower pace than before. Motor skills attain their maximal precision in the performances of athletes, artists, and musicians, whose peak development is at maturity (age 18 to 21). Intelligence and the capacity for reflective thought and the manipulation of mathematical symbols become possible only in adolescence and later. Emotional control, precarious in the school age and all through adolescence, stabilizes in adulthood. We tend to think of all these phenomena as being achieved through the stresses of human relations, which are conditioned and habituated by the powerful influences of social approval. In this extensive and pervasive interaction between the individual and the environment, which is the preoccupation of the child psychiatrist, it is well to remember that the processes of extrinsic and intrinsic organization can be separated only for the purpose of analytic discussion. There is always interdependence rather than conflict between them.

Motor Development

As indicated above (and in Table 28-3), the wide variety and seemingly random movements displayed by the healthy neonate are from birth, and certainly within days, firmly organized into reflexive-instinctual patterns called *automatisms*. The most testable of the automatisms are blinking in response to light, tonic deviation of the eyes in response to labyrinthine stimulation (turning of the head), prehensile and sucking movements of the lips in response to labial contact, swallowing, avoidance movements of the head and neck, startle reaction (Moro response) in response to loud noise or dropping of the head into an extended position, grasp reflexes, and support, stepping, and placing movements. This repertoire of movements, as mentioned earlier, depends on reflexes organized at the spinal and brainstem levels. Only the placing reactions, ocular fixation, and following movements (the latter are established by the third month) are

Table 28-3
Neurologic functions and disturbances in infancy

Age	*Normal functions*	*Pathologic signs*
Newborn period	Blinking, tonic deviation of eyes on turning head, sucking, rooting, swallowing, yawning, grasping, brief extension of neck in prone position, incurvation response, Moro response, flexion postures of limbs Biceps reflexes present and others variable; infantile type of flexor plantar reflex; stable temperature, respirations, and blood pressure; periods of sleep and arousal: vigorous cry	Lack of arousal (stupor or coma) High-pitched or weak cry Abnormal (incomplete or absent) Moro response Opisthotonus Flaccidity or hypertonia Convulsions Tremulous limbs Failure of tonic deviation of eyes on passive movement of head or of head and body
2–3 months	Supports head Smiles Makes vowel sounds Adopts tonic asymmetrical neck postures (tonic neck reflexes) Large range of movements of limbs, tendon reflexes usually present Fixates on and follows a dangling toy Suckles vigorously Period of sleep sharply differentiated from awake periods Support and stepping unelicitable Vertical suspension—legs flex, head up Optokinetic nystagmus elicitable	Absence of any or all of the normal functions Convulsions Hypotonia or hypertonia of neck and limbs Vertical suspension—legs extend and adduct
4 months	Good head support, minimal head lag Coos and chuckles Inspects hands Tone of limbs moderate or diminished Turns to sounds Rolls over from prone to supine Grasping, sucking, and tonic neck reflexes subservient to volition	Lack of head support Motor deficits Hypertonia Lack of social reactions Tonic neck reflexes present Strong Moro response Absence of symmetrical attitude
5–6 months	Babbles Reaches and grasps Vocalizes in social play Discriminates between family and strangers Moro and grasp reflexes disappear Tries to recover lost object Begins to sit; no head lag on pull to sit Positive support reaction Tonic neck reflexes gone Landau response (holds head above horizontal, arches back when held horizontally) Begins to grasp objects with one hand; holds bottle	Altered tone Obligatory postures Cannot sit or roll over Hypo- or hypertonia Persistent Moro and grasp Persistent tonic neck reflexes No Landau response

Table 28-3 *(Continued)*
Neurologic functions and disturbances in infancy

Age	*Normal functions*	*Pathologic signs*
9 months	Creeps and pulls to stand; stands holding on Sits securely Babbles "Mama," "Dada," or equivalent Sociable; plays "pat-a-cake," seeks attention Drinks from cup Landau response present Parachute response present Grasps with thumb to forefinger	Fails to attain these motor, verbal, and social milestones Persistent automatisms and tonic neck reflexes or hypo- or hypertonia
12 months	Stands alone May walk, or walks if led Tries to feed self May say several single words, echoes sounds Plantar reflexes definitely flexor Throws objects	Failure to attain 12-month milestones Persistence of automatisms
15 months	Walks independently (9–16 months), falls easily Moves arms steadily Says several words; scribbles with crayon Requests by pointing Interest in sounds, music, pictures, and animal toys	Retardation in reaching milestones expected at this age Persistent abnormalities of tone and posture Sensory discriminations defective
18 months	Says at least 6 words Feeds self; uses spoon well May obey commands Runs stiffly; seats self in chair Hand dominance Throws ball Plays several nursery games Uses simple tools in imitation Removes shoes and stockings Points to two or three parts of body, common objects, and pictures in book	Cannot walk No words
24 months	Says 2- or 3-word sentences Scribbles Runs well; climbs stairs one at a time Bends over and picks up objects Kicks ball; turns knob Organized play Builds tower of 6 blocks Sometimes toilet trained	Retarded in all motor, linguistic, and social adaptive skills

Source: Modified from Gesell et al., by permission.

thought to depend on emerging cortical connections, but even this is debatable. In the neonatal period, when little of the cerebrum has begun to function, extensive cerebral lesions may cause no derangement of motor function and may pass unnoticed unless special methods of examination—sensory evoked potentials, EEG, CT, and MRI—are used. Of clinically testable neurologic phenomena in the neonatal period, disturbances of ocular movement, seizures, tremulousness of the arms, impaired arousal reactions and muscular tone—all of which relate essentially to upper brainstem and diencephalic mechanisms—provide the most reliable clues to the presence of neurologic disease. Prechtl and associates have documented the importance of disturbances of these neurologic functions at this early age as predictors of retarded development.

During early infancy, the motor system undergoes a variety of differentiations as visual-, auditory-, and tactile-motor mechanisms develop. Bodily postures are modified to accommodate these complex sensorimotor acquisitions. In the normal infant, these emerging motor differentiations and elaborations follow a time schedule prescribed by the maturation of neural connections. Normalcy is expressed by the age of the organism at which each of these appear, as shown in Table 28-3 and Fig. 28-4. It is also evident from this table that reflex and instinctual motor activities are the most important means of evaluating early development. Moreover, in the normally developing infant, some of these activities disappear as others appear. For example, the grasp reflex, extension of the limbs without a flexor phase, Moro response, tonic neck reflexes, and crossed adduction in response to eliciting the knee jerk gradually become less prominent and are usually not elicitable by the sixth month. *The absence of these reflexes in the first few months of life and their persistence beyond this time indicate a defect in cerebral development*, as described further on, under "Delays in Motor Development." By contrast, neck-righting reflexes, support reactions, the Landau reaction (extending neck and legs when held prone), the parachute maneuver (page 621), and the pincer grasp, which are absent in the first 6 months, begin to appear by the seventh to eighth month and are present in all normal infants by the twelfth month (Fig. 28-4).

Since many functions that are classified as mental at a later period of life have a different anatomic basis than motor functions, it is not surprising that early motor achievements do not correlate closely with childhood intelligence. The converse does not apply, however; delay in the acquisition of motor milestones often correlates with mental retardation. Most mentally retarded children sit, stand, walk, and run at a later age than normal children, and deviations from this rule are exceptional.

In the period of early childhood, the reflexive-instinctual activities are no longer of help in evaluating cerebral development, and one must turn to the examination of language functions and learned sensory and motor skills. These are outlined in Tables 28-4 and 28-5.

Table 28-4
Developmental achievements of the normal preschool child

Age	*Observed items*	*Useful clinical tests*
2 years	Runs well Goes up and down stairs, one step at a time Climbs on furniture Opens doors Helps to undress Feeds well with spoon Puts three words together Listens to stories with pictures	Pencil-paper test: scribbles, imitates horizontal stroke Folds paper once Builds tower of six blocks
2½ years	Jumps on both feet; walks on tiptoes if asked Knows full name; asks questions Refers to self as "I" Helps put away toys and clothes Names animals in book, knows one to three colors Can complete three-piece form board	Pencil-paper test: copies horizontal and vertical line Builds tower of eight blocks
3 years	Climbs stairs, alternating feet Talks constantly; recites nursery rhymes Rides tricycle Stands on one foot momentarily Plays simple games Helps in dressing Washes hands Identifies five colors	Builds nine-cube tower Builds bridge with three cubes Imitates circle and cross with pencil
4 years	Climbs well; hops and skips on one foot; throws ball overhand; kicks ball Cuts out pictures with scissors Counts four pennies Tells a story; plays with other children Goes to toilet alone	Copies cross and circle Builds gate with five cubes Builds a bridge from model Draws a human figure with two to four parts other than head Distinguishes short and long line
5 years	Skips Names four colors; counts ten pennies Dresses and undresses Asks questions about meaning of words	Copies square and triangle Distinguishes heavier of two weights More detailed drawing of a human figure

Table 28-5
Useful psychometric tests for evaluating learning and behavioral disabilities in children[a]

Deficit	*Test*
Development	Denver Developmental Test; Vineland Social Maturity Test; Leiter International Performance Scale; Otis Group Intelligence Test
Achievement	Wide Range Achievement Test; Gates Primary Reading Test
Attentiveness	Dehoit Test of hearing aptitude
Calculation	Key Math Diagnostic Arithmetic Test
Vocabulary	Peabody Picture Vocabulary
Developmental Gerstmann syndrome (finger agnosia, right-left disorientation)	Finger Order Tests; Benton Right-Left Discrimination Test
Figure copying	Visual-Motor Integration Test
Visual memory	Benton Visual Retention Test
Error patterns	Boder Test of Reading-Spelling Patterns
Impulsiveness	Matching Familiar Figures Test

[a] For descriptions of individual tests, see Kinsbourne, 1995.

Quite apart from the early stage of motor development, one observes in later childhood and adolescence a remarkable variation in levels of muscular activity, strength, and coordination. Motor acquisitions of later childhood—such as hopping on one foot, kicking a ball, jumping over a line, walking gracefully, dancing, certain skills in sports—are linked to age. Ozeretzkii has combined these in a scale that often discloses arrests in motor development in the mentally retarded. Also in later childhood, precocity in learning complex motor skills as well as skill in games and the development of an all-around interest in athletic activity become evident. By adolescence, high individual physical achievement is well recognized. At the other end of the spectrum are instances of motor underachievement, ineptitude, and intrinsic awkwardness; a member of this group will easily stand out and be designated as "an awkward child." Such awkwardness is to be clearly distinguished from the motor impairment that is associated with a number of cerebral diseases.

Sensory Development

Under normal circumstances, sensory development keeps pace with motor development, and at every age sensorimotor interactions are apparent. However, under conditions of disease, this generalization may not hold; i.e., motor development may remain relatively normal in the face of a sensory defect, or vice versa. The sense organs are fully formed at birth. The neonate is crudely aware of visual, auditory, tactile, and olfactory stimuli, which elicit only low-level reflex responses. Moreover, any stimulus-related response is only to the immediate situation; there is no evidence that previous experience with the stimulus has influenced the response, i.e., that the newborn can learn and remember. The capacity to attend to a stimulus, to fixate upon it for any period of time, also comes later. Indeed, the length of fixation time is a quantifiable index of perceptual development in infancy.

Information is available about the time at which the infant makes the first interpretable responses to each of the different modes of stimulation. The most nearly perfect senses in the newborn are those of touch and pain. A series of pinpricks causes distress, whereas an abrasion of the skin seems not to do so. The sense of touch clearly plays a role in feeding behavior. Newborn infants react vigorously to irritating odors such as ammonia and acetic acid, but discrimination between olfactory stimuli is not evident until much later. Sugar solutions initiate and maintain sucking from birth on, whereas quinine (bitter) solutions seldom do, and the latter stimulus elicits avoidance behavior. Hearing in the newborn is manifest within the first few postnatal days. Sharp, quick sounds elicit responsive blinking and sometimes startle. In some infants, the human voice appears to cause similar reactions by the second week. Strong light and objects held before the face evoke reactions in the neonate; later, visual searching is an integrating factor in most projected motor activities.

Sensation in the newborn infant must be judged largely by motor reactions, so that sensory and motor developments seem to run in parallel; but there are discernible maturational stages that constitute sensory milestones, so to speak. This is most apparent in the visual system, which is more easily studied than the other senses. Sustained ocular fixation on an object is observable at term and even in preterm infants; at these ages it is essentially a reflexive phototropic reaction. However, it has been observed that the neonate will consistently gaze at some stimuli more often than others, suggesting that there must already be some elements of perception and differentiation (Fantz). This type of selective attention to stimuli is spoken of as *differential fixation*. So-called voluntary fixation (i.e., following a moving object) is a later development. Horizontal following occurs at about 50 days; vertical following, at 55 days; and following an object that is moving in a circle, at 2.5 months. Preference for a colored stimulus over a gray one was recorded by Staples by the end of the third month. By 6 months the infant discriminates between colors, and saturated colors can be matched at 30 months. Perception of form, judged by the length of time spent in looking at different visual presentations, is evident at 2 or 3 months of age (Fantz). At this time infants are attracted more to certain patterns than to colors. At 3 months, most infants have discovered their hands and spend considerable time watching their movements. The ages at which infants begin to observe color, size, shape, and numbers can be determined by means of the Terman-Merrill and Stutzman intelligence tests (see Gibson and Olum). Perception of size becomes increasingly accurate in the preschool years. An 18-month-old child discriminates among pictures of familiar animals and recognizes them equally well if they are upside down.

Visual discrimination is reflected in manual reactions, just as auditory discrimination is reflected in vocal responses. Much of early visual development (first year) involves peering at objects, judging their position, reaching for them, and seizing and manipulating them. The inseparability of sensory and motor functions is never more obvious. Sensory deprivation impedes not only the natural sequences of perceptual awareness of the child's surroundings but also the development of all motor activities. *Auditory discrimination*—reflected in vocalizations such as babbling and, later, in word formation—is discussed further on in connection with language development.

The Development of Intelligence

The subject of intellectual endowment and the development and testing of intelligence have already been touched upon in Chap. 21. There, it was pointed out that although intelligence is modifiable by training, practice, and schooling, it is much more a matter of native endowment. Intelligent parents tend to beget intelligent children, and unintelligent parents, unintelligent children; this seems to be not simply a question of environment and providing the stimulus to learn. It is evident early in life that some individuals have a superior intelligence; they clearly maintain this superiority all through life, and the opposite pertains in others.

Much of the uncertainty about the relative influence of heredity and environment relates to our imprecise views of what constitutes intelligence. We view intelligence as a general mental capability, embracing a number of primary abilities: the capacity to comprehend complex ideas, learn from experience, think abstractly, reason, plan, draw analogies, and solve problems. Thus intelligence includes a multiplicity of abilities, which probably accounts for a lack of consensus about its mechanism(s). Kurt Goldstein argued that intelligence is a unitary mental capacity, impairment of which gives rise to a fundamental disorder (*Grundstörung*)—a loss of "abstract attitude." By this he meant an incapacity to deal with objects at a conceptual level and an undue tendency to respond to their immediate, concrete attributes. Everyday experience, however, teaches us that it is not always abstract tasks that suffer most when intelligence is impaired. Indeed, as Zangwill has pointed out, even abstraction may not be a unitary function. Other theoreticians, like Carl Spearman, believed that intelligence comprises a general (*g*), or core, factor and a series of special (*s*) factors. In contrast, Thurstone conceived of intelligence as a mosaic of special factors such as drive and curiosity, verbal and arithmetic ability, memory, capacity for abstract thinking, practical skills in manipulating objects, geographic or spatial sense, and athletic and musical ability—each of which appears to be genetically determined. These and other theorizations about intelligence, such as those of Eysenck and of Gardner and particularly those of Piaget, concerning intellectual development in the child, have been considered in Chap. 21, which should be read together with this section.

The origins of the development of intelligence are difficult to discern. The first hints of something beyond simple sensorimotor reactions and reflex patterns emerge at 8 to 9 months of life, when the infant begins to crawl and explore. For the first time the infant separates itself from the mother. Now, learning proceeds rapidly, as the mother attaches names to objects and helps the baby manipulate them. Gradually the child acquires verbal facility (learning what words mean), memory, color and spatial perception, a concept of number, and the practical use of tools, each at a particular time according to a schedule set largely by the maturational state of the brain. Nevertheless, in these early achievements individuals differ considerably, reflecting to some extent the influence of their parents and others around them. The young child exhibits elementary modes of thinking but is highly suggestible and often incapable of separating imagination from reality.

Neurologists who need a quick and practical method of ascertaining whether an infant or preschool child is measuring up to normal standards for a particular age will find Table 28-4 useful. The main items are drawn from Gesell and Amatruda and from the Denver Developmental Test. In addition, a variety of intelligence tests have been designed to measure the child's special abilities and increasing success in learning in accordance with age (these are listed in Table 28-5). Starting at 6 to 7 years, there is a steady improvement in scores that parallels chronologic age up to about 13 years; thereafter the rate of advance diminishes. By 16 to 17 years, performance reaches a plateau, but this is probably an artifact of the commonly used tests, which are designed to predict success in school. Only late in life do test scores begin to diminish, in a manner that is described in the next chapter. Individuals with high or low IQs at 6 years of age tend to maintain their rank at 10, 15, and 20 years unless the early scores were impaired by anxiety, poor motivation, or a gross lack of opportunity to acquire the skills that are necessary to take such tests (language skill in particular). Even then, performance tasks, which largely eliminate verbal and mathematical skills, will disclose similar individual differences. Effective performance on tests of whatever type obviously requires sustained interest and motivation on the part of the subject.

The reliability of intelligence tests and their validity as predictive measures of scholastic, occupational, and economic success have been heatedly debated for many years. This aspect of the subject is also discussed in Chap. 21 and need not be repeated here. The most persuasive argument for these tests as an index of native abilities is that individuals drawn from a fairly homogeneous environment tend to maintain the same rating on the intelligence scale throughout their lives. Native endowment appears to set the limits of learning and achievement; opportunity and other factors determine how nearly the individual's full potential is realized.

The Development of Language

Closely tied to the development of intelligence is the acquisition of language. Indeed, facility with language is one of the best indices of intelligence (Lenneberg). The acquisition of speech and language by the infant and child has been observed methodically by a number of eminent investigators, and their findings provide a background for the understanding of a number of derangements in the development of these functions (Ingram; Rutter and Martin; Minifie and Lloyd).

First, there are the *babbling*, *cooing*, and *lalling stages*, during which the infant, a few weeks old, emits a variety of cooing and then, at about 6 months, babbling sounds in the form of vowel-consonant (labial and nasoguttural) combinations. Later, babbling becomes interspersed with pauses, inflections, and intonations drawn from what the infant hears. At first this appears to be a purely self-initiated activity, being the same in normal and deaf infants. However, study of the latter shows that auditory modifications begin within a period of 2 to 3 months; without an auditory sense, babblers do not produce the variety of random sounds of the normal infant, nor do they begin to imitate the sounds made by the mother. Thus motor speech is stimulated and reinforced mainly by auditory sensations, which become linked to the kinesthetic ones arising from the speech musculature. It is not clear whether the capacity to hear and understand the spoken word precedes or follows the first motor speech. Perhaps it varies from one infant to another, but the dependence of motor speech development on hearing is undeniable. Comprehension seems to postdate the first verbal utterance in most infants.

Soon babbling merges with *echo speech*, in which short sounds are repeated parrot-like; gradually longer syllable groups are repeated correctly as the praxic function of the speech apparatus develops. As a general rule, the first recognizable words appear by the end of 12 months. Initially these are attached directly to persons and objects and then are used increasingly to designate objects. The word then becomes the symbol, and this substitution greatly facilitates speaking and later thinking about people and objects. Nouns are learned first, then verbs and other parts of speech. Exposure to and correction by parents and siblings gradually shapes vocal behavior, including the development of a distinctive accent, to conform with that of the social group in which the child is raised.

During the second year of life, the child begins to use word combinations. They form the propositions which, according to Hughlings Jackson, are the essence of language. On average, at 18 months the child can combine an average of 1½ words; at 2 years, 2 words; at 2½ years, 3 words, and at 3 years, 4 words. Pronunciation of words undergoes a similar progression; 90 percent of children can articulate all vowel sounds by the age of 3 years. At a slightly later age the consonants *p*, *b*, *m*, *h*, *w*, *d*, *n*, *t*, and *k* are enunciated; *ng* by the age of 4 years; *y*, *j*, *zh*, and *wh* by 5 to 6 years; and *f*, *l*, *v*, *sh*, *ch*, *s*, *v*, and *th* by 7 years. Girls tend to acquire articulatory facility somewhat earlier than boys. The vocabulary increases, so that at 18 months the child knows 6 to 20 words; by 24 months, 50 to 200 words; by 3 years, 200 to 400 words. By 4 years, the child is normally capable of telling stories, but with little distinction between fact and fancy. By 6 years, the average child knows several thousand words. Also by that age, children can indicate spatial and temporal relationships and start to inquire about causality. The understanding of spoken language always exceeds the child's speaking vocabulary; that is to say, most children understand more than they can say.

The next stage of language development is reading. Here there must be an association of graphic symbols with the auditory, visual, and kinesthetic images of words already acquired. Usually the written word is learned by associating it with the spoken word rather than with the seen object. The integrity of the superior gyrus of the temporal lobe (Wernicke's area) and contiguous parieto-occipital areas of the dominant hemisphere are essential to the establishment of these *cross-modal associations*. Writing is learned soon after reading, the audiovisual symbols of words being linked to cursive movements of the hand. The tradition of beginning grade school at 6 years is based not on an arbitrary decision but on the empirically determined age at which the nervous system of the average child is ready to learn and execute the tasks of reading, writing, and—soon thereafter—calculating.

Once language is fully acquired, it is integrated into all aspects of complex action and behavior. Movements of volitional type are activated by a spoken command or the individual's inner phrasing of an intended action. Every plan for the solution of a problem must be cast into language, and the final result is analyzed in verbal terms. Thinking and language are therefore inseparable.

Anthropologists see in all this a grander scheme wherein the individual recapitulates the language development of the human race. They point out that in primitive peoples, language consisted of gestures and the utterance of simple sounds expressing emotion and that, over periods of time, movements and sounds became the conventional signs and verbal symbols of objects. Later these sounds came to designate the abstract qualities of objects. Historically, signs and spoken language were the first means of human communication; graphic records appeared much later. American Indians, for instance, never reached the level of syllabic written language. Writing commenced as pictorial representation, and only much later were alphabets devised. The reading and writing of words are comparatively late achievements.

For further details concerning communicative and cognitive abilities and methods of assessment, the reader should consult the monograph by Minifie and Lloyd.

Sexual Development

The terms *sexual* and *sexuality* have several meanings in medical and nonmedical writings. The most obvious one relates to the functions of the male and female sexual organs through which procreation occurs and the survival of the species is assured as well as to behaviors that serve to attract the opposite sex and ultimately lead to mating. The terms refer also to a person's concern or preoccupation with sex or his erotic desires or activities. A more ambiguous meaning has been proposed by some psychologists, for whom the term is equated with all growth and development, the experience of pleasure, and survival.

Without question, the sexual instinct is one of the most powerful forces in human behavior. Much of adolescent and adult activity is engaged in seeking to satisfy sexual impulses and contending with a society that imposes certain restrictions on their free and irresponsible expression. Much of Freudian psychoanalytic theory centers on the sexual development of the child and—on the basis of questionable observations—espouses the view that repression of the sexual impulse and the psychic conflicts resulting therefrom are the main sources of neurosis and possibly psychosis.

The following are the main chronological steps in sexual development, taken from the observations of Gesell and colleagues and itemized in de Ajuriaguerra's monograph:

18 months	Infant applies term *baby* to both boys and girls.
30 months	Sexual organs noticed and touched when naked. Boy knows his penis is same as father's. Uses terms *boy* and *girl*.
3 years	Gives verbal expression to differences between sexes and their different postures in urination. Likes to touch adults, especially mother's breasts.
4 years	Some pleasure in exhibitionism.

5 years	Conscious of sexual organs of others. Asks why father does not have breasts or sister a penis.
6 years	Boys and girls interested in mutual examination of sexual organs. Ask how babies come out of mother and where they came from.
7 years	First hint of attraction to opposite sex.
8 years	Teases and jokes about sexual matters.
9 years	Interested in details of sexual organs. Becomes shy in appearing nude before father and mother. In groups, each sex prefers to be separate.
Prepubertal	In this period, attachments formed with older person of same sex (girlhood crushes); in boys, attachments to members of same sex (gang formation). One observes here homosexual tendencies.
Puberty	Sexes clearly separated. In girls, menstruation and breast development are added characteristics.
Adolescence	Emergence of increasing display of heterosexual behaviors in school, at dances, and in other social activities.

Penile erections occur intermittently in both infantile and childhood periods. In later childhood, erection is self-initiated and still later is carried to the point of ejaculation and orgasm. It is a natural prelude to heterosexual intercourse but later may be a substitute for it.

The timetable of the menarche and other aspects of sexual development is not uniform; and there is considerable variation. If sexuality is not allowed natural expression, it often becomes a source of worry and preoccupation. Some 10 percent of the population fails to gain the biologically necessary heterosexual orientation.

Derangements of psychosexual function are discussed on pages 545 and 1603.

Homosexuality The homosexual is motivated in adult life by a preferential erotic attraction to members of the same sex. Most psychiatrists exclude from the definition of homosexuality those patterns of behavior that are not motivated by specific preferential desire, such as the incidental homosexuality of adolescents and the situational homosexuality of prisoners.

Figures on incidence are difficult to secure. According to the early reports of Kinsey and colleagues, approximately 4 percent of American males are exclusively homosexual and 8 percent have been "more or less exclusively homosexual for at least three years, sometime between the ages of 16 and 65." For females, the incidence is lower, perhaps half that for males. It was estimated, on the basis of the examination of large numbers of military personnel during World War II, that 1 to 2 percent of servicemen were exclusively or predominantly homosexual. More recent estimates, both in men and women, range from 1 to 5 percent (see LeVay and Hamer). These widely variable figures share a problem with all estimates derived from surveys and questionnaires: they cannot count people who do not wish to be counted.

The origins of homosexuality are obscure. We favor the hypothesis that differences or variations in genetic patterning of the immature nervous system (probably of the hypothalamus) set the sexual predilection during early life. Several morphologic studies of the hypothalamus are significant in this regard. Swaab and Hofman have reported that the preoptic zone is three times larger in heterosexual males than it is in females, but it is about the same size in homosexual males as it is in females. As mentioned in Chap. 27, LeVay found that an aggregate of neurons in the suprachiasmatic nucleus of the hypothalamus is two to three times larger in heterosexual men than it is in women, and also two and three times larger in heterosexual than in homosexual men. These findings, which have been disputed by Byne, if confirmed, would support the view that homosexuality has a biologic basis. Genetic studies point in the same direction. Pooled data from five studies in men have shown that about 57 percent of identical twins (and 13 percent of brothers) of homosexual men are also homosexual. The figures for lesbians are much the same. The inheritance pattern of male homosexuality comes from the maternal side, implicating a gene on the X chromosome (LeVay and Hamer).

Psychoanalytic explanations of homosexuality have never been substantiated. Attempts to demonstrate an endocrine basis for homosexuality have also failed. The most widely held current view is that homosexuality is not a mental or a personality disorder, though it may at times lead to secondary reactive neurotic disturbances. The studies of Kinsey and colleagues indicate that a homosexual orientation cannot be traced to a single social or psychologic root. Instead, as indicated above, homosexuality seems to arise from a deep-seated predisposition, probably biologic in origin and as ingrained as heterosexuality. The status of bisexuality is undetermined.

The Development of Personality and Social Adaptation

Personality is the most inclusive of all psychologic terms. It encompasses all the physical and psychologic traits that distinguish one individual from every other. The notion that one's physical characteristics are determined by inheritance is a fundamental tenet of biology. One has but to observe the resemblances between parent and child to confirm this view. Only the extent of human variation causes surprise. Just as no two persons are physically identical, not even monozygotic twins, so too do they differ in body chemistry or any other quality one chooses to measure. These differences, together with certain predilections to disease, explain why any one person may have an unpredictable reaction to a pathogenic agent. Strictly speaking, the normal person is an abstraction, just as is a typical example of any disease.

However, it is in other, seemingly nonphysical attributes that individuals display the greatest differences. Here reference is made to their variable place on a scale of energy, capacity for effective work, intellectual endowment (which largely determine their educability and capacity to learn), sensitivity, temperament, emotional responsivity, aggressivity or passivity, character, and tolerance to change and stress. The composite of these qualities constitutes the human personality.

In the formation of personality, especially the part concerned with feeling and emotional sensitivity, basic temperament surely plays a part. By nature, some children from the beginning seem to be happy, cheerful, and unconcerned about immediate frustrations; others are the opposite. By the third month of life, Birch and Belmont recognized individual differences in activity-passivity, regularity-irregularity, intensity of action, approach-withdrawal, adaptivity-unadaptivity, high-low threshold of response to stimulation, positive-negative mood, high-low selectivity, and high-low distractibility. Ratings at this early age were found to correlate with the results of examinations made at 5 years. Kagan and Moss recognized the trait of timidity as early as 6 months of age and noted that it persists lifelong. Not all psychologists agree with these observations; some insist that the mother's behavior is of crucial importance in teaching such patterns. The problem is made even more complicated by the possibility that the character of the infant may influence the mother's reactions. The more common aspects of personality—i.e., worry about one's health and other matters, anxiety or serenity, timidity or boldness, the power of instinctual drives and need of satisfaction, sympathy for others, sensitivity to criticism, and degree of disorganization resulting from adverse circumstances—are presumed to be genetically determined. Identical twins raised apart are remarkably alike in these and many other personality traits and have the same IQs, within a few points (Moser et al). The strong genetic influence on personality development has also been demonstrated by Scarr and associates. The related subject of the development of a moral sense that can be said to be part of an individual's personality has been subject to several competing theories. The interested reader is referred to Damon's summary of the topic.

Disorders of personality and the genetic predisposition to certain personality traits are discussed further in Chap 56.

Social behavior, like other neurologic and psychologic functions in general, depends to a great extent on the development and maturation of the brain. Involved also are genetic and environmental factors, for one cannot adapt to society except in the presence of other people; i.e., social interaction is necessary for the emergence of many basic biologic traits. One must think of personality as a series of intrinsic forces continuously emerging and being altered by maturation of the nervous system and by the force of social demands. Thus, the roots of social behavior are traceable to certain instinctive patterns that are progressively elaborated by conditioned emotional reactions. In the long series of human interactions—first with parents, then with siblings and other children, and finally with a widening circle of individuals in the classroom and community—the capacity to cooperate, to subjugate one's own egocentric needs to those of the group, and to lead or be led appear as secondary modes of response (i.e., secondary to some of the basic impulses of anger, fear, self-protection, love, and pleasure). The sources of these social reactions are even more obscure than those of temperament, character, and intelligence.

In children, difficulty in social adaptation tends first to be manifest by an inability to take their places in a classroom. However, the greatest demands and frustrations in social development are likely to occur in late childhood and adolescence. Adolescents, half emancipated from family ties, may become troubled as they seek the recognition and respect of their peers. For the first time, they think seriously of what they are and what they will be. In search of personal identity, they become more critical of their parents and turn increasingly to interaction with larger social groups. If the relationship with their parents is firmly established and the parents respond to their child's doubts and criticisms with sympathetic understanding, this unsettled state is temporary and is followed by a resynthesis of the child's relationship with the family on a firm and lasting basis. The development of adult gonadal function and the further evolution of psychosexual impulses create a bewildering array of new challenges in social adaptation. These types of social adjustment continue as long as life continues. As social roles change, as intellectual and physical capacities first advance and later recede, new challenges demand new adaptations.

At the highest level of social interaction between an individual and the family unit and community, we see more clearly the workings of another principle—that biologic evolution merges with and is finally superseded by cultural evolution. The latter event is uniquely human. Of the primate family, only human beings are able to alter their environment in a systematic fashion, to anticipate and plan for the future, and to think and communicate by symbols. Language enables us to think through the consequences of an action before attempting it, to abstract from the concrete to the general situation, and to analyze the relationship between the elements of a problem without the necessity of actually manipulating the elements. Language is also the agency whereby the experiences of the past are made available for understanding current problems. Thus, we build continuously on our cultural heritage.

DELAYS AND FAILURES OF NORMAL NEUROLOGIC DEVELOPMENT

Delays in Motor Development

A delay in motor development is often accompanied by mental retardation, in which case both are parts of a developmental lag or immaturity of the entire cerebrum. The most severe forms of delayed motor development, associated with spasticity and athetosis, are usually manifestations of particular prenatal and paranatal diseases of the brain; these are discussed in Chap. 38.

In assessing developmental abnormalities of the motor system in the neonate and young infant, the following maneuvers, which elicit certain postures and reflexive movements, are particularly useful:

1. The *Moro response* is the infant's reaction to startle and can be evoked by suddenly withdrawing support of the head and allowing the neck to extend. A loud noise, slapping the bed, or jerking one leg will have the same effect—causing an elevation and abduction of the arms followed by a clasping movement to the midline. This response is present in all newborns and infants up to 4 or 5 months of age, and its absence indicates a profound disorder of the motor system. An absent or inadequate Moro response on one side is found in infants with hemiplegia, brachial plexus palsy, or a fractured clavicle. Persistence of the Moro response beyond 4 or 5 months of age is noted only in infants with severe neurologic defects.

2. The asymmetrical *tonic neck reflex* (extension of the arm and leg on the side to which the head is passively turned and flexion of the opposite limbs), if obligatory and sustained, is a sign at any age of pyramidal or extrapyramidal motor abnormality. Barlow reports that he has obtained this reflex in 25 percent of mentally retarded infants at 9 to 10 months of age. Fragments of the reflex, such as a brief extension of one arm, may be elicited in 60 percent of normal infants at 1 to 2 months of age and may be adopted spontaneously by the infant up to 6 months of age.

3. The *placing reaction* (described earlier, under "Physiologic and Psychologic Development") is present in all normal newborns. Its absence or asymmetry under 6 months of age indicates a motor abnormality.

4. In the *Landau maneuver*, the infant, if suspended horizontally in the prone position, will extend the neck and trunk and will break the trunk extension when the neck is passively flexed. This reaction is present by 6 months; its delayed appearance in a hypotonic child is indicative of a faulty motor apparatus.

5. If an infant is held prone in the horizontal position and is then dropped toward the bed, an extension of the arms is evoked, as if to break the fall. This is known as the "*parachute response*" and is elicitable in most 9-month-old infants. If it is asymmetrical, it indicates a unilateral motor abnormality.

The detection of gross delays or abnormalities of motor development in the neonatal or early infantile period of life is aided little by tests of tendon and plantar reflexes. Arm reflexes are always rather difficult to obtain in infants, and a normal neonate may have a few beats of ankle clonus. The plantar response tends to be wavering and uncertain in pattern. However, a consistent extension of the great toe and fanning of the toes on stroking the side of the foot is abnormal at any age.

The early detection of "cerebral palsy" is hampered by the fact that the corticospinal tract is not fully myelinated until 18 months of age, allowing only quasi-voluntary movements up to this time. For this reason, a *congenital hemiparesis* may not be evident until many months after birth. Even then it is manifest only by subtle signs, such as holding the hand in a fisted posture or clumsiness in reaching for objects and in transferring them from one hand to the other. Later, the leg is seen to be less active as the infant crawls, steps, and places the foot. Early hand dominance should always raise the suspicion of a motor defect on the opposite side. In the upper limb, the characteristic catch and yielding resistance of spasticity is most evident in passive abduction of the arm, extension of the elbow, dorsiflexion of the wrist, and supination of the forearm; in the leg, the change in tone is best detected by passive flexion of the knee. However, the time of appearance and degree of spasticity are variable from patient to patient. The stretch reflexes are hyperactive, and the plantar reflex may be extensor on the affected side. With bilateral hemiplegia, the same abnormalities are detectable, but there is a greater likelihood of pseudobulbar manifestations, with delayed, poorly enunciated speech. Later, intelligence is likely to be impaired (in 40 percent of hemiplegias and 70 percent of quadriplegias). In *diparesis* or *diplegia*, hypotonia gives way to spasticity and the same delay in motor development except that it predominates in the legs. Aside from the hereditary spastic paraplegias, which may become evident in the second and third years, the common causes of weak spastic legs are prematurity and matrix hemorrhages.

Developmental motor delay and other abnormalities are present in a large proportion of infants with *hypotonia*. When the "floppy" infant is lifted and its limbs are passively manipulated, there is little muscle reactivity. In the supine position, the weakness and laxity result in a "frog-leg" posture, along with an increased mobility at the ankles and hips. Hypotonia, if generalized and accompanied by an absence of tendon reflexes, is most often due to Werdnig-Hoffmann disease, although the range of possible diagnoses is large and includes diseases of muscle, nerve, and the central nervous system (see Chaps. 48 and 52). The other causes of this type of neonatal and infantile hypotonia—muscular dystrophies and congenital myopathies, maternal myasthenia gravis, polyneuropathies, Down syndrome, Prader-Willi syndrome, and spinal cord injuries—are described in their appropriate chapters. Sometimes hypotonia is accompanied by congenital fixed contractures of the joints, termed *arthrogryposis* (page 1530).

Infants who will later manifest a central motor defect can sometimes be recognized by the briskness of their tendon reflexes and by the postures they assume when lifted. In the normal infant, the legs are flexed and slightly rotated externally, and associated with vigorous kicking movements. The hypotonic infant with a defect of the motor projection pathways may extend the legs or rotate them internally, with dorsiflexion of the feet and toes. Exceptionally, the legs are firmly flexed, but in either instance relatively few movements are made.

When hypotonia is a forerunner of an extrapyramidal motor disorder (e.g., double athetosis), the first hint of abnormality may be an opisthotonic posturing of the head and neck. However, involuntary choreic movements usually do not appear in the upper limbs before 5 to 6 months of age and often are so slight as to be overlooked. They worsen as the infant matures and by 12 months assume a more athetotic character, often combined with tremor. Tone in the affected limbs is by then increased but may be interrupted during passive manipulation.

When hypotonia is a prelude to a cerebellar motor defect, the ataxia becomes apparent when the infant makes the first reaching movements. Tremulous, irregular movements of the trunk and head are seen when the infant attempts to sit without support. Still later, as the infant attempts to stand, there is unsteadiness of the entire body.

In distinction to the gross deficits in motor development described above, there is a relatively small but distinct group of young children who exhibit only mild abnormalities of muscle tone, clumsiness or unusual postures of the hands, tremor, and ataxia ("fine motor deficit"). Such low-severity developmental deficits in the somewhat older child are referred to as "clumsiness" or "soft signs" and have been extensively described by Gubbay and colleagues in what they called "the clumsy child." Like speech delay and dyslexia, fine motor deficits are more frequent in males. Tirosh found that intranatal problems were increased among children with fine motor deficits (compared to those with gross motor deficits), as were minor physical anomalies and seizures.

Systemic diseases in infancy pose special problems in evaluation of the motor system. The achievement of motor milestones is delayed by illnesses such as congenital heart disease (especially cyanotic forms), cystic fibrosis, renal and hepatic diseases, infections, and surgical procedures. Under such conditions one does well to deal with the immediate illnesses and defer pronouncements about the status of cerebral function. The brain proves to be simultaneously affected in 25 percent of patients with congenital heart disease and an even higher proportion of patients with rubella and Coxsackie B viral infections. In a disease such as cystic fibrosis, where the brain is not affected, it is advisable to depend more on the analysis of language development than of locomotion, because muscular activity may be enfeebled.

Delays in Sensory Development

Failure to see and to hear are the most important sensory defects affecting the infant and child. When *both* senses are affected, a severe cerebral defect is usually responsible; only at a later age, when the child is more testable, does it become apparent that the trouble is not with the peripheral sensory apparatus but with the central integrating mechanisms of the brain.

Failure of development of visual function is usually revealed by a disorder of ocular movements. Any defect of the refractive apparatus or the acuity of the central visual pathways results in wandering, jerky movements of the eyes. The optic discs may be atrophic in such cases, but it should be pointed out that the discs in infants tend naturally to be paler than those of an older child. In congenital hypoplasia of the optic nerves, the nerve heads are extremely small. Defects in the retina and choroid are detectable by funduscopy. Faulty vision becomes increasingly apparent in older infants when the normal sequences of hand inspection and visuomanual coordination fail to emerge. Retention of pupillary light reflexes in a sightless child signifies a defect in the geniculocalcarine tracts or occipital lobes—conditions that may be confirmed by CT scanning and testing of visual evoked responses.

With respect to hearing, again there is the difficulty in evaluating this function in an infant. Normally, after a few weeks of life, alert parents notice a brisk startle to loud noises and a response to other sounds. A tinkling bell brought from behind the infant usually results in hearkening or head turning and visual searching, but a lack of these responses warns only of the most severe hearing defects. The elicitation of slight degrees of deafness, enough to interfere with auditory learning, requires special testing. To make the problem even more difficult, both a peripheral and a central disorder may be present in some conditions, such as kernicterus. Brainstem auditory-evoked responses (BAER) are particularly helpful in confirming peripheral abnormalities in the infant and young child. After the first few months, impaired hearing becomes more obvious and interferes with language development, as described further on.

RESTRICTED DEVELOPMENTAL ABNORMALITIES

A considerable portion of neuropediatric practice is committed to the diagnosis and management of children with a learning disability. It usually comes to light in the school-age child (hence the term *school dysfunction*), whose aptitude for classroom learning is thought to be inferior to his general intelligence. The medical referral may be from a parent, teacher, or psychologist. The clinician's objective is to determine by history and examination whether there is (1) a general congenital developmental abnormality impairing intelligence or (2) a specific deficit in reading, writing, arithmetic, or attention, any one of which may interfere with the child's ability to learn.

Once diagnosis is achieved, the goal of management, undertaken in collaboration with psychologists and educators, is to fashion a program of remedial exercises that will maximize the child's skills, commensurate with his talent and aptitude, and restore his self-confidence (see Rosenberger).

Disorders in the Development of Speech and Language

In the pediatric age period and extending into adult life, one encounters an interesting assortment of developmental disorders of speech and language. Many patients with such disorders come from families in which similar speech defects, ambidexterity, and left-handedness are frequent. Males predominate; in some series, male-to-female ratios as high as 10:1 have been reported.

Developmental disorders of speech and language are far more frequent than acquired disorders, i.e., aphasia. The former include developmental speech delay, congenital deafness with speech delay, cleft-palate speech, developmental word deafness, dyslexia (special reading disability), cluttered speech, infantilisms of speech, and stuttering or stammering. Often in these disorders, the various stages of language development, described in an earlier section of this chapter, are not attained at the usual age and may not be achieved even by adulthood. Disorders of this type, restricted to the language areas, are far more likely to be due to slowness in the normal processes of maturation than to an acquired disease. With the possible exception of developmental dyslexia (see further on), cerebral lesions have not been described in these cases, though it must be emphasized that only a small number of brains of such individuals become available for study and of these only a few have been thoroughly studied by proper methods.

In discussing the developmental disorders of speech and language, we have adopted the conventional classification. Not included in such a classification are the many mundane peculiarities of speech and language that are usually accepted without comment—lack of fluency, inability to speak uninterruptedly in complete sentences, and lack of proper intonation, inflection, and melody of speech (dysprosody). The pathophysiology of such disorders is not at all understood and is not discussed further in this chapter (see Chap. 23).

Developmental Speech Delay Fully two-thirds of children say their first words between 9 and 12 months of age and their first word combinations before their second birthday; when this does not happen, it becomes a matter of parental concern. Children who fail to reach these milestones at the stated times fall into two general categories. In one group there is no clear evidence of mental retardation or impairment of neurologic or auditory function. In a second group, the speech delay has an overt pathologic basis.

The first group, comprising *otherwise normal children who talk late* (they deviate from their age norm well beyond 2 SD), is the more puzzling. It is virtually impossible to predict whether such a child's speech will eventually be normal in all respects and just when this will occur. Prelanguage speech continues into the period when words and phrases should normally be used in propositional speech. The combinations of sounds are close to the standard of normal vowel-consonant combinations of the 1- to 2-year-old, and they may be strung together as in a sentence. Yet, as time passes, the child may utter only a few understandable words, even by the third or fourth year. Often one discovers a family history of delayed speech, and three out of four such patients will be boys. When finally the child begins to talk, he may skip the early stages of spoken language and progress rapidly to speak in full sentences and to develop fluent speech and language. During the period of speech delay, the understanding of words and general intelligence develop normally, and communication by gestures may be remarkably facile. In such children, motor speech delay does not presage mental backwardness. (It is said that Albert Einstein did not speak until the age of 4 and lacked fluency at age 9.)

Nevertheless, the eventual acquisition of fluent speech is no guarantee of normality (Rutter and Martin). Many such children have later educational difficulties, mainly because of dyslexia and dysgraphia, a combination that is sometimes inherited as an autosomal dominant trait—again, more frequently in boys. In a smaller subgroup, articulation remains infantile and the content of speech is impoverished semantically and syntactically. Yet others, as they begin to speak, express themselves fluently, but with distortions, omissions, and cluttering of words (see below); such patients usually recover.

A second broad group of children with speech delay or retarded speech development (no words by 18 months, no phrases by 30 months) comprises those in whom an overt pathologic basis is evident. In clinics where children of the latter type are studied systematically, 35 to 50 percent of cases occur in those with mental retardation or "cerebral palsy." Hearing deficit explains many of the other cases, as discussed below, and a few represent what appears to be a slowness in the maturation of the motor speech areas or an acquired lesion in these parts. Only in this small latter group is it appropriate to refer to the language disorder as aphasia—i.e., a derangement or loss of language due to a cerebral lesion. Aphasia, when it occurs as the result of an acquired lesion (vascular, traumatic), is essentially motor and lasts but a few months. It may be accompanied by a right-sided hemiplegia. An interesting example of acquired aphasia, possibly encephalitic, has been described by Landau and Kleffner in association with seizures and bitemporal focal discharges in the EEG (see page 353).

Congenital Deafness Speech delay due to congenital deafness, whether peripheral (loss of pure-tone acuity) or central (pure-tone threshold normal by audiogram), may at first be difficult to discern. One suspects that faulty hearing is causal when there is a history of familial deaf mutism, congenital rubella, erythroblastosis fetalis, meningitis, chronic bilateral ear infections, or the administration of ototoxic drugs to the pregnant mother or newborn infant—the well-known antecedents of deafness. It is estimated that approximately 3 million American children have hearing defects; 0.1 percent of the school population are deaf and 1.5 percent are hard of hearing. The parents' attention may be drawn to a defect in hearing when the infant fails to heed loud noises, to turn the eyes to sound sources outside the immediate visual fields, and to react to music; but in other instances it is the delay in speaking that calls attention to it.

The deaf child makes the transition from crying to cooing and babbling at the usual age of 3 to 5 months.

After the sixth month, however, the child becomes much quieter, and the usual repertoire of babbling sounds becomes stereotyped and unchanging, though still uttered with pleasant voice. A more conspicuous failure comes somewhat later, when babbling fails to give way to word formation. Should deafness develop within the first few years of life, the child gradually loses such speech as had been acquired but can be retaught by the lipreading method. Speech, however, is harsh, poorly modulated, and unpleasant and accompanied by many peculiar squeals and snorting or grunting noises. Social and other acquisitions appear at the expected times in the congenitally deaf child, unlike the mentally retarded child. The deaf child seems eager to communicate and makes known all his needs by gesture or pantomime—often very cleverly. The deaf child may attract attention by vivid facial expressions, motions of the lips, nodding, or head shaking. The Leiter performance scale, which makes no use of sounds, will show that intelligence is normal. Deafness can be demonstrated at an early age by careful observation of the child's responses to sounds and by free-field audiometry, but the full range of hearing cannot be accurately tested before the age of 3 or 4 years. Recording of auditory-evoked brainstem potentials and testing of the labyrinths, which are frequently unresponsive in deaf mutes, may be helpful. Early diagnosis is important in order to fit the child with a hearing aid, if possible, and to begin appropriate language training.

In contrast to the child in whom deafness is the only abnormality, the mentally retarded child is generally defective and talks little because he or she has nothing to say. Autistic children may also be mute; if they speak, echolalia is prominent and the personal "I" is avoided. Blind children of normal intelligence tend to speak slowly and fail to acquire imitative gestures.

Congenital Word Deafness This disorder—also called *developmental receptive dysphasia*, *verbal auditory agnosia*, or *central deafness*—is rare and may be difficult to distinguish from peripheral deafness. Usually the parents have noted that the word-deaf child responds to loud noises and music, but obviously this does not assure perfect hearing, particularly for high tones. The word-deaf child does not understand what is said, and delay and distortion of speech are evident.

Presumably, in this disorder, the receptive auditory elements of the dominant temporal cortex fail to discriminate the complex acoustic patterns of words and to associate them with visual images of people and objects. Despite intact pure-tone hearing, the child does not seem to hear word patterns properly and fails to reproduce them in natural speech. In other ways the child may be bright, but more often this auditory imperception of words is associated with hyperactivity, inattentiveness, bizarre behavior, or other perceptual defects incident to focal brain damage, particularly of the temporal lobes. Word-deaf children may chatter incessantly and often adopt a language of their own design, which the parents come to understand. This peculiar type of speech is known as *idioglossia*. It is also observed in children with marked articulatory defects.

Speech rehabilitation of the bright word-deaf child follows along the same lines as that of the congenitally deaf one. Such a child learns to lip-read quickly and is clever at acting out his or her own ideas.

Congenital Inarticulation In this developmental defect the child seems unable to coordinate the vocal, articulatory, and respiratory musculature for the purpose of speaking. Again, boys are affected more often than girls, and there is often a family history of the disorder, although the data are not quite sufficient to establish the pattern of inheritance. The incidence is 1 in every 200 children. The motor, sensory, emotional, and social attainments correspond to the norms for age, although in a few cases, a minority in the authors' opinion, there has been some indication of cranial nerve abnormality in the first months of life (ptosis, facial asymmetry, strange neonatal cry, and altered phonation).

In children with congenital inarticulation, the prelanguage sounds are probably abnormal, but this aspect of the speech disorder has not been well studied. Babbling tends to be deficient, and, in the second year, in attempting to say something, the child makes noises that do not sound at all like language; in this way the child is unlike the late talker already described. Again, the understanding of language is entirely normal; the comprehension vocabulary is average for age, and the child can appreciate syntax, as indicated by correct responses to questions by nodding or shaking the head and by the execution of complex spoken commands. Usually such patients are shy but otherwise quick in responding, cheerful, and without other behavioral disorders. Most are bright, but a combination of congenital inarticulation and mild mental dullness is not uncommon. If many of the spontaneous utterances are intelligible, speech correction should be attempted (by a trained therapist). However, if the child makes no sounds that resemble words, the therapeutic effort should be directed toward a modified school program, and speech habilitation should wait until some words are acquired.

Studies of the cerebra of such patients are not available, and it is doubtful if they would show any abnormality by the usual techniques of neuropathologic examination. Occasionally, suspicion of a lesion is raised by focal changes in the EEG or a slight widening of the temporal horn of the left ventricle. All manner of delayed speech is often attributed to "tongue-tie," i.e., a short lingual frenulum, but we have never been convinced of this causal relationship. Also, psychologists have attributed speech retardation to overprotectiveness or excessive pressure by the parents. We are inclined to believe that these are the result rather than the cause of the delay.

A fuller review of this subject can be found in the text *The Child with Delayed Speech*, edited by Rutter and Martin.

Stuttering and Stammering These difficulties occur in an estimated 1 to 2 percent of the school population. Often such conditions disappear in late childhood and adolescence; by adulthood, only about 1 in every 300 individuals suffers from a persistent stammer or stutter. Mild degrees are to some extent cultivated and permit a pause in speech for collecting one's thoughts, and stammering tends to be imitated in certain social circles, as among educated Englishmen (and some Americans).

Stammering and stuttering are difficult to classify. In some respects they belong to and are customarily included in the developmental language disorders, but they differ in being largely centered in articulation. Essentially they represent a disorder of rhythm—an involuntary, repetitive prolongation of speech—due to an insuppressible *spasm of the articulatory muscles*. The spasm may be tonic and result in a complete blocking of speech (at one time referred to as stammering) or clonic, i.e., a rapid series of spasms interrupting the emission of consonants, usually the first letter or syllable of a word (stuttering). There is no valid reason to distinguish between these two forms of the disorder, since they are intermingled, and the terms *stammer* and *stutter* are now used synonymously. Certain sounds, particularly *p* and *b*, offer greater difficulty than others; *paperboy* comes out *p-p-paper b-b-boy*. The severity of the stutter is increased by excitement and stress, as when speaking before others, and is reduced when the stutterer is relaxed and alone or when singing in a chorus. When severe, the spasms may overflow into other groups of muscles, mainly of the face and neck and even of the arms. The muscles involved in stuttering show no fault in actions other than speaking, and all gnostic and semantic aspects of receptive language are intact.

Males are affected four times as often as females. The time of onset of stuttering is mainly at two periods in life—between 2 and 4 years of age, when speech and language are evolving, and between 6 and 8 years, when these functions extend to reciting and reading aloud in the classroom. However, there may be a later onset. Many afflicted children have an associated difficulty in reading and writing. If stuttering is mild, it tends to develop or to be present only during periods of emotional stress, and in four out of five children it disappears entirely or almost so during adolescence or the early adult years (Andrews and Harris). If severe, it persists throughout life regardless of treatment but tends to improve as the patient grows older.

Theories of causation are legion. Slowness in developing hand and eye preference, ambidexterity, or an enforced change from left- to right-hand use have been popular explanations, of which Orton and Travis were leading advocates. According to this theory, stuttering results from a lack of the necessary degree of unilateral control in the synchronization of bilaterally innervated speech mechanisms. Fox and Ingham lend support to the theory of a failure of left hemisphere dominance. By performing PET studies while the subject was reading, they found that the auditory and motor areas of the right hemisphere are activated instead of those of the left hemisphere. However, these explanations apply to only a minority of stutterers (Hécaen and de Ajuriaguerra). The disappearance of mild stuttering with maturation has been attributed incorrectly to all manner of treatment (hypnosis, progressive relaxation, speaking in rhythms, etc.) and used to bolster particular theories of causation. Since stuttering may reappear at times of emotional strain, a psychogenesis has been proposed, but—as pointed out by Orton and by Baker and colleagues—if there are any neurotic tendencies in the stutterer, they are secondary rather than primary. We have observed that many stutterers, probably as a result of this impediment to free social interaction, do become increasingly fearful of talking and develop feelings of inferiority. By the time adolescence and adulthood are reached, emotional factors are so prominent that many physicians have mistaken stuttering for neurosis. Usually there is little or no evidence of any personality deviation before the onset of stuttering, and psychotherapy has not in our experience had a significant effect on the underlying defect. A strong family history in many cases and male dominance point to a genetic origin, but the inheritance does not follow a readily discernible pattern.

Stuttering is not associated with any detectable weakness or ataxia of the speech musculature. The muscles of speech go into spasm *only* when called upon to perform the specific act of speaking. The spasms are not invoked by other actions (which may not be as complex or voluntary as speaking), differing in this way from an apraxia and the intention spasm of athetosis. Also, palilalia is a different condition in which a word or phrase, usually the last one in a sentence, is repeated many times with decreasing volume. In fact, stuttering may represent a special category of movement disorder, much like writer's cramp, which is a selective craft or occupational spasm (page 116). We regard both as highly restricted extrapyramidal motor disorders, bearing some of the characteristics of focal dystonia.

Rarely, in adults as well as in children, stuttering may be acquired as a result of a lesion in the motor speech areas. A distinction has been drawn between developmental and acquired stuttering. The latter is said to interfere with the enunciation of any syllable of a word (not just the first), to favor involvement of grammatical and substantive words, and to be unaccompanied by anxiety and facial grimacing. Such distinctions are probably illusory. The reported lesion sites in acquired stuttering are so variable (right frontal, corpus striatum, left temporal, left parietal) as to be difficult to reconcile with proposed theories of developmental stuttering (Fleet and Heilman).

Another form of acquired stuttering is manifestly an expression of an extrapyramidal disorder. Here there occurs a prolonged repetition of syllables (vowel and consonant), which the patient cannot easily interrupt. The abnormality involves throat-clearing and other vocalizations. We have observed it in some patients with Parkinson disease and in progressive supranuclear palsy.

The therapy of stuttering is difficult to evaluate. As remarked above, all speech-fluency disturbances are modifiable by environmental circumstances. Thus a certain proportion of stutterers will become more fluent under certain conditions, such as reading aloud; others will stutter more severely at this time. Again, a majority of stutterers will be adversely affected by talking on the telephone; a minority are helped by this device. Some stutterers are more fluent under conditions of mild alcohol intoxication. Nearly every stutterer is fluent while singing.

On the whole, the therapy of speech-fluency disorders has been a frustrating effort. Schemes such as the encouragement of associated muscular movements ("penciling," etc.) and the adoption of a "theatrical" approach to speaking have been advocated. Common to all such efforts has been the difficulty of achieving carryover into the natural speaking environment. Progressive relaxation, hypnosis, delayed auditory feedback, loud noise that masks speech sounds, and many other ancillary measures may help temporarily.

Cluttering, or Cluttered, Speech This is another special developmental disorder. It is characterized by uncontrollable speed of speech, which results in truncated, dysrhythmic, and often incoherent utterances. Omissions of consonants, elisions, improper phrasing, and inadequate intonation occur. It is as though the child were too hurried to take the trouble to pronounce each word carefully and to compose sentences. Cluttering is frequently associated with other motor speech impediments. Speech therapy (elocutionary) and maturation are usually attended by a restoration of more normal rhythms.

Other Articulatory Defects These are most common in preschool children, having an incidence of 15 percent. There are several varieties. One is *lisping*, in which the *s* sound is replaced by *th*, e.g., *thimple* for *simple*. Another common condition, *lallation*, or *dyslalia*, is characterized by multiple substitutions or omissions of consonants. Milder degrees consist of difficulty in pronouncing one or two consonants. For example, the letter *r* may be incorrectly pronounced, so that it sounds like *w* or *y*; *running a race* becomes *wunning a wace* or *yunning a yace*. In severe forms, speech may be almost unintelligible. The child seems to be unaware that his or her speech differs from that of others and is distressed at not being understood. These and similar abnormalities of speech are often present in otherwise normal children and are referred to as "infantilisms." Why they persist in some individuals is not understood. More important is the fact that in more than 90 percent of cases, these articulatory abnormalities disappear by the age of 8 years, either spontaneously or in response to speech therapy. The latter is best started if these conditions persist into the fifth year. Presumably the natural cycle of motor speech acquisition has only been delayed, not arrested. Such abnormalities are more frequent among the feebleminded than in normal children; with mental defect, many consonants are persistently mispronounced.

Worster-Drought has described a congenital form of spastic bulbar speech in which words are spoken slowly, with stiff labial and lingual movements, hyperactive jaw and facial reflexes, and sometimes mild dysphagia and dysphonia. The limbs may be unaffected, in contrast to those of most children with cerebral palsy.

The speech disorder resulting from *cleft palate* is easily recognized. Many of these patients also have a harelip; the two abnormalities together interfere with sucking and later in life with the enunciation of labial and guttural consonants. The voice has an unpleasant nasality; often, if the defect is severe, there is an audible escape of air through the nose.

The aforementioned developmental abnormalities of speech are sometimes associated with disturbances of higher-order language processing. Rapin and Allen have described a number of such disturbances. In one, which they call the "semantic pragmatic syndrome," a failure to comprehend complex phrases and sentences is combined with fluent speech and well-formed sentences that are, however, lacking in content. The syndrome resembles Wernicke or transcortical sensory aphasia (Chap. 23). In another, "semantic retrieval-organization syndrome," a severe anomia blocks word finding in spontaneous speech. A mixed expressive-receptive disorder may also be seen as a developmental abnormality; it contains many of the elements of acquired Broca aphasia (pages 505–508).

Developmental Dyslexia (Congenital Word Blindness) This condition, first described by Hinshelwood in 1896, becomes manifest in an older child who lacks the aptitude for one or more of the specific skills necessary to derive meaning from the printed word (Rosenberger). Also defined as a significant discrepancy between "measured intelligence" and "reading achievement" (Hynd et al), it has been found in 3 to 6 percent of all schoolchildren. There are several excellent writings on the subject, to which the interested reader is referred for a detailed account (Orton; Critchley and Critchley; Rutter and Martin; Kinsbourne; Shaywitz).

The main problem is an inability to read words and also to spell and to write them, despite the ability to see and recognize letters. There is no loss of the ability to recognize the meaning of objects, pictures, and diagrams. According to Shaywitz, these children lack an awareness that words can be broken down into individual units of sound ("phonemic unawareness") and that each segment of sound is represented by a letter or letters. In addition to the visuoperceptual defect, some individuals also manifest a failure of sequencing ability, lack of phonemic segmentation, and altered cognitive processing. De Renzi and Luchelli have also noted a deficit of verbal and visual memory. A defect in the decoding of acoustic signals is another postulated mechanism. Often, before the child enters school, reading failure can be anticipated by a delay in attending to spoken words, difficulty with rhyming games, and speech that is characterized by frequent mispronunciations and punctuated by hesitations and dysfluency, or there may be a delay in learning to speak or in attaining clear articulation. In the early school years there are difficulties in copying, color naming, and formation of number concepts as well as the persistent reversal of letters. Writing appears to be defective because of faulty perception of form and a kind of constructional and directional apraxia. Not infrequently, there is an associated vagueness about the serial order of letters in the alphabet and months in the year, as well as difficulty with numbers (acalculia) and an inability to spell and to read music. The complex of symptoms of dyslexia, dyscalculia, finger agnosia, and right-left confusion, found in a few of these children, is interpreted as a developmental form of the Gerstmann syndrome (page 485).

Lesser degrees of dyslexia are more common than the severe ones and are found in a large segment of the school population. Some 10 percent of schoolchildren have some degree of this disability, but the problem is complex because the condition is unquestionably influenced by the way reading is taught. This disorder is stable and persistent; however, as a result of effective methods of training, only a few children are unable to read at all after many years in school.

This form of language disorder, unattended by other neurologic signs, is strongly familial, being almost in conformity with an autosomal dominant or sex-linked recessive pattern. Loci on chromosomes 6 and 15 have been implicated but not confirmed. There is a statistically higher incidence of left-handedness among these persons and members of their families. Shaywitz et al have suggested that the reported predominance of reading disabilities in boys (male-to-female ratios of 2:1 to 5:1) represents a bias in subject selection—many more boys than girls being identified because of associated hyperactivity and other behavioral problems. Our casual clinical experience suggests that there is a genuine gender difference. An estimated 12 to 24 percent of dyslexic children will also have an attention-deficit disorder (see further on).

The steady drilling (many hours per week) of a cooperative and motivated child by a skillful teacher over an extended period slowly overcomes the handicap and enables an otherwise intelligent child to read at grade level and to follow a regular program of education successfully. The Orton phonologic method is one of the most successful (for details, see Rosenberger). Secondary school and college students with reading deficits often resort to tape recorders, tutorial aid, and laptop computers.

In the study of dyslexic and dysgraphic children, a number of other apparently congenital developmental abnormalities have been documented, such as inadequate perception of space and form (poor performance on form boards and in tasks requiring construction); inadequate perception of size, distance, and temporal sequences and rhythms; and inability to imitate sequences of movements gracefully, as well as extreme degrees of clumsiness and reduced proficiency in all motor tasks and games (the *clumsy-child syndrome* as described by Gubbay et al and alluded to earlier in the chapter under "Delays in Motor Development"). These disorders may also occur in brain-injured children; hence there may be considerable difficulty in separating simple delay or arrest in development from a pathologic process in the brain.

Galaburda and associates have studied the brains of four males (ages 14 to 32 years) with developmental dyslexia. In each case there were developmental anomalies of the cerebral cortex, consisting of neuronal ectopias and architectonic dysplasias, located mainly in the perisylvian regions of the left hemisphere. Also, all of the brains were characterized by relative symmetry of the planum temporale, in distinction to the usual pattern of cerebral asymmetry, favoring the planum temporale of the left side. Similar changes have been described in three women with developmental dyslexia (Humphreys et al). CT scanning of larger numbers of dyslexic patients (as well as some patients with autism and developmental speech delay) have demonstrated an increased prevalence of relative symmetry (reversed or "atypical" asymmetry) of the temporal planes of the two hemispheres (Rosenberger; Hynd et al). It is important to note, however, that not all patients with developmental dyslexia (or autism) show this anomalous anatomic asymmetry (Rumsey et al).

Leonard and colleagues, using MRI, have demonstrated several other gyral anomalies in dyslexic subjects. They found, in the planum temporale and neighboring parietal operculum of both hemispheres, that some gyri were missing and others were duplicated. Also, in some dyslexic individuals, the visual evoked responses to rapid low-contrast stimuli are diminished. The latter abnormality may be related to a deficit of large neurons in the lateral geniculate bodies (see Livingstone et al). Stein et al has found that 20 percent of dyslexic children have unstable ocular fixation and that monocular occulsion improves both binocular control and reading.

Developmental Dysgraphia Developmental writing disorders differ from dyslexia in having both linguistic and motor (orthographic) aspects. As indicated earlier, dysgraphias are present in many dyslexic children and may be combined with difficulty in calculation (so-called developmental Gerstmann syndrome). Two forms of dysgraphia have been distinguished. In one there is good handwriting and formation of letters and spacing but many misinterpretations of dictated words (*linguistic dysgraphia*). In the other, there are reversals of letters and letter order and poor alignment (*mechanical dysgraphia*).

Specific *spelling difficulty* probably represents another developmental language disorder, distinct from dyslexia.

Developmental Dyscalculia This disorder, like dyslexia, usually becomes evident in the first few years of grade school, when the child is challenged by tasks of adding and subtracting and, later, multiplying and dividing. In some instances there is an evident disorder in the spatial arrangements of numbers (supposedly a right hemispheral fault); in others, there is a lexical-graphical abnormality (naming and reading the names of numbers) akin to aphasia.

Probably all that has been said about developmental dyslexia applies to the kindred states of *acalculia* and *agraphia*, and the usual type of classroom work does nothing to increase the child's proficiency in writing and arithmetic. All of these impairments are often associated with hyperactivity and attentional defects, as described below (Denckla et al).

Precocious Reading and Calculating In contrast to the foregoing disorders, precocious reading and calculation abilities have also been identified. A 2- or 3-year old child may read with the skill of an average adult. Extraordinary facility with numbers (mathematical prodigies) and memorization ability (eidetic imagery) are comparable traits. Here, one observes a remarkable overdevelopment of these single faculties. Occasionally, one of these special abilities will be observed in a child with a mild form of autism (Asperger syndrome, see Chap. 38). Such a child may exhibit great skill in performing a mathematical trick but be unable to solve simple arithmetical problems or to understand the meaning of numbers (a kind of "idiot savant"). In the child with *Williams syndrome*, language and sometimes musical skills are not so much precocious as relatively normal in comparison to the overall mental deficiency, indicating that not all forms of mental retardation involve language.

Hyperactivity-Inattention Disorders (Attention Deficit–Hyperactivity Disorder, ADHD)

Another large portion of ambulatory pediatric neurology consists of children who are referred because of failure in school, seemingly related to overactivity, impulsivity, and inattentiveness. The question asked is whether they have an identifiable brain disease or the sequela of some brain injury that has altered their behavior. When a large number of such cases is analyzed, fully 80 to 85 percent prove to have no major signs of neurologic disease (Barlow). Perhaps 5 percent are mentally subnormal and another 5 percent show some evidence of minimal brain disorder. Many are clumsy. In the group without neurologic signs, the IQ is normal, though there are a larger number of borderline cases than in the general population. Boys are found to be more hyperactive and inattentive than girls, just as they have more trouble in learning to read and write. Dyslexia is frequently associated, as noted above. Girls tend to have more trouble with numbers and arithmetic.

Human infants exhibit astonishing differences in amount of activity almost from the first days of life. Some babies are constantly on the move, wiry, and hard to hold; others are placid and slack as a sack of meal. Irwin, who studied motility in the neonate, found a difference of 290 times between the most and least active in terms of amount of movement per 24 h.

Once walking and running begin, children normally enter a period of extreme activity, more so than at any other period of life. The degree of activity, which again varies widely from one child to another, seems not to be correlated with the age of achieving motor milestones or with motor skill at a later time. The male is more active than the female, and the Afro-American child tends to be more active and precocious in motor development than the white. Children with cerebral defects tend to exhibit apathy or hyperactivity more often than children without recognizable defects.

Again, two groups of overactive children can be discerned. In one, infants are overactive from birth, sleeping less and feeding poorly; by the age of 2 years, the syndrome is obvious. In the other group, an inability to sit quietly only becomes apparent at the preschool age (4 to 6 years). Seldom do such children remain in one position for more than a few seconds, even when watching television. Attention to any task cannot be sustained, hence the term *attention deficit–hyperactivity disorder*. As a rule, there is also an abnormal impulsivity and often an intolerance of all measures of restraint. Mild degrees of mental retardation and epilepsy and other disabilities are conjoined in some patients.

Once the child is in school, the attention deficit becomes more troubling. Now these children must sit still, watch and listen to the teacher when she speaks to another child, and not react to distracting stimuli. They cannot stay at their desks, take turns in reciting, be quiet, or control their impulsivity. The teacher finds it difficult to discipline them and often insists that the parents seek medical consultation. Some children are so hyperactive that they cannot attend regular school. Their behavior verges on the "organic drivenness" that has been known to occur in children whose brains have been injured by encephalitis. In certain families the disorder is probably inherited (Biederman et al). In about half the patients, the hyperactivity subsides gradually by puberty or soon thereafter, but in the remainder the symptoms persist in modified form into adulthood (Weiss et al). It has also become clear that a group of children exist who have difficulty sustaining concentration but do not manifest hyperactivity or behaviors that betray the attention deficit. It is presumed that they share a similar core problem with hyperkinetic children, and it has been observed that they may be helped in studying and school performance by the same stimulant drugs that are used for more overt ADHD.

For a number of years there was a tendency to consider children with the hyperkinetic syndrome as having minimal brain disease. "Soft neurologic signs" such as right-left confusion, mirror movements, minimal "choreic" instability, awkwardness, finger agnosia, tremor, and borderline hyperreflexia were said to be more frequent. These signs, however, are seen so often in normal children that their attribution to disease is invalid. Schain and others therefore substituted the term *minimal brain dysfunction*, which is no more accurate and simply restates the problem. Lacking altogether are accurate clinicoanatomic and clinicopathologic correlative data.

However, in an MRI study of the brains of 10 children with hyperactivity–attention deficit disorder, Hynd and colleagues found the width of the right frontal lobe to be smaller than normal; also fairly consistently, there was smallness of the dorsolateral, cingulate, and striatal regions. Unlike dyslexics, in whom the planum temporale tends to be equal in the two hemispheres, the left planum was larger in the attention deficit cases, as it is in normals. Also, functional imaging studies have suggested that the inability of these children to block impulsive reactions and the improvement that is seen with methylphenidate are accompanied by functional changes in the striatum. Another approach to understanding the process has been to study a strain of mice that have been genetically altered to eliminate a dopamine transporter gene. These animals display behavioral symptoms that are said to replicate those of ADHD in children and also to respond to stimulants. These observations implicate an abnormality of dopamine and serotonin; the idea is provocative because several genetic linkage studies have suggested an association between ADHD and a polymorphism of the gene that codes for the same dopamine transporter gene.

Apart from the reports of parents and teachers and observation of the child, one is aided in the diagnosis of the attention deficit disorder (and other learning disabilities) by psychometry. An observant psychologist, in performing intelligence tests, notes distractibility and difficulty in sustaining any activity. Erratic performance that is not due to an intellectual or comprehension defect is characteristic.

The treatment of the hyperactive child can proceed intelligently only after medical and psychologic explorations have elucidated the context in which the hyperactivity occurs. If the child is hyperactive and inattentive mainly in school and less so in an unstructured environment, it may be that mental retardation or dyslexia, which prevents scholastic success, is a source of frustration and boredom; the child then turns to other activities that may happen to disturb the classroom. Or the hyperactive child may have failed to acquire self-control because of a disorganized home life, and the overactivity may be but one manifestation of anxiety or intolerance of constraint. Clearly problems such as these require a modification of the educational program.

For overactive children of normal intelligence who have failed to control their impulses, even with parental assistance, who at all times have boundless energy, require little sleep, exhibit a wriggling restlessness (the choreiform syndrome of Prechtl and Stemmer), and who manifest incessant exploratory activity that repeatedly gets them into mischief, even to their own dismay, medical therapy is in order. Paradoxically, stimulants have a quieting effect on these children, whereas phenobarbital and other sedatives may have the opposite effect. Methylphenidate is the drug of choice. Children under 30 kg are given 5 mg each morning on school days for 2 weeks, after which the dose can be raised to 5 mg morning and noon. Children weighing less than 30 kg can be given a single 20-mg sustained-release tablet each morning. If methylphenidate proves ineffective after several weeks or cannot be tolerated, dextroamphetamine 2.5 to 5 mg three times daily is a suitable substitute. Pemoline is a weaker but sometimes better-tolerated stimulant than the others. If these agents control the activity and improve school performance (they can be continued for a number of years), there is no need to alter the child's school program. If stimulants are ineffective, tricyclic antidepressants, particularly desipramine, should be tried. Classroom behavioral conditioning techniques and psychotherapy may be needed for brief periods. Remedial education is reserved for recalcitrant cases.

Certainly the disease is a lifelong problem for a proportion of children, although it is just as clear that many or most "outgrow" it. Hill and Schoener estimate that there is a 50 percent decline in prevalence with each 5 years of growth. In addition to the child with ADHD who grows to adulthood with persistent problems, there has recently emerged an interest in adults who present for the first time with features that they or their physicians attribute to ADHD. Most often these adults realize they have had lifelong problems that are similar to the motor restlessness and wandering attention that led to the diagnosis of ADHD in their children. The efficacy and safety of stimulant drugs in this group is not known with certainty, but this class of medications as well as antidepressants have been tried with some success. In relation to persistent traits of ADHD, several psychiatrists have pointed out that there may be an increase in drug and alcohol dependence among adolescents with the disorder (Zametkin and Ernst) and a connection to tic disorders such as Tourette syndrome (page 117). However, it can be said from general clinical experience that these problems do not arise in the great majority of such children.

Enuresis

Voluntary sphincteric control develops according to a predetermined time scale. Usually normal children stop soiling themselves before they can remain dry, and day control precedes night control. Some children are toilet-trained by their second birthday, but many do not acquire full sphincteric control until the fourth year. Constant dribbling usually indicates spina bifida or another form of dysraphism, but in the boy one must look also for obstruction of the bladder neck and in the girl for an ectopic ureter entering the vagina.

When a child 5 years of age or older wets the bed nearly every night and is dry by day, the child is said to have *nocturnal enuresis*. This condition afflicts approximately 10 percent of children between 4 and 14 years of age, boys more than girls, and continues in many cases to be a problem even into adolescence and adulthood. Although mentally retarded children are notably late in acquiring sphincter control (some never do), the majority of enuretic individuals are normal in other respects.

The cause of this condition is disputed. Often there is a family history of the same complaint. Some psychiatrists have insisted that overzealous parents "pressure" the child until he develops a complex about his bedwetting. Punishment, shaming, rewards, etc., doubtless have this effect, but the underlying condition is believed by most neurologists to be a delay in the maturation of higher control of spinal reflex centers during sleep. These and other abnormalities of bladder function in the enuretic child, as well as treatment, are discussed in the chapter on sleep (page 425).

Sociopathy and Neurosis

Extremes of egocentricity—lack of understanding of the feelings, needs, and actions of other members of one's social group—and an inability to judge one's own strengths and weaknesses stand as the central issues in the development of neurosis and borderline personality disorder. Such difficulties usually become manifest by adolescence. The complete detachment of the child with psychosis, the amorality of the constitutional sociopath, the major disturbances in thinking of the schizophrenic, and the mood swings of the manic-depressive also express themselves in many instances by adolescence and sometimes in late childhood. Here one confronts a key problem in psychiatry—the extent to which neurosis, sociopathy, and psychosis have their roots in genetically determined personality traits or in derangements in the affective and social life of the individual, consequent to a harmful environment. In other words, in what measure are the neuroses and other psychiatric disorders determined by early life experiences and to what extent are they genetically determined?

The answers to these questions cannot be given with finality. Experienced clinicians tend to believe that genetic factors are more important than environmental ones. The discovery that unusually tall males with severe acne vulgaris and aggressive sociopathic behavior may have a karyotype of XYY chromosomes is an example of a possible genetic relationship. The patient with Turner syndrome in whom competent social adaptation is linked closely to an X chromosome of paternal origin is another example. Further, there is no critical evidence to show that deliberate alteration of the familial and social environment or the mental hygienic measures now so popular have ever prevented a neurosis, psychosis, or sociopathy.

It is during the period of late childhood and adolescence, when the personality is least stable, that transient symptoms, many resembling the psychopathologic states of adult life, are most frequent and difficult to interpret. Some of these disorders represent the early signs of autism, schizophrenia, or manic-depressive disease. Others are forerunners of sociopathy. But many of the borderline personality traits have a way of disappearing as adult years are reached, so that one can only surmise that they represented either a maturational delay in complex social behavior or were expressions of adolescent turmoil or what has been called "adolescent adjustment reaction."

Many issues that have been touched upon in the preceding discussion are considered more fully in the section on psychiatric disorders (Chaps. 56 to 58).

MENTAL RETARDATION

The symptom complex of incomplete or insufficient development of mental capacities and associated behavioral abnormalities (variously referred to as *mental retardation*, *mental subnormality*, or *oligophrenia*) combines many of the developmental abnormalities already discussed. Mental retardation stands as the single largest neuropsychiatric disorder in every civilized society. The overall frequency of mental retardation cannot be stated precisely. Rough estimates are that in a group of children between 9 and 14 years of age, about 2 percent or slightly more will be unable to profit from public education or to adapt socially and, when grown up, to live independently. Using any one of a number of indices of social and psychologic failure, two somewhat overlapping groups are recognized: (1) The mildly impaired (IQ 45 to 70), corresponding to what had been called *high-grade imbecile* and *feeble minded*, and (2) the *severely impaired*, corresponding to the categories of *idiot* (IQ below 20) and *low-grade imbecile* (IQ 20 to 45) in older classifications. The second group, also called the *pathologic mentally retarded*, makes up approximately 10 percent of the subnormal population. The first group is now referred to as the *subcultural*, *physiologic*, or *familial mentally retarded* and is much larger than the second. Apart from these two groups, there are the borderline cases previously called "simpletons," "debiles," or "borderline defectives." Because of the opprobrious implications of the terms *idiot*, *imbecile*, and *moron*, the American Association on Mental Deficiency proposed that the mentally retarded be grouped instead into four categories: (1) those with *profound deficiency*, incapable of self-care (IQ below 25); (2) those with *severe deficiency*, incapable of living an independent existence and essentially untrainable (IQ 25 to 39); (3) those with *moderate deficiency*, trainable to some extent (IQ 40 to 54), and (4) those with *mild deficiency*, who are impaired but trainable and to some extent educable.

The above terms, while in common use, satisfy neither neurologists nor psychologists because of their generality, embracing as they do any lifelong global deficit in mental capacities. The terms convey no information of the particular type(s) of intellectual impairment, their causes and mechanisms, or their anatomic and pathologic bases. Moreover, they express only one aspect of impaired mental function—the cognitive—and ignore the inadequate development of personality, social adaptation, and behavior. Specific critical studies, comprising all measurable psychologic functions—such as attention, learning, memory, verbalization, calculation, transmodal sensory associations, etc.—are just now being undertaken. Such handicapped persons present an immense challenge to neurologists, psychologists, and neuropathologists.

It is important to emphasize that only a small proportion of cases of mental retardation—representing those with profound and severe deficiency—can presently be traced to the congenital abnormalities of development and diseases that are reviewed in Chap. 38. When the brains of the severely retarded are examined by conventional histopathologic methods, gross lesions are found in approximately 90 percent of cases, and in fully three-quarters an etiologic diagnosis is possible. Noteworthy is the fact that among the remaining 10 percent of the severely ("pathologic") retarded, the brains are grossly and microscopically normal. In other words, in this 10 percent of retarded, current technology does not enable the neuropathologist to expose a lesion that had caused lifelong severe retardation. Furthermore, the vast majority of the less severely retarded also lack a recognizable tissue pathology and have not exhibited the conventional signs of cerebral disease. For this reason, some physicians have not regarded them as having disease of the brain, even though most informed individuals adhere to the idea that the brain, which is the organ of the mind, must be functionally incompetent.

The most acceptable view of the mildly affected group of retarded persons is that it represents the proportion of the population that is the opposite of genius. On the Gaussian curve of human intelligence, they constitute the lowest 3 percent, the group that falls between 2 to 3 standard deviations below the mean (see Fig. 28-4).

Figure 28-4

Gaussian, or bell-shaped, curve of intelligence and its skewing by the group of mental retardates with diseases of the brain. The shaded areas indicate the two groups of mentally retarded. The hump representing the pathologically retarded is purely diagrammatic, illustrating its overlap with the physiologically retarded. When the population plotted is limited to "mental defectives," a truly bimodal distribution is seen, segregating the two groups of retarded.

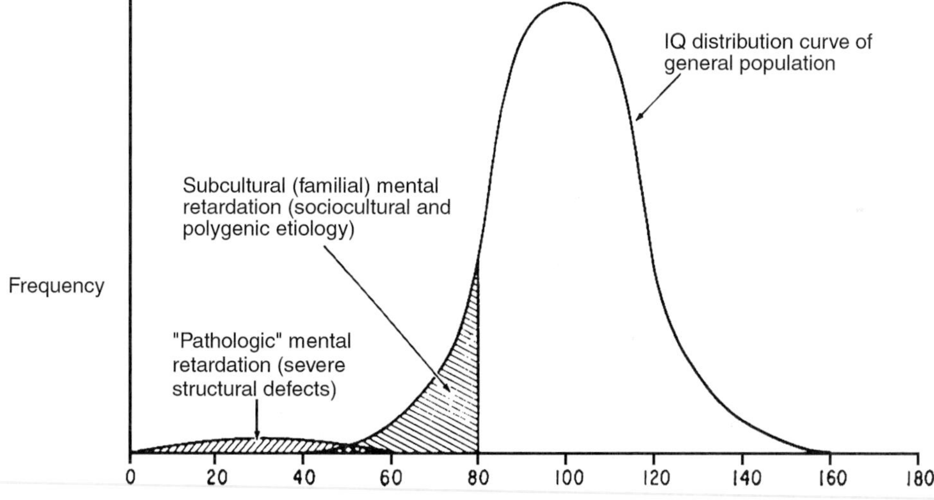

Lewis was one of the first to call attention to this large group of simple mental retardates; he referred to them by the ambiguous term *subcultural*. The term *familial retardation* has also been applied to this group, since in many of the families other members of the same and previous generations are feeble-minded or have other mental disorders. There are several types of hereditary mental retardation, but they have not been fully differentiated clinically or pathologically. There being no visible neuropathology, the cases fall into the category of mental retardation without morphologic changes, discussed below.

As an aid to the neurologist, pediatrician, and child neurologist who must assume responsibility for the diagnosis and management of these backward children, the following descriptions may be of value. The more severe forms of mental retardation and the developmental abnormalities and diseases that cause them will be found in Chap. 38 (page 1093). Here only the milder subcultural forms—i.e., mental retardation without morphologic change—are considered.

Subcultural (Familial) Mental Retardation

Clinical Features Two clinical types can be recognized based on the adequacy of motor skills that are acquired in parallel with cognitive skills. *In the first type*, the essential characteristic is that, almost from birth, the infant is backward in all aspects of development. There is a tendency to sleep more, to be less demanding of nourishment, to move less than normal, and to suck poorly and regurgitate. Parents often comment on how good their baby is, how little he troubles them by crying. As the months pass, every expected achievement is late. The baby is usually more hypotonic and turns over, sits unsupported, and walks later than the normal infant. Yet despite these obvious motor delays, there is later no sign of paralysis, ataxia, chorea, or athetosis. These babies do not smile at the usual time and take little notice of the mother or other persons or objects in their environment. They are inattentive to visual and often to auditory stimuli, to the point where questions are raised about blindness or deafness. Certain phases of normal development, such as hand regard, may persist beyond the sixth month, when they are normally replaced by other activities. Mouthing (putting everything in the mouth) and slobbering, which should end by 1 year of age, also persist. There are only fleeting signs of interest in toys, and the impersistence of attention becomes increasingly prominent. Vocalizations are scant, often guttural, piercing, or high-pitched and feeble. Babbling is not replaced by attempts at word formation at the usual time.

In the second type, early motor milestones (supporting the head, rolling over, sitting, standing, and walking) may be attained at their normal times, yet the infant is inattentive and slow in learning the usual nursery tricks. It seems as though motor development had somehow escaped the retardation process. There may, however, be aimless overactivity and persistence of rhythmic movements, grinding of the teeth (bruxism), and hypotonia.

Because the developmental sequence of motor function and speech may be normal, even to the point where the baby acquires a few words by the end of the first year, the examiner may be misled into thinking that the mentally retarded infant was at first normal and had then deteriorated. In such infants it can even be shown that various test procedures yield lower scores with progressing age (from 3 years onward); this is due not to a decline in ability but to the fact that the tests are not comparable. In the first 3 years, the tests are weighted toward sensorimotor functions and after that toward perception, memory, and concept formation. Interestingly, the development of language depends upon both groups of functions, needing a certain maturation of the auditory and motor apparatus at the start and highly specialized cognitive skills for continued development. These and other aspects of development of speech and language have been considered earlier in this chapter and are commented on further in Chaps. 23 and 38.

Members of both groups of these subcultural retardates exhibit a number of noteworthy features that have medical and social implications. They have a high incidence of minor congenital anomalies of the eyes, face, mouth, ears, and hands; they tend to be sickly, and the more severely retarded among them have poor physiques and are often undersized. Deviant behavior occurs frequently (in 6.6 percent of nonretarded children, in 28.6 percent of the retarded, and in 58.3 percent of the epileptic retarded, according to Rutter and Martin). Most often, this behavior takes the form of poor self-control and aggressiveness, especially pronounced in children with temporal lobe epilepsy. Other behavioral disturbances are restlessness, repetitive activity, explosive rage reactions and tantrums, stereotyped play, and the seeking of sensory experiences in unusual ways (Chess and Hassibi). Pica (the compulsive ingestion of nonnutritive substances) is a problem between ages 2 and 4 years but is also seen in normal neglected children. The parents of a large proportion of children with deviant behavior fall into the lowest segment of the population socially and economically; in other words, the parents may lack the competence to maintain stable homes and to find work. Abandonment, neglect, and child abuse are frequent in this group. The majority of children with deviant behavior need to be placed in special classes or schools, and special measures must be taken to reduce the tendency to truancy, sociopathy, and criminality.

An endless debate is centered on matters of causation—whether the so-called subcultural or physiologic retardates are products of a faulty genetic influence, which prevents successful competition and adaptation, or of societal discrimination and lack of training and education coupled with the effects of malnutrition, infections, or other exogenous factors. Surely both environmental and genetic factors are at work, although the relative importance of each has proved difficult to measure (Moser et al).

Pathologic Features As mentioned earlier, a pathologic basis for subcultural mental retardation has not been established. No visible lesions have been discerned in the brains of this group, unlike those of the severely retarded (pathologic) group, in which malformations and a variety of destructive lesions are obvious in all but 5 to 10 percent of cases. Admittedly, the brains of some such individuals are about 10 percent underweight, but one cannot presently interpret what this means. It is certain that new methodologies, perhaps relating to neuronal connectivity, will be needed if the cerebra of subcultural retardates and the subnormal extreme of the general population (the part that falls more than 2 to 3 SD below the mean) are to be differentiated from the cerebra of highly superior individuals (more than 2 to 3 SD above the mean). Differences might be expected in terms of the number of neurons in thalamic nuclei and cortex, in dendritic-axonal connectivity, or in synaptic surfaces, elements that are not being assayed by the conventional techniques of tissue neuropathology. The observations of Huttenlocher, who found a marked sparsity of dendritic arborization in Golgi-Cox preparations, and of Purpura, who found an absence of short, thick spines on dendrites of cortical neurons and other abnormalities of dendritic spines, are the first steps in this direction.

Sex linkage is a notable feature of some types of mental retardation. Renpenning and colleagues reported a series of 21 males in three generations of a Canadian family, all free of any congenital malformations and with normal head size, and Turner and coworkers have described a similar Australian series (page 1098). No chromosomal abnormality has been found. The fragile-X syndrome (pages 1067 and 1097) predominates in males, accounting for about 10 percent of male retardates. They may be physically normal except for large testicles. Other X-linked forms of mental retardation besides Renpenning and fragile-X syndromes include the Lowe, Lesch-Nyhan, and Menkes syndromes and adrenoleukodystrophy, discussed in Chap. 37.

Diagnosis Infants should be considered at risk for mental subnormality when there is a family history of mental deficiency, low birth weight in relation to the length of gestation (small-for-date babies), marked prematurity, maternal infection early in pregnancy (especially rubella), and toxemia of pregnancy. In the first few months of life, certain of the behavioral characteristics described above are of value in predicting mental retardation. Prechtl and associates have found that a low Apgar score (especially at 5 min after delivery), flaccidity, underactivity, and asymmetrical neurologic signs are the earliest indices of subnormality in the infant. Slow habituation of orienting reactions to novel auditory and visual stimuli and the presence of "fine motor deficits" (as previously discussed under "Delays in Motor Development") are other early warnings of mental retardation.

In the first year or two of life, suspicion of mental retardation is based largely on clinical impression, but it should always be validated by psychometric procedures. Most pediatric neurologists utilize some of the criteria laid down by Gesell and Amatruda or the Denver Developmental Screening Scale, from which a developmental quotient (DQ) is calculated.

For testing of preschool children, the Wechsler Preschool and Primary Scale of Intelligence is used, and for school-age children, the Wechsler Intelligence Scale for Children. IQ tests for preschoolers must be interpreted with caution, since they have had less predictive validity for school success than the tests that are used after 6 years of age. In general, normal scores for age eliminate mental retardation as a cause of poor school achievement and learning disabilities, but special cognitive defects may be revealed by low scores on particular subtests. Retarded children not only have low scores but exhibit more scatter of subtest scores. Also, they achieve greater success with performance than with verbal items. It is essential that the physician know the conditions of testing, for poor scores may be due to fright, inadequate motivation, lapses in attention, dyslexia, or a subtle auditory or visual defect rather than a developmental lag.

Surprisingly, in this group of retarded children without other neurologic or physical signs, analyses by neurobehavioral and psychologic methods have not disclosed the basic fault in nervous functioning. This is particularly frustrating to the neurologist, who approaches such cases with knowledge of the anatomy and clinical expressions of amnesic states, aphasias, apraxias, dyscalculias, visuospatial and other agnosias; such knowledge seemingly fails to be applicable. Is there one domain of faulty psychologic function—such as failure of learning, inattentiveness, or faulty perception—that underlies all forms of mental retardation? Or are there several domains, differing from one case to another or one disease to another? Only by the most innovative and sophisticated neuropsychologic studies will answers to such questions be obtained.

The EEG, in addition to exposing asymptomatic seizure activity, shows a high incidence of other abnormalities in the mentally retarded. Presumably, this is due to a greater degree of immaturity of the cerebrum at any given age. However, a normal EEG is of relatively little help. Moreover, CT scanning and MRI have been singularly unhelpful in revealing abnormalities in this group of children.

In the diagnosis of milder grades of retardation, the possible effects of severe malnutrition, neglect and deprivation, chronic systemic disease, iodine deficiency, impaired hearing and vision, and possibly childhood psychosis must always be considered. Of particular importance is the differentiation of a group of patients who are normal for a variable period after birth and then manifest a progressive decline from disease of the nervous system. This type of disorder is representative of the group of hereditary metabolic and degenerative diseases discussed in Chap. 37. Of importance also is seizure disorder (and anticonvulsant medications), which can impair cerebral function in this group of patients (Chap. 16).

Management Since there is little or no possibility of treating the condition(s) underlying mental retardation and there is no way of restoring function to a nervous system that is developmentally subnormal, the medical objective is to assist in planning for the patient's training, education, and social and occupational adjustments. As Voltaire remarked long ago, guidance is needed more than education. The parents must be guided in forming realistic attitudes and expectations. Psychiatric and social counseling may help the family to maintain gentle but firm support of the patient so that he can acquire, to the fullest extent possible, self-help skills, self-control, good work habits, and a congenial personality.

Most individuals with an IQ above 60 and no other handicaps can be trained to live an independent life. Special schooling may enable such patients to realize their full potential. Social factors that contribute to underachievement must be sought out and eliminated if possible. Later, there is need for advice about possible occupational attainments.

Great care must be exercised in deciding about institutionalization. Whereas severe degrees of retardation are all too apparent by the first or second year, less severe degrees are difficult to recognize early. As stated above, psychologic tests alone are not trustworthy. The method of assessment suggested many years ago by Fernald still has a ring of soundness. It includes (1) physical examination, (2) family background, (3) developmental history, (4) school progress (grade achieved), (5) performance in schoolwork (tests of reading, arithmetic, etc.), (6) practical knowledge, (7) social behavior, (8) industrial efficiency, (9) moral reactions, and (10) intelligence as measured by psychologic tests. All these data except (5) and (10) can be obtained by a skillful physician during the initial medical and neurologic examination.

REFERENCES

ANDERSON LD: The predictive value of infancy tests in relation to intelligence at five years. *Child Dev* 10:203, 1939.

ANDRÉ-THOMAS, CHESNI Y, DARGASSIES SAINT-ANNES S: *The Neurological Examination of the Infant.* London, Medical Advisory Committee, National Spastics Society, 1960.

ANDREWS G, HARRIS M: *Clinics in Developmental Medicine*: No 17. *The Syndrome of Stuttering.* London, Heinemann, 1964.

ASPERGER H: Die autistischen Psychopathie in Kindesalter. *Arch Psychiatr Nervenkr* 117:76, 1944.

BAKER L, CANTWELL DP, MATTISON RE: Behavior problems in children with pure speech disorders and in children with combined speech and language disorders. *J Abnorm Child Psychol* 8:245, 1980.

BARLOW C: *Mental Retardation and Related Disorders.* Philadelphia, Davis, 1977.

BAYLEY H: Comparisons of mental and motor test scores for age 1–15 months by sex, birth order, race, geographic location and education of parents. *Child Dev* 36:379, 1965.

BENDER L: *A Visual-Motor Gestalt Test and Its Use.* New York, American Orthopsychiatric Association, 1938.

BENTON AL: Right-left discrimination. *Pediatr Clin North Am* 15:747, 1968.

BENTON AL: *Revised Visual Retention Test.* New York, Psychological Corporation, 1974.

BIEDERMAN J, MUNIR K, KNEE D, et al: A family study of patients with attention deficit disorder and normal controls. *J Psychiatr Res* 20:263, 1986.

BIRCH HG, BELMONT L: Auditory-visual integration in normal and retarded readers. *Am J Orthopsychiatry* 34:852, 1964.

BYNE W: The biological evidence challenged, in *The Scientific American Book of the Brain*, New York, Lyons Press, 1999, pp 181–194.

Capute AJ, Accardo PJ: *Developmental Disabilities in Infancy and Childhood*. Baltimore, Brookes, 1991.

Chess S: Diagnosis and treatment of the hyperactive child. *NY State J Med* 60:2379, 1960.

Chess S, Hassibi M: Behavioral deviations in mentally retarded children. *J Am Acad Child Psychiatry* 9:282, 1970.

Chugani HT: Functional brain imaging in pediatrics. *Pediatr Clin North Am* 39:777, 1992.

Conel J: *The Postnatal Development of the Human Cerebral Cortex*: Vols 1–8. Cambridge, MA, Harvard University Press, 1939–1967.

Cowan WM: The development of the brain. *Sci Am* 241:112, 1979.

Critchley M, Critchley EA: *Dyslexia Defined*. Springfield, IL, Charles C Thomas, 1978.

Damon W: The moral development of children. *Sci Am*, August 1999, pp 72–79.

Dargassies Saint-Anne S: *Neurological Development in the Full-Term and Premature Neonate*. New York, Excerpta Medica, 1977.

De Ajuriaguerra J: *Manuel de psychiatrie de l'enfant*, 2nd ed. Paris, Masson, 1974.

Denckla MB, Rudel RG, Chapman C, et al: Motor proficiency in dyslexic children with and without attentional disorders. *Arch Neurol* 42:228, 1985.

De Renzi E, Luchelli F: Developmental dysmnesia in a poor reader. *Brain* 113:1337, 1990.

Ellingson RG: The incidence of EEG abnormality among children with mental disorder of apparently nonorganic origin. *Am J Psychiatry* 111:263, 1954.

Fantz RL: The origin of form perception. *Sci Am* 204:66, 1961.

Feess-Higgins A, Larroche J-C: *Development of the Human Fetal Brain*. Paris, Masson, 1987.

Fernald WE: Standardized fields of inquiry for clinical studies of borderline defectives. *Ment Hyg* 1:211, 1917.

Fleet WS, Heilman KM: Acquired stuttering from a right hemisphere lesion in a right hander. *Neurology* 35:1343, 1985.

Fox P, Ingham R: Commentary on stuttering. *Science* 270:1438, 1995.

Frankenberg WK, Dodds JB, Fandal AW: *Denver Developmental Screening Test*, rev ed. Denver, University of Colorado Medical Center, 1970.

Galaburda AM, Kemper TL: Cytoarchitectonic abnormalities in developmental dyslexia: A case study. *Ann Neurol* 6:94, 1979.

Galaburda AM, Sherman CF, Rosen GD, et al: Developmental dyslexia: Four consecutive patients with cortical anomalies. *Ann Neurol* 18:222, 1985.

Gastaut H, Broughton R: A clinical and polygraphic study of episodic phenomena during sleep, in Wortis J (ed): *Recent Advances in Biological Psychiatry*. New York, Plenum Press, 1965, pp 197–221.

Gesell A (Ed): *The First Five Years of Life: A Guide to the Study of the Pre-School Child*. New York, Harper & Row, 1940.

Gesell A, Amatruda CS: *Developmental Diagnosis: Normal and Abnormal Child Development*, 2nd ed. New York, Hoeber-Harper, 1954.

Gibson EJ, Olum V: Experimental methods of studying perception in children, in Mussen P (ed): *Handbook of Research Methods in Child Development*. New York, Wiley, 1960, pp 311–373.

Goldstein K: *Language and Language Disturbances: Aphasic Symptom Complexes and Their Significance for Medicine and Theory of Language*. New York, Grune & Stratton, 1948.

Gubbay SS, Ellis E, Walter JN, Court SDM: Clumsy children: A study of apraxic and agnosic defects in 21 children. *Brain* 88:295, 1965.

Hécaen N, de Ajuriaguerra J: *Left-Handedness*. New York, Grune & Stratton, 1964.

Hinshelwood J: A case of dyslexia—A peculiar form of word blindness. *Lancet* 2:1454, 1896.

Hill JC, Schoener EP: Age-dependent decline of attention deficit hyperactivity disorder. *Am J Psychiatry* 153:1143, 1996.

Humphreys P, Kaufmann WE, Galaburda AM: Developmental dyslexia in women: Neuropathological findings in three patients. *Ann Neurol* 28:727, 1990.

Huttenlocher PR: Dendritic development in neocortex of children with mental defect and infantile spasms. *Neurology* 24:203, 1974.

Hynd GW, Semrud-Clikeman M, Lorys AR, et al: Brain morphology in developmental dyslexia and attention deficit disorder/hyperactivity. *Arch Neurol* 47:919, 1990.

Illingworth RS: *The Development of the Infant and Young Child, Normal and Abnormal*, 3rd ed. Edinburgh, Churchill Livingstone, 1966.

Ingram TTS: Developmental disorders of speech, in Vinken PJ, Bruyn W (eds): *Handbook of Clinical Neurology*. Vol 4: *Disorders of Speech, Perception and Symbolic Behavior*. Amsterdam, North-Holland, 1969, chap 22, pp 407–442.

Irwin OC: Can infants have IQ's? *Psychol Rev* 49:69, 1942.

Kagan J, Moss HA: *Birth to Maturity: A Study of Psychological Development*. New York, Wiley, 1962.

Kanner I: Early infantile autism. *J Pediatr* 25:211, 1944.

Kinsbourne M: Developmental Gerstmann's syndrome: A disorder of sequencing. *Pediatr Clin North Am* 15:771, 1968.

Kinsbourne M: Disorders of mental development, in Menkes JH (ed): *Textbook of Child Neurology*, 5th ed. Baltimore, Williams & Wilkins, 1995, pp 924–964.

Kinsey A, Pomeroy W, Martin C, Gebhard P: *Sexual Behavior in the Human Female*. Philadelphia, Saunders, 1948.

Landau WM, Kleffner FR: Syndrome of acquired aphasia with convulsive disorder in children. *Neurology* 7:523, 1957.

Lenneberg EH: *Biological Foundations of Language*. New York, Wiley, 1967.

Leonard CM, Voeller KKS, Lombardino LJ, et al: Anomalous cerebral structure in dyslexia revealed with magnetic resonance imaging. *Arch Neurol* 50:461, 1993.

LeVay S: A difference in hypothalamic structure between heterosexual and homosexual men. *Science* 253:1034, 1991.

LeVay S, Hamer DH: Evidence for a biological influence in male homosexuality. *Sci Am* 270:44, 1994.

Lewis EO: Types of mental differences and their social significance. *J Ment Sci* 79:298, 1933.

Livingstone MS, Rosen GD, Drislane FW, Galaburda AM: Physiological and anatomical evidence for a magnocellular defect in developmental dyslexia. *Proc Natl Acad Sci USA* 88:7943, 1991.

LOWREY GH: *Growth and Development of Children*, 8th ed. Chicago, Year Book, 1986.

MACKINTOSH NJ: *IQ and Human Intelligence*. Oxford, Oxford University Press, 1998.

MINIFIE FD, LLOYD LL: *Communicative and Cognitive Abilities—Early Behavioral Assessment*. Baltimore, University Park Press, 1978.

MOSER HW, RAMEY CT, LEONARD CO: Mental retardation, in Emery AE, Rimoin DL (eds): *Principles and Practice of Medical Genetics*. Edinburgh, Churchill Livingstone, 1984, pp 352–366.

ORTON ST: *Reading, Writing and Speech Problems in Children*. New York, Norton, 1937.

OZERETZKII NI: Technique of investigating motor function, in Gurevich M, Ozeretzkii NI (eds): *Psychomotor Function*. Moscow, 1930. Quoted by Luria AR: *Higher Cortical Functions in Man*. New York, Basic Books, 1966.

PIAGET J: *The Psychology of Intelligence*. London, Routledge & Kegan Paul, 1950.

PRECHTL HFR: Prognostic value of neurological signs in the newborn. *Proc R Soc Med* 58:3, 1965.

PRECHTL HFR, BEINTEMA D: *The Neurological Examination of the Full Term Newborn Infant*. Little Club Clinics in Developmental Medicine, no 12. London, Heinemann, 1964.

PRECHTL HFR, STEMMER CJ: The choreiform syndrome in children. *Dev Med Child Neurol* 4:119, 1962.

PURPURA D: Dendritic spine "dysgenesis" in mental retardation. *Science* 186:1126, 1974.

RABINOWICZ T: The differential maturation of the cerebral cortex, in Falkner F, Tanner JM (eds): *Human Growth*. New York, Plenum Press, 1986.

RAPIN I, ALLEN DA: Developmental language disorders: Nosologic considerations, in Kirk U (ed): *Neuropsychology of Language, Reading and Spelling*. New York, Academic Press, 1983, pp 155–184.

Raven's Colored Progressive Matrices. New York, Psychological Corporation, 1947–1963.

REISSMAN F: *The Culturally Deprived Child*. New York, Harper & Row, 1962.

RENPENNING H, GERRARD JW, ZALESKI WA, et al: Familial sex-linked mental retardation. *Can Med Assoc J* 87:924, 1962.

ROSENBERGER PB: Morphological cerebral asymmetries and dyslexia, in Pavlidis GT (ed): *Perspectives on Dyslexia*. Vol 1. New York, Wiley, 1990, pp 93–107.

ROSENBERGER PB: Learning disorders, in Berg B (ed): *Principles of Child Neurology*. New York, McGraw-Hill, 1996, pp 335–369.

RUMSEY JM, DONOHUE BC, BRADY DR, et al: A magnetic resonance imaging study of planum temporale asymmetry in men with developmental dyslexia. *Arch Neurol* 54:1481, 1997.

RUTTER M, GRAHAM P, YULE W: *Clinics in Developmental Medicine*. Nos 35 and 36. *A Neuropsychiatric Study in Childhood*. London, Heinemann, 1970.

RUTTER M, MARTIN JAM (eds): *Clinics in Developmental Medicine*. No 43. *The Child with Delayed Speech*. London, Heinemann, 1972, pp 48–51.

SCARR S, WEBBER RA, CUTTING MA: Personality resemblance among adolescents and their parents in biologically related and adoptive families. *J Pers Soc Psychol* 40:885, 1981.

SCHAIN RJ: *Neurology of Childhood Learning Disorders*, 2nd ed. Baltimore, Williams & Wilkins, 1977.

SHAYWITZ SE: Dyslexia. *N Engl J Med* 338:307, 1998.

SHAYWITZ SE, SHAYWITZ BA, FLETCHER JM, et al: Prevalence of reading disabilities in boys and girls. *JAMA* 264:998, 1990.

SPEARMAN C: *Psychology Down the Ages*. London, Macmillan, 1937.

STAPLES R: Responses of infants to color. *J Exp Psychol* 15:119, 1932.

STEIN JF, RICHARDSON AJ, FOWLER MS: Monocular occlusion can improve binocular control and reading in dyslexics, *Brain* 123:164, 2000.

SWAAB DF, HOFMAN MA: An enlarged suprachiasmatic nucleus in homosexual men. *Brain Res* 537:141, 1990.

THURSTONE LL: *The Vectors of the Mind*. Chicago, University of Chicago Press, 1953.

TIROSH E: Fine motor deficit: An etiologically distinct entity. *Pediatr Neurol* 10:213, 1994.

TRAVIS LE: *Speech Therapy*. New York, Appleton-Century, 1931.

TURNER G, TURNER B, COLLINS E: X-linked mental retardation without physical abnormality: Renpenning's syndrome. *Dev Med Child Neurol* 13:71, 1971.

WEISS G, HECHTMAN L, MILROY T, PERLMAN T: Psychiatric status of hyperactives as adults: A controlled prospective 15-year follow-up of 63 hyperactive children. *J Am Acad Child Adolesc Psychiatry* 24:211, 1985.

WORSTER-DROUGHT C: Congenital suprabulbar paresis. *J Laryngol Otol* 70:453, 1956.

YAKOVLEV PI, LECOURS AR: The myelogenetic cycles of regional maturation of the brain, in Minkowski A (ed): *Regional Development of the Brain in Early Life*. Oxford, Blackwell, 1967, pp 3–70.

ZAMETKIN AJ, ERNST M: Problems in the management of attention-deficit hyperactivity disorder. *N Engl J Med* 340:40, 1999.

ZAMETKIN AJ, NORDAHL TE, GROSS M, et al: Cerebral glucose metabolism in adults with hyperactivity of childhood onset. *N Engl J Med* 323:1361, 1990.

Chapter 29

THE NEUROLOGY OF AGING

As indicated in the preceding chapter, standards of growth, development, and maturation provide a frame of reference against which every pathologic process in early life must be viewed. It has been less appreciated, however, that at the other end of the life cycle, neurologic deficits must be judged in a similar way, against a background of normal aging changes (senescence). The earliest of these changes begins long before the acknowledged period of senescence and continues throughout the remainder of life. For some reason, perhaps because of the human yearning for lifelong youthfulness and immortality, there is a reluctance to accept aging and involution as normal and inevitable phases of life. Not a few medical scientists and physicians believe that all changes in senescence are but the cumulative effects of injury and disease.

As a first generalization, it may be said that the length of life itself, the span of the natural life cycle, is one of the organism's most integral characteristics, genetically programmed in some mysterious way by a kind of biologic death clock. Each species has a characteristic average life span. For the mouse, this is 2 to 4 years; for the rhesus monkey, 20 to 25 years; for the seagull, 50 years; for the African elephant, 70 to 75 years; for the Galapagos tortoise, 100 years; and for human beings, about 85 years. Many years ago, the German physiologist Max Rubner pointed out that the total number of calories burned per gram of body weight and the total number of heartbeats in the lifetime of each of these vertebrate species, including humans, are about the same, despite the great differences in their size and life span. Other authors have contended that the life span of humans and other animals correlates roughly with the size of the brain. These observations are intriguing, but there are so many exceptions to these simple rules as to make them almost irrelevant to the aging process.

The common belief that medical science has greatly lengthened life is a misconception, arising from a failure to distinguish between life span and life expectancy. *Life span* is the average duration of life in persons who have avoided all disease and accidents (i.e., who have a "natural death"). As stated above, this span of life is fixed biologically and has been so for millennia. For most persons, the clock runs down by about the eighty-fifth year, and it seems to make little difference whether one inhabits a luxurious urban apartment or a primitive hut. Only a small proportion of individuals survive beyond this period. Popular tales about people who are tucked away in the remote regions of the Himalayas, Ecuador, or the Caucasus and live active lives for as long as 120 years or more have proved to be mythical. Actually, in 1998, the longest verified survival in a human being was 122 years, and the oldest living person at that time was 119 years old. To date, there have been fewer than five fully authenticated instances of a human being having survived to 120 years. From data on documented centenarians, actuaries have shown that a life span of even 115 years is an extreme rarity, occurring only once in 2.1 billion lives.

Life expectancy is something quite different; it refers to the number of years of life that an individual may statistically expect from birth onward. In contrast to the more or less fixed life span, life expectancy has increased remarkably in the past century. Mainly, this has come about through the elimination of fatal infectious diseases in infancy and childhood, allowing an ever-increasing number of individuals to reach adulthood. Thus, in the United States, the life expectancy of a newborn infant has increased from 50 years in 1900 to 75 years in 1987 and to more than 79 years in 1997; in the case of a newborn white female, this is a figure approaching the life span. Nevertheless, life expectancy must always fall short of the life span because, with advancing age, there is a steadily increasing susceptibility to fatal disease. After maturation, the death rate doubles about every 8 years. Demographers have estimated that if all coronary heart disease were eliminated, life expectancy would be extended by only 3.1 years for 35-year-old males (and 3.3 years for females). And if cancer were eliminated completely, life expectancy would be extended only an additional 2.5 years (Kaplan).

That the incidence of death increases with age hardly requires comment, but the particular relationship of one to the other was first recognized in 1825 by the English actuary Benjamin Gompertz. His formulation—that the mortality rate increases exponentially after the age of 30—is conventionally displayed as a survival curve, in which cumulative survival (percentage of the population remaining alive) is plotted against the age of death. Figure 29-1 displays several such curves—an "ideal" curve, representing the estimated survival if death were due only to physiologic aging and accidental trauma, and the life expectancy curves for 1900 and 1980 based on U.S. Bureau of Health statistics. The figure portrays the dramatic increase in life expectancy in this century. The changing configuration of the life expectancy curve as it comes to approximate the ideal curve is spoken of as *rectangularization of the survival curve*.

To the biologist and physician, death is not the main consideration. What is more meaningful are indices of vitality, resistance to disease, and organ efficiency. In fact, *senescence* is defined in just such terms, i.e., the progressive diminution of biologic efficiency and capacity of the organism to maintain itself as an effective machine. Most authors use the terms *aging* and *senescence* interchangeably, but some draw a fine semantic distinction between the purely passive and chronologic process of aging and the composite of bodily changes that characterize this process (senescence). The state of being aged, or senescent, is referred to as *senility*. The process of decline or decay that occurs in all organ systems of the body after middle life is also called *involution*; the unanticipated premature decay of any given tissue or cell population has been termed *abiotrophy*.

The composite of changes that characterize senescence—both bodily changes such as wrinkling of the skin, thinning and graying of the hair, loss of teeth, atrophy of gonads, blunting of visual and auditory acuity, stooped posture, diminution of muscular strength and endurance, and certain psychologic changes, such as rigidity of thinking and a tendency to repetitiveness and forgetfulness—are known to every observant person. Biologists have measured many of these changes. Estimates of the structural and functional decline that accompanies aging from 30 to 80 years are given in Table 29-1. It appears that all structures and functions share in the aging process. However, the time at which senescent changes become manifest and the rate at which these changes progress in different organs vary greatly.

Figure 29-1

Correlation of mortality rate and age. For details see text. (From Fries JF, Crapo LM: Vitality and Aging. San Francisco, Freeman, 1981. Copyright © 1981, by permission. All rights reserved.)

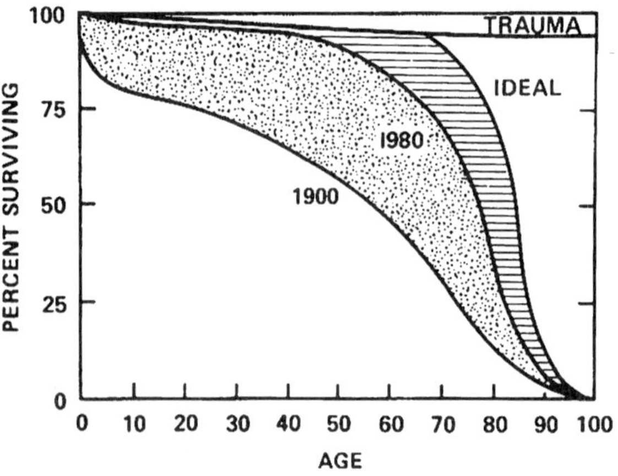

Table 29-1
Physiologic and anatomic deterioration at 80 years of age

	Percent decrease
Brain weight	10–15
Blood flow to brain	20
Speed of return of blood acidity to equilibrium after exercise	83
Cardiac output at rest	35
Number of glomeruli in kidney	44
Glomerular filtration rate	31
Number of fibers in nerves	37
Nerve conduction velocity	10
Number of taste buds	64
Maximum O_2 utilization with exercise	60
Maximum ventilation volume	47
Maximum breathing capacity	44
Power of hand grip	45
Maximum work rate	30
Basal metabolic rate	16
Body water content	18
Body weight (males)	12

Source: Adapted from Shock by permission.

Individual variations are also striking. Some persons withstand the onslaught of aging far better than others, and this constitutional resistance to the effects of aging seems to be familial. It can also be said that such changes are unrelated to Alzheimer disease and other degenerative diseases and that in general the changes of aging reduce the ability of the organism to recover from virtually any illness or trauma.

EFFECTS OF AGING ON THE NERVOUS SYSTEM

Of all the age-related changes, those in the nervous system are of paramount importance. Actors portray old people as being feeble, idle, obstinate, and given to reminiscing and as having tremulous hands, quavering voices, stooped posture, and slow, shuffling steps. In so doing, they have selected some of the most obvious effects of aging on the nervous system. The lay observer, as well as the medical one, often speaks glibly of the changes of advanced age as a kind of second childhood. “Old men are boys again,” said Aristophanes. This view of old age derives from the few resemblances, superficial at best, of the senile dement and the helpless young child.

Neurologic Signs of Aging

Critchley, in 1934, drew attention to a number of neurologic abnormalities that he had observed in octogenarians and for which no cause could be discerned other than the effects of aging itself. Several reviews of this subject have appeared subsequently (see, in particular, those of Jenkyn, of Benassi, and of Kokmen and their associates). The most consistent of the neurologic signs of aging are the following:

1. Neuro-ophthalmic signs: progressive smallness of pupils, decreased reactions to light and on accommodation, farsightedness (hyperopia) due to impairment of accommodation (presbyopia), insufficiency of convergence, restricted range of upward conjugate gaze, frequent loss of Bell’s phenomenon, diminished dark adaptation, and increased sensitivity to glare.

2. Progressive perceptive hearing loss (presbycusis), especially for high tones, and commensurate decline in speech discrimination. Mainly these changes are due to a diminution in the number of hair cells in the organ of Corti.

3. Diminution in the sense of smell and, to a lesser extent, of taste (see Chap. 12).

4. Motor signs: reduced speed and amount of motor activity, slowed reaction time, impairment of fine coordination and agility, reduced muscular power (legs more than arms and proximal muscles more than distal ones) and thinness of muscles, particularly the dorsal interossei, thenar, and anterior tibial muscles. A progressive decrease in the number of anterior horn cells is responsible for these changes, as described further on.

5. Changes in tendon reflexes: A depression of tendon reflexes at the ankles in comparison with those at the knees is observed frequently in persons more than 70 years of age, as is a loss of Achilles reflexes in those above 80 years. The snout or palmomental reflexes, which can be detected in mild form in a small proportion of healthy adults, is a frequent finding in the elderly (in as many as half of normal subjects over 60 years of age, according to R. K. Olney). However, other so-called cortical release signs, such as suck and grasp reflexes, are indicative of frontal lobe disease and are not to be expected simply as a result of aging.

6. Impairment or loss of vibratory sense in the toes and ankles. Proprioception, however, is impaired very little or not at all. Thresholds for the perception of cutaneous stimuli increase with age but require the use of refined methods of testing for their detection. These changes correlate with a loss of sensory fibers on sural nerve biopsy and reduced amplitude of sensory nerve action potentials and probably loss of dorsal root ganglion cells.

7. The most notable aging changes—those of stance, posture, and gait—are fully described in Chap. 7 and further on in this chapter.

The incidence of certain neurologic signs of aging has been determined by Jenkyn and colleagues, based on their examinations of 2029 individuals, aged 50 to 93 years. These data are summarized in Table 29-2.

Effects of Aging on Memory and Other Cognitive Functions

Probably the most detailed information as to the effects of age on the nervous system comes from the measurement of cognitive functions. In the course of standardization of the original Wechsler-Bellevue Intelligence Scale (1955), cross-sectional studies of large samples of the population indicated that there was a steady decline in cognitive function starting at 30 years of age and progressing into the senium. Apparently all forms of cognitive function partake of this decline—although in general certain elements of the verbal scale

Table 29-2
Frequency of certain neurologic signs in uncomplicated aging (in percent)

Sign	*65–69 years*	*70–74 years*	*75–79 years*	*>80 years*
Glabellar sign (inability to inhibit blink)	10	15	27	37
Snout reflex	3	8	7	26
Limited upgaze	6	15	27	29
Limited downgaze	8	15	26	34
Abnormal visual tracking	8	18	22	32
Paratonic rigidity	6	10	12	21
Unable to recall 3 words	24	28	25	55
Unable to spell "world" backward	10	12	18	21

Source: Adapted from Jenkyn et al. by permission.

(vocabulary, fund of information, and comprehension) withstand the effects of aging better than those of the performance scale (block design, reversal of digits, picture arrangement, object assembly, and the digit symbol task).

However, the concept of a linear regression of cognitive function with aging has had to be modified in the light of subsequent longitudinal studies. If the same individual is examined over a period of many years, there is virtually no decline in his performance as measured by tests of verbal function until 60 years of age. Beyond this age, verbal intelligence does decline, but very slowly—by an average of less than 5 percent through the seventh decade and less than 10 percent through the eighth decade (Schaie and Hertzog). Also, in a series of 460 community-dwelling individuals (55 to 95 years of age) studied by Smith and coworkers at the Mayo Clinic, there was no significant decline with age in verbal memory and in registration-attention. The most definite effects of age were in learning and memory and in problem solving—cognitive impairments probably attributable to a progressive reduction in the speed of processing information. The latter can be judged by the measurement of event-related evoked potentials and by a number of special psychologic tests (see Verhaeghen et al).

As regards these latter functions, it hardly needs to be pointed out that the ability to memorize, acquire and retain new information, recall names, and avoid distraction once set on a course of action diminishes with advancing age, particularly in those more than 70 years old. Moreover, memory function may be disturbed in this way despite the relative intactness of other intellectual abilities. Characteristically, there is difficulty with recall of a name or the specific date of an experience ("episodic" memory) despite a preservation of memory for the experience itself or for the many features of a person whose name is momentarily elusive ("tip-of-the-tongue syndrome"). Also characteristic is an inconsistent retrieval of the lost name or information at a later date. Kral, who first wrote informatively on this type of memory disturbance, referred to it as *benign senescent forgetfulness*. He pointed out that such a memory disturbance, in distinction to that of Alzheimer disease, worsens very little or not at all over a period of many years and does not interfere significantly with the person's work performance or activities of daily living. More recently, Crook and coworkers have refined the diagnostic criteria for senescent forgetfulness and have proposed a new term—*age-associated memory impairment* (AAMI). The diagnostic criteria for the latter disorder include age of 50 years or older, a subjective sense of decline in memory, impaired performance on standard tests of memory function (at least one SD below the mean), and absence of any other signs of dementia.

The changes of benign senescent forgetfulness, present in varying degree in most elderly individuals, may sometimes pose a clinical problem—how to decide whether they are part of the aging process per se or the early manifestations of Alzheimer disease. The differentiation can usually be made by careful testing of the mental status, along the lines already described in Chap. 21. Several abbreviated tests of mental status have been developed and are of practical value (Kokmen et al; Folstein et al) in that they can be given at the bedside in 5 to 10 min. Repetition of spoken items, such as a series of digits, orientation as to place and time, capacity to learn and to retain several items, tests of arithmetic and calculation (concentration), and specific tests for memory (particularly tests of delayed recall or forgetfulness) reveal that normal aging persons invariably perform at a significantly higher level than patients with Alzheimer disease and these tests readily discriminate between the two groups (Larrabee et al).

The foregoing effects of age on mental abilities are extremely variable. Some 70-year-olds perform better on psychologic testing than some "normal" 20-year-olds. And a few individuals retain exceptional mental power and perform creative work until late life. Verdi, for example, composed *Otello* at the age of 73 and *Falstaff* at 79. Humboldt wrote the five volumes of his *Kosmos* between the ages of 76 and 89 years; Goethe produced the second part of Faust when he was more than 70 years old; Galileo, Laplace, and Sherrington continued to make scientific contributions in their eighth decades; and Picasso continued to paint in his nineties. It must be pointed out, however, that these accomplishments were essentially continuations of lines of endeavor that had been initiated in early adult life. Indeed, little that is new and original is started after the fortieth year. High intelligence, well-organized work habits, and sound judgment compensate for many of the progressive deficiencies of old age.

Personality Changes in the Aged These are less easily measured than cognitive functions, but certain trends are nevertheless observable and may seriously disturb the lives of aged persons and those around them. Many old people become more opinionated, repetitive, self-centered, and rigid and conservative in their thinking; the opposite qualities—undue pliancy, vacillation, and the uncritical acceptance of ideas—are observed in others. Often these changes can be recognized as exaggerations of lifelong personality traits. Elderly persons tend to become increasingly cautious; many of them seem to lack self-confidence and require a strong probability of success before undertaking certain tasks. These changes may impair their performance on psychologic testing. Kallman's studies of senescent monozygotic twins suggest that genetic factors are more important than environmental ones in molding these traits. Aggressive individuals with much energy and a diversity of interests, leading to a wide range of social interactions, appear to resist the ravages of age better than those with the opposite traits. But this may be effect rather than cause. Those with depressive tendencies are more easily overwhelmed by prospects of the senium and adopt an attitude of hopelessness, fear, suspicion, and worry. This may explain the threefold increase in suicides in late middle life and old age. *Certainly an agitated depression is the most frequent psychiatric disease in these periods of life.*

One of the weaknesses of studies of the aged has been the bias in selection of patients. Many of the reported observations have been made in cohorts of individuals residing in nursing homes. Studies of functionally intact old people of comparable age and living independently, such as those of Kokmen and of Benassi and their colleagues, reveal fewer deficits, consisting mainly of forgetfulness of names, smallness of pupils, restriction of convergence and upward conjugate gaze, diminished Achilles reflexes and vibratory sense in the feet, stooped posture, and impairments of balance, agility, and gait (see below).

Effects of Aging on Stance and Gait and Related Motor Impairments

As noted earlier, these are among the most conspicuous manifestations of the aging process. Motor agility actually begins to decline in early adult life, even by the 30th year; it seems related to a gradual decrease in neuromuscular control as well as to changes in joints and other structures. The reality of this motor decrement is best appreciated by professional athletes who retire at age 35 or thereabout because their legs give out and cannot be restored to their maximal condition by training. They cannot run as well as younger athletes, even though the strength and coordination of their arms is relatively preserved. More subtle and imperceptibly evolving changes in stance and gait are ubiquitous features of aging (Chap. 7). Gradually the steps shorten, walking becomes slower, and there is a tendency to stoop. The old soldier must repeatedly remind himself to maintain an erect bearing. The older person becomes less confident and more cautious in walking and habitually touches the handrail in descending stairs, to prevent a misstep.

Concomitantly, all movements become less graceful, more inelastic. Donning trousers while standing alternately on one leg and then the other becomes difficult. Handwriting tends to worsen, and all arm and hand movements become more clumsy. Choking on food is more frequent. Urinary incontinence, defined as a state in which "involuntary loss of urine is a social or hygienic problem and is objectively demonstrated," is a surprisingly common occurrence in the elderly (Wells and Diokno). Doubtless this complex of motor impairments is based on the aforementioned neuronal losses in the spinal cord, cerebellum, and cerebrum.

To be distinguished from the ubiquitous and subtle changes in gait of the "normal" aged population is a more rapidly evolving and inordinate deterioration of gait that afflicts a small proportion of the aging population while they remain relatively competent in other ways. In all likelihood, this latter disorder represents an age-linked degenerative disease of the brain, since most instances of it are sooner or later accompanied by mental changes. The basis of this gait disorder is probably a combined frontal lobe-basal ganglionic degeneration, the anatomy of which has never been fully clarified.

In the analysis of gait disorders, one should search for evidence of *posterior column or vestibular disorder, cerebellar ataxia, and the spastic ataxia of cervical spondylosis*, all of which may unbalance the patient. *Normal-pressure hydrocephalus*, correctable by a ventriculoperitoneal shunt, accounts for the gait disorder of a sizable group of these elderly patients (Fisher). One recognizes in this latter gait disorder several elements of the Parkinson syndrome, and, of course, Parkinson disease is yet another potentially treatable cause of walking difficulty. These problems are discussed in detail in Chaps. 7 and 39. Obesity and hypertrophic arthritis of the spine, hips, and knees or an old hip fracture add to any gait difficulty.

Falls in the Elderly Among elderly persons without apparent neurological disease, falls constitute a major health problem. Among such persons living in the community, about 30 percent suffer one or more falls each year; this figure rises to 40 percent among those over the age of 80 and to more than 50 percent among elderly persons living in nursing homes (Tinetti et al). According to these authors, 10 to 15 percent of falls in the elderly result in fractures and other serious injuries; they are reportedly an underlying cause of about 9500 deaths annually in the United States.

Several factors, some mentioned above in regard to deterioration of gait, are responsible for the inordinately high rate of falling among older persons. Impairment of visual function and particularly of vestibular function with normal aging are important contributors. In a group of 34 elderly patients who were free of neurologic disease, postural hypotension, and leg deformities, Weiner and colleagues found a severe degree of postural reflex impairment in 15 and moderate impairment in 8. The failure to make rapid postural adjustments, which is a product of aging alone, accounts for the occurrence of falls in the course of usual activities such as walking, changing position, or descending stairs. Postural hypotension, often due to antihypertensive agents and the use of sedative drugs, is another important cause of falling in the elderly.

Of course, falling is an even more prominent feature of certain age-related neurologic diseases: stroke, Parkinson disease, normal-pressure hydrocephalus, and progressive supranuclear palsy, among others.

Other Restricted Motor Abnormalities in the Aged These are too numerous to be more than catalogued. They inform us of the many ways in which the motor system can deteriorate. Compulsive, repetitive movements are the most frequent: mouthing movements, stereotyped grimacing, protrusion of the tongue, side-to-side or to-and-fro tremor of the head, odd vocalizations such as sniffing, snorting, and bleating. In some respects these disorders resemble tics (quasi-voluntary movements to relieve tension), but careful observation shows that they are not really voluntary. Haloperidol and other drugs of this class have an unpredictable therapeutic effect, seeming at times to benefit the patient only by the superimposition of a drug-induced rigidity. The differential diagnosis must raise for consideration one of the phenothiazine-induced faciobuccal dyskinesias.

Old age is thought always to carry a liability to tremulousness, and, indeed, one sees this association with some frequency. The head, chin, or hands tremble and the voice quavers, yet there is not the usual slowness and poverty of movement, facial impassivity, or flexed posture that would stamp the condition as parkinsonian. Some instances are clearly familial, having appeared or worsened only late in life. The relation of tremulousness to senility is always open to doubt. Charcot, in a review of over 2000 elderly inhabitants of the Sâlpètriere, could find only about 30 with tremor.

Spastic, or spasmodic, dysphonia, a disorder of middle and late life characterized by spasm of all the throat muscles on attempted speech, is discussed on page 519. Blepharoclonus, or blepharospasm, an involuntary movement of the eyelids, is also described on page 114.

Classification of these restricted motor abnormalities—as the effects of aging alone or of age-related neurologic diseases—is presently not possible and must await such time as more is learned about their pathologic and genetic bases.

Morphologic and Physiologic Changes in the Aging Nervous System

These have never been fully established. From the third decade of life to the beginning of the tenth decade, the average decline in weight of the male brain is from 1394 to 1161 g, a loss of 233 g. The pace of this change, very gradual at first, accelerates during the sixth or seventh decades. The loss of brain weight, which correlates roughly with enlargement of the lateral ventricles and widening of the sulci, is presumably the result of neuronal degeneration and replacement gliosis, although this has not been proved. The counting of cerebrocortical neurons is fraught with technical difficulties, even with the use of computer-assisted automated techniques (see the critical review of neuron-counting studies by Coleman and Flood). Most studies, point to a depletion of the neuronal population in the neocortex, most evident in the seventh, eighth, and ninth decades.

Cell loss in the limbic system (hippocampus, parahippocampal and cingulate gyri) is of special interest. Ball, who measured the neuronal loss in the hippocampus, recorded a linear decrease of 27 percent between 45 and 95 years of age. Dam reported a similar degree of cell loss and replacement gliosis. These changes seem to proceed without relationship to Alzheimer neurofibrillary changes and senile plaques (Kemper).

Mueller et al have utilized quantitative volumetric MRI techniques to examine a cohort of 46 nondemented elderly individuals. They found small, constant rates of loss of brain volume with aging. Moreover, the rates of volume loss in the last decades of life were no greater than in the immediately preceding decades—suggesting that large changes in brain volume in the elderly are attributable to the dementing diseases common to this age period.

Among lumbosacral anterior horn cells, sensory ganglion cells, and putaminal and Purkinje cells, neuronal loss amounts to approximately 25 percent between youth and old age. Not all neuronal groups are equally susceptible. For example, the locus ceruleus and substantia nigra lose about 35 percent of their neurons, whereas the vestibular nuclei and inferior olives maintain a fairly constant number of cells throughout life. A progressive loss, decade by decade, of the major systems of nerve cells and myelinated fibers of the spinal cord has been convincingly demonstrated by Morrison.

Scheibel and coworkers have described a loss of neuronal dendrites in the aging brain, particularly the horizontal dendrites of the third and fifth layers of the neocortex. However, the Golgi method, which was used in these studies, is difficult to interpret because of artifacts. The careful morphometric studies of Buell and Coleman have shown that the surviving neurons actually exhibit expanded dendritic trees, suggesting that even aging neurons have the capacity to react to cell loss by developing new synapses.

With advancing age, there is an increasing tendency for neuritic ("senile") plaques to appear in the brains of nondemented individuals. At first the plaques appear in the hippocampus and parahippocampus, but later they become more widespread. These are loose aggregates of amorphous argentophilic material containing amyloid. They occur in increasing numbers with advancing age; by the end of the ninth decade of life, few brains are without them. However, as shown by Tomlinson and colleagues, relatively few plaques are present in the brains of mentally intact old people, in contrast to the large numbers in those with Alzheimer disease. Even more impressive is the correlation of neurofibrillary tangles and Alzheimer disease. Very few such tangles are found in the brains of mentally sound individuals, and such as are found are essentially confined to the hippocampus and adjacent entorhinal cortex. By contrast, neurofibrillary tangles are far more abundant and diffusely distributed in patients with Alzheimer disease.

The view is often expressed that neuritic plaques and Alzheimer type of neurofibrillary changes simply represent an acceleration of the natural aging process in the brain. We are more inclined to the idea that the plaques and neurofibrillary changes represent an *acquired age-linked disease*, analogous in this respect to certain cerebrovascular diseases. In support of this latter view are several observations: first, *Homo sapiens* is the only animal species in which Alzheimer neurofibrillary changes and neuritic plaques are regularly found in the aging brain. A few plaque-like structures (but no neurofibrillary changes) have been seen occasionally in old dogs and monkeys but not in mice or rats. It seems unbiologic that human aging should differ from that of all other animal species. Second, some of the most severe forms of Alzheimer disease occur in middle adult life, long before the senium. Third, these histopathologic changes in variable proportion occur in a number of other diseases unrelated to aging, such as dementia pugilistica ("punch-drunk" state), Down syndrome, postencephalitic Parkinson disease, and progressive supranuclear palsy. Fourth, neurofibrillary tangles can be reproduced in the experimental animal by such toxins as aluminum, vincristine, vinblastine, and colchicine. Finally, a small proportion of Alzheimer cases are definitely familial. Alzheimer disease is therefore more appropriately considered under degenerative diseases (see Chap. 39), where the entire subject is discussed further.

Increasing accumulation of lipofuscin granules in the cytoplasm of neurons (see further on, under "Life Span and Aging of Specialized Cells"), sometimes extreme in degree, accompanies advancing age. Also, there is an age-related neuronal accumulation of iron and other pigment bodies. Granulovacuolar changes are a regular finding in aging hippocampi, regardless of the mental state of the individual. The accumulation of amyloid-containing concretions (corpora amylacea) around nerve roots and diffusely in the subpial space is yet another aging effect. In addition, slight thickening and hyalinization of the walls of small blood vessels and pericapillary gliosis (cribriform state) become evident in the aging brain. Many of the small arteries contain amyloid in their walls. Some of the vascular changes are probably not primary but secondary to reduced circulatory need (the so-called vascular atrophy of involuting organs). There is no evidence that the aforementioned aging changes, which are often loosely referred to as arteriosclerotic, depend on any recognized form of vascular disease.

Cerebral blood flow has been extensively investigated in the elderly population. Most studies have shown that flow declines with age and that the cerebral metabolic rate declines in parallel. There is also an age-related increase in cerebrovascular resistance. Declines in flow are somewhat greater in the cortex than in white matter and greater in prefrontal regions than in other parts of the hemispheres. Obrist demonstrated a 28 percent reduction in cerebral flow by age 80. It is noteworthy, however, that every cohort of elderly persons tested in this way contained a significant proportion in which cerebral blood flow was equivalent to that in young control subjects. In fact, in a group of 72-year-old men rigorously selected on the basis of freedom from disease, Sokoloff demonstrated that cerebral blood flow and oxygen consumption did not differ from those of normal men 22 years of age. Cerebral glucose metabolism was reduced in all the elderly subjects, however.

With advancing age there is a general tendency for the electroencephalogram (EEG) to show a slowing of the alpha rhythm, an increase in beta activity, a decline in the percentage of slow-wave sleep, and an increasing intrusion of theta rhythms, particularly over the temporal lobes. There are large individual differences, however.

Many biochemical studies have been made of the effects of aging on cerebral tissues. In general, deoxyribonucleic acid (DNA), ribonucleic acid (RNA), cerebrosides, and other components of myelin diminish in the brains of aged, mentally intact humans and old animals; intracellular enzymes also diminish. The results of these studies are far from consistent, and the problem raised by all of them is whether the changes reflect a primary effect of aging or merely the loss of essential cellular substances in proportion to the loss of neurons and their medullated fibers.

With respect to the neurotransmitters, it is generally agreed that the concentrations of acetylcholine, norepinephrine, and dopamine decline in the course of normal aging. Also, the concentration of gamma-aminobutyric acid (GABA) has been shown to decline with age, particularly in the frontal cortex (Spokes et al). Analyses of postmortem human and animal brains have failed to demonstrate a decline with age in the concentration of serotonin or its metabolites (McEntee and Crook). Accurate assessment of other neurotransmitters has been more difficult because of their marked lability in postmortem material. Data from experiments in rats suggest that the glutamate content of the brain and the number of *N*-methyl-D-aspartate (NMDA) receptors diminish with age, but the functional significance of this finding is unclear. Unlike the case in Alzheimer disease, normal aging is associated with only slight and inconsistent abnormalities of cholinergic innervation of the hippocampus and cortex. This is true also of the acetylcholine content and the activity of choline acetyltransferase (the synthesizing enzyme of acetylcholine) in these regions and the number of cholinergic neurons in the nucleus basalis of Meynert (substantia innominata) and other nuclei of the basal forebrain (Decker). Again, the significance of these changes is difficult to judge. They may simply reflect the depletion of cells that occurs with aging. The topics of cholinergic and glutamatergic function in the aging brain have been critically reviewed by McEntee and Crook.

To what extent the normal neurons in the aging brain can compensate for neurologic deficits by producing new neurons from latent precursor (pluripotential) cells in the cortex, elaborating new dendrites or axonal sprouting is a topic of interest, but only speculations are possible (see Rose and Johnson). The conventional teaching that the cerebral neurons with which we are born are post-mitotic, i.e., lack the capacity to regenerate, remains essentially unchallenged.

Aging Changes in Muscles and Nerves

With advancing age, skeletal muscles lose cells (fibers) and undergo a gradual reduction in their weight more or less parallel to that of the brain. Atrophy of muscles and diminution in peak power and endurance are clinical expressions of these changes. Our own studies indicate that the wasting involves several processes, some principally myopathic and others relating to disuse or denervation, from loss of motor neurons. In this material, denervation atrophy of the gastrocnemius muscles was found in 80 percent of individuals over 70 years of age.

The lost muscle fibers are gradually replaced by endomysial connective tissue and fat cells. The surviving fibers are generally thinner than normal (possibly due to disuse atrophy), but some enlarge, resulting in a wider than normal range of fiber size. Groups of fibers all at the same stage of atrophy undoubtedly relate to loss of motor innervation. The reduction in conduction velocity and decrease in amplitude of motor nerve potentials and, to a greater extent, of sensory nerves in the aged may be taken as other indices of loss of motor and sensory axons. All these changes are more marked in the legs than elsewhere. However, when Roos and colleagues examined the contractile speed and firing rates of the quadriceps muscle in young men and compared them to those of men close to 80 years old, they found little difference despite a 50 percent reduction in the maximum voluntary contraction force developed by the muscle in the older men.

As already mentioned, it has been observed that age is an important prognostic factor in a large number of human diseases. This effect is very evident, for example, in the markedly slower and less complete recovery from Guillain-Barré polyneuropathy in older age groups compared with younger ones. One presumes that structural aging changes in peripheral nerves limit the degree of myelin regeneration and lower the threshold for failure of electrical transmission.

The Cellular Basis of Aging

Many mechanisms are presumed to be involved in the aging process of cellular constituents and structural protein (collagen) of the various bodily organs. Investigations of these mechanisms have been directed along several lines: (1) the failure of cell multiplication and of mitosis in tissues composed of *dividing cells*; (2) the decline in functional efficiency and finally the deterioration and death of highly *specialized nondividing cells* such as the neurons and to some extent the muscle fibers; and (3) the progressive alteration of the structural protein collagen, which constitutes about 40 percent of the body protein and serves as the binding substance of the skin, muscle, bones, and blood vessels.

The Aging Process in Dividing Cells The studies of Hayflick and colleagues on the innate capacity of cells to divide in tissue culture may shed light on the problem of aging. They found that fibroblasts can divide only a finite number of times (contrary to Alexis Carrel's original claim that chicken heart cells, nourished in tissue cultures, could continue to live and divide forever). The fibroblasts of a human infant are capable of dividing about 50 times, those of a 20-year-old about 30 times, and those of an 80-year-old about 20 times. Fibroblasts from patients with progeria, in whom the signs of aging occur in the first decade of life, undergo premature senescence (Hutchinson-Gilford and Werner syndromes). They die after 2 to 12 doublings in cell culture. Toward the end of the life cycle of cultured cells, chromosomal aberrations and peculiarities of cell division appear in some cells. Whether these types of abnormalities are a characteristic feature of human aging has not been settled. Only if neoplastic transformation takes place do cells approach the immortality postulated early in the century by Carrel.

Hayflick saw in this aging process and finite lifetime of normal cells a deterioration of the genetic program that "orchestrates" the development of cells. He postulated that with increasing age the DNA, RNA, and protein-synthesizing apparatus of the *dividing cells* falls prey to an ever-increasing number of copying errors (similar to that which occurs with radiation). The distorted templates serve as faulty models for the production of more faulty enzymes, leading eventually to an "error catastrophe," i.e., to death of the cell. A related line of observation has connected the aging of mammalian cells to a progressive loss of telomeres at the ends of chromosomes. With each cell division, these ends are shortened until their loss no longer permits cell replication. This hypothesis is probably not applicable to the nervous system, considering the fact that cell division does not take place there.

Life Span and Aging of Specialized Cells As was said, nerve cells that cease to divide early in life and are near their maximum number at birth must last the lifetime of the individual. Once destroyed, whether by aging or disease, they are never replaced. Obviously the life span is not the same for every cell; some survive longer than others. If a significant number die early, functional deficits result. Outfall of neurons is a prominent feature during embryogenesis (apoptosis or programmed cell death, see below) and then occurs again at variable times and at a much slower rate during adult life. The point at which functional deficits appear varies for each system, depending upon its "safety factor," i.e., the protective excess of cells that must be lost before symptoms appear. Whether cells falter functionally before their final disintegration is unknown. Possibly they do, in view of the shrinkage of their dendritic surfaces, noted by Scheibel and coworkers.

The cytologic events that lead to the death of nondividing cells are little understood. In humans as well as in animals, accumulation of lipofuscin in the cytoplasm is a phenomenon of such constancy that it can be used as a reliable cytologic index of aging. Called "wear and tear" or "age" pigment, these yellow granules of lipochrome, or lipofuscin, form in the cytoplasm of both nerve and muscle cells, in close relation to lysosomes. Simultaneously, the cell diminishes in volume, due presumably to the loss of other cytoplasmic components such as Nissl bodies (the main cytoplasmic RNA of neurons) and mitochondria. The nucleus becomes smaller, with infolding of the nuclear membrane and alteration of the nucleolus. This process in the past was called "chronic neuronal atrophy" by German neuropathologists. The currently popular term is *apoptosis*, meaning a "dropping off" and is quite inappropriate. The term was used originally to designate the massive programmed cell death that occurs over a brief period during embryogenesis, leaving no trace. The chronic neuronal atrophy of later life is of quite a different nature, being characterized by marked condensation and fragmentation of chromatin and membrane-bound fragments, and ultimately fragmentation of nuclear DNA. Histochemical stains reveal a depletion of oxidative as well as phosphorylative and presumably other enzymes. Neurons are said to lose dendrites and thereby reduce their synaptic surface (Scheibel et al), as described earlier in this chapter. All these changes have been observed in cultured cells.

Considering the ubiquitous nature of these morphologic changes, it is remarkable that we know so little of their pathogenesis. They have been attributed to progressive exhaustion of cell catalysts (enzymes and coenzymes), but this explanation only restates the problem in rather speculative biochemical terms. It is generally believed that the accumulation of lipofuscin is the result of oxidation of lipids, which are polymerized with protein and unsaturated peptides and released when a cell ages or undergoes catabolic changes for any reason. According to this view, any factor (e.g., hemorrhage into fatty tissue) that increases the ratio of tissue oxidant to antioxidant favors the accumulation of lipofuscin. Biologic antioxidants such as vitamins C and E, glutathione, cysteine, and sulfhydryl proteins are said to counteract the process. The neuronal accumulation of lipofuscin may simply represent a stage in a degenerative process or, as appears more likely, the sequestration of lysosomes and lipofuscin may serve as a protective mechanism against neuronal degeneration.

A topic of current research interest, in respect to the mechanisms of neuronal aging and death, is the role of several endogenous amino acids. These amino acids, particularly glutamate and aspartate, which normally act as putative excitatory neurotransmitters, can, under certain conditions, also be neurotoxic. In cell culture and animal experiments, sustained exposure of neurons to toxic concentrations of excitatory neurotransmitters results in acute neuronal swelling (presumably by opening sodium channels). A slower process of neuronal degeneration is possibly dependent upon brief exposure to glutamate or related agonists and the influx of calcium ions that follows (Choi; J. W.Olney). Another currently popular theory implicates a potentially damaging effect of oxygen free radicals (the by-products of oxidative metabolism), particularly on mitochondrial DNA. These and other biologic factors that might be operative in the aging process and cell death have been reviewed by Drachman.

Finally, it should be mentioned that tissue collagen, like nondividing cells, undergoes aging changes in its molecular structure, which progressively diminish its elasticity and contractility.

Age-Related Diseases

The fundamental processes of aging, outlined above, operate during all of adult life; if the person survives long enough, he will succumb to the ultimate failure of normal cells to divide or function. However, relatively few people die of old age alone. Most of them die of diseases, to which they are rendered increasingly susceptible by the aging processes. The most common of the age-related diseases are neoplasia, vascular diseases of the heart and brain, fractures of the hip, infections (chiefly pulmonary), Alzheimer disease, and other degenerative diseases of the nervous system. Not only do these diseases increase in frequency with advancing age, but they do so exponentially, like death itself. Each of these disease processes is considered in its appropriate chapter and only their age-related aspects are mentioned here.

Among the *age-linked degenerative diseases of the nervous system*, the nonhereditary form of Alzheimer disease is the most common and important. The reason for believing that the Alzheimer changes represent an acquired degenerative disease and not simply an acceleration of the aging process have been presented on page 645. Dementia as a cardinal manifestation of cerebral disease is considered in Chap. 21; Alzheimer disease and other age-linked degenerative diseases are described in Chap. 39.

Cerebral atherosclerosis is, of course, a frequent finding in the elderly, but it does not parallel aging with any degree of precision, being severe in some 30- to 40-year-old individuals and practically absent in some octogenarians. In the normotensive individual it tends to occur in scattered, discrete plaques mostly in the aorta and cervical arteries (carotid sinus and higher segments) and at the vertebrobasilar junction and basilar portions of the cerebral arterial system. In the hypertensive and diabetic, it is more diffuse and extends into finer branches of the cerebral and cerebellar arteries. One or more cerebral ischemic softenings are found in about 25 percent of all individuals more than 70 years of age who have been carefully examined postmortem. In addition to atherosclerotic disease, the basilar arteries become somewhat larger and more tortuous and opaque in the elderly.

The *skull* thickens with age. A special form, known as *hyperostosis frontalis interna*, is said to be exclusive to women and joined with obesity and hirsutism. Its neurologic implications are vague, and there has always been a temptation to ascribe more to it than it deserves. At autopsy, aside from close attachments of the dura and opacity of the underlying pia-arachnoid ("milk spots"), we have observed no consistent neuropathologic lesion in the cerebrum itself.

Most *neoplasms of the nervous system* occur with increasing frequency in early and middle adult life. Only in old age does the incidence tend to fall. The cytoplasmic events leading to neoplasia must relate to the process of cell division; postmitotic neurons rarely give rise to tumors. One evidence of this relationship is the tendency of tumors to develop in many organs in experimental animals exposed to gamma radiation; moreover, there is a linear relationship between the intensity of exposure and frequency of tumor formation. One class of endocrine tumors appears to form during periods of intensified functional demands, e.g., hypophysial adenomas with atrophy of gonads and adrenals during late adult life. Reference has already been made to the chromosomal aberrations that appear in older dividing cells. An example is the trisomy of the Down syndrome, which occurs with increasing frequency as the oocyte ages in the later part of reproductive life.

As to increased vulnerability of the older person to infection, it may relate to a diminished capacity of the aging organism to adapt to change rather than to any failure of the inflammatory reaction per se. Older people are slower in adjusting to high and low atmospheric temperatures, but their levels of antibodies and production of leukocytes and the vigor of their cellular immune response are all surprisingly well maintained. Nonetheless, changes in immune function that occur with aging may result in the synthesis of abnormal immune products, which contribute to neurologic disease or increase the susceptibility to infection; or, possibly, age-dependent changes in the nervous system may in some way impair immune regulation (Antel and Minuk).

The high incidence of *adverse drug reactions* in the elderly is related to several factors—the increased duration and severity of disease, the frequent failure to adjust drug dosage to diminished body weight, a reduction in hepatic detoxification and in renal clearance, and, most importantly, the unmasking by certain drugs, sedatives in particular, of an underlying mild dementia.

Often in the elderly, the exigencies of disease cannot be met efficiently because of a combination of organ inadequacies, no single one of which is of sufficient severity to be manifest clinically. The sum total of these organ deficits constitutes a kind of gestalt of senility. The long list of diseases found in the elderly at autopsy reflects the increasing susceptibility to disease with aging. However, the contributing effects of the aging processes are relatively inapparent, which is why the medical student so often asks, after the autopsy of an elderly person, "But what was the cause of death?"

GERONTOLOGIC NEUROLOGY

Gerontology is defined as the study of aging and *gerontologic neurology* as the study of the effects of aging—both of aging itself and of the age-related diseases—on the nervous system. *Geriatrics* and *geriatric medicine* refer to the health and medical care of the elderly. In comparison to pediatric neurology, these disciplines have not aroused much interest. The young physician is more excited by disease than by the seemingly immutable changes due to aging and is inclined to question whether medicine has a significant role to play in treating the neurologic disorders of the elderly. The authors would answer this question affirmatively for the simple reason that a majority of all neurologic patients seen in practice are elderly, especially if one includes those with vascular diseases of the brain. Furthermore, many of their diseases are preventable or therapeutically controllable. Since aging changes do not involve all organs and tissues simultaneously, patients need help and advice about certain of these effects at a time when most of their organs are functionally intact. Some of the age-related chemical deficiencies (i.e., vitamin B deficiencies, diabetes mellitus) and many of the common restricted involutional changes (presbyopia, etc.) can be corrected. Others can even be turned into assets; the forgetfulness of the aged and their deafness may serve to excuse many of their shortcomings and to spare them effort and annoyance. And always, there is the need to counsel the elderly patient on matters pertaining to health and daily activities. This was appreciated even in the time of Cicero, who in his *De Senectute* urged the practice of moderation in exercise and giving due attention to the mind, which must be kept active—or, like a lamp that is not supplied with oil, it will grow dim.

Some physicians hesitate to interpret any change as involutional until the patient is past the biblical three score years and ten—or they may avoid the diagnosis altogether because it implies an incurable condition. Their reasoning is faulty in both instances. Many involutional changes, such as presbyopia, can be demonstrated in their incipient states in the twenties; by the mid-forties, failing visual accommodation is almost universal. Insulin resistance, osteoporosis, and the disorder of uric acid metabolism causing gout are manifest in the forties in an appreciable percentage of all those afflicted. Many restricted forms of involution or abiotrophy, after progressing for a few years, become arrested or progress very slowly and are compensated for in many ways.

In a more general sense, geriatric medicine should present the physician's view of what is needed for the ideal care of the elderly. Obviously the primary concern of the physician is with the diagnosis and management of the patient's illnesses. But once this has been accomplished, attention should turn to the multitude of functional impairments that afflict the elderly patient—the simple matters of dressing, bathing, shopping, cooking, management of money, and so forth. In the end, it is upon these functional incapacities that the physician must focus to decide what help the patient requires and to involve the family and appropriate social agencies in providing this help. The decision as to whether a patient can function independently in an apartment or requires care in a nursing home may depend on so mundane a matter as whether he can get from his bed to the bathroom.

In the past, when America's population was predominantly rural, elderly individuals were cared for by their relatives in their own homes, but this is often difficult or undesirable in present-day urban society. Also, in the past, the younger generation was often spared much of the responsibility for the care of aging parents because of the previously higher mortality among the elderly from vascular disease, neoplasia, and particularly infection. In the nineteenth century, when pneumonia was far more frequently lethal than it is now, Osler referred to it as the "old man's friend," for, as in Ecclesiastes, he considered death as a kindness to the old and feeble. As medical science and public health measures brought these and other diseases under control, the number of elderly persons increased, and it will continue to do so. The U.S. Census Bureau has estimated that in the year 2000 there were 31 million persons over the age of 65 in the United States and that 13 million of them were more than 75 years old. As the number of elderly increases, the need to look after them will occupy more and more of the energies of physicians and the resources of society at large.

Once an old person declines physically and mentally to a vegetative state, the issue of euthanasia and all the ethical problems it entails will arise from time to time. The authors reject this solution while committing themselves fully to measures that prevent pain and suffering.

REFERENCES

Albert ML, Knoefel JE (Eds): *Clinical Neurology of Aging*, 2nd ed. New York, Oxford University Press, 1994.

Antel JP, Minuk J: Neuroimmunology of aging, in Albert ML, Knoefel JE (eds): *Clinical Neurology of Aging*, 2nd ed. New York, Oxford University Press, 1994, pp 121–135.

Ball MJ: Neuronal loss, neurofibrillary tangles and granulovacuolar degeneration in the hippocampus with aging and dementia. *Acta Neuropathol* 27:111, 1977.

Benassi G, D'Alessandro R, Gallassi R, et al: Neurological examination in subjects over 65 years: An epidemiological survey. *Neuroepidemiology* 9:27, 1990.

Blessed G, Tomlinson BE, Roth M: The association between quantitative measures of dementia and of senile change in the cerebral grey matter of elderly subjects. *Br J Psychiatry* 114:797, 1968.

Buell SJ, Coleman PD: Dendritic growth in the aged human brain and failure of growth in senile dementia. *Science* 206:854, 1979.

Carrel A: On the permanent life of tissues outside of the organism. *J Exp Med* 15:516, 1912.

Choi DW: Glutamate neurotoxicity and diseases of the nervous system. *Neuron* 1:623, 1988.

Coleman PD, Flood DG: Neuron numbers and dendritic extent in normal aging and Alzheimer's disease. *Neurobiol Aging* 8:521, 1987.

Comfort A: *The Biology of Senescence*, 3rd ed. New York, Elsevier, 1979.

Critchley M: Neurologic changes in the aged. *J Chronic Dis* 3:459, 1956.

Crook T, Bartus RT, Ferris SH, et al: Age-associated memory impairment: Proposed diagnostic criteria and measures of clinical change—Report of a National Institute of Mental Health Work Group. *Dev Neuropsychol* 2:261, 1986.

Dam AM: The density of neurons in the human hippocampus. *Neuropathol Appl Neurobiol* 5:249, 1979.

Decker MW: The effects of aging on hippocampal and cortical projections of the forebrain cholinergic system. *Brain Res* 434:423, 1987.

Drachman DA: Aging and the brain: A new frontier. *Ann Neurol* 42:819, 1997.

Fisher CM: Hydrocephalus as a cause of disturbances of gait in the elderly. *Neurology* 32:1358, 1982.

Folstein MF, Folstein SE, McHugh PR: "Mini-mental state": A practical method for grading the cognitive state of patients for the clinician. *J Psychiatr Res* 12:189, 1975.

Fries JF: Aging, natural death, and the compression of morbidity. *N Engl J Med* 303:130, 1980.

Fries JF, Crapo LM: *Vitality and Aging*. San Francisco, Freeman, 1981.

Gompertz B: On the nature of the function expressive of the law of human mortality and a new mode of determining the value of life contingencies. *Phil Trans R Soc Lond* 115:513, 1825.

Hartroft WS, Porta EA: Ceroid. *Am J Med Sci* 250:324, 1965.

Hayflick L: The cell biology of human aging. *N Engl J Med* 295:1302, 1976.

Hazzard WR, Blass JP, Ettinger WH, et al (eds): *Principles of Geriatric Medicine and Gerontology*, 4th ed. New York, McGraw-Hill, 1999.

Jenkyn LR, Reeves AG, Warren T, et al: Neurologic signs in senescence. *Arch Neurol* 42:1154, 1985.

Johansson B, Zarit SH, Berg S: Changes in cognitive functioning in the oldest old. *J Gerontol* 47:75, 1992.

Kallman FJ: Genetic factors in aging: Comparative and longitudinal observations on a senescent twin population, in Hoch PH, Zubin J (eds): *Psychopathology of Aging*. New York, Grune & Stratton, 1961.

Kaplan RM: Imagine no coronary heart disease. *Circulation* 83:1452, 1991.

Kemper TL: Neuroanatomical and neuropathological changes during aging and dementia, in Albert ML, Knoefel JE (eds): *Clinical Neurology of Aging*, 2nd ed. New York, Oxford University Press, 1994, pp 3–67.

Kokmen E, Bossemeyer RW Jr, Barney J, Williams WJ: Neurologic manifestations of aging. *J Gerontol* 32:411, 1977.

Kokmen E, Smith GE, Petersen RC, et al: The short test of mental status: Correlations with standardized psychometric testing. *Arch Neurol* 48:725, 1991.

Kral VA: Senescent forgetfulness: Benign and malignant. *J Can Med Assoc* 86:257, 1962.

Larrabee GH, Levin HS, High WM: Senescent forgetfulness: A quantitative study. *Dev Neuropsychol* 2:373, 1986.

McEntee WJ, Crook TH: Serotonin, memory, and the aging brain. *Psychopharmacology* 103:143, 1991.

McFarland D: The aged in the 21st century: A demographer's view, in Jarvik LF (ed): *"Aging into the 21st Century": Middle-Agers Today*. New York, Gardner Press, 1978, pp 5–22.

Medawar PB: The definition and measurement of senescence, in Wolstenholme GEW, Cameron MP (eds): *Ciba Foundation Colloquia on Aging*. Vol 1. Boston, Little, Brown, 1955, pp 4–15.

Morrison LR: *The Effect of Advancing Age upon the Human Spinal Cord*. Cambridge, MA, Harvard University Press, 1959.

Mueller EA, Moore MM, Kerr DC, et al: Brain volume preserved in healthy elderly through the eleventh decade. *Neurology* 51:1555, 1998.

Obrist WD: Cerebral circulatory changes in normal aging and dementia, in Hoffmeister F, Muller C (eds): *Brain Function in Old Age*. Berlin, Springer-Verlag, 1979, pp 278–287.

Olney JW: Excitatory amino acids and neuropsychiatric disorders. *Biol Psychiatry* 26:505, 1989.

Olney RK: The neurology of aging, in Aminoff MJ (ed): *Neurology and General Medicine*, 2nd ed. New York, Churchill Livingstone, 1994, pp 947–962.

Poon LW: Differences in human memory with aging: Nature, causes, and clinical implications, in Birren JE, Schaie KW (eds): *Handbook of the Psychology of Aging*. New York, Van Nostrand Reinhold, 1985, pp 427–462.

Roos MR, Rice CL, Connelly DM, Vandervoort AA: Quadriceps muscle strength, contractile properties, and motor unit firing rates in young and old men. *Muscle Nerve* 22:1094, 1999.

Rose FW, Johnson DA: *Recovery from Brain Damage*. New York, Plenum Press, 1992.

Roth M, Tomlinson BE, Blessed G: Correlation between scores for dementia and counts of senile plaques in cerebral grey matter of elderly subjects. *Nature* 209:109, 1966.

Schaie KW, Hertzog C: Fourteen-year cohort-sequential analyses of adult intellectual development. *Dev Psychol* 19:531, 1983.

Scheibel M, Lindsay RD, Tomiyasu U, Scheibel AB: Progressive dendritic changes in aging human cortex. *Exp Neurol* 47:392, 1975.

Shock MW: System integration, in Finch CE, Hayflick L (eds): *Handbook of the Biology of Aging*. New York, Van Nostrand Reinhold, 1977.

Smith GE, Malec JF, Ivnik RJ: Validity of the construct of nonverbal memory: A factor-analytic study in a normal elderly sample. *J Clin Exp Neuropsychol* 14:211, 1992.

Sokoloff L: Effects of normal aging on cerebral circulation and energy metabolism, in Hoffmeister F, Muller C (eds): *Brain Function in Old Age*. Berlin, Springer-Verlag, 1979, pp 367–380.

Spokes EGS, Garrett NJ, Rossor MN, et al: Distribution of GABA in postmortem brain tissue from control, psychotic, and Huntington's chorea subjects. *J Neurol Sci* 48:303, 1980.

Tinetti ME, Speechley M: Prevention of falls among the elderly. *N Engl J Med* 320:1055, 1989.

Tinetti ME, Speechley M, Ginter SF: Risk factors for falls among elderly persons living in the community. *N Engl J Med* 319:1701, 1988.

Tomlinson BE, Blessed G, Roth M: Observations on the brains of nondemented old people. *J Neurol Sci* 7:331, 1968.

Tomlinson BE, Blessed G, Roth M: Observations on the brains of demented old people. *J Neurol Sci* 11:205, 1970.

Verhaeghen P, Marcoen A, Goossens L: Facts and fiction about memory aging: A quantitative integration of research findings. *J Gerontol* 48:157, 1993.

Verzar F: The aging of collagen. *Sci Am* 208:104, 1963.

Wechsler D: *Manual for the Wechsler Adult Intelligence Scale*. New York, The Psychological Corporation, 1955.

Weiner WJ, Nora LM, Glantz RH: Elderly inpatients: Postural reflex impairment. *Neurology* 34:945, 1984.

Wells TJ, Diokno AC: Urinary incontinence in the elderly. *Semin Neurol* 9:60, 1989.

Part 4

THE MAJOR CATEGORIES OF NEUROLOGIC DISEASE

Chapter 30

DISTURBANCES OF CEREBROSPINAL FLUID AND ITS CIRCULATION, including Hydrocephalus, Pseudotumor Cerebri, and Low-Pressure Syndromes

In many chapters to follow, reference will be made to the ways in which the cerebrospinal fluid (CSF) reflects the basic pathologic processes in a wide variety of inflammatory and infectious, metabolic, neoplastic, demyelinative, and degenerative diseases. The CSF alterations in these varied circumstances raise so many interesting and important problems that we consider it worthwhile to discuss in one place the mechanisms involved in the formation, circulation, and absorption of the CSF, particularly as they pertain to increased intracranial pressure (ICP). Also to be considered in this chapter are hydrocephalus, pseudotumor cerebri, and syndromes produced by greatly reduced pressure in the CSF compartment. In all of these conditions, the primary abnormalities are those of the CSF and its circulation. Examination of the CSF as a diagnostic aid in neurology was discussed in Chap. 2; the primary infective and noninfective inflammatory reactions of the pia-arachnoid (leptomeninges) and ependyma of the ventricles are considered in Chap. 32.

A few historical points call to mind that our knowledge of the physiology, chemistry, and cytology of the CSF is relatively recent. Although the lumbar puncture was introduced by Quincke in 1891, it was not until 1912 that Mestrezat made the first correlations between disease processes and the cellular and chemical changes in the CSF. In 1937, Merritt and Fremont-Smith published their classic monograph on the CSF changes in all types of disease. Most of our knowledge of CSF cytology has accumulated since the late 1950s, when membrane filtration techniques (particularly the cellulose ester, or Millipore, filter) were introduced. The studies of Dandy (1919) and of Weed (1935) provided the basis of our knowledge of CSF formation, circulation, and absorption. There followed the important studies of Pappenheimer and of Ames and their colleagues, and the monographs of Fishman and of Davson and coworkers, which are important recent contributions. The cytology of the CSF is informatively summarized in the monographs of Dufresne and Den Hartog-Jager (see Chap. 2 for references).

PHYSIOLOGY OF THE CEREBROSPINAL FLUID

The primary function of the CSF appears to be a mechanical one; it serves as a kind of water jacket for the spinal cord and brain, protecting them from potentially injurious blows to the spinal column and skull and acute changes in venous pressure. Also, it provides the brain with buoyancy. As pointed out by Fishman, the 1500-g brain, which has a water content of approximately 80 percent, weighs only 50 g when suspended in CSF, so the brain virtually floats in its CSF jacket. Many of the physiologic and chemical mechanisms described below are committed to maintaining the relatively constant volume-pressure relationships of the CSF. Since the brain and spinal cord have no lymphatic channels, the CSF, through its "sink action" (see below), serves to remove the waste products of cerebral metabolism, the main ones being CO_2, lactate, and hydrogen ions. The composition of the CSF is maintained within narrow limits, despite major alterations in the blood; thus the CSF, along with the intercellular fluid of the brain, helps to preserve a stable chemical environment for neurons and their medullated fibers. There is no reason to believe that the CSF is actively involved in the metabolism of the cells of the brain and spinal cord.

In the adult, the average intracranial volume is 1700 mL; the volume of the brain is from 1200 to 1400 mL, CSF volume ranges from 70 to 160 mL (mean, 104), and that of blood is about 150 mL. In addition, the spinal subarachnoid space contains 10 to 20 mL of CSF. Thus, at most, the CSF occupies somewhat less than 10 percent of the intracranial and intraspinal spaces. The proportion of CSF in the ventricles and cisternae and in the subarachnoid spaces between the cerebral hemispheres and the sulci varies with age. These variations have been plotted in CT scans by Meese and coworkers; the distance between the caudate nuclei at the anterior horns gradually widens by approximately 1.0 to 1.5 cm, and the width of the third ventricle increases from 3 to 6 mm (by age 60).

Formation The introduction of the ventriculocisternal perfusion technique by Pappenheimer and colleagues made possible accurate measurement of the rates of formation and absorption of the CSF. It is now established that the average rate of CSF formation is 21 to 22 mL/h (0.35 mL/min), or approximately 500 mL/day. The CSF as a whole is renewed four or five times daily.

The choroid plexuses, located in the floor of the lateral, third, and fourth ventricles, are the main sites of CSF formation (some CSF is formed even after the choroid plexuses are removed). The thin-walled vessels of the plexuses allow passive diffusion of substances from the blood plasma into the extracellular space surrounding choroid cells. Also, the choroidal epithelial cells, like other secretory epithelia, contain organelles, indicating their capacity for an energy-dependent secretory function, i.e., "active transport." The blood vessels in the subependymal regions and the pia also contribute to the CSF, and some substances enter the CSF as readily from the meninges as from the choroid plexuses. Thus, electrolytes equilibrate with the CSF at all points in the ventricular and subarachnoid spaces, and the same is true of glucose. The transport of sodium, the main cation of the CSF, is accomplished by the action of a sodium-potassium-ion exchange pump at the apical surface of the choroid plexus cells, the energy for which is supplied by adenosine triphosphate; drugs that inhibit this system reduce CSF formation (Cutler and Spertell). Electrolytes enter the ventricles more readily than the subarachnoid space (water does the opposite). The penetration of certain drugs and metabolites is in direct relation to their lipid solubility. Ionized compounds, such as hexoses and amino acids, being relatively insoluble in lipids, enter the CSF slowly unless facilitated by a membrane transport system. This type of facilitated (carrier) diffusion is stereospecific; i.e., the carrier (a specific protein or proteolipid) binds only with a solute having a specific configuration and then carries it across the membrane and releases it in the CSF and intercellular fluid.

Diffusion gradients appear to determine the entry of serum proteins into the CSF and also the exchanges of CO_2. Water and sodium diffuse as readily from blood to CSF and intercellular spaces as in the reverse direction. This explains the rapid effects of intravenously injected hypotonic and hypertonic fluids.

Studies using radioisotopic tracer techniques have shown that the various constituents of the CSF (see Table 2-1) are in dynamic equilibrium with the blood. Similarly, CSF in the ventricles and subarachnoid spaces is in equilibrium with the intercellular fluid of the brain, spinal cord, and olfactory and optic nerves. Certain structures that were thought to maintain this equilibrium—namely, *the blood-CSF barrier and brain CSF barrier*—are now subsumed under the term *blood-brain barrier*, which is used to designate all of the interfaces between blood, brain, and CSF. The site of the barrier varies for the different plasma constituents. One is the endothelium of the choroidal and brain capillaries; another is the plasma membrane and adventitia (Rouget cells) of these vessels; a third is the pericapillary foot processes of astrocytes. Large molecules such as albumin are prevented from entry by the capillary endothelium, and this is the barrier also for such molecules as are bound to albumin, e.g., aniline dyes (trypan blue), bilirubin, and most drugs used in neurologic practice. Other smaller molecules are blocked from entering the brain by the capillary plasma membrane or astrocytes. The various substances formed in the nervous system during its metabolic activity diffuse rapidly into the CSF. Thus, the CSF has a kind of "sink action," to use Davson's term, by which the products of brain metabolism are removed into the bloodstream as CSF is absorbed.

Circulation Harvey Cushing aptly termed the CSF the "third circulation," comparable to that of the blood and lymph. From its principal site of formation in the lateral ventricles, the CSF flows downward through the third ventricle, aqueduct, fourth ventricle, and foramens of Magendie (medially) and Luschka (laterally), to the perimedullary and perispinal subarachnoid spaces, thence around the brainstem and rostrally to the basal and ambient cisterns, through the tentorial aperture, and finally to the lateral and superior surfaces of the cerebral hemispheres, where most of it is absorbed. The pressure is highest in the ventricles and diminishes successively along the subarachnoid pathways. Arterial pulsations of the choroid plexuses help drive the fluid from the ventricular system.

The spinal fluid is everywhere in contact with the extracellular fluid of the brain and spinal cord, but the extent of bulk flow through the brain parenchyma is small under normal conditions. The periventricular tissues offer resistance to the entrance of CSF, and although this so-called transmantle pressure is only slightly above zero, the open ventricular-foraminal-subarachnoid conduit directs the bulk of CSF flow in this direction. Only if this conduit is obstructed does the transmantle pressure rise, compressing the periventricular tissues and leading to ventricular enlargement and transependymal flow of CSF.

Absorption The absorption of CSF is through the arachnoid villi. These are microscopic excrescences of arachnoid membrane that penetrate the dura and protrude into the superior sagittal sinus and other venous structures. Multiple villi are aggregated in these locations to form the pacchionian granulations, or bodies, some of them large enough to indent the inner table of the calvarium. The arachnoid villi, most numerous over the sagittal margin of the cerebral hemispheres on both sides of the superior sagittal sinus, are present at the base of the brain and around the spinal cord roots and have been thought to act as functional valves that permit "bulk flow" of CSF into the vascular lumen, unidirectionally. However, electron microscopic studies have shown that the arachnoid villi have a continuous membranous covering. The latter is extremely thin, and CSF passes through the villi at a linearly increasing rate as CSF pressures rise above 68 mmH_2O. The resistance to the passage of CSF into the venous system has been termed R_0 and can be expressed in terms similar to Ohm's law ($E = IR$); the voltage (E) reflects the difference in pressure between the CSF and the venous system, which drives CSF into the veins, and the current, termed I_f, represents the flow rate of CSF, which in the steady state is equal to the rate of CSF production. R_0 is approximately 2.5 and understandably rises in circumstances that block the CSF circulation and lead to an elevation in ICP.

Tripathi and Tripathi, in serial electron micrographs, found that the mesothelial cells of the arachnoid villus continually form giant cytoplasmic vacuoles that are capable of transcellular bulk transport. Certain substances such as penicillin and organic acids and bases are also absorbed by cells of the choroid plexus; the bidirectional action of these cells resembles that of the tubule cells of the kidneys. Some substances have been shown in pathologic specimens to pass between the ependymal cells of the ventricles and to enter subependymal capillaries and venules.

Volume and Pressure In the recumbent position ICP, and consequently CSF pressure measured by lumbar puncture, is normally about 8 mmHg or 110 mmH_2O (1 mmHg equals 13.7 mmH_2O). As the head and trunk are progressively elevated, the weight of the column of CSF is added incrementally to the pressure in the lumbar subarachnoid space, but the ICP drops correspondingly, so that it is close to zero in the standing position. It must be emphasized that, under normal conditions, the cerebral venous pressure, not the resistance to the outflow of CSF, is the main determinant of CSF pressure. Normally the CSF pressure is in equilibrium with the capillary or prevenous pressure, which is influenced mainly by circulatory changes that alter arteriolar tone. Rises in arterial pressure cause little or no increase of pressure at the capillary level (because of autoregulation) and hence no increase in CSF pressure. The inhalation or retention of CO_2 raises the blood P_{CO_2} and correspondingly decreases the pH of the CSF. By a mechanism that is not fully understood, this acidification of the CSF acts as a potent cerebral vasodilator, causing an increase in cerebral blood flow and leading to intracranial hypertension. Hyperventilation, which reduces P_{CO_2}, has the opposite effect—i.e., it increases the pH and the cerebral vascular resistance and thereby decreases CSF pressure; the maneuver of lowering the arterial CO_2 content by hyperventilation is utilized in the treatment of acutely raised ICP.

In contrast to arterial blood pressure, increased venous pressure exerts an immediate effect on CSF pressure by increasing the volume of blood in the veins, venules, and dural sinuses. Compression of the jugular veins causes an immediate rise of intracranial CSF pressure, which is rapidly transmitted to the lumbar subarachnoid space unless there is a spinal subarachnoid block (Queckenstedt test). In the latter case, pressure on the abdominal wall, which compresses the lower spinal veins below the point of subarachnoid block, will increase the lumbar CSF pressure. The Valsalva maneuver—as well as coughing, sneezing, and straining—causes an increased intrathoracic pressure, which is transmitted to the jugular and then to the cerebral and spinal veins. The ICP rises in heart failure, when central and jugular venous pressures becomes elevated. Mediastinal tumors, by obstructing the superior vena cava, have the same effect. When the heart stops, the CSF pressure falls to zero.

DISTURBANCES OF CEREBROSPINAL FLUID PRESSURE, VOLUME, AND CIRCULATION

Increased Intracranial Pressure

The intact cranium and vertebral canal together with the relatively inelastic dura form a rigid container, such that an increase of any of its contents—brain, blood, or CSF—will elevate the intracranial pressure (ICP). Moreover, an increase in volume of any one of these three components must be at the expense of the other two, a relationship that is known as the Monro-Kellie doctrine and is depicted diagrammatically in Fig. 30-1. Of the three intracranial components, the brain is the least compressible. A relatively small increment in brain volume does not immediately raise the ICP, because the increased volume is accommodated for a time by displacement of CSF from the cranial cavity into the spinal canal and to a lesser extent by deformations of the brain and by limited stretching of the infoldings of the unyielding dura (falx cerebri between the hemispheres, tentorium between the hemispheres and cerebellum). Once these buffers have been exhausted, there is displacement, or "herniation of brain" from one dural compartment into another. A further increment in brain size necessarily reduces the volume of intracranial blood contained in the veins and dural sinuses. Also, there is some evidence that the CSF is formed more slowly in these circumstances of raised ICP. These accommodative volume-pressure relationships occur simultaneously and are subsumed under the term *intracranial compliance* (the change in ICP for a given change in intracranial volume). As the brain, blood, or CSF volumes continue to increase, the accommodative mechanisms fail and ICP then rises exponentially.

Besides the aforementioned brain tissue shifts, which are discussed more fully in Chap. 17, greatly raised ICP eventually causes a reduction in cerebral blood flow throughout the brain. In its most severe form, this widespread ischemia produces brain death. Lesser degrees of increased ICP and reduced blood flow can cause correspondingly less severe but still extensive cerebral infarction, of a type quite similar to what arises from reversible cardiac arrest. The numerical difference between raised ICP and mean blood pressure within the cerebral vessels, termed *cerebral perfusion pressure* (CPP), and the duration of its reduction are the main determinants of cerebral damage.

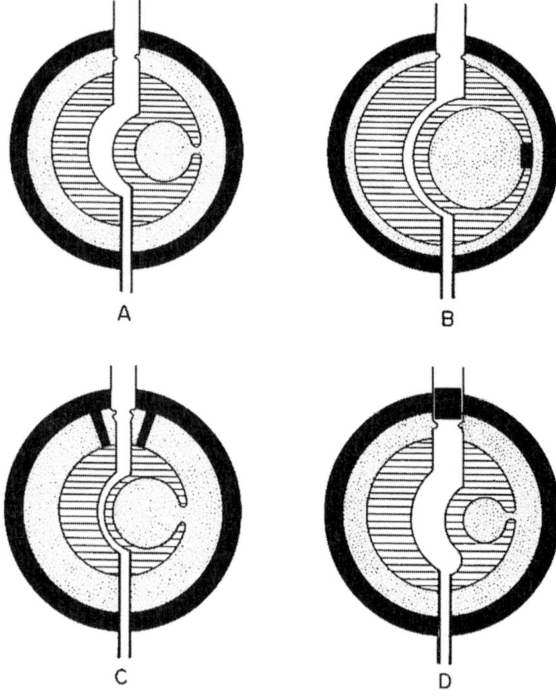

Figure 30-1

A. *Schematic representation of the three components of the intracranial contents: the incompressible brain tissue* (shaded)*; the vascular system; and the CSF* (dotted). B. *With ventricular obstruction.* C. *With obstruction at or near the points of outlet of the CSF.* D. *With obstruction of the venous outflow. (Redrawn from Foley by permission.)*

Several common mechanisms are involved at different times in the genesis of elevated ICP:

1. *A cerebral or extracerebral mass* (tumor; massive infarction with edema; contusion; parenchymal, subdural, or extradural hemorrhage; or abscess) causes increased pressure and deformation of the nearby brain. The deformation is greatest locally, being compartmentalized to a varying degree by dural partitions, as already noted.

2. *Generalized brain swelling*, as occurs in anoxic states, acute hepatic failure, hypertensive encephalopathy, and the Reye syndrome. Here the increase in pressure is widely distributed and reduces cerebral perfusion pressure, but tissue shifts are minimal.

3. An *increase in venous pressure* due to heart failure, obstruction of the superior mediastinal or jugular veins, or cerebral venous thrombosis.

4. *Obstruction to the flow and absorption of CSF*. If the obstruction is within the ventricles or in the subarachnoid space at the base of the brain, hydrocephalus results. Meningitis from one of a number of causes (infectious, carcinomatous, granulomatous, hemorrhagic) is the usual cause. If the block is at the absorptive sites adjacent to the superior sagittal sinus, the ventricles generally remain normal in size or enlarge only slightly because the pressure over the convexities approximates and balances the pressure within the lateral ventricles.

5. A *process that expands the volume of CSF* (meningitis, subarachnoid hemorrhage) or, less commonly, increases CSF production (choroid plexus tumor is a rare mechanism).

Conditions are somewhat different in infants and small children, whose cranial sutures have not closed. Here, increased ICP is manifest by enlargement of the head and by hydrocephalus. The latter must be distinguished from a constitutional macrocrania or enlarged brain and from megalencephaly (as in Krabbe disease, Alexander disease, Tay-Sachs disease, Canavan spongy degeneration of the brain), subdural hematoma or hygroma, neonatal matrix hemorrhage, and cysts or tumors.

Each of these several types of increased ICP has its special mechanism(s) and clinical and pathologic features, as elaborated below.

Elevated ICP due to Intracranial Masses and Brain Swelling

Cranial trauma, cerebral hemorrhage and infarction, tumor, hypoxic and ischemic states, encephalitis and meningitis, and acute generalized brain swelling are associated with elevated ICP. It has been demonstrated repeatedly that the high mortality and morbidity of these intracranial catastrophes is in large part related to uncontrolled rises in ICP. In a normal adult reclining with the head and trunk elevated to 45 degrees, the ICP is between 2 and 5 mmHg. Levels up to 15 mmHg are not considered hazardous; in fact adequate cerebral perfusion can be maintained even at an ICP of 40 mmHg, provided that blood pressure (BP) remains normal. A higher ICP or a lower BP may combine to cause diffuse ischemic damage, as indicated above.

The usual clinical manifestations of increased ICP in children and adults are headache, nausea and vomiting, drowsiness, ocular palsies, papilledema, visual obscurations, and eventual blindness. The practice of monitoring ICP with a pressure device has permitted approximate correlations to be made between these clinical signs and the levels of ICP. However, it should be kept in mind that the usual neurologic signs of a large intracranial mass (pupillary dilatation, abducens palsies, drowsiness, and the Cushing response) are due to displacement of brain tissue and therefore do not bear a strict relationship to ICP. As a rule, patients with normal blood pressure retain normal mental function with ICPs of 25 to 40 mmHg until there is a lateral shift and compression of diencephalic-mesencephalic structures. Stated another way, in most clinical situations, coma cannot be attributed to raised ICP alone. Only beyond the ICP range of 40 to 50 mmHg is the cerebral perfusion pressure (CPP) and cerebral blood flow diminished to a degree that causes a loss of consciousness. The latter is then solely on the basis of a reduction in cerebral perfusion. When this happens, global ischemia and brain death may follow within a short period of time. Nonetheless, high levels of ICP are often associated with a number of signs of tissue distortion, as listed above, and with stupor and coma, as discussed in Chap. 17, and in Chap. 35, in the context of head injury.

From what few correlations have been made, it appears that not until the ICP reaches 28 to 34 mmHg is there a brain shift that causes the pupil to dilate on the side of a mass lesion; exceptions occur when the mass is close to the third nerve, as with lesions of the temporal lobe, in which case pupillary dilation occurs at lower pressures. Likewise, unilateral or bilateral abducens palsies do not bear a strict relationship to the degree of elevation of ICP. This sign is more frequent when raised ICP is due to diffusely distributed brain swelling, hydrocephalus, or pseudotumor states.

Lundberg recorded intraventricular pressures over long periods of time in patients with brain tumors and found them to be subject to periodic spontaneous fluctuations. He described three types of pressure waves, which he designated as A, B, and C. Only the A waves proved to be separable from arterial and respiratory pulsations and were of clinical significance. They coincided with rhythmic rises of pressure, up to 50 mmHg, occurring every 15 to 30 min, or with similar but more protracted elevations. These large *plateau waves* in most instances coincide with an increase in intracranial blood volume, presumably because of a temporary failure of cerebrovascular autoregulation. Rosner and Becker have observed that a plateau wave may sometimes be preceded by mild systemic hypotension. In their view, this leads to cerebral vasodilation as an attempt to maintain normal blood flow; however, the recovery of cerebrovascular tone is delayed after the blood pressure returns to normal; this allows intracranial blood volume to accumulate in the dilated vascular bed, thus raising ICP. In support of this idea is the observation that a brief elevation of blood pressure may paradoxically restore the normal cerebrovascular tone and lead to an abrupt cessation of the plateau waves.

Monitoring of Raised ICP

Considerable evidence has accumulated that the outcome in patients with intracranial mass lesions is favorably influenced by keeping the intracranial pressure below approximately 20 mmHg. Unfortunately, the direct measurement of ICP and aggressive measures to counteract high pressures have not yielded uniformly beneficial results, and—after two decades of popularity—the routine use of ICP monitoring remains controversial. The problem may be partly a matter of the timing of monitoring and the proper selection of patients for aggressive treatment of raised ICP. Only if the ICP measurements are to be used as a guide to medical therapy and the timing of surgical decompression is the insertion of a monitor justified. Therefore the approach of the neurosurgeon involved in the case has a bearing on the decision to undertake monitoring. Also figuring in the decision to institute monitoring are the prospects of ameliorating the underlying lesion, the patient's age, and the associated medical disease(s). Our practice has been to measure ICP with an indwelling fiberoptic monitor or intraventricular drain in younger patients in whom a traumatic or other intracranial mass has caused a shift of intracranial structures. The monitor is generally placed on the same side as the mass. Based on our experience, we have found monitoring not to be particularly helpful in cases of massive cerebral hemorrhage.

The emergency management of raised ICP is considered in detail in Chaps. 34 and 35, in relation to stroke and cerebral trauma. A comprehensive discussion can also be found in the monograph on intensive care (Ropper) listed in the references.

Obstructive (Tension) Hydrocephalus

Essentially, this is a condition in which there is an obstruction to the flow of CSF at some point in its ventricular pathway or aqueduct, at the medullary foramens of exit (Luschka and Magendie) or in the basal subarachnoid space. Because of the obstruction, CSF accumulates within the ventricles under increasing pressure, enlarging the ventricles and expanding the hemispheres. As stated above, in the infant or young child, the head increases in size because of separation of the sutures of the cranial bones; this is called *manifest* or *overt hydrocephalus*.

Unfortunately, the term *hydrocephalus* (literally, "water brain") is frequently but incorrectly applied to passive enlargement of the ventricles consequent to cerebral atrophy, i.e., *hydrocephalus ex vacuo*, and to ventricular enlargement due to failure of development of the brain, a state known as *colpencephaly*. Reference to these conditions as hydrocephalic is so common that it is unlikely to change; hence the authors believe it preferable to use the term *tension hydrocephalus* for the obstructive types in which the CSF is or has been under increased pressure.

In 1914, Dandy and Blackfan introduced the also somewhat inaccurate terms *communicating* and *noncommunicating (obstructive) hydrocephalus*. The concept of a communicating hydrocephalus was based on the observations that dye injected into a lateral ventricle would diffuse readily into the lumbar subarachnoid space and that air injected into the lumbar subarachnoid space would pass into the ventricular system; in other words, the ventricles are in communication with the spinal subarachnoid space. If the lumbar spinal fluid remained colorless after the injection of dye, the hydrocephalus was assumed to be obstructive or non-communicating. The distinction between these two types is not fundamental. All forms of tension hydrocephalus are obstructive, and the obstruction is never complete. Acute and complete aqueductal occlusion is incompatible with survival for more than a few days. The authors suggest that a more appropriate terminology is one in which a prefix indicates the site of the presumed obstruction, e.g., *meningeal-obstructive, aqueductal-obstructive*, or *third ventricular-obstructive tension hydrocephalus*.

Pathogenesis of Obstructive Hydrocephalus

There are several sites of predilection of obstruction to the flow of CSF. One foramen of Monro may be blocked by a tumor or by the horizontal shift that results from a large unilateral hemispheral mass, resulting in expansion of one lateral ventricle or a portion of one. Large tumors of the third ventricle (e.g., colloid cyst) may block both foramina of Monro, leading to dilation of both lateral ventricles. The aqueduct of Sylvius, normally narrow to begin with, may be occluded by a number of developmental or acquired lesions with periaqueductal gliosis (genetically determined atresia or forking, ependymitis, hemorrhage, tumor), and lead to dilation of the third and both lateral ventricles. If the obstruction is in the fourth ventricle, the dilation includes the aqueduct. Other sites of obstruction of the CSF pathways are at the foramina of Luschka and Magendie (e.g., congenital failure of opening of the foramina—Dandy-Walker syndrome) or, as most commonly occurs, in the subarachnoid space around the brainstem due to postinflammatory or posthemorrhagic fibrosing meningitis. The latter forms of obstruction result in enlargement of the entire ventricular system, including the fourth ventricle. An old but still useful adage, attributed to Ayer, is that the ventricle closest to the obstruction enlarges the most; for example, occlusion of the basal CSF pathways causes a disproportionate enlargement of the fourth ventricle, and a mass that obstructs the fourth ventricle leads to a greater dilatation of the third than of the lateral ventricles.

A matter of considerable practical as well as theoretical interest is whether a meningeal obstruction over the cerebral hemispheres, at the site of the arachnoidal villi, or a blockage of the dural sinuses into which the CSF is absorbed can result in tension hydrocephalus. Russell, in her extensive neuropathologic material and her review of the world's literature, could not find a well-documented example of either of these suggested etiologies, and the authors' experience has been similar. Moreover, experiments in animals in which all draining veins had been occluded resulted in a tension hydrocephalus with enlarging lateral ventricles in only a few cases. Yet Gilles and Davidson have stated that tension hydrocephalus in children may be due to a congenital absence or deficient number of arachnoidal villi, and Rosman and Shands have reported an instance that they attributed to increased intracranial venous pressure. Our hesitation in accepting such examples stems from the difficulty that the pathologist has in judging the patency of the basilar subarachnoid space. The latter is much more reliably visualized by radiologic than by neuropathologic means. Theoretically, as alluded to earlier, if the obstruction is high, near (or in) the superior sagittal sinus, the CSF should accumulate under pressure outside as well as inside the brain, and the ventricles should not enlarge at all or only slightly and only after a prolonged period; this has been our experience.

The rarely encountered radiologic picture of enlarged subarachnoid spaces over and between the cerebral hemispheres coupled with modest enlargement of the lateral ventricles has been referred to as an *external hydrocephalus*. Although such a condition does exist, many of the cases so designated have proved to be examples of sporadic or familial subdural hygromas or meningeal cysts.

Processes such as subarachnoid hemorrhage and cerebral hemorrhage that ruptures into the ventricles and rapidly expand the volume of CSF produce the most dramatic form of *acute hydrocephalus*; the obstruction of the CSF pathways may lie within the ventricular system or at the basal meninges. The corresponding clinical syndrome is described below.

An increase in the rate of formation or decrease in the rate of absorption would be expected to cause an accumulation of CSF and increased ICP. The only known cause of overproduction of CSF is a papilloma of the choroid plexus, but even in this circumstance there is usually an associated ventricular obstruction, either of the third or fourth ventricle or of one lateral ventricle. Characteristically, in these cases, there is both a generalized dilatation of the ventricular system and basal cisterns (possibly due to increased CSF volume) and an asymmetrical enlargement of the lateral ventricles due to obstruction of one foramen of Monro.

Clinical Picture of Chronic Hydrocephalus This varies with the age of the patient and acuteness of onset. Four main clinical syndromes are recognized—one that occurs very early in life and causes enlargement of the head (*overt tension hydrocephalus*) and another in which the hydrocephalus becomes symptomatic after the cranial sutures have fused and the head remains normal in size (*occult* hydrocephalus). A special a form of the latter is arrested or compensated hydrocephalus of late adult life (*normal-pressure hydrocephalus*). Yet another syndrome is that of acute hydrocephalus; this form of hydrocephalus is accorded a separate section, below.

Overt Congenital or Infantile Hydrocephalus The cranial bones fuse by the end of the second year; for the head to enlarge, the tension hydrocephalus must develop before this time, sometimes in utero but usually in the first few months of life. Even up to 5 years of age (and very rarely beyond this time), a marked increase of ICP, particularly if it evolves rapidly, may separate the newly formed sutures (diastasis). Tension hydrocephalus, even of mild degree, also molds the shape of the skull in early life, and in radiographs the inner table is unevenly thinned, an appearance referred to as "beaten silver" or as convolutional or digital markings. The frontal regions are unusually prominent (bossed) and the skull tends to be brachicephalic except in the Dandy-Walker syndrome, where, because of bossing of the occiput from enlargement of the posterior fossa, the head is dolichocephalic. With marked enlargement of the skull, the face looks relatively small and pinched and the skin over the cranial bones is tight and thin, revealing prominent distended veins.

The usual causes of this disorder are (1) matrix hemorrhages in premature infants, (2) fetal and neonatal infections, (3) type II Chiari malformation, (4) aqueductal atresia and stenosis, and (5) the Dandy-Walker syndrome.

In this type of hydrocephalus, the head usually enlarges rapidly and soon surpasses the 97th percentile. The anterior and posterior fontanels are tense even when the patient is in the upright position. The infant is fretful, feeds poorly, and may vomit frequently. With continued enlargement of the brain, torpor sets in and the infant appears languid, uninterested in his surroundings, and unable to sustain activity. Later it is noticed that the upper eyelids are retracted and the eyes tend to turn down; there is paralysis of upward gaze, and the sclerae above the irises are visible. This is the so-called setting-sun sign and has been incorrectly attributed to downward pressure of the frontal lobes on the roofs of the orbits. The fact that it disappears on shunting the lateral and third ventricles indicates that it is due to hydrocephalic pressure on the mesencephalic tegmentum. Gradually the infant adopts a posture of flexed arms and flexed or extended legs. Signs of corticospinal tract affection are usually elicitable. Movements are feeble and sometimes the arms are tremulous. There is no papilledema, but later the optic discs become pale and vision is reduced. If the hydrocephalus becomes arrested, the infant or child is retarded but often surprisingly verbal. The head may be so large that the child cannot hold it up and must remain in bed. If the head is only moderately enlarged, the child may be able to sit but not stand or stand but not walk. If ambulatory, the child is clumsy. Acute exacerbations of hydrocephalus or an intercurrent febrile illness may cause vomiting, stupor, or coma.

The special features of congenital hydrocephalus that are associated with the Chiari malformation, aqueductal atresia and stenosis, and the Dandy-Walker syndrome are discussed in Chap. 38.

Occult Tension Hydrocephalus Here the hydrocephalus becomes evident only after the cranial sutures have closed (Fig. 30-2). The causes of obstruction to the flow of CSF are diverse and some are clearly congenital, but symptoms may be delayed as late as adolescence or early adult life, and most commonly even later in life. In some instances the condition gives rise to a *normal-pressure hydrocephalus*, as discussed further on. The clinical features of occult hydrocephalus and the course of the illness are quite variable. Some instances of arrested hydrocephalus are truly occult in that the disease is unrecognized during life or is discovered only by chance imaging of the brain, or on postmortem examination. In other cases, the symptoms are intermittent and relatively mild; in still others, they are slowly or rapidly progressive, in the latter instance giving the clinical impression of an acute disease.

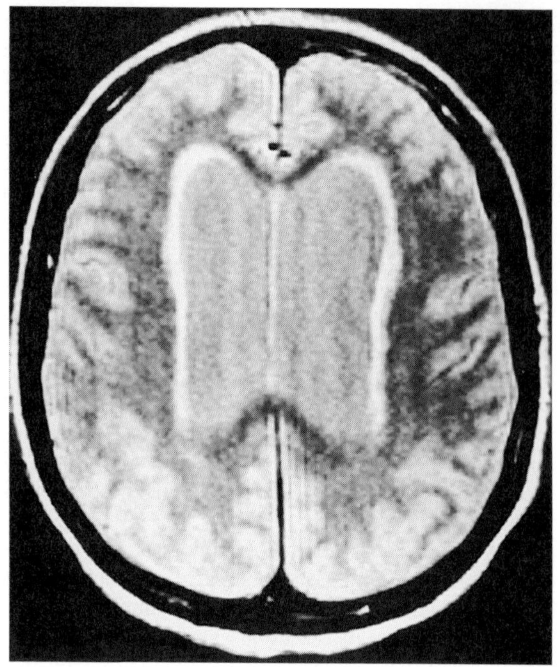

Figure 30-2

MRI of adult tension hydrocephalus from a congenital stenosis of the cerebral aqueduct. There is transependymal movement of water that appears as a T2 signal rimming the lateral ventricles. The third ventricle, but not the fourth, was enlarged.

The patient may complain of bifrontal or bioccipital headaches may be complaints but often these are not present. Other symptoms and signs are predominantly those of a frontal lobe disorder of mentation or of gait. Slowness of mental response, inattentiveness, distractibility, perseveration, and inability to plan activity or to sustain any type of complex cognitive function are characteristic. The immediate responses to verbal and other stimuli are normal, though memory may be slightly impaired. Conspicuous by their absence are apraxia, agnosia, or aphasia. Gait deteriorates early in the course of hydrocephalus, and such deterioration may be present for years before other symptoms become manifest. At first the gait is only slightly uncertain, with reduced speed; later there is a shortening of step and a mild clumsiness that sometimes looks suspiciously parkinsonian or, if more incoordinate, like cerebellar ataxia (see further on, in the description of normal-pressure hydrocephalus in adults). We have seen a few cases in adults in which the gait disturbance appeared abruptly and gave the impression of a cerebellar stroke. Yet rigidity, tremor, or ataxia of leg movements are absent. Falls are frequent, particularly backward falls. Later still, the patient cannot walk without assistance. There is continuous activity in antigravity muscles, and eventually help is needed even in standing. A suck reflex and grasp reflexes of the hands and feet are variably present; plantar reflexes are sometimes extensor. Last, there may be sphincteric incontinence, often without the patient's awareness.

Occult hydrocephalus due to tumor growth is discussed in Chap. 31.

Acute Hydrocephalus Surprisingly little has been written about this syndrome, despite its frequency in clinical practice. It is seen most often following subarachnoid hemorrhage from a ruptured aneurysm, less often with bleeding from an arteriovenous malformation, or from deep hemispheral hemorrhage that dissects into the ventricles; it may also occur as the result of obstruction of the CSF pathways in the fourth ventricle by a tumor or cerebellar-brainstem hemorrhage or within the basal cisterns by neoplastic infiltration of the meninges, although this last process tends to evolve more subacutely. The patient complains of a severe headache and often of visual obscuration, may vomit, and then becomes drowsy or stuporous over a period of minutes or hours. Bilateral Babinski signs are the rule, and in the advanced stages, which are associated with coma, there is increased tone in the lower limbs and extensor posturing. Early in the process, the pupils are normal in size and the eyes may rove horizontally; as the ventricles continue to enlarge, the pupils become miotic, the eyes cease roving and assume an orthotopic position, or there may be bilateral abducens palsies and limitation of upward gaze. The speed with which hydrocephalus develops determines whether there is accompanying papilledema. If left untreated, the pupils eventually dilate symmetrically, the eyes no longer respond to oculocephalic maneuvers, and the limbs become flaccid. Rarely, there occurs an unanticipated cardiac arrest, even at an early stage of evolution of the hydrocephalus; this complication is seen particularly in children and may be presaged by brain compression at the level of the perimesencephalic cisterns, detectable by imaging studies.

Treatment is by drainage of CSF, usually effected by a ventricular catheter or, if there is undoubted communication between all the CSF compartments, by lumbar puncture. The latter may pose some risk if spinal fluid is withdrawn rapidly, by creating a pressure gradient between the cerebral and spinal regions.

Neuropathologic Effects of Tension Hydrocephalus Ventricular expansion tends to be maximal in the frontal horns, explaining the hydrocephalic impairment of frontal lobe functions and of basal ganglionic-frontal motor activity. The central white matter yields to pressure, while the cortical gray matter, thalami, basal ganglia, and brainstem structures remain relatively unaffected. There is an increase in the content of interstitial fluid in the tissue adjacent to the lateral ventricles, readily detected by MRI (Fig. 30-2). Myelinated fibers and axons are injured, but not to the extent that one might expect from the degree of compression; minor degrees of astrocytic gliosis and loss of oligodendrocytes in the affected tissue are present to a decreasing extent away from the ventricles and represent a hydrocephalic atrophy of the brain. The ventricles are characteristically denuded of ependyma and the choroid plexuses are flattened and fibrotic. The lumens of cerebral capillaries in biopsy preparations are said to be narrowed—a finding that is difficult to evaluate.

Normal-Pressure Hydrocephalus

In nonprogressive meningeal and ependymal diseases, hydrocephalus may develop and reach a stable stage. It is said to "compensate," in the sense that formation of CSF equilibrates with absorption. The formation of CSF diminishes slightly, perhaps because of compression of the choroid plexuses; absorption increases in proportion to CSF pressure, but beginning at a higher threshold. Once equilibrium is attained, the ICP gradually falls, though it still maintains a slightly higher gradient from ventricle to basal cistern to cerebral subarachnoid space. A stage is reached where the *CSF pressure reaches a high normal level of 150 to 180 mm*H_2O while the patient still manifests the cerebral effects of the hydrocephalic state. The name given to this condition by Hakim and Adams was *normal-pressure hydrocephalus* (NPH).

A *triad of clinical findings* is characteristic of NPH—a slowly progressive gait disorder, impairment of mental function, and sphincteric incontinence. Grasp reflexes in the feet and falling attacks may also occur.

Headaches are no longer a complaint and may never have been present, and there is no papilledema.

The *gait disturbance* is of several different types, some of them difficult to classify. Most often it takes the form of unsteadiness and impairment of balance, with the greatest difficulty being encountered on stairs and curbs (Fisher). Weakness and tiredness of the legs are also frequent complaints, although examination discloses no paresis or ataxia. The gait in NPH may convey an impression of Parkinson disease, with short steps and stooped, forward-leaning posture, but there is no rigidity, slowness of alternating movement, or tremor. Other patients present with unexplained falls, often backward, but on casual inspection the gait may betray no abnormality at all. When the condition remains untreated, the steps become shorter, with frequent shuffling and falls; eventually standing and sitting and even turning over in bed become impossible. Fisher refers to this advanced state as "hydrocephalic astasia-abasia." (See also page 128.)

The *mental symptoms*, when they occur, are difficult to distinguish from those of early Alzheimer disease. *Urinary symptoms* appear relatively late in the illness. Initially, they consist of urgency and frequency. Later, the urgency is associated with incontinence, and ultimately there is "frontal lobe incontinence," in which the patient is indifferent to his lapses of continence.

This syndrome of NPH may follow subarachnoid hemorrhage from ruptured aneurysm or head trauma, a resolved acute meningitis or a chronic meningitis (tubercular, syphilitic, or other), Paget disease of the base of the skull, mucopolysaccharidosis of the meninges, and achondroplasia. However, in most of our cases, the cause cannot be established; presumably it is due to an asymptomatic fibrosing meningitis.

Verification of the diagnosis of NPH and the selection of patients for ventriculoatrial or ventriculoperitoneal shunt has presented difficulties. A lumbar puncture should be performed for diagnostic purposes. As alluded to, the large ventricles, even at a normal pressure, continue to exert a force against the tracts in the cerebral white matter. In most cases of NPH, the CSF pressure is above 155 mmH_2O, but the disorder occurs infrequently with lower pressures, in rare instances as low as 130 mmH_2O or even less.The CT scan, as shown in Fig. 30-3 (enlarged ventricles without convolutional atrophy), radionuclide cisternography (reflux into ventricles and delayed pericerebral diffusion), and the clinical

Figure 30-3

CT scan of a patient with normal-pressure hydrocephalus. There is enlargement of all the ventricles, particularly of the frontal horns of the lateral ventricles (left), *which is disproportionate to the cortical atrophy* (right).

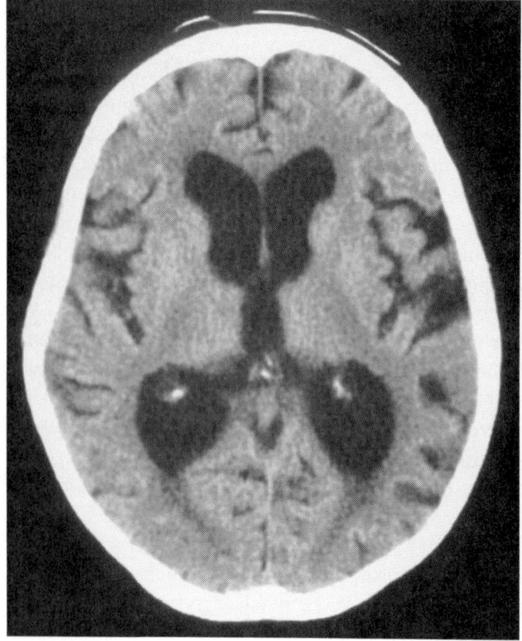

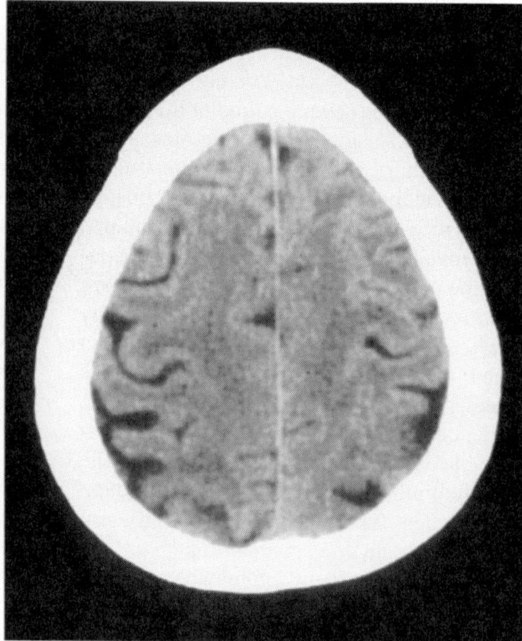

response to the removal of CSF have been the most helpful ancillary examinations (see below), but the findings are not always clear-cut. The span of the frontal horns of the lateral ventricles by CT scanning has also been used as a rough guide to the likelihood of success from ventricular shunting (see below), but an absolute dimension that reliably indicates the presence of NPH has not been determined. More relevant is a disproportionate enlargement of the ventricular system in comparison to the degree of cortical atrophy judged by the CT and MRI appearance. Various formulas designed to assess this ratio have been unwieldy, but some rough guidelines relating the ventricular span to the outcome of treatment are given below. MRI may show some degree of transependymal egress of water surrounding the ventricles, but this is not always the case, and this sign is sometimes difficult to differentiate from the periventricular white matter change that is ubiquitous in the elderly. Monitoring of CSF pressure over a prolonged period may show intermittent rises of pressure, possibly corresponding to the A waves of Lundberg, but this is not practical in most cases. According to Katzman and Hussey, the infusion of normal saline into the lumbar subarachnoid space at a rate of 0.76 mL/min for 30 to 60 min provokes a rise in pressure (300 to 600 mmH_2O) that is not observed in normal individuals. Theoretically, this test should quantitate the adequacy of CSF absorption, but it has yielded unpredictable results.

Drainage of large amounts of CSF (20 to 30 mL or more) by lumbar puncture often results in clinical improvement in stance and gait for a few days, although this change may not be evident for hours or more after the spinal tap. Objective improvement in gait after spinal drainage is one practical way to select patients for shunt operations when the clinical picture is not entirely clear but the test is by no means infallible. It is worthwhile to quantify the speed and facility of gait two or three times before the lumbar puncture and to perform this testing at periodic intervals for several days after the procedure in order to be certain that improvement is genuine.

As a group, patients who have a sustained response to drainage of CSF by shunting, as described below, have had the first two elements of the clinical triad (only half of our successfully treated patients were incontinent), and their lateral ventricular span at the level of the anterior horns was in excess of 50 mm (a true dimension calculated from CT scans), equivalent to approximately 18 mm on the usual CT film, but with relatively little cerebral atrophy.

Treatment of Hydrocephalus in Adults The development of ventricular shunt tubing with one-way valves opened the way to successful treatment of hydrocephalus. The valve can be set at a desired opening pressure, allowing the CSF to escape directly into the bloodstream (ventriculoatrial shunt) or peritoneal cavity (ventriculoperitoneal shunt) whenever the pressure level is exceeded. Gratifying success can be obtained, often a complete or nearly complete restoration of mental function and gait, by the placement of such shunts.

Regarding NPH, the most consistent improvement has been attained in that minority of patients in whom a cause could be established (subarachnoid hemorrhage, chronic meningitis, or tumor of the third ventricle). As already noted, other predictors of success are considerable enlargement of the ventricles in comparison to the degree of cortical atrophy, CSF pressures above 155 mmH_2O, and improvement after spinal puncture, but none of these is entirely dependable. Deviations from the characteristic syndrome—such as the occurrence of dementia without gait disorder or the presence of apraxias, aphasias, and other focal cerebral signs—should lead one to a diagnosis other than NPH. Fisher, on analyzing successfully shunted cases, noted that almost without exception gait disturbance was an early and prominent symptom. Uncertainties of diagnosis increase with advancing age owing to the frequent association of senile dementia and vascular lesions. However, age alone does not exclude the existence of NPH as a cause of gait disorder, and long duration of symptoms does not preclude a salutary outcome from shunting (Fisher). In patients who are averse to the shunting procedure or who have medical conditions that make the surgery inadvisable, it is sometimes possible to produce a reasonable improvement in gait for several months or more by repeating the spinal puncture and drainage of large amounts of fluid every few weeks or months.

The potential failures of shunting must be anticipated in patients who do not conform to the typical syndrome, or whose disease has advanced to the stage of long-standing incontinence or dementia. In some instances, a lack of improvement is explained by inadequate decompression, and this situation justifies a revision of the shunt with a valve that drains at lower pressures. Overdrainage, in contrast, causes headaches that may be chronic or orthostatic and may be associated with small subdural collections of fluid. These fluid collections, or hygromas consisting of CSF and proteinacious fluid derived from blood products, are generally innocuous and do not require drainage unless they enlarge or cause focal neurologic symptoms or, rarely, seizures.

Although shunting is relatively simple as a surgical procedure, it is associated with potential complications, the main ones being a postoperative subdural hygroma or hematoma (if the ventricular pressure is reduced too rapidly, the bridging dural veins may stretch and rupture); infection of the valve and catheter, sometimes with septicemia; occlusion of the tip of the catheter in the ventricle; and, particularly in infants and children, the "slit ventricle syndrome" (see below). Orthostatic headaches can be overcome by raising the opening pressure of the shunt valve and, if the headaches persist, by utilizing an externally programmable valve. Misplacement of the catheter may rarely transect tracts in the deep hemispheral white matter and cause serious neurologic deficits. It is our impression that this occurs more often when the catheter is inserted from the back rather than through the frontal or parietal regions. The incidence of complications may be reduced by placing the catheter in the anterior horn of the right ventricle, where there is no choroid plexus, and by using the latest types of valves, some of which permit extracranial control of valve pressure. Meticulous aseptic technique and the preoperative and postoperative administration of antibiotics have apparently reduced the incidence of shunt infections.

Once the CSF is shunted, the ventricles diminish in size within 3 or 4 days even when the hydrocephalus has been present for a year or more. This indicates that the so-called hydrocephalic compression of the cerebrum is largely reversible. Indeed, in Black's series, the ventricles failed to return to normal in only 1 of his 11 shunted patients, and in that patient there was no clinical improvement. Clinical improvement occurs within a few weeks, the gait disturbance being slower to reverse than the mental disorder. Symptoms of cerebral atrophy due to Alzheimer disease and related conditions are not altered by ventriculoatrial shunting. Of course, if the hydrocephalus is caused by an operable tumor, surgical removal of the obstructing mass is the procedure of choice and only if this is not possible is a shunt placed.

Treatment of Infantile and Childhood Hydrocephalus Here one encounters more difficulties than in the treatment of the adult disorder. The ventricular catheter may wander or become obstructed and require revision. Peritoneal pseudocysts may form (most shunts in children are ventriculoperitoneal). Another unexpected complication of shunting has been coaptation of the ventricles, the so-called slit ventricle syndrome. This occurs more frequently in young children, though we have observed it in adults. These patients may develop a low-pressure syndrome with severe generalized headaches, often with nausea and vomiting, whenever they sit up or stand. Some children become ataxic, irritable, or obtunded or may vomit repeatedly. The CSF pressure in such patients is extremely low and the volume of CSF much reduced. In babies, the cranium may fail to grow even though the brain is of normal size. In most shunted patients, the ICP in the upright position is diminished to -30 mmH_2O, but in patients with the low-pressure shunt syndrome it may reach -100 to -150 mmH_2O. To correct the condition, one would imagine that replacing the shunt valve with another that opens under a higher pressure would suffice. Indeed, this may be successful. But once the condition is established, the most effective measure has been the placement of an antisiphon device, which prevents valve flow when the patient stands. (See further on for a discussion of intracranial hypotension in adults.)

Whether to shunt all hydrocephalic infants soon after birth is a controversial issue. In several large series of cases that have been treated in this way, the number surviving with normal mental function has been small (see review of Leech and Brumback). The series of Dennis and associates is representative. They examined 78 shunted hydrocephalic children and found that 56 (72 percent) had full-scale IQs between 70 and 100; in 22 patients, the IQ was between 100 and 115; in 3 patients, it was below 70, and in 3 others, it was above 115. Mental functions improved unevenly and performance scores lagged behind verbal ones at all levels. The use of the carbonic anhydrase inhibitor acetazolamide or other diuretics to inhibit CSF formation has not been successful in the hands of our colleagues, but several authors believe that by giving 250 to 500 mg of acetazolamide orally daily, shunting can be avoided in both normal-pressure and infantile hydrocephalus (Aimard et al; Shinnar et al).

Increased Intracranial Pressure due to Venous Obstruction

Occlusion of the major dural venous sinuses (superior longitudinal and lateral) results in increased ICP. This is not surprising in view of the direct effect of venous obstruction on CSF pressure. One form of such intracranial hypertension, due to lateral sinus thrombosis, was referred to by Symonds as "otitic hydrocephalus"—a name that he later conceded was inappropriate insofar as the ventricles are not enlarged in this clinical circumstance. As indicated earlier, venous congestion that complicates heart failure and superior mediastinal obstruction also raises the CSF pressure, again without enlargement of the ventricles. This may happen as well with large, high-flow arteriovenous malformations of the brain. The effects of cerebral venous occlusion are considered further in the discussion of pseudotumor cerebri (below) and in Chap. 34, on cerebrovascular disease (page 910).

Pseudotumor Cerebri

The term *pseudotumor cerebri* was coined by Nonne in 1914 and has remained a useful means of designating a common and highly characteristic syndrome of headache, papilledema (unilateral or bilateral), minimal or absent focal neurologic signs, and normal CSF composition, all occurring in the absence of enlarged ventricles or an intracranial mass on CT scanning or MRI. Being a syndrome and not a disease, pseudotumor cerebri has a number of causes or pathogenetic associations (Table 30-1). Actually, the most common form of the syndrome has no firmly established cause—i.e., it is idiopathic and is now generally referred to as *benign* or *idiopathic intracranial hypertension.*

Idiopathic Intracranial Hypertension This syndrome was first described in 1897 by Quincke, who called it "serous meningitis." It is particularly frequent in overweight adolescent girls and young women, attaining an incidence of 19 to 21 per 100,000 in this group, as compared with 1 to 2 per 100,000 in the general population (Radhakrishnan et al). Increased ICP develops over a period of weeks or months. Headache, described as dull or a feeling of pressure, is the cardinal symptom; it can be mainly occipital, generalized, or somewhat asymmetrical. Other less frequent complaints are blurred vision, a vague dizziness, minimal horizontal diplopia, transient visual obscurations that often coincide with the peak intensity of the headache, or a trifling numbness of the face on one side. Rarely, the presenting feature may be a nasal CSF leak, as pointed out by Clarke and colleagues. Self-audible bruits have been reported by many of our patients; this has been attributed to turbulence created by differences in pressure between the cranial and jugular veins. The patient is then discovered to have flagrant papilledema (Figs. 13-8 and 13-9), immediately raising the specter of a brain tumor (rarely, papilledema is only minimally developed or absent). The risk of visual loss and the severity of headache in many instances make the formerly used term of benign intracranial hypertension less acceptable.

The CSF pressure is elevated, usually in the range of 250 to 450 mmH_2O, but it is still not clear whether the brain itself is swollen or, as is more likely, the increased pressure is entirely due to a change in the pressure within the CSF and venous compartments. When the CSF pressure is monitored for many hours, it can be seen to fluctuate. There are irregularly occurring plateau waves of increased pressure lasting 20 to 30 min and then falling abruptly nearly to normal, as though an increased volume of CSF had been vented (Johnston and Paterson) or cerebrovascular tone was unstable.

Table 30-1
Causes and pathogenetic associations of pseudotumor cerebri

I. Idiopathic ("benign") intracranial hypertension
II. Cerebral venous hypertension (diagnosis by imaging of cerebral vasculature)
   A. Occlusion of superior sagittal or lateral venous sinus:
      1. Hypercoagulable states (cancer, birth control pills, dehydration, antiphospolipid antibody, etc.)
      2. Traumatic
      3. Postsurgical
      4. Infectious (mainly of transverse venous sinus due to mastoiditis)
   B. Increased blood volume due to high flow arteriovenous malformation and other vascular anomalies
III. Meningeal diseases (diagnosis by examination of CSF)
   A. Carcinomatous and lymphomatous meningitis
   B. Chronic infectious and granulomatous meningitis (fungal, tuberculous, spirochetal, sarcoidosis, etc.)
IV. Gliomatosis cerebri
V. Toxic
   A. Hypervitaminosis A (especially isotretinoin, used for the treatment of acne)
   B. Lead
   C. Tetracycline
   D. As an infrequent idiosyncratic effect of various drugs (amiodarone, quinolone antibiotics, estrogen, phenothiazines, etc.)
VI. Metabolic disturbances
   A. Administration or withdrawal of corticosteroids
   B. Hyper- and hypoadrenalism
   C. Myxedema
   D. Hypoparathyroidism
VII. Associated with greatly elevated protein concentration in the CSF
   A. Guillain-Barré syndrome
   B. Spinal oligodendroglioma
   C. Systemic lupus erythematosus

Aside from papilledema, there is remarkably little to be found on neurologic examination—perhaps a unilateral or bilateral abducens palsy, fine nystagmus on far lateral gaze, or a minor sensory change. Visual field testing usually shows slight peripheral constriction with enlargement of the blind spots. As vision diminshes, more severe constriction of the fields, with greater nasal or inferior nasal loss, is found. Exceptionally, particularly in children, an otherwise typical Bell's palsy may be associated (Chutorian et al). Mentation and alertness are preserved, and the patient seems surprisingly well. Examinations by CT and MRI have shown the ventricles to be normal in size or small. The sella may be enlarged and filled with CSF ("empty sella," page 716). There is no MRI evidence of change in the water density of the brain and the ventricles are of normal size or small.

As remarked above, most of the patients are young women, often with menstrual irregularities, but the condition may also occur in children or adolescents, in whom there is no clear sex predominance, and in men (Digre and Corbett). We have had experience with several familial instances—e.g., affecting mother and daughter. Practically all of the women with this disease are obese and so are the men, but to a lesser degree (Durcan et al). In obese women without the pseudotumor syndrome, CSF pressure usually does not differ from that of normal persons (Corbett and Mehta). All forms of endocrine and menstrual abnormalities (particularly amenorrhea) and use of oral contraceptives have been postulated as causative factors, but none has been substantiated.

The mechanism of increased CSF pressure in this disorder remains elusive. Using the method of constant infusion manometrics, Mann and coworkers studied a group of patients with pseudotumor and demonstrated an increased resistance to CSF outflow, due presumably to an impaired absorptive function of the arachnoid villi. They showed also that CSF production was reduced in these patients. But except for the few cases that were found to have dural venous obstruction, the cause of impeded absorption remained obscure. Karahalios et al found the cerebral venous pressure to be consistently elevated in pseudotumor cerebri; half of their patients had dural venous outflow obstruction demonstrated by venography (this has not been our experience). These authors proposed that venous hypertension increases the resistance to CSF absorption and is the universal mechanism underlying pseudotumor. However, it is not clear whether the rise in venous pressure is the passive result of increased ICP and whether the venous pressure is high enough to explain the pseudotumor state. Other authors have attributed intracranial hypertension to raised intra-abdominal and cardiac filling pressures, the result of obesity (Sugerman et al). A related finding in some cases, pointed out to us by Fishman, is one of partial obstruction of the lateral sinuses by enlarged pacchionian granulations (seen during the venous phase of conventional angiography). It is unclear if this is a secondary cause of venous obstruction that additionally raises ICP, but it certainly causes diagnostic confusion when the physician views the radiologic studies. Others, on inconclusive evidence, have attributed benign intracranial hypertension to an increase in brain volume secondary to an excess of extracellular fluid or blood volume within the cranium (Sahs and Joynt, Raichle et al). An interesting finding has been an elevated level of vasopressin in the CSF but not in the blood (Seckl and Lightman). In the goat, this peptide causes a rise in ICP and a reduction in CSF absorption. This raises the possibility that pseudotumor is due to an aberration of the transit of water in the cerebrum. Finally, Jacobson and colleagues have made the provocative observation that serum vitamin A levels (in the form of retinol) are 50 percent higher than expected, on average, in patients with pseudotumor, a difference that is not explained by obesity. Because the levels they found were considerably lower than in cases of hypervitaminosis A with pseudotumor, the meaning of these findings is uncertain.

Differential Diagnosis of Pseudotumor Cerebri
The main consideration in cases of generalized elevation of ICP and papilledema in the absence of an intracerebral mass is to distinguish idiopathic pseudotumor cerebri from the following conditions: covert occlusion of the dural venous sinuses, gliomatosis cerebri, occult arteriovenous malformation, and carcinomatous, infectious, or granulomatous meningitis (Table 30-1). Although occlusion of the dural venous sinuses and their large draining veins is sometimes equated with pseudotumor, these are not, strictly speaking, idiopathic instances. When papilledema occurs in the context of a persistent headache that has had an abrupt onset, particularly if the pain is centered near the vertex or medial parietal areas, or if there are seizures, venous occlusion is likely. Venous sinus thrombosis can be detected in most instances by careful attention to the appearance of the superior sagittal and lateral sinuses on the T1-weighted MRI or on the contrast-enhanced CT scans, as discussed in Chap. 34 (page 910).

A large cerebral arteriovenous malformation (AVM), by causing an increase both of venous pressure and cerebral blood volume, can also give rise to a pseudotumor syndrome. In a few of our cases, the changes in the physiology of the cerebral circulation were made evident by the appearance of early venous flow on the angiogram or by thrombosis of the superior sagittal sinus.

Several diseases associated with raised CSF protein concentration have given rise to a pseudotumor syndrome, the commonest being the Guillain-Barré syndrome, systemic lupus, and spinal tumors, particularly oligodendroglioma (Table 30-1). Elevated spinal fluid pressure has been attributed to a blockage of CSF absorption by the proteinaceous fluid, but this mechanism has never been validated and fails to explain those few instances in which the Guillain-Barré and pseudotumor syndromes have been associated with a near normal protein content of the CSF. This explanation is even less appealing if one recalls that the protein concentration of the fluid within the cerebral spaces is considerably lower than in the spinal sac. Also, as Ropper and Marmarou have pointed out, neither the resistance to CSF absorption nor the colloid osmotic effect attributable to an increased protein content in the spinal fluid is adequate to explain the pressure elevation. The mechanism of this type of pseudotumor syndrome is presently unknown.

In addition to mechanical factors, a number of toxic and metabolic disturbances may give rise to a pseudotumor syndrome (Table 30-1). In children, as they are withdrawn from chronic corticosteroid therapy, there may be a period of headache, papilledema, and elevated ICP with only modest enlargement of the lateral ventricles. Lead toxicity in children is marked by brain swelling and papilledema. Excessive doses of tetracycline and vitamin A (particularly in the form of isotretinoin, an oral vitamin A derivative for the treatment of severe acne) have also been shown to cause intracranial hypertension in children and adolescents. Isolated instances of hypo- or hyperadrenalism, myxedema, and hypoparathyroidism have developed increased CSF pressure and papilledema, and occasionally the administration of estrogens, phenothiazines, the antiarrhythmic drug amiodarone, and quinolone antibiotics has the same effect, for reasons not known.

The first step in diagnosis is to exclude an underlying tumor or the other nontumorous cause of raised ICP, discussed above. This can be accomplished by CT and MRI, although it should be borne in mind that certain chronic meningeal reactions (e.g., those due to sarcoidosis or to tuberculous or carcinomatous meningitis), which give rise to headache and papilledema, may sometimes elude detection by these imaging procedures; in these cases, however, lumbar puncture will always disclose the diagnosis. It should not need to be emphasized that *the diagnosis of pseudotumor cerebri should not be accepted when the CSF content is abnormal.*

Treatment Most patients with idiopathic intracranial hypertension will be found initially to have minor visual changes aside from the papilledema, and the headache and lumbar puncture pressure then guide treatment. At least one-third of our patients have recovered within 6 months after repeated lumbar punctures and drainage of sufficient CSF to maintain the pressure at normal or near-normal levels (less than 200 mmH_2O). The lumbar punctures were performed daily or on alternate days at first and then at longer intervals, according to the level of pressure. Evidently this was sufficient to restore the balance between CSF formation and absorption for at least several months. In the larger group of patients, the CSF pressure remains elevated and the papilledema becomes chronic (Fig. 13-10). It is the management of this group of patients that is most difficult and controversial. Weight reduction is always advised but is difficult to accomplish. In two pathologically obese patients, we have resorted to surgical gastric plication, which had a beneficial effect on the pseudotumor but left the patient for a time with the severe gastrointestinal disturbances that commonly complicate this procedure. Sugerman et al (1995) studied eight morbidly obese women who had similar operations and found the results to be satisfactory over several years. Prednisone (40 to 60 mg/day), oral hyperosmotic agents such as glycerol (15 to 60 mg four to six times daily), or carbonic anhydrase inhibitors (acetazolamide 500 mg twice or thrice daily; furosemide 20 to 80 mg twice daily) to reduce CSF formation all have their advocates. We have occasionally observed a gradual recession of papilledema and a lowering of CSF pressure in response to each of these measures, but such responses were not consistent or sustained and it was always difficult to decide whether they represented the effect of treatment or the natural course of the disease. Greer, who has reported on 110 patients, 11 of whom were treated with these agents, decided that they were of no value. Moreover, in patients whose papilledema seems to recede under the influence of corticosteroids, there is always a danger that papilledema will recur when the drug is tapered. Considering the potential for undesirable effects of corticosteroids, we have used them very sparingly and only for brief periods of time while preparing the patient for more definitive treatment.

Careful evaluations of the visual fields and of acuity are required soon after the diagnosis of idiopathic pseudotumor is settled. Repeated examination of visual function, preferably in collaboration with an ophthalmologist, is essential in detecting early and potentially reversible visual loss. However, it must be acknowledged that measurements of visual acuity (and of visual evoked potentials) are relatively insensitive means of detecting early visual field loss; abnormalities in these tests indicate that serious damage to the optic nerve head has already occurred. Quantitative perimetry, using the kinetic Goldmann technique, has been more informative. Fundus photographs are also a reliable means of assessing the course of papilledema. A reduction in previously normal acuity to less than 20/100, an enlargement of the blind spot, or the appearance of sector field defects is an indication for prompt and aggressive treatment.

If intracranial hypertension and papilledema are left untreated or fail to respond to the measures outlined above, the one great danger is loss of vision from compressive damage to the optic nerve fibers. Corbett and associates, who described a group of 57 patients followed for 5 to 41 years, found severe visual impairment in 14, and Wall and George, using highly refined perimetric methods, have reported an even higher incidence of visual loss. Moreover, children with pseudotumor share the same visual risks as adults (Lessell and Rosman). Sometimes vision is lost abruptly, either without warning or following one or more episodes of visual obscuration.

In patients who are unresponsive to the usual therapeutic measures, one alternative that may be considered is a lumbar-peritoneal shunt. Not more than 10 percent of our patients have undergone this surgical procedure. The shunting procedure has been relatively safe and effective, but because of a tendency for the shunt to close or to be dislodged in obese patients, sometimes causing back or sciatic pain, the procedure has fallen out of favor. However, Burgett et al, who treated 30 patients in this way, reported success in reducing headache in almost all and in improving vision in 70 percent. We have not had to resort to subtemporal decompression, a procedure that was formerly used when vision was threatened.

For patients who are progressively or rapidly losing vision, the procedure currently favored by ophthalmologists is unilateral fenestration of the optic nerve sheath. According to Corbett and colleagues, this procedure—which consists of partial unroofing of the orbit and intraorbital incision of the dural-arachnoid sheaths surrounding the optic nerve—effectively preserves or restores vision in 80 to 90 percent of patients. Even when this procedure is performed on only one side, its effect on vision is often bilateral, and about two-thirds of patients have some relief of headache as well. The operation carries a small risk of vascular obstruction and unilateral visual loss, as was the case in two of our patients.

We have been impressed with the persistence of a complex migraine- or tension-like headache in some patients whose spinal fluid pressure has been adequately reduced by repeated lumbar punctures or shunting. After it has been confirmed that the pressure is not elevated, these headaches may be treated in a manner similar to the usual types of chronic headaches, as outlined in Chap. 10. Therapeutic lumbar puncture in pseudotumor may be followed transiently by the type of low-pressure headache described further on; it generally does not warrant treatment in these circumstances.

Pneumocephalus and Pneumocranium These disorders, in which air enters the ventricular system or the subarachnoid spaces, are discussed in relation to cranial injury and the postoperative state (page 928 and Fig. 35-3). In the case of pneumocranium, the collection of air may act as a mass that compresses adjacent brain tissue and requires relief by aspiration.

Ventricular Dilatation without Raised Pressure or Brain Atrophy The wide application of CT and MRI reveals cases of mild to moderate ventricular enlargement in which there is no evidence of parenchymal lesions of the cerebrum. This has been reported in patients with anorexia nervosa and Cushing disease and in those receiving corticosteroids for a long period of time. It has also been observed in children with protein malnutrition and in some schizophrenics and chronic alcoholics; in the latter patients, there is usually no associated neurologic or mental abnormality. In all of the aforementioned conditions, slight widening of the cerebral sulci accompanies the ventricular enlargement. After a prolonged period without steroids or of abstinence from alcohol, the ventricles become smaller and the sulcal widening is less apparent. This change in ventricular size is probably related to a shift of tissue fluids, though not of the usual types of cerebral edema.

Intracranial Hypotension

Lumbar Puncture Headache (See also page 194.) This is a well-known phenomenon, attributable to a lowering of ICP by leakage of CSF through the needle track into the paravertebral muscles and other tissues. Once begun, the headache may last for days or rarely, even for weeks. Actually the syndrome includes more than headache. There may be pain at the base of the skull posteriorly and in the back of the neck and upper thoracic spine, stiffness of the neck, and nausea and vomiting. At times the signs of meningeal irritation are so prominent as to raise the question of postlumbar puncture meningitis, although lack of fever usually excludes this possibility. In addition to a low or unmeasurable CSF pressure if another spinal tap is performed, there are occasionally a few to a dozen white cells in the CSF, which may further raise concern of meningitis. In the infant or young child, stiffness of the neck may be accompanied by irritability, unwillingness to move, and refusal of food. Most characteristic is the relation of the headache to upright posture and its relief within moments after assuming the recumbent position. If the headache is protracted, recumbency still reduces the head pain, but a feeling of dull pressure may remain, which the patient continues to report as a headache. Many patients also report that rapidly turning the head produces a cephalic pain. Occasionally there will be a sixth nerve palsy or a self-audible bruit from turbulence in the intracranial venous system.

It has been recognized that low spinal fluid pressure is associated on the MRI with prominent dural enhancement by gadolinium (Fig. 30-4)—and, when the syndrome is protracted and severe, there may be subdural effusions and mass effect (see below, under "Spontaneous Intracranial Hypotension"). The dural enhancement is thought to be the result of neovascularization of the pachymeninges and perhaps venous dilation in response to the lowered subarachnoid pressure.

The use of a 22- to 24-gauge needle and the performance of a single clean (atraumatic) tap seemingly reduces the likelihood of a post-lumbar puncture headache. A period of enforced recumbency, though widely practiced as a means of preventing headache, probably does not lessen its incidence (Carbaat and van Crevel). The CSF pressure is in the range of 0 to 60 mmH_2O. The ingestion of large volumes of fluids and the infusion of 1000 to 2000 mL of 5% glucose are usually recommended but are of uncertain benefit. The most dependable treatment is a "blood patch" (spinal epidural injection of a few milliliters of the patient's own blood). The headache is often relieved almost immediately even if the blood is injected at some distance from the original puncture (although the procedure is usually done at the same level as the previous spinal tap). The mechanism of this rapid improvement may not simply be the plugging of a dural leak. A number of patients fail to benefit or have only transient effects, and it is then unclear whether repeating the procedure is helpful. The administration of caffeine-ergotamine preparations or intravenous caffeine may also have a salutary though temporary effect on the headache. The addition of analgesic medication is required only if the patient must get up to care for himself or to travel. In protracted cases, patience is called for, since most headaches will resolve in 2 weeks or less.

Panullo and colleagues have shown that there is a vertical descent of the upper brainstem and posterior fossa contents with the low-pressure headache that follows lumbar puncture; but, as pointed out in Chap. 17, there are rarely associated neurologic signs of brain herniations, the exceptions being some of the curious cases discussed below.

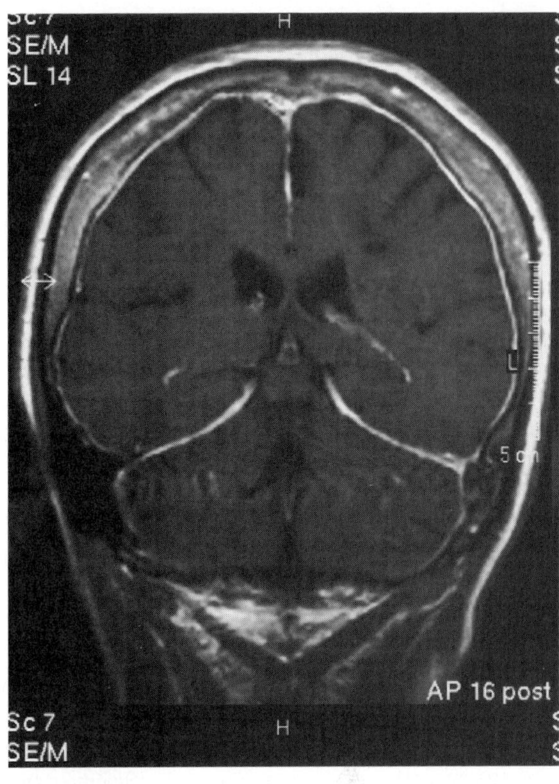

Figure 30-4

MRI after gadolinium infusion (T1 sequence) showing the widespread dural enhancement that is typical of low CSF pressure after lumbar puncture, spontaneous CSF leakage, or shunt overdrainage. Similar changes may be found in the spinal dura.

Aside from this condition, there are few adverse effects of lumbar puncture; these are described in Chap. 2.

Spontaneous Intracranial Hypotension This is a less well known syndrome, in which the same problem as the one that follows lumbar puncture occurs after straining, a nonhurtful fall, or for no known reason. The cardinal feature is orthostatic headache and only rarely are there other neurologic complaints such as diplopia from sixth nerve palsy or a self-audible bruit. In these cases the CSF pressure is low (60 mmH_2O or less) or not measurable; the fluid may contain 20 or more mononuclear cells per milliliter but is most often normal. A few cases have presented with stupor as a result of downward transtentorial displacement of the diencephalic region (Pleasure et al) or an upper cervical myelopathy caused by downward deformation and displacement of the spinal cord (Miyazaki et al).

Presumably in such patients, there has been a tear in the delicate arachnoid surrounding a nerve root, with continuous leakage of CSF. The site of the leak is difficult to ascertain except when it occurs into the paranasal sinuses (CSF rhinorrhea). In a series of 11 patients with spontaneous intracranial hypotension, a putative leak was found by radionuclide cisternography or CT myelography (the preferred procedure) in the cervical region or at the cervicothoracic junction in five patients, in the thoracic region in five, and the lumbar region in one (Schievink et al). In the patients who underwent surgical repair, a leaking meningeal diverticulum (a so-called Tarlov cyst) was found and could be ligated. This seems to be the most common cause. A blood patch, as described above, may also be useful and should be attempted before resorting to surgery. Recumbency for a few days thereafter permits the pressure to build up, and there has been no recurrence in the cases that we have encountered. Others have reported repeated episodes of orthostatic headache.

As noted above, a helpful diagnostic sign is prominent dural enhancement with gadolinium on the MRI (Fig. 30-4), a phenomenon attributed by Fishman and Dillon to dural venous dilatation, and this finding may extend to the pachymeninges of the posterior fossa and the cervical spine. According to Mokri and colleagues, biopsy of the dura and underlying meninges in these cases shows fibroblastic proliferation and neovascularity with an amorphous subdural fluid. There may be subdural effusions and mass effect, either on the cerebral convexities, temporal lobes, optic chiasm, or cerebellar tonsils. Using ultrasound, Chen and colleagues have also described an enlarged superior ophthalmic vein and increased blood flow velocity in this vessel, both of which normalize after successful treatment. Rarely, a case of intracranial hypotension becomes chronic; the headache is then no longer responsive to recumbency. Mokri and colleagues have also made the point that orthostatic headache and diffuse pachymeningeal enhancement on MRI may occur in the presence of normal CSF pressures, and these characteristic features of a CSF leak should prompt a search for the site of leakage despite the normal pressure.

The use of a one-way valve and a ventriculoatrial or ventriculoperitoneal shunt may be complicated by a low-pressure syndrome. Reference has already been made to this syndrome and to the "slit ventricle syndrome" in children being treated for hydrocephalus. Usually the valve setting is too low, and readjustment to maintain a higher pressure is corrective.

SPECIAL MENINGEAL AND EPENDYMAL DISORDERS

The effects of bacterial invasion of the pia-arachnoid, cerebrospinal subarachnoid space, ventricles, and ependyma are described in Chap. 32 and summarized in Table 32-1. The point being made here is that these structures may also be involved in a number of noninfective processes, some of obscure origin.

Since the ventricular and subarachnoid spaces are in continuity, one would expect that a noxious agent entering any one part would extend throughout the CSF pathway. Such is not always the case. The lower spinal roots or spinal cord alone may be implicated in "spinal arachnoiditis." A similar process may affect the optic nerves and chiasm exclusively ("opticochiasmatic arachnoiditis"). It may be accompanied by a pachymeningitis, and the latter may also be restricted to the cervical dura. A predominant localization to these basal or cervical structures may be apparent even in cases of diffuse cerebrospinal meningeal reactions, perhaps because of an uneven concentration of the noxious agent. In other instances, the primary disease appears to have arisen in the dura, with extension only to the adjacent pia-arachnoid. In yet other instances, the ependyma of the aqueduct or fourth ventricle is primarily involved.

The mechanisms by which these meningeal reactions affect parenchymal structures are not fully understood. The most obvious sequela is an obstruction to the flow of CSF in hydrocephalus; here, simple fibrotic narrowing of the CSF circulatory pathway is operative. Progressive constriction of nerve roots and spinal cord, literally a strangulation of these structures, is another plausible mechanism, but in this instance it is difficult to separate vascular factors from the mechanical ones. Since any toxic agent introduced into the subarachnoid space has free access, via Virchow-Robin spaces, to the superficial parts of the brain and spinal cord, direct parenchymal injury may follow. Perivascular reactions of subpial vessels, as in postinfectious degenerative processes, would be a plausible mechanism of injury to optic nerves and spinal cord, where long stretches of myelinated fibers abut the pia.

Regional Arachnoiditis Often arachnoiditis is limited to the lumbosacral roots and has followed ruptured discs, myelograms, and spinal surgery. Chronic neuropathic pain in the back and lower extremities with variable sensorimotor and reflex changes in the legs constitute the clinical picture. Myelography discloses loculated pockets of imaging media (Fig 11-6). This condition is discussed further in Chap. 11, under "The Failed-Back Syndrome."

Another form of spinal arachnoiditis, in which both the spinal cord and roots are entrapped in thickened pia-arachnoid, sometimes with arachnoid-dural adhesions, is another well-known entity. An account of this condition is included with the spinal cord diseases (see Chap. 44). The etiologic factors have been singularly elusive. A subacute and chronic meningitis accounts for a few of the cases. The condition may be accompanied by cranial basilar meningeal fibrosis with optic nerve involvement and hydrocephalus (see below). The most familiar form of spinal arachnoiditis was, in the past, that which followed the use of chemically contaminated spinal anesthetics. The authors saw more than 40 cases of this type, now rare, dating from the time when vials of anesthetic were stored in detergent sterilizing solutions. Instillation of the anesthetic agent was followed immediately by back pain and a rapidly progressive lumbosacral root syndrome (areflexic paralysis, anesthesia of the legs, and paralysis of sphincters). Several cases have, in our recent experience, followed prolonged spinal anesthesia with the patient in a decubitus position, usually for orthopedic procedures, but it is then difficult to separate a direct toxic effect of the anesthetic from local inflammatory changes. The CSF protein rose rapidly in these cases, but pleocytosis was minimal. In other instances, protracted back pain lasting days to weeks was the only immediate effect but was followed, after a period of months or years, by a progressive myeloencephalopathy. This could take the form of some combination of spinal arachnoiditis with ataxic paraparesis and sensory disturbance, hydrocephalus, or opticochiasmatic arachnoiditis. On rare occasions, similar neurologic disorders had formerly followed the instillation of iophendylate (Pantopaque) for myelography and corticosteroids (for pain or multiple sclerosis). The point to be made is that there is always some risk attached to the subarachnoid instillation of any foreign agent.

Opticochiasmatic Arachnoiditis This condition was well known to neurologists during the period when neurosyphilis was a common disease. It occurs after years of chronic syphilitic meningitis, sometimes in conjunction with tabes dorsalis or meningomyelitis. However, there were always nonsyphilitic cases, the cause of which was never ascertained. A constriction of visual fields, usually bilateral and asymmetrical (rarely scotomas), developed insidiously and progressed. Pathologically, the optic nerves were found to be enmeshed in thickened, opaque pia-arachnoid.

Pachymeningitis The term *pachymeningitis* refers to a chronic, circumscribed, inflammatory thickening of the dura. The term is somewhat confusing insofar as the pia and arachnoid are equally involved in the inflammatory thickening and all three membranes are bound together by dense fibrous adhesions. This type of meningeal reaction, which is now exceedingly uncommon, was first described by Charcot and Joffroy. It occurred mainly in the cervical region (hence the name *pachymeningitis cervicalis hypertrophica*) and was attributed to syphilis. Indeed, in some instances there was a gummatous thickening of the dura. Implication of cervical roots and compression of the spinal cord gave rise to variable degrees of paraparesis in association with root pain, paresthesias, sensory loss, and amyotrophy of the upper limbs. In the modern era, rheumatoid arthritis, sarcoidosis and chronic local infection (fungal, tuberculous) have been the main causes, but many cases remain unexplained.

The subdural space and dura can be involved by extension of a pathologic process from the arachnoid, especially in infants and children, in whom subdural hygromas regularly follow meningitis. The fibrous connective tissue of which the dura is composed may undergo pronounced thickening in the course of a mucopolysaccharidosis, especially in cases where fibroblasts are implicated. The basal pia-arachnoid may also be involved and lead to obstructive hydrocephalus. Older medical writings often made reference to syphilitic cranial pachymeningitis, which later proved to be the thickened membranes of subdural hematomas. The neovascular response and fibrosis of the dura and meninges that result from low CSF pressures and give the same appearance as pachymeningitis on enhanced CT scans and MRI have been discussed above.

Other Abnormalities of the Ependyma and Meninges

Although the ependyma may be involved as part of any chronic meningeal reaction, it may also be the site of a relatively isolated process. In experimental animals, Johnson and colleagues found that the mumps virus could localize in and destroy ependymal cells. This results in activation of subependymal astrocytes, which may bury the remaining ependymal cells and, by overgrowth, narrow the aqueduct of Sylvius. Ependymitis with similar consequences may be the dominant change in infantile toxoplasmosis and cytomegalic encephalitis. Spinal fluid and meningeal reactions to degradation products released from tumors that are in contact with the cerebrospinal spaces, particularly dermoid and craniopharyngioma, are discussed in Chap. 32.

Hemosiderosis (Superficial Siderosis) of the Meninges Sometimes mistaken by neuropathologists for hemochromatosis, which has entirely different effects on the nervous system, hemosiderosis is clearly the consequence of repeated contamination of the meninges by blood (McDougal and Adams). An oozing vascular malformation or tumor has been the usual cause in our experience, although there are cases in which the source of the blood could not be found. The red blood corpuscles are phagocytosed, with the formation of hemosiderin, and gradually both iron pigment and ferritin are released into the CSF. The cerebellum, spinal cord, hippocampi, and olfactory bulbs are stained orange-brown. Iron pigments and ferritin, which are toxic, gradually diffuse through the pia into superficial parts of the cerebellum, eighth cranial nerve, and spinal cord, destroying nerve cells and exciting a glial reaction. In microscopic sections stained for iron, the histiocyte-microglial cells contain iron and ferritin, and particles of iron can be seen studding nerve and glial cells for a distance of several millimeters beneath the pia.

The clinical syndrome of siderosis of the meninges consists essentially of a progressive ataxia and nerve deafness; sometimes a spastic paraparesis is added and, rarely, mental impairment. The hemosiderin and iron-stained meninges are readily visualized by MRI, since iron is strongly paramagnetic. All the iron-impregnated tissues are hypointense in T2-weighted images. Koeppen and associates attributed the vunerability of the acoustic nerves to their extended meningeal exposure before acquiring a fibroblastic perineurium and epineurium. There is no treatment other than finding the source of the meningeal blood and preventing further hemorrhage.

REFERENCES

Adams RD, Fisher CM, Hakim S, et al: Symptomatic occult hydrocephalus with "normal" cerebrospinal fluid pressure: A treatable syndrome. *N Engl J Med* 273:117, 1965.

Aimard G, Vighetto A, Gabet JY, et al: Acetazolamide: An alternative to shunting in normal pressure hydrocephalus? Preliminary results. *Rev Neurol* 146:437, 1990.

Ames A, Sakanoue M, Endo S: Na, K, Ca, Mg and Cl concentrations in choroid plexus fluid and cisternal fluid compared with plasma ultrafiltrate. *J Neurophysiol* 27:672, 1964.

Barrows LJ, Hunter FT, Banker BQ: The nature and clinical significance of pigments in the cerebrospinal fluid. *Brain* 78:59, 1955.

Black PM: Idiopathic normal pressure hydrocephalus: Results of shunting in 62 patients. *J Neurosurg* 53:371, 1980.

Burgett RA, Purvin VA, Kawasaki A: Lumboperitoneal shunting for pseudotumor cerebri. *Neurology* 49:734, 1997.

Carbaat P, van Crevel H: Lumbar puncture headache: Controlled study on the preventive effect of 24 hours' bed rest. *Lancet* 2:1133, 1981.

Chen CC, Luo CL, Wang SJ, et al: Colour Doppler imaging for diagnosis of intracranial hypotension. *Lancet* 354:826, 1999.

Chutorian AM, Gold AP, Braun CW: Benign intracranial hypertension and Bell's palsy. *N Engl J Med* 296:1214, 1977.

Clarke D, Bullock P, Hui T, Firth J: Benign intracranial hypertension: A cause of CSF rhinorrhea. *J Neurol Neurosurg Psychiatry* 57:847, 1994.

Corbett JJ: Problems in the diagnosis and treatment of pseudotumor cerebri. *Can J Neurol Sci* 10:221, 1983.

Corbett JJ, Mehta MP: Cerebrospinal fluid pressure in normal obese subjects and patients with pseudotumor cerebri. *Neurology* 33:1386, 1983.

Corbett JJ, Savino PJ, Thompson HS, et al: Visual loss in pseudotumor cerebri. *Arch Neurol* 39:461, 1982.

Corbett JJ, Nerad JA, Tse DT, Anderson RL: Results of optic nerve sheath fenestration for pseudotumor cerebri. *Arch Ophthalmol* 106:1391, 1988.

Corbett JJ, Thompson HS: The rational management of idiopathic intracranial hypertension. *Arch Neurol* 46:1049, 1989.

Cutler RWP, Spertell RB: Cerebrospinal fluid: A selective review. *Ann Neurol* 11:1, 1982.

Dandy WE: Experimental hydrocephalus. *Ann Surg* 70:129, 1919.

Dandy WE, Blackfan KD: Internal hydrocephalus: An experimental, clinical, and pathological study. *Am J Dis Child* 8:406, 1914.

Davson H, Welch K, Segal MB: *Physiology and Pathophysiology of the Cerebrospinal Fluid.* New York, Churchill Livingstone, 1987.

Dennis M, Fritz CR, Netley CT, et al: The intelligence of hydrocephalic children. *Arch Neurol* 38:607, 1981.

Digre KB, Corbett JJ: Pseudotumor cerebri in men. *Arch Neurol* 45:866, 1988.

Durcan FJ, Corbett JJ, Wall M: The incidence of pseudotumor cerebri. *Arch Neurol* 45:875, 1988.

Fisher CM: Hydrocephalus as a cause of disturbances of gait in the elderly. *Neurology* 32:1358, 1982.

Fishman RA: *Cerebrospinal Fluid in Diseases of the Nervous System*, 2nd ed. Philadelphia, Saunders, 1992.

Fishman RA: Superficial siderosis. *Ann Neurol* 34:635, 1993.

Fishman RA: The pathophysiology of pseudotumor cerebri: An unsolved puzzle (editorial). *Arch Neurol* 41:257, 1984.

Fishman RA, Dillon WP: Dural enhancement and cerebral displacement secondary to intracranial hypotension. *Neurology* 43:609, 1993.

FOLEY J: Benign forms of intracranial hypertension—"Toxic" and "otitic" hydrocephalus. *Brain* 78:1, 1955.

GILLES FH, DAVIDSON RI: Communicating hydrocephalus associated with deficient dysplastic parasagittal arachnoid granulations. *J Neurosurg* 35:421, 1971.

GREER M: Benign intracranial hypertension, in Vinken PJ, Bruyn GW (eds): *Handbook of Clinical Neurology*. Vol 16. Amsterdam, North-Holland, 1974, pp 150–166.

HAKIM S, ADAMS RD: The special clinical problem of symptomatic hydrocephalus with normal cerebrospinal fluid pressure. *J Neurol Sci* 2:307, 1965.

HUSSEY F, SCHANZER B, KATZMAN R: A simple constant-infusion manometric test for measurement of CSF absorption: II. Clinical studies. *Neurology* 20:665, 1970.

JACOBSON DM, BERG R, WALL M, et al: Serum vitamin A concentration is elevated in idiopathic intracranial hypertension. *Neurology* 53:1114, 1999.

JOHNSON RT, JOHNSON DP, EDMONDS CS: Virus-induced hydrocephalus: Development of aqueductal stenosis in hamsters after mumps infection. *Science* 157:1066, 1967.

JOHNSTON I, PATERSON A: Benign intracranial hypertension. *Brain* 97:289, 301, 1974.

KARAHALIOS DG, REKATE HL, KHAYATA MH, APOSTOLIDES PJ: Elevated intracranial venous pressure as a universal mechanism in pseudotumor cerebri of varying etiologies. *Neurology* 46:198, 1996.

KATZMAN R, HUSSEY F: A simple constant-infusion manometric test for measurement of CSF absorption: I. Rationale and method. *Neurology* 20:534, 1970.

KOEPPEN AH, DICKSON AC, CHU RC, THACH RE: The pathogenesis of superficial siderosis of the nervous system. *Ann Neurol* 34:646, 1993.

LEECH RW, BRUMBACK RA: *Hydrocephalus: Current Clinical Concepts*. St. Louis, Mosby-Year Book, 1990, pp 86–90.

LESSELL S, ROSMAN P: Permanent visual impairment in childhood pseudotumor cerebri. *Arch Neurol* 43:801, 1986.

LUNDBERG N: Continuous recording and control of ventricular fluid pressure in neurosurgical practice. *Acta Psychiatr Scand* 36(suppl 149):1960.

MANN JD, JOHNSON RN, BUTLER AB, BASS NH: Impairment of cerebrospinal fluid circulatory dynamics in pseudotumor cerebri and response to steroid treatment. *Neurology* 29:550, 1979.

MCDOUGAL WB, ADAMS RD: The neurological changes in hemochromatosis. *Trans Am Neuropathol Soc* 9:117, 1950.

MERRITT HH, FREMONT-SMITH F: *The Cerebrospinal Fluid*. Philadelphia, Saunders, 1937.

MESTREZAT W: *Le Liquide cephalo-rachidien normal et pathologique*. Paris, Maloine, 1912.

MIYAZAKI T, CHIBA A, NISHINA H, et al: Upper cervical myelopathy associated with low CSF pressure: A complication of vertriculoperitoneal shunt. *Neurology* 50:1864, 1866.

MOKRI B, HUNTER SF, ATKINSON JL, PIEPGRAS DG: Orthostatic headaches caused by CSF leak but with normal CSF pressures. *Neurology* 51:786, 1998.

MOKRI B, PARISI JE, SCHEITHAUER BW, et al: Meningeal biopsy in intracranial hypotension: Meningeal enhancement on MRI. *Neurology* 45:1801, 1995.

PANULLO SC, REICH JB, KROL G, et al: MRI changes in intracranial hypotension. *Neurology* 43:919, 1993.

PAPPENHEIMER JR, HEISEY SR, JORDAN EF, DOWNER J: Perfusion of the cerebral ventricular system in unanesthetized goats. *Am J Physiol* 203:763, 1962.

PLEASURE SJH, ABOSCH A, FRIEDMAN, et al: Spontaneous intracranial hypotension resulting in stupor caused by diencephalic compression. *Neurology* 50:1854,1998.

QUINCKE H: Die Lumbarpunktion des Hydrocephalus. *Klin Wochenschr* 28:929, 965, 1891.

RADHAKRISHNAN K, AHLSKOG JE, GARRITY JA, KURLAND LT: Idiopathic intracranial hypertension. *Mayo Clin Proc* 69:169, 1994.

RAICHLE ME, GRUBB RL, PHELPS ME, et al: Cerebral hemodynamics and metabolism in pseudotumor cerebri. *Ann Neurol* 4:104, 1978.

ROPPER AH (ed): *Neurological and Neurosurgical Intensive Care*, 3rd ed. New York, Raven Press, 1993.

ROPPER AH, MARMAROU A: Mechanism of pseudotumor in Guillain-Barré syndrome. *Arch* Neurol 41:259, 1984.

ROSMAN NP SHANDS KN: Hydrocephalus caused by increased intracranial venous pressure: A clinicopathological study. *Ann Neurol* 3:445, 1978.

ROSNER MJ, BECKER DP: Origin and evolution of plateau waves. *J Neurosurg* 60:312, 1984.

RUSSELL DS: *Observations on the Pathology of Hydrocephalus*. London, His Majesty's Stationery Office, 1949.

SAHS A, JOYNT RJ: Brain swelling of unknown cause. *Neurology* 6:791, 1956.

SCHIEVINK WI, MEYER, FB, ATKINSON JL, MOKRI B: Spontaneous spinal cerebrospinal fluid leaks and intracranial hypotension. *J Neurosurg* 84:598, 1996.

SECKL J, LIGHTMAN S: Cerebrospinal fluid neurohypophysial peptides in benign intracranial hypertension. *J Neurol Neurosurg Psychiatry* 51:1538, 1988.

SHINNAR S, GAMMON K, BERGMAN EW JR, et al: Management of hydrocephalus in infancy: Use of acetazolamide and furosemide to avoid cerebrospinal fluid shunts. *J Pediatr* 107:31, 1985.

SUGERMAN HJ, DEMARIA EJ, FELTON WL, et al: Increased intraabdominal pressure and cardiac filling pressures in obesity-associated pseudotumor cerebri. *Neurology* 49:507, 1997.

SUGERMAN HJ, FELTON WL, SALVANT JB, et al: Effects of surgically induced weight loss on idiopathic intracranial hypertension in morbid obesity. *Neurology* 45:1655, 1995.

SYMONDS CP: Otitic hydrocephalus. *Brain* 54:55, 1931.

TRIPATHI BS, TRIPATHI RC: Vacuolar transcellular channels as a drainage pathway for CSF. *J Physiol (Lond)* 239:195, 1974.

VAN CREVEL H: Papilledema, CSF pressure, and CSF flow in cerebral tumours. *J Neurol Neurosurg Psychiatry* 42:493, 1979.

WALL M, GEORGE D: Visual loss in pseudotumor cerebri. *Arch Neurol* 44:170, 1987.

WEED LH: Certain anatomical and physiological aspects of the meninges and cerebrospinal fluid. *Brain* 58:383, 1935.

Chapter 31

INTRACRANIAL NEOPLASMS AND PARANEOPLASTIC DISORDERS

Speaking generally, tumors of the central nervous system constitute a bleak but vitally important chapter of neurologic medicine. Their importance derives from the facts that they occur in great variety; produce numerous neurologic symptoms because of their size, location, and invasive qualities; usually destroy the tissues in which they are situated and displace those around them; are a frequent cause of increased intracranial pressure; and, most of all, are often lethal. Slowly this dismal state of affairs is changing, however, thanks to advances in anesthesiology, stereotactic and microneurosurgical techniques, radiation therapy, and the use of chemotherapeutic agents.

For the clinician, the most important facts to assimilate are the following:

1. Many types of tumor, both primary and secondary, occur in the cranial cavity and spinal canal, and certain ones are much more frequent than others.

2. Some of these tumors—such as the craniopharyngioma, meningioma, and schwannoma—have a disposition to grow in particular parts of the cranial cavity, thereby producing certain characteristic neurologic syndromes.

3. The presence of certain diseases such as AIDS, an inherited disorder such as neurofibromatosis, or some systemic cancers predisposes to the development of tumors of the nervous system.

4. The growth rates and invasiveness of tumors vary; some, like the glioblastoma, are highly malignant, invasive, and rapidly progressive and others, like the meningioma, are benign, slowly progressive, and compressive. These pathologic peculiarities are important, for they have valuable clinical implications, frequently providing the explanation of slowly or rapidly evolving clinical states and determining a good or poor prognosis after surgical excision.

5. Systemic neoplasms, by poorly understood mechanisms, may have a remote effect on the nervous system, quite apart from their compressive, infiltrative, or metastatic effects. Moreover, these remote effects, referred to as "paraneoplastic" may constitute the initial or only clinical manifestation of the underlying neoplasm.

Incidence of CNS Tumors and Their Types In 1996 there were an estimated 400,000 deaths from cancer in the United States. Of these, the number of patients who died of primary tumors of the brain seems comparatively small (about 18,000, half of them malignant gliomas), but in roughly another 100,000 patients the brain was affected at the time of death by metastases. Thus, in approximately 25 percent of all the patients with cancer, the brain and its coverings were involved by neoplasm at some time in the course of the illness. By comparison, there were 190,000 new cases of breast cancer in 1996. Among causes of death from intracranial disease, tumor is exceeded in frequency only by stroke. In children, primary tumors of the brain constitute the most common solid tumor and represent 22 percent of all childhood neoplasms, second in frequency only to leukemia. Viewed from another perspective, in the United States the yearly incidence of all tumors that involve the brain is 46 per 100,000, and of primary brain tumors, 15 per 100,000.

It is difficult to obtain accurate statistics as to the types of intracranial tumors, for most of them have been obtained from university hospitals with specialized neurosurgical centers, which attract the more easily diagnosed and treatable forms. From the figures of Posner and Chernick, one can infer that secondary tumors of the brain greatly outnumber primary ones; yet in the large series reported in the past (those of Cushing, Olivecrona, Zülch, and Zimmerman), only 4 to 8 percent were of this type. In the autopsy statistics of municipal hospitals, where one would expect a more natural selection of cases, the figures for metastatic tumors vary widely, from 20 to 42 percent (Russell and Rubinstein). Even these figures probably err on the low side, since the brain is frequently not examined in cancer patients, and many of the patients with more benign tumors may have found their way to specialized neurosurgical services.

With these qualifications, the figures in Table 31-1 might be taken as representative. In broad terms, most primary brain tumors are of glial cell origin—i.e., gliomas—a category that includes astrocytomas (which occur in several grades of malignancy), oligodendrogliomas, ependymomas (which may have characteristics of both glia and of epithelium), and a number of rarer types. Other tumors arise from ectodermal structures related to the brain (meningioma); an increasingly important group arise from lymphocytes or their progenitor histiocytes (central nervous system lymphoma); a varied constellation is derived from neuronal elements (neuroblastoma, medulloblastoma), germ cells (germinoma, craniopharyngioma, teratoma, etc.), or endocrine elements (pituitary adenoma). The only important change that has occurred since the first edition of this book (1977) is the increase in incidence of primary CNS lymphomas. When Table 31-1 was first composed, the incidence of this tumor, formerly called reticulum cell sarcoma, was almost negligible. In the last 25 years, the number in our hospitals has more than tripled; at the Memorial Sloan-Kettering Cancer Center, the increase in incidence has been even more dramatic (DeAngelis). In most institutions, one in five or six primary brain tumors is now of this type. In large part, this increase is attributable to improved immunopathologic diagnostic techniques and to the rise in number of immunosuppressed individuals, particularly of those with AIDS, but the incidence of this tumor also appears to be increasing even in those with ostensibly normal immune function.

Table 31-1
Types of intracranial tumor in the combined series of Zülch, Cushing, and Olivecrona, expressed in percentage of total (approximately 15,000 cases)[a]

Tumor	*Percent of total*
Gliomas[b]	
Glioblastoma multiforme	20
Astrocytoma	10
Ependymoma	6
Medulloblastoma	4
Oligodendrocytoma	5
Meningioma	15
Pituitary adenoma	7
Neurinoma (schwannoma)	7
Metastatic carcinoma	6
Craniopharyngioma, dermoid, epidermoid, teratoma	4
Angiomas	4
Sarcomas	4
Unclassified (mostly gliomas)	5
Miscellaneous (pinealoma, chordoma, granuloma, lymphoma)[c]	3
Total	100

[a] In the large Latin American series reported by Polak, the frequency of tumor types is much the same except for a somewhat higher proportion of metastatic tumors (see also comments in text).

[b] In *children*, the proportions differ: astrocytoma, 48 percent; medulloblastoma, 44 percent; ependymoma, 8 percent. Seventy percent of gliomas in children are infratentorial; in adults, 70 percent are supratentorial.

[c] Incidence of lymphoma was negligible when these series were collected, but has increased markedly since then (see text).

Classification of Nervous System Tumors Revisions in the classification and grading systems of intracranial tumors abound. Combining recent refinements in histopathologic study of gliomas, the numerical grading system of Daumas-Duport and coworkers (known as the St. Anne–Mayo system), the three-tiered system of Ringertz (which correlates more closely with clinical survival), and the newer classification of the World Health Organization (incorporating the Ringertz system) may be summarized as follows. The diffuse *astrocytic tumors*, the most common forms of glioma, have been subdivided into grade 2 astrocytoma, grade 3 anaplastic astrocytoma, and grade 4 glioblastoma multiforme. These represent a spectrum in terms of growth potential (degree of nuclear atypia, cellularity, mitoses, and vascular changes) and prognosis. Tumors formerly classified as grade 1, or benign, astrocytomas, which are rare and difficult to distinguish from hamartomas, are omitted or, in the WHO system, are reserved for the relatively benign pilocytic astrocytomas. The glioblastomas with the added feature of vascular proliferation, resulting in hemorrhage and necrosis and sometimes sarcomatous changes, are set apart from high-grade (anaplastic, grade 3) astrocytomas on the basis of earlier age of onset and greater clinical and histopathologic malignancy. The pilocytic astrocytomas (well-differentiated tumors mostly of children and young adults), the pleomorphic xanthoastrocytomas (with lipid-filled cells), and the subependymal giant-cell astrocytomas (usually associated with tuberous sclerosis) have been set apart because of their different growth patterns, pathologic features, and prognosis. The *ependymomas* are subdivided into cellular, myxopapillary, clear-cell, and mixed types; the anaplastic myxopapillary tumor and the subependymoma are given separate status. The pathologic criteria of malignant astrocytoma do not apply to *oligodendroglioma*, for reasons elaborated further on. Tumors derived from the choroid plexus are divided into two classes—papillomas and carcinomas. *Meningiomas* are classified on the basis of their cytoarchitecture and genetic origin into three catergories: the usual meningothelial or syncytial type, the anaplastic or malignant type, and atypical forms. Tumors of the pineal gland, which were not included in earlier classifications, comprise pineocytomas, pineoblastomas, and embryonal forms. The *medulloblastoma* has been reclassified with the other tumors of presumed neuroectodermal origin: the neuroblastomas, retinoblastomas, and ependymoblastomas. Tumors of cranial and peripheral nerves are believed to differentiate into three main types: schwannomas, neurofibromas, and neurofibrosarcomas. Given separate status are the intracranial midline germ-cell tumors, such as germinoma, teratoma, choriocarcinoma, and endodermal sinus carcinoma. A miscellaneous group comprises lymphoma, hemangioblastoma, chordoma, hemangiopericytoma, spongioblastoma, and ganglioneuroma.

Biology of Nervous System Tumors In considering the biology of primary nervous system tumors, one of the first problems is with the definition of neoplasia. It is well known that a number of lesions may simulate brain tumors in their clinical manifestations and histologic appearance but are really hamartomas and not true tumors. A hamartoma is a "tumor-like formation that has its basis in maldevelopment" (Russell) and undergoes little change during the life of the host. The difficulty one encounters in distinguishing it from a true neoplasm, which is an evolving blastomatous lesion whose constituent cells multiply without restraint, is well illustrated by tuberous sclerosis and von Recklinghausen neurofibromatosis; in these diseases, both hamartomas and neoplasms can be found. In a number of mass lesions—such as certain cerebellar astrocytomas, bipolar astrocytomas of the pons and optic nerves, von Hippel-Lindau cerebellar cysts, and pineal teratomas—a clear distinction between neoplasms and hamartomas is often not possible.

The many studies of the *pathogenesis of brain tumors* have gradually shed light on their origin. Johannes Muller (1838), in his atlas *Structure and Function of Neoplasms*, first enunciated the appealing idea that tumors might originate in embryonic cells left in the brain during development. This idea was elaborated by Cohnheim (1878), who postulated that the cause of tumors was an anomaly of the embryonic anlage. They would be expected to form, he stated, at sites where there are rapid differentiations of germ layers and complex migrations of cells. Ribbert, in 1918, extended this hypothesis by postulating that the potential for differentiation of these stem cells would favor blastomatous growth. Also implicit in this histogenetic theory is the idea that the degree of anaplasia, or its opposite, differentiation, depends on the status of the cell rests. This Cohnheim-Ribbert theory seems most applicable to tumors that arise from vestigial tissues, such as craniopharyngiomas, teratomas, lipomas, and chordomas, some of which are more like hamartomas than neoplasms. Possibly the embryonic rest theory might account for cerebral gliomas that arise in the course of certain genetic diseases, such as von Recklinghausen neurofibromatosis, tuberous sclerosis, or hemangioblastomatosis; or it might account for certain midline tumors at sites of closure of the neural tube (polar spongioblastoma; retinoblastoma; gliomas of optic nerve, hypothalamus, periaqueductal region, cerebellum, and spinal cord). However, even in the case of medulloblastoma, where the embryonic rest theory is invoked most often, one cannot be sure that the neoplasm arises, as postulated, from primitive neuroblasts of the posterior medullary velum.

For many years, thinking about the pathogenesis of primary CNS tumors was dominated by the *histogenetic theory* of Bailey and Cushing, (1926), which is based on the known or assumed embryology of nerve and glial cells. Now it is generally accepted that certain tumors may arise from neoplastic transformation of maturing adult elements (*dedifferentiation theory*). A normal astrocyte, oligodendrocyte, microgliocyte, or ependymocyte is transformed into a neoplastic cell and, as it multiplies, the daughter cells become variably anaplastic, the more so as the degree of malignancy increases. (*Anaplasia* refers to the primitive undifferentiated state of the constituent cells.) The factor of age is also important in the biology of brain tumors. Medulloblastomas, polar spongioblastomas, optic nerve gliomas, and pinealomas occur mainly before the age of 20 years, and meningiomas and glioblastomas are most frequent in the sixth decade. Heredity figures importantly in the genesis of certain tumors, particularly retinoblastomas, neurofibromas, and hemangioblastomas. The rare familial disorders of multiple endocrine neoplasia and multiple hamartomas are associated with an increased incidence of anterior pituitary tumors and meningiomas, respectively. Glioblastomas and cerebral astrocytomas have also been reported occasionally in more than one member of a family, but the study of such families has not disclosed the operation of an identifiable genetic factor. Only in the gliomas associated with neurofibromatosis and tuberous sclerosis and in the cerebellar hemangioblastoma of von Hippel–Lindau disease is there significant evidence of a hereditary determinant.

All of these ideas have been expanded greatly by studies of the human genome, which have led to the identification of certain chromosomal aberrations that are linked to tumors of the nervous system. Deletions and translocations of parts of chromosomes are associated with the presence of either proto-oncogenes or suppressor genes that regulate cellular division and contribute to malignant transformation. Several studies have elucidated the role of specific oncogenes in the genesis of tumors. For example, Martuza has traced the embryogenesis of some tumor types, the retinoblastomas in particular, to mutations of normal genes (see further on and also Chap. 38 for details). A deletion of inhibitory oncogenes has been identified in the genesis of hemangioblastomas.

Although there has been no direct evidence for an association between viruses and primary tumors of the nervous system, epidemiologic and experimental data—drawn from studies of the human papillomavirus, and the hepatitis B, Epstein-Barr, and human T-lymphotropic viruses—indicate that viruses are a major risk factor in certain human cancers. In transgenic mice, certain viruses are capable of inducing olfactory neuroblastomas and neurofibromas. Each of these viruses possesses a small number of genes that are incorporated in a cellular component of the nervous system (usually a dividing cell such as an astrocyte, oligodendrocyte, ependymocyte, endothelial cell, or lymphocyte). The virus is believed to thrive on the high levels of nucleotides and amino acid precursors and at the same time to force the cell out of its normal reproductive cycle into an unrestrained replicative cycle (Levine). Because of this capacity to transform the cellular genome, the virus product is called an *oncogene*; such oncogenes are capable of immortalizing, so to speak, the stimulated cell to form a tumor.

Aberrations in another family of genes, called *antioncogenes* or *suppressor genes*, have also been implicated in tumor genesis. These genes are inherited in autosomal dominant pattern and are thought to act, in normal proliferating cells, as negative regulators of cell growth; i.e., they suppress the ability of cells to produce tumors. The most relevant of these to human cancers and to gliomas is the p53 gene on chromosome 17p, which encodes a nuclear protein and transcriptional factor that is involved in cell cycle proliferation. Mutations in the normal "wild-type" gene, by some unexplained mechanism, permit the autonomous replication of cells and the development of neoplasm. This proclivity is evident in the cells of malignant astrocytomas; over 50 percent of these tumors and a much smaller number of low-grade gliomas have deletions of the short arm of chromosome 17, which contains the p53 gene. Involvement of this gene is further suggested by the observation that expansion of clones of the transformed astrocytes containing the p53 gene accompanies, and perhaps causes, progression from a low-grade to a malignant glioma. Even more frequent in high-grade gliomas, appearing in 80 to 90 percent of cases, is the entire loss of chromosome 10, suggesting the presence of a tumor suppressor gene on that chromosome as well. Mutations of the retinoblastoma (Rb) gene, a well-characterized tumor suppressor gene, are found not only in retinoblastomas but also in 30 percent of malignant gliomas. The normal Rb form is required to prevent cells from entering the mitotic phase of replication. However, it is not yet clear if any of these chromosomal changes are causative or simply reflect the emergent properties of gliomas, i.e., are part of the aberrant genetic processes that accompany tumor growth and progression.

In about 50 percent of gliomas, there is also an overexpression or mutant form of epidermal growth factor and transforming growth factor, suggesting a role for these trophic factors in the development of this tumor type.

On the basis of this new molecular information, our views of the pathogenesis of neoplasia are being cast along new lines. The specifics of these new data are presented in the following discussions of particular tumor types.

Pathophysiology of Brain Tumors

The production of symptoms by tumor growth is governed by certain principles of mechanics and physiology, some of which were discussed in Chaps. 17 and 30. There it was pointed out that the cranial cavity has a restricted volume, and the three elements contained therein—the brain (about 1200 to 1400 mL), cerebrospinal fluid (CSF; 70 to 140 mL), and blood (150 mL)—are relatively incompressible, particularly the brain substance, and each is subject to displacement by a mass lesion. According to the Monro-Kellie doctrine, the total bulk of the three elements is at all times constant, and any increase in the volume of one of them must be at the expense of one or both of the others (see Fig. 30-1). A tumor growing in one part of the brain compresses brain tissue and displaces CSF and blood; once the limit of this accommodation is reached, the intracranial pressure (ICP) rises. The elevation of the ICP and perioptic pressure impairs axonal transport in the optic nerve and the venous drainage from the optic nerve head and retina, manifesting itself by papilledema.

It must be pointed out, however, that only some brain tumors cause papilledema and that many others—often quite as large—do not. Thus one may question whether the Monro-Kellie doctrine, and its simple implied relationships of intracranial volume and CSF pressure, adequately explains the development of raised ICP and papilledema with brain tumors. In fact, in a slow process such as tumor growth, brain tissue is to some degree compressible, as one might suspect from the large indentations of brain produced by meningiomas.

Presumably, with tumor growth, the venules in the cerebral tissue adjacent to the tumor are compressed, with resulting elevation of capillary pressure, particularly in the cerebral white matter. The slow growth of most tumors permits accommodation of the brain to changes in cerebral blood flow and ICP. Only in the advanced stages of tumor growth do the compensatory mechanisms fail, and CSF pressure and ICP rise, with consequences described in Chap. 30. Once pressure is raised in a particular compartment of the brain, the tumor begins to displace tissue; eventually there is a displacement of tissue at a distance from the tumor, resulting in the *false localizing* signs described in Chap. 17. Indeed, the transtentorial herniations, the paradoxical corticospinal signs of Kernohan and Woltman, sixth and third nerve palsies, and secondary hydrocephalus were all originally described in tumor cases (see further on, under "Brain Displacements and Herniations").

Brain Edema This is a most important aspect of tumor growth, but it also assumes importance in cerebral trauma, massive infarction, hemorrhage, abscess, hypoxia, and other toxic and metabolic states. Brain edema is such a prominent feature of cerebral neoplasm that this is a suitable place to summarize what is known about it.

For a long time it has been recognized that conditions leading to peripheral edema, such as hypoalbuminemia and increased systemic venous pressure, do not have a similar effect on the brain. By contrast, lesions that alter the blood-brain barrier cause rapid swelling of brain tissue. Klatzo specified two categories of edema, *vasogenic* and *cytotoxic*. Fishman accepts these two categories but adds a third, which he calls *interstitial.* An example of the latter is the edema that occurs with obstructive hydrocephalus, in which CSF seeps into the periventricular tissues and occupies the space between cells. Most neuropathologists use the term *interstitial* to refer to any increase in the extravascular intercellular compartment of the brain; this would include both vasogenic and Fishman's interstitial edema.

Vasogenic edema is the type seen in the vicinity of tumor growths and other localized processes as well as in more diffuse injury to the blood vessels (e.g., lead encephalopathy, malignant hypertension). It is practically limited to the white matter and is evidenced by decreased attenuation on CT scanning and by hyperintensity on T2-weighted MR images. Presumably there is increased permeability of the capillary endothelial cells, so that plasma proteins enter the extracellular spaces (Fig. 31-1*A*). This heightened permeability has been attributed to a defect in the tight endothelial cell junctions, but current evidence indicates that increased vesicular transport across the endothelial cells is a more important factor. Microvascular transudative factors, such as proteases released by tumor cells, contribute to the predominantly vasogenic edema by weakening the blood-brain barrier and allowing passage of blood proteins. The small protein fragments that are generated by this protease activity exert osmotic effects as they spread through the white matter of the brain. This is the postulated basis of the regional swelling, also called *localized cerebral edema*, that surrounds the tumor. Experimentally, the increase in permeability has been shown to vary inversely with the molecular weight of various markers; for example, inulin (molecular weight 5000) enters the intercellular space more readily than albumin (molecular weight 70,000).

The particular vulnerability of white matter to vasogenic edema is not well understood; probably its loose structural organization offers less resistance to fluid under pressure than the gray matter. Possibly also, it is related to the special morphologic characteristics of white matter capillaries. The accumulation of plasma filtrate, with its high protein content, in the extracellular spaces and between the layers of myelin sheaths would be expected to alter the ionic balance of nerve fibers, impairing their function.

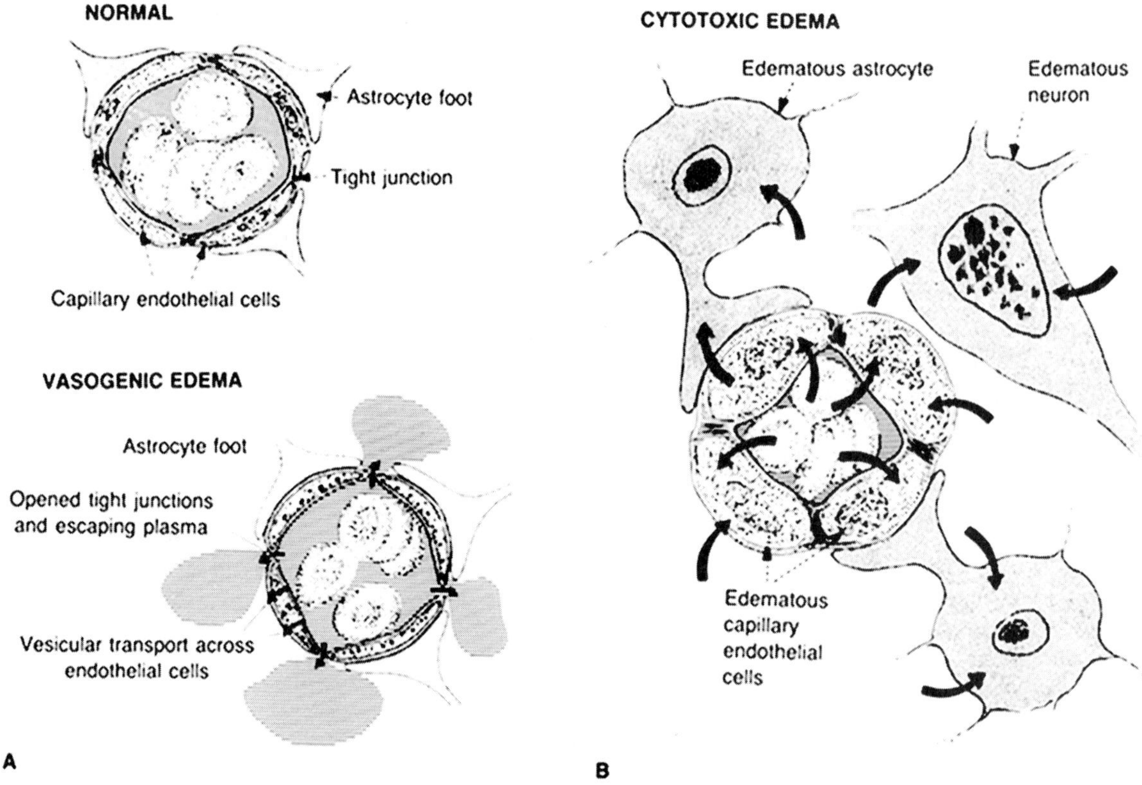

Figure 31-1

A. *Schematic representation of the astrocytes and endothelial cells of the capillary wall in the normal state (above) and in vasogenic edema (below). Heightened permeability in vasogenic edema is due partly to a defect in tight endothelial junctions but mainly to active vesicular transport across endothelial cells.* B. *Cellular (cytotoxic) edema, showing swelling of the endothelial, glial, and neuronal cells at the expense of the extracellular fluid space of the brain. (From Fishman by permission.)*

By contrast, in *cytotoxic edema*, all the cellular elements (neurons, glia, and endothelial cells) imbibe fluid and swell, with a corresponding reduction in the extracellular fluid space. This type of edema occurs typically with hypoxic-ischemic injury. The effect of oxygen deprivation is to cause a failure of the ATP-dependent sodium pump within cells; sodium accumulates in the cells, and water follows (Fig. 31-1*B*). The term *cellular edema* is preferable to *cytotoxic edema* because it emphasizes the cellular swelling rather than a toxic factor in the genesis of the brain edema. When it occurs in pure form, it is most often due to hypoxia, but it may also complicate acute hypo-osmolality of the plasma, as occurs with dilutional hyponatremia, acute hepatic encephalopathy, inappropriate secretion of antidiuretic hormone, or the osmotic disequilibrium syndrome that occurs with hemodialysis (page 1189). It is notable that several other common metabolic and nutritional encephalopathies—such as normotensive uremia and thiamine and vitamin B_{12} deficiencies—are attended by neither vasogenic nor cytotoxic edema. Presumably, both cellular and vasogenic edema occur with cerebral infarction.

So-called *interstitial (hydrocephalic) edema* of Fishman is a recognizable condition but is probably of less clinical significance than cytotoxic or cellular edema. Pathologically, in the former condition, the edema extends for only 2 to 3 mm from the ventricular wall. However, MRI suggests that the periventricular edema is more extensive than what is observed pathologically. Also, there are experimental data to show that the transependymal or periventricular route is utilized for absorption of CSF in hydrocephalus (Rosenberg et al). We would refer to this state as periventricular interstitial edema in association with tension hydrocephalus.

Treatment of Brain Edema and Raised ICP (See also page 948) The definitive treatment of any given case (excision of a tumor, treatment of intracranial infection, placement of a shunt, etc.) will, of course, be governed by the underlying disease. Here we consider only the therapeutic measures that can be directed against the edema itself and the raised ICP that it causes in cases of brain tumor.

The use of high-potency glucocorticosteroids has a beneficial effect upon the vasogenic edema associated with tumors, both primary and metastatic, sometimes beginning within hours. Probably these steroids act directly upon the endothelial cells, reducing their permeability. Steroids also shrink normal brain tissue, thus reducing overall intracranial pressure. In addition, drugs such as dexamethasone reduce the vasogenic edema associated with brain abscess and head injury; their usefulness in cases of large cerebral infarctions, contusions, and hemorrhage is less clear. Possibly the swelling of necrotic tissue is reduced, but there is no evidence that cytotoxic or cellular edema responds to administration of glucocorticoids.

For patients with brain tumor, it is common practice to use doses of dexamethasone of approximately 4 mg every 6 h, or the equivalent dose of methyprednisolone (Solu-Medrol), but only a few patients require a rigid schedule; a dose with meals and at bedtime usually suffices to suppress headache and focal neurologic symptoms. In patients with large tumors and marked secondary edema, further benefit is sometimes achieved by the administration of extremely high doses of dexamethasone, to a total of 100 mg per day or more. Always to be kept in mind are the serious side effects of sustained steroid administration, even at standard dose levels. Therefore the schedule should be carefully titrated to the desired clinical effect. It is also recognized that these drugs interfere with the metabolism of certain anticonvulsants commonly used in brain tumor patients.

In patients who require intravenous fluids, solutions containing water not matched by equivalent amounts of sodium ("free water") should be avoided. Normal saline is preferable and lactated Ringer's solution is acceptable, but dextrose solutions alone, in any concentration, are to be avoided.

The parenteral administration of hypertonic solutions (mannitol, hypertonic saline, urea, glycerol), by shifting water from brain to plasma, is also an effective means, in the short term, of reducing brain volume and lowering ICP. Edema, however, is little affected by these agents. Mannitol is the most widely used of these osmotic solutes. A 25% solution is administered parenterally in a dose of 0.5 to 1.0 g/kg body weight over a period of 2 to 10 min. Hypertonic saline solutions (3% or 1.5%) are equally effective. Urea is used less often. Glycerol is not much favored in the United States because of its high caloric content, but it is used in Europe, largely because it can be taken orally on an outpatient basis. A single administration of these solutes has only a short-lived effect, a matter of several hours, as it gains an equilibrium concentration in the brain; but repeated use on a regular schedule can lead to a reduction in headache and stabilization of the deleterious effects of a mass. Certain diuretic drugs, notably acetazolamide and furosemide, are said to be helpful in special instances (interstitial edema, pseudotumor cerebri) by virtue of creating a hyperosmolar state and by reducing the formation of CSF. However, their effects are usually transient.

The net effect of hyperosmolar therapy is reflected roughly by the degree of hypernatremia that is attained. Aside from a diuresis, which may raise serum osmolality, highly permeable solutes such as glucose offer little advantage in reducing brain volume, since they do not create an osmolar gradient that moves water from the brain to the vasculature. Moreover, with repeated administration of hyperosmolar solutions or diuretics, the brain gradually increases its osmolality—the result of added intracellular solute; these agents are therefore not suitable for long-term use. The notion that hyperosmolar agents might exaggerate tissue shifts by their predominant effect on normal brain tissue has not been borne out.

Controlled hyperventilation is a time-honored method of reducing brain volume by producing respiratory alkalosis and vasoconstriction; it is used mainly in brain trauma with high ICP, during intracranial surgery, and in the management of patients who have become acutely comatose from the mass effect of a tumor, but its effect is of limited duration.

Brain Displacements and Herniations

The problem of brain displacements and herniations is of vital importance in all mass lesions, and the underlying principles are particularly relevant to enlarging brain tumors. Several aspects of this problem, particularly the coma-producing mechanisms, have been considered on page 375. Brain displacements and herniations become possible because the cranial cavity is subdivided into several compartments by sheets of relatively rigid dura (the falx cerebri, which divides the supratentorial space into right and left halves, and the tentorium, which separates the cerebellum from the occipital lobes). The pressure from a mass within any one compartment, therefore, causes shifts or herniations of brain tissue from one compartment where the pressure is high to another where it is lower. There are three well-known herniations, the *subfalcial*, *temporal lobe–tentorial*, and *cerebellar–foramen magnum* (see Fig. 17-1) as well as several less familiar ones (*cerebellar-tentorial*, *diencephalic–sella turcica*, and *orbital frontal–middle cranial* fossa). Herniation of swollen brain through an opening in the calvarium, in relation to craniocerebral injury or operation, is yet another (transcalvarial) type.

Subfalcial herniation, in which the cingulate gyrus is pushed under the falx, occurs frequently, but little is known of its clinical manifestations. The most important herniation is the *temporal lobe–tentorial* one, which was described originally by Adolf Meyer and the clinical significance of which was first appreciated by Kernohan and Woltman and by Jefferson (see Table 31-2). Here the medial part of one temporal lobe (uncus and parahippocampus) is forced into the oval-shaped tentorial opening through which the midbrain passes. The uncal hernia pushes the midbrain and subthalamus against the opposite free edge of the tentorial opening, exerting pressure on the midbrain and subthalamus and on the vessels that encircle and enter these structures. The herniated uncal gyrus may compress the ipsilateral third nerve, causing the pupil to enlarge, and it may intermittently compromise the circulation to the occipital lobes, which results in hemorrhagic infarction of these regions. The hemiparesis that results from compression of the cerebral peduncle against the opposite edge of the tentorium is ipsilateral to the cerebral lesion and thus constitutes a false localizing sign (crus phenomenon, or Kernohan-Woltman sign). This and the coma-producing effects of transtentorial herniation are considered in Chap. 17. The extent to which the clinical disturbances are due to the compressive effects of the prolapsing brain tissue or to lateral shift of central (diencephalic-mesencephalic) structures is, in our view, still unsettled, and both or either mechanism may be operative in an individual case (page 376). Comparison of MR images with pathologic

Table 31-2
Clinicopathologic features of temporal lobe–tentorial herniation

Pathologic change	*Mechanism*	*Clinical disorders*
Injury to outer fibers of ipsilateral oculomotor nerve	Strangulation of nerve between herniating tissue and medial petroclinoid ligament; less often, downward pressure and entrapment of nerve between posterior cerebral and superior cerebellar arteries	Ptosis and pupillary dilatation (Hutchinson pupil), ophthalmoplegia later
Creasing of contralateral cerebral peduncle (Kernohan's notch)	Pressure of laterally displaced midbrain against sharp edge of tentorium	Hemiplegia ipsilateral to herniation (*false localizing sign*) and bilateral corticospinal tract signs
Lateral flattening of midbrain and zones of necrosis and secondary hemorrhages in tegmentum and base of subthalamus, midbrain, and upper pons (Duret hemorrhages)	Crushing of midbrain between herniating temporal lobe and opposite leaf of tentorium and vascular occlusion (hemorrhages around arterioles and veins)	Cheyne-Stokes respirations; stupor-coma; bipyramidal signs; decerebration; dilated, fixed pupils and alterations of gaze (facilitated oculocephalic reflex movement giving way to loss of all response to head movement and labyrinthine stimulation)
Unilateral or bilateral infarction (hemorrhagic) of occipital lobes	Compression of posterior cerebral artery against the tentorium by herniating temporal lobe	Usually none detectable during coma; homonymous hemianopia (unilateral or bilateral) with recovery
Rising intracranial pressure and hydrocephalus	Lateral flattening of aqueduct and third ventricle and blockage of perimesencephalic subarachnoid space	Increasing coma, rising blood pressure, bradycardia

specimens suggests that early symptoms, particularly impaired consciousness and the Kernohan-Woltman phenomenon, result more often from lateral displacement, and that frank herniation sometimes develops later (Ropper).

The *cerebellar-foramen magnum herniation* or *pressure cone*, first described by Cushing in 1917, consists of downward displacement of the inferior mesial parts of the cerebellar hemispheres (mainly the ventral paraflocculi or tonsillae) through the foramen magnum, behind the cervical cord. The displacement may be bilateral or, in the case of a one-sided cerebellar lesion, ispilateral. Bilateral displacement may result from a centrally placed callosal–frontal tumor or from general swelling of the brain and is accompanied by downward displacement of the brainstem. It may also be accompanied by bilateral temporal lobe–tentorial herniations (see above.

The clinical manifestations of downward cerebellar herniation are less well delineated than those of the temporal lobe–tentorial herniation. Cushing considered the typical signs of cerebellar herniation to be episodic tonic extension and arching of the neck and back and extension and internal rotation of the limbs, with respiratory disturbances, cardiac irregularity (bradycardia or tachycardia), and loss of consciousness. Other signs with subacutely evolving masses include pain in the neck, stiff neck, head tilt, paresthesias in the shoulders, dysphagia, and loss of tendon reflexes in the arms. It is difficult to determine which signs are due to the cerebellar herniation per se and which to the attendant effects of ICP and hydrocephalus. We would suggest that head tilt, stiff neck, arching of the neck, and paresthesias over the shoulders are attributable to the herniation, and that tonic extensor spasms of the limbs and body (so-called cerebellar fits) and coma are due to the compressive effects of the cerebellar lesion on medullary structures or of hydrocephalus on upper brainstem structures. *Respiratory arrest* is the most feared and often a fatal effect of medullary compression. It may occur suddenly, without the aforementioned signs. The herniated parts of the inferior cerebellum may undergo infarct necrosis and swelling, adding to the medullary compression.

With cerebellar mass lesions there may also be *upward herniation* of the cerebellum through the notch of the tentorium. Its clinical effects have not been clearly determined, but Cuneo and colleagues have attributed decerebrate posturing and pupillary changes—initially both pupils are miotic but still reactive, progressing to anisocoria and enlargement—to this type of brain displacement.

An understanding of the effects of elevated intracranial pressure, localized vasogenic edema, and displacements of tissue and herniations are absolutely essential to understanding the clinical behavior of intracranial tumors and mass lesions of any type. Often the symptoms of intracranial tumors are related more to these effects than to invasion of neurologic structures per se. The several false localizing signs (unilateral or bilateral abducens palsy, pupillary changes, ipsilateral or bilateral corticospinal tract signs, etc.) are also attributable to these mechanical changes and tissue displacements. This subject is discussed further on pages 375–377.

CLINICAL AND PATHOLOGIC CHARACTERISTICS OF BRAIN TUMORS

It should be stated at the outset that tumors of the brain may exist with hardly any symptoms. Often a slight bewilderment, slowness in comprehension, or loss of capacity for sustained mental activity is the only deviation from normal, and signs of focal cerebral disease are wholly lacking. In some patients, on the other hand, there is early indication of cerebral disease in the form of a progressive hemiparesis, a seizure occurring in a previously well person, or some other dramatic symptom, but until imaging studies are performed, the evidence may not be clear enough to warrant the diagnosis of a cerebral tumor. In a third group, the existence of a brain tumor can be assumed because of the presence of increased intracranial pressure with or without localizing signs of the tumor. In a fourth group, the symptoms are so definite as to make it likely that not only is there an intracranial neoplasm but that it is of a certain type and is located in a particular region. These localized growths may create certain syndromes seldom caused by any other disease.

In the further exposition of this subject, intracranial tumors are considered in relation to these common modes of clinical presentation.

1. Patients who present with general impairment of cerebral function, headaches, or seizures.

2. Patients who present with evidence of increased intracranial pressure.

3. Patients who present with specific intracranial tumor syndromes.

Patients Who Present with General Impairment of Cerebral Function, Headaches, or Seizures

Until the advent of modern imaging procedures, these were the patients who presented the greatest difficulty in diagnosis and about whom decisions were often made with a great degree of uncertainty. Their initial symptoms are vague, and not until some time has elapsed will signs of focal brain disease appear; when they do, they are not always of accurate localizing value. Altered mental function, headache, dizziness, and seizures are the usual manifestations in this group of patients.

Changes in Mental Function The early symptoms may be subtle. A lack of persistent application to everyday tasks, undue irritability, emotional lability, mental inertia, faulty insight, forgetfulness, reduced range of mental activity (judged by inquiring about the patient's introspections and manifested in his conversation), indifference to common social practices, lack of initiative and spontaneity—all of which may incorrectly be attributed to anxiety or depression—make up the mental abnormalities seen in this clinical circumstance. Inordinate drowsiness, apathy, equanimity, or stoicism may be prominent features of this state. We have sought a convenient term for this complex of symptoms, which is the most common type of mental disturbance encountered with neurologic disease, but none seems entirely appropriate. There is both a reduction in the amount of thought and action and a slowing of reaction time. MacCabe refers to this condition as "mental asthenia," which has the merit of distinguishing it from depression. We prefer to call it *psychomotor asthenia*. Much of this change in behavior is accepted by the patient with forbearance; if any complaint is made, it is of being weak, tired, or dizzy (nonrotational). Within a few weeks or months, these symptoms become more prominent. When the patient is questioned, a long pause precedes each reply; at times the patient may not respond at all. Or, at the moment the examiner decides that the patient has not heard the question and prepares to repeat it, an appropriate answer is given, usually in few words. Moreover, the responses are often more intelligent than one would expect, considering the patient's torpid mental state. There are, in addition, patients who are overtly confused or demented. If the condition remains untreated, dullness and somnolence increase gradually and, finally, as increased intracranial pressure supervenes, the patient progresses to stupor or coma.

Mental symptoms of this type cannot be ascribed to disease in any particular part of the brain, but tumors that cause them are more likely to involve central structures, i.e., they are situated deep in the brain, so as to impair the function of the thalamocortical mechanisms underlying attention and alertness, and the long association fiber systems of the cerebral white matter (affecting frontal and temporal areas and the corpus callosum).

Headaches These are an early symptom in fewer than one-third of patients with brain tumor and are variable in nature. In some the pain is slight, dull in character, and episodic; in others it is severe and either dull or sharp but also intermittent. If there are any characteristic features of the headache, they would be its nocturnal occurrence or presence on first awakening and perhaps its deep, nonpulsatile quality. However, these are not specific attributes, since migraine, hypertensive vascular headaches, etc., may also begin in the early morning hours or on awakening. Tumor patients do not always complain of the pain even when it is present but may betray its existence by placing their hands to their heads and looking distressed. When headache appears in the course of the psychomotor asthenia syndrome, it serves to clarify the diagnosis, but not nearly as much as does the occurrence of a seizure.

The mechanism of the headache is not fully understood. In the majority of instances, the CSF pressure is normal during the first weeks when the headache is present, and one can attribute it only to local swelling of tissues and to distortion of blood vessels in or around the tumor. Later the headache appears to be related to increases in intracranial pressure. Tumors above the tentorium cause headache on the side of the tumor and in its vicinity, in the orbital-frontal, temporal, or parietal region; tumors in the posterior fossa usually cause ipsilateral retroauricular or occipital headache. With elevated intracranial pressure, bifrontal or bioccipital headache is the rule regardless of the location of the tumor.

Vomiting and Dizziness Vomiting appears in a relatively small number of patients with a tumor syndrome and usually accompanies the headache when the latter is severe. It is more frequent with tumors of the posterior fossa. The most persistent vomiting (lasting several weeks) that we have observed have been in patients with low brainstem gliomas, fourth ventricular ependymomas, and subtentorial meningiomas. Some patients may vomit unexpectedly and forcibly, without preceding nausea (projectile vomiting), but others suffer both nausea and severe discomfort. Usually the vomiting is not related to the ingestion of food; often it occurs before breakfast.

No less frequent is the complaint of *dizziness*. As a rule it is not described with accuracy and consists of an unnatural sensation in the head, coupled with feelings of strangeness and insecurity when the position of the head is altered. Frank positional vertigo may be a symptom of a tumor in the posterior fossa (see Chap. 15).

Seizures The occurrence of focal or generalized seizures is the other major manifestation besides slowing of mental functions and signs of focal brain damage. Convulsions have been observed, in various series, in 20 to 50 percent of all patients with cerebral tumors. *A first seizure during adulthood is always suggestive of brain tumor and, in the authors' experience, has been the most common initial manifestation.* The localizing significance of seizure patterns has been discussed on pages 337–339. Seizures due to brain tumor most often have a focal onset, i.e., are partial and then become generalized. There may be one seizure or many, and they may follow the other symptoms or precede them by weeks or months or—exceptionally, in patients with low-grade astrocytoma, oligodendroglioma, or meningioma—by several years. Status epilepticus as an early event is rare but has occurred in a few of our patients. As a rule the seizures respond to standard anticonvulsant medications and may also improve after surgery.

Regional or Localizing Symptoms and Signs Sooner or later, in patients with psychomotor asthenia, headaches, and seizures, focal cerebral signs will be discovered; some patients may present with such signs. Nearly always, however, the focal signs are at first slight and subtle. Signs of increased ICP may become manifest and establish the diagnosis of tumor even before focal or lateralizing signs are detectable. Frequently, CT scanning or MRI will have disclosed the presence of a tumor before either focal cerebral signs or the signs of increased intracranial pressure have become evident.

The cerebral tumors that are most likely to produce the syndrome described above are glioblastoma multiforme, astrocytoma, oligodendroglioma, ependymoma, metastatic carcinoma, meningioma, and primary lymphoma of the brain.

Glioblastoma Multiforme and Anaplastic Astrocytoma (High-Grade Gliomas) These tumors account for about 20 percent of all intracranial tumors, or about 55 percent of all tumors of the glioma group, and for more than 90 percent of gliomas of the cerebral hemispheres in adults. Although predominantly cerebral in location, they may also arise in the brainstem, cerebellum, or spinal cord. The peak incidence is in middle adult life (mean age for the occurrence of glioblastoma is 56 to 60 years and 46 years for anaplastic astrocytoma), but no age group is exempt. The incidence is higher in men (ratio of approximately 1.6:1). Almost all of the high-grade gliomas occur sporadically, without a familial predilection.

The glioblastoma, known since the time of Virchow, was definitively recognized as a glioma by Bailey and Cushing and given a place in their histogenetic classification. Most arise in the deep white matter and quickly infiltrate the brain extensively, sometimes attaining enormous size before attracting medical attention. The tumor may extend to the meningeal surface or the ventricular wall, which probably accounts for the increase in CSF protein (more than 100 mg/dL in many cases) as well as for an occasional pleocytosis of 10 to 100 cells or more, mostly lymphocytes. The CSF may be normal, however. Malignant cells, carried in the CSF, may form distant foci on spinal roots or cause a widespread meningeal gliomatosis. Extraneural metastases, involving bone and lymph nodes, are very rare; usually they occur only after a craniotomy has been performed. About 50 percent of glioblastomas occupy more than one lobe of a hemisphere or are bilateral; between 3 and 6 percent show multicentric foci of growth.

The tumor has a variegated appearance, being a mottled gray, red, orange, or brown, depending on the degree of necrosis and presence of hemorrhage, recent or old. The imaging appearance is usually that of a nonhomogeneous mass, often with a center that is hypointense in comparison to adjacent brain and demonstrating an irregular thick or thin ring of enhancement, and surrounded by edema. Part of one lateral ventricle is often distorted, and both lateral and third ventricles may be displaced contralaterally (Fig. 31-2).

The characteristic histologic findings of glioblastoma are great cellularity with pleomorphism of cells and nuclear atypia; identifiable astrocytes with fibrils in combination with primitive forms in many cases; tumor giant cells and cells in mitosis; hyperplasia of endothelial cells of small vessels; and necrosis, hemorrhage, and thrombosis of vessels. This variegated appearance distinguishes glioblastoma from the lower-grade anaplastic gliomas, which show frequent mitoses and atypical cytogenic features but no grossly necrotic or hemorrhagic areas. It is the necrotic and sometimes cystic areas that appear hypointense on imaging studies. The vascu-

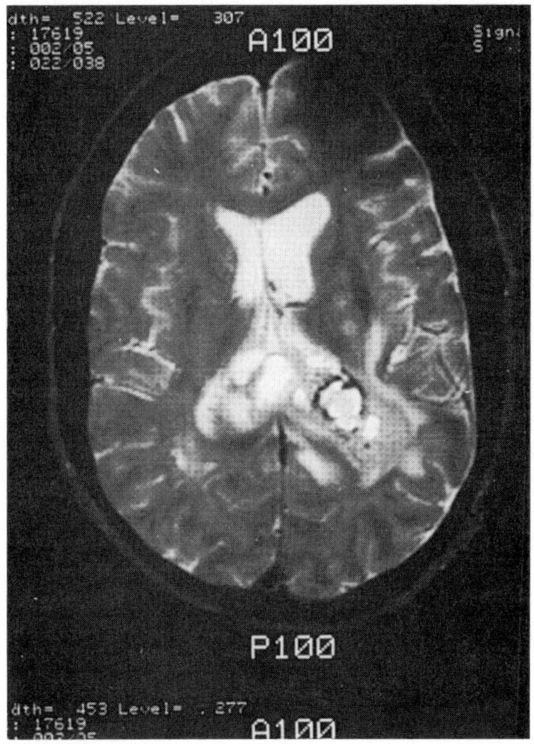

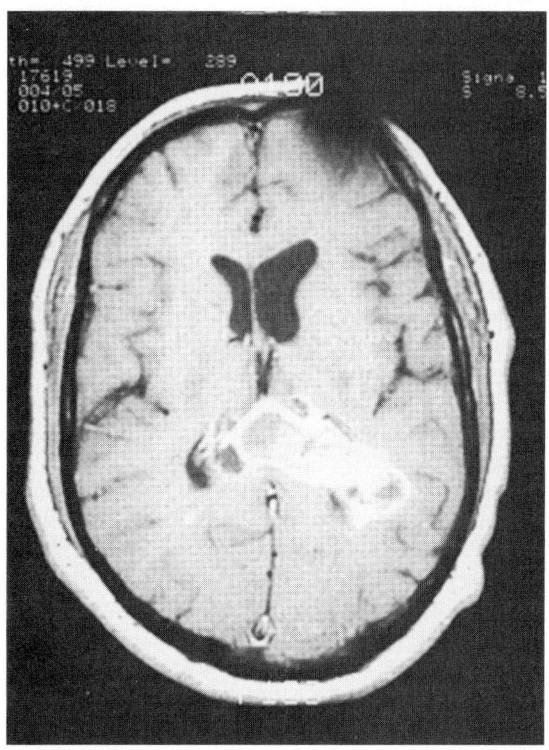

Figure 31-2

Malignant astrocytoma (glioblastoma multiforme). T2-(left) and enhanced T1-weighted (right) MRI illustrate a large tumor deep within the left cerebral hemisphere and extending through the corpus callosum to the right hemisphere. The black rim around a portion of the tumor (left) represents hemorrhage. The patient was a 59-year-old male who presented with seizures.

lature may undergo a sarcomatous transformation with a prominent reticulin and collagen interstitium. The vascular and connective tissue changes suggest the elaboration of a growth factor by the tumor tissue. Originally, the glioblastoma was thought to be derived from and composed of primitive embryonal cells, but it is now generally thought to arise through anaplasia of maturing astrocytes. For these reason, Kernohan and Sayre suggested that the term *glioblastoma* be replaced by *malignant astrocytoma, grade 3 or 4*. Currently, however, the favored terms for the two tumor types are *anaplastic astrocytoma* and *glioblastoma multiforme* (Daumas-Duport et al).

The natural history of glioblastoma is well known. Less than one-fifth of all patients survive for 1 year after the onset of symptoms, and only about 10 percent live beyond 2 years (Shapiro). Age is the most important prognostic factor in this group of tumors; fewer than 10 percent of patients over age 60 survive for 18 months, in comparison to two-thirds of patients under age 40. Cerebral edema and increased intracranial pressure are usually the immediate causes of death.

Treatment Except for palliation, little can be done to alter the course of glioblastoma. For a brief period, corticosteroids, usually dexamethasone in doses of 4 to 10 mg every 4 to 6 h, are helpful if there are symptoms of mass effect such as headache or drowsiness; local signs and surrounding edema tend to improve as well. Anticonvulsants are not required unless there have been seizures, but some neurologists and neurosurgeons administer them in order to preempt a convulsion. Serious skin reactions (erythema multiforme and Stevens-Johnson syndrome) may occur in patients receiving phenytoin at the same time as cranial radiation (Delattre et al). The diagnosis must usually be confirmed by a stereotactic biopsy or by a craniotomy that aims to remove as much tumor as is feasible at the same time. At operation, only part of the tumor can be removed; its multicentricity and diffusely infiltrative character defy the scalpel. Partial resection of the tumor ("debulking"), however, seems to prolong survival marginally. Usually a maximally feasible resection is combined with external beam radiation and chemotherapy. Total cranial irradiation (4500 cGy), boosted with a dose to the region of the tumor (1500 to 2000 cGy), increases survival by 5 months on average (see below). The addition of the chemotherapeutic agent carmustine (BCNU) increases survival only modestly. Somewhat longer survival can be achieved when a combination of drugs—procarbazine, lomustine (CCNU), and vincristine (a combination termed PLV)—is given (Levin et al). Cisplatin and carboplatin provide similar marginal improvement in survival beyond that obtained by debulking and radiation therapy. Brachytherapy (implantation of iodine-125 or iridium-193 beads or needles) and high-dose focused radiation (stereotactic radiosurgery) have so far not significantly altered survival times.

The treatment of recurrent tumor is controversial and must be guided by the location and pattern of tumor growth, the patient's age, and his relative state of health. Almost all glioblastomas recur within 2 cm of their original site and 10 percent develop additional lesions at distant locations. Reoperation is sometimes undertaken for local recurrences, as is brachytherapy, both with uncertain results. The most aggressive approach, a second surgery and chemotherapy, is generally utilized in patients under age 40 who had been treated originally many months earlier.

With aggressive surgical removal and radiotherapy, as described above, median survival for patients with glioblastoma is 12 months, compared to 7 to 9 months without such treatment. The median survival in cases of anaplastic astrocytoma is considerably longer, 2 to 4 years. Viewed from another perspective, in a recent large series, the 18-month postoperative survival was 15 percent in patients with glioblastoma and 62 percent in those with anaplastic astrocytoma.

Astrocytoma Grade 1 and 2 astrocytomas, which constitute between 25 and 30 percent of cerebral gliomas, may occur anywhere in the brain or spinal cord. Favored sites are the cerebrum, cerebellum, hypothalamus, optic nerve and chiasm, and pons. In general, the location of the tumor appears to be influenced by the age of the patient. Astrocytomas of the cerebral hemispheres arise mainly in adults in their third and fourth decades; astrocytomas in other parts of the nervous system, particularly the posterior fossa and optic nerves, are more frequent in children and adolescents. These tumors are classified further according to their histologic characteristics: anaplastic or well-differentiated (protoplasmic or fibrillary); gemistocytic (enlarged cells distended with hyaline and eosinophilic material); pilocytic (elongated, bipolar cells); and mixed astrocytoma-oligodendroglioma types. Many cerebral astrocytomas present as mixed astrocytomas and glioblastomas. The tumor cells contain glial fibrillary protein (GFAP), which is a useful diagnostic marker in biopsy specimens. These distinctions influence the biologic behavior of the astrocytomas and have prognostic importance.

Cerebral astrocytoma is a slowly growing tumor of infiltrative character with a tendency to form large cavities or pseudocysts. Other tumors of this category are noncavitating and appear grayish white, firm, and relatively avascular, almost indistinguishable from normal white matter, with which they merge imperceptibly. Fine granules of calcium may be deposited in parts of the tumor, but this finding in a slow-growing intracerebral tumor is more characteristic of an oligodendroglioma. The CSF is acellular; the only abnormalities in some cases are the increased pressure and protein content. The tumor may distort the lateral and third ventricles and displace the anterior and middle cerebral arteries (seen in CT scans and arteriograms; see Fig. 31-3). Microscopi-

Figure 31-3

Astrocytoma of the left frontal lobe; the T2-weighted MRI shows an infiltrating tumor with minimal mass effect and slight edema. The degree of enhancement varies.

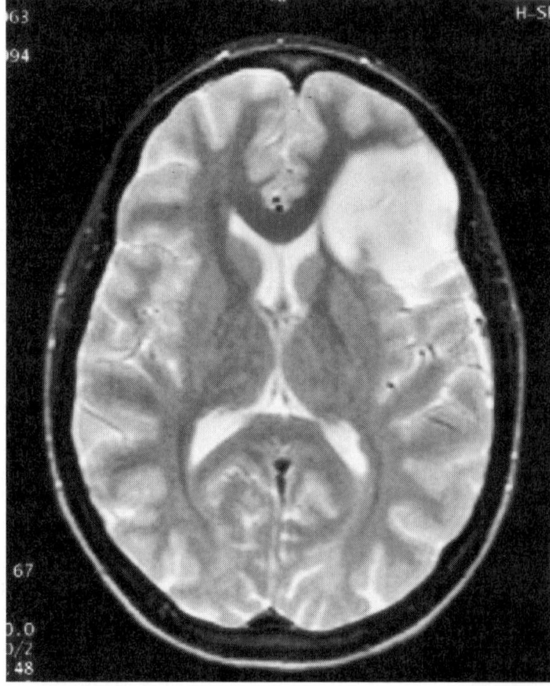

cally, most tumors are composed of well-differentiated astrocytes of fibrillary type.

In about half the patients with astrocytoma, the opening symptom is a focal or generalized seizure, and between 60 and 75 percent of patients have recurrent seizures in the course of their illness. Other subtle cerebral symptoms follow after months, sometimes after years. Headaches and signs of increased intracranial pressure are relatively late occurrences.

In children, the tumor is usually in the cerebellum (Fig. 31-4) and declares itself by some combination of gait unsteadiness, unilateral ataxia, and increased intracranial pressure (headaches, vomiting). In contrast to glioblastoma, the average survival period after the first symptom is 5 to 6 years in cerebral astrocytomas and 8 years or more in cerebellar ones (see also page 718).

MRI may be helpful in distinguishing fibrillary from pilocytic astrocytomas. Pilocytic types are sharply demarcated, with smooth borders and little edema. On T1-weighted MRI they are isointense or hypointense and on T2 sequences, hyperintense. There tends to be marked enhancement of the tumors after gadolinium infusion. Cyst formation and small amounts of calcium are common, especially in cerebellar tumors. The more frequent fibrillary tumors have a less stereotyped appearance, generally taking the form of a hypodense mass with less well defined borders and little or no contrast enhancement.

Figure 31-4

Cystic astrocytoma of the cerebellum. MRI demonstrates the large cystic component of the tumor (smaller arrow) and the solid tissue component (larger arrow). (From Bisese JH: Cranial MRI. New York, McGraw-Hill, 1991 by permission.)

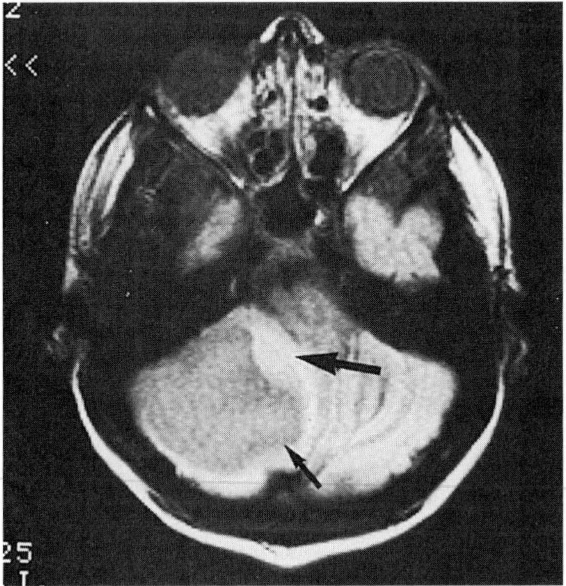

Excision of part of the cerebral astrocytoma, particularly the cystic part, may allow survival in a functional state for many years. The cystic astrocytoma of the cerebellum is particularly benign in its overall behavior. In such cases, resection of the tumor nodule is of particular importance in preventing a recurrence. In recent series, the rate of survival 5 years after successful surgery has been over 90 percent (Pencalet et al). The outcome is less assured when the tumor also involves the brainstem and cannot be safely resected.

The natural history of low-grade gliomas is to grow slowly and eventually undergo malignant transformation. The duration of progression and the latency of recurrence with modern treatment may extend for 3 to 7 years. A survey of the outcome of these low-grade supratentorial tumors showed that 10-year survival after operation was from 11 to 40 percent provided that 5300 cGy was given postoperatively (Shaw et al). In younger patients, particularly if the neurologic examination is normal or nearly so, radiation can be delayed and the course of the tumor evaluated by frequent imaging procedures. *Delaying radiation in younger patients may avoid the dementia and hypopituitarism that it sometimes produces.* An increase in seizures or worsening neurologic signs then presses one to turn to radiation or further surgery. Although repeated operations prolong life in some patients, chemotherapy has as yet no established place in the treatment of low-grade pure astrocytomas. However, tumors with an oligodendroglial component may respond to combination chemotherapy that is used for the treatment of anaplastic oligodendroglioma as descried below.

The special features of astrocytomas of the pons, hypothalamus, optic nerves, and chiasm are discussed further on in this chapter.

Gliomatosis Cerebri In this variant of high-grade glioma there is a diffuse infiltration of neoplastic glial cells, involving much of one cerebral hemisphere or both, with sparing of neuronal elements and without a discrete tumor mass being identified. Whether this gliomatosis represents neoplastic transformation of multicentric origin or direct spread from one or more small neoplastic foci is not known. For these reasons, the tumor is impossible to classify (or to grade) using the conventional brain tumor schemes.

Many small series of gliomatosis cerebri have been reported since Nevin introduced this term in 1938, but no distinctive clinical picture has emerged (Dunn and Kernohan). Impairment of intellect, headache, seizures, and papilledema are the major manifestations and do not set these cases apart on a clinical basis from the malignant astrocytoma, in which the tumor may also be more widespread than the macroscopic picture suggests. CT scans and MRI reveal small ventricles and one or more large confluent areas of signal change (Fig. 31-5). Imaging studies characteristically show the tumor crossing and thickening the corpus callosum. Contrast infusion and gadolinium enhancement tend to be scant, differentiating the tumor from cerebral lymphoma, which otherwise may give a similar appearance. The spinal fluid is acellular, with slight elevation of protein. Corticosteroids have little clinical effect, possibly because of a paucity of edema, and the benefit of radiation is uncertain. When a large region is infiltrated, particularly in the temporal lobe, surgical debulking may be temporarily life-prolonging, but otherwise surgery is futile.

Figure 31-5

Gliomatosis cerebri invading both hemispheres. FLAIR MRI shows large confluent areas of involvement. There is slight enhancement at the edges of the lesions after gadolinium infusion, and the corpus callosum is thickened. The patient was mentally slow but had no other neurologic signs.

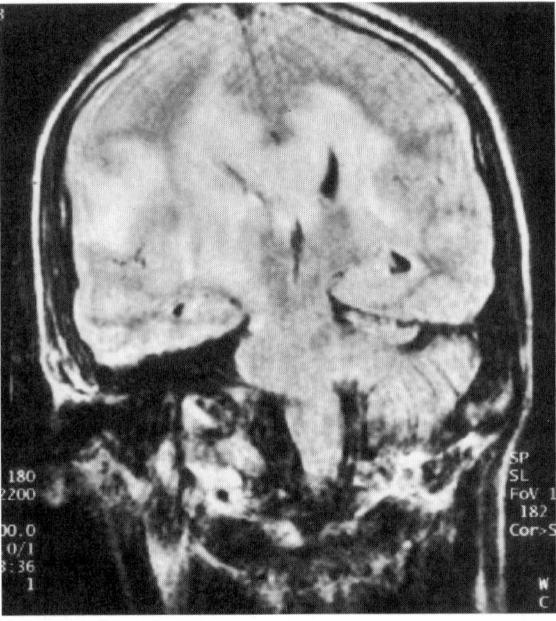

Oligodendroglioma This tumor was first identified by Bailey and Cushing in 1926 and described more fully by Bailey and Bucy in 1929. The tumor is derived from oligodendrocytes or their precursor cells and may occur at any age, most often in the third and fourth decades, with an earlier peak at 6 to 12 years. It is relatively infrequent, constituting about 5 to 7 percent of all intracranial gliomas. Males outnumber females 2:1. In some cases the tumor may be recognized at surgery by its pink-gray color and multilobular form, its relative avascularity and firmness (slightly tougher than surrounding brain), and its tendency to encapsulate and form calcium and small cysts. Most oligodendrogliomas, however, are grossly indistinguishable from other gliomas, and a proportion—up to half in some series—are mixed oligoastrocytomas, suggesting that their precursor cell is pluripotential.

The neoplastic oligodendrocyte has a small round nucleus and a halo of unstained cytoplasm ("fried egg" appearance). The cell processes are few and stubby, visualized only with silver carbonate stains. Some of the gliofibrillary oligodendrocytes have intense immunoreactivity to glial fibrillary acidic protein (GFAP), similar to normal myelin-forming oligodendrocytes. Microscopic calcifications are observed frequently, mainly in relation to zones of necrosis.

The most common sites of this tumor are the frontal and temporal lobes (40 to 70 percent), often deep in the white matter, with a streak of calcium but little or no surrounding edema (Fig. 31-6). Sometimes the tumor presents in a lateral ventricle. Rarely it occurs in other parts of the nervous system. By extending to the pial surface or ependymal wall, the tumor may metastasize distantly in ventricular and subarachnoid spaces, accounting for 11 percent of the Polmeteer and Kernohan series of gliomas with meningeal dissemination (less frequent than medulloblastoma and glioblastoma; see also Yung et al). The tumor does not lend itself to the glioma grading scale, but malignant degeneration, evidenced by greater cellularity and by numerous and abnormal mitoses, and endothelial proliferation occur in about one-third of the cases. Such anaplastic tumors are sometimes called *oligodendroblastomas*. In the oligoastrocytomas, either cell type may be anaplastic.

The typical oligodendroglioma grows slowly. As with astrocytomas, the first symptom in more than half the patients is a focal or generalized seizure; seizures often persist for many years before other symptoms develop. Approximately 15 percent of patients enter the hospital with early symptoms and signs of increased intracranial pressure; an even a smaller number have

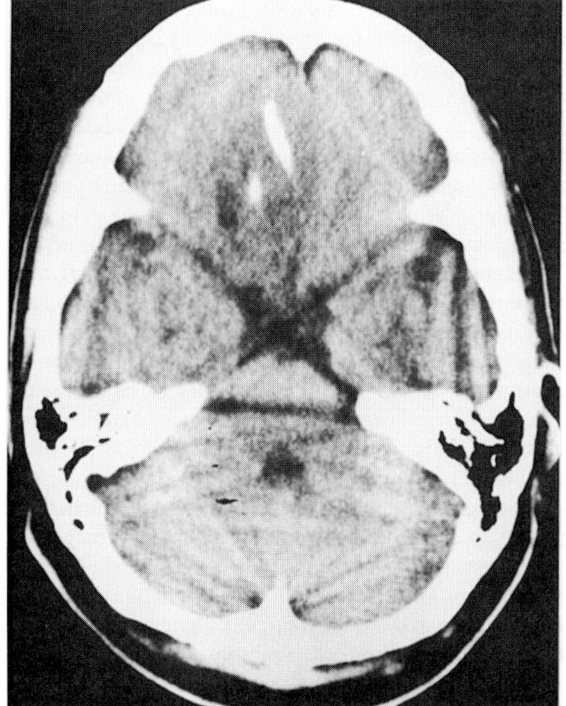

Figure 31-6

An indolent oligodendroglioma of the frontal lobe with typical calcification.

focal cerebral signs (hemiparesis). Much less frequent are unilateral extrapyramidal rigidity, cerebellar ataxia, Parinaud syndrome, intratumoral hemorrhage, and meningeal oligodendrogliosis (cranial-spinal nerve palsies, hydrocephalus, lymphocytes and tumor cells in CSF).

The appearance on imaging studies is variable, but the most typical is a hypodense mass near the cortical surface with relatively well-defined borders. Calcium is seen in CT scans in more than half the cases and is a helpful diagnostic sign (Fig. 31-6), but it should also raise the possibility of an arteriovenous malformation, a low-grade astrocytoma, or a meningioma. Oligodendrogliomas generally do not demonstrate contrast enhancement, but anaplastic ones and the mixed tumors may do so.

Surgical excision followed by radiation therapy has been the conventional treatment for oligodendroglioma. However, because of uncertainty as to the histologic classification of many of the reported cases, it is not clear whether radiation therapy is attended by longer survival. Well-differentiated oligodendrogliomas should probably not receive radiation. Most oligodendrogliomas, especially anaplastic ones, both newly discovered and recurrent, often respond impressively to chemotherapeutic agents, particularly to PCV—a combination of procarbazine, lomustine (CCNU), and vincristine given in approximately six cycles (Cairncross and MacDonald). Mixed oligodendrogliomas and astrocytomas should generally be treated like astrocytomas, with the addition of chemotherapy as recommended in some centers.

Ependymoma (See also page 703) This tumor proves to be more complex and variable than other gliomas. Correctly diagnosed by Virchow as early as 1863, its origin from ependymal cells was first suggested by Mallory, who found the typical blepharoplasts (small, darkly staining cytoplasmic dots related to the ciliation of these cells). Two types were recognized by Bailey and Cushing: one was the ependymoma, and the other, with more malignant and invasive properties, was the ependymoblastoma. More recently a myxopapillomatous type, localized exclusively in the filum terminale of the spinal cord, has been identified (see Chap. 44).

Ependymomas are derived from relatively differentiated ependymal cells—i.e., the cells lining the ventricles of the brain and the central canal of the spinal cord. These cells have both glial and epithelial characteristics. As one might expect, the tumors grow either into the ventricle or adjacent brain tissue. The most common cerebral site is the fourth ventricle; less often, they occur in the lateral or third ventricles (page 703). In the spinal cord, most ependymomas originate in the lumbosacral regions, from the conus or filum terminale. Grossly, those in the fourth ventricle are grayish pink, firm, cauliflower-like growths; those in the cerebrum, arising from the wall of the lateral ventricle, may be large (several centimeters in diameter), reddish gray, and softer and more clearly demarcated from adjacent tissue than astrocytomas, but they are not encapsulated. The tumor cells tend to form canals (rosettes) or circular arrangements around blood vessels (pseudorosettes). Some ependymomas, called epithelial, are densely cellular and anaplastic; others are better differentiated and form papillae. Some of the well-differentiated fourth ventricular tumors are probably derived from subependymal astrocytes (see later in chapter and Fig. 31-12).

Anaplastic ependymomas are identified by their high mitotic activity and endothelial proliferation, nuclear atypia, and necrosis. The correlations between histopathologic features and clinical outcomes have not been well defined, however.

Approximately 6 percent of all intracranial gliomas are ependymomas; the percentage is higher in children (8 percent). About 40 percent of the infratentorial ependymomas occur in the first decade of life, a few as early as the first year. The supratentorial ones are more evenly distributed among all age groups, but in general the age incidence is lower than in other malignant gliomas.

The *symptomatology* depends on the location of the growth. The clinical manifestations of fourth ventricular tumors are described further on in this chapter; the point to be made here is the frequent occurrence of hydrocephalus and signs of raised intracranial pressure (manifest in children by lethargy, nausea, vomiting, and papilledema). Cerebral ependymomas otherwise resemble the other gliomas in their clinical expression. Seizures occur in approximately one-third of the cases.

The imaging characteristics are rather different from those of other tumors. In the CT scan one observes a well-demarcated heterogeneous hyperdense mass with contrast enhancement. Calcification and some degree of cystic change are common in supratentorial tumors but less common in infratentorial ones. There are mixed signal characteristics on MRI, generally hypointense on T1 sequences and hyperintense on T2. *An intraventricular location supports the diagnosis of ependymoma*, but meningioma and a number of other tumors may be found in this location.

The interval between the first symptom to diagnosis ranges from 4 weeks, in the most malignant types, to 7 to 8 years. In a follow-up study of 101 cases in Norway, where ependymomas made up 1.2 percent of all primary intracranial tumors (and 32 percent of intraspinal tumors), the postoperative survival was poor. Within a year, 47 percent of the patients had died, although 13 percent were alive after 10 years. Doubtless the prognosis depends on the degree of anaplasia (Mørk and Løken) and whether the tumor is operable. Surgical removal is supplemented by radiation therapy, particularly to address the high rate of seeding of the ventricles and spinal axis. In the treatment of cerebral ependymoblastomas, antitumor drugs are often used in combination with radiation therapy.

Meningioma (See also page 717) This is a benign tumor, first illustrated by Matthew Bailie in his *Morbid Anatomy* (1787) and first recognized by Bright, in 1831, as originating from the dura mater or arachnoid. It was analyzed from every point of view by Harvey Cushing and was the subject of one of his most important monographs. Meningiomas represent about 15 percent of all primary intracranial tumors; they are more common in women than in men (2:1) and have their highest incidence in the sixth and seventh decades. Some are familial. There is evidence that persons who have undergone radiation therapy to the scalp or cranium are particularly vulnerable to the development of meningiomas and that the tumors appear at an earlier age (Rubinstein et al). There are a number of reports of a meningioma developing at the site of previous trauma, such as a fracture line, but the association is uncertain. Many meningiomas are associated with a karyotype abnormality—a loss of the long arm of chromosome 22 or a deletion of part of it. A number of familial syndromes are associated with meningiomas, the most important being neurofibromatosis type 2, the gene for which is also located on chromosome 22p. Some meningiomas, like many other neoplasms, contain estrogen and progesterone receptors. The implications of these findings are not yet clear but may relate to the increased incidence of the tumor in women, its tendency to enlarge during pregnancy, and an association with breast cancer.

The precise origin of meningiomas is still not settled. According to Rubinstein, they may arise from dural fibroblasts, but, in our opinion, more clearly from arachnoidal (meningothelial) cells, in particular from those forming the arachnoid villi. Since the clusters of arachnoidal cells penetrate the dura in largest number in the vicinity of venous sinuses, these are the sites of predilection. Grossly, the tumor is firm, gray, and sharply circumscribed, and it takes the shape of the space in which it grows; thus, some tumors are flat and plaque-like, others are round and lobulated. They may indent the brain and acquire a pia-arachnoid covering as part of their capsule, but they are clearly demarcated from the brain tissue (extra-axial) except in the unusual circumstance of an invasive meningioma. Rarely, they arise from arachnoidal cells within the choroid plexus, forming an intraventricular meningioma. Microscopically, the cells are relatively uniform, with round or elongated nuclei, visible cytoplasmic membrane, and a characteristic tendency to encircle one another, forming whorls and *psammoma bodies* (laminated calcific concretions). A notable electron microscopic characteristic is the formation of membranous interdigitations between cells and the presence of desmosomes (Kepes). Cushing and Eisenhardt and, more recently, the World Health Organization (Lopes et al) have divided meningiomas into many subtypes depending on their mesenchymal variations, the character of the stroma, and their relative vascularity, but the value of such classifications is debatable. Currently neuropathologists recognize the meningothelial (syncytial) form as being the most common. It is readily distinguished from other nonmeningothelial tumors such as hemangiopericytomas, fibroblastomas, and chondrosarcomas.

The usual sites are the sylvian region, superior parasagittal surface of the frontal and parietal lobes, olfactory groove, lesser wing of the sphenoid bone, tuberculum sellae, superior surface of the cerebellum, cerebellopontine angle, and spinal canal. Some meningiomas—such as those of the olfactory groove, sphenoid wing, and tuberculum sellae—may express themselves by highly distinctive syndromes that are diagnostic in themselves; these are described further on in this chapter. Rarely they are multiple. Inasmuch as they extend to the dural surface, they often invade and erode the cranial bones or excite an osteoblastic reaction. Sometimes they give rise to an exostosis on the external surface of the skull. The following remarks apply to meningiomas of the parasagittal, sylvian, and other surface areas of the cerebrum.

Small meningiomas, less than 2.0 cm in diameter, are often found at autopsy in middle-aged and elderly persons without having caused symptoms. Only when they exceed a certain size and indent the brain do they alter function. The size that must be reached before symptoms appear varies with the size of the space in which the tumor grows and the surrounding anatomic arrangements. Focal seizures are often an early sign of meningiomas that overlie the cerebrum. The parasagittal frontal-parietal meningioma may cause a slowly progressive spastic weakness or numbness of one leg and later of both legs, and incontinence in the late stages. The sylvian tumors are manifest by a variety of motor, sensory, and aphasic disturbances in accord with their location, and by seizures.

In the past, before brain imaging techniques became available, the meningioma often gave rise to neurologic signs for many years before the diagnosis was established, attesting to their slow rate of growth. Even now some tumors reach enormous size, to the point of causing papilledema, before the patient comes to medical attention. A few may be detected in plain films or in CT scans in individuals with unrelated neurologic diseases. Increased intracranial pressure eventually occurs, but it is less frequent with meningiomas than with gliomas.

As mentioned above, the diagnosis of meningiomas is greatly facilitated by their ready visualization with contrast-enhanced CT and MRI (Figs. 31-7 and 31-8) and by arteriography, all of which reveal their tendency to calcify and their prominent vascularity, changes that are reflected by homogeneous contrast enhancement on CT and MRI or by "tumor blush" on angiography. They characteristically take the form of smoothly contoured masses, sometimes lobulated, with one edge abutting the inner surface of the skull or the falcine or tentorial dura. On the CT scan they are isointense or slightly hyperintense unless enhanced by contrast infusion; calcification at the outer surface or heterogeneously through the mass is common. Except for the mass effect they cause, they may be difficult to appreciate on MRI scans that are performed without gadolinium. The amount of edema surrounding the tumor is variable. The CSF protein is usually elevated.

Surgical excision should afford permanent cure in all accessible surface tumors. Recurrence is likely if removal is incomplete, but for some the growth rate is so slow that there may be a latency of many years. A few show malignant qualities—i.e., a high mitotic index, nuclear atypia, marked nuclear and cellular pleomorphism, and invasiveness of brain. Their regrowth is then rapid if they are not completely excised. Tumors that lie beneath the hypothalamus, along the medial part of the sphenoid bone and parasellar region, or anterior to the brainstem are the most difficult to remove surgically. By invading adjacent bone, they may become impossible to remove totally. Carefully planned radiation therapy is beneficial in cases that are inoperable and when the tumor is incompletely removed or shows malignant characteristics (Kornblith et al). Smaller tumors at the base of the skull can be obliterated or greatly reduced in size by focused radiation, probably with less risk than surgery would pose (Chang et al). Conventional chemotherapy is probably ineffective; hormonal therapy with the antiprogestin agent mifepristone (RU 486) has been used with variable results but is still under study (McCutcheon). More recently it has been suggested that hydroxyurea has the capacity to shrink unresectable and recurrent meningiomas (Schrell et al); this mode of treatment is still being evaluated.

Primary Cerebral Lymphoma As mentioned earlier, this tumor has assumed increasing significance in the last two decades because of its frequency in the AIDS and other immunosuppressed populations. However, it is also occurring with increased frequency in immunocompetent persons. The latter finding has no evident explanation, although theories abound. There is a preponderance of men with the peak incidence in the fifth through seventh decades, or in the third and fourth decades in patients with AIDS.

For many years it was taught that this tumor is a histiocytic sarcoma, originating in the reticuloendothelial

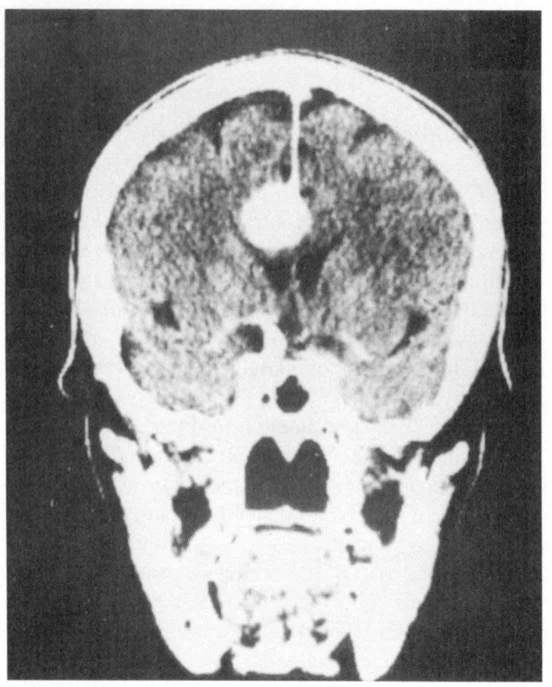

A

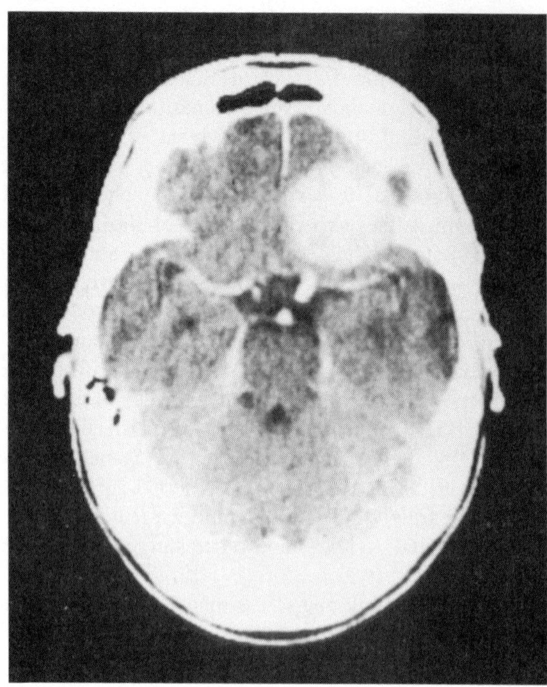

B

Figure 31-7

Contrast-enhanced CT scans. A. *Falx meningioma; coronal image.* B. *Sphenoid wing meningioma.*

system, and that the meningeal and perivascular histiocytes and the microgliocytes, the representatives of this system in the brain, are its sources. Confusion as to the cell type came in part from failure to distinguish tumor from stromal cells. Hence the older terms *reticulum cell sarcoma* and *microglioma.* Now it is postulated, on the basis of immunocytochemical studies, that the tumor cells are B lymphocytes, and that the tumor corresponds histologically to what Rappaport called a large-cell or histiocytic type of malignant lymphoma. As matters now stand, most pathologists believe that the B lymphocyte or lymphoblast is the tumor cell, whereas the fine reticulum and "microgliacytes" are secondary interstitial reactions derived from fibroblasts and microglia or histiocytes. T-cell lymphomas of the nervous system are rare but do occur in both immunocompetent patients and in immunosuppressed patients with AIDS. Since the brain is devoid of lymphatic tissue, it is uncertain how this tumor arises; one theory holds that it represents a systemic lymphoma with a particular and strong proclivity to metastasize to the nervous system. However, systemic lymphomas of the usual kind only rarely metastasize, as discussed further on, under "Involvement of the Nervous System in Systemic Lymphoma."

The tumor may arise primarily in any part of the cerebrum, cerebellum, or brainstem, with 60 percent being in the cerebral hemispheres; they may be either monofocal or multifocal. Periventricular localization is common. Vitreous, uveal, and retinal (ocular) involvement occurs in 20 percent of cases; here vitreous biopsy may be diagnostic, but it is not often performed. Two-thirds of patients with ocular lymphoma alone will have cerebral involvement within a year. The pia-arachnoid may be infiltrated, and a purely meningeal form that involves peripheral and cranial nerves is also known. Most such cases of what has been termed *neurolymphomatosis* present with painful, predominantly motor polyradiculopathies. One of our patients presented with a flaccid paraparesis and back and sciatic pain; MRI showed tumor infiltrating the cauda equina nerve roots and contiguous meninges.

The tumor forms a pinkish gray, soft, ill-defined, infiltrative mass, difficult at times to distinguish from a malignant glioma. Perivascular and meningeal spread results in shedding of cells into the CSF, accounting perhaps for the multifocal appearance of the tumor in almost half of the cases. The tumor is highly cellular, with little tendency to necrosis. The nuclei are oval or bean-shaped

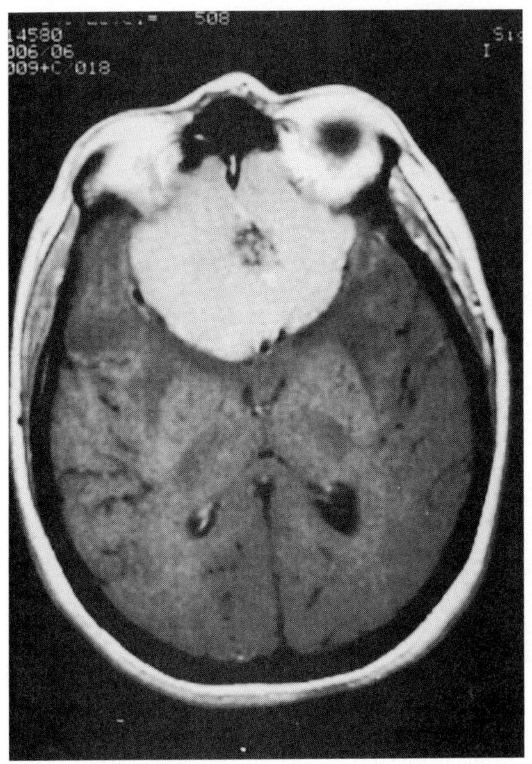

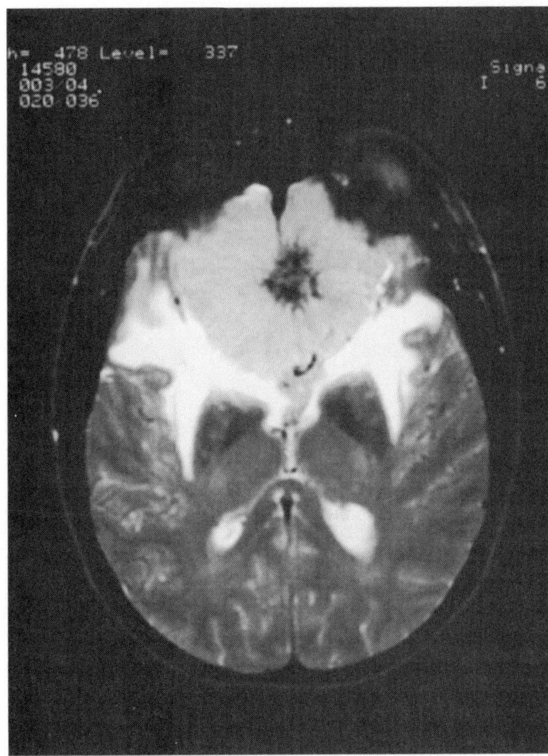

Figure 31-8

Meningioma. MRI with and without gadolinium enhancement showing a large subfrontal mass with central calcification and prominent surrounding vasogenic edema.

with scant cytoplasm, and mitotic figures are numerous. B-cell markers applied to fixed tissue define the cell population as monoclonal and identify the tumor cell type. The stainability of reticulum and microglial cells, the latter by silver carbonate, also serves to distinguish this tumor microscopically.

Primary lymphoma involving the cerebral hemispheres pursues a clinical course somewhat similar to that of the glioblastoma but with a vastly different response to treatment. The interval between the first symptom and operation has been approximately 3 months. Behavioral and personality changes, confusion, dizziness, and focal cerebral signs predominate over headache and other signs of increased intracranial pressure as presenting manifestations. Most cases occur in adult life, but some have been observed in children, in whom the tumor may simulate the cerebellar symptomatology of medulloblastoma. The finding on CT and MRI of one or several dense, homogeneous, and enhancing periventricular masses is characteristic (Fig. 31-9). However, nodular, ring-like enhancement also occurs, and any part of the brain may be involved. The radiologic appearance in AIDS patients is less predictable and may be difficult to distinguish from that of toxoplasmosis or another process with which lymphoma often coexists. Characteristic is the disappearance of the lesions or complete but transient resolution of contrast enhancement in response to corticosteroids. Lymphocytic and mononuclear pleocytosis of CSF is more frequent than with gliomas and metastatic tumors. The immunohistochemical demonstration in CSF of monoclonal lymphocytes or an elevated beta microglobulin points to leptomeningeal spread of the tumor (Li et al), but frequently the diagnosis is not possible from CSF cytologic examination alone.

As already indicated, patients with acquired immunodeficiency syndrome (AIDS) and less common immunodeficiency states, such as the Wiskott-Aldrich syndrome and ataxia-telangiectasia, and those receiving immunosuppressive drugs for long periods, such as patients undergoing renal transplantation, are particularly liable to develop this type of primary cerebral

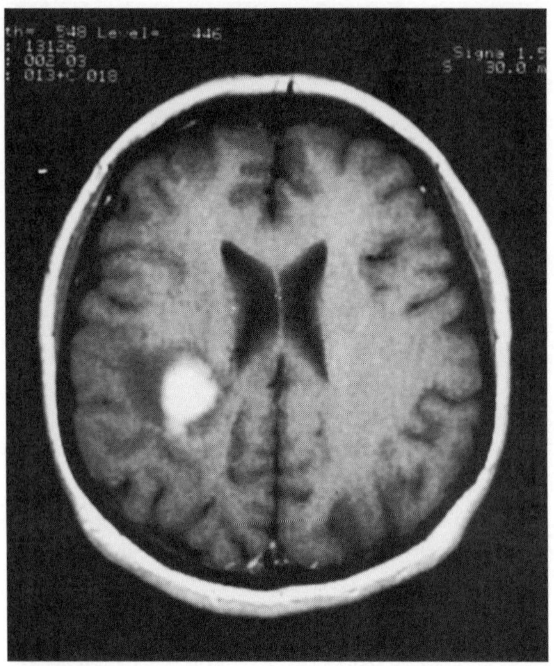

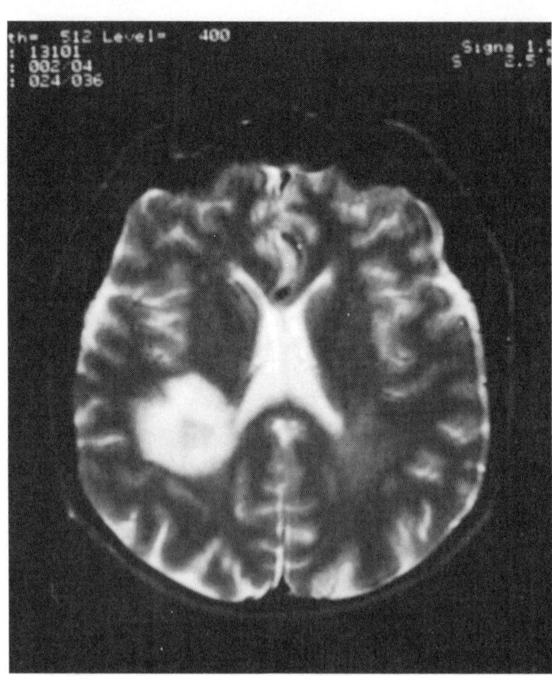

Figure 31-9

Cerebral lymphoma. T1-weighted MR image after gadolinium infusion (left) *and T2-weighted image* (right) *demonstrating a solitary enhancing mass deep within the right hemisphere.*

lymphoma. Eighty percent of the tumors in immunosuppressed patients contain the Epstein-Barr virus (EBV) genome, suggesting a pathogenetic role for the virus (Bashir and colleagues). The EBV genome has been found in the lymphoma cells in both immunocompetent and immunosuppressed patients (Hochberg and Miller). Sometimes this tumor appears as a complication of an obscure medical condition such as salivary and lacrimal gland enlargement (Mikulicz syndrome). In only a few patients is there systemic lymphoma (usually of the lungs).

Because the tumors are deep and often multicentric, surgical resection is ineffective except in rare instances. Stereotactic needle biopsy is the preferred method of establishing the histologic diagnosis. Treatment with cranial irradiation and corticosteroids often produces a partial, or rarely, complete response, as remarked above, but the tumor recurs in more than 90 percent of patients. Until recently the median survival of patients treated in this way has been 10 to 18 months, but less in those with AIDS or in individuals who are otherwise immunocompromised. In immunocompetent patients, the addition of intrathecal methotrexate and intravenous cytosine arabinoside increases median survival to more than 3 years (DeAngelis), and apparent cure is not unknown. However, this combined treatment is associated with a high risk of leukoencephalopathy (see further on and Fig. 31-22) and causes considerable unpleasant systemic side effects.

More recent regimens as outlined by Glass and colleagues, consist of several cycles of intravenous methotrexate (3.5 g/m^2) and citrovorum, administered at 2- to 3-week intervals and at times continued indefinitely, if tolerated. The side effects of these treatments are minimal and there is no need for repeated lumbar punctures or the placement of an Ommaya reservoir. Most of our patients have not developed mucositis or the other side effects of chemotherapy. Radiation treatment may be used subsequently, but there is a high incidence of delayed leukoencephalopathy and dementia. Ocular lymphoma is eradicated only by radiation. Corticosteroids are added at any point as needed to control prominent neurologic symptoms. The median survival time has been in the range of 3.5 years with intravenous methotrexate alone and 4 years or more if radiation is given subsequently. Some patients are alive at 10 years.

Metastatic Carcinoma Among secondary intracranial tumors, only metastatic carcinoma occurs with high frequency. Occasionally one encounters a rhabdomyosarcoma, Ewing tumor, carcinoid, etc., but these tumors are so infrequent that their cerebral metastases seldom become a matter of diagnostic concern. The pathophysiology of metastatic carcinoma—the complex biologic mechanisms that govern the detachment of tumor cells from the primary growth, their transport to distant tissues, and their implantation on the capillary endothelium of the particular organ in which they will eventually grow—have been capably reviewed by Rusciano and Burger and by Posner.

Autopsy studies disclose intracranial metastases in approximately 25 percent of patients who die of cancer (Posner). About 80 percent of the metastases are in the cerebral hemispheres and 20 percent in posterior fossa structures, corresponding roughly to the relative size and weights of these portions of the brain and their blood flow. Cancers of the pelvis and colon are exceptional in this respect, tending to spread to the posterior fossa. Intracranial metastases assume three main patterns—those to the skull and dura, those to the brain itself, and those spreading diffusely through the craniospinal meninges (meningeal carcinomatosis).

Metastases to the skull and dura can occur with any tumor that metastasizes to bone, but they are particularly common with carcinoma of the breast and prostate and with multiple myeloma. These secondary deposits usually occur without metastases to the brain itself and reach the skull either via the systemic circulation (as in carcinoma of the breast) or via Batson's vertebral venous plexus—a valveless system of veins that runs the length of the vertebral column from the pelvic veins to the large venous sinuses of the skull, bypassing the systemic circulation (as in carcinoma of the prostate). Metastatic tumors of the convexity of the skull are usually asymptomatic, but those at the base may involve the cranial nerve roots or the pituitary body. Bony metastases are readily recognized on bone and CT scans and most are evident in plain films. Occasionally, a carcinoma metastasizes to the subdural surface and compresses the brain, like a subdural hematoma.

Apart from the above, carcinomas reach the brain by hematogenous spread. Almost one-third of them originate in the lung and half this number in the breast; melanoma is the third most frequent source, and the gastrointestinal tract (particularly the colon and rectum) and kidney are the next most common. Carcinomas of the gallbladder, liver, thyroid, testicle, uterus, ovary, pancreas, etc., account for the remainder. Carcinomas of the prostate, esophagus, oropharynx, and skin (except for melanoma) almost never metastasize to the substance of the brain. From a somewhat different point of view, certain neoplasms are particularly prone to metastasize to the brain—75 percent of melanomas do so, 57 percent of testicular tumors, and 35 percent of bronchial carcinomas, of which 40 percent are small-cell tumors (Posner and Chernick). According to these authors, the cerebral metastasis is solitary in 47 percent of cases, a somewhat higher figure than that observed in our practice and reported by others (see Henson and Urich). The metastatic tumors most likely to be single come from kidney, breast, thyroid, and lung (adenocarcinoma). Small-cell carcinomas and melanomas tend to be multiple.

Generally the cerebral metastasis forms a circumscribed mass, usually solid but sometimes in the form of a ring (i.e., cystic), and excites rather little glial reaction but much regional vasogenic edema. Often edema alone is evident on imaging studies until administration of contrast exposes small tumor nodules (Fig. 31-10). Metastases from melanoma and chorioepithelioma are

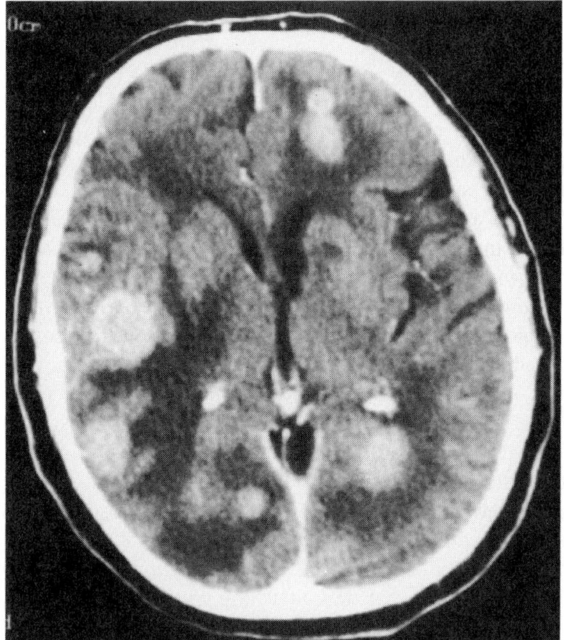

Figure 31-10

Contrast-enhanced CT scan showing multiple metastases from bronchogenic carcinoma. Each lesion is surrounded by edema.

ususlly hemorrhagic, but some from the lung, thyroid, and kidney have this characteristic as well.

The usual clinical picture of *metastatic carcinoma of the brain* is much like that of glioblastoma multiforme. Headache, seizures, focal weakness, mental and behavioral abnormalities, ataxia, aphasia, and signs of increased intracranial pressure—all inexorably progressive over a few weeks or months—are the common clinical manifestations. Also, a number of unusual syndromes may occur. One that presents particular difficulty in diagnosis is a syndrome of diffuse cerebral disturbance with headache, nervousness, depressed mood, trembling, confusion, and forgetfulness, resembling a relatively rapid dementia from degenerative disease. *Cerebellar metastasis*, with headache, dizziness, and ataxia (the latter being brought out only by having the patient walk) is another condition that is difficult to recognize.

Sometimes the onset of symptoms from brain metastases is abrupt or "stroke-like" rather than insidious. Some cases of sudden onset can be explained by bleeding into the tumor and others perhaps by tumor embolism, causing cerebral infarction with early regression of symptoms and later progression from the metastasis left in its wake. Also, marantic endocarditis with cerebral embolism must be suspected when a stroke-like event occurs in a tumor patient. It is not unusual for one or other of these neurologic manifestations to precede those of lung carcinoma.

When any of the several clinical syndromes due to metastatic tumor is fully developed, diagnosis is relatively easy. If only headache and vomiting are present, a common error is to explain these symptoms on a psychologic basis or to attribute them to migraine or tension headache. One should invoke such explanations only if the patient has the standard symptoms of one of these conditions. CT scanning, with and without contrast, will detect practically all sizable (>1 cm) metastases. In addition, MRI will expose associated leptomeningeal disease and is more sensitive to small cerebellar deposits. *Multiple nodular deposits of tumor in the brain on imaging studies most clearly distinguish metastatic cancer from other tumors* but at the same time raises the possibility, on radiologic grounds, of brain abscesses.

Metastatic disease must be distinguished from a primary tumor of the brain and not be confused with certain neurologic syndromes that sometimes accompany carcinoma but are not due to the invasion or compression of the nervous system by tumor. The latter, referred to as *paraneoplastic disorders*, include polyneuropathy (especially with carcinoma of the lung), polymyositis, cerebellar degeneration (ovarian and other carcinomas), necrotizing myelopathy (rare) and certain cerebral disorders (progressive multifocal leukoencephalopathy and "limbic encephalitis"). These latter syndromes are discussed further on, under "Remote Effects of Neoplasia on the Nervous System."

In addition to the aforementioned conditions, there are many patients with cancer who exhibit symptoms of an altered mental state without evidence of metastases or a recognizable paraneoplastic disorder. These mental symptoms probably arise on the basis of systemic metabolic disturbances, drugs, and psychologic reactions and have yet to be clearly delineated. Problems of this type were noted in a high percentage of cancer patients seen in consultation at the Memorial Sloan-Kettering Cancer Center (Clouston et al).

The treatment of secondary (metastatic) tumors of the nervous system is undergoing change. The typical program utilizes various combinations of corticosteroids, brain irradiation, surgical intervention, and chemotherapy (see review by O'Neill et al). Corticosteroids produce prompt improvement, but sustained use is restricted by their many side effects and eventual loss of efficacy. Most patients also benefit from the use of whole-brain irradiation, usually administered over a 2-week period, in 10 doses of 300 cGy each. Focused radiotherapy ("gamma knife") is a suitable alternative.

In patients with a single parenchymatous metastasis (shown to be single by gadolinium-enhanced MRI), surgical extirpation may be undertaken provided that growth of the primary tumor and its systemic metastases is under good control and the cerebral metastasis is accessible to the surgeon and not located in a strategic motor or language area of the brain; usually excision is followed by radiation therapy. Patchell and coworkers have shown that survival and the interval between treatment and recurrence are longer and that the quality of life is better in patients treated in this way than in comparable patients treated with radiation alone. Single or dual metastases from hypernephroma, melanoma, and adenocarcinoma of the gastrointestinal tract lend themselves best to surgical removal, sometimes repeatedly. Several clinical trials of patients with small-cell carcinoma of the lung (Nugent et al) suggest that prophylactic irradiation of the neuraxis decreases the occurrence of metastases but does not prolong survival. Also, there is growing evidence that some metastatic brain tumors are quite sensitive to certain chemotherapeutic agents, especially if the primary tumor is also sensitive. Intrathecal and intraventricular chemotherapy are not thought to be of value in the treatment of parenchymal metastases. Immunotherapy has not yet been widely employed. The prophylactic use of anticonvulsants is still controversial. The balance of evidence favors their use, but—as mentioned earlier—the incidence of severe skin reactions is increased when phenytoin is employed and radiation is given.

Despite these therapeutic measures, survival is only slightly prolonged. The average period of survival, even with therapy, is about 6 months. Between 15 and 30 percent of patients live for a year and 5 to 10 percent for 2 years; with certain radiosensitive tumors (lymphoma, testicular carcinoma, choriocarcinoma, some breast cancers), survival can be much longer. Patients with bone metastases tend to live longer than those with parenchymatous and meningeal metastases.

Meningeal Carcinomatosis ("Carcinomatous Meningitis") Widespread dissemination of tumor cells throughout the meninges and ventricles has been the pattern in about 4 percent of neurologic metastases in our cases of adenocarcinoma of breast, lung, and gastrointestinal tract, melanoma, childhood leukemia, and systemic lymphoma. Headache, backache, polyradiculopathies (particularly of the cauda equina), multiple cranial nerve palsies, and a confusional state have been the principal manifestations. Focal neurologic signs and seizures may be associated, and about half the patients develop hydrocephalus. The diagnosis can be established in most cases by identifying tumor cells in the CSF using flow cytometry, cytospin, centrifugation, or millipore filtering. More than one examination, using generous amounts of CSF, may be needed. Increased pressure, elevation of protein and low glucose levels, and lymphocytic pleocytosis are other common CSF findings. Nevertheless, in a few patients, the CSF remains persistently normal. Measuring the CSF for certain biochemical markers of cancer—such as lactate dehydrogenase, β-glucuronidase, β_2-microglobulin, and carcinoembryonic antigen—offers another means of making the diagnosis and following the response to therapy. These markers are most likely to be abnormal in hematologic malignancies but may also be altered in some cases of intracranial infection and parenchymal metastases (Kaplan et al). In a number of cases of meningeal carcinomatosis, there are also parenchymal metastases.

Treatment consists of radiation therapy to the symptomatic areas, followed by the intraventricular administration of methotrexate, but these measures rarely stabilize neurologic symptoms for more than a few weeks. The methotrexate is administered into the lateral ventricle via an Ommaya reservoir (10 mg diluted in water) or into the lumbar subarachnoid space through a lumbar puncture needle (12 to 15 mg). Several regimens have been devised, including daily instillation for 3 to 4 days followed by radiation, or methotrexate doses on days 1, 4, 8, 11, and 15. Involvement of the cranial nerves or an encephalopathy due to widespread infiltration of the cranial meninges is treated with whole-brain radiation, 3000 cGy, given in fractions of 300 cGy per day for 10 days. Spinal root infiltration responds to spinal radiation, and regional treatments are helpful temporarily for local seeding of the lumbar roots. The median duration of survival after diagnosis of meningeal carcinomatosis was 5.8 months in the large series reported by Wasserstrom and colleagues but only 43 days in the series of Sorenson and coworkers. The leukoencephalopathy that may follow the combined use of intrathecal methotrexate and radiation therapy is described below. The best response to treatment occurs in patients with lymphoma and breast and small-cell lung cancers; cases of meningeal infiltration by melanoma, other lung cancers, and adenocarcinoma do poorly.

Involvement of the Nervous System in Leukemia Almost one-third of all leukemic patients have evidence of diffuse infiltration of the leptomeninges and cranial and spinal nerve roots at autopsy (Barcos et al). The incidence is greater in acute than in chronic leukemia and greater in lymphocytic than in myelocytic leukemia; it is more frequent in children than in adults. The highest incidence is in children with acute lymphocytic (lymphoblastic) leukemia who relapse after treatment with combination chemotherapy (60 to 70 percent at time of death). The clinical and CSF picture of meningeal leukemia is much the same as that of meningeal carcinomatosis, discussed above, with the qualification that leukemic cells are more likely to be found by cytologic examination of the spinal fluid. The treatment of the two disorders is also similar.

The studies of Price and Johnson demonstrated that CNS leukemia is primarily a pial disease. The earliest evidence of leukemia is detected in the walls of pial veins, with or without cells lying freely in the CSF. The leukemic infiltrate in our pathologic material has extended to the deep perivascular spaces, where it is often confined by the pial-glial membrane; at this stage the CSF consistently contains leukemic cells. Depending on the severity of meningeal involvement, transgression of the pial-glial membrane eventually occurs with varying degrees of parenchymal infiltration by collections of leukemic cells. Hemorrhages of varying sizes are other common complications and are sometimes lethal.

Chloroma, a solid green-colored mass of myelogenous leukemic cells, may affect the dura or, less often the brain, but it is distinctly uncommon.

Cranial irradiation, combined with methotrexate given intrathecally or intravenously, has been effective in the prevention and treatment of meningeal involvement in childhood leukemia. However, in a significant number of patients, it has given rise to a distinctive *necrotizing leukoencephalopathy*. This neurologic complication may appear within several days to months after the last administration of methotrexate and several months after completion of radiotherapy (Robain et al). The leukoencephalopathy occurs most frequently and is most severe when all three modalities of treatment, i.e., cranial irradiation and intrathecal and intravenous methotrexate, are used. The initial symptoms—consisting of apathy, drowsiness, depression, and behavioral disorders—evolve over a few weeks to include cerebellar ataxia, spasticity, pseudobulbar palsy, extrapyramidal motor abnormalities, and akinetic mutism. Hypodense areas of varying size appear in the CT scan but—unlike the case with tumor metastases—there is no contrast enhancement. By MRI these methotrexate lesions are hyperintense in T2-weighted images, but compared with pure radiation necrosis (page 728), they have poorly demarcated borders. In some patients the disease stabilizes or improves, with corresponding resolution of the lesions. More often the patient is left with severe persistent sequelae; in most, death occurs within several weeks or months of onset. Throughout the cerebral white matter and to a lesser extent in the brainstem, there are foci of coagulation necrosis of varying size and severity. In the smaller lesions, a perivascular topography of tissue disintegration is evident. The pathogenesis of this disorder is unclear. Radiation injury seems to be the most important factor, coupled with the age of the patient (most are under 5 years of age). It has been speculated that radiation breaks down the blood-brain barrier, allowing methotrexate to injure myelin. Lack of circulation in the necrotic zones prevents the usual liquefaction and eventual cavitation. In this respect it resembles radiation necrosis.

Involvement of the Nervous System in Systemic Lymphoma Extradural compression of the spinal cord or cauda equina is the most common neurologic complication of all types of lymphoma, the result of extension from vertebrae or paravertebral lymph nodes. Treatment is radiation or, if a tissue diagnosis is lacking, surgical decompression. Systemic lymphoma rarely metastasizes to the brain. In a review of more than 10,000 autopsies, our colleague, R. D. Adams, observed only a half-dozen instances where patients with Hodgkin disease had deposits of tumor cells in the brain, and in none of these cases were there intracerebral metastases of multiple myeloma or plasmacytoma (personal communication). In the series of Levitt et al, comprising 592 patients with non-Hodgkin lymphoma, there were only 8 with intracerebral metastases. Much more common is meningeal dissemination of non-Hodgkin lymphoma, the clinical and CSF pictures being similar to those of meningeal leukemia and carcinomatosis. In the rare cases of meningeal involvement with Hodgkin lymphoma, there may be an eosinophilic pleocytosis. Leptomeningeal dissemination occurs most frequently in high-grade lymphomas with diffuse (rather than nodular) changes in the lymph nodes. Cranial nerve palsies are common, with a predilection for the eighth nerve and the cauda equina is involved eventually in most cases. The optimal treatment has not yet been ascertained. Radiotherapy and systemic and intraventricular chemotherapy have all met with some degree of success.

Intravascular Large-Cell Lymphoma (Malignant Angioendotheliomatosis, Angiotropic or Angioblastic Lymphoma, and Lymphomatoid Granulomatosis) These rare and closely related conditions are presented here with other forms of lymphoma, although their clinical behavior is more in keeping with a vasculitic process. The nomenclature is confusing and the original term, *lymphomatoid granulomatosis*, is not universally accepted as equivalent to the more recently elucidated process of intravascular lymphoma; it is more accurate to consider it a prelymphomatous process. As originally described by Liebow and colleagues, lymphomatoid granulomatosis is a systemic disease with prominent pulmonary, dermal, and lymph node changes and, in approximately 30 percent of cases, with involvement of the CNS. In a small proportion of cases, the changes are confined to the nervous system. According to Katzenstein and associates, a systemic malignant lymphoma develops in about 12 percent of such patients, but others have noted this transformation in a considerably higher number.

The *angiocentric, or intravascular, lymphoma*, on the other hand, is regarded as a multifocal neoplasm of large anaplastic lymphocytes that infiltrate the walls of blood vessels and surrounding areas (Sheibani et al) or grow intravascularly and cause occlusion of small and moderate-sized vessels; hence the several alternative designations for the same pathologic process. The tumor typically arises in the nasal cavities or upper respiratory tracts in a pattern similar to that of Wegener granulomatosis. In the brain and spinal cord there are lesions of various sizes that probably represent the combined effects of occlusion of small vessels and concentric infiltration of the adjacent tissue by neoplastic cells. In half of the cases, meningeal vessels are involved and the neoplastic cells have incited an inflammatory response that can be detected in the spinal fluid, although malignant cells are not found. In a few cases, the peripheral nerves have also been involved by the endoneurial neoplasm. Although the lymphoid origin of the anaplastic cells is now clear, not all of them are T cells, as was at one time believed; an equal number have the features of B cells. Moreover, in many cases, portions of the genome of the Epstein-Barr virus (EBV) can be isolated from the malignant B cells within the pleocellular infiltrates. For these reasons it has been proposed that the disorder represents an EBV-induced proliferation of B cells with a prominent inflammatory T-cell reaction (Guinee et al).

Because of the inconsistent location and size of the nervous system lesions, there is no uniform syndrome, but the disease should be suspected in patients with a subacute encephalopathy and indications of focal brain and spinal cord disease. The majority will have nodular or multiple infiltrative pulmonary lesions, skin lesions, or adenopathy, but we have seen three instances that were restricted to the brain and cord. MRI shows multiple variegate abnormalities in T2-weighted images throughout the white matter of the brain. Definitive diagnosis is possible only through a biopsy of radiographically involved lung or nervous tissue that includes numerous intrinsic blood vessels. A helpful diagnostic feature is the presence of antibodies to nuclear cytoplasmic antigens (c-ANCA), which are very frequently present in this disease, as they are in a number of other vasculitic and granulomatous processes.

Like demyelinating and lymphomatous lesions, these abnormalities may recede temporarily in response to treatment with corticosteroids, and some clinical improvement occurs. The course tends to be indolent and relapsing over months or years, although one of our patients died within weeks despite treatment. In a few cases, whole-brain irradiation has been successful in prolonging survival, but the outlook in most instances is poor.

A significant number of these patients have AIDS. The illness must be distinguished from multiple sclerosis, brain lymphoma, gliomatosis cerebri, and the process that simulates it most closely, sarcoidosis (which produces brain and lung lesions) as well as from cerebral vasculitides and Behçet disease.

Sarcomas of the Brain These are malignant tumors composed of cells that are derived from connective tissue elements (fibroblasts, rhabdomyocytes, lipocytes, osteoblasts, smooth muscle cells). They take their names from their histogenetic derivation—namely, fibrosarcoma, rhabdomyosarcoma, osteogenic sarcoma, chondrosarcoma, and sometimes from the tissue of which the cells are a part, such as adventitial sarcomas and hemangiopericytoma.

All these tumors are rare. They constitute from 1 to 3 percent of intracranial tumors, depending on how wide a range of neoplasms one chooses to include in this group (see below). Occasionally one or more cerebral deposits of these types of tumors will occur as a metastasis from a sarcoma in another organ. Others are primary in the cranial cavity and exhibit as one of their unique properties a tendency to metastasize to nonneural tissues, a decidedly rare occurrence with primary glial tumors. It is a disturbing fact that a few sarcomas have developed 5 to 10 years after irradiation or, in one instance of which we are aware, after proton beam irradiation of the brain. Fibrosarcomas have occurred after radiation of pituitary adenomas and osteogenic sarcoma after other types of radiation, all localized to bone or meninges. Our experience with hemangiopericytoma has been limited to two intracranial lesions that simulated meningiomas and two others in the high cervical spinal cord that caused subacute quadriparesis and were initially thought to be polyneuropathies.

A number of other cerebral tumors, described in the literature as sarcomas, are probably tumors of other types. The rapidly growing, highly malignant "monstrocellular sarcoma" of Zülch or "giant-cell fibrosarcoma" of Kernohan and Uihlein, so named for their multinucleated giant cells, have been reinterpreted by Rubinstein as a form of giant cell glioblastoma or mixed glioblastoma and fibrosarcoma. The "hemangiopericytoma of the leptomeninges," also classified by Kernohan and Uihlein as a form of cerebral sarcoma, is considered by Rubinstein to be a variant of the angioblastic meningioma of Bailey and Cushing.

Tumor Patients Who Present Primarily with Signs of Increased Intracranial Pressure

A certain number of patients, when first seen, show the characteristic symptoms and signs of increased intracranial pressure: periodic bifrontal and bioccipital headaches that awaken the patient during the night or are present upon awakening, projectile vomiting, mental torpor, unsteady gait, sphincteric incontinence, and papilledema. Most of these symptoms and the increased ICP are the result of hydrocephalus. Three questions demand immediate answers: (1) Does the patient have a space-occupying intracranial lesion? (2) Where in the cranial cavity is it situated and is it blocking the CSF-ventricular pathways? (3) What is its nature?

The answers to the first two questions are usually provided by the CT scan or MRI, which should be obtained in all patients with symptoms of increased intracranial pressure with or without focal signs. *The tumors most likely to present in this way are medulloblastoma, ependymoma of the fourth ventricle, hemangioblastoma of the cerebellum, pinealoma, colloid cyst of the third ventricle, and less often, craniopharyngioma or a high spinal cord tumor.* In addition, with some of the cerebral gliomas discussed in the preceding section, particularly those of the corpus callosum and frontal lobes and *gliomatosis cerebri*, increased intracranial pressure may occasionally precede focal cerebral signs.

Medulloblastoma, Neuroblastoma, and Retinoblastoma The medulloblastoma is a rapidly growing embryonic tumor that arises in the posterior part of the cerebellar vermis and neuroepithelial roof of the fourth ventricle in children. It accounts for 20 percent of childhood brain tumors. Rarely, it presents elsewhere in the cerebellum or other parts of the brain in adults (Peterson and Walker).

The origin of this tumor remained in doubt for a long time. Bailey and Cushing introduced the name *medulloblastoma*, although medulloblasts have never been identified in the fetal or adult human brain; nevertheless the term is retained for no reason other than its familiarity. The current view of the tumor is that it originates from "stem cells" that have been prevented from maturing and differentiating to their normal growth-arrested state. They retain their capacity to divide ad infinitum. The tumor may differentiate uni- or pluripotentially, varying from case to case. This accounts for the recognized histologic variants, ranging from the undifferentiated medulloblastoma to medulloblastoma with glial, neuronal, or even myoblastic components. Molecular genetic qualities relate the medulloblastoma to retinoblastomas and certain pineal cell tumors and, rarely, to such autosomal dominant diseases as nevoid basal cell carcinoma. The commonest histologic variant, recognized by Hortega in his classic work on the histology of brain tumors, is the "isomorphic glioblastoma," from which both astrocytes and oliogodendrocytes may begin to form. Studies of cell lines from human medulloblastomas reveal a loss of genetic information on the distal part of chromosome 17. Schmidek has proposed that this accounts for the neoplastic transformation of cerebellar stem cells, at various stages of their differentiation, into tumor cells. Another line of research has strongly implicated the JC virus, the same agent that causes "progressive multifocal leukoencephalitis." Genomic sequences from this virus have been found in 72 percent of human tumors by Khalili et al and an experimental transgenic model in which the JC protein is expressed is characterized by a cerebellar tumor that resembles the medulloblstoma. Neuroblastomas differ from medulloblastomas when analyzed for genetic markers, as indicated below.

The majority of the patients are children 4 to 8 years of age, and males outnumber females 3:2 or 3:1 in the many reported series. As a rule, symptoms have been present for 1 to 5 months before the diagnosis is made. The clinical picture is distinctive and derives from the secondary hydrocephalus and raised intracranial pressure. Typically, the child becomes listless, vomits repeatedly, and has a morning headache. The first diagnosis that suggests itself may be gastrointestinal disease or abdominal migraine. Soon, however, a stumbling gait, frequent falls, and diplopia as well as strabismus lead to a neurologic examination and the discovery of papilledema or sixth nerve palsies. Papilledema is present in all except a small proportion of patients by the time they come to the attention of a neurologist except when the tumor is located far laterally in the cerebellum, as it usually is in adults. Dizziness (positional) and nystagmus are frequent. A small proportion of patients have a slight sensory loss on one side of the face and a mild facial weakness. Head tilt, the occiput being tilted back and away from the side of the tumor, indicates a developing cerebellar herniation. Rarely, signs of spinal root and subarachnoid metastases precede cerebellar signs. Extraneural metastases (cervical lymph nodes, lung, liver, bone) may occur, usually after craniotomy, which allows tumor cells to reach scalp lymphatics, but in rare instances they may be blood-borne. Decerebrate attacks ("cerebellar fits") may appear in the late stages of the disease.

The radiologic appearance is also distinctive: high signal intensity on both T-1 and T-2 weighted MRI images, heterogeneous enhancement but of lesser extent than is typical for gliomas, and, of course, the typical location adjacent to and fungating into the fourth ventricle. The tumor frequently fills the fourth ventricle and infiltrates its floor (Fig. 31-11). Seeding of the tumor may occur on the ependymal and meningeal surfaces of

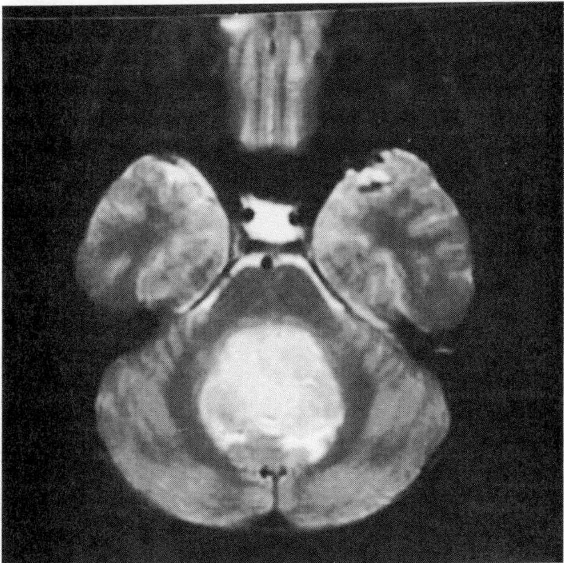

Figure 31-11

Medulloblastoma. MRI in the sagittal (above) *and axial* (below) *planes, illustrating involvement of the cerebellar vermis and neoplastic obliteration of the fourth ventricle.*

the cisterna magna and around the spinal cord. The tumor is solid, gray-pink in color, and fairly well demarcated from the adjacent brain tissue. It is very cellular, and the cells are small and closely packed with hyperchromatic nuclei, little cytoplasm, many mitoses, and a tendency to form clusters and pseudorosettes.

Treatment begins with maximal resection of the tumor. The addition of chemotherapy and radiotherapy of the entire neuraxis improves the rate and length of disease-free survival even for those children with the most extensive tumors at the time of diagnosis (Packer). The combination of surgery, radiation of the entire neuraxis, and chemotherapy permits a 5-year survival in more than 80 percent of cases. The presence of desmoplastic features (i.e., connective tissue formation) is associated with a better prognosis. Brainstem invasion, spinal subarachnoid metastases, incomplete removal, and very early age of onset (younger than 3 years) reduce the period of survival.

Neuroblastoma This, the commonest solid tumor of childhood, is a slightly different tumor of nearly identical histologic type, arising in the adrenal medulla and sometimes metastasizing widely. Usually it remains extradural if it invades the cranial and spinal cavities. *Polymyoclonus with opsoclonus* may occur as a paraneoplastic complication, as discussed further on. A rare form of neuroblastic medulloblastoma in adults tend to be more benign (Rubinstein).

Another closely related tumor is the *retinoblastoma*. This proves to be the most frequent extracranial malignant tumor of infancy and childhood. Eighty percent develop before the fifth year of life. It is a small-cell tumor with neurofibrils and, like the neuroblastoma, has a tendency to form rosettes, which are diagnostic histologic features. The tumor develops within the eye and the blindness that it induces may be overlooked in an infant or small child. The tumor is easily seen ophthalmoscopically, since it arises from cells of the developing retina. The protein encoded by the normal allele of the gene (a growth-suppressor or antioncogene gene, alluded to earlier in the discussion on the genetics of brain tumors) has been identified. It is postulated that an inherited mutation affects one allele of the normal gene, and only if this is accompanied by a mutation that eliminates the function of the second allele will the tumor develop. Early recognition and radiation or surgery effect cure.

Ependymoma and Papilloma of the Fourth Ventricle *Ependymomas*, as pointed out earlier in this chapter, arise from the lining cells in the walls of the ventricles. About 70 percent of them originate in the fourth ventricle, according to Fokes and Earle (Fig. 31-12). Postmortem, some of these tumors if small are found protruding into the fourth ventricle, never having produced symptoms. Whereas the incidence of supratentorial ependymomas is spread evenly throughout life, fourth ventricular ependymomas occur mostly in

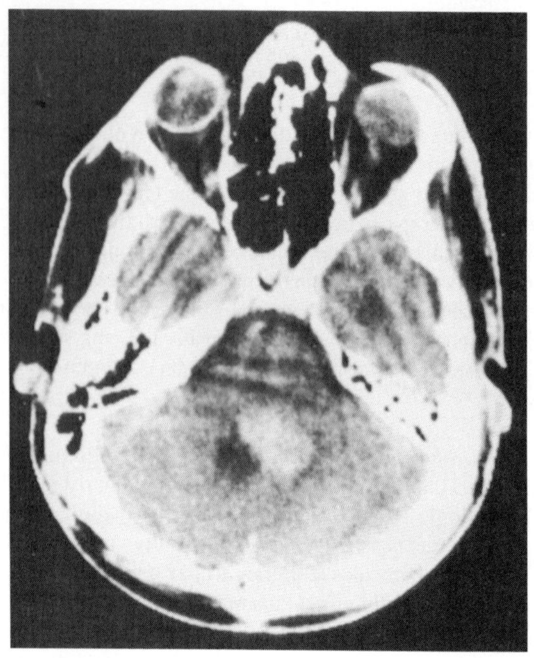

A

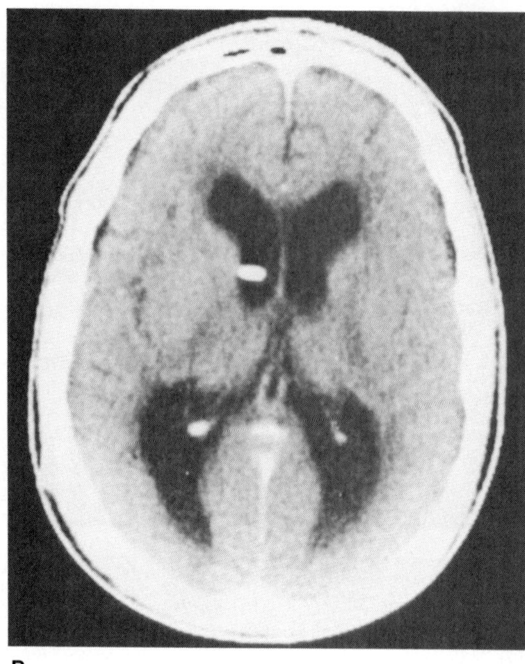

B

Figure 31-12

Ependymoma of the fourth ventricle. A. Ependymoma growing out of the fourth ventricle. B. Contrast-enhanced CT scan in a 4-year-old girl who presented with signs of increased intracranial pressure. Note hydrocephalus and end of shunt tube in right lateral ventricle.

childhood. In the large series of Fokes and Earle (83 cases), 33 occurred in the first decade, 6 in the second, and 44 after the age of 20 years. Males have been affected almost twice as often as females.

Ependymomas usually arise from the floor of the fourth ventricle and extend through the foramina of Luschka and Magendie. They may invade the medulla. These tumors produce a clinical syndrome much like that of the medulloblastoma except for their more protracted course and lack of early cerebellar signs. The histologic features of this tumor have been described earlier in this chapter. The degree of anaplastic change varies and has prognostic significance. The most anaplastic form is the *ependymoblastoma*, a highly aggressive tumor that falls within the spectrum of primitive neuroectodermal tumors (see below).

Symptoms may be present for 1 or 2 years before diagnosis and operation. About two-thirds of the patients come to notice because of increased intracranial pressure; in the remainder, vomiting, difficulty in swallowing, paresthesias of the extremities, abdominal pain, vertigo, and neck flexion or head tilt are prominent manifestations. Some patients with cerebellar herniation are disinclined to sit and have vertical downbeating nystagmus. Surgical removal offers the only hope of survival. The addition of radiation therapy and sometimes ventriculoperitoneal shunting of CSF may prolong life. Myxopapillary ependymoma of the spinal cord and filum are discussed with the spinal cord tumors (page 1331).

Papillomas of the choroid plexus are about one-fifth as frequent as ependymomas. They arise mainly in the lateral and fourth ventricles, occasionally in the third. The two most authoritative studies (Laurence et al; Matson and Crofton) give the ratios of lateral/third/fourth ventricular locations as 50:10:40. The tumor, which takes the form of a giant choroid plexus, has as its cellular element the cuboidal epithelium of the plexus, which is closely related embryologically to the ependyma. An oncogene T (tumor) antigen of the SV40 virus is possibly involved in tumor induction (Schmidek). Essentially these are tumors of childhood. Fully 50 percent cause symptoms in the first year of life and 75 percent in the first decade. In the younger patients, hydrocephalus is usually the presenting syndrome, often aggravated acutely by hemorrhage; there may be papilledema, an unusual finding in a hydrocephalic infant with enlarging head. Headaches, lethargy, stupor, spastic weakness of legs, unsteadiness of gait, and diplopia are more frequent in the older child. Sometimes patients present with a syndrome of the cerebellopontine angle (see further on), where the tumor presumably arises from choroid plexus that projects into the lateral recess of the fourth ventricle. One consequence of the tumor is thought to be increased CSF formation, which contributes to the hydrocephalus. Some of the tumors acquire more malignant attributes (mitoses, atypia of nuclei) and invade surrounding brain. They have the appearance of a carcinoma and may be mistaken for an epithelial metastasis from an extracranial site.

Treatment by surgical excision is usually curative, but palliative ventricular shunting may be needed first if the patient's condition does not permit surgery. The prognosis of the rare choroid plexus carcinomas is poor.

Primitive Neuroectodermal Tumors (PNETs) This term was introduced by Hart and Earle, in 1973, to describe tumors that have the histologic features of medulloblastoma but occur supratentorially. Various poorly differentiated or embryonal tumors of infancy and childhood were included in this group: medulloblastoma, neuroblastoma, retinoblastoma, ependymoblastoma, and pineoblastoma (described further on). Subsequent authors have broadened the category of PNETs to include all CNS neoplasms of neuroectodermal origin. With the advent of immunohistochemical techniques, many of these poorly differentiated neoplasms of infancy came to be recognized as small-cell gliomas (Friede et al), and others could be classified as other types of primitive neoplasms through ultrastructural study. The term *primitive neuroectodermal tumors* has a certain appeal to some pathologists but has added little to our understanding of their undifferentiated embryonal origin. In practical terms—i.e., the prognosis and treatment of all these tumors—regardless of name, is much the same.

Hemangioblastoma of the Cerebellum This tumor is also referred to in connection with von Hippel-Lindau disease (page 1077). Dizziness, ataxia of gait or of the limbs on one side, symptoms and signs of increased intracranial pressure from compression of the fourth ventricle, and in some instances an associated retinal angioma or hepatic and pancreatic cysts (disclosed by CT or MRI) constitute the syndrome. There is a tendency later for the development of malignant renal or adrenal tumors. Many patients have polycythemia due to elaboration of an erythropoietic factor by the tumor.

Age of onset is between 15 and 50 years. Blacks, whites, and Asians are equally affected. Dominant inheritance is well known. Seizinger and coworkers, in cases associated with renal cell carcinoma and pheochromocytoma, have localized a defect in what is probably a tumor suppressor gene on chromosome 3.

The diagnosis can be surmised from the appearance on MRI of a cerebellar cyst containing an enhancing nodular lesion on its wall. Often the associated retinal hemangioma will be disclosed by the same imaging procedure. The angiographic picture is also characteristic: a tightly packed cluster of small vessels forming a mass 1.0 to 2.0 cm in diameter (Fig. 31-13). Craniotomy with opening of the cerebellar cyst and excision of the mural hemangioblastomatous nodule may be curative. There is a high rate of recurrence if the entire tumor, including the nodule, is not completely removed. In the series of Boughey and colleagues, the lesion was successfully excised in 80 percent of their patients. Fifteen percent, in whom an isolated cerebellar lesion had apparently been resected completely, developed recurrent tumors.

Hemangioblastomas of the spinal cord are frequently associated with a syringomyelic lesion (greater than 70 percent of cases); such lesions may be multiple and are located mainly in the posterior columns. A retinal hemangioblastoma may be the initial finding and may lead to blindness if not treated by laser. The children of a parent with a hemangioblastoma of the cerebellum should be examined regularly for an ocular lesion and renal cell carcinoma (another complication). New lesions may form over a period of years while the patient is under observation.

Pinealoma There has been much uncertainty as to the proper classification of pineal tumors. Originally they were all thought to be composed of pineal cells, hence they were regarded as true *pinealomas*, a term suggested by Krabbe. Globus and Silbert believed that the tumors originated from embryonic pineal cells. But later Russell pointed out that some tumors in the pineal region are really atypical teratomas resembling the seminoma of the testicle. Four types of pineal tumor are now recognized—the *germinoma* (atypical teratoma), the *pinealoma* (pineocytoma and pineoblastoma), the true *teratoma* with cellular derivatives of all three germ layers, and the *glioma*.

The germinoma is a firm, discrete mass that usually reaches 3 to 4 cm in greatest diameter. It compresses the superior colliculi and sometimes the superior surface of the cerebellum and narrows the aqueduct of Sylvius. Often it extends anteriorly into the third ventricle and may then compress the hypothalamus. A germinoma may also arise in the floor of the third ventricle; this has

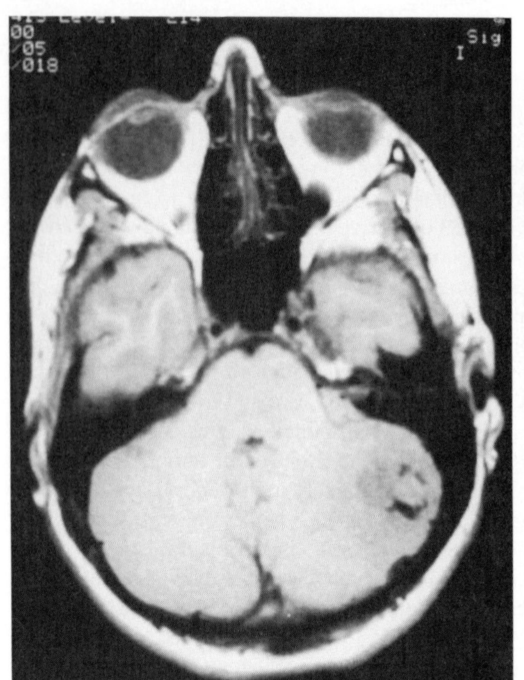

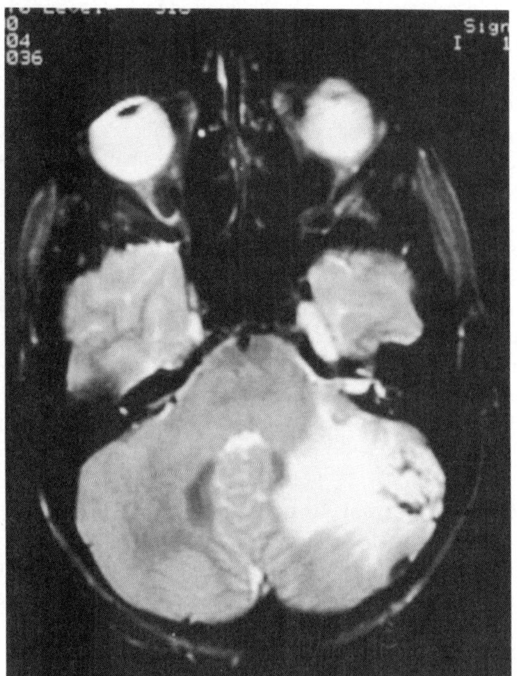

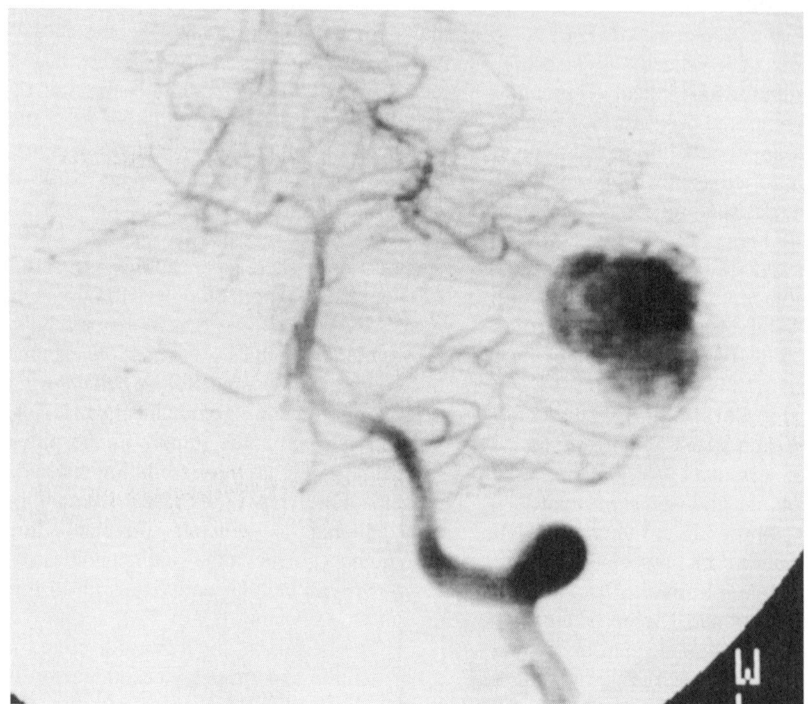

Figure 31-13

Hemangioblastoma. MRI in the axial plane (top) *shows the tumor and the associated edema in the left cerebellar hemisphere. Selective left vertebral angiogram* (bottom) *defines a hypervascular nodule with dilated draining veins.*

been referred to as an ectopic pinealoma or *suprasellar germinoma*. Microscopically, these tumors are composed of large, spherical epithelial cells separated by a network of reticular connective tissue and containing many lymphocytes.

The *pineocytoma* and *pineoblastoma* reproduce the normal structure of the pineal gland. These tumors enlarge the gland, are locally invasive, and may extend into the third ventricle and seed along the neuraxis. Their growth characteristics resemble those of the germinoma. Cytologically, the pineocytoma is a moderately cellular tumor with none of the histologic attributes of anaplasia. The tumor cells tend to form circular arrangements, so-called pineocytomatous rosettes. Pineocytes may be impregnated by silver carbonate methods and some contain the retinal S antigen of photoreceptor cells. Pineoblastomas are highly cellular and composed of small, undifferentiated cells bearing some resemblance to medulloblasts. The *teratoma* and *dermoid* and epidermoid cysts have no special features—some are quite benign. The gliomas have the usual morphologic characteristics of an astrocytoma of varying degrees of malignancy. Of the four groups of pineal tumors, approximately 50 percent are germinomas. True teratomas and gliomas are relatively infrequent. Children, adolescents, and young adults—males more than females—are affected. Only rarely does one see a patient with a pineal tumor that has developed after the thirtieth year of life.

In some cases, the clinical syndrome of the several types of pineal tumors consists solely of symptoms and signs of increased intracranial pressure. Beyond this, the most characteristic localizing signs are an inability to look upward and slightly dilated pupils that react on accommodation but not to light (Parinaud syndrome). Sometimes ataxia of the limbs, choreic movements, or spastic weakness appears in the later stages of the illness. It is uncertain whether the ocular and motor signs are due to neoplastic compression of the brachia conjunctiva and other tegmental structures of the upper midbrain or to hydrocephalus (dilation of the posterior part of the third ventricle). Probably both mechanisms are operative. Precocious puberty occurs in males who harbor a germinoma. Diagnosis is made by CT scanning and MRI (Fig. 31-14). The CSF may contain tumor cells and lymphocytes but may also be entirely normal.

These lesions were formerly judged to be inoperable. However, the use of the operating microscope now makes it possible to excise them by a supracerebellar or transtentorial approach. Operation for purposes of excision and histologic diagnosis is advised, because each type of pineal tumor must be managed differently. Moreover, one may occasionally find an arachnoidal cyst that needs only excision. The germinomas should be removed

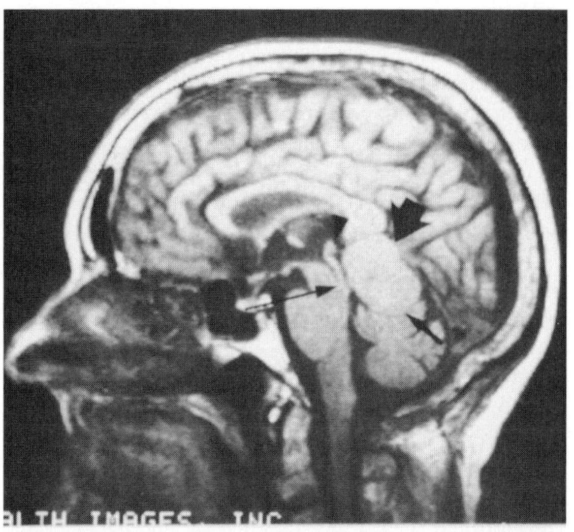

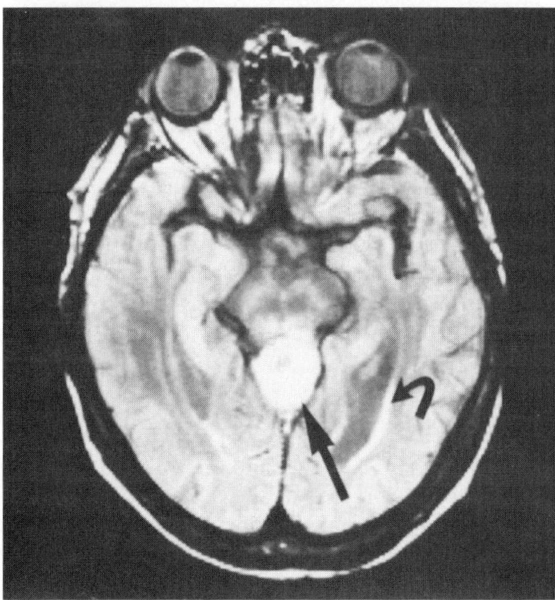

Figure 31-14

Pinealoma. MRI in the sagittal plane (above) *demonstrates the tumor* (large arrow), *which compresses the superior vermis* (smaller arrow) *and the aqueduct* (long-stemmed arrow). *An axial cut* (below) *shows the tumor and evidence of hydrocephalus* (curved arrow), *probably the result of aqueductal compression. (From Bisese JH: Cranial MRI. New York, McGraw-Hill, 1991, by permission.)*

insofar as possible and the whole neuraxis irradiated. The use of chemotherapy in addition to or instead of cranial irradiation is still being evaluated (Allen). Several of our patients have survived more than 5 years after the removal of a pineal glioma.

Other Germinomas, Gangliocytomas, and Mixed Neuronal–Glial Tumors Malignant germ-cell tumors occurring in locations other than the pineal body are usually found in the suprasellar space and rarely in the roof of the third ventricle. Germinoma is the most common of this rare group of neoplasms, which also includes choriocarcinoma, embryonal cell carcinoma, endodermal sinus tumors, and malignant teratomas. Certain biochemical markers of these tumors are of interest and of clinical utility, since they may be detected in samples of the blood and CSF. The β subunit of human chorionic gonadotropin (hCG) is elaborated by choriocarcinoma, and α-fetoprotein, by choriocarcinoma and immature teratomas. Typical germinomas have shown little elevation of either. Most often these markers indicate the presence of complex mixed germ-cell tumors.

Gangliogliomas and mixed neuronal-glial tumors are special tumor types, more frequent in the young and of variable but usually low-grade malignancy. They are composed both of differentiated glial cells, usually astrocytes, and of neurons in various degrees of differentiation. The latter, which may resemble glial cells, can be identified by Nissl stains, silver stains, and immunochemical reactions for cytoskeletal proteins. Some of these developmental tumors are difficult to separate from hamartomas.

The best-known type is called the *gangliocytoma*, one form of which is the dysplastic gangliocytoma of the cerebellum (Lhermitte-Duclos disease). This is a slowly evolving lesion that forms a mass in the cerebellum; it is composed of granule, Purkinje, and glial cells. Reproduced therein, in a disorganized fashion, is the architecture of the cerebellum. The importance of distinguishing this disease from other cerebellar tumors is its lack of growth potential and favorable prognosis. It should be excised if symptomatic.

Other forms of gangliogliomas include the *desmophilic infantile ganglioglioma, some of the xanthoastrocytomas, and the dysembrioplastic neuroepitheliomas.* Often they lie near the ventricles, and they may induce hydrocephalus. Many of these tumors are rare and affect children mostly, for which reasons they are not discussed further here. Good descriptions are to be found in the monographs of Russell and Rubinstein and Levine and Schmidek and in the article by Zentner and coworkers.

Colloid (Paraphysial) Cyst and Other Tumors of the Third Ventricle The most important of these is the colloid tumor, which is derived, it is generally believed, from ependymal cells of a vestigial third ventricular structure known as the *paraphysis*. The cysts formed in this structure are always situated in the anterior portion of the third ventricle between the interventricular foramina and are attached to the roof of the ventricle (Fig. 31-15). They vary from 1 to 4 cm in diameter, are oval or round with a smooth external surface, and are filled with a glairy, gelatinous material containing a vari-

Figure 31-15

MRI in the sagittal and axial planes, showing a colloid cyst of the third ventricle without the usual associated hydrocephalus.

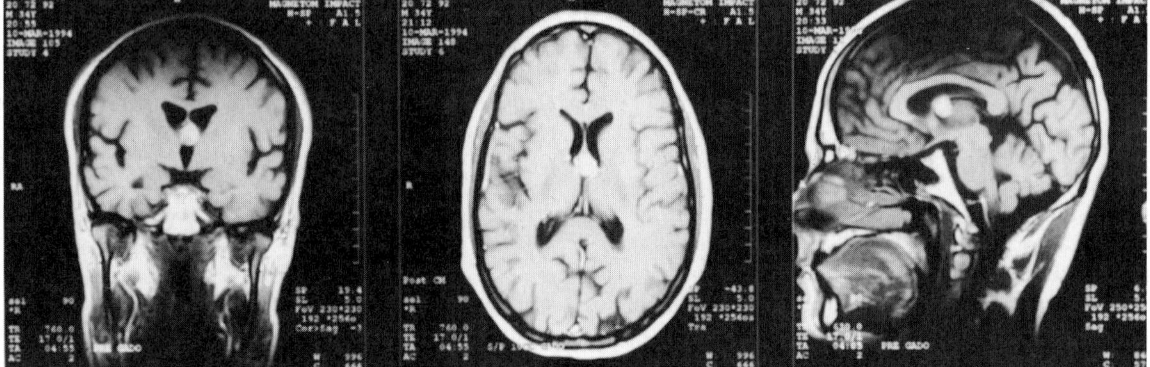

ety of mucopolysaccharides. The wall is composed of a layer of epithelial cells, some ciliated, surrounded by a capsule of fibrous connective tissue. Although congenital, the cysts practically never declare themselves clinically until adult life, when they block the third ventricle and produce an obstructive hydrocephalus.

Suspicion of this tumor is occasioned by intermittent, severe bifrontal-bioccipital headaches, sometimes modified by posture ("ball valve" obstruction of the third ventricle) or with crises of headache and obtundation, incontinence, unsteadiness of gait, bilateral paresthesias, dim vision, and weakness of the legs, with sudden falls but no loss of consciousness ("drop attacks," see page 399). Stooping may result in an increase or onset of headache and loss of balance. However, this intermittent obstructive syndrome has been infrequent in our experience. More often the patient has no headache and presents with the symptoms of normal-pressure hydrocephalus. Subtle behavioral changes are common and a few patients, as emphasized by Lobosky and colleagues, experience mild confusion and changes in personality that may reach the extreme of psychotic behavior. In our experience headache or gait difficulty is usually present by that time.

The treatment for many years has been surgical excision, which always carries some risk, but satisfactory results have also been obtained by ventriculoperitoneal shunting of the CSF, leaving the benign growth untouched. Decompression of the cyst by aspiration under stereotaxic control has also become an increasingly popular procedure.

Other tumors found in the third ventricle and giving rise mainly to obstructive symptoms are craniopharyngiomas (see below), papillomas of the choroid plexus, and ependymomas (discussed earlier).

Supratentorial or Infratentorial Arachnoid Cyst ("Localized Pseudotumor") This lesion, which is probably congenital, presents clinically at all ages but may become evident only in adult life, when it gives rise to symptoms of increased intracranial pressure and sometimes to focal cerebral or cerebellar signs, simulating intracranial neoplasm. In infants and young children, macrocrania and extensive unilateral transillumination are characteristic features. Usually these cysts overlie the sylvian fissure; occasionally they are interhemispheric and lie in the pineal region or under the cerebellum. They may attain a large size, to the point of enlarging the middle fossa and elevating the lesser wing of the sphenoid, but they do not communicate with the ventricle. Rarely, one of these cysts may cover the entire surface of both cerebral hemispheres and create a so-called external hydrocephalus (page 661).The cysts are readily recognized (often accidentally) on the nonenhanced CT scan or MRI, showing a circumscribed tissue defect filled with fluid that has the density of CSF (Gandy and Heier). If these cysts are completely asymptomatic, they should be left alone; if symptomatic, additional (MRI) studies are indicated, so as not to overlook a chronic subdural hematoma, which is often associated and may not be visualized on the unenhanced CT scan. Suprasellar arachnoid cysts are discussed further on (page 716).

Patients Who Present with Specific Intracranial Tumor Syndromes

In this group of tumors, symptoms and signs of general cerebral impairment and increased pressure occur late or not at all. Instead special syndromes referable to particular intracranial loci arise and progress slowly. One arrives at the correct diagnosis by localizing the lesion accurately from the neurologic findings and by reasoning that the etiology must be neoplastic because of the afebrile, steadily progressive nature of the illness. Investigation by CT, MRI, and other special studies will usually confirm the clinical impression.

Tumors that produce these unique intracranial syndromes are *acoustic neuroma* and other tumors of the cerebellopontine angle, *craniopharyngioma*, *pituitary adenomas* and nonneoplastic enlargements of the sella, *meningiomas* of the sphenoid ridge and olfactory groove, *glioma of the optic nerve and chiasm, pontine glioma, chordoma and chondrosarcoma, glomus jugulare and carotid body tumors*, as well as other erosive tumors at the base of the skull.

Acoustic Neuroma (Vestibular Schwannoma) This tumor was first described as a pathologic entity by Sandifort in 1777, first diagnosed clinically by Oppenheim in 1890, and first recognized as a surgically treatable disease around the turn of the century. Cushing's monograph (1917) was a milestone, and the papers of House and Hitselberger and of Ojemann and colleagues provide excellent descriptions of the modern diagnostic tests and surgical treatment as well as comprehensive bibliographies.

Approximately 3000 new cases of acoustic neuroma are diagnosed each year in the United States (incidence rate of 1 per 100,000 per year). The tumor occurs occasionally as part of von Recklinghausen neurofibromatosis, in which case it takes one of two forms. In classic von Recklinghausen disease (peripheral, or type 1, neurofibromatosis, see page 1074), a schwannoma may sporadically involve the eighth nerve, usually in adult life, just as it may involve any other cranial nerve (particularly trigeminal) or spinal nerve root. Rarely if ever do bilateral acoustic neuromas occur in this form of the disease. However, bilateral acoustic neuromas are the hallmark of the genetically distinct neurofibromatosis type 2, in which they practically always occur before the age of 21 and show a strong (autosomal dominant) heredity (Fig. 31-16). Schwannomas are distinguished from neurofibromas (composed of both Schwann cells and fibroblasts) found in peripheral nerves of type 1 von Recklinghausen disease. A small percentage of neurofibromas become malignant, a phenomenon that is highly unusual in schwannomas.

The usual acoustic neuroma in adults presents as a solitary tumor. Being a schwannoma, it originates in nerve. The examination of small tumors reveals that they practically always originate on the vestibular division of the eighth nerve, just within the internal auditory canal (Fig. 31-17). As the eighth nerve schwannoma grows, it extends into the posterior fossa to occupy the angle between the cerebellum and pons (cerebellopontine angle). In this lateral position it is so situated as to compress the seventh, fifth, and less often the ninth and tenth cranial nerves, which are implicated in various combinations. Later it displaces and compresses the pons and lateral medulla and obstructs the CSF circulation; very rarely, it is a source of subarachnoid hemorrhage.

Certain biologic data assume clinical importance. The highest incidence is in the fifth and sixth decades, and the sexes are equally affected. Familial occurrence marks only the tumors that are part of von Recklinghausen disease.

The earliest symptom reported by the patients in the series of Ojemann and coworkers was loss of hearing (33 of 46 patients); headache (4 of 46); disturbed sense of balance (3 of 46); unsteadiness of gait (3 of 46); or facial pain, tinnitus, and facial weakness—each in a single case. Some patients sought medical advice soon after the appearance of the initial symptom, some later, after other symptoms had occurred. Usually, by the time of the first neurologic examination, the clinical picture was quite complex. One-third of the patients were troubled by vertigo associated with nausea, vomiting, and pressure in the ear. The vertiginous symptoms differed from those of

Figure 31-16

Bilateral acoustic schwannomas in neurofibromatosis type 2. MRI in the axial plane, without (left) and with (right) enhancement.

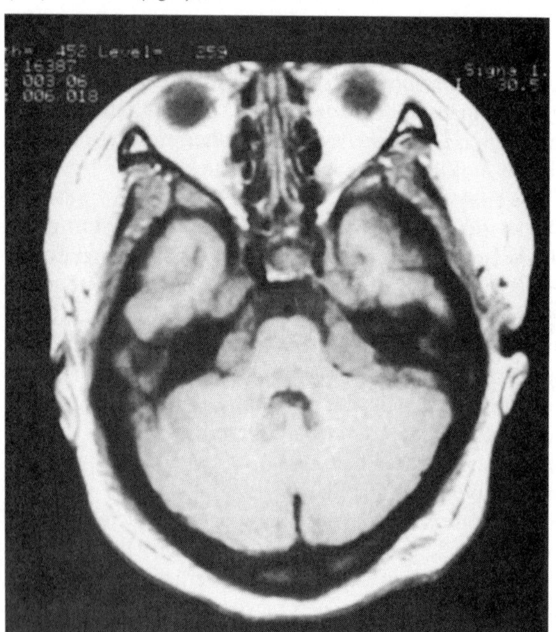

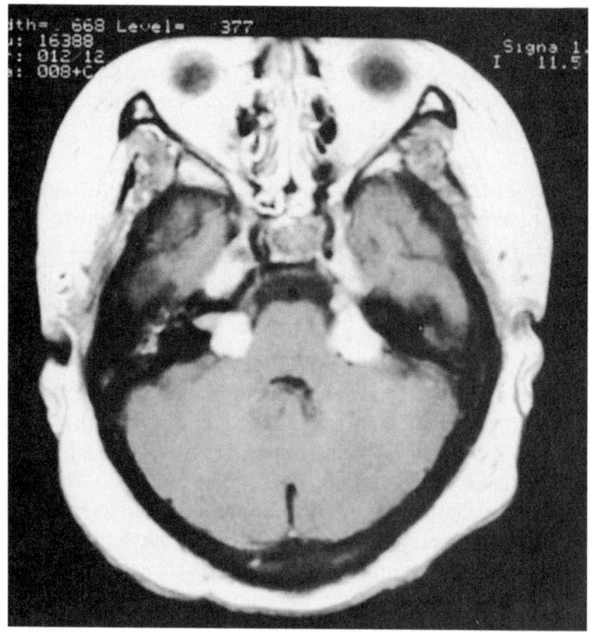

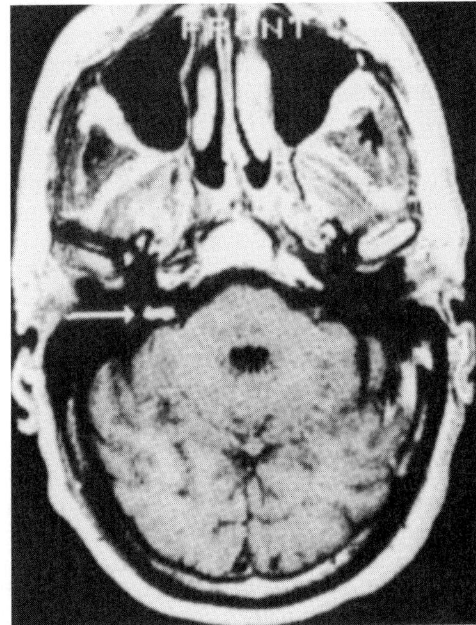

Figure 31-17

T1-weighted axial MR image after gadolinium. Arrow points to an intracanalicular schwannoma.

Ménière disease in that discrete attacks separated by periods of normalcy were rare. The vertigo coincided more or less with hearing loss and tinnitus (most often a unilateral high-pitched ringing, sometimes a machinery-like roaring or hissing sound, like that of a steam kettle). By then, many of the patients were also complaining of unsteadiness, especially on rapid changes of position (e.g., in turning), and this may have interfered with work and other activities. Some of our patients ignored their deafness for many months or years; often the first indication of the tumor in such patients has been their need to use the unaccustomed ear for the telephone. Others neglected these symptoms to a point where they presented with impaired mentation, imbalance, and sphincteric incontinence.

The *neurologic findings* at the time of examination in the series mentioned above were as follows: eighth nerve involvement (auditory and vestibular) in 45 of 46, facial weakness including disturbance of taste (26 of 46), sensory loss over the face (26 of 46), gait abnormality (19 of 46), and unilateral ataxia of the limbs (9 of 46). Inequality of reflexes and 11th and 12th nerve palsies were present in only a few patients. Signs of increased intracranial pressure appear late and have been present in no more than 25 percent of our patients. These findings are comparable to those reported by House and Hitselberger and by Harner and Laws.

The contrast-enhanced CT scan will detect practically all acoustic neuromas that are larger than 2.0 cm in diameter and project further than 1.5 cm into the cerebellopontine angle. Much smaller intracanalicular tumors can be detected reliably by MRI with gadolinium enhancement (Fig. 31-17), a procedure that in general is the most useful in determining the size and anatomic relationships of these tumors. Audiologic and vestibular evaluation includes the various tests described in Chap. 15, the brainstem auditory evoked response probably being the most sensitive one. In combination, they permit localization of the deafness and vestibular disturbance to the cochlear and vestibular nerves rather than to their end organs. The CSF protein is raised in two-thirds of the patients (>100 mg/dL in one-third); a clinically inevident acoustic schwannoma is one of the causes of an unexpectedly high CSF protein when a lumbar puncture is performed for other reasons.

The preferred treatment in most cases is surgical excision. Many neurosurgeons who have had the largest experience with these tumors favor the microsurgical suboccipital transmeatal operation (Martuza and Ojemann). In most instances, the facial nerve can be preserved by intraoperative monitoring of brainstem auditory responses and facial nerve electromyography (EMG); in experienced hands, hearing can be preserved in approximately one-third of patients with tumors smaller than 2.5 cm in diameter. If no attempt is to be made to save hearing, small tumors can be removed safely by the translabyrinthine approach. An alternative is focused gamma or proton radiation, which controls the growth of many of the smaller tumors. In a large series of patients treated with radiosurgery, facial motor and sensory functions were preserved in three-quarters of cases and, after 28 months of observation, no new neurologic deficits were detected (Kondziolka et al). This approach is favored in older patients with few symptoms.

Neurinoma or schwannoma of the trigeminal (gasserian) ganglion or neighboring cranial nerves and meningioma of the cerebellopontine angle may in some instances be indistinguishable from an acoustic neuroma. Fifth nerve tumors should always be considered if deafness, tinnitus, and lack of response to caloric stimulation ("dead labyrinth") are not the initial symptoms of a cerebellopontine angle syndrome. A true *cholesteatoma (epidermoid cyst)* is a relatively rare tumor that is most often located in the cerebellopontine angle, where it may simulate an acoustic neuroma but usually causes more severe facial weakness. Spillage of the contents of the cyst may produce an intense chemical meningitis. Other disorders that enter into the differential diagnosis are glomus jugulare tumor (see below), metastatic cancer, syphilitic meningitis, arachnoid cyst, vascular malformations, and epidural plasmacytoma of the petrous bone. All these disorders may produce a cerebellopontine angle syndrome, but they are more likely to cause only unilateral lower cranial nerve palsies and their temporal course tends to differ from that of acoustic neuroma. Occasionally, a tumor that originates in the pons or in the fourth ventricle (ependymoma, astrocytoma, papilloma, medulloblastoma) or a nasopharyngeal carcinoma may present as a cerebellopontine angle syndrome.

Craniopharyngioma (Suprasellar Epidermoid Cyst, Rathke's Pouch or Hypophysial Duct Tumor, Adamantinoma, Ameloblastoma) These are histologically benign epithelioid tumors, generally assumed to originate from cell rests (remnants of Rathke's pouch) at the junction of the infundibular stem and pituitary. By the time the tumor has attained a diameter of 3 to 4 cm, it is almost always cystic and partly calcified. Usually it lies above the sella turcica, depressing the optic chiasm and extending up into the third ventricle. Less often it is subdiaphragmatic, i.e., within the sella, where it compresses the pituitary body and erodes one part of the wall of the sella or a clinoid process; seldom does it balloon the sella like a pituitary adenoma. Large tumors may obstruct the flow of CSF. The tumor is oval, round, or lobulated and has a smooth surface. The wall of the cyst and the solid parts of the tumor consist of cords and whorls of epithelial cells (often with intercellular bridges and keratohyalin) separated by a loose network of stellate cells. If there are bridges between tumor cells, which have an epithelial origin, the tumor is classed as an *adamantinoma*. The cyst contains dark albuminous fluid, cholesterol crystals, and calcium deposits; the calcium can be seen in plain films or CT scans of the suprasellar region in 70 to 80 percent of cases. The sella beneath the tumor tends to be flattened and enlarged. The majority of the patients are children, but the tumor is not infrequent in adults, and some of our patients have been up to 60 years of age.

The presenting syndrome may be one of increased intracranial pressure, but more often it takes the form of a combined pituitary-hypothalamic-chiasmal derangement. The symptoms are often subtle and of long standing. In children, visual loss and diabetes insipidus are the most frequent findings, followed by adiposity, delayed physical and mental development (Froehlich or Lorain syndrome—see page 595), headaches, and vomiting. The visual disorder takes the form of dim vision, chiasmal field defects, optic atrophy, and papilledema. In adults, waning libido, amenorrhea, slight spastic weakness of one or both legs, headache without papilledema, failing vision, and mental dullness and confusion are the usual manifestations. Later, drowsiness, ocular palsies, diabetes insipidus, and disturbance of temperature regulation—indicating hypothalamic involvement—may occur. Spontaneous rupture of the cystic lesion can incite a severe aseptic meningitis, at times with depressed glucose in the CSF.

In the *differential diagnosis* of the several craniopharyngioma syndromes, a careful clinical analysis is often more informative than laboratory procedures. Among the latter, MRI is likely to give the most useful information. Often, because of the cholesterol content, the tumor gives an increased signal on T1-weighted images. Usually, the cyst itself is isointense, like CSF, but occasionally it may give a decreased T2 signal.

Modern microsurgical techniques, reinforced by corticosteroid therapy before and after surgery, and careful control of temperature and water balance postoperatively permit successful excision of all or part of the tumor in the majority of cases. While smaller tumors can be removed by a transphenoidal approach, attempts at total removal require craniotomy and remain a challenge because of frequent adherence of the mass to surrounding structures (Fahlsbusch et al). Partial removal practically assures recurrence of the tumor mass, usually within 3 years, and the surgical risks of reoperation are considerable (10 percent mortality in large series). In 21 of our 35 patients, only partial removal was possible; of these, 8 died, most in the first postoperative year. Stereotaxic aspiration is sometimes a useful palliative procedure, as are radiation therapy and ventricular shunting in patients with solid, nonresectable tumors. Endocrine replacement may be necessary.

Glomus Jugulare Tumor This tumor is relatively rare but of particular interest nonetheless. It is a purplish red, highly vascular tumor composed of large epithelioid cells, arranged in an alveolar pattern and possessing an abundant capillary network. The tumor is thought to be derived from minute clusters of nonchromaffin paraganglioma cells (glomus bodies) found mainly in the adventitia of the dome of the jugular bulb (*glomus jugulare*) immediately below the floor of the middle ear but also in multiple other sites in and around the temporal bone. These clusters of cells are part of the chemoreceptor system that also includes the carotid, vagal, ciliary, and aortic bodies.

The typical syndrome consists of partial deafness, facial palsy, dysphagia, and unilateral atrophy of the tongue combined with a vascular polyp in the external auditory meatus and a palpable mass below and anterior to the mastoid eminence, often with a bruit that may be audible to the patient ("self-audible bruit"). Other neurologic manifestations are phrenic nerve palsy, numbness of the face, a Horner syndrome, cerebellar ataxia, and temporal lobe epilepsy. The jugular foramen is eroded (visible in basilar skull films) and the CSF protein may be elevated. Women are affected more than men, and the peak incidence is during middle adult life. The tumor grows slowly over a period of many years, sometimes 10 to 20 years or more. Treatment has consisted of radical mastoidectomy and removal of as much tumor as possible, followed by radiation. The combined intracranial and extracranial two-stage operation has resulted in the cure of many cases (Gardner et al). A detailed account of this tumor will be found in the article by Kramer.

Carotid Body Tumor (Paraganglioma) This is a generally benign but potentially malignant tumor originating in a small aggregate of cells of neuroectodermal type. The normal carotid body is small (4 mm in greatest diameter and 10 mg in weight) and is located at the bifurcation of the common carotid artery. The cells are of uniform size, have an abundant cytoplasm, are rich in substance P, and are sensitive to changes in P_{O_2}, P_{CO_2}, and pH (i.e., they are chemoreceptors, not to be confused with baroreceptors). The tumors that arise from these cells are identical in appearance with tumors of other chemoreceptor organs (paragangliomas). Interestingly, they are 12 times more frequent in individuals living at high altitudes.

Clinically the usual presentation is of a painless mass at the side of the neck below the angle of the jaw; thus it must be differentiated from the branchial cleft cyst, mixed tumor of the salivary gland, and carcinomas and aneurysms in this region. As the tumor grows (at an estimated rate of 2.0 cm in diameter every 5 years) it may implicate the sympathetic, glossopharyngeal, vagus, spinal accessory, and hypoglossal nerves (syndrome of the retroparotid space; see Chap. 47). Hearing loss, tinnitus, and vertigo are present in some cases. Tumors of the carotid body have been a source of transient ischemic attacks in 5 to 15 percent of the 600 or more reported cases. One of the most interesting presentations has been with sleep apnea, particularly with bilateral tumors, and respiratory depression as well as lability of blood pressure are common postoperative problems. Malignant transformation occurs in 5 percent of cases.

A similar paraganglioma of the vagus nerve has been reported; it occurs typically in the jugular or nodose ganglion but may arise anywhere along the course of the nerve. These tumors may also undergo malignant transformation, metastasize, or invade the base of the skull.

A carotid body tumor separate from the glomus jugulare tumor has also been seen in combination with von Recklinghausen neurofibromatosis. Familial cases are known, especially with bilateral carotid body tumors (about 5 percent of these tumors are bilateral). The treatment should be surgical excision with or without prior intravascular embolization; radiation therapy is not advised.

Pituitary Adenomas Tumors arising in the anterior pituitary are of considerable interest to neurologists because they often cause visual and other symptoms related to involvement of structures bordering upon the sella turcica. Pituitary tumors are age-linked; they become increasingly numerous with each decade; by the 80th year, small adenomas are found in more than 20 percent of pituitary glands. In some cases, an apparent stimulus to adenoma formation is endocrine end-organ failure, as occurs, for example, with ovarian atrophy that induces a basophilic adenoma. Only a small proportion (6 to 8 percent) enlarge the sella.

On the basis of conventional hematoxylin-eosin staining methods, cells of the normal pituitary gland were for many years classified as chromophobe, acidophil, and basophil, these types being present in a ratio of 5:4:1. Adenomas of the pituitary are most often composed of chromophobe cells (4 to 20 times as common as acidophil-cell adenomas); the incidence of basophil-cell adenomas is uncertain. Histologic study is now based on immunoperoxidase staining techniques that define the nature of the hormones within the pituitary cells—both of the normal gland and of pituitary adenomas. These methods have shown that either a chromophobe or an acidophil cell may produce prolactin, growth hormone (GH), and thyroid-stimulating hormone (TSH), whereas the basophil cells produce adrenocorticotropic hormone (ACTH), β-lipotropin, luteinizing hormone (LH), and follicle-stimulating hormone (FSH).

The development of sensitive (radioimmunoassay) methods for the measurement of pituitary hormones in the serum has made possible the detection of adenomas at an early stage of their development and the designation of several types of pituitary adenomas on the basis of the endocrine disturbance. Hormonal tests for the detection of pituitary adenomas, preferably carried out in an endocrine clinic, are listed in Table 31-3. Between 60 and 70 percent of tumors, in both men and women, are prolactin-secreting. About 10 to 15 percent secrete growth hormone, and a smaller number secrete ACTH. Tumors that secrete gonadotropins and TSH are quite rare. These tumors may be monohormonal or plurihormonal and approximately one-third are composed of nonfunctional (null) cells.

Pituitary tumors usually arise as discrete nodules in the anterior part of the gland (adenohypophysis). They are reddish gray, soft (almost gelatinous), and often partly cystic, with a rim of calcium in some instances. The adenomatous cells are arranged diffusely or in various patterns, with little stroma and few blood vessels; less frequently the architecture is sinusoidal or papillary in type. Variability of nuclear structure, hyperchromatism, cellular pleomorphism, and mitotic figures are interpreted as signs of malignancy, which is exceedingly rare. Tumors less than 1 cm in diameter are referred to as microadenomas and are at first confined to the sella. As the tumor grows, it first compresses the pituitary gland; then, as it extends upward and out of the sella, it compresses the optic chiasm; later, with continued growth, it may extend into the cavernous sinus, third ventricle, temporal lobes, or posterior fossa. Recognition of an adenoma when it is still confined to the sella is of considerable practical importance, since total removal of the tumor by transsphenoidal excision or some form of stereotactic radiosurgery is possible at this stage, with prevention of further damage to normal glandular structure and the optic chiasm. Penetration of the diaphragma sellae by the tumor and invasion of the surrounding structures make treatment more difficult.

Table 31-3
Hormonal tests for detection of pituitary adenomas

Hormone	*Test*
Prolactin	Serum prolactin level Chlorpromazine- or TRH-provocative tests L-dopa suppression
Somatotropin (GH)	Serum GH level Glucagon L-dopa Glucose-GH suppression Somatomicid C
Adrenocorticotropin	Serum cortisol Urinary steroids Metyrapone test Dexamethasone suppression
Gonadotropin	Serum FSH LH Estradiol Testosterone GnRH stimulation
Thyrotropin	TSH T_4 TRH
Vasopressin	Urine and serum osmolality after water restriction for deficiency of hormone; without water restriction for excess of hormone

Key: FSH, follicle-stimulating hormone; LH, luteinizing hormone; GnRH, gonadotropin-releasing hormone; TRH, thyrotropin releasing hormone; T_4, thyroxine; TSH, thyroid-stimulating hormone; GH, growth hormone.

Pituitary adenomas come to medical attention because of endocrine or visual abnormalities. Headaches are present with nearly half of the macroadenomas but are not part of the microadenoma syndrome. The visual disorder usually proves to be a *complete or partial bitemporal hemianopia*, which has developed gradually and may not be evident to the patient. Early on, the upper parts of the visual fields may be affected predominantly. A small number of patients will be almost blind in one eye and have a temporal hemianopia in the other. Bitemporal central hemianopic scotomata are a less frequent finding. A postfixed chiasm may be compressed in such a way that there is an interruption of some of the nasal retinal fibers, which, as they decussate, project into the base of the opposite optic nerve (Wilbrand's knee). This results in a central scotoma on one or both sides (junctional syndrome) as well as a temporal field defect (see Fig. 13-2). If the visual disorder is of long standing, the optic nerve heads are visibly atrophic. *Bitemporal hemianopia with a normal sella* indicates that the causative lesion is probably a saccular aneurysm of the circle of Willis or a meningioma of the tuberculum sellae. In 5 to 10 percent of cases, the pituitary adenoma extends into the cavernous sinus, causing some combination of ocular motor palsies. Other neurologic abnormalities, rare to be sure, are seizures from indentation of the temporal lobe, CSF rhinorrhea, and diabetes insipidus, hypothermia, and somnolence from hypothalamic compression.

The major endocrine syndromes associated with pituitary adenomas are described briefly in the following pages. Their functional classification can be found in the monograph edited by Kovacs and Asa. A detailed discussion of the diagnosis and management of hormone-secreting pituitary adenomas can be found in the reviews of Klibanski and Zervas and of Pappas and colleagues; recommended also is the recent review of the neurologic features of pituitary tumors by Anderson and colleagues.

Amenorrhea-Galactorrhea Syndrome As a rule, this syndrome becomes manifest during the childbearing years. The history usually discloses that menarche had occurred at the appropriate age; primary amenorrhea is rare. A common history is that the patient took birth control pills, only to find, when she stopped, that the menstrual cycle did not reestablish itself. On examination, there may be no abnormalities other than galactorrhea. Serum prolactin concentrations are increased (usually in excess of 100 ng/mL). In general, the longer the duration of amenorrhea and the higher the serum prolactin level, the larger the tumor (prolactinoma). The elevated prolactin levels distinguish this disorder from idiopathic galactorrhea, in which the serum prolactin concentration is normal.

Males with prolactin-secreting tumors rarely have galactorrhea and usually present with a larger tumor and complaints such as headache, impotence, and visual abnormalities. In normal persons, the serum prolactin rises markedly in response to the administration of chlorpromazine or thyrotropin-releasing hormone (TRH); patients with a prolactin-secreting tumor fail to show such a response. With large tumors that compress normal pituitary tissue, thyroid and adrenal function will also be impaired. Large nonfunctioning pituitary adenomas also cause modest hyperprolactinemia by distorting the pituitary stalk and reducing dopamine delivery to prolactin-producing cells.

Acromegaly This disorder consists of acral growth and prognathism in combination with visceromegaly, headache, and several endocrine disorders (hypermetabolism, diabetes mellitus). The highly characteristic facial and bodily appearance, well known to all physicians, is due to an overproduction of growth hormone (GH) after puberty; prior to puberty, an oversecretion of GH leads to gigantism. In a small number of acromegalic patients, there is an excess secretion of both GH and prolactin, derived apparently from two distinct populations of tumor cells. The diagnosis of this disorder, which is often long delayed, is made on the basis of the characteristic clinical changes, the finding of elevated serum GH values ($>$10 ng/mL), and the failure of the serum GH concentration to rise in response to the administration of glucose or TRH.

Cushing Disease Described in 1932 by Cushing, this condition is only about one-fourth as frequent as acromegaly. A distinction is made between *Cushing disease* and *Cushing syndrome*, as indicated in Chap. 27. The former term is reserved for cases that are caused by the excessive secretion of pituitary ACTH, which in turn causes adrenal hyperplasia; the usual basis is a pituitary adenoma. *Cushing syndrome* refers to the effects of cortisol excess from any one of several sources—excessive administration of steroids (the commonest cause), adenoma of the adrenal cortex, ACTH-producing bronchial carcinoma, and very rarely other carcinomas. The clinical effects are the same in all of these disorders and include truncal obesity, hypertension, proximal muscle weakness, amenorrhea, hirsutism, abdominal striae, glycosuria, osteoporosis, and, in some cases, a characteristic psychosis (page 1199).

Although Cushing originally referred to the disease as pituitary basophilism and attributed it to a basophil adenoma, the pathologic change may consist only of hyperplasia of basophilic cells or a nonbasophilic adenoma. Seldom is the sella turcica enlarged: visual symptoms or signs due to involvement of the optic chiasm or nerves or extension to the cavernous sinus are therefore rare. The diagnosis of Cushing disease is made by demonstrating increased concentration of plasma and urinary cortisol; these levels are not suppressed by the administration of relatively small doses of dexamethasone (0.5 mg four times daily), but they are suppressed by high doses (8 mg daily). A low level of ACTH and a high level of cortisol in the blood, increased free cortisol in the urine, and nonsuppression of adrenal function after administration of high doses of dexamethasone are evidence of an adrenal source of the Cushing syndrome—usually a tumor and less often a micronodular hyperplasia of the adrenal gland.

Diagnosis of Pituitary Adenoma This is virtually certain when a chiasmal syndrome is combined with an endocrine syndrome of either hypopituitary or hyperpituitary type. Laboratory data that are confirmatory of an endocrine disorder, as described above, and a ballooned sella turcica in plain films of the skull corroborate the diagnosis. Patients who are suspected of harboring a pituitary adenoma but in whom the plain films are normal should be examined by MRI. The latter procedure will visualize pituitary adenomas as small as 3 mm in diameter and show the relationship of the tumor to the optic chiasm. This also provides the means of following the response of the tumor to therapy (Fig. 31-18).

Tumors other than pituitary adenomas may sometimes expand the sella. Enlargement may be due to an intrasellar craniopharyngioma, carotid aneurysm, or cyst of the pituitary gland. Intrasellar epithelium-lined cysts are rare lesions. They originate from the apical extremity of Rathke's pouch, which may persist as a cleft between the anterior and posterior lobes of the hypophysis. Rarer still are intrasellar cysts that have no epithelial lining and contain thick, dark brown fluid, the product of intermittent hemorrhages. Both types of intrasellar cyst may compress the pituitary gland and mimic the endocrine-suppressive effects of pituitary adenomas. Neoplasms originating in the nasopharynx or sinuses may invade the sella and pituitary gland, and sarcoid lesions at the base of the brain may do the same. Also, the pituitary gland may be the site of metastases, most of them from the lung and breast (Morita et al); they give rise to diabetes insipidus, pituitary insufficiency, or orbital pain and rarely may be the first indication of a systemic tumor.

Figure 31-18

Pituitary tumors. Upper figure: T1-weighted, enhanced coronal MRI. A microadenoma is seen as a nonenhancing nodule (arrow) *within the normally enhancing pituitary gland. The optic chiasm is seen just above the gland. Lower figure: Nonenhanced MRI. Macroadenoma* (arrow) *compressing the optic chiasm.*

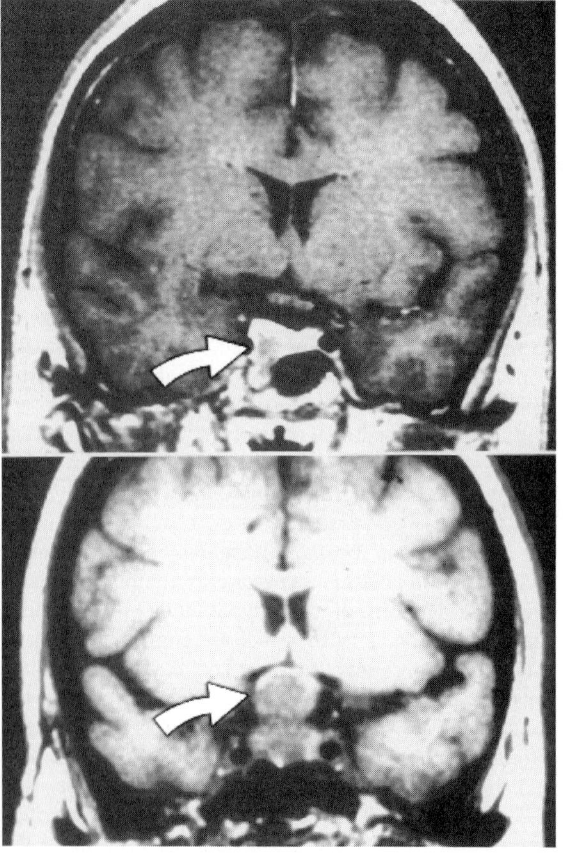

Far more common than the aforementioned conditions is a *nontumorous enlargement of the sella ("empty sella")*. This results from a defect in the dural diaphragm, which may occur without obvious cause or with states of raised intracranial pressure such as pseudotumor cerebri (page 667) or hydrocephalus, or may follow surgical excision of a pituitary adenoma or meningioma of the tuberculum sellae or pituitary apoplexy (see below). The arachnoid covering the diaphragm sellae will bulge downward through the dural defect, and the sella then enlarges gradually, due presumably to the pressure and pulsations of the CSF acting on its walls. In the process, the pituitary gland becomes flattened, sometimes to an extreme degree; however, the functions of the gland are usually unimpaired. Downward herniation of the optic chiasm occurs occasionally and may cause visual disturbances simulating those of a pituitary adenoma (Kaufman et al). As mentioned above, a bitemporal hemianopia with a normal-sized sella is usually due to a primary suprasellar lesion (saccular aneurysm of the distal carotid artery, meningioma, or craniopharyngioma).

Treatment of Intrasellar Pituitary Adenomas This varies with the type and size of the tumor, the status of the endocrine and visual systems, and the age and child-bearing plans of the patient. The administration of the dopamine agonist *bromocriptine* (which inhibits prolactin) in a beginning dosage of 0.5 to 1.25 mg daily with food may be the only therapy needed for small or even large prolactinomas and is a useful adjunct in the treatment of the amenorrhea-galactorrhea syndrome. The dose is slowly increased by 2.5 mg or less every several days until a therapeutic response is obtained. Under the influence of bromocriptine, the tumor decreases in size within days, the prolactin level falls, and the visual field defect improves.

Some cases of acromegaly also respond to the administration of bromocriptine but even better to *octreotide*, an analogue of somatostatin. The initial dose of octreotide is 200 mg/day, increased in divided doses to 1600 mg by increments of 200 mg weekly. In Lambert's series of acromegaly patients, the growth hormone levels returned to normal and the tumor size was reduced in 12 of 15 cases. Treatment with bromocriptine and octreotide must be continuous to prevent relapse. Newer slow-release somatostatin analogues and long-acting dopamine agonists such as cabergoline have been developed for use in patients who do not respond to the conventional agents (Colao and Lombardi).

If the patient is intolerant of bromocriptine (or, in the case of acromegaly, to octreotide and the newer drugs mentioned above), the treatment is surgical, using a transsphenoidal microsurgical approach, with an attempt at total removal of the tumor and preservation of normal pituitary function. Unfortunately, approximately 15 percent of GH-secreting tumors and prolactinomas will recur at 1 year. For this reason, incomplete removal or recurrence of the tumor (or those that are unresponsive to hormonal therapy) should be followed by radiation therapy.

Another alternative treatment is proton beam radiation or some other form of stereotactic radiosurgery *provided that vision is not being threatened and there is no other urgent need for surgery*. These forms of radiation can be focused precisely on the tumor and will destroy it. Kjellberg and colleagues, using proton beam radiation, have treated over 1100 pituitary adenomas without a fatality and with few complications (Kliman et al). A single brief exposure through intact skin and skull was all that was necessary. An endocrine deficit will follow in most instances and must be corrected by hormone replacement therapy. Proton beam therapy is available in only very few centers worldwide, but equivalent methods ("gamma knife," linear accelerator) are readily accessible. The advantage of these radiotherapeutic methods is that tumor recurrence is rare. A disadvantage is that the radiation effect is obtained only after many months. Estrada and colleagues have also reported that external beam radiation therapy may be employed after unsuccessful transsphenoidal surgery for Cushing disease. After approximately 3.5 years, 83 percent of their patients showed no signs of tumor growth. There are reports, however, of a decline in memory ability after radiation treatment of all types.

Large extrasellar extensions of a pituitary growth must be removed by craniotomy, using a transfrontal approach, followed by radiation therapy.

Pituitary Apoplexy This syndrome, described originally by Brougham et al, occurs as a result of infarction of an adenoma that has outgrown its blood supply (see also page 266). It is characterized by the acute onset of headache, ophthalmoplegia, bilateral amaurosis, and drowsiness or coma, with either subarachnoid hemorrhage or pleocytosis and elevated CSF protein. The CT scan or MRI shows infarction of tumor, often with hemorrhage, in and above an enlarged sella. Pituitary apoplexy may threaten life and must be treated by dexamethasone (6 to 12 mg q 6 h); if there is no improvement after 24 to 48 h, transnasal decompression of the sella is indicated. Some pituitary adenomas have been cured by this accident. *Ischemic necrosis of the pituitary*, followed by hypopituitarism, occurs under a wide variety of clinical circumstances, the most common being in the partum or postpartum period (Sheehan syndrome).

Meningioma of the Sphenoid Ridge This tumor is situated over the lesser wing of the sphenoid bone (Fig. 31-8*B*). As it grows, it may expand medially to involve structures in the wall of the cavernous sinus, anteriorly into the orbit, or laterally into the temporal bone. Fully 75 percent of such tumors occur in women and the average age at onset is 50 years. Most prominent among the symptoms are a slowly developing unilateral exophthalmos, slight bulging of the bone in the temporal region, and radiologic evidence of thickening or erosion of the lesser wing of the sphenoid bone. Variants of the clinical syndrome include anosmia, oculomotor palsies, painful ophthalmoplegia (sphenoidal fissure and Tolosa-Hunt syndromes, see Table 47-2), blindness and optic atrophy in one eye, sometimes with papilledema of the other eye (Foster Kennedy syndrome), mental changes, uncinate fits, and increased intracranial pressure. Rarely, a skull bruit can be heard over a highly vascular tumor. Sarcomas arising from skull bones, metastatic carcinoma, orbitoethmoidal osteoma, benign giant-cell bone cyst, tumors of the optic nerve, and angiomas of the orbit must be considered in the differential diagnosis. Scanning by CT and MRI provide the definitive diagnosis. The tumor is resectable without further injury to the optic nerve if the bone has not been invaded.

Meningioma of the Olfactory Groove This tumor originates in arachnoidal cells along the cribriform plate. The diagnosis depends on the finding of ipsilateral or bilateral anosmia or ipsilateral or bilateral blindness—often with optic atrophy and mental changes. The tumors may reach enormous size before coming to the attention of the physician. If the anosmia is unilateral, it is rarely if ever reported by the patient. The unilateral visual disturbance may consist of a slowly developing central scotoma. Abulia, confusion, forgetfulness, and inappropriate jocularity (Witzelsucht) are the usual psychic disturbances (see page 475). The patient may be indifferent to or joke about his blindness. Usually there are radiographic changes along the cribriform plate. The MRI is diagnostic. Except for the largest tumors, extirpation is possible.

Meningioma of the Tuberculum Sella Cushing was the first to delineate the syndrome caused by this tumor. All of his 23 patients were female. The presenting symptoms were visual failure—a slowly advancing bitemporal hemianopia with a sella of normal size. Often the field defects were asymmetrical, indicating a combined chiasm–optic nerve involvement. Usually there are no hypothalamic or pituitary deficits. If the tumor is not too large, complete excision is possible. If removal is incomplete or if the tumor recurs or undergoes malignant changes, radiation therapy is indicated. The outlook is then guarded; several of our patients succumbed within a few years.

Glioma of the Brainstem Astrocytomas of the brainstem are relatively slow-growing tumors that infiltrate tracts and nuclei. They produce a variable clinical picture, depending on their location in the medulla, pons, or midbrain. Most often, this tumor begins in childhood (peak age of onset is 7 years), and 80 percent appear before the 21st year. Symptoms have usually been present for 3 to 5 months before coming to medical notice. In most patients the initial manifestation is a palsy of one or more cranial nerves, usually the sixth and seventh on one side, followed by long tract signs—hemiparesis, unilateral ataxia, ataxia of gait, paraparesis, and hemisensory and gaze disorders. In the remaining patients the symptoms occur in the reverse order—i.e., long tract signs precede the cranial nerve abnormalities. Patients in the latter group survive longer than those whose illness begins with cranial nerve palsies. The combination of a cranial nerve palsy or palsies on one side and motor and/or sensory tract signs on the other always indicates brainstem disease. Headache, vomiting, and papilledema may occur, usually late in the course of the illness, occasionally early. The course is slowly progressive over several years unless some part of the tumor becomes more malignant (anaplastic astrocytoma or glioblastoma multiforme) or spreads to the meninges (meningeal gliomatosis), in which instance the illness may terminate fatally within months.

The main problem in diagnosis is to differentiate this disease from a pontine form of multiple sclerosis, a vascular malformation of the pons (usually a cavernous hemangioma), or a brainstem encephalitis, and to distinguish the focal from the diffuse type of glioma (see below). The most helpful procedure in diagnosis and prognosis is MRI (Fig. 31-19).

A careful imaging and clinical study of 87 patients by Barkovich and coworkers has emphasized the importance of distinguishing between diffusely infiltrating and focal nodular tumors. In the more common diffuse type, there is mass effect with hypointense signal on T1-weighted MRI and heterogeneously increased T2 signal, which reflects edema and tumor spread. The diffusely infiltrating tumors, usually showing an asymmetrical enlargement of the pons, have a poorer prognosis than the focal or nodular tumors, which tend to occur in the dorsal brainstem and often protrude in an exophytic manner. In a few instances of diffuse brainstem glioma, surgical exploration is necessary to establish the diagnosis (inspection and possibly biopsy). However, the histologic characteristics of a minute biopsy specimen of the tumor are not particularly helpful in determining prognosis or treatment and the general practice is to avoid surgery unless the tumor exhibits unusual clinical behavior or does not conform to the typical MRI appearance of the diffuse type. The treatment is radiation, and

Figure 31-19

Pontine glioma. T1-weighted MR images demonstrate a cystic mass with prominent peripheral gadolinium enhancement. The patient was a 3-year-old male with progressive cranial nerve and long tract deficits.

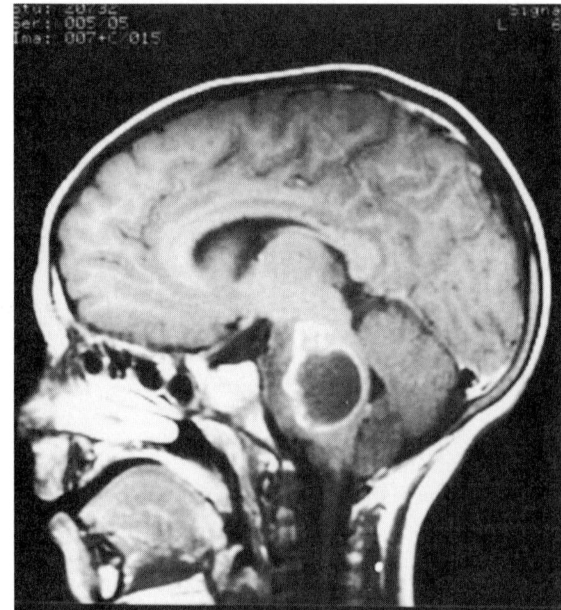

if increased intracranial pressure develops as a result of hydrocephalus, ventricular shunting of CSF becomes necessary. Adjuvant chemotherapy has not been helpful (Kornblith et al). A series of 16 patients treated by Pollack and colleagues emphasizes the fact that the focal and exophytic brainstem tumors are almost all low-grade astrocytomas; these tumors, in contrast to the more diffuse type, usually respond well to partial resection and permit long-term survival because they recur only slowly and do not undergo malignant transformation. Gangliocytomas or mixed astrogangliocytomas are rare imitators of nodular glioma in the brainstem. The rarer cystic glioma of the brainstem (Fig. 31-19), a pilocytic tumor like its counterpart in the cerebellum, is treated by resection of the mural nodule and, as mentioned earlier, has an excellent prognosis. Landolfi et al emphasized the longer survival in adults with pontine glioma (median 54 months) as compared with children. Most of the patients with pontine tumors with which we are familiar proved to have malignant gliomas.

Glioma of the Optic Nerves and Chiasm This tumor, like the brainstem glioma, occurs most frequently during childhood and adolescence. In 85 percent of cases, it appears before the age of 15 years (average 3.5 years), and it is twice as frequent in girls as in boys (see Cogan). The initial symptoms are dimness of vision with constricted fields, followed by bilateral field defects of homonymous, heteronymous, and sometimes bitemporal type and progressing to blindness and optic atrophy with or without papilledema. Ocular proptosis from the orbital mass is the other main symptom. Hypothalamic signs (adiposity, polyuria, somnolence, and genital atrophy) occur occasionally. CT scanning, MRI, and ultrasound will usually reveal the tumor, and radiographs will show an enlargement of the optic foramen (greater than 7.0 mm). This finding and the lack of ballooning of the sella or of suprasellar calcification will exclude pituitary adenoma, craniopharyngioma, Hand-Schüller-Christian disease, and sarcoidosis. In adolescents and young adults, the medial sphenoid, olfactory groove, and intraorbital meningiomas (optic nerve sheath meningioma) are other tumors that cause blindness and proptosis. If the entire tumor is prechiasmatic (the less common configuration), surgical extirpation can be curative. For tumors that have infiltrated the chiasm or are causing regional symptoms and hydrocephalus, partial excision followed by radiation is all that can be offered. Both gliomas and nontumorous gliotic (hamartomatous) lesions of the optic nerves may occur in von Recklinghausen disease; the latter are sometimes impossible to distinguish from optic nerve gliomas.

Chordoma This is a soft, jelly-like, gray-pink growth that arises from remnants of the primitive notochord, located most often along the clivus (from dorsum sellae to foramen magnum) and in the sacrococcygeal region. It affects males more than females, usually in early or middle adult years, and should always be suspected in syndromes involving multiple cranial nerves or the cauda equina. About 40 percent of chordomas occur at each of these two ends of the neuraxis; the rest are found at any point in between. The tumor is made up of cords or masses of large cells with granules of glycogen in their cytoplasm and often with multiple nuclei and intracellular mucoid material. Chordomas are locally invasive, especially of surrounding bone, but they do not metastasize. The cranial neurologic syndrome is remarkable in that all or any combination of cranial nerves from the second to twelfth on one or both sides may be involved. Associated signs in the series of Kendell and Lee were facial pain, conductive deafness, and cerebellar ataxia, the result of pontomedullary and cerebellar compression. A characteristic sign is neck pain radiating to the vertex of the skull on neck flexion. The tumors at the base of the skull may destroy the clivus and bulge into the nasopharynx, causing nasal obstruction and discharge and sometimes dysphagia. Extension to the cervical epidural space may result in cord compression. Thus, chordoma is one of the lesions that may present both as an intracranial and extracranial mass, the others being meningioma, neurofibroma, glomus jugulare tumor, and carcinoma of the sinuses or pharynx. Plain films of the base of the skull, in addition to MRI, are important in diagnosis. Midline (Wegener) granulomas and sarcoidosis must be differentiated. Chondrosarcoma of the clivus produces a similar syndrome.

Treatment of the chordoma is surgical excision and radiation (proton beam or focused gamma radiation). This form of treatment has effected a 5-year cure in approximately 80 percent of patients.

Nasopharyngeal Growths That Erode the Base of the Skull (Transitional Cell Carcinoma, Schmincke Tumor) These are rather common in a general hospital; they arise from the mucous membrane of the paranasal sinuses or the nasopharynx near the eustachian tube, i.e., the fossa of Rosenmüller. In addition to symptoms of nasopharyngeal or sinus disease, which may not be prominent, facial pain and numbness (trigeminal), abducens palsy, and other cranial nerve palsies may occur. Diagnosis depends on inspection and biopsy of a nasopharyngeal mass or an involved cervical lymph node and radiologic evidence of erosion of the base of the skull. Bone and CT scans are helpful in diagnosis. The treatment is surgical resection (in some cases) and radiation. Carcinoma of the ethmoid or sphenoid sinuses and postradiation neuropathy, coming on years after the treatment of a nasopharyngeal tumor, may produce similar clinical pictures and are difficult to differentiate. Special imaging techniques, such as diffusion-weighted imaging, may be useful in separating them. Several syndromes resulting from nasopharyngeal tumors are discussed in Chap. 47 on "Diseases of the Cranial Nerves."

Other Tumors of the Base of the Skull In addition to meningioma and the tumors enumerated above, there are a large number and variety of tumors, rare to be sure, that derive from tissues at the base of the skull and paranasal sinuses, ears, etc., and give rise to certain distinctive syndromes. Included in this category are osteomas, chondromas, ossifying fibromas, giant-cell tumors of bone, lipomas, epidermoids, teratomas, mixed tumors of the parotid gland, and hemangiomas and cylindromas (adenoid cystic carcinomas of salivary gland origin) of the sinuses and orbit (rarely, sarcoid produces the same effect). Most of these tumors are benign, but some have a potential for malignant change. To the group must be added the *esthesioneuroblastoma* (of the nasal cavity) with anterior fossa extension and the malignant tumors that metastasize to basal skull bones (prostate, lung, and breast being the common sources) or involve them as part of a multicentric neoplasia, e.g., primary lymphoma, Ewing sarcoma, plasmacytoma, and leukemic deposits.

Suprasellar arachnoid cysts also occur in this region. CSF flows upward from the interpeduncular cistern but is trapped above the sella by thickened arachnoid (membrane of Liliequist). As the CSF accumulates, it forms a cyst that invaginates the third ventricle; the dome of the cyst may intermittently block the foramina of Monro and cause hydrocephalus (Fox and Al-Mefty). Children with this condition exhibit a curious to-and-fro bobbing and nodding of the head, like a doll with a weighted head resting on a coiled spring. This has been referred to as the "bobble-head doll syndrome" by Benton and colleagues; it can be cured by emptying the cyst.

Details of the pathology, embryogenesis, and symptomatology of these rare tumors are far too varied to include in a textbook devoted to principles of neurology. Table 31-4, on pages 722–723, adapted from Bingas's large neurosurgical service in Berlin, summarizes the known facts about each of them; his authoritative article and the more recent one by Morita and Piepgras, both in the *Handbook of Clinical Neurology*, are recommended references.

Modern imaging techniques now serve to clarify many of the diagnostic problems posed by these tumors. MRI is particularly helpful in delineating structures at the base of the brain and in upper cervical region. CT is also capable of determining the absorptive values of the tumor itself. When the lesion is analyzed in this way, an etiologic diagnosis sometimes becomes possible. For example, the absorptive value of lipomatous tissue is different from that of brain tissue, glioma, blood, and calcium. Bone scans (technetium and gallium) display active destructive lesions with remarkable fidelity, but even when these are seen, it may be difficult to obtain a satisfactory biopsy in some cases.

Tumors of the Foramen Magnum Tumors in the region of the foramen magnum are of particular importance because of the need to differentiate them from diseases such as multiple sclerosis, Chiari malformation, syringomyelia, and bony abnormalities of the craniocervical junction. Failure to recognize these tumors is a serious matter, since the majority are benign and extramedullary, i.e., potentially resectable and curable. If unrecognized, they terminate fatally by causing medullary and spinal cord compression.

Although these tumors are not numerous (about 1 percent of all intracranial and intraspinal tumors), sizable series have been collected by several investigators (see Meyer et al for a complete bibliography). In all series, meningiomas, schwannomas, neurofibromas, and dermoid cysts are the most common types; others, all rare, are teratomas, dermoids, granulomas, cavernous hemangiomas, hemangioblastomas, hemangiopericytomas, lipomas, and epidural carcinomas.

Pain in the suboccipital or posterior cervical region, mostly on the side of the tumor, is usually the first and by far the most prominent complaint. In some instances the pain may extend into the shoulder and even the arm. The latter distribution is more frequent with tumors arising in the spinal canal and extending intracranially than the reverse. For uncertain reasons, the pain may radiate down the back, even to the lower spine. Both spine and root pain can be recognized, the latter due to involvement of either the C2 or C3 root or both. Weakness of one shoulder and arm progressing to the ipsilateral leg and then to the opposite leg and arm ("around the clock" paralysis) is a characteristic but not invariable sequence of events, caused by the encroachment of tumor upon the decussating corticospinal tracts. Occasionally both upper limbs are involved alone; surprisingly, there may be atrophic weakness of the hand or forearm or even intercostal muscles with diminished tendon reflexes well below the level of the tumor, an observation made originally by Oppenheim. Involvement of sensory tracts also occurs; more often it is posterior column sensibility that is impaired on one or both sides, with patterns of progression similar to those of the motor paralysis. Sensation of intense cold in the neck and shoulders has been another unexpected complaint, and also "bands" of hyperesthesia around the neck and back of the head. Segmental bibrachial sensory loss has been demonstrated in a few of the cases and a Lhermitte sign (really a symptom) of electric-like sensations down the spine and limbs on neck flexion has been reported frequently. The cranial nerve signs most frequently seen and indicative of intracranial extension are dysphagia, dysphonia, dysarthria, and drooping shoulder (due to vagal, hypoglossal, and spinal accessory involvement); nystagmus and episodic diplopia; sensory loss over the face and unilateral or bilateral facial weakness; and a Horner syndrome.

Figure 31-20

T1-weighted sagittal MR image demonstrating a meningioma just below the foramen magnum.

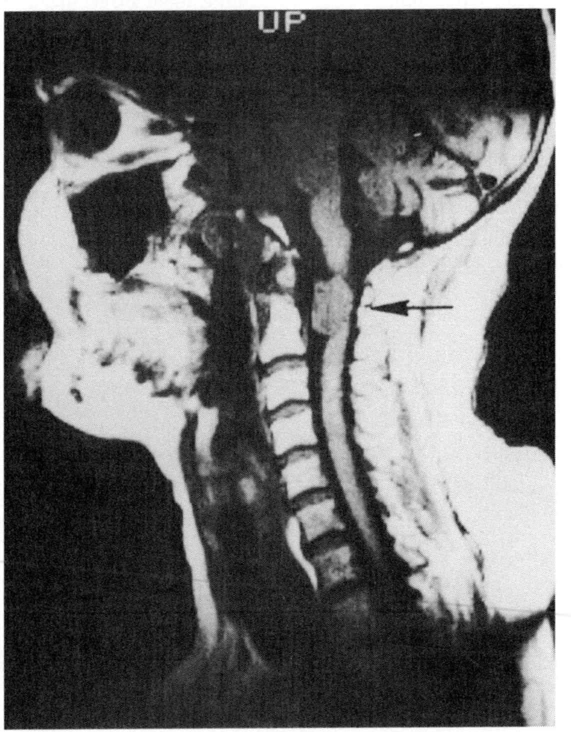

The clinical course of such lesions often extends for 2 years or longer, with deceptive and unexplained fluctuations. With *dermoid cysts* of the upper cervical region, as in the case reported by Adams and Wegner, complete and prolonged remissions from quadriparesis may occur. The important diagnostic procedure is MRI (Fig. 31-20) and, if this is unavailable, CT myelography.

Tumors of the foramen magnum should be suspected in patients with persistent occipital neuralgia or those who carry a diagnosis of spinal or brainstem-cerebellar multiple sclerosis, Chiari malformation, and chronic adhesive arachnoiditis. Treatment is surgical excision (see Hakuba et al).

REMOTE EFFECTS OF NEOPLASIA ON THE NERVOUS SYSTEM (PARANEOPLASTIC DISORDERS)

In the past 50 years there has been delineated a group of neurologic disorders that occur in patients with carcinoma or some other type of neoplasia even though the nervous system is not the site of metastases or direct invasion or compression by the tumor. These so-called paraneoplastic disorders are not specific or confined to cancer, but the two conditions are linked far more frequently than could be accounted for by coincidence. Some of the paraneoplastic disorders that involve nerve and muscle—namely, polyneuropathy, polymyositis, and the myasthenic-myopathic syndrome of Lambert-Eaton—are described on pages 1358 and 1547, respectively. Here we present several other paraneoplastic processes that involve the spinal cord, cerebellum, brainstem, and cerebral hemispheres.

Comprehensive accounts of the paraneoplastic disorders may be found in the writings of Posner and Chernick and of Dropcho. Some of these disorders are associated with IgG autoantibodies (Table 31-5), but it should be remarked that although there are associations of antibodies with specific syndromes, they are not invariably linked to particular cancers. Furthermore, the same syndromes and antibodies occur rarely without an evident tumor, even at autopsy.

The mechanism(s) by which carcinomas produce their remote effects are poorly understood. Perhaps the most plausible theory, as intimated above, is that they have an autoimmune basis. According to this theory, antigenic molecules are shared by certain tumors and central or peripheral neurons. The immune response is

Table 31-4
Clinical syndromes caused by tumors at the base of the skull (see also Tables 47-1 and 47-2)

Site of lesion	*Eponym*	*Clinical symptoms*	*Etiology*[a]
Anterior part of the base of the skull		Olfactory disturbances (uni- or bilateral anosmia), possibly psychiatric disturbances, seizures.	Tumors that invade the anterior part of the base of the skull from the frontal sinus, nasal cavity, or the ethmoid bone, osteomas. Meningiomas of the olfactory groove.
Superior orbital fissure	Rochon-Duvigneau; syndrome of the pterygopalatine fossa (Behr) and the base of the orbit (DeJean) commencing with a lesion of the maxillary and pterygoid rami and evolving into the superior orbital fissure syndrome.	Lesions of the third, fourth, sixth, and first divisions of the fifth nerves with ophthalmoplegia, pain, and sensory disturbances in the area of V_1; often exophthalmos, some vegetative disturbances.	Tumors: meningiomas, osteomas, dermoid cysts, giant-cell tumors, tumors of the orbit, nasopharyngeal tumors, more rarely optic nerve gliomas; eosinophilic granulomas, angiomas, local or neighboring infections, trauma.
Apex of the orbit	Jacod-Rollet (often combined with the syndrome of the superior orbital fissure); infraclinoid syndrome of Dandy.	Visual disturbances, central scotoma, papilledema, optic nerve atrophy; occasional exophthalmos, chemosis.	Optic nerve glioma, infraclinoid aneurysm of the internal carotid artery, trauma, orbital tumors, Paget disease.
Cavernous sinus	Foix-Jefferson; syndrome of the sphenopetrosal fissure (Bonnet and Bonnet) corresponding in part to the cavernous sinus syndrome of Raeder.	Ophthalmoplegia due to lesions of the third, fourth, sixth, and often fifth nerves, exophthalmos, vegetative disturbances. Jefferson distinguished three syndromes: (1) the anterior-superior, corresponding to the superior orbital fissure syndrome; (2) the middle, causing ophthalmoplegia and leasions of V_1 and V_2; (3) the caudal, in addition affecting the whole trigeminal nerve.	Tumors of the sellar and parasellar area, infraclinoid aneurysms of the internal carotid artery, nasopharyngeal tumors, fistulas of the sinus cavernosus and the carotid artery (traumatic), tumors of the middle cranial fossa, e.g., chondromas, meningiomas, and neurinomas.
Apex of the petrous temporal bone	Gradenigo-Lannois	Lesions of the fifth and sixth nerves with neuralgia, sensory, and motor disturbances, diplopia.	Inflammatory processes (otitis), tumors such as cholesteatomas, chondromas, meningiomas, neurinomas of the gasserian ganglion and trigeminal root, primary and secondary sarcomas at the base of the skull.

Table 31-4 *(Continued)*
The most important clinical syndromes caused by tumors at the base of the skull

Site of lesion	*Eponym*	*Clinical symptoms*	*Etiology*[a]
Sphenoid and petrosal bones (petrosphenoidal syndrome)	Jacod	Ophthalmoplegia due to loss of function of the third, fourth, and sixth nerves, amaurosis, trigeminal neuralgia possibly with sensory signs.	Tumors of the sphenoid and petrosal bones and middle cranial fossa, nasopharyngeal tumors, metastases.
Jugular foramen	Vernet	Lesions of ninth, tenth, and eleventh nerves with disturbance of deglutition; curtain phenomenon; sensory disturbances of the tongue, soft palate, pharynx and larynx; hoarseness; weakness of the sternocleidomastoid and trapezius.	Tumors of the glomus jugulare; neurinomas of eighth, ninth, tenth, and eleventh nerves; chondromas, cholesteatomas, meningiomas, nasopharyngeal and ear tumors; infections, angiomas, rarely trauma.
Anterior occipital condyles	Collet-Sicard (Vernet-Sargnon)	Loss of twelfth nerve function (loss of normal tongue mobility) in addition to the symptoms of the jugular foramen.	Tumors of the base of the skull, ear, parotid; leukemic infiltrates; aneurysms, angiomas, and inflammations.
Retroparotid space (retropharyngeal syndrome)	Villaret	Lesions of the lower group of nerves (Collet-Sicard) and Bernard-Horner syndrome with ptosis and miosis.	Tumors of the retroparotid space (carcinomas, sarcomas), trauma, inflammations.
Half of the base of the skull	Garcin (Guillain-Alajouanine-Garcin); also described by Hartmann in 1904.	Loss of function of all twelve cranial nerves of one side; in many cases, isolated cranial nerves spared; rarely signs of raised intracranial pressure or pyramidal tract symptoms.	Nasopharyngeal tumors, primary tumors at the base of the skull, leukemic infiltrates of basal meninges, trauma, metastases.
Cerebellopontine angle		Loss of function of eighth nerve (hearing loss, vertigo, nystagmus); cerebellar disturbances; lesions of the fifth, seventh, and possibly ninth and tenth cranial nerves. Signs of raised intracranial pressure, brainstem symptoms.	Acoustic neuromas (raised protein in CSF), meningiomas, cholesteatomas, metastases, cerebellar tumors, neurinomas of the caudal group of nerves and the trigeminal nerve, vascular processes such as angiomas, basilar aneurysms.

[a] Metastatic deposits may produce any of these syndromes.

Source: Adapted from Bingas.

Table 31-5
The main paraneoplastic disorders and associated autoantibodies[a]

Neurologic disorder	*Clinical features*	*Predominant autoantibody*	*Tumor*
Cerebellar degeneration	Ataxia, subacute	Anti-Yo (anti-Purkinje cell)	Ovary, fallopian tube, lung
Encephalomyelitis	Subacute confusion, brainstem signs, myelitis	Anti-Hu (ANNA 1) Anti-Ma	Small-cell lung, neuroblastoma, prostate, breast, Hodgkin, testicular (Ma)
Opsoclonus-myoclonus-axial ataxia	Ocular movement disorder gait ataxia	Anti-Ri (ANNA 2)	Breast, fallopian tube, small-cell lung
Retinal degeneration	Scotomas, blindness, glare, visual hallucinations	Antirecoverin	Small-cell lung, gynecologic cancers, melanoma
Subacute sensory neuropathy and neuronopathy	Distal or proximal sensory loss	Anti-Hu (ANNA-1)	Small-cell lung, Hodgkin, other lymphomas
Lambert-Eaton myasthenic syndrome	Proximal fatiguing weakness, autonomic symptoms (dry mouth)	Anti-Voltage gated calcium channel	Small-cell lung, Hodgkin, other lymphomas
Stiff-man syndrome	Muscle spasms and rigidity	Antiamphiphysin	Breast

[a] In most cases, a particular autoantibody is associated with a specific tumor type rather than with the clinical syndrome (e.g., small-cell lung cancer and polyneuropathy with ANNA 1, breast cancer with anti-Purkinje cell antibody, testicular tumors with anti Ma). Clinical syndromes similar to each of these may occur with non–small cell lung cancer and lymphoma, most often in the absence of detectable antibodies).

then directed to the shared antigen in both the tumor and the nervous system. The evidence for such an autoimmune response is most clearly exemplified by the Lambert-Eaton syndrome, in which an antibody derived from a tumor binds to voltage-gated calcium channels at neuromuscular junctions (Chap. 53).

Paraneoplastic Cerebellar Degeneration

For many years, this disorder was considered to be quite uncommon. In reviewing this subject in 1970, we were able to find only 41 pathologically verified cases; in a subsequent review (Henson and Urich), only a few more cases were added. The actual incidence is much higher than these figures would indicate. At the Cleveland Metropolitan General Hospital, in a series of 1700 consecutive autopsies in adults, there were five instances of cerebellar degeneration associated with neoplasm. In the experience of Henson and Urich, about half of all patients with nonfamilial, late-onset corticocerebellar degeneration proved sooner or later to be harboring a neoplasm. In recent years, large series of cases have been reported from the Mayo Clinic and the Memorial Sloan-Kettering Cancer Center (Hammock et al; Anderson et al).

In approximately one-third of the cases, the underlying neoplasm has been in the lung (most often a small-cell carcinoma)—a figure reflecting the high incidence of this tumor. However, the association of ovarian carcinoma and lymphoma, particularly Hodgkin disease, accounting for 26 and 16 percent, respectively, is considerably higher than would be expected on the basis of the frequency of these malignancies. Carcinomas of the breast, bowel, uterus, and other viscera have accounted for most of the remaining cases (Posner).

Characteristically, the cerebellar symptoms have an insidious onset and steady progression over a period of weeks to months; in more than half the cases, the cerebellar signs are recognized before those of the associated neoplasm. Ataxia of gait and of the limbs—affecting arms and legs more or less equally, dysarthria, and nystagmus are the usual manifestations. Occasionally, myoclonus and opsoclonus or a fast-frequency myoclonic tremor may be associated. In addition, there are certain symptoms and signs not ordinarily considered to be cerebellar in nature, notably diplopia, vertigo, sensorineural hearing loss, and disorders of ocular motility and sometimes of affect and mentation—findings that serve to distinguish paraneoplastic from alcoholic and other varieties of cerebellar degeneration. The CSF may show a mild pleocytosis and increase of protein, or it may be entirely normal. Early in the course of the disease, CT scanning and MRI may show no abnormality, but after a few months, atrophy of the brainstem and cerebellum may appear. In a few cases, T2-weighted MR images disclose an increased signal of the cerebellar white matter (Hammock et al) but this has not been our experience.

Pathologically, there are diffuse degenerative changes of the cerebellar cortex and deep cerebellar nuclei. Purkinje cells are affected predominantly and all parts of the cerebellar cortex are involved more or less equally. Rarely, there are associated degenerative changes in the spinal cord, involving the posterior columns and spinocerebellar tracts. The cerebellar lesions are frequently associated with perivascular and meningeal clusters of inflammatory cells. Henson and Urich regard the inflammatory changes as an independent process, part of a subacute paraneoplastic encephalomyelitis (see below). This view is supported by the finding that the specific antibodies that are linked to cerebellar degeneration differ from those that are found in paraneoplastic inflammatory lesions in other parts of the nervous system.

Anti–Purkinje cell antibodies (termed anti-Yo) can be found in the sera of about half the patients with paraneoplastic cerebellar degeneration and in the majority of those related to carcinoma of the breast or female genital tract. Thus, in the Mayo Clinic series of 32 patients, 16 had such antibodies; all were women and most of them had mammary or ovarian cancers. Death occurred in 4 to 18 months. In an equal number of cases without antibodies, half were men with lung cancer. Often in this group, in addition to the ataxia, there was vertigo and a disorder of ocular motility, affect, and mentation. Death in these cases occurred in 7 to 120 months.

Whether the antibodies are merely markers of an underlying tumor or the agents of destruction of the Purkinje cells is not known. They have been found to bind to a C-myc protein that is thought to initiate a degeneration of Purkinje cells. Regardless of the pathogenic significance of the antibodies, finding them in a patient with the typical neurologic disorder has considerable diagnostic significance. As mentioned above, the presence of a typical anti–Purkinje cell antibody strongly suggests that there is an underlying breast or ovarian cancer, which may be asymptomatic and small enough to be resected successfully. Other antibodies are found on occasion, such as ones against a glutamate receptor in patients with Hodgkin disease (Smitt et al).

Little can be done to modify the cerebellar symptoms, although there are on record several cases in which there was a partial or complete remission of symptoms after removal of the primary tumor (Paone and Jeyasingham). Further, in some cases associated with Hodgkin disease, there has been spontaneous improvement of the cerebellar symptoms. Preliminary reports of aggressive plasma exchange or intravenous immunoglobulin treatment early in the course suggest some benefit, but it should not be assumed that this approach will succeed in most patients.

Opsoclonus-Myoclonus-Ataxia Syndrome

In children, this syndrome is usually a manifestation of neuroblastoma, but it occurs in adults mainly in relation to breast cancer and small-cell lung cancer. The unique feature is a response to corticosteroids and ACTH in most children and in some adults, and resolution of the neurologic signs when the neuroblastoma is removed. A subgroup of the breast cancer patients produce an antibody that has the neuronal nuclear binding characteristics of the anti-Hu (antineuronal antibody type 1) antibody, but it is directed at a different RNA-binding antigen within the cell. It has therefore been termed *anti-Ri (antineuronal antibody type 2)*. This antibody is not found in the opsoclonus-ataxic syndrome of neuroblastoma and is present only rarely with small cell lung cancer. There have also been a limited number of positive serologic tests in children with opsoclonus, apparently without an underlying tumor. A number of such patients have had a mild pleocytosis; the MRI is usually normal. More complex syndromes have been reported with the anti-Ri antibody involving rigidity and intense stimulus–sensitive myoclonus in addition to the core features of opsoclonus and ataxia.

The neuropathologic findings have not been distinctive; mild cell loss has been described in the Purkinje cell layer, inferior olives, and brainstem, with mild inflammatory changes (Luque et al).

We have seen opsoclonus-myoclonus in a middle-aged woman with bronchial carcinoma and also in a man with gastric carcinoma. Similar cases occur with both cerebellar ataxia and an irregular tremor, which we have interpreted as myoclonic in character. These patients were found to have marked degeneration of the dentate nuclei. The prognosis in this syndrome is somewhat better than that for the other paraneoplastic diseases.

Encephalomyelitis Associated with Carcinoma

The occurrence of regional and bilateral encephalomyelitic changes in association with carcinoma has been described by several authors (Corsellis et al, Henson and Urich, Posner). In most of the reported cases (53 of 69 reviewed by Henson and Urich), the encephalitic process was associated with carcinoma of the bronchus, usually of the small-cell type but all types of neoplasm may be implicated. Histologically, this group of paraneoplastic disorders is characterized by extensive loss of nerve cells, accompanied by microglial proliferation, small patches of necrosis, and marked perivascular cuffing by lymphocytes. Foci of lymphocytic infiltration have been observed in the leptomeninges as well. These pathologic changes may involve the brain and spinal cord diffusely, but more often they predominate in a particular part of the nervous system, notably in the temporal lobes and adjacent nuclei ("limbic encephalitis," Fig. 31-21), the brainstem (particularly in the medulla), the cerebellum (see above), and the gray matter of the spinal cord. The symptoms will, of course, depend on the location and severity of the inflammatory changes and may overlap. Similar syndromes occur occasionally in nontumor cases.

Anxiety and depression, a confusional-agitated state, hallucinations, retentive memory defect (Korsakoff syndrome), and dementia—singly or in various combinations—are the principal manifestations of so-called *limbic encephalitis* (Gultekin et al). Vertigo, nystagmus, ataxia, nausea and vomiting, and a variety of ocular and gaze palsies reflect the presence of *paraneoplastic brainstem encephalitis*. As indicated above, these symptoms may be joined with cerebellar ataxia. We have seen instances of this condition involving only the midbrain and others involving the medulla, the latter with unusual breathing patterns including gasping, inspiratory breath-holding, and vocal-respiratory incoordination. In most of these cases, MRI shows T2 signal changes in affected regions; in severe cases, zones of focal necrosis may be seen. Odd seizures, including epilepsia partialis continua, have been observed with this disorder, but they must be rare. Sensory symptoms may be related to neuronal loss in the posterior horns, but degeneration of the posterior columns can usually be traced to a commonly associated component of the encephalomyelitis discussed in the next section, namely loss of neurons in the dorsal root ganglia (sensory neuronopathy and sensory neuropathy).

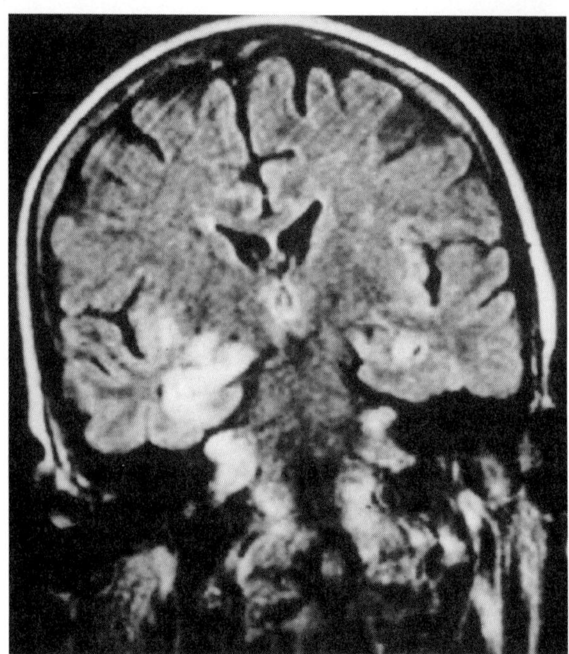

Figure 31-21

Coronal MR FLAIR image from a woman with paraneoplastic "limbic encephalitis" associated with lung cancer and a mild pleocytosis but no detectable autoantibodies. The hippocampi and adjacent regions are involved. Pathologically there proved to be gliosis and a minimal inflammatory infiltrate in these regions.

There may be a slowly progressive, symmetrical or asymmetrical *amyotrophy* of the arms and less often of the legs, related in two of our patients to inflammatory changes in the anterior horns of the spinal gray matter (see further on). A form characterized mainly by corticospinal degeneration is also known but has not been found in our material.

Pathologic studies have not clarified these forms of paraneoplastic disorder. In some cases, no changes were demonstrable in the brain, even though there had been a prominent dementia during life. Contrariwise, widespread inflammatory changes may be found without clinical abnormalities having been recorded during life. We believe that these seemingly paradoxical findings may have to do with the thoroughness of the clinical and pathologic examinations.

Most patients with small-cell lung cancer and paraneoplastic encephalomyelitis have circulating polyclonal IgG antibodies (called *anti-Hu*, or *anti-neuronal antibody, type 1*) that bind to the nuclei of neurons in many regions of the brain and cord, dorsal root ganglion cells, and peripheral autonomic neurons. The antibodies are reactive with certain nuclear RNA binding proteins. Cancers of the prostate and breast and neuroblastoma may rarely produce a similar antibody. As with cerebellar degeneration, the antibody titer is higher in the CSF than in the serum, indicating the production of antibody within the nervous system. Low titers of anti-Hu are found in many patients with small-cell cancer who are neurologically normal, probably because these small-cell tumors have expressed antigens that are recognized by anti-Hu. Several newly discovered antibodies—such as anti-Ma1 and -Ma2, have been detected in cases of brainstem encephalomyelitis and cross react with testicular antigens (Dalmau et al; Voltz et al). While quite rare, the clinical syndromes associated with the anti-Ma antibody and testicular tumors have been diverse: limbic, brainstem, or hypothalamic inflammation and an ataxic-opsoclonic syndrome that is more typical of anti-Ri antibody (see above). The heterogeneity of antibody response to these expressed proteins is thought to account for different clinical manifestations of the presumed immune process, but there is no certain evidence yet of their pathogenetic role.

Despite a few reports of improvement with plasma exchange or intravenous gamma globulin, the results of treatment have been disappointing. However, those few patients who did improve had treatment from the onset of symptoms, and this may be a way of limiting the neuronal loss.

Paraneoplastic Sensory Neuronopathy

This distinctive paraneoplastic syndrome is also associated with the anti-Hu antibody. It was first described by Denny-Brown in 1948 and served to introduce the concept of paraneoplastic neurologic disease. The initial symptoms are numbness or paresthesias, sometimes painful, in a limb or in both feet. There may be lancinating pains at the onset. Over a period of days in some cases, but more typically over weeks, the initially focal symptoms become bilateral and may spread to all limbs and their proximal portions and then to the trunk. This latter distribution, when present, and the affection of the face, scalp, and often the oral and genital mucosa mark the process as a sensory ganglionitis and radiculitis. As the illness progresses, all forms of sensation are greatly reduced, resulting in *disabling ataxia* and pseudoathetoid movements of the outstretched hands. The reflexes are lost but strength is relatively preserved. *Autonomic dysfunction*—including constipation or ileus, sicca syndrome, pupillary areflexia, and orthostatic hypotension—is a common occurrence. Indeed, a virtually pure form of peripheral autonomic failure may occur as a paraneoplastic phenomenon (*paraneoplastic dysautonomia*). One of our patients with sensory neuronopathy had gastric atony with fatal aspiration after vomiting and another died of unexpected cardiac arrhythmia. Very early in the illness, the electrophysiologic studies may be normal, but this gives way to a loss of all sensory potentials, with indications sometimes of a mild motor neuropathy. The spinal fluid often shows an elevated protein and a few lymphocytes. As with paraneoplastic encephalomyelitis, most of the cases that are associated with small-cell lung cancer demonstrate the anti-Hu antibody. The sensory neuronopathy that is related to Sjögren disease and the idiopathic variety do not have this antibody, making the test a reliable marker for lung cancer in patients with sensory neuropathy. The sensory neuronopathy is refractory to all forms of treatment and most patients die within months of onset, but there have been reports of brief remissions with plasma exchange and intravenous gamma globulin utilized early in the illness. Resection of the lung tumor may halt progression of the neurologic illness.

This disorder is discussed further in Chap. 46.

Carcinomatous Necrotizing Myelopathy and Motor Neuronopathy

In addition to the rare instances of subacute degeneration of spinal cord tracts that may be associated with paraneoplastic cerebellar degeneration (see above), there has been described a rapidly progressive form of widespread degeneration of the spinal cord (Mancall and Rosales). The myelopathy has been characterized by a rapidly ascending sensorimotor deficit that terminates fatally in a matter of a week or two and by a roughly symmetrical necrosis of both the gray and white matter of most of the cord. This form of *necrotizing myelopathy* is distinctly rare, being far less common than compression of the spinal cord from cancer and even less frequent than intramedullary metastases as a cause of myelopathy. Indeed, the status of necrotizing myelopathy as a remote effect of carcinoma is uncertain.

Henson and Urich have drawn attention to another rare spinal cord disorder usually associated with carcinoma of the lung. This takes the form of large, wedge-shaped necrotic lesions scattered throughout the cord, affecting mainly the white matter of the posterior and lateral columns. The clinical correlates of this disorder are also unclear.

A *subacute motor neuronopathy* is yet another spinal cord disorder that occurs as a remote effect of bronchogenic carcinoma, Hodgkin disease, and other lymphomas, as mentioned earlier in the section on encephalomyelitis (Schold et al). Clinically, some cases take the form of a relatively benign, purely motor weakness of the limbs, the course and severity of which are independent of the underlying neoplasm. Other cases are progressive, causing respiratory failure and death, thus simulating amyotrophic lateral sclerosis (ALS); some of these will have the anti-Hu antibody (Verma et al, Forsyth et al). The basic neuropathologic change is a depletion of anterior horn cells; also seen are inflammatory changes and neuronophagia, as in chronic poliomyelitis. In addition, the few autopsied cases have shown gliosis of the posterior columns, pointing to an asymptomatic affection of the primary sensory neuron, and a reduction in the number of Purkinje cells.

Forsyth and colleagues have subdivided their cases of *paraneoplastic motor neuron syndromes* into three groups: (1) rapidly progressive amyotrophy and fasciculations with or without brisk reflexes—all of their three patients displayed anti-Hu antibodies, two with small-cell lung cancer and one with prostate cancer; (2) a predominantly corticospinal syndrome that affected the oropharyngeal or limb musculature, without definite evidence of denervation, thus resembling primary lateral sclerosis—all were breast cancer patients but none showed antineuronal antibodies; and (3) a syndrome indistinguishable from ALS in six patients with breast or small-cell lung cancer, Hodgkin disease, or ovarian cancer, none of whom had antineuronal antibodies. In the last two groups one cannot be certain that the idiopathic variety of motor neuron disease was not the cause.

Other Paraneoplastic Disorders

Stiff-Man Syndrome Occasionally this disorder (page 1569) occurs as a paraneoplastic syndrome. Lesser degrees of unexplained mild rigidity are seen from time to time, due perhaps to loss of spinal cord interneurons. In what might be called "stiff-woman syndrome," Folli and associates have described three patients with breast cancer who developed a state of generalized motor hyperexcitability and rigidity. These patients had no antibodies to glutamic acid decarboxylase, as in the "stiff-man syndrome," but presumably there were antibodies to another synaptic protein.

Retinopathy In recent years, there have been several reports of retinopathy as a paraneoplastic syndrome. Small-cell carcinoma of the lung is the most common underlying malignancy. In about half of the reported cases, retinal symptoms preceded the discovery of the tumor by several months. The lesion is in the photoreceptor cells, and antiretinal antibodies have been identified in the serum. Photosensitivity, ring scotomas, and attenuation of the retinal arterioles are the main clinical features; Jacobson and coworkers have suggested that they constitute a diagnostic triad.

The Eaton-Lambert syndrome, probably the commonest paraneoplastic syndrome, is associated with antibodies directed against calcium channels, as mentioned earlier. This disorder is discussed on page 1547. Isolated case reports relating neuromyelitis optica and optic neuritis to neoplasm cannot presently be evaluated.

Radiation Injury of the Brain

Injury to the CNS from radiation is appropriately discussed here, since it occurs mainly in relation to therapy of brain tumors. Three syndromes of radiation damage have been delineated: acute, early delayed, and late delayed, although these stages often blend into one another. The acute reaction may begin during the latter part of a series of fractionated treatments or soon thereafter. There may be a seizure, a transitory worsening of the tumor symptoms, or signs of increased intracranial pressure. The EEG may reveal delta waves but with preserved background activity. Although the condition has been attributed to brain edema, this is not visible in MRI scans. Its basis is unknown. The symptoms subside in days to weeks.

The early delayed syndrome has been more troublesome in our experience. As with the acute syndrome, focal tumor symptoms may increase and, as seen on MRI (Fig. 31-22), the tumor mass enlarges, raising the possibility of further tumor growth, but again the symptoms usually resolve within 6 to 8 weeks. Postmortem examination discloses extensive demyelination, loss of oligodendrocytes beyond the confines of the tumor, and varying degrees of tissue necrosis. Possibly dexamethasone hastens resolution.

The late delayed injury is the most serious of the three complications. Here one finds—in structures adjacent to a cerebral neoplasm, the pituitary gland, or other structures of the head and neck—a coagulation necrosis of the white matter of the brain and occasionally of the brainstem. In some areas, the tissue undergoes softening and liquefaction, with cavitation. With lesser degrees of injury, the process is predominantly a demyelinating one, with partial preservation of axons. Later reactions are thought to be due to vascular changes as a result of radiation energy. Endothelial cells frequently multiply and, since ionization injures dividing cells, the vessels are

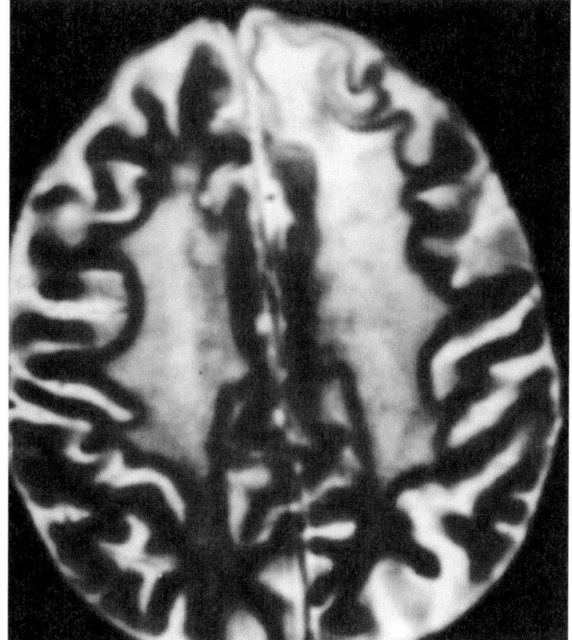

Figure 31-22

MRI showing early delayed radiation change in white matter of both frontal lobes, particularly severe on the right in the region of the treated glioma.

most vulnerable. The result is hyaline thickening of vessels with fibrinoid necrosis and thrombosis. There is a lesser degree of damage to glial cells. Neurons are relatively resistant.

The symptoms, coming on 3 months to many years after radiation therapy, are either those of a subacutely evolving mass, difficult to separate from those of tumor growth, or of a subacute dementia. The clinical pattern varies with the site of the lesion: focal or generalized seizures, impairment of mental function, and sometimes increased intracranial pressure. Whole-brain radiation for tumor or acute lymphoblastic leukemia can lead to multifocal zones of necrosis and holohemispheric spongiform changes in the white matter, with diffuse cerebral atrophy and enlarged ventricles. Progressive dementia, ataxia, and urinary incontinence are the main clinical features of this state (DeAngelis et al). In its mildest form there are no radiographic changes aside from the tumor, but the patient becomes mentally dull, slightly disinhibited, and often sleepy for large parts of the day. Panhypopituitarism is another complication of whole-brain radiotherapy, particularly in children who suffer growth retardation. Radiation necrosis of the spinal cord is further described on page 1302.

In the production of radiation necrosis, the total and fractional doses of radiation and the time over which treatment is administered are obviously important factors, but the exact amounts that produce such damage cannot be stated. Accepted levels of large-field radiation are tolerated in amounts approaching 6000 cGy provided that it is given in small daily doses (200 to 300 cGy) 5 days per week over a period of 6 weeks. Other factors, still undefined, must play a part, since similar courses of radiation treatment may damage one patient and leave another unaffected. CT scans show a low-density contrast-enhancing lesion, and by angiography there is an avascular mass. MRI is somewhat more sensitive in distinguishing radiation necrosis from tumor and peritumor products, but positron emission tomography (PET) is the most reliable way of making this distinction, perhaps obviating the need for biopsy (Glantz et al). Single photon emission tomography (SPECT) can be equally useful for this purpose (Carvalho et al). Treatment has consisted of corticosteroids, which may cause regression of symptoms and of edema surrounding the lesion. Very high doses may be necessary, 40 mg or more of dexamethasone (or its equivalent). Rarely, surgical resection has been attempted, with indifferent results.

Finally, it is known that tumors, usually sarcomas, can be induced by radiation (Cavin et al). While well documented, this occurs rarely and only after an interval of many years. We have also seen two cases of fibrosacroma of the brachial plexus region in the radiation field for breast tumors (Gorson et al). These lesions appeared more than 10 years after the initial treatment and many cases of even longer latency are on record.

Tumors of the spinal cord and peripheral nerves are discussed in Chaps. 44 and 46, respectively.

REFERENCES

Adams RD, Wegner W: Congenital cyst of the spinal meninges as cause of intermittent compression of the spinal cord. *Arch Neurol Psychiatry* 58:57, 1947.

Allen JC: Controversies in the management of intracranial germ cell tumors. *Neurol Clin* 9:441, 1991.

Anderson JR, Antoun N, Burnet N, et al: Neurology of the pituitary gland. *J Neurol Neurosurg Psychiatry* 66:703, 1999.

Anderson NE, Cunningham JM, Posner JB: Autoimmune pathogenesis of paraneoplastic neurological syndromes. *CRC Crit Rev Neurobiol* 3:245, 1987.

Bailey P, Bucy PC: Oligodendrogliomas of the brain. *J Pathol Bacteriol* 32:735, 1929.

Bailey P, Cushing H: *A Classification of Tumors of the Glioma Group on a Histogenetic Basis with a Correlated Study of Prognosis*. Philadelphia, Lippincott, 1926.

Barcos M, Lane W, Gomez GA, et al: An autopsy study of 1,206 acute and chronic leukemias (1958–1982). *Cancer* 60:827, 1987.

Barkovich AJ, Krischer J, Kun LE, et al: Brainstem gliomas: A classification system based on magnetic resonance imaging. *Pediatr Neurosurg* 16:73, 1993.

Bashir RM, Harris NL, Hochberg FH, Singer RM: Detection of Epstein-Barr virus in CNS lymphomas by insitu hybridization. *Neurology* 39:813, 1989.

Bellur SN, Chandra V, McDonald LW: Association of meningiomas with extraneural primary malignancy. *Neurology* 29:1165, 1979.

Benton JW, Nellhaus G, Huttenlocher PR, et al: The bobble-head doll syndrome. *Neurology* 16:725, 1966.

Bigner DD, McLendon RE, Bruner JM (Eds.) *Russell and Rubinstein's Pathology of Tumors of the Nervous System*, 6th Edition. London, Arnold, 1998.

Bingas B: Tumors of the base of the skull, in Vinken PJ, Bruyn GW (eds): *Handbook of Clinical Neurology*. Vol 17. Amsterdam, North-Holland, 1974, pp 136–233.

Boughey AM, Fletcher NA, Harding AE: Central nervous system hemangioblastoma: A clinical and genetic study of 52 cases. *J Neurol Neurosurg Psychiatry* 53:644, 1990.

Brougham M, Heusner AP, Adams RD: Acute degenerative changes in adenomas of the pituitary body—with special reference to pituitary apoplexy. *J Neurosurg* 7:421, 1950.

Burger PC: Malignant astrocytic neoplasms: Classification, pathologic anatomy and response to treatment. *Semin Oncol* 13:16, 1986.

Cairncross JG, MacDonald DR: Chemotherapy for oligodendroglioma: Progress report. *Arch Neurol* 48:225, 1991.

Carvalho PA, Schwartz RB, Alexander E, et al: Detection of recurrent gliomas with quantitative thallium-201/technetium-99m HMPAO single-photon emission computerized tomography. *J Neurosurg* 77:565, 1992.

Cavin LW, Dalrymple GV, McGuire EL, et al: CNS tumor induction by radiotherapy: A report of four new cases and estimate of dose required. *Int J Radiat Oncol Biol Phys* 18:399, 1990.

Chang SD, Alder JR: Treatment of cranial base meningiomas with linear accelerator radiosurgery. *Neurosurgery* 41:1019, 1997.

Clouston PD, DeAngelis LM, Posner JB: The spectrum of neurological disease in patients with systemic cancer. *Ann Neurol* 31:268, 1992.

Cogan DG: Tumors of the optic nerve, in Vinken PJ, Bruyn GW (eds): *Handbook of Clinical Neurology*. Vol 17. Amsterdam, North-Holland, 1974, pp 350–374.

Colao A, Lombardi G: Growth-hormone and prolactin excess. *Lancet* 352:1455,1998.

Corsellis JAN, Goldberg GJ, Norton AR: Limbic encephalitis and its association with carcinoma. *Brain* 91:481, 1968.

Cuneo RA, Caronna JJ, Pitts L, et al: Upward transtentorial herniation. Seven cases and literature review. *Ann Neurol* 36:618, 1979.

Cushing H: Some experimental and clinical observations concerning states of increased intracranial tension. *Am J Med Sci* 124:375, 1902.

Cushing H: *The Pituitary Body and Its Diseases*. Philadelphia, Lippincott, 1912.

Cushing H: *Tumors of the Nervus Acusticus and Syndrome of the Cerebellopontine Angle*. Philadelphia, Saunders, 1917.

Cushing H: *Intracranial Tumors: Notes upon a Series of 2000 Verified Cases with Surgical-Mortality Percentages Pertaining Thereto*. Springfield, IL, Charles C Thomas, 1932.

Cushing H, Eisenhardt L: *Meningiomas*. New York, Hafner, 1962.

Dalmau J, Gultekin H, Voltz R, et al: Ma1, a novel neuron- and testis-specific protein, is recognized by serum of patients with paraneoplastic disorders. *Brain* 122:27, 1999.

Daumas-Duport C, Scheithauer B, O'Fallon J, Kelly P: Grading of astrocytomas: A simple and reproducible method. *Cancer* 62:2152, 1988.

DeAngelis LM: Primary central nervous system lymphoma: A new clinical challenge. *Neurology* 41:619, 1991.

DeAngelis LM: Current management of primary central nervous system lymphoma. *Oncology* 9:63, 1995.

DeAngelis LM, Delattre J-Y, Posner JB: Radiation-induced dementia in patients cured of brain metastases. *Neurology* 39:789, 1989.

Delattre J-Y, Safai B, Posner JB: Erythema multiforme and Stevens Johnson syndrome in patients receiving cranial irradiation and phenytoin. *Neurology* 38:194, 1988.

Dropcho EJ: Autoimmune central nervous system paraneoplastic disorders: Mechanisms, diagnosis and therapeutic options. *Ann Neurol* 37(S1):102, 1995.

Duffner PK, Cohen ME, Myers MH, Heise HW: Survival of children with brain tumors: SEER program, 1973–1980. *Neurology* 36:597, 1986.

Duffner PK, Cohen ME: Primitive neuroectodermal tumors, in Vecht CJ, Vinken PJ, Bruyn GW (eds): *Handbook of Clinical Neurology*. Vol 28. Amsterdam, Elsevier, 1997, pp 221–227.

Dunn J, Kernohan JW: Gliomatosis cerebri. *Arch Pathol* 64:82, 1957.

Estrada J, Boronat M, Mielgo M, et al: The long-term outcome of pituitary irradiation after unsuccessful transsphenoidal surgery in Cushing's disease. *New Engl J Med* 336:172, 1997.

Fahlsbusch R, Honegger J, Paulis W, et al: Surgical treatment of craniopharyngiomas: Experience with 168 patients. *J Neurosurgery* 90:237, 1999.

Feigenbaum L, Ueda H, Jay G: Viral etiology of neurological malignancies in transgenic mice, in Levine AJ, Schmidek HH (eds): *Molecular Genetics of Nervous System Tumors*. New York, Wiley-Liss, 1993, pp 153–161.

Fishman RA: *Cerebrospinal Fluid in Diseases of the Nervous System*, 2nd ed. Philadelphia, Saunders, 1992.

Fokes EC Jr, Earle KM: Ependymomas: Clinical and pathological aspects. *J Neurosurg* 30:585, 1969.

Folli F, Solimena M, Cofiell R, et al: Autoantibodies to a 128-kd synaptic protein in three women with the stiff-man syndrome and breast cancer. *N Engl J Med* 328:546, 1993.

Forsyth PA, Dalmau J, Graus F, et al: Motor neuron syndromes in cancer patients. *Ann Neurol* 41:722, 1997.

Fox JL, Al-Mefty O: Suprasellar arachnoid cysts: An extension of the membrane of Liliequist. *Neurosurgery* 7:615, 1980.

Frankel SA, German WJ: Glioblastoma multiforme: A review of 219 cases with regard to natural history, pathology, diagnostic methods and history. *J Neurosurg* 15:489, 1958.

Friede RL, Janzer RC, Roessmann U: Infantile small-cell gliomas. *Acta Neuropathol* 57:103, 1982.

Gandy SE, Heier LA: Clinical and magnetic resonance features of primary intracranial arachnoid cysts. *Ann Neurol* 21:342, 1987.

Gardner G, Cocke EW Jr, Robertson JT, et al: Combined approach surgery for removal of glomus jugulare tumors. *Laryngoscope* 87:665, 1977.

Glantz MJ, Cole BF, Friedberg MH, et al: A randomized, blinded, placebo-controlled trial of divalproex sodium in adults with newly discovered brain tumors. *Neurology* 46:985, 1996.

Glantz MJ, Hoffman JM, Coleman RE, et al: Identification of early recurrence of primary central nervous system tumors by F18 FDG-PET. *Ann Neurol* 29:347, 1991.

Glass J, Gruber ML, Cher L, Hochberg FH: Preirradiation methotrexate chemotherapy of primary central nervous system lymphoma: Long-term outcome. *J Neurosurg* 81:188, 1994.

Globus JH, Silbert S: Pinealomas. *Arch Neurol Psychiatry* 25:937, 1931.

Gorson KC, Musaphir S, Lathi ES, Wolfe G: Radiation-induced malignant fibrous histiocytoma of the brachial plexus. *J Neurooncol* 26:73, 1995.

Guinee D Jr, Jaffe E, Kingma D, et al: Pulmonary lymphomatoid granulomatosis. *Am J Surg Pathol* 18:753, 1994.

Gultekin SH, Rosenfeld MR, Voltz R, et al: Paraneoplastic limbic encephalitis: Neurologic symptoms, immunological findings and tumor association in 50 patients. *Brain* 123:1481, 2000.

Hakuba A, Hashi K, Fujitani K, et al: Jugular foramen neurinomas. *Surg Neurol* 11:83, 1979.

Hammock JF, Kimmel DW, O'Neill BP, et al: Paraneoplastic cerebellar degeneration: A clinical comparison of patients with and without Purkinje cell antibodies. *Mayo Clin Proc* 65:1423, 1990.

Harner SG, Laws ER: Clinical findings in patients with acoustic neurinoma. *Mayo Clin Proc* 58:721, 1983.

Harper CG, Stewart-Wynne EG: Malignant gliomas in adults. *Arch Neurol* 35:731, 1978.

Henson RA, Urich H: *Cancer and the Nervous System*. Oxford, England, Blackwell, 1982.

Hochberg FH, Miller DC: Primary central nervous system lymphoma. *J Neurosurg* 68:835, 1988.

House WF, Hitselberger WE: Acoustic tumors, in Vinken PJ, Bruyn GW (eds): *Handbook of Clinical Neurology*. Vol 17. Amsterdam, North-Holland, 1974, pp 666–692.

Jacobson DM, Thirkill CE, Tipping SJ: A clinical triad to diagnose paraneoplastic retinopathy. *Ann Neurol* 28:162, 1990.

James CD, Carlbom E, Dumanski JP, et al: Clonal genomic alterations in glioma malignancy stages. *Cancer Res* 48:5546, 1988.

Jefferson G: The tentorial pressure cone. *Arch Neurol Psychiatry* 40:837, 1938.

Kaplan JG, DeSouza TG, Farkash A, et al: Leptomeningeal metastases: Comparison of clinical features and laboratory data of solid tumors, lymphoma, and leukemias. *J Neurooncol* 9:225, 1990.

Katzenstein AA, Carrington CB, Liebow AA: Lymphomatoid granulomatosis. A clinicopathologic study of 12 cases. *Cancer* 43:360, 1979.

Kaufman B, Tomsak RL, Kaufman BA, et al: Herniation of the suprasellar visual system and third ventricule into empty sellae: Morphologic and clinical considerations. *Am J Roentgenol* 152: 597, 1989.

Kendell BE, Lee BCP: Cranial chordomas. *Br J Radiol* 50:687, 1977.

Kepes JJ: *Meningiomas: Biology Pathology, and Differential Diagnosis*. New York, Masson, 1982.

Kernohan JW, Sayre GP: *Tumors of the Central Nervous System*: Fasc 35. *Atlas of Tumor Pathology*. Washington, DC, Armed Forces Institute of Pathology, 1952.

Kernohan JW, Uihlein A: *Sarcomas of the Brain*. Springfield, IL, Charles C Thomas, 1962.

Kernohan JW, Woltman HW: Incisura of the crus due to contralateral brain tumor. *Arch Neurol Psychiatry* 21:274, 1929.

Khalili K, Krynska B, Del Valle L, et al: Medulloblastomas and the human neurotropic polyomavirus JC virus. *Lancet* 353:1152, 1999.

Klatzo I: Neuropathological aspects of brain edema. *J Neuropathol Exp Neurol* 26:1, 1967.

Klibanski A, Zervas NT: Diagnosis and management of hormone-secreting pituitary adenomas. *N Engl J Med* 324:822, 1991.

Kliman B, Kjellberg RN, Swisher B, Butler W: Proton beam therapy of acromegaly: A 20-year experience, in Black PM et al (eds): *Secretory Tumors of the Pituitary Gland*. New York, Raven Press, 1984, pp 191–211.

Kondziolka D, Lunsford D, McLaughlin MR, Flickinger JC: Long-term outcomes after radiosurgery for acoustic neuroma. *New Eng J Med* 339:1426, 1998.

Kornblith PL, Walker MD, Cassady JR: *Neurologic Oncology*. New York, Lippincott, 1987, pp 159–161.

Kovacs K. Asa SL: *Functional Endocrine Pathology*. Boston, Blackwell Scientific, 1991.

Kramer W: Glomus jugulare tumors, in Vinken PJ, Bruyn GW (eds): *Handbook of Clinical Neurology*. Vol 18. Amsterdam, North-Holland, 1975, pp 435–455.

Krouwer HJG, Davis RL, Silver P, Prados M: Gemistocytic astrocytomas: A reappraisal. *J Neurosurg* 74:399, 1991.

Landolfi JC, Thaler HT, DeAngelis LM: Adult brainstem gliomas. *Neurology* 51:1136,1998.

Lamberts SWJ: The role of somatostatin in the regulation of anterior pituitary hormone secretion and the use of its analogs in the treatment of human pituitary tumors. *Endocrinol Rev* 9:417, 1988.

Laurence KM, Hoare RD, Till K: The diagnosis of choroid plexus papilloma of the lateral ventricle. *Brain* 84:628, 1961.

LEVIN VA, EDWARDS MS, WRIGHT DC, et al: Modified procarbazine, CCNU, and vincristine (PCV 3) combination chemotherapy in the treatment of malignant brain tumors. *Cancer Treat Rep* 64:237, 1980.

LEVINE AJ: Tumor suppressor genes, in Levine AJ, Schmidek HH (eds): *Molecular Genetics of Nervous System Tumors*. New York, Wiley-Liss, 1993, pp 137–143.

LEVINE AJ: The oncogenes of the DNA tumor viruses, in Levine AJ, Schmidek HH (eds): *Molecular Genetics of Nervous System Tumors*. New York, Wiley-Liss, 1993, pp 145–151.

LEVITT LJ, DAWSON DM, ROSENTHAL DS, MOLONEY WC: CNS - involvement in the non-Hodgkin's lymphomas. *Cancer* 45:545, 1980.

LI C-Y, WITZIG TE, PHYLIKY RL, et al: Diagnosis of B-cell non-Hodgkin's lymphoma of the central nervous system by immunocytochemical analysis of cerebrospinal fluid lymphocytes. *Cancer* 57:737, 1986.

LIEBOW AA, CARRINGTON CR, FRIEDMAN PJ: Lymphomatoid granulomatosis. *Hum Pathol* 3:457, 1972.

LOBOSKY JM, VANGILDER JC, DAMASIO AR: Behavioural manifestations of third ventricular colloid cysts. *J Neurol Neurosurg Psychiatry* 47:1075, 1984.

LOPES MBS, VANDENBERG SR, SCHEITHAUER BW: The World Health Organization classification of nervous system tumors in experimental neurooncology, in Levine AJ, Schmidek HH (eds): *Molecular Genetics of Nervous System Tumors*. New York, Wiley-Liss, 1993, pp 1–36.

LUDWIG CL, SMITH MT, GODFREY AD, ARMBRUSTMACHER VW: A clinicopathological study of 323 patients with oligodendrogliomas. *Ann Neurol* 19:15, 1986.

LUQUE FA, FURNEAUX HM, FERZIGER R, et al: Anti-Ri: An antibody associated with paraneoplastic opsoclonus and breast cancer. *Ann Neurol* 29:241, 1991.

MACCABE JJ: Glioblastoma, in Vinken PJ, Bruyn GW (eds): *Handbook of Clinical Neurology*. Vol 18. Amsterdam, North-Holland, 1975, pp 49–71.

MCCUTCHEON IE: Management of benign and aggressive intracranial meningiomas. *Oncology* 10:747, 1996.

MANCALL EL, ROSALES RK: Necrotizing myelopathy associated with visceral carcinoma. *Brain* 87:639, 1964.

MARTUZA RL: Genetics of neuro-oncology. *Clin Neurosurg* 21:417, 1984.

MARTUZA RL, OJEMANN RG: Bilateral acoustic neuromas: Clinical aspects, pathogenesis and treatment. *Neurosurgery* 10:1, 1982.

MATSON DD, CROFTON FDL: Papilloma of choroid plexus in childhood. *J Neurosurg* 17:1002, 1960.

MEYER A: Herniation of the brain. *Arch Neurol Psychiatry* 4:387, 1920.

MEYER FB, EBERSOLD MJ, REESE DF: Benign tumors of the foramen magnum. *J Neurosurg* 61:136, 1984.

MORITA A, MEYER FB, LAWS ER: Symptomatic pituitary metastases. *J Neurosurg* 89:69, 1998.

MORITA A, PIEPGRAS DG: Tumors of the base of the skull, in Vinken PJ, Bruyn GW, Vecht C (eds): *Handbook of Clinical Neurology*. Vol 68. Amsterdam, Elsevier 1997, pp 465–496.

MØRK SJ, LØKEN AC: Ependymoma—A follow-up study of 101 cases. *Cancer* 40:907, 1977.

NUGENT JL, BUNN PA, MATTHEWS MJ, et al: CNS metastases in small cell bronchogenic carcinoma. *Cancer* 44:1885, 1979.

OJEMANN RG, MONTGOMERY W, WEISS L: Evaluation and surgical treatment of acoustic neuroma. *N Engl J Med* 287:895, 1972.

OLIVECRONA H: The surgical treatment of intracranial tumors, in *Handbuch der Neurochirurgie*. Vol IV. Berlin, Springer-Verlag, 1967, pp 1–300.

O'NEILL BP, BUCKNER JC, COFFEY RJ, et al: Brain metastatic lesions. *Mayo Clin Proc* 69:1062, 1994.

PACKER RJ: Chemotherapy for medulloblastoma/primitive neuroectodermal tumors of the posterior fossa. *Ann Neurol* 28:823, 1990.

PAONE JF, JEYASINGHAM K: Remission of cerebellar dysfunction after pneumonectomy for bronchogenic carcinoma. *N Engl J Med* 302:156, 1980.

PAPPAS CTE, WHITE WL, BALDREE ME: Pituitary tumors: Anatomy, microsurgery, and management. *Barrows Neurol Inst Q* 6:2, 1990.

PATCHELL RA, TIBBS PA, WALSH JW, et al: A randomized trial of surgery in the treatment of single metastases to the brain. *N Engl J Med* 322:494, 1990.

PENCALET P, MAIXNER W, SAINTE-ROSE C, et al: Benign cerebellar astrocytoma in children. *J Neurosurg* 90:265, 1999.

PETERSON K, WALKER RW: Medulloblastoma/primitive neuroectodermal tumor in 45 adults. *Neurology* 45:440, 1995.

POLAK M: Registro Latino Americano de tumores del sistemo nervioso: Clasificacion sinonimia y estadistica. *Rev Neurol Argentina* 11:97, 1985.

POLLACK IF, HOFFMAN HJ, HUMPHREYS RP, et al: The long-term outcome after surgical resection of dorsally exophytic brain-stem gliomas. *J Neurosurg* 78:859, 1993.

POLLOCK BE, HUSTON J: Natural history of asymptomatic colloid cysts of the third ventricle. *J Neurosurg* 91:364, 1999.

POLMETEER FE, KERNOHAN JW: Meningeal gliomatosis. *Arch Neurol Psychiatry* 57:593, 1947.

POSNER J, CHERNICK NL: Intracranial metastases from systemic cancer. *Adv Neurol* 19:575, 1978.

POSNER JB: Primary lymphoma of the CNS. *Neurol Alert* 5:21, 1987.

POSNER JB: *Neurologic Complications of Cancer*. Philadelphia, Davis, 1995.

PRICE RA, JOHNSON WW: The central nervous system in childhood leukemia: I. The arachnoid. *Cancer* 31:520, 1973.

RIBBERT H: *Geschwulstlehre*. Bonn, Verlag Cohen, 1904.

RINGERTZ N: Grading system of gliomas. *Acta Pathol Microbiol Scand* 27:51, 1950.

ROBAIN O, DULAC O, DOMMERGUES JP, et al: Necrotising leukoencephalopathy complicating treatment of childhood leukaemia. *J Neurol Neurosurg Psychiatry* 47:65, 1984.

ROPPER AH: Lateral displacement of the brain and level of consciousness in patients with an acute hemispheral mass. *N Engl J Med* 314:953, 1986.

ROSENBERG GA, SALAND L, KYNER WT: Pathophysiology of periventricular tissue changes with raised CSF pressure in cats. *J Neurosurg* 59:606, 1983.

RUBINSTEIN AB, SHALIT MN, COHEN ML, et al: Radiation-induced cerebral meningioma: A recognizable entity. *J Neurosurg* 61:966, 1984.

RUBINSTEIN LJ: Embryonal central neuroepithelial tumors and their differentiating potential. *J Neurosurg* 62:795, 1985.

RUBINSTEIN LJ: *Tumors of the Central Nervous System*: Fasc 6, 2nd series. *Atlas of Tumor Pathology*. Washington, DC, Armed Forces Institute of Pathology, 1972.

RULEY HG: Oncogenes, in Levine AJ, Schmidek HH (eds): *Molecular Genetics of Nervous System Tumors*. New York, Wiley-Liss, 1993, pp 89–100.

RUSCIANO D, BURGER MM: Mechanisms of metastasis, in Levine AJ, Schmidek HH (eds): *Molecular Genetics of Nervous System Tumors*. New York, Wiley-Liss, 1993, pp 357–369.

RUSSELL DS: Cellular changes and patterns of neoplasia, in Haymaker W, Adams RD (eds): *Histology and Histopathology of the Nervous System*. Springfield, IL, Charles C Thomas, 1982, pp 1493–1515.

SANBORN GE, SELHORST GB, CALABRESE VP, TAYLOR, GR: Pseudotumor cerebri and insecticide intoxication. *Neurology* 29:1222, 1979.

SCHMIDEK HH: Some current concepts regarding medulloblastomas, in Levine AJ, Schmidek HH (eds): *Molecular Genetics of Nervous System Tumors*. New York, Wiley-Liss, 1993, pp 283–286.

SCHOLD SC, CHO E-S, SOMASUNDARAM M, POSNER JB: Subacute motor neuronopathy: A remote effect of lymphoma. *Ann Neurol* 5:271, 1979.

SEIZINGER BR, ROULEAN GA, OZELIUS LJ, et al: Von Hippel–Lindau disease maps to the region of chromosome 3 associated with renal carcinoma. *Nature* 332:268, 1988.

SHAPIRO WR: Therapy of adult malignant brain tumors: What have the clinical trials taught us? *Semin Oncol* 13:38, 1986.

SHAW EG, DAUMAS-DUPORT C, SCHEITHAUER BS, et al: Radiation therapy in the management of low-grade supratentorial astrocytomas. *J Neurosurg* 70:853, 1989.

SHEIBANI K, BATTIFORA H, WINBERG CD, et al: Further evidence that "malignant angioendotheliomatosis" is an angiotropic large-cell lymphoma. *N Engl J Med* 314:943, 1986.

SMITT PS, KINOSHITA A, LEEUW B, et al: Paraneoplastic cerebellar ataxia due to autoantibodies against a glutamate receptor. *N Engl J Med* 342:21, 2000.

SORENSON SC, EAGAN RT, SCOTT M: Meningeal carcinomatosis in patients with primary breast or lung cancer. *Mayo Clin Proc* 59:91, 1984.

TOMLINSON BE, PERRY RH, STEWART-WYNNE EG: Influence of site of origin of lung carcinomas on clinical presentation and central nervous system metastases. *J Neurol Neurosurg Psychiatry* 42:82, 1979.

VECHT CJ, AVEZAAT CJ, VANPUTTEN WL, et al: The influence of the extent of surgery on the neurological function and survival in malignant glioma: A retrospective analysis in 243 patients. *J Neurol Neurosurg Psychiatry* 53:466, 1990.

VERMA A, BERGER JR, SNODGRASS S, PETITO C: Motor neuron disease: A paraneoplastic process associated with anti-Hu antibody and small-cell lung carcinoma. *Ann Neurol* 40:112, 1996.

VOLTZ R, GULTEKIN SH, ROSENFELD MR, et al: A serologic marker of paraneoplastic limbic and brain-stem encephalitis in patients with testicular cancer. *N Engl J Med* 340:1788, 1999.

WAGA S, MORIKAWA A, SAKAKURA M: Craniopharyngioma with midbrain involvement. *Arch Neurol* 36:319, 1979.

WASSERSTROM WR, GLASS JP, POSNER JB: Diagnosis and treatment of leptomeningeal metastases from solid tumors: Experience with 90 patients. *Cancer* 49:759, 1982.

YUNG WA, HORTEN BC, SHAPIRO WR: Meningeal gliomatosis: A review of 12 cases. *Ann Neurol* 8:605, 1980.

ZENTNER J, WOLF HK, OSTERTUN B, et al: Gangliogliomas: Clinical, radiological, and histopathological findings in 51 patients. *J Neurol Neurosurg Psychiatry* 57:1497, 1994.

ZIMMERMAN HM: Brain tumors: Their incidence and classification in man and their experimental production. *Ann NY Acad Sci* 159:337, 1969.

ZULCH KJ: *Brain Tumors, Their Biology and Pathology*, 3rd ed. New York, Springer-Verlag, 1986.

Chapter 32

INFECTIONS OF THE NERVOUS SYSTEM (BACTERIAL, FUNGAL, SPIROCHETAL, PARASITIC) AND SARCOID

This chapter is concerned mainly with the pyogenic or bacterial infections of the central nervous system (CNS), i.e., bacterial meningitis, septic thrombophlebitis, brain abscess, epidural abscess, and subdural empyema. The granulomatous infections of the CNS—notably tuberculosis, syphilis and other spirochetal infections, and certain fungal infections—are also discussed in some detail. In addition, consideration is given to sarcoid, a granulomatous disease of uncertain etiology, and to the CNS infections and infestations caused by certain rickettsias, protozoa, worms, and ticks.

A number of other infectious diseases of the nervous system are more appropriately discussed elsewhere in this book. Diseases due to bacterial exotoxins—diphtheria, tetanus, botulism—are considered with other toxins that affect the nervous system (Chap. 43). Leprosy, which is essentially a disease of the peripheral nerves, is described in Chap. 46, and trichinosis, mainly a disease of muscle, in Chap. 48. Viral infections of the nervous system, because of their frequency and importance, are allotted a chapter of their own (Chap. 33).

PYOGENIC INFECTIONS OF THE CENTRAL NERVOUS SYSTEM

Pyogenic infections reach the intracranial structures in one of two ways, either by hematogenous spread (emboli of bacteria or infected thrombi) or by extension from cranial structures (ears, paranasal sinuses, osteomyelitic foci in the skull, penetrating cranial injuries, or congenital sinus tracts). In a number of cases, infection is iatrogenic, being introduced in the course of cerebral or spinal surgery, the placement of a ventriculoperitoneal shunt, or rarely by a lumbar puncture needle. Increasingly, infection is nosocomial, i.e., acquired in-hospital; in urban hospitals, nosocomial meningitis is now as frequent as the non-hospital-acquired variety (Durand et al).

Surprisingly little is known about the mechanisms of hematogenous spread, for human autopsy material seldom divulges information on this point, and animal experiments involving the injection of virulent bacteria into the bloodstream have yielded somewhat contradictory results. In most instances of bacteremia or septicemia, the nervous system seems not to be infected; yet in certain cases, a bacteremia due to pneumonia or endocarditis is the only apparent forerunner of meningitis. With respect to the formation of brain abscess, the notable feature is the resistance of cerebral tissue to infection. Direct injection of virulent bacteria into the brain of an animal seldom results in abscess formation. In fact, this condition has been produced consistently only by injecting culture medium along with the bacteria or by causing necrosis of the tissue at the time bacteria are inoculated. In humans, infarction of brain tissue due to arterial occlusion (thrombosis or embolism) or venous occlusion (thrombophlebitis) appears to be a common and perhaps necessary antecedent.

The mechanism of meningitis and brain abscess from infection of the middle ear and paranasal sinuses is easier to understand. The cranial epidural and subdural spaces are practically never the sites of blood-borne infections, in contrast to the spinal epidural space. Furthermore, the cranial bones and the dura mater (which essentially constitutes the inner periosteum of the skull) protect the cranial cavity against the ingress of bacteria. This protective mechanism may fail if suppuration occurs in the middle ear, mastoid cells, or frontal, ethmoid, and sphenoid sinuses. Two pathways from these sources have been demonstrated: (1) infected thrombi may form in diploic veins and spread along these vessels into the dural sinuses (into which the diploic veins flow), and from there, in retrograde fashion, along the meningeal veins into the brain, and (2) an osteomyelitic focus may form, with erosion of the inner table of bone and invasion of the dura, subdural space, pia-arachnoid, and even brain. Each of these pathways has been observed by the authors in some fatal cases of epidural abscess, subdural empyema, meningitis, cranial venous sinusitis and meningeal thrombophlebitis, and brain abscess. However, in many cases coming to autopsy, the pathway of infection cannot be determined.

With a hematogenous infection in the course of a bacteremia, usually a single type of virulent organism gains entry to the cranial cavity. In the adult the most common pathogenic organisms are pneumococcus (*Streptococcus pneumoniae*), meningococcus (*Neisseria meningitides*), *Haemophilus influenzae*, *Listeria monocytogenes*, and staphylococcus; in the neonate, *Escherichia coli* and group B streptococcus; in the infant and child, *H. influenzae*. By contrast, when septic material embolizes from infected lungs, pulmonary arteriovenous fistulae, or congenital heart lesions or extends directly from ears or sinuses, more than one type of bacterial flora common to these sources may be transmitted. Such "mixed infections" pose difficult problems in therapy. Occasionally in these latter conditions, the demonstration of the causative organisms may be unsuccessful, even from the pus of an abscess (mainly because of inadequate culturing techniques for anaerobic organisms and the prior use of antibiotics. Infections that follow neurosurgery or insertion of a cranial appliance are usually staphylococcal; a small number are due to mixed flora, including anaerobic ones, or enteric organisms. In determining the most likely invading organism, the age of the patient, the clinical setting of the infection (community-acquired, postsurgical, or nosocomial), the immune status of the patient, and evidence of systemic and local cranial disease all must be taken into account.

ACUTE BACTERIAL MENINGITIS (LEPTOMENINGITIS)

The Biology of Bacterial Meningitis

The immediate effect of bacteria or other microorganisms in the subarachnoid space is to cause an inflammatory reaction in the pia and arachnoid as well as in the cerebrospinal fluid (CSF). Since the subarachnoid space is continuous around the brain, spinal cord, and optic nerves, an infective agent gaining entry to any one part of the space may spread rapidly to all of it, even its most remote recesses; in other words, meningitis is always cerebrospinal. Infection also reaches the ventricles of the brain, either directly from the choroid plexuses or by reflux through the foramina of Magendie and Luschka.

The first reaction to bacteria or their toxins is hyperemia of the meningeal venules and capillaries and an increased permeability of these vessels, followed shortly by exudation of protein and the migration of neutrophils into the pia and subarachnoid space. The subarachnoid exudate increases rapidly, particularly over the base of the brain; it extends into the sheaths of cranial and spinal nerves and, for a very short distance, into the perivascular spaces of the cortex. During the first few days, mature and immature neutrophils, many of them containing phagocytized bacteria, are the predominant cells. Within a few days, lymphocytes and histiocytes increase gradually in relative and absolute numbers. During this time there is exudation of fibrinogen, which is converted to fibrin after a few days. In the latter part of the second week, plasma cells appear and subsequently increase in number. At about the same time the cellular exudate becomes organized into two layers—an outer one, just beneath the arachnoid membrane, made up of neutrophils and fibrin, and an inner one, next to the pia, composed largely of lymphocytes, plasma cells, and mononuclear cells or macrophages. Although fibroblasts begin to proliferate early, they are not conspicuous until later, when they take part in the organization of the exudate, resulting in fibrosis of the arachnoid and loculation of pockets of exudate.

During the process of resolution, the inflammatory cells disappear in almost the same order as they had appeared. Neutrophils begin to disintegrate by the fourth to fifth day, and soon thereafter, with treatment, no new ones appear. Lymphocytes, plasma cells, and macrophages disappear more slowly, and a few lymphocytes and mononuclear cells may remain in small numbers for several months. The completeness of resolution depends to a large extent on the stage at which the infection is arrested. If it is controlled in the very early stages, there may not be any residual change in the arachnoid; following an infection of several weeks' duration, there is a permanent fibrous overgrowth of the meninges, resulting in a thickened, cloudy, or opaque arachnoid and often in adhesions between the pia and arachnoid and even between the arachnoid and dura.

From the earliest stages of meningitis, changes are also found in the small- and medium-sized subarachnoid arteries. The endothelial cells swell, multiply, and crowd into the lumen. This reaction appears within 48 to 72 h and increases in the days that follow. The adventitial connective tissue sheath becomes infiltrated by neutrophils. Foci of necrosis of the arterial wall sometimes occur. Neutrophils and lymphocytes migrate from the adventitia to the subintimal region, often forming a conspicuous layer. Later there is subintimal fibrosis. This is a striking feature of nearly all types of subacute and chronic infections of the meninges but most notably of tuberculous and syphilitic meningitis (Heubner's arteritis). In the veins, swelling of the endothelial cells and infiltration of the adventitia also occur. Subintimal layering, as occurs in arterioles, is not observed, but there may be a diffuse infiltration of the entire wall of the vessel. It is in veins so affected that focal necrosis of the vessel wall and mural thrombi are most often found. Cortical thrombophlebitis of the larger veins does not usually develop before the end of the second week of the infection.

The unusual prominence of the vascular changes may be related to their anatomic peculiarities. The adventitia of the subarachnoid vessels, both of arterioles and venules, is actually formed by an investment of the arachnoid membrane, which is invariably involved by the infectious process. Thus, in a sense, the outer vessel wall is affected from the beginning by the inflammatory process—an infectious vasculitis. The much more frequent occurrence of thrombosis in veins than in arteries is probably accounted for by the thinner walls and the slower current (possibly stagnation) of blood in the former.

Although the spinal and cranial nerves are surrounded by purulent exudate from the beginning of the infection, the perineurial sheaths become infiltrated by inflammatory cells only after several days. Exceptionally, in some nerves, there is infiltration of the endoneurium and degeneration of myelinated fibers, leading to the formation of fatty macrophages and proliferation of Schwann cells and fibroblasts. More often, there is little or no damage to nerve fibers. Occasionally cellular infiltrations may be found in the optic nerves or olfactory bulbs.

The arachnoid membrane tends to serve as an effective barrier to the spread of infection, but some reaction in the subdural space may occur nevertheless (subdural effusions). This happens far more often in infants than in adults; according to Snedeker and coworkers, approximately 40 percent of infants with meningitis who are less than 18 months of age develop subdural effusions. As a rule, there is no subdural pus, only a yellowish exudate. In an even higher percentage of cases, small amounts of fibrinous exudate are found in microscopic sections that include the cranial and particularly the spinal dura.

When fibrinopurulent exudate accumulates in large quantities around the spinal cord, it blocks off the spinal subarachnoid space. Hydrocephalus is produced by exudate in the foramina of Magendie and Luschka or in the subarachnoid space around the pons and midbrain, interfering with the flow of CSF from the lateral recesses of the fourth ventricle and cisterna magna to the basal cisterns and cerebral convexities. In the later stages, fibrous subarachnoid adhesions are an additional and sometimes the most important factor interfering with the circulation of CSF. An infrequent late sequela of bacterial meningitis is *chronic adhesive arachnoiditis* or *chronic meningomyelitis*.

In the early stages of meningitis, very little change in the substance of the brain can be detected. Neutrophils appear in the Virchow-Robin perivascular spaces but enter the brain only if there is necrosis. After several days, microglia and astrocytes increase in number, at first in the outer zone and later in all layers of the cortex. The associated nerve cell changes may be very slight. Obviously some disorder of the cortical neurons must take place from the beginning of the infection to account for the stupor, coma, and convulsions that are so often observed, but several days must elapse before any change can be demonstrated microscopically. It is uncertain whether these cortical changes are due to the diffusion of toxins from the meninges, to a circulatory disturbance, or to some other factor, such as increased intracranial pressure. The aforementioned changes are not due to invasion of brain substance by bacteria and should therefore be regarded as a noninfectious encephalopathy. When macrophages and astrocytes are exposed to endotoxins in vitro, the cells synthesize and release cytokines, the most important of which are interleukin 1 and tumor necrosis factor. These cytokines are believed to stimulate and modulate the local immune response.

In the early stages of meningitis, there may be little change in the ependyma and the subependymal tissues; but in the later stages, conspicuous changes are invariably found. The most prominent finding is infiltration of the subependymal perivascular spaces and often of the brain tissue with neutrophilic leukocytes and later with lymphocytes and plasma cells. There may be desquamation of ependymal cells. Microglia and astrocytes proliferate, the latter sometimes overgrowing and burying remnants of the ependymal lining. We believe that the bacteria pass through the ependymal lining and set up this inflammatory reaction. This sequence of events is favored by a developing hydrocephalus, which stretches and breaks the ependymal lining. The glial changes are secondary to damage of subependymal tissues. Collections of subependymal astrocytes protrude into the ventricle, giving rise to a granular ependymitis, which, if prominent, may narrow and obstruct the aqueduct of Sylvius. The choroid plexus is at first congested, but within a few days it becomes infiltrated with neutrophils and lymphocytes and eventually may be covered with exudate. As in the case of the meningeal exudate, lymphocytes, plasma cells, and macrophages later predominate. Eventually there is organization of the exudate covering the plexus.

As any meningitis becomes more chronic, the pia-arachnoid exudate tends to accumulate around the base of the brain (basilar meningitis), obstructing the flow of CSF and giving rise to hydrocephalus. The exudate may also encircle cranial nerves and lead to focal neuropathies.

The reader may question this long digression into matters that are more pathologic than clinical, but only a knowledge of the morphologic features of meningitis enables one to understand the clinical state and its sequelae. The meningeal and ependymal reactions to bacterial infection and the clinical correlates of these reactions are summarized in Table 32-1, which should be consulted together with this section.

Types of Bacterial Meningitis

Almost any bacterium gaining entrance to the body may produce meningitis, but, as already noted, by far the most common are *H. influenzae*, *N. meningitidis*, and *Strep. pneumoniae*, which account for about 75 percent of sporadic cases. Infection with *L. monocytogenes* is now the fourth most common type of nontraumatic or nonsurgical bacterial meningitis in adults. The following are less frequent causes: *Staph. aureus* and group A and group D streptococci, usually in association with brain abscess, epidural abscess, head trauma, neurosurgical procedures, or cranial thrombophlebitis; *E. coli* and group B streptococci in newborns; and the other Enterobacteriaceae such as *Klebsiella*, *Proteus*, and *Pseudomonas*, which are usually a consequence of lumbar puncture, spinal anesthesia, or shunting procedures to relieve hydrocephalus. Rarer meningeal pathogens include *Salmonella*, *Shigella*, *Clostridium*, *Neisseria gonorrhoeae*, and *Acinetobacter calcoaceticus*, which may be difficult to distinguish from *Haemophilus* and *Neisseria*. In endemic areas, mycobacterial infections (to be considered further on) are as frequent as those due to other bacterial organisms. They have also assumed greater importance in developed countries as the number of immunosuppressed persons increases.

Epidemiology

Pneumococcal, influenzal (*H. influenzae*), and meningococcal forms of meningitis have a worldwide distribution, occurring mainly during the fall, winter, and spring and predominating in males. Each has a relatively constant yearly incidence, although epidemics of meningococcal meningitis seem to occur roughly in 10-year cycles. Drug-resistant strains appear with varying frequency, and such information, gleaned from national surveillance reports issued by the Centers for Disease Control and Prevention and from reports of local health agencies, are of great practical importance. *H. influenzae* meningitis, formerly encountered mainly in infants and young children, has been nearly eliminated in this age group as a result of vaccination programs in developed countries, It continues to be common in less developed nations and is now occurring with increasing frequency in adults (in the United States there are between 12,000 and 15,000 cases each year). *Meningococcal meningitis* occurs most often in children and adolescents but is also encountered throughout much of adult life, with a sharp decline in incidence after the age of 50. *Pneumococcal meningitis* predominates in the very young and in older adults. Perhaps the greatest change in the epidemiology of bacterial meningitis, aside from the one related to *H. influenzae* vaccination, has been the increasing incidence of nosocomial infections, accounting for 40 percent of cases in large urban hospitals (Durand and colleagues); gram-negative bacilli and staphylococcus account for a large proportion of these. Noteworthy is the report of Schuchat et al, who found that in 1995, some 5 years after the introduction of the conjugate *H. influenzae* vaccine, the overall incidence of bacterial meningitis in the United States had been halved. The yearly incidence rate (per 100,000) of the responsible pathogens now are as follows: *Strep. pneumoniae*, 1.1; *Neisseria meningitidis*, 0.6; group B streptococcus, 0.3; *Listeria monocytogenes*, 0.2; and *H. influenzae*, 0.2.

Pathogenesis

The three most common meningeal pathogens are all inhabitants of the nasopharynx in a significant part of the population and depend upon antiphagocytic capsular or

Table 32-1
Pathologic-clinical correlations in acute, subacute, and chronic meningeal reactions

I. In acute meningeal inflammation:

A. *Pure pia-arachnoiditis*: headache, stiff neck, Kernig and Brudzinski signs. These signs depend on the activation of protective reflexes that shorten the spine and immobilize it. Extension of the neck and flexion of the hips and knees reduce stretch on inflamed spinal structures; resistance to forward flexion of the neck and extension of the legs involves maneuvers that oppose these protective flexor reflexes.

B. *Subpial encephalopathy*: confusion, stupor, coma, and convulsions are related to this lesion. The tissue beneath the pia is not penetrated by bacteria; hence the change is probably toxic (e.g., cytokines). Cerebral infarction due to cortical vein thrombosis may underlie these symptoms in some cases.

C. *Inflammatory or vascular involvement of cranial nerve roots*: ocular palsies, facial weakness, and deafness are the main clinical signs. *Note*: Deafness may also be due to middle ear infection, to extension of meningeal infection to the inner ear, or to toxic effects of antimicrobial agents.

D. *Thrombosis of meningeal veins*: focal seizures, focal cerebral defects such as hemiparesis, aphasia (rarely prominent), etc., may appear on the third or fourth
day after the onset of meningeal infection, but more often after the first week. There may be spinal cord infarction.

E. *Ependymitis, choroidal plexitis*: it is doubtful if there are any recognizable clinical effects aside from those of the associated meningitis and hydrocephalus.

F. *Cerebellar or cerebral hemisphere herniation*: due to swelling (as in B), causing upper cervical cord compression with quadriplegia or signs of midbrain–third nerve compression.

II. In more subacute and chronic forms of meningitis:

A. *Tension hydrocephalus*, due at first to purulent exudate around the base of the brain, later to meningeal fibrosis, and rarely to aqueductal stenosis. In adults, there are variable degrees of impairment of consciousness, decorticate postures (arms flexed, legs extended), grasp and suck reflexes, and sphincteric incontinence. CSF pressure may at first be elevated; as the ventricles enlarge and the choroid plexuses are compressed, it may fall to within limits of normal (normal-pressure hydrocephalus). In infants and young children, the main signs are enlarging head, frontal bossing, inability to look upward (eyes turn down and lids retract on effort to look up—"sunset" sign); in mildest form, there are only psychomotor retardation, unsteadiness of gait, and incontinence.

B. *Subdural effusion*: impaired alertness, refusal to eat, vomiting, immobility, bulging fontanels, and persistence of fever despite clearing of CSF. In infants, the effusion causes an exaggerated transillumination. If fever is present but CSF pressure is normal, and if one-sided cerebral signs are clearly in evidence, thrombophlebitis with infarction of underlying brain is the leading possibility.

C. *Extensive venous or arterial infarction*: unilateral or bilateral hemiplegia, decorticate or decerebrate rigidity, cortical blindness, stupor or coma with or without seizures.

III. Late effects or sequelae:

A. *Meningeal fibrosis around optic nerves or around spinal cord and roots*: blindness and optic atrophy, and spastic paraparesis with sensory loss in the lower segments of the body (opticochiasmatic arachnoiditis and meningomyelitis, respectively).

B. *Chronic meningoencephalitis with hydrocephalus*: dementia, stupor or coma, and paralysis (e.g., general paralysis of the insane). If lumbosacral posterior roots are chronically damaged, a tabetic syndrome results.

C. *Persistent hydrocephalus in the child*: blindness, arrest of all mental activity, bilateral spastic hemiplegia.

---

surface antigens for survival in the tissues of the infected host. To a large extent they express their pathogenicity by extracellular proliferation. It is evident from the frequency with which the carrier state is detected that nasal colonization is not a sufficient explanation of infection of the meninges. Factors that predispose the colonized patient to invasion of the bloodstream, which is the usual route by which bacteria reach the meninges, are obscure but include antecedent viral infections of the upper respiratory passages or, in the case of *Strep. pneumoniae*, infections of the lung. Once blood-borne, it is evident that pneumococci, *H. influenzae*, and meningococci possess a unique predilection for the meninges, although the precise factors that determine this meningeal localization are not known. Whether the organisms enter the CSF via the choroid plexus or meningeal vessels is also unknown. It has been variously postulated that the entry of bacteria into the subarachnoid space is facilitated by disruption of the blood-CSF barrier by trauma, circulating endotoxins, or an initial viral infection of the meninges.

Avenues other than the bloodstream by which bacteria can gain access to the meninges include congenital neuroectodermal defects, craniotomy sites, diseases of the middle ear and paranasal sinuses, skull fractures, and, in cases of recurrent infection, dural tears from remote minor or major trauma. Occasionally a brain abscess may rupture into the subarachnoid space or ventricles, thus infecting the meninges. The isolation of anaerobic streptococci, *Bacteroides*, *Actinomyces*, or a mixture of microorganisms from the CSF should suggest the possibility of a brain abscess with an associated meningitis.

Clinical Features

Adults and Children The early clinical effects of acute bacterial meningitis are fever, severe headache, and stiffness of the neck (resistance to passive movement on forward bending), sometimes with generalized convulsions and a disorder of consciousness (i.e., drowsiness, confusion, stupor, and coma). Flexion at the hip and knee in response to forward flexion of the neck (Brudzinski sign) and inability to completely extend the legs (Kernig sign) have the same significance as stiff neck but are less consistently elicitable. Basically, all of these signs are part of a flexor protective reflex. Stiffness of the neck that is part of paratonic or extrapyramidal rigidity should not be mistaken for that of meningeal irritation. The former is more or less equal in all directions of movement, in distinction to that of meningitis, which is present only or predominantly on forward flexion. Diagnosis of meningitis may be difficult when the initial manifestations consist only of fever and headache, when stiffness of the neck has not yet developed, and when there is only pain in the neck or abdomen or a febrile confusional state or delirium. Also, stiffness of the neck may not be apparent in the deeply stuporous or comatose patient or in the infant, as indicated further on.

The symptoms comprised by the meningitic syndrome are common to the three main types of bacterial meningitis, but certain clinical features and the setting in which each of them occurs correlate more closely with one type than another.

Meningococcal meningitis should always be suspected when the evolution is extremely rapid (delirium and stupor may supervene in a matter of hours), when the onset is attended by a petechial or purpuric rash or by large ecchymoses and lividity of the skin of the lower parts of the body, when there is circulatory shock, and especially during local outbreaks of meningitis. Since a petechial rash accompanies approximately 50 percent of meningococcal infections, its presence dictates immediate institution of antibiotic therapy, even though a similar rash may be observed with certain viral (ECHO-9 and some other enteroviruses and rarely with other bacterial meningitides) as well as *Staph. aureus* infections. *Pneumococcal meningitis* is often preceded by an infection in the lungs, ears, sinuses, or the heart valves. In addition, a pneumococcal etiology should be suspected in alcoholics, in splenectomized patients, in the very elderly, and in those with recurrent bacterial meningitis, dermal sinus tracts, sickle cell anemia ("autosplenectomized"), and basilar skull fracture. *H. influenzae* meningitis usually follows upper respiratory and ear infections in the child.

Other specific bacterial etiologies are suggested by particular clinical settings. Meningitis in the presence of furunculosis or following a neurosurgical procedure should raise the possibility of a coagulase-positive staphylococcal infection. Ventriculovenous shunts, inserted for the control of hydrocephalus, are particularly prone to infection with coagulase-negative staphylococci. HIV infection, myeloproliferative or lymphoproliferative disorders, defects in cranial bones (tumor, osteomyelitis), collagen diseases, metastatic cancer, and therapy with immunosuppressive agents are clinical conditions that favor invasion by such pathogens as Enterobacteriaceae, *Listeria*, *A. calcoaceticus*, *Pseudomonas*, and occasionally by parasites.

Focal cerebral signs in the early stages of the disease, although seldom prominent, are most frequent in pneumococcal and *H. influenzae* meningitides. Some of the transitory focal cerebral signs may represent postictal phenomena (Todd's paralysis); others may be related to an unusually intense focal meningitis—for example, purulent material collected in one sylvian fissure. Seizures are encountered most often with *H. influenzae* meningitis. Although seizures are most frequent in infants and children, it is difficult to judge their significance, since young children may convulse with fever of any cause. Persistent focal cerebral lesions or intractable seizures, which develop most often in the second week of the meningeal infection, are caused by an infectious vasculitis, as described above—usually with occlusion of surface cerebral veins—and infarction of cerebral tissue. Cranial nerve abnormalities are particularly frequent with pneumococcal meningitis, the result of invasion of the nerve by purulent exudate and possibly ischemic damage as the nerve traverses the subarachnoid space.

Infants and Newborns Acute bacterial meningitis during the first month of life is said to be more frequent than in any subsequent 30-day period of life. It poses a number of special problems. Infants, of course, cannot complain of headache, stiff neck may be absent, and one has only the nonspecific signs of a systemic illness—fever, irritability, drowsiness, vomiting, convulsions—and a bulging fontanel to suggest the presence of meningeal infection. Signs of meningeal irritation do occur, but only late in the course of the illness. A high index of suspicion and liberal use of the lumbar puncture needle are the keys to early diagnosis. Lumbar puncture is crucial, and it must be performed before any antibiotics are administered for other neonatal infections. An antibiotic regimen sufficient to control a septicemia may allow a meningeal infection to smolder and to flare up after antibiotic therapy for the systemic infection has been discontinued.

A number of other facts about the natural history of neonatal meningitis are noteworthy. It is more common in males than in females, in a ratio of about 3:1. Obstetric abnormalities in the third trimester (premature birth, prolonged labor, premature rupture of fetal membranes) occur frequently in mothers of infants who develop meningitis in the first weeks of life. The most significant factor in the pathogenesis of the meningitis is maternal infection (usually a urinary tract infection or puerperal fever of unknown cause). The infection in both mother and infant is most often due to gram-negative enterobacteria, particularly *E. coli*, and group B streptococci and less often to *Pseudomonas*, *Listeria*, *Staph. aureus* or *epidermidis* (formerly *albus*), and group A streptococci. Analysis of postmortem material indicates that in most cases infection occurs at or near the time of birth, although clinical signs of infection may not become evident until several days or a week later.

In infants with meningitis, one should be prepared to find a unilateral or bilateral *subdural effusion* regardless of bacterial type. Young age, rapid evolution of the illness, low polymorphonuclear cell count, and markedly elevated protein in the CSF correlate with the formation of effusions, according to Snedeker and coworkers. Also, these attributes greatly increase the likelihood of the meningitis being associated with neurologic signs. Transillumination of the skull is the simplest method of demonstrating the presence of an effusion, but CT scanning and MRI are the definitive diagnostic tests. When aspirated, most of the effusions prove to be sterile if the patient is responding well to antibiotic therapy. If recovery is delayed and neurologic signs persist, a succession of aspirations is required. In our experience and that of others, patients in whom meningitis is complicated by subdural effusions are no more likely to have residual neurologic signs than those without effusions.

Spinal Fluid Examination

As already indicated, *the lumbar puncture is an indispensable part of the examination of patients with the symptoms and signs of meningitis or of any patient in whom this diagnosis is suspected.* Bacteremia is not a contraindication to lumbar puncture. If there is clinical evidence of a focal lesion with increased intracranial pressure, then CT scanning of the head or MRI, looking for a mass lesion, is a prudent first step, but *in most cases this is not necessary and should not delay the administration of antibiotics.*

The dilemma concerning the risk of promoting transtentorial or cerebellar herniation by lumbar puncture, even without a cerebral mass, as indicated in Chaps. 2 and 17, has been settled in favor of performing the tap if there is a reasonable suspicion of meningitis. The highest estimates of risk come from studies such as those of Rennick, who reported a 4 percent incidence of worsening among 445 children undergoing lumbar puncture for the diagnosis of acute meningitis. It must be pointed out that a cerebellar pressure cone may occur in fulminant meningitis independent of lumbar puncture; therefore the risk of the procedure is probably even less than usually stated.

The spinal fluid *pressure* is so consistently elevated (above 180 mmH_2O) that a normal pressure on the initial lumbar puncture in a patient with suspected bacterial meningitis raises the possibility that the needle is partially occluded or the spinal subarachnoid space is blocked. Pressures over 400 mmH_2O suggest the presence of brain swelling and the potential for cerebellar herniation. Many neurologists favor the administration of intravenous mannitol if the pressure is this high, but this practice does not provide assurance that herniation will be avoided.

A *pleocytosis* is diagnostic. The number of leukocytes in the CSF ranges from 250 to 100,000 per cubic millimeter, but the usual number is from 1000 to 10,000. Occasionally, in pneumococcal and influenzal meningitis, the CSF may contain a large number of bacteria but few if any neutrophils for the first few hours. Cell counts of more than 50,000 per cubic millimeter raise the possibility of a brain abscess having ruptured into a ventricle. Neutrophils predominate (85 to 95 percent of the total), but an increasing proportion of mononuclear cells is found as the infection continues, especially in partially treated meningitis. In the early stages, careful cytologic examination may disclose that some of the mononuclear cells are myelocytes or young neutrophils. Later, as treatment takes effect, the proportions of lymphocytes, plasma cells, and histiocytes steadily increase.

The *protein* content is higher than 45 mg/dL in more than 90 percent of the cases; in most it falls in the range of 100 to 500 mg/dL. The *glucose* content is diminished, usually to a concentration below 40 mg/dL, or less than 40 percent of the blood glucose concentration (measured concomitantly) provided that the latter is less than 250 mg/dL. However, in atypical or *culture-negative cases*, other conditions associated with a reduced CSF glucose should be considered. These include hypoglycemia from any cause; sarcoidosis of the CNS; fungal or tuberculous meningitis; and some cases of subarachnoid hemorrhage, meningeal carcinomatosis, chemically induced inflammation from craniopharyngioma or teratoma, or meningeal gliomatosis.

Gram stain of the spinal fluid sediment permits identification of the causative agent in most cases of bacterial meningitis; pneumococci and *H. influenzae* are identified more readily than meningococci. Small numbers of gram-negative diplococci in leukocytes may be indistinguishable from fragmented nuclear material, which may also be gram-negative and of the same shape as bacteria. In such cases, a thin film of uncentrifuged CSF may lend itself more readily to morphologic interpretation than a smear of the sediment. The commonest error in reading Gram-stained smears of CSF is the misinterpretation of precipitated dye or debris as gram-positive cocci or the confusion of pneumococci with *H. influenzae*. The latter organisms may stain heavily at the poles, so that they resemble gram-positive diplococci, and older pneumococci often lose their capacity to take a gram-positive stain.

Cultures of the spinal fluid, which prove to be positive in 70 to 90 percent of cases of bacterial meningitis, are best obtained by collecting the fluid in a sterile tube and immediately inoculating plates of blood, chocolate, and MacConkey agar; tubes of thioglycolate (for anaerobes); and at least one other broth. The advantage of using broth media is that large amounts of CSF can be cultured. The importance of obtaining blood cultures is mentioned below.

The problem of identifying causative organisms that cannot be cultured, particularly in patients who have received antibiotics, may be overcome by the application of several special laboratory techniques. One of these is counterimmunoelectrophoresis (CIE), a sensitive technique that permits the detection of bacterial antigens in the CSF in a matter of 30 to 60 min. It is particularly useful in patients with partially treated meningitis, in whom the CSF still contains bacterial antigens but no organisms detected on a smear or grown in culture. Several more recently developed serologic methods, radioimmunoassay (RIA) and latex particle agglutination (LPA), as well as an enzyme-linked immunosorbent assay (ELISA), may be even more sensitive than CIE. An argument has been made that these procedures are not cost-effective, since—in virtually all instances in which the bacterial antigen can be detected—the Gram stain also shows the organism. Our sense is that the more expensive tests are still of some assistance, particularly if the Gram stain is difficult to interpret and one or more doses of antibiotics render the cultures negative. Gene amplification by the polymerase chain reaction (PCR) is the most recently developed and most sensitive technique. As it becomes more widely available in clinical laboratories, rapid diagnosis may be facilitated (Desforges; Naber), but the use of careful Gram-stain preparations still needs to be encouraged.

Measurements of chloride concentrations in the CSF are not very useful, but they are usually found to be low (less than 700 mg/dL), reflecting dehydration and low serum chloride levels. In contrast, CSF lactate dehydrogenase (LDH), although measured infrequently, can be of diagnostic and prognostic value. A rise in total LDH activity is consistently observed in patients with bacterial meningitis; most of this is due to fractions 4 and 5, which are derived from granulocytes. Fractions 1 and 2 of LDH, which are presumably derived from brain tissue, are only slightly elevated in bacterial meningitis but rise sharply in patients who develop neurologic sequelae or later die. Lysozymal enzymes in the CSF—derived from leukocytes, meningeal cells, or plasma—may also be increased in meningitis, but the clinical significance of this observation is unknown. Levels of lactic acid in the CSF (determined by either gas chromatography or enzymatic analysis) are also elevated in both bacterial and fungal meningitides (above 35 mg/dL) and may be helpful in distinguishing these disorders from viral meningitides, in which lactic acid levels remain normal.

Other Laboratory Findings In addition to CSF cultures, *blood cultures should always be obtained* because they are positive in 40 to 60 percent of patients with *H. influenzae*, meningococcal, and pneumococcal meningitis, and they may provide the only definite clue as to the causative agent. Routine cultures of the oropharynx are as often misleading as they are helpful, because pneumococci, *H. influenzae*, and meningococci are common inhabitants of the throats of healthy persons. In contrast, *cultures of the nasopharynx* may be helpful in diagnosis, though often not in a timely way; the finding of encapsulated *H. influenzae* or groupable meningococci may provide the clue to the etiology of the meningeal infection. Conversely, the absence of such a finding prior to antibiotic treatment makes an *H. influenzae* and meningococcal etiology unlikely. The *leukocyte count* in the blood is generally elevated, and immature forms are usually present. Meningitis may be complicated after several days by severe hyponatremia, the result of inappropriate secretion of antidiuretic hormone (ADH).

Radiologic Studies In patients with bacterial meningitis chest films are essential because they may disclose an area of pneumonitis or abscess. Sinus and skull films may provide clues to the presence of cranial osteomyelitis, paranasal sinusitis, mastoiditis, or cranial osteomyelitis, but these structures are better visualized on CT scans, which have supplanted conventional films in most cases. The CT scan is particularly useful in detecting lesions that erode the skull or spine and provide a route for bacterial invasion, such as tumors or sinus wall defects, as well as in demonstrating a brain abscess or subdural empyema. MRI with gadolinium enhancement may display the meningeal exudate and cortical reaction, and both types of imaging, with appropriate techniques, will demonstrate venous occlusions and adjacent infarctions.

Recurrent Bacterial Meningitis

This is observed most frequently in patients who have had some type of ventriculovenous shunting procedure for the treatment of hydrocephalus or who have an incompletely closed dural opening after surgery. When the recurrence is of inapparent origin, one should always suspect a congenital neuroectodermal sinus or a fistulous connection between the nasal sinuses and the subarachnoid space. The fistula in these latter cases is more often traumatic than congenital in origin (a previous basilar skull fracture), although the interval between injury and the initial bout of meningitis may be several years. The site of trauma is in the frontal or ethmoid sinuses or the cribriform plate, and *Strep. pneumoniae* is the usual pathogen. Often it reflects the predominance of such strains in nasal carriers. These cases usually have a good prognosis; mortality is much lower than in ordinary cases of pneumococcal meningitis.

CSF rhinorrhea is present in most cases of posttraumatic meningitis, but it may be transient and difficult to find. Suspicion of its presence is raised by the recent onset of anosmia or by the occurrence of a watery nasal discharge that is salty to the taste and increases in volume when the head is dependent. One way of confirming the presence of a CSF leak is to measure the glucose concentration of nasal secretions; ordinarily they contain little glucose, but in CSF rhinorrhea the amount of glucose approximates that obtained by lumbar puncture (two-thirds of the serum value). The site of a CSF leak can sometimes be demonstrated by injecting a dye, radioactive albumin, or water-soluble contrast material into the spinal subarachnoid space and detecting its appearance in nasal secretions or its site of exit by CT scanning. This testing is best performed after the acute infection has subsided. Persistence of CSF rhinorrhea requires surgical repair.

Differential Diagnosis

The diagnosis of bacterial meningitis is not difficult provided that one maintains a high index of suspicion. *All febrile patients—even those with low-grade fever and those with only lethargy, headache, or confusion of sudden onset—should be subjected to lumbar puncture*, since a definitive diagnosis of bacterial meningitis can be made only by examination of the CSF. It is particularly important to think of meningitis in drowsy, febrile, and septic patients in an intensive care unit. Overwhelming sepsis itself, or the multiorgan failure that it engenders, may cause an encephalopathy, but if there is a meningitis, it is imperative, in deciding on the choice of antibiotics, to identify it early. The same can be said for the confused alcoholic patient. Too often the symptoms are ascribed to alcohol intoxication or withdrawal, or to hepatic encephalopathy, until examination of the CSF reveals a meningitis. Although this approach may result in many negative spinal fluid examinations, it is preferable to the consequence of overlooking a bacterial meningitis. Viral meningitis (which is far more common than bacterial meningitis), subarachnoid hemorrhage, chemical meningitis (following lumbar puncture, spinal anesthesia, or myelography), and tuberculous, leptospiral, sarcoid, and fungal meningoencephalitis enter into the differential diagnosis as well.

Also, a number of nonbacterial meningitides must be considered in the differential diagnosis when the meningitis recurs repeatedly and all cultures are negative. Included in this group are Epstein-Barr virus (EBV) infections; Behçet disease, which is characterized by recurrent oropharyngeal mucosal ulceration, uveitis, orchitis, and meningitis; so-called Mollaret meningitis, which consists of recurrent episodes of fever and headache in addition to signs of meningeal irritation (due in many cases to herpes simplex, as discussed in Chap. 33); and the Vogt-Koyanagi-Harada syndrome, in which recurrent meningitis is associated with iridocyclitis and depigmentation of the hair and skin. The CSF in these recurrent types may contain large numbers of lymphocytes or polymorphonuclear leukocytes but no bacteria, and the glucose content is not reduced (see discussion of chronic and recurrent meningitis on page 788). Carcinomatous and lymphomatous meningitis rarely present in the fulminant manner of bacterial meningitis, but sometimes they do, and the CSF formulas can be similar. Rarely, a fulminant case of cerebral angiitis or intravascular lymphoma will present with headache, fever, and confusion in conjunction with a meningeal inflammatory reaction.

The other intracranial suppurative diseases and their differentiation from bacterial meningitis are considered further on in this chapter.

Treatment

Bacterial meningitis is a medical emergency. The first therapeutic measures are directed to sustaining blood pressure and treating septic shock (volume replacement, pressor therapy) and choosing an antibiotic that is known to be bactericidal for the established or suspected organism and is able to enter the CSF in effective amounts. *Treatment should begin while awaiting the results of diagnostic tests* and should be changed later in accordance with the findings. Whereas penicillin formerly sufficed to treat almost all meningitides acquired outside the hospital, the initial choice of antibiotic has become increasingly complicated as resistant strains of meningitic bacteria have emerged. The selection of drugs to treat nosocomial infections presents special difficulties.

In recent years, many reports have documented an increasing incidence of pneumococcal isolates that also have a relatively high resistance to penicillin, reaching 50 percent in some European countries. Current estimates are that in some areas of the United States, 15 percent of these isolates are penicillin resistant to some degree (most have a relatively low level of resistance). In the 1970s, the now less frequent *H. influenzae* type B strains producing beta-lactamase, and thus resistant to ampicillin and penicillin, were recognized. Currently 30 percent of *H. influenzae* isolates produce the beta-lactamase enzyme, but almost all remain sensitive to third-generation cephalosporins (cefoxatime, cefoperazone, ceftizoxime, etc.). Isolation from the blood or CSF of a highly resistant organism requires the use of ceftriaxone, with the addition of vancomycin and rifampin. *N. meningitides*, at least in the United States, remains highly susceptible to penicillin and ampicillin. These regional variations and ongoing antibiotic-induced changes in the infecting microorganisms underscore the need for constant awareness of drug resistance in the physician's local area, especially in the case of pneumococcal infections. Throughout the course of treatment, it is necessary to have access to a dependable laboratory that can carry out rapid and detailed drug-resistance testing.

Recommendations for the institution of empiric treatment of meningitis have been reviewed by Quagliarello and Scheld and are summarized in modified form in Table 32-2. In children and adults, third-generation cephalosporins are probably the best initial

Table 32-2
Empiric therapy of bacterial meningitis

Age of patient	*Antimicrobial therapy*[a]
0–4 weeks	Cefotaxime plus ampicillin
4–12 weeks	Third-generation cephalosporin plus ampicillin (plus dexamethasone)
3 months–18 years	Third-generation cephalosporin plus vancomycin (±ampicillin)
18–50 years	Third-generation cephalosporin plus vancomycin (±ampicillin)
>50 years	Third-generation cephalosporin plus vancomycin plus ampicillin
Immunocompromised state	Vancomycin plus ampicillin and ceftazidime
Basilar skull fracture	Third-generation cephalosporin plus vancomycin
Head trauma; neurosurgery	Vancomycin plus ceftazidime
CSF shunt	Vancomycin plus ceftazidime

[a]For all ages from 3 months onward, an alternative treatment is meropenem plus vancomycin. For severe penicillin allergy consider: vancomycin and chloramphenicol (for meningococcus) and trimethoprim/sulfamethoxazole (for *Listeria*). A high failure rate has been reported with chloramphenicol in patients with drug-resistant pneumococcus.

therapy for the three major types of community-acquired meningitides. In areas with substantial or increasing numbers of high-level penicillin-resistant pneumococci, consideration should be given to adding vancomycin and rifampin until the susceptibility of the isolate is established. Ampicillin should be added to the regimen in cases of suspected *Listeria* meningitis. When serious allergy to penicillin and cephalosporins precludes their use, chloramphenicol is a suitable alternative.

In cases of meningitis due to *Staph. aureus*, including those that occur after neurosurgery or major head injury, administration of vancomycin and ceftazidime is a reasonable first approach. Upon determining the sensitivity of the organism, therapy may have to be altered or may be simplified by using vancomycin or nafcillin alone. The recommended dosages of the major antibiotics are given in Table 32-3, and the choice of antibiotic for the optimal treatment of specific bacterial isolates is given in Table 32-4.

Table 32-3
Recommended dosages of antimicrobial agents for bacterial meningitis in adults with normal renal and hepatic function[a]

Antimicrobial agent	*Total daily dose*	*Dosing interval, hours*
Amikacin[b]	15–30 mg/kg	8
Ampicillin	12 g	4
Cefepime	4–6 g	8–12
Cefotaxime	8–12 g	4–6
Ceftazidime	6 g	8
Ceftriaxone	4 g	12–24
Chloramphenicol[c]	4–6 g	6
Ciprofloxacin	800 mg	12
Gentamicin[b]	5 mg/kg	8
Meropenem	3–6 g	8
Nafcillin	9–12 g	4
Oxacillin	9–12 g	4
Penicillin G	24 million units	4
Rifampin[d]	600 mg	24
Tobramycin[b]	5 mg/kg	8
Trimethoprim/ sulfamethoxazole[e]	20 mg/kg	6–12
Vancomycin[b, f]	2–3 g	6–12

[a]Unless indicated, therapy is administered intravenously.
[b]Peak and trough serum concentrations must be monitored.
[c]Higher dose recommended for pneumococcal meningitis.
[d]Oral administration.
[e]Dosage based on trimethoprim component.
[f]CSF concentrations may have to be monitored in severely ill patients.

Duration of Therapy Most cases of bacterial meningitis should be treated for a period of 10 to 14 days except when there is a persistent parameningeal focus of infection. Antibiotics should be administered in full doses parenterally (preferably intravenously) throughout the period of treatment. Treatment failures with certain drugs, notably ampicillin, may be attributable to oral or intramuscular administration, resulting in inadequate concentrations in the CSF. Repeated lumbar punctures are not necessary to assess the effects of therapy as long as there is progressive clinical improvement. The CSF glucose may remain low for many days after other signs of infection have subsided and should occasion concern only if bacteria are present in the fluid and the patient remains febrile and ill.

Prolongation of fever or the late appearance of drowsiness or hemiparesis should raise the suspicion of subdural effusion, mastoiditis, sinus thrombosis, cortical vein or jugular phlebitis, or brain abscess; all require that therapy be continued for a longer period. Bacteriologic relapse after treatment is discontinued requires immediate reinstitution of therapy.

Corticosteroids Early controlled studies demonstrated no beneficial effects of corticosteroids in the treatment of pyogenic meningitis. More recent studies have re-evaluated the therapeutic value of dexamethasone in children with meningitis. Although mortality was not affected, fever subsided more rapidly and the incidence of sensorineural deafness and other neurologic sequelae was reduced, particularly in those with *H. influenzae* meningitis. On these grounds, it is recommended that the treatment of childhood meningitis include dexamethasone in high doses (0.15 mg/kg four times daily for 4 days), instituted as soon as possible. Analogous data in neonates and adults are lacking. Nevertheless, we favor the use of corticosteroids in cases with overwhelming infection at any age (very high CSF pressure or signs of herniation, high CSF bacterial count with minimal pleocytosis, and signs of acute adrenal insufficiency, i.e., the Waterhouse-Friderichsen syndrome).

Other Forms of Therapy There is no evidence that repeated drainage of CSF is therapeutically effective. In fact, increased CSF pressure in the acute phase of bacterial meningitis is largely a consequence of cerebral

Table 32-4
Specific antimicrobial therapy for acute meningitis

Microorganism	*Standard therapy*	*Alternative therapies*
Bacteria		
Haemophilus influenzae		
B-lactamase-negative	Ampicillin	Third-generation cephalosporin[a]; chloramphenicol
B-lactamase-positive	Third-generation cephalosporin[a]	Chloramphenicol; cefepime
Neisseria meningitidis	Penicillin G or ampicillin	Third-generation cephalosporin[a]; chloramphenicol
Streptococcus pneumoniae		
Penicillin MIC <0.1 μg/mL (sensitive)	Penicillin G or ampicillin	Third-generation cephalosporin[a]; chloramphenicol; vancomycin plus rifampin
Penicillin MIC 0.1–1.0 μg/mL (intermediate sensitivity)	Third-generation cephalosporin[a]	Vancomycin; meropenem
Penicillin MIC ≥2.0 μg/mL (highly resistant)	Vancomycin plus third-generation cephalosporin	Meropenem
Enterobacteriaceae	Third-generation cephalosporin[a]	Meropenem; fluoroquinolone; trimethoprim/sulfamethoxazole
Pseudomonas aeruginosa	Ceftazidime[b]	Meropenem; fluoroquinolone[b]
Listeria monocytogenes	Ampicillin or penicillin G[b]	Meropenem; trimethoprim/sulfamethoxazole
Streptococcus agalactiae	Ampicillin or penicillin G[b]	Third-generation cephalosporin[a]; vancomycin
Staphylococcus aureus		
Methicillin-sensitive	Nafcillin or oxacillin	Vancomycin
Methicillin-resistant	Vancomycin	
Staphylococcus epidermidis	Vancomycin[c]	

[a]Cefotaxime or ceftriaxone or cefepime.
[b]Addition of an aminoglycoside should be considered.
[c]Addition of rifampin should be considered.
Key: MIC = Minimal inhibitory concentration.

edema, in which case the lumbar puncture may predispose to cerebellar herniation. Mannitol and urea have been employed with apparent success in some cases of severe brain swelling with unusually high initial CSF pressures (>400 mmH_2O). Acting as osmotic diuretics, these agents enter cerebral tissue slowly, and their net effect is to decrease brain water. However, neither mannitol nor urea has been studied in controlled fashion in the management of meningitis. An adequate but not excessive amount of intravenous normal saline (avoiding fluids with free water) should be given, and anticonvulsants should be prescribed when seizures are present. In children, particular care should be taken to avoid hyponatremia and water intoxication—potential causes of brain swelling.

Anticonvulsants need not be administered routinely but should be given if a seizure has occurred or there is evidence of cortical vein occlusion.

Prophylaxis All household contacts of patients with meningococcal meningitis should be protected. The risk of secondary cases is small for adolescents and adults but ranges from 2 to 4 percent for those less than 5 years of age. A daily oral dose of rifampin—600 mg every 12 h in adults and 10 mg/kg every 12 h in children—for 2 days suffices. If 2 weeks or more have elapsed since the index case was found, no prophylaxis is needed.

Immunization against *H. influenzae* is steadily reducing the incidence of meningitis from this organism. Also, many institutions housing young adults, such as colleges and the military, have instituted programs of immunization against *N. meningitidis*.

Prognosis

Untreated, bacterial meningitis is usually fatal. The overall mortality rate of uncomplicated *H. influenzae* and meningococcal meningitis has remained at about 5 percent for many years; in pneumococcal meningitis, the rate is considerably higher (15 to 30 percent). Fulminant meningococcemia, with or without meningitis, also has a high mortality rate because of the associated vasomotor collapse and infective shock, associated with adrenocortical hemorrhages (Waterhouse-Friderichsen syndrome). A disproportionate number of deaths from meningitis occur in infants and in the aged. The mortality rate is highest in neonates, from 40 to 75 percent in reported series, and at least half of those who recover show serious neurologic sequelae. The presence of bacteremia, coma, seizures, and a variety of concomitant diseases—including alcoholism, diabetes mellitus, multiple myeloma, and head trauma—all worsen the prognosis. The triad of pneumococcal meningitis, pneumonia, and endocarditis has a particularly high fatality rate.

It is often impossible to explain the death of the patient or at least to trace it to a single specific mechanism. The effects of overwhelming infection, with bacteremia and hypotension or brain swelling and cerebellar herniation, are clearly implicated in the deaths of some patients during the initial 48 h. These events may occur in bacterial meningitis of any etiology; however, they are more frequent in meningococcal infection (Waterhouse-Friderichsen syndrome). Some of the deaths occurring later in the course of the illness are attributable to respiratory failure, often consequent to aspiration pneumonia.

Relatively few patients who recover from meningococcal meningitis show residual neurologic defects, whereas such defects are encountered in at least 25 percent of children with *H. influenzae* meningitis and up to 30 percent of child and adults patients with pneumococcal meningitis. Ferry and coworkers, in a prospective study of 50 infants who survived *H. influenzae* meningitis, found that about 50 percent were normal, whereas 9 percent had behavioral problems and about 30 percent had neurologic deficits (seizures and/or impairment of hearing, language, mentation, and motor function). In a report of a personal series of 185 children recovering from bacterial meningitis, Pomeroy and associates found that 69 were still not normal neurologically at the end of a month; however, at the end of a year, only 26 demonstrated neurologic abnormalities; 18 were left with a hearing deficit, 13 with late afebrile seizures, and 8 with multiple deficits. The presence of persistent neurologic deficits was the only independent predictor of late seizures. Dodge and colleagues found that 31 percent of children with pneumococcal meningitis were left with persistent sensorineural hearing loss; for meningococcal and *H. influenzae* meningitis, the figures were 10.5 and 6 percent, respectively. Cranial nerve palsies other than deafness tend to disappear after a few weeks or months. Deafness in these infections is due to suppurative cochlear destruction or to the ototoxic effects of aminoglycoside antibiotics. Bacteria reach the cochlea mainly via the cochlear aqueduct, which connects the subarachnoid space to the scala tympani. This occurs quite early in the course of infection, hearing loss being evident within a day of onset of the meningitis; in about half such cases, the deafness resolves. Hydrocephalus, a rare complication, may become manifest months after treatment and may require shunting if gait or mentation is affected. It may be difficult to determine on clinical grounds whether a residual state of imbalance is the result of hydrocephalus or of eighth nerve damage. We have seen several instances of upper cervical cord infarction, with quadriparesis and respiratory failure, as a result of compression from descent of the cerebellar tonsils (Ropper and Kanis). The role of lumbar puncture in this complication has not been clarified.

The acute complications of bacterial meningitis, the intermediate and late neurologic sequelae, and the pathologic basis of these effects are summarized in Table 32-1. Other aspects of current treatment have been summarized by Lambert.

ENCEPHALITIS DUE TO BACTERIAL INFECTIONS

Quite apart from acute and subacute bacterial endocarditis, which may give rise to cerebral embolism and characteristic inflammatory reactions in the brain (see further on), there are several systemic bacterial infections that may be complicated by a special type of encephalitis or meningoencephalitis. Three common ones are *Mycoplasma pneumoniae* infections, *L. monocytogenes meningoencephalitis*, and *legionnaires' disease*. Probably Lyme borreliosis should be included in this category, but it is more chronic and is described further on in this chapter with the spirochetal infections. The rickettsial encephalitides (particularly Q fever), which mimic bacterial meningoencephalitis, are also addressed later in the chapter. Cat-scratch disease is another rare cause of bacterial meningoencephalitis. Meningoencephalitis due to brucellosis occurs very rarely in the United States. Whipple disease, discussed below, which appears to be a focal invasion of the brain by a novel bacterium, also belongs in this category.

Mycoplasma pneumoniae This organism, which causes10 to 20 percent of all pneumonias, is associated with a number of neurologic syndromes. Guillain-Barré polyneuritis, cranial neuritis, acute myositis, aseptic meningitis, transverse myelitis, global encephalitis, seizures, cerebellitis, acute disseminated (postinfectious) encephalomyelitis, and acute hemorrhagic leukoencephalitis (Hurst disease) have all been reported in association with mycoplasmal pneumonias or with serologic evidence of infection (Westenfelder et al; Fisher et al; Rothstein and Kenny). We have observed several patients with a striking cerebral, cerebellar, brainstem, or spinal syndrome incurred during or soon after a mycoplasmal pneumonia or tracheobronchitis. In addition to the cerebellitis, which is clinically similar to the illness that follows varicella, unusual encephalitic syndromes of choreoathetosis, seizures, delirium, hemiparesis, and acute brain swelling (Reye syndrome) have each been reported in a few cases. The incidence of these complications has been estimated as 1 in 1000 mycoplasmal infections, but it may approach 5 percent when more careful surveillance is carried out during epidemics. A severe prodromal headache has occurred in many of our cases. At the time of onset of the neurologic symptoms, there may be no sign of pneumonia, and in some patients, only an upper respiratory syndrome, mainly a tracheobronchitis, occurs.

The mechanism of cerebral damage that complicates mycoplasmal infections has not been established, but recent evidence suggests that the organism is present in the central nervous system during the acute illness. To our knowledge, the organism has been cultured from the brain in only one fatal case, but polymerase chain reaction (PCR) techniques have detected fragments of mycoplasmal DNA in the spinal fluid from several patients (Narita et al). In other instances, the nature of the neurologic complications and their temporal relationship to the mycoplasmal infection clearly suggest that secondary autoimmune factors are operative; i.e., that these are instances of postinfectious encephalomyelitis (a type of acute disseminated encephalomyelitis described in Chap. 36). Most of the patients with the infectious variety have recovered with few or no sequelae, but rare fatalities are reported.

The CSF usually contains small numbers of lymphocytes and other mononuclear cells and an increased protein content. The diagnosis can be established by culture of the organism from the respiratory tract (which is difficult), by rising serum titers of complement-fixing IgG and IgM antibodies and cold agglutinin antibodies in the CSF, or by specialized DNA detection techniques from the CSF. Erythromycin and tetracycline derivatives reduce morbidity, mainly by eradicating the pulmonary infection; the effects on the nervous system complications are not known.

Listeria monocytogenes Meningoencephalitis from this organism is most likely to occur in immunosuppressed and debilitated individuals and is a well-known and occasionally fatal cause of meningitis in the newborn. Meningitis is the usual neurologic manifestation, but there are numerous recorded instances of a true focal bacterial infectious encephalitis, rarely with a normal CSF. Between 1929, when the organism was discovered, and 1962, when Gray and Killinger collected all the reported cases, it was noted that 35 percent of 467 patients had either meningitis or meningoencephalitis as the primary manifestation. The infection may take the form of a rhombencephalitis—more specifically, several days of headache, fever, nausea, and vomiting followed by asymmetrical cranial nerve palsies, signs of cerebellar dysfunction, hemiparesis, quadriparesis, or sensory loss. Respiratory failure has been reported. Of 62 cases of *Listeria* brainstem encephalitis reported by Armstrong and Fung, 8 percent were in immunosuppressed patients; meningeal signs were present in only half the patients, and the spinal fluid often showed misleadingly mild abnormalities. CSF cultures yielded *Listeria* in only 40 percent of cases (blood cultures were even more often normal). Consistent with our experience, the early CT scan was often normal; MRI, however, has revealed abnormal signals in the parenchyma of the brainstem. The monocytosis, which gives the organism its name, refers to the reaction in the peripheral blood in rabbits and has not been prominent in the blood or CSF of our cases. One of the patients described by Lechtenberg and coworkers had a proven brain abscess; other patients have had multiple abscesses (Uldry et al). Judging from the clinical signs in some cases, the infection appears to affect both the brainstem parenchyma and the extra-axial portion of cranial nerves. Endocarditis is rare. The treatment is ampicillin (1 g intravenously every 4 h) in combination with tobramycin (5 mg/kg intravenously in three divided doses daily). If the condition of the host is compromised, the outcome is often fatal; but most of our patients without serious medical disease have made a full and prompt recovery.

Legionnaires' Disease This potentially fatal respiratory disease, caused by the gram-negative bacillus *Legionella pneumophila*, first came to medical notice in July 1976, when a large number of members of the

American Legion fell ill at their annual convention in Philadelphia. The fatality rate was high. In addition to the obvious pulmonary infection, manifestations referable to the CNS and other organs were observed regularly. Lees and Tyrrell described patients with severe and diffuse cerebral involvement, and Baker et al and Shetty et al described others with cerebellar and brainstem affection. The clinical syndromes have varied. One consisted of headache, obtundation, acute confusion or delirium with high fever, and evidence of pulmonary distress; another took the form of tremor, nystagmus, cerebellar ataxia, extraocular muscle and gaze palsies, and dysarthria. Other neurologic abnormalities have been observed, such as inappropriate ADH secretion, or a syndrome of more diffuse encephalomyelitis or transverse myelitis, similar to that observed with Mycoplasma infections. The CSF is usually normal and CT scans of the brain are negative, a circumstance that makes diagnosis difficult. The neuropathologic abnormalities have not been studied. Suspicion of the disease, based on suspected exposure or the presence of an atypical pneumonia, should prompt tests for serum antibodies to the bacillus, which rise to high levels in a week to 10 days. In most patients the signs of CNS disorder resolve rapidly and completely, although residual impairment of memory and cerebellar ataxia have been recorded. To date the *Legionella* bacillus has not been isolated from the brain. Treatment in adults has consisted of erythromycin, 0.5 to 1.0 g intravenously q 6 h for a 3-week period. The combination of the erythromycin analogue azithromycin and ciprofloxacin (a quinolone) is believed to be more potent.

Cat-Scratch Encephalitis Reports of approximately 100 cases of encephalitis from *cat-scratch disease* have appeared in the medical literature. The causative organism is a gram-negative bacillus now called *Rochalimaea henselae* (formerly *Bartonella henselae*). It usually begins as unilateral axillary or cervical adenopathy occurring after a seemingly innocuous scratch (rarely a bite) from an infected cat. The cases with which we are familiar began with an encephalopathy and high fever, followed by seizures or status epilepticus. The organism has also been implicated in causing a focal cerebral vasculitis in AIDS patients as well as neuroretinitis in both immunocompromised and immune competent patients. Demonstration of elevated complement-fixing titers and detection of the organism by PCR or by silver staining from an excised lymph node are diagnostic. A single high antibody titer is inadequate for this purpose. Erythromycin, chloramphenicol, or doxycycline seem to eradicate the infection; macrolide antibiotics have been recommended in recalcitrant cases. Most patients recover completely, but one of our patients and a few reported by others have died.

Brucellosis This worldwide disease of domesticated livestock is frequently transmitted to humans in areas where the infection is enzootic. In the United States, the disease is distinctly rare, with 200 cases or less being reported annually since 1980. In the 1950s it was a fashionable explanation for chronic fatigue. In the Middle East, infection with *Brucella* is still frequent, attributable to the ingestion of raw milk. In Saudi Arabia, for example, al Deeb and coworkers reported on a series of 400 cases of brucellosis, of which 13 presented with CNS involvement (acute meningoencephalitis, papilledema and increased intracranial pressure, and meningovascular manifestations). The CSF showed a lymphocytic pleocytosis and increased protein content. Blood and CSF titers were greater than 1/640 and 1/128, respectively. Prolonged treatment with rifampin, cotrimoxazole, and doxycycline suppressed the infection.

Whipple Disease This is a rare disorder, predominantly of middle-aged men. Weight loss, fever, anemia, steatorrhea, abdominal pain and distention, arthralgias, lymphadenopathy, and hyperpigmentation are the usual systemic manifestations. Less often, it is associated with a number of neurologic syndromes. It is now known to be caused by a gram-positive bacillus, *Tropheryma whippelii.* Biopsy of the jejunal mucosa, which discloses macrophages filled with the periodic acid–Schiff (PAS)–positive organisms, is diagnostic. PAS-positive histiocytes have also been identified in the CSF as well as in periventricular regions, in the hypothalamic and tuberal nuclei, or diffusely scattered in the brain.

The neurologic manifestations most often take the form of a slowly progressive memory loss or dementia of subacute or early chronic evolution; supranuclear ophthalmoplegia, ataxia, seizures, myoclonus, and a highly characteristic oculomasticatory myorhythmia (which looks more to us like rhythmic myoclonus) have been noted less often. Very rarely, the neurologic symptoms may occur in the absence of gastrointestinal disease (Adams et al). In the extensive review of 84 cases by Louis and colleagues, 71 percent had cognitive changes, half with psychiatric features; 31 percent had myoclonus; 18 percent, ataxia; and 20 percent, the oculomasticatory and skeletal myorhythmias said to be pathognomonic of Whipple disease (Schwartz et al). The latter takes the form of a rhythmic myoclonus or spasm in synchronous bursts in several adjacent regions, mainly the eyes, jaw, and face. Almost always the myorhythmias were accompanied by a supranuclear vertical gaze paresis that sometimes affected horizontal eye movements as well. Presumably, the neurologic complications are the result of infiltration of the brain by the organism, but this has not been satisfactorily established.

Approximately half of the patients have a mild pleocytosis and some of these have PAS-positive material in the CSF. A variety of brain imaging abnormalities have been recorded, none characteristic, but either enhancing focal lesions or a normal scan may be found. The diagnosis is made mainly from PAS staining of an intestinal biopsy, supplemented by PCR testing of the bowel tissue or biopsy material from brain or lymph node. A course of penicillin and streptomycin followed by Bactrim or ceftriaxone and continued for one year is the currently recommended treatment. The current review by Anderson should be consulted for details.

SUBDURAL EMPYEMA

Subdural empyema is an intracranial (rarely intraspinal) suppurative process between the inner surface of the dura and the outer surface of the arachnoid. The term *subdural abscess*, among others, has been applied to this condition, but the proper name is *empyema*, indicating suppuration in a preformed space. Contrary to prevailing opinion, subdural empyema is not a rarity (about one-fifth as frequent as cerebral abscess). It is distinctly more common in males, a feature for which there is no plausible explanation.

The infection usually originates in the frontal or ethmoid or, less often, the sphenoid sinuses and in the middle ear and mastoid cells. As with bacterial meningitis, there has been in the last decade an increasing number of cases that follow surgery of the sinuses and other cranial structures. In infants and children and infrequently in adults, there may be spread from a leptomeningitis. Infection gains entry to the subdural space by direct extension through bone and dura or by spread from septic thrombosis of the venous sinuses, particularly the superior longitudinal sinus. Rarely, the subdural infection is metastatic, from infected lungs; hardly ever is it secondary to bacteremia or septicemia. Occasionally it extends from a brain abscess.

It is of interest that cases of sinus origin predominate in adolescent and young adult men (Kaufman et al). In such cases, streptococci (nonhemolytic and *viridans*) are the most common organisms, followed by anaerobic streptococci (often *Strep. milleri*) or *Bacteroides*. Less often *Staphylococcus aureus*, *E. coli*, *Proteus*, and *Pseudomonas* are causative. In about half the cases unrelated to surgery, no organisms can be cultured or seen on Gram stain. The factors that lead to a subdural empyema rather than to a cerebral abscess are not understood.

Pathology A collection of subdural pus, in quantities of a few milliliters to 100 to 200 mL, lies over the cerebral hemisphere. Pus may spread into the interhemispheric fissure or be confined there; occasionally it is found in the posterior fossa, covering the cerebellum. The arachnoid, when cleared of exudate, is cloudy, and thrombosis of meningeal veins may be seen. The underlying cerebral hemisphere is depressed, and in fatal cases there is often an ipsilateral temporal lobe herniation. Microscopic examination discloses various degrees of organization of the exudate on the inner surface of the dura and infiltration of the underlying arachnoid with small numbers of neutrophilic leukocytes, lymphocytes, and mononuclear cells. The thrombi in cerebral veins seem to begin on the sides of the veins nearest the subdural exudate. The superficial layers of the cerebral cortex undergo ischemic necrosis, which probably accounts for the unilateral seizures and other signs of disordered cerebral function (Kubik and Adams).

Symptomatology and Laboratory Findings Usually the history includes reference to chronic sinusitis or mastoiditis with a recent flare-up causing local pain and increase in purulent nasal or aural discharge. In sinus cases, the pain is usually over the brow or between the eyes; it is associated with tenderness on pressure over these parts and sometimes with orbital swelling. General malaise, fever, and headache—at first localized, then severe and generalized and associated with vomiting—are the first indications of intracranial spread. They are followed in a few days by drowsiness and increasing stupor, rapidly progressing to coma. At about the same time, focal neurologic signs appear, the most important of which are unilateral motor seizures, hemiplegia, hemianesthesia, aphasia, and paralysis of lateral conjugate gaze. Fever and leukocytosis are always present and the neck is stiff. Cases that follow surgery may be more indolent.

The usual CSF findings are an increased pressure, pleocytosis in the range of 50 to 1000/mm^3, polymorphonuclear cells predominating; elevated protein content (75 to 300 mg/dL); and normal glucose values. The fluid is usually sterile. If the patient is stuporous or comatose, there is a risk in performing a lumbar puncture, and one should proceed with other diagnostic procedures (see below).

Diagnosis By CT scanning one can see the ear or sinus lesions or bone erosion. The meninges around the empyema enhance and the collection of pus can be visualized, more dependably with MRI. Empyema that follows meningitis tends to localize on the undersurface of the temporal lobe and may require coronal views in order to be visualized.

Several conditions must be distinguished clinically from subdural empyema—a treated subacute bacterial meningitis, cerebral thrombophlebitis, brain abscess (see further on), herpes simplex encephalitis (page 793), acute necrotizing hemorrhagic leukoencephalitis (page 978), and septic embolism due to bacterial endocarditis (see further on in this chapter).

Treatment Most subdural empyemas, by the time they are recognized clinically, require immediate drainage through multiple enlarged frontal burr holes or through a craniotomy in cases with an interhemispheric, subtemporal, or posterior fossa location. The surgical procedure should be coupled with appropriate antibiotic therapy, which consists of the intravenous administration of 20 to 24 million units of penicillin per day plus a third-generation cephalosporin and metronidazole. Bacteriologic findings or an unusual presumed source may dictate a change to more appropriate drugs, particularly to later-generation cephalosporins. Without such massive antimicrobial therapy and surgery, most patients will die, usually within 7 to 14 days. On the other hand, patients who are treated promptly may make a surprisingly good recovery, including full or partial resolution of their focal neurologic deficits.

As with certain brain abscesses, small subdural collections of pus, which are recognized by CT scanning or MRI before stupor and coma have supervened, may respond to treatment with large doses of antibiotics alone. The resolution (or lack thereof) of the empyema can be followed readily by repeated imaging of the brain (Leys et al).

CRANIAL EPIDURAL ABSCESS

This condition is almost invariably associated with osteomyelitis in a cranial bone and originates from an infection in the ear or paranasal sinuses or from a surgical procedure, particularly if the frontal sinus or mastoid had been opened or a foreign device inserted. Rarely, the infection is metastatic or spreads outward from a dural sinus thrombophlebitis. Pus and granulation tissue accumulate on the outer surface of the dura, separating it from the cranial bone. The symptoms are those of a local inflammatory process: frontal or auricular pain, purulent discharge from sinuses or ear, and fever and local tenderness. Sometimes the neck is slightly stiff. Localizing neurologic signs are usually absent. Rarely, a focal seizure may occur, or the fifth and sixth cranial nerves may be involved with infections of the petrous part of the temporal bone. The CSF is usually clear and under normal pressure but may contain a few lymphocytes and neutrophils (20 to 100 per milliliter) and a slightly increased amount of protein. Treatment consists of antibiotics aimed at the appropriate pathogen(s)—often *Staph. aureus*. Later, the diseased bone in the frontal sinus or the mastoid, from which the extradural infection had arisen, may have to be removed and the wound packed to ensure adequate drainage. Results of treatment are usually good.

Spinal Epidural and Subdural Abscesses These types of abscess possess unique clinical features and constitute important neurologic and neurosurgical emergencies. They are discussed in Chap. 44.

INTRACRANIAL SEPTIC THROMBOPHLEBITIS

The dural sinuses drain blood from all of the brain into the jugular veins. The largest and most important of these sinuses, and the ones usually involved by infection, are the lateral (transverse), cavernous, petrous, and, less frequently, the longitudinal. A complex system of lesser sinuses and cerebral veins connects these large sinuses to one another as well as to the diploic and meningeal veins and veins of the face and scalp. The basilar venous sinuses are contiguous to several of the paranasal sinuses and mastoid cells.

Usually there is evidence that thrombophlebitis of the large dural sinuses has extended from a manifest infection of the middle ear and mastoid cells, the paranasal sinuses, or skin around the upper lip, nose, and eyes. These cases are frequently complicated by other forms of intracranial suppuration, including meningitis, epidural abscess, subdural empyema, and brain abscess. Occasionally infection may be introduced by direct trauma to large veins or dural sinuses. A variety of organisms, including all the ones that ordinarily inhabit the paranasal sinuses and skin of the nose and face, may give rise to intracranial thrombophlebitis. Streptococci and staphylococci are the ones most often incriminated.

Septic Lateral (Transverse) Sinus Thrombophlebitis In lateral sinus thrombophlebitis—which usually follows chronic infection of the middle ear, mastoid, or petrous bone—earache and mastoid tenderness are succeeded, after a period of a few days to weeks, by generalized headache and, in some instances, papilledema. If the thrombophlebitis remains confined to the transverse sinus, there are no other neurologic signs. Spread to the jugular bulb may give rise to the syndrome of the jugular foramen (see Table 47-1) and involvement of the torcula, leading to increased intracranial pressure. One lateral sinus, usually the right, is larger than the other, which may account for an elevated pressure when occluded. Involvement of the superior sagittal sinus causes seizures and focal cerebral signs. Fever, as in all forms of septic intracranial thrombophlebitis, tends to be present and intermittent, and other signs of toxemia may be prominent. Infected emboli may be released into the bloodstream, causing petechiae in the skin and mucous membranes and pulmonary sepsis. The CSF is usually normal but may show a small number of cells and a modest elevation of protein content.

Imaging by MRI and CT has supplanted cerebral venography, arteriography, and the various tests involving compression of the jugular veins. MRI sequences that are appropriate to the slow blood flow in the cerebral venous system must be selected and imaging planes carefully chosen to pass through the venous sinuses. CT and MRI will also exclude abscess and hydrocephalus.

Prolonged administration of high doses of antibiotics is the mainstay of treatment. Anticoagulation, shown to be beneficial in aseptic venous occlusion, is still of uncertain value, but it is usually administered.

Septic Cavernous Sinus Thrombophlebitis This condition is usually secondary to infections of the ethmoid, sphenoid, or maxillary sinuses or the skin around the eyes and nose, sometimes originating in a seemingly innocuous lesion. Occasionally, no antecedent infection can be recognized. In addition to headache, high fluctuating fever, and signs of systemic toxicity, there are characteristic local effects. Obstruction of the ophthalmic veins leads to chemosis, proptosis, and edema of the ipsilateral eyelids, forehead, and nose. The retinal veins become engorged, and this may be followed by retinal hemorrhages and papilledema. More often, however, vision in the affected eye is lost by a yet undefined mechanism, probably an optic neuropathy, as noted below, without visible alterations in the fundus. Involvement of the third, fourth, sixth, and ophthalmic division of the fifth cranial nerves, which lie in the lateral wall of the cavernous sinus, leads to ptosis, varying degrees of ocular palsy, pain around the eye, and sensory loss over the forehead. Within a few days, spread through the circular sinus to the opposite cavernous sinus results in bilateral symptoms. The posterior part of the cavernous sinus may be infected via the superior and inferior petrosal veins without the occurrence of orbital edema or ophthalmoplegia but usually with abducens and facial paralysis. The CSF is usually normal unless there is an associated meningitis or subdural empyema. The only effective therapy in the fulminant variety, associated with thrombosis of the anterior portion of the sinus, is the administration of high doses of antibiotics aimed at coagulase-positive staphylococci and occasionally gram-negative pathogens as well. Anticoagulants have been used, but their value has not been proved. In our cases, the cranial nerve palsies have resolved to a large extent, but visual loss tends to remain, with findings suggestive of infarction of the retro-orbital part of the optic nerve; the mechanism of this complication is not clear. Cavernous sinus thrombosis must be differentiated from mucormycosis infection of the sinuses and orbital cellulitis, which usually occur in patients with uncontrolled diabetes, and from other fungus infections (notably *Aspergillus*), carcinomatous invasion of the sphenoid bone, and sphenoid wing meningioma. (These disorders are described later in this chapter.)

Septic Thrombosis of the Superior Sagittal (Longitudinal) Sinus Occasionally this may be asymptomatic, but more often there is a clinical syndrome of headache, unilateral convulsions, and motor weakness, first on one side of the body, then on the other, due to extension of the thrombophlebitis into the superior cerebral veins. Because of the localization of function in the cortex that is drained by the sinus, the paralysis takes the form of a crural (lower limb) monoplegia, or, less often, of a paraplegia. A cortical sensory loss may occur in the same distribution. Homonymous hemianopia or quadrantanopia, aphasia, paralysis of conjugate gaze, and urinary incontinence (in bilateral cases) have also been observed. Papilledema and increased intracranial pressure almost always accompany these signs. Severe headache is a typical complaint in the awake patient.

As in the case of aseptic thrombosis, loss of the flow void in the superior sagittal sinus in the MRI is diagnostic, and the clot may be visualized if the correct sequences are used. A similar change can be seen on axial images of the contrast-enhanced CT scan by altering the viewing windows so as to show the clot within the posterior portion of the sagittal sinus. The CT scan performed early in the illness without contrast infusion usually shows the high-density clot within cortical veins as well, but only if carefully studied by altering the viewing window at the machine's console.

Treatment consists of large doses of antibiotics and temporization until the thrombus recanalizes. Although not of proven benefit (as it is in bland cerebral vein thrombosis), we have used heparin in these circumstances unless there are large biparietal hemorrhagic infarctions. Because of the high incidence of occlusion of cortical veins that drain into the sagittal sinus and the highly epileptogenic nature of the attendant venous infarction, we have also administered anticonvulsants prophylactically. Recovery from paralysis may be complete, or the patient may be left with seizures and varying degrees of spasticity in the lower limbs.

It should be repeated that all types of thrombophlebitis, especially those related to infections of the ear and paranasal sinuses, may be simultaneously associated with other forms of intracranial purulent infection, namely bacterial meningitis, subdural empyema, or brain abscess. Therapy in these complicated forms of infection must be individualized. As a rule, the best plan is to institute antibiotic treatment of the intracranial disease and to decide, after it has been brought under control, whether surgery on the offending ear or sinus is necessary. To operate on the primary focus before medical treatment has taken hold is to court disaster. In cases complicated by bacterial meningitis, treatment of the latter usually takes precedence over the surgical treatment of complications, such as brain abscess and subdural empyema.

Aseptic thrombosis of intracranial venous sinuses and cerebral veins is discussed in Chap. 34 (page 910) on cerebrovascular disease and in Chap. 30, on CSF circulation.

BRAIN ABSCESS

Pathogenesis With the exception of a small proportion of cases (about 10 percent) in which infection may be introduced from the outside (compound fractures of the skull, intracranial operation, bullet wounds), brain abscess is always secondary to a purulent focus elsewhere in the body. Approximately 40 percent of all brain abscesses are secondary to disease of the paranasal sinuses, middle ear, and mastoid cells. Of those originating in the ear, about one-third lie in the anterolateral part of the cerebellar hemisphere; the remainder occur in the middle and inferior parts of the temporal lobe. The sinuses most frequently implicated are the frontal and sphenoid, and the abscesses derived from them are in the frontal and temporal lobes, respectively. Purulent pulmonary infections (abscess, bronchiectasis) account for a considerable number of brain abscesses.

Otogenic and rhinogenic abscesses reach the nervous system in one of two ways. One is by direct extension, in which the bone of the middle ear or nasal sinuses becomes the seat of an osteomyelitis, with subsequent inflammation and penetration of the dura and leptomeninges by infected material and the creation of a suppurative tract into the brain. Alternatively (or concomitantly), infection may spread along the veins. Also, thrombophlebitis of the pial veins and dural sinuses, by infarcting brain tissue, renders the latter more vulnerable to invasion by infectious material. The close anatomic relationship of the lateral (transverse) sinus to the cerebellum explains the frequency with which this portion of the brain is infected via the venous route. The spread along venous channels also explains how an abscess may sometimes form at a considerable distance from the primary focus in the middle ear or paranasal sinuses.

About one-third of all brain abscesses are metastatic, i.e., hematogenous. A majority of these are traceable to acute bacterial endocarditis or to a primary septic focus in the lungs or pleura, as indicated above. Other metastatic abscesses are traceable to a congenital cardiac defect or pulmonary arteriovenous malformation that permits infected emboli to bypass the pulmonary circulation and reach the brain. Occasional cases are associated with infected pelvic organs, skin, tonsils, abscessed teeth, and osteomyelitis of noncranial bones. Only rarely does an acute bacterial meningitis result in a brain abscess.

In about 20 percent of all cases of brain abscess, the source cannot be ascertained. Metastatic abscesses are usually situated in the distal territory of the middle cerebral arteries, and they are frequently multiple, in contrast to otogenic and rhinogenic abscesses (Fig. 32-1). Almost all deep cerebral abscesses—for example, those within the thalamus—have a systemic source. The clinical and radiologic features of an abscess may mimic those of a brain tumor.

A careful distinction should be made between the neuropathologic effects of subacute and acute bacterial endocarditis. *Subacute bacterial endocarditis* (SBE), i.e., the type caused by the implantation of streptococci of low virulence (alpha and gamma streptococci) or similar

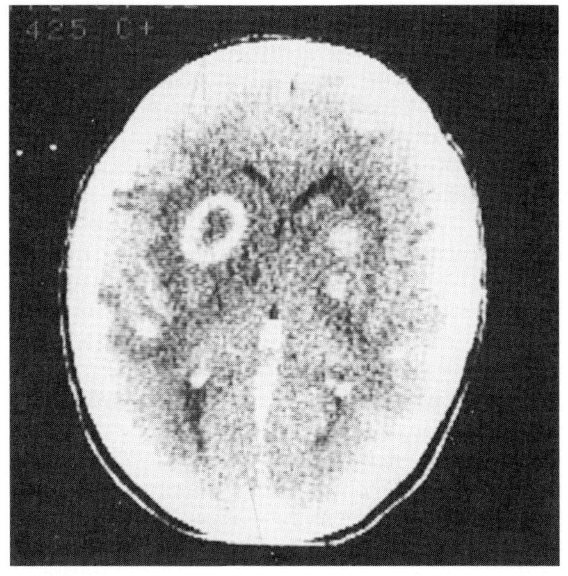

A

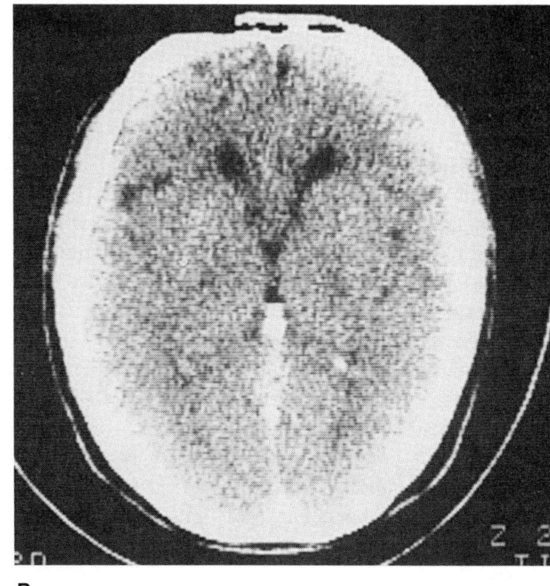

B

Figure 32-1

A. *Multiple brain abscesses associated with bacterial endocarditis (Staphylococcus aureus) in a 55-year-old man. The large abscess in the left hemisphere shows a characteristic ring enhancement.* B. *Contrast-enhanced CT scan 4 months after institution of antibiotic treatment. The abscesses have resolved.*

organisms on valves previously damaged by rheumatic fever or on a patent ductus arteriosus or ventricular septal defect, seldom gives rise to a brain abscess. The cerebral lesions of SBE are due to embolic occlusion of vessels by fragments of vegetations and bacteria, which cause infarction of brain tissue and a restricted inflammatory response around the involved blood vessels and the overlying meninges. The cerebral symptoms of a stroke may be the first clinical manifestations of the disease. The CSF contains a moderate number of polymorphonuclear leukocytes and frequently red cells as well, but the glucose content is not lowered and suppuration in the brain or in the subarachnoid space does not occur. It is theorized that the chronicity of the streptococcal infection allows the body to develop an immunity to the organisms. The meningeal pleocytosis is occassionally associated with headache, stiff neck, and rarely with alterations of consciousness. Over time, the inflamed artery may form an aneurysm that later gives rise to parenchymal or subarachnoid hemorrhage (see page 890).

In contrast to SBE, the more fulminant *acute bacterial endocarditis*—i.e., the type caused by *Staph. aureus*, hemolytic streptococcus, gram-negative organisms, or the pneumococcus (organisms that may involve previously normal valves)—frequently gives rise to multiple small abscesses in the brain and other organs of the body. Purulent meningitis may also develop, or there may be infarcts or meningocerebral hemorrhages and, infrequently, ruptured mycotic aneurysms (page 902). Rarely do the the miliary abscesses progress to large ones, as illustrated in Fig. 32-1. Rapidly evolving cerebral signs in patients with acute endocarditis (delirium, confusional state, mild focal cerebral signs) are nearly always caused by embolic infarction or hemorrhage.

It is estimated that about 5 percent of cases of *congenital heart disease* are complicated by brain abscess (Cohen, Newton). In children, more than 60 percent of cerebral abscesses are associated with congenital heart disease. The abscess is usually solitary; this fact, coupled with the potential correctability of the underlying cardiac abnormality, makes the recognition of brain abscess in congenital heart disease a matter of considerable practical importance. For some unknown reason, brain abscess associated with congenital heart disease is rarely seen before the third year of life; before this time, infarction of the brain due to thrombosis of arteries or veins is the usual neurologic complication. The tetralogy of Fallot is by far the most common anomaly associated with brain abscess, but the latter may occur with any right-to-left shunt that allows venous blood returning to the heart to enter the systemic circulation without first passing through the lungs. Pulmonary emboli, by increasing the back pressure in the right heart, may open (make patent) an occult foramen ovale. A pulmonary arteriovenous malformation has a similar effect. Nearly half of the reported cases of pulmonary arteriovenous fistulas also have Osler-Rendu-Weber telangiectasia and neurologic symptoms. Without telangiectasia, only 18 percent have neurologic symptoms; of these, 5 percent prove to have brain abscesses. When the filtering effect of the lungs is thus circumvented, pyogenic bacteria or infected emboli from a variety of sources may gain access to the brain, where, aided by the effects of venous stasis and perhaps of infarction, an abscess is established. At least this is the current theory of its mechanism.

Etiology The most common organisms causing brain abscess are streptococci, many of which are anaerobic or microaerophilic. These organisms are often found in combination with other anaerobes, notably *Bacteroides* and *Propionibacterium* (diphtheroids), and may be combined with Enterobacteriaceae, such as *E. coli* and *Proteus*. Staphylococci also commonly cause brain abscess, but pneumococci, meningococci, and *H. influenzae* rarely do. In addition, the gram-positive higher bacteria *Actinomyces* and *Nocardia* and certain fungi—notably *Candida*, *Mucor*, and *Aspergillus*—have been isolated in some cases. The type of organism tends to vary with the source of the abscess; staphylococcal abscesses are usually a consequence of accidental or surgical trauma; enteric organisms are almost always associated with otitic infections; and anaerobic streptococci are commonly metastatic from the lung and paranasal sinuses. The organisms associated with acute bacterial endocarditis are mentioned above. Predisposing to nocardial brain abscess is pulmonary nocardial infection, often in immunosuppressed patients; this diagnosis should be in doubt without a pneumonic infiltrate. Thus knowledge of the site of the abscess and the antecedent history enables one to institute appropriate therapy while awaiting the results of bacterial and fungal cultures.

Pathology Localized inflammatory exudate, septic thrombosis of vessels, and aggregates of degenerating leukocytes represent the early reaction to bacterial invasion of the brain. Surrounding the necrotic tissue are macrophages, astroglia, microglia, and many small veins—some of which show endothelial hyperplasia, contain fibrin, and are cuffed with polymorphonuclear leukocytes. There is interstitial edema in the surrounding white matter. At this stage, which is rarely observed postmortem, the lesion is poorly circumscribed and tends to enlarge by a coalescence of inflammatory foci. The term *cerebritis* is loosely applied to this local suppurative encephalitis or immature abscess.

Within several days, the intensity of the reaction begins to subside and the infection tends to become delimited. The center of the abscess takes on the character of pus; at the periphery, fibroblasts proliferate from the adventitia of newly formed blood vessels and form granulation tissue, which is readily identified within 2 weeks of the onset of the infection. As the abscess becomes more chronic, the granulation tissue is replaced by collagenous connective tissue. It has also been noted, both in experimental animals and in humans, that the capsule of the abscess is not of uniform thickness, frequently being thinner on its medial (paraventricular) aspect. These factors account for the propensity of cerebral abscesses to spread deeply into the white matter and to produce daughter abscesses or a chain of abscesses and extensive cerebral edema. In some instances the process culminates in a catastrophic rupture into the ventricles.

Clinical Manifestations Headache is the most frequent initial symptom of intracranial abscess. Other presenting symptoms, roughly in order of their frequency, are drowsiness and confusion; focal or generalized seizures; and focal motor, sensory, or speech disorders. Fever and leucocytosis are not consistently present, depending on the phase of the development of the abscess at the time of presentation (see below). In patients who harbor chronic ear, sinus, or pulmonary infections, a recent activation of the infection frequently precedes the onset of cerebral symptoms. In patients without an obvious focus of infection, headache or other cerebral symptoms may appear abruptly on a background of mild general ill health or congenital heart disease. In some patients, bacterial invasion of the brain may be asymptomatic or may be attended only by a transitory focal neurologic disorder, as might happen when a septic embolus lodges in a brain artery. Sometimes stiff neck accompanies generalized headache, suggesting the diagnosis of meningitis (especially a partially treated one).

These early symptoms may improve in response to antimicrobial agents, but within a few days or weeks, recurrent headache, slowness in mentation, focal or generalized convulsions, and obvious signs of increased intracranial pressure provide evidence of an inflammatory mass in the brain. Localizing neurologic signs become evident sooner or later, but, like papilledema, they occur relatively late in the course of the illness. However, as stated above, some patients present only with focal neurologic signs.

The nature of the focal neurologic defect will, of course, depend on the location of the abscess. In temporal lobe abscess, headache in the early stages is usually on the same side as the abscess and is localized to the frontotemporal region. If the abscess lies in the dominant temporal lobe, there is characteristically an anomic aphasia. An upper homonymous quadrantanopia may be demonstrable owing to interruption of the inferior portion of the optic radiation. This may be the only sign of abscess of the right temporal lobe; contralateral motor or sensory defects in the limbs tend to be minimal, though weakness of the lower face is often observed.

In *cerebellar abscess*, headache in the postauricular or suboccipital region is usually the initial symptom and may at first be ascribed to infection in the mastoid cells. Coarse nystagmus, weakness of conjugate gaze to the side of the lesion, cerebellar ataxia of the ipsilateral arm and leg, and ataxia of gait are the usual signs. The ataxia may be difficult to demonstrate if the patient is very ill and cannot sit up or walk. As a general rule, the signs of increased intracranial pressure are more prominent with cerebellar abscesses than with cerebral ones. Mild contralateral or bilateral corticospinal tract signs are often misleading, being evidence of brainstem compression or hydrocephalus rather than a frontal lobe lesion. In the late stages, consciousness becomes impaired as a result of direct compression of the upper brainstem or from hydrocephalus; both are ominous signs.

In *frontal lobe abscess*, headache, drowsiness, inattention, and general impairment of mental function are prominent. Contralateral hemiparesis with motor seizures and a motor disorder of speech (with dominant hemisphere lesions) are the most frequent neurologic signs. An abscess of the *parietal lobe* will give rise to a series of characteristic focal disturbances (page 483). The main manifestation of an *occipital lobe* lesion is a homonymous hemianopia. All of the aforementioned focal signs may be obscured by inattentiveness, drowsiness, and stupor, and one must be persistent in searching for them. When abscesses are multiple and widely distributed in the cerebral and cerebellar hemispheres, the ultimate syndrome is unpredictable; but most often, in our experience, it has taken the form of a global encephalopathy, like that of a metabolic confusional state, with subtle hemiparesis or seizure.

Although *fever* is characteristic of the invasive phase of cerebral abscess, the temperature may return to normal as the abscess becomes encapsulated. The same is true of leukocytosis. In the early stages of abscess formation, the CSF pressure is moderately increased; the cell count ranges from 20 to 300 per cubic millimeter, occasionally higher or lower, with 10 to 80 percent neutrophils; and the protein content is modestly elevated, rarely more than 100 mg/dL. The sedimentation rate is usually elevated. Glucose values are not lowered and the CSF is sterile unless there is a concomitant bacterial meningitis. As already mentioned, the combination of brain abscess and acute bacterial meningitis occurs only rarely. However, in some patients abscess is combined with subdural empyema; in these instances the clinical picture can be very complicated, although headache, fever, and focal signs again predominate. In a small number of cases there are no spinal fluid abnormalities and the sedimentation rate may be normal.

It is apparent from this overview that the clinical picture of brain abscess is far from stereotyped. Whereas headache is the most prominent feature in most patients, seizures or certain focal signs may predominate in others, and a considerable number of patients will present with only signs of increased intracranial pressure. In some instances the symptoms evolve swiftly over a week, new ones being added day by day. In others, the invasive stage of cerebral infection is inconspicuous, and the course is so indolent that the entire clinical picture does not differ from that of malignant brain tumor. In such cases the abscess may become apparent only when cerebral imaging performed for the evaluation of headache or other symptoms discloses a ring-enhancing mass. Another impressive feature of cerebral abscess is the unpredictability with which the symptoms may evolve, particularly in children. Thus, a patient whose clinical condition seems to have stabilized may be found, in a matter of hours or a day or two, to be in an advanced or irreversible state of coma.

Diagnosis CT and MRI are the most important diagnostic procedures. In the CT scan, the capsule of the abscess enhances and the center of the abscess and surrounding edematous white matter are hypodense (Fig. 32-1). With MRI, in T1-weighted images, the capsule enhances and the interior of the abscess is hypointense; in T2-weighted images, the surrounding edema is apparent and the capsule is hypointense. Suppurative encephalitis (cerebritis) appears as dot-sized areas of decreased density that enhance with gadolinium. Practically all abscesses larger than 1 cm produce positive scans. There is almost no likelihood of cerebral abscess if enhanced CT and MRI studies are negative.

If there is no apparent source of infection and there are only signs and symptoms of a mass lesion, the differential diagnosis includes glioma, metastatic carcinoma, toxoplasmosis, subdural hematoma, subacute infarction of the basal ganglia or thalamus, and resolving cerebral hemorrhage or infarction. Sometimes only surgical exploration will settle the issue, but one must be cautious in interpreting the stereotactic biopsy if only inflammatory and gliotic tissue is obtained, since these changes may appear in the neighborhood of either abscess or tumor.

Treatment During the stage of "cerebritis" and early abscess formation, which is essentially an acute focal purulent encephalitis, intracranial operation accomplishes little and probably adds only further injury and swelling of brain tissue and dissemination of the infection. Some cases can be cured at this stage by the adequate administration of antibiotics. Even before bacteriologic examination of the intracerebral mass, certain antibiotics can be given—20 to 24 million units of penicillin G and either 4 to 6 g of chloramphenicol, or metronidazole, a loading dose of 15 mg/kg followed by 7.5 mg/kg every 6 h. These drugs are given intravenously in divided daily doses. Metronidazole is so well absorbed from the gastrointestinal tract that it can be given orally, 500 mg every 6 h. This choice of antimicrobial agents is based on the fact that anaerobic streptococci and *Bacteroides* are the preponderant causative organisms. Evidence of staphylococcal infection can be presumed if there has been recent neurosurgery or head trauma or a demonstrable bacterial endocarditis with this organism. These circumstances call for the use of a penicillinase-resistant penicillin, such as nafcillin, 1.5 g every 4 h intravenously. In patients sensitive to penicillin, or if methicillin-resistant staphylococci are isolated or known to be common as local nosocomial organisms, the drug of choice is vancomycin 1 g every 12 h, the dose being adjusted to maintain a serum concentration of 20 to 40 mg/mL and trough levels of 10 mg/mL. Abscesses due to bacteria of oral origin do not respond well to any of these regimens because of the frequency of gram-negative organisms; a third- or fourth-generation cephalosporin, such as cefoxatime, 2 g every 4 h intravenously, is then recommended.

The initial elevation of intracranial pressure and threatening temporal lobe or cerebellar herniation should be managed by the use of intravenous mannitol and dexamethasone, 6 to 12 mg every 6 h. If improvement does not begin promptly, it becomes necessary to aspirate the abscess stereotactically or remove it by an open procedure for precise etiologic diagnosis (Gram stain and culture). The decision regarding aspiration or open removal of the abscess is governed by its location and the course of clinical signs and by the degree of mass effect and surrounding edema as visualized by repeated scans.

Only if the abscess is solitary, superficial, and well encapsulated or associated with a foreign body should total excision be attempted; if the abscess is deep, aspiration performed stereotactically and repeated if necessary is the method of choice. If the location of the abscess is such that it causes obstructive hydrocephalus—for example, in the thalamus adjacent to the third ventricle or in the cerebellum—it is advisable to remove or aspirate the mass and to drain the ventricles for a limited time. While it has been our practice to recommend either complete excision for posterior fossa and fungal abscesses, or aspiration if they are deep, there is still a lack of unanimity as to the optimal surgical approach. It is customary to instill antibiotics into the abscess cavity following aspiration.

The combination of antimicrobial therapy and surgery has greatly reduced the mortality from brain abscess. The least satisfactory results are obtained if the patient lapses into coma before treatment is started; more than 50 percent of such patients in the past have died. If treatment is begun while the patient is alert, the mortality is in the range of 5 to 10 percent, and even metastatic abscesses may respond (Fig. 32-1). About 30 percent of surviving patients are left with neurologic residua. Of these, focal epilepsy is one of the most troublesome. Following successful treatment of a cerebral abscess in a patient with congenital heart disease, correction of the cardiac anomaly is indicated to prevent recurrence. One may consider closing a patent foramen ovale if no other explanation for the abscess is apparent.

SUBACUTE AND CHRONIC FORMS OF MENINGITIS (See also Chap. 33)

There are many infectious processes that induce an inflammation of the leptomeninges of lesser intensity than the acute forms described above. Included here are some bacterial and most mycotic infections, tuberculosis, syphilis, Lyme disease, human immunodeficiency virus (HIV) infection, and presumed noninfectious causes, such as lymphoma, sarcoidosis, Wegener granulomatosis, and others. As pointed out by Ellner and Bennett (their experience coincides with that of Swartz and our own), the clinical syndrome comprises cognitive disorders, seizures, absence of lateralizing and focal cerebral signs, with or without headache and mild stiffness of the neck. In some cases there is little or no fever or other manifestation of infection. As with acute bacterial meningitis, the CSF will usually divulge the causative agent, but not so readily as in acute bacterial meningitis, since the organisms are more difficult to detect and culture. The main identifiable forms of subacute and chronic meningitis are described below. The approach to the complicated problem of chronic meningitis (aseptic variety) in which no cause can be found is addressed in Chap. 33.

Tuberculous Meningitis

In the United States and in most western countries, the incidence of tuberculous meningitis, which reflects the incidence of systemic tuberculosis, has until recently decreased steadily since the Second World War. At the Cleveland Metropolitan General Hospital, for example, the incidence of tuberculous meningitis during the years 1959 to 1963 was between 4.4 and 8.4 per 10,000 admissions (a decade earlier it was 5.8 to 12.9 per 10,000 admissions). By contrast, at the K. E. M. Hospital in Bombay during the period 1961 to 1964, the incidence of this disease (in children) was 400 per 10,000 admissions, and similar figures have been reported from other parts of India. Since 1985, however, there has been a significant increase in the incidence of systemic tuberculosis (and tuberculous meningitis) in the United States—a 16 percent annual increase compared to an average annual decline of 6 percent during the preceding 30 years (Snider and Roper). This increase is due mainly though not exclusively to the HIV epidemic. In fact, tuberculosis may be the first clinical manifestation of HIV infection (Barnes et al); among patients with full-blown AIDS, the incidence of tuberculosis is almost 500 times the incidence in the general population (Pitchenik et al). In developing countries, particularly in sub-Saharan Africa, the incidence of tuberculosis is estimated to be more than 25 times that in the United States, again largely because of the prevalence of HIV infection.

Pathogenesis Tuberculous meningitis is usually caused by the acid-fast organism *Mycobacterium tuberculosis* and exceptionally by *Mycobacterium bovis* or *Mycobacterium fortuitum*. The emergence of AIDS has led to a marked increase in cases caused by both the classic organism and these last two atypical mycobacteria. Rich described two stages in the pathogenesis of the meningitis—first a bacterial seeding of the meninges and subpial regions of the brain with the formation of tubercles, followed by the rupture of one or more of the tubercles and the discharge of bacteria into the subarachnoid space. Whether the meningitis always originates in this way is, in our opinion, somewhat uncertain. The meningitis may occur as a terminal event in cases of miliary tuberculosis or as part of generalized tuberculosis with a single focus (tuberculoma) in the brain.

Pathologic Findings Small, discrete white tubercles are scattered over the base of the cerebral hemispheres and to a lesser degree on the convexities. The brunt of the pathologic process falls on the basal meninges, where a thick, gelatinous exudate accumulates, obliterating the pontine and interpeduncular cisterns and extending to the meninges around the medulla, the floor of the third ventricle and subthalamic region, the optic chiasm, and the undersurfaces of the temporal lobes (Fig. 32-2). By comparison, the convexities are little involved, possibly because the associated hydrocephalus obliterates the cerebral subarachnoid space. Microscopically, the meningeal tubercles are like those in other parts of the body, consisting of a central zone of caseation surrounded by epithelioid cells and some giant cells, lymphocytes, plasma cells, and connective tissue. The exudate is

Figure 32-2

MRI in tuberculous meningitis. There is gadolinium enhancement of the basal meninges reflecting intense inflammation that is accompanied by hydrocephalus and cranial nerve palsies.

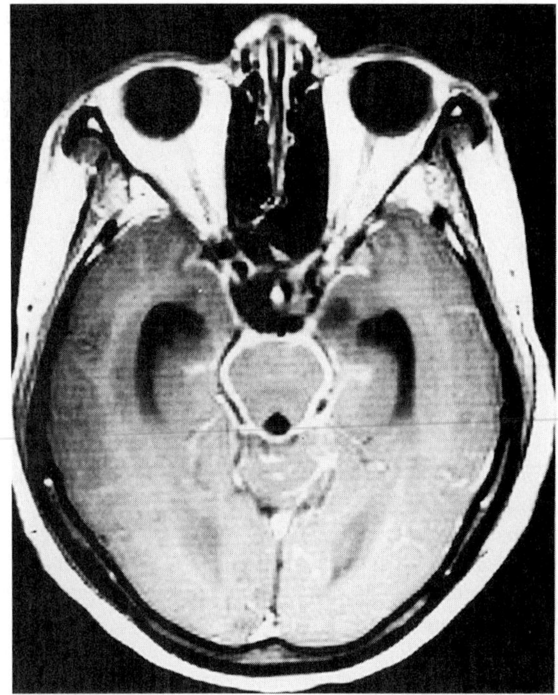

composed of fibrin, lymphocytes, plasma cells, other mononuclear cells, and some polymorphonuclear leukocytes. The ependyma and choroid plexus are studded with minute glistening tubercles. The exudate also surrounds the spinal cord. Unlike the pyogenic meningitides, the disease process is not confined to the subarachnoid space but frequently penetrates the pia and ependyma and invades the underlying brain, so that the process is truly a *meningoencephalitis*.

Other pathologic changes depend upon the chronicity of the pathologic process and recapitulate the changes that occur in the subacute and chronic stages of the pyogenic meningitides (Table 32-1). Cranial nerves are often involved by the inflammatory exudate as they traverse the subarachnoid space. Arteries may become inflamed and occluded, with infarction of brain. Blockage of the basal cisterns frequently results in a meningeal obstructive type of hydrocephalus. Marked ependymitis with blocking of the CSF in the aqueduct or fourth ventricle is a less common cause. The exudate may predominate around the spinal cord, leading to multiple spinal radiculopathies and compression of the cord.

Clinical Features Tuberculous meningitis occurs in persons of all ages. Formerly it was more frequent in young children, but now it is more frequent in adults, at least in the United States. The early manifestations are usually low-grade fever, malaise, headache (more than one-half the cases), lethargy, confusion, and stiff neck (75 percent of cases), with Kernig and Brudzinski signs. Characteristically, these symptoms evolve less rapidly in tuberculous than in bacterial meningitis, usually over a period of a week or two, sometimes longer. In young children and infants, apathy, hyperirritability, vomiting, and seizures are the usual symptoms; stiff neck may not be prominent or may be absent altogether.

Because of the inherent chronicity of the disease, signs of cranial nerve involvement (usually ocular palsies, less often facial palsies or deafness) and papilledema may be present at the time of admission to the hospital (in 20 percent of the cases). Occasionally the disease may present with the rapid onset of a focal neurologic deficit due to hemorrhagic infarction, with signs of raised intracranial pressure, or with symptoms referable to the spinal cord and nerve roots. Hypothermia and hyponatremia have been additional presenting features in several of our cases.

In approximately two-thirds of patients with tuberculous meningitis there is evidence of active tuberculosis elsewhere, usually in the lungs and occasionally in the small bowel, bone, kidney, or ear. In some patients, however, only inactive pulmonary lesions are found, and in others there is no evidence of tuberculosis outside of the nervous system. In the previously mentioned Cleveland series, which comprised 35 patients, active pulmonary tuberculosis was found in 19, inactive in 6, and involvement of the nervous system alone in 9; only 2 of the 35 patients had nonreactive tuberculin tests (Hinman). Among our adult patients, tuberculous meningitis is now seen mainly in those with AIDS, in alcoholics, and in immigrants from the Far East and India. Except for the emergence of drug-resistant organisms, the HIV infection does not appear to change the clinical manifestations or the outcome of tuberculous meningitis. However, others disagree, insisting that the course of the bacterial infection is accelerated in AIDS patients, with more frequent involvement of organs other than the lungs.

If the illness is untreated, its course is characterized by confusion and progressively deepening stupor and coma, coupled with cranial nerve palsies, pupillary abnormalities, focal neurologic deficits, raised intracranial pressure, and decerebrate postures; invariably, a fatal outcome follows within 4 to 8 weeks of the onset.

Laboratory Studies Again, the most important is the lumbar puncture, which preferably should be performed before the administration of antibiotics. The CSF is usually under increased pressure and contains between 50 and 500 white cells per cubic millimeter, rarely more. Early in the disease there may be a more or less equal number of polymorphonuclear leukocytes and lymphocytes; but after several days, lymphocytes predominate in the majority of cases. In some cases, however, *M. tuberculosis* causes a *persistent polymorphonuclear pleocytosis*, the other usual causes of this CSF formula being *Nocardia*, *Aspergillus*, and *Actinomyces* (Peacock). The one case with a persistent polymorphonuclear response in our experience was due to *M. fortuitum*. The protein content of the CSF is always elevated, between 100 to 200 mg/dL in most cases, but much higher if the flow of CSF is blocked around the spinal cord. Glucose is reduced to levels below 40 mg/dL but rarely to the very low values observed in pyogenic meningitis; the glucose falls slowly and a reduction may become manifest only several days after the patient has been admitted to the hospital. The serum sodium and chloride and CSF chloride are often reduced, in most instances because of inappropriate ADH secretion or tuberculosis of the adrenals.

The conventional methods of demonstrating tubercle bacilli in the spinal fluid are inconsistent and often too slow for immediate clinical decisions. The traditional identification of tubercle bacilli in smears of CSF sediment, stained by the Ziehl-Neelsen method, is a function not only of their number but also of the persistence with which they are sought. There are effective means of culturing the tubercle bacilli; but since their quantity is usually small, attention must be paid to proper technique. The amount of CSF submitted to the laboratory is critical; the more that is cultured, the greater the chances of recovering the organism. Unless one of the newer techniques is utilized, growth in culture media is not seen for 3 to 4 weeks. The polymerase chain reaction (PCR), a method of DNA amplification that permits the detection of small amounts of tubercle bacilli, is now widely available for clinical use. There is also a rapid culture technique that allows identification of the organisms in less than 1 week. However, even these new diagnostic methods may give uncertain results or take several days to demonstrate the organism, and they cannot be counted on to exclude the diagnosis. For these reasons, if a presumptive diagnosis of tuberculous meningitis has been made and cryptococcosis and other fungal infections and meningeal neoplasia have been excluded, treatment should be instituted immediately, without waiting for the results of bacteriologic study.

Other diagnostic procedures (CT, MRI) may be necessary in patients who present with or develop raised intracranial pressure, hydrocephalus, or focal neurologic deficits. One or more tuberculomas may also be visualized (see below). MR angiography may demonstrate vascular occlusive disease from granulomatous infiltration of the walls of arteries of the circle of Willis and their primary branches.

Other Forms of Central Nervous System Tuberculosis

Tuberculous Serous Meningitis This condition, which is essentially a self-limited meningitis, is observed with some frequency in countries where tuberculosis is prevalent. The CSF shows a modest pleocytosis in some but not all cases, a normal or elevated protein content, and normal glucose levels. Headache, lethargy, and confusion are present in some cases and there are mild meningeal signs. Lincoln, who was the first to call attention to this syndrome, believed it to be a meningeal reaction to an adjacent tuberculous focus that did not progress to a frank meningitis. This form of meningitis is not always self-limited. In two of our patients who presented with a brainstem tuberculoma, there was a serous meningitis that progressed to a fatal generalized tuberculous meningitis.

Tuberculomas These are tumor-like masses of tuberculous granulation tissue, sometimes multiple, that form in the parenchyma of the brain and range from 2 to 12 mm in diameter (Fig. 32-3). The larger ones may produce symptoms of a space-occupying lesion and periventricular ones may cause obstructive hydrocephalus, but many are unaccompanied by symptoms of focal cerebral disease. In the United States tuberculomas are rarities; but in developing countries they constitute from 5 to 30 percent of all intracranial mass lesions. In some tropical countries, cerebellar tuberculomas are the most frequent intracranial tumors in children. Because of their proximity to the meninges, the CSF often contains a small number of lymphocytes and increased protein (serous meningitis), but the glucose level is not reduced. True tuberculous abscesses of the brain are rare except in AIDS patients.

Myeloradiculitis The spinal cord may be affected in a number of ways in the course of tuberculous infection. In addition to compressing spinal roots and cord, causing

Figure 32-3

A tuberculoma of the deep hemisphere in a Caribbean emigrant to the United States. The mass behaved clinically, and appears on a gadolinium-enhanced MRI, like a primary malignant brain tumor.

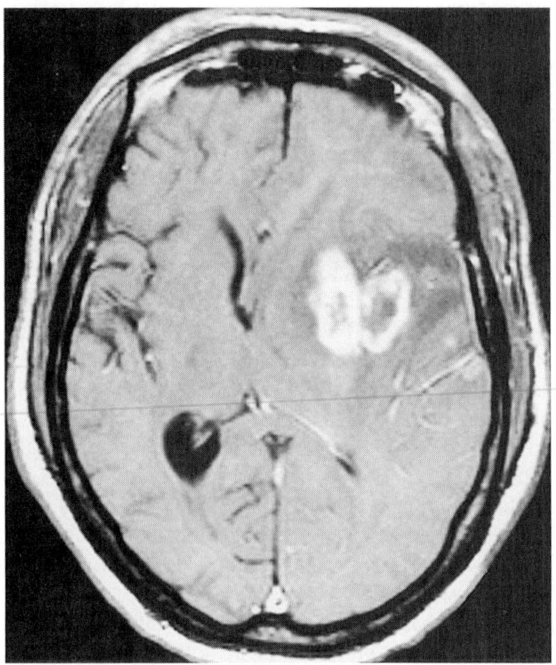

spinal block, the inflammatory meningeal exudate may invade the underlying parenchyma, producing signs of posterior and lateral column and spinal root disease. Spinal cord symptoms may also accompany tuberculous osteomyelitis of the spine with compression of the cord by an epidural abscess, a mass of granulation tissue, or, less frequently, by the mechanical effects of angulation of the vertebral column (Pott's paraplegia).

Treatment of Tuberculous Meningitis

The treatment of tuberculous meningitis consists of the administration of a combination of drugs—isoniazid (INH), rifampin (RMP), and a third and sometimes a fourth drug, which may be ethambutal (EMB), ethionamide (ETA), or preferably pyrazinamide (PZA). All of these drugs have the capacity to penetrate the blood-brain barrier, with INH, ETA, and PZA ranked higher than the others in this respect. Resistant strains are emerging, which require the use of PZA and ETA in addition to the two main drugs (INH and RMP). Antibiotics must be given for a prolonged period, 18 to 24 months as a general rule (although it may not be necessary to give all three or four drugs for the entire period).

Isoniazid is the single most effective drug. It can be given in a single daily dose of 5 mg/kg in adults and 10 mg/kg in children. Its most important adverse effects are neuropathy (see page 1395) and hepatitis, particularly in alcoholics. Neuropathy can be prevented by the administration of 50 mg pyridoxine daily. In patients who develop the symptoms of hepatitis or have abnormal liver function tests, INH should be discontinued. The usual dose of RMP is 600 mg daily for adults, 15 mg/kg for children. Ethambutal is given in a single daily dose of 15 mg/kg. The dosage of ETA is 15 to 25 mg/kg daily for adults; because of its tendency to produce gastric irritation, it is given in divided doses, after meals. The latter two drugs (EMB and ETA) may cause optic neuropathy, so that patients taking them should have regular examinations of visual acuity and red-green color discrimination. Pyrazinamide is given once daily in doses of 20 to 35 mg/kg. Rash, gastrointestinal disturbances, and hepatitis are the main adverse effects. Except for INH, all these drugs can only be given orally or by stomach tube. Isoniazid may be given parenterally, in the same dosage as with oral use. *Corticosteroids* should be used only in patients whose lives are threatened by the effects of subarachnoid block or raised intracranial pressure, and only in conjunction with antituberculous drugs.

Intracranial tuberculoma calls for a similar course of antibiotics, as outlined above. Under the influence of these drugs, the tuberculoma(s) may decrease in size and small ones ultimately disappear or calcify, as judged by the CT scan; if they do not, and especially if there is "mass effect," excision may be necessary. Patients with spinal osteomyelitis (Pott's paraplegia) or localized granulomas with spinal cord compression should also be explored surgically after an initial course of chemotherapy, and an attempt should be made to excise the tuberculous focus. We have, however, dealt successfully with tuberculous osteomyelitis of the cervical spine (without significant abscess) by immbolization in a hard collar and triple drug therapy (at the suggestion of the patient's father, who was a physician in India), once it was established that the spinal column was stable.

The overall mortality of patients with CNS tuberculosis is still significant (about 10 percent), infants and the elderly being at greatest risk. Among HIV-infected patients, the mortality from tuberculous meningitis is considerably higher (21 percent in the series of Berenguer et al)—the result of delays in diagnosis and, more importantly, of resistance to antituberculous drugs in some patients (Snider and Roper). Early diagnosis, as one might expect, enhances the chances of survival. In patients who are treated late in the disease, when coma has supervened, the mortality rate is nearly 50 percent. Between 20 and 30 percent of survivors manifest a variety of residual neurologic sequelae, the most important of which are retarded intellectual function, psychiatric disturbances, recurrent seizures, visual and oculomotor disorders, deafness, and hemiparesis. A detailed account of these has been given by Wasz-Hockert and Donner.

Sarcoidosis

The infectious etiology of sarcoidosis has never been established, but the disease may suitably be considered at this point because of its close resemblance pathologically and clinically to tuberculosis and other granulomatous infections. Indeed, one still credible theory of causation considers sarcoidosis to be a modified form or product of the tubercle bacillus. This has not been proved, and the same is true for various other infectious and noninfectious etiologies that have from time to time been proposed. Current opinion favors the idea that sarcoidosis represents an exaggerated cellular immune response to a limited class of antigens or autoantigens (Crystal).

The essential lesion in sarcoidosis consists of focal collections of epithelioid cells surrounded by a rim of lymphocytes; frequently there are giant cells, but caseation is lacking. The sarcoid tubercles may be found in all organs and tissues including the nervous system, but the most frequently involved are the mediastinal and peripheral lymph nodes, lungs, liver, skin, phalangeal bones, eyes, and parotid glands.

Sarcoidosis is accompanied by nervous system involvement (neurosarcoidosis) in approximately 5 percent of cases, according to the worldwide surveys of Delaney and of Siltzbach and colleagues. It may take any one of several forms. As indicated in Chaps. 46 and 47, isolated sarcoid granulomas may involve peripheral or cranial nerves, giving rise to a subacute or chronic neuropathy or plexopathy of asymmetrical type (Jefferson). Polyneuropathy may occur but is rare (Zuniga et al). Of the cranial nerves, the facial is the most frequently involved, either as part of the uveoparotid syndrome of Heerfordt or independently. The facial palsy may be unilateral or bilateral; if the latter, the nerves may be affected simultaneously or in succession. The occurrence of hyperacusis indicates that the lesion is central to the stylomastoid foramen. Central nervous system sarcoidosis is infrequent; it includes several syndromes that are due to localized involvement of the meninges, brain, and spinal cord. In Scadding's series of 275 patients, for example, only 3 developed CNS lesions; in other large series, the incidence of CNS involvement was greater (10 of 145 patients studied by Mayock et al; 14 of 285, by Chen and McLeod; and 33 of 649, by Stern et al). Delaney, in his review of the literature, found the neurologic involvement in sarcoidosis to be equally divided between the peripheral and central nervous systems. There is also a well-described myopathy associated with sarcoidosis; it is described below and also considered in Chap. 49, and the neuropathy of sarcoidosis is discussed in Chap. 46.

In the CNS, sarcoidosis takes the form of a granulomatous infiltration of the meninges and underlying parenchyma, most prominent at the base of the brain (Fig. 32-4). The disease process is subacute or chronic in nature, mimicking other granulomatous lesions and neoplasms. A number of our patients have presented with a circumscribed lesion of the stalk of the pituitary gland, optic chiasm, and hypothalamus, i.e., with visual disturbances, polydipsia, polyuria, or somnolence. Hydrocephalus, seizures, cranial nerve palsies, and corticospinal and cerebellar signs are other common manifestations. Rarely sarcoid can be a cause of a chronic recurrent meningitis. Also, the spinal meninges and cord may be infiltrated, imparting a picture of adhesive arachnoiditis or an inflammatory myelopathy with more prominent focal contrast enhancement or T2 signal abnormality on MRI than is expected for demyelinating disease and a characteristic enhancement on the surface of the cord at the level of the myelitic lesion (page 1307). There may be a degree of expansion of the cord. We have had experience with several such cases in which the only evidence of sarcoid was a lesion in the thoracic cord; in the absence of systemic manifestations of sarcoid, biopsy of the spinal cord lesion was necessary for diagnosis. In

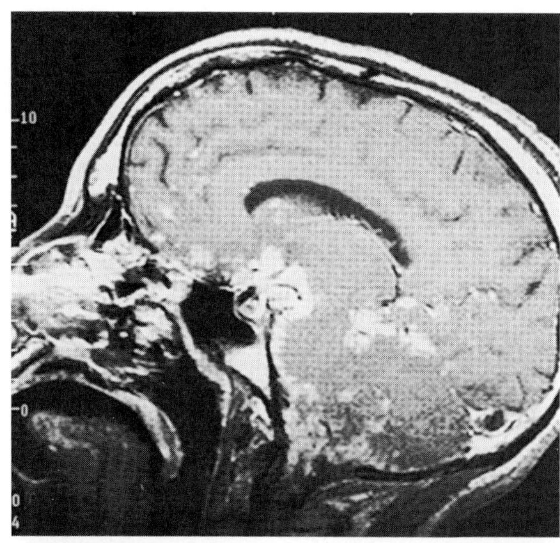

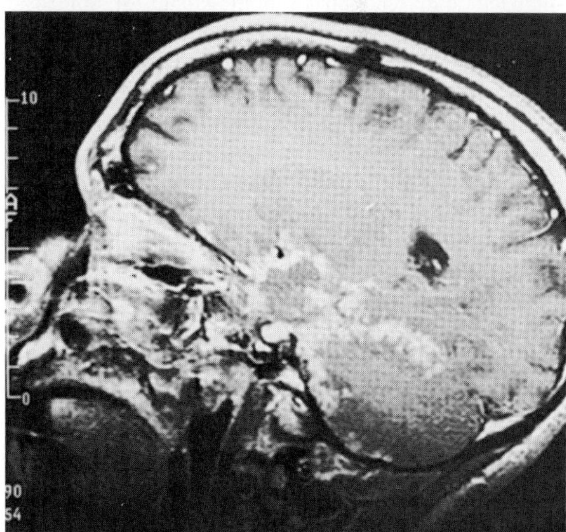

Figure 32-4

Cerebral sarcoid. Gadolinium-enhanced MR image of the brain, in the sagittal plane. Sarcoid lesions coat the base of the brain and cerebellum and surround the pituitary stalk. The patient was a 25-year-old African-American man who presented with pulmonary sarcoid, marked abulia, and panhypopituitarism.

others, focal cerebral signs, including seizures, due presumably to large focal deposits of sarcoid in the brain, are observed. A slight lymphocytic pleocytosis (10 to 200 cells per cubic millimeter) and moderate increase in protein content and gamma globulin, consistent with meningeal involvement, are the usual CSF findings. The glucose content is normal or modestly reduced. The spinal form may be associated with CSF block, the result of enlargement of the cord or adhesive arachnoiditis.

The *diagnosis* of CNS sarcoidosis is made on the basis of the clinical features together with clinical and biopsy evidence of sarcoid granulomas in other tissues (lymph nodes, lungs, bones, uvea, skin, and muscle). The contrast-enhanced CT scan is a useful means of detecting meningeal involvement, and MRI may disclose periventricular and white matter lesions, although the latter pattern is not specific. Test material for the Kveim-Siltzback skin reaction (a homogenate of spleen or lymph node from patients with known sarcoid) is no longer generally available. It has been found that sarcoid can give rise to a noncaseating epithelioid granuloma at the site of a Mantoux test (for tuberculosis) placed on the skin of the forearm. The latency in development of the granuloma (up to 6 weeks), during which time corticosteroids cannot be given, and limited rate of positivity (less than two-thirds of patients) limit the usefulness of this test (see Mankodi et al). Delayed hypersensitivity skin reactions to other antigens are frequently depressed. Mild anemia, lymphocytopenia (occasional eosinophilia), elevated sedimentation rate, hypercalcemia, and hyperglobulinemia are common findings in active disease. Serum levels of angiotensin-converting enzyme (ACE) are increased in two-thirds of the patients. It is not clear if the concentration of ACE is increased in CNS sarcoid.

The differential diagnosis of what has been called "neurosarcoidosis" is quite broad and includes a number of infrequent entities such as Sjögren syndrome, systemic lupus, lymphoma, multiple sclerosis, isolated angiitis of the CNS, intravascular lymphoma, leprosy, cryptococcosis and other fungal infections that cause abscesses and meningitis, toxoplasmosis, brucellosis, syphilis, Wegener granulomatosis, and tuberculosis.

Administration of corticosteroids is the main therapy. Cyclosporine can be used when the patient cannot tolerate steroids, or as adjunctive treatment to reduce the dose of steroid, but other immunosuppressive drugs have not proved to be as effective. The major problem is knowing when to treat the patient, because the disease may remit spontaneously in about half the cases. The recent onset of neurologic symptoms, indicating an active phase of the disease, or a disabling syndrome such as myelopathy are the most certain indications for steroid therapy. Prednisone, in divided daily doses of 40 mg, is given for 2 weeks, followed by 2-week periods in which the dose is reduced by 5 mg, until a maintenance dose of 20 to 10 mg on alternate days is reached. Therapy should be continued for at least 6 months and in many cases is required for several years.

Neurosyphilis

The incidence of neurosyphilis, like that of CNS tuberculosis, declined dramatically in the decades following World War II, with the advent of penicillin. In the United States, for instance, the rate of first admissions to mental hospitals because of neurosyphilis fell from 4.3 per 100,000 population (in 1946) to 0.4 per 100,000 (in 1960). However, in more recent years, the number of reported cases of early syphilis has increased, both in nonimmunocompromised individuals and particularly in HIV-infected ones. One may logically anticipate an increase in late syphilis, including neurosyphilis. Notable also is the shift in clinical presentation of neurosyphilis from parenchymal damage, now quite rare, to one of chronic meningovascular disease, particularly in patients with AIDS.

Etiology and Pathogenesis Syphilis is caused by *Treponema pallidum*, a slender, spiral, motile organism. The biologic characteristics of this organism and the natural history of the disease it produces are described in *Harrison's Principles of Internal Medicine*, which should be read as an introduction to the following discussion. In this chapter, only the basic facts regarding the neurosyphilitic infection are enumerated. These facts have been well established by clinical and postmortem observation, and without knowing them it is not possible to treat patients with syphilis intelligently (Fig. 32-5).

1. *The treponeme usually invades the CNS within 3 to 18 months of inoculation with the organism.* If the nervous system is not involved by the end of the second year, as shown by completely negative CSF, there is only 1 chance in 20 that the patient will develop neurosyphilis as a result of the original infection; if the CSF is negative at the end of 5 years, the likelihood of developing neurosyphilis falls to 1 percent.

2. *The initial event in the neurosyphilitic infection is a meningitis, which occurs in about 25 percent of all cases of syphilis.* Usually the meningitis is asymptomatic and can be discovered only by lumbar puncture. Excep-

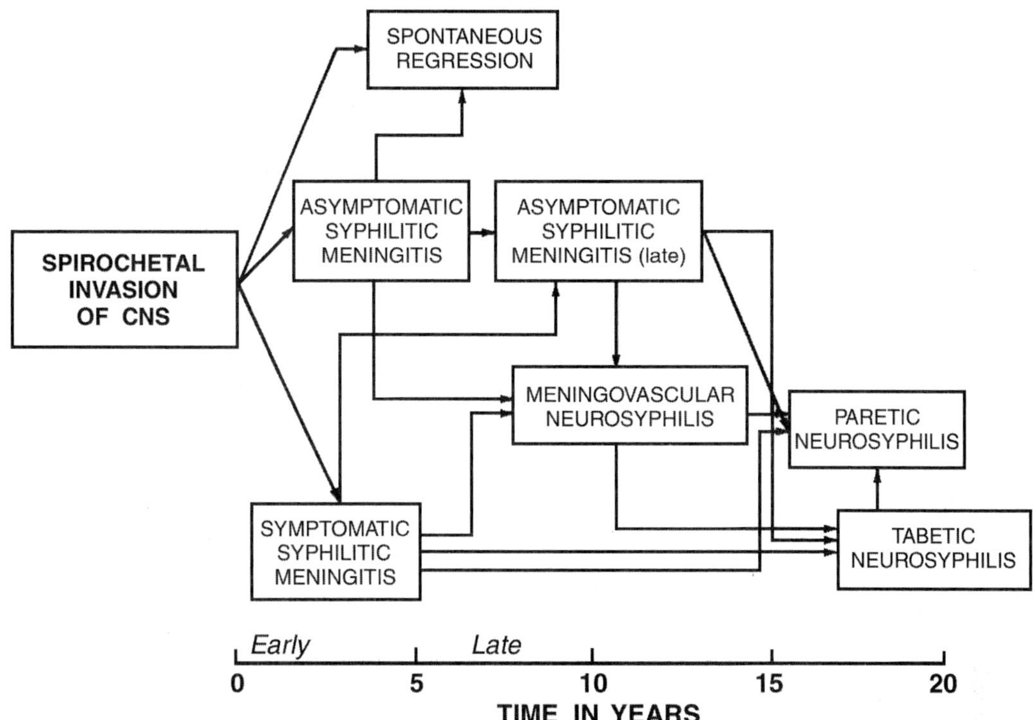

Figure 32-5

Diagram of the evolution of neurosyphillis.

tionally, it is more intense and causes cranial nerve palsies, seizures, apoplectic phenomena (due to associated vascular lesions), and symptoms of increased intracranial pressure. As a corollary, the occurrence of these symptoms in a young adult should always suggest the possibility of neurosyphilis and requires examination of the CSF.

3. *This meningitis may persist in an asymptomatic state and ultimately, after a period of years, cause parenchymal damage*. In some cases, however, there may be a natural subsidence of the meningitis—a spontaneous regression.

4. *All forms of neurosyphilis begin as a meningitis, and a more or less active meningeal inflammation is the invariable accompaniment of all forms of neurosyphilis*. The early clinical syndromes are meningitis and meningovascular syphilis; the late ones are vascular syphilis (1 to 12 years) followed by general paresis, tabes dorsalis, optic atrophy, and meningomyelitis. The latter are pathologic sequences that result from chronic syphilitic meningitis. The intermediate pathologic stages—whether by transformation of a persistent asymptomatic syphilitic meningitis or a relapsing meningitis to the late forms of parenchymal neurosyphilis—are unknown.

5. From a clinical point of view, *asymptomatic neurosyphilis is the most important form of neurosyphilis*. If all cases of asymptomatic neurosyphilis were discovered and adequately treated, the symptomatic varieties would in most instances be prevented. Since asymptomatic neurosyphilis can be recognized only by the changes in the CSF, it is axiomatic that all patients with syphilis should have a lumbar puncture and spinal fluid examination.

6. Clinical syndromes such as syphilitic meningitis, meningovascular syphilis, general paresis, tabes dorsalis, optic atrophy, and meningomyelitis are abstractions, which at autopsy seldom exist in pure form. Since all of them appear to have a common origin in a meningitis, there is usually a combination of two or more syndromes, e.g., meningitis and vascular syphilis, tabes and paresis, etc. Even though the patient's symptoms may have been referable to only one part of the nervous system, postmortem examination usually discloses diffuse changes, in both brain and spinal cord, which were of insufficient severity to be detected clinically.

7. The clinical syndromes and pathologic reactions of *congenital syphilis* are similar to those of the acquired forms, differing only in the age at which they occur. All the aforementioned biologic events are equally applicable to congenital and acquired neurosyphilis.

8. *The CSF is a sensitive indicator of the presence of active neurosyphilitic infection.* The CSF abnormalities consist of (a) a pleocytosis of up to 100 cells per cubic millimeter, sometimes higher, mostly lymphocytes and a few plasma cells and other mononuclear cells (the counts may be lower in patients with AIDS and those with leukopenia); (b) elevation of the total protein, from 40 to 200 mg/dL; (c) an increase in gamma globulin (IgG), usually with oligoclonal banding; and (d) positive serologic tests. The glucose content is usually normal. The earliest changes in the CSF, consisting of pleocytosis and an elevation of protein, may occur in the first few weeks of the infection, before the serologic tests become positive. Later, the CSF changes may vary. With either spontaneous or therapeutic remission of the disease, the cells disappear first; next the total protein returns to normal; and then the gamma globulin concentration is reduced. The positive serologic tests are the last to revert to normal. Frequently the CSF serology remains positive, despite repeated courses of therapy and the subsidence of all signs of inflammatory activity. Once this occurs, it may be safely concluded that the syphilitic inflammation in the nervous system is burned out and that further progression of the disease probably will not occur. If treatment restores the CSF to normal, particularly the cell count and protein, arrest of the clinical symptoms almost always occurs. A return of cells and elevation of protein precedes or accompanies clinical relapse.

Serologic Diagnosis of Syphilis This depends on the demonstration of one of two types of antibodies—nonspecific or nontreponemal (reagin) antibodies and specific treponemal antibodies. The common tests for reagin are the Kolmer, which uses a complement fixation technique, and the Venereal Disease Research Laboratory (VDRL) slide test, which uses a flocculation technique. These reagin tests, if positive *in the CSF*, are diagnostic of neurosyphilis. Serum reactivity alone demonstrates exposure to the organism in the past but does not imply the presence of neurosyphilis. However, serum reagin tests are negative in a significant proportion of patients with late syphilis and in those with neurosyphilis in particular (*seronegative syphilis*). In such patients (and in patients with suspected false-positive reagin tests), it is essential to employ tests for antibodies that are directed specifically against treponemal antigens. The latter are positive in the serum of practically every instance of neurosyphilis. The fluorescent treponemal antibody absorption (FTA-ABS) test is the one in common use. The *T. pallidum* immobilization (TPI) test is the most reliable, but it is expensive, difficult to perform, and available in only a few laboratories.

Principal Types of Neurosyphilis

Asymptomatic Neurosyphilis In this condition, there are no symptoms or physical signs except, in rare cases, abnormal pupils (see page 297). The diagnosis is based entirely on the CSF findings, which vary, as mentioned above.

Meningeal Syphilis Symptoms of meningeal involvement may occur at any time after inoculation but most often within the first 2 years. The commonest symptoms are headache, stiff neck, cranial nerve palsies, convulsions, and mental confusion. Occasionally headache, papilledema, nausea, and vomiting—due to the presence of increased intracranial pressure—are added to the clinical picture. The patient is afebrile, unlike the one with tuberculous meningitis. The CSF is always abnormal, more so than in asymptomatic syphilitic meningitis. Obviously the meningitis is more intense in the symptomatic type and may be associated with hydrocephalus. The prognosis, with adequate treatment, is good. The symptoms usually disappear within days to weeks, but if the CSF remains abnormal, it is likely that some other form of neurosyphilis will subsequently develop.

Meningovascular Syphilis This form of neurosyphilis should always be considered when a young person has one or several cerebrovascular accidents, i.e., the sudden development of hemiplegia, aphasia, sensory loss, visual disturbance, or mental confusion. As indicated earlier, this clinical syndrome is now probably the most common form of neurosyphilis. Whereas in the past strokes accounted for only 10 percent of neurosyphilitic syndromes, their frequency is now estimated to be 35 percent. The commonest time of occurrence of meningovascular syphilis is 6 to 7 years after the original infection, but it may be as early as 6 months or as late as 10 to 12 years.

The CSF almost always shows some abnormality, usually an increase in cells, protein content, and gamma globulin as well as a positive serologic test. However, most patients in middle or late life with stroke and only a positive serologic test will be found at autopsy to have atherothrombotic or embolic infarction rather than meningovascular syphilis. The changes in the latter disorder consist not only of meningeal infiltrates but also of inflammation and fibrosis of small arteries (*Heubner arteritis*), which lead to narrowing and finally occlusion. Most of the infarctions occur in the distal territories of medium- and small-caliber lenticulostriate branches that arise from the stems of the middle and anterior cerebral arteries. Most characteristic perhaps is an internal capsular lesion, extending to the adjacent basal ganglia. The presence of multiple small but not contiguous lesions adjacent to the lateral ventricles is another common pattern. Small, asymptomatic lesions are often seen in the caudate and lenticular nuclei. Several of our patients have had transient prodromal neurologic symptoms.

The neurologic signs that remain after 6 months will usually be permanent, but adequate treatment will prevent further vascular episodes. If repeated cerebrovascular accidents occur despite adequate therapy, one must always consider the possibility of nonsyphilitic vascular disease of the brain.

Paretic Neurosyphilis (General Paresis, Dementia Paralytica, Syphilitic Meningoencephalitis) The general setting of this form of cerebral syphilis is a longstanding meningitis; as remarked above, some 15 to 20 years usually separate the onset of general paresis from the original infection.

The history of the disease is entwined with some of the major historical events in neuropsychiatry. Haslam in 1798 and Esquirol at about the same time first delineated the clinical state. Bayle in 1822 commented on the arachnoiditis and meningitis, and Calmeil, on the encephalitic lesion. Nissl and Alzheimer added details to the pathologic descriptions. The syphilitic nature of the disease was suspected by Lasegue and others long before Schaudinn's discovery of the spirochete; it was finally confirmed by Noguchi in 1913. Kraepelin's monograph *General Paresis* (1913) is one of the classic reviews (see Merritt and colleagues for these and other historical references).

Once a major cause of insanity, accounting for some 4 to 10 percent of admissions to asylums, general paresis is now a rarity. Since syphilis is acquired mainly in late adolescence and early adult life, the middle years (35 to 50) are the usual time of onset of the paretic symptoms. Congenital syphilitic paresis blights early mental development and results in late childhood and adolescent regression in both normal and mentally retarded children.

The clinical picture in its fully developed form includes dementia, dysarthria, myoclonic jerks, action tremor, seizures, hyperreflexia, Babinski signs, and Argyll-Robertson pupils (page 297). However, more importance attaches to diagnosis at an earlier stage, when few of these manifestations are conspicuous. The insidious onset of memory defect, impairment of reasoning, and reduction in critical faculties—along with minor oddities of deportment and conduct, irritability, and lack of interest in personal appearance—are not too different from the syndrome of dementia already outlined in Chap. 21. One can appreciate how elusive the disease may be at any one point in its early evolution. Indeed, with the currently low index of suspicion of the disease, diagnosis at this preparalytic stage is more often accidental than deliberate.

Although classic writings have stressed the development of delusional systems, most dramatically in the direction of megalomania, such symptoms are exceptional in the early or preparalytic phase. More usual has been a simple dementia with weakening of intellectual capacities, forgetfulness, disorders of speaking and writing, and vague concerns about health. In a few patients the first hint of a syphilitic encephalitis, as alluded to earlier, may be facial quivering; tremulousness of the hands; indistinct, hurried speech; myoclonus; and seizures—reminiscent of delirium or acute viral encephalitis. As the deterioration continues into the paralytic stage, intellectual function progressively declines, and aphasias, agnosias, and apraxias intrude themselves.

Physical dissolution progresses concomitantly—impaired station and gait, debility, unsteadiness, dysarthria, and tremor of the tongue and hands. All these disabilities lead eventually to a bedridden state; hence the term *paretic* is quite applicable. Other symptoms are hemiplegia, hemianopia, aphasia, cranial nerve palsies, and seizures with prominent focal signs of unilateral frontal or temporal lobe disease—a syndrome known as Lissauer's cerebral sclerosis. Normal-pressure hydrocephalus may be the basis of some of the cerebral symptoms. Agitated, delirious, depressive, and schizoid psychoses are special psychiatric syndromes that can be differentiated from general paresis by the lack of mental decline, neurologic signs, and CSF findings.

We have elaborated the neuropsychiatric features of this disease, even though rare nowadays, because they are manifest almost uniquely as a chronic frontotemporoparietal meningoencephalitis and create a picture unlike that of most degenerative diseases discussed in Chap. 39 with the possible exception of the newly popularized and imprecise category of "frontotemporal dementia". Also, it is well to remember that many of our ideas about the brain and the mind were shaped historically by this disease.

The blood serology is positive in nearly all cases. The CSF is invariably abnormal, usually with 10 to 200 lymphocytes, plasma cells, and other mononuclear cells per cubic millimeter; a total protein of 40 to 200 mg/dL; an elevated gamma globulin; and strongly positive serologic tests. The elevated gamma globulin in the CSF is produced intrathecally and has been shown to be absorbed to the *T. pallidum* (Vartdal et al). Hence the gamma globulin (oligoclonal IgG) represents a specific antibody response to this organism.

The pathologic changes consist of meningeal thickening, brain atrophy, ventricular enlargement, and granular ependymitis. Microscopically, the perivascular spaces are filled with lymphocytes, plasma cells, and mononuclear cells; nerve cells have disappeared; there are numerous rod-shaped microgliacytes and plump astrocytes in parts of the cortex devastated by neuronal loss; iron is deposited in mononuclear cells; and, with special stains, spirochetes are visible in the cortex. The changes are most pronounced in the frontal and temporal lobes. The ependymal surfaces of the ventricles are studded with granular elevations protruding between ependymal cells (granular ependymitis). Meningeal fibrosis with obstructive hydrocephalus is present in many cases.

The prognosis in early treated cases has in the past been fairly good; 35 to 40 percent of patients will make some occupational readjustment; in another 40 to 50 percent, the disease will be arrested but will leave the patient dependent. Without treatment there is progressive mental enfeeblement, and death occurs within 3 to 4 years.

Tabetic Neurosyphilis (Tabes Dorsalis) This type of neurosyphilis, described by Duchenne in his classic monograph *L'ataxie locomotrice progressive* (1858), usually develops 15 to 20 years after the onset of the infection. The major symptoms are lightning pains, ataxia, and urinary incontinence; the chief signs are absent tendon reflexes at knee and ankle, impaired vibratory and position sense in feet and legs, and a Romberg sign. The ataxia is due purely to the sensory defect. Muscular power, by contrast, is fully retained in most cases. The pupils are abnormal in over 90 percent of cases, usually Argyll-Robertson in type (see page 297), and the majority of patients show ptosis or some degree of ophthalmoplegia. Optic atrophy is frequent. The lancinating or lightning pains (present in over 90 percent of cases) are, as their name implies, sharp, stabbing, and brief, like a flash of lightning. They are more frequent in the legs than elsewhere but roam over the body from face to feet, sometimes playing persistently on one spot "like the repeated twanging of a fiddle string," as Wilson remarked. They may come in bouts lasting several hours or days. "Pins and needles" feelings, coldness, numbness, tingling, and other paresthesias are also present and are associated with variable impairment of tactile, pain, and thermal sensation. The bladder is insensitive and hypotonic, resulting in unpredictable overflow incontinence. Constipation and megacolon as well as impotence are other expressions of dysfunction of the sacral roots and ganglia.

In the established phase of the disease, now seldom seen, ataxia is the most prominent feature. The patient totters and staggers while standing and walking. In mild form it is best seen as the patient walks between obstacles or along a straight line, turns suddenly, or halts. To correct the instability, the patient places his feet and legs wide apart, flexes his body slightly, and repeatedly contracts the extensor muscles of his feet as he sways (*la danse des tendons*). In moving forward, the patient flings his stiffened leg abruptly, and the foot strikes the floor with a resounding thump in a manner quite unlike that seen in the ataxia of cerebellar disease. The patient clatters along in this way with eyes glued to the floor. If his vision is blocked, he is rendered helpless. When the ataxia is severe, walking becomes impossible despite relatively normal strength of the leg muscles. Trophic lesions, perforating ulcers of the feet, and Charcot joints are characteristic complications of the tabetic state.

With regard to the deformity of deafferented *Charcot joints*, they occur in less than 10 percent of tabetics. Most often the hips, knees, and ankles are affected but occasionally also the lumbar spine or upper limbs. The process generally begins as an osteoarthritis which, with repeated injury to the insensitive joint, progresses to destruction of the articular surfaces. Osseous architecture disintegrates, with fractures, dislocations, and subluxations, some of which occasion discomfort. We have observed the arthropathy to occur as frequently in the burned-out as in the active phase of tabes; hence it is only indirectly related to the syphilitic process. Although the basic abnormality appears to be repeated injury to an anesthetic joint, the process need not be painless. Presumably a deep and incomplete hypalgesia and loss of autonomic function are enough to interfere with protective mechanisms. Sherrington reproduced the joint change in animals deprived of pain sensation.

Visceral crises represent another interesting manifestation of this disease, now rarely seen. The gastric ones are the best known. The patient is seized abruptly with epigastric pain that spreads around the body or up over the chest. There may be a sense of thoracic constriction, and nausea and vomiting—the latter repeated until nothing but blood-tinged mucus and bile are raised. The symptoms may last for several days; a barium swallow sometimes demonstrates pylorospasm. The attack subsides as quickly as it came, leaving the patient exhausted, with a soreness of the epigastric skin. Intestinal crises with colic and diarrhea, pharyngeal and laryngeal crises with gulping movements and dyspneic attacks, rectal crises with painful tenesmus, and genitourinary crises with strangury and dysuria are all less frequent but well-documented types.

In most cases that are now being seen, the CSF is normal when the patient is first examined (so-called burned-out tabes). In the remainder it is abnormal, but less often than in general paresis.

Pathologic study reveals a striking thinness and grayness of the posterior roots, principally lumbosacral, and a thinness of the spinal cord due mainly to the degeneration of the posterior columns. Only a slight outfall of neurons is observed in the dorsal root ganglia; the peripheral nerves are therefore essentially normal. For many years there was an argument as to whether the spirochete first attacked the posterior columns of the spinal cord, the posterior root as it pierced the pia, the more distal part of the radicular nerve where it acquires its arachnoid and dural sheaths, or the dorsal root ganglion cell. Our observations of rare active cases have shown the inflammation to be all along the posterior root and the slight dorsal ganglion cell loss and posterior column degeneration to be secondary.

The hypotonia, areflexia, and ataxia relate to destruction of proprioceptive fibers in the sensory roots. The hypotonia and insensitivity of the bladder are due to deafferentation at the S2 and S3 levels; the same is true of the impotence and obstipation. Lightning pains and visceral crises cannot be fully explained but are probably attributable to incomplete posterior root lesions at different levels. Analgesia and joint insensitivity relate to the partial loss of A and C fibers in the roots.

If there is no pleocytosis and the CSF protein content is normal and there is no evidence of cardiovascular or other types of syphilis, no further antisyphilitic treatment is necessary. If the CSF is positive, the patient should be treated with penicillin, as described below. Residual symptoms in the form of lightning pains, gastric crises, Charcot joints, or urinary incontinence frequently continue long after all signs of active neurosyphilitic infection have disappeared. These should be treated symptomatically rather than by antisyphilitic drugs.

Syphilitic Optic Atrophy This takes the form of progressive blindness beginning in one eye and then involving the other (page 266). The usual finding is a constriction of the visual fields, but scotomata may occur in rare cases. The optic discs are gray-white. Other forms of neurosyphilis, particularly tabes dorsalis, not infrequently coexist. The CSF is almost invariably abnormal, though the degree of abnormality may be slight in some cases. The prognosis is poor if vision in both eyes is greatly reduced. If only one eye is badly affected, sight in the other eye can usually be saved. In exceptional cases, visual impairment may progress, even after the CSF becomes negative. The pathologic changes consist of a perioptic meningitis, with subpial gliosis and fibrosis replacing degenerated optic nerve fibers. Exceptionally there are vascular lesions with infarction of central parts of the nerve.

Spinal Syphilis There are several types of spinal syphilis other than tabes. Two of them, *syphilitic meningomyelitis* (sometimes called Erb's spastic paraplegia because of the predominance of bilateral corticospinal tract signs) and *spinal meningovascular syphilis*, are observed from time to time, though less often than tabes. Spinal meningovascular syphilis may occasionally take the form of an anterior spinal artery syndrome. In meningomyelitis, there occurs a subpial loss of myelinated fibers and gliosis as a direct result of the chronic fibrosing meningitis. Gumma of the spinal meninges and cord also occurs but is rare. Progressive muscular atrophy (syphilitic amyotrophy) is a very rare disease of questionable syphilitic etiology. The same is true of syphilitic hypertrophic pachymeningitis or arachnoiditis, which allegedly gives rise to radicular pain, amyotrophy of the hands, and signs of long tract involvement in the legs (*syphilitic amyotrophy with spastic-ataxic paraparesis*). In all these syndromes there is an abnormal CSF unless, of course, the neurosyphilitic infection is burned out. (See Chap. 44, on spinal cord diseases.)

The prognosis in spinal neurosyphilis is uncertain. There is improvement or at least an arrest of the disease process in most instances, though a few patients may progress slightly after treatment is begun. A steady advance of the disease in the face of a negative CSF usually means that there has been a constrictive myelopathy or that the original diagnosis was incorrect and the patient suffers from some other disease, e.g., a spinal form of multiple sclerosis.

Syphilitic Nerve Deafness This may occur in either early or late syphilitic meningitis and may be combined with other syphilitic syndromes. We have had little clinical experience with this disorder and have no pathologic material.

Treatment This consists of the administration of penicillin G, given intravenously in a dosage of 18 to 24 million units daily (3 to 4 million units every 4 h) for 14 days. Erythromycin and tetracycline, in doses of 0.5 g every 6 h for 20 to 30 days, are suitable substitutes in patients who are sensitive to penicillin. The so-called Jarisch-Herxheimer reaction, which occurs after the first dose of penicillin and is a matter of concern in the treatment of primary syphilis, is of little consequence in neurosyphilis; it usually consists of no more than a mild temperature elevation and leukocytosis.

Certain symptoms of neurosyphilis, especially of tabetic neurosyphilis, are unpredictable and often little influenced by treatment with penicillin; they require other measures. Lightning pains may respond to carbamazepine. Analgesics may be helpful, but opiates should be avoided. Neuropathic (Charcot) joints require bracing or fusion. Atropine and phenothiazine derivatives are said to be useful in the treatment of visceral crises.

In all forms of neurosyphilis, the patient should be re-examined every 3 months and the CSF should be retested after a 6-month interval. If after 6 months the patient is free of symptoms and the CSF abnormalities have been reversed (disappearance of cells as well as reduction in protein, gamma globulin, and serology titers), no further treatment is indicated. Follow-up should include clinical examinations at 9 and 12 months and another lumbar puncture as part of the latter examination. Satisfactory progress is judged by absence of symptoms and further improvement in the CSF. These procedures should be repeated every 6 months until the CSF becomes completely negative. In the opinion of most experts, a persistent weakly positive serologic (VDRL) test after the cells and protein levels have returned to normal does not constitute an indication for additional treatment. Such a CSF formula assures that the disease is quiescent or arrested. Others are not convinced of the reliability of this concept and prefer to give more penicillin. If at the end of 6 months there are still an increased number of cells and an elevated protein in the fluid, another full course of penicillin should be given. Clinical relapse is almost invariably attended by recurrence of cells and increase in protein levels. Rapid clinical progression in the face of a negative CSF suggests the presence of a nonsyphilitic disease of the brain or cord.

Finally, it may be said that even with the mild resurgence of the disease due to AIDS, the neurologist finds the various forms of neurosyphilis of more theoretical than practical importance. No other disease has portrayed more vividly the effects of a chronic, continuously active cerebrospinal meningitis on the entire neuraxis.

Lyme Disease (Erythema Chronicum Migrans; the Borrelioses)

Until comparatively recent times, the nonvenereal treponematoses were of little interest to neurologists of the western world. Yaws, pinta, and endemic syphilis rarely if ever affected the nervous system. Leptospirosis was essentially an acute liver disease, with only one variant causing a nonicteric lymphocytic meningitis; tick- and louse-borne relapsing fevers were medical curiosities that did not involve neurologists. However, in the late 1970s, a multisystem disease with prominent neurologic features cropped up in the eastern United States. It was named after the town of Lyme, Connecticut, where a cluster of cases was first recognized in 1975. In 1982, Burgdorfer and colleagues identified the causative spirochetal agent, *Borrelia burgdorferi*. An early skin manifestation of the disease had previously been described in western Europe and referred to as *erythema chronicum migrans*. Later manifestations of the disease—taking the form of acute radicular pain followed by chronic lymphocytic meningitis and frequently accompanied by peripheral and cranial neuropathies—had long been known in Europe as the Bannwarth or Garin-Bujadoux syndrome. The identity of these diseases has been established, as well as their close relationship to relapsing fever—a disease that is also caused by spirochetes of the genus *Borrelia* and transmitted by ticks. The entire group is now classed as the borrelioses.

In humans, all these spirochetoses induce a subacute or chronic illness that evolves in ill-defined stages, with early spirochetemia, vascular damage in many organs, and a high level of neurotropism. As in syphilis, the nervous system is invaded early in the form of an asymptomatic meningitis. Later, neurologic abnormalities appear, but only in a proportion of such cases. The early neurologic complications are mainly derivations of meningitis. In this disease, unlike syphilis, peripheral and cranial nerves may be implicated (see further on and Chap. 46). Immune factors may be important in the later phases of the latent periods and in the development of the neurologic syndromes.

Lyme disease is less acute than leptospirosis (Weil disease) and less chronic than syphilis. It successively involves the skin, the nervous system, the heart, and articular structures over a period of a year and then burns out. The infective organism, as stated above, is the spirochete *B. burgdorferi*, and the vector in the United States is the common ixodid tick. The precise roles of the infecting spirochete, the antibodies it induces, and other features of the human host response in the production of clinical symptoms and signs are not fully understood, but the development of an animal model by Pachner and colleagues suggests that there is a chronic form of *Borrelia* infection in the CNS.

Lyme borreliosis has a worldwide distribution, but the typical neurologic manifestations differ slightly in Europe and America, as emphasized in the review by Garcia-Monco and Benach. In the United States, where approximately 13,000 cases are reported annually, the disease is found mainly in the northeastern and north central states. Most infections are acquired from May to July. In 60 to 80 percent of cases, a skin lesion (erythema chronicum migrans) at the site of a tick bite is the initial manifestation, occurring within 30 days of exposure. It is a solitary, enlarging, ring-like erythematous lesion that may be surrounded by annular satellite lesions. Usually, fatigue and influenza-like symptoms (myalgia, arthralgia, and headache) are associated, and these seem to be more prominent in the North American than in European form of the illness—possibly attributable to a more virulent species of spirochete (Nadelman and Wormser). Weeks to months later, neurologic or cardiac symptoms appear in 15 and 8 percent of the cases, respectively. Still later, if the patient remains untreated, arthritis or, more precisely, synovitis develops in about 60 percent of the cases. Death from this disease does not occur; therefore little is known of the pathology. A long period of disability is to be expected if the disease is not recognized and treated. Diagnosis is not difficult during the summer season in regions where the disease is endemic and when all the clinical manifestations are present. But in some cases, a skin lesion is not observed or may have been forgotten, or there may have been only a few or no secondary lesions and the patient is first seen in the neurologic phase of the illness. Then clinical diagnosis may be difficult.

Neurologic Manifestations The usual pattern of neurologic involvement is one of an aseptic meningitis or a fluctuating meningoencephalitis with cranial or peripheral neuritis, lasting for months (Reik). By the time the neurologic disturbances appear, the systemic symptoms and skin lesions may have long since receded. An infrequent cardiac disorder, which may accompany or occur independently of the neurologic changes, takes the form of myocarditis, a pericarditis, or an atrioventricular block.

The initial nervous system symptoms are rather nonspecific. They consist of headache, mild stiff neck, nausea and vomiting, malaise, and chronic fatigue, fluctuating over a period of weeks to months. These symptoms relate to the meningitis. There is a CSF lymphocytosis with cell counts from 50 to 3000/mL and protein levels from 75 to 400 mg/dL, but both values are typically in the lower range. Polymorphonuclear cells may be prominent in the early part of the illness. Usually the glucose content is normal. Somnolence, irritability, faulty memory, depressed mood, and behavioral changes have been interpreted as marks of encephalitis but are difficult to separate from the effects of meningitis. Seizures, choreic movements, cerebellar ataxia, and dementia have been reported but are infrequent. A myelitic syndrome, causing quadriparesis, is also documented.

In about half the cases, cranial neuropathies become manifest usually within weeks of onset of the illness. The most frequent is a unilateral or bilateral facial palsy, but involvement of other cranial nerves, including the optic nerve, has been observed, usually in association with meningitis. One-third to one-half of the patients with meningitis have multiple radicular or peripheral nerve lesions in various combinations. These are described in Chap. 46. In addition to facial palsies, a severe and painful meningoradiculitis of the cauda equina (Bannwarth syndrome) is particularly characteristic and seems to be more common in Europe than in the United States.

Because of the paucity of autopsy material, knowledge of the nature of Lyme encephalitis is still very imprecise. Such pathologic material as is available has shown a perivascular lymphocytic inflammatory process of the leptomeninges and the presence of subcortical and periventricular demyelinative lesions, like those of multiple sclerosis (Fig. 32-6). Oski and colleagues have recovered *B. burgdorferi* DNA from the involved areas, suggest-ing that the encephalitis is due to direct invasion by the spirochete.

A problematic aspect of Lyme disease relates to the development in some patients of a mild chronic encephalopathy, coupled with extreme fatigue. That such a disorder may occur after a well-documented attack of Lyme disease is undoubted. However, in the absence of a history of the characteristic rash, arthritis, or well-documented aseptic meningitis, the attribution to Lyme disease of fatigue alone or various other vague mental symptoms, such as difficulty in concentration, is almost always erroneous, even if there is serologic evidence of prior exposure to the spirochete.

Serologic tests are of great value but must be interpreted with caution if there has not been an inciting clinical syndrome of erythema chronicum migrans or arthritis. The most valuable initial screening is performed

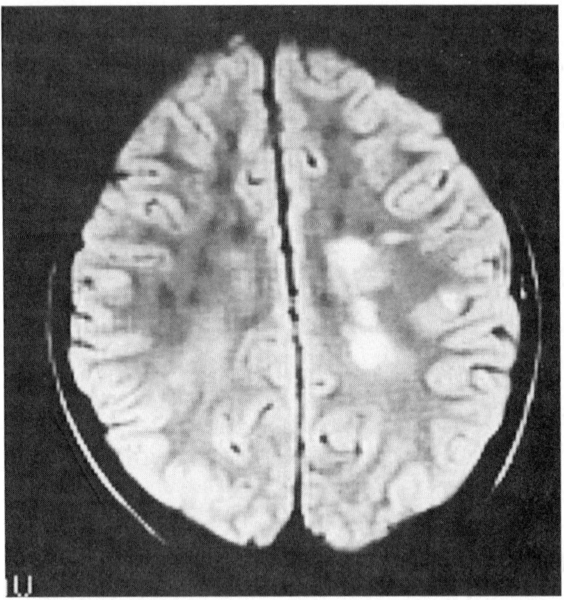

Figure 32-6

Encephalitis in Lyme disease. High-signal areas in the white matter in a patient with Lyme disease arthritis. From JH Bisese: Cranial MRI. New York, McGraw-Hill, 1991 by permission.

by the enzyme-linked immunosorbent assay (ELISA); if both acute and convalescent sera are tested, about 90 percent of patients have a positive IgM response. After the first few weeks, most patients have elevated IgG antibody responses to the spirochete (Berardi et al), and a positive test of this nature may simply reflect prior exposure. False-positive tests do occur in some of the conditions that react to syphilitic reagin *B. burgdorferi*—specific antibodies can also be demonstrated in the CSF. Positive ELISA testing should be pursued with Western blot or immunoblot analysis or other more specific serologies in clinically uncertain cases. Although these latter tests are difficult to carry out and have not been standardized, the presence of both IgG and IgM antibodies is strongly supportive of a recent infection, whereas the IgG is useful in later cases. These complex laboratory issues are discussed by Golightly. In about 30 percent of cases, the organism can be detected in the spinal fluid using PCR techniques. In the chronic phase of the disease, CT and MRI display multifocal and periventricular cerebral lesions (Fig. 32-6).

The recommended treatment in the first stage of the disease is oral tetracycline (250 mg qid) or doxycycline (100 mg bid). Central nervous system cardiac and arthritic disease can thereby be prevented. Once the meninges and nervous system are implicated, high-dose penicillin, 20 million units daily for 10 to 14 days, or, probably more effective, ceftriaxone, 2 g daily, must be given intravenously for a similar period. Tetracycline, 500 mg four times a day for 30 days, is recommended by Reik for patients who are allergic to these intravenous drugs. For late abnormalities, no treatment has proved to be effective. However, most of the symptoms tend to regress regardless of the type of treatment given.

Leptospirosis

This systemic spirochetal infection, caused by *Leptospira interrogans*, is characterized primarily by hepatitis but may include an aseptic meningitis during the second part of a biphasic illness. Initially there is high fever, tender muscles, chest and abdominal pain, and cough. An extreme form (Weil disease) comprises hepatic and renal failure. Prominent conjunctival suffusion and photophobia are typical of leptospirosis and should draw attention to the diagnosis. The CSF during the meningitic stage contains approximately 100 lymphocytes per milliliter, but cell counts in excess of 10,000 have been reported and the protein concentration may reach high levels. Subarachnoid and intracerebral bleeding, probably from inflamed blood vessels, are known to occur. The diagnosis is made by serologic methods (complement fixation screening followed by specific agglutination tests). Antibiotic treatment seems to be effective only if implemented during the initial febrile phase. The meningitis is usually self-limited.

FUNGAL INFECTIONS OF THE NERVOUS SYSTEM

Described in the following pages are a number of infectious diseases, much less common than bacterial ones, in which a systemic infection may secondarily involve the CNS. For the neurologist, the diagnosis rests on two lines of clinical information—one, evidence of infection in the skin, lungs, or other organs, and two, the appearance of a subacute meningeal or multifocal encephalitic disorder. Once demonstrated, the nature of the neurologic disorder is determined by identifying the infective agent in the CSF, by appropriate immunologic tests, and by the biopsy of nonneurologic tissue or brain.

Although a large number of fungal diseases may involve the nervous system, only a few do so with any regularity. Of 57 cases assembled by Walsh and coworkers, there were 27 of candidiasis, 16 of aspergillosis, and 14 of cryptococcosis. Among the opportunistic mycoses (see below), 90 to 95 percent are accounted for by species of *Aspergillus* and *Candida*. Mucormycosis and coccidioidomycosis are far less frequent, and blastomycosis and actinomycosis (*Nocardia*) occur only in isolated instances. These infections, particularly cryptococcal meningitis, are being seen more frequently, mainly in association with AIDS.

General Features

Fungal infections of the CNS may arise without obvious predisposing cause, but frequently they complicate some other disease process, such as AIDS, organ transplantation, severe burns, leukemia, lymphoma or other malignancy, diabetes, collagen vascular disease, or prolonged corticosteroid therapy. The factors operative in these clinical situations are not fully understood, but interference with the body's normal flora and impaired immunologic responses are the most obvious ones. Thus fungal infections tend to occur in patients with leukopenia, inadequate T-lymphocyte function, or insufficient antibodies. For these reasons, patients with AIDS are particularly prone to develop fungal infections. Infections related to impairment of the body's protective mechanisms are referred to as *opportunistic* and include not only fungal infections but also those due to certain bacteria (*Pseudomonas* and other gram-negative organisms, *L. monocytogenes*), protozoa (*Toxoplasma*), and viruses (cytomegalovirus, herpes simplex, and varicella zoster). It follows that these types of infection should always be considered and sought in the aforementioned clinical situations.

Fungal meningitis develops insidiously as a rule, over a period of several days or weeks, as with tuberculous meningitis; the symptoms and signs are also much the same. Involvement of several cranial nerves, arteritis with thrombosis and infarction of brain, multiple cortical and subcortical microabscesses, and hydrocephalus frequently complicate the course of fungal meningitis, just as they do in all chronic meningitides. Often the patient is afebrile or has only intermittent fever.

The spinal fluid changes in fungal meningitis are also like those of tuberculous meningitis. Pressure is elevated to a varying extent, pleocytosis is moderate, usually less than $1000/mm^3$, and lymphocytes predominate. Exceptionally, in acute cases, a pleocytosis above $1000/mm^3$ and a predominant polymorphonuclear response are observed. In patients with AIDS or with leukopenia for other reasons, pleocytosis may be minimal or even absent. Glucose is subnormal, and protein is elevated, sometimes to very high levels.

Specific diagnosis can best be made from smears of the CSF sediment and from cultures and also by demonstrating specific antigens by immunodiffusion, latex particle aggregation, or comparable antigen-recognition tests. The CSF examination should also include a search for tubercle bacilli and abnormal white cells because of the not infrequent concurrence of fungal infection and tuberculosis, leukemia, or lymphoma.

Some of the special features of the more common fungal infections are indicated below.

Cryptococcosis (Torulosis, European Blastomycosis) Cryptococcosis (formerly called *torulosis*) is one of the more frequent fungal infections of the CNS. The cryptococcus is a common soil fungus found in the roosting sites of birds, especially pigeons. Usually the respiratory tract is the portal of entry, less often the skin and mucous membranes. The pathologic changes are those of a granulomatous meningitis; in addition, there may be small granulomas and cysts within the cerebral cortex, and sometimes large granulomas and cystic nodules form deep in the brain. The cortical cysts contain a gelatinous material and large numbers of organisms; the solid granulomatous nodules are composed of fibroblasts, giant cells, aggregates of organisms, and areas of necrosis.

Cryptococcal meningitis has a number of distinctive clinical features as well. Most cases are acquired outside the hospital and evolve subacutely, like other fungal infections or tuberculosis. In the majority of patients, early complaints are headache, nausea, and vomiting; mental changes are present in about half of them. In other cases, however, headaches, fever, and stiff neck are lacking altogether, and the patient presents with symptoms of gradually increasing intracranial pressure due to hydrocephalus (papilledema is present in half such patients) or with a confusional state, dementia, cerebellar ataxia, or spastic paraparesis, usually without other focal neurologic deficit. Cranial nerve palsies are infrequent findings. Rarely, a granulomatous lesion forms in one part of the brain, and the only clue to the etiology of the cerebral mass is a lung lesion and an abnormality of the CSF. Meningovascular lesions, presenting as small deep strokes in an identical manner to meningovascular syphilis, may be superimposed on the clinical picture. A pure motor hemiplegia, like that due to a hypertensive lacune, has been the commonest type of stroke in our experience.

The course of the disease is quite variable. It may be fatal within a few weeks if untreated. More often, the course is steadily progressive over a period of several weeks or months, and in a few patients it may be remarkably indolent, lasting for years, during which there may be periods of clinical improvement and normalization of the CSF. Lymphoma, Hodgkin disease, leukemia, carcinoma, tuberculosis, and other debilitating diseases that alter the immune responses are predisposing factors in as many as half the patients. Patients with AIDS are particularly vulnerable to cryptococcal infection. It is estimated that 6 to 12 percent of such patients are subject to life-threatening meningoencephalitis with the organism.

The principal diseases to be considered in differential diagnosis are tuberculous meningitis (distinguished by fever, distinctive pulmonary lesions, low serum sodium due to inappropriate secretion of ADH, and organisms in CSF); granulomatous cerebral vasculitis (normal glucose values in CSF); multifocal leukoencephalopathy (negative CSF); unidentifiable forms of viral meningoencephalitis (normal CSF glucose values); sarcoidosis; and lymphomatosis or carcinomatosis of meninges (neoplastic cells in CSF). In addition, several forms of granulomatous arteritis need to be considered. One of these is an isolated intracranial vasculitis, which may take several clinical forms including a chronic nonfebrile meningitis with sterile CSF (see page 906). Another is an allergic granulomatous angiitis, which is part of a polyarteritis of the type described by Churg and Strauss (pages 906–910). And yet another is Wegener granulomatosis, in a small number of which cases necrotizing granulomas of the respiratory tracts are associated with a chronic granulomatous meningitis and pronounced dural thickening that is evident in enhanced imaging procedures (Schwartz and Niles).

The spinal fluid shows a variable lymphocytic pleocytosis, usually less than 15 cells/mm^3, but there may be few or no cells in a patient with AIDS. The initial CSF formula may display polymorphonuclear cells, but it rapidly changes to a lymphocytic predominance. The glucose is reduced in three-quarters of cases and the protein may reach high levels. Specific diagnosis depends upon finding *Cryptococcus neoformans* in the CSF. These are spherical cells, 5 to 15 mm in diameter, which retain the Gram stain and are surrounded by a thick, refractile capsule. Large volumes of CSF (20 to 40 mL) may be needed to find the organism in some cases, but in others they are prolific. India-ink preparations are distinctive and diagnostic in experienced hands (debris and talc particles from the gloves used in lumbar puncture may be mistaken for the organism). The carbon particles fail to penetrate the capsule, producing a wide halo around the doubly refractile wall of the organism. In the patients reviewed by Stockstill and Kauffman, the India-ink preparations were positive in 9 of 16 cases. The search for these organisms is particularly important in AIDS patients, in whom the CSF values for cells, glucose, and proteins may be entirely normal. A latex agglutination test for the cryptococcal polysaccharide antigen in the CSF is now widely available and gives rapid results. The latter test, if negative, excludes cryptococcal meningitis with more than 90 percent reliability in AIDS patients but is less reliable in others. In most cases the organisms grow readily in Sabouraud glucose agar at room temperature and at 37°C. Newer enzyme-linked immunoadsorption tests are being evaluated.

Treatment This consists of intravenous administration of amphotericin B, given in a dose of 0.5 to 0.7 mg/kg/day. Intrathecal administration of the drug in addition to the intravenous route appears not to be essential. Administration of the drug should be discontinued if the blood urea nitrogen reaches 40 mg/dL and resumed when it descends to normal levels. Renal tubular acidosis also frequently complicates amphotericin B therapy. The addition of flucytosine (150 mg/kg/day) to amphotericin B results in fewer failures or relapses, more rapid sterilization of the CSF, and less nephrotoxicity than the use of amphotericin B alone because it permits the reduction of the amphotericin dose to 0.3 to 0.5 mg/kg/day. Both medications are usually continued for at least 6 weeks, and longer if CSF cultures remain positive. However, this regimen, which has a success rate of 75 to 85 percent in immunocompetent patients, has proven to be much less effective in patients with AIDS. Such patients are also extremely sensitive to flucytosine and about half of them are forced to discontinue this drug because of neutropenia. Fluconazole, an oral triazole antifungal agent given in a dosage up to 400 mg daily, or oral itraconazole (up to 200 mg per day) are alternatives to flucytosine in AIDS patients and are considerably more effective in preventing relapse if used indefinitely (Saag et al; Powderly et al).

Mortality from cryptococcal meningoencephalitis, even in the absence of AIDS or other disease, is about 40 percent.

Candidiasis (Moniliasis) Candidiasis is probably the most frequent type of opportunistic fungus infection. The commonest antecedents of *Candida* sepsis are severe burns and the use of total parenteral nutrition, especially in children. Urine, blood, skin, and particularly the heart (myocardium and valves) and lungs (alveolar proteinosis) are the usual sites of primary infection. Lipton and colleagues, who reviewed 2631 autopsy records at the Peter Bent Brigham Hospital (1973 to 1980), found evidence of *Candida* infection in 28 cases, in half of which the CNS was infected. The latter infections took the form of scattered intraparenchymal microabscesses, noncaseating granulomas, large abscesses, and meningitis and ependymitis (in that order of frequency). In most of these cases, the diagnosis had not been made during life, possibly because of the difficulty of obtaining the organism from the CSF. Generally the CSF contains several hundred (up to 2000) cells per cubic millimeter. Even with treatment (intravenous amphotericin B), the prognosis is extremely grave. No special features distinguish this fungal infection from others; meningitis, meningoencephalitis, and cerebral abscess, usually multiple, are the modes of clinical presentation.

Aspergillosis In most instances, this fungal infection has presented as a chronic sinusitis (particularly sphenoidal) with osteomyelitis at the base of the skull or as a complication of otitis and mastoiditis. Cranial nerves adjacent to the infected bone or sinus may be involved. We have also observed brain abscesses and cranial and spinal dural granulomas. In one of our patients the *Aspergillus* organisms had formed a granulomatous mass that compressed the cervical spinal cord. Aspergillosis does not present as a meningitis but hyphal invasion of cerebral vessels may occur, with thrombosis, necrosis, and hemorrhage. In some cases the infection is acquired in the hospital, and in most is preceded by a pulmonary infection that is unresponsive to antibiotics. Diagnosis can often be made by finding the organism in a biopsy specimen or culturing it directly from a lesion. Also, specific antibodies are detectable. Amphotericin B in combination with 5-fluorocytosine and imidazole drugs is the recommended treatment, but it is not as effective for aspergillosis as it is for cryptococcal disease. The addition of itraconazole, 200 mg bid, in less immunocompromised patients is recommended. If amphotericin B is given after surgical removal of the infected material, some patients recover.

Mucormycosis (Zygomycosis, Phycomycosis) This is a malignant infection of cerebral vessels with one of the Mucorales. It occurs as a rare complication in patients with diabetic acidosis, in drug addicts, and in patients with leukemia and lymphoma, particularly those treated with corticosteroids and cytotoxic agents.

The cerebral infection begins in the nasal turbinates and paranasal sinuses and spreads from there along infected vessels to the retro-orbital tissues (where it results in proptosis, ophthalmoplegia, and edema of the lids and retina) and then to the adjacent brain causing hemorrhagic infarction. Numerous hyphae are present within the thrombi and vessel wall, often invading the surrounding parenchyma. The cerebral form of mucormycosis is usually fatal in short order. Rapid correction of hyperglycemia and acidosis and treatment with amphotericin B have resulted in recovery in some patients.

Coccidioidomycosis, Histoplasmosis, Blastomycosis, and Actinomycosis *Coccidioidomycosis* is a common infection in the southwestern United States. It usually causes only a benign, influenza-like illness with pulmonary infiltrates that mimic those of nonbacterial pneumonia, but in a few individuals (0.05 to 0.2 percent) the disease takes a disseminated form, of which meningitis may be a part. The pathologic reactions in the meninges and CSF and the clinical features are very much like those of tuberculous meningitis. *Coccidioides immitis* is recovered with difficulty from the CSF but readily from the lungs, lymph nodes, and ulcerating skin lesions.

Treatment consists of the intravenous administration of amphotericin B coupled with implantation of an Ommaya reservoir into the lateral ventricle, permitting injection of the drug for a period of years. Instillation of the drug by repeated lumbar punctures is an alternative, albeit cumbersome, procedure. Even with the most assiduous programs of treatment, only about half the patients with meningeal infections survive.

A similar type of meningitis may occasionally complicate *histoplasmosis*, *blastomycosis*, and *actinomycosis*. These chronic meningitides possesses no specific features except that actinomycosis, like some cases of tuberculosis and nocardiosis, may cause a *persistent polymorphonuclear pleocytosis*. The CSF yields an organism in a minority of patients, so that diagnosis depends upon culture from extraneural sites, biopsy of brain abscesses if present, as well as knowledge of the epidemiology of these fungi. Patients with chronic meningitis in whom no cause can be discovered should also have their CSF tested for antibodies to *Sporothrix schenkii*, an uncommon fungus that is difficult to culture. Several even rarer fungi that must be considered in the diagnosis of chronic meningitis are discussed in the article by Swartz. Penicillin is the drug of choice in actinomycosis; amphotericin B and supplemental antifungal agents are used in the others. Intrathecal amphotericin is administered in patients who relapse.

INFECTIONS CAUSED BY RICKETTSIAS, PROTOZOA, AND WORMS

Rickettsial Diseases

Rickettsias are obligate intracellular parasites that appear microscopically as pleomorphic coccobacilli. The major ones are maintained in nature by a cycle involving an animal reservoir, an insect vector (lice, fleas, mites, and ticks), and humans. Epidemic typhus is an exception, involving only lice and human beings, and Q fever is probably contracted by inhalation. At the time of the First World War, the rickettsial diseases, typhus in particular, were remarkably prevalent and of the utmost gravity. In eastern Europe, between 1915 and 1922, there were an estimated 30 million cases of typhus with 3 million deaths. Now the rickettsial diseases are of minor importance, the result of insect control by DDT and other chemicals and the therapeutic effectiveness of broad-spectrum antibiotics. In the United States these diseases are quite rare, but they assume importance because up to one-third of patients have neurologic manifestations. About 200 cases of Rocky Mountain spotted fever (the most common rickettsial disease) occur each year, with a mortality of 5 percent or less. Neurologic manifestations occur in only a small portion of these cases, and neurologists may not encounter a single instance in a lifetime of practice. For this reason, the rickettsial diseases are simply tabulated here. (A comprehensive account may be found in *Harrison's Principles of Internal Medicine*.)

The following are the major rickettsial diseases:

1. *Epidemic typhus*, small pockets of which are present in many undeveloped parts of the world. It is transmitted from lice to humans and from person to person.

2. *Murine (endemic) typhus*, which is present in the same areas as Rocky Mountain spotted fever (see below). It is transmitted by rat fleas from rats to humans.

3. *Scrub typhus or tsutsugamushi fever*, which is confined to eastern and southeastern Asia. It is transmitted by mites from infected rodents or humans.

4. *Rocky Mountain spotted fever*, first described in Montana, is most common in Long Island, Tennessee, Virginia, North Carolina, and Maryland. It is transmitted by special varieties of ticks.

5. *Q fever*, which has a worldwide distribution (except for the Scandinavian countries and the tropics). It is transmitted in nature by ticks but also by inhalation of dust and handling of materials infected by the causative organism, *Coxiella burnetii*.

With the exception of Q fever, the clinical manifestations and pathologic effects of the rickettsial diseases are much the same, varying only in severity. Typhus may be taken as the prototype. The incubation period varies from 3 to 18 days. The onset is usually abrupt, with fever rising to extreme levels over several days, headache, often severe, and prostration. A macular rash, which resembles that of measles and involves the trunk and limbs, appears on the fourth or fifth febrile day. An important diagnostic sign in scrub typhus is the necrotic ulcer and eschar at the site of attachment of the infected mite. Delirium—followed by progressive stupor and coma, sustained fever, and occasionally focal neurologic signs and optic neuritis—characterizes the untreated cases. Stiffness of the neck is noted only rarely, and the CSF may be entirely normal or show only a modest lymphocytic pleocytosis.

In fatal cases, the rickettsial lesions are scattered diffusely throughout the brain, affecting gray and white matter alike. The changes consist of swelling and proliferation of endothelial cells of small vessels and a microglial reaction, with the formation of so-called typhus nodules.

Q fever, unlike the other rickettsioses, is not associated with an exanthem or agglutinins for the *Proteus* bacteria (Felix-Weil reaction). In the few cases with which we are familiar, the main symptoms were those of a low-grade meningitis. Rare instances of encephalitis, cerebellitis, and myelitis are also reported. There is usually a tracheobronchitis or atypical pneumonia (one in which no organism can be cultured from the sputum) and often a severe prodromal headache. In these respects, the pulmonary and the neurologic illness resembles that of *M. pneumoniae*. The Q fever agent (*Coxiella*) should be suspected if there are concomitant respiratory and meningoencephalitic illnesses and there has been exposure to parturient animals, to livestock, or to wild deer or rabbits. The diagnosis can be made by the finding of a severalfold increase in specific immunofixation antibodies. Patients who survive the illness usually recover completely; a few are left with residual neurologic signs.

Treatment This consists of the administration of chloramphenicol or tetracycline, which are highly effective in all rickettsial diseases. If these drugs are given early, coincident with the appearance of the rash, symptoms abate dramatically and little further therapy is required. Cases recognized late in the course of the disease require considerable supportive care, including the administration of corticosteroids, maintenance of blood volume to overcome the effects of the septic-toxic reaction, and hypoproteinemia.

Protozoal Diseases

Toxoplasmosis This disease is caused by *Toxoplasma gondii*, a tiny (2- to 5-mm) obligate intracellular parasite that is readily recognized in Wright- or Giemsa-stained preparations. It has assumed great importance in recent decades because of the frequency with which it involves the brain in patients with AIDS. Infection in humans is either congenital or acquired. Congenital infection is the result of parasitemia in the mother, who happens to be pregnant at the time of her initial (asymptomatic) *Toxoplasma* infection. (Mothers can be assured, therefore, that there is no risk of producing a second infected infant.) Several modes of transmission of the acquired form have been described—eating raw beef, handling uncooked mutton (in western Europe), and, most often, contact with cat feces, the cat being the natural host of *Toxoplasma*. Most infections in AIDS patients occur in the absence of an obvious source.

The *congenital infection* has attracted attention because of its severe destructive effects upon the neonatal brain. Signs of active infection—fever, rash, seizures, hepatosplenomegaly—may be present at birth. More often, chorioretinitis, hydrocephalus or microcephaly, cerebral calcifications, and psychomotor retardation are the major manifestations. These may become evident soon after birth or only several weeks or months later. Most infants succumb; others survive with varying degrees of the aforementioned abnormalities.

Serologic surveys indicate that the *acquired form of toxoplasmosis* in adults is widespread and frequent (about 40 percent of American city dwellers have specific antibodies); however, cases of clinically evident active infection are rare. It is of interest that in 1975 the medical literature contained only 45 well-documented cases of acquired adult toxoplasmosis (Townsend et al); moreover, in half of them there was an underlying systemic disease (malignant neoplasms, renal transplants, collagen vascular disease) that had been treated intensively with immunosuppressive agents. Now innumerable cases of acquired toxoplasmosis are being seen because it is the most common cause of focal cerebral lesions in patients with AIDS (see Chap. 33). Frequently, the symptoms and signs of infection with *Toxoplasma* are assigned to the primary disease with which toxoplasmosis is associated, and an opportunity for effective therapy is missed.

The clinical picture in patients without AIDS varies. There may be a fulminant, widely disseminated infection with a rickettsia-like rash, encephalitis, myocarditis, and polymyositis. Or the neurologic signs may consist only of myoclonus and asterixis, suggesting a metabolic encephalopathy. More often, there are signs of a meningoencephalitis, i.e., seizures, mental confusion, meningeal irritation, coma, and a lymphocytic pleocytosis and increased CSF protein. The brain in such cases shows foci of inflammatory necrosis (Fig. 32-7) with free and encysted *T. gondii* organisms scattered throughout the white and gray matter. Rarely, large areas of necrosis manifest themselves as one or more mass lesions.

Specific diagnosis depends on the finding of organisms in CSF sediment and occasionally in biopsy specimens of muscle or lymph node. A presumptive diagnosis can be made on the basis of a rising antibody titer or a positive IgM indirect fluorescent antibody or other serologic test. Patients with AIDS and those who are otherwise immunocompromised, however, usually do not display this response (those with lymphoma do have positive serologic tests). In these cases, a clinical syndrome and radiologic features that are consistent with toxoplasmosis and a greatly elevated IgG titer are thought to be diagnostic. In the setting of AIDS, patients with multiple nodular or ring-enhancing brain lesions are treated initially for toxoplasmosis and further evaluation (mainly for cerebral lymphoma) is undertaken only if there is no response. Patients with a presumptive diagnosis should be treated with oral sulfadiazine (4 g initially, then 2 to 6 g daily) and pyrimethamine (100 to 200 mg initially, then 25 mg daily). Leucovorin, 2 to 10 mg daily, should be given to counteract the antifolate action of pyrimethamine. Treatment must be continued for at least 4 weeks. In patients with AIDS, treatment must be lifelong in order to prevent relapses.

Amebic Meningoencephalitis This disease is caused by free-living flagellate amebae, usually of the genus *Naegleria* and less frequently of the genus *Hartmannella* (*Acanthamoeba* and *Balamuthia mandrillaris*). They are acquired by swimming in ponds or lakes where the water is contaminated. One outbreak in Czechoslovakia followed swimming in a chlorinated indoor swimming pool. Most of the cases in this country have occurred in the southeastern states. As of 1989, more than 140 cases of primary amebic meningoencephalitis due to *Naegleria fowleri* and more than 40 cases due to the less virulent *Acanthamoeba* had been reported (Ma et al).

The onset of the illness due to Naegleria is usually abrupt, with severe headache, fever, nausea and vomiting, and stiff neck. The course is inexorably progressive—with seizures, increasing stupor and coma, and focal neurologic signs—and the outcome is practically always

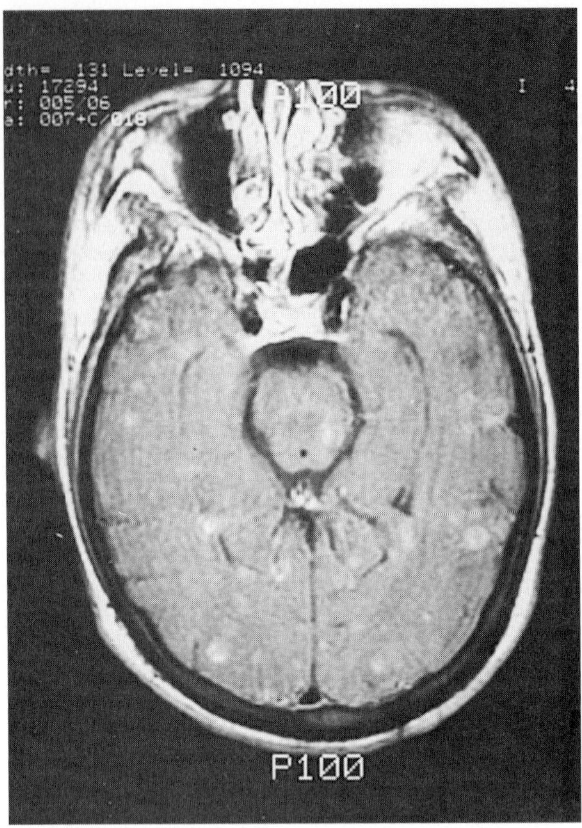

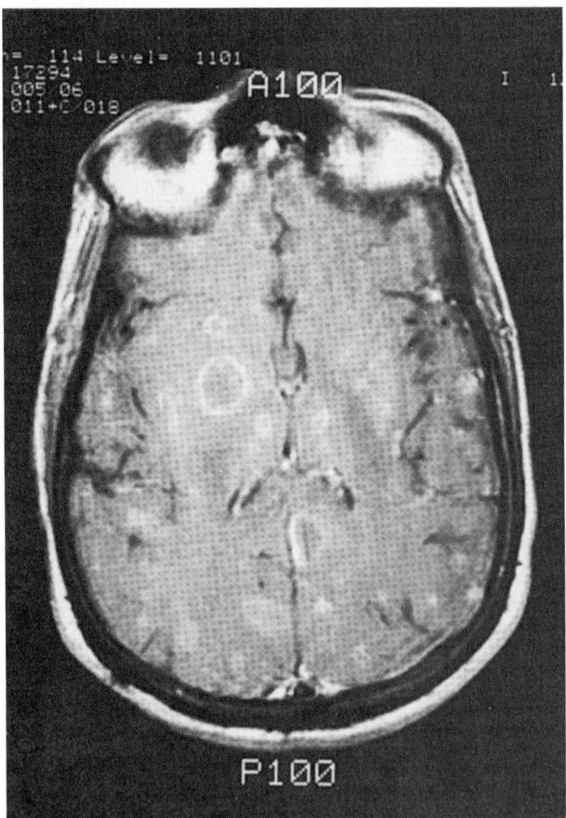

Figure 32-7

Toxoplasmosis. MR images of the brain in the axial plane showing widespread high-signal lesions. In the T1-weighted image (on the right), the lesion shows prominent ring enhancement. The patient was a 28-year-old man with AIDS.

fatal, usually within a week of onset. The reaction in the CSF is like that in acute bacterial meningitis: increased pressure, a large number of polymorphonuclear leukocytes (not eosinophils, as in the parasitic infestations discussed on page 777), and an increased protein and decreased glucose content. The diagnosis depends on eliciting a history of swimming in fresh warm water, particularly of swimming underwater for sustained periods, and on finding viable trophozoites in a wet preparation of unspun spinal fluid. Gram stains and ordinary cultures do not reveal the organism. Autopsy discloses a purulent meningitis and numerous quasi-granulomatous microabscesses in the underlying cortex.

Chronic amebic meningoencephalitis is a rare disease in humans. Isolated instances, due to *Hartmannella* species, have been reported in debilitated and immunosuppressed patients (Gonzalez et al). Usually these patients will have amebic abscesses in the liver and sometimes in the lung and brain. The organism can be cultured from the CSF during periods of recurrent seizures and confusion. In a fatal case of ours, in a leukopenic patient who had been receiving granulocyte-stimulating factor, the illness ran a subacute course over 1 month with headache, mild fever, stupor, and unmeasurably low CSF glucose toward the end of life. Initially, there were scattered, round, enhancing lesions on the MRI that disappeared with corticosteroids; later, there were more irregular confluent white matter lesions. A brain biopsy revealed amebae that could have been easily mistaken for macrophages or cellular debris; the organism proved to be *Balamuthia* (Katz et al).

Treatment with the usual antiprotozoal agents is ineffective. Because of the in vitro sensitivity of *Naegleria* to amphotericin B, this drug should be used, as for cryptococcal meningitis. With such a regimen in combination with rifampin, recovery is sometimes possible.

Malaria A number of other protozoal diseases are of great importance in tropical regions. One is *cerebral malaria*, which complicates about 2 percent of cases of *falciparum malaria*. This is a rapidly fatal disease characterized by headache, seizures, and coma with diffuse cerebral edema and very rarely by hemiplegia, aphasia, hemianopia, cerebellar ataxia, or other focal neurologic signs. Cerebral capillaries and venules are packed with parasitized erythrocytes and the brain is dotted with small foci of necrosis surrounded by glia (Durck nodes). These findings have been the basis of several hypotheses (one of which attributes the cerebral symptoms to mechanical obstruction of the vessels), but none is entirely satisfactory. Also, it seems unlikely that a disorder of immune mechanisms is directly involved in the pathogenesis (see reviews by Roman and by Turner for a discussion of current hypotheses).

Usually the neurologic symptoms appear in the second or third week of the infection, but they may be the initial manifestation. Children in hyperendemic regions are the ones most susceptible to cerebral malaria. Among adults, only pregnant women and nonimmune individuals who discontinue prophylactic medication are liable to CNS involvement (Toro and Roman). Useful laboratory findings are anemia and parasitized RBCs. The CSF may be under increased pressure and sometimes contains a few white blood cells, and the glucose content is normal. With *Plasmodium vivax* infections, there may be drowsiness, confusion, and seizures without invasion of the brain by the parasite. Quinine, chloroquine, and related drugs are curative if the cerebral symptoms are not pronounced, but once coma and convulsions supervene, 20 to 30 percent of patients do not survive. Toro and Roman state that the administration of large doses of dexamethasone, administered as soon as cerebral symptoms appear, may be lifesaving.

Trypanosomiasis This is a common disease in equatorial Africa and in Central and South America. The African type ("sleeping sickness") is caused by *Trypanosoma brucei* and is transmitted by several species of the tsetse fly. The infection begins with a chancre at the site of inoculation and localized lymphadenopathy. Later, episodes of parasitemia occur, and at some time during this stage of dissemination, usually in the second year of the infection, the trypanosomes give rise to a diffuse meningoencephalitis. The latter expresses itself clinically as a chronic progressive neurologic syndrome consisting of a vacant facial expression, ptosis and ophthalmoplegia, dysarthria, and then muteness, seizures, progressive apathy, stupor, and coma.

The South American variety of trypanosomiasis (Chagas disease) is caused by *Trypanosoma cruzi* and is transmitted from infected animals to humans by the bite of reduviid bugs. The sequence of local lymphadenopathy, hematogenous dissemination, and chronic meningoencephalitis is like that of African trypanosomiasis.

Treatment is with pentavalent arsenicals, which are more effective in the African than in the South American form of the disease.

Diseases Caused by Nematodes (See Table 32-5)

Trichinosis This disease is caused by the intestinal nematode *Trichinella spiralis*. Infection in humans results from the ingestion of uncooked or undercooked pork (occasionally bear meat) containing the encysted larvae of *T. spiralis*. The larvae are liberated from their cysts by the gastric juices and develop into adult male and female worms in the duodenum and jejunum. After fertilization, the female burrows into the intestinal mucosa, where she deposits several successive batches of larvae. These make their way—via the lymphatics, regional lymph nodes, thoracic duct, and bloodstream—into all parts of the body. The new larvae penetrate all tissues but survive only in muscle, where they become encysted and eventually calcify. Animals are infected in the same way as humans, and the cycle can be repeated only if a new host ingests the encysted larvae. Gould has written an authoritative review of this subject.

The early symptoms of the disease, beginning a day or two after the ingestion of pork, are those of a mild gastroenteritis. Later symptoms coincide with invasion of muscle by larvae. The latter begin about the end of the first week and may last for 4 to 6 weeks. Low-grade fever, pain and tenderness of muscles, edema of the conjunctivae and eyelids, and fatigue are the usual manifestations. The myopathic aspects of *Trichinella* infestation are considered fully on page 1480.

Particularly heavy infestation is sometimes associated with CNS disorder. Headache, stiff neck, and a mild confusional state are the usual symptoms. Delirium, coma, hemiplegia, and aphasia have also been observed on occasion. The spinal fluid is usually normal but may contain a moderate number of lymphocytes and, rarely, parasites.

An eosinophilic leukocytosis usually appears when the muscles are invaded. Serologic (precipitin) and skin tests become positive early in the third week. The heart is often involved, manifested by tachycardia and electrocardiographic changes; sterile brain embolism

Table 32-5
Parasitic causes of central nervous system lesions

Disease (organism)	*Clinical features*	*Radiographic features*
Cestodes (tapeworms)		
Cysticercosis (*T. solium*) and Coenuriasis (*T. multiceps*)	Seizures with mature lesions, hydrocephalus, ventricular and subarachnoid implantation	Cyst with scolex; late calcification, often multiple
Sparganosis (Spirometra)	Subcutaneous nodule, seizures	Migrating granuloma or mass
Hydatid disease (Echinococcus)	Focal cerebral findings, raised ICP	Large fluid-filled cyst, solid chitinoma
Nematodes (roundworms)		
Trichinosis	Skin lesions, myositis, brain lesions with massive infestation	Granuloma
Angiostrongyloidiasis (*A. cantonensis*)	Meningoencephalitis	Granuloma, nodule, migrating track
Strongyloidiasis (*S. stercoralis*)	Encephalitis, myelitis, seizures	Irregular nodular enhancing lesions, may change position
Visceral larva migrans (*Toxocara canis, cati*)	Eosinophilic meningoencephalitis	
Trematodes (flukes)		
Schistosomiasis (japonicum, mansoni, hematobium)	Myelopathy, seizures, tumor symptoms, swimmer's itch	Single granuloma, may be large
Paragonimiasis	Seizures, meningoencephalitis, pulmonary lesions	Single granuloma
Other tropical and parasitic infections		
Toxoplasmosis (*T. gondii*)	Seizures	Single or multiple enhancing lesions
Amebiasis (*Entamoeba histolytica, Balamuthia mandrallis, Naegleria*)	Hepatosplenic disease, granulomas, encephalopathy, meningoencephalitis, seizures	Abscess, meningoencephalitis
Tuberculoma (*M. Tb.* and *atypical forms*)	Seizure	Granuloma

may follow the myocarditis. These findings may aid in the diagnosis, which can be confirmed by finding the larvae in a muscle biopsy, using the technique of low-power scan of wet tissue pressed between two glass slides.

Trichinosis is seldom fatal. Most patients recover completely, although myalgia may persist for several months. Once recurrent seizures and focal neurologic deficits appear, they may persist indefinitely. The latter are based on the rare occurrence of a trichina encephalitis (the filiform larvae may be seen in cerebral capillaries and in cerebral parenchyma) and emboli from mural thrombi arising in infected heart muscle.

In the *treatment of trichinosis*, thiabendazole, an antihelminthic agent, and corticosteroids are of particular value. Thiabendazole, 25 mg/kg twice daily for 5 to 7 days, is effective in both the enteral and parenteral phases of the disease. This drug prevents larval reproduction and is therefore useful in patients known to have ingested trichinous meat. It also interferes with the metabolism of muscle-dwelling larvae. Fever, myalgia, and eosinophilia respond well to the anti-inflammatory and immunosuppressant effects of prednisone (40 to 60 mg daily), and a salutary effect has been noted on the cardiac and neurologic complications as well.

Other nematodes, mainly toxocara (the cause of visceral larva migrans), strongyloides, and angiostrongyloides may rarely migrate to the brain, but each is characterized by a systemic illness, which is far more common than the neurologic one.

Diseases due to Cestodes (Table 32-5)

Cysticercosis This is the larval or intermediate stage of infection with the pork tapeworm *T. solium*. In Central and South America and in parts of Africa and the Middle

East, cysticercosis is a leading cause of epilepsy and other neurologic disturbances. Because of a considerable emigration from these en-demic areas, patients with cysticercosis are now being seen with some regularity in countries where the disease had previously been unknown. Usually the diagnosis can be made by the presence of multiple calcified lesions in the thigh, leg, and shoulder muscles and in the cerebrum.

The cerebral manifestations of cysticercosis are diverse, related to the encystment and subsequent calcification of the larvae in the cerebral parenchyma, subarachnoid space, and ventricles (Fig. 32-8). The lesions are most often multiple but may be solitary. Before the cyst degenerates and eventually calcifies, CT scanning and MRI may actually visualize the scolex. Most often the neurologic disease presents with seizures, although many patients are entirely asymptomatic, the cysts being discovered radiologically. It is only when the cyst degenerates, many months or years after the initial infestation, that an inflammatory and granulomatous reaction is elicited and focal symptoms arise.

In some patients, a large subarachnoid or intraventricular cyst may obstruct the flow of CSF, in which case the surgical removal of the cyst or a shunt procedure becomes necessary. In a more malignant form of the disease the cysticerci are located in the basilar subarachnoid space, where they induce an intense inflammatory reaction leading to hydrocephalus, vasculitis, and stroke as well as cranial nerve palsies. This so-called racemose form of the illness is little altered by the use of praziquantel or any other form of therapy (Estanol et al).

Figure 32-8

Cysticercosis on MRI scan. Multiple small enhancing cysts and a large cerebellar cyst in a man whose presenting illness was the result of obstructive hydrocephalus. The cysts are in the early stage of degeneration and have not yet calcified.

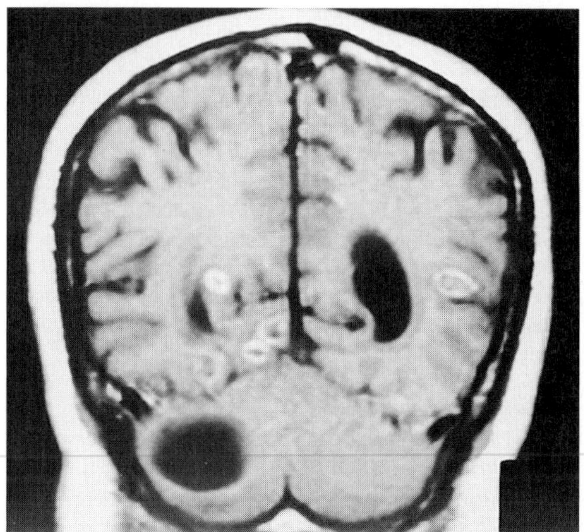

The therapy of this disorder has been greatly improved in recent years by the use of CT and MRI and the administration of praziquantel, an antihelminthic agent that is also active against all species of schistosomes. The usual dose of praziquantel is 50 mg/kg of body weight, given orally daily for 15 to 30 days, depending upon the size and activity of the lesions. Albendazole (5 mg/kg tid for 15 to 30 days), an alternative treatment, is believed by some to be more effective. Initially, treatment may seem to exacerbate neurologic symptoms, with an increase in cells and protein in the CSF, but then the patient improves and may become asymptomatic, with a striking decrease in the size and number of cysts on CT scanning. Corticosteroids may be useful if a large single lesion is causing symptoms by its mass effect.

Other Cestode Infections Infection with *Echinococcus* may occasionally affect the brain. The usual sources of infection are water and vegetables contaminated by canine feces. After they are ingested, the ova hatch and the freed embryos migrate, primarily to lung and liver, but sometimes to brain (approximately 2 percent of cases), where a large solitary (hydatid) cyst may be formed. The typical lesion is a large fluid-filled cyst with the parasite visible by imaging procedures, but a solid nodular brain lesion, a "chitinoma," is also known to occur. We have also observed a compressive spinal cord lesion. Treatment with the drug mebendazole is recommended when surgery is not feasible.

Cerebral coenuriasis (*Coenurus cerebralis*) is an uncommon infestation by larvae of the tapeworm *taenia multiceps*. It occurs mainly in sheep-raising areas where there are many dogs, the latter being the definitive hosts. The larvae form grape-like cysts, most often in the posterior fossa, which obstruct the spinal fluid pathways and cause signs of increased intracranial pressure. Surgical removal is possible.

Another cestode, *Spirometra mansoni*, may migrate within the brain, leaving a visible track as it moves. Subcutaneous nodules are the most common lesions. This parasite is found predominantly in the Far East.

The nervous system may also be invaded directly by certain worms (*Ascaris*, *Filaria*) and flukes (*Schistosoma*, *Paragonimus; see following*). These diseases are virtually non-existent in the United States except among those who have recently returned from endemic areas.

Diseases Caused by Trematodes (Table 32-5)

Schistosomiasis The ova of *trematodes* seldom involve the nervous system, but when they do, the infecting organism is usually *Schistosoma japonicum* or, less often, *Schistosoma haematobium* or *Schistosoma mansoni.* It is said that *Schistosoma japonicum* has a tendency to localize in the cerebral hemispheres and *S. mansoni* in the spinal cord but there have been many exceptions. The cerebral lesions form in relation to direct parasitic invasion of blood vessels and take the form of mixed necrotizing and ischemic parenchymal foci that are infiltrated by eosinophils and giant cells (Scrimgeour and Gajdusek). The lesions do not calcify.

Schistosomiasis is widespread in tropical regions, especially in Egypt; North American neurologists have little contact with it, except in travelers who have bathed in lakes or rivers where the snail hosts of the parasite are plentiful. The initial manifestation is a local skin irritation at the site of entry of the parasite (swimmer's itch). An estimated 3 to 5 percent of patients develop neurologic symptoms several months after exposure. Headaches, convulsions (either focal or generalized), and other cerebral signs appear; with lesions of larger size, papilledema may develop, simulating brain tumor.

Some types of infections due to *Schistosoma* (also called *Bilharzia*), mainly *mansoni*, tend to localize in the spinal cord, causing an acute or subacute myelitis with the clinical picture of a subacutely developing transverse cord lesion. This is one of the most frequent forms of myelitis in Brazil and other parts of South America. We have also observed a few cases in students returning from Africa; their lesions were in the conus. Unless treated immediately, there may be permanent paralysis.

Examination of the CSF in the myelitic form discloses a pleocytosis, often with an increase in eosinophils, increased protein content, and sometimes increased pressure. Biopsy of liver and rectal mucosa, skin tests, and complement fixation tests confirm the diagnosis. Treatment consists of praziquantel orally in a dosage of 20 mg/kg tid. In one series, 8 of 9 patients with epilepsy due to cerebral schistosomiasis became seizure-free after treatment with praziquantel. Surgical excision of spinal granulomatous tumors is sometimes indicated, but the results are unpredictable.

The other major tremstode, *Paragonimus*, has been known rarely to invade the brain, where it creates a solitary granulomatous nodule.

Eosinophilic Meningoencephalitis Due to Parasites An eosinophilic meningoencephalitis with cranial nerve and painful polyradicular findings has been reported with *Angiostrongylus cantonensis*, *Gnathostoma spinigerum*, *Paragonium westernensis*, and *Toxocara canis* and *cati* infections. In the *Strongyloides* infections, snails, freshwater prawns, and unwashed lettuce carry the nematode. The resulting illness may last for weeks to months, with pain, sensorimotor abnormalities, and a confusional state as the main manifestations. Cook has reviewed these and other protozoan and helminthic infections of the CNS. Hodgkin disease, other lymphomas, and cholesterol emboli will also occasionally incite an eosinophilic meningitis.

More detailed descriptions of parasitic diseases of the nervous system can be found in the monographs of Bia and of Gutierrez.

REFERENCES

Adams RD, Kubik CS, Bonner FJ: The clinical and pathological aspects of influenzal meningitis. *Arch Pediatr* 65:354, 1948.

Adams M, Rhyner PA, Day J, et al: Whipple's disease confined to the central nervous system. *Ann Neurol* 21:104, 1987.

Al Deeb SM, Yaqub BA, Sharif HS, Phadke JG: Neurobrucellosis: Clinical characteristics, diagnosis, and outcome. *Neurology* 39:498, 1989.

Anderson M: Neurology of Whipple's disease. *J Neurol Neurosurg Psychiat* 68:1, 2000.

Armstrong RW, Fung PC: Brainstem encephalitis (rhombencephalitis due to *Listeria monocytogenes*: Case report and review. *Clin Infect Dis* 16:689, 1993.

Baker P, Price T, Allen CD: Brainstem and cerebellar dysfunction with legionnaires' disease. *J Neurol Neurosurg Psychiatry* 44:1054, 1981.

Bannwarth A: Chronische lymphocytare Meningitis, entzundliche Polyneuritis und "Rheumatismus." *Arch Psychiatr Nervenkr* 113:284, 1941.

Barnes PF, Bloch AB, Davidson PT, Snider DE Jr: Tuberculosis in patients with human immunodeficiency virus infection. *N Engl J Med* 324:1644, 1991.

Berardi VE, Weeks KE, Steere AC: Serodiagnosis of early Lyme disease: Evaluation of IgM and IgG antibody responses by antibody capture enzyme immunoassay. *J Infect Dis* 158:754, 1988.

Berenguer J, Moreno S, Laguna F, et al: Tuberculous meningitis in patients infected with the human immunodeficiency virus. *N Engl J Med* 326:668, 1992.

Berman PH, Banker BQ: Neonatal meningitis: A clinical and pathological study of 29 cases. *Pediatrics* 38:6, 1966.

Bhandari YS, Sarkari NBS: Subdural empyema: A review of 37 cases. *J Neurosurg* 32:35, 1970.

Bia F (ed): Parasitic diseases of the nervous system. *Semin Neurol* 13(2):1–239, 1993.

BRISSON-NOËL A, AZNAR C, CHUREAU C, et al: Diagnosis of tuberculosis by DNA amplification in clinical practice. *Lancet* 338:364, 1991.

BURGDORFER W, BARBOUR AG, HAYES SF, et al: Lyme disease CA tick-borne spirochetosis. *Science* 216:1317, 1982.

CHEN RC, MCLEOD JG: Neurological complications of sarcoidosis. *Clin Exp Neurol* 26:99, 1989.

COHEN MM: The central nervous system in congenital heart disease. *Neurology* 10:452, 1960.

COOK GC: Protozoan and helminthic infections, in Lambert HP (ed): *Infections of the Central Nervous System*. Philadelphia, Decker, 1991, pp 264–282.

CRYSTAL RG: Sarcoidosis, in Fauci AS, Braunwald E, Isselbacher KJ, et al (eds): *Harrison's Principles of Internal Medicine*, 14th ed. New York, McGraw-Hill, 1998, pp 1922–1928.

DELANEY P: Neurologic manifestations in sarcoidosis: Review of the literature, with a report of 23 cases. *Ann Intern Med* 87:336, 1977.

DESFORGES JA: The use of molecular methods in infectious diseases. *N Engl J Med* 327:1290, 1992.

DISMUKES WE: Cryptococcal meningitis in patients with AIDS. *J Infect Dis* 157:624, 1988.

DODGE PR, DAVIS H, FEIGIN RD, et al: Prospective evaluation of hearing impairment as a sequela of acute bacterial meningitis. *N Engl J Med* 311:869, 1984.

DURAND ML, CALDERWOOD SB, WEBER DJ, et al: Acute bacterial meningitis: A review of 493 episodes. *N Engl J Med* 328:21, 1993.

ELLNER JJ, BENNETT JE: Chronic meningitis. *Medicine (Baltimore)* 55:341, 1976.

ESTANOL B, CORONA T, ABAD P: A prognostic classification of cerebral cysticercosis: Therapeutic implications. *J Neurol Neurosurg Psychiatry* 49:1131, 1986.

FERRY PC, CULBERTSON JL, COOPER JA, et al: Sequelae of *Haemophilus influenzae* meningitis: Preliminary report of a long-term follow-up study, in Sell SH, Wright PF (eds): *Haemophilus Influenzae—Epidemiology, Immunology and Prevention of Disease*. New York, Elsevier, 1982, sec 3, pp 111–116.

FISHER RS CLARK AW, WOLINSKY JS, et al: Postinfectious leukoencephalitis complicating Mycoplasma pneumoniae infection. *Arch Neurol* 40:109, 1983.

GARCIA-MONICO JC, BENACH JL: Lyme neuroborreliosis. *Ann Neurol* 37:691, 1995.

GOLIGHTLY MG: Lyme borreliosis: Laboratory considerations. *Semin Neurol* 17:11,1997.

GONZALEZ MM, GOULD E. DICKINSON G, et al: Acquired immunodeficiency syndrome associated with *Acanthamoeba* infection and other opportunistic organisms. *Arch Pathol Lab Med* 110:749, 1986.

GOULD SE: *Trichinosis in Man and Animals*. Springfield, IL, Charles C Thomas, 1970.

GRAY ML, KILLINGER AH: *Listeria monocytogenes* and *Listeria* infections. *Bacteriol Rev* 30:309, 1966.

GUTIERREZ Y: *Diagnostic Pathology of Parasitic Infections with Clinical Correlations*, 2nd ed., New York, Oxford University Press, 2000.

HINMAN AR: Tuberculous meningitis at Cleveland Metropolitan General Hospital. *Am Rev Respir Dis* 94:465, 1966.

HOOPER DC, PRUITT AA, RUBIN RH: Central nervous system infections in the chronically immunosuppressed. *Medicine* 61:166, 1982.

JEFFERSON M: Sarcoidosis of the nervous system. *Brain* 80:540, 1957.

KATZ DA, BERGER JR: Neurosyphilis in acquired immunodeficiency syndrome. *Arch Neurol* 46:895, 1989.

Katz JD, Ropper AH, Adelman L, et al: A case of *Balamuthia mandrillaris* meningoencephalitis. *Arch Neurol* 57:1210, 2000.

KAUFMAN DM, LITMAN N, MILLER MH: Sinusitis induced subdural empyema. *Neurology* 33:123, 1983.

KUBIK CS, ADAMS RD: Subdural empyema. *Brain* 66:18, 1943.

LAMBERT HP (ed): *Infections of the Central Nervous System*. Philadelphia, Decker, 1991.

LAMBERT HP: Meningitis. *J Neurol Neurosurg Psychiatry* 57:405, 1994.

LECHTENBERG R, STERRA MF, PRINGLE GF, et al: *Listeria monocytogenes*: Brain abscess or meningoencephalitis? *Neurology* 29:86, 1979.

LEES AW, TYRRELL WF: Severe cerebral disturbance in legionnaires' disease. *Lancet* 2:1331, 1978.

LEWIS JL, RABINOVICH S: The wide spectrum of cryptococcal infection. *Am J Med* 53:315, 1972.

LEYS D, DESTEE A, PETIT H, WAROT P: Management of subdural intracranial empyemas should not always require surgery. *J Neurol Neurosurg Psychiatry* 49:635, 1986.

LINCOLN EM: Tuberculous meningitis in children. Serous meningitis. *Ann Rev Tuberculosis* 56:95, 1947.

LIPTON SA, HICKEY WF, MORRIS JH, LOSCALZO J: Candidal infection in the central nervous system. *Am J Med* 76:101, 1984.

LOUIS ED, LYNCH T, KAUFMANN P, FAHN S, ODEL J: Diagnostic guidelines in central nervous system Whipple's disease. *Ann Neurol* 40:561, 1996.

MA P, VISVESVARA GS, MARTINEZ AJ: *Naegleria* and *Acanthamoeba* infections: Review. *Rev Infect Dis* 12:490, 1990.

MANKODI AK, DESAI AD, MATHUR RS, et al: Diagnostic role of Mantoux test site biopsy in neurosarcoidosis. *Neurology* 51: 1216, 1998.

MAYOCK RL, BERTRAND P, MORRISON CE, SCOTT JH: Manifestations of sarcoidosis: Analysis of 145 patients with review of nine series selected from literature. *Am J Med* 35:67, 1963.

MERRITT HH, ADAMS RD, SOLOMON H: *Neurosyphilis*. New York, Oxford University Press, 1946.

NABER SP: Molecular pathology—Diagnosis of infectious disease. *N Engl J Med* 331:1212, 1994.

NADELMAN RB, WORMSER GP: Lyme borreliosis. *Lancet* 352:557, 1998.

NEWTON EM: Hematogenous brain abscess in cyanotic congenital heart disease. *Q J Med* 25:201, 1956.

OSKI J, KALIMO H, MARTTILA RJ, et al: Inflammatory brain changes in Lyme borreliosis. *Brain* 119:2143, 1996.

PACHNER AR, DELANEY E, O'NEILL T: Neuroborreliosis in the nonhuman primate: Borrelia burgdorferi persists in the central nervous system. *Ann Neurol* 38:667, 1995.

PEACOCK JE: Persistent neutrophilic meningitis. *Infect Dis Clin North Am* 4:747, 1990.

PITCHENIK AE, FERTEL D, BLOCH AB: Myobacterial disease: Epidemiology, diagnosis, treatment, and prevention. *Clin Chest Med* 9:425, 1988.

POMEROY SL, HOLMES SJ, DODGE PR, FEIGIN RD: Seizures and other neurologic sequelae of bacterial meningitis in children. *N Engl J Med* 323:1651, 1990.

POWDERLY WG, SAAG MS, CLOUD GA, et al: A controlled trial of fluconazole or amphotericin B to prevent relapse of cryptococcal meningitis in patients with the acquired immunodeficiency syndrome. *N Engl J Med* 326:793, 1992.

QUAGLIARELLO VJ, SCHELD WM: Treatment of bacterial meningitis. *N Engl J Med* 336:708, 1997.

REIK L: Spirochetal infections of the nervous system, in Kennedy PGE, Johnson RT (eds): *Infections of the Nervous System*. Boston, Butterworth, 1987, chap 4, pp 43–75.

RENNICK G: Cerebral herniation during bacterial meningitis in children. *BMJ* 306:953, 1993.

RICH AR: *The Pathogenesis of Tuberculosis*, 2nd ed. Oxford, England, Blackwell, 1951.

ROMAN GC: Cerebral malaria: The unsolved riddle. *J Neurol Sci* 101:1, 1991.

ROPPER AH, KANIS KB: Flaccid quadriplegia from tonsillar herniation in pneumococcal meningitis. *J Clin Neurosci* 7:330, 2000.

ROTHSTEIN TL, KENNY GE: Cranial neuropathy, myeloradiculopathy, and myositis: Complications of *Mycoplasma pneumoniae* infection. *Arch Neurol* 36:476, 1979.

SAAG MS, POWDERLY WG, CLOUD GA, et al: Comparison of amphotericin B with fluconazole in the treatment of acute AIDS-associated cryptococcal meningitis. *N Engl J Med* 326:83, 1992.

SCADDING JG: *SARCOIDOSIS*. London, Eyre and Spottiswoode, 1967.

SCHUCHAT A, ROBINSON K, WENGER JD, et al: Bacterial meningitis in the United States. *N Engl J Med* 337:970, 1997.

SCHWARTZ WJ, NILES JL: Case records of the Massachusetts General Hospital. *N Engl J Med* 340:945, 1999.

SCRIMGEOUR EM, GAJDUSEK DC: Involvement of the central nervous system in *Schistosoma mansoni* and *S. haematobium* infection. *Brain* 108:1023, 1985.

SEIDEL JS, HARMATZ , VISVESVARA GS, et al: Successful treatment of primary amebic meningoencephalitis. *N Engl J Med* 306:346, 1982.

SHETTY KR, CILVO CL, STARR BD, HARTER DH: Legionnaires' disease with profound cerebellar involvement. *Arch Neurol* 37:379, 1980.

SILTZBACH LE, JAMES DG, NEVILLE E, et al: Course and prognosis of sarcoidosis around the world. *Am J Med* 57:847, 1974.

SNEDEKER JD, KAPLAN SL, DODGE PR, et al: Subdural effusion and its relationship with neurologic sequelae of bacterial meningitis in infancy: A prospective study. *Pediatrics* 86:163, 1990.

SNIDER DE, ROPER WL: The new tuberculosis. *N Engl J Med* 326:703, 1992.

SOTELO J, ESCOBEDO F, RODRIGUEZ-CARBAJAL J, et al: Therapy of parenchymal brain cysticercosis with praziquantel. *N Engl J Med* 310:1001, 1984.

STERN BJ, KRUMHOLZ A, JOHN SC, et al: Sarcoidosis and its neurological manifestations. *Arch Neurol* 42:909, 1985.

STOCKSTILL MT, KAUFFMAN CA: Comparison of cryptococcal and tuberculous meningitis. *Arch Neurol* 40:81, 1983.

SWARTZ MN: "Chronic meningitis"—Many causes to consider. *N Engl J Med* 317:957, 1987.

SWARTZ MN, DODGE PR: Bacterial meningitis: A review of selected aspects. *N Engl J Med* 272:725, 779, 842, 898, 1965.

Syphilis: Centers for Disease Control recommended treatment schedules, Venereal Disease Control Advisory Committee. *MMWR* 38(suppl):S-8, 1989.

THOMPSON RA: Clinical features of central nervous system fungus infection, in Thompson RA, Green JR (eds): *Advances in Neurology* Vol 6. New York, Raven Press, 1974, pp 93–100.

TORO G, ROMAN G: Cerebral malaria. *Arch Neurol* 35:271, 1978.

TOWNSEND JJ, WOLINSKY JS, BARINGER JR, JOHNSON PC: Acquired toxoplasmosis. *Arch Neurol* 32:335, 1975.

TURNER G: Cerebral malaria. *Brain Pathol* 7:569, 1997.

TYLER KL, MARTIN JB: *Infectious Diseases of the Nervous System*. Philadelphia, Davis, 1993.

VARTDAL F, VANDVIK B, MICHAELSEN TE, et al: Neurosyphilis: Intrathecal synthesis of oligoclonal antibodies to *Treponema pallidum*. *Ann Neurol* 11:35, 1982.

WALSH TJ, HIER DB, CAPLAN LR: Fungal infections of the central nervous system: Comparative analysis of risk factors and clinical signs in 57 patients. *Neurology* 35:1654, 1985.

WASZ-HOCKERT O, DONNER M: Results of the treatment of 191 children with tuberculous meningitis. *Acta Paediatr* 51(suppl 141):7, 1962.

WATT G, ADAPON B, LONG GW, et al: Praziquantel in treatment of cerebral schistosomiasis. *Lancet* 2:529, 1986.

WESTENFELDER GO, AKEY DT, CORWIN SJ, VICK NA: Acute transverse myelitis due to Mycoplasma pneumoniae infection. *Arch Neurol* 38:317, 1981.

ZUNIGA G, ROPPER AH, FRANK J: Sarcoid peripheral neuropathy. *Neurology* 41:1558, 1991.

Chapter 33

VIRAL INFECTIONS OF THE NERVOUS SYSTEM AND PRION DISEASES

VIRAL INFECTIONS OF THE NERVOUS SYSTEM

The notion that certain viruses are neurotropic is not entirely correct. A more accurate view identifies a number of viruses with a proclivity to invade the nervous system—namely, human immunodeficiency viruses (HIV-1 and HIV-2), herpes simplex viruses (HSV-1 and HSV-2), herpes zoster [or varicella zoster (VZ)] virus, Epstein-Barr virus (EBV), cytomegalovirus (CMV), poliovirus, rabies, and several seasonal arthropod-borne viruses. Nonetheless, there are examples of an innate bond between certain viruses and particular neurons: poliomyelitis viruses and motor neurons, VZ virus and peripheral sensory neurons, rabies virus and Purkinje cells and other neurons. For many of the rest of the neurotropic viruses, the affinity is less selective in that they involve regions of the nervous system—i.e., are neurohistiopathic. Herpes simplex, for example, may devastate the medial parts of the temporal lobes, destroying neurons, glial cells, myelinated nerve fibers, and blood vessels. The acquired immunodeficiency syndrome (AIDS) virus may induce multiple foci of tissue necrosis throughout the cerebrum.

These relationships and many others, which are the subject matter of this chapter, are of wide interest in medicine. In many of these conditions, the systemic effects of the viral infection are negligible; it is the neurologic disorder that brings them to medical attention. In other words, the neural aspects of viral infection may assume a clinical importance that is disproportionate to the systemic illnesses of which they are a part. This aspect of neurology must therefore be familiar to pediatricians and internists, who are likely to be the first to see such patients.

A detailed discussion of viral morphology and cell-virus interactions is beyond the scope of a textbook of neurology. Authoritative overviews of this subject can be found in the current edition of *Harrison's Principles of Internal Medicine* and in the introductory chapters of R. T. Johnson's monograph *Viral Infections of the Nervous System.*

Pathways of Infection

Viruses gain entrance to the body by one of several pathways. Mumps, measles, and varicella enter via the respiratory passages. Polioviruses and other enteroviruses enter by the oral-intestinal route, and HSV, mainly via the oral or genital mucosal route. Other viruses are acquired by inoculation, as a result of the bites of animals (e.g., rabies) or mosquitoes (arthropod-borne or arbovirus infections). The fetus may be infected transplacentally by the rubella virus, CMV, and HIV.

Following entry into the body, the virus multiplies locally and in secondary sites and usually gives rise to a viremia. Most viruses are prevented from entering central nervous system (CNS) tissues, presumably by the blood-brain barrier. However, most antibodies and immunocompetent cells are excluded as well, so that the same mechanism that excludes viruses also deters their clearance. Viral particles are cleared from the blood by the reticuloendothelial system; but if the viremia is massive or other conditions are favorable, they will invade the CNS via the cerebral capillaries and the choroid plexuses.

Another pathway of infection is along peripheral nerves; centripetal movement of virus is accomplished by the retrograde axoplasmic transport system. Herpes simplex, VZ, and rabies viruses utilize this peripheral nerve pathway, which explains why the initial symptoms of rabies and the rare B-virus infection of monkeys occur locally, at a segmental level that corresponds to the animal bite. In animals inoculated subcutaneously with VZ virus, sensitive DNA amplification techniques identify fragments of viral genome only in the dorsal root ganglion or ganglia corresponding to the dermatome(s) containing the site of inoculation. It has been shown experimentally that HSV may spread to the CNS by involving olfactory neurons in the nasal mucosa; the central processes of these cells pass through openings in the cribriform plate and synapse with cells in the olfactory bulb (CNS). Another potential pathway is the trigeminal nerve and gasserian ganglion. However, the role of these pathways in human infection is not certain. Of these different routes of infection, the hematogenous one is by far the most important for the majority of viruses. The steps in the hematogenous spread of infection are illustrated diagrammatically in Fig. 33-1.

Mechanisms of Viral Infections

Viruses, once they invade the nervous system, have diverse clinical and pathologic effects. One reason for this diversity is that different cell populations within the CNS vary in their susceptibility to infection with different viruses. To be susceptible to a viral infection, the host cell must have specific receptor sites on its cytoplasmic membrane, to which the virus attaches. Thus, some infections are confined to meningeal cells, enteroviruses being the most common, in which case the clinical manifestations are those of a benign aseptic meningitis. Other viruses will involve particular classes of neurons of the brain or spinal cord, giving rise to the more serious disorders such as encephalitis and poliomyelitis, respectively. In some viral infections, the susceptibility of particular cell groups is even more specific. In poliomyelitis, for example, motor neurons of cranial and spinal nerves are particularly vulnerable; in rabies, neurons of the trigeminal ganglia, cerebellum, and limbic lobes. The virus or its nucleocapsid must be capable of penetrating the cell, mainly by the process of endocytosis, and of releasing its protective nucleoprotein coating. For virus reproduction to occur, the cell must have the metabolic capacity to transcribe and translate virus-coated proteins, to replicate viral nucleic acid, and, under the direction of the virus's genome, to assemble virions.

Also, the pathologic effects of viruses upon susceptible cells vary greatly. In acute encephalitis, susceptible neurons are invaded directly by virus and the cells undergo lysis. There is an appropriate glial and inflammatory reaction. Neuronophagia (phagocytosis of affected neurons by microglia) is a mark of this phenomenon. In progressive multifocal leukoencephalopathy (PML), there is a selective lysis of oligodendrocytes, resulting in foci of demyelination. With other viral infections, zones of tissue necrosis of gray and white matter occur, and these changes may localize in particular regions, e.g., in the inferomedial parts of the temporal lobes in cases of HSV encephalitis. The VZ virus and HSV may remain latent in neurons of the sensory ganglia for long periods, until some factor triggers reactivation and retrograde spread of virus to cutaneous dermatomes or mucocutaneous epithelium. Only then will the inflammatory reaction to viral replication create symptoms (pain, weakness, sensory loss). In certain congenital infections, e.g., rubella and CMV, the virus persists in nervous tissue for months or years. Differentiating cells of the fetal brain have particular vulnerabilities, and viral incorporation may give rise to malformations and to hydrocephalus (e.g., mumps virus with ependymal destruction and aqueductal stenosis).

In experimental animals, cerebral neoplasms can be induced when the viral genome is incorporated into the DNA of the host cell. There is suggestive evidence of such a mechanism in humans (EBV in B-cell lymphoma). In still other circumstances, a viral infection may exist in the nervous system for a long period before exciting an inflammatory reaction (e.g., progressive multifocal encephalopathy; subacute sclerosing panencephalitis); it may be so indolent as to simulate a degenerative disease.

CLINICAL SYNDROMES

The number of viruses that affect the nervous system is legion. Among the enteroviruses alone, nearly 70 distinct serologic types have been associated with CNS disease, and additional types from this family of viruses and others are still being discovered. There is no need to consider these viruses individually, since there are only a limited number of ways in which they express themselves clinically. Six syndromes recur with regularity and should be familiar to all neurologists: (1) acute aseptic (nonsuppurative or "lymphocytic") or chronic meningitis; (2) acute encephalitis or meningoencephalitis, which may be generalized or focal (cerebral or cerebellar); (3) herpes zoster ganglionitis; (4) chronic invasion of nervous tissue by retroviruses, i.e., the AIDS syndrome and tropical spastic paraparesis (TSP); (5) acute anterior poliomyelitis; and (6) chronic viral infections ("slow infections"). These are presently distinguished from the prion infections, which are discussed later in the chapter.

Figure 33-1

Steps in the hematogenous spread of virus to the central nervous system. (Courtesy of RT Johnson.)

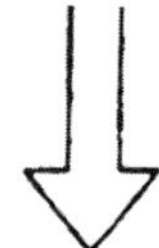

ENTRY INTO HOST
Inoculation
Respiratory
Enteric

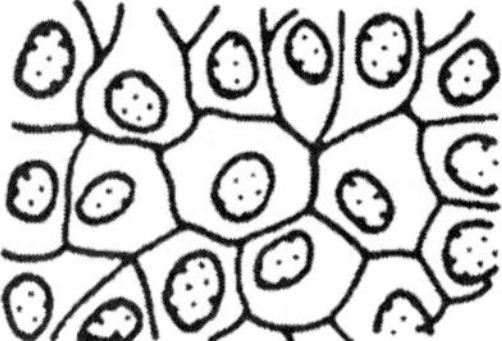

GROWTH IN EXTRANEURAL TISSUES
Primary sites
subcutaneous tissue and muscle, lymph nodes, respiratory or gastrointestinal tracts
Secondary sites
muscle, vascular endothelium, bone marrow, liver, spleen, etc.

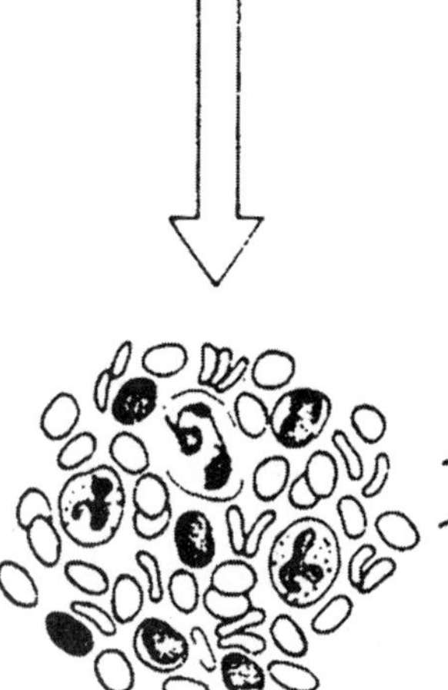

MAINTENANCE OF VIREMIA
Sufficient input
Adsorption to red cells
Growth in white cells
Decreased clearance by RES

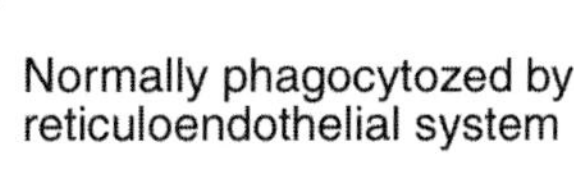

Normally phagocytozed by reticuloendothelial system

CROSSING FROM BLOOD TO BRAIN

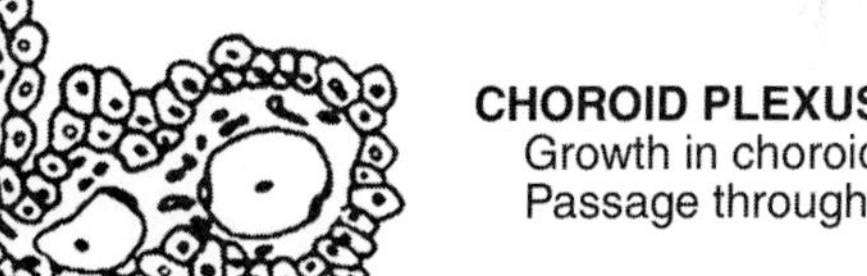

CHOROID PLEXUS TO CSF
Growth in choroid plexus
Passage through choroid plexus

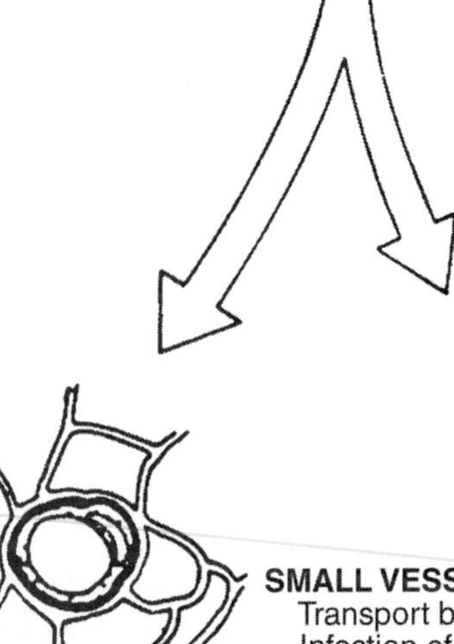

SMALL VESSELS TO BRAIN
Transport by infected leukocytes
Infection of vascular endothelium
Diffusion across normal cells and membranes
Passage through areas of permeability

THE SYNDROME OF ASEPTIC MENINGITIS

The term *aseptic meningitis* was first introduced to designate what was thought to be a specific disease—"aseptic" because bacterial cultures were negative. The term is now applied to a symptom complex that can be produced by any one of numerous infective agents, the majority of which are viral (but a few of which are bacterial—mycoplasma, Q fever, other rickettsial infections, etc.). Since aseptic meningitis is rarely fatal, the precise pathologic changes are uncertain but are presumably limited to the meninges. Conceivably, there may be some minor changes in the brain itself, but these are of insufficient severity to cause neurologic symptoms and signs or to alter the CT scans or MRI.

In outline, the clinical syndrome of aseptic meningitis consists of fever, headache, signs of meningeal irritation, and a predominantly lymphocytic pleocytosis with normal cerebrospinal fluid (CSF) glucose. Usually the onset is acute and the temperature is elevated, from 38 to 40°C. Headache, perhaps more severe than that associated with other febrile states, is the most frequent symptom. A variable degree of lethargy, irritability, and drowsiness may occur; confusion, stupor, and coma are decidedly rare. Photophobia and pain on movement of the eyes are common complaints. Stiffness of the neck and spine on forward bending attests to the presence of meningeal irritation (meningismus), but at first it may be so slight as to pass unnoticed. Here the Kernig and Brudzinski signs help very little, for they are often absent in the presence of a manifest viral meningitis. When there are accompanying neurologic signs, they too tend to be mild or fleeting: paresthesias in an extremity, isolated strabismus and diplopia, a slight inequality of reflexes, or a wavering Babinski sign. Other symptoms and signs are infrequent and depend mainly on the systemic effects of the invading virus; these include sore throat, nausea and vomiting, vague weakness, pain in the back and neck, conjunctivitis, cough, diarrhea, vomiting, rash, adenopathy, etc. In general, the symptoms are mild, and at times the meningitis is entirely asymptomatic. The childhood exanthems that are associated with meningitis and encephalitis (varicella, rubella, mumps) produce well-known eruptions or other characteristic signs. An erythematous papulomacular, nonpruritic rash, confined to the head and neck or generalized, may also be a prominent feature (particularly in children) of certain echoviruses and Coxsackie viruses. An enanthem (herpangina), taking the form of a vesiculoulcerative eruption of the buccal mucosa, may also occur with these viral infections.

The CSF findings consist of a pleocytosis (mainly mononuclear except in the first days of the illness, when more than half the cells may be neutrophils), and a small and variable increase in protein. In milder cases, in the first hours or day of the illness, there may be no abnormalities of the spinal fluid, and the patient may erroneously be thought to have migraine or a headache induced by a systemic infectious illness. Microorganisms cannot be demonstrated by conventional smear or bacterial culture. As a rule, the glucose content of the CSF is normal; this is important because a low glucose concentration in conjunction with a lymphocytic or mononuclear pleocytosis usually signifies tuberculous or fungal meningitis or certain noninfectious disorders such as metastatic carcinoma, lymphoma, or sarcoid of the meninges. Infrequently, a mild depression of the CSF glucose (never below 25 mg/dL) has been reported with the meningitis caused by mumps, herpes simplex virus type 2 (HSV-2), lymphocytic choriomeningitis, or the VZ virus. Since the CSF glucose level may be normal or near normal in the early stages of tuberculous or cryptococcal meningitis, this determination should be repeated at intervals until the diagnosis is established or the patient is definitely convalescent.

Causes of Aseptic Meningitis

Aseptic meningitis is a common occurrence, with an annual incidence rate of 11 to 27 cases per 100,000 population (Beghi et al; Ponka and Pettersson). A majority of cases are due to viral infections. Of these, the most common are the enteroviral infections—echovirus and Coxsackie virus. These make up 80 percent of cases of aseptic meningitis in which a specific viral cause can be established. Mumps is perhaps next in frequency, followed by HSV-2, lymphocytic choriomeningitis (LCM), and adenovirus infections. EBV (infectious mononucleosis), CMV, leptospirosis, HSV-1, and the bacterium *Mycoplasma pneumoniae* (see Chap. 32) may also produce what appears to be an aseptic meningitis. Influenza virus, adenoviruses, and numerous sporadic and otherwise innocuous agents have at times been isolated from the spinal fluid in cases of aseptic meningitis. The California virus, which is an arthropod-borne ("arbo") virus, is responsible for a small number of cases (usually the arboviruses cause an encephalitis or meningoencephalitis, as discussed further on). Rarely, the icteric stage of infectious hepatitis is preceded by mild meningitis, the nature of which becomes evident when the jaundice appears. All these viral infections, particularly those due to the enteroviruses—together with mycoplasmal infection, leptospirosis, and Lyme borreliosis—make up about 95 percent of cases of aseptic meningitis in which the etiology can be established. The chronic and recurrent meningitides constitute a special problem, discussed below.

It is now well recognized that infection with HIV may present as an acute, self-limited aseptic meningitis with an infectious mononucleosis-like clinical picture. While HIV has been obtained from the CSF in the acute phase of the illness, seroconversion occurs only later, during convalescence (see further on in this chapter). Herpes simplex virus type 1 has been isolated from the CSF of patients with recurrent bouts of benign aseptic meningitis (so-called Mollaret meningitis), but not consistently (Steel et al). As discussed in Chap. 47, it is now believed that this virus also underlies many if not most cases of what has been traditionally considered idiopathic Bell's palsy (Murakami et al).

It should be noted that in every published series of cases from virus isolation centers, a specific cause cannot be established in one-third or more of cases of presumed viral origin.

Differential Diagnosis of Viral Meningitis

Clinical distinctions between the many viral causes of aseptic meningitis cannot be made with a high degree of reliability, but useful leads can be obtained by attention to certain details of the clinical history and physical examination. It is important to inquire about recent respiratory or gastrointestinal symptoms, immunizations, past history of infectious disease, family outbreaks, insect bites, contact with animals, and areas of recent travel. The presence or absence of an epidemic, the season during which the illness occurs, and the geographic location are other helpful data.

As already mentioned, the enteroviruses (echo, Coxsackie and, in underdeveloped countries, polio) are by far the commonest causes of viral meningitis. Because these organisms grow in the intestinal tract and are spread mainly by the fecal-oral route, family outbreaks are usual and the infections are most common among children. A number of echovirus and Coxsackie virus (particularly group A) infections are associated with exanthemata and may, in addition, be associated with the grayish vesicular lesions of herpangina. Pleurodynia, brachial neuritis, pericarditis, and orchitis are characteristic of some cases of group B Coxsackie virus infections. Pain in the back and neck and in the muscles should always suggest poliomyelitis. Lower motor neuron weakness may occur with echo and Coxsackie virus infections, but it is usually mild and transient in nature. The peak incidence of enteroviral infections is in August and September. This is true also of infections due to arboviruses, but as a rule the latter cause encephalitis rather than meningitis.

Mumps meningitis occurs sporadically throughout the year, but the highest incidence is in late winter and spring. Males are affected three times more frequently than females. Other manifestations of mumps infection—parotitis, orchitis, mastitis, oophoritis, and pancreatitis—may or may not be present. It should be noted that orchitis is not specific for mumps but occurs occasionally with group B Coxsackie virus infections, infectious mononucleosis, and lymphocytic choriomeningitis. A definite past history of mumps aids in excluding the disease, since an attack confers lifelong immunity.

The natural host of the lymphocytic choriomeningitis (LCM) virus is the common house mouse, *Mus musculus*. Humans acquire the infection by contact with infected hamsters or with dust that is contaminated by mouse excreta. Laboratory workers who handle rodents may be exposed to LCM. The meningitis may be preceded by respiratory symptoms (sometimes with pulmonary infiltrates). The infection is particularly common in late fall and winter, presumably because mice enter dwellings at that time.

The infectious agent in leptospirosis is a spirochete, but the clinical syndrome that it produces is indistinguishable from viral meningitis (discussed in Chap. 32). Infection is acquired by contact with soil or water contaminated by the urine of rats and also of dogs, swine, and cattle. Although leptospirosis may appear in any season, its incidence in the United States shows a striking peak in August. The presence of conjunctival suffusion, a transient blotchy erythema, severe leg and back pain, and pulmonary infiltrates should suggest leptospiral infection.

A far more common spirochetal cause of aseptic meningitis (and meningoencephalitis) is Lyme borreliosis. This is now the most common vector (tick)-borne disease in the United States. Most cases occur in the northeastern states, Minnesota, and Wisconsin during the months of May to July—the questing time among nymphal ixodid ticks. In 60 to 80 percent of patients, a bright-red annular skin lesion at the site of the tick bite, often with secondary annular lesions, precedes the onset of meningeal signs (as discussed more extensively on pages 768–769). There may be associated facial palsies, cauda equina symptoms such as urinary retention and sacral numbness, or a sensory neuropathy (see Chap. 46).

The atypical pneumonia agents *M. pneumoniae* and Q fever (*Coxiella burnetti*) can produce an aseptic meningitis that is indistinguishable from the viral form.

Wild rodents may also be the source of encephalomyocarditis virus infection, and cats, of course, of cat-scratch disease. The latter usually takes the form of a benign febrile adenopathy but occasionally of an encephalitis or a localized cranial arteritis (see page 748).

The presence of sore throat, generalized lymphadenopathy, transient rash, and mild icterus is suggestive of infectious mononucleosis or, at times, of CMV infection. Icterus is a prominent manifestation of viral hepatitis and some serotypes of leptospirosis and of Q fever.

A mononucleosis type of infection (fever, rash, arthralgias, lymphadenopathy) in an individual with recent sexual exposure to a potentially infected partner or a known carrier of HIV—or with exposure to contaminated blood—should always raise the possibility of HIV infection. As with Lyme and HSV, HIV meningitis may be associated with a cauda equina neuritis, as discussed in Chap. 46. In the case of HSV, there is often a preceding genital infection with the virus.

Aside from viral isolation and serologic tests and, more recently, polymerase chain reaction (see further on), few laboratory examinations are helpful. The peripheral white cell count is usually normal but may sometimes be slightly elevated or depressed with a mild lymphocytosis. Eosinophilia should suggest a parasitic infection. Most cases of infectious mononucleosis can be identified by the blood smear and specific serologic tests (heterophile or others). LCM should be suspected if there is an intense pleocytosis. Counts above 1000 mononuclear cells per cubic millimeter in the spinal fluid are most often due to LCM but may occur occasionally with mumps or echovirus 9; in the latter, neutrophils may predominate in the CSF for a week or longer. Serologic reactions of CSF for syphilis should be interpreted with caution, because inflammation of many types, including infectious mononucleosis, can produce a false-positive reaction. Liver function tests are abnormal in many patients with EBV infection, leptospiral infections, and anicteric hepatitis. In the majority of patients with *M. pneumoniae* infections, cold agglutinins appear in the serum toward the end of the first week of the illness. Panels of serologic tests for the main viruses that cause aseptic meningitis are available; most use complement fixation or enzyme-linked immunosorbent assay (ELISA) techniques; an infection is demonstrated by a fourfold increase in titer from acute to convalescent serum drawn at least 10 days apart. In the last few years, the polymerase chain reaction (PCR) has been applied to the diagnosis of viral infections of the nervous system, among them CMV and HSV. The test detects portions of the viral DNA in the spinal fluid and is most sensitive during the active stage of viral replication, in contrast to serologic tests, which are more accurate later in the course of the infection. There are numerous false-negative and fewer false-positive PCR tests for CMV, but they are nonetheless useful in some circumstances, such as the early diagnosis of fulminant infection in AIDS patients (see later in this chapter).

Other Causes of Aseptic, Chronic, and Recurrent Meningitis

Six other categories of disease may cause an apparently sterile, predominantly lymphocytic or mononuclear reaction in the leptomeninges: (1) foci of bacterial infection lying adjacent to the meninges; (2) partially treated bacterial meningitis; (3) specific meningeal infections in which the organism is difficult or impossible to isolate—fungal and tuberculous meningitis should always be considered in these circumstances, and the group also includes parasitic infections; (4) neoplastic invasion of the leptomeninges (lymphoma or carcinoma); (5) granulomatous, vasculitic, or other inflammatory diseases such as sarcoidosis, Behçet disease, and granulomatous angiitis; (6) acute or chronic recurrent inflammatory meningitides of unusual or obscure origin. The latter constitute a vexing group in which no cause can be found, but, as indicated further on, careful follow-up and repeated CSF investigation, or in some cases meningeal biopsy, will reveal a cause in a few, and many others will resolve spontaneously. They are described below, under "Chronic Persistent and Recurrent Meningitis." Other occasional causes include an aseptic chemical meningitis incited by rupture of a craniopharyngioma or other cystic structure containing proteinaceous fluid or the introduction of a foreign substance to the subarachnoid space, but the cause in these instances is usually obvious. Also, an idiosyncratic, presumably immunologic, meningitis has resulted from the use of nonsteroidal anti-inflammatory medications, intravenous immune globulin (actually, a carrier chemical in the solution), and, rarely, from other drugs.

In respect to the first two categories, a smoldering paranasal sinusitis or mastoiditis may produce a CSF picture of aseptic meningitis because of intracranial extension (epidural or subdural infection). Or a brain abscess, the localizing signs of which are minimal or absent, may deceive the clinician into making a diagnosis of aseptic meningitis. It must also be remembered that antibiotic therapy given for a systemic or pulmonary infection may suppress a bacterial meningitis to the point where mononuclear cells predominate, glucose is near normal, and organisms are not detected in the CSF. A mistaken diagnosis of aseptic meningitis may then be made on the basis of the CSF examination. The true state of affairs becomes evident only when the illness worsens, the CSF glucose decreases, and bacteria again appear in the CSF. Careful attention to the history of recent antimicrobial therapy permits recognition of these cases. Rarely, children with scarlet fever or streptococcal pharyngitis have been noted to develop meningeal signs and pleocytosis, the result of a sterile serous inflammation that does not involve invasion of the meninges by organisms. The same may occur in subacute bacterial endocarditis. A number of cases of recurrent bacterial meningitis, as discussed further on and in the previous chapter, result from a CSF leak after head trauma.

Syphilis, cryptococcosis, and tuberculosis are the important members of the third group, as detailed in Chap. 32. Acute syphilitic meningitis may be asymptomatic or symptomatic; in the latter case, both the clinical and CSF features of aseptic meningitis will be present except that the patient is usually afebrile. In the past, acute syphilitic meningitis was likely to develop as a neurorecurrence after inadequate therapy, but now it may be the first manifestation of a syphilitic infection. Tuberculous meningitis, in its initial stages, may occasionally masquerade as an innocent aseptic meningitis; the diagnosis may be delayed because the tubercle bacillus is frequently difficult to find in stained smears, and cultures may require several weeks. Cranial nerve palsies are characteristic of chronic tuberculous meningitis (see below) and the CSF glucose is then severely depressed, although it may be only slightly reduced early in the illness. Similarly, the diagnosis of cryptococcosis, other fungal infection, or nocardiosis is occasionally missed because the organisms may be present in such low numbers as to be overlooked in smears. Brucellosis (Mediterranean fever, Malta fever) is a rare disease, practically confined to the Middle East, that may present as an acute meningitis or meningoencephalitis, with the CSF findings of an aseptic meningitis. *Brucella melitensis* can rarely be cultured from blood or CSF; more often diagnosis depends upon the detection of high serum antibody titers and *Brucella*-specific immunoglobulins, using the ELISA. Lymphocytic meningitis may occur as a complication of Q fever, a rickettsial disease.

In the fourth (neoplastic) group, leukemias and lymphomas are the most common sources of meningeal reactions. In children, a leukemic "meningitis" with cells (lymphoblasts or myeloblasts) in the CSF numbering in the thousands occurs frequently in the late stages of the illness. In adults, a marked lymphocytic or lymphoblastic pleocytosis may complicate non-Hodgkin lymphomas with or without leukemia. In these disorders and in meningeal carcinomatosis (from lung, breast, colon, or other source), great numbers of neoplastic cells may extend throughout the leptomeninges and involve cranial and spinal nerve roots, producing a picture of meningoradiculitis with normal or low CSF glucose values. As already mentioned, lymphocytic meningitis that is accompanied by cranial nerve palsies most often turns out to be tuberculous if the patient is febrile and the CSF glucose is low, and neoplastic if the patient is afebrile and the CSF glucose is normal or mildly decreased. Infiltration of the meninges by a glioma or pinealoma may have the same effect. Concentrated cytologic preparations usually permit identification of the tumor cells. These diseases are discussed in detail in Chap. 31.

There are several inflammatory, granulomatous, and vasculitic disorders that give rise to an aseptic meningitis syndrome, either by infiltrating the leptomeninges or as a reaction to inflammation of small vessels. Sarcoidosis, Behçet disease, intravascular lymphoma, and granulomatous angiitis are the best-known examples of this group. Occlusion of many small cerebral blood vessels by cholesterol emboli may also excite a reaction in meningeal vessels and a pleocytosis that includes eosinophils. Each of these conditions sometimes presents with a clinical picture of meningitis alone, but more often they are seen with signs of both meningeal and parenchymal involvement, i.e., with a meningoencephalitis.

Chronic Persistent and Recurrent Meningitis

Chronic and recurrent meningitides of obscure etiology always pose diagnostic problems. Such patients may have a low-grade fever, headache of varying severity, and stiff neck and a predominantly mononuclear pleocytosis sometimes with raised CSF pressure. There may also be minor focal neurologic signs. A viral or some other type of infective inflammation is always suspected, but a search by culture methods and serology usually yields negative results. Herpesvirus has been presumed to be the cause of a few cases as in the recurrent Mollaret type noted below. Sometimes the process resolves over a period of months or a year or more. In other cases, the cause is eventually found. A few end fatally. In a series of such patients studied at the Mayo Clinic, 33 of 39 underwent a natural resolution and 2 died within 3½ years; 14 were still symptomatic at the time of the report (Smith and Aksamit). In a series from New Zealand of 83 such patients, Anderson et al found tuberculosis to be the single most common identifiable cause, a smaller number being accounted for by neoplastic and cryptococcal meningitis; in fully one-third of the patients, no cause could be established. Charleston and colleagues reported a subgroup of these patients who were responsive to steroids; in 7 of 17 patients, medication could eventually be withdrawn without recurrence; four patients required treatment indefinitely; the remaining six died many months or years after onset of treatment. The outcome and response to steroids in our cases and other reported series has been much the same.

The special problem of *chronic neutrophilic meningitis* has been mentioned on page 758. It is ususally due to *Nocardia*, *Aspergillus*, *Actinomyces*, or certain *Mycobacterium* species (see Peacock, cited in the preceding chapter).

Our practice in the management of such patients is to repeat the lumbar puncture several times to obtain cultures and cytology of CSF, using markers for B and T lymphocytes and tumor cells, a marker for neoplastic meningitis such as β_2-microglobulin, PCR for amplification of herpesviruses, and HIV testing. MRI of the brain and spinal cord with gadolinium should be performed. If the CSF pressure is elevated or there is clinical or radiologic evidence of an angiitis, treatment with steroids should be tried and is sometimes successful. If hydrocephalus develops, it should be managed along the lines described in Chap. 30. A trial of antiviral agents and broad spectrum antibiotics seems reasonable, although we have had no success with them in our last several patients. We resort to a biopsy of the meninges if the diagnosis has not been clarified in 6 to 12 months or if a febrile meningitis persists for more than several weeks, but this practice has also proved to be of limited value. In Andersen's series, which was mentioned above, biopsy yielded a diagnosis in 5 of 25 patients. Finally, if bacterial infection has been reasonably excluded, we try corticosteroids for several weeks or longer and then attempt to taper the dose while observing the patient and rechecking the CSF formula.

Finally, in a number of other chronic or acutely recurring diseases of obscure origin, the CSF formula corresponds to that of aseptic meningitis: (1) The Vogt-Koyanagi-Harada syndrome, which is characterized by various combinations of iridocyclitis, depigmentation of a hair strand (poliosis circumscripta) and skin around the eyes, loss of eyelashes, dysacusis, and deafness. The course is quite benign, and the pathologic basis of the syndrome is not known. (2) Mollaret recurrent meningitis, some instances of which have been associated with HSV-1 (Steel) and some with HSV-2 infection (Cohen et al). These episodes of acute meningitis, with severe headache and sometimes low-grade fever, usually lasting for about 2 weeks, may recur for a period of several months or many years. In a few of our patients, in whom no virus could be identified in the CSF, antiviral therapy met with little success, although corticosteroids seemed to reduce the severity of acute episodes, as mentioned above. (3) Allergic or hypersensitivity meningitis, occurring in the course of serum sickness and of connective tissue diseases, such as lupus erythematosus, and in relation to certain medications such as nonsteroidal anti-inflammatory drugs and intravenously administered immunoglobulin; and (4) Behçet disease, which is an important acute, recurrent inflammatory CNS disease. It is essentially a diffuse inflammatory disease of small blood vessels and is more appropriately considered with the vasculitides (page 909).

In summary, the history of the illness, the associated clinical findings, and the laboratory tests usually provide the clues to the diagnosis of nonviral and chronic forms of aseptic meningitis. It is always important to keep in mind the possibility of neoplasia, HIV, tuberculosis, cryptococcosis, sarcoidosis, syphilis, borreliosis, and inadequately treated bacterial meningitis—each of which may simulate aseptic meningitis and each of which presents an urgent diagnostic problem. By contrast, the various viral forms of aseptic meningitis are usually self-limited and benign; establishing a specific etiologic diagnosis is usually not necessary.

THE SYNDROME OF ACUTE ENCEPHALITIS

From the foregoing discussion it is evident that the separation of the clinical syndromes of aseptic meningitis and encephalitis is not always easy. In some patients with aseptic meningitis, drowsiness or confusion may be present, suggesting cerebral involvement. Conversely, in some patients with encephalitis, the cerebral symptoms may be mild or inapparent, and meningeal symptoms and CSF abnormalities predominate. These facts make it difficult to place complete reliance on statistical data from various virus laboratories about the relative incidence of meningitis and encephalitis. The common practice is to assume that viral meningitis causes only fever, headache, stiff neck, and photophobia, and, if any other CNS symptoms are added, to call the condition meningoencephalitis. It appears that the same spectrum of viruses gives rise to both meningitis and encephalitis. It is our impression that many cases of enteroviral and practically all cases of mumps and LCM encephalopathy are little more than examples of intense meningitis. Rarely have they caused death with postmortem demonstration of cerebral lesions, and surviving patients seldom have residual neurologic signs. Conversely, several agents, notably the arboviruses, may cause encephalitic lesions with only mild meningeal symptoms.

The core of the *encephalitis syndrome* consists of an acute febrile illness with evidence of meningeal involvement, added to which are various combinations of the following symptoms and signs: convulsions, delirium, confusion, stupor, or coma; aphasia or mutism; hemiparesis with asymmetry of tendon reflexes and Babinski signs; involuntary movements, ataxia, and myoclonic jerks; nystagmus, ocular palsies, and facial weakness. The spinal fluid invariably shows a cellular reaction and the protein is slightly elevated. Imaging studies of the brain are most often normal but may show diffuse edema or enhancement of the cortex and, infrequently in certain infections, subcortical and deep nuclear involvement and, in the special case of herpes simplex encephalitis, selective damage of the inferomedial temporal and frontal lobes. One or another of these groups of findings predominates in certain types of encephalitis, as pointed out below, but the clinical diagnosis, in the setting of a febrile aseptic meningitis, always rests on the demonstration of derangement of the function of the cerebrum, brainstem, or cerebellum.

The acute encephalitis syndrome described above may take two forms: the more common direct invasion of brain and meninges (true viral encephalitis) and a postinfectious encephalomyelitis that is based on an autoimmune reaction to the systemic viral infection but in which virus is not present in neural tissue. The distinction between postinfectious disseminated encephalomyelitis (ADEM, page 975) and infectious encephalitis may be difficult, especially in younger patients who appear to have a proclivity to develop the postinfectious variety. ADEM occurs after a latency of several days, as the infectious illness is subsiding. It is expressed by a low-grade fever and cerebral symptoms such as confusion, seizures, coma, ataxia, etc. The spinal fluid shows slight inflammation and elevation of protein—sometimes a more intense reaction, and there are usually characteristic confluent bilateral lesions in the white matter in imaging studies, findings that differ from those of viral encephalitis. When there is no coexistent epidemic of encephalitis to suggest the diagnosis or the systemic illness is absent or obscure, a differentiation may not be possible on clinical grounds alone. Since ADEM is essentially a demyelinative process, we only mention it in this chapter and discuss it more fully in Chap. 36. We have also placed in a special category the now rare postinfectious acute encephalopathy and hepatic failure of Reye-Johnson that follows influenza and other viral infections.

Etiology

Whereas numerous viral, bacterial, fungal, and parasitic agents are listed as causes of the encephalitis syndrome, only the viral ones are considered here, for it is to these that one usually refers when the term *encephalitis* is used. The nonviral forms of encephalitis (mycoplasmal, rickettsial, Lyme, etc.) are considered in Chap. 32. According to the Centers for Disease Control and Prevention, about 20,000 cases of acute viral encephalitis are reported annually in the United States. Death occurs in 5 to 20 percent of these patients and residual signs such as mental deterioration, amnesic defect, personality change, recurrent seizures, and hemiparesis are seen in about another 20 percent. However, these overall figures fail to reflect the widely varying incidence of mortality and residual neurologic abnormalities that follow infection by different viruses. In herpes simplex encephalitis, for example, more than 50 percent of patients die or are left with severe impairment, and in eastern equine encephalitis, the figures are even higher. On the other hand, death and serious neurologic sequelae have been observed in only 5 to 15 percent of those with western equine infections and in even lesser numbers of patients with Venezuelan, St. Louis, and LaCrosse encephalitides.

As with aseptic meningitis, the number of viruses that can cause an encephalitis or a postinfectious autoimmune reaction is large, and one might suppose that the clinical problems would be infinitely complex. However, the types of viral encephalitis that occur with sufficient frequency to be of diagnostic importance are relatively few. HSV is by far the commonest sporadic cause of encephalitis and has no seasonal or geographic predilections. Its age distribution is slightly skewed and biphasic, affecting persons mainly between ages 5 and 30 years and those over 50.

Many other viruses, exemplified by the arboviral encephalitides, have a characteristic geographic and seasonal incidence. In the United States, eastern equine encephalitis, as the name implies, has been observed mainly in the eastern states and on both the Atlantic and

Gulf coasts. Western equine encephalitis is fairly uniformly distributed west of the Mississippi. St. Louis encephalitis, another arthropod-borne late-summer encephalitis, occurs nationwide but especially along the Mississippi River; outbreaks occur in August through October, slightly later than is customary for the other arboviruses. Venezuelan equine encephalitis is common in South and Central America; in the United States it is practically confined to Florida and the southwestern states. California virus encephalitis predominates in the northern Midwest and northeastern states. The LaCrosse variety is perhaps the most frequent identifiable arbovirus encephalitis in the United States. It affects children mainly, causing fever, seizures, and focal neurologic signs, but is otherwise benign, with full recovery. Rabies infections occur worldwide, but in the United States they are seen mostly in the Midwest and along the West Coast. Japanese B encephalitis (the most common encephalitis outside of North America), Russian spring–summer encephalitis, Murray Valley encephalitis (Australian X disease), West Nile fever, and several less common viral encephalitides are virtually unknown in the United States or, in the case of West Nile fever, are just beginning to appear. With the ease and rapidity of travel, many of these will undoubtedly appear in North America and parts of Europe where, hitherto, they have not been seen.

Infectious mononucleosis, which is a primary infection with EBV, may be complicated by meningitis, encephalitis, facial palsy, or polyneuritis of the Guillain-Barré type. Each of these neurologic complications can occur in the absence of the characteristic fever, pharyngitis, and lymphadenopathy of infectious mononucleosis. The same is true of *M. pneumoniae*; in the case of these two diseases, there is uncertainty as to whether these are true infectious encephalitides or postinfectious complications. Recent evidence from PCR testing of spinal fluid is consistent with a direct infection in some cases. Varicella zoster and CMV are other herpes-type viruses that may cause encephalitis. They are discussed in relation to the particular clinical settings in which they occur—with VZ and CMV, as congenital or neonatal infections, and as complications of AIDS (see further on). And, of course, HIV itself causes a subacute encephalitic process thought to be the cause of a progressive dementia.

Definite cases of epidemic (lethargic) encephalitis have not been observed in acute form since 1930, though an occasional patient with residual symptoms (Parkinson syndrome) is still seen in neurology clinics.

The relative frequency of the various viral infections of the nervous system can be gleaned from the following studies. An early study from the Walter Reed Army Institute, comprising 1282 patients, is particularly noteworthy in that a positive laboratory diagnosis was achieved in more than 60 percent of cases (Buescher et al)—a higher rate than in any subsequent study of comparable size. Aside from the poliovirus (some of the data were gathered before 1959), the common infective agents in cases of both aseptic meningitis and encephalitis were group B Coxsackie virus, echovirus, mumps virus, lymphocytic choriomeningitis virus, arboviruses, herpes simplex virus, and *Leptospira*, in that order. In a later prospective virologic study of all children examined at the Mayo Clinic during the years 1974 to 1976, a diagnosis of aseptic meningitis, meningoencephalitis, or encephalitis was entertained in 42 cases and an infectious agent was identified in 30 of them (Donat et al). The California virus was isolated in 19 cases and one of the enteroviruses (echovirus types 19, 16, 21, or Coxsackie virus) in 8 cases; mumps, rubeola, HSV, adenovirus 3, and *M. pneumoniae* were isolated in individual cases (several patients had combined infections). In another more contemporary and particularly large series of viral infections of the nervous system from the United Kingdom involving more than 2000 patients, viral identification in the CSF was attempted by means of PCR, with positive results in only 7 percent, half of which were various enteroviruses (Jeffery et al). The other organisms commonly identified were HSV-1, followed by VZ, EBV, and other herpesviruses. In patients with AIDS, however, relative frequencies of the organisms that cause meningoencephalitis are quite different and include special clinical presentations; this applies particularly to CMV infection of the nervous system, as discussed further on under "Opportunistic Infections and Neoplasms of the Central Nervous System in AIDS" (page 804). Our personal experience has been heavily biased toward simplex encephalitis, outbreaks of eastern equine encephalitis, and AIDS-related encephalitis.

Arboviral Encephalitis

The common arthropod-borne viruses (arboviruses) that cause encephalitis in the United States and their geographic range have been listed earlier. There are alternating cycles of viral infection in mosquitoes and vertebrate hosts; the mosquito becomes infected by taking a blood meal from a viremic host (horse or bird) and injects virus into the host, including humans. The seasonal incidence of these infections is limited to the summer and early fall, when mosquitoes are biting. In the equine encephalitides, regional deaths in horses usually precede human epidemics. In St. Louis encephalitis, the urban bird or animal or possibly the human becomes the intermediate host. West Nile outbreaks are preceded by illness in common birds. California virus infections are endemic because of the cycle of infection in small rodents.

The clinical manifestations of the various arbovirus infections are almost indistinguishable from one another, although they do vary with the age of the patient. In infants, there may be only an abrupt onset of fever and convulsions. In older children, the onset is usually less abrupt, with complaints of headache, listlessness, nausea or vomiting, drowsiness, and fever for several days before medical attention is sought; convulsions, confusion, stupor, and stiff neck then become prominent. Photophobia, diffuse myalgia, and tremor (of either action or intention type) may be observed in this age group and in adults. Reflex asymmetry, hemiparesis, extensor plantar signs, myoclonus, chorea, and sucking and grasping reflexes may also occur.

The CSF findings are much the same as in aseptic meningitis. Recovery of virus from blood or CSF is usually not possible and PCR testing has not been routinely applied. However, antiviral IgM is present within the first days of symptomatic disease and can be detected and quantified by means of ELISA. The fever and neurologic signs subside after 4 to 14 days unless death supervenes or destructive CNS changes have occurred. No antiviral agents are known to be effective in the treatment of arboviral encephalitis; one must rely entirely on supportive measures; on occasion, brain swelling reaches a degree that requires specific therapy, as outlined on pages 682 and 948.

The pathologic changes consist of widespread degeneration of single nerve cells, with neuronophagia as well as scattered foci of inflammatory necrosis involving both the gray and white matter. The brainstem is relatively spared. In some cases of eastern equine encephalitis, the destructive lesions may be massive, involving the major part of a lobe or hemisphere and readily displayed by MRI, but in the other arbovirus infections the foci are microscopic in size. Perivascular cuffing by lymphocytes and other mononuclear leukocytes and plasma cells as well as a patchy infiltration of the meninges with similar cells are the usual histopathologic hallmarks of viral encephalitis.

Of the arbovirus infections in the United States, eastern equine encephalitis is the most serious, since a large proportion of those infected develop encephalitis; of the latter, about one-third die and a similar number, more often children, are left with disabling abnormalities—mental retardation, emotional disorders, recurrent seizures, blindness, deafness, hemiplegia, extrapyramidal motor abnormalities, and speech disorders. Fortunately, eastern equine encephalitis is among the least frequent of the arbovirus infections. The mortality rate in other arbovirus infections varies from 2 to 12 percent in different outbreaks, and the incidence of serious sequelae is about the same.

Herpes Simplex Encephalitis

This is the commonest and gravest form of acute encephalitis. About 2000 cases occur yearly in the United States, accounting for about 10 percent of all cases of encephalitis in this country. Between 30 and 70 percent of these are fatal, and the majority of patients who survive are left with serious neurologic abnormalities. Herpes simplex encephalitis occurs sporadically throughout the year and in patients of all ages and in all parts of the world. It is due almost always to HSV-1, which is also the cause of the common herpetic lesions of the oral mucosa; rarely, however, do the oral and encephalitic lesions coincide. The type 2 virus may also cause acute encephalitis, usually in the neonate and in relation to genital herpetic infection in the mother. Type 2 infection in the adult may cause an aseptic meningitis and sometimes a polyradiculitis or myelitis, again in association with a recent genital herpes infection. Exceptionally, the localized adult type of encephalitis is caused by the type 2 virus and the diffuse neonatal encephalitis by type 1.

Clinical Features The symptoms, which evolve over several days, are in most cases like those of any other acute encephalitis—namely, fever, headache, seizures, confusion, stupor, and coma. In some patients these manifestations are preceded by symptoms and findings that betray the predilection of this disease for the inferomedial portions of the frontal and temporal lobes. The latter manifestations include olfactory or gustatory hallucinations, anosmia, temporal lobe seizures, personality change, bizarre or psychotic behavior or delirium, aphasia, and hemiparesis. Although several seizures at the onset of illness are a common presentation, status epilepticus is rare. Infrequently, an affection of memory can be recognized, but usually this becomes evident only later, in the convalescent stage of the illness, as the patient awakens from stupor or coma. Swelling and herniation of one or both temporal lobes through the tentorium may occur, leading to deep coma and respiratory arrest during the first few days of the illness.

The CSF is often under increased pressure and almost invariably there is a pleocytosis (range, 10 to 500 cells per cubic millimeter, usually less than 200). Mainly the cells are lymphocytes, but occasionally there is a significant number of neutrophils. In a few cases, 3 to 5 percent in some series, the spinal fluid has been normal in the first days of the illness, only to become abnormal when re-examined. In a minority of cases, red cells, sometimes numbering in the thousands, and xanthochromia are found, reflecting the hemorrhagic nature of the lesions; but more often red cells are few in number or may be absent. The protein content is increased in most cases. Rarely, the CSF glucose levels may be reduced to slightly less than 40 mg/dL, creating confusion with tuberculous and fungal meningitides.

Pathology The lesions take the form of an intense hemorrhagic necrosis of the inferior and medial parts of the temporal lobes and the medial-orbital parts of the frontal lobes. They extend upward along the cingulate gyri and sometimes to the insula or the lateral parts of the temporal lobes or caudally into the midbrain. The temporal lobe lesions are usually bilateral but not symmetrical. This distribution of lesions is so characteristic that the diagnosis can be made by gross inspection or by their location and appearance on imaging studies. Cases described in past years as "acute necrotizing encephalitis" and "inclusion body encephalitis" were probably instances of HSV encephalitis. In the acute stages of the disease, intranuclear eosinophilic inclusions are found in neurons and glial cells, in addition to the usual microscopic abnormalities of acute encephalitis.

The unique localization of the lesions in this disease could possibly be explained by the virus's route of entry into the CNS. Two such routes have been suggested (Davis and Johnson). The virus is thought to be latent in the trigeminal ganglia and, with reactivation, to infect the nose and then the olfactory tract. Alternatively, with activation in the trigeminal ganglia, the infection may spread along fibers that innervate the leptomeninges of the anterior and middle fossae. The lack of lesions in the olfactory bulbs in as many as 40 percent of fatal cases (Esiri) is a point in favor of the second pathway.

Diagnosis Acute herpes simplex encephalitis must be distinguished from other types of viral encephalitis, from acute hemorrhagic leukoencephalitis of Weston Hurst (page 978), and from subdural empyema, cerebral abscess, cerebral venous thrombosis, and septic embolism (Chap. 32). When aphasia is the initial manifestation of the illness, it may be mistaken for a stroke. Spinal fluid that contains a large number of red cells may be attributed to a ruptured saccular aneurysm. The EEG changes, consisting of lateralized periodic high-voltage sharp waves in the temporal regions and slow-wave complexes at regular 2- to 3-per-second intervals, are highly suggestive in the appropriate clinical context, though not specific for the disease. CT scans show hypodensity of the affected areas in 50 to 60 percent of cases and MRI shows signal changes in almost all (increased signal in T2-weighted images; Fig. 33-2). T1-weighted images demonstrate areas of low signal intensity, with surrounding edema and sometimes with scattered areas of hemorrhage occupying the inferior parts of the frontal and temporal lobes. Almost always the lesions enhance with contrast infusion or with gadolinium, indicating cortical and pial abnormalities of the blood-brain barrier. A rising titer of neutralizing antibodies can be demonstrated from the acute to the convalescent stage, but this is not of diagnostic help in the acutely ill patient and may not be etiologically significant in patients with recurrent herpes infections of the oral mucosa. More recently developed tests for the detection of HSV antigen in the CSF by the application of PCR are useful in diagnosis while the virus is replicating in the first few days of the illness and enable one to avoid brain biopsy (Rowley et al). A refinement in this technique (a nested PCR assay), reported by Aurelius and coworkers, has a sensitivity of 95 percent and gives virtually no false-positive tests in the first 3 weeks of illness. In the experience of Lakeman et al, the test was 98 percent positive in cases proven by cultures of brain biopsy material and gave 6 percent false positives. Antiviral treatment did not appear to affect the test. The only other absolute way to establish the diagnosis of acute HSV encephalitis is by fluorescent antibody study and by viral culture of cerebral tissue obtained by brain biopsy; the approach to biopsy as a diagnostic test varies among centers. We find it necessary to perform biopsy in only a minority of cases, preferring to treat the patient with antiviral agents based on compatible clinical, radiologic, and CSF findings.

Treatment Until the late 1970s, there was no specific treatment for HSV encephalitis. A collaborative study sponsored by the National Institutes of Health and also a Swedish study indicated that the antiviral agent acyclovir significantly reduces both the mortality and morbidity from HSV encephalitis (Whitley et al; Sköldenberg et al). Acyclovir is given intravenously in a dosage of 30 mg/kg per day and continued for 10 to 14 days in order to prevent relapse. Acyclovir carries little risk and can be discontinued if further clinical or laboratory fea-

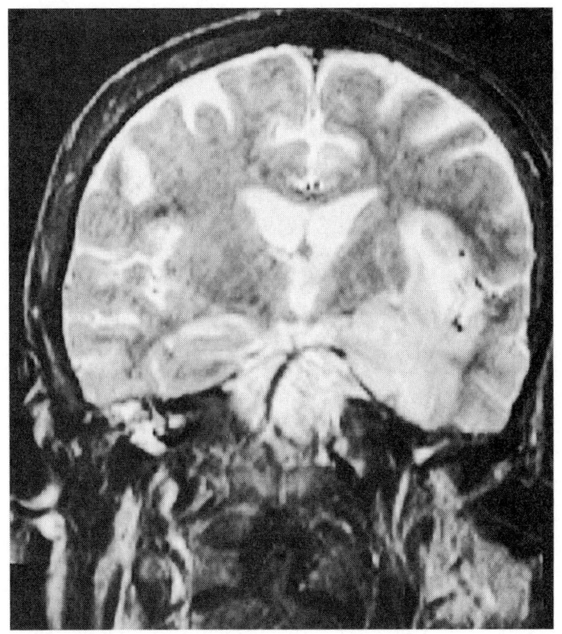

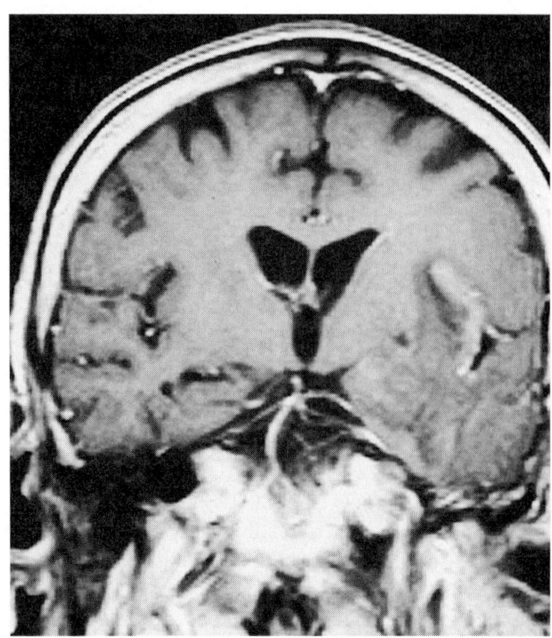

Figure 33-2

Herpes simplex encephalitis. Left: a T2-weighted coronal MR image in the axial plane, taken during the acute stage of the illness. There is increased signal from practically all of the inferior and deep temporal lobe and the insular cortex. Right: a T1-weighted image after gadolinium infusion showing enchancement of the left insular and temporal cortices and early involvement of the right temporal lobe.

tures point to another diagnosis. The main problems with acyclovir are local irritation of the veins used for infusion, mild elevation of hepatic enzymes, or transient impairment of renal function. Nausea, vomiting, tremor, or an encephalopathy that is difficult to distinguish from the encephalitis occur in a very few patients.

When a large volume of brain tissue is involved, the hemorrhagic necrosis and surrounding edema act as an enlarging mass that requires separate attention. Coma and pupillary changes should not be attributed to the mass effect unless compression of the upper brainstem is evident on brain imaging, since the infection is capable of spreading to the mesencephalon from the contiguous deep temporal lobe, thus causing coma by a direct destructive effect. All measures used in the management of brain edema due to mass lesions should be applied, but there are insufficient data by which to judge their effectiveness. The concern that corticosteriods may aggravate the infection has not been borne out by clinical experience, but a subtle detrimental effect cannot be discounted. Our experience (reported by Barnett et al) and that of Schwab and colleagues has been that the presence of raised intracranial pressure early in the illness presages a poor outcome. Seizures are usually brought under control by high doses of conventional anticonvulsants.

The outcome of this disease, both the mortality and morbidity, is governed to a large extent by the patient's age and state of consciousness at the time of institution of acyclovir therapy. If the patient is unconscious (except immediately after a convulsion) the outcome is uniformly poor. However, if treatment is begun within 4 days of onset of the illness in awake patients, survival is greater than 90 percent (Whitley). Evaluation of these patients 2 years after treatment showed 38 percent to be normal or nearly normal, whereas 53 percent were dead or severely impaired. The neurologic sequelae are often of the most serious type, consisting of a Korsakoff amnesic defect or a global dementia, seizures, and aphasia (Drachman and Adams). If there were seizures during the acute illness, it is advisable to continue anticonvulsants for a year or more and then judge the advisability of discontinuing them on the basis of further seizures, the EEG, and the patient's exposure to situations that pose a danger, such as driving. The illness does not recur.

Rabies

This disease also stands apart from other acute viral infections by virtue of the latent period that follows inoculation with the virus and its distinctive clinical and pathologic features. Human examples of this disease are rare in the United States; between 1980 and 1997, only 34 such cases are known to have occurred; since 1960, there have never been more than 5 or so cases in any one year. In some areas (Australia, Hawaii, Great Britain, and the Scandinavian peninsula), no indigenous cases have ever been reported; in India, however, there is a high incidence. The importance of this disease derives from two facts: it has been almost invariably fatal once the characteristic clinical features appear; hence the survival of the infected individual depends upon the institution of specific therapeutic measures before the infection becomes clinically evident. Furthermore, each year 20,000 to 30,000 individuals are treated with rabies vaccine, having been bitten by animals that possibly were rabid, and although the incidence of complications with the newer rabies vaccination is much lower than before, a few serious reactions continue to be encountered (see below and also Chap. 36).

Etiology Practically all cases of rabies are the result of transdermal viral inoculation by an animal bite. In undeveloped countries, where rabies is relatively common, the most frequent source is the rabid dog. In western Europe and the United States, the most common rabid species are raccoons, skunks, foxes, and bats among wild animals and dogs and cats among domestic ones. Because rabid animals commonly bite without provocation, the nature of the attack should be determined. Also, the prevalence of animal rabies virus varies widely in the United States, and local presence of the disease is useful in assessing risk. As indicated earlier, the virus spreads along peripheral nerves to reach the nervous system. Rare cases have been caused by inhalation of the virus shed by bats. The epidemiology and public health aspects of rabies have been reviewed by Fishbein and Robinson.

Clinical Features The incubation period is usually 20 to 60 days but may be as short as 14 days, especially in cases involving multiple deep bites around the face and neck. Tingling or numbness at the site of the bite, even after the wound has healed, is characteristic. This is thought to reflect an inflammatory response that is incited when the virus reaches the sensory ganglion. The main neurologic symptoms (following a 2- to 4-day prodromal period of fever, headache, and malaise) consist of severe apprehension, dysarthria, and psychomotor overactivity, followed by dysphagia (hence salivation and "frothing at the mouth"), spasms of throat muscles induced by attempts to swallow water or in rare cases by the mere sight of water (hence hydrophobia), dysarthria, numbness of the face, and spasms of facial muscles. This localization indicates the involvement of the tegmental medullary nuclei in the rabid form of the disease. Generalized seizures, confusional psychosis, and a state of agitation may follow. A less common paralytic form ("dumb" rabies of older writings, in distinction to the above described "furious" form), due to spinal cord affection, may accompany or replace the state of excitement. The paralytic form is most likely to follow bat bites or postexposure rabies vaccination. Coma gradually follows the acute encephalitic symptoms and death ensues within 4 to 10 days, or longer in the paralytic form. With modern intensive care techniques, there have been a number of survivors. In addition to mechanical respiratory support, several secondary abnormalities must be addressed, including raised intracranial pressure, excessive release of antidiuretic hormone, diabetes insipidus, and extremes of autonomic dysfunction, especially hyper- and hypotension.

Pathologic Features The disease is distinguished by the presence of cytoplasmic eosinophilic inclusions, the Negri bodies. They are most prominent in the pyramidal cells of the hippocampus and the Purkinje cells but have been seen in nerve cells throughout the CNS. In addition there may be widespread perivascular cuffing and meningeal infiltration with lymphocytes and mononuclear cells and small foci of inflammatory necrosis, such as those seen in other viral infections. The inflammatory reaction is most intense in the brainstem. The focal collections of microglia in this disease are referred to as "Babes nodules" (named for Victor Babes, a Romanian microbiologist).

Treatment Bites and scratches from a potentially rabid animal should be thoroughly washed with soap and water and, after all soap has been removed, cleansed with benzyl ammonium chloride (Zephiran), which has been shown to inactivate the virus. Wounds that have broken the skin also require tetanus prophylaxis.

After a bite by a seemingly healthy animal, surveillance of the animal for a 10-day period is necessary. Should signs of illness appear in the animal, it should be killed and the brain sent, under refrigeration, to a government-designated laboratory for appropriate diagnostic tests. Wild animals, if captured, should be killed and the brain examined in the same way.

If the animal is found by fluorescent antibody or other tests to be rabid or if the patient was bitten by a wild animal that escaped, the patient should receive *postexposure prophylaxis*. Human rabies immune globulin (HRIG) should be given in a dose of 20 units per kilogram of body weight (one-half infiltrated around the wound and one-half intramuscularly). This provides passive immunization for 10 to 20 days, allowing time for active immunization. In the recent past, duck embryo vaccine (DEV) was used for the latter purpose and greatly reduced the danger of serious allergic reactions in the CNS (encephalomyelitis) from about 1 in 1000 cases (with equine vaccine) to 1 in 25,000 cases. The more recently developed rabies vaccine grown on a human diploid cell line (HDCV) has reduced the doses needed to just 5 (from the 23 needed with DEV); these are given as 1-mL injections on the day of exposure and then on days 3, 7, 14, and 28 after the first dose. The HDCV vaccine has increased the rate of antibody response and reduced even further the allergic reactions by practically eliminating foreign protein. A thorough trial of the new antiviral agents on patients already symptomatic has not been undertaken. Persons at risk for rabies, such as animal handlers and laboratory workers, should receive pre-exposure vaccination with HDCV. A preventative DNA rabies vaccine has been genetically engineered and tested for use in animal handlers and others at high risk.

Acute Cerebellitis (Acute Ataxia of Childhood)

A special comment should be made here concerning the dramatic syndrome of acute ataxia that occurs in the context of an infectious illness. The syndrome was originally described by Westphal in 1872 following smallpox and typhoid fever in adults, but Batten should be credited with defining the more common ataxic illness that occurred after certain childhood infections such as measles, pertussis, and scarlet fever. Currently, acute ataxia of childhood is most often associated with chickenpox (one-quarter of 73 consecutive cases reported by Connolly et al), but it can occur during or after any of the childhood exanthems, as well as in association with infections due to enteroviruses (mainly Coxsackie), EBV, *Mycoplasma*, CMV, Q fever, vaccinia, a number of vaccinations, rarely with HSV, and also after nondescript respiratory infections (see Weiss and Guberman). In adults, the most common preceding organisms are probably EBV and *Mycoplasma*. The syndrome, which is essentially a "meningocerebellitis," appears relatively abruptly, over a day or so, and consists of limb and gait ataxia and often dysarthria and nystagmus. Additional signs include increased limb tone, Babinski signs, or confusion. As a rule, there is a mild pleocytosis; the CSF protein is elevated or may be normal. The MRI is normal in the majority of cases. Most patients make a slow recovery, but permanent residua are known to follow. Because the benign nature of the illness has precluded extensive pathologic study, there is still uncertainty regarding the infectious or postinfectious nature of these ataxic illnesses. Some cases have shown an inflammatory pathology suggesting a postinfectious process (see Chap. 36), but the finding of fragments of VZ and *Mycoplasma* genomes in the spinal fluid by means of DNA amplification techniques favors a primary infectious encephalitis, at least in some instances.

Syndromes of Herpes Zoster

Herpes zoster ("shingles," zona) is a common viral infection of the nervous system occurring at an overall rate of 3 to 5 cases per 1000 persons per year, with higher rates in the elderly. Shingles is distinctly rare in childhood. It is characterized clinically by radicular pain, a vesicular cutaneous eruption, and, less often, by segmental sensory and motor loss. The pathologic changes consist of an acute inflammatory reaction in isolated spinal or cranial sensory ganglia and lesser degrees of reaction in the posterior and anterior roots, the posterior gray matter of the spinal cord, and the adjacent leptomeninges.

The neurologic implications of the segmental distribution of the rash were recognized by Richard Bright as long ago as 1831. The inflammatory changes in the corresponding ganglia and related portions of the spinal nerves were first described by von Barensprung in 1862 and were later studied extensively. The concept that varicella and zoster are caused by the same agent was introduced by von Bokay in 1909 and was subsequently established by Weller and his associates (1954, 1958). The common agent, referred to as varicella or varicella zoster (VZ) virus, is a DNA virus that is similar in structure to the virus of herpes simplex. These and other historical features of herpes zoster have been reviewed by Denny-Brown and by Weller and their colleagues.

Pathology and Pathogenesis The pathologic changes in VZ are unique and consist of one or more of the following: (1) an inflammatory reaction in several unilateral adjacent sensory ganglia of the spinal or cranial nerves, frequently of such intensity as to cause necrosis of all or part of the ganglion, with or without hemorrhage; (2) an inflammatory reaction in the spinal roots and peripheral nerve contiguous with the involved ganglia; (3) a poliomyelitis that closely resembles acute anterior poliomyelitis but is readily distinguished by its unilaterality, segmental localization, and greater involvement of the dorsal horn, root, and ganglion; and (4) a relatively mild leptomeningitis, largely limited to the involved spinal or cranial segments and nerve roots. These pathologic changes are the substratum of the neuralgic pains, the pleocytosis, and the local palsies that may attend and follow the zoster infection. There may also be a delayed cerebral vasculitis (see further on).

As to *pathogenesis*, herpes zoster represents a spontaneous reactivation of VZ virus infection, which becomes latent in the neurons of sensory ganglia following a primary infection with chickenpox (Hope-Simpson). This hypothesis is consistent with the differences in the clinical manifestations of chickenpox and herpes zoster, even though both are caused by the same virus. Chickenpox is highly contagious, has a well-marked seasonal incidence (winter and spring), and tends to occur in epidemics. Zoster, on the other hand, is not communicable (except to a person who has not had chickenpox), occurs sporadically throughout the year, and shows no increase in incidence during epidemics of chickenpox. In patients with zoster, there is practically always a past history of chickenpox. Such a history may be lacking in rare instances of herpes zoster in infants, but in these latter cases there has usually been prenatal maternal contact with the VZ virus.

Varicella zoster viral DNA is localized primarily in trigeminal and thoracic ganglion cells, corresponding to the dermatomes in which chickenpox lesions are maximal and that are most commonly involved by VZ (Mahalingam et al). The supposition is that in both zoster and varicella infections the virus makes its way from the cutaneous vesicles along the sensory nerves to the ganglion, where it remains latent until activated, at which time it progresses down the axon to the skin. Multiplication of the virus in epidermal cells causes swelling, vacuolization, and lysis of cell boundaries, leading to the formation of vesicles and so-called Lipschutz inclusion bodies. Alternatively, the ganglia could be infected during the viremia of chickenpox, but then one would have to explain why only one or a few sensory ganglia become infected. Reactivation of virus is attributed to waning immunity, which would explain the increasing incidence of zoster with aging and with lymphomas, administration of immunosuppressive drugs, AIDS, and radiation therapy.

The subject of pathogenesis of herpes zoster has been reviewed by Gilden and colleagues, and a monograph by Rentier describes the recent molecular and immune investigation pertaining to VZ virus.

Clinical Features As indicated above, the incidence of herpes zoster rises with age. Hope-Simpson has estimated that if a cohort of 1000 people lived to 85 years of age, half would have had one attack of zoster and 10 would have had two attacks. The notion that one attack of zoster provides lifelong immunity is incorrect, although recurrent attacks are rare and most repeated herpetic eruptions are due to the simplex virus. The sexes are equally affected, as is each side of the body. Herpes zoster occurs in about 10 percent of patients with lymphoma and 25 percent of patients with Hodgkin disease—particularly in those who have undergone splenectomy and received radiotherapy. Conversely, about 5 percent of patients who present with herpes zoster are found to have a concurrent malignancy (about twice the number that would be expected), and the proportion appears to be even higher if more than two dermatomes are involved.

The vesicular eruption is usually preceded for several days by itching, tingling, or burning sensations in the involved dermatome(s), and sometimes by malaise and fever as well. Or there is severe localized or radicular pain that may be mistaken for pleurisy, appendicitis, cholecystitis, or ruptured intervertebral disc, until the diagnosis is clarified by the appearance of vesicles (nearly always within 72 to 96 h). The rash consists of clusters of tense clear vesicles on an erythematous base, which become cloudy after a few days (due to accumulation of inflammatory cells) and dry, crusted, and scaly after 5 to 10 days. In a small number of patients, the vesicles are confluent and hemorrhagic, and healing is delayed for several weeks. In most cases pain and dysesthesia last for 1 to 4 weeks; but in the others (7 to 33 percent of cases in different series) the pain persists for months or, in different forms, even for years and presents a difficult problem in management. Impairment of superficial sensation in the affected dermatome(s) is common, and segmental weakness and atrophy are added in about 5 percent of patients. In the majority of patients the rash and sensorimotor signs are limited to the territory of a single dermatome, but in some, particularly those with cranial or limb involvement, two or more contiguous dermatomes are involved. Rarely (and usually in association with malignancy) the rash is generalized, like that of chickenpox, or altogether absent. The CSF frequently shows a mild increase in cells, mainly lymphocytes, and a modest increase in protein content. The diagnosis can be confirmed by direct immunofluorescence of a biopsied skin lesion, using antibody to VZ virus, or inferred by finding multinucleated giant cells in scrapings from the base of an early vesicle.

Virtually any dermatome may be involved in zoster, but some regions are far more frequently involved than others. The thoracic dermatomes, particularly T5 to T10, are the most common sites, accounting for more than two-thirds of all cases, followed by the craniocervical regions. In the latter cases the disease tends to be more severe, with greater pain, more frequent meningeal signs, and involvement of the mucous membranes.

There are two rather characteristic cranial herpetic syndromes—ophthalmic herpes and so-called geniculate herpes. In *ophthalmic herpes*, which accounts for 10 to 15 percent of all cases of zoster, the pain and rash are in the distribution of the first division of the trigeminal nerve, and the pathologic changes are centered in the gasserian ganglion. The main hazard in this form of the disease is herpetic involvement of the cornea and conjunctiva, resulting in corneal anesthesia and residual scarring. Palsies of extraocular muscles, ptosis, and mydriasis are frequently associated, indicating that the third, fourth, and sixth cranial nerves are affected in addition to the gasserian ganglion.

A less common cranial nerve syndrome consists of a facial palsy in combination with a herpetic eruption of the external auditory meatus, sometimes with tinnitus, vertigo, and deafness. Ramsay Hunt attributed this syndrome to herpes of the geniculate ganglion. R.D. Adams found the geniculate ganglion to be only slightly affected in a man who died 64 days after the onset of a so-called Ramsay Hunt syndrome (during which time the patient had recovered from the facial palsy); there was, however, inflammation of the facial nerve, a finding that provided an explanation for the facial palsy (see Denny-Brown et al).

Herpes zoster of the palate, pharynx, neck, and retroauricular region (*herpes occipitocollaris*) depends upon herpetic infection of the upper cervical roots and the ganglia of the vagus and glossopharyngeal nerves. Herpes zoster in this distribution may also be associated with the Ramsay Hunt syndrome.

Encephalitis and *cerebral angiitis* are rare but well-described complications of cervicocranial zoster, as discussed below, and a restricted myelitis is a similarly rare complication of thoracic zoster. Devinsky and colleagues reported their findings in 13 patients with zoster myelitis (all of them immunocompromised) and have reviewed the literature on this subject. The signs of spinal cord involvement appeared within 5 to 21 days after the rash (median 12 days) and then progressed for a similar period of time. Asymmetrical paraparesis and sensory loss, sphincteric disturbances, and, less often, a Brown-Séquard syndrome were the usual clinical manifestations. The CSF findings are more abnormal than in uncomplicated zoster but otherwise similar. The pathologic changes, which take the form of a necrotizing inflammatory myelopathy and vasculitis, involve not just the dorsal horn but also the contiguous white matter, predominantly on the same side and at the same segment(s) as the affected dorsal roots, ganglia, and posterior horns. Early therapeutic intervention with acyclovir appeared to be beneficial. Another rare complication of zoster, taking the form of a subacute amyotrophy of a portion of a limb, may be linked to a restricted form of VZ myelitis.

Many of the writings on *zoster encephalitis* leave the impression of a severe illness that occurs temporally remote from the attack of shingles in an immunosuppressed patient. Indeed, such instances have been reported in patients with AIDS and may be concurrent with the small vessel vasculitis described below. Our experience is more in keeping with that of Jemsek and colleagues and of Peterslund, who have described a less severe form of encephalitis in patients with normal immune systems. Several of our patients, mostly elderly women, have developed a self-limited encephalitis during the latter stages of an attack of shingles. Confusion and drowsiness, with low-grade fever but little meningismus and a few limited seizures, were characteristic. Recovery was complete and the MRI was normal, in distinction to the vasculitic syndromes. Varicella zoster has been isolated from the CSF in some cases and specific antibody to VZ membrane antigen (VAMA) has been a regular finding in the CSF and serum, though hardly needed for purposes of diagnosis. The differential diagnosis in these elderly patients also includes a drowsy-confusional state induced by narcotics that are given for the control of pain. *Varicella cerebellitis* is discussed above.

The *cerebral angiitis* that occasionally complicates VZ is histologically similar to granulomatous angiitis (page 907). Typically, 2 to 10 weeks after the onset of ophthalmic zoster, the patient develops an acute hemiparesis, hemianesthesia, aphasia, or other focal neurologic or retinal deficits associated with a mononuclear pleocytosis and elevated IgG indices in the CSF. CT scans have demonstrated small, deep infarcts in the hemisphere ipsilateral to the zoster infection. Angiograms have shown narrowing or occlusion of the internal carotid artery adjacent to the ganglia; but in some cases, vasculitis is more diffuse, even involving the contralateral hemisphere. Whether the angiitis results from direct spread of the viral infection from neighboring nerves as postulated by Linnemann and Alvira or represents an allergic reaction during convalescence from zoster has not been ascertained. Varicella zoster-like particles have been found in the vessel walls, suggesting direct infection, and viral DNA has been extracted from affected vessels. Since the exact pathogenetic mechanism is uncertain, treatment with both intravenous acyclovir and corticosteroids is justified.

An entirely different type of delayed *vasculitis that affects small vessels* is being reported increasingly in patients with AIDS and other forms of immunosuppression. In this condition, weeks or months after one or more attacks of zoster, a subacute encephalitis ensues, including fever and focal signs. Some cases arise without a rash but viral DNA and antibodies to VZ are found in the CSF. The MRI shows multiple cortical and white matter lesions, the latter being smaller and less confluent than in progressive multifocal leukoencephalopathy. There is usually a mild pleocytosis. Almost all cases have ended fatally. The vasculitic and other neurologic complications of zoster are reviewed by Gilden and colleagues.

It must be conceded that a facial palsy or pain in the distribution of a trigeminal or intercostal nerve, due to herpetic ganglionitis, may occur very rarely without involvement of the skin (zoster sine herpete). In a few such cases, an antibody response to the VZ virus has been found (Mayo and Booss), and Dueland and associates have described an immunocompromised patient who developed a pathologically and virologically proved zoster infection in the absence of skin lesions. Also, Gilden et al recovered VZ virus DNA from two otherwise healthy immunocompetent men who had experienced chronic radicular pain without a zoster rash. But practically no instances of Bell's palsy, tic douloureux, and intercostal neuralgia are associated with serologic evidence of activation of the VZ virus (Bell's palsy has been associated with herpes simplex virus, as indicated on page 1452).

Treatment During the acute stage, analgesics and drying and soothing lotions, such as calamine, help to blunt the pain. Nerve root blocks provide relief, but only temporarily. After the lesions have dried, the repeated application of capsaicin ointment (derived from hot peppers) may relieve the pain in some cases by inducing a cutaneous anesthesia. When applied soon after the acute stage, capsaicin may actually increase the pain in some patients and should be used cautiously. Acyclovir (800 mg orally five times daily for 7 days) also shortens the duration of acute pain and speeds the healing of vesicles provided that treatment is begun within 48 h of the appearance of the rash (McKendrick et al).

All patients with ophthalmic zoster should receive acyclovir orally; in addition, acyclovir applied topically to the eye, in either a 0.1% solution every hour or a 0.5% ointment four or five times a day, is recommended by some ophthalmologists. Patients who are immunocompromised or have disseminated zoster (lesions in more than three dermatomes) should receive intravenous acyclovir for 10 days. It should be noted, however, that neither acyclovir nor vidarabine decreases the incidence of postherpetic neuralgia (see below). There is now available from the state health agencies a VZ immune globulin (VZIG) that shortens the course of the cutaneous disease and may protect against its dissemination in immunosuppressed patients. However, it does not prevent or ameliorate nervous system complications.

Postherpetic Neuralgia The management of *postherpetic pain* and dysesthesia can be a trying matter for both the patient and the physician. It would appear that incomplete interruption of nerves results in a hyperpathic state, in which every stimulus excites pain. In a number of controlled studies, amitriptyline proved to be an effective therapeutic measure. Initially, it is given in doses of approximately 50 mg at bedtime; if needed, the dosage can be increased gradually to 125 mg daily. Addition of carbamazepine, gabapentin, or valproate may further moderate the pain, particularly if it is of lancinating type. Capsaicin ointment can be applied to painful skin, as noted above. A salve of two aspirin tablets, crushed and mixed with cold cream or chloroform (15 mL) and spread on the painful skin, is reported to be successful in relieving the pain for several hours (King). It should be emphasized that postherpetic neuralgia eventually subsides even in the most severe and persistent cases. Until this happens, the physician must exercise skill and patience in the medical management of chronic pain (see page 150) and avoid the temptation of subjecting the patient to one of the many surgical measures that have been advocated for this disorder. Excision or undercutting the involved region of skin, section of the spinal nerves or roots, and cordotomy have generally proved ineffective or at best have given only temporary relief. Many of the patients with the most persistent complaints have all the major symptoms of a depressive state and will be helped by appropriate antidepressive medications.

NEUROLOGIC DISEASES INDUCED BY RETROVIRUSES AND RESULTANT OPPORTUNISTIC INFECTIONS

Retroviruses are a large group of RNA viruses, so called because they contain the enzyme reverse transcriptase, which permits the reverse flow of genetic information from RNA to DNA. Two families of retroviruses are known to infect humans: (1) the *lentiviruses*, the most important of which is the human immunodeficiency virus (HIV), the cause of AIDS, and (2) the oncornaviruses, which include the human T-cell lymphotropic viruses, i.e., the agents that induce chronic T-cell leukemias and lymphomas (HTLV-II) and tropical spastic paraparesis (HTLV-I).

In the following pages, we consider the major neurologic syndromes induced by the two main human retroviruses—AIDS, a constellation of neurologic diseases caused by HIV, and tropical spastic paraparesis caused by HTLV-I. These diseases are now the subjects of great public interest and laboratory investigation. A current and most comprehensive account of the neurobiology, pathology, and clinical features of these infections can be found in the review by Fauci and Lane in *Harrison's Principles of Internal Medicine.*

The Acquired Immunodeficiency Syndrome (AIDS)

In 1981, physicians became aware of the frequent occurrence of otherwise rare opportunistic infections and neoplasms—notably *Pneumocystis carinii* pneumonia and Kaposi sarcoma—in otherwise healthy young homosexual men. The study of these patients led to the recognition of a new viral disease, AIDS. In 1983, Montagnier and his colleagues isolated a retrovirus from a homosexual patient with lymphadenopathy and named it "lymphadenopathy-associated virus" (LAV). Shortly thereafter, Gallo and associates described a retrovirus in the blood of AIDS patients, which they called "human T-cell lymphotropic virus" (now HTLV-III). These two viruses, LAV and HTLV-III, were shown to be identical, and an international commission changed the name to *human immunodeficiency virus (HIV)*—sometimes referred to as HIV-1 to separate it from a similar virus (HIV-2) that is associated with AIDS predominantly in West Africa and elsewhere in persons of West African origin.

Human immunodeficiency virus infection is characterized by an acquired and usually profound depression of cell-mediated immunity, as manifested by cutaneous anergy, lymphopenia, reversal of the T-helper/T-suppressor cell ratio—more accurately, CD4+/CD8+ lymphocytes—and depressed in vitro lymphoproliferative response to various antigens and mitogens. It is this failure of immune function that explains the development of a wide range of opportunistic infections and unusual neoplasms. Virtually all organ systems are vulnerable, including all parts of the CNS, the peripheral nerves and roots, and muscle. Moreover, the nervous system is susceptible not only to diseases that are due to immunosuppression but also to the AIDS virus per se.

Epidemiology In a span of 20 years, HIV infection and AIDS have spread worldwide, attaining immense pandemic proportions. At the time of writing it was estimated by the World Health Organization (WHO) that approximately 34,000,000 adults were infected worldwide and that about 850,000 adults in the United States were seropositive for the virus. By all accounts, the incidence will continue to increase in the immediate future. Particularly startling are the statistics from sub-Saharan Africa and Southeast Asia, where the WHO estimated that about 25,000,000 adults, or almost 9 percent of the adult population, were infected. In some areas of East Africa, 20 to 30 percent of adults are infected with the virus.

In the United States, AIDS affects mainly homosexual and bisexual males (53 percent of all cases) and male and female drug users (30 percent). Somewhat less than 3 percent of patients at risk are hemophiliacs and others who receive infected blood or blood products, and the disease has occurred in infants born of mothers with AIDS or at risk for AIDS. Moreover, this virus may be transmitted by asymptomatic and still immunologically competent mothers to their offspring. Spread of the disease by heterosexual contact accounts for about 5 percent of cases, but this number is gradually increasing, mainly through the activities of intravenous drug users. (By contrast, an estimated 80 percent of African AIDS patients acquire their disease through heterosexual contact.)

Clinical Features Infection with HIV produces a spectrum of disorders, ranging from *clinically inevident seroconversion* to widespread lymphadenopathy and other relatively benign systemic manifestations ranging from diarrhea, malaise, and weight loss (the so-called *AIDS-related complex*, or *ARC*) to full-blown AIDS, which comprises the direct effects of the virus on all organ systems as well as the complicating effects of a multiplicity of parasitic, fungal, viral, and bacterial infections and a number of neoplasms (all of which require cell-mediated immunity for containment). Until the recent advent of multiple antiviral drug therapy, once the manifestations of AIDS had become established, one-half of the patients died by 1 year and most by 3 years. Clinically, neurologic abnormalities are noted in only about one-third of patients with AIDS, but at autopsy the nervous system is affected in nearly all of them. The infections and neoplastic lesions of the nervous system that complicate AIDS are listed in Table 33-1. Details of their pathology are to be found in the articles by Sharer and by Bell.

It has already been mentioned that HIV infection may present as an acute *asymptomatic meningitis*, with a mild lymphocytic pleocytosis and modest elevation of CSF protein. The acute illness may also take the form of a *meningoencephalitis* or even a *myelopathy* or *neuropathy* (see below). Most patients recover from the acute neurologic illnesses; the relationship to AIDS may pass unrecognized, since these illnesses are quite nonspecific clinically and may precede seroconversion. Once seroconversion has occurred, the patient becomes vulnerable to all the late complications of HIV infection. In adults, the interval between infection and the development of clinical AIDS ranges from several months to 15 years or even longer (the mean latency is 8 to 10 years and 1 year or less in infants). It is believed that practically all seropositive individuals will sooner or later develop AIDS, although new drugs are constantly lengthening the latent period.

Table 33-1
Neurologic complications in patients infected with HIV-1

Brain
- Predominantly nonfocal
  - AIDS dementia complex (subacute-chronic HIV encephalitis)
  - Acute HIV-related encephalitis
  - Cytomegalovirus encephalitis
  - Varicella-zoster virus encephalitis
  - Herpes simplex virus encephalitis
  - Metabolic encephalopathies
- Predominantly focal
  - Cerebral toxoplasmosis
  - Primary CNS lymphoma
  - Progressive multifocal leukoencephalopathy
  - Cryptococcoma
  - Brain abscess/tuberculoma
  - Neurosyphilis (meningovascular)
  - Vascular disorders—notably nonbacterial endocarditis and cerebral hemorrhages associated with thrombocytopenia

Spinal cord
- Vacuolar myelopathy
- Herpes simplex or zoster myelitis

Meninges
- Aseptic meningitis (HIV)
- Cryptococcal meningitis
- Tuberculous meningitis
- Syphilitic meningitis
- Metastatic lymphomatous meningitis

Peripheral nerve and root
- Infectious
- Herpes zoster
- Cytomegalovirus lumbar polyradiculopathy

Virus- or immune-related
- Acute and chronic inflammatory HIV polyneuritis
- Mononeuritis multiplex
- Sensorimotor demyelinating polyneuropathy
- Distal painful sensory polyneuritis

Muscle
- Polymyositis and other myopathies (including drug-induced)

Source: Brew B, Sidtis J, Petito DK, Price RW: The neurologic complications of AIDS and human immunodeficiency virus infection, in Plum F (ed): *Advances in Contemporary Neurology*. Philadelphia, Davis, 1988, Chap 1, by permission.

AIDS Dementia Complex In the later stages of HIV infection, the commonest neurologic complication is a subacute or chronic HIV encephalitis presenting as a form of dementia; formerly it was called *AIDS encephalopathy* or *encephalitis*, but it is now generally referred to as the *AIDS dementia complex*, or *ADC* (Navia and Price). It has been estimated that only 3 percent of AIDS cases present in this manner, but the frequency is far higher, close to two-thirds, after the constitutional symptoms and opportunistic infections of AIDS are established. In children with AIDS, dementia is more common than all opportunistic infections, over 60 percent of children eventually being affected.

This disorder takes the form of a slowly or rapidly progressive dementia (loss of retentive memory, inattentiveness, language disorder, and apathy) accompanied by abnormalities of motor function. Patients complain of being unable to follow conversations, taking longer to complete daily tasks, and becoming forgetful. Incoordination of the limbs, ataxia of gait, and impairment of smooth pursuit and saccadic eye movements are usually early accompaniments of the dementia. Heightened tendon reflexes, Babinski signs, grasp and suck reflexes, weakness of the legs progressing to paraplegia, bladder and bowel incontinence reflecting spinal cord or cerebral involvement, and abulia or mutism are prominent in the later stages of the disease. The dementia evolves relatively rapidly, over a period of weeks or months; survival after the onset of dementia is generally 3 to 6 months but may be considerably longer. Tests of psychomotor speed seem to be most sensitive in the early stages of dementia (e.g., trail-making, pegboard, and symbol-digit testing).

Epstein and colleagues have described a similar disorder in children, who develop a progressive encephalopathy as the primary manifestation of AIDS. The disease in children is characterized by an impairment of cognitive functions and spastic weakness, and secondarily by impairment of brain growth.

The CSF in patients with AIDS dementia (but no other manifestations of AIDS) may be normal or show only a slight elevation of protein content and, less frequently, a mild lymphocytosis. Human immuno-deficiency virus can be isolated from the CSF. In the CT scan there is widening of the sulci and enlargement of the ventricles; MRI may show patchy but confluent or diffuse white matter changes with ill-defined margins (Fig. 33-3). These findings are particularly useful in diagnosis, although CMV infection of the brain in AIDS patients produces a similar MRI appearance, as described further on.

The pathologic basis of the dementia appears to be a diffuse and multifocal rarefaction of the cerebral white matter, accompanied by scanty perivascular infiltrates of lymphocytes and clusters of a few foamy macrophages, microglial nodules, and multinucleated giant cells (Navia et al). Evidence of CMV infection may be added, but accumulating virologic evidence indicates that the AIDS dementia complex is due to direct infection with HIV. Which of these changes, or the cortical atrophy, correspond most closely to the presence and severity of dementia has not been settled. The pathologic changes in AIDS dementia are also not uniform. In one group of patients, there is a diffuse pallor of the cerebral white matter, most obvious with myelin stains, accompanied by reactive astrocytes and macrophages; the myelin pallor seems to reflect a breakdown of the blood-brain barrier. In another form of this process, referred to as "diffuse poliodystrophy," there is widespread astrocytosis and microglial activation in the cerebral cortex, with little recognizable neuronal loss. In yet other patients, small or large perivascular foci of demyelination, like those of postinfectious encephalomyelitis, are observed; the nature of this diffuse lesion is not understood. These forms of pathologic change may occur singly or together and all correlate poorly with the severity of the dementia.

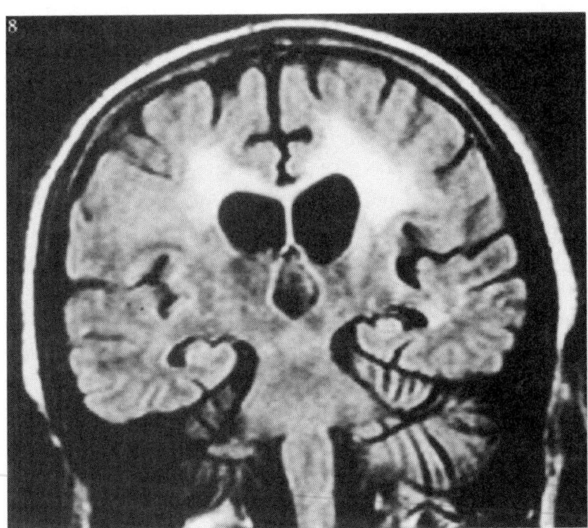

Figure 33-3

MRI of AIDS leukoencephalopathy. There are large areas of white matter change that underlie one form of AIDS dementia; cortical atrophy and ventricular enlargement are evident.

AIDS Myelopathy, Peripheral Neuropathy, and Myopathy A *myelopathy*, taking the form of a vacuolar degeneration that bears a striking resemblance to subacute combined degeneration due to vitamin B_{12} deficiency, is frequently associated with the AIDS dementia complex; or the myelopathy may occur in isolation, as the leading manifestation of the disease (Petito et al). This spinal cord disorder is discussed further on page 1306.

Also, AIDS may be complicated by several forms of *peripheral neuropathy*. Of 50 such patients reported by Snider and coworkers, 8 had a distal, symmetrical, axonal polyneuropathy, predominantly sensory and dysesthetic in type. This has been the most common neuropathic pattern. The HIV virus has been isolated from the peripheral nerves. In fact, this stands as the first proven viral polyneuritis. In other patients, a painful *mononeuropathy multiplex* occurs, seemingly related to a focal vasculitis, or there may be a subacute inflammatory cauda equina syndrome (a *polyradiculitis*) that is due to an accompanying *CMV* infection (Eidelberg et al). Cornblath and colleagues have documented the occurrence of an *inflammatory demyelinating peripheral neuropathy*, of both the acute (Guillain-Barré) and chronic types, in otherwise asymptomatic patients with HIV infection. Most of these patients had a mild pleocytosis in addition to an elevated CSF protein content. Also, all of the patients with inflammatory demyelinating neuropathy recovered—either spontaneously or in response to plasma exchange—suggesting an immunopathogenesis similar to that of the Guillain-Barré syndrome. Cornblath and associates have suggested that all patients with inflammatory demyelinating polyneuropathies should now be tested for the presence of HIV infection, but this is probably appropriate only in groups of patients or in geographic areas where the disease is prevalent. *Facial palsy* is being reported with increasing frequency as a feature of AIDS; its relationship to the generalized polyneuritis of AIDS is uncertain. In the rare complication of AIDS called *diffuse infiltrative lymphocytosis syndrome* (DILS), a variety of clinical syndromes has been described, including all of the usual AIDS polyneuropathies. Some instances of polyneuropathy in AIDS patients are probably due to the nutritional depletion that characterizes advanced stages of the disease and to the effects of therapeutic agents. These AIDS-related neuropathies are discussed in Chap. 46 and are well summarized by Wulff and Simpson.

A primary *myopathy*, taking the form of an inflammatory polymyositis, has been described in AIDS patients, occurring at any stage of the disease (Simpson and Bender). In some of these cases, the myopathy has improved with corticosteroid therapy. The original anti-AIDS drug, zidovudine (AZT), has been said to cause a myopathy, probably due to its effect on mitochondria, but some workers disagree and find almost all such cases to be attributable to the AIDS virus itself (see page 1481).

Opportunistic Infections and Neoplasms of the CNS in AIDS In addition to the direct neurologic effects of HIV infection, a variety of opportunistic disorders, both focal and nonfocal, occur in such patients, as outlined in Table 33-1. Interestingly, there appears to be a predilection for certain ones—CMV infection, primary B-cell lymphoma, cryptococcosis, toxoplasmosis, and progressive multifocal leukoencephalopathy (page 812), in this order of frequency (Johnson). The focal encephalitis and vasculitis of varicella zoster infection, considered earlier in this chapter and unusual types of tuberculosis and syphilis are other common opportunistic infections. Usually *P. carinii* infection and Kaposi sarcoma do not spread to the nervous system.

Toxoplasmosis Of the focal complications, cerebral toxoplasmosis is the most frequent (and treatable, see page 775). In the autopsy series of AIDS reported by Navia and colleagues, areas of inflammatory necrosis due to *Toxoplasma* were found in approximately 13 percent (see Fig. 32-7). Lumbar puncture, contrast-enhanced CT scanning, and MRI are useful in diagnosis. The spinal fluid usually shows an elevation of protein in the range of 50 to 200 mg/dL, and one-third have a lymphocytic pleocytosis. Since the disease represents reactivation of a prior *Toxoplasma* infection, it is important to identify seropositive patients early in the course of AIDS and to treat them vigorously with oral pyrimethamine (100 mg initially and then 25 mg daily) and a sulfonamide (4 to 6 g daily in four divided doses). Curiously, the toxoplasmosis infection, so common in the brains of AIDS patients, is not a frequent cause of myositis.

CNS Lymphoma In the Johns Hopkins study (see Johnson), about 11 percent of AIDS patients developed a *primary CNS lymphoma*, which may in some cases be difficult to distinguish from toxoplasmosis clinically and radiologically. If the cytologic study of the CSF is negative and there has been no response to antibiotics, stereotaxic brain biopsy may be necessary for diagnosis. The prognosis in such patients is considerably less favorable than in non-AIDS patients; the response to radiation therapy, methotrexate, and corticosteroids is short-lived, and survival is usually measured in months.

In the face of enhancing focal brain lesions in AIDS, the current approach should be to initially assume the presence of toxoplasmosis, which is treatable. Antibody tests for toxoplasmosis should be obtained; the absence of IgG antibodies mandates that treatment be changed in order to address the problem of brain lymphoma. Also, if antitoxoplasmal therapy with pyrimethamine and sulfadiazine fails to reduce the size of the lesions within several weeks, another cause should be sought, again mainly lymphoma. In those patients who cannot tolerate the frequent side effects of pyrimethamine or sulfonamides (rash or thrombocytopenia), clindamycin may be of value. Recently it has been suggested that thallium isotope single photon emission computed tomography (SPECT) and positron emission tomography (PET) can confidently exclude lymphoma as the cause of a mass lesion in an AIDS patient. The less frequent possibilities of tuberculous or bacterial brain abscess should be kept in mind if none of the other avenues allow a confident diagnosis.

Cytomegalovirus Among the nonfocal neurologic complications of AIDS, the most common are CMV and *cryptococcal* infections. At autopsy, about one-third of AIDS patients are found to be infected with CMV. However, the contribution of this infection to the total clinical picture is often uncertain. Despite this ambiguity, certain features have emerged as typical of CMV encephalitis in the AIDS patient. According to Holland and colleagues, late in the course of AIDS and usually concurrent with CMV retinitis, the encephalopathy evolves over 3 to 4 weeks. Its clinical features include an acute confusional state or delirium combined, in a small proportion of cases, with cranial nerve signs including ophthalmoparesis, nystagmus, ptosis, facial nerve palsy, or deafness. In one of our own cases, there were progressive oculomotor palsies that began with light-fixed pupils. Pathologic specimens and MRI show the process to be concentrated in the ventricular borders, especially evident as T2 signal hyperintensity in these regions. It may be seen to extend more diffusely through the adjacent white matter and be accompanied by meningeal enhancement by gadolinium in a few cases. Extensive destructive lesions have been also been reported, and this has been true in several of our own cases. Such lesions may be associated with hemorrhagic changes in the CSF in addition to showing an inflammatory response. The diagnosis of CMV infection during life is often difficult. Cultures of the CSF are usually negative and IgG antibody titers are nonspecifically elevated. Newer PCR methods may prove useful for diagnosis. Where the diagnosis is strongly suspected, treatment with the antiviral agents ganciclovir and foscarnet has been recommended, but, as pointed out by Kalayjian and colleagues, the disease may develop and progress while patients are taking these medications as a form of maintenance therapy.

Cryptococcal Infection *Meningitis* with this organism and less often *solitary cryptococcoma* are the most frequent fungal complications of HIV infection. Flagrant symptoms of meningitis or meningoencephalitis may be lacking, however, and the CSF may show little abnormality with respect to cells, protein, and glucose. For these reasons, evidence of cryptococcal infection of the spinal fluid should be actively sought with India-ink preparations, antigen testing, and fungal cultures. Treatment is along the lines outlined (on page 772).

Varicella Zoster Infections with this virus are less common complications of AIDS, but when they do occur, they tend to be severe. They take the form of multifocal lesions of the cerebral white matter, somewhat like those of progressive multifocal leukoencephalopathy, a cerebral vasculitis with hemiplegia (usually in association with ophthalmic zoster), or rarely a myelitis. Encephalitis due to herpes simplex virus types 1 and 2 has also been identified in the brains of AIDS patients, but the clinical correlates are unclear. There is no evidence that acyclovir or other antiviral agents are effective in any of these viral infections.

Tuberculosis Two particular types of mycobacterial infection tend to complicate AIDS—*Mycobacterium tuberculosis* and *Mycobacterium avium-intracellulare*. Tuberculosis predominates among drug abusers and AIDS patients in underdeveloped countries. Diagnosis and treatment are along the same lines as in non-AIDS patients (page 760). Atypical mycobacterial infections are usually associated with other destructive cerebral lesions and respond poorly to therapy.

Neurosyphilis *Syphilitic meningitis* and *meningovascular syphilis* appear to have an increased incidence in AIDS patients. Cell counts in the CSF are unreliable as signs of luetic activity, and diagnosis depends entirely upon serologic tests. It seems unlikely that AIDS causes false-positive tests for syphilis, but this remains to be settled.

Other rare organisms, such as *Rochalimaea henselae* (formerly *Bartonella*), the cause of cat-scratch fever, are found with unexpectedly high frequencies in AIDS patients and have been implicated in an encephalopathy. Progressive multifocal leukoencephalopathy, now closely linked with the immunosuppressed state of AIDS, is discussed further on in this chapter.

Diagnostic Tests for HIV Infection Many screening tests are now available for the detection of antibodies to HIV. All of them are based on an enzyme-linked immunoassay (ELISA or EIA), which has proved to be highly sensitive. However, there is a small incidence of false-positive reactions, particularly when these tests are used to screen persons at low risk for HIV infection. All positive EIA tests should therefore be repeated.

The Western blot test, which identifies antibodies to specific viral proteins, is more specific than EIA tests and should be used to confirm a positive screening test. Indeterminate Western blot tests should be repeated monthly for several months to detect a rising concentration of antibodies. Newer tests, using purified antigens, are being developed and should be more specific than those currently available.

Treatment The treatment of HIV infection/AIDS, as is true for any chronic, life-threatening disease, is difficult. Patients and their families require counseling and education, and frequently, psychiatric support in addition to complex drug regimens. Drug therapy for HIV infection continues to change rapidly. A combination of three drugs, including the reverse transcriptase inhibitors (AZT and 3-TC or lamivudine, which act synergistically and cross the blood-brain barrier) and the newer protease inhibitors (such as indinavir) render 90 percent of patients free of detectable virus for over a year. It is believed that this approach will prolong survival, but it might be expected also to increase the prevalence of neurologic complications of AIDS, each of which needs to be treated symptomatically as it is recognized. For all these reasons, referral to a specialist or a center devoted to the management of this disease is usually required.

Tropical Spastic Paraparesis and HTLV-I Infection

Tropical spastic paraparesis (TSP) is an endemic neurologic disorder in many tropical and subtropical countries. Its cause was overlooked until 1985, when Gessain and coworkers found IgG antibodies to human T-lymphotropic virus type I (HTLV-I) in the sera of 68 percent of TSP patients in Martinique. The same antibodies were then identified in the CSF of Jamaican and Colombian patients with TSP and in patients with a similar neurologic disorder in the temperate zones of southern Japan. The latter disorder was originally called HTLV-I–associated myelopathy (HAM), but it is now considered to be identical to HTLV-I–positive TSP (Roman and Osame). However, only a small proportion of HTLV-I–infected persons (estimated at 2 percent) develop a myelopathy. Sporadic instances of this disease have been reported from many parts of the western world. It is transmitted in one of several ways—from mother to child, either across the placenta or in breast milk; by intravenous drug use or blood transfusions; or by sexual contact. The age of onset is in mid–adult life, and it is more common in females than in males, in a ratio of 2.5 to 3:1.

The clinical and pathologic features of the disease are described in Chap. 44, on spinal cord disorders, and in several reviews (Rodgers-Johnson et al); its differentiation from the progressive spinal form of multiple sclerosis, with which it is most likely to be confused, is discussed on page 1306. No form of treatment has proved effective in reversing this disorder, although there are anecdotal reports that the intravenous administration of immune globulin may halt its progress.

HTLV-II is less common than HTLV-I but the two are difficult to distinguish. There is a high rate of infection with HTLV-II among drug users who are coinfected with HIV. A few cases of myelopathy have been reported in HTLV-II–infected patients, similar in all respects to HTLV-I–associated myelopathy (Lehky et al).

Viral Infections of the Developing Nervous System

Viral infections of the fetus, notably rubella and CMV, and HSV infection of the newborn are important causes of CNS abnormalities. They are considered in Chap. 38, under "Developmental Diseases of Infancy and Childhood."

SYNDROME OF ACUTE ANTERIOR POLIOMYELITIS

In the past, this syndrome was almost invariably the result of infection by one of the three types of poliovirus. Illnesses that clinically resemble poliovirus infections can be caused by other enteroviruses, such as Coxsackie viruses groups A and B and Japanese encephalitis virus. Epidemics of hemorrhagic conjunctivitis (caused by enterovirus 70 and formerly common in Asia and Africa) are also, in a small percentage of cases, associated with a lower motor neuron paralysis resembling poliomyelitis (Wadia et al). In countries with successful poliomyelitis vaccination programs, these other enteroviruses are now the most common causes of the anterior poliomyelitis syndrome. However, the illnesses caused by these viruses are generally benign and the associated paralysis is only rarely significant.

Of course, the important (paralytic) disease in this category is poliomyelitis. Although no longer a scourge in areas where vaccination is practiced, its lethal and crippling effects are still fresh in memory. As recently as the summer of 1955, when New England experienced its last epidemic, 3950 cases of acute poliomyelitis were reported in Massachusetts alone, and 2771 of these were paralytic. Now approximately 15 cases of paralytic poliomyelitis are reported annually in the United States—about equally divided between unvaccinated children and unvaccinated adults, the latter exposed to a recently vaccinated infant. The paralytic residua of previous epidemics can still be seen everywhere. In these cases, progression of muscle weakness may sometimes seem to appear many years after the acute paralytic illness (postpolio syndrome, page 1305). Acute poliomyelitis is still a frequent illness in regions of the world where vaccines are not available. For these reasons, and also because it stands as a prototype of a neurotropic viral infection, it is necessary to review the main features of the disease.

Etiology and Epidemiology The disease is caused by small RNA viruses that are members of the enterovirus group of the picornavirus family. Three antigenically distinct types have been defined, and infection with one does not protect against the others. The disease has a worldwide distribution; the peak incidence of infection in the northern hemisphere was in the months of July through September.

Poliomyelitis is a highly communicable disease. The main reservoir of infection is the human intestinal tract (humans are the only known natural hosts), and the main route of infection is fecal-oral, i.e., hand to mouth, as with other enteric pathogens. The virus multiplies in the pharynx and intestinal tract. During the incubation period, which is from 1 to 3 weeks, the virus can be recovered from both of these sites. In only a small fraction of infected patients is the nervous system invaded. Between 95 and 99 percent of infected patients are asymptomatic or experience only a nonspecific illness. It is the latter type of patient—the carrier with inapparent infection—who is most important in the spread of the virus from one person to another.

Clinical Manifestations As mentioned above, the large majority of infections are *inapparent*, or there may be only mild systemic symptoms with pharyngitis or gastroenteritis (so-called *minor illness* or *abortive poliomyelitis*). The mild symptoms of poliomyelitis correspond to the period of viremia and dissemination of the virus and give rise in most cases to an effective immune response—a feature that accounts for the failure to cause meningitis or poliomyelitis. In the relatively small proportion of patients in whom the nervous system is invaded, the illness still has a wide range of severity, from a mild attack of aseptic meningitis (nonparalytic or preparalytic poliomyelitis) to the most severe forms of paralytic disease (paralytic poliomyelitis).

Nonparalytic, or Preparalytic, Poliomyelitis The prodromal symptoms consist of listlessness, generalized, nonthrobbing headache, fever of 38 to 40°C, stiffness and aching in the muscles, sore throat in the absence of upper respiratory infection, anorexia, nausea, and vomiting. The symptoms may subside to a varying extent, to be followed after 3 to 4 days by recrudescence of headache and fever and by symptoms of nervous system involvement; more often the second phase of the illness blends with the first. Tenderness and pain in the muscles, tightness of the hamstrings (spasm), and pain in the neck and back become increasingly prominent. Other manifestations of nervous system involvement include irritability, restlessness, and emotional instability; these are frequently a prelude to paralysis. Added to these symptoms are stiffness of the neck on forward flexion, Kernig and Brudzinski signs, and the characteristic CSF findings of aseptic meningitis. These symptoms may constitute the entire illness; alternatively, the preparalytic symptoms may be followed by paralytic ones. The weakness becomes manifest while the fever is at its height, or, just as frequently, as the temperature is falling and the general clinical picture seems to be improving.

Paralytic Poliomyelitis Muscle weakness may develop rapidly, attaining its maximum severity in 48 h or even less; or it may develop more slowly or in stuttering fashion, over a week, rarely even longer. As a general rule, there is no progression of weakness after the temperature has been normal for 48 h. The distribution of spinal paralysis is quite variable; rarely there may be an acute symmetrical paralysis of the muscles of the trunk and limbs, as occurs in the Guillain-Barré syndrome. Excessive physical activity and local injections during the period of asymptomatic infection are thought to favor the development of paralysis of the exercised muscles or injected limbs.

Coarse fasciculations are seen frequently as the muscles weaken; they are transient as a rule, but occasionally they persist. Tendon reflexes are diminished and lost as the weakness evolves and paralyzed muscles become flaccid. Patients frequently complain of paresthesias in the affected limbs, but objective sensory loss is seldom demonstrable. Retention of urine is a common occurrence in adult patients but does not persist. Atrophy of muscle can be detected within 3 weeks of onset of paralysis, is maximal at 12 to 15 weeks, and is permanent.

Bulbar paralysis is more common in young adults, but usually such patients have spinal involvement as well. The most frequently involved cranial muscles are those of deglutition, reflecting involvement of the nucleus ambiguus. The other great hazards of bulbar disease are the disturbances of respiration and vasomotor control—hiccough, shallowness and progressive slowing of respiration, cyanosis, restlessness and anxiety (air hunger), hypertension, and ultimately hypotension and circulatory collapse. When these disturbances are added to paralysis of diaphragmatic and intercostal musculature, the patient's survival is threatened and the institution of respiratory assistance and intensive care becomes urgent.

Pathologic Changes and Clinicopathologic Correlations In fatal infections, lesions are found in the precentral (motor) gyrus of the brain (usually of insufficient severity to cause symptoms), brainstem, and spinal cord. The brunt of the disease is borne by the hypothalamus, thalamus, motor nuclei of the brainstem and surrounding reticular formation, vestibular nuclei and roof nuclei of the cerebellum, and the neurons of the anterior and intermediate gray matter of the spinal cord. In these areas, nerve cells are destroyed and phagocytized by microgliacytes (neuronophagia). A leukocytic reaction is present for only a few days, but mononuclear cells persist as perivascular accumulations for many months. Nuclear or cytoplasmic inclusion bodies are not seen. The earliest histopathologic changes are central chromatolysis of the nerve cells, along with an inflammatory reaction. These changes correlate with a multiplication of virus in the CNS and, in the infected monkey, they precede the onset of paralysis by one or several days (Bodian).

In Bodian's experimental material, the infected motor neurons continued to function until a stage of severe chromatolysis was reached. Moreover, if damage to the cell had attained only the stage of central chromatolysis, complete morphologic recovery could be expected—a process that takes a month or longer. After this time, the degree of paralysis and atrophy are closely correlated with the number of motor nerve cells that have been destroyed; where limbs remain atrophic and paralyzed, less than 10 percent of neurons survive in corresponding cord segments.

Lesions in the motor nuclei of the brainstem are associated with paralysis in corresponding muscles, but only if severe in degree. The disturbances of swallowing, respiration, and vasomotor control are related to neuronal lesions in the medullary reticular formation, centered in the region of the nucleus ambiguus.

Atrophic, areflexic paralysis of muscles of the trunk and limbs relates, of course, to destruction of neurons in the anterior and intermediate horns of the corresponding segments of the spinal cord gray matter. Stiffness and pain in the neck and back, attributed to "meningeal irritation," are probably related to the mild inflammatory exudate in the meninges and to the generally mild lesions in the dorsal root ganglia and dorsal horns. Probably these lesions also account for the muscle pain and paresthesias in parts that later become paralyzed. Abnormalities of autonomic function are attributable to lesions of autonomic pathways in the reticular substance of the brainstem and in the lateral horn cells in the spinal cord.

It is of interest that poliovirus has been readily isolated from CNS tissue of fatal cases but can rarely be recovered from the CSF during clinical disease. This is in contrast to the closely related Coxsackie and echo picornaviruses, which have been isolated frequently from the CSF during the neurologic illness.

Treatment Patients in whom acute poliomyelitis is suspected require careful observation of swallowing function, vital capacity, pulse, and blood pressure, in anticipation of respiratory and circulatory complications. With paralysis of limb muscles, foot boards, hand and arm splints, and knee and trochanter rolls prevent foot drop and other deformities. Frequent passive movement prevents contractures and ankylosis.

Respiratory failure, due to paralysis of the intercostal and diaphragmatic muscles or to depression of the respiratory centers in the brainstem, calls for the use of a positive-pressure respirator and, in most patients, for a tracheostomy as well. The management of the pulmonary and circulatory complications does not differ from their management in diseases such as myasthenia gravis and the Guillain-Barré syndrome and is best carried out in special respiratory intensive care units.

The authors know of no systematic study of the potency of antiviral agents in this disease.

Prevention *Prevention*, of course, has proved to be the most significant aspect of treatment and one of the outstanding accomplishments of modern medicine. The cultivation of poliovirus in cultures of human embryonic tissues and monkey kidney cells—the achievement of Enders and associates—made possible the development of effective vaccines. The first of these was the injectable Salk vaccine, containing formalin-inactivated virulent strains of the three viral serotypes. This has been replaced to a large extent by the Sabin vaccine, which consists of attenuated live virus, administered orally in two doses 8 weeks apart; boosters are required at 1 year of age and before starting school. Since 1965, the reported annual incidence rate of poliomyelitis has been less than 0.01 per 100,000 (compared to a rate of 24 cases per 100,000 during the years 1951 to 1955). Very rarely, poliomyelitis may follow vaccination (0.02 to 0.04 cases per million doses). The only obstacle to complete prevention of the disease is inadequate utilization of the vaccine. Significant segments of the population in areas with low public health standards are not being immunized; conceivably, with an increasing lack of immunity, outbreaks of poliomyelitis could occur once again.

Prognosis Mortality from acute paralytic poliomyelitis is between 5 and 10 percent—higher in the elderly and very young. If the patient survives the acute stage, paralysis of respiration and deglutition usually recovers completely; in only a small fraction of such patients is chronic respirator care necessary. Many patients also recover completely from muscular weakness, and the most severely paralyzed improve to some extent. The return of muscle strength occurs mainly in the first 3 to 4 months and is probably the result of morphologic restitution of partially damaged nerve cells. Branching of axons of intact motor cells with collateral reinnervation of muscle fibers of denervated motor units may also play a part. Slow recovery of slight degree may then continue for a year or more, the result of hypertrophy of undamaged muscle. The so-called post–polio syndrome is discussed on page 1305.

Nonpoliovirus Poliomyelitis

As indicated earlier, a number of RNA viruses that cause mundane upper respiratory or enteric infections are now the main, although still rare, causes of a sporadic poliomyelitic syndrome. Fifty-two cases were recorded by the Centers for Disease Control and Prevention over a 4-year period. Most of these have been due to one of the echoviruses and a lesser number to Coxsackie enteroviruses, particularly strains 70 and 71. The former leave little residual paralysis, but the Coxsackie viruses, which have been studied in several outbreaks in the United States, Bulgaria, and Hungary, have been more variable in their effects. Enterovirus 70 causes acute hemorrhagic conjunctivitis in limited epidemics and is followed by a poliomyelitis in 1 of every 10,000 cases. European outbreaks of enterovirus 71, known in the United States as a cause of hand-foot-and-mouth disease and aseptic meningitis, have resulted in poliovirus-type paralysis including fatal bulbar cases (Chumakov et al). In a recent outbreak of enterovirus 71 in Taiwan, Huang et al described a brainstem encephalitis with myoclonus and cranial nerve involvement in a high proportion of the patients.

Our own experience with this form of poliomyelitis has been with five patients who were referred for paralyzing illnesses initially thought to be Guillain-Barré syndrome. In each case, the illness began with fever and active aseptic meningitis (50 to 150 lymphocytes per cubic millimeter in the CSF), followed by backache and widespread, relatively symmetrical paralysis, including the oropharyngeal muscles, except for two cases in which the weakness was asymmetrical and limited to the arms. There were no sensory changes. One patient had a concurrent encephalitic illness. The evolving EMG changes suggested that the paralysis was due to a loss of anterior horn cells rather than to a motor neuropathy or to a purely motor radiculopathy, but this distinction was not always certain. MRI was remarkable in showing distinct changes in the gray matter of the cord, mainly ventrally (Fig. 33-4). No virus could be isolated from the CSF and serologic tests in two patients failed to implicate any of the encephalitic RNA viruses, including poliovirus. The patients had been immunized against the poliomyelitis viruses.

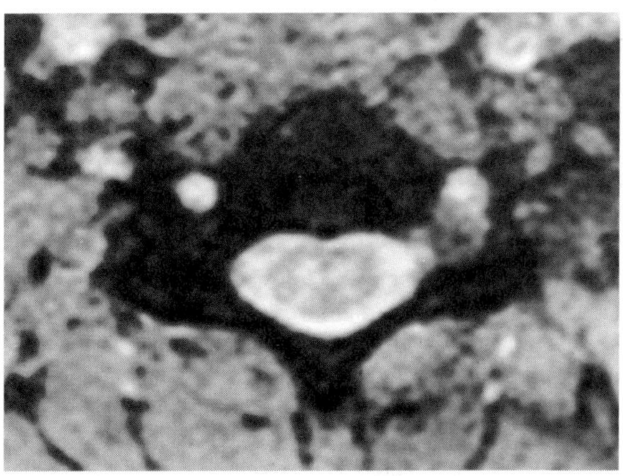

Figure 33-4

MRI of the cervical cord MRI in a patient with nonpoliovirus poliomyelitis and an asymmetrical, flaccid, bibrachial paralysis. There is T–2 signal change in the anterior regions of the gray matter.

SUBACUTE AND CHRONIC VIRAL INFECTIONS SIMULATING DEGENERATIVE DISEASE

The idea that viral infections may lead to chronic disease, especially of the nervous system, had been entertained since the 1920s, but only in relatively recent years was it firmly established. The following indirect and direct evidence supported this view: (1) the demonstration of a slowly progressive noninflammatory degeneration of nigral neurons long after an attack of encephalitis lethargica; (2) the finding of inclusion bodies in cases of subacute and chronic sclerosing encephalitis; (3) the discovery of chronic neurologic disease in sheep caused by a conventional RNA virus (visna)—it was in relation to this disease in sheep that Sigurdsson first used the term "slow infection" to describe the long incubation periods during which the animals appeared well; (4) the demonstration by electron microscopy of viral particles in the lesions of multifocal leukoencephalopathy and, later, isolation of the virus from the lesions. The suggestion that the late onset of progressive weakness after poliomyelitis ("post-polio syndrome") might represent a slow infection has never been verified. Claims have also been made for a viral causation of multiple sclerosis, amyotrophic lateral sclerosis, and other degenerative diseases, but the evidence is questionable.

The slow infections of the nervous system due to conventional viruses include subacute sclerosing panencephalitis (measles), progressive rubella panencephalitis, progressive multifocal leukoencephalopathy (JC virus), and visna in sheep. These slowly progressive diseases except for progressive multifocal leukoencephalopathy (PML) are decidedly rare. They are caused by conventional viruses and are not to be confused with a group of chronic neurologic diseases that also are sometimes referred to as "slow infections" but are due to nonconventional transmissible agents, now called *prions*. The latter are accorded a separate section later in this chapter.

Subacute Sclerosing Panencephalitis (SSPE)

This disease was first described by Dawson in 1934 under the title "inclusion body encephalitis" and extensively studied by Van Bogaert, who renamed it *subacute sclerosing panencephalitis*. It is now recognized to be the result of chronic measles infection. Never a common disease, the condition occurred until recently at a rate of about one case per million children per year. With the introduction and widespread use of measles vaccine, it has practically disappeared in the United States. This has been one of the important advances in preventative neuropediatrics.

Subacute sclerosing panencephalitis affects children and adolescents for the most part, rarely appearing beyond the age of 10 years. Typically there is a history of primary measles infection at a very early age, often before 2 years, followed by a 6- to 8-year asymptomatic period. The illness evolves in several stages. Initially there is a decline in proficiency at school, temper outbursts and other changes in personality, difficulty with language, and loss of interest in usual activities. These soon give way to a severe and progressive intellectual deterioration in association with focal or generalized seizures, widespread myoclonus, ataxia, and sometimes visual disturbances due to progressive chorioretinitis. As the disease advances, rigidity, hyperactive reflexes, Babinski signs, progressive unresponsiveness, and signs of autonomic dysfunction appear. In the final stage the child lies insensate, virtually "decorticated." The course is usually steadily progressive, death occurring within 1 to 3 years. In about 10 percent of cases the course is more prolonged, with one or more remissions. In a similar number the course is fulminant, leading to death within months of onset. Exceptionally, the disease occurs in young adults. In two reported cases in pregnant women, blurred vision and weakness of limbs developed before they became akinetic and mute, without a trace of myoclonus or cerebellar ataxia. Nevertheless, the ataxic-myoclonic chronic dementia was so typical that bedside diagnosis was usually possible.

The EEG shows a characteristic abnormality consisting of periodic (every 5 to 8 s) bursts of 2- to 3-per-second high-voltage waves, followed by a relatively flat pattern. The CSF contains few or no cells, but the protein is increased, particularly the gamma globulin, and agarose gel electrophoresis discloses oligoclonal bands of IgG. These have been shown to represent measles virus–specific antibody (Mehta et al). Both the serum and CSF contain high concentrations of neutralizing antibody to measles (rubeola) virus, but the virus has been recovered from the brain tissue only with difficulty in a few instances. The MRI changes have been shown to begin in the subcortical white matter and spread to the periventricular region (Anlar et al).

Histologically the lesions involve the cerebral cortex and white matter of both hemispheres and the brainstem. The cerebellum is usually spared. Destruction of nerve cells, neuronophagia, and perivenous cuffing by lymphocytes and mononuclear cells indicate the viral nature of the infection. In the white matter there is degeneration of medullated fibers (myelin and axis cylinders), accompanied by perivascular cuffing with mononuclear cells and fibrous gliosis (sclerosing encephalitis). Eosinophilic inclusions, the histopathologic hallmark of the disease, are found in the cytoplasm and nuclei of neurons and glial cells. Virions, thought to be measles nucleocapsids, have been observed in the inclusion-bearing cells examined electron microscopically.

How a ubiquitous and transient viral infection in a seemingly normal young child allows the development, many years later, of a rare encephalitis is a matter of speculation. Sever believes that there is a delay in the development of immune responses during the initial infection and later development of immune responses that are incapable of clearing the suppressed infection. An alternative explanation is that certain brain cells fail to synthesize a so-called M protein, which is essential for the assembly of the viral membrane, and that this limitation of host-cell capability is related to the extent of viral seeding of the brain during the initial infection (Hall et al).

The differential diagnosis includes the childhood and adolescent dementing diseases such as lipid storage diseases (Chap. 37) and Schilder disease (page 967). In presumptive clinical cases of SSPE, the findings of periodic complexes in the EEG, elevated gamma globulin in the CSF, and elevated measles antibody titers in the serum and CSF are sufficient to make the diagnosis.

No effective treatment is available. The administration of amantadine and inosiplex was found by some authors to lead to improvement and prolonged survival but others did not corroborate these effects. The therapeutic value of intrathecal administration of alpha interferon is still to be determined.

Subacute Measles Encephalitis with Immunosuppression Whereas SSPE occurs in children who were previously normal, another rare type of measles encephalitis has been described, affecting both children and adults with defective cell-mediated immune responses (Wolinsky et al). In this latter type, measles or exposure to measles precedes the encephalitis by 1 to 6 months. Seizures (often epilepsia partialis continua), focal neurologic signs, stupor, and coma are the main features of the neurologic illness and lead to death within a few days to a few weeks. The CSF may be normal, and levels of measles antibodies do not increase. Aicardi and colleagues have isolated measles virus from the brain of such a patient. The lesions are similar to those of SSPE (eosinophilic inclusions in neurons and glia, with varying degrees of necrosis) except that inflammatory changes are lacking. In a sense this subacute measles encephalitis is an opportunistic infection of the brain in an immunodeficient patient. The relatively short interval between exposure and onset of neurologic disease, the rapid course, and lack of antibodies distinguish this form of subacute measles encephalitis from both SSPE and postmeasles encephalomyelitis (Chap. 36).

Progressive Rubella Panencephalitis Generally the deficits associated with congenital rubella infection are nonprogressive at least after the second or third year of life. There are, however, descriptions of children with the congenital rubella syndrome in whom a progressive neurologic deterioration occurred after a stable period of 8 to 19 years (Townsend et al; Weil et al). In 1978, Wolinsky described 10 cases of this syndrome, a few of them apparently related to acquired rather than to congenital rubella. Since then, this late-appearing progressive syndrome seems to have disappeared, no new cases having been reported in the past 20 years.

The clinical syndrome has been quite uniform. On a background of the fixed stigmata of congenital rubella, there occurs a deterioration in behavior and school performance, often associated with seizures, and, soon thereafter, a progressive impairment of mental function (dementia). Clumsiness of gait is an early symptom, followed by a frank ataxia of gait and then of the limbs. Spasticity and other corticospinal tract signs, dysarthria, and dysphagia ensue. Pallor of the optic discs, ophthalmoplegia, spastic quadriplegia, and mutism mark the final phase of the illness. The CSF shows a mild increase of lymphocytes and elevation of protein and a marked increase in the proportion of gamma globulin (35 to 52 percent of the total protein), which assumes an oligoclonal pattern on agarose gel electrophoresis. The CSF and serum rubella-antibody titers are elevated.

Pathologic examination of the brain has shown a widespread, progressive subacute panencephalitis mainly affecting the white matter. No inclusion-bearing cells were seen. Thus it appears that rubella virus infection, acquired in utero or in the postnatal period, may persist in the nervous system for years before rekindling a chronic active infection.

Progressive Multifocal Leukoencephalopathy (PML) This disorder, first observed clinically by Adams and colleagues in 1952, was described morphologically by Åstrom and coworkers (1958) and then with a larger material by Richardson. It is characterized by widespread demyelinative lesions, mainly of the cerebral hemispheres but sometimes of the brainstem and cerebellum and rarely of the spinal cord. The lesions vary greatly in size and severity—from microscopic foci of demyelination to massive multifocal zones of destruction of both myelin and axis cylinders involving the major part of a cerebral or cerebellar hemisphere (Fig. 33-5). The abnormalities of the glial cells are distinctive. Many of the reactive astrocytes in the lesions are gigantic and contain deformed and bizarre-shaped nuclei and mitotic figures, changes that are seen otherwise only in malignant glial tumors. Also, at the periphery of the lesions, the nuclei of oligodendrocytes are greatly enlarged and contain abnormal inclusions. Many are destroyed, accounting for the demyelination. Vascular changes are lacking, and inflammatory changes are present but usually insignificant.

Clinical Features An uncommon disease of late adult life, PML usually develops in a patient with a neoplasm or chronic immunodeficiency state. The large majority of cases are now observed in patients with AIDS, in whom the incidence of PML approaches 5 percent. Other important associations are with chronic neoplastic disease (mainly chronic lymphocytic leukemia, Hodgkin disease, lymphosarcoma, myeloproliferative disease) and, less often, with nonneoplastic granulomatosis, such as tuberculosis or sarcoidosis. Some cases occur in patients receiving immunosuppressive drugs for renal transplantation or for other reasons. Personality changes and intellectual impairment may introduce the neurologic syndrome, which evolves over a period of several days to weeks. Any one or some combination of hemiparesis progressing to quadriparesis, visual field defects, cortical blindness, aphasia, ataxia, dysarthria, dementia, confusional states, and coma are the typical manifestations. Seizures and cerebellar ataxia are rare. In most cases death occurs in 3 to 6 months from the onset of neurologic symptoms and even more rapidly in patients with AIDS unless aggressive antiretroviral treatment is undertaken. The CSF is usually normal. CT and MRI localize the lesions with striking clarity (Fig. 33-5).

Pathogenesis Waksman's original suggestion (quoted by Richardson) that PML could be due to viral infection of the CNS in patients with impaired immunologic responses proved to be correct. ZuRhein and Chou (1965), in an electron microscopic study of cerebral lesions from a patient with PML, demonstrated crystalline arrays of particles resembling papovaviruses in the inclusion-bearing oligodendrocytes. Since then, a human polyomavirus, designated "JC virus" or JCV (ini-

Figure 33-5

Progressive multifocal leukoencephalitis. MRI in the axial plane demonstrates multiple nonenhancing white matter lesions in a 31-year-old male with AIDS.

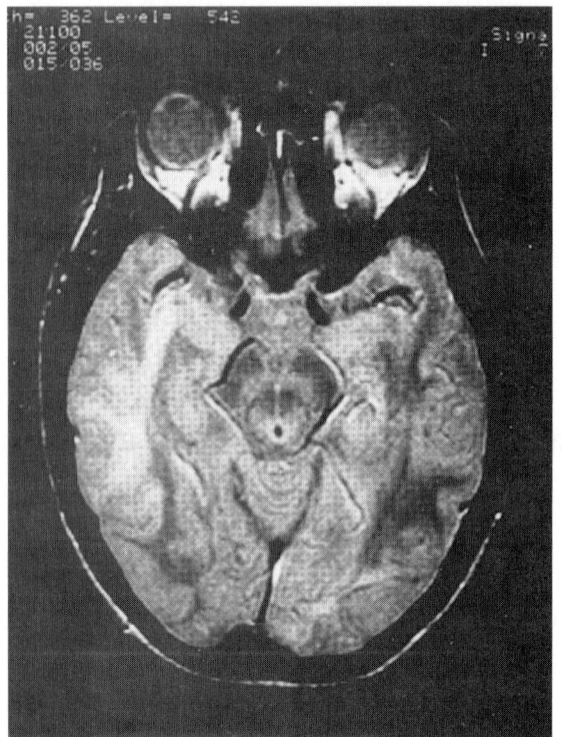

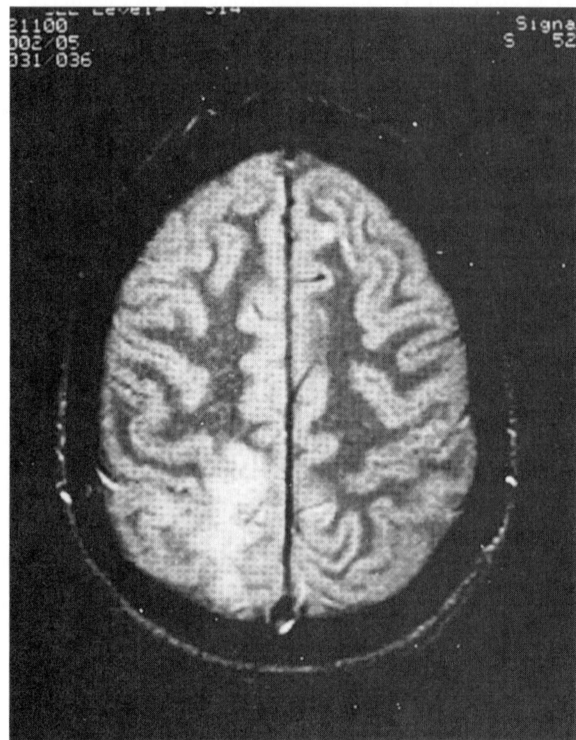

tials of the patient from whom the virus was originally isolated), has repeatedly been shown to be the causative agent. JCV is ubiquitous, as judged by the presence of antibodies to the virus in approximately 70 percent of the normal adult population. It is thought to be dormant until an immunosuppressed state permits its active replication. The virus has been isolated from the urine, blood lymphocytes, and kidney, but there is no clinical evidence of damage to extraneural structures.

Treatment The disease is generally believed to be untreatable in the non-AIDS patient. Several anecdotal reports of the efficacy of cytosine arabinoside have appeared, but a controlled trial has failed to demonstrate an increased survival in AIDS patients with this disease. Interferon alpha has been thought to be beneficial in a few cases. In AIDS patients, aggressive treatment using antiretroviral drug combinations, including protease inhibitors, greatly slows the progression of PML and has even led to its apparent remission.

Encephalitis Lethargica (Von Economo Disease, Sleeping Sickness) Although examples of a somnolent-ophthalmoplegic encephalitis dot the early medical literature (e.g., nona, fébre lethargica, Schlafkrankheit), it was in the wake of the influenza pandemic of World War I that this disease burst on the medical horizon and continued to reappear for about 10 years. The viral agent was never identified, but the clinical and pathologic features were typical of viral infection.

The importance of encephalitis lethargica relates to (1) the unique clinical syndromes and sequelae and (2) its place as the first recognized "slow virus infection" of the nervous system in human beings. The unique symptoms were ophthalmoplegia and pronounced somnolence, from which the disease took its name. Some patients were overly active, and a third group manifested a disorder of movement in the form of bradykinesia, catalepsy, mutism, chorea, or myoclonus. Lymphocytic pleocytosis was found in half the patients, together with variable elevation of the CSF protein content. More than 20 percent of the victims died within a few weeks, and many survivors were left with varying degrees of impairment of mental function. Also, after an interval of weeks or months (occasionally years), a high proportion of survivors developed a parkinsonian syndrome. This is the only form of encephalitis known to cause a delayed extrapyramidal syndrome of this type (a similar though not identical syndrome may follow Japanese B encephalitis). Myoclonus, dystonia, oculogyric crises (page 278) and other muscle spasms, bulimia, obesity, reversal of the sleep pattern, and, in children, a change in personality with compulsive behavior were other distressing sequelae.

The pathology was typical of a viral infection, localized principally to the midbrain, subthalamus, and hypothalamus. In the patients who died years later with a Parkinson syndrome, the main findings were depigmentation of the substantia nigra and locus ceruleus due to nerve cell destruction. Neurofibrillary changes in the surviving nerve cells of the substantia nigra and the oculomotor and adjacent nuclei were also described, indistinguishable from those of progressive supranuclear palsy. Lewy bodies were not seen, in contrast to idiopathic Parkinson disease (paralysis agitans), where they are consistently present. Few new cases of postencephalitic type have been seen in the United States and western Europe since 1930. Sporadic cases such as the four reported by Howard and Lees may be examples of this disease, but there is no way of proving their identity.

Other Forms of Subacute Encephalitis A number of uncommon conditions not covered above are characterized by regional inflammation in the cerebrum. Among these, *Rasmussen encephalitis*, which causes intractable focal seizures and progressive hemiparesis, has been connected to infections by CMV and HSV-I in various studies that used PCR techniques. However, a specific immune reaction consisting of antibodies to glutamate receptor antibodies has been implicated more consistently and immunosupressive treatments may be effective. It is not clear whether this process can be classed with the infectious encephalitides; it is discussed in detail with other epileptic diseases on page 352. Similarly, the restricted inflammatory conditions called *limbic encephalitis* and "brainstem encephalitis"—most often a distant effect of lung cancer—have some characteristics of a subacute viral encephalitis, but no agent has been consistently isolated and they are also best considered immunologic reactions. They are included in the discussion of paraneoplastic illnesses in Chap 31.

THE TRANSMISSIBLE SPONGIFORM ENCEPHALOPATHIES (PRION DISEASES)

This category includes a quartet of human diseases—so-called Creutzfeldt-Jakob disease (and a variant that infects cows and may be rarely transmitted to humans), the Gerstmann-Sträussler-Scheinker syndrome, kuru, and probably fatal familial insomnia.

Although this group of diseases has been included for discussion in the chapter on viral diseases of the nervous system, it has been evident for some time that the cause of these slow infections is neither a virus nor a viroid (nucleic acid alone, without a capsid structure). During the past 20 years, Prusiner and colleagues have presented compelling evidence that the transmissible pathogen is a proteinaceous infectious particle which is devoid of nucleic acid, resists the action of enzymes that destroy RNA and DNA, fails to produce an immune response, and electron microscopically does not have the structure of a virus. To distinguish this pathogen from viruses and viroids, Prusiner introduced the term *prion.* The prion protein (PrP) is encoded by a gene on the short arm of chromosome 20. The discovery of mutations in the PrP genes of patients with familial Creutzfeldt-Jakob disease and Gerstmann-Straüssler-Scheinker syndrome (described below) attests to the fact that prion diseases are both genetic and infectious. In this respect, prions are unique among all infectious pathogens. It is now possible to detect inherited prion disease during life, using DNA extracted from leukocytes. How prions arise in sporadic forms of spongiform encephalopathy is not fully understood; probably the conversion of the normal cellular protein to the infectious form involves a conformational change in the protein structure (see further on).

There remains a simmering skepticism concerning the validity of the prion hypothesis among some microbiologists, who continue to search for virus-like particles or other conventional agents to explain the transmission of the disease. However, to date, evidence that would definitively refute the prion concept has not been forthcoming.

A description of the human prion diseases follows, the most important by far being Creutzfeldt-Jakob disease.

Subacute Spongiform Encephalopathy (Creutzfeldt-Jakob Disease)

These terms refer to a distinctive cerebral disease in which a rapidly progressive and profound dementia is associated with cerebellar ataxia, diffuse myoclonic jerks, and a variety of other visual and other neurologic abnormalities. The major neuropathologic changes are in the cerebral and cerebellar cortices; the outstanding features are widespread neuronal loss and gliosis accompanied by a striking vacuolation or spongy state of the affected regions—hence the designation *subacute spongiform encephalopathy (SSE).* Less severe changes in a patchy distribution are found in cases with a brief clinical course.

These changes, both clinical and pathologic, occur with such uniformity from case to case that they doubtless form a nosologic entity. It is generally referred to as Creutzfeldt-Jakob disease, an inappropriate eponym, since it is most unlikely that the patient described by Creutzfeldt and at least 3 of the 5 patients described by Jakob had the same disease that we now recognize as subacute spongiform encephalopathy (SSE). It is advisable that they be kept distinct from one another, or at least, whenever one speaks of Creutzfeldt-Jakob disease, to specify what is meant—either SSE or the slower progressive dementia with signs of pyramidal and extrapyramidal affection originally described by Creutzfeldt and Jakob (the latter condition is discussed on page 1126). Precision in definition of these states is of greater importance than before, since it was shown by Gibbs and Gajdusek that brain tissue from patients with SSE, injected into chimpanzees, can transmit the disease after an incubation period of a year or longer. However, decades of use makes the term *Creutzfeld-Jakob disease* and its acronym, *CJD*, virtually impossible to displace.

Epidemiology and Pathogenesis The disease appears in all parts of the world and in all seasons, with an annual incidence of 1 to 2 cases per million of population. The incidence is higher in Israelis of Libyan origin, in immigrants to France from North Africa, and in Slovakia, for reasons that are not understood. Although the reported incidence of SSE is somewhat higher in urban than in rural areas, temporospatial clustering of cases has not been observed, at least in the United States. A small proportion of all series of cases is familial—varying from 5 percent reported by Cathala and associates to 15 percent of 1435 cases analyzed by Masters and coworkers. The occurrence of familial cases, not in the same household, suggests a genetic susceptibility to infection, although the possibility of common exposure to the transmissible agent cannot be dismissed. A small number of conjugal cases have been reported. The only clearly demonstrated mechanism of spread of SSE is iatrogenic, having occurred in a few cases after transplantation of corneas or dural grafts from infected individuals, after implantation of infected depth electrodes, and after the injection of human growth hormone or gonadotropins that had been prepared from pooled cadaveric sources of these hormones. At least one neurosurgeon is known to have acquired the disease. Individuals exposed to scrapie-infected sheep and to patients with SSE are not disproportionately affected.

Recently, a great deal of attention has been drawn to an epidemic of prion disease among cows in the British Isles ("mad cow disease"). The epidemic began in 1985, with putative transmission of the disease to some two dozen humans. These patients have been younger (average age of onset, 27 years) than those with typical SSE (65 years) and manifested curious psychiatric and sensory symptoms as the first sign of illness; they did not exhibit the usual EEG findings even as the illness advanced to its later stages (Zeidler et al). This has been called "new variant Creutzfeldt-Jakob disease." It has recently been shown that the prion strain in these patients is identical to the one from affected cattle. The mode of transmission, presumed to be the ingestion of infected meat, is somewhat reminiscent of the propagation of kuru by ceremonial ingestion of brain tissue from infected individuals.

Spongiform encephalopathy has now been fairly firmly associated with the conversion of a normal cellular protein, PrPc to an abnormal isoform, PrPSc. The conversion involves a change in physical conformation in which the α-helical proportion of the protein diminishes and the proportion of the β pleated sheet increases (see reviews by Prusiner). Current theory holds that the "infectivity" of prions and their propagation in brain tissue may result from the susceptibility of the native prion protein to alter its shape as a result of physical exposure to the abnormal protein, a so-called conformational disease. Conformationally altered prions have a tendency to aggregate, and this may be the mode of cellular destruction that leads to disease. In contrast, transmission in familial cases of prion disease is thought to be the result of one of several gene aberrations residing in the region that codes for PrPc.

Clinical Features Transmissible SSE is in most cases a disease of late middle age, although it can occur in young adults. The sexes are affected equally. In the large series of pathologically verified cases reported by Brown and coworkers, prodromal symptoms—consisting of fatigue, depression, weight loss, and disorders of sleep and appetite lasting for several weeks—were observed in about one-third of the patients.

The early stages of the disease are characterized by a great variety of clinical manifestations, but the most frequent are changes in behavior, emotional response, and intellectual function, together with ataxia and abnormalities of vision, such as distortions of the shape and alignment of objects or actual impairment of visual acuity. In many instances the early phase of the disease is dominated by symptoms of confusion, with hallucinations, delusions, and agitation. In some instances, cerebellar ataxia (Brownell-Oppenheimer variant) or visual disturbances (Heidenhain variant) precede the mental changes and may be the most prominent features for several months. Headache, vertigo, and sensory symptoms are features in some patients but become quickly obscured by dementia and muteness.

As a rule, the disease progresses rapidly, so that obvious deterioration is seen from week to week and even day to day. Sooner or later, in almost all cases, myoclonic contractions of various muscle groups appear, perhaps unilaterally at first but later becoming generalized. Or, infrequently, the myoclonus may not appear for weeks or even months after the initial mental changes. These are associated with a striking startle response, mainly to a loud noise. In a few patients, a startle response, which is elicitable for a brief period of time, is the only manifestation of myoclonus. In general, the myoclonic jerks are evocable by sensory stimuli of all sorts, but they occur spontaneously as well. Twitches of individual fingers are typical. Ataxia and dysarthria are likewise prominent in many cases during the first few weeks of the illness. These changes gradually give way to a mute state, stupor, and coma, but the myoclonic contractions may continue to the end. Signs of degeneration of the pyramidal tracts or anterior horn cells, palsies of convergence and upgaze, and extrapyramidal signs occur in a small number of patients as the disease advances.

The diagnosis during life rests mostly on the recognition of one of the clusters of typical clinical features, particularly the unique syndrome of dementia—which progresses much more quickly than that of common degenerative diseases—coupled with stimulus-sensitive myoclonus and the characteristic EEG changes that occur in most patients (see below).

The disease is invariably fatal, usually in less than a year from the onset. In about 10 percent of patients, the illness begins with almost stroke-like suddenness and runs its course rapidly, in a matter of a few weeks or months. A small number of patients have reportedly survived for 2 to 10 years, but these cases should be accepted with caution; in some of them, SSE appears to have been superimposed on Alzheimer or Parkinson disease or some other chronic condition.

Laboratory Diagnosis The CSF and other laboratory tests are normal—useful findings in excluding a number of chronic inflammatory causes of dementia. In many patients, the EEG pattern is distinctive, changing over the course of the disease from one of diffuse and nonspecific slowing to one of stereotyped high-voltage slow- (1- to 2-Hz) and sharp-wave complexes on an increasingly slow and low-voltage background (see Fig. 2-3*G*, page 30). The high-voltage sharp waves, which give the appearance of periodicity (pseudoperiodic), are synchronous with the myoclonus but may persist in its absence. Imaging studies of the brain had been thought until recently to be of little value, but up to 80 percent of cases show a subtle hyperintensity of the lenticular nuclei on T2-weighted images when the disease is fully established (Fig. 33-6).

There are now helpful confirmatory diagnostic tests. Hsich and colleagues have described a highly sensitive test of CSF—the finding by immunoassay of a particular peptide fragments of normal brain proteins, termed "14-3-3," This test is particularly useful in separating SSE from other chronic noninflammatory dementing diseases. A number of other tests are emerging from specialized laboratories that detect the abnormal PrPSc isoform of the prion protein in the spinal fluid. Prusiner's laboratory can detect eight prion strains by fluorescence immunoassay. Also, enolase and neopterin concentrations in CSF are elevated in most cases, but the release of these chemicals may also be found with other types of brain lesions, particularly infarction.

Figure 33-6

MRI showing T2 signal changes in the lenticular nuclei in a patient with Creutzfeldt-Jakob disease of 1 month's duration.

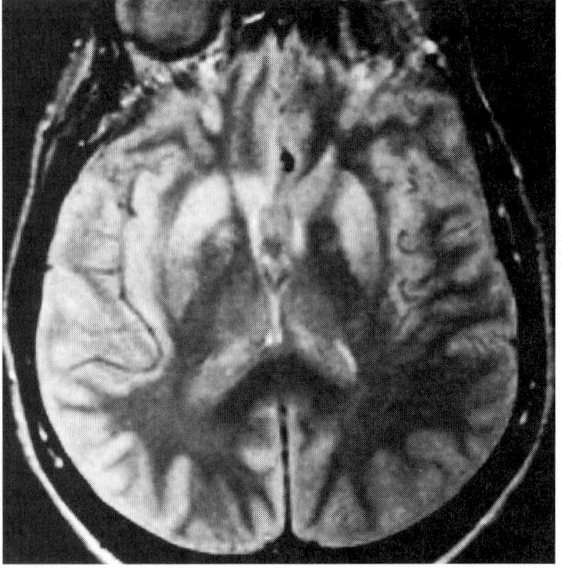

Tonsillar material from patients with new variant Creutzfeldt-Jakob disease ("mad cow disease") stains with antibodies against abnormal prion protein, but this technique does not appear to be applicable to the early diagnosis of the sporadic disease (Hill).

Pathology The disease affects principally the cerebral and cerebellar cortices, generally in a diffuse fashion, although in some cases the occipitoparietal regions are almost exclusively involved, as in those described by Heidenhain. In others, such as the cases of Brownell and Oppenheimer, the cerebellum has been most seriously affected, with early and prominent ataxia. The degeneration and disappearance of nerve cells is associated with extensive astroglial proliferation; ultrastructural studies have shown that the microscopic vacuoles, which give the tissue its typically spongy appearance, are located within the cytoplasmic processes of glial cells and dendrites of nerve cells. Despite the fact that the disease is due to a transmissible agent, the lesions show no evidence of an inflammatory reaction and no viral particles are seen.

Differential Diagnosis The diagnosis of most cases of SSE presents no difficulty. Not infrequently, however, we have been surprised by a "typical" case that proves to be some other disease. Lithium intoxication, Hashimoto encephalopathy (page 1200), Whipple disease (page 748), angiocentric lymphoma, carcinomatous meningitis—all of them characterized by myoclonus and dementia—may mimic SSE in the early weeks of the illness. Contrariwise, the early mental changes of SSE may be misinterpreted as an atypical or unusually intense emotional reaction, as one of the major psychoses, as an unusual form of Alzheimer disease with myoclonus, or as Lewy-body disease. Despite the designation of SSE as a progressive dementia, the similarities to even rapidly developing Alzheimer disease are superficial. Also, diagnosis may be difficult in patients who present with vertigo, gait disturbance, diplopia, or visual disturbances until the rapidly evolving clinical picture clarifies the issue. Subacute sclerosing panencephalitis (see above), in its fully developed form, may resemble SSE, but the former is chiefly a disease of children or young adults, and the CSF shows elevation of gamma globulin (IgG), whereas the latter is essentially a disease of middle age and the presenile period, and the CSF is normal. Limbic-brainstem-cerebellar encephalitis in patients with an occult tumor and AIDS dementia (discussed earlier) also figure in the differential diagnosis. Cerebral lipidosis in children or young adults can result in a similar combination of myoclonus and dementia, but the clinical course in such cases is extremely chronic and there are retinal changes that do not occur in SSE.

Management No specific treatment is known. Antiviral agents have been ineffective. In view of the transmissibility of the disease from humans to primates and iatrogenically from patient to patient, certain precautions should be taken in the medical care of and handling of materials from patients with SSE. Special isolation rooms are not necessary, and the families of SSE patients and nursing staff can be reassured that casual contact poses no risk. Needle punctures and cuts are not thought to pose a risk but some uncertainty remains. The transmissible agent is resistant to boiling, treatment with formalin and alcohol, and ultraviolet radiation but can be inactivated by autoclaving at 132°C and 15 lb per square inch for 1 h or by immersion for 1 h in 5% sodium hypochlorite (household bleach). Workers exposed to infected materials (butchers, abattoir workers, health care workers) should wash thoroughly with ordinary soap. Needles, glassware, needle electrodes, and other instruments should be handled with great care and immersed in appropriate disinfectants and autoclaved or incinerated. The performance of a brain biopsy or autopsy requires that a set of special precautions be followed, as outlined by Brown (see references). Obviously such patients or any others known to have been demented should not be donors of organs for transplantation.

Gerstmann-Sträussler-Scheinker Syndrome This is a rare, strongly familial disease, inherited as an autosomal dominant trait. It begins insidiously in midlife and runs a chronic course (mean duration, 5 years). It is characterized clinically by a progressive cerebellar ataxia, corticospinal tract signs, dysarthria, and nystagmus. Dementia is often associated but is relatively mild. There are characteristic spongiform changes, as in SSE.

Brain tissue from patients with this disease, inoculated into chimpanzees, has produced a spongiform encephalopathy (Masters et al). Molecular genetic studies of affected members consistently demonstrate a mutation of the prion protein gene. This syndrome should be considered as a small familial subset of SSE of slowly progressive type.

Fatal Familial Insomnia This very rare familial disease is characterized by intractable insomnia, sympathetic overactivity, and dementia, leading to death in 7 to 15 months (see also page 414). The pathologic changes, consisting of neuronal loss and gliosis, are found mainly in the medial thalamic nuclei. Studies of a few families have shown a mutation of the prion protein gene, and brain material was found to contain the protease-resistant form of the gene. Transmission of the disease by inoculation of infected brain material has not been accomplished (Medori et al).

Kuru This disease, which occurs exclusively among the Fore linguistic group of natives of the New Guinea highlands, was the first slow infection, due to a nonconventional transmissible agent, to be documented in human beings. Clinically the disease takes the form of an afebrile, progressive cerebellar ataxia, with abnormalities of extraocular movements, weakness progressing to immobility, incontinence in the late stages, and death within 3 to 6 months of onset. The remarkable epidemiologic and pathologic similarities between kuru and scrapie were pointed out by Hadlow (1959), who suggested that it might be possible to transmit kuru to subhuman primates. This was accomplished in 1966 by Gajdusek and coworkers; inoculation of chimpanzees with brain material from affected humans produced a kuru-like syndrome in chimpanzees after a latency of 18 to 36 months. Since then the disease has been transmitted from one chimpanzee to another and to other primates by using both neural and nonneural tissues. Histologically there is a noninflammatory loss of neurons and spongiform change throughout the brain but predominantly in the cerebellar cortex, with astroglial proliferation and PAS-positive stellate plaques of amyloid-like material ("kuru plaques"). The transmissible agent has not been visualized, however.

Kuru has gradually disappeared, apparently because of the cessation of ritual cannibalism, by which the disease had been transmitted. In this ritual, infected tissue was ingested and rubbed over the body of the victim's kin (women and young children of either sex), permitting absorption of the infective agent through conjunctivae, mucous membranes, and abrasions in the skin.

REFERENCES

Adams H, Miller D: Herpes simplex encephalitis: A clinical and pathological analysis of twenty-two cases. *Postgrad Med J* 49:393, 1973.

Aicardi J, Gouthieres F, Arsenio-Nunes HL, Lebon P: Acute measles encephalitis in children with immunosuppression. *Pediatrics* 55:232, 1977.

Anderson NE, Willoughby EW: Chronic meningitis without predisposing illness—A review of 83 cases. *Q J Med* 63:283, 1987.

Anderson NE, Willoghby EW, Synek BK: Leptomeningeal and brain biopsy in chronic meningitis. *Aust N Z J Med* 26:703, 1995.

Anlar B, Saatçi I, Köse, et al: MRI finding in subacture sclerosing panencephalitis. *Neurology* 47:1278, 1996.

Åstrom KE, Mancall EL, Richardson EP Jr: Progressive multifocal leukoencephalopathy. *Brain* 81:93, 1958.

Aurelius E, Johansson B, Sköldenberg B, et al: Rapid diagnosis of herpes simplex encephalitis by nested polymerase chain reaction assay of cerebrospinal fluid. *Lancet* 337:189, 1991.

Barnett GH, Ropper AH, Romeo J: Intracranial pressure and outcome in adult encephalitis. *J Neurosurg* 68:585, 1988.

Beghi E, Nicolosi A, Kurland LT, et al: Encephalitis and aseptic meningitis, Olmstead County, Minnesota, 1950–1981: Epidemiology. *Ann Neurol* 16:283, 1984.

Bell JE: The neuropathology of adult HIV infection. *Rev Neurol* 154:816, 1998.

Bodian D: Histopathologic basis of clinical findings in poliomyelitis. *Am J Med* 6:563, 1949.

Brown P: Guidelines for high risk autopsy cases: Special precautions for Creutzfeldt-Jakob disease, in *Autopsy Performance and Reporting*. Northfield, IL, College of American Pathologists, 1990, chap 12, pp 67–74.

Brown P, Cathala F, Castaigne P, et al: Creutzfeldt-Jakob disease: Clinical analysis of a consecutive series of 230 neuropathologically verified cases. *Ann Neurol* 20:597,1986.

Brownell B, Oppenheimer DR: An ataxic form of subacute presenile polioencephalopathy (Creutzfeldt-Jakob disease). *J Neurol Neurosurg Psychiatry* 20:350, 1965.

Cathala F, Brown P, Chatelain J, et al: Maladie de Creutzfeldt-Jacob en France: Intérêt des formes familiales. *Presse Med* 15:379, 1986.

Charleston AJ, Anderson NE, Willoughby EW: Idiopathic steroid responsive chronic lymphocytic meningitis-Clinical features and long term outcome in 17 patients. *Aust N Z J Med* 28:784, 1998.

Chesebro B: BSE and prions: uncertainties about the agent. *Science* 279:42, 1998.

Chumakov M, Voroshilova M, Shindarov L, et al: Enterovirus 71 isolated from cases of epidemic poliomyelitis-like disease in Bulgaria. *Arch Virology* 60:329, 1979.

Cohen BA, Rowley AH, Long CM: Herpes simplex type 2 in a patient with Mollaret's meningitis: Demonstration by polymerase chain reaction. *Ann Neurol* 35:112, 1994.

Connolly AM, Dodson WE, Prensky AL, Rust RS: Cause and outcome of acute cerebellar ataxia. *Ann Neurol* 35:673, 1994.

Cornblath DR, McArthur JC, Kennedy PGE, et al: Inflammatory demyelinating peripheral neuropathies associated with human T-cell lymphotropic virus type III infection. *Ann Neurol* 21:32, 1987.

Davis LE, Johnson RT: An explanation for the localization of herpes simplex encephalitis. *Ann Neurol* 5:2, 1979.

Dawson JR: Cellular inclusions in cerebral lesions of epidemic encephalitis. *Arch Neurol Psychiatry* 31:685, 1934.

Denny-Brown D, Adams RD, Fitzgerald PJ: Pathologic features of herpes zoster: A note on "geniculate herpes." *Arch Neurol Psychiatry* 51:216, 1944.

Deresiewicz RL, Thaler SJ, Hsu L, et al: Clinical and neuroradiologic manifestations of eastern equine encephalitis. *N Engl J Med* 336:1867, 1997.

Devinsky O, Cho E-S, Petito CK, Price RW: Herpes zoster myelitis. *Brain* 114:1181, 1991.

Donat JF, Rhodes KH, Groover RV, et al: Etiology and outcome in 42 children with acute nonbacterial encephalitis. *Mayo Clin Proc* 55:156, 1980.

Drachman DA, Adams RD: Herpes simplex and acute inclusion-body encephalitis. *Arch Neurol* 7:45, 1962.

Dueland AN, Devlin M, Martin JR, et al: Fatal varicella-zoster virus meningoradiculitis without skin involvement. *Ann Neurol* 29:569, 1991.

Eidelberg D, Sotrel A, Vogel H, et al: Progressive polyradiculopathy in acquired immune deficiency syndrome. *Neurology* 36:912, 1986.

Enders JF, Weller TH, Robbins FC: Cultivation of Lansing strain of poliomyelitis virus in cultures of various human embryonic tissues. *Science* 109:85, 1949.

Epstein LG, Sharer LR, Choe S, et al: HTLV-III/LAV-like retrovirus particles in the brains of patients with AIDS encephalopathy. *AIDS Res* 1:447, 1985.

Esiri MM: Herpes simplex encephalitis: An immunohistological study of the distribution of viral antigen within the brain. *J Neurol Sci* 54:209, 1982.

Fauci AS, Lane HC: Human immunodeficiency virus (HIV) disease: AIDS and related disorders, in Braunwald E, et al (eds), *Harrison's Principles of Internal Medicine*, 2001, Chap. 309.

Fishbein DB, Robinson LE: Rabies. *N Engl J Med* 329:1632, 1993.

Gajdusek DC, Gibbs CJ Jr, Alpers M: Experimental transmission of a kuru-like syndrome to chimpanzees. *Nature* 209:794, 1966.

Gallo RC, Salahuddin SZ, Popovic M, et al: Frequent detection and isolation of cytopathic retroviruses (HTLV-III) from patients with AIDS and at risk for AIDS. *Science* 224:500, 1984.

Gessain A, Barin F, Vernant JC, et al: Antibodies to human T-lymphotropic virus type-I in patients with tropical spastic paraparesis. *Lancet* 2:407, 1985.

Gibbs CJ Jr, Gajdusek DC, Asher DM, Alpers MP: Creutzfeldt-Jakob disease (spongiform encephalopathy): Transmission to the chimpanzee. *Science* 161:388, 1968.

Gibbs CJ, Joy A, Heffner R, et al: Clinical and pathological features and laboratory confirmation of Creutzfeldt-Jakob disease in a recipient of pituitary derived growth hormone. *N Engl J Med* 313:734, 1985.

Gilden DH, Beinlich BR, Rubinstein EM, et al : Varicella-zoster virus myelitis: An expanding spectrum. *Neurology* 44:1818, 1994.

Gilden DH, Klein Schmidt-DeMasters BK, Laguardia JS, et al: Neurologic complications of the reactivation of varicella-zoster virus. *N Engl J Med* 342:635, 2000.

Gilden DH, Wright RR, Schneck SA, et al: Zoster sine herpete, a clinical variant. *Ann Neurol* 35: 530, 1994.

Hadlow WJ: Scrapie and kuru. *Lancet* 2:289, 1959.

Hall WW, Lamb RA, Choppin PW: Measles and SSPE virus proteins: Lack of antibodies to the M protein in patients with subacute sclerosing panencephalitis. *Proc Natl Acad Sci USA* 76:2047, 1979.

Heidenhain A: Klinische und anatomische Untersuchungen uber eine eigenartige organische Erkrankung des Zentralnervensystems im Praesenium. *Z Gesamte Neurol Psychiatry* 118:49, 1929.

Henson RA, Urich H: *Cancer and the Nervous System.* Oxford, Blackwell Scientific, 1982, pp 319–322.

Hill AF, Butterworth J, Joiner S, et al: Investigation of variant Creutzfeldt-Jakob disease and other human prion diseases with tonsil biopsy samples. *Lancet* 353:183, 1999.

Hilt DC, Buchholz D, Krumholz A, et al: Herpes zoster ophthalmicus and delayed contralateral hemiparesis caused by cerebral angiitis: Diagnosis and management approaches. *Ann Neurol* 14:543, 1983.

Hsich G, Kenney K, Gibbs CJ, et al: The 14-3-3 brain protein in cerebrospinal fluid as a marker for transmissable spongiform encephalopathies. *N Engl J Med* 335:924, 1996.

Holland NR, Power C, Mathews VP, et al: Cytomegalovirus encephalitis in acquired immunodeficiency syndrome (AIDS). *Neurology* 44:507, 1994.

Hope-Simpson RE: The nature of herpes zoster: A long-term study and a new hypothesis. *Proc R Soc Med* 58:9, 1965.

Howard RS, Lees AJ: Encephalitis lethargica: A report of four cases. *Brain* 110:19, 1987.

Huang CC, Liu CC, Chang YC, et al: Neurologic complications in children with enterovirus 71 infection. *N Engl J Med* 341:936, 2000.

Jeffery KJ, Read SJ, Petro TE, et al: Diagnosis of viral infections of the central nervous system: Clinical interpretation of PCR results. *Lancet* 349:313, 1997.

Jemsek J, Greenberg SB, Taber L, et al: Herpes zoster associated encephalitis: Clinicopathologic report of 12 cases and review of the literature. *Medicine* 62:81, 1983.

Johnson RT: Arboviral encephalitis, in Warren KS, Mahmoud AAF (eds): *Tropical and Geographical Medicine.* New York, McGraw-Hill, 1990, pp 691–699.

Johnson RT: Selective vulnerability of neural cells to viral infections. *Brain* 103:447, 1980.

Johnson RT: *Viral Infections of the Nervous System*, 2nd ed. Philadelphia, Lippincott-Raven, 1998.

Kalayjian RC, Coehn ML, Bonomo RA, et al: Cytomegalovirus ventriculoencephalitis in AIDS: A syndrome with distinct clinical and pathological features. *Medicine* 72:67, 1993.

King RB: Concerning the management of pain associated with herpes zoster and of post-herpetic neuralgia. *Pain* 33:73, 1988.

Lakeman FD, Whitley RJ, et al: Diagnosis of herpes simplex encephalitis: Application of polymerase chain reaction to cerebrospinal fluid from brain-biopsied patients and correlation with disease. *J Infect Dis* 171:857, 1995.

Linnemann CC Jr, Alvira MM: Pathogenesis of varicella-zoster angiitis in the CNS. *Arch Neurol* 37:239, 1980.

Mahalingam R, Wellis M, Wolf W, et al: Latent varicella-zoster viral DNA in human trigeminal and thoracic ganglia. *N Engl J Med* 323:627, 1990.

Masters CL, Gajdusek DC, Gibbs CJ Jr: Creutzfeldt-Jakob disease virus isolations from the Gerstmann-Sträussler syndrome. *Brain* 104:559, 1981.

Masters CL, Harris JO, Gajdusek C, et al: Creutzfeldt-Jakob disease: Patterns of worldwide occurrence and the significance of familial and sporadic clustering. *Ann Neurol* 5:177, 1979.

Mayo DR, Booss J: Varicella zoster-associated neurologic disease without skin lesions. *Arch Neurol* 46:313, 1989.

McKendrick MW, McGill JI, White JE, Wood MJ: Oral acyclovir in acute herpes zoster. *BMJ* 293:1529, 1986.

McKendrick MW, McGill JI, Wood MJ: Lack of effect of acyclovir on postherpetic neuralgia. *BMJ* 298:431, 1989.

Medori R, Tritschler HJ, LeBlanc A, et al: Fatal familial insomnia: A prion disease with a mutation at codon 178 of the prion protein gene. *N Engl J Med* 326:444, 1992.

Mehta PD, Patrick BA, Thormar H: Identification of virus-specific oligoclonal bands in subacute sclerosing panencephalitis by immunofixation after isoelectric focusing and peroxidase staining. *J Clin Microbiol* 16:985, 1982.

Murakami S, Mizobuchi M, Nakashiro Y, et al: Bell's palsy and herpes simplex virus: Identification of viral DNA in endoneural fluid and muscle. *Ann Intern Med* 124:27, 1996.

Navia BA, Chos E-S, Petito CK, et al: The AIDS dementia complex: II. Neuropathology. *Ann Neurol* 19:525, 1986.

Navia BA, Jordan BD, Price RW: The AIDS dementia complex: I. Clinical features. *Ann Neurol* 19:517, 1986.

Navia BA, Petito CK, Gold JWM, et al: Cerebral toxoplasmosis complicating the acquired immune deficiency syndrome: Clinical and neuropathological findings in 27 patients. *Ann Neurol* 19:224, 1986.

Navia BA, Price RW: The acquired immunodeficiency syndrome dementia complex as the presenting or sole manifestation of human immunodeficiency virus infection. *Arch Neurol* 44:65, 1987.

Padgett BL, Walker DL, ZuRhein GM, Eckroade RJ: Cultivation of papova-like virus from human brain with progressive multifocal leukoencephalopathy. *Lancet* 1:1257, 1971.

Peterslund NA: Herpes zoster associated encephalitis: Clinical findings and acyclovir treatment. *Scand J Infect Dis* 20:583, 1988.

Petito CK, Navia BA, Cho E-S, et al: Vacuolar myelopathy pathologically resembling subacute combined degeneration in patients with acquired immunodeficiency syndrome (AIDS). *N Engl J Med* 312:874, 1985.

Ponka A, Pettersson T: The incidence and aetiology of central nervous system infections in Helsinki in 1980. *Acta Neurol Scand* 66:529, 1982.

Price RW: Neurological complications of HIV infection. *Lancet* 348:445, 1996.

Prusiner SB: Genetic and infectious prion disease. *Arch Neurol* 50:1129, 1993.

Prusiner SB, Hsiao KK: Human prion disease. *Ann Neurol* 35:385, 1994.

Prusiner SB: Prion diseases and the BSE crisis. *Science* 278: 245,1997.

RENTIER B: Second International Conference on the varicella-zoster virus. *Neurology* 45(suppl 8), 1995.

RICHARDSON E: JR: Progressive multifocal leukoencephalopathy. *N Engl J Med* 265:815, 1961.

RODGERS-JOHNSON PE: Tropical spastic paraparesis HTLV-1 associated myelopathy: Etiology and clinical spectrum. *Mol Neurobiol* 8:175, 1994.

ROMAN GC, OSAME M: Identity of HTLV-I associated tropical spastic paraparesis and HTLV-I associated myelopathy. *Lancet* 1:651, 1988.

ROSENBLUM ML, LEVY RM, BREDESEN DE (eds): *AIDS and the Nervous System*. New York, Raven Press, 1988.

ROWLEY AH, WHITLEY RJ, LAKEMAN FD, WOLINSKY SM: Rapid detection of herpes-simplex-virus DNA in cerebrospinal fluid of patients with herpes simplex encephalitis. *Lancet* 335:440, 1990.

SCHWAB S, JUNGER E, SPRANGER M, et al: Craniectomy: An aggressive treatment approach in severe encephalitis. *Neurology* 48:413, 1997.

SELBY G, WALKER GL: Cerebral arteritis in cat-scratch fever. *Neurology* 29:1413, 1979.

SEVER JL: Persistent measles infection in the central nervous system. *Rev Infect Dis* 5:467, 1983.

SHARER LR: Pathology of HIV-1 infection of the central nervous system: A review. *J Neuropathol Exp Neurol* 51:3, 1992.

SIGURDSSON B: RIDA: A chronic encephalitis of sheep, with general remarks on infections which develop slowly and some of their special characteristics. *Br Vet J* 110:341, 1954.

SIMPSON DM, BENDER AN: HTLV-III associated myopathy (abstr). *Neurology* 37(suppl):319, 1987.

SKÖLDENBERG B, FORSGREN M, ALESTIG K, et al: Acyclovir versus vidarabine in herpes simplex encephalitis: Randomised multicentre study in consecutive Swedish patients. *Lancet* 2:707, 1984.

SMITH JE, AKSAMIT AJ: Outcome of chronic idiopathic meningitis. *Mayo Clin Proc* 69:548, 1994.

SNIDER WD, SIMPSON DM, NIELSEN S, et al: Neurological complications of acquired immune deficiency syndrome: Analysis of 50 patients. *Ann Neurol* 14:403, 1983.

SOLOMON J, DUNG NM, KNEEN R, et al: Japanese encephalitis. *J Neurol Neurosurg Psychiatry* 68:405, 2000.

STEEL JG, DIX RD, BARINGER JR: Isolation of herpes simplex virus type I in recurrent Mollaret meningitis. *Ann Neurol* 11:17, 1982.

TOWSEND JJ, BARINGER JR, WOLINSKY JS, et al: Progressive rubella panencephalitis: Late onset after congenital rubella. *N Engl J Med* 292:990, 1975.

TWYMAN RE, GAHRING LC, SPIESS J, ROGERS SW: Glutamate receptor antibodies activate a subset of receptors and reveal agonist binding sites. *Neuron* 14:755, 1995.

VON ECONOMO C: *Encephalitis Lethargica*. New York, Oxford University Press, 1931.

WADIA NH, KATRAK SM, MISRA VP, et al: Polio-like motor paralysis associated with acute hemorrhagic conjunctivitis in an outbreak in 1981 in Bombay, India: Clinical and serologic studies. *J Infect Dis* 147:660, 1983.

WEIL ML, ITABASHI HH, CREMER NE, et al: Chronic progressive panencephalitis due to rubella virus simulating subacute sclerosing panencephalitis. *N Engl J Med* 292:994, 1975.

WEISS S, GUBERMAN A: Acute cerebellar ataxia in infectious disease, in Vinken PJ, Bruyn GW (eds): *Handbook of Clinical Neurology*. Vol 34. Amsterdam, North-Holland, 1978, pp 619–639.

WELLER TH, WITTON HM, BELL EJ: Etiologic agents of varicella and herpes zoster. *J Exp Med* 108:843, 1958.

WHITLEY RJ: The frustrations of treating herpes simplex virus infections of the central nervous system. *JAMA* 259:1067, 1988.

WHITLEY RJ: Viral encephalitis. *N Engl J Med* 323:242, 1990.

WHITLEY RJ, ALFORD CA, HIRSCH MS, et al: Vidarabine versus acyclovir therapy in herpes simplex encephalitis. *N Engl J Med* 314:144, 1986.

WOLINSKY JS: Progressive rubella panencephalitis, in Vinken PJ, Bruyn GW (eds): *Handbook of Clinical Neurology*. Vol 34. Amsterdam, North-Holland, 1978, pp 331–342.

WOLINSKY JS, SWOVELAND P, JOHNSON KP, BARINGER JR: Subacute measles encephalitis complicating Hodgkin's disease in an adult. *Ann Neurol* 1:452, 1977.

WULFF EA, SIMPSON DM: Neuromuscular complications of the human immunodeficiency virus type 1 infection. *Semin Neurol* 19:157, 1999.

ZEIDLER M, STEWART GE, BARRACLOUGH CR, et al: New variant Creutzfeldt-Jakob disease: Neurological features and diagnostic tests. *Lancet* 350:903, 1997.

ZERR I, BODEMER M, OTTO M, et al: Diagnosis of Creutzfeldt-Jakob disease by two-dimensional gel electrophoresis of cerebrospinal fluid. *Lancet* 348:846, 1996.

ZURHEIN GM, GHOU SM: Particles resembling papova-viruses in human cerebral demyelinative disease. *Science* 148:1477, 1965.

Chapter 34

CEREBROVASCULAR DISEASES

Among all the neurologic diseases of adult life, the cerebrovascular ones clearly rank first in frequency and importance. At least 50 percent of the neurologic disorders in a general hospital are of this type. At some time or other, every physician will be required to examine patients with cerebrovascular disease and should at least know something of the common types—particularly those in which there is a reasonable prospect of successful medical or surgical intervention or the prevention of recurrence. There is another advantage to be gained from the study of this group of diseases—namely, that they have traditionally provided one of the most instructive approaches to neurology. As our colleague C. M. Fisher has aptly remarked, house officers and students learn neurology literally "stroke by stroke." Moreover, the focal ischemic lesion has divulged some of our most important ideas about the function of the human brain.

The last decade or two have witnessed a departure from the methodical clinicopathologic studies that have been the foundation of our understanding of cerebrovascular disease. Increasingly, randomized studies involving several hundred and even thousands of patients and conducted simultaneously in dozens of institutions have come to dominate investigative activity in this field. These multicenter trials have yielded highly valuable information about the natural history of a variety of cerebrovascular disorders, both symptomatic and asymptomatic. And many of these studies are providing guidance in the management of these disorders, notably in the use of anticoagulant drugs, antiplatelet agents, surgical measures, and, most recently, acute thrombolytic therapy. However, these trials suffer from a number of inherent weaknesses, the most important of which is that multicenter trials and the homogenized data derived from an aggregate of studies (metanalysis) are not necessarily applicable to a specific subgroup of patients or to a particular case at hand. Moreover, there are often inconsistencies in the results of studies designed to test the same premise, and many large studies show only marginal differences between treated and control groups—differences that would be changed by a slight alteration in the study design, or differences that, when translated into general practice, would have no real meaning for an individual patient. Furthermore, the results of these studies probably reflect the application of an improved system of clinical care rather than simply the effect of some tested drug. Each of these multicenter studies is therefore critically appraised at appropriate points in the ensuing discussion.

Incidence of Cerebrovascular Diseases

Stroke, after heart disease and cancer, is the third most common cause of death in the United States. Every year there are in this country approximately 500,000 cases of stroke—roughly 400,000 infarctions and 100,000 hemorrhages, intracerebral or subarachnoid—with 175,000 fatalities from these causes. Since 1950, coincident with the introduction of effective treatment for hypertension, there has been a significant reduction in the frequency of stroke. Among the residents of Rochester, Minnesota, Broderick and colleagues documented a reduction of 46 percent in cerebral infarction and hemorrhage when the period 1975–1979 was compared with 1950–1954; Nicholls and Johansen reported a 20 percent decline in the United States between 1968 and 1976. Both sexes shared in the reduced incidence. During this period, the incidence of coronary artery disease and malignant hypertension also fell significantly. By contrast, there has been no change in the frequency of aneurysmal rupture. Interestingly, despite the continued improvement in the treatment of hypertension, the incidence rate of stroke for the period 1980–1984 was 17 percent higher than that for 1975–1979, a feature attributed by Broderick and coworkers to the widespread use of computed tomography (CT), which increased the detection of less severe strokes.

Definition of Terms

The term *cerebrovascular disease* designates any abnormality of the brain resulting from a pathologic process of the blood vessels. *Pathologic process* is given an inclusive meaning—namely, occlusion of the lumen by embolism or thrombus, rupture of a vessel, any lesion or altered permeability of the vessel wall, and increased viscosity or other change in the quality of the blood. The pathologic process may be considered not only in its grosser aspects—embolism, thrombosis, dissection, or rupture of a vessel—but also in terms of the more basic or primary disorder, i.e., atherosclerosis, hypertensive arteriosclerotic change, arteritis, aneurysmal dilation, and developmental malformation. Equal importance attaches to the secondary parenchymal changes in the brain. These are of two main types—ischemia, with or without infarction, and hemorrhage—and unless one or the other occurs, the vascular lesion usually remains silent. The only exceptions to this statement are the local pressure effects of an aneurysm, vascular headache (migraine, hypertension, temporal arteritis), multiple small vessel disease with progressive encephalopathy (as in malignant hypertension or cerebral giant cell arteritis), and increased intracranial pressure (as occurs in hypertensive encephalopathy and venous sinus thrombosis). The many types of cerebrovascular diseases are listed in Table 34-1, and the predominant types during each period of life, in Table 34-2.

More than any other organ, the brain depends from minute to minute on an adequate supply of oxygenated blood. Constancy of the cerebral circulation is assured by a series of baroreceptors and vasomotor reflexes under the control of centers in the lower brainstem. In Stokes-Adams attacks, for example, unconsciousness occurs within 10 s of the beginning of asystole; in animal experiments, the complete stoppage of blood flow for longer than 4 to 5 min produces irreversible damage. Brain tissue deprived of blood undergoes *ischemic necrosis* or *infarction* (also referred to as a zone of *softening* or *encephalomalacia*). Obstruction of an artery by thrombus or embolus is the usual cause of focal ischemic damage, but failure of the circulation and hypotension from cardiac decompensation or shock, if severe and prolonged, can produce focal as well as diffuse ischemic changes.

Cerebral infarcts vary greatly in the amount of congestion and hemorrhage found within the softened tissue. Some infarcts are devoid of blood and therefore pallid (*pale infarction*); others show mild congestion (dilatation of blood vessels and escape of red blood cells), especially at their margins; still others show an extensive extravasation of blood from many small vessels in the infarcted tissue (red or *hemorrhagic infarction*). Some infarcts are all of one type, either pale or hemorrhagic; others are mixed. The reason for the occurrence of red infarction—almost always, it seems, in

Table 34-1
Causes of cerebral abnormalities from alterations of arteries and veins

1. Atherosclerotic thrombosis
2. Transient ischemic attacks
3. Embolism
4. Hypertensive hemorrhage
5. Ruptured or unruptured saccular aneurysm or AVM
6. Arteritis
   a. Meningovascular syphilis, arteritis secondary to pyogenic and tuberculous meningitis, rare infective types (typhus, schistosomiasis, malaria, mucormycosis, etc.)
   b. Connective tissue diseases (polyarteritis nodosa, lupus erythematosus), necrotizing arteritis. Wegener arteritis, temporal arteritis, Takayasu disease, granulomatous or giant-cell arteritis of the aorta, and giant-cell granulomatous angiitis of cerebral arteries
7. Cerebral thrombophlebitis: secondary to infection of ear, paranasal sinus, face, etc.; with meningitis and subdural empyema; debilitating states, postpartum, postoperative, cardiac failure, hematologic disease (polycythemia, sickle cell disease), and of undetermined cause
8. Hematologic disorders: anticoagulants and thrombolytics, clotting factor disorders, polycythemia, sickle cell disease, thrombotic thrombocytopenic purpura, thrombocytosis, intravascular lymphoma, etc.
9. Trauma and dissection of carotid and basilar arteries
10. Amyloid angiopathy
11. Dissecting aortic aneurysm
12. Complications of arteriography
13. Neurologic migraine with persistent deficit
14. With tentorial, foramen magnum, and subfalcial herniations
15. Miscellaneous types: fibromuscular dysplasia, with local dissection of carotid, middle cerebral, or vertebral-basilar artery, x-irradiation, unexplained middle cerebral infarction in closed head injury, pressure of unruptured saccular aneurysm, complication of oral contraceptives
16. Undetermined cause in children and young adults: moyamoya disease and others

Table 34-2
Cerebrovascular diseases characteristic of each age period

1. Prenatal circulatory diseases leading to
   a. Porencephaly
   b. Hydranencephaly
   c. Hypoxic-ischemic damage
   d. Unilateral cerebral infarction
2. Perinatal and postnatal circulatory disorders resulting in
   a. Cardiorespiratory failure and generalized ischemia—*état marbre*
   b. Periventricular infarcts
   c. Matrix hemorrhages and ischemic foci in premature infants
   d. Hemorrhagic disease of the newborn
3. Infancy and childhood: vascular diseases associated with
   a. Ischemic infarction
   b. Congenital heart disease and paradoxical embolism
   c. Moyamoya
   d. Bacterial endocarditis, rheumatic fever, lupus erythematosus
   e. Sickle cell anemia
   f. Mitochondrial disorders (MELAS)
   g. Homocystinuria and Fabry's angiokeratosis
4. Adolescence and early adult life: vascular occlusion or hemorrhage with
   a. Pregnancy and puerperium
   b. Estrogen-related stroke
   c. Migraine
   d. Vascular malformations
   e. Premature atherosclerosis
   f. Arteritis
   g. Valvular heart disease
   h. Sickle cell anemia
   i. Antiphospholipid arteriopathy, plasma C-protein deficiency, etc.
   j. Moyamoya, Takayasu disease
   k. Arterial dissections
   l. Amyloid angiopathy
5. Middle age
   a. Atherosclerotic thrombosis and embolism
   b. Cardiogenic embolism
   c. Primary (hypertensive) cerebral hemorrhage
   d. Ruptured saccular aneurysm
   e. Dissecting aneurysm
   f. Fibromuscular dysplasia
6. Late adult life
   a. Atherosclerotic thrombotic occlusive disease
   b. Embolic occlusive disease
   c. Lacunar state
   d. Brain hemorrhage (multiple causes)
   e. Multi-infarct dementia
   f. Binswanger disease

Source: Salam-Adams and Adams by permission.

cases of cerebral embolism—is not fully understood. The explanation most consistent with our observations is that embolic material, after occluding an artery and causing ischemic necrosis of brain tissue, then fragments and migrates distally from its original site. This allows at least partial restoration of the circulation to the infarcted zone, and blood seeps through the damaged small vessels (Fisher and Adams). In such cases, one usually cannot find the embolus by arteriography or postmortem examination, or one finds only a few fragments proximal to the pale ischemic zones.

In cerebral hemorrhage, blood leaks from the vessel (usually a small artery) directly into the brain, forming a hematoma in the brain substance and spreading into the ventricles and then to the subarachnoid space. Once the leakage is arrested, the blood slowly disintegrates and is absorbed over a period of weeks and months. The mass of clotted blood causes physical disruption of the tissue and pressure on the surrounding brain. Blood within the subarachnoid space, if large in quantity, may in addition cause cerebral ischemia through a mechanism of constriction of the vessels of the circle of Willis and their primary branches (vasospasm).

The Stroke Syndrome

So distinctive is the clinical presentation of cerebrovascular disease that the diagnosis is seldom in doubt. The common mode of expression is the *stroke*, defined as the sudden occurrence of a nonconvulsive, focal neurologic deficit. In its most severe form the patient becomes hemiplegic and even comatose—an event so dramatic that it has been given its own designations, namely *apoplexy*, *cerebrovascular accident (CVA)*, or shock (colloquial). However, *stroke* is the preferred term. In its mildest form it may consist of a trivial neurologic disorder insufficient even to demand medical attention. There are all gradations of severity between these two extremes, but in all forms of stroke the denotative feature is the *temporal profile* of neurologic events. It is the abruptness with which the neurologic deficit develops—a matter of seconds, minutes, hours, or at most a few days—that stamps the disorder as vascular. Embolic strokes characteristically occur suddenly, and the deficit reaches its peak almost at once. Thrombotic strokes may have a similarly abrupt onset, but many of them evolve somewhat more slowly over a period of several minutes or hours and occasionally days; in the latter case, the stroke usually progresses in a saltatory fashion, i.e., in a series of steps rather than smoothly. In hypertensive cerebral hemorrhage, the deficit, from the moment of onset, may be virtually static or, more often, is steadily progressive over a period of minutes or hours.

The other important aspect of the temporal profile is the arrest and then regression of the neurologic deficit in all except the fatal strokes. Not infrequently, an extensive deficit from embolism reverses itself dramatically within a few hours or days. More often, and this is the case in most thrombotic strokes, improvement occurs gradually over weeks and months, and the residual disability is considerable. A gradual downhill course over a period of several days or weeks will usually be traced to a nonvascular disease. The only exceptions are the additive effects of multiple vascular occlusions (platelet thrombosis, lupus erythematosus, and other arteritides; see Table 34-1) and the progressive brain edema surrounding large infarctions and cerebral hemorrhages.

The neurologic deficit reflects both the location and the size of the infarct or hemorrhage. Hemiplegia stands as the classic sign of all cerebrovascular diseases, whether in the cerebral hemisphere or brainstem, but there are many other manifestations as well, occurring in an almost infinite number of combinations. These include mental confusion, numbness and sensory deficits of many types, aphasia, visual field defects, diplopia, dizziness, dysarthria, and so forth. The neurovascular syndromes that they form enable the physician to locate the lesion—sometimes so precisely that the affected arterial branch can be specified—and to indicate whether the lesion is an infarct or a hemorrhage. The many neurovascular syndromes are described in the section that follows.

It would be incorrect to assume that every cerebrovascular illness expresses itself as a clearly delineated stroke. Some cerebrovascular lesions are clinically silent or cause disorders of function so mild as to concern the patient little if at all. Neither the patient nor the family can then date the onset of the illness. Other small incidents may become sources of complaint only when their cumulative effects become manifest. Sometimes, stenosis of the common or internal carotid or middle cerebral arteries results in a chronic marginally low blood flow, which, by fluctuating during physical activity, may diminish vision or induce a defect in sensory or motor function or an abnormality of movement. Another problem is that certain dominant hemispheric lesions cause aphasic disturbances, which hamper history taking, and nondominant ones cause anosognosia, in which the patient is unaware of his deficits or denies them—hence his descriptions are useless.

Imaging techniques for the demonstration of both the cerebral lesion and the affected blood vessel continue to enhance the clinical study of stroke patients. CT scanning demonstrates and accurately localizes small hemorrhages, hemorrhagic infarcts, subarachnoid blood, clots in and around aneurysms, regions of infarct necrosis, arteriovenous malformations, and ventricular deformities. Magnetic resonance imaging (MRI) also demonstrates these lesions and, in addition, reveals flow voids in vessels, hemosiderin and iron pigment, and the alterations resulting from ischemic necrosis and gliosis. Of the two procedures, MRI is particularly advantageous in demonstrating small lacunar lesions deep in the hemispheres and abnormalities in the posterior fossa (a region obscured by adjacent bone in CT scans), and in the early detection of an ischemic lesion (within minutes with special diffusion-weighted techniques, but more conventionally within hours)—i.e., considerably earlier than CT.

Other ancillary procedures for the investigation of cerebrovascular disease include Doppler ultrasound flow studies, which demonstrate atheromatous plaques and stenoses of large vessels, particularly of the carotid but also the vertebrobasilar arteries. The transcranial Doppler technique has reached a degree of precision whereby occlusion or spasm of the main vessels of the circle of Willis can be seen. Arteriography, now enhanced by digital processing of images, most accurately demonstrates stenoses and occlusions of the larger vessels as well as aneurysms, vascular malformations, and other blood vessel diseases such as arteritis. More and more, magnetic resonance angiography (MRA) and venography (MRV) are being used to visualize large intracranial arteries and veins; these have the advantage of safety but do not yet give refined images of the smaller vessels and are not as accurate as angiography in measuring the severity of stenosis of a vessel. New CT techniques called *spiral CT* offer images of better resolution, often comparable to conventional arteriograms. They have the additional benefit of demonstrating soft tissues and bone adjacent to these vessels, thus providing the surgeon with important anatomic information (see Chap. 2). Lumbar puncture indicates whether blood has entered the subarachnoid space (from aneurysm, vascular malformation, hypertensive hemorrhage, and some instances of hemorrhagic infarction). The cerebrospinal fluid (CSF) is clear in cases of "pale" infarction from thrombosis and embolism. In most stroke cases, the CT scan or MRI, neither of which entails any risk to the patient, precludes the need for lumbar puncture and conventional angiography.

The electroencephalogram (EEG) is probably underutilized as a readily available and inexpensive means of detecting cortical infarction in the wake of ischemia of a region of one hemisphere. It allows a distinction to be made between occlusion of a small and a large vessel because focal EEG abnormalities are sparse or absent with a deep lacunar stroke. The EEG is most useful soon after the stroke, when the available alternative is the CT scan, which often does not visualize the infarct until several days have passed.

Risk Factors

Several factors are known to increase the liability to stroke. The most important of these are hypertension, heart disease, atrial fibrillation, diabetes mellitus, cigarette smoking of long duration, and hyperlipidemia. Others, such as systemic diseases associated with a hypercoagulable state and the use of birth control pills, also contribute, but to a lesser degree. Hypertension is the most readily recognized factor in the genesis of primary intracerebral hemorrhage. Furthermore, it appears that the stroke-producing potential of hypertension is as much the product of heightened systolic pressure as of diastolic pressure (Fisher; Rabkin et al). The cooperative studies of the Veterans Administration (see Freis et al) and the report by Collins and associates (collating 14 randomized trials of antihypertensive drugs) have convincingly demonstrated that the long-term control of hypertension decreases the incidence of both atherothrombotic infarction and intracerebral hemorrhage. The presence of congestive heart failure and coronary atherosclerosis greatly increase the probability of stroke. As for embolic strokes, the most important risk factors are structural cardiac disease and arrhythmias, particularly atrial fibrillation. Bacterial and nonbacterial (marantic) endocarditis and right-to-left shunts between the cardiac chambers or in the lung also predispose to embolic stroke. Diabetes hastens the atherosclerotic process in both large and small arteries; Weinberger and colleagues and Roehmholdt and coworkers have found diabetic patients to be twice as liable to stroke as age-matched nondiabetic groups. Also, Homer and Ingall and their colleagues have documented the importance of long-duration cigarette smoking in the development of carotid atherosclerosis. The interactions between diabetes and hypertension on the one hand and intracerebral hemorrhage and atherothrombotic infarction on the other as well as the association of cardiac disease and cerebral embolism are considered further on in this chapter, in relation to each of these categories of cerebrovascular disease. Numerous clinical trials have shown a reduction in stroke incidence with the use of cholesterol-lowering drugs, and public health measures designed to detect and reduce the aforementioned risk factors provide the most intelligent long-range approach to the prevention of cerebrovascular disease.

The Ischemic Stroke

Focal cerebral ischemia differs from global ischemia. In the latter state, if absolute, there is no collateral flow and irreversible destruction of neurons occurs within 4 to 8 min at normal body temperature. In focal ischemia there is nearly always some degree of circulation (via collateral vessels), permitting to a varying extent the delivery of oxygenated blood and glucose, which cannot be properly metabolized under anaerobic conditions.

The effects of arterial occlusion on brain tissue vary depending upon the location of the occlusion in relation to available collateral and anastomotic channels. If the obstruction lies proximal to the circle of Willis (toward the heart), the anterior and posterior communicating arteries of the circle are often adequate to prevent infarction. In occlusion of the internal carotid artery in the neck, there may be retrograde anastomotic flow from the external carotid artery through the ophthalmic artery or via other smaller external-internal connections (Fig. 34-1). With blockage of the vertebral artery, the anastomotic flow may be via the deep cervical, thyrocervical, or occipital arteries or retrograde from the other vertebral artery. If the occlusion is in the stem portion of one of the cerebellar arteries or one of the cerebral arteries, i.e., distal to the circle of Willis, then a series of meningeal interarterial anastomoses may carry sufficient blood into the compromised territory to lessen (rarely to prevent) ischemic damage (see Figs. 34-1 and 34-2). There is also a capillary anastomotic system between adjacent arterial branches, and although it may reduce the size of the ischemic field, particularly of the penetrating arteries, it is usually not significant in preventing infarction. Thus, in the event of occlusion of a major arterial trunk, the extent of infarction ranges from none at all to the entire vascular territory of that vessel. Between these two extremes are all degrees of variation in the extent of infarction and its degree of completeness.

Additional *ischemia-modifying factors* determine the extent of necrosis. The speed of occlusion assumes importance; gradual narrowing of a vessel allows time for collateral channels to open. The level of blood pressure may influence the result; hypotension at a critical

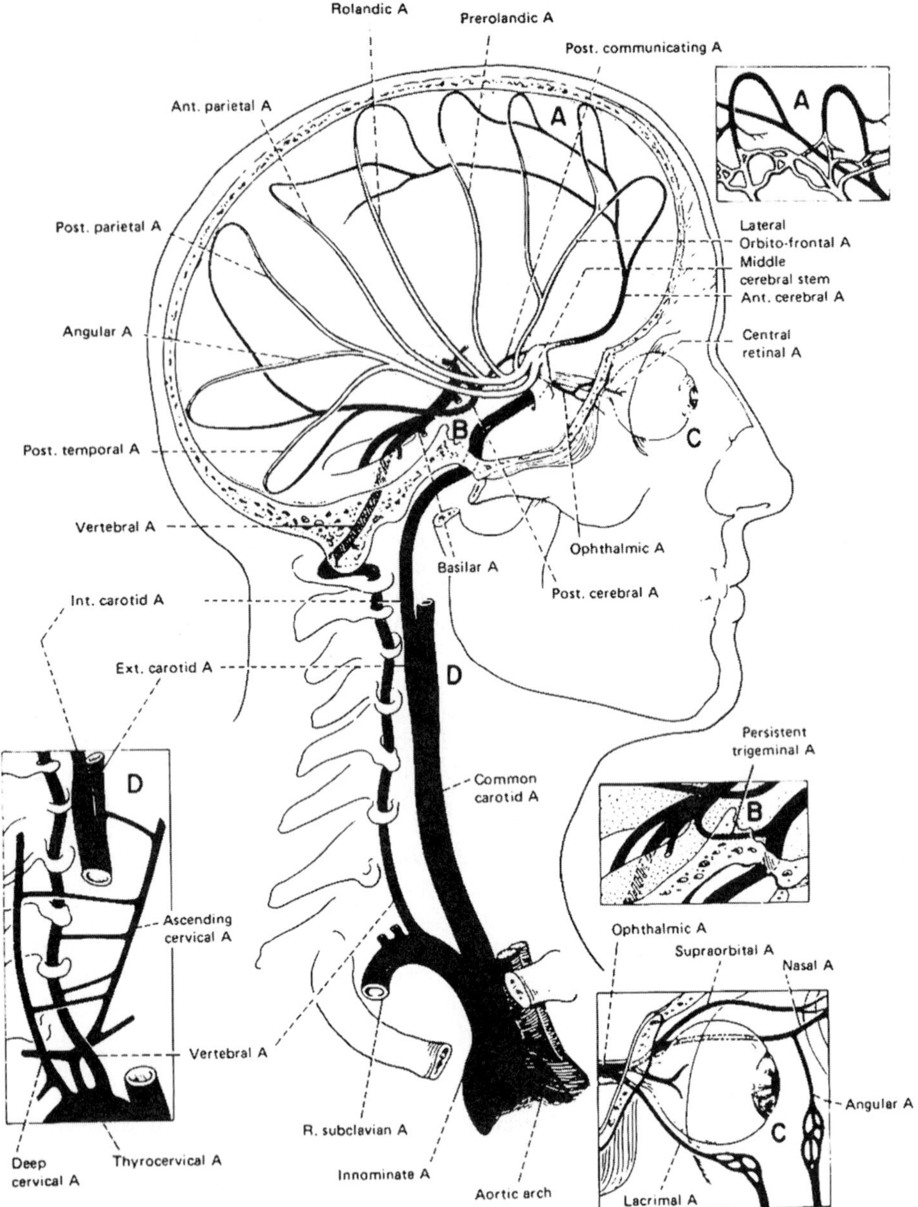

Figure 34-1

Arrangement of the major arteries on the right side carrying blood from the heart to the brain. Also shown are collateral vessels that may modify the effects of cerebral ischemia. For example, the posterior communicating artery connects the internal carotid and the posterior cerebral arteries and may provide anastomosis between the carotid and basilar systems. Over the convexity, the subarachnoid interarterial anastomoses linking the middle, anterior, and posterior cerebral arteries are shown, with insert A *illustrating that these anastomoses are a continuous network of tiny arteries forming a border zone between the major cerebral arterial territories. Occasionally a persistent trigeminal artery connects the internal carotid and basilar arteries proximal to the circle of Willis, as shown in insert* B. *Anastomoses between the internal and external carotid arteries via the orbit are illustrated in insert* C. *Wholly extracranial anastomoses from muscular branches of the cervical arteries to vertebral and external carotid arteries are indicated in insert* D.

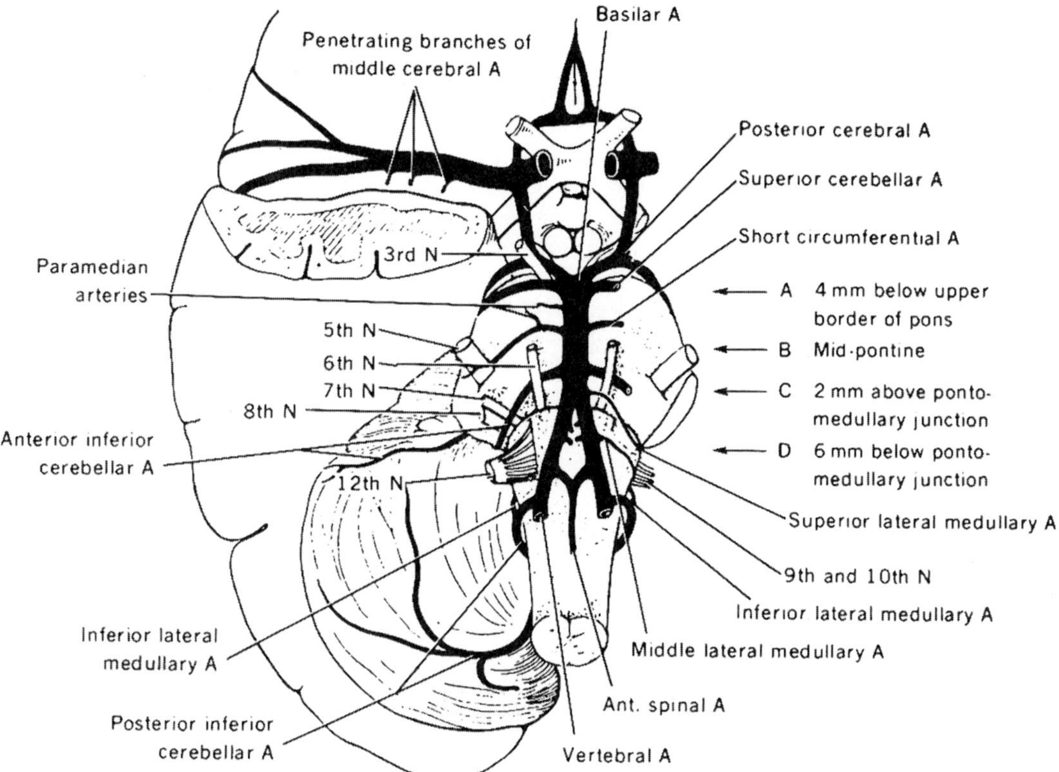

Figure 34-2

Diagram of the brainstem showing the principal vessels of the vertebral-basilar system. The letters and arrows on the right indicate the levels of the four cross sections following: A = *Fig. 34-15;* B = *Fig. 34-14;* C = *Fig. 34-13;* D = *Fig. 34-12.*

Although vascular syndromes of the pons and medulla have been designated by sharply outlined shaded areas, one must appreciate that since satisfactory clinicopathologic studies are scarce, the diagrams do not always represent established fact. The frequency with which infarcts fail to produce a well-recognized syndrome and the special tendency for syndromes to merge with one another must be emphasized.

moment may render anastomotic channels ineffective. Hypoxia and hypercapnia are presumed to have deleterious effects. Altered viscosity and osmolality of the blood and hyperglycemia are potentially important factors but difficult to evaluate. Finally, anomalies of vascular arrangement (of neck vessels, circle of Willis, and surface arteries) and the existence of previous vascular occlusions must influence the outcome.

The specific neurologic deficit obviously relates to the location and size of the infarct or focus of ischemia. The territory of any artery, large or small, deep or superficial, may be involved. When an infarct lies in the territory of a carotid artery, unilateral signs predominate, as would be expected: hemiplegia, hemianesthesia, hemianopia, aphasia, and agnosias of certain types are the usual consequences. In the territory of the basilar artery, the signs of infarction are frequently bilateral; quadriparesis, hemiparesis, and/or unilateral or bilateral sensory impairment occur in conjunction with cranial nerve palsies and other segmental brainstem or cerebellar signs.

Pathophysiology of Cerebral Ischemia and Ischemic Infarction

Cerebral infarction basically comprises two pathophysiologic processes—one, a loss in the supply of oxygen and glucose secondary to vascular occlusion, and two, an array of changes in cellular metabolism consequent upon the collapse of energy-producing processes, with disintegration of cell membranes. Of potential therapeutic importance are the observations that some of the cellular processes leading to neuronal death are not irrevocable and may be reversed by early intervention, either through restoration of blood flow or prevention of the influx of calcium into the cell.

As mentioned above, certain major vessels (carotid, vertebral, and less often a cerebral artery at its origin) can sometimes be occluded with little or no disturbance of neurologic function, and at autopsy there may be complete integrity of the tissue in the territory of the occluded vessel. Moreover, if infarction has occurred, it usually involves a zone that is smaller than the anatomic territory of supply of the artery in question. The margins of the infarct are hyperemic, being nourished by meningeal collaterals, and here there is only minimal or no parenchymal damage. The necrotic tissue swells rapidly, mainly because of excessive intracellular and intercellular water content. Since anoxia also causes necrosis and swelling of cerebral tissue (although in a different distribution), oxygen lack must be a factor common to both infarction and anoxic encephalopathy. Obviously the effects of ischemia, whether functional and reversible or structural and irreversible, depend on its degree and duration.

If the brain is observed at the time of arterial occlusion, the venous blood is first seen to darken, owing to an increase in reduced hemoglobin. The viscosity of the blood and resistance to flow both increase, and there is sludging of formed elements within vessels. The tissue becomes pale. Arteries and arterioles become narrowed, especially in the pale areas. Upon re-establishing flow in the occluded artery, the sequence is reversed and there may be a slight hyperemia. If the ischemia is prolonged, sludging and endothelial damage prevent normal reflow.

These flow factors have been studied in experimental animals by Heiss and by Siesjo and their colleagues and are reviewed in detail by Hossman. They have determined the critical threshold of cerebral blood flow (CBF), measured by xenon clearance, below which functional impairment occurs. In several animal species, including macaque monkeys and gerbils, the critical level was 23 mL/100 g per minute (normal 55 mL); if, after short periods of time, CBF was restored to levels above 23 mL, the impairment of function was reversed. Reduction of CBF below 10 to 12 mL/100 g per minute caused infarction, regardless of its duration. The critical level of hypoperfusion that abolishes function and leads to tissue damage is therefore a CBF between 12 and 23 mL/100 g per minute. At this level of blood flow the EEG was slowed, and below this level it was isoelectric. In the region of marginal perfusion ("ischemic penumbra"), the K level increased (efflux from injured depolarized cells) and the ATP and creatine phosphate were depleted, but these biochemical abnormalities were reversible if the circulation was restored to normal. Disturbance of calcium ion homeostasis and accumulation of free fatty acids interfered with full recovery. A CBF of 6 to 8 mL/100 g per minute with marked ATP depletion, increase in extracellular K, increase in intracellular Ca, and cellular acidosis was invariably associated with histologic signs of necrosis, though these did not become apparent for several hours. Free fatty acids (appearing as phospholipases) are activated and destroy the phospholipids of neuronal membranes. Prostaglandins, leukotrienes, and free radicals accumulate, and intracellular proteins and enzymes are denatured. Cells then swell (cellular edema; see page 681).

In the past decade, interest has focused on the role of excitatory neurotransmitters, particularly glutamate and aspartate, which are formed from glycolytic intermediates of the Krebs cycle. It has been found that these neurotransmitters, released by ischemic cells, excite neurons and produce an intracellular influx of Na and Ca. These changes are said to be responsible for irreversible cell injury. This is presently a subject of active biochemical and clinical research. Most of the current attempts at therapy are directed at limiting the extent of infarction by utilizing blockers of a particular glutamate receptor, the NMDA (*N*-methyl-D-aspartate) channel—one of several calcium channels that open under conditions of ischemia and set in motion a cascade of cellular events, eventuating in neuronal death. However, even complete blockade of the NMDA channels has so far not prevented cellular death, presumably because dysfunction of several other types of calcium channels continues. Novel strategies have been suggested to prevent calcium influx, but the drugs that block the various calcium channels seem to work only if given before the stroke, making them impractical clinically except perhaps in preventing a stroke that might follow cardiac or carotid surgery. Furthermore, with profound ischemic damage, the cell membranes may be disrupted acutely and the neurons cannot be salvaged. There is evidence that additional biochemical events are induced by ischemia, including the production of free radicals, which leads to peroxidation and disruption of the outer cell membrane.

The accumulation of lactic acid in cerebral tissue (and the biochemical changes consequent to the cellular acidosis) may also be of importance in determining the extent of cell damage (see reviews of Raichle and of Plum). Myers and Yamaguchi showed that monkeys infused with glucose before the induction of cardiac arrest suffered more brain damage than did either fasted or saline-infused animals. They suggested that the high cerebral glucose level under anaerobic conditions led to increased glycolysis during the ischemic episode and that the accumulated lactate was neurotoxic. On the basis of such observations, Plum has suggested that scrupulous control of the blood glucose might reduce the risk of cerebral infarction in diabetic and other stroke-prone patients and during conditions of potential hyperglycemia. Clinical implementation of this idea is difficult and its advantages remain to be established.

Morphologic changes may also occur in the ischemic penumbra. In this partially ischemic region (CBF between 12 and 23 mL/100 g per minute), the critical factor is not a particular CBF value but the duration of the ischemia in combination with the residual flow and perhaps other factors. The curve expressing the two functions—the CBF and the duration of ischemia—tends toward infinity at 18 mL/100 g per minute. Also of interest is the fact that not all neurons in marginally necrotic areas are destroyed. Some survive and later undergo degeneration. These differences in vulnerability are not understood.

Olsen and colleagues have studied CBF in patients with middle cerebral artery occlusion; they confirmed the presence of hypoperfusion in zones shown by CT scan to be infarcted and of hyperperfusion in the border zones. In some hypoperfused regions in patients with impaired function, the blood flow measurements fell in the ischemic penumbra. "Steal" phenomena from surrounding normal brain, claimed to occur in response to CO_2 inhalation in cases of infarction, was not demonstrable. Blood flow through collaterals was increased when CO_2 was inhaled and the systolic blood pressure was raised by 30 to 40 mm.

Ames and Nesbett have studied the rabbit retina in an immersion chamber in which O_2 and various substrates could be altered directly rather than through the vasculature. They found that cells could withstand complete absence of O_2 for 20 min. After 30 min of anoxia, there was extensive irreversible damage, reflected by an inability of the tissue to utilize glucose and to synthesize protein. Hypoglycemia further reduced the tolerance to hypoxia, whereas the tolerance could be prolonged by reducing the energy requirements of cells (increasing Mg in the medium). Ames suggested that the long period of tolerance of retinal neurons to complete ischemia in vitro, in comparison to that in vivo, is related to what he has called the no-reflow phenomenon (swelling of capillary endothelial cells, which prevents the restoration of circulation). Body temperature is yet another important factor. A reduction of even 2 to 3°C, by reducing the metabolic requirements of neurons, increases their tolerance to hypoxia by 25 to 30 percent.

The relevance to stroke of these biochemical, cellular, and cerebral blood flow findings relates to the possibility of salvaging brain tissue by maintaining blood flow within the marginally hypoperfused zone. In fact, we know that under conditions of partial ischemia, cerebral tissue may survive for periods of 5 to 6 h or even longer.

NEUROVASCULAR SYNDROMES

For reasons already given, the clinical picture that results from an occlusion of any one artery differs in minor ways from one patient to another. There is sufficient uniformity, however, to justify the assignment of a typical syndrome to each of the major arteries. The following descriptions apply particularly to the clinical effects of ischemia and infarction due to embolism and thrombosis. Although hemorrhage within a specific vascular territory may give rise to many of the same effects, the total clinical picture is different because it usually involves the territory of more than one artery and, by its deep extension and pressure effects, causes secondary features of headache, vomiting, and hypertension as well as a series of falsely localizing signs, as described in Chaps. 17 and 31.

The Carotid Artery

The carotid system consists of three major arteries—the common carotid, internal carotid, and external carotid. As indicated in Fig. 34-1, the right common carotid artery arises at the level of the sternoclavicular notch from the innominate (brachiocephalic) artery, and the left common carotid stems directly from the aortic arch. The common carotids ascend in the neck to the C4 level, just below the angle of the jaw, where each divides into external and internal branches (sometimes the bifurcation is slightly above or below this point).

Common carotid occlusion accounts for less than 1 percent of cases of carotid artery syndrome—the remainder being due to disease of the internal carotid artery itself. Nevertheless, the common carotid can be occluded by an atheromatous plaque at its origin, more often on the left side. Atherosclerotic stenosis or occlusion of the midportion of the common carotid may also occur years after radiation therapy for laryngeal or other head and neck cancer. If the bifurcation is patent, few if any symptoms result, in some cases because retrograde flow from the external carotid maintains internal carotid flow and perfusion of the brain. Because the syndromes caused by common carotid occlusion are identical to those of its internal branch, the remainder of this discussion is concerned with disease of the *internal carotid artery*. The territory supplied by this vessel and its main branches is shown in Figs. 34-3, 34-4, and 34-5. The clinical manifestations of atherosclerotic thrombotic disease of this artery are the most variable of any cerebrovascular syndrome. Unlike other cerebral vessels, the internal carotid artery is not an end vessel, by virtue of its continuity with the vessels of the circle of Willis and those of the orbit, and no part of the brain is completely dependent on it. Therefore occlusion, which occurs most frequently in the first part of the internal carotid artery (immediately beyond the carotid bifurcation), is often silent (30 to 40 percent of cases).

There are two mechanisms by which strokes arise from thrombotic occlusion of the internal carotid artery. First, an embolus arising from the thrombus may cause a stroke in the territory of any of the tributary vessels of the internal carotid artery (middle and anterior cerebral arteries and their branches, as described further on). This has been termed "artery-to-artery" embolism. Second, occlusion of the carotid artery may lead to ischemia in the distal field (watershed or border zone) in the region of lowest perfusion between major branch vessels. Failure of distal perfusion may involve all or part of the middle cerebral territory; when the anterior communicating artery is very small, the ipsilateral anterior cerebral territory is affected as well. In extreme instances where the circle of Willis provides no communication to the side of an occluded carotid artery, thus isolating the hemisphere from other blood flow, massive infarction may result,

Figure 34-3

*Diagram of a cerebral hemisphere, lateral aspect, showing the branches and distribution of the **middle cerebral artery** and the principal regions of cerebral localization. Below is a list of the clinical manifestations of infarction in the territory of this artery and the corresponding regions of cerebral damage. (Continued on the facing page.)*

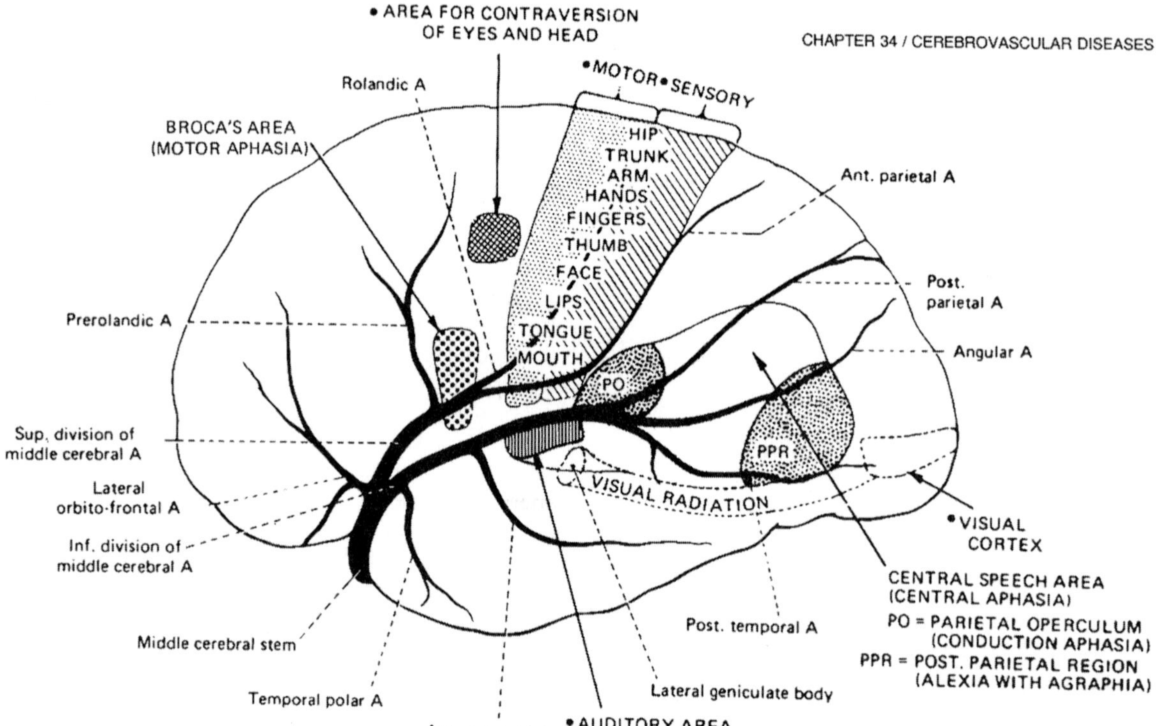

Figure 34-3 (*continued*)

Signs and symptoms	*Structures involved*
Paralysis of the contralateral face, arm, and leg	Somatic motor area for face and arm and the fibers descending from the leg area to enter the corona radiata
Sensory impairment over the contralateral face, arm, and leg (pinprick, cotton touch, vibration, position, two-point discrimination, stereognosis, tactile localization, baragnosis, cutaneographia)	Somatosensory area for face and arm and thalamoparietal projections
Motor speech disorder	Broca and adjacent motor area of the *dominant* hemisphere
"Central" aphasia, word deafness, anomia, jargon speech, alexia, agraphia, acalculia, finger agnosia, right-left confusion (the last four comprise the Gerstmann syndrome)	Central language area and parieto-occipital cortex of the *dominant* hemisphere
Apractagnosia (amorphosynthesis), anosognosia, hemiasomatognosia, unilateral neglect, agnosia for the left half of external space, "dressing apraxia," "constructional apraxia," distortion of visual coordinates, inaccurate localization in the half field, impaired ability to judge distance, upside-down reading, visual illusions	Usually *nondominant* parietal lobe. Loss of topographic memory is usually due to a nondominant lesion, occasionally to a dominant one
Homonymous hemianopia (often superior homonymous quadrantanopia)	Optic radiation deep to second temporal convolution
Paralysis of conjugate gaze to the opposite side	Frontal contraversive field or fibers projecting therefrom
Avoidance reaction of opposite limbs	Parietal lobe
Miscellaneous:	
Ataxia of contralateral limb(s)	Parietal lobe
So-called Bruns ataxia or apraxia of gait	Frontal lobes (bilateral)
Loss or impairment of optokinetic nystagmus	Supramarginal gyrus or inferior parietal lobe
Limb-kinetic apraxia	Premotor or parietal cortical damage
Mirror movements	Precise location of responsible lesions not known
Cheyne-Stokes respiration, contralateral hyperhidrosis, mydriasis (occasionally)	Precise location of responsible lesions not known
Pure motor hemiplegia	Upper portion of the posterior limb of the internal capsule and the adjacent corona radiata

involving the anterior two-thirds or all of the cerebral hemisphere, including the basal ganglia. If the two anterior cerebral arteries arise from a common stem on one side, infarction may occur in the territories of both vessels. The territory supplied by the posterior cerebral artery will also be included in the infarction when this vessel is supplied by the internal carotid rather than the basilar artery (a residual fetal configuration of the origin of the posterior cerebral artery). If one internal carotid artery was occluded at an earlier time, occlusion of the other may cause bilateral cerebral infarction. The clinical effects in such cases may include coma with quadriplegia and continuous horizontal "metronomic" conjugate eye movements.

Occlusion of the intracranial portion of the internal carotid artery—for example by an embolus to its distal part—produces a clinical picture like that of middle cerebral artery occlusion: contralateral hemiplegia,

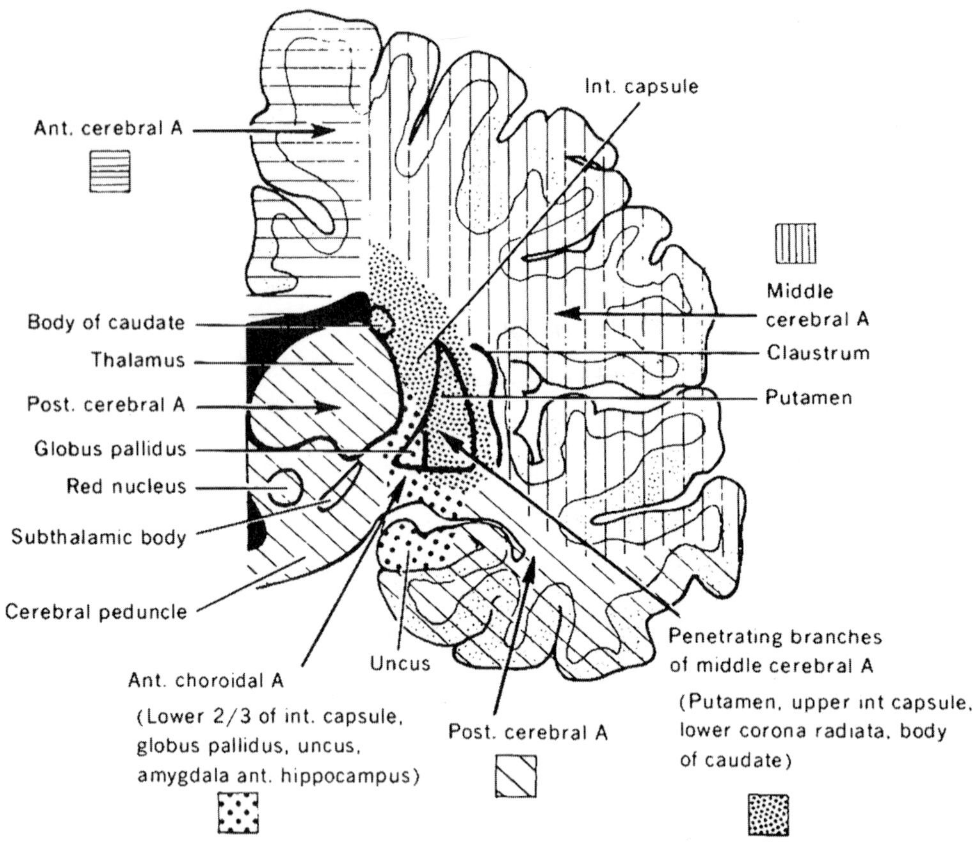

Figure 34-4

Diagram of a cerebral hemisphere, coronal section, showing the territories of the major cerebral vessels.

hemihypesthesia, and aphasia (with involvement of the dominant hemisphere). When the anterior cerebral territory is included, there will be added some or all of the clinical features of the latter (see further on). Patients with such large infarctions are usually immediately drowsy or stuporous because of an ill-defined effect on the reticular activating system. Headache—located, as a rule, above the eyebrow—may occur with thrombosis or embolism of the carotid artery. The headache associated with occlusion of the middle cerebral artery tends to be more lateral, at the temple; that of posterior cerebral occlusion is in or behind the eye.

When the circulation of one carotid artery has been compromised, reducing blood flow in both the middle and anterior cerebral territories, the zone of maximal ischemia lies between the two vascular territories ("cortical watershed") or, alternatively, in the deep portions of the hemisphere, between the territories of the lenticulostriate branches and the penetrating vessels from the convexity ("internal or deep watershed"). The infarction in the first instance occupies a region in the high parietal and frontal cortex and subcortical white matter. Its size depends upon the adequacy of collateral vessels. The weakness that results tends to involve the shoulder and hip more than the hand and face. With long-standing carotid stenosis, the cortical watershed zone tends to shift downward toward the perisylvian portions of the middle cerebral artery territory, even to the extent of affecting facial movement or causing a motor aphasia. The frequent sparing of the posterior part of the hemisphere is reflected in the low incidence of Wernicke types of aphasia and of persistent homonymous hemianopia. With impaired perfusion of the so-called internal watershed, infarctions of varying size are situated in the subfrontal and subparietal portions of the centrum semiovale.

The situation is somewhat different in cases of circulatory collapse, usually from cardiac arrest, in which perfusion fails not only in the watershed areas between

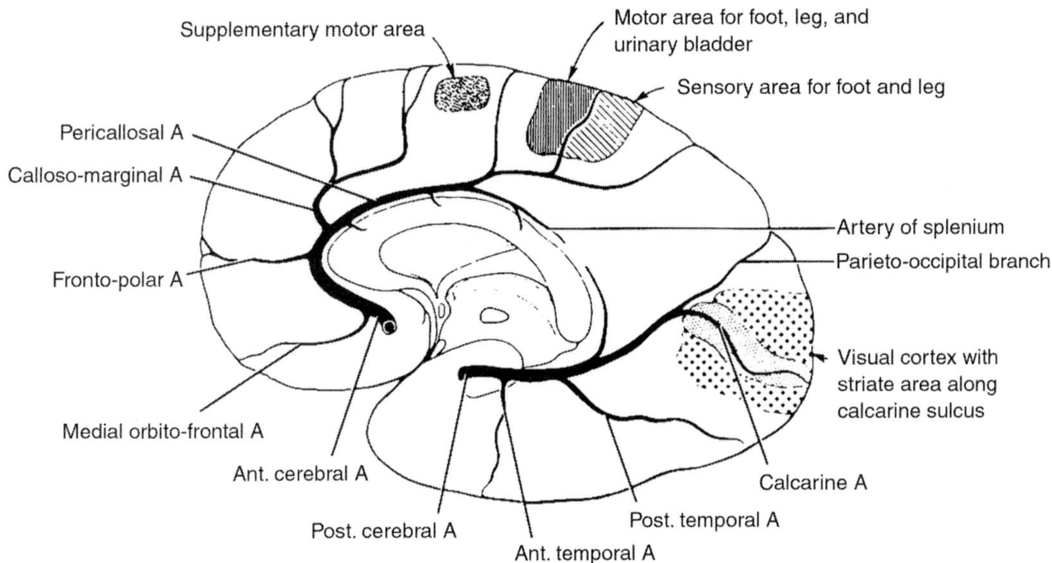

Figure 34-5

*Diagram of a cerebral hemisphere, medial aspect, showing the branches and distribution of the **anterior cerebral artery** and the principal regions of cerebral localization. Below is a list of the clinical manifestations of infarction in the territory of this artery and the corresponding regions of cerebral damage.*

Signs and symptoms	*Structures involved*
Paralysis of opposite foot and leg	Motor leg area
A lesser degree of paresis of opposite arm	Involvement of arm area of cortex or fibers descending therefrom to corona radiata
Cortical sensory loss over toes, foot, and leg	Sensory area for foot and leg
Urinary incontinence	Posteromedial part of superior frontal gyrus (bilateral)
Contralateral grasp reflex, sucking reflex, gegenhalten (paratonic rigidity), "frontal tremor"	Medial surface of the posterior frontal lobe (?)
Abulia (akinetic mutism), slowness, delay, lack of spontaneity, whispering, motor inaction, reflex distraction to sights and sounds	Uncertain localization—probably superomedial lesion near subcallosum
Impairment of gait and stance (gait "apraxia")	Inferomedial frontal–striatal (?)
Mental impairment (perseveration and amnesia)	Localization unknown
Miscellaneous: dyspraxia of left limbs	Corpus callosum
Tactile aphasia in left limbs	Corpus callosum
Cerebral paraplegia	Motor leg area bilaterally (due to bilateral occlusion of anterior cerebral arteries)

Note: Hemianopia does not occur; transcortical aphasia occurs rarely (page 512).

the middle and anterior cerebral arteries but also between the middle and posterior cerebral arteries. The infarction is then situated within a zone that extends as a sickle-shaped strip of variable width from the cortical convexity of the frontal lobe, through the high parietal lobe, to the occipitoparietal junction. Deeper infarctions also occur, but they more often take the form of contiguous extensions of the cortical infarction into the subjacent white matter. Also there may, on occasion, appear to be two or more separate infarctions after hypoperfusion states, but these turn out to be radiographically visible portions of a larger border-zone lesion.

The internal carotid artery nourishes the optic nerve and retina as well as the brain. *Transient monocular blindness* occurs as an intermittent symptom prior to the onset of stroke in 10 to 25 percent of cases of symptomatic carotid occlusion. Yet central retinal artery ischemia is a relatively rare manifestation of carotid artery occlusion, presumably because of efficient collateral supply.

Whereas most cerebral arteries can be evaluated only indirectly, by analysis of the clinical effects of occlusion, more direct means are available for the evaluation of the common and internal carotid arteries in the neck. With severe atherosclerotic stenosis at the level of the carotid sinus, with or without a superimposed thrombus, auscultation frequently discloses a *bruit*, best heard with the bell of the stethoscope. Occasionally the bruit is due to stenosis at the origin of the external carotid artery or is a radiated murmur from the aortic valve and can then be misleading. If the bruit is heard at the angle of the jaw, the stenosis usually lies in the carotid sinus; if heard lower in the neck, it is in the common carotid or subclavian artery. The duration and quality of the bruit are important—bruits that extend into diastole and are high-pitched are almost invariably associated with a tight stenosis (lumen < 1.5 mm). An additional though infrequent sign of carotid occlusion is the presence of a bruit over the opposite carotid artery, heard best by placing the bell of the stethoscope over the eyeball; presumably this murmur is due to augmented circulation through the patent vessel. Pulsation may be palpably reduced or absent in the common carotid artery in the neck, in the external carotid artery in front of the ear, and in the internal carotid artery in the lateral wall of the pharynx, but these are among the least dependable signs of carotid disease. In the presence of a unilateral internal carotid occlusion, compression of the normal common carotid should be avoided because it may precipitate neurologic symptoms. *Central retinal artery pressure* is reduced on the side of a carotid occlusion or severe stenosis, and this can be appreciated by gentle pressure on the globe while viewing the vessels emanating from the optic nerve head. A diastolic retinal pressure (determined by ophthalmic dynamometry) of less than 20 mmHg usually means that the common or internal carotid artery is occluded. These and other tests for measuring carotid flow have been largely supplanted by direct insonation or MRI imaging of the carotid artery.

The occurrence of *emboli* within retinal arteries, either shiny white or reddish in appearance, is another important sign of carotid disease (crystalline cholesterol may be sloughed from an atheromatous ulcer).

Other signs of carotid occlusion include pulseless arms (as in Takayasu disease, see page 908); faintness on arising from the horizontal position or recurrent loss of consciousness when walking; headache and sometimes ocular, retro-orbital, and neck pain; transient blindness, either unilateral or bilateral; unilateral visual loss or dimness of vision with exercise, after exposure to bright light, or on assuming an upright position; retinal atrophy and pigmentation; atrophy of the iris; heterochromia of the iris (differing coloration on the two sides), which is a sign of carotid occlusion early in life; leukomas (corneal scars); peripapillary arteriovenous anastomoses in the retinae; optic atrophy; and claudication of jaw muscles.

Stenoses, ulcerations, and dissections of the internal carotid artery near its origin from the common carotid artery (the bulb, or sinus) may be a source of fibrin platelet emboli or may cause a reduction in blood flow, resulting in transient ischemic attacks (TIAs). These are fully discussed further on, but here it can be stated that severe stenosis of the vessel represents an important risk factor for stroke.

Middle Cerebral Artery

This artery, through its *cortical branches*, supplies the lateral part of the cerebral hemisphere (Fig. 34-3). Its territory encompasses (1) cortex and white matter of the lateral and inferior parts of the frontal lobe—including motor areas 4 and 6, contraversive centers for lateral gaze—and motor speech area of Broca (dominant hemisphere); (2) cortex and white matter of the parietal lobe, including the sensory cortex and the angular and supramarginal convolutions; and (3) superior parts of the temporal lobe and insula, including the sensory language areas of Wernicke. The *penetrating branches* of the middle cerebral artery supply the putamen, part of the head and body of the caudate nucleus, the outer globus pallidus, the posterior limb of the internal capsule, and the corona radiata (Fig. 34-4). The size of both the middle cerebral artery and the territory that it supplies is larger than those of the anterior and posterior cerebral arteries.

The middle cerebral artery may be occluded in its stem, blocking the flow in deep penetrating as well as superficial cortical branches, or the two divisions in the sylvian sulcus and their major branches may be occluded separately. The classic picture of total occlusion of the stem is contralateral hemiplegia (face, arm, and leg), hemianesthesia, and homonymous hemianopia (due to infarction of the lateral geniculate body), with deviation of the head and eyes toward the side of the lesion; in addition, there is a global aphasia with left hemispheric lesions and anosognosia and amorphosynthesis with right-sided ones (see page 484). In the beginning the patient is dull or stuporous because of an ill-defined effect of widespread paralysis of function. Once fully established, the motor, sensory, and language deficits remain static or improve very little as months and years pass. If the patient is globally aphasic for a prolonged period of time, he seldom ever again communicates effectively. Occlusion of branches of the middle cerebral artery gives rise to only parts of the symptom complex.

Occlusion of the stem of the middle cerebral artery by a thrombus, contrary to conventional teaching, is relatively infrequent (2 to 5 percent of middle cerebral artery occlusions). Pathologic studies have shown that most carotid occlusions are thrombotic, whereas most middle cerebral occlusions are embolic (Fisher, 1975; Caplan, 1989). The emboli tend to drift into superficial cortical branches; not more than 1 in 20 will enter deep penetrating branches. As indicated earlier, the distal territory of the middle cerebral artery may also be rendered ischemic by failure of the systemic circulation, especially if the carotid artery is stenotic; this may simulate embolic branch occlusions.

An embolus entering the middle cerebral artery most often lodges in one of its two main divisions, the superior division (supplying the rolandic and prerolandic areas) or the inferior division (supplying the lateral temporal and inferior parietal lobes). Major infarction in the territory of the *superior division* causes a dense sensorimotor deficit in the contralateral face, arm, and, to a lesser extent, leg as well as ipsilateral deviation of the head and eyes; i.e., it mimics the syndrome of stem occlusion except that the foot is spared and the leg is less involved than the arm and face ("brachiofacial paralysis"); there is no impairment of alertness. If the occlusion is lasting (not merely transient ischemia with disintegration of the embolus), there will be slow improvement; after a few months, the patient will be able to walk with a spastic leg, while the motor deficits of the arm and face remain. The sensory deficit may be profound, resembling that of a thalamic infarct (pseudothalamic syndrome of Foix), but more often it is less severe than the motor deficit, taking the form of stereoanesthesia, agraphesthesia, impaired position sense, tactile localization, and two-point discrimination as well as variable changes in touch, pain, and temperature sense. A rare pseudoradicular pattern of sensory loss in the hand and forearm (radial or ulnar half) from a parietal infarct was originally described by Déjerine. With left-sided lesions there may initially be a global aphasia, which changes gradually to a predominantly motor (Broca) aphasia, with improvement in comprehension of spoken and written words and the emergence of an effortful, hesitant, grammatically simplified, and dysmelodic speech (Chap. 23).

Embolic occlusion limited to one of the *branches of the superior division* produces a more circumscribed infarct that further fractionates the syndrome. With occlusion of the ascending frontal branch, the motor deficit is limited to the face and arm with little affection of the leg, and the latter, if weakened at all, soon improves; with left-sided lesions, an initial mutism and mild comprehension defect give way, within days to weeks, to slightly dysfluent and agrammatic speech, with normal comprehension (page 505). Embolic occlusion of the rolandic branches results in sensorimotor paresis with severe dysarthria but little evidence of aphasia. A cortical-subcortical branch occlusion may give rise to a brachial monoplegia. Embolic occlusion of ascending parietal and other posterior branches of the superior division may cause no sensorimotor deficit but only a conduction aphasia (page 510) and bilateral ideomotor apraxia. There are many other limited stroke syndromes or combinations of the aforementioned syndromes relating to small regions of damage in the frontal, parietal, or temporal lobes. Most of these are discussed in Chap. 22, on lesions in particular parts of the cerebrum. Improvement can be expected within a few weeks to months.

Occlusion of the *inferior division* of the middle cerebral artery is less frequent than occlusion of the superior one, but again is nearly always due to cardiogenic embolism. The usual result in left-sided lesions is a Wernicke aphasia which generally remains static for weeks or a month or two, after which some improvement can be expected (page 509). In less extensive infarcts from branch occlusions (superior parietal, angular, or posterior temporal), the deficit in comprehension of spoken and written language may be especially severe. Again, after a few months, the deficits usually improve, often to the point where they are evident only in self-generated efforts to read and copy visually presented words or phrases. With either right- or left-hemispheric lesions, there is usually a superior quadrantanopia or homonymous hemianopia and, with right-sided ones, a left visual neglect and other signs of amorphosynthesis; rarely, an agitated confusional state, presumably from temporal lobe damage, may be a prominent feature of dominant hemispheral lesions and sometimes of nondominant ones as well.

Deep (Striatocapsular) Infarctions A number of interesting syndromes occur with deep lesions in the territory of the penetrating vessels of the middle cerebral artery. Most are attributable to emboli from stem occlusions of the middle cerebral artery, although imaging studies show a patent vessel in half of the cases; a few are presumably atherothrombotic, but these judgments have been made from an analysis of imaging, not pathologic studies. Although centered in the deep white matter, most of these lesions are fragments of the cortical-subcortical stroke patterns described above. The most common type in our experience has been a large *striatocapsular infarction*, similar to that described by Weller and colleagues. Of their 29 patients, all had some degree of hemiparesis and 6 had aphasia or hemineglect. Aphasia, when it occurs, tends to be a limited form of the Broca type or anomia and, in our experience, has been short-lived. We have most often encountered incomplete pure motor syndromes affecting only the arm and hand without language disturbance or neglect; these are quite difficult to differentiate from small embolic cortical strokes. The lesions in the corona radiata are larger than typical lacunes but probably have a similar pathophysiology.

Foix and Levy, who described the clinical effects of deep capsular-basal ganglionic lesions and of superficial cortical-subcortical ones, found few important differences in the degree and pattern of the hemiplegia and sensory disorder. Homonymous hemianopia may occur with posterior capsular lesions, but it must be distinguished from visual hemineglect of contralateral space. Bilateral cerebral infarctions involving mainly the insular-perisylvian (anterior opercular) regions manifest themselves by a facio-glosso-pharyngo-masticatory diplegia (anarthria without aphasia; see Mao et al).

The middle cerebral artery may become stenotic rather than occluded. In several series of such cases, some of the permanent deficiencies were preceded by TIAs, producing a picture resembling that of carotid stenosis (Day; Caplan).

Anterior Cerebral Artery

This artery, through its cortical branches, supplies the anterior three-quarters of the medial surface of the cerebral hemisphere, including the medial-orbital surface of the frontal lobe, the frontal pole, a strip of the lateral surface of the cerebral hemisphere along the superior border, and the anterior four-fifths of the corpus callosum. Deep branches, arising near the circle of Willis (proximal or distal to the anterior communicating artery), supply the anterior limb of the internal capsule, the inferior part of the head of the caudate nucleus, and the anterior part of the globus pallidus (Figs. 34-4, 34-5, and 34-6). The largest of these deep branches is the artery of Heubner.

Again, the clinical picture will depend on the location and size of the infarct, which, in turn, relates to the site of the occlusion, the pattern of the circle of Willis, and the other ischemia-modifying factors mentioned earlier. Well-studied cases of infarction in the territory of the anterior cerebral artery are not numerous; hence the syndromes have not been completely elucidated (see Brust and also Bogousslavsky and Regli for a review of the literature and description of developmental abnormalities of the artery).

Occlusion of the stem of the anterior cerebral artery, proximal to its connection with the anterior com-

Figure 34-6

Corrosion preparations with plastics demonstrating penetrating branches of the anterior and middle cerebral arteries. (1) *Lateral lenticulostriate arteries.* (2) *Heubner artery and medial lenticulostriate arteries.* (3) *Anterior cerebral artery.* (4) *Internal carotid artery.* (5) *Middle cerebral artery. (From Krayenbühl and Yasargil by permission.)*

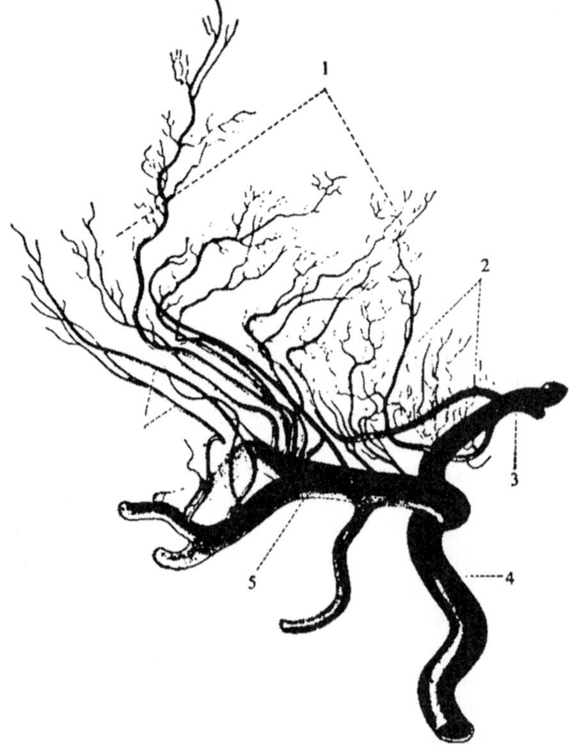

municating artery, is usually well tolerated, since adequate collateral flow will come from the artery of the opposite side. Maximal disturbance occurs when both arteries arise from one anterior cerebral stem, in which case occlusion of the stem will cause infarction of the anterior and medial parts of both cerebral hemispheres and result in paraplegia, incontinence, abulic and motor aphasic symptoms, and frontal lobe personality changes (Chap. 22). Occlusion of the anterior cerebral arteries may also be embolic or surgical (following operations on anterior communicating aneurysms).

Complete infarction due to occlusion of one anterior cerebral artery distal to the anterior communicating artery results in a sensorimotor deficit of the opposite foot and leg and, to a lesser degree, of the shoulder and arm, with sparing of the hand and face. The motor disorder is more in the foot and leg than in the thigh. Sensory loss is mainly of the discriminative modalities and is mild or absent in some cases. The head and eyes may deviate to the side of the lesion. Urinary incontinence and a contralateral grasp reflex and paratonic rigidity (gegenhalten) may be evident. With a left-sided occlusion, there may be a sympathetic apraxia of the left arm and leg or involuntary misdirected movements of the left arm (alien arm or hand). Also, transcortical motor aphasia may occur with occlusions of Heubner's branch of the left anterior cerebral artery. Alexander and Schmitt cite cases in which a right hemiplegia (predominant in the leg) with grasping and groping responses of the right hand and buccofacial apraxia are accompanied by a diminution or absence of spontaneous speech, agraphia, labored telegraphic speech, and a limited ability to name objects and compose word lists but with a striking preservation of the ability to repeat spoken and written sentences (transcortical motor aphasia). Disorders of behavior that may be overlooked are abulia, presenting as slowness and lack of spontaneity in all reactions; muteness or a tendency to speak in whispers; and distractibility. Branch occlusions of the anterior cerebral artery produce only fragments of the total syndrome, usually a spastic weakness or cortical sensory loss in the opposite foot and leg.

With occlusion of *penetrating branches of the anterior cerebral artery* on one or both sides, the anterior limb of the internal capsule is usually involved as well. In a series of 18 unilateral cases of caudate region infarcts collected by Caplan and associates, a transient hemiparesis was present in 13. Dysarthria and either abulia or agitation and hyperactivity were also common. Stuttering and language difficulty occurred with two of the left-sided lesions and visuospatial neglect with three of the right-sided ones. To what extent these symptoms were due to disorder of neighboring structures is difficult to decide. With bilateral caudate infarctions, a syndrome of inattentiveness, abulia, forgetfulness, and sometimes agitation and psychosis was observed. Transitory choreoathetosis and other dyskinesias have also been attributed to ischemia of basal ganglia occurring sometimes under conditions of prolonged standing and exercise (Caplan and Sergay; Margolin and Marsden).

Anterior Choroidal Artery

This is a long, narrow artery that springs from the internal carotid, just above the origin of the posterior communicating artery. It supplies the internal segment of the globus pallidus and posterior limb of the internal capsule and various contiguous structures including (in some patients) the optic tract; then it penetrates the temporal horn of the lateral ventricle, where it supplies the choroid plexus and anastomoses with the posterior choroidal artery.

Only a few complete clinicopathologic studies have been made of the syndrome caused by occlusion of this artery. It was found by Foix and colleagues to consist of contralateral hemiplegia, hemihypesthesia, and homonymous hemianopia due to involvement of the posterior limb of the internal capsule and white matter posterolateral to it, through which the geniculocalcarine tract passes. Cognitive function is notably spared. Decroix and colleagues reported 16 cases (identified by CT) in which the lesion appeared to lie in the vascular territory of this artery. In most of their cases the clinical syndrome fell short of what was expected on anatomic grounds. With right-sided lesions there may be left spatial neglect and constructional apraxia; slight disorders of speech and language may accompany left-sided lesions. Hupperts and colleagues have discussed the controversy regarding the effects of occlusion of the anterior choroidal artery and in particular the variability of its supply to the posterior paraventricular area of the corona radiata and adjacent regions. They concluded, also from a CT survey, that there was no uniform syndrome attributable to occlusion of this vessel and that in most cases its territory of supply was overlapped by small surrounding vessels. Of course, in both these studies, the lesions may have extended beyond the territory of this artery, since postmortem confirmation was lacking. It should be remembered that for a time the anterior choroidal artery was being surgically ligated in order to abolish the tremor and rigidity of unilateral Parkinson disease, without these ischemic effects having been produced.

Vertebrobasilar and Posterior Cerebral Arteries

Posterior Cerebral Artery In about 70 percent of persons, both posterior cerebral arteries are formed by the bifurcation of the basilar artery, and only thin posterior communicating arteries join this system to the internal carotids. In 20 to 25 percent, one posterior cerebral artery arises from the basilar in the usual way, but the other arises from the internal carotid; in the remainder, both arise from the corresponding carotids.

The configuration and branches of the *proximal segment of the posterior cerebral artery* are illustrated in Figs. 34-7 and 34-8. The *interpeduncular branches*, which arise just above the basilar bifurcation, supply the red nuclei, the substantia nigra bilaterally, medial parts of the cerebral peduncles, oculomotor and trochlear nuclei and nerves, reticular substance of the upper brainstem, decussation of the brachia conjunctivae (superior cerebellar peduncles), medial longitudinal fasciculi, and medial lemnisci. The portion of the posterior cerebral artery giving rise to the interpeduncular branches (the portion between the bifurcation of the basilar artery and the ostium of the posterior communicating artery) is also referred to as the *mesencephalic artery* or the *basilar communicating artery*.

The *thalamoperforate branches* (also called *paramedian thalamic arteries*) arise more distally, near the junction of the posterior cerebral and posterior communicating arteries, and supply the inferior, medial, and anterior parts of the thalamus. As pointed out by Percheron (whose name is often applied to these vessels), the arterial configuration of the thalamoperforate arteries varies considerably: in some cases they arise symmetrically, one from each side; in others, both arteries arise from the same posterior cerebral stem, either separately or by a common trunk, which then bifurcates. In the latter case, one posterior cerebral stem supplies the medial thalamic territories on both sides, and an occlusion of this artery or one common paramedian trunk produces a bilateral butterfly-shaped lesion in the medial parts of the diencephalon. The *thalamogeniculate* branches arise still more distally, opposite the lateral geniculate body, and supply the geniculate body and the central and posterior parts of the thalamus. Medial branches from the posterior cerebral, as it encircles the midbrain, supply the lateral part of the cerebral peduncle, lateral tegmentum and corpora quadrigemina, and pineal gland. Posterior choroidal branches run to the posterosuperior thalamus, choroid plexus, posterior parts of the hippocampus, and psalterium (decussation of fornices).

The terminal or *cortical branches of the posterior cerebral artery* supply the inferomedial part of the temporal lobe and the medial occipital lobe, including the lingula, cuneus, precuneus, and visual areas 17, 18, and 19 (see Figs. 34-5, 34-7, and 34-8).

Occlusion of the posterior cerebral artery can produce a greater variety of clinical effects than occlusion of any other artery, because both the upper brainstem,

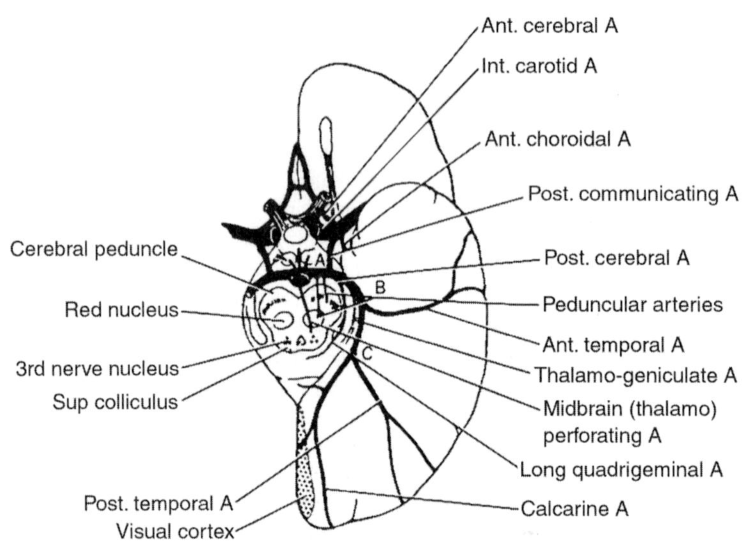

Figure 34-7

Inferior aspect of the brain showing the branches and distribution of the ***posterior cerebral artery*** *and the principal anatomic structures supplied. On the facing page are listed the clinical manifestations produced by infarction in its territory and the corresponding regions of damage. (Continued on the facing page.)*

Figure 34-7 *(continued)*

Signs and symptoms	*Structures involved*
	Central territory
Thalamic syndrome: sensory loss (all modalities), spontaneous pain and dysesthesias, choreoathetosis, intention tremor, spasms of hand, mild hemiparesis	Ventral posterolateral nucleus of thalamus in territory of thalamogeniculate artery. Involvement of the adjacent subthalamic nucleus or its pallidal connections results in hemiballismus and choreoathetosis.
Thalamoperforate syndrome: (1) superior, crossed cerebellar ataxia; (2) inferior, crossed cerebellar ataxia with ipsilateral third nerve palsy (Claude syndrome)	Dentatothalamic tract and issuing third nerve
Weber syndrome—third nerve palsy and contralateral hemiplegia	Issuing third nerve and cerebral peduncle
Contralateral hemiplegia	Cerebral peduncle
Paralysis or paresis of vertical eye movement, skew deviation, sluggish pupillary responses to light, slight miosis and ptosis (retraction nystagmus and "tucked-in" eyelids may be associated)	Supranuclear fibers to third nerve, high midbrain tegmentum ventral to superior colliculus (nucleus of Cajal, nucleus of Darkschevich, rostral interstitial nucleus of the MLF, and posterior commissure)
Contralateral ataxic or postural tremor	Dentatothalamic tract (?) after decussation. Precise site of lesion unknown.
Decerebrate attacks	Damage to motor tracts between red and vestibular nuclei
	Peripheral territory
Homonymous hemianopia	Calcarine cortex or optic radiation; hemiachromatopsia may be present. Macular or central vision is preserved if posterior striate area is spared.
Bilateral homonymous hemianopia, cortical blindness, unawareness or denial of blindness; achromatopsia, failure to see to-and-fro movements, inability to perceive objects not centrally located, apraxia of ocular movements, inability to count or enumerate objects	Bilateral occipital lobe, possibly with involvement of parieto-occipital region
Dyslexia without agraphia, color anomia	Dominant calcarine lesion and posterior part of corpus callosum
Memory defect	Lesion of inferomedial portions of temporal lobe bilaterally; occasionally of the dominant side only
Topographic disorientation and prosopagnosia	Nondominant calcarine and lingual gyri, usually bilateral
Simultagnosia	Dominant visual cortex, sometimes bilateral
Unformed visual hallucinations, metamorphopsia, teleopsia, illusory visual spread, palinopsia, distortion of outlines, photophobia	Calcarine cortex

Note: Tremor in repose has been omitted because of the uncertainty of its occurrence in the posterior cerebral artery syndrome. Peduncular hallucinosis may occur in thalamic-subthalamic ischemic lesions, but the exact location of the lesion is unknown.

which is crowded with important structures, and the inferomedial parts of the temporal and occipital lobes lie within its domain. Obviously the site of the occlusion and the arrangement of the circle of Willis will in large measure determine the location and extent of the resulting infarct. For example, occlusion proximal to the posterior communicating artery may be asymptomatic or have only transitory effects if the collateral flow is adequate (Fig. 34-7; see also Fig. 34-8). Even distal to the posterior communicating artery, an occlusion may cause relatively little damage if the collateral flow through border-zone collaterals from anterior and middle cerebral arteries is sufficient.

In the series of posterior cerebral artery strokes studied by Milandre and coworkers, the causes were in general similar to those of strokes in other vascular territories except that there was a surprisingly high incidence of atherosclerotic occlusion (35 patients) in contrast to cardioembolic types (15 patients). Two of their stroke cases were attributed to migraine. Our experience has differed in that the proportion of presumed embolic occlusions has been greater.

For convenience of exposition, it is helpful to divide the various posterior cerebral artery syndromes into three groups: (1) anterior and proximal (involving interpeduncular, thalamic perforant, and thalamogeniculate branches), (2) cortical (inferior temporal and medial occipital), and (3) bilateral.

Anterior and Proximal Syndromes (See Figs. 34-8 and 34-9.) *The thalamic syndrome of Déjerine and Roussy* (page 172) follows infarction of the sensory relay nuclei in the thalamus, the result of occlusion of thalamogeniculate branches. There is both a deep and cutaneous sensory loss, usually severe in degree, of the opposite side of the body, accompanied by a transitory hemiparesis. A homonymous hemianopia may be conjoined. In some instances there is a dissociated sensory loss—pain and thermal sensation being more affected than touch, vibration, and position—or only one part of the body may be anesthetic. After an interval, sensation begins to return, and the patient may then develop pain, paresthesia, and hyperpathia in the affected parts. The painful paresthetic syndrome may persist for years. There may also be distortion of taste, athetotic posturing of the hand, and alteration of mood. Mania and depression have occasionally been observed with infarction of the diencephalon and adjacent structures, but the data are usually incomplete. The patient may be left with a severe amnesia, even with a unilateral lesion (see below).

Central midbrain and subthalamic syndromes are due to occlusion of the interpeduncular branches. The clinical syndromes include oculomotor palsy with contralateral hemiplegia (*Weber syndrome*), palsies of vertical gaze, stupor or coma, and movement disorders, most often an ataxic tremor that may be contralateral, i.e., on the side of the hemiparesis (see below). A persistent hemiplegia from infarction of the cerebral peduncle is rare.

Anteromedial-inferior thalamic syndromes follow occlusion of the thalamoperforant branches. Here the most common effect is an extrapyramidal movement disorder (hemiballismus or hemichoreoathetosis). Deep sensory loss, hemiataxia, or tremor may be added in various combinations. Hemiballismus is usually due to occlusion of a small branch to the subthalamic nucleus (of Luys) or its connections with the pallidum. Occlusion of the paramedian thalamic branch(es) to the mediodorsal nuclei or to the dominant (left) mediodorsal nucleus is the recognized substrate of the vascular amnesic (Korsakoff) syndrome.

Cortical Syndromes Occlusion of branches to the temporal and occipital lobes gives rise to a homonymous

Figure 34-8

The posterior cerebral and basilar arteries. (From Krayenbühl and Yasargil by permission.) (Continued on the facing page.)

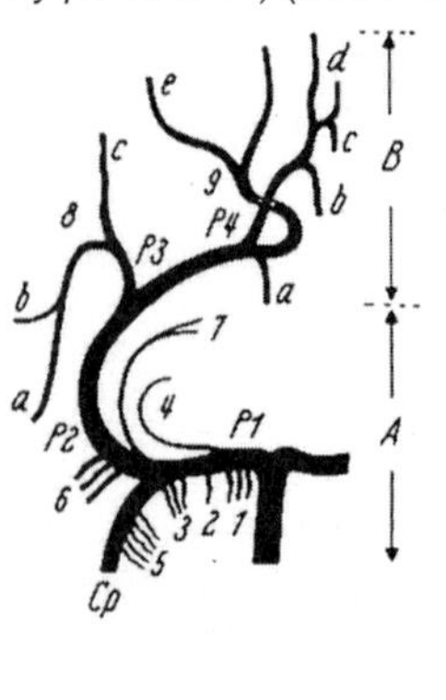

A

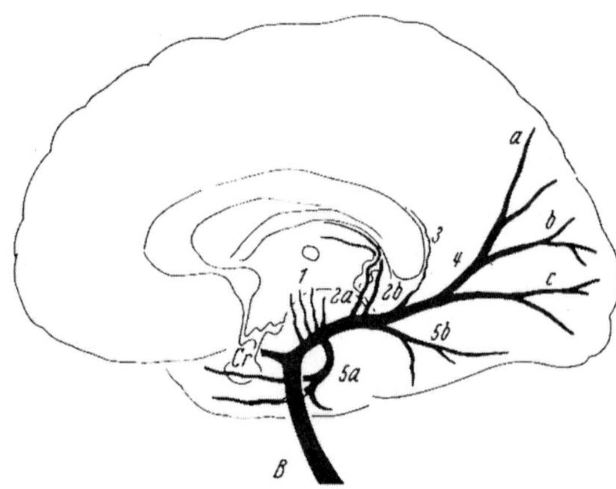

B

Figure 34-8 *(Continued)*

Figure 34-8A: Posterior cerebral artery	*Regions of vascular supply*
A Circular or proximal segment	
(1) Paramedian arteries (interpeduncular, intercrural, perforating)	Substantia nigra, red nucleus, mammillary body, oculomotor nerve, trochlear nerve
(2) Quadrigeminal arteries	Quadrigeminal bodies
(3) Thalamic arteries (medial and lateral)	Central nucleus, medial nucleus, ventrolateral nucleus of the thalamus, pulvinar, lateral geniculate body, internal capsule (posterior portion)
(4) Medial posterior choroidal arteries	
(5) Premammillary arteries (of the posterior communicating artery)	Epithalamus, thalamus, choroid plexus, pineal gland
(6) Peduncular artery	Tuber cinereum, cerebral peduncle, ventral nuclei of the thalamus, nuclei of the hypothalamus, optic chiasm
(7) Lateral posterior choroidal arteries (anterior and posterior)	Hippocampal gyrus, lateral geniculate body, pulvinar, dentate fascia, hippocampus, anterior basal cortex of the temporal lobe, choroid plexus of the temporal horn, trigone, dorsolateral nuclei of the thalamus
B Cortical or distal segment	
(8) Lateral occipital artery	
(a) Anterior temporal arteries	Laterobasal aspects of the temporal and occipital lobe
(b) Middle temporal arteries	
(c) Posterior temporal arteries	
(9) Medial occipital artery	
(a) Dorsal callosal artery	Splenium
(b) Posterior parietal artery	Cuneus, precuneus
(c) Occipitoparietal artery	
(d) Calcarine arteries	Calcarine gyrus, occipital pole
(e) Occipitotemporal artery	Laterobasal occipital lobe

Figure 34-8B: Basilar artery

B Basilar artery
Cr Posterior communicating artery
(1) Thalamic arteries
(2a) Medial posterior choroidal artery
(2b) Lateral posterior choroidal artery
(3) Dorsal callosal artery
(4) Medial occipital artery
(a) Posterior parietal arteries
(b) Occipitoparietal arteries
(c) Calcarine arteries
(5a) Anterior and middle temporal arteries
(5b) Posterior temporal artery

hemianopia because of involvement of the primary visual receptive area (calcarine or striate cortex) or of the converging geniculocalcarine fibers. It may be incomplete and then involves the upper quadrants of the visual fields more than the lower ones (see Chap. 13). Macular or central vision may be spared because of collateralization of the occipital pole from distal branches of the middle (or anterior) cerebral arteries. There may be visual hallucinations in the blind parts of the visual fields (Cogan) or metamorphopsia and palinopsia (Brust and Behrens). Posterior cortical infarcts of the dominant hemisphere cause alexia (with or without agraphia), anomia (amnesic aphasia), a variety of visual agnosias, and rarely some degree of impaired memory. The anomias (dysnomias) are most severe for colors, but the naming of other visually presented material such as pictures, musical notes, mathematical symbols, and manipulable objects may also be impaired. The patient

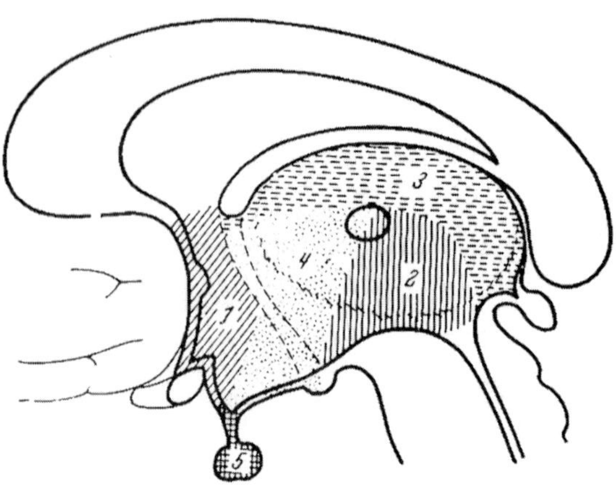

Figure 34-9

Diagram of the vascularization of the diencephalon. Distribution of (1) *the anterior cerebral artery,* (2) *the posterior cerebral artery,* (3) *the anterior and posterior choroidal arteries,* (4) *the posterior communicating artery, and* (5) *the internal carotid artery. (From Krayenbühl and Yasargil by permission.)*

may treat objects as familiar—that is, describe their functions and use them correctly—but be unable to name them. Color dysnomia and amnesic aphasia are more often present in this syndrome than is alexia. The defect in retentive memory is of varying severity and may or may not improve with the passage of time.

A complete proximal arterial occlusion leads to a syndrome that combines cortical and anterior-proximal syndromes in part or totally. The vascular lesion may be either an embolus or an atherosclerotic thrombus.

Bilateral Cortical Syndromes These may occur as a result of successive infarctions or from a single embolic or thrombotic occlusion of the upper basilar artery, especially if the posterior communicating arteries are unusually small.

Bilateral lesions of the occipital lobes, if extensive, cause total blindness of the *cortical* type, i.e., a bilateral homonymous hemianopia, sometimes accompanied by unformed visual hallucinations. The pupillary reflexes are preserved, and the optic discs appear normal. Sometimes the patient is unaware of being blind and may deny it even when it is pointed out to him (Anton syndrome). More frequently the lesions are incomplete, and a sector of the visual fields, usually on one side, remains intact. When the intact remnant is small, vision may fluctuate from moment to moment as the patient attempts to capture the image in the island of intact vision, in which case hysteria may be suspected. The Balint syndrome (page 491) is another effect of bilateral occipitoparietal border-zone lesions. In bilateral lesions confined to the occipital poles, there may be a loss of central vision only (homonymous central scotomas). With more anteriorly placed lesions of the occipital pole, there may be homonymous paracentral scotomas, or the occipital poles may be spared, leaving the patient with only central vision. Horizontal or altitudinal field defects are usually due to lesions affecting the upper or lower banks of the calcarine sulci.

With bilateral lesions that involve the inferomedial portions of the temporal lobes, the impairment of memory may be severe, simulating the Korsakoff amnesic state. In several of our patients, a solely left-sided infarction of the inferomedial temporal lobe impaired retentive memory. The amnesic state and its accompaniments are fully described in Chaps. 21 and 22. Bilateral mesiotemporal-occipital lesions may be accompanied by a lack of recognition of faces (prosopagnosia). These and other effects of temporal and occipital lesions are discussed in Chaps. 13 and 22.

Vertebral Artery The vertebral arteries are the chief arteries of the medulla; each supplies the lower three-fourths of the pyramid, the medial lemniscus, all or nearly all of the retro-olivary (lateral medullary) region, the restiform body, and the posterior inferior part of the cerebellar hemisphere (Figs. 34-10 and 34-11). The relative sizes of the vertebral arteries vary considerably, and in approximately 10 percent of cases, one vessel is so small that the other is essentially the only artery of supply to the brainstem. In the latter cases, if there is no collateral flow from the carotid system via the circle of Willis, occlusion of the one functional vertebral artery is equivalent to occlusion of the basilar artery or both vertebral arteries. The posteroinferior cerebellar artery is usually a branch of the vertebral artery but can have a common origin with the anteroinferior cerebellar artery from the basilar artery. It is necessary to keep these anatomic variations in mind in considering the effects of vertebral artery occlusion.

Since the vertebral arteries have a long extracranial course and pass through the transverse processes of C6 to C1 vertebrae before entering the cranial cavity, one might expect them to be subject to trauma, spondylotic compression, and a variety of other vertebral diseases. In our experience this happens only infrequently. We have not seen convincing examples of spondylotic occlusion.

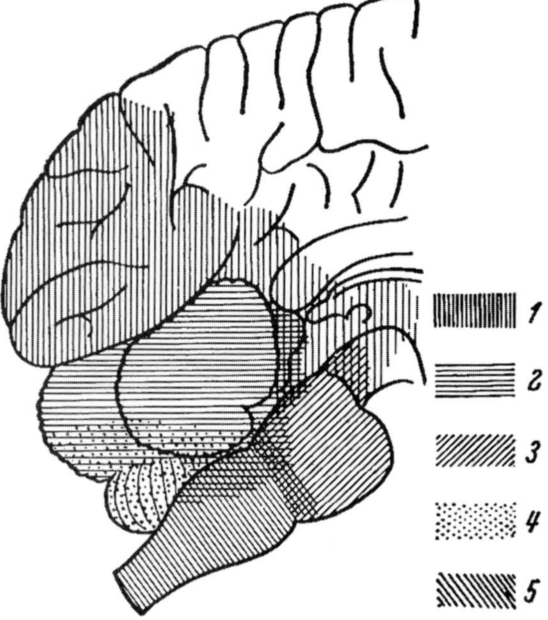

Figure 34-10

Regions of supply by the posterior segment of the circle of Willis, lateral view: (1) *posterior cerebral artery;* (2) *superior cerebellar artery;* (3) *basilar artery and superior cerebellar artery;* (4) *posterior inferior cerebellar artery;* (5) *vertebral artery (posterior inferior cerebellar artery, anterior spinal artery, posterior spinal artery).*

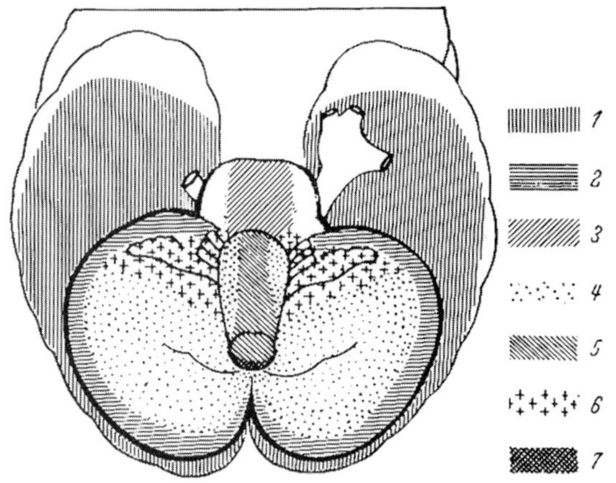

Figure 34-11

Regions supplied by the posterior segment of the circle of Willis, basal view: (1) *posterior cerebral artery;* (2) *superior cerebellar artery;* (3) *paramedian branches of the basilar artery and spinal artery;* (4) *posterior inferior cerebellar artery;* (5) *vertebral artery;* (6) *anterior inferior cerebellar artery;* (7) *dorsal spinal artery. (From Krayenbühl and Yasargil by permission.)*

Neck rotation (chiropractic or other) of extreme degree has been reported as a cause of brainstem ischemia in more than 50 cases (Caplan). Extreme extension of the neck, as occurs in women having their hair washed in beauty parlors, may give rise to transient symptoms in the territories of the vertebral arteries. Dissection of the vertebral artery is well documented; it declares itself by cervico-occipital pain and deficits of brainstem function, usually bilateral. It may be precipitated by vigorous and protracted bouts of coughing or by trauma to the neck or head. Examples of "posterior circulation" stroke in children have been reported in association with odontoid hypoplasia and other atlantoaxial dislocations, causing the vertebral arteries to be stretched or kinked in their course through the transverse processes of C1-C2 (Phillips et al).

The results of vertebral artery occlusion are quite variable. When there are two good-sized arteries, occlusion of one may cause no recognizable symptoms and signs or pathologic changes. If the subclavian artery is blocked proximal to the origin of the left vertebral artery, exercise of the arm on that side may draw blood from the right vertebral and basilar arteries, down the left vertebral and into the distal left subclavian artery—sometimes resulting in the symptoms of basilar insufficiency. This phenomenon, described in 1961 by Reivich and colleagues, was referred to by Fisher as the "*subclavian steal.*" Its most notable feature is transient weakness of the left arm on exercise. There may also be headache and claudication or pain of the arm. If the occlusion of the vertebral artery is so situated as to block the branches supplying the lateral medulla, a characteristic syndrome may result; in this configuration, vertigo may be a prominent symptom (see below). When the vertebral branch to the anterior spinal artery is blocked, flow from the other (corresponding) branch is usually sufficient to prevent infarction of the cervical cord. If the branch to the pyramid is occluded, part of the pyramidal tract may be infarcted, depending on the adequacy of collateral flow. Any of these branches may become occluded in its course as well as at its origin from the vertebral artery, with similar effects.

Rarely, occlusion of the vertebral artery or one of its medial branches produces an infarct that involves the medullary pyramid, the medial lemniscus, and the emergent hypoglossal fibers; the resultant syndrome consists of a contralateral paralysis of arm and leg (with sparing of the face), contralateral loss of position and vibration sense, and ipsilateral paralysis and later atrophy of the tongue. A more limited lesion, from occlusion of one spinal artery arising from the vertebral artery, gives rise to a contralateral hemiplegia (rarely a quadriplegia) that spares the face. This is a fragment of the *medial medullary syndrome* (Fig. 34-12). Occlusion of a vertebral artery low in the neck is usually compensated by anastomotic flow to the upper part of the artery via the thyrocervical, deep cervical, and occipital arteries or reflux from the circle of Willis.

Lateral Medullary Syndrome Known also as the syndrome of Wallenberg (who described a case in 1895), this common syndrome (Fig. 34-12) is produced by infarction of a wedge of lateral medulla lying posterior to the inferior olivary nucleus. The complete syndrome, as outlined by Fisher and colleagues (1961), reflects the involvement of the vestibular nuclei (nystagmus, oscillopsia, vertigo, nausea, vomiting); spinothalamic tract (*contralateral* impairment of pain and thermal sense over half the body); descending sympathetic tract (ipsilateral Horner syndrome—miosis, ptosis, decreased sweating); issuing fibers of the ninth and tenth nerves (hoarseness, dysphagia, ipsilateral paralysis of the palate and vocal cord, diminished gag reflex); otolithic nucleus (vertical diplopia and illusion of tilting of vision); olivocerebellar and/or spinocerebellar fibers and, sometimes, restiform body and inferior cerebellum (*ipsilateral* ataxia of limbs, falling or toppling to the ipsilateral side, or lateropulsion); descending tract and nucleus of the fifth nerve (pain, burning, and impaired sensation over ipsilateral half of the face); nucleus and tractus solitarius (loss of taste); and rarely cuneate and gracile nuclei (numbness of *ipsilateral* limbs). Fragmentary syndromes occur frequently at the onset of the stroke: vertigo and ptosis, toppling and vertical diplopia, hoarseness and disequilibrium, etc. Vertigo alone, however, is not an indication of lateral medullary infarction. The smallest infarction we have studied gave rise only to symptoms of lateropulsion and mild ipsilateral limb ataxia.

The eye signs of lateral medullary infarction may be difficult to interpret. Often there is a fragment of an internuclear ophthalmoplegia or a skew deviation (the globe on the affected side usually higher). Direction changing nystagmus (with different head positions) is said to be the most useful feature that distinguishes vestibular nucleus infarction from labyrinthine disease, but some variants of benign positional vertigo also show this sign (see also Chap. 15).

Figure 34-12

Transverse section through the upper medulla. (Continued on the facing page.)

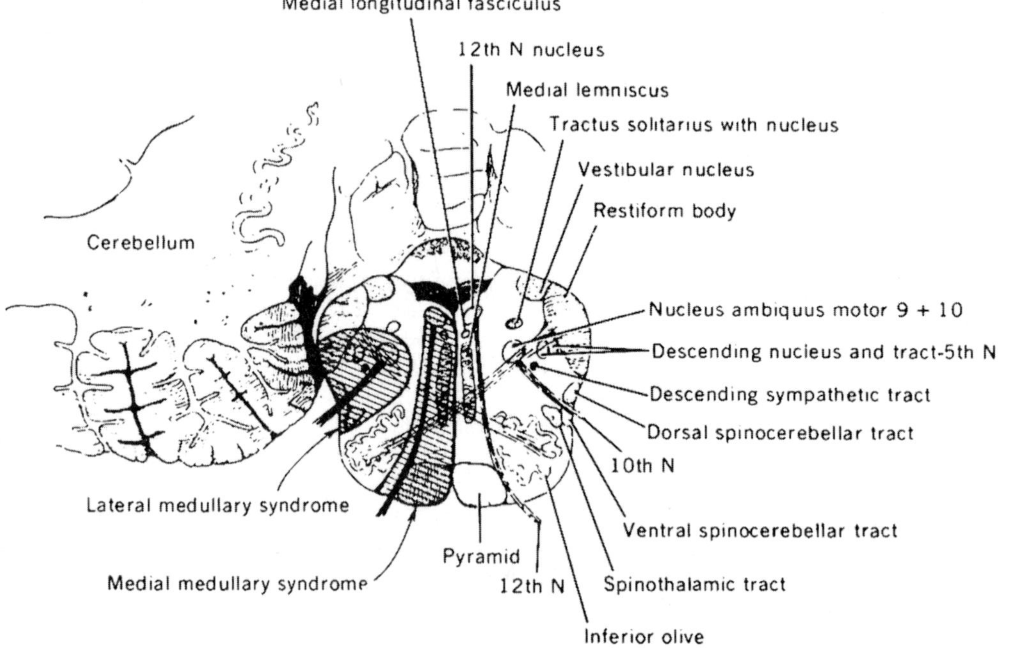

Figure 34-12 *(continued)*

Signs and symptoms	*Structures involved*
1. Medial medullary syndrome (occlusion of vertebral artery or branch of vertebral or lower basilar artery)	
a. On side of lesion	
(1) Paralysis with later hemiatrophy of the tongue	Issuing twelfth nerve
b. On side opposite lesion	
(1) Paralysis of arm and leg sparing face	Pyramidal tract
(2) Impaired tactile and proprioceptive sense over half the body	Medial lemniscus
2. Lateral medullary syndrome (occlusion of any of five vessels may be responsible—vertebral, posterior inferior cerebellar, or superior, middle, or inferior lateral medullary arteries)	
a. On side of lesion	
(1) Pain, numbness, impaired sensation over half the face	Descending tract and nucleus of fifth nerve
(2) Ataxia of limbs, falling to side of lesion	Uncertain—restiform body, cerebellar hemisphere, olivocerebellar fibers, spinocerebellar tract (?)
(3) Vertigo, nausea, vomiting	Vestibular nuclei and connections
(4) Nystagmus, diplopia, oscillopsia	Vestibular nuclei and connections
(5) Horner syndrome (miosis, ptosis, decreased sweating)	Descending sympathetic tract
(6) Dysphagia, hoarseness, paralysis of vocal cord, diminished gag reflex	Issuing fibers ninth and tenth nerves
(7) Loss of taste (rare)	Nucleus and tractus solitarius
(8) Numbness of ipsilateral arm, trunk, or leg	Cuneate and gracile nuclei
(9) Hiccup	Uncertain
b. On side opposite lesion	
(1) Impaired pain and thermal sense over half the body, sometimes face	Spinothalamic tract
3. Total unilateral medullary syndrome (occlusion of vertebral artery); combination of medial and lateral syndromes	
4. Lateral pontomedullary syndrome (occlusion of vertebral artery); combination of medial and lateral syndromes	
5. Basilar artery syndrome (the syndrome of the lone vertebral artery is equivalent); a combination of the various brainstem syndromes plus those arising in the posterior cerebral artery distribution. The clinical picture comprises bilateral long-tract signs (sensory and motor) with cerebellar and cranial nerve abnormalities.	
a. Paralysis or weakness of all extremities, plus all bulbar musculature	Corticobulbar and corticospinal tracts bilaterally
b. Diplopia, paralysis of conjugate lateral and/or vertical gaze, internuclear ophthalmoplegia, horizontal and/or vertical nystagmus	Ocular motor nerves, apparatus for conjugate gaze, medial longitudinal fasciculus, vestibular apparatus
c. Blindness, impaired vision, various visual field defects	Visual cortex
d. Bilateral cerebellar ataxia	Cerebellar peduncles and the cerebellar hemispheres
e. Coma	Tegmentum of midbrain, thalami
f. Sensation may be strikingly intact in the presence of almost total paralysis. Sensory loss may be syringomyelic or the reverse or involve all modalities	Medial lemniscus, spinothalamic tracts or thalamic nuclei

The entire lateral medullary syndrome, one of the most striking in neurology, is almost always due to infarction, with only a small number of cases being the result of hemorrhage or tumor. Although it was traditionally attributed to occlusion of the posterior inferior cerebellar artery (PICA), careful studies have shown that in 8 out of 10 cases it is the vertebral artery that is occluded; in the remainder, either the posterior inferior cerebellar artery or one of the lateral medullary arteries is occluded.

In recent years, we have become aware from our own cases that although most of those with lateral medullary infarction do well and make a considerable recovery, sudden and unexpected death may occur from respiratory or cardiac arrest in the absence of cerebellar swelling or basilar artery thrombosis. Cases of this nature are reviewed by Norving and Cronqvist. The related and important issue of recognizing cerebellar swelling after vertebral or PICA occlusion and the subsequent need for surgery is discussed under "Treatment of Cerebral Edema and Raised Intracranial Pressure" later in the chapter.

Basilar Artery The branches of the basilar artery may be conveniently grouped as follows: (1) paramedian, 7 to 10 in number, supplying a wedge of pons on either side of the midline; (2) short circumferential, 5 to 7 in number, supplying the lateral two-thirds of the pons and the middle and superior cerebellar peduncles; (3) long circumferential, 2 on each side (the superior and anterior inferior cerebellar arteries), which run laterally around the pons to reach the cerebellar hemispheres (Figs. 34-10 and 34-11); and (4) several paramedian (interpeduncular) branches at the bifurcation of the basilar artery supplying the high midbrain and medial subthalamic regions. The interpeduncular and other branches of the posterior cerebral artery have been described above.

The picture of basilar occlusion due to thrombosis may arise in several ways: (1) occlusion of the basilar artery itself, usually in the lower third at the site of an atherosclerotic plaque; (2) occlusion of both vertebral arteries; and (3) occlusion of a single vertebral artery when it is the only one of adequate size. It must be emphasized that thrombosis more frequently involves a branch of the basilar artery than the trunk (*basilar branch occlusion*). When the obstruction is embolic, the embolus usually lodges at the upper bifurcation of the basilar or in one of the posterior cerebral arteries, since the embolus, if it is small enough to pass through the vertebral artery, easily traverses the length of the basilar artery, which is of greater diameter than either vertebral artery.

The syndrome of *basilar artery occlusion*, as delineated by Kubik and Adams, reflects the involvement of a large number of structures: corticospinal and corticobulbar tracts, cerebellum, middle and superior cerebellar peduncles, medial and lateral lemnisci, spinothalamic tracts, medial longitudinal fasciculi, pontine nuclei, vestibular and cochlear nuclei, descending hypothalamospinal sympathetic fibers, and the third through eighth cranial nerves (the nuclei and their segments within the brainstem).

The *complete basilar syndrome* comprises bilateral long tract signs (sensory and motor) with variable cerebellar, cranial nerve, and other segmental abnormalities of the brainstem. Often the patient is comatose because of ischemia of the high midbrain reticular activating system. Others are mute and quadriplegic but conscious, reflecting interruption of motor pathways but sparing of the reticular activating system ("locked-in" syndrome; see page 370). In the presence of the full syndrome, it is usually not difficult to make the correct diagnosis. The aim should be, however, to recognize basilar insufficiency long before the stage of total deficit has been reached. The early manifestations (some in the form of transient ischemic attacks) occur in many combinations, described in detail further on (page 860).

Occlusion of branches at the bifurcation (top) of the basilar artery results in a remarkable number of complex syndromes that include, in various combinations, somnolence, memory defects, akinetic mutism, visual hallucinations, ptosis, disorders of ocular movement (convergence spasm, paralysis of vertical gaze, retraction nystagmus, pseudoabducens palsy, retraction of upper eyelids, skew deviation of the eyes), an agitated confusional state, and visual defects. These have been reviewed by Petit and coworkers and Castaigne and associates as paramedian thalamic, subthalamic, and midbrain infarctions and by Caplan as "top of the basilar" syndromes.

The main signs of occlusion of the *superior cerebellar artery* are ipsilateral cerebellar ataxia (middle and/or superior cerebellar peduncles); nausea and vomiting; slurred (pseudobulbar) speech; and loss of pain and thermal sensation over the opposite side of the body (spinothalamic tract). Partial deafness, static tremor of the ipsilateral upper extremity, an ipsilateral Horner syndrome, and palatal myoclonus have also been reported.

With occlusion of the *anteroinferior cerebellar artery*, the extent of the infarct is extremely variable, since the size of this artery and the territory it supplies vary inversely with the size and territory of supply of the posteroinferior cerebellar artery. The principal findings are vertigo; nausea; vomiting; nystagmus; tinnitus and sometimes unilateral deafness; facial weakness; ipsilateral cerebellar ataxia (inferior or middle cerebellar peduncle); an ipsilateral Horner syndrome and paresis of conjugate lateral gaze; and contralateral loss of pain and temperature sense of the arm, trunk, and leg (lateral spinothalamic tract). If the occlusion is close to the origin of the artery, the corticospinal fibers may also be involved, producing a hemiplegia; if distal, there may be cochlear and labyrinthine infarction. Cerebellar swelling herniation has not been seen in our cases or in the 20 cases collected by Amarenco and Hauw.

The most important manifestation of all these brainstem infarcts is the "crossed" cranial nerve and long tract sensory or motor deficit. These crossed syndromes, which may involve cranial nerves III through XII, are listed in Table 47-2. Although the finding of bilateral neurologic signs strongly suggests brainstem involvement, it must be emphasized that in many instances of infarction within the basilar territory, the signs are limited to one side of the body, with or without cranial nerve involvement, indicating occlusion of a branch of the basilar artery, not of the main trunk.

It is impossible to distinguish a hemiplegia of pontine origin from one of cerebral origin on the basis of motor signs alone. With brainstem lesions as with cerebral ones, a flaccid paralysis gives way to spasticity after a few days or weeks, and there is no satisfactory explanation for the variability in this period of delay or for the occurrence in some cases of spasticity from the onset of the stroke. There may also be a combined hemiparesis and ataxia of the limbs on the same side. Localization of the level of the brainstem lesion depends upon coexisting neurologic signs. With a hemiplegia of pontine origin, the eyes may deviate to the side of the paralysis, i.e., the opposite of what occurs with supratentorial lesions. The pattern of sensory disturbance may be helpful. A dissociated sensory deficit over the ipsilateral face and contralateral half of the body usually indicates a lesion in the lower brainstem, while a hemisensory loss including the face and involving all modalities indicates a lesion in the upper brainstem, in the thalamus, or deep in the white matter of the parietal lobe. When position sense, two-point discrimination, and tactile localization are affected relatively more than pain or thermal and tactile sense, a cerebral lesion is suggested; the converse indicates a brainstem localization. Bilaterality of both motor and sensory signs is almost certain evidence that the lesion lies infratentorially. When hemiplegia or hemiparesis and sensory loss are coextensive, the lesion usually lies supratentorially. Additional manifestations that point unequivocally to a brainstem site are rotational dizziness, diplopia, cerebellar ataxia, a Horner syndrome, and deafness. The several brainstem syndromes illustrate the important point that the cerebellar pathways, spinothalamic tract, trigeminal nucleus, and sympathetic fibers can be involved at different levels, and "neighboring" phenomena must be used to identify the exact site.

A myriad of proper names have been applied to the brainstem syndromes, as noted in Table 47-2. Most of them were originally described in relation to tumors and other nonvascular diseases. The diagnosis of vascular disorders in this region of the brain is not greatly facilitated by a knowledge of these eponymic syndromes; it is much more profitable to memorize the anatomy of the brainstem. The principal syndromes to be recognized are the full basilar, vertebral, posteroinferior cerebellar, anteroinferior cerebellar, superior cerebellar, pontomedullary, and medial medullary. Figures 34-12 to 34-15 (supplied by Dr. C. M. Fisher and used in all previous editions of this book) present both medial and lateral syndromes at four levels of the medulla and pons. Other syndromes can usually be identified as fragments or combinations of the major ones.

Lacunar Syndromes

As one might surmise, small penetrating branches of the cerebral arteries may become occluded, and the resulting infarcts may be so small or so situated as to cause no symptoms whatsoever. As the softened tissue is removed, it leaves a small cavity, or lacune. Early in the twentieth century, Pierre Marie confirmed the occurrence of multiple deep small cavities of this type, first described by Durant-Fardel in 1843. Marie referred to the condition as *état lacunaire*. Marie distinguished these lesions from a fine loosening of tissue around thickened vessels that enter the anterior and posterior perforated spaces, a change to which he gave the name état criblé. Pathologists have not always agreed on these distinctions, but Fisher and Adams have taken the position that the lacunar state is always due to occlusion of small arteries, 50 to 200 mm in diameter, and the cribriform state to mere thickening of vessels and slight fraying of the surrounding tissue.

In our clinical and pathologic material, there has always been a strong correlation of the lacunar state with a combination of hypertension and atherosclerosis and, to a lesser degree, with diabetes. Sacco and colleagues, in a population-based study in Rochester, Minnesota, found hypertension in 81 percent of patients with lacunar

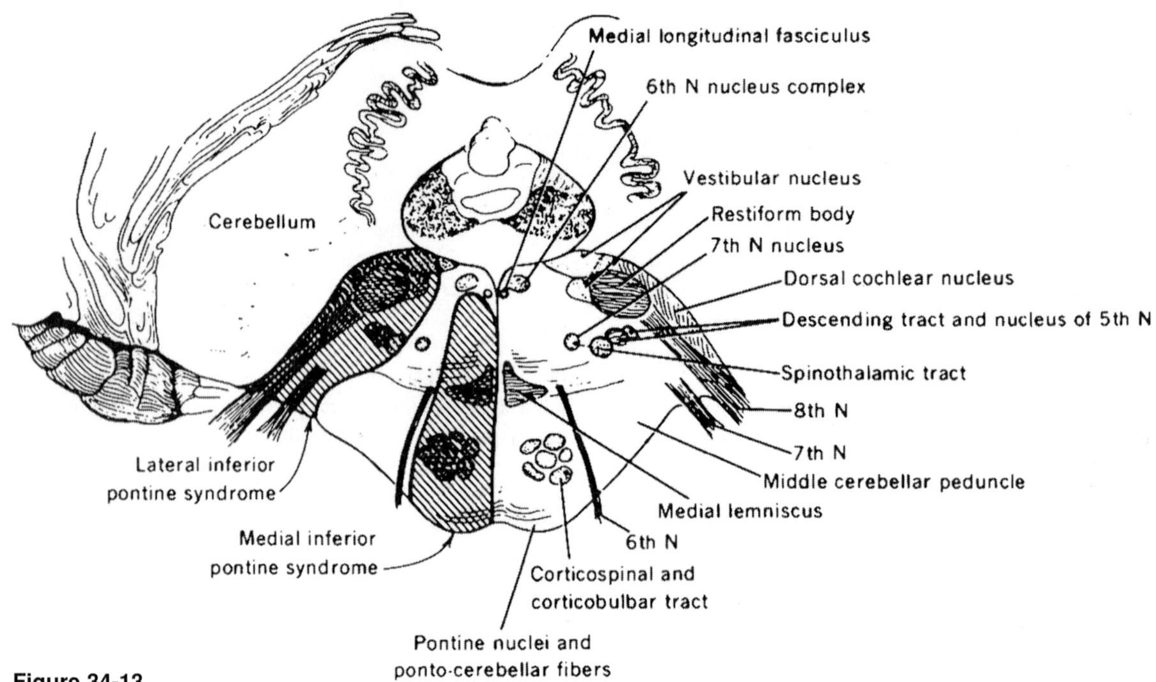

Figure 34-13

Transverse section through the lower pons.

Signs and symptoms	*Structures involved*
1. Medial inferior pontine syndrome (occlusion of paramedian branch of basilar artery)	
a. On side of lesion	
(1) Paralysis of conjugate gaze to side of lesion (preservation of convergence)	Pontine "center" for lateral gaze (PPRF)
(2) Nystagmus	Vestibular nuclei and connections
(3) Ataxia of limbs and gait	Middle cerebellar peduncle (?)
(4) Diplopia on lateral gaze	Abducens nerve or nucleus; PPRF
b. On side opposite lesion	
(1) Paralysis of face, arm, and leg	Corticobulbar and corticospinal tract in lower pons
(2) Impaired tactile and proprioceptive sense over half of the body	Medial lemniscus
2. Lateral inferior pontine syndrome (occlusion of anterior inferior cerebellar artery)	
a. On side of lesion	
(1) Horizontal and vertical nystagmus, vertigo, nausea, vomiting, oscillopsia	Vestibular nerve or nucleus
(2) Facial paralysis	Seventh nerve or nucleus
(3) Paralysis of conjugate gaze to side of lesion	Pontine "center" for lateral gaze (PPRF)
(4) Deafness, tinnitus	Auditory nerve or cochlear nuclei
(5) Ataxia	Middle cerebellar peduncle and cerebellar hemisphere
(6) Impaired sensation over face	Main sensory nucleus and descending tract of fifth nerve
b. On side opposite lesion	
(1) Impaired pain and thermal sense over half the body (may include face)	Spinothalamic tract
3. Total unilateral inferior pontine syndrome (occlusion of anterior inferior cerebellar artery); lateral and medial syndromes combined	

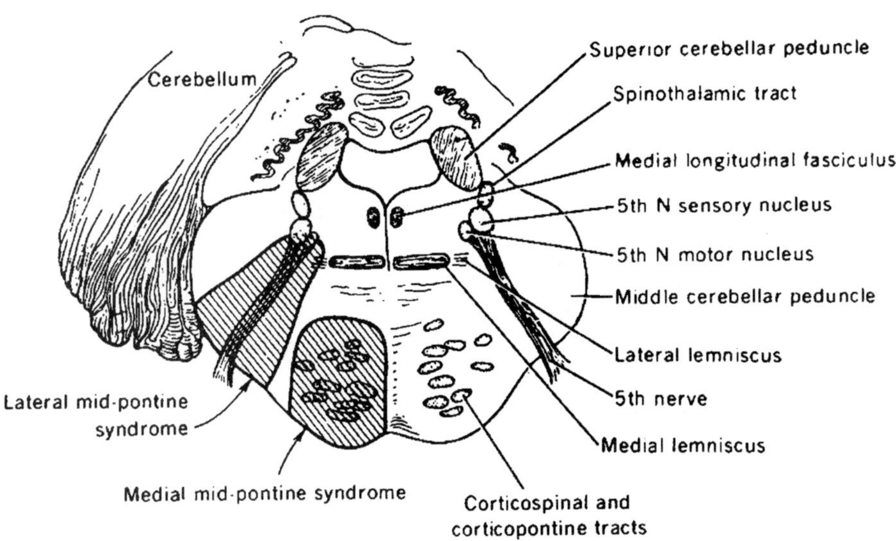

Figure 34-14

Transverse section through the midpons.

Signs and symptoms	*Structures involved*
1. Medial midpontine syndrome (paramedian branch of midbasilar artery)	
a. On side of lesion	
(1) Ataxia of limbs and gait (more prominent in bilateral involvement	Middle cerebellar peduncle
b. On side opposite lesion	
(1) Paralysis of face, arm, and leg	Corticobulbar and corticospinal tract
(2) Deviation of eyes	
(3) Variably impaired touch and proprioception when lesion extends posteriorly. Usually the syndrome is purely motor.	Medial lemniscus
2. Lateral midpontine syndrome (short circumferential artery)	
a. On side of lesion	
(1) Ataxia of limbs	Middle cerebellar peduncle
(2) Paralysis of muscles of mastication	Motor fibers or nucleus of fifth nerve
(3) Impaired sensation over side of face	Sensory fibers or nucleus of fifth nerve

infarctions. One may hypothesize that the basis of the lacunar state is unusually severe atherosclerosis that has not just involved the large arteries, as it usually does, but has extended into their finest branches.

When Fisher examined a series of such lesions in serial sections, from a basal parent artery up to and through the lacune, he found atheroma and thrombosis and less often embolic occlusion of small vessels to be the basic abnormality in some (usually the larger) lacunes, and a lipohyalin degeneration and occlusion of small vessels in the smaller ones. In some instances the latter changes had resulted in false aneurysm formation, resembling the Charcot-Bouchard aneurysms that underlie brain hemorrhage (see further on). Usually 4 to 6 and sometimes up to 10 to 15 lacunes are found in any given brain specimen. They are situated, in descending order of

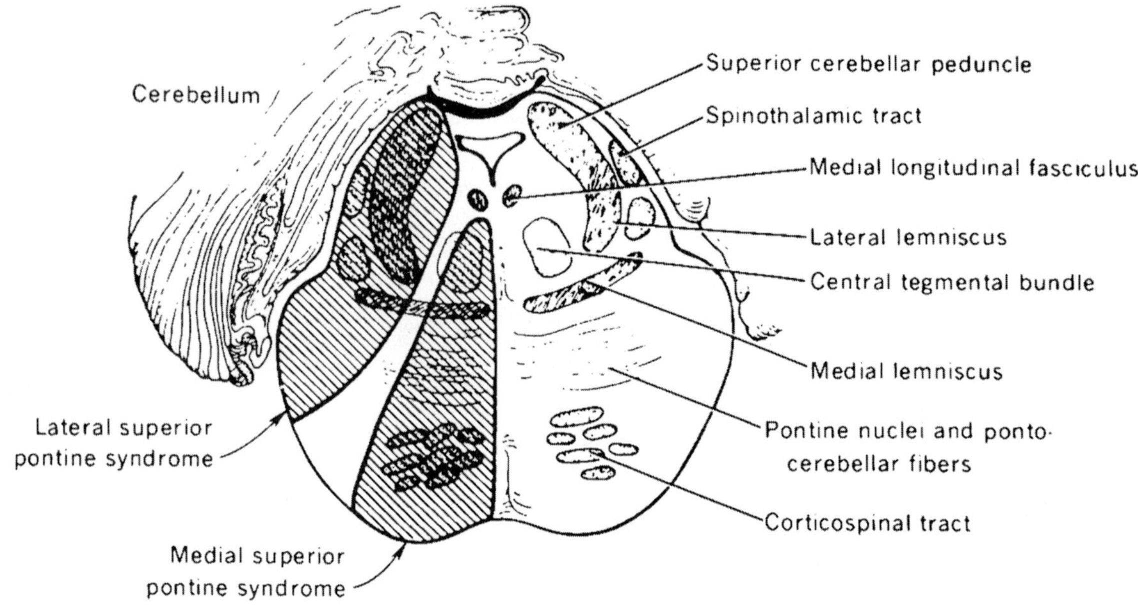

Figure 34-15

Transverse section through the upper pons.

Signs and symptoms	*Structures involved*	
1. Medial superior pontine syndrome (paramedian branches of upper basilar artery)		
a. On side of lesion		
(1) Cerebellar ataxia	Superior and/or middle cerebellar peduncle	
(2) Internuclear ophthalmoplegia	Medial longitudinal fasciculus	
(3) Rhythmic myoclonus of palate, pharynx, vocal cords, respiratory apparatus, face, oculomotor apparatus, etc.	Central tegmental bundle	
b. On side opposite lesion		
(1) Paralysis of face, arm, and leg	Corticobulbar and corticospinal tract	
(2) Rarely touch, vibration, and position senses are affected	Medial lemniscus	
2. Lateral superior pontine syndrome (syndrome of superior cerebellar artery)		
a. On side of lesion		
(1) Ataxia of limbs and gait, falling to side of lesion	Middle and superior cerebellar peduncles, superior surface of cerebellum, dentate nucleus	
(2) Dizziness, nausea, vomiting	Vestibular nuclei	Territory of descending branch to middle cerebellar peduncle (occlusion of superior cerebellar artery)
(3) Horizontal nystagmus	Vestibular nuclei	
(4) Paresis of conjugate gaze (ipsilateral)	Uncertain	
(5) Loss of optokinetic nystagmus	Uncertain	
(6) Skew deviation	Uncertain	
(7) Miosis, ptosis, decreased sweating over face (Horner syndrome)	Descending sympathetic fibers	
b. On side opposite lesion		
(1) Impaired pain and thermal sense on face, limbs, and trunk	Spinothalamic tract	
(2) Impaired touch, vibration, and position sense, more in leg than in arm (there is a tendency to incongruity of pain and touch deficits)	Medial lemniscus (lateral portion)	

frequency, in the putamen and caudate nuclei, thalamus, basis pontis, internal capsule, and convolutional white matter. The cavities range from 3 to 15 mm in diameter, and whether they cause symptoms depends entirely on their location. In a series of 1042 consecutive adults whose brains were examined postmortem, Fisher observed one or more lacunes in 11 percent.

Fisher has delineated some of the more frequent symptomatic forms. If the lacune lies in the territory of a lenticulostriate artery, i.e., in the internal capsule or adjacent corona radiata, it may cause a *pure motor hemiplegia*. Symptoms may be abrupt in onset or evolve over several hours, but in some instances (10 of 34 lacunar syndromes, according to Weisberg) the neurologic deficit evolves stepwise and relatively slowly, over as long a period as 2 to 3 days, simulating a small hemorrhage. CT scanning shows the lesions in about two-thirds of cases, and MRI, in probably a higher proportion. The weakness in pure motor hemiplegia involves the face, arm, and leg. Sometimes the motor disorder takes the form of a dysarthria, with or without hemiplegia. Recovery, which may begin within hours, days, or weeks, is often nearly complete.

Similarly, a lacune of the lateral thalamus or parietal white matter presents as a pure hemisensory defect (*pure sensory stroke*). The incidence, course, and outcome are much the same as in a pure hemiplegia. In the basis pontis, the syndrome may be one of pure motor hemiplegia, mimicking that of internal capsular infarction except for relative sparing of the face and the presence of an ipsilateral paresis of conjugate gaze in some cases; or there may be a combination of *dysarthria and clumsiness* of one hand. Occasionally a lacunar infarction of the pons, midbrain, internal capsule, or parietal white matter gives rise to a *hemiparesis with ataxia* on the same side as the weakness (Fisher; Sage and Lepore). Some of the brainstem syndromes may blend with basilar branch syndromes. There are many other, less frequent syndromes, too numerous to tabulate here. Multiple lacunar infarcts, involving the corticospinal and corticobulbar tracts, are by far the most common cause of pseudobulbar palsy.

In all these cases of lacunar infarction, the diagnosis depends essentially on the occurrence of the aforementioned certain unique stroke syndromes of limited proportions. As mentioned above, CT scanning is less reliable than MRI in demonstrating the lacunes. The EEG may be helpful in a negative sense; in the case of lacunes in the pons or the internal capsule, there is a notable discrepancy between the unilateral paralysis or sensory loss and the negligible electrical changes over the affected hemisphere.

THE MAJOR TYPES OF CEREBROVASCULAR DISEASE

In classifying the cerebrovascular diseases, it is most practical, from the clinical viewpoint, to preserve the classic division into thrombosis, embolism, and hemorrhage. The causes of each of the "big three," along with the criteria for diagnosis and the confirmatory laboratory tests for each, are considered here in separate sections. This classification has the disadvantage of not providing for disorders such as reversible ischemia, hypertensive encephalopathy, and venous thrombosis; these are considered in separate sections later in the chapter.

The frequency of the different types of cerebrovascular disease has been difficult to ascertain. Obviously clinical diagnosis is not always correct, and clinical services are heavily weighted with acute strokes and nonfatal cases of uncertain type. An autopsy series inevitably includes many old vascular lesions, particularly infarcts, whose exact nature cannot always be determined, and there is a bias also toward large fatal lesions (usually hemorrhages). Table 34-3 summarizes

Table 34-3
Major types of cerebrovascular diseases and their frequency

	Harvard stroke series[a] (756 successive cases)	*BCH autopsy series[b] (179 cases)*
Atherosclerotic thrombosis	244 (32%)	21 (12%)
Lacunes	129 (18%)	34 (18.5%)
Embolism	244 (32%)	57 (32%)
Hypertensive hemorrhage	84 (11%)	28 (15.5%)
Ruptured aneurysms and vascular malformations	55 (7%)	8 (4.5%)
Indeterminate		17 (9.5%)
Other[c]		14 (8%)

[a]Compiled by J. Mohr, L. Caplan, D. Pessin, P. Kistler, and G. Duncan at Massachusetts General Hospital and Beth Israel Hospital, Boston.
[b]Compiled by C. M. Fisher and R. D. Adams in an examination of 740 brains during the year 1949 at Mallory Institute of Pathology, Boston City Hospital.
[c]Hypertensive encephalopathy, cerebral vein thrombosis, meningovascular syphilis, and polyarteritis nodosa.

the findings of the Harvard Cooperative Stroke Registry, tabulated in 1978 and comprising 756 successive patients, each of whom was examined by a physician knowledgeable about strokes and subjected when necessary to appropriate ancillary examinations (four-vessel arteriography, CT scan, lumbar puncture). For comparison, we have included an autopsy series of 740 cases, examined during the year 1949 by Fisher and Adams; of these, 179 (nearly 25 percent) had some form of cerebrovascular disease. Interestingly, in both series the ratio of infarcts to hemorrhages was 4:1 and embolism accounted for approximately one-third of all strokes. The above studies correspond reasonably well with more recent data collated in the Stroke Data Bank of the National Institute of Neurological Disorders (NINCDS) (Sacco et al).

Atherothrombotic Infarction

Most cerebrovascular disease can be attributed to atherosclerosis and chronic hypertension; until ways are found to prevent or control them, vascular disease of the brain will continue to be a major cause of morbidity. Hypertension and atherosclerosis interact in a variety of ways. Atherosclerosis, by reducing the resilience of large arteries, induces hypertension. Atherosclerotic stenosis of the renal arteries, by causing ischemia of the kidneys, does the same. In turn, sustained hypertension worsens atherosclerosis, seemingly "driving" it into the walls of small branch arteries (0.5 mm or less). All the coats of the vessel become impregnated with a hyaline-lipid material, a process that Fisher has called *lipohyalinosis*. The segment so affected may weaken and allow the formation of a small dissecting aneurysm (Charcot-Bouchard aneurysm), which some neuropathologists hold responsible for the hypertensive brain hemorrhage. Lipohyalinosis also results in thrombosis of small penetrating arteries, leading to the aforementioned lacunar state.

The atheromatous process in brain arteries is identical to that in the aorta, coronary, and other large arteries. In general the process in the cerebral arteries runs parallel to but is somewhat less severe than that in the aorta, heart, and lower limbs. There are many exceptions to this rule, however, and not infrequently a brain artery becomes occluded when there is no clinical evidence of coronary or peripheral vascular disease. Although atheromatosis is known to have its onset in childhood and adolescence, only in the middle and late years of life is it likely to have clinical effects. Hypertension, hyperlipidemia, and diabetes aggravate the process. As with coronary and peripheral atherosclerosis, individuals with low blood levels of high-density-lipoprotein (HDL) cholesterol and high levels of low-density-lipoprotein (LDL) cholesterol are particularly disposed to cerebral atherosclerosis (Nubiola et al). Long-duration cigarette smoking, an important factor in the genesis of atherosclerosis, decreases both HDL cholesterol and cerebral blood flow (Homer et al, Ingall et al). Added to these well-established risk factors is the possible role of an excess of homocystine and a speculative role for chronic inflammation, particularly with *Chlamydia pneumoniae*. Clinical experience indicates that there are families with a predilection for the development of cerebral atherosclerosis, independent of these well-defined risk factors.

There is a tendency for atheromatous plaques to form at branchings and curves of the cerebral arteries. *The most frequent sites are* in the *internal carotid artery*, at its origin from the common carotid; in the *cervical part of the vertebral arteries and at their junction to form the basilar artery*; in the *stem or at the main bifurcation of the middle cerebral arteries*; in the *posterior cerebral arteries* as they wind around the midbrain; and in the *anterior cerebral arteries* as they curve over the corpus callosum. It is rare for the cerebral arteries to develop plaques beyond their first major branching. Also, it is unusual for the cerebellar and ophthalmic arteries to show atheromatous involvement except in conjunction with hypertension. The common carotid and vertebral arteries at their origins from the aorta are frequent sites of atheromatous deposits, but because of abundant collateral arterial pathways, occlusions at these sites are not commonly associated with cerebral ischemia.

The atheromatous lesions develop and grow silently for 20, 30, or more years; only in the event of a thrombotic complication do they become symptomatic. Although atheromatous plaques may narrow the lumen of an artery, causing stenosis, *complete occlusion is nearly always the consequence of superimposed thrombosis*. In general, the more severe the atheromatosis, the more likely the thrombotic complication, but the two processes do not always run in parallel. A patient with only scattered atheromatous plaques may thrombose a vessel, whereas another with marked atherosclerosis may have only a few thrombosed vessels or none at all. Atheromatous lesions may regress to some extent under the influence of diet and certain drugs. Hennerici and colleagues followed a series of patients with carotid stenoses for a period of 18 months and observed regression in nearly 20 percent of the lesions. In the large majority of cases, however, atherosclerosis is a progressive disease.

Degeneration of or hemorrhage into the wall of a sclerotic vessel (from rupture of the vasa vasorum) may damage the endothelium. This is known to occur particularly in the walls of the internal carotid arteries. Platelets and fibrin then adhere to the damaged part of the wall and form delicate, friable clots, or a subintimal atheromatous deposit may slough, spewing crystalline cholesterol emboli into the lumen and occluding small distal vessels. In contrast to an embolus, a thrombus presumably does not occlude the lumen completely from the first moment of its formation; total blockage may occur only after several hours. In some instances thrombotic particles may form and break off repeatedly, thus becoming an important source of *artery-to-artery* cerebral embolism. Once the lumen of the artery has been completely occluded, the thrombus may propagate distally and proximally to the next branching points and block an anastomotic channel.

These several events in the atherosclerotic-thrombotic process probably account for the prodromal ischemic attacks—intermittent blockage of the circulation and variable impairment of function in the vascular territory, often proceeding to permanent ischemic effects and later progression (after several days). Not infrequently several arteries are affected by stenosis and thrombosis over a period of months or years; then it becomes difficult to decipher the interplay of factors that lead to either transitory or persistent symptoms. Some of the possibilities have been outlined by Adams and colleagues (1961). The evolution of the thrombotic process may be sufficiently prolonged to explain the clinical state known as *stroke in evolution*; when the hemodynamic disturbance stabilizes, the stage of *completed stroke* is reached. These different stages acquire significance in relation to therapy and prognosis.

Pathophysiology of Thrombosis The process of thrombus formation involves an interplay between three components: the endothelium, circulating platelets, and a series of biochemical events known as the "coagulative cascade."

When atherosclerosis is the primary condition, thrombus formation usually begins with a localized injury to the endothelium. As indicated earlier, the overlying endothelium suffers damage from hemorrhage or necrosis of the vessel wall, secondary to an alteration of the vasa vasorum. Thrombus forms from fibrin and platelets and the vessel becomes partly or completely occluded. In the process, regional blood vessels dilate and aggregates of platelets are attracted to the site, partly through the action of prostacyclin (derived from arachidonic acid); the accumulation of nitric oxide (derived from relaxing factor of vessel wall) then leads to vasoconstriction. Also, a substance called vasomodulin on the surface of the endothelium—which, with protein C, normally inhibits the formation of fibrin through its interaction with thrombin—is reduced at the injured site and induces clotting. Homocystine (as in homocystinuria) has a similar effect and is believed thereby to promote thrombosis.

Circulating platelets increase in number locally, enlarge, and become more adherent to one another and to the injured vessel. As they aggregate, they discharge their granules. The latter process is stimulated by thromboxane A_2, which is synthesized in the injured vessel wall. This substance also releases coagulation proteins (including thrombin and Willebrand factor and other elements of the coagulative cascade).

The third component—i.e., the coagulative cascade—involves the complex interplay of a series of factors that leads to the formation of thrombin and the conversion of fibrinogen to fibrin. Involved in this process are changes in a number of natural anticoagulative factors such as heparin cofactor 2, antithrombin III, protein C, and protein S. Some of these are extrinsic to the blood vessels and hence may result in thrombosis in one or in multiple sites without prior vascular injury. Protein C is a vitamin K–dependent protease which, in combination with its cofactors protein S and antithrombin III, inhibits coagulation. A deficiency of any of these may predispose to in situ thrombosis within either the arterial or venous systems. Protein C deficiency (heterozygous in one of every 16,000 individuals) is a cause of thrombosis of both veins and arteries; a resistance to activated protein C has also been described (causing venous thrombosis almost exclusively). Antiphospholipid antibody formation is another possible cause of vascular occlusion that is not incited by damage to the vessel wall (see further on). The metabolic disturbances in Fabry disease also favor clotting. Persons with certain inflammatory bowel diseases (ulcerative colitis, Crohn disease) are prone to develop thrombotic strokes.

These factors should be sought when thrombotic disease in cerebral arteries or veins occurs in children or young adults with unexplained strokes, in families with strokes, in pregnant or parturient women, and in women who are migraineurs or "on the pill" (see further on). According to Markus and Hambley, whose review of this subject is recommended, screening for lupus anticoagulant, anticardiolipin antibodies, deficiency of proteins C and S, and antithrombin III is probably justified only under these special conditions.

Clinical Picture In general, evolution of the clinical phenomena in relation to cerebral thrombosis is more variable than that of embolism and hemorrhage. In more than half of our patients, the main part of the stroke (paralysis or other deficit) is preceded by minor signs or one or more transient attacks of focal neurologic dysfunction, called *transient ischemic attacks* or *TIAs* (Table 34-4). In a sense, these herald the oncoming vascular catastrophe. *A history of such prodromal episodes is of paramount importance in establishing the diagnosis of cerebral thrombosis.* Only rarely and for unclear reasons are embolism and cerebral hemorrhage preceded by a transient neurologic disorder. In carotid and middle cerebral artery disease, the transient attacks consist of monocular blindness or of hemiplegia, hemianesthesia, disturbances of speech and language, confusion, etc. In the vertebrobasilar system, the prodromal spells most often take the form of episodes of dizziness, diplopia, numbness, impaired vision in one or both visual fields, and dysarthria. These TIA syndromes are described more fully further on. Such attacks last from a few minutes to several hours; in most instances the duration is less than 10 min. Those of several hours' duration have a different connotation, since they are usually due to demonstrable embolism. The final stroke may be preceded by one or two attacks or a hundred or more brief TIAs, and the stroke may follow the onset of the attacks by hours, weeks, or, rarely, months. When there are no prodromal ischemic attacks, one must use other criteria to establish the diagnosis of atherosclerotic thrombosis.

Table 34-4
Development of the clinical picture in 125 cases of cerebral thrombosis (C. M. Fisher)

Clinical development	*No. of cases*	*Percent*
Transient ischemic attacks progressing to a major or minor persistent neurologic deficit	53	42
Stepwise development of a stroke, with or without transient ischemic attacks	23	18
Stroke developing as a single event:		
Abrupt (hours), with or without fluctuations	14	11
Slow, gradual (a few days), with or without minor fluctuations	7	6
Transient ischemic attacks only	17	14
Development of a limited stroke followed by transient ischemic attacks	11	9

The thrombotic stroke, whether or not it is preceded by warning attacks, develops in one of several ways. Most often there is a single episode and the whole illness evolves within a few hours. More telling diagnostically is a "stuttering" or intermittent progression of neurologic deficits extending over several hours or a day or longer. Again, a partial stroke may occur and even recede temporarily for several hours, after which there is rapid progression to the completed stroke—or several fleeting episodes may be followed by a longer one and, hours or a day or two later, by a major stroke. Several parts of the body may be affected at once or only one part, such as a limb or one side of the face, the other parts becoming involved serially in steplike fashion until the stroke is fully developed. Sometimes the deficit is episodic; involuntary movement of a hand or arm or dimness of vision, lasting 5 to 10 min, occurs spontaneously or is brought on by standing or walking. Each of the transient attacks and the abrupt episodes of progression reproduces the profile of the stroke in miniature. The principle of intermittency seems to characterize the thrombotic process from beginning to end.

Even more frequent than the modes of onset outlined above is the occurrence of the thrombotic stroke during sleep; the patient awakens paralyzed, either during the night or in the morning. Unaware of any difficulty, he may arise and fall helplessly to the floor with the first step. This is the story in fully 60 percent of our patients with thrombotic strokes and in a certain number with embolic ones as well.

Most deceptive of all are the relatively few patients in whom the neurologic disorder has evolved over several days or even longer, in a slow, gradual fashion ("slow stroke"). One's first impulse is to make a diagnosis of brain tumor, abscess, or subdural hematoma. This error can usually be avoided by a careful analysis of the course of the illness, which will disclose an uneven, saltatory progression; if the clinical data are incomplete, observation for a few days will reveal the stroke profile more clearly. Actually there are a few cases—and these are usually instances of pure motor hemiplegia—in which the evolution of a thrombotic stroke is evenly progressive over a period of days.

In addition to these several modes of evolution of atherothrombotic stroke, thrombotic stenosis or occlusion of certain large vessels may lead instead to the generation of embolic fragments (*artery-to-artery embolus*), thereby precipitating a new stroke in a region distal to the occlusion. This is most likely to occur during the period of clinical fluctuation and active thrombus formation. The most common occurrence of artery-to-artery embolism is with carotid artery thrombosis, the embolus passing to branches of the ipsilateral middle or anterior cerebral artery. With atherothrombotic blockage of the vertebral or lower basilar artery, the embolus lodges in the posterior cerebral artery or the top of the basilar artery (Koroshetz and Ropper).

Arterial thrombosis is not usually accompanied by headache, but the latter does occur in some cases. Usually the pain is located on one side of the head in carotid occlusion, at the back of the head or simultaneously in forehead and occiput in basilar occlusion, and behind the ipsilateral ear or above the eyebrow in vertebral occlusion. The headache is less severe and more regional than that of intracerebral or subarachnoid hemorrhage, and there is no stiffness of the neck. The mechanism is unclear. Presumably it is related to the disease process within the vessel wall, since it may antedate the other manifestations of the stroke by days or even weeks.

Hypertension is more often present than not in patients with atherothrombotic infarction. Diabetes mellitus is common also, or the patient is a smoker or hyperlipidemic. Often there is evidence of vascular disease in other parts of the body: a history of coronary occlusion or angina pectoris, an electrocardiographic (ECG) abnormality reflecting a previous myocardial infarction or left ventricular hypertrophy, intermittent claudication, or an absence of one or several pulses in the lower limbs. The retinal arteries may show uniform or focal narrowing, increase and irregularity of the light reflex, and arteriovenous "nicking," but these findings correlate with hypertension rather than atherosclerosis. The patient is more often elderly but may be in the fourth decade of life or even younger.

Laboratory Findings These have been discussed at various points in the preceding pages and need only be recapitulated briefly. In the laboratory investigation of atherothrombotic infarction, one relies greatly on noninvasive techniques. Ultrasonography will reveal with fair accuracy the cervical and intracranial segments of the internal carotid and vertebrobasilar arteries. MRI is more sensitive to ischemic brain damage than is the CT scan. While the latter reveals hemorrhage immediately after it occurs, softened tissue cannot be seen until several days have elapsed. On the other hand, MRI reveals ischemic damage within a few hours, in both white and gray matter, and diffusion-weighted MRI techniques do so even earlier. By MR angiography, one can see all the major cervical and intracranial arteries and may detect the irregular lumen or occlusion of atherosclerosis and even embolic occlusions in more distal vessels (Fig. 34-16). This method has to a large extent replaced conventional angiography, which is reserved for cases in which the diagnosis is in doubt (e.g., suspected angiitis) or when surgical intervention or long-term anticoagulant therapy is contemplated.

Lumbar puncture is now performed only sparingly in patients with stroke. Cerebral thrombosis does not cause blood to enter the CSF. Frequently the CSF protein is slightly elevated (usually 50 to 80 mg/dL); rarely is it in excess of 100 mg/dL. A small number of polymorphonuclear leukocytes (3 to 8 per cubic millimeter) is not exceptional in the first few days; very rarely, and for unexplained reasons, a brisk, transient pleocytosis (400 to 1000 polymorphonuclear leukocytes per cubic millimeter) occurs on about the third day. A persistent pleocytosis, however, suggests a chronic meningitis (syphilis, tuberculosis, cryptococcosis), granulomatous arteritis, septic embolism, thrombophlebitis, or a nonvascular process as the cause of vascular occlusion.

Serum cholesterol, triglycerides, or both are elevated in many cases, but normal values are not helpful. The EEG is of value in distinguishing large strokes from lacunes, as already mentioned. The EEG changes over a cortical infarct may normalize over several months.

Course and Prognosis When the patient is seen early in the course of cerebral thrombosis, it is difficult to give an accurate prognosis. One must ask where the patient stands in the stroke process at the time of the examination. Is worsening to be anticipated or not? No rules have yet been formulated that allow one to predict the early course with confidence. A mild paralysis today may become a disastrous hemiplegia tomorrow, or the patient's condition may worsen only temporarily for a day or two. In basilar artery occlusion, dizziness and dysphagia may progress in a few days to total paralysis and deep coma. The course of cerebral thrombosis is so often progressive that a cautious attitude on the part of the physician in what first appears to be a mild stroke is justified.

As indicated above, progression of the stroke is due most often to increasing stenosis and occlusion of the involved artery by mural thrombus. In some instances, extension of the thrombus along the vessel may block side branches and hinder anastomotic flow. In the basilar artery, thrombus may gradually build up along its entire length. In the carotid system, thrombus at times propagates distally from the site of origin in the neck to the supraclinoid portion and possibly into the anterior

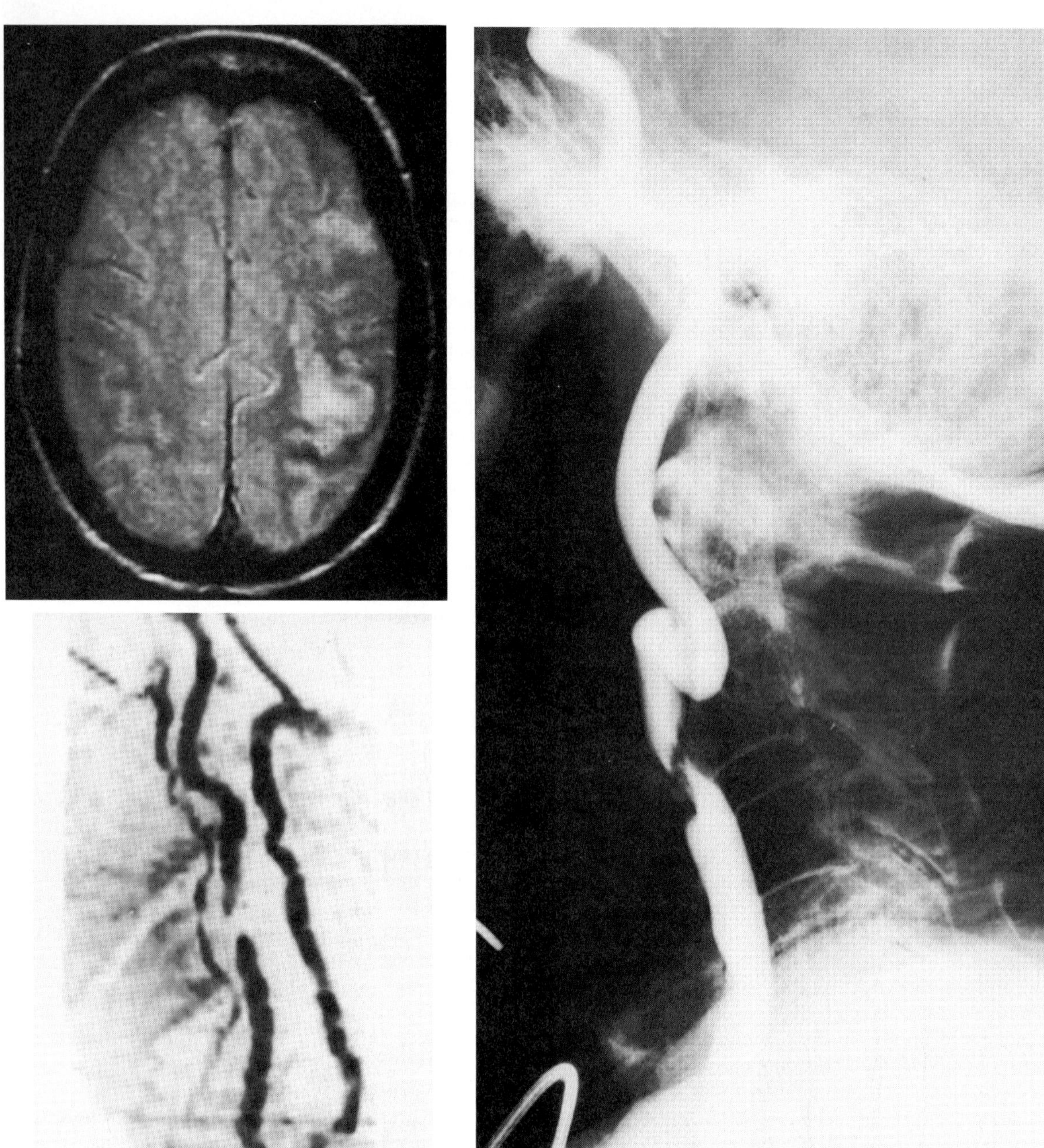

Figure 34-16

Left carotid stenosis with border zone infarction demonstrated by MRI. Magnetic resonance angiography (lower left) *and conventional angiography* (right) *show almost complete stenosis of the left internal carotid artery. The patient was a 72-year-old woman with acute onset of right hemiplegia.*

cerebral artery, preventing collateral flow from the opposite side. In middle cerebral occlusion, retrograde thrombosis may extend to the mouth of the anterior cerebral, perhaps secondarily leading to infarction of the territory of that vessel. And finally, abrupt progression of a stroke may be the result of artery-to-artery embolism, as described above.

Several other circumstances influence the *immediate prognosis* in cerebral thrombosis. In the case of very large infarcts, swelling of the infarcted tissue may occur, followed by displacement of central structures, tentorial herniation, and death of the patient after several days (Fig. 34-17). This can be anticipated by the sheer volume of the infarct and is usually evident on the CT scan within a day of the stroke. Smaller infarcts of the inferior surface of the cerebellum may also cause a fatal herniation into the foramen magnum. Milder degrees of swelling and increased intracranial pressure may progress slightly for 2 to 3 days but do not prove fatal. In extensive brainstem infarction associated with deep coma, due to basilar artery occlusion, the mortality rate approaches 40 percent. In any type of stroke, if coma or stupor is present from the beginning, survival is largely determined by success in keeping the airway clear, controlling brain swelling, preventing aspiration pneumonia, and maintaining fluid and electrolyte balance, as described further on under "Treatment of Cerebral Edema and Raised Intracranial Pressure." With smaller thrombotic infarcts, the mortality is 3 to 6 percent, much of it from myocardial infarction and aspiration pneumonia.

As for the *eventual or long-term prognosis* of the neurologic deficit, there are many possibilities. Improvement is the rule if the patient survives. The patient with a lacunar infarct and pure motor hemiparesis usually fares well. With other small infarcts, recovery may start within a day or two, and restoration may be complete or nearly complete within a week. In cases of severe deficit, there may be no significant recovery; after months of assiduous efforts at rehabilitation, the patient may remain bereft of speech and understanding, with the upper extremity still useless and the lower extremity serving only as an uncertain prop during attempts to walk.

Figure 34-17

Massive ischemic infarct of left cerebral hemisphere in the distribution of the middle cerebral artery. CT scans taken 24 h (left) *and 72 h* (right) *following the onset of neurologic symptoms. The second scan demonstrates marked swelling of the infarcted tissue and displacement of central structures.*

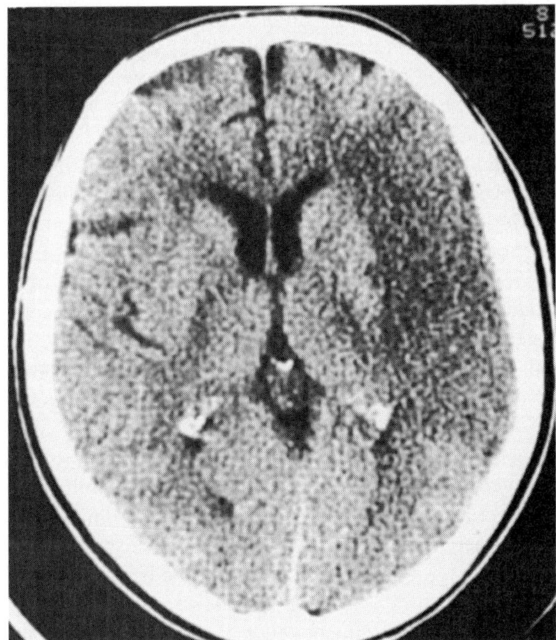

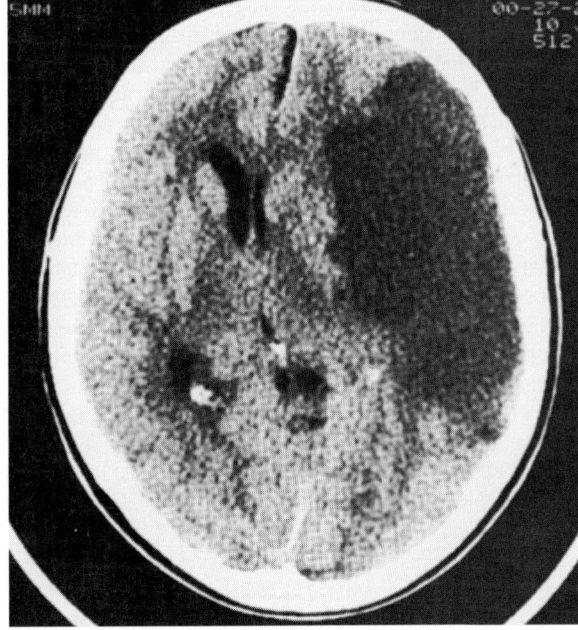

Between these two extremes there is every gradation of recovery. In general, the longer the delay in onset of recovery, the poorer the prognosis. Measurement of central motor conduction by magnetic stimulation has been helpful in predicting recovery and survival. If there is no response within the first few days, the prospect of recovery of function is poor. If clinical recovery does not begin in 1 or 2 weeks, the outlook is gloomy for both motor and language functions. Constructional apraxia, uninhibited anger (with left and rarely with right temporal lesions), nonsensical logorrhea and placidity, unawareness of the paralysis and neglect (with nondominant parietal lesions), and confusion and delirium (with nondominant temporal lesions) all tend to diminish and may disappear within a few weeks. A hemianopia that has not cleared in a few weeks will usually be permanent, although reading and color discrimination may continue to improve. In lateral medullary infarction, difficulty in swallowing may be protracted, lasting 4 to 8 weeks or longer; yet relatively normal function is finally restored in nearly every instance. Aphasia, dysarthria, cerebellar ataxia, and walking may improve for a year or longer, but for all practical purposes it may be said that whatever motor and language deficits remain after 5 to 6 months will be permanent.

Characteristically, the paralyzed muscles are flaccid in the first days or weeks following a stroke; the tendon reflexes are usually unchanged but may be slightly increased or decreased. Gradually spasticity develops, and the tendon reflexes become brisker. The arm tends to assume a flexed adducted posture and the leg an extended one. Function is rarely if ever restored after the slow evolution of spasticity. Conversely, the early development of spasticity in the arm or the early appearance of a grasp reflex may presage a favorable outcome. In some patients with extensive temporoparietal lesions, the hemiplegia remains flaccid; the arm dangles and the slack leg must be braced to stand. The physiologic explanation of this remains obscure. If the internal capsule is not interrupted completely in a stroke that involves the lenticular nucleus or thalamus, the paralysis may give way to hemichoreoathetosis, hemitremor, or hemiataxia, depending upon the particular anatomy of the lesion. Bowel and bladder control usually returns; sphincteric disorders persist in only a few cases. Often the hemiplegic limbs are at first tender and ache on manipulation. Nevertheless, physiotherapy should be initiated early in order to prevent pseudocontracture of muscles and periarthritis at the shoulder, elbow, wrist, knuckles, knee, and ankle. These are frequent complications and often the source of pain and added disability, particularly of the shoulder. Occasionally, atrophy of bone and pain in the hand may accompany the shoulder pain (shoulder-hand syndrome). An annoying feeling of dizziness and unsteadiness often persists after damage to the vestibular system in brainstem infarcts.

Recurrent convulsive (epileptic) seizures are relatively uncommon sequelae of thrombotic strokes in comparison to embolic cortical infarcts, which are followed by seizures in 10 to 20 percent of patients. Most often in our experience, the EEG in these cases had never normalized and showed sharp activity over the region of the infarct even many months after the stroke.

Many patients complain of fatigability and are depressed, possibly more so after strokes that involve the left frontal lobe (Starkstein et al). The explanation of these symptoms is uncertain; some are expressions of a reactive depression. Only a few patients develop serious behavior problems or are psychotic after a stroke, but paranoid trends, confusion, ill temper, stubbornness, and peevishness may appear, or an apathetic state ensues.

Finally, in regard to prognosis, it must be mentioned that having had one thrombotic stroke, the patient is at risk in the ensuing months and years of having a stroke at the same or another site, especially if there is hypertension or diabetes mellitus. When multiple infarcts occur over a period of months or years, special types of dementia may develop, in addition to focal cerebral deficits. These conditions are referred to as *multi-infarct dementia* (page 451). In some of these cases, the major lesions involve the white matter, with relative sparing of the cortex and basal ganglia. This type of lesion is often referred to as *Binswanger subcortical leukoencephalopathy*, which probably equates with multiple white matter infarcts and lacunes (page 878) (see Mohr and Mast). The parts of the white matter that are destroyed tend to lie in the border zones between the penetrating cortical and basal ganglionic arteries. The large patches of subcortical myelin loss and gliosis, in combination with small cortical and subcortical infarcts, produce a special radiologic image. This still incompletely understood process and the inherited infarctive and gliotic condition of white matter termed *CADASIL* are discussed further on.

During the period 1970–1974 in Rochester, Minnesota, 94 percent of patients with ischemic strokes survived for 5 days and 84 percent for 1 month (Garraway et al). The *survival rate* was 54 percent at 3 years and 40 percent at 7 years. In each of these groups, survival was significantly greater than it had been during the period 1965–1969. Among long-term survivors, heart disease is a more frequent cause of death than additional strokes. These figures, which were gathered retrospectively, are comparable to more recent ones reported by Bamford and colleagues. The mortality rate following cerebral infarcts in general (no separation being made between thrombotic and embolic types) at the end of 1 month was 19 percent and at the end of 1 year, 23 percent. Of the survivors, 65 percent were capable of an independent existence.

Transient Ischemic Attacks

As has already been emphasized, when transient ischemic attacks (TIAs) precede a stroke, they almost always stamp the underlying process as atherothrombotic. There is little doubt that they are due to transient focal ischemia. Their mechanism is not fully understood (see further on), but they might be thought of as temporary strokes that fortunately reverse themselves. They belong, therefore, under the heading of atherosclerotic thrombotic disease but are discussed separately here because of their clinical importance.

Current opinion holds that TIAs are brief, reversible episodes of focal, nonconvulsive ischemic neurologic disturbance. Consensus has been that their duration should be less than 24 h, an idea introduced 30 years ago by a committee assigned to the problem. It is more useful clinically to separate attacks that last only a few minutes (up to 1 h) and leave no permanent signs from those of longer duration, which are more likely to be due to embolism. *In any clinical analysis of TIAs, it is also important to separate a single transient episode from repeated ones of uniform type*. The latter are more often a warning sign of impending vascular occlusion, while the former, especially when prolonged, are sometimes due to an embolus that leaves no lasting effect.

In a prospective study of 390 patients with focal TIAs caused by atherosclerotic vascular disease, the 5-year cumulative rate of fatal or nonfatal cerebral infarction was 23 percent (Heyman et al). Interestingly, the rate of myocardial infarction in this group of patients, particularly in those with carotid lesions, was almost as high (21 percent). Thus the occurrence of carotid TIAs is a predictor not only of cerebral infarction but also of myocardial infarction. About two-thirds of all patients with TIAs are men or hypertensive or both, reflecting the higher incidence of atherosclerosis in hypertensives and in males. Occasionally, in younger adults, TIAs may occur as benign phenomena, without recognizable features of or risk factors for atherosclerosis. Migraine is suspect in such patients (see page 184).

Clinical Picture Transient ischemic attacks can reflect the involvement of virtually any cerebral artery: common or internal carotid; middle, posterior, or anterior cerebral; ophthalmic; vertebral, basilar, or cerebellar; or a penetrating branch to the basal ganglia and brainstem. If the posterior cerebral arteries are included in the vertebrobasilar system, transient ischemic episodes are slightly more common in this system than in the carotid one. Transient ischemic attacks may precede, accompany, or infrequently follow the development of a stroke, or they can occur by themselves without leading to a stroke—a fact that makes any form of therapy difficult to evaluate.

As just noted, TIAs may last a few seconds or up to 12 to 24 h, the longer ones almost certainly being due to embolic infarction. Most of them last 2 to 15 min. There may be only a few attacks or several hundred. Between attacks, the neurologic examination may disclose no abnormalities. A stroke may occur after the first or second episode or only after numerous attacks have occurred over a period of weeks or months. Not infrequently the attacks gradually cease and no important paralysis occurs. So far it has not been possible to distinguish those individuals in whom a stroke will develop from those in whom it will not except in a general way. Many attacks over a long period tend to be less likely to lead to thrombosis. Prolonged, fluctuating TIAs are the most ominous. About 20 percent of infarcts that follow TIAs occur within a month after the first attack, and about 50 percent within a year (Whisnant et al, 1973).

Hemispheric Transient Ischemic Attacks (Carotid Artery Territory) The neurologic features of the transient episode indicate the territory or artery involved and are fragments borrowed from the stroke that may be approaching. In the carotid system, the attacks indicate involvement of one cerebral hemisphere or eye. The visual disturbance is ipsilateral; the sensorimotor disturbance is contralateral. Individual attacks tend to involve either the eye or the brain; only rarely are the two involved simultaneously. In the hemispheric attacks, ischemia occurs mainly in the distal territory of the middle cerebral artery and adjacent border zone, producing weakness or numbness of the opposite hand and arm. However, many different combinations may be seen: face and lips, lips and fingers, fingers alone, hand and foot, etc. Rather than being paralyzed or weak, the arm may shake irregularly, simulating a seizure ("limb-shaking TIA") or rarely display other movement disorders (Yanagihara et al). Less common manifestations include confusion, aphasia and difficulty in calculation (when the dominant hemisphere is involved), apractagnosia (nondominant hemisphere), and other temporoparietal disturbances. Headache is not a feature of TIAs.

In ocular attacks, *transient monocular blindness* is the usual symptom (*amaurosis fugax*). Many of the latter episodes evolve swiftly and are described as a shade falling (or rising) smoothly over the visual field until the eye is completely but painlessly blind. The attack clears slowly and uniformly. Sometimes it takes the form of a wedge of visual loss, sudden generalized blurring, or, rarely, a bright light. Transient attacks of monocular blindness are usually more stereotyped than hemispheric attacks. TIAs consisting of a homonymous hemianopia and paresthesias of the hand and arm should suggest a stenosis of the posterior cerebral artery.

The implications of amaurosis fugax have been evaluated by several investigators and found not to be as ominous as those of hemispheral TIAs, particularly in younger patients. Poole and Ross Russell observed a group of 110 medically treated patients for periods of 6 to 19 years following an episode of amaurosis fugax (exclusive of the type caused by cholesterol emboli). At the end of 6 years, the mortality rate (due mainly to heart disease) had risen to 21 percent and the incidence of stroke to 13 percent (compared to expected figures of 15 and 3 percent, respectively, in an age-matched population). Of the patients who were alive at the end of the observation period, 43 percent had had no further attacks of amaurosis fugax following the initial episode. Noteworthy also was the finding that among patients with normal carotid arteriograms, only 1 of 35 had had a stroke during the follow-up period, whereas stroke had occurred in 8 of 21 patients in whom the internal carotid artery was occluded or stenotic. These figures are in keeping with those of Ackerman; in a series of 139 patients with amaurosis fugax and normal lumens of the common and internal carotid arteries, only 3 had a subsequent hemispheric stroke (personal communication). The age of onset of amaurosis fugax is of particular significance. In the series of Poole and Ross Russell, the youngest patient to have a stroke after onset of amaurosis fugax was 57 years old. Tippin and coworkers reviewed the records of 83 patients with onset of amaurosis fugax before the age of 45 years and found evidence of stroke in none of them; moreover, 42 of these patients were examined after a mean period of 5.8 years during which no stroke had occurred. It is evident that in this early-onset, good-prognosis group, a mechanism other than atherosclerosis was operative, such as migraine or an antiphospholipid antibody (discussed further on).

Brainstem Transient Ischemic Attacks (Vertebrobasilar Circulation) Recurrent TIAs referable to vertebrobasilar disease tend to be less stereotyped and more prolonged than those related to the carotid circulation. They are also more likely to culminate in a stroke. The clinical picture of TIAs in the vertebrobasilar territory is diverse, since this circulation sustains such a varied sensorimotor traffic. Vertigo, diplopia (vertical or horizontal), dysarthria, bifacial numbness, ataxia, and weakness or numbness of part or all of one or both sides of the body (i.e., a disturbance of the long motor or sensory tracts bilaterally) are the hallmarks of vertebrobasilar involvement. Transient vertigo, diplopia, or headache occurring as solitary symptoms should not be interpreted as a TIA. Also, in some patients, the complaint of dizziness will prove to be part of a carotid TIA; hence this symptom, in our experience and that of Ueda et al, is not a totally reliable indicator of the vascular territory involved. Other manifestations, in their approximate order of frequency, include staggering, veering to one side, a feeling of cross-eyedness, dark vision, blurred vision, tunnel vision, partial or complete blindness, pupillary change, ptosis, paralysis of gaze, dysarthria, and dysphagia. Less common symptoms include hemiplegia, noise or pounding in the ear or in the head, pain in the head or face or other peculiar head sensations, vomiting, hiccups, sense of tilting, lapse of memory, confused behavior, drowsiness, transient unconsciousness (rare), impaired hearing, deafness, a feeling of movement of a part, hemiballismus, peduncular hallucinosis (page 489), and forced deviation of the eyes. So-called drop attacks (page 399), according to Ross Russell, have been recorded in 10 to 15 percent of patients with vertebrobasilar insufficiency, but we have not observed such attacks as a recurrent ischemic phenomenon or a manifestation of other forms of cerebrovascular disease.

Vertebrobasilar TIAs may be identical from one episode to another, or they may vary in detail while maintaining the same basic pattern, the latter occurrence being more typical of basilar than of carotid TIAs. For example, weakness or numbness may involve fingers and face in some episodes and only the fingers in others; or dizziness and ataxia may occur in some attacks, while in others diplopia is added to the picture. In basilar artery disease, each side of the body may be affected alternately. All the involved parts may be affected simultaneously, or a march or spread from one region to another may occur over a period of 10 s to a minute or a few minutes—much slower than the spread of a seizure.

The individual attack may cease abruptly or fade gradually.

Lacunar Transient Ischemic Attacks It has been recognized that strokes due to occlusion of small penetrating vessels of the brain have a proclivity to be intermittent ("stuttering") at their onset and to allow virtually complete restitution of function between discrete episodes. Whether this constitutes a lacunar TIA has been debated, but it seems to us that the problem is our inability to distinguish a transitory occlusion of a small vessel from that of a larger vessel. Donnan and colleagues speak of a "capsular warning syndrome," which we have seen a number of times, consisting of escalating episodes of weakness in the face, arm, and leg and culminating in a capsular lacunar lesion.

Mechanism of Transient Ischemic Attacks Ophthalmoscopic observations of the retinal vessels made during episodes of transient monocular blindness show either an arrest of blood flow in the retinal arteries and breaking up of the venous columns to form a "boxcar" pattern or scattered bits of white material temporarily blocking the retinal arteries. These observations indicate that in some cases of ischemic attacks involving the retinal vessels, a temporary, complete, or relatively complete cessation of blood flow occurs locally and that it is sometimes associated with microembolism.

Transient ischemic attacks have been attributed to cerebral vasospasm or to transient episodes of systemic arterial hypotension with resulting compromise of the intracranial circulation, but neither of these mechanisms has been established. Although dropping the systolic blood pressure to 80 mmHg or less by tilting the patient from a horizontal to an upright position may cause EEG changes, it has not, in the authors' experience, reproduced the attacks in either the carotid or basilar territory. Nevertheless, a small proportion of patients with carotid or basilar artery stenosis have clearly related the onset of their attacks to standing up after lying or sitting. In the majority of cases, attacks bear no relation to position or activity, although in general they are likely to occur when the patient is up and around rather than lying down. Transient symptoms present on awakening from sleep usually indicate that a stroke is impending. Rarely, TIAs have been experienced in relation to exercise, outbursts of anger or joy, and bouts of coughing.

In states of anemia, polycythemia, thrombocythemia, extreme hyperlipidemia, hyperviscosity from macroglobulinemia, sickle cell anemia, and hypoglycemia, there may be transient neurologic deficits related to rheologic changes in blood. In some of these cases, stenosis in a large or small vessel appears to have accounted for a restricted neurologic deficit, but just as often the vasculature is normal. Patients with antiphospholipid antibodies may have TIAs, the mechanism of which is undefined.

Whatever the exact cause of the attacks, they are in most cases intimately related to vascular stenosis and ulceration due to atherosclerosis and to thrombus formation. Embolization of fibrin-platelet material from atherosclerotic sites is frequently proposed as an explanation of TIAs. This may indeed be the cause of attacks in some cases, but it is difficult to understand, in attacks of identical pattern, how successive emboli from a distance would enter the same arterial branch each time. Moreover, one would expect the involved cerebral tissue to be at least partially damaged, leaving some residual signs. When a single transient episode has occurred, the factor of recurrence does not enter into the diagnosis, and cerebral embolism must then be strongly considered. In some cases of documented embolism, the neurologic state fluctuates from normal to abnormal repeatedly for as long as 36 h, giving the appearance of TIAs ("accelerated TIAs"); in others, a deficit of several hours' duration occurs, fulfilling the traditional criterion of TIAs. As already noted, the same sequence of events can precede lacunar infarction. *A single transitory episode, especially if it lasts longer than 1 h, and multiple episodes of different pattern suggest embolism and must be clearly distinguished from brief (2- to 10-min) recurrent attacks of the same pattern, which suggest atherosclerosis and thrombosis.*

The use of noninvasive imaging techniques and contrast arteriography has shed some light on the problem. Usually the internal carotid or vertebrobasilar arteries are stenotic, and sometimes an atheromatous ulcer is seen. In some instances the TIAs begin after the artery has been occluded by thrombus. As shown by Barnett, emboli may arise from the distal end of the thrombus or enter the upper part of the occluded vessel through a collateral artery. However, almost one-fifth of "carotid TIAs" (Pessin et al) and a somewhat larger proportion of the Winston-Salem series (Ueda et al) had neither stenosis nor ulceration of the carotid arteries. However, in most of the cases with arteriographically normal carotids, the ischemic attacks exceeded 1 h in duration, suggesting embolism from the heart or great vessels including the aortic arch; but there were also a small number of brief ischemic attacks that were unexplained by arteriography. The majority of those with carotid bruits had stenoses with more than 50 percent reduction in the lumen. In general, hemodynamic changes in the retinal or cerebral circulation make their appearance when the lumen of the internal carotid artery is reduced to 1.5 mm or less (normal size, 7.0 mm; range, 5 to 10 mm). This corresponds to a reduction in cross-sectional area of more than 95 percent. The degree of stenosis associated with TIAs and the risk of stroke is controversial and is addressed further on.

Differential Diagnosis of TIAs Transient focal neurologic symptoms are ubiquitous in neurologic practice. They may be due to seizures, migraine, or transient global amnesia (page 457), and they occur occasionally in patients with multiple sclerosis. Almost always the clinical setting in which they occur indicates the nature of the attack. Transient episodes, indistinguishable from TIAs, are also known to occur occasionally in patients with meningioma, glioblastoma, metastatic brain tumors situated in or near the cortex, and even with subdural hematoma. Although infrequent, these attacks are important mainly because the use of anticoagulants is relatively contraindicated in these circumstances. The episodes that we have seen with meningiomas and subdural hematomas have consisted mainly of transient aphasia or speech arrest lasting from 2 min to several hours, but sensory symptoms with or without spread over the body, arm weakness, and hemiparesis have also been reported. Some remarkable cases of meningioma have involved repeated transient attacks for decades. Seizures are always suspected but cannot be proved. It has been speculated that a local vascular disturbance of some kind is operative, but the mechanism is not understood.

Treatment of Atherothrombotic Infarction and Transient Ischemic Attacks

The main objective in these forms of cerebrovascular disease is the prevention of stroke. Ideally this should be accomplished by finding patients in the asymptomatic stage of atherosclerosis. However, the medical profession has no efficient means of screening large populations at risk of developing stroke and only limited methods for altering the progression of the atherosclerotic process, even if discovered in its early stages. For all practical purposes, treatment is directed to patients who have already begun to have symptoms, either TIAs or ischemic lesions that are reversible to some extent.

The current treatment of atherothrombotic disease may be divided into four parts: (1) management in the acute phase, (2) measures to restore the circulation and arrest the pathologic process, (3) physical therapy and rehabilitation, and (4) measures to prevent further strokes and progression of vascular disease.

Management in the Acute Phase The relative advantages of placing the seriously ill acute stroke patient in a neurologic special care or "stroke" unit have been the subject of many articles and are discussed in a monograph by one of the authors. Patients with impaired consciousness require special care of skin, eyes, mouth, bladder, and bowel. These measures are best provided in a unit with trained clinical staff and the technology to monitor blood pressure, pulmonary function, blood gases, and intracranial pressure when appropriate. It is our impression that the outcome—in terms of morbidity and mortality in the seriously ill stroke patient—is improved, though admittedly this is difficult to document (for details, see Ropper and also Brott and Reed). Like the well-organized coronary care unit, stroke units have the capability of expediting the evaluation and early rehabilitation of these patients.

Measures to Restore the Circulation and Arrest the Pathologic Process Once a thrombotic stroke has developed fully (i.e., the completed stroke), none of the therapeutic measures so far devised has proved to be consistently effective in restoring the damaged cerebral tissue or its function. The influence of anticoagulants and thrombolysis at an early stage of stroke are discussed below. One's efforts must be directed to making a diagnosis of thrombosis at the earliest possible stage and circumventing the full catastrophe by all means available without risking the safety of the patient. Even when the symptoms and signs have become persistent, it is conceivable that some of the affected tissue, particularly at the edges of the infarct (the "ischemic penumbra"), has not been irreversibly damaged and will survive if perfusion can be re-established. On the assumption that cerebral perfusion might be diminished by assuming the upright position, patients with a major stroke as the result of ischemic infarction should remain nearly horizontal in bed for the first day. When sitting and walking begin, special attention should be given to maintenance of normal blood pressure (patients should avoid standing quietly or sitting with the feet down for prolonged periods, etc.).

Several studies have confirmed the prevalence of hypertension following an ischemic stroke and its tendency to decline, without medications, during the first few hospital days. The treatment of previously unappreciated hypertension is preferably deferred until the neurologic deficit has stabilized. We agree with Britton and colleagues that it is prudent to avoid antihypertensive drugs in the first few days unless there is active myocardial ischemia or unless the blood pressure is high enough to pose a risk to other organs, particularly the kidneys.

Thrombolytic Agents Tissue plasminogen activators (recombinant t-PA and streptokinase), when administered intravenously, convert plasminogen to plasmin, the latter being a proteolytic enzyme capable of hydrolyzing fibrin, fibrinogen, and other clotting proteins. These drugs are effective in the treatment of coronary artery occlusion (but are associated with a 1 percent risk of cerebral hemorrhage), and they also have a role in the treatment of stroke. Thrombolytics injected intra-arterially can in some instances dissolve occlusions of the middle cerebral and basilar arteries and, if administered within hours, reduce the neurologic deficit. However, intra-arterial injection of thrombolytics into infarcted tissue has produced an unacceptably high incidence of cerebral hemorrhage, approaching 20 percent in some studies and leaving the overall morbidity about the same in treated and untreated patients. The exception, in our experience, has been basilar artery thrombosis without large cerebellar infarctions, where large neurologic deficits are at times reversed with fewer complications. Treatment even several hours after the first symptoms may stop progression, but the lack of a systematic study of this approach makes it difficult to endorse without reservation.

In contrast to these earlier observations, the 1995 multicenter study organized by the National Institute of Neurological Disorders (see the NINCDS and Stroke rt-PA Stroke Study Group in the References) has provided evidence of benefit from *intravenous t-PA*. Treatment within 3 h of the onset of symptoms led to a 30 percent increase in the number of patients who remained with little or no neurologic deficit when reexamined 3 months later and when assessed 1 year later by Kwiatkowski et al. It has not been easily understood why the benefits extended to all types of ischemic stroke, including those apparently due to occlusion of small vessels (lacunes), and why improvement was not apparent in the days following treatment. The t-PA was administered in a dose of 0.9 mg/kg, 10 percent of which was given as a bolus, followed by an infusion of the remainder over 1 h. A dose of 90 mg was not exceeded, this being lower than the dose used for myocardial infarction. The relative improvement in neurologic state came at the expense of a 6 percent risk of symptomatic cerebral hemorrhage, i.e., a far lower rate than in most previous studies (some of the hemorrhages were into the area of infarction without causing symptomatic worsening). Patients with massive infarcts (thought to encompass more than two-thirds of the territory of the middle cerebral artery), those with uncontrolled hypertension or who were, more than 80 years of age, and patients who had recently received anticoagulants (except aspirin) were excluded from these studies.

Comparable data from the randomized European Cooperative Acute Stroke Study (ECASS—see Hacke et al), which included 620 patients, identified two situations in which t-PA administered intravenously within 6 h, but at a slightly higher dose than in the NINCDS trial (1.1 mg/kg, to a total of 100 mg), improved neurologic outcome, but the overall results of this trial were considered to be unfavorable. In a second trial (ECASS II) in 800 patients, using the same dose as in the NINCDS-sponsored trial but giving the thrombolytic drug up to 6 h after the stroke, no benefit could be confirmed and the rate of symptomatic hemorrhage was 8.8 percent (compared with 3.4 percent in untreated patients). Yet a subgroup of patients with carotid–middle cerebral artery strokes of moderate severity—specifically those with moderate-sized infarcts from occlusion of vessels distal to the carotid artery and adequate collateral circulation through surface vessels—did appear to benefit. In patients with basilar artery occlusion with coma of only brief duration and those without extensive thrombosis, prompt t-PA treatment also resulted in an overall improvement in neurologic function, but with numerous exceptions. Patients with large cerebral infarctions in all these trials had a poor outcome and suffered a high incidence of cerebral hemorrhage. It has been concluded that the presence of any amount of blood in the first CT scan and evidence of extensive infarction, occupying most of the MCA territory, precludes this mode of therapy. In two similar trials conducted by the European MAST-I groups (see the Multicentre Acute Stroke Trial in References) using streptokinase within 6 h of stroke, there was an adverse outcome—the treated group having an excess of early deaths; this trial had a 21 percent incidence of symptomatic cerebral hemorrhage and an 18 percent incidence of hemorrhagic infarctions.

At the present time the use of intravenous t-PA therapy can be advocated only in patients who arrive in the emergency department and can be fully evaluated within 3 h of the onset of a stroke (thus excluding those who awaken from a night's sleep with the symptoms because of the uncertain time of onset) and have no hemorrhage by CT scan. Generally excluded are those in whom the deficit is either very small (e.g., hand affected only, dysarthria alone, minor aphasia) or, more importantly, so large as to implicate the entire middle cerebral artery territory. Although seemingly a promising approach to acute stroke, the use of acute thrombolytic therapy depends upon the very early identification of a restricted group of patients—for which reason this therapy is applicable to only a limited proportion of stroke patients who present to the emergency department or who have strokes while under observation in the hospital. It is also noteworthy that attempts to reproduce the beneficial effects of t-PA in a community setting have been disappointing because of deviations from treatment guidelines and an excess number of hemorrhages (Katzan et al). Public health education should increase the numbers of stroke patients who seek early attention and thus raise the proportion who are eligible for t-PA.

Acute Surgical Revascularization Rarely is the patient who has had a stroke brought to medical attention within a few minutes of onset, although this may happen when a patient is in the hospital for another reason. If the common or internal carotid artery has just become thrombosed, intravenous or preferably intra-arterial t-PA may be effective, but we have had more experience with immediate surgical removal of the clot or the performance of a bypass to restore function. Ojemann and colleagues operated on 55 such cases as an emergency procedure; 26 of them had stenotic vessels and 29 acutely thrombosed vessels. Of the latter, circulation was restored in 21, with an excellent or good result in 16. In 19 of the 26 cases with stenotic carotid arteries, an excellent or good result was obtained. Usually several hours will have elapsed before the diagnosis is established. If the interval is longer than 12 h, opening the occluded vessel is usually of little value and may present additional dangers.

Treatment of Cerebral Edema and Raised Intracranial Pressure In the first few days following massive cerebral infarction, edema (both vasogenic and cellular) of the necrotic tissue may threaten life. Most often this occurs with a massive infarction in the territory of the middle cerebral artery and when some degree of mass effect is already evident on a CT scan in the first 24 h. Additional infarction in the anterior cerebral artery territory (total carotid occlusion) worsens the situation. The clinical deterioration occurs within several days of onset (usually worst on the third day, sometimes later) but may evolve in as brief a period as several hours after the onset of the stroke (Fig. 34-17). The signs of worsening—drowsiness, a fixed (but not necessarily enlarged) pupil, and a Babinski sign on the side of the infarction—are all due to secondary tissue shifts, as extensively described in Chaps. 17 and 30. In such instances, controlled hyperventilation may be useful as a temporizing maneuver. Frank has shown that clinical deterioration is not always associated with an initial elevation of intracranial pressure. It may therefore be advisable in selected cases to measure the ICP directly before embarking on an aggressive medical regimen to lower the pressure.

Intravenous mannitol, in doses of 1 g/kg, then 50 g every 2 or 3 h, may forestall further deterioration, but most of these patients, once comatose, are likely to die unless drastic measures are undertaken. Corticosteroids are probably of little value; several trials have failed to demonstrate their efficacy.

In the past several years there has been renewed interest in *hemicraniectomy* as a means of reducing the mass effect and intracranial pressure in these extreme circumstances. Our success in salvaging several patients even after a 14-h period of coma with fixed pupils—similar to reported series by Schwab, Carter, Delshaw, and Rengarchary and coworkers—leads us to believe that hemicraniectomy combined with an overlying duraplasty may appropriately be undertaken while the patient is progressing from a stuporous state to coma and imaging studies show increasing mass effect. Of the 63 patients with severe brain swelling and coma in the series of Schwab et al, 46 survived and none remained chairbound. But there is no question that a number of such patients will remain severely disabled. An anterior temporal lobectomy was added to the craniotomy in some cases, but its effect was not clear. A few surgeons have undertaken sizable "strokectomy," removing infarcted tissue and replacing the cranial bone flap. The value of surgical decompression is not limited to patients with right-hemispheric strokes; those with initially limited degrees of aphasia may also be appropriate candidates, but the family must understand the risks involved and the likelihood that the stroke deficits will persist. After long periods of coma with bilaterally enlarged pupils or with evidence on MRI that the midbrain has been irrevocably damaged, the procedure is futile. Many in the field remain skeptical of these aggressive approaches, and a randomized trial is under way to settle the issue. Whether intracranial pressure monitoring adds much to the management of these patients is still open to question; clinical signs and imaging data on shift of brain tissue are probably more useful in judging the need for osmotic treatment and hemicraniectomy.

In the case of large *cerebellar infarctions*, usually from occlusion of a vertebral artery (see earlier), there may be swelling that compresses the lower brainstem. It carries the risk of sudden clinical decompensation and respiratory arrest. Hydrocephalus invariably develops as a prelude to this event and is manifest as drowsiness and stupor, increased tone in the legs, and Babinski signs; other sentinel signs are gaze paresis, sixth nerve palsy, or hemiparesis ipsilateral to the ataxia (Kanis and Ropper). At times it may be difficult to differentiate the effects of increasing hydrocephalus from those of thrombus propagation in the basilar artery, but the former is in our experience more common (Lehrich et al). Cerebellar swelling may occur with or without an associated lateral medullary syndrome, being the result solely of the infarction and edema of the inferior part of the cerebellum. The situation is comparable to the cerebellar swelling and medullary compression caused by cerebellar hemorrhage (page 885). As in the case of hemorrhage, ventricular drainage alone is usually inadequate and becomes unnecessary if the pressure is relieved by craniectomy and resection of infarcted tissue. Surgical decompression is undertaken almost as soon as cerebellar edema becomes clinically apparent by the appearance of hydrocephalus or brainstem signs, since further swelling can be anticipated. This complication can usually be expected in the first 3 or 4 days after the cerebellar stroke. A brief period of observation before committing to surgery, however, is not unreasonable if the fourth ventricle and peribrainstem cisterns are patent and the patient is awake. Mannitol may be used to prepare the patient for surgery or if a period of observation is anticipated.

Anticoagulant Drugs Warfarin and heparin have been used extensively to prevent TIAs and an impending stroke. These anticoagulants may also halt the advance of a progressive thrombotic stroke, but not in all cases. In deciding whether to use anticoagulants, one faces the question of where in the course of the stroke the patient stands when first examined. One fact seems definite—that the administration of anticoagulants is not of great value once the stroke is fully developed, whether in a patient with a lacunar infarct or one with a massive infarction and hemiplegia. It is as yet uncertain whether the long-term use of anticoagulants prevents the recurrence of a thrombotic stroke; in these cases, the incidence of complicating hemorrhage probably outweighs the value of anticoagulants (atrial fibrillation is an exception—see further on).

The two situations in which the immediate administration of heparin has drawn the most support from clinical practice are a fluctuating basilar artery thrombosis and an impending carotid artery occlusion from thrombosis or dissection (see further on). The diagnosis must be inferred from the clinical presentation, but an ultrasound or MRA study is used to corroborate the diagnosis. In these situations, the administration of heparin may be initiated while the nature of the illness is being clarified and discontinued if contraindicated by new findings. It must be acknowledged that satisfactory clinical studies in support of this approach have not been carried out. The issue of heparinization in cases of cardioembolic cerebral infarction is addressed further on in this chapter, under "Embolic Infarction."

In the case of suspected atherothrombotic occlusion of a major cerebral vessel, if t-PA has not been used in the preceding 24 h, heparin is given intravenously, beginning with a bolus of 100 U/kg followed by a continuous drip (1000 U/h) and adjusted according to the partial thromboplastin time (PTT). Heparin therapy is maintained for several days while warfarin therapy is instituted. The latter may be continued for several months depending on the circumstances (see below). Bleeding into any organ may occur when the PTT is much greater than 2.5 times the preheparin level. When the PTT exceeds approximately 100 s, it is preferable to discontinue the heparin, check the blood clotting values, and then reinstitute the infusion at a lower rate. In circumstances of fluctuating basilar artery ischemia, it has been our practice to permit higher values of PTT.

The use of low-molecular-weight heparin (anti–factor Xa or nadoheparin), which is given subcutaneously within the first 48 h of the onset of symptoms, has been shown to improve outcome from stroke when measured at 6 months. In a randomized study, there was no apparent increase in the frequency of hemorrhagic transformation of the ischemic region when compared to placebo treatment (Kay et al). Because the outcome measures in this study were coarse (death or dependence), further investigations need to be carried out. We can only state that the use of low-molecular-weight heparin (approximately 4000 U subcutaneously, twice daily) appears to be safe and is possibly beneficial.

Whether anticoagulant therapy is effective in preventing strokes in patients with TIAs is a question that has never been answered satisfactorily. Swanson's review of several trials evaluating heparin (including the "International Stroke Trial" and the "TOAST" study) suggested that there was no net benefit from heparin in acute stroke because of an excess of cerebral hemorrhages. However, there was in these series a low incidence, estimated to be 2 percent, of recurrent stroke in the first weeks after a cerebral infarction in the untreated groups. An early recurrent stroke rate this low almost precludes demonstrating a benefit from the use of heparin or heparinoid drugs. Moreover, in none of the large trials mentioned above was anticoagulation adminstered in the manner or dosages that are conventionally employed. Weksler and Lewin reviewed the results obtained with oral anticoagulant therapy in four prospective randomized studies with a total of 93 treated patients and 85 controls. They found no evidence of stroke prevention over a period of more than 20 months. There were 15 deaths in the treated patients (6 from hemorrhage) and 10 deaths in the untreated ones (1 from hemorrhage).

Despite these unencouraging results, heparin and warfarin are still widely used. Of course, the planned use of anticoagulant drugs makes an accurate diagnosis imperative. Intracranial hemorrhage must be excluded by CT scan. Estimation of prothrombin activity and coagulation time is desirable before therapy is started, but if this is not feasible, the initial doses of anticoagulant drugs can usually be given safely if there is no clinical evidence of bleeding anywhere in the body and no recent surgery. Warfarin therapy, beginning with a dose of 5 to 10 mg daily, is relatively safe provided that the international normalized ratio (INR) is brought to 2 to 3 (formerly measured as a time between 16 and 19 s) and the level is determined regularly (once a day for the first 5 days, then two or three times a week for a week or two, and finally once every several weeks). There is no reliable evidence that complications are more frequent in the presence of hypertension if the INR is not allowed to exceed two to three times normal; therefore the authors have not withheld anticoagulant therapy in these patients. However, when the blood pressure is greater than 220/120 mmHg, an attempt is made at the same time to lower it gradually. Numerous drugs may alter the anticoagulant effects of the coumarins or increase the risk of bleeding—aspirin, cholestyramine, alcohol, barbiturates, carbamazepine, cephalosporin and quinolone antibiotics, sulfa drugs, and high-dosage penicillin being the most important. The INR must be determined frequently if administration of one of these drugs is essential. Hemorrhagic skin necrosis is a rare but treacherous side effect of warfarin therapy. It is due to a paradoxical microthrombosis of skin vessels and is liable to occur in patients with unsuspected deficiencies of endogenous clotting proteins (S and C). Although the disseminated form of skin necrosis occurs within days of initiating warfarin therapy, we have seen patients with a limited form of this lesion following local skin injury.

Any type of bleeding from warfarin overdosage demands immediate administration of fresh plasma and vitamin K. An INR above 5 in a patient who must remain anticoagulated—for example, one with a prosthetic heart valve—may be corrected with small doses of vitamin K (0.5 to 2 mg), preferably given intravenously.

The long-term use of warfarin in patients with cerebral and coronary atherosclerosis is still under critical analysis. To date it seems to be of some value in the prevention of further thrombosis and embolism. There are data to suggest that the greatest usefulness of warfarin is in the first 2 to 4 months following the onset of ischemic attack(s); after that the risk of intracranial hemorrhage may exceed the benefits of anticoagulant therapy, since the latter are less clear (Sandok et al). The problem that continues to plague all attempts to use anticoagulants, as already noted for heparin in the acute situation, is the risk of hemorrhage, which approaches 10 percent with a mortality of 1 percent. The risk of intracranial hemorrhage has been estimated by Whisnant and colleagues to be 5 percent overall and considerably higher in elderly patients who have been treated for more than 1 year. Thus, it would appear that with long-term administration of anticoagulants, the risk of hemorrhage outweighs the benefit from prevention of stroke.

Antiplatelet Drugs Apart from warfarin, *aspirin* (325 mg daily) has proved to be the most useful drug in the prevention of thrombotic and embolic strokes (and myocardial infarction). The acetyl moiety of aspirin combines with the platelet membrane and inhibits platelet cyclo-oxygenase, thus preventing the production of thromboxane A_2, a vasoconstricting prostaglandin, and also prostacyclin, a vasodilating prostaglandin. In patients who cannot tolerate aspirin, the platelet aggregate inhibitor clopidogrel or a similar drug can be substituted, or the two may be used together (see below).

A number of controlled studies from different parts of the world have attested to the therapeutic value of aspirin and ticlopidine, clopidogrel, or dipyridamole, but it is important not to exaggerate the magnitude of their effects. These studies have been critically reviewed by Tijssen and by Algra et al. With few exceptions, it can be concluded that aspirin is beneficial in preventing stroke; whether low doses (50 to 100 mg) and high doses (1000 to 1500 mg) provide equivalent protection is still uncertain. From a review of these studies, it appears that both dosages are effective and that the addition of dipyridamole further reduces the risk of stroke by a small amount. Dipyridamole in high doses has not been well tolerated in our patients because of induced dizziness.

Ticlopidine and clopidogrel are believed by some, on the basis of clinical trials, to be marginally more effective than aspirin for the prevention of stroke, but they are far more expensive, and ticlopidine is potentially toxic (neutropenia). The combined use of these drugs with aspirin has not been extensively examined, but such trials are ongoing.

These studies notwithstanding, the therapeutic effectiveness of aspirin is still rather slight. The cumulative evidence from trials with aspirin alone indicates that a dose of aspirin of at least 30 mg/day prevents only 13 percent at most of serious vascular complications (Algra et al). Moreover, in each of the trials, a significant number of ischemic strokes actually occurred in patients while they were receiving aspirin.

Other Forms of Medical Treatment Treatment by hemodilution was popularized by the studies of Wood and Fleischer, which showed a high incidence of short-term improvement when the hematocrit was reduced to approximately 33 percent. That lowering blood viscosity improves regional blood flow in the heart had been known for some time, and a similar effect on the brain has been demonstrated by cerebral blood flow studies. Earlier observations had shown a reduction in the overall neurologic deficit, but almost all larger randomized trials—which included patients in many settings who were treated at various times up to 48 h after stroke—failed to confirm any such benefit, and the use of this treatment has been virtually abandoned. Nevertheless, we continue to see a few patients whose hemiparesis and aphasia have improved during and just after removal of a unit or more of blood and replacement with albumin and saline. While this treatment cannot be recommended as a routine approach, it may have some merit in selected situations such as fluctuating stroke. Therapies aimed at improving blood flow by enhancing cardiac output (aminophylline, pressor agents) or by enhancing the microcirculation (mannitol, glycerol, dextran) or by use of a large number of vasodilating drugs (see below) have failed to show consistent benefits. Hyperbaric oxygen may reduce ischemic deficits temporarily but has no sustained effect.

Calcium channel blockers of the types administered for cardiac disease have also been found to increase cerebral blood flow and to reduce lactic acidosis in stroke patients. However, several multicenter clinical trials that compared calcium channel blockers with placebo did not establish a difference in outcome in the two groups. There has also been interest, as noted earlier in the chapter, in drugs that inhibit excitatory amino acid transmitters and free-radical scavengers such as dimethyl sulfoxide (DMSO) and growth factors, but so far none of these has been successfully applied to humans.

Despite some experimental evidence that certain vasodilators such as CO_2 and papaverine increase cerebral blood flow, none has proved beneficial in carefully studied human stroke cases at the stage of TIAs, thrombosis in evolution, or established stroke. Vasodilators may actually be harmful, at least on theoretical grounds, since by lowering the systemic blood pressure or dilating vessels in normal brain tissue (the autoregulatory mechanisms are lost in vessels within the infarct), they may reduce the intracranial anastomotic flow. Moreover, the vessels in the margin of the infarct (border zone) are already maximally dilated. New discoveries regarding the role of nitric oxide in vascular control will probably give rise to new pharmacologic agents that will have to be evaluated.

Surgery for Symptomatic Carotid Stenosis Arterial stenosis or an ulcerating arterial plaque in the neck and thorax of patients with recurrent ischemic attacks is usually amenable to surgical management, employing endarterectomy or angioplasty with stenting. The region that most often lends itself to such therapy is the carotid sinus (the bulbous expansion of the internal carotid artery just above its origin from the common carotid). Other sites suitable for surgical management include the common carotid, innominate, and subclavian arteries. Operation on the vertebral artery at its origin has proved successful only in exceptional circumstances. In recent years balloon angioplasty and stenting of the carotid artery have become increasingly popular. The final decision as to the effectiveness of this procedure awaits direct comparison with surgical endarterectomy, but it can be recommended at the moment for patients who are too ill to undergo surgery but are at great risk of stroke if the stenosis is not corrected.

Surgery and angioplasty, in our opinion, are as yet applicable only to the group of symptomatic carotid artery cases (the asymptomatic ones are discussed below) with substantial extracranial stenosis but not complete and established occlusion, and, in special instances, in those with obvious ulcerated plaques. This group constitutes less than 20 percent of all patients with TIAs (Marshall); but from the perspective of surgical therapy, the term *symptomatic* encompasses both TIAs and small strokes ipsilateral to the stenosis. There is now convincing evidence that well-executed surgery in appropriately chosen cases arrests the TIAs and diminishes the risk of future strokes. These views have received strong affirmation from two well-designed randomized studies—the North American Symptomatic Carotid Endarterectomy Trial (NASCET) and the European Carotid Surgery Trial (ECST). The conclusion was reached, in each of these studies, that carotid endarterectomy for symptomatic lesions causing severe degrees of stenosis (>70 to 80 percent reduction in diameter) is effective in reducing the incidence of ipsilateral hemispheral strokes. There was a difference between these two trials in the method of estimating the degree of stenosis, but when adjustments are made, the results are concordant (Donnan et al). Patients in the European study with mild or moderate stenosis (up to 70 percent) did not benefit from endarterectomy. In the North American study, however, they did so, but to a lesser extent than the group with severe stenosis. Further analysis of the North American trial by Gasecki and colleagues indicated that the risk of infarction on the side of the symptomatic stenosis is increased if there is a contralateral carotid stenosis but that operated patients (on the side of symptomatic stenosis) still had fewer strokes than those treated with medication alone. In the latter group, the risk of stroke after 2 years was 69 percent, and if operated on, 22 percent. In the final analysis, *the relative benefits of surgery or medical treatment (anticoagulation or aspirin) depend mainly upon the true surgical risk*—i.e., on the record of an individual surgeon. If the surgeon, by an independent audit of his procedures, has an operative complication rate of no more than 4 to 5 percent, and preferably lower, then surgery can be recommended.

Before operation or angioplasty, the existence of the lesion and its extent must be determined. Arteriography, the procedure that yields the best images and measurements of the residual lumen, carries in itself a small risk of worsening the stroke or producing new focal signs. Increasingly the diagnosis of carotid stenosis is being made by noninvasive methods in order to avoid this small but significant morbidity.

If the patient is in good medical condition, has normal vessels on the contralateral side, and has normal cardiac function (no heart failure, uncontrolled angina, or recent infarction), these lesions can usually be dealt with safely by endarterectomy. However, the procedure is not always innocuous. It is sometimes followed by a new *hemiplegia or aphasia that becomes evident immediately or soon after endarterectomy*, when the patient arrives in the recovery room. Or a carotid occlusion is detected by ultrasound soon after the procedure. In general, surgeons prefer to return the patient to the operating room and open the artery. An intimal flap at the distal end of the endarterectomy and varying amounts of fresh clot proximal to it are usually encountered; but after its removal, the effects of the stroke, if one has occurred, are not usually improved. Where the initial dissection was difficult because the distal site of the atheroma was located under the mandible or otherwise inaccessible, it is prudent to begin anticoagulation.

A less common *hyperperfusion syndrome* presents a similar clinical problem but arises several days to a week after carotid endarterectomy. Headache, focal deficits, seizures, brain edema, or cerebral hemorrhage are thought to reflect an abrupt loss of autoregulatory ability of the cerebral vasculature in the face of hypertension and increased perfusion on the side of the recently opened artery. Unilateral headache is the commonest symptom and may be the only manifestation. On occasion the edema is so massive as to lead to death (Breen et al).

For intracranial internal carotid stenosis or for thrombi that extend into the siphon and stem of the middle cerebral artery, a transcranial (superficial temporal–middle cerebral) anastomosis was devised. Though this operation is technically feasible, its therapeutic value has been discounted by the careful worldwide study of Barnett and his collaborators, who found that the bypass did not produce a reduction in TIAs, strokes, or deaths.

Asymptomatic Carotid Stenosis Finally, there is the problem of the asymptomatic carotid bruit or incidentally discovered stenosis. The population study by Heyman and associates has shed some light on this. They found that cervical bruits in men constituted a risk for death from ischemic heart disease. They also noted that the presence of asymptomatic bruits in men (but not in women) does carry a slightly increased risk of stroke but, more importantly, that the subsequent stroke often does not coincide with its angioanatomic locus and laterality with the cervical bruit. Similar findings have been reported by Ford and coworkers and by Chambers and Norris. On the other hand, Wiebers and colleagues found that patients with asymptomatic carotid bruits who were followed for 5 years were approximately three times more likely to have ischemic strokes than an age- and sex-matched population sample without carotid bruits. The findings of the more recent Asymptomatic Carotid Atherosclerotic Study (ACAS), as reported by their Executive Committee, also suggest that the number of strokes can be reduced from 11 to 5 percent over 5 years by removing the plaque in asymptomatic patients in whom there is a stenosis greater than 60 percent (diameter). These findings have been tempered by a reanalysis of the ACAS data, pointing out that almost half of the strokes in these patients were lacunar or cardioembolic in origin (Inzitari et al). Recent data from a European trial, encompassing 2295 patients, cast the matter in a different light. The latter study indicates that asymptomatic carotid stenosis of less than 70 percent carries only a 2 percent risk of stroke over a 3-year period and that the risk is not much greater (5.7 percent) if the stenosis is more than 70 percent. It was concluded that endarterectomy is not justified for asymptomatic carotid stenosis.

We counsel caution until a more definite consensus on this matter has been reached. Also, as already noted, the neurologist's advice should be tempered by the documented surgical risk in his particular institution. Our practice with asymptomatic cases has been to evaluate the lumen of the internal carotid artery (by ultrasound) at 6- to 12-month intervals. Only if the lumen is decreasing in size and becomes narrowed to 1.5 mm or less with diminished blood flow, or if there is an event that could be construed as a TIA referable to the stenotic side, is surgery considered. In the former case of an asymptomatic but progressive stenosis, there is still considerable controversy about treatment; anticoagulation or antiplatelet agents are reasonable alternatives to surgery. Severe stenosis is reflected in conventional angiography by filling of the distal branches of the external carotid artery before the branches of the middle cerebral artery are opacified—a reversal of the usual filling pattern, indicating low flow in the distal carotid circulation.

We generally agree with the guidelines for carotid endartectomy set down by the American Heart Association as reported by Moore and colleagues, but there must be a careful evaluation of the circumstances in each patient and particular caution exercised in operating on asymptomatic patients.

Physical Therapy and Rehabilitation In all but the most seriously ill patients, beginning within a few days of the stroke, the paralyzed limbs should at intervals be carried through a full range of passive movement many times a day. The purpose is to avoid contracture (and periarthritis), especially at the shoulder, elbow, hip, and ankle. Soreness and aching in the paralyzed limbs should not be allowed to interfere with exercises. Patients should be moved from bed to chair as soon as the illness permits. Nearly all hemiplegics regain the ability to walk to some extent, usually within a 3- to 6-month period, and this should be a primary aim in rehabilitation. The presence of deep sensory loss or anosognosia in addition to hemiplegia is the main limiting factor. A short or long leg brace is often required. By teaching patients with cerebellar ataxia new strategies, balance and gait disorders can be made less disabling. As motor function improves and if mentality is preserved, instruction in the activities of daily living and the use of various special devices can assist the patient in becoming at least partly independent in the home. What little research is available on the effectiveness of stroke rehabilitation suggests that a greater intensity of physical therapy does indeed achieve better scores on some measures of walking ability and dexterity. In a randomized trial, Kwakkel and colleagues achieved these results by applying an additional 30 min per day beyond conventional physical therapy of focused treatments to the leg or arm, 5 days per week, for 20 weeks. Other studies have demonstrated clearly the undesirable effects of immobilizing a limb in a splint after a stroke.

The neural substrates of improvement after stroke are just beginning to be studied. Experimental work in monkeys suggests that the cortical motor and sensory representations of the affected limb are lost after focal damage, and this can be prevented with retraining of the limb. In some cases the motor representations can be seen to expand into adjacent undamaged cortical areas, thus indicating the potential for some degree of reorganization that may correspond to clinical recovery.

Speech and language therapy should be given in appropriate cases, if for no other reason than to improve the morale of the patient and family. Further comments on the value of such therapy can be found in Chap. 23, on language disturbances.

Preventive Measures Since the primary objective in the treatment of atherothrombotic disease is prevention, efforts to control the risk factors must continue. The carotid vessels, being readily accessible, must always be studied for the presence of a bruit; the latter quite reliably indicates a stenosis, though not all stenoses cause a bruit. Ultrasound examination of the carotid is justified in almost all patients with TIAs and ischemic stroke. While a *self-audible bruit* occasionally indicates carotid stenosis, dissection, or fibromuscular dysplasia, it is usually benign and in some instances associated with an enlarged, superiorly displaced jugular bulb—a benign anatomic variant that can be discerned on CT scan (Adler and Ropper). The management of patients with asymptomatic carotid bruits has been considered above.

For patients who have had a stroke from atherothrombotic disease and are functional, preventive measures consist of avoiding situations in which strokes are likely to occur. Such measures include the following: (1) aspirin—it has been shown to reduce the risk of second stroke, but its effect, as already noted, should not be overestimated (see page 866); (2) hypotensive agents—whether given therapeutically or for diagnostic procedures, these should be administered with caution; (3) in the elderly patient in whom deep sleep might contribute to a state of cerebral ischemia, oversedation should be avoided; (4) systemic hypotension, severe anemia, and polycythemia should be treated promptly; (5) rapid diuresis may be contraindicated; and (6) particular care should be taken to maintain the systemic blood pressure, oxygenation, and intracranial blood flow during surgical procedures, especially in elderly patients.

The ultimate solution of the problems of ischemic infarction and TIAs lies in more fundamental fields—namely, the prevention or alleviation of hypertension and atherosclerosis. We strongly advise patients to discontinue smoking. Low-cholesterol, low-fat diets, antilipidemic agents, and the use of cholesterol lowering drugs may possibly have a place.

Embolic Infarction

As already stated, this is the commonest cause of stroke. In most cases of cerebral embolism, the embolic material consists of a fragment that has broken away from a thrombus within the heart. Somewhat less frequently the source is intra-arterial, from the distal end of a thrombus within the lumen of an occluded carotid or vertebral artery or the distal end of a carotid dissection, or from an atheromatous plaque that has ulcerated into the lumen of the carotid sinus. Single or sequential emboli may also arise from large atheromatous plaques in the ascending aorta. Embolism due to fat, tumor cells, fibrocartilage, amniotic fluid, or air is a rare occurrence and seldom enters into the differential diagnosis of stroke.

The embolus usually becomes arrested at a bifurcation or other site of natural narrowing of the lumen of an intracranial vessel, and ischemic infarction follows. The infarction is pale, hemorrhagic, or mixed; hemorrhagic infarction nearly always indicates embolism, though most embolic infarcts are pale. Any region of the brain may be affected, the territory of the middle cerebral artery, particularly the superior division, being the most frequently involved. The two cerebral hemispheres are approximately equally affected. Large embolic clots can block large vessels (sometimes the carotids in the neck or at their termination intracranially), while tiny fragments may reach vessels as small as 0.2 mm in diameter. The embolic material may remain arrested and plug the lumen solidly, but more often it breaks into fragments that enter smaller vessels and disappear, so that even careful pathologic examination fails to reveal their final location. In the latter instance, the clinical effects may clear in hours. The anatomic diagnosis must then be made by inference, e.g., absence of a vascular occlusion at the proper site to explain the infarct; absence of atherosclerosis or other cause of occlusion in the offending cerebral vessel; presence of a source of emboli, atrial fibrillation, or infarcts in other organs such as the kidneys and spleen; the occurrence of hemorrhagic infarction; and finally the clinical history, which is characterized by an absolutely abrupt onset, as described below.

Because of the rapidity with which embolic occlusion develops, there is not much time for collateral influx to become established. Thus, sparing of the territory distal to the site of occlusion is not as evident as in thrombosis. However, the *ischemia-modifying factors* mentioned above, under "The Ischemic Stroke," are still operative and influence the size and severity of the infarct.

Brain embolism is predominantly a manifestation of heart disease, and fully 75 percent of cardiogenic emboli lodge in the brain. The commonest identifiable cause is *chronic atrial fibrillation*, the source of the embolus being a mural thrombus within the atrial appendage (Table 34-5). Patients with chronic atrial fibrillation are many times more liable to stroke than an age-matched population with normal cardiac rhythm (Wolf et al). Embolism may also occur during paroxysmal atrial fibrillation or flutter. Mural thrombus deposited on the damaged endocardium overlying a myocardial infarct in the left ventricle, particularly if there is an aneurysmal sac, is an important source of cerebral emboli, as is a thrombus associated with severe mitral stenosis without atrial fibrillation. Emboli tend to occur in the first few weeks after an acute myocardial infarction, but Loh and colleagues found that a lesser degree of risk persists for up to 5 years. *Cardiac catheterization or surgery*, especially valvuloplasty, may disseminate fragments from a thrombus or a calcified valve. *Mitral and aortic valve prostheses* are additional important sources of embolism.

Another source of embolism is the carotid or vertebral artery, where clot forming on an ulcerated atheromatous plaque may be detached and carried to an intracranial branch (artery-to-artery embolism). A similar phenomenon may occur with arterial dissections and sometimes with fibromuscular disease of the carotid or vertebral arteries.

Atheromatous plaques in the ascending aorta are an important source of embolism; Amarenco et al have reported that as many as 38 percent of a group of patients

Table 34-5
Causes of cerebral embolism

1. Cardiac origin
   a. Atrial fibrillation and other arrhythmias (with rheumatic, atherosclerotic, hypertensive, congenital, or syphilitic heart disease)
   b. Myocardial infarction with mural thrombus
   c. Acute and subacute bacterial endocarditis
   d. Heart disease without arrhythmia or mural thrombus (mitral stenosis, myocarditis, etc.)
   e. Complications of cardiac surgery
   f. Valve prostheses
   g. Nonbacterial thrombotic (marantic) endocardial vegetations
   h. Prolapsed mitral valve
   i. Paradoxical embolism with congenital heart disease (e.g., patent foramen ovale)
   j. Myxoma
2. Noncardiac origin
   a. Atherosclerosis of aorta and carotid arteries (mural thrombus, atheromatous material)
   b. From sites of dissection and/or fibromuscular dysplasia of carotid and vertebrobasilar arteries
   c. Thrombus in pulmonary veins
   d. Fat, tumor, or air
   e. Complications of neck and thoracic surgery
   f. Pelvic and lower extremity venous thrombosis in presence of right-to-left cardiac shunt
3. Undetermined origin

with no discernible cause for embolic stroke had echogenic atherosclerotic plaques in the aortic arch that were greater than 4 mm in thickness, a size thought to be associated on a statistical basis with strokes. Disseminated cholesterol emboli are known to occur in the cerebral circulation and may be dispersed in other organs as well; rarely, this is sufficiently severe to cause an encephalopathy and pleocytosis.

Paradoxic embolism can occur when an abnormal communication exists between the right and left sides of the heart (particularly a patent foramen ovale) or when both ventricles communicate with the aorta; thus embolic material arising in the veins of the lower extremities or pelvis or elsewhere in the systemic venous circulation can bypass the pulmonary circulation and reach the cerebral vessels. Pulmonary hypertension (often from previous pulmonary embolism) favors the occurrence of paradoxic embolism, but this may occur with a patent foramen ovale even in the absence of pulmonary hypertension. Of 30 patients in whom a patent foramen ovale could be demonstrated, 17 had evidence of a right-to-left shunt; brain infarction was associated with positive phlebography of the legs and abnormal pulmonary scintigraphy (Itoh et al). Subendocardial fibroelastosis, idiopathic myocardial hypertrophy, cardiac myxomas, and cardiac lesions of trichinosis are rare causes of embolism.

The vegetations of acute and subacute bacterial endocarditis give rise to several different lesions in the brain (pages 752–753). Mycotic aneurysm is a rare complication of septic embolism and may be a source of intracerebral or subarachnoid hemorrhage. *Marantic* or *nonbacterial endocarditis* is a frequently overlooked cause of cerebral embolism; at times it produces a baffling clinical picture, especially when associated, as it often is, with carcinomatosis, cachexia from any cause, or lupus erythematosus. This subject is discussed further on.

Mitral valve prolapse (MVP) may be a source of emboli, especially in young patients, but its frequency has been overestimated. The initial impetus for considering MVP as an important source of embolus came from the study of Barnett and colleagues of a group of 60 patients who had TIAs or partial strokes and were under 45 years of age; MVP was detected (by echocardiography and a characteristic midsystolic click) in 24 patients but in only 5 of 60 age-matched controls. However, in several subsequent large studies (Sandok and Giuliani and Jones et al), only a very small proportion of strokes in young patients could be attributed to prolapse; even then, the connection was only inferred by the exclusion of other causes of stroke. Indeed, in a recent study using stringent criteria for the echocardiographic diagnosis of prolapse, Gilon and colleagues could not establish any relation to stroke. Rice and colleagues have described a family with premature stroke in association with MVP and a similar relationship has been reported in twins; the same may occur in Ehlers-Danlos disease.

The *pulmonary veins* are a potential if infrequent source of cerebral emboli, as indicated by the occurrence of cerebral abscesses in association with pulmonary suppurative disease and by the high incidence of cerebral deposits secondary to pulmonary carcinoma. In Osler-Weber-Rendu disease, pulmonary shunts serve as a conduit for emboli. As remarked above, surgery of the neck and thorax can be complicated by cerebral embolism. A rare type is that which follows thyroidectomy, where thrombosis in the stump of the superior thyroid artery extends proximally until a section of it, protruding into the lumen of the carotid, is carried into the cerebral arteries.

During *cerebral arteriography*, emboli may arise from the tip of the catheter, or manipulation of the catheter may dislodge atheromatous material from the aorta or carotid or vertebral arteries and account for some of the accidents during this procedure. Transcranial Doppler insonation has suggested that small emboli frequently arise during these procedures, and a study by Bendszus and colleagues found that 23 of 100 consecutive patients had new cortical lesions shown on diffusion-weighted MRI just after cerebral arteriography; however, none of these were symptomatic.

Cerebral embolism must always have occurred when secondary tumor is deposited in the brain, and cerebral embolism regularly accompanies septicemia, but a mass of tumor cells or bacteria is seldom large enough to occlude a cerebral artery and produce the picture of stroke. Nevertheless, tumor embolism with stroke has been reported secondary to cardiac myxomas and occasionally to other tumors. It must be distinguished from the marantic endocarditis and embolism (discussed further on) that occasionally complicate neoplasm. Cerebral *fat embolism* is related to severe bone trauma. As a rule, the emboli are minute and widely dispersed, giving rise first to pulmonary symptoms and then to multiple cerebral petechial hemorrhages; accordingly the clinical picture is not strictly focal, as it is in a stroke, although in some instances it may have focal features. Cerebral *air embolism* is a rare complication of abortion, scuba diving, or cranial, cervical, or thoracic operations involving large venous sinuses; it was formerly encountered as a complication of pneumothorax therapy. Clinically, this condition may be difficult to separate from the deficits following hypotension or hypoxia, which frequently coexist. Hyperbaric treatment may be effective if instituted early.

Despite the large number of established sources of emboli, the point of origin cannot be determined in about 30 percent of presumed embolic infarctions. In such cases, emboli may have originated from thrombi in the cardiac chambers but have left behind no residual clot or may be undetectable by even sophisticated methods, such as transesophageal echocardiography and the newer MR techniques. Others may be due to atheromatous material arising from the aorta. If extensive evaluation fails to disclose the origin, the odds still favor a source in the left heart. Not infrequently the diagnosis of cerebral embolism is made at autopsy without finding a source. The search for a thrombotic nidus may not have been sufficiently thorough in these cases, and small thrombi in the atrial appendage, endocardium (between the papillary muscles of the heart), aorta and its branches, or pulmonary veins may have been overlooked. Nevertheless, in some cases studied carefully postmortem, no source of embolic material can be discovered.

Clinical Picture Of all strokes, those due to cerebral embolism develop most rapidly, "like a bolt out of the blue." As a rule, the full-blown picture evolves within seconds, exemplifying most strikingly the temporal profile of a stroke. With rare exceptions, there are no warning episodes. The embolus strikes at any time of the day or night. Getting up to go to the bathroom is a time of danger. Only occasionally and for unclear reasons, the clinical picture unfolds more gradually, over many hours, with some fluctuation of symptoms. Possibly, in these cases, the embolus initiates a thrombotic process in the occluded vessel.

The neurologic picture will depend on the artery involved and the site of obstruction. The syndromes related to each angioanatomic territory are the same as those outlined earlier in this chapter, under "Neurovascular Syndromes." A large embolus may plug the distal internal carotid artery or the stem of the middle cerebral artery, producing the full-blown syndromes that follow occlusion of these arteries. More often the embolus is smaller and passes into one of the branches of the middle cerebral artery, producing a strikingly focal disorder such as a motor speech disorder, a monoplegia, or a receptive type of aphasia with little or no motor paralysis. In fact, most patients with a diagnosis of middle cerebral artery thrombosis prove to have embolic occlusion of the middle cerebral artery (or an atherosclerotic thrombosis of the internal carotid artery).

Embolic material entering the vertebrobasilar system occasionally stops in the vertebral artery just below its union with the basilar; more often it traverses the vertebral and also the basilar artery, which is larger, and is not arrested until it reaches the upper bifurcation, where it produces the abrupt onset of coma and total paralysis or one of the related "top of the basilar" syndromes, described earlier in the chapter. Or the embolus may enter one or both posterior cerebral arteries and, by infarction of the visual cortex, cause a unilateral or bilateral homonymous hemianopia. The medial temporal lobe or thalamus and subthalamus may be affected as a consequence of occlusion of the temporal branches or of small penetrating vessels that arise from the posterior cerebral artery, resulting in a number of disorders of memory, sensation, and movement. Embolic infarction of the undersurface of the cerebellum is not infrequent (Fig. 34-18); in addition to ataxia, there are often telltale signs of lateral medullary ischemia. Embolic material rarely enters the penetrating branches of the pons.

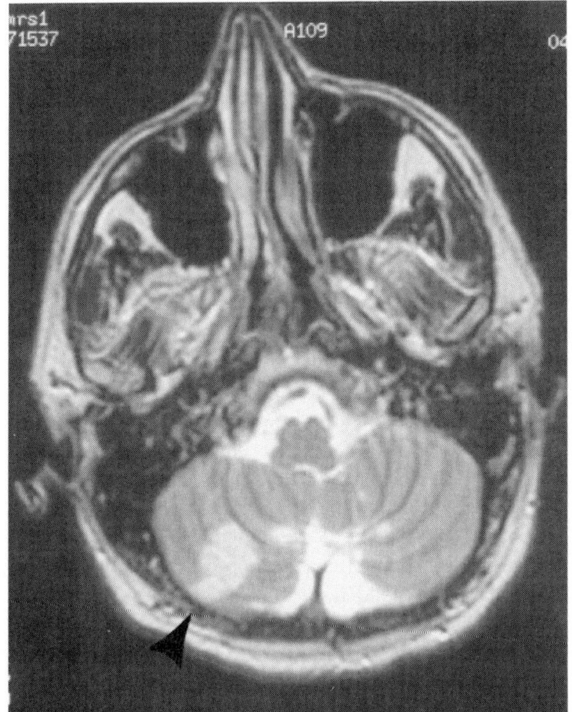

Figure 34-18

*Early inferior cerebellar cortical infarction (*arrowhead*). T2-weighted MRI showing the result of an embolic stroke in the territory of the right posterior inferior cerebellar artery. There are small infarctions on the undersurface of the left cerebellum as well.*

It is important to repeat that an embolus may produce a severe neurologic deficit that is only temporary; symptoms disappear as the embolus fragments. In other words, embolism is a common cause of a single evanescent stroke that may reasonably be called a prolonged TIA. Also, as already pointed out, several emboli can give rise to two or three transient attacks of differing pattern or, rarely, of almost identical pattern.

Also of interest are the symptoms caused by an embolus as it traverses a large vessel. This "*migrating*, or *traveling*, *embolus syndrome*" is most evident in cases of posterior cerebral artery occlusion, either from a cardiogenic source or from a thrombus in the vertebral artery ("artery-to-artery" embolism, see above). Minutes or more before the hemianopia develops, the patient may report fleeting dizziness or vertigo, diplopia, or dysarthria, the result of transient occlusion of the origins of small penetrating vessels as the embolus traverses the basilar artery. Small residual areas of infarction within the brainstem or cerebellum can sometimes be seen on MRI or found at autopsy.

Although the abruptness with which the stroke develops and the lack of prodromal symptoms point strongly to embolism, it is the total clinical picture upon which the diagnosis is based. The presence of atrial fibrillation, a history of myocardial infarction (recent or in the preceding months), cardiac valvular disease or a prosthetic valve, or the occurrence of embolism to other vascular territories of the brain or to other regions of the body all support the diagnosis of embolism. This diagnosis always merits careful consideration in young persons, in whom atherosclerosis is unlikely.

Laboratory Findings Not infrequently the first sign of myocardial infarction is the occurrence of embolism; therefore it is advisable that an *ECG and echocardiogram be obtained in all patients with stroke of uncertain origin*, particularly since about 20 percent of myocardial infarctions are of the "silent" variety; if the ECG does not yield relevant information, prolonged study of heart rhythm with Holter monitoring should be undertaken. Also, as indicated earlier, it is advisable in the elderly or in patients with severe atherosclerosis to image the aortic arch with ultrasound or MRA, looking for plaques greater than 4 mm in thickness (Amarenco et al).

Transesophageal echocardiography, which has a higher sensitivity than transthoracic echocardiography, is an important test in the evaluation of stroke in younger patients, in whom a patent foramen ovale may be a mechanism for paradoxical embolism, and in older patients with arteriopathy, in whom an atrial clot or an aortic plaque may be responsible. In a study of 824 patients at the Cleveland Clinic (Leung and associates), transesophageal echocardiography detected a potential source of embolism in 50 percent, an atrial clot in 7 percent, and a complex aortic atheroma in 13 percent of those with normal transthoracic studies. The precise indications for this test, however, have not been clearly determined.

In some 30 percent of cases, cerebral embolism produces a hemorrhagic infarct. CT scanning or MRI may be helpful in showing the more intense hemorrhagic infarcts, particularly if the scan is repeated on the second or third day. Only in a minority of these instances do red cells enter the CSF (rarely as many as 10,000 red cells per cubic millimeter). In the milder cases of hemorrhagic infarction, a slight xanthochromia may appear after a few days.

In septic embolism resulting from *subacute bacterial endocarditis*, the white blood cells in the CSF may be increased, usually up to 200 per cubic millimeter but occasionally much higher; the proportion of lymphocytes and polymorphonuclear cells varies with the acuteness of the septic process. There may also be an equal number of red blood cells and a faint xanthochromia. The protein content is elevated, but the glucose content is within normal limits. No bacteria are seen or obtained by culture. By contrast, the CSF formula in septic embolism from *acute bacterial endocarditis* may be that of a purulent meningitis.

Course and Prognosis The remarks concerning the *immediate prognosis* of atherothrombotic infarction apply to embolic infarction as well. Most patients survive the initial insult, and in many the neurologic deficit may recede relatively rapidly, as indicated above. Progressive brain swelling occurs in a small proportion, less than 5 percent, of patients with embolic occlusion of the distal carotid or the stem and major branches of the middle cerebral artery and in a larger proportion of sizable cerebellar infarcts. In the case of massive cerebral edema, management follows along the same lines as that for atherosclerotic thrombotic infarction (page 864). The *eventual prognosis* is determined by the occurrence of further emboli and the gravity of the underlying illness—cardiac failure, myocardial infarction, bacterial endocarditis, malignancy, and so on. In a small number of cases, the first episode of cerebral embolism will be followed by another, frequently with severe consequences if the second episode affects the opposite hemisphere. Furthermore, there is no certain way of predicting when the second embolus will strike. However, the incidence of this second event, once thought to be as high as 20 percent, has been revised downward, to perhaps 2 percent, based on several large trials treated by anticoagulation (see the review of Swanson).

Treatment and Prevention Three phases of therapy—(1) general medical management in the acute phase, (2) measures directed to restoring the circulation, and (3) physical therapy and rehabilitation—are much the same as described above under "Atherothrombotic Infarction." Issues pertaining to the prevention of recurrent embolism are discussed below. Thrombolysis has been successful to the extent indicated previously under "Thrombolytic Therapy." There is no evidence that the risk of symptomatic hemorrhage (6 to 20 percent) from this treatment is any higher than in other types of stroke. Embolectomy at the bifurcation of the common carotid artery has usually failed, for which reason it is rarely attempted. If pulsation in the temporal artery in front of the ear is present, the embolus has passed beyond that bifurcation into the internal carotid system. Similarly, embolectomy of the middle cerebral artery has been successful only in rare cases and is no longer undertaken.

Of prime importance is the *prevention of cerebral embolism*, and this applies both to patients who have had an episode of embolism and to those who have not but are at risk of doing so. The long-term use of anticoagulants has proved to be effective in the prevention of embolism in cases of atrial fibrillation, myocardial infarction, and valve prosthesis. In patients with atrial fibrillation of recent onset, an attempt should be made to restore normal sinus rhythm by the use of electrical cardioversion or, for several days before, a trial of antiarrhythmic drugs and anticoagulants; if these fail, prophylactic anticoagulant therapy is recommended. Before attempting cardioversion of more longstanding atrial fibrillation, anticoagulation for several days or longer is recommended.

The most convincing evidence of the efficacy of anticoagulants in the prevention of embolism has been presented by the Boston Area Anticoagulant Trial for Atrial Fibrillation. Patients at risk for stroke were maintained for 2 years on warfarin (INR of 1.5 to 2). There were 212 anticoagulated patients and 208 controls. Recurrent strokes were reduced by 86 percent in the warfarin group and the death rate was also lower. There was one fatal hemorrhage in each group; minor hemorrhages occurred in 38 of the warfarin group and in 21 of the control group. In a similar study from Copenhagen, the incidence of stroke in a group receiving warfarin was calculated to be 2 percent per year, in comparison to 5.5 percent per year in a control group. Several subsequent trials have attested to the efficacy of warfarin in the prevention of stroke in patients with nonrheumatic atrial fibrillation (Singer). It should be pointed out, however, that in the absence of additional risk factors such as diabetes or hypertension, patients younger than 65 years in these trials did not benefit from prophylactic anticoagulation. Aspirin does not afford the same protective benefit in these circumstances.

There is no unanimous opinion about the use and timing of anticoagulation after an embolic stroke, since the risk of recurrent stroke in the first days is low (see comments on pages 865–866). On the basis of recent large trials of acute anticoagulation that show a 2 percent frequency of early recurrent stroke, many clinicians prefer to start warfarin and avoid heparin. Once a firm diagnosis of embolic occlusion has been made, our customary practice has been to begin heparin on the same or the next day, generally without a loading dose, followed by the institution of warfarin on the same or the two following days. However, many of our colleagues no longer use heparin in this setting, and others even forgo the use of warfarin unless a definite source of embolism is detected by echocardiography. It is our impression that the recent trend has been to avoid heparin and simply start warfarin if it is indicted. Whether the newer low-molecular-weight heparin (nadoheparin), mentioned previously, yields an advantage over conventional heparin treatment is not known. In patients with very large cerebral infarcts that have a component of deep (basal ganglionic) tissue damage and especially those who are also hypertensive, there is a distinct risk of anticoagulant-related hemorrhage into the acute infarct (Shields et al). In these patients, anticoagulation therapy should perhaps be avoided in the acute setting.

Also in our opinion, the use of anticoagulant therapy is desirable in most patients with acute myocardial infarction, especially if the left side of the heart is involved. In cerebral embolism associated with subacute bacterial endocarditis, anticoagulant therapy is used cautiously because of the danger of intracranial bleeding, and one proceeds instead to the use of antibiotics. We have generally not anticoagulated these patients.

Valvuloplasty, removal of verrucous lesions in endocarditis, and amputation of the atrial appendage have substantially reduced the incidence of embolism in the now infrequent rheumatic heart disease. The need for special care in preventing emboli that arise from the cardiac chambers or the aortic arch from entering the carotid arteries during the performance of valvuloplasty is appreciated by all cardiac surgeons.

Lacunar Infarction (See page 847)

LESS COMMON CAUSES OF OCCLUSIVE CEREBROVASCULAR DISEASE (See also pages 906–910)

Fibromuscular Dysplasia

This is a segmental, nonatheromatous, noninflammatory arterial disease of unknown etiology. It is uncommon (0.5 percent of 61,000 arteriograms in the series of So et al), but it is being reported with increasing frequency because of improved arteriographic techniques and as an incidental finding in asymptomatic individuals undergoing aortic angiography.

First described in the renal artery by Leadbetter and Burkland in 1938, fibromuscular dysplasia is now known to affect other vessels, including cervicocerebral ones. Of the latter, the internal carotid artery is involved most frequently, followed by the vertebral and cerebral arteries. The radiologic alteration consists of a series of transverse constrictions, giving the appearance of an irregular string of beads or a tubular narrowing; it is observed bilaterally in 75 percent of cases. Usually only the extracranial part of the artery is involved. In the series of Houser and colleagues, 42 of 44 patients were women, and 75 percent were over 50 years of age. All of the patients reported by So and coworkers were women, ranging in age from 41 to 70 years. Cerebral ischemia may complicate the lesion; between 7 and 20 percent of affected individuals have intracranial saccular aneurysms (rarely a giant aneurysm), which may be a source of subarachnoid hemorrhage, and 12 percent develop arterial dissections, as described below.

The pathology of this disease has been described by Schievink et al. The narrowed arterial segments show degeneration of elastic tissue and irregular arrays of fibrous and smooth muscle tissue in a mucous ground substance. The dilatations are due to atrophy of the coat of the vessel wall. There is atherosclerosis in some and arterial dissection in others. Usually vascular occlusion is not present, though there may be marked stenosis. In some instances the mechanism of the cerebral ischemic lesion is unexplained. Possibly thrombi form in the pouches or in relation to intraluminal septa.

So and colleagues have recommended excision of the affected segments of the carotid artery if the neurologic symptoms are related to them and conservative therapy if the fibromuscular dysplasia is an incidental arteriographic finding in an asymptomatic patient. In one group of 79 untreated asymptomatic patients followed for an average of 5 years, 3 had a cerebral infarct 4 to 18 years after the initial diagnosis (Corrin et al). It is now possible to dilate the affected vessel by means of endovascular techniques, and several case reports have suggested that benefit is achieved at lower risk in this way than with excision. Associated intracranial saccular aneurysms should be sought by arteriography and surgically obliterated if their size warrants it (page 895).

Dissection of the Cervical and Intracranial Vessels

Internal Carotid Artery Dissection It has long been appreciated that the process known as Erdheim's medionecrosis aortica cystica may extend into the common carotid arteries, occluding them and causing massive infarction of the cerebral hemispheres. Examples of such an occurrence were cited by Weisman and

Adams in 1944 in their study of the neurology of dissecting aneurysms of the aorta. In more recent years, attention has been drawn to the occurrence of spontaneous dissection of the internal carotid artery and the fact that it is an important cause of hemiplegia in young adults. Several large series of such cases have been reported by Ojemann, Mokri, and Bogousslavsky and their colleagues.

Traumatic or apparently spontaneous carotid dissection is a not uncommon cause of stroke. Bogousslavsky and colleagues found 30 instances (both sexes) in 1200 consecutive patients with a first stroke (2.5 percent). It should be suspected in young adult women (typically in their late thirties or early forties), who seem especially susceptible to the condition, either as a spontaneous occurrence or in relation to severe whiplash injury, bouts of violent coughing, or direct trauma to the head or neck, which need not be severe—e.g., being struck in the neck by a golf or tennis ball. We have also encountered cases that occurred during pregnancy and immediately after delivery. Indeed, it is questionable if cervical arterial dissections are truly "spontaneous," since most can be connected to some inciting event. A small number of patients have fibromuscular disease, as discussed above, and the Ehlers-Danlos and Marfan's syndromes are associated with a particularly high risk of vascular dissection.

It is of interest that most of the patients have had warning attacks of unilateral cranial or facial pain, followed, within minutes to days, by signs of ischemia in the internal carotid artery territory. The pain is nonthrobbing and centered most often in and around the eye; less often, it is in the frontal or temporal regions, angle of the mandible, or high neck. Rapid and marked relief of the pain after the administration of corticosteroids is virtually a diagnostic feature (see below). The ischemic manifestations consist of transient attacks in the territory of the internal carotid, followed frequently by the signs of hemispheral stroke, which may evolve smoothly over a period of a few minutes to hours or over several days in a fluctuating or stepwise fashion. A unilateral Horner syndrome may be conjoined. A new cervical bruit—sometimes audible to the patient, amaurosis fugax, faintness and syncope, and facial numbness are less common symptoms. Most of the patients described by Mokri and coworkers presented with one of two distinct syndromes: (1) unilateral headache associated with an ipsilateral Horner syndrome or (2) unilateral headache and delayed focal cerebral ischemic symptoms. In some patients, there is evidence of involvement of the vagus, spinal accessory, or hypoglossal nerve; these nerves lie in close proximity to the carotid artery and are nourished by small branches from it.

In most cases, dissection of the internal carotid artery can be detected by ultrasound and confirmed by MRI, which shows a double lumen, and MRA. These procedures may obviate the need for arteriography. The latter procedure reveals an elongated, irregular, narrow column of dye, beginning 1.5 to 3 cm above the carotid bifurcation and extending to the base of the skull, a picture that Fisher has called the *string sign*. There may be a tapered occlusion or an outpouching at the upper end of the string. Less often the dissection is confined to the midcervical region, and occasionally it extends into the middle cerebral artery or involves the opposite carotid artery or the vertebral and basilar arteries.

The usual treatment has been immediate anticoagulation to prevent embolism—using first heparin, then warfarin—but it must be acknowledged that this approach has not been demonstrated to be more successful than careful observation. It is of interest, and of therapeutic value, that corticosteroids may relieve the acute pain of cervical and intracranial dissection. Most neurologists take the approach that warfarin, if used, may be discontinued in several months or a year, when angiography or MRA shows the lumen of the carotid artery to be patent, to at least 50 percent of the normal diameter, and smooth-walled. The important study of Mokri and colleagues showed that a complete or excellent recovery occurred in 85 percent of patients with the angiographic signs of dissection; mainly, these were patients without stroke. The outcome in cases complicated by stroke is far less benign. About one-quarter of such patients succumb and one-half of the survivors are seriously impaired (Bogousslavsky et al). In the remainder, early recanalization of the occluded artery occurs (as determined by ultrasonography), with good functional recovery. Pseudoaneurysms form in a small proportion of patients and generally do not require surgical repair; they also do not preclude cautious anticoagulation.

The pathogenesis of spontaneous carotid dissection is undetermined. In most of the recently reported cases, cystic medial necrosis has not been found on microscopic examination of the involved artery. In some, there was a disorganization of the media and internal elastic lamina, but the specificity of these changes is in doubt, since Ojemann and colleagues noted similar changes in some of their control cases. In a small proportion of cases there are the changes of fibromuscular dysplasia, as noted earlier. A more thorough study of these vessels in routine autopsy material is needed.

Vertebral Artery Dissection Dissection of these arteries is less common than dissection of the extracranial carotid artery but is being recognized with increasing frequency. It may originate in the neck and extend into the intracranial portion of the vessel or remain isolated to either of these segments. In both instances there is a tendency to form pseudoaneurysms, more likely with the intracranial type, but only in the latter is there a risk of rupture through the adventitia, leading to a subarachnoid hemorrhage. Rapid and extreme rotational movement of the neck is the most common identifiable cause, chiropractic manipulation being one precipitant, but turning the head to back up a car, extending the neck to have one's hair washed, and swinging a golf club have also led to dissection. Also forceful coughing may cause dissection, as in the carotid vessels. There is no female predominance, but the previously cited intrinsic weaknesses of the vascular wall from Ehlers-Danlos disease and fibromuscular dysplasia are risk factors.

The dissection usually originates in the C1-2 segment of the vessel, where it is mobile but tethered as it leaves the transverse foramen of the axis and turns sharply to enter the cranium. The symptoms, mainly vertigo, derive from the lateral medullary syndrome, often with additional features referable to the pons or midbrain, particularly diplopia and dysarthria. The symptoms in our experience have fluctuated slowly over minutes and hours, quite unlike the usual vertebrobasilar TIA. Less common strokes include artery- to-artery embolism to the posterior cerebral territory or infarction of the rostral spinal cord from occlusion of the anterior spinal artery.

The diagnosis of vertebral dissection should be suspected if occipitonuchal pain is prominent and follows one of the known precipitants—such as chiropractic manipulation of the neck, head trauma, or Valsalva straining or coughing activities—but it may otherwise escape detection until the full-blown medullary or cerebellar stroke is established. The latter may follow the inciting event by several days or weeks or even longer. Axial MRI images, particularly the T1-weighted sequences, show a double lumen in the dissected vessel, and skillful ultrasound investigation documents the same. Treatment is usually with heparin anticoagulation followed for a period by warfarin, but the precise duration of treatment is difficult to determine and the same uncertainties as to effectiveness mentioned in regard to carotid dissection pertain here. Whether there is an inordinate risk of subarachnoid hemorrhage with intracranial dissection has not been settled. The usual practice is to repeat an imaging or ultrasound study several months after the dissection and discontinue the anticoagulation if the vessel lumen has been re-established sufficiently to allow good blood flow. Pseudoaneurysms in the cervical portions of the vessels generally do not require specific treatment.

Mokri et al have found that some patients have evidence of spontaneous or traumatic dissection of multiple extracranial vessels; this also occurs as a consequence of dissection of the aortic arch from chest trauma. As with other dissections, corticosteroids may relieve the associated cranial pain.

Intracranial Arterial Dissection Dissections of intracranial arteries are less common than extracranial dissections and present in several ways. A number of times we have misinterpreted the arteriographic appearance of a short segment of narrowing of the basilar or proximal middle cerebral arteries, assuming these changes to represent embolism or arteritis, when in fact they proved (by axial MRI imaging) to be dissections of the vessel wall. In the case of purely intracranial dissection of the middle cerebral or basilar arteries, there is usually no preceding trauma, but a few patients have had minor head injuries, extreme coughing, or other Valsalva-producing events (e.g., after delivery)—or they had used cocaine. The typical picture is of fluctuating symptoms referable to the affected circulation and severe cranial pain on the side of the occlusion—retro-orbital in the case of middle cerebral dissection, occipital in the case of basilar dissection, occipital combined with supraorbital in the case of vertebral dissection (see above). A few have had sudden strokes that suggested embolic infarction, and a small number present with subarachnoid hemorrhage. Treatment is with anticoagulation and follow-up arteriography; corticosteroids have relieved the cranial and retro-orbital pain in our cases.

Moyamoya Disease

Moyamoya is a Japanese word for a "cloud of smoke" or "haze," and it has been used in recent years to refer to an *extensive basal cerebral rete mirabile*—a network of small anastomotic vessels at the base of the brain around and distal to the circle of Willis, seen in carotid arteriograms, along with segmental stenosis or occlusion of the terminal parts of both internal carotid arteries.

Nishimoto and Takeuchi have reported on 111 cases that were selected on the basis of these two radiologic criteria. The condition was observed mainly in infants, children, and adolescents (more than half the patients were less than 10 years of age, and only 4 of the 111 were older than 40 years). All their patients were Japanese; both males and females were affected, and 8 were siblings. The symptom that led to medical examination was usually weakness of an arm, leg, or both on one side. The weakness tended to clear rapidly but recurred in some instances. Headache, convulsions, impaired mental development, visual disturbance, and nystagmus occurred less frequently. In older patients, subarachnoid hemorrhage was the most common initial manifestation. Other symptoms and signs were speech disturbance, sensory impairment, involuntary movements, and unsteady gait. Only 6 of the entire series became worse after the initial illness, and 4 died. Characteristics noted by others include prolonged TIAs, characteristically induced by hyperventilation or hyperthermia, parenchymal rather than subarachnoid hemorrhages (most are situated in the basal ganglia or thalamus), and an unusual "rebuildup" EEG phenomenon in which high-voltage slow waves reappear 5 min after the end of hyperventilation.

Postmortem examination of these cases has yielded a reasonably clear picture of the distal carotid lesion. The adventitia, media, and internal elastic laminae of the stenotic or occluded arteries were normal, but the intima was greatly thickened by fibrous tissue. No inflammatory cells or atheromata were seen. In a few cases, hypoplasia of the vessel with absent muscularis has been described. The rete mirabile consists of a fine network of vessels over the basal surface (in the pia-arachnoid) which, according to Yamashita and coworkers, reveal microaneurysm formation due to weakness of the internal elastic lamina and thinness of the vessel wall. The latter lesion may be the source of subarachnoid hemorrhage. Thus one part of the symptomatology is traced to the distal carotid stenosis and another to the rupture of the vascular network.

This form of cerebrovascular disease is not limited to the Japanese. The authors have periodically observed such patients, as have others, in the United States, western Europe, and Australia. Opinion is divided as to whether the basal rete mirabile represents a congenital vascular malformation (i.e., a persistence of the embryonal network) or a rich collateral vascularization, secondary to a congenital hypoplasia, acquired stenosis, or occlusion of the internal carotid arteries early in life. The association between moyamoya, Down syndrome, and certain HLA types favors a hereditary basis (Kitahara et al).

The treatment of moyamoya is far from satisfactory. Certain surgical measures have been employed, including application of a vascular muscle flap, omentum, or pedicle containing the superficial temporal artery to the pial surface of the frontal lobe, with the idea of creating neovascularization of the cortical convexity. These measures have reportedly reduced the number of ischemic attacks, but whether they alter the natural history of the illness cannot be stated.

Binswanger Disease

Binswanger disease has been mentioned briefly in the discussion of the course and prognosis of atherothrombotic infarction. The term has come to denote a widespread degeneration of cerebral white matter having a vascular causation and observed in the context of hypertension, atherosclerosis of the small blood vessels, and multiple strokes. Hemiparesis, dysarthria, TIAs, and typical lacunar or cortical strokes are admixed in many cases. The process has been associated with a particular radiologic appearance that reflects the confluence of areas of white matter changes. The term *leukoareosis*, meant to describe the less intense appearance of periventricular tissues in imaging studies, complicates the matter, since this condition is also assumed to have a vascular basis, and the term has been used indiscriminately, particularly by some radiologists, as equivalent to *Binswanger disease*.

Dementia, a pseudobulbar state, and a gait disorder, the main features of Binswanger cases, have been attributed to the cumulative effects of the ischemic changes and specifically to the white matter degeneration, but the existence of such a clinical and pathologic entity has not been well delineated. More importantly, the gliosis that is found in white matter has been assumed to represent a special type of ischemic change, but the vessels in these regions have not been adequately studied (by serial sections). Yet another problem is to distinguish such a state from deficits produced by the cumulative effect of numerous larger lacunes, which have for a century been known to cause the aforementioned syndromes of dementia, gait disturbance, and so on. From time to time, imaging studies of the brain disclose large regions of white matter change or the occurrence of multiple infarctions in the absence of hypertension, and it is not clear how such cases should be classified. Some prove to be areas of demyelination or metabolic dysmyelination, others are mitochondrial disorders, and perhaps some are related to the familial syndrome discussed below. Readers should consult the reviews by Babikian and Ropper, by Caplan, and by Mohr and Mast.

Familial Subcortical Infarction (CADASIL)

A process similar to Binswanger leukoencephalopathy but without hypertension has been identified as an autosomal dominant familial trait linked in several European families to a mutation on chromosome 19. It had been described previously under a number of names, including hereditary multi-infarct dementia. The acronym *CADASIL* has been applied (cerebral autosomal dominant arteriopathy with subcortical infarcts and leukoencephalopathy). In these patients recurrent small strokes, often beginning in early adulthood, culminate in a subcortical dementia. Migraine headaches, often with neurologic accompaniments, may precede the strokes by several years, as may numerous and varied TIAs that are typically attributed to the migraine. The familial nature of the process may not be appreciated because penetrance is not complete until 60 years of age. On MRI scans, clinically unaffected family members may show substantial changes in the white matter well before strokes or dementia arise. In some cases, particularly in Japan, early alopecia and lumbar spondylosis have been associated with CADASIL.

The MRI and CT appearance of multiple confluent white matter lesions of various sizes, many quite small and concentrated around the basal ganglia and periventricular areas, is similar to that in Binswanger disease. When these are asymmetric and periventricular, they are difficult to distinguish from the lesions of multiple sclerosis. In the autopsy cases studied by Jung and colleagues, numerous partially cavitated infarctions were found in the white matter and basal ganglia. In the regions of these infarctions were small vessels, 100 to 200 mm diameter, in which the media contained basophilic granular deposits with degeneration of the smooth muscle fibers. Attribution of the white matter degeneration to these vascular changes presents the same problems as in Binswanger disease, particularly in view of patency of most of the many small vessels in the material. Again, the relation of the vascular changes to lesions in the brain has not been studied in serial sections. Nevertheless, there may be a relationship between the familial cases and sporadic instances of Binswanger disease that occur without hypertension.

A mutation of the Notch 3 gene, in the same locus as the gene for familial hemiplegic migraine, has been found by Joutel and colleagues, and this provides a possible diagnostic test. However, the mechanism by which this leads to the white matter changes is not clear. The diagnosis is said to be confirmable by finding eosinophilic inclusions in the arterioles of a skin biopsy (osmophilic with electron microscopy). Awareness of this apparently vascular form of white matter degeneration adds to the list of inherited leukoencephalopathies.

Strokes in Children and Young Adults

As indicated in Table 34-2, it is probable that ischemic necrosis of cerebral tissue can occur in utero. However, very little is known about the underlying vascular lesions, so that nothing further is said about them here.

The occurrence of acute hemiplegia in infants and children is a well-recognized phenomenon. In a series of 555 consecutive postmortem examinations at the Children's Medical Center in Boston, there were 48 cases (8.7 percent) of occlusive vascular disease of the brain (Banker). The occlusions were both embolic (mainly associated with congenital heart disease) and thrombotic, and the latter were actually more common in veins than in arteries. Similarly, stroke is not an uncommon event in young adults (15 to 45 years). This group accounts for an estimated 3 percent of cerebral infarctions. In terms of causation, this group is remarkably heterogeneous. In a series of 144 such patients, more than 40 possible etiologies were identified (H. P. Adams et al). Nevertheless, 78 percent of the group could be accounted for by three categories, more or less equal in size: atherosclerotic thrombotic infarction (usually with a recognized risk factor); cardiogenic embolism (particularly in association with rheumatic heart disease, bacterial and verrucous endocarditis, paradoxic embolism from patent foramen ovale, and prosthetic valves); and nonatherosclerotic vasculopathies (arterial trauma, "spontaneous" dissection of the carotid artery, moyamoya, lupus erythematosus, drug-induced, etc.). Hematologically related disorders—use of oral contraceptives (see further on), the postpartum state, and hypercoagulable states—were the probable causes in 15 percent of the 144 patients. The presence of antiphospholipid or anticardiolipin antibodies (lupus anticoagulant) appears to explain some of these cases and is discussed further under "Stroke as a Complication of Hematologic Disease"; the majority of these patients are women in their thirties without manifest lupus.

Despite the attention they have received, the thrombophilic disorders that are due to inherited deficiencies of naturally occurring anticoagulant factors (antithrombin, proteins S and C) and those due to disturbances of clotting balance (resistance to activated protein C, or factor V Leiden mutation, and prothrombin mutations as well as excess factor VIII) are only infrequent causes of arterial strokes in young adults; mainly they cause venous clotting, including cerebral venous thrombosis (see discussion by Brown and Bevan). In some series of children with strokes, such as the one of Becker and colleagues, up to half of the cases of cerebral infarction had one of these disorders, the commonest being the factor V Leiden mutation, but others have found this mutation to be much less frequent. In children with unexplained stroke, especially if there has been a previous venous thrombosis or if the strokes are recurrent, it is advisable to carry out an extensive hematologic investigation, including testing for antiphospholipid antibody, as described on page 912. In adults this is far less fruitful, and it should be kept in mind that the levels of protein C and S and antithrombin are depressed after stroke, so that any detected abnormalities must be confirmed months later.

Persistent cerebral ischemia and infarction may occasionally complicate migraine in young persons. The combination of migraine and "the pill" is particularly hazardous, as detailed below. Similarly, despite the common occurrence of mitral valve prolapse in young adults, it is probably only rarely a cause of stroke (see comments on page 184). Stroke due to either arterial or venous occlusion occurs occasionally in association with ulcerative colitis and to a lesser extent with regional enteritis. Evidence points to a hypercoagulable state during exacerbations of inflammatory bowel disease, but a precise defect in coagulation has not been identified. Meningovascular syphilis and other forms of chronic basal meningitis are always considerations in this age group. The uncertain role of mitral valve prolapse in stroke in the young has already been mentioned.

Sickle cell anemia is a rare but important cause of stroke in children of African ancestry; acute hemiplegia is the most common manifestation, but all types of focal cerebral disorders have been observed. The pathologic findings are those of infarction, large and small, and their basis is assumed to be vascular obstruction associated with the sickling process. Intracranial bleeding (subdural, subarachnoid, and intracerebral) and cerebral venous thrombosis may also complicate sickle cell anemia, and—perhaps because of autosplenectomy—there is an increased incidence of pneumococcal meningitis in this disease. Treatment of the cerebral circulatory disorder, based presumably on sludging of red blood cells, is with intravenous hydration and transfusion.

Certain hereditary metabolic diseases (*homocystinuria and Fabry's angiokeratosis*) and the mitochondrial disorder *MELAS*, discussed in Chap. 37, may give rise to strokes in children or young adults.

Oral Contraceptives, Estrogen, and Cerebral Infarction The early studies of Longstreth and Swanson and of Vessey et al clearly indicated that women who take oral contraceptives in the childbearing years—particularly if they are older than 35 years of age and also smoke, are hypertensive, or have migraine—are at increased risk of cerebral infarction as well as ischemic heart disease and subarachnoid hemorrhage. Cerebral infarction in these cases is due to arterial occlusion, occurring in both the carotid–middle cerebral and vertebrobasilar territories. In most of the reported fatal cases, the thrombosed artery has been free of atheroma or other disease. This has been taken to indicate that embolism is responsible for the strokes, but the source of embolism can rarely be demonstrated. Cerebral and noncerebral venous thromboses are other relatively rare complications of "the pill." These observations, coupled with evidence that estrogen alters the coagulability of the blood, suggest that a state of hypercoagulability is an important factor in the genesis of contraceptive-associated infarction.

Mainly at increased risk of stroke are women taking high-dose (0.50 mg) estrogen pills. Lowering the estrogen content has substantially reduced this risk. The use of progestin-only pills (POPs) or of Norplant (subcutaneously implanted capsules of progestin) has not been associated with an increased risk of stroke (Petitti et al).

It is also clear that mutations of the prothrombin gene are far more frequent in patients who acquire cerebral venous thrombosis while on oral contraceptive pills. These genetic abnormalities are thought by Martinelli and associates to account for 35 percent of idiopathic cases of cerebral vein thrombosis; they also contend that contraceptives increase the risk 20-fold.

The vascular lesion underlying cerebral thrombosis in women taking oral contraceptives has been studied by Irey and colleagues. It consists of intimal hyperplasia of nodular eccentric topography with increased acid mucopolysaccharides and replication of the internal elastic lamina. Similar changes have been found in pregnancy and in humans and animals receiving exogenous steroids, including estrogens.

Stroke in Pregnancy and the Postpartum Period
There is also an increased incidence of cerebrovascular events during pregnancy and the postpartum period. The increased risk of both cerebral infarction and intracerebral hemorrhage appears to be mainly in the 6-week period after delivery rather than during the pregnancy itself (Kittner et al). Fisher has reviewed the literature and has himself analyzed 12 postpartum, 9 puerperal,

and 14 contraceptive cases, as well as 9 patients receiving estrogen therapy; arterial thrombosis was demonstrated in half of the group. Most of the focal vascular lesions during pregnancy were due to arterial occlusion, occurring in the second and third trimesters and the first week after delivery. Venous occlusion tended to occur 1 to 4 weeks postpartum. In Rochester, New York, the incidence rate of stroke during pregnancy was 6.2 per 100,000, but it doubled with each advance in age from 25 to 29, 30 to 39, and 40 to 49 years. Included in most series are cases of cardiac disease, particularly valve-related embolism. It is perhaps surprising that subarachnoid hemorrhage is not more frequent during the Valsalva activity of childbirth. Carotid artery dissection may also be encountered late in pregnancy or soon after delivery.

The occurrence of paradoxical embolus is always a consideration in pregnancy because of a tendency to form clots in the pelvic and leg veins, coupled with increased right heart pressures. Amniotic fluid embolus may also cause stroke in this manner and should be suspected in multiparous women who have had uterine tears. There are almost invariably signs of acute pulmonary disease from simultaneous occlusion of lung vessels. A rare peripartum cardiomyopathy is yet another source of embolic stroke.

Stroke with Cardiac Surgery

Incident to cardiac arrest and bypass surgery there is risk of both generalized and focal hypoxia-ischemia of the brain. Improved operative techniques have lessened the incidence of these complications, but they are still distressingly frequent. Fortunately, most of these cerebral disorders are transient. Atherosclerotic plaques may be dislodged during cross-clamping of the proximal aorta and are an important source of cerebral emboli. In the last decade the incidence of stroke related to cardiac surgery has dropped to between 2 and 3 percent in large series numbering thousands of patients (Libman et al, Algren and Aren). Advanced age, congestive heart failure, and more complex surgeries have been listed as risk factors for stroke in various reports. In a retrospective study by Dashe and colleagues, 2.2 percent had strokes, and the risk was greatly increased (greater than 70 percent) on the side of a carotid stenosis. Curiously, almost one-fifth of postoperative strokes have been lacunar. In one prospective study of 2108 patients who underwent coronary operations in several institutions, 3 percent had strokes or TIAs and the same number had a deterioration of cognitive function; mostly the adverse effects occurred in older patients and were transient (Roach et al).

Mohr and coworkers examined 100 consecutive cases pre- and postoperatively and observed two types of complications—one occurring immediately after the operation and the other after an interval of days or weeks. The immediate neurologic disorder consisted of a delay in awakening from the anesthesia, a slowness in thinking, disorientation, agitation, combativeness, visual hallucinations, and poor registration and recall of what was happening. These symptoms, sometimes verging on delirium or psychosis, usually cleared within 5 to 7 days, although some patients were not entirely normal mentally some weeks later. As the confusion cleared, about half of the patients were found to have small visual field defects, dyscalculia, oculomanual ataxia, alexia, and defects of perception suggestive of lesions in the parieto-occipital regions. The immediate effects were attributed to hypotension and various types of embolism (air, silicon, fat, platelets). The delayed effects were more clearly embolic and were especially frequent in patients having prosthetic valve replacements, but they also occurred subsequent to arterial homografts. In addition to overt and covert strokes, a degree of cognitive decline and depression is to be expected in a large proportion of patients undergoing coronary artery bypass grafting. The frequency of these changes is reported to be between 40 and 70 percent (see page 441). It is our impression that these neurologic complications, both small strokes and cognitive abnormalities, pass unnoticed in many cardiac surgical units.

The use of Doppler insonation of the middle cerebral arteries is being studied to detect transient signals called "HITs" (high-intensity transients) as a manifestation of small emboli during surgery—but, as in cerebral arteriography, the clinical importance of these emboli is not known.

The special stroke problems relating to prosthetic heart valves—mainly infective endocarditis causing embolic strokes and anticoagulant-related cerebral hemorrhage—are described in appropriate sections of this chapter.

INTRACRANIAL HEMORRHAGE

This is the third most frequent cause of stroke. Although more than a dozen causes of nontraumatic intracranial hemorrhage are listed in Table 34-6, primary or hypertensive ("spontaneous") intracerebral hemorrhage, ruptured saccular aneurysm and vascular malformation, hemorrhage associated with the use of anticoagulants or

Table 34-6
Causes of intracranial hemorrhage (including intracerebral, subarachnoid, ventricular, and subdural)

1. Primary (hypertensive) intracerebral hemorrhage
2. Ruptured saccular aneurysm
3. Ruptured AVM; less often, venous and dural vascular malformations
4. Cavernous angioma
5. Trauma including posttraumatic delayed apoplexy
6. Hemorrhagic disorders: leukemia, aplastic anemia, thrombocytopenic purpura, liver disease, complication of anticoagulant or thrombolytic therapy, hypofibrinogenemia, hemophilia, Christmas disease, etc.
7. Hemorrhage into primary and secondary brain tumors
8. Septic embolism, mycotic aneurysm
9. With hemorrhagic infarction, arterial or venous
10. With inflammatory and infectious disease of the arteries and veins
11. With arterial amyloidosis
12. Miscellaneous rare types: vasopressor drugs, cocaine, moyamoya, herpes simplex encephalitis, vertebral artery dissection, acute necrotizing hemorrhagic encephalitis (Hurst disease), tularemia, anthrax, etc.

thrombolytic agents, cerebrovascular amyloidosis, and bleeding disorders account for almost all of the hemorrhages that present as strokes. The small brainstem hemorrhages secondary to temporal lobe herniation and compression (Duret hemorrhages), hypertensive encephalopathy, and brain purpura do not simulate a stroke.

Primary (Hypertensive) Intracerebral Hemorrhage

This is the common, well-known "spontaneous" brain hemorrhage. It is due predominantly to chronic hypertension and degenerative changes in cerebral arteries. In recent decades, with increased awareness of the need to control blood pressure, the proportion of cases attributable to hypertension has been greatly reduced; more than one-third such hemorrhages now occur in normotensive individuals, and the hemorrhages more often than previously arise in locations that are not typical for hypertension. Nevertheless, the hypertensive cerebral hemorrhage serves as a paradigm for understanding and managing the nonhypertensive types.

The bleeding occurs within brain tissue, and rupture of arteries lying in the subarachnoid space is practically unknown apart from aneurysms. The extravasation forms a roughly circular or oval mass that disrupts the tissue and grows in volume as the bleeding continues (Fig. 34-19). Adjacent brain tissue is distorted and compressed. If the hemorrhage is large, midline structures are displaced to the opposite side and reticular activating and respiratory centers are compromised, leading to coma and death in the manner described in Chap. 17. The size and location of the clot determine the degree of upper brainstem compression (Andrew et al). Rupture or seepage into the ventricular system usually occurs, and the CSF becomes bloody in more than 90 percent of cases. A hemorrhage of this type almost never ruptures through the cerebral cortex, the blood reaching the subarachnoid space via the ventricular system. When the hemorrhage

Figure 34-19

An unenhanced CT scan showing the typical picture of a massive primary (hypertensive) hemorrhage in the basal ganglia. The third ventricle and ipsilateral lateral ventricle are compressed and displaced by the expanding mass (12 h after onset of stroke).

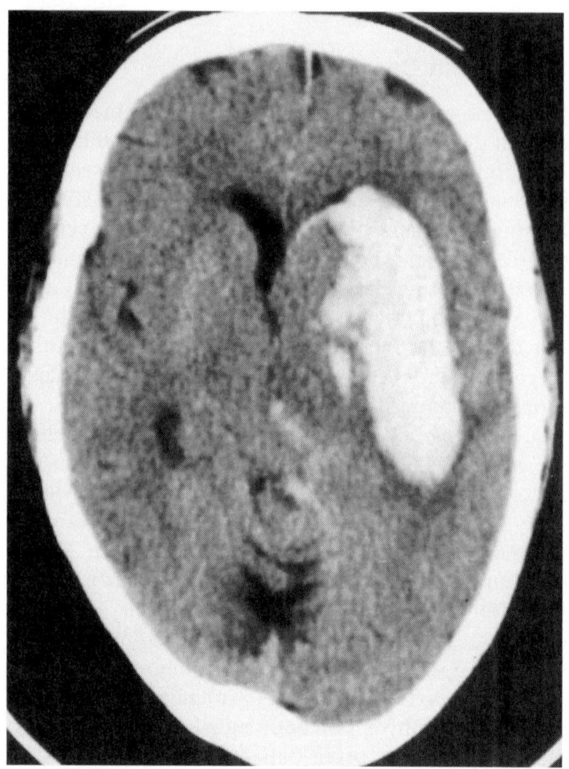

is small and located at a distance from the ventricles, the CSF may remain clear even on repeated examinations. In the first hours and days following the hemorrhage, edema accumulates around the clot and adds to the mass effect. Hydrocephalus may occur as a result of bleeding into the ventricular system or basal cisterns or compression of the third ventricle.

Extravasated blood undergoes a predictable series of changes. At first fluid, it clots within hours. Before the blood clots, red cells may settle in the dependent part of the hematoma and form a meniscus with the plasma above; this is particularly prone to occur in cases of anticoagulant-induced hemorrhage. Only masses of red blood cells (RBCs) and proteins are found within the hematoma; rarely one sees a few remnants of destroyed brain tissue. The hematoma is surrounded by petechial hemorrhages from torn arterioles and venules. Within a few days, hemoglobin products, mainly hemosiderin and hematoidin, begin to appear. The hemosiderin forms within histiocytes that have phagocytized RBCs and takes the form of ferritin granules, which stain positively for iron. As oxyhemoglobin is liberated from the RBCs and becomes deoxygenated, methemoglobin is formed. This begins within a few days and imparts a brownish hue to the periphery of the clot. Phagocytosis of RBCs begins within 24 h, and hemosiderin is first observed around the margins of the clot in 5 to 6 days. The clot changes color gradually, over a few weeks, from dark red to pale red, and the border of golden-brown hemosiderin widens. The edema disappears over many days or weeks. In 2 to 3 months, larger clots are filled with a chrome-colored mush, which is slowly absorbed, leaving a smooth-walled cavity (slit hemorrhage) or a yellow-brown scar. The iron pigment (hematin) becomes dispersed and studs adjacent astrocytes and neurons. It may persist well beyond the border of the hemorrhage for years.

In CT scans, fresh blood is visualized as a white mass as soon as it is shed. The mass effect and the surrounding extruded serum and edema are hypodense. After 2 to 3 weeks, the surrounding edema begins to recede and the density of the hematoma decreases, first at the periphery. Gradually the clot becomes isodense with brain. There may be a ring of enhancement from the hemosiderin-filled macrophages and the reacting cells forming the capsule of the hemorrhage. By MRI, either in T1- or T2-weighted images, the hemorrhage is not easily visible in the 2 or 3 days after bleeding, since oxyhemoglobin is diamagnetic or, at most, is slightly hypointense, so that only the mass effect is evident. After several days the surrounding edema is hyperintense in T2-weighted images. As deoxyhemoglobin and methemoglobin form, the hematoma signal becomes bright on T1-weighted images and dark on T2. As the hematoma becomes subacute, the dark images gradually brighten. When methemoglobin disappears and only hemosiderin remains, the entire remaining mass is hypodense on T2-weighted images, as are the surrounding deposits of iron.

Hemorrhages may be described as massive, moderate, small, slit, and petechial. *Massive* refers to hemorrhages several centimeters in diameter; *small* applies to those 1 to 2 cm in diameter and less than 20 mL in volume; a moderate-sized hemorrhage, of course, falls between these two, both in diameter and in volume. *Slit* refers to an old collapsed hypertensive or traumatic hemorrhage that lies just beneath the cortex. In order of frequency, the most common sites of a primary cerebral hemorrhage are (1) the putamen and adjacent internal capsule (50 percent of cases); (2) the central white matter of the temporal, parietal, or frontal lobes (lobar hemorrhages); (3) the thalamus; (4) a cerebellar hemisphere; and (5) the pons (see Weisberg et al). The vessel involved is usually a penetrating artery. About 2 percent of primary hemorrhages are multiple. Rarely the bleeding is solely intraventricular, possibly from the choroid plexus. Nontraumatic midbrain and medullary hemorrhages are relatively rare, most of them being due to hypertension or a vascular malformation.

Pathogenesis The nature of the hypertensive vascular lesion that leads to arterial rupture is not fully known, but in the few cases studied by serial sections, the hemorrhage appeared to arise from an arterial wall altered by the effects of hypertension, i.e., the change referred to in a preceding section as segmental lipohyalinosis and the false aneurysm (microaneurysm) of Charcot-Bouchard. Ross Russell has affirmed the relationship of these aneurysms to hypertension and hypertensive hemorrhage and their frequent localization on penetrating small arteries and arterioles of the basal ganglia, thalamus, pons, and subcortical white matter. However, in the few hemorrhages examined in serial sections, the bleeding could not be traced to Charcot-Bouchard aneurysms (C. M. Fisher). Takebayashi and coworkers, in an electron microscopic study, found breaks in the elastic lamina at multiple sites, almost always at bifurcations of the small vessels. Possibly these represent sites of secondary rupture from tearing by an expanding hematoma. However, we have also seen this type of change in normal vessels.

Clinical Picture Of all the cerebrovascular diseases, brain hemorrhage is the most dramatic and from ancient times has been surrounded by "an aura of mystery and inevitability." It has been given its own name, "apoplexy." The prototype is an obese, plethoric, hypertensive male who, while sane and sound, falls senseless to the ground—impervious to shouts, shaking, and pinching—breathes stertorously, and dies in a few hours. A massive blood clot escapes from the brain as it is removed postmortem. With smaller hemorrhages, the clinical picture conforms more closely to the usual temporal profile of a stroke, i.e., an abrupt onset of symptoms that evolve gradually and steadily over minutes, hours, or a day or two, depending on the size of the ruptured artery and the speed of bleeding. Headache and vomiting are cardinal features. Very small hemorrhages in "silent" regions of the brain may escape clinical detection. Hemorrhages that complicate the administration of anticoagulants, like those from some vascular malformations, may evolve at a slower pace. Usually there are no warnings or prodromal symptoms; headache, dizziness, epistaxis, or other symptoms do not occur with any consistency. There is no age predilection except that the average age of occurrence is lower than in thrombotic infarction, and neither sex is more disposed. The incidence of hypertensive cerebral hemorrhage is higher in African Americans than in whites and seems recently to have been reported with increasing frequency in Japanese. In the majority of cases, the hemorrhage has its onset while the patient is up and active; onset during sleep is a rarity.

There has long been a notion that acute hypertension precipitates the hemorrhage in some cases. This is based on the occurrence of apoplexy at moments of extreme fright or anger or intense excitement, presumably as the blood pressure rises abruptly beyond its chronically elevated level. The same has been described in relation to taking sympathomimetic medications or cocaine and to numerous other circumstances. However, in fully 90 percent of instances, the hemorrhage occurs when the patient is calm and unstressed (Caplan, 1993). The level of blood pressure rises early in the course of the hemorrhage, but the preceding chronic hypertension is usually of the "essential" type. Other causes of hypertension must always be considered—renal disease, renal artery stenosis, toxemia of pregnancy, pheochromocytoma, aldosteronism, adrenocorticotropic hormone or corticosteroid excess.

There is ordinarily only one episode of hypertensive hemorrhage; recurrent bleeding from the same site, as happens with saccular aneurysm and arteriovenous malformation is infrequent. However, it is now recognized by serial CT scanning that in many instances, as the patient's condition worsens over a few hours, there may be enlargement of the hematoma. Blood that has extravasated into cerebral tissue is removed slowly, over a period of months, during which time symptoms and signs recede. Hence the neurologic deficit is never transitory in intracerebral hemorrhage, as it so often is in embolism; for the same reason, one does not expect rapid improvement in the neurologic deficit from one examination to another.

Putaminal Hemorrhage The most common syndrome is the one due to *putaminal hemorrhage*, usually with extension to the adjacent internal capsule (Fig. 34-19). The neurologic symptoms and signs vary somewhat with the precise site and size of the extravasation, but hemiplegia from interruption of the adjacent internal capsule is a consistent feature of medium-sized and large clots. Vomiting occurs in about half the patients. Headache is frequent but not invariable. With large hemorrhages, patients lapse almost immediately into stupor and coma with hemiplegia, and their condition visibly deteriorates as the hours pass. More often, however, the patient complains of headache or of some other abnormal cephalic sensation. Within a few minutes the face sags on one side, speech becomes slurred or aphasic, the arm and leg gradually weaken, and the eyes tend to deviate away from the side of the paretic limbs. These events, occurring gradually over a period of a few minutes to a half hour, are strongly suggestive of intracerebral bleeding. The paralysis may worsen; a Babinski sign appears, at first unilaterally and then bilaterally; the affected limbs become flaccid; painful stimuli are not appreciated; speaking becomes impossible; and confusion gives way to stupor. The most advanced stages are characterized by signs of upper brainstem compression (coma); bilateral Babinski signs; deep, irregular, or intermittent respiration; dilated, fixed pupils, first on the side of the clot; and occasionally decerebrate rigidity.

The widespread use of CT scanning has disclosed the frequent occurrence of small putaminal hemorrhages, which in former times would have been misdiagnosed as embolic or thrombotic ischemic strokes (especially if the CSF was clear). With hemorrhages confined to the anterior segment of the putamen, the hemiplegia and hyperreflexia tend to be less severe and to clear more rapidly (Caplan). Also there is prominent abulia, motor impersistence, temporary unilateral neglect, and—with left-sided lesions—nonfluent aphasia and dysgraphia. With posterior lesions, weakness is also less and is attended by sensory loss, hemianopia, impaired visual pursuit to the opposite side, Wernicke-type aphasia (left-sided lesions), and anosognosia (right-sided).

Caplan has also analyzed the effects of relatively pure caudate hematomas. Those extending laterally and posteriorly into the internal capsule behave much like large putaminal hemorrhages. Those extending medially into the lateral ventricle give rise to drowsiness, stupor, and either confusion and underactivity or restlessness and agitation.

Thalamic Hemorrhage If large or moderate in size, thalamic hemorrhage also produces a hemiplegia or hemiparesis by compression or destruction of the adjacent internal capsule (Fig. 34-20). The sensory deficit is usually severe and involves all of the opposite side, including the trunk, and may exceed the motor weakness. A fluent aphasia may be present with lesions of the dominant side, and amorphosynthesis and contralateral neglect (page 484) with nondominant lesions. A homonymous field defect, if present, usually clears in a few days.

Thalamic hemorrhage, by virtue of its extension into the subthalamus and high midbrain, may cause a series of ocular disturbances—pseudo-abducens palsies with the eyes turned asymmetrically inward and slightly downward, palsies of vertical and lateral gaze, forced deviation of the eyes downward, inequality of pupils with absence of light reaction, skew deviation with the eye ipsilateral to the hemorrhage assuming a higher position than the contralateral eye, ipsilateral ptosis and miosis (Horner syndrome), absence of convergence, retraction nystagmus, and tucking in (retraction) of the upper eyelids. Extension of the neck may be observed. Compression of the adjacent third ventricle leads to enlargement of the lateral ventricles, and this requires temporary drainage in a small proportion of patients. Small and moderate-sized hemorrhages that rupture into the third ventricle are seemingly associated with fewer neurologic deficits and better outcomes, but early hydrocephalus is almost invariable.

Figure 34-20

CT scan of a left thalamic hemorrhage that caused hemiplegia and hemisensory loss in a hypertensive patient.

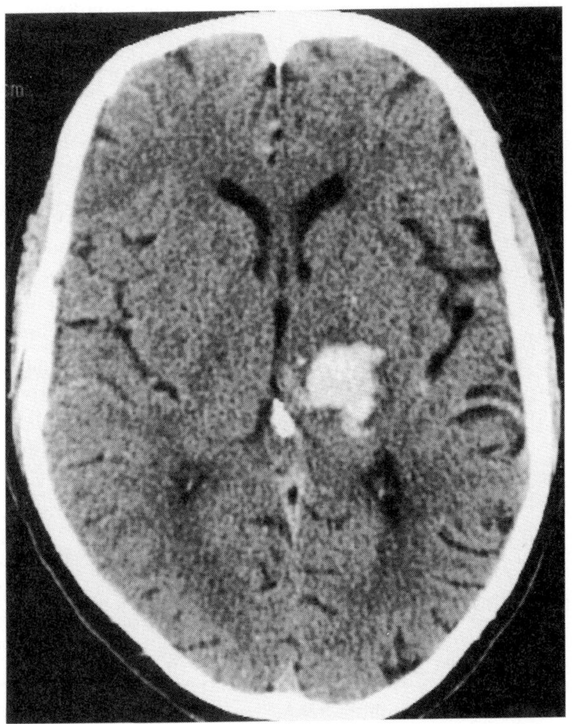

Pontine Hemorrhage Here deep coma usually ensues in a few minutes, and the clinical picture is dominated by total paralysis, decerebrate rigidity, and small (1-mm) pupils that react to light. Lateral eye movements, evoked by head turning or caloric testing, are impaired or absent. Death usually occurs within a few hours, but there are rare exceptions in which consciousness is retained and the clinical manifestations indicate a smaller lesion in the tegmentum of the pons (disturbances of lateral ocular movements, crossed sensory or motor disturbances, small pupils, and cranial nerve palsies) in addition to signs of bilateral corticospinal tract involvement. A small number of our patients with small tegmental hemorrhages and blood in the CSF have survived, with good functional recovery. In a series of 60 patients with pontine hemorrhage reviewed by Nakajima, 19 survived (8 of these had remained alert). Similarly, Wijdicks and St. Louis reported that 21 percent made a good recovery—mostly those who were alert on admission.

Cerebellar Hemorrhage This usually develops over a period of one to several hours, and loss of consciousness at the onset is unusual. Repeated vomiting is a prominent feature, along with occipital headache, vertigo, and inability to sit, stand, or walk. Often these are the only abnormalities, making it imperative to have the patient attempt to stand and walk; otherwise the examination may be falsely normal. In the early phase of the illness, other clinical signs of cerebellar disease may be minimal or lacking; only a minority of cases show nystagmus or cerebellar ataxia of the limbs, although these signs must always be sought. A mild ipsilateral facial weakness and a diminished corneal reflex are common. Dysarthria and dysphagia may be prominent in some cases but usually are absent. Contralateral hemiplegia and facial weakness do not occur unless there is displacement of the medulla against the clivus. There is often paresis of conjugate lateral gaze to the side of the hemorrhage, forced deviation of the eyes to the opposite side, or an ipsilateral sixth nerve weakness. Vertical eye movements are retained. Other ocular signs include blepharospasm, involuntary closure of one eye, skew deviation, "ocular bobbing," and small, often unequal pupils that continue to react until very late in the illness.

Occasionally, at the onset, there is a spastic paraparesis or a quadriparesis with preservation of consciousness. The plantar reflexes are flexor in the early stages but extensor later. When these signs occur, hydrocephalus is present and may require drainage. In the series of St. Louis et al, those with vermian clots and hydrocephalus were at the highest risk for deterioration. As the hours pass, and occasionally with unanticipated suddenness, the patient becomes stuporous and then comatose or suddenly apneic as a result of brainstem compression, at which point reversal of the syndrome, even by surgical therapy, is seldom successful.

Lobar Hemorrhage In a series of 26 cases of lobar hemorrhage, Ropper and Davis found 11 to lie within the occipital lobe (with pain around the ipsilateral eye and a dense homonymous hemianopia); 7 in the temporal lobe (with pain in or anterior to the ear, partial hemianopia, and fluent aphasia); 4 in the frontal lobe (with frontal headache and contralateral hemiplegia, mainly of the arm); and 3 in the parietal lobe (with anterior temporal headache and hemisensory deficit contralaterally). The smaller hematomas simulate an ischemic stroke in the same territory. The occurrence of a progressively worsening headache, vomiting, and drowsiness in conjunction with any one of these syndromes was said to be diagnostic, and, of course, the presence of lobar hemorrhage is readily corroborated by an unenhanced CT scan. Of these 26 patients, 14 had had normal blood pressure, and in several of the fatal cases there was amyloidosis of the affected vessels (see further on). Also, 2 patients were receiving anticoagulants, 2 had an arteriovenous malformation, and 1 had a metastatic tumor. In 22 patients with lobar clots reported by Kase and colleagues, 55 percent were normotensive; metastatic tumors, arteriovenous malformations, and blood dyscrasias were found in 14, 9, and 5 percent of the patients, respectively. The possible role of amyloid angiopathy in lobar hemorrhage is discussed further on.

In summary, several general features of intracerebral hemorrhage should be emphasized. *Acute reactive hypertension*, far exceeding the patient's chronic hypertensive level, is a feature that should always suggest hemorrhage; it is seen with moderate and large clots situated in deep regions. *Vomiting* at the onset of intracerebral hemorrhage occurs much more frequently than with infarction and should always suggest that bleeding is the cause of an acute hemiparesis. Severe headache is generally considered to be an accompaniment of intracerebral hemorrhage and in many cases it is, but in almost 50 percent of our cases headache has been absent or mild in degree. *Nuchal rigidity* is found frequently, but again it is so often absent that failure to find it should by no means detract from the diagnosis. Stiffness of the neck characteristically disappears as coma deepens. It should also be noted that the patient is often alert and responding accurately when first seen. This is true even when the CSF is grossly bloody; thus the adage that hemorrhage into the ventricular system always precipitates coma is quite incorrect. Only if bleeding into the ventricles is massive will coma result. *Seizures*, usually focal, occur in the first few days in some 10 percent of cases of supratentorial hemorrhage, rarely at the time of the ictus, but more commonly as a delayed event, months or even years after the hemorrhage, in association with subcortical slit hemorrhages. The fundi often show hypertensive changes in the arterioles. Rarely, white-centered retinal hemorrhages (Roth spots) or fresh preretinal (subhyaloid) hemorrhages occur; the latter are much more common with ruptured aneurysm, arteriovenous malformation, or severe trauma.

In the localization of intracerebral hemorrhages, ocular signs are particularly important. In putaminal hemorrhage, the eyes are deviated to the side opposite the paralysis; in thalamic hemorrhage, the commonest ocular abnormality is downward deviation of the eyes and the pupils may be unreactive; in pontine hemorrhage, the eyeballs are fixed and the pupils are tiny but reactive; and in cerebellar hemorrhage, the eyes are deviated laterally to the side opposite the lesion and ocular bobbing may occur.

Although the proper interpretation of this array of clinical data allows the correct diagnosis to be established in most cases, the ancillary examinations described below are definitive, especially in the diagnosis of small hemorrhages.

Laboratory Findings Among laboratory methods for the diagnosis of intracerebral hemorrhage, the CT scan occupies the foremost position. This procedure has proved totally reliable in the detection of hemorrhages that are 1.0 cm or more in diameter. Smaller pontine hemorrhages are visualized with less certainty. At the same time, coexisting hydrocephalus, tumor, cerebral swelling, and displacement of the intracranial contents are readily appreciated. MRI is particularly useful for demonstrating brainstem hemorrhages and residual hemorrhages, which remain visible long after they can no longer be seen by the CT scan (after 4 to 5 weeks). Hemosiderin and iron pigment have their own characteristic appearances, as described earlier.

In general, lumbar puncture is ill advised, for it may precipitate or aggravate an impending shift of central structures and herniation. The white cell count in the peripheral blood may rise transiently to 15,000 per cubic millimeter, a higher figure than in thrombosis. Also, the sedimentation rate is mildly elevated in some patients.

Course and Prognosis The immediate prognosis for large and medium-sized cerebral clots is grave; some 30 to 35 percent of patients die in 1 to 30 days. Either the hemorrhage extends into the ventricular system or intracranial pressure is elevated to levels that preclude normal perfusion of the brain. Sometimes the hemorrhage itself seeps into vital centers such as the hypothalamus or midbrain. A formula that predicts outcome of hemorrhage based on clot size has been devised by Broderick and coworkers; it is mainly applicable to putaminal and thalamic hemorrhages. They classified hematomas by size and found a close correlation with outcome. A volume of 30 mL or less, calculated from the CT scan, predicted a generally favorable outcome; only 1 of their 71 patients with clots larger than 30 mL had regained independent function at 1 month. In patients with clots of 60 mL or larger and an initial Glasgow Coma Scale score of 8 or less, the mortality was 90 percent. As remarked earlier, it is the location of the hematoma, not simply its size, that determines the clinical effects. A clot 60 mL in volume is almost uniformly fatal if situated in the basal ganglia but may be relatively benign if located in the frontal or occipital lobe. From the studies of Diringer and colleagues, it appears that hydrocephalus is also an important predictor of poor outcome, and this accords with our experience.

In patients who survive—i.e., in those with smaller hemorrhages—there can be a surprising degree of restoration of function, since, in contrast to infarction, the hemorrhage has to some extent pushed brain tissue aside rather than destroyed it. Function may return very slowly, however, because extravasated blood takes time to be removed from the tissues. Also, since rebleeding from the same site is unlikely, the patient may live for many years. In some instances of medium-sized cerebral and cerebellar hemorrhages, the patient survives but papilledema appears after several days of increased intracranial pressure. This does not mean that the hemorrhage is increasing in size or swelling—only that papilledema is slow to develop. Healed scars impinging on the cortex are liable to be epileptogenic.

The poor prognosis of all but the smallest pontine hemorrhages has already been mentioned. Cerebellar hemorrhages present special problems that are discussed below.

Treatment The management of patients with large intracerebral hemorrhages and coma includes the maintenance of adequate ventilation, use of controlled hyperventilation to a P_{CO_2} of 25 to 30 mmHg, monitoring of intracranial pressure in some cases and its control by the use of tissue-dehydrating agents such as mannitol (osmolality kept at 295 to 305 mosmol/L and Na at 145 to 150 meq), and limiting intravenous infusions to normal saline.

Virtually all patients with intracerebral hemorrhage are hypertensive immediately after the stroke because of a generalized sympathoadrenal response. The natural trend is for the blood pressure to diminish over several days, but active treatment in the acute stages has been a matter of controversy. Rapid reduction in blood pressure, in the hope of reducing further bleeding, is not recommended, since it risks compromising cerebral perfusion in cases of raised intracranial pressure. On the other hand, sustained mean blood pressures of greater than 110 mmHg may exaggerate cerebral edema and risk extension of the clot. It is at approximately this level of acute hypertension that the use of beta-blocking drugs (esmolol, labetalol) or angiotensin-converting enzyme inhibitory drugs is recommended. The major calcium channel blocking drugs are used less often for this purpose because of reports of adverse effects on intracranial pressure, although this information derives mainly from patients with brain tumors. Hayashi and associates have shown that blood pressure is lowered with nifedipine after cerebral hemorrhage, but intracranial pressure is raised, resulting in an unfavorable net reduction in cerebral perfusion pressure. We have, nevertheless, used this class of medication in patients with small and medium-sized clots without adverse effects. Diuretics are helpful in combination with any of the antihypertensive medications. More rapidly acting and titratable agents such as nitroprusside may be used in extreme situations, recognizing that they may further raise intracranial pressure.

Surgical evacuation of a hemispheral clot in the acute stage may occasionally be lifesaving, and we have referred numerous patients for such treatment when hemispheral hemorrhages were larger than 3 cm in diameter and the clinical state was deteriorating. The most successful surgical results have been in patients with lobar or moderate-sized putaminal hemorrhages. Although selected patients may be saved from progression to brain death, the focal neurologic deficit is not altered. Even this modest result requires that operation be carried out before or very soon after coma supervenes. Once the patient becomes deeply comatose with dilated fixed pupils, the chance of any recovery is negligible. Finally, it must be acknowledged, on the basis of several small studies, that surgical results have not been superior to those from medical measures alone (Waga and Yamamato, Batjer et al, Juvela et al). In comatose patients with large hemorrhages, we have found that the placement of a device for constant monitoring of intracranial pressure enables the clinician to use medical measures with greater precision, as outlined in Chap. 17, but there is no evidence that outcome is significantly improved (Ropper and King).

In contrast to cerebral hemorrhage, the *surgical evacuation of cerebellar hematomas* is a generally accepted treatment and is a more urgent matter because of the proximity of the mass to the brainstem and the risk of abrupt progression to coma and respiratory failure. Also, hydrocephalus from compression of the fourth ventricle more often complicates the clinical picture and further raises intracranial pressure (St. Louis et al). As a rule, a cerebellar hematoma of less than 2 cm in diameter leaves most patients awake and infrequently leads to deterioration. Hematomas that are 4 cm or more in greatest diameter, especially if located in the vermis, pose the greatest risk, and some surgeons have recommended evacuation of lesions of this size no matter what the clinical state. In determining the need for surgical evacuation, we have been guided by the clinical state, the mass effect caused by the clot as visualized on CT scan (particularly the degree of compression of the quadrigeminal cistern, as pointed out by Taneda and colleagues), and the presence of hydrocephalus. Often this requires daily or even more frequent CT scans. The patient who is stuporous or displays arrhythmic breathing is best intubated and brought to the operating room within hours. Once coma and pupillary changes supervene, few patients survive, even with surgery; however, rapid medical intervention with mannitol and hyperventilation, followed by surgical evacuation of the clot and drainage of the ventricles very soon after the onset of coma, have been successful in a few cases. Patients who are drowsy and those with hematomas of 2 to 4 cm in diameter pose the greatest difficulty. If the level of consciousness is fluctuating or if there is obliteration of the perimesencephalic cisterns, particularly if coupled with hydrocephalus, we believe that the risk of surgery is less than that of a sudden deterioration. In very few patients have we found it practical to perform only drainage of the enlarged ventricles, although some groups still favor this procedure and eschew a posterior fossa operation. Ultimately, in our experience, evacuation of the clot is more important than reduction of hydrocephalus.

Spontaneous Subarachnoid Hemorrhage (Ruptured Saccular Aneurysm)

This is the fourth most frequent cerebrovascular disorder—following atherothrombosis, embolism, and primary intracerebral hemorrhage. Saccular aneurysms are also called "berry" aneurysms; actually they take the form of small, thin-walled blisters protruding from arteries of the circle of Willis or its major branches. Their rupture causes a flooding of the subarachnoid space with blood under high pressure. As a rule, the aneurysms are located at bifurcations and branchings (Fig. 34-21) and are generally presumed to result from developmental defects in the media and elastica. An alternate theory holds that the aneurysmal process is initiated by focal destruction of the internal elastic membrane, which is produced by hemodynamic forces at the apices of bifurcations (Ferguson). As a result of the local weakness, the intima bulges outward, covered only by adventitia; the sac gradually enlarges and may finally rupture. Saccular aneurysms vary in size from 2 mm to 2 or 3 cm in diameter, averaging 7.5 mm (Wiebers et al). Those that rupture usually have a diameter of 10 mm or more (by angiography), but rupture also occurs in those of lesser size. Aneurysms vary greatly in form. Some are round and connected to the parent artery by a narrow stalk, others are broad-based without a stalk, and still others take the form of narrow cylinders. The site of rupture is usually at the dome of the aneurysm, which may have one or more secondary sacculations. A review of this subject by Schievink is recommended.

In routine autopsies, the incidence of ruptured aneurysms is 1.8 percent; of unruptured ones, 2.0 percent—excluding minor outpouchings of 3 mm or less. Aneurysms are multiple in 20 percent of patients. It has been estimated that 400,000 Americans harbor unrup-

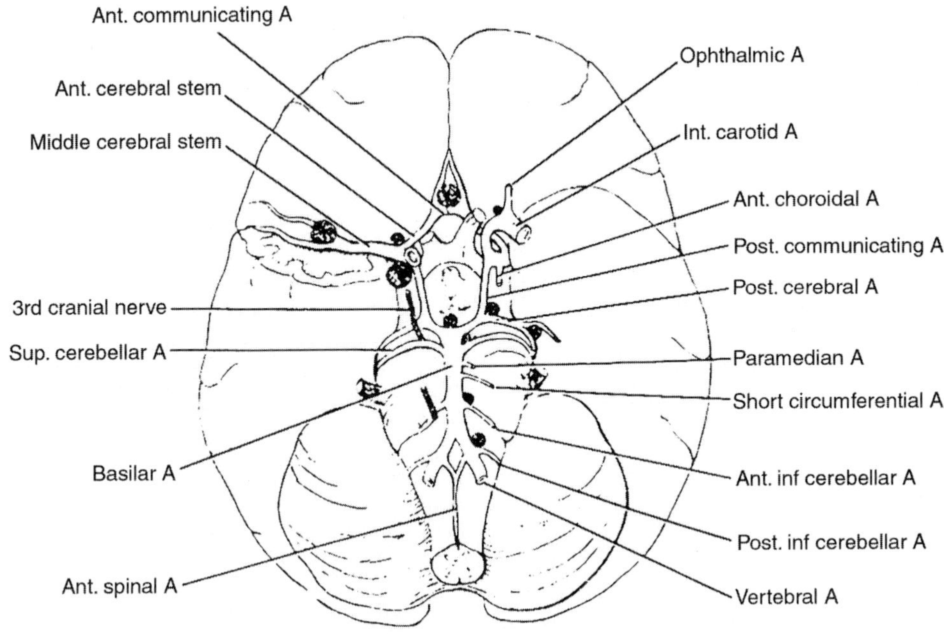

Figure 34-21

Diagram of the circle of Willis to show the principal sites of saccular aneurysms. Approximately 90 percent of aneurysms are on the anterior half of the circle.

tured aneurysms and that there are an estimated 26,000 subarachnoid hemorrhages from them per year (Sahs et al). In childhood, rupture of saccular aneurysms is rare, and they are seldom found at routine postmortem examination; beyond childhood, they gradually increase in frequency to reach their peak incidence between 35 and 65 years of age. Therefore they cannot be regarded as fully formed congenital anomalies; rather, they appear to develop over the years on the basis of either a developmental or acquired arterial defect. There is an increased incidence of congenital polycystic kidneys, fibromuscular dysplasia of the extracranial arteries, moyamoya, and coarctation of the aorta among persons with saccular aneurysms. Numerous reports have documented a familial occurrence of saccular aneurysms, lending support to the idea that genetic factors play a role in their development. The number of first-degree relatives found to harbor an unsuspected aneurysm has been about 4 percent in most series. According to the Magnetic Resonance Angiography in Relatives of Patients with Subarachnoid Hemorrhage Study Group, this low rate, the finding that half of the discovered aneurysms are small, and the complications of surgery make screening of siblings, children, and parents of patients with ruptured aneurysms impractical. A saccular aneurysm occurs in approximately 5 percent of cases of arteriovenous malformation, usually on the main feeding artery of the malformation. Hypertension is more frequently present than in the general population, but aneurysms most often occur in persons with normal blood pressure. Pregnancy does not appear to be associated with an increased incidence of aneurysmal rupture, although there is always concern about the possibility of rupture during the straining of natural delivery. Atherosclerosis, though present in the walls of some saccular aneurysms, probably plays no part in their formation or enlargement.

Approximately 90 to 95 percent of saccular aneurysms lie on the anterior part of the circle of Willis (Fig. 34-21). The four most common sites are (1) in relation to the anterior communicating artery, (2) at the origin of the posterior communicating artery from the stem of the internal carotid, (3) at the first major bifurcation of the middle cerebral artery, and (4) at the bifurcation of the internal carotid into middle and anterior cerebral arteries. Other sites include the internal carotid artery in the cavernous sinus, the origin of the ophthalmic artery, the junction of the posterior communicating and posterior cerebral arteries, the bifurcation of the basilar artery, and the origins of the three cerebellar arteries. Aneurysms that rupture in the cavernous sinus may give rise to an arteriovenous fistula (page 928).

There are several types of aneurysm other than saccular, e.g., mycotic, fusiform, diffuse, and globular. The mycotic aneurysm is caused by a septic embolus that weakens the wall of the vessel in which it lodges (page 902); the others are named for their predominant morphologic characteristics and consist of enlargement or dilatation of the entire circumference of the involved vessels, usually the internal carotid, vertebral, or basilar arteries. The latter are also referred to as arteriosclerotic aneurysms, since they frequently show atheromatous deposition in their walls, but it is likely that they are at least partly developmental in nature. Some are gigantic and press on neighboring structures or become occluded by thrombus; they rupture only infrequently.

Clinical Picture Prior to rupture, saccular aneurysms are usually asymptomatic. Exceptionally, if sufficiently large to compress pain-sensitive structures, they may cause localized cranial pain. With a cavernous or anterolaterally situated aneurysm on the first part of the middle cerebral artery, the pain may be localized to the orbit. An aneurysm on the posteroinferior or anteroinferior cerebellar artery may cause unilateral occipital or cervical pain. The presence of a partial oculomotor palsy with dilated pupil may be indicative of an aneurysm of the posterior communicating–internal carotid junction (less often posterior communicating–posterior cerebral junction). Occasionally, large aneurysms just anterior to the cavernous sinus may compress the optic nerves or chiasm, third nerve, hypothalamus, or pituitary gland. In the cavernous sinus they may compress the third, fourth, or sixth nerve or the ophthalmic division of the fifth nerve. A monocular visual field defect may also develop with a supraclinoid aneurysm near the anterior and middle cerebral bifurcation or the ophthalmic-carotid bifurcation.

Whether a small leak of blood from an aneurysm may serve as a warning sign of rupture has been disputed. We have seen several cases where an exertional headache was found to be associated with a small subarachnoid hemorrhage, discovered by lumbar puncture. There may be a transitory unilateral weakness or numbness or a speech disturbance. Occasionally a severe prodromal headache may occur without evidence of bleeding.

With rupture of the aneurysm, blood under high pressure is forced into the subarachnoid space (where the circle of Willis lies), and the resulting clinical events assume one of three patterns: (1) the patient is stricken with an excruciating generalized headache and vomiting and falls unconscious almost immediately; (2) headache develops in the same manner but the patient remains relatively lucid—the usual syndrome; (3) rarely, consciousness is lost quickly without any preceding complaint. Decerebrate rigidity may occur at the onset of the hemorrhage, in association with unconsciousness. If the hemorrhage is massive, death may ensue in a matter of minutes or hours, so that *ruptured aneurysm must be considered in the differential diagnosis of sudden death.* A considerable proportion of such patients never reach a hospital. Persistent deep coma is accompanied by irregular respirations, attacks of extensor rigidity, and finally respiratory arrest and circulatory collapse. In these rapidly fatal cases, the subarachnoid blood has greatly increased the intracranial pressure to a level that approaches arterial pressure and caused a marked reduction in cerebral perfusion. In some instances the hemorrhage has dissected intracerebrally and entered the ventricular system.

Rupture of the aneurysm usually occurs while the patient is active rather than during sleep, and in some instances sexual intercourse, straining at stool, lifting heavy objects, or other sustained exertion precipitates the ictus. Momentary Valsalva maneuvers, as in coughing or sneezing, have generally not caused aneurysmal rupture (they may cause arterial dissection). In patients who survive the initial rupture, the most feared complication is rerupture, an event that may occur at any time from minutes up to 2 or 3 weeks later.

In less severe cases, consciousness, if lost, may be regained within a few minutes or hours, but a residuum of drowsiness, confusion, and amnesia accompanied by severe headache and stiff neck persists for several days. It is not uncommon for the drowsiness and confusion to last 10 days or longer. Since the hemorrhage is confined to the subarachnoid space, there are few or no focal neurologic signs. That is to say, gross lateralizing signs in the form of hemiplegia, hemiparesis, homonymous hemianopia, or aphasia are absent in the majority of cases. They may occur, however, in the acute stages as the result of an intracerebral clot or ischemia in the territory of the aneurysm-bearing artery. Usually this occurs several days after a large subarachnoid hemorrhage. The pathogenesis of such manifestations is not fully understood, but a transitory fall in pressure in the circulation distal to the aneurysm is postulated in early cases and vasospasm is responsible for the late focal signs. Transient deficits are not common but constitute reliable indicators of the site of the ruptured aneurysm (see below).

Convulsive seizures, usually brief and generalized, occur in 10 to 25 percent of cases according to Hart et al (but far less often in our experience) in relation to acute bleeding or rebleeding. These early seizures do not correlate with the location of the aneurysm and do not appear to alter the prognosis.

Vasospasm *Delayed hemiplegia* or other focal deficit usually appears 3 to 12 days after rupture and rarely before or after this period. These delayed accidents and the focal narrowing of a large artery or arteries, seen on angiography, are referred to as *vasospasm*. Fisher and coworkers have shown that spasm is most frequent in arteries surrounded by the largest collections of subarachnoid blood. The vasospasm appears to be a direct effect of blood or some blood product, possibly hematin or a platelet product, on the adventitia of the artery. Areas of ischemic infarction in the territory of the vessel bearing the aneurysm, usually without atherosclerosis or thrombosis of the vessel, is the usual finding at autopsy in such cases. These ischemic lesions are often multiple and occur with great frequency, according to Hijdra and associates (57 of 176 prospectively studied patients). After a few days, arteries in chronic spasm undergo a series of morphologic changes. The smooth muscle cells of the media become necrotic, and the adventitia is infiltrated with neutrophilic leukocytes, mast cells, and red blood corpuscles, some of which migrate to a subendothelial position (Chyatte and Sundt). We favor the idea that these changes are caused by products of hemolyzed blood seeping inward from the adventitia (the pia-arachnoid coat) of the artery.

The clinical features of cerebral vasospasm depend upon the blood vessel that has been affected but typically include a fluctuating hemiparesis or aphasia and increasing confusion that must be distinguished from the effects of hydrocephalus (see below). In the past, an arteriogram was required to verify the diagnosis, although it was not often performed because of the associated risk and the ease with which the condition can be recognized by its clinical presentation. Transcranial Doppler measurements are an indirect but safer way of following, by observations of blood flow velocity, the caliber of the main vessels at the base of the brain. Almost all patients have a greatly increased velocity of blood flow that can be detected by this method in the days after hemorrhage. Progressive elevation of flow velocity in any one vessel (especially if more than 175 cm/s) suggests that focal vasospasm is occurring. There is a reasonable correlation between these findings and the radiographic appearance of vasospasm, but clinical manifestations of ischemia depend on additional factors such as collateral blood supply and the cerebral perfusion pressure.

Hydrocephalus If a large amount of blood ruptures into the ventricular system or floods the basal subarachnoid space, it may find its way into the ventricles through the foramina of Luschka and Magendie. The patient then may become confused or unconscious as a result of *acute hydrocephalus*. The clinical signs are greatly improved by draining the ventricles, either by external ventriculostomy or, in selected cases, by lumbar puncture. A *subacute hydrocephalus* due to blockage of the CSF pathways by blood may appear after 2 to 4 weeks.

Anatomic-Clinical Correlations In most patients the neurologic manifestations do not point to the exact site of the aneurysm, but it can often be inferred from the location of the main clot on CT scan. A collection of blood in the anterior interhemispheric fissure indicates rupture of an anterior communicating artery aneurysm; in the sylvian fissure, a middle cerebral artery aneurysm; in the anterior perimesencephalic cistern, a posterior communicating or distal basilar artery aneurysm; and so on. In some instances clinical signs do provide clues to the localization, as follows: (1) Third nerve palsy (ptosis, diplopia, dilatation of pupil, and divergent strabismus), as stated above, usually indicates an aneurysm at the junction of the posterior communicating artery and the internal carotid artery; the third nerve passes immediately lateral to this point. (2) Transient paresis of one or both of the lower limbs at the onset of the hemorrhage suggests an anterior communicating aneurysm that has interfered with the circulation in the anterior cerebral arteries. (3) Hemiparesis or aphasia points to an aneurysm at the first major bifurcation of the middle cerebral artery. (4) Unilateral blindness indicates an aneurysm lying anteromedially in the circle of Willis (at the origin of the ophthalmic artery or at the bifurcation of the internal carotid artery). (5) A state of retained consciousness with akinetic mutism or abulia (sometimes associated with paraparesis) favors a location on the anterior communicating artery, with ischemia of or hemorrhage into one or both of the frontal lobes or hypothalamus. (6) The side on which the aneurysm lies may be indicated by a unilateral preponderance of headache or preretinal hemorrhages, the occurrence of monocular pain, or, rarely, lateralization of an intracranial sound heard at the time of rupture of the aneurysm. Sixth nerve palsy, unilateral or bilateral, is usually attributable to raised intracranial pressure and is seldom of localizing value.

In summary, the clinical sequence of sudden severe headache, collapse, relative preservation of consciousness with few or no lateralizing signs, and neck stiffness is diagnostic of subarachnoid hemorrhage due to a ruptured saccular aneurysm.

Other clinical data may be of assistance in reaching a correct diagnosis. Almost all patients are hypertensive for one or several days following the bleed, but preceding hypertension is only slightly more common than in the general population. Levels of 200 mmHg systolic are seen occasionally just after rupture, but usually the pressure is elevated only moderately and fluctuates with the degree of head pain. Spontaneous intracranial bleeding with normal blood pressure should also suggest ruptured aneurysm or arteriovenous malformation and, rarely, hemorrhage into a cerebral tumor. Nuchal rigidity is usually present but occasionally absent, and the main complaint of pain may be referable to the interscapular region or even the low back rather than to the head. Examination of the fundi frequently reveals smooth-surfaced, sharply outlined collections of blood that cover the retinal vessels—the so-called preretinal or subhyaloid hemorrhages; Roth spots are seen occasionally. Bilateral Babinski signs are found in the first few days following rupture if there is hydrocephalus. Fever up to 39°C may be seen in the first week, but most patients are afebrile. Rarely, escaping blood enters the subdural space and produces a hematoma, evacuation of which may be lifesaving.

Laboratory Findings A CT scan will detect blood locally or diffusely in the subarachnoid spaces or within the brain or ventricular system in more than 90 percent of cases and in practically all cases in which the hemorrhage has been severe enough to cause momentary or persistent loss of consciousness (Fig. 34-22). This should therefore be the initial investigative procedure. The blood may appear as a subtle shadow along the tentorium

Figure 34-22

Subarachnoid hemorrhage due to rupture of a basilar artery aneurysm. Left. *Axial CT scan image at the level of the lateral ventricles showing widespread blood in the subarachnoid spaces and layering within the ventricles with resultant hydrocephalus.* Right. *At the level of the basal cisterns blood can be seen surrounding the brainstem, in the anterior sylvian fissures and the anterior interhemispheric fissure. The temporal horns of the lateral ventricles are again enlarged, reflecting acute hydrocephalus.*

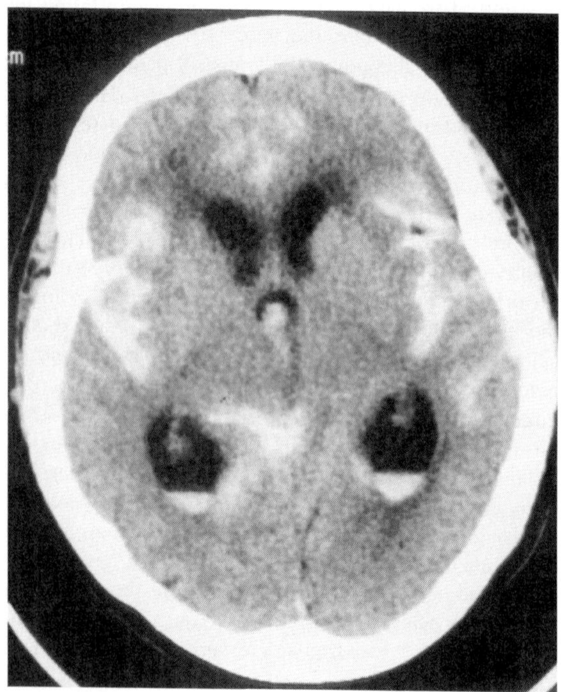

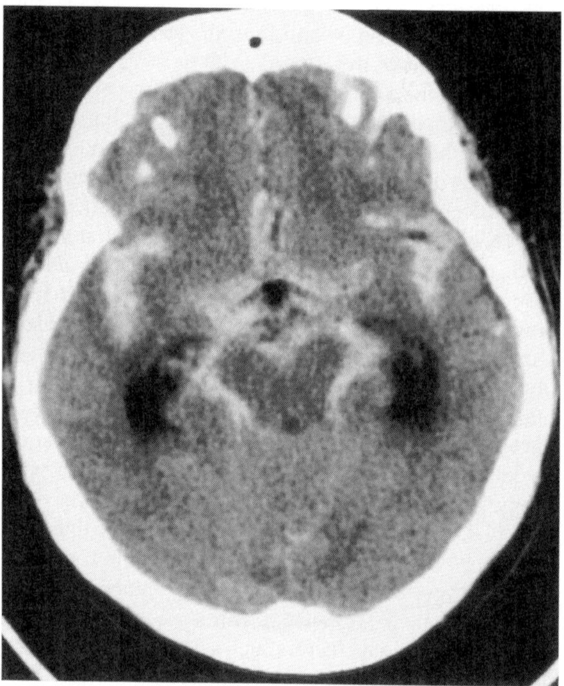

or in the sylvian or adjacent fissures. A large localized collection of subarachnoid blood or a hematoma in brain tissue or within the sylvian fissure indicates the adjacent location of the aneurysm and the likely region of subsequent vasospasm, as already noted. When two or more aneurysms are visualized by arteriography, the CT scan may identify the one that had ruptured by the clot that surrounds it. Also, coexistent hydrocephalus will be demonstrable. If the CT scan documents subarachnoid blood with certainty, a spinal tap is not necessary.

In all other cases a lumbar puncture should be undertaken when the clinical features suggest a subarachnoid hemorrhage. Usually the CSF is grossly bloody within 30 min of the hemorrhage, with RBC counts up to 1 million per cubic millimeter or even higher. With a relatively mild hemorrhage, there may be only a few thousand cells. It is unlikely that an aneurysm can rupture entirely into brain tissue without some leakage of blood into the subarachnoid fluid, so that the diagnosis of ruptured saccular aneurysm (by lumbar puncture) is essentially excluded if blood is not present in the CSF. Xanthochromia is found after centrifugation if several hours have elapsed from the moment of the ictus. In a patient who reports a headache that is consistent with subarachnoid hemorrhage but the occurrence was several days earlier, the CT scan will usually be normal and xanthochromia is the diagnostic finding. The CSF in the first days is under increased pressure, as high as 500 mmH_2O—an important finding in differentiating spontaneous subarachnoid hemorrhage from a traumatic tap. The level of CSF pressure correlates roughly with the initial level of consciousness. The proportion of WBCs to RBCs in the CSF is usually the same as in the circulating blood (approximately 1:1000), but in some patients a brisk CSF leukocytosis appears within 48 h, sometimes reaching more than 1000 cells per cubic millimeter. The protein is slightly or moderately elevated and in some instances glucose is mildly reduced.

Carotid and vertebral angiography is the only certain means of demonstrating an aneurysm and does so in some 85 percent of patients in whom the correct diagnosis of spontaneous subarachnoid hemorrhage is made on clinical grounds. MRI and MRA detect most aneurysms of the basal vessels but are as yet of insufficient sensitivity to replace conventional angiography. Even when MRA or "CT angiography" demonstrates the aneurysm, the surgeon usually requires the kind of anatomic definition that can only be obtained by conventional angiography.

Acute subarachnoid hemorrhage is associated with several characteristic responses in the systemic circulation, water balance, and cardiac function. The ECG changes include symmetrically large peaked T waves and other alterations suggesting subendocardial or myocardial ischemia. Also there is a tendency to develop hyponatremia; the latter abnormality and its relationship to intravascular volume depletion play key roles in treatment. Albuminuria and glycosuria may be present for a few days. Rarely, diabetes insipidus occurs in the acute stages, but water retention or a natriuresis is more frequent. These systemic abnormalities are discussed further on. There may be a leukocytosis of 15,000 to 18,000 cells per cubic millimeter, but the sedimentation rate is usually normal.

Course and Prognosis The outstanding characteristic of this condition is the tendency for the hemorrhage to recur from the same site. This threat colors all prognostications and dominates modern treatment strategies, but unfortunately there appears to be no way of determining reliably which cases will bleed again. The cause of recurrent bleeding is not understood but may be related to naturally occurring mechanisms of clot formation and lysis.

Patients with the typical clinical picture of spontaneous subarachnoid hemorrhage in whom an aneurysm or arteriovenous malformation cannot be demonstrated angiographically have a distinctly better prognosis than those in whom the lesion is visualized (Nishioka et al). In a series of 323 angiographically negative cases followed for an average of 10 years, only 12 rebled (Hawkins et al). After 22 years, 69 percent had survived (expected survival, 89 percent); in 30 cases, death was due to cardiovascular disease. It is customary in most centers to repeat the arteriogram in several weeks, because it has been proposed (with little documentation) that vascular spasm may have earlier obscured the aneurysm. It is advantageous to obtain x-rays in several different planes in order to expose aneurysms that were obscured by adjacent overlying vessels. If the first study involves all cerebral vessels and utilizes several views of the basal circulation, it has been our experience that the second arteriogram is seldom revealing.

Another clinical circumstance with a favorable outcome is *perimesencephalic hemorrhage*, described by van Gijn and colleagues. The cisterns surrounding the midbrain and upper pons are symmetrically filled with blood, the headache is mild, and signs of vasospasm do not develop. No aneurysm is found at the expected site for blood in this region, i.e., at the top of the basilar artery. The patient usually does well and a second arteriogram is probably not required. It has been speculated that the bleeding has a venous source.

McKissock and colleagues found that the patient's state of consciousness at the time of arteriography was the single best index of prognosis. Their data, representative of the status of aneurysm management in the 1950s and consonant with the natural history before the advent of modern surgical and intensive care techniques, indicated that of every 100 patients reaching a hospital and coming to arteriography, 17 were stuporous or comatose and 83 appeared to be recovering from the ictus. At the end of the following 6 months, 8 of every 100 patients had died of the original hemorrhage and 59 had had a recurrence (with 40 deaths), making a total of 48 deaths and 52 survivors. Of the survivors, 36 returned to full work, 12 were partly disabled, and 4 were totally disabled. In regard to recurrence of bleeding, it was found that of 50 patients seen on the first day of the illness, 5 rebled in the first week (all fatal), 8 in the second week (5 fatal), 6 in the third and fourth weeks (4 fatal), and 2 in the next 4 weeks (2 fatal), making a total of 21 recurrences (16 fatal) in 8 weeks.

The most comprehensive long-term analysis of the natural history of the disease is contained in the report of the Cooperative Study of Intracranial Aneurysms and Subarachnoid Hemorrhage (Sahs et al). This study was based on long-term observations of 568 patients who sustained an aneurysmal bleed between 1958 and 1965 and were managed only by a conservative medical program. A follow-up search in 1981 and 1982 disclosed that 378, or two-thirds of the patients, had died; 40 percent of the deaths had occurred within 6 months of the original bleed. For the patients who survived the original hemorrhage for 6 months, the chances of survival during the next two decades were significantly worse than those of a matched normal population. Rebleeding occurred at a rate of 2.2 percent per year during the first decade and 0.86 percent per year during the second decade. Rebleeding episodes were fatal in 78 percent of cases. These statistics, however, also reflect the outcome prior to the modern era of neurologic intensive care management and microsurgery.

Interestingly, these figures have changed very little in recent years. In a prospective clinical trial conducted by the International Cooperative Study and based on observations of 3521 patients (surgery performed in 83 percent), it was found, at the 6-month evaluation, that 26 percent of the patients had died and 58 percent had made a good recovery (Kassell et al). Vasospasm and rebleeding were the leading causes of morbidity and mortality in addition to the initial bleed. In respect to rebleeding, Aoyagi and Hayakawa found that this occurred within 2 weeks in 20 percent of patients, with a peak incidence in the 24 h after the initial bleed.

Treatment This is influenced by the neurologic and general medical state of the patient as well as by the location and morphology of the aneurysm. Ideally, all patients should have the aneurysmal sac surgically obliterated, but the mortality is high if the patient is stuporous or comatose (grade IV or V, see below). Before deciding on a course of action, it has been useful to assess the patient with reference to the widely employed scale introduced by Botterell and by Hunt and Hess, as follows:

Grade I. Asymptomatic or with slight headache and stiff neck

Grade II. Moderate to severe headache and nuchal rigidity but no focal or lateralizing neurologic signs

Grade III. Drowsiness, confusion, and mild focal deficit

Grade IV. Persistent stupor or semicoma, early decerebrate rigidity and vegetative disturbances

Grade V. Deep coma and decerebrate rigidity

The general medical management in the acute stage includes the following, in all or part: bed rest, fluid administration to maintain above-normal circulating volume and central venous pressure, use of elastic stockings and stool softeners; administration of beta-blockers, calcium channel blockers, intravenous nitroprusside, or other medication to reduce greatly elevated blood pressure and then maintain systolic blood pressure at 150 mmHg or less; and pain-relieving medication for headache (this alone will often reduce the hypertension). The prevention of systemic venous thrombosis is critical, usually accomplished by the use of cyclically inflated whole-leg compression boots. The use of anticonvulsants is controversial; many neurosurgeons administer them early, with a view of preventing a seizure-induced risk of rebleeding. We have generally avoided them unless a seizure has occurred.

Calcium channel blockers are being used extensively to reduce the incidence of stroke from vasospasm. Nimodipine 60 mg, administered orally every 4 h, is currently favored. Although calcium channel blockers do not alter the incidence of angiographically demonstrated vasospasm, they have reduced the number of strokes in each of five randomized studies, beginning with the one conducted by Allen and colleagues. Several groups have been using angioplasty techniques to dilate vasospastic vessels and reporting symptomatic improvement, but there are as yet insufficient controlled data to judge the merits and safety of this procedure.

Notable advances in the techniques for the obliteration of aneurysms, particularly the operating microscope, and the management of circulatory volume have significantly improved the outcome of patients with ruptured aneurysms. Wijdicks and colleagues have shown that, in the majority of patients, intravascular volume is depleted in the days after subarachnoid hemorrhage. This, in turn, increases the chances of ischemic infarction from vasospasm, though it does not alter the incidence or severity of vasospasm. In part, this volume contraction can be attributed to bed rest, but sodium loss, probably resulting from the release of atrial natriuretic factor (ANF), a potent oligopeptide stimulator of sodium loss in renal tubules, may also be a factor. Hyponatremia develops in the first week after hemorrhage, but it is unclear whether this also results from the natriuretic effects of ANF or from the effects of antidiuretic hormone, causing water retention. The work of Diringer and colleagues suggests that both mechanisms are operative.

Both the risk of rerupture of the aneurysm and some of the secondary problems that arise because of the massive amount of blood in the subarachnoid space can be obviated by early obliteration of the aneurysm. Because of the changes in water balance and the risk of delayed stroke from vasospasm, there has been an emphasis on early volume expansion and sodium repletion by the intravenous infusion of crystalloids. As Solomon and Fink have pointed out, this can be accomplished with relative safety and without fear of aneurysmal rupture if blood pressure is allowed to rise only minimally. Fluid replacement and a modest elevation of blood pressure become completely safe if the aneurysm has been surgically occluded. Thus the most common current approach is to operate early, within 36 h, on all grades I and II patients and then to increase intravascular volume and maintain normal or above-normal blood pressures. This reduces the risk of rebleeding, with its high mortality, and helps prevent the second important cause of morbidity, stroke from vasospasm. The timing of surgery for grade III patients is still controversial, but if their medical condition allows, they too probably benefit from the same aggressive approach. In grade IV patients, the outcome is generally dismal, no matter what course is taken, but we have usually avoided early operation. The insertion of ventricular drains into both frontal horns has occasionally permitted the raising of a patient with severe hydrocephalus to a better grade and facilitated early operation. In the hands of experienced anesthesiologists and cerebrovascular surgeons using microdissection, the operative mortality, even in grades III and IV patients, has now been reduced to 2 to 3 percent. For a detailed account of the operative approach to each of the major classes of saccular aneurysm, the reader is referred to the monograph by Ojemann and colleagues.

Several alternative therapeutic measures are still being studied. Among these, endovascular obliteration of the lumen of the aneurysm holds the most promise. This has become the preferred approach to aneurysms that are surgically inaccessible—for example, those in the cavernous sinus—or for patients whose medical state does not allow an operation. The infusion of vasodilators to prevent vasospasm has been disappointing, but drugs such as nitroglycerin and treatment along the lines of hemodilution to improve perfusion in the small collateral vessels are still used in selected circumstances.

Because of continuing improvements in imaging techniques and early surgery, the use of antifibrinolytic agents as a means of impeding lysis of the clot at the site of aneurysmal rupture has been generally abandoned. Repeated drainage of the CSF by lumbar puncture is no longer practiced as a routine. One lumbar puncture is carried out for diagnostic purposes if the CT scan is inconclusive; thereafter this procedure is performed only for the relief of intractable headache, to detect recurrence of bleeding, or to measure the intracranial pressure prior to surgery. As mentioned earlier, patients with stupor or coma who have massive hydrocephalus often benefit from decompression of the ventricular system. This is accomplished initially by external drainage and may require permanent shunting if the hydrocephalus returns. The risk of infection of the external shunt tubing is high if it is left in place for much more than 3 days.

Unruptured Intracranial Aneurysms Not infrequently, cerebral angiography, MRI, MRA, or CT scanning discloses the presence of an unruptured saccular aneurysm, invariably raising the problem of management. There is only limited information about the natural history of these lesions. Wiebers and colleagues observed 65 patients with one or more unruptured aneurysms for at least 5 years after their detection. The only clinical feature of significance relative to rupture was aneurysmal size. None of 44 aneurysms smaller than 10 mm in diameter had ruptured, whereas 8 of 29 aneurysms 1 cm or larger eventually did so, with a fatal outcome in 7 cases. In the Cooperative Study of Intracranial Aneurysms, none of the aneurysms less than 7 mm in diameter "had further trouble." A sizable cooperative study that included 2621 patients, conducted by the

International Study of Unruptured Intracranial Aneurysms Investigators, found an extremely low rate of rupture (0.05 percent yearly) for aneurysms smaller than 10 mm in diameter and an annual risk of 1 percent for aneurysms between 10 and 25 mm; the rates were higher if there had been prior bleeding from another site. The location of the lesion also had a bearing on the risk of rupture, as did increasing age; vertebrobasilar and posterior cerebral aneurysms bled at a rate 13.8 times higher than that of the others. Unruptured giant aneurysms, discussed below, bled at a rate of 6 percent in 1 year.

Giant Aneurysms As has been stated, these are believed to be congenital anomalies even when there is considerable atherosclerosis in their walls. They may become enormous in size, by definition greater than 2.5 cm in diameter. Most are located on the carotid, basilar, anterior, or middle cerebral artery. They grow slowly by accretion of blood clot within their lumens or by the organization of surface blood clots from small leaks. At a certain point they may compress adjacent structures, e.g., those in the cavernous sinus, optic nerve, or lower cranial nerves. The giant fusiform aneurysm of the midbasilar artery, with signs of brainstem ischemia and lower cranial nerve palsies, is a relatively common form. Clotting within the aneurysm may cause ischemic infarction in its territory of supply. Giant aneurysms may rupture and cause subarachnoid hemorrhage, but not nearly with the frequency of saccular aneurysms. This clinical observation has been confirmed statistically by the International Study, referred to above.

Treatment is surgical if the lesion is accessible or with endovascular techniques if the lesion is in the vertebral or midbasilar artery. Obliteration of the lumen, coupled with vascular bypass procedures, has been successful in the hands of a few cerebrovascular neurosurgeons, but the morbidity is high. Some aneurysms can be ligated at their necks, others by trapping or by the use of an intravascular detachable balloon. Drake has summarized his experience in the treatment of 174 such cases. Ojemann and colleagues have also had singular success in treating these lesions by a combination of surgical techniques; in more than 40 cases, half of them trapped and half obliterated, there was not a single fatality.

Arteriovenous Malformations of the Brain

An arteriovenous malformation (AVM) consists of a tangle of dilated vessels that form an abnormal communication between the arterial and venous systems, really an arteriovenous fistula. It is a developmental abnormality, representing persistence of an embryonic pattern of blood vessels, and is not a neoplasm, but the constituent vessels may proliferate and enlarge with the passage of time. Arteriovenous malformations have been designated by a number of other terms, such as *angioma* and *arteriovenous aneurysm*, but these are less appropriate; *angioma* suggests a tumor, and the term *aneurysm* is generally reserved for the lesions described in the preceding section. Venous malformations, consisting purely of distended veins deep in the white matter, are a separate entity; they may be the cause of seizures and headaches but seldom of hemorrhage. When bleeding occurs in relation to a venous malformation, it is usually due to an associated cavernous malformation.

Vascular malformations vary in size from a small blemish a few millimeters in diameter lying in the cortex or white matter to a huge mass of tortuous channels constituting an AV shunt of sufficient magnitude, in rare instances, to raise cardiac output. Hypertrophic dilated arterial feeders can be seen approaching the main lesion and to break up into a network of thin-walled blood vessels that connect directly with draining veins. The latter often form greatly dilated, pulsating channels, carrying away arterial blood. The tangled blood vessels interposed between arteries and veins are abnormally thin and do not have the structure of normal arteries or veins. Arteriovenous malformations occur in all parts of the cerebrum, brainstem, and cerebellum, but the larger ones are more frequently found in the central part of a cerebral hemisphere, commonly forming a wedge-shaped lesion extending from the cortex to the ventricle.

When hemorrhage occurs, blood may enter the subarachnoid space almost exclusively, producing a picture identical to that of ruptured saccular aneurysm; but since the AVM lies within cerebral tissue, bleeding is likely to be intracerebral as well, causing a hemiparesis, hemiplegia, and so forth or even death.

Arteriovenous malformations are about one-tenth as common as saccular aneurysms and about equally frequent in males and females. The two lesions—AVM and saccular aneurysm (on the main feeding artery of the AVM)—are associated in about 5 percent of cases; the frequency increases with the size of the AVM and the age of the patient (Miyasaka et al). Rarely, AVMs occur in more than one member of a family in the same generation or successive ones.

Clinical Features Most AVMs are clinically silent for a long time, but sooner or later they bleed. The first hemorrhage may be fatal, but in more than 90 percent of cases the bleeding stops and the patient survives. The rate of hemorrhage in untreated patients is 2 to 4 percent per year. The mortality rate in two major series of cases (Crawford et al, Ondra et al) has been 1 to 2 percent per year. The matter of an increased risk of AVM rupture during pregnancy has been disputed. The weight of evidence suggests that the risk is not raised by pregnancy alone, but—as with saccular aneurysm—parturition and Valsalva activity could precipitate bleeding. Before rupture, chronic, recurrent headache may be a frequent complaint. Usually the headache is of a nondescript type, but a typical neurologic type of migraine occurs in about 10 percent of patients—that is, with greater frequency than it does in the general population. Most of the lesions associated with migraine-like headaches lie in the parieto-occipital region of one cerebral hemisphere, and about two-thirds of such patients have a family history of migraine.

Huge AVMs may produce a slowly progressive neurologic deficit because of compression of neighboring structures by the enlarging mass of vessels and shunting of blood through greatly dilated vascular channels ("intracerebral steal"), resulting in hypoperfusion of the surrounding brain (Homan et al). When the vein of Galen is enlarged as a result of drainage from an adjacent AVM, hydrocephalus may result, but more often this is caused by the meningeal fibrosing effect of subarachnoid hemorrhage in the posterior fossa. Not infrequently one or both carotid arteries pulsate unusually forcefully in the neck. A systolic bruit heard over the carotid in the neck or over the mastoid process or the eyeballs in a young adult is almost pathognomonic of an AVM. Such bruits have been heard in about 25 percent of our patients. Exercise that increases the pulse pressure may bring out a bruit if none is present at rest.

The blood pressure may be elevated or normal; it is axiomatic that the occurrence of intracranial bleeding with a previously normal blood pressure should raise the suspicion of an AVM but also ruptured saccular aneurysm, bleeding diathesis, cerebral vessel amyloidosis, or hemorrhage into a tumor. Rarely, inspection of the eye grounds discloses a retinal vascular malformation, which is coextensive with a similar lesion of the optic nerve and basal portions of the brain. Cutaneous, orbital, and nasopharyngeal AVMs may occasionally be conjoined. Rarely, skull films show crescentic linear calcifications in the larger malformations.

Fully 95 percent of AVMs are disclosed by CT scans if enhanced and an even larger number by MRI (Fig. 34-23). Arteriography establishes the diagnosis with certainty and will demonstrate AVMs larger than 5 mm in diameter. Small ones may be obscured by hemorrhage; even at autopsy, a careful search under the dissecting microscope may be necessary to find them.

The natural history of AVMs has been studied by Ondra and colleagues, who have presented data on all such untreated malformations in Finland over a 30-year period (see further on), and by Crawford and coworkers in Great Britain. In the latter study, comprising 343 patients, 217 were managed without surgery and observed for many years (mean, 10.4 years). Hemorrhage occurred in 42 percent and seizures in 18 percent. By 20 years after diagnosis, 29 percent had died and 27 percent of the survivors had a neurologic handicap. Although the lesion is present from birth, onset of symptoms is most common between 10 and 30 years of age; occasionally it is delayed to age 50 or even beyond. In almost half the patients, the first clinical manifestation is a cerebral subarachnoid hemorrhage; in 30 percent, a seizure is the first and only manifestation; and in 20 percent, the only symptom is headache. Progressive hemiparesis or other focal neurologic deficit is present in about 10 percent of patients. In a series of 1000 patients referred mainly for proton beam radiation of an AVM and studied by our colleague R. D. Adams, 464 had a hemorrhage as the first manifestation and 218 had a seizure; frontal and frontoparietal lesions had a proclivity to cause seizures. In 139, the lesion came to attention as a result of a progressive neurologic deficit; most of these were situated in the posterior fossa or axially in the cerebrum. Headaches were an early symptom in 212, but only 59 of these patients had a subsequent hemorrhage. The combination of headaches, seizures, and a progressive deficit almost always indicated a large malformation.

Treatment The preferred approach in most centers is surgical excision. Some 20 to 40 percent of AVMs are amenable to block dissection, with an operative mortality rate of 2 to 5 percent and a morbidity of 5 to 25 percent. In the others, attempts have been made to obliterate the malformed vessels by ligation of feeding arteries and the use of endovascular embolization and rapidly setting plastics; the latter are injected via a balloon catheter that has been navigated into a feeding vessel. Complete obliteration of large AVMs is usually impossible by these methods, but they have been effective in reducing the size of the AVM prior to surgery. Kjellberg and Chapman pioneered the treatment of AVMs using a single dose of sterotactically directed proton radiation. This technique of radiosurgery has been adopted by others using gamma- and x-ray radiation as an accepted alternative to operative treatment of AVMs

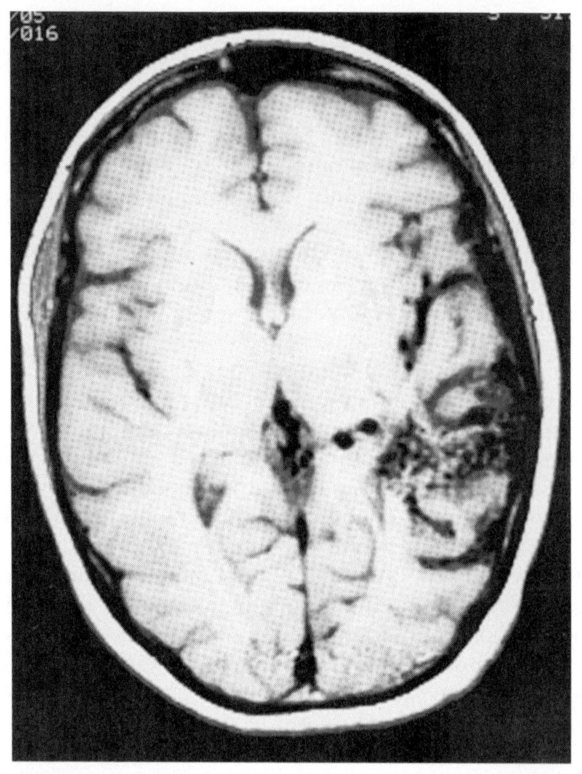

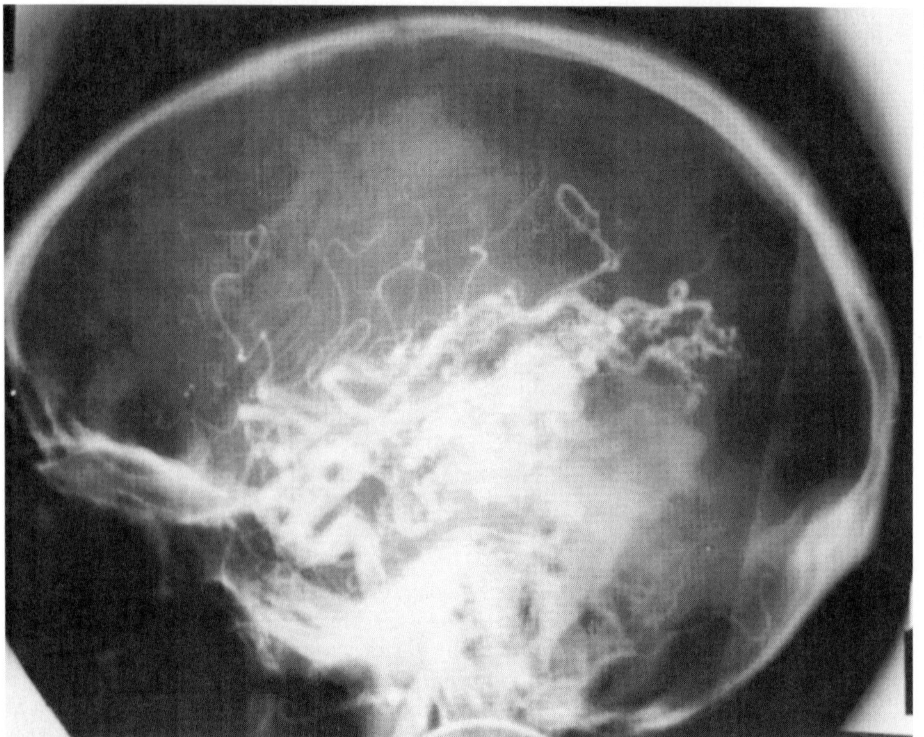

Figure 34-23

Left temporal arteriovenous malformation (AVM), demonstrated by MRI (above), *and angiography* (below). *The patient was a 59-year-old woman with longstanding complaints of headache.*

situated in deep regions, including the brainstem, or in so-called "eloquent" areas of the cortex. Radiosurgical obliteration of AVMs occurs in a delayed manner, usually occurring at least 18 to 24 months after treatment. During this early period the patient is unprotected from rebleeding. The likelihood of successful treatment and the nature of the risks depend on the location and size of the AVM, the radiation dose delivered. After 2 years, 75 to 80 percent of AVMs smaller than 2.5 cm in diameter will be obliterated. Even for those AVMs which have not been totally eliminated, the radiation effect appears to confer some long-term protection from bleeding (Fig. 34-24). Of the larger ones, a majority are shrunken or appear less dense. The rest have shown no change at this low dose level, but even in this group, the morbidity and mortality are lower than in the untreated group.

Kjellberg, Chapman and coworkers have treated more than 2000 AVMs with a low-dose (subnecrotizing) focused proton beam. A single treatment is given, and the patient is sent home the following day. Among more than 250 patients whose AVMs disappeared following proton beam therapy, there has been no recurrence of hemorrhage for up to 10 years; in approximately the last 1000 cases treated in this way, the frequency and severity of hemorrhage have been significantly reduced. The results of treatment of small AVMs (130 mm) with focused gamma radiation at the Karolinska Institute and elsewhere have been about the same as those in our patients treated by proton beam radiation.

These forms of "radiosurgery" have particular significance for brainstem and cerebellar, which in general are not amenable to surgical treatment. In many circumstances, using endovascular techniques (see below) to shrink the malformation prior to radiosurgery raises the likelihood of obliterating the lesion.

The treatment of AVMs by endovascular techniques is increasingly popular but has not been fully evaluated. Nearly every AVM has several feeding arteries, some not reachable by catheter, and some part of the AVM remains. In most series, 25 percent or more of AVMs, mostly of small and medium size, could be completely obliterated, with a mortality rate below 3 percent and morbidity of 5 to 7 percent, which compares favorably with surgical outcomes. The technique is particularly well suited to the treatment of an AVM in which there is an aneurysm on the feeding vessel.

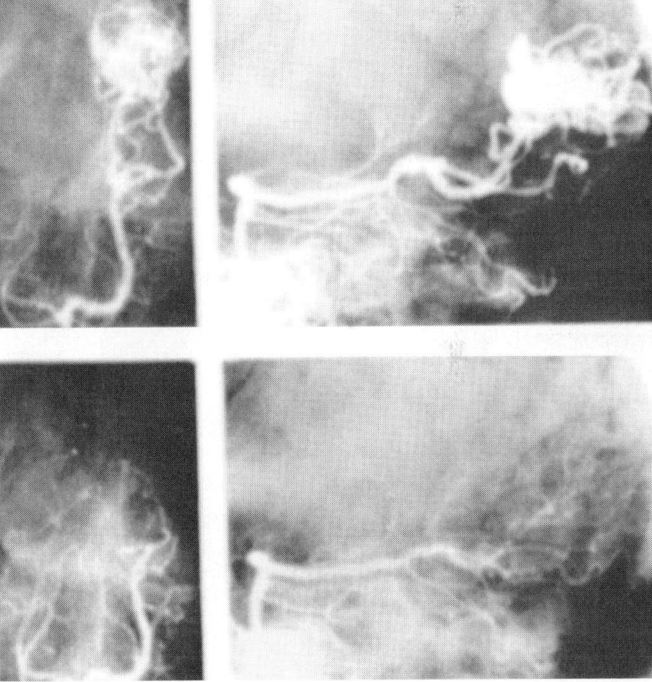

Figure 34-24

Top: *Parieto-occipital AVM, fed by the posterior cerebral artery, in a 50-year-old woman. The AVM had bled and caused small intracerebral and subdural hematomas, with a visual field defect.* Bottom: *Arteriograms taken 2 years after proton beam treatment. The patient was then asymptomatic.*

Dural Arteriovenous Fistulas and Malformations

These vascular abnormalities occur in both the cranial and spinal dura but have different presentations at each site; the latter form is discussed with other diseases of the spinal cord in Chap. 46. The cranial type is being detected with increasing frequency as refinements continue to be made in imaging of the cerebral vessels, but its true incidence and pathogenesis are not fully known. The defining features are radiologic—a nidus of abnormal arteries and veins with arteriovenous shunting contained entirely within the leaflets of the dura. The lesion is fed by dural arterial vessels that are derived from the internal cranial circulation and often, more prolifically, from the external cranial circulation (external carotid artery and muscular branches of the vertebral artery). The venous drainage is complex and is largely into the dural venous sinuses (Fig. 34-25). The rapid transit of injected angiographic dye through these fistulas accounts for the early opacification of the draining venous structures; in the case of high-flow connections, this may not be appreciated unless images are taken almost immediately after the injection. A number of potential feeding vessels must be injected to demonstrate all the conduits into the lesion. On CT scanning and MRI, the malformation is sometimes detected as a thickening or enhancement of a region of dura, generally close to a large dural venous sinus. In other cases the dilated draining vessels may be seen only with the injection of dye or gadolinium.

Figure 34-25

Cerebral angiogram of an intracerebral dural arteriovenous malformation. The nidus is located just above the orbit (arrow). There is rapid filing of the cerebral venous system after injection of dye into one middle cerebral artery.

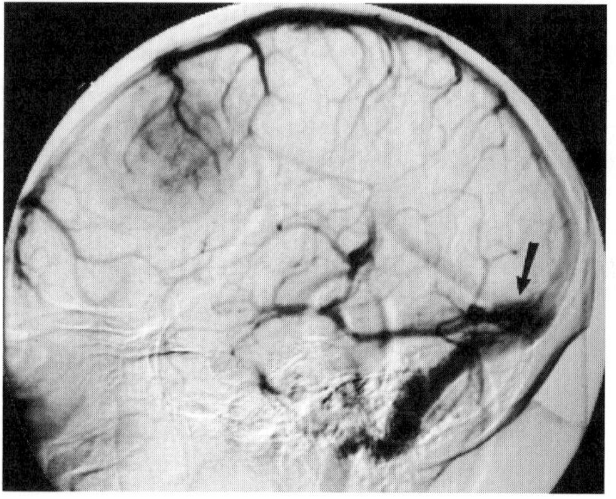

The origin of these vascular lesions has not been settled—several mechanisms may be involved. Existing evidence suggests that some of these lesions, unlike conventional cerebral AVMs and aneurysms, are not developmental in origin. The best-defined such examples are ones that arise in association with an adjacent venous sinus thrombosis or atresia, most often in the transverse sigmoid sinus or adjacent to the cavernous sinus. However, it is not clear whether the abnormality of the dural sinus is the cause or the result of the dural fistula. In a number of other cases, the fistula has appeared after a forceful head injury, often remote from the site of impact. A small group is associated with the Klippel-Trenaunay or Osler-Weber-Rendu syndromes, diseases in which the frequent conjunction with AVMs is well known. Usually, all of these causes can be excluded and the largest group remains idiopathic.

A major obstacle to our understanding of dural AVMs has been the varied and confusing ways in which this lesion presents clinically. Subdural hemorrhage is an infrequent mode of presentation, sometimes creating a large and fatal clot; another mode is cerebral-subarachnoid hemorrhage, although this occurs with not nearly the frequency of bleeding from brain AVMs. However, our knowledge of the risk of bleeding from dural fistulas and the evolution of the lesions is far less precise than it is for cerebral AVMs. It appears that the dural lesions most at risk of bleeding are located in the anterior cranial fossa and at the tentorial incisura. Seizures are distinctly uncommon. A special syndrome linked to dural AVMs, although it may occur also with high-flow cerebral malformations, is of headache, vomiting, and papilledema—namely, *pseudotumor cerebri*. A cranial bruit, often self-audible, is more frequent than with cerebral AVMs. In small children, the high-flow lesions may shunt so much blood as to cause congestive heart failure, similar to malformations of the vein of Galen.

Treatment is by surgical extirpation or endovascular embolization, a painstaking procedure because of the multitude of potential feeding vessels. Surgery seems preferable for the smaller lesions and embolization for larger and inaccessible ones. The issue of anticoagulation, when there is slowed flow in a venous sinus draining a malformation, is unsettled.

Cavernous Malformations

Vascular malformations composed mainly of clusters of thin-walled veins without important arterial feeders and little or no intervening nervous tissue make up a significant group, some 7 to 8 percent of our series of AVMs. Conventional subdivisions into cavernous, venous, and telangiectatic types have not proven useful. We have put all of them into one group, roughly designated as *cavernous*. They have several attributes that set them apart. Their tendency to bleed is probably no less than that of the more common AVMs, but more often the hemorrhages are small and clinically silent. The exact incidence of bleeding is uncertain but is estimated to be less than 1 percent per year per lesion. Often there are multiple lesions. They are generally not seen in arteriograms. The diagnosis is based on their clinical manifestations and MRI, which discloses a cluster of vessels surrounded by a large zone of hypodense ferritin in the T1-weighted images (Fig. 34-26), the product of previous small episodes of bleeding. Some cavernous angiomas are associated with adjacent venous malformations, visualized by imaging studies. The lack of formation of a mass over a long period of time separates this lesion from a malignant tumor that has bled. About one-half of all cavernous angiomas lie in the brainstem, and in the past (before the availability of MRI), many of them were misdiagnosed as multiple sclerosis because of a stepwise accumulation of neurologic deficits with each hemorrhage.

About 10 percent of angiomas are multiple and 5 percent are familial. In one of our families, of Italian-American origin, there were 29 affected members in three generations. The inheritance followed an autosomal dominant pattern; Marchuk and coworkers have localized the abnormal gene to the long arm of chromosome 7. The follow-up of some of our patients has documented the later appearance of new lesions. Angiomas on the surface of the brain, within reach of the neurosurgeon, even those in the brainstem, can be plucked out, like clusters of grapes, with low morbidity and mortality. Kjellberg and colleagues have treated 89 deeply situated cavernous angiomas with low-dose proton radiation. Insufficient time has elapsed to permit a final statement as to the efficacy of this form of therapy, but our initial impression is that these vascular malformations, like the hemangioblastoma, respond poorly to radiation and are not amenable to treatment by endovascular techniques. Lesions that cause recurrent bleeding and are surgically accessible with little risk are often removed, but incidentally discovered angiomas may be left alone.

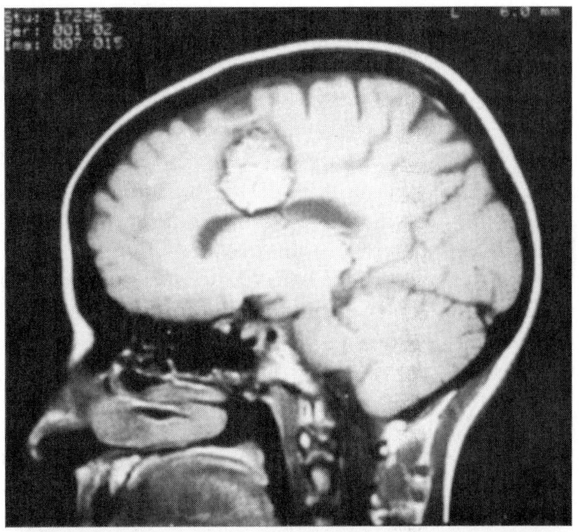

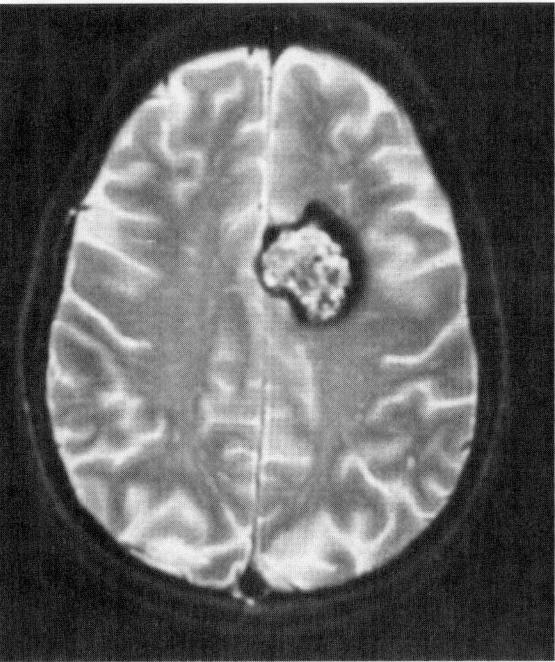

Figure 34-26

Cavernous vascular malformation. MRI in the sagittal (above) *and axial* (below) *planes demonstrates a medial left frontal lesion with a prominent rim of hemosiderin-laden macrophages and no associated edema.*

Other Causes of Intracranial Bleeding

Next to hypertension, *anticoagulant therapy* is the most common cause of cerebral hemorrhage. The hemorrhages that develop, though sometimes situated in the sites of predilection of hypertensive hemorrhage, are more likely to occur elsewhere, mainly in the lobes of the brain. When the bleeding is precipitated by warfarin therapy, treatment with fresh-frozen plasma and vitamin K is recommended; when bleeding is associated with aspirin therapy or other agents that affect platelet function, fresh platelet infusion, often in massive amounts, is required to control the hemorrhage. The use of *thrombolytics* in the treatment of stroke is complicated by intracranial hemorrhage in 6 to 20 percent of cases, depending on the dose and timing of drug administration after the onset of symptoms, as discussed on page 863.

In the elderly, *amyloid angiopathy* appears to be a major cause of lobar hemorrhages, especially if they appear in succession or are multiple. Several of our patients have had minor head injuries in the weeks before hemorrhage. In our own material, only severe impregnation of vessels with amyloid and fibrinoid change in the vessel wall were associated with hemorrhage (Vonsattel et al). Greenberg and colleagues have found that apolipoprotein E4, the same marker that is overrepresented in Alzheimer disease, is associated with severe amyloid angiopathy and intracerebral hemorrhage, but others have found an association with the E2 allele. Contrary to previous notions, there is probably no more risk in evacuating these clots surgically than in the case of other cerebral hemorrhages, but most are of a size that allows conservative management.

Several *primary hematologic disorders* are also complicated by hemorrhage into the brain. The most frequent of these are leukemia, aplastic anemia, and thrombocytopenic purpura. Often there are multiple intracranial hemorrhages, some in the subdural and subarachnoid spaces. As a rule, this complication signals a fatal issue. Other, less common causes of intracerebral bleeding are advanced *liver disease*, uremia being treated with dialysis, and *lymphoma*. Usually several factors are operative in these cases: reduction in prothrombin or other clotting elements (fibrinogen, factor V), bone marrow suppression by antineoplastic drugs, and disseminated intravascular coagulation. Any part of the brain may be involved, and the hemorrhagic lesions are usually multiple. Frequently there is also evidence of abnormal bleeding elsewhere (skin, mucous membranes, kidney) by the time cerebral hemorrhage occurs. Plasma exchange, used in the treatment of myasthenia gravis and Guillain-Barré disease, also lowers the serum fibrinogen to a marked degree, but we have not observed a single instance of intracerebral hemorrhage in more than 500 patients treated in this way.

Acute extradural and subdural hemorrhage must always be considered in the patient who, under unknown circumstances, has rather abruptly developed a neurologic deficit such as hemiparesis or confusion, with or without bloody CSF. In *chronic subdural hemorrhage*, which can occur without known trauma, the indefinite picture of drowsiness, headache, confusion, and mild hemiparesis may erroneously be attributed to a stroke, especially in elderly persons. There should be no hesitation in subjecting patients to CT scanning whenever the diagnosis of subdural hemorrhage cannot readily be excluded on clinical grounds. In the patient who falls and strikes his head at the onset of a stroke, it may be difficult or impossible to decide if blood in the CSF is due to the stroke or to cerebral contusion. These disorders are discussed more fully in the next chapter.

Occasionally the origin of intracranial hemorrhage cannot be determined clinically or pathologically. In some postmortem cases, a careful search under the dissecting microscope discloses a small arteriovenous malformation (AVM); this is the basis for suspecting that an overlooked lesion of this type may be the cause of cerebral hemorrhage in other cases. *Primary intraventricular hemorrhage*, a rare event, can sometimes be traced to a vascular malformation or neoplasm of the choroid plexus; more often, such a hemorrhage is the result of periventricular bleeding, in which blood enters the ventricle immediately, without producing a large parenchymal clot.

Hemorrhage into primary and secondary brain tumors is not rare; when this is the first clinical manifestation of the neoplasm, diagnosis may be difficult. Choriocarcinoma, melanoma, renal cell and bronchogenic carcinoma, pituitary adenoma, thyroid cancer, glioblastoma multiforme, and medulloblastoma may present in this way. Careful inquiry will usually disclose that neurologic symptoms compatible with intracranial tumor growth had preceded the onset of hemorrhage. Needless to say, a thorough search should be made in these circumstances for evidence of intracranial tumor or of secondary tumor deposits in other organs, particularly the lungs.

The term *mycotic aneurysm* designates an aneurysm caused by a localized bacterial or fungal inflammation of an artery (Osler introduced the term *mycotic* to describe endocarditis, but its proper current use is to describe fungal infection). With the introduction of antibiotics, mycotic aneurysms have become less frequent, but they are still being seen in patients with bacterial endocarditis and in intravenous drug abusers. Peripheral arteries are involved more often than intracranial ones; about two-thirds of the latter are associated with subacute bacterial endocarditis due to streptococcal infections. In recent years, the number of mycotic aneurysms due to staphylococcal infections appears to have increased. The usual pathogenic sequence is an embolic occlusion of a small artery, which may announce itself clinically by an ischemic stroke, with cells in the CSF. Later, or as the first manifestation, the weakened vessel wall gives way and causes a subarachnoid or brain hemorrhage. The mycotic aneurysm may appear on only one artery or several arteries, and the hemorrhage may recur. A consensus regarding the treatment of mycotic aneurysm has not been reached. The underlying endocarditis or septicemia mandates appropriate antibiotic therapy and, in at least 30 percent of cases, healing of the aneurysm can be observed in successive arteriograms. Treatment should continue for at least 6 weeks. Some neurosurgeons believe in excising an accessible aneurysm if it is solitary and the systemic infection is under control. Some mycotic aneurysms do not bleed, and in our view medical therapy always takes precedence over surgical therapy.

Brain purpura (pericapillary encephalorrhagia), incorrectly referred to as "hemorrhagic encephalitis," consists of multiple petechial hemorrhages scattered throughout the white matter of the brain. The clinical picture is that of a diffuse encephalopathy, but diagnosis is essentially pathologic. Blood does not appear in the CSF, and the condition should not be confused with a stroke. It is virtually impossible to establish the diagnosis during life, but the pathologic appearance is unique and highly characteristic. The lesions in brain purpura are always small, 0.1 to 2.0 mm in diameter, and are confined to the white matter, particularly the corpus callosum, centrum ovale, and middle cerebellar peduncles. Each lesion is situated around a small blood vessel, usually a capillary. In this para-adventitial area, both the myelin and axis cylinders are destroyed, and the lesion is usually though not always hemorrhagic. Fibrin exudation, perivascular and meningeal infiltrates of inflammatory cells, and widespread necrosis of tissue are not observed. In these respects brain purpura differs fundamentally from acute necrotizing hemorrhagic encephalitis. Usually the patient has become stuporous and comatose without focal neurologic signs, and the CSF is normal. The etiology of brain purpura is quite obscure. It may complicate viral pneumonia, uremia, arsenical intoxication, and, rarely, metabolic encephalopathy and sepsis, or there may be no associated disease.

Inflammatory diseases of arteries and veins, especially polyarteritis nodosa, lupus erythematosus, and moyamoya disease, are occasionally associated with cerebral hemorrhage. Rupture of a vessel in these circumstances may be on the basis of hypertension or local vascular disease, and bleeding nearly always occurs into brain tissue rather than into the subarachnoid space. Rarely, intracranial dissection of an artery (usually the vertebral) may allow some blood to escape into the subarachnoid space.

The other rare types of hemorrhage, listed in Table 34-6, are self-explanatory.

Hemorrhages of *intraspinal* origin, all of them rare, may be the result of trauma, AVM (the usual cause of nontraumatic hematomyelia), anterior spinal artery aneurysms, or bleeding into tumors. Spinal subarachnoid hemorrhage from an AVM may simulate an intracranial subarachnoid hemorrhage, causing a stiff neck, headache, and even subhyaloid hemorrhages. Subarachnoid hemorrhage in which interscapular or neck pain predominates should raise the suspicion of an aneurysm of the anterior spinal artery or of a spinal AVM or cavernous angioma. Angiographic study of the radicular spinal vessels and the origins of the anterior spinal arteries from the vertebral arteries may disclose the source of bleeding. Extradural and subdural spinal extravasations may be *spontaneous* (sometimes in relation to rheumatoid arthritis) but are far more often due to trauma, anticoagulants, or both. Extradural spinal hemorrhage causes the rapid evolution of paraplegia or quadriplegia; diagnosis must be prompt if function is to be salvaged by surgical drainage of the hematoma. These are discussed further in Chap. 44.

HYPERTENSIVE ENCEPHALOPATHY

Clinical Features This is the term applied to a relatively rapidly evolving syndrome of severe hypertension in association with headache, nausea and vomiting, visual disturbances, confusion, and—in advanced cases—stupor and coma. Multiple seizures are frequent and may be more marked on one side of the body than the other. These symptoms of diffuse cerebral disturbance may be accompanied by focal or lateralizing neurologic signs, either transitory or lasting, which should always suggest cerebral hemorrhage or infarction, i.e., the more common cerebrovascular complications of severe chronic hypertension. A clustering of multiple microinfarcts and petechial hemorrhages (the basic neuropathologic changes in hypertensive encephalopathy) in one region may rarely result in a mild hemiparesis, aphasic disorder, or rapid failure of vision (usually due to

retinal lesions). By the time the neurologic manifestations appear, the hypertension has usually reached the malignant stage, with diastolic pressures above 125 mmHg, retinal hemorrhages, exudates, papilledema (*hypertensive retinopathy* grade IV), and evidence of renal and cardiac disease. However, we have seen instances of encephalopathy at lower pressures, especially if the hypertension has been abrupt in onset (see below). The term *hypertensive encephalopathy* should be reserved
for the above syndrome and should not be used to refer to chronic recurrent headaches, dizziness, epileptic seizures, TIAs, or strokes, which often occur in association with high blood pressure.

Hypertensive encephalopathy may complicate hypertension from any cause (chronic renal disease, renal artery stenosis, acute glomerulonephritis, acute toxemia, pheochromocytoma, Cushing syndrome), cocaine, or administration of drugs such as aminophylline or phenylephrine, but it occurs most often in patients with rapidly worsening "essential" hypertension. In *eclampsia and acute renal disease* and particularly in children, encephalopathic symptoms may develop at blood pressure levels considerably lower than those of hypertensive encephalopathy of "essential" type. In eclampsia, the retinal and cerebral lesions are the same as those that complicate malignant nephrosclerosis; in both there is also failure of autoregulation of the cerebral arterioles. In the pathogenesis of pre-eclampsia, inhibition of an endothelium-derived relaxing factor by hemoglobin has been postulated by Sarrel and colleagues.

Laboratory Features In many but not all the cases, the CSF pressure and protein values are elevated, the latter to more than 100 mg/dL in some instances. Lowering of the blood pressure with hypotensive drugs may reverse the picture in a day or two. In the past, when effective antihypertensive drugs were not available, the outcome was often fatal. The BUN is only slightly elevated except in cases of renal failure, and the usual patient is not uremic.

Hypertensive encephalopathy is marked by characteristic changes on CT scanning and MRI. The radiologic findings are often misinterpreted as large areas of infarction or demyelination, but their tendency to normalize over several weeks is remarkable. As summarized by Hauser and coworkers, the main change is bilaterally increased T2 signal intensity in the white matter on MRI and reduced density (edema) on CT, usually concentrated in the posterior part of the hemispheres (Fig. 34-27). These imaging characteristics are due to an accumulation of fluid, but—unlike the edema in trauma, neoplasm, or stroke—there is little or no mass effect and the water does not tend to course along white matter tracts such as the corpus callosum. In addition, scattered cortical lesions occur in a watershed distribution and probably correspond to small infarctions. These same CT findings in the white matter and cortex also occur in eclampsia, which is a special form of hypertensive encephalopathy (Fig. 34-28).

Pathophysiology Neuropathologic examination may reveal a rather normal-looking brain, but in some cases cerebral swelling, hemorrhages of various sizes, or both will be found. A cerebellar pressure cone reflects an increased volume of tissue and increased pressure in the posterior fossa; in some instances lumbar puncture appears to have precipitated fatalities. Microscopically there are widespread minute infarcts in the brain (with a predilection for the basis pontis), the result of fibrinoid necrosis of the walls of arterioles and capillaries and occlusion of their lumens by fibrin thrombi (Chester et al). This is often associated with zones of cerebral edema. Similar vascular changes are found in other organs, particularly in the retinae and kidneys.

Volhard originally attributed the symptoms of hypertensive encephalopathy to vasospasm. This notion was reinforced by Byrom, who demonstrated, in rats, a segmental constriction and dilatation of cerebral and retinal arterioles in response to severe hypertension. However, the observations of Byrom and of others indicate that overdistention of the arterioles (which have lost their adaptive capacity), rather than excessive constriction, may be responsible for the necrosis of the vessel wall (see reviews of Auer and of Chester et al). The brain edema appears to be the result of active exocytosis of water rather than simply a passive leak from vessels subjected to high pressures.

Treatment The standard treatment consists of measures that promptly reduce arterial blood pressure, but they must be used cautiously; a safe target would be 150/100 mmHg. One may use intravenous sodium nitroprusside, 0.5 to 0.8 μg/kg per minute; a calcium channel blocker such as nifedipine, 10 to 20 mg sublingually; or intravenous beta-adrenergic blockers (labetalol, 20 to 40 mg intravenously followed by an infusion at 2 mg/min, and esmolol are favored). These must be followed by a longer-acting antihypertensive agent such as an angiotensin-converting enzyme inhibitor or a calcium channel blocker. If there is already evidence of brain edema and increased intracranial pressure, dexametha-

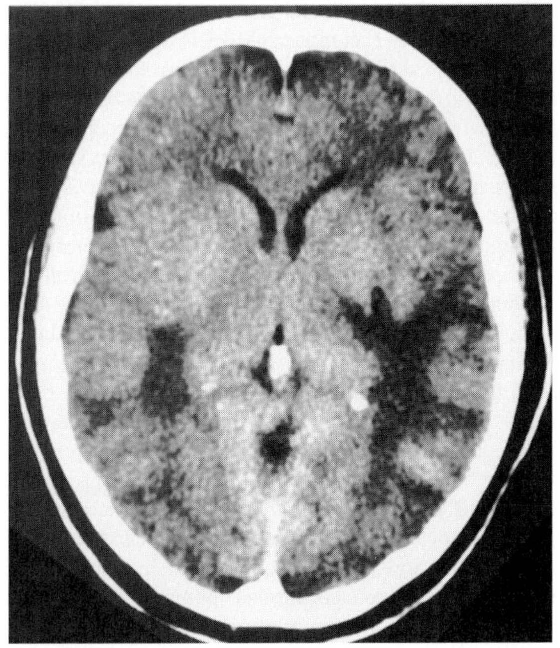

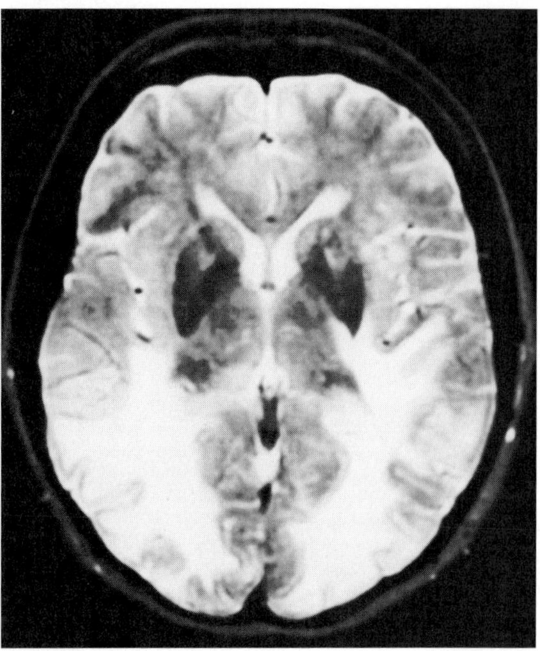

Figure 34-27

Hypertensive encephalopathy in a 55-year-old woman with headache and a single seizure. The characteristic changes of excess water in large regions of the white matter are seen on the CT scan (left panel) *and in T-2 weighted MRI image* (right panel). *The areas of signal change are associated with little mass effect and tend to be concentrated in the posterior regions of the brain. Other small cortical and subcortical lesions are common in watershed areas. The same change may occur in eclampsia.*

sone, 4 to 6 mg every 6 h, is usually added, but its effect and the use of hyperosmolar therapy have not been studied systematically; our clinical impression is that they have little effect.

Diffuse and Focal Cerebral Vasospasm A reduction in the caliber of the basal vessels and their proximal branches is a well-known complication of subarachnoid hemorrhage as described on page 891. Vasospasm has also been implicated in migraine and migrainous stroke and as an explanation for TIAs, but with little supportive evidence. Some degree of attenuation of large cerebral vessels is observed in hypertensive encephalopathy, in eclampsia, and with adrenergic drug use (e.g., phenylpropanolamine, cocaine), but the role of the vascular changes in causing strokes has never been clear. The problem of stroke with migraine, which has an uncertain relationship to vasospasm, is discussed on page 184.

In addition, Call and colleagues have described an idiopathic widespread segmental vasospasm of cerebral vessels that is characterized by severe headache and fluctuating TIA-like episodes. The middle cerebral artery and its branches are mainly affected; the angiographic appearance may be mistaken for arteritis. A number of similar cases have been described, and we have seen several that result in strokes, at times with a posterior leukoencephalopathy that is similar to hypertensive encephalopathy. Sometimes the headache is minimal. The nature of this condition and of a similar state of diffuse vasospasm is unknown. A relationship to hypertensive encephalopathy or to delayed postpartum eclampsia has been suggested, because of the aforementioned white matter changes and the observation of widespread vasospasm in eclamptic women. The patients we have seen with this process, after several weeks of fluctuating focal neurological symptoms and headache, have recovered completely or nearly so. In all likelihood, several disorders cause this type of vasculopathy. Calcium channel blockers or corticosteroids have been prescribed, but their effectiveness cannot be determined.

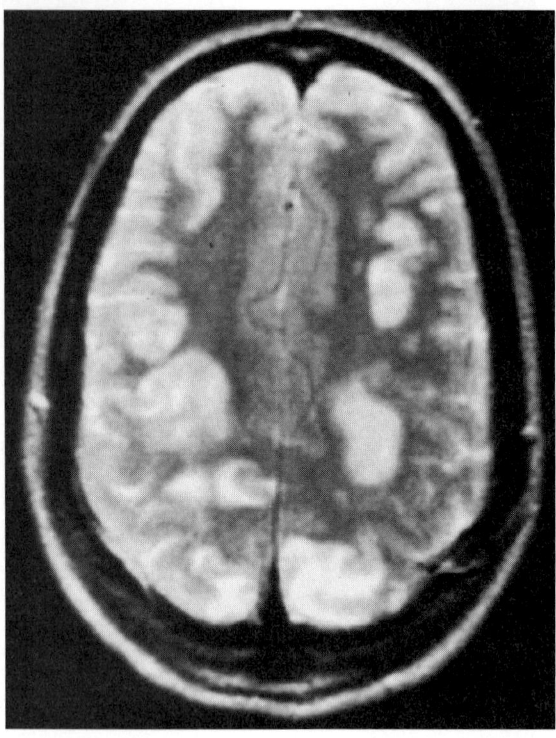

Figure 34-28

MRI T2 signal changes in eclampsia. Most of the vascular changes and edema are situated in the cortical watershed distributions between the middle and an anterior cerebral arteries. These imaging findings were transient as was mild signal change in the occipital subcortical regions, the latter being typical of hypertensive encephalopathy, as in Fig. 34-27.

INFLAMMATORY DISEASES OF BRAIN ARTERIES

Infectious Vasculitis

Inflammatory diseases of the blood vessels of infectious origin and their effects upon the nervous system have been considered in detail in Chap. 32. There it was pointed out that meningovascular syphilis, tuberculous meningitis, fungal meningitis, and the subacute (untreated or partially treated) forms of bacterial meningitis may be accompanied by inflammatory changes and occlusion of the cerebral arteries or veins. Occasionally, in syphilitic, cryptococcal, and tuberculous meningitis, a stroke may be the first clinical sign of meningitis, but more often it develops well after the meningeal symptoms are established. The nature of the cerebral vasculitis that may rarely accompany AIDS is unknown.

Typhus, schistosomiasis, mucormycosis, malaria, and trichinosis are rare causes of inflammatory arterial disease which, unlike the above, are not secondary to meningeal infections. In *typhus and other rickettsial diseases*, capillary and arteriolar changes and perivascular inflammatory cells are found in the brain; presumably they underlie the seizures, acute psychoses, cerebellar syndromes, and coma that characterize the neurologic disorder in these diseases. The internal carotid artery may be occluded in diabetic patients as part of the orbital and cavernous sinus infections with *mucormycosis*. In *trichinosis*, the cause of the cerebral symptoms has not been established. Parasites have been found in the brain; in one of our cases the cerebral lesions were produced by bland emboli arising in the heart and related to a severe myocarditis. In *cerebral malaria*, convulsions, coma, and sometimes focal symptoms appear to be due to the blockage of capillaries and precapillaries by masses of parasitized red blood corpuscles. Schistosomiasis may implicate cerebral or spinal arteries. These diseases are discussed further in Chap. 32.

Noninfectious Inflammatory Diseases of Cranial Arteries

Included under this heading is a diverse group of arteritides that have little in common except their tendency to involve the cerebral vasculature. One subgroup includes the *giant-cell arteritides*—extracranial (temporal) arteritis; granulomatous arteritis of the brain; and aortic branch arteritis, one form of which is known as Takayasu disease, all discussed on the following pages.

A second group includes polyarteritis nodosa, the Churg-Strauss type of arteritis, Wegener granulomatosis, systemic lupus erythematosus, Behçet disease, postzoster arteritis, and AIDS arteritis, as already mentioned. Immunologic studies have shown that in most of these diseases there is an abnormal deposit of complement-fixing immune complex on the endothelium, leading to inflammation, vascular occlusion, or rupture with hemorrhage. The initial event is thought in some cases to be evoked by a virus, bacterium, or drug. It is postulated by some immunologists that in the *granulomatous arteritides*, a different mechanism is operative—that an exogenous antigen induces antibodies that attach to the primary target (the vessel wall) as immune complexes, damage it, and attract lymphocytes and mononuclear cells. The giant cells form around remnants of the vessel wall (elastic tissue, etc.). An acute necrotizing cerebral angiitis—which may be idiopathic, sometimes complicates ulcerative colitis, and responds to treatment with prednisone and cyclophosphamide—may also belong in this category. The special case of angiocentric lymphoma (neoplastic angioendotheliosis), which simulates a cerebral vasculitis, is discussed in Chap. 31.

Temporal Arteritis (Giant-Cell Arteritis, Cranial Arteritis; See also pages 193–194**)** In this affliction, not uncommon among elderly persons, arteries of the external carotid system, particularly the temporal branches, are the sites of a subacute granulomatous inflammatory exudate consisting of lymphocytes and other mononuclear cells, neutrophilic leukocytes, and giant cells. The most severely affected parts of the artery usually become thrombosed. The sedimentation rate is characteristically elevated above 80 mm/h and sometimes exceeds 120 mm/h, but a few cases occur with values below 50 mm/h.

Headache or head pain is the chief complaint, and there may be severe pain, aching, and stiffness in the proximal muscles of the limbs associated with a markedly elevated sedimentation rate. Thus the clinical picture overlaps that of *polymyalgia rheumatica* (pages 230 and 1572). Other less frequent systemic manifestations include fever, anorexia and loss of weight, malaise, anemia, and a mild leukocytosis. Instances of dementia and other neurologic illnesses that have been described in the literature seem to us coincidental.

Occlusion of branches of the ophthalmic artery, resulting in blindness in one or both eyes, is the main complication, occurring in over 25 percent of patients. In the most extreme form, the optic nerve head can be seen to be infarcted, with papilledema and visual loss. In a few cases this is preceded by transient visual loss simulating a TIA. Occasionally the arteries of the ocular nerves are involved, causing an ophthalmoplegia. Rarely, an arteritis of the aorta and its major branches—including the carotid, subclavian, coronary, and femoral arteries—is found at postmortem examination. Significant inflammatory involvement of intracranial arteries is uncommon, perhaps because of a relative lack of elastic tissue, but strokes do occur rarely on the basis of occlusion of the internal carotid or vertebral arteries.

The diagnosis should be suspected in elderly patients who develop severe, persistent headache and elevation of the sedimentation rate; it depends on finding a tender, thrombosed, or thickened cranial artery and demonstration of the lesion in a biopsy. The procedure is innocuous and the diagnosis may require that both sides be sampled because of the patchy distribution of granulomatous lesions. Schmidt and colleagues have reported that the diagnosis can often be made with duplex ultrasonography. In 22 of 30 cases, a dark halo, probably reflecting edema, surrounded the temporal artery; 6 cases showed either occlusion or stenosis of the artery; there were no false-positive tests. A considerable length of the temporal artery can be insonated by this technique, a particularly useful feature in a process that affects the vessel segmentally. From our limited experience, this test can be recommended before resorting to a biopsy. The arteritic changes may also be revealed by arteriography of the external carotid arteries.

The administration of prednisone, 50 to 75 mg/day, provides striking relief of the headache and polymyalgic symptoms within days and sometimes within hours and also prevents blindness. The medication must be given in very gradually diminishing doses for at least several months or longer, guided by the symptoms and the sedimentation rate. The latter begins to drop within days but seldom falls below 25 mm/h.

Intracranial Granulomatous Arteritis Scattered examples of a small-vessel giant-cell arteritis of undetermined etiology in which only brain vessels are affected have come to our notice over the years. The clinical state has taken diverse forms, sometimes presenting as a low-grade, nonfebrile meningitis with sterile CSF, followed by infarction of one or several parts of the cerebrum or cerebellum. In other cases it has masqueraded as a cerebral tumor, evolving over a period of weeks, or as a viral encephalitis or an unusual dementia. Severe headaches, focal cerebral or cerebellar signs of gradual (seldom stroke-like) evolution, confusion with memory loss, pleocytosis and elevated CSF protein, and papilledema as a result of increased intracranial pressure (in about half the cases) constitute the most frequently encountered syndrome. The symptoms usually persist for several months.

In only about half the patients can the diagnosis be made by angiography, which demonstrates an irregular narrowing and blunt ending of small cerebral arteries. CT scanning and MRI show multiple irregular white matter changes and small cortical lesions. Occasionally the white matter abnormalities become confluent and the radiologic appearance simulates Binswanger disease or hypertensive encephalopathy. Tissue excised during an operation (or brain biopsy) for a suspected brain tumor, lymphoma, or white matter disease has clarified the problem in some cases, and in others the diagnosis has been made only at autopsy, the findings coming as a distinct surprise.

The affected vessels are in the 100- to 500-μm range and are surrounded and infiltrated by lymphocytes, plasma cells, and other mononuclear cells; giant cells are distributed in small numbers in the media, adventitia, or perivascular connective tissue. Infarction of tissue can be traced to thrombosis. The meninges are variably infiltrated with inflammatory cells. Sometimes only a part of the brain has been affected—in one of our cases the cerebellum, in another a frontal lobe and the opposite parietal lobe.

The disease raises the question of sarcoidosis, which is sometimes limited to the nervous system, of intravascular lymphoma, or of the polyarteritis (allergic granulomatous angiitis) described by Churg and Strauss. Unlike these diseases, however, the lungs and other organs are spared; there is no eosinophilia, increase in sedimentation rate or in antineutrophil cytoplasmic antibodies (ANCA), or anemia. Brain lymphoma of the intravascular type and multiple sclerosis are also diagnostic considerations, from both a clinical and a radiologic perspective. Some patients with isolated central nervous system (CNS) angiitis (those presenting as an aseptic meningitis with multiple infarcts) have responded dramatically to corticosteroid and cyclophosphamide therapy (Moore).

Aortic Branch Disease (Takayasu Disease, Occlusive Thromboaortopathy) This is a nonspecific arteritis involving mainly the aorta and the large arteries arising from its arch. It is similar in many ways to giant-cell arteritis except for its propensity to involve the proximal rather than the distal branches of the aorta. Most of the patients have been young Asian women, but there are scattered reports of cases from the United States, Latin America, and eastern Europe. The exact etiology has never been ascertained, but an autoimmune mechanism is suspected.

Constitutional symptoms such as malaise, fever, anorexia, weight loss, and night sweats usually introduce the disease. The erythrocyte sedimentation rate is elevated in the early and active stages. Later there is evidence of occlusion of the innominate, subclavian, carotid, vertebral, and other arteries. The affected arteries no longer pulsate, hence the alternative term *pulseless disease*. However, it should be noted that the Occidental pulseless disease is usually due to atherosclerosis. When renal arteries are involved, hypertension may result, and coronary occlusion is often fatal. Involvement of the pulmonary artery may lead to pulmonary hypertension. Coolness of the hands and weak radial pulses are common indicators of the disease and headaches are frequent. Blurring of vision, especially upon activity, dizziness, and hemiparetic and hemisensory syndromes are the usual neurologic manifestation (Lupi-Herrera et al). Several authors have emphasized the frequency of postural symptoms as well as the relative infrequency of major strokes, despite multiple TIA-like spells.

Pathologic studies disclose a periarteritis, often with giant cells and reparative fibrosis. Many of the patients die in 3 to 5 years. According to Ishikawa and colleagues, the administration of corticosteroids in the acute inflammatory stage of the disease improves the prognosis. Reconstructive vascular surgery has helped some of the patients in the later stages of the disease.

Polyarteritis (Periarteritis) Nodosa In this disorder there is an inflammatory necrosis of arteries and arterioles throughout the body. The lungs are usually spared, however, which is the basis of distinguishing this form of vasculitis from the allergic granulomatous angiitis of Churg and Strauss, mentioned above. The vasa nervorum are frequently involved by the lesions of polyarteritis, giving rise to a mononeuropathy multiplex or to a symmetrical axonal type of polyneuropathy (see page 1400). Involvement of the CNS is unusual (occurring in fewer than 5 percent of cases) and takes the form of widespread microinfarcts; macroscopic infarction is a rarity. The clinical manifestations vary: included are headache, confusion and fluctuating cognitive disorders, convulsions, hemiplegia, and brainstem signs. We have also observed acute spinal cord lesions. The CNS lesions and brain hemorrhage are rare and usually occur in a setting of renal hypertension.

Wegener Granulomatosis This is a rare disease of unknown cause, affecting adults as a rule and predominating slightly in males. A subacutely evolving vasculitis with necrotizing granulomas of the upper and lower respiratory tracts followed by necrotizing glomerulonephritis are its main features. Neurologic complications come later in one-third to one-half of cases and take two forms: (1) a peripheral neuropathy either in a pattern of polyneuropathy or, far more frequently, in a pattern of mononeuropathy multiplex (page 1427) and (2) multiple cranial neuropathies as a result of direct extension of the nasal and sinus granulomas to upper cranial nerves and of pharyngeal lesions to the lower nerves (see page 1460). The basilar parts of the skull may be eroded, with spread of granuloma to the cranial cavity and more remote parts. Cerebrovascular events, seizures, and cerebritis are less common neurologic complications. Spastic paraparesis, temporal arteritis, Horner syndrome, and papilledema have been observed but are rare (see Nishino et al). The orbits are involved in 20 percent of patients, and lesions here simulate the clinical and radiologic appearance of orbital pseudotumor, cellulitis, or lymphoma. Pulmonary granulomas, usually asymptomatic but evident on a chest film, are also common. The vasculitis implicates both small arteries and veins. There is a fibrinoid necrosis of their walls and an infiltration by neutrophils and histiocytes. The sedimentation rate is elevated, as are the rheumatoid and antiglobulin factors. The presence in the blood of antineutrophil cytoplasmic antibodies (c–ANCA) has been found to be relatively specific and highly sensitive for Wegener disease (it may also be found in intravascular lymphoma).

A high degree of therapeutic success in this formerly fatal disease has been achieved by the use of cyclophosphamide, chlorambucil, or azathioprine. Cyclophosphamide in oral doses of 1 to 2 mg/kg per day has cured 90 to 95 percent of the cases. In acute cases, rapidly acting steroids—prednisolone, 50 to 75 mg/day —should be given in conjunction with the immunosuppressant drug(s).

Systemic Lupus Erythematosus Involvement of the nervous system is an important aspect of this disease. In the series reported by Johnson and Richardson, the CNS was involved in 75 percent of cases. Disturbances of mental function including alteration of consciousness, seizures, and signs referable to cranial nerves are the usual neurologic manifestations; most often they develop in the late stages of the disease, but they may occur early and may be mild and transient. Hemiparesis, paraparesis, aphasia, homonymous hemianopia, movement disorders (chorea), and derangements of hypothalamic function occur but have been infrequent in our experience. Larger infarcts are usually traceable to emboli from Libman-Sacks endocarditis. In some instances the CNS manifestations resemble multiple sclerosis, especially when there is an optic neuritis and myelopathy. The presence of serum antinuclear antibodies is of help in the diagnosis of lupus erythematosus but in itself does not establish the diagnosis. The CSF is entirely normal or shows only a mild lymphocytic pleocytosis and increase in protein content, although in some patients—primarily those with peripheral neuropathy and myelopathy—the protein content may be greatly increased.

Most of the neurologic manifestations can be accounted for by widespread microinfarcts in the cerebral cortex and brainstem; these, in turn, are related to destructive and proliferative changes in arterioles and capillaries. The acute lesion is subtle; it is not a typical fibrinoid necrosis of the vessel wall, like that in hypertensive encephalopathy, and there is no cellular infiltration. Attachment of immune complexes to the endothelium is the postulated mechanism of vascular injury. Thus, the changes do not represent a vasculitis in the strict sense of the word. Other neurologic manifestations are related to hypertension, which frequently accompanies the disease and may precipitate cerebral hemorrhage; to endocarditis, which may give rise to cerebral embolism; to thrombotic thrombocytopenic purpura, which commonly complicates the terminal phase of the disease (Devinsky et al); and to treatment with corticosteroids, which may precipitate or accentuate muscle weakness, seizures, and psychosis. In other cases, steroids appear to improve these neurologic manifestations.

Arteritis Symptomatic of Underlying Systemic Disease Both AIDS and drug abuse (mainly cocaine) have been associated with a cerebral vasculitis that is similar to polyarteritis nodosa. With respect to the former, if deep infarctions have occurred, a basal meningitis due to tuberculosis, cryptococcosis, or syphilis with occlusion of penetrating vessels must always be entertained. Drug-induced vasculitis is difficult to distinguish from a more common state of focal vasospasm that may also be induced by these same agents. Finally, a true cerebral or spinal cord vasculitis can rarely be found in association with systemic lymphoma, particularly with Hodgkin disease. The nature of this process is indeterminate but may be related to the deposition of circulating immune complexes in the walls of cerebral vessels.

Another type of small-vessel arteritis occurs as a hypersensitivity phenomenon. Often it is associated with an allergic skin lesion (Stevens-Johnson vasculopathy or a leukocytoclastic vasculitis). The clinical picture does not resemble that of polyarteritis nodosa, but the central or peripheral nervous system is affected in rare instances. The response to corticosteroids is excellent.

Yet another ill-defined form of vasculitis has been described by Susac and colleagues. This is a microangiopathy affecting mainly the brain and retina. Psychiatric symptoms, dementia, sensorineural deafness, and impairments of vision are the clinical manifestations. Funduscopy (multiple retinal artery branch occlusions) and arteriography provide evidence of vasculopathy. The patients seem to respond to steroid therapy. Only biopsy material has been examined.

Behçet Disease This disorder may suitably be considered here, since it is essentially a chronic, recurrent vasculitis, involving small vessels, with prominent neurologic manifestations. It is most common in Turkey, where it was first described, in other Near East countries, and in Japan, but it occurs throughout Europe and North America, affecting men more often than women. The disease was originally distinguished by the triad of relapsing iridocyclitis and recurrent oral and genital ulcers, but it is now recognized to be a systemic disease with a much wider range of symptoms, including erythema nodosum, thrombophlebitis, polyarthritis, ulcerative colitis, and a number of neurologic manifestations, some of them encephalitic or meningitic in nature. The most reliable diagnostic criteria, according to an International Study Group that assembled data on 914 cases from 12 medical centers in 7 countries, were recurrent aphthous or herpetiform oral ulceration, recurrent genital ulceration, anterior or posterior uveitis, cells in the vitreous or retinal vasculitis, and erythema nodosum or papulopustular lesions.

The nervous system is affected in about 30 percent of patients with Behçet disease (Chajek and Fainaru); the main manifestations are recurrent meningoencephalitis, cranial nerve (particularly abducens) palsies, cerebellar ataxia, and corticospinal tract signs. There may be episodes of diencephalic and brainstem dysfunction resembling minor strokes. A few postmortem examinations have related these stroke-like episodes to small, appropriately placed foci of necrosis along with perivascular and meningeal infiltration of lymphocytes. There may also be cerebral venous thrombosis. The neurologic symptoms usually have an abrupt onset and are accompanied by a brisk pleocytosis (lymphocytes or neutrophils may predominate), along with elevated protein but normal glucose values (one of our cases had 3000 neutrophils per cubic millimeter at the onset of an acute meningitis). As a rule, neurologic symptoms clear completely in several weeks, but they have a tendency to recur, and some patients are left with persistent neurologic deficits. Rarely, the clinical picture is that of a progressive confusional state and dementia (see the reviews of Alema and of Lehner and Barnes for detailed accounts).

The cause of Behçet disease is unknown. We have been unable to detect virus particles in the margins of an ulcerative mouth lesion. A pathergy skin test—the formation of a sterile pustule at the site of a needle prick—is listed as an important diagnostic test by the International Study Group, but we have found it to be of questionable value. Administration of corticosteroids has been the usual treatment, on the assumption of an autoimmune etiology. Since the episodes of disease naturally subside and recur, evaluation of treatment is difficult.

OTHER FORMS OF CEREBROVASCULAR DISEASE

Thrombosis of Cerebral Veins and Venous Sinuses

Thrombosis of the cerebral venous sinuses, particularly of the superior sagittal or lateral sinus and the tributary cortical and deep veins, gives rise to a number of important neurologic syndromes. Cerebral vein thrombosis may develop in relation to infections of the adjacent ear and paranasal sinuses or to bacterial meningitis, as described in Chap. 32. More common is bland venous occlusion resulting from one of the many hypercoagulable states that are listed below.

Occlusion of cortical veins that are tributaries of the dural sinuses takes the form of a venous infarctive stroke. Diagnosis is difficult except in certain clinical settings known to favor the occurrence of venous thrombosis, such as the taking of birth control pills or postpartum and postoperative states, which are often characterized by thrombocytosis and hyperfibrinogenemia; hypercoagulable states in cancer, cyanotic congenital heart disease; cachexia in infants; sickle cell disease; antiphospholipid antibody syndrome, factor V Leiden mutation, protein S or C deficiency, antithrombin III deficiency, resistance to activated protein C; primary or secondary polycythemia and thrombocythemia; and paroxysmal nocturnal hemoglobinuria. The study by Martinelli and colleagues, alluded to earlier in the chapter, attributes 35 percent of cases to a mutation in the factor V or the prothrombin gene. A few cases will follow head injury or remain unexplained.

A stroke in a patient suffering from any one of these conditions should suggest venous thrombosis, though in some instances—e.g., postpartum strokes—arteries are occluded as often as veins. The somewhat slower evolution of the clinical syndrome, the presence of multiple cerebral lesions not in typical arterial territories, and its greater epileptogenic and hemorrhagic tendency favor venous over arterial thrombosis. Averback, who reported seven cases of venous thrombosis in young adults, has emphasized the diversity of the clinical causes. Two of his patients had carcinoma of the breast and one had ulcerative colitis.

Nevertheless, certain syndromes occur with sufficient regularity to suggest thrombosis of a particular vein or sinus. The signature features of *thrombosis of cortical veins* are the presence of large superficial (cortex and subjacent white matter) hemorrhagic infarctions and a marked tendency to seizures. In the case of *sagittal sinus thrombosis*, intracranial hypertension with headache, vomiting, and papilledema may constitute the entire syndrome or may be conjoined with hemorrhagic infarction; indeed, this is the main consideration in the differential diagnosis of pseudotumor cerebri (Chap. 30). The characteristic CT appearance of sagittal sinus thrombosis is described below. To the extent that most cortical vein thromboses originate from clots in the sagittal sinus, the hemorrhagic infarctions tend to be parasagittal, characteristically biparietal, and less often bifrontal, with headache, paraparesis or hemiparesis predominantly of the leg, or aphasia. The variable location of the infarctions reflects the inconstant location of the main surface cerebral veins (named for Labbé and for Trolard). Isolated cortical vein thrombosis is far less frequent and, according to Jacobs and colleagues, causes partial seizures and headache without signs of intracranial hypertension.

As pointed out in Chap. 13, marked chemosis and proptosis—with affection of cranial nerves III, IV, VI, and the ophthalmic division of V—are indicative of *anterior cavernous sinus thrombosis* (see Fig. 34-29). *Posterior cavernous sinus thrombosis*, spreading to the inferior petrosal sinus, may cause palsies of cranial nerves VI, IX, X, and XI without proptosis, and involvement of the *superior petrosal sinus* may be accompanied by a fifth nerve palsy. Increased intracranial pressure without ventricular dilatation occurs with thrombosis of the superior sagittal sinus, the main jugular vein, and the lateral sinus or torcula.

The common radiologic picture that results from occlusion of the superior sagittal sinus is of superficial paramedian parietal hemorrhagic infarction, often bilateral. In the case of CT scan with contrast infusion, a lack of dye in the posterior empty sagittal sinus can be observed with careful adjustment of the viewing window ("empty delta sign"). The spinal fluid pressure is increased and the fluid may be slightly sanguinous. Lateral sinus thrombosis causes hemorrhagic infarction of the temporal lobe convexity, usually with considerable vasogenic edema. The enhanced CT scan, arteriography (venous phase), and MR venography greatly facilitate diagnosis by directly visualizing the venous occlusion. Once a venous thrombosis becomes established, the tributary veins take on a "corkscrew" appearance.

Anticoagulant therapy beginning with heparin for several days, followed by warfarin, and combined with antibiotics if the venous occlusion is infectious (it rarely is in recent times), has been lifesaving in some cases, but the overall mortality rate remains high due to large hemorrhagic venous infarctions in 10 to 20 percent of cases. The trial by Einhaupl and colleagues has settled the question of therapy in favor of aggressive anticoagulation. Thrombolytic therapy by local venous or systemic infusion has also been successful in small series of cases, such as the 5 patients treated with urokinase and heparin by DiRocco and colleagues, but this has not been subjected to a systematic study. We have reserved

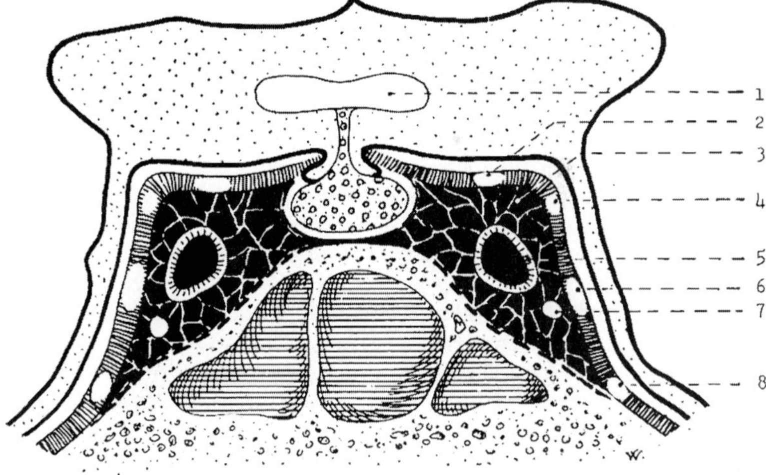

Figure 34-29

Diagram of the cavernous sinus: (1) *optic chiasm;* (2) *oculomotor nerve;* (3) *cavernous sinus;* (4) *trochlear nerve;* (5) *internal carotid artery;* (6) *ophthalmic nerve;* (7) *abducens nerve;* (8) *maxillary nerve. (From Krayenbühl and Yasargil by permission.)*

thrombolysis for extreme cases with stupor or coma and greatly raised CSF pressure.

Marantic Endocarditis and Cerebral Embolism

Sterile vegetations, referred to also as *terminal or non-bacterial thrombotic endocarditis*, consist of fibrin and platelets and are loosely attached to the mitral and aortic valves and contiguous endocardium. They are a common source of cerebral embolism (almost 10 percent of all instances of cerebral embolism according to Barron et al, but lower in the experience of others). In almost half the patients, the vegetations are associated with a malignant neoplasm; the remainder occur in patients debilitated by other diseases (Biller et al). Except for the setting in which it occurs, marantic embolism has no distinctive clinical features that permit differentiation from cerebral embolism of other types. The apoplectic nature of marantic embolism distinguishes it from the usual forms of tumor metastases. The hazards of using anticoagulants in gravely ill patients with widespread malignant disease probably outweigh the benefits from this treatment, but drugs that prevent platelet aggregation have not been studied systematically for this condition.

The lesions of small cerebral arteries formerly observed in patients with rheumatic heart disease and referred to as *rheumatic arteritis* have not been well characterized clinically or pathologically. The vascular lesions and the microinfarcts that accompany them are probably manifestations of diffuse cerebral embolism. Any relationship to the lesion of Sydenham chorea is entirely speculative.

Stroke as a Complication of Hematologic Disease

The brain is involved in the course of many hematologic disorders, some of which have already been mentioned. A number of the better-characterized ones are discussed here.

Antiphospholipid Antibodies This condition, in which migraine, thrombocytopenia, TIAs, or stroke occurs in young adults, has already been alluded to under "Strokes in Children and Young Adults." It is in some instances related to lupus erythematosus vasculopathy. The most frequent neurologic abnormality is a TIA, usually taking the form of amaurosis fugax, with or without retinal arteriolar or venous occlusion (Digre et al). Stroke-like phenomena are more frequent in patients who also have migraine, hyperlipidemia, and antinuclear antibodies and in those who smoke or take birth control pills. Almost one-third of the 48 patients reported by Levine and associates had thrombocytopenia and 23 percent had a false-positive VDRL test. Some of the phospholipids with which the antibodies react are shared with clotting factors, particularly prothrombin or annexin, as well as with the "lupus anticoagulant" (a cardiolipin-glycoprotein complex). These antibodies are circulating serum polyclonal immunoglobulins (IgG, IgM, IgA). The vascular lesions are mainly in the cerebral white matter and are infarcts, seen well with MRI. Angiography reveals occlusions of arteries at unusual sites (Brey et al). The mechanism of stroke is not entirely clear and may derive from emboli originating on mitral valve leaflets similar to nonbacterial thrombotic (Libman-Sacks) endocarditis; alternatively, and more likely in our view, these are due to noninflammatory in situ thrombosis of medium-sized cerebral vessels as suggested by limited pathologic material (Briley et al).

The *Sneddon syndrome* consists of deep blue-red lesions of livedo reticularis and livedo racemosa in association with multiple strokes; 126 cases had been reported up to 1992. Most but not all patients have high titers of antiphospholipid antibodies. Although the skin lesions show a noninflammatory vasculopathy with intimal thickening, the pathology of the occlusive disease has not been adequately studied. In a report of 17 such patients by Stockhammer and coworkers, 8 had strokes and MRI showed lesions in 16 of 17 patients. The age of patients with strokes was 30 to 35 years, hence this condition must always be considered in young adults with cerebrovascular disease. Many of the lesions on MRI were small, deep, and multiple. Although there is a tendency for strokes to recur, many of the patients have remained well for years after their stroke. Skin biopsy aids in diagnosis.

Anticoagulants have been used with some benefit in both of these conditions, and Khamashta and colleagues have found that the INR must be maintained close to 3 for effective prevention of stroke. Plasma exchange may be useful in fulminant cases. Aspirin and heparin are favored in women with recurrent fetal loss related to antiphosphalipid antibody (Lockshin and Sammaritano).

Thrombotic Thrombocytopenic Purpura (TTP, Moschcowitz Syndrome) This is yet another uncommon but serious disease of the small blood vessels, observed mainly in young adults. It is characterized pathologically by widespread occlusions of arterioles and capillaries involving practically all organs of the body, including the brain. The nature of the occluding material has not been completely defined. Fibrin components have been identified by immunofluorescent techniques; some investigators have demonstrated disseminated intravascular platelet aggregation rather than fibrin thrombi. TTP arises because of an inhibitor of von Willebrand factor–cleaving protease; the rarer familial form is caused by a constitutional deficiency of the protease.

Clinically, the main features of this disease are fever, anemia, symptoms of renal and hepatic disease, and thrombocytopenia—the latter giving rise to the common hemorrhagic manifestations (petechiae and ecchymoses of the skin, retinal hemorrhages, hematuria, gastrointestinal bleeding, etc.). Neurologic symptoms are practically always present and are the initial manifestation of the disease in about half the cases. Confusion, delirium, seizures, and altered states of consciousness—sometimes remittent or fluctuating in nature—are the usual manifestations of the nervous system disorder and are readily explained by the widespread microscopic ischemic lesions in the brain. Gross infarction was not observed. The recommended treatment is plasma exchange or plasma infusion.

Thrombocytosis and Thrombocythemia These terms refer to an increase of platelets above 800,000 per cubic millimeter. The condition is generally considered to be a form of myeloproliferative disease. In some patients there is an enlarged spleen, polycythemia, chronic myelogenous leukemia, or myelosclerosis. In several of our patients no explanation of the thrombocytosis was found. They presented with recurrent cerebral and systemic thrombotic episodes, often of minor degree and transient. Cytopheresis, to reduce the platelets, and antimitotic drugs (hydroxyurea) to suppress megakaryocyte formation, are helpful in preventing the neurologic symptoms.

Polycythemia Vera This is a myeloproliferative disorder of unknown cause, characterized by a marked increase in red cell mass (7 to 11 million per cubic millimeter) and blood volume and often by an increase in white cells and platelets as well. This condition must be distinguished from the many secondary or symptomatic forms of polycythemia (erythrocytosis), in which the platelets and white cells remain normal. The slightly increased incidence of thrombosis in primary polycythemia is attributed to the high blood viscosity, engorgement of vessels, and reduced rate of blood flow. The majority of patients with cerebrovascular manifestations have TIAs and small strokes, but on rare occasions we have seen a sagittal sinus thrombosis. The cause of cerebral hemorrhage in this disease is less clear, although a number of abnormalities of platelet function and of coagulation have been described (see Davies-Jones et al).

A wide variety of bleeding disorders—such as *leukemia, aplastic anemia, thrombocytopenic purpura, and hemophilia*—may also give rise to cerebral hemorrhage. Many rare forms of bleeding disease may be complicated by hemorrhagic manifestations; these have been reviewed by Davies-Jones and colleagues.

Sickle Cell Disease This inherited disease is related to the presence of the abnormal hemoglobin S in the red corpuscles. Clinical abnormalities occur only in patients with sickle cell disease, i.e., with the homozygous state, and not in those with the sickle cell trait, which represents the heterozygous state. The disease, which is practically limited to blacks, begins early in life and is characterized by "crises" of infections (particularly pneumococcal meningitis), pain in the limbs and abdomen, chronic leg ulcers, and infarctions of bones and visceral organs. Ischemic lesions of the brain, both large and small, are the most common neurologic complications, but cerebral, subarachnoid, and subdural hemorrhage may also occur and the vascular occlusions may be either arterial or venous.

Disseminated Intravascular Coagulation (DIC) This is perhaps the commonest and most serious disorder of coagulation affecting the nervous system. The basic process depends on the release of thromboplastic substances from damaged tissue, resulting in the activation of the coagulation process and the formation of fibrin, in the course of which clotting factors and platelets are consumed. Virtually any mechanism that produces tissue damage can result in the release of tissue thromboplastins into the circulation. Thus, DIC complicates a wide variety of clinical conditions—overwhelming sepsis, massive trauma, cardiothoracic surgery, heat stroke, burns, incompatible blood transfusions and other immune complex disorders, diabetic ketoacidosis, leukemia, obstetric complications, cyanotic congenital heart disease, and shock from many causes.

The essential pathologic change in DIC is the occurrence of widespread fibrin thrombi in small vessels, resulting in numerous small infarctions of many organs, including the brain. Sometimes DIC is manifest by a hemorrhagic diathesis in which petechial hemorrhages are situated around small penetrating vessels. In some cases the cerebral hemorrhage is quite extensive, similar to a primary hypertensive hemorrhage. The main reason for the hemorrhage is the consumption of platelets and various clotting factors that occurs during fibrin formation; in addition, fibrin degradation products have anticoagulant properties of their own.

The diffuse nature of the neurologic damage may suggest a metabolic rather than a vascular disorder of the brain. In the absence of a clear metabolic, infective, or neoplastic cause of an encephalopathy, the onset of acute and fluctuating focal neurologic abnormalities or a generalized and sometimes terminal neurologic deterioration during the course of a severe illness should arouse suspicion of DIC, and coagulation factors and fibrin split products should be measured. Platelet counts are invariably depressed and there is evidence of consumption of fibrinogen and other clotting factors, indicated by prolonged prothrombin and partial thromboplastin times.

DIFFERENTIATION OF VASCULAR DISEASE FROM OTHER NEUROLOGIC ILLNESSES

The diagnosis of a vascular lesion rests essentially on recognition of the stroke syndrome; without evidence of this, the diagnosis must always be in doubt. The three criteria by which the stroke is identified should be re-emphasized: (1) the temporal profile of the clinical syndrome, (2) evidence of focal brain disease, and (3) the clinical setting. Definition of the temporal profile requires a clear history of the premonitory phenomena, the mode of onset, and the evolution of the neurologic disturbance in relation to the patient's medical status. An inadequate history is the most frequent cause of diagnostic error. If these data are lacking, the stroke profile may still be determined by extending the period of observation for a few days or weeks, thus invoking the clinical rule that the physician's best diagnostic tool is a second and third examination.

There are few categories of neurologic disease whose temporal profile mimics that of the cerebrovascular disorders. Migraine may do so (see page 184), but the history usually provides the diagnosis. A seizure may be followed by a prolonged focal deficit (Todd's paralysis) but is rarely the initial event in a stroke; the setting in which these symptoms occur and their subsequent course clarify the clinical situation. Stroke-like episodes appear in the course of certain hereditary metabolic disorders (Fabry disease, homocystinuria, mitochondrial disease). Differentiation is not difficult because of the associated myopathic and neurologic signs and characteristic metabolic defects. Tumor, infection, inflammation, degeneration, and nutritional deficiency are not likely to manifest themselves precipitously, although rarely a brain metastasis produces a focal deficit of abrupt onset (see below). Trauma, of course, occurs abruptly but usually offers no problem in diagnosis. In multiple sclerosis and other demyelinative diseases, there may be an abrupt onset or exacerbation of symptoms, but for the most part they occur in a different age group and clinical setting. Conversely, a stroke-like onset of cerebral symptoms in a young adult should always raise a suspicion of demyelinative disease. A stroke developing over a period of several days usually progresses in a stepwise fashion, increments of deficit being added abruptly from time to time. A slow, gradual, downhill course over a period of 2 weeks or more indicates that the lesion is probably not vascular but rather neoplastic, demyelinative, infectious (abscess) or granulomatous, or a subdural hematoma.

In regard to the *focal neurologic deficits* of cerebrovascular disease, many of the nonvascular diseases may produce symptoms that are much the same, and the diagnosis cannot rest solely on this aspect of the clinical picture. Nonetheless, certain combinations of neurologic signs, if they conform to a neurovascular pattern—e.g., the lateral medullary syndrome—confidently mark the disease as vascular- occlusive in nature.

Many thrombotic strokes are preceded by TIAs, which, if recognized, are diagnostic of this form of vascular disease. It is essential that TIAs be differentiated from seizures, syncope, panic attacks, neurologic migraine, and attacks of labyrinthine vertigo, since a failure to do so may result in unnecessary arteriographic studies and even a surgical operation.

With very few exceptions, the presence of *blood in the CSF* points to a cerebrovascular (rarely spinal vascular) lesion provided that trauma and a *traumatic* tap can be excluded. *Headache* is common in cerebrovascular disease; it occurs not only with hemorrhage but also with thrombosis, arterial dissections, and rarely with embolism. Seizures are almost never the premonitory, first, or only manifestation of a stroke but can occur in the first few hours after infarction or intracranial bleeding. *Brief unconsciousness* (5 to 10 min) is rare in stroke, being seen only with basilar artery insufficiency and as an initial event in ruptured aneurysm or primary intracerebral hemorrhage. In the latter case, a depression in the state of consciousness soon reasserts itself and is then progressive. Certain neurologic disturbances are hardly ever attributable to stroke—e.g., diabetes insipidus, fever, bitemporal hemianopia, parkinsonism, generalized myoclonus, and isolated cranial nerve palsies—and their presence may be of help in excluding vascular disease.

Finally, the diagnosis of cerebrovascular disease should always be made on positive data, not by exclusion.

A *few conditions are so often confused with cerebrovascular diseases that they merit further consideration.* When a history of trauma is absent, the headache, drowsiness, mild confusion, and hemiparesis of subdural hematoma may be ascribed to a "small stroke," and the patient may fail to receive immediate surgical therapy. In subdural hematoma, the symptoms and signs usually develop gradually over a period of days or weeks. The degree of headache, obtundation, and confusion is disproportionately greater than the focal neurologic deficit, which tends to be indefinite and variable until late in the evolution of the hematoma. The CSF may be blood-tinged or xanthochromic when the type of stroke under suspicion would not be expected to show this. If the patient has fallen and injured his head at the onset of the stroke, it may be impossible to rule out a complicating subdural hematoma on clinical grounds alone, in which case CT scanning and MRI are usually diagnostic.

The reverse diagnostic error will not be made if one remembers that patients with subdural hematoma rarely exhibit a total hemiplegia, monoplegia, hemianesthesia, homonymous hemianopia, or aphasia. If such focal signs are present and particularly if they developed suddenly, subdural hematoma is not likely to be the explanation.

A brain tumor, especially a rapidly growing glioblastoma multiforme or lymphoma, may produce a severe hemiplegia within a week or two. Also, the neurologic deficit due to metastatic carcinoma may evolve rapidly. Moreover, in rare cases, the hemiplegia may be preceded by transitory episodes of neurologic deficit, indistinguishable from TIAs. In such cases, a tumor could be mistaken for a stroke. However, in both conditions, a detailed history will indicate that the evolution of symptoms was gradual; if it was saltatory, seizures will usually have occurred. A number of standard ancillary examinations should never be omitted in these circumstances. A chest film frequently discloses a primary or secondary tumor, and an increased blood sedimentation rate suggests that a concealed systemic disease process is at work. A lack of detailed history may also be responsible for the opposite diagnostic error, i.e., mistaking a relatively slowly evolving stroke (usually due to internal carotid artery or basilar occlusion) for a tumor. Again, CT scanning and MRI will usually settle the problem. A brain abscess or inflammatory necrotic lesion, e.g., toxoplasmosis, may develop without an evident focus of infection and may escape consideration, especially if the patient is elderly.

Senile dementia of the Alzheimer type is often ascribed, on insufficient grounds, to the occurrence of multiple small strokes. If vascular lesions are responsible, evidence of an apoplectic episode or episodes and of focal neurologic deficit to account for at least part of the syndrome will almost invariably be disclosed by history and examination. In the absence of a history of episodic development or of focal neurologic signs, it is unwarranted to attribute senile dementia to cerebrovascular disease—in particular to small strokes in silent areas. *Cerebral arteriosclerosis* is another term that has often been used carelessly to explain such mental changes, the implication (incorrect) being that arteriosclerosis itself causes ischemic damage to the nervous system, producing loss of intellectual function but no other neurologic signs. If cerebral arteriosclerosis (atherosclerosis) is actually responsible, there should be evidence of it in the form of strokes at some time in the course of the illness and often in the heart (myocardial infarction, angina pectoris) or legs (intermittent claudication, loss of pulses). Frequently the lesions of both vascular and Alzheimer disease are present, in which case there may be difficulty in determining to what extent each of them is responsible for the neurologic deficit.

Recurrent seizures as the result of stroke occur in some 10 to 20 percent of cases (*postinfarction epilepsy*). When evidence, by history or examination, of the original stroke is lacking, as it often is, or if the seizures are not observed or leave behind a temporary increase in the neurologic deficit (Todd's paralysis), the diagnosis of another stroke or a tumor may be made in error.

Fear, anxiety, and depression in patients who have had one stroke may lead to additional symptoms—such as generalized weakness, paresthesias, headache, impaired memory, or disequilibrium—and suggest to the patient and physician that further vascular lesions have occurred or threaten.

Miscellaneous conditions occasionally taken to be a stroke are Bell's palsy; Stokes-Adams attacks; a severe attack of labyrinthine vertigo; diabetic ophthalmoplegia; acute ulnar, radial, or peroneal palsy; embolism to a limb; and temporal arteritis associated with blindness.

Contrariwise, certain manifestations of stroke may be incorrectly interpreted as manifestations of some other neurologic disorder. In lateral medullary infarction, *dysphagia* may be the outstanding feature; if the syndrome is not kept in mind, a fruitless radiologic search for a local esophageal or pharyngeal cause may be undertaken. Similarly, *facial pain or a burning sensation*, due to involvement of the trigeminal spinal nucleus, may be misattributed to sinus disease. *Headache*, at times severe, often occurs as a prodrome of a thrombotic stroke or subarachnoid hemorrhage; unless this is appreciated, a diagnosis of migraine may be made. *Dizzy spells or brief intermittent* lapses of equilibrium due to vascular disease of the brainstem may be ascribed to vestibular neuronitis, Ménière disease, Stokes-Adams syncope, or paroxysmal tachycardia. A detailed account of the attack will usually avert this error. A strikingly focal monoplegia of cerebral origin, causing only weakness of the hand or arm or foot drop, is not infrequently misdiagnosed as a peripheral neuropathy.

In the presence of coma, the differentiation of vascular from other neurologic diseases offers special problems. If the patient is comatose when first seen and an adequate history is not available, cerebrovascular lesions have to be differentiated from all the other causes of coma described in Chap. 17. Among cerebrovascular diseases, cerebral or subarachnoid hemorrhage and basilar artery occlusion are usually responsible. In most cases there will be some historical data and focal or lateralizing neurologic signs to direct the series of necessary diagnostic deductions; ancillary examinations, particularly CT scanning and MRI, assume special importance.

COMMON CLINICAL PROBLEMS IN CEREBROVASCULAR DISEASE

Inevitably, most patients are seen first by clinicians who may not be expert in all the fine points of cerebrovascular disease. Situations arise in which critical decisions must be made regarding anticoagulation, further laboratory investigation, and the advice and prognosis given to the family. The following are some of the situations which the authors have encountered that may be of value to students and residents and to nonspecialists in the field.

The patient with a history of an ischemic attack or small stroke in the past The patient may be functioning normally when examined, but it has been ascertained by the history or radiologic procedures that a stroke or TIA occurred in the past. The problem is what measures should be taken to reduce the risk of further strokes. This is particularly problematic if a surgical procedure is planned. A brief focal TIA, several minutes or less in duration, or many stereotyped spells usually represent severe stenosis of the internal carotid artery on the side of the affected cerebral hemisphere. If the symptoms have occurred recently, these may be forerunners of complete occlusion. If the TIA was distant in the past—more than several weeks previously—the immediate risks of occlusion are reduced. The initial approach is to establish the patency of the carotid arteries by ultrasound or MRA. If there is a reduction in diameter of greater than 70 percent when compared with an adjacent normal segment of vessel, and probably if there is a severely ulcerated but not critically stenotic plaque, carotid surgery (or angioplasty) is advisable. If a single TIA lasted more than an hour or the neurologic examination discloses minor signs referable to the region of the hemisphere affected by the TIA, a search for a source of embolus is indicated. Appropriate diagnostic studies include ECG, a transesophageal echocardiogram, monitoring for cardiac arrhythmia, ultrasound of the carotid arteries, and a CT scan or MRI if it has not already been performed. Preventive anticoagulation (warfarin) is instituted if a source of clot within the cardiac chambers is found or if there is atrial fibrillation. Aspirin is appropriate but not imperative if no abnormality is found. Control of elevated blood pressure and perhaps addressing high cholesterol levels are ancillary steps. The mistake is to ignore the potential significance of a small stroke.

Patients with a recent stroke that may not be complete Here the basic problem is whether a thrombotic infarction (venous or arterial) will spread and involve more brain tissue, or if embolic, whether the ischemic tissue will become hemorrhagic or another embolus will occur, or if there is an arterial dissection, whether it will give rise to emboli. Therapies are controversial in most of these circumstances. In some centers it is the practice to try to prevent propagation of a thrombus by administering heparin (or low-molecular-weight heparin) followed by warfarin, as discussed earlier. Thrombolytic agents are an alternative if the stroke has occurred within the previous 2 or 3 h and is not too large. Except perhaps in cases of recent myocardial infarction, atrial fibrillation, or carotid disease, it is not imperative to begin heparin immediately while awaiting the effects of warfarin.

The inevident or misconstrued syndromes of cerebrovascular disease Although hemiplegia is the classic type of stroke, cerebrovascular disease may manifest itself by signs that spare the motor pathways but have the same serious diagnostic and therapeutic implications. The following stroke syndromes tend to be overlooked.

Sometimes disregarded is a leaking aneurysm presenting as a sudden and intense generalized headache lasting hours or days and unlike any headache in the past. Examination may disclose no abnormality except for a slight stiff neck and raised blood pressure. Failure to investigate such a case by imaging procedures and examination of the CSF may permit the occurrence of a later massive subarachnoid hemorrhage. Small cerebral hemorrhages, subdural hematomas, or brain tumors figure into the differential diagnosis, which is usually settled by a CT scan or MRI.

A second inobvious stroke is one caused by occlusion of the posterior cerebral artery, usually embolic. This may not be recognized unless the visual fields are routinely tested at the bedside. The patient himself may not be aware of the difficulty or will complain only of blurring of vision or the need for new glasses. Accompanying deficits are inability to name colors or recognize manipulable objects or faces, difficulty in reading, etc. MRI or CT scanning usually corroborates the clinical diagnosis, and therapy is directed against further emboli or extension of the thrombosis.

Another inapparent or confounding stroke that may be mistaken for psychiatric disease is an attack of paraphasic speech from embolic occlusion of a branch of the left middle cerebral artery. The patient talks in nonsensical phrases, appears confused, and does not fully comprehend what is said to him. He may perform satisfactorily at a superficial level and make socially appropriate greetings and gestures. Only scrutiny of language function and behavior will lead to the correct diagnosis. Infarction (or trauma) of the dominant or nondominant temporal lobe and rarely of the caudate may produce an agitated delirium with few focal findings. This may be mistaken for a toxic or withdrawal state.

Parietal infarctions on either side (usually nondominant hemisphere) are often missed because the patient is entirely unaware of the problem or the symptoms create only a subtle confusional state, drowsiness, or only subtle problems with calculation, dialing a phone, reaching accurately for objects, or loss of ability to write. Extinction of bilaterally presented visual or tactile stimuli gives a clue; marked asymmetry of the optokinetic nystagmus response is sometimes the only definite sign.

A cerebellar hemorrhage may at first be difficult to recognize as a stroke. An occipital headache and complaint of dizziness with vomiting may be interpreted as a labyrinthine disorder, gastroenteritis, or myocardial infarction. A slight ataxia of the limbs, inability to stand, and mild gaze paresis may not have been properly tested or have been overlooked. Early intervention by surgery may be lifesaving; but once the syndrome has progressed to the point of coma and pupillary abnormalities with bilateral Babinski signs, surgery is most often useless.

Periventricular white matter changes (leukoareosis) correlate poorly with cerebrovascular disease and we prefer to ignore them.

The comatose stroke patient The most common causes of vascular coma are intracranial hemorrhage—usually deep in the hemisphere, less often in the cerebellum or brainstem, extensive subarachnoid hemorrhage, and basilar artery occlusion. After several days, brain edema surrounding a large infarction in the territory of the middle cerebral artery or adjacent to a hemorrhage may produce the same effect. Certain remedial surgical measures are still available in these circumstances: drainage of blood from the ventricles, shunting of the ventricles in cases of secondary hydrocephalus due to obstruction of the third ventricle or aqueduct, evacuation of a cerebral hemorrhage in cases of recent decline into stupor and coma, and hemicraniectomy in the case of massive stroke edema. Also, thrombolytic therapy and anticoagulants are sometimes successful in reversing the progression of basilar artery thrombosis. These procedures are best carried out in centers with experience in cerebrovascular intensive care. If coma persists or is deep and sudden, only supportive treatment is possible.

REFERENCES

Adams HP Jr, Butler MJ, Biller J, Toffol GN: Nonhemorrhagic cerebral infarction in young adults. *Arch Neurol* 43:793, 1986.

Adams RD: Mechanisms of apoplexy as determined by clinical and pathological correlation. *J Neuropathol Exp Neurol* 13:1, 1954.

Adams RD, Torvik A, Fisher CM: Progressing stroke: Pathogenesis, in Siekert RG, Whisnant JP (eds): *Cerebral Vascular Diseases, Third Conference*. New York, Grune & Stratton, 1961, pp 133–150.

Adams RD, Vander Eecken HM: Vascular disease of the brain. *Annu Rev Med* 4:213, 1953.

Adler JR, Ropper AH: Self-audible venous bruits and high jugular bulb. *Arch Neurol* 43:257, 1986.

Alema G: Behçet's disease, in Vinken PJ, Bruyn GW (eds): *Handbook of Clinical Neurology*: Vol. 34. *Infection of the Nervous System*. Part II. Amsterdam, North-Holland, 1978, pp 475–512.

Alexander MP, Schmitt MA: The aphasia syndrome of stroke in the left anterior cerebral artery territory. *Arch Neurol* 37:97, 1980.

ALGRA A, VANGIJN J, ALGRA A, KOUDSTALL PJ: Secondary prevention after cerebral ischemia of presumed arterial origin: Is aspirin still the touchstone? *J Neurol Neurosurg Psychiatry* 66:557, 1999.

ALGREN E, AREN C: Cerebral complications after coronary artery bypass surgery and heart valve surgery: Risk factors and onset of symptoms. *J Cardiothorac Vascr Anesth* 12:270, 1998.

ALLEN GS, AHN HS, PREZIOSI TJ, et al: Cerebral arterial vasospasm: A controlled trial of nimodipine in patients with subarachnoid hemorrhage. *N Engl J Med* 308:619, 1983.

AMARENCO P, COHEN A, TZOURIO C, et al: Atherosclerotic disease of the aortic arch and the risk of ischemic stroke. *N Engl J Med* 331:1474, 1994.

AMARENCO P, HAUW J-J: Cerebellar infarction in the territory of the anterior and inferior cerebellar artery: A clinicopathological study of 20 cases. *Brain* 113:139, 1990.

AMES A, NESBETT FB: Pathophysiology of ischemic cell death: I. Time of onset of irreversible damage: Importance of the different components of the ischemic insult. *Stroke* 14:219, 1983.

AMES A, NESBETT FB: Pathophysiology of ischemic cell death: II. Changes in plasma membrane permeability and cell volume. *Stroke* 14:227, 1983.

AMES A, NESBETT FB: Pathophysiology of ischemic cell death: III. Role of extracellular factors. *Stroke* 14:233, 1983.

AMES A, WRIGHT RL, KOWADA M, et al: Cerebral ischemia: II. The no-reflow phenomenon. *Am J Pathol* 52:437, 1968.

ANDREW BT, CHILES BW, OLSEN WL, et al: The effects of intracerebral hematoma location on the risk of brainstem compression and clinical outcome. *J Neurosurg* 69:518, 1988.

AOYAGI N, HAYAKAWA I: Analysis of 223 ruptured intracranial aneurysms with special reference to rerupture. *Surg Neurol* 21:445, 1984.

AUER LM: The pathogenesis of hypertensive encephalopathy. *Acta Neurochir Suppl* 27:1, 1978.

AVERBACK P: Primary cerebral venous thrombosis in young adults: The diverse manifestations of an unrecognized disease. *Ann Neurol* 3:81, 1978.

BABIKIAN V, ROPPER AH: Binswanger's disease: A review. *Stroke* 18:2, 1987.

BAMFORD J, SANDERCOCK P, DENNIS M, et al: A prospective study of acute cerebrovascular disease in the community: The Oxfordshire Community Stroke Project. 1981–1986. *J Neurol Neurosurg Psychiatry* 51:1373, 1988; also 53:16, 1990.

BANKER BQ: Cerebral vascular disease in infancy and childhood: I. Occlusive vascular disease. *J Neuropathol Exp Neurol* 20:127, 1961.

BARNETT HJM: The EC/IC Bypass Study Group. Failure of extracranial-intracranial arterial bypass to reduce the risk of ischemic stroke: Results of an international randomized trial. *N Engl J Med* 313:1191, 1985.

BARNETT HJM, BOUGHNER GR, COOPER PF: Further evidence relating mitral-valve prolapse to cerebral ischemic events. *N Engl J Med* 302:139, 1980.

BARNETT HJM, MOHR JP, STEIN BM, YATSU FM (eds): *Stroke: Pathophysiology, Diagnosis, and Management*, 3rd ed. New York, Churchill Livingstone, 1998.

BARRON KD, SIQUEIRA E, HIRANO A: Cerebral embolism caused by nonbacterial thrombotic endocarditis. *Neurology* 10:391, 1960.

BATJER HH, REISCH JW, ALLEN BC, et al: Failure of surgery to improve outcome in hypertensive putaminal hemorrhage. *Arch Neurol* 47:1103, 1990.

BECKER S, HELLER CH, GROPP F, et al: Thrombophilic disorders in children with cerebral infarction. *Lancet* 352:1756, 1998.

BENDSZUS M, KOLTZENBERG M, BURGER R, et al: Silent embolism in diagnostic cerebral angiography and neurointerventional procedures: A prospective study. *Lancet* 354:1594, 1999.

BILLER J, CHALLA VR, TOOLE JF, HOWARD VJ: Nonbacterial thrombotic endocarditis. *Arch Neurol* 39:95, 1982.

BOGOUSSLAVSKY J, DESPLANT P-A, REGLI F: Spontaneous carotid dissection with acute stroke. *Arch Neurol* 44:137, 1987.

BOGOUSSLAVSKY J, REGLI F: Anterior cerebral artery territory infarction in the Lausanne Stroke Registry: Clinical and etiologic patterns. *Arch Neurol* 47:144, 1990.

BOSTON AREA ANTICOAGULATION TRIAL FOR ATRIAL FIBRILLATION INVESTIGATORS: The effect of low-dose warfarin in the risk of stroke in patients with nonrheumatic atrial fibrillation. *N Engl J Med* 323:1505, 1990.

BOTTERELL EH, LOUGHEED WM, SCOTT JW, VANDEWATER SL: Hypothermia, and interruption of carotid or carotid and vertebral circulation, in the surgical management of intracranial aneurysms. *J Neurosurg* 13:1, 1956.

BREEN JC, CAPLAN LR, DEWITT D, et al: Brain edema after carotid surgery. *Neurology* 46:175, 1996.

BREY RL, HART RG, SHERMAN DG, TEGELER CH: Antiphospholipid antibodies and cerebral ischemia in young people. *Neurology* 40:1190, 1990.

BRILEY DP, COULL BM, GOODNIGHT SH: Neurological disease associated with antiphospholipid antibodies. *Ann Neurol* 25:221, 1989.

BRITTON M, DEFAIRE U, HELMERS C: Hazards of therapy for excessive hypertension in acute stroke. *Acta Med Scand* 207:352, 1980.

BRODERICK JP, BROTT TG, BULDNER JE, et al: Volume of intracerebral hemorrhage. A powerful and easy-to-use predictor of 30-day mortality. *Stroke* 24:987, 1993.

BRODERICK JP, PHILLIPS SJ, WHISNANT JP, et al: Incidence rates of stroke in the eighties: The end of the decline in stroke? *Stroke* 20:577, 1989.

BROTT T, REED RL: Intensive care for acute stroke in the community hospital setting: The first 24 hours. *Stroke* 20:694, 1989.

BROWN MM, BEVAN D: Is inherited thrombophilia a risk factor for arterial stroke? *J Neurol Neurosurg Psychiatry* 65:617, 1998.

BRUST JCM: Anterior cerebral artery disease, in Barnett HJM, Mohr JP, Stein BM, Yalsu FM (eds): *Stroke: Pathophysiology, Diagnosis, and Management*, 2nd ed. New York, Churchill Livingstone, 1992, pp 337–360.

BRUST JCM, BEHRENS MM: "Release hallucinations" as the major symptom of posterior cerebral artery occlusion: A report of 2 cases. *Ann Neurol* 2:432, 1977.

BYROM FB: The pathogenesis of hypertensive encephalopathy. *Lancet* 2:201, 1954.

CALL G, FLEMING M, SEALFON S, et al: Reversible cerebral segmental vasoconstriction. *Stroke* 19:1159, 1988.

CAPLAN LR: Binswanger's disease—revisited. *Neurology* 45:626, 1995.

CAPLAN LR: Intracranial branch atheromatous disease: A neglected, understudied, and overused concept. *Neurology* 39:1246, 1989.

CAPLAN LR: *Stroke: A Clinical Approach*, 2nd ed. Boston, Butterworth-Heinemann, 1993.

CAPLAN LR: "Top of the basilar" syndrome. *Neurology* 30:72, 1980.

CAPLAN LR, SCHMAHMANN JD, KASE CS, et al: Caudate infarcts. *Arch Neurol* 47:133, 1990.

CAPLAN LR, SERGAY S: Positional cerebral ischemia. *J Neurol Neurosurg Psychiatry* 39:385, 1976.

CARLBERG B, ASPLUND K, HAAG E: Factors influencing admission blood pressure levels in patients with acute stroke. *Stroke* 22:527, 1991.

CARTER BS, OGILVY CS, CANDIA GJ, et al: One-year outcome after decompressive surgery for massive nondominant hemispheric infarction. *Neurosurgery* 40:1168, 1997.

CASTAIGNE P, LHERMITTE F, BUGE A, et al: Paramedian thalamic and midbrain infarcts: Clinical and neuropathological study. *Ann Neurol* 10:127, 1981.

CHAJEK T, FAINARU M: Behçet's disease: Report of 41 cases and a review of the literature. *Medicine* 54:179, 1975.

CHAMBERS BR, NORRIS JW: Outcome in patients with asymptomatic neck bruits. *N Engl J Med* 315:860, 1986.

CHESTER EM, AGAMANOLIS DP, BANKER BQ, VICTOR M: Hypertensive encephalopathy: A clinicopathologic study of 20 cases. *Neurology* 28:928, 1978.

CHURG J, STRAUSS L: Allergic granulomatosis, allergic angiitis and periarteritis nodosa. *Am J Pathol* 27:277, 1951.

COGAN DG: Visual hallucinations as release phenomena. *Graefes Arch Clin Exp Ophthalmol* 188:139, 1973.

COLLINS R, PETO R, MACMAHON S, et al: Blood pressure, stroke, and coronary heart disease. *Lancet* 335:827, 1990.

CORRIN LS, SANDOK BA, HOUSER W: Cerebral ischemic events in patients with carotid artery fibromuscular dysplasia. *Arch Neurol* 38:616, 1981.

CRAWFORD PM, WEST CR, CHADWICK DW, et al: Arteriovenous malformations of the brain: Natural history in unoperated patients. *J Neurol Neurosurg Psychiatry* 49:1, 1986.

DASHE JF, PESSIN MS, MURPHY RE, PAYNE DD: Carotid occlusive disease and stroke risk in coronary artery bypass graft surgery. *Neurology* 49:678, 1997.

DAVIES-JONES GAB, PRESTON FE, TIMPERLEY WR: *Neurological Complications in Clinical Haematology*. Oxford, England, Blackwell Scientific Publications, 1980.

DAY AL: Anatomy of extracranial vessels, in Smith RR (ed): *Stroke and Extracranial Vessels*. New York, Raven Press, 1984, pp 9–22.

DECROIX JP, GRAVELEAU R, MASSON M, CAMBIER J: Infarction in the territory of the anterior choroidal artery. *Brain* 109:1071, 1986.

DÉJERINE J: Sémiologie d'affections du système nerveux. Paris, Masson, 1914.

DELSHAW JB, BROADDUS WC, KASSELL NF, et al: Treatment of right hemisphere cerebral infarction by hemicraniectomy. *Stroke* 21: 874, 1990.

DEVINSKY O, PETITO CK, ALONSO DR: Clinical and neuropathological findings in systemic lupus erythematosus: The role of vasculitis, heart emboli, and thrombotic thrombocytopenic purpura. *Ann Neurol* 23:380, 1988.

DIGRE KB, DURCAN FJ, BRANCH DW, et al: Amaurosis fugax associated with antiphospholipid antibodies. *Ann Neurol* 25:228, 1989.

DIRINGER MN, EDWARDS DF, ZAZULIA AR: Hydrocephalus: A previously unrecognized predictor of poor outcome from supratentorial intracerebral hemorrhage. *Stroke* 29:1352, 1998.

DIRINGER MN, LADENSON PW, STERN BJ, et al: Plasma atrial natriuretic factor and subarachnoid hemorrhage. *Stroke* 19:1119, 1988.

DIROCCO C, IANELLI A, LEONE G, et al: Heparin-urokinase treatment in aseptic dural sinus thrombosis. *Arch Neurol* 38:431, 1981.

DONNAN GA, DAVIS SM, CHAMBERS BR, GATES PC: Surgery for prevention of stroke. *Lancet* 351:1372, 1998.

DONNAN GA, O'MALLEY HM, QUANG L, et al: The capsular warning syndrome: Pathogenesis and clinical features. *Neurology* 43:957, 1993.

DRAKE CG: Giant fusiform intracranial aneurysms: Review of 120 patients treated surgically from 1965 to 1992. *J Neurosurg* 87:141, 1997.

EINHAUPL KM, VILLRINGER A, MEISTER W: Heparin treatment in sinus venous thrombosis. *Lancet* 358:597, 1971.

EUROPEAN CAROTID SURGERY TRIALISTS' COLLABORATIVE GROUP: Risk of stroke in the distribution of an asymptomatic carotid artery. *Lancet* 345:209, 1995.

EUROPEAN CAROTID SURGERY TRIALISTS' COLLABORATIVE GROUP: Randomised trial of endarterectomy for recently symptomatic carotid stenosis: Final results of the MRC European Carotid Surgery Trial (ECST). *Lancet* 351:1379, 1998.

EXECUTIVE COMMITTEE FOR THE ASYMPTOMATIC CAROTID ATHEROSCLEROSIS STUDY: Endarterectomy for asymptomatic carotid artery stenosis. *JAMA* 273:1421, 1995.

FERGUSON GG: Physical factors in the initiation, growth, and rupture of human intracranial saccular aneurysms. *J Neurosurg* 37:666, 1972.

FISHER CM: A lacunar stroke: The dysarthria-clumsy hand syndrome. *Neurology* 17:614, 1967.

FISHER CM: Capsular infarct: The underlying vascular lesions. *Arch Neurol* 36:65, 1979.

FISHER CM: Cerebral ischemia—Less familiar types. *Clin Neurosurg* 18:267, 1971.

FISHER CM: Cerebral thromboangiitis obliterans. *Medicine* 36:169, 1957.

FISHER CM: Lacunar strokes and infarcts: A review. *Neurology* 32:871, 1982.

FISHER CM: Late-life migraine accompaniments as a cause of unexplained transient ischemic attacks. *Can J Neurol Sci* 7:9, 1980.

FISHER CM: The anatomy and pathology of the cerebral vasculature, in Meyer JS (ed): *Modern Concepts of Cerebrovascular Disease*. New York, Spectrum, 1975, pp 1–41.

FISHER CM: The pathologic and clinical aspects of thalamic hemorrhage. *Trans Am Neurol Assoc* 84:56, 1959.

FISHER CM, ADAMS RD: Observations on brain embolism with special reference to hemorrhagic infarction, in Furlan AJ (ed): *The Heart and Stroke: Exploring Mutual Cerebrovascular and Cardiovascular Issues*. Berlin, Springer-Verlag, 1987, pp 17–36.

FISHER CM, KARNES WE, KUBIK CS: Lateral medullary infarction—The pattern of vascular occlusion. *J Neuropathol Exp Neurol* 20:323, 1961.

FISHER CM, KISTLER JP, DAVIS JM: Relation of cerebral vasospasm to subarachnoid hemorrhage visualized by CT scanning. *Neurosurgery* 6:1, 1980.

FOIX C, CHAVANEY JA, LEVY M: Syndrome pseudothalamique d'origine parietale. *Rev Neurol* 35:68, 1927.

FOIX C, LEVY M: Les ramollisemente sylvien. *Rev Neurol* 11:51, 1927.

FORD CS, FRYE JL, TOOLE JF, LEFKOWITZ D: Asymptomatic carotid bruit and stenosis. *Arch Neurol* 43:219, 1986.

FRANK JI: Large hemispheric infarction, deterioration, and intracranial pressure. *Neurology* 45:1286, 1995.

FREIS ED, CALABRESI M, CASTLE CH, et al: Veterans Administration Cooperative Study Group on Antihypertensive Agents: Effects of treatment on morbidity in hypertension II: Results in patients with diastolic blood pressure averaging 90 through 114 mm Hg. *JAMA* 213:1143, 1970.

GARRAWAY WM, WHISNANT JP, DRURY I: The changing pattern of survival following stroke. *Stroke* 14:699, 1983.

GARRAWAY WM, WHISNANT JP, DRURY I: The continuing decline in the incidence of stroke. *Mayo Clin Proc* 58:520, 1983.

GASECKI AP, ELIASZIW M, FERGUSON GG, et al: Long-term prognosis and effect of endarterectomy in patients with symptomatic severe carotid stenosis and contralateral carotid stenosis or occlusion: Results from NASCET. *J Neurosurg* 83:778, 1995.

GILON D, BUONANO FS, JOFFE MM, et al: Lack of evidence of an association between mitral-valve prolapse and stroke in young patients. *N Engl J Med* 3:41, 1999.

GREENBERG SM, REBECK GW, VONSATTEL JP, et al: Apolipoprotein E ϵ4 and cerebral hemorrhage associated with amyloid angiopathy. *Ann Neurol* 38:254, 1995.

HACKE W, KASTE M, FIESCHI C, et al: Intravenous thrombolysis with recombinant tissue plasminogen activator for acute hemispheric stroke: The European Cooperative Acute Stroke Trial (ECASS). *JAMA* 274:1017, 1995.

HACKE W, KASTE M, FIESCHI C, et al: Randomised double-blind placebo-controlled trial of thrombolytic therapy with intravenous aleptase in acute ischaemic stroke. *Lancet* 352:1245, 1998.

HART RG, BYER JA, SLAUGHTER JR, et al: Occurrence and implications of seizures in subarachnoid hemorrhage due to ruptured intracranial aneurysms. *Neurosurgery* 8:417, 1981.

HART RG, COULL BM, HART D: Early recurrent embolism associated with nonvalvular atrial fibrillation: A retrospective study. *Stroke* 14:688, 1983.

HAUSER RA, LACEY M, KNIGHT R: Hypertensive encephalopathy: Magnetic resonance imaging demonstration of reversible cortical and white matter lesions. *Arch Neurol* 45:1078, 1988.

HAWKINS TD, SIMS C, HANKA R: Subarachnoid haemorrhage of unknown cause: A long-term follow-up. *J Neurol Neurosurg Psychiatry* 52:230, 1989.

HAYASHI M, KOBAYASHI H, KANANO H, et al: Treatment of systemic hypertension and intracranial hypertension in cases of brain hemorrhage. *Stroke* 19:314, 1988.

HEISS WD: Flow thresholds of functional and morphological damage of brain tissue. *Stroke* 14:329, 1983.

HENNERICI M, TROCKEL U, RAUTENBERG W, et al: Spontaneous progression and regression of carotid atheroma. *Lancet* 1:1415, 1985.

HEYMAN A, WILKINSON WE, HEYDEN S, et al: Risk of stroke in asymptomatic persons with cervical arterial bruits. *N Engl J Med* 302:838, 1980.

HEYMAN A, WILKINSON WE, HURWITZ BJ, et al: Risk of ischemic heart disease in patients with TIA. *Neurology* 34:626, 1984.

HIJDRA A, VANGIJN, STEFANKO S, et al: Delayed cerebral ischemia after aneurysmal subarachnoid hemorrhage: Clinicoanatomic correlations. *Neurology* 36:329, 1986.

HOMAN RW, DEVOUS MD, STOKELY EM, BONTE FJ: Quantification of intracerebral steal in patients with arteriovenous malformation. *Arch Neurol* 43:779, 1986.

HOMER D, INGALL TJ, BAKER HL JR, et al: Serum lipids and lipoproteins are less powerful predictors of extracranial carotid artery atherosclerosis than are cigarette smoking and hypertension. *Mayo Clin Proc* 66:259, 1991.

HOSSMAN K-A: Pathophysiology of cerebral infarction, in Vinken PJ, Bruyn GW, Klawans HL (eds): *Handbook of Clinical Neurology*: Vol 53. *Vascular Diseases*. Part I. Amsterdam, Elsevier, 1988, pp 27–46.

HOUSER OW, BAKER HL JR, SANDOK BA, HOLLEY KE: Fibromuscular dysplasia of the cephalic arterial system, in Vinken PJ, Bruyn GW (eds): *Handbook of Clinical Neurology*: Vol 11. *Vascular Disease of the Nervous System*. Part 1. Amsterdam, North-Holland, 1972, pp 366–385.

HUPPERTS RMM, LODDER J, MEUTS-VAN RAAK EPM, et al: Infarcts in the anterior choroidal artery territory: Anatomical distribution, clinical syndromes, presumed pathogensis, and early outcome. *Brain* 117:825, 1994.

INGALL TJ, HOMER D, BAKER HL JR, et al: Predictors of intracranial carotid artery atherosclerosis: Duration of cigarette smoking and hypertension are more powerful than serum lipid levels. *Arch Neurol* 48:687, 1991.

INTERNATIONAL STUDY OF UNRUPTURED INTRACRANIAL ANEURYSMS INVESTIGATORS: Unruptured intracranial aneurysms—Risk of rupture and risks of surgical intervention. *N Engl J Med* 339:1725, 1998.

INZITARI D, ELIASZIW, M, GATES P, et al: The causes and risks of stroke in patients with asymptomatic internal-carotid-artery stenosis. *N Engl J Med* 342:1693, 2000.

IREY NS, MCALLISTER HA, HENRY JM: Oral contraceptives and stroke in young women: A clinicopathologic correlation. *Neurology* 28:1216, 1978.

ISHIKAWA K, UYAMA M, ASAYAMA K: Occlusive thrombo-aortopathy (Takayasu's disease): Cervical arterial stenoses, retinal arterial pressure, retinal microaneurysms and prognosis. *Stroke* 14:730, 1983.

Itoh T, Matsumoto M, Handa N, et al: Paradoxical embolism as a cause of ischemic stroke of uncertain etiology: A transcranial Doppler sonographic study. *Stroke* 25:771, 1994.

Jacobs K, Moulin T, Bogousslavsky J, et al: The stroke syndrome of cortical vein thrombosis. *Neurology* 47:376, 1996.

Johnson RT, Richardson EP: The neurological manifestations of systemic lupus erythematosus. *Medicine* 47:337, 1968.

Jones HR, Naggar CZ, Seljan MP, Downing LL: Mitral valve prolapse and cerebral ischemic events: A comparison between a neurology population with stroke and a cardiology population with mitral valve prolapse observed for five years. *Stroke* 13:451, 1982.

Joutel A, Vahedi K, Corpechot C, et al: Strong clustering and stereotyped nature of Notch3 mutations in CADASIL patients. *Lancet* 350:1511, 1997.

Jung HH, Bassetti C, Tourier-Lasserve E: Cerebral autosomal dominant arteriopathy with subcortical infarcts and leukoencephalopathy: A clinicopathologic and genetic study of a Swiss family. *J Neurol Neurosurg Psychiatry* 59:138, 1995.

Junque C, Pujol J, Vendrell P, et al: Leuko-araiosis on magnetic resonance imaging and speed of mental processing. *Arch Neurol* 47:151, 1990.

Juvela S, Helskanen O, Poranen A, et al: The treatment of spontaneous intracerebral hemorrhage. *J Neurosurg* 70:755, 1989.

Kanis K, Ropper AH: Homolateral hemiparesis as an early sign of cerebellar mass effect. *Neurology* 44:2194, 1994.

Kase CS, Caplan LR: *Intracerebral Hemorrhage*. Boston, Butterworth-Heinemann, 1994.

Kase CS, Williams JP, Wyatt DA, Mohr JP: Lobar intracerebral hematomas: Clinical and CT analysis of 22 cases. *Neurology* 32:1146, 1982.

Kassell NF, Torner JC, Haley EC Jr, et al: The International Cooperative Study on the Timing of Aneurysm Surgery: Part 1. Overall management results. *J Neurosurg* 73:18, 1990; Part 2: Surgical results. *J Neurosurg* 73:37, 1990.

Katzan IL, Furlan AJ, Lloyd LE, et al: Use of tissue-type plasminogen activator for acute ischemic stroke: The Cleveland area experience. *JAMA* 288:1151, 2000.

Kay R, Wong KS, Ling YL, et al: Low-molecular-weight heparin for the treatment of acute ischemic stroke. *N Engl J Med* 333:1588, 1995.

Khamashta MA, Cuadro MJ, Mujic F, et al: The management of thrombosis in the antiphospholipid syndrome. *N Engl J Med* 332: 993, 1995.

Kistler JP, Buonanno FS, Gress DR: Carotid endarterectomy—Specific therapy based on pathophysiology. *N Engl J Med* 325: 505, 1991.

Kitahara T, Okumura K, Semba A, et al: Genetic and immunologic analysis on moya-moya. *J Neurol Neurosurg Psychiatry* 45:1048, 1982.

Kittner SJ, Stern BJ, Feeser BR, et al: Pregnancy and the risk of stroke. *N Engl J Med* 335:768, 1996.

Kjellberg RN, Hanamura T, Davis KR, et al: Bragg-peak proton-beam therapy for arteriovenous malformations of the brain. *N Engl J Med* 309:269, 1983.

Koroshetz WJ, Ropper AH: Artery to artery embolism causing stroke in the posterior circulation. *Neurology* 37:292, 1987.

Krayenbühl H, Yasargil MG: Radiological anatomy and topography of the cerebral arteries, in Vinken PJ, Bruyn GW (eds): *Handbook of Clinical Neurology*: Vol 11. *Vascular Diseases of the Nervous System*. Part 1. Amsterdam, North-Holland, 1972, pp 65–101.

Kubik CS, Adams RD: Occlusion of the basilar artery—A clinical and pathological study. *Brain* 69:73, 1946.

Kwakkel G, Wagenaar RC, Twisk JW, et al: Intensity of leg and arm training after primary middle-cerebral-artery stroke: A randomised trial. *Lancet* 354:191, 1999.

Kwiatkowski TG, Libman RB, Frankel M, et al: Effects of tissue plasminogen activator for acute ischemic stroke at one year. *N Engl J Med* 340:1781, 1999.

Lehner T, Barnes CG (eds): *Behçet's Syndrome: Clinical and Immunological Features*. New York, Academic Press, 1980.

Lehrich J, Winkler G, Ojemann R: Cerebellar infarction with brainstem compression: Diagnosis and surgical treatment. *Arch Neurol* 22:490, 1970.

Leung DY, Black IW, Cranney GB, et al: Selection of patients for transesophageal echocardiography after stroke and systemic embolic events. *Stroke* 26:1820, 1995.

Levine SR, Brust JCM, Futrell N, et al: Cerebrovascular complications of the use of the "crack" form of alkaloidal cocaine. *N Engl J Med* 323:699, 1990.

Levine SR, Deegan MJ, Futrell N, Welch KMA: Cerebrovascular and neurologic disease associated with antiphospholipid antibodies: 48 cases. *Neurology* 40:1181, 1990.

Libman RB, Wirkowski E, Neystat M, et al: Stroke associated with cardiac surgery: Determinants, timing, and stroke subtypes. *Arch Neurol* 54:83, 1997.

Lockshin MD, Sammaritano LR: Antiphospholipid antibodies and fetal loss. *N Engl J Med* 326:951, 1992.

Locksley HB: Natural history of subarachnoid hemorrhage, intracranial aneurysms and arteriovenous malformations—Based on 6368 cases in the cooperative study. *J Neurosurg* 25:219, 1966.

Lodder J, van der Lugt PJM: Evaluation of the risk of immediate anticoagulant treatment in patients with embolic stroke of cardiac origin. *Stroke* 14:42, 1983.

Loh E, Sutton M, Wun C, et al: Ventricular dysfunction and the risk of stroke after myocardial infarction. *N Engl J Med* 336:251, 1997.

Longstreth WT, Swanson PD: Oral contraceptives and stroke. *Stroke* 15:747, 1984.

Lupi-Herrera E, Sanchez-Torres G, Marcushamer J, et al: Takayasu's arteritis: Clinical study of 107 cases. *Am Heart J* 93:94, 1977.

MacMahon S, Peto R, Cutler J, et al: Blood pressure, stroke, and coronary heart disease: Part I. Prolonged differences in blood pressure: Prospective observational studies corrected for the regression dilution bias. *Lancet* 335:765, 1990.

Mao C-C, Coull BM, Golper LAC, Rau MT: Anterior operculum syndrome. *Neurology* 39:1169, 1989.

Marchuk DA, Gallione CJ, Morrison LA, et al: A locus for cerebral cavernous malformations maps to chromosome 7q in two families. *Genomics* 28:31, 1995.

Margolin DI, Marsden CD: Episodic dyskinesias and transient cerebral ischemia. *Neurology* 32:1379, 1982.

Markus HS, Hambley H: Neurology and the blood: Haematological abnormalities in ischaemic stroke. *J Neurol Neurosurg Psychiatry* 64:150, 1998.

Marshall J: Angiography in the investigation of ischemic episodes in the territory of the internal carotid artery. *Lancet* 1:719, 1971.

Martinelli I, Sacchi E, Landi G, et al: High-risk of cerebral-vein thrombosis in carriers of a prothrombin gene mutation and in users of oral contraceptives. *N Engl J Med* 338:1793, 1998.

McKissock W, Paine KW, Walsh LS: An analysis of the results of treatment of ruptured intracranial aneurysms: A report of 722 consecutive cases. *J Neurosurg* 17:762, 1960.

Milandre L, Brosset C, Botti G, Khawl R: A study of 82 cerebral infarctions in the area of posterior cerebral arteries. *Rev Neurol* 150:133, 1994.

Miyasaka K, Wolpert SM, Prager RJ: The association of cerebral aneurysms, infundibula, and intracranial arteriovenous malformations. *Stroke* 13:196, 1982.

Mohr JP, Caplan LR, Melski JW, et al: The Harvard Cooperative Stroke Registry: A prospective registry of patients hospitalized with stroke. *Neurology* 28:754, 1978.

Mohr JP, Mast H: Binswanger's disease, in Barnett HJM et al (eds): *Stroke: Pathophysiology, Diagnosis, and Management*, 3rd ed. New York, Churchill Livingstone, 1998, pp 921–931.

Mokri B, Houser W, Sandok BA, Piepgras DG: Spontaneous dissections of the vertebral arteries. *Neurology* 38:880, 1988.

Mokri B, Sundt TM Jr, Houser W, Piepgras DG: Spontaneous dissection of the cervical internal carotid artery. *Ann Neurol* 19:126, 1986.

Moore PM: Diagnosis and management of isolated angiitis of the central nervous system. *Neurology* 39:167, 1989.

Moore PM (ed): Vasculitis. *Semin Neurol* 14:291, 1994.

Moore WS, Barnett HJ, Beebe HG, et al: Guidelines for carotid endarterectomy: A multidisciplinary consensus statement from the ad hoc committee, American Heart Association. *Stroke* 25:188, 1995.

Multicenter Acute Stroke Trial—Europe Study Group: Thrombolytic therapy with streptokinase in acute stroke. *N Engl J Med* 335:145, 1996.

Multicentre Acute Stroke Trial—Italy (MAST-I) Group: Randomised controlled trial of streptokinase, aspirin, and combination of both in treatment of acute ischaemic stroke. *Lancet* 346:1509, 1995.

Myers RE, Yamaguchi S: Nervous system effects of cardiac arrest in monkeys. *Arch Neurol* 34:65, 1977.

Nakajima K: Clinicopathological study of pontine hemorrhage. *Stroke* 14:485, 1983.

National Institute of Neurological Disorders and Stroke rt-PA Stroke Study Group: Tissue plasminogen activator for acute ischemic stroke. *N Engl J Med* 333:1581, 1995.

Nelson J, Barron MM, Riggs JE, et al: Cerebral vasculitis and ulcerative colitis. *Neurology* 36:719, 1986.

Nicholls ES, Johansen HL: Implications of changing trends in cerebrovascular and ischemic heart disease mortality. *Stroke* 14:153, 1983.

Nishimoto A, Takeuchi S: Moyamoya disease, in Vinken PJ, Bruyn GW (eds): *Handbook of Clinical Neurology*: Vol 12. *Vascular Diseases of the Nervous System*. Part 2. Amsterdam, North-Holland, 1972, pp 352–383.

Nishino H, Rubino FA, DeRemee RA, et al: Neurological involvement in Wegener's granulomatosis: An analysis of 324 consecutive patients at the Mayo Clinic. *Ann Neurol* 33:4, 1993.

Nishioka H, Torner JC, Graf CJ, et al: Cooperative study of intracranial aneurysms and subarachnoid hemorrhage: A long-term prognostic study: II. Ruptured intracranial aneurysms managed conservatively. *Arch Neurol* 41:1142, 1984.

North American Symptomatic Carotid Endarterectomy Trial Collaborators: Beneficial effect of carotid endarterectomy in symptomatic patients with high-grade carotid stenosis. *N Engl J Med* 325:445, 1991.

Norving B, Cronqvist S: Lateral medullary infarction: Prognosis in an unselected series. *Neurology* 41:244, 1991.

Nubiola AR, Masana L, Masdeu S, et al: High-density lipoprotein cholesterol in cerebrovascular disease. *Arch Neurol* 38:468, 1981.

Ojemann RG, Fisher CM, Rich JC: Spontaneous dissecting aneurysms of the internal carotid artery. *Stroke* 3:434, 1972.

Ojemann RG, Ogilvy CS, Crowell RM, Heros RC: *Surgical Management of Neuro-vascular Disease*, 3rd ed. Baltimore, Williams & Wilkins, 1995.

Olsen TS, Larsen B, Herning M, et al: Blood flow and vascular reactivity in collaterally perfused brain tissue. *Stroke* 14:332, 1983.

Ondra SL, Troupp H, George ED, Schwab K: The natural history of symptomatic arteriovenous malformations of the brain: A 24-year follow-up assessment. *J Neurosurg* 73:387, 1990.

Percheron G: Les artères du thalamus humain: II. Artères et territoires thalamiques paramédians de l'artère basilaire communicante. *Rev Neurol* 132:309, 1976.

Pessin MS, Duncan GW, Mohr JP, Poskanzer DC: Clinical and angiographic features of carotid transient ischemic attacks. *N Engl J Med* 296:358, 1977.

Pessin MS, Hinton RC, Davis KR, et al: Mechanisms of acute carotid stroke. *Ann Neurol* 6:245, 1979.

Petit H, Rousseaux M, Clarisse J, Delafosse A: Troubles oculocephalomoteurs et infarctus thalamo-sous-thalamique bilateral. *Rev Neurol* 137:709, 1981.

Petitti DB, Sidney S, Bernstein A, et al: Stroke in users of low-dose oral contraceptives. *N Engl J Med* 335:8, 1996.

Phillips PC, Lorentsen KJ, Shropshire LC, Ahn HS: Congenital odontoid aplasia and posterior circulation stroke in childhood. *Ann Neurol* 23:410, 1988.

Plum F: What causes infarction in ischemic brain? The Robert Wartenberg lecture. *Neurology* 33:222, 1983.

Poole CMJ, Ross Russell RW: Mortality and stroke after amaurosis fugax. *J Neurol Neurosurg Psychiatry* 48:902, 1985.

Rabkin SW, Mathewson FAL, Tate RB: Long-term changes in blood pressure and risk of cerebrovascular disease. *Stroke* 9:319, 1978.

RAICHLE ME: The pathophysiology of brain ischemia. *Ann Neurol* 13:2, 1983.

RAUH R, FISCHEREDER M, SPENGEL FA: Transesophageal echocardiography in patients with focal cerebral ischemia of unknown cause. *Stroke* 27:691, 1996.

REIVICH M, HOLLING HE, ROBERTS B, TOOLE JF: Reversal of blood flow through the vertebral artery and its effect on cerebral circulation. *N Engl J Med* 265:878, 1961.

RENGARCHARY SS, BATNITZKY S, MORANTZ R, et al: Hemicraniectomy for acute massive cerebral infarction. *Neurosurgery* 8:321, 1981.

RICE GPA, BOUGHNER DR, STILLER C, EBERS GC: Familial stroke syndrome associated with mitral valve prolapse. *Ann Neurol* 7:130, 1980.

RICHARDSON AE, JANE JA: Long-term prognosis in untreated cerebral aneurysms: I. Incidence of late hemorrhage in cerebral aneurysm: Ten-year evaluation of 364 patients. *Ann Neurol* 1:358, 1977.

RIEKE K, SCHWAB S, KRIEGER D, et al: Decompressive surgery in space occupying hemispheric infarction: Results of an open, prospective trial. *Crit Care Med* 23:1567, 1995.

ROACH GW, KANCHUGER M, MANGANO CM, et al: Adverse cerebral outcomes after coronary bypass surgery. *N Engl J Med* 335:1857, 1996.

ROEHMHOLDT ME, PALUMBO PJ, WHISNANT JP, ELVEBACK LR: Transient ischemic attack and stroke in a community-based diabetic cohort. *Mayo Clin Proc* 58:56, 1983.

ROPPER AH: Neurologic intensive care, in Vinken PJ, Bruyn GW, Klawans HL (eds): *Handbook of Clinical Neurology*. Vascular Diseases. Part III. Vol 55. Amsterdam, Elsevier, 1990, pp 203–232.

ROPPER AH, DAVIS KR: Lobar cerebral hemorrhages: Acute clinical syndromes in 26 cases. *Ann Neurol* 8:141, 1980.

ROPPER AH, KING RB: Intracranial pressure monitoring in comatose patients with cerebral hemorrhage. *Arch Neurol* 41:725, 1984.

ROSS RUSSELL RW: *Vascular Disease of the Central Nervous System*, 2nd ed. Edinburgh, Churchill Livingstone, 1983, pp 206–207.

SACCO RL, ELLENBERG JH, MOHR JP, et al: Infarcts of undetermined cause: The NINCDS stroke data bank. *Ann Neurol* 25:382, 1989.

SACCO SE, WHISNANT JP, BRODERICK JP, et al: Epidemiological characteristics of lacunar infarcts in a population. *Stroke* 22:1236, 1991.

SAGE JI, LEPORE FE: Ataxic hemiparesis from lesions of the corona radiata. *Arch Neurol* 40:449, 1983.

SAHS AL, NIBBELIN KDW, TORNER JC (eds): *Aneurysmal Subarachnoid Hemorrhage*. Baltimore, Urban & Schwarzenberg, 1981.

SAHS AL, NISHIOKA H, TORNER JC, et al: Cooperative study of intracranial aneurysms and subarachnoid hemorrhage: A long term prognostic study. *Arch Neurol* 41:1140, 1142, 1147, 1984.

SALAM-ADAMS M, ADAMS RD: Cerebrovascular disease by age group, in Vinken PJ, Bruyn GW, Klawans HL (eds): *Handbook of Clinical Neurology*: Vol 53. *Vascular Diseases*. Part I. Amsterdam, Elsevier, 1988, pp 27–46.

SANDOK BA, FURLAN AJ, WHISNANT JP, SUNDT TM JR: Guidelines for the management of transient ischemic attacks. *Mayo Clin Proc* 53:665, 1978.

SANDOK BA, GIULIANI ER: Cerebral ischemic events in patients with mitral valve prolapse. *Stroke* 13:448, 1982.

SARREL PM, LINDSAY DC, POOLE-WILSON PA, COLLINS P: Hypothesis: Inhibition of endothelium-derived relaxing factor by haemoglobin in the pathogenesis of pre-eclampsia. *Lancet* 336:1030, 1990.

SCHIEVINK WI: Intracranial aneurysms. *N Engl J Med* 336:28, 1997.

SCHIEVINK WI, BJORNSSON J, PARISI JE, PRAKASH UB: Arterial fibromuscular dysplasia associated with severe alpha 1-antitrypsin (alpha 1-AT) deficiency. *Mayo Clin Proc* 69:1040, 1994.

SCHMIDT WA, KRAFT HE, VORPAHL K, et al: Color duplex ultrasonography in the diagnosis of temporal arteritis. *N Engl J Med* 337:1336, 1997.

SCHWAB S, STEINER T, ASCHOFF A, et al: Early hemicraniectomy in patients with complete middle cerebral artery infarction. *Stroke* 29:1888, 1998.

SHIELDS RW JR, LAURENO R, LACHMAN T, VICTOR M: Anticoagulant-related hemorrhage in acute cerebral embolism. *Stroke* 15:426, 1984.

SIESJO BK: Historical overview: Calcium, ischemia, and death of brain cells. *Ann NY Acad Sci* 522:638, 1988.

SIGSBEE B, DECK MDF, POSNER JB: Nonmetastatic superior sagittal sinus thrombosis complicating systemic cancer. *Neurology* 29: 139, 1979.

SINGER DE: Randomized trials of warfarin for atrial fibrillation. *N Engl J Med* 327:1451, 1992.

SNEDDON JB: Cerebrovascular lesions and livedo reticularis. *Br J Dermatol* 77:180, 1965.

SO EL, TOOLE JF, DALAL P, MOODY DM: Cephalic fibromuscular dysplasia in 32 patients: Clinical findings and radiologic features. *Arch Neurol* 38:619, 1981.

SOLOMON RA, FINK ME: Current strategies for the management of aneurysmal subarachnoid hemorrhage. *Arch Neurol* 44:769, 1987.

STARKSTEIN SE, ROBINSON RG, PRICE TR: Comparison of cortical and subcortical lesions in the production of post-stroke mood disorders. *Brain* 110:1045, 1987.

STEWART RM, SAMSON D, DIEHL J, et al: Unruptured cerebral aneurysms presenting as recurrent transient neurologic deficits. *Neurology* 30:47, 1980.

ST LOUIS, WIJDICKS EF, LI H: Predicting neurologic deterioration in patients with cerebellar haematomas. *Neurology* 51:1364, 1998.

STOCKHAMMER G, FELBER SR, ZELGER B, et al: Sneddon's syndrome: Diagnosis by skin biopsy and MRI in 17 patients. *Stroke* 24:685, 1993.

STRAND T, ASPLUND K, ERIKSSON S, et al: A randomized control trial of hemodilution therapy in acute ischemic stroke. *Stroke* 15:980, 1984.

SUSAC JO, HARDMAN JM, SELHORST JB: Microangiopathy of the brain and retina. *Neurology* 29:313, 1979.

SWANSON RA: Intravenous heparin for acute stroke: What can we learn from the megatrials? *Neurology* 52:1746, 1999.

TAKAYASU M: A case with peculiar changes of the central retinal vessels. *Acta Soc Ophthalmol Jpn* 12:554, 1908.

Takebayashi S, Sakata N, Kawamura A: Reevaluation of miliary aneurysm in hypertensive brain: Recanalization of small hemorrhage? *Stroke* 21(suppl):1–59, 1990.

Taneda M, Hayakawa T, Mogami H: Primary cerebellar hemorrhage: Quadrigeminal cistern obliteration as a predictor of outcome. *J Neurosurg* 67:545, 1987.

Taomoto K, Asada M, Kamazawa Y, Matsumoto S: Usefulness of the measurement of plasma-thromboglobulin (b-TG) in cerebrovascular disease. *Stroke* 14:518, 1983.

The Magnetic Resonance Angiography in Relatives of Patients with Subarachnoid Hemorrhage Study Group: Risks and benefits of screening for intracranial aneurysms in first-degree relatives of patients with sporadic subarachnoid hemorrhage. *N Engl J Med* 341:1344, 1999.

Tijssen JG: Low-dose and high-dose acetylsalicylic acid, with and without dipyrimadole: A review of clinical trial results. *Neurology* 51(suppl 3):15, 1998.

Tippin J, Corbett JJ, Kerber RE, et al: Amaurosis fugax and ocular infarction in adolescents and young adults. *Ann Neurol* 26:69, 1989.

Ueda K, Toole JF, McHenry LC: Carotid and vertebral transient ischemic attacks: Clinical and angiographic correlation. *Neurology* 29:1094, 1978.

vander Eecken HM, Adams RD: Anatomy and functional significance of meningeal arterial anastomoses of human brain. *J Neuropathol Exp Neurol* 12:132, 1953.

van Gijn J, Van Donegen KJ, Vermeulen M, et al: Perimesencephalic hemorrhage: A nonaneurysmal and benign form of subarchnoid hemorrhage. *Neurology* 30:493, 1985.

Vessey MP, Lawless M, Yeates D: Oral contraceptives and stroke: Findings in a large prospective study. *Br Med J* 289:530, 1984.

Volhard F: Clinical aspects of Bright's disease, in Berglund H, et al (eds): *The Kidney in Health and Disease*. Philadelphia, Lea & Febiger, 1935, pp 665–688.

Vonsattel JP, Myers RH, Hedley-Whyte ET, et al: Cerebral amyloid angiopathy without and with cerebral hemorrhages: A comparative histological study. *Ann Neurol* 30:637, 1991.

Waga S, Yamamoto Y: Hypertensive putaminal hemorrhage—Treatment and results: Is surgical treatment superior to conservative? *Stroke* 14:486, 1983.

Weinberger J, Biscarra V, Weisberg MK: Factors contributing to stroke in patients with atherosclerotic disease of the great vessels: The role of diabetes. *Stroke* 14:709, 1983.

Weisberg LA: Lacunar infarcts. *Arch Neurol* 39:37, 1982.

Weisberg LA, Stazio A, Shamsnia M, Elliott D: Nontraumatic parenchymal brain hemorrhages. *Medicine* 69:277, 1990.

Weisman AD, Adams RD: The neurological complications of dissecting aortic aneurysm. *Brain* 67:69, 1944.

Weksler BB, Lewin M: Progress in cerebrovascular disease: Anticoagulation in cerebral ischemia. *Stroke* 14:658, 1983.

Weller C, Ringlestein B, Reiche W, et al: The large striatocapsular infarct. A clinical and pathophysiological entity. *Arch Neurol* 47:1085, 1990.

Whisnant JP, Matsumoto N, Elveback LR: Transient cerebral ischemic attacks in a community: Rochester, Minnesota, 1955 through 1969. *Mayo Clin Proc* 48:194, 1973.

White HD, Simes JS, Anderson NE, et al: Pravastatin therapy and the risk of stroke. *N Engl J Med* 343:317, 2000.

Wiebers DO: Ischemic cerebrovascular complications of pregnancy. *Arch Neurol* 42:1106, 1985.

Wiebers DO, Whisnant JP, O'Fallon WM: The natural history of unruptured intracranial aneurysms. *N Engl J Med* 304:696, 1981.

Wiebers DO, Whisnant JP, Sandok BA, O'Fallon WM: Prospective comparison of a cohort with asymptomatic carotid bruit and a population-based cohort without carotid bruit. *Stroke* 21:984, 1990.

Wiebers DO, Whisnant JP, Sundt TM, O'Fallon WM: The significance of unruptured intracranial saccular aneurysms. *J Neurosurg* 66:23, 1987.

Wijdicks EF, St Louis E: Clinical profiles predictive of outcome in pontine hemorrhage. *Neurology* 49:1342, 1997.

Wijdicks EFM, Ropper AH, Hunnicut EJ, et al: Atrial natriuretic factor and salt wasting after subarachnoid hemorrhage. *Stroke* 22:1519, 1991.

Wijdicks EFM, Vermeulen M, Hudra A, et al: Hyponatremia and cerebral infarction in patients with ruptured intracranial aneurysms: Is fluid restriction harmful? *Ann Neurol* 17:137, 1985.

Wolf PA, Kannel WB, McGee DL, et al: Duration of atrial fibrillation and imminence of stroke: The Framingham Study. *Stroke* 14:664, 1983.

Wood JH, Fleischer AS: Observations during hypervolemic hemodilution of patients with acute focal cerebral ischemia. *JAMA* 248:2999, 1982.

Yamashita M, Oka K, Tanaka K: Histopathology of the brain vascular network in moyamoya disease. *Stroke* 14:50, 1983.

Yanagihara P, Piepgras DG, Klass DW: Repetitive involuntary movement associated with episodic cerebral ischemia. *Ann Neurol* 18:244, 1985.

Chapter 35

CRANIOCEREBRAL TRAUMA

Among the vast array of neurologic diseases, cerebral trauma ranks high in order of frequency and gravity. In the United States, in persons up to 44 years of age, trauma is the leading cause of death, and more than half of these deaths are due to head injuries. Each year, according to the American Trauma Society, an estimated 500,000 Americans are admitted to hospitals following cerebral trauma; of these, 75,000 to 90,000 die and even larger numbers, most of them young and otherwise healthy, are left permanently disabled.

The basic problem in craniocerebral trauma is at once both simple and complex: simple because there is usually no difficulty in determining causation—namely, a blow to the head—complex because of a number of delayed effects that may complicate the injury. As for the trauma itself, nothing medical can be done, for it is finished before the physician arrives on the scene. At most there can be an assessment of the full extent of the immediate cerebral injury, an evaluation of factors conducive to complications and further lesions, and the institution of measures to avoid such additional problems. But of the disastrous intracranial phenomena that can be initiated by head injury, several fall within the purview of the neurologist, for they are secondary effects that evolve during the period of medical observation, offering possibilities of treatment.

It is a common misconception that craniocerebral injuries are matters that concern only the neurosurgeon and not the general physician or neurologist. Actually, some 80 percent of head injuries are first seen by a general physician in an emergency department, and probably fewer than 20 percent ever require neurosurgical intervention of any kind—even this number is decreasing. Often neurologists must take charge of the head-injured patient, or their opinion is sought in consultation. To enact their role effectively, they must be familiar with the clinical manifestations and the natural course of the primary brain injury and its complications and have a sound grasp of the underlying physiologic mechanisms. Such knowledge must be up to date and immediately applicable, particularly as it relates to the interpretation of computed tomography (CT) scans and magnetic resonance imaging (MRI), both of which have greatly enhanced our ability to deal with head trauma and its complications. The present chapter reviews the salient facts concerning craniocerebral injuries and outlines a clinical approach that the authors have found useful over the years. Matters pertaining to spinal injury are considered in Chap. 44.

DEFINITIONS AND MECHANISMS

The very language that one uses to discuss certain types of head injury divulges a number of misconceptions inherited from previous generations of physicians. Certain words have crept into the medical vocabulary and have often been retained long after the ideas for which they stood have been refuted—attesting to the disadvantage of premature adoption of explanatory terms rather than descriptive ones. The word *concussion*, for example, implies a violent shaking or jarring of the brain and a resulting transient functional impairment. Yet despite numerous postulates of physical changes within nerve cells, axons, or myelin sheaths (vibration effects, formation of intracellular vacuoles, etc.), little convincing confirmation of their existence has been possible in humans or in experimental animals. Similarly the word *contusion*, meaning a bruising of cerebral tissue without interruption of its architecture, is applied rather indiscriminately to a variety of clinical states, some of which could not depend on a pathologic change of this type, e.g., "minor contusion state or syndrome"—an expression introduced by Wilfred Trotter, who was himself most critical of words that "embalm a fallacious theory."

In all attempts to analyze the mechanisms of *closed*, or *blunt* (*nonpenetrating*), head injury, one fact stands pre-eminent—that there must be the sudden application of a physical force of considerable magnitude to the head. Unless the head is struck, the brain suffers no injury—except in the rare instances of violent flexion-extension (whiplash) of the neck and somewhat controversial cases of crush injury to the chest or explosive injury with a sudden extreme increase of intrapulmonary pressure. The factors of particular importance in brain injury are the differential mobility of the head and brain, the tethering of the cerebral hemispheres at the upper brainstem, and the differing densities of the gray and white matter. As pointed out below, all concussive injuries involve a physical force that imparts motion to the stationary head or a hard surface that arrests the motion of the moving head. This is the basis of most civilian head injuries, and they are notable in two respects: (1) they frequently induce at least a temporary loss of consciousness and (2) even though the skull is not penetrated, the brain may suffer gross damage, i.e., contusion, laceration, hemorrhage, and swelling. A theory that would bring into plausible form these gross neuropathologic changes and the transient loss of consciousness (concussion) or prolonged coma has been formulated only in relatively recent years.

By contrast, high-velocity missiles may penetrate the skull and cranial cavity or, rarely, the skull may be compressed between two converging forces that crush the brain without causing significant displacement of the head or the brain. In these circumstances the patient may suffer severe and even fatal injury without immediate loss of consciousness. Hemorrhage, destruction of brain tissue, and, if the patient survives for a time, meningitis or abscess are the principal pathologic changes created by injuries of these types. They offer little difficulty to our understanding. These various types of head injuries are illustrated in Fig. 35-1.

The relation of *skull fracture* to brain injury has been viewed in changing perspective throughout the history of this subject. In the first half of the century, fractures dominated the thinking of the medical profession, and cerebral lesions were regarded as secondary. Later, it became known that the skull, though rigid, is

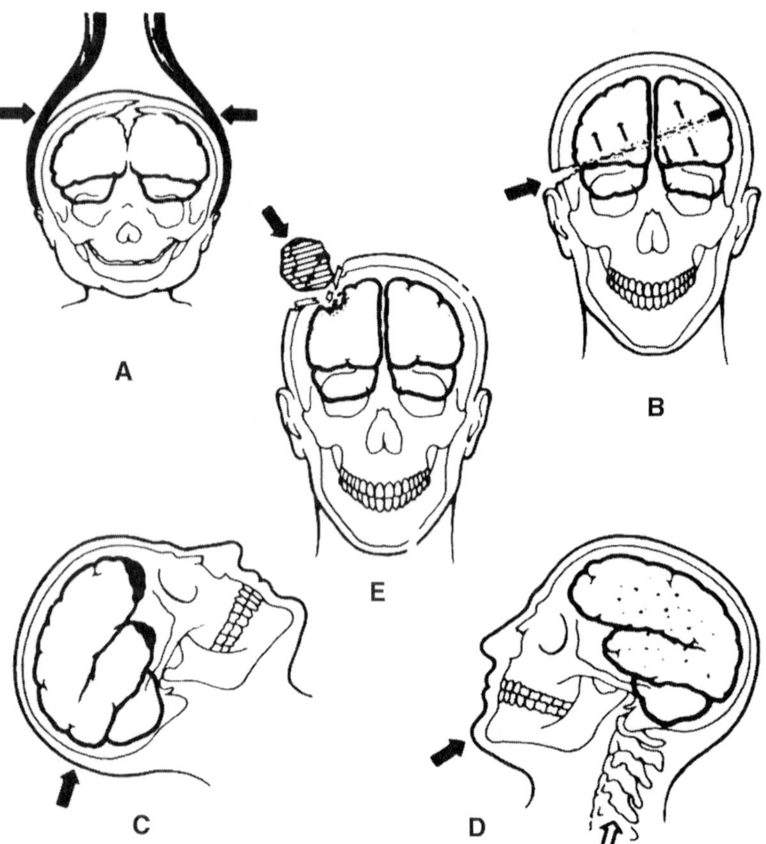

Figure 35-1

Mechanisms of craniocerebral injury. A. *Cranium distorted by forceps (birth injury).* B. *Gunshot wound of the brain.* C. *Falls (also traffic accidents).* D. *Blows on the chin ("punch drunk").* E. *Injury to skull and brain by falling objects. [From Courville (a study based upon a survey of lesions found in a series of 15,000 autopsies). By permission.]*

still flexible enough to yield to a blow that could injure the brain without causing fracture. Therefore, the presence of a fracture, although a rough measure of the force to which the brain has been exposed, is no longer considered an infallible index of the presence of cerebral injury. Even in fatal head injuries, autopsy reveals an intact skull in some 20 to 30 percent of cases (see also page 933). Contrariwise, many patients suffer skull fractures without serious or prolonged disorder of cerebral function, in part because the energy of a blow is dissipated in the fracture.

The modern trend is to be concerned primarily with the presence or absence of brain injury rather than with the fracture of the skull itself. Nevertheless, fractures cannot be dismissed without further comment for several reasons. The presence of a fracture always warns of the possibility of cerebral injury. Overall, brain injury is estimated to be 5 to 10 times more frequent with skull fracture than without and perhaps 20 times more frequent with severe injuries. Moreover, fractures assume importance in indicating the site and possible severity of brain damage, in providing an explanation for cranial nerve palsies, and in creating potential pathways for the ingress of bacteria and air or the egress of cerebrospinal fluid (CSF). In all these respects, fractures through the base of the skull are of special significance (more so than those of the cranial vault) and are considered below.

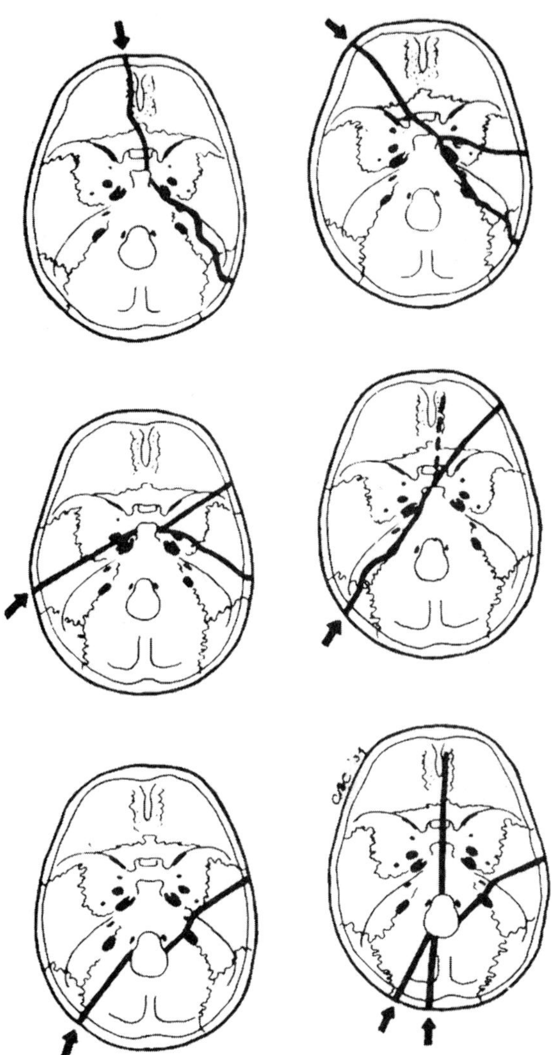

Figure 35-2

The course of fracture lines through the base of the skull. Arrows indicate point of application and direction of force. (From Courville by permission.)

Basal Skull Fractures and Cranial Nerve Injuries

Some of the major sites and directions of basilar skull fractures are indicated in Fig. 35-2. One can readily perceive the possibilities of injury to cranial nerves in relation to such fractures. Fractures of the base are often difficult to detect in plain skull films, but their presence should always be suspected if any one of a number of characteristic clinical signs is in evidence. Fracture of the petrous pyramid often deforms the external auditory canal or tears the tympanic membrane, with leakage of CSF (otorrhea); or, blood may collect behind an intact tympanic membrane and discolor it. If the fracture extends more posteriorly, damaging the sigmoid sinus, the tissue behind the ear and over the mastoid process becomes boggy and discolored (Battle sign). Basal fracture of the anterior skull may cause blood to leak into the periorbital tissues, imparting a characteristic "raccoon" or "panda bear" appearance. The presence of any of these signs calls for CT scanning of the skull base using bone window settings.

Commonly the existence of a basal fracture is indicated by signs of cranial nerve damage. The olfactory, facial, and auditory nerves are the ones most liable to injury, but any one, including the twelfth, may be damaged. *Anosmia and an apparent loss of taste* (actually a loss of perception of aromatic flavors, since the elementary modalities of taste—salt, sweet, bitter, sour—are unimpaired) are frequent sequelae of head injury, especially with falls on the back of the head. In the majority of cases the anosmia is permanent. If unilateral, it will not be noticed by the patient. The mechanism of these disturbances is thought to be a displacement of the brain and tearing of the olfactory nerve filaments in or near the cribriform plate, through which they course.

A fracture in or near the sella may tear the stalk of the pituitary gland, with resulting *diabetes insipidus*, impotence and reduced libido, and amenorrhea. Rarely such a fracture may cause bleeding from a pre-existing pituitary adenoma and produce the syndrome of pituitary apoplexy (page 717). A fracture of the sphenoid bone may lacerate the optic nerve, with blindness from the beginning. The pupil is unreactive to a direct light stimulus but still reacts to a light stimulus to the opposite eye (consensual reflex). The optic disc becomes pale, i.e., atrophic, after an interval of several weeks. Partial injuries of the optic nerve may result in scotomas and a troublesome blurring of vision.

Complete *oculomotor nerve injury* is characterized by ptosis, a divergence of the globes with the affected eye resting in an abducted and elevated position, loss of medial and vertical movements of the eye, and a fixed, dilated pupil. Diplopia—worse on looking down—and compensatory tilting of the head suggest *trochlear nerve* injury. In a series of 60 patients with recent head injury, Lepore found that fourth nerve palsy was the commonest cause of diplopia, occurring unilaterally twice as often as bilaterally, followed in frequency by damage to one or both third nerves, then, least frequently, to the sixth nerves. Five of his patients had palsies that reflected damage to more than one nerve, and seven had supranuclear disorders of convergence. These optic and ocular motor nerve disorders must be distinguished from those due to displacement of the globe by direct injury to the orbit and the oculomotor muscles.

Injury to the *ophthalmic and maxillary divisions of the trigeminal nerve* may be the result of either a basal fracture across the middle cranial fossa or a direct extracranial injury to the branches of the nerves. Numbness and paresthesias of the skin supplied by the nerve(s) or a neuralgia can be troublesome sequelae of these injuries.

The *facial nerve* may be involved in one of two ways. In one, associated with transverse fractures through the petrous bone, there is an immediate facial palsy, probably due to transection of the nerve. Surgical anastomosis has sometimes been successful in this circumstance. In the second, more common type, associated with longitudinal fractures of the petrous bone, the facial palsy is delayed for several days—a sequence that may be misinterpreted as progression of the intracranial traumatic lesion. The second type is usually transitory, and its mechanism is not known.

Injury to the *eighth cranial nerve*, due to petrous fractures, results in a loss of hearing or in postural vertigo and nystagmus coming on immediately after the trauma. Deafness due to nerve injury must be distinguished from the high-tone hearing loss due to *cochlear* injury and from deafness caused by bleeding into the middle ear, with disruption of the ossicular chain (conduction deafness). Also, vertigo must be distinguished from posttraumatic giddiness. A fracture through the hypoglossal canal causes weakness of one side of the tongue. It should be kept in mind that blows to the upper neck may also cause lower cranial nerve palsies, either by direct injury to their peripheral extensions or as a result of *carotid artery dissection*, either of its cervical or intracranial segment.

Carotid-Cavernous Fistula

A basal fracture through the sphenoid bone may lacerate the internal carotid artery or one of its intracavernous branches, where it lies in the cavernous sinus. Within hours or a day or two, a disfiguring pulsating exophthalmos develops as arterial blood enters and distends the superior and inferior ophthalmic veins that empty into the sinus. The orbit feels tight and painful, and the eye may become partially or completely immobile because of pressure on the oculomotor nerves, which traverse the sinus (Fig. 14-3). The sixth nerve is affected most often and the third and fourth nerves less frequently. Also, there may be a loss of vision, due to ischemia of the optic nerve and retina; congestion of the retinal veins and glaucoma are additional factors in the visual failure. Some 5 to 10 percent of fistulas resolve spontaneously, but the remainder must be obliterated by interventional radiologic means (by a detachable balloon inserted via a catheter transfemorally) or by a direct surgical repair of the fistula (Stern).

Not all carotid-cavernous fistulas are traumatic. They may occasionally occur with rupture of an intracavernous saccular aneurysm or in Ehlers-Danlos disease, where the connective tissue is defective; or the cause may be unexplained.

Pneumocephalus, Aerocele, and Rhinorrhea (Cerebrospinal Fluid Leak)

If the skin over a skull fracture is lacerated and the underlying meninges are torn, or if the fracture passes through the inner wall of a paranasal sinus, bacteria may enter the cranial cavity, with resulting meningitis or abscess. Also, CSF may leak into the sinus and present as a watery discharge from the nose (*CSF rhinorrhea*). The nasal discharge can be identified as CSF by testing it for glucose with diabetic test tape (mucus has no glucose) or for the presence of fluorescein or iodinated water-soluble dye that is injected into the lumbar subarachnoid space and then absorbed by pledgets placed in the nasal cavity. Most cases of acute CSF rhinorrhea heal by themselves. If the condition is persistent or is complicated by an episode of meningitis, repair of the torn dura mater is indicated. The prophylactic use of antibiotics to prevent meningitis from a CSF leak is not favored, but many neurosurgeons continue this practice, particularly in children (see page 743).

A collection of air in the cranial cavity (aerocele) is a common occurrence following skull fracture or an extended neurosurgical procedure. It is usually found (by CT scan) in the epidural or subdural space over the convexities or between the hemispheres and serves only to warn of a potential route for the entry of bacteria into the cranium. Small collections of air are usually absorbed without incident, but a large collection of air may act as a mass and cause clinical deterioration after injury (tension pneumocranium; Fig. 35-3). Inhalation of 100% oxygen has a transient salutary effect, but needle aspiration of the air is required if it is causing clinical signs (Fig. 35-3).

Depressed ("derby hat") fractures are of significance only if the underlying dura is lacerated or the brain is compressed by indentation of bone. They should then be surgically repaired, preferably within the first 24 to 48 h.

Figure 35-3

CT of postoperative tension pneumocranium (aerocele) that caused progressive drowsiness and required removal by aspiration. The air is apparent as a very low density collection that compresses the frontal lobes.

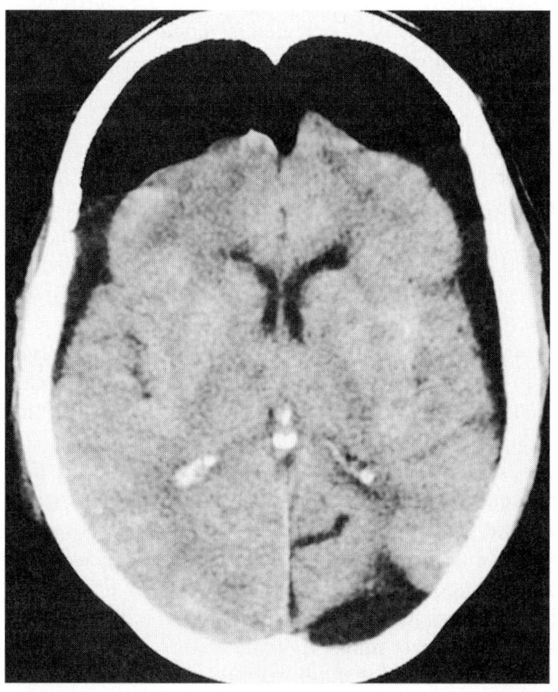

Cerebral Concussion

Mechanisms of Concussion Much has been written about the mechanisms of concussion and coma in closed, or blunt, head injury. Certain facts concerning these conditions stand out: (1) Concussion, meaning a *reversible traumatic paralysis of nervous function*, is always immediate (not delayed even by seconds). (2) The effects of concussion on brain function may last for a variable time (seconds, minutes, hours, or longer). To set arbitrary limits on the duration of loss of consciousness—i.e., to consider a brief loss as indicative of concussion and a prolonged loss as indicative of contusion or other traumatic cerebral lesion, as proposed in some medical writings—is illogical and unsound physiologically. As pointed out by Symonds, any such difference is quantitative, not qualitative. Admittedly, in the more prolonged states of coma, there is a greater chance of finding hemorrhage and contusion, which undoubtedly contribute to the persistence of coma and the likelihood of irreversible change. (3) The optimal condition for the production of concussion, demonstrated originally by Denny-Brown and Russell, is a change in the momentum of the head; i.e., either movement is imparted to the head by a blow or movement of the head is arrested by a hard, unyielding surface. These two types of blunt (nonpenetrating) head injury are called *accelerative* and *decelerative*, respectively.

The mechanism of concussive cerebral paralysis has been interpreted in various ways throughout medical history in light of the state of scientific knowledge at a particular time. The favored hypotheses for the better part of a century were "vasoparalysis" (suggested by Fischer in 1870) or an arrest of circulation by an instantaneous rise in intracranial pressure (proposed by Strohmeyer in 1864 and popularized by Trotter in 1932). Jefferson, in his essay on the nature of concussion (1944), convincingly refuted these vascular hypotheses; later, Shatsky and coworkers, by the use of high-speed cineangiography, showed displacement of vessels but no arrest of circulation immediately after impact.

Beginning with the work of Denny-Brown and Russell in 1941, the physical factors involved in head and brain injury have been subjected to careful analysis. These investigators demonstrated, in the monkey and cat, that concussion resulted when the freely moving head was struck by a heavy mass. If the head was prevented from moving at the moment of impact, the same degree of force invariably failed to produce concussion. More recently, the importance of head motion per se was verified by Gennarelli and colleagues, who were able to induce concussion in primates by rapid acceleration of the head without impact, a condition that rarely occurs in humans.

Holbourn (1943), a Cambridge physicist, from a study of gelatin models under conditions simulating head trauma, deduced that when the head is struck, movement of the partly tethered but suspended brain always lags (inertia); but inevitably the brain moves also, and when it does it must rotate, for it occupies a round skull whose motions (because of attachment to the neck) usually describe an arc. Pudenz and Sheldon and later Ommaya and coworkers (1974) proved the correctness of this assumption by photographing the brain through a transparent (Lucite) calvarium at the moment of impact. The brain is thus subjected to shearing stresses set up by rotational forces centered at its point of tethering in the high midbrain and subthalamus. The torque at the level of the upper reticular formation would explain the immediate loss of consciousness, as described below. Also, these rotational movements of the brain provide a reasonable explanation for the occurrence of surface injuries in certain places, i.e., where the swirling brain comes into contact with bony prominences on the inner surface of the skull (petrous and orbital ridges, sphenoid wings), and of injuries to the corpus callosum, which is flung against the falx.

These views on the site and mechanism of concussion were supported by a number of additional observations. Foltz and Schmidt, in 1956, suggested that the reticular formation of the upper brainstem was the anatomic site of concussive injury. They showed that in the concussed monkey, lemniscal sensory transmission through the brainstem was unaltered but its effect in activating the high reticular formation was blocked. They also demonstrated that the electrical activity of the medial reticular formation was depressed for a longer time and more severely than that of the cerebral cortex.

In 1956 and again in 1961, Strich described the neuropathologic findings in patients who died months after severe closed head injuries that had caused immediate and protracted coma. In all of her cases—in which there were no signs of skull fracture, raised intracranial pressure, or gross subarachnoid hemorrhage—she observed an uneven but diffuse degeneration of the cerebral white matter. In cases of shorter survival (up to 6 weeks), she observed ballooning and interruption of axis cylinders. These findings were subsequently confirmed by Nevin, by J. H. Adams and colleagues, and by Gennarelli et al, the last of these groups working with monkeys. It is noteworthy that in most of these cases and subsequent ones reported by Jellinger and Seitelberger, there were also lesions in the region of the reticular activating system and small hemorrhagic softenings in the corpus callosum, superior cerebellar peduncles, and dorsolateral tegmentum of the midbrain. Strich interpreted the extensive white matter lesions, both in the hemispheres and in the brainstem, to represent a primary degeneration of nerve fibers that had been stretched or torn by the shear stresses set up during rotational acceleration of the head (*diffuse axonal injury*), as had been postulated earlier by Holbourn. She suggested that if nerve fibers are stretched rather than torn, the lesions may be reversible and may play a part in the production of concussion. Symonds elaborated this view. He saw in the shearing stresses—which are maximal at the point where the cerebral hemispheres rotate on the relatively fixed brainstem (i.e., at the midbrain-subthalamic level)—the explanation of concussion.

Clinical Manifestations of Concussion The immediate abolition of consciousness, suppression of reflexes (falling to the ground if standing), transient arrest of respiration, a brief period of bradycardia, and fall in blood pressure following a momentary rise at the time of impact are the characteristic clinical signs of concussive injury. Rarely, if these abnormalities are sufficiently intense, death may occur at this moment, presumably from respiratory arrest. Usually the vital signs return to normal and stabilize within a few seconds while the patient remains unconscious. The plantar reflexes are extensor. Then, after a variable period of time, the patient begins to stir and opens his eyes but is unseeing. Corneal, pharyngeal, and cutaneous reflexes, originally depressed, return, and the limbs are withdrawn from painful stimuli. Gradually contact is made with the environment, and the patient begins to obey simple commands and respond slowly and inadequately to simple questions. Memories are not formed during this period; the patient may even carry on a conversation which, later on, he cannot recall. Finally there is full recovery, corresponding to the time when the patient can form consecutive memories of current experiences. The time required for the patient to pass through these stages of recovery may be only a few seconds or minutes, several hours, or possibly days; but again, between these extremes there are only quantitative differences, varying with the intensity of the process. To the observer, such patients are comatose only from the moment of injury until they open their eyes and begin to speak; for the patient, the period of unconsciousness extends from a point before the injury occurred (*retrograde amnesia*) until the time when he is able to form consecutive memories—namely, at the end of the period of anterograde amnesia. The duration of the amnesic period, particularly of *anterograde amnesia*, is the most reliable index of the severity of the concussive injury. If there is no disturbance or loss of consciousness, none of the lesions described below are to be found.

Pathologic Changes Associated with Severe Head Injury

In fatal cases of head injury, the brain is often bruised, swollen, and lacerated and there may be hemorrhages, either meningeal or intracerebral, and hypoxic-ischemic lesions. The prominence of these pathologic findings were responsible for the long-prevailing view that cerebral injuries are largely a matter of bruises (*contusions*), hemorrhages, and the need for urgent operations. That this can hardly be the case is indicated by the fact that some patients survive and make an excellent recovery from head injuries that are clinically as severe or almost as severe as the fatal ones. One can only conclude, therefore, that most of the immediate symptoms of severe head injury depend on invisible and highly reversible changes, i.e., the changes underlying concussion.

The effects of bruises, lacerations, hemorrhages, localized swellings, white matter necroses, and herniations of tissue should not be minimized, since they are probably responsible for or contribute to many of the fatalities that occur 12 to 72 h or more after the injury. As pointed out by Jennett, a majority of patients who remain in coma for more than 24 h after a head injury are found to have intracerebral hematomas. Of these lesions, the most important are contusions of the surface of the brain beneath the point of impact (*coup lesion*) and the more extensive lacerations and contusions on the side opposite the site of impact (*contrecoup lesion*) as shown in Fig. 35-4. Blows to the front of the head produce mainly coup lesions, whereas blows to the back of the head

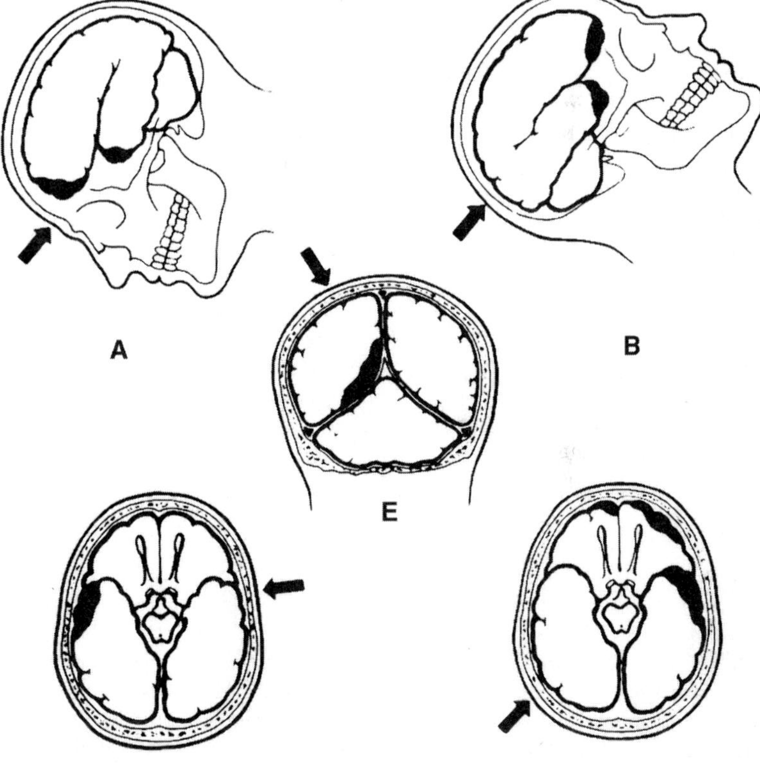

Figure 35-4

Mechanisms of cerebral contusion. Arrows indicate point of application and direction of force; black areas indicate location of contusion. A. *Frontotemporal contusion consequent to frontal injury.* B. *Frontotemporal contusion following occipital injury.* C. *Contusion of temporal lobe due to contralateral injury.* D. *Frontotemporal contusion due to injury to opposite temporo-occipital region.* E. *Diffuse mesial temporo-occipital contusion due to blow on vertex. (From Courville by permission.)*

cause mainly contrecoup lesions (sometimes coup lesions as well). Blows to the side of the head produce either coup or contrecoup lesions or both. Irrespective of the site of the impact, the common sites of cerebral contusions are in the frontal and temporal lobes, as illustrated in Figs. 34-4 and 35-5. The inertia of the malleable brain—which causes it to be flung against the side of the skull that was struck, to be pulled away from the contralateral side, and to rotate against bony promontories within the cranial cavity—explains these coup-contrecoup contusions. As noted, the experimental studies of Ommaya and others indicate that the effects of linear acceleration of the head are much less significant than those due to rotation. Relative sparing of the occipital lobes in coup-contrecoup injury is explained by the smooth inner surface of the occipital bones and tentorium.

The contused area of cortex is diffusely swollen and hemorrhagic, most of the blood being found around parenchymal vessels. On CT scanning, the contusions appear as edematous regions of cortex and subcortical white matter admixed with areas of increased density representing leaked blood (Fig. 35-5). The bleeding points may coalesce and give the appearance of a clot in the cortex and immediately subjacent white matter. The predilection of these lesions for the crowns of convolutions attests to their traumatic origin (being thrown against the overlying skull) and distinguishes them from cerebrovascular and other cerebral lesions.

Figure 35-5

CT scan without contrast infusion showing areas of hemorrhagic contusion adjacent to bony prominences.

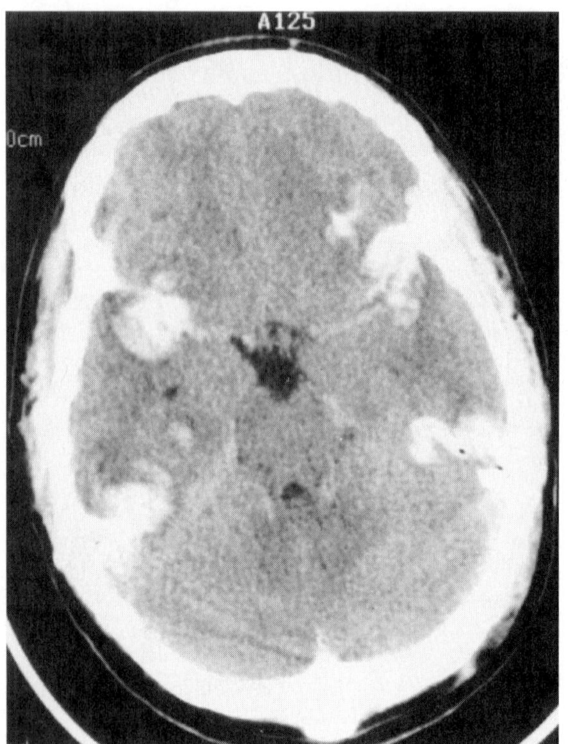

In nearly all cases of severe head injury there is damage to the corpus callosum by impact with the falx; necrosis and hemorrhage are sometimes visible by CT scanning and can be seen to spread to adjacent white matter. Also, there may be scattered hemorrhages in the white matter along lines of force from the point of impact. Areas of white matter degeneration of the type described by Strich may also be present. In the authors' pathologic material, these white matter lesions tend to be focal, some in regions near hemorrhages, contusions, and ischemic lesions and others at a distance, along transcallosal and ascending and descending tracts that had been interrupted by such lesions. As indicated earlier, the degeneration of white matter can be remarkably diffuse, with no apparent relationship to focal destructive lesions. This *diffuse axonal injury*, as it is now generally designated, and the callosal and midbrain injuries are the predominant abnormalities in many cases of severe head injury. Recent investigations using MRI, such as the one by Kampfl and colleagues, indicate that diffuse injury of this type is a common substrate of the persistent vegetative state. They found a pattern of damage in the corpus callosum, corona radiata, and the dorsolateral midbrain tegmentum that conformed closely to pathologic changes in cases of diffuse axonal injury. But in all of our cases of severe cranial injury and protracted coma, there were zones of ischemia and old hemorrhages in the midbrain and subthalamus—i.e., in the zones subjected to the greatest torque—and we continue to favor these as the critical lesions in cases of persistent coma (Ropper and Miller). This was true also of the cases of persistent coma described by Jellinger and Seitelberger. It should be pointed out that in the aforementioned study by Kampfl there were MRI lesions in the thalamic region in only 40 percent of cases. Notable again is the fact that these deep lesions coincide with the postulated locus of reversible concussive paralysis.

Primary brainstem hemorrhages, as described above, are to be distinguished from the secondary so-called Duret hemorrhages resulting from the effects of downward and lateral displacement of the brainstem (transtentorial herniations). Duret originally emphasized the medullary location of these hemorrhages, but the term *Duret hemorrhage* has come to signify any secondary brainstem hemorrhage.

In addition to contusions and extradural, subdural, subarachnoid, and intracerebral hemorrhages, there are variable degrees of vasogenic edema, which increases in the first 24 to 48 h, and zones of infarction, apparently due to vascular spasm from subarachnoid blood surrounding basal vessels, similar to the situation that pertains in aneurysmal subarachnoid hemorrhage. Marmarou et al have convincingly demonstrated that *brain swelling* after head injury is essentially the result of edema and not of an increase in cerebral blood volume, as has long been postulated. In children and in some cases in adults, the cerebral edema may be massive and lead to secondary brainstem compression (see page 941).

APPROACH TO THE PATIENT WITH HEAD INJURY

The physician first called upon to attend a patient who has had a closed (blunt) head injury will generally find the patient in one of three clinical conditions, each of which must be dealt with differently. Usually it is possible to categorize the patient in this way by assessing his mental and neurologic status when first seen and at intervals after the accident. In many emergency wards and intensive care units, the *Glasgow Coma Scale* is used as a rapid and effective means to accomplish this purpose (Table 35-1). The scores provided by this scale have been found to correspond roughly with outcome of the head injury, as discussed further on.

Table 35-1
Glasgow Coma Scale
(Total score is used for serial assessment and prognosis)

Eyes open	
Never	1
To pain	2
To verbal stimuli	3
Spontaneously	4
Best verbal response	
No response	1
Incomprehensible sounds	2
Inappropriate words	3
Disoriented and converses	4
Oriented and converses	5
Best motor response	
No response	1
Extension (decerebrate rigidity)	2
Flexion abnormal (decorticate rigidity)	3
Flexion withdrawal	4
Localizes pain	5
Obeys	6
Total	3–15

Patients Who Are Conscious or Are Rapidly Regaining Consciousness (Minor Head Injury)

This is the most frequently encountered clinical situation. Roughly, two degrees of disturbed function can be recognized within this category. In one, the patient was not unconscious at all but only stunned momentarily or "saw stars." This injury is insignificant when judged in terms of life or death and brain damage—though, as we point out further on, there is always the possibility of a skull fracture or the later development of an epidural or subdural hematoma. Moreover, the patient is still liable to a troublesome posttraumatic syndrome—consisting of headache, giddiness, fatigability, insomnia, and nervousness—which may appear soon after or within a few days of the injury. In the second instance, consciousness was temporarily abolished for a few seconds or minutes, i.e., the patient was concussed. When such a patient is first seen, recovery may already be complete, or he may be in one of the stages of recovery described earlier under "Clinical Manifestations of Concussion." Even though mentally clear, the patient may have an amnesia for events immediately preceding and following the injury. Thereafter, headache and other symptoms of the posttraumatic syndrome or compensation neurosis may develop.

In most cases of this type, there is little need of a neurologic consultation, and hospitalization is not required provided that a responsible family member is available to report any change in the clinical state. In only a small group of these patients, mainly in those who are slow in regaining consciousness or have a skull fracture, is there significant risk of ongoing hemorrhage or other delayed complications. Whether to obtain films of the head routinely in such patients is an unresolved problem. In our litigious society, the physician is inclined to do so. If there is no fracture and the patient is mentally clear, Jennett estimates that there is only one chance in a thousand of developing an intracranial (extradural) hemorrhage. He states that this increases to 1 in 30 in patients with a fracture; but most studies, such as the one by Lloyd and colleagues, have found that the presence of a skull fracture in children is a relatively poor indicator of intracranial injury.

These minor and seemingly trivial head injuries may sometimes be followed by a number of puzzling and worrisome clinical phenomena, some insignificant, others serious and indicative of a pathologic process other than concussion. The latter are described below. When they occur, a neurologic or neurosurgical evaluation is indicated.

Delayed Fainting after Head Injury Following an accident, the injured person, after walking about and seeming to be normal, may turn pale and fall unconscious to the ground. Recovery occurs within a few seconds or minutes. This is a vasodepressor syncopal attack, related to pain and emotional upset and differing in no way from the syncope that follows pain and fright without injury. Such syncopal attacks also occur with injuries that spare the head, but with head injury they become more difficult to interpret.

Denny-Brown described a more severe type of delayed posttraumatic collapse that we have seen only rarely. Again, the patient appears to be recovering from a blow to the head, which may simply have dazed him or caused a brief period of unconsciousness, when suddenly, after a period of several minutes to hours, he collapses and becomes unresponsive. The most disquieting feature of this clinical state is a marked bradycardia, which, coupled with the lucid interval, raises the specter of an evolving epidural hemorrhage (actually, bradycardia is a late and inconstant sign of epidural bleeding). However, intracranial pressure is not raised, the disorder fails to develop further, and—following a brief period of restlessness, vomiting, and headache—the patient recovers completely over a period of several days. Denny-Brown suggested that this form of delayed posttraumatic collapse was due to a contusion of the medulla, but how this explains the sequence of clinical events is not clear. The authors believe it to be a severe form of vasodepressor syncope.

A more serious form of delayed collapse after head injury is described further on under "Concussion Followed by a Lucid Interval."

Drowsiness, Headache, and Confusion This syndrome occurs most often in children, who, after a concussive or nonconcussive head injury, seem not to be themselves. They lie down, are drowsy, complain of headache, and may vomit—symptoms that suggest the presence of an epidural or subdural hemorrhage. Mild focal edema near the point of impact may be seen on MRI. There is usually no skull fracture. The symptoms subside after a few hours, attesting to the benign nature of the condition.

Transient Traumatic Paraplegia, Blindness, and Migrainous Phenomena With falls or blows on top of the head, both legs may become temporarily weak and numb, with bilateral Babinski signs and sometimes with sphincteric incontinence. Blows to the occiput may cause temporary blindness. The symptoms disappear after a few hours. It seems unlikely that these transient symptoms represent a direct localized concussive effect, caused either by indentation of the skull or by impact of these parts of the brain against the inner table of the skull. A concussion of the cervical portion of the spinal cord is another suggested but improbable mechanism of transient paraplegia. The blindness and paraplegia are usually followed by a throbbing vascular type of headache. Transient migrainous visual phenomena, aphasia, or hemiparesis, followed by a headache, are observed sometimes in athletes who participate in competetive contact sports. Probably all of these phenomena are due to an attack of migraine or migraine equivalent induced by a blow to the head. This can be perplexing for a few hours, especially if it is the first such attack of migraine in a child. Another clinical possibility, particularly in acute quadriplegic cases, is cartilagenous embolism of the cervical cord (page 1321).

Delayed Hemiplegia In our experience, most examples of these disorders have occurred in male adolescents or young adults who, some hours after a relatively minor athletic or road injury, developed a massive hemiplegia, homonymous hemianopia, or aphasia (with left-sided lesions). Imaging or ultrasound may reveal a *dissection of the internal carotid artery*. The dissection may occur in the intracranial portion of the carotid artery and should be sought by MR angiography or arteriography if the hemiparesis has no other explanation. In other instances, particularly after a blow to the neck, a mural thrombus forms in the carotid, which, in turn, may shed an embolus to the anterior or middle cerebral artery. In yet other instances, the hemiplegia has no explanation other than the blow to the head.

Other causes of delayed hemiplegia are a late evolving epidural or subdural hematoma and, in more severe injuries, an intracerebral hemorrhage (occasionally from a pre-existent arteriovenous malformation).

Most of these are associated with a diminution in the level of consciousness.

Fat Embolism With fractures of large bones, there may be, after 24 to 72 h, an acute onset of pulmonary symptoms (dyspnea and hyperpnea) followed by coma with or without focal signs; this sequence is due to systemic fat embolism, first of the lungs and then of the brain. In some cases the onset of pulmonary symptoms is associated with a petechial rash over the thorax, and one in three cases is said to show fat globules in the urine. Respiratory distress is the most important and often the only feature of the fat embolism syndrome, evident in the chest film as fluffy infiltrates in both lungs. In the brain, the fat emboli cause widespread petechial hemorrhages, involving both white and gray matter and a few larger infarcts. Most cases of fat embolism recover spontaneously in 3 or 4 days, although a mortality rate of up to 10 percent is quoted, usually related to the underlying injuries.

Patients Who Have Been Comatose from the Time of Head Injury

Here the central problem, so ably set forth by Symonds, is the relationship between concussion and contusion. Since consciousness is abolished at the moment of injury, one can hardly doubt the existence of concussion in such cases; but when hours and days pass without consciousness being regained, the second half of the usual definition of concussion—namely, that the paralysis of cerebral function be transitory—is not satisfied. Careful pathologic examination of such cases usually discloses evidence of increased intracranial pressure and of cerebral contusions, lacerations, subarachnoid hemorrhage, zones of infarction, and scattered intracerebral hemorrhages—both at the point of injury (coup) and on the opposite side (contrecoup), in the corpus callosum, and between these points, along the *line of force* of the injury. In some patients, the diffuse axonal type of injury is the most prominent abnormality; in others, there are separate but strategically placed ischemic and hemorrhagic lesions in the upper midbrain and lower thalamic region, as already mentioned. The tissue around the contusions is swollen, and in postmortem preparations the white matter in these regions appears pale in myelin stains. Varying amounts of blood in the subdural space are usually present. A major shift of the thalamus and midbrain is frequently present, the latter with compression of the opposite cerebral peduncle against the free margin of the tentorium as well as secondary midbrain hemorrhages and zones of necrosis; in some cases, there is frank transtentorial herniation.

It should be kept in mind that severe head injury is associated with an immediate arrest of respiration and sometimes with bradyarrhythmia and cardiac arrest. The effects on the brain of these systemic changes may in themselves be sufficiently profound to cause coma. Also, head injury often complicates alcohol and drug ingestion, so that the possibility of a toxic or metabolic encephalopathy as the cause (or a contributing cause) of stupor must always be considered.

Within this category of severe head injury and protracted coma, three clinical subgroups can be recognized: one in which cerebral and other bodily injuries are incompatible with survival; *a second* in which improvement sets in within a few days or a week or two, followed by variable degrees of recovery but leaving the patient with residual neurologic signs; and *a third* and relatively small group in which the patients remain permanently comatose, stuporous, or profoundly reduced in their cerebral capacities. Of course there are many degrees of injury that fall between these three arbitrary subgroups. In all of these patients, following the initial period of stabilization, the matters of interest are the clinical and radiologic assessment, with the purpose of uncovering a surgically remediable lesion—namely a subdural or epidural hematoma—or a treatable intraparenchymal hematoma. In most cases, the discovery of such a mass lesion mandates surgical removal. But unless it is the only lesion, the procedure often proves to be insufficient and coma is likely to persist because of the associated cerebral damage. The recognition and management of these hematomas are described further on in this section.

The *first subgroup* comprises patients who are so severely injured that their lives are obviously endangered. When first seen, such a patient may be in shock (possibly from rupture of a visceral organ or injury of the cervical cord), with hypotension, hypothermia, fast, thready pulse, and pale, moist skin. If this state persists along with deep coma, widely dilated fixed pupils, absent eye movements and corneal and pharyngeal reflexes, flaccid limbs, stertorous and irregular respirations or respiratory failure, death usually follows in a short time. Once respiration ceases and the EEG becomes isoelectric, the clinical state corresponds to brain death, as described on page 371. However, the diagnosis of brain death should not be made immediately after injury, in order to allow time to exclude the effects of anoxia, drug or alcohol intoxication, and hypotension. In some of these patients, the blood pressure and respirations stabilize, and the degree of cerebral injury can then be evaluated over a period of hours by observing the depth of coma and the temperature, pulse, and blood pressure. Deep coma with subnormal temperature and rising pulse rate are grave prognostic signs, as are a rapidly rising temperature and pulse rate with rapid, irregular respirations. In some fatal cases, the temperature continues to rise until the end, when there is circulatory collapse.

Small linear or rounded hemorrhages are seen in a nonenhanced CT scan. These hemorrhages are evidently consequent upon rotational forces acting on the upper brainstem and corpus callosum (Fig. 35-6).

In this category of severe cerebral injury, where the patients survive for only a few hours or days, postmortem examination commonly discloses cerebral contusion and focal hemorrhage, necrosis of tissue, and brain swelling. In the Traumatic Coma Data Bank, which included 1030 gravely injured patients with Glasgow Coma Scale scores of 8 or less, 21 percent had subdural hematomas, 11 percent had intracerebral clots, and 5 percent had epidural hematomas. Notable, however, is the fact that half the patients had no mass lesions on the CT scan. On the basis of CT criteria, these patients were thought to have diffuse axonal injury, although it coexisted with mass lesions in many cases. In 50 consecutive autopsies of such severely injured patients, summarized in an earlier era by Rowbotham, all but two showed macroscopic changes. The lesions in these cases consisted of surface contusions (48 percent), lacerations of the cerebral cortex (28 percent), subarachnoid hemorrhage (72 percent), subdural hematoma (15 percent), extradural hemorrhage (20 percent), and skull fractures (72 percent). As these figures indicate, several of these changes were found in the same patient. Moreover, trauma of extracranial organs and tissues is frequent and obviously contributes to the fatal outcome.

Figure 35-6

CT scan from a patient with diffuse axonal injury. There are multiple small hemorrhagic areas (one of which is circled) in the cerebral white matter and corpus callosum.

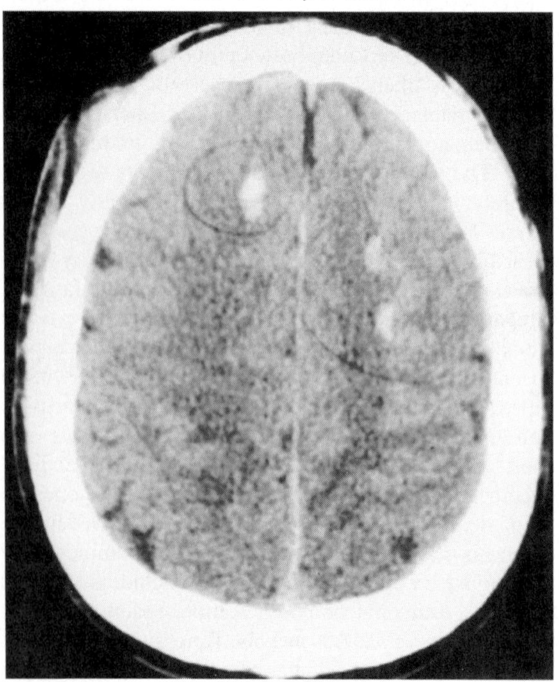

In respect to *the second subgroup*, i.e., the relatively less severe and seldom fatal head injuries, all gradations in tempo and degree of recovery can be observed. In the least severely injured of this group, recovery of consciousness begins in a few hours, although there may be a relapse within the first day or two as a result of swelling of the contused brain tissue, enlargement of a subdural hematoma, brain hemorrhage, or infarction, the last provoked by arterial spasm in relation to subarachnoid hemorrhage. The CSF is usually bloody. Eventually, recovery may be nearly complete, but the period of traumatic amnesia covers a span of several days or even weeks. It should be repeated that occasionally penetrating types of injuries and depressed fractures may seriously damage the brain without causing concussion at all, but here we are considering only the blunt, nonpenetrating head injuries.

In this second subgroup, the sequence of clinical events is the same as that described in relation to concussion except that their duration is more protracted. Stupor gives way to a confusional state that may last for weeks, and it may for a variable period be associated with aggressive behavior and uncooperativeness (traumatic delirium). The period of traumatic amnesia is proportionately longer than in the less severely injured. It is during the period of recovery of consciousness that focal neurologic signs (hemiparesis, aphasia, abulia, etc.) become more obvious, though some unilateral signs may have been discerned during the comatose period. Once the patient improves to the point of being able to converse, he is demonstrably slow in thinking, with few mental associations; unstable in emotional reactions; and faulty in judgment—a state sometimes referred to as "traumatic dementia."

Finally there is that relatively small, distressing group of *severely brain-injured patients in whom the vital signs become normal but who never regain full con-*

sciousness. As the weeks pass, the prospects become more bleak. Such a patient, especially if young, may still emerge from coma after 6 to 12 weeks and make a surprisingly good though usually an incomplete recovery, but such instances are decidedly rare. Some of those who survive for long periods open their eyes and move their heads and eyes from side to side but betray no evidence of seeing or recognizing even the closest members of their families. They do not speak and are capable of only primitive postural or reflex withdrawal movements. Jennett and Plum referred to this as the "persistent vegetative state" (see page 369). Fourteen percent of the patients in the Traumatic Coma Data Bank were left in this state. Hemiplegia or quadriplegia with varying degrees of decerebrate or decorticate posturing is usually demonstrable. Life is mercifully terminated after several months or years by some medical complication. Our colleague, R. D. Adams, has examined the brains of 14 patients who remained in coma and in vegetative states from one to 14 years. All showed extensive zones of necrosis and hemorrhage in the upper brainstem.

In generalizing about this category of head injury, i.e., patients who are and have been comatose from the time of injury, the effects of contusion, hemorrhage, and brain swelling often become evident within 18 to 36 h after the injury and then may progress for several days. If the patients survive this period, their chances of dying from complications of these effects—such as increased intracranial pressure, herniations of the temporal lobe, subdural hemorrhage, hypoxia, and pneumonia—are greatly reduced. The mortality rate of those who reach the hospital in coma is about 20 percent, and most of the deaths occur in the first 12 to 24 h as a result of direct injury to the brain in combination with other nonneurologic injuries. Of those alive at 24 h, the overall mortality falls to 7 to 8 percent; after 48 h, only 1 to 2 percent succumb. There is some evidence that transfer of such patients to an intensive care unit, where they can be monitored by personnel experienced in the handling of head injury, improves the chances for survival (see further on).

Concussion Followed by a Lucid Interval and Serious Cerebral Damage

This group is smaller than the other two but is of great importance because it includes a disproportionate number of patients who are in urgent need of surgical treatment. The initial coma may have lasted only a few minutes or, exceptionally, there may have been none at all—in which instance one might wrongly conclude that since there was no concussion, there is no possibility of traumatic hemorrhage or other type of brain injury.

Patients who display this serious sequence of events, referred to as "talk and die" by Marshall and associates, deteriorate because of the delayed expansion of a small subdural hematoma, a worsening brain edema, or occasionally the late appearance of an epidural clot. Among 34 such patients in the Traumatic Coma Data Bank (Marshall et al), the majority showed substantial degrees of midline shift on the initial CT scan, reflecting the presence of brain edema and contusion. A similar condition of delayed intracerebral hematoma discussed further on (*Spätapoplexie*) is a feature of a severe initial head injury that engenders coma from the onset and places the patient at great risk. The following conditions must be considered in all cases of these delayed types.

Acute Epidural Hemorrhage As a rule, this condition is due to a temporal or parietal fracture with laceration of the middle meningeal artery or vein. Less often, there is a tear in a dural venous sinus. The injury, even when it fractures the skull, may not have produced coma initially, or it may be part of a devastating craniocerebral injury. A far more typical example is that of a child who has fallen from a bicycle or swing or has suffered some other hard blow to the head and was unconscious only momentarily. A few hours or a day later (exceptionally, with venous bleeding, the interval may be several days or a week), headache of increasing severity develops, with vomiting, drowsiness, confusion, aphasia, seizures (which may be one-sided), hemiparesis with slightly increased tendon reflexes, and a Babinski sign. As coma develops, the hemiparesis may give way to bilateral spasticity of the limbs and Babinski signs. When the patient remains untreated, the respirations become deeper and stertorous, then shallow and irregular; finally, they cease. The pulse is often slow (below 60 beats per minute) and bounding, with a concomitant rise in systolic blood pressure (Cushing effect). The pupil may dilate on the side of the hematoma. Physicians need not be reminded that lumbar puncture is contraindicated in this setting, now that CT and MRI are available. Death, which is almost invariable if the clot is not removed surgically, comes at the end of a comatose period and is due to respiratory arrest. The visualization of a fracture line across the groove of the middle meningeal artery and knowledge of which side of the head was struck (the clot is usually on that side) are of aid in diagnosis and lateralization of the lesion. However, meningeal vessels may be torn without fracture. The CT scan reveals a lens-shaped clot with a smooth inner margin (Fig. 35-7). The surgical procedure consists of placement of burr holes or, preferably, a craniotomy, drainage of the hematoma, and identification and ligation of the bleeding vessel. The operative results are excellent except in the cases with extended fractures and laceration of the dural venous sinuses, in which the epidural hematoma may be bilateral rather than unilateral, as it ordinarily is. If coma, bilateral Babinski signs, spasticity, or decerebrate rigidity supervene before operation, it usually means that displacement of central structures and crushing of the midbrain have already occurred; prognosis for life is then poor. Small epidural hemorrhages, followed by serial CT scanning, will be seen to enlarge gradually for a week or two and then be absorbed.

Acute and Chronic Subdural Hematomas The problems created by acute and chronic subdural hematomas are so different that they must be discussed separately. In *acute subdural hematoma*, which may be unilateral or bilateral, there may be a brief lucid interval between the blow to the head and the advent of coma. Or, more often, the patient is comatose from the time of the injury and the coma deepens progressively. Frequently the acute subdural hematoma is combined with epidural hemorrhage, cerebral contusion, or laceration. The clinical effects of these several lesions are difficult to distinguish; there are some patients in whom it is impossible to state before operation whether the clot is epidural or subdural in location. Subdural clots more than 5 mm thick can be accurately visualized by the CT scan in more than 90 percent of cases (Fig. 35-8). A large acute clot causes a pineal shift as well as marked compression of one lateral ventricle; but if the lesion is bilateral, there may be no shift and the ventricles appear symmetrical.

Acute, rapidly evolving subdural hematomas are due to tearing of bridging veins, and symptoms are caused by compression of the brain by an expanding clot of fresh blood. Unlike epidural arterial hemorrhage, which is steadily progressive, venous bleeding is usually arrested by the rising intracranial pressure.

Exceptionally, *the subdural hematoma forms in the posterior fossa* and gives rise to headache, vomiting, pupillary inequality, dysphagia, cranial nerve palsies, and, rarely, stiff neck and ataxia of the trunk and gait if the patient is well enough to be tested for these functions. Because of their apposition to bone or their axial orien-

Figure 35-7

Acute epidural hematoma; unenhanced CT scan showing a typical lenticular-shaped frontal epidural clot.

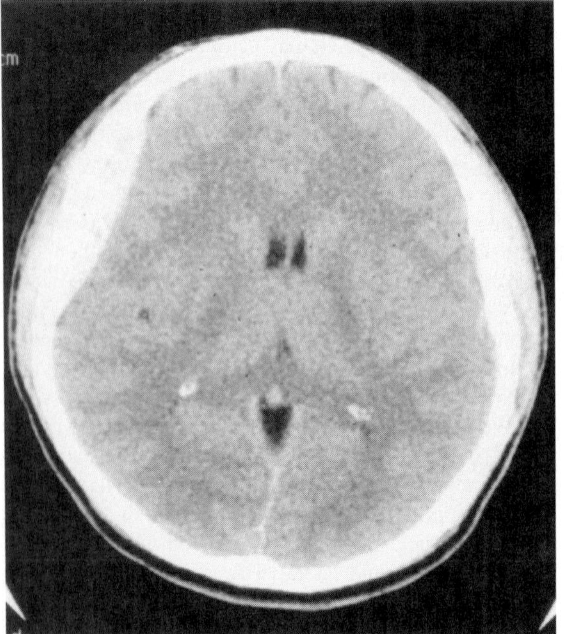

Figure 35-8

Acute subdural hematoma over the right convexity, with substantial mass effect (displacement) of brain tissue, but little edema.

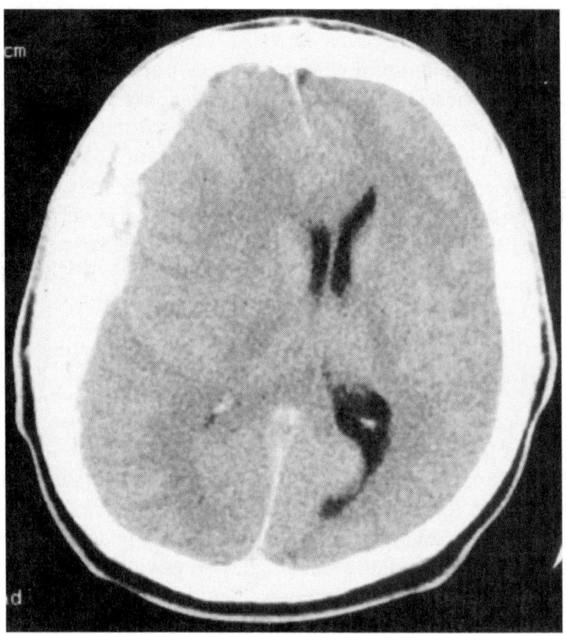

tation along the tentorial dura, posterior fossa clots are more likely to be missed in CT scans than clots over the cerebral convexities.

In *chronic subdural hematoma*, the traumatic etiology is often less clear. The head injury, especially in elderly persons and in those taking anticoagulant drugs, may have been trivial and may even have been forgotten. A period of weeks then follows when headaches (not invariable), light-headedness, slowness in thinking, apathy and drowsiness, and occasionally a seizure or two are the main symptoms. The initial impression may be that the patient has a vascular lesion or brain tumor or is suffering from drug intoxication, a depressive illness, or Alzheimer disease. As with acute subdural hematoma, the disturbances of mentation and consciousness (drowsiness, inattentiveness, incoherence of thinking, and confusion) are more prominent than focal or lateralizing signs, and they may fluctuate. The focal signs usually consist of hemiparesis and rarely of an aphasic disturbance. Homonymous hemianopia is seldom observed, probably because the geniculocalcarine pathway is deep and not easily compressed; similarly, hemiplegia, i.e., complete paralysis of one arm and leg, is usually indicative of a lesion within the cerebral hemisphere rather than a compressive lesion on its surface. An important feature of the hemiparesis is that it may sometimes be ipsilateral, depending on whether the contralateral cerebral peduncle has been compressed against the free edge of the tentorium by horizontal displacement (Kernohan-Woltman false localizing sign; see page 367). If the condition progresses, the patient becomes stuporous or comatose but often with striking fluctuations of awareness.

Dilatation of the ipsilateral pupil is a more reliable indicator of the side of the hematoma than the hemiparesis, though the side of pupillary abnormality may also be misleading (occurring on the opposite side in 10 percent of cases, according to Pevehouse and coworkers). Convulsions are seen occasionally, most often in alcoholics or in patients with cerebral contusions, but they cannot be regarded as a cardinal sign of subdural hematoma. Rare cases of internuclear ophthalmoplegia and of chorea have been reported but have not occurred in our material. Presumably they are a result of distortion of deep structures. Also, transient disturbances of neurologic function simulating transient ischemic attacks (TIAs) may occur. In infants and children, enlargement of the head, vomiting, and convulsions are prominent manifestations of subdural hematoma (see page 1053).

CT scanning with contrast infusion and MRI are the most reliable diagnostic procedures. On CT scans, the clot is initially hyperdense but becomes isodense after a period of time (Fig. 35-9), during which it may be difficult to detect except by the tissue shifts it causes; It then becomes progressively hypodense (with respect to the cortex) over the first 2 to 6 weeks. The evolution of signal changes in the MRI are similar to the sequential changes of parenchymal hematomas. The acute clot is hypointense on T2-weighted images, reflecting the presence of deoxyhemoglobin. Over the subsequent weeks, all image sequences show it as hyperintense as a result of methemoglobin formation. Eventually the chronic clot again becomes hypointense on the T1-weighted images. With contrast infusion, both imaging procedures usually reveal the vascular and reactive border surrounding the clot. Usually, by the fourth week, sometimes later, the hematoma becomes hypodense, typical of a chronic subdural hygroma.

Other formerly used investigative measures are seldom necessary but are mentioned here for completeness and in the event that the diagnosis is made in the course of evaluating some other neurologic problem.

Figure 35-9

Subacute subdural hematoma. CT scans after administration of intravenous contrast material. The lesion is isodense, but its margin can be appreciated with contrast enhancement. Note displacement of cerebral structures.

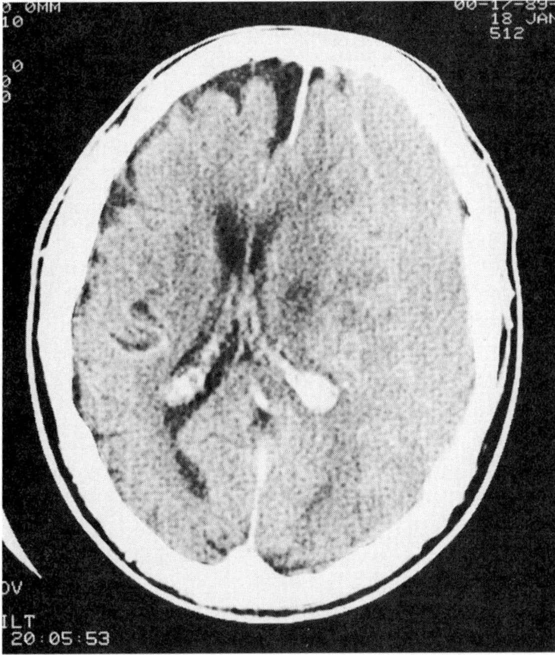

Skull films are helpful when there is calcification surrounding a chronic hematoma, a calcified pineal that is shifted to one side, or an unexpected fracture line is found. The EEG is usually abnormal bilaterally, sometimes with reduced voltage or electrical silence over the hematoma and high-voltage slow waves over the opposite side, because of the damping effects of the clot and displacement of the brain, respectively. In an arteriogram, the cortical branches of the middle cerebral artery are separated from the inner surface of the skull, and the anterior cerebral artery may be displaced contralaterally. The CSF may be clear and acellular, but more often is bloody or xanthochromic, depending on the presence or absence of recent or old contusions and subarachnoid hemorrhage; the pressure may be elevated or normal. A xanthochromic fluid with relatively low protein content should always raise the suspicion of chronic subdural hematoma.

The chronic subdural hematoma becomes encysted by fibrous membranes (pseudomembranes) that grow from the dura. Some hematomas—probably the ones in which the initial bleeding was slight (see below)—resorb spontaneously. Others expand slowly and act as space-occupying masses (Fig. 35-10). Gardner, in 1932, first postulated that the gradual enlargement of the hematoma was due to the accession of fluid, particularly CSF—which was drawn into the hemorrhagic cyst by its increasing osmotic tension—as red blood cells hemolyzed and protein was liberated. This hypothesis, which came to be widely accepted, is not supported by the available data. Rabe and colleagues demonstrated that the breakdown of red cells contributes little if at all to the accumulation of fluid in the subdural space. According to the latter authors, the most important factor in the accumulation of subdural fluid is a pathologic permeability of the developing capillaries in the outer pseudomembrane. The CSF plays no discernible role in this process, contrary to the original view of Munro and Merritt. In any event, as the hematoma enlarges, the compressive effects increase. Severe cerebral compression and displacement with temporal lobe–tentorial herniation are the usual causes of death.

Why somewhat less than one-half of all subdural hematomas remain solid and nonenlarging and the remainder liquefy and then enlarge is not known. The experimental observations of Labadie and Glover suggest that the volume of the original clot is a critical factor: the larger its initial size, the more likely that it will enlarge. An inflammatory reaction, triggered by the breakdown products of blood elements in the clot, appears to be an additional stimulus for growth as well as for neomembrane formation and its vascularization.

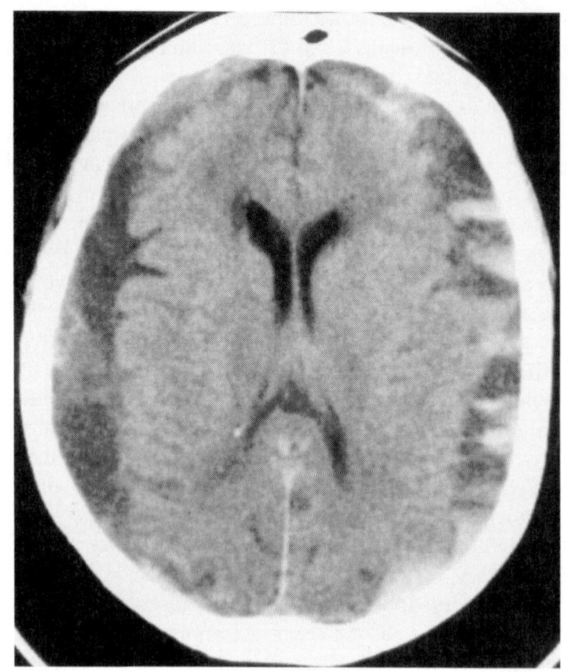

Figure 35-10

Chronic subdural hematomas over both cerebral hemispheres, without shift of the ventricular system. Chronicity results in hypodense appearance of the clots. Some old blood can still be seen on the right side. The bilaterally balanced masses result in an absence of horizontal displacement, but they may compress the upper brainstem.

Subdural hygroma (an encapsulated collection of xanthochromic fluid in the subdural space) may form after an injury as well as after meningitis (in an infant or young child). More often subdural hygromas appear without infection, presumably due to a ball-valve effect of an arachnoidal tear that allows fluid to collect in the space between the arachnoid and the dura; brain atrophy is conducive to this process. Occasionally a hygroma originates from a tear in an arachnoidal cyst. It may be difficult to differentiate a long-standing subdural hematoma from hygroma, and some chronic subdural hematomas are probably the result of repeated small hemorrhages that arise from the membranes of hygromas. In the past, subdural hygroma also occurred as a complication of pneumoencephalography. Shrinkage of the hydrocephalic brain after ventriculoperitoneal shunting is also conducive to the formation of a subdural hematoma or hygroma, in which case drowsiness, confusion, irritability, and low-grade fever are relieved when the subdural fluid is aspirated or drained. In adults, hygromas are usually asymptomatic and do not require treatment.

Treatment of Subdural Hematoma In most cases of acute hematoma, it is sufficient to place burr holes and evacuate the clot before deep coma has developed. Treatment of larger hematomas consists of wide craniotomy to permit control of the bleeding and removal of the clot. As one would expect, the interval between loss of consciousness and the surgical drainage of the clot is perhaps the most important determinant of outcome in serious cases. Thin, crescentic clots can be observed over several weeks and surgery undertaken only if focal signs develop or indications of increasing intracranial pressure arise (headache, vomiting, and bradycardia). Small subdural hematomas causing no symptoms and followed by CT scans will self-absorb, leaving only a deep yellow, sometimes calcified membrane attached to the inner dural surface.

The surgical results are less certain than in chronic subdural hematoma. If the clot is too small to explain the coma or other symptoms, there is probably extensive contusion and laceration of the cerebrum. In other, more chronic hematomas, a craniotomy must be performed and an attempt made to strip the membranes that surround the clot. This diminishes the likelihood of reaccumulation of fluid but is not always successful. Other causes of operative failure are swelling of the compressed hemisphere or failure of the hemisphere to expand after removal of a large clot. Elderly patients may be slow to recover after removal of the hematoma or may have a prolonged period of confusion. Postoperative expansion of the brain can be followed by serial CT scans.

Although no longer a common practice, the administration of corticosteroids is an alternative to surgical removal of subacute and chronic subdural hematomas in patients with minor symptoms or with some contraindication to surgery. Headache and other symptoms such as gait difficulty or limb clumsiness may resolve satisfactorily after several weeks of medication and may remain abated when the steroids are slowly reduced.

Cerebral Contusion Severe closed head injury is almost universally accompanied by cortical contusions and surrounding edema. The mass effect of contusional swelling, if sufficiently large, is a major factor in the genesis of tissue shifts and raised intracranial pressure. The CT appearance of contusion has already been described (page 931; see also Figs. 35-4 and 35-5). In the first few hours after injury, the bleeding points in the contused area may appear small and innocuous. The main concern, however, is the tendency for a contused area to swell or to develop a hematoma. This may give rise to clinical deterioration hours to days after the injury, sometimes abrupt in onset and concurrent with the appearance of swelling of the damaged region on the CT scan. It has been claimed, on uncertain grounds, that the swelling in the region of an acute contusion is precipitated by excessive administration of intravenous fluids (fluid management is considered further on in this chapter).

Traumatic Intracerebral Hemorrhage One or several intracerebral hemorrhages may be apparent immediately after head injury or hemorrhage may be delayed in its development by several days (*Spätapoplexie*). It may occur in the subcortical white matter of one lobe of the brain or in deeper structures, such as the basal ganglia or thalamus. The injury is nearly always severe; blood vessels as well as cortical tissue are torn.

The clinical picture is similar to that of hypertensive brain hemorrhage (deepening coma with hemiplegia, a dilating pupil, bilateral Babinski signs, stertorous and irregular respirations). It may be manifest by an abrupt rise in intracranial pressure. In elderly patients, it is sometimes difficult to determine whether a fall was the cause or the result of an intracerebral hemorrhage. Craniotomy with evacuation of the clot has given a successful result in a few cases, but the advisability of surgery is governed by several factors, including the level of consciousness, the time from the initial injury, and the associated damage that is shown by imaging studies. The wider application of intracranial pressure monitoring and of CT scans at intervals after the injury should facilitate diagnosis and perhaps help to elucidate the pathogenesis of the delayed hemorrhage(s).

Acute Brain Swelling in Children This condition is seen in the first hours after injury and may prove rapidly fatal. The CT scan shows enlargement of both hemispheres and compression of the basal cisterns. There is usually no papilledema in the early stages, during which the child hyperventilates, vomits, and shows extensor posturing. The presumption has been that this represents a loss of regulation of cerebral blood flow and a massive increase in the blood volume of the brain. The administration of excessive water in intravenous fluids may contribute to the problem and should be avoided. We have not observed this complication in head-injured adults.

Penetrating Wounds of the Head

Missiles and Fragments All the descriptions in the preceding pages apply to blunt, nonpenetrating injuries of the skull and their effects on the brain. The disorders included in this section are more the concern of the neurosurgeon than the neurologist. In the past, the care of penetrating craniocerebral injuries was mainly the preoccupation of the military surgeon, but—with the increasing amount of violent crime in western society—such cases have become commonplace on the emergency wards of general hospitals.

In civilian life, *missile injuries* are essentially caused by bullets fired from rifles or handguns at high velocities. Air is compressed in front of the bullet so that it has an explosive effect upon entering tissue and causes damage for a considerable distance around the missile track. *Missile fragments*, or *shrapnel*, are pieces of exploding shells, grenades, or bombs and are the usual causes of penetrating cranial injuries in wartime. The cranial wounds that result from missiles and shrapnel have been classified by Purvis as (1) tangential injuries, with scalp lacerations, depressed skull fractures, and meningeal and cerebral lacerations; (2) penetrating injuries with in-driven metal particles, hair, skin, and bone fragments; and (3) through-and-through wounds.

If the brain is penetrated at the lower levels of the brainstem, death is instantaneous because of respiratory and cardiac arrest. Even through-and-through wounds at higher levels, as a result of energy dissipated in the brain tissue, damage vital centers sufficiently to cause death immediately or within a few minutes in 80 percent of cases. If vital centers are untouched, the immediate problem is intracranial bleeding and rising intracranial pressure from swelling of the traumatized brain tissue.

Once the initial complications are dealt with, the surgical problems, as outlined by Meirowsky, are reduced to three: (1) prevention of infection by rapid and radical (definitive) debridement, accompanied by the administration of broad-spectrum antibiotics; (2) control of increased intracranial pressure and shift of midline structures by removal of clots of blood and the vigorous administration of mannitol or other dehydrating agents as well as dexamethasone; and (3) the prevention of life-threatening systemic complications.

When first seen, the majority of patients with penetrating cerebral lesions are comatose. A small metal fragment may penetrate the skull without causing concussion, but this is not true of high-velocity missiles. In a series of 132 cases of the latter type analyzed by Frazier and Ingham, consciousness was lost in 120. The depth and duration of coma seemed to depend upon the degree of cerebral necrosis, edema, and hemorrhage. In the Traumatic Coma Data Bank Series, the mortality rate in 163 patients who were initially comatose from a cranial gunshot wound was 88 percent—more than twice the mortality that results from severe blunt head injury. Upon emerging from coma, the patient passes through states of stupor, confusion, and amnesia, not unlike those of severe closed head injuries. Headache, vomiting, vertigo, pallor, sweating, slowness of pulse, and elevation of blood pressure are other common findings. Focal or focal and generalized seizures occur in the early phase of the injury in some 15 to 20 percent of cases.

Recovery may take many months. Frazier and Ingham comment on the "loss of memory, slow cerebration, indifference, mild depression, inability to concentrate, sense of fatigue, irritability, vasomotor and cardiac instability, frequent seizures, headaches and giddiness, all reminiscent of the residual symptoms from severe closed head injury with contusions." Every possible combination of focal cerebral symptoms may be caused by such lesions. The classic articles by Feiring and Davidoff and also by Russell and by Teuber, listed at the end of this chapter, are still very useful references on this subject.

Epilepsy is the most troublesome sequela and is described below. Ascroft and also Caviness, in reviewing World War II cases, found that approximately half of all patients with wounds that had penetrated the dura eventually developed epilepsy, most often focal in nature; the figures reported by Caveness for Korean War veterans are about the same (see discussion below).

CSF rhinorrhea, discussed earlier and in Chap. 30, may occur as an acute manifestation of a penetrating injury that produces a fracture through the frontal, ethmoid, or sphenoid bones. Cairns listed these acute cases as a separate group in his classification of CSF rhinorrheas, the others being (1) a delayed form after craniocerebral injury, (2) a form that follows sinus and cranial surgery, and (3) a spontaneous variety. *Pneumoencephalocele (aerocele)*—i.e., air entering the cerebral subarachnoid space or ventricles spontaneously or as a result of sneezing or blowing the nose—is evidence of an opening from the paranasal sinus through the dura.

Crushing Injuries of the Skull Aside from the absence of concussion, these relatively rare cerebral lesions present no special clinical features or neurologic problems not already discussed.

Birth Injuries These involve a unique combination of physical forces and circulatory-oxygenation factors and are discussed separately in Chap. 38.

SEQUELAE OF HEAD INJURY

Posttraumatic Epilepsy Epilepsy is the most common delayed sequela of craniocerebral trauma, with an overall incidence of about 5 percent in patients with closed head injuries and 50 percent in those who had sustained a compound skull fracture and wound of the brain. The basis is nearly always a contusion or laceration of the cortex. As one might expect, the risk of developing posttraumatic epilepsy is related to the severity of the head injury. In a civilian cohort of 2747 head-injured patients described by Annegers and colleagues, the risk of seizures after severe head injury (loss of consciousness or amnesia for more than 24 h, including subdural hematoma and brain contusion) was 7 percent within 1 year and 11.5 percent in 5 years. If the injury was only moderate (unconsciousness or amnesia for 30 min to 24 h or causing only a skull fracture), the risk fell to 0.7 and 1.6 percent, respectively. After mild injury (loss of consciousness or amnesia of less than 30 min) the incidence of seizures was not significantly greater than in the general population. In a subsequent study (1998), Annegers et al expanded the original cohort to include 4541 children and adults with cerebral trauma. The results were much the same as those of the first study except that in patients with mild closed head injuries, there was only a slight excess risk of developing seizures—a risk that remained elevated only until the fifth year after injury. The likelihood of epilepsy is said to be greater in parietal and posterior frontal lesions, but it may arise from lesions in any area of the cerebral cortex. Also, the frequency of seizures is considerably higher after penetrating cranial injury, as cited above.

The interval between the head injury and the first seizure varies greatly. A small number of patients have a generalized seizure within moments of the injury (*immediate epilepsy*). Usually this amounts to a brief tonic extension of the limbs, with slight shaking movements immediately after concussion, followed by awakening in a mild confusional state. Whether this represents a true epileptic phenomenon or, as appears more likely, is the result of arrest of cerebral blood flow is unclear. Some 4 to 5 percent of hospitalized head-injured individuals are said to have one or more seizures within the first week of their injury (*early epilepsy*). Immediate seizures have a good prognosis; on the other hand, late epilepsy is significantly more frequent in patients who had experienced early epilepsy (Jennett). In medical writings, the term *posttraumatic epilepsy* usually refers to late epilepsy, i.e., to seizures that develop several weeks or months after the head injury (1 to 3 months in most cases). Approximately 6 months after injury, half the patients who will develop epilepsy have had their first attack, and by the end of 2 years the figure rises to 80 percent (Walker). The interval between head injury and development of seizures is said to be longer in children. The longer the interval, the less certain one is of its relation to the traumatic incident. Data derived from a 15-year study of military personnel with severe (penetrating) brain wounds indicate that patients who escape seizures for 1 year after injury can be 75 percent certain of remaining seizure-free; patients without seizures for 2 years can be 90 percent certain; and for 3 years, 95 percent certain. For the less severely injured (mainly closed head injuries), the corresponding times are 2 to 6 months, 12 to 17 months, and 21 to 25 months (Weiss et al).

Posttraumatic seizures (both focal and generalized) tend to decrease in frequency as the years pass, and a significant number of patients (10 to 30 percent, according to Caveness) eventually stop having them. Individuals who have early attacks (within a week of injury) are more likely to have a complete remission of their seizures than those whose attacks begin a year or so after injury. A low frequency of attacks is another favorable prognostic sign. Alcoholism has an adverse effect on this seizure state. We have observed some 25 patients with posttraumatic epilepsy in whom seizures had ceased altogether for several years, only to recur in relation to drinking. In these patients the seizures were precipitated by a weekend or even one evening of heavy drinking and occurred, as a rule, not when the patient was intoxicated but in the "sobering-up" period.

The Nature of the Epileptogenic Lesion This has been elusive. From the examination of old cortical contusions (*plaques jaunes*), one cannot, on morphologic grounds, determine whether the lesion had been epileptogenic. Electrocorticograms of the brain in regions adjacent to old traumatic foci reveal a number of electrically active zones adjacent to the scars. Microscopically these foci show neuronal loss and an increase of astrocytes. It is postulated that abnormalities of dendritic branching provide the groundwork for the excitatory focus. Other investigators favor deafferentation of residual cortical neurons as the cause of their increased irritability.

Treatment and Prophylaxis Usually the seizures can be controlled by a single anticonvulsant medication, and relatively few are recalcitrant to the point of requiring excision of the epileptic focus. The surgical results vary according to the methods of selection and techniques of operation. Under the best of neurosurgical conditions three decades ago, with careful selection of cases, Rasmussen (also Penfield and Jasper) was able to eradicate seizures in 50 to 75 percent of cases by excision of the focus, and the results currently are even better.

The use of anticonvulsant drugs to prevent the first seizure and subsequent epilepsy has its proponents and opponents. In one study, patients taking phenytoin developed fewer seizures at the end of the first year than a placebo group, but a year after medication was discontinued, the incidence was the same in the two groups. In another prospective double-blind study, one group of patients was given 60 mg phenobarbital and 200 mg phenytoin daily for 18 months and another group was untreated; at the end of 3- and 6-year periods, there was no significant difference in the occurrence of seizures between treated and untreated groups (Penry et al). Also, in a study of a large number of patients with penetrating head injuries, the prophylactic use of anticonvulsants was ineffective in preventing early seizures (Rish and Caveness).

Autonomic Dysfunction Syndrome in Traumatic Coma A troublesome consequence of severe head injury, observed most often in comatose patients and in those with the persistent vegetative state, is the occurrence of episodic violent extensor posturing, profuse diaphoresis, hypertension, and tachycardia lasting minutes to an hour. A slight fever may accompany the spells. Families and staff are greatly disturbed by the display, particularly when accompanying grimacing suggests suffering. These spells of hypersympathetic activity and posturing may be precipitated by painful stimuli or distension of a viscus, but often they arise spontaneously. The syndrome is often identified as a seizure and in many texts is still incorrectly referred to as "diencephalic epilepsy," but it is more likely the result of decortication, allowing the hypothalamus to function independently of normal inhibitory mechanisms. A survey of 35 such patients by Baugley and colleagues identified diffuse axonal injury and a period of hypoxia as being the main associated forms of injury, and this has been our experience as well. Narcotics and diazepines have a slight beneficial effect, but bromocriptine, which may be used in combination with sedatives or with small doses of morphine, has been most effective (Rossitch and Bullard).

Extrapyramidal and Cerebellar Disorders Following Trauma The question of a causative relationship between cerebral trauma and the development of Parkinson disease has been a controversial issue for many years—usually with the conclusion that it does not exist and that any apparent relationship is superficial and coincidental. Most such patients probably had early symptoms of Parkinson disease, brought to light by the head injury. There are, however, rare cases, such as the one reported by Doder and colleagues, in which traumatic necrosis of the lenticular and caudate nuclei was followed, after a period of 6 weeks, by the onset of predominantly contralateral parkinsonian signs, including tremor, which progressed slowly and were unresponsive to L-dopa. An exception to these statements may be a parkinsonian syndrome in ex-boxers, as a manifestation of the "punch-drunk" syndrome (see below). Cerebellar ataxia is a rare consequence of cranial trauma unless the latter was complicated by cerebral anoxia or a hemorrhage strategically placed in the deep midbrain or cerebellum. When cerebellar ataxia is due to the trauma itself, it is frequently unilateral and the result of injury to the superior cerebellar peduncle. An ataxia of gait may also reflect the presence of a communicating hydrocephalus.

"Punch-Drunk Encephalopathy" (Dementia Pugilistica) The cumulative effects of repeated cerebral injuries, observed in boxers who had engaged in many bouts over a long period of time, constitute a type of head injury that is difficult to classify. What is referred to is the development, after many years in the ring (sometimes toward the end of the boxer's career, more often within a few years of retirement), of dysarthric speech and a state of forgetfulness, slowness in thinking, and other signs of dementia. Movements are slow, stiff, and uncertain, especially those involving the legs, and there is a shuffling, wide-based gait. Often a parkinsonian syndrome emerges (found in 20 of the 52 cases that Roberts and coworkers abstracted from the literature up to 1969) and sometimes a moderately disabling ataxia. The plantar reflexes may be extensor on one or both sides. The EEG contains slow waves of theta and sometimes of delta type. The clinical syndrome was reanalyzed by Roberts and colleagues, who found it present to some degree in 37 of the 224 professional boxers they examined. More recent studies have shown that in about one-half of all professional boxers, both active and retired, the CT scan discloses ventricular dilatation and/or sulcal widening and a cavum septi pellucidi (why the latter, which is a developmental anomaly, would be overrepresented in boxers is unclear). These abnormalities had been demonstrated many years before, by pneumoencephalography, and were found to be related to the number of bouts (Ross et al; Casson et al).

A thorough pathologic study of this disorder has been made by Corsellis and associates. They examined the brains of 15 retired boxers who had shown the punch-drunk syndrome and identified a group of cerebral changes that appear to explain the clinical findings. Mild to moderate enlargement of the lateral ventricles and thinning of the corpus callosum were present in all cases. Also, practically all of them showed a greatly widened cavum septi pellucidi and fenestration of the septal leaves. Readily identified areas of glial scarring were situated on the inferior surface of the cerebellar cortex. In these areas and well beyond them, Purkinje cells were lost and the granule cell layer was somewhat thinned. Surprisingly, cerebral cortical contusions were found in only a few cases. Notably absent, also, was evidence of previous hemorrhage. Of the 15 cases, 11 showed varying degrees of loss of pigmented cells of the substantia nigra and locus ceruleus, and many of the cells that remained showed the Alzheimer neurofibrillary change; Lewy bodies were not observed, however. The neurofibrillary changes were scattered diffusely through the cerebral cortex and brainstem but were most prominent in the medial temporal gray matter. Noteworthy was the absence of discrete senile plaques in this material; however, all cases showed extensive immunoreactive deposits of β-amyloid ("diffuse plaques"). In three boxers who developed a parkinsonian syndrome, Davie and colleagues found a reduction of *N*-acetylaspartate in the putamen and pallidum by protein magnetic resonance spectroscopy. This probably reflected a loss of neurons in these regions and differentiated the process from idiopathic Parkinson disease. The pathogenesis of the punch-drunk state remains unclear.

Posttraumatic Hydrocephalus This is an uncommon complication of severe head injury. Intermittent headaches, vomiting, confusion, and drowsiness are the initial manifestations. Later there are mental dullness, apathy, and psychomotor retardation, by which time the CSF pressure may have fallen to a normal level (normal-pressure hydrocephalus). Postmortem examinations have demonstrated an adhesive basilar arachnoiditis. Since a similar syndrome is observed occasionally after the rupture of a saccular aneurysm with subarachnoid hemorrhage, the same mechanisms, i.e., blocking of the aqueduct and fourth ventricle by blood clot and basilar meningeal fibrosis, may also be operative in traumatic hydrocephalus. Response to ventriculoperitoneal shunt may be dramatic. Zander and Foroglou have had extensive experience with this condition and have written informatively about it.

Posttraumatic Nervous Instability (Postconcussion Syndrome) This troublesome and frequent sequela of head injury has been alluded to above as well as in the chapter on headache (page 192). It has also been called the *posttraumatic* or *postconcussion syndrome*, *posttraumatic headache*, *traumatic neurasthenia* (Symonds), and *traumatic psychasthenia*, among many other names. Headache is the central symptom, either generalized or localized to the part that had been struck. The headache is variously described as aching, throbbing, pounding, stabbing, pressing, or band-like and is remarkable for its variability. The intensification of the headache and other symptoms by mental and physical effort, straining, stooping, and emotional excitement has already been mentioned; rest and quiet tend to relieve it. Such headaches may present a major obstacle to convalescence. Dizziness, another prominent symptom, is usually not a true vertigo but a giddiness or light-headedness. The patient may feel unsteady, dazed, weak, or faint. However, a certain number of patients describe symptoms that are consonant with labyrinthine disorder. They report that objects in the environment move momentarily, and that looking upward or to the side may cause a sense of unbalance; labyrinthine tests may show hyporeactivity; far more often they disclose no abnormalities. McHugh found a high incidence of minor abnormalities by electronystagmography both in concussed patients and in those suffering from whiplash injuries of the neck, but some of the data we find difficult to interpret. Exceptionally, vertigo is accompanied by diminished excitability of both the labyrinth and the cochlea (deafness), and one may assume the existence of direct injury to the eighth nerve or end organ.

The patient with posttraumatic nervous instability is intolerant of noise, emotional excitement, and crowds. Tenseness, restlessness, fragmentation of sleep, inability to concentrate, feelings of nervousness, fatigue, worry, apprehension, and an inability to tolerate the usual amount of alcohol complete the clinical picture. The resemblance of these symptoms to those of anxiety and depression is quite apparent. In contrast to this multiplicity of subjective symptoms, memory and other intellectual functions show little or no impairment, although this has been disputed. Leininger et al, for example, found that most of their 53 patients who suffered minor head injury in traffic accidents performed less well than controls on psychologic tests (category test, auditory verbal learning, copying of complex figures). The fact that those who were merely dazed did as poorly as those who were concussed and that litigation was involved in some cases would lead one to question these results.

The syndrome of posttraumatic nervous instability complicates all types of head injury, mild and severe. Once established, it may persist for months or even years, and it tends to resist all varieties of treatment. Eventually, the symptoms lessen. Strangely, this syndrome is almost unknown in children. Characteristic also is the augmentation of both the duration and intensity of this syndrome by problems with compensation and litigation, suggesting a psychologic factor. In countries where these matters are a less prominent part of the social fabric, the occurrence of posttraumatic syndrome is far less frequent. In respect to the syndrome of posttraumatic nervous instability, the constitution of the patient appears to be important. Stable, athletic, tough-fibered individuals take a concussive injury in stride, while the sensitive, nervous, complaining types may be so overwhelmed by such an accident that they are unable to expel it from their minds. Environmental stress assumes importance as well, for if too much is demanded of the patient soon after injury, irritability, insomnia, and anxiety are enhanced. In this connection, an interesting experiment has been conducted by Mittenberg and colleagues. A group of subjects with no personal experience or knowledge of head injury were asked to select from a list those symptoms that they would expect after a concussive head injury. They chose a cluster of symptoms virtually identical to that of the postconcussion syndrome.

An approach to such patients is given further on, in the section on treatment under "Patients with Only Transient Unconsciousness."

Other Posttraumatic Cognitive and Psychiatric Disorders

In all patients with cerebral concussive injury, there remains a gap in memory (traumatic amnesia) spanning a variable period from before the accident to some point following it. This gap is permanent and is filled in only by what the patient is told. In addition, as stated in the introduction to this section, some degree of impairment of higher cortical function may persist for weeks (or be permanent) after moderate to severe head injuries, even after the patient has reached the stage of forming continuous memories. During the period of deranged mentation, the memory disorder is the most prominent feature, so that the state resembles the alcoholic form of the Korsakoff amnesic state. It has been repeatedly asserted that this amnesic state is a constant feature of every prolonged traumatic mental disorder, but to the authors it reflects in part the ease with which memory can be tested. With more careful testing, other cognitive disorders are evident. Concussed patients, during the period of posttraumatic amnesia, rarely confabulate and usually have an impaired ability to register events and information, an abnormality not ordinarily observed in patients entering the chronic phases of Korsakoff psychosis. Apart from disorientation in place and time, the head-injured patient also shows defects in attention, distractibility, perseveration, and an inability to synthesize perceptual data. Judgment is impaired, sometimes severely. A perseverative tendency interferes with both action and thought.

As a general rule, the lower the score on the Glasgow Coma Scale (Table 35-1) and the longer the posttraumatic gap in the formation of memories (anterograde amnesia), the more likely the patient is to suffer permanent cognitive and personality changes. Abnormalities in these spheres were found in 12 percent of head-injured patients who had been in coma for longer than 24 h (Sazbon et al). If respiration and motor function were normal (except for early decorticate posturing) and there was no extraneural trauma, 94 percent of the patients recovered. According to Jennett and Bond, patients with good recovery achieved their maximum degree of improvement within 6 months. Others have found that detailed and repeated psychologic testing over a prolonged period, even in patients with relatively minor cerebral injuries, discloses measurable improvement for as long as 12 to 18 months.

There are other mental and behavioral abnormalities of a more subtle type that remain as sequelae to cerebral injury. As the stage of posttraumatic dementia recedes, the patient may find it impossible to work or to adjust to the family situation. Such patients continue to be abnormally abrupt, argumentative, stubborn, opinionated, and suspicious. Unlike the traumatic mental disorder described above, in which there is a certain uniformity, these traits vary with the patient's age, constitution, past experience, and the environmental stresses to which he is subjected. Extremes of age are important. The most prominent behavioral abnormality in children, described by Bowman et al is a change in character. They become impulsive, heedless of the consequences of their actions, and lacking in moral sense—much like those who had recovered from encephalitis lethargica. Some adolescents or young adults show the general lack of inhibition and impulsivity that one associates with frontal lobe disease. In the older person it is the impairment of intellectual functions that assumes prominence.

The tendency is for all such symptoms to subside slowly though not always completely, even in those in whom an accident has provoked a frank outburst of psychosis (as may happen to a manic-depressive, paranoid schizophrenic, or neurotic patient). These forms of "traumatic insanity" were carefully analyzed for the first time by Adolf Meyer.

Hysterical symptoms that develop after head injury appear to be more common than those following injury to other parts of the body. These symptoms are discussed in Chap. 56.

TREATMENT

Patients with Only Transient Unconsciousness

Patients with an uncomplicated concussive injury who have already regained consciousness by the time they are seen in a hospital pose few difficulties in management. They should not be discharged until the appropriate examinations (CT scans, skull films, etc.) have been made and the results prove to be negative. Also, the patient should not be released until the capacity for consecutive memories has been regained and arrangements have been made for observation by the family of signs of possible though unlikely delayed complications (subdural and epidural hemorrhage, intracerebral bleeding, and edema).

The patients with persistent complaints of headache, dizziness, and nervousness, the syndrome that we have designated as *posttraumatic nervous instability*, are the most difficult to manage. Three subgroups of this latter syndrome can be discerned. *In the first group*, the accident has provoked anxiety or an anxious depression. Compensation factors loom large in this group, especially for the patient whose circumstances are marginal and who is uncertain of a job and must care for dependents. Such a person is often willing to persist in illness, even if compensated at a level considerably below his earning capacity, if it provides a modicum of security. Obviously, we are often dealing here with matters that have little to do with the purely physical factors involved in cerebral trauma. The *second group* consists of patients in whom the *premorbid personality* was of a neurotic or depressive type. The injury to the brain is but one more factor in decompensating a tenuous social and occupational adjustment. The *third and smallest number of patients*, obviously the more severely injured, are found, upon close examination, to be *still suffering from a personality change* and *subtle impairments of cognitive function*, i.e., traumatic psychosis or dementia. The anxiety and depression reflect an awareness of their inability to cope with environmental stress.

A treatment program must be planned in accordance with the basic problem. If there is mainly an anxious depression, antidepressants—such as fluoxetine, paroxetine, or a tricyclic—are often useful. Simple analgesics, such as aspirin or acetaminophen or nonsteroidal anti-inflammatory drugs, should be prescribed for the headache. Litigation should be settled as soon as possible. To delay settlement usually works to the disadvantage of the patient. Long periods of observation, repetition of a multitude of tests, and waiting only reinforce the patient's worries and fears and reduce the motivation to return to work.

Severe Head Injury

If the physician arrives at the scene of the accident and finds an unconscious patient, a quick examination should be made before the patient is moved. First it must be determined whether the patient is breathing and has a clear airway and obtainable pulse and blood pressure, and whether there is dangerous hemorrhage from a scalp laceration or injured viscera. Severe head injuries that arrest respiration are soon followed by cessation of cardiac function. Injuries of this magnitude are often fatal; if resuscitative measures do not restore and sustain cardiopulmonary function within 4 to 5 min, the brain is usually irreparably damaged. The likelihood of a cervical fracture-dislocation, which is occasionally associated with head injury, is the reason for taking the precautions, outlined on page 1300, in moving the patient. It is best to assume that all such patients have had a neck injury and immobilize the cervical spine. Bleeding from the scalp can usually be controlled by a pressure bandage unless an artery is divided, and then a suture becomes necessary. Resuscitative measures (artificial respiration and cardiac compression) should be continued until they are taken over by ambulance personnel.

In the hospital the first step is to clear the airway and ensure adequate ventilation by endotracheal intubation if necessary. A careful search for other injuries must be made, particularly of the abdomen, chest, spine, and long bones. Although the hypotension that follows some injuries is a vasodepressor response and usually comes under control without pressor drugs, a large, unimpeded intravenous line should be inserted. Persistent hypotension due to head injury alone is an uncommon occurrence and should always raise the suspicion of a ruptured viscus or thoracic or abdominal internal bleeding, extensive fractures, or trauma to the cervical cord.

The profound effects of sustained hypotension on outcome are commented upon below. Hypertension is a more common finding immediately after severe head injury (see further on). Initially, infused fluid should be normal saline, avoiding the administration of excessive free water because of its adverse effect on brain edema. Cervical spine films and a cranial CT scan should be obtained en route to the intensive care unit once vital functions are stable. If films of the cervical spine are negative, there is no longer a need to immobilize the neck.

A rapid survey can now be made, with attention to the depth of coma, size of the pupils and their reaction to light, ocular movements, corneal reflexes, facial movements during grimace, swallowing, vocalization, gag reflexes, muscle tone and movements of the limbs, predominant postures, reactions to pinch, and reflexes. Bogginess of the temporal or postauricular area (Battle sign), bleeding from the nose or ear, and extensive conjunctival edema and hemorrhage are useful signs of an underlying basal skull fracture. However, it should be remembered that rupture of an eardrum or a blow to the nose may also cause bleeding from these parts. Fracture of the orbital bones may displace the eye, with resulting strabismus; fracture of the jaw results in malocclusion and discomfort on attempting to open the mouth. If urine is retained and the bladder is distended, a catheter should be inserted and kept there. Temperature, pulse, respiration, blood pressure, and state of consciousness should be checked and charted every hour.

The *Glasgow Coma Scale*, mentioned above, provides a practical means by which the state of impaired consciousness can be evaluated at frequent intervals (Table 35-1), but it should not be considered a substitute for a more complete neurologic examination. It registers three aspects of neurologic functions: (1) eye opening (spontaneously, in response to command, and in response to pain); (2) verbal responsiveness (in terms of orientation, confusion, inappropriateness, and incomprehensibility); (3) motor responsiveness (to command, to a localized stimulus, flexion and extension responses to pressure on the limb). This scale requires little training of ward personnel. It is useful in following the course and predicting the outcome of severe head injuries (a score of less than 8 is associated with a poor prognosis). A deteriorating scale dictates a change in management.

CT scanning is of central importance at this juncture. A sizable epidural, subdural, or intracerebral blood clot is an indication for immediate surgery. The presence of contusions, brain edema, and displacement of central structures calls for measures to monitor progression of these lesions and to control intracranial pressure. These measures are best carried out in a critical care unit.

Management of Raised Intracranial Pressure It is the practice in some hospitals to insert one of several available devices that permits continuous recording of intracranial pressure (ICP) after moderate and severe head injury (Narayan et al). Pressure measurements through a lumbar puncture needle do not accurately reflect the ICP and increase the risk of a cerebellar or temporal lobe herniation. Nor do the neurologic signs that constitute the Glasgow Coma Scale reflect the pressure in the cranium. The arguments for and against monitoring the ICP have been addressed earlier (page 660). Our impression is that, in comatose patients, at a minimum, monitoring the ICP prevents errors in fluid administration and refines other details of management, including the appropriate use of osmotic diuretics and the correct level of hyperventilation. In these respects, monitoring can be helpful. However, there are few critical data to support the routine use of ICP monitoring; certainly the patient who is only drowsy or shows only minimal mass effect on CT scanning is not likely to benefit. In the absence of data to guide the decision regarding the insertion of these devices, we favor their use to guide therapy and warn of impending deterioration from brain edema or hemorrhage. The current generation of ICP monitors employs fiberoptic strain gauges that can be inserted directly into the cerebral cortex without apparent damage. While the risk of infection is low, prolonged use may be complicated by bacterial meningitis.

The first step in lowering high ICP is to control the secondary factors that are known to raise the pressure, such as hypoxia, hypercarbia, hyperthermia, awkward head positions, and high mean airway pressures (Ropper). If the intracranial pressure exceeds 15 to 20 mmHg, several measures can be instituted, such as inducing hypocarbia by controlled ventilation (maintaining P_{CO_2} at 28 to 33 mmHg) and by hyperosmolar dehydration (0.25 to 1.0 g of 20% mannitol every 3 to 6 h or 0.75 to 1 mg/kg of furosemide) to maintain serum sodium above 138 meq/L and osmolality at 290 to 300 mosmol/L. Even if ICP monitoring is not utilized, an attempt should be made to maintain this level of osmolality for the first days if contusion and brain swelling are detected on the CT scan. Elevations in osmolality that are due to excessive concentrations of solutes such as glucose are not useful in reducing intracranial volume because they do not provide a water gradient across the cerebral vasculature. For this reason, the measurement of serum sodium is in some ways a more accurate reflection of free water depletion. An initial sodium level of 136 to 141 meq/L is adequate. Intravenous fluids with free water should be avoided so as not to intensify cerebral edema. This poses a particular danger in children who, because of inappropriate secretion of antidiuretic hormone, easily develop water intoxication. With this exception, however, restriction of the overall volume of fluid is less of a concern than effecting a reduction in free water. Fluids such as 5% dextrose in water, 0.5% saline, and 5% dextrose in 0.5% saline are therefore avoided; lactated Ringer's solution is permissible but normal saline, with or without added dextrose, is ideal.

Hyperventilation is effective in reducing ICP for only a limited time since the pH of the spinal fluid equilibrates over hours and returns cerebral blood volume to its previous level. A single-step reduction in P_{CO_2} typically lowers ICP for approximately 20 to 40 min. In a few cases the effect may persist for hours. Attempts to prolong the effect of hypocarbia and alkalosis of the spinal fluid by the administration of ammonium buffers have met with mixed success. It has even been suggested that hyperventilation may be harmful to some head-injured patients, but the risk, if any, appears to be minimal.

If the ICP continues to rise and brain swelling to progress despite these measures, the outlook for survival is bleak. Hypothermia and barbiturate anesthesia to reduce ICP have been used, but relatively few patients respond to such measures. A randomized controlled trial of cooling patients with severe closed head injury (Glasgow Coma Scale scores of 3 to 7) to 33°C for 24 hours appeared to hasten neurologic recovery and may have modestly improved outcome (Marion et al). Barbiturates, while they lower ICP, may lower the blood pressure as well, which worsens the situation, though Marshall and coworkers claim a high rate of good survival even in cases where the ICP exceeded 40 mmHg. The more definitive randomized study by Eisenberg and associates showed no benefit from barbiturate anesthesia. Several large controlled studies have established that the administration of high-dose steroids does not significantly affect the clinical outcome of severe head injuries (Gudeman et al; Dearden et al; Braakman et al; Saul et al). The use of decompression craniectomy in cases of intractable brain swelling is commented upon below.

The management of posttraumatic systemic hypertension can be a difficult problem. Immediately after head injury there is a sympathoadrenal response and elevation of blood pressure which recede spontaneously in a matter of a few hours or days. Unless the blood pressure elevation is severe (greater than 180/95 mmHg), it can be disregarded in the early stages. In animal experiments, it has been found that severe hypertension leads to increased perfusion of the brain and an augmentation of the edema surrounding contusions and hemorrhages. As mentioned earlier, edema is the main element in the genesis of brain swelling and raised ICP in head-injured patients (Marmarou et al). This sequence reflects a failure of autoregulatory vascular mechanisms, with resulting transudative edema in damaged areas of the brain. The control of high blood pressure must be balanced against the risk of reducing cerebral perfusion pressure and the observation that even a brief period of mild hypotension may provoke a cycle of cerebral vasodilation, increased cerebral blood volume, and elevated ICP in the form of a plateau wave (Rosner and Becker). Data such as these emphasize the need for immediate and vigorous management of hypotension in severely head-injured patients. Chestnut et al, in a study of patients from the Traumatic Coma Data Bank, found that sustained early hypotension (systolic BP<90 mmHg) was associated with a doubling of mortality. If shock was present on admission to the emergency ward, the mortality was 65 percent.

Since most therapies for elevated ICP dehydrate the patient or reduce cardiac filling pressures, leading to hypotension, a middle course, of avoiding both severe hypertension and hypotension, seems the best compromise. In lowering high levels of blood pressure, diuretics, beta-adrenergic blocking agents, or angiotensin converting enzyme inhibitors should be used, rather than agents that dilate the cerebral vasculature (nitroglycerin and nitroprusside, hydralazine, and some of the calcium channel blockers). Hypotension should be corrected by vasopressor agents such as neosynephrine. The precise level of blood pressure that requires treatment must be judged in the context of the ICP and the presence of plateau waves (the goal being to maintain normal cerebral perfusion), the patient's previous blood pressure level, and evidence of end-organ failure such as cardiac ischemia.

General Medical Measures If coma persists for more than 48 h, a nasogastric tube should be passed and fluids and nutrition given by this route. Agents that reduce gastric acid production—or the equivalent, antacids by stomach tube to keep gastric acidity at a pH above 3.5—are of value in preventing gastric hemorrhage. The prophylactic use of anticonvulsant drugs, as discussed earlier under "Posttraumatic Epilepsy," is not generally favored. Only if there has been a seizure are conventional anticonvulsants given.

Restlessness is controlled by diazepam or a similar sedative, but only if careful nursing fails to quiet the patient and provide sleep for a few hours at a time. Haloperidol is usually avoided in the acute stage. Fever is counteracted by antipyretics such as acetaminophen, and, if necessary, by a cooling blanket.

Surgical Measures The need for surgical intervention during the acute posttraumatic period is decided by two factors: the clinical status of the patient and CT scanning. The presence of a subdural or epidural clot that is causing a shift of central brain structures calls for its immediate evacuation. The approach to subdural hematomas has been discussed earlier in the chapter. Should the elevated ICP not respond to this procedure or to the standard osmotic agents and other medical measures outlined above, or should the condition of the patient and vital signs then begin to deteriorate (pulse rising, temperature rising or falling below normal, state of consciousness worsening, hemiplegia more obvious, plantar reflexes more clearly extensor), a renewed search must be undertaken for a late-occurring cerebral mass. Usually, in these clinical circumstances, CT scanning will disclose an epidural, subdural, or intracerebral hematoma, marked cerebral edema, and a lateral shift of central cerebral structures. *If death or severe disability is to be avoided, operation in these cases must be undertaken before the advanced signs of brainstem compression—decerebrate or decorticate posturing, hypertension, bradycardia—have appeared.*

The use of *decompressive craniectomy* in patients with progressive and intractable traumatic brain swelling has been a subject of renewed interest in recent years, after having been practically abandoned several decades ago. Guerra and colleagues have reported on 57 such patients, mostly young adults, who underwent wide frontotemporal craniectomy, unilateral in 31 and bilateral in 26. Of these, 11 patients died, 5 remained in a persistent vegetative state, and 6 survived in a severely damaged condition; however, 33 patients (58 percent) attained surprisingly good states of rehabilitation. The authors were of the opinion that these results represented a significant improvement over the expected outcome in this particular category of patients. Similar results in children have been reported by Polin et al.

The treatment of other problems attendant upon protracted coma has been outlined in Chap. 17. Every patient presents certain unique problems that must be dealt with individually.

PROGNOSIS

In respect to severe head injury, as has been intimated, the outcome is particularly discouraging. In the large European Brain Injury Consortium survey, comprising 10,005 adult patients, the injury proved fatal in 31 percent; 3 percent were left in a persistent vegetative state, and 16 percent remained severely neurologically disabled (Murray et al). Data from the Traumatic Coma Data Bank are comparable (Marshall et al). The signs of focal brain disease, whether due to closed head injuries or to open and penetrating ones, tend always to ameliorate as the months pass. A hemiplegia is often reduced to a minimal hemiparesis or to an ineptitude of voluntary motor function with exaggerated reflexes and an equivocal Babinski sign on that side, and an aphasia is gradually transformed into a stuttering or hesitant paraphasia or dysnomia that is not disabling except to a professional person, speaker, or writer. Many of the signs of brainstem disease (cranial nerve dysfunction and ataxia) improve also, usually within the first 6 months after injury (Jennett and Bond), and often to a surprising extent. Most patients who had been in coma for many hours or days, i.e., those with severe brain injuries, are left with memory impairment and other cognitive defects and with personality changes. These may be the only lasting sequelae. According to Jennett and Bond, these mental and personality changes are a greater handicap than focal neurologic ones as far as social adjustment is concerned. In open head wounds and penetrating brain injuries, Grafman and coworkers found that the magnitude of tissue loss and location of the lesion were the main factors affecting the outcome.

The prognosis of head injury is influenced by several other factors. The *age of the patient* is the most important of these (Vollmer et al). Increasing age reduces the chances of survival and of good recovery. Older patients often remain disabled, especially when compensation is involved. Young and middle-aged ones do better, particularly if they are not entitled to compensation. Russell has pointed out that the severity of the injury as measured by the duration of *traumatic amnesia* is a useful prognostic index. Of patients with a period of amnesia lasting less than 1 h, 95 percent were back at work within 2 months; if the amnesia lasted longer than 24 h, only 80 percent had returned to work within 6 months. However, about 60 percent of the patients in his very large series still had symptoms at the end of 2 months, and 40 percent at the end of 18 months. Of the most severely injured (those comatose for several days), many remained permanently disabled. However, the degree of recovery was often better than one had expected; the motor impairment, aphasia, and dementia tended to lessen and sometimes cleared. Improvement could continue over a period of 3 or more years. Children seemed to recover more completely than adults.

REFERENCES

ADAMS JH, GRAHAM DI, MURRAY LS, SCOTT G: Diffuse axonal injury due to nonmissile head injury in humans: An analysis of 45 cases. *Ann Neurol* 12:557, 1982.

ANNEGERS JF, GRABOW JD, GROOVER RV, et al: Seizures after head trauma: A population study. *Neurology* 30:683, 1980.

ANNEGERS JF, HAUSER A, COAN SP, ROCCA WA: A population-based study of seizures after traumatic brain injuries. *N Engl J Med* 338:20, 1998.

ASCROFT RB: Traumatic epilepsy after gunshot wounds of the head. *BMJ* 1:739, 1941.

BAUGLEY IJ, NICHOLLS JL, FELMINGHAM KL, et al: Dysautonomia after traumatic brain injury: A forgotten syndrome. *J Neurol Neurosurg Psychiatry* 67:39, 1999.

BOWMAN KM, BLAU A, REICH R: Psychiatric states following head injury in adults and children, in Feiring EH (ed): *Brock's Injuries of the Brain and Spinal Cord and Their Coverings*, 5th ed. New York, Springer, 1974, pp 570–613.

BRAAKMAN R, SCHOUTEN HJA, BLAAUW-VAN DISHOECK, MINDERHOUD JM: Megadose steroids in severe head injury: Results of a prospective double-blind clinical trial. *J Neurosurg* 58:326, 1983.

BRITISH MEDICAL JOURNAL: A group of neurosurgeons: Guidelines for initial management after head injury in adults. *BMJ* 288:983, 1984.

CAIRNS H: Injuries of frontal and ethmoid sinuses with special reference to CSF rhinorrhea and aerocele. *J Laryngol Otol* 52: 289, 1937.

CASSON IR, SHAM RAJ, CAMPBELL EA, et al: Neurological and CT evaluation of knocked-out boxers. *J Neurol Neurosurg Psychiatry* 45:170, 1982.

CAVENESS WF: Onset and cessation of fits following craniocerebral trauma. *J Neurosurg* 20:570, 1963.

CAVENESS WF: Post-traumatic sequelae, in Caveness WF, Walker AE (eds): *Head Injury*. Philadelphia, Lippincott, 1966, chap 17, pp 209–219.

CAVINESS VS JR: Epilepsy and craniocerebral injury of warfare, in Caveness WF, Walker AE (eds): *Head Injury*. Philadelphia, Lippincott, 1966, pp 220–234.

CHESTNUT RM, MARSHALL SB, PIEK J, et al: Early and late systemic hypotension as a frequent and fundamental source of cerebral ischaemia following severe brain injury in the Traumatic Coma Data Bank. *Acta Neurochir* (Suppl)59:121, 1993.

CORSELLIS JAN, BRUTON CJ, FREEMAN-BROWNE D: The aftermath of boxing. *Psychol Med* 3:270, 1973.

COURVILLE CB: *Pathology of the Central Nervous System*: Part 4. Mountain View, CA, Pacific, 1937.

DAVIE CA, PIRTOSEKZ, BARKER GJ, et al: Magnetic resonance spectroscopic study of parkinsonism related to boxing. *J Neurol Neurosurg Psychiatry* 58:688, 1995.

DEARDEN NM, GIBSON JS, MCDOWALL DG, et al: Effect of high-dose dexamethasone on outcome from severe head injury. *J Neurosurg* 64:81, 1986.

DENNY-BROWN D: Delayed collapse after head injury. *Lancet* 1:371, 1941.

DENNY-BROWN D, RUSSELL WR: Experimental cerebral concussion. *Brain* 64:93, 1941.

DODER M, JAHANSHAHI M, TURJANSKI N, et al: Parkinson's syndrome after closed head injury: a single case report. *J Neurol Neurosurg Psychiatry* 66:380, 1999.

EISENBERG HM, FRANKOWSKI HF, CONANT LP, et al: High dose barbiturate control of elevated intracranial pressure in patients with severe head injury. *J Neurosurg* 69:15, 1988.

FEIRING EH, DAVIDOFF LM: Gunshot wounds of the brain and their complications, in Feiring EH (ed): *Brock's Injuries of the Brain and Spinal Cord and Their Coverings*, 5th ed. New York, Springer, 1974, pp 283–335.

FOLTZ EL, SCHMIDT RP: The role of reticular formation in the coma of head injury. *J Neurosurg* 13:145, 1956.

FRAZIER CH, INGHAM SD: A review of the effects of gunshot wounds of the head based on the observation of 200 cases at US Army General Hospital, No 11, Cape May, NJ. *Trans Am Neurol Assoc* 45:59, 1919.

GENNARELLI TA, THIBAULT LE, ADAMS JH, et al: Diffuse axonal injury and traumatic coma in the primate. *Ann Neurol* 12:564, 1982.

GRAFMAN J, JONES BS, MARTIN A, et al: Intellectual function following penetrating head injury in Vietnam veterans. *Brain* 3:169, 1988.

GRAHAM DI, ADAMS JH, DOYLE D: Ischemic brain damage in fatal nonmissile injuries. *J Neurol Sci* 39:213, 1978.

GUDEMAN JK, MULLA JD, BECKER DP: Failure of high-dose steroid therapy to influence intracranial pressure in patients with severe head injury. *J Neurosurg* 51:301, 1979.

GUERRA WK, GAAB MR, DIETZ H, et al: Surgical decompression for traumatic brain swelling: indications and results. *J Neurosurg* 90:187, 1999.

HOLBOURN AHS: Mechanics of head injury. *Lancet* 2:438, 1943.

JEFFERSON G: The nature of concussion. *BMJ* 1:1, 1944.

JELLINGER K, SEITELBERGER F: Protracted post-traumatic encephalopathy: Pathology, pathogenesis and clinical implications. *J Neurol Sci* 10:51, 1970.

JENNETT B: *Epilepsy after Non-missile Head Injuries*, 2nd ed. London, Heinemann, 1975.

JENNETT B: Head trauma, in Asbury AK, McKhann GM, McDonald WI (eds): *Diseases of the Nervous System*, 2nd ed. Philadelphia, Saunders, 1992, pp 1229–1237.

JENNETT B, BOND M: Assessment of outcome after severe brain damage. *Lancet* 1:480, 1975.

JENNETT B, TEASDALE G: *Management of Head Injuries: Contemporary Neurology*, no 20. Philadelphia, Davis, 1981.

KAMPFL A, FRANZ G, AICHNER F, et al: the persistent vegetative state after closed head injury: clinical and magnetic resonance imaging findings in 42 patients. *J Neurosurg* 88:809,1998.

Labadie EL, Glover D: Physiopathogenesis of subdural hematomas. *J Neurosurg* 45:382, 393, 1976.

Leininger BE, Gramling SE, Farrell AD, et al: Neuropsychological deficits in symptomatic minor head injury patients after concussion and mild concussion. *J Neurol Neurosurg Psychiatry* 53:293, 1990.

Lepore FE: Disorders of ocular motility following head trauma. *Arch Neurol* 52:924, 1995.

Lloyd DA, Carty H, Patterson M, et al: Predictive value of skull radiography for intracranial injury in children with blunt head injury. *Lancet* 349,821, 1997.

Marion DW, Penrod LE, Kelsey SF, et al: Treatment of traumatic brain injury with moderate hypothermia. *N Engl J Med* 336:540, 1997.

Marmarou A, Fatouros PP, Barzo P, et al: Contribution of edema and cerebral blood volume to traumatic brain swelling in head-injured patients. *J Neurosurg* 93:183, 2000.

Marshall LF, Smith RW, Shapiro HM: The outcome with aggressive treatment in severe head injury: Part II. Acute and chronic barbiturate administration in the management of head injury. *J Neurosurg* 50:26, 1979.

Marshall LF, Toole BM, Bowers SA: The National Traumatic Coma Data Bank: Part 2. Patients who talk and deteriorate: Implications for treatment. *J Neurosurg* 59: 285, 1983.

McHugh HE: Auditory and vestibular disorders in head injury, in Caveness WF, Walker AE (eds): *Head Injury*. Philadelphia, Lippincott, 1966, pp 97–105.

Meirowsky AM: Penetrating craniocerebral trauma, in Caveness WF, Walker AE (eds): *Head Injury*. Philadelphia, Lippincott, 1966, pp 195–202.

Meyer A: The anatomical facts and clinical varieties of traumatic insanity. *Am J Insanity* 60:373, 1904.

Mittenberg W, DiGiulio DV, Perrin S, Bass AE: Symptoms following mild head injury: Expectations as aetiology. *J Neurol Neurosurg Psychiatry* 55:200, 1992.

Munro D, Merritt HH: Surgical pathology of subdural hematoma based on a study of 105 cases. *Arch Neurol Psychiatry* 35:64, 1936.

Murray GD, Teasdale GM, Braakman, et al: The European Brain Injury Consortium survey of head injuries. *Acta Neurochir* 141:223, 1999.

Narayan RK, Kishore PRS, Becker DP, et al: Intracranial pressure: To monitor or not to monitor? A review of our experience with severe head injury. *J Neurosurg* 56:650, 1982.

Narayan RK, Wildberger JE, Povlishock JT: *Neurotrauma*. New York, McGraw-Hill, 1996.

Nevin NC: Neuropathological changes in the white matter following head injury. *J Neuropathol Exp Neurol* 26:77, 1967.

Ommaya AK, Gennarelli TA: Cerebral concussion and traumatic unconsciousness: Correlations and experimental and clinical observations on blunt head injuries. *Brain* 97:633, 1974.

Ommaya AK, Grubb RL, Naumann RA: Coup and contre-coup injury: Observations on the mechanics of visible brain injuries in the rhesus monkey. *J Neurosurg* 35:503, 1971.

Penfield W, Jasper HH: *Epilepsy and Functional Anatomy of the Human Brain*. Boston, Little, Brown, 1954.

Penry JK, White BG, Brackett CE: A controlled prospective study of the pharmacologic prophylaxis of post-traumatic epilepsy. *Neurology* 29:600, 1979.

Pevehouse BC, Blom WH, McKissock KW: Ophthalmologic aspects of diagnosis and localization of subdural hematoma. *Neurology* 10:1037, 1960.

Polin RS, Shaffrey ME, Bogaev CA, et al: Decompressive bifrontal craniectomy in the treatment of severe refractory posttraumatic cerebral edema. *Neurosurgery* 41:84,1997.

Pudenz RH, Sheldon CH: The lucite calvarium—Method for direct observation of the brain. *J Neurosurg* 3:487, 1946.

Purvis JT: Craniocerebral injuries due to missiles and fragments, in Caveness WF, Walker AE (eds): *Head Injury*. Philadelphia, Lippincott, 1966, pp 133–141.

Rabe EF, Flynn RE, Dodge PR: A study of subdural effusions in an infant. *Neurology* 12:79, 1962.

Rabe EF, Young GF, Dodge PR: The distribution and fate of subdurally instilled human serum albumin in infants with subdural collections of fluid. *Neurology* 14:1020, 1964.

Rasmussen T: Surgical therapy of post-traumatic epilepsy, in Walker AE, Caveness WF, Critchley M (eds): *Late Effects of Head Injury*. Springfield, IL, Charles C Thomas, 1969, pp 277–305.

Rish BL, Caveness WR: Relation of prophylactic medication to the occurrence of early seizures following craniocerebral trauma. *J Neurosurg* 38:155, 1973.

Roberts AJ: *Brain Damage in Boxers: A Study of Prevalence of Traumatic Encephalopathy among Ex-professional Boxers*. London, Pitman, 1969.

Roberts GW, Allsop D, Bruton C: The occult aftermath of boxing. *J Neurol Neurosurg Psychiatry* 53:373, 1990.

Ropper AH (ed): *Neurological and Neurosurgical Intensive Care*, 3rd ed. New York, Raven Press, 1993.

Ropper AH, Miller D: Acute traumatic midbrain hemorrhage. *Ann Neurol* 18:80, 1985.

Rosner MJ, Becker DP: Origin and evolution of plateau waves. *J Neurosurg* 60:312, 1984.

Ross RJ, Cole M, Thompson JS, Kim KH: Boxers—Computed tomography, EEG, and neurological evaluation. *JAMA* 249:211, 1983.

Rossitch E Jr, Bullard DE: The autonomic dysfunction syndrome: Aetiology and treatment. *Br J Neurosurg* 2:471, 1988.

Rowbotham GF (ed): *Acute Injuries of the Head*, 4th ed, Baltimore, Williams and Wilkins, 1964.

Russell WR: *The Traumatic Amnesias*. London, Oxford, 1971.

Saul TG, Ducker TB, Salcman M, Carro E: Steroids in severe head injury: A prospective randomized clinical trial. *J Neurosurg* 54:596, 1981.

Sazbon L, Fuchs C, Costeff H: Prognosis for recovery from prolonged posttraumatic unawareness: Logistic analysis. *J Neurol Neurosurg Psychiatry* 54:149, 1991.

Shatsky SA, Evans DE, Miller F, Martins AN: High speed angiography of experimental head injury. *J Neurosurg* 41:523, 1974.

Stern WE: Carotid-cavernous fistula, in Vinken PJ, Bruyn GW (eds): *Handbook of Clinical Neurology*. Vol 24. Amsterdam, North-Holland, 1975, pp 399–440.

STRICH SJ: Diffuse degeneration of the cerebral white matter in severe dementia following head injury. *J Neurol Neurosurg Psychiatry* 19:163, 1956.

STRICH SJ: The pathology of severe head injury. *Lancet* 2:443, 1961.

SYMONDS CP: Concussion and its sequelae. *Lancet* 1:1, 1962.

SYMONDS CP: Concussion and contusion of the brain and their sequelae, in Feiring EH (ed): *Brock's Injuries of the Brain and Spinal Cord and Their Coverings*, 5th ed. New York, Springer, 1974, pp 100–161.

TEASDALE G, JENNETT B: Assessment of coma and impaired consciousness: A practical scale. *Lancet* 2:81, 1974.

TEUBER H-L: Effects of brain wounds implicating right or left hemisphere in man, in Mountcastle VB (ed): *Interhemispheric Relations and Cerebral Dominance*. Baltimore, Johns Hopkins, 1962, pp 131–157.

TROTTER W: Certain minor injuries of the brain. *Lancet* 1:935, 1924.

VOLLMER DG, TORNER JC, JANE JA, et al: Age and outcome following traumatic coma: Why do older patients fare worse? *J Neurosurg* 75(suppl):s37, 1991.

WALKER AE: Post-traumatic epilepsy, in Rowbotham GF (ed): *Acute Injuries of the Head*, 4th ed, Baltimore, Williams and Wilkins, 1964, pp 486–509.

WEIR B: The osmolality of subdural hematoma fluid. *J Neurosurg* 34:528, 1971.

WEISS GH, SALAZAR AM, VANCE SC, et al: Predicting posttraumatic epilepsy in penetrating head injury. *Arch Neurol* 43:771, 1986.

ZANDER E. FOROGLOU G: Post-traumatic hydrocephalus, in Vinken PJ, Bruyn GW (eds): *Handbook of Clinical Neurology*. Vol 24. Amsterdam, North-Holland, 1976, pp 231–253.

Chapter 36

MULTIPLE SCLEROSIS AND ALLIED DEMYELINATIVE DISEASES

It has long been the practice to set apart a group of diseases of the brain and spinal cord in which destruction of myelin (demyelination) is a prominent feature. To define these diseases precisely is difficult, for the simple reason that there is probably no disease in which myelin destruction is the exclusive pathologic change. The idea of a demyelinative disease is, more or less, an abstraction that serves primarily to focus attention on one of the more striking and distinctive features of the pathologic process.

The commonly accepted pathologic criteria of a demyelinative disease are (1) destruction of the myelin sheaths of nerve fibers; (2) *relative* sparing of the other elements of nervous tissue, i.e., of axis cylinders, nerve cells, and supporting structures; (3) infiltration of inflammatory cells in a perivascular distribution; (4) a particular distribution of lesions, often perivenous and primarily in white matter, either in multiple small disseminated foci or in larger foci spreading from one or more centers; and (5) a relative lack of wallerian, or secondary, degeneration of fiber tracts (an expression of the relative integrity of the axis cylinders in the lesions).

A classification of the demyelinative diseases is presented in Table 36-1. The diseases included in this classification conform approximately to the criteria enumerated above. Like all classifications that are not based on etiology, this one has its shortcomings in that it is somewhat arbitrary and inconsistent. In some of the diseases here classified as demyelinative, notably Schilder disease and necrotizing hemorrhagic leukoencephalitis and even multiple sclerosis, there can be a severe degree of damage to axis cylinders as well as to myelin. Contrariwise, a number of diseases in which demyelination is a prominent feature are not included. In some cases of anoxic encephalopathy, for example, the myelin sheaths of the radiating nerve fibers in the deep layers of the cerebral cortex or in ill-defined patches in the convolutional and central white matter are destroyed, while most of the axis cylinders are spared. A relatively selective degeneration of myelin may also occur in some small ischemic foci due to vascular occlusion or in larger confluent areas as in Binswanger disease (see Chap. 34). In subacute combined degeneration (SCD) of the spinal cord associated with pernicious anemia and in tropical spastic paraparesis (TSP), a demyelinating spinal cord disease, myelin may be affected earlier and to a greater extent than axis cylinders; the same is true of progressive multifocal leukoencephalopathy (PML), adrenoleukodystrophy (ADL), central pontine myelinolysis, and Marchiafava-Bignami disease. Some of these disorders and several others are no longer classified as demyelinative because their etiology has become known. PML is a viral infection of oligodendrocytes in immune-deficient subjects, ADL is a hereditary disease related to a defect in peroxisomal enzymes, SCD is due to vitamin B_{12} defi-

Table 36-1
Classification of the demyelinative diseases

I. Multiple sclerosis (disseminated sclerosis)
   A. Chronic relapsing encephalomyelopathic form
   B. Acute multiple sclerosis
   C. Diffuse cerebral sclerosis (encephalitis periaxialis diffusa) of Schilder and concentric sclerosis of Balo

II. Neuromyelitis optica (Devic)

III. Acute disseminated encephalomyelitis
   A. Following measles, chickenpox, smallpox, mumps, rubella, influenza, and other viral and some bacterial infections (*Mycoplasma*, *Rickettsia*, etc.)
   B. Following rabies or smallpox and rarely other types of vaccination (postvaccinal)

IV. Acute and subacute necrotizing hemorrhagic encephalitis
   A. Acute encephalopathic form (hemorrhagic leukoencephalitis of Hurst)
   B. Subacute necrotic myelopathy

ciency, and TSP is caused by a retrovirus, for which reasons these disorders are more appropriately included with the viral and nutritional diseases. Other diseases are not categorized as demyelinative because they lack the characteristic perivascular inflammatory changes and exhibit pathologic features that are judged to be more fundamental than the demyelination. Also, for reasons that will become clear in subsequent discussion, the chronic progressive leukodystrophies of childhood and adolescence (e.g., globoid body, metachromatic, and adrenal leukodystrophies), while clearly diseases of myelin, are set apart because of their unique genetic and morphologic features and are discussed in Chap. 37. Occupying an uncertain place in this nosology are demyelinative lesions associated with connective tissue diseases or merely with autoantibodies directed against DNA or phospholipids. The central nervous system (CNS) lesions may be multiple and cannot easily be distinguished radiologically from multiple sclerosis (MS), but, as noted further on, their nature is uncertain and some are due to vasculitis. Excluded from discussion in this chapter are demyelinative diseases of the peripheral nerves, although they share a number of pathologic features with demyelinating diseases of the CNS; they are described in Chap. 46.

In the language of neurology, therefore, the term *demyelination* has acquired a special meaning; if it is to retain its value, it should be used in the restricted sense indicated above and not as a synonym for complete degeneration of nerve fibers or necrosis of white matter, even though the lesions may look alike in a section stained for myelin.

MULTIPLE SCLEROSIS

Multiple sclerosis, referred to by the British as *disseminated sclerosis* and by the French as *sclerose en plaques*, is among the most venerable of neurologic diseases and one of the most important by virtue of its frequency, chronicity, and tendency to attack young adults. It is characterized clinically by episodes of focal disorder of the optic nerves, spinal cord, and brain, which remit to a varying extent and recur over a period of many years. The neurologic manifestations are protean, being determined by the varied location and extent of the demyelinative foci; nevertheless, the lesions have a predilection for certain portions of the CNS, resulting in complexes of symptoms and signs and radiologic appearances that can often be recognized as characteristic of MS.

Classic features include motor weakness, paraparesis, paresthesias, impaired vision, diplopia, nystagmus, dysarthria, intention tremor, ataxia, impairment of deep sensation, and bladder dysfunction. Diagnosis may be uncertain at the onset and in the early years of the disease, when symptoms and signs point to a lesion in only one locus of the nervous system. Later, as the disease recurs and disseminates throughout the cerebrospinal axis, diagnostic accuracy approaches 100 percent. A long period of latency (1 to 10 years or longer) between a minor initial symptom, which may not even come to medical attention, and the subsequent development of more characteristic symptoms and signs may delay the diagnosis. In most cases the initial manifestations improve partially or completely, to be followed after a variable interval by the recurrence of the same abnormalities or the appearance of new ones in other parts of the nervous system. In as many as half the patients, the disease takes the form of an intermittently progressive illness and sometimes of a steadily progressive one, especially in patients more than 40 years of age. A rule that has guided clinicians for many years is that the diagnosis of MS is not secure unless there is a history of remission and relapse and evidence on examination of more than one discrete lesion of the CNS. The advent of certain ancillary procedures—notably evoked potentials and magnetic resonance imaging (MRI)—and their capacity to identify clinically inevident lesions has obviated the exclusive dependence on clinical criteria for the diagnosis.

Pathologic Findings

Before being sectioned, the brain generally shows no evidence of disease, but the surface of the spinal cord may appear and feel uneven. Sectioning of the brain and cord discloses numerous scattered patches where the tissue is slightly depressed below the cut surface and stands out from the surrounding white matter by virtue of its pink-gray color (due to loss of myelin). The lesions may vary in diameter from less than a millimeter to several centimeters; they affect principally the white matter of the brain and spinal cord and do not extend beyond the root entry zones of the cranial and spinal nerves. It is because of their sharp delineation that they were called *plaques* by French pathologists.

The topography of the lesions is noteworthy. A periventricular localization is characteristic, but only where subependymal veins line the ventricles (mainly adjacent to the bodies and atria of the lateral ventricles). Other favored structures are the optic nerves and chiasm (but rarely the optic tracts) and the spinal cord, where pial veins lie next to the white matter (see Figs. 36-1 and 36-2; see also page 969 on "MRI in MS"). The lesions are distributed randomly throughout the brainstem, spinal cord, and cerebellar peduncles without reference to particular systems of fibers. In the cerebral cortex and central nuclear and spinal structures, the lesions destroy myelin sheaths but leave the nerve cells essentially intact.

The histologic appearance of the lesion depends on its age. Relatively recent lesions show a partial or complete destruction and loss of myelin throughout a zone formed by the confluence of many small, predominantly perivenous foci; the axis cylinders are relatively spared. There is a variable but slight degeneration of oligodendroglia, a neuroglial (astrocytic) reaction, and perivascular and para-adventitial infiltration with mononuclear cells and lymphocytes. Later, large numbers of microglial phagocytes (macrophages) infiltrate the lesions, and astrocytes in and around the lesions increase in number and size. Long-standing lesions, on the other hand, are composed of thickly matted, relatively acellular fibroglial tissue, with only occasional perivascular lymphocytes and macrophages; in such lesions, a few intact axis cylinders may still be found. Sparing of axis cylinders (axons) prevents wallerian degeneration. However, in old lesions with interruption of axons, there may be descending and ascending degeneration of long fiber tracts in the spinal cord. Partial remyelination is believed to take place on undamaged axons and to account for the partially demyelinated "shadow patches" (Prineas and Connell). Exceptionally, a few of the older lesions undergo cavitation, indicating that the disease process has affected not only myelin and axons but also supporting tissues and blood vessels as well. All gradations of histopathologic change between these two extremes may be found in lesions of diverse size, shape, and age, consistent with the extended clinical course.

Figure 36-1

Multiple sclerosis. T2-weighted MR images demonstrating multiple plaques in the periventricular white matter (left) *and cervical spinal cord* (right).

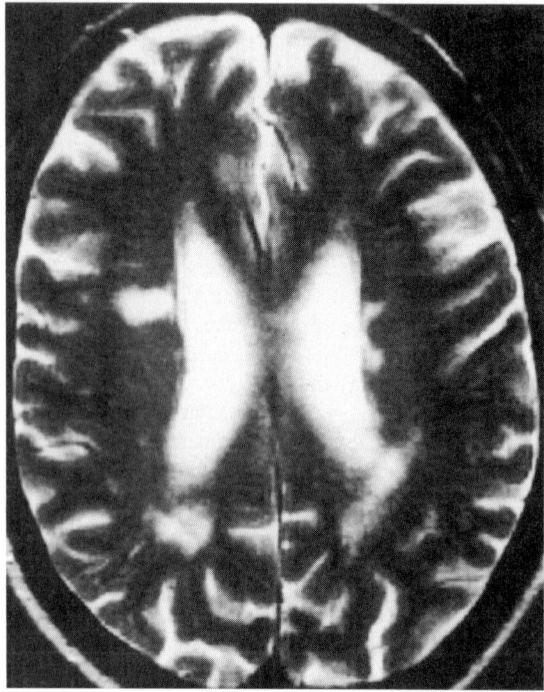

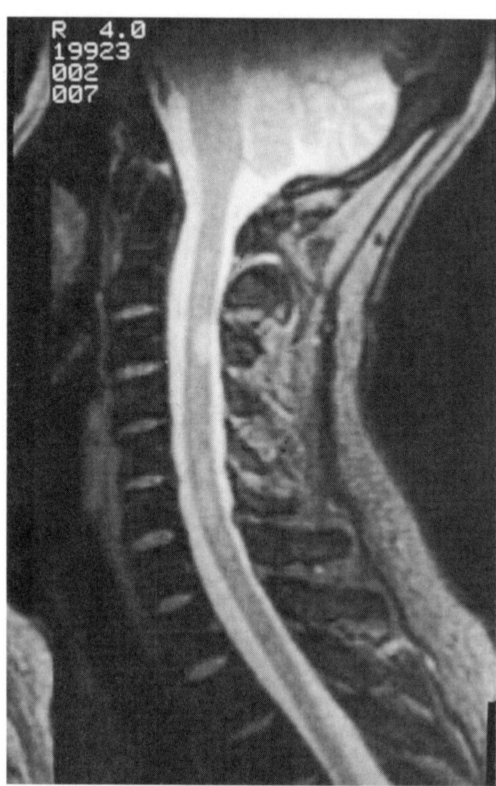

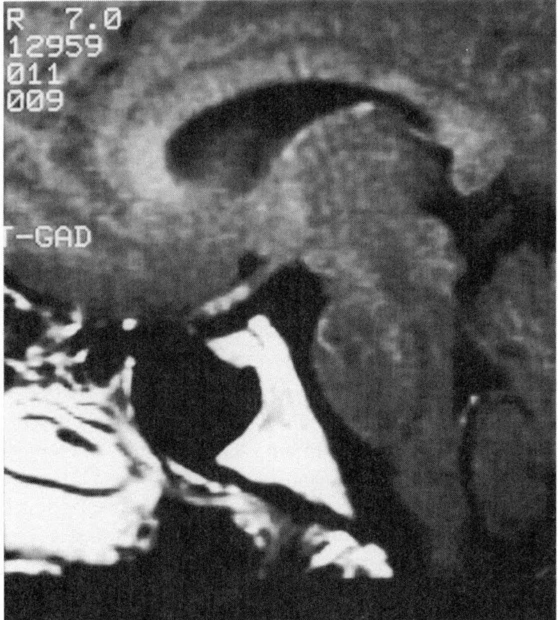

Figure 36-2

Multiple sclerosis. Gadolinium-enhanced MRI in a 36-year-old male with subacute evolution of diminished visual acuity. Enhancing plaques are seen in the optic chiasm and floor of the lateral ventricle.

Etiology and Epidemiology

Cruveilhier (circa 1835), in his original description of the disease, attributed it to suppression of sweat, and since that time there has been endless speculation about the etiology. Many of the early theories appear ludicrous in the light of present-day concepts, and others are of only historical interest. There is no point in enumerating them here; complete accounts are to be found in the reviews of DeJong (1970), Prineas (1970), R. T. Johnson (1978), and McDonald (1986).

Although the precise cause of MS remains undetermined, a number of epidemiologic facts have been clearly established and will eventually have to be incorporated in any etiologic hypothesis. The disease has a prevalence of less than 1 per 100,000 in equatorial areas; 6 to 14 per 100,000 in the southern United States and southern Europe; and 30 to 80 per 100,000 in Canada, northern Europe, and the northern United States. A less well defined gradient exists in the Southern Hemisphere. Kurland's studies indicate that there is a threefold increase in prevalence and a fivefold gradient in mortality rate between New Orleans (30 degrees north latitude) on the one hand, and Boston (42 degrees north) and Winnipeg (50 degrees north) on the other. In Japan there is a similar though less distinct geographic gradient; however, the prevalence of MS there is much lower than in corresponding latitudes of North America and northern Europe.

The increasing risk of developing MS with increasing latitude has been confirmed by Kurtzke and associates, who studied a series of unprecedented size (5305 undoubted cases of MS and matched controls). Their study showed that in the United States, African Americans are at lower risk than whites at all latitudes, but both races show the same south-to-north gradient in risk, indicating the importance of an environmental factor regardless of race. Supporting this view are the descriptions, by Kurtzke and Hyllested, of an "epidemic" of MS in the Faroe Islands of the North Atlantic. They found a much higher than expected incidence of the disease, occurring as three separate outbreaks of decreasing extent between the years 1943 and 1973. It is their contention that the disease was introduced by British troops who occupied the islands in large numbers in the years immediately preceding the outbreak. Kurtzke and colleagues have also described a similar postwar epidemic in Iceland.

Several studies indicate that persons who migrate from a high-risk to a low-risk zone carry with them at least part of the risk of their country of origin, even though the disease may not become apparent until 20 years after migration. Such a pattern has been demonstrated in both South Africa and Israel. Dean determined that the prevalence in native-born white South Africans was 3 to 11 per 100,000, whereas the rate in immigrants from northern Europe was about 50 per 100,000, only slightly less than in the nonimmigrating natives of those countries. The data of Dean and Kurtzke indicate further that in persons who had immigrated before the age of 15, the risk was similar to that of native-born South Africans; whereas in persons who had immigrated after that age, the risk was similar to that of their birthplace. Alter and colleagues found that in the descendants of European immigrants born in Israel, the risk of MS was low, similar to that of other native-born Israelis, whereas among recent immigrants the incidence in each national group approached that of the land of birth. Again, the critical age of immigration appeared to be about 15 years. These epidemiologic studies and others have shown that MS is associated with particular localities rather than with a particular ethnic group in those localities and emphasize the importance of environmental factors in the genesis of the disease.

Also, a familial aggregation of MS is now well established. About 15 percent of MS patients have an affected relative, with the highest risk of concurrence (5 percent) being observed in the patient's siblings (Ebers, 1983). In a large population-based study carried out in British Columbia by Sadovnick and colleagues, it was found that almost 20 percent of index cases had an affected relative, again with the highest risk in siblings. In a subsequent study, Sadovnick and colleagues studied the heritability of MS by comparing the risk of disease in the half-sibs (one biologic parent in common) of affected individuals with the risk in full sibs. They found that the risk for full sibs was two to three times greater than for half-sibs and they interpreted these results to mean that the difference is largely genetic.

The case for heritability is supported also by studies of twins in whom one of each pair is known to have MS. In the most careful of these studies (Ebers et al), the diagnosis was verified in 12 of 35 pairs of monozygotic twins (34 percent) and in only 2 of 49 pairs of dizygotic twins (4 percent). Notable also was the observation that in two additional sets of monozygotic twins who were clinically normal, lesions were detected by MRI. The concordance rate in dizygotic pairs is similar to that in nontwin siblings. However, within families with more than one affected member, no consistent pattern of mendelian inheritance has emerged. Of course, one must not assume that all diseases with an increased familial incidence are hereditary, for instances of the same condition in several members of a family may simply reflect an exposure to a common environmental agent. Paralytic poliomyelitis, for example, was about eight times more common in immediate family members than in the population at large.

Further suggestive of a genetic factor in the causation of MS is the finding that certain histocompatibility antigens (HLAs) are more frequent in patients with multiple sclerosis than in control subjects. The strongest association is with the DR locus on the sixth chromosome. Other HLAs that are overrepresented in MS (HLA-DR2 and, to a lesser extent, -DR3, -B7, and -A3) are thought to be markers for an MS "susceptibility gene"—possibly an immune response gene. The presence of one of these markers is said to increase the risk that an individual will develop MS by a factor of 3 to 5. These antigens may indeed prove to be related to the frequency of the disease, but their presence is not invariable and their exact role is far from clear (see Compston).

The low conjugal incidence of MS supports the view that common exposure to this disease must occur early in life. In order to test this hypothesis, Schapira and coworkers determined the periods of common exposure (common habitation periods) in members of families with two or more cases. From this they calculated the mean common exposure to have happened before 14 years of age, with a latency of about 21 years—figures that are in general agreement with those derived from the migration studies quoted above.

The incidence of MS is two or three times higher in women than in men, but the significance of this fact is unclear. The incidence in children is very low; only 0.3 to 0.4 percent of all cases appear during the first decade. In an analysis of three childhood-onset cases, Hauser and colleagues found no phenotypic differences between childhood and adult cases. Beyond childhood, the risk of first developing symptoms of the disease rises steeply with age, reaching a peak at about 30 years, remaining high in the fourth decade, then falling off sharply and becoming low in the sixth decade. It has been pointed out that MS has a unimodal age-specific onset curve, similar to the age-specific onset curves of many infectious diseases.

About two-thirds of cases of MS have their onset between 20 and 40 years of age. Of the remainder, most cases begin before the age of 20; in a smaller number, the disease appears to develop in late adult life (late fifties and sixties). In the latter patients, early symptoms may have been forgotten or may never have declared themselves clinically (we have several times found the typical lesions of MS in autopsied individuals who had no history of neurologic illness). Gilbert and Sadler report five such cases and from their pathologic findings declare that the true incidence of MS may be three times higher than stated figures.

Several studies from northern Europe and Canada have suggested that the likelihood of developing MS is somewhat greater among rural than among urban dwellers; studies of American army personnel indicate the opposite (Beebe et al). A number of surveys in Great Britain have intimated that the disease is more frequent in the higher socioeconomic groups than in the lower ones. Yet in the United States, no clear relationship has been established to the poverty or social deprivations that are part of a low socioeconomic status. Numerous other environmental factors (surgical operations, trauma, anesthesia, exposure to household pets, mercury in silver amalgam fillings in teeth) have been proposed but are unsupported by firm evidence.

Pathogenesis

All these epidemiologic data point to a relationship between MS and some environmental factor that is encountered in childhood and, after years of latency, either evokes the disease or contributes to its causation. In recent years, speculation has grown that this factor is an infection, most often viral. A large body of indirect evidence has been marshaled in support of this idea, based on the demonstration, in patients with MS, of alterations in humoral and cell-mediated immunity to viral agents (see reviews of R. T. Johnson, Lampert, K. P. Johnson et al, McFarlin and McFarland, and Antel and Cashman). However, to this day no virus (including all known members of the human retrovirus family) has been seen in or isolated from the tissues of patients with MS despite innumerable attempts to do so, and no satisfactory viral model of MS has been produced experimentally. Nevertheless, the fact that a retrovirus produces tropical spastic paraparesis (a demyelinating disease) and the experimental production of a demyelinating disease in transgenic mice that express a T-cell receptor for myelin basic protein (but not in mice that are kept in a sterile environment; Goverman et al) continue to spur the search for a viral causation of MS. Recently, the bacterial agent *Chlamydia pneumoniae* and herpesvirus type 6 have been similarly implicated by the finding of their genomic material in MS plaques, but the evidence for their direct participation in the disease is no more compelling than that for any other infectious agent.

If indeed the initial event in the genesis of MS is a viral or other infection of the nervous system, then some secondary factor must be operative in later life to activate the neurologic disease and cause exacerbations. The most popular view is that this secondary mechanism is an autoimmune reaction, attacking some components of myelin and, in its most intense form, destroying all tissue elements, including axons. Several lines of argument have been advanced in support of this view. One is to draw an analogy between the lesions of MS and those of disseminated encephalomyelitis, which is almost certainly an autoimmune disease of delayed hypersensitivity type (see further on). Another is that antibodies to specific myelin proteins—e.g., myelin basic protein (MBP)—have been found in both the serum and cerebrospinal fluid (CSF) of MS patients, and these antibodies, along with T cells that are reactive to MBP and to other myelin proteolipids, increase with disease activity; moreover, MBP cross-reacts to some extent with measles virus antibodies. The arguments that a chronic viral infection reactivates and perpetuates the disease are, however, less convincing than those proposing a role for viruses in the initiation of the process in susceptible individuals.

A possible way in which viral infections and autoimmune reactions in the nervous system might be linked to the abnormal expression of autoantigens on CNS cells has been suggested by R. T. Johnson. He found that several different viruses (rubeola, rubella, varicella) could cause autoimmunization of T lymphocytes against myelin basic protein. This means that the T lymphocyte recognizes an identical structure in the virus and myelin sheath. Once the autoimmune process is initiated by a virus in childhood, it can later be reactivated by any of the common viral infections to which the individual is exposed, particularly in the higher northern and southern latitudes. This phenomenon of molecular mimicry (a shared antigen between the virus and CNS myelin or the oligodendrocyte) has been invoked as a mechanism in several diseases, notably in rheumatic fever, certain paraneoplastic diseases, and Guillain-Barré syndrome.

The role of humoral and cellular factors in the production of MS plaques is not fully understood. That the humoral immune system is involved is evident from the presence in the CSF of most patients of oligoclonal immune proteins, which are produced by B lymphocytes within the CNS. Sera from patients with MS (and some normal controls), when added to organotypic cultures of nervous system tissue from newborn mice in the presence of complement, can damage myelin, inhibit remyelination, and block axonal conduction. Antibodies to oligodendrocytes are present in the serum of up to 90 percent of patients in some studies, but far less in others.

In respect to cellular factors, the focus of attention in recent years has been on the pathogenetic role of T lymphocytes, which regulate humoral immune responses either as potentiators (T-helper cells) or as inhibitors (T-suppressor cells) of immunoglobulin production by the B lymphocytes. So-called helper (CD4+) T cells are found in abundance within MS plaques and surrounding venules (perivascular cuffing). It has been demonstrated that T-cell receptors respond to antigens presented by (major histocompatibility complex, or MHC) class II molecules on macrophages and astrocytes. This interaction is thought to stimulate T-cell proliferation and a cascade of related cellular events, including the activation of B cells and macrophages and the secretion of cytokines (one of which is interferon beta and another interferon gamma; see further on). These cellular events are accompanied by a breakdown of the blood-brain barrier and, if sufficiently intense, by destruction of oligodendrocytes and myelin (see review by Ffrench-Constant). These findings strongly support the concept of a T-cell-mediated autoimmune inflammatory reaction, at least as a mechanism for sustaining the inflammation. A reduction in the blood of suppressor T lymphocytes was originally thought to characterize clinical relapse but has proved to be an inconstant feature. However, a reduction in T cells, both helper and suppressor subsets, or an increase in helper-suppressor ratios, does appear to be associated with increasing disability in patients with MS.

Many immunologists subscribe to the notion that MS is a T-cell-mediated disease. The idea is supported by evidence that T cells initiate the lesions of experimental allergic encephalomyelitis (EAE), which is repeatedly invoked as the animal model of MS. Although the entry of autoreactive T cells into the CNS results in a perivascular inflammatory reaction, the relationship to the main feature of MS, demyelination, is unclear. Conceivably, intense T-cell stimulation is in itself sufficient to induce demyelination, but it is also possible that the primary target of the immune reaction is the oligodendrocyte itself or its myelin processes and that the T-cell infiltration is the result of the demyelination. Other investigators believe that an additional insult is required, as illustrated by the EAE animal model, in which myelin and an adjuvant immune stimulus of portions of the tubercle bacilli are required. But EAE may be an imperfect model; it is not a naturally occurring disease but one in which a demyelination of the CNS is induced in susceptible animals by immunization with autologous myelin antigens. In other words, the inducing antigen in EAE is well defined, whereas *the antigen in MS is not known*. Nor, in broader terms, is the autoimmune hypothesis of MS beyond challenge. It is noteworthy that the prevalence of other diseases of presumed autoimmune origin is no higher in MS patients than in the general population (De Keyser). Moreover, the course of MS has been altered only inconsistently and to a slight extent by the administration of any of the nonspecific immunosuppressive therapies (Goodkin et al, 1992).

In summary, the immune mechanisms that are operative in the genesis of MS cannot as yet be specified.

Also worthy of comment is the relatively ineffective remyelination of the MS plaque. When remyelination occurs, thinly myelinated fibers are produced, creating areas of so-called shadow plaques. Histologic evidence suggests not only that some of the oligodendrocytes are destroyed in areas of active demyelination but also that the remaining ones have little ability to proliferate. Instead, there is an influx of oligodendroglial precursor cells, which mature into oligodendrocytes and provide the remaining axons with new myelin. Probably, the astrocytic hyperplasia in regions of damage and the persistent inflammatory response account for the inadequacy of the reparative process (see Prineas et al).

Physiologic Effects of Demyelination

The main physiologic effect of demyelination is to impede saltatory electrical conduction from one node of Ranvier, where sodium channels are concentrated, to the next node. The resulting failure of electrical transmission is thought to underlie most of the abnormalities of function resulting from demyelinating disease of both the central and peripheral nerve fibers. The delay in electrical conduction in the optic nerve (found by using pattern-shifting visual stimuli in MS patients with normal visual acuity and normal visual fields) raises a number of points about the pathophysiology of demyelination. When the demyelinative process is acute and reversible within a few days, the block in nerve fiber conduction is obviously physiologic rather than pathologic; in such a brief period, recovery is unlikely to have been due to remyelination. More likely, recovery is due to subsidence of the edema and acute inflammatory changes in and around the lesion. Remyelination probably does occur, as described above, but it is a slower process and partial at best, and its functional effects in the CNS are unknown. A slowing of optic nerve conduction, if it is present in an eye with normal vision, may account for the reduction in flicker fusion and in perception of multiple visual stimuli (Halliday and McDonald). It also explains one of the classic symptoms of optic neuritis—a reduction in the intensity (desaturation) of the color red. It is clear, however, that many of the plaques visualized on MRI are unaccompanied by corresponding symptoms; in some cases as well, there is no electrophysiologic abnormality, as tested with evoked responses. Either there has been remyelination in these plaques, sufficient to support clinical functioning, or, in the acute stage, the plaque may represent edema rather than demyelination.

Another classic feature of MS is the temporary induction, by heat or exercise, of symptoms such as unilateral visual blurring (the Uhthoff phenomenon) or tingling and weakness of a limb (the basis of the hot-tub test used in previous years). This has been shown experimentally to represent an extreme sensitivity of conduction in demyelinated nerve fibers to an elevation in temperature. A rise of only 0.5°C can block electrical transmission in some demyelinated fibers. Likewise, hyperventilation slows conduction of the visual evoked response, an effect that is rarely perceived by the patient. The remarkable sensitivity of demyelinated and remyelinated regions to subtle metabolic and environmental changes provides an explanation for the rapid onset of symptoms in some patients and the apparent fluctuations of MS that show no laboratory evidence of active inflammatory changes in the CNS. Smoking, fatigue, hyperventilation, and a rise in environmental temperature are all capable of briefly worsening neurologic functioning and are easily confused with relapses of disease.

Precipitating Factors

A variety of events occurring immediately before the initial symptoms or exacerbations of MS have been invoked as precipitating factors. The most common are infection, trauma, and pregnancy. However, in our view, none of these has been convincingly related to an increased risk of new attacks of MS, and there are no adequately controlled studies that would contradict this view. The incidence of respiratory or gastrointestinal viral infections that precede the onset or exacerbations of the disease varies greatly in different series, from 5 to 50 percent. The swine influenza vaccine, which was given to 45 million persons in the United States in late 1976, caused a slight increase in the incidence of Guillain-Barré disease but not of MS (Kurland et al). On the other hand, in an occasional individual an endogenous infection, such as labial or genital herpes, has regularly preceded an attack of MS.

The possible role of trauma in precipitating MS is more difficult to assess. McAlpine and Compston found that the incidence of trauma within a 3-month period preceding the onset of MS was slightly greater than in a random control group of hospital patients. Furthermore, there appeared to be a relationship between the site of the injury and the site of initial symptoms, particularly in patients who developed symptoms within a week of injury. We do not find this evidence convincing. Other forms of trauma (including lumbar puncture and general surgical procedures) that occur after the onset of the neurologic disorder have not been shown to have an adverse effect on the course of the illness. Matthews, who has extensive personal experience with survivors of penetrating head wounds, did not find a single instance of MS among them. One of the most meaningful prospective studies of the relation of physical injury to MS is that of Sibley and colleagues. They followed 170 MS patients and 134 controls for an average of 5 years, during which they recorded all (1407) instances of trauma and measured their effects on exacerbation rate and progression of the disease. With the possible exception of a case or two of electrical injury, there was no significant correlation between traumatic episodes and exacerbations.

Certain other epidemiologic data have a bearing on this subject. There are, in the United States, 250,000 to 350,000 cases of physician-diagnosed MS (Anderson et al). Also, a study from the National Center for Health Statistics has determined that trauma sufficiently severe to be recalled at a periodic health examination occurs in one-third of the population of the United States (some 83 million persons) each year. Moreover, MS patients suffer physical injuries two or three times more often than normal persons (Sibley et al). In light of these data, it is hardly surprising that a traumatic event and an exacerbation should sometimes coincide, quite by chance.

Clinical Manifestations

The conventional view of MS as a disease that strikes young people at a time when they are enjoying perfect health is not altogether correct. In some patients, the history discloses that fatigue, lack of energy, weight loss, and vague muscle and joint pains had been present for several weeks or months before the onset of neurologic symptoms. Nor is it generally appreciated that the neurologic disorder may have an acute, almost apoplectic onset. In fact, McAlpine and coworkers (1972), who analyzed the mode of onset in 219 patients, found that in about 20 percent the neurologic symptoms were fully developed in a matter of minutes, and in a similar number, in a matter of hours. In about 30 percent the symptoms evolved more slowly, over a period of a day or several days, and in another 20 percent more slowly still, over several weeks to months. In the remaining 10 percent the symptoms had an insidious onset and slow, steady, or intermittent progression over months and years. The relapsing-remitting pattern of disease is more likely to appear in patients who are less than 40 years of age. The inflammatory process of MS affects no organ system except the CNS.

Early Symptoms and Signs Weakness or numbness, sometimes both, in one or more limbs is the initial symptom in about half the patients. Symptoms of tingling of the extremities and tight band-like sensations around the trunk or limbs are commonly associated and are probably the result of involvement of the posterior columns of the spinal cord. The resulting clinical syndromes vary from a mere dragging or poor control of one or both legs to a spastic or ataxic paraparesis. The tendon reflexes are retained and later become hyperactive with extensor plantar reflexes; disappearance of the abdominal reflexes and varying degrees of deep and superficial sensory loss may be associated. It is a useful adage that the patient with MS presents with symptoms in one leg but with signs in both; the patient will complain of weakness, incoordination, or numbness and tingling in one lower limb and prove to have bilateral Babinski signs and other evidence of bilateral corticospinal and posterior column disease.

Passive flexion of the neck may induce a tingling, electric-like feeling down the shoulders and back and, less commonly, down the anterior thighs. This phenomenon is known as a *Lhermitte sign*, although it is more a symptom than a sign and was originally described by Babinski in a case of cervical cord trauma. Lhermitte's contribution was to draw attention to the frequent occurrence of this phenomenon in MS. It is the manifestation of increased sensitivity of demyelinated axons to the stretch or pressure on the spinal cord induced by neck flexion.

Dull, aching *pain* in the low back is a common complaint, but its relation to the lesions of MS is uncertain. Sharp, burning, poorly localized, or characteristic lancinating-radicular pain, localized to a limb or discrete part of the trunk, occurs but is infrequent. Nevertheless, these types of pain, presumably caused by demyelinative foci involving the root entry zones, have a few times been the presenting feature of the disease or have appeared at any time in established cases of the disease (Ramirez-Lassepas et al).

Other common modes of onset are optic neuritis, transverse myelitis, cerebellar ataxia, brainstem symptoms (vertigo, facial pain or numbness, dysarthria, diplopia), paresthesias in one limb, and disorders of micturition. These modes of presentation are often features of the established disease as well. They may pose diagnostic questions that at least have only conjectural answers, since they may represent disease other than MS. The more common presentations of MS are considered in the following paragraphs.

Optic Neuritis In about 25 percent of all MS patients (and in a larger proportion of children), the initial manifestation is an episode of *retrobulbar* or *optic neuritis*. Characteristically, over a period of several days, there is partial or total loss of vision in one eye. Some patients, for a day or two before the visual loss, experience pain within the orbit, worsened by eye movement or palpation of the globe. Rarely, the visual loss is steadily progressive for several weeks, mimicking a compressive lesion or intrinsic tumor of the optic nerve (Ormerod and McDonald). Usually a scotoma involving the macular area and blind spot (cecocentral) can be demonstrated, but a wide variety of other field defects may occur, rarely even hemianopic ones (sometimes homonymous). In some patients, both optic nerves are involved, either simultaneously or, more commonly, within a few days or weeks of one another, and at least 1 in 8 patients will have repeated attacks. Serial examinations may disclose evidence of swelling, or edema, of the optic nerve head (papillitis) in about half the patients. The occurrence of papillitis depends upon the proximity of the demyelinating lesion to the nerve head. Papillitis can be distinguished from the papilledema of increased intracranial pressure by the severe and acute visual loss that accompanies only the former. Subtle manifestations of optic nerve affection—such as atrophy of retinal nerve fibers or sheathing of retinal veins (page 261) and abnormalities of the visual evoked response (page 36)—should be sought in patients who have no visual complaints but are suspected of having MS. Only in cases of substantial visual loss is there a diminished pupillary response to light, but the pupil is said never to be dilated in ambient light. (Demyelination of the third nerve in its brainstem course, however, may be associated with a fixed enlargement of the pupil.) It will be recalled that the optic nerve is in fact a tract of the brain, and involvement of the optic nerves is therefore consistent with the rule that lesions of MS are confined to the CNS.

About one-third of patients with optic neuritis recover completely, and most of the remaining ones improve significantly, even those who present initially with profound visual loss and, later, pallor of the optic disc (Slamovitis et al). In a cohort of 397 patients enrolled in the Optic Neuritis Treatment Trial and examined 5 years after the initial attack of optic neuritis, visual acuity had returned to 20/25 or better in 87 percent of patients, and to 20/40 or better in 94 percent—even if there had been a recurrence of optic neuritis during the 5-year period. Moreover, the mode of treatment did not appear to influence the outcome. Dyschromatopsia, generally taking the form of a perceived desaturation of colors, is a frequent persistent finding. When improvement occurs, it begins usually within 2 weeks of onset, as is true of most acute manifestations of MS, perhaps sooner with corticosteroid treatment. Once improvement in neurologic function begins, it may continue for several months.

One-half or more of adult patients who present with optic neuritis alone will eventually develop other signs of MS. The prospective investigation of Rizzo and Lessell showed that MS developed in 74 percent of women and 34 percent of men by the 15th year after onset of visual loss. The risk is much lower if the initial attack of optic neuritis occurs in childhood (26 percent after 40 years of follow-up; Lucchinetti et al); this suggests that some instances of the childhood disease are of a different type. The longer the period of observation and the greater the care given to detection of mild cases, the greater the proportion of patients who are found to develop other signs of MS; however, most do so within 5 years of the original attack (Ebers, Hely et al). In fact, in many patients with clinically isolated optic neuritis, MRI has disclosed lesions of the cerebral white matter—suggesting that dissemination, albeit asymptomatic, had already occurred (Jacobs et al, Ormerod et al). The Optic Neuritis Study Group has made the point, well known to neurologists, that the recurrence of optic neuritis greatly increases the chances of developing MS.

It is unclear whether optic neuritis that occurs alone and is not followed by other evidence of demyelinating disease is simply a restricted form of MS or a manifestation of some other disease process, such as postinfectious encephalomyelitis. By far the most common pathologic basis for optic neuritis is demyelinative disease, though it is known that a vascular lesion or compression of an optic nerve by a tumor or mucocele may cause a central or cecocentral scotoma.

Uveitis and sheathing of the retinal veins are other ophthalmic disorders that have a higher than expected incidence in patients with MS. The retinal vascular sheathing is due to T-cell infiltration, identical to that in typical plaques, but this is an anomalous finding, since the retina usually contains no myelinated fibers (Lightman et al).

The treatment of optic neuritis is discussed further on.

Acute Myelitis (Transverse Myelitis) This is the common designation for an acutely evolving inflammatory-demyelinative lesion of the spinal cord, which proves in most instances to be an expression of MS, of either monophasic or chronic (polyphasic) type. In this sense the myelitic lesion is analogous to that of optic neuritis. The term *transverse* in relation to the myelitis is somewhat imprecise, implying that all of the elements in the cord are involved in the transverse plane, usually over a short vertical extent. Instead, in MS, the spinal cord signs are asymmetrical and incomplete and involve only the long ascending and descending tracts.

Clinically, the illness is characterized by a rapidly evolving (several hours or days) symmetrical or asymmetrical paraparesis, a sensory level on the trunk, sphincteric dysfunction, and bilateral Babinski signs. The CSF shows a modest increase in lymphocytes and total protein but may be normal early in the illness. As many as one-third of patients report an infectious illness in the weeks preceding the onset of neurologic symptoms, in which case a monophasic postinfectious demyelinating disease is the likely cause of the myelitis. We have found that fewer than half the patients have evidence of an asymptomatic demyelinative lesion elsewhere in the nervous system or develop clinical evidence of dissemination within 5 years of the initial attack (Ropper and Poskanzer). Thus, acute transverse myelitis is somewhat less often an initial expression of MS than is optic neuritis. An alternative view is that the majority of cases of transverse myelitis will ultimately develop MS and that only lengthy follow-up will uncover the association. Other aspects of transverse myelitis are discussed in Chap. 44, "Diseases of the Spinal Cord," and under "Acute Disseminated Encephalomyelitis" later in this chapter.

A special problem is presented by patients with *recurrent myelitis* at one level of the spinal cord but in whom no other signs of demyelinative disease can be found by careful clinical examination or MR imaging. Some of them may even have oligoclonal bands in the CSF, which are commonly associated with MS (see further on). Enough cases of this limited nature have come to our attention to permit the conclusion that there is a recurrent form of spinal cord MS, in which cerebral dissemination is infrequent (Tippet et al). It should be mentioned that isolated recurrent myelitis occurs occasionally with lupus erythematosus, mixed connective tissue disease, or antiphospholipid antibody syndrome, or in the presence of other autoantibodies. An analogous situation pertains in respect to some instances of optic neuritis—repeated attacks that remain confined to the optic nerve.

Other Patterns of Multiple Sclerosis (See also "variants of MS", page 965) Like the modes of onset cited above, other early manifestations of MS, in descending order of frequency, are unsteadiness in walking, brainstem symptoms (diplopia, vertigo, vomiting, etc.), paresthesias or numbness of an entire arm or leg, facial pain, and disorders of micturition. In our experience, vertigo of central type has been a frequent initial sign of MS. Discrete manifestations—such as hemiplegia, trigeminal neuralgia or other pain syndromes, facial paralysis, deafness, or seizures—occur in a small proportion of cases. Most often the disease presents with more than one of the aforementioned symptoms. Another syndrome of note, occurring mainly in elderly women, is a slowly progressive cervical myelopathy with weakness and ataxia. This is particularly difficult to differentiate from cervical spondylosis.

Not infrequently a prominent feature of the disease is *nystagmus and ataxia*, with or without weakness and spasticity of the limbs—a syndrome that reflects involvement of the cerebellar and corticospinal tracts. Ataxia of cerebellar type can be recognized by scanning speech, rhythmic instability of the head and trunk, intention tremor of the arms and legs, and incoordination of voluntary movements and gait, as described in Chap. 5. The combination of nystagmus, scanning speech, and intention tremor is known as *Charcot's triad*; while this group of symptoms is often seen in the advanced stages of the disease, most neurologists would agree that it is not a common mode of presentation. The most severe forms of cerebellar ataxia, in which the slightest attempt to move the trunk or limbs precipitates a violent and uncontrollable ataxic tremor, are observed among patients with long-standing MS. The responsible lesion probably lies in the tegmentum of the midbrain and involves the dentatorubrothalamic tracts and adjacent structures. Cerebellar ataxia may be combined with sensory ataxia, owing to involvement of the posterior columns of the spinal cord or medial lemnisci of the brainstem. In most cases of this type the signs of spinal cord involvement ultimately predominate; in others, the cerebellar signs are more prominent.

Diplopia is another common presenting complaint. It is due most often to involvement of the medial longitudinal fasciculi, producing an internuclear *ophthalmoplegia* (see page 289). The latter is characterized by paresis of the medial rectus on attempted lateral gaze, with a coarse nystagmus in the abducting eye; in MS, this abnormality is usually bilateral (unlike small pontine infarcts, which cause a unilateral internuclear ophthalmoplegia). As a corollary, *the presence of bilateral internuclear ophthalmoplegia presenting in a young adult is virtually diagnostic of MS*. Occasionally, internuclear ophthalmoplegia in one direction is combined with a horizontal gaze paresis in the other, although this "one-and-a-half syndrome" is more typical of brainstem stroke (see also page 289). Other palsies of gaze (due to interruption of supranuclear connections) or palsies of individual ocular muscles (due to involvement of the ocular motor nerves in their intramedullary course) also occur, but less frequently. Additional manifestations of brainstem involvement include myokymia or paralysis of facial muscles, deafness, tinnitus, unformed auditory hallucinations (because of involvement of cochlear connections), vertigo—as noted above, vomiting (vestibular connections), and rarely stupor and coma. The occurrence of *transient facial hypesthesia or anesthesia or of trigeminal neuralgia* in a young adult should always suggest the diagnosis of MS, with involvement of the intramedullary fibers of the fifth cranial nerve.

Symptoms and Signs in the Established Stage of the Disease When the diagnosis of MS has become virtually certain, a number of clinical syndromes are observed to occur with regularity. Approximately one-half of the patients will manifest a clinical picture of *mixed* or *generalized type* with signs pointing to involvement of the optic nerves, brainstem, cerebellum, and spinal cord. Another 30 to 40 percent will exhibit varying degrees of spastic ataxia and deep sensory changes in the extremities, i.e., essentially a *spinal form of the disease*. In either case, an asymmetrical spastic paraparesis is probably the most common manifestation of progressive MS. A predominantly *cerebellar* or *pontobulbar-cerebellar form* will be noted in only about 5 percent of cases and an *amaurotic form* in a like number. Thus the mixed and spinal forms together have made up at least 80 percent of our clinical material.

Traditional teaching has overemphasized the frequency of *euphoria*, a pathologic cheerfulness or elation that seems inappropriate in the face of the obvious neurologic deficit. (Charcot spoke of this phenomenon as "stupid indifference" and Vulpian as "morbid optimism.") Some patients do show this mental abnormality, always in association with other signs of cerebral impairment. In some instances it is manifestly a part of the syndrome of pseudobulbar palsy. A much larger number of patients, however, are *depressed*, irritable, and short-tempered as a reaction to the disabling features of the disease. Dalos and coworkers, in comparing MS patients with a group of traumatic paraplegics, found a significantly higher incidence of *emotional disturbance* in the former group, especially during periods of relapse. Other mental disturbances—such as a loss of retentive memory, a global *dementia*, or a confusional-psychotic state—also occur with some regularity in the advanced stages of the disease. The cognitive impairment is more in keeping with what has been ascribed to "subcortical dementia" (pages 450).

Symptoms of *bladder dysfunction*—including hesitancy, urgency, frequency, and incontinence—occur commonly with spinal cord involvement. Urinary retention, due to affection of sacral segments, is less frequent (Fig. 26-5). In males, these symptoms are often associated with impotence, a symptom that the patient may not report unless specifically questioned in this regard.

Abrupt attacks of neurologic deficit, lasting a few seconds or minutes and sometimes recurring many times daily, are a relatively infrequent but well-recognized feature of MS (see Osterman and Westerbey). Usually the attacks occur during the relapsing and remitting phase of the illness, rarely as an initial manifestation. These clinical phenomena are referable to any part of the CNS but tend to be stereotyped in an individual patient. The most common of these consist of dysarthria and ataxia, paroxysmal pain and dysesthesia in a limb, flashing lights, paroxysmal itching, or tonic seizures, taking the form of flexion (dystonic) spasm of the hand, wrist, and elbow with extension of the lower limb. The paroxysmal symptoms, particularly the tonic spasms, may be triggered by sensory stimuli or can be elicited by hyperventilation. The cause of paroxysmal phenomena is uncertain. They have been attributed by Halliday and McDonald to ephaptic transmission ("cross-talk") between adjacent demyelinated axons within a lesion. Carbamazepine is usually effective in controlling the attacks.

These transitory symptoms appear suddenly, may recur frequently for several days or weeks, sometimes longer, and then remit completely, i.e., they exhibit the temporal profile of a relapse or an exacerbation. It is sometimes difficult to determine whether they represent an exacerbation or a new lesion. Years ago, Thygessen pointed out, in an analysis of 105 exacerbations in 60 patients, that there were new symptoms in only 19 percent; in the remainder there was only a recurrence of old symptoms. Another problem is that the original lesion may have been asymptomatic. For example, many of the patients found to have impaired visual evoked responses have never had symptomatic visual changes. Thus, new symptoms and signs may be manifestations of previously formed but asymptomatic plaques. However, the observations of Prineas and Connell indicate that symptoms and signs may progress without the appearance of new plaques. These and other factors need to be taken into consideration in evaluating the clinical course of the illness and the effects of a therapeutic program (Poser).

Unusually severe *fatigue* is another peculiar symptom of MS; it is often transient and more likely to occur when there is fever or other evidence of disease activity, but it can be a persistent complaint and a source of considerable distress. Depression may play a role in these recalcitrant cases.

A number of interesting manifestations of MS have come to our attention over the years and have given rise to difficulties in diagnosis. The occurrence of typical tic douloureux in young patients has already been mentioned; only their young age and the bilaterality of the pain in some of them raised the suspicion of MS, confirmed later by sensory loss in the face and other neurologic signs. Brachial, thoracic, or lumbosacral pain consisting mainly of thermal and algesic dysesthesias was a source of puzzlement in several other patients until additional lesions developed. Not infrequently the relatively acute occurrence of a right hemiplegia and aphasia first raised the probability of a cerebrovascular lesion; in still others, a more slowly evolving hemiplegia had led to the diagnosis of a cerebral glioma.

Approximately 3 percent of patients have focal seizures, usually in relation to an obvious cerebral lesion. Several times we have seen coma during relapse, and in each instance it continued to death. In one case it occurred in a 64-year-old woman who had had two previous episodes of nondisabling spinal MS at 30 and 44 years of age. A confusional psychosis with drowsiness was the initial syndrome in another patient whom we saw later with a relapse involving the cerebellum and spinal cord. Another unusual syndrome is one of slow intellectual decline with slight cerebellar ataxia. A 10-year, slowly progressive cerebellar ataxia in an adolescent girl was another perplexing variant until she later developed internuclear ophthalmoplegia. A rapid onset of ascending paralysis of legs, bladder and bowel, and trunk with severe pain in sacral parts, areflexia, and a mononuclear pleocytosis of 1600 cells per cubic millimeter occurred in another of our patients and lasted 2 years before she began to walk again; earlier she had had diplopia and retrobulbar neuritis.

Repeatedly, seemingly more in recent years, we have observed patients whose illness satisfied all the clinical criteria for the diagnosis of MS except for the onset of symptoms in the sixth or seventh decade. Presumably we were witnessing the late deteriorative phase of the illness, earlier symptoms having been forgotten or having never been recognized. As mentioned in the chapter on spinal cord disease, some instances of MS in late adult life take the form of a slowly progressive cervical myelopathy.

Variants of MS

Several variants of MS merit more extended discussion. They are acute MS, neuromyelitis optica, acquired Schilder disease, and the conjunction of MS and polyneuropathy.

Acute Multiple Sclerosis Rarely, MS takes a rapidly progressive and highly malignant form. A combination of cerebral, brainstem, and spinal manifestations evolves over a few weeks, rendering the patient stuporous, comatose, or decerebrate, with prominent cranial nerve and corticospinal abnormalities. Death may end the illness within a few weeks to months without any remission having occurred. At autopsy the lesions (unlike those of acute disseminated encephalomyelitis) are of macroscopic dimensions, typical of the acute plaques of MS. The only difference from the usual form of MS is that many plaques are of the same age and the confluence of many perivenous zones of demyelination is more obvious. Two of our most striking examples of this rapidly fatal form were in a 6-year-old girl and a 16-year-old boy, both of whom died within 5 weeks of the onset of symptoms. Another was a 30-year-old man who lived 2 months. In none of them had there been a preceding exanthem or inoculation or any symptoms suggestive of demyelinative disease. Usually the CSF shows a brisk cellular response.

Nonfatal clinical cases of similar type in children, adolescents, and young adults are admitted to our hospitals once or twice a year. Some have responded to high doses of intravenous corticosteroids; others worsened while receiving this medication. We have also had experience with two patients who improved rapidly after the institution of plasma exchange treatments, similar to the report by Rodriquez and coworkers. However, it is clear that most patients with acute myelitis do not respond to this treatment. Some have made an astonishing recovery after several months, and a few have then remained well for 25 to 30 years. Others have relapsed, and the subsequent clinical course was typical of MS.

Most neurologists are familiar with similar episodes of acute deterioration that punctuate otherwise typical cases of MS. These aggressive relapses occur most often in the first year of illness and in middle-aged patients and take the form of an exacerbation of a preexisting myelopathy in combination with a new brainstem syndrome. After a severe episode of this sort or multiple ones, a few of the lesions are cavitating rather than demyelinative.

It seems to the authors that more than one disease is being included in the clinical category of acute MS. One type conforms in its temporal profile to a rather protracted form of acute disseminated encephalomyelitis—an acute monophasic illness extending over 4 to 8 weeks akin to some of the Japanese post–rabies inoculation cases (Shiraki and Otani). Others subsequently prove to be typical polyphasic MS. The main consideration in differential diagnosis is a CNS vasculitis.

Neuromyelitis Optica (Devic Disease, Necrotic Myelopathy; see also Chap. 46) The simultaneous or successive involvement of optic nerves and spinal cord has been convincingly documented. The combination was remarked upon by Clifford Albutt in 1870, and Gault (1894), stimulated by his teacher Devic, devoted his thesis to the subject. Devic endeavored to crystallize medical thought about a condition that has come to be known as neuromyelitis optica. Its principal features are the acute to subacute onset of blindness in one or both eyes, preceded or followed within days or weeks by a transverse or ascending myelitis (Mandler et al). The spinal cord lesions in cases of neuromyelitis optica are often necrotizing rather than purely demyelinative in type, leading eventually to cavitation; as would be expected, the clinical effects are more likely to be permanent than those of demyelination. A few of the patients have been children; in a number of instances, they suffered only a single episode of neurologic illness.

Although it is true that cases corresponding to this prototype are seen on occasion in every large medical center and at all age periods, the isolation of such an entity on clinical grounds alone has been unsatisfactory. Most of our patients have proved by subsequent clinical developments, and in a few instances by autopsy, to have chronic relapsing MS. In one notable example, where hemiplegia and aphasia were followed within 2 weeks by a necrotizing myelitis from which there was no recovery, the patient later developed typical attacks of MS, including retrobulbar neuritis. At autopsy, more than 15.0 cm of the spinal cord had been destroyed, reducing it to a collapsed membranous tube. Elsewhere the lesions were typically demyelinative.

One might conclude from cases such as these that neuromyelitis optica is but a variant form of MS (or some other type of demyelinative disease). Many cases of neuromyelitis optica, however, stand apart from MS by virtue of a number of distinctive clinical and pathologic features—namely, failure to develop brainstem, cerebellar, or cerebral demyelinative lesions and normality on MRI of the cerebral white matter, even after several years of illness; almost uniform absence of oligoclonal bands and other abnormalities of IgG in the spinal fluid; and finally the necrotizing and cavitary nature of the spinal cord lesion, affecting white and gray matter alike, with prominent thickening of vessels but without inflammatory infiltrates. On the basis of these differences, Mandler and O'Riordan and their colleagues and others have favored the separation of Devic disease from MS. For reasons mentioned above, we are uncertain that the distinction is quite so clear. Insofar as the cause neither of MS nor of Devic disease is known, uncertainties about the relationship of these diseases cannot be resolved with finality. Also, acute disseminated encephalomyelitis may occasionally present as neuromyelitis optica.

There also exists a progressive and saltatory *subacute necrotic myelopathy* without optic neuritis that shares all the myelopathic features of Devic disease and, in our view, probably represents the same entity (Katz and Ropper). The differential diagnosis is broader and includes arteriovenous malformation and infarction of the cord.

The treatment of neuromyelitis optica and of subacute necrotic myelopathy has been largely unsuccessful, most cases progressing despite aggressive therapy, including high-dose corticosteroids and cyclophosphamide.

Diffuse Cerebral Sclerosis of Schilder (Schilder Disease, Encephalitis Periaxialis Diffusa) Exceptionally the cerebrum is the site of massive demyelination, occurring in multiple foci or as a single large focus. Such cases are more frequent in childhood and adolescence than in adult life.

The term *diffuse sclerosis* was probably first used by Strumpell (1879) to describe the hard texture of the freshly removed brain of an alcoholic; later the term was applied to widespread cerebral gliosis of whatever cause. In 1912, Schilder described an instance of what he considered to be "diffuse sclerosis." The case was that of a 14-year-old girl with progressive mental deterioration and signs of increased intracranial pressure, terminating fatally after 19 weeks. Postmortem examination disclosed large, well-demarcated areas of demyelination in the white matter of both cerebral hemispheres as well as a number of smaller demyelinative foci, resembling the common lesions of MS. Because of the similarities of the pathologic changes to those of MS (prominence of the inflammatory reaction and relative sparing of axis cylinders), Schilder called this disease *encephalitis periaxialis diffusa*, bringing it in line with *encephalitis periaxialis scleroticans*, a term that Marburg had used to describe a case of acute MS. Unfortunately, in subsequent publications, Schilder used the same term for two other conditions of different type. One appears to have been a familial leukodystrophy (adrenoleukodystrophy) in a boy, and the other, quite unlike either of the first two cases, was suggestive of an infiltrative lymphoma. The last two reports seriously confused the subject, and for many years the terms *Schilder's disease* and *diffuse sclerosis* were indiscriminately attached to many different conditions.

One group of diseases of the cerebral white matter, which can be readily culled from the overall category of diffuse sclerosis, is the leukodystrophies, including adrenoleukodystrophy of boys and young men; globoid-cell leukodystrophy of Krabbe; sudanophilic leukodystrophy; and metachromatic leukodystrophy—all of which may involve peripheral nerves as well as the CNS tissue. The leukodystrophies (discussed in detail in Chap. 37) are characterized clinically by progressive visual failure, mental deterioration, and spastic paralysis and pathologically by massive and more or less symmetrical destruction of the white matter of the cerebral hemispheres. In each of them there is a specific inherited biochemical defect in the metabolism of myelin proteolipids.

If one sets aside the hereditary metabolic leukodystrophies and other childhood disorders of cerebral white matter that were incorrectly included under the rubric of "Schilder's disease" or "diffuse sclerosis," there remains a characteristic group of cases that does indeed correspond to Schilder's original description. These cases are nonfamilial and are most frequently encountered in children or young adults. As with the case reported by Ellison and Barron, the disease may follow the course of MS. Clinically these cases run a progressive course, either steady and unremitting or punctuated by a series of episodes of rapid worsening. In rare instances the disease may become arrested for many years, or the patient may even improve for a time. Dementia, homonymous hemianopia, cerebral blindness and deafness, varying degrees of hemiplegia and quadriplegia, and pseudobulbar palsy are the usual clinical findings. Optic neuritis may occur before or after the cerebral symptoms. The CSF may show changes similar to those in chronic relapsing MS, but often there are no oligoclonal bands; instead, myelin basic protein is found in large quantity in the CSF. Death occurs in most patients within a few months or years, but some survive for a decade or longer. In the differential diagnosis, a diffuse cerebral neoplasm, adrenoleukodystrophy, and progressive multifocal leukoencephalopathy (Chap. 33) are the main considerations.

The characteristic lesion in these cases is a large, sharply outlined, asymmetrical focus of myelin destruction often involving an entire lobe or cerebral hemisphere, typically with extension across the corpus callosum and affection of the opposite hemisphere (Fig. 36-3). In some cases both hemispheres may be symmetrically involved. A careful examination of the optic nerves, brainstem, and spinal cord often discloses the typical discrete lesions of MS. Histologically, the large single focus as well as the smaller disseminated ones show the characteristic features of MS.

Poser's review of the literature in 1957 uncovered 105 cases that could be designated as the Schilder type of diffuse sclerosis in the original sense of the term. In 33

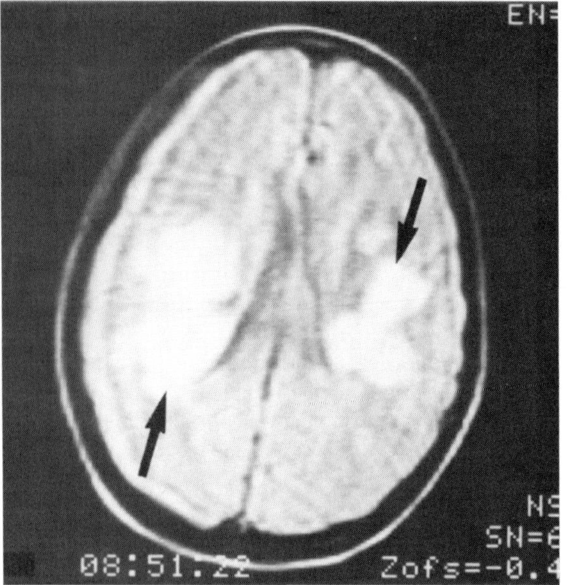

Figure 36-3

Diffuse cerebral sclerosis (Schilder disease). MR image showing large asymmetrical foci of involvement of white matter in a 12-year-old boy, 2 1/2 months after onset of symptoms. The clinical picture was one of rapidly worsening episodes of bilateral hemiplegia and hemianopia. (From Bisese JH, Cranial MRI, New York, McGraw-Hill, 1991, by permission.)

of these, the only lesions were the extensive areas of demyelination involving the centrum ovale; most of the patients in this group were children, and the disease had a tendency to take a subacute progressive course. In 72 patients, in addition to the large foci in the cerebral white matter, isolated demyelinative plaques were found in other parts of the CNS; the age of onset in this latter group was similar to that of chronic, relapsing MS; frequently, the illness ran a protracted and remitting course. These findings were elaborated by Poser and colleagues in a subsequent (1986) review of this subject. It is apparent that diffuse cerebral sclerosis of this type must be closely related to MS and may indeed be a variant of it, as Schilder originally proposed.

The *concentric sclerosis of Balo* is probably a variety of Schilder disease, which it resembles in its clinical aspects and in the overall distribution of its lesions. The distinguishing feature is the occurrence of alternating bands of destruction and preservation of myelin in a series of concentric rings. The occurrence of lesions in this pattern suggests the centrifugal diffusion of some factor that is damaging to myelin. A similar pattern of lesions, although far less extensive, is seen in occasional cases of chronic relapsing MS.

Multiple Sclerosis in Conjunction with Peripheral Neuropathy From time to time there have been patients with MS who also have a polyneuropathy or mononeuropathy multiplex. This relationship always invites speculation and controversy. The rarity of the combination suggests a purely coincidental occurrence, perhaps with an underlying disease as an explanation (e.g., Lyme disease, AIDS). Another view, expressed by Thomas et al and by Mendell et al, is that an autoimmune demyelination has been incited in both spinal cord and peripheral nerve, the latter taking the form of a chronic inflammatory polyradiculoneuropathy. Of course, radicular and neuropathic symptoms, motor and/or sensory, can result from the involvement of myelinated fibers in the root entry zone of the cord or fibers of exit in the ventral white matter. And in the late stages of MS there is always the possibility of vitamin deficiency polyneuropathy or multiple pressure palsies.

Laboratory Findings

Cerebrospinal Fluid In about one-third of all MS patients, particularly those with an acute onset or exacerbation, there may be a slight to moderate mononuclear pleocytosis (usually less than 50 cells per cubic millimeter). In rapidly progressive cases of neuromyelitis optica (see above) and in certain instances of severe demyelinative disease of the brainstem, the total cell count may reach or exceed 100 and rarely 1000 cells per cubic millimeter; the greater proportion of these in the hyperacute cases may be polymorphonuclear leukocytes. This pleocytosis may in fact be the only measure of activity of the disease. Other laboratory tests (except perhaps for myelin basic protein, see below) do not reflect the activity of the disease.

Also, in about 40 percent of patients, the total protein content of the CSF is increased. The increase is slight, however, and a concentration of more than 100 mg/dL is so unusual that the possibility of another diagnosis should be entertained. More importantly, the proportion of gamma globulin (essentially IgG) is increased (greater than 12 percent of the total protein) in about two-thirds of patients. Another less frequently used diagnostic measure is the IgG index, which is obtained by measuring albumin and gamma globulin in both the serum and CSF and using the following formula:

$$\frac{\text{CSF IgG/serum IgG}}{\text{CSF alb/serum alb}}$$

A ratio of more than 1.7 indicates the probability of MS.

It has been shown that the gamma globulins in the CSF of patients with MS are synthesized in the CNS (Tourtellotte and Booe) and that they migrate in agarose electrophoresis as abnormal discrete populations, so-called *oligoclonal bands*. A simple method for demonstrating these bands uses readily available commercial reagents and apparatus. Determination of the IgG index and testing for oligoclonal IgG bands is done in most commercial and hospital laboratories and will show CSF abnormalities in more than 90 percent of cases of MS. Such bands also appear in the CSF of patients with syphilis and subacute sclerosing panencephalitis—disorders that should not be difficult to distinguish from MS on clinical grounds. The demonstration of oligoclonal bands in the CSF and not in the blood is particularly helpful in confirming the diagnosis of MS, but these are not always found with the first attack or even in the later stages of the disease. The presence of such bands in a first attack of MS is predictive of chronic relapsing MS, according to Moulin and coworkers and others.

It has also been shown, by the use of a sensitive radioimmunoassay, that the CSF of many patients contains high concentrations of myelin basic protein (MBP) during acute exacerbations of MS and that these levels are lower or normal in slowly progressive MS and normal during remissions of the disease (Cohen et al). Other lesions that destroy myelin (e.g., infarction) can also increase the level of MBP in the spinal fluid. Thus the assay is not particularly useful as a diagnostic test. The method is not simple but is available commercially.

When cells, total protein, gamma globulin, and oligoclonal bands are all taken into account, some abnormality of the spinal fluid will be found in the great majority of patients with MS. At present the measurement of gamma globulins as a fraction of total protein and oligoclonal bands in the CSF are the most reliable of the chemical tests for MS. We are not convinced that other, more complicated laboratory procedures, such as CSF measurements of globulin production or MBP, provide additional diagnostic sensitivity.

MRI in MS It is now widely appreciated that MRI is the most helpful ancillary examination in the diagnosis of MS, by virtue of its ability to reveal asymptomatic plaques in the cerebrum, brainstem, optic nerves, and spinal cord (see Figs. 36-1 and 36-2). Our experience accords with that of Stewart and coworkers, who found multifocal lesions in 80 percent of their established cases. In a series of 114 patients with clinically definite MS, Ormerod and colleagues recorded T2-intense periventricular MRI abnormalities in all but 2 patients and discrete cerebral white matter lesions in all but 12. It is remarkable that even when there are a multitude of cerebral lesions, they tend to be asymptomatic; the opposite is generally the case with spinal cord lesions.

It should be stressed that foci of periventricular hyperintensity are observed with a variety of pathologic processes and even in normal persons, particularly older ones; in the latter cases, the periventricular changes are usually milder in degree and smoother in outline than the lesions of MS. The signal characteristics of MS lesions vary somewhat depending on the field strength of the magnet and the ratio of T1 and T2 weighting—but, curiously, not on the age of the lesions. In general, MS plaques that are hypointense (white) on T2-weighted images may be even more strikingly obvious on FLAIR images. Lesions that have undergone some degree of cavitation, as happens only occasionally, are hypointense on T1-weighted images. The discrete cerebral lesions of MS do not always impart a specific MR imaging appearance; but the finding, on T2-weighted images, of several asymmetrical, well-demarcated lesions immediately adjacent to the ventricular surface usually denotes MS. These areas typically extend into the centrum semiovale and may reach the convolutional white matter. In advanced cases the lesions become confluent, usually at the poles of the ventricles. *Especially diagnostic are oval or linear regions of demyelination, oriented perpendicularly to the ventricular surface and corresponding to the radially oriented fiber bundles of the white matter and periventricular veins.* When viewed in sagittal images, they extend outward from the corpus callosum and have been called "Dawson fingers." Some lesions display contrast enhancement when acute; these can be brought out by administration of double or triple the usual dose of gadolinium. The spectrum of these changes has been commented upon by Berry and colleagues. Infrequently, a large acute lesion may have a mass effect and a ring-like contrast-enhancing border, resembling a glioblastoma or an infarct, and the correct diagnosis may be made only by biopsy. A series of focal tumor-like lesions of the brain, the demyelinative nature of which only became evident after biopsy, has been reported by Kepes. Serially performed MRI can demonstrate the progress of the disease. As with other laboratory procedures, MRI changes assume diagnostic significance only if they are consistent with the clinical findings.

Evoked Potentials and Other Tests When the clinical data point to only one lesion in the CNS, as often happens in the early stages of the disease or in the spinal form, a number of other sensitive physiologic and radiologic tests may establish the existence of additional asymptomatic lesions. These tests include visual, auditory, and somatosensory evoked responses and the less easily available perceptual delay on visual stimulation; electro-oculography; altered blink reflexes; and a change in flicker fusion of visual images. Halliday and McDonald reported abnormalities in one or more of these tests in 50 to 90 percent of a series of MS patients. At our hospitals, abnormal visual evoked responses have been found in 70 percent of patients with the clinical features of definite MS and 60 percent of patients with probable or possible MS. The corresponding figures for somatosensory evoked responses were 69 percent and 51 percent, and for brainstem auditory evoked responses (usually prolonged interwave latency or decreased amplitude of wave 5), 47 percent and 20 percent, respectively (see Chap. 2).

CT scanning may also demonstrate cerebral lesions, often unexpectedly. Doubling the dose of contrast material and delaying the scan for an hour postinfusion increases the yield of lesions during exacerbations of MS. Two points worth noting about the CT scan are that acute plaques can appear as contrast-enhanced ring lesions, simulating abscess or tumor, and that some contrast-enhanced periventricular lesions become radiologically inevident after steroid treatment, as occurs also with CNS lymphoma.

As mentioned earlier, the ancillary examinations in common use—MRI, evoked potentials, and oligoclonal bands in the CSF—have broadened the criteria for the diagnosis of MS. Often these procedures disclose the presence of multiple plaques when clinical examination has failed to do so. Stated differently, the time-honored rule that the diagnosis of MS requires evidence of "lesions scattered in time and space" is still valid, but the evidence now includes certain laboratory findings as well as purely clinical ones. Finally, it should be noted that no single laboratory procedure—including MRI, altered blood-brain barrier, immunoglobulin synthesis, and MBP in CSF—when viewed alone or at a single time is a totally reliable marker for MS.

Clinical Course and Prognosis

The intermittency of the clinical manifestations—the disease advancing in a series of attacks, each permitting less and less remission—is perhaps the most important clinical attribute of MS. Some patients will have a complete clinical remission after the initial attack, or, rarely, there may be a series of exacerbations, each with complete remission; such exacerbations may be severe enough to have caused quadriplegia and pseudobulbar palsy. The relapse rate is 0.3 to 0.4 attacks per year according to the calculations of McAlpine and Compston, but the interval between the opening symptom and the first relapse is highly variable. It occurred within 1 year in 30 percent of McAlpine's cases and within 2 years in another 20 percent. A further 20 percent relapsed in 5 to 9 years, and another 10 percent in 10 to 30 years. Not only the length of this latent interval is remarkable, but also the fact that the pathologic process can remain potentially active for such a long time.

Weinshenker and colleagues, on the basis of observations in 1099 MS patients over a 12-year period, have identified a number of features of the early clinical course that are predictive, in a general way, of the outcome of the illness. Perhaps not surprisingly, they found that a high degree of disability, as measured by the Kurtzke Disability Status Scale (DSS 6, indicating assistance required for walking), was reached earlier in patients with a higher number of attacks, a shorter first interattack interval, and a shorter time to reach a state of moderate disability (DSS 3). Kurtzke had earlier reported that the feature most predictive of long-term disability was the degree of disability at 5 years from the first symptom.

After a number of years there is an increasing tendency for the patient to enter a phase of slow, steady, or fluctuating deterioration of neurologic function, attributable to the cumulative effect of increasing numbers of lesions. However, in about 10 percent of cases the clinical course is almost evenly progressive from the beginning (primary progressive multiple sclerosis; see Thompson et al). In these latter cases the disease usually takes the form of a chronic asymmetrical spastic paraparesis and probably represents the most frequent type of obscure myelopathy observed by the authors. In Thompson's review of such cases, there was an absence of progression of the MRI findings, a negligible response to therapy, and a poor outcome.

Few if any factors are known to affect the course of the disease. Contrary to commonly held opinion, pregnancy does not have an adverse effect on MS. In fact, pregnancy is typically associated with clinical stability or even with improvement, as it is in a number of autoimmune diseases. The average relapse rate in established cases declines in each trimester, reaching a level less than one-third of the expected rate by the third trimester. However, there appears to be an increased risk of exacerbations, up to twofold, in the first few months postpartum (Birk and Rudick). An extensive study of 269 pregnancies by Confavreux and colleagues established a rate of relapse of 0.7 per woman per year before pregnancy and rates of 0.5 in the first, 0.6 in the second, and 0.2 in the third trimester, the rate then increasing substantially to 1.2 in the first three postpartum months.

The duration of the disease is exceedingly variable. A small number of patients die within several months or years of the onset, but the average duration is in excess of 30 years. A 60-year appraisal of the resident population of Rochester, Minnesota, disclosed that 74 percent of patients with MS survived 25 years, as compared with 86 percent of the general population. At the end of 25 years, one-third of the surviving patients were still working and two-thirds were still ambulatory (Percy et al). Other statistical analyses have given a far less optimistic prognosis; these have been reviewed by Matthews. Patients with mild and quiescent forms of the disease are, of course, less likely to be included in such surveys.

Differential Diagnosis

In the usual forms of MS—that is, in those with a relapsing and remitting course and evidence of disseminated lesions in the CNS—the diagnosis is rarely in doubt. Only meningovascular syphilis, certain rare forms of cerebral arteritis, vascular malformations (cavernous angiomas) of the brainstem or spinal cord with multiple episodes of bleeding, lupus erythematosus, and Behçet disease could possibly simulate relapsing MS, and each of these has its own characteristic diagnostic features. The list can be stretched by inclusion of corticosteroid-responsive cerebral lymphoma, intravascular lymphoma, and the numerous causes of multiple, well-demarcated white matter abnormalities on MRI, such as embolic infarcts, progressive multifocal leukoencephalopathy, Lyme disease, tumors, etc. Difficulties are most likely to arise when the standard clinical criteria for the diagnosis of MS are lacking, as occurs in the acute initial attack of the disease and in cases with an insidious onset and slow, steady progression. Other *features that call for caution in diagnosis of MS are an absence of symptoms and signs of optic neuritis, the presence of amyotrophy, entirely normal eye movements, a hemianopic field defect, pain as the predominant symptom, and a progressive nonremitting illness that begins in youth.*

As has been stated, *the initial attack of MS* may mimic acute labyrinthine vertigo or tic douloureux (trigeminal neuralgia). Careful neurologic examination of such patients usually discloses other signs of a brainstem lesion; the CSF examination may be particularly helpful in these circumstances. Extensive brainstem demyelination of subacute evolution, involving tracts and cranial nerves sequentially, may be mistaken for a pontine glioma. With brainstem symptoms of acute onset, there may be difficulty in distinguishing an MS plaque from a small infarction due to a basilar branch occlusion. In several patients that we have observed, recurrent bleeding from multiple cavernous vascular malformations and small brainstem arteriovenous malformations simulated MS. With MRI, visualization of blood products surrounding the small vascular lesions clarifies the diagnosis (see Fig. 34-26). Sequential MRI and the course of the illness settle the matter; symptoms of brainstem MS remit as a rule, and to a surprisingly complete degree in many cases.

Disseminated encephalomyelitis (see further on) is an acute illness with widely scattered small demyelinative lesions, but it is self-limited and monophasic; furthermore, fever, stupor, and coma, which are characteristic, rarely occur in MS.

In systemic lupus erythematosus and rarely in other autoimmune diseases (mixed connective tissue disease, Sjögren syndrome, scleroderma, primary biliary cirrhosis), there may be multiple lesions of the CNS white matter. These may parallel the activity of the underlying immune disease or the level of autoantibodies, such as those against native DNA or phospholipids, but myelitis or lesions in the cerebral hemispheres are known to occur before other organ systems are affected. Conversely, between 5 and 10 percent of MS patients have antinuclear or anti-double-stranded DNA antibodies without signs of lupus. In addition, it has been pointed out that the relatives of patients with MS have a higher than expected incidence of autoantibodies of various types, suggesting an as yet unproved connection between autoimmune disease and MS. On MRI, the lesions of lupus appear similar to plaques, and both the optic nerve and the spinal cord may be involved, even repeatedly, in a succession of attacks resembling MS. Nevertheless, in our pathologic material, the lesions represent small zones of infarct necrosis rather than demyelination and are traceable to small-vessel vasculitis or cardiogenic embolism. In a few instances, inflammatory demyelination without vascular changes may be seen. It is best for the moment to consider these as special manifestations of lupus or related diseases that mimic MS.

Periarteritis nodosa or vasculitis confined to the nervous system may produce multifocal lesions simulating MS. The distinction may be particularly difficult in rare instances of the vasculitic process in which the neurologic manifestations take the form of a relapsing or steroid-responsive myelitis. In these cases, the CSF may contain 100 or more white blood cells per cubic millimeter and there may be no evidence of disease elsewhere in the nervous system. Occassionally, a young individual with Lyme disease may have complaints of inordinate fatigue and vague neurologic symptoms coupled with T-2 bright lesions on the cranial MRI. Close attention to the characteristic history (rash, arthritis, etc.) and serologic findings should permit the distinction of the two diseases.

The distinguishing features of Behçet disease are recurrent iridocyclitis and meningitis, mucous membrane ulcers of mouth and genitalia, and symptoms of articular, renal, lung, and multifocal cerebral disease. The chronic forms of brucellosis in the Mediterranean regions and Lyme borreliosis throughout North America and Europe may cause myelopathy or encephalopathy with multiple white matter lesions on imaging studies, but in each case the history and other features of the disease help to identify the infectious illness (see Chap. 32).

The *purely spinal form of MS*, presenting as a progressive spastic paraparesis, hemiparesis, or—in several of our cases—spastic monoparesis of a leg with varying degrees of posterior column involvement, is a special source of diagnostic difficulty. A tendency to affect older women has already been mentioned. Such patients require careful evaluation for the presence of spinal cord compression due to neoplasm or cervical spondylosis. Radicular pain at some point in the illness is a frequent manifestation of these disorders and is much less frequent in MS. Pain in the neck, restricted mobility of the cervical spine, and severe muscle wasting due to spinal root involvement, as is sometimes seen in spondylosis, are almost unknown in MS. Moderate atrophy of the first dorsal interosseus muscles has, however, been commented on as a common finding in MS. As a general rule, loss of abdominal reflexes, impotence in males, and disturbances of bladder function occur early in the course of demyelinative myelopathy but late or not at all in cervical spondylosis. The CSF protein in the latter condition is apt to be significantly elevated, but the other typical protein abnormalities of MS are absent. The definitive tests are MRI and CT myelography and perhaps electromyography (EMG), which is sensitive to the radicular features of spondylosis. Every patient with progressive spastic paraparesis in whom the neurologic signs are limited to the spinal cord should be investigated by these methods. A special problem arises when imaging procedures reveal a regional swelling of the spinal cord, which happens occasionally with an episode of myelitis and suggests a tumor. In several of our patients this finding has led to fruitless laminectomy.

The problem of differentiating MS from tropical spastic paraparesis (human lymphotropic virus, myelitis of the HTLV 1 type) and progressive familial spastic paraplegia may also arise occasionally. Amyotrophic lateral sclerosis (ALS) and subacute combined degeneration (SCD) of the cord should not be confused with MS. Amyotrophic lateral sclerosis can be identified by the presence of muscle wasting, fasciculations, and the absence of sensory involvement, while SCD is characterized by symmetrical involvement of the posterior and then lateral columns of the spinal cord, low serum levels of vitamin B_{12}, gastric achlorhydria, the presence of multilobed polymorphonuclear cells, megaloblastic marrow and macrocytic anemia in many cases, high serum concentrations of methylmalonic acid and homocystine, and defective absorption of vitamin B_{12} as determined by the Schilling test (page 1122).

Platybasia and basilar impression of the skull should also be considered in the differential diagnosis, but patients with these conditions have a characteristic shortening of the neck; careful radiographs of the base of the skull will be diagnostic. Neurologic syndromes resulting from the Chiari malformation, syringomyelia, and tumors of the foramen magnum, cerebellopontine angle, clivus, and other parts of the posterior fossa have been misdiagnosed as MS. In each of these instances, a solitary, strategically placed lesion may give rise to a variety of neurologic symptoms and signs referable to the lower brainstem and cranial nerves, cerebellum, and upper cervical cord and may give the impression of dissemination of lesions. It is an excellent clinical rule that a diagnosis of MS should not be made when all the patient's symptoms and signs can be explained by a single lesion in one region of the neuraxis.

Occasionally MS may be confused with the hereditary ataxias, particularly the spinocerebellar types. The latter are generally distinguished by their familial incidence and other associated genetic traits; by their insidious onset and slow, steady progression; and by their symmetry and stereotyped clinical pattern. Intactness of abdominal reflexes and sphincteric function and the presence of pes cavus, kyphoscoliosis, and cardiac disease are other features that favor the diagnosis of a heredodegenerative disorder (see Chap. 39). Finally, as mentioned above, the periventricular lesions of cerebral lymphoma—an increasingly common tumor—and angiocentric lymphoma (page 700) may closely resemble

MS plaques on MRI and may also produce a multifocal, relapsing, steroid-responsive illness of the CNS. This last disease has been associated at times with oligoclonal bands in the spinal fluid.

Careful clinical appraisal will usually lead to accurate diagnosis, but the label of MS should not be attached to a patient until the evidence is unequivocal. Once such a label is applied, it tends to stick, and since the diagnosis of MS will explain almost any subsequent neurologic event, attention may be directed away from consideration of another, perhaps treatable disease.

Treatment

As one might expect, numerous forms of treatment have been proposed over the years, and many were thought to be successful, no doubt because of the remitting naure of the disease. To enumerate them all here would serve no useful purpose. The many therapeutic trials of recent years, utilizing mainly anti-inflammatory and immunosuppressive drugs, have been critically reviewed by Matthews and by Ebers and more recently by Rudick and colleagues. On the basis of controlled clinical trials, only adrenocorticotropic hormone (ACTH), methylprednisolone, prednisone, cyclophosphamide, and beta-interferon have proved to have a beneficial effect on the disease and on MRI lesions. Under the influence of the anti-inflammatory agents, recovery from an attack, including an attack of optic neuritis, appears to be hastened. However, a substantial group of patients with acute exacerbations fail to respond; in others, benefit is not apparent for a month or longer after the course of treatment has been completed. Also, there is no evidence that steroids have a significant effect upon the ultimate course of this disease or that they prevent recurrences, so there is little justification for steroid treatment over a period of many months or years.

Corticosteroids As to the dosage of corticosteroids for an acute attack, it has seemed to us important that a high dose be used initially to be effective, but this has been disputed, as noted below. The intravenous administration of massive doses of methylprednisolone (a bolus of 500 to 1000 mg daily for 3 to 5 days), followed by high oral doses of prednisone (beginning with 60 to 80 mg daily and tapering this dosage over a 12-day period) is generally effective in aborting or shortening an acute or subacute exacerbation of MS or of optic neuritis and is probably as effective as but far less cumbersome than the administration of ACTH, which was popular during the 1970s and 1980s. When it is impractical to administer parenteral methylprednisolone, one may substitute oral methylprednisolone—48 mg in a single daily dose for 1 week, followed by 24 mg daily for 1 week, and finally 12 mg daily for 1 week (Barnes et al). This has the advantage of avoiding hospitalization, but we have the impression that severe attacks, especially of myelitis, respond more quickly to high-dose intravenous medication. However, a randomized trial of oral and intravenous methylprednisolone in acute relapses of MS demonstrated no clear advantage of the intravenous regimen (Barnes et al).

We attempt to limit the period of corticosteroid administration to less than 2 weeks but prolong the period of tapering the drug if neurologic signs return. This brief period of corticosteroid administration generally produces few adverse effects, but some patients complain of insomnia and a few will develop depressive or manic symptoms. Patients who, because of clinical relapse upon withdrawal of the medication, require treatment for more than several weeks are subject to the effects of hypercortisolism, including the facial and truncal cosmetic changes of Cushing syndrome, hypertension, hyperglycemia and erratic diabetic control, osteoporosis, aseptic necrosis of the acetabulum, and cataracts; less often, there may be gastrointestinal hemorrhage and activation of tuberculosis. Modest potassium replacement is advisable. Alternate-day steroid treatment offers little benefit, in our experience. However, pulses of high-dose intravenous steroids, administered once each month, seem to keep some patients from having relapses and are better tolerated than the continuous administration of oral medication. It must be acknowledged that the corticosteroid regimens and dosages in common use are derived from anecdotal experience (the Optic Neuritis Treatment Trial being an exception) and that certain patients appear, at least for a period of time, to respond better to one or another method of treatment.

Treatment of Optic Neuritis The Optic Neuritis Treatment Trial, reported by Beck and colleagues, cautioned against the use of oral prednisone in the treatment of acute optic neuritis (see also Lessell). In this randomized, controlled study involving 457 patients with acute optic neuritis, it was found that the use of intravenous methylprednisolone followed by oral prednisone did indeed speed the recovery from visual loss, although at 6 months there was little difference between patients treated in this way and those treated with placebo. However, treatment with oral prednisone alone increased the risk of new episodes of optic neuritis. In a subsequent randomized trial conducted by Sellebjerg and colleagues, it was found that methylprednisolone 500 mg orally for

5 days had a beneficial effect on visual function at 1 and 3 weeks. However, at 8 weeks no effect could be shown (compared with the placebo-treated group), nor was there an effect on the subsequent relapse rate.

Interferon Beta and Copolymer I These are more recently introduced forms of treatment for patients with relapsing-remitting multiple sclerosis and give promise of modestly altering the natural history of the disease. Interferon beta-1b (Betaseron), a nonglycosylated bacterial cell product with an amino acid sequence identical to that of natural interferon beta, was the first of these agents to be tested (see Arnason). Several trials have now shown that the subcutaneous injection of this agent, every second day for up to 5 years, decreases the frequency and severity of relapses by almost one-third and also the number of new or enlarging lesions ("lesion burden") in serial MR images. A more recent large-scale trial (European Study Group) has extended the observations with interferon beta-1b to patients with the secondarily progressive type of MS; progression of the disease was delayed for 9 to 12 months in a study period of 2 to 3 years.

The treatment of relapsing-remitting MS with interferon beta-1a (a glycosylated mammalian-cell product, Avonex) is equally effective; it may be taken once weekly as an intramuscular injection (PRISMS Study Group). The dose currently used is 30 μg, or 6.6 million units. Copolymer I (glatiramer acetate), which was synthesized to mimic the actions of MBP, a putative autoantigen in multiple sclerosis, is given daily in subcutaneous doses of 20 mg. Glatiramer acetate (Copaxone) may be particularly useful in patients who become resistant, i.e. develop serum antibodies to interferon beta (Rudick et al).

Overall, the side effects of these agents have been modest, consisting mainly of flu-like symptoms, sweating, and malaise that begin several hours after the injection and persist for up to 14 h; they tend to abate with continued use of the agents, but some patients cannot tolerate them. The salutary effects of treatment are definite though not overwhelming, and difficulties in judging the clinical trials remain; these have been summarized by Hughes and Sharrack. Treatment is somewhat tedious and quite expensive. The long-term effects remain to be clarified, particularly the significance of neutralizing antibodies and the reducation in MRI changes, and the extent to which the latter translate into clinical benefit.

Immunosuppressive Drugs A number of experimental agents that modify immune reactivity have been tried, with limited success. Drugs such as azathioprine and cyclophosphamide, as well as total lymphoid irradiation, have been given to small groups of patients and seem to have improved the clinical course of some (Aimard et al, Hauser et al, Cook et al). However, the risks of prolonged use of immunosuppressive drugs, including a risk of neoplastic change, will probably preclude their widespread use. Moreover, the careful study by the British and Dutch Multiple Sclerosis Azathioprine Trial Group attributed no significant advantage to treatment with this drug. For the chronic, progressive phase of the disease, an MS study group has reported a modest delay in the advance of the disease after a 2-year trial of prednisolone and cyclophosphamide. They caution, however, that the "burdensome and potentially serious toxicity must temper one's consideration of its use in this disease." At least one subsequent blinded, placebo-controlled study with cyclophosphamide has failed to show any benefit. In one trial involving patients with chronic progressive MS, weekly, low-dose oral methotrexate has made a slight clinical difference and produced some reduction in the volume of cerebral lesions on the MRI compared with control cases (Goodkin et al). Because this regimen is well tolerated, it may still have some use in otherwise untreatable progressive cases.

Other Therapies There are no valid studies to substantiate claims that have been made for the value of synthetic polypeptides, hyperbaric oxygen, low-fat and gluten-free diets, or linoleate supplementation of the diet. As mentioned under "Acute Multiple Sclerosis," there may be a role for plasma exchange (Rodriquez et al) and perhaps immunoglobulin in fulminant cases, but these have not been tested rigorously. One trial has shown some benefit, in patients with relapsing-remitting disease, of monthly infusions of intravenous immunoglobulin (0.2 g/kg) for 2 years (Fazekas et al).

General Measures These include the provision of an adequate period of bed rest and convalescence to ensure maximum recovery from the initial attack or exacerbation, prevention of excessive fatigue and infection, the use of all possible rehabilitative measures to postpone the bedridden stage of the disease (braces, chairs, ramps, lifts, cars with manual controls, etc.), and meticulous attention to the prevention of bedsores in the bedridden patient by the use of alternating-pressure mattresses, silicone gel pads, and other special devices.

Fatigue, a common complaint of MS patients, particularly in relation to acute attacks, responds to some extent to amantadine (100 mg morning and noon), modafinil (200 to 400 mg/day), or pemoline (20 to 75 mg each morning).

Disorders of bladder function may raise serious problems in management. Where the major disorder is one of urinary retention, bethanechol chloride may be helpful. In this situation, monitoring and reducing the residual urinary volume is an important means of preventing infection; volumes up to 100 mL are generally well tolerated. Some patients with severe bladder dysfunction, particularly those with urinary retention, benefit from intermittent catheterization, which they can learn to do themselves and which lessens the constant risk of infection from an indwelling catheter. More often the problem is one of urinary urgency and frequency (spastic bladder), in which case the use of propantheline (Pro-Banthine) or oxybutynin (Ditropan) may serve to relax the detrusor muscle (Chap. 26). These drugs are best used intermittently. Severe constipation is best managed with properly spaced enemas. Often a program of bowel training can be successfully undertaken.

In patients with severe spastic paralysis and painful flexor spasms of the legs, intrathecal infusion of baclofen through an indwelling catheter and implanted pump, as in other spastic states, is sometimes of value. The selective injection of botulinum toxin into the most hypertonic muscles may help some patients. Some patients with lesser degrees of spasticity have benefited from the oral administration of baclofen. Failing this measure, one of several surgical procedures—dorsal rhizotomy, myelotomy, crushing of the obturator nerves, and, most useful of all in severe cases, intrathecal baclofen infusion by pump—may give relief for a prolonged period.

The very severe and disabling tremor that is brought out by the slightest movement of the limbs, if unilateral, can be managed surgically by ventrolateral thalamotomy. Most surgical series report that about two-thirds of patients achieve a satisfactory reduction in their intention tremor (Critchley and Richardson; Geny et al). In the experience of others, the results have not been quite this reliable. In the series of Hooper and Whittle, only three of ten MS patients who underwent thalamotomy for a severe tremor had sustained improvement. Hallett and colleagues have reported that severe postural tremor of this type can be improved by the administration of isoniazid (300 mg daily, increased by weekly increments of 300 mg to a dose of 1200 mg daily) in combination with 100 mg pyridoxine daily. How isoniazid produces its beneficial effects is not known. Variable success may also be achieved with carbamazepine or clonazepam.

The importance of an understanding and sympathetic physician in the care of patients with a chronic incapacitating neurologic disease of this kind cannot be overemphasized. Enlisting the support of physical and occupational therapists, visiting nurses, and social workers can be equally important. From the beginning, when the patients first inquire about the nature of their illness, they require advice about their daily routine, marriage, pregnancy, the use of drugs, inoculations, and so on. As indicated earlier, the term *multiple sclerosis* should not be introduced until the diagnosis is certain, and then it should be qualified by a balanced explanation of the symptoms, stressing always the optimistic aspects of the disease. Most patients desire an honest appraisal of their condition and prognosis; some consider the uncertainty of their prognosis worse than their actual disability.

ACUTE DISSEMINATED ENCEPHALOMYELITIS (ADEM)

Postinfectious, Postexanthem, Postvaccinal Encephalomyelitis

Some of these terms, used originally to refer to the neurologic sequelae of infectious fevers, were introduced into medicine in the late nineteenth century, but it was not until the late 1920s that Perdrau, Pette, Greenfield, and others identified a type of pathologic reaction common to a number of exanthems and vaccines. The current view of this entity is that it represents an acute demyelinative disease, distinguished pathologically by numerous foci of demyelination scattered throughout the brain and spinal cord; some are restricted to the cerebellum or spinal cord. These foci vary from 0.1 to several millimeters (when confluent) in diameter and invariably surround small and medium-sized veins. The axons and nerve cells are more or less intact. Equally distinctive is the perivenular inflammatory reaction; the perivascular spaces are infiltrated with lymphocytes and mononuclear cells and the adjacent regions of white matter are invaded by pleomorphic microglia corresponding to the zones of demyelination. Multifocal meningeal infiltration is another invariable feature but is rarely severe in degree.

An acute encephalitic, myelitic, or encephalomyelitic process of this type is observed in a number of clinical settings. In the originally described form, it occurred within a few days of onset of the exanthem of measles, rubella, smallpox, and chickenpox. Prior to widespread immunization against measles, an epidemic in a large city might have resulted in 100,000 cases of measles and clinically evident neurologic complications in 1 in 800 to 1 in 2000 cases. The mortality among patients with such complications ranged from 10 to 20 percent; about an equal number were left with persistent neurologic damage. The neurologic complications of measles alone provide sufficient justification for immunization against the disease. The incidence of encephalomyelitis was less following chickenpox and rubella and much less following mumps (the latter never seen in our material). In the past, a similar illness was observed to follow vaccination against rabies and smallpox and, reportedly, after administration of tetanus antitoxin (rare), as discussed further on. Now, however, most cases, clinically and pathologically indistinguishable from these two categories of acute disseminated encephalomyelitis, appear to develop after seemingly banal respiratory infections and after documented infections with Epstein-Barr, cytomegalovirus, and *Mycoplasma pneumoniae*; occasionally there is no clearly defined preceding illness or inoculation. Many instances of predominantly unifocal and nonrelapsing acute transverse myelitis may represent the same postinfectious process. The neurologic illness may coincide with the respiratory manifestations of the infection, in which case the term *parainfectious* may be appropriate. Rarely, it occurs after influenza and mumps (to be distinguished from the more common mumps meningitis).

Irrespective of the clinical setting in which it occurs, disseminated encephalomyelitis in its severe form is of grave import, because of the significant rate of neurologic defects in patients who survive. In children, recovery from the acute stage is sometimes followed by a permanent disorder of behavior, mental retardation, or epilepsy; paradoxically, most adults make good recoveries. The *cerebellitis* and acute ataxia that follow chickenpox and other infections are more benign and normally clear over several months as discussed further on.

Pathogenesis The pathogenesis of disseminated encephalomyelitis is still unclear despite its obvious association with viral infections. In the exanthem cases, a definite interval usually separates the onset of disseminated encephalomyelitis from the onset of the rash; also, the pathologic changes are quite different from those of viral infections and virus is rarely if ever recovered from the CSF or brains of patients with disseminated encephalomyelitis. For these reasons it is believed that the disorder represents an immune-mediated complication of infection rather than a direct infection of the CNS. However, as discussed in Chap. 33, new molecular techniques have been able to detect fragments of DNA from varicella zoster virus, *Mycoplasma*, and other organisms, so that the question of pathogenesis cannot be answered with finality. Nevertheless, Waksman and Adams found the pathologic changes in these two circumstances—postinfectious demyelination and direct viral infection of the CNS—to be different.

A laboratory model of the disease, experimental allergic encephalomyelitis (EAE), has been produced by inoculating animals with a combination of sterile brain tissue and adjuvants. The experimental disease appears most commonly between the eighth and fifteenth days after sensitization (see below) and is characterized by the same perivenular demyelinative and inflammatory lesions that one observes in the human disease. Presumably the lesions are the result of a T-cell-mediated immune reaction to components of myelin or oligodendrocytes.

The notion that EAE and disseminated encephalomyelitis have a similar pathogenesis has received strong support from the observations of R. T. Johnson and colleagues. They studied 19 patients with postinfectious encephalomyelitis complicating natural measles virus infections. Early myelin destruction was demonstrated by the presence of MBP in the CSF, and lymphocyte proliferative responses to MBP were found in 8 of 17 patients tested. Similar responses were observed in patients with encephalomyelitis after rabies vaccine and after varicella and rubella virus infections, suggesting a common immune-mediated pathogenesis. Moreover, the patients with postmeasles encephalomyelitis showed a lack of intrathecal synthesis of antibody against measles virus, indicating that the neurologic disease was not dependent on virus replication within the CNS.

Clinical Features In the encephalitic form, as the acute infectious illness resolves or after a latency of several days or longer, there is the abrupt onset of confusion, somnolence, and often convulsions with headache, fever, and varying degrees of neck stiffness. Ataxia, myoclonic movements, and choreoathetosis are observed less frequently. In the more severe cases, stupor, coma, and at times decerebrate rigidity may occur in rapid succession. In the myelitic form (*postinfectious myelitis, acute transverse myelitis*), there is partial or complete paraplegia or quadriplegia, diminution or loss of tendon reflexes, sensory impairment, and varying degrees of paralysis of bladder and bowel. A syndrome that simulates anterior spinal artery occlusion (spastic paraplegia and loss of pain sensation below a level on the trunk, but tending to spare large-fiber sensibility) is not uncommon in our experience. Also, we have cared for a few patients with a limited sacral form of myelitis. Midline back pain may be a prominent symptom at the onset. There is generally no fever, and the peripheral white blood cell count is normal if the underlying infection has resolved. These features serve to distinguish a postinfectious disseminated encephalomyelitis from a viral meningoencephalitis. Either process may be associated with an aseptic meningitis.

In the case of postexanthem encephalomyelitis, the syndrome generally begins 2 to 4 days after the appearance of the rash. Usually the rash is fading and other symptoms are improving when the patient, usually a child, suddenly develops a recrudescence of fever, convulsions, stupor, and sometimes coma. Less commonly, the patient may develop hemiplegia or a virtually pure cerebellar syndrome, as noted below (particularly after chickenpox), and occasionally a transverse myelitis, sphincteric disturbance, or other signs of spinal cord involvement. Choreoathetotic movements are seen infrequently. In many cases the disease is much less severe and the patient suffers a transient encephalitic illness with headaches, confusion, and signs of meningeal irritation. The CSF usually shows an increase in lymphocytes and protein content, but these are highly variable, a few cases having no cells and others up to several hundred. The MRI scan shows bilateral confluent white matter lesions in both cerebral hemispheres early in the course of acute disseminated encephalomyelitis (Fig. 36-4); when these are large and numerous, the diagnosis is more certain, but some instances of viral encephalitis display subcortical changes in the white matter as well.

A variant of postinfectious encephalomyelitis that involves solely or predominantly the cerebellum deserves special comment. Typically, a mild ataxia with variable corticospinal or other signs appears within days of one of the childhood exanthems as well as after Epstein-Barr virus, *Mycoplasma*, *Legionella*, and cytomegalovirus infections and after a number of vaccinations and nondescript respiratory infections. It is described in detail on page 797 because it has a close relationship to certain viruses, particularly varicella, suggesting that some if not most cases are due to an infectious meningoencephalitis. Others—for example, following mycoplasmal infection—occur after a long latency and show pathologic changes that are consistent with a postinfectious demyelination. Thus it appears that there may be two types of acute cerebellitis, one para- or postinfectious and the other due to a direct infection of the brain and meninges. The benign nature of the illness has precluded adequate pathologic examination, hence some of these statements are speculative.

Differential Diagnosis It must be re-emphasized that not all the neurologic complications of measles and other exanthems and acute viral infections are examples of postinfectious encephalomyelitis. As already noted, the illness is at times difficult to distinguish from viral meningoencephalitis. Infectious mononucleosis, herpes simplex, mycoplasmal infection, and other forms of encephalitis may all mimic the postinfectious variety. In some cases cerebrovascular disease (particularly thrombophlebitis), hypoxic encephalopathy, or acute toxic hepatoencephalopathy (Reye syndrome) is responsible for these complications. The Reye syndrome is usually not difficult to separate from postinfectious encephalomyelitis, even when it follows chickenpox or viral influenza, because of the normal CSF and high serum concentrations of liver enzymes and ammonia (see page 1187). In a child, the first attack of febrile seizures in the course of an exanthematous illness may raise the suspicion of encephalitis or postinfectious encephalomyelitis.

Postvaccinal Encephalomyelitis Since late in the nineteenth century, it has been known that a severe form

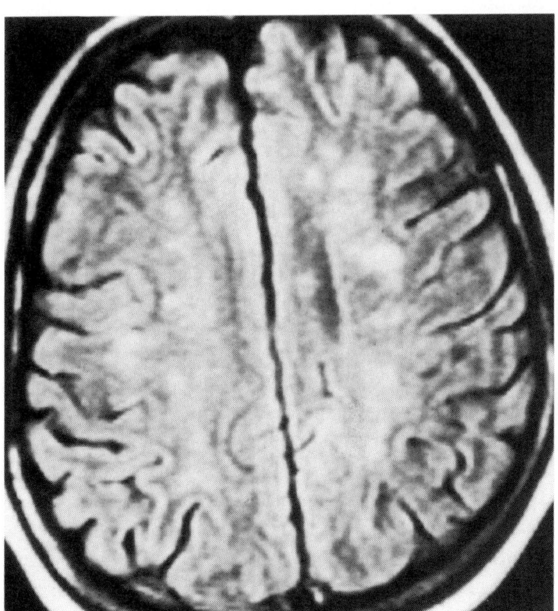

Figure 36-4

FLAIR MRI of acute (postinfectious) disseminated encephalomyelitis, showing numerous lesions of varying size throughout the white matter of both hemispheres.

of encephalomyelitis may complicate the injection of rabies vaccine ("neuroparalytic accident"). Until quite recently, the vaccine in common use consisted of killed virus that had been grown in rabbit brain tissue. Encephalomyelitis occurred in about 1 in 750 patients inoculated with this vaccine, and about 25 percent of cases with this complication proved fatal. Alternative vaccines, made from embryonated duck eggs (and later from human diploid cells) infected with fixed viruses, contain very little or no nerve tissue and are almost free of neurologic complications. In developing countries, where less expensive brain-based vaccines are still in use, neuroparalytic accidents continue to occur. The observations of Hemachudha and colleagues indicate that the altered immune mechanism that is operative in the neuroparalytic accident is the same as that in post-measles encephalomyelitis and experimental allergic encephalomyelitis.

There are numerous recorded instances in which the old rabies vaccine (with neural tissue) induced an attack of what appeared to be MS. Shiraki and Otani reported such examples from Japan. The evolution of symptoms was subacute, over a period of 2 to 4 weeks, and the demyelinative lesions were macroscopic—up to 1 to 2.0 cm in diameter—but composed of confluent perivenous lesions. The disease could be reproduced in dogs—persuasive evidence that one form of acute MS is a variant of ADEM.

Encephalomyelitis following vaccination against smallpox has been known since 1860, having occurred about once in 4000 vaccinations. This disease is now of historical interest only, insofar as smallpox has disappeared as a human illness worldwide. In the United States, there have been no new cases for years, and smallpox vaccination is no longer included as part of immunization schedules.

The association of the neurologic disorder with vaccination usually leaves the diagnosis in little doubt, and the characteristic combination of encephalitic and myelitic features will help to distinguish the condition from meningitis, viral encephalitis, and poliomyelitis. Rarely, an atypical case may mimic any one of these disorders. On occasion, the disease may suggest involvement of nerve roots and peripheral nerves and may resemble acute inflammatory polyneuritis (Guillain-Barré syndrome). In fact, the rabies vaccine produced in South America from suckling mouse brain causes this type of peripheral nerve disease more often than encephalomyelitis.

The mortality rate of postvaccinal encephalomyelitis is high, between 30 and 50 percent. If recovery occurs, it may be surprisingly complete. However, a significant proportion of patients show residual neurologic signs, intellectual impairment, and behavioral abnormalities.

With regard to *treatment* of ADEM, the use of high-potency steroids appears to be the best choice, although controlled trials of this treatment have not been carried out. Steroids, given before or immediately upon the appearance of neurologic signs, modify the severity of experimental allergic encephalomyelitis; this provides the logic for their use in the human counterpart of this disease. However, the pathologic process cannot be altered once the first signs appear. Plasma exchange and intravenous immune globulin have also been anecdotally successful in some fulminant cases (Kanter et al; Stricker et al) but not in four of our own.

Acute Necrotizing Hemorrhagic Encephalomyelitis (Acute Hemorrhagic Leukoencephalitis of Weston Hurst)

This, the most fulminant form of demyelinative disease, affects mainly young adults but also children. It is almost invariably preceded by a respiratory infection of variable duration (1 to 14 days), sometimes due to *M. pneumoniae* but more often of indeterminate cause. The neurologic symptoms appear abruptly, beginning with headache, fever, stiff neck, and confusion. These are followed in short order by signs of disease of one or both cerebral hemispheres and brainstem—focal seizures, hemiplegia or quadriplegia, pseudobulbar paralysis, and progressively deepening coma. Leukocytosis is usually present, sometimes reaching 30,000 cells per cubic millimeter, and the sedimentation rate is elevated. The CSF is often under increased pressure; cells vary in number from a few lymphocytes to a polymorphonuclear pleocytosis of up to 3000 cells per cubic millimeter; red cells may be present in variable numbers; protein content is increased, but glucose values are normal. Diagnosis is greatly facilitated by CT scanning and MRI, which reveal bilateral but asymmetrical large, confluent edematous lesions in the cerebral white matter (Fig. 36-5). The size of the lesions and the extent of the surrounding edema are beyond what is seen in the usual case of postinfectious ADEM. Many cases terminate fatally in 2 to 4 days, but in others survival is longer. Patients with a similar clinical picture who are thought to have the same disease on the basis of brain biopsy examinations have recovered with almost no residual symptoms. In one of the fatal cases reported by Adams et al, the illness evolved more slowly—over a period of 2 to 3 weeks—

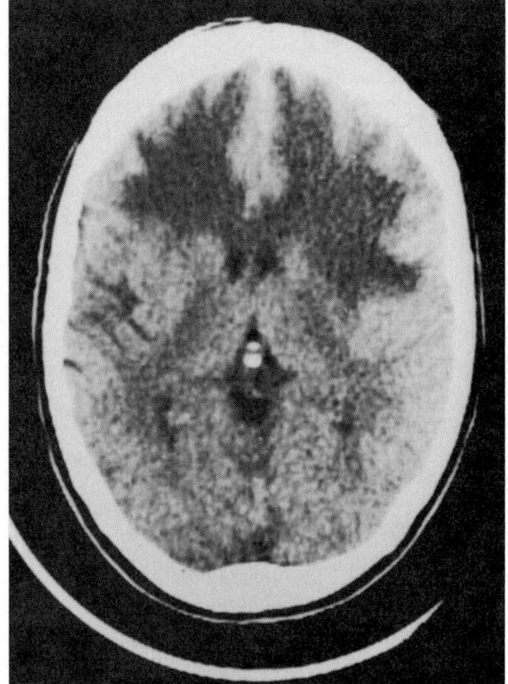

Figure 36-5

Acute necrotizing hemorrhagic leukoencephalitis, mainly bifrontal.

while another patient died with temporal lobe herniation within 12 h. A single recurrence of the disease was observed in one of our cases.

Brain abscess, subdural empyema, focal embolic encephalomalacia, and acute encephalitis due especially to type 1 herpes simplex virus are the important considerations in the differential diagnosis.

The *pathologic findings* are distinctive. On sectioning of the brain, the white matter of one or both hemispheres is seen to be destroyed almost to the point of liquefaction. The involved tissue is pink or yellow-gray and flecked with multiple small hemorrhages. Similar changes are often found in the brainstem and cerebellar peduncles and probably in the spinal cord (acute necrotizing myelitis and Devic disease). On histologic examination one finds widespread necrosis of small blood vessels and brain tissue around the vessels, with intense cellular infiltration, multiple small hemorrhages, and an inflammatory reaction in the meninges of variable intensity. The pathologic picture resembles that of disseminated encephalomyelitis in its perivascular distribution, with the added features of a more widespread necrosis and a tendency of lesions to form large foci in the cerebral hemispheres. The vascular lesions result in a characteristic exudation of fibrin into the vessel wall and surrounding tissue. It is possible that certain patients showing an explosive myelitic illness are suffering from a necrotizing lesion of similar type, but pathologic evidence in support of this view has been difficult to obtain. Fibrin exudation in an acute fatal myelitis was present in a case examined by Adams and colleagues.

The *etiology* of this condition remains obscure, but the resemblance to other demyelinating diseases should be emphasized. The similarities of the histologic changes to those of disseminated encephalomyelitis, noted above, suggest that the two diseases are related forms of the same fundamental process. In fact, cases combining both types of pathologic change have been described (Fisher et al). The observations of Behan and colleagues—that the lymphocytes of a patient with postinfectious encephalomyelitis and of another patient with acute necrotizing hemorrhagic encephalitis underwent transformation to lymphoblasts in response to a pure encephalitogenic MBP—support the view that delayed hypersensitivity mechanisms are operative in both diseases. Earlier, Waksman and Adams had demonstrated that the vascular lesions of experimental allergic encephalomyelitis could be converted to those of necrotizing encephalomyelitis by inducing a Schwartzman reaction (by intravenous injection of meningococcal toxin). It is also noteworthy that among the small number of patients who have recovered from what appeared to be a typical necrotizing hemorrhagic encephalitis, a few have gone on to develop typical MS. These points of similarity are sufficient to suggest that corticosteroids should be used in the treatment of acute necrotizing hemorrhagic encephalopathy; in several personally observed patients, we had the impression that they produced a favorable result. The use of plasma exchange and intravenous immunoglobulin, as for acute disseminated encephalomyelitis, is being explored and has had success in single reported cases when instituted early.

REFERENCES

Adams RD, Cammermeyer J, Denny-Brown D: Acute hemorrhagic encephalopathy. *J Neuropathol Exp Neurol* 8:1, 1949.

Adams RD, Kubik CS: The morbid anatomy of the demyelinative diseases. *Am J Med* 12:510, 1952.

Aimard G, Confavreux C, Ventre JJ, et al: Etude de 213 cas de sclerose en plaques traites par l'azathiaprine de 1967–1982. *Rev Neurol* 139:509, 1983.

ALLEN IV, MILLER JHD, SHILLINGTON RKA: Systemic lupus erythematosus clinically resembling multiple sclerosis and with unusual pathological ultrastructural features. *J Neurol Neurosurg Psychiatry* 42:392, 1979.

ALTER M, HALPERN L, KURLAND LT, et al: Multiple sclerosis in Israel. *Arch Neurol* 7:253, 1962.

ANDERSON DW, ELLENBERG JH, LEVENTHAL CM, et al: Revised estimate of the prevalence of multiple sclerosis in the United States. *Ann Neurol* 31:333, 1992.

ANTEL JP, CASHMAN NR: Human retrovirus and multiple sclerosis. *Mayo Clin Proc* 66:752, 1991.

ARNASON BGW: Interferon beta in multiple sclerosis. *Neurology* 43:641, 1993.

BARNES D, HUGHES RAC, MORRIS RW, et al: Randomised trial of oral and intravenous methylprednisolone in acute relapses of multiple sclerosis. *Lancet* 349:902, 1997.

BATTEN FE: Ataxia in childhood. *Brain* 28:484, 1905.

BECK RW, CLEARY PA, ANDERSON MM JR, et al: A randomized controlled trial of corticosteroids in the treatment of acute optic neuritis. *N Engl J Med* 326:581, 1992.

BEEBE GW, KURTZKE JF, KURLAND LT, et al: Studies on the natural history of multiple sclerosis: 3. Epidemiologic analyses of the Army experience in World War II. *Neurology* 17:1, 1967.

BEHAN PO, GESCHWIND N, LAMARCHE JB, et al: Delayed hypersensitivity to encephalitogenic protein in disseminated encephalomyelitis. *Lancet* 2:1009, 1968.

BERRY I, RANJEVA J-P, MANELFE C, CLANET M: Visualisation I.R.M. des lésions de S.E.P. *Rev Neurol* 154:607, 1998.

BIRK K, RUDICK R: Pregnancy and multiple sclerosis. *Arch Neurol* 43:719, 1986.

BORNSTEIN MB, MILLER A, SLAGLE S, et al: A pilot trial of COP I in exacerbating-remitting multiple sclerosis. *N Engl J Med* 317: 408, 1987.

COHEN SR, HERNDON RM, MCKHANN GM: Radioimmunoassay of myelin basic protein in spinal fluid. *N Engl J Med* 295:1455, 1976.

COMPSTON DAS: Genetic susceptibility to multiple sclerosis, in Compston A et al (eds): *McAlpine's Multiple Sclerosis*, 3rd ed. New York, Churchill Livingstone, 1991, pp 301–319.

CONFAVREUX C, HUTCHINSON M, HOURS MM, et al: Rate of pregnancy related relapse in multiple sclerosis. *N Engl J Med* 339:285, 1998.

COOK SD, DEVEREUX C, TROIANO R, et al: Effect of total lymphoid irradiation in chronic progressive multiple sclerosis. *Lancet* 1:1405, 1986.

COXE WS, LUSE SA: Acute hemorrhagic leukoencephalitis. *J Neurosurg* 20:584, 1963.

CRITCHLEY GR, RICHARDSON PL: Vim thalamotomy for the relief of the intention tremor of multiple sclerosis. *Br J Neurosurg* 12:559, 1998.

DALOS NP, ROBINS PV, BROOKS BR, et al: Disease activity and emotional state in multiple sclerosis. *Ann Neurol* 13:573, 1983.

DEAN G: The multiple sclerosis problem. *Sci Am* 233:40, 1970.

DEAN G, KURTZKE JF: On the risk of multiple sclerosis according to age at immigration to South Africa. *Br Med J* 3:725, 1971.

DEJONG RN: Multiple sclerosis: History, definition and general considerations, in Vinken PJ, Bruyn GW (eds): *Handbook of Clinical Neurology*. Vol 9. Amsterdam, North-Holland, 1970, pp 45–62.

DE KEYSER J: Autoimmunity in multiple sclerosis. *Neurology* 38: 371, 1988.

EBERS GC: Genetic factors in multiple sclerosis. *Neurol Clin* 1:645, 1983.

EBERS GC: Optic neuritis and multiple sclerosis. *Arch Neurol* 42: 702, 1985.

EBERS GC, BULMAN DE, SADOVNICK AD: A population-based study of multiple sclerosis in twins. *N Engl J Med* 315:1638, 1986.

ELLISON PH, BARRON KD: Clinical recovery from Schilder's disease. *Neurology* 29:244, 1979.

European Study Group on Interferon β-1b in Secondary Progressive MS. *Lancet* 352:1491, 1998.

FAZEKAS F, DEISENHAMMER F, STRASSER-FUCHS S, et al: Randomised placebo-controlled trial of monthly intravenous immunoglobulin in relapsing-remitting multiple sclerosis. *Lancet* 349:589, 1997.

FISHER RS, CLARK AW, WOLINSKY JS, et al: Post-infectious leukoencephalitis complicating *Mycoplasma pneumoniae* infection. *Arch Neurol* 40:109, 1983.

FFRENCH-CONSTANT C: Pathogenesis of multiple sclerosis. *Lancet* 343:271, 1994.

GENY C, NGEYEN JP, POLLIN B, et al: Improvement in severe postural cerebellar tremor in multiple sclerosis by thalamic stimulation. *Mov Disord* 11:489, 1996.

GILBERT JJ, SADLER M: Unsuspected multiple sclerosis. *Arch Neurol* 40:533, 1983.

GOODKIN DE, RANSOHOFF RM, RUDICK RA: Experimental therapies for multiple sclerosis: Current status. *Cleve Clin J Med* 59:63, 1992.

GOODKIN DE, RUDICK RA, MEDENDORP V, et al: Low-dose oral methotrexate in chronic progressive multiple sclerosis. *Neurology* 47:1153, 1996.

GOVERMAN J, WOODS A, LARSON L, et al: Transgenic mice that express a myelin basic protein-specific T cell receptor develop spontaneous autoimmunity. *Cell* 72:551, 1993.

HALLETT M, LINDSEY JW, ADELSTEIN BD, RILEY PO: Controlled trial of isoniazid therapy for severe postural cerebellar tremor in multiple sclerosis. *Neurology* 35:1314, 1985.

HALLIDAY AM, MCDONALD WI: Pathophysiology of demyelinating disease. *Br Med Bull* 33:21, 1977.

HAUSER SL, BRESNAN MJ, REINHERZ EL, WEINER HL: Childhood multiple sclerosis: Clinical features and demonstration of changes in T-cell subsets with disease activity. *Ann Neurol* 11:463, 1982.

HAUSER SL, DAWSON DM, LEHRICH JR: Intensive immune suppression in progressive multiple sclerosis: A randomized three arm study of high-dose intravenous cyclophosphamide, plasma exchange and ACTH. *N Engl J Med* 308:173, 1983.

HELY MA, MCMANIS PG, DORAN TJ, et al: Acute optic neuritis: A prospective study of risk factors for multiple sclerosis. *J Neurol Neurosurg Psychiatry* 49:1125, 1986.

HEMACHUDHA T, GRIFFIN DE, GIFFELS JJ, et al: Myelin basic protein as an encephalitogen in encephalomyelitis and polyneuritis following rabies vaccination. *N Engl J Med* 316:369, 1987.

HOOPER J, WHITTLE IR: Long-term outcome after thalamotomy for movement disorders in multiple sclerosis. *Lancet* 352:1984, 1998.

HUGHES RAC, SHARRACK B: More immunotherapy for multiple sclerosis. *J Neurol Neurosurg Psychiatry* 61:239, 1996.

JACOBS L, KINKEL PR, KINKEL WR: Silent brain lesions in patients with isolated idiopathic optic neuritis. *Arch Neurol* 43:452, 1986.

JACOBS L, O'MALLEY JA, FREEMAN A, et al: Intrathecal interferon in the treatment of multiple sclerosis: Patient follow-up. *Arch Neurol* 42:841, 1985.

JOHNSON KP, ARRIGO SC, NELSON BS, GINSBERG A: Agarose electrophoresis of cerebrospinal fluid in multiple sclerosis. *Neurology* 27:273, 1977.

JOHNSON KP, LIKOSKY WH, NELSON BJ, FINE G: Comprehensive viral immunology of multiple sclerosis: I. Clinical, epidemiological, and CSF studies. *Arch Neurol* 37:537, 610, 616, 1980.

JOHNSON RT: Current knowledge of multiple sclerosis. *South Med J* 71:2, 1978.

JOHNSON RT: The virology of demyelinating diseases. *Ann Neurol* 36(suppl):S54, 1994.

JOHNSON RT, GRIFFIN DE, HIRSCH RL, et al: Measles encephalomyelitis: Clinical and immunologic studies. *N Engl J Med* 310:137, 1984.

KANTER DS, HORENSKY D, SPERLING RA, et al: Plasmapheresis in fulminant acute disseminated encephalomyelitis. *Neurology* 45:824, 1995.

KATZ J, ROPPER AH: Progressive necrotic myelopathy: Clinical course in 9 patients. *Arch Neurol* 57:355, 2000.

KEPES JJ: Large focal tumor-like demyelinating lesions of the brain: Intermediate entity between multiple sclerosis and acute disseminated encephalomyelitis: A study of 31 patients. *Ann Neurol* 33:18, 1993.

KURLAND LT: The frequency and geographic distribution of multiple sclerosis as indicated by mortality statistics and morbidity surveys in the United States and Canada. *Am J Hyg* 55:457, 1952.

KURLAND LT, MOLGAARD CA, KURLAND EM, et al: Swine flu vaccine and multiple sclerosis. *JAMA* 251:2672, 1984.

KURTZKE JF: On the evaluation of disability in multiple sclerosis. *Neurology* 11:686, 1961.

KURTZKE JF: Optic neuritis or multiple sclerosis. *Arch Neurol* 42:704, 1985.

KURTZKE JF, BEEBE GW, NAGLER B, et al: Studies on the natural history of multiple sclerosis: Early prognostic features of the later course of the illness. *J Chronic Dis* 30:819, 1977.

KURTZKE JF, BEEBE GW, NORMAN JE JR: Epidemiology of multiple sclerosis in U.S. veterans: I. Race, sex, and geographic distribution. *Neurology* 29:1228, 1979.

KURTZKE JF, GUDMUNDSSON KR, BERGMANN S: Multiple sclerosis in Iceland: I. Evidence of a post-war epidemic. *Neurology* 32:143, 1982.

KURTZKE JF, HYLLESTED K: Multiple sclerosis in the Faroe Islands: II. Clinical update, transmission, and the nature of MS. *Neurology* 36:307, 1986.

LAMPERT PW: Autoimmune and virus-induced demyelinating diseases. *Am J Pathol* 91:176, 1978.

LESSELL S: Corticosteroid treatment of acute optic neuritis. *N Engl J Med* 326:634, 1992.

LIGHTMAN S, MCDONALD WI, BIRD AC, et al: Retinal venous sheathing in optic neuritis. *Brain* 110:405, 1987.

LUCCHINETTI CF, KIERS L, O'DUFFY A, et al: Risk factors for developing multiple sclerosis after childhood optic neuritis. *Neurology* 49:1413, 1997.

MANDLER RN, DAVIS LE, JEFFREY DR, KORNFELD M: Devic's neuromyelitis optica: A clinicopathologic study of 8 patients. *Ann Neurol* 34:162, 1993.

MATTHEWS WB (ed): *McAlpine's Multiple Sclerosis*, 2nd ed. New York, Churchill Livingstone, 1991, pp 41–298.

MCALPINE D, COMPSTON MD: Some aspects of the natural history of disseminated sclerosis. *Q J Med* 21:135, 1952.

MCALPINE D, LUMSDEN CE, ACHESON ED: *Multiple Sclerosis: A Reappraisal*, 2nd ed. Edinburgh, Churchill Livingstone, 1972.

MCDONALD WI: The mystery of the origin of multiple sclerosis. *J Neurol Neurosurg Psychiatry* 49:113, 1986.

MCDONALD WI, HALLIDAY AM: Diagnosis and classification of multiple sclerosis. *Br Med Bull* 33:4, 1977.

MCFARLIN DE, MCFARLAND HF: Multiple sclerosis. *N Engl J Med* 307:1246, 1982.

MENDELL JR, KOLKIN S, KISSEL JT, et al: Evidence for central nervous system demyelination in chronic inflammatory demyelinating polyradiculoneuropathy. *Neurology* 37:1291, 1987.

MOULIN D, PATY DW, EBERS GC: The predictive value of CSF electrophoresis in "possible" multiple sclerosis. *Brain* 106:809, 1983.

THE MULTIPLE SCLEROSIS STUDY GROUP: Efficacy and toxicity of cyclosporine in chronic progressive multiple sclerosis: A randomized, double-blinded, placebo-controlled clinical trial. *Ann Neurol* 27:591, 1990.

NATIONAL CENTER FOR HEALTH STATISTICS, COLLINS JG: *Types of Injuries and Impairments Due to Injuries*. United States Vital Statistics. Series 10, no 159, DHHS, no (PHS) 871587. Public Health Service. Washington, DC, U.S. Government Printing Office, 1986.

OPTIC NEURITIS STUDY GROUP: The five-year risk of MS after optic neuritis. *Neurology* 49:1404, 1997.

O'RIORDAN JI, GALLAGHER HL, THOMPSON AJ, et al: Clinical, CSF, and MRI findings in Devic's neuromyelitis optica. *J Neurol Neurosurg Psychiatry* 60:382, 1996.

ORMEROD IEC, MCDONALD WI: Multiple sclerosis presenting with progressive visual failure. *J Neurol Neurosurg Psychiatry* 47:943, 1984.

ORMEROD IEC, MCDONALD WI, DUBOULAY GH, et al: Disseminated lesions at presentation in patients with optic neuritis. *J Neurol Neurosurg Psychiatry* 49:124, 1986.

OSTERMAN PO, WESTERBEY CE: Paroxysmal attacks in multiple sclerosis. *Brain* 98:189, 1975.

PANITCH HS: Systemic α-interferon in multiple sclerosis: Long-term patient follow-up. *Arch Neurol* 44:61, 1987.

PANITCH HS, HALEY AS, HIRSCH RLA, et al: A trial of gamma interferon in multiple sclerosis: Clinical results. *Neurology* 36(suppl 1):285, 1986.

PERCY AK, NOBREGA FT, OKAZAKI H: Multiple sclerosis in Rochester, Minnesota: A 60-year appraisal. *Arch Neurol* 25:105, 1971.

POSER CM: Diffuse-disseminated sclerosis in the adult. *J Neuropathol Exp Neurol* 16:61, 1957.

POSER CM: Exacerbations, activity and progression in multiple sclerosis. *Arch Neurol* 37:471, 1980.

POSER CM, GOUTIERES F, CARPENTIER M: Schilder's myelinoclastic diffuse sclerosis. *Pediatrics* 77:107, 1986.

POSER CM, ROMAN GC, VERNANT J-C: Multiple sclerosis or HTLV-1 myelitis? *Neurology* 40:1020, 1990.

POSER CM, VAN BOGAERT L: Natural history and evolution of the concept of Schilder's diffuse sclerosis. *Acta Psychiatr Neurol Scand* 31:285, 1956.

POSKANZER DC, SCHAPIRA K, MILLER H: Multiple sclerosis and poliomyelitis. *Lancet* 2:917, 1963.

PRINEAS JW: The etiology and pathogenesis of multiple sclerosis, in Vinken PJ, Bruyn GW (eds): *Handbook of Clinical Neurology.* Vol 9. Amsterdam, North-Holland, 1970, pp 107–160.

PRINEAS JW, BARNARD RO, KWON EE, et al: Multiple sclerosis: Remyelination of nascent lesions. *Ann Neurol* 33:137, 1993.

PRINEAS JW, CONNELL F: The fine structure of chronically active multiple sclerosis plaques. *Neurology* 28:68, 1978.

PRISMS STUDY GROUP: Randomized double-blind placebo-controlled study of interferon β-1a in relapsing/remitting multiple sclerosis. *Lancet* 352:1498, 1998.

RAMIREZ-LASSEPAS M, TULLOCK JW, QUINONES MR, SNYDER BD: Acute radicular pain as a presenting symptom in multiple sclerosis. *Arch Neurol* 49:255, 1992.

RIZZO JF III, LESSELL S: Risk of developing multiple sclerosis after uncomplicated optic neuritis: A long-term prospective study. *Neurology* 38:185, 1988.

RODRIQUEZ M, KARNES WE, BARTELSON JD, PINEDA AA: Plasmapheresis in acute episodes of fulminant inflammatory demyelination. *Neurology* 43:1100, 1993.

ROPPER AH, POSKANZER DC: The prognosis of acute and subacute transverse myelitis based on early signs and symptoms. *Ann Neurol* 4:51, 1978.

RUDICK RA, COHEN JA, WEINSTOCK-GUTTMAN B, et al: Management of multiple sclerosis. *N Engl J Med* 337:1604, 1997.

SADOVNICK AD, BAIRD PA, WARD RH: Multiple sclerosis: Updated risks for relatives. *Am J Med Genet* 29:533, 1988.

SADOVNICK AD, EBERS GC, DYMENT DA, et al: Evidence for a genetic basis for multiple sclerosis. *Lancet* 347:1728, 1996.

SCHAPIRA K, POSKANZER DC, MILLER H: Familial and conjugal multiple sclerosis. *Brain* 86:315, 1963.

SCHIFFER RB, SLATER RJ: Neuropsychiatric features of multiple sclerosis: Recognition and management. *Semin Neurol* 5:127, 1985.

SCHILDER P: Zur Kenntniss der sogenannten diffusen Sklerose. *Z Gesamte Neurol Psychiatry* 10:1, 1912.

SEARS ES, MCCAMMON A, BIGELOW R, HAYMAN LA: Maximizing the harvest of contrast enhancing lesions in multiple sclerosis. *Neurology* 32:815, 1982.

SELLEBJERG F, NIELSEN S, FREDERIKSON JL, et al: A randomized controlled trial of oral high-dose methylprednisolone in acute optic neuritis. *Neurology* 52:1479, 1999.

SHIRAKI H, OTANI S: Clinical and pathological features of rabies postvaccinal encephalomyelitis in man, in Kies MW, Alvord EC Jr (eds): *"Allergic" Encephalomyelitis.* Springfield, IL, Charles C Thomas, 1959, pp 58–129.

SIBLEY WA, BAMFORD CRF, CLARK K, et al: A prospective study of physical trauma and multiple sclerosis. *J Neurol Neurosurg Psychiatry* 54:584, 1991.

SLAMOVITIS S, ROSEN CE, CHENG KP, et al: Visual recovery in patients with optic neuritis and visual loss to no light perception. *Am J Ophthalmol* 111:209, 1991.

STEWART JM, HOUSER GW, BAKER HL: Magnetic resonance imaging and clinical relationships in multiple sclerosis. *Mayo Clin Proc* 62:174, 1987.

STRICKER RD, MILLER RG, KIPROV DO: Role of plasmapheresis in acute disseminated (postinfectious) encephalomyelitis. *J Clin Apheresis* 7:173, 1992.

THOMAS PK, WALKER RWH, RUDGE P, et al: Chronic demyelinating peripheral neuropathy associated with multifocal central nervous system demyelination. *Brain* 110:53, 1987.

THOMPSON AJ, POLMAN CH, MILLER DH, et al: Primary progressive multiple sclerosis. *Brain* 120:1085, 1997.

THYGESSEN P: *The Course of Disseminated Sclerosis: A Close-Up of 105 Attacks.* Copenhagen, Rosenkilde and Bagger, 1953.

TIPPET DS, FISHMAN PS, PANITCH HS: Recurrent transverse myelitis. *Neurology* 41:703, 1991.

TOURTELLOTTE WW, BOOE IM: Multiple sclerosis: The blood-brain barrier and the measurement of de novo central nervous system IgG synthesis. *Neurology* 28(suppl):76, 1978.

WAKSMAN BH, ADAMS RD: Studies of the effect of the Schwartzman reaction on the lesions of experimental allergic encephalomyelitis. *Am J Pathol* 33:131, 1957.

WEINSHENKER BG, RICE GP, NOSEWORTHY JH, et al: The natural history of multiple sclerosis: A geographically based study: 2. Predictive value of the early clinical course. *Brain* 112:1419, 1989.

Chapter 37

THE INHERITED METABOLIC DISEASES OF THE NERVOUS SYSTEM

Advances in biochemistry and molecular genetics have led to the discovery of such a large number of metabolic diseases of the nervous system that it taxes the mind just to remember their names. Standard laboratory methods—utilizing paper chromatography, gas-liquid chromatography, mass spectroscopy, and electron microscopy of tissue samples—are currently being supplemented by definitive nuclear and mitochondrial DNA gene analyses. Many of these techniques are now available in teaching hospitals and commercial laboratories and have significantly advanced our understanding of inherited disease. The problem for the neurologist is to know when and how to use them.

Since the causes and mechanisms of the diseases included in this chapter (and in several that follow) are increasingly being expressed in terms of molecular genetics, it seems appropriate, by way of introduction, to consider briefly some basic facts pertaining to the genetics of neurologic disease. A complete account of this subject may be found in the three-volume text edited by Scriver and colleagues.

One must be reminded that the biochemistry of every human organism is unique and that every person, in some particular way, has an inborn tendency to develop certain diseases. This constitutional predisposition, or diathesis, lies in the DNA of the chromosomes of each cell. Knowledge of the molecular basis of the constitutional predisposition will ultimately provide the means of diagnosis, prevention, and care of most human diseases.

The diseases grouped in this chapter and the next represent four particular categories of genetic abnormality: (1) monogenic disorders that are determined by a single mutant gene and follow a mendelian pattern of inheritance; (2) multifactorial disorders, again following a mendelian pattern of inheritance but in which intrinsic (i.e., genetic) factors interact with exogenous environmental ones; (3) nonmendelian chromosomal aberrations, characterized by an excess, a lack, or a structural alteration of one or more of the 23 pairs of chromosomes (these are considered in the next chapter, with the developmental disorders); and (4) mitochondrial transmission of disease in a nonmendelian, mainly maternal pattern.

As to the frequency of these types of genetic abnormality (reported in the monograph of Scriver et al), 6 to 8 percent of diseases in hospitalized children are attributable to single gene defects and 0.4 to 2.5 percent to a chromosomal abnormality. Another 22 to 31 percent have a disease thought to be gene-influenced. In the general population, when multifactorial inheritance of late-onset diseases is included, the latter figure rises to about 60 percent. Mitochondrial inheritance is much less frequent and has unusual patterns of transmission, mostly through maternal lines.

The nervous system is more frequently affected by a genetic abnormality than any other organ system, probably because of the large number of genes implicated in its development (an estimated one-third of all the genes in the human genome). Approximately one-third of all inherited diseases are neurologic to some extent; if one adds the inherited diseases affecting the musculature, skeleton, eye, and ear, the number rises to 80 to 90 percent.

Of the almost 6000 entities itemized in the 1998 edition of McKusick's catalogue of inherited diseases, about 500 are identified as enzymopathies, i.e., mendelian disorders with a demonstrated primary enzyme defect. The latter constitute only one-third of the known recessive (autosomal and X-linked) disorders. Most of the enzymopathies become manifest in infancy and childhood; only a few appear as late as adolescence or adult life. Many damage the nervous system so severely that survival to adult years and reproduction are impossible. As a group, these diseases—along with congenital anomalies (Chap. 38), birth injuries, epilepsy, disharmonies of development, and learning disabilities (Chap. 28)—make up the bulk of the clinical problems with which the pediatric neurologist must contend.

Autosomal and Sex-Linked Patterns of Inheritance

Traditionally, the recognition of these broad categories of genetically determined diseases has rested on their pattern of occurrence in families, segregated according to mendelian inheritance into autosomal dominant, autosomal recessive, and sex-linked types. Mutations of nuclear DNA account for the majority of heritable autosomal and sex-linked diseases described in this chapter, and they are remarkably diverse in nature. Some are lethal and are therefore not transmitted to successive generations; others are less harmful and may conform to one of the classic mendelian patterns. The mutation may be large and may result in duplication or deletion of a major part of a chromosome or even of the entire genome (diploidy), or it may create a third copy of the entire complement of genes (triploidy). Other mutations are very small, involving only a single base pair ("point mutation"). Between these two extremes are deletions or duplications that include a portion of a gene, an entire gene, or contiguous genes.

Factors that are conducive to mutations are poorly understood. Increasing age of the parent is important in inducing some mutations; the size, structure, and placement of the gene on the chromosome are important in others. A mutation of the DNA of a germ cell leaves the somatic phenotype of the individual in whom it occurs normal, but it may have a devastating effect on the descendants. Conversely, a DNA mutation of a somatic cell affecting only part of the cell population may change the individual harboring it but may not be passed on to the descendants. Such an individual, with both normal cells and cells containing the mutant gene, is referred to as a *mosaic*. Mutations of somatic cells appear to be most relevant to cancer and aging.

In the monogenic inheritance of all three mendelian patterns, the mutation usually causes an abnormality of a single protein molecule. It may involve an enzyme, peptide hormone, immunoglobulin, collagen, or coagulation factor. Such abnormalities of single genes have been isolated in more than 300 diseases, but little is known of their products. About one-quarter of these diseases are apparent soon after birth and more than 90 percent by puberty. More than half of them affect more than one organ. As to their patterns of inheritance, of the 10 in every 1000 live births with genetic diseases, 7 are dominant, 2.5 are recessive, and the remainder are sex-linked.

Autosomal dominant genes usually cause manifest disease in heterozygotes, but variations in the size of the gene abnormality can produce any one of the several phenotypes. This poses a challenge to current clinical and pathologic classifications of disease. Moreover, an identical clinical syndrome may be traced to a gene on two different chromosomes. Even more surprising, an estimated 28 percent of all gene loci have polymorphic rather than monomorphic effects—that is, the same mutation has several different phenotypic expressions. Another problem is that of differentiating dominant from recessive inheritance. In small families, in which only one descendant is afflicted and the parent is seemingly normal, one may mistakenly conclude that the inheritance is recessive. Variable degrees of penetrance and expressivity are characteristic features of dominant patterns of inheritance but not of recessive ones. There is a general tendency for dominantly inherited disease to appear long after birth.

Autosomal recessive diseases, in contrast to dominant ones, occur only in the homozygous state (both alleles abnormal). They are characterized by a more uniform phenotypic expression and an onset soon after birth. The basic abnormality is more often an enzyme deficiency than an abnormality of some other protein.

In disorders of X-linked genes, in which the mutant gene affects mainly one sex, the female will suffer the same fate as the male if one X chromosome is inactivated in most cells during embryonic development (Lyon phenomenon). However, even if the abnormal X chromosome is not widely expressed, the female carrier may still exhibit minor abnormalities. In the latter case, sex-linked inheritance becomes difficult to distinguish from dominant inheritance. Also, sex linkage is deceptive when a disease is lethal to one sex. The biochemical abnormality has more often been one of a basic protein than an enzyme deficiency.

Multifactorial genetic diseases and their associated birth defects are by nature familial. They may present as constitutional disorders with gene abnormalities located on several chromosomes (polygenic). The precise number of such genes required to produce a given abnormality is not known, making the risk of inheritance difficult to calculate. Here also the relative contributions of "risk genes" and environmental influences are highly variable. The methodology for identifying this category of genetic disease has usually required the analysis of large families and the comparison between progeny living with their biologic parents and those adopted by normal families at an early age. Monozygotic and dizygotic twin comparisons provide essential information about "risk genes."

The Genetics of Mitochondrial Disease

In the past several years, an entirely new type of genetic transmission relating to the DNA that lies in the mitochondria has been discovered. Mitochondria contain their own, extrachromosomal DNA, distinct from nuclear DNA. Mitochondrial DNA ("the other human genome") is a double-stranded, circular molecule that encodes the protein subunits required mainly for translation of the proteins located on the mitochondrial inner membrane. Of the 37 mitochondrial genes, small in number by comparison with nuclear DNA, 13 partake in the cellular processes of oxidative phosphorylation and the production of adenosine triphosphate (ATP). A smaller number of genes in the cell's nucleus also code for some oxidative enzymes of the mitochondria, but their inheritance follows a mendelian pattern.

Each mitochondrion contains up to 10 DNA molecules, and each cell contains numerous mitochondria. Mutant genes may exist next to normal ones (*heteroplasmy*), a state that permits an otherwise lethal mutation to persist (Johns). The presence of either completely normal or completely mutant mitochondrial DNA is termed *homoplasmy*. The essential feature of mitochondrial genes and any of the mutations to which they are subject is that they are inherited from the maternal genome. Moreover, mitochondrial DNA does not recombine, thus permitting the accumulation of mutations through the maternal lines. Also, the replication and distribution of mitochondrial DNA during cell division does not follow the nuclear mitotic cycle. Instead, there are contributions during cell division from the genes of various mitochondria to the progeny of dividing cells. The combination of a heteroplasmic state and the capricious dispersion of mitochondria to daughter cells (replicative segregation) explains the variable expression of mitochondrial mutations in different regions of the nervous system as well as variations in the age of onset of the mitochondrial diseases.

The genetic error in each of the mitochondrial diseases is most often a single point mutation of an amino acid, but there may also be single or multiple deletions or duplications of mitochondrial genes that tend to be homoplasmic and do not conform to maternal inheritance or are caused by nuclear DNA defects. The Kearns-Sayre syndrome and some instances of progressive external ophthalmoplegia are of this type. Another of the general rules of mitochondrial inheritance is exemplified by an infantile myopathy (cytochrome oxidase deficiency) that is usually fatal but may also occur in a less severe form and have a later onset. In cases of earlier onset, there is less of the normal mitochondrial DNA than in the cases of later onset. It is important to note that about 85 percent of the protein components of the respiratory chain are coded in nuclear DNA and are then imported into the mitochondrion; as mentioned above, this allows for a mitochondrial disease with a mendelian pattern of inheritance rather than a maternal one.

Since the unique function of mitochondria is the production of ATP by oxidative phosphorylation, it is not surprising that most of the genes contained in mitochondria code for proteins in the respiratory chain. However, there is not always concordance between the error in the mitochondrial genome and the enzymatic defect that leads to disease. Of the five complexes that make up the respiratory chain, cytochrome-*c* oxidase (complex IV) is the one most often disordered, and its deficient function gives rise to lactic acidosis, a feature common to many of the mitochondrial disorders (see further on). In keeping with the mutable nature of this class of disorders, it is thought that some cases of complex IV defect are autosomally transmitted. Complex I defects, which originate in mitochondrial mutations, are seen in Leber optic atrophy. A more complete account of the disorders of the mitochondrial respiratory chain can be found in the recent review by Leonard and Schapira.

As one would expect, aberrant function of the ubiquitous energy-producing mitochondria results in disease of many organs. Nevertheless, most of the mitochondrial disorders affect the nervous system prominently and at times exclusively. Certain fairly well defined conditions traceable to mitochondrial abnormalities include those with a particular change in muscle fibers termed "ragged red fibers" and others having in common a lactic acidosis. The most common of these syndromes are the so-called MELAS and MERFF syndromes (acronyms described further on), Leber hereditary optic atrophy, progressive external ophthalmoplegia, and the Leigh syndrome. These diseases and syndromes are described in the last part of this chapter.

Diagnostic Features of Hereditary Metabolic Diseases

In clinical practice, one should consider the possibility of a hereditary metabolic disease when presented with the following lines of evidence:

1. A neurologic disorder of similar type in a sibling or close relative
2. Recurrent nonconvulsive episodes of impaired consciousness
3. Some combination of unexplained spastic weakness, cerebellar ataxia, extrapyramidal disorder, deafness, or blindness
4. Progression of a neurologic disease measured in weeks, months, or a few years
5. Mental retardation in a sibling or close relative
6. Mental retardation in an individual, particularly if there are no congenital somatic abnormalities
7. Intractable seizures
8. Infantile spasms and progressive myoclonic seizures with microcephaly, in the absence of neonatal hypoxia-ischemia

In the face of such clinical information, one should request appropriate biochemical analyses of blood, urine, and cerebrospinal fluid (CSF); magnetic resonance imaging (MRI) of the brain; and, in certain instances, chromosome-genetic studies.

The array of available genetic and biochemical tests has made practical the mass screening of newborns for inborn metabolic defects. In addition, innovative tests have led to the discovery of a number of previously unknown diseases and have clarified the basic biochemistry of old ones. As a consequence, the neurologist's role is changing. No longer must he wait until a disease of the nervous system has declared itself by conventional symptoms and signs, by which time the lesion may have become irreversible. Now it is possible to find patients who, though asymptomatic, are at risk and to introduce dietary and other measures to prevent injury to the nervous system. This is especially important to families who have already had an affected infant. To assume this new responsibility intelligently requires some knowledge of genetics, biochemical screening methods, and public health measures.

The many clinical syndromes by which these inborn errors of metabolism declare themselves vary in accordance with the nature of the biochemical defect and the stage of maturation of the nervous system at which it acts. In phenylketonuria, for example, there is a specific effect on the cerebral white matter, mainly during the period of active myelination; once the maturational processes are complete, the biochemical abnormality becomes relatively harmless. Even more important is the level of function that has been achieved by the developing nervous system when the disease strikes. A derangement of function in a neonate or infant, in whom much of the cerebrum is not fully developed, is much less obvious than one in an older child; as the disease evolves, the clinical manifestations are always influenced by the continuing maturation of the untouched elements in the nervous system. The separation of metabolic-genetic from degenerative diseases (here accorded separate chapters) may disquiet the reader, for there are many seemingly illogical overlaps between the two groups. The current division is tenable only until such time as all the degenerative diseases will have been shown to have a metabolic basis.

Because of the overriding importance of the age factor and the tendency of certain pathologic processes to appear in particular epochs of life, it has seemed to the authors logical to group the inherited metabolic diseases not according to their major syndromes of expression, as we have done in other parts of the book, but in relation to the periods of life at which they are most likely to be encountered: the neonatal period, infancy (1 to 12 months), early childhood (1 to 4 years), late childhood, adolescence, and adult life. Only in the last two age periods do we return to a syndromic ordering of diseases.

In adopting this chronological subdivision, we realize that *certain hereditary metabolic defects that most typically manifest themselves at a particular period in life are not necessarily confined to that epoch and may appear, sometimes in variant form, at a later stage.* Such variations are noted at appropriate points in the discussion.

THE NEUROLOGY OF NEONATAL METABOLIC DISEASES

A small number of progressive metabolic diseases become manifest in the first few days of life. The importance of these diseases relates not to their frequency (they constitute only a small fraction of diseases that compromise nervous system function in the neonate) but to the fact that they must be recognized promptly if the infant is to be prevented from dying or from suffering a worse fate, that of a lifelong severe mental deficiency. This inherent threat introduces an element of urgency into neonatal neurology. Recognition of these diseases is also important for purposes of family and prenatal testing.

Two approaches to the neonatal metabolic disorders are possible—one, to screen every newborn, using a battery of biochemical tests of blood and urine, and the other, to undertake in the days following birth a detailed neurologic assessment that will detect the earliest signs of these diseases. Unfortunately, not all the biochemical tests have been simplified to the point where they can be adapted to a mass screening program, and many of the commonly used clinical tests at this age have yet to be validated as markers of disease. Moreover, the tests are costly, and practical issues such as cost-effectiveness insinuate themselves, to the distress of the pediatrician. The recent introduction of tandem mass spectrometry has allayed some of the latter concerns.

The Neurologic Assessment of Neonates with Metabolic Disease

As pointed out in Chap. 28, the neonate's nervous system functions essentially at a brainstem-spinal level. The pallidum and visuomotor cortices are only beginning to be myelinated and their contribution to the totality of neonatal behavior cannot be very great. Neurologic examination, to be informative, must therefore be directed to evaluating diencephalic-midbrain, cerebellar–lower brainstem, and spinal functions. The integrity of these functions in the neonate is most reliably assessed by noting the following, as described in Chap. 28:

1. Control of respiration and body temperature; regulation of thirst, fluid balance, and appetite-hypothalamus-brainstem mechanisms
2. Certain elemental automatisms, such as sucking, rooting, swallowing, grasping—brainstem-cerebellar mechanisms
3. Movements and postures of the neck, trunk, and limbs, such as reactions of support, extension of the neck and trunk, flexion movements and steppage—lower brainstem (reticulospinal), cerebellar, and spinal mechanisms
4. Muscle tone of limbs and trunk—spinal neuronal and neuromuscular function
5. Reflex eye movements—tegmental midbrain and pontine mechanisms (a modified optokinetic nystagmus can be recognized by the third day of life)
6. The state of alertness and attention (stimulus responsivity and capacity of the examiner to make contact) as well as sleep-waking and electroencephalographic patterns—diencephalic mechanisms
7. Certain reflexive reactions such as the startle (Moro) response and placing reactions of the foot and hand—upper brainstem–spinal mechanisms with cortical facilitation

Derangements of these functions are manifest as impairments of alertness and arousal, hypotonia, disturbances of ocular movement (oscillations of the eyes, nystagmus, loss of tonic conjugate deviation of the eyes in response to vestibular stimulation, i.e., to rotation of the upright infant), failure to feed, tremors, clonic jerkings, tonic spasms, opisthotonos, diminution or absence of limb movements, irregular or chaotic breathing, hypothermia or poikilothermia, bradycardia, circulatory difficulties, poor color, and seizures.

In most instances of neonatal metabolic disease, the pregnancy and delivery proceed without mishap. Birth at full term is usual. The infant is of a size and weight expected for the duration of pregnancy, and there are no signs of a developmental abnormality (in a few instances the infant is somewhat small, and in G_{M1} gangliosidosis there may be a pseudo-Hurler appearance; see further on). Furthermore, function continues to be normal in the first few days of life. The first hint of trouble may be the occurrence of feeding difficulties: food intolerance, diarrhea, and vomiting. The infant becomes fretful and fails to gain weight and thrive—all of which should suggest a disorder of amino acid, ammonia, or organic acid metabolism.

The first definite indication of disordered nervous system function is likely to be the occurrence of seizures. These usually take the form of unpatterned clonic or tonic contractions of one side of the body or independent bilateral contractions, sudden arrest of respiration, turning of the head and eyes to one side, or twitching of the hands and face. Some of the seizures may become generalized. They occur singly or in clusters, and in the latter instance are associated with unresponsiveness, immobility, and arrest of respiration. While seizures are occurring, certain automatic activities such as sucking, grasping, steppage, and the Moro and support reactions are suppressed.

The other clinical abnormalities, according to authorities such as Prechtl and Beintema, can be subdivided roughly into three groups, each of which constitutes a kind of syndrome: (1) hyperkinetic-hypertonic, (2) apathetic-hypotonic, or (3) unilateral or hemisyndromic. Prechtl and Beintema, from a study of more than 1500 newborns, found that if clinical examination consistently discloses any one of the three syndromes, the chances are two out of three that by the seventh year the child will be abnormal neurologically. They found also that certain neurologic signs—such as facial palsy, lack of grasping, excessive floppiness, and impairment of sucking—while sometimes indicative of serious disease of the nervous system, are less dependable; also, being rare, these signs will identify but few brain-damaged infants. It is not the single neurologic sign but groups of them that are held to be the most reliable indices of brain abnormality, and the three syndromes mentioned above are the important ones, even though their anatomic and physiologic bases are not completely known.

In our observations of the neonatal metabolic diseases, we have endeavored to determine if particular ones consistently manifest themselves by one or another of the three syndromes; this we are able to affirm to some degree. In cases of hypocalcemia-hypomagnesemia, the hyperkinetic-hypertonic syndrome prevails. Although most of the other diseases tend to induce the apathetic-hypotonic state, the hyperactive-hypertonic syndrome may represent the initial phase of the illness and always carries a less ominous prognosis than the apathetic-hypotonic state, which represents a more severe and potentially dangerous condition regardless of cause. We have been least confident in the recognition of the third putative group of unilateral abnormalities in the metabolic diseases. Even more discouraging has been the frequent overlapping of the two other syndromes and the fact that seizures may occur in all of them. The anatomic correlate for some of these neurologic abnormalities can be provided by MRI. Clearly what is needed is a new neonatal neurologic semiology utilizing every possible type of stimulus-response test, including visual, auditory, and somatosensory evoked potentials; also needed are ways of accurately quantifying more of the natural activities of this age period. Even the brain death syndrome, in which all brainstem-spinal reflexes are abolished, has not been fully defined in the neonate (Adams et al).

The Neonatal Metabolic Diseases and Their Estimated Frequency

In New England, screening of all newborns for metabolic disorders has been in operation for almost 40 years. Current data on the diseases with neurologic implications have been collated by our colleague, H. L. Levy, and are summarized in Table 37-1. Some of these disorders can be recognized by simple color reactions in the urine; these are listed in Table 37-2.

To this group should be added the inherited hyperammonemic syndromes and vitamin-responsive aminoacidopathies (such as pyridoxine dependency and biopterin deficiency) as well as certain nonfamilial metabolic disorders that make their appearance in the neonatal period—hypocalcemia, hypothyroidism and cretinism, hypomagnesemia with tetany, and hypoglycemia.

It is important to note that the three most frequently identified hereditary metabolic diseases—phenylketonuria (PKU), hyperphenylalaninemia, and congenital hypothyroidism—do not become clinically manifest in the neonatal period and are therefore discussed in a later portion of this chapter and in Chap. 40 (in the discussion of congenital hypothyroidism, page 1200). This is fortunate, for it allows time to introduce preventive measures before the first symptoms appear. A number of others, which can be recognized either by screening or by early signs, are synopsized below.

Vitamin-Responsive Aminoacidopathies Included under this heading is a group of diseases that respond not to dietary restriction of a specific amino acid but to the oral supplementation of a specific vitamin. Some 30 vitamin-responsive aminoacidopathies are known (the more common ones are listed in Table 41-3), and many of them result in injury to the central nervous system. Pyridoxine dependency is the classic example. This is a rare disease, inherited as an autosomal recessive trait. It is characterized by the early onset of convulsions, sometimes in utero; failure to thrive; hypertonia-hyperkinesia; irritability; tremulous movements ("jittery baby"); exaggerated auditory startle (hyperacusis); and later, if untreated, by psychomotor retardation. The specific laboratory abnormality is an increased excretion of xanthurenic acid in response to a tryptophan load. There are decreased levels of pyridoxal-5-phosphate and gamma-aminobutyric acid (GABA) in brain tissue. The neuropathology has been studied in only a few cases. In one of our patients, a 13 1/2-year-old boy with mental retardation, pale optic discs, and spastic legs, the brain weight was 350 g below normal. There was a decreased amount of central white matter in the cerebral hemispheres and a depletion of neurons in the thalamic nuclei and cerebellum, with gliosis (Lott et al). The administration of 50 to 100 mg of vitamin B_6 suppresses the seizure state, and daily doses of 40 mg permit normal development.

Table 37-1
Estimated frequency of metabolic disorders with neurologic implications among newborn infants in New England (1999)

Disorder	*Total screened*	*Total detected*	*Frequency*
Congenital hypothyroidism	3,105,000	948	1:3,300
Phenylketonuria	4,738,789	336	1:14,000
Atypical PKU	4,738,789	286	1:17,000
Hartnup disorder	1,028,581	46	1:22,000
Histidinemia	1,028,581	38	1:27,000
Methylmalonic acidemia	1,028,581	19	1:54,000
Galactosemia	3,888,716	63	1:62,000
Argininosuccinic acidemia	1,028,581	13	1:80,000
Biotinidase deficiency	1,319,123	14	1:94,000
Homocystinuria	3,300,000	16	1:200,000
Maple syrup urine disease	4,599,373	19	1:240,000
Prolidase deficiency	1,028,581	3	1:350,000
Hyperprolinemia (type II)	1,028,581	2	1:500,000
Short-chain acyl-CoA dehydrogenase deficiency	1,028,581	1	1:1000,000

Source: Data compiled by Harvey L. Levy, MD, and Cecelia Walraven, BS.

Biopterin Deficiency Some patients with increased concentrations of serum phenylalanine in the neonatal period are unresponsive to measures that lower phenylalanine. They are usually found to have a defect in biopterin metabolism. If this condition is unrecognized and not treated promptly, seizures of both myoclonic and later grand mal types combined with a poor level of responsiveness and generalized hypotonia develop. Swallowing difficulty is another prominent symptom. Within a few months, developmental delay becomes prominent. Unlike in PKU, phenylalanine hydroxylase enzyme levels are normal, but there is a lack of tetrahydrobiopterin, which is a cofactor of phenylalanine hydroxylase. Treatment consists of administration of tetrahydrobiopterin in a dosage of 7.5 mg/kg per day in combination with a low-phenylalanine diet. It is important

Table 37-2
Urinary screening tests for metabolic defects

Disease	*Ferric chloride*	*DNPH*[a]	*Benedict reaction*	*Nitroprusside reaction*
Phenylketonuria	Green	+	−	−
Maple syrup urine disease	Navy blue	+	−	−
Tyrosinemia	Pale green (transient)	+	−	
Histidinemia	Green-brown	±	−	−
Propionic acidemia	Purple	+	−	−
Methylmalonic aciduria	Purple	+	−	−
Homocystinuria	−	−	−	+
Cystinuria		−	−	+
Galactosemia	−	−	+	−
Fructose intolerance	−	−	+	−

[a] Diaminophenylhydrazine.

to recognize this condition early in life by the measurement of urine pterins and to institute appropriate therapy before irreversible brain injury occurs.

Galactosemia Inheritance of this disorder is autosomal recessive. The biochemical abnormality consists of a defect in galactose-1-phosphate uridyl transferase (GALT), the enzyme that catalyzes the conversion of galactose-1-phosphate to uridine diphosphate galactose. Several forms of galactosemia have been described, based on the degree of completeness of the metabolic block. In the classic (severe) form, the onset of symptoms is in the first days of life, after the ingestion of milk; vomiting and diarrhea are followed by a failure to thrive. Drowsiness, inattention, hypotonia, and diminution in the vigor of neonatal automatisms then become evident. The fontanelles may bulge, the liver and spleen enlarge, the skin becomes yellow (in excess of neonatal jaundice), and anemia develops. Rarely there is thrombocytopenia with cerebral bleeding. Cataracts may form due to the accumulation of galactitol in the lens. Surviving infants show retarded psychomotor development, visual impairment, and residual cirrhosis, sometimes with splenomegaly and ascites. In one such patient, who died at 8 years, the main change in the brain was slight microcephaly with fibrous gliosis of the white matter and some loss of Purkinje and granule cells in the cerebellum, also with gliosis (Crome). The diagnostic laboratory findings are an elevated blood galactose level, low glucose, galactosuria, and deficiency of GALT in red and white blood cells and in liver cells. The treatment is essentially dietary, using milk substitutes; if this is instituted early, the brain is protected from injury.

A late-onset neurologic syndrome has also been observed by Friedman and colleagues in galactosemic patients who survived the infantile disease. By late adolescence, they are found to be subnormal intellectually and socially maladjusted; some have shown cerebellar ataxia, dystonia, and apraxia. One of these patients was middle-aged.

Organic Acidurias of Infancy These have been divided into ketotic and nonketotic types. Among the *ketotic types*, the main one is *propionic acidemia*. It is an autosomal recessive disease due to a primary defect in organic acid metabolism that is expressed clinically by episodes of vomiting, lethargy, coma, convulsions, hypertonia, and respiratory difficulty. The onset is in the neonatal or early infantile period; in time, psychomotor retardation becomes evident. Death usually occurs within a few months. Propionic acid, glycine, various forms of fatty acids, and butanone are elevated in the serum. High protein intake induces ketotic attacks.

A number of other ketotic acidurias also occur in infancy. The most important of these are *methylmalonic acidemia, isovaleric acidemia, beta-keto acidemia*, and *lactic acidemia*. Each of these disorders can present with profound metabolic acidosis and intermittent lethargy, vomiting, tachypnea, and coma, with early death in about half the patients and developmental retardation in those who survive. Rare subtypes of methylmalonic acidemia respond to vitamin B_{12}. Isovaleric acidemia is characterized by a striking odor of stale perspiration, which has given it the sobriquet "sweaty foot syndrome." Marked restriction of dietary protein (specifically leucine) may prevent attacks of ketoacidosis and permit relatively good psychomotor development. Numerous metabolic defects, most commonly of pyruvate decarboxylase and pyruvate dehydrogenase, are responsible for the accumulation of lactic and pyruvic acids. The enzymatic defect of isovaleric acidemia has also been demonstrated in a recurrent form of episodic cerebellar ataxia and athetosis and in a persistent form in mitochondrial encephalopathies (Leigh disease), as described further on in this chapter.

Type II glutaric acidemia has also been observed in the neonatal period and causes episodes of acidosis with vomiting and hyperglycemia. Multiple congenital anomalies of brain and somatic structures and cardiomyopathy are conjoined. A diet low in the specific toxic amino acid and supplements of carnitine and riboflavin are recommended, but the effects are unclear.

In the *nonketotic form of hyperglycinemia*, there are high levels of glycine but no acidosis. The notable diagnostic finding is an elevation of the CSF glycine, several times higher than that of the blood. The effects on the nervous system are more devastating than in the ketotic form. In reported cases (the authors have seen several), the neonate is hypotonic, listless, and dyspneic, with dysconjugate eye movements, opisthotonic posturing, myoclonus, and seizures. A few such neonates survive to infancy but are extremely retarded and helpless. Spongy degeneration of the brain has been reported both in this disease and in the ketotic form (Shuman et al). No treatment has been effective in severe cases. In an atypical milder form with neurologic abnormalities that appear in later infancy or childhood, reduction of dietary protein and administration of sodium benzoate in doses up to 250 mg/kg per day have been beneficial. The use of dextromethorphan, which blocks glycine receptors, is effective in preventing seizures and coma.

Inherited Hyperammonemias These are a group of six diseases caused by inborn deficiencies of the enzymes of the Krebs-Henseleit urea cycle; they are designated as *N-acetyl glutamate synthetase, carbamyl phosphate synthetase* (CPS), *ornithine transcarbamylase* (OTC), *argininosuccinic acid synthetase (citrullinemia), argininosuccinase deficiency*, and *arginase deficiency*. Hyperornithemia-hyperammonemia-homocitrurlinemia (HHH) and intrinsic protein intolerance are closely related disorders. A detailed account of these inherited hyperammonemic syndromes is contained in the review by Brusilow and Horwich.

The pattern of inheritance of each of these disorders is autosomal recessive except for OTC deficiency, which is X-linked dominant. Their clinical manifestations are a common expression of an accumulation of ammonia or of urea cycle intermediates in the brain; they differ only in severity, in accordance with the degree of completeness of the enzymatic deficiency and with the age of the affected individual. The one exception is arginase deficiency, which commonly presents during later childhood as a progressive spastic paraplegia with mental retardation. Clinically it has been convenient to divide the hyperammonemias into two groups—one that presents in the neonatal period and another that presents in the weeks or months thereafter. This division is somewhat artificial, the clinical presentation being more in the nature of a continuous spectrum governed by the biologic factors mentioned above.

In the most severe forms of the hyperammonemic disorders, the infants are asymptomatic at birth and during the first day or two of life, after which they refuse their feedings, vomit, and rapidly become inactive and lethargic, soon lapsing into an irreversible coma. Profuse sweating, focal or generalized seizures, rigidity with opisthotonos, and hypothermia and hyperventilation have been observed in the course of the illness. These symptoms constitute a medical emergency, and even with measures to reduce ammonium, the disease is usually fatal.

In less severely affected infants, hyperammonemia develops some months later, when protein feeding is increased. There is a failure to thrive, and attempts to enforce feeding or periods of constipation (both of which increase ammonia production in the bowel) may be accompanied by bouts of vomiting, hyperirritability, and screaming. Respiratory alkalosis is a consistent feature. Other manifestations are episodes of alternating hypertonia and hypotonia, seizures, ataxia, blurred vision, and periods of confusion, stupor, and coma. During episodes of stupor, often precipitated by dehydration, an alimentary protein load, or minor surgery, brain edema may be seen by CT and MRI; with repeated relapses, the brain edema gives way to atrophy, which appears as symmetrical areas of decreased attenuation in the cerebral white matter. Between attacks, some patients with partial deficiency may be normal or show only a slight hyperbilirubinemia (diMagno et al, Rowe et al). With decompensation, the bilirubin rises, as does ammonia, but neither reaches exceedingly high levels. After repeated attacks, signs of motor and mental retardation become evident, and the patient is vulnerable to recurrent infections. Two adult male patients in our care, who were married (azoospermia is common) and working at technically demanding jobs, came to medical attention because of bouts of visual blurring followed by stupor that evolved over hours. They had displayed an aversion to protein and milk products as children; in later life, after meals high in protein, they became encephalopathic, one with severe brain swelling (Shih et al). There are few phenotypic differences among the late-onset hyperammonemias except for *argininosuccinic aciduria*, in which excessive dryness and brittleness of the hair (trichorrhexis nodosa) are notable features.

Diagnosis is established by the finding of hyperammonemia, often as high as 1500 mg/dL. The precise biochemical diagnosis requires testing of blood and urine for amino acids or assays for specific enzymes in red cells, liver, or jejunal biopsies. The primary hyperammonemias must be distinguished from the organic acidurias, including *methylmalonic aciduria* (see above), in which hyperammonemia can occur as a secondary metabolic abnormality.

In all the neonatal hyperammonemic diseases, the liver is often enlarged and liver cells appear to be inadequate in their metabolic functions, but how the enzymatic deficiencies or other disorders of amino acid metabolism affect the brain remains uncertain. It must be assumed that in some the saturation of the brain by ammonia impairs the oxidative metabolism of cerebral neurons, and when blood levels of ammonium increase (from protein ingestion, constipation, etc.), episodic coma or a more chronic impairment of cerebral functions occurs—as it does in adults with cirrhosis of the liver and portal-systemic encephalopathy. When the hyperammonemia is abrupt in onset and severe, the resulting combination of encephalopathy, brain swelling, and respiratory alkalosis simulates the *Reye syndrome*. As in all forms of liver disease, valproic acid and other hepatic toxins may cause hepatic coma by further impairing the urea cycle enzymes. In a few cases, a hyperammonemic disease has come to light after the administration of one of these drugs.

Ornithine Transcarbamylase Deficiency and Argininosuccinic Aciduria These are episodic diseases in which hyperammonemia develops usually later in childhood, but they may become manifest in the neonatal period. The main clinical features are episodic stupor, ataxia, and seizures. They are discussed above.

Treatment of the Hyperammonemic Syndromes The *treatment* of acute hyperammonemic syndromes is directed to the lowering of ammonium by hemodialysis, exchange transfusions, and administration of arginine and certain organic acids. With subsidence of the acute symptoms, a systematic form of management (as outlined by Brusilow et al and by Msall et al) should be undertaken. Sodium benzoate should be given in doses up to 250 mg/day, supplemented by sodium phenylacetate or sodium phenylbutyrate, which on theoretical grounds should divert nitrogen from the ureagenesis cycle. Arginine (50 to 150 mg/kg) should be added to the diet, since a deficiency of this substance may be responsible for the mental retardation and skin rashes. In more chronic cases, treatment consists of decreasing the ammonium load (by dietary protein restriction and by administration of oral antibiotics and lactulose). In infants with inborn errors of ureagenesis, there is a constant danger of recurrent episodes of hyperammonemia and coma, particularly in response to infections. In a few instances, careful management of the metabolic error has resulted in normal psychomotor development.

Liver transplantation may prove to be a therapeutic option.

Branched Chain Aminoacidopathies (Maple Syrup Urine Disease and Its Phenotypes) These conditions are caused by a deficiency of α-ketoacid dehydrogenase, resulting in the accumulation of the branched chain amino acids leucine, isoleucine, and valine and the corresponding branched chain α-keto acids. Maple syrup urine disease may be taken as the prototype. The pattern of inheritance is autosomal recessive. The infant appears normal at birth, but toward the end of the first week, intermittent hypertonicity, opisthotonos, and respiratory irregularities appear. These are followed by diminished neonatal automatisms, convulsions, severe ketoacidosis, and often coma and death toward the end of the second to fourth week. This disease is one of the causes of the malignant epileptic syndrome of early infancy (Brett). Milder forms of the disease present with feeding difficulties that begin somewhat later in the early infantile period, followed by recurrent infections, episodic acidosis, coma, and retarded psychomotor development. Some of these patients, toward the end of the first year, may become quadriparetic or ataxic; or there may be only a nonspecific mental retardation. The urine smells like maple syrup and gives a positive test for 2,4-dinitrophenylhydrazine (DNPH).

Other important laboratory findings are increased plasma and urine concentrations of leucine, isoleucine, valine, and keto acids. Secondary accumulation of a derivative of α-hydroxybutyric acid probably accounts for the maple syrup odor. The neuropathologic findings are uncertain. In the first acute case described, only interstitial edema was observed; in more chronic cases, pallor and loss of myelin and gliosis of the cerebral white matter are found. Treatment by restriction of foods containing branched chain amino acids (leucine, isoleucine, and valine) allows reasonably normal mental development, but only if such restriction is begun in the neonatal period. A thiamine-responsive variant with a slightly different pattern of ketoacids has been described by Prensky and Moser.

Other Organic Acidemias In addition to maple syrup urine disease, there are a number of other metabolic disturbances, some of them of mitochondrial origin, that appear in the neonatal period or later and are marked by an organic acidemia. If they are severe, the infant manifests a metabolic (lactic) acidosis soon after birth, with lethargy, feeding problems, rapid respirations, and vomiting. Or there may be irritability, jerky limb movements, and hypertonia. Later presentations take the form of feeding difficulties, repeated vomiting, hypotonia, and failure to thrive; with the passage of time, psychomotor retardation and drug-resistant seizures become evident. Metabolic stress—e.g., intercurrent infection or surgical procedures—may precipitate an episode of lactic or ketoacidosis.

Biochemical studies may disclose a biotinidase deficiency, methylmalonic aciduria, glutaric acidemia, methylglutagonic acidemia, or any number of other organic acid abnormalities. The precise abnormality is determined by measuring enzyme activity in white blood cells or cultured skin fibroblasts. As remarked above, some of these enzymes act in conjunction with a specific vitamin cofactor, so that exact diagnosis is imperative. The biotinidase deficiency may respond to 10 mg of biotin per day; the methylmalonic acidemia to 1 to 2 mg of vitamin B_{12} per day; maple syrup urine disease to 10 to 20 mg of thiamine per day; and glutaric acidemia types I and II to 300 mg of riboflavin per day. The administration of carnitine may increase the elimination of toxic metabolites.

The care of these patients during an acute illness is of extreme importance. See Lyon and colleagues for a more complete description.

Sulfite Oxidase Deficiency (See also page 1038) This is an extremely rare disorder of sulfur metabolism, manifest clinically during the neonatal period by seizures, reduced level of responsivity, and spasms with opisthotonos. With survival into infancy, episodic confusion and stupor give way to seizures, mental retardation, and ataxia. In one of our cases described by Shih and colleagues, a stroke-like syndrome of hemiplegia and aphasia appeared during a relapse at the age of 4.5 years, and in a Belgian case, subluxation of the lenses and choreoathetosis appeared at 8 months of age.

Shih and colleagues have identified sulfite, thiosulfite, and S-sulfocysteine in the urine. Cerebral atrophy with loss and destruction of white matter and gray matter (cerebral cortex, basal ganglia, and cerebellar nuclei) has been observed in one postmortem examination. Increasing the intake of molybdenum or lowering the dietary intake of sulfur amino acids are therapeutic possibilities, not yet fully tried.

Diagnosis of Neonatal Metabolic Diseases

An important clue, of course, is provided by the history of a neonatal disease or unexplained death earlier in the same sibship or in a male maternal relative. A history that protein foods are rejected by the infant, or even a history among relatives of a dislike of protein or feeding difficulties in infancy, should raise the suspicion of an inherited hyperammonemic disorder or an organic acidemia. Measurements of blood ammonia and lactate and of the urine for ketones and reducing substances are the key laboratory tests. A wide-spectrum screening program may disclose a biochemical abnormality; this is the optimal state of affairs, especially when this type of screening provides the information before symptoms appear.

A number of nonhereditary metabolic diseases must be distinguished from the hereditary ones in this period of life. *Hypocalcemia* is one of the most frequent causes of neonatal seizures; tetany, spasms, and tremulous movements are usually present. Its cause is unknown, but the disorder is easily corrected, with excellent prognosis. Symptomatic *hypoglycemic* reactions are frequent in neonates. Premature infants are the most susceptible. With blood sugar levels of less than 30 mg/dL in the mature infant and less than 20 mg/dL in the premature, there are seizures, tremulousness, and drowsiness. Maternal toxemia and diabetes mellitus also predispose to hypoglycemia. Other causes of hypoglycemia are adrenal insufficiency, galactosemia, an idiopathic pancreatic islet-cell hyperplasia, the treatable fatty acid beta oxidation disorders, and the recently reported congenital deficiency of CSF glucose transport—causing persistent hypoglycorachia and refractory seizures unless blood glucose levels are kept high. The damaging effects of untreated hypoglycemia have been well documented by Koivisto and colleagues. There is also a recently recognized disorder of CSF serine transport causing failure to thrive, severe developmental disability and spasticity, and intractable epilepsy. Diagnosis is made by measuring CSF amino acids; treatment is with high-dose oral serine. *Cretinism* and *idiopathic hypercalcemia* are other recognizable entities at this age period.

Aicardi has described a neonatal myoclonic syndrome and Ohtahara, a malignant neonatal seizure disorder. In some of the cases, the neonatal syndrome merged later with the West type of infantile spasm disorder and the Lennox-Gastaut syndrome. Some of the cases had developmental abnormalities of the cerebrum, and severe mental retardation was the outcome. In other cases of this type, a familial coincidence was a feature; a metabolic defect was suspected in these cases but never proved.

The hereditary metabolic diseases must also be distinguished from a number of other catastrophic disorders that occur at or soon after birth, such as asphyxia, perinatal ventricular hemorrhage with the respiratory distress syndrome of hyaline membrane disease, other hypotensive-hypoxic states, erythroblastosis fetalis with kernicterus, neonatal bacterial meningitis, meningoencephalitis (herpes simplex, cytomegalic inclusion disease, listeriosis, rubella, syphilis, and toxoplasmosis), and hemorrhagic disease of the newborn. These are described in Chap. 38.

THE HEREDITARY METABOLIC DISEASES OF INFANCY

The hallmark of all the hereditary metabolic diseases is *psychosensorimotor regression*. However, those that have their onset in the first year of life pose extraordinary problems in neurologic diagnosis. If the onset is in the first postnatal months, before the infant has had time to develop the normal complex repertoire of behavior, the first signs of disease may take the form of subtle delays in maturation rather than of psychomotor regression. Departures from normalcy include a lack of interest in the surroundings, a lack of visual engagement, continued poor head control, an inability to sit up at the usual time, poor hand-eye coordination, and persistence of infantile automatisms. Of course, embryologic maldevelopment of the brain may have similar effects, and systemic diseases and other visceral malformations—such as cystic fibrosis, renal disease, biliary atresia and congenital heart disease, chronic infection, malnutrition, and seizures (with drug therapy)—may appear to impede psychomotor development. Diagnosis becomes somewhat easier in the second half of the first year, especially if development in the first half had proceeded normally. Then an observant mother can perceive a loss of certain early acquisitions, attesting to the progressive nature of a disease.

The most distinctive members of this category of neurologic disease are the *leukodystrophies* and the so-called *lysosomal storage diseases*. The leukodystrophies are a group of inherited metabolic diseases of the nervous system, characterized by progressive, symmetrical, and usually massive destruction of the white matter of the brain and sometimes of the spinal cord; each type of leukodystrophy is distinguished by a particular abnormal product of degeneration of myelinated fibers. In the *lysosomal storage diseases*, there is a genetic deficiency of the enzymes (usually one or more of the acid hydrolases) necessary for the degradation of specific glycosidic or peptide linkages in the intracytoplasmic lysosomes, causing nerve cells to become engorged with material that they would ordinarily degrade. These metabolites eventually damage the nerve cell or myelin sheath. Most of these diseases are classed as sphingolipidoses. It was Brady in 1966 who made the observation that in each of these disorders an increased quantity of sphingolipid accumulated in the brain and other tissues. The sphingolipids are a class of intracellular lipids that all have ceramide as their basic structure, but each has a different attached oligosaccharide or phosphorylcholine. The rate of synthesis of the sphingolipids is normal and their accumulation results from a defect of a specific lysosomal enzyme that normally degrades each of the glycoproteins, glycolipids, and mucopolysaccharides by removing a monosaccharide or sulfate moiety. It is the type of enzyme deficiency and accumulated metabolite, as well as the tissue distribution of the undegradable substrate, that impart a distinctive biochemical and clinical character to each of the diseases in this category.

The concept of lysosomal storage diseases, introduced by Hers in 1965, excited great interest among neurologists because it provided the potential for prenatal diagnosis and detection of carriers. The diagnosis of this group of diseases has also been facilitated by the use of CT scanning, MRI, and evoked response techniques, which confirm the existence of leukodystrophies, and by the electron microscopic examination of skin, rectal, or conjunctival biopsies, circulating lymphocytes, and cultured amniotic fluid cells, which discloses the lysosomal storage material in nonneural cells. The activity of most lysosomal enzymes can be determined by exposing them to artificial chromogenic or fluorogenic substrates.

There are now more than 40 lysosomal storage diseases in which the biochemical abnormalities have been determined. They are listed in Table 37-3, which was adapted originally from the review of Kolodny and Cable and recently updated by Kolodny. In addition to the sphingolipidoses, which are the lysosomal storage diseases most likely to be encountered in the first year of life, the table includes the storage diseases encountered in childhood and adolescence, to be considered later in the chapter.

The inherited metabolic diseases of infancy occur at an estimated frequency of one in every 5000 births. The more frequent ones are listed below:

1. Tay-Sachs disease (G_{M2} gangliosidosis) and variants such as Sandhoff disease
2. Infantile Gaucher disease
3. Infantile Niemann-Pick disease
4. Infantile G_{M1} generalized gangliosidosis
5. Krabbe globoid-body leukodystrophy
6. Farber lipogranulomatosis
7. Pelizaeus-Merzbacher and other sudanophilic leukodystrophies
8. Spongy degeneration (Canavan-Van Bogaert-Bertrand)
9. Alexander disease
10. Alpers disease
11. Zellweger encephalopathy
12. Lowe oculorenalcerebral disease
13. Kinky-hair, or steely-hair, disease
14. Congenital lactic acidosis

In the following descriptions, we have summarized the clinical and pathologic features of each of the diseases listed above and have italicized the characteristic clinical signs and the corroborative laboratory tests.

Table 37-3 Lysosomal storage diseases

Disorder	*Primary deficiency*	*Accumulated metabolite*
	Sphingolipidoses	
G_{M1} gangliosidosis	β-Galactosidase	G_{M1} ganglioside, galactosyl oligosaccharides, keratan sulfate
G_{M2} gangliosidosis		
Tay-Sachs disease	α-*N*-acetylhexosaminidase α subunit	G_{M2} ganglioside
Sandhoff disease	β-*N*-acetylhexosaminidase β subunit	G_{M2} ganglioside, oligosaccharides, glycosaminoglycans
Activator deficiency	G_{M2} activator	G_{M2} ganglioside
Metachromatic leukodystrophy	Arylsulfatase A (sulfatidase), sulfatide activator (saposin B)	Galactosylsulfatide, lactosylsulfatide
Krabbe disease	Galactocerebrosidase	Galactosylceramide
Fabry disease	α-Galactosidase A	Ceramide trihexoside
Gaucher disease	Glucocerebrosidase	Glucosylceramide, glycopeptides
Niemann-Pick disease		
Types A and B	Sphingomyelinase	Sphingomyelin, cholesterol
Type C	Cholesterol esterification	Free cholesterol, *bis*-monoacylglycerophosphate
Farber disease	Ceramide	Ceramide
Schindler disease	α-Galactosidase B	α-*N*-acetylgalactosaminyl oligosaccharides and glycopeptides
	Neuronal ceroid lipofuscinoses	
Infantile form (Haltia-Santavuori)	Palmitoyl-protein thioesterase	Granular osmiophilic deposits
Late infantile form (Jansky-Bielschowsky)	Tripeptidyl peptidase I	Curvilinear bodies, subunit C of mitochondrial ATP synthase
Juvenile form (Spielmeyer-Sjögren)	438-amino acid membrane protein	Curvilinear and laminated (fingerprint) bodies, subunit C of mitochondrial ATP synthase
Adult form (Kufs disease)	Unknown	Mixed type osmiophilic deposits and lamellar inclusions
	Glycoproteinoses	
Aspartylglucosaminuria	Aspartylglucosaminidase	Aspartylglucosamine
Fucosidosis	α-L-Fucosidase	Fucosyloligosaccharides, fucosylglycosphingolipids
Galactosialidosis	Protective protein (β-galactosidase and α-neuraminidase)	Sialyloligosaccharides, galactosyloligosaccharides
α-Mannosidosis	α-Mannosidase	α-Mannosyl-oligosaccharides
β-Mannosidosis	β-Mannosidase	β-Mannosyl-oligosaccharides
	Mucolipidoses	
Sialidosis (mucolipidosis I)	α-Neuraminidase	Sialyloligosaccharides, sialylglycopeptides
Mucolipidosis II (I-cell disease)	UDP-*N*-acetylglucosamine: lysosomal enzyme, *N*-acetylglucosamine-1-phosphotransferase	Sialyloligosaccharides, glycoproteins, glycolipids
Mucolipidosis III (pseudo-Hurler polydystrophy)	Same phosphotransferase as above	Sialyloligosaccharides, glycoproteins, glycolipids
Mucolipidosis IV	Unknown	Gangliosides, phospholipids, mucopolysaccharides
	Other lysosomal diseases	
Acid lipase deficiency		
Wolman disease	Acid lipase	Cholesterol esters, triglycerides
Cholesterol ester storage disease	Acid lipase	Cholesterol esters, triglycerides
Glycogenosis type II (Pompe disease)	α-Glucosidase (acid maltase)	Glycogen
Sialic acid storage disease		
Infantile form	Sialic acid transport	Free sialic acid
Salla disease	Sialic acid transport	Free sialic acid
	Mucopolysaccharidoses (see Table 37-6)	

Leigh disease, which may appear in this age group, is described with the mitochondrial diseases, further on in this chapter.

Tay-Sachs Disease (G_{M2} Gangliosidosis, Hexosaminadase A Deficiency)

This is an autosomal recessive disease, mostly of Jewish infants of eastern European background. It was described by Tay, a British ophthalmologist, in 1881, and Sachs, an American neurologist, in 1887. They called it amaurotic family idiocy. The disease becomes apparent in the first weeks and months of life, almost always by the fourth month. The first manifestations are an abnormal startle to acoustic stimuli, listlessness, irritability, and poor reactions to visual stimuli, followed by a *delay in psychomotor development* or regression (by 4 to 6 months), with inability to roll over and sit. At first axial hypotonia is prominent, but later spasticity and other corticospinal tract signs develop, as does visual failure. Degeneration of the macular cells exposes the underlying red vascular choroid surrounded by a whitish gray ring of retinal cells distended with ganglioside. The resulting appearance is of *cherry-red spots* with optic atrophy (Fig. 37-1). These are observed in the retinas in more than 90 percent of patients. In the second year, there are tonic-clonic or minor motor seizures and an increasing size of the head (diastasis of sutures) with relatively normal ventricles; in the third year, the clinical picture is one of dementia, decerebration, blindness. Cachexia and death occur at 3 to 5 years. The electroencephalogram (EEG) becomes abnormal in the early stages (paroxysmal slow waves with multiple spikes). Occasionally one observes basophilic granules in leukocytes and vacuoles in lymphocytes. There are no visceral, skeletal, or bone marrow abnormalities by light microscopy.

Figure 37-1

Retinal cherry-red spot in a patient with Tay-Sachs disease. The whitish ring surrounds the dark (red) macula. (From Lyon et al by permission.)

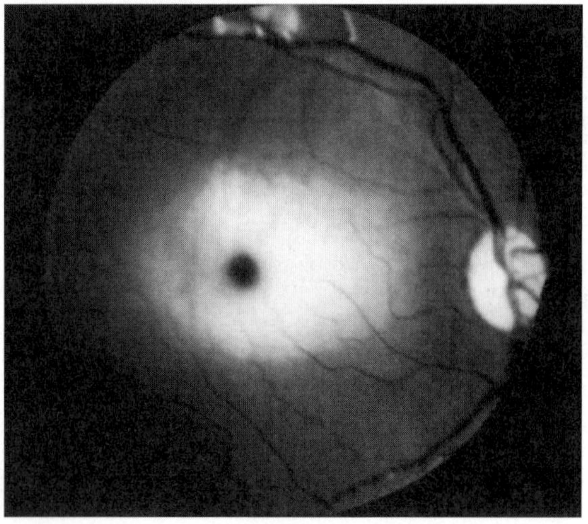

The basic enzymatic abnormality is a *deficiency of hexosaminidase A*, which normally cleaves the *N*-acetylgalactosamine from gangliosides. As a result of this deficiency, G_{M2} ganglioside accumulates in the cerebral cortical neurons, Purkinje cells, retinal ganglion cells, and, to a lesser extent, larger neurons of the brainstem and spinal cord. The enzymatic defect can be found in the serum, white blood cells, and cultured fibroblasts from the skin or amniotic fluid, giving parents the option of abortion to prevent a presently untreatable and fatal disease. Testing for hexosaminidase A also permits the detection of heterozygote carriers of the gene defect. Detection of this enzyme defect is complicated by the fact that more than 50 mutations of the alpha subunit of the beta hexosaminidases have been isolated and the enzyme itself is normal in one form of activator enzyme deficiency. Fortunately, only three mutations account for 98 percent of the form that is common in Jews.

The brain is large, sometimes twice the normal weight. In addition, there is a loss of neurons and a reactive gliosis; remaining nerve cells throughout the central nervous system (CNS) are distended with glycolipid. Biopsies of the rectal mucosa disclose glycolipid distention of the ganglion cells of the Auerbach plexus, but the need for this procedure has been obviated by enzyme analysis of white blood cells. Under the electron microscope, the particles of stored material appear as membranous cytoplasmic bodies. Retinal ganglion cells are distended with the same material and, together with fat-filled histiocytes, cause the whitish gray rings around the fovea, where there are no nerve cells, as noted above.

The same neuropathologic process has been found in a few congenital cases in which there was a rapidly progressive decline of a microcephalic infant. Kolodny and Raghavan have described two other, probably allelic variants of the hexosamine A defect. One presents as a childhood spinocerebellar degeneration, the other as a progressive spinal muscular atrophy in juveniles and young adults, due presumably to widespread involvement of spinal motor neurons (see further on).

Tay-Sachs disease is untreatable but can be prevented by testing all individuals of Jewish origin for the recessive trait. Since this screening was instituted at the

E. K. Shriver Center in 1968, there has not been a single case known to us in Massachusetts.

In *Sandhoff disease*, which affects non-Jewish infants, there is a deficiency of both hexosaminidase A and B, moderate hepatosplenomegaly, and coarse granulations in bone marrow histiocytes. The clinical and pathologic picture is the same as in Tay-Sachs disease except for the additional signs of visceral lipid storage. Occasionally these visceral organs are not enlarged.

Infantile Gaucher Disease (Type II Neuronopathic Form, Glucocerebrosidase Deficiency)

This is an autosomal recessive disease without ethnic predominance, first described by Gaucher in 1882. The onset of the neuronopathic form is usually before 6 months and frequently before 3 months. The clinical course is more rapid than that of Tay-Sachs disease (most patients with infantile Gaucher disease do not survive beyond 1 year and 90 percent, not beyond 2 years). There is rapid loss of head control, of ability to roll over and sit, and of purposeful movements—along with apathy, irritability, frequent crying, and difficulty in sucking and swallowing. In some cases progression is slower, with acquisition of single words by the first year, bilateral corticospinal signs (Babinski signs and hyperactive tendon reflexes), *persistent retroflexion of the neck*, and *strabismus*. Laryngeal stridor and trismus, diminished reaction to stimuli, smallness of the head, rare seizures, normal optic fundi, *enlarged spleen* and slightly enlarged liver, poor nutrition, yellowish skin and scleral pigmentation, osteoporosis, vertebral collapse and kyphoscoliosis, and sometimes lymphadenopathy complete the clinical picture. The CSF is normal; the EEG is abnormal but nonspecifically so.

The important laboratory findings are an *increase in serum acid phosphatase and characteristic histiocytes* (*Gaucher cells*) in marrow smears and liver and spleen biopsies. A *deficiency of glucocerebrosidase* in leukocytes and hepatocytes is diagnostic; glucocerebroside accumulates in the involved tissues. The characteristic pathologic feature is the Gaucher cell, 20 to 60 μm in diameter, with a wrinkled appearance of the cytoplasm and eccentricity of the nucleus. These cells are found in the marrow, lungs, and other viscera; neuronal storage is seldom evident. In the brain, the main abnormality is a loss of nerve cells, particularly in the bulbar nuclei, and a reactive gliosis.

Type I Gaucher disease, by contrast, is nonneuronopathic and relatively benign. A type III Gaucher disease is neuropathic. It expresses itself in late childhood or adolescence by a slowly progressive mental decline, seizures, and ataxia, and, later, by spastic weakness and splenomegaly. Vision and retinae remain normal. Highly diagnostic is a defect in voluntary lateral gaze, with full movements on the oculocephalic ("doll's head") maneuver. These signs help to differentiate Gaucher from Niemann-Pick disease, in which vertical eye movements are lost. The nucleotide sequence of the cloned glucocerebrosidase of type I Gaucher disease was found by Tsuji and associates to be different from that of types II and III. There is no treatment for the latter types.

Infantile Niemann-Pick Disease (Sphingomyelinase Deficiency)

This is also an autosomal recessive disease. Two-thirds of the affected infants have been of Ashkenazi Jewish parentage. The onset of symptoms in the usual type A disease is between 3 and 9 months of age, frequently with marked *enlargement of liver, spleen, and lymph nodes and infiltration of the lungs*; rarely there is jaundice and ascites. Cerebral abnormalities are definite by the end of the first year, often earlier. The usual manifestations are loss of spontaneous movements, lack of interest in the environment, axial hypotonia with bilateral corticospinal signs, blindness and amaurotic nystagmus, and a macular cherry-red spot (in about one-quarter of the patients). Seizures may occur but are relatively late. There is no acoustic myoclonus, and head size is normal or slightly reduced. Loss of tendon reflexes and slowed conduction in peripheral nerves have been reported but are rare. Protuberant eyes, mild hypertelorism, slight yellowish pigmentation of oral mucosa, and dysplasia of dental enamel have also been reported but are rare. Most patients succumb to an intercurrent infection by the end of the second year.

Vacuolated histiocytes ("foam cells") in the bone marrow and vacuolated blood lymphocytes are the important laboratory findings. A *deficiency of sphingomyelinase* in leukocytes, cultured fibroblasts, and hepatocytes is diagnostic. Neurons are decreased in number, and many of the remaining ones are pale and ballooned, and have a granular cytoplasm. The most prominent neuronal changes are seen in the midbrain, spinal cord, and cerebellum. The white matter is little affected. The retinal nerve cell changes are similar to those in the brain. The foamy histiocytes (Niemann-Pick cells) that fill the viscera contain sphingomyelin and cholesterol; the distended nerve cells contain mainly sphingomyelin.

There are also less severe late infantile and juvenile forms of Niemann-Pick disease, types C and D. These are discussed in a later section of this chapter.

Infantile, Generalized G_{M1} Gangliosidosis (Type I, β-Galactosidase Deficiency, Pseudo-Hurler Disease)

This is probably an autosomal recessive disease without ethnic predominance. The infants appear abnormal at birth. They have *dysmorphic facial features*, like those of the mucopolysaccharidoses: depressed and wide nasal bridge, frontal bossing, hypertelorism, epicanthi, puffy eyelids, long upper lip, gingival and alveolar hypertrophy, macroglossia, and low-set ears. These features, with the bone changes mentioned below, account for the term "pseudo-Hurler." Other indications of the disease are the onset of impaired awareness and reduced responsivity in the first days or weeks of life; lack of *psychomotor development* after 3 to 6 months; hypotonia, and later hypertonia with lively tendon reflexes and Babinski signs. Seizures are frequent. The head size is variable (microcephaly more often than macrocephaly). *Loss of vision, coarse nystagmus and strabismus, macular cherry-red spots* (in half the cases), flexion pseudocontractures of elbows and knees, kyphoscoliosis, and enlarged liver and sometimes enlarged spleen are the other important clinical findings. Radiographic abnormalities include subperiosteal bone formation, midshaft widening and demineralization of long bones, and hypoplasia and beaking of the thoracolumbar vertebrae. Vacuoles are seen in 10 to 80 percent of blood lymphocytes and foam cells in the urinary sediment.

A partial or complete deficiency of β-galactosidase and accumulation of G_{M1} ganglioside in the viscera and in neurons and glial cells throughout the CNS are the specific biochemical abnormalities. In addition, the epithelial cells of renal glomeruli, histiocytes of the spleen, and liver cells contain a modified keratan sulfate and a galactose-containing oligosaccharide. The changes in the bone are also like those in the Hurler form of mucopolysaccharidosis. The disease should be suspected in an infant who has the facial features of mucopolysaccharidosis and severe early-onset neurologic abnormalities.

A remarkably benign variant, also inherited as an autosomal recessive trait, begins later in childhood but may advance so slowly as to allow attainment of adult life. Dystonia, myoclonus, seizures, visual impairment, and macular red spots were features of the two cases described by Goldman and coworkers.

Globoid Cell Leukodystrophy (Krabbe Disease, Galactocerebrosidase Deficiency)

This is an autosomal recessive disease without ethnic predilection, first described by Krabbe, a Danish neurologist, in 1916. The onset is usually before the sixth month and often before the third month (10 percent after 1 year). Early manifestations are *generalized rigidity*, loss of head control, diminished alertness, frequent vomiting, irritability and bouts of inexplicable crying, and spasms induced by stimulation. With increasing muscular tone, *opisthotonic* recurvation of neck and trunk develop. Later signs are adduction and extension of the legs, flexion of the arms, clenching of the fists, hyperactive tendon reflexes, and Babinski signs. Later still the tendon reflexes are depressed or lost but Babinski signs remain, an indication that *neuropathy* is added to corticospinal damage. This finding, shared with some of the other leukodystrophies, is of diagnostic value. Blindness and optic atrophy supervene. Convulsions occur but are rare and difficult to distinguish from tonic spasms. Myoclonus in response to auditory stimuli is present in some cases. The head size is normal or, rarely, slightly increased. In the last stage of the disease, which may occur from one to several months after the onset, the child is blind and usually deaf, opisthotonic, irritable, and cachectic. Most patients die by the end of the first year and survival beyond 2 years is unusual, although a considerable number of cases of later onset have been reported (see below).

The EEG shows nonspecific slowing without spikes, and the CSF protein is usually elevated (70 to 450 mg/dL). CT scanning and MRI reveal symmetrical nonenhancing areas of increased density in the internal capsules and basal ganglia. As the disease advances, more of the cerebral white matter and brainstem become involved (Fig. 37-2). Clinical signs of neuropathy may be difficult to detect except for a decrease or loss of tendon reflexes, but *electromyographic (EMG) evidence of denervation and slowed motor and sensory nerve conduction velocities*, reflecting a demyelinating type of polyneuropathy, are frequent findings.

The deficient enzyme in Krabbe disease is *galactocerebrosidase* (also called galactosylceramide β-galactosidase, or GALC). It results in the accumulation of galactocerebroside, particularly in the cerebral white matter. The gene mutation is located on chromosome 14q. Gross examination of the brain discloses a marked reduction in the cerebral white matter, which feels firm and rubbery. Microscopically, there are wide-

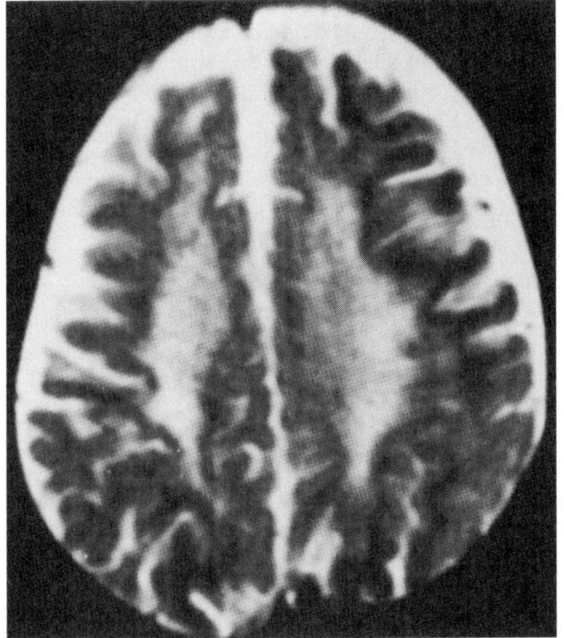

Figure 37-2

Krabbe disease. T2-weighted MRI in the axial plane demonstrating an abnormal high signal in the periventricular white matter. Arcuate fibers are spared. The patient was a 14-month-old boy with severe generalized rigidity. Diagnosis was proved postmortem (4 months after the MRI). (From Lee SH, Rao K, Zimmerman RA: Cranial MRI and CT, 3rd ed. New York, McGraw-Hill, 1992, by permission.)

spread myelin degeneration and gliosis in the cerebrum, brainstem, spinal cord, and nerves. The characteristic globoid cells are large histiocytes containing the accumulated metabolite. Schwann cells have tubular or crystalloid inclusions under electron microscopy.

About a dozen variants of globoid cell leukodystrophy have been reported, many of them allowing survival for years. In these, neurologic regression begins in the 2- to 6-year period. Visual failure with optic atrophy and normal electroretinogram is an early finding. Later there is ataxia as well as spastic weakness of the legs, mental regression, and finally decerebration. In three patients observed by R. D. Adams, a progressive quadriparesis with mild pseudobulbar signs, slowly progressive impairment of memory and other mental functions, dystonic posturing of the arms, and preserved sphincteric control constituted the clinical picture. The patients were alive at ages 9, 12, and 16 years. We have observed another rare variant, beginning in adult years, with spastic quadriparesis (asymmetrical) and optic atrophy. Mentation was essentially normal and, on CT scanning and MRI, the cerebral lesion was restricted. Unlike typical Krabbe disease, these CNS abnormalities are unaccompanied by any change in the spinal fluid. The nerve conduction velocities in the late-onset form may be either normal or abnormal.

Kolodny and colleagues have reported 15 cases of even later onset (ages 4 to 73 years); pes cavus, optic pallor, progressive spastic quadriparesis, a demyelinating sensorimotor neuropathy, and symmetrical parieto-occipital white matter changes (on imaging studies) were the main features. Galactocerebrosidase levels were not as much reduced as in the infantile form; possibly these late-onset variants represent a structural mutation of the enzyme (see Farrell and Swedberg).

In this disease, as well as others described in this chapter, it has become clear that different mutations involving the same enzyme or metabolic pathway can produce strikingly different phenotypes and that there is a wide range in the age of onset in what had been considered, until relatively recently, a disease confined to infancy and early childhood.

Lipogranulomatosis (Farber Disease, Ceramidase Deficiency)

This is a very rare disorder that is probably genetic, affecting both sexes and without a particular racial predilection. The onset is in the first weeks of life, with a hoarse cry due to fixation of laryngeal cartilage, respiratory distress, and sensitivity of the joints, followed by characteristic *periarticular and subcutaneous swellings* and *progressive arthropathy* leading finally to ankylosis. Usually there is severe psychomotor retardation, but a few patients have appeared neurologically normal. Inanition and recurrent infections lead to death in the first 2 years. The diagnostic abnormality is a *deficiency of ceramidase*, leading to accumulation of ceramide. There is widespread lipid storage in neurons, granulomas of the skin, and accumulation of periodic acid–Schiff (PAS)-positive macrophages in periarticular and visceral tissues.

Sudanophilic Leukodystrophies and Pelizaeus-Merzbacher Disease

These are a heterogeneous group of disorders that have in common a defective myelination of the cerebrum, brainstem, cerebellum, spinal cord, and peripheral nerves. Morphologic peculiarities and genetic features separate a certain group called *Pelizaeus-Merzbacher disease*; other types have been artificially delineated; as a result, a relatively meaningless terminology has been introduced.

Pelizaeus-Merzbacher Disease This is predominantly an X-linked disease of infancy, childhood, and adolescence and includes other closely related pathologic entities with different modes of inheritance. The gene is the same as the one that encodes proteolipid protein, one of the two myelin basic proteins; Koeppen and associates have offered evidence of a defective synthesis of this protein.

The onset of symptoms is most often in the first months of life; other cases begin later in childhood. The first signs are *abnormal movements of the eyes* (rapid, irregular, often asymmetrical pendular nystagmus), jerk nystagmus on extremes of lateral movements, upbeat nystagmus on upward gaze, and hypometric saccades (Trobe et al). There is spastic weakness of the limbs, ataxia, optic atrophy, intention tremor, choreiform or athetotic movements of the arms, and slow psychomotor development with delay in sitting, standing, and walking. Seizures occur occasionally. In later-developing cases, pendular nystagmus, choreoathetosis, corticospinal signs, dysarthria, cerebellar ataxia, and mental deterioration are the major manifestations. CT scanning and MRI confirm the white matter involvement. Patients may survive to the second and third decades. One group of cases resembles the Cockayne syndrome (page 1018), with photosensitivity of skin, dwarfism, cerebellar ataxia, corticospinal signs, cataracts, retinitis pigmentosa, and deafness. Pathologically, islands of preserved myelin impart a tigroid pattern of degenerated and intact myelin in the cerebrum. Seitelberger has obtained pathologic verification of this lesion in cases beginning as late as adult years. *This disease and Cockayne syndrome are the only leukodystrophies in which nystagmus has been an invariable finding.*

Unclassifiable Sporadic and Familial Sudanophilic Leukodystrophies There are two types of disorder, one with early and the other with late onset. In the former, onset is before 3 months with survival of less than 2 years; in the latter type, onset is from 3 to 7 years and the course is chronic. *Psychomotor regression; spastic paralysis; incoordination; blindness* and optic atrophy; seizures (rare); *severe microcephaly*; and absence of skeletal, visceral, and hematologic evidence of the metabolic abnormality are the main features. No characteristic laboratory abnormalities are known. Diffuse degeneration of medullated fibers with phagocytosis of *sudanophilic degeneration products of myelin* (visible by MRI) and gliosis are the major changes. In two cases followed by R. D. Adams, a brother and sister living to adolescence, the destroyed white matter was widely cavitated.

Spongy Degeneration of Infancy (Canavan-Van Bogaert-Bertrand Disease)

This is an autosomal recessive disease first described by Canavan as Schilder disease in 1931 but later categorized as a spongy degeneration of the brain by Van Bogaert and Bertrand in 1949. Of 48 affected families reported by Banker and Victor, 28 were Jewish. Onset is early, often recognizable in the first 3 months of life. There is either a lack of development or rapid *regression of psychomotor function, loss of sight and optic atrophy*, lethargy, difficulty in sucking, irritability, reduced motor activity, hypotonia followed by spasticity of the limbs with corticospinal signs, and an *enlarged head* (macrocephaly). There are no visceral or skeletal abnormalities. Seizures occur in some cases. An interesting but unexplored aspect of the disease is the occurrence of blond hair and light complexion in affected members, in contrast to the darker hair and complexion of their normal siblings (Banker and Victor).

The CSF is usually normal, but the protein is slightly elevated in some cases. The disease is characterized by an increased urinary excretion of *N*-acetyl-L-aspartic acid (NAA), which may be used as a biochemical marker. It reflects the basic enzyme abnormality, a deficiency of aspartoacylase (Matalon et al). On CT scans there is *attenuation of cerebral and cerebellar white matter in an enlarged brain with relatively normal ventricles*. The MRI appearance (Fig. 37-3) is that of diffuse high signal intensity on T2-weighted images. A leukodystrophy with behavioral regression, an enlarging head, a characteristic MRI abnormality, and a marked elevation of urinary NAA should leave little doubt about the diagnosis.

The characteristic pathologic changes are an increase in brain volume (and weight), spongy degeneration in the deep layers of the cerebral cortex and subcortical white matter, widespread loss of myelin involving the convolutional more than the central white matter, loss of Purkinje cells, and hyperplasia of Alzheimer type II astrocytes throughout the cerebral cortex and basal ganglia. Adachi and coworkers have demonstrated an abnormal accumulation of fluid in astrocytes and between split myelin lamellae; they have

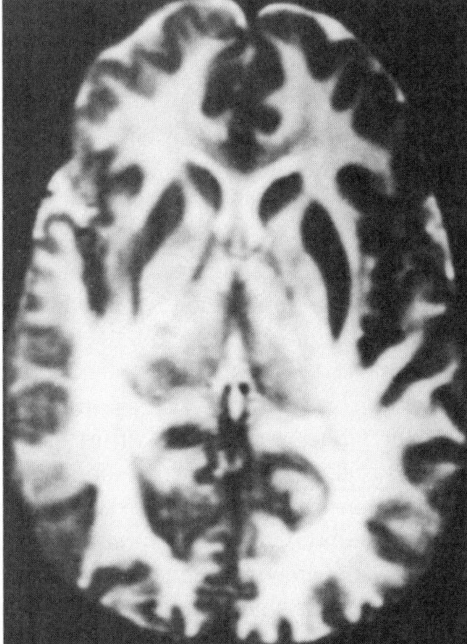

Figure 37-3

Spongy degeneration of infancy (Canavan–van Bogaert disease). T2-weighted axial MR image from an infant with a positive urine assay for N-acetyl aspartic acid. The abnormal white matter appears hyperintense and extends to the cortex without sparing of the arcuate fiber. (From Lee SH, Rao K, Zimmerman RA: Cranial MRI and CT, 3rd ed. New York, McGraw-Hill, 1992, by permission.)

suggested that the loss of myelin is secondary to these changes.

The disease must be distinguished clinically from G_{M2} gangliosidosis, Alexander disease, Krabbe disease, and nonprogressive megalocephaly and pathologically from a variety of disorders characterized by vacuolation of nervous tissue.

Alexander Disease

The classification of this rare disease is uncertain. A familial incidence has not been reported, and no metabolic fault has been defined. It shares certain features with the leukodystrophies and gray matter diseases (poliodystrophies), both clinically and pathologically. The onset is in infancy with a *failure to thrive, psychomotor retardation, and seizures*. An early and progressive macrocephaly has been a consistent feature. Pathologically, there are severe destructive changes in the cerebral white matter, most intense in the frontal lobes. Distinctive eosinophilic hyaline bodies, most prominent just below the pia and around blood vessels, are seen throughout the cerebral cortex, brainstem, and spinal cord. These have been identified as *Rosenthal fibers* and probably represent glial degradation products.

Alpers Disease This is a progressive disease of the cerebral gray matter, known also as *progressive cerebral poliodystrophy or diffuse cerebral degeneration in infancy*. A familial form (probably autosomal recessive) and some sporadic cases are known. In both groups there is a certain uniformity of clinical features—loss of smile and disinterest in the surroundings, sweating attacks, *seizures and diffuse myoclonic jerks* from early infancy, followed by incoordination of movements; progressive spasticity of limb, trunk, and cranial muscles; blindness and optic atrophy; growth retardation and *increasing microcephaly*; and finally, virtual decortication. In some instances, the late onset of jaundice and fatty degeneration or cirrhosis of the liver have been described (Alpers-Huttenlocher syndrome); the hepatic changes are distinctive and probably not related to the use of anticonvulsant drugs (Harding et al). By the age of 4 years these patients are hypotonic, anemic, and thrombopenic; they also show hair changes (trichorrhexis).

The nature of this combined hepatic-cerebral degeneration remains unexplained, but some instances have been connected to the mitochondrial disorders, as noted below. EEG abnormalities, progressive atrophy (particularly occipital) on the CT scan, loss of visual evoked potentials, and abnormal liver function tests are diagnostically useful. Neuropathologic examination shows marked atrophy of the cerebral convolutions and cerebellar cortex, with loss of nerve cells and fibrous gliosis ("walnut brain"). The cerebral white matter and basal ganglia are relatively preserved. In some cases, the spongiform vacuolization of the gray matter of the brain resembles that seen in Creutzfeldt-Jakob disease. Hypoglycemic, hypoxic, and hypotensive encephalopathies must always be considered in the diagnosis but can usually be eliminated by knowledge of the clinical circumstances at the onset of the illness.

A number of biochemical abnormalities have been identified in patients with Alpers disease, including pyruvate dehydrogenase deficiency, decreased pyruvate utilization, dysfunction of the citric acid cycle, and decreased cytochromes *a* and aa_3. The biochemical and pathologic changes suggest a relationship to Leigh encephalomyelopathy and a mitochondrial transmission. Many authoritative texts classify it with the mitochondrial diseases, but the nosologic place of the disease is in our opinion still uncertain (Shaffner and Wallace; see further on).

Congenital Lactic Acidosis

This is an uncommon disease of the neonatal period or early infancy, of many biochemical etiologies. The symptoms have consisted of *psychomotor regression* and *episodic hyperventilation*, *hypotonia*, and *convulsions*, with intervening periods of normalcy. *Choreoathetosis* has been observed in a few cases. Death often occurs before the third year. The important laboratory findings are *acidosis with an anion gap and high serum lactate levels* and hyperalaninemia. Defects can be found in the pyruvate dehydrogenase complex of enzymes and the electron transport chain complexes, which function in the oxidative decarboxylation of pyruvate to acetyl CoA—relating the disease to defects in the mitochondrial respiratory chain enzymes. Indeed, lactic acidosis is a feature of several of the mitochondropathies discussed later in the chapter. Cases that have been examined postmortem have shown necrosis and cavitation of the globus pallidus and cerebral white matter. Possibly this is a variant of Leigh disease (page 1042). It must be distinguished from the several diseases of infancy that are complicated secondarily by lactic acidosis, especially the organic acidopathies. Cases of benign transient infantile lactic acidosis have been reported, but their etiology is unclear.

Cerebrohepatorenal (Zellweger) Disease (Peroxisomal Disorder)

This disease, estimated to occur once in every 100,000 births, is inherited as an autosomal recessive trait. It has its onset in the neonatal period or early infancy and as a rule leads to death within a few months. Motor inactivity and hypotonia, *dysmorphic alterations of the skull and face* (high forehead, shallow orbits, hypertelorism, high arched palate, abnormal helices of ears, retrognathia), poor visual fixation, multifocal seizures, swallowing difficulties, fixed flexion posture of the limbs, cataracts, abnormal retinal pigmentation, optic atrophy, cloudy corneas, hepatomegaly, and hepatic dysfunction are the usual manifestations. *Stippled, irregular calcifications of the patellae and greater trochanters are highly characteristic*. Pathologically, there is dysgenesis of the cerebral cortex and degeneration of white matter as well as a number of visceral abnormalities—cortical renal cysts, hepatic fibrosis, intrahepatic biliary dysgenesis, agenesis of the thymus, and iron storage in the reticuloendothelial system.

As to the biochemical abnormality, A. B. Moser and coworkers have demonstrated a fivefold increase of very long chain fatty acids, particularly hexacosanoic acid, in the plasma and cultured skin fibroblasts from 35 patients with Zellweger disease. A similar abnormality was found in cultured amniocytes of women at risk of bearing a child with Zellweger disease, thus permitting prenatal diagnosis. The findings of Moser and colleagues are in keeping with current notions about the basic abnormality in Zellweger syndrome—namely, that it is due to a lack of liver peroxisomes (oxidase-containing, membrane-bound cytoplasmic organelles), in which the very long chain fatty acids are normally oxidized (Goldfischer et al).

Currently, a spectrum of at least 10 disorders of peroxisomal function is recognized, all of them characterized by deficiencies in the peroxisomal enzyme of fatty acid oxidation—a veritable peroxisomal assembly. The Zellweger cerebrohepatorenal syndrome is the prototype. Each variant can be identified by its characteristic profile of elevated long and very long chain fatty acids and the specific diagnosis confirmed by enzymology of cultured fibroblasts or amniocytes.

The Oculocerebrorenal (Lowe) Syndrome

Here the mode of inheritance is probably X-linked recessive, although sporadic cases have been reported in girls. The clinical abnormalities comprise *bilateral cataracts* (which may be present at birth), glaucoma, large eyes with megalocornea and buphthalmos, corneal opacities and blindness, pendular nystagmus, hypotonia and absent or depressed tendon reflexes, corticospinal signs without paralysis, slow movements of the hands, high-pitched cry, occasional seizures, and psychomotor regression. Later the frontal bones become prominent and the eyes sunken. The characteristic biochemical abnormality is a *renal tubular acidosis*, and death is usually from *renal failure*. Additional laboratory findings include demineralization of bones and typical rachitic deformities, anemia, metabolic acidosis, and generalized aminoaciduria. The neuropathologic changes are nonspecific; inconstant atrophy and poor myelination have been described in the brain and tubular abnormalities in the kidneys. The main diagnostic distinction is from Zellweger disease.

Kinky- or Steely-Hair Disease (Menkes Disease; Trichopoliodystrophy)

This is a rare disorder, inherited as a sex-linked recessive trait. In most of our cases, birth was premature. Poor feeding and failure to gain weight, instability of temperature (mainly *hypothermia*), and seizures become apparent in early infancy. The hair is normal at birth, but the secondary growth is lusterless and depigmented and feels like steel wool; strands of hair break easily; under the microscope they appear twisted (*pili torti*). Radiologic examination shows *metaphyseal spurring*, mainly of the femurs, and subperiosteal calcifications of the shafts. Arteriography discloses *tortuosity and elongation of the cerebral and systemic arteries* and occlusion of some of them. The combination of intracerebral hemorrhage and metaphysial bone spurs, which may be interpreted as "corner fractures," has led in some cases to the erroneous diagnosis of child abuse. There is no discernible neurologic development, and rarely does the untreated child survive beyond the second year. Treated with copper histidine, patients may survive to adolescence, but they remain profoundly impaired and hypotonic and require gastric feeding; seizures may abate. Three of our cases have been examined postmortem (Williams et al). There was a diffuse loss of neurons in the relay nuclei of the thalamus, the cerebral cortex, and the cerebellum (granule and stellate cells) and of dendritic arborizations of residual neurons of the motor cortex and Purkinje cells.

The manifestations of this disease are attributable to a deficiency of several copper-dependent enzymes, including cytochrome oxidase, resulting in a *failure of absorption of copper from the gastrointestinal tract* and a profound deficiency of tissue copper (Danks et al). Further, since copper fails to cross the placenta, a severe reduction of copper in the brain and liver is evident from birth. In this sense, the abnormality of copper metabolism is the opposite of that in Wilson disease. Parenteral administration of cupric salts restores the serum and hepatic copper but does not materially influence the neurologic symptoms, as noted above.

Diagnosis of Inherited Metabolic Diseases of Infancy

It will be recognized from the foregoing synopses that many of the neurologic manifestations of the inherited metabolic diseases of infancy are nonspecific and are common to most or all of the diseases in this group. In general, in the early stages of all these diseases there is a loss of postural tone and a paucity of movement without paralysis or loss of reflexes; later there is spasticity with hyperreflexia and Babinski signs. Equally nonspecific are features such as irritability and prolonged crying; poor feeding, difficulty in swallowing, inanition, and retarded growth; failure of fixation of gaze and following movements of the eyes (often misinterpreted as blindness); and tonic spasms, clonic jerks, and focal and generalized seizures.

The differentiation of the inherited metabolic diseases of infancy rests essentially upon four types of data: (1) a few highly characteristic neurologic and ophthalmic signs; (2) the presence of an enlarged liver and/or spleen; (3) special dysmorphic features of the face; and (4) the results of certain relatively simple laboratory tests, such as radiographs of the thoracolumbar spine, hips, and long bones, smears of the peripheral blood and bone marrow, CSF examination, and certain urinary tests and other biochemical estimations (serum lactate, glucose, ammonia, and urinary ketones, amino acids, and organic acids). For purposes of differential diagnosis, we have found the flowcharts constructed by our colleague Kolodny to be most serviceable. One such schematic, illustrated in Fig. 37-4, is based on the subdivision of patients into three groups: (1) dysmorphic, (2) visceromegalic, and (3) purely neurologic. Only rarely does an inherited metabolic disease fall into more than one of these categories. There is also considerable value in classifying the process as a leukodystrophy or poliodystrophy, although this distinction is easier to make in the older child.

Once the patient is placed in one of these major categories, correct diagnosis then depends on the recognition of particular clinical and laboratory features, tabulated below (see also Tables 37-4 and 37-5).

Neurologic signs that are more or less specific for certain metabolic diseases are as follows:

1. Acousticomotor obligatory startle: Tay-Sachs disease

2. Abolished tendon reflexes with definite Babinski signs: globoid cell (Krabbe) leukodystrophy, occasionally Leigh disease, and (beyond infancy) metachromatic leukodystrophy

3. Peculiar eye movements, pendular nystagmus, and head rolling: Pelizaeus-Merzbacher disease, Leigh disease; later, hyperbilirubinemia and Lesch-Nyhan hyperuricemia (see further on)

4. Marked rigidity, opisthotonos, and tonic spasms: Krabbe, Alpers disease, or infantile Gaucher disease (classic triad: trismus, strabismus, opisthotonos.)

5. Intractable seizures and generalized or multifocal myoclonus: Alpers disease

6. Intermittent hyperventilation: Leigh disease and congenital lactic acidosis (also nonprogressive familial agenesis of vermis)

7. Strabismus, hypotonia, seizures, lipodystrophy: carbohydrate deficient glycoprotein syndrome

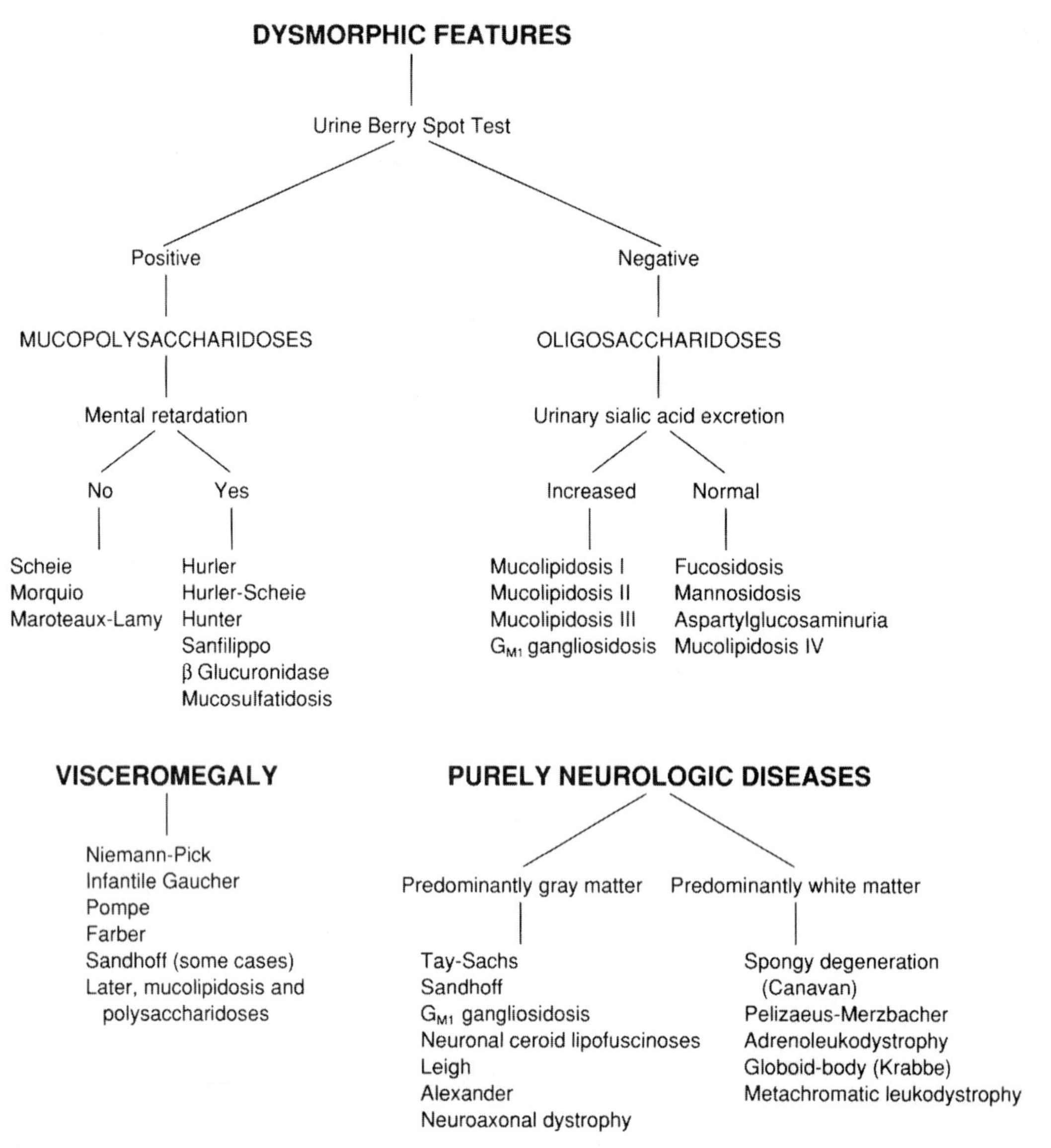

Figure 37-4

A schematic for diagnosis of the inherited metabolic diseases of infancy. Courtesy of Dr. Edwin Kolodny.

Ocular abnormalities of specific diagnostic value:

1. Rapid pendular nystagmus: Pelizaeus-Merzbacher disease, rarely Krabbe leukodystrophy

2. Macular cherry-red spots: Tay-Sachs disease and Sandhoff variant, some cases of infantile Niemann-Pick disease, and rarely lipofuscinosis

3. Corneal opacification: Lowe disease, infantile G_{M1} gangliosidosis; later, the mucopolysaccharidoses

4. Cataracts: galactosemia, Lowe disease, Zellweger disease (also congenital rubella)

Other medical findings of specific diagnostic value:

1. Dysmorphic facies: generalized G_{M1} gangliosidosis, Lowe and Zellweger syndromes, and some early cases of mucopolysaccharidosis and mucolipidosis

Table 37-4
Differential diagnosis of poliodystrophies of infancy

	Tay-Sachs	*Niemann-Pick*	*Gaucher*	*Alpers*	*Subacute necrotizing encephalopathy*
Age of onset	4–6 months	Under 6 months	Under 6 months	Under 1 year	Under 1 year, rarely late childhood
Rate of progression	Rapid Death 2–3 years	Rapid Death before 3 years	Very rapid Death before 2 years	Rapid Death before 3 years	Usually rapid Death before 3 years
Ethnic group	Almost all Jewish	50% Jewish			
Genetic	Recessive	Recessive	Recessive		Recessive
Head size	Enlarges late	Normal	Normal	Reduces late	Normal
Skin and/or systemic lesions	Normal	Hepatosplenomegaly Xanthoma of skin, rare	Hepato-splenomegaly	Normal	Normal
Eye	Cherry-red macula Optic atrophy	Cherry-red macula Optic atrophy	Normal	Normal	Optic atrophy
Seizures	Frequent, but late	Rare	Rare	Onset with seizures Myoclonus and other types	Seizures late and rare
Neurologic signs	Early: flaccid paresis Late: spastic paralysis Dementia: early hyperacusis with myoclonus	Spastic paralysis Early: dementia	Early: retroflexion of head, dementia Strabismus Bulbar palsy Spastic paralysis	Spastic paralysis Dementia Cortical blindness and deafness	Bulbar palsy Weak, infrequent cry Flaccid paresis with immobility
Blood	Absent fructose-l-phosphate-aldolase ↑ SGOT ↑ Vacuolated lymphocytes	↑ Serum lipids ↑ SGOT ↑ Vacuolated lymphocytes	↑ Total acid phosphatase (prostatic acid phophatase is normal)	Normal	Normal
Urine	Normal	Normal	Normal	Normal	Normal
CSF	Normal	Normal		Normal	Normal
Biopsy	Rectal	"Foam cells" in bone marrow	Gaucher cells in bone marrow		
X-ray		Diffuse pulmonary infiltrates Demineralization of bone			
Electroretinogram	Normal				
Diagnostic biochemical abnormality	See text				

Source: Adapted from Drew AL, Jr, with permission.

Table 37-5
Differential diagnosis of leukodystrophies of infancy

	Krabbe	*Metachromatic leukodystrophy*	*Spongy degeneration*	*Pelizaeus-Merzbacher*	*Schilder disease; sudanophilic and adrenoleukodystrophy*
Age of onset	3–6 months	1–2 years, rarely late childhood	0–4 months	6–24 months	5–10 years
Rate of progression	Rapid Death by 2 years Some later and slow	Slow Death by 3–5 years	Rapid Death by 3 years	Slow May survive to adult life	Abrupt onset Death in months to years
Sex or ethnic group			Most Jewish	Predominantly males	
Genetic	Recessive	Recessive	Recessive	Sex-linked recessive	Adrenoleukodystrophy form—X-linked recessive
Head size	Normal	Enlarges late	Enlarges early	Normal	Normal
Skin or systemic lesions	Normal	Normal	Normal	Normal	Bronzing with adrenal atrophy
Eye	Late: optic atrophy	Late: optic atrophy	Optic atrophy, blindness	Slow optic atrophy	Optic neuritis or optic atrophy
Seizures	Tonic spasms	Rare	Uncommon	Late	Rare, late
Neurologic signs	Spastic paralysis Nystagmus Head retraction Bulbar palsy Dementia	Changes in gait Ataxia Combined upper and lower motor neuron signs Bulbar palsy, Blindness, Deafness, Dementia } late	Hypotonia→ spastic diplegia→ decerebrate rigidity	Pendular nystagmus Titubation of head and other cerebellar signs in early childhood Spastic diplegia, late childhood Slow dementia	Early spastic paralysis Dementia Late: cortical blindness, deafness, aphasia, pseudobulbar palsy
Miscellaneous	Slowed nerve conduction (rare)	Slowed nerve conduction			EEG diffuse delta waves
Blood	Normal	Normal	↓ *N*-acetyl-L-aspartic acid (NAA)	Normal	Normal or ↓ cortisol
Urine	Normal	Metachromatic bodies	Normal	Normal	Normal
CSF:	↑ Protein (150–300 mg/dL)	Normal or ↑ protein up to 200 mg/dL	↑ Pressure Normal or ↑ protein up to 200 mg/dL	Normal	Normal or ↑ gamma globulin
Biopsy	Brain	Sural nerve	Brain		
X-ray		Nonfilling of gallbladder	Suture separation		
Diagnostic biochemical abnormality See text					

Source: Adapted from Drew AL Jr, with permission.

2. Enlarged liver and spleen: infantile Gaucher disease and Niemann-Pick disease; one type of hyperammonemia; Sandhoff disease; later, the mucopolysaccharidoses and mucolipidoses

3. Enlarging head without hydrocephalus (macrocephaly): Canavan spongy degeneration of infancy, some cases of Tay-Sachs disease, Alexander disease

4. Beaking of vertebral bodies in radiographs: G_{M1} gangliosidosis (and, at a more advanced age, the mucopolysaccharidoses, fucosidosis, mannosidosis, and the mucolipidoses)

5. Multiple arthropathies and raucous dysphonia: Farber disease

6. Storage granules and vacuolated lymphocytes: Niemann-Pick disease, generalized G_{M1} gangliosidosis

7. Abnormal histiocytes in marrow smears: Gaucher cells, foamy histiocytes in Niemann-Pick disease, generalized G_{M1} gangliosidosis and closely related diseases, Farber disease

8. Colorless, friable hair: Menkes disease

INHERITED METABOLIC DISEASES OF EARLY CHILDHOOD

Included here are the diseases that become manifest between the ages of 1 and 4 years. Diagnosis is less difficult than in the neonate and young infant. A morbid process in the nervous system is reliably ascertained by the obvious progression of a neurologic disorder, such as a loss of ability to walk and to speak, which usually parallels a regression in other high-level (quasi-intellectual) functions. Embryologic anomalies, prenatal diseases, and birth injuries can be excluded with relative certainty if psychomotor development was normal in the first year or two. Diseases characterized by seizures and myoclonus may prove more difficult to interpret, for the seizures may occur at any age from a variety of distant or immediate neurologic causes and, if frequent, may cause a significant impairment of psychomotor function. The effects of anticonvulsant medications may add to the impairment of cortical function. Unfortunately, most of the slowly advancing metabolic diseases of the second year may be so subtle in their effects that for a time the physician cannot be sure whether a regression of intellectual functions is taking place or mental retardation is becoming apparent for the first time. To distinguish the two is more difficult if the parents have been unobservant. Repeated examinations and testing will usually settle the matter. Suspicion of a progressive encephalopathy is heightened by the presence of certain ocular, visceral, and skeletal abnormalities, as described below.

Once a neurologic syndrome is clearly established, there is an advantage in determining whether its main characteristics reflect a disorder of the cerebral white matter (oligodendrocytes and myelin) or of gray matter (neurons). Indicative of predominantly white matter affection (*leukodystrophy* or leukoencephalopathy) are early onset of spastic paralysis of the limbs, with or without ataxia, and visual impairment with optic atrophy but normal retinae. Seizures and intellectual deterioration are late events. MRI usually confirms the involvement of white matter. Indicative of gray matter disease (poliodystrophy or polioencephalopathy) are the early onset of seizures, myoclonus, blindness with retinal changes, and mental regression. Choreoathetosis and ataxia, spastic paralysis, and signs of sensorimotor tract involvement occur later. On MRI, only a generalized atrophy and ventricular enlargement may be seen.

Neuronal storage diseases, such as those described in the previous section, as well as neuroaxonal dystrophy and the lipofuscinoses, conform to the pattern of gray matter diseases (Table 37-4). Metachromatic, globoid-body, sudanophilic leukodystrophy and spongy degeneration of infancy exemplify white matter diseases (Table 37-5). Although this mode of categorization is helpful, there is some degree of overlap; for example, Tay-Sachs disease, a poliodystrophy, also causes white matter changes, and metachromatic leukodystrophy may be accompanied by some degree of neuronal storage.

The following are inherited metabolic diseases that occur most frequently in late infancy and early childhood:

1. Many of the milder disorders of amino acid metabolism
2. Metachromatic leukodystrophy
3. Late infantile G_{M1} gangliosidosis
4. Late infantile Gaucher disease and Niemann-Pick disease
5. Neuroaxonal dystrophy
6. The mucopolysaccharidoses
7. The mucolipidoses
8. Fucosidosis
9. The mannosidoses
10. Aspartylglycosaminuria
11. Ceroid lipofuscinosis (Jansky-Bielschowsky)
12. Cockayne syndrome

The Aminoacidopathies (Aminoacidurias)

In a group of 48 inherited aminoacidopathies, tabulated by Rosenberg and Scriver, at least one-half were associated with recognizable neurologic abnormalities. Twenty other aminoacidopathies result in a defect in the renal transport of amino acids, and some of the latter may secondarily damage the nervous system. Usually, when the nervous system is involved, the only clinical manifestation is simply a lag in psychomotor development which, if mild, does not become evident until the second and third years or later. Like other inherited metabolic disorders, the aminoacidurias do not impair growth, development, and maturation in utero or interfere with parturition. No physical sign betrays their presence in the early months of life. The only possible means of detection is by screening all newborns. The relative frequency of these diseases is indicated in Table 37-1, and the practical tests for their identification are summarized in Table 37-2.

Three aminoacidopathies of the late infantile and early childhood period—phenylketonuria (PKU), tyrosinemia, and Hartnup disease—are described here because of their clinical importance and because they exemplify different types of biochemical defect. Reference is also made to certain other aminoacidurias, described in the first part of this chapter, which, like Hartnup disease, are associated with intermittent ataxia. Only passing comments are made about the other aminoacidurias, which are exceedingly rare or have only an uncertain effect upon the nervous system. A detailed and current account of these disorders can be found in the monograph of Scriver and coworkers.

The Phenylketonurias (PKU, Phenylalanine Hydroxylase Deficiency) Apart from being the most frequent of the aminoacidurias, this entity has a special historical significance. Since its discovery by Følling in 1934, it has remained the classic example of an aminoaciduria, illustrating three principles of medical genetics: first, it is inherited as an autosomal recessive trait; second, PKU exemplifies Garrod's cardinal principle of gene action, in which genetic factors specify chemical reactions as well as biochemical individuality; third, PKU is a disease, and hyperphenylalaninemia is a phenotype only when the allele is expressed in an environment that contains an abundance of L-phenylalanine. Thus, as predicted by Galton, the ultimate phenotype is a product of "nature and nurture" (Scriver and Clow).

One must refer to the phenylketonurias in the plural, for there are (1) the usual type and several mild and severe variants thereof, in all of which mental retardation is invariable if the disease is not treated early in life, and (2) other types, presumably allelic mutations, in which there is hyperphenylalaninemia without PKU and without effect on the nervous system. Also there are a small number of patients (3 percent in our series) in whom a lowering of the hyperphenylalaninemia does not prevent the progression of the neurologic lesion.

At birth, the typical PKU infant is believed to have a normal nervous system. The disease appears later, only after long exposure of the nervous system to PA, because the homozygous infant lacks the means of protecting the nervous system. However, if the mother is homozygous with high PA levels in the blood, the CNS is damaged in utero and the heterozygous infant is mentally defective from birth.

In the classic form of PKU, the *impairment of psychomotor development* can usually be recognized in the latter part of the first year, when expected performances lag. By 5 to 6 years in an untreated child, when the IQ can be estimated, it is usually less than 20, occasionally 20 to 50, and exceptionally above 50. *Hyperactivity*, aggressivity, self-injurious behavior, including severe injury to the eyes, clumsy gait, fine tremor of the hands, poor coordination, odd posturings, *repetitious digital mannerisms* and other so-called rhythmias, and slight corticospinal tract signs stand out as the main clinical manifestations. Athetosis, dystonia, and frank cerebellar ataxia have been described but must be exceedingly rare. Also, seizures are said to occur in 25 percent of severely retarded patients, taking the form at first of flexor spasms and later of absence and grand mal attacks. However, of more than 30 of our PKU patients at the Fernald School, none had seizures or extrapyramidal signs. The majority are blue-eyed and fair in skin and hair color, and their skin is rough and dry and subject to eczema. A musty body odor (due to phenylacetic acid excretion) can often be detected. Two-thirds are slightly microcephalic. The fundi are normal, and there is no visceral enlargement or skeletal abnormality.

The finding of *high levels of serum phenylalanine* (above 15 mg/dL) and of *phenylpyruvic acid in the blood, CSF, and urine* are diagnostic of PKU. The level is normal at birth and rises only after the first few days. Screening by the Guthrie (ferric chloride) test then identifies the patient at risk: the addition of 3 to 5 drops of 10% ferric chloride to 1 mL of urine yields an emerald-green color that reaches a peak intensity in 3 to 4 min and fades in 20 to 40 min. In contrast, the green-brown color in the urine of patients with histidinemia is permanent. In maple syrup urine disease, the ferric chloride test gives a navy-blue color; propionic and methylmalonic acidemia and ketones or salicylates in the urine yield a purple color.

The fundamental biochemical abnormality is a deficiency of the hepatic enzyme PA hydroxylase; the failure of conversion of PA to tyrosine results in the excretion of phenylpyruvic acid by affected individuals. The precise step that is faulty in the complex phenylalanine hydroxylating reaction is still unknown. The mutant gene has been localized on chromosome 12. Pathologic examination shows poor staining of myelin in the cerebral hemispheres. The usually pigmented nuclei (substantia nigra, locus ceruleus, dorsal vagal motor) fail to acquire dark coloration because of a block in the production of melanin. Reduction in size of cortical neurons and their dendritic arborizations is said to be demonstrable in some cases.

If instituted in infancy, diets low but not totally lacking in PA can improve intellectual development (blood level should be maintained at 5 to 10 mg/dL). Once the neurologic picture unfolds, diet has little or no effect on the mental status but may improve behavior. Prolonged dietary treatment has many untoward effects and should be supervised by physicians experienced in its use; if too restricted, it may retard growth. This is particularly important, since it has been shown that intellectual impairment is greatest among children who were the earliest to abandon their diets, permitting the PA concentration to rise above 15 mg/dL, and least in children who maintained dietary control the longest (Holtzman et al). Continued dietary treatment is necessary. In children with hyperphenylalaninemia but without PKU, dietary treatment is not indicated. With the widespread screening for PKU and the initiation of dietary control during early postnatal life, this metabolic brain disease has virtually disappeared in our states. Treated women who reach childbearing age should be particularly careful about dietary restriction, since high levels of phenylalanine are harmful to the normal fetus.

The late forms of maple syrup urine disease, histidinemia, and hydroxyprolinemia evolve in much the same fashion as PKU and raise similar problems in diagnosis and therapy.

A small number of infants have a variant of PKU in which a restricted PA diet does not prevent neurologic involvement. In some such infants, a dystonic extrapyramidal rigidity ("stiff-baby syndrome") has been present as early as the neonatal period, and, according to Allen and coworkers, it responds to biopterin. Such infants have normal levels of PA hydroxylase in the liver. The defect is a failure to synthesize the active cofactor tetrahydrobiopterin, because of either an insufficiency of dihydropteridine reductase or an inability to synthesize biopterin (see page 989). The urinary metabolites of catecholamines and serotonin are reduced and are not responsive to low-PA diets. There is some evidence that the underlying neurotransmitter fault can be corrected by L-dopa and 5-hydroxytryptophan (Scriver and Clow).

Hereditary Tyrosinemia (Richner-Hanhart Disease) This is a rare, predominantly dermatologic aminoacidopathy, but in approximately one-half of the infants there is a mild to moderate degree of mental retardation. Also, there may be self-mutilation and incoordination of limb movements. Language defects are prominent. Toward the end of the first or second year of life, lacrimation, photophobia, and redness of the eyes (due to corneal erosions) appear. Neovascularization of the corneas and opacification follow. Palmar and plantar keratosis with hyperhydrosis and pain are frequently present as a result of an inflammatory reaction to deposits of crystalline tyrosine (also the cause of the corneal changes). Elevated tyrosine in the blood (>0.18 mM) and urine are diagnostic. The disease is due to a defect on chromosome 15 that codes for the enzyme fumarylacetoacetate hydrolase, a deficiency of which results in the accumulation of tyrosine and its metabolites.

A low-tyrosine and low-PA diet, optimized to allow growth and development, has resulted in rapid amelioration of symptoms but must be started early. Retinoids given orally improve the skin lesions. Neonatal tyrosinemia can cause liver failure and early death.

Hartnup Disease This disease, named after the family in which it was first observed, is probably transmitted as an autosomal recessive trait. Women carrying this trait deliver babies who are normal at birth. The onset of symptoms is in late infancy or early childhood. The clinical features consist of an *intermittent red, scaly rash over the face, neck, hands, and legs*, resembling that of pellagra; growth failure and developmental delay; episodic personality disorder in the form of *emotional lability*, uncontrolled temper, and confusional-hallucinatory psychosis; *episodic cerebellar ataxia* (unsteady gait, intention tremor, and dysarthria); and occasionally spasticity, vertigo, nystagmus, ptosis, and diplopia. Attacks of disease are triggered by exposure to sunlight, emotional stress, and sulfonamide drugs and last for about 2 weeks, followed by variable periods of relative normalcy. The frequency of attacks diminishes with maturation, but some children are left with a mild persistent mental retardation.

The metabolic faults are due to a *transport error of neutral amino acids across renal tubules, with excretion of greatly increased amounts of these amino acids in the urine and feces*. In particular, there is the excretion of large amounts of indicans, mainly indoxyl sulfate, particularly after oral L-tryptophan loading; and an abnormally high excretion of nonhydroxylated indole metabolites. Loss of tryptophan in the urine reduces its availability for the synthesis of niacin and accounts for the pellagrous skin changes. The pathologic basis of the disease is undetermined. Differential diagnosis includes a large number of intermittent and progressive cerebellar ataxias of childhood, described below.

Treatment consists of avoiding exposure to sunlight and to sulfonamide drugs. Because of the similarities between pellagra and Hartnup disease, the usual practice is to give nicotinamide in doses of 50 to 300 mg daily. The skin lesions disappear and there are reports of subsidence of ataxia and psychotic behavior. However, the results of treatment are inconsistent. Possibly a better response is obtained by the administration of L-tryptophan ethyl ester in doses of 20 mg/kg tid.

Other Metabolic Diseases with Intermittent or Persistent Ataxia, Seizures, and Mental Retardation

In addition to Hartnup disease, a number of other metabolic diseases give rise to episodic ataxias during early childhood. These are (1) mild forms of maple syrup urine disease and the congenital hyperammonemias (type II hyperammonemia, citrullinemia, argininosuccinic aciduria, hyperornithinemia), described in an earlier part of the chapter; (2) necrotizing encephalomyelopathy (Leigh), described further on; (3) hyperalaninemia and hyperpyruvic acidemia (Lonsdale et al, Blass et al); and (4) autosomal dominant, acetazolamide-responsive ataxia that may have its onset in childhood but usually appears later (page 1022).

In all these conditions the ataxia, which is of cerebellar type, is highly variable from time to time and may follow a burst of seizures (as in argininosuccinic aciduria). The seizures are treated with anticonvulsant drugs, which may at first be held responsible for the ataxia. In time, however, it becomes apparent that the ataxia lasts a week or two and bears no relationship to the medicine. Indeed, seizures and ataxia are both due to the common biochemical abnormality. Between attacks, in all the intermittent ataxias, the patient's movements are relatively normal, but most of the affected children are slow in learning and remain backward mentally to a varying degree.

The Problem of Progressive Cerebellar Ataxia of Early Childhood

The differentiation of the childhood ataxias is difficult. The problem is twofold—first, to be certain that ataxia exists, and, second, to differentiate cerebellar ataxia from the sensory ataxia of peripheral nerve disease and from generalized tremor and polymyoclonus. Since cerebellar ataxia is more a disorder of voluntary than of postural movements, its presence usually cannot be determined with certainty until intentional (projected) movements become part of the child's repertoire of motor activity. As indicated in Chap. 28, the earliest signs become manifest in the arms when the infant reaches for an object and brings it to his mouth or transfers it from hand to hand. A jerky, wavering, tremulous movement then appears; in sitting, a titubation of the head and a tremor of the trunk may be apparent. Once walking begins, apart from the usual clumsiness of the toddler, there is a similar incoordination of movement. Sensory ataxia is always difficult to distinguish but is rare at this age and usually accompanied by weakness and absence of tendon reflexes. By the fourth or fifth year, when more detailed sensory testing becomes possible, the presence or absence of a proprioceptive disturbance can be demonstrated.

The group of persistent and progressive cerebellar ataxias is heterogeneous and of varied etiology; some of them merge with Friedreich ataxia, Levy-Roussy neuropathy, and other adolescent-adult hereditary ataxias. These disorders are discussed in the chapter on degenerative diseases, since, apart from their hereditary nature, neither their cause nor their pathogenesis is known. There are many other childhood ataxias that probably belong in the category of degenerative disease, some in which cerebellar ataxia is the most prominent abnormality and some in which other neurologic abnormalities are more prominent. To describe each in detail would be impractical in a book on the principles of neurology, for which reason they are only tabulated here.

1. The disequilibrium and dyssynergia syndrome of Hagberg and Janner: early-life onset of relatively pure cerebellar ataxia, with psychomotor retardation.

2. Cerebellar ataxia with diplegia, hypotonia, and mental retardation (also called *atonic diplegia* of Foerster); this is either a fetal disease or birth injury and the neuropathology is uncertain.

3. Agenesis of the cerebellum: early cerebellar ataxia (with or without mental retardation) and episodic

hyperventilation (Norman's family with granule-cell degeneration falls into this category).

4. Cerebellar ataxia with cataracts and oligophrenia: onset from childhood (mainly) to as late as adult years (Marinesco-Sjögren disease).

5. Familial cerebellar ataxia and retinal degeneration.

6. Familial cerebellar ataxia with cataracts and ophthalmoplegia or with cataracts and mental as well as physical retardation.

7. Familial cerebellar ataxia with mydriasis.

8. Familial cerebellar ataxia with deafness and blindness and a similar combination, called retinocochleodentate degeneration, referring to loss of neurons in these three structures.

9. Familial cerebellar ataxia with choreoathetosis, corticospinal tract signs, and mental and motor retardation.

In none of the syndromes mentioned above has a biochemical abnormality been established, so their metabolic nature is a matter of speculation. However, disorders of the electron transport chain can, on occasion, present as the Marinesco-Sjögren phenotype, mentioned above.

The persistent cerebellar ataxias of childhood in which a metabolic fault or gene defect has been demonstrated are (1) Refsum disease, (2) abetalipoproteinemia (Bassen-Kornzweig syndrome), (3) ataxia-telangiectasia, (4) galactosemia, and (5) possibly Friedreich ataxia. Refsum disease is discussed with the hereditary polyneuropathies (page 1421). The Bassen-Kornzweig syndrome more often has its onset in late than in early childhood and is more appropriately described in the following section of this chapter. Ataxia-telangiectasia is described below. Galactosemia has been described on page 990 and Friedreich ataxia on page 1145. Generally, it is not difficult to differentiate these diseases from the acquired postinfectious variety that occurs predominantly in children.

Ataxia-Telangiectasia This disease, sometimes referred to as the *Louis-Bar syndrome*, was first described by Sylaba and Henner in 1926, long before Louis-Bar's report in 1941. Like xeroderma pigmentosum and the Cockayne syndrome, ataxia-telangiectasia has been attributed to defective repair of DNA. The inheritance pattern is autosomal recessive. The disorder first presents as an ataxic-dyskinetic syndrome in children who appear to have been normal in the first few years of life. The onset of the disease coincides more or less with the acquisition of walking, which is awkward and unsteady. Later, by the age of 4 to 5 years, the limbs become ataxic, and choreoathetosis, grimacing, and dysarthric speech are added. The eye movements become jerky, with slow and long-latency saccades, and there is also apraxia for voluntary gaze (the patient turns the head but not the eyes on attempting to look to the side). Optokinetic nystagmus is lost. By the age of 9 to 10 years, slight intellectual decline sets in and signs of mild polyneuropathy are evident. Muscle power is reduced little if at all until late in the illness, but tendon reflexes may disappear. The characteristic telangiectatic lesions, which are mainly transversely oriented subpapillary venous plexuses, appear at 3 to 5 years of age or later and are most apparent in the outer parts of the bulbar conjunctivae (Fig. 37-5), over the ears, on exposed parts of the neck, on the bridge of the nose and cheeks in a butterfly pattern, and in the flexor creases of the forearms. Vitiligo, café-au-lait spots, loss of subcutaneous fat, and premature graying of hair are observed in some patients. Many of

Figure 37-5

Ocular appearance of ataxia-telangiectasia. (From Lyon et al by permission.)

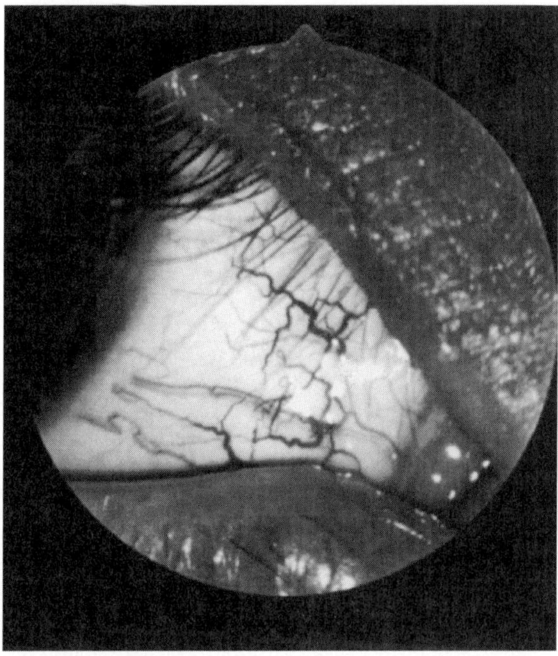

the patients have endocrine alterations (absence of secondary sexual development, glucose intolerance). The disease is progressive, and death usually occurs in the second decade from intercurrent bronchopulmonary infection or neoplasia—usually lymphoma, less often glioma (Boder and Sedgwick).

The significant abnormalities in the CNS are severe degeneration in the cerebellar cortex; loss of myelinated fibers in the posterior columns, spinocerebellar tracts, and peripheral nerves; degenerative changes in the posterior roots and cells of the sympathetic ganglia; and loss of anterior horn cells at all levels of the spinal cord. In a few cases, vascular abnormalities, like the mucocutaneous ones, have been found scattered diffusely in the white matter of the brain and spinal cord, but they are of questionable significance. Also, there may be a loss of pigmented cells in the substantia nigra and locus ceruleus, and cytoplasmic inclusions (Lewy bodies) in the cells that remain (Agamanolis and Greenstein). Intranuclear inclusions and bizarre nuclear formations have also been found in the satellite cells (amphicytes) of dorsal root ganglion neurons (Strich).

An absence or decrease in several immunoglobulins—IgA, IgE and isotypes, IgG_2, IgG_4—has been found in practically every patient. These deficiencies, shown by McFarlin and associates to be due to decreased synthesis, are associated with hypoplasia of the thymus, loss of follicles in lymph nodes, failure of delayed hypersensitivity reactions, lymphopenia, and slow formation of circulating antibodies. There are breaks in chromosome 14 and, the abnormal gene has now been identified. After radiation, there is faulty repair of DNA. Probably this immunodeficient state accounts for the striking susceptibility of these patients to recurrent pulmonary infections and bronchiectasis. Transplantation of normal thymus tissue into the patient and administration of thymus extracts have been of no therapeutic value. The only therapy centers on the control of infections.

Metachromatic Leukodystrophy (Aryl Sulfatase Deficiency)

This is another of the lysosomal (sphingolipid) storage diseases (Table 37-3). The basic abnormality, localized in chromosome 22, is the absence of the enzyme aryl sulfatase A, a deficiency of which prevents the conversion of sulfatide to cerebroside (a major component of myelin) and results in an accumulation of the former. The disease is transmitted as an autosomal recessive trait and usually becomes manifest between the first and fourth years of life (variants have their onset in the congenital period, in late childhood, and even in adult life). Variability of gene mutation accounts for the different forms. The disease is characterized clinically by *progressive impairment of motor function* (gait disorder, spasticity) in combination with reduced output of speech and *mental regression.* At first the tendon reflexes are usually brisk, but later, as the peripheral nerves become more involved, the *reflexes are decreased and eventually lost.* Or, there may be variable hypotonia and areflexia from the beginning, or spasticity may be present throughout the illness, but with hyporeflexia and slowed conduction velocities. Signs of mental regression may be apparent from the onset or appear after the motor disorder has become established. Later there is impairment of vision, sometimes with squint and nystagmus; intention tremor in the arms and dysarthria; dysphagia and drooling; and optic atrophy (one-third of patients), sometimes with grayish degeneration around the maculae. Seizures are rare, and there are no somatic abnormalities. The head size is usually normal, but rarely there is macrocephaly. Progression to a bedridden quadriplegic state without speech or comprehension occurs over a 1- to 3-year period, somewhat more slowly in late-onset types. The CSF protein is elevated.

There is widespread degeneration of myelinated fibers in the cerebrum (Fig. 37-6), cerebellum, spinal cord, and peripheral nerves. The presence of metachromatic granules in glial cells and engorged macrophages is characteristic and enables the diagnosis to be made from a biopsy of a peripheral nerve. The stored material, *sulfatide*, stains brown-orange rather than purple with aniline dyes. Sulfatides are also PAS-positive in frozen sections.

The diagnostic laboratory findings, in addition to the MRI and histologic changes, are an elevated CSF protein (75 to 250 mg/dL) and a *marked increase in sulfatide in urine and an absence of aryl sulfatase A* in white blood cells, in serum, and in cultured fibroblasts. Assays of aryl sulfatase A activity in cultured fibroblasts and amniocytes permit the identification of carriers and prenatal diagnosis of the disease.

Treatment with enzyme replacement or bone marrow transplantation is being tried. Marrow transplant appears to be of no benefit once the patient becomes symptomatic, but it may be useful in the treatment of an asymptomatic sibling of an index case.

The differential diagnosis of this leukodystrophy is from neuroaxonal dystrophy (see below), cases of early-onset inherited polyneuropathy, late-onset Krabbe disease, and childhood forms of Gaucher disease and Niemann-Pick disease. A *variant of metachromatic*

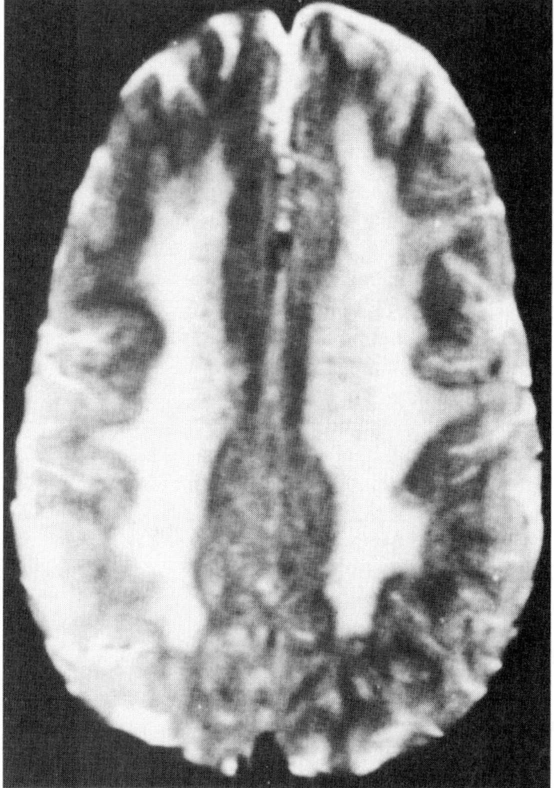

Figure 37-6

Metachromatic leukodystrophy. T2-weighted axial MRI of a 3-year-old boy. Abnormal high signal intensity involves the entire centrum ovale but spares the subcortical arcuate fibers. (From Lee SH, Rao K, Zimmerman RA: Cranial MRI and CT, 3rd ed. New York, McGraw-Hill, 1992, by permission.)

leukoencephalopathy, due to a deficiency of the isoenzymes of aryl sulfatase A, B, and C, was described by Austin in 1973. He called it "multiple sulfatase deficiency." The neurologic manifestations resemble those of metachromatic leukodystrophy, but, in addition, there are facial and skeletal changes similar to those of a mucopolysaccharidosis. Deafness, hepatic enlargement, ichthyosis, and beaking of lumbar vertebrae are additional findings in some cases. Metachromatic material is found in the urinary sediment. Pathologically, in addition to metachromasia of degenerating white matter in cerebrum and peripheral nerve, there may be storage material, like that found in the gangliosidoses in neurons. Granules are demonstrable in neutrophilic leukocytes. There has also been described a state of "aryl sulfatase pseudo-deficiency," which exists as a polymorphism in about 7 percent of Europeans and makes the point that low enzyme levels alone are insufficient to express a phenotype of metachromatic leukodystrophy.

Forms of metachromatic leukodystrophy developing in adult years are discussed further on.

Neuroaxonal Dystrophy (Degeneration)

This is a rare disease, inherited as an autosomal recessive trait. In the largest group of cases (77 collected by Aicardi and Castelein), the onset was near the beginning of the second year in 50 patients and before the third year in all instances. The clinical constellation comprised psychomotor deterioration (loss of ability to walk, stand, sit, and speak), marked hypotonia but brisk reflexes and Babinski signs, and progressive blindness with optic atrophy but normal retinae. Seizures, myoclonus, and extrapyramidal signs were rare. Loss of sensation was found later in some cases. Terminally, bulbar signs, spasticity, and decerebrate rigidity often supervened. The course was relentlessly progressive, with fatal issue in a decorticate state in 3 to 8 years. There were no abnormalities of the liver and spleen and no facial or skeletal changes.

Pathologic examination reveals eosinophilic spheroids of swollen axoplasm in the posterior columns and nuclei of Goll and Burdach and in Clarke's column, substantia nigra, subthalamic nuclei, central nuclei of brainstem, and cerebral cortex. There is cerebellar atrophy, affecting the granule cell layer predominantly, and increased iron-containing pigment in the basal ganglia (like that observed in Hallervorden-Spatz disease).

The CT scans and CSF are normal, and there are no biochemical or blood cell abnormalities. After the age of 2 years, however, the EEG shows characteristic high-amplitude fast rhythms (16 to 22 Hz). Evoked responses may be abnormal. Nerve conduction velocities are normal despite EMG evidence of denervation. The diagnosis can be reliably established during life by electron microscopic examination of skin and conjunctival nerves, which show the characteristic spheroids within axons.

There is a later-onset form of the disease in which the course is more protracted and the neurologic manifestations (rigidity and spasticity, cerebellar ataxia, and myoclonus) are more pronounced. In these cases the mental regression is slow. Vision may be retained but tapetoretinal degeneration has been documented. Some of the late-onset cases are indistinguishable from Hallervorden-Spatz disease (page 1029).

Late Infantile and Early Childhood Gaucher Disease

As stated earlier (page 997), Gaucher disease usually develops in early infancy, but some cases, so-called Gaucher disease type III, may begin in childhood, between 3 and 8 years of age. The clinical picture is variable and combines features of infantile Gaucher disease—such as abducens palsies, dysphagia, trismus, rigidity of the limbs, and dementia—with features of the late childhood–early adult form, such as palsies of horizontal gaze, diffuse myoclonus, generalized seizures, and a chronic course (Winkelman et al). The diagnosis is established by the finding of splenomegaly, Gaucher cells, glucocerebroside storage, and deficient activity of glucocerebrosidase in leukocytes or cultured fibroblasts.

Late Infantile–Early Childhood Niemann-Pick Disease

A number of cases of subacute or chronic neurovisceral storage diseases with early signs of hepatosplenomegaly and later signs (2 to 4 years) of neurologic involvement have been described. Crocker and Farber classified them as types III and IV Niemann-Pick disease. Others have classified them as types C and D, although it is now generally agreed that they are best considered a single entity.

The neurologic disorder consists of progressive dementia, dysarthria, ataxia, rarely extrapyramidal signs (choreoathetosis), and *paralysis of horizontal and vertical gaze*, the latter being a distinguishing feature. On attempting to look to the side, some of the patients make head-thrusting movements of the same type that one observes in ataxia-telangiectasia (page 1011) and the oculomotor apraxia of Cogan (page 1080). Lateral eye movements are full on passive movement of the head (oculocephalic maneuver). Convergence is also deficient. A special syndrome called *juvenile dystonic lipidosis* is characterized by extrapyramidal symptoms and paralysis of vertical eye movements. The syndrome of the "sea-blue histiocyte" (liver, spleen, and bone marrow contain histiocytes with sea-blue granules)—in which there is retardation in mental and motor development, grayish macular degeneration, and, in one of our cases, posterior column and pyramidal degeneration—may be another variant.

The diagnosis is made by bone marrow biopsy, which discloses vacuolated macrophages and sea-blue histiocytes, and by measuring the defect in cholesterol esterification in cultured fibroblasts.

Late Infantile–Childhood G_{M1} Gangliosidosis

In type 2 or so-called juvenile G_{M1} gangliosidosis, the onset is between 12 and 24 months, with survival for 3 to 10 years. The first sign is usually *difficulty in walking*, with frequent falls, followed by awkwardness of arm movements, loss of speech, severe mental regression, gradual development of spastic quadriparesis and pseudobulbar palsy (dysarthria, dysphagia, drooling), and seizures. Retinal changes are variable—usually they are absent, but macular red spots may be seen at the age of 10 to 12 years; vision is usually retained, but squints (comitant) are common. There is a facial dysmorphism resembling that of the Hurler syndrome, and the liver and spleen are enlarged. Important laboratory findings are hypoplasia of the thoracolumbar vertebral bodies, mild hypoplasia of the acetabula, and the presence in the bone marrow of histiocytes with clear vacuoles or wrinkled cytoplasm. As noted on page 998, leukocytes and cultured skin fibroblasts show a *deficiency* or absence of β-*galactosidase* activity. G_{M1} ganglioside accumulates in the cerebral neurons.

The Neuronal Ceroid Lipofuscinoses (Batten Disease)

As a group, the lipofuscinoses have been the most frequent of the neurodegenerative diseases of infancy and childhood diagnosed at the Lysosomal Enzyme Laboratory of the E. K. Shriver Center. Four types have been identified: Santavuori-Haltia Finnish type, Jansky-Bielschowsky early-childhood type, Vogt-Spielmeyer juvenile type, and Kufs adult type. All except a few adult cases are autosomal recessive. The storage material in neuronal cytoplasm consists of two pigmented lipids, presumably ceroid and lipofuscin, which are cross-linked polymers of polyunsaturated fatty acids and have the property of autofluorescence. Mole has published a useful review of the genetics of these diseases and points out that at least eight gene loci are implicated, four of which have been identified. All the infantile forms and one juvenile form of the disease are due to mutations affecting the lysosomal enzyme, palmitoyl-protein thioesterase. Other lysosomal enzymes are abnormal in the remaining juvenile and in the adult forms.

In the Finnish form of the disease, infants from 3 to 18 months of age, after a normal period of development, undergo psychomotor regression with ataxia, hypotonia, and *widespread myoclonus*. There are retinal changes with extinction of the electroretinogram, slowing of the EEG with spike and slow-wave discharges, and eventually an isoelectric record. Within a few years these patients become blind, develop spastic quadriplegia and microcephaly, and succumb.

In the *Jansky-Bielschowsky type*, the onset of symptoms is between 2 and 4 years, after normal or slightly retarded earlier development, with survival to 4 to 8 years of age. Usually the first neurologic manifestations are seizures (petit mal or grand mal) and *myoclonic jerks* evoked by proprioceptive and other sensory stimuli, including voluntary movement and emotional excitement. Incoordination, tremor, ataxia, and spastic weakness with lively tendon reflexes and Babinski signs, deterioration of mental faculties, and dysarthria proceed to dementia and eventually to mutism. In patients with relatively late onset, dementia is the cardinal manifestation. Visual failure may occur early in some cases because of *retinal degeneration* (of rods and cones) and pigmentary deposits, but in others vision is normal. The electroretinogram becomes isoelectric if vision is affected. Abnormal inclusions (translucent vacuoles) are seen in 10 to 30 percent of circulating lymphocytes, and azurophilic granules in neutrophils. High-voltage EEG spikes are induced by photic stimuli. Only in early-onset cases is there microcephaly.

Pathologic examination shows neuronal loss in the cerebral and cerebellar cortices (granule and Purkinje cells), and curvilinear storage particles and osmiophilic granules are seen in the neurons. Inclusions are also observed in cutaneous nerve twigs and endothelial cells, which permits diagnosis during life (electron microscopy of skin, conjunctival, or rectal mucosal biopsies). In many patients with lipofuscinoses, *diagnosis* can be confirmed by demonstrating the presence of one of several recently identified gene mutations. There are no definite markers for the group in blood or urine, but in some patients a structural component of mitochondria is excreted in excess (the so-called C-fragment). In the differential diagnosis, one must consider late infantile G_{M1} gangliosidosis, idiopathic epilepsy, Alpers disease, and other forms of neuronal ceroid-lipofuscinosis (page 1024).

The lipofuscinoses of later onset—the Vogt-Spielmeyer (juvenile) type and the Kufs (adult) type—are discussed further on in this chapter.

Mucopolysaccharidoses

This is a group of diseases in which a storage of lipid in neurons is combined with that of polysaccharides in connective tissues. As a consequence there is a conjunction of neurologic and skeletal abnormalities that is virtually unique. The nervous system may also be involved secondarily as a result of skeletal deformities and thickening and hyperplasia of connective tissue at the base of the brain, leading to obliteration of the subarachnoid space and obstructive hydrocephalus or compression of the cervical cord. Depending on the degree of visceral-skeletal and neurologic changes, at least seven distinct clinical subtypes are recognized (see Table 37-6).

The basic abnormality is an enzymatic defect that prevents the degradation of acid mucopolysaccharides (now called *glycosaminoglycans*). They can be measured in excess in serum, leukocytes, or cultured fibroblasts. The storage is, again, within lysosomes in the brain, spinal cord, heart, viscera, bone, and connective tissue. All forms of the disease except the Hunter syndrome, which is sex-linked, are inherited in an autosomal recessive pattern. The studies of Neufeld and Muenzer indicate that each type of mucopolysaccharidosis is caused by a defect in a different enzyme.

Hurler Disease This, the classic form, known as MPS IH, begins clinically toward the end of the first year. *Mental retardation* is severe, and *skeletal abnormalities* are prominent (dwarfism, gargoyle facies, large head with synostosis of longitudinal suture, kyphosis, broad hands with short, stubby fingers, flexion contractures at knees and elbows). Conductive deafness and corticospinal signs are usually present. Protuberant abdomen, hernias, *enlarged liver and spleen*, valvular heart disease, chronic rhinitis, recurrent respiratory infections, and *corneal opacities* are the common systemic findings. The biochemical abnormalities consist of the accumulation of *dermatan* and *heparan sulfate* (polyglycosaminoglycans) in the tissues and their *excretion in the urine*, due probably to absence of activity of α-L-iduronidase. Also, there is an increase in the ganglioside content in nerve cells of the brains of these patients. In the Scheie (MPS IS) variant of Hurler disease, intelligence and life span are normal. Enzyme replacement therapy is now becoming available.

Hunter Disease Unlike the Hurler and other types, the Hunter form (MPS II) is transmitted as an *X-linked trait*. The Hurler and Hunter syndromes are clinically alike except that the Hunter form is milder: mental retardation is less severe than in the Hurler type, deafness is less common, and *corneal clouding is usually absent*. Probably there are two forms of the syndrome—a more severe one, in which the patients do not survive beyond their midteens, and a less severe form, with relatively normal intelligence and survival to middle age. Excessive amounts of dermatan and heparan sulfate are excreted in the urine. The basic abnormality is a *deficiency of iduronate sulfatase*.

Table 37-6
Classification of the mucopolysaccharidoses

Number	*Eponym*	*Clinical manifestations*	*Enzyme deficiency*	*Glycosaminoglycan*
MPS I[a]	Hurler	Corneal clouding, severe skeletal changes and MR,[b] organomegaly, heart disease	α-L-Iduronidase	Dermatan sulfate, heparan sulfate
MPS II	Hunter	Dysostosis, normal corneas, MR, joint stiffness, hydrocephalus, short stature, organomegaly	Iduronate sulfatase	Dermatan sulfate, heparan sulfate
MPS III	Sanfilippo	MR, mild or absent somatic changes, hyperactivity, hepatosplenomegaly	Heparan *N*-sulfatase	Heparan sulfate
MPS IV	Morquio	Distinctive skeletal abnormalities, slight corneal clouding, odontoid hypoplasia, normal intelligence, hepatomegaly	Galactose 6-sulfatase	Keratan sulfate, chondroitin 6-sulfate
MPS V	No longer used			
MPS VI	Maroteaux-Lamy	Dysostosis, corneal clouding, normal intelligence, spinal cord compression, organomegaly	*N*-acetylgalactos-amine, 4-sulfatase (aryl sulfatase B)	Dermatan sulfate
MPS VII	Sly	Dysostosis, hepato-splenomegaly, wide range of severity, corneal clouding	β Glucoronidase	Dermatan sulfate, heparan sulfate, chondroitin 4-sulfate

[a] Less severe phenotypes are known as Scheie or Hurler-Scheie syndromes.

[b] MR = mental retardation.

Source: Modified from Neufeld and Muenzer, with permission.

Sanfilippo Disease This form, or MPS III, expresses itself clinically between 2 and 3 years of age, with progressive intellectual deterioration. The patients are of short stature, but in other respects the physical changes are fewer and less severe than in the Hunter and Hurler syndromes. Three and possibly four types of Sanfilippo disease, designated A, B, C, and D, are distinguished on the basis of their enzymatic defects (Neufeld and Muenzer). All subtypes are phenotypically similar, and all of them may excrete excessive amounts of heparan sulfate in the urine.

Morquio Disease This form of the disease, MPS IV, is characterized by marked *dwarfism* and *osteoporosis*. Skeletal deformity and compression of the spinal cord and medulla are constant threats, because of hypoplasia of the odontoid process and atlantoaxial dislocation and thickening of the dura around the cervical cord and inferior surface of the cerebellum. Intelligence is affected only slightly or not at all. *Corneal opacities may be present.* Patients excrete large amounts of keratan sulfate in the urine; two types of enzymatic deficiency have been identified (Neufeld and Muenzer).

Maroteaux-Lamy Disease This syndrome, MPS VI, includes severe skeletal deformities (short stature, anteriorly beaked vertebrae) but *normal intelligence*. Several of our cases have had a cervical pachymeningitis with spinal cord compression and hydrocephalus during adult life. Spinal cord function improved with cervical decompression and the hydrocephalus with ventriculoatrial shunting (Young et al). Hepatosplenomegaly is often present. Large amounts of dermatan sulfate are excreted in the urine, as a result of an *aryl sulfatase B deficiency*.

β-Glucuronidase Deficiency (Sly Disease) This (MPS VII) is a rare type of mucopolysaccharidosis, the clinical features of which have yet to be sharply delineated. Short stature, progressive thoracolumbar gibbus, hepatosplenomegaly, and the bony changes of dysostosis multiplex (as in the Hurler type) are the main clinical features. There is excessive excretion of dermatan and heparan sulfate, the result of a deficiency of β-glucuronidase.

Attempts to treat the mucopolysaccharidoses by replacement therapy (plasma and leukocytes), bone marrow transplantation, and gene transfer are in progress.

Mucolipidoses and Other Diseases of Complex Carbohydrates (Sialidoses; Oligosaccharidoses)

In recent years several new diseases have been described in which there is an abnormal accumulation of mucopolysaccharides, sphingolipids, and glycolipids in visceral, mesenchymal, and neural tissues, due to an α-*N*-acetylneuraminidase defect. In some types there is an additional deficiency of β-galactosidase. All are autosomal recessive diseases that manifest many of the clinical features of Hurler disease, but—in contrast to the mucopolysaccharidoses—normal amounts of mucopolysaccharides are excreted in the urine. Frequently, G_{M1} gangliosidosis, described above, is also classified with the mucolipidoses. The other members of this category are synopsized below and in Table 37-3.

Mucolipidoses At least three and possibly four closely related forms have been described. In mucolipidosis I (*lipomucopolysaccharidosis*), the morphologic features are those of gargoylism, with slowly progressive mental retardation. Cherry-red spots in the maculae, corneal opacities, and ataxia have been noted in some patients. Vacuolation of lymphocytes, marrow cells, hepatocytes, and Kupffer cells in the liver and metachromatic changes in the sural nerve have been described.

In *mucolipidosis II ("I-cell" disease)*, the most common of the mucolipidoses, there is usually an early onset of psychomotor retardation, but often this does not appear until the second or third decade. *Abnormal facies* and *periosteal thickening (dysostosis multiplex*, like that of G_{M1} gangliosidosis and Hurler disease) are characteristic. *Gingival hyperplasia* is prominent, and the *liver* and *spleen are enlarged*; but deafness is not found and corneal opacities are slower to develop. Tonic-clonic seizures are frequent in older patients. In most cases, death from heart failure occurs by the third to eighth year. There is a typical vacuolation of lymphocytes, Kupffer cells, and cells of the renal glomeruli. Bone marrow cells are also vacuolated and contain refractile cytoplasmic granules (hence the designation *inclusion-cell*, or *I-cell, disease*). A deficiency of several lysosomal enzymes required for the catabolism of mucopolysaccharides, glycolipids, and glycoproteins has been described.

In *mucolipidosis III (pseudo-Hurler polydystrophy)*, the biochemical abnormalities are like those of I-cell disease, but there are clinical differences. In the pseudo-Hurler type, symptoms do not appear until 2 years of age or later and are relatively mild. Retardation of growth, fine corneal opacities, and valvular heart disease are the major manifestations.

Yet another variant, so-called mucolipidosis IV, has been described (see Tellez-Nagel et al). Here, clouding of the corneas is noticed soon after birth, and profound retardation is evident by 1 year of age. Skeletal deformities, enlargement of liver and spleen, seizures, or other neurologic abnormalities are notably lacking. Ultrastructural examination of conjunctival and skin fibroblasts has demonstrated lysosomal inclusions of material similar to lipids and mucopolysaccharides which remain to be further characterized.

Mannosidosis This is another rare hereditary disorder with poorly differentiated symptomatology. The onset is in the first 2 years, with *Hurler-like facial* and *skeletal deformities*, *mental retardation*, and slight motor disability. Corticospinal signs, loss of hearing, variable degrees of gingival hyperplasia, and spoke-like opacities of the lens (but no diffuse corneal clouding) may be present. The liver and spleen are enlarged in some cases. Radiographs show beaking of the vertebral bodies and poor trabeculation of long bones. Vacuolated lymphocytes and granulated leukocytes are present and aid in diagnosis. The urinary mucopolysaccharides are normal.

Mannosiduria is diagnostic, caused by a defect in α-mannosidase. Mannose-containing oligosaccharides accumulate in nerve cells, spleen, liver, and leukocytes (Kistler et al).

Fucosidosis This also is a rare autosomal recessive disorder, with neurologic deterioration beginning usually at 12 to 15 months and progressing to spastic quadriplegia, decerebrate rigidity, severe psychomotor regression, and death within 4 to 6 years. *Hepatomegaly*, splenomegaly, enlarged salivary glands, thickened skin, excessive sweating, normal or typical gargoyle facies, *beaking of the vertebral bodies*, and vacuolated lymphocytes are the main features. A variant of this disease has been described with slower progression and survival into late childhood and adolescence and even into adult life (Ikeda et al). The latter type is characterized by mental and motor retardation, along with the corneal opacities, coarse facial features, skeletal deformities of gargoylism, and dermatologic changes of Fabry disease (angiokeratoma corporis diffusum), but no hepatosplenomegaly. The basic abnormality in both types is a lack of lysosomal L-fucosidase, resulting in accumulation of fucose-rich sphingolipids, glycoproteins, and oligosaccharides in cells of the skin, conjunctivae, and rectal mucosa.

Aspartylglycosaminuria This disease is characterized by the early onset of psychomotor regression; delayed, inadequate speech; severe behavioral abnormalities (*bouts of hyperactivity* mixed with apathy and hypoactivity or psychotic manifestations); progressive dementia; clumsy movements; corticospinal signs; corneal clouding (rare); retinal abnormalities and cataracts; coarse facies including low bridge of the nose, epicanthi, thickening of the lips and skin; enlarged liver; and abdominal hernias in some. Radiographs show minimal *beaking of the vertebral bodies*, and vacuolated lymphocytes are seen in the blood.

The pattern of inheritance in this entire group of diseases is, as already stated, probably autosomal recessive. Diagnostic methods applicable to amniotic fluid and cells are being developed so that prenatal diagnosis will be possible, prompted often by the occurrence of the disease in an earlier child. Neurons are vacuolated rather than stuffed with granules, much like the lymphocytes and liver cells. The specific biochemical abnormalities, as far as they are known, are indicated in Table 37-3.

Cockayne Syndrome

This disorder is probably inherited as an autosomal recessive trait. The onset is in late infancy, after apparently normal earlier development. The main clinical findings are *stunting of growth*, evident by the second and third years; *photosensitivity of the skin*; microcephaly; *retinitis pigmentosa*, *cataracts*, blindness, and pendular nystagmus; nerve deafness; *delayed psychomotor* and speech development; spastic weakness and *ataxia of limbs* and gait; occasionally athetosis; amyotrophy with abolished reflexes and reduced nerve conduction velocities; wizened face, sunken eyes, prominent nose, prognathism, anhydrosis, and poor lacrimation (resembling progeria and bird-headed dwarfism). Some cases show calcification of the basal ganglia. The CSF is normal, and there are no diagnostic biochemical findings.

Pathologic examination reveals a small brain, striatocerebellar calcifications, leukodystrophy like that of Pelizaeus-Merzbacher disease, and a severe cerebellar cortical atrophy. The peripheral nerve changes are those of a primary segmental demyelination. The pathogenesis is unknown. The variability in clinical and pathologic manifestations of reported cases suggests that not all of them are representative of the same disease.

Rett Syndrome

This syndrome is mentioned here because for many years, on the basis of psychomotor regression after a period of normal development, it was presumed to have a metabolic basis (urea cycle defect). However, neither this metabolic defect nor any other has ever been substantiated. Recently, the responsible gene mutation has been discovered. The syndrome is discussed fully in Chap. 38, with other forms of developmental mental retardation and autism.

Other Diseases of Late Infancy and Early Childhood

Globoid cell leukodystrophy (Krabbe), subacute necrotizing encephalomyelopathy (Leigh), and Gaucher disease may also begin in late infancy or early childhood. They have been described in the preceding section of this chapter. Familial striatocerebellar calcification (Fahr disease) and Lesch-Nyhan disease may also become manifest in this age period, but they usually have a later onset and are therefore described with the diseases of later childhood in the section that follows.

Diagnosis of Metabolic Diseases of Late Infancy and Early Childhood

This group of metabolic disorders presents many of the same diagnostic problems as those of early infancy. The flowchart (Fig. 37-4), which divides these disorders into dysmorphic, visceromegalic, and purely neurologic groups, is equally serviceable in the differential diagnosis of both groups. Also, as with the early infantile diseases, certain clusters of neurologic, skeletal, dermal, ophthalmic, and laboratory findings are highly distinctive and often permit the identification of a particular disease. These signs are listed below:

1. Evidence of involvement of peripheral nerves (weakness, hypotonia, areflexia, sensory loss, reduced conduction velocities) in conjunction with lesions of the central nervous system—metachromatic leukodystrophy, Krabbe leukodystrophy, neuroaxonal dystrophy, and Leigh disease (rare)
2. Ophthalmic signs
   a. Corneal clouding—several of the mucopolysaccharidoses (Hurler, Scheie, Morquio, Maroteaux-Lamy), mucolipidoses, tyrosinemia, aspartylglycosaminuria (rare)
   b. Cherry-red macular spot—G_{M2} gangliosidosis, G_{M1} gangliosidosis (half the cases), lipomucopolysaccharidosis, occasionally Niemann-Pick disease
   c. Retinal degeneration with pigmentary deposits—Jansky-Bielschowsky lipid storage disease, G_{M1} gangliosidosis, syndrome of sea-blue histiocytes
   d. Optic atrophy and blindness—metachromatic leukodystrophy, neuroaxonal dystrophy
   e. Cataracts—Marinesco-Sjögren syndrome, Fabry disease, mannosidosis
   f. Telangiectasia and ocular apraxia—ataxia-telangiectasia, Niemann-Pick disease
   g. Impairment of vertical eye movements—late infantile Niemann-Pick disease, juvenile dystonic lipidosis, sea-blue histiocyte syndrome, Wilson disease
   h. Jerky eye movements, limited abduction—late infantile Gaucher disease
3. Extrapyramidal signs—late-onset Niemann-Pick disease (rigidity, abnormal postures), juvenile dystonic lipidosis (dystonia, choreoathetosis), Rett, ataxia-telangiectasia (athetosis), Sanfilippo mucopolysaccharidosis, type I glutaric acidemia, Wilson disease, Segawa dopa-responsive dystonia
4. Facial dysmorphism—Hurler, Scheie, Morquio, and Maroteaux-Lamy forms of mucopolysaccharidosis, aspartylglycosaminuria, mucolipidoses, G_{M1} gangliosidosis, mannosidosis, fucosidosis (some cases), multisulfatase deficiencies (Austin), some mitochondrial disorders
5. Dwarfism, spine deformities, arthropathies—Hurler, Morquio, and other mucopolysaccharidoses, Cockayne syndrome
6. Enlarged liver and spleen—Niemann-Pick disease, Gaucher disease, all mucopolysaccharidoses, fucosidosis, mucolipidoses, G_{M1} gangliosidosis
7. Alterations of skin—photosensitivity (Cockayne syndrome and one form of porphyria); papular nevi and angiokeratoma (Fabry disease, fucosidosis); telangiectasia of ears, conjunctiva, chest (ataxia-telangiectasia); ichthyosis (Sjögren-Larsen disease, caused by fatty alcohol dehydrogenase deficiency); plaque-like lesions in Hunter syndrome
8. Beaked thoracolumbar vertebrae—all mucopolysaccharidoses, mucolipidoses, mannosidosis, fucosidosis; aspartylglycosaminuria, multiple sulfatase deficiencies
9. Deafness—mucopolysaccharidoses, mannosidosis, Cockayne syndrome
10. Hypertrophied gums—mucolipidoses, mannosidosis
11. Vacuolated lymphocytes—all mucopolysaccharidoses, mucolipidoses, mannosidosis, fucosidosis
12. Granules in neutrophils—all mucopolysaccharidoses, mucolipidoses, mannosidosis, fucosidosis, multiple sulfatase deficiencies

In our experience the most difficult diagnostic problems in this age period are raised by neuroaxonal dystrophy, metachromatic leukodystrophy, the mitochondrial disorder subacute necrotizing encephalomyelopathy (Leigh disease), some cases of lipofuscinosis, and the late form of G_{M1} gangliosidosis. In none of these diseases is the clinical picture entirely stereotyped. Most helpful in the clinical diagnosis of neuroaxonal dystrophy is the onset, at 1 to 2 years of age, of severe hypotonia with retained reflexes and Babinski signs, early visual involvement without retinal changes, lack of seizures, normal CSF, physiologic evidence of denervation of muscles, fast-frequency EEG, normal CT scan, and *N*-acetylgalactosaminidase deficiency in cultured fibroblasts. Metachromatic leukodystrophy can be excluded if the CSF protein is normal and if nerve conduction velocities and enzymatic studies of leukocytes and fibroblasts are normal. Similar criteria enable one to rule out G_{M1} gangliosidosis. Leigh disease may begin at the same age, with hypotonia and optic atrophy, but abnormalities of ocular movement and respiration appear early; in many cases the lactic acidosis and pyruvate decarboxylase defect will corroborate the diagnosis. Also in Leigh disease, CT scanning and MRI may disclose hypodense lesions in the basal ganglia and brainstem, in contrast to the normal CT scan in neuroaxonal dystrophy. In metachromatic leukodystrophy, the cerebral white matter shows a diffusely decreased attenuation and the MR images are striking (Fig. 37-6). Lipofuscinosis cannot always be diagnosed accurately; curvilinear bodies in nerve twigs, endothelial cells in skin biopsies, and the recently discovered gene mutations are the best laboratory tests.

INHERITED METABOLIC ENCEPHALOPATHIES OF LATE CHILDHOOD AND ADOLESCENCE

Unavoidably, one must refer here to certain inherited metabolic diseases already described that permit survival into late childhood and adolescence as well as to diseases that begin in adolescence or adult life after a normal childhood. There is a tendency for them to be less severe and less rapidly progressive, an attribute shared by many diseases with a dominant mode of inheritance. Nonetheless, there are diseases, such as Wilson disease, in which the onset of neurologic symptoms occurs after the 10th year and in rare instances after the 30th year, and the mode of inheritance is recessive in type. However, in the latter instance, the basic abnormality has existed since early childhood in the form of a ceruloplasmin deficiency with early cirrhosis and splenomegaly; only the neurologic disorder is of late onset. This brings us to another principle—that the pathogenesis of the cerebral lesion may involve a factor or factors once removed from the underlying biologic abnormality, in this case cirrhosis of the liver.

Genetic heterogeneity poses another problem with respect to both the clinical and biochemical findings. It is well established that a single clinical phenotype such as the one seen in Hurler disease can be the expression of a number of different alleles of a given gene mutation. Conversely, a number of different clinical phenotypes may be based on different degrees of the same enzyme deficiency. One must, therefore, not rely solely on clinical appearances for diagnosis but always combine them with biochemical tests and molecular genetic studies for confirmation. No one of these lines of data is sufficient for classification of disease.

The diseases in this category are probably of greater interest to neurologists than the preceding ones, for they more consistently cause familiar neurologic abnormalities such as epilepsy, polymyoclonus, dementia, cerebellar ataxia, choreoathetosis, dystonia, tremor, spastic-ataxic paraparesis, blindness, deafness, and stroke. These manifestations appear much the same in late childhood and adolescence as they do in adult life, and the neurologist whose experience has been mainly with adult patients feels quite comfortable with them.

Diseases in this age period have a diversity of manifestations, yet each disease tends to have a certain characteristic pattern of neurologic expression, as though the pathogenetic mechanism were acting selectively on particular systems of neurons. Such affinities between the disease process and certain anatomic structures raise the question of *pathoclisis*, i.e., specific vulnerability of particular neuronal systems to certain morbid agents. Stated another way, for each disease there is a common and relatively stereotyped clinical syndrome and a small number of variants; conversely, certain other symptoms and syndromes are rarely observed with a given disease. At the same time, however, it is clear that more than one disease may cause the same syndrome.

In deference to these principles, *the diseases in this section are grouped according to their most common mode of clinical expression*, as follows:

1. The progressive cerebellar ataxias of childhood and adolescence
2. The familial polymyoclonias and epilepsies
3. Extrapyramidal syndromes of parkinsonian type
4. The syndrome of dystonia and generalized choreoathetosis
5. The syndrome of bilateral hemiplegia, cerebral blindness and deafness, and other manifestations of focal cerebral disorder
6. Strokes in association with inherited metabolic diseases
7. Metabolic polyneuropathies
8. Personality changes and behavioral disturbances as manifestations of inherited metabolic diseases

It is advantageous to be familiar with these groupings, for a knowledge of them, like the age of onset and gray and white matter distinctions in diseases of earlier onset, facilitates clinical diagnosis. Variants seen personally by the authors are mentioned in the descriptions of the diseases themselves. One word of caution—it is a mistake to assume that the diseases in these categories affect one and only one particular part of the nervous system or to assume that they are exclusively neurologic. Once the biochemical abnormality is discovered, it is usually found to implicate cells of certain nonneurologic tissues as well; whether or not the effects of such involvement become symptomatic is often a quantitative matter. Also, one encounters mixed neurologic syndromes in which tremor, myoclonus, cerebellar ataxia, and choreoathetosis are present in various combinations; sometimes it is difficult to decide whether a movement disorder is of one type or another.

The Progressive Cerebellar Ataxias of Late Childhood and Adolescence

In the preceding section it was pointed out that there is a large group of diseases, some with (but most without) a known metabolic basis, in which an acute, episodic, or chronic cerebellar ataxia becomes manifest in early childhood. Here the discussion of the cerebellar ataxias is continued, with reference to those forms that begin in late childhood and adolescence. In these later age periods the number of ataxias of proven metabolic type diminishes markedly. Most of them, of chronic progressive type, are part of the late-onset lipid storage diseases. Of the other cerebellar ataxias of late childhood and adolescence, only the Bassen-Kornzweig acanthocytosis and a genetic fault in vitamin E metabolism fall into the category of a truly metabolic disease—and one could perhaps add late-onset G_{M2} gangliosidosis (page 1024), Refsum disease, ataxia-telangiectasia, and prolonged vitamin E deficiency. Refsum disease is so clearly a polyneuropathy (cerebellar features only in exceptional cases) that it is presented in Chap. 46. Ataxia-telangiectasia is usually encountered in late childhood, but the ataxia may begin as early as the second year of life; therefore it has been described in the preceding section with the ataxias of early childhood. The effect of vitamin E deficiency on the nervous system is described on page 1224.

Doubtless, many of the progressive forms of cerebellar ataxia now classified as degenerative and described in Chap. 39 will soon be proved to have an underlying biochemical pathogenesis and will logically be placed here, with the metabolic diseases. At present, when faced with a progressive ataxia of cerebellar type, the reader should consult both this chapter and Chap. 39.

The *acute forms of cerebellar ataxia* that occur in late childhood and adolescence are essentially nonmetabolic, being observed as part of postinfectious encephalomyelitis (page 797); in postanoxic, postmeningitic, and posthyperthermic states; and with certain drug intoxications. And with pure cerebellar ataxias of this age period, postinfectious cerebellitis, cerebellar tumors (medulloblastomas, astrocytomas, hemangioblastomas, and ganglioneuromas of Lhermitte-Duclos) must always be considered. MRI usually establishes the correct diagnosis.

Bassen-Kornzweig Acanthocytosis (Abetalipoproteinemia) This disease, first described by Bassen and Kornzweig in 1950, excited great interest, for it gave promise of a breakthrough into a hitherto obscure group of "degenerative" disorders. In the 15-year period that followed the original report, less than a dozen cases were recorded, and several of the reports were based on the study of the same case. In our experience, it is a rare disease. We have seen only three cases. The resemblance to Friedreich ataxia is not so close that an experienced clinician would be likely to confuse the two.

The inheritance of this disease is autosomal recessive in type. The initial symptoms, occurring between 6 and 12 years (range, 2 to 17 years), are weakness of the limbs with areflexia and an ataxia of sensory (tabetic) type, to which a cerebellar component is added later (see also page 1421). Steatorrhea, raising the suspicion of celiac disease, often precedes the weak, unsteady gait. Later, in more than half the patients, vision may fail because of retinal degeneration (similar to retinitis pigmentosa). Kyphoscoliosis, pes cavus, and Babinski signs are other elements in the clinical picture. The neurologic disorder is relatively slowly progressive—by the second to third decade, the patient is usually bedridden.

The diagnostic laboratory findings are spiky or thorny red blood cells (acanthocytes), low sedimentation rate, and a marked reduction in the serum of low-density lipoproteins (cholesterol, phospholipid, and β-lipoprotein levels are all subnormal). Pathologic study has revealed the presence of foamy, vacuolated epithelial cells in the intestinal mucosa (causing absorption block); diminished numbers of myelinated nerve fibers in sural nerve biopsies, depletion of Purkinje and granule cells in all parts of the cerebellum; loss of fibers in the posterior columns and spinocerebellar tracts; loss of anterior horn and retinal ganglion cells; muscle fiber loss; and fibrosis of the myocardium. It has been proposed that the basic defect is an inability of the body to synthesize the proteins of cell membranes, because of the impaired absorption of fat through the mucosa of the small intestine. Vitamin E deficiency may be a pathogenic factor, since the administration of a low-fat diet and high doses of vitamins A and E may prevent progression of the neurologic disorder (Illingworth et al).

Familial Hypobetalipoproteinemia This is a well-described disease, resembling abetalipoproteinemia, in which there is hypocholesterolemia, acanthocytosis of red blood corpuscles, retinitis pigmentosa, and a pallidal atrophy (HARP syndrome). Inheritance is autosomal dominant, and heterozygotes may exhibit some part of the syndrome. Fat droplets may be seen in the jejunal mucosa, indicating malabsorption. Cases have been reported from Europe, Asia, and the United States. Treatment consists of restriction of dietary fat and supplements of vitamin E.

An adult form of acanthocytosis and hereditary chorea and dystonia has also been recognized, but evidence of lipid malabsorption is lacking. This disease is described in Chap. 39.

There are doubtless many other conditions of metabolic type in which cerebellar ataxia figures importantly in the clinical picture. Some of these are associated with polymyoclonus and cherry-red macular spots (sialidosis or neuraminodosis; see below). Cerebellar ataxia is a prominent feature of Unverricht-Lundborg (Baltic) disease and Lafora-body disease. The Cockayne syndrome and Marinesco-Sjögren disease, already described under "Inherited Metabolic Diseases of Late Infancy and Early Childhood," persist into later childhood and adolescence or may even have their onset in this later period. In cerebrotendinous xanthomatosis (see further on), spastic weakness and pseudobulbar palsy are combined with cerebellar ataxia. Prader-Willi children have a broad-based gait and are clumsy in addition to being obese, genitally deficient, and diabetic. One family of five males with a syndrome of hyperuricemia, spinocerebellar ataxia, and deafness has been reported by Rosenberg and colleagues, and several other variants of defective purine and pyrimidine metabolism fit into this category; the enzymatic defect of Lesch-Nyhan disease was not present, however. Marsden and coworkers have observed cerebellar ataxia beginning in late childhood, as an expression of adrenoleukodystrophy (see below). The familial syndrome of neurodegeneration, ataxia, and retinitis pigmentosa (NARP, page 1043) caused by a mitochondrial genome mutation that impairs ATP synthase can closely mimic the Marinesco-Sjögren syndrome.

Hereditary Paroxysmal Cerebellar Ataxia This not uncommon syndrome of periodic ataxia, akin to the familial paroxysmal choreoathetosis and periodic dystonia described in Chap. 4, is inherited as an autosomal dominant trait. The gene for hereditary paroxysmal ataxia, which codes for a portion of the calcium channel, maps to chromosome 19p (Vahedi et al). It has its onset in childhood or early adult life and takes the form of disabling episodic attacks of ataxia, nystagmus, and dysarthria, each attack lasting a few minutes or a few hours. Between attacks the patients are asymptomatic or show only a mild nystagmus or minimal clumsiness. The attacks can be prevented by the administration of acetazolamide, 250 mg tid, as had been noted originally by Griggs et al. These characteristics apply to what is now termed *familial episodic ataxia* type 2; a rarer type 1 is related to a mutation in the voltage-gated potassium channel and is associated with myokymia and epilepsy.

The Familial Polymyoclonias

As stated in Chap. 6, the term *myoclonus* is applied to many conditions that are not at all alike but share a single clinical feature—a multitude of exceedingly brief, random, arrhythmic twitches of parts of muscles, entire muscles, or groups of muscles. Myoclonic jerks differ from chorea by virtue of their brevity (15 to 50 ms). Notably, both phenomena are considered to be symptomatic of "gray matter" diseases.

Myoclonus or polymyoclonus may, in certain conditions, stand alone as a relatively pure syndrome. In other cases, it is mixed with epilepsy or athetosis and dystonia, discussed further on. Most often, myoclonus is associated with cerebellar ataxia, for which reason it is being considered here, juxtaposed with the progressive cerebellar ataxias. The many acquired forms of polymyoclonus, such as subacute sclerosing panencephalitis, have been mentioned in Chap. 6. In this chapter we are concerned only with those of known or presumed metabolic origin.

Myoclonic Encephalopathy of Infants Under this title Kinsbourne originally described a form of widespread, continuous myoclonus (except during deep sleep) affecting male and female infants whose development had been normal until the onset of the disease at the age of 9 to 20 months. The myoclonus evolves over a week or less, affects all the muscles of the body, and interferes seriously with all the natural muscular activities of the child. The eyes are notably affected by rapid (up to 8 per second), irregular conjugate movements ("dancing eyes" of an opsoclonic type). The child is irritable and speech may cease. All laboratory tests are normal.

Adrenocorticotropic hormone and dexamethasone, the latter in doses of 1.5 to 4.0 mg/day, suppress the myoclonus and permit developmental progress. Some patients have recovered from the myoclonus and have been mentally slow and mildly ataxic afterward. Others have required corticosteroid therapy for 5 to 10 years, with relapse whenever it is discontinued. Ordinary anticonvulsants seem to have no effect. The pathologic basis of the polymyoclonus has not been defined.

A similar syndrome has been observed in conjunction with neuroblastoma, rarely with bronchogenic and other occult carcinomas, and as a transient illness of unknown (possibly viral) cause in young adults (Baringer et al; see page 1087).

In a broader survey of the pediatric opsoclonus-myoclonus syndrome, Pranzatelli and associates reported their experience with 27 cases, some with neural crest tumors, others with viral infections or hypoxic injury (intention myoclonus). In nearly all of their patients there was cerebellar ataxia and mental disorder, and 10 percent had seizures. The CSF was normal. The investigators emphasize the pathogenetic heterogeneity and define a serotoninergic type (low levels of 5-hydroxytryptophan and homovanillic acid in the CSF) that responds to 5-hydroxyindole acetic acid.

Familial Progressive Myoclonus Five major categories of familial polymyoclonus of late childhood and adolescence have been delineated: (1) Lafora- or amyloid-body type, (2) juvenile cerebroretinal degeneration, (3) cherry-red spot-myoclonus (sialidosis or neuraminidosis), (4) mitochondrial encephalopathy, and (5) a more benign degenerative disease (dyssynergia cerebellaris myoclonica of Hunt). Familial myoclonus may also be a prominent feature of two other diseases—G_{M2} gangliosidosis and Gaucher disease—which occasionally have their onset in this age period.

Lafora-Body Polymyoclonus with Epilepsy This disease, which is inherited as an autosomal recessive trait, was first identified by Lafora in 1911 on the basis of the large basophilic cytoplasmic bodies that were found in the dentate, brainstem, and thalamic neurons. They have been shown by Yokoi and colleagues to be composed of a glucose polymer (polyglycosan) that is chemically but not structurally related to glycogen. Possibly some of the cases of familial myoclonus epilepsy reported by Unverricht and by Lundborg were of this type, but since these authors provided no pathologic data, one cannot be sure.

Beginning in late childhood and adolescence (11 to 18 years) in a previously normal individual, the disease announces itself by a seizure, a burst of myoclonic jerks, or both. In about half the cases there are focal (often occipital) seizures. The illness may at first be mistaken for ordinary epilepsy, but within a few months it becomes evident that it is far more serious. The myoclonus becomes widespread and can be evoked by noise, startle, an unexpected tactile stimulus (even the tap of a reflex hammer), excitement, or certain sustained motor activities. An evoked train of myoclonic jerks may progress to a generalized seizure with loss of consciousness. As the disease advances, the myoclonus interferes increasingly with the patient's motor activities until function is seriously impaired. Speech may be marred, much as it is in chorea. Close examination may also reveal an alteration in muscle tone and a slight degree of cerebellar ataxia. At this time, or even before the onset of myoclonus and seizures, the patient may experience visual hallucinations or exhibit irritability, odd traits of character, uninhibited or impulsive behavior, and, ultimately, progressive failure in all cognitive functions. Deafness has been an early sign in a few cases. Rigidity or hypotonia, impaired tendon reflexes, acrocyanosis, and rarely corticospinal tract signs are late findings. Finally the patient becomes cachectic and bedfast and succumbs to intercurrent infection. Most do not survive beyond their 25th birthday. Nonetheless there are isolated reports of Lafora-body disease in which symptoms began as late as 40 years, with death as late as 50 years. These late cases may constitute a separate genetic type.

No abnormalities of the blood, urine, or CSF have been detected. The EEG shows diffuse slow waves and spikes as well as focal or multifocal discharges. Altered hepatocytes with homogeneous PAS-positive bodies that displace the nuclei have been observed in both the presymptomatic and symptomatic stages of the disease. These inclusions have been seen in skin and liver biopsies even though liver function tests were normal. Neuropathologic examinations have shown a slight loss of granule and Purkinje cells and loss of neurons in the dentate nuclei, inner segment of globus pallidus, and cerebral cortex in addition to the Lafora bodies. The latter may also be seen in the retina, cerebral cortex, myocardium, and striated muscles. Anticonvulsant drugs, especially methsuximide and valproic acid, help in the control of the seizures but have no effect on the basic process.

Polyglycosan Body Disease This is another closely related disease, reviewed by Robitaille and coworkers, in which glycosamine bodies are found in the central and peripheral nervous system. The clinical syndrome included dementia, chorea, and amyotrophy with or without sensory loss in the limbs. Similar bodies were found in liver and heart. This progressive disease beginning in adult life was attributed to the accumulation of polymers of glucose. Diagnosis is confirmed by the finding of these bodies in the axons of peripheral nerves or liver cells.

Juvenile Cerebroretinal Degeneration (Ceroid Lipofuscinosis) As stated earlier, this is one of the most variable forms of the lipidoses. The salient clinical features of the later-onset types are severe myoclonus, seizures, and visual loss. In the juvenile type, the first lesions are seen in the maculae; they appear as yellow-gray areas of degeneration and stand in contrast to the cherry-red spot and the encircling white ring of Tay-Sachs disease. At first the particles of pigment are fine and dust-like; later they agglomerate to resemble more the bone-corpuscular shapes of retinitis pigmentosa. The liver and spleen are not enlarged, and there are no osseous changes. The usual development of these and other manifestations of the disease was outlined by Sjögren, who studied a large number of the late infantile and juvenile types of cases in Sweden. He divided the illness into five stages:

1. Visual impairment, sometimes preceding retinal changes by months.

2. After approximately 2 years, the onset of generalized seizures and myoclonus, often with irritability, poor control of emotions, and stuttering, jerky speech.

3. Gradual intellectual deterioration (poor memory, reduced mental activity, inattentiveness). By this stage the movements have usually become slow, stiff, and tremulous, resembling somewhat those of Parkinson disease—to which are added elements of cerebellar ataxia and intention tremor, coming in this way to resemble Wilson disease.

4. Stage of severe dementia in which the patient needs assistance to walk, no longer speaks, and may scream when disturbed or forced to move. The muscles are wasted, though the tendon reflexes are lively and the plantar reflexes are extensor.

5. Finally the patient lies curled up in bed, blind and speechless, with strong extensor plantar reflexes, occasionally adopting dystonic postures. Mercifully the illness ends in 10 to 15 years.

In the early stages the EEG picture of random, high-voltage, triphasic waves is diagnostic; later, as the seizures and myoclonic jerks become less frequent and finally cease, only delta waves remain. The electroretinographic waveforms are lost once the retina is affected. The lateral ventricles are slightly dilated in CT scans and on MRI. The CSF is normal. Diagnosis can be confirmed by electron microscopic study of biopsy material, particularly of the eccrine sweat glands of the skin. A defective membrane protein has been identified that shows a curvilinear "fingerprint" pattern of the inclusion material in the commonest, or classic, juvenile phenotype. A gene mutation has been identified on chromosome 16p.

The *Kufs type of ceroid lipofuscinosis*, which develops later (15 to 25 years), is often unattended by visual or retinal changes and is even slower in its evolution. Personality change and seizures, usually with some degree of myoclonus, are the principal abnormalities. As the disease progresses, cerebellar ataxia, spasticity and rigidity or athetosis, or mixtures thereof, are combined with dementia. Van Bogaert (personal communication) noted that relatives of these patients may have retinal changes without neurologic accompaniments.

Of all the lipidoses, these cerebroretinal degenerations have defied biochemical definition. In a few of the early childhood types, mutations of one of several lysosomal enzymes have been identified, as summarized by Mole. As mentioned earlier, Zeman and coworkers have shown that the cytoplasmic inclusions are autofluorescent and give a positive histochemical reaction for ceroid and lipofuscin, but this has not been biochemically differentiated from the similar lipid substance that accumulates in aging cells. In addition to the presence of curvilinear bodies in the cytoplasm of neurons, some in a fingerprint pattern, there is a reduction in type II synapses in the distal parts of the axon. All these changes precede nerve cell loss.

Childhood or Juvenile G_{M2} Gangliosidosis Rarely, instances of the recessive type of G_{M2} gangliosidosis have their onset at this age period. Twenty-four such cases (from 20 kindreds) were found in the medical literature by Meek and coworkers. Ataxia and dysarthria were frequently the presenting symptoms, followed by dementia, dysphagia, spasticity, dystonia, seizures, and myoclonus. Degeneration of anterior horn cells with progressive muscular atrophy may be a feature, although this is more characteristic of the adult-onset variety (see further on). Atypical cherry-red spots are observed in some patients. The biochemical abnormality, i.e., a deficiency of hexosaminidase A, is the same as in Tay-Sachs disease but not as severe or as extensive. Progression of the disease is slow, over a period of many years. Some of our patients are alive at 40 years, the disease having begun in adolescence.

Late Gaucher Disease with Polymyoclonus A type of Gaucher disease is occasionally encountered in which seizures, severe diffuse myoclonus, supranuclear gaze disorders (slow saccades, saccadic and pursuit horizontal gaze palsies), and cerebellar ataxia begin in late childhood, adolescence, or adult life. The course is slowly progressive. The intellect is relatively spared. The spleen is enlarged. The pathologic and biochemical abnormalities are the same as those of Gaucher disease of earlier onset (Winkelman et al).

Cherry-Red Spot–Myoclonus Syndrome This is a relatively new and genetically distinct class of disease characterized by the storage of sialidated glycopeptides in tissues; it is due to a neuraminidase deficiency. In some of the patients the onset has been in late childhood or adolescence and in others even later. In addition to the patients reported by Rapin and coworkers, 24 similar cases have been reported in the medical literature, and we have personally observed several such instances.

In the cases of Rapin and colleagues and in two of our own, the first findings were visual impairment with cherry-red macular spots, similar to those seen in Tay-Sachs disease and less consistently in G_{M1} gangliosidosis, Niemann-Pick disease, and metachromatic leukodystrophy. In one case there was severe episodic pain in the hands, legs, and feet during hot weather, reminiscent of Fabry disease. Polymyoclonus followed within a few years and, together with cerebellar ataxia, disabled the patients. Mental function remained relatively normal. Liver and spleen were not enlarged, but storage material was found in the Kupffer cells, neurons of the myenteric plexus, and cerebral neurons, and presumably in cerebellar and retinal ones.

The cases of Thomas and colleagues were young adults, all members of one generation, who had developed dysarthria, intention myoclonus, cerebellar ataxia, and cherry-red macular lesions. Like the cases of Rapin and coworkers, the heredity was autosomal recessive. There was urinary excretion of sialilated oligosaccharides and a sialidase deficiency in cultured fibroblasts. The two patients described by Tsuji and associates are noteworthy insofar as they were aged 50 and 30 years, respectively. In addition to the macular lesions, polymyoclonia, and cerebellar ataxia, there were gargoyle-like facial features, corneal opacities, and vertebral dysplasia. These patients also had a neuraminidase (partial β-galactosidase) deficiency.

Dentatorubral Cerebellar Atrophy with Polymyoclonus This progressive degeneration of the cerebellar-dentatal efferent system was originally described by Ramsay Hunt under the title of *dyssynergia cerebellaris myoclonica*. The onset is in late childhood; both sexes are vulnerable, and it probably has more than one cause. In Hunt's case, a progressive ataxia was accompanied by a striking degree of action myoclonus. Seizures are infrequent and the intellect is relatively preserved. The neurons of the dentate nuclei and their ascending and descending brainstem axons gradually disappear. Berkovic and associates have studied 84 cases of polymyoclonus, 13 of which conformed to the Hunt syndrome. Of these, 9 proved to have a mitochondrial encephalomyopathy. However, there are other reports (Tassinari et al) in which muscle biopsies showed no mitochondrial abnormalities. In the series of 30 cases reported by Marsden and coworkers, the onset was usually before the age of 21 years. There were cortical discharges preceding each myoclonic twitch. A clinical or biochemically supported diagnosis could not be made in nearly half of their cases.

We have observed restricted, extremely chronic forms of rhythmic myoclonus that involved only the facial and bulbar muscles. Although this benign familial polymyoclonia has not been associated with any biochemical abnormalities, its association with cellular mitochondrial abnormalities in some cases justifies its inclusion in this chapter rather than with the degenerative diseases. Another mitochondrial disorder, the myoclonic epilepsy ragged red fiber disease (MERRF), begins in the second decade or later with myoclonus and ataxia and enters into the differential diagnosis of this group of diseases. The mitochondrial diseases as a group are considered in the last part of this chapter.

Epilepsies of Hereditary Metabolic Disease

Convulsive seizures may complicate nearly all hereditary metabolic diseases. The seizures may occur at all ages but more frequently in the neonate, infant, or young child than in the older child or adolescent. The seizures take many forms, as discussed in Chap. 16. Most often they are generalized grand mal or partial types; typical petit mal probably does not occur. Some diseases may cause focal seizures, simple or complex partial, before becoming generalized. The combination of series of polymyoclonic jerks progressing to a generalized motor seizure is always highly suggestive of one of the hereditary metabolic diseases. Another highly significant form of presentation is with sensory evoked seizures. The subject of epilepsy and the hereditary metabolic diseases has recently been reviewed by Sansaricq and colleagues.

Extrapyramidal Syndromes with Hereditary Metabolic Disease

Reference is made here to the distinctive motor disorders described in Chap. 4. In the typical parkinsonian syndrome, with features of rigidity, tremor, and bradykinesia, strength remains relatively intact and corticospinal signs are absent, but effectiveness of movement is nonetheless impaired by the patient's disinclination to use the affected parts (hypo- or akinesia), by slowness (bradykinesia), and by rigidity and tremor. Other clinical syndromes include choreoathetosis, dystonia, and spasms of gaze.

When the parkinsonian syndrome or some component thereof has its onset in middle or late adult life, it usually indicates Parkinson disease or related multisystem forms of striatonigral degeneration. The development of such an extrapyramidal motor disorder in late childhood and adolescence should always suggest Wilson disease, Hallervorden-Spatz disease, and the Segawa type of L-dopa-responsive dystonia.

Hepatolenticular Degeneration (Wilson Disease, Westphal-Strümpell Pseudosclerosis) Wilson's classic description of "progressive lenticular degeneration: a familial nervous disease associated with cirrhosis of the liver" appeared in 1912. A similar neurologic disorder had been described previously by Gowers (1906) under the title of "tetanoid chorea" and by Westphal (1883) and Strümpell (1898), as "pseudosclerosis." None of these authors, however, recognized the association with cirrhosis. The clinical studies of Hall (1921) and the histopathologic studies of Spielmeyer (1920), who reexamined sections from the liver and brain of Westphal's and Strümpell's cases, clearly established that the pseudosclerosis described by these authors was the same disease as the one that had been described by Wilson. Interestingly, none of these authors, including Wilson, noticed the golden-brown (Kayser-Fleischer) corneal ring, the one pathognomonic sign of the disease. The corneal abnormality was first described by Kayser in 1902, and in the following year Fleischer related it to pseudosclerosis. Rumpell had demonstrated the greatly increased copper content of the liver and brain as early as 1913, but this discovery was generally ignored until Mandelbrote (1948) found, quite by chance, that the urinary excretion of copper was greatly increased in patients with Wilson disease, and that it was increased even more after the intramuscular administration of the chelating agent British antilewisite (BAL). In 1952, Scheinberg and Gitlin discovered that ceruloplasmin, the serum protein that binds copper, is consistently reduced in this disease (see reviews by Scheinberg and Sternlieb for a full historical account and references).

The prevalence of the disease cannot be stated exactly but is on the order of 1 per 50,000 to 1 per 100,000 of the general population. Siblings of a patient with Wilson disease have a 1 in 4 risk of developing the disease. The disease is transmitted as an autosomal recessive trait, and the abnormal gene has been assigned, by linkage analysis, to chromosome 13, in the region 13q14. One of the curious aspects of the genetics of the disease is the multitude of mutations that give rise to the disease within this particular segment of the gene, akin to an allelic variant at a normal site; no one mutation accounts for more than 30 percent of cases. The gene, called ATP7B (homologous with the ATP7A gene, which is defective in Menkes disease), codes for a membrane-bound, copper-binding ATPase. Inadequate functioning of this enzyme in some way reduces excretion of copper in the bile. As noted further on, liver transplantation halts progression of the disease, indicating that the primary effect of the mutation is on the liver rather than the nervous system.

The genetic defect gives rise to two fundamental disturbances of copper metabolism—a reduced rate of incorporation of copper into ceruloplasmin and a reduction in biliary excretion of copper. The deposition of copper in tissues is the cause of virtually all the manifestations of the disease—cirrhosis, hemolytic anemia, degeneration of the basal ganglia, and Kayser-Fleischer rings—as discussed below.

Clinical Features The onset of neurologic symptoms is usually in the second and less often in the third decade, rarely beyond that time. Half of patients are symptomatic by age 15. Exceptional cases, including two with which we are familiar, had their first clinical manifestations as late as their mid-fifties. In all instances, the initial event is a deposition of copper in the liver, leading to an acute or chronic hepatopathy and eventually to multilobular cirrhosis and splenomegaly (Scheinberg and Sternlieb). In childhood, the liver disorder often takes the form of attacks of jaundice, unexplained hepatosplenomegaly, or hypersplenism with thrombocytopenia and bleeding. The hepatitis may be symptomatic (except for elevated serum transaminases), in which case the initial clinical presentation is neurologic. In some instances, a hemolytic anemia may first draw attention to the disease.

The first neurologic manifestations are almost invariably extrapyramidal and with a proclivity to affect the oropharyngeal musculature. The typical presentations are tremor of a limb or of the head and generalized slowness of movement (i.e., a parkinsonian syndrome); or slowness of movement of the tongue, lips, pharynx, larynx, and jaws, resulting in dysarthria, dysphagia, and hoarseness; or there may be slowness of finger movement and occasionally choreic movements or dystonic postures of the limbs. Often the mouth is held slightly open in the early stage of the disease. Exceptionally, an abnormality of behavior (argumentativeness, impulsiveness, excessive emotionality) or a gradual impairment of intellectual faculties precedes other neurologic signs (Starosta-Rubinstein et al). As the disease progresses, the "classic syndrome" evolves: dysphagia and drooling, rigidity and slowness of movements of the limbs; flexed postures; fixity of facial muscles with mouth constantly agape, giving an appearance of grinning or a "vacuous smile"; virtual anarthria (bulbar extrapyramidal syndrome); and a tremor in repose that increases when the limbs are outstretched (coarse, "wing-beating" tremor). Slowed saccadic eye movements and limitation of upgaze are also characteristic. Usually elements of cerebellar ataxia and intention tremor of variable degree are added at some stage of the disease. *A notable feature is the tendency for the motor disorders to be concentrated in the bulbar musculature* and to spread caudally. Thus, the syndrome differs from classic parkinsonism. Approximately 6 percent of patients develop seizures (Dening et al).

With progression of the neurologic disease, the *Kayser-Fleischer rings* become more evident (Fig. 37-7). They take the form of a crescentic rusty-brown discoloration of the deepest layer of the cornea (Descemet's membrane). In the purely hepatic stage of the disease, the rings may not be evident (in 25 percent of cases), but *they are invariably present once the neurologic signs become manifest.* A slit-lamp examination may be necessary for their detection, particularly in brown-eyed patients, but in the majority of patients with neurologic signs the rings can be visualized with the naked eye or with the aid of an indirect ophthalmoscope focused on the limbus. Gradually the disability increases because of increasing rigidity and tremor. The patient becomes mute, immobile, extremely rigid, dystonic, and slowed mentally (late and variable effect).

The diagnosis is virtually certain when there is a similar syndrome in a sibling or when an extrapyramidal motor disorder of this type is conjoined with liver disease and the corneal rings. Variants of the above syndrome that the authors have seen are an early choreoathetosis (like Sydenham chorea); prominent dystonic postures; a cerebellar ataxia with minimal rigidity; a syndrome of coarse action or action and intention tremor resembling that of dentatorubral degeneration; an immobile mute state with profound rigidity; and, a dementia, character change, or psychosis with relatively few extrapyramidal signs. Action myoclonus as a prominent early manifestation has also been described.

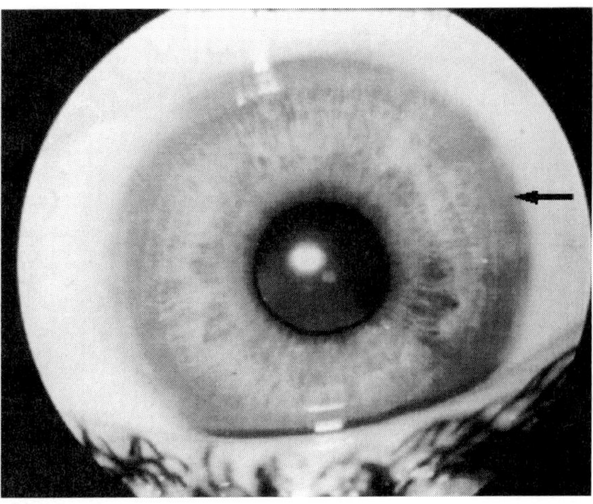

Figure 37-7

Kayser-Fleischer corneal ring (arrow) in Wilson disease. (From Lyon et al by permission.)

Laboratory Findings In both the typical and variant forms of the disease, the finding of a low serum ceruloplasmin level (less than 20 mg/dL in 80 to 90 percent of patients), low serum copper (3 to 10 μM/L; normal 11 to 24 μM/L), and increased urinary copper excretion (more than 100 mg Cu/24 h) corroborate the diagnosis. Because 90 percent of copper is carried by ceruloplasmin, and the latter is generally reduced in Wilson disease, serum copper values alone may be misleadingly normal or low. Early in the course of the illness, the most reliable diagnostic findings are a high copper content in a biopsy of liver tissue (more than 200 mg Cu/g dry weight) and a failure to incorporate labeled ^{64}Cu into ceruloplasmin. The latter test, however, fails to dependably differentiate asymptomatic carriers from affected individuals. Measurement of increased cupruresis after the administration of pencillamine has not been shown to be more sensitive than an unenhanced

24-h urine collection for copper. Persistent aminoaciduria, reflecting a renal tubular abnormality, is present in most but not all patients. Liver function tests are usually abnormal; some patients are jaundiced and other signs of liver failure may appear late in the illness. In these patients, the serum ammonia may be elevated and the symptomatology may worsen with increases in dietary protein. The cirrhosis may not always be evident in a liver biopsy (some regenerative nodules are large, and the biopsy may be taken from one of them). As mentioned earlier, the large number of mutations that give rise to the disease makes it impractical to use genetic analysis for diagnosis, but once the gene abnormality has been established in a given family, linkage studies may be used to identify other affected sibs.

In studies of large groups of patients, it has been established that copper deposition in the liver is the initial disturbance; over time it leads to cirrhosis. The hepatic stage of the disease precedes neurologic involvement. Cranial CT scans are abnormal even in the hepatic stage, and are invariably so when the neurologic disorder supervenes. The lateral ventricles and often the third ventricle are slightly enlarged, the cerebral and cerebellar sulci are widened, the brainstem appears shrunken, and the posterior parts of the lenticular nuclei, red nuclei, and dentate nuclei become hypodense (Ropper et al). With treatment, these radiologic changes become less marked (Williams and Walshe). Magnetic resonance imaging is an even more sensitive means of visualizing the structural changes, particularly those in the subcortical white matter, midbrain, pons, and cerebellum (Starosta-Rubinstein et al). In the MRI survey by Saatci and colleagues, the putamen was involved most frequently (though not invariably), showing a symmetrical T2 signal change in a laminar pattern; there was also an increase in T1 signal throughout the basal ganglia, particularly in the pallidum. Signal changes are almost universally found in the claustrum and also in the midbrain (pars compacta of the substantia nigra), dentate nucleus of the cerebellum, pons, and thalami. We have been impressed with a glassy diffuse and confluent signal abnormality on T2-weighted and FLAIR images in the hemispheral white matter in some cases—findings that were mistaken for multiple sclerosis.

Neuropathologic Changes These vary with the rate of progress of the disease. Exceptionally, in the rapidly advancing and fatal form, there is frank cavitation in the lenticular (putaminal and pallidal) nuclei, as observed in Wilson's original cases. In the more chronic form there is only shrinkage and a light-brown discoloration of these structures. Nerve cell loss and some degree of degeneration of myelinated fibers in lenticular nuclei, substantia nigra, and dentate nuclei are usually apparent. Subcortical myelin degeneration is found in some cases. More striking, however, is a marked hyperplasia of protoplasmic astrocytes (Alzheimer type II cells) in the cerebral cortex, basal ganglia, brainstem nuclei, and cerebellum.

Treatment Ideally treatment should be started before the appearance of neurologic signs; if this can be effected, the neurologic abnormalities can be prevented to a large extent. Treatment consists of (1) reduction of dietary copper to less than 1 mg/day, which can usually be accomplished by avoidance of copper-rich foods (liver, mushrooms, cocoa, chocolate, nuts, and shellfish), and (2) administration of the copper chelating agent D-penicillamine (1 to 3 g/day) by mouth, in divided doses. Pyridoxine 25 mg/day should be added in order to prevent anemia. The use of D-penicillamine is associated with a number of problems. Sensitivity reactions to the drug (rash, arthralgia, fever, leukopenia) develop in 20 percent of patients and require a temporary reduction of dosage or a course of prednisone to bring them under control. Reinstitution of drug therapy should then be undertaken, using low dosages (250 mg daily) and, later, small, widely spaced increases. If the patient is still sensitive to D-penicillamine or if severe reactions (lupus-like or nephrotic syndromes) occur, the drug should be discontinued and another chelating agent, triethylene tetramine (trientene) or ammonium tetrathiomolybdate, substituted. Zinc, which blocks the intestinal absorption of copper, is also a suitable substitute. It is given as zinc acetate, 100 to 150 mg daily in three to four divided doses at least 1 h before meals (Hoogenraad et al). The appropriate drug must then be continued for the patient's lifetime. Some women report improvement in neurologic symptoms during pregnancy, although there is no apparent change in copper metabolism during this time. In most patients, neurologic signs improve in response to decoppering agents. The Kayser-Fleischer rings disappear and liver function tests may return to normal, although the abnormalities of copper metabolism remain unchanged. In moderately severe and advanced cases, clinical improvement may not begin for several weeks or months despite full doses of D-penicillamine, and it is important to resist discontinuing the drug during this latent period. One of our patients had a complete remission of neurologic symptoms with penicillamine treatment and has remained symptom-free for 30 years.

It is also well known that the institution of treatment with penicillamine may induce an abrupt worsening of neurologic signs, and we have witnessed several such instances, including one that culminated fatally. Furthermore, in many of these patients, the lost function is never retrieved. Presumably this deterioration is due to the rapid mobilization of copper from the liver and its redistribution to the brain. The slow introduction of penicillamine may avoid this complication. The use of zinc or one of the newer agents mentioned above should be instituted as soon as neurologic deterioration becomes evident. In at least one reported case, new lesions of Wilson disease (shown by MRI) developed while the patient was receiving full doses of D-penicillamine and excellent decoppering of the liver had occurred (Brewer et al). In the few patients who develop epilepsy, the seizures become apparent soon after therapy is begun.

Many wilsonian patients with advanced liver disease have been subjected to liver transplantation, which is curative for the underlying metabolic defect. The degree of neurologic improvement varies; in some it has been remarkable and sustained, confirming that the hepatic defect is primary and that the brain is involved secondarily. According to Schilsky and coworkers, the main indication for transplantation is severe and progressive liver damage, but the operation has been used successfully in some patients with intractable neurologic deterioration and only mild signs of liver disease.

An important aspect of treatment is the screening of potentially affected relatives for abnormalities of serum copper and ceruloplasmin; if any relative is found to have the disease, penicillamine should be given indefinitely to prevent the emergence of neurologic symptoms. A full explanation of the dangers of ceasing the medication must be given, and compliance may need to be monitored.

Hereditary Deficiency of Ceruloplasmin This is a rare illness, quite similar to Wilson disease, occurring in patients with a recessively inherited deficiency of ceruloplasmin that is not simply a heterozygous form of Wilson disease (the mutation involves a different gene). Cirrhosis and Kayser-Fleischer rings are not features of the disease, but diabetes is common and extrapyramidal signs may or may not arise. Rather than copper, iron is deposited in the brain and liver (see discussion by Logan).

Hallervorden-Spatz Disease This disease is also known as *pigmentary degeneration of the globus pallidus, substantia nigra, and red nucleus*. It is inherited as an autosomal recessive trait. The onset is in late childhood or early adolescence, and it progresses slowly over a period of 10 or more years. The early signs are highly variable but are predominantly motor, both corticospinal (spasticity, hyperreflexia, Babinski signs) and extrapyramidal (rigidity, dystonia, and choreoathetosis). General deterioration of intellect is conjoined. In individual cases, ataxia and myoclonus have appeared at some phase of the illness. The spasticity and rigidity are most prominent in the legs, but in some instances they begin in the bulbar muscles, interfering with speech and swallowing, as happens in Wilson disease. We have observed patients who, over a period of years, exhibited only dystonia of the tongue or blepharospasm or arching of the back. The relationship of this restricted form to the complete syndrome remains unsettled. Eventually, the patient becomes almost completely inarticulate and unable to walk or use his arms. Optic atrophy has been mentioned in a few reports, but we have not observed it.

No known biochemical test corroborates the diagnosis. The characteristic deposits of iron in the basal ganglia have not been associated with a demonstrable abnormality of serum iron or of iron metabolism. It has, however, been reported that there is a high uptake of radioactive iron in the region of the basal ganglia following intravenous injection of labeled ferrous citrate (Vakili et al, Szanto and Gallyas). This technique may prove to be useful in diagnosis. CT scanning reveals hypodense zones in the lenticular nuclei, resembling those of hepatolenticular degeneration, sulfite oxidase deficiency, glutaric acidemia, and Leigh disease, although high-density lesions have been described in one autopsy-proven case of this disease (Tennison et al). The MRI findings are striking (Fig. 37-8). In T2-weighted images, the pallidum appears intensely black, with a small white area in its medial part ("eye of the tiger" sign; see also Savoiardo et al).

The neuropathology proves to be the most distinctive attribute of the disease. There is an intense brown pigmentation of the globus pallidus, substantia nigra (especially the anteromedial parts), and red nucleus. Granules and larger amorphous deposits of iron mixed with calcium stud the walls of small blood vessels or lie free in the tissue. A loss of neurons and medullated fibers occurs in the most affected regions. Another unique feature is the presence of swollen axon fragments, which resemble those of neuroaxonal dystrophy; for this reason, some neuropathologists regard Hallervorden-Spatz disease as a juvenile form of neuroaxonal dystrophy. Iron deposits are less conspicuous in the latter disease, leaving this interpretation in doubt. The significance of iron deposition is difficult to judge. To some extent, there is an increase of iron in the basal ganglia in other degenerative

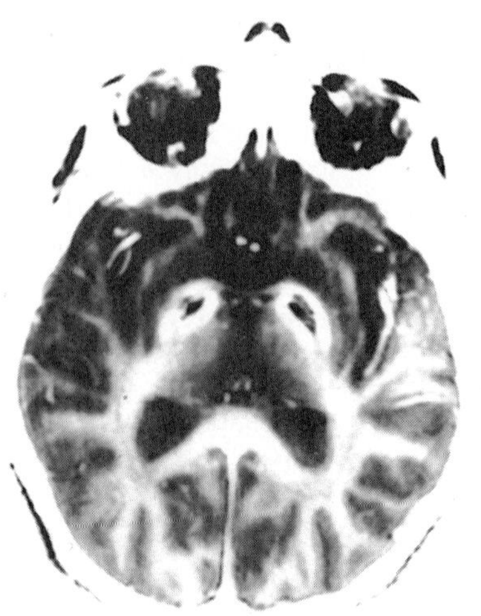

Figure 37-8

Hallervorden-Spatz disease. T2-weighted MR image showing areas of decreased signal intensity of the pallidum bilaterally (corresponding to iron deposition) and a central high signal area due to necrosis ("eye of the tiger" sign).

diseases. In Parkinson disease and striatonigral degeneration, for example, the deposition of iron is two to three times normal, presumably the result of degeneration of those tissues that are known to be rich in iron.

No treatment is known to be effective. Some of our patients responded temporarily to L-dopa, but the effect was slight. The use of chelating agents to reduce iron storage has not helped.

Differential Diagnosis of Wilson and Hallervorden-Spatz Diseases Disorders that must be differentiated from Wilson and Hallervorden-Spatz diseases are tardive dyskinesia, restricted forms of dystonia, adult and juvenile Parkinson disease and the related Segawa type of L-dopa-responsive dystonia, early-onset rigid form of Huntington chorea, status dysmyelinatus, Fahr disease (see below), Lafora-body disease, Leigh subacute necrotizing encephalomyelopathy, multiple sclerosis, dentatorubropallidoluysian degeneration, ceroid lipofuscinosis, polyglucosan disease, and other rare, presumably biochemical disorders of unknown type. Several of these have come to our attention, simulating at least some components of the extrapyramidal picture of Wilson disease but without evidence of liver involvement or copper abnormality. Difficult to categorize are diseases such as the one reported by Willvonseder and colleagues—in which a mild dementia, spastic dysarthria, paresis of vertical eye movements, gait disturbance, and splenomegaly came on during early adult life. Here abnormalities of copper metabolism were found (slightly decreased serum ceruloplasmin, copper turnover values in the range of those in heterozygous carriers of Wilson disease, but no increase in urinary copper excretion). The authors have seen several such patients. One such individual in her fifties with the subacute onset of parkinsonism, severe dysarthria, wilsonian facies, mild ataxia, and exaggerated facial and limb reflexes had symmetrical signal changes in the pallidum and dentate nucleus and diffusely through the white matter. She had some degree of improvement without treatment.

In families known to have Huntington chorea, children and some adults may be afflicted with a predominantly rigid-parkinsonian form (Westhpal variant). About 5 percent of all cases of Huntington chorea are of this "juvenile type." Rather than a movement disorder, this condition is marked by a slow decay in intellect, slurred speech, rigidity of the limbs, short-stepped gait, and flexion hypertonia of the limbs and trunk. Nevertheless, choreoathetosis does eventually appear in some cases. Ocular movements are full except for upward gaze. The disease is inexorably progressive, and eventually the patient becomes mute and rigidly immobile, with mouth agape, limbs flexed, and hands fisted in fixed, dystonic postures. Progressive supranuclear palsy may for a considerable period of time lack the characteristic limitation of vertical gaze, or it may be minimal. The main features are then axial rigidity, extension dystonia of the neck, and some rigidity and dystonia of the limbs. This differentiation has presented problems in diagnosis in a few of our patients whose illness began in their late forties or fifties. See Chap. 39 for discussion of the neuropathology and treatment of these two diseases.

Juvenile paralysis agitans was described by Ramsay Hunt in 1917. Judging by the descriptions, the resemblance to adult Parkinson disease is close. The course is slowly progressive. A familial incidence (two brothers aged 10 and 19) was reported by van Bogaert, but most cases have been sporadic. Postmortem examination has reportedly shown a shrinkage of the lenticular nuclei and a loss of large cells in the pallidum, but in an anatomic specimen from van Bogaert's laboratory (the age of onset was 7 years), cell loss was noted in the substantia nigra and pallidum. There was no evidence of encephalitis lethargica, and the pathologic findings differed from those of paralysis agitans, Wilson disease, Hallervorden-Spatz disease, and Huntington chorea. The authors are puzzled about this entity and have had no personal experience with it upon which to base an opinion.

It may be linked with the early-onset type of parkinsonism-dystonia that is responsive to L-dopa.

The status dysmyelinatus of Vogt and Vogt represents another obscure disease in which all myelinated fibers and nerve cells in the lenticular nuclei (both striatofugal and pallidofugal) disappear. The principal clinical features are extrapyramidal rigidity and, later, athetosis. Eventually the child becomes helpless, with limbs in weird postures and contorted by spasms. At one stage it is said to resemble Parkinson disease.

In isolated late-life cases of Lafora-body disease (discussed earlier in this chapter), there may be rigidity, akinesia, and tremor; but usually myoclonus, seizures, and dementia dominate the picture. Rarely, Leigh disease (described later in the chapter) gives rise to a slowly evolving extrapyramidal rigidity in late childhood or adolescence with bilateral cavitation of the putamen in CT scans.

The differential diagnosis of the aforementioned diseases presents certain difficulties. The recognition of Hallervorden-Spatz disease was for many years a problem for want of a satisfactory laboratory test, but this has been simplified by MRI, as noted above. The similarities between the diseases included under the rubric of the Parkinson syndrome are in general smaller than the differences. Wilson disease, for example, shares certain signs with Parkinson disease, yet the appearance of each is in general distinctive. The special qualities of the facial expression in Wilson disease—as well as the dysarthria, severe ataxic tremor, rigidity, and dystonia—are not readily confused with Parkinson disease. Furthermore, in several of the diseases in this category, there may be myoclonus and extrapyramidal signs such as choreoathetosis, dystonia, and so on, which are essential parts of the next category of syndromes. Therefore one must not insist that each disease conform strictly to a unique clinical syndrome.

The Syndrome of Dystonia and Generalized Chorea and Athetosis

As indicated in Chap. 4, we do not find the differences between dystonia and choreoathetosis to be fundamental. If one examines many patients with these involuntary movements, every gradation between the two is seen; not infrequently, the quicker, unpatterned involuntary movements of chorea and ballismus are seen as well. Even tremor and myoclonus may complicate the composite movement disorder. With reference to muscular tone in patients with athetosis and dystonia, there are unpredictable associations of hypertonia and hypotonia.

A number of inherited metabolic diseases, all of them rare, express themselves by the syndrome of chorea, athetosis, and dystonia.

The Lesch-Nyhan Syndrome and Hyperuricemia

This rare metabolic disease is inherited as an X-linked recessive trait. Although it carries the names of Lesch and Nyhan (1964), the occurrence of uricemia in association with spasticity and choreoathetosis in early childhood had been described earlier by Catel and Schmidt. Essentially it is a hereditary choreoathetosis with self-mutilation and hyperuricemia. The affected children appear normal at birth and usually develop on schedule up to 3 to 6 months of age. Maturational delay then sets in, initially with hypotonia that later gives way to hypertonia. Also, the patients' behavior becomes abnormal, with aggressiveness and compulsive actions. The compulsive self-mutilation, mainly of the lips, occurs early (during the second and third year), and spasticity, choreoathetosis, and tremor come later. Most of the children learn to walk. Speech is delayed and, once attained, it is dysarthric throughout life. Mental retardation is moderately severe. In patients more than 10 years of age, gouty tophi appear on the ears, and there is increasing risk from gouty nephropathy. The serum levels of uric acid are in the range of 7 to 10 mg/dL.

A deficiency of the enzyme hypoxanthine-guanine-phosphoribosyl transferase (HPRT) has been found in all typical cases of this disease. The HPRT gene lies on the X chromosome (Xq 26-q 27), and accurate diagnosis of affected males and carriers can be made by DNA analysis. As a result of this deficiency, hypoxanthine is either excreted or catabolized to xanthine and uric acid. The details of the biochemical abnormality responsible for CNS dysfunction are unclear.

In the differential diagnosis, one must consider nonspecific mental retardation with hand biting and other self-mutilations, athetosis from birth trauma, and encephalopathies with chronic renal disease. Hyperuricemia has also been reported in a family with spinocerebellar ataxia and deafness and in another with autism and mental retardation, neither of them with the enzymatic defect of Lesch-Nyhan disease. As mentioned earlier, there are several other disorders of purine and pyrimidine metabolism, some of them with hyperuricemia, that present with a neurologic syndrome like that of Lesch-Nyhan.

Treatment with the xanthine oxidase inhibitor allopurinol, which blocks the last steps of uric acid synthesis, reduces the uric acid in Lesch-Nyhan disease and prevents the uricosuric nephropathy, but it seems to have no effect on CNS symptoms. Guanosine 5-monophosphate and inosine 5-monophosphate, both of which are deficient in Lesch-Nyhan disease, have been replaced without benefit to the patient. Transitory success has been reported with the administration of 5-hydroxytryptophan in combination with L-dopa. Fluphenazine (Prolixin) is reported to have eliminated the self-mutilation after haloperidol (Haldol) had failed to do so. Behavior modification programs may be of some value.

Calcification of Vessels in Basal Ganglia and Cerebellum (Hypoparathyroidism and Fahr Syndrome)

Ferruginization and calcification of vessels in the basal ganglia occur to a slight degree in many elderly persons (and in other mammals) who are otherwise normal. The widespread use of CT scans and MRI has brought the condition to light with increasing frequency (Fig. 37-9). Usually it may be dismissed as an aging phenomenon of no clinical significance. When it occurs early in life and is of such degree as to be visible in plain films of the skull, it must always be regarded as abnormal. An adult case of this type was described by Fahr, so that his name is sometimes attached to this disorder, but it was known long before his publication appeared, and his account added little to our knowledge of the condition.

Many authors have called attention to a form of calcification of the basal ganglia and cerebellum in which choreoathetosis and rigidity are prominent. The clinical state may also take the form of a parkinsonian syndrome or bilateral athetosis. In several of our patients there was a unilateral choreoathetosis, which was replaced gradually by a parkinsonian syndrome. In two of our sporadic cases, the initial abnormality was a unilateral dystonia, responsive to L-dopa. Some patients have been mentally retarded, others intellectually intact. We have observed a familial form of basal ganglionic–cerebellar calcification inherited as an autosomal recessive trait. Its onset was in adolescence and early adult life and it presented clinically as a complex syndrome of choreoathetosis, tremor, ataxia, and dementia. The serum calcium levels in the aforementioned types of cases are usually normal, and there is no explanation of the calcification. This was also true of our cases. In a family described by Martinelli and colleagues, there was autosomal dominant inheritance and abnormal vitamin D metabolism.

In hypoparathyroidism (idiopathic or acquired) and pseudohypoparathyroidism (a rare familial disease characterized by the symptoms and signs of hypoparathyroidism in association with distinctive skeletal and developmental abnormalities), the diminution in ion-

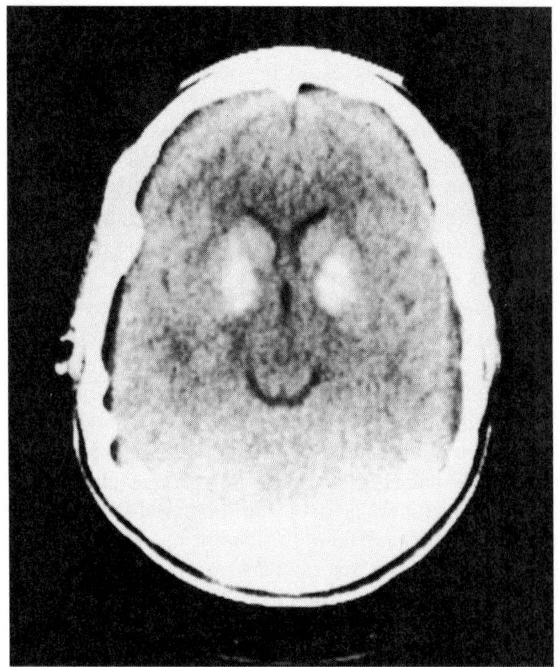

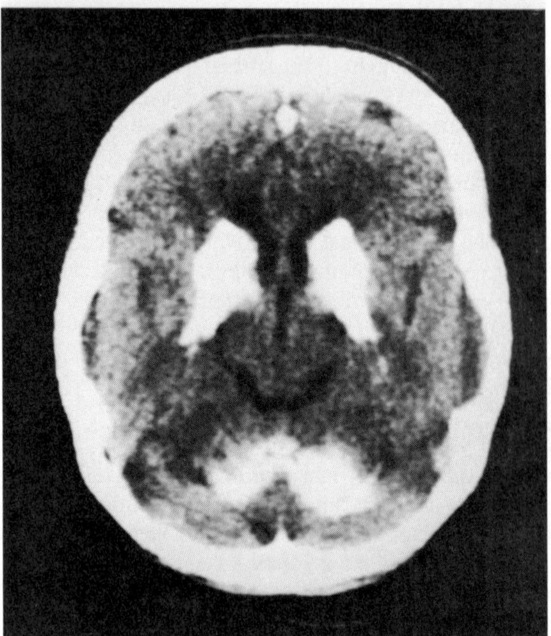

Figure 37-9

Above: *Idiopathic basal ganglionic calcification in a 25-year-old woman without symptoms or signs of cerebral disease.* Below: *Idiopathic basal ganglionic and cerebellar calcification, discovered 5 years after the onset of a slowly progressive rigid Parkinson syndrome in a 54-year-old woman.*

ized serum calcium induces not only tetany and seizures but sometimes choreoathetosis as well. This last symptom is presumably due to calcification of the basal ganglia, which occurs in about one-half of the patients. Also, in some instances there are signs of a cerebellar lesion.

Sly and colleagues have described the familial occurrence (21 cases in 12 families) of calcification in the caudate and lenticular nuclei, thalami, and frontal lobe white matter in association with osteopetrosis ("marble bones") and renal tubular acidosis. Clinically there were multiple cranial nerve palsies—including optic atrophy as well as psychomotor delay and learning disabilities—but no extrapyramidal signs. The cranial nerve palsies, which are due to bony encroachment in neural foramina, were much less severe than in the lethal form of osteopetrosis. The pattern of inheritance of this disease is autosomal recessive, and the basic abnormality was found to be a deficiency in carbonic anhydrase II in red blood corpuscles and probably in kidney and brain.

Other Metabolic Disorders Associated with Choreoathetosis and Dystonia Exceptionally, ceroid-lipofuscinosis of the Kufs type, G_{M1} gangliosidosis, late-onset metachromatic leukodystrophy, Niemann-Pick disease (type C), Hallervorden-Spatz disease, and Wilson disease may present with a syndrome of which dystonia or athetosis is an important component. Usually, other elements in the clinical picture are detectable, so that the correct diagnosis is seldom in doubt for long. Dal Canto and colleagues have described a variant of *neuronal ceroid-lipofuscinosis* in which a boy and girl of unrelated non-Jewish parents developed severe choreoathetosis and dystonia at 6 to 7 years of age. Intellectual deterioration, gait abnormality, and seizures were the other clinical features. Cerebral biopsy showed intraneuronal inclusions consisting of curvilinear bodies. These observations support the notion of nosologic heterogeneity among the nonglycolipid neuronal storage disorders.

Glutaric acidemia (type I) is another rare metabolic disorder, in which progressive choreoathetosis and dystonia are added to an intermittent acidemia. In some cases, ataxia of movement and a variable degree of mental retardation are also present. Glutaric acid is present in the urine, as are its metabolites 3-OH glutarate and glutamate. The basic defect is in glutaryl CoA dehydrogenase, which has been found in leukocytes, hepatocytes, and fibroblasts. Neuropathologically, there is loss of neurons in the caudate, putamen, and pallidum, with gliosis. A spongy change is said to affect the white matter.

Infants with glutaric acidemia often present with sudden episodes of acidosis, coma, and flaccidity, associated with a signal change on MRI, corresponding to the acute necrosis of nerve cells in the basal ganglia. These crises can be prevented and the infants can develop normally if the diagnosis is made before the development of neurologic signs (as in a sibling of an older affected child) and treatment is undertaken with a diet low in protein, particularly in tryptophan and lysine (Cho et al).

Finally, in regard to extrapyramidal motor disorders, it should be pointed out that those of acquired type are much more common than inherited ones. A prototype of athetosis is known to follow hypoxic encephalopathy of birth, leading to *état marbré* of the basal ganglia. This is the basis of the double athetosis syndrome that usually becomes manifest only after the first year of life and persists thereafter (page 1085). The Rh and ABO blood incompatibilities that induce erythroblastosis fetalis and *kernicterus* may also be the cause of a bilateral athetosis at about the same period of life, but this syndrome is distinguished by deafness and paralysis of upward gaze (page1085). The same is true of the Crigler-Najjar form of hereditary hyperbilirubinemia, in which kernicterus (with ataxia or athetosis) may rarely appear as late as childhood or adolescence; the defect is one of glucuronide-bilirubin conjugation.

A number of other rare diseases, which can only be classified as heredofamilial degenerations, must also figure in the differential diagnosis of choreoathetotic or dystonic syndromes. Torsion dystonia is the best-known example (page 1141). One familial variant with certain features of Parkinson disease and responsive to L-dopa (Segawa disease) is described in Chap. 39. A nonprogressive familial choreoathetosis with onset in early childhood has been reported by Pincus and Chutorian; here, cerebellar signs were usually conjoined but the intellect was spared. This syndrome is thought to be inherited as an autosomal recessive trait. We have also encountered families with an uncomplicated choreoathetosis, which is inherited as an autosomal dominant trait. A paroxysmal and sometimes kinesogenic form of *familial choreoathetosis* was recognized by Mount and Reback in 1940 and subsequently elaborated by Lance (page 83). One wonders in retrospect if some of these patients were dopamine-responsive. We have observed attacks of this kind in children with "cerebral palsy" as a manifestation of phenytoin (or carbamazepine) toxicity; lowering the dose of the drug terminated the attacks.

Sethi and coworkers have described an adult with dementia and choreoathetosis, simulating Huntington chorea, in whom episodic nausea, vomiting, and lethargy during childhood were due to propionic aciduria. The movement disorder did not appear until the patient was 28 years old. In others, the chorea begins in infancy and persists despite treatment. The authors have added this disease to the other inherited choreas (Huntington disease, neuroacanthocytosis, familial calcification of basal ganglia, Hallervorden-Spatz disease, dentatorubrothalamic atrophy).

Several of the above-mentioned diseases are presently classified as degenerative and are discussed in Chap. 39.

Bilateral Hemiplegia, Cerebral Blindness, and Other Manifestations of Decerebration (the Leukodystrophies)

Embodied in this heading are the features that characterize the aforementioned "white matter syndrome" by which most of the familial leukodystrophies are expressed. Of the several varieties of late-onset leukodystrophy, some are of unquestionable metabolic origin and others of uncertain status. As emphasized earlier, all differ from the cerebral gray matter diseases (poliodystrophies), which have a different mode of presentation—seizures, myoclonus, chorea, choreoathetosis, and tremor being prominent. Categorization of the entire group of leukodystrophies is based on the identification of symptoms and signs attributable to the interruption of tracts (corticospinal, corticobulbar, cerebellar peduncular, sensory, medial longitudinal fasciculi) and visual pathways (optic nerve, optic tract, geniculocalcarine), and the infrequency or absence of seizures, myoclonus, and spike-and-wave abnormalities in the EEG. However, this distinction is not always reliable, particularly in the later stages of the disease. The terms *metachromatic*, *sudanophilic*, *orthochromic*, etc., refer to the distinctive products of myelin degeneration and staining characteristics of the white matter in the individual leukodystrophies.

The syndrome of progressive spasticity and rigidity with spastic dysarthria and pseudobulbar palsy poses a difficult diagnostic problem. One's first impulse is to assume the presence of a corticospinal disorder, especially if tendon reflexes are brisk, but frequently the plantar reflexes are flexor and the facial reflexes are not enhanced. The opposite combination of Babinski signs and reduced or absent tendon reflexes, signifying a combination of corticospinal and peripheral nerve lesions, is highly characteristic of metachromatic leukoencephalopathy, adrenomyeloneuropathy, or subacute combined degeneration of the spinal cord (vitamin B_{12} deficiency). Unusual postures and a more plastic type of rigidity are consistent with an extrapyramidal condition. Such combinations, with mental backwardness and dementia, characterize the mild and late forms of *metachromatic leukodystrophy*—which may be taken as a paradigm of the leukoencephalopathies.

The leukodystrophies that become apparent only in later life pose another problem—the clinical and radiologic differentiation from multiple sclerosis. In cases of early onset, in which myelin has yet to be normally formed, the metabolic disturbance may result in hypomyelination (e.g., Pelizaeus-Merzbacher disease); by contrast, the process in adolescent or adult-onset cases is one of destruction of myelin already formed. In identifying the metabolic diseases, one is helped by the relative symmetry and steady progression of the clinical signs; the early onset of cognitive impairment (which is uncharacteristic of multiple sclerosis); and the symmetrical and massive degeneration of the cerebral white matter (in distinction to the asymmetrical and often multiple lesions of demyelinative disease).

Adrenoleukodystrophy (Sudanophilic Leukodystrophy with Bronzing of Skin and Adrenal Atrophy)

This combination of leukodystrophy and Addison disease, originally included under the rubric of Schilder disease, is now set apart as an independent metabolic encephalopathy. It is transmitted as an X-linked recessive trait with an incidence of 1 in 20,000 male births. The fundamental defect is an impairment in peroxisomal oxidation of very long chain fatty acids (VLCFA), leading to their accumulation in the brain and adrenal glands (Igarashi and associates). The deficient membrane protein is encoded by a gene that maps to chromosome X28, close to the gene for color vision.

The onset is usually between 4 and 8 years, sometimes later; in the commonest form of this disorder, only males are affected (probably sex-linked recessive). The signs of either the adrenal insufficiency or the cerebral lesion may be the first to appear. In the case of Siemerling and Creutzfeldt, the first recorded example of this disorder, bronzing of the skin of the hands appeared at 4 years of age; quadriparesis, with dysarthria and dysphagia (i.e., pseudobulbar palsy), became evident at 7 years; a single seizure occurred at 8 years; and by 9 years, shortly before death, the patient was *decerebrate* and unresponsive. In personally observed cases, the first abnormalities appeared at 9 to 10 years and took the form of episodic vomiting, decline in scholastic performance, and change in per-

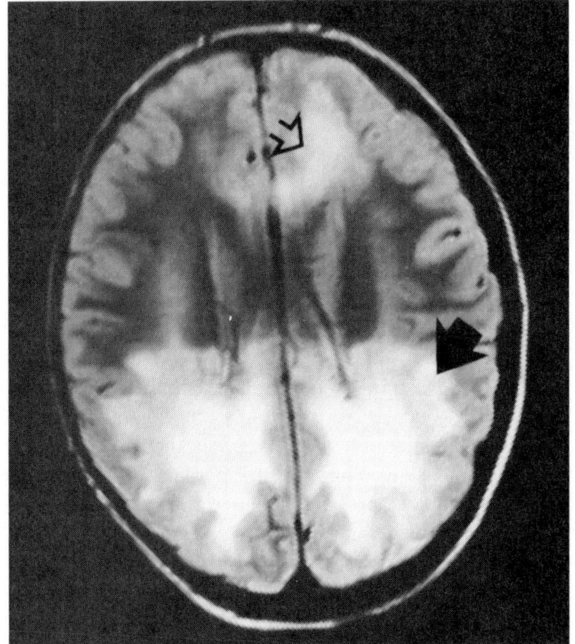

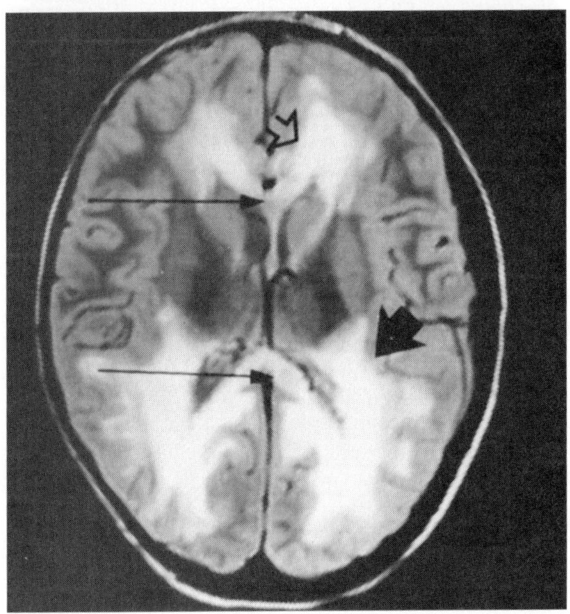

Figure 37-10

Adrenal leukodystrophy in a 7-year-old male. A confluent area of increased signal involves the occipital and parietal white matter; there is also asymmetrical involvement of the white matter in the frontal lobes. The lower image demonstrates the changes on a lower cut, including involvement of both the anterior and posterior portions of the corpus callosum (long-stemmed arrows). (From Bisese JH: Cranial MRI. New York, McGraw-Hill, 1991, by permission.)

sonality, with silly, inappropriate giggling and crying. After a time, severe vomiting and even an episode of circulatory collapse occurred, following which the gait became unsteady and arms ataxic, with an action or intention tremor. Only then did increasing pigmentation of the oral mucosa and the skin around nipples and over elbows, knees, and scrotum become evident. *Cortical blindness* followed in some instances. The late stages were marked by bilateral hemiplegia (at first asymmetrical), pseudobulbar paralysis, blindness, deafness, and impairment of all higher cerebral functions. The severity of the disease varies. We are caring for several adult men in whom the cerebral symptoms have been mild, allowing for high-level cognitive function, the main manifestations consisting of personality quirks, spastic gait, urinary difficulty, testicular insufficiency, and baldness. Two of the men related the characteristic history of a male sibling who died in childhood, ostensibly of Addison disease.

Griffin and coworkers have described a spinal-neuropathic form of the disease (adrenomyeloneuropathy). In their patients, evidence of adrenal insufficiency was present since early childhood, but only in the third decade of life did a progressive spastic paraparesis and a relatively mild polyneuropathy develop. The spasticity is occasionally asymmetrical, and the gait may have an ataxic component. This neurologic picture, in mild form and without adrenal insufficiency, is the manner in which the disease may present in female carriers of the gene abnormality.

Moser and colleagues, using clinical and biochemical criteria, have identified the following subtypes: (1) familial instances of Addison disease without neurologic involvement in males, but with a mild spastic paraparesis in females; (2) progressive degeneration of cerebral white matter in young males, often with cortical blindness—the classic type (Fig. 37-10); (3) an intermediate form in juvenile or young adult males with cerebral and spinal involvement; (4) a progressive spinal cord tract degeneration in adult males; (5) a chronic nonprogressive spastic paraparesis in *heterozygous females*; and (6) possibly, in male infants, a form originating at birth (e.g., Zellweger disease).

Illustrating the variability in presentation among kindreds, Marsden and colleagues and, subsequently, Kobayashi and colleagues described a familial spinocerebellar syndrome, and Ohno and associates have reported a sporadic instance of adrenoleukodystrophy presenting as olivopontocerebellar atrophy. Moser found cerebral forms alone in 30 percent, adrenomyeloneuropathy alone in 20 percent, and combined childhood cerebral and myelopathic forms in the remaining half. Regarding the heterozygotes, neurologic manifestations have been said to develop in up to 50 percent, but in our experience with siblings of affected patients, the figure has been lower. The onset of a spastic paraparesis tends to occur later, usually in the third or fourth decade, and progression tends to be slow, but an explosive onset has been reported. As already mentioned, multiple sclerosis is the main consideration in differential diagnosis, particularly since 20 percent of heterozygotes have white matter changes on cerebral MRI. Overt adrenal insufficiency is rare in female carriers, but scalp hair may be scant as a subtle manifestation of adrenal dysfunction.

The specific laboratory marker of the disease is an excess of VLCFAs, in particular hexacosanoic acids, in plasma, erythrocytes, leukocytes, or cultured fibroblasts; this reflects the basic biochemical fault in this disease, namely defective fatty acid oxidation within the peroxisomes. If skin fibroblasts and plasma testing are both performed, 93 percent of female carriers will show the abnormal VLCFA. Cranial MRI is abnormal in the majority of patients with cerebral symptoms and in a proportion of others.

Other important laboratory findings are low serum sodium and chloride levels and elevated potassium levels—reflecting the atrophy of the adrenal glands. The latter results in reduced excretion of corticosteroids, low serum cortisol levels, and lack of rise in 17-hydroxyketosteroids after ACTH stimulation. Adrenal insufficiency may be the only manifestation of the disease. The CSF protein may be elevated.

In classic instances, massive degeneration of the myelin occurs, often asymmetrically in various parts of the cerebrum, brainstem, optic nerves, and sometimes spinal cord (Fig. 37-10). Degradation products of myelin are visible in macrophages in recent lesions—namely, sudanophilic demyelination. Axis cylinders are damaged, but to a lesser degree. The cortex of the adrenal glands is atrophic, and the cells and invading histiocytes contain an abnormal lipid material. The testes show marked interstitial fibrosis and atrophy of the seminiferous tubules. Electron microscopically, the macrophages of the brain and adrenals and the Leydig cells of the testes contain characteristic lamellar cytoplasmic inclusions.

Adrenal replacement therapy prolongs life and occasionally effects a partial neurologic remission. A diet enriched with monounsaturated fatty acids and devoid of long-chain fatty acids appears to slow the progress of the disease in some cases. Bone marrow transplantation, to date performed in over 50 children, has been the only treatment shown to stabilize the disease and reverse some of the MRI changes. The review by van Geel and colleagues, summarizing current diagnosis and treatment, is recommended.

Metachromatic Leukodystrophy (MLD) This form of leukodystrophy has already been described in relation to the inherited metabolic disorders of late infancy and early childhood (page 1012). It is mentioned here again to emphasize the point that the disease may have its onset at almost any age. Juvenile forms may begin between 4 and 12 years and adult forms between the mid teens and the seventh decade. Some of the sporadic cases reported in the adult have probably been examples of cerebral multiple sclerosis, but we have seen, as have others, cases of MLD appearing as late as middle adult life. In all cases, the clinical picture is one of intellectual decline with spastic weakness, hyperreflexia, Babinski signs, and stiff, short-stepped gait. As the disease progresses over a period of 3 to 5 years, there is a loss of vision and speech, then of hearing, and finally a state of virtual decerebration.

In some of these cases it is impossible to distinguish the white matter disease from that of Pelizaeus-Merzbacher and of Cockayne, described in the preceding section.

Cerebrotendinous Xanthomatosis This rare disease is probably transmitted by an autosomal recessive gene. It usually begins in late childhood, with cataracts and xanthomata of tendon sheaths and lungs. As it progresses, difficulty in learning, impairment of retentive memory, and deficits in attention and visuospatial perception (the earliest neurologic manifestations) give way to dementia, ataxic or ataxic-spastic gait, dysarthria and dysphagia, and polyneuropathy. In the late stages (after 5 to 15 years), the patient becomes bedfast and helpless; death occurs at 20 to 30 years of age. In other cases the clinical course is much more benign. Neuropathologic examination shows masses of crystalline cholesterol in the brainstem and cerebellum and sometimes in the spinal cord, with symmetrical destruction of myelin in the same areas. The lesions are visible by CT scanning and MRI.

The basic defect is in the synthesis of primary bile acids, leading to an increased hepatic production of cholesterol and cholestanol, which accumulate in brain and tendons. The serum cholesterol levels are normal in most cases but as high as 450 mg/dL in others. The tendon xanthomas contain cholesterol, of which 4 to 9 percent is cholestanol (dihydrocholesterol). Cholestanol levels in the serum and red cells are increased. The same elevated levels are found in heterozygotes.

In response to long-term treatment with chenodeoxycholic acid, 750 mg daily, the corticospinal and cerebellar signs and dementia receded in 10 of 17 patients followed by Berginer and coworkers. This drug corrects the defective synthesis of bile acids and restores the low level of chenodeoxycholic acid. Ideally treatment should begin before the neurologic symptoms appear (Meiner et al).

Strokes in Association with Inherited Metabolic Diseases

In Chap. 34 it was remarked that strokes occur from time to time in children and young adults, often due to inherited disorders of the clotting system typified by protein C deficiency, but also due to a number of other metabolic derangements. Among the many causes, three metabolic diseases must always be considered in the diagnosis of such cases: homocystinuria, Fabry disease, and sulfite oxidase deficiency. Other less common ones are Tangier disease and familial hypercholesterolemia. Stroke in young persons is also a central feature of the mitochondrial disorder MELAS, discussed further on in this chapter.

Homocystinuria This aminoaciduria is inherited as an autosomal recessive trait and simulates Marfan disease. Tall, slender habitus, great length of limbs, sometimes scoliosis and arachnodactyly (long, spidery fingers and toes), thin and rather weak muscles, knock-knees, highly arched feet, and kyphosis are the typical skeletal features. Sparse, blond, brittle hair, malar flush, and livedo reticularis are common dermal manifestations, and a dislocation of one or both lenses (usually downward) may occur, imparting a tremulous appearance to the irides (iridodenesis). The only neurologic abnormality is mental retardation, usually of mild degree, which sets this syndrome apart from Marfan disease, in which intellect is unimpaired.

Blood vessel changes—thickening and fibrosis of the coronary, cerebral, and renal arteries—tend to appear later in the illness. An abnormality of platelets favoring clot formation and thrombosis of cerebral arteries has been observed. Some patients have died of coronary occlusions during adolescence, and a myocardial lesion may be the source of emboli to cerebral arteries.

Homocystine is elevated in the blood, CSF, and urine. This is due to an inherited cystathionine synthase deficiency that results in an inadequacy of cystathionine formation, a substance essential to many tissues including the brain. This may be the explanation of the mental retardation. Plasma methionine levels are also elevated. The infarcts in the brain are clearly related to thrombotic and embolic arterial occlusions. The administration of a low-methionine diet and large doses (50 to 500 mg) of pyridoxine (a cystathionine synthase coenzyme) reduces the excretion of homocystine. If vascular lesions have occurred, anticoagulants probably prevent further occlusions.

Homocystinuria may also be an expression of 5,10-methylenetetrahydrofolate reductase deficiency. Again, the clinical manifestations consist of multiple cerebrovascular lesions, dementia, epilepsy, and polyneuropathy. The last is believed to be due to a coincidental folic acid deficiency, but in some cases it may have been caused by chronic phenytoin administration (Nishimura et al).

Fabry Disease (Anderson-Fabry Disease, Hereditary Dystopic Lipidosis) This disease, also known as *angiokeratoma corporis diffusum*, is inherited as an X-linked recessive trait. It occurs in complete form in men and in incomplete form in female carriers. The primary deficit is in the enzyme α-galactosidase A, the result of which is the accumulation of ceramide trihexoside in endothelial, perithelial, and smooth muscle cells of the blood vessels as well as in renal tubular and glomerular cells and other viscera and in nerve cells in many parts of the nervous system (hypothalamic and amygdaloid nuclei, substantia nigra, reticular and other nuclei of the brainstem, anterior and intermediolateral horns of the spinal cord, sympathetic and dorsal root ganglia). The disease becomes manifest clinically in childhood or adolescence, with intermittent lancinating pains and dysesthesias of the extremities. A notable feature of these pains is their evocation by fever, hot weather, and vigorous exercise. Usually there is no sensory loss, but autonomic disturbances have been recorded in a series of our cases. Later, the diffuse vascular involvement leads to hypertension, renal damage, cardiomegaly, and myocardial ischemia. Thrombotic infarctions occur in the brain during early adult years. The characteristic angiokeratomas tend to be most prominent periumbilically and resemble small angiomas that obliterate slightly with pressure. Enzyme replacement is now available. Desnick and colleagues have reviewed the neurologic, neuropathologic, and biochemical findings in this disease. Its painful neuropathic features are discussed on page 1422.

Sulfite Oxidase Deficiency This disorder was discussed briefly with the neonatal metabolic disorders (page 933). The occurrence of stroke as a complication of this disorder was placed on record by Shih and colleagues. A child 4.5 years of age, whose development had been retarded since birth (seizures and opisthotonos had been present), became hemiplegic. Another unrelated child, supposedly normal until 2 years of age, entered the hospital with fever, confusion, generalized seizures, right hemiplegia, and aphasia (infantile hemiplegia); subluxation of the lenses (upward) was discovered later. There was an increased level of sulfite and thiosulfite and an abnormal amino acid, S-sulfocysteine, in the blood. One child appeared to respond to a low-sulfur–amino acid diet.

Changes in Behavior and Intellect as Manifestations of Inherited Metabolic Disease

Although rare among the large numbers of maladjusted, sociopathic, and psychotic adolescents, certain metabolic diseases may cause serious disturbances of mental life and behavior. The diagnosis and management of these metabolic diseases are so special that some special remarks are appropriate.

All the metabolic diseases of late childhood and adolescence may share to some degree the property of deranging behavior, thinking, feeling, and emotional reactions. The most obvious and easily detectable of these derangements are in the cognitive sphere, i.e., reduction in the capacity to learn and remember, to calculate, to solve problems, and to exercise verbal skills. Impulsivity, loss of self-control, and antisocial behavior are the most troubling behavioral abnormalities. Certain forms of these impairments are attributable to integrated systems of modules of cerebral neurons and are recognized as special neurologic deficits, such as the amnesic state, aphasia, dyscalculia, and visual-perceptual disorientation. Each of these phenomena has its own cerebral anatomy, as pointed out in Chap. 22, and the state known as dementia comprises various degrees and combinations of these abnormalities.

Intellectual functions are little developed in early childhood; it is therefore difficult to decide upon normal qualities of the mind for this age group. Slowness in learning, in acquiring language functions, and so on may be interpreted loosely as mental retardation. At this age these intellectual functions have not developed sufficiently to permit recognition of their regression. Only in late childhood do mental retardation and dementia become clearly distinguishable. Far less tangible are subtle changes in personality and behavior that must always be judged against the standards of the cultural group of which the patient is a member.

The principle that most neuropsychiatrists follow in selecting from the large mass of maladjusted adolescents those with a metabolic brain disease is that such a condition will sooner or later cause a *regression in cognitive and intellectual functions*. Schizophrenia and manic-depressive psychosis and the sociopathies and character disorders do so little or not at all. This is not to say that personality changes and emotional disturbances do not occur in the metabolic encephalopathies; of course they do. However, their recognition depends more on the demonstration of failing memory, impaired thinking, inability to learn, and loss of verbal and arithmetic abilities, many of which are measured quantitatively by intelligence tests.

If one reviews all the diseases described in this chapter and selects those that may demonstrate *early regression of cognitive function in association with personality change and alteration of behavior*—diseases that may for a time be unaccompanied by other neurologic abnormalities—the following merit special consideration:

1. Wilson disease
2. Hallervorden-Spatz pigmentary degeneration
3. Lafora-body myoclonic epilepsy
4. Late-onset neuronal ceroid-lipofuscinosis (Kufs form)
5. Juvenile and adult Gaucher disease (type III)
6. Some of the mucopolysaccharidoses
7. Adrenoleukodystrophy
8. Metachromatic leukodystrophy
9. Adult G_{M2} gangliosidosis
10. Mucolipidosis I (type I sialidosis)
11. Nonwilsonian copper disorder (hereditary ceruloplasmin deficiency)

In each of the above diseases, dementia and personality disorder may gradually develop and persist for many months, even a year or two, before other neurologic signs appear. One must look carefully for the earliest signs of movement disorders and other neurologic abnormalities, which greatly clarify the diagnostic problem. A safe rule is to assume that if there are mental and personality changes in each of the above diseases, other subtle neurologic disorders coexist. The common use of neuroleptic drugs, causing tardive dyskinesia, is the major obstacle to applying this rule.

ADULT FORMS OF INHERITED METABOLIC DISEASES

The increasing range and precision of biochemical and cytologic tests has brought to light a number of inherited metabolic diseases that sometimes have their onset in adult life. Such disorders, while uncommon, nevertheless are important because they must be considered in the differential diagnosis of degenerative diseases and atrophies, for which explanations are beginning to be found. Also to be considered in the differential diagnosis is an array of mitochondrial disorders, to be discussed further on in this chapter.

In the last decade or two, the authors have personally observed or have otherwise come to know of examples of the following metabolic diseases, the onset of which was in late adolescence or adult life:

1. Metachromatic leukoencephalopathy
2. Adrenoleukodystrophy
3. Globoid body leukodystrophy (Krabbe disease)
4. Kufs form of lipid storage disease
5. G_{M2} gangliosidosis
6. Wilson disease
7. Leigh disease
8. Gaucher disease
9. Niemann-Pick disease
10. Mucopolysaccharide encephalopathy
11. Mucolipidosis type I
12. Polyneuropathies (Andrade disease, Fabry disease, porphyria, Refsum disease)
13. Mitochondrial diseases, particularly progressive external ophthalmoplegia and Leigh disease
14. CADASIL (see page 879)

In the encephalopathic forms of the metabolic and mitochondrial diseases (described below), the diagnosis is usually made only after symptoms have been present for months or years, the disease having been mistaken for some other condition. For example, one of our patients with metachromatic leukodystrophy, a 30-year-old man, began failing in college years and was later unsuccessful in holding a job because of carelessness and mistakes in his work and indifference, irritability, and stubborness (clearly traceable to a mild dementia). Only when Babinski signs and loss of tendon reflexes in the legs were detected was the diagnosis entertained for the first time. By then he had been ill for nearly 10 years. Bosch and Hart described a patient with the onset of dementia at 62 years of age and drew attention to 27 other cases of adult-onset metachromatic leukoencephalopathy. Overt signs of neuropathy are usually lacking in adult-onset cases, but EMG and sural nerve biopsy will disclose the characteristic abnormalities. One of our adult patients with Wilson disease had been committed to a psychiatric hospital because of his paranoid tendencies and fighting with his family; the presence of a tremor and mild rigidity of the limbs had been attributed at first to phenothiazine drugs. In some of Griffin's cases of adrenomyeloneuropathy, a spastic weakness of the legs and sensory ataxia, progressing over several years, were the main clinical manifestations; a spinocerebellar degeneration was suspected. One of our patients with Kufs lipid storage disease began to deteriorate mentally in early adult life and only later showed an increasing rigidity with athetotic posturing of limbs and difficulty in walking; he succumbed to his disease after more than 10 years.

Cerebellar ataxia, polymyoclonus, and progressive blindness have been observed in several adolescents and adults with a variant of G_{M2} gangliosidosis; cherry-red macular spots provided the clue to diagnosis. Several such cases have been reported in the last decade, particularly among the Japanese (Miyatake et al). We have observed two adult patients with progressive spinal muscular atrophy who proved to have the hexosaminidase deficiency of Tay-Sachs disease; the process was clinically indistinguishable from motor neuron disease (Kugelberg-Welander disease in adolescents) but might have the additional features of ataxia and an intermittent and atypical psychosis.

Dementia, optic atrophy, mild cerebellar ataxia, and corticospinal signs have been features of several personally observed patients with Leigh disease who survived in a relatively helpless state for nearly 20 years. Kalimo and associates have reported a similar family. An asymmetrical corticospinal syndrome with areflexia had advanced so slowly in one of our cases of Krabbe disease that she was not disabled until past her sixtieth year.

Another of our patients, an adolescent with severe diffuse myoclonus and seizures and slight intellectual deterioration, was found after several years to have one of the rare variants of Gaucher disease. Another with dementia, rigidity, choreoathetosis, slight cerebellar ataxia, and Babinski signs had a variant of Niemann-Pick disease. For many years we had under observation a family with Gaucher disease, several members of which developed seizures, generalized myoclonus, supranuclear gaze palsies, and cerebellar ataxia in early adult life (Winkelman et al). Rarely, Gaucher disease may be associated with an early and severe parkinsonian syndrome.

We have had the experience of finding laboratory evidence of adrenal insufficiency in several young men with white matter lesions of the frontal lobes and other parts of the cerebrum; there was no bronzing of the skin, and earlier a diagnosis of multiple sclerosis or Schilder disease had been made. Eldridge and coworkers have described a large kindred with widespread noninflammatory degeneration of the cerebral and cerebellar white matter; individual members were thought to have multiple sclerosis before a pattern of autosomal dominant inheritance became evident (possibly CADASIL, page 879). Such cases are likely to be found in multiple sclerosis clinics. Adrenoleukodystrophy presenting in adult life as a spinocerebellar or olivopontocerebellar syndrome has already been mentioned.

These rare forms of inherited metabolic disease are notable for their chronicity and for the early prominence of a particular neurologic symptom or syndrome. Once the disease is established, however, there is nearly always evidence of involvement of multiple neuronal systems, reflected in a subtle or overt dementia, character disorder, or signs referable to cerebellar, pyramidal, extrapyramidal, visual, and peripheral nerve structures. *This multiplicity of neuronal system involvement is much more a feature of heritable metabolic disease than of degenerative disease, and the finding of such involvement should always provoke a search for an inherited metabolic disorder.* The dictum that tract involvement (corticospinal, cerebellar, peduncular, sensory, optic nerve) indicates a leukodystrophy and that "gray matter" signs (seizures, myoclonus, dementia, retinal lesions) indicate a poliodystrophy is useful mainly in the early stages of a disease. Some of the lysosomal storage diseases affect both galactolipids (galactocerebrosides and sulfatides) and gangliosides; hence both white and gray matter are involved.

In concluding this discussion, which classifies the inherited monogenetic metabolic diseases in accordance with their salient clinical characteristics, the careful reader will appreciate its artificiality. Nearly every one of the diseases of each category may present some neurologic abnormality other than the ones we have emphasized, so that the potential number of variations is almost limitless. However, it is hoped that the plan presented here—of thinking of these diseases in reference to age periods and syndromic relationships—will be of heuristic value and facilitate clinical study of this extremely difficult part of neurologic medicine.

MITOCHONDRIAL DISORDERS

The diseases included under this heading are so diverse and involve so many parts of the nervous system that the clinical entities by which they are identified cannot be easily addressed in any one part of the book. In their heterogeneity and complex overlapping relationships, these diseases are unlike the more common, discrete clinical entities that are caused by nuclear genetic mutations. As stated in the introduction to this chapter, the neural damage in the mitochondrial diseases appears to derive from defects in the energy-producing systems of many cells and organs. This diversity is evident not only in the details of clinical presentation but also in the age at which symptoms first become apparent and the presence or absence of dysmorphic features, and—what is most intriguing—sometimes in the abrupt onset of illness. Most of this variability is understandable from the principles of mitochondrial genetics already outlined. Fortunately for the clinician, the most important of these diseases are expressed in several recognizable core syndromes and a few variants thereof. It is this perspective that we have found to be most useful clinically. A number of acronyms formed from the initial letters of the main clinical features have been used to designate these syndromes (MERRF, MELAS, PEO, NARP, etc.), as summarized in Table 37-7. The addition of certain dysmorphic features, including short stature, endocrinopathies, particularly diabetes, and a number of other systemic abnormalities discussed further on, aids in diagnosis (see page 1045).

The best-characterized member of this group of diseases is a symmetrical proximal myopathy that can occur in isolation or in combination with CNS dysfunction. In 1966, Shy and coworkers described the histochemical and electron-microscopic abnormalities of the muscle mitochondria in a childhood myopathy, which they called *megaconial* (meaning marked enlargement of the mitochondria) or *pleoconial* (an abundance of mitochondria). Later this change came to be known as "ragged red fibers," so named because of the subsarcolemmal and intermyofibrillar collections of membranous (mitochondrial) material in many of the type 1 (red) fibers, visualized in Gomori trichrome–stained sections of frozen muscle. This change in muscle, sometimes asymptomatic, is a manifestation of several of

Table 37-7
The major categories of mitochondrial disorders

Syndrome	*Common mitochondrial gene mutation*	*Ragged red fibers*	*Lactic acidosis*
Ragged red fiber polymyopathy	Point mutation at 3250	+	−
Progressive external ophthalmoplegia (PEO) and Kearns-Sayre variants	Heteroplasmic deletions or point mutation at 3243	−	−
Leigh syndrome, fatal lactic acidosis and NARP	Point mutation at 8993	−	+
Myoclonic epilepsy and ragged red fibers in muscle (MERRF)	Point mutation at 8344	+ (usually)	+/−
Mitochondrial encephalomyopathy, lactic acidosis, and stroke (MELAS)	Point mutation at 3243	+	+
Leber optic neuropathy	Point mutation at 3460, 4160, or 11778	−	−
Myoneural-gastrointestinal encephalopathy	Unknown (maternal inheritance)	+	−

Key: + = present; − = absent; NARP = neuropathy with proximal weakness, ataxia, and retinitis pigmentosa.

the mitochondrial diseases of the nervous system as well. At the same time, it should be understood that most neurologic disorders designated as "mitochondrial" show no histologic or ultrastructural abnormalities in muscle mitochondria. Many patients with mitochondrial abnormalities show elevations of lactate or lactate-to-pyruvate ratios in the blood and CSF as a result of the respiratory chain abnormalities. These elevations are most prominent after exercise, infection, or alcohol ingestion, and—in some conditions—are capable of inducing recurrent ketoacidotic coma, which may be the main manifestation of a mitochondrial disease. Leigh syndrome and MELAS also have a marked tendency to exhibit elevations of lactate; however, the diagnosis of either cannot be excluded in the presence of normal levels, even after provocation by exercise. Using phosphorus MRI scans, one can compare levels of inorganic phosphate to phosphocreatine levels in muscle; in genetic muscle diseases of several types, this ratio increases but it is highest in those of mitochondrial origin.

Although the mitochondrial diseases are considered here as a group, individual ones are of necessity mentioned in other chapters. Thus, the syndrome that combines epilepsy, deafness, and developmental delay with ragged red muscle fibers (myoclonic epilepsy with ragged red fibers, or MERRF) has already been discussed in Chap. 16, on epilepsy. The syndrome of progressive external ophthalmoplegia (PEO) was discussed with other abnormalities of eye movement (Chap. 14); lactic acidosis and stroke-like episodes (MELAS) was considered in Chap. 34, with the cerebrovascular diseases; and Leber hereditary optic neuropathy, with other causes of visual loss (Chap. 13). The Leigh syndrome, a symmetrical subacute necrotizing encephalomyelopathy, usually with lactic acidosis, also has a number of complex relationships—in this instance, different degrees of a mitochondrial abnormality cause several disparate clinical presentations. For each of the aforementioned core syndromes, a wider clinical experience will bring to light an individual or a family in whom some other mitochondrial disorder is associated. Also, fragmentary subsyndromes of each of the main types are known to occur, with onset from childhood to early adult life. It serves little purpose, therefore, to catalogue all of these linkages. Only the main and best characterized syndromes listed in Table 37-7 are described. The most common combinations have been of Kearns-Sayre syndrome with MELAS or with MERRF, progressive ophthalmoplegia with MERRF, and MERRF with MELAS.

We prefer to avoid the issue of what best defines a mitochondrial disorder—its genetic defect, the biochemical disorder, or the clinical syndrome. The clinician assigns this term to particular combinations of a genetic mutation of mitochondrial DNA and certain clinical features that define syndromes; the biochemical changes are best viewed as markers of the inadequate energy-producing mechanisms of the mitochondrial machinery.

Mitochondrial Myopathies

The mildest form of mitochondrial myopathy may cause only a benign proximal weakness that tends to be more severe in the arms. Exercise intolerance is reported in half or more of these patients. There are adult-onset variants, but careful questioning usually elicits a lifelong exercise intolerance (weakness, discomfort, exertional dyspnea, and tachycardia), which is so slowly progressive that the patient can lead a relatively normal life for decades. Rare patterns include a fascioscapulohumeral or limb-girdle pattern of weakness as well as a recurrent exertional myoglobinuria. Some patients develop progressive external ophthalmoplegia (PEO) several years after the weakness becomes evident. Several mutations have been associated with a pure or predominant myopathy syndrome, the most common being located at position 3250 of the mitochondrial genome. Variants such as combined skeletal weakness and cardiomyopathy are referable to other loci.

At the more severe end of the spectrum is an infantile myopathy in which weakness and lactic acidosis become evident in the first week of life and are fatal by 1 year. Many of these patients and some families have a history of renal dysfunction combined with weakness of early onset. The muscle tissue shows numerous ragged red fibers, and cytochrome oxidase activity is virtually absent. DiMauro and others have described an apparently reversible form, which requires ventilatory support and gastric feeding but improves clinically with increasing age of the patient; the lactic acidosis is lost by age 2 or 3 years. In the childhood cases, the deficiencies in cytochrome oxidase suggest a defect in mitochondrial genes, but none has been found.

The histologic feature that unites the mitochondrial myopathies is the presence of so-called ragged red fibers. This finding in other mitochondrial diseases, such as PEO and MERRF, gives added credibility to the diagnosis of a mitochondrial disorder in any case where weakness is coupled with exercise intolerance, excess lactate, and a family history of similar problems. Also, the presence of ragged red fibers differentiates the mitochondrial myopathies from the glycogenoses. It bears repeating, however, that ragged red fibers are rare in infants and young children, even in those with confirmed mitochondrial disease.

Progressive External Ophthalmoplegia and Kearns-Sayre Syndrome

The combination of progressive ptosis and ophthalmoplegia is a common manifestation of mitochondrial disease. Usually there is no diplopia or strabismus or at most only transient diplopia, despite slightly dysconjugate gaze. We have been impressed at how long the illness can exist before it brings the patient to a physician.

Progressive external ophthalmoplegia bears a close relationship to the Kearns-Sayre syndrome of retinitis pigmentosa (onset before age 20), ataxia, heart block, and elevated CSF protein; sensorineural deafness, seizures, or pyramidal signs may be added (page 1502). The CNS syndromes of MELAS or MERRF (see further on) may also be combined occasionally with PEO.

Subacute Necrotizing Encephalomyelopathy (Leigh Disease; SNE)

This is a familial or sporadic mitochondrial disorder with a wide range of clinical manifestations. Some cases display a maternal pattern of inheritance. The onset in more than half the cases is in the first year of life, mostly before the sixth month, but late-onset varieties, with an even greater heterogeneity of presentation in young adulthood, are also known. As with some of the other mitochondrial diseases, the onset of neurologic symptoms is usually subacute or abrupt, sometimes precipitated by a febrile episode or a surgical operation.

In infants, loss of head control and other recent motor acquisitions, hypotonia, poor sucking, anorexia and vomiting, irritability and continuous crying, generalized seizures, and myoclonic jerks constitute the usual clinical picture. If the onset is in the second year, there are difficulties in walking, ataxia, dysarthria, psychomotor regression, tonic spasms, characteristic respiratory disturbances (episodic hyperventilation, especially during infections, and periods of apnea, gasping, and quiet sobbing), external ophthalmoplegia, nystagmus, and disorders of gaze (like those of Wernicke disease), paralysis of deglutition, and abnormal movements of the limbs (particularly dystonia but also jerky, choreiform movements and ataxia). Mild cases, showing developmental delay, have been mistaken for cerebral palsy. Peripheral nerves are involved in some cases (areflexia, weakness, atrophy, and slowed conduction velocities); in a few, autonomic failure is the most prominent feature. In some children the disease is episodic; in others it is intermittently progressive and quite protracted, with exacerbation of neurologic symptoms in association with nonspecific infections. The CSF is usually normal, but the protein content may be increased.

The pathologic changes take the form of bilaterally symmetrical foci of spongy necrosis with myelin degeneration, vascular proliferation, and gliosis in the thalami, midbrain, pons, medulla, and spinal cord. The basal ganglia are characteristically but not invariably affected. Also, there may be a demyelinative type of peripheral neuropathy. In their distribution and histologic appearance, the CNS lesions resemble those of Wernicke disease (athiaminosis) except that the lesions of SNE tend to be more extensive—sometimes involving the striatum—and they tend to spare the mammillary bodies. The lesions, particularly those of the lenticular nuclei and brainstem, may be seen in CT scans and are strikingly demonstrated by MRI. The histochemical appearance of muscle is normal, although electron microscopy may show an increased number of mitochondria.

The clinical boundaries of Leigh disease have not been defined precisely. A familial disorder of infancy and early childhood—referred to as bilateral striatial necrosis and associated with dystonia, visual failure, and other neurologic defects—is probably a variant of Leigh disease. The same may be true for an obscure adult-onset syndrome of progressive dementia from a thalamic lesion, showing necrosis, vascular proliferation, and gliosis.

The mitochondrial gene mutation most often associated with the Leigh syndrome is also considered in relation to the NARP syndrome discussed below. The close relationship between the two syndromes re-emphasizes the point that several mitochondrial mutations appear to give rise to the same clinical and pathologic picture of a subacute necrotizing encephalopathy.

Neuropathy, Ataxia, Retinitis Pigmentosa Syndrome (NARP) Leigh syndrome exemplifies to a remarkable degree the heterogeneity of abnormalities that may be associated with cytochrome oxidase deficiency due to a single mitochondrial gene mutation. A minor transversion error, the substitution of one amino acid in the mitochondrial DNA at position 8993, also gives rise to a maternally inherited syndrome of sensory neuropathy, ataxia, and retinitis pigmentosa (NARP). It may include developmental delay, seizures, and proximal muscle weakness. This gene abnormality creates an error in the ATPase-6 of complex V of the mitochondrial respiratory chain. The severity of the NARP syndrome corresponds to the amount of aberrant DNA in the mitochondrial genome; when the mutation involves over 90 percent of mitochondrial DNA, it produces the more severe phenotype of the Leigh syndrome (SNE). Santorelli and colleagues found that 12 of 50 patients with Leigh syndrome from 10 families displayed the 8993 point mutation. Within one kindred, the mitochondrial aberration may manifest itself as mild developmental delay, NARP, the full-blown Leigh syndrome, or early death with lactic acidosis. These differences in severity are thought to result from the protective effect of even small amounts of the normal mitochondrial genome. The first manifestations of disease may not appear until adulthood, although it begins only rarely after age 20. The similarities to Refsum disease are discussed on page 1421.

Further confounding the understanding of this disease complex is the observation that many patients with the Leigh syndrome have a pyruvate dehydrogenase (usually X-linked) or pyruvate decarboxylase deficiency, whereas others have the cytochrome oxidase deficiency, which is common to many mitochondrial disorders and inherited usually as an autosomal recessive trait. But Leigh syndrome patients with the 8993 mutation tend to have neither of these enzymatic deficiencies. Bridging these complex cases are children with cytochrome oxidase deficiency who have psychomotor retardation, slowed growth, and lactic acidosis, some with and others without the striatal or brainstem spinal necroses of Leigh syndrome.

Congenital Lactic Acidosis and Recurrent Ketoacidosis

Certain types of organic acidemia, occurring in early infancy and of unproved genetic etiology, have already been mentioned (page 992). Here reference is made to those few cases that are associated with deletions of mitochondrial DNA. The syndrome has consisted of *psychomotor regression* and *episodic hyperventilation, hypotonia, and convulsions* with intervening periods of normalcy. Choreoathetosis or progressive ophthalmoplegia have been added in a few cases. Some children are also dysmorphic, with a broad nasal bridge, micrognathia, posteriorly rotated ears, short arms and fingers, and other features. A synopsis of such cases is given by De Vivo and coworkers. Death usually occurs before the third year. The important laboratory findings are acidosis with high lactate levels and hyperalalinemia. The few cases that have been examined postmortem are found to have necrosis and cavitation of the globus pallidus and cerebral white matter, as occurs in SNE. Probably most cases of this type are due to disorders of the mitochondrial respiratory chain, particularly of the pyruvate-decarboxylase complex. The diagnosis can be made by the finding of ragged red fibers in muscle or by measurement of the enzyme activity. It must be distinguished from the several diseases of infancy that are complicated by lactic acidosis.

Myoclonic Epilepsy with Ragged Red Fiber Myopathy (MERRF)

This is perhaps the most distinctive mitochondrial disease, presenting as it does with progressive myoclonic epilepsy or myoclonic ataxia. These cases, as was noted in Chap. 6, must be differentiated from several entities with a predictable clinical course, such as juvenile myoclonic epilepsy, Unverricht-Lundborg disease, Lafora-body disease, Baltic myoclonus, and neuronal ceroid-lipofuscinosis, discussed earlier in this chapter. Tsairis and colleagues were the first to describe the connection between familial myoclonic epilepsy and mitochondrial changes in muscle, and numerous variants of this core syndrome have been described since their report.

In our limited experience with this disease, myoclonus in a child or young adult is the most typical feature and is elicited by startle or by movement of the limbs. The nature of the seizures varies but includes drop attacks, focal epilepsy, or tonic-clonic types, some of which are photosensitive. Ataxia tends to worsen progressively, eclipsing the myoclonus and seizures in some instances and remaining a minor feature in others. The myopathy is usually inapparent or mild. The presence of mitochondrial muscle abnormalities is necessary for clinical diagnosis. To this constellation may be added any of the other elements of the mitochondrial diseases that have already been cited, including deafness (present in the cases we have seen), mental decline, optic atrophy, ophthalmoplegia, cervical lipomas, short stature, or neuropathy.

Most cases are familial and display maternal inheritance, but the age of onset may vary and affected individuals have been reported with symptoms beginning as late as the sixth decade. Almost always the latter represent the mildest cases, with only myoclonic epilepsy. Those with onset in the first decade tend to be more severely affected and die before the third decade. As with the other mitochondrial processes, the quantitative burden of mutant DNA has been related to the time of onset and severity of the disease. Eighty percent of patients with MERRF have a point mutation of the mitochondrial genome at locus 8344, which codes for a transfer RNA, and, conversely, most patients with this mutation will have MERRF, including those with crossover features of the Leigh syndrome.

Mitochondrial Myopathy, Encephalopathy, Lactic Acidosis, and Stroke-Like Episodes (MELAS)

In patients with this syndrome, normal early development is followed by poor growth, focal or generalized seizures, and recurrent acute episodes that resemble strokes or prolonged transient ischemic attacks. The stroke deficits often improve but in some cases lead to a progressive encephalopathy. Some patients have hemicranial headaches that cannot be distinguished from migraine, and others suffer repetitive vomiting or episodic lactic acidosis. If there are any characteristic features, they take the form of an unusual clinical pattern of focal seizures, sometimes prolonged, which herald a stroke and have a unique radiographic pattern involving the cortex and immediate subcortical white matter. The CT may show numerous low-density regions that have no clinical correlates. Most patients have ragged red muscle fibers, but only rarely is there weakness or exercise intolerance.

As with the MERRF syndrome, approximately 80 percent of MELAS cases are related to a mitochondrial mutation occurring at the 3243 site, or, in a few instances, at an alternative locus that also codes for a segment of transfer RNA. Maternal inheritance is common but sporadic cases are well known. In the survey conducted by Hammans and coworkers, only half of the instances of the 3243 mutation were associated with the MELAS syndrome. The finding of an abnormal mitochondrial genome in the endothelium and smooth muscle of cerebral vessels has been suggested as a basis for the strokes and migraine headaches.

The Diagnosis of Mitochondrial Disorders

If there are any characteristic neurologic signs of a mitochondrial disorder, they fall into four broad groups: (1) combinations of ataxia, seizures, and myoclonus, typified by the MERRF syndrome; (2) migraine-like headaches, recurrent small strokes, and preceding seizures, typified by the MELAS syndrome; (3) ophthalmoplegia and retinitis pigmentosa with polyneuropathy, optic atrophy (Leber type), or deafness (Kearns-Sayre syndrome); and (4) a myopathy that is slowly progressive or fluctuating in severity. These may be combined with dementia, lactic acidosis, short stature, ptosis, pigmentary retinal degeneration, and cardiac conduction defects (as in the Kearns-Sayre syndrome) as well as with multiple symmetrical lipomas. Peripheral nerve involvement, although common in these disorders, is usually asymptomatic; autonomic failure may be a manifestation. A panoply of visceral dysfunctions may be associated with the mitochondrial disorders—including bone marrow changes of sideroblastic anemia, renal tubular defects, endocrinopathies (diabetes, hypothyroidism, deficiency of growth hormone), hepatopathy, cardiomyopathy, and recurrent vomiting with intestinal pseudo-obstruction. Diabetes has been a marker in several of the early-onset MELAS and MERRF cases that we have seen, but less often when the first manifestations were in adulthood.

The investigation of a suspected case of mitochondrial disease begins with an exploration of the family history for childhood diseases, including neonatal death, unexplained seizure disorders, and progressive neurologic deficits of the types already described. Unexplained deafness or diabetes in family members should also raise the suspicion of a mitochondrial disorder. Commercial tests of leukocytes for the more frequent mitochondrial point mutation sites (3243, 8993, and 8344 are the usual ones) are useful but reveal mutations in only about 15 percent of patients, even in those whose muscles contain an abundant amount of mutant mitochondrial genome. Resting and postexercise lactate and pyruvate determinations are also helpful. A muscle biopsy is probably the next step and may disclose several basic abnormalities; ragged red fibers can be recognized by use of the modified Gomori stain on frozen material, and the absence of succinate dehydrogenase and cytochrome oxidase, by appropriate histochemical staining. In cases of suspected Leigh syndrome or MELAS, the CT or MRI may show some of the characteristic lesions; in the other mitochondrial disorders there are often focal nondescript hyperintensities on T2-weighted MRI, atrophy, lucencies, or calcification. Sampling of chorionic villi for prenatal diagnosis may show mutant mitochondrial DNA, but this information is not entirely dependable.

It should be evident from the foregoing discussion that normal findings in any of these tests, including the muscle biopsy, do not exclude mitochondrial disease. In the final analysis, it is the clinical syndrome, family history, and any corroborating evidence of a mitochondrial disorder or its genetic representation that is diagnostic. The review of Jackson and coworkers suggests that isolated phenomena such as dementia, muscle weakness, epilepsy, nerve deafness, migraine with strokes, small stature, myoclonic epilepsy, and cardiomyopathy should prompt consideration of a mitochondrial disorder when no other explanation is evident.

REFERENCES

Adachi M, Torii J, Schneck L, Volk BW: Electron microscopic and enzyme histochemical studies of the cerebellum in spongy degeneration. *Acta Neuropathol* 20:22, 1972.

Adams RD, Prod'holm LS, Rabinowicz TH: Intrauterine brain death. *Acta Neuropathol* 40:41, 1977.

Agamanolis DP, Greenstein JI: Ataxia-telangiectasia. *J Neuropathol Exp Neurol* 38:475, 1979.

Aicardi J: Early myoclonic encephalopathy, in Roger J, Dravet C, Bureau M, et al (eds): *Epileptic Syndromes in Infancy, Childhood, and Adolescence*. New York, Demos, 1985.

Aicardi J, Castelein P: Infantile neuroaxonal dystrophy. *Brain* 102:727, 1979.

Allen RJ, Young W, Bonacci J, et al: Neonatal dystonic parkinsonism, a "stiff baby syndrome," in biopterin deficiency with hyperprolactinemia detected by newborn screening for hyperphenylalaninemia, and responsiveness to treatment. *Ann Neurol* 28:434, 1990.

Alpers BJ: Diffuse progressive degeneration of cerebral gray matter. *Arch Neurol Psychiatry* 25:469, 1931.

Auborg P, Scotto J, Richicioli F: Neonatal adrenoleukodystrophy. *J Neurol Neurosurg Psychiatry* 49:77, 1986.

Austin J: Studies in metachromatic leukodystrophy: XII. Multiple sulfatase deficiency. *Arch Neurol* 28:258, 1973.

Banker BQ, Victor M: Spongy degeneration of infancy, in Goodman RM, Motulsky AG (eds): *Genetic Diseases among Ashkenazi Jews*. New York, Raven Press, 1979, pp 210–216.

Baringer JR, Sweeney VP, Winkler GF: An acute syndrome of ocular oscillations and truncal myoclonus. *Brain* 91:473, 1968.

Bassen FA, Kornzweig AL: Malformation of the erythrocytes in a case of atypical retinitis pigmentosa. *Blood* 5:381, 1950.

Baumann RJ, Kocoshis SA, Wilson D: Lafora disease: Liver histopathology in presymptomatic children. *Ann Neurol* 14:86, 1983.

Berginer VM, Salen G, Shefer S: Long-term treatment of cerebrotendinous xanthomatosis with chenodeoxycholic acid. *N Engl J Med* 311:1649, 1984.

Berkovic SF, Andermann F, Carpenter S, et al: Progressive myoclonus epilepsies and specific causes and diagnosis. *N Engl J Med* 315:296, 1986.

Blass JP, Avigan J, Uhlendorf BW: A defect in pyruvate decarboxylase in a child with intermittent movement disorder. *J Clin Invest* 49:423, 1970.

Boder E, Sedgwick RP: Ataxia-telangiectasia: A familial syndrome of progressive cerebellar ataxia, oculocutaneous telangiectasia and frequent pulmonary infection. *Pediatrics* 21:526, 1958.

Bosch EP, Hart MN: Late adult onset metachromatic leukodystrophy. *Arch Neurol* 35:475, 1978.

Brady RO: The sphingolipidoses. *N Engl J Med* 275:312, 1966.

Brett EM (ed): *Paediatric Neurology*, 3rd ed. London, Churchill Livingstone, 1991.

Brewer GJ, Terry CA, Aisen AM, Hill GM: Worsening of neurologic syndrome in patients with Wilson's disease with initial penicillamine therapy. *Arch Neurol* 44:490, 1987.

Brusilow SW, Danney M, Waber LJ, et al: Treatment of episodic hyperammonemia in children with inborn errors of urea synthesis. *N Engl J Med* 310:1630, 1984.

Brusilow SW, Horwich AL: Urea cycle enzymes, in Scriver CR, Beaudet AL, Sly WS, Valle D (eds): *The Metabolic Basis of Inherited Disease*, 7th ed. New York, McGraw-Hill, 1995, pp 1187–1232.

Burton BK, Nadler HL: Clinical diagnosis of the inborn errors of metabolism in the neonatal period. *Pediatrics* 61:398, 1978.

Cho CH, Mamourian AC, Filiano J, Nordgren RE: Glutaric aciduria: Improved MR appearance after aggressive therapy. *Pediatr Radiol* 25:484, 1995.

Cowen D, Olmstead EV: Infantile neuroaxonal dystrophy. *J Neuropathol Exp Neurol* 22:175, 1963.

Crocker AC, Farber S: Niemann-Pick disease: A review of 18 patients. *Medicine* 37:1, 1958.

Crome L: A case of galactosaemia with the pathological and neuropathological findings. *Arch Dis Child* 37:415, 1962.

dal Canto MC, Rapin I, Suzuki K: Neuronal storage disorder with chorea and curvilinear bodies. *Neurology* 24:1026, 1974.

Danks DM, Cartwright E, Stevens BJ, Townley RRW: Menkes' kinky-hair disease: Further definition of the defect in copper transport. *Science* 179:1140, 1973.

Dening TR, Berrios GE, Walshe JM: Wilson's disease and epilepsy. *Brain* 111:1139, 1988.

Desnick RJ, Ioannou YA, Eng CM: α-Galactosidase A deficiency: Fabry disease, in Scriver CR, Beaudet AL, Sly WS, Valle D (eds): *The Metabolic and Molecular Bases of Inherited Disease*, 7th ed. New York, McGraw-Hill, 1995, pp 2741–2784.

De Vivo DC, Haymond MW, Obert KA, et al: Defective activation of the pyruvate dehydrogenase complex in subacute necrotizing encephalomyelopathy (Leigh disease). *Ann Neurol* 6:483, 1979.

DiMagno EP, Lowe JL, Snodgrass PJ, et al: Ornithine transcarbamalase deficiency: A cause of bizarre behavior in a man. *N Engl J Med* 315:744, 1986.

DiMauro S, Nicholson JF, Hays A, et al: Benign infantile mitochondrial myopathy due to reversible cytochrome c oxidase deficiency. *Ann Neurol* 14:226, 1983.

Drew AL Jr: The degenerative and demyelinating diseases of the nervous system, in Carter S, Gold AP (eds): *Neurology of Infancy and Childhood.* New York, Appleton-Century-Crofts, 1974, pp 57–89.

Eldridge R, Anayiotos CP, Schlesinger S, et al: Hereditary adult-onset leukodystrophy simulating chronic progressive multiple sclerosis. *N Engl J Med* 311:948, 1984.

Elfenbein LB: Dystonic juvenile idiocy without amaurosis. *Johns Hopkins Med J* 123:205, 1968.

Fahr T: Idiopathische Verkalkung der Hirngefasse. *Zentralbl Allg Pathol* 50:129, 1930–1931.

Farrell DF, Swedberg K: Clinical and biochemical heterogeneity of globoid cell leukodystrophy. *Ann Neurol* 10:364, 1981.

Følling A: Über Ausscheidung von Phenylbrenztraubensaure in den Harn als Stoffwechselanomalie in Verbindung mit Imbezilitat. *Hoppe-Seyler's Z Physiol Chem* 227:169, 1934.

Friedman JH, Levy HL, Boustany R-M: Late onset of distinct neurologic syndromes in galactosemic siblings. *Neurology* 39:741, 1989.

Frydman M, Bonne-Tamir B, Farber LA, et al: Assignment of the gene for Wilson disease to chromosome 13: Linkage to the esterase D locus. *Proc Natl Acad Sci USA* 82:1819, 1985.

Goldfischer S, Moore CL, Johnson AB, et al: Peroxisomal and mitochondrial defects in the cerebro-hepato-renal syndrome. *Science* 182:62, 1973.

Goldman JE, Katz O, Rapur I, et al: Chronic G_{M1} gangliosidosis presenting as dystonia: Clinical and pathological features. *Ann Neurol* 9:465, 1981.

Griffin JW, Goren E, Schaumburg H, et al: Adrenomyeloneuropathy: A probable variant of adrenoleukodystrophy. *Neurology* 27: 1107, 1977.

Griggs RC, Moxley RT, LaFrance RA, McQuillen J: Hereditary paroxysmal ataxia: Response to acetazolamide. *Neurology* 28: 1259, 1978.

Hammans SR, Sweeny MG, Hanna MG, et al: The mitochondrial DNA transfer RNA Leu (44R) A_G (3243) mutation: A clinical and genetic study. *Brain* 118:721, 1995.

Harding BN, Egger J, Portmann B, Erdohazi M: Progressive neuronal degeneration of childhood with liver disease. *Brain* 109:181, 1986.

Hers HG: Inborn lysosomal diseases. *Gastroenterology* 48:625, 1965.

Holmes LB, Moser HW, Halldorsson S, et al: *Mental Retardation: An Atlas of Diseases with Associated Physical Abnormalities*. New York, Macmillan, 1972.

Holtzman NA, Kronmal RA, van Doorninck W, et al: Effect of age and loss of dietary control on intellectual performance and behavior of children with phenylketonuria. *N Engl J Med* 314:593, 1986.

Hoogenraad TU, Van Hattum J, Van Den Hamer CSA: Management of Wilson's disease with zinc sulfate: Experience in a series of 27 patients. *J Neurol Sci* 77:137, 1987.

HUNT JR: Dyssynergia cerebellaris myoclonica. *Brain* 44:490, 1921.

IGARASHI M, SCHAUMBURG HH, POWERS J, et al: Fatty acid abnormality in adrenoleukodystrophy. *J Neurochem* 26:851, 1976.

IKEDA S, KONDO K, OGUCHI K, et al: Adult fucosidosis: Histochemical and ultrastructural studies of rectal mucosa biopsy. *Neurology* 34:451, 1984.

ILLINGWORTH DR, CONNOR WE, MILLER RG: Abetalipoproteinemia: Report of two cases and review of therapy. *Arch Neurol* 37:659, 1980.

JACKSON MJ, SCHAEFER A, JOHNSON MA: Presentation and clinical investigation of mitochondrial respiratory chain disease. *Brain* 118:339, 1995.

JOHNS DR: Mitochondrial DNA and disease. *N Engl J Med* 333:638, 1995.

JOHNSON RC, MCKEAN CM, SHAH SN: Fatty acid composition of lipids in cerebral myelin and synaptosomes in phenylketonuria and Down syndrome. *Arch Neurol* 34:288, 1977.

KALIMO H, LUNDBERG PO, OLSSON Y: Familial subacute necrotizing encephalomyelopathy of the adult form (adult Leigh syndrome). *Ann Neurol* 6:200, 1979.

KENDALL BE, KINGSLEY DPE, LEONARD JV, et al: Neurological features and computed tomography of the brain in children with ornithine carbamyl transferase deficiency. *J Neurol Neurosurg Psychiatry* 46:28, 1983.

KINSBOURNE M: Myoclonic encephalopathy in infants. *J Neurol Neurosurg Psychiatry* 25:271, 1962.

KISTLER JP, LOTT IT, KOLODNY EH, et al: Mannosidosis. *Arch Neurol* 34:45, 1977.

KOBAYASHI T, NODA S, UMEZAKI H, et al: Familial spinocerebellar degeneration as an expression of adrenoleukodystrophy. *J Neurol Neurosurg Psychiatry* 49:1438, 1986.

KOEPPEN AH, RONCA NA, GREENFIELD EA, HANS MB: Defective biosynthesis of proteolipid protein in Pelizaeus-Merzbacher disease. *Ann Neurol* 21:159, 1987.

KOIVISTO M, BLENCO-SEQUIROS M, KRAUSE U: Neonatal symptomatic hypoglycemia: A follow-up of 151 children. *Dev Med Child Neurol* 14:603, 1972.

KOLODNY EH, CABLE WJL: Inborn errors of metabolism. *Ann Neurol* 11:221, 1982.

KOLODNY EH, RAGHAVAN SS: G_{M2} gangliosidosis hexosaminidase mutations not of the Tay-Sachs type produce unusual clinical variants. *Trends Neurol Sci* 6:16, 1983.

KOLODNY EH, RAGHAVAN SS, KRIVIT W: Late-onset Krabbe disease (globoid cell leukodystrophy): Clinical and biochemical features in 15 cases. *Dev Neurosci* 13:232, 1991.

LANCE JW: Familial paroxysmal dystonic choreoathetosis and its differentiation from related syndromes. *Ann Neurol* 2:285, 1977.

LEONARD JV, SCHAPIRA AHV: Mitochondrial respiratory chain disorders I and II. *Lancet* 355:299, 389, 2000.

LESCH M, NYHAN WL: A familial disorder of uric acid metabolism and central nervous system function. *Am J Med* 36:561, 1964.

LEVY HL: Screening of the newborn, in Tausch HW, Ballard RA, Avery ME (eds): *Diseases of the Newborn.* Philadelphia, Saunders, 1991, pp 111–119.

LOGAN JI: Hereditary deficiency of ferroxidase (aka ceruloplasmin). *J Neurol Neurosurg Psychiatry* 61:431,1996.

LONSDALE D, FAULKNER WR, PRICE JW, SMEBY RR: Intermittent cerebellar ataxia associated with hyperpyruvic acidemia, hyperalininemia and hyperalininuria. *Pediatrics* 43:1025, 1969.

LOTT IT, COULOMBE T, DIPAOLO RV, et al: Vitamin B_6-dependent seizures: Pathology and chemical findings in brain. *Neurology* 28:47, 1978.

LOUIS-BAR D: Sur un syndrome progressif comprenant des télangiectasies capillaires cutanée et conjonctivales symetrique a disposition naevoide et des troubles cérébelleux. *Confin Neurol* 4:32, 1941.

LUNDBORG H: *Die progressive Myoklonus-epilepsie (Unverricht's Myoklonie).* Uppsala, Sweden, Almqvist and Wiksell, 1903.

LYON G, ADAMS RD, KOLODNY EH: *Neurology of Hereditary Metabolic Diseases of Children*, 2nd ed. New York, McGraw-Hill, 1996.

MAESTRI NE, BRUSILOW SW, CLISSOLD DB, et al: Long-term treatment of girls with ornithine transcarbamylase deficiency. *N Engl J Med* 335:855, 1996.

MARSDEN CD, HARDING AE, OBESO JA, LU C-S: Progressive myoclonic ataxia (the Ramsay Hunt syndrome). *Arch Neurol* 47:1121, 1990.

MARSDEN CD, OGESO JA, LANG AE: Adrenoleukomyeloneuropathy presenting as spinocerebellar degeneration. *Neurology* 32:1031, 1982.

MARTINELLI P, GUILIANI S, IPPOLITO N, et al: Familial idiopathic striato-pallido-dentate calcifications with late onset extrapyramidal syndrome. *Mov Disord* 8:220, 1993.

MATALON R, MICHALS K, SEBESTA D, et al: Aspartoacylase deficiency and *N*-acetylaspartic aciduria in patients with Canavan disease. *Am J Med Genet* 29:463, 1988.

MCFARLIN DE, STROBER W, BARLOW M, et al: The immunological deficiency state in ataxia-telangiectasia. *Res Publ Assoc Res Nerv Ment Dis* 49:275, 1971.

MCKUSICK VA: *Mendelian Inheritance in Man: A Catalog of Human Genes and Genetic Disorders*, 12th ed. Baltimore, Johns Hopkins University Press, 1998.

MEEK D, WOLFE LS, ANDERMANN E, ANDERMANN F: Juvenile progressive dystonia: A new phenotype of G_{M2} gangliosidosis. *Ann Neurol* 15:348, 1984.

MEINER V, MEINER Z, RESHEF A, et al: Cerebrotendinous xanthomatosis: Molecular diagnosis enables presymptomatic detection of a treatable disease. *Neurology* 44:288, 1994.

MELCHIOR JC, BENDA CE, YAKOVLEV PI: Familial idiopathic cerebral calcifications in childhood. *Am J Dis Child* 99:787, 1960.

MIYATAKE T, ATSUMI T, OBAYASHI T, et al: Adult type neuronal storage disease with neuraminidase deficiency. *Ann Neurol* 6:232, 1979.

MOLE SE: Batten's disease: Eight genes and still counting? *Lancet* 354:443, 1999.

MOSER AB, SINGH I, BROWN FR III, et al: The cerebrohepatorenal (Zellweger) syndrome. *N Engl J Med* 310:1141, 1984.

MOSER HW: Adrenoleukodystrophy: Phenotype, genetics, pathogenesis and therapy. *Brain* 120:1485, 1997.

Moser HW: Therapy of genetically determined metabolic disorders, in Fukuyama Y, Suzuki Y, Kamoshita S, Casaer P (eds): *Fetal and Perinatal Neurology*. Basel, Karger, 1992, pp 93–107.

Moser HW, Moser AB, Kawamura N, et al: Adrenoleukodystrophy: Elevated C26 fatty acid in cultured skin fibroblasts. *Ann Neurol* 7:542, 1980.

Mount LA, Reback S: Familial paroxysmal choreoathetosis: Preliminary report on a hitherto undescribed clinical syndrome. *Arch Neurol Psychiatry* 44:841, 1940.

Msall M, Batshaw ML, Suss R, et al: Neurologic outcome in children with inborn errors of urea synthesis. *N Engl J Med* 310:1500, 1984.

Neufeld EF, Muenzer J: The mucopolysaccharidoses, in Scriver CR, Beaudet AL, Sly WS, Valle D (eds): *The Metabolic and Molecular Bases of Inherited Disease*, 7th ed. New York, McGraw-Hill, 1995, pp 2465–2494.

Nishimura M, Yoshimo K, Tomita Y: Central and peripheral nervous system pathology due to methylenetetrahydrofolate reductase deficiency. *Pediatr Neurol* 1:375, 1985.

Nygaard TG, Marsden CD, Fahn S: Dopa-responsive dystonia: Long-term treatment response and prognosis. *Ann Neurol* 35:396, 1994.

Ohno T, Tsuchida H, Fukuhara N, et al: Adrenoleukodystrophy: A clinical variant presenting as olivopontocerebellar atrophy. *J Neurol* 231:167, 1984.

Ohtahara S: Seizure disorders in infancy and childhood. *Brain Dev* 6:509, 1984.

Pavlakis SG, Phillips PC, DiMauro S, et al: Mitochondrial myopathy, encephalopathy, lactic acidosis, and stroke-like episodes: A distinctive clinical syndrome. *Ann Neurol* 16:481, 1984.

Pincus JH, Chutorian A: Familial benign chorea with intention tremor: A clinical entity. *J Pediatr* 70:724, 1967.

Prader A, Labhart A, Willi H: Ein Syndrom von Adipositas, Kleinwuchs, Kryptorchismus und Oligophrenie nach myatonieartigem Zustand im Neugeborenenalter. *Schweiz Med Wochenschr* 86:1260, 1956.

Pranzatelli MR, Huang Y, Tate E, et al: Cerebrospinal fluid 5-hydroxy indoleacetic acid in the pediatric opsoclonus-myoclonus syndrome. *Ann Neurol* 37:189, 1995.

Prechtl H, Beintema D: *The Neurological Examination of the Full-Term Newborn Infant*. London, Spastics Society, 1964.

Prensky AL, Moser HW: Brain lipids, proteo-lipids and free amino acids in maple syrup urine disease. *J Neurochem* 13:863, 1966.

Rapin I, Goldfischer S, Katzman R, et al: The cherry-red spot-myoclonus syndrome. *Ann Neurol* 3:134, 1978.

Robitaille Y, Carpenter S, Karpati G, et al: A distinct form of adult polyglycosan body disease with massive involvement of central and peripheral neuronal processes and astrocytes. *Brain* 103:315, 1980.

Ropper AH, Hatten HP, Davis KR: Computed tomography in Wilson disease: Report of two cases. *Ann Neurol* 5:102, 1979.

Rosenberg AL, Bergstrom L, Troost BT, Bartholomew BA: Hyperuricemia and neurologic deficits: A family study. *N Engl J Med* 282:992, 1970.

Rosenberg LE, Scriver CR: Disorders of amino acid metabolism, in Bondy PK, Rosenberg LE (eds): *Metabolic Control and Disease*, 8th ed. Philadelphia, Saunders, 1980, pp 583–776.

Rowe PC, Newman SL, Brusilow SW: Natural history of symptomatic partial ornithine transcarbamylase deficiency. *N Engl J Med* 314:541, 1986.

Saatci I, Topcu M, Baltaoglu FF, et al: Cranial MRI findings in Wilson's disease. *Acta Radiol* 38:250, 1997.

Salem M: Metabolic ataxias, in Vinken PJ, Bruyn GW (eds): *Handbook of Clinical Neurology*. Vol 21. Amsterdam, North-Holland, 1975, pp 573–585.

Sansaricq C, Lyon G, Kolodny EH: Seizures in hereditary metabolic disease: Evaluation of suspected hereditary metabolic disease in the etiology of seizures, in Kotogal P, Luders H (eds): *The Epilepsies: Etiologies and Prevention*. San Diego, Academic, 1999, pp 457–464.

Santavuori P, Haltia M, Rapola J, Raitta C: Infantile type of so-called neuronal ceroid-lipofuscinosis: Part 1. A clinical study of 15 patients. *J Neurol Sci* 18:257, 1973.

Santorelli F, Shanske S, Macay A, et al: The mutation at nt 8993 of mitochondrial DNA is a common cause of Leigh's syndrome. *Ann Neurol* 34:827, 1994.

Savoiardo M, Halliday WC, Nardocci N, et al: Hallervorden-Spatz disease: MR and pathologic findings. *AJNR* 14:155, 1993.

Schapira AH, DiMauro S (eds): *Mitochondrial Disorders in Neurology*. Oxford, England, Butterworth-Heinemann, 1994.

Scheinberg IH, Gitlin D: Deficiency of ceruloplasmin in patients with hepatolenticular degeneration (Wilson's disease). *Science* 116:484, 1952.

Scheinberg IH, Sternlieb I: *Wilson's Disease: Major Problems in Internal Medicine*. Vol 23. Philadelphia, Saunders, 1984.

Schilsky ML, Scheinberg IH, Sternlieb I: Liver transplantation for Wilson's disease: Indications and outcome. *Hepatology* 19:583, 1994.

Scriver CR, Beaudet AL, Sly WS, Valle D (eds): *The Metabolic and Molecular Bases of Inherited Disease*, 7th ed. New York, McGraw-Hill, 1995.

Scriver CR, Clow CL: Phenylketonuria: Epitome of human biochemical genetics. *N Engl J Med* 303:1335, 1980.

Seitelberger F: Pelizaeus-Merzbacher disease, in Vinken PJ, Bruyn GW (eds): *Handbook of Clinical Neurology*, vol 10. Amsterdam, North-Holland, 1970, pp 150–202.

Sethi KD, Ray R, Roesel RA, et al: Adult-onset chorea and dementia with propionic acidemia. *Neurology* 39:1343, 1989.

Shaffner JM, Wallace DC: Oxidative phosphorylation diseases, in Scriver CR, Beaudet AL, Sly WS, Valle D (eds): *The Metabolic and Molecular Bases of Inherited Disease*, 7th ed. New York, McGraw-Hill, 1995, pp 1535–1609.

Shih VE, Abrams IF, Johnson JL, et al: Sulfite oxidase deficiency. *N Engl J Med* 297:1022, 1977.

SHIH VE, SAFRAN AP, ROPPER AH, TUCHMAN M: Ornithine carbamoyl transferase deficiency: Unusual clinical findings and novel mutation. *J Inherit Met Dis* 22:672, 1999.

SHUMAN RM, LEECH RW, SCOTT CR: The neuropathology of the nonketotic and ketotic hyperglycinemias: Three cases. *Neurology* 28:139, 1978.

SHY GM, GONATAS NK, PEREZ M: Two childhood myopathies with abnormal mitochondria: I. Megaconial myopathy. II. Pleoclonial myopathy. *Brain* 89:133, 1966.

SIEMERLING E, CREUTZFELDT HG: Bronzekrankheit und sklerosierende Encephalomyelitis (Diffuse Sklerose). *Arch Psychiatr Nervenkr* 68:217, 1923.

SJÖGREN T: Die juvenile amaurotische Idiotie: Klinische und erblichkeitsmedizinische Untersuchungen. *Hereditas* 14:197, 1931.

SLY WS, WHYTE MP, SUNDERAM V: Carbonic anhydrase II deficiency in 12 families with the autosomal recessive syndrome of osteopetrosis with renal tubular acidosis with cerebral calcification. *N Engl J Med* 313:139, 1985.

STAROSTA-RUBINSTEIN S, YOUNG AB, KLUIN K, et al: Clinical assessment of 31 patients with Wilson's disease. *Arch Neurol* 44:365, 1987.

STRICH SJ: Pathological findings in three cases of ataxia-telangiectasia. *J Neurol Neurosurg Psychiatry* 29:489, 1966.

SZANTO J, GALLYAS F: A study of iron metabolism in neuropsychiatric patients: Hallervorden-Spatz disease. *Arch Neurol* 14:438, 1966.

TASSINARI CA, MICHELUCCI R, GENTON P, et al: Dyssynergia cerebellaris myoclonica (Ramsay Hunt syndrome): A condition unrelated to mitochondrial encephalomyopathies. *J Neurol Neurosurg Psychiatry* 52:262, 1989.

TELLEZ-NAGEL I, RAPIN I, IWAMOTO T, et al: Mucolipidosis IV. *Arch Neurol* 33:828, 1976.

TENNISON MB, BOULDIN TW, WHALEY RA: Mineralization of the basal ganglia detected by CT in Hallervorden-Spatz syndrome. *Neurology* 38:155, 1988.

THOMAS PK, ABRAMS JD, SWALLOW D, STEWART G: Sialidosis type I: Cherry-red spot-myoclonus syndrome with sialidase deficiency and altered electrophoretic mobilities of some enzymes known to be glycoproteins. *J Neurol Neurosurg Psychiatry* 42:873, 1979.

TROBE JD, SHARPE JA, HIRSCH DK, GEBARSKI SS: Nystagmus of Pelizaeus-Merzbacher disease: A magnetic search-coil study. *Arch Neurol* 48:87, 1991.

TSAIRIS P, ENGEL WK, KARK P: Familial myoclonic epilepsy syndrome associated with skeletal muscle abnormalities. *Neurology* 23:408, 1973.

TSUJI S, CHOUDARY PV, MARTIN BM, et al: A mutation in the human glucocerebrosidase gene in neuronopathic Gaucher's disease. *N Engl J Med* 311:570, 1987.

TSUJI S, YAMADA T, TSUTSUMI A, MIYATAKE T: Neuraminidase deficiency and accumulation of sialic acid in lymphocytes in adult type sialidosis with partial β-galactosidase deficiency. *Ann Neurol* 11:541, 1982.

VAHEDI K, JOUTEL A, VAN BOGAERT P, et al: A gene for hereditary paroxysmal ataxia maps to chromosome 19p. *Ann Neurol* 37:289, 1995.

VAKILI S, DREW AL, VON SCHUCHING S, et al: Hallervorden-Spatz syndrome. *Arch Neurol* 34:729, 1977.

VAN BOGAERT L: Contribution clinique et anatomique a l'etude de la paralysie agitante juvenile primitive. *Rev Neurol* 2:315, 1930.

VAN BOGAERT L: Le cadre des xanthomatoses et leurs differents types: Xanthomatoses secondaires. *Rev Med* 17:433, 1962.

VAN BOGAERT L, BERTRAND I: Sur une idiotie famaliale avec dégénérescence spongieuse du neuraxe. *Acta Neurol Belg* 49:572, 1949.

VAN GEEL MB, ASSIES J, WANDERS RJ, BARTH P'G: X linked adrenoleukodystrophy: Clinical presentation, diagnosis and therapy. *J Neurol Neurosurg Psychiatry* 63:4, 1997.

VOGT C, VOGT O: Zur Lehre der Erkrankungen des striaren Systems. *J Psychol Neurol* 25:627, 1920.

WALSH PJ: Adrenoleukodystrophy. *Arch Neurol* 37:448, 1980.

WILLIAMS FJB, WALSHE JM: Wilson's disease: An analysis of the cranial computerized tomographic experiences found in 60 patients and the changes in response to treatment with chelating agents. *Brain* 104:735, 1981.

WILLIAMS RS, MARSHALL PC, LOTT IT, et al: The cellular pathology of Menkes steely hair syndrome. *Neurology* 28:575, 1978.

WILLVONSEDER R, GOLDSTEIN NP, MCCALL JT, et al: A hereditary disorder with dementia, spastic dysarthria, vertical eye movement paresis, gait disturbance, splenomegaly, and abnormal copper metabolism. *Neurology* 23:1039, 1973.

WILSON SAK: Progressive lenticular degeneration: A familial nervous disease associated with cirrhosis of the liver. *Brain* 34:295, 1912.

WINKELMAN MD, BANKER BQ, VICTOR M, MOSER HW: Non-infantile neuronopathic Gaucher's disease: A clinico-pathologic study. *Neurology* 33:994, 1983.

YOKOI S, NAKAYAMA H, NEGESHI T: Biochemical studies on tissues from a patient with Lafora disease. *Clin Chim Acta* 62:415, 1975.

YOUNG RR, KLEINMAN G, OJEMANN RG, et al: Compressive myelopathy in Maroteaux-Lamy syndrome: Clinical and pathological findings. *Ann Neurol* 8:336, 1980.

ZEMAN W, DONAHUE S, DYKEN P, GREEN J: The neuronal ceroid-lipofuscinoses (Batten-Vogt syndrome), in Vinken PJ, Bruyn GW (eds): *Handbook of Clinical Neurology*. Vol 10. Amsterdam, North-Holland, 1970, pp 588–679.

Chapter 38

DEVELOPMENTAL DISEASES OF THE NERVOUS SYSTEM

Subsumed under this broad heading is a diversity of developmental malformations and diseases acquired during the intrauterine period of life. They number in the hundreds, according to the tabulation of Dyken and Krawiecki, although many of them are very rare. Taxonomically they include many unrelated pathologic processes of different origins: some stem from germplasm abnormalities; others are associated with triplication, deletion, and translocations of chromosomes; and probably some are inherited on a polygenic basis. Still others are due to the effects of a variety of noxious agents acting at different times on the immature nervous system, i.e., during the embryonal, fetal, and paranatal periods of life.

It would be intellectually satisfying if all the states that originate in the intrauterine period could be separated into genetic (hereditary) or nongenetic (congenital) forms, but in many instances the biologic information and the pathologic changes in the brain at this early age do not allow such a division. For example, among the many diseases in which the neural tube fails to close (rachischisis), more than one member of a family may be affected; but it cannot be stated whether a genetic factor is operative or an exogenous factor, such as folic acid deficiency, has acted upon several members during a succession of pregnancies of one mother. Even what appears to be an outright malformation of the brain may be no more than a reflection of the timing of a pathologic process that has affected the nervous system and other organs early in the embryonal period, derailing later processes of development. *Teratology*, the scientific study of neurosomatic malformations, is replete with such examples.

The authors do not wish to imply that medical and biologic ideas about these conditions are completely unsettled, for there are diseases, transmitted from one generation to another, that affect both of the identical (monovular) twins and only one of the fraternal (biovular) twins. In these, a genetic determinant cannot be questioned, for the unaffected fraternal twin shares the same intrauterine environment as the twin sibling. Then, too, a few diseases destroy parts of the brain in utero in specific ways; others affect it in nonspecific ways but leave little doubt as to the action of an exogenous pathogen.

As to the frequency of developmental disorders, Smith (see K. L. Jones) points out that a single malformation, usually of no clinical significance, occurs in 14 percent of newborns. Two malformations appear in 0.8 percent, and in this group, a major defect is five times more frequent than in the normal population. Three or more malformations are found in 0.5 percent of newborns, and in this latter group, more than 90 percent have one or more major abnormalities (defined as structural abnormalities of prenatal origin that seriously interfere with viability or physical well-being). The figures for major congenital malformations, compiled by Kalter and Warkany, are somewhat higher. What is most important for the neurologist is the fact that the nervous system is involved in most of these infants with major malformations. In fact, about 40 percent of deaths during the first postnatal year are in some manner related to prenatal malformations of the central nervous system (CNS).

A perusal of the following pages makes it evident that there is a great variety of structural defects of the nervous system in early life; in fact, every part of the brain, spinal cord, nerves, and musculature may be affected. However, certain principles are applicable to the entire group. *First*, the abnormality of the nervous system is frequently accompanied by an abnormality of some other structure or organ (eye, nose, cranium, spine, ear, and heart), which relates them chronologically to a certain period of embryogenesis. Conversely, the presence of these malformations of nonnervous tissues suggests that an associated abnormality of the nervous system is developmental in nature. However, this principle is not inviolable; in certain maldevelopments of the brain, which must have originated in the embryonal period, all other organs are normal. One can only assume that the brain is more vulnerable than any other organ to prenatal as well as natal influences. Perhaps this occurs because the nervous system, of all organ systems, requires the longest time for its development and maturation, during which it is susceptible to disease. *Second*, a maldevelopment of whatever cause should be present at birth and remain stable thereafter, i.e., be nonprogressive; again, this principle requires qualification—the abnormality may have affected parts of the brain that are not functional at birth, so that an interval of time must elapse postnatally before the defect can express itself. *Third*, birth should have been nontraumatic and the pregnancy uncomplicated by infection or other injurious event. However, the occurrence of a traumatic birth is not proof of a causative relationship between the injury (or infection) and the abnormality, because a defective nervous system may itself interfere with the birth or the gestational process. *Fourth*, if the birth abnormality has occurred in other members of the family of the same or previous generations, it is usually genetic—although, as noted above, this does not exclude the possible adverse effects of exogenous agents. *Fifth*, many of the teratologic conditions that cause birth defects pass unrecognized because they end in spontaneous abortions. For example, defects due to chromosomal abnormalities occur in about 0.6 percent of live births, but such defects are found in more than 5 percent of spontaneous abortions at 5 to 12 weeks gestational age. *Sixth*, low birth weight and gestational age, indicative of premature birth, increase the risk of mental subnormality, seizures, cerebral palsy, and death.

Regarding *etiology*, which is really the crux of the problem of birth defects, some order and classification have emerged. In general, malformations may be subdivided into four groups: (1) one in which a single mutant gene is responsible (2.25 per 1000 live births); (2) one in which birth defects are associated with chromosomal aberrations; (3) a group comprising defects attributable solely to exogenous factors (a virus or other infectious agent, irradiation, or toxin); and (4) the largest group of all (60 percent of cases), in which no cause can be identified. It has been stated that true malformations are due to fundamental endogenous disturbances of cytogenesis and histogenesis occurring in the first half of gestation, and that exogenous factors, which destroy brain tissue but do not cause malformations, operate in the second half. The potential fallacy of this division is obvious. An exogenous lesion occurring during the embryonal period may not only destroy tissue but derail the neuronal migrations of normal development.

A textbook on principles of neurology is not the place in which to present a detailed account of all the hereditary and congenital developmental abnormalities that might affect the nervous system. For such details, the interested reader should refer to several excellent monographs. Three that the authors recommend are Brett's *Pediatric Neurology*, Berg's *Principles of Child Neurology*, and Lyon and Evrard's *Neuropediatrie*. In this chapter we sketch only the major groups and discuss in detail a few of the more common disease entities. The classification in Table 38-1 adheres to a *grouping in accordance with the main presenting abnormality or abnormalities*. Represented here are the common problems that lead families to seek consultation with the pediatric neurologist: (1) structural defects of the cranium, spine, and limbs, and of eyes, nose, ears, jaws, and skin; (2) disturbed motor function—taking the form of retarded development or abnormal movements; (3) epilepsy; and (4) mental retardation. The following discussion focuses on each of these clinical states.

NEUROLOGIC DISORDERS ASSOCIATED WITH CRANIOSPINAL DEFORMITIES

A majority of the disorders in this group are due to a genetic error, including those with a specific chromosomal abnormality, or to some unknown factor. One has only to walk through an institution for the mentally retarded to appreciate the remarkable number and diversity of physical disfigurements that attend abnormalities of the nervous system. Smith, in the third edition of his monograph on the patterns of human malformations, listed 345 distinctive syndromes; in the fourth edition (edited by K. L. Jones, 1988), many new ones were added. Indeed, a normal-appearing individual stands out in such a crowd and will frequently be found to have an inherited metabolic defect or birth injury.

The intimate relationship between the growth and development of the cranium and that of the brain deserves comment. In embryonic life the most rapidly growing parts of the neural tube induce special changes in and at the same time are influenced by the overlying mesoderm (a process known as *induction*); hence abnormalities in the formation of skull, orbits, nose, and spine are regularly associated with anomalies of the brain and spinal cord. During early fetal life the cranial bones and vertebral arches enclose and protect the developing brain and spinal cord; throughout the period of rapid brain growth, as pressure is exerted on the inner table of the skull, the latter accommodates to the increasing size of the brain. This adaptation is facilitated by the membranous fontanels, which remain open until maximal brain growth has been attained; only then do they ossify (close).

In addition, stature is controlled by the nervous system, as shown by the fact that a majority of mental retardates are also stunted physically to a varying degree. Thus disorders of craniovertebral development assume importance not merely because of the physical disfigurement but also because they often reflect an abnormality of the underlying brain and spinal cord, i.e., they become diagnostic signs.

Cranial Malformations at Birth and in Early Infancy

Certain alterations in size and shape of the head in the infant, child, or even adult always signify a pathologic process that affected the brain before birth or in early infancy. The size of the cranium reflects the size of the brain; therefore the tape measure is one of the most useful tools in pediatric neurology; no examination in a neurologically affected child is complete without a measurement of the circumference of the head. Graphs of the head circumference in males and females, from birth to 18 years of age, have been compiled by Nellhaus. A newborn whose head circumference is below the third percentile for age and sex and whose fontanelles are

Table 38-1
Classification of congenital neurologic disorders

I. Neurologic disorders associated with craniospinal deformities
   A. Enlarged head
      1. Hydrocephalus
      2. Hydranencephaly
      3. Macrocephaly
   B. Craniostenoses
      1. Turricephaly
      2. Scaphocephaly
      3. Brachycephaly
   C. Disturbances of neuronal formation and migration
      1. Anencephaly
      2. Lissencephaly, holoprosencephaly, and gyral malformations
   D. Microcephaly
      1. Primary (vera)
      2. Secondary to cerebral disease
   E. Combinations of cerebral, cranial, and other anomalies
      1. Syndactylic craniocerebral anomalies
      2. Other craniofacial anomalies
      3. Oculoencephalic defects
      4. Oculoauriculocephalic anomalies
      5. Dwarfism
      6. Dermatocephalic anomalies
   F. Rachischisis
      1. Cephalic and spinal meningocele, meningoencephalocele, Dandy-Walker syndrome, meningomyelocele
      2. Chiari malformation
      3. Platybasia and cervical-spinal anomalies (Chap. 45)
   G. Chromosomal abnormalities

II. The phakomatoses
   A. Tuberous sclerosis
   B. Neurofibromatosis
   C. Cutaneous angiomatosis with CNS abnormalities

III. Restricted developmental abnormalities of the nervous system
   A. Focal cortical dysgenesis
   B. Möbius syndrome
   C. Congenital apraxia of gaze
   D. Other restricted congenital abnormalities (Horner syndrome, unilateral ptosis, anisocoria, etc.)

IV. Congenital abnormalities of motor function *(cerebral palsy)*
   A. Subependymal (matrix) hemorrhage
   B. Cerebral spastic diplegia
   C. Infantile hemiplegia, double hemiplegia, and quadriplegia
   D. Congenital extrapyramidal disorders (double athetosis; erythroblastosis fetalis and kernicterus)
   E. Congenital ataxias
   F. The flaccid paralyses

V. Prenatal and paranatal infections
   A. Rubella
   B. Cytomegalic inclusion disease
   C. Congenital neurosyphilis
   D. HIV infection and AIDS
   E. Toxoplasmosis
   F. Other viral and bacterial infections

VI. Epilepsies of infancy and childhood

VII. Mental retardation

closed may be judged to have a developmental abnormality of the brain. A head that is normal in size at term but fails to keep pace with body length reflects a later failure of growth and maturation of the cerebral hemispheres (microcephaly and microencephaly).

Enlargement of the Head (Macrocephaly) This can be due to hydrocephalus, hydranencephalus (as defined below), or excessive brain growth (megalo- or macroencephaly). The *hydrocephalic head* is distinguished by several features—frontal protruberance, or bossing, a tendency for the eyes to turn down so that the sclerae are visible between the upper eyelids and iris (sunset sign), thinning of the scalp and prominence of scalp veins, separation of the cranial sutures, and a "cracked pot" sound on percussion of the skull. Hydrocephalus usually comes to medical attention because of an expanding cranium that exceeds normal dimensions for age. The usual causes are type II Chiari malformation, hereditary aqueductal stenosis, and prenatal infections, e.g., toxoplasmosis. These disorders are discussed further on and in Chap. 30.

The *hydranencephalic head* (hydrocephalus and destruction or failure of development of parts of the cerebrum) is often associated with enlargement of the skull. When it is transilluminated with a strong flashlight in a darkened room, the fluid-filled region of the cranium glows like a jack-o'-lantern. Hydranencephaly is not a well-defined entity. It can be caused by intrauterine vascular occlusion or diseases such as toxoplasmosis and cytomegalovirus (CMV) disease, which destroy parts of each cerebral hemisphere. The lack of brain tissue reduces resistance to intraventricular pressure, permitting great enlargement of both lateral ventricles; it is especially marked if there is an added hydrocephalic state due to interference with cerebrospinal fluid (CSF) circulation. This type of destruction of the cerebral mantle in the embryonal period may lead to the formation of huge defects, with apposition of ventricular and pial surfaces (*porencephaly*) and subsequent failure of development (evagination) of the brain. Yakovlev and Wadsworth referred to the localized failure of evagination as *schizencephaly* and postulated that it was the result of a focal developmental defect in the wall of the cerebral mantle. They based their interpretation on the finding of malformed cortex in the margins of the defect, but this might indicate only that the lesion preceded neuronal migration. Levine and coworkers have attributed it to a destructive, possibly ischemic lesion occurring in the first few weeks of gestation, at a time when neuronal migration was incomplete. We favor the latter explanation and describe it further in relation to the cerebral palsies. In either event, the lack of resistance of the defective cerebral mantle to ventricular pressure expands the brain and cranium.

The *macrocephalic head* (a large head with normal or only slightly enlarged ventricles) may be indicative of an advancing metabolic disease that enlarges the brain, as in *Alexander disease, spongy degeneration of infancy, and later phases of Tay-Sachs disease. Subdural hematomas* may also enlarge the head and cause bulging of the fontanelles and separation of the sutures. In the latter condition, the infant is usually irritable and listless, taking nourishment poorly. Infants and children with neurofibromatosis, osteogenesis imperfecta, and achondroplasia also have enlarged heads; in the last condition some degree of hydrocephalus appears to be responsible. Ultrasonography, which can be performed in the prenatal and neonatal periods, is usually diagnostic in all these cranial enlargements. Also MRI and CT scanning will disclose the size of the ventricles and the presence of subdural blood or fluid (hygroma).

Finally, *agenesis of the corpus callosum*, a common congenital defect, may be associated with macrocephaly and varying degrees of mental impairment, optic defects, and seizures. In a series of 56 patients with agenesis of the corpus callosum, Taylor and David reported the presence of epilepsy in 32 and varying degrees of mental retardation in 28; only 9 had no recognizable neurologic defects. Also noted was a high incidence of psychiatric disturbances in these patients. In such cases, CT scans and MRI reveal the characteristic "bat-wing" deformity of the ventricles. There is also asynchrony of electrical activity of the two cerebral hemispheres on the electroencephalogram (EEG). In a few of these patients, an autosomal dominant inheritance has been found (Lynn et al). Agenesis of the corpus callosum is also part of the Aicardi syndrome (see further on), the Andermann syndrome, and nonketotic hyperglycinemia.

Apart from patients with these pathologic states, there are individuals whose head and brain are enlarged but who are normal in all other respects. Many of these individuals come from families with large heads; Schreier and colleagues, who traced this condition through three generations of some families, declared it to be an autosomal dominant trait. This group represented 20 percent of 557 children referred to a clinic because of cranial enlargement (Lorber and Priestley).

Hemimegalencephaly This term refers to a marked enlargement of one cerebral hemisphere as a result of a developmental abnormality. The cortical gray matter and sometimes the basal ganglia are greatly increased in volume and weight. The cerebellum, brainstem, and spinal cord retain their normal dimensions. The cranium may be misshapen or enlarged but is normal in size in some cases. Rarely, the face and body are enlarged on the side of the enlarged hemisphere. The cortex of the giant hemisphere is thick and disorganized. Neurons are in disarray and some are enlarged; in some places the natural lamination of the cortex is effaced. Nothing is known about causation, but apparently embryogenesis has been deranged at the stage of neuroblast formation.

Clinically, most affected individuals have been mentally retarded and some are epileptic. A degree of hemiparesis may be present, but severe hemispheral neurologic deficits are generally not reported. The hemimegalencephaly has been discovered at autopsy in a few individuals who had no mental or neurologic deficits.

Craniostenoses Some of the most startling cranial deformities are caused by premature closure of the cranial sutures (membranous junctions between bones of the skull). Such conditions are estimated to occur in 1 of every 1000 births, with a predominance in males (Lyon and Evrard). The growth of the cranium is inhibited in a direction perpendicular to the involved suture(s), with a compensatory enlargement in other dimensions, as allowed by the patent sutures. For example, when the lambdoid and coronal sutures are both affected, the thrust of the growing brain enlarges the head in a vertical direction (*tower skull*, or *oxycephaly*, also referred to as *turricephaly* and *acrocephaly*). The orbits are shallow, the eyes bulge, and skull films show islands of bone thinning (*Lückenschadel*). When only the sagittal suture is involved, the head is long and narrow (*scaphocephalic*), and the closed suture projects, keel-like, in the midline. With premature closure of the coronal suture, the head is excessively wide and short (*brachycephalic*). The nervous system is usually normal in these restricted craniostenoses. If this condition is recognized before 3 months of age, the surgeon can make artificial sutures that may permit the shape of the head to become more normal (Shillito and Matson). Once brain growth has been completed, nothing can be done. When several sutures (usually coronal and sagittal) are closed, so as to diminish the cranial capacity, intracranial pressure may increase, impairing cerebral function and causing headache, vomiting, and papilledema. Obviously an operation is then needed to increase the capacity of the skull. In craniostenoses that are combined with syndactyly (acrocephalosyndactyly or Apert syndrome), there are often added complications—mental retardation, deafness, convulsions, and loss of sight secondary to papilledema. The so-called clover-shaped skull is the most severe and lethal of the craniostenoses because of the associated developmental anomalies of the brain (see further on).

When, for any reason, an infant lies with the head turned constantly to one side (because of a shortened sternomastoid muscle or hemianopia, for example), the occiput on that side becomes flattened, as does the opposite frontal bone. The other occipital and frontal bones bulge, so that the maximum length of the skull is not in the sagittal but in the diagonal plane. This condition is called *plagiocephaly*, or *wry head*. Craniostenosis of one-half of a coronal suture may also distort the skull in this way.

Disturbances of Neuronal Migration

Neuroembryologic studies have identified several milestones of neuroblast formation, migration, cortical organization, neuron differentiation, and connectivity. Certain developmental anomalies have been traced to one or another of these stages of cytogenesis and histogenesis in the first trimester of gestation and to the growth and differentiation that take place in the second and third trimesters. Originally there is an excess of neurons, many of which degenerate during development—a process called apoptosis. There are recorded instances in which the full complement of neuroblasts and neurons fails to be generated. Or the emergence of two separate cerebral hemispheres may not occur (*holoprosencephaly*), or the bihemispheral brain may remain small (*microcephaly*). In other described specimens, a diminished number of neurons is less obvious than their failure to migrate to the cortical surface; they remain scattered through the mantle zone in sheets and heterotopic aggregates. One type of focal band-shaped subcortical heterotopia ("double-cortex") with *micropolygyria* (an excessive number of abnormally small gyri) is X-linked, occurring only in females. It is expressed by a syndrome of mental retardation, seizures, delayed speech, and motor abnormalities. The cortex may fail to become sulcated—i.e., it is *lissencephalic* or may be defectively convoluted, forming microgyric and *pachygyric* (broad gyral) patterns. In yet other specimens, neuronal migration is normal for the most part, but small groups of neurons in particular regions may lag or present in regional *heterotopias* (focal dysgeneses) (Fig. 38-1). These are just now being recognized by MRI and are

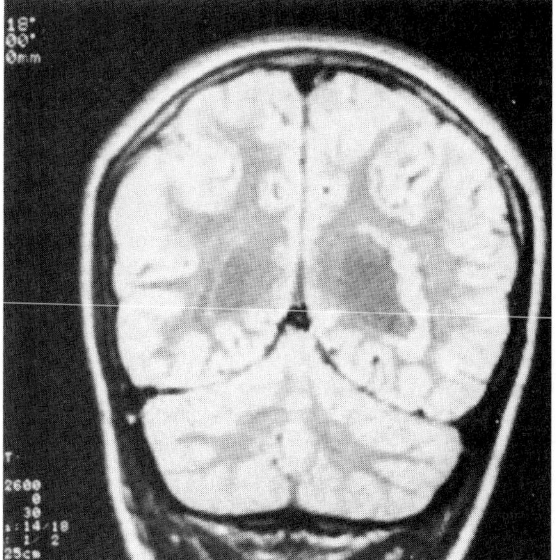

Figure 38-1

Magnetic resonance imaging in the coronal plane in an infant with seizures. Deep in the white matter, adjacent to the lateral ventricle, is a large heterotopic aggregate of gray matter. Also, there appears to be an increased infolding of the cerebral cortex (polymicrogyria).

found to have a possible functional significance in such states as mental retardation, epilepsy, and dyslexia. Finally, the cortex may be normally formed and structured but there is a failure of differentiation of intra- and intercortical and interhemispheral connections, the most obvious one being agenesis of the corpus callosum.

Since each phase of cerebral development is believed to be under genetic control, it comes as no surprise that aberrant development might also be genetic. Indeed, certain cases of lissencephaly have been traced to a defect on chromosome 17, double cortex to xq21, and periventricular heterotopias to x28. Some of the aforementioned cranial abnormalities, of which microcephaly is the most frequent, are secondary to anomalies of cerebral growth. Others—such as abnormalities of the eyes, root of nose, upper lip, ears, and limbs—may represent part of the basic developmental disorder.

The conjunction of cardiac, limb, gut, and bladder abnormalities with neurologic disorder indicates the time at which the insult takes place: cardiac abnormalities occur between the fifth and sixth week; extroversion of the bladder at less than 30 days; duodenal atresia, before 30 days; syndactyly, before 6 weeks; meningomyelocele, before 28 days; anencephaly, before 28 days; cleft lip, before 36 days; syndactyly, cyclopia, and holoprosencephaly, before 23 days.

With these elementary facts of neuroembryology in mind, the bases of the following clinical states are readily conceptualized: anencephaly, lissencephaly, holoprosencephaly, polymicrogyria and pachygyria, microcephaly, and special cranial and somatic abnormalities; each is described below.

There are also special types of tumors, thought to be the consequence of abnormal neuronal or glial development, and they should be mentioned here. They are variously termed gangliomas, dysembryoblastic neuroepitheliomas, and low-grade astrocytomas. Often they become manifest in the first year of life or even before birth. Their relatively slow growth and benign character suggest that some of them represent hamartomas rather than true neoplasms (see Chap. 31).

Anencephaly This is one of the most frequent and also most appalling congenital malformations of the brain. Its incidence is 0.1 to 0.7 per 1000 births, and females predominate in ratios of 3:1 to 7:1. The concordance rate is low, being the same in identical and fraternal twins, but the incidence of the malformation is several times the expected rate if one child in the sibship has already been afflicted. Anencephaly is more frequent in certain geographic areas, e.g., Ireland. Lacking are large portions of scalp, cranial bones, and brain, both cerebral cortex and white matter. All that is seen is a hemorrhagic nubbin of nerve, glial, and connective tissue. Brainstem, cerebellum, and spinal cord are present, but often they too are malformed, as are the heart and other organs (15 to 40 percent of cases). In anencephalics who survive for a few days (65 percent die in utero and almost 100 percent before the end of the first postnatal week), startle reactions may be observed, as well as movements of limbs, spontaneous respirations, pupillary light reactions, ocular movements, and corneal reflexes. In a few, avoidance reactions, crying, and feeding reflexes can be elicited.

This condition can be anticipated if the mother's serum levels of α-fetoprotein and acetylcholine esterase are elevated—even more reliably if testing is done on amniotic fluid. Positive tests should lead to ultrasound imaging of the fetus. Hydramnios is common. Apparently, the causes of anencephaly are multiple and include chromosomal abnormalities, maternal hyperthermia, and deficiencies of folate, zinc, and copper (see Medical Task Force on Anencephaly in the References). There is fairly secure evidence that supplemental intake of folic acid during the first trimester of pregnancy (i.e., from the time of conception) greatly reduces the incidence of anencephaly and myelomeningocele.

There are additional comments on anencephaly further on in this chapter, in the section on rachischisis.

Lissencephaly (Agyria), Holoprosencephaly, and Gyral Malformations Included under this heading are several forms of neuronal migratory defects. In the lissencephalies, cortical convolutions may be absent altogether and there is morphologic evidence of several types of neuroblast deficiency resulting from either generalized or restricted problems in neuronal migration. Such cases are of particular interest to neonatologists because of their associated physical abnormalities. The degree of impairment of neurologic function seldom allows longevity, so that relatively few examples are to be found in institutions for the mentally retarded. Seizures, poor temperature regulation, failure to accept nourishment, and apneic attacks combine to shorten life. The failures of migration are of varying degrees of severity. There may be a failure of neurons to form or migrate along glial guidelines to reach the more superficial layers of the cortex (Bielschowsky type); or the cortex, meninges, and eyes may fail to differentiate normally except for the dentate gyrus and hippocampus (Walker-Warburg type); or there may be relatively minor focal derangements of cortical migrations and lamination with heterotopias of neurons in the white matter.

In the complete lissencephalies, the cerebral ventricles enlarge due to a lack of the normal quantities of surrounding cerebral tissue. The cerebellar cortex is also abnormal. In some lissencephalic brains, there is slight sulcation presenting as abnormally broad or narrow convolutions, with thick, poorly laminated cortex; these are called *pachygyria* or *microgyria*, respectively, but the migratory abnormality is basically the same. The cerebellum is also abnormal with hypoplasia or aplasia involving the vermis or neocerebellum. In the *Dandy-Walker syndrome*, there is vermian hypoplasia with or without hydrocephalus, agenesis of the corpus callosum, and cerebral cortical dysgeneses (Landrieu). This defect, which is identified by the cystic enlargement of the fourth ventricle, is discussed further on, with the dysraphic neural tube defects. That some instances of lissencephaly have a genetic basis (a defect in chromosome 17) has already been mentioned.

In the severe migratory defects, the cranium is small at birth. In one type, which is inherited as an autosomal recessive trait, there are subtle craniofacial features (short nose, small mandible, ear abnormalities, congenital heart disease). In another group, there is an associated familial congenital muscular dystrophy, placing the case between the Fukuyama and Walker-Warburg syndromes (see page 1507). Most cases are sporadic, and the infants seldom survive for long.

Alobar and lobar *holoprosencephalies* are other examples of neuronal migratory defects with craniofacial abnormalities in which development has gone awry in the fifth and sixth weeks of gestation (see Volpe). In these subtypes, the two cerebral hemispheres, either totally or only in part, form as a single telencephalic mass. In nearly every case the cerebral defect is expressed by a single eye (cyclopia) and absence of nose, imparting an astonishing but diagnostic appearance.

In a few of the foregoing malformations, a congenital infection with cytomegalovirus of rubella has been implicated (Hayward et al).

Microcephaly In the above-mentioned cerebral dysplasias, the cranium and brain are small, but there is also a primary form of hereditary microcephaly, called *microcephaly vera*, in which the head is astonishingly reduced in size (circumference less than 45 cm in adult life—i.e., 5 standard deviations below the mean). In contrast, the face is of normal size, the forehead is narrow and recedes sharply, and the occiput is flat. Stature is only moderately reduced. Such individuals can be recognized at birth by their anthropoid appearance and later by their lumbering gait, extremely low intelligence, and lack of communicative speech. Vision, hearing, and cutaneous sensation are spared. In one of our cases, by laborious effort using operant conditioning, it was possible to teach the patient the shapes of simple figures. His sister's brain, examined by R. D. Adams, was malformed and weighed only 280 g. Tendon reflexes in the legs are brisk, and the plantar reflexes may be extensor. Skull films show that the cranial sutures are present, as are convolutional markings on the inner table. There are two types of inheritance of microcephaly vera, autosomal recessive and sex-linked. The brain often weighs less than 300 g (normal adult range, 1100 to 1500 g) and shows only a few primary and secondary sulci. The cerebral cortex is thick and unlaminated and grossly deficient in neurons. In a few reported cases, there has been an associated cerebellar hypoplasia or an infantile muscular atrophy. Lesser degrees of microencephaly have been associated with progressive motor neuron disease and degeneration of the substantia nigra (Halperin et al).

Evrard and associates have described a rare, special type of microcephaly which they call "radial microbrain." Birth is at term, but the infant dies in the first month of postnatal life. The sulcal pattern is normal, and neuronal arrangements in the cerebral cortex are normal as well. The defect appears to be in the small number of neurons that are generated, not in their migration.

Combined Cerebral, Cranial, and Somatic Abnormalities

As has been remarked, many diseases that interfere with cerebral development also deform the cranial and facial bones, eyes, nose, and ears. Such somatic stigmata therefore assume significance as indicators of altered cerebral structure and function. Moreover, they constitute irrefutable evidence that the associated neural abnormality is in the nature of a maldevelopment, either hereditary or the result of a disease acquired during the intrauterine period.

There are so many cerebrosomatic anomalies that one can hardly retain visual images of them, much less recall all the physicians' names by which they are known. Of necessity one turns to atlases, one of the best of which has been compiled by Holmes and colleagues and is based on clinical material drawn from the Fernald School and Eunice K. Shriver Center in Massachusetts. The reader may turn to this book or to the ones by Gorlin and colleagues and by Jones for specific information. Ford's *Diseases of the Nervous System in Infancy, Childhood, and Adolescence* is still a valuable reference, as is Jablonski's *Dictionary of Syndromes and Eponymic Diseases*.

There is some advantage in grouping these anomalies according to whether the extremities, face, eyes, ears, and skin are associated with a cerebral defect. The sheer number and variety of these anomalies permit only an enumeration of the more common ones and their most obvious physical characteristics. To identify a particular anomaly, one has recourse to the specialized monographs and atlases mentioned above. Unfortunately, apart from certain genetic linkages, no useful leads as to their origin have been forthcoming.

The Syndactylic-Craniocerebral Anomalies Commonly, fusion of two fingers or two toes or the presence of a tab of skin representing an extra digit may be seen at birth in an otherwise normal individual. However, as pointed out above, when syndactylism is of more severe degree and is accompanied by premature closure of cranial sutures, the nervous system usually proves to be abnormal as well. The general term *acrocephalosyndactyly* is used to describe the several combinations of craniostenotic and facial deformities and fusion of digits. The following descriptions include only the major features; most have, in addition, distinctive malformations of the orbits, ears, and palate.

1. *Acrocephalosyndactyly types I and II (typical and atypical Apert syndrome).* Turribrachycephalic skull, syndactyly of hands and feet ("mitten hands," "sock feet"), moderate to severe mental retardation.

2. *Acrocephalosyndactyly III (Saethre-Chotzen syndrome).* Transmission as an autosomal dominant trait, various types of craniostenosis, proximally fused and shortened digits, moderate degree of mental retardation; autosomal dominant.

3. *Acrocephalosyndactyly IV (Pfeiffer syndrome).* Turribrachycephaly; broad, enlarged thumbs and great toes; partially flexed elbows (radiohumeral or radioulnar synostoses); mild and variable mental retardation; autosomal dominant inheritance.

4. *Acrocephalopolysyndactyly (Carpenter syndrome).* Premature fusion of all cranial sutures with acrocephaly, flat bridge of nose, medial canthi displaced laterally, excess digits and syndactyly, subnormal intelligence.

5. *Acrocephalosyndactyly with absent digits.* High, bitemporally flattened head; absent toes and syndactylic fingers; moderate mental retardation.

6. *Acrocephaly with cleft lip and palate, radial aplasia, and absent digits.* Microbrachycephaly due to craniostenosis, cleft lip and palate, absent radial bones, severe mental retardation.

7. *Dyschondroplasia, facial anomalies, and polysyndactyly.* Keel-shaped skull and ridge through center of forehead (metopic suture), short arms and legs, postaxial polydactyly and short digits, moderate mental retardation.

In all the foregoing types of syndactylism and cranial abnormality, which may be regarded as variants of a common syndrome, the diagnosis can be made at a glance because of the deformed head, protuberant eyes, and abnormal hands and feet. The mental retardation proves to be variable, usually moderate to severe, but occasionally intelligence is normal or nearly so. The brain has been examined in only a few instances and not in a fashion to display fully the developmental abnormality.

Other Craniocephalic-Skeletal Anomalies Members of this group have distinctive anomalies of the cranium, face, and other parts, but craniostenosis is not a consistent feature.

1. *Craniofacial dysostosis (Crouzon syndrome).* Autosomal dominant inheritance; variable degrees of craniosynostosis; broad forehead with prominence in the anterior fontanel region; shallow orbits with proptosis; midline facial hypoplasia and short upper lip; malformed auditory canals and ears; high, narrow palate; moderate mental retardation. A genetic defect of the fibroblast growth factor receptor, located on chromosome 4, is apparently responsible for about one-third of cases that are not associated with other deformities (Moloney et al).

2. *Median cleft facial syndrome (frontonasal dysplasia; hypertelorism of Greig).* Widely spaced eyes, broad nasal root, cleft nose and premaxilla, V-shaped frontal hairline, heterotypic anterior frontal fontanel (midline cranial defect); mild to severe mental retardation.

3. *Chondrodystrophia calcificans congenita (chondrodysplasia punctata, Conradi-Hünerman syndrome).* Prominent forehead; flat nose; widely separated eyes; short neck and trunk with kyphoscoliosis; dry, scaly, atrophic skin; cicatricial alopecia; irregularly deformed vertebral bodies; mental retardation infrequent. Severe shortening of limbs in some cases.

4. *Orofaciodigital syndrome.* All the patients are female. Pseudoclefts involving the mandible, tongue, maxilla, and palate; hypertrophied buccal frenuli; hamartomas of tongue; sparse scalp hair; subnormal intelligence in one-half of cases.

5. *Pyknodysostosis.* Large head and frontal-occipital bossing, underdeveloped facial bones, micrognathia, unerupted and deformed teeth, dense and defective long bones with shortened limbs, short and broad terminal digits of fingers and toes, mental retardation in one-quarter.

6. *Craniotubular bone dysplasias and hyperostoses.* Included under this title are several different genetic disorders of bone, characterized by modeling errors of tubular and cranial bones. Frontal and occipital hyperostosis, overgrowth of facial bones, and widening of long bones occur in various combinations. Hypertelorism, broad nasal root, nasal obstruction, seizures, visual failure, deafness, prognathism, and retardation of growth are the major features.

Oculoencephalic (Cranio-ocular) Defects In this category of anomalies, there is simultaneous failure or imperfect development of eye and brain. One member of this group, the oculocerebrorenal syndrome of Lowe, has already been mentioned on page 1002, and, of course, a number of the mucopolysaccharidoses are characterized by corneal opacities, skeletal changes, and psychomotor regression. Also, congenital syphilis, rubella, toxoplasmosis, and CMV inclusion disease may affect retina and brain; hypoxia at birth requiring treatment with oxygen may injure the brain and lead to *retrolental fibrodysplasia.*

1. *Anophthalmia with mental retardation.* Sex-linked recessive. Absent eyes; orbits and maxillae remain underdeveloped, but adnexal tissues of eyes (lids) are intact; subnormal intelligence.

2. *Norrie disease.* Also, sex-linked recessive; some sight may be present at birth; later, eyes become shrunken and recessed (phthisis bulbi); some have short digits, outbursts of anger, hallucinations, and possibly regression of psychomotor function.

3. *Oculocerebral syndrome with hypopigmentation.* Autosomal recessive with absence of pigment of hair and skin; small, cloudy, vascularized corneas and small globes (microphthalmia); marked mental retardation; athetotic movements of limbs.

4. *Microphthalmia with corneal opacities, eccentric pupils, spasticity, and severe mental retardation.*

5. *Aicardi syndrome with ocular abnormality.* Chorioretinopathy, retinal lacunae, staphyloma, coloboma of optic nerve, microphthalmos, mental retardation, infantile spasms and other forms of epilepsy, agenesis of corpus callosum, and cortical heterotopias. The "bat-wing" deformity of the third and lateral ventricles on MRI images and asynchronous burst-suppression discharges and sleep spindles are diagnostic. The condition is found only in females.

6. *Lissencephaly of the Walker-Warburg type.* Autosomal recessive inheritance. Ocular lesions are constant but variable (retinal dysplasia, microphthalmia, coloboma, cataracts, corneal opacities). There may be hydrocephalus, and by CT scans or MRI, the lack of cerebral sulci (lissencephaly) is disclosed. The abnormal eyes and orbits and absence of cerebellar vermis are diagnostic.

7. *Congenital tapetoretinal degeneration (Leber amaurosis).* Visual loss from birth, moderate to severe mental retardation, and microcephaly. Early onset of

blindness and absent electrical potentials on the electroretinogram (ERG) distinguish it from later-onset Leber optic atrophy.

8. *Septo-optic dysplasia (de Morsier syndrome).* Diminished visual acuity, small optic discs, absence of septum pellucidum, and precocious puberty. Varying degrees of pituitary insufficiency may be present, requiring endocrine replacement.

Oculoauriculocephalic Anomalies These are less important from the neurologic standpoint and mental retardation is present only in some cases.

1. *Mandibulofacial dysostosis (Treacher-Collins syndrome,* Franceschetti-Zwahlen-Klein syndrome).

2. *Oculoauriculovertebral dysplasia (Goldenhar syndrome).*

3. *Oculomandibulodyscephaly with hypotrichosis (Hallermann-Streiff syndrome).*

Dwarfism Midgets are abnormally small but perfectly formed people of normal intelligence; they differ from dwarfs, who are not only very small but whose bodily proportions are markedly abnormal. A majority of mentally retarded patients fall below average for height and weight, but there is a small group whose fully attained height is well below 135 cm (4 1/2 ft) and who stand apart by this quality alone (see K. L. Jones for Smith's classification of dwarfs).

1. *Nanocephalic dwarfism (Seckel bird-headed dwarfism).* The uncomplimentary term *bird head* has been applied to individuals with a small head, large-appearing eyeballs, beaked nose, and underdeveloped chin. Such a physiognomy is not unique to any disease, but when combined with dwarfism it includes a few more or less specific syndromes. Up to 1976, approximately 25 cases had been reported, some with other skeletal and urogenital abnormalities, such as medial curvature of middle digits; occasional syndactyly of toes; dislocations of elbow, hip, and knee; premature closure of cranial sutures; and clubfoot deformity. These individuals are short at birth and remain so, living until adolescence or adulthood. Retardation is severe. A recessive autosomal type of inheritance is probable. At autopsy the brain is found to have a simplified convolutional pattern; one of our patients had a type of myelin degeneration similar to that of Pelizaeus-Merzbacher disease.

2. *Russell-Silver syndrome.* Possibly an autosomal dominant pattern of inheritance, with short stature of prenatal onset, craniofacial dysostosis, short arms, congenital hemihypertrophy (arm and leg on one side larger and longer), pseudohydrocephalic head (normal-sized cranium with small facial bones), abnormalities of genital development in one-third of cases, delay in closure of fontanels and in epiphyseal maturation, elevation of urinary gonadotropins.

3. *Smith-Lemli-Opitz syndrome.* Autosomal recessive inheritance with microcephaly, broad nasal tip and anteverted nares, wide-set eyes, epicanthal folds, ptosis, small chin, low-set ears, enlarged alveolar maxillary ridge, cutaneous syndactyly, hypospadias in boys, short stature, subnormal neonatal activity, normal amino acids and serum immunoglobulins. Older survivors are bereft of language and paraparetic, with increased reflexes and Babinski signs. The hips are usually dislocated. The karyotype is normal. The brain is small but has not been fully examined. Two of our patients are sibling girls.

4. *Rubinstein-Taybi syndrome.* Microcephaly but no craniostenosis, downward palpebral slant, heavy eyebrows, beaked nose with nasal septum extending below alae nasi, mild retrognathia, "grimacing smile," strabismus, cataracts, obstruction of nasolacrimal canals, broad thumbs and toes, clinodactyly, overlapping digits, excessive hair growth, hypotonia, lax ligaments, stiff gait, seizures, hyperactive tendon reflexes, absence of corpus callosum, mental retardation, and short stature.

5. *Pierre Robin syndrome.* Possible autosomal recessive pattern of inheritance with microcephaly but no craniostenosis, small and symmetrically receded chin ("Andy Gump" appearance), glossoptosis (tongue falls back into pharynx), cleft palate, flat bridge of nose, low-set ears, mental deficiency, and congenital heart disease in half the cases. Camptomelia (bent bones), diastrophic dwarfism (short limbs) common.

6. *DeLange syndrome.* The phenotype shows some degree of variability, but the essential diagnostic features are intrauterine growth retardation and stature falling below the third percentile at all ages, microbrachycephaly, generalized hirsutism and eyebrows that meet across the midline (synophrys), anteverted nostrils, long upper lip, and skeletal abnormalities (flexion of elbows, webbing of second and third toes, clinodactyly of fifth fingers, transverse palmar crease). All are severely retarded mentally, which, with craniofacial abnormalities, is diagnostic. It has been said, and it has been our experience, that these patients are prone to have a bad disposition, manifest as by biting and spitting. There are no chromosomal abnormalities. A polygenic inheritance has been postulated, but most cases are sporadic.

Neurocutaneous Anomalies with Mental Retardation

It is not surprising that skin and nervous system should share in pathologic states that impair development, since both have a common ectodermal derivation. Nevertheless, it is difficult to find a common theme in the diseases that affect both organs. In some instances, it is clear that ectoderm has been malformed from early intrauterine life; in others, a number of acquired diseases of skin may have been superimposed. For reasons to be elaborated later, neurofibromatosis, tuberous sclerosis, and Sturge-Weber encephalofacial angiomatosis must be set apart as a different category of disease.

Hemangiomas of the skin are without doubt the most frequent cutaneous abnormalities present at birth, and usually they are entirely innocent. Many recede in the first months of life. On the other hand, an extensive vascular nevus located in the territory of the trigeminal nerve—and sometimes in other parts of the body as well—causes permanent disfigurement and usually portends an associated cerebral lesion.

Other neurocutaneous diseases are summarized below. A more complete review of these diseases will be found in the article by Short and Adams and the monograph edited by Gomez, listed in the References. The related category of phakomatoses is discussed on pages 1069–1077. The importance of recognizing the cutaneous abnormalities relates to the fact that the nervous system is usually abnormal, and often the skin lesion appears before the neurologic symptoms are detectable. Thus the skin lesion becomes a predictor of potential neurologic involvement.

1. *Basal-cell nevus syndrome*. This condition is transmitted as an autosomal dominant trait and is characterized by superficial pits in the palms and soles; multiple solid or cystic tumors over the head, face, and neck appearing in infancy or early childhood; mental retardation in some cases; frontoparietal bossing; hypertelorism; and kyphoscoliosis.

2. *Congenital ichthyosis, hypogonadism, and mental retardation*. This disorder is inherited as a sex-linked recessive trait. Aside from the characteristic triad of anomalies, there are no special features.

3. *Xeroderma pigmentosum*. The pattern of inheritance is autosomal recessive. Skin lesions appear in infancy, taking the form of erythema, blistering, scaling, scarring, and pigmentation on exposure to sunlight; old lesions are telangiectatic and parchment-like, covered with fine scales; skin cancer may develop later; loss of eyelashes, synblepharon, dry bulbar conjunctivae; microcephaly, hypogonadism, and mental retardation (50 percent of cases). Kanda and associates classify this disease with the DeSanctis-Cacchione syndrome of xerodermic idiocy and believe the basic mechanism to be a faulty repair of DNA. These authors described two young adults with low intelligence, evidence of spinal cord degeneration, and peripheral neuropathy. The peripheral nerve lesions resembled those of amyloidosis, Riley-Day syndrome, and Fabry disease in that there was a predominant loss of small fibers. Other variants are described.

4. *Sjögren-Larssen syndrome*. Autosomal recessive with congenital ichthyosiform erythroderma, normal or thin scalp hair, sometimes defective dental enamel, pigmentary degeneration of retinae, spastic legs, and mental retardation.

5. *Poikiloderma congenitale (Rothmund-Thompson syndrome)*. Autosomal recessive heredity; appearance of skin changes from the third to sixth months of life; diffuse pink coloration of cheeks spreading to ears and buttocks, later replaced by macular and reticular pattern of skin atrophy mixed with striae, telangiectasia, and pigmentation; sparse hair in half of the cases; cataracts; small genitalia; abnormal hands and feet; short stature; and mental retardation.

6. *Linear sebaceous nevus syndrome*. Genetics uncertain, linear organoid nevus of one side of face and trunk, lipodermoids on bulbar conjunctivae, vascularization of corneas, mental retardation, focal seizures, and spike and slow waves in the EEG.

7. *Incontinentia pigmenti (Bloch-Sulzberger syndrome)*. Only females affected; appearance of dermal lesions in first weeks of life; vesicles and bullae followed by hyperkeratoses and streaks of pigmentation, scarring of scalp, and alopecia; abnormalities of dentition; hemiparesis; quadriparesis; seizures; mental retardation; up to 50 percent eosinophils in blood. The status of this disease is uncertain.

8. *Focal dermal hypoplasia*. Also, a disease limited to females. Areas of dermal hypoplasia with protrusions of subcutaneous fat, hypo- and hyperpigmentation, scoliosis, syndactyly in a few, short stature, thin body habitus, intelligence occasionally subnormal.

Other rare entities are neurocutaneous melanosis, neuroectodermal melanolysosomal disease with mental retardation, progeria, Cockayne syndrome, ataxia telangiectasia (Chap. 37; see also Gomez).

Dysraphism or Rachischisis (Encephaloceles and Spina Bifida)

Included under this heading are the large number of disorders of fusion of dorsal midline structures of the primitive neural tube, a process that takes place during the first 3 weeks of postconceptual life. Exogenous factors are presumed to be operative. The entire cranium may be missing at birth, and the undeveloped brain lies in the base of the skull, a small vascular mass without recognizable nervous structures. This state, *anencephaly*, has been discussed in the section "Disturbances of Neuronal Migration," above, and is the most frequent of the rachischises. It has many associations with other conditions in which the vertebral laminae fail to fuse.

An eventration of brain tissue and its coverings through an unfused midline defect in the skull is called an *encephalocele*. Frontal encephaloceles may deform the forehead or remain occult. Associated defects of the frontal cortex, anterior corpus callosum, and optic-hypothalamic structures and CSF leakage into frontal or ethmoid sinuses pose a risk of meningitis. Some of these children are relatively normal mentally. Far more severe are the posterior encephaloceles, some of which are enormous and are attended by grave neurologic deficits. However, lesser degrees of the defect are well known and may be small or hidden, such as a *meningoencephalocele* connected with the rest of the brain through a small opening in the skull. Small nasal encephaloceles may cause no neurologic signs, but if they are mistaken for nasal polyps and snipped off, CSF fistulae may result. The larger occipital ones are associated with blindness, ataxia, and mental retardation.

A failure of development of the midline portion of the cerebellum, referred to earlier, forms the basis of the *Dandy-Walker syndrome* (Fig. 38-2). A cyst-like structure, representing the greatly dilated fourth ventricle,

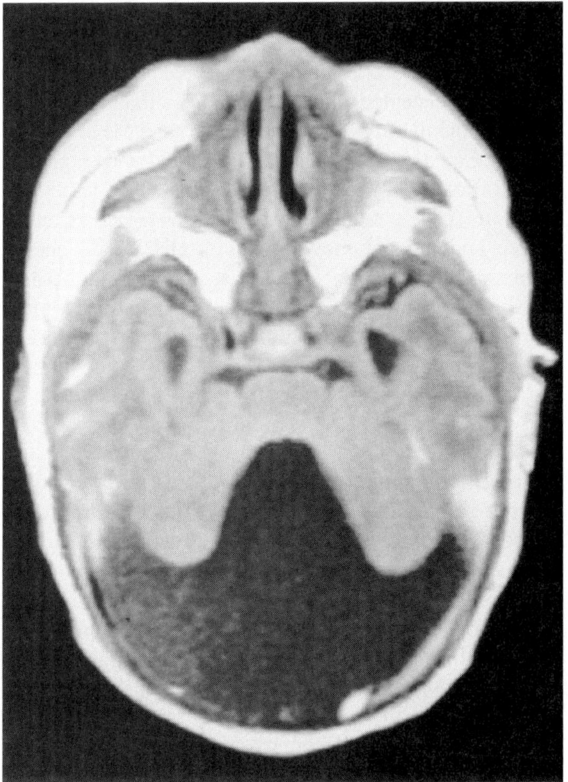

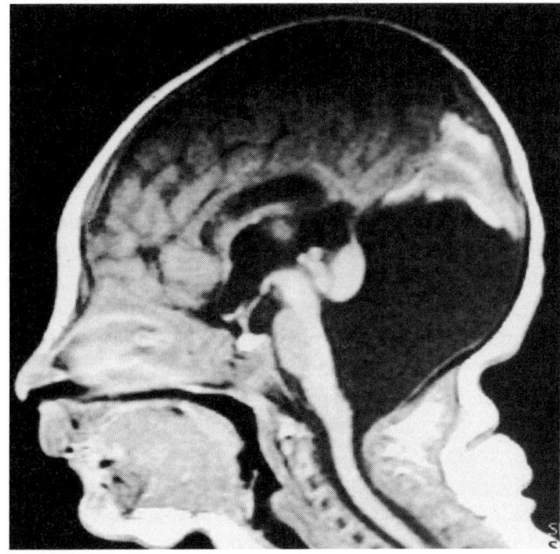

Figure 38-2

Dandy-Walker syndrome. MRI showing agenesis of the midline cerebellum and large midline cyst, representing the greatly dilated fourth ventricle, which occupies the posterior fossa. A. *Axial view,* B. *Sagittal view.*

expands in the midline, causing the occipital bone to bulge posteriorly and to displace the tentorium and torcula upward. In addition, the cerebellar vermis is aplastic, the corpus callosum may be deficient or absent, and there is dilatation of the aqueduct as well as the third and lateral ventricles.

Even more frequent are abnormalities of closure of the vertebral arches. These take the form of a *spina bifida occulta*, *meningocele*, and *meningomyelocele* of the lumbosacral or other regions.

In *spina bifida occulta*, the cord remains inside the canal and there is no external sac, although a subcutaneous lipoma or a dimple or wisp of hair on the overlying skin may mark the site of the lesion. In *meningocele*, there is a protrusion of only the dura and arachnoid through the defect in the vertebral laminae, forming a cystic swelling usually in the lumbosacral region; the cord remains in the canal, however. In *meningomyelocele*, which is 10 times as frequent as meningocele, the cord (more often the cauda equina) is extruded also and is closely applied to the fundus of the cystic swelling.

The incidence of spinal dysraphism (myeloschisis), like that of anencephaly, varies widely from one locale to another, and the disorder is more likely to occur in a second child if one child has already been affected (the incidence rises from 1 per 1000 to 40 to 50 per 1000). Exogenous factors (e.g., potato blight in Ireland) have been implicated in the genesis of both myeloschisis and anencephaly. Vitamin A and especially folic acid, given before the 28th day of pregnancy, can be protective. As with anencephaly, the diagnosis can often be inferred by the presence of α-fetoprotein in the amniotic fluid (sampled at 15 to 16 weeks of pregnancy) and the deformity confirmed by ultrasound in utero; blood contamination is a source of error in the fetoprotein test (Milunsky). Acetylcholinesterase immunoassay, done on amniotic fluid, is another reliable means of confirming the presence of neural tube defects. Some parents, on receiving this information, request abortion.

In the case of meningomyelocele, the child is born with a large externalized lumbosacral sac covered by delicate, weeping skin. It may have ruptured in utero or during birth, but more often the covering is intact. Stroking of the sac may elicit involuntary movements of the legs. As a rule the legs are motionless; urine dribbles, keeping the patient constantly wet; there is no response to pinprick over the lumbosacral zones; and the tendon reflexes are absent. In contrast, craniocervical structures are normal unless a Chiari malformation is associated (see further on). The neurologic abnormalities of the legs prove that the sac contains elements of spinal cord or cauda equina. Differences are noted in the neurologic picture depending on the level of the lesion. If it is entirely sacral, bladder and bowel sphincters are affected but legs escape; if lower lumbar and sacral, the buttocks, legs, and feet are more impaired than hip flexors and quadriceps; if upper lumbar, the feet and legs are sometimes spared and ankle reflexes retained, and there may be Babinski signs. The dreaded complications of these severe spinal defects are meningitis and progressive hydrocephalus from a Chiari malformation, which is often associated (see below). The subject of neural tube defects has recently been reviewed by Botto and colleagues.

Treatment Opinions as to proper management are not entirely settled. Excision and closure of the coverings of the meningomyelocele in the first few days of life is advised if the objective is to prevent a fatal meningitis. After a few weeks or months, as hydrocephalus reveals its presence by rapid increase in head size and enlargement of the ventricles on the CT scan, a ventriculoatrial or ventriculoperitoneal shunt is required. Patients with high spinal lesions and total paraplegia, kyphosis, hydrocephalus, and other major congenital anomalies are usually not accepted for treatment. Less than 30 percent of such patients survive beyond 1 year, and the long-term results of treating these patients have not been encouraging. Lorber and others report that 80 to 90 percent of their surviving patients are mentally retarded to some degree and are paraplegic—thus totally dependent on others for their care. The decision to undertake rather formidable surgical procedures is being questioned more and more frequently. Exceptionally, the patient with meningomyelocele and most of those with lumbar meningocele are mentally normal. Clinical differentiation of these two lesions is important.

Other Developmental Spinal Defects and Delayed Effects of Failure of Midline Fusion, Including Tethered Cord The problems of meningomyelocele and its complications are so strictly pediatric and surgical that the neurologist seldom becomes involved except in the initial evaluation of the patient, in the treatment of meningeal infection, or in the case of shunt failure with decompensation of hydrocephalus. Of greater interest to the neurologist are a series of closely related abnormalities that produce symptoms for the first time in late childhood, adolescence, or even adult life. These include sinus tracts with recurrent meningeal infections, lumbosacral lipomas, and myeloschisis with low tethering of the spinal cord ("tethered cord") and a delayed radicular or spinal cord syndrome; diastematomyelia, cysts, or tumors with spina bifida and a progressive myeloradiculopathy; and a Chiari malformation and syringomyelia that first present in adolescence or adult life. These abnormalities are described below.

Another class of disorders involves an occult lumbosacral dysraphism that is not inherited but is due to faulty development of the cell mass that lies caudal to the posterior neuropore (normally this undergoes closure by the 28th day of embryonic life). Occult spinal dysraphism of this type is also associated with meningoceles, lipomas, and sacrococcygeal teratomas. Another well-recognized anomaly is agenesis of the sacrum and sometimes the lower lumbar vertebrae (*caudal regression syndrome*). Interestingly, in 15 percent of such cases, the mother is diabetic (Lyon and Evrard). Here there is flaccid paralysis of legs, often with arthrogrypotic contractures and urinary incontinence. Sensory loss is less prominent, mental function develops normally, and there is no hydrocephalus.

Sinus tracts in the lumbosacral or occipital regions are of importance, for they may be a source of bacterial meningitis at any age. They are often betrayed by a small dimple in the skin or by a tuft of hair along the posterior surface of the body in the midline. (The pilonidal sinus should not be included in this group.) The sinus tract may lead to a terminal myelocystocele and be associated with dermoid cysts or fibrolipomas in the central part of the tract. Cloacal defects (no abdominal wall and no partition between bladder and rectum) may be combined with anterior meningoceles. Evidence of sinus tracts should be sought in every instance of meningitis, especially when the infection has recurred.

There are, in addition, other *congenital cysts* and *tumors*, particularly lipoma and dermoid, that arise in the filum terminale and attach (tether) the cord to the sacrum; progressive symptoms and signs are produced as the spine elongates during development, stretching the caudally fixed cord (Fig. 38-3). Some of these children have bladder and leg weakness soon after birth. Others deteriorate neurologically at a later age (generally between 1.5 to 16 years, sometimes later). According to Chapman and Davis, it is not the myelolipoma but the tethering of the cord that gives rise to symptoms; removal of the tumor is of little benefit unless the cord is untethered at the same time. This may be difficult, for the lipoma may be fused with the dorsal surface of the spinal cord).

Diastematomyelia is another unusual abnormality of the spinal cord often associated with spina bifida. Here a bony spicule or fibrous band protrudes into the spinal canal from the body of one of the thoracic or upper lumbar vertebrae and divides the spinal cord in two halves for a variable vertical extent. Or the division of the cord may be complete, each half with its own dural sac and complete set of nerve roots. This longitudinal fissuring and doubling of the cord are spoken of as *diplomyelia*. With growth, it leads to a *traction myelopathy*, presenting with pain and progressive sensory, motor, and bladder symptoms, sometimes as late as adult life. Removal of the fibrous-bony spicule and untethering of the spinal cord have been beneficial in some cases.

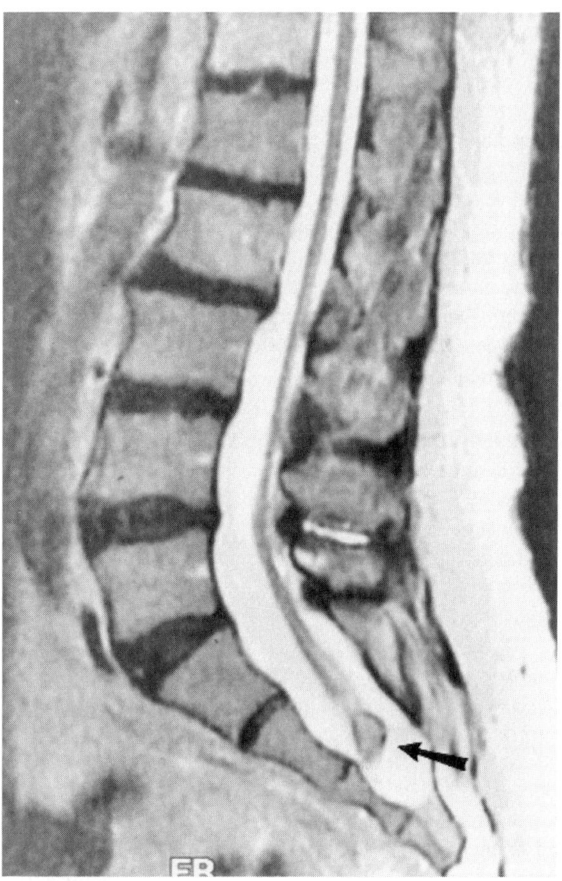

Figure 38-3

Magnetic resonance image of an adult with tethered cord and the typical lipoma at its caudal extent (arrow). *The conus lies behind the lower lumbar vertebra. No dystraphism is present. The main features were a flaccid bladder, asymmetrical weakness and atrophy of the forelegs, and a degree of spasticity in the legs.*

Several clinical *syndromes of delayed progressive disease* (adolescents or adults), due mainly to a tethered cord, have been delineated:

1. *Progressive cauda equina syndrome* with lesions in the lumbosacral region. In our experience this has been the commonest presentation of the *tethered cord* syndrome, with or without a lipoma or dermoid. Complex disturbances of bladder function that produce urgency and incontinence beginning in the second or third decade may be the only manifestation, or the bladder symptoms may be combined with impotence (in the male) and numbness of the feet and legs or foot drop (Pang and Wilberger). Several of our adult patients have had unusual visceral reflex reactions, such as involuntary defecation or priapism with stimulation of the abdomen or perineum.

2. *Progressive spastic weakness* in some of the weak muscles of the legs in a patient known to have had a meningocele or meningomyelocele. Presumably the spinal cord, which is securely attached to the lumbar vertebrae, is stretched during the period of rapid lengthening of the vertebral column.

3. *An acute cauda equina syndrome*, following some unusual activity or accident (e.g., rowing, or a fall in a sitting position), in patients who have had an asymptomatic or symptomatic spina bifida or meningocele. The implicated sensory and motor roots are believed to be injured by sudden or repeated stretching.

4. *Syringomyelia* (page 1337).

Also, there are a variety of neurologic problems associated with spinal abnormalities in the high cervical region [fusion of atlas and occiput or of cervical vertebrae (Klippel-Feil syndrome), congenital dislocation of the odontoid process and atlas, platybasia and basilar impression]. These abnormalities are reviewed in Chap. 45, with other diseases of the spinal cord.

Chiari Malformation

Encompassed by this term are a number of congenital anomalies at the base of the brain, the most consistent of which are (1) extension of a tongue of cerebellar tissue, posterior to the medulla and spinal cord, into the cervical canal and (2) displacement of the medulla into the cervical canal, along with the inferior part of the fourth ventricle. These and associated anomalies were first clearly described by Chiari (1891, 1896). Arnold's name is often attached to the syndrome (Arnold-Chiari malformation), but his contribution to our understanding of these malformations was relatively insignificant. However, use of the double eponym is so entrenched that a dispute over its aptness will not alter its usage. Chiari recognized four types of abnormality. In recent years the term has come to be restricted to Chiari's types I and II—i.e., to the cerebellomedullary malformation without and with a meningomyelocele, respectively. Type III Chiari malformation is no more than a high cervical or occipitocervical meningomyelocele with cerebellar herniation, and type IV consists only of cerebellar hypoplasia.

Several other morphologic features are characteristic. The medulla and pons are elongated and the aqueduct is narrowed. The displaced tissue (medulla and cerebellum) occludes the foramen magnum; the remainder of the cerebellum, which is small, is also displaced so as to obliterate the cisterna magna. The foramens of Luschka and Magendie open into the cervical canal, and the arachnoidal tissue around the herniated brainstem and cerebellum is fibrotic. All these factors are probably operative in the production of hydrocephalus, which is always associated. Just below the herniated tail of cerebellar tissue there is a kink or spur in the spinal cord, pushed posteriorly by the lower end of the fourth ventricle. In this type of malformation, a meningomyelocele is nearly always found. It should also be emphasized that *hydromyelia or syringomyelia of the cervical cord are commonly associated findings.*

Developmental abnormalities of the cerebrum (particularly polymicrogyria) may coexist, and the lower end of the spinal cord (i.e., filum terminale) may extend as low as the sacrum. There are usually bony abnormalities as well. The posterior fossa is small; the foramen magnum is enlarged and grooved posteriorly. Nishikawa et al have suggested that smallness of the posterior fossa, with overcrowding, is the primary abnormality, leading to the brain malformation. Often the base of the skull is flattened or infolded by the cervical spine (basilar impression).

Clinical Manifestations In type II Chiari malformation (with meningomyelocele), the problem is essentially one of progressive hydrocephalus. Cerebellar signs cannot be discerned in the first few months of life. However, lower cranial nerve abnormalities—laryngeal stridor, fasciculations of the tongue, sternomastoid paralysis (head lag), facial weakness, deafness, bilateral abducens palsies—may be present in varying combinations. If the patient survives to later childhood or adolescence, one of the syndromes that occurs with the type I malformation may become manifest.

In type I Chiari malformation (without meningocele or other signs of dysraphism), neurologic symptoms may not develop until adolescence or adult life. The symptoms may be those of (1) increased intracranial pressure, mainly headache, (2) progressive cerebellar ataxia, (3) progressive spastic quadriparesis, (4) downbeating nystagmus, or (5) syringomyelia (segmental amyotrophy and sensory loss, with or without pain). Or the patient may show a combination of disorders of the lower cranial nerves, cerebellum, medulla, and spinal cord (sensory and motor tract disorders), usually in conjunction with headache that is mainly occipital. This combination of symptoms is often mistaken for multiple sclerosis or a foramen magnum tumor. The symptoms may have an acute onset after sustained extension of the neck, as, for example, after a long session of dental work, hairdressing in women, or chiropractic manipulation. The physical habitus of such patients may be normal, but about 25 percent have signs of an arrested hydrocephalus or a short "bull neck." When basilar impression and a Chiari malformation coexist, it may be impossible to decide which of the two is responsible for the clinical findings.

Diagnosis and Treatment Until the advent of MRI, myelography, performed with the patient supine, was the most reliable means of corroborating the clinical diagnosis. The tongue of cerebellar tissue and the kinked cervical cord obstructed the upward flow of dye and gave a highly characteristic radiologic profile. This procedure and several others have been superseded by MRI because of the clarity with which the latter exposes abnormalities of the craniocervical region (Fig. 38-4). Inspection of the axial sections of CT scans at the level of the foramen magnum also demonstrate crowding of the upper cervical canal by inferiorly displaced cerebellar tissue, but one must be aware of the variations in the normal position of the cerebellar tonsils at this level. The low-pressure CSF syndrome may also lead to a slight descent of the cerebellar tonsils that is reversible and is not indicative of a Chiari malformation. The CSF is usually normal but may show an elevated pressure and protein level in some cases.

The treatment of Chiari malformation (and basilar impression) is far from satisfactory. If clinical progression is slight or uncertain, it is probably best to do nothing. If progression is certain and disability is increasing, upper cervical laminectomy and enlargement of the foramen magnum are indicated. Often this procedure halts the progress of the neurologic illness, arrests the hydrocephalus, or results in some improvement. The outcome, in our experience, has been unsatisfactory when decompression was performed mainly for intractable headache. The surgical procedure must be done cautiously. Opening of the dura and extensive manipulation of the malformation or excision of herniated cerebellum may aggravate the symptoms or even cause death. The treatment of an associated syringomyelia and other developmental abnormalities in this region is discussed further on page 1337.

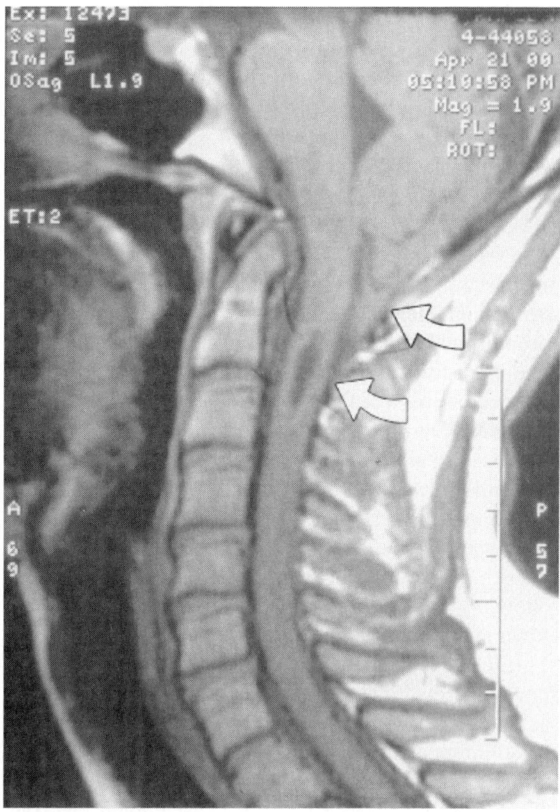

Figure 38-4

Chiari type malformation and developmental syringomyelia. T1-weighted MRI the low-lying cerebellar tonsils below the foramen magnum and behind the upper cervical cord (upper arrow) and the syrinx cavity in the upper cord (lower arrow).

Chromosomal Abnormalities (Chromosomal Dysgeneses)

A mid-twentieth-century discovery of outstanding significance was the recognition of a group of developmental anomalies of the brain and other organs associated with a demonstrable abnormality of an autosomal or sex chromosome. Jacobs and Lejeune almost simultaneously were the first to note a triplication of the twenty-first chromosome in the Down syndrome, and there followed the discovery of a number of other trisomies as well as deletions or translocations of other autosomal chromosomes and a lack or excess of one of the sex chromosomes. By recent count, 24 chromosomal abnormalities had been identified. Such an event must take place sometime after the formation of the oocyte, during the long period that it lies fallow in the aging ovary or during the process of conception or germination and first cell divisions. Thus, all the cells in the embryo may be affected or only some of them, the latter condition being called *mosaicism*.

The manner in which triplication or some other imperfection of a chromosome is able to derail the pathways of ontogenesis is a mystery. In some instances, a chromosomal imperfection may result from the lack of a gene or distortion or fragmentation of a gene or by an enlarged or unstable DNA nucleotide sequence, as in the fragile-X syndrome.

Certain chromosomal abnormalities are incompatible with life, and it has been found that the cells of many unexplained abortuses and stillborns show abnormal karyotypes. On the other hand, the organism may survive and exhibit any one of many syndromes, of which the following are the best known and most frequent: (1) Down syndrome (mongolism, trisomy 21); (2) one type of arrhinencephaly (trisomy 13, Patau syndrome); (3) trisomy 18 (Edwards syndrome); (4) cri-du-chat syndrome (deletion of short arm of chromosome 5); (5) monosomy 21 (antimongolism); (6) ring chromosomes; (7) Klinefelter syndrome (XXY); (8) Turner syndrome (XO); (9) others (XXXX, XXX, XYY, YY, XXYY); (10) the fragile-X syndrome, the most common form of inherited mental retardation; (11) Williams syndrome; (12) Prader-Willi and Angelman syndromes; and (13) Rett syndrome. The overall frequency of chromosomal abnormalities in live births is 0.6 percent (Kalter and Warkany). See Lemieux for a comprehensive account of the chromosome-linked disorders.

Down Syndrome Described first in 1866 by Langdon Down, this is the best known of the chromosomal dysgeneses. The frequency is 1 in 600 to 700 births, and this condition accounts for approximately 10 percent of all reported series of cases of severe mental retardation. Familiarity with the condition permits its recognition at birth, but it becomes more obvious with advancing age. The round head, open mouth, stubby hands, slanting palpebral fissures, and short stature impart an unmistakable clinical picture. The ears are low-set and oval, with small lobules. The palpebral fissures slant slightly upward and outward owing to the presence of medial epicanthal folds that partly cover the inner canthi (hence the old term "mongolism"). The bridge of the nose is poorly developed and the face is flattened (hypoplasia of the maxillae). The tongue is usually enlarged, heavily fissured, and protruded. Gray-white specks of depigmentation are seen in the irides (Brushfield spots). The little fingers are often short (hypoplastic middle phalanx) and incurved (clinodactyly). The fontanels are patent but slow to close. The hands are broad, with a single transverse (simian) palmar crease and other characteristic dermal markings. Lenticular opacities and congenital heart lesions (septal and other defects) as well as gastrointestinal abnormalities (stenosis of duodenum) are frequent. Hypotonia of limbs is a prominent finding. At first the Moro response is reduced or absent, and feeding is difficult. The patient with Down syndrome is slightly below average size at birth and is characteristically short at later periods of life. The height attained in adult life seldom exceeds that of a 10-year-old child. Most affected children do not walk until 3 to 4 years of age; their acquisition of speech is delayed, but over 90 percent talk by 5 years. The intelligence quotient (IQ) is variable, and that of a large group follows a Gaussian curve; the median IQ is 40 to 50, and the range is 20 to 70. A placid, docile, and affectionate personality characterizes most Down patients. A high incidence of atlantoaxial instability puts them at risk of spinal cord compression in athletic ventures. Also, an increased incidence of myelocytic and lymphocytic leukemia takes its toll. A number of patients have had embolic strokes and brain abscesses secondary to cardiac abnormalities. Life expectancy is later shortened by the almost universal development of Alzheimer disease by the 40th year of life.

One cannot distinguish the Down syndrome with a triplication of chromosome 21 from that with a translocation. There is a strong correlation between each of these types and the age of the mother. Whereas the triplication is found in the offspring of older mothers, the less frequent translocation is found equally in the offspring of young and old. In other subtypes of the Down syndrome, referred to as *mosaics*, some cells share in the chromosomal abnormality and others are normal. Mosaics have atypical forms of the syndrome, and some such individuals are of normal intelligence. Laboratory tests are not helpful in clarifying the mechanism of the disorder; abnormalities include decreased serotonin, increased alkaline phosphatase in the white cells, increased glucose diphosphate in red cells, and a 50 percent increase in superoxide dismutase. The latter enzyme derives from a gene located on the long arm of chromosome 21 and is a convenient marker of the trisomy, but it is not thought to be responsible for the dysmorphism or mental retardation. (This enzyme assumes importance in the familial form of amyotrophic lateral sclerosis.)

Pathologic Findings Brain weight is approximately 10 percent less than average. The convolutional pattern is rather simple. The frontal lobes are smaller than normal, and the superior temporal gyri are thin. There are claims of delayed myelination of cerebral white matter and also of immature and poorly differentiated cortical neurons. Alzheimer neurofibrillary changes and neuritic plaques are practically always found in Down cases beyond 40 years of age. As Alzheimer disease develops, the usual clinical picture is marked by inattentiveness, reduced speech, impairment of visuospatial orientation, loss of memory and judgment, and seizures.

It is possible to make the diagnosis of Down syndrome by demonstrating the chromosomal abnormalities in cells of the amniotic fluid. About one-third of pregnant mothers (in the second trimester) also have an abnormal elevation of serum α-fetoprotein. Other independent predictors of fetal Down syndrome are elevated serum chorionic gonadotropin and decreased estriol (Haddow et al). One can uncover a considerable proportion of the Down population by prenatal screening for these serum markers and doing amniocentesis on all pregnant women with positive tests to search for the chromosomal abnormality.

Other Chromosomal Dysgeneses

1. *Trisomy 13 (Patau syndrome)*. Frequency 1:2000 live births, more female than male, average maternal age 31 years, microcephaly and sloping forehead, microphthalmos, coloboma of iris, corneal opacities, anosmia, low-set ears, cleft lip and palate, capillary hemangiomata, polydactyly, flexed fingers, posterior prominence of heels, dextrocardia, umbilical hernia, impaired hearing, hypertonia, severe mental retardation, death in early childhood.

2. *Trisomy 18*. Frequency 1:4000 live births, more in females, average maternal age 34 years, slow growth, occasional seizures, severe mental retardation, hypertonia, ptosis and lid abnormalities, low-set ears, small mouth, mottled skin, clenched fists with index fingers over third finger, syndactyly, rocker-bottom feet, shortened big toe, ventricular septal defect, umbilical and inguinal hernias, short sternum, small pelvis, small mandible, death in early infancy.

3. *Cri-du-chat syndrome* (deletion in short arm of chromosome 5). Abnormal cry, like a kitten, severe mental retardation, hypertelorism, epicanthal folds, brachycephaly, moon face, antimongoloid slant of palpebral fissures, micrognathia, hypotonia, strabismus.

4. *Ring chromosomes*. Mental retardation with variable physical abnormalities.

5. *Klinefelter syndrome (XXY)*. Only males. Eunuchoid appearance, wide arm span, sparse facial and body hair, high-pitched voice, gynecomastia, small testicles, usually mentally retarded but not severely so; high incidence of psychosis, asthma, and diabetes.

6. *Turner syndrome (XO)*. Only females. Triangular face, small chin, occasionally hypertelorism and epicanthal folds, widely spaced nipples, clinodactyly, cubitus valgus, hypoplastic nails, short stature, webbed neck, delayed sexual development, mild mental retardation.

7. *Colpocephaly*. A rare type of malformation of the brain consisting of marked dilatation of the occipital horns of the lateral ventricles, thickening of the overlying rim of cortical gray matter, and thinning of the white matter. The associated clinical picture comprises mental retardation, spasticity, seizures, and visual abnormalities (due to optic nerve hypoplasia). This disorder is probably of diverse causation, but it is listed with the chromosomal abnormalities because some cases have been associated with the mosaicism for trisomy 8 (Herskowitz et al). The term colpocephaly is often used incorrectly to apply to all forms of ventricular enlargement associated with abnormal development of the brain.

8. *Fragile-X syndrome* (see also page 1097). With the advent of new markers for the detailed structure of chromosomes, Lubs observed an unusual site of frequent breakage ("fragility") on the X chromosome and related it to a syndrome that includes mental retardation, flaring ears, elongated facies, slightly reduced cranial perimeter, normal stature, and enlarged testes. *This chromosomal abnormality appears to be the most common inherited form of mental retardation* (estimated to cause 1 case of retardation in every 1500 male births). Females, with their two X chromosomes, are affected about half as frequently, and then only to a slight degree. It is estimated that 10 percent of severely retarded males harbor the fragile-X chromosome. In the Fernald School population, this figure seems correct. The fragility appears to be due to a heritable, CGG-unstable repeating sequence. Affected individuals have over 200 repeats and normal carriers have 43 to 200 repeats. The prolonged sequence inactivates a gene (FMR1) that codes for an RNA-binding protein. Rousseau and colleagues have described a simple and sensitive test, using DNA analysis, for the diagnosis of the syndrome both prenatally and after birth.

Because the length of the triplet repeat relates to the degree of expression of retardation, the fragile-X alteration occasionally turns up in mentally normal males, and in some instances the male children of their daughters have the disease. In some of our cases, the intellectual deficit has been moderate in degree; the main abnormalities have taken the form of troublesome behavior, logorrhea, an autistic type of gaze aversion, and asociality. These and other peculiar features of the syndrome and its unique pattern of inheritance (it is neither recessive nor dominant) have been discussed by Shapiro. At first, it was assumed that the fragile-X syndrome was only an example of the Renpenning syndrome (hereditary feeble-mindedness in males with X-linked chromosomal disorder—see pages 635 and 1098), until it was pointed out that in this latter condition, stature was reduced, as was the cranial circumference, and that the X chromosomes of the Renpenning patients were not fragile.

9. *Williams syndrome*. Described by J. C. P. Williams of Australia from the perspective of a supravalvular aortic stenosis and later by Beuren and colleagues, this unique combination of cerebral maldevelopment and cardiovascular abnormalities has been traced in most patients to a microdeletion on chromosome 7 in the region of the gene that codes for elastin. Its frequency is 1:20,000 newborns. Further discussion of clinical features of this syndrome will be found on page 1098.

10. *Prader-Willi and Angelman syndromes*. The Prader-Willi syndrome has already been mentioned in relation to the hyperphagia of hypothalamic disorders (page 595). It is a not uncommon syndrome (one in 20,000 births) and affects both sexes equally. Hypotonia, areflexia, small stature, dysmorphic facies, and hypoplastic genitalia are evident and arthrogryposis may be present at birth; after the first year, mental retardation becomes obvious and obesity, due to hyperphagia, becomes prominent. Patients are identified by the H3O mnemonic, referring to hypomentia, hypotonia, hypogonadism, and obesity. The disorder is associated with a deletion at 15q11-q13, which can be identified by a combination of cytogenetic and DNA analyses. In 70 percent of cases the disease is due to a noninherited deletion from the paternal X chromosome. The Angelman syndrome, another cause of severe mental retardation, is associated with the identical chromosomal abnormality that is found in the Prader-Willi syndrome, i.e., a deletion at 15q11-q13, but in the case of Angelman syndrome there is usually a maternally inherited single gene defect. The difference in phenotype derives from a complex genetic phenomenon termed *spatially restricted imprinting*. Phenotypically, however, the two disorders are quite distinct. The Angelman syndrome, in addition to mental retardation, is characterized by microcephaly, the early development of seizures that are refractory to antiepileptic drugs, and an unusual marionette-like stance and movement disorder coupled with a persistent tendency to laugh and smile (hence the old name "happy puppet syndrome").

11. *Rett syndrome*, discussed more fully on page 1098, is due to a dominant defect on the X chromosome. It affects one of every 10,000 to 15,000 girls. After 6 to 18 months of normal development, motor skills and mental abilities slowly regress. Certain hand-wringing and other stereotyped hand movements are characteristic as the disease progresses.

Several generalizations can be made about these chromosomal dysgeneses. First, the autosomal ones are often lethal, and they almost always have a devastating effect on cerebral growth and development, whether the infant survives or not. Anomalies of nonneural structures are regularly present—an association so constant that one may safely predict that a normally formed infant will not have a detectable chromosomal defect. However, only in the Down syndrome and trisomy 13 (and possibly trisomy 18) are the physiognomy and bodily configuration of predictive value. Surprisingly, some of the most grotesque disfigurements, such as anencephaly and multiple congenital anomalies, are not related to a morphologic abnormality of chromosomes. By contrast, an insufficiency of sex chromosomes does induce subtle effects on the brain, affecting intellect, and personality; to some extent this is true of supernumerary sex chromosomes (XYY, for example).

The basic abnormality of the brain underlying the mental retardation in many of these chromosomal dysgeneses has not been ascertained. The cerebra are slightly small, but only minor changes are seen in the convolutional pattern and cortical architecture in conventional microscopic preparations. Neurocellular methodologies are not sufficiently advanced to reveal the abnormalities.

Environmental Teratologic Factors

A number of observations have repudiated the belief that the human embryo is shielded against exogenous causes of maldevelopment. Irradiation during the first trimester, rubella and CMV infections, severe hypothyroidism of the mother during this same period, and the action of aminopterin, alcohol, vitamin A, and thalidomide all give rise to serious disorders of development. Also, the offspring of mothers receiving anticonvulsant drugs during the early months of pregnancy have a slightly increased risk of developing birth defects (approximately 5 percent, compared to 3 percent for the general population). The greatest risk is with trimethadione, but phenytoin, carbamazepine, valproate, and phenobarbital have also been implicated. Cleft lip and palate are the most common anomalies attributable to anticonvulsant drugs; other craniofacial defects, spina bifida, and dysraphisms have also been reported (Janz et al). Concerning other teratogens, there is much controversy. Claims and counterclaims have been made concerning the pathogenicity of the substances listed in Table 38-2. Mainly, the data are from animals given amounts far in excess of any possible therapeutic doses in humans. The data are so meager that they are not discussed here. The reader may refer to the article by Kalter and Warkany for further information.

Table 38-2
Environmental substances suspected of causing congenital malformations in human beings

A. Contaminants and food additives
- Cadminium
- Cyclamates
- Dioxin
- Dichlorodiphenyl trichloroethane
- Food coloring
- Hair dyes
- Lead
- Mercury
- Monosodium glutamate
- Nitrates
- Polyhalogenated biphenyls
- Saccharin
- Sodium fluoride

B. Natural substances
- Blighted potatoes
- Cyanide in cassava
- Goitrogens in brassicae

C. Habituating and addicting drugs
- Alcohol
- Cigarettes
- Coffee
- Gasoline sniffing
- Lysergic acid diethylamide
- Marijuana
- Methadone
- Phencyclidine
- Tea
- Tobacco chewing
- Toluene sniffing

D. Occupational exposure
- Anesthetic gases
- Fat solvents
- Hair-spray adhesives
- Hexachlorophene
- Hydrocarbons
- Organic solvents
- Substances used in smelting and printing industries and chemical laboratories

E. Antiepileptic drugs (trimethadione, phenytoin, and others)

Source: Adapted from Kalter and Warkany, with permission.

THE PHAKOMATOSES (CONGENITAL ECTODERMOSES)

As stated earlier, there are two broad categories of neurocutaneous diseases. In one, the infant is born with a special type of skin disease or develops it in the first weeks of life; in the other, particular forms of cutaneous abnormality, though often present in minor degree at birth, later evolve as quasi-neoplastic disorders. The latter, to which van der Hoeve (1920) applied the term *phakomatoses* (from the Greek *phakos*, meaning "mother spot," "mole," or "freckle"), include tuberous sclerosis, neurofibromatosis, and cutaneous angiomatosis with central nervous system (CNS) abnormalities. These diseases have many features in common—hereditary transmission, involvement of organs of ectodermal origin (nervous system, eyeball, retina, and skin), slow evolution of lesions in childhood and adolescence, tendency to form hamartomas (benign tumor-like formations due to maldevelopment), and a disposition to fatal malignant transformation. These disorders are discussed below.

Tuberous Sclerosis (Bourneville Disease)

Tuberous sclerosis is a congenital disease of hereditary type in which a variety of lesions, due to a limited hyperplasia of ectodermal and mesodermal cells, appear in the skin, nervous system, heart, kidney, and other organs. It is characterized clinically by the triad of adenoma sebaceum, epilepsy, and mental retardation.

It is stated that Virchow had recognized scleromas of the cerebrum in the 1860s and that von Recklinghausen had reported a similar lesion combined with multiple myomata of the heart in 1862, but Bourneville's articles, appearing between 1880 and 1900, presented the first systematic accounts of the disease and related the cerebral lesions to those of the skin of the face. Vogt (1890) fully appreciated the significance of the neurocutaneous relationship and formally delineated the triad of *facial adenoma sebaceum, epilepsy, and mental retardation*. "Epiloia," a term for the disease introduced by

Sherlock in 1911, never gained general acceptance. These and other historical aspects are reviewed in Gomez's monograph on tuberous sclerosis.

Epidemiology This disease has been described in all parts of the world and is equally frequent in all races and both sexes. Heredity is evident in only a minority of cases—50 percent in some series and as little as 14 percent in the series of Bundag and Evans (cited by Brett). It is determined by a single autosomal dominant gene, the estimated prevalence of which is 1:50,000 to 1:300,000. The remaining cases are attributed to a gene mutation, the frequency of which is calculated to be 1:20,000 to 1:50,000. The disease involves many organs in addition to the skin and brain, and it may assume a diversity of forms, the least severe of which (i.e., the forme fruste) is difficult to diagnose; hence, one cannot be precise about the incidence of the disease. Tuberous sclerosis accounts for about 0.66 percent of the mentally retarded in institutions and 0.32 percent of epileptics. The medical literature contains a number of reports of patients whose mentality is preserved and who have never had convulsions. It is likely that data drawn from mental hospital populations have exaggerated the overall frequency of mental retardation (Gomez).

Etiology and Pathogenesis The abnormal gene has been localized to one of two sites—the long arm of chromosome 9, designated as TSC 1, and the short arm of chromosome 16, TSC 2. The former site is linked closely to the ABO blood group genes. The mutations are at loci of tumor-suppressor genes that are inactivated and this may, in part, explain the proclivity to develop various growths and hamartomas. Several hypotheses relating to neuronal migration or to the excessive secretion of growth factors have been proposed to link the inactivation of these genes with the pathogenesis of the characteristic lesions. The cellular elements within the lesions are abnormal in both number and size. The tumor-like growths in different organs may include cells of more than one type (e.g., fibroblasts, cardiac myoblasts, angioblasts, glioblasts, and neuroblasts), and their number is locally excessive. Something appears to have gone awry with the proliferative process during embryologic development, yet it is usually kept under control, in the sense that only rarely do the growths undergo malignant transformation. Highly specialized cells within the lesions may attain giant size; neurons three to four times normal size may be observed in the cerebral scleroses. These facts emphasize the potentially blastomatous character of the process.

Clinical Manifestations The disease may be present at the time of birth (the diagnosis has been made by CT scan in neonates), but more often the infant is judged at first to be normal. In approximately 75 percent of cases, attention is drawn to the disease initially by the occurrence of focal or generalized seizures or by retarded psychomotor development. As with any condition that leads to mental retardation, the first suspicion is raised by delay in reaching normal maturational milestones. Whatever the initial symptom, the convulsive disorder and mental retardation become more prominent within 2 to 3 years. The facial cutaneous abnormality, the so-called adenoma sebaceum, appears later in childhood, usually between the fourth and tenth years, and is progressive thereafter.

As the years pass, the seizures change pattern. In the first year or two they take the form of massive flexion spasms with hypsarrhythmia (irregular dysrhythmic bursts of high-voltage spikes and slow waves in the EEG). As many as 25 percent of our patients with these types of seizures have been found to have tuberous sclerosis. Later, the seizures change to more typical generalized motor and psychomotor attacks or atypical petit mal. Any one of the seizure types may be brief, especially if the patient is receiving anticonvulsant medication. Seizures are always the most reliable index of the cerebral lesions; focal neurologic abnormalities, which one might expect to occur from the size and location of the lesions, are distinctly uncommon.

Mental function continues to deteriorate slowly. Exceptionally there is a spastic weakness or mild choreoathetosis of the limbs and in a few cases an obstructive hydrocephalus. As in any state of severe mental retardation, a variety of nonspecific motor peculiarities—such as constant crying, muttering, stereotypical rocking and swaying movements, and digital mannerisms—may be observed. In nearly half of the cases, affective and behavioral derangements, often of hyperkinetic and aggressive type, are added to the intellectual deficiency.

The lack of parallelism in the severity of the epilepsy, mental deficit, and cutaneous abnormalities has been noted by all clinicians who have had a wide experience with this disease. Some patients are subject to recurrent seizures while retaining relatively normal mental function; in others, trivial skin lesions or a retinal phakoma may suggest the diagnosis in a mentally normal person with few seizures. In such cases, recognition may elude competent neurologists and dermatologists. As a general rule, early onset of seizures is predictive of mental retardation. Gomez and colleagues have suggested that the seizures damage the brain, a point with which we agree. However, it seems likely that both the epilepsy and mental retardation are the product of severe involvement of the brain by the lesions of tuberous sclerosis.

Limitation of space allows no more than a catalogue of other visceral abnormalities. In about half the cases, gray or yellow plaques (in reality gliomatous tumors) may be found in the retina in or near the optic disc or at a distance from it. It is from this lesion, called a *phakoma*, that van der Hoeve derived the term that is applied to all neurocutaneous diseases of this class. About half of all benign rhabdomyomas of the heart are associated with tuberous sclerosis, and, if located in the wall of the atrium, they may cause conduction defects. Other benign tumors of mixed cell type (angiomyolipomas) have been found in the kidneys, liver, lungs, thyroid, testes, and gastrointestinal tract. Cysts of the pleura or lungs, bone cysts in digits, and zones of marbling or densification in bones are some of the less common abnormalities.

In approximately 90 percent of patients with tuberous sclerosis, congenital hypomelanotic macules (formerly mistaken for "partial albinism" or "vitiligo") appear before any of the other skin lesions (Fitzpatrick et al). They are arranged in linear fashion over the trunk or limbs and range in size from a few millimeters to several centimeters; their configuration is oval, with one end round and the other pointed, in the shape of an ash leaf. A Wood's lamp, which transmits only ultraviolet rays, facilitates the demonstration of the ash leaf lesions because of the absence of melanoblasts, which normally absorb light in the ultraviolet range (360-nm wavelength). These lesions become pink when rubbed and contain sweat glands; they are not usually present on the face or head. There is occasionally a white tuft of hair (poliosis). Electron microscopic examination shows a normal or reduced number of melanocytes, but their dopa reaction is reduced and melanosomes are small. Gold and Freeman as well as Fitzpatrick and colleagues have emphasized the frequency of these leukodermic lesions and their value in the diagnosis of tuberous sclerosis during infancy, before the appearance of other cutaneous lesions.

The well-developed facial lesions (adenomas of Pringle), pathognomonic of tuberous sclerosis, are present in 90 percent of patients over 4 years of age. Typically they are red to pink nodules with a smooth, glistening surface, and they tend to be limited to the nasolabial folds, cheeks, and chin; sometimes they also involve the forehead and scalp. Although called "adenoma sebaceum," these nodules are actually angiofibromas; the sebaceous glands are only passively involved (Fig. 38-5). The earliest manifestation of facial angiofibromatosis may be a mild erythema over the cheeks and forehead, intensified by crying. The occurrence of large plaques of connective tissue on the forehead is usually expressive of a severe form of the disease.

On the trunk, the diagnostic lesion is the "shagreen patch" (in reality a plaque of subepidermal fibrosis) found most often in the lumbosacral region. It appears as a flat, slightly elevated, flesh-colored area of skin 1 to 10 cm in diameter, with a "pigskin," "elephant hide," or "orange peel" appearance (Fig. 38-6). Another common site of fibromatous involvement is the nail bed; subungual fibromas usually appear at puberty and continue to develop with age. Other common skin changes, not in themselves diagnostic, include fibroepithelial tags (soft fibromas), café au lait spots, and port-wine hemangiomas.

Pathology The brain exhibits a number of diagnostic anomalies. Broadening, unnatural whiteness, and firmness of parts of some of the cerebral convolutions are simulated by no other disease. These are the tubers after which the disease is named. On the surface of the brain, they range in width from 5 mm to 2 or 3 cm. Their cut surface reveals a lack of demarcation from cortex and white matter and the presence of white flecks of

Figure 38-5

Adenoma sebaceum of tuberous sclerosis.

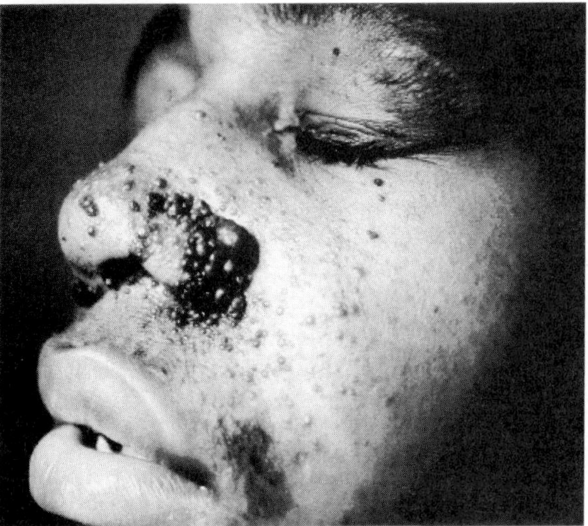

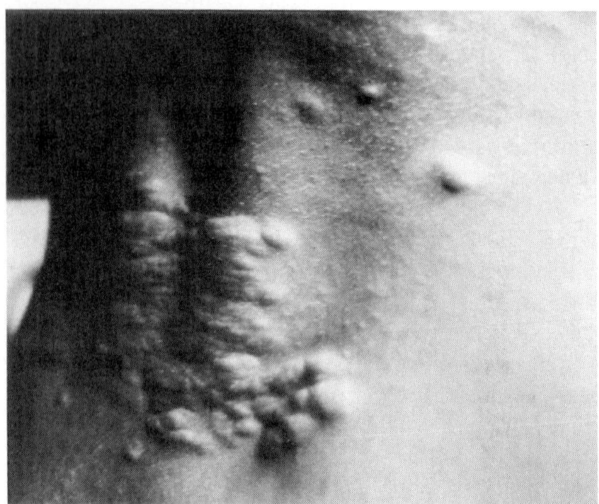

Figure 38-6

Shagreen patch on the skin of the lower back in a young patient with tuberous sclerosis.

calcium; the latter, which are readily seen on CT scans and MRI, are called *brain stones* (see below). The walls of the lateral ventricles may be encrusted with white or pink-white masses resembling candle getterings. When calcified, they appear in radiographs as curvilinear opacities that follow the outline of the ventricle. Rarely, nodules of abnormal tissue are observed in the basal ganglia, thalamus, cerebellum, brainstem, and spinal cord.

Under the microscope the tubers are seen to be composed of interlacing rows of plump, fibrous astrocytes (much like an astrocytoma, though lacking in glial fibrillar protein). In the cerebral cortex and ganglionic structures, derangements of architecture result from the presence of abnormal-appearing cells; greatly enlarged "monstrous" neurons and glial cells—often difficult to distinguish from one another, and displaced normal-sized neurons contribute to the chaotic histologic appearance. Gliomatous deposits may obstruct the foramina of Monro or the aqueduct or floor of the fourth ventricle, causing hydrocephalus. Neoplastic transformation of abnormal glial cells, a not infrequent occurrence, usually takes the form of a large-cell astrocytoma, less often of a glioblastoma or meningioma.

The phakomas of the retina are composed mainly of neuronal and glial components, but occasionally there is an admixture of fibrous tissue.

Diagnosis When the full combination of seizures and mental and dermal abnormalities are conjoined, the diagnosis is self-evident. It is the early stage of the disease and the *forme fruste* that give trouble, and here the experienced dermatologist can be of great help. Epilepsy—i.e., flexion spasms in infancy—and delay in psychomotor development are by no means diagnostic of tuberous sclerosis, since they occur in many diseases. It is in these cases and also in every sizable population of the epileptic or mentally retarded, especially when the family history is unrevealing, that a search for the dermal equivalents of the disease—the hypomelanotic ash-leaf spots, adenoma sebaceum, collagenous patch, phakoma of the retina, or subungual or gingival fibromas—is so rewarding. The finding of any one of these lesions provides confirmation of the partial and atypical case. Adenoma sebaceum may occasionally occur alone and is easily confused with acne vulgaris in the adolescent. The history of epilepsy and/or the demonstration of a dull mentality are helpful, but neither is a requisite for the diagnosis of tuberous sclerosis (Gomez).

The most useful laboratory measures for corroborating the disease are CT scanning and MRI (Fig. 38-7). The periventricular calcific lesions are particularly well shown on the CT scan, whereas MRI is more sensitive in detecting cortical lesions. A striking feature is an absence of edema in the surrounding tissue. An increasing number of cortical lesions demonstrated with MRI appears to correlate with an increased impairment of neurologic function (Roach et al).

Treatment Nothing can be offered in the way of prevention other than genetic counseling. Anticonvulsant therapy of the standard type suppresses the convulsive tendency more or less effectively and should be applied assiduously. Adrenocorticotropic hormone (ACTH) suppresses the flexor spasms and tends to normalize the EEG abnormality. It is pointless to attempt the excision of tumors, especially in severely affected individuals (with the exception of renal hamartomas that impair function). However, there are patients who are not mentally impaired and who have benefited from dermabrasion of the facial lesions, with the knowledge that these slowly regrow; and neurosurgeons have partially excised brain tumors that were causing recalcitrant epilepsy or shunted the lateral ventricular in patients with increased intracranial pressure.

Course and Prognosis In general, the disease advances so slowly that years must elapse before one can be sure of progression. Of the severe cases, approximately 30 percent die before the fifth year, and 50 to 75 percent before attaining adult age. Worsening is

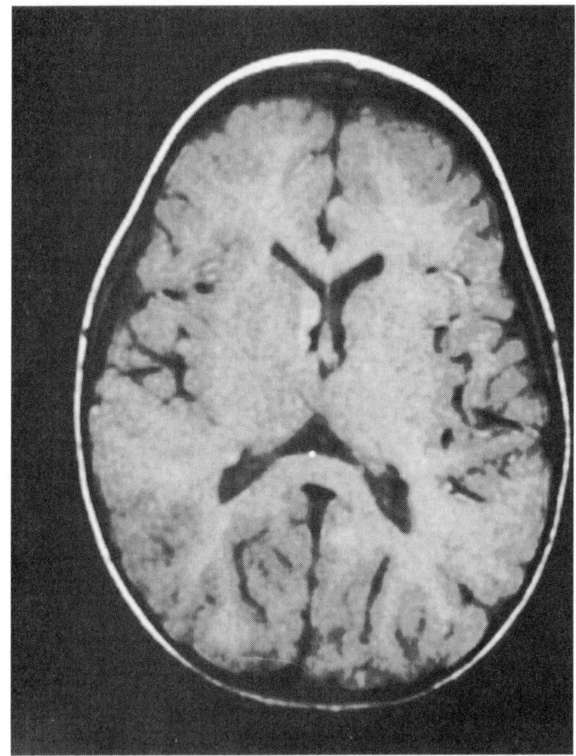

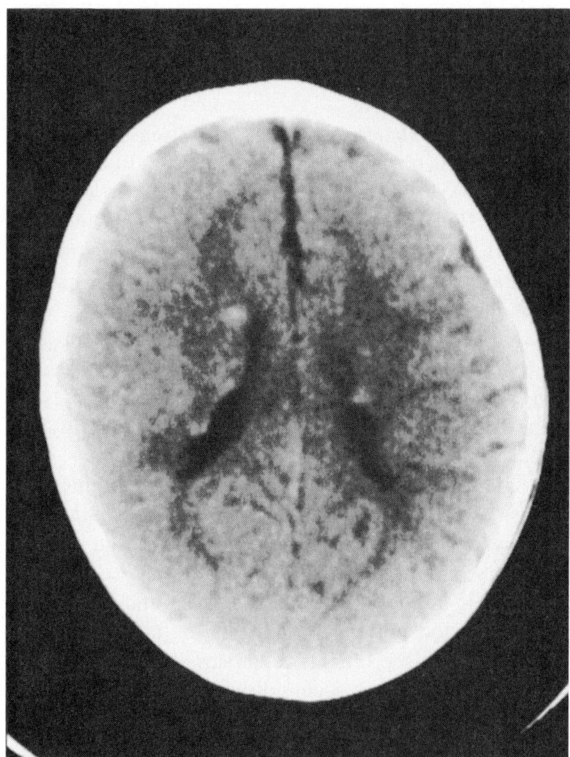

Figure 38-7

Tuberous sclerosis. Subependymal nodules ("brain stones") are demonstrated on both MRI (left) *and CT* (right).

mainly in the mental sphere. Status epilepticus accounted for many deaths in the past, but improved anticonvulsant therapy has reduced this hazard. Neoplasias take their toll; the authors have had several such patients who died of malignant gliomas arising in striatothalamic regions.

Neurofibromatosis of von Recklinghausen

Neurofibromatosis (NF) is a comparatively common hereditary disease in which the skin, nervous system, bones, endocrine glands, and sometimes other organs are the sites of a variety of congenital abnormalities, often taking the form of benign tumors. The typical clinical picture, usually identifiable at a glance, consists of multiple circumscribed areas of increased skin pigmentation accompanied by dermal and neural tumors of various types.

The condition known as multiple idiopathic neuromas was the subject of a monograph by R. W. Smith in 1849; even at that time, he referred to examples recorded by other writers. It was von Recklinghausen, however, who in 1882 gave the definitive account of its clinical and pathologic features. The subsequent studies of the disease by Yakovlev and Guthrie, Lichtenstein, Riccardi, and Martuza and Eldridge, and most recently by Créange et al and the comprehensive monographs of Crowe and Riccardi and their colleagues have provided a complete analysis of the clinical, pathologic, and genetic data pertaining to the disease.

Epidemiology Crowe and associates have calculated the prevalence of the disease to be 30 to 40 per 100,000 and expect one case in every 2500 to 3300 births. Approximately half of their cases had affected relatives, and in all instances the distribution of cases within a family was consistent with an autosomal dominant mode of inheritance. The disease has been observed in all races in different parts of the world, and males and females are about equally affected.

Cause and Pathogenesis The hereditary nature of NF has been appreciated for many years. More recently it has been established that NF comprises two distinct disorders, the genes for which are located on two separate chromosomes. The classic form of the disease, described below, has been shown by linkage analysis to be caused by a mutation located near the centromere on chromosome 17 (Barker et al). The second type, in which the main feature is bilateral acoustic nerve neuromas, described further on, has been linked to a DNA marker on chromosome 22 (Rouleau et al). These two forms of NF have been loosely referred to as peripheral and central, respectively, but the terms *neurofibromatosis type 1* and *neurofibromatosis type 2* are less confusing (Martuza and Eldridge) and are used in the following discussion.

The pathogenesis remains obscure. Cellular elements derived from the neural crest (i.e., Schwann cells, melanocytes, and endoneurial fibroblasts, the natural components of skin and nerves) proliferate excessively in multiple foci, and the melanocytes function abnormally; but the hormones and growth factors that are involved in this proliferative process and the mechanism(s) by which it is accomplished are as unclear as in tuberous sclerosis.

Neurofibromatosis Type 1 (Classic, or Peripheral, NF) In the majority of patients, spots of hyperpigmentation and cutaneous and subcutaneous neurofibromatous tumors are the basis of clinical diagnosis. Pigmentary changes in the skin are nearly always present at birth, but neurofibromas are infrequent at that age. Both lesions increase in number and size during late childhood and adolescence. There may be a spurt of new lesions at puberty or during pregnancy. Exceptionally, a neurofibroma of a cranial nerve or a spinal root (sometimes with compression of the cord), disclosed during neurosurgical intervention, may be the initial manifestation of the disease. In the study of a large series of patients with neurofibromatosis (Crowe et al), approximately one-third were found to have the cutaneous manifestations while being examined for symptoms of some other disease; that is to say, the NF was asymptomatic. Usually these are the cases with the slightest degree of cutaneous abnormality. Of the remaining two-thirds, most consulted a physician because of the disfigurement produced by the tumors or because some of the neurofibromas were producing symptoms.

The patches of cutaneous pigmentation, appearing shortly after birth and occurring any place on the body, constitute the most striking clinical expression of the disease. They vary in size from a millimeter or two to many centimeters and in color from a light to dark brown (café au lait) and are rarely associated with any other pathologic state (Fig. 38-8). They do not appear to change in number as the patient ages but they do become more pigmented. In a survey of pigmented spots in the skin, Crowe and associates found that 10 percent of the normal population had one or more spots of this type; however, anyone with more than six such spots, some exceeding 1.5 cm in diameter, nearly always proved to have von Recklinghausen disease. Of their 223 patients with NF, 95 percent had at least one spot, and 78 percent had more than six large ones. Freckle-like or diffuse pigmentation of the axillae and other intertriginous areas (groin, under breast), and small, round, whitish spots are characteristic and almost pathognomonic of the syndrome.

The appearance of multiple cutaneous and subcutaneous tumors in late childhood or early adolescence is the other principal feature of the disease. The cutaneous tumors are situated in the dermis and form discrete, soft or firm papules varying in size from a few millimeters to a centimeter or more (molluscum fibrosum; Fig. 38-9). They assume many shapes—flattened, sessile, pedunculated, conical, lobulated, and so on. They are flesh-colored or violaceous and often topped with a comedo. When pressed, the soft tumors tend to invaginate through a small opening in the skin, giving the feeling of a seedless raisin or a scrotum without a testicle. This phenomenon, spoken of as "buttonholing," is useful in distinguishing the lesions of this disease from other tumors, e.g., multiple lipomas. A patient may have anywhere from a few of these dermal tumors to hundreds.

Figure 38-8

Typical large café au lait spot. The presence of six or more hyperpigmented lesions, each over 1.5 cm, is diagnostic of neurofibromatosis type 1.

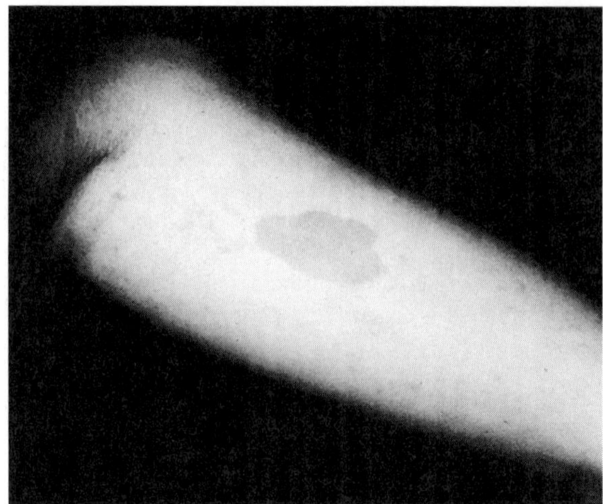

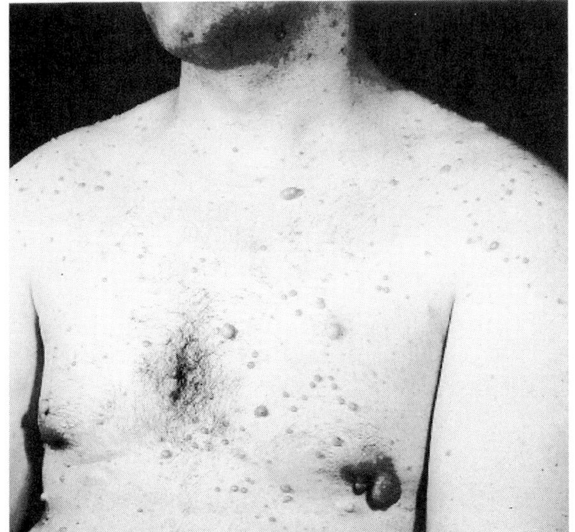

Figure 38-9

Molluscum fibrosum non-neural skin tumors of von Recklinghausen disease.

The subcutaneous neural tumors, which are also multiple, take two forms: (1) firm, discrete nodules attached to a nerve or (2) an overgrowth of subcutaneous tissue, sometimes reaching enormous size. The latter, which are called *plexiform neuromas* (also pachydermatocele, elephantiasis neuromatosis, *la tumeur royale*), occur most often in the face, scalp, neck, and chest and may cause hideous disfigurement. When palpated, they feel like a bag of worms or strings; the bone underlying the tumor may thicken. Neurofibromas are easily distinguished from lipomas, which are soft, unattached to the skin or nerve, and not accompanied by any neurologic disorder. The only exceptions to this statement are rare cases of multiple symmetrical lipomatosis with axonal polyneuropathy (Launois-Beusaude disease). As a rule, congenital neurofibromas tend to be highly vascular and invasive and are especially prominent in the orbital, periorbital, and cervical regions. They are often accompanied by hypertrophy of a segment of the body. When the hyperpigmentation overlies a plexiform neurofibroma and extends to the midline, one should suspect an intraspinal tumor at that level.

Other abnormalities associated with type 1 (peripheral) NF include bone cysts, pathologic fractures (pseudoarthrosis), cranial bone defects with pulsating exophthalmos (sphenoid bone dysgenesis), bone hypertrophy, precocious puberty, pheochromocytoma, scoliosis, syringomyelia, nodules of abnormal glial cells in brain and spinal cord, and macrocephaly, rarely with obstructive hydrocephalus due to overgrowth of glial tissue around the sylvian aqueduct and fourth ventricle. Some degree of intellectual impairment is common (40 percent of Riccardi's series of 133 patients); but in our experience the figure is much less, and the impairment is usually not profound. Learning difficulty, developmental disorder, or hyperactivity have been more frequent abnormalities, occurring in almost 40 percent of patients. Rosman and Pearce have ascribed mental retardation in NF to congenital malformation of the cerebral cortex (cortical dysgenesis). The incidence of seizures is about 20 times higher than that in the general population. Headache, hydrocephalus, and tumors involving the optic pathways, meningiomas, gliomas, and malignant peripheral nerve tumors are common, even among adults, according to the survey of 158 patients by Créange and colleagues; also, pain was a common symptom in adults and often related to a malignant peripheral nerve sheath tumor.

Another unique finding is the Lisch nodule. This is a small whitish spot (hamartoma) in the iris (Fig. 38-10), present in 94 percent of Riccardi's type 1 cases but not found in patients with type 2 NF (bilateral acoustic neuromas) or in normal individuals (see below). Exceptionally, NF has been associated with peroneal muscular atrophy, congenital deafness, and partial albinism (Bradley et al).

In childhood, progressive blindness is a particularly troublesome complication. One or both optic nerves are involved in a tumor mass composed mainly of astrocytes. The diagnosis comes to mind at once in a child

Figure 38-10

Hamartomas of the iris (Lisch nodules), typical of neurofibromatosis, type 1.

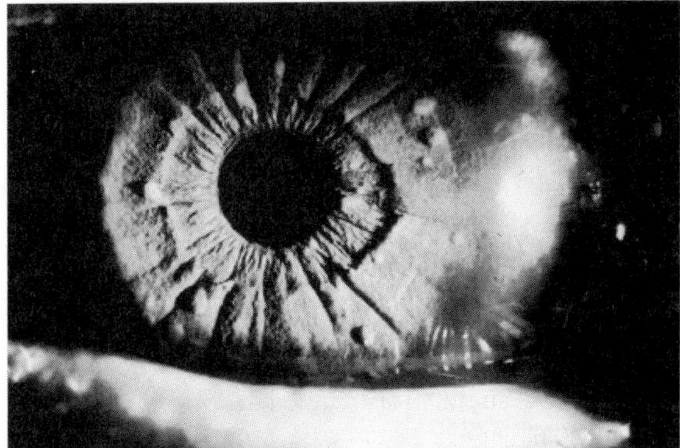

with any of the cutaneous manifestations of NF. Uncertainty as to its nature arises from the fact that the neuropathologist may be unable to decide between a benign hamartoma and a grade 1 astrocytoma. Enlargement in a succession of MRI scans may be needed to affirm its blastomatous nature.

Neurofibromatosis Type 2 (Acoustic, or Central, NF) In type 2 neurofibromatosis, as mentioned above, there is an absence or paucity of cutaneous lesions. Progressive deafness and the demonstration by enhanced CT or MRI of *bilateral acoustic neuromas* affords accurate diagnosis (Fig. 31-16). Other cranial or spinal neurofibromas, meningioma (sometimes multiple), and glioma may be added to the syndrome of deafness. This condition is considerably less frequent than type 1 NF.

Pathology of NF1 and NF2 The cutaneous tumors are characterized by a rather thin epidermis whose basal layer may or may not be pigmented. The collagen and elastin of the dermis is replaced by a loose arrangement of elongated connective tissue cells. It lacks the compactness of the normal dermal collagen, which accounts for the palpable opening in the skin.

The pigmented (café au lait) lesions contain only the normal numbers of melanocytes; the dark color of the skin is due instead to an excess of melanosomes in the malpighian cells. Abnormally large melanosomes, measuring up to several microns in diameter, appear in some of the basal cells of the epidermis.

The nerve tumors are composed of a mixture of fibroblasts and Schwann cells (except the optic nerve tumors, which contain a combination of astrocytes and fibroblasts). Predominance of one or the other of these cells is the basis of the diagnosis of neurofibroma or schwannoma. Palisading of nuclei, sometimes encircling arrangements (Verocay bodies), is a feature of both. Occasionally, along spinal roots or sympathetic chains, one may find a tumor made up of partially or completely differentiated nerve cells (a typical ganglioneuroma). Clusters of abnormal glial cells may be found in the brain and spinal cord, and, according to Bielschowsky, they form a link with tuberous sclerosis. Clinically and genetically, however, the two diseases are quite independent.

Malignant degeneration of the tumors is found in 2 to 5 percent of cases; peripherally they become sarcomas, and centrally, astrocytomas or glioblastomas (Fig. 38-11).

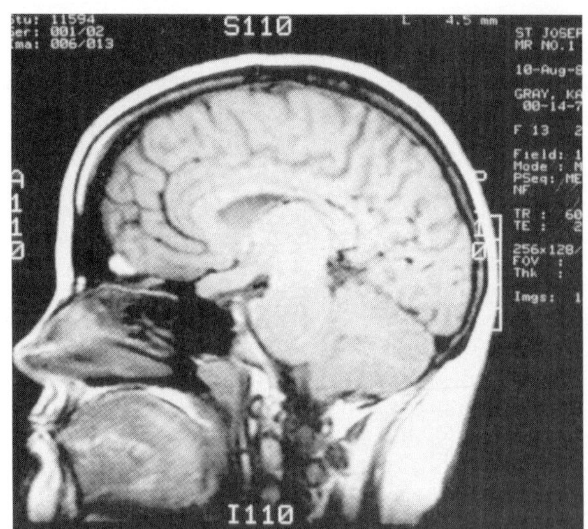

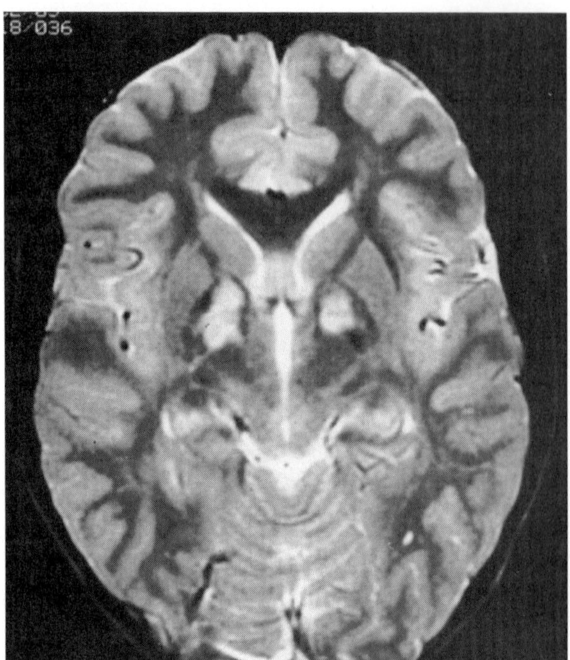

Figure 38-11

Neurofibromatosis, type 1. T1-weighted MR image in the sagittal plane demonstrating a glioma involving the optic chiasm and brainstem (above). *T2-weighted axial image showing multiple foci of hyperintensity, presumably hamartomas* (below).

Diagnosis If skin tumors and café au lait spots are numerous and Lisch nodules are present in the iris, the identification of the disease as type 1 neurofibromatosis offers no difficulty. A history of the illness in antecedent and collateral family members makes diagnosis even more certain. Uncertainty arises most frequently in patients with bilateral acoustic neuromas or other cranial or spinal neurofibromas or schwannomas with no skin lesions or only a few random ones although the tendency for these forms of NF to be accompanied by a paucity of skin lesions is well recognized. Plexiform neuromas with muscle weakness, due to nerve involvement, and abnormalities of underlying bone may be confused with other tumors, especially in young children, who tend to have few café au lait spots and few cutaneous tumors. Hypertrophy of a limb, which may also occur, requires differentiation from other developmental anomalies.

As already mentioned, Crowe and coworkers believe that 80 percent of patients with von Recklinghausen disease can be diagnosed by the presence of more than six café au lait spots. Of the remaining 20 percent, those over 21 years of age will be found to have multiple cutaneous tumors, axillary freckling, and a few pigmented spots; in those under 21 with no dermal tumors and only a few café au lait patches, a positive family history and radiographic demonstration of bone cysts will be helpful in some instances. Café au lait spots and cutaneous tumors should always be sought, for they may help the neurologist diagnose an otherwise obscure progressive spinal syndrome, a cerebellopontine angle syndrome, bilateral deafness, progressive blindness, and an occasional case of precocious puberty, hydrocephalus, or mental retardation.

Because of the many conditions that accompany classic neurofibromatosis and because they are potentially dangerous, the initial clinical evaluation should be supplemented by a number of ancillary examinations: measurement of IQ, EEG, slit-lamp examination of irides, radiography of optic foramens and internal auditory meati, visual and auditory evoked responses, and CT scans or MRI of cranium and sometimes of spine and mediastinum. In the series of Duffner and colleagues, 74 percent of cases had abnormal signals in T2-weighted images of the basal ganglia, thalamus, hypothalamus, brainstem, and cerebellum. The EEG in their cases was abnormal in 25 percent. If there is suspicion of a pheochromocytoma, a 24-h urine should be tested for metabolites of epinephrine. Each of these tests not only is an aid to diagnosis but is essential to the intelligent management of the illness.

Treatment The skin tumors should not be excised unless they are cosmetically objectionable or show an increase in size, suggesting malignant change. The effects of radiotherapy are so insignificant that they do not justify the risk of exposure. Plexiform neuromas about the face offer especially difficult problems. Here one must resort to plastic surgery, but the results are not always satisfactory because the growths may involve cranial nerves superficially (with risk of greater paralysis after surgical excision) or alter the underlying bone, the latter being either eroded from pressure or hypertrophied from increased blood supply. Cranial and spinal neurofibromas are amenable to excision, and the gliomas and meningiomas usually demand surgical measures as well. Here the differentiation of hamartomas from gliomas of structures such as the optic nerves, hypothalamus, or pons may be difficult. Bilateral optic nerve gliomas are usually treated with radiation; unilateral ones are excised. Peripheral nerve tumors that have undergone malignant (sarcomatous) degeneration pose special surgical problems.

Affected individuals should be advised not to have children—a precaution that may not be necessary, because fertility, especially in males, seems to be reduced by the disease. Prognosis varies with the grade of severity, being most favorable in those with only a few lesions. But the disease is always progressive, and the patient should remain under continuous surveillance.

Cutaneous Angiomatosis with Abnormalities of the Central Nervous System

There are seven diseases in which a cutaneous or ocular vascular anomaly is associated with an abnormality of the nervous system: (1) meningo- or encephalofacial (encephalotrigeminal) angiomatosis with cerebral calcification (Sturge-Weber syndrome); (2) dermatomal hemangiomas and spinal vascular malformations (sometimes with limb hypertrophy, as in Klippel-Trenaunay-Weber syndrome); (3) the epidermal nevus (linear sebaceous nevus) syndrome; (4) familial telangiectasia (Osler-Rendu-Weber disease); (5) hemangioblastoma of cerebellum and retina (von Hippel-Lindau disease); (6) ataxia-telangiectasia (Louis-Bar disease); and (7) angiokeratosis corporis diffusum (Fabry disease). The last three disorders are considered elsewhere: ataxia-telangiectasia and Fabry disease with the inherited metabolic disorders (pages 1011 and 1037, respectively) and von Hippel-Lindau disease with intracranial neoplasms (page 705).

Meningo- or Encephalofacial Angiomatosis with Cerebral Calcification (Sturge-Weber Syndrome)

A vascular nevus is observed at birth to cover a large part of the face and cranium on one side (in the territory of the ophthalmic division of the trigeminal nerve). In one-quarter of the cases the nevus is bilateral. The lesions vary in extent, the most limited being an involvement of only the upper eyelid and forehead and the most extensive being the entire head and even other parts of the body. The nevus is deep red (port-wine nevus), and its margins may be raised or flat; soft or firm papules, evidently composed of vessels, cause surface elevations and irregularities. Orbital tissue, especially the upper eyelid, is almost invariably involved; congenital buphthalmos may enlarge the eye before birth and glaucoma may develop later in that eye, causing blindness. The choroid is implicated in some cases. The increased cutaneous vascularity may result in an overgrowth of connective tissue and underlying bone, giving rise to a deformity like that of the Klippel-Trenaunay-Weber syndrome. Indications of cerebral affection appear as early as the first year of life or later in childhood; the most frequent clinical manifestations are unilateral seizures followed by increasing degrees of spastic hemiparesis with smallness of the arm and leg, hemisensory defect, and homonymous hemianopia, all on the side contralateral to the trigeminal nevus. Skull films (usually normal just after birth) taken after the second year reveal a characteristic "tramline" calcification, which outlines the convolutions of the parieto-occipital cortex. CT scanning and MRI show the abnormalities of the involved cortex at an earlier age.

This condition is generally referred to as the Sturge-Weber syndrome, since it was W. Allen Sturge, in 1879, who originally described a child with sensorimotor seizures contralateral to a facial "port-wine mark," and Parkes Weber (1922, 1929), who gave the first radiographic demonstration of the atrophy and calcification of the cerebral hemisphere homolateral to the skin lesion. This eponym overlooks the important intervening contributions of Kalischer (1897, 1901), who first described the meningeal angioma in conjunction with the facial one; of Volland (1913), who demonstrated the intracortical calcific deposits; and of Dimitri (1923), who described the characteristic double-contoured radiographic shadows. Krabbe (1932, 1934) showed conclusively that the calcification lay not in the blood vessels (as Dimitri and many others had concluded) but in the second and third layers of the cortex (see Wohlwill and Yakovlev for historical review and bibliography).

It must not be thought that all cranial hemangiomas affect the cerebrum; facial nevi, especially the flat midline ones and the elevated strawberry nevi, are of no neurologic significance. And a cerebral meningeal angiomatosis may be present without skin lesions. The involvement of the upper eyelid is of greatest importance; nearly all such cases are associated with cerebral lesions (Barlow). There seems to be a close correlation between the persistence or maldevelopment of the embryonic vascular plexus of the eyelid and forehead and that of the occipitoparietal parts of the brain. When the nevus lies entirely below the upper eyelid or high on the scalp, a cerebral lesion is usually absent, although in a few instances such an angioma has been associated with a vascular malformation of the meninges overlying the brainstem and cerebellum. In angiograms, the abnormal meningeal vessels, which are largely veins, are not well seen; thus they can be distinguished from arteriovenous malformations. Meningeal nevi are rarely the source of subarachnoid or cerebral hemorrhage, and they do not enlarge to form a "mass lesion." The cortical lesion is destructive in type; lost neurons are replaced by glial tissue that calcifies. Possibly diversion of blood to the meninges during seizures causes the progressive ischemia of the cerebral cortex. Barlow believes the seizures to be responsible for the progressive neurologic deficits and that a special effort should be made to prevent them by carefully regulated medical therapy. Occasionally surgical excision of intractable discharging foci may be necessary, but often this may not be feasible in view of the magnitude of the cerebral lesion. Radiotherapy is unsuccessful in reducing the skin blemish; sensitive individuals usually try to hide it with cosmetics.

Although the encephalotrigeminal syndrome is of congenital origin, its cause and pathogenesis are unknown. Familial coincidence has been observed but is exceptional. No chromosomal abnormality has been demonstrated.

Dermatomal Hemangiomas with Spinal Vascular Malformations A hemangioma of the spinal cord may rarely be accompanied by a vascular nevus in the corresponding dermatome, as first pointed out by Cobb. Such nevi are most frequent on the arm and trunk. When the cutaneous lesion involves an arm or leg, there may be enlargement of the entire limb or fingers in combination with underdevelopment of certain other parts (Klippel-Trenaunay-Weber syndrome). Some of these angiomatous syndromes, as well as those described by Wyburn-Mason, combine a spinal or retinodiencephalic arteriovenous malformation (AVM) with a nevus of the trunk or face, respectively. Such cases provide a link to the common AVMs described in Chap. 34.

The Epidermal Nevus Syndrome This is a closely related congenital neurocutaneous disorder in which a specific skin lesion (epidermal nevus or linear sebaceous nevus) is associated with a variety of hemicranial and neurologic abnormalities. The skull and brain abnormalities are ipsilateral to the nevus. One-sided thickening of the bones of the skull is characteristic. Mental retardation, seizures, and hemiparesis are the usual neurologic manifestations and have their basis in a wide variety of cerebral lesions—unilateral cerebral atrophy, porencephalic cyst, leptomeningeal hemangioma, arteriovenous malformation, and atresia of cerebral arteries and veins. The somatic and neurologic abnormalities have been comprehensively reviewed by Solomon and Esterley and by Baker and associates.

Familial Telangiectasia (Osler-Rendu-Weber Disease) This, a vascular anomaly transmitted as an autosomal dominant trait, affects the skin, mucous membranes, gastrointestinal and genitourinary tracts, and occasionally the nervous system. The basic lesion is probably a defect in the vessel wall, and bleeding is thought to be due to the mechanical fragility of the vessel. The lesions range from the size of a pinhead to 3 mm or more; they are bright red or violaceous and blanch under pressure. Located sparsely in the skin of any part of the body, they first appear during childhood, enlarge during adolescence, and may assume spidery forms, resembling the cutaneous telangiectases of cirrhosis in late adult life. The significance of the lesions lies in their hemorrhagic tendency. During adult years they may give rise to severe and repeated epistaxis or gastric, intestinal, or urinary tract bleeding and result in an iron-deficiency anemia. Pulmonary fistulas constitute another important feature of the generalized vascular dysplasia; patients with such lesions are particularly subject to brain abscesses and less so to bland embolic strokes.

The angiomas of this disease may form in either the spinal cord or brain, where they can produce apoplectic syndromes; or as in one of our patients, an intermittently progressive focal thalamic syndrome resulting from enlargement of the vascular lesions (or possibly from a succession of small hemorrhages). An unexplained gastrointestinal, genitourinary, intracranial, or intraspinal hemorrhage warrants a search for small cutaneous lesions, which are easily overlooked. Cautery eradicates a bleeding lesion, but satellite lesions tend to form.

Restricted Developmental Abnormalities of the Nervous System

In the course of clinical practice, one encounters a remarkable number of restricted disorders of the nervous system, many of which are transmitted from generation to generation as a mendelian dominant trait. Only a few of the more striking examples are described here. The reader may turn to books on genetics or teratology for an account of such oddities as hereditary unilateral ptosis, hereditary Horner syndrome, pupillary inequalities, jaw winking, absence of a particular muscle, etc.

Bifacial and Abducens Palsies (Möbius Syndrome) The syndrome of congenital facial diplegia with convergent strabismus is generally referred to as *Möbius syndrome*, although it had been described earlier by von Graefe. Its presence at birth is disclosed by the lack of facial movements and full eye closure. The most complete review of the subject in the English literature is that of Henderson. In his analysis of 61 cases of the congenital facial diplegia syndrome, there were 45 instances of abducens palsy, 15 of complete external ophthalmoplegia, 18 of lingual palsy, 17 of clubfeet, 13 of brachial disorders, 6 of mental defect, and 8 of an absent pectoral muscle. Thus the overlap with other neuromuscular and CNS abnormalities is evident. Early in life the mouth hangs open, the lower lip is everted, and there is difficulty in sucking. Usually this syndrome can be distinguished from the facial palsy of forceps or birth injury by its bilaterality and the other associated weaknesses. Occasionally more than one family member is affected (usually autosomal dominant inheritance). The cause of this peculiar condition is not known. The few adequate pathologic studies have shown a lack of nerve cells in the motor nuclei of the brainstem, changes that also characterize the Fazio-Londe syndrome (page 1162). Rarely, there may be an aplasia of facial muscles. The Möbius syndrome is also referred to on page 1531 in relation to restricted palsies of myopathic and nuclear origin.

Partial paralysis of facial muscles that dates from birth and cannot be attributed to obstetric trauma is not infrequent. In a common type, the lower lip on the involved side remains immobile when the child smiles or cries; the lip on the unaffected side is drawn downward and outward, resulting in a prominent asymmetry of the lower face. Often it is not appreciated that the side that droops during crying is the normal side (Hoefnagel and Penry).

Congenital Lack of Lateral Gaze (Oculomotor Apraxia of Cogan; See page 278**)** Children with this congenital defect are unable to turn their eyes to either side volitionally or on command. Attempting to look to the right, the child turns the head to the right (there is no associated apraxia of head turning, as in the acquired condition), but the eyes lag and turn to the left. As a result, the patient has to overshoot the mark with the head in order to attain ocular fixation. Once the eyes fixate, the head returns to the primary position. To compensate for the deficiency of eye movements, the patient develops jerky thrusting movements of the head, which characterize all attempts at voluntary gaze. Caloric stimulation of the labyrinth causes tonic movement of the eyes but not nystagmus, as in the normal person. Also, optokinetic nystagmus cannot be induced. Vertical movements are normal, however. A similar ocular condition may occur in conjunction with ataxia-telangiectasia and Gaucher disease. These children are slow to walk, and Ford observed one such child whose sibling had an absence of the vermis of the cerebellum. Aside from this observation, the anatomic basis of this condition has not been studied.

CONGENITAL ABNORMALITIES OF MOTOR FUNCTION

In this group of congenital disorders, a major disturbance of motor function, usually nonprogressive, has been present since infancy or early childhood. The popular terms for these conditions have been *infantile cerebral paralysis* (Freud) and *cerebral palsy*. The latter name is not appropriate, nor is it useful from the physician's viewpoint, collocating, as it does, diseases of widely differing etiologic and anatomic types, wherein the hereditary and acquired and the intrauterine, natal, and postnatal diseases lose their identity. Unfortunately the name has been adopted as a slogan for fund-raising societies and for all manner of rehabilitation clinics throughout the United States, so that it will not soon disappear from medical terminology. The term often abbreviated ("CP") is still being used indiscriminately by laymen and many physicians to designate every conceivable cognitive and motor disorder of corticospinal, extrapyramidal, cerebellar, and even neuromuscular type in infants and children.

Etiology of the Congenital Cerebral Motor Disorders

Motor abnormalities that have had their onset early in life are numerous and diverse in their clinical manifestations. Marked prematurity is a determining factor in a large proportion of cases. Each year, about 50,000 infants weighing less than 1500 g are born in the United States. Approximately 85 percent survive, and of these, 5 to 15 percent have a motor disorder of cerebral origin and 25 to 30 percent are mentally impaired at school age (Volpe; see also Hack et al). To ascertain the etiologic and pathogenic factor(s), it is helpful to categorize a given case according to the extent and nature of the motor abnormality. A careful history of possible prenatal, perinatal, or postnatal insults to the developing nervous system must always be sought; certain correlations of these factors with the resulting pattern of neurologic deficit are outlined below. Most patients with these motor abnormalities of infancy and childhood reach adult years. Many of them have some degree of mental retardation and epilepsy in addition to the motor abnormalities, and there is an unavoidable overlapping in any consideration of the mechanisms of these three clinical states.

The following discussion of these problems is centered on three major etiologic syndromes—matrix hemorrhages in the immature infant, hypoxic-ischemic encephalopathy (Little disease), and certain developmental motor abnormalities.

Matrix (Subependymal) Hemorrhage in Premature Infants In low-weight immature infants (20 to 35 weeks gestational age), there often occurs, within a few days after birth, a catastrophic decline in cerebral function, usually preceded by respiratory distress (hyaline-membrane disease), with cyanosis and apneic spells. Also seen are failure of brainstem automatisms (sucking and swallowing), bulging of the fontanels, and appearance of sanguineous CSF. Once the infant becomes completely unresponsive, death usually ensues within a few days. Autopsy discloses a small lake of blood in each cerebral hemisphere (often asymmetrical), occupying the highly cellular (subependymal) germinal matrix, near the caudate nucleus at the level of the foramen of Monro. This region is supplied by the lenticulostriate, choroidal, and Heubner's recurrent arteries and is drained by deep veins, which enter the vein of Galen. In about 25 percent of cases, the blood remains loculated in the matrix zone, while in the others it ruptures into the lateral ventricle or adjacent brain tissue. In a series of 914 consecutive autopsies in newborns, subependymal hemorrhage was found in 284 (31 percent); practically all of these neonates were of low birth weight (Banker and Bruce-Gregorios).

Lesser degrees of this complex of cerebral lesions are now being identified by ultrasonography (Fig. 38-12) and CT scans, and it is apparent that many infants with lesions of lesser magnitude survive. Some rapidly develop an obstructive hydrocephalus and require a ventricular shunt. In others, the hydrocephalus stabilizes and there is clinical improvement. Several series of surviving cases have now been followed for many years. Those in whom the hemorrhage was relatively more extensive are often left with motor and intellectual handicaps. In the Swedish series of Hagberg and Hagberg, 55 percent of the patients with spastic diplegia had preterm births and the neuropathologic basis was believed to be matrix hemorrhage, leukomalacia (see further on), or both. Congenital hemiplegia or quadriplegia are observed at lower frequency. In another series of 20 cases of posthemorrhagic hydrocephalus (Chaplin et al), 40 percent had significant motor deficits and over 60 percent had IQ scores of less than 85. In a personal experience with 12 less severe cases (mean birth weight 1.8 kg and gestational age of 32.3 weeks), only one had a residual spastic diplegia and 9 of the 12 had IQs in the low-normal or normal range. The average age of the children at the time of the last evaluation was 8.5 years.

The cause of this unique form of matrix hemorrhage is unsettled. In all probability it is related to greatly increased pressure in the thin-walled veins of the germinal matrix, coupled with a lack of adequate supporting tissue in these zones. The increased blood pressure or venous pressure is, in turn, manifestly related to the pulmonary disorders that occur in immature infants. These infants are also prone to the development of characteristic lesions of the cerebral white matter (periventricular leukomalacia, see below), and the residual neurologic deficits are the result of these lesions, added to the deficits due to the subependymal hemorrhage (mainly hydrocephalus). Acetazolamide and furosemide, which reduce the formation of spinal fluid and have been widely used in the treatment of posthemorrhagic ventricular dilatation, have been shown, in a large-scale controlled study, to be of little value in reducing the need for shunt placement (see International PHVD Drug Trial Group in the References).

Figure 38-12

Ultrasound demonstration of subependymal matrix hemorrhage in a premature infant (arrow).

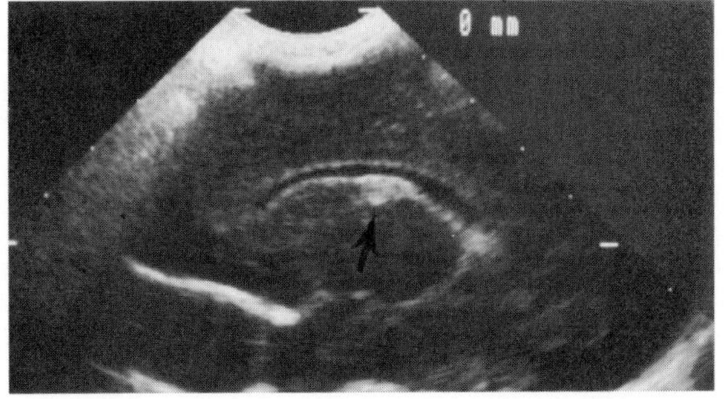

Periventricular Leukomalacia These are zones of necrosis of white matter in the deep watershed territories of cortical and central arteries. They lie lateral and posterolateral to the lateral ventricles, in a position to involve the occipital radiations and the sensorimotor fibers in the corona radiata (Banker and Larroche; Shuman and Selednik). These white-matter lesions occur in about one-third of cases of subependymal hemorrhage, but they may develop independently in both premature and full-term infants who have suffered hypotension and apnea. In a study of 753 preterm infants, those born at 28 weeks gestation were at highest risk of this complication; the combination of intrauterine infection and premature rupture of membranes carried a 22 percent risk (Zupan et al). Survivors often manifest cerebral diplegia and mental impairment. The motor disorder is usually more severe than the cognitive and language impairment.

Control of respiratory distress may reduce the incidence of matrix hemorrhages and periventricular leukomalacia. Claims have been made that the administration of indomethacin ethamsylate, a drug that reduces capillary bleeding, and the intramuscular injection of vitamin E for the first 3 days after birth and possibly the use of betamethasone reduce the incidence of periventricular hemorrhage (Benson et al; Sinha et al; see also Volpe for discussion of control of cerebral hemodynamics and effects of drugs in the neonatal period.)

Hypoxic-Ischemic Damage Little's conception of the hypoxic-ischemic form of "birth injury," enunciated in 1862, has been subjected to scrutiny over the years. While it is evident that many newborns suffer some degree of perinatal asphyxia, relatively few of them seem to manifest brain damage. Moreover, many infants with a variety of cerebral motor syndromes appear to have passed the parturitional (perinatal) period without mishap, indicating the greater importance of other prenatal and postnatal causative factors. Nonetheless, severe neonatal asphyxia of term or preterm babies is an important cause of spastic-dystonic-ataxic syndromes, often accompanied by seizures and mental subnormality.

One has the impression that the CNS tolerates hypoxia and reduced blood flow in the postnatal period better than at any other time in life. Indeed, animal experimentation supports this view. Not until the arterial O_2 tension is reduced to 10 to 15 percent of normal does brain damage occur, and even then the impaired function of other organs contributes to the damage; nearly always there are irregularities of the heart and hypotension from myocardial damage as well as hepatic and renal failure. Thus it is more correct to think of the encephalopathy in terms of both hypoxia and ischemia, which usually occur in utero and are expressed postnatally by recognizable clinical syndromes.

As regards the cerebral syndromes that do follow an obviously difficult birth (reflected by low 5-min Apgar scores and the need of resuscitative measures), Fenichel finds it helpful to divide them into three groups, according to their severity: (1) In newborns with mild hypoxic-ischemic encephalopathy, the symptoms are maximal in the first 24 h and take the form of hyperalertness and tremulousness of the limbs and jaw (the "jittery baby") and a low threshold of the Moro reaction. The tone of the limbs is normal except for a mild increase in head lag during traction. The reflexes are brisk and there may be ankle clonus. The anterior fontanel is soft. The EEG is normal. Recovery is complete and the risk of handicap is extremely low. (2) Newborns with moderate hypoxic-ischemic encephalopathy are lethargic, obtunded, and hypotonic, with normal movements. After 48 to 72 h, the neonate may improve (having passed through a jittery hyperactive phase) or worsen, becoming less responsive in association with convulsions, cerebral edema, hyponatremia, and hyperammonemia from liver damage. The EEG is abnormal; Fenichel associates epileptiform activity and voltage suppression with an unfavorable outcome. Abnormal visual and auditory evoked potentials are other poor prognostic signs. (3) In neonates with severe hypoxic-ischemic encephalopathy, stupor or coma are present from birth; respirations are irregular, requiring mechanical ventilation. There are usually convulsions within the first 12 h. The limbs are hypotonic and motionless even in attempts to elicit the Moro response. Sucking and swallowing are depressed, but pupillary reactions and eye movements may at first be retained, only to be lost as the coma deepens.

It is in the second and third categories, i.e., the states of moderate to severe encephalopathy, where correction of the respiratory insufficiency and the metabolic abnormalities permits survival, that a number of motor abnormalities (corticospinal, extrapyramidal, and cerebellar) and mental retardation eventually emerge. Included in the category of severe hypoxic-ischemic encephalopathy are also newborns with a variety of developmental anomalies of the brain and other organs. In addition, they may have been exposed to certain prenatal risk factors (toxemia of pregnancy, antepartum uterine hemorrhage), or their growth may have been abnormal (small-for-date babies). Some are born at term; others are premature, and the birth process may or may not have been abnormal. One must then consider the possibility, originally pointed out by Sigmund Freud, that the abnormality of the birth process, instead of being causal, was actually the consequence of prenatal pathology. The latter might include preterm intrauterine hypoxia-ischemia.

Other evidence of multifactorial etiology in the "causation" of cerebral palsy has been provided by Nelson and Ellenberg, who found that maternal mental retardation, birth weight below 2000 g, and fetal malformation were among the leading predictors. Breech presentation was another factor, and one-third of these cases also had a noncerebral malformation. Twenty-one percent of the 189 children in their series had also suffered some degree of asphyxia. Additional determinants were maternal seizures, a motor deficit in an older sibling, two or more prior fetal deaths, hyperthyroidism in the mother, pre-eclampsia, and eclampsia. In children with cerebral diplegia born at term, likely contributory factors that were operative in nearly half of them included toxemia of pregnancy, low birth weight for age (indicating undernutrition), placental infarction, and intrauterine asphyxia.

The factors enumerated above are involved to different degrees in the outcome of pregnancies but are informative because they bring to light the significant proportion of cases of cerebral birth injury in which hypoxia-ischemia, matrix hemorrhages, and leukomalacia were not operative. In this last group, we would also include the symmetrical porencephalies and hydranencephalies (see also page 1053). The porencephalic cerebral defect, if unilateral, is usually in the frontal lobe and is a cause of congenital hemiplegia. If the defect is bilateral, there is bilateral hemiplegia as well as severe impairment of mental development. In hydranencephaly, the greater part of both cerebral hemispheres is replaced by a membrane. Only the inferior temporal and occipital lobes remain, along with the thalamus and basal ganglia. The cranium may be full-sized or enlarged. Such children survive for only a short time (weeks, months, or a few years), functioning essentially as brainstem preparations. CT scanning and MRI facilitate the recognition of both of these disorders.

Clinical Syndromes of Congenital Motor Disorders

With reference to the types of motor disorder evolving from the four major categories of cerebral disease—matrix hemorrhage, periventricular leukomalacia, hypoxic-ischemic encephalopathy, kernicterus (discussed further on)—the most frequent is spastic diplegia; i.e., motor disturbances are severe in the lower limbs and mild in the upper. In addition to diplegia, hypoxic-ischemic injury occurring in the term or preterm infant may take the form of a hemiplegia, double hemiplegia (quadriplegia), or a mixed pyramidal-extrapyramidal or spastic-ataxic syndrome.

A second form of motor disorder is characterized by the development of severe spastic quadriplegia and mental retardation. The major insult is intrapartum asphyxia and attendant fetal distress. Usually such infants will have required resuscitation and will have had low 5-min Apgar scores, which in this circumstance have important predictive value. The pathologic lesions of the brain in this second group consist of hypoxic-ischemic infarction in distal fields of arterial flow, primarily in the cortex and white matter of parietal and posterior frontal lobes, leaving a ulegyric sclerotic cortex.

A third group, also discussed below, is characterized mainly by extrapyramidal abnormalities, combining athetosis, dystonia, and ataxia in various proportions. In summarizing several large series of congenital and neonatal motor disorders, spastic diplegia occurred in 10 to 33 percent of cases, spastic quadriplegia 19 to 43 percent, extrapyramidal forms in 10 to 22 percent, and mixed forms in 9 to 20 percent.

Spastic Diplegia (Cerebral Spastic Diplegia; Little Disease) The pattern of paralysis is more variable than the term *spastic diplegia* implies; actually, several subtypes may be distinguished: the paraplegic, diplegic, quadriplegic, pseudobulbar, and generalized. Pure paraplegic and pseudobulbar types are relatively rare. Usually all four extremities are affected, but the legs much more than the arms, which is the real meaning of *diplegia*. Hypotonia—with retained tendon reflexes and hypoactivity—is usually present initially. Only after the first few months will evident weakness and spasticity appear, first in the adductors of the legs. The plantar reflexes, which are often ambiguous in the normal infant, here are clearly extensor, a finding that is pathologic at any later age. Also, stiff, awkward movements of the legs, which are maintained in an extended, adducted posture when the infant is lifted by the axillae, often do not attract attention until several weeks or months have passed. Seizures occur in approximately one-third of the cases, and it is not uncommon to observe a delay in all developmental sequences, especially those that depend on the motor system. Once walking is attempted, usually at a much later date than normal, the characteristic stance and gait become manifest. The slightly flexed legs are advanced stiffly in short steps, each describing part of an arc of a circle; adduction of the thighs is often so strong that the legs may actually cross (scissors gait); the feet are flexed and turned in with the heels not touching the ground. In the adolescent and adult, the legs tend to be short and small, but the muscles are not markedly atrophic, as in spinal muscular atrophy. Passive manipulation of the limbs reveals spasticity in the extensors and adductors and slight shortening of the calf muscles. The arms may be affected only slightly or not at all, but there may be awkwardness and stiffness of the fingers and, in a few, pronounced weakness and spasticity. In reaching for an object, the hand may overpronate. Speech may be well articulated or noticeably slurred, and in some instances the face is set in a spastic smile. The deep tendon reflexes are exaggerated, those in the legs more than the arms; the plantar reflexes are extensor in the majority of cases. Scoliosis is frequent and may secondarily give rise to spinal cord and root compression and impaired respiratory function. As a rule, there is no disturbance of sphincteric function, though delay in acquiring voluntary control is usual. Athetotic postures and movements of the face, tongue, and hands are present in some patients and may actually conceal the spastic weakness; ataxic and hypotonic forms also exist (see further on).

One subtype of spastic diplegia is associated with a relatively slight diminution in head size and intelligence. As indicated above, there is no unifying neuropathology; the condition occurs independently of matrix hemorrhages and periventricular leukomalacia as well as with them. The frequency of cerebral spastic diplegia, which is closely related to the degree of prematurity, has declined significantly since the introduction of neonatal intensive care facilities, and there is reason to believe that heredogenetic factors are of importance.

Infantile Hemiplegia, Paraplegia, and Quadriplegia Hemiplegia is a common condition of infancy and early childhood. The functional difference between the two sides may be noticed soon after birth, but more often it is not perceived by the mother until after the first 4 to 6 months of life. In a second group, the child is in excellent health for a year or longer before the abrupt onset of hemiplegia (see below). In hemiplegia that dates from earliest infancy—i.e., congenital hemiplegia—the parents first notice that movements of prehension and exploration are carried out with only one arm. A manifest hand preference at an early age should always raise the suspicion of a unilateral motor defect. The affection of the leg is usually recognized later, i.e., during the first attempts to stand and walk. Sitting and walking are usually delayed by a few months. In the older child, there is evident hyperactivity of tendon reflexes and usually a Babinski sign. The arm is held flexed, adducted, and pronated, and the foot assumes an equinovarus posture. Sensory and visual field defects are present in some patients. Mental defect may be associated with infantile hemiplegia but is less common and lesser in degree than with cerebral diplegia and much less common than with bilateral hemiplegia. There may also be speech delay, regardless of the side of the lesion; when this is present, one should look for mental retardation and expect to find a bilaterality of motor abnormality. Convulsions occur in 35 to 50 percent of children with congenital hemiplegia, and these may persist throughout life. They may be generalized but are frequently unilateral and limited to the hemiplegic side. Often, after a series of seizures, the weakness on the affected side will be increased for several hours or longer (Todd's paralysis). Gastaut and associates have described a hemiconvulsive-hemiplegic syndrome in which the progressive paralysis and cerebral atrophy are attributed to the convulsions. As months and years pass, the osseous and muscular growth of the hemiplegic limbs is retarded, leading to an obvious hemiatrophy.

With respect to the causation of congenital hemiplegia, it is generally agreed that perinatal asphyxia is only one of the possibilities. In the series of 681 children with "cerebral palsy" collected by Hagberg and Hagberg, there were 244 with hemiplegia. Of the latter, 189 were full-term babies and 55 preterm. Prenatal risk factors were identified in only 45 percent, and they were mostly in the infants born prematurely. In nearly half of the cases, there was no clue as to the time in the intrauterine period when the cerebral lesion occurred.

In the second group—*acquired infantile hemiplegia*—a normal infant or young child, usually between the ages of 3 to 18 months, develops a massive hemiplegia, with or without aphasia, within hours. The disorder often begins with seizures, and the hemiplegia may not be recognized until the seizures have subsided. In Banker's autopsy series, there was arterial or venous thrombosis in some cases, but in many no occlusions were found. Some of the latter cases, in which arteriography had been negative, may have been embolic, possibly of cardiac origin. If the stroke occurs at an early age, the recovery of speech may be complete, though reduced scholastic capacity remains. The degree of recovery of motor function varies. Often, as the deficit recedes, the arm becomes involved by athetotic, tremulous, or ataxic movements. There may be an interval of months or years between the hemiplegia and the athetosis.

Encephaloclastic (destructive) lesions underlie most of the cases of infantile hemiplegia and some cases of bilateral hemiplegia. The pathologic change is essentially that of ischemic necrosis. In many cases, the lesions must have been incurred in utero. (Precipitant delivery, fetal distress, and prepartum uterine hemorrhage may be indications of the process.) The lesions reflect not only the effects of anoxia but also those of circulatory insufficiency (ischemia), the result of hypotension or circulatory failure. The ischemia of circulatory failure tends to affect the tissues lying in arterial border zones, and there may also be venous stasis with congestion and hemorrhage (occurring particularly in the deep central structures such as the basal ganglia and periventricular matrix zones). If they are purely hypoxic, the lesions should be bilateral. Myers has reproduced such lesions in the neonatal monkey by reducing the maternal circulation over a period of several hours. As the lesions heal, the monkeys develop the same ulegyric sclerotic changes in the cortex and white matter of the cerebrum (lobar sclerosis) and the "marbling" (état marbré) that characterize the brains of patients with spastic diplegia and double athetosis (see below).

The quadriplegic state differs from bilateral hemiplegias in that the bulbar musculature is often involved in the latter and mental retardation is more severe. The condition is relatively rare and is usually due to a bilateral cerebral lesion. However, one should also be alert to the possibility of a high cervical cord lesion. In the infant, this is usually the result of a fracture-dislocation of the cervical spine incurred during a difficult breech delivery. Similarly, in paraplegia, with weakness or paralysis limited to the legs, the lesion may be either a cerebral or a spinal one. Sphincteric disturbances and a loss of somatic sensation below a certain level on the trunk always point to a spinal localization. Congenital cysts, tumors, and diastematomyelia are more frequently causes of paraplegia than of quadriplegia. Another recognized cause of infantile paraplegia is spinal cord infarction from thrombotic complications of umbilical artery catheterization.

Extrapyramidal Syndromes The spastic cerebral diplegias discussed above shade almost imperceptibly into the congenital extrapyramidal syndromes. Patients with these latter syndromes are found in every cerebral palsy clinic, and ultimately they reach adult neurology clinics as well. Corticospinal tract signs may be completely absent, and the student, familiar only with the syndrome of pure spastic diplegia, is always puzzled as to their classification. Some cases of extrapyramidal type are undoubtedly attributable to severe perinatal hypoxia and others to diseases such as erythroblastosis fetalis with kernicterus. In order to state the probable pathologic basis and future course of these illnesses, it is desirable to separate the extrapyramidal syndromes of prenatal-natal origin (which usually become manifest during the first year of life) from the acquired or hereditary postnatal syndromes, such as familial athetosis, Wilson disease, dystonia musculorum deformans, and the hereditary cerebellar ataxias, which become manifest later.

Double Athetosis This is probably the most frequent of the congenital extrapyramidal disorders. In our clinical material and in reported series of cases, two types stand out—one that is due to hyperbilirubinemia or Rh incompatibility (kernicterus, see below) and the other due to hypoxic-ischemic encephalopathy. With control of neonatal hyperbilirubinemia (by use of anti-Rh immune globulin, exchange transfusions, and phototherapy), kernicterus has almost disappeared, whereas the other, more severe hypoxic-ischemic form regularly continues to be seen. Rarely, a congenital, nonhemolytic icterus or a glucose-6-phosphate dehydrogenase deficiency produces the same syndrome.

Like the spastic states, double athetosis may not be recognized at birth but only after several months or a year have elapsed. In some cases the appearance of choreoathetosis is delayed for several years, and it may seem to progress during adolescence and even early adult life. It must then be differentiated from some of the inherited metabolic and degenerative extrapyramidal diseases. Chorea and athetosis dominate the clinical picture, but bewildering combinations of involuntary movements—including dystonia, ataxic tremor, myoclonus, and even hemiballismus—may be found in a single case. At times, we have been unable to classify the movement disorder because of its complexity. It should be noted that practically all instances of double athetosis are also associated with a defect in voluntary movement.

Choreoathetosis in infants and children varies greatly in severity. In some, the abnormal movements are so mild as to be misinterpreted as restlessness or "the fidgets"; in others, every attempted voluntary act provokes violent involuntary movements, leaving the patient nearly helpless. The clinical appearance of choreoathetosis and other involuntary movements is discussed in Chap. 4.

An early hypotonia, followed by retardation of motor development, is the rule in these cases. Erect posture and walking may be delayed until the age of 3 to 5 years and may never be attained in some patients. Tonic neck reflexes or fragments thereof tend to persist well beyond their usual time of disappearance. The plantar reflexes are usually flexor, though they may be difficult to interpret because of the continuous flexion and extension of the toes. Sensory abnormalities are not elicited. Because of the motor and speech impairment, patients are often erroneously thought to be mentally defective. In some, this conclusion is doubtless correct, but in others intellectual function is adequate, and a few can be educated to a high level.

A variety of rehabilitative measures have been tried: physiotherapy, surgery, sensory integrative therapy, progressive patterned movement, and neuromuscular facilitation. We agree with Hur, who has critically reviewed this subject, that properly controlled studies provide no proof of the success of any of these measures. Surely, with growth and development, new postures and motor capacities are acquired. The less severely affected patients can even make successful occupational adjustments. The more severely affected ones rarely achieve a degree of motor control that permits them to live independently. One sees some of these unfortunate persons bobbing and twisting laboriously as they make their way in public places.

Imaging studies are seldom of diagnostic value. Mild cerebral atrophy and loss of volume of the basal ganglia are seen in some cases, and cavitary lesions are present in some of the severe anoxic encephalopathies. The EEG is rarely helpful unless there are seizures.

The most frequent pathologic finding in the brain has been a whitish, marble-like appearance of the putamen, thalamus, and border zones of the cerebral cortex. These whitish strands represent foci of nerve cell loss and gliosis with condensation of adjacent transversing myelinated fibers—so-called *status marmoratus (état marbré)*. This lesion does not develop after infancy, i.e., after the myelination glia have completed their developmental cycle.

Kernicterus This is now a rare cause of extrapyramidal motor disorder in children and adults. Such cases raise the broader question of the neurologic sequelae of erythroblastosis fetalis secondary to Rh and ABO blood incompatibilities or to a deficiency of the hepatic enzyme glucuronosyltransferase. The symptoms of kernicterus appear in the jaundiced neonate on the second or third postnatal day. The infant becomes listless, sucks poorly, develops respiratory difficulties as well as opisthotonos (head retraction), and becomes stuporous as jaundice intensifies. The serum bilirubin is usually greater than 25 mg/dL. In acidotic and hypoxic infants (e.g., those with low birth weight and hyaline membrane disease), the kernicteric lesions develop with much lower levels of serum bilirubin.

The majority of infants with this disease die within the first week or two of life. Many of those who survive are mentally retarded, deaf, hypotonic, totally unable to sit, stand, or walk, and spend their lives in homes for the feebleminded. There are exceptional patients, however, obviously less damaged, who are mentally normal or at most only slightly backward. These are the ones who develop a variety of persistent neurologic sequelae—choreoathetosis, dystonia, and rigidity of the limbs—a picture not too different from that of cerebral spastic diplegia with involuntary movements. Kernicterus should always be suspected if an extrapyramidal syndrome is accompanied by bilateral deafness and palsy of upward gaze. Later there may be a greenish pigmentation of the dental enamel.

Neonates who die in the acute stage of kernicterus show a unique yellow staining (icterus) of nuclear masses (Kern nuclei) in the basal ganglia, brainstem, and cerebellum. In surviving patients the pathologic changes consist of a symmetrically distributed nerve cell loss and gliosis in the subthalamic nucleus of Luys, the globus pallidus, the thalamus, and the oculomotor and cochlear nuclei; these lesions are the result of the hyperbilirubinemia. The immature cerebral cortex is usually spared. In the newborn, unconjugated bilirubin can pass through the poorly developed blood-brain barrier into these nuclei, where it is directly toxic. Acidosis and hypoxia exacerbate the effect. Also in the newborn, the development of hyperbilirubinemia is enhanced by a transient deficiency of the enzyme glucuronosyltransferase, essential for the conjugation of bilirubin. *Hereditary hyperbilirubinemia*, due to lack of this enzyme (*Crigler-Najjar syndrome*), may have the same effect on the nervous system at a later period of infancy or childhood as hyperbilirubinemia due to Rh incompatibility.

Immunization, phototherapy, and exchange transfusions with female blood, designed to prevent high levels of unconjugated serum bilirubin, have been shown to protect the nervous system. If the blood bilirubin level can be held to less than 20 mg/dL (10 mg/dL in prematures), the nervous system may escape damage. The effective use of these measures has practically eradicated this dreaded disease.

Both kernicterus and ischemic état marbré must be differentiated clinically from hereditary choreoathetosis, the Lesch-Nyhan syndrome, and—later in life—from ataxia-telangiectasia and Friedreich ataxia.

Congenital and Neonatal Ataxias In these patients, difficulty in standing and walking cannot be attributed to spasticity or paralysis. Again, hypotonia and poverty of movement are the initial motor abnormalities; the cerebellar deficit becomes manifest at a later time, when the patient begins to sit, stand, and walk. There may or may not be a delay in reaching "motor milestones." Attempts to attain sitting balance will first reveal an unsteadiness that is not soon overcome, even with practice. Reaching for a proffered toy is accomplished by jerky, incoordinated movements. The first steps are unsteady, as would be expected, with many tumbles, but the gait remains clumsy. Instability of the trunk may be accompanied by similar, more or less rhythmic movements of the head, so-called titubation. Despite the severity of the ataxia, the muscles are of normal size, and voluntary movements, though weak in some patients, are possible in all the limbs. The tendon reflexes are present, and the plantar reflexes are either flexor or extensor. In some cases, the ataxia is associated with spasticity rather than hypotonia (spastic-ataxic diplegia). Relative improvement may occur in later years. In the older child, a cerebellar gait, ataxia of limb movements, nystagmus, and uneven articulation of words are readily distinguished from myoclonus, chorea, athetosis, dystonia, and tremor.

In only a few cases have the pathologic changes been studied. Aplasia or hypoplasia of the cerebellum has been observed, but sclerotic lesions of the cerebellum are more common. The CT scan or MRI verifies the cerebellar atrophy. A cerebral and cerebellar lesion may coexist in patients with congenital ataxia, which is the reason for the term *cerebrocerebellar diplegia.*

Several risk factors have been identified in the congenital ataxias. A genetic factor is operative in some cases (Hagberg and Hagberg). Radiation of the maternal abdomen during the first trimester of pregnancy is said to have resulted in cerebellar hypoplasia. Mercury poisoning in utero is another cause of congenital ataxia. Most importantly, cerebellar ataxia may be the most prominent or sole effect of neonatal ischemia-hypoxia.

Pontocerebellar Hypoplasias Aside from the congenital ataxia described above, there are several rare familial forms in which a failure of cerebellar development is associated with mental retardation. Joubert reported a family in which there was dysgenesis of the vermis of the cerebellum, mental retardation, episodic hyperpnea, irregular, jerky eye movements, and unsteady gait. The syndrome appeared in 4 of 6 siblings. In other reports, choroidal-retinal colobomas, polydactyly, cryptorchidism, and prognathism have been mentioned. Detailed examination of the cerebra of such cases is needed. In the *Gillespie syndrome*, a combination of aniridia, cerebellar ataxia, and mental retardation are the denominating features. In the *Paine syndrome*, a familial disorder with developmental delay and mental retardation, there is microcephaly, spasticity, optic hypoplasia, and myoclonic ataxia, the last presumably related to the cerebellar hypoplasia. These dysgeneses and the disequilibrium syndrome reported from Sweden are brought together by the cerebellar ataxia; in the past, they fell into the group of ataxic cerebral palsies. Imaging studies demonstrate the cerebellocerebral abnormality. Genetic factors are operative in some, but matters pertaining to etiology remain obscure (see Harding for details). A pure congenital cerebellar hypoplasia has been mapped to a gene locus on chromosome Xq (Illarioshkin et al). The ataxia was inherited as an X-linked recessive trait and was nonprogressive beyond early childhood.

Differential Diagnosis of the Congenital Ataxias The congenital ataxias must be distinguished from the progressive hereditary ataxias. The latter are likely to begin at a later age than the congenital ones. Some hereditary ataxias are intermittent or episodic. They are discussed in page 1010. Several forms of childhood ataxia are neither congenital nor hereditary; they have an acute onset and may persist during childhood, adolescence, and adult life.

Also to be distinguished from the ataxias of congenital and neonatal origin is an *acute cerebellar ataxia of childhood*, which can usually be traced to a viral infection or a postinfectious encephalitis, particularly after chickenpox. The *opsoclonus-myoclonus ("dancing eyes") syndrome* of Kinsbourne is another postinfectious disease peculiar to childhood (see pages 977 and 1097). The cerebellar ataxia in this disease may be overshadowed by polymyoclonus, which marks every attempted movement. With improvement, under the influence of corticosteroids, a cerebellar disorder of speech and movement becomes evident. A majority of the cases in which the disease becomes chronic (16 of the 26 cases followed by Marshall et al) were found later to be mentally backward. The cause of the disease has never been established. An occult neuroblastoma or other tumor is uncovered occasionally.

Yet another form of cerebellar ataxia, which is inherited as an autosomal dominant trait, occurs in discrete attacks. It usually begins in childhood and persists through adult life. In two of our patients, it began in mid-adult life; one form is improved by the administration of acetazolamide (see page 1022).

In the differential diagnosis of these acute forms of cerebellar ataxia, one must not overlook intoxication with phenytoin, barbiturates, or similar drugs.

The Flaccid Paralyses The cerebral form, first described by Foerster and called *cerebral atonic diplegia*, has already been mentioned. It can usually be distinguished from the paralysis of spinal and peripheral nerve origin and congenital muscular dystrophy by the retention of postural reflexes (flexion of the legs at the knees and hips when the infant is lifted by the axillae), preservation of tendon reflexes, and coincident failure of mental development.

The syndrome of *infantile spinal muscular atrophy (Werdnig-Hoffmann disease)* is the leading example of flaccid paralysis of lower motor neuron type. Perceptive mothers may be aware of a paucity of fetal movements in utero, and in most cases the motor defect becomes evident soon after birth or the infant is born with arthrogrypotic deformities. Several other types of familial progressive muscular atrophy have been described in which the onset is in early or late childhood, adolescence, or early adult life. Weakness, atrophy, and reflex loss without sensory change are the main features and are discussed in detail in Chap. 39. A few patients suspected of having infantile or childhood muscular atrophy prove, with the passage of time, to be merely inactive "slack" children, whose motor development has proceeded at a slower rate than normal. Others may remain weak throughout life, with thin musculature. These and several other congenital myopathies—*central core, rod-body, nemaline, mitochondrial, myotubular, and fiber type disproportion and predominance*—are described in Chap. 52. Unlike Werdnig-Hoffmann disease, the effects of many of them tend to ameliorate as the natural growth of muscle proceeds. Rarely, polymyositis and acute idiopathic polyneuritis manifest themselves as a syndrome of congenital hypotonia.

Infantile muscular dystrophy and lipid and glycogen storage diseases may also produce a clinical picture of progressive atrophy and weakness of muscles. The diagnosis of *glycogen storage disease* (usually the Pompe form) should be suspected when progressive muscular atrophy is associated with enlargement of the tongue, heart, liver, or spleen. The motor disturbance in this condition may be related in some way to the abnormal deposits of glycogen in skeletal muscles, though it is more likely due to degeneration of anterior horn cells that are also distended with glycogen and other substances. Certain forms of *muscular dystrophy* (myotonic dystrophy and several types of congenital dystrophy) may also be evident at birth or soon thereafter. The latter may have led to arthrogryposis and club foot (see page 1530). All of these disorders are described in detail in the chapters on muscle diseases.

Brachial plexus palsies, well-known complications of dystocia, usually result from forcible extraction of the fetus by traction on the shoulder in a breech presentation or from traction and tipping of the head in a shoulder presentation. The effects of such injuries are sometimes lifelong. Their neonatal onset is betrayed later by the small size and inadequate osseous development of the affected limb. Either the upper brachial plexus (fifth and sixth cervical roots) or the lower brachial plexus (seventh and eighth cervical and first thoracic roots) suffer the brunt of the injury. Upper plexus injuries (Erb) are about 20 times more frequent than lower ones (Klumpke). Sometimes the entire plexus is involved (page 1427).

Facial paralysis, due to forceps injury to the facial nerve immediately distal to its exit from the stylomastoid foramen, is another common (usually unilateral) peripheral nerve affection in the newborn. Failure of one eye to close and difficulty in sucking make this condition easy to recognize. It must be distinguished from the congenital facial diplegia that is often associated with abducens palsy, i.e., the Möbius syndrome discussed earlier in the chapter. In most cases of facial paralysis due to physical injury, function is recovered after a few weeks; in some, the paralysis is permanent and may account for lifelong facial asymmetry.

In summary, it can be said that all these forms of disabling motor abnormalities rank high as important issues in neuropediatrics. Steps have been taken in most hospitals to identify and eliminate risk factors in attempts at prevention. Indeed, better prenatal care, reduction in premature births, and control of respiratory problems in critical care wards have reduced their incidence and prevalence. Physical and mental therapeutic measures appear to be helpful, but many of the methods have been difficult to evaluate in a nervous system undergoing maturation and change. The neurologist can contribute most by segregating groups of cases of identical pattern and etiology and in differentiating the congenital groups of delayed expressivity from the treatable acquired diseases of this age period. Woefully lacking are critical neuropathologic studies.

INTRAUTERINE AND NEONATAL INFECTIONS

Throughout the intrauterine period the embryo and fetus are subject to particular infections. Since the infective agent must reach the fetus through the placenta, it is evident that the permeability of the latter at different stages of gestation and the immune status of the maternal organism are determinative. We are including a discussion of these intrauterine infections here because some of them may lead to malformations of the brain and, later in life, must be distinguished from developmental abnormalities.

Until the third to fourth month of gestation, the large microbial organisms—such as bacteria, spirochetes, protozoa, and fungi—cannot invade the embryo, even though the mother harbors the infection. Viruses may do so, however—specifically rubella, cytomegalovirus (CMV), human immunodeficiency virus (HIV), and possibly others. The rubella virus enters embryonal tissues during the first trimester, *Treponema pallidum* in the fourth to fifth postconceptional month, and *Toxoplasma* after that period. Bacterial meningitis (except for that due to *Listeria monocytogenes*, described below) is essentially a paranatal infection contracted during or immediately after parturition. Neonatal herpes simplex encephalitis, due to the type 2 (genital) virus, is also usually acquired by passage through an infected birth canal. Some cases of HIV infection may be acquired during delivery, but most are due to transplacental transmission.

The main neonatal infections—toxoplasmosis, rubella, cytomegalovirus and herpes—are commonly designated by the acronym TORCH. With the persistence of *Listeria*, the rise of AIDS infections, and a marked reduction in rubella infections, the mnemonic LATCH, which includes *Listeria* and AIDS, might be more appropriate. Infants with all these infections share certain common features, such as low birth weight, prematurity, congenital heart disease, purpura, jaundice, anemia, microcephaly or hydrocephaly, cerebral calcifications, choreoretinitis, cataracts, microphthalmia, and pneumonitis; as a corollary, if any combination of these features is manifest, one should suspect one of these infectious agents and take measures to identify it. However, in none of the types of infections are all these clinical manifestations likely to be present, and in the cases of rubella and cytomegalovirus, only a small percentage of infected infants will show major systemic signs or symptoms.. Nevertheless, on clinical grounds alone, certain of these infections can be identified and others excluded. For example, cerebral calcifications are present mainly in toxoplasmosis and CMV encephalopathy, being rare in rubella and absent in HSV encephalitis; the calcifications are widely disseminated in toxoplasmosis and have a periventricular distribution in CMV infection. Cardiac lesions are present only with rubella, and deafness occurs only with CMV and rubella. Thus, there are clinical signposts to guide the clinician in selecting the appropriate diagnostic tests. Most importantly, in considering neonatal infections, one must also search for other, non-LATCH infections (see Chaps. 32 and 33).

Added difficulty in the diagnosis of embryonal and fetal infections arises when the mother has been entirely asymptomatic. Isolation of the organism from fetal and neonatal tissues is possible, but usually they are inaccessible, and it may be impossible to demonstrate antibodies or other immune responses because of the early stage of the infection or limitations of the infant's immune response.

Rubella

Gregg, in 1941, first reported the association of maternal rubella and congenital cataracts in the neonate. His observations were quickly verified, and soon it became widely known that cataracts, deafness, congenital heart disease, and mental retardation constituted a kind of tetrad diagnostic of this disease. That a virus could affect so many tissues, causing in essence a noninflammatory developmental disorder of multiple organs, was a novel concept, and it raised the interesting prospect that other viruses might have similar effects. Surprisingly, however, only CMV and possibly herpes simplex viruses (HSV) have been incriminated in embryonal neuropathology. A large number of other viruses (e.g., influenza, Epstein-Barr, hepatitis) have been implicated in human teratogenesis, but in none is the relationship beyond doubt.

It is now well established that most instances of congenital rubella infection occur in the first 10 weeks of gestation, and that the earlier the infection occurs, the greater the risk to the fetus. However, there is considerable risk beyond the first trimester, up to the 24th week (Hardy).

Following the massive rubella epidemics of 1964 and 1965, the congenital rubella syndrome has been expanded to include low birth weight; sensorineural deafness, sometimes unilateral (the most common complication); microphthalmia; pigmentary degeneration of the retina (salt-and-pepper chorioretinitis); glaucoma, cloudy corneas, and cataracts of special type (the latter two abnormalities usually cause visual impairment); hepatosplenomegaly, jaundice, and thrombocytopenic purpura; and patent ductus arteriosus or interventricular septal defect. There may be one, a few, or many of these abnormalities, in various combinations. The mental retardation is severe and may be accompanied by seizures and motor defects such as hemiplegia or spastic diplegia and rarely by seizures. Psychiatric symptoms, some resembling autism, are not infrequent.

Infection of the fetus after the first trimester results in a less impressive neonatal syndrome. The infant may seem lethargic and fail to thrive. The cranium is abnormally small. Only a cardiac abnormality, deafness, or chorioretinitis may provide clues to the diagnosis. The CSF shows an increase of mononuclear cells and an elevated protein. The infection may persist for a year or longer. Foci of calcification are rare and CT scanning and MRI are of little help in diagnosis. The maternal infection may be so mild that it is passed off as minor; but even when it is evident, the fetus is spared in about 50 percent of cases. Diagnosis can be verified in the neonate by demonstrating IgM antibodies to the virus or by the isolation of the virus from the throat, urine, stool, or CSF. Also, the virus has been obtained from cells in the amniotic fluid.

The *neuropathology* is of considerable interest. In the nervous system of abortuses (the abortion performed because of proven maternal rubella in the first trimester), R. D. Adams found no visible lesions by light microscopy, even though the virus had been isolated from the brain by Enders. At this period of development there is no inflammatory reaction because of the absence of polymorphonuclear leukocytes, lymphocytes, and other mononuclear cells in the fetus. At birth the brain is usually of normal size, and there may be no discernible lesions. In a few, a mild meningeal infiltration of lymphocytes as well as a few zones of necrosis and vasculitis with later calcification of vessels are seen, as are small hemorrhages, presumably related to the thrombocytopenia. Smallness of the brain and delay in myelination have been observed in children dying at 1 to 2 years of age. None of the brains in our series have been malformed. Rubella virus continues to be recoverable from the CSF for at least 18 months after birth. A delayed progressive rubella encephalitis in childhood has also been described (page 811).

Since there is no treatment for the active infection, the obvious approach to the problem of congenital rubella infection is to make sure that every woman has been vaccinated against rubella or has had the infection prior to pregnancy. The widespread use of rubella vaccine has reduced the chance of major outbreaks, but sporadic infections continue to be seen, and outbreaks of epidemic proportions continue to occur in developing countries.

Cytomegalovirus Infection

For many years it was known that, in the tissues of some infants who died in the first weeks and months of life, there were swollen cells containing intranuclear and cytoplasmic inclusions. This cytologic change seemed related to the fatalities. In 1956 and 1957, three different laboratories isolated what has come to be called the *human cytomegalovirus*, or CMV (see Weller). This has proved to be the most frequent intrauterine viral infection.

Cytomegalovirus disease is caused by a DNA virus, a member of the herpes group, and is widespread in the general population. Although cervicitis is common, the virus is probably transmitted to the fetus transplacentally. Infection of the fetus usually occurs in the first trimester of pregnancy, sometimes later, by way of an inapparent maternal viremia and active infection of the placenta. The newborn can also be infected in the course of delivery or afterward by the mother's milk or by transfusions. However, only a small proportion of women known to harbor the virus give birth to infants with active infection. The likelihood of the fetus being infected is much greater if the seronegative mother becomes infected for the first time during pregnancy. Eighteen percent of infants born to such mothers were symptomatic at birth, and 25 percent became blind, deaf, or feebleminded within a few years (Fowler et al). In mothers with recurrent CMV infection, the infants were asymptomatic at birth, and only a few of them developed serious sequelae. Evidently, the presence of maternal antibodies before conception protects against congenital CMV infection.

Early infection of the fetus may result in a malformation of the cerebrum; later, there is only inflammatory necrosis in parts of the normally formed brain. In the low-birth-weight or full-term infant, the clinical picture is one of jaundice, petechiae, hematemesis, melena, direct hyperbilirubinemia, thrombocytopenia, hepatosplenomegaly, microcephaly, mental defect, and convulsions. Cells in the urine may show cytomegalic changes. There is a pleocytosis and an increased protein in the CSF. Disseminated inflammatory foci involve the cerebrum, brainstem, and retinae. In the centers of aggregates of lymphocytes, mononuclear cells, and plasma cells are microglial cells containing inclusion bodies; some astrocytes are similarly affected. The granulomas later calcify, particularly in the periventricular regions. Often there is hydrocephalus.

Congenital CMV infections pose a much greater problem than rubella. There is no way of identifying the infected fetus prior to birth or to prevent inapparent infections in the pregnant woman. As indicated above, if the pregnant woman has measurable titers of antibodies to CMV at the time of conception, her infant is relatively protected. Moreover, some infected infants (with viruria) may appear normal at birth but develop neural deafness and mental retardation several years later. Virus replication in infected organs continues after the first year and health workers are at risk. A second child may be infected.

There is no known treatment. The difficulties in prenatal diagnosis of maternal infection preclude planned abortion. Routine serologic testing should be done on every young woman of childbearing age. Until an effective vaccine becomes available, pregnancy should be avoided if a sexual partner is infected.

Childhood HIV Infection and AIDS

In the United States, about 10 percent of cases of acquired immunodeficiency syndrome (AIDS) have occurred in women, almost all of them of childbearing age, and the rate of new cases is increasing at a faster rate among them than among men. In children, practically all instances of AIDS come from an HIV-infected mother ("vertical transmission"). The infection may be acquired in utero, during delivery, or from breast feeding. The relative importance of each of these modes of transmission has not been settled.

It is estimated that HIV infection and AIDS occur in 15 to 30 percent of infants born to HIV-seropositive mothers (see Prober and Gerson). Infected infants present special difficulties in diagnosis, and the infection runs a more accelerated course in them than in adults. In the perinatal period, infected and noninfected infants can only rarely be distinguished clinically, and laboratory diagnosis is hampered by the presence of maternally derived antibody to HIV. The initial clinical signs usually appear within a few months after birth; practically all infected infants become ill before their first birthday, and very few are asymptomatic beyond 3 years of age. Early signs consist of lymphadenopathy, splenomegaly, hepatomegaly, failure to thrive, oral candidiasis, and parotitis. In the European Collaborative Study, comprising 600 children born to HIV-infected mothers, 83 percent of infected children showed laboratory or clinical features of HIV infection by 6 months of age. By 12 months, 26 percent had AIDS and 17 percent had died of HIV-related diseases. Once AIDS is established in children, it does not differ materially from the syndrome in adults (Chap. 33).

With reference to the involvement of the nervous system, there is often a delay in the attainment of psychomotor milestones. In others, after a period of normal development, a psychomotor decline begins, with corticospinal or peripheral nerve signs, often with pleocytosis. The typical giant-cell AIDS encephalitis, neuritis, and myelitis is easily distinguished from CMV encephalitis and toxoplasmosis.

Infected children are also subject to a variety of opportunistic infections, including bacterial meningitis, toxoplasmosis, CMV encephalitis, fungal infections (cryptococcosis, aspergillosis, candidiasis, herpes simplex and zoster, and mycobacterial meningitis). There may also be vascular lesions, with infarction or hemorrhage and lymphoid neoplasia. These are discussed in Chaps. 32 and 33. There is little to be done for these children, but this may be changing with the current use of three-drug antiretroviral therapy, as described in Chap. 33.

Toxoplasmosis

This tiny protozoan, *Toxoplasma gondii*, occurring freely or in pseudocyst form, is a frequent cause of meningoencephalitis in utero or in the perinatal period of life. The disease exists in all parts of the United States but is more frequent in western European countries, particularly in hot, humid climates. The mother is most often infected by exposure to cat feces, handling uncooked infected mutton or other meat, or eating partially cooked meat, but she is nearly always asymptomatic or has only a mild fever and cervical lymphadenopathy.

The precise times of placental and fetal invasion are not known, but presumably they are late in the gestational period. The clinical syndrome usually becomes manifest in the first days and weeks of postnatal life, when seizures, impaired alertness, hypotonia, weakness of the extremities, progressive hydrocephalus, and chorioretinitis appear. The retinal lesions consist of large, pale areas surrounded by deposits of pigment. If the infection is severe, the maculae are destroyed; optic atrophy and microphthalmos follow. In older infants, we have several times observed hemiplegias, first on one side and then on the other, followed by hydrocephalus. The latter is present in about one-third of the cases. The CSF contains a moderate number of white blood cells, mostly lymphocytes and mononuclear cells, and the protein content is in the range of 100 to 400 mg/dL (i.e., a higher protein content than all other neonatal infections except bacterial meningitis). The glucose values are normal. Less than 10 percent of infected children recover; the others are mentally retarded, with seizures and paralysis. In those without symptoms of infection at birth, the outcome is better.

Granulomatous masses and zones of inflammatory necrosis abut the ependyma and meninges. The organisms, 6 to 7 mm in length and 2 to 4 mm in width, are visible in and near the lesions. Microcysts may also be found, lying free in the tissues without surrounding inflammatory reaction. The necrotic lesions calcify rapidly and, after several weeks or months, are readily visible in plain films of the skull. These appear in periventricular and other regions of the brain as multiple nodular densities.

In adults, mainly in patients with AIDS, the disease takes the form of a rapidly evolving meningitis and multifocal encephalitis in conjunction with myocarditis, hepatitis, and polymyositis. This syndrome is described on page 775, as are the diagnostic tests and treatment. In the infant, infections such as rubella, syphilis, CMV disease, and herpes simplex must be considered in the differential diagnosis. The most reliable means of diagnosis is the IgM indirect fluorescent antibody test, performed on umbilical cord blood. Passive transfer of IgG antibody from mother to fetus takes place, but its presence in the latter is not proof of active infection.

In women who develop antibodies in the first 2 or 3 months of pregnancy, treatment with spiramycin (Rovamycin) prevents fetal infection. Once the fetus is infected, pyrimethamine and sulfadiazine must be used. A later second pregnancy is not affected.

Congenital Neurosyphilis

The clinical syndromes and pathologic reactions of congenital neurosyphilis of the newborn are similar to those of the adult, as described on pages 762 to 768. Such differences as exist are determined principally by the immaturity of the nervous system at the time of spirochetal invasion.

The syphilitic infection may be transmitted to the fetus at any time from the fourth to the seventh months. The fetus may die, with resulting miscarriage or stillbirth, or may survive only to be born with florid manifestations of secondary syphilis. The dissemination of the spirochetes throughout the body, the time of appearance of the secondary manifestations, and the time of formation of antisyphilitic antibodies (reagin) in the blood are all governed by the same biologic principles that apply to adult syphilis.

At birth the spirochetemia may not have had time to cause syphilitic reagin or antibodies to appear; hence a negative Venereal Disease Research Laboratories (VDRL) reaction in umbilical cord blood does not exclude syphilis. In unselected groups of syphilitic mothers, 25 to 80 percent of fetuses are infected, and in 20 to 40 percent of those infected, the CNS is invaded, as judged by the finding of abnormal CSF. The types of congenital neurosyphilis (asymptomatic and symptomatic meningitis, meningovascular disease, hydrocephalus, general paresis, and tabes dorsalis) are the same as those in the adult except for the great rarity of tabes dorsalis. The Hutchinson triad (dental deformities, interstitial keratitis, and bilateral deafness) is infrequently observed in complete form. The sequence of neurologic syndromes is also the same as in the adult, all stemming basically from a chronic spirochetal meningitis. The latter may become symptomatic in the first weeks and months of postnatal life, meningovascular lesions and hydrocephalus reaching maximal frequency during the 9-month to 6-year period; congenital paresis and tabes usually appear between the ninth to fifteenth years. The pathologic basis of each neurosyphilitic syndrome is, respectively, meningoarteritis (vascular syphilis), meningoencephalitis (general paresis), and meningoradiculitis (tabes dorsalis).

All neurologists have observed fewer and fewer cases of congenital neurosyphilis as the years pass, but there may be a recrudescence of the disease. If the syphilitic mother is treated before the fourth month of pregnancy, the fetus will not be infected. The infant may be normal at birth or exhibit only mucocutaneous lesions, hepatosplenomegaly, lymphadenopathy, and anemia. There are in the neonatal period no signs of meningeal invasion, or there may be only an asymptomatic meningitis. If the latter is actively treated until the CSF is normal, vascular lesions of brain and spinal cord, hydrocephalus, general paresis, and tabes dorsalis will not develop. If cases of meningovascular syphilis, general paresis, and tabes dorsalis are treated for 3 to 4 weeks with penicillin until the CSF is rendered acellular and the protein reduced to normal, the neurologic disorder will be arrested and often there is functional improvement.

The various neurosyphilitic syndromes are described fully in Chap. 32, as mentioned above.

Congenital syphilis must be considered a potential albeit rare cause of epilepsy and mental retardation. Once the syphilitic infection has been treated in early life and rendered inactive (acellular CSF, normal protein), the occurrence of a congenital luetic infection can only be substantiated by an accurate history; the finding of the syphilitic stigmata in the eyes, teeth, and ears; or a positive serologic reaction in the CSF.

Treatment of syphilis in the child follows along the same lines as treatment of the syphilitic adult (page 767), with appropriate adjustment of dosage in accordance with the child's weight.

Other Viral and Bacterial Infections

Several other infections of late fetal life or the neonatal period are only mentioned here, for to describe them all would be tedious and would elucidate no new neurologic principles. Meningitis due to the small gram-positive rod *Listeria monocytogenes* may be acquired in the usual way, at the time of passage through an infected birth canal or in utero, as a complication of maternal and fetal septicemia due to this organism. In the latter case, it causes abortion or premature delivery. Neonatal meningitis is a particularly devastating and often fatal type of bacterial infection, not easily diagnosed unless the pediatrician is alert to the possibility of a silent meningitis in every case of neonatal infection (page 740).

Herpes simplex virus (HSV) encephalitis may destroy large parts of the brain, particularly of the temporal lobes, and is frequently fatal. Coxsackie B, polioviruses, other enteroviruses, and arboviruses (western equine) seem to be able to cross the placental barrier late in pregnancy and cause encephalitis or encephalomyelitis in the fetus at term—indistinguishable from the disease in the very young infant.

Epstein-Barr virus is another and not infrequent cause of meningoencephalitis. In some instances it may present as an aseptic meningitis or a Guillain-Barré type of acute polyneuritis. This infection is more apt to affect the nervous system of children than that of adults. It is estimated that approximately 2 percent of children and adolescents with this infection have some type of neurologic dysfunction; rarely this will be the only manifestation of the disease. Stupor, chorea, and aseptic meningitis were the main neurologic findings in the case reported by Friedland and Yahr, and acute cerebellar ataxia and deafness in the case of Erzurum and associates (see also Chaps. 32 and 33). Herpes zoster may occur in utero, leaving cutaneous scars and retarding development. Or zoster may appear soon after birth, the infection having been contracted from the mother. Later in childhood, varicella may induce an autoimmune perivenous demyelination and possibly a direct infection, affecting predominantly the cerebellum (pages 797 and 977), or the now rare Reye syndrome.

EPILEPSIES OF INFANCY AND CHILDHOOD

The major types of seizure disorder have already been discussed in some detail in Chap. 16. In bringing them up again here, attention is drawn to the fact that epilepsy is mainly a disease of infancy and childhood. Approximately 75 percent of epileptics fall into these age periods, and some of the most interesting and unique types of seizure are peculiar to these epochs of life. Epilepsies that are observed exclusively in infants and children are benign neonatal convulsions, benign myoclonic epilepsy of infancy, febrile seizures (both genetic and acquired), infantile spasms of West, absence seizures, the Lennox-Gastaut syndrome, rolandic and occipital paroxysms and other benign focal epilepsies, and the juvenile myoclonic epilepsies.

One principle that emerges is that the form taken by seizures in early life is in part age-linked. Neonatal seizures are predominantly partial or focal; infantile seizures take the form of myoclonic flexor (sometimes extensor) spasms; and the various forms of petit mal are essentially diseases of childhood (4 to 13 years). The motor phenomena of epilepsy in young children are often termed *myoclonic*, but this should not be confused with other, later-occurring epilepsies that are endowed with the same name. Further, certain epileptic states tend to occur during certain epochs of life—one type of febrile seizures from 6 months to 6 years and generalized or temporal spike-wave activity with benign motor and complex partial seizures from 6 to 16 years, and juvenile myoclonic epilepsy in the mid- and late-adolescent years. In general, idiopathic epilepsy, so called because the cause cannot be determined, is predominantly a pediatric neurologic problem. This is not to say that seizures of unknown cause do not occur for the first time in adult life but rather that the onset of such seizures is far more frequent in childhood and tends to diminish once adulthood is reached.

The clinical characteristics of infantile and childhood seizures are fully described in Chap. 16.

MORE SEVERE FORMS OF MENTAL RETARDATION

The subject of mental retardation was introduced in Chap. 28, where it was pointed out that two major categories of this disorder have been delineated. In one, and by far the more common group, the mental retardation is relatively mild, allowing the individual to benefit from training and education; it is often familial (called subcultural) and is featured by a lack of definite neurologic abnormalities (except possibly a slightly higher incidence of seizures) and the absence of neuropathologic changes. A large part of this group, falling between 2 and 3 standard deviations from the normal mean IQ, probably are the lower end of the Gaussian curve of intelligence, the converse of which is genius. In the second group, the degree of mental retardation is usually more severe, most are nonfamilial, and a wide variety of neuropathologic changes are in evidence. The division is not absolute, for there are a few metabolic and developmental diseases in which mental retardation is profound, but with no somatic or neurologic abnormalities and no well-defined neuropathologic changes—e.g., Rett syndrome, autism, and the X-linked mental retardation syndromes such as the Renpenning and fragile-X types. In this chapter only these major types of *severe mental retardation* are described.

The overall frequency of severe mental retardation cannot be stated precisely. Rough estimates would place the figure at 0.2 to 0.4 percent of the general population and at about 10 percent of the retarded segment of society. It is important to emphasize that severe mental retardation in a large proportion of individuals can presently not be traced to particular congenital anomalies of development or to any of the disorders reviewed in the preceding pages. When groups of such severely retarded patients are *studied clinically, a reasonably accurate etiologic determination of the underlying brain disease can be made in only slightly more than half of them.* According to Penrose, chromosome abnormalities account for 15 percent, single-gene disorders for 7 percent, and environmental agents for 20 percent. Recent studies of the subtelomeric parts of chromosomes reportedly find abnormalities in another 7 percent of severely retarded children (Knight et al). No cause is found for the remaining cases. Males outnumber females 3:1. For purposes of comparison, our figures, obtained from a study of 1372 patients at the Walter E. Fernald School, are presented in Table 38-3.

From the neuropathologic standpoint, *the examination of the brains of the severely retarded by conventional histopathologic methods discloses lesions in approximately 90 percent, and in fully three-quarters an etiologic diagnosis can be determined.* Many of the remaining 10 percent of the "pathologically retarded"

Table 38-3
Causes of severe and mild mental retardation in 1372 patients at the W. E. Fernald State School

Disease category	*Number of patients* IQ<50	IQ>50	*Percent of all patients*
Acquired destructive lesions	278	79	26.0
Chromosomal abnormalities	247	10	18.7
Multiple congenital anomalies	64	16	5.8
Developmental abnormality of brain	49	16	4.7
Metabolic and endocrine diseases	38	5	3.1
Progressive degenerative disease	5	7	0.9
Neurocutaneous diseases	4	0	0.3
Psychosis	7	6	1.0
Mentally retarded (cause unknown)	385	156	39.5

actually lack definite pathologic changes, but their brains are lighter in weight by 10 to 15 percent than age-matched normal brains. Interestingly, the proportion of vascular, hypoxic-ischemic, metabolic, and genetic lesions in this group of severely retarded is much the same as is found in a group selected on the basis of "cerebral palsy."

Here it is important to repeat a point made earlier and in Chap. 28, that a few of the severely disabled and a large majority of the mildly retarded do not have a recognizable cerebral pathology or exhibit any of the familiar and conventional signs of cerebral disease. Although the milder forms of mental retardation tend to be familial, this does not by itself separate them from the severe forms of mental retardation. There are several types of hereditary mental retardation, in which the retardation may be severe and in some of which there may be maldevelopment of the cerebral cortex. These are discussed further on.

Clinical Characteristics of the Severely Retarded

In one large group of severely retarded, designated the *dysmorphic retardates*, a variety of physical deformities, particularly microcephaly, is common. In a second group, *multiple system retardation*, the mental retardation is linked to nonskeletal abnormalities (hepatosplenomegaly as well as hematologic and skin disorders), which provide reliable clues to the underlying somatic disease. In a third group, the *neurologic retardates*, somatic abnormalities are lacking; the configuration of neurologic signs often leads to the diagnosis. And in a fourth and most difficult group, the *uncomplicated retardates*, there are no or minimal somatic, visceral, and neurologic abnormalities. One is then forced to turn to special features of the mental retardation itself for identification of the underlying disease. Table 38-4 elaborates our classification of the types of mental retardation.

The profoundly retarded infant with a virtually untestable IQ (idiot level in the older classifications) is identified early in life because he does not sit, stand, or walk. If any one of these motor activities is acquired, it appears to be late and is imperfectly performed. Language never develops; at most a few spoken words or phrases are understood and fewer are uttered, or the patient only vocalizes in a meaningless way. Such a person may not even indicate bodily needs for food, drink, excretion, and so on. Usually the patient is continuously idle and interacts little with people and objects in his surroundings. Only the most primitive emotional reactions are exhibited, often without connection to an appropriate stimulus. Physical growth is usually retarded, nutrition may be poor, and susceptibility to infections is increased. Sphincteric control may never be attained, and if attained is precarious.

If the mental defect is less severe than the one described above, falling into the IQ range of 20 to 45, or 45 to 70, there may still be somatic neurologic abnormalities; if specific motor defects do not coexist, then sitting, standing, and walking are achieved but not at the expected times. The existence of a mental defect is most clearly evidenced by psychomotor delay and a failure to speak by the second or third postnatal year. The patient does not acquire the usual household and play activities as well as other children. However, delay in speech development must not, by itself, be taken as a mark of mental retardation, for in some children a unique delay in speech can be an isolated abnormality (see Chap. 28), with subsequent normal development of speech. Toilet training may be difficult to accomplish in the retarded child, but, again, bed wetting may be a problem in an otherwise normal child. Also, the deaf child may have to be considered separately; the problem becomes apparent by an indifference to noise and reduced vocalization (stereotypy of babbling).

More searching analyses of cognitive functions in the moderately retarded child have been undertaken by

O'Connor and Hermelin, by Pulsifer, and by others. These authors have attempted to measure efficiency of visual and auditory perception, adequacy of communication, relations between language development and thought, cross-modal sensory encoding, alertness, attention, and memory. It was concluded that none of these functions was specifically impaired. Instead, the retarded child could not properly encode new information because the memory systems and stock of assimilated knowledge were insufficient to provide a framework of items and categories with which new information could be integrated. Some also seem unable, perhaps because of this, to extract from perceived material selective features that can be interpreted. Further, they were unable to deal with an array of sensory experiences like normal children. The complexity of these operations, which the authors would reduce to a global failure of the normal processes of apperception and integration, has been called by Piaget a failure of assimilation and accommodation. This type of inadequacy is common to many different diseases, but in each one there are other subtle differences not yet fully analyzed by neuropsychologists.

Within the spectrum of mental retardation, apart from cognitive impairments, there are differences in behavior and personality, even in those with more or less the same IQ. Some moderately severe retardates are pleasant and amiable and achieve a rather satisfactory social adjustment. This is particularly notable in patients with Down and Williams syndromes. At the opposite end of the behavioral scale is the syndrome of autism, in which the individual fails to manifest normal interpersonal social contact, including communicative language. The phenylketonuric retardate is usually irritable, unaffectionate, and implacable, and the same is said of other retardates, such as those with the DeLange syndrome, discussed earlier in the section on retardation with dwarfism.

Regarding activity levels, many retarded individuals are slow, clumsy, and relatively akinetic. Others, as many as half of them, display an incessant hyperactivity characterized by a restless, seemingly inquisitive searching of the environment. When thwarted, they have a low frustration tolerance. They may be destructive and recklessly fearless and impervious to the risk of injury. Some exhibit a peculiar anhedonia that renders them indifferent to both punishment and reward. Other aberrant types of behavior, such as violent aggressiveness and self-mutilation, are common. Rhythmic rocking, head banging, incessant arm movements—so-called rhythmias or movement stereotypies—are observed in the majority of severe retardates. They are maintained hour after hour without fatigue and may be accompanied by breathing sounds, squeals, and other exclamations. Self-stimulation, even hurtful—such as striking the forehead or ears or biting the fingers and forearms—seems compulsive or perhaps provides satisfaction. It is not that these rhythmias are by themselves abnormal, for some of them occur for brief periods in normal babies, but that they persist. Some moderately retarded persons, when assigned to a simple task such as putting envelopes in a box, can continue this activity under supervision for several hours.

It is impossible to list all the varieties of mental retardation here; the point to be made is that all aspects of intellectual life, personality, and deportment are affected in differing degrees and that these effects have a neurologic basis. There is more than a hint that in particular diseases, because of their anatomy, the cognitive experience, affective life, and behavior are affected in special ways. The group of moderately retarded, like the severely retarded, is divisible into groups with somatic systemic and neurologic abnormalities, though the proportions are not the same. There are fewer of the dysmorphic type and more of the nondysmorphic, nonneurologic group.

Etiology of Severe Mental Retardation From Table 38-3 it is obvious that many diseases can blight the development and maturation of the brain, leaving it in an arrested state. Some of them are acquired and some are congenital and hereditary. Some affect all parts of the organism, giving rise to associated dermal, skeletal, and visceral abnormalities, while others affect only the nervous system in particular patterns. With respect to the *milder degrees of mental retardation*, in all populations thus far studied, extreme low-birth-weight infants are more likely to have disabilities, brain abnormalities, and poorer language development and scholastic achievement. This correlates with lower social status, which must relate in some manner to biological factors (Scottish Low-Birth-Weight Study). Viral and spirochetal infections and parturitional accidents are common causes. They act acutely and are theoretically preventable. The factor of malnutrition during the fetal or infantile period of life as a cause of severe mental retardation has received considerable attention because it is worldwide. Animal experiments (by Winick and others) have demonstrated that severe undernutrition in early life leads to behavioral abnormalities and biochemical and morphologic changes in the brain, which may be permanent (see Chap. 41). Galler studied a group of infants in Barbados who were malnourished during the first year of life and then given an adequate diet. These children were followed to adulthood and compared with normally nourished siblings. Galler observed no effect on physical growth, but there were persistent attention deficits in 60 percent of the undernourished group and in only 15 percent of controls. The IQ scores of the former were also lower. Unfortunately, genetic factors were not completely controlled. In general, it may be said that the data showing mental retardation to be caused by malnutrition, while suggestive, are far from convincing.

Severe protein-calorie malnutrition in the first 8 months of life, which induces kwashiorkor, does seem to retard mental development. However, such patients are said to regain mental function when fed. The authors have been impressed with the ability of the nervous system to withstand the effects of nutritional deficiency, perhaps better than any other organ.

The action of exogenous toxins during pregnancy is another factor to be considered. Severe maternal alcoholism has been linked to a dysgenetic syndrome, including mental retardation, but the findings of several studies have not been consistent (see Chap. 42). Surprisingly, maternal addiction to opiates, while causing an opiate withdrawal in infants for weeks or even months (Wilson et al), seems not to result in permanent injury to the nervous system. The exposure to small amounts of environmental lead is also controversial.

The effect of psychologic deprivation has been of interest. Following the observations that complete isolation of young female monkeys had a devastating effect on their later sexual and nurturing behavior, the idea became popular that sensory deprivation might cause faulty mental development in humans. Orphaned and neglected babies were found to be inactive, apathetic, and backward in comparison with those who were constantly stimulated by caring mothers. But surprisingly, when nurtured properly at a later time, these babies soon caught up with their peers. This general idea of psychologic deprivation was the basis of many interesting head-start programs for poor and neglected children. To this day, however, it has not been proven that sensory, emotional, and psychologic deprivations are the causes of severe mental retardation or repeated scholastic failure. However, the problem is a complex one, and the arguments pro and con have been carefully elaborated by Haywood and Wachs. The controversies regarding the effects of prematurity, maternal hypertension, and eclampsia, which are often associated with retarded psychomotor development, were described earlier in this chapter.

The genetic types of severe mental retardation, including the novel type associated with subtelomeric abnormalities, have already been mentioned.

Differentiation of Types of Retardation: Clinical Approach

As a particular guide to the pediatrician and neurologist who must assume responsibility for the diagnosis and management of backward children harboring a wide array of diseases and maldevelopments of the nervous system, the following clinical approach is suggested. First, as already described, there is an advantage in setting aside as one large group those who are only mildly retarded from those who have been severely delayed in psychomotor development since early life. With regard to the former group, having no obvious neurologic signs or physical stigmata, the only medical problems they present are in the spheres of behavioral, educational, and psychosocial adjustments. One should nevertheless initiate a search for the common metabolic, chromosomal, and infective diseases. In this large group one must be sure that their deficit is a general one and not one of hearing, poor sight, or the special language and attention deficits described in Chaps. 23 and 28.

For patients with the moderately severe and very severe deficits, one begins always with a careful physical examination, searching for somatic stigmata and neurologic signs. Abnormalities of eyes, nose, lips, ears, fingers, and toes are particularly important, as are a variety of neurologic abnormalities, as outlined in Table 38-4. Data so obtained allow classification into one of three categories, as follows.

In one group, *those with somatic abnormalities* (with or without obvious neurologic signs), one assumes the presence of a maldevelopment of the brain, possibly caused by a chromosomal abnormality. The psychomotor retardation is usually severe and often nongenetic and, as as a rule, has a well-defined neuropathology. Diagnosis is determined by the gestalt of physical signs. The possible maldevelopments are numerous and diverse and have been summarized in Tables 38-1 and 38-4; some of the main ones have been described earlier in the chapter. One inevitably turns to the several atlases to denominate the syndromes (Holmes et al; Jones).

In the second group, in which the *abnormalities are confined to the nervous system*, attention is focused on a larger number of diseases, many due to exogenous factors such as perinatal hypoxia-ischemia, pre- or postnatal infections, trauma, and so on. There are usually conspicuous neurologic signs. The degree of mental retardation is variable, depending on the location and extent of a demonstrable neuropathology. Usually the

Table 38-4
Types of severe mental retardation

I. Dysmorphic defect with somatic developmental abnormalities in nonnervous structures
   A. Those affecting cranioskeletal structures
      1. Microcephaly
      2. Macrocephaly
      3. Hydrocephalus (including myelomeningocele with Chiari malformation and associated cerebral anomalies)
      4. Down syndrome
      5. Cretinism (congenital hypothyroidism)
      6. Mucopolysaccharidoses (Hurler, Hunter, and Sanfilippo types)
      7. Acrocephalosyndactyly (craniostenosis) and other craniosomatic abnormalities
      8. Arthrogryposis multiplex congenita (in certain cases)
      9. Rare specific syndromes: De Lange
      10. Dwarfism, short stature: Russel-Silver dwarf, Seckel bird-headed dwarf, Rubinstein-Taybi dwarf, Cockayne-Neel dwarf, etc.
      11. Hypertelorism, median cleft face syndromes, agenesis of corpus callosum
   B. Those affecting nonskeletal structures
      1. Neurocutaneous syndromes: tuberous sclerosis, Sturge-Weber, neurofibromatosis
      2. Congenital rubella syndrome (deafness, blindness, congenital heart disease, small stature)
      3. Chromosomal disorders: Down syndrome, some cases of Klinefelter syndrome (XXY), XYY, Turner (XO) syndrome (occasionally), and others
      4. Laurence-Moon-Biedl syndrome (retinitis pigmentosa, obesity, polydactyly)
      5. Eye disorders: toxoplasmosis (chorioretinitis), galactosemia (cataract), congenital rubella
      6. Prader-Willi syndrome (obesity, hypogenitalism)

II. Nondysmorphic mental defect without somatic anomalies but with cerebral and other neurologic abnormalities
   A. Cerebral spastic diplegia
   B. Cerebral hemiplegia, unilateral or bilateral
   C. Congenital choreoathetosis or ataxia
      1. Kernicterus
      2. Status marmoratus
   D. Congenital ataxia
   E. Congenital atonic diplegia
   F. Syndromes resulting from hypoglycemia, trauma, meningitis, and encephalitis
   G. Associated with other neuromuscular abnormalities (muscular dystrophy, cerebellar ataxia, etc.)
   H. Cerebral degenerative diseases (lipidoses)
   I. Associated with inborn errors of metabolism (phenylketonuria, other aminoacidurias, organic acidurias, Lesch-Nyhan syndrome)
   J. Congenital infections (some cases of congenital syphilis, cytomegalic inclusion disease)

III. Genetic mental defect of indeterminate type without signs of somatic abnormality or neurologic disorder
   A. Infantile autism, Renpenning, Williams, fragile X, and Rett syndromes.

family history is negative, but careful questioning of parents regarding the pregnancy, delivery, and early postnatal period, and examination of older hospital records may disclose the nature of the neurologic insult.

The third category of retardates is one in which *neither somatic anomalies nor focal neurologic signs* are present. The more severely retarded of this third group are represented by the following disease states: autism (Asperger-Kanner syndrome), the Rett and Williams syndromes, and the fragile-X and Renpenning syndromes. The last three have a genetic basis and are described together below.

The practical importance of this clinical approach is that it directs the intelligent use of laboratory procedures for confirmation of the diagnosis. CT scanning and MRI are useful in clarifying maldevelopment and neurologic diseases but are seldom helpful in the third group. EEG confirms seizure discharges when there is uncertainty as to the nature of episodic neural dysfunction. Karyoptyping and genetic studies are useful in group 1 and rarely in group 2 patients.

The major pitfall to be avoided in this clinical approach is in mistaking a hereditary metabolic disease for a developmental one. Here one is helped by the fact that manifestations of the metabolic diseases are not usually present in the first days and weeks of life; they appear later and are progressive and often associated with visceral abnormalities. However, some metabolic diseases are of such slow progression that they appear stable, especially the late-onset ones, such as one type of metachromatic leukodystrophy, late-onset Krabbe leukodystrophy, adult adrenoleukodystrophy, and adult hexoseaminidase deficiency (see Chap. 37).

Hereditary Mental Retardations

Fragile-X Syndrome There is now great interest in this syndrome, which some geneticists hold accountable, at least in part, for the preponderance of males among institutionalized retarded individuals. The subject is discussed earlier in this chapter, particularly as it relates to other chromosomal abnormalities (page 1067). A large kindred in which mental retardation was inherited in an X-linked pattern was first reported by Martin and Bell in 1943. It was in such a family, with X-linked mental retardation, that Lubs, in 1969, discovered a fragile site at the distal end of the long arm of the X chromosome; subsequently it was established that there is an unstable inherited CGG repeating sequence at this site, as discussed previously.

Fully 10 percent of mentally retarded males have this fragile X chromosomal abnormality. Females are sometimes affected, but their mental function is only slightly reduced. Affected males have only mild dysmorphic features (large ears, broad forehead, elongated face, and enlarged testes) that may not become obvious until puberty. Others are somatically normal. Behavioral problems of one sort or another are almost universal. Pulsifer, whose review of the neuropsychologic aspects of mental retardation is recommended, lists self-injurious, hyperactive, and impulsive behaviors as the most common. The hand flapping that is characteristic of autism may also be seen.

Renpenning Syndrome A similar type of hereditary, male sex-linked mental retardation has been described by Renpenning. The family comprised 21 males in two generations of Mennonites in western Canada whose IQs ranged from 30 to 40. As with the fragile-X syndrome, female siblings may show slight degrees of retardation. Affected members were small in stature and slightly microcephalic but otherwise free of somatic and neurologic abnormalities. They did not have the fragile-X abnormality.

Rett Syndrome This is yet another hereditary form of mental retardation, but affecting only girls. None of the cases reported by Hagberg and coworkers were male. Recently the responsible spontaneous mutation has been shown to be a dominant defect at chromosomal site Xq28. A fatal outcome in boys explains the expression of the disease only in girls, who are mosaics for the mutation. The involved gene, MECP2, is responsible for suppressing various other genes at critical stages of development.

The syndrome is characterized clinically by withdrawn behavior that simulates autism, dementia, ataxia, loss of purposeful hand movements, and respiratory irregularities, all of which appear and progress after a period of 6 to 18 months of normal development. Spasticity, muscle wasting, scoliosis, and lower limb deformities may become evident in late stages of the illness. Hand waving, hand wringing, and similar stereotypes are very characteristic features (and are subtly different from the hand flapping of autistic children).

Armstrong and Naidu, who have reviewed the neuropathology, have drawn attention to a number of subtle cortical abnormalities, most of which are consistent with disruption of the dynamic phase of brain development postnatally; however, not all cases showed these abnormalities. While most cases appear to be sporadic, there is a high familial incidence and concordance in twins. However, this is still a matter of contention.

Williams Syndrome This inherited form of mental retardation has also been mentioned earlier, on page 1068, in relation to the chromosomal abnormalities. It is characterized by only mild mental retardation but with striking retention and even precocity of musical aptitude, social amiability, and in some instances a retained facility for writing, permitting the production of long written descriptions; at the same time these subjects are barely able to draw simple objects. The child is physically retarded and has minor but distinctive somatic changes (wide mouth, almond-shaped eyes, upturned nose, small pointed ears), together described as "elfin." He is usually sensitive to auditory stimuli. There is a delay in the acquisition of communicative speech and defects in visual, spatial, and motor skills, making these children seem more backward than they actually are. Striking sociability and empathy sets them apart; they represent virtually the converse of autism in this respect. Memory for musical scores—such as memorizing a complete symphony after one hearing—may be prodigious. By the use of high-resolution cytogenetics, the disease has been traced in 90 percent of cases to a microdeletion on chromosome 7 in the region of the gene that controls the production of elastin (Nickerson et al). This is of interest because an index feature of these cases is a supravalvular aortic stenosis. It is not known whether there is a characteristic brain pathology, but a recent case of Golden and colleagues, examined at 35 years of age, showed no cerebral abnormalities except for Alzheimer changes, mainly plaque deposition in the entorhinal cortex and amygdala.

Autism (Kanner-Asperger Syndrome; Autistic Spectrum Disorders)

This condition was described almost simultaneously by Kanner in Baltimore (in 1943) and Asperger in Vienna (in 1944). Among the large group of retarded children, Kanner observed exceptional children who appeared to be *asocial, lacking in communicative skills both verbal and nonverbal, and committed to repetitive ritualistic behaviors.* At the same time certain intellectual capacities—such as retentive memory, skilled sensory and motor aptitudes, and capacity for visual spatial perception—were retained. In other words, the disorder did not pervade all aspects of mental development. It is the gestalt of negative and positive aptitudes that sets this syndrome apart from other types of retardation. Kanner incorrectly ascribed the condition to psychosocial factors—such as a cold, aloof parent—and regarded it as an autistic psychopathy. The implication that these children are literally "autistic"—i.e., that they have a rich inner psychic life or dream world out of relation to reality—is an assumption wholly without foundation. Asperger, whose observations included somewhat older children, less completely disabled, ascribed it to a special metabolic disease, possibly related to hyperammonemia. Opinion varied as to the relationship between the severe Kanner syndrome and the less severe Asperger syndrome. The authors have taken the position that these forms of autism represent a single syndrome of varying severity, with similar pathologic underpinnings but possibly of multiple etiologies, including genetic.

For reasons mentioned above, the term *autism*, drawn from psychiatry, is inappropriate but is firmly embedded in the medical lexicon. Despite many claims to the contrary, there is absolutely no evidence of a psychogenesis. However, as Rapin points out, behavioral modification and special education are beneficial for the less severely affected. At one time the disorder was referred to as childhood schizophrenia, but the afflicted individuals do not resemble schizophrenics, even when they reach adult years. The very early onset (preschool) onset of autism, the lack of delusional thinking, and different inheritance patterns are other points against this being a type of childhood schizophrenia. Moreover, the manifestations of autism change to some extent in the course of development—a characteristic of what is called, for lack of a better label, a neurodevelopmental disorder.

The overall prevalence of the autistic state has been calculated at 4.5 to 20 per 10,000. Although there is said to be no familial tendency to autism, this is almost certainly incorrect; we have seen the disease in both of identical twins and in brothers, and a small familial subgroups are known to exist. Autistic traits, without the full syndrome, are being found with increasing frequency in sibs and other family members, suggesting a polygenic inheritance. DeMyer found that 4 out of 11 monozygotic twins were concordant for autism and that siblings have a 50 times greater risk of developing the disorder. Bailey and also LeCouteur and associates have reported a concordance rate in monozygotic twins of 71 percent for the autistic spectrum disorder and 92 percent for an even broader phenotype of disordered social communication and stereotypic or obsessive behaviors. DeLong finds a surprisingly high incidence of manic-depressive disease in the families of one group of autistic children.

Clinical Features The autistic child is ostensibly normal at birth and may continue to be normal in achieving early behavioral sequences until 18 to 24 months of age. Then an alarming regression occurs. In some instances, however, the abnormality appears even before the first birthday and is identified as different from normal by the mother; or, if there had been a previously autistic child, she recognizes the early behavioral characteristics. The level of activity is reduced or increased. There may be less crying and an apparent indifference to surroundings. Toys are ignored or held tenaciously. Cuddling may be resisted. Motor developments, on the other hand, proceed normally and may even be precocious. Later there may be an unusual sensitivity to all modes of sensory stimulation. Occasionally the onset appears to have a relationship to an injury or an upsetting experience.

Regardless of the time of and rapidity of onset, the autistic child exhibits a disregard for other persons; this is typically quite striking but in milder cases is more subtle. Little or no eye contact is made, and the child is no more interested in another person than in an article of furniture. Proferred toys are manipulated cleverly, placed in varying lines, or rejected. Insistence on constancy of environment may reach a point where the patient becomes distraught if even a single one of his possessions is moved from its original place and remains distraught until it is replaced. If speech develops at all, it is highly automatic (echolalic) and not used effectively to communicate. A repertoire of elaborate stereotyped movements—such as whirling of the body, manipulating an object, toe walking and particularly hand flapping are characteristic. Spinning toys or running water may have a strange fascination for these children.

It is important to point out, however, that in any sizable group of autistic children *there is a wide range of deficits in sociability, drive, affect, and communicative (verbal and gestural behavior) ability*, ranging from the averbal negativistic, completely isolated state to one showing considerable language skill and some capacity for attachment to certain people and for scholastic achievement. In this higher-functioning group, taken to typify the Asperger syndrome, the child may be unusually adept in reading, calculating, drawing, or memorizing while still having difficulty in adjusting socially and emotionally to others. Many are clumsy and inept in athletic activities. The least degree of deficit allows success in a professional field but with handicap in the social sphere. We take the current emphasis on the term *autistic spectrum disorders* to reflect a concept that each of the core elements of autism (in social, language, cognitive, and behavioral domains) may occur in widely varying degrees of severity. This view permits a syndromic diagnosis of autism in patients with coexisitng elements of other disorders, such as attention deficit disorder and manic-depressive or obsessive-compulsive disorders and expands the diagnosis to many children who are highly functional except for gaze aversion and other "soft signs" (Filipek).

Rapin, drawing on a large clinical experience with autism, has carefully documented its linguistic, cognitive, and behavioral features. She uses the term *semantic-pragmatic disorder* to designate the characteristic affection of language and behavior and to distinguish it from other forms of developmental disorders and mental retardation.

Elements of autism, but not the whole syndrome with its positive and negative attributes, may appear in other diseases that interfere with brain development, specifically fragile-X and Rett syndromes, and fragmentary similarities are found in a few children with phenylketonuria, tuberous sclerosis, Angleman syndrome, and, rarely, Down syndrome—but these patients are easily distinguished from those with the far more common type of autism. Bolton and Griffiths have made the intriguing observation that autistic traits in patients with tuberous sclerosis correspond to the finding of tubers in the temporal lobe, and DeLong and Heinz point out that patients with seizures from bilateral (but not unilateral) hippocampal sclerosis may fail to develop (or may lose) language ability as well as to acquire social skills after a period of normal development, in a manner similar to idiopathic autism. The IQ of the majority is below 70.

Etiology and Pathology of Autism The basis of childhood autism is as much a mystery today as it was when Kanner and Asperger described it. Most of these children are physically normal except for a larger than average head size, but with no other somatic anomalies. The EEG is normal, as is CT or MRI. The significance of cerebellar vermal changes, reported originally by Courchesne et al, remains to be determined (Filipek).

In the few brains examined postmortem, no lesions of any of the conventional types were found. In five brains studied in serial sections by Bauman and Kemper, smallness of neurons and increased packing density were observed in the medial temporal areas (hippocampus, subiculum, entorrhinal cortex), amygdala and septal nuclei, and mammillary bodies. In a subsequent review of the neuropathology, Kemper and Bauman concluded that three changes stand out: a curtailment of the normal development of neurons in the limbic system; a decrease in the number of Purkinje cells that appears to be congenital; and—in contrast to this—age-related changes in the size and number of the neurons in the diagonal band of Broca (located in the basal frontal septal region) as well as in the cerebellar nuclei and inferior olive. The age-related changes were inferred from studying the brains of autistic children who died at different ages, and they gave the appearance of a progressive or ongoing pathology that continues into adult life. These findings are in keeping with the concept of autism as a neurodevelopmental disorder, but they allow only speculation regarding the derivation of the clinical features of the disease. An increased concentration of platelet serotonin and low serum serotonin is detected in many but not all patients with autism; the biologic significance of these findings is unclear.

Course and Prognosis The disease is essentially nonprogressive, although some patients, as they grow older, begin to manifest additional visuoperceptive or auditory defects. The outcome is bleak, although a group of lesser affected children may show improvement in social relationships and schoolwork with the use of serotonin reuptake inhibitors, sometimes in very small doses (DeLong; Filipek, personal communication). The peptide secretin has produced a number of anecdotal successes, but this outcome could not be reproduced in a controlled study (Sandler et al). According to Eisenberg, who reviewed many of Kanner's original cases and followed many other cases into adult life, one-third never spoke and remained social isolates, one-third acquired a rudimentary language devoid of communicative value, and the remainder were functional to various degrees with an affected, stilted, colorless speech. It is in the latter group, representing the mildest degrees of autism, that one finds the eccentrics, the mirthless, flat personalities, unable to adapt socially and habitually avoiding eye contact but sometimes possessing certain unusual aptitudes in memory, mathematics, factual knowledge, history, and science. Rutter, who has written extensively on the subject, says that the degree of language impairment and lowered intelligence predicts outcome; those who do not speak by 5 years of age never learn to speak well.

Management of Mental Retardation

Since there is little or no possibility of treating most of the diseases underlying mental retardation and there is no way of restoring function to a nervous system that is developmentally subnormal, the objective is to assist in planning for the patient's care, training, education, and social adjustment. The parents must be guided in forming realistic attitudes and expectations. Psychiatric and social counseling may help the family to maintain gentle but firm support of the patient so that he or she can acquire, to the fullest extent possible, good work habits and a congenial personality.

Most individuals with an IQ above 60 and no other handicaps can be trained to live an independent life: special schooling may enable them to learn skills useful in a vocation. Social factors that contribute to underachievement must be sought and eliminated if possible.

If the IQ is below 20, institutionalization is almost inevitable, for few families can provide the long-term custodial care that is needed. Well-run institutions are usually better than community homes because they offer many more facilities (medical, educational, recreational). Often institutional care is necessary for individuals with IQs of 20 to 50. Patients in this group, if stable in temperament and relatively well adjusted to society, can work under supervision, but they rarely become vocationally independent. For the more severely retarded, special training in hygiene and self-care is the most that can be expected.

Great care must be exercised in recommending institutionalization. Whereas the need will be all too apparent in the gravely retarded by the first or second year of life, the less severely affected are difficult to evaluate at an early age. As stated earlier, psychologic tests alone are not altogether trustworthy. It is best to observe the patient over a period of time. The method of evaluation suggested long ago by Fernald has a ring of soundness, albeit in dated terms. As noted in Chap. 28, the final decision about optimal care is determined by (1) the physical, medical, and neurologic findings; (2) the family background; (3) the developmental history; (4) school progress or lack thereof; (5) performance tests; (6) social behavior; (7) industrial efficiency; (8) what was called in Fernald's time, moral behavior (for example, masturbation); and (9) intelligence as measured by psychological tests.

REFERENCES

Aicardi J: *Epilepsy in Children*. New York, Raven Press, 1986.

Aicardi J, LeFebvre J, Lerique-Koechlin A: A new syndrome: Spasm in flexion, callosal agenesis, ocular abnormalities. *Electroencephalogr Clin Neurophysiol* 19:609, 1965.

Armstrong DD: Review of Rett syndrome. *J Neuropath Exp Neurol* 56:843,1997.

Asperger H: Die "Autistischen Psychopathen" im Kindesalter. *Arch Psychiatr Nervenkrankh* 117:76, 1944.

Baker RS, Ross PA, Bauman RJ: Neurologic complications of the epidermal nevus syndrome. *Arch Neurol* 44:227, 1987.

Banker BQ: Cerebral vascular disease in infancy and childhood: 1. Occlusive vascular disease. *J Neuropathol Exp Neurol* 20:127, 1961.

Banker BQ, Bruce-Gregorios J: A neuropathologic study of diseases of the nervous system in the first year of life, in Thompson GH, Rubin IL, Bilenker RM (eds): *Comprehensive Management of Cerebral Palsy*. New York, Grune & Stratton, 1982, pp 25–31.

Banker BQ, Larroche J-C: Periventricular leukomalacia of infancy. *Arch Neurol* 7:386, 1962.

Bailey A, LeCouteur A, Gottesman A, et al: Autism as a strongly genetic disorder: evidence from a British twin study. *Psychol Med* 25:63, 1995.

Barker E, Wright K, Nguyen K, et al: Gene for von Recklinghausen neurofibromatosis in the pericentromeric region of chromosome 17. *Science* 236:1100, 1987.

Barlow CF: *Mental Retardation and Related Disorders*. Philadelphia, Davis, 1978.

Bauman M, Kemper TL: Histoanatomic observations of the brain in early infantile autism. *Neurology* 35:866, 1985.

Benson JWI, Hayward C, Osborne J, et al: Multicentre trial of ethamsylate for prevention of periventricular hemorrhage in very low birth weight infants. *Lancet* 2:1297, 1986.

Berg BO (ed): *Principles of Child Neurology*. New York, McGraw-Hill, 1996.

Beuren AJ, Apitz J, Harmjanz D: Supravalvular aortic stenosis in association with mental retardation and a certain facial appearance. *Circulation* 26:1235, 1962.

Bielschowsky M: Über tuberose Sklerose and ihre Beziehungen zur Recklinghausenschen Krankheit. *Z Gesamte Neurol Psychiatr* 26:133, 1914.

Bolton PF, Griffiths PD: Association of tuberous sclerosis of temporal lobes with autism and atypical autism. *Lancet* 349:392, 1997.

Botto LD, Moore CA, Khoury MJ, Erickson JD: Neural-tube defects. *N Engl J Med* 341:1509, 1999.

BRADLEY WG, RICHARDSON J, FREW IJC: The familial association of neurofibromatosis, peroneal muscular atrophy, congenital deafness, partial albinism and Axenfeld's defect. *Brain* 97:521, 1974.

BRETT EM (ed): *Paediatric Neurology*, 3rd ed. New York, Churchill Livingstone, 1997.

CHAPLIN ER, GOLDSTEIN GW, MYERBERG DZ, et al: Posthemorrhagic hydrocephalus in the preterm infant. *Pediatrics* 65:901, 1980.

CHAPMAN PH: Congenital intraspinal lipomas: Anatomic considerations and surgical treatment. *Childs Brain* 9:37, 1982.

CHAPMAN PH, DAVIS KR: Surgical treatment of spinal lipomas in childhood, in Raimondi AJ (ed): *Concepts in Pediatric Neurosurgery*. Munich, Karger, 1983.

COBB S: Haemangioma of the spinal cord associated with skin naevi of the same metamere. *Ann Surg* 62:641, 1915.

COGAN DC: A type of congenital ocular motor apraxia presenting jerky head movements. *Trans Am Acad Ophthalmol* 56:853, 1952.

COURCHESNE E, YEUNG-COURCHESNE R, PRESS GA, et al: Hypolplasia of cerebellar vermal lobules VI and VII in autism. *N Engl J Med* 318:1349, 1988.

CRÉANGE A, ZELLER J, ROSTAING-RIGATTIEREI S, et al: Neurologic complications of neurofibromatosis type 1 in adulthood. *Brain* 122:473, 1999.

CROWE FW: Axillary freckling as a diagnostic aid in neurofibromatosis. *Ann Intern Med* 61:1142, 1964.

CROWE FW, SCHULL WJ, NEEL JV: *A Clinical, Pathological and Genetic Study of Multiple Neurofibromatosis*. Springfield, IL, Charles C Thomas, 1956.

DELONG GR, HEINZ ER: The clinical syndrome of early-life bilateral hippocampal sclerosis. *Ann Neurol* 42:11, 1997.

DELONG GR: Autism: new data suggest a new hypothesis. *Neurology* 52:911, 1999.

DEMYER MK: Infantile autism: Patients and families. *Curr Probl Pediatr* 12:1, 1982.

DENNIS J: Neonatal convulsions: Aetiology, late neonatal status and long-term outcome. *Dev Med Child Neurol* 20:143, 1978.

DUFFNER PK, COHEN ME, SEIDEL G, SHUCARD DW: The significance of MRI abnormalities in children with neurofibromatosis. *Neurology* 39:373, 1989.

DYKEN P, KRAWIECKI N: Neurodegenerative diseases of infancy and childhood. *Ann Neurol* 13:351, 1983.

EISENBERG L: The autistic child in adolescence. *Am J Psychiatry* 112:607, 1965.

ELDRIDGE R: Central neurofibromatosis with bilateral acoustic neuroma, in Riccardi VM, Mulvihill JJ (eds): *Advances in Neurology*. Vol 29: *Neurofibromatosis (Von Recklinghausen Disease)*. New York, Raven Press, 1981, pp 57–65.

ERZURUM S, KALAVSKY SM, WATANAKUNAKORN C: Acute cerebellar ataxia and hearing loss as initial symptoms of infectious mononucleosis. *Arch Neurol* 40:760, 1983.

EUROPEAN COLLABORATIVE STUDY: Children born to women with HIV-1 infection: Natural history and risk of transmission. *Lancet* 337:253, 1991.

EVRARD PH, DE SAINT-GEORGES P, KADHIM H, et al: Pathology of prenatal encephalopathies, in French JH, Harel S, Casaer P (eds): *Child Neurology and Developmental Disabilities*. Baltimore, Brookes, 1989.

FENICHEL GM: Hypoxic-ischemic encephalopathy in the newborn. *Arch Neurol* 40:261, 1983.

FENICHEL GM: *Neonatal Neurology*, 3rd ed. New York, Churchill Livingstone, 1990.

FILIPEK PA: Quantitative magnetic resonance imaging in autism: The cerebellar vermis. *Curr Opin Neurol* 8:134, 1995.

FITZPATRICK TB, SZABO G, HORI Y, et al: White leaf-shaped macules, earliest visible sign of tuberous sclerosis. *Arch Dermatol* 98:1, 1968.

FORD FR: *Diseases of the Nervous System in Infancy, Childhood and Adolescence*, 6th ed. Springfield, IL, Charles C Thomas, 1973.

FOWLER KB, STAGNO S, PASS RF, et al: The outcome of congenital cytomegalovirus infection in relation to maternal antibody status. *N Engl J Med* 326:663, 1992.

FREUD S: *Infantile Cerebral Paralysis*. Russin LA (trans). Coral Gables, FL, University of Miami Press, 1968.

FRIEDLAND R, YAHR MD: Meningoencephalopathy secondary to infectious mononucleosis: Unusual presentation with stupor and chorea. *Arch Neurol* 34:186, 1977.

FRITH U (ed): *Autism and Asperger Syndrome*. Cambridge, England, Cambridge University Press, 1991.

GALLER JR: Malnutrition: A neglected cause of learning failure. *Postgrad Med* 80:225, 1986.

GARCIA CA, DUNN D, TREVOR R: The lissencephaly (agyria) syndrome in siblings. *Arch Neurol* 35:608, 1978.

GASTAUT H, POIRIER F, PAYAN H, et al: HHE syndrome: Hemiconvulsion, hemiplegia, epilepsy. *Epilepsia* 1:418, 1960.

GELLIS SB, FEINGOLD M, RUTMAN JY: Mental Retardation Syndromes. Washington, DC, U.S. Department of Health, Education, and Welfare, 1968.

GILLBERG C: Asperger syndrome in 23 Swedish children. *Dev Med Child Neurol* 31:520, 1989.

GOLD AP, FREEMAN JM: Depigmented nevi, the earliest sign of tuberous sclerosis. *Pediatrics* 35:1003, 1965.

GOLDEN JA, NIELSEN GP, POBER BR, et al: The neuropathology of Williams syndrome; Report of a 35 year old man with presenile beta/A4 amyloid plaques and neurofibrillary tangles. *Arch Neurol* 52:209, 1995.

GOMEZ MR: *Tuberous Sclerosis*. New York, Raven Press, 1979.

GOMEZ MR: *Neurocutaneous Disease (A Practical Approach)*. Boston, Butterworth, 1987.

GOMEZ MR, KUNTZ NL, WESTMORELAND BF: Tuberous sclerosis, early onset of seizures, and mental subnormality: Study of discordant homozygous twins. *Neurology* 32:604, 1982.

GORLIN RS, PINDBORG JJ, COHEN MM JR: *Syndromes of the Head and Neck*. New York, McGraw-Hill, 1976.

GREGG NM: Congenital cataract following German measles in the mother. *Trans Ophthalmol Soc Austr* 3:35, 1941.

HACK M, TAYLOR G, KLEIN N, et al: School-age outcomes in children with birth weight under 750 g. *N Engl J Med* 331:753, 1994.

HADDOW JE, PALOMAKI GE, KNIGHT GJ, et al: Prenatal screening for Down's syndrome with use of maternal serum markers. *N Engl J Med* 327:588, 1992.

Hagberg B: Rett syndrome: clinical and biological mysteries. *Acta Paediatr* 84:971, 1995.

Hagberg B, Aicardi J, Dias K, et al: A progressive syndrome of autism, dementia, ataxia and loss of purposeful hand movements in girls: Rett's syndrome. *Ann Neurol* 14:471, 1983.

Hagberg B, Hagberg G: Prenatal and perinatal risk factors in a survey of 681 Swedish cases, in Stanley FJ, Alberman ED (eds): *The Epidemiology of the Cerebral Palsies*. Vol 10. London, Spastics International, 1984.

Hagberg B, Hagberg G, Olow I: The changing panorama of cerebral palsy in Sweden, 1954–1976: II. Analysis of the various syndromes. *Acta Paediatr Scand* 64:193, 1975.

Halperin JJ, Williams RS, Kolodny EH: Microcephaly vera, progressive motor neuron disease and nigral degeneration. *Neurology* 32:317, 1982.

Harding AE: *The Hereditary Ataxias and Related Disorders*. New York, Churchill Livingstone, 1984.

Hardy JB: Clinical and developmental aspects of congenital rubella. *Arch Otolaryngol* 98:230, 1973.

Harper JR: True myoclonic epilepsy in childhood. *Arch Dis Child* 43:28, 1968.

Hayward JC, Titelbaum DS, Clancy RC, et al: Lissencephaly-pachygryia associated with congenital cytomegalovirus infection. *J Child Neurol* 6:109, 1991.

Haywood HC, Wachs TD: Intelligence, cognition, and individual differences, in Begal MJ, Haywood HC, Garber HL (eds): *Psychosocial Influences in Retarded Performance*. Vol I. Baltimore, University Park Press, 1981.

Henderson JL: The congenital facial diplegia syndrome: Clinical features, pathology and etiology. *Brain* 62:381, 1939.

Herskowitz J, Rosman P, Wheller CB: Colpocephaly: Clinical, radiologic and pathogenetic aspects. *Neurology* 35:1594, 1985.

Hoefnagel D, Penry JK: Partial facial paralysis in young children. *N Engl J Med* 262:1126, 1960.

Holmes LB, Moser HW, Halldrósson S, et al: *Mental Retardation: An Atlas of Diseases with Associated Physical Abnormalities*. New York, Macmillan, 1972.

Hur JJ: Review of research on therapeutic interventions for children with cerebral palsy. *Acta Neurol Scand* 91:427, 1995.

Huttenlocher PR, Hapke RJ: A follow-up study of intractable seizures in childhood. *Ann Neurol* 28:699, 1990.

Hutto C, Parks WP, Lai S, et al: A hospital-based prospective study of perinatal infection with human immunodeficiency virus type 1. *J Pediatr* 118:347, 1991.

Illarioshkin SN, Tanaka H, Markova ED, et al: X-linked nonprogressive congenital cerebellar hypoplasia: Clinical description and mapping to chromosome Xq. *Ann Neurol* 40:75, 1996.

International PHVD Drug Trial Group: *Lancet* 352:433, 1998.

Jablonski S: *Dictionary of Syndromes and Eponymic Diseases*, 2nd ed. Malabar, FL, Krieger, 1991.

Janz D, Dam M, Richens A, et al (eds): *Epilepsy, Pregnancy, and the Child*. New York, Raven Press, 1982.

Johnson KP: Viral infections of the developing nervous system, in Thompson RA, Green JR (eds): *Advances in Neurology*. Vol 6. New York, Raven Press, 1974, pp 53–67.

Jones KL: *Smith's Recognizable Patterns of Human Malformation*, 4th ed. Philadelphia, Saunders, 1988.

Kalter H, Warkany J: Congenital malformations: Etiologic factors and their role in prevention. *N Engl J Med* 308:424, 1983.

Kanda T, Oda M, Yonezawa M, et al: Peripheral neuropathy in xeroderma pigmentosum. *Brain* 113:1025, 1990.

Kanner L: Autistic disturbances of affective contact. *Nervous Child* 2:217, 1943.

Kemper TL, Bauman M: Neuropathology of autism. *J Neuropathol Exp Neurol* 57:645, 1998.

Kinsbourne M: Myoclonic encephalopathy of infants. *J Neurol Neurosurg Psychiatry* 25:271, 1962.

Kline MW, Shearer WT: Impact of human immunodeficiency virus infection on women and infants. *Infect Dis Clin North Am* 6:1, 1992.

Knight SJ, Regan R, Nicod A, et al: Subtle chromosomal rearrangements in children with unexplained mental retardation. *Lancet* 354:1676, 1999.

Krishnamoorthy KS, Kuehnle KJ, Todres ID, DeLong GR: Neurodevelopmental outcome of survivors with posthemorrhagic hydrocephalus following grade II neonatal intraventricular hemorrhage. *Ann Neurol* 15:201, 1984.

Landrieu P: Approches de la pathologic cerebelleuse chronique chez l'enfant. *Rev Neurol (Paris)* 149:776, 1993.

LeCouteur A, Bailey A, Goode S, et al: A broader phenotype of autism: the clinical spectrum in twins. *J Child Psychology Psychiatry* 37:785, 1996.

Lemieux BG: Chromosome-linked disorders, in Swaiman K (ed): *Pediatric Neurology: Principles and Practice*, 2nd ed. St. Louis, Mosby, 1994, pp 357–419.

Levene MI, Grindulis H, Sands C, Moore JR: Comparison of two methods of predicting outcome in perinatal asphyxia. *Lancet* 1:67, 1986.

Levine DN, Fisher MA, Caviness VS Jr: Porencephaly with microgyria: A pathologic study. *Acta Neuropathol (Berl)* 29:99, 1974.

Lewis EO: Types of mental deficiency and their social significance. *J Ment Sci* 79:298, 1933.

Lichtenstein BW: Neurofibromatosis (Von Recklinghausen's disease of the nervous system). *Arch Neurol Psychiatry* 62:822, 1949.

Lorber J: Spina bifida cystica: Results of treatment of 270 cases with criteria for selection in the future. *Arch Dis Child* 47:854, 1972.

Lorber J, Priestley BL: Children with large heads: A practical approach to diagnosis in 557 children with special reference to 109 children with megalencephaly. *Dev Med Child Neurol* 23:494, 1981.

Lubs HA: A marker X chromosome. *Am J Hum Genet* 21:231, 1969.

Lynn RB, Buchanan DC, Fenichel GM, Freeman FR: Agenesis of the corpus callosum. *Arch Neurol* 37:444, 1980.

Lyon G, Evrard PH: *Neuropediatrie*. Paris, Masson, 1987.

Marshall PC, Brett EM, Wilson J: Myoclonic encephalopathy of childhood (the dancing eye syndrome): A long-term follow-up study. *Neurology* 28:348, 1978.

MARTIN JP, BELL JA: A pedigree of mental defect showing sex linkage. *J Neurol Neurosurg Psychiatry* 6:154, 1943.

MARTUZA RL, ELDRIDGE R: Neurofibromatosis 2 (bilateral acoustic neurofibromatosis). *N Engl J Med* 318:684, 1988.

MEDICAL TASK FORCE ON ANENCEPHALY: The infant with anencephaly. *N Engl J Med* 322:669, 1990.

MILUNSKY A: Prenatal detection of neural tube defects: VI. Experience with 20,000 pregnancies. *JAMA* 244:2731, 1980.

MOLONEY DM, WALL SA, ASHWORTH GJ, et al: Prevalence of Pro250Arg mutation of fibroblast growth factor receptor in coronal craniosynostosis. *Lancet* 349:1059,1997.

MYERS RE: Experimental models of perinatal brain damage: Relevance to human pathology, in Glueck L (ed): *Intrauterine Asphyxia and the Developing Fetal Brain*. Bethesda, MD, Year Book, 1977, pp 37–97.

NAIDU S: Rett syndrome: a disorder affecting early brain growth. *Ann Neurol* 42:3, 1997.

NELLHAUS G: Head circumference from birth to 18 years. *Pediatrics* 41:106, 1968.

NELSON KB, ELLENBERG JH: Antecedents of cerebral palsy. *N Engl J Med* 315:81, 1986.

NICKERSON E, GREENBERG F, KEATING MT, et al: Deletions of the elastin gene at 7q11.23 occur in approximately 90% of patients with Williams syndrome. *Am J Hum Genet* 56:1156, 1995.

NISHIKAWA M, SAKAMOTO H, HAKURA A, et al: Pathogenesis of Chiari malformation; a morphometric study of the posterior cranial fossa. *J Neurosurg* 86:40, 1997.

O'CONNOR N, HERMELIN B: Cognitive defects in children. *Br Med Bull* 27:227, 1971.

OHTAHARA S: Seizure disorders in infancy and childhood. *Brain Dev* 6:509, 1984.

OUNSTED C, LINDSAY J, RICHARDS P (eds): *Temporal Lobe Epilepsy, 1948–1986: A Biological Study*. London, Keith Press, 1987.

PANG D, WILBERGER JE: Tethered cord syndrome in adults. *J Neurosurg* 57:32, 1982.

PRNROSE LS: *The Biology of Mental Defect*. New York, Grune & Stratton, 1949.

PIAGET J: *The Origins of Intelligence in Children*. New York, International Universities Press, 1952.

PROBER CG, GERSON AA: Medical management of newborns and infants born to human immunodeficiency virus-seropositive mothers. *Pediatr Infect Dis J* 10:684, 1991.

PULSIFER MB: The neuropsychology of mental retardation. *J Int Neuropsychol Soc* 2:159, 1996.

PURPURA DP: Normal and aberrant neuronal development in the cerebral cortex of human fetus and young infant, in Buchwald NA, Brazier MA (eds): *Brain Mechanisms in Mental Retardation*. New York, Academic Press, 1975, pp 141–171.

RAPIN I: Autism. *N Engl J Med* 337:97, 1997.

RENPENNING H, GERARD JW, ZALESKI WA, et al: Familial sex-linked mental retardation. *Can Med Assoc J* 87:954, 1962.

RICCARDI VM: Von Recklinghausen neurofibromatosis. *N Engl J Med* 305:1617, 1981.

RICCARDI VM, MULVIHILL JJ (eds): *Advances in Neurology*. Vol 29: *Neurofibromatosis (Von Recklinghausen Disease)*. New York, Raven Press, 1981.

ROACH ES, WILLIAMS OP, LASTER DW: Magnetic resonance imaging in tuberous sclerosis. *Arch Neurol* 44:301, 1987.

ROSMAN NP, PEARCE J: The brain in neurofibromatosis. *Brain* 90:829, 1967.

ROULEAU GA, WERTELECKI W, HAINES JL, et al: Genetic linkage of bilateral acoustic neurofibromatosis to a DNA marker on chromosome 22. *Nature* 329:246, 1987.

ROUSSEAU F, HEITZ D, BIANCALANA V, et al: Direct diagnosis by DNA analysis of the fragile X syndrome of mental retardation. *N Engl J Med* 325:1674, 1991.

RUTTER M: Infantile autism and other pervasive developmental disorders, in Rutter M, Taylor EA, Hersov LA (eds): *Child and Adolescent Psychiatry: Modern Approaches*, 3rd ed. Oxford, England, Blackwell, 1994.

SANDLER AD, SUTTON KA, DEWEESE J, et al: Lack of benefit of a single dose of synthetic human secretin in the treatment of autism and pervasive developmental disorder. *N Engl J Med* 341:1801, 1999.

SCHREIER H, RAPIN I, DAVIS J: Familial megalencephaly or hydrocephalus? *Neurology* 24:232, 1974.

SCOTTISH LOW BIRTHWEIGHT STUDY: II. Language attainment, cognitive status and behavioral problems. *Arch Dis Child* 67:682, 1992.

SHAPIRO LR: The fragile X syndrome: A peculiar pattern of inheritance. *N Engl J Med* 325:1736, 1991.

SHILLITO J JR, MATSON DD: Craniosynostosis: A review of 519 surgical patients. *Pediatrics* 41:829, 1968.

SHORT MP, ADAMS RD: Neurocutaneous diseases, in Fitzpatrick TB, et al (eds): *Dermatology in General Medicine*, 4th ed. New York, McGraw-Hill, 1993, pp 2249–2290.

SHUMAN RM, SELEDNIK LJ: Periventricular leukomalacia. *Arch Neurol* 37:231, 1980.

SINHA S, DAVIES J, TONER N, et al: Vitamin E supplementation reduces frequency of periventricular hemorrhage in very premature babies. *Lancet* 1:466, 1987.

SMITH DW: Recognizable patterns of human malformation: Genetic, embryologic, and clinical aspects. *Major Probl Clin Pediatr* 7:1, 1970.

SOLOMON LM, ESTERLEY NB: Epidermal and other congenital organoid nevi. *Curr Probl Pediatr* 6:1, 1975.

TAYLOR M, DAVID AS: Agenesis of the corpus callosum: a United Kingdom series of 56 cases. *J Neurol Neurosurg Psychiatry* 64:131, 1998.

THOMAS GH: High male : female ratio of germ line mutations: An alternative explanation for postulated gestational lethality in males with X-linked dominant disorders. *Am J Hum Genet* 58:1364, 1996.

VAN DER HOEVE J: Eye symptoms of tuberous sclerosis of the brain. *Trans Ophthalmol Soc UK* 40:329, 1920.

VOLKMAR FR, COHEN DJ: Neurobiologic aspects of autism. *N Engl J Med* 318:1390, 1988.

VOLPE JJ: *Neurology of the Newborn*, 3rd ed. Philadelphia, Saunders, 1995.

Volpe JJ: Intraventricular hemorrhage in the premature infant: Current concepts, parts I and II. *Ann Neurol* 25:3, 109, 1989.

Weber F, Parkes R: Association of extensive haemangiomatous naevus of skin with cerebral (meningeal) haemangioma, especially cases of facial vascular naevus with contralateral hemiplegia. *Proc R Soc Med* 22:25, 1929.

Weller TH: Cytomegaloviruses: The difficult years. *J Infect Dis* 122:532, 1970.

Weller TH: The cytomegaloviruses: Ubiquitous agents with protean clinical manifestations. *N Engl J Med* 285:267, 1971.

Williams JC, Barratt-Boyes BG, Lowe JB: Supravalvular aortic stenosis. *Circulation* 24:1311, 1961.

Wilson GS, Desmond MM, Verniand W: Early development of infants of heroin-addicted mothers. *Am J Dis Child* 126:457, 1973.

Winick M: *Malnutrition and Brain Development*. New York, Oxford University Press, 1976.

Wohlwill FJ, Yakovlev PI: Histopathology of meningofacial angiomatosis (Sturge-Weber's disease). *J Neuropathol Exp Neurol* 16:341, 1957.

Wyburn-Mason R: *Vascular Abnormalities and Tumors of the Spinal Cord and Its Membranes*. St Louis, Mosby, 1944.

Yakovlev PI, Guthrie RH: Congenital ectodermoses (neurocutaneous syndromes) in epileptic patients. *Arch Neurol Psychiatry* 26:1145, 1931.

Yakovlev PI, Wadsworth RC: Schizencephalies: A study of the congenital clefts in the cerebral mantle. *J Neuropathol Exp Neurol* 5:116, 169, 1946.

Zupan V, Gonzalez P, Lacaze-Masmonteil T, et al: Periventricular leukomalacia: Risk factors revisited. *Dev Med Child Neurol* 38:1061, 1996.

Chapter 39

DEGENERATIVE DISEASES OF THE NERVOUS SYSTEM

The adjective *degenerative* has no great appeal to the modern neurologist. For one thing, it has an unpleasant non-medical connotation, referring as it does to a state of moral turpitude or deviant behavior as the consequence of a sociopathic tendency. More important, it is not a satisfactory term medically, since it implies an inexplicable decline from a previous level of normalcy to a lower level of function—an ambiguous conceptualization of disease that satisfies neither theoretician nor scientist.

It is becoming increasingly evident that many of the diseases included in this category depend on genetic factors, or at least they appear in more than one member of the same family, in which case they are more properly designated as *heredodegenerative*. Even more diseases, not differing in any fundamental way from the heredodegenerative ones, occur sporadically, i.e., as isolated instances in given families. For diseases of this type, Gowers in 1902 suggested the term *abiotrophy*, by which he meant a lack of "vital endurance" of the affected neurons, resulting in their premature death. This concept embodies an untested, unproven hypothesis—that aging and degenerative changes of cells are based on the same process. Understandably, contemporary neuropathologists are reluctant to attribute to simple aging the diverse processes of cellular diseases that are constantly being revealed by ultrastructural and molecular genetic techniques.

The reader may be perplexed by the inconsistent use of the terms *atrophy* and *degeneration*, both of which are applied to diseases of this category. Spatz argued that on purely histopathologic grounds they are different. *Atrophy* specifies a gradual wasting and loss of a system of neurons, leaving in their wake no degradative products and only a sparsely cellular, fibrous gliosis. *Degeneration* refers to a more rapid process of neuronal, myelin, or tissue breakdown, the degradative products of which evoke a more vigorous reaction of phagocytosis and cellular gliosis. The difference lies in both the speed and the type of breakdown. It is of some interest that many of the diseases that are characterized by degeneration, in Spatz's sense of the term, are now known to be of metabolic origin, while very few of the purely atrophic ones have been shown to have a metabolic basis.

The new and fashionable pathologic term for the wasting and dissolution of neurons, in both the system atrophies and the degenerative diseases, is *apoptosis*. This term has been borrowed from embryology, where it refers to the naturally occurring cell death in the central nervous system during development and probably involves the expression of genes that cause a dissolution of neurons over a short period of time ("programmed" cell death), leaving no trace of a pathologic reaction. The process of neuronal degeneration is quite different; it refers to a series of changes in mature neurons, occurring over a relatively protracted period of time and leaving a discrete glial scar.

There are also, within recent memory, several examples of diseases that were formerly classed as degenerative but are now known to have a metabolic, toxic, or nutritional basis or to be caused by a "slow virus" or by a nonviral transmissible agent. It seems reasonable to expect that with increasing knowledge, more and more diseases whose causes are now unknown will find their way into these categories. Until such time as the causation of all neurologic diseases is known, there must be a name and a place for a group of diseases that have no known cause and are united only by the common attribute of gradually progressive disintegration of part or parts of the nervous system. In deference to traditional practice, they are collected here under the rubric *degenerative diseases*.

General Clinical Characteristics

The diseases included in the degenerative category *begin insidiously, after a long period of normal nervous system function, and pursue a gradually progressive course that may continue for many years, often a decade or longer.* In this respect they differ from most of the metabolic diseases. Frequently it is impossible to assign a date of onset. Sometimes, the patient or the patient's family gives a history of abrupt appearance of disability, particularly if some injury, infection, surgical procedure, or other memorable event coincided with the initial symptoms. Often a skillfully taken history will reveal that the patient or family had been aware of a pre-existent condition, the subtle symptoms of which had been present for some time but had attracted little attention. Whether trauma or other stress can actually evoke or aggravate a degenerative disease is a question that cannot be answered with absolute certainty, but it seems highly improbable. Anyone who states otherwise must offer evidence that at present is purely anecdotal. Instead, these degenerative disease processes by their very nature appear to develop de novo, without relation to known antecedent events, and their symptomatic expressions are late events in the pathologic process, occurring only when the degree of neuronal loss reaches or exceeds the "safety factor" for a particular neuronal system.

The *familial occurrence* of disease is of great importance, but it must be emphasized that such information is often difficult to obtain on first contact with the patient. The family may be small or widely scattered, so that the patient is unaware of the health of other members. The patient or the patient's relatives may be ashamed to admit that a neurologic disease has "tainted" the family. Furthermore, it may not be realized that an illness is hereditary if other members of the family have a much more or much less severe form of the disorder than the patient. Sometimes, in the latter case, only the careful examination of other family members will disclose the presence of a hereditary disease. It should be remembered, however, that familial occurrence of a disease does not necessarily mean that it is inherited but may indicate instead that more than one member of a family had been exposed to the same infectious or toxic agent.

As a rule, the degenerative diseases of the nervous system run a *ceaselessly progressive course* and with few exceptions are uninfluenced by any medical or surgical measures, so that dealing with a patient with this type of illness may be an anguishing experience for all concerned. However, some of these diseases are characterized by long periods of stability; moreover, some symptoms (e.g., those of Parkinson disease) can be alleviated by skillful management, and the physician's interest and advice may be of great help.

The bilateral symmetry of the clinical manifestations and lesions is another noteworthy feature of the degenerative diseases; it alone may distinguish members of this group from many other diseases of the nervous system. Again, this principle requires qualification, for in the earliest stages of some degenerative diseases (e.g., Parkinson disease, amyotrophic lateral sclerosis) there may be greater involvement of one limb or one side of the body. Sooner or later, however, despite the asymmetrical beginning, the inherently symmetrical nature of the process asserts itself.

General Pathologic Features

Many of the degenerative diseases are characterized by the *selective involvement of anatomically and physiologically related systems of neurons.* This feature is exemplified by amyotrophic lateral sclerosis, in which the pathologic process is limited to motor neurons of the cerebral cortex, brainstem, and spinal cord, and by certain forms of progressive ataxia, in which only the Purkinje cells of the cerebellum are affected. Many other examples could be cited (e.g., Friedreich ataxia) in which several discrete neuronal systems disintegrate, leaving others unscathed. These degenerative diseases have therefore been called *system atrophies* or *systemic neuronal atrophies*, and many of them turn out to be strongly hereditary. The selective vulnerability of certain systems of neurons is not an exclusive property of the degenerative diseases, however: several disease processes of known cause have similarly circumscribed effects on the nervous system. Diphtheria toxin, for instance, selectively affects the myelin of the peripheral nerves near the spinal ganglia, and triorthocresyl phosphate affects both the corticospinal tracts of the spinal cord and the spinal motor neurons. Other examples are the special vulnerability of the Purkinje cells to hyperthermia, the cerebellar granule cells to methyl mercury compounds, the basal ganglionic neurons to manganese, and the hippocampal neurons to anoxia. Conversely, in Alzheimer disease and most other degenerative diseases, the pathologic changes are somewhat less selective and eventually more diffuse.

As one would expect of any pathologic process that is based on the slow wasting and loss of neurons, not only the cell bodies but also their dendrites, axons, and myelin sheaths disappear—unaccompanied by an intense tissue reaction or cellular response. The cerebrospinal fluid (CSF), therefore, shows little if any change—at most a slight increase in protein content. Moreover, since these diseases invariably result in tissue loss (rather than in new tissue formation, as occurs with neoplasms or inflammations), *radiologic examination shows either no change or a volumetric reduction (atrophy)* with a corresponding enlargement of the CSF compartments. These radiologic findings help distinguish the neuronal atrophies from other large classes of progressive disease of the nervous system—namely, tumors, infections, and other processes of inflammatory type.

CLASSIFICATION

Since grouping of the degenerative diseases in terms of etiology is not possible (except that in many a hereditary, or genetic, factor can be recognized), we resort, for practical purposes, to a division based on the presenting clinical syndromes and their pathologic anatomy. Although this is the most elementary mode of classification of naturally occurring phenomena, it is a necessary prelude to diagnosis and scientific study and preferable to a haphazard listing of diseases by the names of the neurologists or neuropathologists who first described them.

I. **Syndrome of progressive dementia, other neurologic signs being absent or inconspicuous**
   - A. Diffuse cerebral atrophy
     1. Alzheimer disease
     2. Diffuse cerebral cortical atrophy of non-Alzheimer type
     3. Some cases of Lewy body dementia
   - B. Circumscribed cerebral atrophy
     1. Pick disease (lobar sclerosis)
     2. Frontotemporal dementia
     3. Thalamic degeneration

II. **Syndrome of progressive dementia in combination with other neurologic abnormalities**
   - A. Huntington chorea
   - B. Other (nonhuntingtonian) types of chorea and dementia
   - C. Cortical-striatal-spinal degeneration (Jakob) and the dementia–Parkinson–amyotrophic lateral sclerosis complex (Guamanian and others)
   - D. Dentatorubropallidoluysian degeneration (DRPLA)
   - E. Cerebrocerebellar degeneration
   - F. Familial dementia with spastic paraparesis, amyotrophy, or myoclonus
   - G. Lewy body disease
   - H. Some cases of Parkinson disease
   - I. Corticobasal ganglionic degeneration
   - J. Polyglucosan body disease

III. **Syndrome of disordered posture and movement**
   - A. Parkinson disease (paralysis agitans)
   - B. Striatonigral degeneration with or without autonomic failure (Shy-Drager syndrome) and olivopontocerebellar atrophy (multiple system atrophy)
   - C. Progressive supranuclear palsy (Steele-Richardson-Olszewski)
   - D. Dystonia musculorum deformans (torsion spasm)
   - E. Hallervorden-Spatz disease
   - F. Corticobasal ganglionic degeneration
   - G. Restricted dystonias, including spasmodic torticollis and Meige syndrome
   - H. Familial tremors
   - I. Multiple tic disease (Gilles de la Tourette syndrome)
   - J. Acanthocytic chorea

IV. **Syndrome of progressive ataxia**
   - A. Spinocerebellar ataxias (early onset)
     1. Friedreich ataxia
     2. Non-Friedreich, early-onset ataxia (with retained reflexes, hypogonadism, myoclonus, and other disorders)
   - B. Cerebellar cortical ataxias
     1. Holmes type of familial pure cerebellar-olivary atrophy
     2. Late-onset cerebellar atrophy of Marie, Foix, and Alajouanine
   - C. Complicated cerebellar ataxia (later-onset ataxia with brainstem and other neurologic disorders)
     1. Olivopontocerebellar degenerations (OPCA)
        - a. Clinically pure (Déjerine-Thomas type)
        - b. With extrapyramidal and autonomic degeneration (multiple system atrophy)
        - c. Conjoined with spinocerebellar degeneration (Menzel type)
     2. Dentatorubral degeneration (Ramsay Hunt type)
     3. Dentatorubropallidoluysian atrophy
     4. Machado-Joseph-Azorean disease
     5. Other complicated late-onset, autosomal dominant ataxias (including Harding's types 1, 2, and 3) with pigmentary retinopathy, ophthalmoplegia, slow eye movements (Wadia), neuropathy, optic atrophy, deafness, extrapyramidal features, and dementia

V. **Syndrome of slowly developing muscular weakness and atrophy (nuclear amyotrophy)**
   - A. *Motor disorders with amyotrophy: motor system disease*
     1. Amyotrophic lateral sclerosis
     2. Progressive spinal muscular atrophy
     3. Progressive bulbar palsy
     4. Hereditary forms of progressive muscular atrophy and spastic paraplegia
   - B. *Spastic paraplegia without amyotrophy*
     1. Primary lateral sclerosis
     2. Hereditary spastic paraplegia

VI. **Sensory and sensorimotor disorders (neuropathies)**
   - A. Hereditary sensorimotor neuropathies—peroneal muscular atrophy (Charcot-Marie-Tooth); hypertrophic interstitial polyneuropathy (Déjerine-Sottas); Refsum disease; etc.

VII. **Syndrome of progressive blindness or ophthalmoplegia with or without other neurologic disorders**
   - A. Hereditary optic neuropathy (Leber)
   - B. Pigmentary degeneration of retina (retinitis pigmentosa)
   - C. Stargardt disease

D. Progressive external ophthalmoplegia with or without deafness or other system atrophies (Kearns-Sayre syndrome)

VIII. **Syndromes characterized by neurosensory deafness**
   A. Pure neurosensory deafness
   B. Hereditary hearing loss with retinal diseases
   C. Hereditary hearing loss with system atrophies of the nervous system

DISEASES CHARACTERIZED MAINLY BY PROGRESSIVE DEMENTIA

Alzheimer Disease

This is the most common and important degenerative disease of the brain, incurring to an increasing degree an immense societal impact. Some aspects of the intellectual deterioration that characterizes this disease have already been described in Chap. 21, under "The Neurology of Dementia," and the relationship of this disease to the aging process has been fully discussed in Chap. 29. There it was pointed out that some degree of shrinkage in size and weight of the brain, i.e., "atrophy," is an inevitable accompaniment of advancing age, but that these changes alone are of slight clinical significance and their structural basis is uncertain (e.g., slight loss of brain weight or simple depletion of neurons). By contrast, severe degrees of diffuse cerebral atrophy that evolve over a few years are invariably associated with dementia, and the underlying pathologic changes in these cases most often prove to be those of Alzheimer disease. For this reason it is usual to speak of the clinical syndrome as *dementia of the Alzheimer type* (DAT) or *probable Alzheimer disease*, if the diagnosis is uncertain. The traditional practice of giving Alzheimer disease and senile dementia the status of separate diseases was probably attributable to the relatively young age (51 years) of the patient originally studied by Alois Alzheimer in 1907. Such a division is illogical, since the two conditions, except for their age of onset, are clinically and pathologically indistinguishable. There is a smooth, exponential, age-dependent increase in incidence after 40 years of age.

Epidemiology Although Alzheimer disease has been described at every period of adult life, the majority of patients are in their sixties or older; a relatively small number have been in their late fifties or younger. It is one of the most frequent mental illnesses, making up some 20 percent of all patients in psychiatric hospitals and an even larger proportion in nursing homes. In the United States, in 17 series comprising 15,000 persons over the age of 60 years, the mean incidence of moderate to severe dementia was calculated to be 4.8 percent (Wang). In Rochester, Minnesota, the incidence rate for dementia in general is 187 cases per 100,000 population per year, and for Alzheimer disease, 123 cases per 100,000 annually (Schoenberg et al).

These staggering statistics may be viewed from another perspective. The incidence rate of clinically diagnosed Alzheimer disease is similar throughout the world, and it increases comparably with age, approximating 3 new cases yearly per 100,000 persons below age 60 and 125 new cases per 100,000 of those over 60. The prevalence of the disease per 100,000 population is near 300 in the group aged 60 to 69; it is 3200 in the 70-to-79 group and 10,800 in those over age 80. In the year 2000, there were an estimated 2 million persons with Alzheimer disease in the United States. Prevalence rates, which depend also on overall mortality, are three times higher in women, although it does appear that the incidence of new cases is only slightly disproportionate in women. The survival of patients with Alzheimer disease is reduced to half of the expected rate, most of the deaths occurring ultimately from respiratory and cardiovascular causes.

Several putative epidemiologic risk factors for Alzheimer disease—such as birth order, mother's age at birth, family history of Down syndrome, or head injury—seem marginal at best and in some instances may be due to selection bias. Whether low educational attainment is a risk factor for the development of Alzheimer disease or, conversely, whether cognitively demanding occupations protect against dementia has not been settled (Katzman; Cobb et al).

The *familial occurrence* of Alzheimer disease, accounting for less than 1 percent of all cases, has been well established, most of the pedigrees being consistent with an autosomal dominant inheritance (Nee et al, Goudsmit et al; see further on, in the section on pathogenesis). Reports of a substantial familial aggregation of dementia without a specific pattern of inheritance also suggest the operation of more than one genetic factor. Several studies have documented a significant increase in the risk of apparently sporadic Alzheimer disease among first-degree relatives of patients with this disorder. Again, this risk is disproportionately greater in females, adding to the evidence that women in general are at slightly higher risk for Alzheimer disease (Silverman et al). Li and coworkers have provided evidence that patients with an earlier age of onset of Alzheimer disease (before age 70) are more likely to have relatives with the disease than are patients with later onset. Genetic studies are difficult because the disease does not appear at the same age in a given proband. Even in identical twins, it may develop at the age of 60 years in one of the pair and at 80 years in the other. Death from other diseases may prevent its detection.

Clinical Features The onset of mental changes is usually so insidious that neither the family nor the patient can date the time of its beginning. Occasionally, however, it is brought to attention by an unusual degree of confusion in relation to a febrile illness, an operation, mild head injury, or the taking of medication. Other patients may present with complaints of dizziness, nondescript headaches, or other vaguely expressed and changeable somatic symptoms.

The gradual development of forgetfulness is the major symptom. Small day-to-day happenings are not remembered. Seldom-used names are particularly elusive. Little-used words from an earlier period of life also tend to be lost. Appointments are forgotten and possessions misplaced. Questions are repeated again and again, the patient having forgotten what was just discussed. It is said that remote memories are preserved and recent ones lost (Ribot's law of memory), but this is only relatively true; it is difficult to check the accuracy of ancient memories. Albert and associates, who tested the patient's recognition of dated political events and pictures of prominent people past and present, found that some degree of memory loss extends to all decades of life (specific neuropsychological testing is discussed further on).

Once the memory disorder has become pronounced, other failures in cerebral function become increasingly apparent. The patient's speech is halting because of failure to recall the needed word. The same difficulty interrupts writing. Vocabulary becomes restricted, and expressive language stereotyped and inflexible. Comprehension of spoken words seems at first to be preserved, until it is observed that the patient does not carry out a complicated request; even then it is uncertain whether the request was not understood because of inattention or was forgotten. Almost imperceptible at first, these disturbances of language become more apparent as the disease progresses. Finally, there is a failure to speak in full sentences; the finding of words requires a continuous search; and little that is said or written is fully comprehended. There is a tendency to repeat a question before answering it, and later there may be a rather dramatic repetition of every spoken phrase (*echolalia*). The deterioration of verbal skills has by then progressed beyond a groping for names and common nouns to an obvious anomic aphasia. Other elements of receptive and executive aphasia are later added, but discrete aphasias of the Broca or Wernicke type are characteristically lacking.

Skill in arithmetic suffers a similar deterioration. Faults in balancing the checkbook, mistakes in figuring the price of items and in making the correct change—all these and others progress to a point where the patient can no longer carry out the simplest calculations (*acalculia* or *dyscalculia*).

In some patients, visuospatial orientation becomes defective. The car cannot be parked; the arms do not find the correct sleeves of the dressing gown; the corners of the tablecloth cannot be oriented with the corners of the table; the patient turns in the wrong direction on the way home or becomes lost. The route from one place to another cannot be described, nor can given directions be understood. As this state worsens, the simplest of geometric forms and patterns cannot be copied.

Late in the course of the illness, the patient forgets how to use common objects and tools while retaining the necessary motor power and co-ordination for these activities. The razor is no longer correctly applied to the face; the latch of the door cannot be unfastened; and eating utensils are no longer used properly. Finally, only the most habitual and virtually automatic actions are preserved. Tests of commanded and demonstrated actions cannot be executed or imitated. *Ideational* and *ideomotor apraxia* are the terms applied to the advanced forms of this motor incapacity (pages 59 and 486).

As these many amnesic, aphasic, agnosic, and apraxic deficits declare themselves, the patient at first seems unchanged in overall motility, behavior, temperament, and conduct. Social graces, whatever they were, are retained in the initial phase of the illness, but troublesome alterations gradually appear in this sphere as well. Imprudent business deals may be made. Restlessness and agitation or their opposites—inertia and placidity—become evident. Dressing, shaving, and bathing are neglected. Anxieties and phobias, particularly fear of being left alone, may emerge. A disturbance of the normal day and night sleep patterns is prominent in some patients. A poorly organized paranoid delusional state, sometimes with hallucinations, may become manifest. The patient may suspect his elderly wife of having an illicit relationship or his children of stealing his possessions. A stable marriage may be disrupted by the patient's infatuation with a younger person or by sexual indiscretions, which may astonish the community. The patient's affect coarsens; he is more egocentric and indifferent to the feelings and reactions of others. A gluttonous appetite sometimes develops, but more often eating is neglected, with gradual weight loss. Later, grasping and sucking reflexes and other signs of frontal lobe disorder are readily elicited (Neary et al), sphincteric continence fails, and the patient sinks into a state of relative akinesia and mutism, as described in Chap. 21.

Difficulty in locomotion, a kind of unsteadiness with shortened steps but with only slight motor weakness and rigidity, frequently supervenes. Elements of parkinsonian akinesia and rigidity and a fine tremor can be perceived in patients with advanced motor disability. Ultimately the patient loses the ability to stand and walk, being forced to lie inert in bed and having to be fed and bathed, and the legs may curl into a fixed posture of paraplegia in flexion (persistent vegetative state; page 369).

The symptomatic course of this tragic illness usually extends over a period of 5 or more years but, judging from studies of Down cases, the pathologic course has a much longer asymptomatic duration. This concept is supported by the detailed studies of Linn and colleagues, who found that a lengthy "preclinical" period (7 years or more) of stepwise decline in memory and attention span preceded the clinical diagnosis. Surprisingly, throughout this period, corticospinal and corticosensory functions, visual acuity, ocular movements, and visual fields remain relatively intact. If there is hemiplegia, homonymous hemianopia, etc., either the diagnosis of Alzheimer disease is incorrect or the disease has been complicated by a stroke, tumor, or subdural hematoma. Exceptions to this statement are rare. The tendon reflexes are little altered and the plantar reflexes almost always remain flexor. There is no true sensory or cerebellar ataxia. Convulsions are rare until late in the illness, when up to 5 percent of patients reportedly have infrequent seizures. Occasionally, widespread myoclonic jerks or mild choreoathetotic movements are observed late in the illness. Eventually, with the patient in a bedfast state, an intercurrent infection such as aspiration pneumonia or some other disease mercifully terminates life.

The sequence of neurologic disabilities may not follow this described order, and one or another deficit may take precedence, presumably because the disease process, after becoming manifest in the memory cortex of the temporal lobes, may affect one particular part of the associative cortex earlier or more severely in one patient than in another. This allows a relatively restricted deficit to become the source of early medical complaint long before the full syndrome of dementia has declared itself. We have observed four limited deficits of this type, as follows:

1. *Korsakoff amnesic state*. The early stages of Alzheimer disease may be dominated by a disproportionate failure of retentive memory, with integrity of other cognitive abilities. In such patients, immediate memory (essentially a measure of attention), tested by the capacity to repeat a series of numbers or words, is essentially intact; it is the short- and long-term (retentive) memory that fails. Retentive memory may become impaired to the point where the patient can recall nothing of what he had learned a minute or two previously. Yet as a business executive, for example, he may continue to make acceptable decisions if the work utilizes long-established habit patterns and practices. In such cases, the temporal horns tend to be enlarged more than the rest of the ventricular system, reflecting the disproportionate atrophy of the inferomedial temporal lobes.

2. *Dysnomia*. The forgetting of words, especially proper names, may first bring the patient to a neurologist. Later the difficulty involves common nouns and progresses to the point where fluency of speech is seriously impaired. Every sentence is broken by a pause and search for the wanted word; if this is not found, a circumlocution is substituted or the sentence is left unfinished. When the patient is given a choice of words, including the one that was missed, there may be a failure of recognition. Repetition of the spoken words of others, at first flawless, later brings out a lesser degree of the same difficulty. A useful test for the failure to find names (*dysnomia*), which is probably the most common abnormality of language in this disease, is the category-fluency test. The patient is given 1 min to name as many items as possible in each of four categories—vegetables, vehicles, tools, and clothing. Alzheimer patients fall below a score of 50 items. The naming defect may be evident with even simpler tests, e.g., asking the patient to generate a list of farm animals—a test that may elicit only three or four responses. Other components of language may be relatively intact, but before long it is evident that the patient does not understand all that he hears or reads. In contrast, nonverbal memory and the ability to calculate and make simple judgments may still be preserved. Duplicating our own experience, Mesulam and Chawluk and their colleagues have described patients in whom an aphasic disorder began with anomia and eventually affected reading, writing, and comprehension without the additional intellectual and behavioral disturbances of dementia. In our own observation of such patients, if observed for a sufficiently long period, develop a more

general dementia, sometimes as long as 5 years or more after the onset of aphasia. Rarely, this syndrome represents a focal degenerative disorder (lobar atrophy of Pick or frontotemporal dementia), distinct from Alzheimer disease (Lippa et al, Kirshner et al). Usually the electroencephalogram (EEG) is normal or shows only a mild degree of slowing, but magnetic resonance imaging (MRI) may disclose a focal atrophy of the language areas (Caselli et al).

3. *Visuospatial disorientation.* Parieto-occipital functions are sometimes deranged in the course of Alzheimer disease and may fail while other functions are relatively preserved. As remarked above and in Chap. 22, prosopagnosia, losing one's way in familiar surroundings or inability to interpret a road map, to distinguish right from left, or to park or garage a car, and difficulty in setting the table or dressing are all manifestations of a special failure to orient the schema of one's body with that of surrounding space. Exceptionally there is a neglect of stimuli in one visual field.

4. *Paranoia and other personality changes.* Frequently, at some point in the development of senile dementia, the most prominent event is the occurrence of paranoia or bizarre behavior. The patient becomes convinced that relatives are stealing his possessions or that an elderly and even infirm spouse is guilty of infidelity. He may hide his belongings, even relatively worthless ones, and go about spying on family members. Hostilities arise, and wills may be altered irrationally. Many of these patients are constantly worried, tense, and agitated. Of course, paranoid delusions may be part of a depressive psychosis and of other dementias, but most of the senile patients in whom paranoia is the presenting problem seem not to be depressed, and their cognitive functions are for a time relatively well preserved. It is tempting to think that a very early senile change of the limbic cortices has exposed a lifelong trait of suspiciousness, but this is purely hypothetical.

Sometimes other oddities of behavior will announce the oncoming dementia. Social indiscretions, rejection of an old friend, embarking on an imprudent financial venture, or an amorous pursuit that is out of character are examples of these types of behavioral change.

Some clinicians attempt to subdivide the Alzheimer–senile dementia syndrome into subtypes. Amnesic defect without lexical-semantic abnormalities represents more than 50 percent of cases. Chin and coworkers observed more prevalent and severe language disorder and more rapid progression in early-onset familial cases. Others point to a disproportionately severe defect in praxic functions and a greater tendency to abnormal EEG findings in such cases. Whether such distinctions represent fundamental differences in the disease process is questionable.

It has been our impression that each of the restricted cerebral disorders described above is only *relatively pure*. Careful testing of mental function—and this is of diagnostic importance—frequently discloses subtle abnormalities in several cognitive spheres. Initially, most patients have a disproportionate affection of the temporoparietal cortices, hence the earlier impairment on the performance parts of the Wechsler Adult Intelligence Scale. Within several months to a year or two, the more generalized aspects of mental deterioration become apparent, and the aphasic-agnosic-apraxic aspects of the syndrome become increasingly prominent. If one of the foregoing restricted deficits remains uncomplicated over a period of years, one is justified in suspecting some cause other than Alzheimer disease, such as Binswanger disease, hydrocephalus, frontotemporal dementia (see further on), or embolic infarction of one part of the temporal or parietal lobe (pages 451 and 878). Also, as stated earlier, a hemianopic visual field defect, cortical sensory loss, or hemiparesis is seldom if ever due to Alzheimer disease alone. However, more complex disturbances of visual perception, taking the form of impaired recognition of objects (*object agnosia*) or faces (*prosopagnosia*), visual scanning, color identification, stereoacuity, separation of figures from background, and hand-eye coordination, are frequent in the more advanced stages (Mendez et al). Rarely there is a partial or even a complete Balint syndrome (page 491).

While it is true that most patients with Alzheimer disease walk normally until relatively late in their illness, infrequently a short-stepped gait and imbalance draw attention to the disease and worsen slowly for several years before cognitive manifestations become evident.

For research purposes and to establish certain inclusive and exclusive criteria for the diagnosis of Alzheimer disease, a work group of the National Institute of Neurological and Communicative Disorders and Stroke (NINCDS) and the Alzheimer's Disease and Related Diseases Association (ADRDA) have proposed the following diagnostic criteria: (1) dementia defined by clinical examination, the Mini-Mental Scale, the Blessed Dementia Scale, or similar mental status examination; (2) age of patient (over 40 years); (3) deficits in two or more areas of cognition and progressive worsening of memory and other cognitive functions—such as language, perception, and motor skills (praxis); (4) absence of disturbed consciousness; and (5) exclusion of other brain diseases (McKhann et al; Tierney et al). Using these criteria, the correct diagnosis is achieved in more than 85 percent of patients.

Pathology In the advanced stages of the disease, the brain presents a diffusely atrophied appearance and brain weight is usually reduced by 20 percent or more (Fig. 39-1). Cerebral convolutions are narrowed and sulci are widened. The third and lateral ventricles are symmetrically enlarged to a varying degree. Usually the atrophic process involves the frontal, temporal, and parietal lobes, but cases vary considerably. The extreme atrophy of the hippocampus—the most prominent finding, visible on coronal MRI—is believed to be diagnostic. Microscopically, there is widespread loss of nerve cells, most marked in the cerebral cortex. In addition to pronounced neuronal loss in the hippocampus, adjacent parts of the medial temporal cortex—namely, the entorhinal cortex, parahippocampal gyri, and subiculum—are affected. The anterior nuclei of the thalamus, septal nuclei and diagonal band of Broca, the amygdala, and particular brainstem parts of the monoaminergic systems are also depleted. The cholinergic neurons of the nucleus basalis of Meynert (the substantia innominata) and locus ceruleus are also reduced in number, a finding that at one time aroused great interest because of its putative role in memory loss (see below). In the cerebral cortex, the cell loss affects both large pyramidal neurons and smaller interneurons. Residual neurons are observed to have lost volume and ribonucleoprotein and their dendrites are diminished and crowd upon one another owing to the loss of synapses and neuropil. Astrocytic proliferation follows as a compensatory or reparative process, most prominent in layers III and V.

In addition, three microscopic changes give this disease its distinctive character: (1) the presence within the nerve cell cytoplasm of thick, fiber-like strands of silver-staining material, often in the form of loops, coils, or tangled masses (Alzheimer neurofibrillary change, or "tangles"). The strands are composed of a hyperphosphorylated form of the microtubular protein "tau" and appear as pairs of helical filaments when studied ultrastructurally; (2) spherical deposits of amorphous material scattered throughout the cerebral cortex and most easily seen with periodic acid–Schiff (PAS) and silver-staining methods; the core of the aggregates is the protein amyloid, surrounded by degenerating nerve terminals (*senile* or *neuritic plaques*). Amyloid is also scattered throughout the cerebral cortex in a nascent "diffuse" form, without organization or core formation and appreciated mainly by immunohistochemical methods, as well as in the walls of small blood vessels near the plaques—

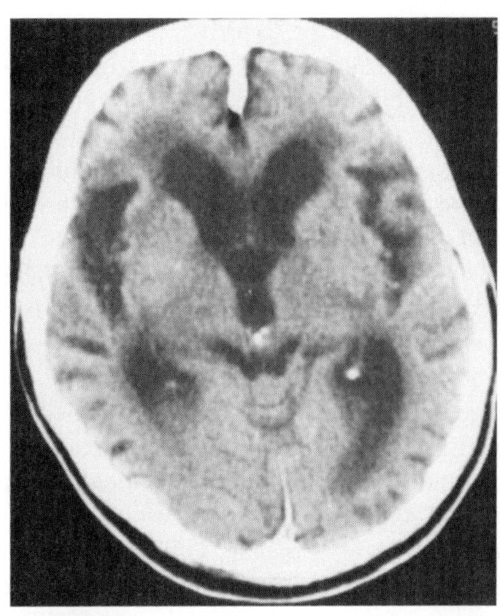

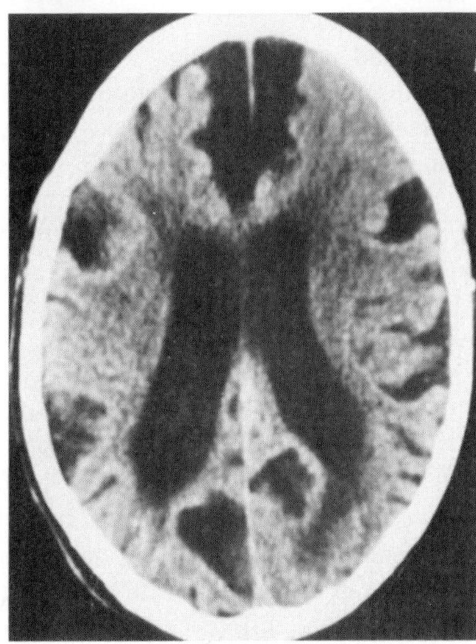

Figure 39-1

Top: Alzheimer disease. Axial CT section demonstrating severe generalized cerebral cortical atrophy and moderately severe ventricular enlargement. Bottom: Pick disease. Pronounced selective atrophy of the frontal and temporal lobes. (From Lee SH, Rao KCVG, Zimmerman RA: Cranial MRI and CT. New York, McGraw-Hill, 1992, by permission.)

so-called congophilic angiopathy; (3) *granulovacuolar degeneration* of neurons, most evident in the pyramidal layer of the hippocampus.

Neuritic plaques and neurofibrillary changes are found in all the association areas of the cerebral cortex, but it is the neurofibrillary tangles and neuronal alterations and loss, not the plaques, that correlate best with the severity of the dementia (Arriagada et al). If any part of the brain is disproportionately affected, it is the hippocampus, particularly the CA1 and CA2 zones (of Lorente de Nó) and the entorhinal cortex, subiculum, and amygdala. These parts have abundant connections with other parts of the temporal lobe cortex and dentate nucleus of the hippocampus and undoubtedly account for the amnesic component of the dementia. The parietal lobes are another favored site. Only a few tangles and plaques are found in the hypothalamus, thalamus, periaqueductal region, pontine tegmentum, and granule-cell layer of the cerebellum.

Experienced neuropathologists recognize a form of Alzheimer disease, particularly in older patients ($>$75 years), in which there are senile plaques but few or no neuronal tangles (20 percent of 150 cases reported by Joachim et al). [In general, senile (neuritic) plaques are found to be more diffusely distributed than the fibrillary changes.] Another problem for the neuropathologist is to distinguish between the normal aged brain and that of Alzheimer disease. It is not unusual to find a scattering of senile plaques in individuals who were thought to be mentally normal during life. Henderson and Hubbard studied 27 demented individuals aged 64 to 92 years and 20 age-matched, nondemented controls. In the former, 3 to 38 percent of the hippocampal neurons contained neurofibrillary tangles; in all but 2 of the controls, the number of hippocampal neurons with tangles fell below 2.5 percent. Hence, the difference between plaques and tangles in the aging brain and in Alzheimer disease is largely quantitative.

Of interest also is the observation of Joachim and associates that 18 percent of their Alzheimer cases had sufficient neuronal loss and Lewy bodies in the substantia nigra to justify a diagnosis of Parkinson disease. Leverenz and Sumi found that 25 percent of their Alzheimer patients showed the pathologic (and clinical) changes of Parkinson disease—a much higher incidence than can be attributed to chance. Also, of 11 patients with progressive supranuclear palsy reported by Gearing and coworkers, 10 were demented and 5 had Alzheimer disease. These mixed cases, including those with Pick disease, present problems not only of classification, but also in understanding the neurobiology of these degenerative diseases. This subject is discussed further on in the section on Parkinson disease.

It is of historical interest that Alzheimer was not the first to describe plaques, one of the hallmarks of this pathologic state. These miliary lesions ("*Herdchen*") had been observed in senile brains by Blocq and Marinesco in 1892 and were named *senile plaques* by Simchowicz in 1910. In 1907, Alzheimer described the case of a 51-year-old woman who died after a 5-year illness characterized by progressive dementia. Throughout the cerebral cortex he found the characteristic plaques, but he also noted—thanks to the use of Bielschowsky's silver impregnation method—a clumping and distortion of fibrils in the neuronal cytoplasm, the neurofibrillary change which now, appropriately, carries Alzheimer's name.

Pathogenesis Careful analyses of the senile plaques and neuronal fibrillary changes have been made in recent years in an attempt to elucidate the mechanism of Alzheimer disease. Several new histologic techniques have been devised and put to service in this endeavor—refinements of the silver impregnation method, which stains both amyloid and its main constituent (amyloid β protein, or Aβ); immunoreactive methods, using antibodies raised to rabbit thymus (ubiquitin), to demonstrate neuronal tau protein and amyloid β protein; and thioflavine S and Congo red with ultraviolet and polarized light to identify amyloid β protein and amyloid. Tau is a discrete cytoskeletal protein that is thought to promote the assembly of microtubules and to stabilize their structure as well as to participate in synaptic plasticity in a yet to be defined manner. In the pathologic circumstances of Alzheimer disease, progressive supranuclear palsy, and frontotemporal dementia (see further on), tau is hyperphosphorylated and aggregates, resulting in an overloading of the perikarya and neurites with paired helical filaments which constitute neurofibrillary tangles. Electrophoretically, tau moves with the $beta_2$ globulins and is thought to function as a transferrin, i.e., it binds iron and delivers it to the cell. Tau can be measured in the CSF and serum.

The Aβ protein is a small portion of a set of amino acids collectively referred to as the *amyloid β-protein precursor* (APP), which is normally bound to neuronal membranes. The Aβ protein is cleaved from the APP by the action of proteases termed α, β, and δ secretase. A current hypothesis, favored by Selkoe, focuses on the manner in which APP is cleaved by these enzymes to give rise to different-length residues of Aβ, normally secreted as a 40–amino acid product, $A\beta_{40}$, and as a longer 42–amino acid form, $A\beta_{42}$. The latter assumes a nonfibrillar amorphous form, the main ingredient in the diffuse plaque, and in theory is believed to be toxic to neurons. It may be the δ form of secretase that is largely responsible for creating the longer $A\beta_{42}$ fragment. This might offer a potential method of treatment by blocking the activity this enzyme.

Several pieces of evidence favor this hypothesis. It appears that the diffuse deposition of $A\beta_{42}$ precedes the formation of neurofibrils and plaques. The fact that the gene coding for APP is located on chromosome 21, one of the regions linked to familial Alzheimer disease, and that this chromosome is the one duplicated in the Down syndrome (see further on), suggests a causative connection between the overproduction of amyloid and all its Aβ residues and the disease. Another suggestive connection between these mechanisms has been the finding that the gene errors in several forms of familial Alzheimer disease code for a category of endosomal proteins termed *presenilins*, which interact with, or may indeed be, the δ secretase enzyme that produces $A\beta_{42}$. Transgenic mice with mutations for APP or for human presenilins develop plaques with $A\beta_{42}$ but not neurofibrillary tangles. Also, there is a provocative relationship between certain circulating proteins, particularly lipoproteins, and amyloid; this is discussed further on. It should be noted in this regard that mutations of the APP gene, detailed below, are associated with fewer than 0.1 percent of Alzheimer patients (Terry).

It must be conceded that there is still considerable uncertainty about the relationship of these changes to the loss of nerve cells and brain atrophy. The finding of a reduced number and enlargement of synapses in affected cortex by DeKosky and Scheff and others could be interpreted as either the first sign of neuronal death or the result of the neuronal loss. Amyloid deposition would then be a secondary phenomenon. The primary role of neurofibrillary tangles has also been questioned, and the manner in which amyloid deposition relates to tangle formation is unclear. Unexplained also is the prominent senile plaque formation in some cases and neurofibrillary tangles in others. Nonetheless, the amyloid hypothesis is currently the strongest, and all the more interesting insofar as APP and its Aβ products seem to have no useful purpose in the organism and conceivably could be reduced in quantity without harm.

Vascular changes do not have an important role in the pathogenesis of Alzheimer disease. It is definite that Alzheimer disease is not related to any of the usual types of arteriosclerosis. There are, however, small-vessel changes, accounting for the reduced cerebral blood flow reported by many investigators. This small-vessel change is probably secondary to the cerebral atrophy, since a lesser degree of reduction in cerebral blood flow is found in mentally intact old individuals. Probably the deposition of amyloid in cerebral vessels is a secondary phenomenon as well. The initial reports of the transmissibility of Alzheimer disease (Goudsmit et al) have not been corroborated.

No relationship to premorbid personality traits or to the level of cognitive functioning earlier in life has been established, but an intriguing finding from what has become known as the "nun study" suggests that poor linguistic ability early in life corresponds to the later development of Alzheimer disease (DA Snowden et al). In this study, the autobiographies of 93 nuns, written in their twenties, were rated for linguistic and ideational complexity. Of 14 sisters who died in late life, deterioration of cognitive function and neuropathologically proven Alzheimer disease occurred in 7 who had low "idea density" in their writings and in none of 7 whose writings were cognitively more complex. Obviously this correlation requires further study.

Neurotransmitter Abnormalities Considerable interest was created in the late 1970s by the finding of a marked reduction in choline acetyltransferase (ChAT) and acetylcholine in the hippocampus and neocortex of patients with Alzheimer disease. This loss of cholinergic synthetic capacity was attributed to the loss of cells in the basal forebrain nuclei (nucleus basalis of Meynert), from which the major portion of neocortical cholinergic terminals originate (Whitehouse et al). As is often true in medical science, the early enthusiasm for the cholinergic hypothesis proved less justified in the light of subsequent research. A 50 percent reduction in ChAT activity has been found in regions such as the caudate nucleus, which show neither plaques nor tangles (see review of Selkoe). The specificity of the nucleus basalis-cholinergic-cortical changes was questioned for other reasons as well. Also, the Alzheimer brain shows a loss of monoaminergic neurons in addition to cholinergic ones and a diminution of noradrenergic, GABAergic, and serotoninergic functions in the affected neocortex. The concentration of amino acid transmitters, particularly of glutamate, is also reduced in cortical and subcortical areas (Sasaki et al). The Alzheimer cortex shows a decreased concentration of several neuropeptide transmitters—notably substance P, somatostatin, and cholecystokinin—but it has not been determined whether any of the aforementioned biochemical abnormalities, including the cholinergic ones, are primary or are secondary to heterogeneous neuronal loss. Finally, the administration of cholinomimetics—whether they be acetylcholine precursors (e.g., choline or lecithin), degradation inhibitors (e.g., physostigmine), or muscarinic agonists that act directly on postsynaptic receptors—has not had a sustained therapeutic effect.

Chase and associates have demonstrated a 30 percent reduction in cerebral glucose metabolism in Alzheimer disease, greatest in the parietal lobes, but again the meaning of this, whether it is due to loss or to hypofunction of neurons, remains to be decided. The significance of aluminum in the genesis of neurofibrillary tangles, as once proposed, has never been determined. Recently it has been suggested that the use of estrogen by postmenopausal women delays the onset of the disease and might reduce its frequency (Tang et al). Carefully constructed, prospective studies are needed to test this idea and the long-term safety of the drug.

Genetic Aspects of Alzheimer Disease Of great interest and potential importance was the discovery, in patients with the clearly inherited form of Alzheimer disease, of a defective gene localized to a region of chromosome 21, near the β-amyloid gene that codes for an errant amyloid precursor protein (APP) (St. George-Hyslop et al). This also provided a possible explanation for the Alzheimer changes that characterize practically all patients with the trisomy 21 defect (Down syndrome) after their 20th year, but the gene defect on chromosome 21, as already noted, is responsible for only a tiny percentage of proved familial cases. Other kindreds with familial Alzheimer disease have been linked to gene mutations of chromosome 14 (Sherrington et al), accounting for up to 50 percent of familial cases, and on chromosome 1, which may account for many of the remaining inherited cases (Levy-Lahad et al). These genes and their protein products are now termed presenilin-1 and presenilin-2, respectively, to distinguish them from the APP mutations on chromosome 21; numerous mutations at these sites have been determined. The age of onset of the disease in these familial forms, as in the Down cases, is earlier than that in sporadic forms; asynchronous myoclonus, epilepsy, aphasia, and paratonia are more prominent in the familial disease.

Apolipoprotein E, a regulator of lipid metabolism that has an affinity for the β-amyloid protein in Alzheimer plaques, has been found to be another genetic marker that greatly modifies the risk of acquiring Alzheimer disease. Of the several isoforms of apolipoprotein E, the presence of E4 (and its corresponding gene allele ϵ4 on chromosome 19) is associated with a tripling of the risk of developing sporadic Alzheimer disease (Roses, Strittmatter et al, and Polvikoski et al). (This is the same allele that contributes to an elevated low-density lipoprotein fraction in the serum.) Possession of two ϵ4 alleles virtually assures the development of disease in those who survive to their eighties. The ϵ4 allele also modifies the age of onset of some of the familial forms of the disease. In contrast, the ϵ2 allele is underrepresented among Alzheimer patients. For these reasons it has been proposed that apolipoprotein E, by interacting with APP or tau protein in some way, modifies the formation of plaques.

These findings have led to interest in using the ϵ4 genotype as a marker for the risk of Alzheimer disease, but it must be pointed out that these are statistical relationships that do not invariably connect the allele to the disease in a particular individual. Therefore the results of such testing must be interpreted with caution. The ϵ4 allele does not act as a mendelian trait but as a susceptibility (risk) factor. It follows that many individuals without the allele also develop Alzheimer disease.

Studies of the molecular genetics of Alzheimer disease are yielding new information at such an astonishing rate that much of the foregoing text will soon be outdated. Useful basic reviews of this subject are those of Martin and of Selkoe, listed in the references.

Diagnostic Studies The most important ancillary tests in routine use are CT scanning and MRI (Fig. 39-1). In patients with advanced Alzheimer disease, the lateral and third ventricles are enlarged to about twice normal size and the cerebral sulci are widened. As stated previously, fine-section coronal MRI of the medial temporal lobes reveals a disproportionate atrophy of the hippocampi and a corresponding enlargement of the temporal horns of the lateral ventricles. Early in the disease, however, the changes do not exceed those found in many mentally intact old persons. For this reason, one cannot rely on imaging procedures alone for diagnosis. They are most valuable in excluding brain tumor, subdural hematoma, multi-infarct dementia, and obstructive hydrocephalus. The EEG undergoes a diffuse slowing, to the theta and delta range, but only late in the course of the illness. The CSF is also normal, though occasionally the total protein is slightly elevated. Using the constellation of clinical data, CT scanning, and MRI—along with the age of the patient and time course of the disease—the diagnosis of senile dementia of Alzheimer type is being made correctly in 85 to 90 percent of cases.

Neuropsychologic tests show a deterioration in memory and verbal access skills. Testing is particularly useful when there is a serial decline in ability. The use of these examinations is described in Chap. 21. Certain aspects of attention and executive function in Alzheimer disease have recently been reviewed by Perry and Hodges.

There is no available biologic marker of Alzheimer disease with the exception of an imprecise association with the disease-modifying ϵ4 apolipoprotein allele, as mentioned earlier. The specificity of certain pupillary reactions has been negated. Interest in this subject followed a report that Alzheimer patients show an enhanced pupillary sensitivity (mydriasis) to instillation of tropicamide eyedrops. Subsequent studies have failed to replicate these observations. The measurement of amyloid protein and its derivatives in the spinal fluid and blood are being investigated as diagnostic tests.

Differential Diagnosis Formerly, when virtually all forms of presenile and senile dementia were untreatable, there was little advantage to either the patient or the family in ascertaining the cause of the cerebral disease. Such patients were customarily left at home or committed to an institution for care of the psychiatrically or chronically ill. Now that a number of dementing diseases are treatable, a great premium attaches to correct diagnosis. The physician is compelled to exercise care in their detection even though they may be relatively infrequent.

The treatable forms of dementia are those due to neurosyphilis (general paresis) and other chronic meningitides, normal-pressure hydrocephalus, chronic subdural hematoma, nutritional deficiencies (Wernicke-Korsakoff syndrome, Marchiafava-Bignami disease, pellagra, vitamin B_{12} deficiency with subacute degeneration of the spinal cord and brain), chronic drug intoxication (e.g., alcohol, sedatives), certain endocrine-metabolic disorders (myxedema, Hashimoto thyroiditis encephalopathy, Cushing disease, chronic hepatic encephalopathy), some types of frontal and temporal lobe tumors, cerebral vasculitis, and, above all, the pseudodementia of depression. The dementia of AIDS and paraneoplastic limbic encephalitis may be partially amenable to treatment. Exclusion of these several diseases is most readily accomplished by sequential outpatient evaluations or by a brief admission to a hospital, where examinations of blood and CSF, EEG, CT, MRI, and neuropsycholgic testing can be undertaken.

The most difficult problem in differential diagnosis, in the authors' experience, has been the distinction between a late-life depression and a dementia, especially when some degree of both is present. Multi-infarct dementia may be difficult to separate from Alzheimer dementia, since patients with the latter illness may have had one or more clinically inevident infarcts. The dementia of normal-pressure hydrocephalus may also be confused with Alzheimer dementia. The differential diagnosis of these several treatable conditions is discussed in Chaps. 21, 30, 34, and 49. From time to time, we have been confident on clinical grounds that a patient had Alzheimer disease, only to have revealed at autopsy that progressive supranuclear palsy, Lewy body disease, Pick disease or another non-Alzheimer degeneration of the frontal lobes, or cortical-basal ganglionic degeneration was the cause. All of these are discussed later in this chapter.

Treatment There is no certain evidence that any of the proposed forms of therapy for Alzheimer disease—cerebral vasodilators, stimulants, L-dopa, massive doses of vitamins B, C, and E, and many others—has any salutary effect. Trials of oral physostigmine, choline, and lecithin have yielded mostly negative or uninterpretable results, and the same can be said for currently popular cholinergic precursors and agonists and acetylcholinesterase inhibitors, such as tacrine and donepezil, although there is some evidence of mild effect. The use of trazodone, haloperidol, thioridazine, risperidone, and related drugs may suppress some of the aberrant behavior and hallucinations when these are problems, making life more comfortable for both patient and family. Small doses of diazepines, such as lorazepam, are useful when sleep is severely disturbed.

The general management of the demented patient should proceed along the lines outlined in Chap. 21, keeping in mind that the physician's counsel is often the family's main resource for medical and social issues.

Associated Pathologic States As indicated earlier, the histologic changes of Alzheimer disease have a number of interesting associations. The changes are far more common in the brains of patients with Parkinson disease than in the brains of age-matched controls (Hakim and Mathieson). As a corollary, large numbers of Lewy bodies (a characteristic feature of Parkinson disease) have been found in 10 percent of patients who had been diagnosed as having Alzheimer disease (Woodard). These findings at least partly explain the high incidence of dementia in patients with Parkinson disease (see further on, in the sections regarding Parkinson disease and Lewy body dementia), yet not more than 20 to 30 percent of patients with Parkinson disease have plaques and tangles. Another association between the two diseases is apparent in the *Guamanian Parkinson-dementia complex*, which is also discussed below. In this entity, the symptoms of dementia and parkinsonism are related to neurofibrillary changes in the cerebral cortex and substantia nigra, respectively; senile plaques and Lewy bodies are unusual findings.

There are rare instances, such as those reported by Malamud and Lowenberg and by Loken and Cyvin, in which dementia begins in late childhood, with the finding at postmortem examination of the typical Alzheimer lesions in the cerebral cortex and basal ganglia. The clinical picture in these juvenile and early adult cases has been more varied than in the older ones. In some, paucity of speech, mutism, tremor, stooped posture, marked grasp and suck reflexes, and pyramidal and cerebellar signs leading to inability to stand or walk have appeared at various stages of the disease.

The finding of neurofibrillary changes (and to a lesser extent of plaques) in boxers ("*punch-drunk*" *syndrome*, or "*dementia pugilistica*") is another interesting ramification of the Alzheimer disease process (page 944). Hydrocephalus is present also, but there is insufficient information to determine whether it is a normal-pressure tension hydrocephalus from multiple subarachnoid hemorrhages or a hydrocephalus ex vacuo from cerebral atrophy.

Alzheimer disease in relation to the Down syndrome, first noted and reported by Jervis, is now widely recognized. The characteristic plaques and neurofibrillary tangles appear in the third decade; they increase with age and are present in practically all patients with the Down syndrome after 40 years of age.

The lobar sclerosis of Pick (see further on) has in some cases been associated with the histologic alterations of Alzheimer disease. A close relationship between Pick, Alzheimer, and Parkinson diseases has been demonstrated in a large family with dysphasic dementia (Morris et al). Other isolated combinations, wherein Alzheimer disease, hypothyroidism, hypopituitarism, or neurosyphilis were conjoined, were probably a matter of chance and prove nothing. From time to time other unusual associations come to light, such as *dementia with motor neuron disease* or the cases of *familial dementia with spastic paraplegia* reported by Worster-Drought and by van Bogaert and their associates (see further on in this chapter).

Lobar Atrophy (Pick Disease)

In 1892, Arnold Pick of Prague first described a special form of cerebral degeneration in which the atrophy is circumscribed (most often in the frontal and/or temporal lobes), with involvement of both gray and white matter—hence the term *lobar* rather than *cortical* sclerosis. In 1911, Alzheimer presented the first careful study of the microscopic changes. The most complete analyses of the pathologic changes are those of Spatz, van Mansvelt, Morris and coworkers, and Tissot and associates. Since the recognition of Pick disease rests more on pathologic than on clinical criteria, they are described first.

In contrast to Alzheimer disease, in which the atrophy is relatively mild and diffuse, the pathologic change in lobar atrophy is more circumscribed and sometimes asymmetrical. The atrophy may extend to the island of Reil and the amygdaloid-hippocampal structures. The parietal lobes are involved less frequently than the frontal and temporal lobes. The affected gyri become paper-thin; these parts of the brain resemble the kernel of a dried walnut. The cut surface reveals not only a markedly thinned cortical ribbon but a grayish appearance and reduced volume of the white matter. The corpus callosum and anterior commissure share in the atrophy. The overlying pia-arachnoid is thickened, and the ventricles are enlarged. The pre- and postcentral, superior temporal, and occipital convolutions are relatively unaffected and stand out in striking contrast to the wasted parts. Pick insisted that the disease essentially involves the association areas of Flechsig. In some instances, atrophy of the caudate nuclei has been pronounced, almost to the degree seen in Huntington chorea. The thalamus, subthalamic nucleus, substantia nigra, and globus pallidus may also be affected, but only to a slight degree.

The salient histologic feature of Pick disease is a loss of neurons, most marked in the first three cortical layers. Surviving neurons are often swollen, and some of them contain argentophilic (Pick) bodies within the cytoplasm. Ultrastructurally, the Pick bodies are made up of straight fibrils, thus differing from the paired helical filaments that characterize Alzheimer disease. These bodies predominate in the medial parts of the temporal lobes, especially in the atrophic hippocampi. "Ballooning" of cortical neurons is found mainly in the frontal cortex; in such cases, according to Tissot and others, atrophy of the basal ganglia and substantia nigra is especially frequent. There is a loss of myelinated fibers in the white matter beneath the atrophic cortex. A heavy astrocytic gliosis is seen in both the cortex and subcortical white matter. Most neuropathologists consider the loss of myelinated fibers to be consequent to neuronal loss. Senile plaques and Alzheimer neurofibrillary changes are seen in the atrophic zones in some of the cases (mixed Alzheimer and Pick disease), alluded to earlier, and there is granulovacuolar degeneration of neurons in the hippocampus, but not to the degree seen in Alzheimer disease.

The striking lobar cortical atrophy and changes in the white matter are readily visualized by CT scanning and MRI.

Clinical Features Whether the diagnosis of Pick disease can be made on purely clinical grounds is doubtful. Our predictions as to the existence of the pathologic changes and their differentiation from those of Alzheimer disease and the recently defined entity of "frontotemporal dementia" (described below) have been erratic, although they should improve with the use of stricter clinical criteria, CT scanning, and MRI. In our experience, the gradual onset of mental confusion with respect to place and time, anomia, slowness of comprehension, inability to cope with unaccustomed problems, loss of tact, deterioration of work habits, neglect of personal hygiene and grooming, apathy, and alterations of personality and behavior have been prominent features. In addition to personality changes, inability to perform sequences of motor tasks, motor perseveration, apathy (emotional indifference), inattention, abulia, impairment of gait and upright stance, and prominent grasp and suck reflexes are attributable to predominant affection of the frontal lobes.

Focal disturbances, particularly aphasia and apraxia, are said to occur early and to be prominent in patients with Pick disease, pointing to a lesion in the left frontal and temporal lobes. Early language disorder has been reported in two-thirds of all patients with temporal lobe atrophy. At first the patient speaks less but language is intact; later, he may forget and misuse words and soon fails to understand much of what is heard or read. Speech becomes a "medley of disconnected words and phrases" and eventually is reduced to an incomprehensible jargon. Finally, the patient is mute, seemingly without impulse to speak, and he loses the ability to form words (Snowden et al). Verbal perseveration, palilalia, and echolalia are frequent. Bulimia and alterations in sexual behavior occur to a distressing degree in some patients (Tissot et al).

Wilson distinguished two patterns of abnormal behavior: in one, the patient is talkative, lighthearted, cheerful or anxious, constantly on the move, occupied with trifles, and attentive to every passing incident; in the other, the patient is taciturn, inert, emotionally dull, and lacking in initiative and impulse. Probably these two patterns represent predominantly temporal and frontal types, respectively. According to Tissot and colleagues, the frontal, temporal, and parietal lobes are all affected in 75 percent of patients by the time the disease terminates.

The cause of Pick disease is unknown. Sjögren and associates concluded from a genetic survey of the cases in Stockholm that Pick disease was probably transmitted as a dominant trait with polygenic modification. A Dutch family with almost 100 percent penetrance over several generations has been reported by Schenk. Women seem to be affected more often than men. No chemical, vascular, traumatic, or other factor of possible causal importance has been identified.

The course of the illness is usually 2 to 5 years, occasionally longer, and nothing can be done therapeutically except to postpone the end by careful nursing.

Frontotemporal Dementia

This descriptive term has long been used by neurologists and neuropathologists to refer to any dementia that is associated with degeneration of the frontal and temporal lobes. Most such instances have proved to be examples of Alzheimer disease and, in lesser numbers, to Pick disease, as noted above. Also for many years, neuropathologists have been aware of instances of dementia that are identical clinically and in their gross pathology (gyral atrophy) to the Alzheimer and Pick types but do not show the characteristic histologic changes of either of these diseases. They do, however, exhibit tau-staining material in neurons of the affected regions. One source of abnormal (i.e., hyperphosphorylated) tau is from a mutation of the tau gene on chromosome 17; indeed, an abnormality of this gene is associated with such a frontotemporal dementia (Basun et al). But abnormal aggregates of tau have been identified in practically all neurodegenerative diseases and form the main constituent of the paired helical filaments (neurofibrillary tangles) of Alzheimer disease.

It appears from the observations of Brun and of Neary and their associates that pure tau-reactive cases actually outnumber Pick disease as strictly defined by the Pick inclusion, but the distinctions between the two have not always been clear from writings on the subject. Some of the clinical aspects are discussed in Chap. 21, but, broadly speaking, the patients under discussion present the personality and behavioral abnormalities that would be expected from frontal and anterior temporal lobe dysfunction, such as apathy, perseveration, poor judgment and abstraction, bizarre affect, and a general disengagement. An initial diagnosis of depression is common. Other psychiatric symptoms—such as sociopathic and disinhibited behavior with aspects of hyperorality and hyperphagia—may predominate. (All of Wilson's comments, noted above in relation to Pick disease, pertain here as well.) Alternatively, aphasic or word-finding syndrome corresponding to a lateral temporal lobe degeneration may be the initial presenting and predominant feature, sometimes for several years, before other manifestations of dementia become evident.

In recent writings on this subject, the term *frontotemporal dementia* has come to be used in a highly restricted sense, being arbitrarily assigned to cases that show only tau-staining material in neurons. More such cases are sporadic, but an inherited variety linked to chromosome 17 has been described, in which parkinsonism is prominent; it is in these cases that the intraneural deposition of tau is most striking, in both the frontotemporal cortex and the substantia nigra.

Noteworthy also is the observation that a dementia identical to that of the tau-reactive cases occurs without any tau staining of neurons. Also, some of the frontally predominant cases have shown only marked vacuolation (microcavitation) of the affected cortex; cases of the latter type have been described in patients with amyotrophic lateral sclerosis (where tau staining has reportedly been found in the anterior horn cells).

The relationship between Pick disease and frontotemporal dementia is still uncertain. The clinical and gross pathologic findings—a regional frontotemporal atrophy of the cerebrum—are nearly identical in the two disorders. The main distinction is the presence or absence of Pick bodies or tau-staining material in neurons of the affected regions and greater affection of the white matter in Pick disease. If indeed the Pick and tau inclusions are shown in the future to be clearly distinctive biological changes, they can be considered to represent separate diseases, but many reported cases of sporadic lobar atrophy demonstrate both types of change, or what is even more confusing, neither type—making it impossible at this time to be certain of the purity of each type.

Other Degenerative Dementias

Diffuse Cerebral Atrophy of Non-Alzheimer Type

There are other forms of progressive, diffuse brain atrophy leading to dementia that show none of the pathologic features of either Alzheimer or Pick disease or any of the other diseases that are sometimes associated with a dementing illness (Parkinson or Lewy body disease, amyotrophic lateral sclerosis, progressive supranuclear palsy, etc.).

In Sweden, for example, Sjögren has found familial cases of this type, as have Schaumburg and Suzuki in this country, and we have seen occasional sporadic examples. The clinical picture in these cases has been indistinguishable or has varied slightly from that of Alzheimer disease, and autopsy has disclosed widespread cerebral atrophy, most pronounced in the frontal lobes. Microscopically these cases are characterized by a diffuse neuronal loss, slight glial proliferation, and secondary demyelination of the white matter, like that observed with the frontal lobe atrophy of Pick disease. Other instances of sporadic and familial presenile dementia have shown subcortical gliosis or nonspecific cellular changes (atrophy of nerve cells and nuclei, loss of Nissl substance). Some examples of the latter type have in the past been described under the rubric of "Kraepelin disease" and more recently as "dementia lacking distinctive histologic features" (Knopman et al). Perhaps some or all of these cases will turn out to be a variant of the "tau" form of frontotemporal dementia, as discussed above.

Lewy Body Disease Another syndrome in which the dementia may be clinically indistinguishable from Alzheimer disease is one in which the cortical neurons contain Lewy bodies and in which neurofibrillary changes or senile plaques are less conspicuous or absent. Reports of Lewy body dementia have been increasing steadily since the original communication by Okazaki and others in 1961; many of these have been from Japan (see Kosaka's review). To some extent this is due to improved histologic techniques, particularly the immunoreactive ubiquitin and, more recently, synuclein stains, which enable one to visualize Lewy bodies in the cerebral cortex more clearly than before (see the discussion of Parkinson disease, which follows). The fact that aggregated α-synuclein makes up most of the Lewy body will undoubtedly prove important in relation to both Parkinson disease and Lewy body dementia. Next to Alzheimer disease and diffuse (non-Alzheimer) cerebral atrophy, diffuse Lewy body disease is thought to be the most common form of diffuse cerebral cortical atrophy with dementia.

Burkhardt and colleagues, in an analysis of 34 cases of diffuse Lewy body disease, found that the most characteristic syndrome was one of progressive dementia in an elderly patient with late onset of parkinsonian signs in some cases. For this reason, the disease also properly belongs in the category of dementias that are accompanied by other prominent neurologic features (page 1108). The movement disorder may be mild or prominent and may occur as an early or a late manifestation. In Lennox's summary of 75 cases published up to 1990, parkinsonism, particularly a limb and axial rigidity, was a prominent feature in 90 percent, and almost half had tremor. The parkinsonian features respond favorably to

L-dopa, but for a limited time and sometimes at the expense of delirium or hallucinations (Hely et al). Some patients have orthostatic hypotension corresponding to cell loss and Lewy bodies in the intermediolateral cell column of the spinal cord or sympathetic ganglia.

Byrne and associates noted that episodic increases in confusion, hallucinations, and paranoid delusions were a feature of the Lewy body dementia; these psychotic features are generally uncharacteristic of Alzheimer and lobar dementias. In Lennox's review, one-third of patients with Lewy body dementia had these swings in behavior, but as the illness advanced, the amnesia, dyscalculia, visuospatial disorientation, aphasia, and apraxia did not differ from those of Alzheimer disease. In the cases of Fearnley and coworkers, there was a supranuclear gaze palsy simulating that of progressive supranuclear palsy. In our limited experience with Lewy body disease, the parkinsonian symptoms have been more prominent than in progressive supranuclear palsy; the most characteristic feature besides the movement disorder has indeed been intermittent psychotic or delirious behavior. Others have commented on an extreme sensitivity to neuroleptic drugs, including increased confusion and greatly worsening parkinsonism or the development of the neuroleptic malignant syndrome.

Thalamic Dementia A relatively pure degeneration of thalamic neurons has been described in relation to a progressive dementia (Stern; Schulman). The dementia in these cases evolved relatively rapidly (several months) and was associated with choreoathetosis. Garcin and colleagues described five cases of subacutely developing dementia, which they considered to be examples of Creutzfeldt-Jakob disease; in each of them the pathologic changes consisted primarily of neuronal loss and gliosis of the thalamus. A large kindred of such cases, characterized by subacute dementia and myoclonus and inherited as an autosomal trait, has been reported by Little and coworkers. In members of this family, the clinical presentation was also very similar to that of Creutzfeldt-Jakob disease; however, the pathologic changes were confined to the thalami, particularly to the mediodorsal and other medial thalamic nuclei. Transmission of the disease to primates was unsuccessful.

In the *diagnosis* of this large category of chronic dementias, one must consider several nondegenerative disorders in which dementia may predominate and focal neurologic abnormalities may be minimal. Several of the treatable ones are listed in the discussion of Alzheimer disease, above, and a larger group is reviewed in Chap. 21. Also to be considered, particularly in dementias with onset at an early age, are the inherited metabolic diseases discussed in Chap. 37, the chief among which are the leukodystrophies—metachromatic, adrenal, globoid body (Krabbe disease)—and the poliodystrophies—neuronal ceroid lipofuscinosis (Kuf disease), GM_2 gangliosidosis, and Wilson disease (see page 1026). Each of these displays characteristic neurologic features, but each may present in the early stages with a decline in intellectual function and a behavioral disorder.

Finally, a brief comment is required regarding the group of diseases called "vascular dementia," listed in many classifications as the second most common cause of mental decline after Alzheimer disease. As discussed in Chap. 34, multiple cortical strokes may cause increasing deficits that cumulatively qualify as a dementia, but each element of focal cerebral disease that contributes to the cognitive decline can be identified, and a stepwise decline that corresponds to the abrupt onset of each stroke is evident. A more difficult problem arises in a limited number of patients who have a multitude of deep lacunar infarctions. Their mental capacities may appear to decline slowly, although memory is not involved disproportionately, and usually a pseudobulbar state or one of the other characteristic lacunar stroke syndromes can be identified, so there is little trouble in differentiation from the degenerative dementias. The subcortical white matter change of Binswanger disease causes similar diagnostic problems, as discussed on pages 451 and 878. Beyond these vascular diseases and the familial CADASIL disease (cerebral autosomal dominant arteriopathy with subcortical infarcts, page 878), which is of uncertain cause, the authors are dubious of the category of vascular dementia. Most cases turn out to be Alzheimer disease with one or more visible infarctions.

DISEASES IN WHICH DEMENTIA IS ASSOCIATED WITH OTHER NEUROLOGIC ABNORMALITIES

Huntington Chorea

This disease, distinguished by the triad of dominant inheritance, choreoathetosis, and dementia, commemorates the name of George Huntington, a medical practitioner of Pomeroy, Ohio. In 1872, in a paper read before the Meigs and Mason Academy of Medicine and published later that year in the *Medical and Surgical*

Reporter of Philadelphia, Huntington gave a succinct and graphic account of the disease, based on observations of patients that his father and grandfather had made in the course of their practice in East Hampton, Long Island. Reports of this disease had appeared previously (see DeJong, in the References, for historical background), but they lacked the accuracy and completeness of Huntington's description. Vessie, in 1932, was able to show that practically all the patients with this disease in the eastern United States could be traced to about six individuals who had emigrated in 1630 from the tiny East Anglian village of Bures, in Suffolk, England. One remarkable family was traced for 300 years through 12 generations, in each of which the disease had expressed itself.

To quote Huntington, the rule has been that "When either or both of the parents have shown manifestations of the disease . . . one or more of the offspring invariably suffer of the disease, if they live to adult life. But if by any chance these children go through life without it, the thread is broken and the grandchildren and great-grandchildren of the original shakers may rest assured that they are free from disease." Davenport, in a review of 962 patients with Huntington chorea, found only 5 who had descended from unaffected parents. Possibly, in these latter patients, a parent had the trait, but in very mild form. Or, one or more of these patients represented rare sporadic instances of Huntington chorea, i.e., individuals in whom a mutation had occurred from a normal gene to the mutant, disease-producing form.

In university hospital centers, this is one of the most frequently observed types of hereditary nervous system disease. Its overall frequency is estimated at 4 to 5 per million, and 30 to 70 per million among whites of northern European ancestry. The usual age of onset is in the fourth and fifth decades, but 3 to 5 percent begin before the 15th year and some even in childhood. In about 30 percent, symptoms become apparent after 50 years. The progression of the disease is slower in older patients. Once begun, the disease progresses relentlessly, until only a restricted existence in a nursing home or psychiatric hospital is possible and some other disease terminates life.

Exhaustive genealogic documentation has established the cause to be an autosomal dominant gene with complete penetrance (see below). Martin has made the observation that young patients usually inherit the disease from their fathers and older patients from their mothers. It has been observed beginning at almost the same age in identical twins.

Until recently, it had not been possible to foretell which of the children of a patient will be stricken with the disease. Caudate glucose metabolism—measured by positron emission tomography (PET) in earlier studies—although reduced in most presymptomatic patients, proved not to be a sufficiently dependable indicator of persons at risk for Huntington disease. The most important achievement in respect to the presymptomatic detection of Huntington disease was the discovery, by Gusella and colleagues, of a marker linked to the Huntington gene, localized to the short arm of chromosome 4. Subsequently these investigators and others identified the gene abnormality as an excessively long repeat of trinucleotides (CAG), the length of which determines not only the presence of the disease but also the age of onset. This discovery has made possible the development of a test for the detection of the defective gene in asymptomatic individuals. In view of the fact that there is no treatment for the disease, testing raises certain ethical considerations that need to be resolved before its widespread utilization.

Clinical Features *The mental disorder* assumes several subtle forms long before the more obvious deterioration of cognitive functions becomes evident. In approximately half the cases, slight and often annoying alterations of character are the first to appear. Patients begin to find fault with everything, to complain constantly, and to nag other members of the family; they may be suspicious, irritable, impulsive, eccentric, untidy, or excessively religious, or they may exhibit a false sense of superiority. Poor self-control may be reflected in outbursts of temper, fits of despondency, alcoholism, or sexual promiscuity. Disturbances of mood, particularly depression, are common (almost half of the patients in some series) and may constitute the most prominent symptoms early in the disease. Invariably, sooner or later, the intellect begins to fail. The patient becomes less communicative and more socially withdrawn. These emotional disturbances and changes in personality may reach such proportions as to constitute a virtual psychosis (with persecutory delusions or hallucinations).

Diminished work performance, inability to manage household responsibilities, and disturbances of sleep may prompt medical consultation. There is difficulty in maintaining attention, in concentration, and in assimilating new material. Mental flexibility lessens. There is loss of fine manual skills (see further on). The performance parts of the Wechsler Adult Intelligence Scale show greater loss than the verbal parts. Memory is relatively spared. This gradual dilapidation of intellectual function has been characterized as a "subcortical dementia" (page 450), i.e., elements of aphasia, agnosia, and apraxia are observed only rarely and memory loss is not profound. Often the process is so slow that some degree of intellectual capacity is retained for many years.

The *abnormality of movement* is at first slight and most evident in the hands and face; often the patient is merely considered to be fidgety, restless, or "nervous." Slowness of movement of the fingers and hands, a reduced rate of finger tapping, and difficulty in performing a sequence of hand movements are early motor signs. Gradually these abnormalities become more pronounced until the entire musculature is implicated. The frequency of blinking is increased (the opposite of parkinsonism), and voluntary protrusion of the tongue is constantly interrupted by unwanted darting movements. In the advanced stage of the disease, the patient is seldom still for more than a few seconds. The movements are slower than the brusque jerks and postural lapses of Sydenham chorea, and they involve many more muscles. They tend to recur in stereotyped patterns yet are not as stereotyped as tics. In more advanced cases, they acquire an athetoid or dystonic quality. Muscle tone is usually decreased until late in the illness, when there may also be some degree of rigidity, tremor, and bradykinesia, elements suggestive of Parkinson disease (Westphal or "rigid" variant, which is more common with a childhood onset). Tendon reflexes are exaggerated in one-third of patients, but only a few have Babinski signs. Voluntary movements are initiated and executed more slowly than normal, but there is no weakness and no real ataxia, although speech, which becomes dysarthric and explosive due to incoordination between tongue and diaphragm, may convey the impression of a cerebellar disorder. There is poor control of the tongue and diaphragm. Denny-Brown pointed out that when the Huntington patient is suspended, the upper limbs assume a flexed posture and the legs an extended one, a posture that he considered to be expressive of the striatal syndrome. The disorder of movement that characterizes Huntington chorea is described more fully in Chap. 4. Oculomotor function is affected in most patients (Leigh et al; Lasker et al). Particularly characteristic are impaired initiation and slowness of pursuit and volitional saccadic movements and an inability to make a volitional saccade without movement of the head. Excessive distractibility may be noticed during attempted ocular fixation. The patient feels compelled to glance at extraneous stimuli even when specifically instructed to ignore them. Upward gaze is often impaired.

As Wilson stated, the relation of the choreic to the mental symptoms "abides by no general rule." Most often the mental symptoms precede the chorea, but they may accompany or follow it, sometimes by many years. In our own material, with two exceptions of late onset with rigidity rather than chorea, once the movement disorder was fully established, there was nearly always some degree, perhaps slight, of cognitive abnormality. Exceptional cases have been reported, in which the movement disorder existed for 10 to 30 years without mental changes in patients with the gene abnormality of Huntington disease (Britton et al). After 10 to 15 years, most patients deteriorate to a vegetative state, unable to stand or walk and eating little; in this late stage, a mild amyotrophy may appear. Noteworthy is the high suicide rate in huntingtonians, as pointed out by Huntington (Schoenfeld et al). Also, there is a high incidence of trauma; chronic subdural hematoma is a common finding at autopsy.

The first signs of the disease may appear in childhood, before puberty (even under the age of 4), and several series of such cases have been described (Farrer and Conneally; van Dijk et al). Mental deterioration at this early age is more often accompanied by cerebellar ataxia, behavior problems, seizures, bradykinesia, rigidity, and dystonia than by chorea (Byers et al). However, this rigid form of the disease (Westphal variant) is known also to occur occasionally in adults, as mentioned above. Functional decline is much faster in children than it is in adults (Young et al).

Earlier onset in successive generations (*anticipation*) is well described in the early writings on the subject and is now known to be attributable to increasing lengths of the CAG repeat sequence, as already pointed out. The dementia is generally more severe in cases of early onset (15 to 40 years) than in those of later onset (55 to 60 years).

At the gene locus implicated in Huntington disease there are normally 11 to 34 (median 19) consecutive repetitions of the CAG triplet that codes for glutamine; individuals with more than 35 to 39 triplets may have the disease and those with more than 42 invariably acquire the signs of disease if they live long enough. As already noted, the CAG repeat length correlates with disease severity, the early-onset cases having the largest number of repeats. Furthermore, in adult patients with early onset of the disease, the emotional disturbance tends to be initially prominent and precedes the chorea and intellectual loss by many years; with older age of onset, choreiform movements and progressive dementia are more often the initial components and have their onset at nearly the same age.

Pathology and Pathogenesis Gross atrophy of the head of the caudate nucleus and putamen bilaterally is the characteristic abnormality, usually accompanied by a moderate degree of gyral atrophy in the frontal and temporal regions. The caudatal atrophy alters the configuration of the frontal horns of the lateral ventricles; the inferolateral borders do not show the usual bulge formed by the head of the caudate nucleus; in addition, the ventricles are diffusely enlarged (Fig. 39-2). In CT scans, the bicaudate-cranial ratio is increased in the majority of patients. This finding corroborates the clinical diagnosis in the moderately advanced case.

The early articles of Alzheimer and Dunlap and the more recent one of Vonsattel and DiFiglia contain the most authoritative descriptions of the microscopic changes. The latter authors have graded the disease into early, moderately advanced, and far advanced stages. In five genetically verified early cases, no striatal lesion was found, which suggests that the first clinical manifestations are based on a biochemical disorder without visible structural change, at least by light microscopy. This view is supported by the observation that Huntington patients studied with PET show a characteristic decrease in glucose metabolism, which appears early in the disease and precedes the loss of tissue (Hayden et al). The striatal degeneration begins in the medial part of the caudate nucleus and spreads, tending to spare the nucleus accumbens. Of the six cell types in the striatum (differentiation based on size, dendritic arborizations, spines, and axon trajectories), the smaller cells are affected before the larger ones. Loss of dendrites of the small spiny neurons has been an early finding. The large cells are relatively preserved and exhibit no special alterations. The lost cells are replaced by fibrous astrocytes. With neuronal loss, the myelinated fibers also disappear. The anterior parts of the putamen and caudatum are more affected than the posterior parts. In our own cases we have not been impressed with changes in the globus pallidus, subthalamic nucleus, red nucleus, or cerebellum, but others have observed slight changes in these parts and in the pars reticulata of the substantia nigra. In the cerebral cortex, there is said to be slight neuronal loss in layers 3, 5, and 6, with replacement gliosis. Cases are reported with typical striatal lesions but normal cortices, in which only chorea had been present during late life. In our early to moderately advanced cases, even quantitative analyses of the cortex have not disclosed a significant loss of neurons. Several neuropathologists have observed marked cell loss and gliosis in the subthalamic nuclei in children or young adults with chorea and behavior disorders.

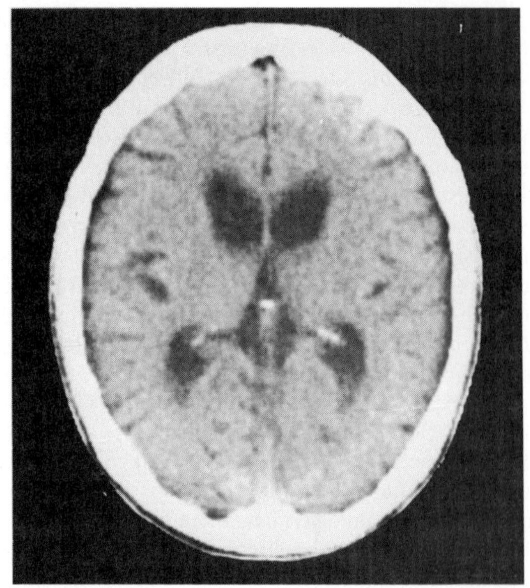

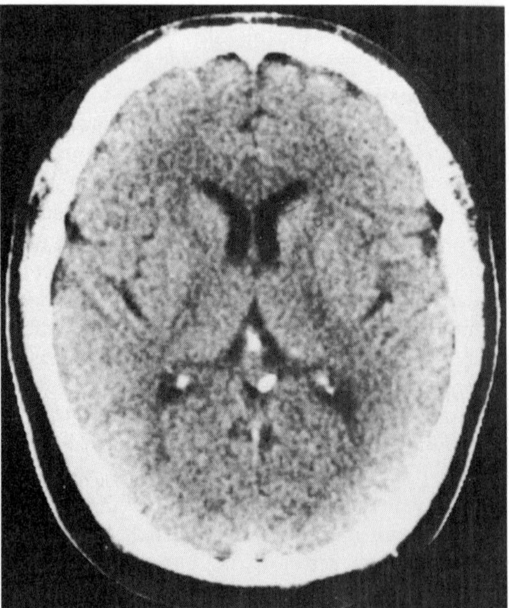

Figure 39-2

The upper CT scan is from a 54-year-old mildly demented woman with a 10-year history of Huntington chorea. The bulge in the inferolateral border of the lateral ventricle, normally created by the head of the caudate nucleus (lower scan from a patient of the same age for comparison), has been obliterated. There is also a diffuse enlargement of the lateral ventricles.

The biochemical defects in Huntington chorea are only beginning to be understood. The impaired glucose metabolism in the caudate nucleus, preceding visible atrophy, has already been mentioned. Since at least a partial explanation for L-dopa–induced involuntary movements is an excess of dopamine (in contrast to Parkinson disease, in which there is a decrease), it has been postulated that the abnormal movements of Huntington chorea represent a heightened sensitivity of striatal dopamine receptors. There are disturbances in the metabolism of other putative neurotransmitters (norepinephrine, glutamic acid decarboxylase, choline acetyltransferase, GABA, acetylcholine, and somatostatin), but the significance of these biochemical disturbances is unknown.

The product of the Huntington gene locus has been termed *huntingtin* and its mutated form contains an excessive number of glutamine residues as a result of the excess copies of the CAG nucleotide. Although the function of the protein is not known, an excess of huntingtin accumulates in the nuclei of neurons in human disease and in transgenic mice with an increased number of CAG repeats. Moreover, the protein accumulates in cells of the striatum and parts of the cortex affected in Huntington disease.

Diagnostic Problems Once the disease has been observed in its fully developed form, its recognition requires no great clinical acumen. The main difficulty arises with patients who lack a family history but in whom the progressive chorea, emotional disturbance, and dementia with onset in adult life are typical. This difficulty has been largely overcome since the mutation causing Huntington disease was identified. It is now possible to confirm or exclude the diagnosis by analysis of DNA from a blood sample, the presence of greater than 39 to 42 CAG repeats at the Huntington locus essentially confirming its presence; lesser numbers leave room for equivocation. Sometimes it is learned later that the family history was incomplete or falsified or that an illness in a parent had been misinterpreted. Chorea that begins in late life, with only mild or questionable intellectual impairment and without a family history of similar disease, is another source of difficulty; referring to it as senile chorea does not solve the problem. Indeed, senile chorea may have more than one cause. We have seen it appear with infections, drug therapy, and thyrotoxicosis, only to disappear after a few weeks. *Chorea in early adult life* always raises the question of a late form of Sydenham chorea or of lupus erythematosus with antiphospholipid antibodies, but neither familial occurrence nor mental deterioration is part of these diseases. Other progressive neurologic disorders that are inherited as autosomal dominant traits and begin in adolescence or adult life (e.g., polymyoclonus with or without ataxia, acanthocytosis with progressive chorea, and especially dentatorubropallidoluysian degeneration) can closely mimic Huntington disease, as described further on, and sometimes only the pathologic picture settles the matter.

Other problems in differential diagnosis include bilateral thalamic degeneration with dementia and chorea, referred to earlier; paroxysmal choreoathetosis (page 83); Wilson disease (page 1026); acquired hepatocerebral degeneration (page 1195); and, most often, schizophrenia or manic-depressive psychosis complicated by tardive dyskinesia (page 1264). Many drugs in addition to L-dopa occasionally cause chorea (amphetamines, tricyclic antidepressants, lithium, isoniazid).

Therapy The dopamine antagonist haloperidol, in daily doses of 2 to 10 mg, is probably the most effective agent in suppressing the movement disorder. Because of the danger of superimposing tardive dyskinesia on the chronic disorder, the chorea should be treated only if it is functionally disabling, using the smallest possible dosages and providing numerous drug holidays. Haloperidol may also help alleviate abnormalities of behavior or emotional lability, but it does not alter the progress of the disease. The authors have not been impressed with the therapeutic effectiveness of other currently available drugs. Levodopa and other dopamine agonists make the chorea worse and, in the rigid form of the disease, evoke chorea. Drugs that deplete dopamine or block dopamine receptors—such as reserpine, clozapine, and tetrabenazine—suppress the chorea to some degree, but their side effects (drowsiness, akathisia, and tardive dyskinesia) outweigh their desired effects. The juvenile (rigid) form of the disease is probably best treated with antiparkinsonian drugs. Huntington disease pursues a steadily progressive course and death occurs, on an average, 15 to 20 years after onset, sometimes much earlier or later. The psychologic and social consequences of the disease require supportive therapy, and genetic counseling is essential.

Acanthocytosis with Chorea

A few reports of a slowly progressive familial chorea and dementia in association with an abnormality of erythrocytes have appeared in English, American, and Japanese journals. The disease has the following characteristics: (1) onset in adolescence or early adult life of generalized involuntary movements (described as chorea but including dystonia and tics), usually beginning as an orofacial dyskinesia and spreading to other parts of the body; (2) mild to moderate mental deterioration in some but not all of the cases; (3) decreased or absent tendon reflexes and evidence of chronic axonal neuropathy and denervation atrophy of muscles; (4) atrophy and gliosis of the caudate nuclei and putamens but no neuronal loss in the cerebral cortex or other parts of the brain; and (5) acanthocytosis (thorny or spiky appearance of erythrocytes). The last change, according to Sakai and coworkers, is due to an abnormal composition of covalently (tightly) bound fatty acids in erythrocyte membrane proteins (palmitic and docosahexanoic acids increased and stearic acid decreased). The pattern of inheritance has been autosomal recessive but was dominant in one New England family. The acanthocytosis may be overlooked when it is mild but can be detected by scanning electron microscopy. In the series of 19 cases reported by Hardie and colleagues, the manifestations included dystonia, tics, vocalizations, rigidity, and lip and tongue biting; more than half had cognitive impairment or psychiatric features. The average age of onset was 32 years; 7 of the 19 cases were sporadic. The disease has been linked in almost all families to chromosome 9q. The so-called McLeod phenotype differs hematologically in that there is an abnormal expression of Kell surface antigens on the erythrocyte.

Several *other rare degenerative disorders with chorea*, some of which have already been mentioned, fall into this category. Midlife progressive chorea without dementia (after more than 25 years follow-up) has been reported. There was no abnormality of chromosome 4. *Dentatorubropallidoluysian atrophy*, diagnosed clinically as Huntington chorea, was found in four European families by Warner and associates and is described further on in the section on cerebellar degenerations. The extrapyramidal manifestations included chorea, myoclonus, and rigidity. Adult-onset chorea and dementia have been described with *propionic acidemia*; propionic acid was elevated in the plasma, urine, and CSF. This disorder must be added to other metabolic diseases described in Chap. 37 as causes of chorea and dyskinesia—such as glutaric acidemia, keratin sulfaturia, calcification of basal ganglia, and Hallervorden-Spatz disease (Hagberg et al).

Corticostriatospinal Degenerations

Included in this category are a number of degenerative diseases in which the symptoms of dementia, parkinsonism, and amyotrophic lateral sclerosis present in various combinations. Some of the diseases that make up this group have not been sharply delineated and are difficult to separate from one another (see also page 1140).

Under the title "spastic pseudosclerosis," Jakob, in 1921, described a chronic disease of middle to late adult life, characterized by abnormalities of behavior and intellect; weakness, ataxia, and spasticity of the limbs (chiefly the legs); extrapyramidal symptoms such as rigidity, slowness of movement, tremors, athetotic postures, and hesitant, dysarthric speech; and normal spinal fluid. The pathologic changes were diffuse and consisted mainly of an outfall of neurons in the frontal, temporal, and central motor gyri, corpus striatum, ventromedial thalamus, and bulbar motor nuclei. In one of Jakob's cases, there were also prominent changes in the anterior horns and corticospinal tracts in the spinal cord like those of amyotrophic lateral sclerosis (ALS). The latter finding gave rise to Wilson's concept of the disease as a *corticostriatospinal degeneration*. A degenerative and probably familial disorder that had been described earlier by Creutzfeldt was considered by Spielmeyer to be sufficiently similar to the one of Jakob to warrant the designation Creutzfeldt-Jakob disease.

As discussed in Chap. 33, the disorder described by Creutzfeldt and Jakob has been a source of endless controversy because of its indeterminate character. On the one hand, it has been confused with the subacutely evolving myoclonic dementia, "subacute spongiform encephalopathy," which is now known to be an infection due to an unconventional transmissible agent (prion). The authors believe that the latter disease, which is described on page 814, bears at best only a superficial resemblance to the one described by Creutzfeldt and Jakob, and that the two disorders should be clearly separated. Unfortunately, the eponym is so entrenched in medical usage that any attempt to remove it stands little chance of success. On the other hand, sporadic and familial cases that are not transmissible and lack a prominent spongiform change merge with a rather heterogeneous but overlapping group of degenerative disorders, all rare, including progressive dementia and spastic paraplegia, progressive dementia and ALS, the Parkinson-dementia-ALS complex of Guam, and the corticopallidospinal degeneration of Davison.

Other variants of this category of disease continue to appear. The authors have observed several patients in whom extreme rigidity, corticospinal signs, and evidence of ALS have developed over a period of several years. In the later stages of the disease, the patient, while alert, is totally helpless—unable to speak, swallow, or move the limbs. Only eye movements are retained, and even these are hampered by supranuclear gaze palsies in advanced cases. Intellectual functioning appears to be better preserved than movement but is difficult to assess. Other bodily functions are intact. The course is slowly progressive and ends fatally in 5 to 10 years. There is no family history of similar disease, and there are no clues as to causation. Gilbert and colleagues have described similar cases with signs of Parkinson disease, motor neuron disease, and dementia; in their cases, there were no senile plaques or Lewy bodies. The concurrence of typical motor neuron disease and Parkinson disease may be coincidental, but Qureshi and colleagues described 13 patients in whom both disease processes began within a brief time of one another and considered them to be related. In the variant described by Tandan and colleagues, an autosomal dominant syndrome of Charcot-Marie-Tooth polyneuropathy was combined with ptosis, Parkinson syndrome, and dementia, again without Lewy bodies or senile plaques. Yet other variants have been described by Schmitt and coworkers and by Mata and colleagues. Hudson has reviewed 42 sporadic cases in which ALS-parkinsonism-dementia were combined (see References).

The *Guamanian Parkinson-dementia-ALS* complex deserves separate comment because it constitutes a large number of carefully studied cases with almost uniform clinical and pathologic features. The disease occurs in the indigenous Chamorro peoples of Guam and the Mariana islands, predominantly in men between ages 50 and 60. Progressive parkinsonism and dementia are combined with upper or lower motor neuron disease (ALS is also common among the Chamorro), leading to death in 5 years. The pathologic changes, described by Hirano and others, consist of severe cortical atrophy with neurofibrillary tangles but, conspicuously, no plaques are detectable, even with sensitive neurochemical staining. As in Parkinson disease, the substantia nigra and to a lesser extent other pigmented nuclei are depopulated of nerve cells but contain no Lewy bodies. Cases with amyotrophy show an appropriate anterior horn cell loss.

One is tempted to conclude that the spastic pseudosclerosis of Jakob should not be considered as a disease type, and certainly everyone agrees that the term *pseudosclerosis* (also used for the Westphal-Strümpell form of hepatolenticular degeneration) is meaningless.

Familial Dementia with Spastic Paraparesis

From time to time the authors have encountered families in which several members developed a spastic paraparesis and a gradual failure of intellect during the middle adult years. The mental horizon of the patient narrowed gradually, and the capacity for high-level thinking diminished; in addition, the examination showed appropriately exaggerated tendon reflexes, clonus, and Babinski signs. In one such family the illness had occurred in two generations; in another, three brothers in a single generation were afflicted. Skre described two recessive types of hereditary spastic paraplegia in Norway, one with onset in childhood, the other in adult life. In contrast to the dominant form (see further on), the recessive types displayed evidence of more widespread involvement of the nervous system, including dementia, cerebellar ataxia, and epilepsy. Also, Cross and McKusick have observed a recessive type of paraplegia accompanied by dementia beginning in adolescence. They named it the *Mast syndrome*, after the afflicted family.

Worster-Drought and others have reported the pathologic findings in two cases of this type. In addition to senile plaques and neurofibrillary changes, there was demyelination of the subcortical white matter and corpus callosum and a "patchy but gross swelling of the arterioles," which gave the staining reactions for amyloid ("Scholz's perivascular plaques"). Van Bogaert and associates published an account of similar cases that showed the characteristic pathologic features of Alzheimer disease.

Adult forms of metachromatic leukodystrophy and adrenoleukodystrophy may present with a similar clinical picture (Chap. 37). Another interesting association of familial spastic paraplegia is with progressive cerebellar ataxia. Fully one-third of the cases that we have seen with such a spastic weakness were also ataxic and would fall into the category of spinocerebellar degenerations. Yet another variant of this group of diseases has been described by Farmer and colleagues; the inheritance in their cases was autosomal dominant, and the main clinical features were deafness and dizziness, ataxia, chorea, seizures, and dementia, evolving in that order. Postmortem examinations of two patients disclosed calcification in the globus pallidus, neuronal loss in the dentate nuclei, and destruction of myelinated fibers in the centrum semiovale.

Adult Polyglucosan Body Disease

Under this title Robitaille and colleagues described a distinct type of progressive neurologic disease in adults, characterized clinically by spasticity, chorea, dementia, and a predominantly sensory polyneuropathy. Structures that closely resembled Lafora bodies and corpora amylacea were found in large numbers in both central and peripheral neural processes (mainly in axons) and also in astrocytes. These basophilic, periodic acid–Schiff (PAS)–positive structures, up to 40 mm in size, were made up of glucose polymers (polyglucosans) and were readily apparent in sural nerve biopsies. Some were found in the heart and liver.

More recently, Rifal and associates have reviewed the findings in 25 cases of this disease—one observed personally and 24 that had been reported previously. The dementia appears to be relatively mild, consisting of impairment of retentive memory, dysnomia, dyscalculia, and sometimes expressive dysphasia and deficits of "visual integration"; this is overshadowed by the rigidity and spasticity of the limbs and the peripheral nerve disorder. Nerve conduction velocities are diminished and leg muscles are denervated. Moderate degrees of generalized cerebral atrophy, multifocal areas of white matter rarefaction, and increased iron deposition in the putamina are disclosed by MRI. The finding of polyglycosan axon inclusion in biopsied nerve confirms the diagnosis. The disease was sometimes misdiagnosed as adrenoleukodystrophy.

DISEASES CHARACTERIZED BY ABNORMALITIES OF POSTURE AND MOVEMENT

Parkinson Disease (Paralysis Agitans)

This common disease, known since ancient times, was first cogently described by James Parkinson in 1817. In his words, it is characterized by "involuntary tremulous motion, with lessened muscular power, in parts not in action and even when supported; with a propensity to bend the trunk forward, and to pass from a walking to a running pace, the senses and intellect being uninjured." Strangely, his essay contains no reference to rigidity or to slowness of movement, and it stresses unduly the reduction in muscular power. The same criticism can be leveled against the term *paralysis agitans*, which appeared for the first time in 1841, in Marshall Hall's textbook *Diseases and Derangements of the Nervous System*.

Certain aspects of the natural history of the disease are of interest. As a rule, it begins between 40 and 70 years of age, with the peak age of onset in the sixth decade. It is infrequent before 30 years of age (only 4 of 380 cases in one series), and most series contain a somewhat larger proportion of men. Trauma, emotional upset, overwork, exposure to cold, "rigid personality," and so on, among many other factors, have been suggested as predisposing to the disease, but there is no convincing evidence to support any such claims. The possible relationship to repeated cerebral trauma and to the "punch-drunk" syndrome (dementia pugilistica, page 944) has been particularly problematic and is unresolved despite the documentation provided by several celebrated cases (Lees). Idiopathic Parkinson disease is observed in all countries, all ethnic groups, and all socioeconomic classes, although the incidence in blacks is only one-quarter that in whites; in Asians, the incidence is one-third to one-half that in whites. A lack of concordance of Parkinson disease in twins appears to negate the role of genetic factors, but a study of dopamine metabolism utilizing PET scanning has shown that 75 percent of asymptomatic twins of Parkinson patients had evidence of striatal dysfunction and only a small portion of dizygotic twins showed these changes (Piccini et al). These data suggest a more substantial role for an inherited trait in cases of ostensibly sporadic disease. Also, Krüger and colleagues have reported a 13-fold increased susceptibility to the disease in patients who harbor a combination of α-synuclein and apolipoprotein E genotypes (see below).

While familial cases are decidedly rare, Golbe and colleagues have described two large kindreds (probably related and originating from a small town in southern Italy) in which 41 patients in four generations were affected. The illness in their cases was characteristic of Parkinson disease both clinically and pathologically, the only unusual features being a somewhat earlier onset (mean age 46 years), a relatively rapid course (10 years from onset to death), and a reported incidence of tremor in only 8 of the 41 patients. The dominantly inherited parkinsonism described by Dwork and others also differed clinically (onset in third decade, prominence of dystonia) and pathologically (absence of Lewy bodies) from classic Parkinson disease. It was in the latter kindred and in three Greek families that Polymeropoulos et al identified a locus on chromosome 4q that contained a mutation for α-synuclein, a main component of the Lewy body. Other families in which there have been mendelian patterns of inheritance are associated with gene defects at other sites (but still mostly on chromosome 4). These genetic data have been reviewed by Dunnett and Björklund.

The disease is common. In North America there are approximately 1 million patients, constituting about 1 percent of the population over the age of 65 years. The incidence in all countries where vital statistics are kept is similar. Considering its frequency, coincidence in a family on the basis of chance occurrence might be as high as 5 percent.

Clinical Features The core syndrome of expressionless face, poverty and slowness of voluntary movement, "resting" tremor, stooped posture, axial instability, rigidity, and festinating gait has been fully described in Chap. 4, and only certain diagnostic problems and variants in the clinical picture need to be considered here. The early symptoms may be difficult to perceive and are often overlooked. Advancing years have a way of rendering the spine and limbs less pliable and elastic, and in the senium the gait may become short-stepped and then reduced to a shuffle. The voice tends to become soft and monotonous. Hence it is all too easy to attribute the early symptoms of Parkinson disease to the effects of aging. For a long time the patient may not be conscious of the inroads of the disease; at first the only complaints may be of aching of the back, neck, shoulders, or hips and of vague weakness. A slight stiffness and slowness of movement or a reduction in the natural swing of one arm during walking are ignored, until one day it occurs to the physician or to a member of the family that the patient has Parkinson disease. Infrequency of blinking, as pointed out originally by Pierre Marie, is often a helpful early sign. The usual rate (12 to 20 blinks per minute) is reduced in the parkinsonian patient to 5 to 10. And with it there is a slight widening of the palpebral fissures, creating a stare (Stellwag sign). A reduction in movements of the small facial muscles imparts the characteristic expressionless ("masked") appearance (hypomimia). When seated, the patient makes fewer small shifts and adjustments of position than the normal person (hypokinesia), and the fingers straighten and assume a flexed and adducted posture at the metacarpophalangeal joints.

The characteristic tremor, which usually involves a hand, is often listed as the initial sign; but in at least half the cases, observant family members will have remarked earlier on the patient's relative immobility and poverty of movement. Moreover, in 20 to 25 percent of cases the tremor is mild and intermittent or evident in only one finger or one hand. The tremor of the fully developed case takes several forms, as was remarked in Chap. 6. The 4-per-second "pill-rolling" tremor of the thumb and fingers is seen in only a small proportion of patients and is typically present when the hand is motionless, i.e., not used in voluntary movement (hence the term *resting tremor*). Complete relaxation, however, greatly reduces or abolishes the tremor, and a volitional movement usually but not always dampens it momentarily. The rhythmic beat coincides with an alternating burst of activity in agonists and antagonists in the electromyogram (EMG). The arm, jaw, tongue, eyelids, and foot are less often involved. The least degree of tremor is felt during passive movement of a rigid part (cogwheel phenomenon or Negro's sign). The tremor shows surprising fluctuations in severity and is aggravated by walking and excitement, but tremor frequency remains constant (Hunker and Abbs). *One side of the body is typically involved before the other*, and the tremor then remains asymmetrical as the illness advances.

Lance and associates have called attention to another common type of tremor in Parkinson disease—a fine, 7- to 8-per-second, slightly irregular action tremor of the outstretched fingers and hands. This tremor, unlike the slower one, persists throughout voluntary movement, is not evident with the limb in a resting position, and is more easily suppressed by relaxation. Electromyographically, it lacks the alternating bursts of action potentials seen in the more typical tremor. The patient may have either type of tremor or both.

We have been less impressed with rigidity and hypertonus as important early findings. They tend to appear in the more advanced stages of the disease. Once rigidity develops, it is constantly present; it can be felt by the palpating finger and seen as a salience of muscle groups even when the patient relaxes. When the examiner passively moves the limb, a mild resistance appears from the start (without the short free interval that characterizes spasticity), and it continues evenly throughout the movement, in both flexor and extensor groups, being interrupted only by the cogwheel phenomenon. Both the rigidity and its cogwheel feature can be elicited by having the patient occupy the opposite limb with a motor task requiring some degree of concentration, such as tracing circles in the air or touching each finger to the thumb. Postural hypertonus predominates in the flexor muscles of trunk and limbs and confers upon the patient the characteristic flexed posture. Particulars of the parkinsonian disorders of muscle tone, stance, and gait are discussed further in Chaps. 4 and 7.

Regarding the quality of volitional and postural movements, a few additional points should be made. The patient is slow and ineffective in attempts to deliver a quick hard blow; he cannot complete a quick (ballistic) movement by a single burst of agonist-antagonist-agonist sequence of energizing activity, like the normal person; several bursts are needed (Hallett and Khoshbin). Alternating movements, at first successful, become progressively impeded and finally are blocked completely or adopt the rhythm of the patient's tremor. Also, the patient has difficulty in executing two motor acts simultaneously. Originally the impaired facility of movement was attributed to rigidity, but the observation that appropriately placed surgical lesions can abolish rigidity without affecting the disorder of movement refutes this interpretation. Thus the difficulty is not one of rigidity but one of *bradykinesia* (slowness in both the initiation and execution of movement), the extreme degree of which is akinesia. The latter deficits underlie the characteristic poverty of movement, shown by infrequency of swallowing, slowness of chewing, a limited capacity to make postural adjustments of the body and limbs in response to displacement of these parts, a lack of small "movements of cooperation" (as in arising from a chair without first adjusting the feet), absence of arm swing in walking, etc. Despite a perception of muscle weakness, the patient is able to generate normal or near-normal power, especially in the large muscles; however, in the small ones, strength is slightly diminished.

As the disorder of movement worsens, all customary activities show the effects. Handwriting becomes small (micrographia), tremulous, and cramped, as first noted by Charcot. The voice softens and the speech seems hurried and monotonous; the voice becomes less audible and finally the patient only whispers. Exceptionally, "mumbling" is an early complaint. Caekebeke and coworkers refer to the speech disorder as a "hypokinetic dysarthria"; they attribute it to respiratory, phonatory, and articulatory dysfunction. The consumption of a meal takes an inordinately long time. Each morsel of food must be swallowed before the next bite is taken. Walking becomes reduced to a shuffle; the patient frequently loses his balance, and in walking forward or backward must "chase the body's center of gravity" with a series of short steps in order to avoid falling (festination). Defense and righting reactions are faulty. Falls do occur, but surprisingly infrequently given the degree of postural instability. Gait is typically improved by sensory guidance, as by holding the patient at the elbow, whereas obstacles have the opposite effect, at times causing the patient to "freeze" in place. Difficulty in turning over in bed is a characteristic feature as the illness advances, but the patient rarely volunteers this information. Shaving or applying lipstick becomes difficult, as the facial muscles become more immobile and rigid.

Persistent extension or clawing of the toes, jaw clenching, and other fragments of dystonia may enter the picture but rarely are early findings.

As noted above, these various motor impediments and tremor characteristically begin in one limb (more often the left) and spread to one side and later to both sides, until the patient is quite helpless. Yet in the excitement of some unusual circumstance (a fire, for example), the patient is capable of brief but remarkably effective movement (*kinesis paradoxica*).

Regarding other elicitable neurologic signs, there is an inability to inhibit blinking in response to a tap over the bridge of the nose or glabella (Myerson sign), but grasp and suck reflexes are not present and buccal and jaw jerks are rarely enhanced. Commonly there is an impairment of upward gaze and convergence; if noted early in the disease, this raises the possibility of progressive supranuclear palsy. The bradykinesia may extend to eye movements, in that patients may show a delay in the initiation of gaze to one side, slowing of conjugate movements (decreased maximal saccadic velocity), hypometric saccades, and breakdown of pursuit movements into small saccades. There are no sensory changes. Drooling is troublesome; an excess flow of saliva has been assumed, but actually the problem is one of failure to swallow with normal frequency. Seborrhea and excessive sweating are probably secondary as well, the former due to failure to cleanse the face sufficiently, the latter to the effects of the constant motor activity. Postural instability can be elicited by tugging at the patient's shoulders from behind and noting the lack of a small step backward to maintain balance. The tendon reflexes vary, as they do in normal individuals, from being barely elicitable to brisk. Even when parkinsonian symptoms are confined to one side of the body, the reflexes are usually equal on the two sides, and the plantar responses are flexor. Exceptionally, the reflexes on the affected side are slightly more brisk, which raises the question of corticospinal involvement; but the plantar reflex remains flexor. In these respects, the clinical picture differs from that of corticobasal ganglionic degeneration, in which rigidity, hyperactive tendon reflexes, and Babinski signs are combined with apraxia (see further on). There is a tendency to syncope in some cases; this was found by Rajput and Rozdilsky to be related to cell loss in the sympathetic ganglia. However, syncope is never as prominent as in striatonigral degeneration.

At times, Parkinson disease is complicated by a dementia, a feature that had been commented upon by Charcot. The reported frequency of this combination varies considerably, based on the selection of patients and type of testing. An estimate of 10 to 15 percent (Mayeux et al) is generally accepted and matches our experience. The incidence increases with advancing age, approaching 65 percent in Parkinson patients above 80 years of age. In some instances of Parkinson disease with dementia, MRI reveals lesions in the cerebral white matter (in T1-weighted images) not seen in parkinsonians without dementia. The pathologic basis of the dementia in Parkinson disease is discussed below.

The overall course of the disease is quite variable. In the majority of patients, the mean period of time from inception of the disease to a chairbound state is 7.5 years (Hoehn and Yahr; Martilla and Rinne). On the other hand, as many as one-third of cases are relatively mild and remain stable for 10 years or more.

Diagnosis Early in the course of Parkinson disease, when only a slight asymmetry of stride or an ineptitude of one hand is present and tremor has yet to appear and impart the unmistakable stamp of the disease, a number of small signs already alluded to may be helpful in diagnosis. These include a reduced blink rate, the Myerson glabellar sign, a lack of arm swing, digital impedance (a tendency for rapid alternating movements to be slowed, to assume a tremor rhythm, or to be blocked altogether) and perceptible rigidity of one arm when the opposite limb is occupied in a motor task such as tracing circles in the air. Lack of a Babinski sign or of increased tendon reflexes in the affected limbs eliminates a corticospinal lesion as the cause of slowed movements, and lack of a grasp reflex helps to exclude a premotor cerebral disorder.

The main difficulty in diagnosis is to distinguish Parkinson disease from the many parkinsonian syndromes, some caused by other degenerative diseases and some by medications or toxins. Parkinson disease is far more common than any of the syndromes that resemble it. Bradykinesia and rigidity of the limbs and axial musculature are shared symptoms, but only in Parkinson disease is "resting" tremor an early sign, and it remains prominent even late in the illness.

The typical signs of Parkinson disease, when present in their entirety, impart an unmistakable clinical picture. When not all the signs are evident, there is no alternative but to re-examine the patient at several-month intervals until it is clear that Parkinson disease is present or until the signature of another degenerative process becomes evident (e.g., vertical gaze impairment in progressive supranuclear palsy; dysautonomia with fainting, bladder, or vocal cord signs in striatonigral degeneration; early and rapidly evolving dementia or psychosis in Lewy body disease, or apraxia in corticobasal ganglionic degeneration). If the patient's symptoms warrant, a beneficial response to levodopa also gives a reasonably secure although not entirely conclusive indication of the presence of Parkinson disease. The other parkinsonian syndromes are for the most part unchanged by the drug.

As pointed out on page 813, the epidemic of encephalitis lethargica (von Economo encephalitis) that spread over western Europe and the United States after the First World War left great numbers of parkinsonian cases in its wake. No definite instance of this form of encephalitis had been recorded before the period 1914–1918, and virtually none has been seen since 1930; hence postencephalitic parkinsonism is no longer a diagnostic consideration. Rarely, a Parkinson-like syndrome has been described with other forms of encephalitis (particularly with Japanese B virus and eastern equine encephalitis).

In England and Europe an "arteriopathic" or "arteriosclerotic" form of Parkinson disease was at one time much diagnosed, but we have never been convinced of its reality. Pseudobulbar palsy from a series of lacunar infarcts or from Binswanger disease (page 878) can cause a clinical picture simulating certain aspects of Parkinson disease, but unilateral and bilateral corticospinal tract signs, hyperactive facial reflexes, spasmodic crying and laughing, and other characteristic features distinguish spastic bulbar palsy from Parkinson disease. Of course, the parkinsonian patient in advancing years is not impervious to cerebrovascular disease, and the two conditions then overlap.

Normal-pressure hydrocephalus can create a syndrome that resembles Parkinson disease, particularly in regard to gait and postural instability and at times to bradykinesia; but rigid postures, slowness of alternating movements, hypokinetic ballistic movements, and resting tremor are not part of the clinical picture.

Senile (familial or essential) tremor is distinguished by its fine, quick quality, its tendency to become manifest during volitional movement and to disappear when the limb is in a position of repose, and the lack of associated slowness of movement, flexed postures, etc. The head is more often involved in senile tremor than in Parkinson disease. Some of the slower, alternating forms of essential tremor are difficult to distinguish from parkinsonian tremor, and one can only wait to see whether it is the first manifestation of Parkinson disease.

Progressive supranuclear palsy (see further on) is characterized by rigidity and dystonic postures of the neck and shoulders, a staring and immobile countenance, and a tendency to topple when walking—all of which are suggestive of Parkinson disease. Inability to produce vertical saccades and, later, paralysis of upward and downward gaze and eventually of lateral gaze with retention of reflex eye movements establish the diagnosis in most cases. Strict adherence to the diagnostic criteria for Parkinson disease also permits its differentiation from corticostriatospinal, striatonigral, and corticobasal ganglionic degeneration and Machado-Joseph disease—all of which are discussed in other parts of this chapter.

Paucity of movement, unchanging attitudes and postural sets, and a slightly stiff and unbalanced gait may be observed in patients with an anergic or hypokinetic ("retarded") type of depression. Since as many as 25 to 30 percent of parkinsonian patients are depressed, the separation of these two conditions may then be difficult (see page 1612). The authors have seen patients who were called parkinsonian by competent neurologists but whose movements became normal when antidepressant medication or electroconvulsive therapy was given.

The rapid onset of the Parkinson syndrome, especially in conjunction with other medical diseases, should always raise the suspicion of drug effects; phenothiazines, haloperidol, and the neuroleptics pimozide and metoclopramide, used at times as antiemetics, all cause a slight masking of the face, stiffness of the trunk and limbs, lack of arm swing, fine tremor of the hands, and mumbling speech. They may also evoke an inner restlessness, a "muscular impatience," an inability to sit still, and a compulsion to move about much like that which occurs at times in the parkinsonian patient (akathisia; page 118). Spasms of the neck, face, and jaw muscles (open mouth, protruded tongue, retrocollis or torticollis, grimacing) may also be provoked by such drugs. A mild, localized rigidity of an arm due to local tetanus was studied by R. D. Adams) in a patient who had been referred as a case of acute parkinsonism.

All in all, if one adheres to the strict definition of Parkinson disease—bradykinesia, "resting" tremor, postural changes and instability, cogwheel rigidity, and response to L-dopa—errors in diagnosis are few. Yet in a series of 100 cases, studied clinically and pathologically by Hughes and associates, the diagnosis was inaccurate in 25 percent. The reasons are that about this number of Parkinson patients do not have the characteristic tremor and about 10 percent do not respond to L-dopa. These authors noted that early dementia and autonomic disorder and the presence of ataxia and corticospinal signs were reliable exclusion criteria.

Pathology and Pathogenesis It is now accepted that a loss of pigmented cells in the substantia nigra and other pigmented nuclei (locus ceruleus, dorsal motor nucleus of the vagus) is the most constant finding in both idiopathic and postencephalitic Parkinson disease. The substantia nigra is visibly pale to the naked eye; microscopically, the pigmented nuclei show a marked depletion of cells and replacement gliosis, findings that enable one to state with confidence that the patient must have suffered from Parkinson disease. Also, many of the remaining cells of the pigmented nuclei contain eosinophilic cytoplasmic inclusions with a faint halo, called Lewy bodies. These are seen in practically all cases of idiopathic Parkinson disease. They were present in a few postencephalitic cases as well, but in the latter neurofibrillary tangles were more usual. However, both of these cellular abnormalities appear occasionally in the substantia nigra of aging, nonparkinsonian individuals. Possibly the individuals with Lewy bodies would have developed Parkinson disease if they had lived a few more years. Noteworthy is the finding by McGeer et al that nigral cells normally diminish with age, from a maximal complement of about 425,000 to 200,000 at age 80. Tyrosine-hydroxylase, the rate-limiting enzyme for dopamine, diminishes correspondingly. These authors found that in patients with Parkinson disease, the number of pigmented neurons was reduced to about 30 percent of that in age-matched controls. Using more refined counting techniques, Pakkenberg and coworkers estimated the average total number of pigmented neurons to be 550,000 and to be reduced by 66 percent in Parkinson patients. The number of nonpigmented neurons in their control subjects was 260,000 and again was reduced in patients by 24 percent. Thus, aging contributes importantly to nigral cell loss, but the cell depletion is so much more marked in Parkinson disease that some factor other than aging must also be operative.

Other depletions of cells are widespread, but they have not been quantitatively evaluated and their significance is less clear. There is neuronal loss in the mesencephalic reticular formation, near the substantia nigra. These cells project to the thalamus and limbic lobes. In the sympathetic ganglia, there is slight neuronal loss and Lewy bodies are seen; this is also true of the pigmented nuclei of the lower brainstem as well as of the putamen, caudatum, pallidum, and substantia innominata. Dopaminergic neurons that project to cortical and limbic structures, to caudate nucleus and nucleus accumbens, and to periaqueductal gray matter and spinal cord are affected little or not at all. The lack of a consistent lesion in either the striatum or the pallidum is noteworthy in view of the reciprocal connections between the striatum and the substantia nigra and the depletion of striatal dopamine that characterizes the parkinsonian state.

The statistical data relating Parkinson and Alzheimer diseases are difficult to assess because of different methods of examination from one reported series to another (Quinn et al). Nevertheless, the overlap of the two diseases is more than fortuitous, as indicated in an earlier part of this chapter. In our own pathologic material, the majority of the demented Parkinson patients showed Alzheimer-type changes, but there were several in whom few plaques or neurofibrillary changes could be found or in whom the cortical neuronal loss was accompanied by a widespread distribution of Lewy bodies (Lewy body dementia, discussed earlier, on page 1120).

Of great interest in recent years has been the observation, both in human opiate addicts and in monkeys, that a neurotoxin (known as MPTP) can produce irreversible signs of parkinsonism and selective destruction of cells in the substantia nigra (as described on page 105). The toxin, ingested by persons who self-administered an analogue of meperidine, was shown to bind with high affinity to an extraneural enzyme, monoamine oxidase, which transformed it to a toxic metabolite, pyridinium MPP+. The latter is bound by the melanin in the dopaminergic nigral neurons in sufficient concentration to destroy the cells. The precise mechanism by which MPTP produces the Parkinson syndrome is unsettled. One hypothesis is that the inner segment of the globus pallidus is rendered hyperactive because of reduction of the GABA influence of the subthalamic nucleus. The theory of an environmental toxin as a cause of Parkinson disease has been greatly stimulated by the MPTP findings. (Uhl et al; see also the review by Snyder and D'Amato). The disease is more frequent in industrialized countries and agrarian areas in which toxins are commonly used, but its universal occurrence would militate against any one toxin. To date, no chemical toxin, heavy metal, etc., has been incriminated in the causation of Parkinson disease.

Provocative recent discoveries have involved the synaptic protein alpha-synuclein, the main component of Lewy bodies in both the sporadic and inherited forms of Parkinson disease as well as in Lewy body disease. Synuclein normally exists in a soluble unfolded form, but in high concentrations it forms aggregates of neurofilaments to form the Lewy body. Immunostaining techniques have also disclosed less specific proteins, such as ubiquitin and tau, within the Lewy bodies. Furthermore, as noted earlier, in four unrelated families with the rare autosomal dominant form of Parkinson disease, a mutation on chromosome 4 has been found that codes for an aberrant form of synuclein (Polymeropoulos et al). However, no gene error relating to synuclein has been found in patients with sporadic Parkinson disease and the misfolding of synuclein as a cause of the common sporadic disease is only a speculation.

Treatment Although there is no known treatment that will halt or reverse the neuronal degeneration that presumably underlies Parkinson disease, methods are now available that afford considerable relief from symptoms. Treatment can be medical or surgical, although reliance is placed mainly on drugs, particularly on L-dopa.

At present, L-dihydroxyphenylalanine (L-dopa) is unquestionably the most effective agent for the treatment of Parkinson disease, and the therapeutic results, even in those with far-advanced disease, are much better than have been obtained with other drugs, even newer ones that act as dopamine agonists. As mentioned earlier, some degree of response is so nearly universal that many neurologists use it as a diagnostic criterion. The theoretical basis for the use of this compound rests on the observation that striatal dopamine is depleted in patients with Parkinson disease but that the remaining nigral cells are capable of producing dopamine by taking up its precursor, L-dopa. The neurons of the striatum that are targets of nigral projections are not depleted and remain receptive to any dopamine released by nigral cells. Over time, however, the number of remaining nigral neurons that convert L-dopa to dopamine becomes inadequate and the receptivity to dopamine of the striatal target neurons becomes excessive, possibly as a result of denervation hypersensitivity; this results in both a reduced response to L-dopa and to paradoxical and excessive movements (dyskinesias) with each dose.

By combining a decarboxylase inhibitor (carbidopa or benserizide), which is unable to penetrate the central nervous system (CNS), with L-dopa, the decarboxylation of L-dopa to dopamine is greatly diminished in peripheral tissues. This permits a greater proportion of L-dopa to reach nigral neurons and, at the same time, a reduction in the peripheral side effects of L-dopa and dopamine (nausea, hypotension, etc.). Combinations of levodopa-carbidopa are available in a 10:1 or 4:1 ratio and the benserizide combination in a 4:1 ratio. The initial dose of levodopa-carbidopa is typically one-half of a 100-mg/25-mg tablet given two or three times daily and increased slowly until optimum improvement is achieved, usually up to a maximum of two tablets administered four times daily, or a similar dose of the 250-mg/25-mg combination. A newer class of catechol-*O*-methyltransferase (COMT) inhibitors, typified by tolcapone, extends the plasma half-life and the duration of L-dopa effect by preventing its breakdown (as opposed to increasing its bioavailability as with carbidopa). But these drugs require further study, for there have been several complications and rare unexplained deaths after their use.

Long-acting preparations of levodopa-carbidopa may reduce dyskinesias in some patients (Hutton and

Morris) in the advanced stages of disease, but our experience with these drugs given earlier in the course has been less impressive. In transferring a patient from conventional L-dopa/carbidopa preparations to the long-acting formulation, the frequency of administration can be roughly halved while the total amount of L-dopa initially remains unchanged. The absorption of the long-acting drug, however, is approximately 70 percent, often necessitating a slight increase in total dose. To facilitate the treatment of morning rigidity and tremor, the long-acting tablet can be broken in half to speed absorption or a small dose of conventional medication can be given at the same time. Often some degree of dyskinesia must be accepted as the price to be paid for the therapeutic effect.

Bromocriptine, *pergolide*, and *lisuride* are synthetic ergot derivatives whose action in Parkinson disease is explained by their direct stimulating effect on dopamine (D_2) receptors, which are located on corticostriate neurons, thus bypassing the depleted nigral neurons. The newer nonergot dopamine agonists *ropinirole* and *pramipexole* seem to be tolerated well and have a duration of effectiveness similar to that of other D_2 agonists; these agents are very helpful in supplementing L-dopa and are now increasingly popular as the sole therapeutic agent before L-dopa is instituted. Rascol and colleagues have reported that the use of ropinirole during the first 5 years of the parkinsonian illness controlled the symptoms satisfactorily and, in addition, reduced the incidence of dyskinesias, compared to treatment with L-dopa. Why dyskinesias are less frequent with ropinirole than with L-dopa is not known. Bromocriptine should be introduced cautiously, 7.5 to 10 mg daily in three to four divided doses, and the dosage increased very slowly to an optimal level of 40 to 60 mg daily; levodopa-carbidopa should be reduced concomitantly by 50 percent. A dose of 5 to 10 mg of bromocriptine has about the equivalent effect of 100/25 mg levodopa/carbidopa. It has a longer duration of action than L-dopa and causes nausea and vomiting less often, but otherwise the action and side effects of the two drugs are much the same. Even small doses of these drugs, when first introduced, may induce a prolonged episode of hypotension. Our observations are in agreement with those of Marsden, who found that of 263 patients, all but 82 had abandoned one of the ergot dopamine agonists after 6 months because of lack of effect or adverse reactions. Nevertheless, a proportion of patients continue to benefit for up to 3 years. Ropinirole and pramipexole are useful in smoothing the effects of L-dopa and allowing a reduction in its dose. As with the ergot-based dopamine agonists, they can be utilized in some patients as the sole treatment for a limited time. They may produce sudden and unpredictable sleepiness, similar to narcolepsy, and patients should be warned of this possibility in relation to driving. More data are required to judge the efficacy of initiating therapy with a dopamine agonist rather than with L-dopa combinations.

Because of the side effects of levodopa and of dopaminergic agents, particularly in older patients, some neurologists avoid all types of pharmacotherapy if the patient is in the early phase of the disease and the parkinsonian symptoms are not troublesome. When the symptoms become more annoying, initial therapy with either amantadine 100 mg bid or an anticholinergic medication may be advised. Only when the symptoms begin to interfere with work and social life or falling becomes a threat is a carbidopa/levodopa preparation introduced, and then at the lowest possible dose—10/100 mg bid or tid. This dose is slowly increased until maximal benefit is achieved.

Another approach, now controversial, has been to initiate the treatment of new cases of Parkinson disease with the monoamine oxidase inhibitor selegiline, 5 mg bid, and to continue its use until symptoms become disabling, at which point L-dopa or a dopamine agonist is introduced. Selegiline inhibits the intracerebral metabolic degradation of dopamine, and clinical trials conducted by the Parkinson Study Group have suggested that it slows progression of the disease in its early stages. Subsequent observations, however, have not confirmed the view that selegiline markedly alters the natural course of the disease, and we use it infrequently.

As already mentioned, L-dopa is not without significant side effects, so that its use is limited in some circumstances. Approximately two-thirds of patients tolerate the drug initially and experience few serious adverse effects; one-third will show dramatic improvement, especially in hypokinesia and tremor. Many patients are at first troubled by nausea, especially if the medication is not taken with meals, and a few have orthostatic hypotensive episodes. Nausea usually disappears after several weeks of continued use or can be allayed by the specific dopaminergic chemoreceptor antagonist domperidone. Coincident psychiatric symptoms may also present problems and are to be expected in 15 to 25 percent of patients, particularly in the elderly. Depression is occasionally a serious problem, even to the point of suicide; delusional thinking may occur in these circumstances. This combination of movement and psychiatric disorders is difficult to treat, and one must institute an antidepressant regimen or one of the newer class of antipsychotic medications that are associated with few extrapyramidal side effects, as described below and in Chap. 50. Trazodone has been helpful in treating depression and insomnia, which may be a major problem. The selective serotonin reuptake inhibitors are useful in apathetic depressions, but some patients report worsening of parkinsonian symptoms. Excitement and aggressiveness appear in a few. A return of libido may lead to sexual assertiveness.

Confusion and outright *psychosis* (hallucinations and delusions), seen in advanced cases of Parkinson disease when high doses of L-dopa are required, is first treated by attempting to reduce the dose of the drug. If this is not possible, the atypical neuroleptics olanzapine, clozapine, risperidone, or quetiapine in low doses are often successful (Friedman and Lannon). The side effects of these drugs include sleepiness, orthostatic hypotension, sialorrhea, and the most serious, agranulocytosis, requiring regular monitoring of the blood count. Clozapine has been said to provide an additional benefit of suppressing dyskinesias in advanced Parkinson disease (Bennett et al), but it requires weekly surveillance of the blood count because of the idiosyncratic occurrence of agranulocytosis in up to 2 percent of patients. Although useful in the treatment of frankly psychotic patients, these drugs tend to be far less effective once dementia has supervened. The anticonvulsant valproate is also said to be useful in this circumstance, but our experience with this drug has not been as favorable as with clozapine. Despite their lesser tendency to produce rigidity, olanzapine and probably the other similar agents in high doses eventually worsen motor disability.

The most common and troublesome effects of L-dopa, requiring individualization of therapy, are end-of-dose failure, the "on-off" phenomenon, and the induction of involuntary movements—restlessness, head wagging, grimacing, lingual-labial dyskinesia, and choreoathetosis and dystonia of the limbs, neck, and trunk. *The on-off phenomenon* refers to an unpredictable change in the patient, in a matter of minutes or from one hour to the next, from a state of relative mobility to one of complete or nearly complete immobility. These disorders eventually appear in about 75 percent of patients within 5 years. Above a certain daily dose, which varies from patient to patient, very few patients escape these effects, forcing a reduction in dosage.

If involuntary movements are induced by relatively small doses of L-dopa, the therapeutic effect may be enhanced to some extent by the addition of other dopaminergic agents, such as pergolide, bromocriptine, or the newer nonergot preparations, such as ropinirole and pramipexole (see below) and, to some extent, amantadine. The use of long-acting preparations of L-dopa may also be helpful in reducing dyskinesias, as mentioned above. *Amantadine*, an antiviral agent, is thought to act by releasing dopamine from striatal neurons; it also has an anticholinergic property. It is given in doses of 50 to 100 mg three times daily. Its benefit appears almost immediately but tends to be slight. In addition to anticholinergic symptoms (dry mouth, etc.), the side effects are similar to those of L-dopa but are much milder. Edema of the legs has been troublesome in some patients. However, amantadine is effective in combination with L-dopa and may reduce the dyskinesias and motor fluctuations associated with advanced disease (Verhagen Metman et al). Given alone or in combination with L-dopa, it offers a modest alternative treatment for patients with early Parkinson disease or those who are having untoward effects with standard doses of L-dopa.

The notion that the administration of L-dopa early in the disease might reduce the period over which it remains effective has been largely dispelled, but some experts continue to adhere to this idea. Cedarbaum et al, who reviewed the course of the illness in 307 patients over a 7-year period, found no evidence that the early initiation of L-dopa treatment predisposes to the development of motor response fluctuations, dyskinesia, and dementia. Also, the large multicenter study reported by Diamond et al indicated that patients who were given L-dopa early in the disease actually survived longer and with less disability than those who were started late.

Anticholinergic agents have long been in use and are still given occasionally, either in conjunction with L-dopa or to patients who cannot tolerate the latter drug. Several synthetic preparations are available, the most widely used being trihexyphenidyl (Artane) and benztropine mesylate (Cogentin) and amantadine (see above). When tremor is the most prominent symptom, we have had success with the related drug ethopropazine (Parsidol, Parsitan in Canada). In order to obtain maximum benefit from the use of these drugs, they should be given in gradually increasing dosage to the point where toxic effects appear: dryness of the mouth (which can be beneficial when drooling of saliva is a problem), blurring of vision from pupillary mydriasis (for which corrective glasses may be indicated), constipation, and sometimes urinary retention (especially with prostatism). Unfortunately, mental slowing, confusional states, hallucinations, and impairment of memory—especially in patients with already impaired mental function—are frequent side effects of these drugs and sharply limit their usefulness. Ethopropazine, 50 to 200 mg daily, is given in divided doses. We have effectively managed cases of isolated parkinsonian tremor in young patients using anticholinergic drugs alone. The optimum dosage level is the point at which the greatest relief from tremor is achieved within the limits of tolerable side effects. Occasionally, further benefit may accrue from the addition of one of the antihistaminic drugs, such as diphenhydramine or phenindamine. An important note of warning: anticholinergic agents or L-dopa should not be discontinued abruptly in advanced cases. If this is done, the patient may become totally immobilized by a sudden and severe increase of tremor and rigidity; rarely, a neuroleptic syndrome has been induced by such withdrawal.

Long-term treatment with L-dopa or dopamine receptor agonists has not prevented the slow advance of the disease. With progressive loss of nigral cells, there is an increasing inability to store L-dopa and periods of drug effectiveness become shorter. In some instances, the patient becomes so sensitive to L-dopa that as slight an excess as 50 to 100 mg will precipitate choreoathetosis; if the dose is lowered by the same amount, the patient may develop disabling rigidity. With the end-of-dose loss of effectiveness and on-off phenomenon, which with time become increasingly frequent and unpredictable, the patient may experience pain, respiratory distress, akathisia, depression, anxiety, and even hallucinations. Some patients function quite well in the morning and much less well in the afternoon, or vice versa. In such cases, and for end-of-dose and on-off phenomena, one must titrate the dose of L-dopa and utilize more frequent doses during the 24-h day; combining it with a dopamine agonist or use of the long-acting preparations may be helpful. Sometimes temporarily withdrawing L-dopa and at the same time substituting other medications will control the on-off phenomenon.

Based on the hypothesis that alimentary-derived amino acids antagonize the clinical effects of L-dopa, the use of a low-protein diet has been advocated as a means of controlling the motor fluctuations described above (Pincus and Barry). Symptoms can often be reduced by the simple expedient of eliminating dietary protein from breakfast and lunch. Moreover, this dietary regimen may permit the patient to reduce the total daily dose of L-dopa. Such dietary manipulation is worth trying in appropriate patients; it is not harmful, and most of our patients who have persisted with this diet have reported improvement in their symptoms or an enhanced effect of L-dopa.

Surgical Measures Until recently, success with L-dopa had practically replaced the use of ablative surgical therapy. The latter involves the stereotactic placement of lesions in either the globus pallidus, ventrolateral thalamus, or subthalamic nucleus, contralateral to the side of the body chiefly affected. The best results have been obtained in relatively young patients, in whom unilateral tremor or rigidity, rather than akinesia, are the predominant symptoms. The symptoms that have responded least well to operation (or to treatment with L-dopa) are postural imbalance and instability, paroxysmal akinesia, bladder and bowel disturbances, dystonia, and speech difficulties.

In the last decade, through the work of Laitinen and others, this mode of therapy has been revived and expanded. Under precise stereotactic control and with placement of a lesion in the posterior and ventral (medial) part of the globus pallidus, improvement of contralateral parkinsonian symptoms has been effected more reliably than in the past. Also, postoperatively, there is an enhanced responsiveness to L-dopa and a reduction of drug-induced dyskinesias, To what extent the improvement will be sustained remains to be determined, since the disease process continues to advance. In patients who have been studied for more than a few years, the beneficial effects on dyskinesias contralateral to the operation are sustained to some extent, but not in the ipsilateral limbs. The improvement in "off-state" bradykinesia is lost after 2 or so years and any betterment in axial rigidity and imbalance is lost in many patients within a year of operation, as summarized by Gregory and by Lang et al. In the only randomized trial to date that has compared pallidotomy to continued medical treatment of patients with dyskinesias, bradykinesia, or severe fluctuations in response to L-dopa, de Bie and colleagues demonstrated a clear improvement in motor function after surgery, while the group treated with medication continued to worsen. Using patient diaries, they estimated that dyskinesias were reduced 50 percent contralateral to the operated side and that parkinsonian symptoms during the "off phase" were improved by 30 to 50 percent. These improvements do not persist indefinitely and are in part due to the ability to reduce the dose of L-dopa. It should be mentioned that most groups have abandoned the pallidum as a surgical target in favor of the subthalamic nucleus.

Recently, through the use of implanted electrodes, the sites that are the targets of ablative procedures have been subjected to high-frequency stimulation—with virtually identical if not better results. In particular, high-frequency stimulation of the subthalamic nucleus has produced impressive improvement in all features of the disease (Limousin et al). Long-term studies are in progress to determine the persistence of these effects and their merits in comparison to ablative lesions.

The cerebral implantation of adrenal medullary tissue from 8- to 10-week-old human fetuses has provided a modest but undeniable improvement in motor function (Spencer et al), and some patients also appear to have benefited from the striatal implantation of human fetal and porcine nigral cells and autologous adrenal cells. These procedures are hampered by many difficulties, mainly in obtaining tissue and the failure of grafts to survive. Much of the original enthusiasm for these procedures has subsided, and it seems unlikely that they will have wide applicability in the treatment of Parkinson disease in the near future. Investigation into their possible usefulness continues.

Finally, in the management of the patient with Parkinson disease, one must not neglect the maintenance of optimum general health and neuromuscular efficiency by a planned program of exercise, activity, and rest; expert physical therapy and exercises such as those performed in yoga may be of help in achieving these ends. Sleep may be aided by the soporific antidepressants. Postural imbalance can be greatly mitigated by the use of a cane or walking frame. Hypotensive episodes respond to 0.5 mg of fludrocortisone (Florinef) each morning. In addition, the patient often needs much emotional support in dealing with the stress of the illness, in comprehending its nature, and in carrying on courageously in spite of it.

Striatonigral Degeneration and Multiple System Atrophy

Closely related to Parkinson disease clinically but with a different pathologic basis is a state designated by Adams and colleagues as *striatonigral degeneration*. The pathologic changes were found by chance in four middle-aged patients, none with a family history of similar disease, in three of whom a parkinsonian syndrome had been described clinically. In one of the three, who had been examined clinically, the typical rigidity, stiffness, and akinesia had begun on one side of the body, then spread to the other, and progressed over a 5-year period, but with little or none of the characteristic tremor of idiopathic Parkinson disease. A flexed posture of the trunk and limbs, slowness of all movements, poor balance, mumbling speech, and a tendency to faint when standing were other elements in the clinical picture. Mental function was intact, and there were no reflex changes, no suck and grasp reflexes, and no cerebellar signs or involuntary movements. The other two patients had been seen by competent neurologists who had made a diagnosis of Parkinson disease. Some of the symptoms had been partially relieved by anticholinergic drugs. There was an early-onset cerebellar ataxia in the fourth patient, later obscured by a Parkinson syndrome.

In each case the postmortem examination disclosed extensive loss of neurons in the zona compacta of the substantia nigra, but notably there were no Lewy bodies or neurofibrillary tangles in the remaining cells. Even more striking were the degenerative changes in the putamina and to a lesser extent in the caudate nuclei. These structures were greatly reduced in size and had lost most of their neurons—more of the small than the large ones and more on the side opposite the first clinical symptoms. The findings were suggestive of the striatal lesions of Huntington chorea except that the cell loss was greater in the putamen than in the caudatum. Secondary pallidal atrophy (mainly a loss of striatopallidal fibers) was present. In the fourth patient there was, in addition, an advanced olivopontocerebellar degeneration.

Following the original report, in 1964, many patients were recognized in whom the changes of striatonigral and olivopontocerebellar degeneration (page 1148) were combined and in some of whom the symptoms and signs of cerebellar ataxia actually preceded the parkinsonian manifestations. Equally frequent is a predominantly extrapyramidal syndrome accompanied by autonomic dysfunction, as described below.

Shy-Drager Syndrome Nearly half of the patients with striatonigral degeneration are handicapped by *orthostatic hypotension*, which proves at autopsy to be associated with loss of intermediolateral horn cells and pigmented nuclei of the brainstem. This combined parkinsonian and autonomic disorder, generally referred to as the Shy-Drager syndrome, has already been mentioned in the chapters on fainting and the autonomic nervous system (pages 396 and 564). In addition to orthostatic hypotension, symptoms include impotence, loss of sweating, dry mouth, miosis, and urinary retention or incontinence. Vocal cord palsy is an important and sometimes the initial manifestation of the autonomic disorder, causing dysphonia or even stridor and airway obstruction, and requiring tracheostomy (see page 565).

Multiple System Atrophy Because of the recognition that the clinical and pathologic features of sporadic striatonigral degeneration, with or without autonomic failure, and those of olivopontocerebellar atrophy often coexist, each component expressing itself variably in any individual, Graham and Oppenheimer, in 1969, proposed the term *multiple system atrophy* (MSA), which has gained wide acceptance. Several large series of cases of this complex syndrome have now been published, providing a perspective on the frequency and nature of its components.

In the Brain Tissue Bank of the Parkinson Disease Society of Great Britain, MSA accounted for 13 percent of cases that had been identified during life as idiopathic Parkinson disease. All of the patients with MSA had one or more symptoms of autonomic failure (postural hypotension, urinary urgency or retention, urinary or fecal incontinence, impotence, and dysphonia or stridor). Babinski signs were present in half of the patients and cerebellar ataxia in one-third. Tremor was rare. Males were affected more often than females.

In a series of 100 patients (67 men and 33 women) studied by Wenning and coworkers, the disease began with a striatonigral-parkinsonian syndrome in 46 percent; often it was asymmetrical to begin with. Mild tremor was detected in 29 percent, but in very few was it of the "resting" Parkinson type. In another 41 percent the illness began with autonomic manifestations; orthostatic hypotension occurred eventually in almost all patients, but it was disabling in only a few. Cerebellar features dominated the initial stages of the disease in only 5 percent, but ataxia was eventually obvious in half of the group. The illness, on the whole, was more severe than Parkinson disease, since more than 40 percent of patients were confined to a wheelchair or otherwise severely disabled within 5 years. These observations generally match the findings in a group of 188 patients described by Quinn and colleagues. In that series, parkinsonism was evident at some time in 89 percent of patients and was conjoined with cerebellar signs in half, pyramidal signs in 60 percent, and autonomic features in 77 percent. The other main presentation was with ataxia of gait, and this was accompanied by pyramidal signs in 69 percent; one-quarter of the patients had parkinsonism alone.

Colosimo and colleagues, who reviewed the clinical findings in 16 pathologically verified cases of multiple system atrophy, found that several signs—namely, the relative symmetry of the signs and rapid course, the lack of response to L-dopa and absence of tremor, and the presence of autonomic disorders—reliably distinguished this syndrome from Parkinson disease. These observations are in keeping with our own. It is noteworthy that levodopa has had little or no effect or has made these patients worse early in the disease. This is probably attributable to the loss of striatal dopamine receptors.

The diagnosis of MSA has been enhanced by imaging techniques. Both MRI and CT scans frequently show atrophy of the cerebellum and pons. The putamina are hypodense on T2-weighted MR images and may show an increased deposition of iron. Studies with PET have disclosed an impairment of glucose metabolism in the striatum and to a lesser extent in the frontal cortex—a reflection, no doubt, of the loss of functioning neuronal elements in these parts. Finally, it must be repeated that despite the frequent concurrence of striatonigral degeneration, olivopontocerebellar degeneration, and the Shy-Drager syndrome, *each of these disorders may occur in pure form*, for which reason we prefer to retain their original designations. Indeed, in a series of 51 patients with olivopontocerebellar atrophy followed by Gilman et al for up to 10 years, only 17 had acquired a parkinsonian syndrome or autonomic failure.

In recent years, attention has been drawn to the presence of argyrophilic staining material in glial cells of patients with the MSA complex and to its possible relevance in the pathogenesis of this syndrome. The abnormal staining material is most prominent in the cytoplasm of oligodendrocytes but is found in other glial cells and in neurons as well. These cytoplasmic aggregates have been referred to as "oligodendroglial cytoplasmic inclusions" (Papp et al), although morphologically they bear little resemblance to the discrete rounded inclusions that have come to be accepted as characteristic of other degenerative CNS diseases (e.g., Lewy bodies). It has been proposed that the glial accumulations of argyrophilic material represent a reliable histopathologic hallmark of sporadic cases of MSA (Chin and Goldman; Lantos). These aggregates, however, are far from specific; they have been identified in practically every degenerative disease that has been subjected to sensitive silver impregnation stains (Gallyas silver technique). Moreover, appropriate control studies to determine whether the argyrophilic glial inclusions are found in *nondegenerative* lesions in brain (at the edge of an infarct, for example) are lacking. Another serious deficiency is the lack of any systematic information about the argyrophilic staining properties of glia in relation to the aging brain. The fundamental question remains unanswered: Do the cytoplasmic glial aggregates play a central role in the genesis of the degenerative diseases, or are they simply some form of detritus that accumulates in glia as a reaction to or a by-product of the basic abnormality—namely, the wasting and loss of neurons?

Progressive Supranuclear Palsy

In 1963 Richardson, Steele, and Olszewski crystallized medical thought about a clinicopathologic entity—progressive supranuclear palsy, or PSP—to which there had been only ambiguous reference in the past. The condition is not rare or unusual. By 1972, when Steele reviewed the subject, 73 cases (22 with postmortem examinations) had been described in the medical literature, and several examples are to be found in every large neurologic center; the present authors encounter approximately five new cases yearly, most of them not previously diagnosed. Rare familial clusters have been described in which the pattern of inheritance is compatible with autosomal dominant transmission (Brown et al; de Yébenes et al). No toxic, encephalitic, racial, or geographic factor has been incriminated as a possible cause.

Clinical Features Characteristically the disease has its onset in the sixth decade (range 45 to 75 years) with some combination of difficulty in balance, abrupt falls, visual and ocular disturbances, slurred speech, dysphagia, and vague changes in personality, sometimes with an apprehensiveness and fretfulness suggestive of an agitated depression. The commonest early complaint is unsteadiness of gait and unexplained falling. At first the neurologic and ophthalmologic examinations may be unrevealing, and it may take a year or longer for the characteristic syndrome—comprising supranuclear ophthalmoplegia, pseudobulbar palsy, and axial dystonia—to develop fully.

Difficulty in voluntary vertical movement of the eyes, often downward but sometimes upward and involving voluntary saccades first, is a characteristic and relatively early feature in more than half of the cases. A related but more subtle sign has been the finding of hypometric saccades in response to an optokinetic drum or striped cloth moving vertically in one direction (usually best seen with stripes moving downward) compared to the saccades with the targets moving in the opposite direction or horizontally. Later, both the ocular pursuit and refixation movements deteriorate and eventually all voluntary eye movements are lost, first the vertical ones and then the horizontal ones as well. However, if the eyes are fixated on a target and the head is turned, full movements can be obtained, proving the supranuclear, nonparalytic character of the gaze disorder. Other prominent oculomotor signs are sudden jerks of the eyes during fixation, cogwheel pursuit movements, and hypometric saccades of long duration (Troost and Daroff). Bell's phenomenon (reflexive upturning of eyes on forced closure of the eyelids) and ability to converge are also lost, and the pupils then become small. The upper eyelids may be retracted, and the wide-eyed, unblinking stare, imparting an expression of perpetual surprise, is highly characteristic. Blepharospasm and involuntary eye closure are prominent in some cases. In the late stages, the eyes may be fixed centrally, and all oculocephalic and vestibular reflexes may be lost as well. It should be emphasized, however, that *a proportion of patients do not demonstrate these eye signs for a year or more* after the onset of the illness.

The *gait disturbance* and *repeated falling* have proved difficult to analyze. Walking becomes more and more awkward and tentative; the patient has a tendency to totter and fall repeatedly but has no ataxia of the limbs or Romberg sign. Some patients tend to lean and fall backward (retropulsion). One of our patients, a large man, fell repeatedly, wrecking household furniture as he went down, yet careful examination provided no clue as to the basic defect in this "toppling phenomenon."

Along with the oculomotor and balance disorders, there is a gradual stiffening and extension of the neck (in one of our cases it was sharply flexed), but this is not an invariable finding. The face acquires a staring, "worried" expression with a furrowed brow and staring demeanor, made more striking by the paucity of eye movements. A number of our patients have displayed mild dystonic postures of a hand or foot, especially as the illness advanced but occasionally early on. The limbs may be slightly stiff, with Babinski signs in a few cases.

The stiffness, slowness of movement, difficulty in turning and sitting down, and hypomimia may suggest a diagnosis of Parkinson disease. However, the facial expression of the PSP patient is more a matter of tonic grimace than of lack of movement, and the lack of tremor, erect rather than stooped posture, and prominence of oculomotor abnormalities also serve to distinguish the two disorders. The signs of pseudobulbar palsy are eventually prominent. The face becomes less expressive ("masked"), speech is slurred, the mouth tends to be held open, and swallowing is difficult. Forced laughing and crying, said to be infrequent, have been present in about half of our cases. Many patients complain of sleep disturbances. The total sleep time and rapid-eye-movement (REM) sleep are reduced, and spontaneous awakenings during the night are more frequent and longer than in normal individuals of the same age. Features such as focal limb dystonia, palilalia, myoclonus, chorea, orofacial dyskinesias, and disturbances of vestibular function are observed in some cases. Finally the patient becomes anarthric, immobile, and quite helpless. Some patients do eventually become forgetful and appear apathetic and slow in thinking; a few are irritable and at times euphoric. Complaints of urinary frequency and urgency are very frequent in advanced cases. Dementia of some degree is probably present in many cases but is mild in most.

By MRI, one can, in advanced cases, visualize the atrophy of the mesencephalon (superior colliculi, red nuclei) giving rise to a "mouse ears" configuration. The CSF remains normal.

Although most cases of PSP are sporadic, the disease can be familial. Rojo and coworkers have described 12 pathologically confirmed pedigrees. The mode of inheritance is thought to be autosomal dominant with incomplete penetrance. The authors made note of the variable phenotypical expression of the disease even within a single pedigree.

Postmortem examinations have disclosed a bilateral loss of neurons and gliosis in the periaqueductal gray matter, superior colliculus, subthalamic nucleus of Luys, red nucleus, pallidum, dentate nucleus, and pretectal and vestibular nuclei, and to some extent in the oculomotor nucleus. The neurons of the cerebral cortex have been involved in some cases (shown by staining of tau protein), but these changes apparently do not correlate with dementia. The cerebellar cortex is usually spared. Loss of the medullated fiber bundles arising from these nuclear structures has been observed. A remarkable finding has been the neurofibrillary degeneration of many of the residual neurons. The neurofibrillary tangles are thick and often composed of single strands, either twisted or in parallel arrangement. We have followed several patients who had no disorder of eye movement during life but in whom the typical pathologic changes of PSP were found unexpectedly. In one such case there was a subcortical type of dementia, and in another, focal limb dystonia and parkinsonism.

The cause and nature of this disease are quite obscure. Attempts to transmit it to primates by the inoculation of fresh brain tissue have failed. Conceivably, some cases originally considered to be instances of postencephalitic parkinsonism were examples of PSP. Studies with PET have demonstrated a decrease in blood flow—most marked in the frontal lobes—and a lesser extent of oxygen utilization in central structures (Leenders et al). Striatal dopamine formation and storage have been significantly decreased compared with control values.

Progressive supranuclear palsy should be suspected whenever an older adult inexplicably develops a state of imbalance, frequent falls with preserved consciousness, and variable extrapyramidal symptoms, particularly dystonia of the neck, ocular palsies, or a picture resembling pseudobulbar palsy. When only a parkinsonian syndrome without tremor is present, the main diagnostic consideration is striatonigral degeneration or the cortical-basal-ganglionic syndrome, described below.

L-Dopa has been of slight but unsustained benefit in some of our patients, and combinations of L-dopa and anticholinergic drugs have been entirely ineffective in others. A marked response to these drugs should, of course, suggest the diagnosis of Parkinson disease. Recently, the drug zolpidem, a GABAergic agonist of benzodiazepine receptors, has been reported to ameliorate the akinesia and rigidity of PSP (Daniele et al); however, these observations require corroboration.

Cortical-Basal-Ganglionic Syndromes

Over the years, the authors have observed several elderly patients, both men and women, in whom the essential abnormality was a progressive extrapyramidal rigidity, combined with signs of corticospinal disease. Sometimes a mild postural action tremor (beginning unilaterally and suggestive in some respects of Parkinson disease) was added. The relation of such cases to corticostriatospinal degeneration, described earlier, is indeterminate. The patients, though able to exert considerable muscle power, cannot effectively direct their voluntary actions. Attempts to move a limb to accomplish some purposeful act might result in a totally inappropriate movement, always with great enhancement of rigidity in the limb and in other affected parts, or the limb may drift off and assume an odd posture, such as a persistent elevation of the arm without the patient's awareness—a kind of involuntary catalepsy. The disorder of limb function has some of the attributes of an apraxia, but the hand postures, involuntary movements, and changes in tone are at times more reminiscent of what has been described as "the alien hand." Some patients exhibit an anosognosia.

With progression of the disease, the limbs—first on one side, then on both sides of the body—and the cranial muscles become involved; apraxia and variable combinations of rigidity, bradykinesia, hemiparesis, sensory ataxia, and postural and action tremor and sometimes myoclonic jerking finally render the patient helpless—unable to sit, stand, speak, or take care of his basic needs. Apraxias of gaze, eyelid opening and closure, and stimulus-sensitive myoclonus appear in some cases. Mental deterioration occurs late and only in some cases. In a few cases, there is some involvement of lower motor neurons with resulting amyotrophy. The condition progresses for 5 years or more before some medical complication overtakes the patient. Wenning and colleagues have described a series of 14 such patients in whom the diagnosis was confirmed at postmortem examination. The most common early symptom was an asymmetrical clumsiness of the limbs, in half of the patients with rigidity and in one-fifth with tremor; as the illness progressed, almost all the patients developed an asymmetrical or unilateral akinetic-rigid syndrome, various forms of gait disorder, and dysarthria. Stimulus-induced myoclonus and pyramidal signs, mentioned in other reports, were not prominent, and fewer than half the patients exhibited an alien-hand phenomenon; limitations of vertical gaze and frontal lobe release signs eventually became apparent in half of the patients.

Postmortem examination of several of our cases, reported by Rebeiz and colleagues, has disclosed a combination of findings that stamps the disease process as unique. Cortical atrophy (mainly in the frontal motor-premotor and anterior parietal lobes) is associated with degeneration of the substantia nigra and, in one instance, of the dentatorubrothalamic fibers. The loss of nerve cells is fairly marked, but there is no gross lobar atrophy, as occurs in Pick disease. The neuronal degeneration may be more on one side than the other. There is moderate gliosis in the cortex and underlying white matter. Many of the residual nerve cells are swollen and chromatolyzed with eccentric nuclei, a state that was called *achromasia* by Rebeiz and colleagues; it resembles the central chromatolysis of axonal reaction. More recently, the affected neurons and adjacent glia have been shown to be filled with tau protein, but no Pick bodies, Alzheimer fibrillary changes, senile plaques, granulovacuolar changes, amyloid deposits, or Lewy bodies are seen. Both CT and MRI have demonstrated asymmetrical cerebral and pontine atrophy, and PET studies have shown thalamoparietal metabolic asymmetries—a greater reduction of glucose metabolism on the side of the most extensive lesion (Riley et al).

Many investigators have searched unsuccessfully for clues as to the cause and pathogenesis of this disease. There is no family history. No organ other than the CNS is affected. The progression is relentless. None of the drugs in common use for spasticity, rigidity, and tremor has been helpful. We know of no attempt to transfer the disease to primates.

Marinescu has described a rather different state resembling more a severe form of Alzheimer disease, but with signs of both pyramidal and extrapyramidal disease (rigidity, tremor, nystagmus, incoordination, confusion, disorientation, and loss of memory). There was amyloidosis of blood vessels (so-called Scholz's perivascular plaques) in the cerebral white matter as well as in the liver and kidney. The disease bears some resemblance to the corticostriatospinal degeneration ("spastic pseudosclerosis") of Jakob discussed on page 1126. The relation of this disease to the corticopallidospinal and the pallidopyramidal syndromes first described by Davison (1932, 1954) is also uncertain. The features of eight such cases ("pallido-pyramidal" syndrome) have more recently been summarized by Tranchant and associates.

Dystonic Disorders

Dystonia Musculorum Deformans (Torsion Dystonia) Dystonia as a symptom has been discussed on pages 79 and 112. Here we are concerned with a disease or diseases of which dystonia is the major manifestation. Schwalbe's account, in 1908, of three siblings of a Jewish family who were afflicted with progressive involuntary movements of trunk and limbs probably represents the first description of the disease. In 1911, Oppenheim contributed other cases and coined the term *dystonia musculorum deformans* in the mistaken belief that the disorder was primarily one of muscle and always associated with deformity. Flatau and Sterling, in the same year, first suggested that the disease might have a hereditary basis and gave it the more accurate name *torsion dystonia of childhood.* At first thought to be a manifestation of hysteria, it gradually came to be established as a morbid entity with a preference for Russian and Polish Jews. Soon thereafter, a second hereditary form of torsion dystonia, affecting non-Jews, was defined. The epidemiologic study of Eldridge, who analyzed all reported primary cases up to 1970, revealed two patterns of inheritance, one autosomal recessive, the other dominant. The recessive form begins in early childhood, is progressive over a few years, and is restricted to Jewish patients with normal and often even superior intelligence. The dominant form begins later, usually in late childhood and adolescence, progresses more slowly, and is not limited to any ethnic group.

With widening clinical experience, the spectrum of dystonic syndromes has been greatly expanded to include an array of hereditary and nonhereditary forms, both generalized and restricted, as well as symptomatic (secondary) types due to vascular, metabolic (Wilson and Hallervorden-Spatz disease), and other degenerative forms (Huntington chorea among many others.)

As indicated in Chap. 6, most instances of idiopathic (primary) dystonias that come to our attention, particularly the segmental or restricted types, do not conform to the classic hereditary types as defined above. In general, these more restricted types have a later onset and a relatively milder, more slowly progressive course, with a tendency to involve the axial or the distal musculature alone; only the paravertebral, cervical, or cranial muscles may be involved (focal dystonia including torticollis and writer's cramp), with little change from year to year. The clinical classification of the predominantly adult-onset dystonias is made more complex by the fact that both the restricted and generalized forms may be sporadic or familial in type. Bressman et al, for example, have described a restricted (cervicocranial) adult-onset form of dystonia in four generations of a non-Jewish family. The symptomatology included cervical dystonia, facial grimacing, dysarthria, and dysphonia. In one of our familial cases, a dystonia of the foot appeared during adolescence and later disappeared; we have also observed this to happen in spasmodic torticollis, which is another form of restricted or segmental dystonia, described further on.

In a survey of idiopathic torsion dystonia in the United Kingdom by Fletcher and associates, both generalized and restricted varieties were included. The investigators concluded that approximately 85 percent of these cases were due to an autosomal dominant gene of low penetrance and that a small proportion represented new mutations. They could not confirm the existence of autosomal recessive or X-linked patterns of inheritance in their patients. The risk of the disease in a first-degree relative of a familial case is about 25 percent.

Molecular genetic studies, though still incomplete, hold the promise of clarifying the classification of the heritable dystonias (see Korf). An abnormal gene (DYT1), which codes for the protein torsin A, has been mapped to the long arm of chromosome 9q in both Jewish and non-Jewish families and is inherited in an autosomal dominant pattern. This gene probably accounts for the majority of inherited cases of generalized dystonia. Although the penetrance of the clinical trait in these families is low, PET scanning demonstrates hypermetabolism in the cerebellum, lenticular nuclei, and supplementary motor cortex in all carriers of the mutated gene. German Mennonite families with restricted adult-onset dystonia (torticollis and spasmodic dysphonia) have a mutation at 18p, and an X-chromosome mutation has also been described. The unique dopa-responsive dystonia, described below, has been mapped to chromosome 14q (Nygaard et al).

The relationship of the childhood and adolescent inherited varieties of generalized dystonia to the more common sporadic and restricted dystonias has not been settled, but a few individuals in affected families demonstrate only the most localized forms (e.g., writer's cramp), arising in adulthood. The general rule stated above, however, still holds—namely, that the inherited variety that is tied to chromosome 9q begins early in life in one limb, followed by generalization of the dystonic movements, while in other types, some of which are heritable and some not, the craniocervical or another region is affected early and the condition does not spread.

Clinical Features The first manifestations of the idiopathic generalized disease may be rather subtle. The patient (usually a child between 6 and 14 years of age, less often an adolescent) begins intermittently and usually after activity (late in the day) to invert one foot, to extend one leg and foot in an unnatural way, or to hunch one shoulder, raising the question of a nervous tic. As time passes, however, the motor peculiarity becomes more persistent and interferes increasingly with the patient's activities. Soon the muscles of the spine and shoulder or pelvic girdles become implicated in involuntary spasmodic twisting movements. The spasms are intermittent at first, and in free intervals muscular tone and volitional movements are normal. Indeed, in some instances the muscles are hypotonic. Gradually the spasms become more frequent; finally they are continuous, and the body may become grotesquely contorted. Lateral and rotatory scoliosis are regular secondary deformities. For a time recumbency relieves the spasms, but later position has no influence. The hands are seldom involved, though at times they may be fisted. Cranial muscles do not escape, and in a few instances a slurring, staccato-type speech has even been the initial manifestation. Uncontrollable blepharospasm was the initial disorder in one of our cases; in two others, severe dysarthria and dysphagia were the first signs of the disease, caused by dystonia of the tongue, pharyngeal, and laryngeal muscles. Other manifestations of the movement disorder include torticollis, tortipelvis, dromedary gait, propulsive gait, action tremor, myoclonic jerks during voluntary movement, and mild choreoathetosis of the limbs. Excitement worsens the condition and sleep abolishes it; but as the years pass the postural distortion may become fixed to the point where it does not disappear even in sleep. Tendon reflexes are at all times normal; corticospinal signs are absent; there is no ataxia, sensory abnormality, convulsive disorder, or dementia. Several subgroups have been defined—one type is responsive to L-dopa, another is sex-linked (in the Philippines), and others are associated with parkinsonian symptoms or myoclonus.

Pathology No agreement has been reached concerning the pathologic substrate of the disease. In several reported cases the ferrocalcinosis of Hallervorden-Spatz disease, the lesions of Wilson disease or of kernicterus, the état marbré of neonatal hypoxia, or the CT lucencies of familial striatal necrosis were observed in the basal ganglia. Obviously in these cases the dystonia was symptomatic of another disease. However, in the hereditary forms, which are the subject of this section, one cannot be certain of any specific lesions that would account for the clinical manifestations. The brain is grossly normal, and the ventricular size is not increased. According to Zeman, who reviewed all the reported autopsy studies up to 1970, there are no significant changes in the striatum, pallidum, or elsewhere. This does not mean that there are no lesions, only that the techniques being used (qualitative analysis of random sections by light microscopy) are inadequate for their demonstration. Newer methods of identification of striatal cell types have probably not been adequately utilized. Dopamine β-hydroxylase is elevated in the plasma of patients with the autosomal dominant form of the disease and the plasma norepinephrine levels are also raised, but the meaning of these findings is not clear; PET scan changes have already been mentioned.

Treatment Early in the course of the illness, several drugs—including L-dopa, bromocriptine, carbamazepine, diazepam, and tetrabenazine—seem to be helpful, but only in a few patients, and the benefit is not lasting. Intrathecal baclofen has been somewhat more successful in children. The rare hereditary form of dystonia-parkinsonism (described below) responds well to small doses of L-dopa and dopamine agonists and is exceptional in this respect. Burke and coworkers advocate the use of very high doses (30 mg daily or more) of trihexyphenidyl (Artane). Apparently dystonic children can tolerate these high doses if they are raised gradually, by 5-mg increments weekly. In adults, high-dose anticholinergic treatment is less successful but worthy of a trial. Clonazepam is beneficial in some patients with segmental myoclonus. The most impressive results have been obtained by the use of stereotactic techniques to make lesions that are centered in the ventrolateral nuclei of the thalamus or in the pallidum–ansa lenticularis region. Some frightfully deformed children, unable to sit or stand, have been restored to near normalcy for a time. Approximately 70 percent of the patients in Cooper's series were moderately to markedly improved by unilateral or bilateral operations, and, based on a 20-year follow-up study, the improvement was usually sustained. More recent studies have reported a somewhat less favorable but nonetheless clear-cut improvement (Tasker et al; Andrew et al). The main risk of operation has been a corticospinal tract lesion, produced inadvertently by damaging the internal capsule.

Hereditary Dystonia-Parkinsonism (Segawa Syndrome, Dopa-Responsive Dystonia) Following the description of this disease by Segawa and colleagues in 1976, several other reports have drawn attention to this unique form of hereditary dystonia (Allen and Knopp; Deonna; Nygaard and Duvoisin). The pattern of inheritance in this disease is probably autosomal dominant, and there is no ethnic predilection. Nygaard and colleagues have found a linkage to chromosome 14q. The dystonic manifestations become evident in childhood, usually between 4 and 8 years of age; females outnumber males in a ratio of 3:2. Often the legs are first affected by intermittent stiffening, with frequent falls and peculiar posturing, sometimes assuming an equinovarus position. The arms become involved as well as the truncal muscles; retrocollis or torticollis may appear. Within 4 to 5 years, all parts of the body including the bulbar muscles are involved. Sometimes parkinsonian features (rigidity, bradykinesia, postural instability) can be detected early in the course of the illness, but characteristically they are added to the clinical picture several years later. Among our own patients and in those of Deonna, there was in some instances a rigidity of the limbs as well as slowness of movement and tremor at rest, all aspects more parkinsonian than dystonic. In still others, the clinical picture has been one of cerebral spastic diplegia. Usually the symptoms disappear after a period of sleep and worsen as the day progresses. This diurnal variation has been a notable feature in some but not all cases. Fluctuations of symptoms with exercise and menses and in the first month of pregnancy are features of some cases.

In one autopsied case, there was a reduction in the amount of tyrosine hydroxylase in the striatum and depigmentation but no cell loss in the substantia nigra (Rajput et al). The enzyme was also reduced in the striatum, as was the level of dopamine.

The unique feature of this *juvenile dystonia-parkinsonism syndrome*, as it has been called, is the dramatic response of both the dystonic and parkinsonian symptoms to treatment with L-dopa. As little as 10 mg/kg per day may eliminate the movement disorder and permit normal functioning. In this condition, unlike Parkinson disease, the medication can be continued indefinitely without the development of tolerance or wearing-off effects. Segawa disease accounts for some cases that had been reported in the past as juvenile Parkinson disease.

Torticollis and Other Restricted Dyskinesias and Dystonias With advancing age, a large variety of degenerative movement disorders come to light. Supposedly there is loss of neurons in certain parts of the basal ganglia, but this has not been verified by appropriate pathologic studies. Groups of muscles begin to manifest arrhythmic involuntary spasms. The patient's inability to suppress the dystonia and the recognition that it is for the most part beyond voluntary control distinguishes it from the common tics, habit spasms, and mannerisms described in Chap. 6. If the muscle contraction is frequent and prolonged, it is accompanied by an aching pain that may mistakenly be blamed for the spasm and the involved muscle may gradually undergo hypertrophy. Worsening under conditions of excitement and stress and improvement during quiet and relaxation are typical of this group of disorders and contributed in the past to the mistaken notion that the spasms had a psychogenic origin.

The most frequent and familiar type is *torticollis*, wherein an adult, more often a woman, becomes aware of a turning of the head to one side while walking. Usually this condition worsens gradually to a point where it may be more or less continuous, but in some patients it remains mild for years on end. When followed over the years, the condition is observed to remain limited to the same muscles (mainly the scalene, sternocleidomastoid, and upper trapezius). Occasionally torticollis is combined with dystonia of the arm and trunk, tremor, facial spasms, or dystonic writer's cramp.

Other restricted dyskinesias involve the neck in combination with facial muscles, the orbicularis oculi (*blepharospasm* and *blepharoclonus*), the throat and respiratory muscles ("*spastic dysphonia*," *orofacial dyskinesia*, and *respiratory* and *phonatory spasms*), the hand as in writer's cramp (*graphospasm*) or musician's dystonia, and proximal leg and pelvic girdle muscles, where dyskinesia is elicited by walking. *All these conditions and their treatment are discussed fully in Chap. 6.*

Other Forms of Hereditary Dystonia Several familial movement-induced (kinesogenic) dystonic syndromes and a type that is not kinesogenic and arises suddenly in adolescence, at times with parkinsonian features, have been described (see page 83). There are other degenerative diseases that combine hereditary dystonia with neural deafness and intellectual impairment (Scribanu and Kennedy) and with amyotrophy in a paraplegic distribution (Gilman and Romanul).

Two other important diseases that fall into the category of hereditary dystonia have been described in Chap. 37. These are Hallervorden-Spatz disease and calcification of the basal ganglia—and, of course, Wilson disease may have dystonia as a central feature.

SYNDROME OF PROGRESSIVE ATAXIA

This topic was introduced in Chap. 5, and some of the congenital and acute acquired varieties are mentioned on pages 1010, 1021, and 1197. Here we consider only the *chronic progressive forms of cerebellar disease*, many of which are familial and which are more or less confined to this part of the nervous system, although a number of other systems may be involved to a varying degree. Many of these diseases are so chronic that one would expect a close correspondence between their symptomatology and anatomic pathology, yet attempts to determine these relationships have generally been disappointing. Traditionally, the classic examples of chronic progressive cerebellar disease are subsumed under the system atrophies, but no one classification designed to bring precise order to these diseases has proved entirely satisfactory. Wilson wrote that "The group of degenerative conditions strung together by the common feature of ataxia is one for which no very suitable classification has yet been devised"—a statement that is as appropriate today as when it was written almost 60 years ago. Even recent insights provided by the tools of molecular genetics have not fully resolved the problem of classification, mainly because a single gene abnormality may be expressed by a number of different phenotypic syndromes.

Nevertheless, largely through the clinical and pathologic studies of Greenfield and the subsequent studies of Harding, a semblance of order has been brought to the classification of the hereditary ataxias. The classification proposed by Harding represents the most thorough and scholarly effort to meet this goal. Setting aside those of congenital type and those with an underlying metabolic disorder, she has grouped them by age of onset, pattern of heredity, and associated features. A modification of the classifications of Greenfield and of Harding, which is included in the introductory classification of the degenerative diseases (page 1108), is used here. It divides the progressive cerebellar ataxias into three groups—the spinocerebellar ataxias, with unmistakable involvement of the spinal cord (Romberg sign, sensory loss, diminished tendon reflexes, Babinski signs); the pure cerebellar ataxias, with no other associated neurologic disorders; and the complicated cerebellar ataxias, with a variety of retinal, optic nerve, oculomotor, auditory, pyramidal, extrapyramidal, peripheral nerve, and cerebrocortical accompaniments. Inherited ataxias of early onset (before the age of 20 years) are usually of autosomal recessive type; those of later onset may be autosomal recessive but are usually autosomal dominant.

In the approach to a patient with a heritable ataxia, we find such a classification—based on well-established clinical and pathologic features and patterns of mendelian inheritance—to be the most useful. The molecular genetic revolution of recent years is transforming our understanding of the inherited ataxias and has already disclosed a large number of unexpected relationships between specific genetic defects and other neural and nonneural disorders. These data are incorporated at appropriate points in the following discussion and are summarized at the end of the section.

Early-Onset Spinocerebellar Ataxias (Predominantly Spinal)

Friedreich Ataxia This is the prototype of all forms of progressive spinocerebellar ataxia and accounts for about half of all cases of hereditary ataxia in most large series (86 of 171 cases in Sjögren's series). Friedreich, of Heidelberg, began in 1861 to report on a form of familial progressive ataxia that he had observed among nearby villagers. It was already known through the writings of Duchenne in Paris that locomotor ataxia was the prominent feature of spinal cord syphilis, i.e., tabes dorsalis, and it was Friedreich who demonstrated that a nonsyphilitic hereditary type also existed. This concept was greeted with some skepticism, but soon Duchenne himself affirmed the existence of the new disease and other case reports appeared in England, France, and the United States. In 1882, in a thesis on this subject by Brousse of Montpelier, Friedreich's name was attached to the new entity.

As new cases appeared, it was noted that in about half of them the disease had its onset before the tenth year and sometimes as early as the second or third; Mollaret could find no examples with onset after the age of 25 years. The disease is invariably and steadily progressive; within 5 years of onset, walking is no longer possible in many cases. Genetic linkage studies of 22 families with three or more affected siblings have led to the assignment of the gene mutation to chromosome 9q13-2 (Chamberlain et al). A form of Friedreich ataxia of later onset (between 20 and 30 years) and slower progression has been recorded (DeMichele et al). The gene abnormality, like that of the more classic Friedreich ataxia, is also in the centromeric region of chromosome 9. The gene error related to the chromosome 9 mutation is an expanded repetition of the trinucleotide GAA that codes for a protein called *frataxin*. The current hypothesis is that frataxin is a mitochondrium-associated protein and that the cellular dysfunction is in some way the result of a failure of energy metabolism. Clinical and neuropathologic phenotypes in Friedreich ataxia are associated with diminution or absence of frataxin. Thus despite the variability of the clinical picture, current evidence favors a single gene locus for the disease. The incidence rate among Europeans and North Americans is 1.5 per 100,000 per year.

Clinical Features Ataxia of gait is nearly always the initial symptom. Occasionally the ataxia begins rather abruptly after a febrile illness, and one leg may become clumsy before the other. This "hemiplegic" pattern is exceptional; usually both legs are affected simultaneously. Difficulty in standing steadily and in running are early symptoms, and Wilson has commented on fatigability, leg pains, and postexertional cramps—symptoms that we have seldom elicited. The hands usually become clumsy months or years after the gait disorder, and dysarthric speech appears after the arms are involved (rarely is this an early symptom).

In some patients, pes cavus and kyphoscoliosis precede the neurologic symptoms; in others, they follow by several years. The characteristic foot deformity takes the form of a high plantar arch with retraction of the toes at the metatarsophalangeal joints and flexion at the interphalangeal joints (hammer toes).

A cardiomyopathy is demonstrable in more than half of the patients. The myocardial fibers are hypertrophic and may contain iron-reactive granules (Koeppen). Many of the patients die as a result of cardiac arrhythmia or congestive failure. Kyphoscoliosis and restricted respiratory function are also important contributory causes of death. Harding observed that about 10 percent of these patients have diabetes mellitus and a similar percentage have impaired glucose tolerance.

In the fully developed state, the abnormality of gait is of mixed sensory and cerebellar type, aptly called *tabetocerebellar* by Charcot. According to Mollaret, the author of an authoritative monograph on this disease, the cerebellar component predominates, but in our relatively small series we have been impressed almost as much with the sensory (tabetic) aspect. The patient stands with feet wide apart, constantly shifting position to maintain balance. Friedreich referred to the constant teetering and swaying on standing as static ataxia. In walking, as with all sensory ataxias, the movements of the legs tend to be brusque, the feet resounding unevenly and irregularly as they strike the floor. Closure of the eyes causes the patient to fall (Romberg sign). This reflects the spinal component (posterior columns). Attempts to correct the imbalance may result in abrupt, wild movements. Often there is a rhythmic tremor of the head. The arms are grossly ataxic, and both action and intention tremors are manifest. Speech is slow, slurred, explosive, and finally almost incomprehensible. Breathing, speaking, swallowing, and laughing may be so incoordinate that the patient nearly chokes while speaking. Holmes remarked upon an ataxia of respiration that causes "curious short inspiratory whoops." Facial, buccal, and arm muscles may display tremulous and sometimes choreiform movements.

Mentation has been preserved in all of our patients. However, emotional lability has been sufficiently prominent to provoke comment by others. Horizontal nystagmus may be present in the primary position and is increased on lateral gaze. Rotatory and vertical nystagmus are rare. Deafness has been recorded, along with vertigo and, more rarely, with inexcitability of the labyrinths and blindness with optic atrophy. Ocular movements usually remain full, and pupillary reflexes are normal. The facial muscles may seem slightly weak, and deglutition may become impaired. Amyotrophy occurs late in the illness and is usually slight, but it may be extreme in patients with an associated neuropathy (see below). The tendon reflexes are abolished in nearly every case; rarely, they may be obtainable when the patient is examined early in the illness. Plantar reflexes are extensor, and flexor spasms may occur even with complete absence of tendon reflexes, indicating that the areflexia is sensory in origin. The abdominal reflexes are usually retained until late in the illness. Loss of vibratory and position sense is invariable from the beginning; later, there may be some diminution of tactile, pain, and temperature sensation as well. Sphincter control is usually preserved.

In one important *variant of Friedreich ataxia* the tendon reflexes are preserved or even hyperactive and the limbs may be spastic. Some of these cases are associated with hypogonadism. The finding of the aberrant gene in these cases on chromosome 9 links them to Friedreich ataxia. Harding found 20 such cases among her 200 familial ataxias at the National Hospital, London. Nevertheless, the distinction between classic Friedreich ataxia and ataxia with retained tendon reflexes is an important one clinically, insofar as kyphoscoliosis and heart disease do not occur in the latter group and the prognosis is better. In other cases, some familial, a spastic paraparesis and optic atrophy are combined with ataxia (Behr). We would also include here cases of the type described by Hogan and Bauman, in which a progressive cerebellar ataxia was associated with spasticity and other corticospinal tract signs of the legs. Cerebellar atrophy has not been a prominent feature of these cases, and we would adopt the position that they are forms of spinocerebellar degeneration that are transitional between Friedreich ataxia and some of the other heredoataxias with cerebellar atrophy. In the few autopsied cases, the main abnormality has been in the spinal cord and the spinocerebellar (cerebellopetal) tracts, but some in addition show corticospinal tract degeneration.

Other abortive and atypical forms are numerous. Peroneal muscular atrophy is sometimes associated with Friedreich ataxia, as is true of the areflexic dystasia (sensory neuropathy) of Roussy and Levy. These disorders are discussed with the hereditary neuropathies on page 1420. Hereditary forms of optic atrophy, retinitis pigmentosa, deafness, and myoclonus are occasionally combined with Friedreich ataxia as well, but we agree with Skre that they probably represent genetically independent entities. Two of our Friedreich patients had occasional seizures.

Laboratory tests of diagnostic value are sensory nerve conduction velocities and amplitudes, electrocardiography, and chest and spine films (to show heart size and kyphoscoliosis). The CT scans and MRI seldom show a significant degree of cerebellar atrophy; the spinal cord is small, and there is no consistent abnormality of blood or CSF. Visual evoked potentials are abnormal only in patients with associated optic atrophy.

Pathology The spinal cord is thin. The posterior columns and the corticospinal and spinocerebellar tracts are all depleted of medullated fibers, and there is a fibrous gliosis that does not replace the bulk of the lost fibers. The nerve cells in Clarke's column and the large neurons of the dorsal root ganglia, especially lumbosacral ones, are reduced in number—but perhaps not to a degree that would fully explain the posterior column degeneration. The posterior roots are thin. Betz cells are also diminished in some cases, but the corticospinal tracts are relatively intact down to the medullary-cervical junction. Beyond this point, the corticospinal tracts are degenerated, but to a lesser degree than the posterior columns. The nuclei of cranial nerves VIII, X, and XII all exhibit a reduction of cells. Slight to moderate neuronal loss is seen also in the dentate nuclei, and the middle and superior cerebellar peduncles are reduced in size. Some depletion of Purkinje cells in the superior vermis and neurons in corresponding parts of the inferior olivary nuclei can be seen.

Many of the myocardial muscle fibers degenerate and are replaced by fibrous connective tissue. No consistent biochemical abnormalities have been demonstrated.

By way of exploring the anatomic basis of the clinical findings, pes cavus is not different from that seen in other diseases with mild hypertonus of the long extensors and flexors of the feet and in the early-onset hereditary polyneuropathies. These also cause amyotrophy of intrinsic foot muscles when the bones of the feet are still malleable. The kyphoscoliosis is probably due to imbalance of the paravertebral muscles. The tabetic aspects of the disease are explained by the degeneration of large cells in the dorsal root ganglia and the large sensory fibers in nerves, dorsal roots, and the columns of Goll and Burdach. The loss of large neurons in the sensory ganglia also causes abolition of tendon reflexes. The cerebellar ataxia is attributable to a degeneration of the spinocerebellar tracts, the superior vermis, and the dentatorubral pathways in various combinations. Corticospinal lesions account for the weakness and Babinski signs and the pes cavus as well.

Diagnosis Friedreich disease and its variants must be distinguished from the familial cerebellar cortical atrophy, described next, and familial spastic paraparesis with ataxia, as well as from peroneal muscular atrophy and the Levy-Roussy syndrome, which are discussed with the hereditary neuropathies in Chap. 46. Vitamin E deficiency causes a spinocerebellar syndrome with areflexia in children, as detailed in Chap. 41, but it is distinguishable from Friedreich ataxia by the absence of dysarthria and skeletal or cardiac abnormalities. A form of chronic inflammatory demyelinating polyneuropathy has long overtaken tabes dorsalis as the most frequent type of areflexic ataxia; it bears a superficial resemblance to Friedreich ataxia when its onset is in childhood but lacks cerebellar dysarthria and Babinski signs. In late-onset cases, a form of spinocerebellar degeneration related to human T-cell lymphotrophic virus type I (HTLV-I), causing so-called tropical spastic paraparesis as well as the vacuolar myelopathy of AIDS, also needs to be included in the differential diagnosis.

Treatment In a double-blind crossover study by Trouillas and associates, the administration of oral 5-hydroxytryptophan was found to significantly modify the cerebellar symptoms. This drug is serotoninergic and is known to suppress posthypoxic action myoclonus. Apart from this form of treatment, with which we have had no experience, no therapeutic measures are known to alter the course of the neurologic disease. Heart failure, arrhythmias, and diabetes mellitus are treated by the usual means. Surgery for scoliosis and foot deformities may be helpful in selected cases.

Predominantly Cerebellar (Cortical) Forms of Hereditary Ataxia

Soon after the publication of Friedreich's descriptions of a spinal type of hereditary ataxia, reports began to appear of somewhat different diseases in which the ataxia was related to degenerative changes in the cerebellum and brainstem rather than the spinal cord. Claims of their independence from the spinal type were based largely on a later age of onset, a more definite hereditary transmission—usually of autosomal dominant type, the persistence or hyperactivity of tendon reflexes, and the more frequent concurrence of ophthalmoplegia, retinal degeneration, and optic atrophy. Several of these clinical features, particularly briskness of tendon reflexes, are alien to the classic form of Friedreich ataxia.

By 1893 Pierre Marie thought it desirable to create a new category of hereditary ataxia that would embrace all of the non-Friedreich cases. He collated the familial cases of progressive ataxia that had been described by Fraser, Nonne, Sanger Brown, and Klippel and Durante (see Greenfield and Harding for references) and proposed that all of them were examples of an entity to which he applied the name *heredoataxie cerebelleuse*. Marie's proposition was based almost entirely on clinical observations—not his own but those made by the aforementioned authors. Later, as members of these families died, postmortem examinations disclosed that Marie's hereditary cerebellar ataxia included not one but several disease entities. Indeed, as pointed out by Holmes (1907) and later by Greenfield, in three of the four families the cerebellum showed no significant lesions at all. Yet there was by then no doubt of a separate class of predominantly cerebellar atrophies, some purely cortical and others associated with a variety of noncerebellar lesions.

Pure Cerebellar Cortical Atrophy Holmes in 1907 described a family of 8 siblings, of whom 3 brothers and 1 sister were affected by a progressive ataxia, beginning with a reeling gait and followed by clumsiness of the hands, dysarthria, tremor of the head, and a variable nystagmus. The ataxia began insidiously in the fourth decade and progressed slowly over many years. The late cortical cerebellar atrophy of Marie, Foix, and Alajouanine, reported in 1922, is probably the same disease. In their patients also, the onset was in later life (average age 57 years). The onset was usually insidious, rarely abrupt, and the progress was extremely slow (survival 15 to 20 years). Ataxia of gait, instability of the trunk, tremor of the hands and head, and slightly slowed, hesitant speech conformed to the usual clinical picture of a progressive cerebellar ataxia. Nystagmus was rare. Intelligence was usually preserved. The patellar reflexes were increased in many cases, the ankle jerks were often absent, and the plantar reflexes were said to be of extensor type in some. The last finding, in the absence of hyperreflexia and spasticity, must be accepted with caution, since withdrawal responses are often mistaken for extensor reflexes. In our own practices, sporadic forms of pure cerebellar degeneration have been as common as inherited ones. The differential diagnosis in the nonfamilial cases is quite broad, as discussed at the end of this section.

Postmortem examination of the Holmes-type cases disclosed a symmetrical atrophy of the cerebellum, involving mainly the anterior lobe and vermis, the latter being more affected than the hemispheres. The Purkinje cells were absent in the lingula, centralis, and pyramis of the superior vermis and reduced in number in the quadrangularis, flocculus, biventral, and pyramidal lobes. The other cerebellar cortical neurons and granule cells were diminished in number, but the latter less so. The white matter was slightly pale in myelin stains. The roof nuclei and pontine nuclei were normal. There was cell loss in the dorsal and medial parts of the inferior olivary nuclei. A questionable pallor was noted in the corticospinal and spinocerebellar tracts in myelin stains of the spinal cord. The vermian atrophy and that of adjacent parts of the cerebellum can be visualized with great clarity in MR images (Fig. 39-3).

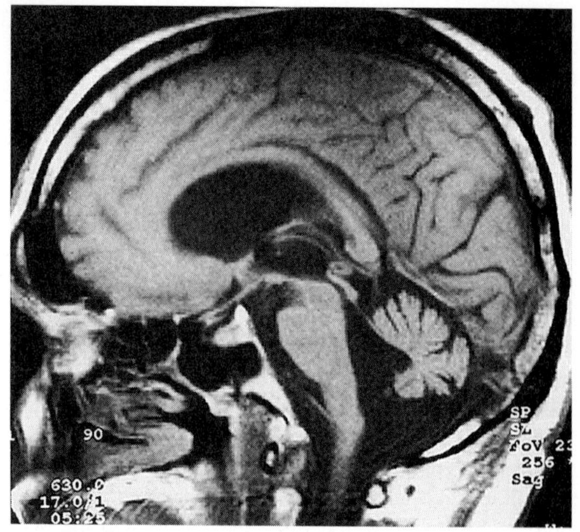

Figure 39-3

Familial cortical cerebellar atrophy. T1-weighted MR image in the sagittal plane showing marked atrophy of vermis and enlargement of fourth ventricle. The brainstem is only mildly atrophic. Compare with Fig. 39-4.

The pathologic findings in the cases of Marie, Foix, and Alajouanine were essentially the same. In further reports, both familial and sporadic cases of this type have been collected. The similarity of the pathologic (and clinical) changes to those of *alcoholic cerebellar degeneration* is at once apparent and should always raise the question of an alcoholic-nutritional cause in sporadic cases (Chap. 41).

Cerebellar Atrophy with Prominent Brainstem Lesions

Sporadic and Familial Olivopontocerebellar Atrophy A sporadically occurring instance of a disorder closely resembling the Holmes type of cortical cerebellar degeneration but with additional features of brainstem atrophy was described in 1900 by Déjerine and André-Thomas, who named it olivopontocerebellar atrophy (OPCA). The onset of symptoms was in the fifth decade of life, and the main manifestations were ataxia—first in the legs, then in the arms and hands and the bulbar musculature—a symptomatology common to all the cerebellar atrophies. As more and more cases of this type were collected (by 1943, Rosenhagen had collected 45 from the literature, to which he added 11 of his own), a *hereditary pattern* (autosomal dominant) was evident in some, and one or more long tracts in the spinal cord were found to have degenerated. About half the cases later developed the symptoms of Parkinson disease with degeneration of nigral cells and, in a few, of striatal cells as well.

Notable findings in both the sporadic (Menzel and Déjerine-Thomas types) and the familial forms of OPCA are the extensive degeneration of the middle cerebellar peduncles, the cerebellar white matter, and the pontine, olivary, and arcuate nuclei; loss of Purkinje cells has been variable (Fig. 39-4). Most likely this degeneration represents a terminal "dying back" of axons of the pontine and olivary nuclei with secondary myelin degeneration.

The boundaries of the entity of hereditary OPCA have gradually been extended; Konigsmark and Weiner subdivided them into the following types: (1) hereditary (dominant) type of Menzel; (2) hereditary (recessive) type of Fickler-Winkler; (3) hereditary (dominant) type with retinal degeneration; (4) hereditary (dominant) type of Shut-Haymaker, with spastic paraplegia and areflexia;

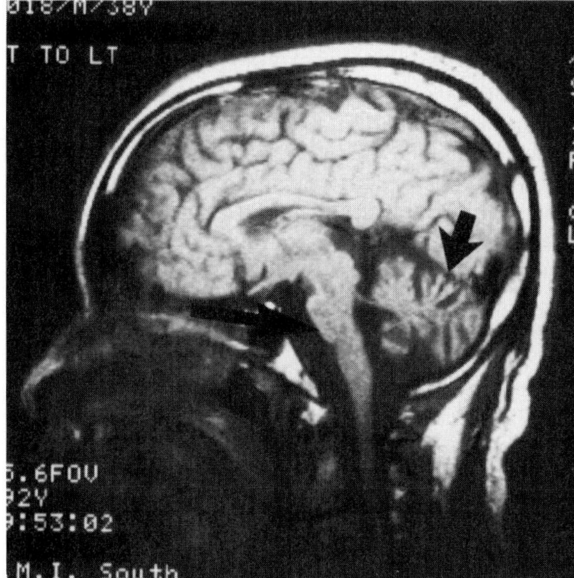

Figure 39-4

Olivopontocerebellar atrophy. MRI in the sagittal plane demonstrating both vermian atrophy (short arrow) *and smallness of the pons* (long arrow). *(From Bisese JH: Cranial MRI. New York, McGraw-Hill, 1991, by permission.)*

and (5) hereditary (dominant) type with dementia, ophthalmoplegia, and extrapyramidal signs. But even this classification does not do justice to the variable presentations. To these can be added two additional types: (6) inherited cases of OPCA with neuropathy and slowed eye movements (described by Wadia) and (7) cases with dystonia and a variety of other clinical findings, most of them in single cases (hemiballismus, athetosis, contractures of the legs, fixed pupils, ophthalmoplegia, ptosis, gaze palsy, deafness, retinal degeneration, mental retardation and epilepsy, claw foot and scoliosis, incontinence, parkinsonian symptoms and signs, dementia). Even a neonatal type is known. Some are detailed further on, under "Other Complicated Hereditary Cerebellar Ataxias."

Cases of *sporadic olivopontocerebellar atrophy* are more common and tend to occur at an older age than the familial ones, and nystagmus, optic atrophy, retinal degeneration, ophthalmoplegia, and urinary incontinence are generally not observed. However, there are numerous variants that include mild extrapyramidal and neuropathic signs, slow eye movements, dystonia, impairment of vertical saccadic eye movements (thus simulating progressive supranuclear palsy), a vocal cord paralysis that is typical of multiple system atrophy, and deafness, of each of which we have seen examples. The relationship of olivopontocerebellar atrophy to *multiple system atrophy* has already been discussed (page 1137), but we would emphasize again that OPCA occurs most often independent of extrapyramidal degeneration. The same uncertainty regarding the significance of cytoplasmic and neuronal inclusions expressed in the discussion of multiple system atrophy pertains to OPCA.

Machado-Joseph-Azorean Disease Aside from the Andrade type of amyloid polyneuropathy, a special form of hereditary ataxia has been described in patients mainly but not exclusively of Portuguese-Azorean origin. One such case was described by Woods and Schaumburg in 1972 under the name *nigrospinodentatal degeneration with nuclear ophthalmoplegia*. The disorder was characterized by an autosomal dominant pattern of inheritance and by a slowly progressive ataxia beginning in adolescence or early adult life, in association with hyperreflexia, extrapyramidal (parkinsonian) rigidity, dystonia, bulbar signs, distal motor weakness, and ophthalmoplegia. There was no impairment of intellect, and in the examples the authors have seen, the extrapyramidal symptoms were mainly rigidity and slowness of movement. There were no signs of corticospinal involvement. The conjunction of a Parkinson syndrome with cerebellar ataxia was reminiscent of certain cases of *multiple system atrophy* except for an earlier age of onset and the prominence of dystonia, amyotrophy, and ophthalmoplegia. Postmortem examination disclosed a degeneration of the dentate nuclei and spinocerebellar tracts and a loss of anterior horn cells and neurons of the pons, substantia nigra, and oculomotor nuclei. The heredoataxia was unaccompanied by signs of polyneuropathy, which was an important feature of the disease in Portuguese emigrants, described earlier by Nakano and colleagues as Machado disease, this being the name of the progenitor of the afflicted family.

A similarly affected Azorean family named Joseph was described by Rosenberg and colleagues (1976) under the name of *autosomal dominant striatonigral degeneration*. The disease had its onset in early adult life and was characterized by progressive ataxia of gait, followed by dysarthria, nystagmus, slowness of eye movements, reduced facial mobility, slow lingual movements, fasciculations of face and tongue, dystonic postures, rigidity of the limbs, cerebellar tremor, hyperreflexia, and Babinski signs. Rosenberg and coworkers considered the disorder to be a striatonigral degeneration on the basis of their findings in one autopsied case. The choice of this designation was unfortunate, insofar as the clinical and pathologic picture was quite unlike that of the striatonigral degeneration reported by Adams and associates. The diagnosis of striatonigral degeneration was also disputed by Nielsen and by Romanul, who were able to study the brain of the patient reported by Rosenberg and colleagues.

Under the name *Azorean disease of the nervous system*, Romanul and colleagues described yet another family of Portuguese-Azorean descent, many members of which were affected by a syndrome comprising a progressive ataxia of gait, parkinsonian features, limitation of conjugate gaze, fasciculations, areflexia, nystagmus, ataxic tremor, and extensor plantar responses; the pathologic changes closely resembled those described by Woods and Schaumburg. Romanul and coworkers compared the genetic, clinical, and pathologic features of their cases with those described in other Portuguese-Azorean families and concluded that all of them represent a single genetic entity with variable expression. This concept of the disease has been corroborated by the further observations of Rosenberg and of Fowler, who studied 20 patients with the Machado-Joseph-Azorean disease over a 10-year period.

This disease is not limited to Azoreans. Cases conforming to the above descriptions have now been observed among black, Indian, and Japanese families (Sakai et al, Yuasa et al, Bharucha et al). Cancel and colleagues have found an unstable number of CAG repeating sequences on chromosome 14 and named the disorder, which corresponds to Machado-Joseph disease, type 3 spinocerebellar ataxia (SCA 3).

There is no treatment. Early diagnosis of patients at risk is possible by the examination of ocular movements. In asymptomatic patients, Hotson and associates found dysmetric horizontal and vertical saccades similar to those in symptomatic ones. In fully developed cases, the MRI findings are characteristic—reduced width of the superior and middle cerebellar peduncles, atrophy of the frontal and temporal lobes, and smallness of the pons and globus pallidus (Murata et al).

Dentatorubropallidoluysian Atrophy (DRPLA) This is a rare familial disorder, described mostly in Japan and in small European pockets, in which symptoms of cerebellar ataxia are coupled with those of choreoathetosis and dystonia, but including, in isolated instances, myoclonus, parkinsonism, epilepsy, or dementia. Pathologically there is degeneration of the dentatorubral and pallidoluysian systems (Smith; Iizuka et al). The main diagnostic consideration when chorea is prominent is the separation of this disorder from Huntington disease (Warner et al). The gene defect in four European families has been identified as an unstable CAG trinucleotide repeat on chromosome 12 (Warner et al). As with Huntington chorea, this disease is inherited as an autosomal dominant trait and there is an inverse correlation between the age of onset and the size of the expansion repeat. Diagnosis can be confirmed by means of DNA analysis.

Dentatorubral Degeneration In 1921, Ramsay Hunt published an account of 6 patients (2 of whom were twin brothers) in whom myoclonus was combined with progressive cerebellar ataxia. The age of onset in the 4 nonfamilial cases was between 7 and 17 years, and the cerebellar ataxia followed the myoclonus by an interval of 1 to 20 years. Hunt named this disorder *dyssynergia cerebellaris myoclonica*. In the twin brothers there were signs of Friedreich ataxia; postmortem examination of one of them showed a degeneration of the posterior columns and spinocerebellar tracts but not of the corticospinal tracts. The only lesion in the cerebellum was an atrophy and sclerosis of the dentate nuclei with degeneration of the superior cerebellar peduncles. Louis-Bar and van Bogaert in 1947 reported a similar case, and they noted, in addition to the above findings, degeneration of the corticospinal tracts and loss of fibers in the posterior roots. Thus the pathology was identical to that of Friedreich ataxia except for the more severe atrophy of the dentate nuclei.

Earlier (1914), under the title of *dyssynergia cerebellaris progressiva*, Hunt had drawn attention to a progressive disease in young individuals manifest by what he considered to be a pure cerebellar syndrome. One of the three patients described in this paper died 13 years after the onset of her illness, and necropsy disclosed cavitary lesions in the lenticular nuclei, cerebellum, and pons and a diffuse increase of Alzheimer (type 2) glial cells, associated with nodular cirrhosis of the liver—i.e., findings typical of progressive lenticular degeneration (Wilson disease). Hunt's reports emphasize the hazard of classifying cerebellar ataxias on the basis of clinical findings alone, a point made effectively by Holmes in relation to the hereditary cerebellar ataxia of Marie (see earlier).

Other Complicated Hereditary Cerebellar Ataxias In addition to the ones enumerated earlier, briefly mentioned here are the hereditary ataxias, all rare, with optic atrophy; the autosomal recessive syndrome of cerebellar ataxia with pigmentary retinal degeneration and congenital deafness; an autosomal dominant hereditary ataxia with muscular atrophy, retinal degeneration, and diabetes mellitus; Friedreich ataxia with juvenile parkinsonism; the autosomal recessive ataxia with total albinism; the autosomal recessive ataxia with cataracts, oligophrenia, pyramidal signs, and stunting of growth; and an essential (familial) tremor complicated in later years by cerebellar ataxia. Details regarding these rare ataxias and appropriate references can be found in the monograph on the inherited ataxias edited by Kark et al. Pollock and Kies have described yet another late-life form of hereditary cerebellar ataxia with near global loss of pain and temperature sensation (due to loss of primary sensory afferents).

One adult form of hereditary cerebellar ataxia is paroxysmal in nature; the episodes occur without explanation and last several hours, leaving the patient normal between episodes or with only minimal ataxia of the limbs and nystagmus (Griggs et al). It is the only cerebellar ataxia that responds to oral acetazolamide (see Chap. 5 and page 1021). Of related interest is spinocerebellar atrophy type 6, in which a mutation occurs on chromosome 19 in the gene that codes for a voltage-gated calcium channel, resulting in progressive ataxia, dysarthria, and loss of proprioception. This gene is also implicated in the acetazolamide-responsive paroxysmal ataxia.

Genetics of the Heredodegenerative Ataxias Probably the many ataxic disorders just described are genetically distinct. As indicated above, *autosomal recessive* Friedreich ataxia is due to an expanded GAA repeat on chromosome 9q (Campuzano et al). Larger GAA expansions correlate with an earlier age of onset. The direct molecular test for the GAA expansion is useful for diagnosis, particularly for atypical cases with late onset (Dürr et al). The rarer recessive type that is precipitated by vitamin E deficiency shows GAA repeats on chromosome 8q, which codes for an α-tocopherol transport gene (see page 1224).

Among the *autosomal dominant* cerebellar ataxias of later onset, molecular-gene studies have identified mutant genes at seven chromosomal loci. Five of these eight forms of autosomal dominant ataxia are known to be caused by expanded CAG-trinucleotide repeats (SCA types 1, 3, 6, and 7 and dentatorubropallidoluysian atrophy, or DRPLA). However, the mechanism by which the resultant increase in glutamine components affects cell dysfunction remains speculative. Tabulated below are the chromosomal loci of the cerebellar atrophies and their genetic terminology and related neural abnormalities:

6p: SCA 1; ophthalmoparesis, pyramidal and extrapyramidal signs; included in this group are most of the olivopontocerebellar atrophies

12q: SCA 2; slowed saccades

12p: Dentatorubropallidoluysian atrophy

14q: SCA 3; the Machado-Joseph phenotype with several allelic variants

16q: SCA 4; sensory neuropathy and pyramidal signs

11centromeric: SCA 5

3p: SCA 7; retinal degeneration

19p: SCA 6; related to the alpha subunit of a voltage-dependent calcium channel; a different mutation at the same locus causes the acetazolamide-responsive episodic ataxia

In addition, several types of autosomal dominant episodic ataxia have been analyzed and found to be linked to chromosomes 12p (a potassium channel gene) and 19p (a calcium channel gene), as mentioned earlier.

Differential Diagnosis Sporadic forms of cerebellar ataxia in adults are in some instances traceable to strokes involving cerebellar pathways (Safe et al). Some are alcoholic-nutritional in origin, and a few are related to abuse of drugs (especially anticonvulsants, which may in a few cases cause a permanent ataxia). The paraneoplastic variety of cerebellar degeneration enters into the differential diagnosis; as a rule it occurs mostly in women with breast or ovarian cancers and evolves much more rapidly than any of the heredodegenerative forms. The more rapid onset of ataxia and the presence of anti-Purkinje cell antibodies (anti-Yo; page 724) are central to making the distinction. From time to time one observes an idiopathic variety of subacute cerebellar degeneration, particularly in women; clinically this disorder is indistinguishable from the paraneoplastic variety except that no relationship to neoplasm can be discerned (Ropper). Rare cases of ataxia have been associated with celiac disease and Whipple disease. The ataxias caused by transmissible agents are discussed in Chap. 33, and the metabolic ataxias are discussed further in Chap. 37. Of these, late-onset GM_2 gangliosidosis may simulate a cerebellar degeneration in adults (page 1021).

Treatment has been unsatisfactory and is limited largely to devising strategies to prevent falling. Amantadine 200 mg daily for several months has shown limited benefit in some studies (Boetz et al).

Hereditary Polymyoclonus

The syndrome of quick, arrhythmic, involuntary single or repetitive twitches of a muscle or group of muscles was described in Chap. 6, where it was pointed out that the condition has many causes. Those due to hereditary metabolic diseases are presented in Chap. 37. Familial forms are known, one of which, associated with cerebellar ataxia, was discussed earlier (dyssynergia cerebellaris myoclonica of Ramsay Hunt). But there is another disease, known as *hereditary essential benign myoclonus*, that occurs in relatively pure form unaccompanied by ataxia (page 108). In the latter condition, it may at times be difficult to evaluate coordination because willed movement is interrupted by the myoclonus and may be mistaken for intention tremor. Only by slowing the voluntary movement can the myoclonus be reduced or eliminated. This myoclonic disease is inherited as an autosomal dominant trait. It becomes manifest early in life; once established, it persists with little or no change in severity throughout life, often with rather little disability. It can, by its natural course, be differentiated from some of the hereditary metabolic diseases such as the Unverricht and Lafora types of myoclonic epilepsy, the lipidoses, tuberous sclerosis, and myoclonic disorders that follow certain viral infections and anoxic encephalopathy. Of interest is the response of this form of movement disorder, just as in the cases of acquired postanoxic myoclonus, to certain pharmacologic agents, notably clonazepam, valproic acid, and 5-hydroxytryptophan, the amino acid precursor of serotonin, particularly when these agents are used in combination.

SYNDROME OF MUSCULAR WEAKNESS AND WASTING WITHOUT SENSORY CHANGES

Motor System Disease

This general term is used to designate a progressive degenerative disorder of motor neurons in the spinal cord, brainstem, and motor cortex, manifest clinically by muscular weakness, atrophy, and corticospinal tract signs in varying combinations. It is a disease of middle life, for the most part, and progresses to death in a matter of 2 to 6 years or longer in exceptional cases.

Customarily, motor system disease is subdivided into several types on the basis of the particular grouping of symptoms and signs. The most frequent form, in which amyotrophy and hyperreflexia are combined, is called *amyotrophic lateral sclerosis*, or *ALS* (*amyotrophy* is the term applied to denervation atrophy and weakness of muscles). Less frequent are cases in which weakness and atrophy occur alone, without evidence of corticospinal tract dysfunction; for these the term *progressive spinal muscular atrophy* is used. When the weakness and wasting predominate in muscles innervated by the motor nuclei of the lower brainstem (i.e., muscles of the jaw, face, tongue, pharynx, and larynx), it is customary to speak of *progressive bulbar palsy* (*bulb* being the old name for the medulla oblongata). In a small proportion of patients the clinical state is dominated for a time by spastic weakness, hyperreflexia, and Babinski signs, lower motor neuron affection becoming apparent at a later stage of the illness. *Primary lateral sclerosis* designates a rare form of motor system disease in which the degenerative process remains confined to the corticospinal pathways (Pringle et al). The present authors believe that the pure spastic paraplegias without amyotrophy represent a special class of disease, hence they are described separately. There is also a relatively common familial form of spastic paraplegia in which the disease process may be confined to the corticospinal tracts or, in some cases, combined with posterior column or other neurologic signs.

Special types of spinal muscular atrophy are particularly frequent in infancy and childhood. Indeed, they are the leading cause of heritable infant mortality and, after cystic fibrosis, the most frequent form of serious autosomal recessive disease (Pearn). The best known is the Werdnig-Hoffmann type of *infantile spinal muscular atrophy* (SMA type I); but there are other familial forms beginning in later childhood, adolescence, or adult life (SMA types II and III, or the Wohlfart-Kugelberg-Welander type). Despite the clinical heterogeneity of the heritable childhood spinal muscular atrophies, they all map to a single locus on chromosome 5q—i.e., they are genetically homogeneous (Gilliam et al; Brzustowicz et al). This group of early-onset spinal muscular atrophies is genetically distinct from familial ALS, in which linkage analysis has identified a gene defect on chromosome 21 (Siddique et al). In respect to the more common nonfamilial forms, there is no reason to believe that the subgroups are anything other than variants of a single pathologic process—an upper and lower motor neuron degeneration or atrophy of unknown etiology.

History Credit for the original delineation of amyotrophic lateral sclerosis is appropriately given to Charcot. With Joffroy in 1869 and Gombault in 1871, he studied the pathologic aspects of the disease. In a series of lectures given from 1872 to 1874, he gave a lucid account of the clinical and pathologic findings. Although called Charcot disease in France, amyotrophic lateral sclerosis (the term recommended by Charcot) has been preferred in the English-speaking world. Duchenne had earlier (1858) described *labioglossolaryngeal paralysis*, a term that Wachsmuth in 1864 changed to *progressive bulbar palsy*. In 1869 Charcot called attention to the nuclear origin of progressive bulbar palsy, and in 1882 Déjerine established its relationship to amyotrophic lateral sclerosis. Most authors credit Aran and Duchenne with the earliest descriptions of progressive spinal muscular atrophy, which they believed to be of myogenic origin. This interpretation was, of course, incorrect; Cruveilhier, a few years later, noted the slender anterior roots, and soon thereafter the disease was brought into line with ALS as a myelopathic or spinal muscular atrophy.

Amyotrophic Lateral Sclerosis This is a common disease, with an annual incidence rate of 0.4 to 1.76 per 100,000 population. Men are affected somewhat more frequently than women. Most patients are more than 50 years old at the onset of symptoms, and the incidence increases with each decade of life (Mulder). The disease occurs in a random pattern throughout the world except for a dramatic clustering of patients among inhabitants of the Kii peninsula in Japan and in Guam, where ALS is often combined with dementia and parkinsonism. In about 5 percent of cases the disease is familial, being inherited as an autosomal dominant trait with age-dependent penetrance. The familial cases do not differ in their symptoms and clinical course from nonfamilial ones, although as a group the former have a somewhat earlier age of onset, an equal distribution in men and women, a slightly shorter survival, and a greater tendency for the weakness to begin in the legs.

In the most typical form of ALS, awkwardness in tasks requiring fine finger movements (difficulty with buttons and automobile ignition keys), stiffness of the fingers, and slight weakness or wasting of the hand muscles are the first indications of the disease. Cramping beyond what seems natural and fasciculations of the muscles of the forearm, upper arm, and shoulder girdle also appear. As the weeks and months pass, the other hand and arm may be similarly affected. Before long, the triad of atrophic weakness of the hands and forearms, slight spasticity of the arms and legs, and generalized hyperreflexia—all in the absence of sensory change—leaves little doubt as to the diagnosis. Muscle strength and bulk diminish in parallel; yet despite the amyotrophy, the tendon reflexes are notable for their liveliness. Babinski signs are variably present early in the illness. Abductors, adductors, and extensors of fingers and thumb tend to become weak before the long flexors, on which the handgrip depends, and the dorsal interosseous spaces become hollowed, giving rise to the "cadaveric," or "skeletal," hand. The muscles of the upper arm and shoulder girdles are involved later. All this occurs while the thigh and leg muscles seem relatively normal, and there may come a time in some cases when the patient walks about with useless, dangling arms. Later the atrophic weakness spreads to the neck, tongue, pharyngeal, and laryngeal muscles, and eventually those in the trunk and lower extremities yield to the onslaught of the disease.

The affected parts may ache and feel cold, but true paresthesias, except from poor positioning and pressure on nerves, do not occur. Sphincteric control is said to be usually well maintained even after both legs have become weak and spastic, but many of our patients have acquired urinary and sometimes fecal urgency in the advanced stages of the disease. The abdominal reflexes may be elicitable even when the plantar reflexes are extensor. Extreme spasticity is rarely seen. Coarse fasciculations are usually evident in the weakened muscles but may not be noticed by the patient until the physician calls attention to them. Fasciculations are almost never the sole presenting feature of ALS—a clinical truism with which one can reassure physicians and medical students who fear, on the basis of persistent focal muscle twitching, that they are developing the disease.

Other Patterns of Evolution In addition to the special configurations discussed further on, there are many patterns of neuromuscular involvement other than the one just described. A leg may be affected before the hands. A foot drop with weakness and wasting of the pretibial muscles may be incorrectly attributed to peroneal nerve compression until weakness of the gastrocnemius and other muscles betrays a more widespread involvement of lumbosacral neurons. In our experience this crural amyotrophy is nearly as frequent as the brachial-manual type. Another variant is the early involvement of thoracic, abdominal, or posterior neck muscles, the last being one of the main causes of head lolling in older individuals. Yet another pattern is of early diaphragmatic weakness; such cases come to attention because of respiratory failure. The pattern of proximal limb or shoulder girdle amyotrophy with onset at an early age is also well known and simulates muscular dystrophy (Wohlfart-Kugelberg-Welander disease—page 1161). On several occasions we have observed a pattern involving the arm and leg on the same side, first with spasticity and then with some degree of amyotrophy; this is sometimes called the *hemiplegic*, or *Mills*, *variant*. (More often this condition turns out to be due to multiple sclerosis.) The first manifestations may be a spastic weakness of the legs; a diagnosis of primary lateral sclerosis may be made (discussed further on), and only after a year or two do the hand and arm muscles weaken, waste, and fasciculate. It is cases of this type that led to the inclusion of spastic paraparesis as a variant of ALS. Exceptionally, cramps or fasciculations of the limb muscles may precede recognizable weakness and wasting by a month or two. From time to time, as the disease advances, very mild distal sensory loss is observed in the feet without explanation, but perhaps corresponding to abnormalities of the somatosensory evoked potentials, as noted below; if the sensory loss is definite and an early feature, the diagnosis must remain in doubt. Rarely in North America, ALS has been observed in conjunction with a frontotemporal dementia and with Parkinson disease (page 1126), a complex similar to that observed among the natives of Guam.

The course of this illness, irrespective of its particular mode of onset and pattern of evolution, is inexorably progressive. Half the patients succumb within 3 years of onset and 90 percent within 6 years (Mulder et al). The variants of motor neuron disease that occur with regularity and have distinguishing clinical features are described below.

Progressive Muscular Atrophy This type of motor system disease is more common in men than in women, in a ratio of 3.6:1 (Chio et al). In about half the patients, progressive muscular atrophy (PMA) takes the form of a symmetrical (sometimes asymmetrical) wasting of intrinsic hand muscles, slowly advancing to the more proximal parts of the arms; less often, the legs and thighs are the sites of onset of atrophic weakness; less often still, the proximal parts of the limbs are affected before the distal parts. These purely nuclear amyotrophies tend to progress at a slower pace than the usual case of ALS, some patients surviving for 15 years or longer. Chio and colleagues, who analyzed the factors affecting life expectancy in 155 patients with PMA, found that younger patients had a more benign course—the 5-year survival was 72 percent in patients with onset of PMA before age 50 and 40 percent in patients with onset after age 50. Some of the most chronic varieties of PMA are familial. Otherwise they differ from ALS only in that the tendon reflexes are diminished or absent and signs of corticospinal tract disease cannot be detected. Fascicular twitchings and cramping are variably present. The main disease to be distinguished from PMA is the rare immune-mediated motor neuropathy that occurs with or without multifocal block of electrical conduction (page 1411). The presence of a paraproteinemia, specifically IgM with antibodies against the GM_1 ganglioside, or the finding of focal conduction block or sensory nerve abnormalities on the EMG implies the presence of an immune neuropathic disease rather than one of the motor neuron type.

Progressive Bulbar Palsy Here reference is made to a condition in which the first and dominant symptoms relate to weakness of muscles innervated by the motor nuclei of the lower brainstem, i.e., muscles of the jaw, face, tongue, pharynx, and larynx. This weakness gives rise to an early defect in articulation, in which there is difficulty in the pronunciation of lingual (*r*, *n*, *l*), labial (*b*, *m*, *p*, *f*), dental (*d*, *t*), and palatal (*k*, *g*) consonants. As the condition worsens, syllables lose their clarity and run together until finally speech becomes unintelligible. In other patients, slurring is due to spasticity of the tongue, pharyngeal, and laryngeal muscles or to a combination of atrophic and spastic weakness, as indicated below. Defective modulation of the voice with variable degrees of rasping and nasality is another characteristic. The pharyngeal reflex is lost, and the palate and vocal cords move imperfectly or not at all during attempted phonation. Mastication and deglutition also become impaired; the bolus of food cannot be manipulated and may lodge between the cheek and teeth; and the pharyngeal muscles do not force it properly into the esophagus. Liquids and small particles of food find their way into the trachea or the nose. The facial muscles, particularly of the lower face, weaken and sag. Fasciculations and focal loss of tissue of the tongue are usually early manifestations; eventually the tongue becomes shriveled and lies useless in the floor of the mouth. The chin may also quiver from fascicular twitchings, but diagnosis of the disease should not be made on the basis of fasciculations alone, i.e., in the absence of weakness or atrophy. Fasciculations in themselves may be entirely benign or a part of the syndrome of myokymia or of "continuous muscular activity" (page 1568).

The jaw jerk may be present or exaggerated at a time when the muscles of mastication are markedly weak. In fact, spasticity of the jaw muscles may be so pronounced that the slightest tap on the chin will evoke clonus and blinking; rarely, attempts to open the mouth elicit a "bulldog" reflex (jaws snap shut involuntarily). Spastic weakness of the oropharyngeal muscles may be the initial manifestation of bulbar palsy and may at times surpass signs of atrophic weakness; pseudobulbar signs (pathologic laughter and crying) may reach extreme degrees. This is the only common clinical situation in which spastic and atrophic bulbar palsy coexist. Strangely, the ocular muscles always escape.

As with other forms of motor system disease, the course of bulbar palsy is inexorably progressive. Eventually the weakness spreads to the respiratory muscles and deglutition fails entirely; the patient dies of inanition and aspiration pneumonia, usually within 2 to 3 years of onset. About 25 percent of cases of motor system disease begin with bulbar symptoms, but rarely if ever does the sporadic form of progressive bulbar palsy run its course as an independent syndrome (pure heredofamilial forms of progressive bulbar palsy in the adult are known but are rare). Practically always, after a few months, the other manifestations of ALS become evident. In general, the earlier the onset of the bulbar involvement in the course of ALS, the shorter the course of the disease.

Primary Lateral Sclerosis This entity, like ALS, is a form of motor neuron disease, although we consider it to be a separate process. Virtually all patients in whom the signs of corticospinal tract degeneration betray the presence of ALS will develop indications of lower motor neuron disease within 1 year, usually earlier. Those who remain with restricted bilateral signs of upper motor neuron disease often turn out to have multiple sclerosis, a slow compression of the spinal cord by spondylosis or meningioma, or the myelopathic form of adrenoleukodystrophy (affected males or female carriers); in a few, tropical spastic paraplegia, HIV myelopathy, or a family history of spastic paraplegia (Strümpell-Lorrain disease, described further on) is uncovered. Approximately 20 percent of these patients, however, have a slowly progressive corticospinal tract disorder that begins with a pure spastic paraparesis; later, and to a lesser degree, the arms and oropharyngeal muscles become involved. These cases have distinctive neuropathologic features and are designated as *primary lateral sclerosis*, a term originally suggested by Erb in 1875. A historical review of the subject appears in the article by Pringle and colleagues.

The typical case begins insidiously in the fifth or sixth decade with a stiffness in one leg, then the other; there is a slowing of gait, with spasticity predominating over weakness as the years go on. Walking is still possible with the help of a cane for many years after the onset, but eventually this condition acquires the characteristic features of a severe spastic paraparesis. Over the years, finger movements become slower, the arms become spastic, and, if the illness persists for decades, speech takes on a pseudobulbar tone. In some patients the illness evolves over a few years. There are no sensory symptoms or signs. Power in the legs is often found to be surprisingly good, the difficulty in locomotion being attributable mainly to rigid spasticity. About half the patients acquire spasticity of the bladder. Pringle and associates suggest that an important diagnostic criterion of the disease is progression for 3 years without evidence of lower motor neuron dysfunction. A rare type of spasticity begins in the oropharyngeal muscles, as mentioned above.

Pathologic studies have disclosed a relatively stereotyped pattern of reduced numbers of Betz cells in the frontal and prefrontal motor cortex, degeneration of the corticospinal tracts, and preservation of motor neurons in the spinal cord and brainstem (Beal and Richardson, Pringle et al). The corticospinal tract lesions are identical to those in typical ALS, described further on. Whether some of these cases are examples of late-onset familial spastic paraplegia (see further on) has not been explored with molecular techniques.

As to treatment, an attempt can be made to reduce the spasticity with medications such as baclofen or tizanidine, or subarachnoid infusions of baclofen. Initial intrathecal test doses are given to predict a response to pump infusions of baclofen, but this test may fail; in severe cases, it may be advisable to proceed with a constant infusion for several days. Some degree of improved comfort from a reduction in the extreme rigidity is usually the most that can be expected.

Laboratory Features of Motor Neuron Disease Laboratory investigation of the patient with motor system disease provides useful confirmatory evidence even in the presence of the typical clinical pictures. The EMG, as expected, displays widespread fibrillations and fasciculations (evidence of active denervation and reinnervation), and motor nerve conduction studies reveal only a slight slowing. If the atrophic paresis is restricted to an arm or hand, raising the question of cervical spondylosis, evidence of denervation over many somatic segments favors the diagnosis of ALS. In questionable cases, it is good practice to insist that denervation be demonstrated in at least three limbs before concluding that the process is ALS. Widespread denervation of the paraspinal muscles and genioglossus or facial muscles is also a strong indicator of the disease, but testing of these muscles and interpretation of the tests demands considerable experience. Sensory nerve action potentials should be normal; tests of motor nerve conduction show a normal velocity, but the amplitudes become progressively lower as the disease progresses—in the earliest stages, they too may be normal. The CSF protein is usually normal or marginally elevated. Serum creatine kinase is slightly or moderately elevated in cases with rapidly progressive atrophy and weakness but is just as often normal.

It has become clear that sensory evoked potentials are abnormal in a proportion of patients, but the explanation for this finding is obscure in a disease that clinically and pathologically affects solely the motor system. When the amplitudes of sensory nerve action potentials are reduced, there is usually an underlying entrapment neuropathy or late-life neuropathy. Sensory complaints and minimal sensory loss have been commented on above. Motor evoked potentials that are elicited from the cortex are also prolonged in those with prominent corticospinal signs. In this group, the MRI may show slight atrophy of the motor cortices and wallerian degeneration of the motor tracts (Fig. 39-5). These changes may be diagnostically useful and appear as subtly increased T2 signal intensity in the posterior limb of the internal capsule, brainstem, and spinal cord, all of which can be missed because of their symmetry.

Pathology The principal finding in ALS is a loss of nerve cells in the anterior horns of the spinal cord and motor nuclei of the lower brainstem. Large neurons tend to be affected before small ones. Lost cells are replaced by fibrous astrocytes. Many of the surviving nerve cells are small, shrunken, and filled with lipofuscin. Occasionally, an ill-defined cytoplasmic inclusion body is seen. According to some reports, swelling of the proximal axon is an early finding, presumably antedating visible changes in the cell body itself. The anterior roots are thin, and there is a disproportionate loss of large myelinated fibers in motor nerves (Bradley et al). The muscles show typical denervation atrophy of different ages. Whitehouse and coworkers found a depletion of muscarinic, cholinergic, glycinergic, and benzodiazepine receptors in regions of the spinal cord where motor neurons had disappeared.

The corticospinal tract degeneration is most evident in the lower parts of the spinal cord, but it can be traced up through the brainstem to the posterior limb of the internal capsule and corona radiata by means of fat stains, which show the macrophages that accumulate in response to the myelin degeneration. There is a loss of Betz cells in the motor cortex; this is evident as frontal lobe atrophy on the MRI in primary lateral sclerosis, but it is not a prominent finding in most cases of ALS (Kiernan and Hudson). Other fibers in the ventral and lateral funiculi are depleted, imparting a characteristic pallor in

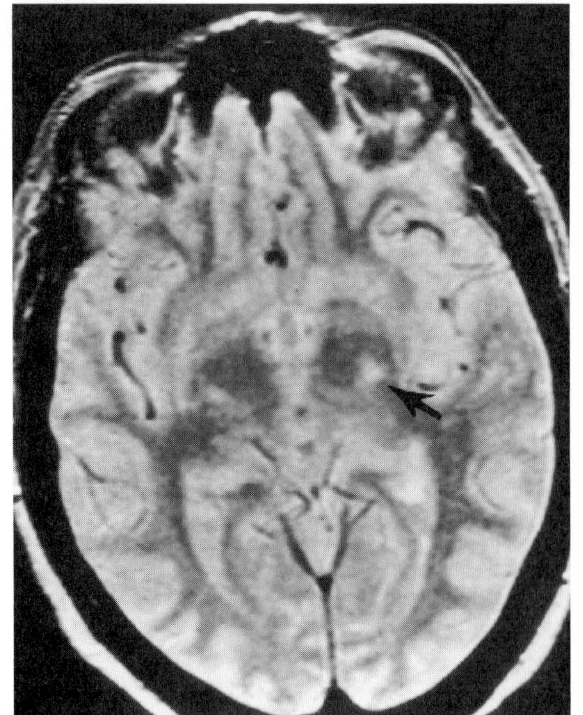

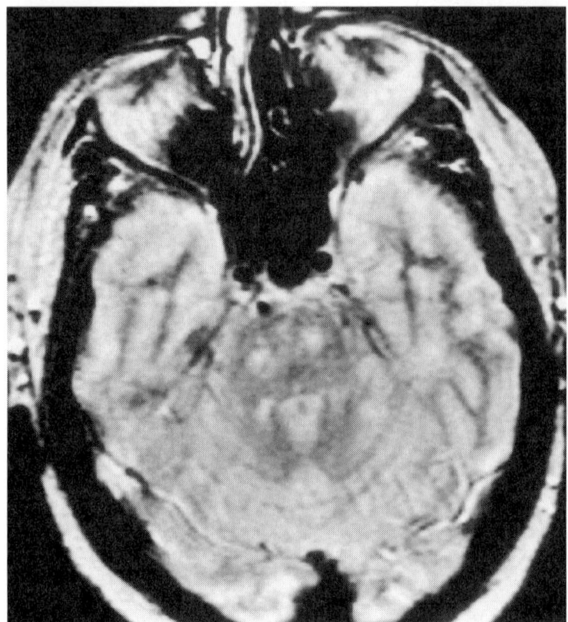

Figure 39-5

T2-weighted MR image showing signal changes that reflect wallerian change in the corticospinal tracts at the level of the internal capsule (top, arrow) *and the pons* (bottom) *in a case of ALS.*

myelin stains. Some pathologists have interpreted this as evidence of involvement of nonmotor neurons and hence object to the term *motor system disease*. However, we regard this condition as due to a loss of collaterals of motor neurons that contribute to the lamina propria. One observes the same effect in severe, long-standing poliomyelitis.

Neuropathologic studies of cases of ALS with dementia are few in number. In addition to the usual affection of motor neurons, these cases have shown an extensive neuronal loss, gliosis, and vacuolation involving the premotor area, particularly the superior frontal gyri and the inferolateral cortex of the temporal lobes. The histologic changes of Alzheimer or Pick disease have not been seen in our cases; neurofibrillary degeneration has been observed but is inconsequential in comparison to that seen in the Guamanian Parkinson-dementia-ALS complex (Finlayson et al; Mitsuyama). Attempts to transmit this ALS-dementia syndrome to subhuman primates have been unsuccessful.

Diagnosis Motor system disease may be simulated by a central spondylotic bar or ruptured cervical disc, but with these latter conditions there is usually pain in the neck and shoulders, limitation of neck movements, and sensory changes; the lower motor neuron affection is restricted to one or two spinal segments. Electromyography is helpful if not decisive in differentiating these disorders, as indicated above. Already mentioned in the diagnosis of ALS is the finding of active denervation in three limbs and in paraspinal, facial, and tongue muscles. A mild hemiparesis or monoparesis due to multiple sclerosis may for a time be difficult to distinguish from early ALS. Progressive spinal muscular atrophy may be differentiated from peroneal muscular atrophy (Charcot-Marie-Tooth neuropathy) by the lack of family history, the complete lack of sensory change, and different EMG patterns. Motor system disease beginning in the proximal limb muscles may be misdiagnosed as a limb-girdle type of muscular dystrophy. The main considerations in relation to progressive bulbar palsy are myasthenia gravis and, less often, polymyositis, muscular dystrophy, and especially the inherited (Kennedy) type of bulbospinal atrophy, which is discussed further on. The spastic form of bulbar palsy may suggest the pseudobulbar palsy of lacunar disease. A crural form of progressive muscular atrophy may be confused with diabetic polyradiculopathy or polymyositis.

As mentioned earlier, a major consideration is the differentiation of progressive muscular atrophy from chronic motor polyneuropathy with or without multifocal conduction block and related disorders, in which there is an idiopathic motor axonopathy. These distinctions are made by careful, extensive conduction studies and needle EMG examinations (Chap. 45); they are discussed with the peripheral neuropathies (Chap. 46). There is also a rare form of subacute poliomyelitis (possibly viral) in patients with lymphoma or carcinoma; it leads to an amyotrophy that progresses to death over a period of several months.

Over the years, the authors have occasionally encountered a patient with a localized amyotrophy of the leg or arm that became arrested and did not advance over a decade or two. Several reports of such a partial spinal amyotrophy have appeared in recent years (Hirayama et al; Moreno Martinez et al). In a familial variety of pure restricted amyotrophy, only the vocal cords became paralyzed over a period of years in adult life; only later were the hands affected.

Some patients who have recovered from paralytic poliomyelitis may develop progressive muscular weakness 30 or 40 years later; the nature of this relationship is quite obscure. We favor the explanation that atrophy of anterior horn cells with aging brings to light a critically depleted motor neuron population (see further on).

An observation of interest is the finding of a form of progressive spinal muscular atrophy in patients with GM_2 gangliosidosis, the storage disease that presents in infancy as Tay-Sachs disease (Kolodny and Raghavan). The onset is in late adolescence and early adult life and the atrophic paralysis is progressive, so that this condition is often mistaken for Wohlfart-Kugelberg-Welander disease or ALS. A number of cases of this type have been uncovered in Ashkenazi Jews by the use of lysosomal enzyme analysis.

All these caveats notwithstanding, ALS or the more discrete forms of motor system disease rarely offer any difficulty in diagnosis.

Pathogenesis The pathogenesis of sporadic motor system disease is not known. Of considerable interest has been the discovery of a mutant gene that codes for the enzyme Cu-Zn superoxide dismutase (SOD) in some familial cases of ALS (Rosen et al), and of an abnormality of the gene for a subunit of the neurofilament protein in others (Figlewicz et al). Both dominant and rarer recessive forms have been described (Siddique et al, 1996). The former is reflected in a 20 to 50 percent reduction in SOD enzyme activity in affected patients and has led to speculation that an excess of free radicals attributable to the enzyme deficiency allows a slow destruction of neurons. This explanation is probably an oversimplification. An enhancement of excitotoxic glutaminergic activity due to the SOD defect has been proposed as an alternative explanation and is supported by a putative response to treatment with certain glutamate blockers (see further on). Whether these enzymatic and biochemical abnormalities extend to the sporadic type of ALS is unknown, but this approach is providing the most provocative avenues for research.

Trauma, particularly traction injury of an arm, has been reported from time to time as an antecedent event in patients with ALS, but a causative relationship has not been established. Younger and coworkers have reported a higher incidence of paraproteinemia in patients with motor system disease than can be accounted for by chance. Many other examples of disordered immune function have been described in patients with motor system disease, but a coherent explanation of ALS as an autoimmune disease has not emerged. It has never been proved that intoxication with heavy metals (lead, mercury, aluminum) can cause motor system disease. Rare instances of PMA and ALS have been described in patients who had suffered a remote attack of poliomyelitis; these probably represent chance occurrences. There is little evidence that such cases represent a reactivation of the virus or the presence of some other infectious agent. The progressive weakness that occurs some 30 to 40 years after recovery from polio should not be confused with PMA, as indicated above.

Treatment There is no specific treatment for any of the motor neuron diseases; only supportive measures can be utilized. It has been our practice to give the patient some idea of the seriousness of the condition but not to make the devastating statement that it is invariably fatal. Usually it is advisable to give medication of some type "to try to slow the progress of the disease," even though none is known to be definitely effective. Guanidine hydrochloride and injections of cobra venom, gangliosides, interferons, high-dose intravenous cyclophosphamide, and thyrotropin-releasing hormone are but some of a long list of agents that have been said to arrest the process, but these claims either have been discredited or remain uncorroborated. Bensimon and colleagues have reported that the antiglutamate agent riluzole appears to slow the progression of ALS and improve survival in patients with disease of bulbar onset, but add, at best, only 3 months to life expectancy. This claim requires confirmation but is supported by the slight beneficial effects of riluzole and gabapentin, another glutamate inhibitor, on a model of the familial disease in which a mutant superoxide dismutase has been produced in mice.

In the early stages of ALS, physical therapy is useful in maintaining mobility, but overwork of the muscles generally leads to fatigue and cramps. In the early stages of respiratory failure, nasally applied positive pressure is helpful in assisting sleeping and avoiding daytime somnolence in patients who are able to tolerate the device. Food should be cut into small pieces and dry foods, such as toast, avoided; milk shakes may be tolerated best. A mechanized bed and structural accommodations in the home that facilitate entry of a wheelchair and use of the bath or shower as well as thick-handled utensils make life easier for the patient. The treatment of spasticity, the main concern in primary lateral sclerosis and occasionally a source of difficulty in ALS, is discussed on page 1155.

Complex and sometimes unresolvable decisions must be made by the patient regarding the level of treatment desired as the disease progresses. When the time is appropriate and the patient is receptive or—as often happens with the availability of information on the Internet—the patient raises these issues, we broach the subject of tracheostomy, respiratory support, and feeding tubes and reassure the patient that under no circumstances will he be allowed to suffocate or suffer physically in any other way. In a survey by Albert and colleagues, a surprisingly small number of patients with ALS chose to have a tracheostomy or gastrostomy, and their views early in the illness tended to hold true later. Free access to the neurologist and, if desired by the patient, regular visits for advice can be very reassuring to the patient and family. Hospice-type care is often needed in the last weeks of illness in patients who can otherwise be cared for at home, and morphine or similar drugs as well as antianxiety agents should be used liberally to ease discomfort, respiratory distress, and anxiety in the final days.

Heredofamilial Forms of Progressive Muscular Atrophy and Spastic Paraplegia

Infantile Spinal Muscular Atrophy (Werdnig-Hoffmann Disease) This is the classic form of spinal muscular atrophy of hereditary type. It was first described by Werdnig in 1891 and 1894, by Hoffman in 1893, and, at about the same time, by Thomsen and Bruce. The cases described by these authors all involved infants. Further clinical analyses, however, indicated the inadequacy of this narrow grouping. Brandt, in his study of 112 Danish patients, found that in about one-third the weakness was present at birth, and in 97 the onset was in the first year of life; in 9 patients, the disease was not recognized until after the first year of life. Of the patients with early-onset disease, 53 had died by the end of the first year, but 8 of those with a later onset survived for 4 to 10 years. In 1956 Walton, and later Wohlfart and colleagues and Kugelberg and Welander (see below), identified milder forms of spinal muscular atrophy in which the onset was between 2 and 17 years and walking was still possible in adult life. Byers and Banker, in a study of 52 patients, subdivided them into three groups on the basis of age of onset; in one group the disease was recognized at birth or in the first month or two of life; in a second, between 6 and 12 months; and in a third, after the first year. Again, in their last group, it was not unusual for the patient to survive into adolescence and adult life. In a few of the late-onset types, signs of corticospinal tract involvement are conjoined, and Bonduelle has also included some patients with areflexia, pes cavus, Babinski signs, choreiform movements, and mental retardation in this group. More recently, the designations SMA I, II, and III have been introduced, based largely on the age of onset (Table 39-1).

Familial spinal muscular atrophy that begins in infancy and childhood is inherited mainly as an autosomal recessive trait. Autosomal dominant and X-linked patterns of inheritance have been reported, usually in adults. All of these phenotypes in children have been mapped to the same chromosome: 5q11.2-13.3 (Brzustowicz et al; Gilliam et al; Munsat et al). Several different mutations have been found in the gene at what has been termed the "survival of motor neuron" (SMN) site. Although the gene product is not known, it has been proposed that the amount of this product may determine the severity of disease. Affected siblings demonstrate very similar clinical patterns of disease, but the same gene error gives rise to very different phenotypes in different families, so that modifying nongenetic attributes must be playing a role.

Finally, it should be reiterated that clinical disorders more or less similar to the spinal muscular atrophies may occur occasionally in certain hereditary metabolic diseases. For example, Johnson and coworkers have described a patient who began experiencing weakness of the legs, cramping, and fasciculations during adolescence in what proved to be a variant of hexosaminidase

Table 39-1
Classification of the spinal muscular atrophies

Type	*Inheritance*	*Age of onset*	*Clinical features*	*Prognosis*
SMA I (infantile, Werdnig-Hoffman)	Autosomal recessive	Preterm to 6 months	Neonatal hypotonia (floppy baby), weakness of sucking and swallowing, may have arthrogryposis, unable to sit	Few survive 1 year
SMA II (intermediate type)	Autosomal recessive	6 to 15 months	Proximal weakness, fasciculation, fine hand tremor, unable to stand	Variable; death from respiratory complications
SMA III (Wohlfart-Kugelberg-Welander)	Autosomal recessive or dominant	1 year to adolescence	Delayed motor development, proximal leg weakness	Slowly progressive, variable outcome
Kennedy syndrome (bulbospinal atrophy)	X-linked (CAG repeat expansion), less often autosomal dominant	Early adulthood	Scapuloperoneal or distal atrophy, oropharyngeal weakness, gynecomastia, oligospermia	Slowly progressive
Fazio-Londe disease	Autosomal recessive, rarely dominant	Childhood to early adolescence	Progressive bulbar and respiratory failure	Survival for years, respiratory failure

A (GM_2) deficiency, and biopsy of rectal mucosa showed nerve cells with the typical membranous cytoplasmic bodies of Tay-Sachs disease. Others have reported similar cases. A progressive motor neuron or motor nerve disorder has also been observed in glycogen storage disease affecting anterior horn cells. Motor nerve fibers also suffer damage in metachromatic and globoid body leukoencephalopathies, and, as mentioned, this may occur in adults, in association with paraproteinemia and multiple myeloma and as a paraneoplastic process.

Clinical Manifestations (Early-Onset Classic Type; SMA I) The most frequent form of these spinal muscular atrophies, the severe infantile type, is a common disease, occurring once in every 20,000 live births. After cystic fibrosis, it is the most common cause of death from a recessively inherited disease. Characteristically the infant, usually born normally, is noted from birth to be unnaturally weak and limp ("floppy"). Some mothers report that fetal movement in utero had been less than expected or lacking altogether. In severe cases, arthrogryposis at ankles and wrists or dislocation of the hips is noted at birth (page 1530). The muscle weakness in these children is generalized from the beginning, and death comes early, usually within the first year. Other infants seem to develop normally for several months before the weakness becomes apparent. In these, the trunk, pelvic, and shoulder-girdle muscles are at first disproportionately affected, while the fingers and hands, toes and feet, and cranial muscles retain their mobility. *Hypotonia* accompanies the weakness, and since passive displacement of articulated parts in testing muscle tone is easier to judge than power of contraction at this early age, it may be singled out as the dominant clinical characteristic. As a rule the tendon reflexes are unobtainable. Volume of muscle is diminished but is difficult to evaluate because of the coverings of adipose tissue. Fasciculations are seldom visible except sometimes in the tongue. Perception of tactile and painful stimuli is undiminished, and emotional and social development measure up to age.

As the months pass, the weakness and hypotonia progress gradually and spread to all of the skeletal muscles except the ocular ones. Intercostal paralysis with a degree of collapse of the chest is the rule. Respiratory movements become paradoxical (abdominal protrusion with chest retraction). The cry becomes feeble, and sucking and swallowing are less efficient. Such infants are unable to sit unless propped, and they cannot hold up their heads without support. They cannot roll over or support their weight when placed on their feet. Their posture is characteristic: arms abducted and flexed at the elbow, legs in the "frog position" with external rotation and abduction at hips and flexion at hips and knees. If the effects of gravity are removed, all muscles continue to contract; i.e., there is paresis, not paralysis. Until late in the illness, these children appear bright-eyed, alert, and responsive.

The disease runs a steadily downhill course. Infants in whom the disease becomes apparent only after several months of life run a less precipitous course than those affected in utero or at birth. Some of the former become able to sit and creep and even to walk with support; those with later onset may survive for several years and even into adolescence or early adult life, as already mentioned.

Laboratory data of confirmatory value are few. Muscle enzymes in the serum are usually normal, rarely elevated. The EMG, if performed at a late enough stage of development, displays fibrillations, proving the denervative basis of the weakness. Motor unit potentials are diminished in number and, in the more slowly evolving cases, some are larger than normal (giant or polyphasic potentials reflecting reinnervation). Motor nerve conduction velocities are normal or fall in the low-normal range (these are normally slower in infants than in adults). Early electrophysiologic studies may also give ambiguous results.

Pathologic Findings Muscle biopsy after 1 month of age reveals a typical picture of group atrophy; shortly after birth this change is difficult to discern. Aside from denervative atrophy, the essential abnormalities are in the anterior horn cells in the spinal cord and the motor nuclei in the lower brainstem. Nerve cells are greatly reduced in number, and many of the remaining ones are in varying stages of degeneration; a few are chromatolytic and contain cytoplasmic inclusions. It is not unusual to see figures of neuronophagia. There is replacement gliosis and secondary degeneration in roots and nerves. Other systems of neurons, including the corticospinal and corticobulbar, remain intact.

Differential Diagnosis *The major problem in diagnosis is to distinguish Werdnig-Hoffmann disease from an array of other diseases that cause hypotonia and delayed motor development in the neonate and infant.* The congenital myopathies (as described in Chap. 52), the glycogenoses, and disorders of fatty acid metabolism frequently present in this way. The preservation of tendon reflexes and relative lack of progression of muscle weakness distinguish these latter disorders. The muscle biopsy, if studied properly, usually yields the correct diagnosis. Because of the gravity of the diagnosis, muscle biopsy should be performed if there is any suspicion of spinal muscular atrophy. If studied properly, the biopsy usually yields the correct diagnosis.

Certain forms of muscular dystrophy, notably myotonic dystrophy, which is about twice as frequent as Werding-Hoffman disease, may become manifest in the neonatal period and interfere with sucking and motor development (Chap. 52). As a rule, the weakness is not as severe or diffuse as that in Werdnig-Hoffmann disease. Also, a number of polyneuropathies may cause a serious degree of weakness in early childhood. Unfortunately, in respect to the latter, adequate sensory testing is not possible because of the patients' age, but the CSF protein is often elevated. Again, diagnosis is greatly facilitated by nerve-muscle biopsy and measurement of nerve conduction velocities. The latter are reduced but must be interpreted with caution because of incomplete development of axons and of myelination in the first months of life. The needle EMG examination shows subtle signs of denervation that cannot be easily distinguished from the finding in the spinal muscular atrophies. Examination of parents and siblings may disclose a clinically inapparent neuropathy. Polymyositis of childhood may also simulate both muscular dystrophy and motor neuron disease (page 1482).

Mental retardation with a flaccid rather than spastic weakness of the limbs is another major category of disease that must be distinguished. Also, certain of the polioencephalopathies and leukodystrophies may weaken muscles and abolish tendon reflexes, but usually there is evidence of cerebral involvement. The same may be said of the Down syndrome, cretinism, and achondrodysplasia. Finally, very sick children with celiac disease, cystic fibrosis, and other chronic diseases may be hypotonic to the point of simulating neuromuscular disease. Usually speech is not delayed and tendon reflexes are preserved in these purely medical states, and strength returns as the medical problem is corrected.

There remains, after the assiduous study of the "floppy infant," a group of cases of hypotonia and motor underdevelopment that cannot be classified. The term *amyotonia congenita* (Oppenheim) was once applied to all of this group but is now obsolete. Walton devised the term *benign congenital hypotonia* to designate patients who manifest limp and flabby limbs in infancy and a delay in sitting up and walking and who improve gradually, some completely and others incompletely. Neither of these terms serves the purpose of precise diagnosis, and so they should be abandoned. It is likely that among this group there are other examples of congenital myopathy that await differentiation by application of modern histochemical, ultrastructural, and genetic techniques.

Chronic Childhood and Juvenile Proximal Spinal Muscular Atrophy (Wohlfart-Kugelberg-Welander Syndrome) This is a somewhat different form of heredofamilial spinal muscular atrophy which, as the name indicates, involves the proximal muscles of the limbs predominantly and is only slowly progressive. It was first clearly separated from other forms of motor system disease and from muscular dystrophy by Wohlfart and by Kugelberg and Welander in the mid-1950s. In about one-third of the cases, the onset is before 2 years of age, and in half, between 3 and 18 years. Males predominate, especially among patients with juvenile and adult onset. The usual form of transmission is by an autosomal recessive gene, but families with dominant and sex-linked inheritance have also been described.

The disease begins insidiously, with weakness and atrophy of the pelvic girdle and proximal leg muscles, followed by involvement of the shoulder girdle and upper arm muscles. Unlike the sporadic form of spinal muscular atrophy, the Wohlfart-Kugelberg-Welander variety is bilaterally symmetrical from the beginning, and fasciculations are observed in only half the cases. Ultimately the distal limb muscles are involved and tendon reflexes are lost. Bulbar musculature and corticospinal tracts are spared, although Babinski signs and an associated ophthalmoplegia (presumably neural) have been reported in rare instances.

The presence of fasciculations and the EMG and muscle biopsy findings—all of which show the characteristic abnormalities of neural atrophy—permit distinction from muscular dystrophy. Cases that have been examined postmortem have shown loss and degeneration of the anterior horn cells.

The disease progresses very slowly, and some patients survive to old age without serious disability. In general, the earlier the onset, the less favorable the prognosis; however, even the most severely affected patients retain the ability to walk for at least 10 years after the onset. Admittedly, it is difficult to make a sharp distinction between these cases of Wohlfart-Kugelberg-Welander disease and certain milder instances of Werdnig-Hoffmann disease with onset in late infancy and early childhood and prolonged survival (Byers and Banker).

Kennedy Syndrome (Bulbospinal Atrophy) An unusual pattern of *distal atrophy with prominent bulbar signs* and, less often, ocular palsies was first described by Kennedy. The time of onset has varied from childhood to adult age, but most patients have been in their third decade when neurologic symptoms arise. Most cases have shown an X-linked pattern of inheritance and a lesser number an autosomal dominant pattern. The proximal shoulder and hip musculature are involved first by weakness and atrophy, followed by dysarthria and dysphagia in about half of patients. Often muscle cramps or twitching appears before weakness becomes evident. Facial fasciculations are said to be characteristic. The tendon reflexes become depressed and may be absent; a mild sensory neuropathy is almost universal. In the family described by Kaeser, in which 12 members in five generations were affected, the pattern of weakness was shoulder-shank, i.e., scapuloperoneal, for which reason it may be mistaken for muscle dystrophy. The muscular atrophy is associated in two-thirds of patients with gynecomastia (this feature may first identify affected men in a kindred), oligospermia, and sometimes diabetes. The CK level is elevated, sometimes tenfold, and physiologic studies reveal denervation and reinnervation as well as indications of a mild sensory neuropathy.

The fundamental defect is a CAG expansion in the gene that codes for the androgen receptor on the short arm of the X chromosome (La Spada et al). Lengthened sequences are associated with an earlier age of onset (anticipation, as in Huntington disease) but have no relation to the severity of disease. Androgen receptors have been found on motor neurons of the spinal cord, but the degeneration of motor neurons seems to be independent of this finding. Neuronal inclusions have recently been described, the presumption being that they are aggregations of the abnormally long polyglutamine protein sequences that correspond to the CAG expansion. A family with the bulbospinal phenotype but without the CAG expansion has also been reported (Paradiso et al). Other features, such as optic atrophy and sensory neuronopathy, were present in some members. The diagnosis can be confirmed by genetic testing for the lengthened repeat trinucleotide sequence. Prenatal diagnosis and identification of female carriers is also possible by genetic testing.

Progressive Bulbar Palsy (Fazio-Londe Syndrome) Fazio in 1892 and Londe in 1893 described the development of a progressive bulbar palsy in children, adolescents, and young adults. There is progressive paralysis of the facial, lingual, pharyngeal, laryngeal, and sometimes ocular muscles. The illness usually presents with stridor and respiratory symptoms, following which facial diplegia, dysarthria, dysphagia, and dysphonia are observed. These become increasingly pronounced until the time of death some years after onset. In a few patients there is a late development of corticospinal signs and sometimes ocular palsies. Also jaw and oculomotor weakness appears occasionally, and in one case there was progressive deafness. The disease is rare, only 24 well-described examples having been recorded in the medical literature by 1992 (McShane et al). Inheritance may be autosomal dominant, as in Fazio's original case, and rarely X-linked, but it is more likely to be autosomal recessive. Pathologic examination has shown a loss of motor neurons in the hypoglossal, ambiguus, facial, and trigeminal motor nuclei. In a few cases, the nerve cells in the ocular motor nuclei were also diminished. This disease, the few times we have encountered it, had to be differentiated from myasthenia gravis, a pontomedullary glioma, and brainstem multiple sclerosis.

Hereditary Spastic Paraplegia or Diplegia (Strümpell-Lorrain Disease) This disease was described by Seeligmuller in 1874 and later by Strümpell in Germany and Lorrain in France; it has now been identified in nearly every part of the world. The pattern of inheritance is usually autosomal dominant, less often recessive (one family has shown X-linked inheritance), and the onset may be at any age from childhood to the senium. Harding divided the disease into two groups, the more common one beginning before age 35 with a very protracted course and the other with a late onset (40 to 60 years); the latter type often shows sensory loss, urinary symptoms, and kinetic tremor. The clinical picture is that of a gradual development of spastic weakness of the legs with increasing difficulty in walking. The tendon reflexes are hyperactive and the plantar reflexes extensor. In the pure form of the disease, sensory and other nervous functions are entirely intact. If the onset is in childhood, as many cases are, a common orthopedic problem arises of arched and shortened feet and there is a shortening (pseudocontracture) of calf muscles, forcing the child or adolescent to "toe-walk." In children, the legs appear to be underdeveloped, and they are rather thin in both children and adults. Sometimes the knees are slightly flexed; at other times the legs are fully extended (genu recurvatum) and adducted. Weakness is variable and difficult to estimate. Sphincteric function is usually retained. Subtle sensory loss in the feet has been reported. The arms are variably involved. In some patients, the arms appear to be spared even though the tendon reflexes are lively. In others, the hands are stiff, movements are clumsy, and speech is mildly dysarthric. Conjoined findings such as nystagmus, ocular palsies, optic atrophy, pigmentary macular degeneration, ataxia (both cerebellar and sensory), sensorimotor polyneuropathy, ichthyosis, patchy skin pigmentation, epilepsy, and dementia have all been described in isolated families (see further on).

The few available pathologic studies have shown that, in addition to degeneration of the corticospinal tracts throughout the spinal cord, there is thinning of the columns of Goll, mainly in the lumbosacral regions, and of the spinocerebellar tracts, even when no sensory abnormalities had been detected during life. These were the pathologic findings described by Strümpell in his original (1880) report of two brothers with spastic paraplegia; one of them, in addition, had a cerebellar syndrome, but again there were no sensory abnormalities. A reduction in the number of Betz and anterior horn cells has also been reported.

Inheritance and Pathogenesis Several genetic mutations have given rise to this disease. The uncomplicated autosomal dominant variety has been linked so far to chromosomes 2p, 8q, 14q, and 15q, the 2q variety being most frequent and most often associated with dementia; the recessive variety has been linked to 8p, 15q (the most frequent recessive type), and 16q. The recessive type has the unusual feature of thinning of the corpus callosum. As is true with many similar genetic diseases, the common variety associated with a mutation on 2p shows great variability in clinical presentation within and among families, as has been pointed out by Nielsen and colleagues. Rare X-linked types have been associated with two sites on the long arm of the chromosome, one of which is an allelic variant of the Pelizaeus-Merzbacher gene. In only a few of these kindreds have the genes responsible for disease been identified. A protein called *paraplegin*, a metalloprotease of the mitochondrial inner membrane, has been related to the 16q mutation. A defect in oxidative phosphorylation has been demonstrated in these patients and in theory is related to the abnormal gene product. The genetics of the hereditary spastic paraplegias has recently been reviewed by Figlewicz and Bird.

Differential Diagnosis In the diagnosis of this disorder, one must always consider an indolent spinal cord or foramen magnum tumor, cervical spondylosis, multiple sclerosis (this was the clinical diagnosis in Strümpell's original cases), Chiari malformation, compression of the cord by a variety of congenital bony malformations at the craniocervical junction, and a number of chronic myelitides—Lyme disease, lupus erythematosus, sarcoidosis, acquired immune deficiency syndrome (AIDS), adrenomyeloneuropathy, primary lateral sclerosis (described earlier in this chapter), and tropical spastic paraparesis.

Variants of Familial Spastic Paraplegia The neurologic literature contains a large number of descriptions of familial spastic paraplegia combined with other neurologic abnormalities. Some of the syndromes had developed early in life, in conjunction with moderate degrees of mental retardation. Nevertheless the rest of the neurologic picture appeared many years after birth and was progressive. Some idea of the number of these "hereditary paraplegia-plus" syndromes and the diverse combinations in which they may present is conveyed in the recent review by Gout and colleagues. Again, it is hardly possible to describe each of these symptoms in any degree of detail. The following list includes the best-known entities. But if the term *hereditary spastic paraplegia* is to have any neurologic significance, it should be applied only to the relatively rare, pure form of the progressive syndrome. The more common "atypical" cases—with amyotrophy, cerebellar ataxia, tremors, dystonia, athetosis, optic atrophy, retinal degeneration, amentia, and dementia—should be put in separate categories and their identity retained for nosologic purposes until such time as some biochemical and genetic data related to pathogenesis are forthcoming. Separable also are all the congenital nonprogressive types of spastic diplegia and athetosis. The following list includes the best-known entities:

1. *Hereditary spastic paraplegia with spinocerebellar and ocular symptoms (Ferguson-Critchley syndrome).* This syndrome is characterized by a disorder of gaze, optic atrophy, cerebellar ataxia, and spastic paraparesis. Most impressive are the manifestations of spinocerebellar ataxia beginning during the fourth and fifth decades of life accompanied by weakness of the legs, alterations of mood, pathologic crying and laughing, dysarthria and diplopia, dysesthesias of limbs, and poor bladder control. The tendon reflexes are lively, with bilateral Babinski signs. Sensation is diminished distally in the limbs. The whole picture resembles multiple sclerosis. In other cases, running through several generations of a family, the extrapyramidal features were more striking; such cases overlap with the following syndromes.

2. *Hereditary spastic paraplegia with extrapyramidal signs.* Action and static tremors, parkinsonian rigidity,

dystonic tongue movement, and athetosis of the limbs have all been found in combination with spastic paraplegia. Gilman and Romanul have reviewed the literature on this subject. The picture of parkinsonism with spastic weakness and other corticospinal signs has been the most frequent combination, in the authors' experience.

3. *Hereditary spastic paraplegia with optic atrophy*. This is known as *Behr syndrome* or *optic atrophy-ataxia syndrome*, since cerebellar signs are usually conjoined. Some of the members of the large family reported by Bruyn and Went also had athetosis. The syndrome is transmitted as an autosomal recessive trait, with onset in infancy and slow progression.

4. *Hereditary spastic paraplegia with macular degeneration (Kjellin syndrome)*. Spastic paraplegia with amyotrophy, oligophrenia, and central retinal degeneration constitutes the syndrome described in 1959 by Kjellin. While the mental retardation is stationary, the spastic weakness and retinal changes are of late onset and progressive. When ophthalmoplegia is added, it is called the *Barnard-Scholz syndrome*.

5. *Hereditary spastic paraplegia with mental retardation or dementia*. Many of the children with progressive spastic paraplegia either have been mentally retarded since early life or have appeared to regress mentally as other neurologic symptoms developed. Examples of this syndrome and its variants are too numerous to be considered here but are contained in the review of Gilman and Romanul. The autosomal *recessive syndrome of Sjögren-Larsson*, with the onset in infancy of spastic weakness of the legs in association with mental retardation, stands somewhat apart because of the associated ichthyosis.

6. *Hereditary spastic paraplegia with polyneuropathy*. We have observed several patients in whom a sensorimotor polyneuropathy was combined with unmistakable signs of corticospinal disease. The age of onset was in childhood or adolescence, and the disability progressed to the point where the patient was chairbound by early adult life. In two of the cases, a sural nerve biopsy revealed a typical hypertrophic polyneuropathy; in a third case there was only a depletion of large myelinated fibers. The syndrome resembles the myeloneuropathy of adrenoleukodystrophy.

7. *Spastic paraparesis with distal muscle wasting (Broyer syndrome)*. This disorder is transmitted as an autosomal recessive trait. Onset is in childhood with amyotrophy of the hands, followed by spasticity and contractures of the lower limbs. Cerebellar signs (mild), athetosis, and deafness may be added.

SYNDROME OF PROGRESSIVE BLINDNESS

There are two main classes of progressive blindness in children, adolescents, and adults: progressive optic neuropathy and retinal (pigmentary or tapetoretinal) degeneration. Of course there are many congenital anomalies and retinal diseases beginning in infancy that result in blindness and microphthalmia. Some of those of neurologic interest were already described briefly in connection with the hereditary spastic paraplegias and in Chap. 13.

Hereditary Optic Atrophy of Leber

Athough familial amaurosis was known in the early eighteenth century, it was Leber in 1871 who gave the definitive description of this disease and traced it through many genealogies. The family studies of Nikoskelainen and coworkers indicate that all daughters of carrier mothers become carriers themselves, a type of transmission that is determined by inheritance of defective mitochondrial DNA from the mother (Wallace et al). In an extensive review of Leber hereditary optic atrophy by the National Hospital group in London, some of the clinical variations are described. Common to all their cases was the presence of a pathogenic mitochondrial DNA abnormality (Riordan-Eva et al), but this may occur at one of several sites (page 1140). Thus, Leber optic atrophy has been added to the growing list of mitochondrial diseases, which, as a group, are discussed in detail in Chap. 37.

In most patients, the visual loss begins between 18 and 25 years, but the range of age of onset is much broader. Usually the visual loss has an insidious onset and a subacute evolution, but it may evolve rapidly, so as to suggest a retrobulbar neuritis; moreover, in these latter instances, aching in the eye or brow may accompany the visual loss. Subjective visual phenomena are reported by some. Usually both eyes are affected simultaneously, though in some one eye is affected first, followed by the other after an interval of several weeks or months. In practically all cases, the second eye is affected within a year of the first. In the unimpaired eye, abnormalities of visual evoked potentials may precede impairment of visual acuity (Carroll and Mastaglia).

Once started, the visual loss progresses over a period of weeks to months. Characteristically, central vision is affected before peripheral, and there is a stage in which bilateral central scotomata are readily demonstrated. Early on, perception of blue-yellow is deficient, while that of red and green is relatively preserved. In the more advanced stages, however, the patients are totally color-blind. Constriction of the fields may be added later. At first there may be swelling and hyperemia of the discs, but soon they become atrophic. Peripapillary vasculopathy, consisting of tortuosity and arteriovenous shunting, is the primary structural change, and this has been present also in asymptomatic offspring of carrier females.

As visual symptoms develop, fluorescein angiography shows shunting in the abnormal vascular bed, with reduced filling of the capillaries of the papillomacular bundle. Although patients are left with dense central scotomata, it is of some importance that the visual impairment is seldom complete; in some patients, relative stabilization of visual function occurs. In a few, there may be a surprising improvement.

Examination of the optic nerve lesion shows the central parts of the nerves to be degenerated from papillae to the lateral geniculate bodies, i.e., the papillomacular bundles are particularly affected. Presumably axis cylinders and myelin degenerate together, as would be expected from the loss of nerve cells in the superficial layer of the retina. Both astrocytic glial and endoneurial fibroblastic connective tissue are increased.

Congenital optic atrophy (of which recessive and dominant forms are known), retrobulbar neuritis, and nutritional optic neuropathy are the main considerations in differential diagnosis.

Retinitis Pigmentosa

This remarkable retinal abiotrophy, known since Helmholtz first invented the ophthalmoscope in 1851, usually begins in childhood and adolescence. Unlike the optic atrophy of Leber, which affects only the third neuron of the visual neuronal chain, retinitis pigmentosa affects all the retinal layers, both the neuroepithelium and pigment epithelium (see Fig. 13-1). For this combination, Leber proposed the term *tapetoretinal degeneration*, thinking it preferable to *retinitis pigmentosa*, since there is no evidence of inflammation. The incidence of this disorder is two or three times greater in males than in females. Inheritance is more often autosomal recessive than dominant; in the former, consanguinity plays an important part, increasing the likelihood of the disease by approximately 20 times. Sex-linked types are also known. It is estimated that 100,000 Americans are afflicted with this disease.

One form of retinitis pigmentosa is linked to chromosome 3, where the gene for the photosensitive rod-cell protein opsin (which, in combination with vitamin A, forms rhodopsin) is located. When light strikes rhodopsin in the normal eye, the opsin releases vitamin A, and this initiates the sequence of changes that activate the rods. As a consequence of the gene abnormality, the quantity of opsin and rhodopsin in retinitis pigmentosa is reduced; one amino acid building block (proline) in the protein is substituted by histidine (Dryja et al).

The first symptom is usually an impairment of twilight vision (nyctalopia). Under dim light, the visual fields tend to constrict; but slowly, as the disease progresses, there is permanent visual impairment in all degrees of illumination. The perimacular zones tend to be the first and most severely involved, giving rise to partial or complete ring scotomata. Peripheral loss sets in later. Usually both eyes are affected simultaneously, but cases are on record where one eye was affected first and more severely. Color vision is lost relatively late. The electrical activity of the retina (measured by the electroretinogram) is extinguished, in contrast to the Leber type of optic atrophy, in which it is retained.

Ophthalmoscopic examination shows the characteristic triad of pigmentary deposits that assume the configuration of bone corpuscles, attenuated vessels, and pallor of the optic discs. The pigment is due to clumping of epithelial cells that migrate from the pigment layer to the superficial parts of the retina as the rod cells degenerate. The pigmentary change spares only the fovea, so that eventually the world is perceived by the patient as though he were looking through narrow tubes.

Syndromes to which retinitis pigmentosa may be linked are oligophrenia, obesity, syndactyly, and hypogonadism (Bardet-Biedl syndrome); hypogenitalism, obesity, and mental deficiency (Laurence-Moon syndrome); Friedreich and other types of spinocerebellar and cerebellar ataxia; spastic paraplegia and quadriplegia with Laurence-Moon syndrome; neurogenic amyotrophy, myopia, and color blindness; polyneuropathy and deafness (Refsum disease); deaf mutism; Cockayne syndrome and Bassen-Kornzweig disease; and several mitochondrial diseases—particularly progressive external ophthalmoplegia and Kearns-Sayre syndromes.

Differential diagnosis includes the Batten form of cerebroretinal degeneration, Pelizaeus-Merzbacher disease, and Gaucher disease as well as the various forms of ceroid lipofuscinosis and retinal infections such as syphilis, toxoplasmosis, and cytomegalic inclusion disease.

Virtual blindness is the outcome in many cases, but in others the visual failure stops short of that. It is doubtful whether any of the many proposed modes of therapy (sympathectomy, steroids, vitamins A and E) have any effect in halting the progress of the disease.

Stargardt Disease

This is a bilaterally symmetrical, slowly progressive macular degeneration, differentiated from retinitis pigmentosa by Stargardt in 1909. In essence it is a hereditary (usually autosomal recessive) tapetoretinal degeneration or dystrophy (the latter term being preferred by Waardenburg), with onset between 6 and 20 years, rarely later, and leading to a loss of central vision. The macular region becomes gray or yellow-brown with pigmentary spots, and the visual fields show central scotomata. Later the periphery of the retina may become dystrophic. The lesion is well visualized by fluorescein angiography, which discloses a virtually pathognomonic "dark choroid" pattern. Activity in the electroretinogram is diminished or abolished. Both dominantly inherited Stargardt disease and the closely related cone-rod dystrophy have been linked to a defect on chromosome 6p in some families and 13q in others; the less common recessive variety has been mapped to 1p. In the former type, several gene errors code for a transporter protein (termed ABCR) of the photoreceptor.

This disease, with its selective loss of cone function, is in a sense the inverse of retinitis pigmentosa. According to Cohan and associates, it may be associated with epilepsy, Refsum syndrome, Kearns-Sayre syndrome, Bassen-Kornzweig syndrome, or Sjögren-Larsson syndrome, or with spinocerebellar and other forms of cerebellar degeneration and familial paraplegia.

SYNDROME OF PROGRESSIVE DEAFNESS
(See pages 296–299)

There is an impressive group of hereditary, progressive cochleovestibular atrophies that are linked to atrophies and degenerations of the nervous system. These are the subject of an informative review by Konigsmark. Such neuro-otologic syndromes must be set alongside a group of five diseases that affect the auditory and vestibular nerves exclusively: dominant progressive nerve deafness; dominant, low-frequency hearing loss; dominant midfrequency hearing loss; sex-linked, early-onset neural deafness; and hereditary episodic vertigo and hearing loss. The last of these is of special interest to neurologists because both balance and hearing are affected.

It should be pointed out that in 70 percent of cases of hereditary deafness, there are no other somatic or neurologic abnormalities. To date, three separate autosomal mutations have been identified that are associated with this pure "nonsyndromic" type of hereditary deafness. In one such family from Costa Rica, the gene codes for protein that regulates the polymerization of actin, the major cytoskeletal component of the hair cells of the inner ear (see review by Pennisi). More recently, a number of mitochondrial disorders have been associated with deafness alone as well as with a number of the better-characterized mitochondrial syndromes (see Chap. 37). The age of onset of hearing loss in the pure forms has been variable, extending well into adulthood.

Hereditary Hearing Loss with Retinal Diseases

Konigsmark has separated this overall category into three subgroups: patients with typical retinitis pigmentosa, those with Leber optic atrophy, and those with other retinal changes.

With respect to retinitis pigmentosa, four syndromes are recognized. Retinitis pigmentosa in combination with congenital hearing loss is referred to as the Usher syndrome. Retinitis pigmentosa and hereditary hearing loss may also be combined with polyneuropathy (Refsum syndrome); with hypogonadism and obesity (Alstrom syndrome); and with dwarfism, mental retardation, premature senility, and photosensitive dermatitis (Cockayne syndrome).

Hereditary hearing loss with optic atrophy forms the core of four syndromes: dominant optic atrophy, ataxia, muscle wasting, and progressive hearing loss (Sylvester disease); recessive optic atrophy, polyneuropathy, and neural hearing loss (Rosenberg-Chutorian syndrome); optic atrophy, hearing loss, and juvenile diabetes mellitus (Tunbridge-Paley syndrome); and opticocochleodentate degeneration with optic atrophy, hearing loss, quadriparesis, and mental retardation (Nyssen–van Bogaert syndrome).

Hearing loss has also been observed with other retinal changes, two of which might be mentioned: Norrie disease, with retinal malformation, hearing loss, and mental retardation (oculoacousticocerebral degeneration), and Small disease, with recessive hearing loss, mental retardation, narrowing of retinal vessels, and muscle atrophy. In the former, the infant is born blind, with a white vascularized retinal mass behind a clear lens; later the lens and cornea become opaque. The eyes are small and the iris is atrophied. In the latter, the optic fundi show tortuosity of vessels, telangiectases, and retinal detachment. The nature of the progressive generalized muscular weakness has not been ascertained.

Hereditary Hearing Loss with Diseases of the Nervous System There are several conditions in which hereditary deafness accompanies degenerative disease of the peripheral or central nervous system. Those associated with mitochondrial encephalopathies have already been mentioned. The other main ones with autosomal inheritance include the following:

1. *Hereditary hearing loss with epilepsy.* The seizure disorder is mainly one of myoclonus. In one dominantly inherited form, photomyoclonus is associated with mental deterioration, hearing loss, and nephropathy (Hermann disease). In May-White disease, also inherited as an autosomal dominant trait, myoclonus and ataxia accompany hearing loss. Congenital deafness and mild chronic epilepsy of recessive type have also been observed (Latham-Monro disease).

2. *Hereditary hearing loss and ataxia.* Here Konigsmark was able to delineate five syndromes, the first two of which show a dominant pattern of heredity, the last three a recessive pattern: piebaldism, ataxia, and neural hearing loss (Telfer syndrome); hearing loss, hyperuricemia, and ataxia (Rosenberg-Bergstrom syndrome); ataxia and progressive hearing loss (Lichtenstein-Knorr syndrome); ataxia, hypogonadism, mental deficiency, and hearing loss (Richards-Rundles syndrome); ataxia, mental retardation, hearing loss, and pigmentary changes in the skin (Jeune-Tommasi syndrome).

3. *Hereditary hearing loss and other neurologic syndromes.* These include dominantly inherited sensory radicular neuropathy (Denny-Brown); progressive polyneuropathy, kyphoscoliosis, skin atrophy, eye defects (myopia, cataracts, atypical retinitis pigmentosa), bone cysts, and osteoporosis (Flynn-Aird syndrome); chronic polyneuropathy and nephritis (Lemieux-Neemeh syndrome); congenital pain asymbolia and auditory imperception (Osuntokun syndrome); and bulbopontine paralysis (facial weakness, dysarthria, dysphagia, and atrophy of the tongue with fasciculations) with progressive neural hearing loss. The onset of the last syndrome occurs at 10 to 35 years of age; the pattern of inheritance is autosomal recessive. The disease progresses to death. It resembles the progressive hereditary bulbar paralysis of Fazio-Londe except for the progressive deafness and loss of vestibular responses. Regrettably, in most of these syndromes, there are no data regarding labyrinthine function.

The details of these many syndromes are contained in Konigsmark's review. The syndromes are listed in Table 15-1 and have been summarized here in order to increase awareness of the large number of hereditary neurologic diseases for which the clue is provided by the detection of impaired hearing and labyrinthine functions.

REFERENCES

Adams RD, van Bogaert L, van der Eecken H: Striato-nigral degeneration. *J Neuropathol Exp Neurol* 23:584, 1964.

Albert MS, Butters N, Brandt J: Patterns of remote memory in amnesic and demented patients. *Arch Neurol* 38:495, 1981.

Albert SM, Murphy L, Del Bene ML, Rowland LP: A prospective study of preferences and actual treatment choices on ALS. *Neurology* 53:278, 1999.

Allen N, Knopp W: Hereditary parkinsonism-dystonia with sustained control by L-dopa and anticholinergic medication, in Eldridge R, Fahn S (eds): *Advances in Neurology*. Vol 14. *Dystonia*. New York, Raven Press, 1976, pp 201–215.

Alzheimer A: Uber eine eigenartige Erkrankung der Hirnrinde. *Allg Z Psychiatr* 64:146, 1907.

Alzheimer A: Uber eigenartige Krankheitsfalle des spateren Alters. *Z Gesamte Neurol Psychiatr* 4:356, 1911.

Andrew J, Fowler CJ, Harrison MJ: Stereotaxic thalamotomy in 55 cases of dystonia. *Brain* 106:981, 1983.

Arriagada PV, Growdon JH, Hedley-Whyte ET, Hyman BT: Neurofibrillary tangles but not senile plaques parallel duration and severity of Alzheimer's disease. *Neurology* 42:631, 1992.

Bannister R, Oppenheimer DR: Degenerative diseases of the nervous system associated with autonomic failure. *Brain* 95: 457, 1972.

Basun H, Almkvist O, Axelman K, et al: Clinical characteristics of a chromosome 17-linked rapidly progressive familial frontotemporal dementia. *Ann Neurol* 54:539, 1997.

Beal MF, Richardson EP Jr: Primary lateral sclerosis: A case report. *Arch Neurol* 38:630, 1981.

Behr C: Die komplizierte, hereditar-familiare Optikusatrophie des Kindesalters: Ein bisher nicht beschriebener Symptomkomplex. *Klin Monatsbl Augenheilkd* 47(pt 2):138, 1909.

Bennett JP, Landow ER, Schuh LA: Suppression of dyskinesias in advanced Parkinson's disease: II. Increasing daily clozapine doses suppress dyskinesias and improve Parkinsonism symptoms. *Neurology* 43:1551, 1993.

Bensimon G, Lacomblez L, Meininger V: A controlled trial of riluzole in amyotrophic lateral sclerosis: ALS/Riluzole Study Group. *N Engl J Med* 330:585, 1994.

Bharucha NE, Bharucha EP, Bhabha SR: Machado-Joseph-Azorean disease in India. *Arch Neurol* 43:142, 1986.

Boetz MI, Boetz-Marquard T, Elie R, et al: Amantadine hydrochloride treatment in heredodegenerative ataxias: A double blind study. *J Neurol Neurosurg Psychiatry* 61:259, 1996.

Bonduelle M: Amyotrophic lateral sclerosis, in Vinken RT, Bruyn GW (eds): *Handbook of Clinical Neurology*. Vol 29. Amsterdam, North Holland, 1975, pp 281–338.

Bradley WG, Good P, Rasool CG, et al: Morphometric and biochemical studies of peripheral nerves in amyotrophic lateral sclerosis. *Ann Neurol* 14:267, 1983.

Brandt S: *Werdnig-Hoffmann's Infantile Progressive Muscular Atrophy*. Thesis: Vol 22. Copenhagen, Munksgaard, 1950.

BRESSMAN SB, HEIMAN GA, NYGAARD TG, et al: A study of idiopathic torsion dystonia in a non-Jewish family. *Neurology* 44:283, 1994.

BRITTON JW, UITTI RJ, AHLSKOG JE, et al: Hereditary late-onset chorea without significant dementia. *Neurology* 45:443, 1995.

BROOKS DJ: Dopamine agonists: Their role in the treatment of Parkinson's disease. *J Neurol Neurosurg Psychiatry* 68:685, 2000.

BROWN J, LANTOS P, STRATTON M, et al: Familial progressive supranuclear palsy. *J Neurol Neurosurg Psychiatry* 56:473, 1993.

BRUN A, PASSANT U: Frontal lobe degeneration of non-Alzheimer type: Structural characteristics, diagnostic criteria, and relation to frontotemporal dementia. *Acta Neurol Scand* 168:28, 1996.

BRZUSTOWICZ LM, LEHNER T, CASTILLA LH, et al: Genetic mapping of chronic childhood-onset spinal muscular atrophy to chromosome 5q11.2-13.3. *Nature* 344:540, 1990.

BURKE RE, FAHN S, MARSDEN CD: Torsion dystonia: A double-blind, prospective trial of high-dosage trihexyphenidyl. *Neurology* 36:160, 1986.

BURKHARDT CR, FILLEY CM, KLEINSCHMIDT-DEMASTERS BK, et al: Diffuse Lewy body disease and progressive dementia. *Neurology* 38:1520, 1988.

BYERS RK, BANKER BQ: Infantile muscular atrophy. *Arch Neurol* 5:140, 1961.

BYERS RK, GILLES FH, FUNG C: Huntington's disease in children: Neuropathologic study of four cases. *Neurology* 23:561, 1973.

BYRNE EJ, LENNOX G, LOWE J, GODWIN-AUSTEN RB: Diffuse Lewy body disease: Clinical features in 15 cases. *J Neurol Neurosurg Psychiatry* 52:709, 1989.

CAEKEBEKE JFV, JENNEKENS-SCHINKEL A, VAN DER LINDEN ME, et al: The interpretation of dysprosody in patients with Parkinson's disease. *J Neurol Neurosurg Psychiatry* 54:145, 1991.

CAMPUZANO V, MONTERMINI L, MOLTÒ MD, et al: Friedreich's ataxia: Autosomal recessive disease caused by an intronic GAA triplet repeat expansion. *Science* 271:1423, 1996.

CANCEL G, ABBAS N, STEVANIN G, et al: Marked phenotypic heterogeneity associated with expansion of a CAG repeat sequence at the spinocerebellar ataxia/3 Machado-Joseph disease locus. *Am J Hum Genet* 57:809, 1995.

CARROLL WM, MASTAGLIA FL: Leber's optic neuropathy. *Brain* 102:559, 1979.

CASELLI RN, JACK CR, PETERSEN RC, et al: Asymmetric cortical degenerative syndromes: Clinical and radiologic correlations. *Neurology* 42:1462, 1992.

CEDARBAUM JM, GANDY SE, MCDOWELL FH: "Early" initiation of levodopa treatment does not promote the development of motor response fluctuations, dyskinesias, or dementia in Parkinson's disease. *Neurology* 41:622, 1991.

CHAMBERLAIN S, SHAW J, ROWLAND A, et al: Mapping of mutation causing Friedreich's ataxia to human chromosome 9. *Nature* 334:248, 1988.

CHASE TN, FOSTER NL, MANSI L: Alzheimer's disease and the parietal lobe. *Lancet* 2:225, 1983.

CHAWLUK JB, MESULAM M-M, HURTIG H, et al: Slowly progressive aphasia without generalized dementia: Studies with positron emission tomography. *Ann Neurol* 19:68, 1986.

CHIN HC, TENG EC, HENDERSON EL, et al: Clinical subtypes of dementia of Alzheimer type. *Neurology* 35:1544, 1985.

CHIN SS-M, GOLDMAN JE: Glial inclusions in CNS degenerative diseases. *J Neuropathol Exp Neurol* 55:499, 1996.

CHIO A, BRIGNOLIO F, LEONE M, et al: A survival analysis of 155 cases of progressive muscular atrophy. *Acta Neurol Scand* 72:407, 1985.

COBB JL, WOLF PA, AU R, et al: The effect of education on the incidence of dementia and Alzheimer's disease in the Framingham study. *Neurology* 45:1707, 1995.

COHAN SL, KATTAH JC, LIMAYE SR: Familial tapetoretinal degeneration and epilepsy. *Arch Neurol* 36:544, 1979.

COHEN J, LOW P, FEELEY R: Somatic and autonomic function in progressive autonomic failure and multiple system atrophy. *Ann Neurol* 22:692, 1987.

COLOSIMO C, ALBANESE A, HUGHES AJ, et al: Some specific clinical features differentiate multiple system atrophy (striatonigral variety) from Parkinson's disease. *Arch Neurol* 52:294, 1995.

COOPER IS: 20-year follow-up study of the neurosurgical treatment of dystonia musculorum deformans, in Eldridge R, Fahn S (eds): *Advances in Neurology*: Vol 14. *Dystonia*. New York, Raven Press, 1976, pp 423–453.

CREUTZFELDT HG: Uber eine eigenartige herdformige Erkrankung des Zentralnervensystems. *Z Gesamte Neurol Psychiatr* 57:1, 1920.

CROSS HE, MCKUSICK VA: The mast syndrome. *Arch Neurol* 16:1, 1967.

DANIELE A, MORO E, BENTIVOGLIO AR: Zolpidem in progressive supranuclear palsy. *N Engl J Med* 341:543, 1999.

DAVENPORT CG: Huntington's chorea in relation to heredity and eugenics. *Proc Natl Acad Sci USA* 1:283, 1915.

DAVISON C: Spastic pseudosclerosis (cortico-pallido-spinal degeneration). *Brain* 55:247, 1932.

DAVISON C: Pallido-pyramidal disease. *J Neuropathol Exp Neurol* 13:50, 1954.

DE BIE RAM, DE HAAN RJ, NIJSSEN PCG, et al: Unilateral pallidotomy in Parkinson's disease: A randomized, single-blind multicentre trial. *Lancet* 354:1665, 1999.

DÉJERINE J, ANDRE-THOMAS: L'atrophie olivo-ponto-cérebélleuse. *Nouv Icon Salpét* 13:330, 1900.

DEJONG RN: The history of Huntington's chorea in the United States of America, in Barbeau A, et al (eds): *Advances in Neurology*. Vol 1. *Huntington's Chorea, 1872–1972*. New York, Raven Press, 1973, pp 19–27.

DEKOSKY ST, SCHEFF SW: Synapse loss in frontal cortex biopsies in Alzheimer's disease: Correlation with cognitive severity. *Ann Neurol* 27:457, 1990.

DEMICHELE G, FILLA A, BARBIERI F, et al: Late onset recessive ataxia with Friedreich's disease phenotype. *J Neurol Neurosurg Psychiatry* 52:1398, 1989.

DEONNA T: DOPA-sensitive progressive dystonia of childhood with fluctuations of symptoms—Segawa's syndrome and possible variants. *Neuropediatrics* 17:81, 1986.

DE YÉBENES JG, SARASA JL, DANIEL SE, LEES AJ: Familial progressive supranuclear palsy. *Brain* 118:1095, 1995.

DIAMOND SG, MARKHAM CH, HOEHN MM, et al: Multi-center study of Parkinson mortality with early versus late dopa treatment. *Ann Neurol* 22:8, 1987.

DRYJA TP, MCGEE TL, REICHEL E, et al: A point mutation of the rhodopsin gene in one form of retinitis pigmentosa. *Nature* 343:364, 1990.

DUNLAP CB: Pathologic changes in Huntington's chorea, with special reference to corpus striatum. *Arch Neurol Psychiatry* 18:867, 1927.

DUNNETT SB, BJÖRKLUND A: Prospects for the new restorative and neuroprotective treatments in Parkinson's disease. *Nature* 399(suppl 24):A32, 1999.

DÜRR A, COSSEE M, AGID Y, et al: Clinical and genetic abnormalities in patients with Friedreich's ataxia. *N Engl J Med* 335:1169, 1996.

DWORK AJ, BALMACEDA C, FAZZINI EF, et al: Dominantly inherited, early-onset parkinsonism: Neuropathology of a new form. *Neurology* 43:69, 1993.

ELDRIDGE R: The torsion dystonias: Literature review and genetic and clinical studies. *Neurology* 20(11, pt 2):1, 1970.

EMERY AEH: The nosology of progressive muscular atrophy. *J Med Genet* 8:481, 1971.

FARMER TW, WINGFIELD MS, LYNCH SA, et al: Ataxia, chorea, seizures, and dementia. *Arch Neurol* 46:774, 1989.

FARRER LA, CONNEALLY M: Predictability of phenotype in Huntington's disease. *Arch Neurol* 44:109, 1987.

FEARNLEY JM, REVESZ T, BROOKS DJ, et al: Diffuse Lewy body disease presenting with a supranuclear gaze palsy. *J Neurol Neurosurg Psychiatry* 54:159, 1991.

FIGLEWICZ DA, BIRD TD: "Pure" hereditary spastic paraplegias. *Neurology* 53:5, 1999.

FIGLEWICZ DA, KRIZUS A, MARTOLINI MG, et al: Variants of the heavy neurofilament subunit are associated with the development of amyotrophic lateral sclerosis. *Hum Mol Genet* 3:1757, 1994.

FINLAYSON MH, GUBERMAN A, MARTIN JB: Cerebral lesions in familial amyotrophic lateral sclerosis and dementia. *Acta Neuropathol* 26:237, 1973.

FLATAU E, STERLING W: Progressiver Torsionsspasmus bei Kindern. *Z Gesamte Neurol Psychiatr* 7:586, 1911.

FLETCHER NA, HARDING AE, MARSDEN CD: A genetic study of idiopathic torsion dystonia in the United Kingdom. *Brain* 113:379, 1990.

FOWLER HL: Machado-Joseph-Azorean disease: A ten-year study. *Arch Neurol* 41:921, 1984.

FRIEDMAN JH, LANNON MC: Clozapine in the treatment of psychosis in Parkinson's disease. *Neurology* 39:1219, 1989.

GARCIN R, BRION S, KNOCHNEIVISS AA: La syndrome de Creutzfeldt-Jakob et les syndromes cortico-stries du presenium (ã l'occasion de 5 observations anatomo cliniques. *Rev Neurol* 109:419, 1963.

GEARING M, OLSON DA, WATTIS RL, MIRRA S: Progressive supranuclear palsy: Neuropathologic and clinical heterogeneity. *Neurology* 44:1015, 1994.

GILBERT JJ, KISH SJ, CHANG LJ, et al: Dementia, parkinsonism, and motor neuron disease: Neurochemical and neuropathological correlates. *Ann Neurol* 24:688, 1988.

GILLIAM TC, BRZUSTOWICZ LM, CASTILLA LH, et al: Genetic homogeneity between acute and chronic forms of spinal muscular atrophy. *Nature* 345:823, 1990.

GILMAN S, LITTLE R, JOHANNS J, et al: Evolution of sporadic olivopontocerebellar atrophy into multiple system atrophy. *Neurology* 55:527, 2000.

GILMAN S, ROMANUL FCA: Hereditary dystonic paraplegia with amyotrophy and mental deficiency: Clinical and neuropathological characteristics, in Vinken PJ, Bruyn GW (eds): *Handbook of Clinical Neurology*. Vol 22. Amsterdam, North-Holland, 1975, pp 445–465.

GOLBE LI, DIIORIO G, BONAVITA V, et al: A large kindred with autosomal dominant Parkinson's disease. *Ann Neurol* 27:276, 1990.

GOUDSMIT J, MORROW CH, ASHER DM, et al: Evidence for and against the transmissibility of Alzheimer's disease. *Neurology* 30:945, 1980.

GOUDSMIT J, WHITE BJ, WEITKAMP LR, et al: Familial Alzheimer's disease in two kindreds of the same geographic and ethnic origin. *J Neurol Sci* 49:79, 1981.

GOUT O, FONTAINE B, LYON-CAEN O: Paraparesis spastique de l'adulte orientation diagnostiques. *Rev Neurol* 150:809, 1994.

GRAHAM JG, OPPENHEIMER DR: Orthostatic hypotension and nicotine sensitivity in a case of multiple system atrophy. *J Neurol Neurosurg Psychiatry* 32:28, 1969.

GREENFIELD JG: *The Spino-Cerebellar Degenerations*. Springfield, IL, Charles C Thomas, 1954.

GREGORY R: Unilateral pallidotomy for advanced Parkinson's disease. *Brain* 122:382, 1999.

GRIGGS RC, MOXLEY RT, LAFRANCE RA, et al: Hereditary paroxysmal ataxia: Response to acetazolamide. *Neurology* 28:1259, 1978.

GUSELLA JF, WEXLER NS, CONNEALLY PM, et al: A polymorphic DNA marker, genetically linked to Huntington's disease. *Nature* 306:234, 1983.

HAGBERG B, KYLLERMAN M, STEEN G: Dyskinesia and dystonia in neurometabolic disorders. *Neuropaediatrie* 10:305, 1979.

HAKIM AM, MATHIESON G: Basis of dementia in Parkinson's disease. *Lancet* 2:729, 1978.

HALLETT M, KHOSHBIN S: A physiological mechanism of bradykinesia. *Brain* 103:301, 1980.

HARDIE RJ, PULLON HW, HARDING AE, et al: Neuroacanthocytosis: A clinical, haematological, and pathological study of 19 cases. *Brain* 114(pt 1A):13, 1991.

HARDING AE: Early onset cerebellar ataxia with retained tendon reflexes: A clinical and genetic study of a disorder distinct from Friedreich's ataxia. *J Neurol Neurosurg Psychiatry* 44:503, 1981.

HARDING AE: Clinical features and classification of inherited ataxias, in Harding AE, Deufel T (eds): *Inherited Ataxias*. New York, Raven Press, 1993, pp 1–14.

HAYDEN MR, MARTIN WRW, STOESSI AJ, et al: Positron emission tomography in the early diagnosis of Huntington's disease. *Neurology* 36:888, 1986.

HELY MA, REID WGJ, HALLIDAY GM, et al: Diffuse Lewy body disease: Clinical features in nine cases without coexistent Alzheimer's disease. *J Neurol Neurosurg Psychiatry* 60:531, 1996.

Henderson JM, Hubbard BM: Definition of Alzheimer disease. *Lancet* 1:408, 1985.

Hirano A, Kurland LT, Krooth RS, Lessell S: Parkinsonism-dementia complex, an endemic disease on the Island of Guam: I. Clinical features. *Brain* 84:642, 1961.

Hirano A, Malamud M, Kurland LT: Parkinsonism-dementia complex on the Island of Guam: II. Pathological features. *Brain* 84:662, 1961.

Hirayama K, Tomonaga M, Kitano K, et al: Focal cervical poliopathy causing juvenile muscular atrophy of distal upper extremity: A pathological study. *J Neurol Neurosurg Psychiatry* 50:285, 1987.

Hoehn MM, Yahr MD: Parkinsonism: Onset, progression, and mortality. *Neurology* 17:427, 1967.

Hogan GW, Bauman ML: Familial spastic ataxia: Occurrence in childhood. *Neurology* 27:520, 1977.

Holmes GM: A form of familial degeneration of the cerebellum. *Brain* 30:466, 1907.

Holmes GM: An attempt to classify cerebellar disease with a note on Marie's hereditary cerebellar ataxia. *Brain* 30:545, 1907.

Hotson JR, Langston EB, Louis AA: The search for a physiologic marker of Machado-Joseph disease. *Neurology* 37:112, 1987.

Hudson AJ: Amyotrophic lateral sclerosis and its associations with dementia, parkinsonism and other neurologic disorders. *Brain* 104:217, 1981.

Hughes AJ, Daniel SE, Kilford L, Less AJ: Accuracy of clinical diagnosis of idiopathic Parkinson's disease: A clinico-pathological study of 100 cases. *J Neurol Neurosurg Psychiatry* 55:181, 1992.

Hunker CJ, Abbs JH: Frequency of parkinsonian resting tremor in the lips, jaw, tongue, and index finger. *Mov Disord* 5:71, 1990.

Hunt JR: Dyssynergia cerebellaris progressiva: A chronic progressive form of cerebellar tremor. *Brain* 37:247, 1914.

Hunt JR: Progressive atrophy of the globus pallidus. *Brain* 40:58, 1917.

Hunt JR: Dyssynergia cerebellaris myoclonica—Primary atrophy of the dentate system: A contribution to the pathology and symptomatology of the cerebellum. *Brain* 44:490, 1921.

Hunt JR: The striocerebellar tremor. *Arch Neurol Psychiatry* 8:664, 1922.

Huntington G: On chorea. *Med Surg Rep* 26:317, 1872.

Hutton JT, Morris JL: Long-acting carbidopa-levodopa in the management of moderate and advanced Parkinson's disease. *Neurology* 42(suppl 1):51, 1992.

Iizuka R, Hirayama K, Maehara K: Dentato-rubro-pallido-luysian atrophy: A clinico-pathological study. *J Neurol Neurosurg Psychiatry* 47:1288, 1984.

Jakob A: Uber eigenartige Erkrankungen des Zentralnervensystems mit bemerkenswertem anatomischen Befunde (spastische Pseudosclerose-Encephalomyelopathie mit disseminierten Degenerationsherden). *Z Gesamte Neurol Psychiatr* 64:147, 1921.

Jakob A: Uber eine der multiplen Sklerose klinisch nahestehende Erkrankung des Zentralnervensystems (spastische Pseudosklerose) mit bemerkenswertem anatomischen Befunde. *Med Klin* 17:382, 1921.

Jervis GA: Early senile dementia in mongoloid idiocy. *Am J Psychiatry* 105:102, 1948.

Joachim CL, Morris JH, Selkoe DJ: Clinically diagnosed Alzheimer disease: Autopsy results in 150 cases. *Ann Neurol* 24:50, 1988.

Johnson WG, Wigger J, Karp HR: Juvenile spinal muscular atrophy: A new hexosamine deficiency phenotype. *Ann Neurol* 11:11, 1982.

Kaeser HE: Scapuloperoneal muscular dystrophy. *Brain* 88:407, 1965.

Kark RAP, Rosenberg RN, Schut LJ (eds): *Advances in Neurology*. Vol 21. *The Inherited Ataxias*. New York, Raven Press, 1978.

Katzman R: Education and the prevalence of dementia and Alzheimer's disease. *Neurology* 43:13, 1993.

Kennedy WR, Alter M, Sung JH: Progressive proximal spinal and bulbar muscular atrophy of late onset: A sex-linked recessive trait. *Neurology* 18:617, 1968.

Kiernan JA, Hudson AJ: Frontal lobe atrophy in motor neuron diseases. *Brain* 117:747, 1994.

Kirby R, Fowler C, Gosling J, Bannister R: Urethrovesical dysfunction in progressive autonomic failure with multiple system atrophy. *J Neurol Neurosurg Psychiatry* 49:554, 1986.

Kirshner HS, Tanridag O, Thurman L, Whetsell WO Jr: Progressive aphasia without dementia: Two cases with focal spongiform degeneration. *Ann Neurol* 22:527, 1987.

Kjellin KG: Hereditary spastic paraplegia and retinal degeneration (Kjellin syndrome and Barnard-Scholz syndrome), in Vinken PJ, Bruyn GW (eds): *Handbook of Clinical Neurology*. Vol 22. Amsterdam, North-Holland, 1975, pp 467–473.

Knopman DS, Mastri AR, Frey II, et al: Dementia lacking distinctive histologic features: A common non-Alzheimer degenerative dementia. *Neurology* 40:251, 1990.

Koeppen AH: The hereditary ataxias. *J Neuropathol Exp Neurol* 57:531, 1998.

Kolodny EH, Raghavan SS: GM_2-gangliosidosis hexosaminidase mutations not of the Tay-Sachs type produce unusual clinical variants. *Trends Neurosci* 6:16, 1983.

Konigsmark BW: Hereditary diseases of the nervous system with hearing loss, in Vinken PJ, Bruyn GW (eds): *Handbook of Clinical Neurology*. Vol 22. Amsterdam, North-Holland, 1975, pp 499–526.

Konigsmark BW, Weiner LP: The olivopontocerebellar atrophies: A review. *Medicine* 49:227, 1970.

Korf BR: The hereditary dystonias: An emerging story with a twist. *Ann Neurol* 44:4, 1998.

Kosaka K: Diffuse Lewy body disease in Japan. *J Neurol* 237:197, 1990.

Krüger R, Vieira-Saecker AM, Kuhn W, et al: Increased susceptibility to sporadic Parkinson's disease by a certain combined α-synuclein/apolipoprotein E genotype. *Ann Neurol* 45:611, 1999.

Kugelberg E: Chronic proximal (pseudomyopathic) spinal muscular atrophy: Kugelberg-Welander syndrome, in Vinken PJ, Bruyn GW (eds): *Handbook of Clinical Neurology*. Vol 22. Amsterdam, North-Holland, 1975, pp 67–80.

Kugelberg E, Welander L: Heredofamilial juvenile muscular atrophy simulating muscular dystrophy. *Arch Neurol Psychiatry* 5:500, 1956.

Laitinen LV: Leksell's posteroventral pallidotomy in the treatment of Parkinson's disease. *J Neurosurg* 76:53, 1992.

Lance JW, Schwab RS, Peterson EA: Action tremor and the cogwheel phenomenon in Parkinson's disease. *Brain* 86:95, 1963.

Lang AE, Lozano AM, Montgomery E: Posteroventral medial pallidotomy in advanced Parkinson's disease: Second of two parts. *N Engl J Med* 337:1036, 1997.

Lantos P: The definition of multiple system atrophy: A review of recent developments. *J Neuropathol Exp Neurol* 57:1099, 1998.

Lasker AG, Zee DS, Hain TC, et al: Saccades in Huntington's disease: Initiation defects and distractibility. *Neurology* 37:364, 1987.

La Spada AR, Wilson EM, Lubahn DB: Androgen receptor mutation in X-linked spinal and bulbar muscular atrophy. *Nature* 352:77, 1991.

Leber T: Ueber hereditare und congenital angelegte Sehnervenleiden. *Graefes Arch Clin Exp Ophthalmol* 17:249, 1871.

Leenders KL, Frackowiak SJ, Lees AJ: Steele-Richardson-Olszewski syndrome. *Brain* 111:615, 1988.

Lees AJ: Trauma and Parkinson's disease. *Rev Neurol* 153:541, 1997.

Leigh RJ, Newman SA, Folstein SE, et al: Abnormal ocular motor control in Huntington's disease. *Neurology* 33:1268, 1983.

Lennox G: Lewy body dementia. *Baillieres Clin Neurol* 1:653, 1993.

Leverenz J, Sumi SM: Parkinson's disease in patients with Alzheimer's disease. *Arch Neurol* 43:662, 1986.

Levy-Lahad E, Wasco W, Poorkaj P, et al: Candidate gene for the chromosome familial Alzheimer's disease locus. *Science* 269:973, 1995.

Li G, Silverman JM, Smith CJ, et al: Age at onset and familial risk in Alzheimer's disease. *Am J Psychiatry* 152:424, 1995.

Limousin P, Krack P, Pollak P, et al: Electrical stimulation of the subthalamic nucleus in advanced Parkinson's disease. *N Engl J Med* 339:1105, 1998.

Linn RT, Wolf PA, Bachman DL: Preclinical phase of Alzheimer's disease. *Arch Neurol* 52:485, 1995.

Lippa CF, Cohen R, Smith TW, Drachman DA: Primary progressive aphasia with focal neuronal achromasia. *Neurology* 41:882, 1991.

Little BW, Brown PW, Rodgers-Johnson P, et al: Familial myoclonic dementia masquerading as Creutzfeldt-Jakob disease. *Ann Neurol* 20:231, 1986.

Loken H, Cyvin K: Case of clinical juvenile amaurotic idiocy with histological picture of Alzheimer's disease. *J Neurol Neurosurg Psychiatry* 17:211, 1954.

Louis-Bar D, van Bogaert L: Sur la dyssynergie cérébelleuse myoclonique (Hunt). *Monatschr Psychiatr Neurol* 113:215, 1947.

Malamud W, Lowenberg K: Alzheimer's disease: Contributions to its etiology and classification. *Arch Neurol Psychiatry* 21:805, 1929.

Marie P: Sur l'hérédo-ataxie cérébelleuse. *Semin Med* 13:444, 1893.

Marie P, Foix C, Alajouanine T: De l'atrophie cérébelleuse tardive à prédominance corticale. *Rev Neurol* 38:849, 1082, 1922.

Marinescu G: Sur une affection particulière simulant, au point de vue clinique, la sclérose en plaques et ayant pour substratum des plaques du type senile spécial. *Arch Roum Pathol Exp Microbiol* 4:41, March 1931 (*Rev Neurol* 2:453, October 1931).

Marsden CD: Parkinson's disease. *J Neurol Neurosurg Psychiatry* 57:672, 1994.

Martilla PJ, Rinne UK: Disability and progression in Parkinson's disease. *Acta Neurol Scand* 56:159, 1967.

Martin JB: Genetic testing in Huntington's disease. *Ann Neurol* 16:511, 1984.

Martin JB: Molecular basis of the neurodegenerative disorders. *N Engl J Med* 340:1970, 1999.

Mata M, Dorvovini-Zis K, Wilson M, Young AB: New form of familial Parkinson dementia syndrome: Clinical and pathologic findings. *Neurology* 33:1439, 1983.

Mayeux R, Chen J, Mirabello E, et al: An estimate of the incidence of dementia in idiopathic Parkinson's disease. *Neurology* 40:1513, 1990.

McGeer PL, McGeer EG, Suzuki J, et al: Aging, Alzheimer disease and the cholinergic system of the basal forebrain. *Neurology* 34:741, 1984.

McKhann G, Drachman D, Folstein M, et al: Clinical diagnosis of Alzheimer's disease. *Neurology* 34:939, 1984.

McShane MA, Boyd S, Harding B, et al: Progressive bulbar paralysis of childhood: A reappraisal of Fazio-Londe disease. *Brain* 115:1889, 1992.

Mendez MF, Adams NL, Lewandowski KS: Neurobehavioral changes associated with caudate lesions. *Neurology* 39:349, 1989.

Mendez MF, Mendez MA, Martin R, et al: Complex visual disturbances in Alzheimer's disease. *Neurology* 40:439, 1990.

Mesulam M-M: Slowly progressive aphasia without generalized dementia. *Ann Neurol* 11:592, 1982.

Mitsuyama Y: Presenile dementia with motor neuron disease in Japan: Clinico-pathological review of 26 cases. *J Neurol Neurosurg Psychiatry* 47:953, 1984.

Mollaret P: *La Maladie de Friedreich*. Paris, Legrand, 1929.

Moreno Martinez JM, Garcia de la Rocha ML, Martin Araquez A: Monomelic segmental amyotrophy: A Spanish case involving the leg. *Rev Neurol (Paris)* 146:443, 1990.

Morris JC, Cole M, Banker BQ, Wright D: Hereditary dysphasic dementia and the Pick-Alzheimer spectrum. *Ann Neurol* 16:458, 1984.

Mulder DW, Kurland LT, Offord KP, Beard CM: Familial adult motor neuron disease: Amyotrophic lateral sclerosis. *Neurology* 36:511, 1986.

Munsat TL, Skerry L, Korf B, et al: Phenotypic heterogeneity of spinal muscular atrophy mapping to chromosome 5q11.2-13.3 (SMA 5q). *Neurology* 40:1831, 1990.

Murata Y, Yamaguchi S, Kawakami H: Characteristic magnetic resonance imaging findings in Machado-Joseph disease. *Arch Neurol* 55:33, 1998.

NAKANO KK, DAWSON DM, SPENCE A: Machado disease: A hereditary ataxia in Portuguese emigrants to Massachusetts. *Neurology* 22:49, 1972.

NEARY D: Non-Alzheimer's disease forms of cerebral atrophy. *J Neurol Neurosurg Psychiatry* 53:929, 1990.

NEARY D, SNOWDEN JS, BOWDEN DM: Neuropsychological syndromes in presenile dementia due to cerebral atrophy. *J Neurol Neurosurg Psychiatry* 49:163, 1986.

NEE LE, ELDRIDGE R, SUNDERLAND T, et al: Dementia of the Alzheimer type: Clinical and family study of 22 twin pairs. *Neurology* 37:359, 1987.

NIELSEN JE, KRABBE K, JENNUM P, et al: Autosomal dominant pure spastic paraplegia: A clinical, paraclinical and genetic study. *J Neurol Neurosurg Psychiatry* 64:61, 1998.

NIELSEN SL: Striatonigral degeneration disputed in familial disorder. *Neurology* 27:306, 1977.

NIKOSKELAINEN E, SAVONTAUS ML, WANNE OP, et al: Leber's hereditary optic neuroretinopathy—A maternally inherited disease: A genealogic study in four pedigrees. *Arch Ophthalmol* 105:665, 1987.

NYGAARD TG, DUVOISIN RC: Hereditary dystonia-parkinsonism syndrome of juvenile onset. *Neurology* 36:1424, 1986.

NYGAARD TG, WILHELMSEN KC, RISCH NJ, et al: Linkage mapping of dopa-responsive dystonia (DRD) to chromosome 14q. *Nature Genet* 5:386, 1993.

OKAZAKI H, LIPKIN LE, ARONSON SM: Diffuse intracytoplasmic ganglionic inclusions (Lewy type) associated with progressive dementia and quadriparesis in flexion. *J Neuropathol Exp Neurol* 20:237, 1961.

OPPENHEIM H: *Textbook of Nervous Diseases* (A. Bruce, transl). Edinburgh, Schulze, 1911, p 512.

PAKKENBERG B, MOLLER A, GUNDERSEN HJG, et al: The absolute number of nerve cells in substantia nigra in normal subjects and in patients with Parkinson's disease estimated with an unbiased stereological method. *J Neurol Neurosurg Psychiatry* 54:30, 1991.

PAPP MI, KAHN JE, LANTOS PL: Glial cytoplasmic inclusions in the CNS of patients with multiple system atrophy (striatonigral degeneration, olivopontocerebellar atrophy and Shy-Drager syndrome). *J Neurol Sci* 94:79, 1989.

PARADISO G, MICHELI F, TARATUTO AL, PARERA IC: Familial bulbospinal neuronopathy with optic neuropathy: A distinct entity. *J Neurol Neurosurg Psychiatry* 61:196, 1996.

PEARN J: Classification of spinal muscular atrophies. *Lancet* 1:919, 1980.

PENNISI E: The architecture of hearing. *Science* 278:1223, 1997.

PERRY RJ, HODGES JR: Attention and executive deficits in Alzheimer's disease. *Brain* 122:383, 1999.

PICCINI P, BURN DJ, CERAVOLO R, et al: The role of inheritance in sporadic Parkinson's disease: Evidence from a longitudinal study of dopaminergic function in twins. *Ann Neurol* 45:577, 1999.

PICK A: Uber die Beziehungen der senilen Hirnatrophie zur Aphasie. *Prager Med Wochenschr* 17:165, 1892.

PILLON B, DUBOIS B, PLASKA A, AGID Y: Severity and specificity of cognitive impairment in Alzheimer's, Huntington's, and Parkinson's diseases and progressive supranuclear palsy. *Neurology* 41:634, 1991.

PINCUS JH, BARRY K: Influence of dietary protein on motor fluctuations in Parkinson's disease. *Arch Neurol* 44:270, 1987.

POLLOCK M, KIES B: Benign hereditary cerebellar ataxia with extensive thermoanalgesia. *Brain* 113:857, 1990.

POLVIKOSKI T, SULKAVA R, HALTIA M, et al: Apolipoprotein E, dementia, and cortical deposition of β-amyloid protein. *N Engl J Med* 333:1242, 1995.

POLYMEROPOULOS MH, LAVEDAN C, LEROY E, et al: Mutation in the alpha-synuclein gene identified in families with Parkinsons disease. *Science* 276:2045, 1997.

PRINGLE CE, HUDSON AS, MUNOZ DG, et al: Primary lateral sclerosis: Clinical features, neuropathology, and diagnostic criteria. *Brain* 115:495, 1992.

QUINN NP, ROSSOR MN, MARSDEN CD: Dementia and Parkinson's disease: Pathological and neurochemical considerations. *Br Med Bull* 42:86, 1986.

QURESHI AI, WILMOT G, DIHENIA B, et al: Motor neuron disease with Parkinsonism. *Arch Neurol* 53:987, 1996.

RAJPUT AH, GIBB WRG, ZHONG XH, et al: Dopa-responsive dystonia: Pathological and biochemical observations in a case. *Ann Neurol* 35:396, 1994.

RAJPUT AH, ROZDILSKY B: Dysautonomia in parkinsonism: A clinicopathologic study. *J Neurol Neurosurg Psychiatry* 39:1092, 1976.

RASCOL O, BROOKS DJ, KORCZYN AD, et al: A five-year study of the incidence of dyskinesias in patients with early Parkinson's disease who were treated with ropinirole or levodopa. *N Engl J Med* 342:1484, 2000.

REBEIZ JJ, KOLODNY EH, RICHARDSON EP: Corticodentatonigral degeneration with neuronal achromasia. *Arch Neurol* 18:20, 1968.

RICHARDSON JC, STEELE J, OLSZEWSKI J: Supranuclear ophthalmoplegia, pseudobulbar palsy, nuchal dystonia and dementia. *Trans Am Neurol Assoc* 88:25, 1963.

RIFAL Z, KLITZKE M, TAWIL R, et al: Dementia of adult polyglucosan body disease. *Arch Neurol* 51:90, 1994.

RILEY DE, LANG AE, LEWIS A, et al: Cortical-basal ganglionic degeneration. *Neurology* 40:1203, 1990.

RIORDAN-EVA P, SANDERS MD, GOVAN GG, et al: The clinical features of Leber's hereditary optic neuropathy defined by the presence of a pathogenic mitochondrial DNA mutation. *Brain* 118:319, 1995.

ROBITAILLE Y, CARPENTER S, KARPATI G, DIMAURO S: A distinct form of adult polyglucosan body disease with massive involvement of central and peripheral neuronal processes and astrocytes. *Brain* 103:315, 1980.

ROJO A, PERNAUTE RS, FONTAN A, et al: Clinical genetics of familial progressive supranuclear palsy. *Brain* 122:1233, 1999.

ROMANUL FCA: Azorean disease of the nervous system. *N Engl J Med* 297:729, 1977.

ROMANUL FCA, FOWLER HL, RADVANY J, et al: Azorean disease of the nervous system. *N Engl J Med* 296:1505, 1977.

ROPPER AH: Seronegative, non-neoplastic acute cerebellar degeneration. *Neurology* 43:1602, 1993.

ROSEN DR, SIDDIQUE T, PATTERSON D, et al: Mutations in Cu, Zn superoxide dismutase gene are associated with familial amyotrophic lateral sclerosis. *Nature* 362:59, 1993.

ROSENBERG RN: Joseph disease: An autosomal dominant motor system degeneration, in Duvoisin RC, Plaitakis A (eds): *The Olivopontocerebellar Atrophies*. New York, Raven Press, 1984, pp 179–183.

ROSENBERG RN: DNA-triplet repeats and neurologic disease. *N Engl J Med* 335:1222, 1996.

ROSENBERG RN, NYHAN WL, BAY C, SHORE P: Autosomal dominant striatonigral degeneration: A clinical, pathologic and biochemical study of a new genetic disorder. *Neurology* 26:703, 1976.

ROSENHAGEN H: Die primäre Atrophie des Brächenfusses und der unteren Oliven. *Arch Psychiatr Nervenkr* 116:163, 1943.

ROSES AD: Apolipoprotein E gene typing in the differential diagnosis, not prediction, of Alzheimer's disease. *Ann Neurol* 38:6, 1995.

ROUSSY G, LEVY G: Sept cas d'un maladie familiale particulaire. *Rev Neurol* 1:427, 1926.

SAFE AF, COOPER S, WINDSOR ACM: Cerebellar ataxia in the elderly. *Proc R Soc Med* 85:449, 1992.

SAKAI T, ANTOKU Y, IWASHITA H, et al: Chorea-acanthocytosis: Abnormal composition of covalently bound fatty acids of erythrocyte membrane proteins. *Ann Neurol* 29:664, 1991.

SAKAI T, OHTA M, ISHINO H: Joseph disease in a non-Portuguese family. *Neurology* 33:74, 1983.

SASAKI H, MURAMOTO A, KANAZAWA I, et al: Regional distribution of amino acid transmitters in postmortem brains of presenile and senile dementia of Alzheimer type. *Ann Neurol* 19:263, 1986.

SCHAUMBURG HH, SUZUKI K: Non-specific familial presenile dementia. *J Neurol Neurosurg Psychiatry* 31:479, 1968.

SCHENK VWD: Re-examination of a family with Pick's disease. *Ann Hum Genet* 23:325, 1959.

SCHMITT HP, ESMER W, HEIMES C: Familial occurrence of amyotrophic lateral sclerosis, parkinsonism, and dementia. *Ann Neurol* 16:642, 1984.

SCHOENBERG BS, KOKMEN E, OKAZAKI H: Alzheimer's disease and other dementing illnesses in a defined United States population: Incidence rates and clinical features. *Ann Neurol* 22:724, 1987.

SCHOENFELD M, MYERS RH, CUPPLES LA, et al: Increased rate of suicide among patients with Huntington's disease. *J Neurol Neurosurg Psychiatry* 47:1283, 1984.

SCHULMAN S: Bilateral symmetrical degeneration of the thalamus: A clinicopathological study. *J Neuropathol Exp Neurol* 16:446, 1957.

SCRIBANU N, KENNEDY C: Familial syndrome with dystonia, neural deafness and possible intellectual impairment: Clinical course and pathologic features, in Eldridge R, Fahn S (eds): *Advances in Neurology*. Vol 14. *Dystonia*. New York, Raven Press, 1976, pp 235–245.

SEGAWA M, HOSAKA A, MIYAGAWA F, et al: Hereditary progressive dystonia with marked diurnal fluctuation. *Adv Neurol* 14:215, 1976.

SEGAWA M, NOMURA Y, TANAKA S, et al: Hereditary progressive dystonia with marked diurnal fluctuation: Consideration on its pathophysiology based on the characteristics of clinical and polysomnographical findings. *Adv Neurol* 50:367, 1988.

SELKOE DJ: Translating cell biology into therapeutic advances in Alzheimer's disease. *Nature* 399(suppl 24):A23, 1999.

SHERRINGTON R, ROGAEV EI, LIANG Y, et al: Cloning of a gene bearing missense imitations in early-onset familial Alzheimer's disease. *Nature* 375:754, 1995.

SIDDIQUE T, NIJHAWAN D, HENTATI A: Molecular genetic basis of familial ALS. *Neurology* 47(suppl 2):S27, 1996.

SILVERMAN JM, RAIFORD K, EDLAND S, et al: The consortium to establish a registry for Alzheimer's disease (CERAD). *Neurology* 44:1253, 1994.

SJÖGREN T: Klinische und erbbiologische Untersuchungen über die Heredoataxien. *Acta Psychiatr (Kbh)* suppl 27, 1943.

SKRE H: Hereditary spastic paraplegia in western Norway. *Clin Genet* 6:165, 1974.

SMITH JK: Dentatorubropallidoluysian atrophy, in Vinken PJ, Bruyn GW (eds): *Handbook of Clinical Neurology*. Vol 21. Amsterdam, North-Holland, 1975, pp 519–534.

SNOWDEN DA, KEMPER SJ, MORTIMER JA, et al: Linguistic ability in early life and cognitive function and Alzheimer's disease in late life: Findings from the Nun study. *JAMA* 275:528, 1996.

SNOWDEN JS, NEARY D, MANN DMA: Progressive language disorder due to lobar atrophy. *Ann Neurol* 31:174, 1992.

SNYDER SH, D'AMATO RJ: MPTP: A neurotoxin relevant to the pathophysiology of Parkinson's disease. *Neurology* 36:250, 1986.

SPATZ H: Die Systematischen Atrophien. *Arch Psychiatry* 108:1, 1938.

SPENCER DD, ROBBINS RJ, NAFTOLIN F, et al: Unilateral transplantation of human fetal mesencephalic tissue into the caudate nucleus of patients with Parkinson's disease. *N Engl J Med* 327:1541, 1992.

SPIELMEYER W: *Histopathologie des Nervensystems*. Berlin, Springer-Verlag, 1922, pp 223–229.

ST. GEORGE-HYSLOP PH, TANZI RE, POLINSKY RJ, et al: The genetic defect causing familial Alzheimer's disease maps on chromosome 21. *Science* 235:885, 1987.

STARGARDT K: Uber familiare, progressive Degeneration in der Maculagegend. *Graefes Arch Clin Exp Ophthalmol* 71:534, 1909.

STEELE JC: Progressive supranuclear palsy. *Brain* 95:693, 1972.

STERN K: Severe dementia associated with bilateral symmetrical degeneration of the thalamus. *Brain* 61:339, 1938.

STRITTMATTER WJ, SAUNDERS AM, SCHMECHEL D, et al: Apolipoprotein E: High avidity binding to β-amyloid and increased frequency of type 4 allele in late-onset familial Alzheimer disease. *Proc Natl Acad Sci USA* 90:1977, 1993.

TANDAN R, TAYLOR R, ADESINA A, et al: Benign autosomal dominant syndrome of neuronal Charcot-Marie-Tooth disease, ptosis, parkinsonism, and dementia. *Neurology* 40:773, 1990.

TANG M-X, JACOBS D, STERN Y, et al: Effect of oestrogen during menopause on risk and age at onset of Alzheimer's disease. *Lancet* 348:429, 1996.

TASKER RR, DOORLY T, YAMASHIRO K: Thalamotomy in generalized dystonia. *Adv Neurol* 50:615, 1988.

TERRY RD: The pathogenesis of Alzheimer disease: An alternative to the amyloid hypothesis. *J Neuropathol Exp Neurol* 55:1023, 1996.

Terry RD, Katzman R: Senile dementia of the Alzheimer type. *Ann Neurol* 14:497, 1983.

Tierney MC, Fisher RH, Lewis AJ, et al: The NINCDS-ADRDA Work Group criteria for the clinical diagnosis of probable Alzheimer's disease: A clinicopathological study of 57 cases. *Neurology* 38:359, 1988.

Tierney MC, Snow WG, Reid DW, et al: Psychometric differentiation of dementia. *Arch Neurol* 44:720, 1987.

Tissot R, Constantinidis J, Richard J: *La Maladie de Pick*. Paris, Masson, 1975.

Tranchant C, Boulay C, Warter JM: Pallido-pyramidal syndrome: An unrecognized entity. *Rev Neurol* 147:308, 1991.

Troost BT, Daroff RB: The ocular motor defects in progressive supranuclear palsy. *Ann Neurol* 2:397, 1977.

Trouillas P, Serratrice G, Laplane D, et al: Levorotatory form of 5-hydroxytryptophan in Friedreich's ataxia. *Arch Neurol* 52:456, 1995.

Uhl JA, Javitch JA, Snyder SN: Normal MPTP binding in Parkinson substantia nigra. *Lancet* 1:956, 1985.

van Bogaert L, van Maere M, Desmedt E: Sur les formes familiales precoces de la maladie d'Alzheimer. *Monatsschr Psychiatr Neurol* 102:249, 1940.

van Dijk JG, van der Velde EA, Roos RAC, et al: Juvenile Huntington's disease. *Hum Genet* 73:235, 1986.

van Mansvelt J: Pick's disease: A syndrome of lobar cerebral atrophy: Clinicoanatomical and histopathological types. Thesis, Utrecht, 1954.

Verhagen Metman L, Del Dotto van den Munckhof P, et al: Amantadine as treatment for dyskinesias and motor fluctuations in Parkinson's disease. *Neurology* 50:1323, 1998.

Vessie PR: On the transmission of Huntington chorea for 300 years: The Bures family group. *J Nerv Ment Dis* 76:553, 1932.

Victor M, Adams RD, Mancall EL: A restricted form of cerebellar degeneration occurring in alcoholic patients. *Arch Neurol* 1:577, 1959.

Vonsattel JP, DiFiglia M: Huntington disease. *J Neuropathol Exp Neurol* 57:369, 1998.

Waardenburg PJ: Uber familiar-erbliche Falle von seniler Maculadegeneration. *Genetica* 18:38, 1936.

Wadia NH: A variety of olivopontocerebellar atrophy distinguished by slow eye movements and peripheral neuropathy. *Adv Neurol* 41:149, 1984.

Wallace DC, Singh G, Lott MT, et al: Mitochondrial DNA mutation associated with Leber's hereditary optic neuropathy. *Science* 242:1427, 1988.

Wang HS: Dementia in old age, in Smith LW, Kinsbourne M (eds): *Aging and Dementia*. New York, Spectrum, 1977, pp 1–4.

Warner TT, Williams LD, Walker RW, et al: A clinical and molecular genetic study of dentatorubropallidoluysian atrophy in four European families. *Ann Neurol* 37:452, 1995.

Wenning GK, Ben-Shlomo Y, Magalhaes M, et al: Clinical features and natural history of multiple system atrophy: An analysis of 100 cases. *Brain* 117:835, 1994.

Wenning GK, Ben-Shlomo Y, Magalhaes M, et al: Clinicopathologic study of 35 cases of multiple system atrophy. *J Neurol Neurosurg Psychiatry* 58:160, 1995.

Wenning GK, Litvan I, Jankcovic J, et al: Natural history and survival of 14 patients with corticobasal degeneration confirmed at postmortem examination. *J Neurol Neurosurg Psychiatry* 64:184, 1998.

Whitehouse PJ, Hedreen JC, White CL, et al: Basal forebrain neurons in the dementia of Parkinson disease. *Ann Neurol* 13:243, 1983.

Whitehouse PJ, Price DL, Clark AW, et al: Alzheimer disease: Evidence for loss of cholinergic neurons in nucleus basalis. *Ann Neurol* 10:122, 1981.

Wilson SAK: *Neurology*. Baltimore, Williams & Wilkins, 1940.

Wohlfart G, Fex J, Eliasson S: Hereditary proximal spinal muscular atrophy: A clinical entity simulating progressive muscular dystrophy. *Acta Psychiatr Neurol Scand* 30:395, 1955.

Woodard JS: Concentric hyaline inclusion body formation in mental disease. Analysis of twenty-seven cases. *J Neuropathol Exp Neurol* 21:442, 1962.

Woods BT, Schaumburg HH: Nigrospinodentatal degeneration with nuclear ophthalmoplegia, in Vinken PJ, Bruyn GW (eds): *Handbook of Clinical Neurology*. Vol 22. Amsterdam, North-Holland, 1975, pp 157–176.

Worster-Drought C, Greenfield JG, McMenemey WH: A form of familial progressive dementia with spastic paralysis. *Brain* 67:38, 1944.

Young AB, Shoulson I, Penney JB, et al: Huntington's disease in Venezuela: Neurologic features and functional decline. *Neurology* 36:244, 1986.

Young RR: The differential diagnosis of Parkinson's disease. *Int J Neurol* 12:210, 1977.

Younger DS, Rowland LP, Latov N, et al: Motor neuron disease and amyotrophic lateral sclerosis: Relation of high CSF protein content to paraproteinemia and clinical syndromes. *Neurology* 40:595, 1990.

Yuasa T, Ohama E, Harayama H, et al: Joseph's disease: Clinical and pathological studies in a Japanese family. *Ann Neurol* 19:152, 1986.

Zeman W: Pathology of the torsion dystonias (dystonia musculorum deformans). *Neurology* 20(no 11, pt 2):79, 1970.

Chapter 40

THE ACQUIRED METABOLIC DISORDERS OF THE NERVOUS SYSTEM

An important segment of neurologic medicine, and one that is seen with great frequency in general hospitals, consists of disorders in which a global disturbance of cerebral function (encephalopathy) results from failure of some other organ system—heart and circulation, lungs and respiration, kidneys, liver, pancreas, and the endocrine glands. Unlike the diseases considered in Chap. 37, in which a genetic abnormality affects many organs and tissues, including the brain, the cerebral disorders discussed in this chapter are strictly secondary to derangements of the visceral organs themselves. They stand at the interface of internal medicine and neurology.

Relationships of this type, between an acquired disease of some thoracic or abdominal organ and the brain, have rather interesting implications. In the first place, recognition of the neurologic syndrome may be a guide to the diagnosis of the systemic disease; indeed, the neurologic symptoms may be more informative and significant than the symptoms referable to the organ primarily involved. Moreover, these encephalopathies are often reversible if the systemic dysfunction is brought under control. Neurologists must therefore have an understanding of the underlying medical disorder, for this may provide the means of controlling the neurologic part of the disease. In other words, the therapy for what appears to be a neurologic disease lies squarely in the field of internal medicine—a clear reason why every neurologist should be well trained in internal medicine. Of more theoretical importance, the investigation of the acquired metabolic diseases provides new insights into the chemistry and pathology of the brain. To select a single example, the discovery of an episodic encephalopathy that is associated with advanced liver disease and portocaval shunts opened a vast new area in brain chemistry, pertaining to the effect of ammonia on glutamine metabolism, and has brought to light an intriguing histopathologic change—a relatively pure hyperplasia of protoplasmic astrocytes. Each visceral disease affects the brain in a somewhat different way, and since the pathogenic mechanism is not completely understood in any of them, the study of these metabolic diseases promises rich rewards to the scientist.

In Table 40-1 the acquired metabolic diseases of the nervous system are classified according to their most common modes of clinical expression. Not included are the diseases due to nutritional deficiencies and those due to exogenous drugs and toxins, which can be considered metabolic in the broad sense; these are presented in the following chapters.

METABOLIC DISEASES PRESENTING AS A SYNDROME OF CONFUSION, STUPOR, OR COMA

The *syndrome of impaired consciousness*, its general features, the terms used to describe it, and the mechanisms involved in its genesis are discussed in Chap. 17, which serves as an introduction to this section. There it is pointed out that metabolic disturbances are frequent causes of impaired consciousness and that their presence must always be considered when there are no focal signs of cerebral disease and both the imaging studies and the cerebrospinal fluid (CSF) are normal. Intoxication with alcohol and other drugs figures prominently in the differential diagnosis. *The main features of the reversible metabolic encephalopathies are mental confusion, typified by disorientation and inattentiveness and accompanied in certain instances by asterixis, tremor, and myoclonus, usually without signs of focal cerebral disease such as hemiparesis, hemianopia, hemianesthesia, or a disorder of the cranial nerves.* This state may progress in stages to one of stupor and coma. Slowing of the background rhythms in the electroencephalogram

Table 40-1
Classification of the acquired metabolic disorders of the nervous system

I. Metabolic diseases presenting as a syndrome of confusion, stupor, or coma
   A. Ischemia-hypoxia
   B. Hypercapnia
   C. Hypoglycemia
   D. Hyperglycemia
   E. Hepatic failure
   F. Reye syndrome
   G. Azotemia
   H. Disturbances of sodium, water balance, and osmolality
   I. Hypercalcemia
   J. Other metabolic encephalopathies: acidosis due to diabetes mellitus or renal failure (see also inherited forms of acidosis in Chap. 37); Addison disease; bismuth subgallate intoxication
II. Metabolic diseases presenting as a progressive extrapyramidal syndrome
   A. Acquired hepatocerebral degeneration
   B. Hyperbilirubinemia and kernicterus
   C. Hypoparathyroidism
III. Metabolic diseases presenting as cerebellar ataxia
   A. Hypothyroidism
   B. Hyperthermia
   C. Celiac-sprue disease
IV. Metabolic diseases causing psychosis or dementia
   A. Cushing disease and steroid encephalopathy
   B. Thyroid psychosis and hypothyroidism
   C. Hyperparathyroidism
   D. Pancreatic encephalopathy (?)

(EEG) reflects the severity of the metabolic disturbance. With few exceptions, usually pertaining to cerebral edema, imaging studies are normal.

Laboratory examinations are highly informative in the investigation of the acquired metabolic diseases. In every patient with symptoms suggestive of a metabolic encephalopathy, the following determinations should be made: serum Na, K, Ca, glucose, BUN, NH_3, and osmolality. If there is evidence of hypoxia or the patient is known to have chronic obstructive airway disease, determination of arterial pH, P_{CO_2} and P_{O_2} are carried out as well. Serum osmolality can be measured directly or calculated from the values of Na (in meq/L), K (in meq/L), glucose (in mg/dL), and BUN (in mg/dL), using the following formula:

$$\text{Serum osmolality} = 2[(\text{Na}) \times (\text{K})] + \frac{\text{glucose}}{18} + \frac{\text{BUN}}{3}$$

When there is a discrepancy between the calculated and the directly measured osmolalities, it can be assumed that additional circulating ions are present. Most often they are derived from an exogenous toxin or drug such as mannitol, but renal failure, ketonemia, and an increase of serum lactate may also result in the accumulation of small molecules that contribute to the serum osmolality.

Where an exogenous toxin is suspected of causing an encephalopathy and in all cases where the cause is unknown, a "toxic screen" of blood and urine, using high-pressure liquid chromatography, should be obtained. A point to be remembered is that the brain may be damaged, even to an irreparable degree, by a disturbance of blood chemistry (e.g., hypoglycemia, hypoxia) that is no longer present when the patient is first seen.

Ischemic-Hypoxic Encephalopathy

Here the basic disorder is a lack of oxygen to the brain, the result of failure of the heart and circulation or of the lungs and respiration. Often both are responsible and one cannot say which predominates; hence the ambiguous allusion in clinical records to "cardiorespiratory failure."

Ischemic-hypoxic encephalopathy in various forms and degrees of severity is one of the most frequent and disastrous cerebral accidents encountered in the emergency departments and recovery rooms of every general hospital. The medical conditions that most often lead to it are (1) myocardial infarction or ventricular arrhythmia, external or internal hemorrhage, and septic or traumatic shock—in all of which cardiac function fails before that of respiration; (2) suffocation from drowning, strangulation, aspiration of vomitus, food, or blood, compression of the trachea by a mass or hemorrhage, or tracheal obstruction by a foreign body; (3) carbon monoxide (CO) poisoning, in which respiration fails first and then the cardiovascular system; (4) diseases that paralyze the respiratory muscles (Guillain-Barré syndrome, amyotrophic lateral sclerosis, myasthenia, and, in the past, poliomyelitis) or damage the CNS diffusely but the medulla specifically, again with respiratory failure being the initial factor, followed by cardiac failure; and (5) a general anesthesia accident during which the patient is exposed to inspired gas that is oxygen-deficient.

The terms *anoxic*, *anemic*, and *stagnant*, introduced by Barcroft to designate the various forms of anoxia, are now little used in clinical medicine, since the ultimate effect of all three is the same—namely, to deprive the brain and other organs of their critical oxygen supply.

The oxygen content of the blood is the product of hemoglobin concentration and the oxygen saturation of the hemoglobin molecule. At normal temperature and pH, hemoglobin is 90 percent saturated at an oxygen partial pressure of 60 mmHg and still 75 percent saturated at 40 mmHg, i.e., the oxygen saturation curve is not linear.

Reduced to the simplest formulation, a deficient supply of oxygen to the brain is due either to a failure of cerebral perfusion (ischemia) or to a reduced amount of circulating arterial oxygen, the result of diminished oxygen saturation or insufficiency of hemoglobin. The neurologic effects of these two are subtly different.

Physiology of Ischemic and Hypoxic Damage

Physiologic mechanisms of a homeostatic nature protect the brain under conditions of both ischemia and hypoxia. When the cerebral perfusion pressure is reduced, there is a compensatory dilatation of resistance vessels, which maintains blood flow at a constant rate (autoregulation). When the cerebral blood pressure falls below 60 to 70 mmHg, increased oxygen extraction still allows normal energy metabolism to continue. In total ischemia, the tissue is depleted of its sources of energy in about 5 min, although longer periods are tolerated under conditions of barbiturate coma and hypothermia. Energy failure due to hypoxia is counteracted by an autoregulatory increase in cerebral blood flow; at a P_{O_2} of 25 mmHg, the increase is approximately 400 percent. A similar increase in flow occurs with a decrease in hemoglobin to 20 percent of normal, but here a decrease in viscosity also facilitates the circulatory response.

Ischemic injury from systemic hypotension differs from that due to pure anoxia. In ischemia, the main damage takes the form of incomplete infarctions in the border zones between major cerebral arteries. With anoxia, neurons in parts of the hippocampus and deep folia of the cerebellum are particularly vulnerable. With more severe degrees of either ischemia or hypoxia, there is first selective damage to certain layers of cortical neurons, and later, generalized damage of all the cerebral cortex, deep nuclei, and cerebellum. Nuclei of the brainstem are relatively resistant to anoxia and hypotension and stop functioning only after the cortex has been badly damaged.

In most of the clinical situations in which the brain is deprived of adequate oxygen, there is a combination of ischemia and hypoxia, but one or the other usually predominates. The cellular pathophysiology of neuronal and tissue damage in cerebral and cerebellar cortices and pallidum under conditions of ischemia is discussed in Chap. 34. Essentially, the mechanism in hypoxic-ischemic injury is an arrest of all aerobic metabolic processes necessary to sustain the Krebs (tricarboxylic acid) cycle and the electron transport system. The neurons, if completely deprived of their source of energy, proceed to catabolize themselves in an attempt to maintain their activity, and in so doing are damaged to a degree that does not permit their survival, i.e., they undergo necrosis. The accumulation of catabolic products (particularly lactic acid) in the interstitial tissue contributes to the parenchymal damage. Also, there is some experimental evidence that excitatory neurotransmitters, particularly glutamate, contribute to the rapid destruction of neurons under conditions of anoxia and ischemia (Choi and Rothman); how this pertains to clinical situations is uncertain. Ultimately, massive calcium influx through a number of different membrane channels is thought to participate in the process of cellular destruction.

There is also a phenomenon of delayed neurologic deterioration after anoxia that is not understood but may be due to the blockage or exhaustion of some enzymatic process during the period when brain metabolism is restored or even increased (as it is in hyperthermia or possibly with seizures or increased motor activity).

Clinical Features of Anoxic Encephalopathy *Mild degrees of hypoxia without loss of consciousness* induce only inattentiveness, poor judgment, and motor incoordination; in our experience there have been no lasting clinical effects in such cases, though Hornbein and colleagues found, on psychologic testing, a slight decline in visual and verbal long-term memory and mild aphasic errors in Himalayan mountaineers who had ascended to altitudes of 18,000 to 29,000 ft. These observations make the point that profound anoxia may be well tolerated if arrived at gradually. We have seen several patients with advanced pulmonary disease who were fully awake when their arterial oxygen pressure was in the range of 30 mmHg. This level, if it occurs abruptly, causes coma. *An important clinical rule is that degrees of hypoxia that at no time abolish consciousness rarely if ever cause permanent damage to the nervous system.*

In the circumstances of *severe global ischemia with prolonged loss of consciousness*, the clinical effects can be quite variable. With cardiac arrest, for example, consciousness is lost within seconds, but recovery will be complete if breathing, oxygenation of blood, and cardiac action are restored within 3 to 5 min. Beyond 5 min there is usually permanent injury. As shown in experimental models, one of the reasons for the irreversibility of the lesion is swelling of the endothelium and blockage of circulation into the ischemic cerebral tissues (no-reflow phenomenon; Ames et al). Clinically, however, it is difficult to judge the precise degree of hypoxia, since slight heart action or an imperceptible blood pressure may have served to maintain the circulation to some extent. Hence some individuals have made an excellent recovery after cerebral hypoxia that allegedly lasted 8 to 10 min or longer. Subnormal body temperatures, as might occur when the body is immersed in ice-cold water, greatly prolong the tolerable period of hypoxia. Generally speaking, anoxic patients who demonstrate intact brainstem function (as indicated by normal pupillary light and ciliospinal responses, "doll's-head" eye movements, and oculovestibular reflexes) have a more favorable outlook for recovery of consciousness and perhaps all of their faculties. Conversely, absence of these brainstem reflexes even after circulation and oxygenation have been restored, particularly fixed pupils to light, implies a grave outlook in most circumstances, as elaborated further on.

Most patients who have suffered severe but lesser degrees of hypoxia will have stabilized their breathing and cardiac activity by the time they are first examined; yet they may be profoundly comatose, with the eyes slightly divergent and motionless but with reactive pupils, the limbs inert and flaccid or intensely rigid, and the tendon reflexes diminished. Within a few minutes after cardiac action and breathing have been restored, generalized convulsions and also isolated or grouped myoclonic twitches of muscles may supervene. The seizures, if severe and recurrent, double or treble the oxygen need of cerebral tissues. If the damage is severe, coma persists, decerebrate postures may be present or may occur in response to painful stimuli, and bilateral Babinski signs can be evoked. In the first 24 to 48 h, death may terminate this state in a setting of rising temperature, deepening coma, and circulatory collapse. Tragically, however, the individual may survive for an indefinite period in a state that is variously referred to as cortical death, irreversible coma, or *persistent vegetative state* (see Chap. 17).

With this severe degree of injury, the cerebral and cerebellar cortices and parts of the thalami are partly or completely destroyed but most often brainstem-spinal structures survive. Some patients remain mute, unresponsive, and unaware of their environment for weeks, months, or years. Long survival is usually attended by some degree of improvement, but the patient appears to know nothing of his present situation and to have lost all past memories, power of reasoning, and capacity for meaningful social interaction and independent existence. One has only to observe such patients and their families to appreciate the gravity of the problem, the heartache, and the tremendous expense of medical care. The only person who does not appear to suffer is the patient.

With lesser degrees of anoxic-ischemic injury, the patient improves after a period of coma. Some of these patients quickly pass through this acute posthypoxic phase and proceed to make a full recovery; others are left with varying degrees of permanent disability.

Brain Death Syndrome (See also Chap. 17.) This represents the most severe degree of oxygen lack, usually caused by circulatory arrest (ischemic anoxia), and is manifest by a state of complete unawareness and unresponsiveness with abolition of all brainstem reflexes. Natural respiration cannot be sustained; only cardiac action and blood pressure are maintained. No electrical activity is seen in the EEG (it is isoelectric). This is the *brain death syndrome* (see page 371). At autopsy one finds that most if not all the gray matter of cerebral, cerebellar, and brainstem structures, and in some instances even of the spinal cord, has been severely damaged.

One must exercise caution in concluding that a patient has irreversible brain damage, because anesthesia, intoxication with certain drugs, and hypothermia may also cause deep coma and an isoelectric EEG but permit recovery. Therefore it is advisable to repeat the clinical and laboratory tests after an interval of a day or two, during which time the results of toxic screening also become available. Such cases have been brought increasingly to public attention because of ethical and moral issues pertaining to discontinuation of medical therapy. The authors' experience corroborates the general notion that the vital functions of patients with the brain death syndrome usually cannot be sustained for more than several days; in other words, the problem settles itself. In exceptional cases, however, the provision of adequate fluid, vasopressor, and respiratory support allows preservation of the somatic organism in a comatose state for longer periods.

Posthypoxic Neurologic Syndromes The permanent neurologic sequelae or *posthypoxic syndromes* observed most frequently are (1) *persistent coma or stupor*, described above, and, with lesser degrees of cerebral injury, (2) *dementia* with or without extrapyramidal signs, (3) *extrapyramidal (parkinsonian) syndrome with* *cognitive impairment* (discussed in relation to CO poisoning), (4) *choreoathetosis*, (5) *cerebellar ataxia*, (6) *intention or action myoclonus*, and (7) *a Korsakoff amnesic state*. If *ischemic hypoperfusion* dominates, the patient may also display the manifestations of watershed infarctions, situated between the end territories of the major cerebral vessels, the main syndromes being (8) *visual agnosias and "cortical blindness"* and (9) *proximal arm and shoulder weakness*, sometimes accompanied by hip weakness (referred to as a "man in the barrel syndrome"). *Seizures* may or may not continue to be a problem. These sequelae rarely occur in pure form; usually they overlap in various combinations, although any one of them may predominate.

Delayed Postanoxic Encephalopathy This is a relatively uncommon and unexplained phenomenon. Initial improvement, which appears to be complete, is followed after a variable period of time (1 to 4 weeks in most instances) by a relapse, characterized by apathy, confusion, irritability, and occasionally agitation or mania. Most patients survive this second episode, but some of them are left with serious mental and motor disturbances (Choi; Plum et al). In still other cases there appears to be progression of the initial neurologic syndrome, with additional weakness, shuffling gait, diffuse rigidity and spasticity, sphincteric incontinence, coma, and death after 1 to 2 weeks. Exceptionally, there is yet another chronic syndrome in which an episode of hypoxia is followed by slow deterioration, which progresses for weeks to months until the patient is mute, rigid, and helpless. In such cases the basal ganglia are affected more than the cerebral cortex and white matter (Dooling and Richardson).

Prognosis of Hypoxic-Ischemic Brain Injury Several logistic models have been developed to predict the outcome of anoxic-ischemic coma. All of them utilize certain simple criteria, involving loss of motor, verbal, and pupillary functions in various combinations. The most often cited and extensive such study, by Levy and colleagues, based on 150 patients who remained in coma for at least 6 h after cardiac arrest, has provided the following guidelines. Mortality from this state is high: 20 percent on the first day and 64 percent at the end of 1 week. Most patients destined to recover awaken within a brief period of time; thus, 17 percent of their patients who recovered were conscious by 3 days, and by 2 weeks the number of conscious patients had risen only by 2 percent. At the other extreme were 31 percent of patients who appeared to be in the vegetative state at 1 day; of this group, 70 percent survived for 1 week, and only 3 patients in all recovered.

Once intoxication is excluded, the presence of fixed dilated pupils and paralysis of eye movement for 24 to 48 h, along with absence of motor responses to painful stimuli, signify irreversible cerebral damage. We have never observed deep coma of this type lasting 5 days or more to be attended by full recovery. The question of what to do with such cases of protracted coma is a societal and not a medical problem. The most that can be expected of the neurologist is to state the level and degree of brain damage, its cause, and the prognosis based on his own and published experience. One prudently avoids heroic, lifesaving therapeutic measures once the nature of this state has been determined with certainty.

Treatment of Hypoxic-Ischemic Encephalopathy Treatment is directed mainly to the prevention of an initial critical degree of hypoxic injury. After a clear airway is secured, the use of cardiopulmonary resuscitation, a cardiac defibrillator, or pacemaker has its place, and every second counts in their prompt utilization. Once cardiac and pulmonary function are restored, there is experimental evidence that reducing cerebral metabolic requirements by hypothermia and by barbiturates or glutamate-blocking medication may prevent the delayed worsening referred to above. However, attempts to demonstrate any of these beneficial effects by controlled trials have failed. Vasodilator drugs and calcium channel blockers are also of no proven benefit. Oxygen may be of value during the first hours but is probably of little use after the blood becomes well oxygenated. Corticosteroids theoretically help to allay brain (possibly cellular) swelling, but again their therapeutic benefit has not been corroborated by clinical trials or practice.

Seizures should be controlled by the methods indicated in Chap. 16. If they are severe, continuous, and unresponsive to the usual anticonvulsant drugs, controlled respiration, continuous infusion of a drug such as midazolam, and eventually neuromuscular blocking agents may have to be used. Often the seizures cease after a few hours and are replaced by polymyoclonus. For the latter; clonazepam, 8 to 12 mg daily in divided doses, may be useful, but the commonly used anticonvulsants have little effect in our experience. This state of spontaneous and stimulus-sensitive myoclonus as well as persistent limb posturing usually presages a poor outcome. The delayed movement-induced myoclonus and ataxic tremor that appear after the patient awakens, described by Lance and Adams, is a special issue that is discussed on page 110. Its treatment requires the use of multiple medications.

Carbon Monoxide Poisoning

Strictly speaking, carbon monoxide (CO) is an exogenous toxin, but it is considered here because it produces a special type of anoxia and one that is frequently associated with delayed neurologic deterioration. The extreme affinity of CO for hemoglobin (over 200 times that of oxygen) drastically reduces the oxygen content of blood and subjects the brain to prolonged hypoxia and acidosis. Cardiac toxicity and hypotension generally follow. Whether CO also has a direct toxic action on neuronal components is not settled. The effects on the brain appear to simulate those caused by cardiac arrest. Neurologists are likely to encounter instances of CO poisoning in burn units and in patients who have attempted suicide or have been exposed accidentally to a faulty furnace or to car exhaust in a closed garage.

Early symptoms include headache, nausea, dyspnea, confusion, dizziness, and clumsiness. These occur when the carboxyhemoglobin level reaches 20 to 30 percent. Exposure to relatively low levels of CO from faulty furnaces and gasoline engines should be suspected as the cause of recurrent headaches and confusion that clear upon hospitalization or other change of venue. A cherry-red color of the skin may appear but is actually an infrequent finding; cyanosis is more common. At slightly higher levels of carboxyhemoglobin, blindness, visual field defects, and papilledema develop, and levels of 50 to 60 percent are associated with coma, decerebrate or decorticate posturing, seizures in a few patients, and generalized slowing of the EEG rhythms. CT scanning is normal or shows mild cerebral edema, or, if hypotension has been profound, the same types of border-zone infarctions that are seen after cardiac arrest.

Delayed neurologic deterioration 1 to 3 weeks (sometimes much longer) after CO exposure occurs more frequently with CO poisoning than with other forms of cerebral hypoxia. In Choi's survey, this feature was observed in 3 percent of 2360 cases of CO poisoning and in 12 percent of those ill enough to be admitted to a hospital. Extrapyramidal features (parkinsonian gait and bradykinesia) predominated. Three-quarters of such patients were said to recover within a year. Discrete lesions centered in the globus pallidus bilaterally and sometimes the inner portion of the putamina are characteristic of CO poisoning that had produced coma (Fig. 40-1), but similar lesions may be seen after drowning, strangulation, and other forms of anoxia. The common feature among the delayed-relapse patients seems to be a prolonged period of pure anoxia (before the occurrence of ischemia). The basal ganglia lesions may be quite prominent on CT scans even when delayed neurologic sequelae do not occur, but they are almost invariably present between 1 and 4 weeks in patients who develop a delayed extrapyramidal syndrome. In less affected patients, we have seen such lesions resolve.

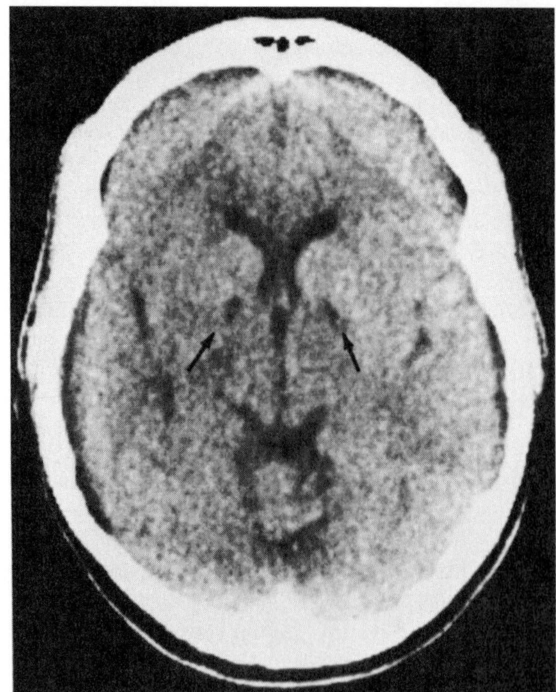

Figure 40-1

Unenhanced CT scan of brain of a 30-year-old woman who attempted suicide by carbon monoxide inhalation. The only neurologic residua were a mild defect in retentive memory and areas of decreased attenuation in the pallidum bilaterally (arrows).

Because the half-life of CO is greatly reduced by the administration of hyperbaric oxygen at 2 or 3 atmospheres, this treatment is recommended when the carboxyhemoglobin concentration is greater than 40 percent or if the patient is comatose or having seizures (Myers et al). It is not known whether this treatment reduces the incidence of neurologic sequelae.

High-Altitude (Mountain) Sickness

Acute mountain sickness is another special form of cerebral hypoxia. It occurs when a sea-level inhabitant abruptly ascends to a high altitude. Headache, anorexia, nausea and vomiting, weakness, and insomnia appear at altitudes above 8000 ft; even modest physical exertion at this level causes dyspnea in unconditioned individuals. On reaching higher altitudes, there may be ataxia, tremor, abnormal behavior, drowsiness, and hallucinations. At 16,000 ft, according to Griggs and Sutton, 50 percent of individuals develop asymptomatic retinal hemorrhages, and it is suggested that such hemorrhages may also occur in the cerebral white matter. With more prolonged stays at these altitudes or with further ascent, affected individuals show mental impairment that may progress to coma. Hypoxemia is intensified during sleep, as ventilation diminishes. Reference was made earlier to the observation of Hornbein et al of a mild but possibly lasting memory impairment in even acclimated mountaineers who had been exposed to even higher altitudes for several days.

Chronic mountain sickness, sometimes called Monge disease, is observed in long-term inhabitants of high-altitude mountainous regions. Pulmonary hypertension, cor pulmonale, and secondary polycythemia are the main features. There is usually hypercarbia as well, with the expected mental dullness, slowness, fatigue, nocturnal headache, and sometimes papilledema (see below).

Sedatives, alcohol, and a slightly elevated P_{CO_2} in the blood all reduce one's tolerance to high altitude. Dexamethasone and acetazolamide prevent and counteract mountain sickness to some extent. The most effective preventive measure is acclimatization by a 2- to 4-day stay at intermediate altitudes of 6000 to 8000 ft.

Hypercapnic Pulmonary Disease

Chronic emphysema, chronic fibrosing lung disease, neuromuscular weakness, and in some instances an inadequacy of the respiratory centers lead to chronic respiratory acidosis, with an elevation of P_{CO_2} and a reduction in arterial P_{O_2}. The clinical syndrome described by Austen et al comprises *headache, papilledema, mental dullness, drowsiness, confusion, stupor and coma, and asterixis*. Some patients have a degree of superimposed fast-frequency tremor. The headache tends to be generalized, frontal, or occipital in location and intense, persistent, steady, and aching in type; nocturnal occurrence is a feature in some cases. The papilledema is bilateral but may be slightly greater in one eye than in the other, and hemorrhages may encircle the choked disc (a late finding). Visual acuity is undiminished and visual fields are full. Tendon reflexes are lively and plantar reflexes may be extensor. Intermittent drowsiness, indifference to the environment, inattentiveness, reduction of psychomotor activity, inability to perceive all the items in a sequence of events, and forgetfulness constitute the more subtle manifestations of this syndrome and may prompt the family to seek medical help. Such symptoms may last only a few minutes or hours, and one cannot count on their presence at the time of a particular examination. In fully developed cases, the CSF is under increased pressure. P_{CO_2} may exceed 75 mmHg and the O_2 saturation of arterial blood ranges from 85 percent to as low as 40 percent. The EEG shows slow activity in the delta or theta range, which is sometimes bilaterally synchronous.

The mechanism of the cerebral disorder is said to be CO_2 narcosis, but the biochemical details are not all known. Normally the CSF is slightly acidotic in comparison to the blood, and the P_{CO_2} of the CSF is about 10 mmHg higher than that of the blood. With respiratory acidosis, the pH of the CSF falls (in the range of 7.15 to 7.25) and cerebral blood flow increases because of cerebral vasodilatation. However, the brain rapidly adapts to respiratory acidosis through the generation and secretion of bicarbonate by the choroid plexuses. Brain water also increases, mainly in the white matter. In animal models of hypercarbia, NH_3 is elevated, which may explain the similarity of the syndrome to that of hyperammonemia (Herrera and Kazemi).

The most effective therapeutic measures are ventilation with a positive-pressure device, using oxygen if there is hypoxia; treatment of heart failure; phlebotomy to reduce the viscosity of the blood; and antibiotics to suppress pulmonary infection. Often these measures result in a surprising degree of improvement, which may be maintained for months or years. The danger of administering morphine, which depresses the respiratory center (now insensitive to CO_2), and the danger of oxygen inhalation, which in these circumstances removes the major stimulus to the respiratory center, are now widely recognized; patients treated with oxygen have lapsed into coma.

Unlike pure hypoxic encephalopathy, prolonged coma due to hypercapnia is relatively rare and in our experience has not led to irreversible brain damage. Papilledema and jerky, intermittent lapses of sustained muscular contraction (asterixis) are important diagnostic features. The syndrome is apt to be mistaken for a brain tumor, confusional psychosis of other type, or a disease causing chorea or myoclonus. In the latter case, hypercapnia must be distinguished from other metabolic diseases presenting as chronic extrapyramidal syndromes, as described later in this chapter.

Hypoglycemic Encephalopathy

This condition is relatively infrequent but is an important cause of confusion, convulsions, stupor, and coma; as such, it merits separate consideration as a metabolic disorder of the brain. The essential biochemical abnormality is a critical lowering of the blood glucose. At a level of about 30 mg/dL, the cerebral disorder takes the form of a confusional state, and one or more seizures may occur; at a level of 10 mg/dL, there is profound coma that may result in irreparable injury to the brain if not corrected immediately by the administration of glucose.

The normal brain has a glucose reserve of 1 to 2 g (30 mmol per 100 g of tissue), mostly in the form of glycogen. Since glucose is utilized by the brain at a rate of 60 to 80 mg/min, the glucose reserve will sustain cerebral activity for only about 30 min once blood glucose is no longer available. Glucose is transported from the blood to the brain by a carrier system. When glucose enters the brain, it either undergoes glycolysis or is stored as glycogen. During normal oxygenation (aerobic metabolism), glucose is converted to pyruvate, which enters the Krebs cycle; during anaerobic metabolism, lactate is formed. The oxidation of 1 mol of glucose requires 6 mol of O_2. Of the glucose taken up by the brain, 85 to 90 percent is oxidized; the remainder enters an amino acid pool and is utilized in the formation of proteins and other substances—notably neurotransmitters, and particularly gamma-aminobutyric acid (GABA).

The brain is the only organ, besides the heart, that suffers severe functional and structural impairment under conditions of hypoglycemia. The pathophysiology of the cerebral disorder has not been fully elucidated. It is known that hypoglycemia reduces O_2 uptake and increases cerebral blood flow. As with anoxia and ischemia, there is experimental evidence that the excitatory amino acid glutamate is ultimately involved in the destruction of neurons. The levels of several brain phospholipid fractions decrease when animals are given large doses of insulin. However, the suggestion that hypoglycemia results in a rapid depletion and inadequate production of high-energy phosphate compounds has not been corroborated; some other glucose-dependent biochemical process must be implicated.

When blood glucose falls, the CNS can utilize nonglucose substrates to a variable extent for its metabolic needs, especially keto acids and intermediates of glucose metabolism such as lactate, pyruvate, fructose, and other hexoses. In the neonatal brain, which has a higher glycogen reserve, keto acids provide a considerable proportion of cerebral energy requirements; this also happens after prolonged starvation. Hypoglycemia also acts on the adrenal glands and the autonomic nervous system to induce a corrective gluconeogenesis. However, in the face of severe and sustained hypoglycemia, these nonglucose substrates are not adequate to preserve the structural integrity of cerebral neurons, and eventually adenosine triphosphate (ATP) is depleted as well. If convulsions occur, they usually do so during a period of mental confusion; the convulsions have been attributed to an altered integrity of neuronal membranes and to elevated NH_3 and depressed GABA and lactate levels (Wilkinson and Prockop).

Etiology The most common causes of hypoglycemic encephalopathy are (1) accidental or deliberate overdose of insulin or an oral diabetic agent; (2) islet cell, insulin-secreting tumor of the pancreas; (3) depletion of liver glycogen that occasionally follows a prolonged alcoholic binge, starvation, or some form of acute liver disease such as acute nonicteric hepatoencephalopathy of childhood (Reye syndrome); (4) glycogen storage disease of infancy; and (5) an idiopathic hypoglycemia in the neonatal period and sometimes in infancy. Moderate degrees of hypoglycemia (50 mg/dL) may be observed with chronic renal insufficiency (Fisher et al). In the past, hypoglycemic encephalopathy was a not infrequent complication of "insulin shock" therapy for schizophrenia. In functional hyperinsulinism, as occurs in anorexia nervosa and in dietary faddism, the hypoglycemia is rarely of sufficient severity or duration to damage the CNS.

Clinical Features When the level of blood glucose has descended to about 30 mg/dL, the initial symptoms appear—nervousness, hunger, flushed facies, sweating, headache, palpitation, trembling, and anxiety; these gradually give way to confusion and drowsiness and occasionally to excitement, overactivity, and bizarre behavior. Many of the early and mild symptoms relate to adrenal and sympathetic overactivity, and therefore some of the manifestations may be muted in diabetic patients with neuropathy. In the next stage, forced sucking, grasping, motor restlessness, muscular spasms, and decerebrate rigidity occur, in that sequence. Myoclonic twitching and convulsions develop in some patients but are by no means the rule. Rarely there are focal cerebral deficits, the pathogenesis of which remains unexplained. Hemiplegia, corrected by intravenous glucose, was observed in 3 of 125 patients who presented with symptomatic hypoglycemia (Malouf and Brust).

Blood glucose levels of approximately 10 mg/dL are associated with deep coma, dilatation of pupils, pale skin, shallow respiration, slow pulse, and hypotonia of limb musculature—the so-called medullary phase of hypoglycemia. If glucose is administered before this level has been attained, the patient can be restored to normalcy, retracing the aforementioned steps in reverse order. However, once the "medullary phase" is reached, and particularly if it persists for a time before the hypoglycemia is corrected by intravenous glucose or spontaneously as a result of the gluconeogenic activities of the adrenal glands and liver, recovery is delayed for a period of days or weeks and may be incomplete.

The EEG is altered as the blood glucose falls, but the correlations are inexact. There is diffuse slowing in the theta or delta range. During recovery, sharp waves may appear and coincide in some cases with seizures.

A large dose of insulin, which produces intense hypoglycemia, even of relatively brief duration (30 to 60 min), is more dangerous than a series of less severe hypoglycemic episodes from smaller doses of insulin, possibly because the former impairs or exhausts essential enzymes—a condition that cannot then be overcome by large quantities of intravenous glucose.

The major clinical differences between hypoglycemic and hypoxic encephalopathy lie in the setting and the mode of evolution of the neurologic disorder. The effects of hypoglycemia usually unfold more slowly, over a period of 30 to 60 min, rather than in a few seconds or minutes. The recovery phase and sequelae of the two conditions are quite similar. A severe and prolonged episode of hypoglycemia may result in permanent impairment of intellectual function as well as other neurologic residua, like those that follow severe anoxia. We have also observed states of protracted coma as well as relatively pure Korsakoff amnesia. However, one should not be hasty in *prognosis*, for we have observed slow improvement to continue for 1 to 2 years. *Recurrent hypoglycemia*, as with an islet cell tumor, may masquerade for some time as an episodic confusional psychosis or convulsive illness, and diagnosis then awaits the demonstration of low blood glucose or hyperinsulinism in association with the neurologic symptoms.

Lesser degrees and more chronic forms of low blood glucose may produce two other distinct but not mutually exclusive syndromes, according to Marks and Rose, who have written an authoritative monograph on the subject. One of these syndromes, termed *subacute hypoglycemia*, is characterized by drowsiness and lethargy, diminution in psychomotor activity, deterioration of social behavior, and confusion. Oral or intravenous glucose will immediately alleviate the symptoms. In the other syndrome, termed *chronic hypoglycemia*, there is a gradual deterioration of intellectual functions, raising the question of dementia; in some reported instances, tremor, chorea, rigidity, cerebellar ataxia, and rarely signs of lower motor neuron involvement (*hypoglycemic amyotrophy*) are added. The latter feature has not been seen by the authors, who can only refer the reader to the report by Tom and Richardson.

These subacute and chronic forms of hypoglycemia have been observed in conjunction with islet cell hypertrophy and islet cell tumors of the pancreas, carcinoma of the stomach, fibrous mesothelioma, carcinoma of the cecum, and hepatoma. Supposedly an insulin-like substance is elaborated by these nonpancreatic tumors.

Functional or reactive hypoglycemia is the most ambiguous of all syndromes related to low blood glucose. This condition is usually idiopathic but may precede the onset of diabetes mellitus. The rise of insulin in response to a carbohydrate meal is delayed but then causes an excessive fall in blood glucose, to 30 to 40 mg/dL. The symptoms are malaise, fatigue, nervousness, headache, tremor, and so on, which may be difficult to distinguish from anxious depression. Not surprisingly, the term *functional hypoglycemia* has been much abused, being applied indiscriminately to a variety of complaints that would now be called chronic fatigue syndrome. In fact, the syndrome of functional or reactive hypoglycemia is rare and its diagnosis requires the finding of an excessive reaction to insulin, a low blood glucose during the symptomatic period, and a salutary response to oral glucose. Treatment, which consists of a high-protein, low-carbohydrate diet, should be reserved for patients whose symptom complex correlates with pronounced hypoglycemia as documented by a 5-h glucose tolerance test.

Pathologically, in all forms of hypoglycemic encephalopathy, the major damage is to the cerebral cortex. Cortical nerve cells degenerate and are replaced by microgliacytes and astrocytes. The distribution of lesions is similar, though probably not identical to that in hypoxic encephalopathy. (It appears that the cerebellar cortex is less vulnerable to hypoglycemia than to hypoxia.) Auer has described the ultrastructural changes in neurons resulting from experimental hypoglycemia; with increasing duration of hypoglycemia and EEG silence, there are mitochondrial changes, first in dendrites and then in nerve cell soma, followed by nuclear membrane disruption leading to cell death.

Treatment of all forms of hypoglycemia obviously consists of correction of the hypoglycemia at the earliest possible moment. It is not known whether hypothermia or other measures will increase the safety period in hypoglycemia or alter the outcome.

Hyperglycemia

Two syndromes have been defined, mainly in diabetics: (1) hyperglycemia with ketoacidosis and (2) hyperosmolar nonketotic hyperglycemia.

In *diabetic acidosis* the familiar picture is one of dehydration, fatigue, weakness, headache, abdominal pain, dryness of the mouth, stupor or coma, and Kussmaul type of breathing. Usually the condition has developed over a period of days in a patient known or proven to be diabetic. Insulin has often been omitted. The blood glucose level is found to be more than 400 mg/dL, the pH of the blood less than 7.20, and the bicarbonate less than 10 meq/L. Ketone bodies and β-hydroxybutyric acid are elevated in the blood and urine, and there is a marked glycosuria. The prompt administration of insulin and repletion of intravascular volume correct the clinical and chemical abnormalities over a period of hours.

Of considerable interest is a small group of patients with diabetic ketoacidosis, such as those reported by Young and Bradley, in whom deepening coma and cerebral edema develop as the elevated blood level of glucose is corrected. This condition, which is indicated by rising CSF pressure, has been attributed by Prockop to an accumulation of fructose and sorbitol in the brain. The latter substance, a polyol that is formed during hyperglycemia, crosses membranes slowly, but once it does so is said to cause a shift of water into the brain and an intracellular edema. However, according to Fishman, the increased polyols in the brain in hyperglycemia are not present in sufficient concentration to be important osmotically; they may induce other metabolic effects related to the encephalopathy. These are matters of conjecture, since the increase of polyols has never been found. The edema in this condition is probably due to reversal of the osmolality gradient from blood to brain, which occurs with rapid correction of hyperglycemia. The pathophysiology of the cerebral disorder in diabetic ketoacidosis is not fully understood. No consistent cellular pathology of the brain has been identified in the cases we have examined. Factors such as ketosis, tissue acidosis, hypotension, hyperosmolality, and hypoxia have not proved to be causative. Attempts at therapy by the administration of urea, mannitol, salt-poor albumin, and dexamethasone are usually unsuccessful, though recoveries are reported.

In *hyperosmolar nonketotic hyperglycemia*, the blood glucose is extremely high, over 600 mg/dL, but ketoacidosis does not develop or is mild. Osmolality is usually around 350 mosmol. There is also hemoconcentration and prerenal azotemia. Appreciation of the neurologic syndrome is generally credited to Wegierko, who published descriptions of it in 1956 and 1957. Most of the patients are elderly diabetics, but some were not previously known to have been diabetic. An infection, enteritis, pancreatitis, or a drug known to upset diabetic control (thiazides, prednisone, phenytoin) leads to polyuria, fatigue, confusion, stupor, and coma. Often the syndrome arises in conjunction with the combined use of corticosteroids and phenytoin (which inhibits insulin release), for example, in elderly patients with brain tumors. The use of osmotic diuretics enhances the risk. If the patient is seen before coma supervenes, seizures and focal signs such as a hemiparesis, a hemisensory defect, or a homonymous visual field defect erroneously suggest the possibility of a stroke. The mortality rate has been as high as 40 percent. Fluids should be replaced cautiously, using isotonic saline and potassium. Correction of the markedly elevated blood glucose requires relatively small amounts of insulin, since these patients often do not have a high degree of insulin resistance.

Hepatic Stupor and Coma (Hepatic or Portal-Systemic Encephalopathy)

Chronic hepatic insufficiency with portocaval shunting of blood is often punctuated by episodes of stupor, coma, and other neurologic symptoms—a state that is referred to as *hepatic stupor*, *coma*, or *acute hepatic encephalopathy*. This state complicates all varieties of liver disease. Less widely known is the fact that a surgical portal-systemic shunt (Eck fistula) is attended by the same clinical picture, in which case the liver itself may be little affected. Also, there are a number of hereditary hyperammonemic syndromes, usually presenting in infancy or childhood (see Chap. 37), that lead to episodic coma with or without seizures. In all these states, it is common for an excess of protein, derived from the diet or gastrointestinal hemorrhage, to induce or worsen the encephalopathy. Additional predisposing factors are hypoxia, hypokalemia, metabolic alkalosis, excessive diuresis, use of sedative hypnotic drugs, and constipation. Reye syndrome, a special type of acute nonicteric hepatic encephalopathy of children, is also associated with very high levels of ammonia in the blood (see further on in this chapter).

Clinical Features The clinical picture of subacute or chronic hepatic encephalopathy consists essentially of a derangement of consciousness, presenting first as mental confusion with decreased psychomotor activity, occasionally with hyperactivity, followed by progressive drowsiness, stupor, and coma. The confusional state, before coma supervenes, is frequently combined with a characteristic intermittency of sustained muscle contraction; this phenomenon, which was originally described in patients with hepatic stupor by Adams and Foley and called *asterixis* (from the Greek *sterixis*, a "fixed position"), is now recognized as a sign of various metabolic encephalopathies (page 107). It is conventionally demonstrated by having the patient hold his arms outstretched with the wrists extended, but the same tremor can be elicited by any sustained posture, including that of the protruded tongue. A variable, fluctuating rigidity of the trunk and limbs, grimacing, suck and grasp reflexes, exaggeration or asymmetry of tendon reflexes, Babinski signs, and focal or generalized seizures round out the clinical picture.

The EEG is a sensitive and reliable indicator of impending coma, becoming abnormal during the earliest phases of the disordered mental state. The usual EEG abnormality consists of paroxysms of bilaterally synchronous slow or triphasic waves, in the delta range, which at first predominate frontally and are interspersed with alpha activity and later, as the coma deepens, displace all normal activity (Fig. 2-3*H*, page 30). A small number of patients show only random high-voltage asynchronous slow waves.

This syndrome of hepatic encephalopathy is remarkably diverse in its clinical presentation. It usually evolves over a period of days to weeks and often terminates fatally; or, with appropriate treatment, the symptoms may regress completely or only partially and then fluctuate in severity for several weeks or months. Persistent hepatic coma of the latter type proves fatal in about half of the patients (Levy et al). In many patients, the syndrome is relatively mild and does not evolve beyond the stage of mental dullness and confusion, with asterixis and EEG changes. In yet others, a subtle disorder of mood, personality, and intellect may be protracted over a period of many months or even years; this chronic but nevertheless reversible mental disturbance need not be associated with overt clinical signs of liver failure (mainly jaundice and ascites) or other neurologic signs. Characteristically in these patients an extensive portal-systemic collateral circulation can be demonstrated (hence the term *portal-systemic encephalopathy*) and an association established between the mental disturbance and an intolerance to dietary protein and raised blood ammonia levels (Summerskill et al).

Finally, there is a group of patients (most of whom have experienced repeated attacks of hepatic coma) in whom an *irreversible* mild dementia and a disorder of posture and movement (grimacing, tremor, dysarthria, ataxia of gait, choreoathetosis) gradually appear. This condition of *chronic acquired hepatocerebral degeneration* must be distinguished from other dementing and extrapyramidal syndromes (see further on). A few cases of isolated spastic-ataxic paraplegia (so-called *hepatic myelopathy*) have also been described (page 1329).

The concentrations of blood NH_3, particularly if measured repeatedly in arterial blood samples, usually are well in excess of 200 mg/dL, and the severity of the neurologic and EEG disorders is roughly parallel to the ammonium levels. With treatment, the fall in the NH_3 levels precedes clinical improvement. If the diagnosis remains uncertain, an intolerance to ammonium can be demonstrated by the administration of an oral dose of 6.0 g of NH_3Cl, which raises the blood NH_3 and sometimes produces mild symptoms of hepatic encephalopathy. In a normal person, this dosage does not alter the blood NH_3 concentrations.

Neuropathologic Changes The striking finding in patients who die in a state of hepatic coma is a diffuse increase in the number and size of the protoplasmic astrocytes in the deep layers of the cerebral cortex, lenticular nuclei, thalamus, substantia nigra, cerebellar cortex, and red, dentate, and pontine nuclei, with little or no visible alteration in the nerve cells or other parenchymal elements. With periodic acid–Schiff (PAS) staining, the astrocytes are seen to contain characteristic glycogen inclusions. These abnormal glial cells are generally referred to as Alzheimer type II astrocytes, having been described originally in 1912 by von Hosslin and Alzheimer in a patient with Westphal-Strümpell pseudosclerosis (familial hepatolenticular degeneration, or Wilson disease). These astrocytes have been studied electron microscopically in rats with surgically created portocaval shunts (Cavanagh; Norenberg); the astrocytes showed a number of striking abnormalities—swelling of their terminal processes, cytoplasmic vacuolation (distended sacs of rough endoplasmic reticulum), formation of folds in the basement membrane around capillaries, diminution in glycogen, and an increase in the number of mitochondria and in enzymes that catabolize ammonia. Also, some degeneration in myelinated nerve fibers in the neuropil and increase in the cytoplasm of oligodendrocytes were seen. In chronic cases, we have found neuronal loss in the deep layers of the cerebral and cerebellar cortex and in the lenticular nuclei as well as a vacuolization of tissue (possibly astrocyte vacuolation) resembling the lesions of Wilson disease.

The ubiquitous astrocytic alterations occur to some degree in all patients who die of progressive liver failure, and the degree of this glial abnormality corresponds roughly to the intensity and duration of the neurologic disorder. Presumably the astrocytic changes affect the synaptic activities of the neurons. The clinical and EEG features of hepatic encephalopathy as well as the astrocytic hyperplasia, though highly characteristic, are not specific features of this metabolic disorder. Nevertheless, taken together in a setting of liver failure, these manifestations constitute a distinctive clinicopathologic entity.

Pathogenesis of Hepatic Encephalopathy The most plausible hypothesis relates hepatic coma to an abnormality of nitrogen metabolism, wherein ammonia (NH_3), which is formed in the bowel by the action of urease-containing organisms on dietary protein, is carried to the liver in the portal circulation but fails to be converted into urea, because of either hepatocellular disease, portal-systemic shunting of blood, or both. As a result, excess amounts of NH_3 reach the systemic circulation, where they interfere with cerebral metabolism in a way that is not yet fully understood. Certainly the ammonia theory best explains the basic neuropathologic change. Norenberg has proposed that the hypertrophy of the astrocytic cytoplasm and proliferation of the mitochondria and endoplasmic reticulum, as well as the increase in the astroglial glutamic dehydrogenase activity, reflect the heightened metabolic activity associated with ammonia detoxification. Removal of brain ammonia depends upon the formation of glutamine, a reaction that is catalyzed by the ATP-dependent enzyme glutamine synthetase, which is localized in the astrocytes. It has been shown in experimental animals that hyperammonemia leads to a depletion of ATP in midbrain reticular nuclei. Whether this is the primary cause of coma has not been resolved.

Numerous alternative theories have been suggested. One is that CNS function in cirrhotic patients is impaired by phenols or short-chain fatty acids (from the diet or from bacterial metabolism of carbohydrate). Another suggestion is that biogenic amines (e.g., octopamine), which arise in the gut and bypass the liver, act as false neurotransmitters, displacing the putative transmitters norepinephrine and dopamine (Fischer and Baldessarini). Zieve has presented evidence that mercaptans (methanethiol, methionine), which are also generated in the gastrointestinal tract and removed by the liver, act in conjunction with NH_3 to produce hepatic encephalopathy. This theory and others have been the subject of reviews by Butterworth and coworkers, by Zieve, by Rothstein and Herlong, and by Jones and Basile, to which the reader is referred for detailed information.

For some time, it has been known that hepatic encephalopathy is associated with increased activity of the inhibitory transmitter GABA. It is also known that increased GABAergic neurotransmission may result from substances that inhibit the binding of endogenous benzodiazepines to their receptors (Basile et al), and these antagonists have some clinical effect (transient awakening) in patients with hepatic encephalopathy. The actions of benzodiazepines are mediated by these receptors—hence the designation *GABA-benzodiazepine theory*. The practicality of using benzodiazepine receptor antagonists (e.g., flumazenil) in the treatment of hepatic encephalopathy remains to be determined (see Mullen).

Until recently, the ammonia and the GABAergic-benzodiazepine hypotheses of the pathogenesis of hepatic encephalopathy have appeared to be unrelated and even mutually exclusive. However, there is a growing body of evidence (recently reviewed by Jones and Basile) that ammonia, even in the modestly elevated concentrations that occur in liver failure, probably enhances GABAergic neurotransmission—a concept that may unify the two hypotheses.

Also in recent years, manganese has emerged as a potential neurotoxin in the pathogenesis of hepatic encephalopathy (Kreiger et al; Pomier-Layrargues et al). In patients with chronic liver diseases and with spontaneous or surgically induced portal-systemic shunts, manganese accumulates in the serum and in the brain, more specifically in the pallidum. This accumulation is readily discernible as a pallidal signal hyperintensity on T1-weighted MRI. Following liver transplantation, there is normalization of the MRI changes and the associated extrapyramidal symptoms. The effects of manganese chelation on such patients have not been studied and the possible mechanisms of accumulated manganese in the pathogenesis of hepatic encephalopathy are not known.

Treatment Despite the incompleteness of our understanding of the role of disordered ammonium metabolism in the genesis of hepatic coma, an awareness of this relationship has provided the few effective means of treating this disorder: restriction of dietary protein; reducing bowel flora by oral administration of neomycin or kanamycin, which suppresses the urease-producing organisms in the bowel; and the use of enemas. The mainstay of treatment has been the use of lactulose, an inert sugar that acidifies the colonic contents and greatly reduces bacterial activity. The sustained use of oral neomycin carries a risk of renal damage and ototoxicity and has therefore been relegated to a second line of therapy. The salutary effects of these therapeutic measures, the common attribute of which is the lowering of the blood NH_3, lend strong support to the theory of ammonia intoxication. Ultimately, in cases of intractable liver failure, transplantation becomes a treatment of last resort.

Other methods of treatment, the value of which still remains to be established, include the use of bromocriptine, flumazenil, and keto-analogues of essential amino acids. Theoretically, the keto-analogues should provide a nitrogen-free source of essential amino acids (Maddrey et al), and bromocriptine, a dopamine agonist, should enhance dopaminergic transmission (Morgan et al). Administration of branched-chain amino acids may result in considerable improvement in mental status, but their effects have been variable and associated with an increased mortality (Naylor et al).

Fulminant Hepatic Failure and Cerebral Edema In *acute hepatitis*, confusional, delirious, and comatose states also occur, but their mechanisms are still unknown. Blood NH_3 may be elevated, but usually not to a degree that would be expected to affect the CNS. Severe acute hepatic failure may cause hypoglycemia, which contributes to the encephalopathy and often presages a fatal outcome.

Cerebral edema is a prominent finding in cases of fulminant hepatic failure from any cause and is the main cause of death in patients awaiting liver transplantation. The cerebral edema that occurs in these circumstances appears to be related to the rapidity of rise of blood ammonia, but it probably depends as well on additional metabolic derangements that complicate acute liver failure. The combination of rapidly evolving hepatic failure and massive cerebral edema is similar to that observed in the Reye syndrome.

CT scanning is an effective means of detecting cerebral edema in patients with fulminant hepatic failure, and the degree of cerebral swelling is roughly proportional to the severity of encephalopathy (Wijdicks et al). Since patients with fulminant hepatic failure can survive liver transplantation with few or no neurologic deficits, it is important to recognize cerebral edema early, before the stages of stupor and coma and greatly increased intracranial pressure have been reached. Short of transplantation, death in these cases may sometimes be prevented by monitoring the intracranial pressure (as outlined by Lidofsky et al) and by the use of osmotic diuretics and hyperventilation, as detailed in Chap. 30. However, some survivors may be left with cerebral damage from raised intracranial pressure.

Reye Syndrome (Reye-Johnson Syndrome) As indicated above, this is a special type of nonicteric hepatic encephalopathy occurring in children and adolescents and characterized by acute brain swelling in association with fatty infiltration of the viscera, particularly of the liver. Although individual cases of this disorder had been described for many years, its recognition as a clinical-pathologic entity dates from 1963, when a large series was reported from Australia by Reye and colleagues and from the United States by Johnson and coworkers. The disorder tends to occur in outbreaks (286 cases were reported to the Centers for Disease Control during a 4-month period in 1974). Mainly, these outbreaks were observed in association with influenza B virus and varicella infections, but a variety of other viral infections have been implicated (influenza A, echovirus, reovirus, rubella, rubeola, herpes simplex, Epstein-Barr virus). In addition, the toxic or adjuvant effects of aspirin given during these infections seem to play a role in producing the disease. Only occasional instances of the Reye syndrome are observed now that the association with aspirin administration has become widely known and its use in children with the above infections has been interdicted.

Most patients are children, boys and girls being equally affected, but rare instances have been observed in infants (Huttenlocher and Trauner) and in young adults. In most cases the encephalopathy is preceded for several days to a week by fever, symptoms of upper respiratory infection, and protracted vomiting. These symptoms are followed by the rapid evolution of stupor and coma, associated in many cases with focal and generalized seizures, signs of sympathetic overactivity (tachypnea, tachycardia, mydriasis), decorticate and decerebrate rigidity, and loss of pupillary, corneal, and vestibulo-ocular reflexes. In infants, respiratory distress, tachypnea, and apnea are the most prominent features. The liver may be greatly enlarged, often extending to the pelvis and providing an important diagnostic clue as to the cause of the cerebral changes. Initially there is a metabolic acidosis, followed by a respiratory alkalosis (rising arterial pH and falling P_{CO_2}). The CSF is usually under increased pressure and is acellular; glucose values may be low, reflecting the hypoglycemia. The serum glutamic-oxaloacetic transaminase (SGOT), prothrombin time, and blood ammonia are increased, sometimes to an extreme degree. The EEG is characterized by diffuse arrhythmic delta activity, progressing to electrocerebral silence in patients who fail to survive.

The major *pathologic findings* are cerebral edema, often with cerebellar herniation, and infiltration of hepatocytes with fine droplets of fat (mainly triglycerides); the renal tubules, myocardium, skeletal muscles, pancreas, and spleen are infiltrated to a lesser extent. There are no inflammatory lesions in the brain, liver, or other organs. There is not full agreement as to the pathogenesis of this disorder.

Prognosis and Treatment In a series of children with blood ammonia levels greater than 500 mg/dL who were treated during the years 1967 to 1974, Shaywitz and colleagues reported a mortality of 60 percent. Once the child became comatose, death was almost inevitable. In more recent years, early diagnosis (elevations of SGOT, prothrombin time, and serum NH_3) and initiation of treatment before the onset of coma have reduced the fatality rate to 5 to 10 percent. Treatment consists of the following measures: temperature control with a cooling blanket; nasotracheal intubation and controlled ventilation to maintain P_{CO_2} above 20 mmHg; intravenous glucose covered by insulin to maintain blood glucose at 150 to 200 mg/dL; administration of neomycin enemas and lactulose; control of intracranial pressure by means of continual monitoring and the use of hypertonic solutions (see Chap. 30); and the maintenance of fluid and electrolyte balance (Trauner). Upon recovery, cerebral function returns to normal unless there had been deep and prolonged coma or protracted elevation of intracranial pressure.

Uremic Encephalopathy

Episodic confusion and stupor and other neurologic symptoms may accompany any form of severe renal disease—acute or chronic. The cerebral symptoms attributable to uremia per se (first described by Addison in 1832) are best discerned in normotensive individuals in whom renal failure develops rapidly. Apathy, fatigue, inattentiveness, and irritability are usually the initial symptoms; later, there is confusion, disturbances of sensory perception, hallucinations, dysarthria, and asterixis. Sometimes this takes the form of a toxic psychosis, with hallucinations, delusions, insomnia, or catatonia (Marshall). Characteristically these symptoms fluctuate from day to day or even from hour to hour. In some patients, especially in those who become anuric, symptoms may come on rather abruptly and progress rapidly to a state of stupor and coma. In others, in whom uremia develops more gradually, mild visual hallucinations and a disorder of attention may persist for several weeks in relatively pure form. The EEG becomes diffusely slow and may remain so for several weeks after the institution of dialysis. The CSF pressure is normal and the protein is not elevated unless there is a uremic or diabetic neuropathy. In several reports, meningismus and a low-grade mononuclear pleocytosis is mentioned, but we have not found this.

In acute renal failure, clouding of the sensorium is practically always associated with a variety of motor phenomena, which usually occur early in the course of the encephalopathy, sometimes when the patient is still mentally clear. The patient begins to twitch and jerk and may convulse. The twitches involve parts of muscles, whole muscles, or limbs and are lightning-quick, arrhythmic, and asynchronous on the two sides of the body; they are incessant during both wakefulness and sleep. At times the movements resemble those of chorea or an arrhythmic tremor, and asterixis is readily evoked. The motor phenomena are often difficult to classify. The authors prefer to describe the condition as the *uremic twitch-convulsive syndrome*.

Because of the similarity of this syndrome to tetany, measurement should be made of serum calcium and magnesium—and, of course, hypocalcemia and hypomagnesemia do occur in uremia. But often the values for these ions are normal or near normal, and the administration of calcium and magnesium salts has little effect. The resemblance of uremic encephalopathy to hepatic and other metabolic encephalopathies has been stressed by Raskin and Fishman, yet we are more impressed with differences than with similarities. We have observed the twitch-convulsive syndrome in association with a variety of diseases such as widespread neoplasia, delirium tremens, diabetes with necrotizing pyelonephritis, and lupus erythematosus, in which the blood urea nitrogen was only modestly elevated; but always the factor of renal failure was ultimately discovered.

As the uremia worsens, the patient lapses into a quiet coma. Unless the accompanying metabolic acidosis is corrected, Kussmaul breathing appears and gives way to Cheyne-Stokes breathing and death.

It is important to keep in mind that encephalopathy and coma in the patient with renal failure may be due to disorders other than uremia itself. The altered excretion of drugs leads to their accumulation, sometimes evoking excessive sedation even though serum concentrations are normal. Subdural and intracerebral hemorrhages may complicate uremia because of clotting defects and hypertension, and chronically azotemic patients are prone to infections, including meningitis.

Since uremia is so frequently associated with hypertension, a major problem also arises in distinguishing the cerebral effects of uremia from those of severe and accelerated hypertension. Volhard was the first to make this distinction; he introduced the term *pseudouremia* to designate the cerebral effects of malignant hypertension and to separate them from true uremia. The term *hypertensive encephalopathy*, by which pseudouremia is now known, was first used by Oppenheimer and Fishberg. The clinical picture of the latter disorder and its pathophysiology are discussed on page 903.

Opinions vary as to the biochemical basis of uremic encephalopathy and the twitch-convulsive syndrome. Restoration of renal function completely corrects the neurologic syndrome, attesting to a functional disorder of subcellular type. Whether caused by the retention of organic acids, elevation of phosphate in the CSF (claimed by Harrison et al), or the action of urea or other toxins has never been settled. The data supporting the causative role of urea are ambiguous, as they are for other endogenous putative agents (see Bolton and Young and the review by Burn and Bates). However, it can be stated that urea itself is not the sole inductive agent, since its infusion does not produce the syndrome in man or animals.

It would appear that every level of the CNS is affected, from spinal cord to cerebrum. The authors have been unable to detect cellular changes in the brain or spinal cord other than a mild hyperplasia of protoplasmic astrocytes in some cases, but never of the degree observed in hepatic encephalopathy. Cerebral edema is notably absent. In fact, CT scans and MRI regularly show an element of cerebral shrinkage, probably on the basis of hyperosmolality. A peripheral neuropathy is also a common complication of uremia and is considered in Chap. 46.

In the *treatment* of uremic encephalopathy, the nature of the renal disease assumes paramount importance; if it is irreversible and progressive, the prognosis is poor without dialysis or renal transplantation. Improvement of encephalopathic symptoms may not be evident for a day or two after institution of dialysis. Convulsions, which occur in about one-third of cases, often preterminally, may respond to relatively low plasma concentrations of anticonvulsants, the reason being that serum albumin is depressed in uremia, increasing the unbound, therapeutically active portion. If there are severe associated metabolic disturbances, such as hyponatremia, the seizures may be difficult to control. One must be cautious in prescribing any of a large number of drugs in the face of renal failure, for inordinately high, toxic blood levels may result. Examples are aminoglycoside antibiotics (vestibular damage); furosemide (cochlear damage); and nitrofurantoin, isoniazid, and hydralazine (peripheral nerve damage).

Dialysis "Disequilibrium Syndrome" This term refers to a group of symptoms that may occur during and following hemodialysis or peritoneal dialysis in association with some degree of cerebral edema. The symptoms include headaches, nausea, muscular cramps, nervous irritability, agitation, drowsiness, and convulsions. The headache, which may be bilateral and throbbing or resemble common migraine, develops in approximately 70 percent of patients, while the other symptoms are observed in 5 to 10 percent, usually in those undergoing rapid dialysis or in the early stages of a dialysis program. The symptoms tend to occur in the third or fourth hour of dialysis and last for several hours. Sometimes they appear 8 to 48 h after the completion of dialysis. Originally these symptoms were attributed to the rapid lowering of serum urea, leaving the brain with a higher concentration of urea than the serum and resulting in a shift of water into the brain to equalize the osmotic gradient (*reverse urea syndrome*). Now it is believed that the shift of water into the brain is akin to water intoxication and is due to the inappropriate secretion of antidiuretic hormone.

The symptoms of subdural hematoma, which in some series have occurred in 3 to 4 percent of patients undergoing dialysis, may be mistakenly attributed to the disequilibrium syndrome.

Dialysis Encephalopathy (Dialysis Dementia) This is a subacutely progressive syndrome, now virtually extinct, that complicated chronic hemodialysis. Characteristically the condition begins with a hesitant, stuttering dysarthria, dysphasia, and sometimes apraxia of speech, to which are added facial and then generalized myoclonus, focal and generalized seizures, personality and behavioral changes, and intellectual decline. The EEG is invariably abnormal, taking the form of paroxysmal and sometimes periodic sharp-wave or spike-and-wave activity (up to 500 mV and lasting 1 to 20 s) intermixed with abundant theta and delta activity. The CSF is normal except, occasionally, for increased protein.

At first the myoclonus and speech disorders are intermittent, occurring during or immediately after dialysis and lasting for only a few hours, but gradually they become more persistent and eventually permanent. Once established, the syndrome is usually steadily progressive over a 1- to 15-month period (average survival of 6 months in the 42 cases analyzed by Lederman and Henry).

The neuropathologic changes are subtle and consist of a mild degree of microcavitation of the superficial layers of the cerebral cortex. Although the changes are diffuse, they have been found, in one study, to be more severe in the left (dominant) hemisphere than in the right and more severe in the left frontotemporal operculum than in the surrounding cortex (Winkelman and Ricanati). The disproportionate affection of the left frontotemporal opercular cortex would explain the distinctive disorder of speech and language.

The current view of the pathogenesis of dialysis encephalopathy is that it represented a form of aluminum intoxication (Alfrey et al), the aluminum being derived from the dialysate or from orally administered aluminum gels. In recent years, this disorder has disappeared, the result, no doubt, of the universal practice of purifying the water used in dialysis and thereby removing aluminum from the dialysate. The subject has been reviewed by Parkinson and coworkers.

Complications of Renal Transplantation The risk, in immunosuppressed persons, of developing a primary lymphoma of the brain or progressive multifocal leukoencephalopathy has already been mentioned (pages 695 and 812). A different encephalopathy that is marked by widespread edema of the cerebral white matter, evident on the MRI and predominantly occipital, occurs after the administration of cyclosporine and other immunosuppressants. The pattern on MRI is not specific, being seen also in patients with hypertensive encephalopathy and other conditions. Systemic fungal infections are found at autopsy in about 45 percent of patients who have had renal transplants and long periods of immunosuppressive treatment; in about one-third of these patients, the CNS is involved. *Cryptococcus*, *Listeria*, *Aspergillus*, *Candida*, *Nocardia*, and *Histoplasma* are the usual organisms. Other CNS infections that have complicated transplantation are toxoplasmosis and cytomegalic inclusion disease.

In some nutritionally depleted uremic patients who are subjected to treatment that involves major shifts of plasma water and electrolytes, diseases unrelated to uremia may develop. In our necropsy material, we have found examples of Wernicke-Korsakoff disease and central pontine myelinolysis. A bleeding diathesis may result in subdural or cerebral hemorrhage.

Encephalopathy Associated with Sepsis and Burns

Bolton and Young have drawn attention to the frequent occurrence, in severely septic patients, of a drowsy or confusional state that is reversible but is not explained by hepatic, pulmonary, or renal failure, electrolyte imbalance, hypotension, drug intoxication, or a primary lesion of the brain. According to their surveys, 70 percent of patients become disoriented and confused within hours of the onset of severe systemic infection; in a few cases, this state may progress to stupor and coma. Notably there are no signs of asterixis, myoclonus, or focal cerebral disorder, but paratonia is common, as is the later development of a polyneuropathy.

The encephalopathic state that occurs with severe systemic infection may also occur independently of sepsis, as a component of a syndrome of multiple organ failure and as a complication of widespread cutaneous burns (Aikawa et al).

It has been useful, in clinical work, to distinguish these encephalopathies of infection and multiorgan failure from those due to isolated hepatic or renal disease. The lack of a biochemical marker and the confounding effects of hypotension during sepsis (septic shock) leave doubt as to pathogenesis. Altered phenylalanine metabolism and circulating cytokines have been proposed as causes, without firm evidence. Of interest in two of our fatal cases was the presence of *brain purpura*, but this has otherwise been an infrequent finding. The white matter of the cerebrum and cerebellum was speckled with myriads of pericapillary hemorrhages and zones of pericapillary necrosis. This pathologic reaction is nonspecific, having also been seen in some of our cases (10 in all) of viral pneumonia, heart failure with morphine overdose, and arsenical intoxication.

Disorders of Sodium, Potassium, and Water Balance

Drowsiness, confusion, stupor, and coma, in conjunction with seizures and sometimes with other neurologic deficits, may have as their basis a more or less pure abnormality of electrolyte or water balance. Only brief reference is made to some of these—such as hypocalcemia, hypercalcemia, hypophosphatemia, and hypomagnesemia—since they are considered in other parts of the text.

Hyponatremia Among the many causes of hyponatremia, the *syndrome of inappropriate antidiuretic hormone secretion (SIADH)* is of special importance, since it may complicate neurologic diseases of many types—head trauma, bacterial meningitis and encephalitis, cerebral infarction, subarachnoid hemorrhage, neoplasm, and Guillain-Barré disease. The diagnosis of SIADH should be suspected in any critically ill neurologic or neurosurgical patient who excretes urine that is hypertonic relative to the plasma. As the hyponatremia develops, there is a decrease in alertness, which progresses through stages of confusion to coma, often with convulsions. *As with many other metabolic derangements, the severity of the clinical effects is related to the rapidity of decline in serum Na.* Lack of recognition of this state may allow the serum Na to fall to dangerously low levels, 100 meq/L or lower. One's first impulse is to administer NaCl intravenously, but this must be done cautiously, because in most of these patients the intravascular volume is already expanded and there is a risk of congestive heart failure. Most cases respond to the restriction of fluid intake—to 500 mL per 24 h if the serum Na is less than 120 meq/L and to 1000 mL per 24 h if less than 130 meq/L. Even when the Na reaches 130 meq/L, the fluid intake should not exceed 1500 mL per 24 h. In extreme cases of hyponatremia with stupor or seizures, infusion of NaCl is necessary. The amount of NaCl to be infused can be calculated from the current and the target levels of serum Na by assuming that the infused sodium load is distributed throughout the total body water content (0.6 × weight in kg):

$$[\text{Target Na} - \text{starting Na}] \times 0.6 \times \text{weight (kg)} = \text{desired infused Na load (meq)}$$

The desired volume of normal saline can then be calculated by keeping in mind that its sodium concentration is 154 meq/L, and that of 3 percent (hypertonic) saline is 462 meq/L. If hypertonic saline is administered, it is usually necessary to simultaneously reduce intravascular volume with furosemide, beginning with a dose of 0.5 mg/kg intravenously, and to increase the dosage until a diuresis is obtained. Guidelines for the rapidity of correction of Na are elaborated further on in relation to central pontine myelinolysis (no more than 10 mmol/L in the first 24 h). Although the syndrome of SIADH is self-limiting, it may continue for weeks or months, depending on the type of associated brain disease.

It must be emphasized that not all patients with intracranial disorders who show hyponatremia and natriuresis have SIADH. In fact, in many of such patients, renal loss of salt is the cause of hyponatremia and, in contrast to SIADH, results in decreased blood volume. The process has been termed "cerebral salt wasting" (Nelson et al). Sodium loss in these circumstances is attributable to the production by the heart or brain of a potent polypeptide, atrial natiuretic factor. As discussed in Chap. 34, under "Subarachnoid Hemorrhage," the distinction between SIADH and cerebral salt wasting is of more than theoretical importance, insofar as fluid restriction to correct hyponatremia may be dangerous in patients with salt wasting, particularly in those with vasospasm after ruptured intracranial aneurysms.

Arieff has emphasized the hazards of *postoperative hyponatremia.* He has reported a series of 15 patients, all of them women, in whom *severe hyponatremia* followed elective surgery. About 48 h after these patients had recovered from anesthesia, their serum Na fell to an average level of 108 meq/L; the urinary sodium was 68 mmol/L, and the urinary osmolality was 501 mosmol/kg. At this point, generalized seizures occurred, followed by respiratory arrest, requiring intubation. Of the 15 women, 5 died; there were no diagnostic pathologic findings, and no lesions of central pontine myelinolysis (see below) were found. Seven patients, whose serum Na was corrected slowly, improved over a period of several days but then developed a rapidly progressive diminution in alertness and increasing nausea, headache, and obtundation, followed by a recurrence of seizures and coma. These patients survived in a persistent vegetative state. We find the syndrome difficult to interpret. The initial hyponatremia was probably the result of SIADH. What happened later could have been the consequence of immediate and delayed hypoxia, but this is speculative.

An important consideration in the management of severe hyponatremia and hyperosmolality is *the rapidity with which these abnormalities are corrected and the danger of provoking central pontine myelinolysis (CPM)* and related brainstem, cerebellar, and cerebral lesions (extrapontine myelinolysis). These issues are considered below, in the section on CPM.

Hypernatremia Severe hypernatremia (Na >155 meq/L) and dehydration are observed in diabetes insipidus, the neurologic causes of which include head trauma with damage to the pituitary stalk (Chap. 27), nonketotic diabetic coma, protracted diarrhea in infants, and the deprivation of fluid intake in the stuporous patient. The last condition is usually associated with a brain lesion that impairs consciousness. Exceptionally, in patients with chronic hydrocephalus, the hypothalamic thirst center is rendered inactive, and severe hypernatremia, stupor, and coma may follow a failure to drink. In hypernatremia from any cause, the brain volume is manifestly reduced in CT scans. Retraction of the cerebral cortex from the dura has been known to rupture a bridging vein and cause a subdural hematoma.

As is true for hyponatremia, the degree of CNS disturbance in hypernatremia is generally related to the rate at which the serum Na rises. Slowly rising values, to levels as high as 170 meq/L, are often well tolerated. Rapid elevations shrink the brain, especially in infants. Extremely high levels cause impairment of consciousness with asterixis, myoclonus, seizures, and choreiform movements. In addition, muscular weakness, rhabdomyolysis, and myoglobinuria have been reported.

It is to be noted that hyponatremia is usually accompanied by hypo-osmolality of the serum, and hypernatremia by hyperosmolality. However, there is no strict correlation between the degree of hypo- or hyperosmolality and neurologic dysfunction. Instead, the rapidity of change, as already emphasized, plays a major role. In hyponatremia plus hypo-osmolality, Fishman finds an increase in intracellular water and a diminution in intracellular K; but in our view it is the dehydration that is more critical and coincides with the neuronal derangement. In hypernatremia plus hyperosmolality, the neurons do not lose water as much as do other cells, a compensatory reaction that Fishman attributes to the presence of "idiogenic osmoles"—probably glucose, glucose metabolites, and amino acids. The impairment of neuronal function in this state is not understood. Theoretically one would expect neuronal shrinkage and possibly alteration of the synaptic surface of the cell.

Hypo- and Hyperkalemia The main clinical effect of *hypokalemia* (K, 2.0 meq/L or less) is generalized muscular weakness (see Chap. 48). A confusional state may also be added but is infrequent. Both conditions are readily corrected by adding K to intravenous fluid and infusing it at no more than 4 to 6 meq/h. *Hyperkalemia* (above 7 meq/L) also may manifest itself by generalized muscle weakness, although the main effects are changes in the electrocardiogram (ECG), possibly leading to cardiac arrest.

Other Metabolic Encephalopathies Limitation of space permits only brief reference to other metabolic disturbances that may present as episodic confusion, stupor, or coma. The most important members of this group are summarized below.

Hypercalcemia This is defined as an elevation of the serum calcium concentration above 10.5 mg/dL. If the serum protein content is normal, Ca levels greater than 12 mg/dL are required to produce neurologic symptoms. However, with low serum albumin levels, an increased proportion of the serum Ca is in the unbound or ionized form (upon which the clinical effects depend), and symptoms may occur with serum Ca levels as low as 10 mg/dL.

In young persons, the most common cause of hypercalcemia is hyperparathyroidism (either primary or secondary); in older persons, osteolytic bone tumors, particularly metastatic carcinoma and multiple myeloma, are often causative. Less common causes are vitamin D intoxication, prolonged immobilization, hyperthyroidism, sarcoidosis, and decreased calcium excretion (renal failure).

Anorexia, nausea and vomiting, fatigue, and headache are usually the *initial symptoms*, followed by confusion (rarely a delirium) and drowsiness, progressing to stupor or coma in untreated patients. Diffuse myoclonus and rigidity occur occasionally, as do elevations of spinal fluid protein (up to 175 mg/100 mL). Convulsions occur uncommonly.

Hypocalcemia The usual manifestations of *hypocalcemia* are tetany and seizures. With severe and persistent hypocalcemia, altered mental status in the form of depression, confusion, dementia, or personality change can occur. Even coma may result, in which case there may be papilledema due to increased intracranial pressure. Aside from the raised pressure, the CSF shows no consistent abnormality. This increase in intracranial pressure may be manifest by headache and papilledema without altered mentation. Hypoparathydroidism is discussed further on.

Metabolic acidosis from any cause produces a typical syndrome of drowsiness, stupor, and coma, with dry skin and Kussmaul breathing. The CNS depression does not correlate with the concentration of ketones. Probably there are associated effects on neurotransmitters, consequent to the increase in osmolality and release of intracellular calcium.

In infants and children, acidosis may occur in the course of hyperammonemia, isovaleric acidemia, maple syrup urine disease, lactic and glutaric acidemia, hyperglycinemia, and other disorders, which are described in detail in Chap. 37. High-voltage slow activity predominates in the EEG, and correction of the acidosis or elevated ammonia level restores CNS function to normal provided that coma was not prolonged or complicated by hypoxia or hypotension. In uncomplicated acidotic coma, we have observed no recognizable neuropathologic change by light microscopy.

Encephalopathy due to *Addison disease* (adrenal insufficiency) may be attended by episodic confusion, stupor, or coma without special identifying features; it is usually precipitated in the addisonian patient by infection or surgical stress. Hemorrhagic destruction of the adrenals is another cause. Hypotension and diminished cerebral circulation and hypoglycemia are the most readily recognized metabolic abnormalities; measures that correct these conditions reverse the adrenal crisis in some instances.

Myxedema is well known to cause a mental dullness, drowsiness, and stupor. We have encountered several instances of an encephalopathy with myoclonus in patients with Hashimoto thyroiditis; some of these patients had nearly normal thyroid function studies, but they had high titers of antithyroglobulin antibodies; the encephalopathy in the latter case is thought to be on an autoimmune basis. These are discussed in a later part of the chapter.

The various neurologic syndrome that are consequent upon electrolytic disorders have been reviewed by Laureno.

Central Pontine Myelinolysis

In 1950, Adams and Victor observed a rapidly evolving quadriplegia and pseudobulbar palsy in a young alcoholic man who had entered the hospital 10 days earlier with symptoms of alcohol withdrawal. Postmortem examination several weeks later disclosed a large, symmetrical, essentially demyelinative lesion occupying the greater part of the basis pontis. Over the next 5 years, three additional cases (two alcoholic patients and one with scleroderma) were studied clinically and pathologically, and in 1959 these four cases were reported by Adams et al under the heading of *central pontine myelinolysis* (CPM). This term was chosen because it denotes both the specific anatomic localization of the disease and its essential pathologic attribute: the remarkably unsystematic dissolution of the sheaths of medullated fibers. Once attention was focused on this distinctive lesion, many other reports appeared. The exact incidence of this disease is not known, but in a series of 3548 consecutive autopsies in adults, the typical lesion was found in 9 cases, or 0.25 percent (Victor and Laureno).

Pathologic Features One is compelled to define this disease in terms of its pathologic anatomy, because this stands as its most certain feature. Transverse sectioning of the fixed brainstem discloses a grayish discoloration and fine granularity in the center of the basis pontis. The lesion may be only a few millimeters in diameter, or it may occupy almost the entire basis pontis. There is always a rim of intact myelin between the lesion and the surface of the pons. Posteriorly it may reach and involve the medial lemnisci and, in the most advanced cases, other tegmental structures as well. Very rarely, the lesion encroaches on the midbrain, but inferiorly it does not extend as far as the medulla. Exceptionally the extensive pontine lesions may be associated with identical myelinolytic foci symmetrically distributed in the thalamus, subthalamic nucleus, striatum, internal capsule, amygdaloid nuclei, lateral geniculate body, white matter of the cerebellar folia, and deep layers of the cerebral cortex and subjacent white matter ("extrapontine myelinolysis"; Wright et al).

Microscopically, the fundamental abnormality consists of destruction of the medullated sheaths throughout the lesion, with relative sparing of the axis cylinders and intactness of the nerve cells of the pontine nuclei. These changes always begin and are most severe in the geometric center of the pons, where they may proceed to frank necrosis of tissue. Reactive phagocytes and glial cells are in evidence throughout the demyelinative focus, but no oligodendrocytes are seen. Signs of inflammation are conspicuously absent.

This constellation of pathologic findings provides easy differentiation of the lesion from infarction and the inflammatory demyelinations of multiple sclerosis and postinfectious encephalomyelitis. Microscopically, the lesion resembles that of Marchiafava-Bignami disease (Chap. 41), with which it is rarely associated. Wernicke disease is not infrequently associated with CPM, but the lesions bear no resemblance to one another in terms of topography and histology.

Clinical Features Central pontine myelinosis occurs only sporadically, with no hint of a genetic factor. The two sexes are affected equally, and the patients do not fall into any one age period. Whereas the cases first reported had occurred in adults, there are now many reports of the disease in children, particularly in those with severe burns (McKee et al).

The outstanding clinical characteristic of CPM is its invariable association with some other serious, often life-threatening disease. In more than half the cases, it has appeared in the late stages of chronic alcoholism, often in association with Wernicke disease and polyneuropathy. Among the other medical conditions and diseases with which CPM has been conjoined are chronic renal failure being treated with dialysis, hepatic failure, advanced lymphoma, carcinoma, cachexia from a variety of other causes, severe bacterial infections, dehydration and electrolyte disturbances, acute hemorrhagic pancreatitis, and pellagra.

In many patients with CPM there are no symptoms or signs that betray the pontine lesion, presumably because it is so small, extending only 2 to 3 mm on either side of the median raphe and involving only a small portion of the corticopontine or pontocerebellar fibers. In others, the presence of CPM is obscured by coma from a metabolic or other associated disease. Probably only a minority of cases, exemplified by the first patient whom we observed, are recognized during life. In this patient, a serious alcoholic with delirium tremens and pneumonia, there evolved, over a period of several days, a flaccid paralysis of all four limbs and an inability to chew, swallow, or speak (thus simulating occlusion of the basilar artery). Pupillary reflexes, movements of the eyes and lids, corneal reflexes, and facial sensation were spared. In some instances, however, conjugate eye movements are limited, and there may be nystagmus. With survival for several days, the tendon reflexes become more active, followed by spasticity and extensor posturing of the limbs on painful stimulation. Some patients are left in a state of mutism and paralysis with relative intactness of sensation and comprehension, i.e., the "locked-in syndrome."

The capacity of CT scanning but especially MRI to visualize the pontine lesion has greatly increased the frequency of premortem diagnoses. The MRI discloses a characteristic "bat wing" lesion of the basis pontis in some cases (Fig. 40-2), although this change may become evident only several days after the onset of symptoms. Brainstem auditory evoked responses also disclose the lesions that encroach upon the pontine tegmentum.

Variants of this syndrome are being encountered with increasing frequency. Two of our elderly patients, with confusion and stupor—but without signs of corticospinal or pseudobulbar palsy—recovered; however, they were left with a severe dysarthria and cerebellar ataxia lasting many months. By CT and MRI, no lesions were observed in the tegmentum of the brainstem and cerebellum. After 6 months, these patients' nervous system function was essentially normal; originally both had serum Na levels of 99 meq/L, but information about the rate of restoration of serum Na was not available. Another of our patients developed a typical locked-in syndrome after the rapid correction of a serum sodium of 104 meq/L. He showed large symmetrical lesions of the frontal cortex and underlying white matter but no pontine lesion (by MRI).

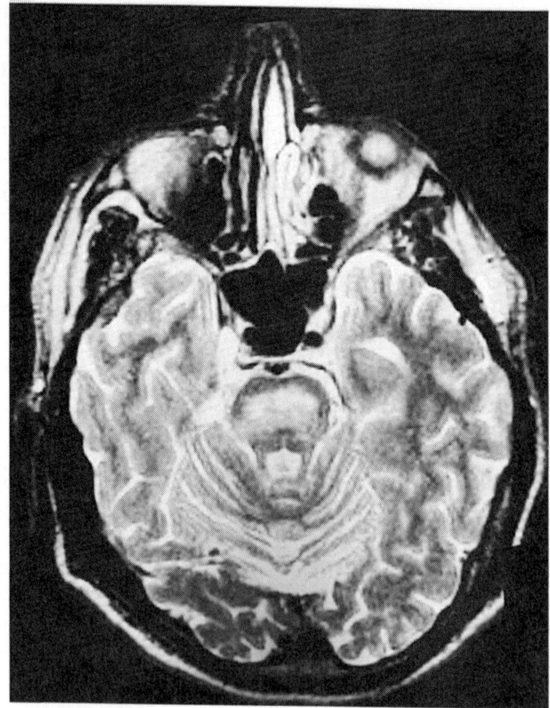

Figure 40-2

T2-weighted MR image showing the typical lesion of central pontine myelinolysis in an alcoholic patient.

Brainstem infarction due to basilar artery occlusion may be a source of confusion to the clinician. Sudden onset or step-like progression of the clinical state, asymmetry of long tract signs, and more extensive involvement of tegmental structures of the pons as well as the midbrain and thalamus are the distinguishing characteristics of vertebrobasilar thrombosis or embolism. Massive pontine demyelination in acute or chronic relapsing multiple sclerosis rarely produces a pure basis pontis syndrome. Other features of this disease provide the clues to correct diagnosis.

Etiology and Pathogenesis Nutritional deficiency is a commonly invoked cause of CPM, because it is observed so frequently in chronic wasting diseases and particularly in malnourished alcoholics, often in association with Wernicke disease. Nevertheless, there are cases in which a nutritional factor cannot be incriminated. As mentioned in the section on hyponatremia, the rapid correction of the serum sodium to normal or higher than normal levels plays an important role in the genesis of CPM. Significant hyponatremia, always less than 130 meq/L and usually much less, has been present in all our patients and in all the patients reported by Burcar and colleagues and by Karp and Laureno. The importance of serum sodium in the pathogenesis of this disease was demonstrated experimentally by Laureno. Dogs were made severely hyponatremic (100 to 115 meq/L) by repeated injections of vasopressin and intraperitoneal infusions of water. The hyponatremia and profound weakness were corrected rapidly by infusion of hypertonic (3%) saline, following which the dogs developed a rigid quadriparesis and showed, at autopsy, pontine and extrapontine lesions that were indistinguishable in their distribution and histologic features from those of the human disease. Hyponatremia alone or slowly corrected hyponatremia (<15 meq/dL in the initial 24 h) did not produce the disease.

McKee and colleagues have adduced evidence that extreme serum hyperosmolality and not necessarily the rapid correction or overcorrection of hyponatremia is the important factor in the pathogenesis of CPM. They found the characteristic pontine and extrapontine lesions in 10 of 139 severely burned patients who were examined after death. Each of their patients with CPM had suffered a prolonged, nonterminal episode of severe serum hyperosmolality, which coincided temporally with the onset of the lesion, as judged by its histologic features. Hyponatremia was not present, and no other independent factors—such as hypernatremia, hyperglycemia, or azotemia—correlated with the development of CPM.

Therapeutic guidelines for the correction of hyponatremia are still being considered. Karp and Laureno, on the basis of their experience and that of Sterns et al, have suggested that the hyponatremia be corrected by no more than 10 meq/L in the initial 24 h and by no more than 21 meq/L in the initial 48 h.

At the present time all one can say is that specific regions or zones of the brain, most often the center of the basis pontis, have a special susceptibility to some acute metabolic fault (possibly rapid correction or overcorrection of hyponatremia, possibly hyperosmolality), analogous perhaps to the selective vulnerability of the corpus callosum and anterior commissure in Marchiafava-Bignami disease (Chap. 41).

METABOLIC DISEASES PRESENTING AS PROGRESSIVE EXTRAPYRAMIDAL SYNDROMES

These syndromes are usually of mixed type—i.e., they include a number of basal ganglionic and cerebellar symptoms in various combinations and may emerge as part of an acquired chronic hepatocerebral degeneration or chronic hypoparathyroidism or as sequels to kernicterus or hypoxic or hypoglycemic encephalopathy. The basal ganglionic-cerebellar symptoms that result from severe anoxia and hypoglycemia have been described in the preceding section and in Chaps. 4 and 5. Kernicterus is considered on page 1085, with the neurologic diseases of infancy and childhood, and calcification of the basal ganglia and cerebellum (due to chronic parathyroid deficiency) on page 1032, with the inherited metabolic disorders, as well as further on in this chapter. It must be realized, however, that acquired hypoparathyroidism may also lead to calcification of the basal ganglia (see below, under "Metabolic Diseases Presenting as Cerebellar Ataxia"). We have observed choreiform movements in patients with hyperosmolar coma and with severe hyperthyroidism, ascribed by Weiner and Klawans to a disturbance of dopamine metabolism.

Chronic Acquired (Non-Wilsonian) Hepatocerebral Degeneration

Patients who survive an episode or several episodes of hepatic coma are sometimes left with residual neurologic abnormalities, such as tremor of the head or arms, asterixis, grimacing, choreic movements and twitching of the limbs, dysarthria, ataxia of gait, or impairment of intellectual function; these symptoms may worsen, with repeated attacks of stupor and coma. In a few patients with chronic liver disease, permanent neurologic abnormalities become manifest in the absence of discrete episodes of hepatic coma. In either event, patients with these abnormalities deteriorate neurologically over a period of years. Examination of the brains of such patients discloses foci of destruction of nerve cells and other parenchymal elements in addition to a widespread transformation of astrocytes—changes that are very much the same as those of Wilson disease.

Probably the first to describe the acquired type of hepatocerebral degeneration was van Woerkom (1914), whose report appeared only 2 years after Wilson's classic description of the familial form. A full account of the cases reported since that time as well as of our own extensive experience with this disorder is contained in the article by Victor, Adams, and Cole, listed in the References.

Clinical Features The first symptom may be a tremor of the outstretched arms, fleeting arrhythmic twitches of the face and limbs (resembling either myoclonus or chorea), or a mild unsteadiness of gait with action tremor. As the condition evolves over months or years, a rather characteristic dysarthria, ataxia, wide-based, unsteady gait, and choreoathetosis—mainly of the face, neck, and shoulders—are joined in a common syndrome. Mental function is slowly altered, taking the form of a simple dementia with a seeming lack of concern about the illness. A coarse, rhythmic tremor of the arms appearing with certain sustained postures, mild corticospinal tract signs, and diffuse EEG abnormalities complete the clinical picture. Other less frequent signs are muscular rigidity, grasp reflexes, tremor in repose, nystagmus, asterixis, and action or intention myoclonus. In essence, each of the neurologic abnormalities that are observed in patients with acute hepatic encephalopathy are also part of chronic hepatocerebral degeneration, the only difference being that the abnormalities are evanescent in the former and irreversible and progressive in the latter.

As a rule, all measurable hepatic functions are altered, but the chronic neurologic disorder correlates best with an elevation of serum ammonia (usually greater than 200 mg/dL). Unlike Wilson disease, where the cirrhosis usually remains occult for a long time, there is no question about its presence in the acquired syndrome; jaundice, ascites, and esophageal varices are manifest in most of the acquired cases. Wilson disease, which enters into the differential diagnosis, is usually not difficult to differentiate on clinical grounds, although the distinction in some cases requires the critical evidence of familial occurrence, Kayser-Fleischer rings (never found in the acquired type), and certain biochemical abnormalities (diminished serum ceruloplasmin, elevated serum copper, and urinary copper excretion—see page 1026).

Pathology The chronic cerebral symptoms, like the transient ones, may occur with all varieties of chronic liver disease. The cerebral lesion is localized more regularly in the cortex than is the case in Wilson disease. In some specimens an irregular gray line of necrosis or gliosis can be observed throughout both hemispheres, and the lenticular nuclei may appear shrunken and discolored. These lesions resemble hypoxic ones and may be concentrated in the vascular border zones, but they tend to spare the hippocampus, globus pallidus, and deep folia of the cerebellar cortex—the sites of predilection in anoxic encephalopathy. Microscopically, a widespread hyperplasia of protoplasmic astrocytes is visible in the deep layers of the cerebral cortex and in the cerebellar cortex as well as in thalamic and lenticular nuclei and other nuclear structures of the brainstem. In the necrotic zones, the medullated fibers and nerve cells are destroyed, with marginal fibrous gliosis; at the corticomedullary junction, in the striatum (particularly in the superior pole of the putamen), and in the cerebellar white matter, polymicrocavitation may be prominent. Protoplasmic astrocytic nuclei contain PAS-positive glycogen granules. Some nerve cells appear swollen and chromatolyzed, taking the form, we believe, of the so-called Opalski cells usually associated with Wilson disease. The similarity of the neuropathologic lesions in the familial and acquired forms of hepatocerebral disease is striking.

Pathogenesis It is evident that a close relationship exists between the acute, transient form of hepatic encephalopathy (hepatic coma) and the chronic, largely irreversible hepatocerebral syndrome; frequently one blends imperceptibly into the other. This relationship is reflected in the pathologic findings as well; the astrocytic hyperplasia and PAS-positive inclusions are identical in both forms of the disease, and the distribution of the destructive lesions follows closely the distribution of the astrocytic change. Also, both disorders are characterized by hyperammonemia, episodic in one and persistent in the other. Reducing the serum ammonia by the measures that are effective in acute hepatic encephalopathy will cause a recession of many of the chronic neurologic abnormalities, not completely but to an extent that permits the patient to function better.

It appears that the parenchymal damage in the chronic disease simply represents the most severe degree of a pathologic process that in its mildest form is reflected in an astrocytic hyperplasia alone.

Kernicterus

Kernicterus, formerly a common cause of congenital choreoathetosis, has now been virtually eliminated. It is discussed on page 1085.

Hypoparathyroidism

This condition and pseudohypoparathyroidism (page 1032) were mentioned in relation to the hereditary metabolic disorders. In the past, the usual cause of hypoparathyroidism was surgical removal of the parathyroid glands during subtotal thyroidectomy, although there were always idiopathic cases as well. With the more widespread use of radiation and drug therapy for thyroid disease, the number of surgically created cases has become small in proportion to nonsurgical ones. The latter may occur in pure form, presumably as an agene-sis of the parathyroid glands with unmeasurable levels of parathyroid hormone in the blood, or as part of the DiGeorge syndrome of agenesis of the thymus and parathyroid glands, organs that are embryologically derived from the third and fourth branchial clefts. Hypoparathyroidism is also part of a familial disorder in which a deficiency of thyroid, ovarian, and adrenal function, pernicious anemia, and other defects are combined, based presumably on a derangement of autoimmune mechanisms. Other causes are intestinal malabsorption, pancreatic insufficiency, and vitamin D deficiency. In all instances the low levels of parathormone and normal responses to injected hormone permit the recognition of a primary defect of the parathyroid glands and distinguish it from all other conditions in which there is hypocalcemia and hyperphosphatemia.

The clinical manifestations, mainly attributable to the effects of hypocalcemia, are tetany, paresthesias, muscle cramps, laryngeal spasm, and convulsions. Children with this disease may be irritable and show personality changes. In adults with chronic hypocalcemia, calcium deposits occur in the basal ganglia, dentate nuclei, and cerebellar cortex. In such patients we have observed unilateral tremor, a restless choreoathetotic hand, bilateral rigidity, slowness of movement and flexed posture resembling Parkinson disease, and ataxia of the limbs and gait—in various combinations. Interestingly, the multiple skeletal and developmental abnormalities that characterize both pseudo- and pseudopseudohypoparathyroidism (short stature, round face, short neck, stocky body build, shortening of metacarpal and metatarsal bones and phalanges from premature epiphyseal closure) are rarely seen in pure hypoparathyroidism.

A similar deposition of ferrocalc in the walls of small blood vessels of the lenticular and dentate nuclei and to a lesser extent in other parts of the brain is a common finding and is similar to that observed in normal older individuals but more severe. It also occurs in animals. Occasionally it reaches a degree of severity that destroys striatal or dentate neurons. In such cases, films of the skull and particularly CT scans will reveal the deposits. Cases of this type have been reported for years (page 1032). The cause of the deposits is unknown. Apparently some protein in the capillary walls has an avidity for both calcium and iron.

METABOLIC DISEASES PRESENTING AS CEREBELLAR ATAXIA

Cerebellar Ataxia Associated with Myxedema

The association of myxedema and cerebellar ataxia has been mentioned sporadically in medical writings since the latter part of the nineteenth century. Interest in this problem was revived in more recent years by Jellinek and Kelly, who described 6 such cases. All of them showed an ataxia of gait; in addition, some degree of ataxia of the arms and dysarthria were present in 4 instances, and nystagmus in 2. Cremer and coworkers have reported a similar clinical experience, based on a study of 24 patients with either primary or secondary hypothyroidism.

There have been only a few reports of the pathologic changes, and these are far from satisfactory. The myxedematous patient described by Price and Netsky had also been a serious alcoholic, and the clinical signs (ataxia of gait and of the legs) and pathologic changes (loss of Purkinje cells and gliosis of the molecular layer, most pronounced in the vermis) cannot be distinguished from those due to alcoholism and malnutrition. Scattered throughout the nervous system of their case were unusual glycogen-containing bodies, similar but not identical to corpora amylacea. These structures, designated myxedema bodies by Price and Netsky, were also observed in the cerebellar white matter of a second case of myxedema; there were no other neuropathologic changes, however, and this patient had shown no ataxia during life. It is difficult to know whether these peculiar bodies have anything to do with myxedema. If they do, it should be possible to demonstrate them in more than two cases. We have not seen them in one carefully studied case of myxedema, nor have they been described by others. Thyroid medication corrects the defect in motor coordination, raising doubt as to whether it could be based on a visible structural lesion.

Other metabolic disorders, some heritable, in which ataxia may be a leading manifestation include Whipple disease (Chap. 33), GM_2 gangliosidosis, sprue (discussed below), and a large number of neonatal and infantile aminoacidopathies. The various causes of cerebellar ataxia, including these, are summarized in Table 5-1 (page 97).

Effects of Hyperthermia on the Cerebellum

The damaging effects of *hyperthermia*, like those of anoxia, involve the brain diffusely. In the case of hyperthermia, however, the changes are disproportionately severe in the cerebellum. The acute manifestations of profound hyperthermia are coma and convulsions, frequently complicated by shock and renal failure. Patients who survive the initial stage of the illness frequently show signs of widespread cerebral affection, such as confusion and pseudobulbar and spastic paralysis. These abnormalities tend to resolve gradually, leaving the patient with a more or less pure disorder of cerebellar function.

The most extensive account of the pathologic effects of hyperthermia is that of Malamud and colleagues. These authors studied 125 fatal cases of heat stroke, but their observations are probably applicable to hyperthermia of other types. In patients who survived less than 24 h, the changes consisted mainly of a loss of some of the Purkinje cells and swelling, pyknosis, and disintegration of those that remained. In cases surviving beyond 24 h, there was almost complete degeneration of the Purkinje cells, with gliosis throughout the cerebellar cortex as well as degeneration of the dentate nuclei. The changes in the cerebellar cortex were equally pronounced in the hemispheres and vermis. The unanswered question is whether high temperature alone is an adequate cause or must be combined with hypoxia and ischemia. It is of interest that we have not seen this syndrome in patients with infective fevers, malignant hyperthermia, or the malignant neuroleptic syndrome—either the neuropathologic changes or the clinical cerebellar syndrome in survivors.

Cerebellar Syndromes Associated with Celiac-Sprue and Jejunoileal Bypass

A progressive cerebellar ataxia of gait and limbs, sometimes with polymyoclonus in association with a gluten-sensitive enteropathy, has been the subject of several reports. The underlying lesion is a villus atrophy of the intestinal mucosa, consistent with celiac disease of children and sprue in adults. The neurologic disorder may appear several years after onset of the enteropathy and, in addition to ataxia, usually includes signs of peripheral neuropathy and, in some cases, myelopathy and encephalopathy (dementia). According to Finelli et al, neurologic abnormalities occur in approximately 10 percent of cases of adult celiac-sprue. This subject has been reviewed by Bhatia et al and recently by Hadjivassiliou et al. The latter authors emphasize the frequent occurrence of ataxia in patients with gluten sensitivity (indicated by circulating antibodies to gliadin) but without overt signs of bowel disease. There is also a strong association (in more than 90 percent of patients) with the HLA DQ8 class II genotype. The few cases that have come to autopsy have shown severe cerebellar atrophy, a finding that may also be disclosed by MRI. Hadjivassiliou et al observed lymphocytic infiltration and perivascular cuffing in the cerebellar cortex and peripheral nerves in one autopsied case but not in another, changes that they took to represent immunologic injury to these parts. The main differential diagnostic considerations are paraneoplastic cerebellar degeneration and Whipple disease.

Vitamin E deficiency may induce a similar syndrome with features of spinocerebellar dysfunction (see page 1224).

Jejunoileal bypass operations, in addition to causing a chronic arthropathy, neuropathy, and vasculitic skin lesions, may give rise to an episodic confusion and cerebellar ataxia associated with a lactic acidosis and abnormalities of pyruvate metabolism. Overfeeding and fasting are provocative factors (Dahlquist et al).

METABOLIC DISEASE PRESENTING AS PSYCHOSIS AND DEMENTIA

The point has been made that milder forms of diseases that cause episodic stupor and coma, if persistent, may present as states of protracted confusion, difficult to distinguish from the dementias. Chronic hepatic encephalopathy and the syndromes of chronic hypoglycemia, chronic hypercalcemia (in multiple myeloma, metastatic cancer, and sarcoidosis), and dialysis encephalopathy all fall within this category. Unlike the common types of dementia described in Chap. 21, the acquired metabolic diseases are nearly always accompanied by drowsiness, inattentiveness, and reduced alertness; i.e., by a clouding of the sensorium and inaccurate perceptions and interpretations—attributes that usually allow an encephalopathic confusional state to be distinguished from a dementia. If the onset of the illness is abrupt rather than gradual and of brief duration and if therapy reverses the condition, restoring full mental clarity, the conclusion is justified that one is dealing with a confusional state; but at any one time in the active phase of the disease the clinical state may resemble dementia.

In general hospitals, an episodic confusional state lasting days and weeks in the course of a medical illness or following an operation should always raise the suspicion of one of the aforementioned metabolic states. Usually, however, all of them can be excluded, and one falls back on a rather unsatisfactory interpretation—that a combination of drugs, fever, toxemia, and unspecifiable metabolic disorders is responsible. The "septic encephalopathy" described earlier in the chapter falls into this category.

In the endocrine encephalopathies, which are described below, the clinical phenomena may be even more abstruse, although they often take the form of a unique psychosis. Confusional states may be combined with agitation, hallucinations, delusions, anxiety, and depression, and the time span of the illness may be in terms of weeks and months rather than days. Certain aspects of the endocrine psychoses are discussed further on page 1641.

Cushing Disease and Corticosteroid Psychoses

Derangements of mental function that followed administration of adrenocorticotropic hormone (ACTH) and then of corticosteroids have become the prototypes of iatrogenic psychoses. The same disturbances of mental function may accompany Cushing disease (page 715).

Our experience with this neuropsychiatric condition was derived originally from observations of patients receiving ACTH and later from patients receiving prednisone for a variety of neurologic and medical diseases. With low doses there is usually no psychic effect other than a sense of well-being and decreased fatigability. At higher doses (60 to 100 mg/day of prednisone), approximately 10 to 15 percent of patients become overly active, emotionally labile, and unable to sleep. Unless the dose is promptly reduced, there follows a progressive shift in mood, usually toward euphoria and hypomania—but sometimes toward depression and then inattentiveness, distractibility, and mild confusion. The EEG becomes less well modulated and slower frequencies appear. A minority of patients experience frank hallucinations and delusions, giving the illness a truly psychotic stamp and raising the suspicion of schizophrenia or manic-depressive disease. In nearly all instances, however, this mixture of confusion and mood change, in association with disordered cognitive function, distinguishes the iatrogenic corticosteroid psychosis. Withdrawal of medication relieves the symptoms, but full recovery may take several days to a few weeks, at which time, as with all confusional states and deliria, the patient has only a fragmentary recollection of events that occurred during the illness.

The neurologic basis of this condition is poorly understood. Its attribution to premorbid personality traits or a disposition to psychiatric illness is plausible but lacks convincing documentation. Part of the difficulty is the lack of knowledge of the role of these endocrine agents in normal cerebral metabolism. We have only incomplete knowledge, for example, as to how they act to reduce the volume of the edematous cerebral tissue around a tumor or to shrink the brain. Critical studies of cellular or subcellular metabolism and morphologic changes are lacking. "Cerebral atrophy" (ventricular enlargement and sulcal widening) has been shown radiologically in patients with Cushing disease and after a prolonged period of corticosteroid therapy, but the basis of this change also is unexplained (Momose et al). In most cases, withdrawal of steroids has led to reversal of symptoms and reduction in ventricular size, documented by repeated CT scans.

In patients with Cushing disease due to adrenal or basophilic pituitary tumors, mental changes suggestive of dementia and enlarged ventricles are not unusual. Here again there is a peculiar combination of mood changes and impaired cognitive function. A frank psychosis may occur. This condition is described more completely in Chap. 57 and the attending polymyopathy, in Chap. 51.

Thyroid Encephalopathies

Hyperthyroidism The neurology of thyrotoxicosis has proved to be particularly elusive. Allusions to psychosis are frequent in the medical literature, and some thyrotoxic patients have been observed with mental confusion, seizures, manic or depressive attacks, and delusions. Tremor is almost universal, and chorea occurs occasionally in various combinations with muscular weakness and atrophy, periodic paralysis, and myasthenia. In descriptions of the chorea, it is often not clear whether it was chorea, tremor, myoclonus, or just fidgetiness that was observed. Treatment of the hyperthyroidism gradually restores the mental state to normal, leaving one with no explanation of what had happened to the CNS.

Thyroid crisis or "storm" refers to a fulminant increase in the symptoms and signs of thyrotoxicosis—extreme restlessness, tachycardia, fever, vomiting, and diarrhea—leading to delirium or coma. In the past, this was a not uncommon postoperative event in patients poorly prepared for thyroid surgery. Now it is seen mainly in patients with inadequately treated or untreated thyrotoxicosis complicated by serious medical or surgical illness.

Hashimoto Encephalopathy Shaw and colleagues have described an encephalopathy consisting of confusion, altered consciousness, and prominent myoclonus, sometimes relapsing, in patients with Hashimoto disease ("Hashimoto encephalopathy"). Curiously, most have had normal thyroid function. There are, however, high titers of several antithyroid antibodies, including antibodies against thyroid peroxidase and thyroglobulin. Seizures—including myoclonic and rarely nonconvulsive status epilepticus—hemiparesis, ataxia, psychosis, and unusual tremors have been reported in individual cases. Often there are others in the family with autoimmune diseases. It has been the myoclonic aspect of the encephalopathy, a feature of all of our cases, that has led to consideration of this diagnosis. We have encountered several such cases, two of which were initially mistaken for Creutzfeldt-Jacob disease (subacute spongiform encephalopathy). Early descriptions included a pleocytosis and white matter lesions, but we have not noted these abnormalities. The encephalopathic symptoms and high titers of antithyroid antibodies responded well to steroid therapy. In the case of Newcomer and associates, a rapid reversal of thyrotoxic coma (and corticospinal signs) was effected by plasma exchange, in parallel with a reduction in T4 and T3 levels. The specific circulating antibodies and the response to corticosteroids and plasma exchange implicate an immune pathogenesis, similar to paraneoplastic "limbic encephalitis" and perhaps to lupus, as well as to the rare encephalopathy that occurs in patients with thymoma.

Hypothyroidism As a rule, the myxedematous patient is slow to react and psychomotor activity is reduced; but only in exceptional cases have we noted a significant change in cerebral function. When such a change has been observed, we have been more impressed with drowsiness, inattentiveness, and apathy. In two personally observed cases, the somnolence was so extreme that the patients could not stay awake long enough to be fed or examined. They were in a state of hypothermic stupor but exhibited no other neurologic abnormality. The extreme somnolence can be reversed within a few days by thyroid medication.

Hypothyroidism is associated with a number of distinctive myopathic disturbances, which are discussed in Chap. 51. The ataxia and peripheral neuropathy that are sometimes observed in patients with myxedema are described in this chapter (above) and in Chap. 46, respectively.

Cretinism and Neonatal Myxedema This form of severe hypothyroidism, occurring during intrauterine life (hypothyroidism in mother and fetus) or postnatally as a hereditary or acquired thyroid disease, is probably the most frequent and potentially preventable and correctable metabolic mental defect in the world. A perspective on its relative frequency among neonatal metabolic disorders is given in Table 37-1. Although the condition is most common in goitrous regions where there is a lack of iodine, it may also be due to any of several genetically determined defects in thyroxin synthesis that have come to light in recent years (Vassart et al). In areas of endemic cretinism, additional factors may be operative, such as the widespread ingestion of cassava, which contains a toxic goitrogen that inhibits the uptake of iodine by the thyroid.

As a rule, the symptoms and signs of congenital thyroid deficiency are not recognizable at birth but become apparent only after a few weeks; more often the diagnosis is first made between the sixth and twelfth months of life. Physiologic jaundice tends to be severe and prolonged (up to 3 months), and this, along with widening of the posterior fontanelle and mottling of the skin, should raise suspicion of the disease.

In general, two types of early life hypothyroidism are recognized—sporadic and endemic. The sporadic type occurs occasionally in developed countries (less than once in 4000 births) and is consequent upon a congenital metabolic or anatomic disorder of the thyroid gland. At birth, the gland is either absent or represented by cysts, indicating a failure of development or a destructive lesion. In the sporadic form, in the latter part of the first year, stunting of growth and delay in psychomotor development become evident. Untreated, the child is severely retarded but placid and good-natured; such children sleep contentedly for longer periods than normal children. Sitting, standing, and walking are delayed. Movements are slow, and if tendon reflexes can be obtained, their relaxation time is clearly delayed. The body temperature is low, and the extremities are cold and cyanotic. Although the head is small, the fontanelles may not close until the sixth or seventh year, and there is delayed ossification. This type of hypothyroidism is preventable by treatment with thyroid hormone.

Endemic cretinism is most common in developing countries, with an estimated incidence in these areas of 5 to 15 percent. DeLong and colleagues, on the basis of epidemiologic surveys in Ecuador, Zaire, and western China, have distinguished two forms of endemic cretinism—neurologic and myxedematous. The occurrence of the two different types is governed by the timing, duration, and severity of the iodine deficiency (Thilly et al).

The *neurologic form of endemic cretinism* is characterized by varying degrees of deaf-mutism or lesser degrees of hearing loss, dysarthria, proximal limb and truncal rigid-spastic motor disorder involving mainly the lower extremities, and mental deficiency of a characteristic type. In the most severely affected, there is also strabismus, kyphoscoliosis, underdevelopment of leg muscles, and frontal lobe release signs. Bone age, head size, and height are normal and there are none of the coarse facial features of the myxedematous form. In the so-called *myxedematous form of endemic cretinism*, short stature, microcephaly, coarse facial features, and retarded psychomotor development are the main features. There is no deafness or spastic rigidity of the limbs. In typical instances, the face is pale and puffy; the skin dry; the hair coarse, scanty, and dry; the eyelids thickened; the heavy lips parted by the enlarged tongue; the forehead low; and the base of the nose broad. There are fat pads above the clavicles and in the axillae. The abdomen is protuberant, often with an umbilical hernia, and the head is small—a physical appearance that prompted William Boyd to remark: "What was intended to be created in the image of God has turned out to be the pariah of nature, all for the want of a little thyroid."

DeLong and others attribute neurologic cretinism to a lack of available iodine in the mother and fetus during the second and third trimesters of pregnancy; neither mother nor fetus elaborate thyroxin. The first and part of the second trimester developmental period, which does not require iodine or thyroxin, passes normally and the general morphology of the brain is normal. It is during the second trimester, when the cochleas and the neuronal population of the cerebral cortex and basal ganglia are forming, that these structures suffer irreparable damage. The effects of this midfetal hypothyroidism and iodine deficiency cannot be corrected by giving thyroid hormone at birth and thereafter. It can be prevented only by providing iodine therapy to the mother before and during the first trimester of pregnancy (Cao et al). The myxedematous form of cretinism is more likely to occur from lack of thyroid hormone in the late second and the third trimesters.

The mental defect ranges from apathy and absence of social interaction to an alert, cooperative state, but a backwardness in higher-order thinking and verbal facility is always evident. Retentive memory and apperception are commensurate with overall intellectual competence as judged by the level of mental associations and capacity for abstract thought. The status of the thyroid gland varies; among neurologic cretins, about half are goitrous or have palpable glands; in the rest, the glands are atrophied; practically all the myxedematous cretins are athyreotic. Although typical examples of neurologic and myxedematous hypothyroidism are readily distinguished, both types may exist in the same endemic area and the stigmata of both forms may be recognized in the same individual. The QRS complex of the electrocardiogram is of low voltage; the EEG is slower than normal, with less alpha activity; the CSF contains an excess of protein (50 to 150 mg/dL); and the serum T3 and T4, protein-bound iodine, and radioactive iodine uptake are all subnormal. Serum cholesterol is increased (300 to 600 mg/dL).

At autopsy the brain of neurologic cretinism, though small, is normally formed, with all central and brainstem structures and cortical sulcation intact. A reduction in number of nerve cells was described by Marinesco, especially in the fifth cortical layer, but others have not confirmed this finding. The use of Golgi and other silver techniques has shown decreased interneuronal distances (packing density is increased, as in the immature cortex) and a deficiency of neuropil. The latter change is due to a poverty of dendritic branchings and crossings, and presumably there is a decrease of the synaptic surfaces of cells (Eayrs). Thyroid hormone appears to be essential, not for neuronal formation and migration but for dendritic-axonic development and organization.

There is fairly substantial evidence that the administration of iodinated oil to hypothyroid women before and during the first trimester of pregnancy prevents sporadic and endemic cretinism. Treatment begun during the second trimester protects the fetal brain to a varying degree. Treatment that is started after the beginning of the third trimester does not improve the neurologic status, although head growth and statural development may improve slightly (Cao et al). In sporadic cretinism, if the condition is recognized early, say at birth, and treated consistently with potent thyroid hormones, statural and mental development can be stimulated to normal or near-normal levels. Extent of recovery depends on the severity and duration of intrauterine hypothyroidism, i.e., its duration before treatment was begun and the adequacy of therapy. In most patients, some degree of mental deficiency persists throughout life.

Pancreatic Encephalopathy

This term was introduced by Rothermich and von Haam in 1941 to describe what they considered to be a fairly uniform clinical state in patients with acute abdominal symptoms referable to pancreatic disease, mainly pancreatitis. The encephalopathy, as they described it, consists of an agitated, confused state, sometimes with hallucinations and clouding of consciousness, dysarthria, and changing rigidity of the limbs—all of which fluctuate over a period of hours or days. Coma and quadriplegia have been reported. At autopsy, a variety of lesions have been described; two cases have had central pontine myelinolysis and others have had small foci of necrosis and edema, petechial hemorrhages, and "demyelination" scattered through the cerebrum, brainstem, and cerebellum. These have been uncritically attributed to the action of released lipases and proteases from the action of pancreatic enzymes (see review of this subject by Sharf and Levy). The term *pancreatic encephalopathy* has also been applied to a depressive illness which seems to occur with disproportionate frequency before the symptoms of a pancreatic tumor become apparent.

The status of this entity, in the authors' opinion, is uncertain. Pallis and Lewis also express reservations and suggest that before such a diagnosis can be seriously entertained in a patient with acute pancreatitis, one must exclude delirium tremens, shock, renal failure, hypoglycemia, diabetic acidosis, hyperosmolality, and hypocalcemia or hypercalcemia—any one of which may complicate the underlying disease. Other cases conform to the encephalopathy of multiorgan failure discussed earlier. Several patients in our care who were thought originally to have pancreatic encephalopathy proved to have sequential strokes from marantic endocarditis.

REFERENCES

Adams RD, Foley JM: The neurological disorder associated with liver disease. *Res Publ Assoc Res Nerv Ment Dis* 32:198, 1953.

Adams RD, Victor M, Mancall EL: Central pontine myelinolysis. *Arch Neurol Psychiatry* 81:154, 1959.

Aikawa N, Shinozawa Y, Ishibiki K, et al: Clinical analysis of multiple organ failure in burned patients. *Burns* 13:103, 1987.

Alfrey AC, Legendre GR, Kaehny WD: The dialysis encephalopathy syndrome: Possible aluminum intoxication. *N Engl J Med* 294:184, 1976.

Ames A, Wright RL, Kowada M, et al: Cerebral ischemia: II. The no-reflow phenomenon. *Am J Pathol* 52:437, 1968.

Arieff AI: Hyponatremia associated with permanent brain damage. *Adv Intern Med* 21:325, 1987.

Arieff AI: Hyponatremia, convulsions, respiratory arrest, and permanent brain damage after elective surgery in healthy women. *N Engl J Med* 314:1529, 1986.

Auer RN: Progress review: Hypoglycemic brain damage. *Stroke* 17:699, 1986.

Austen FK, Carmichael MW, Adams RD: Neurologic manifestations of chronic pulmonary insufficiency. *N Engl J Med* 257:579, 1957.

Barcroft R: *The Respiratory Function of the Blood*. London, Cambridge University Press, 1925.

Basile AS, Hughes RD, Harrison PM, et al: Elevated brain concentrations of 1,4-benzodiazepines in fulminant hepatic failure. *N Engl J Med* 325:473, 1991.

Bhatia MP, Brown P, Gregory R, et al: Progressive myoclonic ataxia associated with coeliac disease. *Brain* 118:1087, 1995.

Bolton CF, Young GB: *Neurological Complications of Renal Disease*. Boston, Butterworth, 1990.

Bolton C, Young GB, Zochodne DW: The neurological complications of sepsis. *Ann Neurol* 33:94, 1993.

Burcar PJ, Norenberg MD, Yarnell PR: Hyponatremia and central pontine myelinosis. *Neurology* 27:223, 1977.

Burn DJ, Bates D: Neurology and the kidney. *J Neurol Neurosurg Psychiatry* 65:810, 1998.

Butterworth RF, Giguiere JF, Michaud J, et al: Ammonia: Key factor in the pathogenesis of hepatic encephalopathy. *Neurochem Pathol* 6:1, 1987.

Cao X-Y, Jian G X-M, Dou Z-H, et al: Timing of vulnerability of the brain to iodine deficiency in endemic cretinism. *N Engl J Med* 331:1739, 1994.

Cavanagh JB: Liver bypass and the glia, in Plum F (ed): Brain dysfunction in metabolic disorders. *Res Publ Assoc Res Nerv Ment Dis* 53:13, 1974.

Choi DW, Rothman SM: The role of glutamate neurotoxicity in hypoxic-ischemic neuronal death. *Annu Rev Neurosci* 13:171, 1990.

Choi IS: Delayed neurologic sequelae in carbon monoxide intoxication. *Arch Neurol* 40:433, 1983.

Cremer GM, Goldstine NP, Paris J: Myxedema and ataxia. *Neurology* 19:37, 1969.

Dahlquist NR, Perrault J, Callaway CW: D-Lactic acidosis and encephalopathy after jejunoileostomy: Response to overfeeding and to fasting in humans. *Mayo Clin Proc* 59:141, 1984.

DeLong GR, Stanbury JB, Fierro-Benitez R: Neurological signs in congenital iodine-deficiency disorder (endemic cretinism). *Dev Med Child Neurol* 27:317, 1985.

DiMauro S, Tonin P, Servidei S: Metabolic myopathies, in Rowland LP, DiMauro S (eds): *Handbook of Clinical Neurology*. Vol 18. New York, Elsevier, 1992, pp 479–526.

Dooling EC, Richardson EP Jr: Delayed encephalopathy after strangling. *Arch Neurol* 33:196, 1976.

EAYRS JT: Influence of the thyroid on the central nervous system. *Br Med Bull* 16:122, 1960.

FERRENDELLI JA: Cerebral utilization of nonglucose substrates and their effect in hypoglycemia, in Plum F (ed): Brain dysfunction in metabolic disorders. *Res Publ Assoc Res Nerv Ment Dis* 53:113, 1974.

FINELLI PF, MCENTEE WJ, AMBLER M, KESTENBAUM D: Adult celiac disease presenting as cerebellar syndrome. *Neurology* 30:245, 1980.

FISCHER JE, BALDESSARINI RJ: Pathogenesis and therapy of hepatic coma, in Popper H, Schaffner F (eds): *Progress in Liver Disease*. New York, Grune & Stratton, 1976, pp 363–397.

FISHER KF, LEES JA, NEWMAN JH: Hypoglycemia in hospitalized patients. *N Engl J Med* 315:1245, 1986.

FISHMAN RA: Cell volume, pumps and neurologic function: Brain's adaptation to osmotic stress, in Plum F (ed): Brain dysfunction in metabolic disorders. *Res Publ Assoc Res Nerv Ment Dis* 53:159, 1974.

FISHMAN RA: *Cerebrospinal Fluid in Diseases of the Nervous System*, 2nd ed. Philadelphia, Saunders, 1992.

GRIGGS RC, SUTTON JR: Neurologic manifestations of respiratory diseases, in Asbury AK, McKhann GM, McDonald WI (eds): *Diseases of the Nervous System*, 2nd ed. Philadelphia, Saunders, 1992, pp 1432–1441.

HADJIVASSILIOU M, GRÜNEWALD RA, CHATOPADHYAY AK, et al: Clinical, radiological, neurophysiological, and neuropathological characteristics of gluten ataxia. *Lancet* 352:1582, 1998.

HARRISON TR, MASON MF, RESNICK H: Observations on the mechanism of muscular twitchings in uremia. *J Clin Invest* 15:463, 1936.

HERRERA L, KAZEMI H: CSF bicarbonate regulation in metabolic acidosis: Role of HCO_3 formation in CSF. *J Appl Physiol* 49:778, 1980.

HORNBEIN TF, TOWNES BD, SCHOENE RB, et al: The cost to the central nervous system of climbing to extremely high altitude. *N Engl J Med* 321:1714, 1989.

HUTTENLOCHER P, TRAUNER D: Reye's syndrome in infancy. *Pediatrics* 62:84, 1978.

JELLINEK EH, KELLY RE: Cerebellar syndrome in myxedema. *Lancet* 2:225, 1960.

JOHNSON GM, SCURLETIS TD, CARROLL NB: A study of sixteen fatal cases of encephalitis-like disease in North Carolina children. *N C Med J* 24:464, 1963.

JONES EA, BASILE AS: Does ammonia contribute to increased GABA-ergic neurotransmission in liver failure? *Metab Brain Dis* 13:351, 1998.

KARP BI, LAURENO R: Pontine and extrapontine myelinolysis: A neurologic disorder following rapid correction of hyponatremia. *Medicine* 72:359, 1993.

KREIGER D, KREIGER S, JANSEN O, et al: Manganese and chronic hepatic encephalopathy. *Lancet* 346:270, 1995.

LANCE JW, ADAMS RD: The syndrome of intention or action myoclonus as a sequel to hypoxic encephalopathy. *Brain* 87:111, 1963.

LAURENO R: Central pontine myelinolysis following rapid correction of hyponatremia. *Ann Neurol* 13:232, 1983.

LAURENO R: Neurologic syndromes accompanying electrolyte disorders, in Goetz CG et al (eds): *Handbook of Clinical Neurology*. Vol 19. Amsterdam, Elsevier, 1993, pp 545–573.

LEDERMAN RS, HENRY CE: Progressive dialysis encephalopathy. *Ann Neurol* 4:199, 1978.

LEVY DE, BATES D, CARONNA JJ: Prognosis in nontraumatic coma. *Ann Intern Med* 94:293, 1981.

LIDOFSKY SD, BASS NM, PRAGER MC, et al: Intracranial pressure monitoring and liver transplantation for fulminant hepatic failure. *Hepatology* 16:1, 1992.

MADDREY WC, WEBER FL JR, COULTER AW, et al: Effects of keto analogues of essential amino acids in portal-systemic encephalopathy. *Gastroenterology* 71:190, 1976.

MALAMUD N, HAYMAKER W, CUSTER RP: Heat stroke: A clinicopathologic study of 125 fatal cases. *Mil Surg* 99:397, 1946.

MALOUF R, BRUST JCM: Hypoglycemia: Causes, neurological manifestations, and outcome. *Ann Neurol* 17:421, 1985.

MARINESCO G: Lesions en myxoedeme congenitale avec idiotie. *L'Encephale* 19:265, 1924.

MARKS R, ROSE FC: *Hypoglycemia*. Oxford, Blackwell, 1965.

MARSHALL JR: Neuropsychiatric aspects of renal failure. *J Clin Psychiatry* 40:181, 1979.

MCKEE AC, WINKELMAN MD, BANKER BQ: Central pontine myelinolysis in severely burned patients: Relationship to serum hyperosmolality. *Neurology* 38:1211, 1988.

MOMOSE KJ, KJELLBERG RN, KLIMAN B: High incidence of cortical atrophy of the cerebral and cerebellar hemisphere in Cushing's disease. *Radiology* 99:341, 1971.

MORGAN MY, JAKOBOVITS AW, JAMES IM, SHERLOCK S: Successful use of bromocriptine in the treatment of chronic hepatic encephalopathy. *Gastroenterology* 78:663, 1980.

MULLEN KD: Benzodiazepine compounds and hepatic encephalopathy. *N Engl J Med* 325:509, 1991.

MYERS RAM, SNYDER SK, EMHOFF TA: Subacute sequelae of carbon monoxide poisoning. *Ann Emerg Med* 14:1163, 1985.

NAYLOR CD, O'ROURKE K, DETSKY AS, BAKER JP: Parenteral nutrition with branched-chain amino acids in hepatic encephalopathy: A meta-analysis. *Gastroenterology* 97:1033, 1989.

NELSON PB, SEIF SM, MAROON JC, ROBINSON AG: Hyponatremia in intracranial disease: Perhaps not the syndrome of inappropriate secretion of antidiuretic hormone (SIADH). *J Neurosurg* 55:038, 1981.

NEWCOMER J, HAIRE W, HARTMAN CR: Coma and thyrotoxicosis. *Ann Neurol* 14:689, 1983.

NORENBERG MD: Astroglial dysfunction in hepatic encephalopathy. *Metab Brain Dis* 13:319, 1998.

OPPENHEIMER BS, FISHBERG AM: Hypertensive encephalopathy. *Arch Intern Med* 41:264, 1928.

PALLIS CA, LEWIS PD: *The Neurology of Gastrointestinal Disease*. London, Saunders, 1974.

PARKINSON IS, WARD MK, KERR DNS: Dialysis encephalopathy, bone disease and anemia: The aluminum intoxication syndrome during regular hemodialysis. *J Clin Pathol* 34:1285, 1981.

PLUM F, POSNER JB: *Diagnosis of Stupor and Coma*, 3rd ed. Philadelphia, Davis, 1980.

PLUM F, POSNER JB, HAIN RF: Delayed neurological deterioration after anoxia. *Arch Intern Med* 110:18, 1962.

POMIER-LAYRARGUES G, ROSE C, SPAHR L, et al: Role of manganese in the pathogenesis of portal-systemic encephalopathy. *Metab Brain Dis* 13:311, 1998.

PRICE TR, NETSKY MG: Myxedema and ataxia: Cerebellar alterations and "neural myxedema bodies." *Neurology* 16:957, 1966.

PROCKOP LD: Hyperglycemia: Effects on the nervous system, in Vinken PJ, Bruyn BW (eds): *Handbook of Clinical Neurology*. Vol 27. *Metabolic and Deficiency Diseases of the Nervous System*. Part I. Amsterdam, North-Holland, 1976, pp 79–99.

RASKIN NH, FISHMAN RA: Neurologic disorders in renal failure. *N Engl J Med* 294:143, 204, 1976.

REYE RDK, MORGAN G, BARAL J: Encephalopathy and fatty degeneration of the viscera: A disease entity in childhood. *Lancet* 2:749, 1963.

ROTHERMICH NO, VON HAAM E: Pancreatic encephalopathy. *J Clin Endocrinol* 1:872, 1941.

ROTHSTEIN JD, HERLONG HF: Neurologic manifestations of hepatic disease. *Neurol Clin* 7:563, 1989.

SHARF B, LEVY N: Pancreatic encephalopathy, in Vinken PJ, Bruyn GW, Klawans H (eds): *Handbook of Clinical Neurology*. Vol 27. *Metabolic and Deficiency Diseases of the Nervous System*. Part I. Amsterdam, North-Holland, 1976, pp. 449–458.

SHAW PJ, WALLS TJ, NEMAN MB, et al: Hashimoto's encephalopathy: A steroid-responsive disorder associated with high anti-thyroid antibody titers—Report of 5 cases. *Neurology* 41:228, 1991.

SHAYWITZ BA, ROTHSTEIN P, VENES JL: Monitoring and management of increased intracranial pressure in Reye syndrome: Results in 29 children. *Pediatrics* 66:198, 1980.

STERNS RH, RIGGS JE, SCHOCHET SS: Osmotic demyelination syndromes following correction of hyponatremia. *N Engl J Med* 314:1555, 1986.

SUMMERSKILL WHJ, DAVIDSON EA, SHERLOCK S, STEINER RE: The neuropsychiatric syndrome associated with hepatic cirrhosis and extensive portal collateral circulation. *Q J Med* 25:245, 1956.

THILLY CH, BOURDOUX PP, DUE DT, et al: Myxedematous cretinism: An indicator of the most severe goiter endemias, in Medeiros-Neto G, Gaitan E (eds): *Frontiers in Thyroidology*. New York, Plenum Press, 1986, pp 1081–1084.

TOM MI, RICHARDSON JC: Hypoglycaemia from islet cell tumor of pancreas with amyotrophy and cerebrospinal nerve cell changes. *J Neuropathol Exp Neurol* 10:57, 1951.

TRAUNER DA: Treatment of Reye syndrome. *Ann Neurol* 7:2, 1980.

VAN WOERKOM W: La cirrhose hepatique avec alterations dans les centres nerveux evoluant chez des sujets d'age moyen. *Nouvelle Iconographie de la Salpêtrière* 27:41, 1914.

VASSART G, DUMONT JE, REFETOFF S: Thyroid disorders, in Scriver CR, Beaudet AL, Sly WS, Valle D (eds): *The Metabolic and Molecular Bases of Inherited Diseases*, 7th ed. New York, McGraw-Hill, 1995, pp 2883–2928.

VICTOR M, ADAMS RD, COLE M: The acquired (non-Wilsonian) type of chronic hepatocerebral degeneration. *Medicine* 44:345, 1965.

VICTOR M, LAURENO R: Neurologic complications of alcohol abuse: Epidemiologic aspects, in Schoenberg BS (ed): *Advances in Neurology*. Vol 19. New York, Raven Press, 1978, pp 603–617.

VICTOR M, ROTHSTEIN J: Neurologic manifestations of hepatic and gastrointestinal diseases, in Asbury AK, McKhann GM, McDonald WI (eds): *Diseases of the Nervous System*, 2nd ed. Philadelphia, Saunders, 1992, pp 1442–1455.

VOLHARD F: Clinical aspects of Bright's disease, in Berglund H et al (eds): *The Kidney in Health and Disease*. Philadelphia, Lea & Febiger, 1935, pp 665–673.

VON HOSSLIN C, ALZHEIMER A: Ein Beitrag zur Klinik und pathologischen Anatomie der Westphal-Strumpellschen Pseudosklerose. *Z Gesamte Neurol Psychiatr* 8:183, 1912.

WEGIERKO J: Typical syndrome of clinical manifestations in diabetes mellitus with fatal termination in coma without ketotic acidemia: So-called third coma. *Pol Tyg Lek* 11:2020, 1956.

WEINER WJ, KLAWANS HL: Hyperthyroid chorea, in Vinken PJ, Bruyn BW (eds): *Handbook of Clinical Neurology*. Vol 27. *Metabolic and Deficiency Diseases of the Nervous System*. Part I. Amsterdam, North-Holland, 1976, pp 279–281.

WIJDICKS EFM, PLEVAK DJ, RAKELA J, WIESNER RH: Clinical and radiologic features of cerebral edema in fulminant hepatic failure. *Mayo Clin Proc* 70:119, 1995.

WILKINSON DS, PROCKOP LD: Hypoglycemia: Effects on the nervous system, in Vinken PJ, Bruyn BW (eds): *Handbook of Clinical Neurology*. Vol 27. *Metabolic and Deficiency Diseases of the Nervous System*. Part I. Amsterdam, North-Holland, 1976, pp 53–78.

WILSON SAK: Progressive lenticular degeneration: A familial nervous disease associated with cirrhosis of the liver. *Brain* 34:295, 1912.

WINKELMAN MD, RICANATI ES: Dialysis encephalopathy: Neuropathologic aspects. *Hum Pathol* 17:823, 1986.

WRIGHT DG, LAURENO R, VICTOR M: Pontine and extrapontine myelinolysis. *Brain* 102:361, 1979.

YOUNG E, BRADLEY RF: Cerebral edema with irreversible coma in severe diabetic ketoacidosis. *N Engl J Med* 276:665, 1967.

ZIEVE L: Pathogenesis of hepatic encephalopathy. *Metab Brain Dis* 2:147, 1987.

Chapter 41

DISEASES OF THE NERVOUS SYSTEM DUE TO NUTRITIONAL DEFICIENCY

Among nutritional disorders, those of the nervous system occupy a position of special interest and importance. The early studies of beriberi, at the turn of the century, were largely responsible for the discovery of thiamine, and consequently for the modern concept of deficiency disease. Despite the notable achievements in the science of nutrition that followed the discovery of vitamins, diseases due to nutritional deficiency—and particularly those of the nervous system—continue to represent a worldwide health problem of serious proportions. In Far Eastern communities, where the diet consists mainly of highly milled rice, there is still a significant incidence of beriberi. In other underdeveloped countries, deficiency diseases are endemic, the result of chronic dietary deprivation. And the ultimate effects on the nervous system of mass starvation, involving entire nations of the African continent, is alarming to contemplate.

It comes as a surprise to many physicians that deficiency diseases are also common in the United States and other parts of the western world. To a large extent this is attributable to the prevalence of alcoholism. Relatively less common causes are dietary faddism and impaired absorption of dietary nutrients (which occurs in patients with celiac sprue, pernicious anemia, or surgical exclusion of portions of the gastrointestinal tract—for treatment of obesity or other reasons). Finally, there are the deficiencies induced by the use of vitamin antagonists or certain drugs, such as isonicotinic acid hydrazide (INH), which is used in the treatment of tuberculosis and interferes with the enzymatic function of pyridoxine.

General Considerations

The term *deficiency* is used throughout this chapter in its strictest sense, to designate disorders that result from *the lack of an essential nutrient(s) in the diet or from a conditioning factor that increases the need for these nutrients.* The most important of these nutrients are the vitamins, more specifically, members of the B group—thiamine, nicotinic acid, pyridoxine, pantothenic acid, riboflavin, folic acid, and cobalamin (vitamin B_{12}). Most deficiency diseases cannot be related to the lack of a single vitamin (subacute combined degeneration of the cord, due to vitamin B_{12} deficiency, is a notable exception). Usually the effects of several vitamin deficiencies can be recognized. This statement should not obscure the fact that particular manifestations of deficiency disease (e.g., the ocular palsies of Wernicke disease) are indeed related to a deficiency of a specific nutrient, nor should it diminish the need to identify such relationships.

Nutritional diseases of the nervous system are not simply a matter of vitamin deprivation, however. Practically always, the general signs of undernutrition, such as circulatory abnormalities and loss of subcutaneous fat and muscle bulk, are associated. Furthermore, a total lack of vitamins, as in starvation, is rarely associated with the classic deficiency syndromes of beriberi or pellagra; a certain amount of food is necessary to produce them. An excessive intake of carbohydrate relative to the supply of thiamine favors the development of a thiamine deficiency state. All deficiency diseases, including those of the nervous system, are influenced by factors such as exercise, growth, pregnancy, and infection, which increase the need for essential nutrients, and by disorders of the liver and the gastrointestinal tract, which may interfere with the synthesis and absorption of these nutrients.

As already mentioned, alcoholism is an important factor in the causation of nutritional diseases of the nervous system. Alcohol acts mainly by displacing food in the diet but also by adding carbohydrate calories (alcohol is burned almost entirely as carbohydrate), thus increasing the need for thiamine. There is some evidence as well that alcohol impairs the absorption of thiamine and other vitamins from the gastrointestinal tract.

In infants and young children, a reduction of protein and caloric intake (so-called protein-calorie malnutrition, or PCM) has a devastating effect upon body growth. Whether or not PCM also hinders the growth of the brain, with consequent effects upon intellectual and behavioral development, cannot be answered as readily. The data bearing on this matter are discussed in the last part of the chapter.

Deficiency diseases of the nervous system may occur in pure form and are so described in the following pages. But more often, the symptoms of other deficiencies are added, i.e., the deficiency diseases occur in various combinations. Characteristic also of the nutritional diseases is the involvement of both the central and peripheral nervous systems, an attribute shared only with certain hereditary metabolic disorders.

The following deficiency diseases are discussed in this chapter:

1. Wernicke disease and Korsakoff psychosis
2. Nutritional polyneuropathy (neuropathic beriberi)
3. Deficiency amblyopia (nutritional optic neuropathy; "tobacco-alcohol" amblyopia)
4. Pellagra (with some remarks on spinal spastic ataxia and nicotinic acid deficiency encephalopathy)
5. The syndrome of amblyopia, painful neuropathy, and orogenital dermatitis (so-called Strachan syndrome)
6. Subacute combined degeneration of the spinal cord (vitamin B_{12} deficiency)
7. Neurologic disorders due to a deficiency of pyridoxine and possibly other B vitamins (pantothenic acid, riboflavin, folic acid)
8. Vitamin E deficiency

In addition, attention is drawn to several distinctive neurologic disorders in which nutritional deficiency may play a role, although this has not been proved: (1) "alcoholic" cerebellar degeneration, (2) central pontine and extrapontine myelinolysis, and (3) primary degeneration of the corpus callosum (Marchiafava-Bignami disease). Also, some comments are made about PCM, the neurologic disorders consequent upon intestinal malabsorption, and the rare, hereditary vitamin-responsive diseases. Deficiencies of trace elements, because of their rarity, are not discussed; only iodine deficiency (cretinism) is of much importance in humans, and it is discussed in the chapter on acquired metabolic disease. Deficiencies of other elements have been reviewed by Fowden and colleagues.

The Wernicke-Korsakoff Syndrome

Wernicke disease and the Korsakoff amnesic state are common neurologic disorders that have been recognized since the 1880s. *Wernicke disease* (originally called polioencephalitis hemorrhagica superioris) is characterized by nystagmus, abducens and conjugate gaze palsies, ataxia of gait, and mental confusion. These symptoms develop acutely or subacutely and may occur singly or, more often, in various combinations. Wernicke disease is due to nutritional deficiency, more specifically to a deficiency of thiamine, and is observed mainly, though far from exclusively, in alcoholics.

The *Korsakoff amnesic state* (Korsakoff psychosis) refers to a unique mental disorder in which retentive memory is impaired out of proportion to other cognitive functions in an otherwise alert and responsive patient. This amnesic disorder, like Wernicke disease, is most often associated with alcoholism and malnutrition, but it may be a symptom of various other diseases that have their basis in lesions of the medial thalami or the inferomedial portions of the temporal lobes, such as infarction in the territory of the temporal lobe branches of the posterior cerebral arteries, hippocampal damage after cardiac arrest, third ventricular tumors, or herpes simplex encephalitis. A Korsakoff type of memory disturbance may also follow lesions that involve the basal septal nuclei of the frontal lobe. Transient impairments of retentive memory of the Korsakoff type may be the salient manifestations of temporal lobe epilepsy, concussive head injury, and a unique disorder known as transient global amnesia; and a permanent abnormality of this sort may be the most prominent feature of anoxic encephalopathy and of Alzheimer disease. The anatomic basis of the Korsakoff syndrome is discussed further in Chap. 21.

In the alcoholic, nutritionally deficient patient, the Korsakoff amnesic state is usually associated with Wernicke disease. Stated another way, *Korsakoff psychosis* is the psychic manifestation of Wernicke disease. For this reason and others elaborated below, the term *Wernicke disease* or *Wernicke encephalopathy* should be applied to a symptom complex of ophthalmoparesis, nystagmus, ataxia, and an acute apathetic-confusional state. If an enduring defect in learning and memory is added, the symptom complex is appropriately designated as the *Wernicke-Korsakoff syndrome*.

Historical Note In 1881, Carl Wernicke first described an illness of sudden onset characterized by paralysis of eye movements, ataxia of gait, and mental confusion. Swelling of the optic discs and retinal hemorrhages were also said to be present. His observations were made in 3 patients, of whom 2 were alcoholics and 1 was a young woman with persistent vomiting following the ingestion of sulfuric acid. In each of these patients there was progressive stupor and coma, culminating in death. The pathologic changes described by Wernicke consisted of punctate hemorrhages, primarily affecting the gray matter around the third and fourth ventricles and aqueduct of Sylvius; he considered these changes to be inflammatory in nature and confined to the gray matter, hence his designation "polioencephalitis hemorrhagica superioris." In the belief that *Gâyet* had described an identical disorder in 1875, the term Gâyet-Wernicke is used frequently by French authors. Such a designation is hardly justified insofar as the clinical signs and pathologic change in Gâyet's patient differed from those of Wernicke's patients in all essential details.

In a similar vein, a number of early writers, beginning with Magnus Huss in 1852, made casual reference to a disturbance of memory in the course of chronic alcoholism. However, the first comprehensive account of this disorder was given by the Russian psychiatrist S. S. Korsakoff in a series of articles published between 1887 and 1891 (for English translation and commentary, see reference by Victor and Yakovlev). Korsakoff stressed the relationship between "neuritis" (a term used at that time for all types of peripheral nerve disease) and the characteristic disorder of memory, which he believed to be "two facets of the same disease" and which he called "psychosis polyneuritica." But he also made the points, generally disregarded by subsequent authors, that neuritis need not accompany the characteristic amnesic syndrome and that both disorders could affect nonalcoholic as well as alcoholic patients. His clinical descriptions were remarkably complete and have hardly been surpassed to the present day.

It is of interest that the relationship between Wernicke disease and Korsakoff polyneuritic psychosis was appreciated neither by Wernicke nor by Korsakoff. Murawieff, in 1897, first postulated that a single cause was responsible for both. The intimate clinical relationship was established by Bonhoeffer in 1904, who stated that in all cases of Wernicke disease he found neuritis and an amnesic psychosis. Confirmation of this relationship on pathologic grounds came much later (for further details, see the monograph by Victor et al).

Clinical Features The incidence of the Wernicke-Korsakoff syndrome cannot be stated with precision, but it is has, until relatively recent years, been a common disorder, judging from our experience. At the Cleveland Metropolitan General Hospital, for example, in a consecutive series of 3548 autopsies in adults (for the period 1963 to 1976), the pathognomonic lesions were found in 77 cases (2.2 percent). The disease affects males only slightly more frequently than females, and the age of onset is fairly evenly distributed between 30 and 70 years. In the past two decades, the incidence of the Wernicke-Korsakoff syndrome has fallen significantly in the alcoholic population. However, it is being recognized with increasing frequency among nonalcoholic patients in a variety of clinical settings, mainly iatrogenic ones.

The triad of clinical features described by Wernicke—ophthalmoplegia, ataxia, and disturbances of mentation and consciousness—is still diagnostically useful provided that the diagnosis is suspected and the signs are carefully sought. Often the disease begins with ataxia, followed in a few days or weeks by mental confusion; or there may be the more or less simultaneous onset of ataxia, nystagmus, and ophthalmoparesis, with or without confusion. Less often, one component of this triad may be the sole manifestation of the disease. A description of each of the major manifestations follows.

Ocularmotor Abnormalities The diagnosis of Wernicke disease is made most readily on the basis of the ocular signs. These consist of (1) nystagmus that is both horizontal and vertical, (2) weakness or paralysis of the lateral rectus muscles, and (3) weakness or paralysis of conjugate gaze. Usually there is some combination of these abnormalities (see Chap. 14).

Next to nystagmus, the most frequent ocular abnormality is lateral rectus weakness, which is bilateral but not necessarily symmetrical and is accompanied by diplopia and internal strabismus. With complete paralysis of the lateral rectus muscles, nystagmus is initially absent in the abducting eyes, but it becomes evident as the weakness improves. The palsy of conjugate gaze varies from merely a nystagmus on extreme gaze to a complete loss of ocular movement in that direction. This applies to both horizontal and vertical movements, abnormalities of the former being somewhat more frequent. Paralysis of downward gaze is an unusual manifestation, but internuclear ophthalmoplegia is common. In advanced stages of the disease there may be a complete loss of ocular movements, and the pupils, which are usually spared, may become miotic and nonreacting. Ptosis, small retinal hemorrhages, involvement of the near-far focusing mechanism, and evidence of optic neuropathy occur occasionally, but we have never observed papilledema in this disease. Although the aforementioned ocular signs are highly characteristic of Wernicke disease, disappearance of nystagmus and an improvement in ophthalmoparesis within hours or a day or two of the administration of thiamine will confirm the diagnosis.

Ataxia Essentially the ataxia is one of stance and gait, and in the acute stage of the disease it may be so severe that the patient cannot stand or walk without support. Lesser degrees are characterized by a wide-based stance and a slow, uncertain, short-stepped gait; the mildest degrees are apparent only in tandem walking. In contrast to the gross disorder of locomotion is the relative infrequency of a limb ataxia and intention tremor; when present, they are more likely to be elicited by heel-to-knee than by finger-to-nose testing. Scanning speech is present only rarely.

Disturbances of Consciousness and Mentation These are present in some form in all but 10 percent of patients. Four types of deranged mentation and consciousness can be recognized. By far the commonest disturbance is a *global confusional state*. The patient is apathetic, inattentive, and indifferent to his surroundings. Spontaneous speech is minimal and many questions are left unanswered, or the patient may suspend conversation and drift off to sleep, although he can be aroused without difficulty. Such questions as are answered by the patient betray disorientation in time and place, misidentification of those around him, and an inability to grasp the immediate situation. Many of the patient's remarks are irrational and lack consistency from one moment to another. If the patient's interest and attention can be maintained long enough to ensure adequate testing, one finds that memory and learning ability are also impaired. In response to the administration of thiamine or an adequate diet, the patient rapidly becomes more alert and attentive and more capable of taking part in mental testing. Then the most prominent abnormality is one of retentive memory (Korsakoff amnesic state).

About 15 percent of patients show the signs of alcohol withdrawal, i.e., hallucinations and other disorders of perception, confusion, agitation, tremor, and overactivity of autonomic nervous system function. These symptoms are evanescent in nature and usually mild in degree.

Although drowsiness is a common feature of the global confusional state, stupor and coma are rare as *initial* manifestations of Wernicke disease. However, if the early signs of the disease are not recognized and the patient remains untreated, there occurs a progressive depression of the state of consciousness, with stupor, coma, and death in a matter of a week or two, just as occurred in Wernicke's original cases. Autopsy series of Wernicke disease are heavily weighted with cases of the latter type, often undiagnosed during life (Harper; Torvik et al).

Some patients are alert and responsive from the time they are first seen and already show the characteristic features of the Korsakoff amnesic state. In a small number of such patients, the amnesic state is the only manifestation of the syndrome, and no ocular or ataxic signs (other than possibly nystagmus) can be discerned. The memory disorder, which constitutes the chronic and truly crippling feature of the Wernicke-Korsakoff syndrome, is described below.

The Amnesic State As indicated in Chap. 21, the core of the amnesic disorder is a defect in learning (*anterograde amnesia*) and a loss of past memories (*retrograde amnesia*). The defect in learning (memorization) can be remarkably severe. The patient may be incapable, for example, of committing to memory three simple facts (such as the examiner's name, the date, and the time of day), despite countless attempts; the patient can repeat each fact as it is presented, indicating that he understands what is wanted of him and that "registration" is intact, but by the time the third fact is repeated, the first may have been forgotten. However, certain subtle learning may take place; for example, with repeated trials, the patient may learn mirror writing or to negotiate a maze, despite no recollection of ever having learned these tasks.

Anterograde amnesia is always coupled with a disturbance of past or remote memory (retrograde amnesia). The latter disorder is usually severe in degree, though rarely complete, and covers a period that antedates the onset of the illness by several years. Characteristically, a few isolated events and information from the past are retained, but these are related without regard for the intervals that separated them or for their proper temporal sequence. Usually the patient "telescopes" events, sometimes the opposite. This aspect of the memory disorder becomes prominent as the initial (global confusional) stage of the illness subsides and some improvement in memory function occurs; this may account for certain instances of confabulation (see below).

It is probably true that memories of the recent past are more severely impaired than those of the remote past

(Ribot's rule); language, computation, knowledge acquired in school, and all habitual actions are preserved. This is not to say that all remote memories are intact. These are not as readily tested as more recent memories, and the two are therefore difficult to compare. It is our impression that there are gaps and inaccuracies in memories of the distant past in practically all cases of the Korsakoff amnesic state and serious impairments in many of them.

It should be emphasized that the cognitive impairment of the Korsakoff patient cannot be explained in terms of memory loss alone, even though this is the most critical functional loss. Psychologic testing discloses that certain cognitive and perceptual functions that depend little or not at all on retentive memory are also impaired. The most consistent failure is with the digit symbol task and, to a lesser degree, with arithmetic and block design. Also, as a rule, the Korsakoff patient has no insight into his illness and is characteristically apathetic and inert, lacking in spontaneity and initiative and indifferent to everything and everybody around him. However, the patient has a relatively normal capacity to reason with data immediately before him.

Confabulation is generally considered to be a specific feature of Korsakoff psychosis. The validity of this view depends largely on how one defines confabulation, and there is no uniformity of opinion on this point. Our observations do not support the oft-repeated statement that the Korsakoff patient fills the gaps in his memory with confabulation. In the sense that gaps in memory exist and that whatever the patient supplies in place of the correct answers fills these gaps, the statement is incontrovertible. It is hardly explanatory, however. The implication that confabulation is a deliberate attempt to hide the memory defect, out of embarrassment or for other reasons, is probably not correct. In fact, the opposite seems to pertain: as the patient improves and become more aware of a defect in memory, the tendency to confabulate becomes less.

In our experience, confabulation is associated with two phases of the Wernicke-Korsakoff syndrome: the initial phase, in which profound general confusion dominates the disease; and the convalescent phase, in which the patient recalls fragments of past experience in a distorted fashion. Events that were separated by long intervals are juxtaposed or related out of sequence, so that the narrative has an implausible or fictional aspect. Whether one designates the latter defect as confabulation or as a particular defect of retentive memory is academic. In the chronic, stable state of the disease, confabulation is usually absent. These and other aspects of confabulation are discussed more fully in the monograph by Victor and colleagues.

Other Clinical Abnormalities Signs of *peripheral neuropathy* are found in more than 80 percent of patients with the Wernicke-Korsakoff syndrome. In most of them the neuropathic disease is mild and does not account for the disorder of gait, but it may be so severe that stance and gait cannot be tested. In a small number, retrobulbar neuropathy is added. Despite the frequency of peripheral neuropathy, overt signs of beriberi heart disease are rare. However, indications of disordered cardiovascular function such as tachycardia, exertional dyspnea, postural hypotension, and minor electrocardiographic abnormalities are frequent; occasionally, the patient dies suddenly, following only slight exertion. These patients may show an elevation of cardiac output associated with low peripheral vascular resistance—abnormalities that revert to normal after the administration of thiamine. *Postural hypotension* and syncope are common findings in Wernicke disease and are probably due to impaired function of the autonomic nervous system, more specifically to a defect in the sympathetic outflow (Birchfield). There may be mild *hypothermia*. Patients with the Korsakoff amnesic state may have a demonstrably *impaired olfactory discrimination*. This deficit, like the notable apathy that is present in most Wernicke patients, is probably attributable to a lesion of the mediodorsal nucleus of the thalamus and its connections and not to a lesion of the peripheral olfactory system (Mair et al).

Ancillary Laboratory Findings Vestibular function, as measured by the response to standard ice-water caloric tests, is universally impaired in the acute stage of Wernicke disease (Ghez). Vertigo is not a complaint, however. To this abnormality of function, which is bilateral and more or less symmetrical, the term *vestibular paresis* has been applied. It probably accounts for the severe disequilibrium in the initial stage of the illness. The CSF in uncomplicated cases of the Wernicke-Korsakoff syndrome is normal or shows only a modest elevation of the protein content. Protein values above 100 mg/dL or a pleocytosis should suggest the presence of a complicating illness—subdural hematoma and meningeal infection being the most common.

Blood pyruvate is elevated in untreated cases of Wernicke disease, but *blood transketolase* activity is a more accurate index of the thiamine deficiency. Transketolase, one of the enzymes of the hexose monophosphate shunt, requires thiamine pyrophosphate (TPP) as a cofactor. In normal adult subjects, transketolase values (expressed as sedoheptulose-7-phosphate produced per milliliter per hour) range from 90 to 140 mg and the TPP effect from 0 to 10 percent, depending upon the degree of vitamin supplementation. Before specific treatment with thiamine, patients with Wernicke disease show a marked reduction in their transketolase activity (as low as one-third of normal values) and a striking TPP effect (up to 50 percent). Restoration of these values toward normal occurs within a few hours of the administration of thiamine, and completely normal values are usually attained within 24 h.

An important abnormality of transketolase has been described by Blass and Gibson. They found that transketolase in cultured fibroblasts from four alcoholics with Wernicke-Korsakoff disease bound TPP less avidly than did the transketolase from control lines. Presumably this defect in transketolase would be insignificant if the diet were adequate but would be deleterious if the diet were low in thiamine. These findings, which have been corroborated by Mukherjee and colleagues, suggest a hereditary factor in the genesis of Wernicke-Korsakoff disease and possibly may explain why only a small proportion of nutritionally deficient alcoholics develop this disease.

Only about half the patients with Wernicke-Korsakoff disease show electroencephalographic (EEG) abnormalities, consisting of diffuse mild to moderate slow activity. Total cerebral blood flow and cerebral oxygen and glucose consumption may be greatly reduced in the acute stages of the disease, and these defects may still be present after several weeks of treatment (Shimojyo et al). These observations indicate that significant reductions in brain metabolism need not be reflected in EEG abnormalities or in depression of the state of consciousness and that the latter is more a function of the location of the lesion than of the overall degree of metabolic defect.

The acute lesions of the Wernicke-Korsakoff syndrome, both the medial thalamic and periaqueductal ones, can be demonstrated by magnetic resonance imaging (Donnal et al, Gallucci et al). This procedure is particularly useful in patients in whom stupor or coma has supervened or in whom ocular and ataxic signs are otherwise inevident (Victor, 1990).

Course of the Illness The mortality rate in the acute phase of Wernicke disease was 17 percent in our series of patients. Mainly the fatalities were attributable to hepatic failure and to infection (pneumonia, pulmonary tuberculosis, and septicemia being the most common). Some deaths were undoubtedly due to the effects of thiamine deficiency that had reached an irreversible stage.

Most patients respond in a fairly predictable manner to the administration of thiamine, as detailed further on. The most dramatic improvement is in the ocular manifestations, as already mentioned. Recovery *begins* often within hours after the administration of thiamine and practically always within several days. This effect is so constant that a failure of the ocular palsies to respond to thiamine should raise doubts about the diagnosis of Wernicke disease. Sixth nerve palsies, ptosis, and vertical gaze palsies recover *completely* within a week or two in most cases, but vertical nystagmus may sometimes persist for several months. Horizontal gaze palsies recover completely as a rule, but in 60 percent of cases a fine horizontal nystagmus remains as a permanent sequela. In this respect, horizontal nystagmus is unique among the ocular signs.

In comparison with the ocular signs, improvement of ataxia is somewhat delayed. About 40 percent of patients recover completely from ataxia. The remainder recover incompletely or not at all and are left with a slow, shuffling, wide-based gait and inability to walk tandem. The residual gait disturbances and horizontal nystagmus provide a means of identifying obscure and chronic cases of dementia as alcoholic-nutritional in origin. Vestibular function improves at about the same rate as the ataxia of gait, and recovery is usually but not always complete.

The early symptoms of apathy, drowsiness, and global confusion invariably recede, and as they do so the defect in memory and learning stands out more clearly. The memory disorder, once established, recovers completely or almost completely in only 20 percent of patients. The remainder are left with varying degrees of permanent disability.

It is apparent from the foregoing account that Wernicke disease and Korsakoff psychosis are not separate diseases but that *the changing ocular and ataxic signs and the transformation of the global confusional state into an amnesic syndrome are simply successive stages in a single disease process*. Of 186 patients in our series who presented with Wernicke disease and survived the acute illness, 157 (84 percent) showed this sequence of clinical events. As a corollary, a survey of alcoholic patients with Korsakoff psychosis in a state mental hospital disclosed that in most the illness had begun with the symptoms of Wernicke disease, and that about 60 percent of them still showed the ocular and/or cerebellar stigmata of Wernicke disease many years after the onset.

Neuropathologic Findings and Clinical-Pathologic Correlation Patients who die in the acute stages of Wernicke disease show symmetrical lesions in the paraventricular regions of the thalamus and hypothalamus, mammillary bodies, periaqueductal region of the midbrain, floor of the fourth ventricle (particularly in the regions of the dorsal motor nuclei of the vagus and vestibular nuclei), and superior cerebellar vermis. Lesions are consistently found in the mammillary bodies and less consistently in other areas. The microscopic changes are characterized by varying degrees of necrosis of parenchymal structures. Within the area of necrosis, nerve cells are lost, but usually some remain; some of these are damaged, but others are intact. Myelinated fibers are more affected than neurons. These changes are accompanied by a prominence of the blood vessels, although in some cases there appears to be a primary endothelial proliferation. In the areas of parenchymal damage there is astrocytic and microglial proliferation. Discrete hemorrhages were found in only 20 percent of our cases, and many of them appeared to be agonal in nature. The cerebellar changes consist of a degeneration of all layers of the cortex, particularly of the Purkinje cells; usually this lesion is confined to the superior parts of the vermis, but in advanced cases the cortex of the most anterior parts of the anterior lobes is involved as well. Of interest is the fact that the lesions of Leigh's encephalomyelopathy, in which a disorder of pyruvate metabolism has been found (page 1042), bear a close resemblance to those of Wernicke disease in both their distribution and their histologic characteristics.

The ocular muscle and gaze palsies are attributable to lesions of the sixth and third nerve nuclei and adjacent tegmentum and the nystagmus to lesions in the regions of the vestibular nuclei. The latter are also responsible for the loss of caloric responses and probably for the gross disturbance of equilibrium that characterizes the initial stage of the disease. The lack of significant destruction of nerve cells in these lesions accounts for the rapid improvement and the high degree of recovery of oculomotor and vestibular functions. The persistent ataxia of stance and gait is due to the lesion of the superior vermis of the cerebellum; ataxia of individual movements of the legs is attributable to an extension of the lesion into the anterior parts of the anterior lobes. Hypothermia, which occurs sometimes as a presenting feature of Wernicke disease, is probably attributable to lesions in the posterior and posterolateral nuclei of the hypothalamus (experimentally placed lesions in these parts have been shown to cause hypothermia or poikilothermia in monkeys).

The topography of the neuropathologic changes in patients who die in the chronic stages of the disease, when the amnesic symptoms predominate, is much the same as the changes in the acute stages of Wernicke disease. Apart from the expected differences in age of the glial and vascular reactions, the only important difference has to do with the involvement or lack of involvement of the medial dorsal and anterior nuclei of the thalamus. The medial parts of these nuclei were consistently involved in our patients who had shown the Korsakoff amnesic state during life; they were not involved in patients who had had no persistent amnesic symptoms. The mammillary bodies were affected in all of the patients, both those with the amnesic defect and those without. These observations suggest that the lesions responsible for the memory disorder are those of the thalami, predominantly of the medial dorsal nuclei (and their connections with the medial temporal lobes and amygdaloid nuclei, i.e., a thalamic amnesic state), and not those of the mammillary bodies, as is frequently stated. It is also notable that the hippocampal formations, the site of damage in many other types of Korsakoff memory loss, are intact.

Treatment of the Wernicke-Korsakoff Syndrome Wernicke disease constitutes a medical emergency, and its recognition (or even the suspicion of its presence) demands the *immediate administration of thiamine*. The prompt use of thiamine prevents progression of the disease and reverses those lesions that have not yet progressed to the point of fixed structural change. In patients who show only ocular signs and ataxia, the administration of thiamine is crucial in preventing the development of an irreversible amnesic state.

Although 2 to 3 mg of thiamine may be sufficient to modify the ocular signs, much larger doses are needed to sustain improvement and replenish the depleted thiamine stores—50 mg intravenously and 50 mg intramuscularly—the latter dose being repeated each day until the patient resumes a normal diet.

It should be standard practice in emergency departments to administer 50 to 100 mg of thiamine simultaneously with intravenous fluids that contain glucose in order to avoid precipitating Wernicke disease. It is also good practice to give B vitamins to all alcoholic patients. The chronic alcoholic (or the nonalcoholic with persistent vomiting) exhausts his body stores of thiamine in a matter of 7 or 8 weeks, at which time the administration of glucose may serve to precipitate Wernicke disease or cause an early form of the disease to progress rapidly. The further management of Wernicke disease involves the use of a balanced diet and all the B vitamins, since the patient is usually deficient in more than thiamine alone.

A problem in management may arise once the patient has recovered from Wernicke disease and the amnesic psychosis becomes prominent. As indicated above, only a minority of such patients (less than 20 percent in our series) recover; moreover, the onset of recovery in such patients may be delayed for several weeks or even months, and then it proceeds very slowly over a period of many months. The extent to which the amnesic symptoms will recover cannot be predicted accurately during the acute stages of the illness; one must guard against the premature commitment of the patient to a mental hospital. Interestingly, the alcoholic Korsakoff patient, once more or less recovered, seldom demands alcohol but will drink it if it is offered.

Infantile Wernicke-Beriberi Disease This term designates an acute and frequently fatal disease of infants, which until recently was very common in rice-eating communities of the Far East. It affects only breast-fed infants, usually in the second to the fifth months of life. Acute cardiac symptoms dominate the clinical picture, but neurologic symptoms (aphonia, strabismus, nystagmus, spasmodic contraction of facial muscles, and convulsions) have been described in many cases. This syndrome can be reversed dramatically by the administration of thiamine, so that some authors prefer to call it *acute thiamine deficiency in infants*. In the few neuropathologic studies that have been made of this disorder, changes like those of Wernicke disease in the adult have been described.

Infantile beriberi bears no consistent relationship to beriberi in the mother. Infants of mothers with overt signs of beriberi may be quite normal. Conversely, mothers of infants with beriberi may themselves be free of the disease. The levels of thiamine in the breast milk of such mothers have not been determined, however. The absence of beriberi in the mothers of affected infants suggests that infantile beriberi might be due to a toxic factor in breast milk, but such a factor, if it exists, has never been isolated.

Rarely, the clinical manifestations of beriberi in infancy represent an inherited (autosomal recessive) thiamine-dependent state, responding to the continued administration of massive doses of thiamine (Mandel et al; see also Table 41-2).

NUTRITIONAL POLYNEUROPATHY (NEUROPATHIC BERIBERI)

Most physicians in the western world have only a dim notion about beriberi, which they recall as an ill-defined, predominantly cardiac disorder occurring among the rice-eating people of the Orient. In fact, beriberi is a distinct clinical entity that is not confined to any particular part of the world. Essentially it is a disease of the heart and of the peripheral nerves (which may be affected separately), with or without edema, the latter feature providing the basis for the classic division into "wet" and "dry" forms. The cardiac manifestations range from tachycardia and exertional dyspnea to acute and rapidly fatal heart failure. This last is the most dramatic manifestation of beriberi, but it is uncommon. Here we are concerned with the affection of the peripheral nerves, or *neuropathic beriberi*, as it is designated.

That beriberi is essentially a degenerative disorder of the peripheral nerves was established in the late nineteenth century by the classic studies of the Dutch investigators Eijkman, Pekelharing and Winkler, and Grijns. Only after beriberi gained acceptance as a nutritional disease (this followed Funk's discovery of vitamins in 1911) was it suspected that the neuropathy of alcoholics was also nutritional in origin. The similarity between beriberi and alcoholic neuropathy was commented upon by several authors, but it was Shattuck, in 1928, who first seriously discussed the relationship of the two disorders. He suggested that "polyneuritis of chronic alcoholism was caused chiefly by failure to take or assimilate food containing a sufficient quantity of vitamin B . . . and might properly be regarded as true beriberi." Convincing evidence that "alcoholic neuritis" is not due to the neurotoxic effect of alcohol was supplied by Strauss. He allowed 10 patients to continue their daily consumption of whiskey while they consumed a well-balanced diet supplemented with yeast and vitamin B concentrates; the peripheral nerve symptoms improved in every case. Our own observations support Strauss's contention that alcoholic polyneuropathy is essentially a nutritional disease.

Clinical Features The symptomatology of nutritional polyneuropathy is diverse. In fact, many patients are asymptomatic, and evidence of peripheral nerve affection is found only on clinical or electromyographic examination. In the latter circumstance the neuropathic signs are mild in degree, consisting of thinness and tenderness of the leg muscles, loss or depression of the Achilles reflexes and perhaps of the patellar reflexes, and at times a patchy blunting of pain and touch sensation over the feet and shins.

The majority of patients, however, are symptomatic—weakness, paresthesias, and pain being the usual complaints. The symptoms are insidious in onset and slowly progressive, but occasionally they seem to evolve or to worsen rapidly, over a matter of days. The initial symptoms are usually referred to the distal portions of the limbs and progress proximally if the illness remains untreated. The lower limbs are always affected earlier and more severely than the upper ones. Most often some aspect of motor disability constitutes the chief complaint, but in about one-quarter of the patients the main complaints are pain and paresthesias. The discomfort takes several forms: a dull, constant ache in the feet or legs; sharp and lancinating pains, momentary in duration, like those of tabes dorsalis; sensations of cramping or tightness in the muscles of the feet and calves; or band-like feelings around the legs. Coldness of the feet is a common complaint but is purely subjective. Far more distressing are feelings of heat or "burning" affecting mainly the soles, less frequently the dorsal aspects of the feet. The dysesthesias fluctuate in severity and characteristically are worsened by contactual stimuli, sometimes to the point where the patient cannot walk or bear the touch of bedclothes, despite the relative preservation of motor power. The term *burning feet* has been applied to this syndrome, but it is not particularly apt, since the patient also complains of other types of paresthesia and pain, and these symptoms may involve the hands as well as the feet.

Examination discloses varying degrees of motor, sensory, and reflex loss. As the symptoms suggest, the signs are symmetrical, usually more severe in distal than in proximal portions of the limbs, and often confined to the legs. The disproportionate affection of motor power may be striking, taking the form of a foot and wrist drop; but even in these patients the proximal muscles are usually affected as well (indicated by difficulty in arising from a squatting position). In other patients, all the leg muscles are affected more or less equally, and in a few, weakness appears to be most severe in the proximal muscles. Absolute paralysis of the legs is observed only rarely; immobility due to contractures at the knees and ankles is a more common occurrence. Tenderness of muscles on deep pressure is a highly characteristic finding, elicited most readily in the muscles of the feet and calves. Deep tendon reflexes in the legs are almost always lost, even when weakness is slight in degree. In the arms, tendon reflexes are sometimes retained despite a loss of strength in the hands. In a small number of patients, particularly those in whom pain and dysesthesias are prominent and motor loss is slight, the reflexes at knee and ankle may be retained or even of greater than average briskness.

Excessive sweating of the soles and dorsal aspects of the feet and of the volar surfaces of the hands and fingers is a common manifestation of alcohol-induced nutritional neuropathy. Postural hypotension is sometimes associated. These symptoms are indicative of involvement of the peripheral sympathetic nerve fibers.

Sensory loss or impairment may involve all the modalities, although one may be affected out of proportion to the others. One cannot predict from the patient's symptoms which mode of sensation might be affected disproportionately. In patients with impairment of superficial sensation (i.e., touch, pain, and temperature), the border between impaired and normal sensation is not sharp but shades off gradually over a considerable vertical extent of the limbs.

Patients in whom pain is the outstanding symptom do not constitute a distinct group in terms of their neurologic signs. Pain and dysesthesias may be prominent in patients with either severe or slight degrees of motor, reflex, and sensory loss. The term *hyperesthetic* is used commonly to designate the exquisitely painful form of neuropathy but is not well chosen; as pointed out on page 145, one is usually able, by using finely graded stimuli, to demonstrate an elevated threshold to painful, thermal, and tactile stimuli in the "hyperesthetic" zone. Once the stimulus is perceived, however, it has a painful and diffuse, unpleasant quality (hyperpathia). Tactile evocation of pain or burning is an example of allodynia.

In most patients with nutritional polyneuropathy, only the limbs are involved; the abdominal, thoracic, and bulbar muscles are usually spared. In the most advanced instances of neuropathy, hoarseness and weakness of the voice and dysphagia due to affection of the vagus nerves may be added to the clinical picture.

Some idea of the incidence of the motor, reflex, and sensory abnormalities and the combinations in which they occur can be obtained from Table 41-1, which is based on our study of 189 nutritionally depleted alcoholic patients. Noteworthy is the fact that only 66 (35 percent) of the 189 patients showed the clinical picture of polyneuropathy in its entirety—i.e., a symmetrical impairment or loss of tendon reflexes, sensation,

Table 41-1
Clinical findings in nutritional polyneuropathy

Neuropathic abnormality	*Legs (189 cases)*	*Arms (57 cases)*
Loss of reflexes alone	45 (24)[a]	6 (10)[b]
Loss of sensation alone	10 (5)	10 (18)
Weakness alone	—	5 (9)
Weakness and sensory loss	2 (1)	10 (18)
Reflex and sensory loss	40 (21)	2 (3)
Sensory, motor, and reflex loss	66 (35)	17 (30)
Data incomplete	26 (14)	7 (12)

[a] Figures in parentheses indicate percent of 189 cases.
[b] Figures in parentheses indicate percent of 57 cases.

and motor power affecting legs more than the arms and the distal more than the proximal segments of the limbs. In the remaining patients, the motor-reflex-sensory signs occurred in various combinations, as indicated in Table 41-1.

Stasis edema and pigmentation, glossiness, and thinness of the skin of the lower legs and feet are common findings in patients with severe forms of neuropathy. Major dystrophic changes, in the form of perforating plantar ulcers and painless destruction of the bones and joints of the feet (ulcero-osteolytic neuropathy; "Charcot forefeet"), have been described but are rare. Repeated trauma to insensitive parts and superimposed infection are thought to be responsible for the neuropathic arthropathy.

The CSF is usually normal, although a modest elevation of protein content is found in a small number of cases. Electromyographic (EMG) findings include mild to moderate degrees of slowing of motor and sensory conduction and a marked reduction of the amplitudes of sensory action potentials; the motor conduction velocities in distal segments of the nerves may be reduced, while conduction in proximal segments is normal. Denervated muscles show fibrillation potentials.

Pathologic Features The essential pathologic change is one of axonal degeneration, with destruction of both axon and myelin sheath. Segmental demyelination may also occur, but only in a small proportion of fibers. This change may be difficult to discern in myelin-stained sections of whole nerve trunks, but it can be observed in teased nerve fibers stained with osmium. The most pronounced changes are observed in the distal parts of the longest and largest myelinated fibers in the crural and, to a lesser extent, brachial nerves. In advanced cases the degenerative changes extend into the anterior and posterior nerve roots. The vagus and phrenic nerves and paravertebral sympathetic trunks may be affected in advanced cases.

Anterior horn and dorsal root ganglion cells undergo chromatolysis, indicating axonal damage. Degenerative changes in the posterior columns are seen in some cases and are probably secondary to the changes in the dorsal spinal roots.

Pathophysiology The nutritional factor(s) responsible for the neuropathy of alcoholism and beriberi have not been defined precisely. Because of the difficulties in producing peripheral neuropathy in Mammalia by means of a thiamine-deficient diet, several investigators in the past questioned the idea that thiamine is the antineuritic vitamin. Very few of the animal experiments undertaken to settle this point are satisfactory from a nutritional and pathologic point of view. Nevertheless, several studies in birds and humans do indeed indicate that uncomplicated thiamine deficiency may result in peripheral nerve disease. The necessity of either accepting or rejecting the specific role of thiamine became less urgent when it was demonstrated, in both animals and humans, that a deficiency of pyridoxine or of pantothenic acid could also result in degeneration of the peripheral nerves (see Swank and Adams).

The question of whether polyneuropathy in the alcoholic patient might be due to the direct toxic effects of alcohol and not to a nutritional deficiency has been raised from time to time (see, for example, Denny-Brown and Behse and Buchthal). The evidence for this view is not compelling, either on clinical or on experimental grounds (see reference to Strauss, in introductory section on nutritional neuropathy). The interested reader will find a detailed critique of this subject in the chapters by Victor and by Windebank in the second and third editions, respectively, of *Peripheral Neuropathy*, edited by Dyck and coworkers.

Treatment and Prognosis The first consideration is to supply adequate nutrition in the form of a balanced diet supplemented with B vitamins. Equally important is to make certain that the patient follows the prescribed diet. If persistent vomiting or other gastrointestinal complications prevent the patient from eating, then parenteral feeding becomes necessary; the vitamins may be given intramuscularly or added to intravenous fluids.

Where pain and sensitivity of the feet are the major complaints, the pressure of bedclothes may be avoided by placing a cradle support over the legs. Aching of the limbs may be related to their immobility, in which case they should be moved passively on frequent occasions. Aspirin or acetaminophen is usually sufficient to control hyperpathia; occasionally codeine in doses of 15 to 30 mg must be added. Obviously, opiates and addicting synthetic analgesics should be avoided. Some of our patients with severe burning pain (similar to causalgia) in the feet have been helped by blocking the lumbar sympathetic ganglia or by epidural injection of analgesics. The response to phenytoin and carbamazepine (Tegretol) has been inconsistent. Adrenergic blocking medication has been of little value.

The regeneration of peripheral nerves, which may take many months, will be of no avail if the muscles have been allowed to undergo contracture and the joints to become fixed. The patient's legs should be positioned so that the soles rest firmly against a footboard, in order to prevent shortening of the heel cords. In cases of severe paralysis, molded splints should be applied to the arms, hands, legs, and feet during periods of rest. Pressure on the heels and elbows can be avoided by padding the splints and by turning the patient frequently or by asking the patient to do so. As soon as the patient's general condition permits, the limbs must be passively moved through a full range of movement several times daily. As function returns, more vigorous physiotherapeutic measures can be undertaken.

Recovery from nutritional polyneuropathy is a slow process. In the mildest cases there may be a considerable restoration of motor function in a few weeks. In severe forms of the disease, several months may pass before the patient is able to walk unaided. The slowness of recovery creates a special problem for the alcoholic patient, in whom the great danger to continued recovery is the resumption of drinking. Suitable arrangements must therefore be made for close supervision during the long and tedious convalescence.

Deficiency Amblyopia (Nutritional Optic Neuropathy)

("Tobacco-Alcohol Amblyopia"; See also Chap. 13)

These terms refer to a characteristic form of visual impairment that results from nutritional deficiency. The defect in vision is due not to an abnormality of the cornea or other parts of the refractive mechanism but to a lesion of the optic nerve, more or less confined to the region of the papillomacular bundle.

Typically, the patient complains of dimness or blurring of vision for near and distant objects, evolving gradually over a period of several days or weeks. Examination discloses a reduction in visual acuity due to the presence of central or centrocecal scotomata, which are larger for colored than for white test objects. Pallor of the temporal portion of the optic disc is observed in some cases. These abnormalities are bilateral and roughly symmetrical and, if untreated, may progress to blindness and irreversible optic atrophy. With nutritious diet and vitamin supplements, improvement occurs in all but the most chronic cases, the degree of recovery depending upon the severity of the amblyopia and particularly upon its duration before therapy is instituted.

Although the precise deficiency responsible cannot be named, the nutritional basis of this disorder was established beyond doubt during World War II and the Korean War, when innumerable instances were observed in prisoners of war who had been confined for prolonged periods under conditions of severe dietary deprivation. Fisher described the optic nerve lesions in 4 such patients who had died of unrelated causes between 8 and 10 years after the onset of amblyopia. The optic nerves in each case showed a loss of myelin and axis cylinders restricted to the region of the papillomacular fibers. Of the 4 cases, 3 also showed demyelination of the posterior columns of the spinal cord, no doubt an expression of the associated sensory polyneuropathy.

In the western world, a visual disorder indistinguishable clinically and pathologically from that observed in prisoners of war is observed infrequently, mainly among undernourished alcoholics. For many years this has been referred to as *tobacco-alcohol amblyopia*, with the implication that the visual loss is due to the toxic effects of alcohol, tobacco, or both. Actually, the evidence is overwhelming that so-called tobacco-alcohol amblyopia is due to nutritional deficiency. A specific nutrient has not been identified, however. There is evidence in humans and in animals that under certain conditions a deficiency of one or more of the B vitamins—thiamine, vitamin B_{12}, and perhaps riboflavin—may cause degenerative changes in the optic nerves, a situation that pertains in the peripheral nerves as well.

In the 1960s, a popular theory held that the combined effects of vitamin B_{12} deficiency and chronic poisoning by cyanide (generated in tobacco smoke) were responsible for "tobacco amblyopia." Vitamin B_{12} deficiency is a rare but undoubted cause of optic neuropathy (page 263), but the notion that cyanide or other substances in tobacco smoke have a damaging effect upon the optic nerves is supported neither by logic nor by experimental data (see reviews of Potts and of Victor). Clinically, instances of Leber's hereditary optic atrophy may be mistaken for "tobacco-alcohol amblyopia"—an error that should no longer be made because the former disorder can now be identified with certainty by mitochondrial DNA testing.

The most recent outbreaks of nutritional optic neuropathy occurred in Cuba during 1991–1993 and in Tanzania. In both outbreaks the optic neuropathy was frequently associated with peripheral neuropathy, for which reason they are considered further on, with the Strachan syndrome.

Pellagra

In the early 1900s, pellagra attained epidemic proportions in the southern United States and in the alcoholic population of large urban centers. Since 1940, the prevalence of pellagra has diminished greatly because of the general practice of enriching bread with niacin. Nevertheless, among the vegetarian, maize-eating people of underdeveloped countries and among the black population of South Africa, pellagra is still a common disease (Bomb et al, Shah et al, Ronthal and Adler). In developed countries, pellagra is practically confined to alcoholics (Ishii and Nishihara, Spivak and Jackson, Serdaru et al).

In its fully developed form, pellagra affects the skin, alimentary tract, and hematopoietic and nervous systems. The early symptoms may be mistaken for those of a neurosis. Insomnia, fatigue, nervousness, irritability, and feelings of depression are common complaints; examination may disclose mental dullness, apathy, and an impairment of memory. Sometimes an acute confusional psychosis dominates the clinical picture. Untreated, these symptoms may progress to a dementia. Pellagra may not only produce insanity but occasionally result from it, by virtue of the anorexia and refusal of food that accompany certain mental illnesses. The *spinal cord* manifestations have not been clearly described; in general, the signs are referable to both the posterior and lateral columns, predominantly the former. Signs of *peripheral nerve affection* are relatively less common and are indistinguishable from those of neuropathic beriberi.

Pathologic Changes These are most readily discerned in the large cells of the motor cortex, the cells of Betz and are seen to a lesser extent in the smaller pyramidal cells of the cortex, the large cells of the basal ganglia, the cells of the cranial motor and dentate nuclei, and the anterior horn cells of the spinal cord. The affected cells appear swollen and rounded, with eccentric nuclei and loss of the Nissl bodies (frequently referred to as "axonal reaction"). In the pathologic material of Hauw and associates, the chromatolytic changes were most pronounced in the brainstem nuclei (upper reticular and pontine) and not in the Betz cells. They concluded that these changes were not due to a retrograde axonal lesion, but did not comment on the status of the spinal cord.

The spinal cord lesions in pellagra take the form of a symmetrical degeneration of the dorsal columns, especially of Goll, and to a lesser extent of the corticospinal tracts. Such a posterior column degeneration, affecting a specific system of fibers, is likely to be secondary to degeneration of the dorsal root ganglion cells or posterior roots. The reason for the corticospinal tract degeneration is not clear. The few studies of the peripheral nerves in pellagra have disclosed changes like those in alcoholics and other patients with nutritional deficiency.

Etiology It has been known since 1937, when Elvehjem and coworkers showed that nicotinic acid cured black tongue, a pellagra-like disease in dogs, that this vitamin is effective in the treatment of pellagra. Many years before, Goldberger had demonstrated the curative effects of dietary protein and proposed that pellagra was caused by a lack of specific amino acids (see Terris). Now it is known that pellagra may result from a deficiency of either nicotinic acid or tryptophan, the amino acid precursor of nicotinic acid. One milligram of nicotinic acid is formed from 60 mg of tryptophan, a process for which pyridoxine is essential. This explains the frequent occurrence of pellagra in persons who subsist mainly on corn, which contains only small amounts of tryptophan and niacin—some of the niacin being in bound form and unavailable for absorption.

It should be pointed out that in experimental subjects, only the cutaneous-gastrointestinal-neurasthenic manifestations of pellagra have been produced by the feeding of tryptophan- or niacin-deficient diets; neurologic abnormalities were not produced by these diets (Goldsmith). As a corollary, only the dermal, gastrointestinal, and neurasthenic manifestations respond to treatment with niacin and tryptophan; neurologic disturbances in pellagrins have proved to be recalcitrant to prolonged treatment with nicotinic acid, although the peripheral nerve disorder may subsequently respond to treatment with thiamine. In monkeys, degeneration of peripheral nerves as well as the unique cerebrocortical changes of pellagra were induced by a deficiency of pyridoxine (Victor and Adams, 1956). Swank and Adams described degeneration of the peripheral nerves in pyridoxine- and pantothenic acid–deficient swine, and Vilter and colleagues produced polyneuropathy in human subjects rendered pyridoxine-deficient; these subjects also showed seborrheic dermatitis and glossitis (indistinguishable from that of niacin deficiency) and the cheilosis and angular stomatitis that are usually attributed to riboflavin deficiency. The foregoing observations indicate that certain lingual and cutaneous manifestations of pellagra may be produced by a deficiency of pyridoxine or other B vitamins and that the neurologic manifestations of pellagra are most likely due to pyridoxine deficiency.

In the special case of Hartnup disease, a niacin deficiency is believed to result from the high excretion of indicans and indole metabolites (see page 1009).

Nutritional Spinal Spastic and Ataxic Syndrome This syndrome is observed occasionally in nutritionally depleted alcoholics. The main clinical signs are spastic weakness of the legs, with absent abdominal and increased tendon reflexes, clonus, extensor plantar responses, and a loss of position and vibratory senses. In our experience, this syndrome is usually associated with other nutritional disorders, such as Wernicke disease and peripheral and optic neuropathy. In prisoner-of-war camps, the "spastic syndrome" was observed in association with mental and emotional changes and dimness of vision, and at times with widespread muscular rigidity, confusion, coma, and death. The latter syndrome has never been studied pathologically, so that it is impossible to state whether the lesions are the same as or different from those of pellagra.

The syndromes of tropical spastic paraparesis and of lathyrism, another form of spastic paraplegia that is common in India and certain parts of Africa, were for many years suspected of being nutritional in origin but are now known to be due to a virus and to a toxin, respectively. These and other types of tropical spastic paraplegia are discussed in greater detail with the spinal cord diseases (Chap. 44). A chronic tropical disease of the peripheral nerves, designated as "ataxic neuropathy of Nigeria," has been attributed to the ingestion of inadequately detoxified cassava (Osuntokun).

Nicotinic Acid Deficiency Encephalopathy Under this title, Jolliffe and coworkers, in 1940, described an acute cerebral syndrome in alcoholic patients consisting of clouding of consciousness, progressing to extrapyramidal rigidity and tremors ("cogwheel" rigidity) of the extremities, uncontrollable grasping and sucking reflexes, and coma. Most of their patients showed overt manifestations of nutritional deficiency, such as Wernicke disease, pellagra, scurvy, and polyneuropathy. These authors concluded that the encephalopathy represented an acute form of nicotinic acid deficiency, since most of their patients recovered when treated with a diet of low vitamin B content supplemented by intravenous glucose and saline and large doses of nicotinic acid. Sydenstricker and colleagues (1938) had previously reported the salutary effects of nicotinic acid on the unresponsive state observed in elderly undernourished patients, and Spillane (1947) described a similar syndrome and response to nicotinic acid in the indigent Arab population of the Middle East.

The status of this syndrome and its relation to pellagra are uncertain. The clinical, nutritional, and pathologic features were never delineated precisely. Serdaru and associates reported 22 presumed examples of this syndrome in the alcoholic population of the Salpêtrière clinic in Paris, all reviewed retrospectively after the finding, in postmortem material, of pellagra-like changes in nerve cells. Prominent were confusional states, oppositional rigidity (gegenhalten), ataxia, and polymyoclonia—a picture somewhat like that described by Jolliffe and coworkers (above). Skin lesions were absent. We have not encountered identical cases among the undernourished patients in the alcoholic populations of Boston and Cleveland.

Syndrome of Amblyopia, Painful Neuropathy, and Orogenital Dermatitis ("Strachan Syndrome")

There remains to be considered a neurologic syndrome that almost certainly is nutritional in origin but does not conform clinically to beriberi and pellagra, the classic deficiency diseases. This syndrome was originally observed by Strachan in 1897 among Jamaican sugar cane workers. The main symptoms in his patients were pain, numbness, and paresthesias of the extremities; objectively there was ataxia of gait, weakness, wasting, and loss of deep tendon reflexes and sensation in the limbs. Dimness of vision and impairment of hearing were common findings, as were soreness and excoriation of the mucocutaneous junctions of the mouth. This disorder, originally known as "Jamaican neuritis," was quickly recognized in other parts of the world, particularly in the undernourished populations of tropical countries. Subsequently, many cases of this syndrome were observed in the besieged population of Madrid during the Spanish Civil War and during World War II among prisoners of war in North Africa and the Far East.

As indicated earlier, a massive outbreak of a similar disorder, affecting more than 50,000 persons, occurred in Cuba from late 1991 through 1993. The association of this epidemic with widespread dietary deprivation and the salutary response of both optic and peripheral nerve symptoms to treatment with B vitamins suggests a nutritional causation (see *Morbidity and Mortality Weekly Report* and the report of the Cuba Neuropathy Field Investigation Team, cited in the References). Shortly thereafter, Plant and colleagues reported on a similar outbreak of optic and peripheral neuropathy from Tanzania.

The clinical descriptions from these varied sources are not entirely uniform, but certain features are common to all of them, and others occur with sufficient frequency to allow the delineation of a neurologic syndrome and its identification with the one described by Strachan. The core disorder is an affection of the peripheral and optic nerves. The former consists mainly of sensory symptoms and signs, and the latter is characterized by the subacute evolution of failing vision, which, if untreated, may go on to complete blindness and pallor of the optic discs. Deafness and vertigo are generally uncommon, but in some outbreaks among prisoners of war these symptoms were frequent enough to earn the epithet "camp dizziness." In all these respects the syndrome differs from beriberi. Along with the neurologic signs there may be varying degrees of stomatoglossitis, corneal degeneration, and genital dermatitis (the orogenital syndrome). These mucocutaneous lesions are unlike those of pellagra.

There have been only a few neuropathologic studies of this syndrome. Aside from the changes in the papillomacular bundle of the optic nerve, the most consistent abnormality has been a loss of medullated fibers in each column of Goll adjacent to the midline. Fisher has interpreted this change to indicate a degeneration of the central processes of the bipolar sensory neurons of the dorsal root ganglia. The fact that the primary sensory neuron is the main site of the neuropathic disorder is consistent with the predominantly sensory symptomatology. The present authors find it difficult to draw a sharp dividing line between the nutritional peripheral (and optic) neuropathy and the Strachan syndrome.

The Neurologic Manifestations of Vitamin B_{12} Deficiency

The spinal cord, brain, optic nerves, and peripheral nerves may all be affected by vitamin B_{12} (cobalamin) deficiency. The spinal cord is usually affected first and often exclusively. The term *subacute combined degeneration* (SCD) is customarily reserved for the spinal cord lesion of vitamin B_{12} deficiency and serves to distinguish it from other types of spinal cord disease that happen to involve the posterior and lateral columns (loosely referred to as *combined system disease*). Whether the peripheral neuropathy is a primary component of the disease or is secondary to damage of the fibers of entry or exit in the cord has been debated, but the available pathologic evidence favors the former.

The hematologic effects of vitamin B_{12} deficiency—i.e., *pernicious anemia*—and its neurologic manifestations are distinctive insofar as they result not from a dietary lack of vitamin B_{12} but from the failure to transfer minute amounts of this nutrient across the intestinal mucosa—"starvation in the midst of plenty," as Castle aptly put it. This failure derives from the chronic absence of an intrinsic factor, which is secreted (along with hydrochloric acid) by the parietal cells of the gastric mucosa and which transports cobalamin (extrinsic factor in the diet) to the ileum, where it is absorbed into the portal system. This is referred to as a *conditioned deficiency*, since it is conditional upon the lack of an intrinsic factor.

The hematologic and neurologic manifestations of vitamin B_{12} deficiency occasionally complicate other malabsorptive disorders: celiac sprue; extensive gastric or ileal resections; overgrowth of intestinal bacteria in "blind loops," anastomoses, diverticula, and other conditions resulting in intestinal stasis; and infestation with cobalamin-metabolizing fish tapeworm (*Diphyllobothrium latum*). Rare instances of vitamin B_{12} deficiency are observed in lactovegetarians, in infants nursed by mothers deficient in vitamin B_{12}, and as a result of nitrous oxide poisoning. Finally, vitamin B_{12} deficiency may be due to a rare genetic defect of methylmalonyl coenzyme A (CoA) mutase (Table 41-2).

Clinical Manifestations Symptoms of nervous system disease occur in the majority of patients with pernicious anemia. The patient first notices general weakness and paresthesias consisting of tingling, "pins and needles" feelings, or other vaguely described sensations. The paresthesias involve the hands and feet, more often the former, and tend to be constant and steadily progressive and the source of much distress. As the illness progresses, the gait becomes unsteady and stiffness and weakness of the limbs, especially of the legs,

Table 41-2
Vitamin-responsive inherited disorders affecting the nervous system

Vitamin	*Disorder*	*Therapeutic dose*	*Enzymatic defect*	*Neurologic manifestations*
Thiamine (B_1)	Branched-chain keto-aciduria	5–20 mg	Branched-chain keto acid decarboxylase	Lethargy, coma
	Lactic acidosis	5–20 mg	Pyruvate carboxylase	Mental retardation
	Pyruvic acidemia	5–20 mg	Pyruvate dehydrogenase	Cerebellar ataxia
	Anemia	50 mg	—	Same as thiamine-deficient beriberi of infancy and childhood
Pyridoxine (B_6)	Homocystinuria	>25 mg	Cystathionine synthase	Mental retardation, cerebrovascular accidents, psychoses
	Infantile convulsions	10–50 mg	Glutamic acid decarboxylase	Seizures
	Xanthurenic aciduria	5–10 mg	Kynureninase	Mental retardation
Cobalamin (B_{12})	Methylmalonic aciduria	1000 g	Methylmalonyl CoA mutase apoenzyme	Lethargy, coma, psychomotor retardation
	Methylmalonic aciduria and homocystinuria	> 500 g	Defects in synthesis of adenosylcobalamin and methylcobalamin	Developmental arrest, cerebellar ataxia
Folic acid	Megaloblastic anemia	<0.05 mg	Folate deficiency	Mental retardation
	Formiminotransferase deficiency	>5 mg	Intestinal malabsorption of formiminotransferase	Mental retardation
	Homocystinuria and hypomethioninemia	>10 mg	N^5, N^{10}-Methylenetetrahydrofolate reductase	Schizophrenic syndrome
Biotin	β-Methylcrotonylglycinuria	↑ 5–10 mg	β-Methylcrotonyl CoA carboxylase	Mental retardation
	Propionic acidemia	↑ 5–10 mg	Propionyl CoA carboxylase	Lethargy, coma
Nicotinamide	Hartnup disease	>400 mg	Intestinal malabsorption of tryptophan	Cerebellar ataxia

Source: Adapted from Rosenberg and from Matsui et al, by permission.

develop. If the disease remains untreated, an ataxic paraplegia evolves, with variable degrees of spasticity and contracture.

Early in the course of the illness, when only paresthesias are present, there may be no objective signs. Later, examination discloses a disorder of the posterior and lateral columns of the spinal cord, predominantly of the former. Loss of vibration sense is by far the most consistent sign; it is more pronounced in the feet and legs than in the hands and arms and frequently extends over the trunk. Position sense is usually impaired as well. The motor signs, usually limited to the legs, include a mild symmetrical loss of strength in proximal limb muscles, spasticity, changes in tendon reflexes, clonus, and extensor plantar responses. At first the patellar and Achilles reflexes are found to be diminished as frequently as they are increased, and they may even be absent. With treatment the reflexes may return to normal or become hyperactive. The gait at first is predominantly ataxic, later ataxic and spastic.

Loss of superficial sensation below a segmental level on the trunk may occur in isolated instances, implicating the spinothalamic tracts, but such a finding should always suggest the possibility of some other disease of the spinal cord. The defect of cutaneous sensation may take the form of impaired tactile, pain, and thermal sensation over the limbs in a distal distribution, implicating the peripheral nerves, but such findings are also relatively uncommon. The Lhermitte phenomenon (paresthesias down the spine or across the shoulders induced by rapid flexion of the neck) is a not uncommon finding if sought.

The nervous system involvement in subacute combined degeneration is roughly symmetrical, and sensory disturbances precede the motor ones; predominantly motor involvement from the beginning and a definite asymmetry of motor or sensory findings maintained over a period of weeks or months should always cast doubt on the diagnosis.

Mental signs are frequent, ranging from irritability, apathy, somnolence, suspiciousness, and emotional instability to a marked confusional or depressive psychosis or intellectual deterioration. Lindenbaum and coworkers have reported cases in which neuropsychiatric symptoms, responsive to vitamin B_{12}, were present without spinal cord or peripheral nerve abnormalities. In our clinical material, symptoms of dementia have not been frequent and always followed the spinal cord disorder. *Visual impairment* due to optic neuropathy may occasionally be the earliest or sole manifestation of pernicious anemia; examination discloses roughly symmetrical centrocecal scotomata and optic atrophy in the most advanced cases (page 263). The fact that visual evoked potentials may be abnormal in vitamin B_{12}-deficient patients without clinical signs of visual impairment suggests that the visual pathways may be affected more often than is evident from the neurologic examination alone. A small number of patients have symptoms of autonomic dysfunction, including urinary sphincteric symptoms and impotence.

The CSF is usually normal; in some cases there is a moderate increase in protein. The EMG shows slowing of sensory conduction or reduced-amplitude sensory potentials. Almost always, according to Hemmer and colleagues, somatosensory evoked potentials show delayed conduction or absent responses; these changes are known to recover with treatment. Quite remarkable, as these authors report, is the finding on MRI of a T2 signal change that demarcates the posterior columns of the cord (Fig. 41-1).

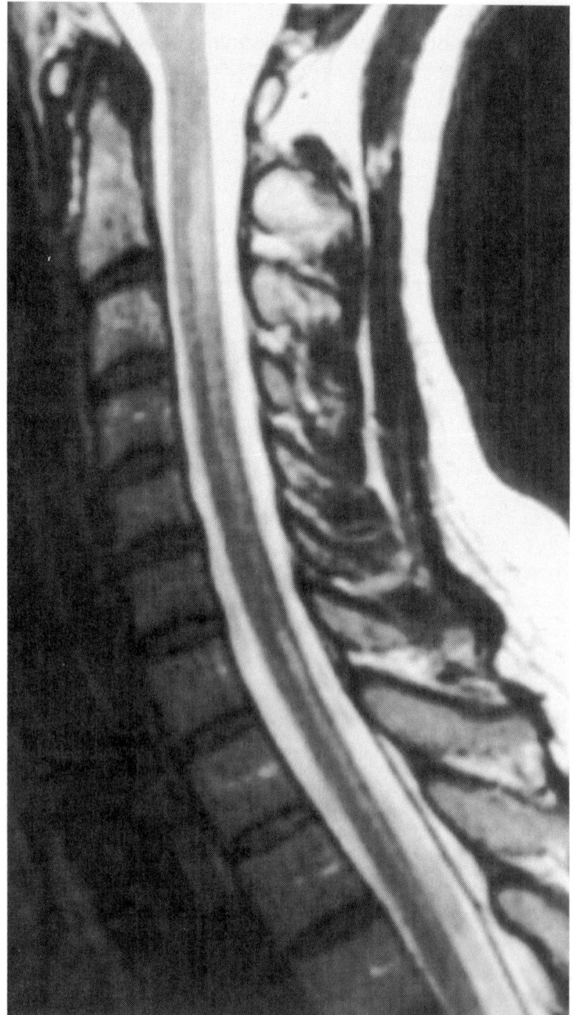

Figure 41-1

Sagittal spinal MRI, T2-weighted image in subacute combined degeneration showing signal changes in the posterior columns. The patient had markedly reduced vibration and position sense and a Romberg sign; the tendon reflexes were preserved and there were no corticospinal tract or peripheral nerve signs. (Courtesy of Dr. James Corbett.)

Neuropathologic Changes The pathologic process takes the form of a diffuse though uneven degeneration of white matter of the spinal cord and occasionally of the brain. The earliest histologic event is a swelling of myelin sheaths, characterized by the formation of intramyelinic vacuoles and separation of myelin lamellae. This is followed by a coalescence of small foci of tissue destruction into larger ones, imparting a vacuolated, sieve-like appearance to the tissue—an appearance also observed commonly in the myelopathy of AIDS and rarely in lupus erythematosus. The myelin sheaths and axis cylinders are both involved in the degenerative process, the former more obviously and perhaps earlier than the latter. There is relatively little fibrous gliosis in the early lesions, but in more chronic ones, particularly those in which considerable tissue is destroyed, the gliosis is pronounced. The changes begin in the posterior columns of the lower cervical and upper thoracic segments of the cord and spread from this region up and down the cord as well as forward into the lateral and anterior columns. The lesions are not limited to specific systems of fibers within the posterior and lateral funiculi but are scattered irregularly through the white matter. For this reason, the term *combined system disease*, which is often used loosely to designate the myelopathy of pernicious anemia, is a less appropriate term than *subacute combined degeneration*.

In rare instances, foci of spongy degeneration are found in the optic nerves and chiasm and in the central white matter of the brain (Adams and Kubik). The peripheral nerves may show a loss of myelin, but there is no unequivocal evidence that axis cylinders are significantly affected.

It has been shown that monkeys who are sustained on a vitamin B_{12}–deficient diet for a prolonged period develop neuropathologic changes indistinguishable from those of subacute combined degeneration in humans (Agamanolis et al). The time required for the production of central nervous system changes in monkeys—33 to 45 months—is comparable to the time required to deplete the vitamin B_{12} stores of patients with pernicious anemia in whom parenteral vitamin B_{12} therapy had been discontinued. It is noteworthy that vitamin B_{12}–deprived monkeys do not become anemic, despite the prolonged period of vitamin B_{12} deficiency. Also, in distinction to the human condition, involvement of the optic nerves is particularly severe in the monkey and probably precedes the degeneration of the spinal cord. The optic nerve lesion appears first in the papillomacular bundles, in the retrobulbar portions of the nerves; it subsequently spreads beyond the confines of this bundle and caudally in the optic nerves, chiasm, and tracts. These changes are much the same as those of "tobacco-alcohol amblyopia" (see above). The peripheral nerves were not affected in the experimentally produced vitamin B_{12} deficiency.

The paresthesias, impairment of deep sensation, and ataxia are due to lesions in the posterior columns, and these may also account for the loss of tendon reflexes. Weakness, spasticity, increased tendon reflexes, and Babinski signs depend on involvement of the corticospinal tracts. The spinothalamic tracts may be involved in the pathologic process, which explains the occasional finding of a sensory level for pain and temperature on the trunk. The distal and symmetrical impairment of superficial sensation and loss of tendon reflexes that occur in some patients are best explained by involvement of peripheral nerves and are reflected in nerve conduction studies (see further on, under "Diagnosis").

Pathogenesis *Methylcobalamin* is an essential cofactor in the conversion of homocysteine to methionine. An impairment of this reaction due to a deficiency of cobalamin is thought to cause a failure of DNA synthesis, accounting for the hematologic abnormalities and particularly for the production of megaloblasts. However, since neurons do not divide, this sequence of chemical events does not explain the central nervous system abnormalities. One of the better-understood functions of vitamin B_{12} is its role as a coenzyme in the methylmalonyl CoA–mutase reaction. In this reaction, which is a key step in propionate metabolism, methylmalonyl CoA is transformed to succinyl CoA, which subsequently enters the Krebs cycle. A lack or failure of the cobalamin-dependent enzyme methylmalonyl CoA mutase leads to the accumulation of methylmalonyl CoA and its precursor, propionyl CoA. According to this theory, propionyl CoA displaces succinyl CoA, which is the usual primer for the synthesis of even-chain fatty acids and results in the anomalous insertion of odd-chain fatty acids into membrane lipids, such as are found in myelin sheaths. Conceivably this biochemical abnormality underlies the lesions of myelinated fibers that characterize this disease. However, Carmel and associates have described a hereditary form of cobalamin deficiency in which the methylmalonyl CoA mutase activity was normal, despite the presence of typical neurologic abnormalities. In their view, the primary failure is one of methylation of homocysteine to methionine, i.e., a failure of the methionine synthetase reaction, for which the coenzyme methylcobalamin is necessary.

Evidence for the latter view comes also from the observations that prolonged administration of nitrous oxide (N_2O) may produce not only megaloblastic changes in the marrow (Amess et al) but also a sensorimotor polyneuropathy, often combined with signs of involvement of the posterior and lateral columns of the spinal cord (Layzer). Probably N_2O produces its effects by inactivating the methylcobalamin-dependent enzyme methionine synthetase. These and other hypotheses are discussed by Jandl, Carmel and colleagues, and Beck.

The role of *folate deficiency* in the genesis of SCD is even less certain. One mistake has been to treat pernicious anemia by giving folic acid; this corrects the anemia but may worsen or even evoke the spinal cord lesions. There are, nevertheless, a few reported examples of cerebral and spinal cord lesions indistinguishable from those due to vitamin B_{12} deficiency in patients with defective folate metabolism—both in adults with acquired deficiency (Pincus) and in children with an inborn metabolic error (Clayton et al).

Diagnosis The main differential diagnostic considerations are cervical spondylosis (page 1322), multiple sclerosis of the cervical cord (page 963), rarities such as the female carrier state of adrenoleukodystrophy (adrenomyeloneuropathy, page 1035), and combined system disease (page 1328). The chief obstacle to *early diagnosis* is the lack of parallelism that may exist between the hematologic and neurologic signs, occurring particularly in patients who have taken dietary or medicinal folate. Anemia may be absent, sometimes for many months, in patients who have not taken folate. In a retrospective study of 141 patients with neuropsychiatric abnormalities due to cobalamin deficiency, there were 19 patients in whom both the hematocrit and mean cell volume were normal (Lindenbaum et al); in these patients, subtle morphologic abnormalities—hypersegmented polymorphonuclear leukocytes and megaloblastosis in bone marrow smears—were almost always found if carefully sought.

Achlorhydria is almost invariably present in patients with pernicious anemia; its presence can be detected by measuring the serum gastrin level. Antibodies to gastric parietal cells are also present in as many as 90 percent of patients with cobalamin deficiency, but this test often yields false-positive results. The finding of serum antibodies against intrinsic factor is diagnostically specific, but unfortunately they are found in only 60 percent of cases.

Serum cobalamin should be measured whenever the diagnosis of vitamin B_{12} deficiency is in question. Microbiologic assay (using *Euglena gracilis*) is the most accurate way to measure vitamin B_{12}, but the method is time-consuming and cumbersome and has been largely replaced by a commercial radioisotope dilution assay (the inexpensive chemiluminescence assay is slightly less dependable). With the radioassay, serum levels of less than 100 pg/mL are usually associated with neurologic symptoms and signs of vitamin B_{12} deficiency. Levels below 200 pg/mL unassociated with symptoms call for further investigation of cobalamin deficiency. Even serum levels of 200 to 300 pg/mL may be associated (in 5 to 10 percent of cases) with cobalamin deficiency. It must be emphasized that the serum cobalamin level is not a measure of total body cobalamin. In a patient who stops absorbing ingested cobalamin, the serum levels may long remain in the normal range despite decreasing tissue reserves. In patients who have received vitamin B_{12} parenterally, the two-stage Schilling test is a reliable indicator of cobalamin deficiency, since it uncovers a defect in absorption of the vitamin. Low cobalamin levels with or without the clinical signs of deficiency may occur in patients with atrophic gastritis or after subtotal gastrectomy. The malabsorption in such cases is thought to be due to a failure to extract cobalamin from food rather than a failure of the intrinsic-factor mechanism ("food-cobalamin malabsorption"); since the absorption of free cobalamin is normal, the Schilling test is unimpaired (Carmel). High serum concentrations of cobalamin metabolites—methylmalonic acid (normal range, 73 to 271 nmol/L) and homocysteine (normal range 5.4 to 16.2 mmol/L) are probably the most reliable indicators of an intracellular cobalamin deficiency and can be used to establish the diagnosis (Allen et al; Lindenbaum et al).

Nerve conduction tests have varied in vitamin B_{12}–deficient patients. Early in the course of SCD, nerve conduction may be normal, but in our experience most patients with neurologic symptoms have slowing of distal sensory conduction; others have found reduced amplitudes and minor signs of denervation, suggestive of axonal change. In patients with normal peripheral nerve studies, the somatosensory evoked potentials show abnormalities that are attributable to central conduction delays, implicating the posterior columns as the cause of the sensory symptoms (Fine and Hallett). In advanced cases, motor conduction and late responses may be affected to a slight degree. These ambiguities reflect the inconsistent and poorly understood role of the peripheral neuropathic component in this disease.

Treatment The diagnosis of subacute combined degeneration demands the administration of vitamin B_{12} and the continuation of treatment for the rest of the patient's lifetime. Initially the patient should be given 1000 mg of cyanocobalamin or hydroxycobalamin intramuscularly each day. Thereafter this dose is repeated weekly for a month and then monthly for the remainder of the patient's life. Although most of the injected cobalamin is excreted, these patients must be flooded with the vitamin, because the repletion of cobalamin stores is a direct function of the dose.

The most important factor influencing the response to treatment is the duration of symptoms before treatment is begun; age, sex, and the degree of anemia are relatively unimportant factors. The greatest improvement occurs in those patients whose disturbance of gait has been present for less than 3 months, and recovery may be complete if therapy is instituted within a few weeks after the onset of symptoms. In practically all instances, there is some degree of improvement after treatment, although sometimes, in cases of longest duration, the best that can be accomplished is an arrest of progression. All neurologic symptoms and signs may improve, mostly during the first 3 to 6 months of therapy, and then, at a slower tempo, during the ensuing year or even longer.

Other Neurologic Disorders due to B Vitamin Deficiencies

Pyridoxine (Vitamin B_6) Deficiency A special type of nutritional polyneuropathy is encountered in tuberculous patients as a complication of treatment with isonicotinic acid hydrazide (INH; isoniazid). In the recent past, a similar neuropathy was observed in hypertensive patients treated with hydralazine.

The occurrence of a neuropathy due to INH was recognized in the early 1950s, soon after the introduction of this drug for the treatment of tuberculosis. The neuropathy was characterized by paresthesias and burning pain of the feet and legs, followed by weakness of these parts and loss of ankle reflexes. Rarely, with continued use of the drug, the hands were affected as well. The nature of INH-induced neuropathy was clarified by Biehl and Vilter. They found that the administration of isoniazid results in a marked excretion of pyridoxine, and that the administration of pyridoxine in conjunction with INH prevents the development of neuropathy. As a result of this simple preventive measure, very few examples of INH-induced neuropathy are now observed. Hydralazine, closely related in structure to INH, causes the formation of pyridoxal-isoniazid complexes (hydrazones), which makes pyridoxal (the main form of vitamin B_6) unavailable to the tissues. The neuropathy responds favorably to discontinuation of the drug and the administration of pyridoxine.

Pyridoxine deficiency in animals and humans also causes *seizures*. This was first observed in swine by Swank and Adams and later in infants who were maintained on a milk formula lacking in pyridoxine.

Paradoxically, the *consumption of large amounts of pyridoxine* (by food and vitamin faddists) may also cause a *peripheral neuropathy* (Schaumburg et al; Albin et al). There is no weakness; the symptoms, including ataxia, are purely sensory and can be quite disabling. Improvement is the rule when the drug is withdrawn. This disorder is probably due to the direct toxic effect of pyridoxine on dorsal root ganglion cells.

Pantothenic Acid Deficiency A predominantly sensory neuropathy has also been induced, again in swine, by Swank and Adams and later in humans by a deficiency of pantothenic acid (a constituent of coenzyme A), as reported by Bean et al. In some patients the administration of pantothenic acid has allegedly reversed the painful dysesthesias of the "burning foot" syndrome.

Riboflavin Deficiency Whether or not riboflavin deficiency leads to neurologic symptoms has been controversial. In the past, there were claims that glossitis, cheilosis, and neuropathy were due to riboflavin deficiency, but its effects were never isolated. Antozzi and coworkers have reported that a metabolic disorder similar to the Reye syndrome can be caused by riboflavin deficiency and corrected by administration of riboflavin alone. The affected infants were hypoglycemic, hypotonic, and episodically weak and unresponsive. Antozzi and colleagues also recorded instances of disease in older children and adults manifesting as a lipid storage polymyopathy due to either a deficiency or malabsorption of riboflavin. Presumably a disorder of flavin metabolism caused an impairment of both beta oxidation of fatty acids and respiratory chain I and II complexes. Serum creatine phosphate was normal in these individuals, but carnitine was reduced. The oral administration of 200 mg of riboflavin and 4 g of carnitine per day relieved the symptoms. We have had no experience with such cases.

In summary, polyneuropathy may be caused by a deficiency of at least four B vitamins—thiamine, pyridoxine, pantothenic acid, and vitamin B_{12}. That a deficiency of riboflavin causes lesions of the central or peripheral nervous system has not been proved. Despite the frequency of folic acid deficiency and its hematologic effects, its role in the pathogenesis of nervous system disease has not been established beyond doubt (see reviews by Crellin et al and by Carney).

The polyneuropathy that occasionally complicates the chronic administration of phenytoin has been attributed, on uncertain grounds, to folate deficiency. Botez and colleagues have described a group of 10 patients with sensorimotor polyneuropathy (4 also had spinal cord disease) presumably due to intestinal malabsorption; all of the patients improved over several months while receiving large doses of folic acid. This experience is unique, however. The possible role of folate deficiency in the pathogenesis of spinal cord disease has been mentioned above in relation to vitamin B_{12} deficiency, and its putative role in psychiatric disease has been discussed by Carney.

Disorders Due to Deficiencies of Fat-Soluble Vitamins

Vitamin E Deficiency A rare neurologic disorder of childhood, consisting essentially of spinocerebellar degeneration in association with polyneuropathy and pigmentary retinopathy, has been attributed to a deficiency of vitamin E consequent upon prolonged intestinal fat malabsorption (Muller et al; Satya-Murti et al). The same mechanism has been proposed to explain the neurologic disorders that sometimes complicate abetalipoproteinemia (page 1021), fibrocystic disease (Sokol et al), celiac-sprue disease (page 1198), and extensive intestinal resections (Harding et al). Vitamin E deficiency has also been observed in young children with chronic cholestatic hepatobiliary disease (Rosenblum et al). Ataxia, loss of tendon reflexes, ophthalmoparesis, proximal muscle weakness with elevated serum creatine kinase, and decreased sensation are the usual manifestations. These symptoms are referable to parts of the nervous system and musculature that are found to be diseased in animals deprived of vitamin E—degeneration of Clark's columns, spinocerebellar tracts, posterior columns, nuclei of Goll and Burdach, and sensory roots (Nelson et al). Local differences in the natural concentration of vitamin E in various parts of the nervous system and musculature may account for the distribution of the lesions. In affected children, neurologic function improves after long-term daily supplementation with high doses of vitamin E.

In recent years there have been several reports of an inherited form of spinocerebellar degeneration attributable to vitamin E deficiency ("familial isolated vitamin E deficiency"). In these patients, absorption and transport of vitamin E to the liver is normal, but hepatic incorporation of α-tocopherol (the active form of vitamin E) into very low density lipoproteins is defective (Traber et al). The α-tocopherol transfer protein, which normally is needed for this transport, is thought to be abnormal in these patients and the cause of spinocerebellar disease. The abnormality has been traced to a mutation in the gene for the α-tocopherol transfer protein, located on chromosome 8q (Gotoda et al). In a sense this is a vitamin deficiency conditioned by genetic mutation.

Vitamins A and D Disorders due to a lack or excess of these fat-soluble vitamins are seen occasionally. Vitamin A deficiency sometimes occurs with malabsorption syndromes, causing impairment of vision. Excess of vitamin A in children may result in the syndrome of *pseudotumor cerebri* (page 667). Vitamin D deficiency is usually associated with hypoparathyroidism or a malabsorption state and leads to proximal muscle weakness and rickets.

DISEASES OF THE NERVOUS SYSTEM OF PROBABLE BUT UNPROVEN NUTRITIONAL ORIGIN

The disorders comprised by this category, as the above title indicates, have only an uncertain causal relationship to nutritional deficiency. They are found mainly in alcoholics, but their relationship to alcohol is probably not fundamental, since each of them has also been observed in nonalcoholic patients. The belief that these disorders are nutritional in origin is based on certain indirect evidence: (1) Usually a prolonged period of undernutrition, associated with a significant loss of weight, precedes the neurologic illness. In such cases as are associated with alcoholism, the amount of alcohol consumed need not be large, but the dietary deprivation is always severe. (2) Examination at the onset of the illness frequently discloses general physical evidence of undernutrition as well as the presence of neurologic disorders of known nutritional etiology. (3) Certain attributes of the neuropathologic changes—namely their subacute evolution, symmetry, and constancy of localization—are precisely the features that characterize neurologic disorders of known nutritional etiology. (4) The same syndromes are observed occasionally in nonalcoholics under conditions of dietary depletion. (5) There is at least a partial response to correction of the nutritional impairment.

"Alcoholic" Cerebellar Degeneration

This term refers to a common and uniform type of cerebellar degeneration in alcoholics. Its incidence is about twice that of Wernicke disease, but, unlike the latter, it is considerably more frequent in men than in women. It is characterized clinically by a wide-based stance and gait, varying degrees of instability of the trunk, and ataxia of the legs, the arms being affected to a lesser extent and often not at all. Nystagmus and dysarthria are infrequent signs. In addition to an ataxic (intention) tremor, there may be a tremor of the fingers or hands resembling one of the two types of parkinsonian tremor but appearing only when the limbs are placed in certain sustained postures. Mauritz and coworkers have demonstrated that the instability of the trunk in these cases consists of a specific 3-Hz rhythmic swaying in the anteroposterior direction; by contrast, patients with lesions of the cerebellar hemispheres show only slight postural instability without directional preponderance.

In most cases, the cerebellar syndrome evolves over a period of several weeks or months, after which it remains unchanged for many years. In others, it develops more rapidly or more slowly, but in these cases also the disease eventually stabilizes. Occasionally, the cerebellar disorder progresses in a saltatory manner, the symptoms worsening in relation to a severe infectious illness or an attack of delirium tremens.

The *pathologic changes* consist of a degeneration of all the neurocellular elements of the cerebellar cortex, but particularly of the Purkinje cells; they are restricted to the anterior and superior aspects of the vermis and, in advanced cases, to the anterior parts of the anterior lobes. The cerebellar atrophy is readily visualized by computed tomography (CT) (Fig. 41-2) and MRI.

Two particular forms of this syndrome have not been emphasized sufficiently. In one, the clinical abnormalities are limited to an instability of station and gait, individual movements of the limbs being unaffected. The pathologic changes in such cases are restricted to the anterosuperior portions of the vermis. A second type is acute and transient in nature. Here, except for their

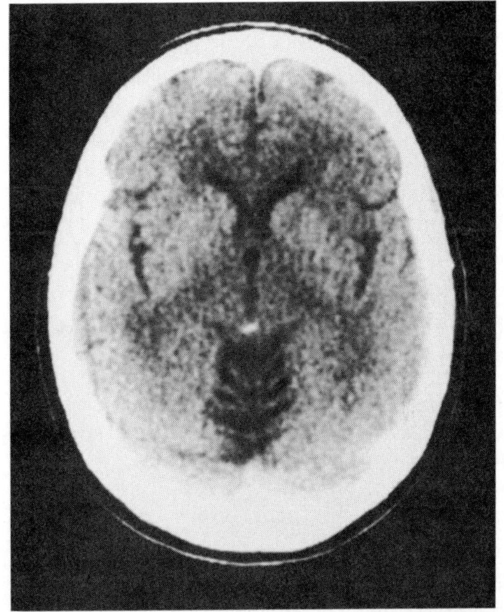

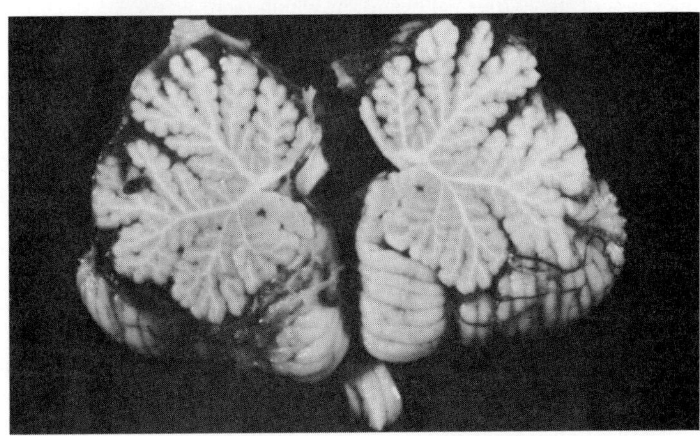

Figure 41-2

CT scan from a 60-year-old alcoholic patient showing prominence of midline cerebellar sulci. A broad-based gait and ataxia of the legs had been present for many years. Death was from myocardial infarction. The cerebellum, cut in the midsagittal plane (below), shows folial atrophy of the anterior-superior vermis, characteristic of alcoholic cerebellar degeneration.

reversibility, the cerebellar symptoms are identical to those that characterize the chronic, fixed form of the disease. In this transient type, the derangement is only one of function ("biochemical lesion") and has probably not progressed to the point of fixed structural changes. These forms of cerebellar disease, and particularly the restricted and reversible varieties, cannot be distinguished from the cerebellar manifestations of Wernicke disease either on pathologic or on clinical grounds. It is our opinion that the cerebellar ataxia of Wernicke disease and that referred to as *alcoholic cerebellar degeneration* represent the same disease process, the former term being applicable when the cerebellar abnormalities are associated with ocular and mental signs and the latter when the cerebellar syndrome stands alone. Alcoholic cerebellar degeneration is in all likelihood due to nutritional deficiency and not to the toxic effects of alcohol or other causes, for reasons already indicated. Insofar as the cerebellar ataxia usually improves to some extent under the influence of thiamine alone (see above, under "Wernicke-Korsakoff Syndrome"), it is likely that a deficiency of this vitamin is responsible for the cerebellar lesion.

Marchiafava-Bignami Disease (Primary Degeneration of the Corpus Callosum)

In 1903, the Italian pathologists Marchiafava and Bignami described a unique alteration of the corpus callosum in three alcoholic patients. In each case, coronal sectioning of the fixed brain disclosed a pink-gray discoloration of the central portion of the corpus callosum throughout the longitudinal extent of this structure. Microscopically, the lesion proved to be confined to the middle lamina (which makes up about two-thirds of the thickness of the corpus callosum), in which there was a loss of myelin with relative preservation of the axis cylinders; macrophages were abundant in the altered zone, and astrocytic proliferation followed. The clinical observations in these patients were few and incomplete. In 1907, Bignami described a case in which the corpus callosum lesion was accompanied by a similar lesion in the central portion of the anterior commissure.

These early reports were followed by a spate of articles that confirmed and amplified the original clinical and pathologic findings. By 1922 about 40 cases of this disorder had been described in the Italian literature (Mingazzini). With one exception, all the reported cases were in males, and all of these men were insatiable drinkers. They drank red wine for the most part but other forms of liquor also. Beginning in 1936, with the report of King and Meehan, the disease came to be recognized throughout the world, and the notions that it had a predilection for drinkers of red wine and a special racial predisposition or geographic restriction were abandoned.

Pathologic Features Marchiafava-Bignami disease is more readily defined by its pathologic than by its clinical features. The principal alteration is in the middle portion of the corpus callosum, which on gross examination appears somewhat rarefied and sunken and reddish or gray-yellow in color, depending on its age. In the anterior portion of the corpus callosum, the lesion tends to be more severe in the midline than in its lateral parts; in the splenium, however, the opposite may pertain. The most chronic lesion takes the form of a centrally placed gray cleft or cavity, with collapse of the surrounding tissue and reduction in thickness of the corpus callosum. Microscopically, corresponding to the gross lesions, one observes clearly demarcated zones of demyelination, with variable involvement of the axis cylinders and an abundance of fatty macrophages with gliosis at the margins. Inflammatory changes are absent.

Infrequently, lesions of a similar nature are found in the central portions of the anterior and posterior commissures and the brachia pontis. These zones of myelin destruction are always surrounded by a rim of intact white matter. The predilection of this disease process for commissural fiber systems has been stressed, but it is certainly not confined to these fibers. Symmetrically placed lesions have been observed in the columns of Goll, superior cerebellar peduncles, and cerebral hemispheres, involving the centrum semiovale and extending, in some cases, into the adjacent convolutional white matter. As a rule, the internal capsule and corona radiata, subcortical arcuate fibers, and cerebellum are spared. In several cases, the lesions of deficiency amblyopia (see above) have been observed, and in others, the lesions of Wernicke disease.

Many of the reported cases, as first pointed out by Jequier and Wildi, have involved cortical lesions of a special type: the neurons in the third layer of the frontal and temporal lobe cortices had disappeared and were replaced by a fibrous gliosis. Morel, who first described this *cortical laminar sclerosis*, did not observe its association with Marchiafava-Bignami disease. However, when Jequier and Adams reviewed his original cases (unpublished), all had Marchiafava-Bignami disease. In a subsequent report by Delay and colleagues comprising 14 cases of cortical laminar sclerosis, the cortical lesion was also consistently associated with a corpus callosum lesion. We believe the cortical lesions to be secondary to the callosal degeneration.

Clinical Features The disease affects persons in middle and late adult life. With few exceptions, the patients have been males and severe chronic alcoholics. The clinical features of the illness are otherwise quite variable, and a clear-cut syndrome of uniform type has not emerged. Many patients have presented in a state of terminal stupor or coma, precluding a detailed neurologic assessment. In others, the clinical picture was dominated by the manifestations of chronic inebriation and alcohol withdrawal—tremor, seizures, hallucinosis, and delirium tremens. In some of these patients, following the subsidence of the withdrawal symptoms, no signs of neurologic disease could be elicited, even in the end stage of the disease, which lasted for several days to weeks. In yet another group, a progressive dementia has been described, evolving slowly over a 3- to 6-year period before death. Emotional disorders leading to acts of violence, marked apathy, moral perversions, and sexual misdemeanors have been noted in these patients; dysarthria, slowing and unsteadiness of movement, transient sphincteric incontinence, hemiparesis, and apractic or aphasic disorders were superimposed. The last stage of the disease is characterized by physical decline, seizures, stupor, and coma. An impressive feature of these varied neurologic deficits in some patients has been their tendency toward remission when nutrition was restored.

In two cases that have come to our attention, the clinical manifestations were essentially those of bilateral frontal lobe disease: motor and mental slowness; apathy; prominent grasping and sucking reflexes; gegenhalten; incontinence; and a slow, hesitant, wide-based gait. In both of these cases, the neurologic abnormalities evolved over a period of about 2 months, and both patients recovered from these symptoms within a few weeks of hospitalization. Death occurred several years later as a result of liver disease and subdural hematoma, respectively. In each case, autopsy disclosed an old lesion typical of Marchiafava-Bignami disease confined to the central portion of the most anterior parts of the corpus callosum, but one had to look closely to see the gray line of gliosis.

In view of the great variability of the clinical picture and the obscuration in many patients of subtle mental and neurologic abnormalities by the effects of chronic inebriation and other alcoholic neurologic disorders, the *diagnosis* of Marchiafava-Bignami disease is understandably difficult. In fact, it is rarely made during life. The occurrence, in a chronic alcoholic, of a frontal lobe syndrome or a symptom complex that points to a diagnosis of frontal or corpus callosum tumor but in whom the symptoms remit should suggest the diagnosis of Marchiafava-Bignami disease. The CT scan and MRI have disclosed some unsuspected instances of this disease (see also Kawamura et al).

Pathogenesis and Etiology Originally, Marchiafava-Bignami disease was attributed to the toxic effects of alcohol, but this is an unlikely explanation in view of the prevalence of alcoholism and the rarity of corpus callosum degeneration. Further, the distinctive callosal lesions have not been observed with other neurotoxins. Very rarely, undoubted examples of Marchiafava-Bignami disease have occurred in abstainers, so that alcohol cannot be an indispensable factor. A nutritional etiology has been invoked, for the reasons given earlier, but the deficient factor has not been defined. The mechanisms involved in the selective necrosis of particular areas of white matter remain to be elucidated. Perhaps, when its mechanism becomes known, Marchiafava-Bignami disease, like central pontine myelinolysis (which it resembles histologically), will have to be considered in a chapter other than one on nutritional disease.

Protein-Calorie Malnutrition (PCM) and Mental Retardation

The reader might gather from the foregoing descriptions that the nervous system is rarely affected by nutritional deficiency except when subjected to the influence of chronic alcoholism, and then the essential problem is one of dietary imbalance—an inadequacy of B vitamins in the face of an adequate or near adequate caloric intake. It is true that the CNS resists the effects of starvation better than other organs. Nonetheless, there is increasing evidence that severe dietary deprivation during critical phases of brain development may result in permanent impairment of cerebral function and in mental retardation. Inasmuch as there are an estimated 100 million children in the world who are undernourished and suffer from varying degrees of protein, calorie, and other dietary inadequacies, this is one of the most pressing problems in medicine and society.

Two overlapping syndromes have been defined in malnourished infants and children: kwashiorkor and marasmus. *Kwashiorkor* is a syndrome of weanling children and is due to protein deficiency; it is manifest by edema (and sometimes ascites), hair changes (sparsity and depigmentation), and stunting of growth. The edema is due to hypoalbuminemia; in addition, there is an abnormal pattern of blood amino acids as well as a fatty liver. Sometimes there are skin changes suggestive of pellagra or riboflavin deficiency. *Marasmus* is characterized by an extreme degree of cachexia and growth failure in early infancy. Infants with marasmus have usually been weaned early or were never breast-fed. Common to both groups of children is an apathy and indifference to the environment combined with irritability when they are handled or moved. The children are underactive; even after an adequate diet has been instituted, their tendency is to follow with the eyes rather than to move. At one stage of early convalescence, some kwashiorkor children pass through a phase of rigidity and tremor for which there has been no explanation.

As a rule, the clinical signs of polyneuropathy or subacute combined degeneration of the cord are lacking in children with PCM. However, electrophysiologic testing may disclose a reduction of motor nerve conduction velocity and abnormalities of sensory conduction (Chopra et al). In children with severe degrees of PCM, it is said that there may be evidence, in sural nerve biopsies, of retarded myelination (persistence of only the small myelinated fibers) and segmental demyelination.

Of great interest is whether the children who are rescued from these states of undernutrition by proper feeding are left with an underdeveloped or damaged brain. This subject has been studied extensively in many species of animals, as well as in humans, by clinical, biochemical, and neuropathologic methods. The literature is too large to review here, but excellent critiques have been provided by Winick, Birch and coworkers, Latham, and Dodge and colleagues.

In contrast to the devastating effect of PCM upon body growth, brain weight is only slightly reduced. Nevertheless, on the basis of experiments in dogs, pigs, and rats, it is evident that prenatal and early postnatal malnutrition retards cellular proliferation in the brain. All cells are affected, including oligodendroglia, with a proportional reduction in myelin. Also, the process of dendritic branching may be retarded by early malnutrition. A limited number of studies in humans suggest that PCM has a similar effect upon the brain during the first 8 months of life. In animals, varying degrees of recovery from the effects of early malnutrition are possible if normal nutrition is reestablished during the vulnerable periods. Presumably this is true for humans as well, although proof is difficult to obtain. In every series of severely undernourished infants and young children who have been observed for a period of many years, a variable proportion has been left scholastically incompetent and mentally backward to a modest degree; the majority recover, however (Galler). Unfortunately, the neurologic and intellectual consequences of PCM have defied accurate assessment because of the difficulty of isolating the effects of severe malnutrition from those of infection, social deprivation, genetic faults, and other factors. The relative importance of these various factors is still under study.

Nutritional Deficiencies Secondary to Diseases of the Gastrointestinal Tract

The vitamins that are known to be essential to the normal functioning of the central and peripheral nervous systems cannot be synthesized by the human organism. Each is ingested as an essential part of the normal diet and absorbed in certain regions of the gastrointestinal tract. Impairment or failure of absorption due to diseases of the gastrointestinal tract gives rise to several malabsorption syndromes. In these diseases, the site of the block in transport from the intestinal lumen varies; it may be at the surface of the enterocytes or at their interface with the lymphatic channels and portal capillaries.

Table 41-3, which is modified from Pallis and Lewis, lists the malabsorptive diseases and their relationships to the intestinal abnormalities. Of all these diseases, celiac sprue (gluten enteropathy) is the most common. The neurologic complications of this disorder, in our experience, have always taken the form of a symmetrical sensory polyneuropathy. However, other complications have been described, notably a progressive cerebellar syndrome with cortical, dentatal, and olivary cell loss (Finelli et al; see also Chap. 40). The cerebellar changes may be coupled with a symmetrical demyelination of the posterior columns, producing a spinocerebellar disorder similar to that of vitamin E deficiency (Cooke and Smith). In the latter case, however, vitamin E supplementation has no consistent effect. Hallert and colleagues have described a high incidence of depression and other psychiatric disturbances in adult patients with celiac sprue. Unexplained seizures are also said to occur.

Polyneuropathy and subacute combined degeneration of the spinal cord manifesting themselves many years after gastrectomy are encountered only rarely.

An important effect of fat malabsorption is a deficiency of vitamin E, which, in turn, may give rise to neurologic symptoms, particularly in young children. This topic is discussed in an earlier part of this chapter.

The neurology of gastrointestinal disease has been reviewed recently by Perkin and Murray-Lyon.

Table 41-3
Mechanisms whereby malabsorption may be related to neurologic disease

Gastrointestinal defect	*Substance malabsorbed*	*Associated neurological disorder*
Localized gastric lesions:		
Pernicious anemia	Vitamin B_{12}	Myelopathy, optic neuropathy, etc.
Congenital lack of intrinsic factor	Vitamin B_{12}	Myelopathy, neuropathy, etc.
Partial gastrectomy	Vitamin B_{12}	Myelopathy, neuropathy, etc.
	Vitamin D	Osteomalacic myopathy
Lesions of small intestine:		
Predominantly proximal	? Water-soluble vitamins	? Hypovitaminosis B
	Vitamin D	? Osteomalacic myopathy
	Folic acid	Probably none
Predominantly distal	Vitamin B_{12}	Neuropathy, myelopathy, etc.
Diffuse		Myoclonus, ataxia, etc.
Bacterial contamination of small bowel (jejunal diverticulosis, blind-loop syndrome, strictures)	Vitamin B_{12}	Neuropathy, myelopathy, etc.
Congenital absorptive defect	"Neutral" amino acids	Hartnup disease
	Tryptophan	"Blue diaper" syndrome
	Methionine	"Oast-house" urine disease
	Folic acid	Mental retardation, seizures, ataxia, choreoathetosis
	Vitamin B_{12}	Neuropathy, myelopathy
Transmucosal transport disorders associated with steatorrhoea:	Fat-soluble vitamins	Xerophthalmia
Endocrine causes		Keratomalacia
Postirradiation		? Osteomalacic myopathy
Drug-induced		
Defective synthesis of chylomicrons with prolonged intestinal malabsorption	Vitamin E (carrier lipoprotein not synthesized in liver)	Bassen-Kornzweig disease spinocerebellar degeneration with polyneuropathy
Infiltration of villous cores	Fats (defective chylomicron release)	Encephalopathy of Whipple disease
Competition for essential nutrients (e.g., fish tapeworm)	Vitamin B_{12}	Neuropathy, myelopathy, etc.

Source: Pallis and Lewis, by permission.

Inherited Vitamin-Responsive Neurologic Diseases (See Also Chap. 37)

Although humans lack the capacity to synthesize essential vitamin molecules, they are nonetheless able to use them in a series of complex chemical reactions involved in intestinal absorption, transport in the plasma, entry into the organelles of many organs, activation of the vitamin into coenzyme, and finally their interaction with certain specific apoenzyme proteins. This compels consideration of another aspect of nutrition wherein one or more of these steps in vitamin utilization may be defective because of a genetic abnormality. Under these circumstances, the signs of vitamin deficiency result not from vitamin deficiency in the diet but from a genetically deranged control mechanism. In some instances the defect is only quantitative, and by loading the organism with a great excess of the vitamin in question the biochemical abnormality can be overcome. The special type of vitamin E deficiency that results from an inherited inability to incorporate the vitamin into lipoproteins also falls into this category—the diseases of which, being of hereditary type, have already been described in Chap. 37, "The Inherited Metabolic Diseases of the Nervous System." Rosenberg has listed the most important of these hereditary vitamin-responsive diseases, which we have simplified for the reader interested in this subject in Table 41-2.

REFERENCES

ADAMS RD, KUBIK CS: Subacute degeneration of the brain in pernicious anemia. *N Engl J Med* 231:2, 1944.

AGAMANOLIS DP, CHESTER EM, VICTOR M, et al: Neuropathology of experimental vitamin B_{12} deficiency in monkeys. *Neurology* 26:905, 1976.

AGAMANOLIS DP, VICTOR M, HARRIS JW, et al: An ultrastructural study of subacute combined degeneration of the spinal cord in vitamin B_{12} deficient rhesus monkeys. *J Neuropathol Exp Neurol* 37:273, 1978.

ALBIN RL, ALBERS JW, GREENBERG HS, et al: Acute sensory neuropathy-neuronopathy from pyridoxine overdosage. *Neurology* 37:1729, 1987.

ALLEN RH, STABLER SP, SAVAGE DG, LINDENBAUM J: Diagnosis of cobalamin deficiencies: I. Usefulness of serum methylmalonic acid and total homocysteine concentrations. *Am J Hematol* 34:90, 1990.

AMESS JAL, BURMAN JF, NANCEKIEVILL DG, MOLLIN DL: Megaloblastic haemopoiesis in patients receiving nitrous oxide. *Lancet* 2:339, 1978.

ANTOZZI C, GARAVAGLIA B, MORA M, et al: Late-onset riboflavin-responsive myopathy with combined multiple acyl coenzyme A dehydrogenase and respiratory chain deficiency. *Neurology* 44:2153, 1994.

BEAN WB, HODGES RE, DAUM KE: Pantothenic acid deficiency induced in human subjects. *J Clin Invest* 34:1073, 1955.

BECK WS: Cobalamin and the nervous system. *N Engl J Med* 318:1752, 1988.

BECK WS: Neuropsychiatric consequences of cobalamin deficiency. *Adv Intern Med* 36:33, 1991.

BEHSE F, BUCHTHAL F: Alcoholic neuropathy: Clinical, electrophysiological, and biopsy findings. *Ann Neurol* 2:95, 1977.

BIEHL JP, VILTER RW: The effect of isoniazid on vitamin B_6 metabolism and its possible significance in producing isoniazid neuritis. *Proc Soc Exp Biol Med* 85:389, 1954.

BIGNAMI A: Sulle alterazione del corpo calloso e della commissura anteriore ritrovate in un alcoolista. *Policlinico* (sez prat) 14:460, 1907.

BIRCH HG, PINEIRO C, ALCADE E, et al: Relation of kwashiorkor in early childhood and intelligence at school age. *Pediatr Res* 5:579, 1971.

BIRCHFIELD RE: Postural hypotension in Wernicke's disease: A manifestation of autonomic nervous system involvement. *Am J Med* 36:404, 1964.

BLASS JP, GIBSON GE: Abnormality of a thiamine-requiring enzyme in patients with Wernicke-Korsakoff syndrome. *N Engl J Med* 297:1367, 1977.

BOMB BS, BEDI HK, BHATNAGAR LK: Post-ischaemic paresthesiae in pellagrins. *J Neurol Neurosurg Psychiatry* 40:265, 1977.

BOTEZ MI, PEYRONNARD J, CHARRON L: Polyneuropathies responsive to folic acid therapy, in Botez MI, Reynolds EH (eds): *Folic Acid in Neurology, Psychiatry, and Internal Medicine*. New York, Raven Press, 1979, pp 401–412.

CARMEL R: Subtle and atypical cobalamin deficiency states. *Am J Hematol* 34:108, 1990.

CARMEL R, WATKINS D, GOODMAN SI, ROSENBLATT DS: Hereditary defect of cobalamin metabolism (cblG mutation) presenting as a neurologic disorder in adulthood. *N Engl J Med* 318:1738, 1988.

CARNEY MWP: Neuropsychiatric disorders associated with nutritional deficiencies. *CNS Drugs* 3:279, 1995.

CARTON H, KAYENBE K, KABEYA, et al: Epidemic spastic paraparesis in Bandundu (Zaire). *J Neurol Neurosurg Psychiatry* 49:620, 1986.

CHOPRA JS, DHAND UK, MEHTA S, et al: Effect of protein calorie malnutrition on peripheral nerves. *Brain* 109:307, 1986.

CLAYTON PT, SMITH I, HARDING B, et al: Subacute combined degeneration of the cord, dementia, and parkinsonism due to an inborn error of metabolism. *J Neurol Neurosurg Psychiatry* 49:920, 1986.

COOKE WT, SMITH WT: Neurological disorders associated with adult coeliac disease. *Brain* 89:683, 1966.

CRELLIN R, BOTTIGLIERI T, REYNOLDS EH: Folate and psychiatric disorder: Clinical potential. *Drugs* 45:623, 1993.

CUBA NEUROPATHY FIELD INVESTIGATION TEAM: Epidemic optic neuropathy in Cuba—Clinical characterization and risk factors. *N Engl J Med* 333:1176, 1995.

DELAY J, BRION S, ESCOUROLLE R, SANCHEZ A: Rapports entre la degenerescence du corps calleux de Marchiafava-Bignami et la sclerose laminaire corticale de Morel. *Encephale* 49:281, 1959.

DENNY-BROWN DE: The neurological aspects of thiamine deficiency. *Fed Proc* 17(suppl 2):35, 1958.

DODGE PR, PRENSKY AL, FEIGIN R: *Nutrition and the Developing Nervous System*. St Louis, Mosby, 1975.

DONNAL JF, HEINZ ER, BURGER PC: MR of reversible thalamic lesions in Wernicke syndrome. *Am J Neuroradiol* 11:893, 1990.

DREYFUS PM, MONIZ R: The quantitative histochemical estimation of transketolase in the nervous system of the rat. *Biochim Biophys Acta* 65:181, 1962.

ELVEHJEM CA, MADDEN RJ, STRONG FM, WOOLLEY DW: Relation of nicotinic acid and nicotinic acid amide to canine black tongue. *J Am Chem Soc* 59:1767, 1937.

FINE EJ, HALLETT M: Neurophysiological study of subacute combined degeneration. *J Neurol Sci* 45:331, 1980.

FINELLI PF, MCENTEE WV, AMBLER M, KESTENBAUM D: Adult celiac disease presenting as cerebellar syndrome. *Neurology* 30:245, 1980.

FISHER CM: Residual neuropathological changes in Canadians held prisoners of war by the Japanese. *Can Serv Med J* 11:157, 1955.

FOWDEN L, GARTON GA, MILLS CF: Metabolic and physiological consequences of trace element deficiency in animals and man. *Philos Trans R Soc Lond [Biol]* 294:1, 1981.

GALLER JR: Malnutrition-A neglected cause of learning failure. *Postgrad Med* 80:225, 1986.

GALLUCCI M, BOZZAO A, SPLENDIANI A, et al: Wernicke encephalopathy: MR findings in five patients. *Am J Neuroradiol* 11:887, 1990.

GHEZ C: Vestibular paresis: A clinical feature of Wernicke's disease. *J Neurol Neurosurg Psychiatry* 32:134, 1969.

GOLDSMITH GA: Niacin-tryptophan relationships in man and niacin requirement. *Am J Clin Nutr* 6:479, 1958.

GOTODA T, ARITA M, ARAI H, et al: Adult-onset spinocerebellar dysfunction caused by a mutation in the gene for the α-tocopherol-transfer protein. *N Engl J Med* 333:1313, 1995.

GREEN R, KINSELLA LJ: Current concepts in the diagnosis of cobalamin deficiency. *Neurology* 45:1435, 1995.

HALLERT C, ASTROM J: Psychic disturbances in adult celiac disease: II. Psychological findings. *Scand J Gastroenterol* 17:21, 1982.

HALLERT C, DEEREFELDT T: Psychic disturbances in adult celiac disease: I. Clinical manifestations. *Scand J Gastroenterol* 17:17, 1982.

HARDING AE, MATHEWS S, JONES S, et al: Spinocerebellar degeneration associated with a selective defect of vitamin E absorption. *N Engl J Med* 313:32, 1985.

HARPER C: The incidence of Wernicke's encephalopathy in Australia—A neuropathological study of 131 cases. *J Neurol Neurosurg Psychiatry* 46:593, 1983.

HAUW J-J, DEBAECQUE C, HAUSSER-HAUW C, SERDARU M: Chromatolysis in alcoholic encephalopathies: Pellagra-like changes in 22 cases. *Brain* 111:843, 1988.

HEMMER B, GLOCKER FX, SCHUMACHER M, et al: Subacute combined degeneration: Clinical, electrophysiologic, and magnetic resonance imaging findings, *J Neurol Neurosurg Psychiatry* 65:822, 1998.

ISHII N, NISHIHARA Y: Pellagra among chronic alcoholics: Clinical and pathological study of 20 necropsy cases. *J Neurol Neurosurg Psychiatry* 44:209, 1981.

JANDL JH: Cobalamin deficiency, in Jandl JH, *Blood: Textbook of Hematology*, 2nd ed. Boston, Little, Brown, 1996, pp 259–270.

JEQUIER M, WILDI E: Le syndrome de Marchiafava-Bignami. *Schweiz Arch Neurol Psychiatr* 77:393, 1956.

JOLLIFFE N, BOWMAN KM, ROSENBLUM LA, FEIN HD: Nicotinic acid deficiency encephalopathy. *JAMA* 114:307, 1940.

KAWAMURA M, SHIOTA J, YAGISHITA T, HIRAYAMA K: Marchiafava-Bignami disease: Computed tomographic scan and magnetic resonance imaging. *Ann Neurol* 18:103, 1985.

KING LS, MEEHAN MC: Primary degeneration of the corpus callosum (Marchiafava's disease). *Arch Neurol Psychiatry* 36:547, 1936.

KOPELMAN MD: Two types of confabulation. *J Neurol Neurosurg Psychiatry* 50:1482, 1987.

LATHAM MC: Protein-calorie malnutrition in children and its relation to psychological development and behavior. *Physiol Rev* 54:541, 1974.

LAYZER RB: Myeloneuropathy after prolonged exposure to nitrous oxide. *Lancet* 2:1227, 1978.

LEVENTHAL CM, BARINGER JR, ARNASON BG, FISHER CM: A case of Marchiafava-Bignami disease with clinical recovery. *Trans Am Neurol Assoc* 90:87, 1965.

LINDENBAUM J, HEALTON EB, SAVAGE DG, et al: Neuropsychiatric disorders caused by cobalamin deficiency in the absence of anemia or macrocytosis. *N Engl J Med* 318:1720, 1988.

MAIR RG, CAPRA C, MCENTEE WJ, ENGEN T: Odor discrimination and memory in Korsakoff's psychosis. *J Exp Psychol* 6:445, 1980.

MANDEL H, BERNAT M, HAZANI A, NAVEH Y: Thiamine-dependent beriberi in the thalamic-reponsive anemia syndrome. *N Engl J Med* 311:836, 1984.

MARCHIAFAVA E, BIGNAMI A: Sopra un alterazione del corpo calloso osservata in soggetti alcoolisti. *Riv Patol Nerv* 8:544, 1903.

MATSUI SM, MAHONEY MJ, ROSENBERG LE: The natural history of inherited methylmalonic acidemias. *N Engl J Med* 308:857, 1983.

MAURITZ KH, DICHGANS J, HUFSCHMIDT A: Quantitative analysis of stance in late cortical cerebellar atrophy of the anterior lobe and other forms of cerebellar ataxia. *Brain* 102:461, 1979.

MINGAZZINI G: *Der Balken*. Berlin, Springer Verlag, 1922.

Morbidity and Mortality Weekly Report (MMWR) 43:183, 189, 1994.

MOREL F: Une forme anatomo-clinique particuliere de l'alcoolisme chronique: Sclerose corticale laminaire alcoolique. *Rev Neurol* 71:280, 1939.

MUKHERJEE AB, SVORONOS S, GHAZANFARI A, et al: Transketolase abnormality in cultured fibroblasts from familial chronic alcoholic men and their male offspring. *J Clin Invest* 79:1039, 1987.

MULLER DPR, LLOYD JK, WOLFF OH: Vitamin E and neurological function. *Lancet* 1:225, 1983.

NELSON JS, FITCH CD, FISHER VW, et al: Progressive neuropathologic lesions in vitamin E deficient rhesus monkey. *J Neuropathol Exp Neurol* 40:166, 1981.

OSUNTOKUN BO: Cassava diet, chronic cyanide intoxication and neuropathy in the Nigerian Africans. *World Rev Nutr Diet* 36:141, 1981.

PALLIS CA, LEWIS PD: *The Neurology of Gastrointestinal Disease*. Philadelphia, Saunders, 1974.

PERKIN CD, MURRAY-LYON I: Neurology and the gastrointestinal system. *J Neurol Neurosurg Psychiatry* 65:291, 1998.

PINCUS JH: Folic acid deficiency: A cause of subacute combined system degeneration, in Botez MI, Reynolds EH (eds): *Folic Acid in Neurology, Psychiatry, and Internal Medicine*. New York, Raven Press, 1979, pp 427–433.

PLANT GT, MTANDA AT, ARDEN GB, JOHNSON GJ: An epidemic of optic neuropathy in Tanzania: Characterization of the visual disorder and associated peripheral neuropathy. *J Neurol Sci* 145:127, 1997.

POTTS AM: Tobacco amblyopia. *Surv Ophthalmol* 17:313, 1973.

RONTHAL M, ADLER H: Motor nerve conduction velocity and the electromyograph in pellagra. *S Afr Med J* 43:642, 1969.

ROSENBERG LE: Vitamin-responsive inherited diseases affecting the nervous system, in Plum F (ed): *Brain Dysfunction in Metabolic Disorders*. Vol 53. New York, Raven Press, 1974, pp 263–270.

ROSENBLUM JL, KEATING JP, PRENSKY AL, NELSON JS: A progressive neurologic syndrome in children with chronic liver disease. *N Engl J Med* 304:503, 1981.

SATYA-MURTI S, HOWARD L, KROHEL G, WOLF B: The spectrum of neurologic disorder from vitamin E deficiency. *Neurology* 36:917, 1986.

SCHAUMBURG H, KAPLAN J, WINDEBANK A, et al: Sensory neuropathy from pyridoxine abuse: A new megavitamin syndrome. *N Engl J Med* 309:445, 1983.

SERDARU M, HAUSSER-HAUW C, LAPLANE D, et al: The clinical spectrum of alcoholic pellagra encephalopathy. *Brain* 111:829, 1988.

Shah DR, Singh SV, Jain IL: Neurological manifestations in pellagra. *J Assoc Physicians India* 19:443, 1971.

Shattuck GC: Relation of beriberi to polyneuritis from other causes. *Am J Trop Med Hyg* 8:539, 1928.

Shimojyo S, Scheinberg P, Reinmuth OM: Cerebral blood flow and metabolism in the Wernicke-Korsakoff syndrome. *J Clin Invest* 46:849, 1967.

Sokol RJ, Butler-Simon N, Neubi JE, et al: Vitamin E deficiency neuropathy in children with fat malabsorption: Studies in cystic fibrosis and chronic cholestasis. *Ann N Y Acad Sci* 570:156, 1989.

Spillane JD: *Nutritional Disorders of the Nervous System.* Baltimore, Williams & Wilkins, 1947.

Spivak JL, Jackson DL: Pellagra: An analysis of 18 patients and a review of the literature. *Johns Hopkins Med J* 140:295, 1977.

Strachan H: On a form of multiple neuritis prevalent in the West Indies. *Practitioner* 59:477, 1897.

Strauss MB: Etiology of "alcoholic" polyneuritis. *Am J Med Sci* 189:378, 1935.

Swank RL, Adams RD: Pyridoxine and pantothenic acid deficiency in swine. *J Neuropathol Exp Neurol* 7:274, 1948.

Sydenstricker VP, Schmidt HL Jr, Fulton MC, et al: Treatment of pellagra with nicotinic acid: Observations in 45 cases. *South Med J* 31:1155, 1938.

Terris M (ed): *Goldberger on Pellagra.* Baton Rouge, LA, Louisiana State University Press, 1964.

Torvik A, Lindboe CF, Rogde S: Brain lesions in alcoholics: A neuropathological study with clinical correlations. *J Neurol Neurosurg Psychiatry* 56:233, 1982.

Traber MG, Sokol RJ, Burton GW, et al: Impaired ability of patients with familial isolated vitamin E deficiency to incorporate α-tocopherol into lipoproteins secreted by the liver. *J Clin Invest* 85:397, 1990.

Victor M: MR in the diagnosis of Wernicke-Korsakoff syndrome. *Am J Neuroradiol* 11:895, 1990.

Victor M: Polyneuropathy due to nutritional deficiency and alcoholism, in Dyck PJ, Thomas PK, Lambert EH, Bunge R (eds): *Peripheral Neuropathy*, 2nd ed. Philadelphia, Saunders, 1984, pp 1899–1940.

Victor M: Tobacco amblyopia, cyanide poisoning and vitamin B_{12} deficiency: A critique of current concepts, in Smith JL (ed): *Miami Neuroophthalmology Symposium.* Vol 5. Hallandale, FL, Huffman, 1970, pp 33–48.

Victor M, Adams RD: Neuropathology of experimental vitamin B_6 deficiency in monkeys. *Am J Clin Nutr* 4:346, 1956.

Victor M, Adams RD: On the etiology of the alcoholic neurologic diseases with special reference to the role of nutrition. *Am J Clin Nutr* 9:379, 1961.

Victor M, Adams RD, Collins GH: *The Wernicke-Korsakoff Syndrome and Related Neurologic Disorders Due to Alcoholism and Malnutrition*, 2nd ed. Philadelphia, Davis, 1989.

Victor M, Adams RD, Mancall EL: A restricted form of cerebellar degeneration occurring in alcoholic patients. *Arch Neurol* 1:577, 1959.

Victor M, Laureno R: Neurologic complications of alcohol abuse: Epidemiologic aspects, in Schoenberg BS (ed): *Advances in Neurology*. Vol 19. New York, Raven Press, 1978, pp 603–617.

Victor M, Mancall EL, Dreyfus PM: Deficiency amblyopia in the alcoholic patient: A clinicopathologic study. *Arch Ophthalmol* 64:1, 1960.

Victor M, Yakovlev PI: SS Korsakoff's psychic disorder in conjunction with peripheral neuritis: A translation of Korsakoff's original article with brief comments on the author and his contribution to clinical medicine. *Neurology* 5:394, 1955.

Vilter RW, Mueller JF, Glazer HS, et al: The effect of vitamin B_6 deficiency induced by desoxypyridoxine in human beings. *J Lab Clin Med* 42:335, 1953.

Windebank AJ: Polyneuropathy due to nutritional deficiency and alcoholism, in Dyck PJ, Thomas PK, et al (eds): *Peripheral Neuropathy*, 3rd ed. Philadelphia, Saunders, 1993, pp 1310–1321.

Winick M: *Malnutrition and Brain Development.* New York, Oxford University Press, 1976.

Chapter 42

ALCOHOL AND ALCOHOLISM

Intemperance in the use of alcohol creates many problems in modern society, the importance of which can be judged by the repeated emphasis they receive in contemporary writings, both literary and scientific. These problems may be divided into three categories: psychologic, medical, and sociologic. The main psychologic problem is why a person drinks excessively, often with full knowledge that such action will result in physical injury and even death. The medical problem embraces all aspects of alcoholic habituation as well as the diseases that result from the abuse of alcohol. The sociologic problem consists of the effects of sustained drinking on the patient's work, family, and community. Some idea of the enormity of these problems can be gleaned from figures supplied by the Secretary of Health and Human Services—which reveal that up to 40 percent of medical and surgical patients have alcohol-related problems and that these patients account for 15 percent of all health care costs (which in 1995 were estimated at 150 billion dollars).

These several problems engendered by excessive drinking cannot be separated from one another; the physician must therefore be conversant with all aspects of this subject. He may be asked to help the patient to overcome his drinking problem or to diagnose and treat the numerous diseases to which such a patient is subject; often he must admit the patient to a "detoxification" unit or a general hospital or to a psychiatric facility, according to the nature of the clinical disorder; and, last, he may be required to enlist the aid of social agencies when their services are needed by either the patient or the patient's family.

Primary alcoholism has been defined as both a chronic disease and a disorder of behavior, characterized in either context by chronic, repetitive, excessive drinking to an extent that interferes with the drinker's health, interpersonal relations, or means of livelihood. Reduced to pharmacologic terms, it is addiction to alcohol. *Secondary alcoholism* refers to excessive drinking in the context of another major psychiatric illness—e.g., manic-depressive disease. The term *alcoholism*, unqualified, refers to the primary variety.

The causation of alcoholism remains obscure, although environmental, cultural, and genetic factors are clearly implicated in certain groups of patients. No single personality type has been shown to predict reliably who will become addicted to alcohol and who will not. Similarly, no particular aspect of alcohol metabolism has been found to account for the development of addiction in some individuals and not in others, with the possible exception of aldehyde dehydrogenase (see below). Some persons drink excessively and become alcoholics in response to some profoundly disturbing personal or family problem, but many do not. Alcoholism may develop in response to a depressive illness, more so in women than in men, but far more often depression is a consequence of drinking. Social and cultural influences are undoubtedly important in the genesis of alcoholism, as evidenced, for example, by the remarkably high incidence of alcoholism and drinking problems in the American Indian and Eskimo populations and by the disparity in the prevalence of alcoholism, within a single community, between the Irish and the Jews. However, no ethnic or racial group and no social or economic class is exempt. Moreover, no particular pattern of child rearing or cultural attitude is universally effective in facilitating or protecting against the development of alcoholism. The writings of Schuckit and of Mello, listed in the references, provide critical overviews of the many etiologic theories.

The importance of genetic factors in the causation of alcoholism is being increasingly recognized. Goodwin and coworkers studied 55 Danish men whose biologic parents were alcoholic and 55 control subjects whose biologic parents were not alcoholic. All of the subjects had been adopted before the age of 5 weeks and had no knowledge of their biologic parentage. Twenty percent of the offspring of biologic alcoholic parents, but only 5 percent of the control subjects, had become alcoholics by the age of 25 to 29 years. A Swedish adoption study (Bohman) and one in the United States (Cadoret et al) have corroborated these findings. Family studies have disclosed a three- to fourfold increased risk for alcoholism in sons and daughters of alcoholics, and twin studies have shown a twofold higher concordance rate for alcoholism in monozygotic than in dizygotic pairs. Details of these studies can be found in the comprehensive reviews of the genetics of alcoholism by Grove and Cadoret and by Schuckit. The search goes on for a biologic trait, or marker, that would identify those who are genetically vulnerable to the development of alcoholism, but to date none has proved to be sufficiently practical or sensitive to identify all such persons (Reich).

As to the frequency of alcoholism, the survey by Grant et al of more than 43,000 households is still an epidemiologic benchmark. They estimated that in 1988, some 15.3 million Americans (8.6 percent of persons 18 years or older) were either alcohol abusers or alcohol-dependent. Of this number, 4.1 million were women. In addition, there were approximately 4.6 million problem drinkers among adolescents (about 20 percent of the persons in this age group). Several more recent surveys have suggested a rate of alcohol dependence of 3 to 5.5 percent of adults. Schuckit has estimated that the lifetime risk for alcoholism is at least 10 percent for men and 3 to 5 percent for women. A minimum of 3 percent of deaths in the United States can be attributed to alcohol-related causes. Alcohol intoxication is responsible for approximately 45 percent of fatal motor vehicle accidents and 22 percent of boating accidents. It requires little imagination to conceive the havoc wrought by alcohol in terms of decreased productivity, increased incidence of suicide, accidents, crime, mental and physical disease, and disruption of family life.

PHARMACOLOGIC AND PHYSIOLOGIC CONSIDERATIONS

Ethyl alcohol, or ethanol, is the active ingredient in beer, wine, whiskey, gin, brandy, and other less common alcoholic beverages. In addition, the stronger spirits contain enanthic ethers, which provide flavor but have no important pharmacologic properties, and impurities such as amyl alcohol (fusel oil) and acetaldehyde, which act like alcohol but are more toxic. Contrary to popular opinion, the content of B vitamins in American beer and other liquors is so low as to have little nutritional value (Davidson).

Absorption, Distribution, and Metabolism of Alcohol Alcohol is absorbed unaltered from the gastrointestinal tract, about 25 percent from the stomach and the rest from the upper small intestine. Its presence may be detected in the blood within 5 min after ingestion, and the maximum concentration is reached in 30 to 90 min. The ingestion of milk and fatty foods impedes and water facilitates its absorption. The rate of absorption increases after gastrectomy; in such cases maximum blood alcohol concentrations are higher and are attained faster than in persons with intact stomachs. In habituated persons, the blood alcohol concentration rises somewhat faster and reaches a higher maximum than in abstainers. Also in this respect, there may be a difference between the sexes. After consuming comparable amounts of alcohol, women develop higher blood alcohol concentrations than men (Frezza et al). This effect has been attributed to a diminished "first-pass" metabolism of alcohol in the gastric mucosa, where the alcohol dehydrogenase activity was found to be less in women than it is in men.

Alcohol is carried chiefly in the plasma and enters the various organs of the body—as well as the cerebrospinal fluid (CSF), urine, and pulmonary alveolar air—in concentrations that bear a constant relationship to the concentration in the blood. Alcohol is metabolized chiefly by oxidation, less than 10 percent being excreted chemically unchanged in the urine, perspiration, and breath. The energy liberated by the oxidation of alcohol (7 kcal/g) can be utilized as completely as that derived from the metabolism of other carbohydrates. However, calories from alcohol are empty of nutrients such as proteins and vitamins and cannot be used in the repair of damaged tissue. Therefore, unless the chronic drinker takes an adequate amount of protein (which he frequently fails to do), muscle bulk is lost and other tissues are subject to damage.

All ingested alcohol except that metabolized by alcohol dehydrogenase in the stomach wall is carried by the portal system to the liver. Here several enzyme systems (located in different subcellular compartments of the hepatocyte) can independently oxidize alcohol to acetaldehyde. The most important of these systems, accounting for 80 to 90 percent of ethanol oxidation in vivo, are alcohol dehydrogenase (ADH) and its isoenzymes; they are found in the soluble fraction of the hepatocyte and utilize nicotinamide adenine dinucleotide (NAD) as the cofactor. This reaction leads to the formation of acetaldehyde and the reduction of NAD to

NADH. A second pathway involves catalase, which is located in the peroxisomes and mitochondria; a third utilizes the "microsomal ethanol oxidizing system" (MEOS), located mainly in the microsomes of the endoplasmic reticulum. The MEOS, which is dependent upon reduced nicotinamide adenine dinucleotide phosphate (NADPH), does not account for much of the alcohol metabolized in normal circumstances, but it may be responsible for the increased rate of alcohol metabolism observed in chronic alcoholics.

The aforementioned shift in the NADH/NAD ratio results in a number of metabolic derangements in carbohydrate and lipid metabolism. The synthesis of glucose declines and there is a conversion of lactic to pyruvic acid. However, a significant lowering of blood glucose will occur only if the hepatic glycogen stores are depleted—as a result of fasting, for example. The levels of serum lactate will be increased occasionally, to the point of lactic acidosis. In certain circumstances alcohol can interfere with the peripheral utilization of glucose, resulting in hyperglycemia. Also, as a result of the changed NADH/NAD ratio, there occurs a depression in the oxidation of fatty acids, the excess of which are converted to triglycerides. This leads, in turn, to a fatty liver. Such changes are related to alcohol per se and are independent of malnutrition.

The details of the process by which acetaldehyde is metabolized are still not settled. Most likely it is converted by aldehyde dehydrogenase to acetate. Acetaldehyde has a number of unique biochemical effects that are not produced by alcohol alone. Persons who flush easily after ingestion of alcohol (Chinese, Japanese, and other Asians) differ from "nonflushers" with respect to the metabolism of acetaldehyde rather than to the metabolism of alcohol. The flushing reaction has been traced to a deficiency of aldehyde dehydrogenase activity (Harada et al). The low rate of alcoholism among Asians is said to be related to the flushing reaction (which is, in effect, a modified alcohol-disulfiram reaction—see further on), but this can hardly be the case, since North American Indians, a group with a high incidence of alcoholism, show the same reaction. There are no valid data to support the claim that acetaldehyde, rather than ethanol itself, is the major intoxicating and addicting agent in alcoholism.

For all practical purposes, it may be accepted that once the absorption of alcohol has ended and an equilibrium has been established with the tissues, *ethanol is oxidized at a constant rate, independent of its concentration in the blood* (about 150 mg alcohol per kilogram of body weight per hour, or about 1 oz of 90-proof whiskey per hour). Actually, slightly more alcohol is metabolized per hour when the initial concentrations are very high, and repeated ingestion of alcohol may facilitate its metabolism, but these increments are of little clinical significance. Neither do agents such as amino acids, insulin, and fructose have any practical value in enhancing ethanol metabolism. On the other hand, the rate of oxidation of acetaldehyde does depend on its concentration in the tissues. This fact is of importance in connection with the drug disulfiram (Antabuse), which acts by raising the tissue concentration necessary for the metabolism of a certain amount of acetaldehyde per unit of time. The patient taking both disulfiram and alcohol will accumulate an inordinate amount of acetaldehyde, resulting in nausea, vomiting, and hypotension, sometimes so pronounced in degree as to be fatal. This pharmacologic principle underlies the treatment of alcoholism with disulfiram. Certain other drugs—notably the sulfonylureas, metronidazole, and furazolidone—have effects like those of disulfiram but are less potent.

The fraction of ingested alcohol that survives first-pass oxidation in the stomach wall and the liver equilibrates rapidly with all bodily tissues and fluids and affects their function to a degree that is governed by the blood alcohol concentration. Only the effects on the nervous system concern us in this chapter. Complete accounts of the nonneurologic effects can be found in the monographs edited by Lieber and by Mendelson and Mello.

Pharmacologic Effects Alcohol acts directly on neuronal membranes in a manner akin to that of the general anesthetics. These agents, as well as barbiturates and benzodiazepines, are lipid-soluble and are thought to produce their effects by dissolving in the cell membranes (in direct relation to the degree of their lipid solubility). This process has a disordering effect on other membrane structures, particularly proteins. With continued ingestion of alcohol, the neuronal membranes rigidify and become resistant to the fluidizing effect of alcohol (Chin and Goldstein; Harris et al).

It is unlikely, however, that these changes in the physical properties of cell membranes are in themselves sufficient to alter cell function. Probably of greater importance are the effects of alcohol on membrane receptor systems, which regulate ion channels, particularly the chloride and calcium channels. One likely site that relates to the acute intoxicating effects of alcohol is a receptor for the inhibitory neurotransmitter gamma-aminobutyric acid (GABA) and its associated chloride-ion channel. Benzodiazepine antagonists appear to block the potentiation by alcohol of GABA-induced chloride flux. Like the GABA-chloride channel, the *N*-methyl-D-aspartate (NMDA) receptors, which transduce signals carried by glutamate (the major excitatory transmitter in brain), are sensitive to extremely low concentrations of alcohol. There is also evidence that alcohol selectively potentiates serotonin 5-HT3 receptor-ion currents, and the activity of this receptor has been implicated in alcohol- and drug-seeking behavior and addiction.

The effect of chronic administration of alcohol is to increase the number of neuronal calcium channels in the cell membrane; moreover, calcium channel blockers, given during chronic administration, prevent both the increase in neuronal calcium channels and the development of tolerance to alcohol (Dolin and Little). The significance of these findings has been demonstrated by Little and colleagues, who showed that calcium channel blockers, given to chronically intoxicated animals after withdrawal, prevent withdrawal convulsions.

The molecular mechanisms involved in the genesis of alcohol intoxication and tolerance are obviously far more complex than the foregoing remarks would indicate (see reviews by Charness and by Samson and Harris). There is now a vast literature on this subject, much of it contradictory. A unified concept of the role of neurotransmitters and their receptors and modulators in the production of alcohol intoxication and tolerance has yet to emerge. The role of internal cellular messengers, which have attracted much attention in the field of addiction, is also currently under investigation.

Physiologic Effects Alcohol functions not as a central nervous system (CNS) stimulant but as a depressant. Some of the early toxic effects of alcohol, such as garrulousness, aggressiveness, excessive activity, and increased electrical excitability of the cerebral cortex—all of them suggestive of cerebral stimulation—are thought to be due to the inhibition of certain subcortical structures (possibly the high brainstem reticular formation) that ordinarily modulate cerebrocortical activity. Similarly, the initial hyperactivity of tendon reflexes may represent a transitory escape of spinal motor neurons from higher inhibitory centers. With increasing amounts of alcohol, however, the depressant action spreads to involve the cortical as well as other brainstem and spinal neurons.

All manner of motor functions—whether the simple maintenance of a standing posture, the control of speech and eye movements, or highly organized and complex motor skills—are adversely affected by alcohol. The movements involved in these acts are not only slower than normal but also more inaccurate and random in character and therefore less well adapted to the accomplishment of specific ends.

Alcohol also impairs the efficiency of mental function by interfering with the speed of perception and the ability to persist in mental processing. The learning process is slowed and rendered less effective. Facility in forming associations, whether of words or of figures, and the ability to focus, sustain attention, and concentrate are reduced. The subject is less versatile in directing thought along new lines appropriate to the problem at hand. Finally, alcohol impairs the faculties of judgment and discrimination and, all in all, the ability to think and reason clearly.

A scale relating various degrees of functional impairment to blood alcohol levels in *nonhabituated* persons was constructed many years ago by Miles. At a blood alcohol level of 30 mg/dL, a mild euphoria was detectable, and at 50 mg/dL, a mild incoordination. At 100 mg/dL, ataxia was obvious; at 200 mg/dL, there was confusion and a reduced level of mental activity; at 300 mg/dL, the subjects were stuporous; and a level of 400 mg/dL—accompanied by deep anesthesia—was potentially fatal. These figures are valid provided that the alcohol content in the blood rises steadily over a 2-h period.

Tolerance It should be emphasized that a scale such as the one described above has virtually no value in the chronic alcoholic patient, for it does not take into account the adaptation of the organism to alcohol, i.e., the phenomenon of tolerance. It is common knowledge that a habituated person can drink more and show fewer effects than the moderate drinker or abstainer. This phenomenon accounts for the surprisingly large amounts of alcohol that the chronic drinker can consume without showing significant signs of drunkenness. Sober-appearing alcoholics may have blood alcohol levels of 400 to 500 mg/dL. The aspect of tolerance must always be considered in judging the significance of a single estimation of the blood alcohol concentration as an index of functional capacity.

The nervous system is capable of adapting to alcohol after a very short exposure. Thus, if the alcohol concentration in the blood is raised very slowly, few symptoms appear, even at quite high levels. Contrariwise, the degree of intoxication is more severe when the blood alcohol level peaks rapidly. As mentioned earlier, the important factor in this rapid adaptability is not so much the height of the blood alcohol concentration as the length of time the alcohol has been present in the body. If the dosage of alcohol that causes blood levels to be high is held constant, the blood alcohol concentration falls gradually and clinical evidence of intoxication disappears. The cause of this fall in alcohol concentration is not clear.

The mechanisms that underlie tolerance and addiction are just beginning to be understood. There is little evidence that an enhanced rate of alcohol metabolism can adequately account for the degree of tolerance observed in alcoholics. An increased degree of neuronal adaptation to alcohol is a more likely explanation. As mentioned earlier, the main factors that are operative in this adaptation are the increasing resistance of neuronal membranes to the "fluidizing" effects of alcohol and an increase in the number of neuronal calcium channels in the cell membrane.

CLINICAL EFFECTS OF ALCOHOL ON THE NERVOUS SYSTEM

A large number of neurologic disorders are associated with alcoholism. The factor common to all of them, of course, is the abuse of alcohol, but the mechanism by which alcohol produces its effects varies widely from one group of disorders to another. The classification that follows is based for the most part on known mechanisms.

I. Alcohol intoxication—drunkenness, coma, excitement ("pathologic intoxication"), "blackouts"
II. The abstinence or withdrawal syndrome—tremulousness, hallucinosis, seizures, delirium tremens
III. Nutritional diseases of the nervous system secondary to alcoholism
   A. Wernicke-Korsakoff syndrome
   B. Polyneuropathy
   C. Optic neuropathy ("tobacco-alcohol amblyopia")
   D. Pellagra
IV. Diseases of uncertain pathogenesis associated with alcoholism
   A. Cerebellar degeneration
   B. Marchiafava-Bignami disease
   C. Central pontine myelinolysis
   D. "Alcoholic" myopathy and cardiomyopathy
   E. Alcoholic dementia
   F. Cerebral atrophy
V. Fetal alcohol syndrome
VI. Neurologic disorders consequent upon cirrhosis and portal-systemic shunts
   A. Hepatic stupor and coma
   B. Chronic hepatocerebral degeneration

Alcohol Intoxication

The usual manifestations of alcohol intoxication are so commonplace that they require little elaboration. They consist of varying degrees of exhilaration and excitement, loss of restraint, irregularity of behavior, loquacity and slurred speech, incoordination of movement and gait, irritability, drowsiness, and, in advanced cases, stupor and coma. There are several *complicated* types of alcohol intoxication, which are considered below.

Pathologic Intoxication Despite what has been said above, on rare occasions, alcohol has an excitatory rather than a sedative effect. This reaction has been referred to in the past as *pathologic*, or *complicated, intoxication* and as *acute alcoholic paranoid state*. Since all forms of intoxication are pathologic, *atypical intoxication* or *idiosyncratic alcohol intoxication* are more appropriate designations. Nevertheless, the term *pathologic intoxication* is still widely used. The boundaries of this syndrome have never been clearly drawn. In the past, variant forms of delirium tremens and epileptic phenomena as well as psychopathic and criminal behavior were indiscriminately included. Now the term is generally used to designate an outburst of blind fury with assaultive and destructive behavior. Often the patient is subdued only with difficulty. The attack terminates with deep sleep, which occurs spontaneously or in response to parenteral sedation; on awakening, the patient has no memory of the episode. Lesser degrees are also known wherein the patient, after several drinks, repeatedly commits gross social indiscretions. Allegedly this reaction may follow the ingestion of a small amount of alcohol, but in our experience the amount has always been substantial. Unlike the usual forms of alcohol intoxication and withdrawal, the atypical form has not been produced in experimental subjects, and the diagnosis depends upon the aforementioned arbitrary anecdotal criteria.

Pathologic intoxication has been ascribed to many factors, the common ones being constitutional differences in the susceptibility to alcohol (idiosyncratic reaction to alcohol), pre-existent craniocerebral trauma or other brain disease, and an underlying "hysterical or epileptoid temperament or sociopathy." There are no meaningful data to support any of these beliefs. However, an analogy may be drawn between pathologic intoxication and the paradoxical reaction that occasionally follows the administration of barbiturates or other sedative drugs.

The diagnosis of pathologic or idiosyncratic intoxication could conceivably have important legal implications. Because of long-held public and legal attitudes, a person suffering from alcoholism or the *usual* forms of drunkenness is considered to be responsible for the consequences of his drinking, whereas a person with pathologic intoxication might be considered insane at the time and therefore not responsible. The main disorders to be distinguished from pathologic intoxication are temporal lobe seizures that occasionally take the form of outbursts of rage and violence and the explosive episodes of violence that characterize the behavior of certain sociopaths. The diagnosis in these cases may be difficult and depends on eliciting the other manifestations of temporal lobe epilepsy or sociopathy.

Alcoholic "Blackouts" In the language of the alcoholic, the term *blackout* refers to an interval of time, during a period of severe intoxication, for which the patient, when sober, has no memory—even though the state of consciousness, as observed by others, was not grossly altered during that interval. However, a systematic assessment of mental function during the amnesic period has usually not been made. A few observations indicate that it is short-term (retentive) memory, rather than immediate or long-term memory, that is impaired; this feature and the subsequent amnesia for the episode are somewhat reminiscent of the disorder known as *transient global amnesia* (page 457).

The nature and significance of such episodes are unclear. It is widely held that the occurrence of blackouts is an early and serious indicator of the development of alcohol addiction. In our experience, blackouts may occur at any time in the course of alcoholism, even during the first drinking experience, and they certainly have happened in persons who never became alcoholics. The salient facts are that there is a degree of intoxication which interferes with the registration of events and the formation of memories during the period of intoxication, and that the amount of alcohol consumed in moderate social drinking will rarely produce this effect.

Alcoholic Stupor and Coma As has been indicated, the symptoms of alcoholic intoxication are the result of the depressant action of alcohol on cerebral and spinal neurons. In this respect alcohol acts on nerve cells in a manner akin to the general anesthetics. Unlike the latter, however, the margin between the dose of alcohol that produces surgical anesthesia and that which dangerously depresses respiration is a narrow one, a fact that adds an element of urgency to the diagnosis and treatment of alcoholic narcosis. One must also be alert to the possibility that barbiturates or other sedative-hypnotic drugs may have potentiated the depressant effects of alcohol.

The signs of alcohol intoxication are distinctive and most forms present no problem in diagnosis or management. On the other hand, coma due to alcohol may present difficulties in differential diagnosis. It should be stressed that the diagnosis of alcoholic coma is made not merely on the basis of a flushed face, stupor, and the odor of alcohol but only after the careful exclusion of all other causes of coma (page 383).

Treatment of Alcohol Intoxication Mild to moderate degrees of intoxication require no special treatment. Certain time-honored forms of stimulation—such as a cold shower, strong coffee, forced activity, or induction of vomiting—may be helpful, but there is no evidence that any of them influences the rate of disappearance of alcohol from the blood. Alcoholic stupor is also a relatively brief, self-limited state; if the vital signs are normal, no special therapeutic measures are necessary. *Pathologic intoxication* may require the use of restraints and the parenteral administration of diazepam (5 to 10 mg) or haloperidol (2 to 5 mg), repeated once after 30 to 40 min if necessary.

Coma due to alcohol intoxication represents a medical emergency. The main object of treatment is to prevent respiratory depression and the complications it engenders. The management of the comatose patient is described in Chap. 17. One would like to lower the blood alcohol level as rapidly as possible, but the administration of fructose or of insulin and glucose for this purpose is of little practical value. Analeptic drugs such as amphetamine and various mixtures of caffeine and picrotoxin are antagonistic to alcohol only insofar as they are powerful cerebrocortical stimulants and overall nervous system excitants; they do not hasten the oxidation of alcohol. The use of hemodialysis should be considered in comatose patients with extremely high blood alcohol concentrations (>500 mg/dL), particularly if accompanied by acidosis, and in those who have concurrently ingested methanol or ethylene glycol or some other dialyzable drug.

Methyl, Amyl, and Isopropyl Alcohols and Ethylene Glycol Poisoning with alcohols other than ethyl alcohol is a relatively rare occurrence. *Amyl alcohol* (fusel oil) and *isopropyl alcohol* are used as industrial solvents and in the manufacture of varnishes, lacquers, and pharmaceuticals; in addition, isopropyl alcohol is readily available as a rubbing alcohol. Intoxication may follow the ingestion of these alcohols or inhalation of their vapors. The effects of both are much like those of ethyl alcohol, but much more toxic.

Methyl alcohol (methanol, wood alcohol) is a component of antifreeze and many combustibles and is used in the manufacture of formaldehyde, as an industrial solvent, and as an adulterant of alcoholic beverages, the latter being the most common source of methyl alcohol intoxication. The oxidation of methyl alcohol to formaldehyde and formic acid proceeds relatively slowly; thus, signs of intoxication do not appear for several hours or may be delayed for a day or longer. Many of the toxic effects are like those of ethyl alcohol, but in addition severe methyl alcohol poisoning may produce serious degrees of acidosis (with an anion gap), damage to retinal ganglion cells—giving rise to scotomata and varying degrees of blindness, dilated unreactive pupils, and retinal edema—and bilateral degeneration of the putamens, readily visible on computed tomography (CT) scans. Survivors may be left blind and parkinsonian (McLean et al). The most important aspect of treatment is the intravenous administration of large amounts of sodium bicarbonate. Hemodialysis may be a useful adjunct because of the slow rate of oxidation of methanol.

Ethylene glycol, an aliphatic alcohol, is a commonly used industrial solvent and the major constituent of antifreeze. In the latter form it is sometimes consumed by skid-row alcoholics (5000 cases of poisoning annually in the United States), with disastrous results. At first the patient merely appears drunk, but after a period of 4 to 12 h, hyperventilation and severe metabolic acidosis develop, followed by confusion, convulsions, coma, and renal failure in rapid succession. Cerebrospinal fluid lymphocytosis is a characteristic feature. The metabolic acidosis is due to the conversion of ethylene glycol by alcohol dehydrogenase into glycolic acid, thus producing an anion gap that reflects the presence of this substance in the blood. The cause of the renal toxicity is less clear—probably it is due to the formation of oxalate from glycolate and the deposition of oxalate crystals. These appear in the urine and sometimes in the CSF and aid in diagnosis. The treatment of ethylene glycol poisoning has, until relatively recently, consisted of hemodialysis and the intravenous infusion of sodium bicarbonate and ethanol, the latter serving as a competitive substrate for alcohol dehydrogenase. However, the use of ethanol in this regimen is problematic. Baud and colleagues and more recently Brent et al and Jacobsen have advocated the use of intravenous 4-methylpyrazole (fomepizole), which is a far more effective inhibitor of alcohol dehydrogenase than is alcohol. They recommend this form of treatment for methanol poisoning as well.

Some of the patients who recover from the acute renal and metabolic effects are left with multiple cranial nerve defects, particularly of the seventh and eighth nerves. The latter abnormalities develop 6 to 18 days after the ingestion of ethylene glycol and have been attributed to the deposition of oxalate crystals along the subarachnoid portions of the affected nerves (Spillane et al).

The Abstinence, or Withdrawal, Syndrome

Included under this title is the symptom complex of tremulousness, hallucinations, seizures, confusion, and psychomotor and autonomic overactivity. Although a sustained period of chronic inebriation is the most obvious factor in the causation of these symptoms, they become manifest only after a *period of relative or absolute abstinence* from alcohol—hence the designation *abstinence*, or *withdrawal*, syndrome. This concept is illustrated in Fig. 42-1. Each of the major manifestations of the withdrawal syndrome may occur in more or less pure form and are so described below, but usually they occur in various combinations. Major withdrawal symptoms are observed mainly in the spree, or periodic, drinker, although the steady drinker is not immune if for some reason he stops drinking. The full syndrome, depicted further on, is called *delirium tremens*.

Figure 42-1

Relation of acute neurologic disturbances to cessation of drinking. The shaded drinking period is greatly foreshortened and not intended to be quantitative. The periodic notching in the baseline represents the tremulousness, nausea, and so on that occur following a night's sleep. The time relations of the various groups of symptoms to withdrawal are explained in the text. (Adapted from Victor M, Adams RD: The effect of alcohol on the nervous system. Res Publ Assoc Res Nerv Ment Dis 32:526, 1953, by permission.)

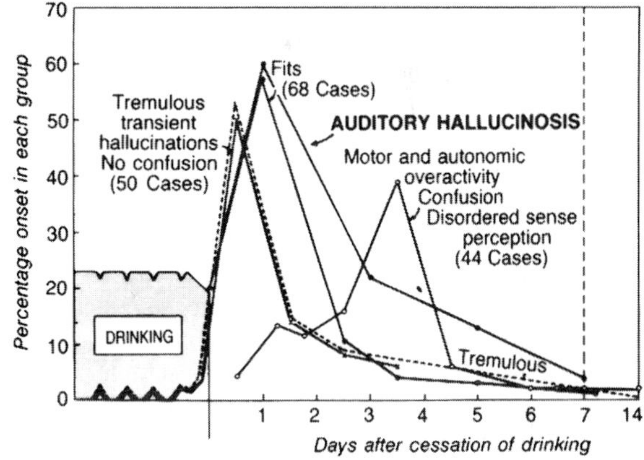

Tremulousness and Associated Symptoms The most common single manifestation of the abstinence syndrome is tremulousness, often referred to as "the shakes" or "the jitters," combined with general irritability and gastrointestinal symptoms, particularly nausea and vomiting. These symptoms first appear after several days of drinking, usually in the morning after a night's abstinence. The patient "quiets his nerves" with a few drinks and is then able to drink for the rest of the day without undue distress. The symptoms return on successive mornings with increasing severity. The duration of drinking of this type varies greatly. It is terminated most often because of increasing severity of the recurrent tremor and vomiting, but for other reasons as well, such as profound general weakness, self-disgust, injury, concurrent illness, a lack of funds, and so forth. The symptoms then become greatly augmented, reaching their peak intensity 24 to 36 h after the complete cessation of drinking.

At this stage, the patient presents a distinctive clinical picture. The face is deeply flushed, the conjunctivae are injected, and there is usually tachycardia, anorexia, nausea, and retching. The patient is fully awake, startles easily, and complains of insomnia. He is inattentive, and disinclined to answer questions, and may respond in a rude or perfunctory manner. The patient may be mildly disoriented in time and have a poor memory for events of the last few days of the drinking spree, but he shows no serious confusion, being generally aware of his immediate surroundings and the nature of his illness.

Generalized tremor is the most obvious feature of this illness. It is of fast frequency (6 to 8 Hz), slightly irregular, and variable in severity, tending to diminish when the patient is in quiet surroundings and to increase with motor activity or emotional stress. The tremor may be so violent that the patient cannot stand without help, speak clearly, or eat without assistance. Sometimes there is little objective evidence of tremor, and the patient complains only of being "shaky inside."

Within a few days, the flushed facies, anorexia, tachycardia, and tremor subside to a large extent, but the overalertness, tendency to startle easily, and jerkiness of movement may persist for a week or longer, and the feeling of uneasiness may not leave the patient completely for 10 to 14 days. These features are suggestive of adrenergic hyperactivity, and indeed the concentrations of norepinephrine and its metabolites are elevated in both the blood and CSF (Hawley et al). According to Porjesz and Begleiter, certain electrophysiologic abnormalities (diminished amplitudes of sensory evoked potentials and prolonged latencies and conduction velocities of auditory brainstem potentials) remain altered long after the clinical abnormalities have subsided.

Hallucinosis Symptoms of disordered perception occur in about one-quarter of hospitalized tremulous patients. The patient may complain of "bad dreams"—nightmarish episodes associated with disturbed sleep—which he finds difficult to separate from real experience. Sounds and shadows may be misinterpreted, or familiar objects may be distorted and assume unreal forms (illusions). Although these are not hallucinations in the strict sense of the term, they represent the most common forms of disordered sense perception in the alcoholic.

Hallucinations may be purely visual in type, mixed visual and auditory, tactile, or olfactory, in this order of frequency. There is little evidence to support the popular belief that certain visual hallucinations (bugs, pink elephants) are specific to alcoholism. Actually, the hallucinations comprise the full range of visual experience. They are more often animate than inanimate; persons or animals may appear singly or in panoramas, shrunken or enlarged, natural and pleasant, or distorted, hideous, and frightening. The hallucinosis may be an isolated phenomenon lasting for a few hours and it may later be attended by other withdrawal signs.

Acute and Chronic Auditory Hallucinosis A special type of alcoholic psychosis, consisting of a more or less pure auditory hallucinosis, has been recognized for many years. Kraepelin referred to it as the "hallucinatory insanity of drunkards," or "alcoholic mania." A report of 75 such cases was made by Victor and Hope. The central feature of the illness, in the beginning, is the occurrence of auditory hallucinations despite an otherwise clear sensorium; i.e., the patients are not disoriented or obtunded, and they have an intact memory. The hallucinations may take the form of unstructured sounds such as buzzing, ringing, gunshots, or clicking (the elementary hallucinations of Bleuler), or they may have a musical quality, like a low-pitched hum or chant. The most common hallucinations, however, are human voices. When the voices can be identified, they are often attributed to the patient's family, friends, or neighbors—rarely to God, radio, or radar. The voices may be addressed directly to the patient, but more frequently they discuss him in the third person. In the majority of cases the voices are maligning, reproachful, or threatening in nature and are disturbing to the patient; a significant proportion, however, are not unpleasant and leave the patient undisturbed. To the patient, the voices are clearly audible and intensely real, and they tend to be exteriorized; i.e., they come from behind a radiator or door, from the corridor, or through a wall, window, or floor. Another feature of auditory hallucinosis (and of visual hallucinosis as well) is that the patient's response is more or less understandable in light of the hallucinatory content. The patient may call on the police for protection or erect a barricade against invaders; he may even attempt suicide to avoid what the voices threaten. The hallucinations are most prominent during the night, and their duration varies greatly: they may be momentary, or they may recur intermittently for days on end and, in exceptional instances, for weeks or months.

While hallucinating, most patients have no appreciation of the unreality of their hallucinations. With improvement, the patient begins to question the reality of his hallucinations and may be reluctant to talk about them and may even question his own sanity. Full recovery is characterized by the realization that the voices were imaginary and by the ability to recall, sometimes with remarkable clarity, some of the abnormal thought content of the psychotic episode.

A unique feature of this alcoholic psychosis is its evolution, in a small proportion of the patients, to a state of *chronic auditory hallucinosis*. The chronic disorder begins like the acute one, but after a short period, perhaps a week or two, the symptomatology begins to change. The patient becomes quiet and resigned, even though the hallucinations remain threatening and derogatory. Ideas of reference and influence and other poorly systematized paranoid delusions become prominent. At this stage the illness may be mistaken for paranoid schizophrenia and indeed was so identified by Bleuler. There are, however, important differences between the two disorders: the alcoholic illness develops in close relation to a drinking bout and the past history rarely reveals schizoid personality traits. Moreover, alcoholic patients with hallucinosis are not distinguished by a high incidence of schizophrenia within their families (Schuckit and Winokur, Scott), and a large number of such patients, whom we evaluated long after their acute attacks, did not show an increased incidence of schizophrenia. There is some evidence that repeated attacks of acute auditory hallucinosis render the patient more susceptible to the chronic state.

Withdrawal Seizures ("Rum Fits") In the setting of alcohol withdrawal (i.e., where relative or absolute abstinence follows a period of chronic inebriation), convulsive seizures are a common occurrence. More than 90 percent of withdrawal seizures occur during the 7- to 48-h period following the cessation of drinking, with a peak incidence between 13 and 24 h. During the period of seizure activity, the electroencephalogram (EEG) is usually abnormal, but it reverts to normal in a matter of days, even though the patient may go on to develop delirium tremens. Also during the period of seizure activity, the patient is unusually sensitive to stroboscopic stimulation; almost half the patients respond with generalized myoclonus or a convulsive seizure (photomyogenic or photoparoxysmal response). By contrast, this type of response to photic stimulation is observed only rarely in nonalcoholic epileptics, and then usually in those with tonic-clonic seizures on awakening.

Seizures occurring in the abstinence period have a number of other distinctive features. There may be only a single seizure, but in the majority of cases the seizures occur in bursts of two to six, occasionally even more; 2 percent of our patients developed status epilepticus. The seizures are grand mal in type, i.e., generalized, tonic-clonic convulsions with loss of consciousness. Focal seizures should always suggest the presence of a focal lesion (most often traumatic) in addition to the effects of alcohol. Twenty-eight percent of our patients with generalized withdrawal seizures went on to develop delirium tremens (the percentage has been less in other series); invariably the seizures preceded the delirium. The postictal confusional state may blend imperceptibly with the onset of the delirium, or the postictal state may clear over several hours or even a day or longer before the delirium sets in. Seizures of this type typically occur in patients whose drinking history has extended over a period of many years and must be distinguished from other forms of seizures that have their onset in adult life.

It is suggested that the term *rum fits*, or *whiskey fits*—i.e., the names sometimes used by alcoholics—be reserved for seizures with the attributes described above. This serves to distinguish the form of seizure activity that occurs only in the immediate abstinence period from seizures that occur in the interdrinking period, long after withdrawal has been accomplished.

It is important to note that the common idiopathic or posttraumatic forms of epilepsy are also influenced by alcohol. In these types of epilepsy, a seizure or seizures may be precipitated by only a short period of drinking (e.g., a weekend, or even one evening of heavy social drinking); interestingly, in these circumstances, the seizures occur not when the patient is intoxicated but usually the morning after, in the "sobering-up" period.

The EEG findings in alcoholic subjects with abstinence seizures do not support the notion that the seizures merely represent latent epilepsy made manifest by alcohol. Instead, the EEG reflects a sequence of changes induced by alcohol itself: a decrease in the frequency of brain waves during the period of chronic intoxication; a rapid return of the EEG toward normal immediately after cessation of drinking; a brief period of dysrhythmia (sharp waves and paroxysmal discharges) that coincides with the flurry of convulsive activity; and again, a rapid return of the EEG to normal. Except for the transient dysrhythmia in the withdrawal period, the incidence of EEG abnormalities in patients who have had rum fits is no greater than in normal persons, in sharp contrast to the EEGs of nonalcoholic patients with recurrent seizures.

Treatment of Withdrawal Seizures Many cases do not require the use of anticonvulsant drugs, since the entire episode of seizure activity—whether a single seizure or a brief flurry of seizures—may have terminated before the patient is brought to medical attention. The parenteral administration of diazepam or sodium phenobarbital early in the withdrawal period could conceivably prevent rum fits in patients with a previous history of this disorder or those who might be expected to develop seizures on withdrawal of alcohol, but this prophylactic plan has never been documented satisfactorily. Recently however, D'Onofrio and colleagues have presented data that support the effectiveness of intravenous lorazepam (2 mg in 2 mL of normal saline) in preventing *recurrent seizures* in the withdrawal period. The long-term administration of anticonvulsants is not practical: if such patients remain abstinent, they will be free of seizures; if they resume drinking, they usually abandon their medicines. Furthermore, it is not certain that continued administration of anticonvulsants dependably prevents abstinence seizures. The rare instances of status epilepticus should be managed like status of any other type (page 361). In alcoholics with a history of idiopathic or posttraumatic epilepsy, the goal of treatment should be abstinence from alcohol, because of the tendency of even short periods of drinking to precipitate seizures. Such patients need to be maintained on anticonvulsant drugs.

Delirium Tremens ("DTs") This is the most dramatic and grave of all the alcoholic illnesses. It is characterized by profound confusion, delusions, vivid hallucinations, tremor, agitation, and sleeplessness as well as by the signs of increased autonomic nervous system overactivity—i.e., dilated pupils, fever, tachycardia, and profuse perspiration. The clinical features of delirium are presented in detail in Chap. 20.

Delirium tremens develops in one of several settings. The patient, an excessive and steady drinker for many years, may have been admitted to the hospital for an unrelated illness, accident, or operation and, after 2 to 4 days, occasionally even later, becomes delirious. Or, following a prolonged drinking binge, the patient may have experienced several days of tremulousness and hallucinosis or one or more seizures and may even be recovering from these symptoms when delirium tremens develops, rather abruptly as a rule.

As to the frequency of delirium tremens, Foy and Kay reported an incidence of 0.65 percent of all patients admitted for other reasons to a large general hospital. Among 200 consecutive alcoholics admitted to a city hospital, Ferguson et al reported that 24 percent developed delirium tremens; of these, 8 percent died—figures that are considerably higher than those recorded in our hospitals. Of course, the reported incidence of delirium tremens will vary greatly, depending on the population served by a particular hospital, the admission policy of the hospital, and the strictness with which delirium tremens is defined and distinguished from lesser forms of alcohol withdrawal.

In the majority of cases delirium tremens is benign and short-lived, ending as abruptly as it begins. Consumed by relentless activity and wakefulness for several days, the patient falls into a deep sleep and then awakens lucid, quiet, and exhausted, with virtually no memory of the events of the delirious period. Somewhat less commonly, the delirious state subsides gradually with intermittent episodes of recurrence. In either event, when delirium tremens occurs as a single episode, the duration is 72 h or less in over 80 percent of cases. Less frequently still, there may be one or more relapses, several episodes of delirium of varying severity being separated by intervals of relative lucidity—the entire process lasting for several days or occasionally for as long as 4 to 5 weeks.

In the past, approximately 15 percent of cases of delirium tremens ended fatally, but the figure now is closer to 5 percent. In many of the fatal cases there is an associated infectious illness or injury, but in others no complicating illness is discernible. Many of the patients die in a state of hyperthermia; in some, death comes so suddenly that the nature of the terminal events cannot be determined. Reports of a negligible mortality in delirium tremens can usually be traced to a failure to distinguish between delirium tremens and the minor forms of the withdrawal syndrome, which are far more common and practically never fatal.

Atypical Delirious-Hallucinatory or Confusional States These are alcohol withdrawal states, closely related to delirium tremens and about as frequent, in which one facet of the delirium tremens complex assumes prominence, to the virtual exclusion of the other symptoms. The patient may simply exhibit a transient state of quiet confusion, agitation, or peculiar behavior lasting several days or weeks. Or there may be a vivid hallucinatory-delusional state and abnormal behavior consistent with the patient's false beliefs. Unlike typical delirium tremens, the atypical states usually present as a single circumscribed episode without recurrences, are only rarely preceded by seizures, and do not end fatally. This may be another way of saying that they are a partial or less severe form of the disease.

Pathology *Pathologic examination* is singularly unrevealing in patients with delirium tremens. Edema and brain swelling have been absent in the authors' pathologic material except when shock or hypoxia had occurred terminally. There have been no significant light-microscopic changes in the brain, which is what one would expect in a disease that is essentially reversible. Abnormalities of the CSF occur unpredictably, as do changes on CT scanning or MRI; they may indicate the presence of some medical or surgical complication. Enlargement of the third and lateral ventricles is a common finding (see below). The EEG findings have been discussed in relation to withdrawal seizures.

Other Laboratory Findings Rarely, blood glucose is seriously depressed in the alcohol withdrawal states, for the reasons given earlier, under "Absorption, Distribution, and Metabolism of Alcohol." Ketoacidosis with normal blood glucose is another infrequent finding. Disturbances of electrolytes are of varying frequency and significance. Serum sodium levels are altered infrequently and are more often increased than decreased. The same is true for chlorides and phosphate. Serum calcium and potassium were found to be lowered in about one-quarter of our patients. Most patients show some degree of hypomagnesemia, low P_{CO_2}, and high arterial pH—abnormalities that are probably important in the pathogenesis of withdrawal symptoms (see below).

Pathogenesis of the Tremulous-Hallucinatory-Delirious Disorders For many years prior to 1950, it was the common belief that these symptoms represented the most severe forms of alcohol intoxication—an idea that fails to satisfy the simplest clinical logic. The symptoms of toxicity—consisting of slurred speech, uninhibited behavior, staggering gait, stupor, and coma—are in themselves distinctive and, in a sense, the opposite of the symptom complex of tremor, fits, and delirium. The former symptoms are associated with an elevated blood alcohol level, whereas the latter become evident only when the blood alcohol has been reduced. Finally, the symptoms of intoxication increase in severity as more alcohol is consumed, whereas tremor and hallucinosis and even full-blown delirium tremens are diminished or nullified by the administration of alcohol. Also, although much discussed in the past, there is no convincing evidence that an endocrine abnormality (other than the central release of norepinephrine) or nutritional deficiency plays a role in the genesis of delirium tremens and related symptoms.

It is evident, from observations in both humans and experimental animals, that the most important and the one indispensable factor in the genesis of delirium tremens and related disorders is the withdrawal of alcohol following a period of sustained chronic intoxication. Further, the emergence of withdrawal symptoms depends upon a *decline* in the blood alcohol level from a previously higher level and not necessarily upon the complete disappearance of alcohol from the blood.

The mechanisms by which the withdrawal of alcohol produces symptoms are only beginning to be understood. In all but the mildest cases, the early phase of alcohol withdrawal (beginning within 7 to 8 h after cessation of drinking) is attended by a drop in serum magnesium concentration and a rise in arterial pH—the latter on the basis of respiratory alkalosis (Wolfe and Victor). Possibly the compounded effect of these two factors, both of which are associated with hyperexcitability of the nervous system, is responsible for seizures and for other symptoms that characterize the early phase of withdrawal. As an explanation of delirium tremens, however, hypomagnesemia is probably not important, since the serum magnesium level has frequently been restored to normal before the onset of the delirium. The respiratory alkalosis can be explained by the fact that, with chronic alcohol intoxication, certain aggregates of respiratory-related neurons in the lateral medullary tegmentum are rendered progressively more insensitive to circulating CO_2; in the "rebound" phase, these cells become more sensitive than normal to CO_2, with resultant hyperventilation and a rise in arterial pH. The molecular mechanisms that are thought to be operative in the genesis of alcohol tolerance and withdrawal have been considered above. The GABAergic system has been most strongly implicated, in part because the receptors for this inhibitory transmitter are downregulated by chronic alcohol use, but the situation is not nearly so simple, insofar as the excitatory glutaminergic system is also inhibited by alcohol.

Treatment of Delirium Tremens and Minor Withdrawal Symptoms The general aspects of management of the delirious and confused patient have been described on page 442. More specifically, the treatment of delirium tremens begins with a careful search for associated injuries (particularly head injury with cerebral lacerations or subdural hematoma), infections (pneumonia or meningitis), pancreatitis, and liver disease. Because of the frequency and seriousness of these complications, chest films and a CT scan should be obtained in most instances, and lumbar puncture should be performed if there is the slightest suspicion of meningitis. In severe forms of delirium tremens, the temperature, pulse, and blood pressure should be noted at frequent intervals in anticipation of peripheral circulatory collapse and hyperthermia, which, added to the effects of injury and infection, are the usual causes of death in this disease. In the case of hypotension, one must act quickly, utilizing intravenous fluids and, if called for, vasopressor drugs. The occurrence of hyperthermia demands the use of a cooling mattress or evaporative cooling in addition to specific treatment for any infection that may be present.

An important element in treatment is the correction of fluid and electrolyte imbalance. Severe degrees of agitation and perspiration may require the administration of up to 5 L of fluid daily, of which at least 1500 to 2000 mL should be normal saline. The specific electrolytes and the amounts that must be administered are governed by the laboratory values for these electrolytes. If the serum sodium is extremely low, one must be cautious in raising the level lest a central pontine myelinolysis be induced (see page 1193). In the rare case of hypoglycemia, the administration of glucose is an urgent matter. Patients who present with severe ketoacidosis and normal or only slightly elevated blood glucose concentrations usually recover promptly, without the use of insulin.

It must be emphasized again that a *special danger attends the use of glucose solutions in alcoholic patients.* The administration of intravenous glucose may serve to consume the last available reserves of thiamine and precipitate Wernicke disease, as discussed in Chap. 41. Typically, these patients have subsisted on a diet disproportionately high in carbohydrate (in addition to alcohol, which is metabolized entirely as carbohydrate) and low in thiamine, and their body stores of B vitamins may have been further reduced by gastroenteritis and diarrhea. For this reason it is good practice to add B vitamins, specifically thiamine (which may also be supplemented by intramuscular injection), in all cases requiring parenterally administered glucose—even though the alcoholic disorder under treatment, e.g., delirium tremens, is not primarily due to vitamin deficiency.

With respect to the use of medications, it is important to distinguish between mild withdrawal symptoms, which are essentially benign and responsive to practically any sedative drug, and delirium tremens, which has a serious mortality and is relatively unresponsive to drugs. In the case of minor withdrawal symptoms, the purpose of medication is to ensure rest and sleep. This can be carried out on a hospital ward or a special "detoxification" unit. However, there is no certain way to predict whether a patient with the early signs of withdrawal will progress to a state of delirium tremens. In the latter state, the object of drug therapy is to blunt the psychomotor overactivity and prevent exhaustion and facilitate the administration of parenteral fluid and nursing care; one should not attempt to suppress agitation at all costs, since doing so requires an amount of drug that might seriously depress respiration.

A wide variety of drugs are effective in controlling withdrawal symptoms. The more popular ones in recent years have been chlordiazepoxide (Librium), diazepam (Valium), meprobamate, hydroxyzine (Vistaril) and the ancillary medications, clonidine and beta-adrenergic blockers, and newer anticonvulsant drugs such as gabapentin, which may reduce the requirement for sedative drugs. There is little to choose among these drugs in respect to their therapeutic efficacy. More importantly, there are few data to indicate that any one of them can prevent hallucinosis or delirium tremens or shorten the duration or alter the mortality rate of the latter disorder (Kaim et al). In general, phenothiazine drugs should be avoided because they reduce the threshold to seizures.

Currently, chlordiazepoxide and diazepam are the most frequently used drugs for treatment of withdrawal symptoms. If parenteral medication is necessary, we prefer 10 mg of diazepam or chlordiazepoxide given intravenously and repeated once or twice at 20- to 30-min intervals until the patient is calm but awake. Virtually equivalent alternatives are sodium phenobarbital in doses of 120 mg or haloperidol (10 mg) repeated at 3- to 4-h intervals intramuscularly (provided there is no serious liver disease). Beta-blocking agents, such as propranolol and atenolol, are helpful in reducing heart rate, blood pressure, and the tremor to some extent. Lofexidine, an $alpha_2$ agonist that blocks autonomic outflow centrally, and clonidine are similarly effective. Corticosteroids have no place in the treatment of the withdrawal syndrome.

Nutritional Diseases of the Nervous System

Alcoholism provides the ideal setting for the development of nutritional diseases of the nervous system. Although only a small proportion of alcoholics develop nutritional diseases, the overall number of these diseases is substantial because of the frequency of alcoholism. The importance of the alcohol-induced deficiency diseases relates to the fact that they are preventable and, if neglected, may lead to permanent disability. These illnesses are discussed fully in the preceding chapter, "Diseases of the Nervous System Due to Nutritional Deficiency."

Disorders of Uncertain Pathogenesis Associated with Alcoholism

Also discussed in Chap. 41 are so-called *alcoholic cerebellar degeneration* and *Marchiafava-Bignami disease*. The former is almost certainly of nutritional origin; in the latter a nutritional-metabolic etiology seems likely but has not been established. Central pontine myelinolysis, though frequently observed in alcoholics, is more appropriately considered with the acquired metabolic disorders (Chap. 40). Certain disorders of skeletal and cardiac muscle associated with alcoholism (*alcoholic myopathy and cardiomyopathy*) are described in Chap. 51, with the myopathies due to drugs and toxins. There remain to be discussed several diverse disorders that have been attributed to alcoholism but whose causal relationship to alcohol abuse, nutritional deficiency, or some other factor is not clear.

Alcoholic Dementia and Cerebral Atrophy The term *alcoholic dementia* is used widely and often indiscriminately to designate a presumably distinctive form of dementia that is attributable to the chronic, direct effects of alcohol on the brain. An immediate problem with this category of alcoholic disease is its definition. A syndrome subsumed under the title of *alcoholic dementia* and its many synonyms (*alcoholic deteriorated state, chronic alcoholic psychosis, chronic or organic brain syndrome due to alcohol*) has never been delineated satisfactorily, either clinically or pathologically. In the *Comprehensive Textbook of Psychiatry*, it has been defined as "a gradual disintegration of personality structure, with emotional lability, loss of control, and dementia" (Sadock and Sadock). To other psychiatrists (Strecker et al), the alcoholic deteriorated state denotes "the common end reaction of all chronic alcoholics who do not recover from their alcoholism or do not die of some accident or intercurrent episode." Purported examples of this state show a remarkably diverse group of symptoms, including jealousy and suspiciousness; coarsening of moral fiber and other personality and behavioral disorders; deterioration of work performance, personal care, and living habits; and disorientation, impaired judgment, and defects of intellectual function, particularly of memory. Some early authors were apparently impressed with similarities between the alcoholic deteriorated state and general paresis, hence the term *alcoholic pseudoparesis*. Mercifully this term no longer appears in medical writings.

In recent years, there have been attempts to redefine alcoholic dementia. Cutting and also Lishman have expressed the view that the term *Korsakoff psychosis* should be limited to patients with a fairly pure disorder of memory of acute onset and that patients with more global symptoms of intellectual deterioration, of gradual evolution, be considered to have alcoholic dementia. These are rather weak diagnostic criteria. As pointed out in Chap. 41, *Korsakoff psychosis* may have an insidious onset and gradual progression, and patients with this disorder, in addition to an amnesic defect, characteristically show disturbances of cognitive functions that depend little or not at all on memory. More importantly, in none of the patients designated by these authors as having alcoholic dementia was there a neuropathologic examination, without which the clinical assessment must remain arbitrary and imprecise.

The pathologic changes that purportedly underlie primary alcoholic dementia are even less precisely defined than the clinical syndrome. Courville, whose writings have been quoted most frequently in this respect, described a series of cerebral cortical changes that he attributed to the toxic effects of alcohol. Some of these changes turn out on close inspection to be quite nonspecific. Many of the cellular changes noted by Courville may have reflected a state of hepatic failure or terminal anoxia, and others reflect nothing more than the effects of aging or the insignificant artifacts of tissue fixation and staining.

More recently, Harper and colleagues have reported that the mean brain weight is decreased in alcoholics and the pericerebral space is increased—findings that do no more than confirm the brain shrinkage that is demonstrable by CT scans in many alcoholics and is reversible with sustained abstinence (see below). Also, using an automated cell-counting method, they reported a reduction in the number of neurons in the superior frontal cortex. Other investigators, using more accurate (stereologic) counting methods, have not duplicated these findings (Hansen et al; Jensen and Pakkenberg), nor have experimental studies in animals settled the problem.

In our experience, the majority of cases that come to autopsy with the label of *alcoholic dementia* or *deteriorated state* prove to have the lesions of the Wernicke-Korsakoff syndrome. Traumatic lesions of varying degrees of severity are commonly added. Other cases show the lesions of anoxic or hepatic encephalopathy, communicating hydrocephalus, Alzheimer disease, ischemic necrosis, or some other disease quite unrelated to alcoholism. Practically always, in our material, the clinical state can be accounted for by one or a combination of these disease processes, and there has been no need to invoke a hypothetical toxic effect of alcohol on the brain. This has also been the experience of Torvik and associates; with a few exceptions, such as coincidental Alzheimer disease, all their cases that had been diagnosed as having alcoholic dementia turned out, on neuropathologic examination, to have the chronic lesions of Wernicke-Korsakoff disease.

In brief, the most serious flaw in the concept of a primary alcoholic dementia is that it lacks a distinctive, well-defined pathology. Until such time as the morphologic basis is established, its status must remain ambiguous. A more detailed discussion of this subject and of so-called alcoholic cerebral atrophy (see below) can be found in the review by one of the present authors (M.V.), listed in the References.

Cerebral Atrophy in Chronic Alcoholism This disorder, like the "alcoholic deteriorated state," does not constitute a well-defined entity. The concept of alcoholic cerebral atrophy was the product originally of pneumoencephalographic studies. Relatively young alcoholics, some with and some without symptoms of cerebral disease, were often found to have enlarged cerebral ventricles and widened sulci, mainly of the frontal lobes (see, for example, reports of Brewer and Perrett and of Haug). Similar findings have been reported in chronic alcoholics examined by CT scanning and MRI (see review by Carlen et al).

The clinical correlates of these radiologic findings are quite unclear. In some patients, so-called cerebral atrophy is associated with an overt complication of alcoholism—e.g., the Wernicke-Korsakoff syndrome (about one-quarter of our autopsied cases). In other patients, there is a history of recurrent seizures or evidence of liver disease, cerebral trauma, or some other event that might have resulted in ventricular enlargement. More often, however, the finding of large ventricles comes as a surprise, no symptoms or signs of neuropsychiatric disease having been noted in the course of the usual neurologic and mental status testing. In this connection, the findings of Wilkinson are of particular importance. He demonstrated that in clinically normal alcoholics, the radiologic measures of "brain atrophy" were age-related; once the age factor was removed, the CT findings in these subjects did not differ significantly from those in nonalcoholic controls.

The term *alcoholic cerebral atrophy* implies that chronic exposure of the brain to alcohol causes an irreversible loss of cerebral tissue. However, this idea is open to criticism, for dilated ventricles have in fact been reversible to a considerable extent when abstinence is maintained (Carlen et al, Lishman, Zipursky et al, Schroth et al). Moreover, a similar ventricular enlargement, or brain shrinkage, also reversible, has been observed in patients with the Cushing syndrome, anorexia nervosa, and Lennox-Gastaut syndrome (treated with ACTH and corticosteroids). This reversibility would suggest that a shift of fluids had occurred in the brain (over many months), rather than loss of tissue. A rapid increase of the alcohol-inhibited antidiuretic hormone or a rise in protein synthesis after alcohol withdrawal are other possible explanations. Until this matter has been studied further, it would be preferable to refer to this condition as an asymptomatic ventricular enlargement and sulcal widening in alcoholics, rather than as cerebral atrophy.

Alcoholic Paranoia and Jealousy These are outmoded terms that were used in the past to designate what was thought to be a special type of paranoid reaction in chronic alcoholics, in which the patient, usually a male, developed ideas of infidelity on the part of his wife. The delusions of jealousy that might occur acutely in the course of alcoholic intoxication or withdrawal, or chronically as part of the "alcoholic deteriorated state," were generally not included under this rubric. The notion that pathologic jealousy merits classification as a distinctive complication of alcoholism is not warranted, since the morbid jealousy that develops in alcoholics differs in no essential way from that in nonalcoholics. Nevertheless, among individuals with the syndrome of morbid jealousy, chronic alcoholism may be an important associated factor (11 of 66 cases reported by Langfeldt). Among the alcoholic patients, the delusions of jealousy may at first be evident only in relation to episodes of acute intoxication, but later they evolve, through a stage of constant suspicion and efforts to detect infidelity, into a fixed morbid reaction that persists during periods of sobriety as well.

Fetal Alcohol Syndrome

That parental alcoholism may have an adverse effect on the offspring has been a recurrent theme in medical lore. Probably the first documented occurrence of such a relationship was that of Sullivan (1899), who reported that the mortality among the children of drunken mothers was more than two times greater than that among children of nondrinking women of "similar stock." This increased mortality was attributed by Sullivan and later by Haggard and Jellinek to postnatal influences such as poor nutrition and a chaotic home environment rather than to the intrauterine effects of alcohol. The idea that maternal alcoholism could damage the fetus was generally rejected and relegated to the category of superstitions about alcoholism or the claims of temperance ideologues.

In the late 1960s, the effects of alcohol abuse on the fetus were rediscovered, so to speak. Lemoine and associates in France and then Ulleland and Jones and Smith in the United States described a distinctive pattern of abnormalities in infants born of severely alcoholic mothers. The affected infants are small in length in comparison to weight, and most of them fall below the third percentile for head circumference. They are distinguished also by the presence of short palpebral fissures (shortened distance between inner and outer canthi) and epicanthal folds; maxillary hypoplasia, micrognathia, indistinct philtrum, and thin upper lip; and longitudinally oriented palmar creases, flexion deformities of the fingers, and a limited range of motion of other joints. Cardiac anomalies (usually spontaneously closing septal defects), anomalous external genitalia, and cleft lip and palate are much more frequent than in the general population. The newborn infants suck and sleep poorly, and many of them are irritable, restless, hyperactive, and tremulous; these last symptoms resemble those of alcohol withdrawal except that they persist.

The first long-term study of children with what has come to be called *fetal alcohol syndrome* (FAS) was reported by Jones and coworkers. Among 23 infants born to alcoholic mothers, there was a neonatal mortality of 17 percent; among the infants who survived the neonatal period, almost half failed to achieve normal weight, length, and head circumference or remained backward mentally to a varying degree, even under optimal environmental conditions. Several large groups of FAS children have now been observed for 20 years or longer (see Streissguth). Distractibility, inattentiveness, hyperactivity, and impairment of fine motor coordination are prominent features in early childhood. Most such children are given the diagnosis of attention-deficit hyperactivity disorder. Slow growth of head circumference is a consistent finding throughout infancy and childhood. The physical stigmata of the syndrome become less distinctive after puberty, but practically all adolescents are left with some degree of mental retardation and behavioral abnormalities.

The pathologic changes that underlie the FAS have been studied in a small number of cases. Clarren and colleagues found extensive leptomeningeal neuroglial heterotopias and an obstructive hydrocephalus. Neuronal ectopias in the cerebral white matter and agenesis of the corpus callosum were also present. Peiffer and colleagues described a broader spectrum of malformations, including cerebellar heterotopias similar to those of the Dandy-Walker syndrome, schizencephaly, agenesis of the corpus callosum, and signs of arrhinencephaly.

Although the relationship of this syndrome to severe maternal alcoholism seems undoubted, the mechanism by which alcohol produces its effects is not fully understood. It is noteworthy that infants born to nonalcoholic mothers who had been subjected to severe dietary deprivation during pregnancy (during World War II) were small and often premature, but these infants did not show the pattern of malformations that characterizes FAS. Alcohol readily crosses the placenta in humans and animals; in the mouse, rat, chick, miniature swine, and beagle dog, alcohol has been shown to have both embryotoxic and teratogenic effects. Thus, the evidence to date favors a toxic effect of alcohol, although a possible toxic effect of acetaldehyde and smoking and a possible contributory role for nutritional deficiency have not been totally excluded. As to the specific mechanisms by which alcohol impairs the growth and development of the fetus, a compromised blood flow to the placenta and an ethanol-induced increase in prostaglandins have been suggested but are as yet unproved hypotheses (Schenker et al).

Unequivocal cases of FAS observed to date have occurred only in infants born to severely alcoholic mothers (many of them with delirium tremens and liver disease) who continued to drink heavily throughout pregnancy. Far less secure is a relationship to lesser degrees of alcohol intake. Data derived from the collaborative study sponsored by the National Institutes of Health indicate that about one-third of the offspring of women who are heavy drinkers have the FAS. Abel and Sokol have estimated that the worldwide incidence of the FAS is 1.9 per 1000 live births and have pronounced it to be the leading known cause of mental retardation in the western world. The degree of maternal alcoholism that is necessary to produce the syndrome and the critical stage in gestation during which it occurs are still vague. The various teratogenic effects described above are estimated to occur in the embryonic period, i.e., in the first 2 months of fetal life. Other nonteratogenic effects appear to be related to periods during gestation when the fetus is exposed to particularly high alcohol levels.

Diagnostic difficulties arise when only certain components of the syndrome occur in association with heavy maternal drinking, in the absence of the fully developed syndrome; these have been termed *fetal alcohol effects*, and their incidence is more difficult to determine. A comprehensive account of alcohol-related birth defects and the controversial issues surrounding this subject is contained in a special issue of *Alcohol Health and Research World*, published by the National Institutes of Health (Vol. 18, 1994).

Neurologic Complications of Alcoholic Cirrhosis and Portal-Systemic Shunts

This category of alcoholic disease is discussed in Chap. 40, in connection with the acquired metabolic disorders of the nervous system.

Treatment of Alcohol Addiction

Following recovery from the acute medical and neurologic complications of alcoholism, the underlying problem of alcohol dependence remains. To treat only the medical complications and leave the management of the drinking problem to the patient alone is shortsighted. Almost always, drinking is resumed, with a predictable recurrence of medical illness. For this reason the physician must be prepared to deal with the addiction or at least to initiate treatment.

The problem of excessive drinking is formidable but not nearly as hopeless as it is generally made out to be (see review of O'Connor and Schottenfeld). A common misconception among physicians is that specialized training in psychiatry and an inordinately large amount of time are required to deal with the addictive drinker. Actually, a successful program of treatment can be initiated by any interested physician, using the standard techniques of history taking, establishing rapport with the patient, and setting up a schedule of frequent visits, though not necessarily for prolonged periods. Our position on this matter was reinforced by a controlled study of problem drinkers in whom treatment was equally successful whether carried out by general practitioners or by specialists (Drummond et al). Useful points at which to undertake treatment are during convalescence from a serious medical or neurologic complication of alcoholism or in relation to loss of employment, arrest, or threatened divorce. Such a crisis may help to convince the patient, more than any argument presented by family or physician, that the drinking problem has reached serious proportions.

The requisite for successful treatment is total abstinence from alcohol; for all practical purposes, this represents the only permanent solution. It is generally agreed that any attempts to curb the drinking habit will fail if the patient continues to drink. There are said to be alcohol addicts who have been able to reduce their intake of alcohol and eventually to drink in moderation, but they must represent only a small proportion of the addict population. Also, it is frequently stated that alcoholics must recognize that they are alcoholics—i.e., that their drinking is beyond their control—and must express willingness to be helped. Undoubtedly there is truth in both these statements, but they should not be interpreted to mean that alcoholic patients must gain this recognition and willingness entirely on their own initiative and that they will be helped only after they have done so. The physician can do a great deal to help such patients understand the nature of their problem and thus to motivate them to accept treatment. The help of family, employer, courts, and clergy should be enlisted in an attempt to convince these patients that abstinence is preferable to chronic inebriety. Alcoholic patients must be made fully aware of the medical and social consequences of continued drinking and must also be made to understand that because of some constitutional peculiarity (like that of the diabetic, who cannot handle sugar), they are incapable of drinking in moderation. These facts should be presented in much the same way as one would explain the essential features of any other disease; there is nothing to be gained from adopting a punitive or moralizing attitude. Yet patients should not be given the idea that they are in no way to blame for their illness; there appears to be an advantage in making them feel that they are responsible for doing something about their drinking.

The prevalent belief that an alcoholic will not stop drinking under duress also requires qualification. In fact, one of the few careful studies of this matter disclosed that relatively few patients would have sought help unless pressure had been exerted by family or employer; furthermore, those who came to the clinic under duress of this sort did just as well as those who came voluntarily.

A number of methods have proved valuable in the short- and long-term management of patients. The more important of these are admission to a detoxification or special hospital unit, rehabilitative therapy, aversion treatment, the use of disulfiram (Antabuse), and the participation in self-help organizations for recovery from alcoholism. Detoxification clinics and special hospital units for the treatment of alcoholism are now widely available. The physician should be fully aware of all the community resources available for the management of this problem and should be prepared to take advantage of them in appropriate cases. Most inpatient programs include individual and group counseling, didactics about the illness and recovery, and family intervention. Outpatient treatment (of individuals or groups) is widely available, either from specialized facilities or from specialized therapists in general mental health facilities; family counseling is usually offered as well and is often beneficial. Most professional alcoholism treatment in the United States includes an introduction to the methods and utilization of Alcoholics Anonymous (AA, see below).

Aversion treatment consists of the simultaneous administration of a drink of alcohol and injection of an emetic. The violent nausea and vomiting that ensue are intended to create in the patient a strong revulsion for alcohol. This form of treatment, as well as other types of conditioned-reflex treatment, have been employed with some success in special clinics. Most of the facilities that offer aversion treatment also incorporate the features of conventional rehabilitation therapy and support involvement with AA.

Disulfiram interferes with the metabolism of alcohol, so that a patient who takes both alcohol and disulfiram accumulates an inordinate amount of acetaldehyde in the tissues, resulting in nausea, vomiting, and hypotension, sometimes pronounced in degree. It is no longer considered necessary to demonstrate these effects to patients; it is sufficient to warn them of the severe reactions that may result if they drink while they have the drug in their bodies. Treatment with disulfiram is instituted only after the patient has been sober for several days, preferably longer. It should never be given to patients with cardiac or advanced liver disease. The drug is taken each morning or at another suitable time daily in a dosage of 250 mg, preferably under supervision. This form of treatment may be of value in the spree or periodic drinker, in whom relapse from abstinence usually represents an impulsive rather than a carefully planned or premeditated act. The patient taking disulfiram, aware of the dangers of mixing liquor and the drug, is "protected" against the impulse to drink, and this protection may be renewed every 24 h by the simple expedient of taking a pill. The willingness with which the patient accepts this form of treatment also serves as a rough test of his willingness to stop drinking. Should the patient drink while taking disulfiram, the ensuing reaction is usually severe enough to require medical attention, and a protracted spree can thus be prevented. Disulfiram may cause a polyneuropathy if continued over a period of months or years, but this is a rare complication.

Several other drugs may be helpful in maintaining abstinence. The opioid antagonist naltrexone (50 mg/day) has been used for this purpose, with mixed results. In Europe, a modicum of success has been achieved with acamprosate (2000 mg daily), but this drug is not yet available in the United States.

Alcoholics Anonymous (AA), an informal fellowship of recovering alcoholics, has proved to be the single most effective force in the rehabilitation of alcoholic patients. The philosophy of this organization is embodied in its "12 steps," a series of principles for sober living that guide the patient to recovery. These steps have been adopted by analogous fellowships for recovery from other addictive states, such as compulsive overeating, gambling, and dependence on narcotics. The AA philosophy stresses in particular the practice of making restitution, the necessity to help other alcoholics, trust in a higher power, the group confessional, and the belief that the alcoholic alone is powerless over alcohol. The AA philosophy also embodies the 24-h plan, in which the alcoholic strives to be abstinent for just a day at a time (a concept inspired by the Sermon on the Mount) as a means of facilitating the maintenance of sobriety. Although accurate statistics are lacking, it is said that about one-third of the members who express more than a passing interest in the program attain a state of long-sustained or permanent sobriety. Although the methods used by AA are not preferred by every patient, most who persist can benefit; in particular, the physician should not accept a patient's initial negative reaction as reason to abandon AA as a mode of treatment.

Finally, it should be noted that alcoholism is frequently associated with psychiatric disease of other type, particularly sociopathy and affective illness. In the latter case, the prevailing mood is far more often one of depression than of mania and is more often encountered in women, who are more apt to drink under these conditions than are men. In these circumstances, expert psychiatric help should be sought, preferably from someone who is also familiar with addictive diseases.

REFERENCES

ABEL EL, SOKOL RJ: Incidence of fetal alcohol syndrome and economic impact of FAS-related anomalies. *Drug Alcohol Depend* 19:51, 1987.

BAUD FJ, GALLIOT M, ASTIER A, et al: Treatment of ethylene glycol poisoning with intravenous 4-methylpyrazole. *N Engl J Med* 319:97, 1988.

BRENT J, MCMARTIN K, PHILLIPS S, et al: Fomepizole for the treatment of ethylene glycol poisoning. *N Engl J Med* 340:832, 1999.

BOHMAN M: Some genetic aspects of alcoholism and criminality. *Arch Gen Psychiatry* 35: 269, 1978.

BREWER C, PERRETT L: Brain damage due to alcohol consumption: An air-encephalographic, psychometric and electroencephalographic study. *Br J Addict* 66(3):170, 1971.

CADORET RJ, CAIN C, GROVE WM: Development of alcoholism in adoptees raised apart from alcoholic biologic relatives. *Arch Gen Psychiatry* 37:561, 1980.

CARLEN PL, WORTZMAN G, HOLGATE RC, et al: Reversible cerebral atrophy in recently abstinent chronic alcoholics measured by computed tomography scans. *Science* 200:1076, 1978.

CHARNESS ME: Molecular mechanisms of ethanol intoxication, tolerance, and physical dependence, in Mendelson JH, Mello NK (eds): *Medical Diagnosis and Treatment of Alcoholism.* New York, McGraw-Hill, 1992, pp 155–199.

CHIN JH, GOLDSTEIN DB: Drug tolerance in biomembranes: A spin label study of the effects of ethanol. *Science* 196:684, 1977.

CLARREN SK, ALVORD EC JR, SUMI SM, et al: Brain malformations related to prenatal exposure to ethanol. *J Pediatr* 92:64, 1978.

COURVILLE CB: *Effects of Alcohol on the Nervous System of Man.* Los Angeles, San Lucas Press, 1955.

CUSHMAN P JR, FORBES R, LERNER WD, STEWART M: Alcohol withdrawal syndrome: Clinical management with lofexidine. *Alcoholism* 9:103, 1985.

CUTTING J: The relationship between Korsakov's syndrome and "alcoholic" dementia. *Br J Psychiatry* 132:240, 1978.

DAVIDSON CS: Nutrient content of beers and ales. *N Engl J Med* 264:185, 1961.

DOLIN SJ, LITTLE HJ: Are changes in neuronal calcium channels involved in ethanol tolerance? *J Pharmacol Exp Ther* 250:985, 1989.

D'ONOFRIO G, RATHLEV NK, ULRICH AS, et al: Lorazepam for the prevention of recurrent seizures related to alcohol. *N Engl J Med* 340:915, 1999.

DRUMMOND DC, THOM B, BROWN C, et al: Specialist versus general practitioner treatment of problem drinkers. *Lancet* 336:915, 1990.

FERGUSON JA, SUELZER CJ, ECJERT GJ, et al: Risk factors for delirium tremens development. *J Gen Intern Med* 11:410, 1996.

FOY A, KAY J: The incidence of alcohol-related problems and the risk of alcohol withdrawal in a general hospital population. *Drug Alcohol Rev* 14:49, 1995.

FREZZA M, DI PADOVA C, POZZATO G, et al: High blood alcohol levels in women: The role of decreased gastric alcohol dehydrogenase activity and first-pass metabolism. *N Engl J Med* 322:95, 1990.

GESSNER PK: Drug therapy of the alcohol withdrawal syndrome, in Majchrowicz E, Noble EP (eds): *Biochemistry and Pharmacology of Ethanol.* Vol 2. New York, Plenum Press, 1979, pp 375–435.

GOLDSTEIN DB: *Pharmacology of Alcohol.* New York, Oxford University Press, 1983.

GOODWIN DW, SCHULSINGER F, MOLLER N, et al: Drinking problems in adopted and nonadopted sons of alcoholics. *Arch Gen Psychiatry* 31:164, 1974.

GRANT BF, HARFORD TC, CHOUP P, et al: Prevalence of DSM-III-R alcohol abuse and dependence: United States, 1988. *Alcohol Health Res World* 15:91, 1991.

GROVE WM, CADORET RJ: Genetic factors in alcoholism, in Kissin B, Begleiter H (eds): *The Biology of Alcoholism.* Vol 7. *The Pathogenesis of Alcoholism.* New York, Plenum Press, 1983, pp 31–56.

HAGGARD HW, JELLINEK EM: *Alcohol Explored.* Garden City, NY, Doubleday Doran, 1942.

HANSEN LA, NATELSON BH, LEMERE C, et al: Alcohol-induced brain changes in dogs. *Arch Neurol* 48:939, 1991.

HARADA S, AGARWAL DP, GOEDDE HW: Aldehyde dehydrogenase deficiency as cause of facial flushing reaction to alcohol in Japanese. *Lancet* 2:982, 1981.

HARPER CG, BLUMBERGS PC: Brain weights in alcoholics. *J Neurol Neurosurg Psychiatry* 45:838, 1982.

HARPER CG, KRIL JJ: Brain atrophy in chronic alcoholic patients: A quantitative pathologic study. *J Neurol Neurosurg Psychiatry* 48:211, 1985.

HARRIS RA, BAXTER DM, MITCHELL MA, et al: Physical properties and lipid composition of brain membranes from ethanol tolerant-dependent mice. *Mol Pharmacol* 25:401, 1984.

HAUG JO: Pneumoencephalographic evidence of brain damage in chronic alcoholics: A preliminary report. *Acta Psychiatr Scand* 203(suppl):135, 1968.

HAWLEY RJ, MAJOR JF, SCHULMAN EA, et al: CSF levels of norepinephrine during alcohol withdrawal. *Arch Neurol* 38: 289, 1981.

ISBELL H, FRASER HF, WIKLER A, et al: An experimental study of the etiology of "rum fits" and delirium tremens. *Q J Stud Alcohol* 16:1, 1955.

JACOBSEN D: New treatment for ethylene glycol poisoning. *N Engl J Med* 340: 879, 1999.

JENSEN GB, PAKKENBERG B: Do alcoholics drink their neurons away? *Lancet* 342:1201, 1993.

JONES KL, SMITH DW: Recognition of the fetal alcohol syndrome in early infancy. *Lancet* 2:999, 1973.

JONES KL, SMITH DW, STREISSGUTH AP, MYRIANTHOPOULOS NC: Outcome in offspring of chronic alcoholic women. *Lancet* 1:1076, 1974.

KAIM SC, KLETT CJ, ROTHFELD B: Treatment of acute alcohol withdrawal state: A comparison of four drugs. *Am J Psychiatry* 125:1640, 1969.

KRIL JJ, HARPER CG: Neuronal counts from four cortical regions in alcoholic brains. *Acta Neuropathol (Berl)* 79:200, 1989.

LANGFELDT G: The erotic jealousy syndrome: A clinical study. *Acta Psychiatr Neurol Scand* 36(suppl 151):7, 1961.

LEMOINE P, HAROUSSEAU H, BORTEYRU JP, MENUET JC: Les enfants de parents alcooliques: Anomalies observées à propos de 127 cas. *Ouest-Med* 25:477, 1968.

LIEBER CS (ed): *Medical and Nutritional Complications of Alcoholism: Mechanisms and Management.* New York, Plenum Press, 1992.

LISHMAN WA: Cerebral disorder in alcoholism: Syndromes of impairment. *Brain* 104:1, 1981.

LITTLE HJ, DOLIN SJ, HALSEY MJ: Calcium channel antagonists decrease the ethanol withdrawal syndrome. *Life Sci* 39:2059, 1986.

MCLEAN DR, JACOBS H, MIELKE BW: Methanol poisoning: A clinical and pathological study. *Ann Neurol* 8:161, 1980.

MELLO NK: Etiological theories of alcoholism, in Mello NK (ed): *Behavioral and Biological Research.* Vol III. *Advances in Substance Abuse.* Greenwich, CT: JAI Press, 1983, pp 271–312.

MENDELSON JH, MELLO NK (eds): *Medical Diagnosis and Treatment of Alcoholism.* New York, McGraw-Hill, 1992.

MILES WR: Psychological effects of alcohol and man, in Emerson H (ed): *Alcohol and Man.* New York, Macmillan, 1932, p 224.

O'CONNOR PG, SCHOTTENFELD RS: Patients with alcohol problems. *N Engl J Med* 338:592, 1998.

PEIFFER J, MAJEWSKI F, FISCHBACH H, et al: Alcohol embryo- and fetopathy: Neuropathology of 3 children and 3 fetuses. *J Neurol Sci* 41:125, 1979.

PORJESZ B, BEGLEITER H: Brain dysfunction and alcohol, in Kissin B, Begleiter H (eds): *The Biology of Alcoholism.* Vol 7. *The Pathogenesis of Alcoholism.* New York, Plenum Press, 1983, pp 415–483.

REICH T: Biologic-marker studies in alcoholism. *N Engl J Med* 318:180, 1988.

SADOCK BJ, SADOCK VA (eds): *Kaplan and Sadock's Comprehensive Textbook of Psychiatry.* Philadelphia, Lippincott Williams & Wilkins, 2000.

SAMSON HH, HARRIS RA: Neurobiology of alcohol abuse. *Trends Pharmacol Sci* 13:206, 1992.

SCHENKER S, BECKER HC, RANDALL CL, et al: Fetal alcohol syndrome: Current status of pathogenesis. *Alcohol Clin Exp Res* 14:635, 1990.

SCHROTH G, NAEGELE T, KLOSE U, et al: Reversible brain shrinkage in abstinent alcoholics, measured by MRI. *Neuroradiology* 30:385, 1988.

SCHUCKIT MA: Genetic aspects of alcoholism. *Ann Emerg Med* 15:991, 1986.

SCHUCKIT MA, WINOKUR G: Alcoholic hallucinosis and schizophrenia: A negative study. *Br J Psychiatry* 119:549, 1971.

SCOTT DF: Alcoholic hallucinosis: An aetiological study. *Br J Addict* 62:113, 1967.

SECRETARY OF HEALTH AND HUMAN SERVICES. *Ninth Special Report to the U.S. Congress on Alcohol and Health.* NIH publication no. 97-4017. Washington, D.C.: Government Printing Office, 1997.

SPILLANE L, ROBERTS JR, MEYER AE: Multiple cranial nerve deficits after ethylene glycol poisoning. *Ann Emerg Med* 20:208, 1991.

STRECKER EA, EBAUGH FG, EWALT JR: *Practical Clinical Psychiatry.* New York, McGraw-Hill, 1951, pp 150–170.

STREISSGUTH AP: A long-term perspective of FAS. *Alcohol Health Res World* 18:74, 1994.

SULLIVAN WC: A note on the influence of maternal inebriety on the offspring. *J Mental Sci* 45:489, 1899.

TORVIK A, LINDBOE CF, ROGDE S: Brain lesions in alcoholics. *J Neurol Sci* 56:233, 1982.

ULLELAND C: The offspring of alcoholic mothers. *Ann N Y Acad Sci* 197:167, 1972.

VICTOR M: Alcoholic dementia. *Can J Neurol Sci* 21:88, 1994.

VICTOR M: Introductory remarks. *Ann N Y Acad Sci* 215:210, 1973.

VICTOR M: The pathophysiology of alcoholic epilepsy. *Res Publ Assoc Res Nerv Ment Dis* 46:431, 1968.

VICTOR M, ADAMS RD: The effect of alcohol on the nervous system. *Res Publ Assoc Res Nerv Ment Dis* 32:526, 1953.

VICTOR M, ADAMS RD, COLLINS GH: *The Wernicke-Korsakoff Syndrome and Other Disorders Due to Alcoholism and Malnutrition.* Philadelphia, Davis, 1989.

VICTOR M, HOPE J: The phenomenon of auditory hallucinations in chronic alcoholism. *J Nerv Ment Dis* 126:451, 1958.

WILKINSON DA: Examination of alcoholics by computed tomographic scans: A critical review. *Alcohol Clin Exp Res* 6:31, 1982.

WOLFE SM, VICTOR M: The relationship of hypomagnesemia and alkalosis to alcohol withdrawal symptoms. *Ann N Y Acad Sci* 162:973, 1969.

ZIPURSKY RB, LIM KO, PFEFFERBAUM A: MRI study of brain changes with short-term abstinence from alcohol. *Alcohol Clin Exp Res* 13:664, 1989.

Chapter 43

DISORDERS OF THE NERVOUS SYSTEM DUE TO DRUGS AND OTHER CHEMICAL AGENTS

Subsumed under this title is a diverse group of disorders of the nervous system that result from introduction into the body of drugs and other injurious or poisonous substances. A drug can be broadly defined as *any chemical agent that affects living processes*, but for purposes of this chapter, the discussion is limited to such drugs as are useful in the prevention and treatment of diseases of the nervous system. In addition, the neurologist must be concerned with the myriad of chemical agents that have no therapeutic utility but may adversely affect the nervous system; they abound in the environment as household products, insecticides, industrial solvents, and other poisons, the toxic effects of which must be recognized and treated. Also included among neurotoxins are those generated by bacteria and other infectious agents as well as several found in nature, such as marine toxins and agents elaborated by living animals. These are designated as *endogenous* if they arise within the body and *exogenous* if introduced from outside. Such a division cannot always be sharply drawn, as in the case of toxins produced by certain bacteria after being introduced from the outside (e.g., tetanus).

It would hardly be possible within the confines of this chapter to discuss with any degree of completeness the innumerable drugs and toxins that affect the nervous system. The interested reader is referred to a number of comprehensive monographs and references listed at the end of this chapter. In addition, an up-to-date handbook of pharmacology and toxicology should be part of the library of every physician.

The scope of this chapter is also limited because the therapeutic and adverse effects of many drugs are considered elsewhere in this volume, in relation to particular symptoms and diseases. Thus, the toxic effects of ethyl, methyl, amyl, and isopropyl alcohol, as well as ethylene glycol, are discussed in Chap. 42, on alcohol. The adverse effects of antibiotics on cochlear and vestibular function and on neuromuscular transmission are discussed in Chaps. 15 and 53, respectively. Many of the undesirable side effects of the common drugs used in the treatment of extrapyramidal motor symptoms, pain, headache, convulsive seizures, sleep disorders, psychiatric illnesses, and so forth are considered in the chapters dealing with each of these disorders. Cyanide and carbon monoxide poisoning are discussed in relation to anoxic encephalopathy (Chap. 40). A number of therapeutic agents that damage the peripheral nerves (e.g., cisplatin, disulfiram, vincristine, dapsone, etc.) are mentioned in this chapter but are discussed further in Chap. 46, and those affecting muscle, in Chap. 51.

The presentation of this subject is introduced by some general remarks on the action of drugs on the nervous system and then focuses on the more common categories of drugs and chemical agents that affect the nervous system selectively or predominantly. The references at the end of the chapter are listed in relation to each of these categories:

1. Action of drugs on the nervous system: general principles
2. The addicting drugs: opiates and synthetic analgesics
3. Sedative-hypnotic drugs
4. Antipsychotic drugs

5. Antidepressant drugs
6. Stimulants
7. Psychoactive drugs
8. Bacterial toxins
9. Plant poisons, venoms, bites, and stings
10. Heavy metals
11. Industrial toxins
12. Antineoplastic and immunosuppressive agents
13. Thalidomide
14. Aminoglycoside antibiotics (ototoxicity) and penicillin derivatives (seizures)
15. Cardioactive agents (beta blockers, digitalis derivatives, amiodarone)

NEUROPHARMACOLOGY: GENERAL PRINCIPLES

Of primary importance is the manner in which a therapeutic agent, specifically its chemical structure, affects the biochemistry and physiology of neurons and their supporting elements (*pharmacodynamics*). The rational use of any drug also requires a knowledge of the best route of administration, the drug's absorption characteristics, its distribution in the nervous system and other organs, and its biotransformations and excretion (*pharmacokinetics*). Since every drug, if given in excess, has some adverse effects, therapeutics and toxicology are inseparable.

Drug–Nervous System Interactions

In no other field of neurology is it more apparent that all systems of neurons are not identical. Each has its own vulnerabilities to particular drugs and toxic agents. This principle, originally enunciated by O. and C. Vogt in their theory termed *pathoclisis*, has been elegantly confirmed by tracing chemical molecules to specific aggregates of neurons. Thus, pathoclisis explains the preferential effects of anesthetics on the neurons of the upper brainstem reticular formation, which, with its diffuse cortical connections, underlies consciousness. There are examples not only of certain groups of nerve cells being destroyed by a particular agent but also of their function and presumably particular parts of their structure being altered. Drugs may be targeted to the terminal axons, dendrites, neurofilaments, or receptors on pre- and postsynaptic surfaces of neurons or to certain of their metabolic activities, whereby they synthesize and release neurotransmitters or maintain their cellular integrity by the synthesis of RNA, DNA, and other proteins. Parkinson disease and the neurotoxin 1-methyl-4-phenyl-1,2,3,6-tetrahydropyridine (MPTP) are excellent examples of pathoclisis, in which a disease process and a synthetic toxin effect a progressive loss of melanin-bearing nigral neurons and a depletion of their neurotransmitter, dopamine. Evidence is also accumulating about the mechanisms by which drugs and toxins can alter particular steps in the formation, storage in presynaptic vesicles, release, uptake, catabolism, and resynthesis of neurotransmitters such as dopamine, serotonin, norepinephrine, acetylcholine, and other catecholamines. Johnston and Silverstein have summarized current views of how these transmitters and modulating agents, by attaching to receptors at neuronal synapses, are able to increase or decrease the permeability of ion channels and stimulate or inhibit second cytoplasmic messengers. Drugs such as L-dopa, tryptophan, and choline are believed to act by enhancing the synthesis of dopamine, serotonin, and acetylcholine, respectively. Baclofen is thought to modulate the release of gamma-aminobutyric acid (GABA), the main inhibitory transmitter in the central nervous system (CNS). Clonidine prevents the release of norepinephrine; botulinus toxin has a similar effect on acetycholine, and tetanus toxin on GABA in Renshaw cells of the spinal cord. Amantadine, an antiviral agent, is thought to promote the release of dopamine, and guanidine, of acetylcholine. Benzodiazepines, bromocriptine, and methylphenidate are viewed as receptor agonists; the phenothiazines and anticholinergics act as receptor antagonists. Certain drugs enhance the activity of neurotransmitters by inhibiting their reuptake, as, for example, the antidepressant class of drugs, which has a relatively selective influence on the reuptake of serotonin. One must not assume that these are the exclusive modes of action of each of these drugs, but these new data are instructive and indicate the future direction of neuropharmacology.

Lacking still is information about the precise mechanisms of even the most common anesthetics. It is assumed that by their lipid solubility they alter the physicochemical properties of the cell membrane and thus impair the activities of the membrane receptor systems that regulate ion channels, particularly the chloride and calcium channels. Antiviral agents such as acyclovir possibly block viral replication in nerve and glial cells once the inactive form of the drug is activated by thymidine kinase in these cells. A similar mode of action is postulated for azidothymidine (AZT), used in the treatment of acquired immunodeficiency syndrome (AIDS).

Bioavailability

A majority of drugs that act on the nervous system are ingested; factors that govern their intestinal absorption must, therefore, be taken into account. Small molecules usually enter the plasma by diffusion, larger ones by pinocytosis. The substances with which the drugs are mixed (excipients); the presence of food, other drugs, or intestinal diseases; and the age of the patient all influence the rate of absorption and blood concentrations. Different calculations are necessary for intramuscular, subcutaneous, and intrathecal routes of administration. To some extent, the solubilities of drugs (in lipid or water) determine the routes by which they can be given; some drugs, such as morphine, can be administered by manifold routes. Carried in the blood, the drug (or toxin) reaches many tissues, including the nervous system; protein binding in the plasma has an important influence on distribution. Many drugs and toxic substances bind to serum albumin and other serum proteins, limiting the availability of the ionized form. The common drug and toxin transformations involve hydroxylation, deamination, oxidation, and dealkylation, which enhance their solubility and elimination by the kidney. Most of these catalytic processes occur in liver cells and utilize multiple enzymes.

To enter the extracellular compartment of the nervous system, the drug or toxic agent in question must transgress the tight capillary endothelial barrier (blood-brain barrier) and the barrier between the blood and cerebrospinal fluid (CSF). Intrathecal injection circumvents these barriers, but then the agent tends to concentrate in the immediate subpial and subependymal regions. The process of movement from plasma to brain is by diffusion through capillaries or by facilitated transport. The solubility characteristics of the drug determine its rate of diffusion.

In the following exposition on neurotoxins, the reader will be repeatedly exposed to a number of novel phenomena: *tolerance* (lessening effect of increasing dose), *dependence* and *addiction* (insatiable need), *habituation*, *drug-seeking behaviors*, and *abstinence* and associated *withdrawal effects*. These were described in Chap. 42 on alcoholism and are further elaborated below. Particularly difficult in reference to drugs such as nicotine is the separation of habituation from addiction, i.e., of psychologic dependence from physical dependence (see further on).

To make intelligent use of any of the pharmacologic agents described below, the neurologist must know about their pharmacodynamic and pharmacokinetic properties. The few examples given above are intended to provide a glimpse of the complex interactions between chemical agents and the cells of the nervous system. For more specific information, the reader is referred to *The Biochemical Basis of Neuropharmacology* by Cooper, Bloom, and Roth, an excellent text that we have consulted through its seven editions. The continued elucidation of the modes of action of the several hundred drugs and toxins that act on the nervous system promises to yield important information about the biochemical physiology of neurons and opens for study an inviting field of experimental neuropharmacology.

OPIATES AND SYNTHETIC ANALGESIC DRUGS

The opiates, strictly speaking, include all the naturally occurring alkaloids in opium, which is prepared from the seed capsules of the poppy *Papaver somniferum*. For clinical purposes, the term *opiate* refers only to the alkaloids that have a high degree of analgesic activity, i.e., morphine and codeine. The terms *opioid* and *narcotic-analgesic* designate drugs with actions similar to those of morphine. Compounds that are chemical modifications of morphine include diacetylmorphine, or heroin (still the most commonly abused opioid), hydromorphone (Dilaudid), codeine, hydrocodone (Hydrocet), oxymorphone (Numorphan), and oxycodone (Percodan). A second class of opioids comprises the purely synthetic analgesics: meperidine (Demerol) and its congeners, notably fentanyl (Sublimaze), methadone (Dolophine), levorphanol (Levo-Dromoran), propoxyphene (Darvon), pentazocine (Talwin), diphenoxylate (the main component of Lomotil), and phenazocine (Prinadol). The synthetic analgesics are similar to the opiates, in both their pharmacologic effects and patterns of abuse, the differences being mainly quantitative.

The clinical effects of the opioids are considered from two points of view: (1) acute poisoning and (2) addiction.

Opioid Overdose

Because of the common and particularly the illicit use of opioids, poisoning is a frequent occurrence. This happens as a result of ingestion or injection with suicidal intent, errors in the calculation of dosage, the use of a substitute or contaminated street product, or unusual sensitivity. Children exhibit an increased susceptibility to opioids, so that relatively small doses may prove toxic. This is true also of adults with myxedema, Addison disease, chronic liver disease, or pneumonia. Acute poisoning may also occur in addicts who are unaware that available opioids vary greatly in potency and that tolerance for opioids declines quickly after the withdrawal of the drug; upon resumption of the habit, a formerly well-tolerated dose can be fatal.

Varying degrees of unresponsiveness, shallow respirations, slow respiratory rate (e.g., two to four per minute) or periodic breathing, pinpoint pupils, bradycardia, and hypothermia are the well-recognized clinical manifestations of acute opioid poisoning. In the most advanced stage, the pupils dilate, the skin and mucous membranes become cyanotic, and the circulation fails. The immediate cause of death is usually respiratory depression, with consequent asphyxia. Patients who suffer a cardiorespiratory arrest are sometimes left with all the known residua of anoxic encephalopathy. Others who recover from coma may occasionally reveal a hemiplegia, presumably due to vascular occlusion. Mild degrees of intoxication are betrayed by anorexia, nausea, vomiting, constipation, and loss of sexual interest.

Treatment This consists of the administration of naloxone (Narcan), a specific antidote to the opiates and also to the synthetic analgesics. The dose of naloxone is 0.7 mg/70 kg body weight *intravenously*, repeated if necessary once or twice at 5-min intervals. In cases of opioid poisoning, the improvements in circulation and respiration and reversal of miosis are usually dramatic. In fact, failure of naloxone to produce such a response should cast doubt on the diagnosis of opioid intoxication. If an adequate respiratory and pupillary response to naloxone is obtained, the patient should be observed carefully for 24 h and further doses of naloxone (50 percent higher than the ones previously found effective) should be given *intramuscularly* as often as necessary. Naloxone has little direct effect on consciousness, however, and the patient may remain drowsy for many hours. This is not harmful provided that respiration is well maintained. Gastric lavage is a useful measure if the drug was taken orally. This procedure may be efficacious many hours after ingestion, since one of the toxic effects of opioids is severe pylorospasm and ileus, which causes much of the drug to be retained in the stomach.

Once the patient regains consciousness, complaints such as pruritus, sneezing, tearing, piloerection, diffuse body pains, yawning, and diarrhea may appear. These are the recognizable symptoms of the opioid abstinence, or withdrawal, syndrome, described below. An antidote therefore must be used with great caution in an addict who has taken an overdose of opioid, because in this circumstance it may precipitate withdrawal phenomena. Nausea and severe abdominal pain, due presumably to pancreatitis (from spasm of the sphincter of Oddi), are other troublesome symptoms of opiate use or withdrawal. Seizures are rare.

Opioid Addiction

Just 30 to 35 years ago there were an estimated 60,000 persons addicted to narcotic drugs in the United States, exclusive of those who were receiving drugs because of incurable painful diseases. This represented a relatively small public health problem in comparison with the abuse of alcohol and barbiturates. Moreover, opioid addiction was of serious proportions in only a few cities—New York, Chicago, Los Angeles, Washington, and Detroit. Since the late 1960s, a remarkable increase in opioid (mainly heroin) addiction has taken place. The precise number of opioid addicts is not known but is currently estimated by the Drug Enforcement Administration to be more than 500,000 (a disproportionate number in New York and a few other large cities). The prevalence and patterns of opioid abuse have been reviewed by Brust.

Etiology and Pathogenesis A number of factors—socioeconomic, psychologic, and pharmacologic—contribute to the genesis of opioid addiction. In our culture, the most susceptible subjects are young men or delinquent youths living in the economically depressed areas of large cities, but significant numbers are now found in the suburbs and in small cities as well. The onset of opioid use is usually in adolescence, with a peak at 17 to 18 years; fully two-thirds of addicts start using the drugs before the age of 21. Almost 90 percent of addicts engage in criminal activity, often to obtain their daily ration of drugs, but most of them have a history of arrests or convictions antedating their addiction. Also, many of them have psychiatric disturbances, conduct disorder and sociopathy being the most common. Monroe and colleagues, using the Lexington Personality Inventory, examined a group of 837 opioid addicts and found evidence of antisocial personality in 42 percent, emotional disturbance in 29 percent, and thinking disorder in 22 percent; only 7 percent were free of such disorders. Obviously, vulnerability to addiction is not confined to one personality type.

Association with addicts is the apparent explanation for beginning addiction. One addict recruits another person into addiction, and the new recruit does likewise. In this sense opioid addiction is contagious, and as a result of this pattern, heroin addiction has attained epidemic proportions. A small, almost insignificant proportion of addicts are introduced to drugs by physicians in the course of an illness. One seldom hesitates, therefore, to prescribe opiates to patients with chronic pain (e.g., cancer pain) because of the risk of addiction.

Opioid addiction consists of three recognizable phases: (1) episodic intoxication, or "euphoria," (2) pharmacogenic dependence or drug-seeking behavior (addiction), and (3) the propensity to relapse after a period of abstinence.

Some of the symptoms of opioid intoxication have already been considered. In patients with severe pain or pain-anticipatory anxiety, the administration of opioids produces a sense of unusual well-being, a state that has traditionally been referred to as *morphine euphoria*. It should be emphasized that only a negligible proportion of such persons continue to use opioids habitually after their pain has subsided. The vast majority of potential addicts are not suffering from painful illnesses at the time they initiate opioid use, and the term *euphoria* is not an apt description of the initial effects. These persons, as indicated above, are mainly teenagers who self-administer opioids under the tutelage of their peers. They learn, after several repetitions, to recognize a "high," despite the subsequent recurrence of unpleasant, or *dysphoric*, symptoms (nausea, vomiting, faintness as the drug effect wanes). The repeated self-administration of the drug ("reinforcement" in the language of operant psychology) is the most important factor in the genesis of *addiction*. Regardless of how one characterizes the state of mind that is produced by episodic injection of the drug, the individual quickly discovers the need to increase the dose in order to obtain the original effects. Although the initial effects may not be fully recaptured, the progressively increasing dose of the drug does relieve the discomfort that arises as the effects of each injection wear off. In this way a new *pharmacogenically induced* need is developed, and the use of opioids becomes self-perpetuating. At the same time a marked degree of *tolerance* is produced, so that enormous amounts of drugs, e.g., 5000 mg of morphine daily, have eventually been administered without the development of toxic symptoms.

The pharmacologic criteria of addiction, as indicated in the chapter on alcoholism, are *tolerance* and *physical dependence*. The latter refers to the symptoms and signs that become manifest when the drug is withdrawn following a period of continued use. These symptoms and signs constitute a specific clinical state, termed *the abstinence* or *withdrawal syndrome* (see below). The mechanisms that underlie the development of tolerance and physical dependence are not fully understood. However, it is known that opioids activate the brain's opioid antinociceptive system (enkephalins, dynorphins, endorphins) and specific opioid receptors, which are located at different levels of the nervous system (these are described in Chap. 8, on pain; see also the review of Fields).

The Opioid Abstinence Syndrome The intensity of the *abstinence* or *withdrawal* syndrome depends on the dose of the drug and the duration of addiction. The onset of abstinence symptoms in relation to the last exposure to the drug, however, is related to the pharmacologic half-life of the agent. With morphine, the majority of individuals receiving 240 mg daily for 30 days or more will show moderately severe abstinence symptoms following withdrawal. Mild signs of opiate abstinence can be precipitated by narcotic antagonists in persons who have taken as little as 15 mg of morphine or an equivalent dose of methadone or heroin three times daily for 3 days.

The abstinence syndrome that occurs in the morphine addict may be taken as the prototype of the opioid group. The first 8 to 16 h of abstinence usually pass asymptomatically. At the end of this period, yawning, rhinorrhea, sweating, piloerection, and lacrimation become manifest. Mild at first, these symptoms increase in severity over a period of several hours and then remain constant for several days. The patient may be able to sleep during the early abstinence period but is restless, and thereafter insomnia remains a prominent feature. Dilatation of the pupils, recurring waves of gooseflesh, and twitchings of the muscles appear. The patient complains of aching in the back, abdomen, and legs and of "hot and cold flashes"; he frequently asks for blankets. At about 36 h the restlessness becomes more severe, and nausea, vomiting, and diarrhea usually develop. Temperature, respiratory rate, and blood pressure are slightly elevated. All these symptoms reach their peak intensity 48 to 72 h after withdrawal and then gradually subside. The opioid abstinence syndrome is rarely fatal (it is life-threatening only in infants). After 7 to 10 days, the clinical signs of abstinence are no longer evident, although the patient may complain of insomnia, nervousness, weakness, and muscle aches for several more weeks, and small deviations of a number of physiologic variables can be detected with refined techniques for up to 10 months (protracted abstinence).

Habituation, also designated as emotional or psychologic *dependence*, refers to the substitution of drug-seeking activities for all other aims and objectives in life and is the essence of addiction. It is this feature (craving or "purposive" abstinence changes) that fosters relapse to the use of the drug long after the physiologic ("nonpurposive") abstinence changes seem to have disappeared. The cause for relapse is not fully understood. Theoretically, fragments of the abstinence syndrome may remain as a conditioned response, and these abstinence signs may be evoked by the appropriate environmental stimuli. Thus, when a "cured" addict is in a situation where narcotic drugs are readily available or in a setting that was associated with the initial use of drugs, the incompletely extinguished drug-seeking behavior may reassert itself.

The characteristics of addiction and of abstinence are qualitatively similar with all drugs of the opiate group as well as the related synthetic analgesics. The differences are quantitative and are related to the differences in dosage, potency, and length of action. Heroin is two to three times more potent than morphine, but the heroin withdrawal syndrome encountered in hospital practice is usually mild in degree because of the low dosage of the drug in the street product. Dilaudid (hydromorphone) is more potent than morphine and has a shorter duration of action; hence the addict requires more doses per day, and the abstinence syndrome comes on and subsides more rapidly. Abstinence symptoms from codeine, while definite, are less severe than those from morphine. The addiction liabilities of propoxyphene are negligible. Abstinence symptoms from methadone are less intense than those from morphine and do not become evident until 3 or 4 days after withdrawal; for these reasons methadone can be used in the treatment of morphine dependency (see further on). Meperidine addiction is of particular importance because of its high incidence among physicians and nurses. Tolerance to the drug's toxic effects is not complete, so that the addict may show tremors, twitching of muscles, confusion, hallucinations, and sometimes convulsions. Signs of abstinence appear 3 to 4 h after the last dose and reach their maximum intensity in 8 to 12 h, at which time they may be worse than those of morphine abstinence.

As to the biologic basis of tolerance and physical dependence, our understanding is still very limited. Experiments in animals have provided the first insights into the neurotransmitter and neuronal systems involved. As a result of microdialysing opiates and their antagonists into central brain structures, it has been tentatively concluded that mesolimbic structures, particularly the nucleus accumbens, ventral tegmentum of the midbrain, and locus ceruleus are activated or depressed under conditions of repeated opiate exposure. Thus, chronic opiate exposure increases the levels of certain intracellular messengers (possibly G proteins) that drive cyclic-AMP activity in the locus ceruleus and in the nucleus accumbens; blocking the expression of these proteins markedly increases the self-administration of opiates by addicted rats. As with alcohol addiction, certain subtypes of the serotonin and dopamine receptors in limbic structures have been implicated. These incipient insights into the neurochemical mechanism of addiction have been reviewed by Hyman and by Nestler and Aghajanian.

Diagnosis of addiction is usually made when the patient admits to using and needing drugs. Should the patient conceal this fact, one relies on collateral evidence such as miosis, needle marks, emaciation, abscess scars, or chemical analyses. Meperidine addicts are likely to have dilated pupils and twitching of muscles. The finding of morphine or opiate derivatives (heroin is excreted as morphine) in the urine is confirmatory evidence that the patient has taken or has been given a dose of such drugs within 24 h of the test. The diagnosis of opiate addiction is at once apparent when the treatment of acute opiate intoxication precipitates a characteristic abstinence syndrome.

Treatment of the Opioid Abstinence Syndrome (Physical Dependence) This consists of substituting methadone for opioid, in the ratio of 1 mg methadone for 3 mg morphine, 1 mg heroin, or 20 mg meperidine. Since methadone is long-acting and effective orally, it need be given only twice daily by mouth—10 to 20 mg per dose being sufficient to suppress abstinence symptoms. After a stabilization period of 3 to 5 days, this dosage of methadone is reduced and the drug is withdrawn over a similar period of time. An alternative but less effective method is to use clonidine, a drug that counteracts most of the noradrenergic withdrawal symptoms (5 mg/kg twice a day for a week); hypotension may be a problem, however (Jasinski et al).

Recently, the use of rapid detoxification under general anesthesia has become popular in a number of centers as a means of treating opiate addiction. The technique consists of administering increasing doses of opioid receptor antagonists (naloxone or naltrexone) over several hours while the autonomic and other features of the withdrawal syndrome are suppressed by the infusion of propofol or a similar anesthetic, supplemented by intravenous fluids. Medications such as clonidine and sedatives are given in the immediate postanesthetic period. The addict is instructed to continue taking naltrexone for several days or weeks, a practice adopted from one of the outpatient treatments for addiction described below. There are substantial risks involved in the procedure, and a few deaths have occurred. Furthermore, a number of patients continue to manifest signs of withdrawal after the procedure and require continued hospitalization. There are as yet no careful studies of the efficacy of this procedure, particularly in regard to conferring long-term abstinence.

Treatment of Habituation (Psychologic Dependence) This is far more demanding than the treatment of opioid withdrawal and can be best accomplished in special facilities and programs that are devoted wholly to the problem and are available in most communities. The most effective facilities have been the ambulatory methadone maintenance clinics, where more than 100,000 former heroin addicts are participating in rehabilitation programs approved by the Food and Drug Administration. Methadone, in a dosage of 60 to 100 mg daily (sufficient to suppress the craving for heroin), is given under supervision day by day (less often with long-acting methadone) for months or years. Various forms of psychotherapy and social service counseling (often by former heroin addicts) are integral parts of the program.

The results of methadone treatment are difficult to assess and vary considerably from one program to another. Even the most successful programs suffer an attrition rate of about 25 percent when they are evaluated after several years. Of the patients who remain, the majority achieve a high degree of social rehabilitation, i.e., they are gainfully employed and no longer engage in criminal behavior or prostitution. Another notable achievement of the methadone maintenance programs has been the reduction in the number of chronic intravenous drug abusers. This is quite important, for one-quarter of the latter group are seropositive for human immunodeficiency virus (HIV) and are the chief source of transmission of AIDS to newborns and to the heterosexual nonaddicted population.

The usual practice of methadone programs is to accept only addicts over the age of 16 years with a history of heroin addiction for at least 1 year. This leaves many adolescent addicts untreated. The number of addicts who can fully withdraw from methadone and maintain a drug-free existence is very small. This means that the large majority of addicts now enrolled in methadone programs are committed to an indefinite period of methadone maintenance, and the effects of such a regimen are uncertain.

An alternative method of ambulatory treatment of the opiate addict involves the use of narcotic antagonists, of which naloxone and naltrexone are the best known. Naltrexone is favored because it has a longer effect than naloxone, is almost free of agonist effects, and can be administered orally. Good results have also been achieved with cyclazocine in a small number of highly motivated patients; this drug is administered orally in increasing amounts until a dosage of 2 mg/70 kg body weight is attained. The drug is taken twice daily (for 2 to 6 weeks) and is then withdrawn slowly.

More recently, interest has centered on the use of buprenorphine for the treatment of heroin (and cocaine) abuse. Buprenorphine is unique in that it has both opioid agonist and antagonist properties; it therefore mutes the effect of withdrawal and serves also as an aversive agent, like naltrexone. In addition, there is evidence, based on animal experiments and the treatment of small numbers of addicts, that it may be useful for the treatment of dual dependence on cocaine and opiates (see Mello and Mendelson). Buprenorphine has the additional advantage of being administered as a sublingual tablet. The FDA has recently approved its use.

Medical and Neurologic Complications of Opioid Use In addition to the toxic effects of the opioid itself, the addict may suffer a variety of neurologic and infectious complications resulting from the injection of contaminated adulterants (quinine, talc, lactose, powdered milk, and fruit sugars) and of various infectious agents (injections administered by unsterile methods). The most important of these is HIV infection, but septicemia and endocarditis and viral hepatitis may also occur. Particulate matter that is injected with heroin or a vasculitis that is induced by chronic heroin abuse may cause *occlusion of cerebral arteries*, with hemiplegia or other focal cerebral signs. *Amblyopia*, due probably to the toxic effects of quinine in the heroin mixtures, has been reported, as well as *transverse myelopathy* and several types of *peripheral neuropathy*. The spinal cord disorder expresses itself clinically by the abrupt onset of paraplegia with a level on the trunk below which motor function and sensation are lost or impaired and by urinary retention. Pathologically, there is an acute necrotizing lesion involving both gray and white matter over a considerable vertical extent of the thoracic and occasionally the cervical cord. In some cases a myelopathy has followed the first intravenous injection of heroin after a prolonged period of abstinence. We have seen several cases of cervical myelopathy from heroin-induced stupor that had led to a prolonged period of immobility with the neck hyperextended over the back of a chair or sofa. We have also observed several instances of a progressive cerebral leukoencephalopathy attributed to heroin use, similar to ones that occurred in Amsterdam in the 1980s, the result of inhalation of heroin pyrolysate or an adulterant thereof (Wolters et al and Tan et al). In our cases the white matter changes were concentrated in the posterior portions of the hemispheres and in the internal capsules. A similar leukoencephalopathy has also been observed in cocaine users, in some of whom a hypertensive encephalopathy or an adrenergic-induced vasculopathy may have played a role. Damage to single peripheral nerves at the injection site and from compression is a relatively common occurrence. Bilateral compression of the sciatic nerves, caused by sitting or lying for a prolonged period in a stuporous state or in the lotus position while "stoned," has been observed in several of our patients. In sciatic compression of this sort, the peroneal branch is more affected than the tibial, causing foot drop with less in the way of weakness of plantar flexion. More difficult to understand is the involvement of other individual nerves, particularly the radial nerve, and painful affection of the brachial plexus, apparently unrelated to compression and remote from the sites of injection.

An acute generalized *myonecrosis* with myoglobinuria and renal failure has been ascribed to the intravenous injection of adulterated heroin. Brawny edema and fibrosing myopathy (Volkmann contracture) are the sequelae of venous thrombosis resulting from the administration of heroin and its adulterants by the intramuscular and subcutaneous routes. Occasionally there may be massive swelling of an extremity into which heroin had been injected subcutaneously or intramuscularly; infection and venous thrombosis appear to be involved in its causation.

The diagnosis of drug addiction or the suspicion of this diagnosis should always raise the prospect of infectious complications, particularly AIDS, syphilis, abscesses and cellulitis at injection sites, septic thrombophlebitis, hepatitis, and periarteritis. Tetanus, endocarditis (due mainly to *Staphylococcus aureus*), spinal epidural abscess, meningitis, brain abscess, and tuberculosis have occurred less frequently.

SEDATIVE-HYPNOTIC DRUGS

This class of drugs, also referred to as depressants, consists of two main groups. The first includes the barbiturates and chloral hydrate. These drugs are now little used, having been largely replaced by a second group, comprising *meprobamate* and other glycerol derivatives and the *benzodiazepines*, the most important of which are chlordiazepoxide (Librium), lorazepam (Ativan), alprazolam (Xanax), and diazepam (Valium). Closely related are the non-benzodiazepine hypnotics, typified by zolpidem (Ambien). The advantages of the benzodiazepine drugs are their *relatively* low toxicity and addictive potential and their minimal interactions with other drugs.

Barbiturates

Despite the marked reduction in the medical use of barbiturates during the past three decades, the improper use of these drugs—particularly their nonmedical and illicit use—still leads to suicide, accidental death, and addiction. In the past, about fifty barbiturates were marketed for clinical use, but only the following are now encountered with any regularity: pentobarbital (Nembutal), secobarbital (Seconal), amobarbital (Amytal), thiopental (Pentothal), barbital (Veronal), and phenobarbital (Luminal). The first three are the ones most commonly abused.

Mechanism of Action All the common barbiturates are derived from barbituric acid; the differences between them depend on variations in the side chains of the parent molecule. The potency of each drug is a function of the ionization constant and lipid solubility. The higher its lipid solubility, the greater the drug's potency and the quicker and briefer its action. The lowering of plasma pH increases the rate of entry of the ionized form into the brain. The action of barbiturates is to suppress neuronal transmission, presumably by enhancing GABA inhibition at pre- and postsynaptic receptor sites, and to reduce excitatory postsynaptic potentials. The major points of action in the CNS are similar to those of alcohol and other coma-producing drugs; impaired consciousness or coma relates to inactivation of neurons in the reticular formation of the upper brainstem. The liver is the main locus of drug metabolism, and the kidney is the locus of elimination. All the barbiturates are similar pharmacologically and differ only in the speed of onset and duration of their action. The clinical problems posed by the barbiturates are different, however, depending on whether the intoxication is acute or chronic.

Acute Barbiturate Intoxication This results from the ingestion of large amounts of the drug, either accidentally or with suicidal intent. The latter is most frequently the act of a depressed person. The hysteric or sociopath may take an overdose as a suicidal gesture and become seriously intoxicated because of miscalculation or ignorance of the toxic dosage. Often the drug is taken while the individual is inebriated—a dangerous situation, since alcohol and barbiturate have an additive effect.

Diagnosis of Barbiturate Intoxication The symptoms and signs vary with the type and amount of drug as well as with the length of time that has elapsed since it was ingested. Pentobarbital and secobarbital produce their effects quickly, and recovery is relatively rapid. Phenobarbital induces coma more slowly, and its effects tend to be prolonged. The duration of action of these drugs can be judged by the hypnotic effect of an average oral dose. In the case of long-acting barbiturates, such as phenobarbital and barbital, the effect lasts 6 h or more; with the intermediate-acting drugs, amobarbital and aprobarbital, 3 to 6 h; and with the short-acting drugs, secobarbital and pentobarbital, less than 3 h. Most fatalities follow the ingestion of secobarbital, amobarbital, or pentobarbital. The ingestion by adults of more than 3.0 g of these drugs at one time will prove fatal unless intensive and skilled treatment is applied promptly. The potentially fatal dose of phenobarbital is 6 to 10 g. The lowest plasma concentration associated with lethal overdosage of phenobarbital or barbital is 60 mg/mL and that of amobarbital and pentobarbital is 10 mg/mL.

In regard to prognosis and treatment, it is useful to recognize three grades of severity of acute barbiturate intoxication. *Mild intoxication* follows the ingestion of approximately 0.3 g pentobarbital (Nembutal; the hypnotic dose in an unhabituated patient is 100 mg) or its equivalent. The patient is drowsy or asleep, although readily roused if called or shaken. The symptoms resemble those of alcohol intoxication. The patient thinks slowly, and there may be mild disorientation, lability of mood, impairment of judgment, slurred speech, drunken gait, and nystagmus. *Moderate intoxication* follows the ingestion of 5 to 10 times the oral hypnotic dose. The patient is stuporous, tendon reflexes are usually depressed or absent, and respirations are slow but not shallow. Corneal and pupillary reflexes are retained, with occasional exceptions. Usually the patient can be roused by vigorous manual stimulation; when awakened, he is confused and dysarthric and, after a few moments, drifts back into stupor. *Severe intoxication* occurs with the ingestion of 10 to 20 times the oral hypnotic dose. The patient cannot be roused by any means. Respiration is slow and shallow or irregular, and pulmonary edema and cyanosis may be present. The tendon reflexes are usually but not invariably absent. Most patients show no response to plantar stimulation, but in those who do, the responses are extensor. With deep coma, the corneal and gag reflexes may also be abolished. Ordinarily the pupillary light reflex is retained in severe intoxication and is lost only if the patient is asphyxiated; but in advanced cases, the pupils become miotic and poorly reactive, simulating opiate intoxication. At this point respiration is greatly depressed and oculocephalic and oculovestibular reflex responses are usually abolished. In the early hours of coma, there may be a phase of flexor or extensor posturing or rigidity of the limbs, hyperactive reflexes, ankle clonus, and extensor plantar signs; persistence of these signs indicates that anoxic damage has been added. The temperature may be subnormal, the pulse is thready and rapid, and the blood pressure is at shock levels.

There are few conditions other than barbiturate intoxication that cause a flaccid coma with small reactive pupils, hypothermia, and hypotension. A pontine hemorrhage may do so, but a hysterical trance or catatonic stupor presents the main problem in differential diagnosis. The use of gas and high-pressure liquid chromatography provides a reliable means of identifying the type and amount of barbiturate in the blood. A patient who has also ingested alcohol may be comatose with relatively low blood barbiturate concentrations. Contrariwise, the addicted (tolerant) patient may show only mild signs of intoxication with very high blood barbiturate concentrations.

The electroencephalogram (EEG) may also be useful in diagnosis. In mild intoxication, the normal activity is replaced by fast (beta) activity, in the range of 20 to 30 cycles per second, and is most prominent in the frontal regions. In more severe intoxication, the fast waves become less regular and interspersed with 3- to 4-per-second slow activity; in still more advanced cases, there are short periods of suppression of all activity, separated by bursts of slow (delta) waves of variable frequency. In extreme overdosage, all electrical activity ceases. This is one instance in which a "flat" EEG cannot be equated with brain death, and the effects are fully reversible unless anoxic damage has supervened.

Management In mild or moderate intoxication, recovery is the rule and vigorous treatment is not required. If the patient is unresponsive, special measures must be taken to maintain respiration and prevent infection. An endotracheal tube should be inserted, with suctioning as necessary. Any risk of respiratory depression or underventilation requires the use of a positive-pressure respirator.

Hemodialysis or hemofiltration with charcoal may be used in profoundly comatose patients who fail to respond to the measures outlined above. They are particularly useful in cases of coma due to long-acting barbiturates and are mandatory if anuria or uremia has developed. Treatment with analeptic drugs (e.g., picrotoxin, pentylenetetrazol), which enjoyed a brief period of popularity, has been generally abandoned, since these drugs do not affect the rate of metabolism or the excretion of barbiturates.

Occasionally, in the case of a barbiturate addict who has taken an overdose of the drug, recovery from coma is followed by the development of abstinence symptoms, as described below.

Barbiturate Addiction (Chronic Barbiturate Intoxication) Chronic barbiturate intoxication, like other drug addictions, tends to develop on a background of some psychiatric disorder, most commonly a depressive illness with symptoms of anxiety and insomnia. Addiction to alcohol or to opiates may predispose to barbiturate addiction. Alcoholics find that barbiturates effectively relieve their nervousness and tremor. They may then continue to take both alcohol and barbiturate, or the barbiturate may replace the alcohol. As with other drug addictions, the incidence of barbiturism is particularly high in individuals with ready access to drugs, such as physicians, pharmacists, and nurses.

The manifestations of barbiturism are much the same as those of alcohol intoxication. The barbiturate addict thinks slowly, exhibits increased emotional lability, and becomes untidy in dress and personal habits. The neurologic signs include dysarthria, nystagmus, and cerebellar incoordination. If the dosage is elevated rapidly, the signs of moderate or severe intoxication, as described above, become manifest.

A characteristic feature of chronic barbiturate intoxication is the development of tolerance, sometimes striking in degree. The average addict ingests about 1.5 g of a potent barbiturate daily and does not manifest signs of severe intoxication unless this amount is exceeded. Tolerance to barbiturates does not develop as rapidly as to opiates. Most persons can ingest 0.4 g daily for as long as 3 months without developing major withdrawal signs (seizures or delirium). With a dosage of 0.8 g daily for a period of 2 weeks to 2 months, abrupt withdrawal will result in serious symptoms in the majority of patients (see below).

Barbiturate Abstinence, or Withdrawal, Syndrome Immediately following withdrawal, the patient seemingly improves over a period of 8 to 12 h, as the symptoms of intoxication diminish. Then a new group of symptoms develops, consisting of nervousness, tremor, insomnia, postural hypotension, and weakness. With chronic phenobarbital or barbital intoxication, withdrawal symptoms may not become apparent until 48 to 72 h after the final dose. Generalized seizures with loss of consciousness may occur, usually between the second and fourth days of abstinence but occasionally as long as 6 or 7 days after withdrawal. There may be a single seizure, several seizures, or, rarely, status epilepticus. Characteristically, in the withdrawal period, there is a greatly heightened sensitivity to photic stimulation, to which the patient responds with myoclonus or a seizure accompanied by paroxysmal changes in the EEG. The convulsive phase may be followed directly by a delusional-hallucinatory state or a full-blown delirium indistinguishable from delirium tremens, or a varying degree of improvement may follow the seizures before the delirium becomes manifest. Death has been reported under these circumstances. The abstinence syndrome may occur in varying degrees of completeness; some patients have seizures and recover without developing delirium, and others have a delirium without preceding seizures. The abrupt onset of seizures or an acute psychosis in adult life should always raise the suspicion of addiction to barbiturates or other sedative-hypnotic drugs.

Treatment of Chronic Barbiturate Intoxication This should always be carried out in the hospital. If the diagnosis of addiction is made before signs of abstinence have appeared, the "stabilization dosage" should first be determined. This is the amount of short-acting barbiturate required to produce mild symptoms of intoxication (nystagmus, slight ataxia, and dysarthria). Usually 0.2 g of pentobarbital given orally every 6 h is sufficient for this purpose. Then a gradual withdrawal of the drug is undertaken, 0.1 g daily, the reduction being stopped for several days if abstinence symptoms appear. In this way, a severely addicted person can be withdrawn in 14 to 21 days. The patient who presents with severe withdrawal symptoms, such as seizures, is given 0.3 to 0.5 g of phenobarbital intramuscularly and then enough to maintain a state of mild intoxication. Most other anticonvulsant medicines are ineffective against barbiturate withdrawal convulsions. Withdrawal should then be carried out as indicated above. If the abstinence symptoms are not severe, it is not necessary to reintoxicate the patient, but treatment can proceed along the lines laid down for other forms of delirium and confusion. After recovery has taken place, whether from acute or chronic intoxication, the psychiatric problem requires evaluation and an appropriate plan of therapy.

Chloral Hydrate

This is the oldest and one of the safest, most effective, and most inexpensive of the sedative-hypnotic drugs. After oral administration, chloral hydrate is reduced rapidly to trichloroethanol, which is responsible for the depressant effects on the CNS. A significant portion of the trichloroethanol is excreted in the urine as the glucuronide, which may give a false-positive test for glucose.

Tolerance and addiction to chloral hydrate develop only rarely; for this reason it is an appropriate medication for the management of insomnia, particularly the type that is associated with depression. Poisoning with chloral hydrate is a rare occurrence and resembles acute barbiturate intoxication except for the finding of miosis, which is said to characterize the former. Treatment follows along the same lines as for barbiturate poisoning. Death from poisoning is due to respiratory depression and hypotension; patients who survive may show signs of liver and kidney disease.

Paraldehyde, another member of this group of sedative drugs, is no longer being manufactured in the United States, and chloral hydrate is now available mainly as an elixir for pediatric use.

Benzodiazepines

With the introduction of chlordiazepoxide in 1960 and the benzodiazepine drugs that followed (particularly diazepam), the older sedative drugs (barbiturates, paraldehyde, chloral hydrate) have become virtually obsolete. Indeed, the benzodiazepines are the most commonly prescribed drugs in the world today. According to Hollister, 15 percent of all adults in the United States use a benzodiazepine at least once yearly and about half this number use the drug for a month or longer. As mentioned earlier, the benzodiazepines, compared with the older sedatives, have *relatively* minor hypnotic effects and low abuse potential and are *relatively* safe when taken in overdose.

The benzodiazepines have been used extensively for the treatment of anxiety and insomnia, and they are especially effective when the anxiety symptoms are severe. Also, they have been used to control overactivity and destructive behavior in children and the symptoms of alcohol withdrawal in adults. Diazepam is particularly useful in the treatment of delirious patients who require parenteral medication. The benzodiazepines possess anticonvulsant properties, and the intravenous use of diazepam, lorazepam, and midazolam is an effective means of controlling status epilepticus, as described on page 361. Diazepam in massive doses has been used with considerable success in the management of muscle spasm in tetanus and in "stiff man" syndrome (page 1569). Diazepam has been far less successful in the treatment of extrapyramidal movement disorders and dystonic spasms. Alprazolam (Xanax) has a central place in the treatment of panic attacks and other anxiety states, as an adjunct in some depressive illnesses, and in the behavioral disturbances in Alzheimer disease. It seems, however, to create more dependence than some of the others in its class.

Other important benzodiazepine drugs are flurazepam (Dalmane), triazolam (Halcion), chlorazepate (Tranxene), temazepam (Restoril), and other newer varieties, all widely used in the treatment of insomnia (page 414), and clonazepam (Klonipin), which is useful in the treatment of myoclonic seizures (pages 357 and 360) and intention myoclonus (page 110). Midazolam (Versed), a short-acting parenteral agent, is used frequently to achieve the brief sedation required for procedures such as MRI or endoscopy and is useful in the treatment of status epilepticus, but it is known to cause respiratory arrest on occasion. Lorazepam (Ativan) and oxazepam (Serax) are said to be preferable to other benzodiazepines in treating the elderly and those with impaired liver function. Many other benzodiazepine compounds have appeared in recent years, but a clear advantage over the original ones remains to be demonstrated (Hollister; Pirodsky and Cohn). Zolpidem (Ambien) differs from the benzodiazepines structurally but is pharmacologically the same.

The benzodiazepine drugs, like barbiturates, have a depressant action on the CNS by binding to specific receptors on GABA inhibitory systems. The benzodiazepines act in concert with GABA to open chloride ion channels and hyperpolarize postsynaptic neurons and reduce their firing rate. The primary sites of their action are the cerebral cortex and limbic system, which accounts for their anticonvulsive and anxiolytic effects. While quite safe in the recommended dosages, they are far from ideal. They frequently cause unsteadiness of gait and drowsiness and at times hypotension and syncope, confusion, and impairment of memory, especially in the elderly. If taken in large doses, the benzodiazepines can produce a depression of the state of consciousness, resembling that of other sedative-hypnotic drugs but with less respiratory suppression and hypotension. *Flumazenil*, a specific pharmacologic antagonist of the CNS effects of benzodiazepines, rapidly but briefly reverses most of the symptoms and signs of benzodiazepine overdose. It acts by binding to CNS diazepine receptors and thereby blocking the activation of inhibitory GABAergic synapses. Flumazenil may also have diagnostic utility in cases of coma of unknown etiology and in hepatic encephalopathy (see page 1186).

Signs of physical dependence and true addiction, though relatively rare, undoubtedly occur in chronic benzodiazepine users, even in those taking therapeutic doses. The withdrawal symptoms are much the same as those that follow the chronic use of other sedative drugs (anxiety, jitteriness, insomnia, seizures) but may not appear until the third day after the cessation of the drug and may not reach their peak of severity until the fifth day (Hollister). In chronic benzodiazepine users, the gradual tapering of dosage over a period of 1 to 2 weeks minimizes the withdrawal effects.

Carbonic Acid Derivatives

These drugs are capable of modest depressant action and are effective in relieving mild degrees of nervousness, anxiety, and muscle tension. Meprobamate (Equanil, Miltown) is the best-known member of this group. It was the first of the new antianxiety drugs, a chemical variant of the weak and ineffective muscle relaxant mephenesin. With average doses (400 mg three or four times a day), the patient is able to function quite effectively; larger doses cause ataxia, drowsiness, stupor, coma, and vasomotor collapse.

Meprobamate has turned out to have the same disadvantages as the barbiturates, including death from overdosage. Addiction to meprobamate may occur, and if four or more times the daily recommended dose is administered over a period of weeks to months, withdrawal symptoms (including convulsions) may appear. Because of this tendency to produce physical dependence and other disadvantages (serious toxic reactions and a high degree of sedation), meprobamate and its congeners are now seldom used except illicitly.

Other Antianxiety Agents A new class of antianxiety agents, exemplified by the selective 5HT-2 serotoninergic agent buspirone (Buspar), is chemically and pharmacologically different from the benzodiazepines, barbiturates, or other sedatives. Because of its apparently reduced potential for abuse and tolerance, it is not a controlled pharmaceutical substance in the United States, but adverse interactions with MAO inhibitors are known; its use with other psychotropic drugs is still under investigation. It does not block the withdrawal syndrome due to other sedative-hypnotic drugs.

ANTIPSYCHOTIC DRUGS

In the mid-1950s, a large series of pharmacologic agents, originally referred to as tranquilizers (later, as psychotropic or neuroleptic drugs), came into prominent use—mainly for the control of schizophrenia, psychotic states associated with "organic brain syndromes," and affective disorders (depression and manic-depressive disease). The mechanisms by which these drugs ameliorate disturbances of thought and affect in psychotic states are not fully understood, but presumably they act by blocking the postsynaptic dopamine receptors (there are four subtypes, termed D_1 through D_4) on neuronal membranes. The D_2 receptors are located mainly in the frontal cortex, hippocampus, and limbic cortex, and the D_1 receptors in the striatum. There is also some adrenergic blocking effect. The blockade of dopamine receptors in the striatum is probably responsible for the parkinsonian side effects of this entire class of drugs, and the blockade of another dopaminergic (tuberoinfundibular) system, for the increased prolactin secretion by the pituitary. The newer "atypical" antipsychotic drugs, typified by clozapine (Clozaril), apparently achieve the same degree of D_2 and D_3 blockade in the temporal lobes while exhibiting substantially less antagonistic activity in the striatum—accounting for their lesser parkinsonian side effects.

Since the introduction, in the 1950s, of the phenothiazine chlorpromazine as an anesthetic agent and its application to schizophrenics as a result of serendipitously discovered antipsychotic activity, a large number of antipsychotic drugs have been marketed for clinical use. No attempt is made here to describe or even list all of them. Some have had only an evanescent popularity, and others have yet to prove their value. Chemically, these compounds form a heterogeneous group; eight of them are of particular clinical importance: (1) the phenothiazines; (2) the thioxanthines; (3) the butyrophenones; (4) the rauwolfia alkaloids; (5) an indole derivative, loxapine (Loxitane), and a unique dihydroindalone, molindone (Moban); (6) a diphenylbutylpiperidine, pimozide (Orap); (7) dibenzodiazepines, typified by clozapine (Clozaril) and olanzapine (Zyprexa); and (8) a benzisoxazole derivative, risperidone (Risperdal). The last four of these drugs were introduced more recently than the others and also have a more limited use. Molindone and loxapine are about as effective as the phenothiazines in the management of schizophrenia, and their side effects are also the same; their main use is in patients who are not responsive to the older drugs or who suffer intolerable side effects from them. The antipsychotic agents in the class of clozapine have attracted great interest, since—as already mentioned—they appear to be relatively free of extrapyramidal side effects. For this reason, they are particularly successful in controlling the confusion and psychosis of parkinsonian patients. The other new class of drugs, of which risperidone is the main example, also has few extrapyramidal side effects and a more rapid onset of action than the traditional antipsychotic medications. Pimozide may be useful in the treatment of haloperidol-refractory cases of Gilles de la Tourette syndrome (page 117); its main danger is its tendency to produce cardiac arrhythmias.

Phenothiazines

This group comprises some of the most widely used tranquilizers, such as the phenothiazines chlorpromazine (Thorazine), promazine (Sparine), triflupromazine (Vesprin), prochlorperazine (Compazine), perphenazine (Trilafon), fluphenazine (Permitil, Prolixin), thioridazine (Mellaril), mesoridazine (Serentil), and trifluoperazine (Stelazine). In addition to their psychotherapeutic effects, these drugs have a number of other actions, so that certain members of this group are used as antiemetics (prochlorperazine) and antihistaminics (promethazine).

The phenothiazines have had their widest application in the treatment of the psychoses (schizophrenia and, to a lesser extent, manic-depressive psychosis). Under the influence of these drugs, many patients who would otherwise be hospitalized are able to live at home and even work productively. In the hospital, the use of these drugs has greatly facilitated the care of hyperactive and combative patients (see Chaps. 57 and 58 for details of the clinical usage of these drugs).

Side effects of the phenothiazines are frequent and often serious. All of them may cause a cholestatic type of jaundice, agranulocytosis, convulsive seizures, orthostatic hypotension, skin sensitivity reactions, mental depression, and, most importantly, immediate or delayed extrapyramidal motor disorders. The neuroleptic malignant syndrome is the most extreme complication and is discussed separately further on. The following types of extrapyramidal symptoms, also discussed on page 1637, have been noted in association with all of the phenothiazines [as well as the butyrophenones and, to a lesser extent, metoclopramide (Reglan) and pimozide, which block dopaminergic receptors]:

1. A parkinsonian syndrome—masked facies, tremor, generalized rigidity, shuffling gait, and slowness of movement. These symptoms may appear after several days of drug therapy but more often after several weeks. Suppression of dopamine in the striatum (similar to the effect of loss of nigral cells) is presumably the basis of the parkinsonian syndrome.

2. Dyskinesia and dystonia, taking the form of involuntary movements of lower facial muscles (mainly around the mouth) and protrusion of the tongue (buccolingual or oral-masticatory syndrome), dysphagia, torticollis and retrocollis, oculogyric crises, and tonic spasms of a limb. These complications usually occur early in the course of administration of the drug, sometimes after the initial dose, in which case they can be improved dramatically by immediate discontinuation of the drug and the intravenous administration of diphenhydramine hydrochloride (Benadryl).

3. An inner restlessness reflected by a persistent shifting of the body and feet and an inability to sit still, such that the patient paces the floor or jiggles the legs constantly (akathisia, see page 118). Of all the phenothiazines, molindone has a special tendency to cause akathisia. This disorder often responds to oral propranolol.

4. A group of *late and persistent complications* of neuroleptic therapy, which may continue after removal of the offending drug, comprises lingual-facial-buccal-cervical dyskinesias, choreoathetotic and dystonic movements of the trunk and limbs, diffuse myoclonus (rare), perioral tremor ("rabbit" syndrome), and dysarthria or anarthria. These movement abnormalities constitute the important group of *tardive dyskinesias*. Snyder has postulated that the movements are due to hypersensitivity of dopamine receptors in the basal ganglia, secondary to prolonged blockade of the receptors by antipsychotic medication. Baldessarini estimates that as many as 40 percent of patients receiving long-term antipsychotic medication develop tardive dyskinesia of some degree. A pathology has never been ascertained.

5. The neuroleptic malignant syndrome, which is discussed separately below.

Butyrophenones Haloperidol (Haldol) is the only member of this group approved for use as an antipsychotic in the United States. It has much the same therapeutic effects as the phenothiazines in the management of the acute psychoses. It also has the same side effects as the phenothiazines but has little or no adrenergic blocking action. It is an effective substitute for the phenothiazines in patients who are intolerant of the latter drugs, particularly of their autonomic effects. It is also one of the drugs of choice in treating Gilles de la Tourette syndrome (the other being pimozide) and the movement disorder of Huntington chorea.

Treatment of Neuroleptic Side Effects As indicated above, acute dystonic spasms usually respond to diphenhydramine (Benadryl). The purely parkinsonian syndrome usually improves as well, but the tardive dyskinesias may persist for months or years and may be permanent. Administration of antiparkinsonian drugs of the anticholinergic type (trihexyphenidyl, procyclidine, and benztropine) may hasten recovery from some of the symptoms. Oral, lingual, and laryngeal dyskinesias are affected relatively little by any antiparkinsonian drugs. Amantadine (Symmetrel) in doses of 50 to 100 mg tid has been useful in some cases of postphenothiazine dyskinesia. Many other drugs have been tried in the treatment of tardive dyskinesia, with uncertain results. No treatment has been uniformly successful in the present authors' experience. Nevertheless, we have noted a tendency for most of the obstinate forms of tardive dyskinesia to subside slowly even after several years of unsuccessful therapy. The use of low doses of antipsychotic drugs and frequent drug holidays, especially in the more susceptible older patients, may help to prevent the development of tardive dyskinesia.

Neuroleptic Malignant Syndrome This is the most dreaded complication of phenothiazine and haloperidol use; its incidence has been calculated to be 0.2 percent of all patients receiving neuroleptics (Caroff and Mann), and its seriousness is underscored by a mortality rate of 15 to 30 percent if not recognized and treated promptly. It may occur days, weeks, or months after neuroleptic treatment is begun. The syndrome consists of catatonic rigidity, stupor, unstable blood pressure, variable hyperthermia, diaphoresis and other signs of autonomic dysfunction, high serum creatine kinase (CK) values (up to 60,000 units), and, in fatal cases, renal failure due to myoglobinuria. The syndrome was first observed in patients being treated with haloperidol, and since then other neuroleptic drugs have been incriminated, particularly the highly potent thioxanthine derivative thiothixine and the phenothiazines—chlorpromazine, fluphenazine, and thioridazine—but also, on rare occasions, the less potent drugs that are used to control nausea, such as promethazine. It has recently become evident that the newer antipsychotic drugs, and specifically olanzapine, are also capable of inducing the syndrome. All of these drugs are thought to act through blockade of dopamine receptors in the basal ganglia and hypothalamus.

The neuroleptic malignant syndrome bears a close relationship to *malignant hyperthermia*, not only in its clinical aspects but also in its response to bromocriptine and dantrolene. Malignant hyperthermia is an inherited disorder that, in susceptible individuals, is triggered by inhalation anesthetics and skeletal muscle relaxants (page 1563). This disorder was described before the introduction of neuroleptic drugs and has recently been related to a mutation of the ryanodine receptor gene on chromosome 19q. A genetic factor is also suspected to underlie the neuroleptic malignant syndrome, possibly provoked by fatigue and dehydration.

If treatment is started early, when consciousness is first altered and the temperature is rising, bromocriptine in oral doses of 5 mg tid (up to 20 mg tid) will terminate the condition in a few hours. Once oral medication can no longer be taken, dantrolene, 0.25 to 3.0 mg intravenously may be lifesaving. Once coma has supervened, shock and anuria may prove fatal or leave the patient in a vegetative state. The rigors during high fever may cause muscle damage and myoglobinuria, and the circulatory collapse may lead to hypoxic-ischemic brain injury.

Meningitis, heat stroke, lithium intoxication, and acute dystonic reactions figure in the differential diagnosis. Of course, neuroleptic medication must be discontinued as soon as any of the severe extrapyramidal reactions are recognized, and it is felt that the offending neuroleptic should not be used in the future; but the risk of using another class of antipsychotic agent has not been fully addressed.

It hardly needs to be pointed out that the antipsychotic drugs have been much overused. This would be suspected just from the frequency with which they are being prescribed. These powerful medications have specific indications, noted above and in Chaps. 56, 57, and 58, and the physician should be certain of the diagnosis before using them. The fact that the neuroleptic drugs can produce tardive dyskinesia in nonpsychotic patients is reason enough not to use them for nervousness, apprehension, anxiety, mild depression, and the many normal psychologic reactions to trying environmental circumstances. These drugs are not curative but only suppress or partially alleviate symptoms, and they should not serve as a substitute for, or divert the physician from, the use of other measures for the relief of abnormal mental states.

ANTIDEPRESSANTS

Four classes of drugs—the monoamine oxidase (MAO) inhibitors, the tricyclic compounds, the serotoninergic drugs, and lithium—are particularly useful in the treatment of depressive illnesses. The adjective *antidepressant* refers to their therapeutic effect and is employed here in deference to common clinical practice. *Antidepressive* or *antidepression* drugs would be preferable, since the term *depressant* still has a pharmacologic connotation that does not necessarily equate with the therapeutic effect. For example, barbiturates and chloral hydrate are depressants in the pharmacologic sense and mood elevators or antidepressants in the clinical sense.

Monoamine Oxidase Inhibitors

The observation that iproniazid, an inhibitor of monoamine oxidase (MAO), had a mood-elevating effect in tuberculous patients initiated a great deal of interest in compounds of this type and led quickly to their exploitation in the treatment of depression. Iproniazid proved exceedingly toxic to the liver and was soon taken off the market, as were several subsequently developed MAO inhibitors; but other drugs in this class, much better tolerated, are still available. These include isocarboxazid (Marplan), phenelzine (Nardil), and tranylcypromine (Parnate), the latter two being the more frequently used. Tranylcypromine, which bears a close chemical resemblance to dextroamphetamine, may produce unwanted stimulation, but the most common adverse effect of all the MAO inhibitors is postural hypotension. Also, interactions with a wide array of other drugs and ingested substances may produce severe hypertension.

Monoamine oxidase is located on the outer surface of the mitochondria in neurons and is utilized in the catabolism of catecholamines (Coyle). In the gut and liver, this enzyme normally serves to deaminate phenethylamine, tyramine, and tryptamine—the products of protein catabolism. Inhibition of MAO allows these dietary amines, which have an amphetamine-like action, to enter the systemic circulation in increased quantities, thus releasing norepinephrine from sympathetic nerve endings and increasing heart rate and blood pressure. Probably more relevant to their action as antidepressants, the MAO inhibitors also have in common the ability to block the intraneuronal oxidative deamination of naturally occurring amines (norepinephrine, epinephrine, and serotonin), and it has been suggested that the accumulation of these substances is responsible for the antidepressant effect. However, many enzymes other than monoamine oxidase are inhibited by MAO inhibitors, and the latter drugs have numerous actions unrelated to enzyme inhibition. Furthermore, many agents with antidepressant effects like those of the MAO inhibitors do not inhibit MAO. One cannot assume that the therapeutic effect of these drugs has a direct relation to the property of MAO inhibition in the brain.

The MAO inhibitors must be dispensed with great caution and constant awareness of their potentially serious side effects. They may at times cause excitement, restlessness, agitation, insomnia, and anxiety, occasionally with the usual dose but more often with an overdose. Mania and convulsions may occur (especially in epileptic patients). Other side effects are muscle twitching and involuntary movements, urinary retention, skin rashes, tachycardia, jaundice, visual impairment, enhancement of glaucoma, impotence, sweating, muscle spasms, paresthesias, and a serious degree of orthostatic hypotension.

Patients taking MAO inhibitors must be warned against the use of phenothiazines, CNS stimulants, tricyclic and serotoninergic antidepressants (see below), and also sympathomimetic amines and tyramine; the combination of an MAO inhibitor and any of these drugs or amines may induce severe hypertension, atrial and ventricular arrhythmia, pulmonary edema, stroke, and even death. Sympathomimetic amines are contained in some commonly used cold remedies, nasal sprays, nose drops, and certain foods—aged cheese, beer, red wine, pickled herring, sardines, sausages, and preserved meat or fish. Exaggerated responses to the usual dose of meperidine (Demerol) and other narcotic drugs have also been observed; respiratory function may be depressed to a serious degree, and hyperpyrexia, agitation, and pronounced hypotension may occur as well, sometimes with fatal issue. Unpredictable side effects may also accompany the simultaneous administration of barbiturates and MAO inhibitors. The abrupt occurrence of severe occipital headache, nausea, vomiting, pupillary dilation, or visual blurring should suggest a hypertensive crisis; treatment is with intravenous phentolamine 5 mg, nitroprusside, or a calcium channel blocker administered slowly to prevent hypotension. Overdosage presents with coma, for which there is no treatment other than supportive care.

The therapeutic use of MAO inhibitors is discussed further in Chaps. 56 and 57.

Tricyclic Antidepressants

Soon after the first successes with MAO inhibitors, a new class of tricyclic compounds appeared. The first was imipramine (Tofranil), soon followed by amitriptyline (Elavil) and then by desipramine (Norpramin) and nortriptyline (Pamelor). Another important dibenzazepine derivative is carbamazepine (Tegretol), which is widely used in the control of seizures but has also found a role in the treatment of lancinating neuropathic and myelopathic pain and possibly of depression and mood instability. Subsequently, a number of additional antidepressant drugs were introduced. Included are variants of the conventional tricyclic drugs (amoxapine, protriptyline, trimipramine, doxepin), tetracyclics (maprotiline), bicyclics (zimeldine), and others (trazodone, buproprion). A full account of these drugs, which cannot be attempted here, will be found in the monographs of Hollister and of Pirodsky and Cohn. The newer drugs seem to be safer than the older ones when taken in overdose, but whether they have a clear therapeutic advantage in depression has not been established.

The mode of action of these agents is not fully understood, but there is evidence that they block the reuptake of amine neurotransmitters, both norepinephrine and serotonin. Blocking this amine pump mechanism (called the presynaptic plasma transporter), which ordinarily terminates synaptic transmission, permits the persistence of neurotransmitter substances in the synaptic cleft and supports the hypothesis that endogenous depression is due to a deficiency of noradrenergic or serotoninergic transmission.

The tricyclic antidepressants and the serotoninergic drugs discussed in the next section, are presently the most effective drugs for the treatment of patients with depressive illnesses, the former being particularly useful for those with anergic depressions associated with hyposomnia, early morning awakening, and decreased appetite and libido. The side effects of the tricyclic drugs are far less frequent and serious than those of the MAO inhibitors.

The tricyclic (dibenzazepine) compounds are potent anticholinergic agents, which accounts for their most prominent and serious side effects—orthostatic hypotension and urinary bladder weakness. They may also produce CNS excitement—leading to insomnia, agitation, and restlessness—but usually these effects are readily controlled by small doses of phenothiazines or benzodiazepines given concurrently or in the evenings. Occasionally they may cause ataxia and blood dyscrasias. As indicated above, the tricyclic drugs should not be given with an MAO inhibitor; serious reactions have allegedly occurred when small doses of imipramine were given to patients who had discontinued the MAO inhibitor 1 week previously. Finally, it must be repeated that both the MAO inhibitors and the tricyclic antidepressants are extremely dangerous drugs when taken in excess.

Tricyclic compounds are a frequent cause of accidental poisoning and a favorite suicidal instrument of depressed patients. It is common for the intoxicated patient to have taken several drugs, in which case chemical analyses of the blood and urine are particularly helpful in determining the drugs involved and in sorting out therapeutic and toxic concentrations. Mortality from overdose is due to cardiac disturbances, particularly tachyarrhythmias and impaired conduction. Treatment consists of gastric aspiration and instillation of activated charcoal and the addition of physostigmine to reverse serious arrhythmias; its short duration of action requires that frequent doses be given. Dialysis is of no value because of the low plasma concentrations of the drug.

Serotonin Reuptake Inhibitors and Related Drugs

The selective serotonin reuptake inhibitors (SSRI) constitute a newer class of antidepressants; paroxetine (Paxil), fluoxetine (Prozac), and sertraline (Zoloft) are the ones most often used, but others are being developed at a rapid pace. They act presumably by inhibiting the reuptake of serotonin and to a slightly lesser extent of norepinephrine, somewhat like the effect of a tricyclic. This results in a potentiation of the actions of these neurotransmitters. Because they do not bind as avidly as tricyclic drugs to the muscarinic and adrenergic receptors in the brain, they produce fewer side effects, but some patients complain of anxiety or insomnia when they are first introduced. *As with the tricyclic agents, the concomitant administration of MAO inhibitors is hazardous.* There should be a period of at least 1 week between the administration of these two classes of drugs to allow for the washout of the last agent used. The symptoms of a "serotonin syndrome" that results from excessive intake or from the concurrent use of MAO inhibitors include confusion, restlessness, myoclonus, shivering, and diaphoresis, as summarized by Sternbach.

The SSRI drugs are well tolerated, may be effective in a shorter time than the tricyclic agents, and are justifiably very popular at the moment, but their long-term therapeutic usefulness in comparison with their predecessors remains to be determined (see review of Richelson). Fluoxetine has also been used with benefit in a group of autistic children (page 1100). Several related drugs such as venlafaxine (Effexor), nefazodone (Serzone), and citalopram (Celexa) have novel structures that are not analogous to those of the other categories of antidepressants. They are believed to act similarly to the SSRI class by inhibiting the reuptake of serotonin and norepinephrine. These newer drugs share most of the side effects of the SSRI drugs, including the danger of concomitant MAO inhibitor administration.

Lithium

The discovery of the therapeutic effects of lithium salts in mania has led to its widespread use in the treatment of manic-depressive disease (bipolar disorder). The drug has proved relatively safe and blood levels are easily monitored. Its value is much more certain in treatment of the manic phase of bipolar disorder and prevention of recurrences of cyclic mood shifts than it is in treatment of anxiety and depression. Guidelines for the clinical use of lithium are given in Chap. 57. Its mechanism of action is unclear, but there is experimental evidence that lithium blocks the stimulus-induced release of norepinephrine and enhances the reuptake of this amine—the opposite, in a sense, of what occurs with the other classes of antidepressants.

With blood levels of lithium in the upper therapeutic range, it is not uncommon to observe a fast-frequency action tremor or asterixis, together with nausea, loose stools, fatigue, polydipsia, and polyuria. These symptoms usually subside with time. Above a level of 1.5 to 2 meq/L, particularly in patients with impaired renal function or in those taking a thiazide diuretic, serious intoxication becomes manifest—clouding of consciousness, confusion, delirium, dizziness, nystagmus, ataxia, stammering, diffuse myoclonic twitching, and nephrogenic diabetes insipidus. Vertical (downbeating) nystagmus and opsoclonus may also be prominent. This clinical state, associated with sharp waves in the EEG, may mimic Creutzfeldt-Jakob disease, but there should be no problem in diagnosis if the setting of the illness and the administration of lithium are known. At a blood lithium concentration of 3.5 meq/L, these symptoms are replaced by stupor and coma, sometimes with convulsions, and may prove fatal.

Discontinuing lithium in the intoxicated patient, which is the initial step in therapy, does not result in immediate disappearance of toxic symptoms. This may be delayed by a week or two, and the diabetes insipidus may persist even longer. Fluids, sodium chloride, aminophylline, and acetazolamide promote the excretion of lithium. Lithium coma may require hemodialysis, which has proved to be the most rapid means of reducing the blood lithium concentration.

STIMULANTS

Drugs that act primarily as CNS stimulants have a relatively limited therapeutic use but assume clinical importance for other reasons. Some members of this group, e.g., the amphetamines, are much abused, and others are not infrequent causes of poisoning.

Amphetamine (Benzedrine, Adderall) This drug and dextroamphetamine, its D-isomer, are powerful analeptics (CNS stimulants) and in addition have significant hypertensive, respiratory-stimulant, and appetite-depressant effects. They are useful in the management of narcolepsy but have been much more widely and indiscriminately used for the control of obesity, the abolition of fatigue, and the treatment of hyperactivity in children. Undoubtedly, they are able to reverse fatigue, postpone the need for sleep, and elevate mood, but these effects are not entirely predictable, and the user must pay for the period of wakefulness with even greater fatigue and often with depression. The intravenous use of a high dose of amphetamine produces an immediate feeling of ecstasy, the "flash."

Because of the popularity of the amphetamines and the ease with which they can be procured, instances of acute and chronic intoxication are observed frequently. The toxic signs are essentially an exaggeration of the analeptic effects—restlessness, excessive speech and motor activity, tremor, and insomnia. Severe intoxication may give rise to hallucinations, delusions, and changes in affect and thought processes—a state that may be indistinguishable from paranoid schizophrenia. Amphetamine vasculitis and intracerebral and subarachnoid hemorrhage are well-recognized but rare complications of chronic intoxication (Harrington et al), and they may occur after acute use as well. Similar cerebrovascular complications occur with sympathomimetic agents contained in over-the-counter cold medications and in dieting aids; phenylpropanolamine has been implicated most often, but ephedrine and similar agents rarely have the same effects and induce a vasculopathy. The pathogenesis of the vascular lesion is unknown (both vasospasm and arteritis have been reported), and the same state occurs with cocaine, as described below.

Chronic use of amphetamines can lead to a high degree of tolerance and psychologic dependence. Withdrawal of the drug after sustained oral or intravenous use is regularly followed by a period of prolonged sleep (a disproportionate amount of which is REM sleep), from which the patient awakens with a ravenous appetite, muscle pains, and feelings of profound fatigue and depression. Treatment consists of discontinuing the use of amphetamine and administering antipsychotic drugs. Nitrites may be useful if the blood pressure is markedly elevated.

Methylphenidate (Ritalin) This drug has much the same type of action as dextroamphetamine and is useful in the treatment of narcolepsy. Paradoxically, like amphetamine, it is useful in the management of attention-deficit hyperactivity disorder in children (see page 629).

HALLUCINOGENS

Included in this category is a heterogeneous group of drugs, the primary effect of which is to alter perception, mood, and thinking out of proportion to other aspects of cognitive function and consciousness. This group of drugs comprises *cocaine*, *lysergic acid derivatives* [e.g., lysergic acid diethylamide (LSD)], *phenylethylamine derivatives* (mescaline or peyote), *psilocybin*, *certain indolic derivatives*, *cannabis* (marijuana), *phencyclidine* (PCP), and a number of less important compounds. They are also referred to as psychoactive and psychotomimetic drugs and as hallucinogens and psychedelics—but none of these names is entirely suitable. The problems raised by the nontherapeutic use of these drugs, which has declined somewhat but is still of serious proportions, have been reviewed by Nicholi and by Peroutka, and by Verebey and their associates.

Cocaine

The conventional use of cocaine as a local anesthetic has for many years been overshadowed by its illicit and widespread use as a stimulant and mood elevator. Originally, cocaine was sold as a white, lactose-adulterated powder that was usually administered intranasally ("snorted"); less often, it was smoked or injected intravenously or intramuscularly. Since 1985 there has been an alarming escalation in the use of cocaine, mainly because a relatively pure and inexpensive form of the free alkaloid base ("crack") became readily available at that time. This form of cocaine is heat-stable and therefore suitable for smoking. According to the National Household Survey on Drug Abuse, there were, in 1998, an estimated 600,000 frequent cocaine users in the United States. (Frequent use was arbitrarily defined as use on 51 or more days during the preceding year.) The number of occasional users (less than 12 days in the preceding year) was 2.4 million. These figures are subject to significant underreporting.

A sense of well-being, euphoria, loquacity, and restlessness are the familiar effects. Pharmacologically, cocaine is thought to act like the tricyclic antidepressants; i.e., it blocks the presynaptic reuptake of biogenic amines, thus producing vasoconstriction, hypertension, and tachycardia and predisposing to generalized tremor, myoclonus, seizures, and psychotic behavior. These actions as well as its immediate mood-elevating and euphoric effects are much the same as those of dextroamphetamine (see above). The cocaine abuser readily develops psychologic dependence or habituation, i.e., an inability to abstain from frequent compulsive use ("craving"). The manifestations of physical dependence are more subtle and difficult to recognize. Nevertheless, abstinence from cocaine following a period of chronic abuse is regularly attended by insomnia, restlessness, anorexia, depression, hyperprolactinemia, and signs of dopaminergic hypersensitivity—a symptom complex that constitutes an identifiable withdrawal syndrome.

With the increasingly widespread use of cocaine, a variety of new complications continues to emerge. The symptoms of severe intoxication (overdose), noted above, may lead to coma and death and require emergency treatment in an intensive care unit, along the lines indicated for the management of barbiturate coma. Seizures often occur in this setting and are treated more effectively with benzodiazepines than with standard anticonvulsant drugs. Spontaneous subarachnoid or intracerebral hemorrhage and cerebral infarction have rarely followed the intranasal use and smoking of cocaine (Levine et al). These complications are presumably the result of vasospasm induced by the sympathomimetic actions of cocaine. Cocaine and amphetamines also, on occasion, produce a state of generalized vasospasm leading to multiple cortical infarctions and posterior white matter changes that are evident on imaging studies, not unlike those seen with hypertensive encephalopathy (page 903). Several cases of a pathologically verified vasculitis and instances of "beading" of cerebral vessels on the arteriogram have been reported. We have seen several instances of vasospasm but have no experience with the vasculitis; however, it would seem that two different types of vasculopathy can result from cocaine and amphetamine use. Roth and colleagues have described 39 patients who developed acute rhabdomyolysis after cocaine use; 13 of these had acute renal failure, severe liver dysfunction, and disseminated intravascular coagulation and 6 of them died. Some reports indicate that cocaine use during pregnancy may cause fetal damage, abortion, or persistent signs of toxicity in the newborn infant.

Anxiety, paranoia, and other manifestations of psychosis may develop within several hours of cocaine use. These complications are best treated with haloperidol.

Marijuana

During the past three decades the prevalence of marijuana use has declined by about half, but it is still the most commonly used illicit drug in the United States. Its effects, when taken by inhaling the smoke from cigarettes, are prompt in onset and evanescent. With low doses, the symptoms are like those of mild alcohol intoxication (drowsiness, euphoria, dulling of the senses, and perceptual distortions). With increasing amounts, the effects are similar to those of LSD, mescaline, and psilocybin (see below); they may be quite disabling for many hours. With even larger doses, severe depression and stupor may occur, but death is rare (for a full account, see Hollister, 1988). No damage to the nervous system has been found after chronic use.

Reverse tolerance to marijuana (i.e., increasing sensitization) may be observed initially, but on continued use, tolerance to the euphoriant effects develops. In one of the few experimental studies of chronic marijuana use, the subjects reported feeling "jittery" during the first 24 h after abrupt cessation of smoking marijuana, although no objective withdrawal signs could be detected.

The mild antiemetic and antinauseant effects of marijuana coupled with euphoria have led to its use as an agent to ameliorate the effects of cancer chemotherapies, and this purported therapeutic effect is the mainstay of the movement for its legalization.

Mescaline, LSD, and Psilocybin

These drugs produce much the same clinical effects if given in comparable amounts. The perceptual changes are the most dramatic: the user describes vivid visual hallucinations, alterations in the shape and color of objects, unusual dreams, and feelings of depersonalization. An increase in auditory acuity has been described, but auditory hallucinations are rare. Cognitive functions are difficult to assess because of inattention, drowsiness, and inability to co-operate in mental testing. The somatic symptoms consist of dizziness, nausea, paresthesias, and blurring of vision. Sympathomimetic effects—pupillary dilation, piloerection, hyperthermia, and tachycardia—are prominent, and the user may also show hyperreflexia, incoordination of the limbs, and ataxia.

Tolerance to LSD, mescaline, and psilocybin develops rapidly, even on a once-daily dosage. Furthermore, subjects tolerant to any one of these three drugs are cross-tolerant to the other two. Tolerance is lost rapidly when the drugs are discontinued abruptly, but no characteristic signs of physical dependence (abstinence syndrome) ensue. In this sense, addiction does not develop, although users may become dependent upon the drugs for emotional support (psychologic dependence or habituation).

Although LSD has no therapeutic value and the use of marijuana is governed by the federal narcotic laws, these drugs are widely used. They are taken by narcotic addicts as a temporary substitute for more potent drugs; by "drugheads" (i.e., individuals who use any agent that alters consciousness); and by many troubled, unhappy college and high school students for social conformity or for reasons that even they cannot ascertain. The use of these drugs is attended by a number of serious adverse reactions taking the form of acute panic attacks, long-lasting psychotic states resembling paranoid schizophrenia, and flashbacks (spontaneous recurrences of the original LSD experience, sometimes precipitated by smoking marijuana and accompanied by panic attacks). Serious physical injury may follow upon impairment of the user's critical faculties. Whether prolonged usage leads to permanent damage to the nervous system is not certain; there are some data to suggest that this may happen, but there is little doubt that the mental state of some psychologically predisposed individuals is permanently altered. The reports claiming that LSD may cause chromosomal damage remain to be validated. Numerous claims have been made that LSD and related drugs are effective in the treatment of mental disease and a wide variety of social ills and that they have the capacity to increase one's intellectual performance, creativity, and self-understanding. To date there have been no acceptable studies that validate any of these claims.

Phencyclidine ("Angel Dust" and "Ecstasy")

During the early 1970s, the abuse of phencyclidine (PCP) and its many analogues was a significant problem. The popularity of these drugs has dropped sharply, but some illicit use continues because they are relatively cheap, easily available, and quite powerful. Phencyclidine is taken illicitly as a granular powder, frequently mixed with other drugs, and is smoked or snorted. It is usually classified as a hallucinogen, although it also has stimulant and depressant properties. The effects of intoxication are like those of LSD and other hallucinogens and resemble those of an acute schizophrenic episode, which may last several days to a week or more. After the ingestion of a large amount (10 mg or more) of phencyclidine, it is present in the blood and urine for only a few hours. Its manufacture as a veterinary anesthetic was stopped in 1979.

Toxicity from the illicit use of "ecstasy" (MDMA) during all-night dance parties (raves) has recently increased as a result of its ill-founded reputation for safety. It appears to cause a release of both serotonin and dopamine in the brain and produces an elated state similar to the effects of cocaine. Seizures, cerebral hemorrhages, and psychosis have been reported in previously healthy individuals (Vereby et al).

A discussion of the legal implications of the illicit use of the aforementioned drugs and their social impact is beyond the scope of this chapter but can be found in the appended references.

DISORDERS DUE TO BACTERIAL TOXINS

The most important diseases in this category are tetanus, botulism, and diphtheria. Each is caused by an extraordinarily powerful bacterial toxin that acts primarily upon the nervous system.

Tetanus

The cause of this disease is the anaerobic, spore-forming rod *Clostridium tetani*. The organisms are found in the feces of some humans and many animals, particularly horses, whence they readily contaminate the soil. The spores may remain dormant for many months or years, but when they are introduced into a wound, especially if a foreign body or suppurative bacteria are present, they are converted into their vegetative forms, which produce the exotoxin tetanospasmin. In developing countries, tetanus is still a common disease, particularly in newborns, in whom the spores are introduced via the umbilical cord (*tetanus neonatorum*). In the United States, the incidence rate of tetanus is about one per million per year. Injection of contaminated heroin is a significant cause. About two-thirds of all injuries leading to tetanus occur from deep scratches and puncture wounds in the home and about 20 percent in gardens and on farms.

Since 1903, when Morax and Marie proposed their theory of centripetal migration of the tetanus toxin, it has been taught that spread to the nervous system occurs via the peripheral nerves, the toxin ascending in the axis cylinders or the perineural sheaths. Modern studies, utilizing fluorescein-labeled tetanus antitoxin, have disclosed that the toxin is also widely disseminated via blood or lymphatics, probably accounting for the generalized form of the disease. However, in local tetanus, the likely mode of spread to the CNS is by retrograde axonal transport.

Mode of Action of Tetanus Toxin Like botulinum toxin, the tetanus toxin is a zinc-dependent protease. It blocks neurotransmitter release by cleaving surface proteins of the synaptic vesicles, thus preventing the normal exocytosis of neurotransmitter. The toxin interferes with the function of the reflex arc by the blockade of inhibitory transmitters, mainly GABA, at presynaptic sites in the spinal cord and brainstem. Elicitation of the jaw jerk, for example, is normally followed by the abrupt suppression of motor neuron activity, manifested in the electromyogram (EMG) as a "silent period" (see further on). In the patient with tetanus, there is a failure of this inhibitory mechanism, with a resulting increase in activation of the neurons that innervate the masseter muscles (*trismus* or lockjaw). Of all neuromuscular systems, the masseter innervation seems to be the most sensitive to the toxin. Not only do afferent stimuli produce an exaggerated effect, but they also abolish reciprocal innervation; both agonists and antagonists contract, giving rise to the characteristic muscular spasm. In addition to its generalized effects on the motor neurons of the spinal cord and brainstem, there is evidence that the toxin acts directly on skeletal muscle at the point where the axon forms the end plate (accounting perhaps for localized tetanus) and also upon the cerebral cortex and the sympathetic nervous system, in the hypothalamus.

The incubation period varies greatly, from a day or two to a month or even longer. Long incubation periods are associated with mild and localized types of the disease.

Clinical Features There are several clinical types of tetanus, usually designated as local, cephalic, and generalized.

Generalized Tetanus This is the most common form. It may begin as local tetanus that becomes generalized after a few days, or it may be diffuse from the beginning. Trismus is frequently the first manifestation. In some cases this is preceded by a feeling of stiffness in the jaw or neck, slight fever, and other general symptoms of infection. The localized muscle stiffness and spasms spread quickly to other bulbar muscles as well as those of the neck, trunk, and limbs. A state of unremitting rigidity develops in all the involved muscles: the abdomen is board-like, the legs are rigidly extended, and the lips are pursed or retracted (*risus sardonicus*); the eyes are partially closed by contraction of the orbicularis oculi or the eyebrows are elevated by spasm of the frontalis. Superimposed on this persistent state of enhanced muscle activity are paroxysms of tonic contraction or spasm of muscles (tetanic seizures or convulsions), which occur spontaneously or in response to the slightest external stimulus. They are agonizingly painful. Consciousness is not lost during these paroxysms. The tonic contraction of groups of muscles results in opisthotonos or in forward flexion of the trunk, flexion and adduction of the arms, clenching of the fists, and extension of the legs. Spasms of the pharyngeal, laryngeal, or respiratory muscles carry the constant threat of apnea or suffocation. Fever and pneumonia are common complications. Large swings in blood pressure and pulse as well as profuse diaphoresis are typical, mainly in response to the intense muscular contractions but also related to the action of the toxin on the CNS. Death is usually attributable to asphyxia from laryngospasm, to heart failure, or to shock, the latter resulting from the action of the toxin on the hypothalamus and sympathetic nervous system.

Generalized spasms and rigidity of trunk and limbs developing in a neonate a few days after birth should always suggest the diagnosis of tetanus. This form of tetanus occurs when there has been inadequate sterile treatment of the umbilical cord stump in a neonate born to an unimmunized mother.

Local Tetanus This is the most benign form. The initial symptoms are stiffness, tightness, and pain in the muscles in the neighborhood of a wound, followed by twitchings and brief spasms of the affected muscles. Local tetanus occurs most often in relation to a wound of the hand or forearm, rarely in the abdominal or paravertebral muscles. Gradually, some degree of continuous involuntary spasm becomes evident. This is referred to as *rigidity*, *hypertonic contractions*, or *tetanic spasticity*, terms that denote the sustained tautness of the affected muscles and resistance of the part to passive movement. Superimposed on this background of more or less continuous motor activity are brief, intense spasms, lasting from a few seconds to minutes and occurring "spontaneously" or in response to all variety of stimulation (Struppler et al). Early in the course of the illness there may be periods when the affected muscles are palpably soft and appear to be relaxed. A useful diagnostic maneuver at this stage is to have the patient perform some repetitive voluntary movements, such as opening and closing the hand, in response to which there occurs a gradual increase in the tonic contraction and spasms of the affected muscles, followed by spread to neighboring muscle groups (recruitment spasm). The phenomenon resembles paradoxical myotonia (page 1559). Even with mild localized tetanus there may be a slight trismus, a useful diagnostic sign.

Symptoms may persist in localized form for several weeks or months. Gradually the spasms become less frequent and more difficult to evoke, and they finally disappear without residue. Complete recovery is to be expected, since there are no pathologic changes in muscles, nerves, spinal cord, or brain, even in the most severe generalized forms of tetanus.

Cephalic Tetanus This form of tetanus follows wounds of the face and head. The incubation period is short, 1 or 2 days as a rule. The affected muscles (most often facial) are weak or paralyzed. Nevertheless, during accessions of tetanic spasm, the palsied muscles are seen to contract. Apparently the disturbance in the facial motoneurons is sufficient to prevent voluntary movement but insufficient to prevent the strong reflex impulses that elicit facial spasm. The spasms may involve the tongue and throat, with persistent dysarthria, dysphonia, and dysphagia. Ophthalmoparesis is known to occur but is difficult to verify because of severe blepharospasm. In a strict sense these cephalic forms of tetanus are examples of local tetanus that frequently becomes generalized. Many cases prove fatal.

Diagnosis This is made from the clinical features and a history of preceding injury. The latter is sometimes disclosed only after careful questioning, the injury having been trivial and forgotten. The organisms may or may not be recovered from the wound by the time the patient receives medical attention; other laboratory tests, apart from the EMG, are of little value. Serum CK may be moderately elevated if the rigidity is generalized. The EMG recorded from muscles in spasm shows continuous discharges of normal motor units like those recorded from a forceful voluntary muscle contraction. Most characteristic of tetanus, as mentioned earlier, is a loss of the silent period that occurs 50 to 100 ms after reflex contraction. This pause, normally effected by the recurrent inhibition of Renshaw cells, is blocked by tetanus toxin. In generalized tetanus the loss of the silent period can almost always be demonstrated in the masseter, and it is found in a muscle affected by local tetanus. Interestingly, the silent period is preserved in the stiff man syndrome (page 1569). Tetany due to hypocalcemia, the spasms of strychnine poisoning or black widow spider bite, trismus due to painful conditions in and around the jaw, the dysphagia of rabies, hysterical spasms, rigidity and dystonic spasms caused by neuroleptic drugs, and the spasms of the stiff man syndrome all resemble the spasms of tetanus but should not be difficult to distinguish when all aspects of these disorders are considered.

The death rate from tetanus is about 50 percent overall; it is highest in newborns, heroin addicts, and patients with the cephalic form of the disease. The patient usually recovers if there are no severe generalized muscle spasms during the course of the illness or if the spasms remain localized.

Treatment This must be directed along several lines. At the outset, a single dose of antitoxin (3000 to 6000 units of tetanus immune human globulin) should be given and a 10-day course of penicillin (1.2 million units of procaine penicillin daily), metronidazole (500 mg every 6 h intravenously or 400 mg rectally), or tetracycline (2 g daily) instituted. These drugs are effective against the vegetative forms of *C. tetani*. Immediate surgical treatment of the wound (excision or debridement) is imperative, and the tissue around the wound should be infiltrated with antitoxin.

Survival depends upon expert and constant nursing in an intensive care unit and may be necessary for weeks. Tracheostomy is a requisite in all patients with recurrent generalized tonic spasms and should not be delayed until apnea or cyanosis has occurred. The patient must be kept as quiet as possible to avoid stimulus-induced spasms. This requires a darkened, quiet room and the judicious use of sedation. The benzodiazepines are the most useful drugs; diazepam 120 mg/day or more can be given in frequent divided doses if ventilatory support is available, or midazolam can be given in a continuous intravenous infusion. Short-acting barbiturates (secobarbital or pentobarbital) and chlorpromazine may also be useful, as is morphine. Intrathecal baclofen and continuous atropine infusions have been used with success in severe cases, and intramuscular injections of botulinus toxin may be used for trismus and local spasm. The aim of therapy is to suppress muscle spasms and to keep the patient drowsy but arousable. All treatments and manipulations should be kept to a minimum; they should be carefully planned and coordinated, and the patient should be sedated beforehand.

Failure of these measures to control the tetanic paroxysms demands that intravenous administration of neuromuscular blocking agents such as pancuronium or vecuronium be used to abolish all muscle activity; appropriate sedative medication is instituted for as long as necessary, breathing being maintained entirely by a positive-pressure respirator. Many units favor the use of neuromuscular paralytic drugs in all but the mildest cases. Further details concerning treatment in the intensive care unit can be found in the recent review by Farrar et al.

All persons should be immunized against tetanus and receive a booster dose of toxoid every 10 years—a practice that is frequently neglected in the elderly. Injuries that carry a threat of tetanus should be treated by an injection of toxoid if the patient has not received a booster injection in the preceding year, and a second dose of toxoid should be given 6 weeks later. If the injured person has not received a booster injection since the original immunization, he or she should receive an injection of both toxoid and human antitoxin; the same applies to the injured person who has never been immunized. An attack of tetanus does not confer permanent immunity, and all persons who recover should be actively immunized.

Diphtheria

Diphtheria, an acute infectious disease caused by *Corynebacterium diphtheriae*, is now quite rare in the United States and western Europe. The faucial-pharyngeal form of the disease, which is the most common clinical type, is characterized by the formation of an inflammatory exudate of the throat and trachea; at this site, the bacteria elaborate an exotoxin, which affects the heart and nervous system in about 20 percent of cases.

The involvement of the nervous system follows a predictable pattern (Fisher and Adams). It begins locally, with *palatal paralysis* (nasal voice, regurgitation, and dysphagia) between the fifth and twelfth days of illness. At this time or shortly afterward, other cranial nerves (trigeminal, facial, vagus, and hypoglossal) may also be affected. *Ciliary paralysis* with loss of accommodation and blurring of vision appears usually in the second or third week. Very rarely the extraocular muscles are involved. The cranial nerve signs may clear without further involvement of the nervous system, or a sensorimotor polyneuropathy may develop between the fifth and eighth weeks of the disease. The latter varies in severity from a mild, predominantly distal affection of the limbs to a rapidly evolving, ascending paralysis, like that of the Guillain-Barré syndrome; CSF findings are similar as well (acellular fluid with elevated protein). The neuropathic symptoms progress for a week or two, and if the patient does not succumb to respiratory paralysis or cardiac failure (cardiomyopathy), these conditions stabilize and then improve slowly and more or less completely.

The early oropharyngeal symptoms, the unique ciliary paralysis, and the subacute evolution of a delayed symmetrical sensorimotor peripheral neuropathy distinguish diphtheritic from all other forms of polyneuropathy.

The long latency between the initial infection and the involvement of the nervous system has no clear explanation. In experimental animals, Waksman and colleagues have shown that the toxin reaches the Schwann cells in the most vascular parts of the peripheral nervous system within 24 to 48 h of infection, but its metabolic effect on cell membranes extends over a period of weeks. As in humans, the toxin produces demyelination in the proximal parts of spinal nerves, in dorsal root ganglia, and in spinal roots. The cardiac musculature and the conducting system of the heart undergo focal necroses.

The source of diphtheritic infection may be extrafaucial—a penetrating wound, skin ulcer, or umbilicus. The systemic and neurologic complications of faucial diphtheria can also be observed in the extrafaucial form of the disease, after a similar latent period. It is probable, therefore, that the toxin reaches its neural site via the bloodstream; but, in addition, some action is exerted locally, as evidenced by palatal paralysis in faucial cases and by initial weakness and sensory impairment in the neighborhood of the infected wound.

There is no specific treatment for any of the neurologic complications of diphtheria. It is generally agreed that the administration of antitoxin within 48 h of the earliest symptoms of the primary diphtheritic infection lessens the incidence and severity of complications.

The polyneuropathy of diphtheria is discussed further in Chap. 46 (page 1389).

Botulism

Botulism is a rare form of food-borne illness caused by the exotoxin of *Clostridium botulinum*. Outbreaks of poisoning are more often due to home-preserved than to commercially canned products, and vegetables and home-cured ham are incriminated more commonly than any other food product. Very rarely, a contaminated wound is the source of infection. Although the disease is ubiquitous, five western states (California, Washington, Colorado, New Mexico, and Oregon) account for more than half of all reported outbreaks in the United States. *Neonatal and infantile forms* of the disease have been reported, due to absorption of the toxin formed by germination of ingested spores (rather than ingestion of preformed toxin), an important source of which is contaminated natural (raw) honey. A few adult cases may have a similar source.

It is now well established, on the basis of observations in both animals and humans, that the primary site of action of botulinus toxin is at the neuromuscular junction, more specifically on the presynaptic endings. The toxin interferes with the release of acetylcholine quanta by a mechanism like that of tetanus toxin (see previous discussion). The physiologic defect is similar to the one that characterizes the myasthenic syndrome of Lambert-Eaton (page 1547) but different from that of myasthenia gravis.

Symptoms usually appear within 12 to 36 h of ingestion of the tainted food. Anorexia, nausea, and vomiting occur in most patients. As a rule, blurred vision and diplopia are the initial neural symptoms; their association with ptosis, strabismus, and extraocular muscle palsies, particularly of the sixth nerve, may at first suggest a diagnosis of myasthenia gravis. In botulism, however, the pupils are often unreactive. Other symptoms of bulbar involvement—nasality of the voice and hoarseness, dysarthria, dysphagia, and an inability to phonate—follow in quick succession, and these, in turn, are followed by progressive weakness of muscles of the face, neck, trunk, and limbs and by respiratory insufficiency. Despite the oropharyngeal weakness, it is not unusual for the gag reflex to be retained. Tendon reflexes are lost in cases of severe weakness. These symptoms and signs evolve rapidly, over 2 to 4 days as a rule, and may be mistaken for those of the Guillain-Barré syndrome. Sensation remains intact, however, and the spinal fluid usually shows no abnormalities. Severe constipation is characteristic of botulism, due perhaps to paresis of smooth muscle of the intestine. Consciousness is retained throughout the illness unless severe degrees of anoxia develop. In the past, the mortality was consistently above 60 percent, but it has declined in recent decades, with improvements in the intensive care of acute respiratory failure and the effectiveness of *C. botulinum* antitoxins.

The clinical diagnosis can be confirmed by electrophysiologic studies (reduced amplitude of evoked muscle potentials and an increase in amplitude with rapid repetitive nerve stimulation). In patients who recover, improvement begins within a few weeks, first in ocular movement, then in other cranial nerve function. Complete recovery of paralyzed limb and trunk musculature may take many months.

The three types of botulinus toxin, A, B, and E, cannot be distinguished by their clinical effects alone, so that the patient should receive the trivalent antiserum as soon as the clinical diagnosis is made. This antitoxin can be obtained from the Centers for Disease Control and Prevention, Atlanta. An initial dose of 10,000 units is given intravenously after intradermal testing for sensitivity to horse serum, followed by daily doses of 50,000 units intramuscularly until improvement begins.

Guanidine hydrochloride (50 mg/kg) has reportedly been useful in reversing the weakness of limb and extraocular muscles. Antitoxin and guanidine probably change the course of the illness relatively little, and recovery, in the final analysis, depends upon the effectiveness of respiratory care, maintenance of fluid and electrolyte balance, prevention of infection, and so on.

The skilled injection of small quantities of botulinus toxin (Botox) into a muscle will weaken or paralyze it for weeks to months. Advantage is taken of this phenomenon in the treatment of the localized dystonias (page 114).

POISONING DUE TO PLANTS, VENOMS, BITES, AND STINGS

Ergotism

Ergotism is the name applied to poisoning with ergot, a drug derived from the rye fungus *Claviceps purpurea*. Ergot is used therapeutically to control postpartum hemorrhage due to uterine atony; one of its alkaloids, ergotamine, is a frequently used drug in the treatment of migraine, and a class of dopamine agonists used in the treatment of Parkinson disease has ergot activity. Chronic overdosage of the drug is the usual cause of ergotism; acute overdosage in the postpartum state or in the treatment of migraine may cause an alarming rise in blood pressure.

Two types of ergotism are recognized: *gangrenous*, due to a vasospastic, occlusive process in the small arteries of the extremities, and *convulsive*, or *neurogenic* ergotism. The latter is characterized by fasciculations, myoclonus, and spasms of muscles, followed by seizures. In nonfatal cases, a tabes-like neurologic syndrome may develop, with loss of knee and ankle jerks, ataxia, and impairment of deep and superficial sensation. The pathologic changes are said to consist of degeneration of the posterior columns, dorsal roots, and peripheral nerves, but they have been poorly described. The relation of these changes to ergot poisoning is not clear, since most of the cases have occurred in areas where malnutrition was endemic. The authors have had no experience with this condition.

Lathyrism

Lathyrism is a neurologic syndrome characterized by the relatively acute onset of pain, paresthesias, and weakness in the lower extremities, progressing to a permanent spastic paraplegia. It is a serious medical problem in India and in some North African countries and is probably due to a toxin contained in the chickling vetch, *Lathyrus*, a legume that is consumed in excess during periods of famine. This disorder is discussed further with the spinal cord diseases (page 1336).

Mushroom Poisoning

The gathering of wild mushrooms, a popular pastime in late summer and early fall, always carries with it the danger of poisoning. As many as one hundred species of mushrooms are poisonous. Most of them cause only transient gastrointestinal symptoms, but some elaborate toxins that can be fatal. The most important of these toxins are the cyclopeptides, which are contained in several species of *Amanita phalloides* and *muscaria* and account for more than 90 percent of fatal mushroom poisonings. These toxins disrupt RNA metabolism, causing hepatic and renal necrosis. Symptoms of poisoning with *Amanita* usually appear between 10 and 14 h after ingestion and consist of nausea, vomiting, colicky pain, and diarrhea, followed by irritability, restlessness, ataxia, hallucinations, convulsions, and coma. There may be added evidence of a polymyopathy presenting as flaccid areflexic paralysis, high serum CK, diminished EMG potentials, and fiber necrosis.

Other important toxins are methylhydrazine (contained in the *cyromitra* species) and muscarine (*inocybe* and *clitocybe* species). The former gives rise to a clinical picture much like that caused by the cyclopeptides. The symptoms of muscarine poisoning, which appear within 30 to 60 min of ingestion, are essentially those of parasympathetic stimulation—miosis, lacrimation, salivation, nausea, vomiting, diarrhea, perspiration, bradycardia, and hypotension. Tremor, seizures, and delirium occur in cases of severe poisoning.

The mushroom toxins have no effective antidotes. If vomiting has not occurred, it should be induced with ipecac, following which activated charcoal should be administered orally in order to bind what toxin remains in the gastrointestinal tract. A local poison control center may help identify the poisonous mushroom and its toxin. Even more important, the gathering and ingestion of field varieties of mushrooms should be left to those absolutely certain of their identity.

Buckthorn Poisoning

A rapidly progressive and sometimes fatal paralysis follows the ingestion of the small fruit of the buckthorn shrub that is indigenous to northern Mexico and the neighboring parts of the United States. The responsible toxin causes a predominantly motor polyneuropathy, probably of axonal type. Except for a normal spinal fluid protein concentration, the disorder closely resembles Guillain-Barré syndrome and tick paralysis, and its recognition depends upon awareness of ingestion of the fruit in endemic areas.

Neurotoxin Fish Poisoning (Ciguatera)

Ingestion of marine toxins that block neural sodium channels is a common form of poisoning throughout coastal areas and islands of the world. It results from eating fish that have fed on toxin-containing microscopic dinoflagelates. Reef fish and shellfish are subject to high concentrations of the organisms during periodic upswings in the population of the dinoflagelates, which may be so profuse as to color the surrounding water (red tide). Although the toxins differ (tetrodotoxin, pufferfish; ciguatoxin, snails; saxitoxin and brevitoxin, shellfish), the neurologic and gastrointestinal symptoms that follow the ingestion of affected fish are similar. The initial symptoms are diarrhea, vomiting, or abdominal cramps coming on minutes to hours after the ingestion of the poisoned fish. These are followed by paresthesias that often begin periorally and then involve the limbs distally. Hot and cold sensory stimuli (e.g., ice cream) are characteristically associated with electrical-like or burning paresthesias. Muscle aches and shooting pains are also mentioned by most patients. In pufferfish poisoning and in advanced stages poisoning from other fish, weakness occurs, and there have been a few reports of coma and of respiratory failure. The recognition of this type of fish poisoning is straightforward in endemic areas, in some of which there is a seasonal clustering of cases. In tourists returning home from endemic areas or in persons consuming imported fish, the illness may be mistaken for the Guillain-Barré syndrome. Prominent perioral paresthesias should suggest the correct diagnosis. Supportive treatment is all that is required, but treatment with intravenous mannitol appears to hasten recovery.

Venoms, Bites, and Stings

These are relatively rare but nonetheless important causes of mortality in the United States. The venoms of certain species of snakes, lizards, spiders (especially the black widow spider), and scorpions contain neurotoxins that may cause a fatal depression of respiration and curare-like failure of neuromuscular transmission. In the United States, there are about 8000 poisonous snake bites per year. Some, such as the coral snake envenomation, are neurotoxic, producing pupillary dilatation, ptosis, ocular palsies, ataxia, and respiratory paralysis. Others (rattlesnakes, water moccasin snakes) cause tissue necrosis and circulatory collapse. The serious effects of *Hymenoptera stings* (bees, wasps, hornets, and fire ants) are due mainly to hypersensitivity and anaphylaxis. All of these disorders are discussed in detail in *Harrison's Principles of Internal Medicine*.

Tick Paralysis

This rare condition is the result of a toxin secreted by the gravid tick. In Canada and the northwestern United States, the wood tick *Dermacentor andersoni* is mainly responsible; in the southeastern United States it is *Dermacentor variabilis*, a dog tick, but various other ticks may occasionally have the same effect. Most cases occur in children because their small body mass makes them susceptible to the effects of only modest amounts of the toxin. The illness arises almost exclusively in the spring, when the mature ticks are most plentiful. The illness requires that the gravid tick be attached to the skin for several days.

The neurotoxin causes a generalized, flaccid, areflexic paralysis, appearing over 1 or 2 days and mimicking the Guillain-Barré syndrome. Often several days of ataxia and areflexia precede the paralysis, but sensory loss tends to be minimal. The external ophthalmoplegia that occurred in 5 of the 6 children described by Grattan-Smith et al has more often been absent in other reports; internal ophthalmoplegia and pharyngeal weakness are also known to occur, thus raising the diagnostic possibility of botulism or diphtheria. The CSF is normal and electrophysiologic studies show reduction in the amplitude of the muscle action potentials but normal or slightly slowed nerve conduction. Prominent ptosis and neck weakness may also raise the question of a neuromuscular process, but repetitive stimulation testing is normal or shows only a slight decrement or increment in some cases.

The ticks tend to attach to the hairlines or in the matted hair of the scalp, neck, and pubis, where a careful search will reveal them (nurses and electroencephalography technicians often are the ones who find them; see Felz et al). The diagnosis is most important in endemic areas and during the tick season, since the removal of the tick results in rapid and dramatic improvement.

From a neurologic point of view, the most notable disorder that follows tick bite is what has come to be known as *Lyme disease*—so named for the Connecticut community in which it was discovered. The causative agent is *Borrelia burgdorferi*, a spirochetal organism transmitted by the tick *Ixodes dammini*. The disorder is discussed fully with other infectious diseases in Chap. 32 and in Chap. 46, with the neuropathies.

HEAVY METALS

Lead

The causes and clinical manifestations of lead poisoning are quite different in children and adults.

Lead Poisoning in Children In the United States, the disease occurs most often in 1- to 3-year-old children who inhabit urban slum areas where old, deteriorated housing prevails. (Lead paint was used in most houses built before 1940 and in many built before 1960.) The chewing of leaded paint, the most common sources of which are windowsills and painted plaster walls, and its compulsive ingestion (pica), are the important factors in the causation of lead poisoning. The development of an acute encephalopathy is the most serious complication, leading to death in 5 to 20 percent of cases and to permanent neurologic and mental sequelae in more than 25 percent of survivors.

Clinical Manifestations These develop over a period of 3 to 6 weeks. The child becomes anorectic, less playful and less alert, and more irritable. These symptoms may be misinterpreted as a behavior disorder or mental retardation. Intermittent vomiting, vague abdominal pain, clumsiness, and ataxia may be added. If these early signs of intoxication are not recognized and the child continues to ingest lead, more flagrant signs of acute encephalopathy may develop—most frequently in the summer months, for reasons that are not understood. Vomiting becomes more persistent, apathy progresses to drowsiness and stupor interspersed with periods of hyperirritability, and finally seizures, papilledema, and coma supervene. This syndrome evolves in a period of a week or less and most rapidly in children under 2 years of age; in older children, it is more likely to develop in recurrent and less severe episodes. This clinical syndrome must be distinguished from tuberculous meningitis, viral meningoencephalitis, and the various conditions causing acute increased intracranial pressure. Usually, in lead encephalopathy, the CSF is under increased pressure and may show a slight lymphocytic pleocytosis and elevated protein, but glucose values are normal. It follows that lumbar puncture should be done with caution and only if it is essential for diagnosis.

In children who die of acute lead encephalopathy, the brain is massively swollen, with herniation of the temporal lobes and cerebellum, multiple microscopic ischemic foci in the cerebrum and cerebellum, and endothelial damage and deposition of proteinaceous material and mononuclear inflammatory cells around many of the small blood vessels.

Diagnosis Since the symptoms of plumbism are nonspecific, the diagnosis depends upon an appreciation of the causative factors, a high index of suspicion, and certain laboratory tests. The presence of lead lines at the metaphyses of long bones and basophilic stippling of red cells are too inconstant to be relied upon, but basophilic stippling of bone marrow normoblasts is uniformly increased. Impairment of heme synthesis, which is exquisitely sensitive to the toxic effects of lead, results in the increased excretion of urinary coproporphyrin (UCP) and of δ-aminolevulinic acid (ALA). These urinary indices and the lead concentrations in the serum bear an imperfect relationship to the clinical manifestations. In the test for UCP, which is readily performed in the clinic and emergency department, a few milliliters of urine are acidified with acetic acid and shaken with an equal volume of ether; if coproporphyrin is present, the ether layer will reveal a reddish fluorescence under a Wood's lamp. This test is strongly positive when the whole blood concentration of lead exceeds 80 μg/dL. The diagnosis can be confirmed by promoting lead excretion with calcium disodium edetate ($CaNa_2$ EDTA), given in three doses (25 mg/kg) at 8-h intervals. Excretion of over 500 mg in 24 h is indicative of plumbism. The measurement of zinc protoporphyrin (ZPP) in the blood is another reliable means of determining the presence and degree of lead exposure. The binding of erythrocyte protoporphyrin to zinc occurs when lead impairs the normal binding of erythrocyte protoporphyrin to iron. Elevated ZPP can also occur when access to iron is limited by other conditions, such as iron deficiency anemia.

Treatment At blood lead concentrations of 70 μg/dL, symptoms may be minimal, but acute encephalopathy may occur abruptly and unpredictably, for which reason the child should be hospitalized for chelation therapy. Some children with a blood lead level of 50 μg/dL may have symptoms of severe encephalopathy, whereas others may be asymptomatic. In the latter case, an attempt should be made to discover and remove the source of lead intoxication and the child should be reexamined at frequent intervals. The seriousness of lead encephalopathy is indicated by the fact that most of the children who become stuporous or comatose remain mentally retarded despite treatment. The physician's aim, therefore, is to *institute treatment before the severe symptoms of encephalopathy have become manifest.*

The plan of therapy includes the following:

1. Establishment of urinary flow, following which intravenous fluid therapy is restricted to basal water and electrolyte requirements.

2. In cases of acute encephalopathy, combined chelation therapy with 2,3-dimercaptopropanol (BAL, 12 to 24 mg/kg) and $CaNa_2$ EDTA (0.5 to 1.5 g/m^2 body surface area) for 5 to 7 days. This is followed by a course of oral penicillamine (40 mg/kg, not exceeding 1 g per day). In acute cases the goal is to reduce the serum lead levels below 40 μg/dL. Once the absorption of lead has ceased, chelating agents remove lead only from soft tissues and not from bone, where most of the lead is stored. Any intercurrent illness may result in a mobilization of lead from bones and soft tissues and an exacerbation of symptoms of lead intoxication.

3. Repeated doses of mannitol for relief of cerebral edema.

4. Microcytic hypochromic anemia is treated with iron once the chelating agents have been discontinued.

5. Seizures are best controlled with intravenous diazepam or midazolam.

Prevention The prevention of reintoxication (or intoxication) demands that the child be removed from the source of lead. Although this is axiomatic, it is often difficult to accomplish, despite the best efforts of local health departments and hospital and city social workers. Nevertheless, an attempt to correct the environmental factor must be made in each case. Such attempts, among other things, have resulted in a marked decrease in the incidence of acute lead encephalopathy in the past two decades. Although florid examples of this encephalopathy are now uncommon, undue exposure to lead (blood levels > 30 μg/dL) remains inordinately prevalent and a continuing source of concern to public health authorities. As to the levels that pose a danger to the child, there is still some uncertainty. Rutter, who reviewed all of the evidence up to 1980, concluded that persistent blood levels above 40 μg/dL may cause slight cognitive impairment and, less certainly, an increased risk of behavioral difficulties. The oral lead chelator *succimer* is approved for outpatient treatment of asymptomatic children with blood lead levels higher than 45 μg/dL. A 3-week course of treatment is given, with weekly monitoring of blood lead levels to identify lead mobilization from bones and soft tissues (Jorgensen).

In 1988, on the basis of epidemiologic and experimental studies in the United States, Europe, and Australia, the Agency for Toxic Substances and Disease Registry set a much lower threshold for neurobehavioral toxicity (10 to 15 μg/dL). They estimated that 3 to 4 million American children have blood levels in excess of this amount. Needleman et al studied the long-term effects of low doses of lead in asymptomatic children, 132 of whom had had demonstrable levels of lead in the dentin of shed teeth (average 24 μg/dL). Eleven years later, the children were found to have behavioral abnormalities proportionate to their early lead levels. In comparison to a normal population, more had dropped out of school and more had lower vocabulary and grammatical reasoning scores, more reading difficulty, poorer hand-eye coordination performance, slower finger-tapping rates, and longer reaction times. The authors claimed to have eliminated other confounding variables such as lower social class and genetic factors. These findings have been confirmed by the long-term studies of Baghurst et al (see also Mahaffey).

Lead Intoxication in Adults This is much less common than in children. The hazards to adults are exposure to dust of inorganic lead salts and to fumes resulting from the burning of lead or processes that require the remelting of lead. Painting, printing, pottery glazing, lead smelting, and storage battery manufacturing are the industries in which these hazards are likeliest to occur. Miners and brass foundry and garage workers (during automobile radiator repair, when soldered joints are heated) are the ones most at risk.

The usual manifestations of lead poisoning in adults are colic, anemia, and peripheral neuropathy. Encephalopathy is decidedly rare; usually it results from consumption of illicit liquor contaminated by lead solder in the pipes of stills. Lead colic, frequently precipitated by an intercurrent infection or by alcohol intoxication, is characterized by severe, poorly localized abdominal pain, often with rigidity of abdominal muscles but without fever or leukocytosis. The pain responds to the intravenous injection of calcium salts, at least temporarily, but very little to morphine. Mild anemia is common. A black line of lead sulfide may develop along the gingival margins. Peripheral neuropathy, usually a bilateral wrist drop, is a rare manifestation and is discussed on page 1393.

The diagnostic tests for plumbism in children are generally applicable to adults, with the exception of bone films, which are of no value in the latter. Also, the treatment of adults with chelating agents follows the same principles as in children.

Intoxication with tetraethyl and tetramethyl (organic) lead, used as additives in gasoline, presents a special problem. It is caused by inhalation of gasoline fumes and has occurred most often in workers who clean gasoline storage tanks. Insomnia, irritability, delusions, and hallucinations are the usual clinical manifestations, and a maniacal state may develop. The hematologic abnormalities of inorganic lead poisoning are not found, and chelating agents are of no value in treatment. Organic lead poisoning is usually reversible, but fatalities have been reported. The pathologic changes have not been well described.

Arsenic

In the past, medications such as Fowler's solution (potassium arsenite) and the arsphenamines, used in the treatment of syphilis, were frequent causes of intoxication, but now the most common cause is the suicidal or accidental ingestion of herbicides, insecticides, or rodenticides containing copper acetoarsenate (Paris green) or calcium or lead arsenate. In rural areas, arsenic-containing insecticide sprays are a common source of poisoning. Arsenic is used also in the manufacture of paints, enamels, and metals; as a disinfectant for skins and furs; and also in galvanizing, soldering, etching, and lead plating. Occasional cases of poisoning are reported in relation to these occupations. Arsenic is still contained in some topical creams that are used in the treatment of psoriasis and other skin disorders.

Arsenic exerts its toxic effects by reacting with the sulfhydryl radicals of certain enzymes necessary for cellular metabolism. The effects on the nervous system are those of an encephalopathy or peripheral neuropathy. The latter may be the product of chronic poisoning or may become manifest between 1 and 2 weeks after recovery from the effects of acute poisoning. It takes the form of a distal axonopathy and is described on page 1393. In our cases of arsenical polyneuropathy a distal sensorimotor areflexic syndrome has developed subacutely. At autopsy there was a dying back pattern of myelin and axons with macrophage and Schwann cell reactions and chromatolysis of motor neurons and sensory ganglion cells. The CNS appeared normal.

The symptoms of encephalopathy (headache, drowsiness, mental confusion, delirium, and convulsive seizures) may also occur as part of acute or chronic intoxication. In the latter case, they are accompanied by weakness and muscular aching, hemolysis, chills and fever (in patients exposed to arsine gas), mucosal irritation, a diffuse scaly desquamation, and transverse white lines, 1 to 2 mm in width, above the lunula of each fingernail (Mees lines). Acute poisoning by the oral route is associated with severe gastrointestinal symptoms, circulatory collapse, and death in a large proportion of patients. The CSF is normal. Examination of the brain in such cases discloses numerous punctate hemorrhages in the white matter. Microscopically, the lesions consist of pericapillary zones of degeneration, which, in turn, are ringed by red cells (brain purpura or encephalorrhagia, incorrectly referred to as hemorrhagic encephalitis). These neuropathologic changes are not specific for arsenical poisoning but have been observed in such diverse conditions as pneumonia, gram-negative bacillary septicemia from urinary tract infections, sulfonamide and phosgene poisoning, dysentery, disseminated intravascular coagulation, and others.

The diagnosis of arsenical poisoning depends upon the demonstration of increased levels of arsenic in the hair and urine. Arsenic is deposited in the hair within 2 weeks of exposure and may remain fixed there for years. Concentrations of more than 0.1 mg arsenic per 100 mg hair are indicative of poisoning. Arsenic also remains within bones for long periods and is slowly excreted in the urine and feces. Excretion of more than 0.1 mg arsenic per liter of urine is considered abnormal; levels greater than 1 mg/L may occur soon after acute exposure. The CSF protein level may be raised (50 to 100 mg/dL).

Acute poisoning is treated by gastric lavage, vasopressor agents, dimercaprol (BAL), maintenance of renal perfusion, and exchange transfusions if massive hemoglobinuria occurs. Once polyneuropathy has occurred, it is little affected by treatment with BAL, but other manifestations of chronic arsenical poisoning respond favorably. There has been a gradual recovery from the polyneuropathy in our cases.

Manganese

Manganese poisoning results from the chronic inhalation and ingestion of manganese particles and occurs in miners of manganese ore and in workers who separate manganese from other ore. Several clinical syndromes have been observed. The initial stages of intoxication may be marked by a prolonged confusional-hallucinatory state. Later, the symptoms are predominantly extrapyramidal. They are often described as parkinsonian in type, but in the patients seen by the authors, the resemblance was not close: an odd gait ("cock walk"), dystonia and rigidity of the trunk, postural instability, and falling backwards were features seen in two South American miners. Others, however, have reported stiffness and awkwardness of the limbs, often with tremor of the hands, "cogwheel" phenomenon, gross rhythmic movements of the trunk and head, and retropulsive and propulsive gait. Corticospinal and corticobulbar signs may be added. Progressive weakness, fatigability, and sleepiness as well as psychiatric symptoms (manganese madness) are other clinical features. Rarely, severe axial rigidity and dystonia, like those of Wilson disease, are said to have been the outstanding manifestations.

Neuronal loss and gliosis, affecting mainly the pallidum and striatum but also the frontoparietal and cerebellar cortex and hypothalamus, have been described, but the pathologic changes have not been carefully studied.

The neurologic abnormalities have not responded to treatment with chelating agents. In the chronic "dystonic form" of manganese intoxication, dramatic and sustained improvement has been reported with the administration of L-dopa; patients with the more common "parkinsonian type" of manganese intoxication have shown only slight if any improvement with L-dopa.

Mercury

Mercury poisoning arises in two forms, one due to inorganic compounds (elemental or mercury salt) and the other, more dangerous, to organic mercury. Among the latter, methyl mercury compounds give rise to a wide array of serious neurologic symptoms that may be delayed for days or weeks after exposure, including tremor of the extremities, tongue, and lips; mental confusion; and a progressive cerebellar syndrome, with ataxia of gait and of the arms, intention tremor, and dysarthria. Choreoathetosis and parkinsonian facies have also been described. Changes in mood and behavior are prominent, consisting at first of subjective weakness and fatigability and later of extreme depression and lethargy alternating with irritability. This *delayed form of subacute mercury poisoning* has been reported in chemical laboratory workers after exposure to methyl mercury compounds. These agents, particularly dimethyl mercury, are extremely hazardous because they are absorbed transdermally and by inhalation, allowing severe toxicity to occur with even brief contact. In a fatal case of a chemist reported by Nierenberg et al, a rapidly progressive ataxia and encephalopathy developed 154 days after exposure; the cerebellum was most severely affected, with loss of all cortical neuronal elements, and the calcarine fissures were affected in a pattern similar to the Minamata cases described below. The pathologic changes are characterized by neuronal loss and gliosis of the calcarine cortex and to a lesser extent of other parts of the cerebral cortex and a striking degeneration of the granular layer of the cerebellar cortex, with relative sparing of the Purkinje cells.

The chronic form of inorganic mercury poisoning occurs in persons exposed to large amounts of the metal used in the manufacture of thermometers, mirrors, incandescent lights, x-ray machines, and vacuum pumps. Since mercury volatilizes at room temperature, it readily contaminates the air and then condenses on the skin and respiratory mucous membranes. Nitrate of mercury, used in the manufacture of felt hats ("mad hatters"), and phenyl mercury, used in the paper, pulp, and electrochemical industries, are other sources of intoxication. Paresthesias, lassitude, confusion, incoordination, and intention tremor are characteristic, and, with continued exposure, delirium occurs. Headache, various bodily pains, visual and hearing symptoms, and corticospinal signs may be added, but their pathologic basis is unknown. The term *erethism* was coined to describe the timidity, memory loss, and insomnia that were said to be characteristic of chronic intoxication. Unless the exposure has been of minimal amounts over a long period of time, gastrointestinal disturbances are prone to occur (anorexia, weight loss) as well as stomatitis and gingivitis with loosening of the teeth. Acute exposure to inorganic mercury in larger amounts is even more corrosive to the gastrointestinal system and produces nausea, vomiting, hematemesis, abdominal pain, and bloody diarrhea as well as renal tubular necrosis.

Isolated instances of polyneuropathy associated with exposure to mercury have also been reported (Albers et al, Agocs et al) and may be responsible for the paresthesias that accompany most cases and the acrodynic syndrome described below. The inhalation of vaporized mercury as a result of extensive dental work has been alleged to affect the peripheral nerves, but the connection is very tenuous.

The presence of mercury in industrial waste has contaminated many sources of water supply and fish, which are ingested by humans and cause mercurial poisoning. So-called Minamata disease is a case in point. Between 1953 and 1956, a large number of villagers living near Minamata Bay in Kyushu Island, Japan, were afflicted with a syndrome of chronic mercurialism, traced to the ingestion of fish that had been contaminated with industrial wastes containing methyl mercury. Concentric constriction of the visual fields, hearing loss, cerebellar ataxia, postural and action tremors, and sensory impairment of the legs and arms and sometimes of the tongue and lips were the usual clinical manifestations. The syndrome evolved over a few weeks. Pathologically there was diffuse neuronal loss in both cerebral and cerebellar cortices, most marked in the anterior parts of the calcarine cortex and granule cell layer of the cerebellum. CT scans in survivors, years after the mass poisoning, disclosed bilaterally symmetrical areas of decreased attenuation in the visual cortex and diffuse atrophy of the cerebellar hemispheres and vermis, especially the inferior vermis (Tokuomi et al).

A painful neuropathy of children (acrodynia) has been traced to mercury exposure from interior latex paint, to calomel (mercurous chloride), to teething powders, and to a mercuric fungicide used in washing diapers (Agocs et al, Clarkson). Albers et al observed the appearance of symptoms (mild decrease in strength, tremor, and incoordination) 20 to 35 years after exposure to elemental mercury. These authors believe that the natural neuronal attrition with aging had unmasked the neurologic disorder.

In the *treatment* of chronic mercury poisoning, penicillamine has been the drug of choice, since it can be administered orally and appears to chelate mercury selectively, with less effect on copper, which is an essential element in many metabolic processes. Dimercaptosuccinic acid (succimer), which is also given orally and has few side effects, will probably prove to be a superior form of treatment (Clarkson). Because it increases the concentration of mercury in the brain, BAL is an unsuitable chelating agent.

Phosphorus and Organophosphate Poisoning

Nervous system function may be deranged as part of acute and frequently fatal poisoning with inorganic phosphorus compounds (found in rat poisons, roach powders, and matchheads). More important clinically is poisoning with organophosphorus compounds, the best known of which is triorthocresyl phosphate (TOCP).

Organophosphates are widely used as *insecticides*. Since 1945, approximately 15,000 individual compounds have come into use. Certain ones, such as tetraethylpyrophosphate, have been the cause of major outbreaks of neurologic disorder, especially in children. These substances have an acute anticholinesterase effect but no delayed neurotoxic action. Chlorophos, which is a 1-hydroxy-2,2,2-trichlorethylphosphonate, has, in addition, a delayed action, as does TOCP.

The *immediate* anticholinesterase effect manifests itself by headache, vomiting, sweating, abdominal cramps, salivation, wheezing secondary to bronchial spasm, miosis, and muscular weakness and twitching. Most of these symptoms can be reversed by administration of atropine and pralidoxine. Some of the patients suffer a *delayed effect*, 2 to 5 weeks following acute organophosphorus insecticide poisoning. This takes the form of a distal symmetrical sensorimotor (predominantly motor) polyneuropathy, progressing to atrophy. Recovery occurs to a variable degree, and then, in patients poisoned with TOCP, signs of corticospinal damage become detectable. The severity of paralysis and its permanence vary with the dosage of TOCP. Whether a polyneuropathy can arise without the preceding symptoms of cholinergic toxicity is debated; however, based on a review of the subject and a study of 11 patients exposed to these agents, 3 of whom later acquired sensory neuropathy, Moretto and Lotti express the view that such an occurrence must be rare.

In addition to the acute and delayed neurotoxic effects of organophosphorus, an *intermediate syndrome* has been described (Senanayake and Karalliedde). Symptoms come on 24 to 96 h after the acute cholinergic phase and consist of weakness or paralysis of proximal limb muscles, neck flexors, motor cranial nerves, and respiratory muscles. Respiratory paralysis may prove fatal. In patients who survive, the paralytic symptoms last for 2 to 3 weeks and then subside. The intermediate and delayed symptoms do not respond to atropine or other drugs.

Several striking outbreaks of TOCP poisoning have been reported. During the latter part of the prohibition era and to a lesser extent thereafter, outbreaks of "jake paralysis" were traced to drinking an extract of Jamaica ginger that had been contaminated with TOCP. The authors have examined several "ginger jake" cases many years later and found only signs of corticospinal disease. Another outbreak occurred in Morocco, in 1959, when lubricating oil containing TOCP was used deliberately to dilute olive oil. Several other outbreaks have been caused by the ingestion of grain and cooking oil that had been stored in inadequately cleaned containers previously used for storing TOCP.

The effect of TOCP on the peripheral nervous system has been studied extensively in experimental animals. In cats, there occurs a dying back from the terminal ends of the largest and longest medullated motor nerve fibers, including those from the annulospiral endings of the muscle spindles (Cavanagh and Patangia). The long fiber tracts of the spinal cord show a similar dying-back phenomenon. Abnormal membrane-bound vesicles and tubules were observed by Prineas to accumulate in axoplasm before degeneration. These effects have been traced to the inhibitory action of TOCP on esterases. There is still uncertainty as to the details of these reactions, and no treatment for the prevention or control of the neurotoxic effects has been devised.

Thallium

In the late nineteenth century, thallium was used medicinally in the treatment of venereal disease, ringworm, and tuberculosis and later in rodenticides and insecticides. Poisoning was fairly common. Sporadic instances of poisoning still occur, usually as a result of accidental or suicidal ingestion of thallium-containing rodenticides and rarely from overuse of depilatory agents. Patients who survive the effects of acute poisoning develop a rapidly progressive and painful sensory polyneuropathy, optic atrophy, and occasionally ophthalmoplegia—followed, 15 to 30 days after ingestion, by diffuse alopecia. The latter feature should always suggest the diagnosis of thallium poisoning, which can be confirmed by finding this metallic element in the urine. Two of our patients had only a severe sensory and mild motor polyneuropathy and alopecia, from which they were recovering a month later. It is not uncommon for the neuropathy to have a painful component involving acral regions. The condition can end fatally. The use of potassium chloride by mouth may hasten thallium excretion.

Other Metals

Iron, antimony, tin, aluminum, zinc, barium, bismuth, copper, silver, gold, platinum, and lithium may all produce serious degrees of intoxication. The major manifestations in each case are gastrointestinal or renal, but certain neurologic symptoms—notably headache, irritability, confusional psychosis, stupor, coma, and convulsions—may be observed in cases of profound poisoning, often as terminal events.

Gold preparations, which are still used occasionally in the treatment of arthritis, may, after several months of treatment, give rise to focal or generalized myokymia and a rapidly progressive, symmetrical polyneuropathy (Katrak et al). The adverse effects of *platinum* are discussed below, with the antineoplastic agents. *Lithium* has been discussed earlier.

Attention has already been drawn to the possible causative role of *aluminum intoxication* in so-called dialysis dementia or encephalopathy (page 1189). Removal of aluminum from the water used in renal dialysis has practically eliminated this disorder. However, the neuropathologic changes in experimental aluminum intoxication (see below) are not those observed in dialysis dementia. Perl and colleagues have reported the accumulation of aluminum in tangle-bearing neurons of patients with Alzheimer disease and in the Guamanian Parkinson–dementia–amyotrophic lateral sclerosis (ALS) complex. However, analysis of neuritic plaques by nuclear microscopy, without using chemical stains, failed to demonstrate the presence of aluminum (Landsberg et al). The significance of these findings remains to be determined. Longstreth and colleagues have described a progressive neurologic disorder consisting of intention tremor, incoordination, and spastic paraparesis in three patients who had worked for more than 12 years in the same pot room of an aluminum smelting plant. Similar cases attributable to aluminum intoxication have not been reported, however.

Organic compounds of *tin* may seriously damage the nervous system. Diffuse edema of the white matter of the brain and spinal cord has been produced experimentally with *triethyltin*. Presumably this was the basis of the mass poisoning produced by a triethyltin-contaminated drug called Stalinon. The illness was characterized by greatly elevated intracranial pressure and by a spinal cord lesion in some cases (Alajouanine et al). *Trimethyltin* intoxication is much rarer; seizures are the main manifestation. Experimental studies in rats have shown neuronal loss in the hippocampus, largely *sparing* the Sommer sector, with later involvement of neurons in the pyriform cortex and amygdala (see review by Le-Quesne).

A stereotyped episodic encephalopathy has been associated with *bismuth intoxication*, usually arising from the ingestion of bismuth subgallate. Large outbreaks have been reported in Australia and France (Burns et al, Buge et al). The onset of the neurologic disturbance is usually subacute, with a mild and fluctuating confusion, somnolence, difficulty in concentration, tremulousness, and sometimes hallucinations and delusions. With continued ingestion of bismuth, there occurs a rapid (24- to 48-h) worsening of the confusion and tremulousness, along with diffuse myoclonic jerks, seizures, ataxia, and inability to stand or walk. These symptoms regress over a period of a few days to weeks when the bismuth is withdrawn, but some patients have died of acute intoxication. High concentrations of bismuth were found in the cerebral and cerebellar cortices and in the nuclear masses throughout the brain. These concentrations can be recognized as hyperdensities in the CT scan (Buge et al).

Industrial Toxins

Some of these, the heavy metals, have already been considered. In addition, a large number of synthetic organic compounds are widely used in industry and are frequent sources of toxicity, and the list is constantly being expanded. The reader is referred to the references at the end of the chapter, particularly to the most current text, edited by Spencer and Schaumburg, for details concerning these compounds; here we can do little more than enumerate the most important ones: chlorinated diphenyls (e.g., DDT) or chlorinated polycyclic compounds (Kepone), used as insecticides; diethylene dioxide (Dioxane); carbon disulfide; the halogenated hydrocarbons (methyl chloride, tetrachloroethane, carbon tetrachloride, trichloroethylene, and methyl bromide); naphthalene (used in moth repellants); benzine (gasoline); benzene and its derivatives [toluene, xylene, nitrobenzene, phenol, and amyl acetate (banana oil)] and the hexacarbon solvents (*n*-hexane and methyl *n*-butyl ketone).

The acute toxic effects of these substances are much the same from one compound to another. In general, the primary effect is on nonneurologic structures. Neural symptoms consist of varying combinations of headache, restlessness, drowsiness, confusion, delirium, coma, and convulsions, which, as a rule, occur late in the illness or preterminally. Some of these industrial toxins (carbon disulfide, carbon tetrachloride and tetrachloroethane, acrylamide, *n*-hexane) may cause polyneuropathy, which becomes evident with recovery from acute toxicity. Extrapyramidal symptoms may result from chronic exposure to carbon disulfide. A syndrome of persistent fatigue, lack of stamina, inability to concentrate, poor memory, and irritability has also been attributed to chronic exposure to solvents, but these symptoms are quite nonspecific, and evidence for such a syndrome is unsupported by convincing experimental or epidemiologic studies.

Of the aforementioned industrial toxins, the ones most likely to cause neurologic disease are *toluene* (methyl benzene) and the *hexacarbons*. The chronic inhalation of fumes containing toluene (usually in glue, contact cement, or certain brands of spray paint) may lead to severe and irreversible tremor and cerebellar ataxia, affecting movements of the eyes (opsoclonus, ocular dysmetria) and limbs as well as stance and gait. Cognitive impairment is usually associated; corticospinal tract signs, progressive optic neuropathy, sensorineural hearing loss, and hyposmia occur in some patients. Generalized cerebral atrophy and particularly cerebellar atrophy are evident in CT scans (Fornazzari et al, Hormes et al). Also, it has become apparent that acute toluene intoxication is an important cause of seizures, hallucinations, and coma in children (King et al).

The prolonged exposure to high concentrations of *n*-hexane or methyl-*n*-butyl ketone may cause a sensorimotor neuropathy, so-called glue-sniffer's neuropathy (page 1394). These solvents are metabolized to 2,5-hexanedione, which is the agent that damages the peripheral nerves. The neuropathy may result from exposure in certain industrial settings (mainly the manufacture of vinyl products) or, more often, from the deliberate inhalation of vapors from solvents, lacquers, glue, or glue thinners containing *n*-hexane (see also Chap. 46). Impure trichloroethylene, through its breakdown product dichloroacetylene, has a predilection for the trigeminal nerve, which can be damaged selectively.

ANTINEOPLASTIC AND IMMUNOSUPPRESSIVE AGENTS

The increasing use of potent antineoplastic agents has given rise to a diverse group of neurologic complications, the most important of which are summarized below. A more detailed account of these agents—as well as the neurologic complications of corticosteroid therapy, immunosuppression, and radiation—can be found in the monograph edited by Rottenberg and in the review of Tuxen and Hansen. The neurotoxic effects of certain agents used in the treatment of brain tumors are also considered in Chap. 31.

Vincristine

This drug is used in the treatment of acute lymphoblastic leukemia, lymphomas, and some solid tumors. Its most important toxic side effect, and the one that limits its use as a chemotherapeutic agent, is a peripheral neuropathy. Paresthesias of the feet, hands, or both may occur within a few weeks of the beginning of treatment; with continued use of the drug, a progressive symmetrical neuropathy evolves (mainly sensory with reflex loss). Cranial nerves are affected less frequently; ptosis and lateral rectus, facial, and vocal cord palsies are the usual manifestations. Autonomic nervous system function may also be affected: constipation and impotence are frequent complications; orthostatic hypotension, atonicity of the bladder, and adynamic ileus are less frequent. The polyneuropathy is described more fully on page 1394. Inappropriate antidiuretic hormone secretion and seizures have been reported but are relatively uncommon.

The neural complications of *vinblastine* are similar to those of vincristine but are usually avoided because bone marrow suppression limits the dose of the drug that can safely be employed. *Vinorelbine* is a more recently introduced semisynthetic vinca alkaloid. It has much the same antitumor activity as vincristine but is said to be less toxic.

Procarbazine

This drug, originally synthesized as an MAO inhibitor, is now an important oral agent in the treatment of Hodgkin disease and other lymphomas, bronchogenic carcinoma, and malignant gliomas. It has proved to be especially effective in the treatment of oligodendrogliomas. Neural complications are infrequent and usually take the form of somnolence, confusion, agitation, and depression. Diffuse aching pain in proximal muscles of the limbs and mild symptoms and signs of polyneuropathy occur in 10 to 15 percent of patients treated with relatively high doses. A reversible ataxia has also been described. Procarbazine, taken in conjunction with phenothiazines, barbiturates, narcotics, or alcohol, may produce serious degrees of oversedation. Other toxic reactions, such as orthostatic hypotension, are related to the MAO inhibitory action of procarbazine.

L-Asparaginase

L-Asparaginase is an enzymatic inhibitor of protein synthesis and is used in the treatment of acute lymphoblastic leukemia. Drowsiness, confusion, delirium, stupor, coma, and diffuse EEG slowing are the common neurologic effects and are dose-related and cumulative. They may occur within a day of onset of treatment and clear quickly when the drug is withdrawn, or they may be delayed in onset, in which case they may persist for several weeks. These abnormalities are at least in part attributable to the systemic metabolic derangements induced by L-asparaginase, including liver dysfunction.

In recent years, increasing attention has been drawn to cerebrovascular complications of L-asparaginase therapy, including ischemic and hemorrhagic infarction and cerebral venous and dural sinus thrombosis. Fineberg and Swenson have analyzed the clinical features of 38 such cases. These cerebrovascular complications are attributable to transient deficiencies in plasma proteins that are important in coagulation and fibrinolysis.

5-Fluorouracil

This is a pyrimidine analogue, used mainly in the treatment of cancer of the breast, ovary, and gastrointestinal tract. A small proportion of patients receiving this drug develop dizziness, cerebellar ataxia of the trunk and the extremities, dysarthria, and nystagmus—symptoms that are much the same as those produced by cytarabine (Ara-C; see page 1285). These abnormalities must be distinguished from metastatic involvement of the cerebellum and paraneoplastic cerebellar degeneration. The drug effects are usually mild and subside within 1 to 6 weeks after discontinuation of therapy. The anatomic basis of this cerebellar syndrome is not known.

Methotrexate

Administered in conventional oral or intravenous doses, methotrexate (MTX) is not neurotoxic. However, given intrathecally to treat meningeal leukemia or carcinomatosis, MTX commonly causes aseptic meningitis, with headache, nausea and vomiting, stiff neck, fever, and cells in the spinal fluid. Very rarely, probably as an idiosyncratic response to the drug, intrathecal administration results in an acute paraplegia that may be permanent. The pathology of this condition has not been studied. The most serious of the neurologic problems associated with chemotherapy is a necrotizing leukoencephalopathy or leukomyelopathy caused by MTX when given in combination with cranial or neuraxis radiation therapy (page 729). This develops several months after repeated intrathecal or high systemic doses of MTX. The full-blown syndrome consists of the insidious evolution of dementia, pseudobulbar palsy, ataxia, focal cerebral cortical deficits, or paraplegia. The brain shows disseminated foci of coagulation necrosis of white matter, usually periventricular, which can be detected with CT and MRI. Yet unsettled is the role of MTX in the development of asymptomatic CT scan abnormalities or of mild neurologic abnormalities in children with acute lymphoblastic leukemia given intrathecal MTX and cranial irradiation as prophylaxis; the same uncertainty pertains to the relation of this white matter change to that seen with the use of cyclosporin, as discussed further on. Mineralizing microangiopathy (fibrosis and calcification of small vessels, mainly in the basal ganglia) is yet another complication of MTX therapy. It may occur with MTX treatment or with cranial irradiation but is particularly common when both forms of treatment are combined. To the present authors these lesions have the features of the coagulative necrosis of radiation encephalopathy.

Cisplatin

Cisplatin, a heavy metal that inhibits DNA synthesis, is effective in the treatment of gonadal and head and neck tumors as well as carcinoma of the bladder, prostate, and breast. The dose-limiting factors in its use are nephrotoxicity and vomiting and a peripheral neuropathy (see also page 1394). The latter manifests itself by numbness and tingling in fingers and toes, sometimes painful—symptoms that are being observed with increasing frequency. This toxic manifestation appears to be related to the total amount administered, and it usually improves slowly after the drug has been discontinued. Biopsies of peripheral nerve have shown a primary axonal degeneration. Approximately one-third of patients receiving this drug also experience tinnitus or high-frequency hearing loss (4000 to 8000 Hz) or both. This otoxicity is also dose-related, cumulative, and only occasionally reversible. Some preventative effect for cisplatin neuropathy has been claimed for the melanocortin compound ACTH (4-9), but the benefits in a trial by Gerristen and colleagues were quite small and probably do not justify its administration on a routine basis. Retrobulbar neuritis occurs rarely. Seizures associated with drug-induced hyponatremia and hypomagnesemia have been reported.

Paclitaxel and Docetaxel

Taxol (paclitaxel) and Taxotere (docetaxel) are new anticancer drugs derived from the bark of the western yew. Both are particularly useful in the treatment of ovarian and breast cancer, but they have a wide range of antineoplastic activities. A purely or predominantly sensory neuropathy is a common complication. These drugs are thought to cause neuropathy by their action as inhibitors of the depolymerization of tubulin, thereby promoting excessive microtubule assembly within the axon. The neuropathy is dose-dependent, occurring with doses greater than 200 mg/m^2 of paclitaxel and at a wide range of dose levels for docetaxel (generally over 600 mg/m^2). Symptoms may begin 1 to 3 days following the first dose and affect the feet and hands simultaneously. Autonomic neuropathy (orthostatic hypotension) may occur as well. The neuropathy is axonal in type, with secondary demyelination, and is at least partially reversible after discontinuation of the drug.

The Nitrosoureas

Carmustine (BCNU) and lomustine (CCNU) are nitrosoureas used to treat malignant cerebral gliomas. They are not neurotoxic when given in conventional intravenous doses, but intracarotid injection of the drugs may cause orbital, eye, and neck pain, focal seizures, confusion, and possibly focal neurologic deficits. Postmortem examinations of patients who had been treated with BCNU have disclosed diffuse foci of swollen axis cylinders and myelin vacuolization and a diffuse vasculopathy characterized by fibrinoid necrosis and microthrombi (Burger et al, Kleinschmidt-de Masters).

Cytarabine (Ara-C)

This drug, long used in the treatment of acute nonlymphocytic leukemia, is not neurotoxic when given in systemic daily doses of 100 to 200 mg/m^2. The administration of very high doses of Ara-C (up to 30 times the usual dose) has been shown to induce remissions in patients refractory to conventional treatment, but it also produces a severe degree of cerebellar degeneration in a considerable proportion of cases (4 of 24 patients reported by Winkelman and Hines). Ataxia of gait and limbs, dysarthria, and nystagmus develop as early as 5 to 7 days after the beginning of high-dose treatment and worsen rapidly. Postmortem examination has disclosed a diffuse degeneration of Purkinje cells, most marked in the depths of the folia, as well as a patchy necrosis of the cerebellar cortex affecting all the cellular elements. Other patients receiving high-dose Ara-C develop a mild, reversible cerebellar syndrome with the same clinical features as the irreversible one. Patients more than 50 years of age are said to be six times more likely to develop cerebellar degeneration than those younger than 50; therefore the former should be treated with a lower dosage than the latter (Herzig et al).

Cyclosporine and Tacrolimus (FK-506)

These immunosuppressive drugs are used to prevent transplant rejection and to treat aplastic anemia and certain intrinsic immune diseases. Tremor is perhaps the most frequent side effect, particularly of tacrolimus, and myoclonus may be added. Sometimes these impart a stuttering character to speech. Headache and insomnia are common. Seizures may be a manifestation of toxicity, but the cause may lie with the other complications of organ transplantation and immunosuppression. The neurologic effects of these drugs have been reviewed by Wijdicks. A syndrome resembling hypertensive encephalopathy—headache, vomiting, confusion, seizures, and visual loss (cortical blindness)—may follow the use of either drug (see page 903). The appearance on CT scans and MRI of symmetrical signal and density changes mainly in the posterior white matter likewise conforms to the pattern that is seen in hypertensive encephalopathy. Lesions may also appear subcortically in the frontal and parietal lobes. Hinchey and colleagues describe several such cases and suggest that cyclosporin alters the blood-brain barrier and that the fluid overload and hypertension that may accompany the use of cyclosporin may cause the syndrome and the radiologic changes. A variety of psychotic syndromes with delusions, paranoia, and visual hallucinations has also been ascribed to the use of these drugs (see Wijdicks).

Thalidomide

Despite the catastrophic effects of thalidomide on the developing fetus (following its introduction as a soporific in 1957), this drug has now found several specific uses in the treatment of immunologic and infectious diseases. It is highly effective in the treatment of leprosy, erythema nodosum, and the oral ulcerations of AIDS and Behçet disease. Experimental uses include suppression of graft-versus-host reactions and inhibition of blood vessel proliferation in vascular tumors. A dose-dependent sensory neuropathy is the limiting factor in its use, and serial electrophysiologic testing is recommended if the medication is to be prescribed for protracted periods. Of course, it must never be given to a woman who is or might be pregnant.

Antibiotics and Other Drugs

Numerous antibiotics, cardioactive medications, and other drugs may have adverse effects on the central or peripheral nervous system. Some of the latter are addressed on page 1395. Here we mention only that penicillin and its derivatives such as imipenem and cephalosporins are capable of causing seizures when high serum concentrations are attained. This occurs most often in patients with renal failure.

Other important examples are optic neuropathy due to ethambutol toxicity; ototoxicity and neuromuscular blockade from aminoglycoside antibiotics (page 1549); neuropathy, encephalopathy, and an Antabuse-like reaction to alcohol in patients taking metronidazole; INH neuropathy and optic neuropathy and possibly peripheral neuropathy due to chloramphenicol.

The most notorious of this group of drugs was *clioquinol*, which was sold as Entero-vioform and used in many parts of the world to prevent traveler's diarrhea and as a treatment for chronic gastroenteritis. In 1971, clinical observations began to appear in medical journals of a subacute myelo-opticoneuropathy (SMON). During the 1960s, more than 10,000 cases of this neurotoxic disease were collected in Japan by Tsubaki et al. Usually the disease began with a gastrointestinal disturbance, followed by ascending numbness and weakness of the legs, paralysis of sphincters, and autonomic disorder. Later, vision was affected. The onset was acute in about two-thirds of the cases and subacute in the remainder. The occurrence of these neurologic complications was related to the prolonged use of clioquinol. In Japan the drug was withdrawn from the market, and the incidence of SMON immediately fell, supporting the theory that it was caused by clioquinol.

Recovery is usually incomplete. Two patients seen by the authors several years after onset of the disease had been left with optic atrophy and a spastic-ataxic paraparesis.

REFERENCES

General

Cooper JR, Bloom FE, Roth RH: *The Biochemical Basis of Neuropharmacology*, 7th ed. New York, Oxford University Press, 1996.

Dickey W, Morrow JI: Drug-induced neurological disorders. *Prog Neurobiol* 34:331, 1990.

Enna SJ, Coyle JT: *Pharmacological Management of Neurological and Psychiatric Disorders*. New York, McGraw-Hill, 1998.

Goldfrank LR (ed): *Goldfrank's Toxicologic Emergencies*, 6th ed. Stamford, CT, Appleton & Lange, 1998.

Harbison RD (ed): *Hamilton and Hardy's Industrial Toxicology*, 5th ed. St. Louis, Mosby, 1998.

Hardman JG, Limbird LE, Molinoff PB, et al (eds): *Goodman and Gilman's The Pharmacological Basis of Therapeutics*, 9th ed. New York, McGraw-Hill, 1996.

Hollister LE: *Clinical Pharmacology of Psychotherapeutic Drugs*, 3rd ed. New York, Churchill Livingstone, 1990.

Johnston MV, Silverstein FS: Fundamentals of drug therapy in neurology, in Johnston MV, MacDonald RL, Young AB (eds): *Principles of Drug Therapy in Neurology*. Philadelphia, Davis, 1992, pp 1–49.

Klaassen CD (ed): *Casarett and Doull's Toxicology: The Basic Science of Poisons*, 5th ed. New York, McGraw-Hill, 1995.

Levy BS, Wegman DH: *Occupational Health: Recognizing and Preventing Work-Related Disease and Injury*, 4th ed. Philadelphia, Lippincott Williams & Wilkins, 1999.

Payne R, Pasternak GW: Pain, in Johnston MV, MacDonald RL, Young AB (eds): *Principles of Drug Therapy in Neurology*. Philadelphia, Davis, 1992, pp 268–301.

Pirodsky DM, Cohn JS: *Clinical Primer of Psychopharmacology*, 2nd ed. New York, McGraw-Hill, 1992.

Rom WN (ed): *Environmental and Occupational Medicine*, 3rd ed. Philadelphia, Lippincott-Raven, 1998.

Rosenberg NL: *Occupational and Environmental Neurology*. Boston, Butterworth-Heineman, 1995.

Spencer PS, Schaumburg HH (eds): *Experimental and Clinical Neurotoxicology*, 2nd ed. New York, Oxford, 2000.

Opiates and Synthetic Analgesics

American Psychiatric Association: Practical guidelines for the treatment of substance use disorders. *Am J Psychiatry* 52(suppl):1, 1995.

Ball J, Ross A: *The Effectiveness of Methadone Maintenance Treatments*. New York, Springer Verlag, 1991.

Brust JCM: The nonimpact of opiate research on opiate abuse. *Neurology* 33:1327, 1983.

Fields HL: *Pain*. New York, McGraw-Hill, 1987.

Hyman SE: Molecular and cell biology of addiction. *Curr Opin Neurol Neurosurg* 6:609, 1993.

Jasinski DR, Johnson RE, Kocher TR: Clonidine in morphine withdrawal. *Arch Gen Psychiatry* 42:1063, 1985.

Mello NK, Mendelson JH: Buprenorphine treatment of cocaine and heroin abuse, in Cowan A, Lewis JW (eds) *Buprenorphine: Combatting Drug Abuse with a Unique Opioid*. Wiley-Liss, 1995, pp 241–287.

Monroe JJ, Ross WF, Berzins JI: The decline of the addict as "psychopath": Implications for community care. *Int J Addict* 6:601, 1971.

Nestler EJ, Aghajanian GK: Molecular and cellular basis of addiction. *Science* 278:58, 1997.

Tan TP, Algra PR, Valk J, Wolters EC: Toxic leukoencephalopathy after inhalation of poisoned heroin: MR findings. *AJNR* 15:175, 1994.

Wikler A: *Opioid Dependence: Mechanisms and Treatment*. New York, Plenum Press, 1980.

Wolters EC, van Wijngaarden GK, Stam FC, et al: Leukoencephalopathy after inhaling "heroin" pyrolysate. *Lancet* 2:1233, 1982.

Barbiturates, Benzodiazepines, Antidepressants, and Neuroleptic Drugs

Baldessarini RJ: Drugs and the treatment of psychiatric disorders: Psychosis and anxiety, in Hardman JG, Limbrin LE, Molinoff PB, et al (eds): *Goodman and Gilman's The Pharmacological Basis of Therapeutics*, 9th ed. New York, McGraw-Hill, 1996, chap 18, pp 399–430.

Baldessarini RJ: Drugs and the treatment of psychiatric disorders: Depression and mania, in Hardman JG, Limbrin LE, Molinoff PB, et al (eds): *Goodman and Gilman's The Pharmacological Basis of Therapeutics*, 9th ed. New York, McGraw-Hill, 1996, chap 19, pp 431–460.

Baldessarini RJ, Frankenburg FR: Clozapine: A novel antipsychotic agent. *N Engl J Med* 324:746, 1991.

Bloomer HA, Maddock RK Jr: An assessment of diuresis and dialysis for treating acute barbiturate poisoning, in Mathew H (ed): *Acute Barbiturate Poisoning*. Amsterdam, Excerpta Medica, 1971, chap 15.

Caroff SN, Mann SC: Neuroleptic malignant syndrome. *Med Clin North Am* 77:185, 1993.

Coyle JT: Psychiatric disorders, in Johnston MV, MacDonald RL, Young AB (eds): *Principles of Drug Therapy in Neurology*. Philadelphia, Davis, 1992, pp 206–225.

Enna SJ, Coyle JT: *Pharmacological Management of Neurological and Psychiatric Disorders*. New York, McGraw-Hill, 1998.

Hobbs WR, Rall TW, Verdoon TA: Hypnotics and sedatives; alcohol, in Hardman JG, Limbrin LE, Molinoff PB, et al (eds): *Goodman and Gilman's The Pharmacological Basis of Therapeutics*, 9th ed. New York, McGraw-Hill, 1996, chap 17, pp 361–398.

Isbell H, Altschul S, Kornetsky CH, et al: Chronic barbiturate intoxication: An experimental study. *Arch Neurol Psychiatry* 64:1, 1950.

Krisanda TJ: Flumazenil: An antidote for benzodiazepine toxicity. *Am Fam Physician* 47:891, 1993.

Marks J: *The Benzodiazepines: Use, Overuse, Misuse, Abuse*, 2nd ed. Boston, MTP Press, 1985.

Richelson E: Pharmacology of antidepressants—Characteristics of the ideal drug. *Mayo Clin Proc* 69:1069, 1994.

Snyder SH: Receptors, neurotransmitters and drug responses. *New Engl J Med* 300: 465, 1979.

Sternbach H: The serotonin syndrome. *Am J Psychiatry* 148:705, 1991.

Stimulants (Including Cocaine and Amphetamines) and Psychomimetic Drugs

Altura BT, Altura BM: Phencyclidine, lysergic acid diethylamide and mescaline: Cerebral artery spasms and hallucinogenic activity. *Science* 212:1051, 1981.

Baldessarini RJ: Drugs and the treatment of psychiatric disorders: Psychosis and anxiety, in Hardman JG, Limbrin LE, Molinoff PB, et al (eds): *Goodman and Gilman's The Pharmacological Basis of Therapeutics*, 9th ed. New York, McGraw-Hill, 1996, chap 18, pp 399–430.

Coyle JT: Psychiatric disorders, in Johnston MV, MacDonald RL, Young AB (eds): *Principles of Drug Therapy in Neurology*. Philadelphia, Davis, 1992, pp 206–225.

Cregler LL, Mark H: Medical complications of cocaine abuse. *N Engl J Med* 315:1495, 1986.

GAWIN FH, ELLINWOOD FH: Cocaine and other stimulants: Actions, abuse, and treatment. *N Engl J Med* 318:1173, 1988.

GREENBLATT DJ, HARMATZ JS, ZINNY MA, SHADER RI: Effect of gradual withdrawal on the rebound sleep disorder after discontinuation of triazolam. *N Engl J Med* 317:722, 1987.

HARRINGTON H, HELLER A, DAWSON D: Intracerebral hemorrhage and oral amphetamine. *Arch Neurol* 40:503, 1983.

HOLLISTER LE: Cannabis. *Acta Psychiatr Scand* 78(suppl 345):108, 1988.

HOLLISTER LE: *Clinical Pharmacology of Psychotherapeutic Drugs*, 3rd ed. New York, Churchill Livingstone, 1990.

HOLLISTER LE, CSERNANSKY JG: Drug-induced psychiatric disorders and their management. *Med Toxicol* 1:428, 1986.

LEVINE SR, BRUST JCM, FUTRELL N, et al: Cerebrovascular complications of the use of the "crack" form of alkaloidal cocaine. *N Engl J Med* 323:699, 1990.

MENDELSON JH, MELLO NK: Management of cocaine abuse and dependence. *N Engl J Med* 334:965, 1996.

NICHOLI AM: The nontherapeutic use of psychoactive drugs. *N Engl J Med* 308:925, 1983.

O'BRIEN CO: Drug addiction and drug abuse, in Hardman JG, Limbrin LE, Molinoff PB, et al (eds): *Goodman and Gilman's The Pharmacological Basis of Therapeutics*, 9th ed. New York, McGraw-Hill, 1996, chap 24, pp 557–578.

PEROUTKA SJ, NEWMAN H, HARRIS H: Subjective effects of 3-4 methylenedioxymethamphetamine in recreational users. *Neuropsychopharmacology* 1:273, 1988.

PETERSON RC, STILLMAN RC: Phencyclidine: An overview, in Peterson RC, Stillman RC (eds): *Phencyclidine (PCP) Abuse, Research.* Monograph Series 21. Washington, DC, National Institute on Drug Abuse, 1978, chap 1.

ROTH D, ALARCON FJ, FERNANDEZ JA, et al: Acute rhabdomyolysis associated with cocaine intoxication. *N Engl J Med* 319:673, 1988.

VEREBEY K, ALRAZI J, JAFFE JH: Complications of "ecstasy" (MDMA). *JAMA* 259:1649, 1988.

Tetanus

FARRAR JJ, YEN LM, COOK T, et al: Tetanus. *J Neurol Neurosurg Psychiat* 69:292, 2000.

GRIFFIN JW: Bacterial toxins: Botulism and tetanus, in Kennedy PGE, Johnson RT (eds): *Infections of the Nervous System.* London, Butterworth, 1987, pp 83–92.

SANFORD JP: Tetanus—Forgotten but not gone. *N Engl J Med* 332:812, 1995.

STRUPPLER A, STRUPPLER E, ADAMS RD: Local tetanus in man. *Arch Neurol* 8:162, 1963.

WEINSTEIN L: Current concepts: Tetanus. *N Engl J Med* 289:1293, 1973.

Diphtheria

FISHER CM, ADAMS RD: Diphtheritic polyneuritis: A pathological study. *J Neuropathol Exp Neurol* 15:243, 1956.

MCDONALD WI, KOCEN RS: Diphtheritic neuropathy, in Dyck PJ, Thomas PK, Griffin JW, et al (eds): *Peripheral Neuropathy*, 3rd ed. Philadelphia, Saunders, 1993, pp 1412–1423.

PAPPENHEIMER AM: Diphtheria toxin. *Annu Rev Biochem* 46:69, 1977.

WAKSMAN BH, ADAMS RD, MANSMANN HC: Experimental study of diphtheritic polyneuritis in the rabbit and guinea pig. *J Exp Med* 105:591, 1957.

Botulism

FERRARI ND, WEISSE ME: Botulism. *Adv Pediatr Infect Dis* 10:81, 1995.

GRIFFIN JW: Bacterial toxins: Botulism and tetanus, in Kennedy PGE, Johnson RT (eds): *Infections of the Nervous System.* London, Butterworth, 1987, pp 76–92.

HATHEWAY CL: Botulism: The present status of disease. *Curr Top Microbiol Immunol* 195:55, 1995.

JANKOVIC J: Botulinium toxin in movement disorders. *Curr Opin Neurol* 7:358, 1994.

MAYER RF: The neuromuscular defect in human botulism, in Locke S (ed): *Modern Neurology.* Boston, Little, Brown, 1969, pp 169–186.

ROBLOT P, ROBLOT F, FAUCHERE JL, et al: Retrospective study of 108 cases of botulism in Poitiers, France. *J Med Microbiol* 40:379, 1994.

Mushroom Poisoning

KOPPEL C: Clinical symptomatology and management of mushroom poisoning. *Toxicon* 31:1513, 1993.

Mushroom poisoning. *Med Lett* 26:67, 1984.

Venoms, Bites, and Stings

FELZ MW, SMITH CD, SWIFT TR: A six year old girl with tick paralysis. *New Eng J Med* 342:90, 2000.

GARCIA-MONCO JC, BENACH J: Lyme neuroborreliosis. *Ann Neurol* 37:691, 1995.

GRATTAN-SMITH PJ, MORRIS JG, JOHNSTON HM, et al: Clinical and neurophysiological features of tick paralysis. *Brain* 120:1975, 1997.

RAHN D, EVANS J (eds): *Lyme Disease*. Philadelphia, American College of Physicians, 1998.

Metals and Industrial Agents—General

DYCK PJ, THOMAS PK, GRIFFIN JW, et al (eds): Neuropathy associated with industrial agents, metals, and drugs, in *Peripheral Neuropathy*, 3rd ed. Vol 2. Philadelphia, Saunders, 1993, pp 1533–1581.

Lead

Agency for Toxic Substances and Disease Registry: *The Nature and Extent of Lead Poisoning in Children in the United States: A Report to Congress*. Atlanta: Department of Health and Human Services, 1988.

Baghurst PA, McMichael AJ, Wigg NR, et al: Environmental exposure to lead and children's intelligence at the age of seven years—The Port Pirie Cohort Study. *N Engl J Med* 327:1279, 1992.

Goldman RH, Baker EL, Hannan M, Kamerow DB: Lead poisoning in automobile radiator mechanics. *N Engl J Med* 317:214, 1987.

Jorgensen FM: Succimer: The first approved oral lead chelator. *Am Fam Physician* 48:1496, 1993.

Mahaffey KR: Exposure to lead in childhood. *N Engl J Med* 327:1308, 1992.

Mahaffey KR, Annest JL, Roberts J, Murphy RS: National estimates of blood lead levels: United States, 1976–1980. *N Engl J Med* 307:573, 1982.

Mortensen ME, Walson PD: Chelation therapy for childhood lead poisoning. The changing scene in the 1990s. *Clin Pediatr* 32:284, 1993.

Needleman HL: Childhood lead poisoning. *Curr Opin Neurol* 7: 187, 1994.

Needleman HL, Schell A, Bellinger D, et al: The long-term effects of exposure to low doses of lead in childhood: An 11-year follow-up report. *N Engl J Med* 322:83, 1990.

Rutter M: Raised lead levels and impaired cognitive/behavioural functioning: A review of the evidence. *Dev Med Child Neurol* 22(suppl 42):1, 1980.

Arsenic

Heyman A, Pfeiffer JB Jr, Willett RW, Taylor HM: Peripheral neuropathy caused by arsenical intoxication. *N Engl J Med* 254:401, 1956.

Jenkins RB: Inorganic arsenic and the nervous system. *Brain* 89:479, 1966.

Moyer TP: Testing for arsenic. *Mayo Clin Proc* 68:1210, 1993.

Manganese

Calne DB, Chu NS, Huang CC, et al: Manganism and idiopathic parkinsonism: Similarities and differences. *Neurology* 44:1583, 1994.

Mena I, Marin O, Fuenzalida S, Cotzias GC: Chronic manganese poisoning: Clinical picture and manganese turnover. *Neurology* 17:128, 1967.

Mercury

Agocs MM, Etzel RA, Parrish RG, et al: Mercury exposure from interior latex paint. *N Engl J Med* 323:1096, 1990.

Albers JW, Kallenbach LR, Fine LJ, et al (The Mercury Workers Study Group): Neurological abnormalities associated with remote occupational elemental mercury exposure. *Ann Neurol* 24:651, 1988.

Clarkson TW: Mercury: An element of mystery. *N Engl J Med* 323:1137, 1990.

Harada M: Minamata disease: Methylmercury poisoning in Japan caused by environmental pollution. *Crit Rev Toxicol* 25:1, 1995.

Kark RAP, Poskanzer DC, Bullock JD, Boylen G: Mercury poisoning and its treatment with *N*-acetyl-*dl*-penicillamine. *N Engl J Med* 285:10, 1971.

Nierenberg DW, Nordgren RE, Chang MB, et al: Delayed cerebellar disease and death after accidental exposure to dimethylmercury. *N Engl J Med* 338:1672, 1998.

Tokuomi H, Uchino M, Imamura S, et al: Minamata disease (organic mercury poisoning): Neuroradiologic and electrophysiologic studies. *Neurology* 32:1369, 1982.

Organophosphates

Cavanagh JB, Patangia GN: Changes in the central nervous system of the cat as a result of tri-*o*-cresyl phosphate poisoning. *Brain* 88:165, 1965.

Jamal GA: Long term neurotoxic effects of organophosphate compounds. *Adverse Drug React Toxicol Rev* 14:85, 1995.

Moretto A, Lotti M: Poisoning by organophosphorus insecticides and sensory polyneuropathy. *J Neurol Neurosurg Psychiatry* 64:463, 1998.

Prineas J: The pathogenesis of the dying-back polyneuropathies. *J Neuropathol Exp Neurol* 28:571, 1969.

Senanayake N, Karalliedde L: Neurotoxic effects of organophosphate insecticide. *N Engl J Med* 316:761, 1987.

Sherman JD: Organophosphate pesticides—Neurological and respiratory toxicity. *Toxicol Ind Health* 11:33, 1995.

Thallium

Bank WJ, Pleasure DE, Suzuki D, et al: Thallium poisoning. *Arch Neurol* 26:456, 1972.

Desenclos JC, Wilder MH, Coppenger GW, et al: Thallium poisoning: An outbreak in Florida, 1988. *South Med J* 85:1203, 1992.

Gold

Katrak SM, Pollock M, O'Brien CP, et al: Clinical and morphological features of gold neuropathy. *Brain* 103:671, 1980.

Aluminum

Landsberg JP, McDonald B, Watt F: Absence of aluminum in neuritic plaque cores in Alzheimer's disease. *Nature* 360:65, 1992.

LeQuesne PM: Toxic substances and the nervous system: The role of clinical observation. *J Neurol Neurosurg Psychiatry* 44:1, 1981.

Longstreth WT, Rosenstock L, Heyer NJ: Potroom palsy? Neurologic disorder in three aluminum smelter workers. *Arch Intern Med* 145:1972, 1985.

Perl DP, Brody AR: Alzheimer's disease: X-ray spectrometric evidence of aluminum accumulation in neurofibrillary tangle-bearing neurons. *Science* 208:297, 1980.

Perl DP, Gajdusek DC, Garruto RM, et al: Intraneuronal aluminum accumulation in amyotrophic lateral sclerosis and parkinsonism-dementia of Guam. *Science* 217:1053, 1982.

Tin

Alajouanine TH, Derobert L, Thieffry S: Etude clinique d'ensemble de 210 cas d'intoxication par les sels organiques d'étain. *Rev Neurol (Paris)* 98:85, 1958.

LeQuesne PM: Metal neurotoxicity, in Asbury AK, McKhann GM, McDonald WI (eds): *Diseases of the Nervous System*, 2nd ed. Philadelphia, Saunders, 1992, pp 1250–1258.

Bismuth

Buge A, Supino-Viterbo V, Rancurel G, Pontes C: Epileptic phenomena in bismuth toxic encephalopathy. *J Neurol Neurosurg Psychiatry* 44:62, 1981.

Burns R, Thomas DQ, Barron VJ: Reversible encephalopathy possibly associated with bismuth subgallate ingestion. *BMJ* 1:220, 1974.

Mendelowitz PC, Hoffman RS, Weber S: Bismuth absorption and myoclonic encephalopathy during bismuth subsalicylate therapy. *Ann Intern Med* 112:140, 1990.

Industrial Toxins and Solvents

Editorial: Hexacarbon neuropathy. *Lancet* 2:942, 1979.

Elofsson SA, Gamberale F, Hindmarsh T, et al: Exposure to organic solvents. *Scand J Work Environ Health* 6:239, 1980.

Fornazzari L, Wilkinson DA, Kapur BM, Carlen PL: Cerebellar, cortical and functional impairment in toluene abusers. *Acta Neurol Scand* 67:319, 1983.

Hormes JT, Filley CM, Rosenberg NL: Neurologic sequelae of chronic solvent vapor abuse. *Neurology* 36:698, 1986.

King MD, Day RE, Oliver JS, et al: Solvent encephalopathy. *BMJ* 283:663, 1981.

Spencer PS, Schaumburg HH: Organic solvent neurotoxicity. *Scand J Work Environ Health* 11(suppl 1):53, 1985.

Antineoplastic and Immunosuppressive Agents and Antibiotics

American Academy of Pediatrics Committee on Drugs: Clioquinol (iodochlorhydroxquin, Vioform) and iodoquinol (diiodohydroxyquin): Blindness and neuropathy. *Pediatrics* 86:797, 1990.

Burger PC, Kamenar E, Schold SC, et al: Encephalomyelopathy following high-dose BCNU therapy. *Cancer* 48:1318, 1981.

Fineberg WM, Swenson MR: Cerebrovascular complications of L-asparaginase therapy. *Neurology* 38:127, 1988.

Gerristen HR, Vecht CJ, Van der Burg MEL, et al: Prevention of cisplatin induced neuropathy with an ACTH (4-9) analogue in patients with ovarian cancer. *N Engl J Med* 322:89, 1990.

Herzig RH, Hines JD, Herzig GP: Cellular toxicity with high-dose cytosine-arabinoside. *J Clin Oncol* 5:927, 1987.

Hinchey J, Chaves C, Appigani B, et al: A reversible posterior leukoencephalopathy syndrome. *N Engl J Med* 334:494, 1996.

Kaplan RS, Wiernik PH: Neurotoxicity of antineoplastic drugs. *Semin Oncol* 9:103, 1982.

Kleinschmidt-de Masters BK: Intracarotid BCNU leukoencephalopathy. *Cancer* 57:1276, 1986.

Postma TJ, Vermorken JB, Liefting AJ, et al: Paclitaxel-induced neuropathy. *Ann Oncol* 6:489, 1995.

Rottenberg DA (ed): *Neurological Complications of Cancer Therapy*. Boston, Butterworth-Heinemann, 1991.

Tsubaki T, Honmay Y, Hoshl M: Neurological syndrome associated with clioquinol. *Lancet* 1:696, 1971.

Tuxen MK, Hansen SW: Neurotoxicity secondary to antineoplastic drugs. *Cancer Treat Rev* 20:191, 1994.

Wijdicks EFM: Neurologic manifestations of immunosuppresive agents, in Wijdicks EFM (ed): *Neurologic Complications in Organ Transplant Recipients*. Boston, Butterworth-Heinemann, 1999.

Winkelman MD, Hines JD: Cerebellar degeneration caused by high-dose cytosine arabinoside: A clinicopathological study. *Ann Neurol* 14:520, 1983.

Part 5

DISEASES OF SPINAL CORD, PERIPHERAL NERVE, AND MUSCLE

Chapter 44

DISEASES OF THE SPINAL CORD

Diseases of the nervous system may be confined to the spinal cord, where they produce a number of distinctive syndromes. The latter relate to special physiologic and anatomic features of the cord, such as its prominent function in sensorimotor conduction and relatively primitive reflex activity; its long, cylindrical shape; its small cross-sectional size; its tight envelopment by meninges; the peripheral location of myelinated fibers, next to the pia; the special arrangement of its blood vessels; and its particular relationships to the vertebral column.

Woolsey and Young estimate that there are about thirty diseases known to affect the spinal cord, of which half are seen with regularity. These diseases express themselves by a number of readily recognized syndromes and, as will be evident, certain ones preferentially evoke one syndrome and not others. The syndromic grouping of the spinal cord disorders, which is in keeping with the general plan of this book, facilitates clinical diagnosis and reduces the number of ancillary examinations needed for confirmation.

The main syndromes to be considered in this chapter are (1) a transverse sensorimotor myelopathy that may be complete or involve most of the ascending and descending tracts; (2) a combined painful radicular and transverse cord syndrome; (3) the hemicord (Brown-Séquard) syndrome and its variants; (4) a ventral cord syndrome, sparing posterior column function; (5) a high cervical–foramen magnum syndrome; (6) a central cord or syringomyelic syndrome; (7) a syndrome of the conus medullaris; and (8) a syndrome of the cauda equina (see also pages 1332 to 1334). It is also useful to distinguish between lesions within the cord (*intramedullary*) and those that compress the cord from without (*extramedullary*). Certain processes have a proclivity to cause one or another of these syndromes, and each of them will be considered in the course of exposition of the major categories of spinal cord disease.

Some of the anatomic and physiologic considerations pertinent to an understanding of disorders of the cord (and of the spine) can be found in Chaps. 3, 9 (particularly Fig. 9-4), and 11, on motor paralysis, somatic sensation, and back pain, respectively.

THE SYNDROME OF ACUTE PARAPLEGIA OR QUADRIPLEGIA DUE TO COMPLETE TRANSVERSE LESIONS OF THE SPINAL CORD

This syndrome is best considered in relation to trauma, its most frequent cause, but it occurs also as a result of infarction or hemorrhage and with rapidly advancing compressive, necrotizing, demyelinative, or inflammatory lesions (myelitis). Each of these categories of acute spinal cord disease is discussed in the following pages. For convenience of exposition we have included radiation myelopathy, which evolves subacutely.

Trauma to the Spine and Spinal Cord

Throughout recorded medical history, signal advances in the understanding of spinal cord disease have coincided with periods of warfare. The first thoroughly documented study of the effects of sudden total cord transection was that of Theodor Kocher in 1896, based on his observations of 15 patients. During World War I, Riddoch—and later Head and Riddoch—gave the classic descriptions of spinal transection in humans; Lhermitte and Guillain and Barré made additional observations. Little could be done for these patients, however. Fully 80 percent died in the first few weeks (from infections), and survival was possible only if the spinal cord lesion was a partial one. World War II marked a turning point in the understanding and management of spinal cord injuries.

The advent of antibiotics and the ability to control skin, bladder, and pulmonary infections permitted the survival of unprecedented numbers of soldiers with spinal cord injuries and provided the opportunity for long-term observation. In special centers, such as the Long Beach, Hines, and West Roxbury Veterans Administration Hospitals in the United States and the Stoke Mandeville National Spinal Injuries Centre in England, the care and rehabilitation of the paraplegic were perfected. Studies conducted in these centers have greatly enhanced our knowledge of the functional capacity of the chronically isolated spinal cord. Kuhn, Munro, Martin and Davis, Guttmann, Pollock, and their associates, listed in the references, have made particularly important contributions to this subject.

Mechanisms of Spine and Spinal Cord Injury

Although trauma may involve the spinal cord alone, the vertebral column is almost invariably injured at the same time. Often there is an associated head injury as well, as pointed out in Chap. 35.

A useful classification of *spinal injuries* is one that divides them into fracture-dislocations, pure fractures, and pure dislocations. The relative frequency of these types is about 3:1:1. Except for bullet, shrapnel, and stab wounds, a direct blow to the spine is a relatively uncommon cause of serious spinal cord injury. In civilian life, most spinal injuries are the result of *force applied at a distance* from the site of spinal fracture and dislocation. All three types of spinal injury mentioned above are produced by a similar mechanism, usually a vertical compression of the spinal column to which anteroflexion is almost immediately added (anterohyperflexion injury); or, the mechanism may be one of vertical compression and retrohyperflexion (commonly referred to as hyperextension). The most important variables in the mechanics of vertebral injury are the nature of the bones at the level of the injury and the intensity, direction, and point of impact of the force.

If the cranium is struck by a hard object at high velocity, a skull fracture occurs, the force of the injury being absorbed mainly by the elastic quality of the skull. If the traumatizing force is relatively soft yet unyielding, the spine, and particularly its most mobile (cervical) portion, will be the part injured. If the neck happens to be rigid and straight and the force is applied quickly to the head, the atlas and the odontoid process of the axis may break. If the force is applied less quickly, an element of flexion or extension is added.

In the case of severe forward *flexion injury*, the head is bent sharply forward when the force is applied. The adjacent vertebrae are forced together at the level of maximum stress. The anteroinferior edge of the upper vertebral body is driven into the one below, sometimes splitting it in two. The posterior part of the fractured body is displaced backward and compresses the cord. Concomitantly, there is tearing of the interspinous and posterior longitudinal ligaments. Less severe degrees of anteroflexion injury produce only dislocation. Vulnerability to the effects of anteroflexion (and to some extent to retroflexion injuries) is increased by the presence of cervical spondylosis or ankylosing spondylitis or a congenital stenosis of the spinal canal.

In *hyperextension injuries*, the mechanism is one of vertical compression with the head in an extended position. Stress is mainly on the posterior elements of the midcervical vertebrae (C4 to C6)—i.e., on their laminae and pedicles, which may be fractured, unilaterally or bilaterally—and on the anterior ligaments. This dual disruption in the spinal architecture allows for displacement of one vertebral body on an adjacent one. The dislocation results in the cord being caught between the laminae of the lower vertebra and the body of the one above. Damage that primarily affects the central cord (as described further on) is usually due to an extension injury.

Finally, it should be pointed out that a hyperextension injury to the spinal cord may occur without apparent damage or misalignment of the vertebrae when viewed radiologically. In these instances the spinal cord damage, which can be nonetheless profound and permanent, is caused by a sudden inward bulge of the ligamentum flavum or a transient vertebral dislocation and then realignment. This type of spinal cord damage, without radiologic evidence of fracture or dislocation, is particularly common in children.

CT, MRI, and plain lateral spine films are all satisfactory means of demonstrating the vertebral injury, but the tearing and bulging of ligaments from vertebral dislocation is dependably demonstrated only by MRI (or by contrast myelography) and can only be inferred from the spinal displacement. Radiologic studies during cautious flexion or extension of the neck are the only way one can demonstrate instability from ligamentous injury alone.

Another mechanism of cord and root injury, involving extremes of extension and flexion of the neck, is so-called *whiplash* or *recoil injury*. This type of injury is most often the result of an automobile accident. When a vehicle is struck sharply from behind, the head of the occupant is flung back uncontrollably; or, if a fast-moving vehicle stops abruptly, there is sudden forward flexion of the neck, followed by retroflexion. Under these conditions occipitonuchal and sternocleidomastoid muscles and other supporting structures of the neck and head are affected much more often than the spinal cord or roots. Nevertheless, in rare instances, quadriparesis, temporary or permanent, results from a violent whiplash injury. The exact mechanism of neural injury in these circumstances is not clear; perhaps there is a transient posterior dislocation of a vertebral body, a momentary buckling of the ligmentum flavum, or retropulsion of the intervertebral disc into the spinal canal. Again, the presence of a congenitally narrow cervical spinal canal or of spinal diseases such as cervical spondylosis, rheumatoid arthritis, or ankylosing spondylitis greatly adds to the hazard of damage to the cord or roots. Preexisting spondylotic symptoms may be aggravated and become the source of chronic pain. Also, there are examples of spinal cord compression that result from the persistent hyperextension of the cervical spine during a protracted period of coma. Arterial hypotension may be an added factor in particular instances. This combination accounts for some of the cases of quadriplegia in opiate or other drug addicts following a period of sustained unresponsiveness (Ell et al).

A special type of spinal cord injury, occurring most often in wartime, is one in which a high-velocity missile penetrates the vertebral canal and damages the spinal cord directly. In some cases the missile strikes the vertebral column without entering the spinal canal but virtually shatters the contents of the dural tube or produces lesser degrees of impairment of spinal cord function. Rarely, the transmitted shock wave will cause a paralysis of spinal cord function that is completely reversible in a day or two (*spinal cord concussion*, described further on).

Acute traumatic paralysis may also be the consequence of a vascular mechanism. Fibrocartilaginous emboli from an intervertebral disc that has ruptured into radicular arteries or veins of the spinal cord may cause infarction. Or, a traumatic dissecting aneurysm of the aorta may occlude the segmental arteries of the spinal cord, as in the cases reported by Weisman and Adams and by Kneisley.

An analysis of 2000 cases of spinal injury collected from the medical literature by Jefferson showed that most vertebral injuries occurred at the levels of the first and second cervical, fourth to sixth cervical, and eleventh thoracic to second lumbar vertebrae. Industrial accidents most often involved the thoracolumbar vertebrae. Impact to the head with the neck flexed or sharply retroflexed, as mentioned above, was the main cause of injuries to the cervical region. These are not only the most mobile portions of the vertebral column but also the regions in which the cervical and lumbar enlargements of the cord greatly reduce the space between neural and bony structures. The thoracic cord is relatively small and its spinal canal is capacious; additional protection is provided by the high articular facets (making dislocation difficult) and limitations in anterior movement imposed by the thoracic cage.

In the authors' experience, the usual circumstances of spinal cord injury have been motor vehicle accidents, falls (mainly during a state of alcoholic intoxication), gunshot or stab wounds, diving accidents, motorcycle accidents, crushing industrial injuries, and birth injury, in that order of frequency. The majority of the fatal cases were associated with fracture-dislocations or dislocations of the cervical spine. Respiration is paralyzed by lesions of the C1, C2, and C3 segments. Among nonfatal cases, fracture-dislocation of the lower cervical spine is the most frequent established mechanism of spinal cord injury in civilian life. In the United States, the annual incidence of spinal cord injury is from 5 to 5.5 cases per 100,000 population. Males predominate (4:1). Each year about 3500 persons die in close relation to their injury, and another 5000 are left with complete or nearly complete loss of spinal cord function.

Pathology of Spinal Cord Injury As a result of squeezing or shearing of the spinal cord, there is destruction of gray and white matter and a variable amount of hemorrhage, chiefly in the more vascular central parts. These changes, best designated as *traumatic necrosis* of the spinal cord, are maximal at the level of injury and one or two segments above and below it. Rarely is the cord cut in two, and seldom is the pia-arachnoid lacerated. Separation of concomitant pathologic entities—such as hematomyelia, concussion, contusion, and hematorrhachis (bleeding into the spinal canal)—is of little value either clinically or pathologically. As a lesion heals, it leaves a gliotic focus or cavitation with variable amounts of hemosiderin and iron pigment. Progressive meningeal fibrosis and cavitation (traumatic syringomyelia) will sometimes develop after an interval of months or years and lead to a delayed central or transverse cord syndrome (see further on).

In most traumatic lesions, the central part of the spinal cord, with its vascular gray matter, suffers greater injury than the peripheral parts. In some instances, the lesion is virtually restricted to the anterior and posterior gray matter, giving rise to segmental weakness and sensory loss in the arms with few long tract signs. This has been called the *central cervical cord syndrome* (or

Schneider syndrome, see further on). Fragments of the syndrome are not uncommon as transient phenomena that reverse over several days.

As with most lesions, the total clinical effect is compounded of an irreversible structural component and a reversible disorder of function, each of which may vary in degree. The extent and permanence of the clinical manifestations are determined by the relative proportions of these two elements.

Experimental Spinal Cord Injury Investigation of the pathophysiology of acute spinal cord injury dates from the experimental studies of Allen, in the early 1900s. His method consisted of dropping graded weights onto the dura-covered thoracic cord of surgically prepared animals. The technique was refined over the years by precise measurements of the velocity, force, and direction of the dropped weights.

This type of impact on the cord, of sufficient severity to render the animal immediately paraplegic and abolish sensory evoked responses from structures below the lesion, indicates that action potentials can no longer be conducted across the injured spinal cord segment. No histologic changes, by either light or electron microscopy, can be detected for several minutes after impact. The earliest tissue alterations consist of hyperemia and small hemorrhages in the central gray matter. By 1 h, the microscopic hemorrhages coalesce and become macroscopically visible and tissue oxygen saturation is diminished in the region. Within 4 h, the central part of the cord is swollen and a spreading edema pervades the surrounding white matter; however, irrevocable white matter necrosis may not be evident for up to 8 h, an observation that has led to numerous strategies designed to spare long tracts. Surgical intervention to minimize white matter edema—such as laminectomy and myelotomy—spinal cord cooling, hyperbaric exposure, and the administration of pharmacologic measures have been tried but appear to have no effects on the evolving lesion. The early administration of high-dose corticosteroids has been a widely used mode of treatment, but the clinical benefits are questionable. Certain mechanisms that are currently thought to be operative in the death of cerebral neurons have also been invoked in spinal cord injury. These include glutamate release and exposure of neurons to calcium and agents that release free radicals. The latter mechanism may explain the salutary effect of high doses of corticosteroids rather than the ostensible effect of these drugs on edema. There are controversies concerning the putative role of accumulated vasoactive amines and opioids on the damaged segments of cord. Osterholm postulated that the initial event in acute impact injury was the release of norepinephrine from injured neurons in the central gray matter and that the subsequent vasoconstriction was responsible for both the central hemorrhagic and lateral white matter lesions. Later experimental work failed to substantiate these suggestions. Also, the contention that opioid release at the moment of trauma plays an important role in tissue damage has not been confirmed experimentally. The main problem with all the experimental work is that it does not truly reproduce the various types of spinal injury in humans.

Clinical Effects of Spinal Cord Injury When the spinal cord is suddenly and completely or almost completely severed, three disorders of function are at once evident: (1) all voluntary movement in parts of the body below the lesion is immediately and permanently lost; (2) all sensation from the lower (aboral) parts is abolished; and (3) reflex functions in all segments of the isolated spinal cord are suspended. The last effect, called *spinal shock*, involves tendon as well as autonomic reflexes; it is of variable duration (1 to 6 weeks as a rule) and is so dramatic that Riddoch used it as a basis for dividing the clinical effects of spinal cord transection into two stages: (1) spinal shock or areflexia and (2) heightened reflex activity. The separation of these two stages is not as sharp as this statement might imply but is nevertheless fundamental. Less complete lesions of the spinal cord may result in little or no spinal shock, and the same is true of any type of lesion that develops slowly.

Stage of Spinal Shock or Areflexia The loss of motor function at the time of injury—quadriplegia (better termed tetraplegia) with lesions of the fourth to fifth cervical segments, paraplegia with lesions of the thoracic cord—is accompanied by atonic paralysis of bladder and bowel, gastric atony, loss of sensation below a level corresponding to the spinal cord lesion, muscular flaccidity, and complete or almost complete suppression of all spinal segmental reflex activity below the lesion. The neural elements below the lesion fail to perform their normal function because of their sudden separation from those of higher levels. Impaired also in the segments below the lesion is the control of autonomic function. Vasomotor tone, sweating, and piloerection in the lower parts of the body are temporarily abolished. Systemic hypotension may be severe and contribute to the spinal cord damage. The lower extremities lose heat if left uncovered, and they swell if dependent. The skin is dry and pale, and ulcerations may develop over bony prominences. The sphincters of the bladder and the rectum remain contracted to some degree due to the loss of inhibitory influence of higher central nervous system (CNS) centers, but the detrusor of the bladder and smooth muscle of the rectum are atonic. Urine accumulates until the intravesicular pressure is sufficient to overcome the sphincters; then driblets escape (overflow incontinence). There is also passive distention of the bowel, retention of feces, and absence of peristalsis (paralytic ileus). Genital reflexes (penile erection, bulbocavernosus reflex, contraction of dartos muscle) are abolished or profoundly depressed.

The duration of the stage of complete areflexia varies considerably. In a small number (5 of Kuhn's 29 patients, for example) it is permanent, or only fragmentary reflex activity is regained many months or years after the injury. In such patients the spinal segments below the level of transection may have themselves been injured—perhaps by a vascular mechanism, although this explanation is unproven. More likely there is a loss of the brainstem-spinal facilitatory mechanisms and an increase in inhibitory activity in the isolated segments as indicated below. In some patients, minimal genital and flexor reflex activity can be detected within a few days of the injury. In the majority of patients, this minimal reflex activity appears within a period of 1 to 6 weeks. Usually the bulbocavernosus reflex is the first to return. Noxious stimulation of the plantar surfaces evokes a tremulous twitching and brief flexion or extension movements of the great toes. Contraction of the anal sphincter can be elicited by plantar or perianal stimulation, and other genital reflexes reappear at about the same time.

The explanation of spinal shock, which is brief in submammalian forms and more lasting in higher mammals, especially in primates, is believed to be the sudden interruption of suprasegmental descending fiber systems that normally keep the spinal motor neurons in a continuous state of subliminal depolarization (ready to respond). In the cat and monkey, Fulton found the facilitatory tracts in question to be the reticulospinal and vestibulospinal. Subsequent studies showed that in monkeys, some degree of spinal shock can result from interruption of the corticospinal tracts alone. This cannot be the significant factor, however, at least in humans, because spinal shock may be very mild or inevident as a result of acute cerebral and brainstem lesions that interrupt the corticospinal tracts. F waves, which reflect the functioning of the motor neurons of a segment of the cord, are suppressed until spasticity supervenes, at which time they become excessively easy to elicit. Interest in recent years has focused on a possible role for neurotransmitters (catecholamines, endorphins, substance P, and 5-hydroxytryptamine). As already indicated, the claim that naloxone and the endogenous opiate antagonist thyrotropin releasing factor might reduce the extent of an acute spinal cord lesion has not been corroborated. Clonidine, a noradrenergic receptor activator, is reported to reduce flexor spasms and spasticity and to restore the balance between excitatory and inhibitory activity, allowing the spinal reflex generator for locomotion to function (Woolsey and Young).

Stage of Heightened Reflex Activity This is the very familiar neurologic state that emerges within several weeks or months after the spinal injury. Usually, after a few weeks, the reflex responses to stimulation, which are initially minimal and unsustained, become stronger and more easily elicitable and come to include additional and more proximal muscles. Gradually the typical pattern of heightened flexion reflexes emerges: dorsiflexion of the big toe (Babinski sign); fanning of the other toes; and later, flexion or slow withdrawal movements of the foot, leg, and thigh with contraction of the tensor fascia lata (triple flexion). Tactile stimulation of the foot may suffice as a stimulus, but a painful stimulus is more effective. The Achilles reflexes and then the patellar reflexes return. Retention of urine becomes less complete, and at irregular intervals urine is expelled by active contractions of the detrusor muscle. Reflex defecation also begins. After several months the withdrawal reflexes become greatly exaggerated, to the point of flexor spasms, and may be accompanied by profuse sweating, piloerection, and automatic emptying of the bladder (occasionally of the rectum). This is the "mass reflex," which is evoked by stimulation of the skin of the legs or by some interoceptive stimulus, such as a full bladder. Varying degrees of heightened flexor reflex activity may last for years. Heat-induced sweating is defective, but reflex-evoked ("spinal") sweating may be profuse (see Kneisley). Presumably, in such cases the lateral horn cells in much of the thoracic cord are still viable and disinhibited. Above the level of the lesion, thermoregulatory sweating may be exaggerated and is accompanied by cutaneous flushing, pounding headache, hypertension, and reflex bradycardia. This syndrome ("autonomic dysreflexia") is episodic and occurs in response to a particular stimulus, such as a distended bladder or rectum. It has been ascribed to the reflex release of adrenalin from the adrenal medulla and of norepinephrine from the disinhibited sympathetic terminals caudal to the lesion.

Extensor reflexes eventually develop in most cases (18 of 22 of Kuhn's patients who survived more than

2 years), but their appearance does not lead to the abolition of the flexor reflexes. The overactivity of extensor muscles may appear as early as 6 months after the injury, but this only happens, as a rule, after the flexor responses are fully developed. Extensor responses are at first manifest in certain muscles of the hip and thigh and later of the leg. In a few patients extensor reflexes are organized into support reactions sufficient to permit *spinal standing*. Kuhn observed that extensor movements were at first provoked most readily by a sudden shift from a sitting to a supine position and later by proprioceptive stimuli (squeezing of the thigh muscles) and tactile stimuli from wide areas. Marshall, in a study of 44 patients with chronic spastic paraplegia of spinal origin, found all possible combinations of flexor and extensor reflexes; the type of reflex obtained was determined by the intensity and duration of the stimulus (a mild prolonged noxious stimulus evoked an ipsilateral extensor reflex; an intense brief stimulus, a flexor response).

From these observations one would suspect that the ultimate posture of the legs—flexion or extension—does not depend solely on the completeness or incompleteness of the spinal cord lesion, as originally postulated by Riddoch. The development of *paraplegia in flexion* relates also to the level of the lesion, being seen most often with cervical lesions and progressively less often with more caudal ones. Repeated flexor spasms, which are more frequent with higher lesions, and the ensuing contractures ultimately determine a fixed flexor posture. Conversely, reduction of flexor spasms by elimination of nociceptive stimuli (infected bladder, decubiti, etc.) favors an extensor posture of the legs (*paraplegia in extension*). According to Guttmann, the positioning of the limbs during the early stages of paraplegia greatly influences their ultimate posture. Thus, prolonged fixation of the paralyzed limbs in adduction and semiflexion favors subsequent paraplegia in flexion. Placing the patient prone or placing the limbs in abduction and extension facilitates the development of predominantly extensor postures. Nevertheless, strong and persistent extensor postures are observed only with partial lesions of the spinal cord.

Of some interest is the fact that many patients report sensory symptoms in segments of the body below the level of their transection. Thus, a tactile stimulus above the level of the lesion may be felt below the transection (synesthesia). Patients describe a variety of paresthesias, the most common being a dull, burning pain in the lower back and abdomen, buttocks, and perineum. We have encountered patients in whom aching testicular or rectal pain was the main problem. The pain may be intense and last for a year or longer, after which it gradually subsides. It may persist after rhizotomy but can be abolished by anesthetizing the stump of the proximal (upper) segment of the spinal cord, according to Pollock and his collaborators. Transmission of sensation over splanchnic afferents to levels of the spinal cord above the lesion, the conventional explanation, is therefore not the most plausible one.

The overactivity of neurons in the isolated segments of the spinal cord has several explanations. One assumes that suprasegmental inhibitory influences have been removed by the transection, so that afferent sensory impulses evoke exaggerated nocifensive and phasic and tonic myotatic reflexes. But isolated neurons also become hypersensitive to neurotransmitters. Since the early experiments of Cannon and Rosenblueth, it has been known that section of sympathetic motor fibers leaves the denervated structures hypersensitive to epinephrine; these authors also found the motor neurons in the isolated spinal segments to be abnormally sensitive to acetylcholine.

Various combinations of residual deficits (of lower and upper motor neurons and sensory neurons) are to be expected. Some of the resulting clinical pictures are complete or incomplete voluntary motor paralysis; a flaccid atrophic paralysis of upper limb muscles (if appropriate segments of gray matter are destroyed) with spastic weakness of the legs (amyotrophy with spastic paraplegia in flexion or extension); a partial or rarely a complete Brown-Séquard syndrome (pages 62 and 161); and each of these with variable sensory impairment in the legs and arms. High cervical lesions may result in extreme and prolonged tonic spasms of the legs due to release of tonic myotatic reflexes. Under these circumstances, attempted voluntary movement may excite intense contraction of all flexor and extensor muscles lasting for several minutes. Segmental damage in the low cervical or lumbar gray matter, destroying inhibitory Renshaw neurons, may release activity of remaining anterior horn cells, leading to spinal segmental spasticity. Any residual symptoms persisting after 6 months are likely to be permanent, although in a small proportion of patients some return of function (particularly sensation) is possible after this time. Loss of motor and sensory function above the lesion, coming on years after the trauma, occurs occasionally and is due to an enlarging cavity in the proximal segment of the cord (see further on, under "Syringomyelia").

Transient Cord Injury (Spinal Cord Concussion)

These terms refer to a transient loss of motor and/or sensory function of the spinal cord that recovers within minutes or hours but sometimes persists for a day or several days. In most instances the symptoms are already diminishing and no neurologic abnormalities are found at the time of the first examination. There are a number of such transient syndromes; bibrachial weakness; quadriparesis (occasionally hemiparesis); paresthesias and dysesthesias in a similar distribution to the weakness; or sensory symptoms alone ("burning hands syndrome"). In the first and last of these the central gray matter of the cervical cord is implicated. It is assumed that the cord undergoes some form of elastic deformation when the head is struck at the vertex or frontally and the cervical spine is compressed or hyperextended; however, the same effects can be produced by direct blows to the spine or forceful falls flat on the back and occasionally by a sharp fall on the tip of the coccyx. Little is known of the pathologic changes or the mechanisms that underlie these transient and reversible syndromes.

Spinal cord concussion is observed most frequently in athletes engaged in contact sports (football, rugby, and hockey). A congenitally narrow cervical canal is thought to predispose to spinal cord concussion and to increase the risk of recurrence. As with cerebral concussion, particularly if there have been previous concussions, a difficult decision arises—whether to allow resumption of competitive sports. There are no reliable data on which to base this decision—only guidelines that favor continued participation if the deficit has been brief. Certainly, it is advisable in most cases to be certain that spinal instability has not been induced by the injury. This can be ascertained by obtaining flexion and extension radiographs of the affected spinal region. The subject is reviewed by Zwimpfer and Bernstein.

Central Cord Syndrome (Schneider Syndrome and "Cruciate Paralysis") In the acute central cord lesion, the loss of motor function is characteristically more severe in the upper limbs than in the lower ones and particularly severe in the hands. Bladder dysfunction with urinary retention occurs in some of the cases, and sensory loss is often slight (hyperpathia over the shoulders and arms may be the only sensory abnormality). Damage of the centrally situated gray matter (motor and sensory neurons) may leave an atrophic, areflexic paralysis and a segmental loss of pain and thermal sensation from interruption of crossing pain and thermal fibers. Retroflexion injuries of the head and neck are the ones most often associated with the central cord syndrome, but hematomyelia, necrotizing myelitis, fibrocartilagenous embolism, and possibly infarction due to compression of the vertebral artery in the medullary-cervical region are other causes (Morse).

According to Dickman and colleagues, approximately 4 percent of patients who survive high cervical cord injuries demonstrate what these authors refer to as "cruciate paralysis." The latter state is similar to the central cord syndrome except that the weakness is even more selective, being practically limited to the arms, a feature that is attributable to the segregation of corticospinal fibers to the arms (rostral) and to the legs (caudal) within the decussation. The patients described in the literature have had injuries, basically contusions, of the C1–C2 region. The arm weakness may be asymmetrical or even unilateral; sensory loss is inconsistent.

Examination of the Spine-Injured Patient The level of the spinal cord and vertebral lesions can be determined from the clinical findings. A complete paralysis of the arms and legs usually indicates a fracture or dislocation at the fourth to fifth cervical vertebrae. If the legs are paralyzed and the arms can still be abducted and flexed, the lesion is likely to be at the fifth to sixth cervical vertebrae. Paralysis of the legs and only the hands indicates a lesion at the sixth to seventh cervical level. Below the cervical region, the spinal cord segments and roots are not opposite their similarly numbered vertebrae (Fig. 44-1). The spinal cord ends opposite the first lumbar vertebra, usually at its rostral border. Vertebral lesions below this point give rise predominantly to cauda equina syndromes; these carry a better prognosis than injuries to the lower thoracic vertebrae, which involve both cord and multiple roots. The level of sensory loss on the trunk, determined by perception of pinprick, is also an accurate guide to the level of the lesion, with a few qualifications. With lesions of the lower cervical cord, even if complete, sensation may be preserved down to the nipple line, because of the contribution of the C3 and C4 cutaneous branches of the cervical plexus, which innervate skin below the clavicle. Rarely, a lesion will involve only the outermost fibers of the spinothalamic pathways, sparing the innermost ones, in which case the sensory level (to pain and temperature) will be below the level of the lesion. In all cases of spinal cord and cauda equina injury, the prognosis for recovery is more favorable if any movement or sensation is elicitable during the first 48 to 72 h.

If the spine can be examined safely, it should be inspected for angulations or irregularities and gently percussed to elicit signs of bony injury. Collateral injury of the thorax, abdomen, and long bones must always be sought.

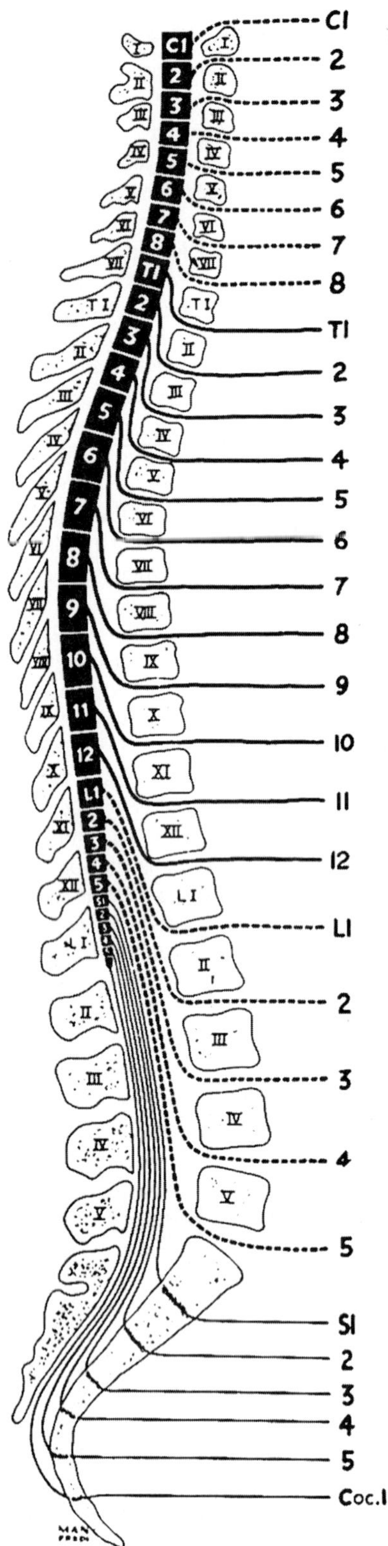

Management of Spinal Injury In all cases of suspected spinal injury, the immediate concern is that there be no movement (especially flexion) of the cervical spine from the moment of the accident. The patient should be placed supine on a firm, flat surface (with one person assigned to keeping the head and neck immobile) and should be transported by a vehicle that can accept the litter. Preferably, the patient should be transported by an ambulance equipped with spine boards, to which the head is rigidly fixed by straps. This provides a more effective means of immobilization than sandbags or similar objects placed on each side of the head and neck. On arrival at the hospital, it is useful to have the patient remain on the backboard until a lateral film or a CT or MRI of the cervical spine have been obtained.

A careful neurologic examination with detailed recording of motor, sensory, and sphincter function is necessary to follow the clinical progress of spinal cord injury. A common practice is to define the injury according to the standards of the American Spinal Injury Association and to assign the injury to a point on the Frankel Scale.

1. Complete: motor and sensory loss below the lesion
2. Incomplete: some sensory preservation below the zone of injury
3. Incomplete: motor and sensory sparing, but the patient is nonfunctional
4. Incomplete: motor and sensory sparing and the patient is functional (stands and walks)
5. Complete functional recovery: reflexes may be abnormal

Obviously, groups 2, 3, and 4 have a more favorable prognosis for recovery of ambulation than does group 1.

Once the degrees of injury to spine and cord have been assessed, the usual practice during the past decade has been to administer methylprednisolone in high dosage (bolus of 30 mg/kg followed by 5.4 mg/kg every hour), beginning within 8 h of the injury and continued for 23 h. This measure, according to the multicenter National Acute Spinal Cord Study (Bracken et al) resulted in a slight but significant improvement in both

Figure 44-1

The relationship of spinal segments and roots to the vertebral bodies and spinous processes. The cervical roots (except C8) exit through foramina above their respective vertebral bodies, and the other roots issue below these bodies. (From Haymaker and Woodhall: Peripheral Nerve Injuries, 2nd ed. Philadelphia, Saunders, 1953, by permission.)

motor and sensory function. Despite its widespread use, the therapeutic value of this measure has not been established beyond doubt, and its value has been questioned after careful re-analysis of the data (Nesathurai; Hurlbert). Also, in a small series of patients, the administration of G_{M1} ganglioside (100 mg intravenously each day from the time of the accident) was found to enhance ultimate recovery to a modest degree (Geisler et al), but again, this finding must be corroborated.

Next, radiologic examinations are undertaken to determine the alignment of vertebral bodies and pedicles, compression of the spinal cord or cauda equina due to malalignment or bone debris in the spinal canal, and the presence of tissue damage within the cord. The MRI is ideally suited to display these processes; but if it is not available and there is uncertainty regarding cord compression, myelography with CT scanning is a useful alternative. Instability of the spinal elements can often be inferred from dislocations or from certain fractures of the pedicles, pars articularis, or transverse processes, but gentle flexion and extension of the injured areas must sometimes be undertaken and plain films obtained in each position.

If a cervical spinal cord injury is associated with vertebral dislocation, traction on the neck is necessary to secure proper alignment and maintain immobilization. This is best accomplished by use of a halo brace, which, of all the appliances used for this purpose, provides the most rigid external fixation of the cervical spine. This type of fixation is usually continued for 4 to 6 weeks, after which a rigid collar may be substituted.

In general, concerning the early surgical management of spinal cord injury, there have been two schools of thought. One, represented by Guttmann and others, advocates reduction and alignment of the dislocated vertebrae by traction and immobilization until skeletal fixation is obtained, and then rehabilitation. The other school, represented by Munro and later by Collins and Chehrazi, proposes early surgical decompression, correction of bony displacements, and removal of herniated disc tissue and intra- and extramedullary hemorrhage; often the spine is fixed at the same time by a bone graft or other form of stabilization. The issue of acute decompressive surgery remains contentious to the present day. Most American neurosurgeons take the less aggressive stance, delaying operation or operating only on patients with compound wounds or those with progression or worsening of the neurologic deficit despite adequate reduction and stabilization. With complete spinal cord lesions, most surgeons do not favor surgery.

The results of the conservative and aggressive surgical plans of management have been difficult to compare and have not been evaluated with modern neurologic techniques. Collins, a participant in the National Institutes of Health (NIH) study of acute management of spinal cord injury, concluded that the survival rate was increased as a result of early surgical stabilization of fractures and fixation of the spine (in addition to the usual measures for the prevention of respiratory, urinary, and cutaneous complications and the early institution of rehabilitation measures). Other neurosurgeons, however, have not been able to document a reduction in neurologic disability as a result of early operation, and they have increasingly inclined toward nonoperative management of both complete and partial spinal cord lesions (Clark; Murphy et al). In any given case, the approach must be guided by the particular features of the patient's injuries. A detailed description of the orthopedic and neurosurgical treatment of spinal fracture-dislocations is beyond the scope of a textbook of neurology but can be found in the account by Ogilvy and Heros and in the book edited by Woolsey and Young, listed in the References.

The greatest risk to the patient with spinal cord injury is in the first week or 10 days, when gastric dilatation, ileus, shock, and infection are the main threats to life. According to Messard and colleagues, the mortality rate falls rapidly after the first 3 months; beyond this time, 86 percent of paraplegics and 80 percent of quadriplegics will survive for 10 years or longer. In children, the survival rate is even higher (DeVivo et al). The latter authors found that the cumulative 7-year survival rate in spinal cord–injured patients (who had survived at least 24 h after injury) was 87 percent. Advanced age at the time of injury and being rendered completely quadriplegic were the worst prognostic factors.

The aftercare of patients with paraplegia is concerned with management of bladder and bowel disturbances, care of the skin, prevention of pulmonary embolism, and maintenance of nutrition. Decubitus ulcers can be prevented by frequent turning to avoid pressure necrosis, use of special mattresses, and meticulous skin care. Deep lesions require debridement and full-thickness grafting. At first continual catheterization is necessary; then, after several weeks, the bladder can be managed by intermittent catheterization once or twice daily, using a scrupulous aseptic technique. Close watch is kept for bladder infection, which is treated promptly should it occur. Bacteruria is common and does not require treatment with antibiotics unless there is associated pyuria. Morning suppositories and periodically spaced enemas are the most effective means of controlling fecal incontinence. Chronic pain (present in 30 to

50 percent of cases) requires the use of nonsteroidal anti-inflammatory medication, injections of local anesthetics, and transcutaneous nerve stimulation. A combination of carbamazepine and either clonazepam or tricyclic antidepressants may be helpful in cases of burning leg and trunk pain. Recalcitrant pain may require more aggressive therapy, such as epidural injections of analgesics or corticosteroids, but often even these measures are ineffective. Spasticity and flexor spasms may be troublesome; oral baclofen, diazepam, or tizanidine may provide some relief. In permanent spastic paraplegia with severe stiffness and adductor and flexor spasms of the legs, intrathecal baclofen, delivered by an automated pump in doses of 12 to 400 mg/day, has reportedly been helpful. The drug is believed to act at the synapses of spinal reflexes (Penn and Kroin). One must always be alert to the threat of pulmonary embolism from deep-vein thrombi, although the incidence is surprisingly low after the first several months. Physiotherapy, muscle reeducation, and the proper use of braces are all important in the rehabilitation of the patient. All this is best carried out in special centers for rehabilitation of spinal cord injuries.

Posttraumatic syringomyelia is described further on (see Fig. 44-12).

Radiation Injury of the Spinal Cord

Delayed necrosis of the spinal cord and brain is a well-recognized sequela of radiation therapy for tumors in these regions and in the thorax and neck. The peripheral nerves are more resistant to this adverse effect, although we have observed, as have others, an early reversible and a late progressive and permanent sensorimotor neuropathy coming on several months or years after irradiation. Finally, a lower motor neuron lesion, presumably due to injury to the gray matter of the spinal cord, may also follow radiation therapy.

Transient Myelopathy The "early" type of radiation myelopathy (appearing 3 to 6 months after radiotherapy) is characterized mainly by paresthesias in the extremities. The paresthesias may be evoked or exacerbated by neck flexion (Lhermitte symptom). In one of our patients there was impairment of vibratory and position sense in the legs but no weakness. The sensory abnormalities disappear after a few months and, according to Jones, are not followed by the delayed progressive radiation myelopathy (see below). The pathology has not been fully elucidated, but there is said to be a spongy appearance of the white matter with demyelination and depletion of oligodendrocytes.

Delayed Progressive Radiation Myelopathy This, the most dreaded complication of radiation therapy, is a progressive myelopathy that follows, after a characteristic latent period, the irradiation of malignant tissues in the vicinity of the spinal cord. The incidence of this complication is difficult to determine because many patients die of their malignant disease before the cord lesion matures, but it is estimated to be between 2 and 3 percent (Palmer). According to Douglas et al, patients who have undergone hyperthermia as a treatment for cancer are particularly vulnerable to radiation myelopathy.

Clinical Features The neurologic disorder first appears many months after the course of radiation therapy, practically always after 6 months and usually between 12 and 15 months (latent periods as long as 60 months or even longer have been reported). The onset is insidious, usually with sensory symptoms—paresthesias and dysesthesias of the feet or a Lhermitte phenomenon, and similar symptoms in the hands in cases of cervical cord damage. Weakness of one or both legs usually follows the sensory loss. Initially, local pain is notably absent, in distinction to the effects of spinal metastases. In some cases, the sensory abnormalities are transitory; more often, additional signs make their appearance and progress, at first rapidly and then more slowly and irregularly, over a period of several weeks or months, with involvement of the corticospinal and spinothalamic pathways. Originally, the neurologic disturbance may take the form of a Brown-Séquard syndrome, but with progression it takes the form of a transverse myelopathy, with a spastic paraplegia, sensory loss below a level on the trunk, and sphincteric disturbance.

Reagan and coworkers, who have had a large experience with radiation myelopathy at the Mayo Clinic (1 percent of all cases of myelopathy were of this type), describe yet another myelopathic radiation syndrome—namely, a slowly evolving amyotrophy, with weakness and atrophy of muscles and areflexia in parts of the body supplied by anterior horn cells of the irradiated spinal segments. Most patients with this form of the disease die within a year of onset. Knowledge of the pathology is incomplete.

The CSF in delayed progressive radiation myelopathy is normal except for a slight elevation of protein content in some cases. MRI demonstrates an abnormal signal intensity, decreased in T1-weighted and increased in T2-weighted images. Early in the course of the myelopathy the cord may be swollen and there is often enhancement with gadolinium infusion. The cord lesion corresponds to the irradiated portal, which can be identified precisely by the radiation effect on the marrow of the vertebral bodies. The spinal cord lesion tends to be more extensive than the usual vascular or demyelinative lesion. These are important points to establish, because a mistaken diagnosis of intraspinal tumor may lead to another operation or further irradiation of an already damaged cord.

Pathologic Findings In the spinal cord, corresponding with the level of the irradiated area and extending over several segments, there is an irregular zone of coagulation necrosis involving both white and gray matter, the former to a greater extent than the latter. Varying degrees of secondary degeneration are seen in the ascending and descending tracts. Vascular changes—necrosis of arterioles or hyaline thickening of their walls, with thrombotic occlusion of their lumens—are prominent in the most severely damaged portions of the cord. Most neuropathologists have attributed the parenchymal lesion to the blood vessel changes; others believe that the degree of vascular change is insufficient to explain the parenchymal change (Malamud et al; Burns et al). Certainly the most severe parenchymal changes in the cord are typical of infarction; but the insidious onset and slow, steady progression of the clinical disorder and the coagulative nature of the necrosis would then have to be explained by a steady succession of vascular occlusions. Exceptional instances, in which a transverse myelopathy has developed within a few hours (as described by Reagan et al), are more readily explained by thrombotic occlusion of a larger spinal artery.

Treatment and Prevention It must be kept in mind that radiation myelopathy is an iatrogenic disease and is therefore largely preventable. The tolerance of the adult human spinal cord to radiation—taking into account the volume of tissue irradiated, the duration of the irradiation, and the total dose—has been determined by Kagan and colleagues. These authors reviewed all of the cases in the literature up to 1980 and concluded that radiation injury could be avoided if the total dose was kept below 6000 cGy and was given over a period of 30 to 70 days, provided that each daily fraction did not exceed 200 cGy and the weekly dose was not in excess of 900 cGy. It is noteworthy that in the cases reported by Sanyal and associates, the amount of radiation surpassed these limits. Forewarned with this knowledge, physicians now have the impression that the incidence of this complication is decreasing.

A number of case reports remark on temporary improvement in neurologic function after the administration of steroids. This therapy should be tried, because in some patients the disease process appears, after a time, to be arrested short of complete destruction of all sensory and motor tracts. Claims have also been made of regression of early symptoms in response to the administration of heparin split products.

Neurologists attached to tumor treatment centers are sometimes confronted with the late development (up to 10 to 15 years after radiation) of a slowly progressive sensorimotor paralysis of a limb (motor weakness predominates). The condition raises questions of recurrent tumor or the development of a local sarcoma, but the absence of a mass lesion and of pain and the signs on neurologic examination are most consistent with a regional interstitial fibrosing neuropathy. Examples that we have seen are multiple cranial neuropathies after radiation of nasopharyngeal tumors, cervical and especially brachial neuropathies after laryngeal and breast cancers, and lumbosacral plexopathies with pelvic tumors. These are discussed further in Chap. 46.

Spinal Cord Injury due to Electric Currents and Lightning

Among acute physical injuries to the spinal cord, those due to electric currents and lightning should be mentioned. They can also injure the brain and peripheral nerves. These effects are noted briefly, since they are infrequent. It is the spinal cord, however, that is most severely damaged.

Electrical Injuries In the United States, inadvertent contact with an electric current causes about 1000 deaths annually and many more nonfatal but serious injuries. About one-third of the fatal accidents result from contact with household currents, indicating the vulnerability of most of the population to this type of injury.

The factor that governs the damage to the nervous system is the amount, or amperage, of the current with which the victim has contact, not simply the voltage, as is generally believed. In any particular case, the duration of contact with the current and the resistance offered by the skin (this is greatly reduced if the skin is moist or a body part is immersed in water) are of critical importance. The physics of electrical injuries is much more complex than these brief remarks indicate (for a full discussion, see reviews by Panse and by Winkelman).

Any part of the peripheral or central nervous system may be injured by electric currents and lightning.

The effects may be immediate, which is understandable, but of greater interest are the instances of neurologic damage that occur after a delay of 1 day to 6 weeks (1 week on the average). The immediate effects are apparently the result of direct heating of the nervous tissue, but the pathogenesis of the delayed effects is not well understood. They have been attributed to vascular occlusive changes induced by the electric current, a mechanism that seems to underlie the delayed effects of radiation therapy (see above). However, the latent period of radiation myelopathy is measured in many months rather than in days and the course is more often progressive than self-limited. Moreover, the few postmortem studies of myelopathy due to electrical injury have disclosed a widespread demyelination of long tracts, to the point of tissue necrosis in some segments, and relative sparing of the gray matter, but no abnormalities of the blood vessels.

A rare syndrome of focal muscular atrophy, occurring after an electric shock, has been described by Panse under the title of *spinal atrophic paralysis*. It occurs when the path of the current, usually of low voltage, is from arm to arm (across the cervical cord) or arm to leg. Pain and paresthesias occur immediately in the involved limb, but these symptoms are transient. Weakness, also unilateral, is immediate as well, followed in several weeks or months by muscle wasting, most often taking the form of segmental muscular atrophy; occasionally the syndrome simulates that of amyotrophic lateral sclerosis or transverse myelopathy (most patients have some degree of weakness and spasticity of the legs). In contrast to injuries due to high-tension current, which affects mainly the spinal white matter (see above), it is mainly the gray matter that is injured in cases of spinal atrophic paralysis, at least as judged from experimental studies.

When the head is one of the contact points, the patient may become unconscious or suffer tinnitus, deafness, or headache for a short period following the injury. In a small number of surviving patients, after an asymptomatic interval of days to months, there has been an apoplectic onset of hemiplegia with or without aphasia or a striatal or brainstem syndrome, presumably due to thrombotic occlusion of cerebral vessels with infarction of tissue.

Lightning Injuries The factors involved in injuries from lightning are less well defined than those from electric currents, but the effects are much the same. The risk of being struck by lightning is about thirty times greater in rural areas than in cities. Direct strikes are often fatal; nearby strikes produce the neurologic damage described below. Prominences such as trees, hills, and towers are struck preferentially, so these should be avoided; a person caught in the open should curl up on the ground, lying on one side with legs close together.

Arborescent red lines or burns on the skin indicate the point of contact of lightning, but the path through the body can be deduced only approximately from the clinical sequelae. Death is due to ventricular fibrillation or to the effects of intense desiccating heat on vital regions of the brain. Lightning that strikes the head is particularly dangerous, proving fatal in 30 percent of cases. Persons struck by lightning are initially unconscious, irrespective of where they are struck. In those who survive, consciousness is usually regained rapidly and completely. Rarely, unconsciousness or an agitated-confusional state may persist for a week or two. There is usually a disturbance of sensorimotor function of a limb or all the limbs, which may be pale and cold or cyanotic. As a rule, these signs are also evanescent, but in some instances they persist, or an atrophic paralysis of a limb or part of a limb makes its appearance after a symptom-free interval of several months. Persistent seizures are surprisingly rare.

MYELITIS

In the nineteenth century, almost every disease of the spinal cord was labeled *myelitis*. Morton Prince, writing in *Dercum's Textbook of Nervous Diseases* in 1895, referred to traumatic myelitis, compressive myelitis, and so on, obviously giving a rather imprecise meaning to the term. Gradually, however, as knowledge of neuropathology advanced, one disease after another was removed from this category until only the truly inflammatory ones remained.

Today the spinal cord is known to be the locus of a limited number of infective and noninfective inflammatory processes, some causing selective destruction of neurons, others affecting primarily white matter (tracts), and yet another group involving the meninges and white matter or leading to a necrosis of both gray and white matter. The currently accepted term for all these inflammatory conditions is *myelitis*. Other special terms are used to indicate more precisely the distribution of the process: if it is confined to gray matter, the proper expression is *poliomyelitis*; if to white matter, *leukomyelitis*. If the whole cross-sectional area of the cord is involved, the process is said to be a *transverse myelitis*; if the lesions are multiple and widespread over a long vertical extent, the modifying adjectives *diffuse* or *disseminated* are used. The term *meningomyelitis* refers to combined inflammation of meninges and spinal cord, and *meningoradiculitis*, to combined meningeal and root involvement. An inflammatory process limited to the spinal dura is called *pachymeningitis*; and if infected material collects in the epidural or subdural space, it is called *epidural spinal abscess* or *granuloma*, as the case may be. The adjectives *acute*, *subacute*, and *chronic* denote the tempo of evolution of myelitic symptoms—more or less within days, 2 to 6 weeks, or more than 6 weeks, respectively.

Classification of Inflammatory Diseases of the Spinal Cord

I. Viral myelitis (Chap. 33)
   A. Enteroviruses (groups A and B Coxsackie virus, poliomyelitis, others)
   B. Herpes zoster
   C. Myelitis of AIDS
   D. Epstein-Barr virus (EBV), cytomegalovirus (CMV), herpes simplex
   E. Rabies
   F. Japanese B virus
   G. HTLV-1 (tropical spastic paraparesis)
II. Myelitis secondary to bacterial, fungal, parasitic, and primary granulomatous diseases of the meninges and spinal cord
   A. *Mycoplasma pneumoniae* (Chap. 32)
   B. Lyme disease
   C. Pyogenic myelitis
      1. Acute epidural abscess and granuloma
      2. Abscess of spinal cord
   D. Tuberculous myelitis (Chap. 32)
      1. Pott's disease with spinal cord compression
      2. Tuberculous meningomyelitis
      3. Tuberculoma of spinal cord
   E. Parasitic and fungal infections producing epidural granuloma, localized meningitis, or meningomyelitis and abscess (Chap. 32)
   F. Syphilitic myelitis (Chap. 32)
      1. Chronic meningoradiculitis (tabes dorsalis)
      2. Chronic meningomyelitis
      3. Meningovascular syphilis
      4. Gummatous meningitis including chronic spinal pachymeningitis
   G. Sarcoid myelitis (Chap. 32)
III. Myelitis (myelopathy) of noninfectious inflammatory type
   A. Postinfectious and postvaccinal myelitis (Chap. 36)
   B. Acute and chronic relapsing or progressive multiple sclerosis (Chap. 36)
   C. Subacute necrotizing myelitis (Chap. 36)
   D. Myelopathy with lupus or other forms of angiitis
   E. Paraneoplastic myelopathy and poliomyelitis (Chap. 31)

From this outline it is evident that many different and totally unrelated diseases are under consideration and that a general description cannot possibly encompass such a diversity of pathologic processes. Many of the myelitides are considered elsewhere in this volume in relation to the diseases of which they are a part. Here it is only necessary to comment on the three principal categories and to describe a few of the common subtypes.

Myelitis due to Viruses

The enteroviruses, of which Coxsackie and poliomyelitis are examples, herpes zoster, and AIDS are the important members of this category. The enteroviruses have an affinity for neurons of the anterior horns of the spinal cord and motor nuclei of the brainstem (i.e., they are poliomyelitides), and herpes zoster virus for the dorsal root ganglia; hence the disturbances of function are in terms of motor and sensory neurons, respectively, not of spinal tracts. The onset of these conditions is acute and features a febrile meningomyelitis (see Chap. 33). Although there are systemic symptoms and sometimes cutaneous ones (in the case of zoster), it is the nervous system disorder that is most significant. The patient suffers the immediate effects of nerve cell destruction, and improvement nearly always follows as altered nerve cells recover. Later in life, possibly as the neuronal loss of aging occurs in the anterior horns and dorsal root ganglia, there may be an increased loss of strength in muscles originally weakened by poliomyelitis ("post-polio syndrome").

The rapid expansion of knowledge of herpesvirus infections has added a new chapter to the viral myelitides. Relatively rare examples of myelitis due to herpes simplex virus (HSV types 1 and 2), varicella-zoster virus (VZV), cytomegalovirus (CMV), Epstein-Barr virus (EBV), and SV70 virus (epidemic conjunctivitis) have been reported, some in patients with immunodeficiency states, particularly HIV infections. The situation is more complex clinically, since most of these agents may also produce a postinfectious variety of myelitis, described further on in this chapter and in Chaps. 33 and 36. In HSV type 2 infections, there may also be an acute lumbosacral radiculitis with urinary retention; and in VZV infections, a sensory ganglionitis, vasculitis, or encephalitis. There is, in a few cases, evidence of an extensive inflammatory necrosis of the spinal cord with involvement of sensory and motor tracts. In other words, these conditions may at times simulate acute paraplegic and quadriplegic transverse or panmyelitis syndromes of nonviral type. However, pleocytosis and isolation of portions of the viral DNA by the polymerase chain reaction or direct culture from the cerebrospinal fluid (CSF) confirm the diagnosis of a primary viral infection, as discussed in Chap. 33 (see Dawson and Potts).

Affection of the white matter, with sensory and motor paralysis below the level of a lesion, has been reported in so-called dumb rabies (in contrast to the usual form of "mad" or "furious" rabies encephalitis), zoster and simplex myelitis, EBV myelitis, and an infection transmitted by the bite of a monkey, called the *B virus*. Each of these is decidedly rare. Far more common is the myelopathy of AIDS; much rarer is the myelopathy of spinal spastic paraparesis (HTLV-1). With these exceptions, one may say that any myelitis that expresses itself by dysfunction of motor and sensory tracts will usually prove not to be viral in origin but due rather to one of the disease processes in category II or III of the preceding classification. The unique vacuolar myelopathy of AIDS and the myelopathy of human HTLV infections are described below and also in Chap. 33.

There are other rare forms of poliomyelitic reactions of unknown, presumably viral etiology. One such condition presents as an acute febrile meningomyelitis and leaves all the limbs paralyzed and flaccid, sparing the brainstem and affecting the diaphragm to a variable extent. Several such patients have harbored a carcinoma or Hodgkin disease, and the pathology proved to be like that of a poliomyelitic viral infection rather than the usual paraneoplastic syndromes. We have cared for several others who have had destruction of anterior horn cells due apparently to an enterovirus other than poliomyelitis virus (see further on and page 809 and Fig. 33-4).

Vacuolar Myelopathy with AIDS As the neurology of AIDS has been elucidated, this new clinical and pathologic entity has emerged. Its frequency is impressive—20 of 89 successive cases of AIDS on whom a postmortem examination was performed (Petito et al). Often the clinical symptoms and signs of spinal cord disease are obscured by a neuropathy or one or more of the cerebral disorders that complicate AIDS—due either to HIV or to an opportunistic infection (CMV disease, toxoplasmosis, etc.). In five cases of severe vacuolar myelopathy in Petito's series, there was leg weakness or leg and arm weakness, often asymmetrical and developing over a period of weeks, to which the signs of sensory tract involvement and sphincteric disorder were added. A sensory ataxia has been a common early feature in our experience. The CSF shows a small number of lymphocytes, a slight elevation of protein, and, occasionally, bizarre giant cells. The white matter of the spinal cord is vacuolated, most severely in thoracic segments. Posterior and lateral funiculi are affected diffusely without confinement to discrete sensory or motor systems. Axons are involved to a lesser degree than myelin sheaths, and lipid-laden macrophages are present in abundance. Similar vacuolar lesions may be seen in the brain in some cases. Although the lesions in the spinal cord resemble those of subacute combined degeneration, levels of vitamin B_{12} and folic acid have been normal. A similar lesion was seen in one of our cases of chronic lupus erythematosus. Often there are coexistent features of AIDS dementia or one of the several neuropathies that occur in the intermediate and advanced stages of the disease (discussed in Chap. 33). The antiretroviral drugs that slow the progress of AIDS seem to have little effect on the myelopathy, and one can only resort to the symptomatic treatment of spasticity.

Tropical Spastic Paraparesis due to Human T-Cell Lymphotropic Virus Type I (HTLV-1) The tropical myeloneuropathies were drawn to the attention of neurologists 45 years ago through the observations and writings of Cruickshank. However, it is only relatively recently that a chronic infective-inflammatory disease of the spinal cord due to the retrovirus HTLV-I has been discovered. The clinical implications of this discovery are broad and extend even to the demyelinative and possibly the degenerative diseases.

Spinal cord disease of this type has been reported from the Caribbean islands, southern United States, southern Japan, South America, and Africa. The clinical picture is one of a slowly progressive paraparesis with increased tendon reflexes and Babinski signs; disorder of sphincteric control is usually an early change. Paresthesias, reduced vibratory and position senses, and ataxia have been described. A few of the patients have had an associated polyneuropathy, as in Cruikshank's early cases. The upper extremities are usually spared (except for lively tendon reflexes), as are cerebral and brainstem structures.

The CSF contains small numbers of lymphocytes of T type (10 to 50 per cubic millimeter), normal concentrations of protein and glucose, and an increased content of IgG with antibodies to HTLV-I. The diagnosis is confirmed by the detection in the serum of the antibodies to the virus. Thinness of the spinal cord is evident on MRI, and subcortical cerebral white matter lesions may be seen as well. Neuropathologic study has documented an inflammatory myelitis with focal spongiform, demyelinative, and necrotic lesions, perivascular and meningeal infiltrates of inflammatory cells, and focal destruction of gray matter. The posterior columns and corticospinal tracts are the main sites of disease, most evident in the thoracic cord. It is strongly suspected but not established that the disease is due to the cytotoxic effect of the viral infection, but an alternative theory of autoimmune damage has been proposed.

The clinical picture can easily be confused with that of progressive spastic paraplegia of the heredofamilial variety, sporadic motor neuron disease, or the chronic phase of multiple sclerosis. There are also similarities with the AIDS myelopathy described above, but the other features of HIV infection are absent. Tropical spastic paraparesis and HTLV-I are also considered in the chapter on viral disease (page 806). There are anecdotal reports of improvement with intravenous administration of gamma globulin.

Myelitis Secondary to Bacterial, Fungal, Parasitic, and Granulomatous Diseases

With few exceptions, this class of spinal cord disease seldom offers any difficulty in diagnosis. The CSF often holds the clue to causation. In most cases, the inflammatory reaction of the spinal meninges is only one manifestation of a generalized (systemic) disease process. The spinal lesion may involve primarily the pia-arachnoid (leptomeningitis), the dura (pachymeningitis), or the epidural space, e.g., taking the form of an abscess or granuloma; in the last circumstance, damage to the spinal cord is due to compression and ischemia. In some acute forms, both the spinal cord and meninges are simultaneously affected, or the cord lesions may predominate. Chronic spinal meningitis may involve the pial arteries or veins; as the inflamed vessels become thrombosed, infarction (myelomalacia) of the spinal cord results. Chronic meningeal inflammation may provoke a progressive constrictive pial fibrosis (so-called spinal arachnoiditis) that virtually strangulates the spinal cord. In certain instances, spinal roots become progressively damaged, especially the lumbosacral ones, which have a long meningeal course. Posterior roots, which enter the subarachnoid space near arachnoidal villi (where CSF is resorbed), tend to suffer greater injury than anterior ones (as happens in tabes dorsalis). Interestingly, there are many cases of chronic cerebrospinal meningitis that remain entirely without symptoms until the spinal cord or roots become involved.

The unique myelitis caused by the atypical pneumonia agent *Mycoplasma pneumoniae* has been conceptualized as a postinfectious immune disease, as discussed on pages 747 and 975. However, portions of the DNA from this organism have been found in the spinal fluid early in the course of illness (using the polymerase chain reaction), suggesting instead a direct bacterial infection of the spinal cord (see Chap. 32). It is not known whether antibiotic treatment alters the course of the illness.

Syphilitic myelitis is discussed on page 787. *Abscess of the spinal cord* (acute bacterial myelitis) is exceedingly rare and is only beginning to be recognized by MRI. At times it stands as a single pyogenic metastasis, but more often there has been spread from a contiguous infected surgical site or a fistulous connection with a superficial abscess or furuncle. *Acute spinal epidural abscess and granuloma* are the more important representatives of this group.

Sarcoid may present as an intramedullary spinal cord mass, as in the cases of Levivier and colleagues. More often the granulomatous lesion, which may be focal or multifocal, simulates demyelinative disease, with respect to its tendency to relapse and remit and an apparent response to corticosteroids (page 761). An asymmetrical ascending paraparesis and bladder disturbance have been the features in our patients. Usually there is evidence of disseminated sarcoidosis and the CSF is abnormal (increase in cells and protein), but we have encountered several instances of sarcoid restricted to the spinal cord before it was clinically evident in the chest (chest CT will generally demonstrate hilar adenopathy). Elevation of the spinal fluid IgG concentration and the presence of oligoclonal bands are typical but not constant in these cases of neurosarcoidosis, and often there are activated histiocytes in the CSF. The use of angiotensin-converting enzyme levels in the CSF to distinguish sarcoidosis from multiple sclerosis suffers from the lack of normative values for this test, but it is said to be elevated in two-thirds of patients. The MRI is invariably abnormal and the conus may show intramedullary lesions, but the most characteristic finding is a nodular enhancement of the meninges adjacent to a lesion of the cord or nerve roots, similar to that observed in neoplastic meningitis. The diagnosis can be confirmed by mediastinal lymph node biopsy or by the less desirable method of biopsy of the spinal meninges and subpial cord.

A number of other rare granulomatous conditions have on occasion caused an intrinsic or, more often, an extrinsic compressive myelopathy, including brucellosis, xanthogranulomatosis, and eosinophilic granuloma. The diagnosis may be suspected if the systemic disease is apparent at the time, but in some instances only the histology of a surgical specimen reveals the underlying process.

Spinal Epidural Abscess This process is worthy of emphasis because the diagnosis is often missed or mistaken for another disease, with disastrous results. Children or adults may be affected. Infection of the epidural space has a wide variety of sources. An injury to the back, often trivial at the time, furunculosis or other skin or wound infection, or a bacteremia may permit seeding of the spinal epidural space or of a vertebral body. This gives rise to osteomyelitis with extension to the epidural space. Occasionally, extension is from an infected disc. An epidural abscess or granuloma may also develop in the course of a septicemia or in an addict following the use of nonsterile needles or the injection of contaminated drugs. In other cases organisms may be introduced into the epidural space during spinal surgery or rarely via a lumbar puncture needle during epidural or spinal anesthesia or epidural injections of steroid or other therapeutic agents. The localization in these latter instances is over lumbar and sacral roots. In the cases of *cauda equina epidural abscess*, back pain may be severe and neurologic symptomatology minimal unless the infection extends upward to the upper lumbar and thoracic segments of the spinal cord. *Staphylococcus aureus* is the most frequent etiologic agent, followed by streptococci, gram-negative bacilli, and anaerobic organisms.

At first, the suppurative process is accompanied only by fever and pain, usually intense, in the back, followed within a day or several days by radicular pain in most cases. Headache and nuchal rigidity are sometimes present; more often there is persistent pain and a disinclination to move the back. After several more days, there is the onset of a rapidly progressive paraparesis and paraplegia or quadriplegia, associated with sensory loss in the lower parts of the body and sphincteric paralysis with urinary and fecal retention. Percussion of the spine elicits tenderness over the site of the infection. Examination discloses all the signs of a complete or partial transverse cord lesion, with elements of spinal shock if paralysis has evolved rapidly. The CSF contains a relatively small number of white cells (usually fewer than 100 per cubic millimeter), both polymorphonuclear leukocytes and lymphocytes, unless the needle penetrates the abscess, in which case pus is obtained. The protein content is relatively high (100 to 400 mg/100 mL or more), but the glucose is normal. An elevation of the sedimentation rate and a peripheral neutrophilic leukocytosis are important clues (often neglected) to the diagnosis (Baker et al).

The foregoing clinical and spinal fluid findings call for immediate MRI imaging or CT, the latter preferably with myelography, to determine the level of the infected mass. If not treated surgically by laminectomy and drainage at the earliest possible time, before the onset of paralysis, the spinal cord lesion, which is due in part to ischemia (compression mainly of veins), becomes more or less irreversible. Antibiotics in large doses must also be given. Cauda equina epidural abscess without neurologic signs may in many cases be treated solely with antibiotics, although some surgeons favor drainage, which must be undertaken in any case if osteomyelitis develops. When osteomyelitis of a vertebral body is the primary abnormality, the epidural extension may implicate only a few spinal sensory and motor roots, leaving long tracts and other intramedullary structures intact. In some cases with cervical epidural abscesses, stiff neck, fever, and deltoid-biceps weakness are the main neurologic abnormalities.

A slowly progressive and then stabilizing syndrome of incomplete cord compression may occur after apparently successful drainage of an epidural abscess. This is usually caused by the formation of a fibrous and granulomatous reaction at the operative site. Distinguishing this inflammatory mass from residual epidural abscess may be quite difficult, even with enhanced MRI, but persistent fever, leukocytosis, and an elevated sedimentation rate should suggest that surgical drainage of the abscess was incomplete.

Spinal subdural bacterial infections also occur and, clinically, are virtually indistinguishable from epidural ones. A clue is provided by the CT myelogram, in which the subdural lesion has a less sharp margin and a greater vertical extent. The difference is also appreciated on axial MRI. The epidural and subdural infections, if they smolder owing to delayed diagnosis or inadequate therapy, may evolve into a chronic adhesive meningomyelitis.

Subacute pyogenic infections and *granulomatous infections* (tuberculous, fungal) may also arise in the spinal epidural space. The clinical picture is less dramatic, and local and radicular pain is slight or absent; the diagnosis depends on the demonstration, in a patient with weakness and sensory loss below a certain level on the trunk, of a partial or complete block by CT myelography and MRI. Osteomyelitis may not be seen for a time in plain films, but bone scans and MRI are revealing. Treatment depends on the nature of the underlying disease and the general condition of the patient.

Spinal Cord Abscess This entity was first described by Hart in 1830 and, although it is rare, 73 cases had been reported by 1994 (Candon and Frerebeau). In some instances the patient was known to have had a systemic bacterial infection, a septicemia, or endocarditis; in others there was a contiguous abscess in the skin or subcutaneous tissues with a fistula to the spinal cord through an intervertebral foramen. Spinal cord abscess is a rare complication of spinal dysraphism or of a developmentally open fistulous tract. The symptoms are indistinguishable from those of epidural abscess—namely, spinal and radicular pain followed by sensory and motor paralysis; the CSF findings are also the same. Woltman and Adson described a patient in whom surgical drainage of an encapsulated intramedullary abscess led to recovery, and Morrison and associates reported a similar case caused by *Listeria monocytogenes*, which was successfully drained and the meningeal infection suppressed by ampicillin and chloramphenicol. MRI is the most useful diagnostic procedure.

Tuberculous Myelitis Solitary tuberculoma of the spinal cord as part of a generalized infection is an extreme rarity. Tuberculous osteitis of the spine with kyphosis (Pott's disease) is more frequent; pus or caseous granulation tissue may extrude from an infected vertebra and gives rise to an epidural compression of the cord (Pott's paraplegia). Occasionally a tuberculous meningitis may result in pial arteritis and spinal cord infarction. The paraplegia may appear before the tuberculous meningitis is diagnosed.

All these forms of tuberculosis have become infrequent in the United States and western Europe. Additional comments can be found on page 759.

Meningomyelitis due to Fungus and Parasitic Diseases A wide variety of fungal and parasitic agents may involve the spinal meninges. Such infections are rare, and some do not occur at all in the United States or are limited to certain geographic areas, particularly among immigrant populations. *Actinomyces*, *Blastomyces*, *Coccidioides*, and *Aspergillus* may invade the spinal epidural space via intervertebral foramina or by extension from a vertebral osteomyelitic focus. *Cryptococcus*, which causes meningoencephalitis and rarely a cerebral granuloma, in our experience seldom causes spinal lesions. Hematogenous metastases to the spinal cord or meninges may occur in both blastomycosis and coccidioidomycosis. Occasionally an echinococcal infection of the posterior mediastinum may extend to the spinal canal (epidural space) via intervertebral foramina and compress the spinal cord.

Schistosomiasis (bilharziasis) is a recognized cause of myelitis in the Far East, Africa, and South America. The spinal cord is a target for all three common forms of *Schistosoma*: *S. haematobium*, *S. japonicum*, and *S. mansoni*, but particularly the last of these (see page 780). The schistosomal ova evoke a granulomatous myelomeningoradiculitis. The lesions are destructive of gray and white matter, with ova in arteries and veins leading to obstruction and ischemia (Scrimgeour and Gajdusek). Less often, a localized granuloma gives rise to a compressive cord syndrome and, rarely, the disease takes the form of an acute transverse myelitis with massive necrosis of cord tissue (Queiroz et al). We have studied two patients in whom the spinal cord in the low thoracic and lumbar region was infected approximately 3 weeks after they swam in contaminated water during an African vacation. The CSF showed only a slight elevation of protein, and there was no abnormality in the myelogram. The administration of praziquantel arrested the course of the illness, but the patients were left disabled.

Myelitis of Noninfectious Inflammatory Type (Acute Transverse Myelitis)

The spinal cord disorders that make up this category take the form of a leukomyelitis based on either demyelination or necrosis of the tracts in the spinal cord. In their pathogenesis, the critical factor appears to be a disordered immune response to an infection rather than the direct effect of an infectious agent. Varied clinical syndromes are induced, and the basic disease is classified in most textbooks under headings such as *acute transverse myelitis*, *postinfectious myelitis*, *postvaccinal myelitis*, *acute multiple sclerosis*, and *necrotizing myelitis*. While each of these conditions may affect other parts of the nervous system (most often the optic nerves or brain), often the only manifestations are spinal. The aforementioned myelitides or myelopathies are sufficiently distinct to justify their separate classification, for in most cases they run true to form; but transitional cases, sharing the clinical and pathologic attributes of more than one disease, are encountered in any large clinical and pathologic material.

Postinfectious and Postvaccinal Myelitides The characteristic features of these diseases are (1) their temporal relationship to certain viral infections or vaccinations (see pages 975 to 979); (2) the development of neurologic signs over the period of a few days; and (3) a monophasic temporal course, i.e., a single attack of several weeks' duration with variable degrees of recovery and no recurrence. These diseases may involve the brain as well as the spinal cord, in which case the process is appropriately designated as *acute disseminated encephalomyelitis* (ADEM); in others cases the spinal cord is affected predominantly or exclusively—an acute myelitis or inflammatory myelopathy. On the basis of the clinical features of disseminated postinfectious encephalomyelitis and the animal model of experimental allergic encephalomyelitis (EAE), postinfectious myelitis is presumed to be immunologic in nature, reflecting an attack that is more or less confined to spinal cord myelin (see Chap. 36).

The usual history in these cases is for weakness and numbness of the feet and legs (less often of the hands and arms) to develop over a few days, sometimes mimicking the pattern of the Guillain-Barré syndrome. However, an asymmetry of the symptoms and signs, a sensory level on the trunk, or a Babinski sign marks the disease as a myelopathy. Sphincteric disturbances and backache are common in the first days. Headache and stiff neck may or may not be present. There may or may not have been a recent infectious illness, such as a mundane upper respiratory syndrome, but the patient is usually afebrile when the myelopathic symptoms begin. Almost invariably the CSF contains lymphocytes and other mononuclear cells in the range of 10 to 100 (sometimes higher) per cubic millimeter, with slightly raised protein and normal glucose content. In milder cases there may be only 3 or 4 cells per cubic millimeter, making the inflammatory aspect less clear but nonetheless representing the same postinfectious immune process. In most instances that have come under our care in recent years, the MRI has shown T2 signal abnormalities and slight gadolinium enhancement extending over two or three spinal segments (the distinction from multiple sclerosis is discussed below); the cord may be swollen in these regions (Fig. 44-2). Several patients with mild and partial myelitis have had normal MRI studies.

Figure 44-2

MRI of acute postinfectious myelitis in the sagittal (A) *and axial* (B) *planes. There is T2 signal change and other images showed mild enhancement after gadolinium infusion. The cord is slightly enlarged at the involved level.*

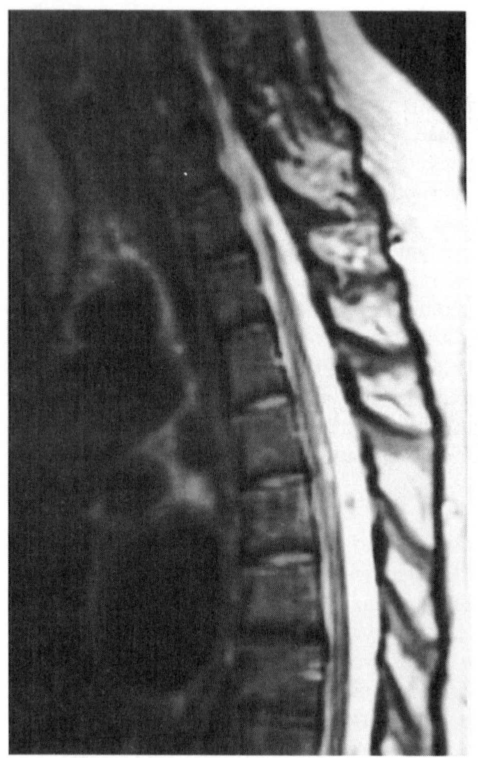

A

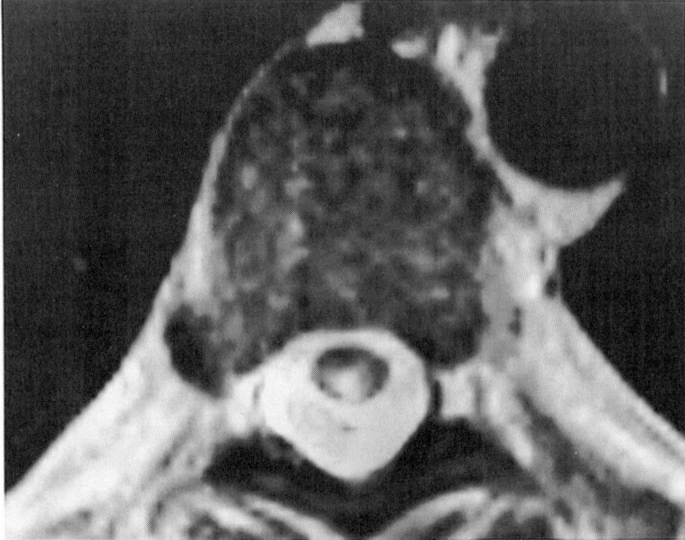

B

These signs evolve over several days, although in a few instances a complete "transverse" involvement of the cord is attained in a matter of hours. More often there is an incomplete corticospinal and spinothalamic syndrome affecting one side more than the other.

Variants in our experience have included an almost pure paresthetic illness with posterior column dysfunction and the converse, a symmetrical paraparesis with analgesia below a level on the trunk but without affection of deep sensation (a syndrome usually associated with cord infarction in the territory of the anterior spinal artery); a variable sensory loss involving the leg and groin on one side or both; a purely lumbosacral or sacral myelopathy (conus syndrome with saddle analgesia and sphincter disturbances); and a Brown-Séquard–like syndrome.

In the past, postinfectious myelitis was most often observed in relation to the common exanthems (rubella, rubeola, varicella), the neurologic signs appearing as the rash was fading, often with a recrudescence of fever. Vaccination against smallpox and rabies was also a frequent cause. The former, of course, is no longer a concern, and rabies vaccine as a cause of myelitic symptoms has virtually disappeared, at least in the United States, with the use of vaccine grown on cultures of human tissue rather than myelinated spinal cord.

In more recent years, practically all human viruses have at one time or another been reported to precede acute myelitis; the large DNA viruses, such as Epstein-Barr and cytomegalovirus, have a proclivity to do so, but hepatitis B, varicella, and entero- and rhinoviruses have been detected when systematically sought. *Mycoplasma* is almost unique as a bacterial trigger of the disease, but—as noted earlier—it may also be capable of causing direct infection, leaving the mechanism uncertain. In many instances the connection to a preceding infection is presumed but cannot be proved. Only the associations with EBV, CMV, and *Mycoplasma* seem certain, based on the regularity of their occurrence. The list of antecedent infections is otherwise much the same as that for the Guillain-Barré syndrome with the notable absence of *Campylobacter jejuni*, which has not led to myelitis. A pharyngitis, respiratory infection, or conjunctivitis, etc., with or without fever, is likely related if it occurred several days or in a 2- to 3-week period before the onset of neurologic symptoms. Severe headache with or before the fever and neurologic signs suggests *Mycoplasma*, influenza, or another atypical pneumonia agent, and abnormal liver function tests or severe pharyngitis with cervical adenopathy usually indicates EBV or, less often, CMV infection.

More difficult to understand are the instances of myelitis, including autopsy proven ones, in which the disease develops without an apparent antecedent infection. There is always uncertainty in such cases as to whether the illness is the opening phase of multiple sclerosis (MS) of the type described below, under "Demyelinative Myelitis." In our cases of transverse myelitis, fewer than half have shown other signs of MS after 20 years (this is a far lower incidence than following a bout of optic neuritis). Also, there is a *relapsing form of myelitis*, sometimes but not always triggered by an infection, that does not manifest lesions elsewhere in the neuraxis and therefore has an ambiguous relationship to multiple sclerosis. Further discussion of acute transverse myelitis in relation to other demyelinating diseases can be found on page 963.

The *pathologic changes* take the form of myriads of subpial and perivenular zones of demyelination, with perivascular and meningeal infiltrations of lymphocytes and other mononuclear cells, and para-adventitial pleomorphic histiocytes and microgliacytes (page 975).

Treatment Once symptoms begin, it is doubtful if any treatment other than supportive therapy is of consistent value. One's first impulse, assuming the mechanism to be an autoimmune disorder, is to administer high doses of corticosteroids—a practice we have followed, but without conviction. Perhaps it is advisable to do so, but there is as yet no evidence that this practice alters the natural course of the illness. We have also tried plasma exchange and intravenous immune globulin in several patients, with uncertain results, although this approach was seemingly helpful in a few patients.

In general, the prognosis is better than the initial symptoms might suggest. Invariably, the purely myelitic disease improves, sometimes to a surprising degree, but there are examples in which the sequelae have been severe and permanent. Pain in the midthoracic region or an abrupt, severe onset usually indicates a poor prognosis (Ropper and Poskanzer). The authors have several times given a good prognosis for long-term recovery and assurance that no relapse will occur, only to witness a recrudescence of other symptoms at a later date, suggesting that the original illness was multiple sclerosis.

Demyelinative Myelitis (Acute Multiple Sclerosis)

The lesions of acute MS presenting as a myelitis share many of the features of the postinfectious type except that the clinical manifestations of the former tend to evolve more slowly, over a period of 1 to 3 weeks or even longer. Also, their relation to antecedent infections is less certain, and in most recorded examples such events were lacking. The difficulty of distinguishing between an attack of demyelinative and postinfectious myelitis was mentioned above and was emphasized by Uchimura and Shiraki in their study of postrabies inoculation in Japan. In most of their cases, the myelitis took the form of acute MS, but the disease did have the monophasic character and some of the pathologic attributes of the postinfectious variety. However, in other cases of similar onset, the occurrence of subsequent attacks indicated that the basic illness was one of chronic recurrent demyelination, identical to the usual type of MS.

The most typical mode of clinical expression of demyelinative myelitis is with numbness that spreads over one or both sides of the body from the sacral segments to the feet, anterior thighs, and up over the trunk, with coincident weakness and then paralysis of the legs. As this process becomes complete, the bladder is also affected. The sensorimotor disturbance may extend to involve the arms, and a sensory level can be demonstrated on the trunk. The CSF usually shows a mild lymphocytosis, as in the postinfectious variety, but it may be normal. Bakshi and colleagues have suggested that in myelitis due to MS, the MRI abnormality occupies only a few adjacent segments and the postinfectious lesions have a longer vertical extent, but this has not been consistent in our experience and we have seen either process to cause expansion of the cord. As a general rule, acute MS is relatively painless and without fever, and the patient usually improves, with variable residual signs.

The differential diagnosis of demyelinative myelitis is fully considered in Chap. 36.

Treatment Corticosteroids, as outlined for MS (page 973), may lead to a regression of symptoms, sometimes with relapse when the medication is discontinued too soon (after 1 to 2 weeks). Other patients, however, show no apparent response, and a few have even continued to worsen while the medication was being given. Plasma exchange and intravenous immune globulin have reportedly been beneficial in individual cases, particularly in those with an explosive onset (see below). Our results with plasma exchange have been too variable to interpret.

Myelitis (Myelopathy) with Systemic Lupus Erythematosus A rapidly evolving or subacute myelopathy in association with systemic lupus erythematosus must always be considered in the differential diagnosis of demyelinative myelitis. It is presumed to arise from a microvasculitis of the spinal cord. Propper and Bucknall presented such a case and reviewed 44 others in which a patient with lupus erythematosus developed a transverse myelitis over a period of days. There was back pain at the level of sensory loss, although the cases we have seen have been painless. Pleocytosis and elevation of CSF protein were characteristic. The MRI revealed a segmental swelling of the spinal cord. Postmortem examinations of such cases have disclosed widespread vasculopathy of small vessels with variable inflammation and myelomalacia, and, rarely, a vacuolar myelopathy.

Many but not all cases have antiphospholipid antibodies; the relationship of these antibodies to the myelopathy is uncertain (see also page 912). The incidence of lupus myelopathy is not known, but one such case comes to our attention every year or two.

Acute and Subacute Necrotizing Myelitis and Devic Disease In every large medical center, occasional examples of this disorder are found among the many patients who present with an acute onset of paraplegia or quadriplegia, sensory loss, and sphincter paralysis. The neurologic signs may erupt so precipitously that a vascular lesion is assumed. In other cases the disease evolves at a somewhat slower pace, over several days or a week or longer. The main clinical features that distinguish necrotizing myelopathy from the more common types of transverse myelitis are a persistent and profound flaccidity of the legs (or arms if the lesion is cervical), areflexia, and atonicity of the bladder—all reflecting a widespread pannecrosis that involves both the gray and white matter over a considerable vertical extent of the spinal cord—or spinal shock.

A small number of such cases are associated with unilateral or bilateral optic neuritis. This combination of spinal cord necrosis and optic neuritis corresponds to the syndrome described by Devic in 1894 and named *neuromyelitis optica* (page 966). But nearly all neurologists agree that a similar clinical syndrome involving the optic nerve and spinal cord (usually without necrosis) may be caused infrequently by postinfectious encephalomyelitis and, more often, by MS.

A few or several hundred mononuclear cells per cubic millimeter and increased protein may be found in the CSF, but oligoclonal banding is usually absent. The MRI shows more dramatic signal changes and gadolinium enhancement than most cases of transverse myelitis, usually extending over several levels (Fig. 44-3). In later imaging studies the involved segments of cord which were initially swollen appear atrophic. The electromyogram (EMG), several weeks or more after the illness has begun, reveals several contiguous denervated myotomes,

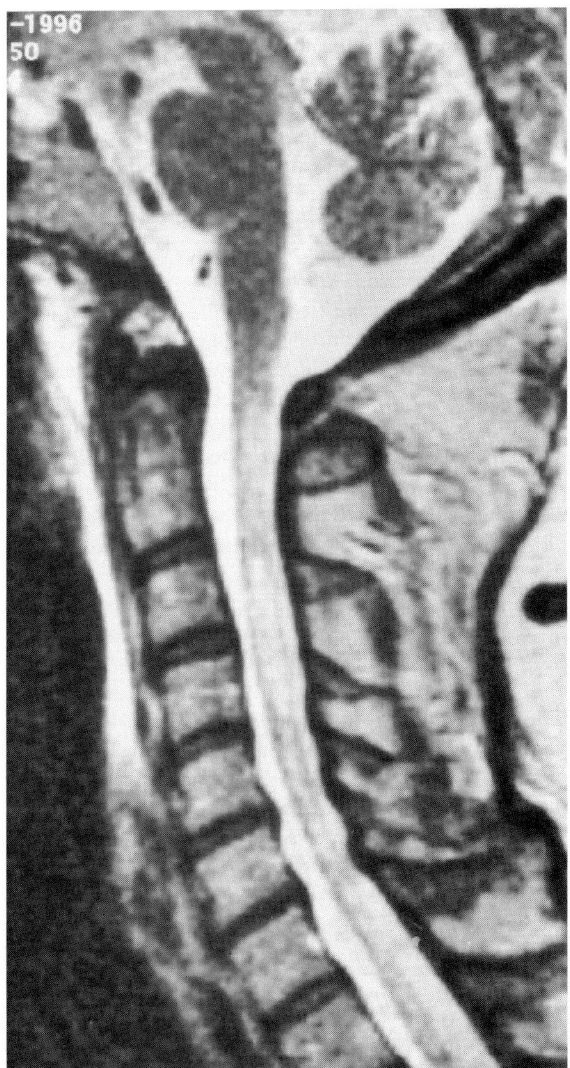

Figure 44-3

MRI of necrotic myelopathy in a patient without optic neuritis.

reflecting damage to the gray matter of those segments. A characteristic feature in most of our cases of necrotic myelopathy without optic neuritis has been a relapsing course, usually with saltatory worsening but occasionally punctuated by brief and limited remissions. Survival has been the rule, but the neurologic deficits of necrotic myelopathy—unlike those of the demyelinative and postinfectious myelitides described above—tend to be profound and lasting; in a few cases, they have been progressive over weeks or months. None of the treatments we have offered seemed to make a noticeable difference, but some authors have the impression that high-dose corticosteroids, cyclophosphamide, or plasma exchange may have been beneficial in individual cases.

In several cases coming to postmortem examination at variable times after the onset, the acute lesion has proved to be a necrotizing myelitis, not essentially different from the hemorrhagic leukoencephalitis of Hurst or an aggressive form of ADEM, described on page 978, but in a pattern that appears infarctive, i.e., not respecting the borders of gray and white matter. However, there are also areas of inflammation and demyelination at the edges of the destructive lesions. For this reason the authors agree with Hughes in classifying this condition with the demyelinative diseases. Older lesions will have left the spinal cord cavitated or collapsed over a vertical extent of 5 to 20 cm, often with conical extensions into the gray matter above and below the main area of necrosis. In one of the cases studied by R. D. Adams, in which death occurred many years after the onset of the myelitis, there was an old cavitated, obviously necrotizing lesion and many cerebral ones, the latter typical of MS. Cases of this type emphasize the overlapping relationship between the necrotizing and demyelinative processes. Also, we have been unable to make a clear distinction between the necrotic myelopathy of Devic disease and an identical process occurring without optic neuropathy. In the cases described by Greenfield and Turner as well as by Hughes and in our own (Katz and Ropper), patients of all ages and both sexes were affected. The optic nerve lesions, when present, tend to be of demyelinative type, much like those of MS.

Under the title "Subacute Necrotic Myelitis," Foix and Alajouanine and later Greenfield and Turner described a disorder of adult men characterized by an amyotrophic paraplegia that ran a progressive course over several months. An early spastic paraplegia evolved after a few weeks or longer into a flaccid, areflexive one. Sensory loss, at first dissociated and then complete, and loss of sphincteric control followed the initial paresis. The CSF protein was considerably elevated but there were no cells. Postmortem examinations in two of the cases of Foix and Alajouanine (11 and 22 months after onset, respectively) and in subsequent ones have shown the lumbosacral segments to be the most severely involved, with progressively less severe affection of the thoracic segments. In the affected areas there was severe necrosis of both gray and white matter with appropriate macrophage and astrocytic reactions. The small vessels seemed to be increased in number; their walls were thickened, cellular, and fibrotic, yet their lumens were not occluded ("angiodysplastic"). The veins were also thickened and surrounded by lymphocytes, mononuclear cells, and macrophages. These findings have been difficult to interpret. The importance of spinal venous thrombosis in the pathogenesis has been emphasized, but in the case of Mair and Folkerts, only one thrombosed anterior spinal vein was seen; in the cases of Foix and Alajouanine, no thrombosed vessels were found. We believe the evidence of venous occlusion to be unconvincing and are inclined to the view of Antoni and of others, who were impressed with the prominence of large arteries and veins and have reinterpreted this pathologic process as an arteriovenous malformation (see further on). However, in most cases of necrotic myelopathy, the vascular abnormality simply reflects the neovascular response to spinal cord necrosis. We suggest that only when enlarged and abnormal vessels involve the surface and adjacent parenchyma of the cord (as they did in the cases of Foix and Alajouanine) does the disorder deserve to be designated as Foix-Alajouanine myelopathy; the remaining cases are of the inflammatory-necrotizing type described above.

Rarely, a similar syndrome is produced by an idiopathic granulomatous or necrotizing angiitis that is confined to the spinal cord (Caccamo et al). In those cases, there has been a persistent and marked pleocytosis and some clinical stabilization with corticosteroids. One of our patients with a similar subacute necrotizing myelitis, seemingly responsive to corticosteroids, persistently had 50 or more cells in the spinal fluid, many of them polymorphonuclear, and died because of inflammatory cerebral hemorrhages; there were multiple occlusions of small vessels surrounding the spinal cord but no well-developed vasculitis. Polyarteritis nodosa and necrotizing arteritis rarely involve the spinal cord.

Paraneoplastic Myelitis A subacute necrotic myelitis developing in conjunction with a bronchogenic carcinoma was first brought to notice by Mancall and Rosales in 1964. Several dozen cases have been recorded, some in association with lymphomas. The clinical syndrome as we have seen it consists of a rapidly progressive painless loss of motor and then sensory tract function, usually with sphincter disorder. Imaging studies demonstrate an area of T2 signal change or may be normal, in distinction to the nodular enhancing appearance of an intramedullary metastasis or of extradural metastatic disease with cord compression. Actually, in cancer patients, intramedullary metastasis is a more common than paraneoplastic disease as a cause of intrinsic myelopathy. A compressive lesion must always be excluded and is, of course, far more frequent than either of these entities, which are discussed in later parts of the chapter.

The CSF may contain a few mononuclear cells and a slightly increased protein, or it may be normal. The lesions are essentially of necrotic type and respect neither gray nor white matter, but the latter is more affected. There is no evidence of an infective-inflammatory or ischemic lesion, for the blood vessels, apart from a modest cuffing with mononuclear cells, are normal. No tumor cells are visible in the CSF, meninges, or spinal cord tissue, and no virus has been isolated. Unlike the case in most of the paraneoplastic neurologic disorders, there is no antineural antibody to act as a diagnostic marker or to connect the neoplasm to the destructive lesion. In particular, this myelopathy does not seem to be a component of the anti-Hu–associated encephalitis-neuropathy spectrum of disease.

In some cases of paraneoplastic myelopathy, the degenerative changes are more chronic, confined to the posterior and lateral funiculi; they are often associated with a diffuse loss of cerebellar Purkinje cells. This latter syndrome has a disproportionately high association with ovarian carcinoma but has been observed with carcinoma of other types and with Hodgkin disease. All of the reported cases of these types have ended fatally; steroids and plasmapheresis were of no value. A special but rare variety of paraneoplastic anterior horn cell destruction is known to occur with lymphomas, which are discussed with the paraneoplastic syndromes in Chap. 31.

Subacute Spinal Neuronitis Whitely and colleagues have drawn attention to a rare but distinctive form of encephalomyelitis of unknown cause, characterized clinically by tonic rigidity and intermittent myoclonic jerking of the trunk and limb muscles and by painful spasms of these muscles evoked by sensory or emotional stimuli. In the late stages of the disease, signs of brainstem involvement appear which are usually progressive over a period of several weeks, months, or a year or longer; consciousness is preserved, however. The CSF may be normal or show a mild lymphocytosis and increase in protein content. This is probably the same disorder that had been described earlier by Campbell and Garland under the title of *subacute myoclonic spinal neuronitis* and later by Howell and coworkers. The disorder under discussion must be differentiated clinically from the syndrome of *continuous muscle fiber activity* of Isaacs and the "*stiff man*" syndrome of Moersch and Woltman (see page 1569).

The brunt of the pathologic process falls on the cervical portion of the spinal cord. Widespread loss of internuncial neurons with relative sparing of the anterior horn cells, neuronophagia of internuncial neurons, reactive gliosis and microglial proliferation, conspicuous lymphocytic cuffing of small blood vessels, and scanty meningeal inflammation are the main findings. Involvement of the white matter is less marked.

The pathophysiology of the rigidity in these cases is not well understood but may be due to the impaired function (or destruction) of Renshaw cells, with the release of tonic myotatic reflexes (Penry et al). The painful spasms and dysesthesias relate in some way to neuronal lesions in the posterior horns of the spinal cord and dorsal root ganglia. We agree with Whitely and with Lhermitte and their coworkers that these cases probably represent a rare and obscure form of viral myelitis. Myoclonic jerking of the trunk and limbs in a focal or segmental distribution is probably due to neuronal damage that is limited to the spinal cord. We have seen several such cases, usually of regional abdominal or thoracic myoclonus, in otherwise healthy patients and have been unable to determine its cause. Anticonvulsants and antispasticity drugs in some combination may partially suppress the myoclonus, and local injection of botulinum toxin has improved the symptoms. Rarely, a similar syndrome complicates vertebral or spinal artery angiography (see below).

VASCULAR DISEASES OF THE SPINAL CORD

In comparison with the brain, the spinal cord is an uncommon site of vascular disease. Blackwood, in a review of 3737 necropsies at the National Hospital for Nervous Diseases, London, in the period 1903 to 1958, found only 9 cases, but in general hospitals such as ours, the incidence is considerably higher. The spinal arteries tend not to be susceptible to atherosclerosis, and emboli rarely lodge there. Of all the vascular disorders of the spinal cord, infarction, bleeding, and arteriovenous malformation are the only ones that occur with any regularity, but they are rare in comparison with demyelinating myelitis. In current practice, most cases occur in relation to operations on the aorta, usually the thoracic portion, where the aorta must be clamped for some period of time. An understanding of these disorders requires some knowledge of the blood supply of the spinal cord.

Vascular Anatomy of the Spinal Cord The blood supply of the spinal cord is derived from a series of segmental vessels arising from the aorta and from branches of the subclavian and internal iliac arteries (Fig. 44-4). The most important branches of the subclavian are the vertebral arteries, the segmental branches of which form the rostral origins of the anterior median and posterior and lateral spinal arteries and constitute the major blood

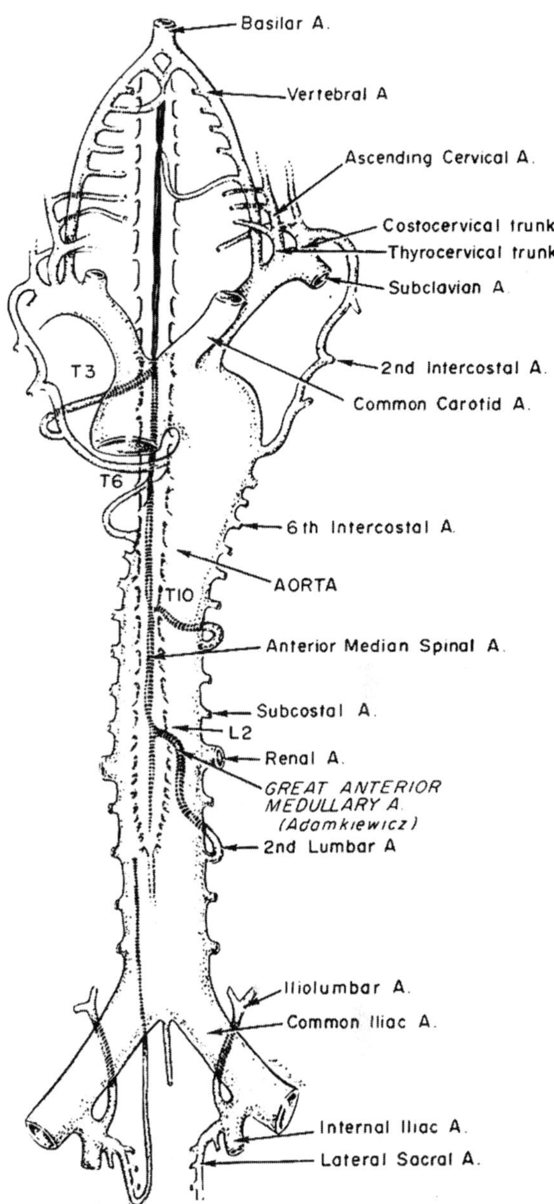

Figure 44-4

Anterior view of spinal cord with its segmental blood supply from the aorta. See text for details. (From Herrick and Mills by permission.)

supply to the cervical cord. The thoracic and lumbar cord is nourished by segmental arteries arising from the aorta and internal iliac arteries; segmental branches of the lateral sacral arteries supply the sacral cord.

A typical segmental artery divides into an anterior and a posterior ramus (Fig. 44-5). Each posterior ramus gives rise to a spinal artery, which enters the vertebral foramen, pierces the dura, and supplies the spinal ganglion and roots through its anterior and posterior radicular branches. Most anterior radicular arteries are small and some never reach the spinal cord, but a variable number (four to nine), arising at irregular intervals, are much larger and supply most of the blood to the spinal cord. Tributaries of the radicular arteries supply blood to the vertebral bodies and surrounding ligaments. The venous drainage of the marrow is into the posterior veins forming the spinal plexus. Their importance relates to the pathogenesis of fibrocartilaginous embolism (see further on).

Lazorthes, in his excellent review of the circulation of the spinal cord, divides the radiculomedullary arteries into three groups: (1) upper or cervicothoracic, which are derived from the anterior spinal arteries and branches of thyrocervical and costovertebral arteries; (2)

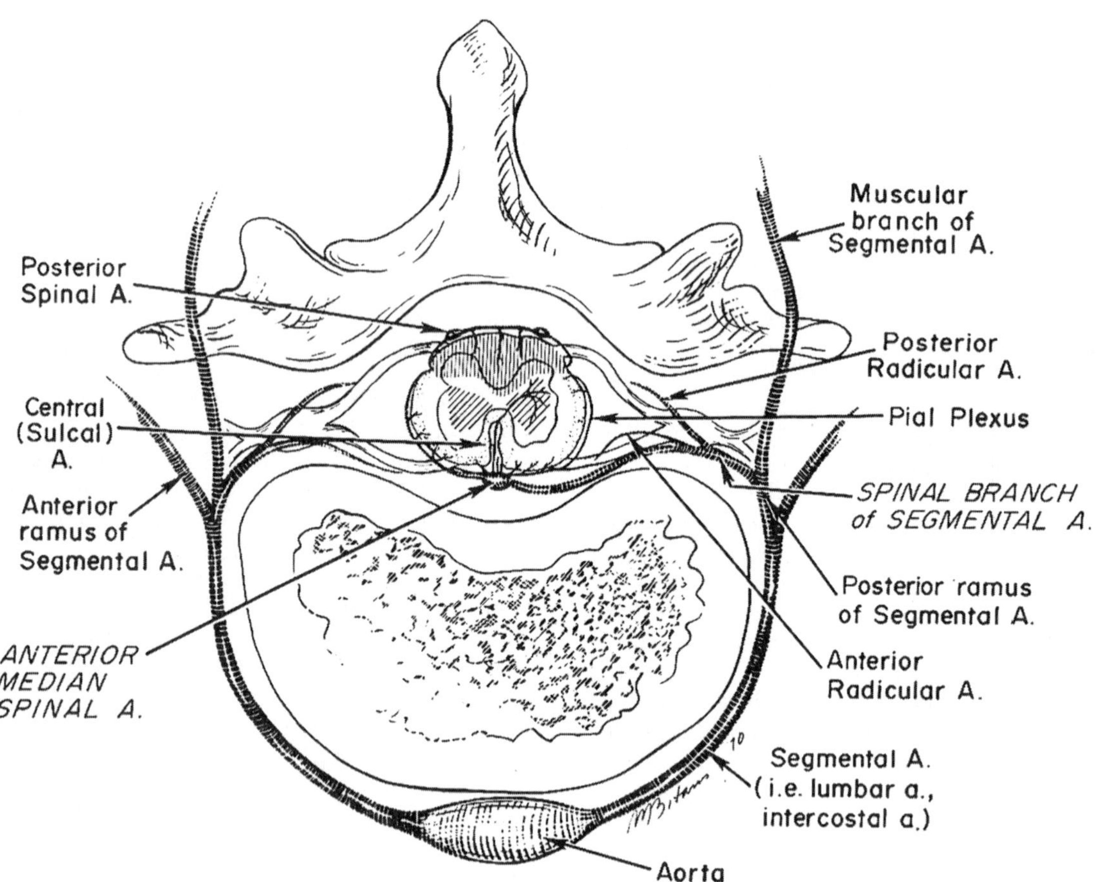

Figure 44-5

Representative cross section of lumbar vertebra and spinal cord with its blood supply at level of an anterior medullary artery. The shaded zones in the posterior part of the cord, ventral part of the cord, and margins of the ventral cord represent the regions of blood supply of the posterior spinal arteries, central (sulcal) arteries, and pial plexus, respectively. Borders of these three zones, appearing between the shaded areas in the diagram, represent watershed areas. (From Herrick and Mills, by permission.)

intermediate or middle thoracic (T3 to T8 cord segments), usually from a single T7 radicular artery; and (3) lower or thoracolumbar, from a large T10 or L1 anterior radicular artery called the *arteria radicularis magna* or the *artery of Adamkiewicz*. This artery may supply the lower two-thirds of the cord, but in any individual one cannot predict the precise area supplied by this or any other anterior radiculomedullary artery or what proportion of cord will be infarcted if one of these vessels is occluded. The junction between the vertebral spinal and aortic circulations typically lies at the T2–T3 spinal segment, but most ischemic lesions lie below this level.

The anterior medullary arteries form the single anterior median spinal artery, which runs the full length of the cord in the anterior sulcus and gives off direct penetrating branches via the central (sulcocommissural) arteries. These penetrating branches supply most of the anterior gray columns and the ventral portions of the dorsal gray columns of neurons (Fig. 44-5). The peripheral rim of white matter of the anterior two-thirds of the cord is supplied from a pial radial network, which also originates from the anterior median spinal artery. Thus, the branches of the anterior median spinal artery supply roughly the ventral two-thirds of the spinal cord. The posterior medullary arteries form the paired posterior spinal arteries that supply the dorsal third of the cord by means of direct penetrating vessels and a plexus of pial vessels (similar to that of the ventral cord, with which it anastomoses freely). Within the cord substance, then, there is a "watershed" area of capillaries where the penetrating branches of the anterior median spinal artery meet the penetrating branches of the posterior spinal arteries and the branches of the circumferential pial network. All spinal segments, because of the variable size of collateral arteries, do not have the same abundance of circulatory protection.

Normally there are 8 to 12 anterior medullary veins and a greater number of posterior medullary veins arranged fairly close to one another at every segmental level. They drain into radicular veins. In addition, a network of valveless veins extends along the vertebral column from the pelvic venous plexuses to the intracranial venous sinuses without passing through the lungs (Batson's plexus) and is considered a route for metastatic disease from the pelvis.

Infarction of the Spinal Cord (Myelomalacia)

Ischemic softening of the spinal cord usually involves the territory of the anterior spinal artery, i.e., a variable vertical extent of the ventral two-thirds of the spinal cord. Infarctions in this territory are relatively uncommon, representing 1.2 percent of all strokes (Sandson and Friedman). The resulting clinical abnormalities are generally referred to as the *anterior spinal artery syndrome*, first described by Spiller in 1909. Atherosclerosis and thrombotic occlusion of the anterior spinal artery itself is quite uncommon, however, and infarction in the territory of this artery is more often secondary to disease of an important extravertebral collateral artery or to disease of the aorta—either advanced atherosclerosis or a dissecting aneurysm—which occludes or shears the important segmental spinal arteries at their origins. We have seen a few instances of myelomalacia in adolescents and young adults in whom no aortic or spinal arterial disease could be demonstrated. An ischemic myelopathy has been reported in cocaine users, including episodes of cord dysfunction resembling transient ischemic attacks. Cardiac and aortic surgery, which requires clamping of the aorta for more than 30 min, and aortic arteriography may occasionally be complicated by infarction in the territory of the anterior spinal artery; more often in these circumstances damage to central neuronal elements is greater than that to anterior and lateral funiculi. Occasionally, polyarteritis nodosa may cause occlusion of a spinal medullary artery. Systemic cholesterol embolism arising from a severely atheromatous aorta may have the same effect. This type of embolism is prone to occur after surgical procedures, angioplasty, or cardiopulmonary resuscitation. Sometimes the operation precedes the spinal cord infarction by up to 3 weeks, as noted in Dahlberg's series. In almost all such patients, other evidence of widespread embolism can be expected. A quite different progressive ischemic necrosis of the cord occurs in the neighborhood of an arteriovenous malformation and is considered later in this chapter (see also the subacute necrotic myelitis of Foix and Alajouanine, described earlier). Infarction of the spinal cord due to fibrocartilagenous embolism is a special type of vascular disease, also discussed further on.

The clinical manifestations of arterial occlusion will, of course, vary with the level and portions of the cord that are infarcted, but common to practically all cases of infarction in the territory of the anterior spinal artery is pain in the neck or back and the development of motor paralysis and loss of pain and thermal sensation below the level of the lesion, accompanied by paralysis of sphincteric function. Rarely, infarction is preceded by transient spinal ischemic attacks. The symptoms may develop instantaneously or over an hour or two, but more rapidly than in the myelitides. Radicular pain is sometimes a complaint, corresponding to the upper level of the lesion. Paralysis is usually bilateral, occasionally unilateral, and rarely complete. Except in high cervical lesions, the sensory changes are dissociated; i.e., pain and temperature sensations are lost (due to interruption of the spinothalamic tracts), but vibration and position sense, two-point discrimination, judgment of degree of pressure, and perception of direction of cutaneous stroking are unimpaired (sparing of posterior columns). In this respect the syndrome differs from the acute transverse myelopathy of trauma, but—as mentioned earlier—a similar syndrome can occasionally be produced by a myelitis. In complete cases, the limbs are initially flaccid and areflexic, as in spinal shock from traumatic lesions, followed after several weeks by the development of spasticity, hyperactive tendon reflexes, clonus and Babinski signs, and some degree of voluntary bladder control (unless sacral segments have been infarcted). Some patients regain substantial motor function, mainly in the first month but extending over a year (Sandson and Friedman; Cheshire et al). Infarction in the territory of the posterior spinal arteries is uncommon and does not give rise to a stereotyped syndrome. It may occur with surgery or trauma of the spine or with vertebral artery dissections.

Most spinal cord infarctions can be detected by MRI. After a few days, there are obvious lesions on the T2 image sequences, presumably reflecting edema, over several levels. There may be slight enhancement after infusion of gadolinium. Incomplete infarctions may not be so evident. After several weeks there is myelomalacia, and in the chronic stages the region collapses and is shown to be attenuated on MRI.

A dissecting aneurysm of the aorta—which is characterized by intense interscapular and/or chest pain (occasionally it is painless), widening of the aorta, and signs of impaired circulation to the legs or arms and various organs—gives rise to a number of neurologic syndromes. The most common of these, according to Weisman and Adams, are (1) paralysis of the sphincters and both legs with sensory loss usually below T6, (2) obstruction of a brachial artery with a sensorimotor neuropathy of the limb, (3) obstruction of a common carotid artery with hemiplegia, and, less commonly, (4) ischemic infarction of the cord confined to the gray matter, in which case there is an abrupt onset of muscle weakness or myoclonus and spasms in the legs but no pain or sensory loss.

In the past, aortography was sometimes complicated by an acute myelopathy; the authors have observed a number of such cases, and Killen and Foster reviewed 43 examples of this accident. The most striking examples, fortunately rare, are now observed as complications of vertebral angiography, resulting in high cervical infarction. The onset of sensorimotor paralysis is immediate, and the effects are often permanent. The syndrome of painful segmental spasms, spinal myoclonus, and rigidity, mentioned above, has also been observed under these conditions. Vascular spasm and occlusion result in infarct necrosis. The frequency of this complication was greatly reduced by the introduction of less toxic contrast media.

Treatment of all forms of spinal cord infarction can only be symptomatic, with attention during the acute stage to the care of bladder, bowel, and skin; after 10 to 14 days, more active rehabilitation measures can be started. Whether the acute effects of infarction can be modified by high-dose corticosteroids or heparinization is not known but seems unlikely.

Vascular Anomalies and Hemorrhage of the Spinal Cord and Spinal Canal

Hemorrhage into the spinal cord is rare, compared with the frequency of cerebral hemorrhage. The apoplectic onset of symptoms that involve tracts (motor, sensory, or both) in the spinal cord, associated with blood and xanthochromia in the spinal fluid, are the identifying features of hematomyelia. Aside from trauma, *hematomyelia is usually traceable to a vascular malformation or a bleeding disease and particularly to the administration of anticoagulants.* The same causes may underlie bleeding into the epidural or subdural space and give rise to a rapidly evolving compressive myelopathy. In some cases, as in those of Leech and coworkers, one cannot ascertain the source of the bleeding, even at autopsy. Epidural or subdural bleeding, like epidural abscess, represents a neurologic emergency and calls for immediate radiologic localization and surgical evacuation. Actually, most vascular malformations of the spinal cord do not cause hemorrhage, but instead produce a progressive, presumably ischemic myelopathy, as described below.

Advances in the techniques of selective spinal angiography and microsurgery have permitted the visualization and treatment of vascular lesions with a precision not imaginable a few decades ago. These angiographic procedures make it possible to distinguish among the several types of vascular malformations, arteriovenous fistulas, and hemangioblastomas and to localize them accurately to the spinal cord, epidural or subdural space, or vertebral bodies.

Vascular Malformations of the Spinal Cord and Overlying Dura These are well-known lesions, occurring not infrequently and causing both ischemic and hemorrhagic lesions. Some are arteriovenous malformations (AVM) and others more limited fistulas, the distinctions being the size of the nidus of communication between an artery and a vein and the size and location of feeding and draining vessels. The classification of spinal AVMs has been confusing, in part because the enlarged draining veins by which the lesions were identified pathologically are probably a secondary feature. The most useful categorization reflects the appearance and location of the malformation by angiography and by surgical examination. We divide these malformations into three groups: (1) true arteriovenous malformations that may be strictly intramedullary or involve the meninges and surrounding structures such as the vertebral bodies; (2) a variety of intradural perimedullary fistulas; and (3) purely dural fistulas. There is not sufficient pathologic material to determine whether these represent distinct pathologic entities or simply differing degrees and configurations of a common developmental process.

The true AVM, previously referred to as *angioma racemosum venosum or dorsal extramedullary arteriovenous malformation*, is typically located on the dorsal surface of the lower half of the spinal cord and occurs most often in middle-aged and elderly men (23 of 25 of Logue's cases were male). However, this lesion may occur at any age and at any location in the cord. In only a few cases has there been an associated dermatomal nevus. The clinical picture has been well described by Wyburn-Mason. Acute cramp-like, lancinating pain, sometimes in a sciatic distribution, is often a prominent early feature. It may occur in a series of episodes over a period of several days or weeks; sometimes it is worse in recumbency. Almost always it is associated with weakness or paralysis of one or both legs and numbness and paresthesias in the same distribution. Wasting and weakness of the legs may introduce the disease in some instances, with uneven progression, sometimes in a series of abrupt episodes. Severe disability of gait is usually present within 6 months, and half of the patients described by Aminoff and Logue were chair-bound within 3 years; the average survival in the past was 5 to 6 years, but the disorder has rarely been fatal in our patients. These lesions infrequently give rise to intramedullary or subarachnoid hemorrhage.

As mentioned, when viewed pathologically, the dorsal surface of the lower cord may be covered with a tangle of veins, some involving roots and penetrating the surface of the cord. The progression of symptoms is due presumably to the chronic venous hypertension and secondary intramedullary ischemic changes, and the abrupt episodes of worsening have been attributed to the thrombosis of vessels. However, angiographic studies sometimes show only a single or a few such dilated draining vessels. Furthermore, there is not sufficient pathologic material to determine whether some of the more prominent venous anomalies represent true venous angiomas (probably they do not). These lesions rarely bleed.

Increasingly, it has been recognized that arteriovenous fistulas that lie *within the dura* overlying the spinal cord or at times at a distance from the cord are capable of causing a myelopathy, sometimes several segments distant from the malformation. The majority of spinal AVMs that we have encountered are of this dural type, usually in the region of the low thoracic cord or the conus and with a limited venous draining system. Some appear to be situated in a dural root sleeve and to drain into the normal perimedullary coronal venous plexus. The clinical effects are also subacute and saltatory in evolution, sometimes painless, although most of our patients have had a spinal ache or sciatica. A claudicatory syndrome has been reported. These lesions bleed only rarely.

The third type, a pial fistulous arteriovenous communication that involves the superficial aspect of the cord to a variable extent, is the least frequent. In contrast to dorsal arteriovenous malformations, these fistulas tend to involve the lower thoracic and upper lumbar segments or the anterior parts of the cervical enlargement. The patients are often younger, and the sexes are equally affected. The clinical syndrome may also take the form of slow spinal cord compression, sometimes with a sudden exacerbation; or the initial symptoms may be apoplectic in nature, due to either thrombosis of a vessel or a hemorrhage from an associated draining vein that dilates to aneurysmal size and bleeds into the subarachnoid space or cord (hematomyelia and subarachnoid hemorrhage); the latter complication occurred in 7 of 30 cases reported by Wyburn-Mason.

Any of these lesions, dural or intradural, may be revealed on CT myelography or MRI by the presence of one or more fortuitously discovered enlarged and serpiginous draining vessels in the subarachnoid space; just as often, they are not visualized by these methods. The diagnosis is established through selective angiography, which shows the fistula in the dura overlying the cord or on the surface of the cord itself, but the most conspicuous finding is often the associated early draining vein (Fig. 44-6). As with other spinal cord malformations, demonstration of the fistula may require the painstaking injection of feeding vessels at numerous levels above and below the suspected lesion, since the main vessel of

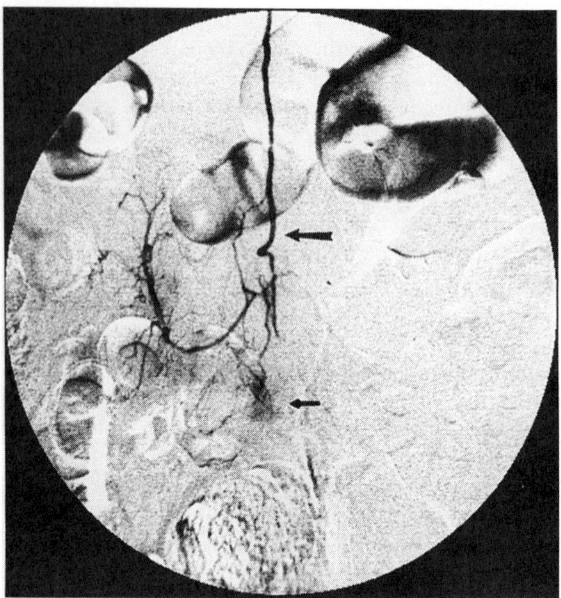

Figure 44-6

Angiographic injection of a low lumbar radicular vessel demonstrating a vascular blush of a fistula in the dura overlying the lumbar cord (small arrow) and a prominent early draining vein (large arrow), which was barely seen on a CT myelogram and was not seen on MRI. This dural arteriovenous malformation caused a subacute myelopathy involving the lumbosacral cord.

origin is often some distance away from the malformation. Also, blood flow through the nidus may be so rapid and brief that it is missed. In rare instances the fistula or high-flow arteriovenous malformation lies well outside the cord—for example, in the kidney—and gives rise to a similar myelopathy, presumably by raising venous pressures within the cord. A comparable lesion may exist in the cranial dura (page 900).

In the *Klippel-Trenaunay-Weber syndrome*, a vascular malformation of the spinal cord is associated with a cutaneous vascular nevus; when the malformation lies in the low cervical region, there may be enlargement of finger, hand, or arm (the hemangiectatic hypertrophy of Parkes Weber). Spinal segmental and tract lesions may occur at any age, but three of our patients were young adults. Vascular occlusion or hemorrhage was responsible. Some of these vascular lesions have been treated by defining and ligating their feeding vessels. In a few reported cases it has been possible to extirpate the entire lesion, especially if it occupied the surface of the cord.

Other vascular anomalies of the spinal cord include *aneurysm of a spinal artery with coarctation of the aorta* (rare) and *telangiectasia*, which may or may not be associated with the hereditary hemorrhagic type of Osler-Rendu-Weber. The authors have had under their care over the years several patients with the latter disease who developed acute hemorrhagic lesions of the spinal cord. Also, we have observed several *cavernous hemangiomas of the spinal cord.* In two of our cases, an angiographically negative solitary cavernous angioma had been the source of an acute partial transverse myelopathy. The lesions were clearly demonstrable only in the T2-weighted MR images. McCormick and associates have reported similar cases. Characteristically, the cord lesions cause partial syndromes and are followed by considerable recovery of function. There may or may not be blood in the CSF. Rarely, the same disease is responsible for one or more hemorrhagic lesions of the brain. The association of cavernous angiomas with arteriovenous fistulas of the lung is a rare finding, and the latter may be a source of brain abscess. In *coarctation of the aorta*, the circulation to the lower part of the spinal cord may be deficient, with resultant paresis of the legs, sensory loss, and sphincteric impairment. Or there may be intracranial subarachnoid hemorrhage from a ruptured saccular aneurysm.

Treatment By occluding the feeding artery, which is often single, and eliminating the pressure in veins, the course of disease can be arrested and pain reduced (Symon et al). In most of our cases, there has been postoperative improvement in the neurologic state over a few weeks or months. In cases of the racemose AVMs, stripping the enlarged veins along the dorsal cord is no longer considered necessary and may be dangerous. Alternatively, one may obliterate a fistula or an AVM that is limited in size by the use of endovascular techniques, using special catheters and one of a number of types of embolic particles. The procedure is long and painstaking, for the radiologist must identify and embolize all the feeding vessels of the malformation; general anesthesia is utilized in most cases. This approach has certain drawbacks; recanalization occurs in many instances, as does distal occlusion of the venous drainage system. For these reasons, surgical ligation of the arterial supply is still preferred for larger AVMs as the initial procedure. Some surgeons advise a staged approach in which the size of the malformation is first reduced by endovascular techniques. This makes the surgery less complicated. Intradural fistulas are usually treated by endovascular methods. Interventional radiologic techniques have also been used to advantage in the intramedullary malformations, either as the sole treatment or in combination with surgery. The results of focused radiation have been difficult to evaluate, since most series are too small to judge its effectiveness.

Fibrocartilaginous Embolism

In 1961, Naiman and coworkers described the case of an adolescent boy who died of sudden paralysis after an athletic injury and was found to have extensive myelomalacia, due to numerous occlusions of spinal vessels by emboli of nucleus pulposus. Many more such cases have now been observed. Bots and colleagues encountered three cases in one year, and we regularly see one or two such cases each year. The clinical picture is essentially one of spinal apoplexy—the patient experiences the abrupt onset of pain in the back or neck, accompanied by the signs of a transverse cord lesion affecting all sensory, motor, and sphincteric functions and evolving over a period of a few minutes to an hour or more. Occasionally, the syndrome spares the posterior columns thus simulating an anterior spinal artery occlusion. The CSF is normal.

In some of the reported instances the patient had not engaged in excessive activity at the time of onset of spinal cord symptoms. However, this has not been true of our patients, who had been participating in some strenuous activity earlier in the day. A few had fallen and injured themselves on the day of the illness or on preceding days; a direct blow to the back, as occurs during contact athletic sports, was a preceding event in several others. Survival has ranged from hours to months, and some patients survived indefinitely.

At autopsy numerous small arteries and veins within the spinal cord are occluded by typical fibrocartilage, with infarct necrosis of the spinal cord. A ruptured disc of the usual type was not found to be evident in these patients, but high-resolution radiographs in a few of them showed a discontinuity of the cortical bone of the vertebral body adjacent to a collapsed disc and herniation of disc tissue into a vertebral body. A reasonable explanation suggested by Yogananden and colleagues is that the high intravertebral pressure forces the nucleus pulposus material into venules and arteries of the marrow of the vertebral body, thence into radicular vessels. This unique lesion can sometimes be diagnosed during life by clinical data and MRI of the vertebrae and spinal cord (Tosi et al). It has probably been overlooked in many cases of acute ischemic myelopathy.

Caisson Disease

Decompression sickness ("the bends"), observed in persons who are subjected to high underwater pressure, affects mainly the upper thoracic spinal cord as a result of nitrogen bubbles that are formed and trapped in spinal vessels. There may be little or no involvement of the brain. Haymaker, who has provided the most complete account of the neuropathologic changes, observed lesions of ischemic type mainly in the white matter of the upper thoracic cord; the posterior columns were more affected than lateral and anterior ones. We have encountered instances in which an almost complete transverse myelopathy was evident soon after the patient resurfaced but improved to some extent, leaving the patient with an asymmetrical and incomplete albeit permanent syndrome. The smallest degree of cord damage is probably a minor myelopathy that affects the anterior or the posterior funiculi, leaving either spasticity of the legs or numbness. Immediate treatment consists of recompression in a hyperbaric chamber; later treatment is symptomatic, with antispasticity drugs and physical therapy.

Spinal Subdural Hemorrhage

We have had experience with a few instances of spinal subdural hemorrhage that presented with excruciating thoracic back pain of such severity as to cause a bizarre, almost psychotic, reaction (Swann et al). The neck becomes slightly stiff and there may be a headache, suggesting subarachnoid hemorrhage. However, signs of a myelopathy do not appear, indicating that the bleeding is confined to the pliable subdural spaces surrounding the cord. This syndrome is rare and not readily recognized. Lumbar puncture yields dark yellow-brown spinal fluid. The color is imparted by methemoglobin and reflects the presence of adjacent, walled-off blood. Usually there are also some red blood cells in the CSF, suggesting seepage into the subarachnoid space from adjacent clot. CT myelography shows a subdural collection, with characteristically smooth borders; when drained operatively, this is found to be blood clot. Usually no vascular malformation is found and the cause remains obscure. Trauma or anticoagulation underlie a few cases. The symptoms resolve in 1 or 2 weeks, after removal of the subdural hematoma. Small collections may be managed without surgery, in which case corticosteroids may be helpful.

THE SYNDROME OF SUBACUTE OR CHRONIC SPINAL PARAPARESIS WITH OR WITHOUT ATAXIA

The gradual development of weakness of the legs is the common manifestation of several diseases of the spinal cord. A syndrome of this type—including ataxia of gait, beginning insidiously in late childhood or adolescence, and progressing steadily—is usually indicative of hereditary spinocerebellar degeneration (Friedreich ataxia) or one of its variants (see Chap. 39). In early adult life, MS is the most frequent cause and AIDS myelopathy is being increasingly recognized; syphilitic meningomyelitis is now quite uncommon. In middle and late adult life, cervical spondylosis, subacute combined degeneration of the cord (vitamin B_{12} deficiency), combined system degeneration of the non–pernicious anemia type, demyelinative myelopathy (MS), radiation myelopathy, tropical spastic paraplegia, spinal arachnoiditis, and spinal tumor, particularly meningioma, are the important diagnostic considerations. In most forms of subacute and chronic spinal cord disease, spastic paraparesis is much more prominent than posterior column ataxia (Friedreich ataxia and myelopathy due to vitamin B_{12} deficiency are notable exceptions).

Spinal Multiple Sclerosis (See also Chap. 36)

Ataxic paraparesis is among the most common manifestations of MS. Asymmetrical affection of the limbs and signs of cerebral, optic nerve, brainstem, and cerebellar involvement usually provide confirmatory diagnostic evidence. Nevertheless, purely spinal involvement may occur, no lesions being found outside the spinal cord even at autopsy. A frequent problem in diagnosis is posed by the older adult patient who is not known to have had MS in earlier life (previous episodes having been asymptomatic or forgotten). The secondary progressive stage in this group is thought to be consequent to recurrent demyelinative attacks. But there is another group in which slowly advancing neurologic deterioration represents the primary manifestation of the disease. The National Hospital Research Group examined 20 cases of the secondary progressive type and 20 of the primary type by gadolinium-enhanced MRI of the spinal cord and brain and found new lesions in only 3 of each group (Kidd et al). They suggest that the progression correlates better with progressive atrophy of the spinal cord than with recurrent demyelinative lesions. In both groups the clinical state must be differentiated from cervical disc disease, spondylosis, and tumor. As previously discussed, the main aids in diagnosis are the CSF findings (minor pleocytosis and oligoclonal IgG abnormalities), present in 70 to 90 percent of cases, the demonstration by evoked potential studies of lesions in the optic nerves or in the auditory and sensory tracts, and particularly MRI, which may disclose unsuspected white matter lesions in the spinal cord and brain.

Cervical Spondylosis with Myelopathy

It has been stated, correctly in our opinion, that this is the most frequently observed myelopathy in general practice. Basically a degenerative disease of the spine involving the lower and midcervical vertebrae, it narrows the spinal canal and intervertebral foramina and causes progressive injury of the spinal cord, roots, or both.

Historical Note Key, in 1838, probably gave the first description of a so-called spondylotic bar. In two cases of compressive myelopathy with paraplegia, he found "a projection of the intervertebral substance, or rather the posterior ligament of the spine, which was thickened and presented a firm ridge which had lessened the diameter of the canal by nearly a third. The ligament, where it passes over the posterior surface of the intervertebral substance, was found to be ossified." In 1892, Horsley performed a cervical laminectomy in such a patient; a "transverse ridge of bone" was found to be compressing the spinal cord at the level of the sixth cervical vertebra. Thereafter, operations were performed in many cases of this sort, and the tissues removed at operation were repeatedly misidentified as benign cartilaginous tumors or "chondromata." In 1928, Stookey described in detail the pathologic effects upon the spinal cord and roots of these "ventral extradural chondromas." Peet and Echols, in 1934, were probably the first to suggest that the so-called chondromata represented protrusions of intervertebral disc material. This idea gained wide credence after the publication, in the same year, of the classic article on ruptured intervertebral disc by Mixter and Barr. Although their names are usually associated with the lumbar disc syndrome, 4 of their original 19 cases were instances of cervical disc disease.

Also of historical importance is Gowers's original account, in 1892, of *vertebral exostoses*, in which he described osteophytes that protrude from the posterior surfaces of the vertebral bodies and encroach upon the spinal canal, causing slow compression of the cord as well as bony overgrowth in the intervertebral foramina, giving rise to radicular pain. Gowers correctly predicted that these lesions would offer a more promising field for the surgeon than other kinds of vertebral tumors.

For some reason, there was little awareness of the frequency and importance of spondylotic myelopathy for many years after these early observations had been made. All the interest was in the acute ruptured disc. Finally it was Russell Brain, in 1948, who put cervical spondylosis on the neurologic map, so to speak. He drew a distinction between acute rupture and protrusion of the cervical disc (often traumatic and more likely to compress the nerve roots than the spinal cord) and chronic spinal cord and root compression consequent upon disc degeneration and associated osteophytic outgrowths (*hard disc*) as well as changes in the surrounding joints and ligaments. In 1957, Payne and Spillane documented the importance of a smaller-than-normal spinal canal in the genesis of myelopathy in patients with cervical spondylosis. These reports were followed by a spate of articles on the subject (see Wilkinson). Rowland's review of the natural history of cervical spondylosis and the results of surgical therapy is a useful modern reference, as is that of Uttley and Monro.

Symptomatology In outline, the characteristic syndrome consists of varying combinations of the following tetrad: (1) painful, stiff neck; (2) pain in the neck, shoulders, and upper arms (brachialgia) that may be aching or radicular (sharp and radiating); (3); spastic leg weakness with Babinski signs and unsteadiness of gait; and (4) numbness and paresthesias. The latter symptoms typically involve the distal limbs, especially the hands, but are infrequently the earliest symptoms. Variations of these symptoms are elaborated below. Each of the components may occur separately, or they may occur in several combinations and sequences.

With reference to the first of these symptoms, in any sizable group of patients beyond 50 years of age, about 40 percent will be found to have some clinical abnormality of the neck, usually crepitus or pain, with restriction of lateral flexion and rotation (less often of extension). Pallis and colleagues, in a survey of 50 patients, all of them over 50 years of age and none with neurologic complaints, found that 75 percent showed radiologic evidence of narrowing of the cervical spinal canal due to osteophytosis of the posterior vertebral bodies or to narrowing of the intervertebral foramina due to osteoarthropathy at the apophyseal joints; thickening of the ligaments (both the ligamentum flavum posteriorly and the posterior longitudinal ligament anteriorly) adds to the narrowing of the canal. About half of the patients with radiologic abnormalities showed physical signs of root or cord involvement (changes in the tendon reflexes in the arms, briskness of reflexes and impairment of vibratory sense in the legs, and sometimes Babinski signs). The occasional finding of a Babinski sign in older individuals who had never had a stroke or complained of neurologic symptoms may be explained by an otherwise silent cervical osteophyte (Savitsky and Madonick).

In patients with only shoulder and arm symptoms as well as those in whom these symptoms are combined with a disorder of the legs, pain is the most frequent symptom. It is centered in the back of the neck, often radiating to an area above the scapula. When brachialgia is also present, it takes several forms: a stabbing pain in the pre- or postaxial border of the limb, extending to the elbow, wrist, or fingers; or a persistent dull ache in the forearm or wrist, sometimes with a burning sensation. Discomfort may be elicited by coughing, Valsalva maneuver, or neck extension, or neck flexion may induce electrical feelings down the spine (Lhermitte symptom). Rarely, the pain is referred substernally. Some patients also complain of numbness or paresthesias, most often in one or two digits, a part of the palm, or a longitudinal band along the forearm. Frequently, patients describe their fingers and hands as feeling constantly swollen. Slight clumsiness or weakness of a hand is another complaint.

The biceps and brachioradial reflexes may be depressed, sometimes in association with an increase in the triceps and finger reflexes. The hand or forearm muscles, if chronically weakened, undergo slight atrophy. In some cases, the atrophy of hand muscles is severe. Interestingly, in such cases, the spondylotic compression, as judged by CT myelography, may be confined to the high cervical cord. In patients with sensory loss, pain and thermal sensation often appear to be affected more than tactile sense.

The third part of the typical syndrome, spastic legs from a compressive myelopathy, most often presents as a complaint of weakness of a leg and slight unsteadiness of gait. The whole leg or the quadriceps feels stiff and heavy and gives out quickly after exercise. Mobility of the ankle may be reduced, and the advancing toe of the shoe scrapes the floor. On examination, spasticity is more evident than weakness, and the tendon reflexes are increased (ankle jerks may not share in this change in the elderly). Although the patient may believe that only one leg is affected, it is commonly found that both plantar reflexes are extensor, the one on the side of the stiffer leg being more clearly so. Less often both legs are equally affected. As the compression continues, walking becomes unsteady because of the addition of sensory ataxia.

As to the sensory disorders (which may occasionally be absent), numbness, tingling, and prickling of the hands and soles of the feet and around the ankles are the most frequent complaints. We have seen a few patients in whom paresthesias in the distal limbs and trunk were present for months before any indication of motor involvement; in advanced cases there may be a vague sensory level just above the clavicles. Impaired vibratory sensation and diminished position sense in the toes and feet (all indicative of a lesion of the posterior columns) as well as the Romberg sign are the most conspicuous sensory findings. This imparts a "tabetic" unsteadiness to the gait. These sensory defects tend also to be asymmetrical. Rarely the sensorimotor pattern takes the form of a Brown-Séquard syndrome. Infrequently, paresthesias and dysesthesias in the lower extremities and trunk may be the principal symptoms; far less often there are sensory complaints on the face, ostensibly corresponding to compression of the trigeminal sensory tract in the upper cervical cord.

As the myelopathy progresses, sometimes intermittently, both legs become weaker and more spastic. Sphincteric control may then be altered; slight hesitancy or precipitancy of micturition are the usual complaints; frank incontinence is infrequent. In the more advanced form of this condition, walking requires the aid of a cane or canes or a walker; in some cases all locomotion ultimately becomes impossible, especially in the elderly patient. Abrupt worsening, even paraplegia or quadriplegia, may follow forceful flexion or extension injuries of the neck, as indicated below.

Pathologic Changes The fundamental lesion is a fraying of the annulus fibrosus, with extrusion of disc material into the spinal canal. The disc becomes covered with fibrous tissue or partly calcified. Another common lesion is bulging of the annulus without extrusion of nuclear material; this may also be associated with the formation of osteophytes and transverse bony ridges. The latter changes, unlike ruptured discs that occur mainly at the C5-6 or C6-7 interspace, often involve higher interspaces and occur at several levels. The adjacent dura mater may be thickened and adherent to the posterior longitudinal ligament. The underlying pia-arachnoid is also thickened and the adjacent ligamentous hypertrophy may contribute to compression of the cord or the nerve roots. This series of pathologic changes is frequently ascribed to hypertrophic osteoarthritis. However, in lesser degree, the osteophyte formation and ridging are so frequently observed in patients who have no other signs of arthritic disease that this explanation is surely incorrect. Subclinical trauma is far more likely, in the authors' opinion.

When a root is compressed by osteophytic overgrowth, the dural sleeve is thickened and occluded and the root fibers are damaged. Usually the fifth, sixth, or seventh cervical roots are affected in this way, both the anterior and posterior or only the anterior, on one or both sides. A small neuroma may appear proximal to the site of anterior root compression.

The dura is ridged and the underlying spinal cord is flattened. The root lesions may lead to secondary wedge-shaped areas of degeneration in the lateral parts of the posterior columns at higher levels. The most marked changes in the spinal cord are at the level(s) of compression. There may be zones of demyelination or focal necrosis at the points of attachment of the dentate ligaments (which tether the spinal cord to the dura) and zones of necrosis in the posterior and lateral columns as well as loss of nerve cells. The latter lesions, often asymmetrical, are attributed by Hughes to ischemia.

Pathogenesis The particular vulnerability of the lower cervical spine to degenerative change has no ready explanation. Most likely it is related in some way to the high degree of mobility of the lower cervical vertebrae, which is accentuated by their situation next to the relatively immobile thoracic spine.

The mechanism of spinal cord injury would seem to be one of simple compression and ischemia. When the spinal canal is diminished in its anteroposterior dimension at one or several points, the space available for the spinal cord is insufficient. However, the presence and degree of cord injury correlate inexactly with the anteroposterior dimensions of the spinal canal, since there is considerable variability in the diameter from individual to individual. The range of narrowing that produces symptomatic cervical spondylosis is from 7 to 12 mm (normal, 17 to 18 mm). One must consider, therefore, several additional mechanisms by which the cord might be damaged. The effects of the natural motions of the spinal cord during flexion and extension of the neck are probably important in this respect. Adams and Logue confirmed the observation of O'Connell that, during full flexion and extension of the neck, the cervical cord and dura move up and down. The spinal cord is literally dragged over protruding osteophytes and hypertrophied ligaments; conceivably it is this type of intermittent trauma that progressively injures the spinal cord. It has also been shown that the spinal cord, displaced posteriorly by osteophytes, will be compressed by the infolding ligamentum flavum each time the neck is extended

(Stoltmann and Blackwood). Segmental ischemic necrosis resulting from intermittent compression of spinal arteries or from compression (possibly spasm) of the anterior spinal artery has also been postulated. Most neuropathologists favor the idea of intermittent cord compression between osteophytes anteriorly and ligamentum flavum posteriorly, with an added vascular element accounting for the scattered lesions deep in the cord. Trauma from sudden extreme extension, as in a fall, severe whiplash injury, or chiropractic manipulation, or from a lesser degree of retraction of the head during myelography, tooth extraction, or a tonsillectomy may be an additional factor, particularly in patients with congenitally narrow canals.

Diagnosis When pain and stiffness in the neck, brachialgia, and sensorimotor-reflex changes in the arms are combined with signs of myelopathy, there is little difficulty in diagnosis. When the neck and arm changes are inconspicuous or absent, the diagnosis becomes more difficult. The myelopathy must then be distinguished from the late, progressive form of spinal MS. Since posterior vertebral osteophytes and other bony alterations are frequent in the sixth and seventh decades, the question that must be answered in any given case is whether the vertebral changes are related to the neurologic abnormality. The finding of some degree of sensorimotor or reflex change corresponding only to the level of the spinal abnormalities is a point that always favors spondylotic myelopathy. A lack of such corresponding changes and the presence of oligoclonal bands and signs of lesions in the optic nerves and brain argue for demyelinative myelopathy. Both MRI and CT myelography become critical in such cases (Fig. 44-7). The MRI tends to overestimate the degree of cord compression by an osteophyte, but clear deformation of the cord into the shape of a bean, obliteration of the surrounding CSF spaces and the signal due to fat surrounding the cord, and T2 signal changes within the cord all support the diagnosis. Contrast myelography with the patient supine and lateral views taken during flexion and extension of the neck are also useful diagnostic procedures. There should be flattening of the cord and considerable encroachment on the CSF space at that level, not simply an impingement or slight deformation of the normal oval shape of the cord.

It is said that spondylotic myelopathy may simulate amyotrophic lateral sclerosis (amyotrophy of arms and spastic weakness of the legs). This has seldom been a diagnostic problem in our experience. We have observed only a few patients with spondylotic myelopathy who exhibited an absolutely pure motor syndrome, i.e., one in which there was no cervical or brachial pain and no sensory symptoms in the arms or impairment of vibratory or position sense in the legs. A pure spastic paraparesis is more likely to be a manifestation of MS, hereditary spastic paraplegia, motor neuron disease

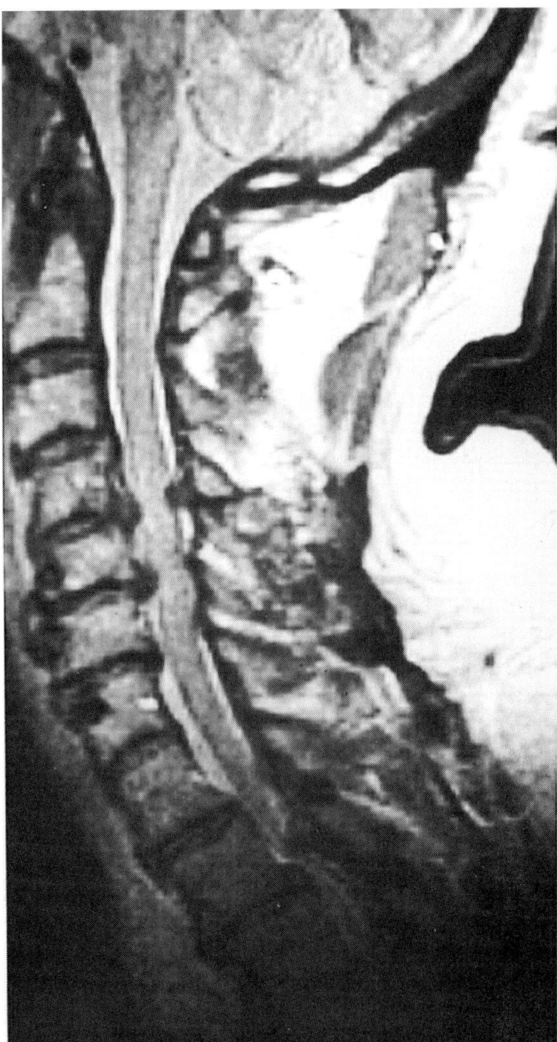

Figure 44-7

MRI in a patient with symptomatic cervical spondylosis. The spinal cord at C4-5 and C5-6 is flattened on its ventral surface by spondylotic bars and on its posterior surface by ligamentous hypertrophy. Axial images are required to confirm that the cord is truly compressed and that the subarachnoid space is nearly or completely obliterated.

(primary lateral sclerosis), HTLV-I myelopathy, or the carrier state of adrenoleukodystrophy.

When imbalance, both perceived by the patient and observed in tests of walking, is a major symptom, spondylosis must be differentiated from a number of acquired large-fiber polyneuropathies, particularly inflammatory or immune types and the more benign sensory neuropathy of the aged (see page 1414). Loss of tactile sensation in the feet and loss of tendon reflexes are characteristic of the latter; examination of the tendon reflexes distinguishes the two. Subacute combined degeneration of the spinal cord due to vitamin B_{12} deficiency, combined system disease of the non–pernicious anemia type, AIDS and HTLV-I myelopathy, ossification of the posterior longitudinal ligament, and spinal cord tumor (discussed further on) are usually listed among the conditions that might be confused with spondylotic myelopathy. Adherence to the diagnostic criteria for each of these disorders and scrutiny of the radiologic studies should eliminate the possibility of error in most instances. The gait abnormality produced by spondylotic myelopathy may be mistaken for that of normal-pressure hydrocephalus; a marked increase of imbalance with removal of visual cues (Romberg sign) is a feature of spondylosis but not of hydrocephalus.

The special problems of spondylotic radiculopathy are discussed on pages 224 and 227.

Treatment The slow, intermittently progressive course of cervical myelopathy with long periods of relatively unchanging symptomatology makes it difficult to evaluate therapy. Assuming that the prevailing opinion of the mechanisms of the cord and root injury is correct, the use of a soft collar to restrict anteroposterior motions of the neck seems reasonable. This form of treatment alone may be sufficient to control the discomfort in the neck and arms. Only exceptionally in our experience has arm and shoulder pain alone been sufficiently severe and persistent to require radicular decompression unless there is a laterally protruded disc.

Many of our patients have been dissatisfied with this passive approach and dislike or refuse to wear a collar for prolonged periods. If posterior osteophytes have narrowed the spinal canal at several interspaces, a posterior decompressive laminectomy with severance of the dentate ligaments helps to prevent further injury. The results of such a procedure are fairly satisfactory (Epstein and Epstein); in fully two-thirds of the patients, improvement in the function of the legs occurs, and in most of the others, progression of the myelopathy is halted. The operation carries some risk; rarely, an acute quadriplegia—due, presumably, to manipulation of the spinal cord and damage to nutrient spinal arteries—has followed the surgical procedure. When one or two interspaces are the site of osteophytic overgrowths, their removal by an anterior approach has given better results and carries less risk. The surgical methods and their relative advantages are reviewed by Braakman.

However, the long-term results after surgical treatment are less than satisfactory. Ebersold and colleagues evaluated the outcome in 84 patients in whom the median duration of follow-up was 7 years. In the group of 33 patients who had undergone anterior decompressive procedures, 18 had improved, 9 were unchanged, and 6 had deteriorated. Of the 51 patients who underwent posterior decompression, 19 had improved, 13 were unchanged, and 19 were worse at their last follow-up examinations. These results, similar to those of most other series, indicate that the long-term outcome is variable and that a significant proportion, even after adequate decompression and initial improvement, have persistent symptoms or undergo later functional deterioration.

Lumbar Stenosis This is another spondylotic abnormality, seen with particular frequency in older individuals, particularly men. Usually it declares itself by numbness and weakness of the legs, sometime with poor control of sphincters. There is generally no pain or only a spine ache that fluctuates from day to day. A notable feature is induction or aggravation of the neurologic symptoms upon standing and walking (neurologic claudication). See page 218 for further discussion.

Ankylosing Spondylitis This rheumatologic condition of the spine is due to inflammation at the sites of ligamentous insertions into bone that leads to an intense calcification at these and adjacent sites. The sacroiliac joints and lumbar spine are most affected, as discussed on page 220, but as the disease advances, the entire spine becomes fused and rigid. The biomechanics of the rigid spine make it susceptible to fracture. The most common complication is a spinal stenosis and cauda equina syndrome. Bartleson and associates described 14 patients (and referred to 30 others in the medical literature) who, years after the onset of spondylitis, developed sensory, motor, reflex, and sphincteric disorders referable to L4, L5, and the sacral roots. Surprisingly, the spinal canal was not narrowed and the caudal sac was actually dilated. Confavreux et al have presented evidence that enlargement of the lumbar dural sac is due to a defect in resorption of the CSF. There are usually arachnoidal diverticulae of the posterior root sleeves, but no other explanation can be given for the radicular symptoms and signs, which can be verified by electromyography. Surgical decompression has not benefited the patients, nor has corticosteroid therapy. This condition occasionally occurs at higher levels and gives rise to a myelopathy. We have observed similar symptoms in the cervical region and also with root-sleeve diverticulae.

The most hazardous complication of ankylosing spondylitis is compression of the cord itself, in which a seemingly minor trauma has resulted in fracture-dislocation. Fox and colleagues from the Mayo Clinic treated 31 such instances in a 5-year period; the majority of unstable fractures that required surgical fixation were in the cervical region, and several patients had fracture-dislocations at two levels. The instability at the upper spinal levels may be difficult to detect radiologically, and caution should be observed in allowing patients to resume full activity after a neck injury if the cervical spine is seen to be involved by spondylitis. Careful flexion and extension x-ray views usually but not always demonstrate the instability.

Multiple arachnoid cysts in the thoracic or lumbar region have been associated with a spinal cord syndrome in ankylosing spondylitis and in *Marfan disease*.

Ossification of the Posterior Longitudinal Ligament (OPLL) Compressive cervical myelopathy due to this process occurs almost exclusively in patients of Japanese extraction and has been demonstrated to us by colleagues in Hawaii. The clinical signs are much the same as those of cervical spondylosis, but the radiologic appearance is unique. The ligamentous calcification can be seen on plain films, CT scan, and MRI, and may be mistaken for spondylotic change. The ossified areas may enlarge to form bone marrow. Laminoplasty with enlargement of the spinal canal has been successful.

Paget Disease (Osteitis Deformans) Enlargement of the vertebral bodies, pedicles, and laminae in Paget disease may result in narrowing of the spinal canal. The clinical picture is one of spinal cord compression. Plasma alkaline phosphatase concentrations are high, and the typical bone changes are seen in radiographs. Usually several adjacent vertebrae of the thoracic spine are affected. Other parts of the skeleton are also involved (see below), which facilitates diagnosis. Posterior surgical decompression, leaving the pedicles intact, is indicated if there is sufficient stability of the vertebral bodies to prevent collapse. Medical management includes the use of nonsteroidal anti-inflammatory drugs for persistent pain; calcitonin to reduce pain and plasma levels of alkaline phosphatase; and cytotoxic drugs such as plicamycin and etidronate disodium to reduce bone resorption (see Singer and Krane).

Other Spinal Abnormalities with Myelopathy

The spinal cord is obviously vulnerable to any vertebral maldevelopment or disease that encroaches upon the spinal canal or compresses its nutrient arteries. Some of the common ones are listed below.

Anomalies at the Craniocervical Junction Of these, congenital *fusion of the atlas and foramen magnum* is the most common. McCrae, who described the radiologic features of more than 100 patients with bony abnormalities at the craniocervical junction, found a partial or complete bony union of the atlas and foramen magnum in 28 cases. He noted also that whenever the anteroposterior diameter of the canal behind the odontoid process was less than 19 mm, there were signs of spinal cord compression. Fusion of the second and third cervical vertebrae is a common anomaly as well but does not seem to be of clinical significance.

Abnormalities of the Odontoid Process These were found in 17 cases of McCrae's series. There may be complete separation of the odontoid from the axis or chronic *atlantoaxial dislocation* (atlas displaced anteriorly in relation to the axis). These abnormalities may be congenital or the result of injury and are known causes of acute or chronic spinal cord compression and stiffness of the neck.

Rheumatoid arthritis is another cause of atlanto-axial dislocation. The ligaments that attach the odontoid to the atlas and to the skull and the joint tissue are weakened by the destructive inflammatory process. The subsequent dislocation of the atlas on the axis may remain mobile or become fixed and give rise to an intermittent or persistent mild to moderate paraparesis or quadriparesis. Similar effects may result from a forward subluxation of C4 on C5 (see Nakano et al). Atlantoaxial dislocation is known to be a cause of collapse and sudden death. If the upper cervical cord is compressed, the odontoid process must be removed and C1–C2 decompressed and stabilized.

In all the congenital anomalies of the foramen magnum and the upper cervical spine there is a high incidence of syringomeylia. McCrae found that 38 percent of all patients with syringomyelia and syringobulbia showed such bony anomalies. All patients whose symptoms might be explained by a lesion in the cervicocranial region (particularly patients in whom multiple sclerosis and foramen magnum tumor are suspected) require careful radiologic examination.

In mucopolysaccharidosis IV, or the Morquio syndrome (page 1016), a typical feature is the absence or severe hypoplasia of the odontoid process. This abnormality, combined with laxity or redundancy of the surrounding ligaments, results in atlantoaxial subluxation and compression of the spinal cord. Affected children refuse to walk or develop spastic weakness of the limbs. Early in life they excrete an excess of keratan sulfate (Chap. 37), but this may no longer be detectable in adult life. In certain of the mucopolysaccharidoses, we have also seen a true pachymeningiopathy—great thickening of the dura in the basal cisterns and high cervical region with spinal cord compression. Surgical decompression and spinal immobilization may be curative.

Achondroplasia This dominantly inherited form of dwarfism is due to a mutant gene on chromosome 4, which causes a failure of conversion of fetal cartilage to bone at the growth plate. It occasionally results in great thickening of the vertebral bodies, neural arches, laminae, and pedicles because of increased periosteal bone formation. The spinal canal is narrowed in the thoracolumbar region, often with kyphosis, leading sometimes to a progressive spinal cord or cauda equina syndrome. Another neurologic complication, which results from a small foramen magnum, is hydrocephalus (internal, with large ventricles, or external, with widened subarachnoid spaces). In young children, a syndrome of central apnea and spasticity of the legs is characteristic. These complications may require ventricular shunting. Narrowing of the lumbar canal tends to present later in life.

Platybasia and Basilar Invagination *Platybasia* refers to a flattening of the base of the skull (the angle formed by intersection of the plane of the clivus and the plane of the anterior fossa is greater than 135 degrees). *Basilar impression* or *invagination* has a somewhat different meaning—namely, an upward bulging of the occipital condyles; if the condyles, which bear the thrust of the spine, are displaced above the plane of the foramen magnum, basilar invagination is present. Each of these abnormalities may be congenital or acquired (as in Paget disease); frequently they are combined. They give rise to a characteristic shortness of the neck and a combination of cerebellar and spinal signs. A normal-pressure hydrocephalus may also develop.

Tethered Cord This developmental anomaly is discussed fully in Chap. 38. A progressive cauda equina syndrome with prominent urinary difficulties, and varying degrees of spasticity are the usual presentations.

Syphilitic Meningomyelitis

Here, as in MS, the degree of ataxia and spastic weakness is variable. A few patients have an almost pure state of spastic weakness of the legs, requiring differentiation from motor system disease and familial spastic paraplegia. Such a syndrome, formerly called Erb's spastic paraplegia and attributed to meningovascular syphilis, is now recognized as being nonspecific. In a minority of patients, sensory ataxia and other posterior column signs predominate, and ventral roots are involved in the chronic meningeal inflammation. There may be signs of segmental amyotrophy, hence the term *syphilitic amyotrophy of the upper extremities with spastic paraplegia*. Confirmation of this diagnosis depends on finding a lymphocytic pleocytosis, an elevated protein and gamma globulin, and a positive serologic reaction in the CSF. Other aspects of this disease and treatment are discussed on page 767.

Subacute Combined Degeneration of the Spinal Cord (SCD)

This form of spinal cord disease is due to vitamin B_{12} deficiency and is fully described in Chap. 41. Almost invariably it begins with bilateral symptoms and signs of posterior column involvement, which, if untreated, is followed within a matter of several weeks or months by spastic paraparesis due to affection of the corticospinal tracts. Of particular importance is the fact that SCD is a treatable disease and that the degree of reversibility is dependent upon the duration of symptoms before specific treatment is begun. There is a premium, therefore, on early diagnosis.

Combined System Disease of Non–Pernicious Anemia Type

This term refers to an intrinsic degenerative disease of the spinal cord, somewhat more common than SCD and affecting the posterior and lateral columns (in this sense, *a combined system disease*). There is no association with vitamin B_{12} or folate deficiency. In this syndrome, in distinction to SCD, signs of corticospinal tract disease usually precede those of the posterior columns and are more prominent throughout the illness, which is slowly and chronically progressive. Little is known of its pathologic basis or cause.

Progressive spastic or spastic-ataxic paraparesis of a chronic, irreversible type may also develop in conjunction with chronic, decompensated liver disease (page 1185); with AIDS; in certain cases of adrenoleukodystrophy, particularly in the symptomatic heterozygote, i.e., the female carrier (page 1035); in tropical spastic paraplegia (HTLV-I); in radiation myelopathy; and in adhesive spinal arachnoiditis, which is discussed below.

Spinal Arachnoiditis (Chronic Adhesive Arachnoiditis)

This is a relatively uncommon spinal cord disorder that was introduced in relation to the subject of low back pain (page 219). It is characterized clinically by a combination of root and spinal cord symptoms that may mimic intraspinal tumor. Pathologically there is opacification and thickening of the arachnoidal membranes and adhesions between the arachnoid and dura—the result of proliferation of connective tissue. The subarachnoid space is unevenly obliterated. In this sense, the term *arachnoiditis* is not entirely appropriate, although it seems likely that the connective tissue overgrowth is a reaction to an antecedent arachnoidal inflammation. Some forms of arachnoiditis can be traced to syphilis or to a subacute, therapeutically resistant meningitis of another type. Still others have followed the introduction of a variety of substances, most no longer used, into the subarachnoid space for diagnostic or therapeutic purposes. These include penicillin and other antibiotics, iophendylate (Pantopaque) and other contrast media and corticosteroids. At one time, many examples of adhesive arachnoiditis were observed following spinal anesthesia, occurring soon afterward or after an interval of weeks, months, or even years. We observed more than 40 such cases. This complication was eventually traced to a detergent that had contaminated vials of procaine. If enough of the contaminant was injected, an areflexic paralysis of the legs and sphincters of bladder and bowel and sensory loss in the legs developed within a few days, along with considerable pain. More pernicious, however, was a delayed meningomyelopathy that developed within a few months to a few years, causing a spastic paralysis, sensory loss, and incontinence of sphincters. Still common is a restricted form of arachnoiditis that complicates a series of operations for lumbar discs (lumbar arachnoiditis). Less convincing are cases of arachnoiditis attributed to closed spinal injuries. In many cases no provocative factor can be recognized. A familial form has been reported by Duke and Hashimoto, but we have had no experience with it.

Clinical Manifestations Spinal arachnoiditis may occur at any age, although the highest incidence of onset of symptoms is between 40 and 60 years; it is rare below the age of 20. Symptoms may occur in close temporal relation to an acute arachnoidal inflammation or may be delayed for weeks, months, or even years. The commonest mode of onset is with pain in the distribution of one or more sensory nerve roots, first on one side, then on both, in the lumbofemoral regions. The pain has a burning, stinging, or aching quality and is persistent. Abnormalities of tendon reflexes are common, but weakness and atrophy, the results of damage to anterior roots, are less frequent findings and tend to occur in cases involving the cauda equina. In thoracic lesions, symptoms of root involvement may antedate those of cord compression by months or years. Sooner or later, however, there is involvement of the spinal cord, manifest by a slowly progressive spastic ataxia with sphincter disturbances.

The localized lumbar arachnoiditis associated with repeated disc surgery (the common variety being seen in chronic pain clinics) is characterized by back and or leg pain with other inconstant signs of radiculopathy (loss of tendon reflexes, weakness, and variable degrees of sensory loss), usually bilateral.

The CSF is abnormal during the acute stage in practically all cases of adhesive arachnoiditis. In some there is a moderate lymphocytic pleocytosis, occurring soon after the inciting event, but the striking finding is a partial or complete obliteration of the spinal subarachnoid space, sometimes extreme in degree. In the localized lumbar arachnoiditis, referred to above, the CSF may be normal or show only a slight increase in protein content. The myelographic appearance of arachnoiditis is characteristic (patchy dispersion of the column of dye and a "candle-guttering" appearance that was most evident with oil-based contrast media); MRI reveals a loss of the normal ring of CSF or localized loculations of CSF (see Fig. 11-6). These ancillary procedures and the CSF formula allow one to make the diagnosis with certainty.

Pathologic Features In advanced cases the subarachnoid space is completely obliterated and the roots and cord are strangulated by the thickened connective tissue. Subpial nerve fibers of the cord are destroyed to a varying extent, and peripherally placed fibers of the posterior and lateral columns undergo secondary degeneration. Where the pathologic process is confined to relatively circumscribed portions of the cord, the subarachnoid space may be occupied by loculated collections of yellowish, high-protein fluid (meningitis serosa circumscripta). The rare association of spinal arachnoiditis and syringomyelic cavitation of the cord is considered further on in this chapter.

Treatment In the early stages of arachnoiditis, corticosteroids have been given systemically to control the inflammatory reaction and to prevent progress of the disease, but their value is questionable. Surgery may be effective in the rare case of localized "cyst" formation and cord compression. Severe radicular pain can be effectively relieved by posterior rhizotomy, but there is a strong tendency for the pain to return after an interval of several months or a year or two. For chronic adhesive lumbar arachnoiditis, in which diffuse back and limb pain is the most distressing symptom, there is no effective surgical or medical treatment, although relief has reportedly been provided in isolated instances by painstaking microsurgical dissection of the lumbar roots. Administration of corticosteroids, systemic and epidural, has not been consistently beneficial but may be tried. Transcutaneous stimulator treatment and gabapentin may also be tried.

Cord Herniation due to Dural Tear

Exceedingly violent trauma to the spinal canal or skull can be associated with arachnoidal and dural tears; the associated neural injury dominates the picture, and the dural tear may require repair in order to minimize the development of a meningitis. More difficult to understand is the occurrence of spinal cord herniation through an apparently spontaneous rent in the adjacent dura with no injury. We have encountered four such instances in a decade, without trauma having occurred. A vertically oriented tear of limited extent occurs in the ventral dura, usually in the mid- or high-thoracic region, and a segment of the spinal cord protrudes into the epidural space. The result is a painless, subacute, and incomplete spinal cord syndrome, which reaches a plateau and leaves the patient with an asymmetrical spastic paraparesis and variable sensory loss. Orthostatic headache of low-CSF pressure is not part of the syndrome. MRI demonstrates the protruded segment of the cord where it buckles through the dura. Presumably the herniation creates a sufficient degree of local ischemia or mechanical disturbance to account for the myelopathic symptoms. Surgical replacement of the cord in its proper position and repair of the tear has resulted in partial return of neurologic function (Vallee et al).

Intraspinal Tumors

Tumors of the spinal cord are considerably less frequent than tumors that involve the brain; in the Mayo Clinic series of 8784 primary tumors of the CNS, only 15 percent were intraspinal (Sloof et al). In distinction to brain tumors, the majority of intraspinal ones are benign and produce their effects mainly by compression of the spinal cord rather than by invasion. Thus, a large proportion of intraspinal tumors are amenable to surgical removal, and their early recognition, before irreversible neurologic changes have occurred, becomes a matter of utmost importance.

Anatomic Considerations Neoplasms and other space-occupying lesions within the spinal canal can be divided into two groups: (1) those that arise within the substance of the spinal cord, either as a primary neural neoplasm or as a metastasis, and invade and destroy tracts and central gray structures (*intramedullary*) and (2) those arising outside the spinal cord (*extramedullary*), either in the vertebral bodies and epidural tissues (extradural) or in the leptomeninges or roots (intradural). In a general hospital, the relative frequency of spinal tumors in these different locations is about 5 percent intramedullary, 40 percent intradural-extramedullary, and 55 percent extradural. This percentage of extradural lesions is higher than that encountered in more specialized neurosurgical services (e.g., Elsberg's figures of 7, 64, and 29 percent, respectively), probably because the latter do not include as many patients with extradural lymphomas, metastatic carcinomas, etc., as are seen in general hospitals.

The commonest *primary extramedullary* tumors are the neurofibromas and meningiomas (Fig. 44-8), which together constitute about 55 percent of all intraspinal neoplasms. They are more often intradural than extradural. Neurofibromas have a predilection for the thoracic region, whereas meningiomas are more evenly distributed over the vertical extent of the cord. The other primary extramedullary tumors are sarcomas, vascular tumors, chordomas, and epidermoid and similar tumors, in that order of frequency.

Primary intramedullary tumors of the spinal cord have the same cellular origins as those arising in the brain (Chap. 31), although the proportions of particular

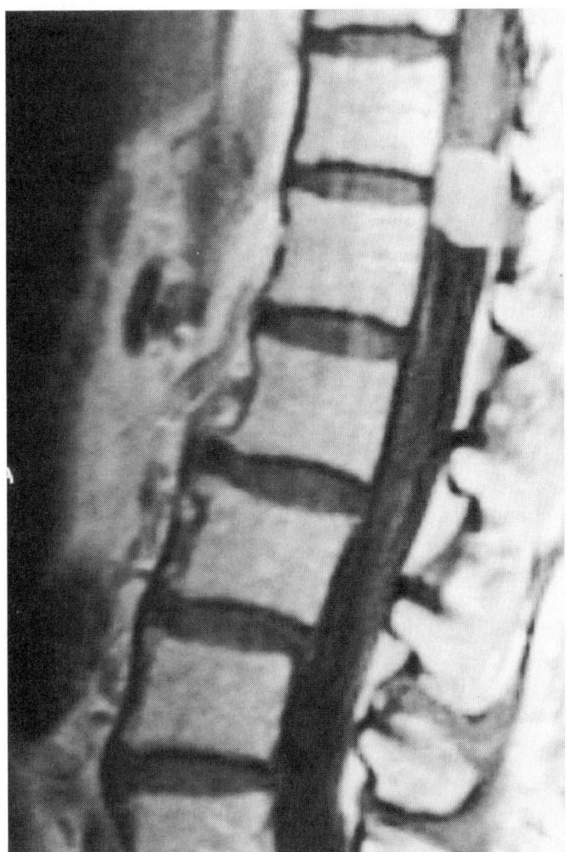

Figure 44-8

Gadolinium enhanced MRI of intraspinal meningioma that caused incontinence and leg weakness, including spastic and flaccid elements (combined conus and cauda syndrome).

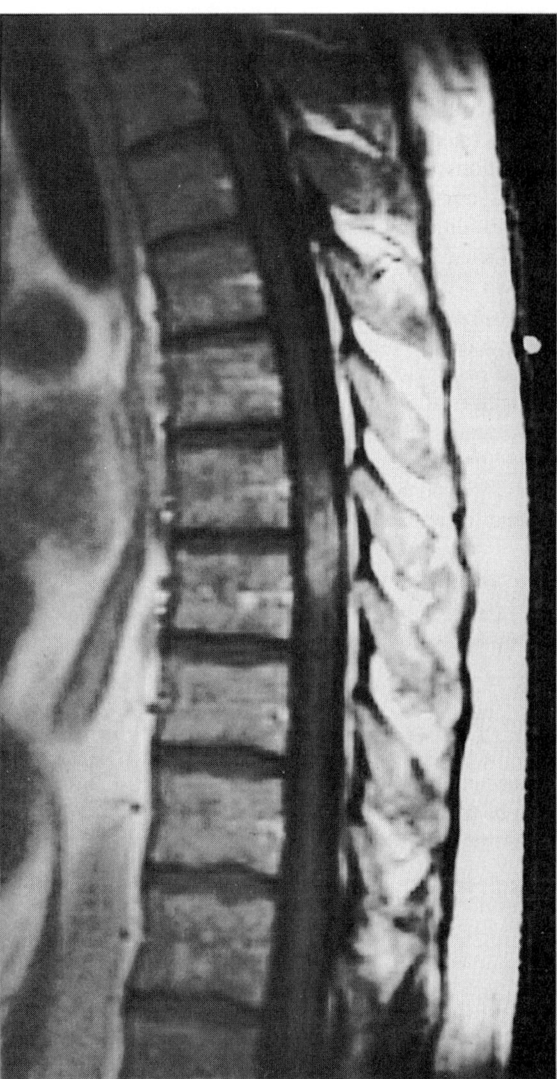

Figure 44-9

T1-weighted MRI of an intramedullary thoracic ependymoma, causing expansion of the cord and edema over several segments. There is faint enhancement of the tumor with gadolinium.

cell types differ. Ependymomas (many of which arise from the filum terminale; page 704) make up 60 percent of the spinal cord cases (Fig. 44-9) and astrocytomas about 25 percent. The astrocytoma is the commonest intramedullary tumor if one excludes tumors arising in the filum terminale. Oligodendrogliomas are much less common. The remainder (about 10 percent) consists of a diverse group of nongliomatous tumors: lipomas, epidermoids, dermoids, teratomas, hemangiomas, hemangioblastomas, and metastatic carcinomas. The hemangioma may be a source of spontaneous hematomyelia. As indicated further on, there is a frequent association between intramedullary tumors (both gliomatous and nongliomatous) and syringomyelia. The basis of this relationship remains obscure.

Intramedullary growths invade as well as compress and distort fasciculi in the spinal cord white matter. As the cord enlarges from the tumor growing within it or is compressed by a tumor from without, the free space around the cord is eventually consumed, and the CSF below the lesion becomes isolated or loculated from the remainder of the circulating fluid above the lesion. This is indicated by a Froin syndrome (xanthochromia and clotting of CSF) and an interruption of flow of contrast medium in the subarachnoid space (by myelogram). The most informative diagnostic procedure is an MRI, which demonstrates both the intramedullary extent of the tumor and the effect on the surrounding subarachnoid space.

Secondary spinal cord tumors can also be subdivided into intramedullary and extramedullary types. *Extradural metastases (carcinoma, lymphoma, myeloma) are the most common of all spinal tumors.* They account for the largest group of patients who develop symptoms of myelopathy while being cared for in hospital and are therefore likely to be encountered in the course of providing neurologic consultations. Extradural metastases arise from hematogenous deposits or extend from tumors of the vertebral bodies or from a paraspinal tumor extending via the intervertebral foramina (Fig. 44-10). Secondary extramedullary tumor growths are far more often extradural than intradural. The intradural type takes the form of a meningeal carcinomatosis or lymphomatosis and is considered in Chap. 31.

Intramedullary metastases are not as rare as is generally believed. In a retrospective autopsy study of 627 patients with systemic cancer, Costigan and Winkelman found 153 cases with CNS metastases, in 13 of which the metastases were located within the cord. In 9 of the 13 cases, the metastasis was deep in the cord, unassociated with leptomeningeal carcinomatosis; in 4 cases, the neoplasm seemed to extend from the pia. Bronchogenic carcinoma was the main source. Diagnosis is difficult but is aided greatly by MRI with gadolinium infusion; there is generally extensive contiguous edema (Fig. 44-11). Differentiation is from meningeal carcinomatosis, radiation myelopathy, and paraneoplastic necrotizing myelopathy, which is the rarest of these entities. Treatment is usually ineffective unless radiation therapy is begun before paraplegia supervenes (Winkelman et al).

Symptomatology Patients with spinal cord tumors are likely to present with one of three clinical syndromes:

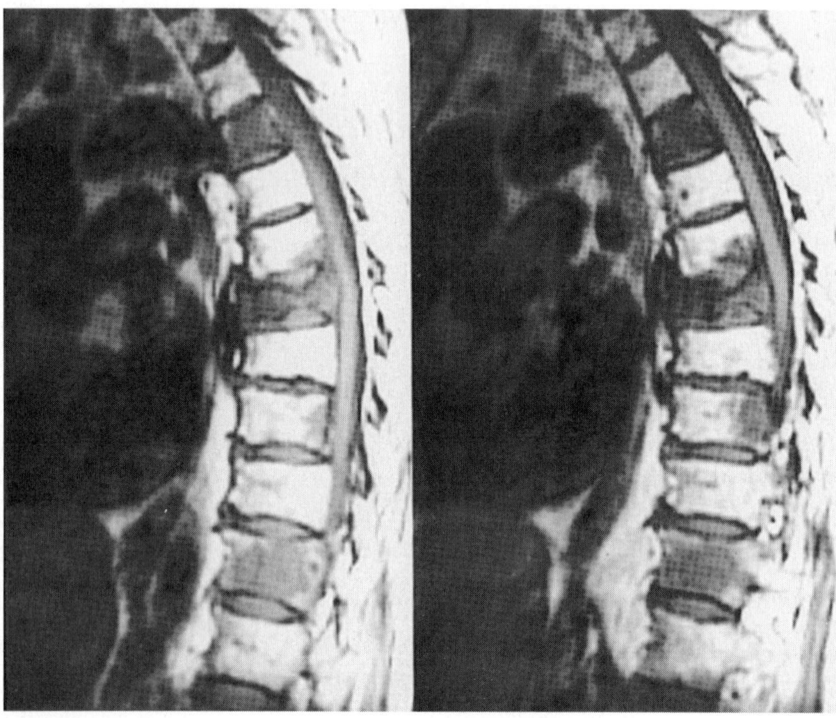

Figure 44-10

MRI of multiple spinal metastases from carcinoma of the lung. The metastases exhibit low signal intensity on T1-weighted images. An epidural mass is present, compressing the cord.

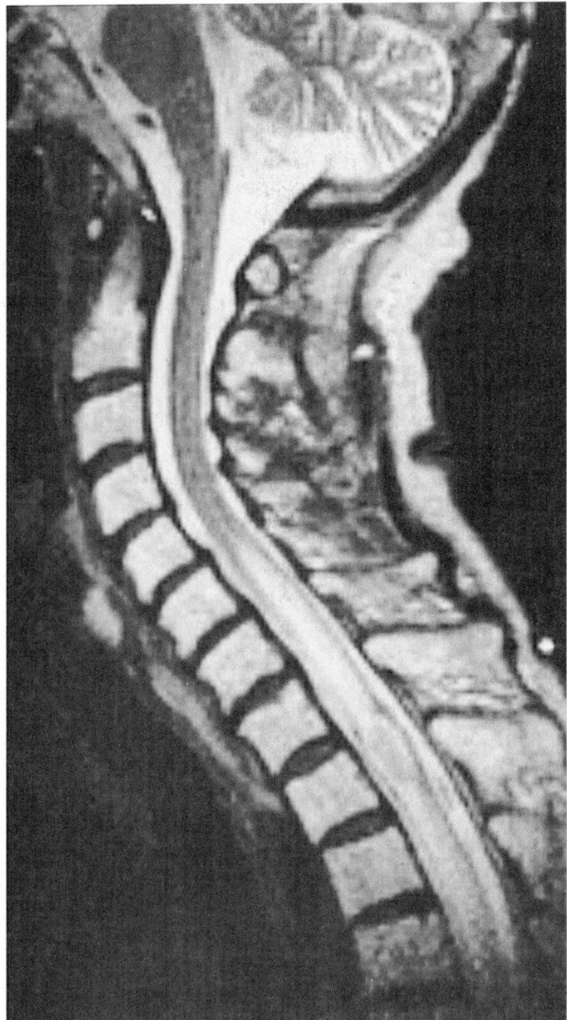

Figure 44-11

MRI of an intramedullary metastasis from breast cancer. The expansile lesion is at C8 and the adjacent edema extends over a great length of the spinal cord.

(1) a sensorimotor spinal tract syndrome, (2) a painful radicular-spinal cord syndrome, or (3) rarely, an intramedullary syringomyelic syndrome.

Pain and stiffness of the back may antedate signs of spinal cord disease or dominate the clinical picture in some cases of extramedullary tumor. The back pain is usually worse when the patient lies down or may become worse after several hours in the recumbent position and be improved by sitting up. *In children*, severe back pain associated with spasm of paravertebral muscles is often prominent initially; scoliosis and spastic weakness of the legs come later. Because of this somewhat unusual clinical presentation and the rarity of intraspinal lesions in childhood, spinal cord tumors in this age group may be overlooked.

Sensorimotor Spinal Tract Syndrome The clinical picture is related predominantly to compression and less often to invasion and destruction of spinal cord tracts. The signs of compression consist of (1) an asymmetrical spastic weakness of the legs with thoracolumbar lesions and of the arms and legs with cervical lesions, (2) a sensory level on the trunk below which perception of pain and temperature is reduced or lost, (3) posterior column signs, and (4) a spastic bladder under weak voluntary control. The onset of the compressive symptoms is usually gradual and the course progressive over a period of weeks and months, frequently with back pain. With extradural tumors, paralysis usually develops over a period of several days to several weeks, but the tempo of progression may be more rapid or more leisurely. The initial disturbance may be motor or sensory and the distribution asymmetrical. With cervical or foramen magnum lesions, a common sequence of motor impairment is first of an arm, followed by the ipsilateral leg, contralateral leg, and finally the remaining arm ("around-the-clock" pattern). With thoracic lesions, one leg usually becomes weak and stiff before the other one. Subjective sensory symptoms of the dorsal column type (tingling paresthesias) assume similar patterns. Pain and thermal senses are more likely to be affected than tactile, vibration, and position senses. Nevertheless, the posterior columns are frequently involved. Initially the sensory disturbance is contralateral to the maximum motor weakness, but a sharply defined Brown-Séquard syndrome is rarely observed. The bladder and bowel usually become paralyzed coincident with paralysis of the legs. If the compression is relieved, there is recovery from these sensory and motor symptoms, often in the reverse order of their appearance; the first part affected is the last to recover, and sensory symptoms tend to disappear before motor ones.

Radicular-Spinal Cord Syndrome The syndrome of spinal cord compression is often combined with radicular pain, i.e., pain in the distribution of a sensory nerve root. It is described as knife-like or as a dull ache with superimposed sharp stabs of pain, which radiate in a distal direction, i.e., away from the spine, and are intensified by coughing, sneezing, or straining. Segmental sensory changes (paresthesias, impaired perception of pinprick and touch) and/or motor disturbances (cramp, atrophy, fascicular twitching, and loss of tendon reflexes) and an ache in the spine, in addition to the radicular pain, are the usual manifestations of a cord compressive-irritative root lesion. Tenderness of spinous processes over the growth is found in about half the patients. These segmental changes, particularly the sensory ones, often precede the signs of spinal cord compression by months if the lesion is benign.

Intramedullary Syringomyelic Syndrome No single symptom is unique to *intramedullary tumors*. Pain is the most common symptom and is almost invariably present with tumors of the filum terminale. Ependymomas and astrocytomas, the two most common intramedullary tumors, usually give rise to a mixed sensorimotor tract syndrome. When the intramedullary tumor involves the central gray matter, a *syringomyelic syndrome* may result. Theoretically, intramedullary tumors that destroy mainly the gray matter should cause a central cord syndrome, with segmental or dissociated sensory loss, amyotrophy, early incontinence, and late corticospinal weakness. Also, on sensory examination, sacral sparing may be found but is of limited value in distinguishing intramedullary from extramedullary lesions. A dissociation of thermal pain and tactile sensory loss over several segments on the trunk is a more dependable sign of an intramedullary lesion. Rarely, for reasons that are difficult to understand, an extramedullary tumor may give rise to a syringomyelic syndrome.

Special Spinal Syndromes Unusual clinical syndromes may be found in patients with *tumors in the region of the foramen magnum*. They may produce a quadriparesis with pain in the back of the head and stiff neck, weakness and atrophy of the hands and dorsal neck muscles, marked imbalance, and variable sensory changes—or, if they spread intracranially, there may be signs of cerebellar and lower cranial nerve involvement. These tumor types are described fully in Chap. 31. Lesions at the level of the lowermost thoracic and the first lumbar vertebrae may result in mixed cauda equina and spinal cord symptoms. A Babinski sign means that the spinal cord is involved above the fifth lumbar segment. *Lesions of the cauda equina* alone, always difficult to separate from those of the lumbosacral plexuses and multiple nerves, are usually attended in the early stages by pain, which is variously combined with a bilaterally asymmetrical, atrophic, areflexic paralysis, radicular sensory loss, and sphincteric disorder. These must be distinguished from *lesions of the conus medullaris* (lower sacral segments of the spinal cord), in which there are early disturbances of the bladder and bowel (urinary retention and constipation), back pain, symmetrical hypesthesia or anesthesia over the sacral dermatomes, a lax anal sphincter with loss of anal and bulbocavernosus reflexes, impotence, and sometimes weakness of leg muscles. Sensory abnormalities may precede motor and reflex changes by many months. Very rarely, for unclear reasons, tumors of the thoracolumbar cord (intramedullary, as a rule) are associated with elevated spinal fluid protein and hydrocephalus; these respond to shunting and removal of the spinal tumor (Feldman et al).

Differential Diagnosis Several problems may arise in the diagnosis of spinal cord tumors in addition to those mentioned above. In their early stages they must be distinguished from other diseases that cause pain over certain segments of the body, i.e., diseases affecting the gallbladder, pancreas, kidney, stomach and intestinal tract, pleura, etc. Localization of the pain to a dermatome; its intensification by sneezing, coughing, and straining, and sometimes by recumbency; and the finding of segmental sensory changes and minor alterations of motor, reflex, or sensory function in the legs will usually provide the clues to the presence of a spinal cord-radicular lesion. Examination of the CSF, CT myelography, and particularly MRI will settle the diagnosis in most instances.

If the symptoms and signs of involvement of sensorimotor tracts are present, there is still the problem of locating the segmental level of the lesion. At first the sensory and motor deficits may be most pronounced in those parts of the body farthest removed from the lesion, i.e., in the feet or lumbosacral segments. Later the levels of the sensory and motor deficits ascend, but they may still be below the lesion. In determining the level of the lesion, the location of the root pain and atrophic paralysis is of greater help than the upper level of hypalgesia.

Once vertebral and segmental levels of the lesion are settled, there remains the necessity of determining whether the lesion is extradural, intradural-extramedullary, or intramedullary and whether it is neoplastic. This is important from the standpoint of etiologic diagnosis. If there is a visible or palpable spinal deformity or radiographic evidence of vertebral destruction, one may confidently assume an extradural localization. Even without these changes, one still suspects an extradural lesion if root pain developed early and is bilateral, if pain and aching in the spine are prominent and percussion tenderness is marked, if motor symptoms below the lesion preceded sensory ones, and if sphincter disturbances were late. However, to distinguish between intradural-extramedullary lesions and intramedullary lesions on clinical grounds alone may be impossible. The findings of segmental amyotrophy and sensory loss of dissociated type (loss of pain and temperature and preservation of tactile sensation) point to an intramedullary lesion.

Extradural tumors, both primary and secondary, must be differentiated from cervical spondylosis, tuberculous granuloma, sarcoidosis, and certain chronic pyogenic or fungal granulomatous lesions, from lipomas in patients receiving corticosteroids for prolonged periods, and from the rare necrotizing myelopathy associated with occult tumors. In the thoracic region, a ruptured disc or dural tear is always a possibility. In the region of the lower back, i.e., over the cauda equina, one must also distinguish between tumor and protruded intervertebral disc. Here, an extradural tumor may produce mainly sciatic and low back pain with little or no motor, sensory, reflex, or sphincteric disturbances. With intradural-extramedullary lesions, the important diagnostic considerations are meningioma, neurofibroma, meningeal carcinomatosis, cholesteatoma, and teratomatous cyst, a meningomyelitic process, or adhesive arachnoiditis. The study of cells in the CSF by centrifugation and Millipore filter and by similar techniques and the use of CT myelography and particularly MRI are the essential laboratory aids. Intramedullary lesions are usually gliomas, ependymomas, or vascular malformations or, in the context of a known carcinoma, intramedullary metastases. The definition of vascular malformations by means of selective spinal angiography has been discussed in an earlier section of this chapter. Normal or relatively low protein in the CSF and negative MRI effectively rule out intramedullary tumors or granulomatous lesions.

Treatment This depends on the nature of the lesion and the clinical condition of the patient. Intradural-extramedullary tumors should be removed as soon as possible after their discovery, and this applies to benign extradural tumors that are symptomatic as well. Laminectomy, decompression, excision in isolated cases, and radiotherapy constitute the treatment of intramedullary gliomas. Such patients may improve and lead useful lives for a decade or longer.

Epidural growths of carcinoma and lymphoma are best managed by the administration of radiation to the region of tumor involvement, endocrine therapy (for carcinoma of breast and prostate), the administration of antineoplastic drugs (for certain lymphomas and myelomas), and the early use of high-dose steroids and analgesics for pain. Seldom is operation necessary as a first resort; Gilbert and his associates have presented convincing evidence that patients who receive high-dose corticosteroids (16 to 60 mg of dexamethasone) and fractionated radiation (500 cGy on each of the first 3 days and then spaced radiation up to 3000 cGy) do as well as surgically treated patients. Sometimes laminectomy and decompression are necessary for diagnosis and, with a rapidly growing tumor, to prevent irreversible compressive effects and infarction of the spinal cord. Cases that have been allowed to progress should probably be operated on if paraplegia has just occurred. If the maximal safe radiation dosage had previously been applied to the spinal column, surgical palliation is also usually undertaken.

The main consideration in the management of epidural metastases is the need for early diagnosis, at a stage when only back pain is present and before neurologic symptoms and signs have appeared. Once neurologic signs appear, the results of treatment are poor. Thus, patients with back pain and vertebral metastases should have MRI or CT myelography and be treated aggressively with radiation (Rodichok et al, Portenoy et al). The management of other forms of spinal cord and cauda equina compression is considered in relation to the specific compressive lesions.

Other Rare Causes of Spinal Cord Compression

Intraspinal lipoma (intra- or extradural) should be suspected when there is a protracted evolution of neurologic symptoms and particularly when there is a palpable subcutaneous soft tissue mass, an associated bony abnormality, and myelographic and MRI evidence of a large dural sac and low-lying conus medullaris. Thomas and Miller found 60 such cases (over a period of 40 years) in the files of the Mayo Clinic. Epidural fat deposition with spinal cord or cauda equina compression occurs in Cushing disease and after the long-term use of corticosteroids but also in the absence of these disorders. The clinical picture may suggest discogenic disease (Lipson et al). Copious amounts of normal adipose tissue are found at laminectomy, and removal of this tissue is curative. Lowering the dose of steroid and caloric restriction will help mobilize the fat and relieve the symptoms.

Arachnoid diverticula—intra- or extradural outpouchings from the posterior nerve root—are very rare causes of a radicular-spinal cord syndrome first described by Bechterew in 1893. They tend to occur in the thoracic or lumbosacral regions. The symptoms, in order of decreasing frequency, are pain, radicular weakness and sensory disorder, gait disorder, and sphincteric disturbances (Cilluffo et al). The frequent association of arachnoid diverticula with osteoporosis, ankylosing spondylitis, and arachnoiditis makes it difficult to interpret the role of the diverticulae themselves. Surgical obliteration of the diverticula has yielded unpredictable results.

Spinal cord compression with paraplegia has also been caused by extramedullary hematopoiesis in cases of myelosclerosis, thalassemia, cyanotic heart disease, myelogenous leukemia, sideropenic anemia, and polycythemia vera (Oustwani et al). A similar phenomenon occurs with ossification of the posterior longitudinal ligament, as mentioned earlier in the chapter.

Solitary osteochondromas of vertebral bodies and multiple exostoses of hereditary type are other reported causes of spinal cord compression. In the case reported by Buur and Morch, the clinical syndrome was one of pure spastic paraparesis of several months' progression.

Lathyrism

From the interesting historical review of Dastur, one learns that this disease was known to Hippocrates, Pliny, and Galen in Europe, to Avicenna in the Middle East, and to the ancient Hindus. The term *lathyrism* was applied by Cantani, in Italy, because of its recognized relationship to the prolonged consumption of *Lathyrus sativus* (chickling vetch, or grass pea).

The disease is still common in some parts of India and Africa. In these districts, during periods of famine, when wheat and other grains are in short supply, the diet may for months consist of flour made of the grass pea. In individuals so exposed there occurs a gradual weakening of the legs accompanied by spasticity and cramps. Paresthesias, numbness, formication in the legs, and frequency and urgency of micturition, impotence, and sphincteric spasms are added. The upper extremities may exhibit coarse tremors and involuntary movements. These symptoms, once established, are more or less permanent but not constantly progressive, and most of the patients live out their natural life span.

Only two reports on the neuropathology of lathyrism were known to Dastur, one by Buzzard and Greenfield in England, the other by Filiminoff in Russia. Both of their patients had been in a stationary paraplegic state for years. Greenfield noted a loss of ascending and descending tracts in the spinal cord, particularly the corticospinal and direct spinocerebellar tracts. Filiminoff observed a loss of myelinated fibers in the lateral and posterior columns. (Unlike the cases of Spencer et al, there had been a loss of pain and thermal sensation in the upper extremities.) The larger Betz cells had disappeared, while anterior horn cells were unaffected. Gliosis and thickening of blood vessels was seen in the degenerated tracts.

The toxic nature of this disease, long suspected, has been confirmed by Spencer and colleagues. They extracted a neuroexcitatory amino acid, beta-*N*-oxalylaminoalanine (BOAA), from grass peas and were able to induce corticospinal dysfunction in monkeys by giving this substance with a nutritious diet. Subsequently, Hugon and coworkers produced a primate model of lathyrism by feeding monkeys a diet of *L. sativus* in addition to an alcoholic extract of this legume. These findings tend to negate the importance of several other factors that until now had been thought to be causative—namely, malnutrition, ergot contamination, and toxins derived from *Vicia sativa*, the common vetch that grows alongside the lathyrus species.

Possibly the more recently described African acute spastic paraplegia called "konzo" has a similar toxic pathogenesis.

Dysraphic and Congenital Tumor Syndromes

See Chap. 38.

Familial Spastic Paraplegia

There are several familial forms of progressive spastic paraplegia, some beginning in childhood, others in adult life. The pattern of inheritance in our adult cases has been autosomal dominant. A lack of sensory symptoms and signs and sparing of sphincteric function until late in the illness are important diagnostic features. A number of adult cases are "complicated" in the sense that the spastic paraplegia is associated with cerebellar ataxia or dementia. By contrast, *primary lateral sclerosis*, a sporadic form of degenerative disease of the motor system, is characterized by a pure spastic paraplegia, the result of changes that are confined to the corticospinal pathways. These disorders are discussed extensively with the heredodegenerative diseases in Chap. 39, and the myelopathy associated with adrenoleukodystrophy in Chap. 37.

SYRINGOMYELIC SYNDROME OF SEGMENTAL SENSORY DISSOCIATION WITH BRACHIAL AMYOTROPHY

This syndrome is most often ascribable to syringomyelia (i.e., a central cavitation of the spinal cord of undetermined cause), but a similar clinical syndrome may sometimes be observed in association with other pathologic states, such as intramedullary cord tumors, traumatic myelopathy, postradiation myelopathy, infarction (myelomalacia), bleeding (hematomyelia), and rarely with extramedullary tumors, cervical spondylosis, spinal arachnoiditis, and cervical necrotizing myelitis.

Syringomyelia (Syrinx)

Syringomyelia (from the Greek *syrinx*, "pipe" or "tube") may be defined as a chronic progressive degenerative or developmental disorder of the spinal cord, characterized clinically by painless weakness and wasting of the hands and arms (brachial amyotrophy) and segmental sensory loss of dissociated type (loss of thermal and painful sensation with sparing of tactile, joint position, and vibratory sense, as described below). Pathologically there is cavitation of the central parts of the spinal cord, usually in the cervical region, but extending upward in some cases into the medulla oblongata and pons (syringobulbia) or downward into the thoracic or even the lumbar segments. Frequently there are associated developmental abnormalities of the vertebral column (thoracic scoliosis, fusion of vertebrae, or Klippel-Feil anomaly), of the base of the skull (platybasia and basilar invagination), and particularly of the cerebellum and brainstem (type I Chiari malformation). Approximately 90 percent of cases of syringomyelia have type I Chiari malformation (descent of cerebellar tonsils, see page 1064); conversely, approximately 50 percent of type I Chiari malformations are associated with syringomyelia. In contrast to the frequency of these developmentally related abnormalities is a less frequent but well-described association of syringomyelia with acquired processes such as intramedullary tumor (astrocytoma, hemangioblastoma, ependymoma) and traumatic necrosis of the spinal cord.

Wider experience with the pathology of syringomyelia and better understanding of the postulated mechanisms have led to the following classification, modified from Barnett et al:

Type I. Syringomyelia with obstruction of the foramen magnum and dilation of the central canal
- *A.* With type I Chiari malformation
- *B.* With other obstructive lesions of the foramen magnum

Type II. Syringomyelia without obstruction of the foramen magnum (idiopathic type)

Type III. Syringomyelia with other diseases of the spinal cord (acquired types)
- *A.* Spinal cord tumors (usually intramedullary)
- *B.* Traumatic myelopathy
- *C.* Spinal arachnoiditis and pachymeningitis
- *D.* Secondary myelomalacia from cord compression (tumor, spondylosis) or infarction (AVM, etc.)

Type IV. Pure hydromyelia (developmental dilatation of the central canal), usually with hydrocephalus

Historical Note Although pathologic cavitation of the spinal cord was recognized as early as the sixteenth century, the term *syringomyelia* was first used to describe this process in 1827 by Ollivier d'Angers (cited by Ballantine et al). Later, following recognition of the central canal as a normal structure, it was assumed by Virchow (1863) and by Leyden (1876) that cavitation of the spinal cord had its origin in an abnormal expansion of the central canal, and they renamed the process *hydromyelia*. Cavities in the central portions of the spinal cord, unconnected with the central canal, were recognized by Hallopeau (1870); Simon suggested in 1875 that the term *syringomyelia* be reserved for such cavities and that the term *hydromyelia* be restricted to simple dilatation of the central canal. Thus, a century ago, the stage was set for an argument about pathogenesis that has not been settled to the present day.

Clinical Features The clinical picture varies in the four pathologic types listed above, the differences depending not only on the extent of the syrinx but also on the associated pathologic changes, particularly those related to the Chiari malformation. In type 1 (idiopathic and Chiari developmental syringomyelia), symptoms usually begin in early adult life (20 to 40 years). Males and females are equally affected. Rarely, some abnormality is noted at birth, and occasionally the first symptom appears in late childhood or adolescence. The onset is usually insidious and the course irregularly progressive. In many instances the symptoms or signs are discovered accidentally (a painless burn or atrophy of the hand), and the patient cannot say when the disease began. Rarely, there is an almost apoplectic onset or worsening; there are cases on record of an aggravation of old symptoms or the appearance of new symptoms after a violent strain or paroxysm of coughing. Once the disease is recognized, some patients remain much the same for years, even decades, but more often there is intermittent progression to the point of being chair-bound within 5 to 10 years. This extremely variable course makes it difficult to evaluate therapy.

The precise clinical picture at any given point in the evolution of the disease depends upon the cross-sectional and longitudinal extent of the syrinx, but certain clinical features are so common that the diagnosis can hardly be made without them. These features are *segmental weakness and atrophy of the hands and arms with loss of tendon reflexes and segmental anesthesia of a dissociated type* (loss of pain and thermal sense and preservation of the sense of touch) over the neck, shoulders, and arms. Finally, there are weakness and ataxia of the legs from involvement of the corticospinal tracts (possibly at their decussation) and posterior columns in the cervical region. Kyphoscoliosis is added in many of the cases, and in nearly one-quarter of them there is an overt cervico-occipital malformation (short neck, low hairline, odd posture of the head and neck, fused or missing cervical vertebrae).

The particular muscle groups that are affected on the two sides may vary. Exceptionally, motor function is spared, and the segmental dissociated sensory loss and/or pain are the only marks of the disease. In a few of the cases, especially those with the Chiari malformation, the reflexes in the arms are preserved or even hyperactive, as might be expected with upper rather than lower motor neuron involvement. Or the shoulder muscles may be atrophic and the hands spastic. In the lower extremities the weakness, if present, is of a spastic (corticospinal) type.

The characteristic segmental sensory dissociation is usually bilateral, but a unilateral pattern is not unknown, and this is true of the amyotrophy as well. The sensory loss has a cape or hemicape distribution, often extending to the face or back of the head and onto the trunk. Although tactile sensation is usually preserved, there are cases in which it is impaired, usually in the region of the most dense analgesia. Exceptionally there is no sensory loss in the presence of amyotrophy, and cases have been recorded in which only a hydrocephalus and hydromyelia were present with spastic paraparesis (type IV). If tactile sensation is affected in the arms, joint position and vibratory sense tend also to be impaired. In the lower extremities there may be some loss of pain and thermal sensation proximally and over the abdomen, but more often there is a loss of vibratory and position sense which is indicative of a posterior column lesion and is the basis of ataxia. A Horner syndrome may result from ipsilateral involvement of the intermediolateral cell column at the C8, T1, and T2 levels.

Pain has been a symptom in about half of our patients with types I and II syringomyelia. The pain is usually unilateral or more marked on one side; it is of a burning, aching quality, mostly in or at the border of areas of sensory impairment. In a few patients it involves the face or trunk. An aching pain at the base of the skull or posterior cervical region—intensified by coughing, sneezing, or stooping (brief exertional pain)—is often present in type I cases. But, as Logue and Edwards point out, pain of this type is often a feature of Chiari malformation without syringomyelia and is probably attributable to compression or stretching of cervical roots.

Syringobulbia is the bulbar equivalent of syringomyelia. Usually the two coexist, but occasionally the bulbar manifestations precede the spinal ones or, rarely, occur independently. The glial cleft or cavity is located most often in the lateral tegmentum of the medulla, but it may extend into the pons and, rarely, even higher. The symptoms and signs are characteristically unilateral and consist of nystagmus, analgesia, and thermoanesthesia of the face (numbness); wasting and weakness of the tongue (dysarthria); and palatal and vocal cord paralysis (dysphagia and hoarseness). Diplopia, episodic vertigo, trigeminal pain or facial sensory loss, and persistent hiccough are less common symptoms. The clinical and pathologic features of syringobulbia have been described in great detail by Jonesco-Sisesti. A most unusual keyhole-shaped syrinx, which was confined to the upper pons and midbrain and communicated with the fourth ventricle, has been described by de la Monte and colleagues.

When a Chiari malformation is associated with syringomyelia and syringobulbia, it may be difficult to separate the effects of the two disorders. Clinical features that favor the diagnosis of type I syringomyelia with Chiari malformation are nystagmus, cerebellar ataxia, exertional head-neck pain, prominent corticospinal and sensory tract involvement in the lower extremities, hydrocephalus, and craniocervical malformations. In type I syringomyelia without a Chiari malformation but with some other type of obstructive lesion at the foramen magnum, the clinical picture is much the same, and the nature of the foramen magnum lesion can be determined only by MRI or surgical exploration.

The association of syringomyelia with an intramedullary tumor (type III) should be suspected when there is a syringomyelic type of sensorimotor abnormality extending over many segments of the body. With Von Hippel-Lindau disease, the diagnosis hinges on the finding of the characteristic hereditary hemangioblastoma in the syrinx and retinal and cerebellar vascular malformations. In the posttraumatic cases, a traumatic necrosis of the spinal cord that has been stable for months or years begins to cause pain and spreading sensory or motor loss, recognizable most easily in segments above the original lesion (Schurch et al). This has occurred in approximately 3 percent of the cases of Rossier and coworkers, more in quadriplegics than in paraplegics. The posttraumatic syrinx is not as well defined as the usual forms of syringomyelia but consists instead of several contiguous areas of glia-lined myelomalacia with differing degrees of cavitation. In some instances of progressive spinal cord symptoms occurring several years after spinal surgery, the lesion has proved to be one of arachnoiditis and cord atrophy and not a syrinx (Avrahami et al).

In the few cases of hydromyelia that have come to our attention, there has sometimes been a long-standing hydrocephalus, often congenital, complicated years later by progressive weakness and atrophy of the shoulders and the muscles of the arms and hands. Segmental sensory loss has been reported in only a few instances. Proof of the existence of this entity in the past has been based on necropsy demonstration of an enormously widened central canal, with or without hydrocephalus. Now it should be easily diagnosable by MRI.

Pathogenesis One theory of the pathogenesis of developmental syringomyelia, of which Gardner was the most persuasive protagonist, is that normal flow of CSF is prevented by a congenital failure of opening of the outlets of the fourth ventricle. As a result, a pulse wave of CSF pressure, generated by systolic pulsations of the choroid plexuses, is transmitted into the cord from the fourth ventricle through the central canal. According to this theory, the syrinx consists essentially of a greatly dilated central canal with a diverticulum that ramifies from the central canal and dissects along gray matter and fiber tracts. The frequency with which syringomyelia is linked to malformations at the craniocervical junction, i.e., to lesions that could interfere with normal flow of CSF, lent credence to this theory.

There are many instances, however, where Gardner's hydrodynamic theory could not explain the syringomyelia. In some cases the foramens of Luschka and Magendie are found to be patent, and other abnormalities of the posterior fossa or foramen magnum are also not in evidence. Cases have been observed in which two well-developed cavities, one at a cervical and another at a lumbar level, were unconnected by any patent channel. Furthermore, in many cases, including several of our own, serial histologic sections have failed to demonstrate a connection between the fourth ventricle and the syrinx in the spinal cord or a widening of the central canal above the syrinx (see also Hughes).

Gardner's theory has been questioned on other grounds. Ball and Dayan calculated the pulse-pressure wave transmitted into the cord to be of so low an order as to be unlikely to produce a syrinx. These authors suggested a somewhat different mechanism, with which we are in accord. In their view, the CSF around the cervical cord, under increased pressure during strain or physical effort because of subarachnoid obstruction at the craniocervical junction, tracks into the spinal cord along the Virchow-Robin spaces or other subpial channels. Over a prolonged period of time, abetted perhaps by traumatic lesions, small pools of fluid coalesce to form a syrinx; originally the syrinx forms independently of the central canal, but eventually the two may become connected, perhaps because of the secondary enlargement of the canal (hydromyelia ex vacuo). The recent findings of Heiss and colleagues, who studied patients with syringomyelia and Chiari malformation, lend strong support to the theory of Ball and Dayan. According to Heiss et al, progression of syringomyelia is produced by the action of the cerebellar tonsils, which partially occlude the subarachnoid space at the foramen magnum and create pressure waves that compress the spinal cord from without and not from within; the pressure waves propagate syrinx fluid caudally with each heartbeat.

A blastomatous formation in the spinal cord, akin to tuberous sclerosis or central von Recklinghausen disease but with a tendency for the abnormal tissue to cavitate, is another suggested explanation of syrinx formation—a view that can be discounted because of the lack of blastomatous tissue in the walls of the syrinx. Still others have suggested that edema is a major pathogenetic factor, induced by angiomatous malformations, neoplasms, trauma, arachnoiditis, etc. This hardly exhausts the list of hypotheses, but none of them is easy to confirm, and there is no point in enumerating them all. The authors favor the view that in the most common type of syringomyelia, a cervical cord lesion, occurring in childhood as part of a Chiari malformation or other developmental abnormality, results in an enlarging cavity in the substance of the spinal cord, with secondary diverticulation of the spinal canal via a hydrodynamic mechanism within a destructive lesion—as postulated originally by Gordon Holmes and elaborated by Ball and Dayan. We are impressed with the relationship between basal cranial, cervical spine, and cerebellospinal malformations and hydrosyringomyelia and with disturbed hydrodynamics of perispinal CSF as important factors in the pathogenesis. Logue and Edwards have documented several cases of syringomyelia in which the foramen magnum was obstructed by a lesion other than a Chiari formation—dural cyst, localized arachnoiditis, atlanto-axial fusion, simple cerebellar cyst, and basilar invagination (see Williams for a review of the numerous hypotheses).

Irrespective of its mode of origin, the syrinx first occupies the central gray matter of the cervical portion of the spinal cord, where it interrupts the crossing pain and temperature fibers in the anterior commissure at several successive cord segments. As the cavity enlarges, it extends symmetrically or asymmetrically into the posterior and anterior horns and eventually into the lateral and posterior funiculi of the cord. It may enlarge the spinal cord and even widen the interpedicular spaces. The cavity is lined with astrocytic glia and a few thick-walled blood vessels, and the fluid in the cavity is clear and has a relatively low protein content, like CSF.

The cavitation is nearly always found in the cervical portion of the cord and only reaches the thoracic and lumbar portions by extension from the cervical region. Either a cavity or a glial septum may extend asymmetrically into the medulla oblongata, usually in the vicinity of the descending tract of the fifth cranial nerve (syringobulbia).

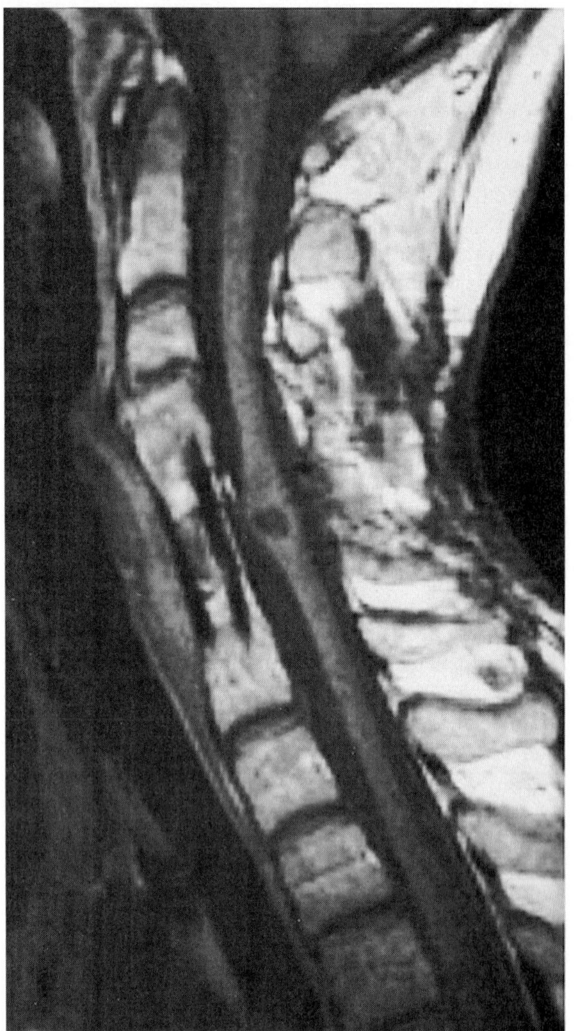

Figure 44-12

T1-weighted sagittal MRI of the cervical cord, showing a posttraumatic syrinx that led to progressive clinical worsening. At operation there proved to be glial septa within the cavity.

Diagnosis The clinical picture of syringomyelia is so characteristic that diagnosis is seldom in doubt. Now one can obtain spectacular demonstrations of the syrinx, Chiari malformations, and other foramen magnum lesions by MRI in the sagittal plane of the brain and spinal cord (see Figs. 38-4 and 44-12). Also, contrast myelography and delayed CT scanning, performed with the patient in the supine, head-down position, will reveal the Chiari malformation and usually expose the syrinx; the contrast material fills the syrinx and the central canal directly, probably from the surface of the cord (Ball and Dayan).

Certain rare neuropathies (amyloid, Tangier disease, and Fabry disease) that preferentially affect small fibers in the nerves of the upper extremities can reproduce the dissociated sensory loss that is characteristic of a syrinx, but syringomyelic motor abnormalities are not found in these cases.

Treatment The only therapy of lasting value for type I syringomyelia (related to Chiari malformation) is surgical decompression of the foramen magnum and upper cervical canal. Headache and neck pain are helped most; ataxia and nystagmus tend to persist. Radiation therapy, which was formerly recommended, is of no benefit. The operation advised by Gardner, of plugging the connection between the fourth ventricle and the central canal of the cervical cord, has been abandoned. There have been complications of this operative procedure, and the results appear to be no better than those obtained from simple decompression. The latter operation also carries some risk, especially if there is an attempt to excise the tonsillar projections of the cerebellum. In the series of Logue and Edwards, comprising 56 cases of type I syringomyelia, the occipitocervical pain was relieved by decompression in most patients, but the shoulder-arm pain usually persisted. Upper motor neuron weakness of the legs and sensory ataxia were often improved, whereas the segmental sensory and motor manifestations of the syringomyelia were not. Hankinson has reported good results from decompression in 75 percent of type I cases of syringomyelia. In the retrospective review of 141 adult patients by Stevens and colleagues, good surgical outcome was achieved in 50 percent of those with minor degrees of descent of the cerebellar tonsils but in only 12 percent of those with major cerebellar ectopia. A distended syrinx also led to a more favorable outcome. Whether the long-term course of these diseases is altered has not been determined.

Syringostomy or shunting of the cavity has been performed in type I and some of the type II (idiopathic) cases, but the results have been unpredictable. Love and Olafson, who performed this procedure in 40 patients of both types (mainly type II), stated that 30 percent had an excellent outcome. Schurch and coworkers obtained improvement of pain and motor weakness in 5 of their 7 cases by stabilization of the spine and syringotomy with placement of a T-tube within the syrinx. In a more recent and comprehensive study of 73 patients with a developmental syrinx operated by Sgouros and Williams, one-half remained clinically stable for a 10-year period; 15 percent had serious complications of the surgery, however. Our experiences with this procedure have not persuaded us of its lasting value; most of our patients, even those who reported some improvement originally, soon relapsed to their preoperative state, and the disease then progressed in the usual way. An enlarged cervical cord with progressive clinical worsening may nonetheless justify shunting of the cavity.

Surgery for the posttraumatic cases has given more favorable results. With incomplete myelopathy, syringostomy relieved the pain in all the 10 patients of Shannon and associates. Where they found the myelopathy to be complete, the cord was transected and the upper stump excised. Sgouros and Williams have also studied 57 such patients and recommend decompressive laminectomy and reconstruction of the subarachnoid space as the most effective of the several procedures that have been used in the management of this complication.

In the cases of syringomyelia with tumor, in which the cyst fluid may be high in protein and viscid (unlike the low-protein fluid of the usual syrinx), the tumor should be excised if possible. This has been done successfully with hemangioblastomas of the posterior columns and occasionally with ependymomas.

The rare symptomatic purely hydromyelic cases should benefit from ventriculoperitoneal shunts of the hydrocephalus, and a few excellent results are reported. This procedure has also been attempted in type I cases, with unimpressive results unless there is an associated hydrocephalus. Draining the central canal by amputation of the tip of the sacral cord has been unsuccessful and can be harmful.

CONCLUDING REMARKS

It is always well to remind oneself that of the more than thirty diseases of the spinal cord, effective means of treatment are available for only a few: spondylosis, extramedullary spinal cord tumors, syphilis (meningomyelitis and tabes), epidural abscess, hematoma and granuloma (tuberculous, fungal, sarcoidosis), perhaps syringomyelia, and subacute combined degeneration and other forms of nutritional myelopathy. Some of the inflammatory myelopathies may respond to immune modulating measures. The physician's major responsibility is to determine whether the patient has one of these treatable diseases.

REFERENCES

Adams CBT, Logue V: Studies in cervical spondylotic myelopathy. *Brain* 94:557, 569, 1971.

Allen AR: Surgery of experimental lesions of the spinal cord equivalent to crush injury of fracture dislocation of the spinal column: A preliminary report. *JAMA* 57:878, 1911.

American Spinal Injury Association: *Standards for Neurological Classification of Spinal Injury Patients*. Chicago, American Spinal Injury Association, 1984.

Aminoff MJ, Logue V: The prognosis of patients with spinal vascular malformations. *Brain* 97:211, 1974.

Antoni N: Spinal vascular malformations (angiomas) and myelomalacia. *Neurology* 12:795, 1962.

Avrahami E, Tadmor R, Cohn DF: Magnetic resonance imaging in patients with progressive myelopathy following spinal surgery. *J Neurol Neurosurg Psychiatry* 52:176, 1989.

Baker AS, Ojemann RG, Swartz MN, Richardson EP Jr: Spinal epidural abscess. *N Engl J Med* 293:463, 1975.

Bakshi R, Kinkel PR, Mechtler LL, et al: Magnetic resonance imaging findings in 22 cases of myelitis: Comparison between patients with and without multiple sclerosis. *Eur J Neurol* 5:35, 1998.

Ball MJ, Dayan AD: Pathogenesis of syringomyelia. *Lancet* 2:799, 1972.

Ballantine HT, Ojemann RG, Drew JH: Syringohydromyelia, in Krayenbuhl H, Maspes PE, Sweet WH (eds): *Progress in Neurological Surgery*. Vol 4. New York, Karger, 1971, pp 227–245.

Barnett JHM, Foster JB, Hudgson P: *Syringomyelia*. Philadelphia, Saunders, 1973.

Bartleson JO, Cohen MD, Harrington TM: Cauda equina syndrome secondary to long-standing ankylosing spondylitis. *Ann Neurol* 14:662, 1983.

Blackwood W: Discussion of vascular disease of the spinal cord. *Proc R Soc Med* 51:543, 1958.

Bots TAM, Wattendorf AR, Buruma OJS: Acute myelopathy caused by fibrocartilagenous emboli. *Neurology* 31:1250, 1981.

Braakman R: Management of cervical spondylotic myelopathy and radiculopathy. *J Neurol Neurosurg Psychiatry* 57:257, 1994.

Bracken MR, Shepard MJ, Collins WF, et al: A randomized controlled trial of methylprednisolone or naloxone in treatment of acute spinal cord injury. *N Engl J Med* 322:1405, 1990.

Bracken MR, Shepard MJ, Collins WF, et al: Methylprednisolone or naloxone treatment after acute spinal cord injury: 1-year follow-up data. *J Neurosurg* 76:23, 1992.

Brain WR: Discussion on rupture of the intervertebral disc in the cervical region. *Proc R Soc Med* 41:509, 1948.

Brain WR, Northfield D, Wilkinson M: The neurological manifestations of cervical spondylosis. *Brain* 75:187, 1952.

Burns RJ, Jones AN, Robertson JS: Pathology of radiation myelopathy. *J Neurol Neurosurg Psychiatry* 35:888, 1972.

Buur T, Morch MM: Hereditary multiple exostoses with spinal cord compression. *J Neurol Neurosurg Psychiatry* 46:96, 1983.

Caccamo DV, Garcia JH, Ho K-L: Isolated granulomatous angiitis of the spinal cord. *Ann Neurol* 32:580, 1992.

Campbell AMG, Garland H: Subacute myoclonic spinal neuronitis. *J Neurol Neurosurg Psychiatry* 19:268, 1956.

Candon E, Frerebeau P: Abcés bacteriens de la moelle épinière. *Rev Neurol* 150:370, 1994.

Cannon WB, Rosenblueth A: *The Supersensitivity of Denervated Structures*. New York, Macmillan, 1949.

Cheshire WP, Santos CC, Massey EW, Howard JF: Spinal cord infarction: Etiology and outcome. *Neurology* 47:321, 1996.

Cilluffo JM, Gomez MR, Reese DF, et al: Idiopathic (congenital) spinal arachnoid diverticula. *Mayo Clin Proc* 56:93, 1981.

Clark K: Injuries to the cervical spine and spinal cord, in Youmans JR (ed): *Neurological Surgery*, 2nd ed. Philadelphia, Saunders, 1982, pp 2318–2337.

Collins WF, Chehrazi B: Concepts of the acute management of spinal cord injury, in Mathews WB, Glaser GH (eds): *Recent Advances in Clinical Neurology*. London, Churchill Livingstone, 1983, pp 67–82.

Confavreux C, Larbre J-P, Lejeune E, et al: Cerebrospinal fluid dynamics in the tardive cauda equina syndrome of ankylosing spondylitis. *Ann Neurol* 29:221, 1991.

Costigan DA, Winkelman MD: Intramedullary spinal cord metastasis. *J Neurosurg* 62:227, 1985.

Creed RS, Denny-Brown D, Eccles JC, et al: *Reflex Activity of the Spinal Cord*. Oxford, Clarendon Press, 1932, p 154.

Cruickshank EK: A neuropathic syndrome of uncertain origin. *West Indian Med* 5:147, 1956.

Dahlberg PJ, Frecentese DF, Cogbill TH: Cholesterol embolism: Experience with 22 histologically proven cases. *Surgery* 10:737, 1989.

Dastur DK: Lathyrism. *World Neurol* 3:721, 1962.

Dawson DM, Potts F: Acute nontraumatic myelopathies, in Woolsey RM, Young RR (eds): *Neurologic Clinics: Disorders of the Spinal Cord*. Philadelphia, Saunders, 1991, p 585.

de la Monte SM, Horowitz SA, Larocque AA, Richardson EP Jr: Keyhole aqueduct syndrome. *Arch Neurol* 43:926, 1986.

DeVivo MJ, Kartus PT, Stover SI: Seven-year survival following spinal cord injury. *Arch Neurol* 44:872, 1987.

Dickman CA, Hadley NM, Pappas CTE, et al: Cruciate paralysis: A clinical and radiologic analysis of injuries to the cervicomedullary spine. *J Neurosurg* 73:850, 1990.

Douglas MA, Parks LC, Bebin J. Sudden myelopathy secondary to therapeutic total-body hyperthermia after spinal-cord irradiation. *N Engl J Med* 304:583, 1981.

Duke RJ, Hashimoto S: Familial spinal arachnoiditis. *Arch Neurol* 30:300, 1974.

Ebersold MJ, Pare MC, Quast LM: Surgical treatment for cervical spondylotic myelopathy. *J Neurosurg* 82:745, 1995.

Elkington J St C: Arachnoiditis, in Feiling A (ed): *Modern Trends in Neurology*. New York, Hoeber-Harper, 1951, pp 149–161.

Ell JJ, Uttley D, Silver JR: Acute myelopathy in association with heroin addiction. *J Neurol Neurosurg Psychiatry* 44:448, 1981.

Elsberg CA: *Surgical Diseases of the Spinal Cord, Membranes and Nerve Roots: Symptoms, Diagnosis and Treatment*. New York, Hoeber-Harper, 1941.

Epstein JA, Epstein NE: The surgical management of cervical spinal stenosis, spondylosis, and myeloradiculopathy by means of the posterior approach, in Cervical Spine Research Society (ed): *The Cervical Spine*. Philadelphia, Lippincott, 1989, pp 625–669.

Feldman E, Bromfield E, Navia B, et al: Hydrocephalic dementia and spinal cord tumor. *Arch Neurol* 43:714, 1986.

Filiminoff IN: Zur pathologisch-anatomischen Charakteristik des Lathyrismus. *Z Ges Neurol Psychiatry* 105:76, 1926.

Foix C, Alajouanine T: La myelite necrotique subaigue. *Rev Neurol* 2:1, 1926.

Folliss AGH, Netzky MG: Progressive necrotic myelopathy, in Vinken PJ, Bruyn GW (eds): *Handbook of Clinical Neurology*. Vol 9. Amsterdam, North-Holland, 1970, pp 452–468.

Fox MW, Onofrio BM, Kilgore JE: Neurological complications of ankylosing spondylitis. *J Neurosurg* 78:871, 1993.

Fulton JF: *Physiology of the Nervous System*. London, Oxford University Press, 1943.

Gardner WJ: Hydrodynamic mechanism of syringomyelia: Its relationship to myelocele. *J Neurol Neurosurg Psychiatry* 28: 247, 1965.

Geisler FH, Dorsey FC, Coleman WP: Recovery of motor function after spinal cord injury: A randomized, placebo-controlled trial with GM1 ganglioside. *N Engl J Med* 324:1829, 1991.

Gilbert RW, Kim J-H, Posner JB: Epidural spinal cord compression from metastatic tumor: Diagnosis and treatment. *Ann Neurol* 3:40, 1978.

Greenberg HS, Kim JH, Posner JB: Epidural spinal cord compression from metastatic tumor. *Ann Neurol* 8:361, 1980.

Greenfield JG, Turner JWA: Acute and subacute necrotic myelitis. *Brain* 62:227, 1939.

Guttmann L: *Spinal Cord Injuries: Comprehensive Management and Research*. Oxford, Blackwell, 1976.

Hankinson J: Syringomyelia and the surgeon, in Williams D (ed): *Modern Trends in Neurology*. Vol 5. London, Butterworth, 1970, pp 127–148.

Haymaker W: Decompression sickness, in Scholz W (ed): *Handbuch der Speziellen Pathologischen Anatomie und Histologie*: vol XIII/1B. Berlin, Springer-Verlag, 1957, pp 1600–1672.

Head H, Riddoch G: The automatic bladder: Excessive sweating and some other reflex conditions in gross injuries of the spinal cord. *Brain* 40:188, 1917.

Heiss JD, Patronas N, DeVroom HL, et al: Elucidating the pathophysiology of syringomyelia. *J Neurosurg* 91:553, 1999.

Herrick M, Mills PE Jr: Infarction of spinal cord. *Arch Neurol* 24:228, 1971.

Holmes G: On the spinal injuries of warfare: Goulstonian lectures. *BMJ* 2:769, 1915.

Howell DA, Lees AJ, Toghill PJ: Spinal internuncial neurones in progressive encephalomyelitis with rigidity. *J Neurol Neurosurg Psychiatry* 42:773, 1979.

Hughes JT: *Pathology of the Spinal Cord*, 2nd ed. Philadelphia, Saunders, 1978.

Hugon J, Ludolph A, Roy DN, et al: Studies on the etiology and pathogenesis of motor neuron diseases: II. Clinical and electrophysiologic features of pyramidal dysfunction in macaques fed *Lathyrus sativus* and IDPN. *Neurology* 38:435, 1988.

Hurlbert RJ: Methylprednisolone for acute spinal cord injury: An inappropriate standard of care. *J Neurosurg* 93:1, 2000.

Jefferson G: Discussion on spinal injuries. *Proc R Soc Med* 21:625, 1927.

Jones A: Transient radiation myelitis. *Br J Radiol* 37:727, 1964.

Jonesco-Sisesti N: *Syringobulbia: A Contribution to the Pathophysiology of the Brainstem*. Translated into English, edited, and annotated by RT Ross. New York, Praeger, 1986.

Kagan RA, Wollin M, Gilbert HA, et al: Comparison of the tolerance of the brain and spinal cord to injury by radiation, in Gilbert HA, Kagan RA (eds): *Radiation Damage to the Nervous System*. New York, Raven Press, 1980.

Katz J, Ropper AH: Progressive necrotic myelopathy: Clinical course in 9 patients. *Arch Neurol* 57:355, 2000.

Kidd D, Thorpe JW, Kiendall BE, et al: MRI dynamics of brain and spinal cord in progressive multiple sclerosis. *J Neurol Neurosurg Psychiatry* 60:15, 1996.

Killen DA, Foster JH: Spinal cord injury as a complication of contrast angiography. *Surgery* 59:962, 1966.

Kneisley LW: Hyperhydrosis in paraplegia. *Arch Neurol* 34:536, 1977.

Kocher T: Die Wirletzungen der Virbelsäule zugleich als Beitrag zur Physiologie des menschlichen Ruckenmarcks. *Mitt Grenzgeb Med Chir* 1:415, 1896.

Kuhn RA: Functional capacity of the isolated human spinal cord. *Brain* 73:1, 1950.

Lazorthes G: Pathology, classification and clinical aspects of vascular diseases of the spinal cord, in Vinken PJ, Bruyn GW (eds): *Handbook of Clinical Neurology*. Vol 12. Amsterdam, North-Holland, 1972, pp 492–506.

Leech RW, Pitha JV, Brumback RA: Spontaneous haematomyelia: A necropsy study. *J Neurol Neurosurg Psychiatry* 54: 172, 1991.

Levivier M, Baleriaux D, Matos C, et al: Sarcoid myelopathy. *Neurology* 41:1529, 1991.

Lhermitte F, Chain F, Escourolle R, et al: Un nouveau cas de contracture tetaniforme distinct du stiff-man syndrome. *Rev Neurol* 128:3, 1923.

Lipson SJ, Naheedy MH, Kaplan MH: Spinal stenosis caused by epidural lipomatosis in Cushing's syndrome. *N Engl J Med* 302:36, 1980.

Logue V: Angiomas of the spinal cord: Review of the pathogenesis, clinical features, and results of surgery. *J Neurol Neurosurg Psychiatry* 42:1, 1979.

Logue V, Edwards MR: Syringomyelia and its surgical treatment: An analysis of 75 cases. *J Neurol Neurosurg Psychiatry* 44:273, 1981.

Love JG, Olafson RA: Syringomyelia: A look at surgical therapy. *J Neurosurg* 24:714, 1966.

Mair WGP, Folkerts JF: Necrosis of spinal cord due to thrombophlebitis (subacute necrotic myelitis). *Brain* 76:563, 1953.

Malamud N, Boldrey EB, Welch WK, Fadell EJ: Necrosis of brain and spinal cord following x-ray therapy. *J Neurosurg* 11:353, 1954.

Mancall EL, Rosales RK: Necrotizing myelopathy associated with visceral carcinoma. *Brain* 87:639, 1964.

Marshall J: Observations on reflex changes in the lower limbs in spastic paraplegia in man. *Brain* 77:290, 1954.

Martin J, Davis L: Studies upon spinal cord injuries: Altered reflex activity. *Surg Gynecol Obstet* 86:535, 1948.

McCormick PC, Michelsen WJ, Post KD, et al: Cavernous malformations of the spinal cord. *Neurosurgery* 23:459, 1988.

McCrae DL: Bony abnormalities in the region of the foramen magnum: Correlation of the anatomic and neurologic findings. *Acta Radiol* 40:335, 1953.

Messard L, Carmody A, Mannarino E, Ruge D: Survival after spinal cord trauma: A life table analysis. *Arch Neurol* 35:78, 1978.

Mixter WJ, Barr JS: Rupture of the intervertebral disc with involvement of the spinal canal. *N Engl J Med* 211:210, 1934.

Morrison RE, Brown J, Gooding RS: Spinal cord abscess caused by *Listeria monocytogenes*. *Arch Neurol* 37:243, 1980.

Morse SD: Acute central cervical spinal cord syndrome. *Ann Emerg Med* 11:436, 1982.

Munro D: The rehabilitation of patients totally paralyzed below the waist. *N Engl J Med* 234:207, 1946.

Murphy KP, Opitz JL, Cabanela ME, Ebersold MJ: Cervical fractures and spinal cord injury: Outcome of surgical and nonsurgical management. *Mayo Clin Proc* 65:949, 1990.

Naiman JL, Donahue WL, Pritchard JS: Fatal nucleus pulposus embolism of spinal cord after trauma. *Neurology* 11:83, 1961.

Nakano KK, Schoene WC, Baker RA, Dawson DM: The cervical myelopathy associated with rheumatoid arthritis: Analysis of 32 patients, with 2 postmortem cases. *Ann Neurol* 3:144, 1978.

Nesathurai S: Steroids and spinal cord injury: Revisiting the NASCIS 2 and NASCIS 3 trials. *J Trauma* 45:1088, 1998.

O'Connell JEA: The clinical signs of meningeal irritation. *Brain* 69:9, 1946.

Ogilvy CS, Heros RC: Spinal cord compression, in Ropper AH (ed): *Neurological and Neurosurgical Intensive Care*, 3rd ed. New York, Raven Press, 1993, pp 437–451.

Osame M, Matsumoto M, Usuku K, et al: Chronic progressive myelopathy associated with elevated antibodies to human T-lymphotropic virus type I and adult T-cell leukemia-like cells. *Ann Neurol* 21:117, 1987.

Osterholm JL: The pathophysiological response to spinal cord injury. *J Neurosurg* 40:3, 1974.

Oustwani MB, Kurtides ES, Christ M, Ciric I: Spinal cord compression with paraplegia in myelofibrosis. *Arch Neurol* 37:389, 1980.

Pallis C, Jones AM, Spillane JD: Cervical spondylosis. *Brain* 77:274, 1954.

Palmer JJ: Radiation myelopathy. *Brain* 95:109, 1972.

Panse F: Electrical lesions of the nervous system, in Vinken PJ, Bruyn GW (eds): *Handbook of Clinical Neurology*. Vol 7. Amsterdam, North-Holland, 1970, pp 344–387.

Payne EE, Spillane JD: The cervical spine: An anatomicopathological study of 70 specimens (using a special technique) with particular reference to the problem of cervical spondylosis. *Brain* 80:571, 1957.

Peet MM, Echols DH: Herniation of nucleus pulposus: Cause of compression of spinal cord. *Arch Neurol Psychiatry* 32:924, 1934.

Penn RD, Kroin JS: Continuous intrathecal baclofen for severe spasticity. *Lancet* 2:125, 1985.

Penry JK, Hoefnagel D, Vanden Noort S, Denny-Brown D: Muscle spasm and abnormal postures resulting from damage to interneurones in spinal cord. *Arch Neurol* 3:500, 1960.

Petito CK, Navia BA, Cho ES, et al: Vacuolar myelopathy pathologically resembling subacute combined degeneration in patients with AIDS. *N Engl J Med* 312:374, 1985.

Pollock LJ: Spasticity, pseudospontaneous spasm, and other reflex activities late after injury to the spinal cord. *Arch Neurol Psychiatry* 66:537, 1951.

Pollock LJ, Brown M, Boshes B, et al: Pain below the level of injury of the spinal cord. *Arch Neurol Psychiatry* 65:319, 1951.

Portenoy RK, Lipton RB, Foley KM: Back pain in the cancer patient: An algorithm for evaluation and management. *Neurology* 37:134, 1987.

Propper DJ, Bucknall RC: Acute transverse myelopathy complicating systemic lupus erythematosus. *Ann Rheum Dis* 48:512, 1989.

Queiroz L de S, Nucci A, Facure NO, Facure JJ: Massive spinal cord necrosis in schistosomiasis. *Arch Neurol* 36:517, 1979.

Reagan TJ, Thomas JE, Colby MY: Chronic progressive radiation myelopathy. *JAMA* 203:128, 1968.

Riddoch G: The reflex functions of the completely divided spinal cord in man, compared with those associated with less severe lesions. *Brain* 40:264, 1917.

Rodichok LD, Harper GR, Ruckdeschell JC, et al: Early diagnosis of spinal epidural metastases. *Am J Med* 70:1081, 1981.

Ropper AH, Poskanzer DC: The prognosis of acute and subacute transverse myelitis based on early signs and symptoms. *Ann Neurol* 4:51,1978.

Rossier AB, Foo D, Shillito J: Post-traumatic cervical syringomyelia. *Brain* 108:439, 1985.

Rowland LP: Surgical treatment of cervical spondylotic myelopathy: Time for a controlled study. *Neurology* 42:5, 1992.

Sandson TA, Friedman SH: Spinal cord infarction: Report of 8 cases and review of the literature. *Medicine* 68:282, 1989.

Sanyal B, Pant GC, Subrahmaniyam K, et al: Radiation myelopathy. *J Neurol Neurosurg Psychiatry* 42:413, 1979.

Savitsky N, Madonick MJ: Statistical control studies in neurology: Babinski sign. *Arch Neurol Psychiatry* 49:272, 1943.

Schneider RC, Cherry G, Pantek H: The syndrome of acute central cervical spinal cord injury. *J Neurosurg* 11:546, 1954.

Schurch B, Wichmann W, Rossier AB: Post-traumatic syringomelia (cystic myelopathy): A prospective study of 449 patients with spinal cord injury. *J Neurol Neurosurg Psychiatry* 60:61, 1996.

Scrimgeour EM, Gajdusek DC: Involvement of the central nervous system in *Schistosoma mansoni* and *S. haematobium* infection. *Brain* 108:1023, 1985.

Sgouros S, Williams B: A critical appraisal of drainage in syringomyelia. *J Neurosurg* 82:1, 1995.

Sgouros S, Williams B: Management and outcome of post-traumatic syringomyelia. *J Neurosurg* 85:197, 1996.

Shannon N, Simon L, Logue V: Clinical features, investigation, and treatment of post-traumatic syringomyelia. *J Neurol Neurosurg Psychiatry* 44:35, 1981.

Singer FR, Krane SM: Paget's disease of bone, in Avioli LV, Krane SM (eds): *Metabolic Bone Disease*. Philadelphia, Saunders, 1990.

Sloof JH, Kernohan JW, MacCarty CS: *Primary Intramedullary Tumors of the Spinal Cord and Filum Terminale*. Philadelphia, Saunders, 1964.

Spencer PS, Roy DN, Ludolph A, et al: Lathyrism: Evidence for role of the neuroexcitatory amino acid BOAA. *Lancet* 2:1066, 1986.

Spiller WG: Thrombosis of the cervical anterior median spinal artery: Syphilitic acute anterior poliomyelitis. *J Nerv Ment Dis* 36:601, 1909.

Stevens JM, Serva WA, Kendall BE, et al: Chiari malformation in adults: Relation of morphologic aspects to clinical features and operative outcome. *J Neurol Neurosurg Psychiatry* 56:1072, 1993.

STOLTMANN HF, BLACKWOOD W: The role of the ligamenta flava in the pathogenesis of myelopathy in cervical spondylosis. *Brain* 87:45, 1964.

STOOKEY B: Compression of the spinal cord due to ventral extradural cervical chondromas. *Arch Neurol Psychiatry* 20:275, 1928.

SWANN KW, ROPPER AH, NEW PFJ, POLETTI CE: Spontaneous spinal subarachnoid hemorrhage and subdural hematoma. *J Neurosurg* 61:975, 1984.

SYMON L, KUYAMA H, KENDALL B: Dural arteriovenous malformations of the spine: Clinical features and surgical results in 55 cases. *J Neurosurg* 60:238, 1984.

THOMAS JE, MILLER RH: Lipomatous tumors of the spinal canal. *Mayo Clin Proc* 48:393, 1973.

TOSI L, RIGOLI G, BELTRAMELLO A: Fibrocartilaginous embolism of the spinal cord: A clinical and pathogenetic consideration. *J Neurol Neurosurg Psychiatry* 60:55, 1996.

UCHIMURA I, SHIRAKI H: A contribution to the classification and pathogenesis of demyelinating encephalomyelitis. *J Neuropathol Exp Neurol* 16:139, 1957.

UTTLEY D, MONRO P: Neurosurgery for cervical spondylosis. *Br J Hosp Med* 42:62, 1989.

VALLEE B, MERCIER P, MENEI P, et al: Ventral transdural herniation of the thoracic cord: surgical treatment in four cases and review of the literature. *Acta Neurochir* 141:907, 1999.

WADIA NH: Myelopathy complicating congenital atlanto-axial dislocation (a study of 28 cases). *Brain* 90:449, 1967.

WEISMAN AD, ADAMS RD: The neurological complications of dissecting aortic aneurysm. *Brain* 67:69, 1944.

WESTENFELDER GO, AKEY DT, CORWIN SJ, et al: Acute transverse myelitis due to *Mycoplasma pneumoniae* infection. *Arch Neurol* 38:317, 1981.

WHITELY AM, SWASH M, URICH H: Progressive encephalomyelitis with rigidity. *Brain* 99:27, 1976.

WILKINSON M: *Cervical Spondylosis*, 2nd ed. Philadelphia, Saunders, 1971.

WILLIAMS B: The cystic spinal cord. *J Neurol Neurosurg Psychiatry* 58:649, 1995.

WINKELMAN MD: Neurological complications of thermal and electrical burns, in Aminoff MJ (ed): *Neurology and General Medicine*. New York, Churchill Livingstone, 1994, pp 915–929.

WINKELMAN MD, ADELSTEIN DJ, KARLINS NL: Intramedullary spinal cord metastases: Diagnostic and therapeutic considerations. *Arch Neurol* 44:526, 1987.

WOLTMAN HW, ADSON AW: Abscess of the spinal cord. *Brain* 49:193, 1926.

WOOLSEY RM, YOUNG RR (eds): *Neurologic Clinics: Disorders of the Spinal Cord*. Philadelphia, Saunders, 1991.

WYBURN-MASON R: *Vascular Abnormalities and Tumors of the Spinal Cord and Its Membranes*. St Louis, Mosby, 1944.

YOGANANDEN N, LARSON SJ, GALLAGHER M: Correlation of microtrauma in the spine with intraosseous pressure. *Spine* 19:435, 1994.

ZWIMPFER TJ, BERNSTEIN M: Spinal cord compression. *J Neurosurg* 72:894, 1990.

Chapter 45

ELECTROPHYSIOLOGIC TESTING AND LABORATORY AIDS IN THE DIAGNOSIS OF NEUROMUSCULAR DISEASE

The clinical suspicion of neuromuscular disease, disclosed by any of the symptoms or syndromes in the succeeding chapters, finds ready confirmation in the laboratory. The intelligent use of ancillary examinations requires some knowledge of the biochemistry and physiology of muscle fiber contraction, nerve action potentials, and neuromuscular conduction. These subjects are therefore reviewed briefly, as an introduction to the descriptions of the laboratory methods and the subject matter of the chapters that follow. The relevant anatomy is presented in later parts of this chapter and in Chap. 3.

Electrolytes and Neuromuscular Activity

It is not possible here to review all the biochemical and biophysical data that explain nerve impulse generation and conduction. Since the early studies of Hodgkin (1951) and of Hodgkin and Huxley (1952), tomes have been written on these subjects. Suffice it to say that the nerve and muscle fibers, like other bodily cells, maintain a fluid internal environment that is distinctly different from the external or interstitial medium. The main intracellular constituents are potassium (K), magnesium (Mg), and phosphorus (P), whereas those outside the cell are sodium (Na), calcium (Ca), and chloride (Cl). In both nerve and muscle the intracellular concentrations of these ions are held within a narrow range by electrical and chemical forces, which maintain the membranes in electrochemical equilibrium ("resting membrane potential"). These forces are the result of selective permeability of the membranes to various ions and the continuous expulsion of intracellular Na through special channels by a pump mechanism ("the sodium pump"). The function of the pump is dependent on the enzyme Na-K-ATPase, which is localized in the membranes. The resulting electrochemical equilibrium is such that the interior of the cell is kept 70 to 90 mV negative with respect to the exterior (the resting membrane potential).

This resting membrane potential is therefore dependent on the differential concentrations of K and Na. The interior of the cell is some 30 times richer in K than the extracellular fluid, and the concentration of Na is 10 to 12 times greater in the extracellular fluid. In the resting state the chemical forces that promote diffusion of K ions out of the cell (down their concentration gradient) are counterbalanced by electrical forces (the external positivity opposes further diffusion of K to the exterior of the cell). At the resting potential, the situation of Na ions is the opposite; they tend to diffuse into the cell, both because of their concentration gradient and because of the relative negativity inside the cell. Because the membrane is less permeable to Na than to K, the amount of K leaving the cell exceeds the amount of Na entering the cell, thus creating the difference in electrical charge across the membrane.

Electrical discharge of neural and muscular tissue is predicated on a special property of excitable membranes—namely, that the permeability of the cell to Na is controlled by the electrical potential of the membrane. As the membrane is depolarized by any slight electrical or chemical change, there is an increased permeability to Na. The subsequent movement of K outward repolarizes the membrane and thereby reduces its permeability to

Na. These slight fluxes of ions in the resting state are known as *passive decay*. If a greater degree of depolarization occurs, a situation arises in which the outward movement of K is unable to stabilize the membrane. At this new threshold, the membrane becomes even more depolarized and progressively more permeable to Na, and an "explosive" regenerative Na current develops; Na rushes down its chemical and electrical gradients into the cell. Eventually a new equilibrium potential is reached where the interior of the cell becomes about 40 mV positive. It is this rapid inward flux of sodium that creates the action potential, which lasts only a millisecond or less before the membrane loses its permeability to Na and becomes much more permeable to K. The resulting efflux of K then repolarizes the membrane to a resting level. During this brief period of repolarization, the nerve and muscle fibers are refractory, at first absolutely then relatively, to another depolarizing stimulus.

Conduction, or propagation of the action potential along excitable membranes, occurs as the current flows into the depolarized zone and the contiguous membrane becomes depolarized. When the depolarization reaches the threshold for development of an action potential and a new zone of increased Na permeability is created, the action potential then spreads in an all-or-none fashion, down the length of the nerve or muscle membrane (see Kuffler et al for further details). The action potentials in individual nerve fibers are too small and brief to be detected by conventional nerve conduction techniques, but a summated volley of all the fibers comprised by a nerve is large enough to be recorded, and it is this property that is utilized to study nerve function in the clinical electromyography (EMG) laboratory.

As the motor nerve impulses pass centrifugally from the parent axon into its terminal branches, transmission may still "break down," especially if the repetition rate is excessive and impulses arrive too frequently at branch points. Impulses may then fail to reach the myoneural junction of these fibers. Or there may be failure of conduction at the myoneural junction, which is what occurs in myasthenia gravis.

In large motor and sensory nerves, contiguous spread of action potentials along a fiber is slow and eventually decays over long distances. In these large fibers, conduction is aided by the myelin sheaths. The sodium channels, which generate the action potential, are concentrated at short exposed segments of the axon, the nodes of Ranvier, lying between longer segments of myelinated axon. The portions of axon that are covered by myelin remain electrically insulated. This creates "flux lines" that are concentrated at the nodes and allows current to be generated repeatedly at each of these gaps in the myelin. The speed of electrical conduction, which jumps in this "saltatory" fashion from node to node, is many times faster than through unmyelinated axons. The largest-diameter fibers, which by reason of their size have the fastest conduction times, also have the thickest myelin sheaths and longest internodal distances.

Conventional laboratory studies of nerve conduction generally measure the speed of these fastest-conducting fibers. This dependence of nerve conduction on the myelin sheath explains a number of abnormalities consequent upon myelin destruction. The most common finding, as one might predict, is a slowing of nerve conduction due to loss of the impulses contributed by the largest-diameter and fastest-conducting fibers. When myelin destruction is severe or a circulating factor impedes the channels that regenerate a sodium current, there is a total block of electrical conduction. An intermediate state of partial demyelination slows and desynchronizes the electrical volley, leading to temporal dispersion of the action potentials that reach the muscle. The cumulative effect of these changes is to reduce the number of nerve fibers that are capable of conducting an electrical volley, leading to a graduated reduction in the amplitude of the muscle action potential as longer segments of nerve are tested. This reduction in amplitude of the compound muscle action potential (CMAP) as the stimulating electrode is moved proximally during electrophysiologic examination is termed *conduction block* (discussed under "Conduction Studies of Nerve," below). Blocked conduction of this nature is the most reliable marker of an acquired demyelinating neuropathy; of all the electromyographic changes, it corresponds most closely to the degree of muscle weakness (see further on).

The Neuromuscular Junction (Motor End Plate)

This is the interface between the finely branched nerve fiber and the muscle fiber, where the electrical activity of the motor nerve is translated into muscle action (Fig. 45-1). The nerve fiber, as it indents the muscle cell membrane, leaves a small space of 50 μm—the *synaptic cleft*, between the axolemma and sarcolemma (Fig. 53-1). In the nerve terminal, a relatively fixed number of packets, or quanta, of acetylcholine (ACh), each packet consisting of about 10,000 molecules, are liberated through an exocytotic process by the arrival of axonal action potentials, but some are also released spontaneously. Arrival of the electrical impulse opens calcium channels in the presynaptic

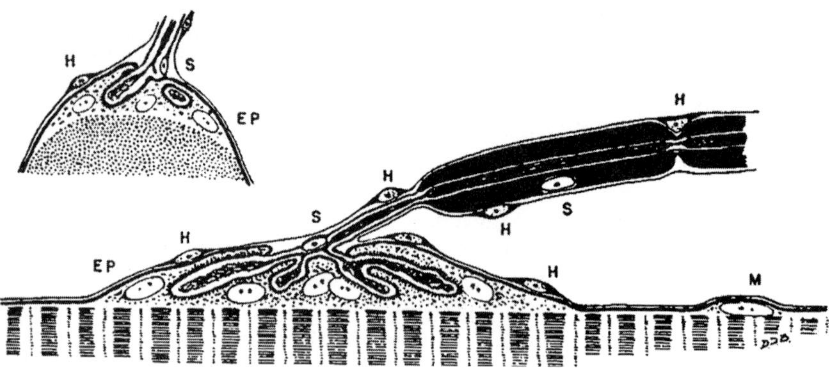

Figure 45-1

Motor end plate showing relationship between various structures in nerve and muscle. Last segment of myelin, with Schwann nucleus (S), terminates abruptly, leaving axis cylinder covered by sheaths of Schwann and Henle. End-plate nuclei (EP) of muscle fiber lie embedded in sarcoplasm and have same staining reactions as sarcolemmal nuclei (M). Ramifications of axis cylinder (teleodendria) lie in grooves or pouches in granular sarcoplasm, each lined by spiny "subneural apparatus" of Couteaux, which is continuous with membranous sarcolemma and also Schwann membrane. Nucleus (S) of sheath of Schwann commonly lies near point of branching of axon. Sheath of Henle has small nuclei (H) and fuses with endomysial sheath of muscle fiber. (Courtesy of Dr. D. Denny-Brown.)

membrane, which serve to bind packets of ACh to the membrane and govern their release. Molecules of ACh diffuse into the synaptic cleft and attach to receptor sites on the postsynaptic membrane. Each impulse triggers the release of approximately 200 quanta of ACh and produces a depolarization of sufficient size to initiate an action potential in the muscle through the same mechanism of a regenerative sodium current described above. Botulinum toxin and a high concentration of Mg ions interfere with the entry of calcium on the presynaptic side and raise the threshold for quantal release. There is also known to be a nonquantal release of ACh through continuous leakage. This appears to play a role in the trophic influence of nerve on muscle.

Each ACh molecule binds to a postsynaptic ACh receptor protein, thereby causing a conformational change in the postsynaptic part of the motor end plate and a local increase in the conductance of Na and K and other small ions. This produces a depolarization known as the *end-plate potential*. Small (miniature) end-plate potentials (MEPPs) are continuously formed and regenerated as the membranes repolarize, much as in the process of passive decay described above. These potentials are too small to be recorded by routine EMG testing, although fortuitous needle placement adjacent to a synapse may detect them. The bound ACh is hydrolyzed by cholinesterase, a glycoprotein enzyme that exists in free form in the cleft; its main function is to terminate the action potential and permit the sequential activation of muscle. The postsynaptic membrane, once depolarized, is refractory to another action potential until it is repolarized.

The calcium that entered the presynaptic nerve terminal is sequestered and then extruded and the choline from the hydrolyzed ACh enters the nerve terminal, where it is resynthesized to ACh near the release sites.

The analysis of a rapid series of electrically elicited muscle contractions is used specifically to analyze the function of the neuromuscular junction. A decrement in the amplitude of muscle action potentials is typical of postsynaptic failure of conduction, and an increment, of presynaptic failure. *Myasthenia gravis* is the principal disease affecting the neuromuscular junction. The fundamental defect is not a deficiency of ACh or its release, but rather its failure to attach to the postsynaptic receptor, being blocked by an antibody at the receptor site. There are several other synaptic disorders—due to botulism, aminoglycoside antibiotics, and the antibodies of the Lambert-Eaton myasthenic syndrome—which impede presynaptic release of ACh. Certain pharmacologic agents interfere with neuromuscular transmission by combining with the cholinergic (nicotinic) receptor on the postsynaptic membrane, thereby competitively blocking the transmitter action of ACh. The curariform drugs, derived from curare and termed *nondepolarizing neuromuscular blockers*, are the main examples. Other drugs, notably succinylcholine and decamethonium, cause neuromuscular blockage by producing direct depolarization of the end plate and adjacent sarcoplasmic membrane (depolarizing neuromuscular blockers). Agents that inactivate cholinesterase have the opposite effect, i.e., they enhance the action of ACh. The ones in clinical use (for the treatment of myasthenia gravis) are the carbamates neostigmine, physostigmine, pyridostigmine, etc., the effects of which are reversible. The organophosphates are irreversible blockers of cholinesterase function, for which reason they are feared weapons of chemical warfare. Atropine is a potent cholinergic antagonist that is active only at muscarinic sites and therefore has no effect at the neuromuscular junction.

Chemistry of Muscle Contraction

The sarcolemma, the transverse tubules, and the sarcoplasmic reticulum each play a role in the control of the activity of muscle fibers. The structural components involved in excitation, contraction, and relaxation of muscle are illustrated in Fig. 45-2. Following nerve stimulation, an action potential is transmitted by the sarcolemma from the motor end-plate region to both ends of the muscle fiber. Depolarization spreads quickly to the interior of the fiber along the walls of the transverse

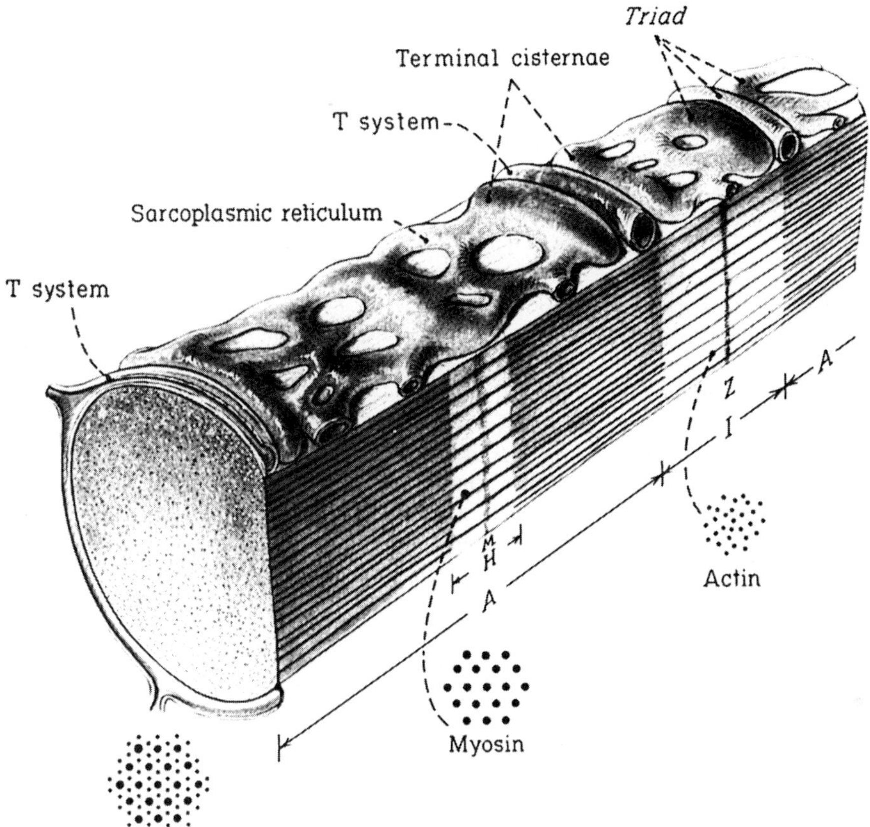

Figure 45-2

Schematic illustration of the major subcellular components of a myofibril. The transverse (T) system, which is an invagination of the plasma membrane of the cell, surrounds the myofibril midway between the Z lines and the center of the A bands; the T system is approximated to, but apparently not continuous with, dilated elements (terminal cisternae) of the sarcoplasmic reticulum on either side. Thus, each sarcomere (the repeating Z-line-to-Z-line unit) contains two "triads," each composed of a pair of terminal cisternae on each side of the T tubule. (From Peter, by permission.)

tubules, probably by a conducted action potential. The transverse tubules and the terminal cisternae of the sarcoplasmic reticulum come into close proximity at points referred to as *triads*. Here, by a mechanism that is not fully understood, depolarization of the transverse tubules is transmitted to the sarcoplasmic reticulum, which releases Ca stored in its interior. Calcium binds to the regulatory protein *troponin*, thereby removing the inhibition exerted by the troponin-tropomyosin system upon the contractile protein *actin*. This allows an interaction to take place between the actin molecules of the thin filaments and the cross bridges of the myosin molecules in the thick filaments and enables myosin adenosine triphosphatase (ATPase) to split adenosine triphosphate (ATP) at a rapid rate, thereby providing the energy for contraction. This chemical change causes the filaments to slide past each other. Relaxation occurs as a result of active (energy-dependent) Ca reuptake by the sarcoplasmic reticulum.

The pyrophosphate bonds of ATP, which supply the energy for muscle contraction, must be replenished constantly by a reaction that involves interchanges with the muscle phosphagen creatine diphosphate, where high-energy phosphate bonds are stored. These interactions, in both contraction and relaxation, require the action of creatine kinase (CK). Myoglobin, another important muscle protein, functions in the transfer of oxygen, and a series of oxidative enzymes are involved in this exchange. The intracellular Ca, as noted above, is released by the muscle action potential and must be reaccumulated within the cisternae of the sarcoplasmic reticulum before actin and myosin filaments can slide back past one another in relaxation. The reuptake of Ca requires the expenditure of considerable energy. When there is defective generation of ATP, the muscle remains shortened, as in the *contracture* of phosphorylase deficiency (McArdle disease) or of phosphofructose kinase deficiency. The same sort of shortening occurs under normal conditions in some of the "catch muscles" of certain mollusks and is the basis of rigor mortis in mammals.

Many glycolytic and other enzymes (transaminases, aldolase, CK) are utilized in the metabolic activity of muscle, particularly under relatively anaerobic conditions. Muscle fibers differ from one another in their relative content of oxidative and glycolytic enzymes; the latter determine the capacity of the muscle fiber to sustain anaerobic metabolism during periods of contraction with inadequate blood flow. Muscle cells rich in oxidative enzymes (type 1 fibers) contain more mitochondria and larger amounts of myoglobin (therefore appearing red), have slower rates of contraction and relaxation, fire more tonically, and are less fatigable than muscle fibers poor in oxidative enzymes. The latter (type 2 fibers) fire in bursts and are utilized in quick phasic rather than sustained reactions. The amount of myosin ATPase activity, which governs the speed of contraction, is low in oxidative-rich fibers and high in glycolytic-rich fibers. The myosin ATPase stain at pH 9.4 has been used to identify these two types of fibers in microscopic sections. Type 1 fibers have a low content of myosin ATPase, and type 2 (phosphorylative-rich) fibers have a high content of this enzyme; hence type 1 fibers stain lightly and type 2 darkly (the reverse reaction occurs at pH 4.6). Other less well differentiated histochemical types have also been identified. All the fibers within one motor unit are of the same type, a feature that is used to advantage to identify the reinnervation of muscle fibers by a single motor neuron (fiber type grouping) after adjacent neurons have died and denervated their constituent muscle fibers.

The chemical energy required to maintain the various activities of the muscle cell is derived mainly from the metabolism of carbohydrate (blood glucose, muscle glycogen) and fatty acids (plasma free fatty acids, esterified fatty acids, and ketone bodies). There is a lesser contribution from branched-chain and other amino acids, but this may increase during prolonged exercise.

The most readily available source of energy is glycogen, which is synthesized and stored in muscle cells. It provides over 90 percent of the energy needs of muscle under conditions of high work intensity and during the early stages of submaximal exercise. Blood glucose and free fatty acids supplement intracellular glycogen as exercise proceeds. The free fatty acids are obtained from endogenous triglycerides (found mostly in type 1 fibers), from the triglycerides released by circulating lipoproteins, and from the lipolysis of adipose tissue. Most of the energy needs of resting muscle are provided by fatty acids.

The enzymatic reactions involved in the transport of these substrates into muscle cells and their intracellular synthesis and degradation during anaerobic and aerobic cell conditions have been thoroughly investigated and most of the enzymes identified. This subject is too complicated to present in a textbook of neurology, but enough is known about these matters to state confidently that there are a number of diseases that can impair the contractile functions of muscle in different ways without destroying the fiber. Specific enzymatic deficiencies under genetic control may affect carbohydrate utilization (myophosphorylase, debrancher enzyme, phosphofructokinase, phosphoglyceromutase, and myoadenylate deaminase), fatty acid utilization (carnitine and carnitine palmitoyl transferase deficiencies), pyruvate metabolism, and cytochrome oxidase activity (in the mitochondrial diseases). These enzymatic disturbances are discussed in later chapters.

Physiology of Muscle Contraction

The contraction of a muscle fiber is to be viewed as both a series of electrochemical events and a mechanical event. The mechanical change far outlasts the electrical one and extends through the period when the muscle fiber is refractory to another action potential. When a second muscle action potential arrives, after the refractory phase of the previous action potential but before the muscle has relaxed, the contraction will be prolonged. Thus, at frequencies of anterior horn cell firing of more than 100 per second, the twitches fuse into a sustained contraction or *fused tetanus*. In most sustained contractions, there is incomplete tetanus, attained by firing rates of 40 to 50 per second. In this fashion the mechanical phenomena are smoothed into a continuous process, even though the electrical potentials present as a series of depolarizations, separated by intervals during which the muscle membrane resumes its resting polarized state.

As pointed out in Chap. 3, the physiology of muscle activity should always be considered in terms of motor units, i.e., the group of muscle fibers within the domain of each anterior horn cell. The strength of muscle contraction is a function of the number and rates of firing of many motor units. The smoothness of contraction depends on the integrated enlistment of motor units of increasing size. The electrical signal of this summated contraction, as recorded at the skin surface over a muscle, is the main feature of the surface EMG and the basis of motor nerve conduction examinations.

Further study involves the insertion into the muscle of a coaxial needle, which samples a multitude of motor units in the vicinity of the electrode. When elicited by a sustained voluntary contraction, the flurry of electrical activity from many units at different distances from the electrodes is referred to as an *interference pattern*. If the motor units are stimulated by a brief electrical stimulus applied to a motor nerve, the effect is a compound muscle action potential (CMAP). The CMAP can be visualized on the screen of an oscilloscope or a computer and utilized to measure the speed of motor nerve conduction and the summated amplitudes produced by all the innervating nerve fibers. It can also be converted into an audible noise (see further on, under "Conduction Studies of Nerve" and "Needle Examination of Muscle").

Biochemical changes may cause not only an impairment of neuromuscular activity (paresis, paralysis) but also excessive irritability, tetany, spasm, and cramp. In the latter instances, spontaneous discharges may occur from an instability of axon polarization; hence a single nerve impulse may initiate a train of action potentials in nerve and muscle, as in the tetany of hypocalcemia and in hemifacial spasm. In tetany, there may also be paresthesias, on the basis of irritability and ectopic discharges of sensory nerve fibers. The common cramps of calf and foot muscles (painful, sustained contractions with motor unit discharges at frequencies up to 200 per second) may be due to increased excitability (or unstable polarization) of the motor axons. Quinine, procainamide, diphenhydramine, and warmth reduce the irritability of nerve and muscle fiber membranes, as do a number of anticonvulsant drugs that act by blocking sodium channels and thereby limiting spontaneous membrane discharges.

To summarize, the muscle fiber, which is wholly dependent on the nerve for its stimulus to contract, may be physiologically activated or paralyzed in a number of ways. The nerve cell may be disinhibited in the anterior horn of the spinal cord, permitting the discharge of continuous action potentials, as in tetanus and the "stiff-man" syndrome (page 1569); the nerve fiber may fail to conduct impulses (demyelinating neuropathies) or the number of fibers may be inadequate to produce a fused and sustained contraction (axonal neuropathies); the neurilemma may not distribute the nerve impulse simultaneously to all parts of the motor unit ("jitter" phenomenon in distal axonal damage or neuromuscular junction diseases); ACh may not be released at the presynaptic region of the neuromuscular junction (as occurs in botulism and in the Eaton-Lambert syndrome) or, once released, ACh may not be inactivated by cholinesterase (physostigmine, organophosphates); the receptor zone on the postsynaptic membrane may be destroyed or blocked by antibodies or pharmacologic agents (myasthenia gravis or curariform drugs); and, finally, the metabolic or contractile elements of the muscle may not react or, once contracted, may not relax. Similarly, the mechanisms involved in fasciculations, cramps, and muscle spasms may be traced to a number of different loci in the neuromuscular apparatus. There may be an unstable polarization of the nerve fibers, as in tetany and in dehydration with salt depletion, or unexplained hyperirritability of the motor unit, as in amyotrophic lateral sclerosis. The threshold of mechanical activation or electrical reactivation of the sarcolemmal membrane may be reduced, as in myotonia, or impairment of an energy mechanism within the fiber may slow the contractile process, as in hypothyroidism; or a deficiency of phosphorylase, which deprives muscle of its carbohydrate energy source, may prevent relaxation, as in the contracture of McArdle disease. Lesions of the most peripheral branches of nerves, which allow nerve regeneration, may give rise to continuous activity of motor units. This is expressed clinically as a rippling of muscle, or *myokymia* (see pages 1467 and 1568).

In recent years, new technologies, such as isolation of complementary DNA, have made it possible to isolate each of the proteins and channels involved in neuromuscular transmission and the excitation-contraction-relaxation of muscle fibers. The amino acid composition of most of these proteins has also been determined. This information is being increasingly applied to the analysis of gene products in the normal state and under conditions of disease. Pertinent references to this subject are found in the chapters that follow.

Effects on Muscle of Abnormalities of Serum Electrolytes

Diffuse muscle weakness or muscle twitching, spasms, and cramps should always raise the question of uremia or an abnormality in serum electrolytes. These disorders reflect the concentrations of electrolytes in the intra- and extracellular fluids. The electrocardiogram (ECG) may reveal alterations of their intracellular levels in the heart. If the plasma concentration of *potassium falls below 2.5 meq/L or rises above 7 meq/L*, weakness of extremity and trunk muscles results; below 2 meq/L or above 9 meq/L, there is almost always flaccid paralysis of these muscles and later of the respiratory ones as well, only the extraocular and other cranial muscles being spared. In addition, the tendon reflexes are diminished or absent. The normal reaction of muscle to direct percussion (idiomuscular irritability) is also reduced or abolished, suggesting impairment of transmission along the sarcolemmal membranes themselves. *Hypocalcemia* of 7 mg/dL or less (as in rickets or hypoparathyroidism) or relative reduction in the proportion of ionized calcium (as in hyperventilation) causes increased muscle irritability and spontaneous discharge of sensory and motor nerve fibers (i.e., tetany) and sometimes convulsions from similar effects upon cerebral neurons; frequent repetitive and finally prolonged spontaneous discharges grouped in couplets or triplets appear in the EMG, and convulsive effects are reflected in the EEG. *Hypercalcemia* above 12 mg/dL (as in vitamin D intoxication, hyperparathyroidism, carcinomatosis, sarcoid, and multiple myeloma) causes weakness and lethargy, perhaps on a central basis. Extreme *hypophosphatemia*, observed most often with intravenous hyperalimentation or bone tumor, can cause acute areflexic paralysis with nerve conduction abnormalities. *Reduction in the plasma concentration of magnesium* also results in tremor, muscle weakness, tetanic muscle spasms, and convulsions; a considerable *increase in magnesium levels* leads to muscle weakness and depression of central nervous function (confusion). The weakness of muscle may be due, in part at least, to reduced release of ACh at the motor end plate.

Changes in Serum Levels of Enzymes Originating in Muscle Cells

In all diseases causing extensive damage to striated muscle fibers, intracellular enzymes leak out of the fiber and enter the blood. Those measured routinely are the transaminases, lactic acid dehydrogenase, aldolase, and creatine kinase (CK). Of these, the concentration of CK in serum has proved to be the most sensitive measure of muscle damage. Since high concentrations of this enzyme are found in heart muscle and brain, raised serum values may be due to myocardial or cerebral infarction as well as to the necrotizing diseases of striated muscle (polymyositis, muscle trauma, muscle infarction, paroxysmal myoglobinuria, and the more rapidly advancing muscular dystrophies). For serum CK levels to be interpretable, one has to be certain that the enzyme being released into the serum is not derived from heart or brain. This can be determined by the quantitation of serum isoenzymes of CK, referred to as MB, MM, and BB (M, muscle; B, brain); their measurement provides a sensitive means for the detection of damage to myocardium (MB), skeletal muscle (MM), and nervous tissue (BB), respectively.

The MM form of CK is found in highest concentration in striated muscle, but there is also 5 to 6 percent MB. Heart contains 17 to 59 percent MB; hence, the diagnosis of myocardial infarction requires that the CK-MB fraction be greater than 6 percent (or that troponin, which is overrepresented in heart muscle, be present in the serum). Embryonic and regenerating muscle contains more CK-MB than mature normal muscle. In patients with destructive lesions of striated muscle, serum values of CK often exceed 1000 units and may reach 40,000 units or more (the upper limit of normal varies from 65 to 200 units, depending on the method). Serum of the normal adult contains only the MM isoenzyme, but in normal children, as much as 25 percent of serum CK may be derived from the MB fraction. Even more interesting is its rise in some children with progressive muscular dystrophy before there is enough destruction of fibers for the disease to be clinically manifest, at least as judged by the relatively crude tests of muscle strength. Moreover, the unaffected female carrier of Duchenne dystrophy may often be identified by an elevated serum level of CK. Alterations of serum enzyme levels are nonspecific for dystrophy since they occur in all types of disease that damage the muscle fiber. Moreover, in the more slowly evolving types of dystrophy, such as that of Landouzy-Déjerine, the serum levels of CK may be normal. It would be expected that the values would always be normal in denervation paralysis with muscular atrophy, but slight elevations are sometimes observed in patients with progressive spinal muscular atrophy and amyotrophic lateral sclerosis. Even vigorous exercise or surgical operations elevate CK, sometimes exceeding 6 percent from the MB fraction. In some individuals, CK may be persistently elevated without evidence of muscle or other diseases. An unexplained alteration of the sarcolemma with high serum CK occurs in hypothyroidism and in alcoholism.

An isolated elevation of aldolase, the serum enzyme other than CK that is derived predominantly from skeletal muscle, generally has less clinical significance. Measurement in the serum of various transaminases or lactate dehydrogenase is not particularly useful for the diagnosis of muscle disease because of their ubiquitous distribution in many mammalian tissues. Nevertheless, the neurologist should be aware that unexplained elevations in all of the muscle-derived enzymes (CK, LDH, SGOT, etc.) can be caused by inevident muscle trauma.

Myoglobinuria

The red pigment myoglobin, responsible for much of the color of muscle, is an iron-protein compound present in the sarcoplasm of striated skeletal and cardiac fibers. Of the total body hematin compounds, about 25 percent is in muscle, the remainder in red blood corpuscles and other cells. Destruction of striated muscle, regardless of the process—whether trauma, ischemia, or metabolic disease—liberates myoglobin, and because of its relatively small size, the molecule filters through the glomeruli and appears in the urine, imparting to it a burgundy red color. Because of the low renal threshold for myoglobin, excretion of this pigment is so rapid that the serum remains uncolored. In contrast, because of the high renal threshold for hemoglobin, destruction of red blood corpuscles colors both the serum and the urine. Myoglobinuria should thus be suspected when the urine is deep red and the serum is normal in color. It is estimated that 200 g of muscle must be destroyed to color the urine visibly (Rowland). As in hemoglobinuria, the guaiac and benzidine tests of urine are positive. The colored urine does not fluoresce, as it does in porphyria. On spectroscopic analysis, myoglobin shows an absorption band at 581 nm, but the most sensitive method for measuring myoglobin in the urine and serum is by radioimmunoassay techniques (Rosano and Kenny). Hyperkalemia, hyperphosphatemia, and hypercalcemia may complicate massive rhabdomyolysis.

Some years ago, the measurement of creatine and creatinine in blood and urine was a standard method of estimating damage to striated muscle. This technique is now seldom used for clinical or research purposes, having been replaced largely by the measurement of CK and its isoenzymes.

Endocrine Myopathies

In a number of disorders of the endocrine glands, muscle weakness may be a prominent feature, and occasionally it may be the chief complaint. Although these diseases are discussed in detail in Chap. 51, it should be noted that such weakness, local or generalized, acute or chronic, may occur in the absence of changes in serum electrolytes or enzymes. Specific hormone assays are then necessary for diagnosis. This is particularly true of patients with thyrotoxicosis or Cushing disease and those receiving prolonged corticosteroid therapy. In thyrotoxicosis, muscle paresis may appear without the classic signs of Graves disease.

ELECTRODIAGNOSIS OF NEUROMUSCULAR DISEASE (ELECTROMYOGRAPHY; EMG)

It was long ago discovered that muscle would contract when a pulse of electric current was applied to the skin, near the point of entrance of the muscular nerve (*motor point*). The electrical pulse required is brief, less than a millisecond, and is most effectively induced by a rapidly alternating (faradic) current. *After denervation*, an electrical pulse of several milliseconds, induced by a constant electrical (galvanic) stimulus, is required to produce the same response. This change, in which the galvanic stimulus remains effective after the faradic one has failed, was the basis of *Erb's reaction of degeneration*, and varying degrees of this change were later plotted in the form of *strength-duration curves*. For decades, this was the standard electrical method for evaluating denervation of muscle. Though still valid, it was replaced long ago by nerve conduction studies and by the needle electrode examination. The latter tests, based on the sherringtonian concept of the "motor unit" (page 47), is accomplished by recording the firing characteristics of evoked motor unit potentials (MUPs and CMAPs) and by the insertion into muscle of needle electrodes to measure spontaneous and voluntarily evoked muscle fiber activity. The terms *electromyography* and *electromyogram* (EMG) were coined originally to describe only the needle electrode examination but are now commonly used to describe the entire electrodiagnostic evaluation, including the *nerve conduction studies*, described below.

Conduction Studies of Nerve

The main laboratory technique for the study of peripheral nerve function involves the percutaneous stimulation of motor or sensory nerves and recording of the elicited muscle and sensory action potentials. The results of these *motor and sensory nerve conduction studies*, expressed as amplitudes, conduction velocities, and distal latencies, yield certain quantitative information and additional qualitative observations regarding the waveform and dispersion of electrical impulses.

Hodes and coworkers in 1948 were the first to perform nerve conduction studies in patients. An accessible nerve is stimulated through the skin by surface electrodes, using a stimulus that recruits all available fibers, and the resulting compound action potential is recorded by electrodes on the skin (1) over the nerve more proximally, using orthodromic techniques for sensory fibers stimulated in the digital nerves, (2) over the nerve more distally, using antidromic techniques for sensory nerve conduction studies (this has many technical advantages over orthodromic techniques), (3) over the muscle more distally in the case of motor fibers stimulated in a mixed or motor nerve, and (4) over the nerve more proximally for mixed nerve conduction studies (Fig. 45-3). The second and third techniques are the ones used most often in clinical work. An alternative but much more demanding technique uses "near nerve" needle electrodes to record action potentials as they course through the nerve.

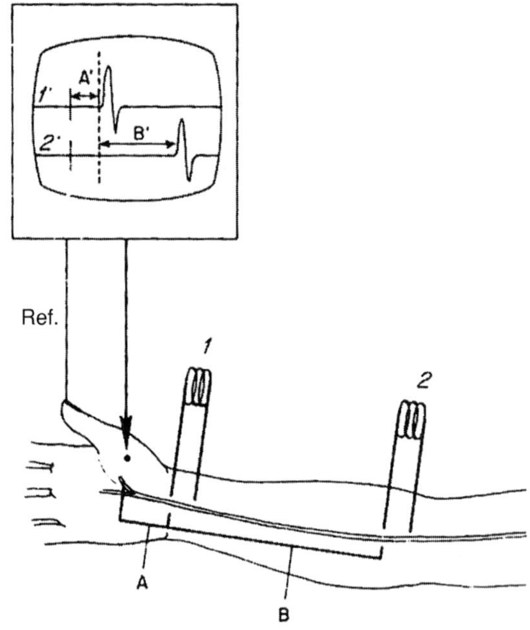

Figure 45-3

The median nerve is stimulated percutaneously (1) at the wrist and (2) in the antecubital fossa with the resultant compound muscle action potential recorded as the potential difference between a surface electrode over the thenar eminence (arrow) and a reference electrode (Ref.) more distally. Sweep 1′ on the display depicts the stimulus artifact followed by the compound muscle action potential. The distal latency, A′, is the time from the stimulus artifact to the take-off phase of the compound muscle action potential and corresponds to conduction over distance A. The same is true for sweep 2′, where stimulation is at 2 and the time from the artifact to the response is A′ + B′. The maximum motor conduction velocity over segment B is calculated by dividing distance B by the time B′.

Distal (Terminal) Latencies, Conduction Times, and Conduction Velocities The conduction times from the most distal stimulating electrode to the recording site, in milliseconds, as determined by measurements from the stimulus artifact to the onset and to the peak of the response, are termed the *distal* (or terminal) and *peak* latencies, respectively. *The distal latency* (the time to the onset of the compound muscle action potential) is used as a measure of the speed of conduction (Fig. 45-4). If a second stimulus is applied to a mixed nerve more proximally (or if recording or stimulating electrodes can be placed more proximally in the case of sensory fibers), a new and longer conduction time can be measured. When the distance (in millimeters) between the two sites of stimulation of motor fibers or recording of sensory fibers is divided by the difference in conduction times (in milliseconds), one obtains a maximal conduction velocity (in meters per second), which describes the velocity of propagation of the action potentials in the largest and fastest nerve fibers. These velocities in normal subjects vary from a minimum of 40 or 45 m/s to a maximum of 65 to 75 m/s, depending upon which nerve is studied (slower in the legs than in the arms; Table 45-1). Values are lower in infants, reaching the adult range by the age of 2 to 4 years and decline again with advancing age. They are diminished also with exposure to cold—a potentially important artifact in these recordings.

Normal values have been established for distal latencies from the distalmost site of stimulation on various mixed nerves to the appropriate muscles; when one stimulates the median nerve at the wrist, for example (electrode 1 and segment A in Fig. 45-3), the latency for motor conduction through the carpal tunnel to the median-innervated thenar muscles is always less than 4.5 ms in normal adults. Similar normal values have been compiled for orthodromic and antidromic sensory conduction velocities and distal latencies (Table 45-1).

Disease processes that preferentially injure the fastest-conducting, large-diameter fibers in peripheral nerves reduce the maximal conduction velocity to some degree because the remaining fibers with smaller diameters conduct more slowly. In most neuropathies, only a part of the axon is affected (either by the "dying-back" phenomenon or by wallerian degeneration), and nerve conduction velocities are then relatively uninformative. This is true for typical alcoholic-nutritional, carcinomatous, uremic, and some diabetic and other metabolic neuropathies, in which conduction velocities range from low normal to mildly slow. On the other hand, the motor and particularly the sensory nerve amplitudes as described below are usually diminished, and there may be fibrillations and changes in motor unit potentials on needle examination of the more distal muscles.

In contrast, demyelinating neuropathies of the acute (Guillain-Barré) and chronic inflammatory types and those associated with diphtheria, metachromatic leukodystrophy, Krabbe disease, and Charcot-Marie-Tooth disease (as it is seen in most kinships) affect Schwann cells primarily and produce *segmental demyelination*, which

Table 45-1
Normal values for representative nerve conduction values at various sites of stimulation (mean values +/− 2 SD for adults 16 to 65 years of age)

Motor Nerve Conduction Studies

Nerve	*Distal Stimulation Site*	*Other Stimulation Sites*	*Recording Site*	*Onset Latency (ms)*	*Amp (mV)*	*CV (m/s)*	*Distance (cm)*	*F-Wave Latency (ms)*
Median	Wrist	Elbow	APB	<4.2	>4.4	>49	6–8	<31
Ulnar	Wrist	BG, AG	ADM	<3.4	>6.0	>49	5.5–7.5	<32
Radial	Forearm	Elbow, SG	EIP	<5.2	>4.0	>50	10	NA
Peroneal	Ankle	BFH, AFH	EDB	<5.8	>2.0	>42	6–11	<58
Peroneal	BFH	AFH	TA	<3.0	>5.0	>42	10	NA
Tibial	Ankle	PF	AH	<6.5	>3.0	>41	6–8	<59[a]

Sensory Nerve Conduction Studies[b]

Nerve	*Stimulation Sites*	*Recording Site*	*Onset Latency (ms)*	*Peak Latency (ms)*	*Amp (μV)*	*CV (m/s)*	*Distance (cm)*
Median	Wrist	Dig2	<2.5	<3.5	>20	>52	13
Ulnar	Wrist	Dig5	<2.1	<3.0	>15	>52	11
Radial	Forearm	Wrist	<1.9	<2.8	>20	>48	10
Sural	Calf	Ankle	<3.2	<4.4	>6	>42	14

Key: AG, above ulnar groove; BG, below ulnar groove; AFH, above fibular head; BFH, below fibular head; SG, spiral groove; TA, anterior tibialis; EDB, extensor digitalis brevis; EIP, extensor indicis proprius; ADM, adductor digiti minimi; APB, abductor pollicis brevis; AH, abductor hallucis; PF, popliteal fossa.

[a] Tibial H reflexes: latency <35 ms; side-to-side difference <1.4 ms.

[b] Sensory studies are performed antidromically; amplitudes are measured from baseline to negative peak of nerve potential.

markedly slows conduction velocities or, in the case of the acquired demyelinating neuropathies, produces dispersion of the action potential and conduction block (see below).

Amplitude of the Compound Muscle Action Potential In addition to the study of distal latency and conduction velocity, the amplitudes of the evoked muscle action potential yield valuable information about peripheral nerve function. A stimulus that provides the maximal-amplitude muscle potential is used. These amplitudes are a semiquantitative measure of the number of nerve fibers that respond to a given stimulus and are conducted to the various recording points, hence allowing the detection of conduction block and axonal loss. In addition, segmental demyelinative lesions or axonal loss affecting the large and fast-conducting fibers may be detected by finding evidence of differential slowing causing a dispersal of the response. Reduction in motor and sensory amplitudes is a far more specific and sensitive indicator of axonal loss than a slowing of conduction velocity or prolongation of distal latencies. Conversely, prolonged distal latencies and slowed motor conduction velocities—as well as conduction blocks and dispersed responses, which reduce amplitudes—are the hallmarks of segmental demyelinative lesions. The range of normal amplitudes for the compound muscle action potentials (CMAPs) that are elicited by stimulation of the main motor nerves is shown in Table 45-1.

It is usually possible to obtain a reliable motor conduction study as long as some functioning nerve fibers remain. These conduction velocities reflect the status of surviving fibers and, if some of the latter are unaffected by the disease process, may be normal despite widespread axonal degeneration. Thus, following incomplete transection of a nerve, the maximal motor conduction velocity may be normal in the few remaining fibers, although the muscle involved is almost paralyzed and the compound muscle potential recorded from it is very low.

Sensory Nerve Action Potentials When motor fibers in a mixed nerve are stimulated, a compound action potential of many hundreds of microvolts can easily be recorded from electrodes on the skin over the muscle. However, when one attempts to measure sensory potentials, where activity must be recorded from nerve fibers themselves, one lacks the "amplification" provided by all the muscle fibers in many motor units, as noted above, and much greater electronic amplification is required. Abnormal sensory potentials are sometimes very small or absent even when powerful computer-averaging techniques are used, and sensory conduction measurements may be difficult or impossible to record, particularly in the lower extremities of elderly patients. Table 45-1 gives the range of normal values for sensory nerve action potential amplitudes and velocities.

Conduction Block By stimulating a motor nerve at multiple sites along its course, it is possible to demonstrate segments in which conduction is partially "blocked" or is differentially slowed. From such data one infers the presence of multifocal demyelinative lesions in motor nerves. This contrasts with the findings in certain of the demyelinating inherited neuropathies, in which all parts of the nerve fiber are altered to more or less the same degree and there is uniform slowing of conduction velocity but no block. Conduction blocks are demonstrated by a reduction in the amplitude of the CMAP that is elicited from proximal nerve stimulation, compared with stimulation at a more distal site, as described earlier. Generally, a 40 percent reduction in amplitude over a short distance, or 50 percent over longer distances, qualifies as a block, the exception being the tibial nerve, in which it is difficult to stimulate all the motor nerve fibers and a drop in amplitude is expected. It is important also to be certain that the reduction in amplitude along the course of the nerve is not due solely to dispersion of the waveform and that the block not be attributable simply to nerve compression at the common sites (fibular head, across the elbow, flexor retinaculum at the wrist, etc.). Conduction block can also be inferred from the finding of poor recruitment of muscle action potentials but no active denervation after weakness has been present for several weeks in the same muscle. The finding of conduction block is a central feature in a number of acquired immune demyelinating neuropathies, including Guillain-Barré syndrome, chronic inflammatory demyelinating neuropathy, and multifocal conduction block associated with the GM_1 antibody, all of which are discussed in Chap. 46.

Focal compression of nerve, as in the entrapment syndromes mentioned above, may produce localized slowing or blocks in conduction, perhaps because of segmental demyelination at the site of compression. The demonstration of such localized changes of conduction affords ready confirmation of nerve entrapment; for example, if the distal latency of the median nerve (A, Fig. 45-3) exceeds 4.5 ms while that of the ulnar nerve remains normal, compression of the median nerve in the carpal tunnel is likely. Similar focal slowing or partial block of conduction may be recorded from the ulnar nerve at the elbow and from the peroneal nerve at the fibular head.

Electrodiagnostic Studies of Nerve Roots and Spinal Segments (Late Responses, Blink Responses, Segmental Evoked Responses)

H Reflex and F Wave Information about the conduction of impulses through the proximal segments of a nerve that is not obtainable by routine nerve conduction techniques may be provided by the study of the H reflex and the F wave. In 1918, Hoffmann, after whom the H reflex was later named, showed that submaximal stimulation of mixed motor-sensory nerves, insufficient to produce a direct motor response, produces a muscle contraction (H wave) after a latency that is much longer than that of the direct motor response. This reflex is based on activation of spindle afferent fibers (those involved in the tendon reflex), and the long delay in muscular response reflects the time required for the impulses to reach the spinal cord along the sensory fibers, synapse with anterior horn cells, and then be transmitted along motor fibers to the muscle (see Fig. 3-1). Thus the H reflex is the electrical representation of the tendon reflex circuit and can be useful because the impulse traverses both the posterior and anterior roots. The H reflex is particularly helpful in the diagnosis of S1 radiculopathy and of polyneuropathies, including predominantly sensory ones, and its presence generally parallels the state of the Achilles reflex. It is, however, difficult to elicit from nerves other than the tibial. Stimuli of increasing frequency but low intensity cause a progressive depression and finally obliteration of H waves. The latter phenomenon has been used to study spasticity, rigidity, and cerebellar ataxia, in which there are differences in the frequency-depression curves of H waves.

The F response, so named because it was initially elicited in the feet, was first described by Magladery and McDougal in 1950. It is evoked by a supramaximal stimulus of a motor-sensory nerve. Again, after a latency longer than that for the direct motor response (latencies of 28 to 32 ms in arms, 40 to 50 ms in legs), a second small muscle action potential is recorded (F wave). The F wave is produced by the stimulation of motor fibers that travel antidromically to the anterior horn cells; a small number of anterior horn cells are activated and produce an orthodromic response that can be recorded in a distal muscle. The F response is a more discerning test than the H wave in that the former traverses only the ventral root and can be elicited from any number of muscles. Normal F responses and absent H reflexes can be seen with disease of sensory nerves and roots. The late responses find their main use as corroborative tests that are interpreted in the context of the entire nerve conduction examination (see Wilbourn in the References). The usually elicited late response latencies are given in Table 45-1.

Electrical Blink Responses This special nerve conduction test may be useful in the diagnosis of certain cases of demyelinating neuropathy and other regional processes that affect the trigeminal or facial nerve. The patient's supraorbital (or infraorbital) nerve is stimulated transcutaneously and the reflex closure of both orbicularis oculi muscles is recorded with surface electrodes. Two EMG bursts are observed: the first (R1) appears ipsilaterally 10 ms after the stimulus and the second (R2) ipsilaterally at 30 ms and contralaterally up to 5 ms later. The amplitudes of the responses vary considerably and are not in themselves clinically important. The first response is not visible as a muscular contraction but may serve some preparatory function by shortening the blink reflex delay. R1 is mediated by an oligosynaptic pontine circuit consisting of one to three neurons located in the vicinity of the main sensory nucleus. It has been established that R1 and R2 share the same facial motor neurons.

The elicitation of blink reflexes confirms the integrity of the afferent trigeminal nerve, the efferent facial nerve, and the interneurons in the pons (R1) and caudal medulla (mainly related to the bilateral R2 response). The test may be helpful in identifying a demyelinating neuropathy when the facial and oropharyngeal muscles are affected and those of the limbs relatively spared, leaving conventional nerve studies normal. In such cases, the blink responses are delayed, ipsilaterally and contralaterally, as a result of conduction block in the proximal facial nerve. Direct facial nerve stimulation often fails to demonstrate this block because only the distal segment of the nerve is amenable to study. Although this test is rarely necessary for diagnosis, most patients with hereditary neuropathy have blink response abnormalities. In Bell's palsy there is a delay or absence of R1 and R2 responses only on the affected side. Large acoustic neuromas may interfere with the trigeminal portion of the pathway and give rise to abnormal responses on the affected side. Diseases of the brainstem have yielded inconsistent responses. It is noteworthy that the test is normal in patients with trigeminal neuralgia.

Segmental Motor, Cranial, and Somatosensory Evoked Potentials These techniques are particularly useful in diseases that affect spinal roots. By applying a magnetic stimulus, which induces an electrical impulse, or an electrical stimulus delivered directly by an electrode, over the cranium or lower cervical or lumbar spine, it is possible to activate motor cortex or motor roots and measure the time required to elicit a muscle contraction. In the latter case, the motor point stimulated is believed to be where the motor axons issue from the spinal cord (Cros and Chiappa). Since these techniques excite central structures in the spinal cord, it is possible to measure both peripheral and central conduction times. These root stimulation tests can be quite uncomfortable for the patient because of the contraction of muscles surrounding the stimulation site.

Transcranial magnetic stimulation of the cerebral cortex permits measurement of the latency of muscle contraction. The integrity of the entire corticospinal system, from the cortical motor neurons through spinal tracts, anterior horn cells, and the peripheral motor nerve, can be determined. This form of testing has its main use in the study of amyotrophic lateral sclerosis and related disorders.

Also, as described in Chap. 2, by applying repetitive electrical stimuli to a peripheral nerve, the sensory evoked responses can be recorded, using a computer, from sites along the nerve and plexus. Other nerve conduction techniques are available as well, but a description of their performance and interpretation is beyond the scope of this text. Detailed information on magnetic stimulation, collision techniques, quantitative EMG, etc., can be found in several monographs, such as the ones by Kimura, by Aminoff, and by Brown and Bolton.

Repetitive Nerve Stimulation (Jolly Test)

This test of the neuromuscular junction is based on Jolly's observation in 1895 that in myasthenics the strength of contractions is progressively diminished during a train of stimuli. By adjusting the amplitude of a stimulus over a nerve to supramaximal range, a maximal CMAP may be obtained for each stimulus; the form of the response will depend on the number of motor units activated and the number of muscle fibers sampled. With repeated stimuli, each response will have the same form and amplitude until fatigue supervenes. A normal response will follow each stimulus even with rates of stimulation up to 25 per second for periods of 60 s or more before a decrement of the CMAP appears. The latter is due to the failure of some muscle fibers to respond, presumably because the nerve impulse is not transmitted through some branching points of the terminal axon.

In certain disorders, notably myasthenia gravis, the initial CMAP produced by electrical stimulation is slightly reduced or normal. After a train of 4 to 10 stimuli at rates of 2 to 5 per second (optimal rate 2 to 3 per second), the amplitude of the potentials decreases by 25 percent or more (though not to zero) and then, after four or five further stimuli, may increase somewhat (Fig. 45-4*A*). A progressive reduction in amplitude is most likely to be found in proximal muscles, but these are not easily stimulated; the locations most commonly tested are the accessory nerve in the posterior triangle of the neck and the trapezius muscle, the ulnar nerve and hypothenar muscle, the median nerve at the wrist and the thenar muscle, and the facial nerve and orbicularis oculi. Any decrement greater than 10 percent denotes a failure of a proportion of the neuromuscular junctions that are being stimulated. The sensitivity of the procedure is improved by first exercising the tested muscle for 30 to 60 s. This induced failure of neuromuscular transmission in myasthenics is similar to the one produced by curare and other nondepolarizing neuromuscular blocking agents, and it can be partially corrected with anticholinesterase drugs such as neostigmine and edrophonium. Similar but

Figure 45-4

Compound action potentials evoked in hypothenar muscles by electrical stimulation of the ulnar nerve at the wrist. A. *Patient with myasthenia gravis—typical pattern of decrement in first four responses followed by slight increment. At this rate of stimulation (4 per second), the decrement in response does not continue to zero.* B. *Patient with Lambert-Eaton syndrome and oat-cell carcinoma—typical marked increase toward normal amplitude with rapid repetitive stimulation (20 per second). Horizontal calibration: 250 ms.*

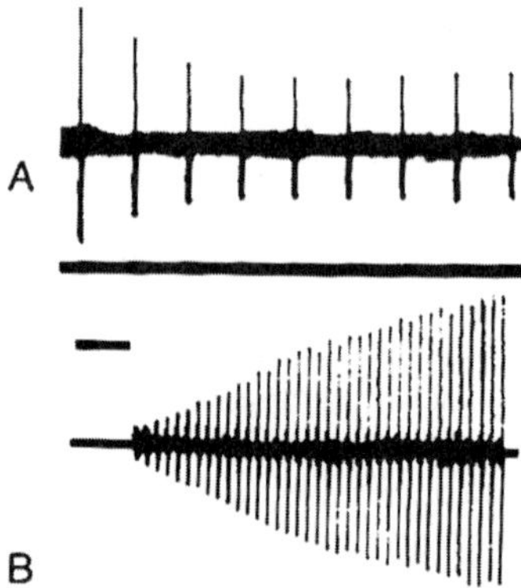

lesser decremental responses may occur in poliomyelitis, amyotrophic lateral sclerosis, and certain other diseases of the motor unit or motor nerve, particularly those with reinnervating nerve twigs following nerve injury.

The presynaptic myasthenic syndrome of Lambert-Eaton, often associated with oat-cell carcinoma of the lung, is characterized by a different type of defect of neuromuscular transmission. During tetanic stimulation (20- to 50-per-second repetitive stimulation of nerve), the muscle action potentials, which are small or practically absent with the first stimulus, increase in voltage with each successive response until a more nearly normal amplitude is attained (Fig. 45-4*B*). Exercising the muscle for 10 s before testing will cause a similar posttetanic facilitation (200-fold increases are not uncommon). A less important decremental response to slow stimulation may occur, but it is difficult to discern because of the greatly diminished amplitude of the initial responses. Neostigmine has little effect on this phenomenon, but it may be reversed by guanidine and 3,4-diaminopyridine, which stimulate the release of ACh. The effects of this myasthenic syndrome are similar to those produced by botulinum toxin or by aminoglycoside antibiotics.

The single-fiber EMG, discussed in a later section, is a more sensitive method of detecting failure of the neuromuscular junction.

Needle Examination of Muscle

This technique requires the use of monopolar or concentric bipolar needle electrodes, which are inserted into the body of the muscle. With concentric needle electrodes, the tip of the wire that runs in the hollow of the needle is in proximity to many muscle fibers belonging to several motor units; this is the active recording electrode. The shaft of the needle, in contact over most of its length with intercellular fluid and many other muscle fibers, serves as the reference electrode. With monopolar electrodes, the uninsulated needle tip is the active electrode, while the reference electrode may be another monopolar needle electrode placed in subcutaneous tissue or a surface electrode on the skin overlying the muscle being tested. Patients almost invariably find this portion of the test uncomfortable and should be prepared by a description of the procedure. Rapid and brief needle insertion by the skilled examiner makes the test more tolerable.

When an electrical impulse travels along the surface of the muscle toward the recording electrode, a positive potential (by convention) is recorded on the oscilloscope, i.e., the recorded signal is deflected downward (at A in Fig 45-5). When the depolarized zone moves under the recording electrode, it becomes relatively negative and the beam is deflected upward (at B). As the depolarized zone continues to move along the sarcolemma, away from the recording electrode, the current begins to flow outward through the membrane toward the distant depolarized region, and the recording electrode becomes relatively positive again (at C). It then returns to its resting isopotential position. The net result is a triphasic action potential, as in Fig. 45-5. This configuration is typical of the firing of a single fiber.

The electrical activity of various muscles is recorded both at rest and during active contraction by the patient. As indicated above, muscle fibers do not discharge in normally innervated muscle until activated together in motor unit activity, which involves the almost simultaneous contraction of all the muscle fibers innervated by a single anterior horn cell. Although the typical configuration of a motor unit potential (MUP) is triphasic, up to 10 percent of normal MUPs consist of four or

Figure 45-5

The shaded area represents the zone of the action potential, which is negative to all other points on the fiber surface. It is shown at three points in its course (from left to right) *along the fiber. At each point, the correspondingly lettered portion of the triphasic muscle-action potential displayed on the display screen reflects the potential difference between the active* (vertical arrow) *and reference (Ref.) electrodes. Polarity in this and subsequent figures is negative upward as depicted. The time calibration is on the screen.*

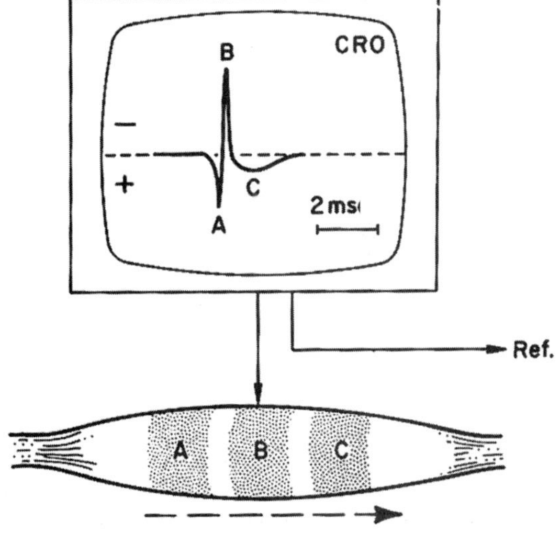

more phases (*polyphasic potentials*); an excess of polyphasic potentials beyond this is pathologic.

Normal muscle in the resting state should be electrically silent; the small tension spoken of as muscle tone has no EMG equivalent. There are, however, two closely related types of normal spontaneous activity and another that is induced by the insertion of the needle itself. One is a low-amplitude, 10- to 20-mV monophasic (negative) potential of very brief (0.5 to 1 ms) duration. These represent single or synchronized MEPPs due to the small number of ACh quanta that are being released at all times. They are normally sparse but are most evident when the recording needle electrode is placed near a motor end plate ("end-plate noise"). Placement of the needle electrode very close to or in contact with the end plate gives rise to a second type of normal spontaneous activity. The latter is characterized by irregularly discharging high-frequency (50- to 100-Hz) biphasic (negative-positive) spike discharges, 100 to 300 mV in amplitude (i.e., large enough to cause an isolated muscle action potential). These potentials have been termed "end-plate spikes" and represent discharges of single muscle fibers excited by activity in nerve terminals. These potentials must be distinguished from fibrillation potentials (see below). Insertion of the needle electrode into the muscle injures and mechanically stimulates many fibers, causing a burst of potentials of short duration (< 300 ms). This is referred to as *normal insertional activity*.

When muscle is voluntarily contracted, the action potentials of motor units begin to appear. One can observe the way force is built up by watching the progressive recruitment of MUPs, the initial ones, representing the activity of smaller motor units of (type 1), firing at rates of 5 to 10 per second. With increased force of contraction, there is recruitment of larger, previously inactive motor units as well as an increased rate of firing (40 to 50 per second; see Fig. 45-6*A*). Since individual MUPs can no longer be distinguished during maximal voluntary contraction, this activity is referred to as a *complete interference pattern* (Fig. 45-6*A*, right). This is not only seen as a summated signal pattern but also heard as a mixed high-frequency clicking when the electrical activity is made audible by the EMG machine. As muscles relax, more and more units drop out. If a muscle is weakened by denervation or if electrical conduction is blocked, there will obviously be fewer MUPs, firing at a moderately rapid rate (reduced recruitment, Fig. 47-6*B*). In contrast, with poor voluntary effort and with upper motor neuron lesions, the MUPs fire in decreased numbers, at slower rates, and often in an irregular pattern (termed *poor activation*).

In the usual EMG examination, a plan for the study is made based on detailed knowledge of muscular

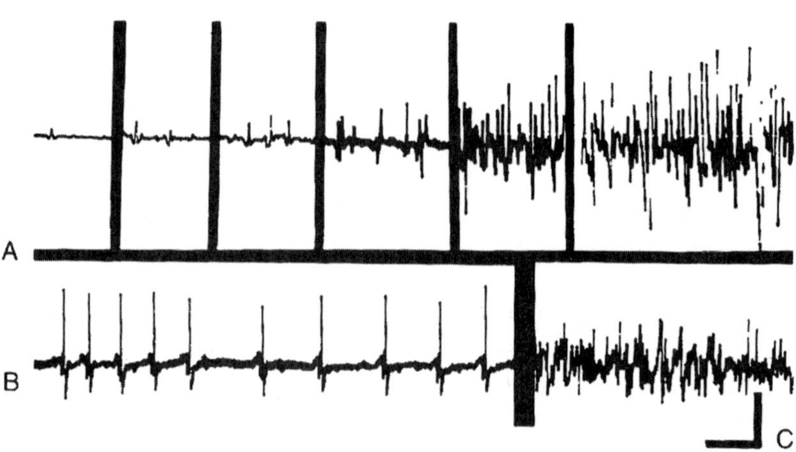

Figure 45-6

Patterns of motor unit recruitment. A. *Normal. With each increment of voluntary effort, more and larger units are brought into play until, with full effort at the extreme right, a complete "interference pattern" is seen in which single units are no longer recognizable.* B. *After denervation, only a single motor unit is recorded despite maximal effort. It is seen to fire repetitively.* C. *With myopathic diseases, a normal number of units is recruited on minimal effort, though the amplitude of the pattern is reduced. Calibrations: 50 ms (horizontal) and 1 mV in* A *and* B*; 200 mV in* C *(vertical).*

innervation and focusing on the regions affected by weakness and by other major clinical features of the illness. In some patients, as in those with motor neuron diseases or polymyositis, a wider sampling of muscles is required to detect changes in asymptomatic regions.

The Abnormal Electromyogram Clinically important deviations from the normal EMG include (1) increased or decreased insertional activity; (2) the occurrence of abnormal "spontaneous" activity during relaxation (fibrillation potentials, positive sharp waves, fasciculation potentials, cramp potentials, myotonic discharges, myokymic potentials); (3) abnormalities in the amplitude, duration, and shape of single MUPs; (4) a decrease in the number of MUPs and changes in their firing pattern; (5) variation in amplitude and number of phases of MUPs during voluntary contraction of muscle; and (6) the demonstration of special phenomena, such as electrical silence during obvious shortening of the muscle (true contracture).

Insertional Activity At the moment the needle is inserted into muscle, there is usually a brief burst of action potentials that ceases once the needle is stable provided that it is not in a position to irritate a nerve terminal. Increased insertional activity is seen in most instances of denervation as well as in many forms of primary muscle disease and in disorders that dispose to muscle cramps. In cases of advanced denervation or myopathy, in which muscle fibers have been largely replaced by connective tissue and fat, insertional activity may be decreased and there may be increased mechanical resistance to insertion of the needle electrode.

Abnormal "Spontaneous" Activity With the muscle at rest, spontaneous activity of single muscle fibers and of motor units, known respectively as *fibrillation* potentials and *fasciculation* potentials, is abnormal. The two phenomena are often confused. *Fibrillation* is the spontaneous contraction of a *single muscle fiber*. It occurs when the muscle fiber has lost its nerve supply and is ordinarily not visible through the skin. *Fasciculation* represents the spontaneous firing of a motor unit, causing contraction of a group of muscle fibers, and may be visible through the skin. The firing irregularly of a number of motor units, seen as a rippling of the skin, is called *myokymia*.

Fibrillation Potentials When a motor neuron is destroyed by disease or its axon is interrupted, the distal part of the axon degenerates, a process that takes several days or more. The muscle fibers formerly innervated by the branches of the dead axon—that is, the motor unit—are disconnected from the nervous system. For reasons that are still obscure, the chemosensitive region of the sarcolemma at the motor end plate "spreads" after denervation to involve the entire surface of the muscle fiber. Then, 10 to 25 days after death of the axon, the denervated fibers develop spontaneous activity; each fiber contracts at its own rate and without relation to the activity of neighboring fibers. This spontaneous activity is associated with a totally random conglomeration of brief di- or triphasic fibrillation potentials (Fig. 45-7*A*), having a duration of 1 to 5 ms and rarely exceeding 300 mV in amplitude. When brief spontaneous potentials of this sort are observed firing regularly at two or three different locations outside the end-plate zone of a resting muscle, one may conclude that the fibers are denervated. Usually, fibrillation potentials discharge at an almost regular rate. In some early lesions (less than 6 to 8 weeks), irregularly firing fibrillation potentials may be observed. Diseases such as poliomyelitis, which damage spinal motor neurons, or injuries of peripheral nerves or anterior spinal roots frequently produce only partial denervation of the involved muscles. In such muscles, one electrode placement may record fibrillation potentials at rest from denervated fibers and normal potentials during voluntary

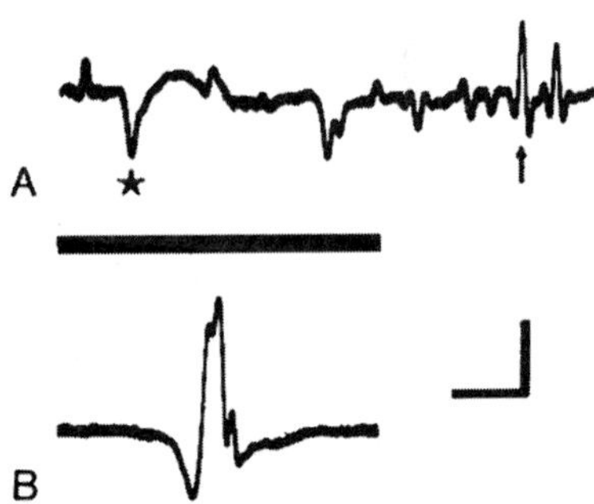

Figure 45-7

A. *Fibrillations and positive sharp waves. This spontaneous activity was recorded from a totally denervated muscle—no motor unit potentials were produced by attempts at voluntary contraction. The fibrillations (above arrow) are 1 to 2 ms in duration, 100 to 300 mV in amplitude, and largely negative (upward) in polarity following an initial positive deflection. A typical positive sharp wave is seen above the star.* B. *Fasciculation. This spontaneous motor unit potential was recorded from a patient with amyotrophic lateral sclerosis. It has a serrated configuration and it fired once every second or two. Calibrations: 5 ms (horizontal) and 200 mV in* A; *1 mV in* B *(vertical).*

contraction from nearby healthy fibers. Fibrillation potentials continue until the muscle fiber is reinnervated by progressive proximal-distal regeneration of the interrupted nerve fiber or by the outgrowth of new axons from nearby healthy nerve fibers (collateral sprouting), or until the atrophied fibers degenerate and are replaced by connective tissue, a process that may take many years. In addition, fibrillation potentials may take the form of positive sharp waves, i.e., spontaneous, initially positive diphasic potentials of longer duration and slightly greater amplitude than the spikes of fibrillation potentials (Fig. 45-7*A*).

Unfortunately, fibrillation potentials, while characteristic of neurogenic denervation, are not altogether specific; for example, they are seen in muscle diseases such as polymyositis and inclusion body myositis, which presumably damage the neural innervation to small regions of muscle or isolate segments of a muscle fiber from its end plate.

Fasciculation Potentials As stated above, a fasciculation is the spontaneous or involuntary contraction of a motor unit or part of a motor unit. Such contractions may cause a visible dimpling or twitching under the skin, though ordinarily they are of insufficient force to move a joint. Large fasciculations, however, can briefly displace a finger or toe; they occur irregularly and infrequently, and prolonged inspection may be necessary to detect them. The form of the accompanying fasciculation potential, like that of an ordinary MUP seen on voluntary contraction, is relatively constant. If the motor unit from which the fasciculation arises is otherwise normal, the accompanying fasciculation potential will have three to five phases, a duration of 5 to 15 ms (somewhat less in the facial muscles), and an amplitude of several millivolts (Fig. 45-7*B*). Fasciculation potentials are evidence of motor nerve fiber irritability, most often the result of reinnervation following nerve or motor neuron damage.

The precise source of fasciculation is still contested. Forster and colleagues, in the 1940s, challenged the original belief that the discharge originated in anterior horn cells by demonstrating that fasciculations persisted after nerve block in amyotrophic lateral sclerosis (ALS) and ceased only with the appearance of fibrillation potentials, signifying wallerian (axonal) degeneration. These observations favored a distal site of generation. Other physiologic and pharmacologic evidence pointed to the first segment of the motor axon, or to the distal axon, or even to the motor point, involving elements of the postsynaptic muscle membrane (particularly in the case of benign fasciculations) as the source of the spontaneous electrical activity. It seems that several regions of the axon are capable of spontaneous impulse generation, depending on the underlying disease; most involve the anterior horn cell or the motor root, but distal sites are operative in cases of nerve compression and polyneuropathy.

Occasional fasciculation potentials—particularly in the calves, hands, and periocular or paranasal muscles—occur in many normal persons. They can be almost constant for days or weeks on end, or even for years in some individuals, without weakness or wasting; therefore they need not be taken as evidence of disease (benign fasciculations). Certain quantitative features of fasciculations, such as brief duration and a consistent pattern of firing, favor benign over pathologic discharges. Shivering induced by low temperature and twitchings associated with low serum calcium levels are other forms of fasciculatory activity.

Fasciculation potentials occur with great frequency in chronic, slowly advancing, destructive diseases of the anterior horn cells, such as ALS and progressive spinal muscular atrophy. In these primary spinal cord diseases, both voluntary MUPs and fasciculation potentials may be of long duration (more than 15 ms) and of increased amplitude, indicating chronic denervation and reinnervation. They are seen often in the early stages of poliomyelitis but only occasionally in the chronic phase of the disease, perhaps because the affected cells die rapidly. When anterior horn cells degenerate once again in older individuals who had had poliomyelitis (postpolio syndrome), fasciculations may return. Occasionally, they are seen with compressive anterior root lesions, such as those caused by a protruded intervertebral disc; large numbers of axons may be affected, with the result that the fasciculations (or even cramps) may be more prominent than with disease of anterior horn cells. Fasciculation potentials in lesser numbers are also observed with chronic nerve entrapments, e.g., ulnar neuropathy at the elbow and other peripheral nerve lesions and some polyneuropathies. In all these cases, the damaged neuron or its axon seems to leave intact axons in a state of hyperirritability. The repetitive axon potentials produce activity in all the muscle fibers that the axon innervates. The blocking of axon conduction by local anesthesia does not abolish the fasciculation, but curare-like drugs do so.

Less Common Types of Spontaneous Activity One of these is *myokymia* (pages 1467 and 1568), a persistent quivering and rippling of muscles at rest ("live flesh"). The EMG picture is distinctive. The spontaneously firing

MUPs are called *myokymic potentials* or *discharges* and consist of groups of repetitive discharging units, each firing at its own rate, quasi-rhythmically, usually several times per second, followed by an even briefer period of silence. The small motor unit discharges may occur singly or as doublets, triplets, or multiplets. The site of generation of this activity has been contested, possibly because it may arise from several sites, but always the site is peripheral, not central, and is believed to correspond to an alteration in the calcium concentration in the microenvironment of the motor axon. Spontaneous discharges arising in large myelinated fibers have been implicated in the genesis of myokymia; indeed, demyelinating polyneuropathies are among the conditions that give rise to this phenomenon. This activity may be blocked by lidocaine infusion around the peripheral nerve and may be diminished by carbamazepine or phenytoin.

In the *syndrome of continuous muscle fiber activity or Isaacs syndrome* (page 1568), which is actually a generalized form of myokymia, EMG discloses high-frequency (up to 300-Hz) repetitive discharges of varying wave forms.

Focal and segmental myokymias are related, as judged by their EMG patterns. They differ in small ways from the generalized form of myokymia with regard to the timing and duration of the discharges. The focal types refer mainly to facial myokymia, seen most often in multiple sclerosis, Guillain-Barré syndrome, or large cerebellopontine angle tumors, but it may follow any peripheral nerve injury and regeneration. The EMG patterns are complex, either high-frequency (30- to 100-Hz) recurrent bursts or brief lower-frequency bursts. Segmental myokymia is a common occurrence in radiation injuries of the brachial plexus. The EMG bursts tend to be longer and less frequent than in generalized myokymia, and the interburst frequency is highly variable. The origin of these discharges (also referred to as *neuromyotonia*) is probably in the distal peripheral nerve, where activity of afferent fibers, possibly via ephaptic transmission, irregularly excites distal motor terminals. This activity persists during sleep and general anesthesia.

The phenomenon of *myotonia* (see page 1553) is characterized by high-frequency repetitive discharges generally having a positive sharp waveform. These myotonic discharges wax and wane in amplitude and frequency, producing a "dive-bomber" sound on the audio monitor. The discharges can be elicited mechanically by percussion of the muscle or movement of the needle electrode and are also seen following voluntary contraction or electrical stimulation of the muscle via its motor nerve. The MUPs may appear normal during voluntary contraction, but they are not followed by the silence that normally occurs on relaxation; instead, there is a "prolonged afterdischarge" consisting of long trains of fibrillation-like potentials that may take as long as several minutes to subside (Fig. 45-8*A*). These EMG findings, which can be seen with any myotonic disorder, correspond to the clinical failure of voluntary relaxation of muscle following a forceful contraction. If the muscle is activated repeatedly at short intervals, the late discharge becomes briefer and briefer and eventually disappears (Fig. 45-8*B*), as the patient becomes able to relax the exercised muscle ("warm-up" effect). In the paradoxical myotonia observed in some cases of von Eulenberg paramyotonia, Nielsen and colleagues have found a decreasing recruitment pattern and increasing activity after each of a succession of voluntary contractions. This is the converse of what happens in congenital myotonia. As shown by the single-fiber EMG studies of Denny-Brown and Nevin, myotonia is generated by single

Figure 45-8

A. *Myotonia congenita (Thomsen disease). The five lines are a continuous record of activity in the biceps brachii following a tap on the tendon. The initial response is within normal limits, but it is followed by a prolonged burst of rapid activity, gradually subsiding over a period of many seconds or minutes.* B. *Same electrode placement as in A. Response to the fifth of a series of tendon taps. "Warm-up" has occurred, and the characteristic prolonged myotonic activity is no longer evident.*

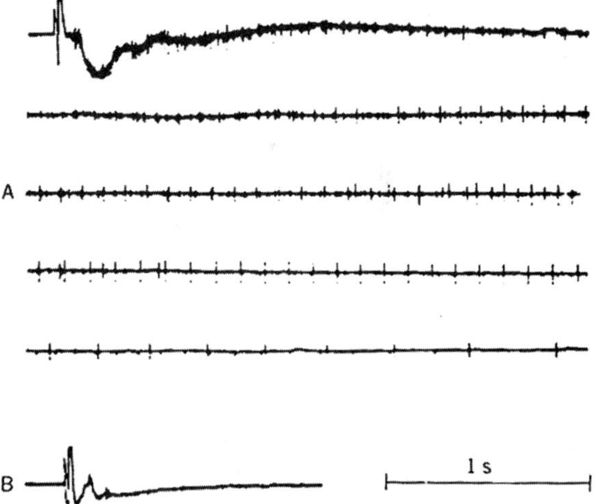

muscle fibers, and the mechanism of the membrane instability, at least in some forms, seems to involve changes in the chloride conductance. In the *stiff-man syndrome*, painful muscle spasms and stiffness are generated by a central mechanism; the EMG potentials resemble normal motor units but are abnormal by virtue of continuous firing at rest.

Complex repetitive discharges—formerly referred to as bizarre high-frequency discharges and, even earlier, as *pseudomyotonia*—consist of repetitive spontaneous potentials often having an erratic configuration and starting and stopping abruptly. They are seen in some myopathies, in hypothyroidism, and in certain denervating disorders and are a mark of chronicity (lesions over 6 months old). High-frequency coupling of action potentials into doublets, triplets, or higher multiples of single units, indicating instability in repolarization of the nerve fiber to a muscle, occurs in tetany and in the early stages of myokymia.

The *cramp-like contracture* of McArdle disease and phosphofructokinase deficiency is associated with electrical silence of contracting muscle. This feature is important in the definition of this syndrome.

Abnormalities in Amplitude, Duration, and Shape of Motor Unit Potentials Figures 45-9 (schematically) and 45-10 depict the ways in which disease processes affect the motor unit and the appearance of the MUP in the EMG.

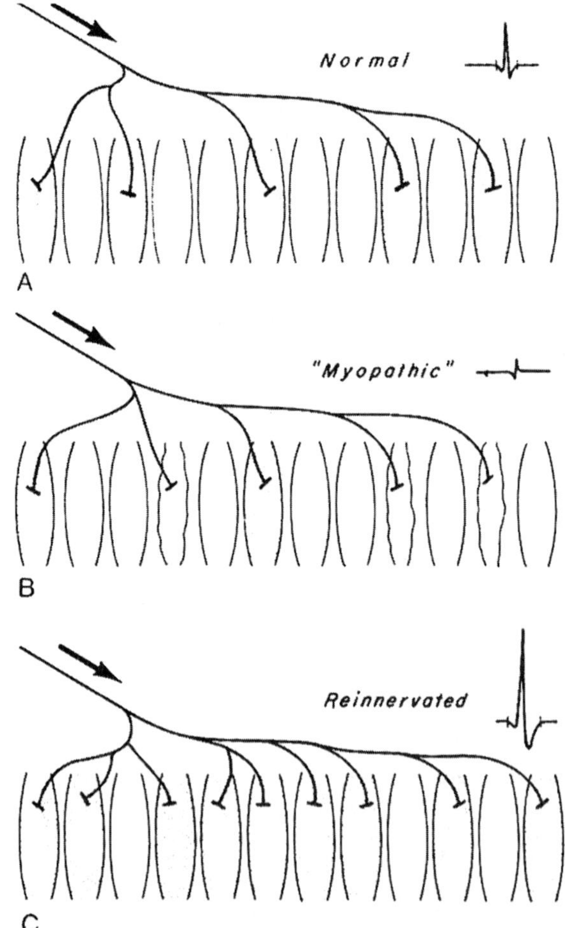

Figure 45-9

The shaded muscle fibers are functional members of one motor unit, whose axon enters from the upper left and branches terminally to innervate the appropriate muscle fibers. The action potential produced by each motor unit is seen in the upper right: its duration is measured between the two vertical lines. The normal-appearing but unshaded fibers belong to other motor units. A. *Hypothetical situation, with five muscle fibers in the active unit.* B. *In this myopathic unit, only two fibers remain active; the other three (shrunken) have been affected by one of the primary muscle diseases.* C. *Four fibers which originally belonged to other motor units and had been denervated have now been reinnervated by terminal sprouting from an undamaged axon. Both the motor unit and its action potential are now larger than normal. Note that only under these abnormal circumstances do fibers in the same unit lie next to one another.*

Motor Unit Potentials in Denervation Early in the course of denervation, many motor units with functional connections to the spinal cord are unaffected, and though the number of MUPs appearing during contraction is reduced, the configurations of the remaining ones are quite normal. In time, the remaining MUPs often increase in amplitude, perhaps two to three times normal, and become longer in duration and sometimes *polyphasic* (more than four phases).

Such large and sometimes *giant potentials* (Figs. 45-9*C* and 45-10*B*) are believed to arise from motor units containing more than the usual number of muscle fibers that are spread out over a greatly enlarged territory within the muscle. Presumably, new nerve twigs have sprouted from nodal points and terminals of undamaged axons and have reinnervated previously denervated muscle fibers, thus adding them to their own motor units. Soon after reinnervation, the MUPs generated will be low in amplitude, extremely prolonged, and polyphasic,

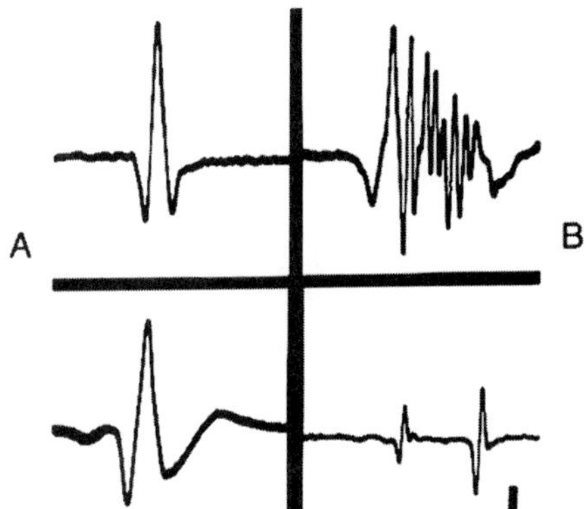

Figure 45-10

Single voluntary motor unit potentials. A. *Normal.* B. *Prolonged polyphasic potential seen with reinnervation.* C. *"Giant unit"—normally shaped but of much greater amplitude than normal.* D. *Brief, low-amplitude "myopathic" units. Calibrations: 5 ms (horizontal) and 1 mV in* A *and* B; *5 mV in* C; *100 mV in* D *(vertical).*

findings that constitute a transitional configuration of early reinnervation. These amplitudes disappear as the motor unit is re-established. Increased amplitude is usually associated with very chronic, proximal axon loss, e.g., with remote poliomyelitis and chronic cervical radiculopathy. These MUPs are to be differentiated from (1) polyphasic potentials of normal duration, which, as was said, make up as much as 10 percent of the total number of MUPs in normal muscle, and (2) polyphasic MUPs of short duration and low amplitude, which are characteristic of most myopathies and of myasthenia gravis and other disorders of neuromuscular transmission.

The Motor Unit Potential in Myopathy Diseases such as polymyositis, the muscular dystrophies, and other myopathies that randomly destroy muscle fibers or render them nonfunctional obviously reduce the population of muscle fibers per motor unit, as in Fig. 45-9*B*. Therefore, when such a unit is activated, its potential is of lower voltage and shorter duration than normal, and it may also appear polyphasic as the compound MUP becomes fragmented into its constituent single-fiber potentials. Slowing of the propagated muscle fiber action potential in affected muscle fibers is also believed to contribute to the changes in the myopathic MUP. When most of the muscle fibers are affected, the MUPs are very small and of short duration and are recruited out of proportion to the tension generated—so-called *increased recruitment.* Both types of alterations produce a characteristic high-pitched crackling sound from the audio monitor that has been likened to rain falling on a tin roof. They occur in all forms of progressive muscular dystrophy and are indistinguishable from those of polymyositis, dermatomyositis, and other chronic myopathies. Identical MUP changes can occasionally be seen with other processes that cause disintegration of the motor unit, e.g., early Guillain-Barré syndrome (due to conduction block along some of the terminal nerve fibers), and rarely with disorders of neuromuscular transmission (myasthenia gravis, other myasthenic syndromes), but they are most characteristic of primary muscle disease. Fibrillation potentials are sometimes seen in the myositides, inclusion-body myopathy, and the rapidly progressive muscular dystrophies, perhaps because of segmental necrosis of muscle fibers, which may isolate a segment of the fiber from its nerve supply. In myasthenia gravis, where transmission of impulse fails at the neuromuscular junction, a single MUP may vary in amplitude during sustained weak contraction. Electromyographic recordings of single muscle fibers belonging to the same motor unit disclose varying interpotential intervals on successive discharges; this phenomenon is called "jitter" and increases to the point of actual block, with deficits in neuromuscular transmission (see below).

Abnormalities of the Interference Pattern Diseases that reduce the population of functional motor neurons or axons within the peripheral nerve obviously decrease the number of motor units that can be recruited in the affected muscles. The decreased number of motor units available for activation now produce an incomplete interference pattern, which is manifest by a decreased number of units firing at a moderate to rapid rate. A severe reduction in the interference pattern may result in the recruitment of only a single unit (Fig. 45-6*B*).

If muscle power is reduced in diseases such as polymyositis or muscular dystrophy, in which individual muscle fibers are affected, there may be little or no reduction in the number of motor units available for recruitment until the process is far advanced and entire MUPs have been lost due to random loss of all their constituent muscle fibers. Nonetheless, each motor unit will consist of fewer muscle fibers than normal, so more motor units must be activated to reach a certain degree of force. A modest effort can thus produce a full interference pattern despite marked weakness (increased recruitment). Because fewer muscle fibers are firing, the amplitude of the pattern will be reduced from normal.

This type of full, highly complex interference pattern of less than usual amplitude in the face of dramatic weakness is the hallmark of myopathy (Fig. 45-6*C*).

Motor Unit Counting This technique, developed by McComas and colleagues, estimates the size of motor units and is thus exquisitely sensitive to changes of denervation and reinnervation. It is carried out by applying a weak stimulus to a motor nerve or motor point and increasing it gradually as the evoked muscle response is recorded. Each quantal increase in the compound evoked response is presumed to be due to the addition of a single motor unit. In reinnervated muscles the additional units are reduced in number and are abnormally large. This technique is used mainly for the investigation of motor neuron disorders. When a normal number and configuration of motor units is found, it has been helpful in distinguishing benign fasciculations from those of serious diseases.

Single-Fiber Electromyography (SF-EMG) This is a special technique for the recording of single-muscle-fiber action potentials and is used to measure fiber density and so-called jitter. *Fiber density* is an index of the number and distribution of muscle fibers within a motor unit. *Jitter* is the variability of the interpotential interval of successive discharges of two single-muscle-fiber action potentials belonging to the same motor unit. Jitter is due largely to the variability of delay at the branch points in the distal axon and synaptic delay at the neuromuscular junction. For this reason, SF-EMG is particularly useful in the detection of disorders of neuromuscular transmission, especially myasthenia gravis. Fiber density and jitter are often markedly increased in neuropathic disorders that cause denervation with reinnervation. They are usually normal or only slightly increased in myopathic disorders.

The testing is carried out with the patient voluntarily contracting a muscle slightly in order to activate only one motor unit (requiring a great deal of cooperation by the patient) or by stimulating an intramuscular nerve twig (requiring great patience on the part of the examiner). The EMG needle is advanced until two muscle fibers from the same motor unit are recorded. By measuring the interval between the activation of the two muscle fibers (the result of slightly differing lengths of the terminal axons), one determines a mean interpeak interval. Approximately 20 fiber pairs are sampled, and an average of the mean consecutive intervals is derived. In a muscle such as the extensor digitorum communis, the average variation should be no more than 34 ms. The acceptable average is lower for large proximal muscles. One muscle fiber in a pair may fail to fire intermittently as a result of a blocking of conduction. If the sweep is triggered by the firing of the first fiber, a fluctuating latency or failure to discharge of the second fiber potential can be seen on the screen as a movement (jitter) of the second peak. Further details of this technique and its clinical applications are discussed fully by Stålberg and Trontelj.

Imaging of Muscle

Imaging techniques—computed tomography (CT), magnetic resonance imaging (MRI), ultrasound—enable one to measure muscle volume and to recognize qualitative changes in muscle structure (see review of deVisser and Reimers). CT scans of dystrophic muscle show foci of decreased attenuation, representing masses of fat cells. The fatty masses spread gradually from multiple foci and eventually replace muscle fibers. The original shape of the muscle is retained; indeed, an enlarged weak muscle containing mostly fat confirms the clinical impression of pseudohypertrophy. In denervative atrophy, the muscles are obviously small and contain multiple punctate areas of decreased attenuation, which represent interstitial fat. Eventually, large portions of chronically denervated muscle may be replaced by fat. Blood, blood products, and calcium deposits are expressed by increased attenuation in CT. This may be helpful in the diagnosis of muscle trauma and polymyositis.

In MR images, fat and bone marrow have a high signal intensity, while fascia, ligaments, and cortical bone lack signal intensity. In T1-weighted images, normal muscle has a low signal and dystrophic muscle, a slightly increased signal; in T2-weighted images, dystrophic muscle has a slightly enhanced signal.

Ultrasonography reveals the volume of muscle and epimysial and perimysial septa, which are diminished in neuromuscular diseases. There has also been interest in the diagnostic value of the sounds that can be recorded from the contraction and relaxation of muscle by a sensitive microphone applied to the skin; this technique is experimental.

Biopsies of Muscle and Nerve

Muscle biopsy can be of great diagnostic value, but both surgical and microscopic techniques must be exacting. The muscle chosen for study should be accessible; there should be evidence that it has been affected but not totally destroyed by the disease in question; it should not have been the site of a recent injection or EMG study, since the trauma of the needles produces focal necrotizing and inflammatory lesions. Muscle biopsy is helpful in distinguishing the following basic disorders in patients with neuromuscular disease.

1. *Denervation atrophy.* Reduction in the size of muscle fibers with enlargement of intact motor units (due to collateral reinnervation) and degenerative changes in some fibers are the main changes of denervation atrophy. *Group atrophy*, which denotes enlarged motor units where all the fibers in the group are reduced to the same size, is typical of denervation. Normally, the fibers of each motor unit are not clustered, so that when grouping occurs it means that some fibers of a denervated unit have been adopted by an adjacent intact motor unit. This change typifies axonal neuropathies and many spinal cord diseases and is particularly well shown in histochemical stains for ATPase, phosphorylase, and oxidases, where the normal mosaic pattern of fiber types is altered, i.e., muscle fibers of similar histochemical type form groups of 15 or more fibers (*fiber-type grouping*), also a specific feature of denervation. The diagnosis of denervation atrophy can usually be made from the clinical and EMG examinations; seldom is biopsy necessary for this purpose, but it is still utilized in cases of possible ALS, for example, where the diagnosis remains uncertain after other testing.

2. *Segmental necrosis of muscle fibers with myophagia and various manifestations of regeneration.* These are the typical changes in idiopathic polymyositis (in combination with infiltrates of inflammatory cells), and infective polymyositis (in the presence of *Trichinella*, *Toxoplasma*, etc.). These changes may also be observed in Duchenne and other rapidly progressive muscular dystrophies.

3. *Inflammation and vasculitis.* Lymphocytic infiltration of the endomysium is most characteristic of polymyositis and in dermatomyositis it may be perimysial in addition. The lymphocytic infiltrate is often florid in these two processes, whereas it tends to be less intense in inclusion body myositis. Lesser degrees of inflammation are common in Sjögren syndrome, mixed connective tissue disease, and scleroderma. Numerous other processes—including the infections mentioned above and some dystrophies (especially the fascioscapulohumeral type)—may be associated with an inflammatory process. There is usually myofibrillar destruction in regions of maximal lymphocytic infiltration.

The muscle is a frequent site of inflammatory vascular destruction (vasculitis) in systemic diseases such as polyarteritis nodosa, and for this reason it is often useful to obtain a small sample of muscle adjacent to a nerve biopsy. The finding of a granulomatous myopathy may indicate the presence of systemic sarcoidosis.

4. *Unusual changes of muscle fibers.* Included here are sarcoplasmic masses and disorganized ring or serpentine collections of myofibrils and myofilaments (*Ringbinden*) in myotonic dystrophy; glycogen masses in glycogen storage diseases, rods (nemaline), central cores, aggregates of lipid bodies, and other cytoplasmic changes (such as aggregation and other abnormalities of mitochondria) in certain congenital myopathies; and nuclear and cytoplasmic inclusions (and other changes) that characterize inclusion-body myositis. Application of histochemical methods and electron microscopy are the important techniques in the diagnosis of these disorders.

5. *Alterations in number and size of fibers as a reflection of abnormalities of growth, maturation, and aging.* Many states of dwarfism and congenital myopathies of myotubular type present principally with numerical or volumetric changes, which must be distinguished from denervation, disuse effects, cachexia, and work hypertrophy.

6. *Disorders of the neuromuscular junctions in which nerve fibers and muscle fibers appear to be intact.* Here the abnormality is revealed by performing the more demanding procedure, motor point biopsy (to include the motor end plate), and using electron microscopy and special staining techniques for nerve terminals, cholinesterase, and the outlining of acetylcholine receptors. Myasthenia gravis, botulism, Lambert-Eaton syndrome, and myasthenic syndrome with motor end-plate cholinesterase deficiency fall into this category. Again, biopsy is rarely necessary for diagnosis.

7. *Alterations in the histochemical composition of muscle fibers* may be shown by special stains for enzymes and structural proteins that are implicated in disease. For example, it has become possible to detect the absence or deficiency of specific structural proteins of the muscle membrane that define each of the muscular dystrophies: dystrophin, sarcoglycan, laminin, etc., as discussed in Chap. 50. These tests require rapid freezing (in a cryostat) rather than formalin fixation. Also, a number of enzymatic deficiencies that lead to weakness and muscle fatigue may be detected by appropriate histochemical staining (Chap. 51).

As a rule, the biopsy procedure requires no more than a cleanly excised block of muscle, 1.0 to 2.0 cm, which is prevented from contracting by a clamp or by tying at full length to a tongue depressor. Percutaneous needle biopsies are now being done frequently and may be adequate for the diagnosis of certain muscle dystrophies and for their study over a period of time. In general, the needle biopsy is far less satisfactory than an open biopsy. The study of the muscle biopsy requires special care in removal, transport, and fixation techniques. These are discussed in detail by Engel.

Sural nerve biopsies, processed for study by thin-section phase and electron microscopy and supplemented by study of teased fiber preparations, can provide valuable histopathologic data. Even with ordinary microscopy, one may find evidence of focal inflammation or angiitis, amyloidosis, leprosy, or sarcoid. These procedures are most valuable in the diagnosis of inflammatory and vasculitic neuropathies. They are helpful, also, in the study of palpably enlarged nerves. In children, the nerve biopsy may reveal the histologic features of metachromatic or globoid leukodystrophy, giant axonopathy, or neuroaxonal dystrophy. Nerve biopsy is relatively unhelpful in most other poly-neuropathies and should be used with prudence because the procedure itself is not without complications, such as the occasional occurrence of wound infections, painful stump pseudoneuromas, persistent dysesthesias of the heel, and thrombophlebitis.

In diseases that involve only the motor nerves, it is sometimes useful to sample a fascicle of the superficial radial nerve or the nerve to the extensor digitorum brevis, which may be taken with the muscle itself. Chronic inflammatory neuropathy and vasculitic neuropathy may be disclosed by this biopsy when the sural nerve sensory action potentials are normal. Also, in selected circumstances we have undertaken biopsy of small radicles of upper lumbar roots (L1 or L2) to establish the diagnosis of an infiltrative lymphoma. Little deficit occurs from the removal of nerves from these three alternative sites if the procedure is done by an experienced neurosurgeon.

Additional techniques that are utilized in the study of muscle biopsies and specific pathologic findings that characterize the many individual diseases, of both muscle and peripheral nerve, are discussed in the chapters that follow.

Laboratory Tests in the Study of Muscle and Nerve Disease None of the results of the diagnostic laboratory procedures described above may be taken as an infallible index of a specific disease of muscle. Each procedure is subject to technical error and the findings to misinterpretation. A biopsy specimen may be excised from an unaffected muscle or portion of a muscle and, because of this sampling error, be negative in the face of clinical evidence of obvious disease.

Rough excision and improper fixation and staining may produce artifacts that may be misinterpreted as marks of disease when, in fact, the muscle (and nerve) is microscopically normal. Similarly, EMG study may fail to record fibrillations in obviously denervated muscle, particularly in slowly progressive disorders. Also, in some of the muscles of the feet, fibrillations and fasciculations may be found in normal asymptomatic older individuals (Falck and Alaranta). As in the study of all disease, laboratory data have significance only if evaluated in the light of the clinical findings.

REFERENCES

Aminoff MJ: *Electrodiagnosis in Clinical Neurology*, 4th ed. New York, Churchill Livingstone, 1999.

Brown WE, Bolton CF: *Clinical Electromyography*, 2nd ed. Boston, Butterworth-Heinemann, 1993.

Buchthal F, Kamieniecka Z: Diagnostic yield of quantified electromyography and quantified muscle biopsy in neuromuscular disorders. *Muscle Nerve* 5:265, 1982.

Cros D, Chiappa K: Cervical magnetic stimulation. *Neurology* 40:1751, 1990.

Denny-Brown D, Nevin A: The phenomenon of myotonia. *Brain* 64:1, 1941.

deVisser M, Reimers CD: Muscle imaging, in Engel AG, Franzini-Armstrong C (eds): *Myology: Basic and Clinical*, 2nd ed. New York, McGraw-Hill, 1994, pp 795–806.

Elmquist D, Lambert EH: Detailed analysis of neuromuscular transmission in a patient with the myasthenic syndrome associated with bronchogenic carcinoma. *Mayo Clin Proc* 43: 689, 1968.

Engel AG: The neuromuscular junction, in Engel AG, Franzini-Armstrong C (eds): *Myology: Basic and Clinical*, 2nd ed. New York, McGraw-Hill, 1994, pp 261–302.

Engel AG: The muscle biopsy, in Engel AG, Franzini-Armstrong C (eds): *Myology: Basic and Clinical*, 2nd ed. New York, McGraw-Hill, 1994, pp 822–831.

Falck B, Alaranta H: Fibrillation potentials, positive sharp waves and fasciculations in the intrinsic muscles of the foot in healthy subjects. *J Neurol Neurosurg Psychiatry* 46:681, 1983.

Fishbeck K: Structure and function of striated muscle, in Asbury AK, McKhann GM, McDonald W (eds): *Diseases of the Nervous System*, 2nd ed. Philadelphia, Saunders, 1992, pp 123–134.

Forster FM, Borkowski WJ, Alpers BJ: Effects of denervation on fasciculations in human muscle. *Arch Neurol Psychiatry* 56:276, 1976.

Franzini-Armstrong C: The sarcoplasmic reticulum and transverse tubules, in Engel AG, Franzini-Armstrong C (eds): *Myology: Basic and Clinical*, 2nd ed. New York, McGraw-Hill, 1994, pp 176–199.

Hodes R, Larrabee MG, German W: The human electromyogram in response to nerve stimulation and conduction velocity of motor axons: Studies on normal and on injured peripheral nerves. *Arch Neurol Psychiatry* 60:340, 1948.

Hodgkin AL: Ionic basis of electrical activity in nerve and muscle. *Biol Rev* 26:339, 1951.

Hodgkin AL, Huxley AF: Currents carried by sodium and potassium ions through the membranes of the giant axon of Loligo. *J Physiol* 116:449, 1952.

Huxley HE: Molecular basis of contraction in cross-striated muscles, in Bourne GH (ed): *The Structure and Function of Muscle*, 2nd ed. Vol 1. *Structure*. New York, Academic Press, 1972, pp 301–387.

Kakulas BA, Adams RD: *Diseases of Muscle: Pathological Foundations of Clinical Myology*, 4th ed. New York, Harper & Row, 1985.

Katz B: *Nerve, Muscle and Synapse*. New York, McGraw-Hill, 1966.

Kimura J: *Electrodiagnosis in Diseases of Nerve and Muscle: Principles and Practice*, 2nd ed. Philadelphia, Davis, 1989.

Kuffler SW, Nicholls JG, Martin AR: *From Neuron to Brain*, 2nd ed. Sunderland, MA, Sinauer, 1984.

Magladery JW, McDougal DB: Electrophysiological studies of nerve and reflex activity in normal man. *Johns Hopkins Med J* 86:265, 1950.

McComas AJ, Fawcett PR, Campbell MJ, et al: Electrophysiologic estimation of the number of motor units within a human muscle. *J Neurol Neurosurg Psychiatry* 34:121, 1971.

Newham DJ, Jones DA, Edwards RHT: Large delayed CK changes after stepping exercise. *Muscle Nerve* 6:380, 1983.

Nielsen VK, Friis ML, Johnsen T: Electromyographic distinction between paramyotonia congenita and myotonia congenita: Effect of cold. *Neurology* 32:827, 1982.

Peter JB: Skeletal muscle: Diversity and mutability of its histochemical, electron-microscopic, biochemical and physiologic properties, in Pearson CM, Mostofi FK (eds): *The Striated Muscle*. Baltimore, Williams & Wilkins, 1973, pp 1–18.

Rosano TG, Kenny MD: A radioimmunoassay for human serum myoglobin: Method development and normal values. *Clin Chem* 23:69, 1977.

Rowland LP: Myoglobinuria. *Can J Neurol Sci* 11:1, 1984.

Stålberg E, Trontelj JV: *Single Fiber Electromyography*. Old Woking, Surrey, UK, Miraville Press, 1979.

Wilbourn AJ: The value and limitations of electromyographic examination in the diagnosis of lumbosacral radiculopathy, in Hardy RW (ed): *Lumbar Disc Disease*. New York, Raven Press, 1982, pp 65–109.

Wilbourn AJ, Aminoff MJ: AAEE Minimonograph 32: The electrophysiologic examination in patients with radiculopathies. *Muscle Nerve* 11:1099, 1988.

Chapter 46

DISEASES OF THE PERIPHERAL NERVES

In this one chapter, an attempt is made to provide an overview of the very large and difficult subject of peripheral nerve disease. Since the structure and function of the peripheral nervous system are relatively simple, one might suppose that our knowledge of its diseases would be complete. Such is not the case. For example, when a group of patients with chronic polyneuropathy were investigated intensively in a highly specialized center for the study of peripheral nerve diseases, a suitable explanation for their condition could not be found in 24 percent (Dyck et al, 1981). Moreover, the physiologic basis of many neuropathic symptoms continues to elude experts in the field, and in many of the neuropathies the pathologic changes have not been fully determined.

In the last few decades there has been a surge of interest in diseases of the peripheral nervous system, which promises to change this state of affairs. Electron-microscopic studies, new quantitative histometric methods, and refined physiologic techniques have already expanded our knowledge of the structure and function of peripheral nerves, and rapidly advancing techniques in the fields of immunology and molecular genetics are beginning to clarify entire categories of neuropathic disease. Also, during the last decade or two, effective forms of treatment for several peripheral neuropathies have been introduced, making accurate diagnosis imperative. For these reasons, clinicians now find the peripheral neuropathies among the most challenging categories of neurologic disease.

GENERAL CONSIDERATIONS

It is important to have a clear concept of the extent of the peripheral nervous system (PNS) and the mechanisms whereby it can be affected by disease. The PNS includes all neural structures lying outside the pial membrane of the spinal cord and brainstem with the exception of the optic nerves and olfactory bulbs, which are but special extensions of the brain. The parts of the PNS within the spinal canal and attached to the ventral and dorsal surfaces of the cord are called the *spinal nerve roots*; those attached to the ventrolateral surface of the brainstem are the *cranial nerve roots*, or just cranial nerves.

The dorsal (afferent or sensory) roots consist of central axonal processes of the dorsal root and cranial ganglion cells. On reaching the spinal cord and brainstem, they extend for variable distances into the dorsal horns and posterior columns (funiculi) of the cord and into the spinal trigeminal and other tracts in the medulla and pons before synapsing with secondary neurons. The peripheral axons of the dorsal root ganglion cells are the sensory nerve fibers. They terminate as freely branching or specialized corpuscular endings—i.e., the sensory receptors—in the skin, joints, and other tissues. The ventral (efferent, or motor) roots are composed of the emerging axons of anterior and lateral horn cells and motor nuclei of the brainstem; they terminate on muscle fibers or in sympathetic or parasympathetic ganglia. From these ganglia also issue the axons that terminate in smooth muscle, heart muscle, and glands. They are thin and lack a myelin covering. Traversing the subarachnoid space, where they lack well-formed epineurial sheaths (Fig. 46-1), the cranial and spinal roots (both sensory and motor) are bathed in and susceptible to substances in the cerebrospinal fluid (CSF), the lumbosacral roots having the longest exposure. The sensory nerve fibers also vary greatly in size and the thickness of their myelin covering; based on these dimensions, they are classified as type A, B, or C (see Chap. 8).

The vast extent of the peripheral ramifications of cranial and spinal nerves is noteworthy, as are their thick protective and supporting sheaths of perineurium and epineurium and their unique vascular supply through longitudinal arrays of richly anastomosing nutrient arterial branches that run in the epineurium and perineurium. The perineurium comprises the connective tissue sheaths that surround and separate bundles of nerve fibers (fascicles) of varying size, each fascicle containing several hundred axons. The sheath that binds all the fascicles of

Figure 46-1

Diagram showing the relationships of the peripheral nerve sheaths to the meningeal coverings of the spinal cord. The epineurium (EP) is in direct continuity with the dura mater (DM). The endoneurium (EN) remains unchanged from the peripheral nerve and spinal root to the junction with the spinal cord. At the subarachnoid angle (SA), the greater portion of the perineurium (P) passes outward between the dura mater and the arachnoid (A), but a few layers appear to continue over the nerve root as part of the root sheath (RS). At the subarachnoid angle, the arachnoid is reflected over the roots and becomes continuous with the outer layers of the root sheath. At the junction with the spinal cord, the outer layers of the root sheath become continuous with the pia mater (PM). (From Haller FR, Low FM: Am J Anat 131:1, 1971, by permission.)

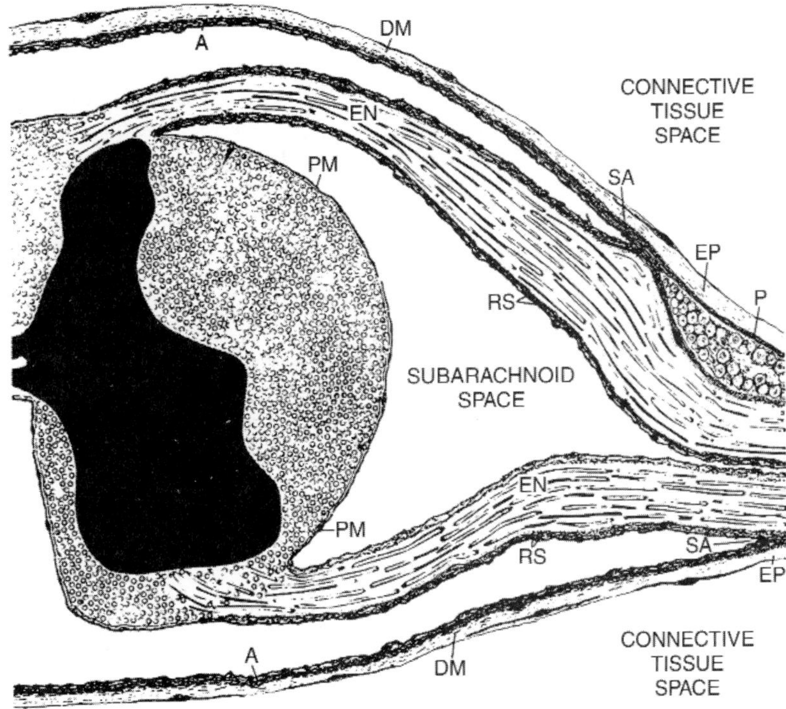

the nerve is the epineurium. As the nerve root approaches the cord, the epineurium blends with the dura (Fig. 46-1). The fine connective tissue covering of individual nerve fibers is the endoneurium. The nerves traverse narrow foramina (intervertebral and cranial) and a number pass through tight channels peripherally (e.g., the median nerve between the carpal ligament and tendon sheaths of flexor forearm muscles; the ulnar nerve in the cubital tunnel). These anatomic features explain the susceptibility of certain nerves to compression and entrapment and to ischemic damage. The axons themselves contain a complex microtubular apparatus for maintaining the integrity of their membranes and transporting substances such as neurotransmitters over long distances between the nerve cell body and the distant reaches of the nerve fiber.

Nerve fibers (axons) are coated with short segments of myelin of variable length (250 to 1000 mm), each of which is enveloped by a satellite cell—i.e., by a Schwann cell and its membrane. In fact, the PNS may be defined as the part of the nervous system that is invested by Schwann cells. Each myelin segment has a symbiotic relationship to the axon but is always morphologically independent. The structure of the axonal membrane in the gaps between segments of the myelin sheaths (nodes of Ranvier) is specialized, containing a high concentration of sodium channels and permitting the saltatory electrical conduction of nerve impulses, as described in Chap. 45. Unmyelinated fibers, more numerous in peripheral nerves than myelinated ones, also arise from cells in dorsal root and autonomic ganglia. Small bundles of naked axons are enveloped by a single Schwann cell. Delicate tongues of Schwann cell cytoplasm partition the bundles and separate individual axons.

Pathogenic Mechanisms in Peripheral Nerve Disease

The anatomic features mentioned above enable one to conceptualize the possible avenues by which disease may affect the peripheral nerves. Pathologic processes may be directed at any one of several groups of nerve cells whose axons constitute the nerves, i.e., the cells of the anterior or lateral horns of the spinal cord, the dorsal root ganglia, or sympathetic and parasympathetic ganglia. Each cell type exhibits specific vulnerabilities to disease processes, and if destroyed—as are the motor nerve cells in poliomyelitis—there results a secondary degeneration of the axons and myelin sheaths of the peripheral fibers of these cells. Neuropathic symptoms may also be induced by alterations of function and structure of the ventral and dorsal columns (funiculi) of the spinal cord, which contain the fibers of exit and entry of anterior horn and dorsal root ganglion cells, respectively.

The myelin of these centrally located fibers is constituted differently from that of the peripheral nerves, being enveloped by oligodendrocytes rather than Schwann cells, and the fibers are supported by astrocytes rather than fibroblasts. Because of the intimate relation of the roots to the CSF and to specialized arachnoidal cells (the arachnoidal villi), a pathologic process in the CSF or leptomeninges may damage the exposed spinal roots. Destruction of anterior roots results in wallerian degeneration (see below) of the motor fibers in peripheral nerves; destruction of posterior roots results in wallerian degeneration of the posterior columns of the spinal cord but not of peripheral sensory nerves. The continuity of the latter is maintained by spinal ganglion cells and their peripheral extensions (the sensory nerves). Disease of the connective tissues may affect the peripheral nerves that lie within their sheaths. Diffuse or localized arterial diseases may injure nerves by occluding their nutrient arteries. In a large category of immune-mediated neuropathies, nerves are damaged by a cellular or humoral attack on various components of myelin. Some of the immune-mediated diseases are also characterized by the binding of circulating antibodies to the specialized regions at the nodes of Ranvier, causing a block of electrical conduction with or without damage of adjacent axons or myelin. Also, a complement-dependent humoral immune reaction against the radicular or peripheral axolemma has been delineated. Toxic agents that selectively damage the Schwann cells or their membranes, which compose the myelin sheaths, cause demyelination of peripheral nerves, leaving axons relatively intact, or a toxin may specifically affect axons by poisoning their cell bodies, the axolemma, or the lengthy and complex axonal transport apparatus. Finally, one might suppose that axons of the motor or sensory nerves, sympathetic fibers of varying diameter and length, or the end organs to which they are attached would each have its own particular liability to disease.

Much of this is theoretical and somewhat speculative. At present we can cite only a few examples of diseases or intoxicants that utilize these potential pathways exclusively: diphtheria, in which the bacterial toxin acts directly on the membranes of the Schwann cells near the dorsal root ganglia and adjacent parts of motor and sensory nerves (the most vascular parts of the peripheral nerve); polyarteritis nodosa, which causes widespread occlusion of vasa nervorum, resulting in multifocal nerve infarction; tabes dorsalis, in which there is a treponemal meningoradiculitis of the posterior roots (mainly of the lumbosacral segments) that lie next to the arachnoidal villi where CSF is resorbed; doxorubicin intoxication, wherein protein synthesis of dorsal root ganglion cells is blocked, with subsequent neuronal destruction; poisoning with arsenic, which combines with the axoplasm of the largest sensory and motor nerves via sulfhydryl bonds; and vincristine toxicity, which damages the microtubular transport system. Analogous anatomic pathways are probably implicated in other diseases by mechanisms that remain to be divulged.

Pathologic Reactions of Peripheral Nerve

Pathologically, several distinct processes are recognized, although they are not disease-specific and may be present in varying combinations in any given patient. The major ones are *segmental demyelination*, *wallerian degeneration*, and *axonal degeneration* (diagrammatically illustrated in Fig. 46-2).

The myelin sheath is the most susceptible element of the nerve fiber, for it may break down as part of a primary process involving the Schwann cells or myelin, or it may be damaged secondarily, consequent to disease affecting its axon. Focal degeneration of the myelin sheath with sparing of the axon is called *segmental demyelination*. Degeneration of myelin secondary to axonal disease has been called *medullary-axonic* and may occur either proximal or distal to the site of axonal interruption (*wallerian degeneration*) or as part of a "dying-back" phenomenon in more generalized, metabolically determined polyneuropathies (*axonal degeneration*). The latter form of degeneration affects distal parts of the axons in peripheral nerves and in some instances the terminal parts of the central axons in the posterior columns of the spinal cord. Destruction of axons results within several days in a degeneration of all the myelin distal to the point of injury. The myelin breaks down into blocks or ovoids in which lie fragments of axons (the digestion chambers of Cajal). Secondary degeneration of myelinated fibers due to destruction of the nerve cells has been called *neuronopathy* rather than neuropathy; here also the myelin breaks up into fragments that are then converted, through the action of macrophages, into neutral fats and cholesterol esters and carried by these cells to the bloodstream. Disease may cause either motor or sensory neuronopathy; in the former case the anterior horn cell is affected primarily (motor neuron disease, or motor neuronopathy), and in the latter, the sensory ganglion cell (ganglionopathy).

These pathologic reactions are more easily understood if one considers certain features of cytoskeletal structure and function of nerve cells and their axons. The axon contains longitudinally oriented neurofilaments and

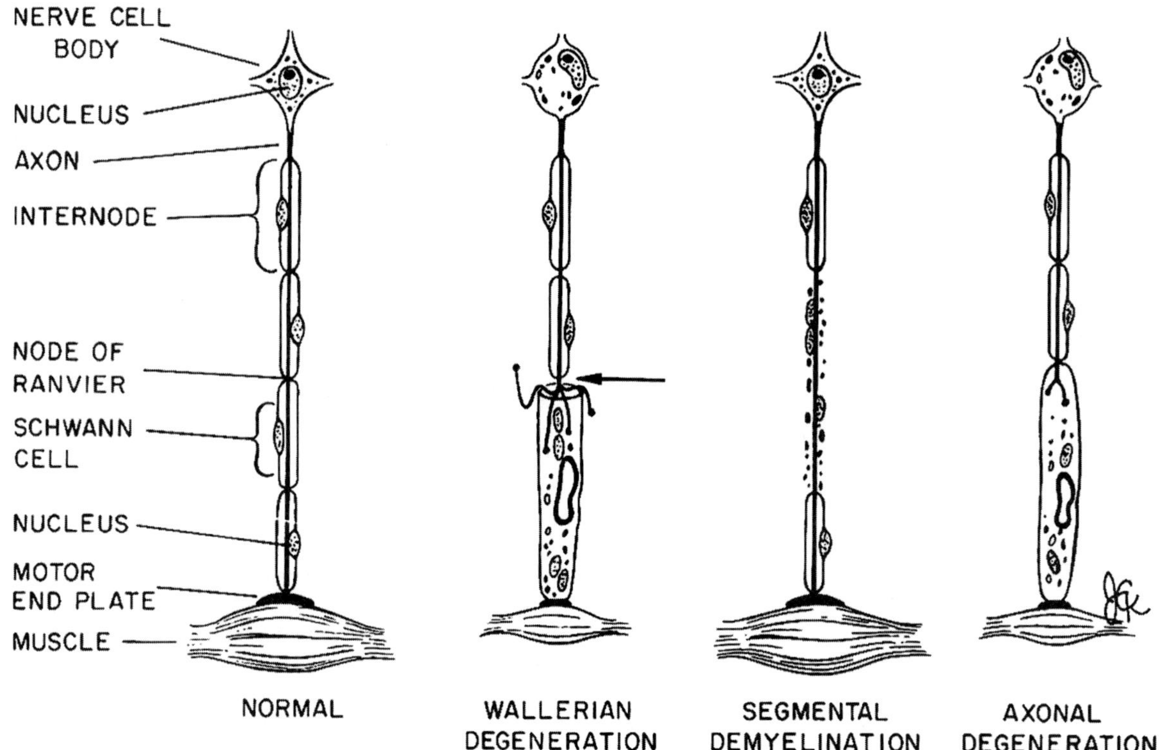

Figure 46-2

Diagram of the basic pathologic processes affecting peripheral nerves. In wallerian degeneration, there is degeneration of the axis cylinder and myelin distal to the site of axonal interruption (arrow), and central chromatolysis. In segmental demyelination, the axon is spared. In axonal degeneration, there is a distal degeneration of myelin and axis cylinder as a result of neuronal disease. Both wallerian and axonal degeneration cause muscle atrophy. Further details in text. (Courtesy of Dr. Arthur Asbury.)

microtubules, which are separated but interconnected by cross bridges. Their main function involves the transport of substances from nerve cell body to axon terminal (anterograde transport) and from the distal axon back to the cell body (retrograde transport). Thus, when the axon is severed, organelles cannot be transmitted to the distal axon for the purpose of renewing membrane and neurotransmitter systems. By means of retrograde axonal transport, the cell bodies receive signals to increase their metabolic activity and to produce growth factors and other materials needed for axonal regeneration. The histopathologic changes in the nerve cell body that are due to axonal interruption (swelling of the cell cytoplasm and marginalization and dissolution of the Nissl substance) are called *chromatolysis* or *axonal reaction*. The important point is that despite the destructive changes in the nerve fibers, the nerve cells, while altered in histologic appearance, are left intact and reactive.

In *segmental demyelination*, recovery of function may be rapid because the intact but denuded axon needs only to become remyelinated. The newly formed internodal segments are thinner than normal and of variable length. By contrast, with wallerian or axonal degeneration, recovery is slower, often requiring months to a year or more, because the axon must first regenerate and then reconnect to muscle, sensory organ, blood vessel, etc., before function returns. When the regenerating axon becomes myelinated, the internodal segments are inappropriately short, one old internode being replaced by three or four new ones. Recurrent demyelination and remyelination lead to "onion bulb" formations and enlargement of nerves, the result of proliferating Schwann cells and fibroblasts that encircle the axon and its thin myelin sheath.

When a nerve is severed by a crude destructive lesion involving nerve fibers and connective tissue sheathing, the continuity is interrupted and may not be reestablished. Regenerating axonic filaments then take aberrant courses and, with fibroblastic scar formation at the end of the central portion of the interrupted nerve, they form a pseudoneuroma. When nerve cells are destroyed, no recovery of their function is possible except by collateral regeneration from axons of intact nerve cells.

These relatively few pathologic reactions cannot in themselves differentiate the hundred or more diseases of the peripheral nerves; but when they are considered in relation to the selective effects on various types and sizes of fibers, the topography of the lesions, and the time course of the process, they furnish a set of criteria whereby many diseases can be distinguished. There are also special pathologic changes that characterize certain diseases of the peripheral nervous system. For example, in acute demyelinative polyneuritis of the Guillain-Barré type, there are endoneurial infiltrations of lymphocytes, plasma cells, and other mononuclear cells in the roots, sensory and sympathetic ganglia, and nerves; frequently the infiltrates and destruction of myelin have a perivenous distribution. In polyarteritis nodosa, a characteristic *necrotizing panarteritis* with thrombotic occlusion of vessels and focal infarction of peripheral nerves—and less often with rupture of vessels and hemorrhage into nerves—are the dominant findings. Deposition of amyloid in the endoneurial connective tissue and walls of vessels, affecting the nerve fibers secondarily by compression or ischemia, are the distinctive features of amyloid polyneuropathy. In one of the inherited polyneuropathies of childhood, the axons are enlarged by tightly packed masses of neurofilaments. The now rare diphtheritic polyneuropathy is typified by the predominantly demyelinative character of the nerve fiber change, the location of this change in and around the roots and sensory ganglia, the subacute course, and the lack of inflammatory reaction. Other polyneuropathies (paraneoplastic, nutritional, porphyric, arsenical, and uremic) are topographically symmetrical but are not presently distinguishable from one another by histopathologic means. The least is known about the familial types of polyneuropathy; although genetic factors are clearly involved, their biochemical mechanisms and pathology are just beginning to be studied.

Concerning the pathology of the *mononeuropathies*, our knowledge is also incomplete. Compression of nerve, producing local or segmental ischemia, violent stretch, and laceration of nerves are understandable mechanisms, and their pathologic changes have been reproduced in animals. Tumor infiltration and vasculitis with ischemic infarction of nerve account for some cases. Of infections localized to single nerves, only leprosy, sarcoid, and herpes zoster represent identifiable disease states. For most of the acute mononeuropathies, the pathologic changes have yet to be defined, since they are usually benign, reversible states that provide no opportunity for complete pathologic examination.

SYMPTOMATOLOGY OF PERIPHERAL NERVE DISEASE

There are a number of motor, sensory, reflex, autonomic, and trophic symptoms and signs that are more or less typical of peripheral nerve disease. Grouping them into syndromes based on their temporal and topographic features has proved to be of value in clinical diagnosis.

Impairment of Motor Function Whereas anesthetic agents, nerve toxins, cooling, and ischemia may temporarily cause weakness or paralysis, persistent impairment of motor function over days, weeks, or months always signifies segmental demyelination, axonal interruption, or destruction of motor neurons. The degree of weakness is proportional to the number of axons or motor neurons affected, although pain and kinesthetic loss may contribute.

Most *polyneuropathies* are marked by a characteristic distribution of the weakness and paralysis. Usually the muscles of the feet and legs are affected earlier and more severely than those of the hands and forearms. In milder form, only the lower legs are involved. Truncal and cranial muscles are usually the last to yield, and then only in severe cases. The main exceptions to this rule are seen in the acute and chronic demyelinating inflammatory neuropathies, where the multifocal nature of lesions and blockage of electrical conduction can lead to weakness of proximal limb and facial muscles before distal parts are weakened. Most of the nutritional, metabolic, and toxic neuropathies assume the more common, predominantly distal pattern. The pathologic changes in such cases begin in the far distal parts of the largest and longest nerves and advance along the affected fibers toward their nerve cell bodies ("dying-back neuropathy," "distal axonopathy"). One possible explanation for this process is that the primary damage is to the neuronal perikaryon, which fails in its function of synthesizing proteins and delivering them to the distal parts of the axon. There is also the possibility that a primary affection of axons impairs anterograde axonal transport to the periphery; the functional impairment would then be proportional to the size and length of the blocked axons.

Another characteristic pattern of neuropathic weakness is one in which all the muscles of the limbs, trunk, and neck are involved, leading often to respiratory paralysis. The vast majority of acute, predominantly motor neuropathies requiring respiratory support are of this type. The best known is the Guillain-Barré syndrome (GBS). Porphyric, diphtheritic, and certain toxic polyneuropathies are far less common causes of such a pattern of paralysis, but fatalities, when they do occur, are usually due to respiratory paralysis.

A predominantly *bibrachial paralysis* is an unusual presentation of neuropathic disease but may occur as an initial event in Guillain-Barré disease as well as in the Sjögren syndrome, chronic immune or paraneoplastic neuropathies, lead neuropathy, Tangier disease, and, rarely, as a familial brachial neuritis. However, the most frequent cause of bibrachial palsy is disease of the motor neurons themselves, specifically, motor system disease, as discussed on page 1153. *Paraparesis* may occur with any of the generalized polyneuropathies, infections and inflammations of the cauda equina, as occurs with Lyme disease, cytomegalovirus, herpes simplex, and with neoplastic nerve root infiltrations. Bifacial and other cranial nerve paralyses are most likely to occur in GBS, with neoplastic invasion, and also with connective tissue diseases, HIV infection, herpes virus, sarcoidosis, Lyme disease, or one of the rare metabolic neuropathies (Refsum, Bassen-Kornzweig, Tangier, and Riley-Day).

Atrophy of weak or paralyzed muscles proceeds slowly over several months, its degree being proportional to the number of damaged motor nerve fibers; the maximum degree of denervation atrophy occurs in 90 to 120 days and reduces muscle volume by 75 to 80 percent. Atrophy is also a consequence of disuse; it occurs over many weeks and in itself does not reduce muscle volume by more than 25 to 30 percent. Atrophy, therefore, does not coincide with or correspond to acute paralysis and is least prominent in the acute demyelinative neuropathies. In chronic axonal neuropathies, the degrees of paralysis and atrophy tend to correspond. Ultimately there is degeneration and loss of the denervated muscle fibers. This process begins in 6 to 12 months; in 3 to 4 years, most of the denervated fibers will have degenerated. If reinnervation takes place within a year, motor function and muscle volume may be restored.

Tendon Reflexes The rule is that diminution or loss of tendon reflexes is an invariable sign of peripheral nerve disease. In the *small-fiber neuropathies*, however, tendon reflexes may sometimes be retained, even with marked loss of perception of painful and thermal stimuli and loss of autonomic function. This discrepancy is attributable to the fact that the afferent arc of the tendon reflexes utilizes the large heavily myelinated fibers. Conversely, reflexes can be diminished out of proportion to weakness because of involvement of the large afferent fibers that innervate the muscle spindles. Slowing of conduction velocities in sensory fibers may impair or abolish the reflex by dispersing the afferent volley of impulses initiated by the tendon tap. This concept is borne out in cases of peripheral neuropathy by the general concordance between areflexia and a loss of proprioceptive and joint-position senses; the large nerve fibers from spindle afferents are of the same type and size as those mediating these forms of sensation, and they tend to be affected together by disease of the nerve or its roots. By contrast, a loss of sensory functions that are dependent on large fibers, in the presence of preserved reflexes, implicates the central projections from the sensory ganglion cells in the posterior columns of the spinal cord. Early in an acute polyneuropathy, the reflexes may be diminished but not absent and may become perceptibly more reduced from day to day.

Sensory Loss (See also pages 167 to 172) Most polyneuropathies cause impairment of both motor and sensory functions, but one may be affected more than the other. In GBS for example, paralysis is more prominent than sensory loss. In most of the toxic and metabolic neuropathies, sensory loss exceeds weakness; and in sensory neuronopathy, there is virtually no motor deficit. These differences are emphasized in the descriptions of individual peripheral nerve diseases.

In the polyneuropathies, sensation, even more than motor function, is affected symmetrically in the distal segments of the limbs, and more in the legs than in the arms (see Chap. 9). In most polyneuropathies, all sensory modalities (touch-pressure, pain and temperature, vibratory, and joint position senses) are impaired or eventually lost, although one modality may seemingly be affected out of proportion to the others, or superficial sensation may be impaired more than deep sensation. Vibratory sense is often affected more than position and tactile senses. As the neuropathy worsens, there is spread of sensory loss from the distal to more proximal parts of the limbs and, rarely, to the lower abdomen and face.

A relatively rare form of sensory loss affects the trunk, scalp, and face; this pattern is characteristic of sensory ganglionopathy. The escutcheon region of the lower abdomen may be involved as part of severe axonal neuropathy and should not be mistaken for the pattern of segmental truncal loss seen with ganglionopathies or a sensory level that occurs with spinal cord disease.

Another pattern of neuropathic sensory loss is notable—namely, a loss of pain and temperature sensation with either sparing or lesser impairment of touch-pressure, vibratory, and position senses. This resembles the dissociated sensory disturbance of syringomyelia except that it is predominantly lumbosacral (originally it was referred to as "lumbosacral syringomyelia"). This *pseudosyringomyelic* dissociation of sensation may extend over the arms, trunk, and even cranial surfaces. Thévenard was the first to question its spinal basis, and it is now generally agreed that most such examples are due to hereditary sensory or certain acquired small-fiber neuropathies, such as primary amyloidosis, congenital absence of pain, Riley-Day syndrome, and Tangier disease. Usually the unmyelinated autonomic fibers are also interrupted. Exceptionally, as in one of the families studied by Adams and associates, all forms of sensation may be lost over the entire body, while motor power and autonomic functions are preserved. More often, *universal sensory loss* is attributable to an acquired disease affecting the sensory ganglia (sensory neuronopathy). Usually this is a paraneoplastic syndrome, but it may also be due to a toxic or immune disease (e.g., in Sjögren disease or scleroderma).

Paresthesias, Pain, and Dysesthesias These abnormalities of sensation have been described in Chap. 9. They tend to be especially marked in the hands and feet. "Pins and needles," stabbing, tingling, prickling, electrical, Novocain-like, and band-like sensations are the adjectives used most frequently to describe these abnormalities. Some sensory neuropathies are attended only by these paresthesias and by numbness; if the symptoms are slight, there may be no objective sensory loss. Others are extremely painful. The pains may be described as burning, aching, sharp and cutting, or crushing, or they may resemble the lightning pains of tabes dorsalis. Perversion of sensation (allodynia) is commonplace—e.g., tingling, burning, or stabbing pain induced by tactile stimuli. Under these conditions, a given stimulus induces not only an aberrant sensation but also one that radiates and persists after the stimulus is withdrawn. As remarked on pages 145 and 163, the patient's reaction may seem to indicate a hypersensitivity ("hyperesthesia"), but more often the sensory threshold is actually raised and only the sensory experience or response is exaggerated (*hyperpathia*).

These paresthesias and dysesthesias are particularly common in certain types of diabetic and alcoholic-nutritional neuropathy. Mainly they affect the feet ("burning feet") and less often the hands; they are confined to limited regions of the body in herpes zoster, in some cases of diabetic and other types of vascular neuropathy, and in certain sensory neuropathies of obscure nature. A particularly intense form of burning pain typifies causalgia, due to a partial lesion (usually traumatic) of the ulnar, median, posterior tibial, peroneal, or occasionally some other nerve (pages 148 and 1438).

The mechanism of thermal and painful dysesthesias is not fully understood. It has been theorized that a loss of large touch-pressure fibers disinhibits the pain-receiving nerve cells in the posterior horns of the spinal cord. An argument against this explanation is the lack of pain in Friedreich ataxia, in which the larger neurons degenerate, and also in certain purely sensory polyneuropathies, where only the perception of tactile stimuli (large fibers) is lost. A more likely explanation, supported by microneurographic recordings after release of tourniquet compression, is that dysesthetic pain results from autogenic ectopic discharges arising at many sites along surviving intact or regenerating nociceptive nerve fibers or their terminal receptors, as described in Chap. 8. In contrast to dysesthetic pain, it has been postulated that the deep, aching pain of sciatica or brachial neuritis (nerve trunk pain) arises from irritation of the normal endings (nervi nervorum) in the sheaths of the nerve trunks themselves (Asbury and Fields).

Sensory Ataxia and Tremor Proprioceptive deafferentation with retention of a reasonable degree of motor function is the basis of ataxia of gait and of limb movement, as discussed in Chap. 9. An action tremor of fast-frequency type may also appear during certain phases of a polyneuropathy. Shahani and coworkers have the impression that it is due to either a loss of input or slowed nerve conduction from some of the muscle-spindle afferents. Corticosteroid therapy enhances the fast tremor. A particularly severe form of slower tremor is combined with clumsiness in certain neuropathies that affect large afferent fibers, specifically in the autoimmune, anti–myelin-associated glycoprotein (MAG) neuropathy and in some cases of chronic inflammatory demyelinating polyneuropathy (CIDP). During action, the tremor may at times be so coarse as to resemble the intention tremor of cerebellar disease.

Ataxia without weakness is characteristic of tabes dorsalis, a purely posterior root affection, but this syndrome can be nearly duplicated by diabetic polyneuropathy, which affects posterior roots as well as nerves (diabetic pseudotabes), by a variant of the Guillain-Barré syndrome (Fisher syndrome as well as a variant that produces almost pure ataxia), and by sensory neuronopathy (ganglionopathy). The ataxia in some instances is virtually indistinguishable from that caused by cerebellar disease, but lacking are other features of cerebellar dysfunction. Several chronic sensory neuropathies have prominent ataxic features, and the movements, though strong, are rendered ineffective by virtue of the deep sensory loss alone. Characteristic of the sensory (tabetic) ataxic gait are the brusque, flinging, slapping movements of the legs.

Deformity and Trophic Changes In a number of chronic polyneuropathies, the feet, hands, and spine become deformed. This is most apt to occur when the disease begins during childhood. Austin pointed out that foot deformity is found in 30 percent of patients with hereditary hypertrophic polyneuropathy and spine curvature in 20 percent. In early life, the feet are pulled into a position of talipes equinus (plantar deviation) because of the disproportionate weakness of the pretibial and peroneal muscles and the unopposed action of the calf muscles. The atrophic paralysis of the intrinsic foot muscles allows the long extensors of the toes to dorsiflex the proximal phalanges and the long flexors to shorten the foot, heighten the arch, and flex the distal phalanges. The result is the *claw foot—le pied en griffe* of the French. The claw hand has a similar basis. In early childhood, unequal weakening of the paravertebral muscles on the two sides of the spine leads to kyphoscoliosis.

Denervation atrophy of muscle is the main trophic disturbance resulting from interruption of the motor nerves. Analgesia of distal parts makes them susceptible to burns, pressure sores, and other forms of injury that are easily infected and heal poorly. In an anesthetic and immobile limb, the skin becomes tight and shiny, the nails curved and ridged, and the subcutaneous tissue thickened. Hair growth is diminished in denervated areas. If the autonomic fibers are interrupted, the limb is warm and pink. Repeated injuries and chronic subcutaneous and osteomyelitic infections may result in a painless loss of digits and the formation of plantar ulcers (*mal perforant du pied*). These are prominent features of the recessive form of hereditary sensory neuropathy, and we have observed them in dominant forms as well. In certain familial and other chronic polyneuropathies, analgesic joints, when chronically traumatized, may disintegrate (Charcot arthropathy), as occurs in tabes dorsalis and syringomyelia.

The pathogenesis of the trophic changes is not fully understood. Apart from analgesia, a critical factor may be inappropriate neural regulation of the distal vasculature, which interferes with normal tissue responses to trauma and infection. Ali and colleagues relate the ulcer formation to loss of C fibers, which mediate both pain and autonomic reflexes. However, paralyzed limbs, even in hysteria, if left dependent, are often cold, swollen, and pale or blue. These are probably secondary disuse effects, as pointed out long ago by Lewis and Pickering. Erythema and edema, burning pain, and cold sensations have been evoked by peripheral nerve irritation, particularly of C and A-δ fibers.

Autonomic Dysfunction Anhidrosis and orthostatic hypotension, the two most frequent manifestations of autonomic dysfunction, may be major features of certain types of polyneuropathy. They occur most frequently in amyloidosis and certain other *hereditary small-fiber polyneuropathies*, diabetic polyneuropathies, and several congenital types. In addition, they are central features of an acute pure autonomic polyneuropathy called pandysautonomia (Young et al, Low et al) and can be a prominent feature of GBS. These conditions are described in detail in Chap. 26.

Other manifestations of autonomic paralysis are small or medium-sized unreactive pupils that are unusually sensitive to certain drugs (pages 296 and 563); lack of sweat, tears, and saliva; sexual impotence; weak bowel and bladder sphincters with urinary retention or overflow incontinence; and weakness and dilatation of the esophagus and colon. Also, the normal variability of heart rate is lost and there may be pain from paralytic ileus or dyscoordinated peristalsis as well as achlorhydria and hyponatremia. Some of these abnormalities are found in diabetic and amyloid polyneuropathy. In general these autonomic disturbances correlate with degeneration of unmyelinated (Remak) fibers in the peripheral nerves. Usually, in any neuropathy involving sensory nerves, there is loss of autonomic function in the same zones as sensory loss. *This is not true of radicular diseases* because the autonomic fibers join the spinal nerves more distally. Such losses may also be demonstrated by special tests, as described in Chap. 26.

Fasciculations, Cramps, and Spasms In most polyneuropathies, fasciculations and cramps are not important findings. Occasionally one observes a state of mild motor polyneuropathy that, upon recovery, leaves the muscles in a state variably referred to as myokymia, continuous muscular activity, and neuromyotonia (see Chaps. 45 and 54). All the affected muscles ripple and quiver and occasionally cramp. Use of the muscles increases this activity, and there is a reduction in their efficiency, which the patient senses as a stiffness and heaviness. In some instances this apparently constitutes the entire neuropathic syndrome and may be gratifyingly relieved by carbamazepine or phenytoin. It raises the question of a terminal nerve conduction abnormality. Other closely related phenomena are spasms (e.g., hemifacial spasm) or involuntary movements of the toes and feet. The latter, referred to by Spillane and colleagues as the syndrome of painful legs and moving toes, is attributed by Nathan to ectopic discharges in sensory roots, ganglia, or nerves, evoking both pain and organized movements. Other possible mechanisms are ephaptic cross transmission, segmental hyperactivity from deafferentation, and neuronal sprouting and reinnervation. In yet other instances, the muscle activity induces odd postures or slow writhing movements that Jankovic and van der Linden have likened to dystonia. The precise pathophysiology of these seemingly spontaneous asynchronous activities of motor neurons is not known. Stimulation of a motor nerve, instead of causing a brief burst of action potentials in the muscle, results in a prolonged or dispersed series of potentials lasting several hundred milliseconds. Also, the distal latencies are prolonged. Evidently, branched axons involved in collateral innervation have an unstable polarization that may last for years.

APPROACH TO THE PATIENT WITH PERIPHERAL NEUROPATHY

The clinician is faced with two problems: (1) establishing the existence of disease of the peripheral nervous system, and (2) ascertaining its nature and the possibilities of treatment. The former is not difficult when one becomes familiar with the symptomatology of peripheral nerve diseases, described above. At the outset it must be determined whether the *pattern* of neurologic findings corresponds to one of the following:

Polyneuropathy

Polyradiculopathy

Neuronopathy—motor or sensory

Mononeuropathy

Multiple mononeuropathies (mononeuropathy multiplex)

Plexopathy (involvement of multiple nerves in a plexus)

A brief definition of each of these neuropathic states follows: (1) In a *polyneuropathy*, weakness is relatively symmetrical from the beginning and progresses bilaterally; reflexes are lost in affected parts, but particularly at the ankles; sensory complaints and loss of sensation are most pronounced distally, in the feet before the hands in most cases. (2) A *polyradiculopathy* (implicating multiple spinal roots) differs from a polyneuropathy in that the pattern of neurologic signs is asymmetrical, causing weakness and sensory loss that may be proximal in one limb and distal in another, and involving muscles and sensory zones that can only be explained on the basis of root disease; pain in the distribution of one or more roots is a common feature. (3) In *sensory neuronopathy*, the sensory ganglion cells rather than the peripheral sensory nerves are predominantly affected. This gives rise to symptoms and signs of sensory loss in both a proximal and distal distribution, often including the scalp, thorax, abdomen, and buttocks as well as the extremities; sensory ataxia is a common accompaniment. *Motor neuronopathy* is essentially a disorder of the anterior horn cells causing weakness, fasciculations, and atrophy in a widespread distribution. (4) A *mononeuropathy* is the most circumscribed form of peripheral nerve disease, reflected by weakness and sensory loss in the territory of a single peripheral nerve. Certain constellations of signs serve to differentiate mononeuropathy from a radiculopathy—for example, weakness in dorsiflexion and eversion of the foot is referable to the peroneal nerve; however, if inversion of the foot, innervated by the tibial nerve, is also affected, then the L5 root is implicated. (5) *Plexopathies* (brachial or lumbosacral) may create the most confusing patterns of involvement; only one limb is affected but not necessarily in a pattern involving several adjacent nerve roots. Knowledge of the innervation of the involved muscles usually clarifies the situation.

Of the multitude of diseases of the peripheral nerves, certain ones almost always manifest themselves by one or another of above-described patterns. *Thus the pattern of the neuropathy sets limits on the etiologic possibilities.* Also, in the analysis of a polyneuropathy it is important to determine whether the process is predominantly motor with less sensory involvement (motor-sensory), or the converse (sensorimotor), or purely sensory, motor, or autonomic (see Table 46-1). The *time course* of the disease is also informative. An acute onset (i.e., rapid evolution) is nearly always diagnostic of an inflammatory, immunologic, toxic, or vascular etiology. The other extreme, a polyneuropathy evolving slowly over many years is indicative of a hereditary or, rarely, a metabolic disease. Most of the toxic, nutritional, and systemic diseases of nerve develop

Table 46-1 Principal neuropathic syndromes

I. Syndrome of acute motor paralysis with variable disturbance of sensory and autonomic function
  A. Guillain-Barré syndrome (GBS; acute inflammatory polyneuropathy; acute autoimmune neuropathy)
  B. Acute axonal form of GBS
  C. Acute sensory neuro(no)pathy syndrome
  D. Diphtheritic polyneuropathy
  E. Porphyric polyneuropathy
  F. Certain toxic polyneuropathies (thallium, triorthocresyl phosphate)
  G. Rarely, paraneoplastic
  H. Acute pandysautonomic neuropathy
  I. Tick paralysis
  J. Critical illness polyneuropathy

II. Syndrome of subacute sensorimotor paralysis
  A. Symmetrical polyneuropathies
    1. Deficiency states: alcoholism (beriberi), pellagra, vitamin B_{12} deficiency, chronic gastrointestinal disease (see Chap. 41)
    2. Poisoning with heavy metals and solvents: arsenic, lead, mercury, thallium, methyl *n*-butyl ketone, *n*-hexane, methyl bromide, ethylene oxide, organophosphates (TOCP etc.), acrylamide (Chap. 43)
    3. Drug toxicity: isoniazid, ethionamide, hydralazine, nitrofurantoin and related nitrofurazones, disulfiram, carbon disulfide, vincristine, cisplatin, paclitaxel, chloramphenicol, phenytoin, pyridoxine, amitriptyline, dapsone, stilbamidine, trichlorethylene, thalidomide, clioquinol, amiodirione, adulterated agents such as L-tryptophan, etc.
    4. Uremic polyneuropathy (Chap. 40)
    5. Subacute inflammatory polyneuropathy
  B. Asymmetrical neuropathies (mononeuropathy multiplex)
    1. Diabetes
    2. Polyarteritis nodosa and other inflammatory angiopathic neuropathies (Churg-Strauss, hypereosinophilic, rheumatoid, lupus, Wegener granulomatosis, isolated peripheral nervous system vasculitis)
    3. Mixed cryoglobulinemia
    4. Sjögren-sicca syndrome
    5. Sarcoidosis
    6. Ischemic neuropathy with peripheral vascular disease
    7. Lyme disease
  C. Unusual sensory neuropathies
    1. Wartenberg migrant sensory neuropathy
    2. Sensory perineuritis
  D. Meningeal based nerve root disease (polyradiculopathy)
    1. Neoplastic infiltration
    2. Granulomatous and infectious infiltration: Lyme, sarcoid, etc.
    3. Spinal diseases: osteoarthritic spondylitis, etc.
    4. Idiopathic polyradiculopathy

III. Syndrome of chronic sensorimotor polyneuropathy
  A. Less chronic, acquired forms
    1. Paraneoplastic: carcinoma, lymphoma, myeloma, and other malignancies
    2. Chronic inflammatory demyelinating polyneuropathy (CIDP)
    3. Paraproteinemias
    4. Uremia (occasionally subacute)
    5. Beriberi (usually subacute)
    6. Diabetes
    7. Connective tissue diseases
    8. Amyloidosis
    9. Leprosy
    10. Hypothyroidism
    11. Benign sensory form in the elderly
  B. Syndrome of more chronic polyneuropathy, genetically determined forms
    1. Inherited polyneuropathies of predominantly sensory type
      a. Dominant mutilating sensory neuropathy in adults
      b. Recessive mutilating sensory neuropathy of childhood
      c. Congenital insensitivity to pain
      d. Other inherited sensory neuropathies, including those associated with spinocerebellar degenerations, Riley-Day syndrome, and the universal anesthesia syndrome
  C. Inherited polyneuropathies of mixed sensorimotor types
    1. Idiopathic group
      a. Peroneal muscular atrophy [Charcot-Marie-Tooth; hereditary motor-sensory neuropathy (HMSN), types I and II]
      b. Hypertrophic polyneuropathy of Déjerine-Sottas, adult and childhood forms
      c. Roussy-Lévy polyneuropathy
      d. Polyneuropathy with optic atrophy, spastic paraplegia, spinocerebellar degeneration, mental retardation, and dementia
      e. Hereditary liability to pressure palsy
    2. Inherited polyneuropathies with a recognized metabolic disorder (see also Chap. 37)
      a. Refsum disease
      b. Metachromatic leukodystrophy
      c. Globoid-body leukodystrophy (Krabbe disease)
      d. Adrenoleukodystrophy
      e. Amyloid polyneuropathy
      f. Porphyric polyneuropathy
      g. Anderson-Fabry disease
      h. Abetalipoproteinemia and Tangier disease

IV. Neuropathy associated with mitochondrial diseases (Chap. 37)

V. Syndrome of recurrent or relapsing polyneuropathy
  A. GBS
  B. Porphyria
  C. Chronic inflammatory demyelinating polyneuropathy
  D. Certain forms of mononeuritis multiplex
  E. Beriberi or intoxications
  F. Refsum disease, Tangier disease

VI. Syndrome of mononeuropathy or plexopathy
  A. Brachial plexus neuropathies
  B. Brachial mononeuropathies
  C. Causalgia
  D. Lumbosacral plexopathies
  E. Crural mononeuropathies
  F. Migrant sensory neuropathy
  G. Entrapment neuropathies

subacutely or "early chronically" over several weeks and months.

The etiologic diagnosis of both polyneuropathy and mononeuropathy multiplex is facilitated further by determining whether the myelin sheath or the axon is primarily involved (*demyelinative disease* or *axonopathy*). Sometimes the neurologic examination is sufficient to make this distinction, but it can be made with greater precision by utilizing nerve conduction studies and needle examination of muscles by electromyography (EMG). The latter also helps to distinguish primary disorders of muscle (myopathies) from disorders that are secondary to denervation and those due to neuromuscular block. The electrical examinations of nerve and muscle are described fully in Chap. 45. In a few instances, the EMG abnormalities are so characteristic as to virtually define a group of neuropathies, e.g., the chronic demyelinative motor neuropathies with multifocal conduction block (page 1411). The EMG and conduction studies refine the diagnosis within each of the main categories of neuropathic disease, at times greatly reducing the number of possible etiologic diagnoses. Other useful laboratory procedures are (1) biochemical tests to identify the metabolic, nutritional, or toxic states that produce neuropathy; (2) CSF examination (increase in protein and in cells that indicate radicular or meningeal involvement); (3) nerve and muscle biopsy; (4) measurement of immunoglobulins and antineural antibodies that relate to immune-mediated neuropathies; and (5) newly available genetic testing for several of the inherited neuropathies.

Once having established that the patient has a disease of the peripheral nerves and having ascertained its clinical and electrophysiologic pattern and time course, one must then attempt to determine its nature. This is accomplished most readily by allocating the case in question to one of the categories in Table 46-1, in which the peripheral nerve diseases are classified syndromically, according to their mode of evolution and clinical presentation. Having categorized the neuropathic syndrome in this way, one then seeks to identify the case in question with a particular disease in that category. These are listed in the sections that follow.

Our use of the terms *acute*, *subacute*, and *chronic* must be explained. By *acute* we mean evolution in terms of days and *subacute*, in weeks. We divide *chronic* into two groups: *early chronic*—in which the neuropathy evolves over a period of several months to a few years, and *late chronic*—more than several years.

Diseases of the peripheral nerves are considered in the most comprehensive fashion in the two-volume monograph *Peripheral Neuropathy*, edited by Dyck and colleagues. Also recommended are more concise monographs on this subject by Schaumburg and associates and by Asbury and Thomas and the recently published atlas on the pathology of peripheral nerve by King.

SYNDROME OF ACUTE MOTOR PARALYSIS WITH VARIABLE DISTURBANCE OF SENSORY AND AUTONOMIC FUNCTION

A number of subtle differences separate the polyneuropathies comprised by this category: (1) acute inflammatory demyelinating or the less frequent axonal, type (Guillain-Barré syndrome), (2) some angiitic polyneuropathies, (3) porphyria, (4) certain toxic polyneuropathies, and (5) acute sensory and autonomic polyneuropathies. Of these various acute polyneuropathic diseases, the Guillain-Barré demyelinative syndrome, because of its frequency and gravity, is most demanding of the physician's attention.

Guillain-Barré Syndrome (Landry-Guillain-Barré-Strohl Syndrome, Acute Inflammatory Polyneuropathy)

This acute polyneuropathy, generally referred to as Guillain-Barré syndrome or GBS, occurs in all parts of the world and in all seasons; it affects children and adults of all ages and both sexes. A mild respiratory or gastrointestinal infection precedes the neuropathic symptoms by 1 to 3 weeks (sometimes longer) in about 60 percent of the patients. In recent years, it has come to be appreciated from serologic studies that the enteric organism *Campylobacter jejuni* is the most frequent identifiable preceding infection. Other, less common antecedent events or associated illnesses include viral exanthems and other viral illnesses [cytomegalovirus (CMV), Epstein-Barr virus (EBV), human immunodeficiency virus (HIV)], bacterial infections other than *Campylobacter* (*Mycoplasma pneumoniae*, Lyme disease), exposure to thrombolytic agents, and lymphoma (particularly Hodgkin disease). The administration of outmoded antirabies vaccines and the A/New Jersey (swine) influenza vaccine, given in late 1976, was associated with a slight increase in the incidence of GBS and at least one subsequent influenza vaccination program has been associated with a marginal increase. Trauma and surgical operations may precede the neuropathy, but a causal association remains uncertain.

Historical Background The earliest description is probably that of Wardrop and Ollivier, in 1834. Other important landmarks are Landry's report (1859) of an acute, ascending, predominantly motor paralysis with respiratory failure, leading to death; Osler's (1892) description of a febrile polyneuritis; the account by Guillain, Barré, and Strohl (1916) of a benign polyneuritis with albuminocytologic dissociation in the CSF (increase in protein without cells); and the elaboration of the clinical picture by many British and American investigators. The first comprehensive account of the pathology of GBS was that of Haymaker and Kernohan (1949), who stressed that edema of the peripheral nerves was the important change in the early stages of the disease. Subsequently, Asbury, Arnason, and Adams (1969) established that the essential lesion, from the beginning of the disease, is a perivascular mononuclear inflammatory infiltration of the roots and nerves. (For details of the historical and other aspects of this disease, see the monographs by Ropper and colleagues and by Hughes.)

Incidence Our experience with this disease has shown it to be nonseasonal and nonepidemic. Year after year, between 15 and 25 patients have been admitted to each of our institutions. Females are only slightly more susceptible. The age range of 160 consecutive, prospectively studied patients was 8 months to 81 years, with attack rates highest in persons 50 to 74 years of age. The reported incidence rate worldwide has varied from 0.4 to 1.7 cases per 100,000 persons per year; the latter figure is probably the more accurate.

Symptomatology The usual case of GBS is readily identified. Paresthesias and numbness are frequent and early symptoms, but occasionally they are absent throughout the illness. The major clinical manifestation is weakness, which evolves more or less symmetrically over a period of several days or a week or two, rarely somewhat longer. Proximal as well as distal muscles of the limbs are involved, usually the lower extremities before the upper ("Landry's ascending paralysis"); the trunk, intercostal, neck, and cranial muscles may be affected later. The weakness can progress to total motor paralysis with death from respiratory failure within a few days. More than half of the patients complain of pain and an aching discomfort in the muscles, mainly those of the hips, thighs, and back. Objective sensory loss occurs to a variable degree during the first days and in a few is barely detectable; when such loss is present, deep sensibility (touch-pressure-vibration) tends to be more affected than superficial (pain-temperature).

Reduced and then absent tendon reflexes are consistent findings. Rarely, only the ankle reflexes are lost during the first week of illness. At an early stage, the arm muscles may be less weak than the leg muscles or are spared entirely. Facial diplegia occurs in about half of all cases, and other cranial nerve palsies, if they occur, usually come later, after the arms are affected; infrequently they are the initial signs. Disturbances of autonomic function (sinus tachycardia and less often bradycardia, facial flushing, fluctuating hypertension and hypotension, loss of sweating or episodic profuse diaphoresis) are common, but rarely do these abnormalities persist for more than a week or two. Urinary retention occurs in about 15 percent of patients soon after the onset of weakness, but catheterization is seldom required for more than a few days.

Variants of the Typical Pattern Portions of the clinical picture frequently appear in isolated or abortive form and cause diagnostic confusion. Whereas in most patients the paralysis ascends from legs to trunk, arms, and cranial muscles and reaches a peak of severity within 10 to 14 days, occasionally the *pharyngeal-cervical-brachial* muscles are affected first, creating difficulty in swallowing as well as neck and proximal arm weakness (Ropper, 1986). Ptosis, sometimes with ophthalmoplegia may be added. Moreover, this pattern may persist without the development of limb weakness. The differential diagnosis is then from myasthenia gravis, diphtheria, and botulism and from a lesion affecting the central portion of the cervical spinal cord and lower brainstem. A syndrome comprising *complete ophthalmoplegia with ataxia* and areflexia and thought to be a variant of GBS was described by Fisher. A *purely ophthalmoplegic* form also exists; it may be coupled with pharyngeal-cervical-brachial weakness, as mentioned above. The ophthalmoplegia, whether occurring alone or with weakness or ataxia of other parts, is uniformly associated with a specific antineural antibody, anti-GQ1B. The ophthalmoplegic pattern raises the possibility of myasthenia gravis, botulism, diphtheria, tick paralysis, and basilar artery disease. Bilateral but asymmetrical *facial and abducens weakness*, coupled with distal paresthesias or with proximal leg weakness, are other fairly common variants in our experience (Ropper, 1994). The tendon reflexes may be absent initially at the ankles or at the knees. Lyme disease and sarcoidosis are then considerations in diagnosis. *Paraparetic*, *ataxic*, and *purely motor* forms of the illness have also been observed.

A few cases will continue to evolve for 3 to 4 weeks or even longer. From this group a chronic form of demyelinative neuropathy (chronic inflammatory demyelinating polyneuropathy, or CIDP) often emerges and is described further on.

Numerous phenomena related to dysautonomia occur, and there are important complications secondary to immobilization and respiratory failure, as discussed further on, under "Treatment." At the onset of illness, the temperature is normal, and lymphadenopathy and splenomegaly, if they occur, are related to a preceding viral infection.

Laboratory Findings The most important laboratory aids are the electrodiagnostic studies and the CSF examination. The CSF is under normal pressure and is acellular or contains only a few lymphocytes in all but 10 percent of patients; in the latter, 10 to 50 cells (rarely more) per cubic millimeter, predominantly lymphocytes, may be found. In the few patients with pleocytosis, the number of cells decreases rapidly, in a matter of 2 to 3 days; a failure to do so should suggest an alternative diagnosis. We have been unable to relate an occasional pleocytosis with any of the clinical features of GBS or their severity. Usually, the protein content is normal during the first few days of symptoms, but then it begins to rise, reaching a peak in 4 to 6 weeks. The increase in CSF protein is probably a reflection of the widespread inflammatory disease of the nerve roots, but high values have no clinical or prognostic significance. In a few patients (10 percent or less), the CSF protein values are normal throughout the illness. Among patients with the Fisher syndrome and other restricted forms of GBS, there is a much higher proportion with normal protein values.

Nerve conduction studies are a dependable and early diagnostic indicator of GBS, and in instances with a typical clinical and EMG presentation, one can dispense with the CSF analysis. Although a limited electrodiagnostic examination may be normal early in the illness, a more thorough study, which includes measurement of late responses, almost invariably shows abnormalities in an affected limb within days of the first symptom. Also early on, features that indicate widespread axonal damage (so-called axonal GBS) portend a poor prognosis for complete recovery of motor function. The most frequent early findings are a reduction in the amplitudes of muscle action potentials, slowed conduction velocity, or conduction block in motor nerves. Prolonged distal latencies (reflecting distal conduction block) and prolonged or absent F responses (indicating affection of proximal parts of nerves) are other important diagnostic findings, all reflecting demyelination. The clinical, CSF, and electrodiagnostic criteria for GBS have recently been reassessed by Asbury and Cornblath and are discussed in detail in the monograph by Ropper et al. We have also found that 20 of 24 patients with acute GBS showed gadolinium enhancement of the cauda equine roots on an MRI of the lumbar spine (Gorson et al).

Abnormalities of liver function occur in less than 10 percent of patients, probably reflecting a recent or ongoing viral hepatitis, usually due to the CMV or Epstein-Barr virus (rarely one of the hepatitis viruses). T-wave and other electrocardiographic changes of minor degree are reported frequently but are evanescent. The sedimentation rate is normal. Hyponatremia occurs in a small proportion of cases after the first week, especially in ventilated patients. This is usually attributable to the syndrome of inappropriate antidiuretic hormone secretion (SIADH), but a natriuretic type also occurs, apparently from an excess of atrial natriuretic factor. Transient diabetes insipidus is a rare and unexplained occurrence.

Pathologic Findings These have had a relatively consistent pattern and form. Even when the disease is fatal within a few days, virtually all cases have shown perivascular lymphocytic infiltrates. Later the characteristic inflammatory cell infiltrates and perivenous demyelination are combined with segmental demyelination and a variable degree of wallerian degeneration. Infiltrates are scattered throughout the cranial nerves, ventral and dorsal roots, and dorsal root ganglia and along the entire length of the peripheral nerves. Sparse infiltrates of inflammatory cells (lymphocytes and other mononuclear cells) may also be found in lymph nodes, liver, spleen, heart, and other organs.

Variations of this pattern of peripheral nerve damage have been observed, each perhaps representing a different immunopathology. Rarely, in a clinically typical case, there may be widespread demyelinative changes and only a paucity of perivascular lymphocytes. In patients whose electrophysiologic tests display severe axonal damage early in the illness (the acute axonal type of GBS, discussed below), the pathologic findings corroborate the predominantly axonal nature of the disease, with secondary myelin damage and little inflammatory response. An occasional case has shown an inflammatory process with primary axonal damage rather than demyelination (Honovar et al). The acute axonal form is described further on.

Pathogenesis and Etiology Most of the evidence suggests that the clinical manifestations of this disorder are the result of a cell-mediated immunologic reaction directed at peripheral nerve. Waksman and Adams demonstrated that a peripheral nerve disease (experimental allergic neuritis or EAN), clinically and pathologically indistinguishable from GBS, develops in animals about 2 weeks after immunization with peripheral nerve homogenate. Brostoff and colleagues suggested that the antigen in this reaction is a basic protein, designated P_2, found only in peripheral nerve myelin. Subsequent investigations by these authors indicated that the neuritogenic factor was a specific peptide in the P_2 protein. It has become evident that there is no unifying antigen-antibody reaction and that any number of myelin and axonal elements may be involved in the immune reaction. The pathologic steps in this proposed reaction are diagrammatically illustrated in Fig. 46-3. Hartung and colleagues have found high levels of soluble interleukin (IL)-2 receptors, shed from activated T cells, and IL-2 itself in the serum of patients with acute GBS, reflecting activation of these cells. As noted below, complement also seems to be a necessary factor in the initial attack on myelin.

Although the transmission of EAN by T cells sensitized to myelin is strong evidence of their role in GBS, antimyelin antibodies probably play a significant part in initiating the disease. The serum from patients with GBS damages myelin in tissue cultures, in which it induces a characteristic ("vesicular") form of myelin destruction. Subepineural injection of serum from GBS patients into the sciatic nerve of rats leads to local demyelination and electrical conduction block. The studies of Koski and associates of complement-dependent myelin damage by IgM antimyelin antibodies in GBS provide the best evidence that antimyelin antibodies are able to initiate myelin destruction even if T cells and macrophages ultimately effect the damage. Indeed, the very earliest change that could be detected by Hafer-Macko and colleagues was the deposition of complement on the abaxonal surface of the Schwann cell (inner layer of myelin). A number of autoantibodies are detected inconsistently in patients with GBS, the most prominent being anti-GQ_1b, which is found in almost all patients with ophthalmoplegia. Approximately 15 percent of patients will have anti-GM_1 antibodies early in their course, corresponding in most instances to a predominantly motor presentation, the highest titers usually being associated with *Campylobacter* infections. It would therefore seem that casting GBS exclusively as a humoral or a cellular immune disease is an oversimplification. Several animal diseases—such as coonhound paralysis, Marek's disease of chickens (a viral neuritis), and cauda equina neuritis of the horse—resemble GBS superficially but do not share its main clinical or pathologic features.

An unanswered question is what initiates the immune reaction in humans. All attempts to isolate a virus or microbial agent from nerves or to demonstrate one by electron microscopy have failed, and it is more likely that a variety of agents—viral, bacterial (particularly *C. jejuni*), certain vaccines, and perhaps neural injury itself—are all capable, in susceptible individuals, of precipitating a response against autologous peripheral myelin. The occurrence of GBS in patients with AIDS or with EBV or CMV infections simply indicates that these agents too might induce such an autoimmune response without implicating a direct viral infection of nerve.

Differential Diagnosis GBS is not only one of the most frequent types of acute polyneuropathy seen in a general hospital but also the most rapidly evolving and potentially fatal form. Any polyneuropathy that brings the patient to the brink of death from respiratory failure within a few days will usually be of this variety. However, several other neurologic conditions must be distinguished from GBS.

The immediate problem is to differentiate GBS from acute spinal cord disease (marked by sensorimotor paralysis below a level on the trunk and sphincteric paralysis). Confusion may occur with acute lesions of the cord in which tendon reflexes are initially lost (spinal shock), or with necrotizing myelopathy, where a permanent loss of tendon reflexes follows destruction of spinal neurons (pages 966 and 1313). Several rules of thumb are useful in distinguishing GBS from a cervical myelopathy: in GBS, the facial and respiratory muscles are usually involved if there is generalized paralysis; the fingertips should be paresthetic once sensory symptoms have ascended to the level of the midcalves; marked sensory loss proximal to the hands or feet is unusual early in the illness; and tendon reflexes are almost invariably lost within 24 h in limbs that are too weak to resist gravity.

Another problem arises in distinguishing generalized GBS or the Fisher variant from basilar artery thrombosis. The presence of reactive pupils, areflexia, and F-wave abnormalities in GBS and of lively reflexes and Babinski signs in the case of brainstem infarction dependably separates the two disorders.

A predominantly motor paralysis is the major characteristic of GBS, for which reason the differential diagnosis also includes poliomyelitis, now usually caused by enteroviruses other than the polio agent; here the infectious agent is marked by fever, meningeal

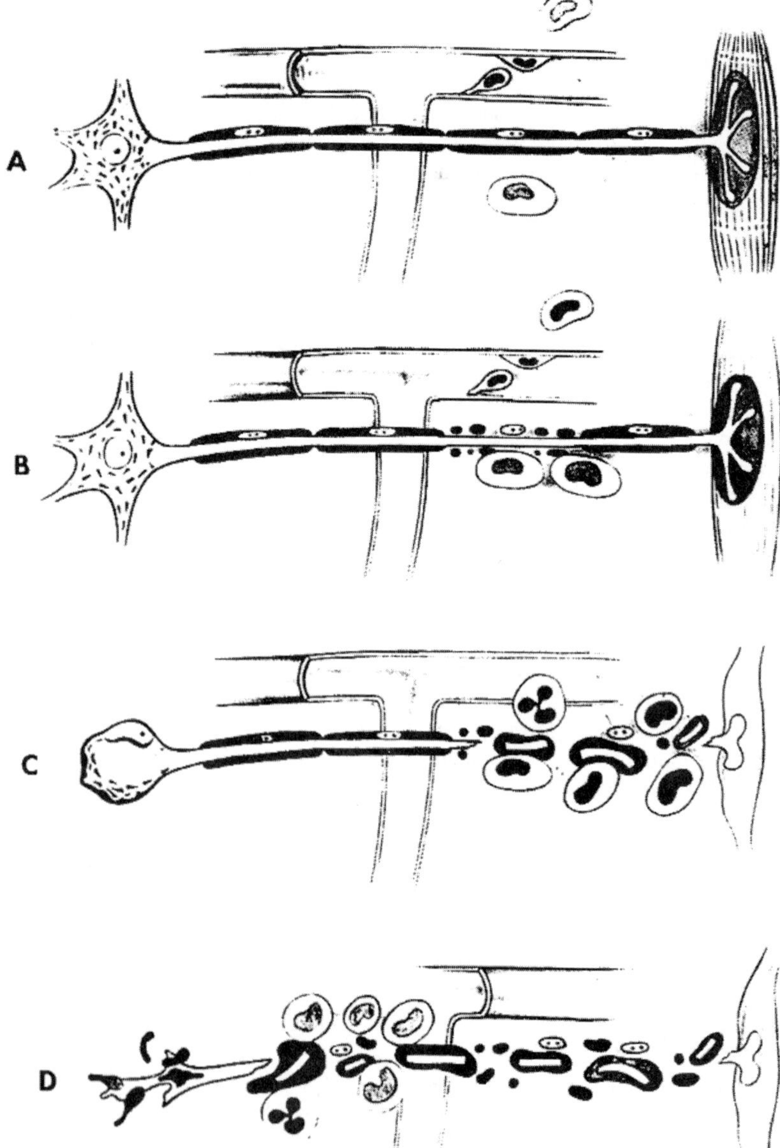

Figure 46-3

Diagram of probable cellular events in acute inflammatory polyneuropathy (GBS). **A.** *Lymphocytes attach to the walls of endoneurial vessels and migrate through the vessel wall, enlarging and transforming as they do so. At this stage no nerve damage has occurred.* **B.** *More lymphocytes have migrated into the surrounding tissue. The first effect upon the nerve is breakdown of myelin, the axon being spared (segmental demyelination). This change appears to be mediated by the mononuclear exudate, but the mechanism is uncertain.* **C.** *The lesion is more intense, polymorphonuclear leukocytes being present as well as lymphocytes. There is interruption of the axon in addition to myelin sheath damage; as a result, the muscle undergoes denervation atrophy and the nerve cell body shows central chromatolysis. If the axonal damage is distal, the nerve cell body will survive, and regeneration and clinical recovery is likely. If, as in* **D**, *axonal interruption has occurred proximally because of a particularly intense root or proximal nerve lesion, the nerve cell body may die and undergo dissolution. In this situation, there is no regeneration, only the possibility of collateral reinnervation of muscle from surviving motor fibers. (From Asbury et al, 1969, by permission.)*

symptoms, early pleocytosis, and purely motor and usually asymmetrical areflexic paralysis.

Ptosis and oculomotor weakness, features of GBS in some cases, may cause confusion with acute myasthenia gravis (MG), but in the latter disease there are no sensory symptoms and tendon reflexes are unimpaired. The mandibular muscles remain relatively strong in GBS, whereas the exercised jaw hangs open in MG. Botulism may also simulate GBS, but pupillary reflexes are lost early in the former (this also occurs in advanced cases of GBS), and there is usually a bradycardia, which is unusual for GBS. Tick paralysis may be nearly impossible to distinguish from GBS unless one finds the tick (page 1277); both cause an acute ascending paralysis. Both also sometimes cause ataxia and may paralyze eye movements, but sensory loss is not usually a feature of tick paralysis and the CSF protein remains normal. Ingestion of shellfish or reef fish contaminated with saxitoxin, ciguatoxin, or tetrodotoxin (ciguatera) is another cause of acute facial-brachial paresthesias, weakness, tachypnea, and iridoplegia lasting a few days—symptoms that resemble the cranial nerve variants of GBS (page1276).

In critically ill patients, a number of neuromuscular disorders may arise that must always to be distinguished from GBS. These include the so-called polyneuropathy of critical illness (page 1388); an accelerated neuropathy of renal failure that is seen mainly in diabetic patients receiving peritoneal dialysis (both discussed further on); acute hypophosphatemia induced by hyperalimentation; polymyopathy produced by the administration of high-dose corticosteroids (page 1522); and the prolonged effects of neuromuscular blocking drugs, resulting in the accumulation of their metabolites in patients with renal failure and acidosis.

Treatment *In severe cases, respiratory assistance and careful nursing are paramount*, since the disease remits naturally and the outlook for recovery is favorable in the majority of cases. About 30 percent of our patients have needed the assistance of mechanical ventilation. However, since the patient's condition may deteriorate unpredictably and rapidly, virtually all cases must initially be admitted to the hospital for observation of respiratory function. Measurement of maximal inspiratory force and expiratory vital capacity suffices for bedside guidance to the adequacy of diaphragmatic strength and the likelihood of respiratory failure. As in poliomyelitis, the strength of the neck muscles and trapezii, which share the same segmental innervation as the diaphragm, tends to parallel respiratory strength. A very rough estimate of breathing capacity may be obtained by having the patient count quickly on one deep breath. The ability to reach 20 generally corresponds to a vital capacity of greater than 1.5 L. If a downward trend in these measurements is recognized and the vital capacity reaches 12 to 15 mL/kg, endotracheal intubation and mechanical ventilation should be considered. There is usually a slight rise in the respiratory rate at this time. This degree of impaired ventilation usually occurs before the first sign of dyspnea appears and before there is any elevation of arterial carbon dioxide content, but it generally coincides with tachypnea and a slight decrease in arterial oxygen tension (P_{O_2} less than 85 mmHg). If respiratory failure arises gradually, over days or longer, there is often slight tachycardia, diaphoresis, restlessness, and tachypnea. Attempts to forestall the need for a positive-pressure ventilator by the use of negative-pressure cuirass-type devices have generally been unsatisfactory. Patients with oropharyngeal weakness may require intubation even earlier to prevent aspiration, but mechanical ventilation is not always required at the same time. These types of treatment demand that the patient be admitted to an intensive care unit staffed by personnel skilled in maintaining ventilation and airway patency.

The other major aspects of the treatment in severely affected patients involve the management of *cardiovascular autonomic instability* and attempts to forestall the many general medical problems that attend any critical illness. Hypotension from *dysautonomia,* which occurs in about 10 percent of severely affected patients, is treated by intravenous volume infusion and the use of vasopressor agents for brief periods. Extremes of hypertension are managed by short-acting and titratable antihypertensive medications, such as intravenous labetalol. This choice of antihypertensive is important, since these episodes may be rapidly succeeded by a precipitous drop in pressure. Prevention of electrolyte imbalance, gastrointestinal hemorrhage, and particularly pulmonary embolism in patients who are bedbound (by the use of subcutaneous heparin or pneumatic compression boots) all require careful attention. Adynamic ileus is a problem in some cases, manifest first by abdominal pain coincident with nasogastric tube feeding and by bloating; it may lead to bowel perforation if feeding is continued. A number of patients become hyponatremic, usually from SIADH but occasionally from a natriuresis, and the drop in sodium may be exaggerated by positive-pressure mechanical ventilation. The distinction between these two conditions determines the course of treatment: fluid restriction or salt replacement.

Failure to effectively clear the tracheobronchial airways and the need for prolonged mechanical ventilation are the usual inidcations for tracheostomy. In most cases this procedure can be postponed until the end of the second third week of intubation. However, in patients who become rapidly quadriplegic and ventilator-dependent, tracheostomy may be needed earlier. Once tracheostomy is performed, careful tracheal toilet and treatment of pulmonary and urinary tract infections by the use of appropriate antibiotics are required. Prophylactic antibiotic treatment is not recommended. Under these conditions the mortality from the disease can be reduced to 3 percent or less (Ropper and Kehne).

The decision to discontinue respiratory aid and to remove the endotracheal or tracheostomy tube is based on the degree of recovery of respiratory function. The weaning process generally begins when the vital capacity reaches approximately10 mL/kg and can be sustained for a few hours. Physical therapy (passive movement and positioning of limbs to prevent pressure palsies and, later, mild resistance exercises) should begin once the patient can comfortably undertake it.

Plasma Exchange and Immune Globulin Specific therapy of GBS includes the use of plasma exchange and intravenous immune globulin (IVIG). Our practice has been to observe the patient closely for several days, even if mildly affected. If the patient becomes unable to walk unaided or if he shows a significant reduction in vital capacity or signs of severe oropharyngeal weakness, plasma exchange or IVIG (not both) is instituted promptly.

Three large randomized trials comprising more than 500 patients have clearly established the usefulness of *plasma exchange* in the evolving phase of GBS. In patients who are treated within 2 weeks of onset, there is a reduction in the period of hospitalization, in the length of time that the patient requires mechanical ventilation, and in the time required to achieve independent ambulation. However, when plasma exchange is delayed for 2 weeks or longer after the onset of the disease, the procedure has, with a few notable exceptions, been of little value. The most important predictors of responsiveness to plasma exchange treatment are the patient's age (responders are younger) and the preservation of motor compound muscle action potential amplitudes prior to instituting treatment (McKhann et al). One study found that the overall condition of patients treated in this way was better at 6 and 12 months after treatment; other studies have been equivocal on this point.

The regimen we use removes a total of 200 to 250 mL/kg of plasma in four to six treatments on alternate days or over a shorter period if there is no coagulopathy. The replacement fluid is saline combined with 5% albumin. The need for large-bore venous access usually requires the insertion of subclavian or internal jugular catheters, and this may be the main source of complications (pneumothorax, infection, hemorrhage). In many patients, however, treatment can be instituted through the antecubital veins. During the procedure, hypotension, hypoprothrombinemia with bleeding (usually epistaxis), and cardiac arrhythmias may occur. Some groups prefer to use the level of fibrinogen, which is greatly reduced by the treatment, as a gauge to the risk of potential hemorrhage before beginning the next exchange. Reactions to the citrate that is used to prevent blood from clotting in the plasma exchange machine are common but can be obviated by the cautious addition of calcium to the intravenous return line. Hepatitis and AIDS are not risks if plasma is replaced with albumin and saline rather than pooled plasma.

The Dutch Study Group has found that the *intravenous administration of immune globulin* (0.4 g/kg per day for 5 consecutive days) is as effective as plasma exchange and is both easier to administer and probably safer because there is no need for large intravenous access (van der Meche et al). Their results have been corroborated by an international study led by Hughes that compared the two main modes of treatment and evaluated their serial use. In the latter trial there was a trend toward a better outcome in patients who received plasma exchange, and results were even better in a group who were treated with plasma exchange followed immediately by 5 days of immune globulin infusions; in both instances, however, the differences failed to attain statistical significance. Most patients tolerate IVIG treatment well. Renal failure, proteinuria, and aseptic meningitis, reflected most often by severe headache, are rare complications. The only serious reactions we have encountered were in those very few patients who congenitally lacked IgA and in whom pooled gamma globulin caused anaphylaxis and inflammatory local venous thrombosis.

After the use of either plasma exchange or IVIG, 5 to 10 percent of patients who initially improve will have a relapse that becomes apparent several days to 3 weeks after completion of treatment. If there was a good response to initial therapy, the same treatment may be repeated or the alternative treatment may be tried; either can be successful. A few such patients relapse repeatedly and have a course more suggestive of chronic inflammatory demyelinating polyneuropathy (see further on). In some such patients under our care the disease stabilized after several months in response to the administration of corticosteroids, either alone with very gradual tapering of the dose over several months, or in combination with repeated courses of IVIG or plasma exchanges.

The value of corticosteroids in the treatment of GBS has been disputed for decades. Many clinicians were persuaded of their benefits. However, two randomized controlled studies, one with conventional-dose prednisolone and the other with high-dose methylprednisolone, have failed to demonstrate any beneficial effect (Hughes et al). Although corticosteroids can no longer be recommended as routine treatment for acute GBS, we have observed a few instances in which the administration of intravenous high-dose corticosteroids seemingly halted the progress of the disease.

Prognosis As already indicated, 3 to 5 percent of patients do not survive the illness, even in the best-equipped hospitals. In the early stages, death is most often due to cardiac arrest, perhaps related to dysautonomia, adult respiratory distress syndrome, or some type of accidental machine failure. Later in the illness, pulmonary embolism and other complications (usually bacterial) of prolonged immobilization and respiratory failure are the main causes.

The majority of patients recover completely or nearly completely (with mild motor deficits in the feet or legs). In about 10 percent of patients, however, the residual disability is pronounced; this occurs in those with the most severe and rapidly evolving form of the disease, when there has been evidence of widespread axonal damage (see below), and in those requiring early and prolonged mechanical ventilatory assistance. A consistent predictor of residual weakness is the EMG finding of severely reduced amplitudes of muscle action potentials and widespread denervation, both indicative of axonal damage. In patients with respiratory failure, the average period of machine-assisted respiration has been 22 days and the period of hospitalization approximately 50 days (these were twice as long prior to the introduction of plasma exchange and IVIG). As a rule, older adults recover more slowly and have more residual weakness.

The commonest residual difficulties are weakness of the lower leg muscles, numbness of the feet and toes, and mild bifacial weakness. A few patients are left with a sensory ataxia; when this occurs, it tends to be severe and has been quite disabling. Distal neuropathic pain and persistent autonomic problems occur but are infrequent. All manner of other late symptoms are attributed with little evidence to the illness and should be addressed on their own merits—fatigue and asthenia, muscle cramps, dizziness, breathlessness, etc.

The speed of recovery varies but its pace is steady. Often it occurs within a few weeks or months; however, if axons have degenerated, their regeneration may require 6 to 18 months or longer. Little or no real improvement can be expected in disabilities that have lasted 2 or 3 years.

Some 5 to 10 percent of patients suffer one or more recurrences of acute polyneuropathy. Also, an illness that in the beginning appeared to be an acute inflammatory polyradiculoneuropathy may fail to stabilize and continue to progress steadily, or there may be an incomplete remission followed by a chronic, fluctuating, slowly progressive neuropathy. These chronic forms of inflammatory neuropathy are described in a later section of this chapter.

Acute Axonal Form of Guillain-Barré Syndrome Feasby and colleagues drew attention to an acute polyneuropathy clinically similar to GBS but characterized pathologically by widespread and severe axonal degeneration. They described five patients, all of them with a particularly rapid evolution of polyneuropathy and poor recovery. Unlike the common form of GBS, muscle atrophy in these patients was apparent relatively early in the disease (weeks), reflecting widespread axonal damage. The defining EMG features are said to be the presence of numerous electrically inexcitable motor nerves and accompanying signs of denervation. Others, however, have noted that the inability to excite a motor nerve is not unique and may signify a distal demyelinating block, from which complete recovery is possible (Triggs et al).

Postmortem examinations in these cases have disclosed severe axonal degeneration in nerves and roots, with minimal inflammatory changes and only minimal demyelination early in the disease. Prominent in some of these cases were deposits of complement and the presence of macrophages in the periaxonal space; axonal degeneration and wallerian degeneration followed. A humoral antibody against some component of the axolemma was postulated by Griffin and associates. Visser and colleagues have reported a similar series of acute motor polyneuropathies from Holland. The outbreaks of motor neuropathy that occur seasonally in rural China have many of the characteristics of axonal GBS. These outbreaks are triggered largely by *C. jejuni* infections and some but not all sporadic instances have been preceded by the same infection. It is noteworthy, however, that the same organism can precede a typical demyelinating form of GBS.

Most experience with the axonal form of GBS indicates that recovery is prolonged and complete resolution of weakness is uncommon. IVIG and plasma exchange have had some beneficial effect, but not of the degree seen in demyelinating cases. Whether this acute axonal polyneuropathy is a distinct entity or a variant of GBS cannot be answered with confidence. This may be largely a semantic issue, depending on one's definition of the clinical, immunologic, and pathologic boundaries of GBS. Certainly, there is a degree of axonal damage in all severe cases, even if the predominant process is demyelinating. At present it is useful to distinguish these cases from typical GBS if only to lower expectations for the response to immune treatments and for the ultimate clinical outcome.

Critical Illness Polyneuropathy

An acute or subacute symmetrical polyneuropathy is a frequent development in critically ill and septic patients, particularly in those with failure of multiple organs (Zochodne et al). This type of neuropathy may pose a major difficulty in weaning the patient from the ventilator as the underlying critical illness comes under control. The neuropathic abnormality, predominantly of motor type, varies in severity from an electrophysiologic abnormality without obvious clinical signs to a profound quadriparesis with respiratory failure. Usually the cranial nerves are spared and there are no overt dysautonomic manifestations. In general, the disease appears after several days or more of profound sepsis and multiple organ failure and is preceded in most instances by a confusional state or a depressed state of consciousness ("septic encephalopathy"). The EMG findings of a primary axonal degeneration and a normal CSF distinguish the neuropathy from the demyelinative form of GBS, and autopsies have usually disclosed no inflammatory changes in the peripheral nerves. The toxic effects of drugs and antibiotics and nutritional deficiency must always be considered in causation, but rarely can they be established. Perhaps some of the many systemic mediators of sepsis are toxic to the peripheral nervous system.

This form of polyneuropathy must be distinguished from a poorly understood *acute quadriplegic myopathy* that sometimes complicates critical illness (page 1522). High doses of corticosteroids, particularly in combination with neuromuscular blocking agents, have been implicated. The acute myopathy, which affects both distal and proximal muscles, is usually heralded by an elevation in the serum creatine kinase (CK) concentration and myopathic potentials in the EMG, and there is a unique degeneration of myofilaments.

Acute Uremic Polyneuropathy

An accelerated neuropathy in chronically uremic patients has been known for some time but has not been generally recognized as a cause of acute and subacute weakness that simulates GBS (Ropper). Most patients are diabetics in stable end-stage renal failure that is being treated with peritoneal dialysis. In contrast to the better-characterized chronic uremic neuropathy (page 1413), generalized weakness and distal paresthesias progress over one or more weeks to a bedbound state. More aggressive dialysis or a change to hemodialysis has little immediate effect, although kidney transplantation is curative. Electrophysiologic studies show some demyelinating features but usually not a conduction block. There is raised CSF protein concentration (not unexpectedly, for there is usually an element of diabetic neuropathy). A few cases have been reported that are clinically indistinguishable from an inflammatory demyelinating polyneuropathy, including, in some of them, a response to plasma exchange or gamma globulin. The cause of this acute neuropathy, like that of the more common chronic form, is not understood.

Acute Sensory Neuronopathy and Neuropathy

Sterman and colleagues described three adult patients with rapidly evolving sensory ataxia, areflexia, numbness, and pain, beginning in the face and spreading to involve the entire body. In each case, the symptoms began within 4 to 12 days following the institution of penicillin therapy for a febrile illness. Mainly proprioceptive sensation was affected, and there was no weakness or muscle atrophy despite areflexia. The sensory deficit attained its maximum severity within a week of onset, after which it stabilized and improved very little. Electrical studies showed absent or slowed sensory conduction but no abnormalities of motor nerve conduction or signs of denervation. In two of these patients, the CSF protein content was elevated to 126 and 175 mg/dL, respectively. Follow-up observations (for up to 5 years) disclosed no neoplastic or immunologic disorder. A toxic disorder, akin to that produced experimentally by doxorubicin and pyridoxine, was postulated. Lacking pathology, it was assumed, from the permanence of the condition, that sensory neurons were destroyed (*sensory neuronopathy*).

A subsequent study by Windebank et al emphasized the asymmetrical and brachial patterns of symptoms in some patients and an initial affection of the face in two. In contrast to Sterman's cases, the CSF was usually normal. Eight patients had a spontaneous resolution of the disease. The authors viewed the process as a neuropathy. In subsequent reports of such cases antibiotics were not implicated. Probably, some instances are immune-postinfectious in nature. The same pattern of sensory loss evolving in a subacute or chronic manner is known to occur as a paraneoplastic phenomenon, described further on in this chapter, or in association with the Sjögren syndrome, scleroderma, or lupus erythematosus, paraproteinemia, and HTLV-I infection. Certain drugs and other agents, especially cisplatin and excessive intake of pyridoxine, also cause a sensory neuronopathy. A process also to be distinguished from sensory neuronopathy is a rare form of the Guillain-Barré syndrome that involves predominantly the large sensory fibers. In the latter there is usually some degree of proximal weakness, and the sensory changes do not extend to the face and trunk.

Diphtheritic Polyneuropathy

Some of the neurotoxic effects of *Corynebacterium diphtheriae* and the mode of action of the exotoxin elaborated by the bacillus are described in Chap. 32. Local action of the exotoxin may paralyze pharyngeal and laryngeal muscles (dysphagia, nasal voice) within 1 or 2 weeks after the onset of the infection and shortly thereafter may also cause blurring of vision due to loss of accommodation, but these and other cranial nerve symptoms may be overlooked. At this stage, the cranial neuropathy must be distinguished from that of GBS and from myasthenia gravis. The polyneuropathy, coming 5 to 8 weeks later, takes the form of an acute to subacute limb weakness with paresthesias and distal loss of vibratory and position sense. The weakness characteristically involves all four extremities at the same time or may descend from arms to legs. After a few days to a week or more, the patient may be unable to stand or walk, and occasionally the paralysis is so severe and extensive as to impair respiration. The CSF protein is usually elevated (50 to 200 mg/dL). Diphtheritic deaths that occur after the pharyngeal infection has subsided are usually due to cardiomyopathy or to polyneuropathy with respiratory paralysis. This type of polyneuropathy should be suspected in the midst of an outbreak of diphtheritic infection, as occurred recently in Russia (Logina and Donaghy).

As indicated earlier, the important pathologic change is a demyelination without inflammatory reaction of spinal roots, sensory ganglia, and adjacent spinal nerves. Anterior horn cells, axons, peripheral nerves distally, and muscle fibers remain normal (Fisher and Adams).

Diphtheria antitoxin, given within 48 h of the onset of the infection, reduces the incidence and severity of neuropathic complications. Antitoxin is probably of no value once the polyneuropathy begins. Thereafter, treatment is purely symptomatic, along the lines indicated for GBS. The prognosis for full recovery is excellent once respiratory paralysis is circumvented.

Porphyric Polyneuropathy

A severe, rapidly advancing, more or less symmetrical polyneuropathy—often with abdominal pain, psychosis (delirium or confusion), and convulsions—may be a manifestation of *acute intermittent porphyria.* This type of porphyria is inherited as an autosomal dominant trait and is not associated with cutaneous sensitivity to sunlight. The metabolic defect is in the liver and is marked by increased production and urinary excretion of porphobilinogen and of the porphyrin precursor δ-amino-levulinic acid. The peripheral and central nervous systems may also be affected in another hepatic type of porphyria (so-called variegate type). In the latter type, the skin is markedly sensitive to light and trauma, and porphyrins are at all times found in the stools. Both of these *hepatic* forms of porphyria are to be distinguished from the rare *erythropoietic* (*congenital photosensitive*) porphyria, in which the nervous system is not affected.

The seminal study of acute intermittent porphyria was made by Waldenstrom in 1937. The initial and often the most prominent symptom is moderate to severe colicky abdominal pain. It may be generalized or localized and is unattended by rigidity of the abdominal wall or tenderness. Radiographs show intestinal distention and spasm. Constipation is frequent. Attacks last for days to weeks and repeated vomiting may lead to inanition. In latent forms, the patient may be asymptomatic or complain only of slight dyspepsia.

The disease is characterized by recurrent attacks, often precipitated by drugs such as sulfonamides, griseofulvin, estrogens, barbiturates, phenytoin, and the succinimide anticonvulsants. The possibility of sensitivity to these drugs must always be kept in mind when convulsions are being treated in the porphyric patient. The first attack rarely occurs before puberty, and the disease is most likely to threaten life during adolescence and early adulthood. An acute polyneuropathy that appears for the first time in mid- or late adult life is not likely to be porphyric.

The neurologic manifestations are usually those of a polyneuropathy involving the motor nerves more severely than the sensory ones; less often both sensory and motor nerves are affected more or less equally, and sometimes autonomic nerves as well. The symptoms may begin in the feet and legs and ascend, or they may begin in the hands and arms (sometimes asymmetrically) and spread in a few days to the trunk and legs. Occasionally the weakness predominates in the proximal muscles of the limbs and limb girdle muscles, in which case there is loss of knee jerks with preservation of reflexes at the ankles. Sensory loss, often extending to the trunk, is present in half the cases. Facial paralysis, dysphagia, and ocular palsies are features of only the most severe cases, then simulating GBS. The CSF protein content is normal or slightly elevated. The course of the polyneuropathy is variable. In mild cases the symptoms may regress in a few weeks. Severe cases may progress to a fatal respiratory or cardiac paralysis in a few days, or the symptoms may advance in a saltatory fashion over a period of several weeks, resulting in a severe sensorimotor paralysis that improves only after many months.

A disturbance of cerebral function (confusion, delirium, visual field defects, and convulsions) is likely to precede the severe rather than the mild forms of polyneuropathy, and it may not appear at all. The cerebral manifestations usually subside in a few days to weeks, though one of our patients was left with a lasting homonymous hemianopia.

Tachycardia and hypertension are frequent in the acute phase of the disease, and fever and leukocytosis also may occur; these are said to reflect the activity of the pathologic process.

In general, the prognosis for ultimate recovery is excellent, though relapse of the porphyria may result in further involvement of the peripheral nervous system (see discussion of *relapsing polyneuropathy*, further on), but death may result from respiratory paralysis or cardiac arrest and sometimes from uremia and cachexia.

In sum, the most characteristic clinical features are acute onset, initial abdominal pain, psychotic symptoms, predominant motor neuropathy, often an early bibrachial distribution of weakness, truncal sensory loss, and tachycardia. Rarely the neuropathy develops without other symptoms.

The pathologic findings in the peripheral nervous system vary according to the stage of the illness at which death occurs. If the patient dies in the first few days, the myelinated fibers may appear entirely normal, despite an almost complete paralysis. If symptoms had been present for weeks, degeneration of both axons and myelin sheaths will be found in most of the peripheral nerves. The relation between the abnormality of porphyrin biosynthesis in the liver and nervous dysfunction has never been explained satisfactorily.

Diagnosis is confirmed by the demonstration of large amounts of porphobilinogen and δ-aminolevulinic acid in the urine. The urine turns dark when standing due to the formation of porphobilin, an oxidation product of porphobilinogen.

Treatment consists of respiratory support, use of beta-blocking agents (propranolol) if tachycardia and hypertension are severe, intravenous glucose to suppress the heme biosynthetic pathway, and pyridoxine (100 mg twice a day) on the supposition that vitamin B6 depletion has occurred. The use of intravenous glucose and intravenous hematin (4 mg/kg daily for 3 to 14 days) is recommended as the most direct and effective therapy (Windebank and Bonkovsky).

Prevention is of the utmost importance, since attacks can be precipitated by porphyrinogenic drugs, the most common of which are the barbiturates.

Acute Toxic Polyneuropathies

As indicated in Chap. 43, the peripheral nerves may be affected by a wide variety of toxins, including metals, drugs, and industrial solvents. As a general rule, the neuropathies induced by these agents fall into the early chronic category (to be discussed further on). Certain drugs, however—notably triorthocresylphosphate (TOCP) and other organophosphates (page 1281), thallium, and rarely arsenic—produce a polyneuropathy that may be fatal in a matter of days. It should be stressed that organophosphate neuropathy almost never occurs without severe anticholinergic effects immediately after exposure. Severe and permanent motor paralysis is caused by TOCP; this ultimately proves to be due to involvement of both upper and lower motor neurons.

Thallium salts, when taken in sufficient amount, may produce a clinical picture resembling that of GBS or an acute sensory polyneuropathy. If the salts are taken orally, there is first abdominal pain, vomiting, and diarrhea, followed within a few days by pain and tingling in the toes and fingertips and then rapid weakening of muscles of the limbs, initially the distal ones. As the weakness progresses, the tendon reflexes diminish. Pain sensation is reduced more than tactile, vibratory, and position sense. Persistent acral pain with allodynia has been a major feature in three of the five cases we have examined; in two patients there was no weakness, only sensory loss and ataxia. All cranial nerves except the first and eighth may be affected; facial palsies, ophthalmoplegia, nystagmus, optic neuritis with visual impairment, and vocal cord palsies are prominent abnormalities, but only in the most severely affected patients. The CSF protein rises to more than 100 mg. Death may occur in the first 10 days, due to cardiac arrest. The early onset of painful paresthesias, sensory loss, and pain localized to joints, back, and chest as well as *rapid loss of hair* (within a week or two) help differentiate this neuropathy from GBS, porphyria, and other acute polyneuropathies. Relative preservation of reflexes is noteworthy, and a rapidly evolving, complete alopecia is a striking feature. Patients with lesser degrees of intoxication may recover completely within weeks or months. Thallium salts act like potassium, and a high intake of potassium chloride hastens the excretion of thallium; chelating agents are of unproven value.

Some cases of *arsenical* and possibly *mercurial* polyneuropathy may develop acutely, and this is true also of the eosinophilia-myalgia syndrome due to intoxication with contamined L-tryptophan. More often these neuropathies evolve subacutely, for which reason they are discussed further on.

In regard to this category of polyneuropathy, it must be pointed out that many instances of neuropathy are imputed with little substantiation to a toxic cause by patients and unskeptical physicians. Before making such an attribution, it is useful to ask whether the clinical features were compatible with the known neurotoxicity of an environmental agent or drug; whether the severity of symptoms was consistent with degree of exposure; whether the associated systemic signs of intoxication were present; if other individuals similarly exposed had been affected; and whether symptoms stabilized or improved once the patient had been removed from the presumed source of exposure. Failure to satisfy these precepts generally signifies some disorder other than exposure to a toxin.

Other Acute Polyneuropathies

On rare occasions, a vasculitic polyneuropathy associated with lupus erythematosus, polyarteritis nodosa, and related disorders may develop as rapidly as GBS, and careful clinical and electrophysiologic testing may be needed to distinguish these disorders. Three of our patients with polyarteritis and one with Churg-Strauss disease became paralyzed within a week, and one died of intestinal perforation. However, most cases of neuropathy due to polyarteritis evolve more slowly, and often the syndrome assumes an asymmetrical distribution, for which reason it is described in the next section.

We have observed a few patients with alcoholism, occult carcinoma, Hodgkin disease, and renal transplantation who developed an acute polyneuropathy, as rapid in its evolution as GBS, and acute episodes of this type have also been described in patients with Refsum disease. Formerly, the use of smallpox and rabies vaccines and injections of antitoxin with foreign protein were sometimes followed by a sensorimotor polyneuritis. The usual picture, however, is a brachial plexitis, and these conditions are more appropriately discussed with the brachial plexus neuropathies (further on in this chapter).

Pure Autonomic Polyneuropathy

Since the first description of such a case by Young and colleagues, a number of similar ones have been recorded (Low et al). The condition is described in detail in Chap. 26. Some success has been achieved by treatment with intravenous immune globulin, similar to that used in GBS.

SYNDROME OF SUBACUTE SENSORIMOTOR PARALYSIS

Subacute Symmetrical Polyneuropathies

Placed in this category are neuropathic conditions that evolve over a period of several weeks to months and, after reaching their peak of severity, tend to persist for a variable period. Admittedly, as intimated earlier, the dividing line between such cases and neuropathies that evolve over a somewhat shorter or longer period is indistinct; there are diseases of nerve that overlap both the acute and the early chronic categories. In contrast to the acute polyneuropathies, most of those that are subacute are of axonal type. However, a subacute inflammatory-demyelinative type, essentially a slow form of GBS, evolving over 4 to 8 weeks, does occur, as documented by Hughes and coworkers. Similarly, some instances of diphtheritic neuropathy evolve subacutely, but most develop rapidly. A symmetrical syndrome of subacute type most often proves to be due to alcoholism and nutritional deficiency, to a remote effect of cancer (paraneoplastic as described below), or to poisoning with arsenic, lead, or to any number of drugs used for therapeutic purposes (cisplatin, nitrofurantoin, isoniazid, etc.). Occasionally other drugs, metals, and industrial solvents can be incriminated; these are discussed in Chap. 43.

Nutritional Deficiency Neuropathy

In the western world, nutritional polyneuropathy is usually associated with alcoholism. As indicated in Chap. 41, all data point to the identity of alcoholic neuropathy and neuropathic beriberi. A nutritional factor is responsible for both, though in any given case it often remains unclear whether the deficiency is one of thiamine, pyridoxine, pantothenic acid, folic acid, or a combination of the B vitamins. We have not been able to define a form of polyneuropathy that is attributable to the direct toxic effect of alcohol, though claims of such an entity have been made. Neuropathic beriberi and other forms of deficiency neuropathy (Strachan syndrome, pellagra, vitamin B_{12} deficiency, and malabsorption syndromes) are described fully in Chap. 41.

Paraneoplastic Polyneuropathy (See also page 727.) Although capable of a number of clinical presentations, most often this takes the form of a predominantly distal, symmetrical sensory or sensorimotor polyneuropathy occurring as a remote effect of carcinoma, lymphoma, or multiple myeloma. Severe weakness and atrophy, ataxia, and sensory loss of the limbs may advance over several months to the point where the patient is confined to a wheelchair or bed; usually the CSF protein content is moderately elevated. All these symptoms may occur several months or even a year or longer before a malignant tumor is found.

A mixed sensorimotor polyneuropathy is four to five times more frequent than a purely sensory one. The latter syndrome, described originally by Denny-Brown, is characterized by a loss of all modalities of sensation spreading from the distal to the proximal segments of the limbs and eventually to the trunk and face. There is severe ataxia and loss of tendon reflexes, but motor power is retained. More recently, it has been appreciated that the sensory loss in the beginning may have a multifocal distribution. The sensory loss reaches its peak in a few months, occasionally in weeks, and in a few instances the development has been as rapid as that of GBS. The pathologic changes are those of an inflammatory and destructive neuronopathy (ganglionopathy) and are part of a more widespread neoplastic affection of the nervous system related to the anti-Hu antibody (also termed *antinuclear neuronal antibody*) that is most typical of small-cell cancer of the lung. In a series of 71 patients with sensory neuronopathy reported by Dalmau and colleagues, more than half were associated with symptomatic inflammatory lesions in the temporal lobes (limbic encephalitis, page 727), the brainstem, and rarely the anterior horn neurons of the spinal cord. Other more distinctive paraneoplastic syndromes such as cerebellar degeneration or Lambert-Eaton myasthenic syndrome were found in isolated cases, and there were signs of dysautonomia in 28 percent. The CSF protein is moderately elevated but acellular and shows high titers of the anti-Hu antibody. Sensory potentials are usually absent in all nerves after a few weeks but may be spared early on. The localization of anti-Hu antibody to the several affected regions of the nervous system and to the tumor itself suggests that the lung tumors are typically small or inevident because the antibody suppresses tumor growth. Clinically, serum anti-Hu testing is useful in distinguishing paraneoplastic varieties of sensory neuropathy and neuronopathy from those due to postinfectious or immune disorders, such as Sjögren syndrome, and from HIV infection. The finding of high antibody titers should lead to detailed radiologic and bronchoscopic examinations.

An unusual assortment of polyneuropathies may be associated with non-Hodgkin lymphomas of both T- and B-cell types and with several related conditions such as Castleman disease (angiofollicular lymphoid hyperplasia), angiocentric T-cell lymphoma (and the related lymphomatoid granulomatosis, page 700), hypersensitivity lymph node hyperplasia (angioimmunoblastic or immunoblastic lymphadenopathy), and Kimura disease (lymphoid hyperplasia with eosinophilia mainly involving skin). In most of these neuropathies, particularly the one associated with Castleman disease, there is a paraproteinemia, often polyclonal, thereby relating this group to the paraproteinemic neuropathies and to osteosclerotic myeloma, discussed below. In several of our cases the neuropathic manifestations have appeared simultaneously with lymph node enlargement in the groin, axilla, or thorax. Clinically, these neuropathies take the form of GBS, chronic demyelinating polyneuropathy, subacute motor polyneuropathy or anterior horn cell disease, lumbar and brachial plexopathies, and polyradiculopathies—each occurring as a paralymphomatous condition separable from cases of meningeal and direct neural infiltration by tumor. Corticosteroids have been helpful in some of our patients with the lymphoid diseases; in others the neuropathy resolves spontaneously or with radiation of the lymph nodes. Plasma exchange and intravenous immune globulin have been suggested in these and in the paraneoplastic neuropathies based on favorable outcomes in single cases but have not been successful in our patients. Vallat and colleagues have summarized their experience with the more conventional types of neuropathy accompanying non-Hodgkin lymphoma.

These various forms of paraneoplastic polyneuropathy are manifest clinically in 2 to 5 percent of patients with malignant disease. The figures are much higher if one includes the mild neuropathies that occur in the terminal stages of cancer and those identified by EMG in asymptomatic patients (Henson and Urich). Carcinoma of the lung accounts for about 50 percent of the cases of paraneoplastic sensorimotor polyneuropathy and for 75 percent of those with pure sensory neuropathy (Croft and Wilkinson); nevertheless, these neuropathies may be associated with neoplasms of all types. As mentioned, other remote neurologic effects of neoplasia may coexist (pages 721 to 728).

The *pathology* of the paraneoplastic polyneuropathies has not been completely defined. In the purely sensory type, there is not only a loss of nerve cells in the dorsal root ganglia but also an inflammatory reaction (Horwich et al), with secondary degeneration of the dorsal nerve roots and posterior columns of the spinal cord—much the same changes as occur with the sensory neuronopathy of Sjögren syndrome. In the mixed sensorimotor polyneuropathy, the degeneration is greater in the distal than in the proximal segments of the peripheral nerves, but it extends into the roots in advanced cases. Dorsal root ganglion cells may be lost in small numbers. If the histologic examination is performed early in the course of the neuropathy, sparse infiltrates of lymphocytes are observed, distributed in foci around blood vessels. Their relation to both segmental demyelination and axonal degeneration of myelinated fibers is unclear. No tumor cells are seen in the nerves or spinal ganglia, unlike the rare instances of carcinomatous and lymphomatous mononeuropathy multiplex, in which tumor cells actually infiltrate nerves. Degeneration of the dorsal columns and chromatolysis of anterior horn cells are probably secondary to changes in the peripheral nerves and roots.

The overall *prognosis* of the paraneoplastic neuropathies is poor. Even though the polyneuropathy may stabilize and not progress or even remit to some extent with therapy, most of the patients succumb to the underlying tumor within a year. If the tumor can be treated effectively, the neuropathy improves, the exception being the pure sensory neuronopathy. Treatment with plasma exchange, gamma globulin, or immunosuppression has only a minimal effect, but there are anecdotal reports of success with very early immune treatment. In the report by Uchuya and colleagues, only 1 of 18 patients with a subacute sensory neuropathy improved and another became dependent for sustained improvement on immune globulin; most of the others stabilized or worsened, and the authors concluded that the treatment was of doubtful value.

Arsenical Polyneuropathy Of the neuropathies caused by metallic poisoning, that due to arsenic is particularly well known. In cases of chronic poisoning, the neuropathic symptoms develop rather slowly, over a period of several weeks or months, and have the same sensory and motor distribution as the nutritional polyneuropathies. Gastrointestinal symptoms, the result of ingestion of arsenic compounds, may precede the polyneuropathy, which is nearly always associated with anemia, jaundice, brownish cutaneous pigmentation, hyperkeratosis of palms and soles, and later with white transverse banding of the nails (Mees' lines). The disease is accompanied by an excess of arsenic in the urine and hair. Pathologically, this form of arsenical neuropathy is of the "dying back" (axonal degeneration) type.

In patients who survive the ingestion of a single massive dose of arsenic, a more rapidly evolving polyneuropathy may appear after a period of 8 to 21 days. The neuropathy may be preceded by severe gastrointestinal symptoms, renal and hepatic failure, and mental disturbances, convulsions, confusion, and coma—i.e., arsenical encephalopathy—the pathologic basis of which is a brain purpura, or pericapillary hemorrhages. Initially, the neuropathy that develops in this setting may resemble GBS, both clinically and electromyographically (partial conduction block, prolonged F responses).

Diagnosis and treatment of arsenical poisoning are discussed further in Chap. 43.

Lead Neuropathy (Plumbism) Lead neuropathy is an uncommon disorder. In adults, as a rule, it occurs following chronic exposure to lead paint or fumes (as occurs in smelting industries or from burning batteries) and ingestion of liquor distilled in lead pipes. Its most characteristic clinical feature is the predominantly motor affection, mainly in the distribution of the radial nerves (wrist and finger drop). In a few personally observed patients, this was the main abnormality, but there was also a slight sensory loss in the radial territory of the hand. Less commonly, foot drop is observed, occurring alone or in combination with weakness of the proximal arm and shoulder girdle muscles. As pointed out in Chap. 43, lead neuropathy seldom occurs in children, in whom lead poisoning usually results in an encephalopathy. Although the neuropathy has been known since ancient times, details of the pathology are obscure. Axonal degeneration with secondary myelin change and swelling and chromatolysis of anterior horn cells has been described. Lead accumulates in the nerve and may be toxic to Schwann cells or to endothelial capillary cells, causing edema.

The diagnosis is established by the history of lead exposure, the predominant and restricted motor involvement, the associated medical findings (anemia, basophilic stippling of red cell precursors in the bone marrow, a "lead line" along the gingival margins, colicky abdominal pain, and constipation), and the urinary excretion of lead and coproporphyrins. Blood lead levels of more than 70 μg/dL are always abnormal. In patients with lower levels, doubling of the 24-h urinary lead excretion following an infusion of the chelating agent $CaNa_2$ EDTA indicates a significant degree of lead intoxication. Coproporphyrin in the urine is abnormal in any amount, but it may be found in porphyria, alcoholism, iron deficiency, and other disorders as well as in lead intoxication.

Treatment consists of terminating the exposure to lead and eliminating lead from the bloodstream and the bones. For this purpose, penicillamine, which is safe and can be administered orally, is preferable to dimercaprol [British antilewisite (BAL)] or EDTA.

Other Metals and Industrial Agents Chronic poisoning with *thallium* and sometimes with *lithium*, *gold*, *mercury*, and *platinum* (in the antineoplastic agent cisplatin) may produce a sensorimotor polyneuropathy similar to arsenical polyneuropathy; these intoxications are discussed in Chap. 43. A predominantly motor neuropathy is known with occupational exposure to metallic mercury and mercury vapor, but the connection to the mercury content in dental amalgam has been vastly overplayed. Exposure to manganese, bismuth, antimony, zinc, and copper may give rise to systemic signs of poisoning; some of them affect the central nervous system, but one cannot be certain that any of them specifically involves the peripheral nerves.

A distal, symmetrical sensorimotor (predominantly sensory) axonopathy may follow exposure to certain hexacarbon industrial solvents. These include *n-hexane* (found in contact cements, thus affecting "glue sniffers" who inhale the vapors); *methyl n-butyl ketone* (used in the production of plastic-coated and color-printed fabrics); dimethylaminopropionitrile (DMAPN), used in the manufacture of polyurethane foam); the fumigant *methyl bromide*; and the gas sterilant *ethylene oxide*. Operating room nurses are affected by the latter when the agent is absorbed through the skin, leaving a characteristic rash at exposed sites (usually the wrists, where a surgical gown ends). A mild peripheral neuropathy and central nervous system changes of memory loss and headaches have been reported by Brashear and colleagues. Also there is a risk to operating room personnel of *nitrous oxide* neurotoxicity; but at the present time the neuropathy has most often resulted from its repeated use as a euphoriant. The process is said to have the clinical and electrophysiologic features of a distal axonopathy but is more likely a myeloneuropathy related to impairment of vitamin B_{12} metabolism. Presumably the neuropathy occurs in marginally vitamin B_{12}–deficient individuals. The associated macrocytic anemia is reversed by the administration of B_{12}, but the neurologic illness is little affected (page 1218).

Detailed accounts of the clinical and experimental neurotoxicology of these agents can be found in the recent monograph of Spencer and Schaumburg.

Drug-Induced Neuropathies A number of medications, the main ones described below, are sources of polyneuropathy of predominantly sensory type. Most are dose-dependent and are therefore more or less predictable after particularly large doses of the drug have been used (e.g., in chemotherapy) or after prolonged administration for other reasons. Often, in the latter case, the patient fails to connect his sensory symptoms to drug toxicity.

Antineoplastic Drugs Among chemotherapeutic agents in current use, *cisplatin* and *carboplatin* are known to evoke a predominantly sensory polyneuropathy, which begins several weeks *after* completion of therapy in at least half of the patients (page 1285). Proprioception and vibratory sensation are most severely impaired, and there may be degeneration in the posterior columns—the basis for a Lhermitte symptom in this form of toxicity. Some patients develop acrodynia and episodic color changes in the fingertips and toes, suggesting that autonomic nerves are also involved. Others exhibit a sensory ataxia and pseudoathetosis. The severity of histopathologic changes in the peripheral nervous system corresponds to the concentration of plantinum in these tissues, the highest concentrations being found in dorsal root ganglia.

The taxanes *paclitaxel* (Taxol) and the more potent *docetaxel* (Taxotere), both cited as inhibitors of the depolymerization of neurotubules, are used mainly in the treatment of ovarian cancer. They produce a sensory polyneuropathy similar to that of cisplatin. The nerve lesion regresses slowly with a reduction in dosage (see also page 1285). Pathologic studies have shown a distal axonopathy affecting mainly large fibers.

Peripheral neuropathy commonly complicates the use of *vincristine*, an antineoplastic agent widely used in treatment of the lymphomas and leukemia (page 1283). Paresthesias are the commonest symptom, but objective sensory loss is uncommon. Loss of ankle jerks is also an early manifestation. Weakness usually precedes objective sensory loss. Weakness is observed in the extensor muscles of the fingers and wrists, later in the dorsiflexors of the toes and feet; if the dosage of vincristine is not reduced, weakness may spread rapidly to involve the proximal muscles of the limbs. In patients receiving large doses of the drug, foot drop may develop. The weakness is usually mild, but in the past occasional patients became quadriparetic and bedbound. Adults are more severely affected than children, as are persons with preexisting polyneuropathies. The neuropathy is strictly dose-related, and reduction in dosage is followed by improvement of neuropathic symptoms, although this may take several months. Many patients are then able to continue the use of vincristine in low dosage, such as 1 mg every 2 weeks, for many months.

Antimicrobial Drugs As mentioned in Chap. 43, *isoniazid*-induced polyneuropathy was a common occurrence in the early 1950s, when this drug was first used for the treatment of tuberculosis. Symptoms of neuropathy appeared between 3 and 35 weeks after treatment was begun and affected about 10 percent of patients receiving therapeutic doses (10 mg/kg daily).

The initial symptoms are a symmetrical numbness and tingling of the toes and feet, spreading, if the drug is continued, to the knees and occasionally the hands. Aching and burning pain in these parts then becomes prominent. In addition to sensory loss, examination discloses a loss of tendon reflexes and weakness in the distal muscles of the legs. Severe degrees of weakness and loss of deep sensation are observed only rarely.

Isoniazid (INH) produces its effects on the peripheral nerves by interfering with pyridoxine metabolism, perhaps by inhibiting the phosphorylation of pyridoxine (the collective name for the B_6 group of vitamins) and decreasing the tissue levels of its active form, pyridoxal phosphate. The administration of 150 to 450 mg of pyridoxine daily, in conjunction with isoniazid, completely prevents the neuropathic disorder. The same mechanism is probably operative in the neuropathies that occasionally complicate the administration of the isoniazid-related substances such as *ethionamide*, used in the treatment of tuberculosis, and the now little-used antihypertensive agent *hydralazine*. Paradoxically, the prolonged administration of *extremely high doses of pyridoxine* may actually cause a disabling, predominantly sensory neuropathy (Schaumburg et al).

A relatively mild sensory neuropathy (acral paresthesia) associated with optic neuropathy occasionally complicates *chloramphenicol* therapy. The chronic administration of *metronidazole* (used in the treatment of Crohn disease and anaerobic infections) may have the same effect. A predominantly motor neuropathy may be induced by the chronic administration of *dapsone*, a sulfone used to treat leprosy and certain dermatologic conditions. *Stilbamidine*, used in the treatment of kala azar, may produce a purely sensory neuropathy, mainly in the distribution of the trigeminal nerves.

The introduction in 1952 of *nitrofurantoin* for the treatment of bladder infections was soon followed by reports of neurotoxicity attributable to this drug. The earliest symptoms are pain and tingling paresthesias of the toes and feet, followed shortly by similar sensations in the fingers. If the drug is not discontinued, this disorder may progress to a severe, symmetrical sensorimotor polyneuropathy. Patients with chronic renal failure and azotemia are particularly prone to neurotoxicity from nitrofurantoin, presumably because diminished excretion results in high tissue levels of the drug. To make matters more difficult, the uremic state itself may be responsible for a clinically similar polyneuropathy, so that the distinction between uremic and nitrofurantoin neuropathy in the presence of chronic renal failure may be impossible. The neuropathologic studies of Lhermitte and colleagues disclosed an axonal degeneration in peripheral nerves and sensory roots.

Cardiac Drugs *Amiodarone*, a drug that is commonly used for treating angina pectoris and ventricular tachyarrhythmias, induces a motor-sensory neuropathy in about 5 percent of patients after several months of treatment. *Perhexiline maleate*, another drug for the treatment of angina pectoris, may also cause a generalized, predominantly sensory polyneuropathy in a small proportion of patients. Affected persons show a striking neuronal lipidosis. Patients taking *niacin* to lower blood cholesterol levels may experience intense distal and truncal paresthesias, but no neuropathy has been identified.

Disulfiram (Antabuse) The development of a sensorimotor neuropathy similar to that produced by isoniazid is sometimes associated with the chronic use of disulfiram in the treatment of alcoholism. Its neurotoxic effects have been attributed to the action of *carbon disulfide*, which is produced during the metabolism of the drug, and is known to produce polyneuropathy and sometimes an optic neuropathy in workers in the viscose rayon industry. Pathologic data, though scant, tend to discredit this notion, insofar as disulfiram produces a wallerian type of axonal degeneration, whereas carbon disulfide neuropathy is characterized by swollen (giant) axons that are filled with neurofilaments (Bouldin et al).

Other Agents Some patients who have taken *phenytoin* for many years may show absence of ankle and patellar reflexes, a mild, distal symmetrical impairment of sensation, a reduced conduction velocity in the peripheral nerves of the legs, and, rarely, weakness of the distal musculature. *Colchicine* has long been known to cause a myopathy, but a few cases of predominantly axonal sensory neuropathy have also been reported. *Triorthocresyl phosphate* and *acrylamide* are potent peripheral nerve poisons. Both of these drugs cause a "dying-back" polyneuropathy (axonal degeneration) and have been used experimentally to produce this effect. *Thalidomide*, which can produce sensory polyneuropathy, had been withdrawn from the market but is now being used again experimentally for graft-versus-host disease and for drug-resistant erythema nodosum, leprous eruptions, and apthous stomatitis, particularly in AIDS patients—also as an experimental anti-neoplastic agent for vascular tumors. The thalidomide polyneuropathy is dose-dependent and can be anticipated at certain levels of administration. Severe *botulinum* poisoning and the prolonged use of *neuromuscular blocking agents* is said to leave some patients with a distal axonopathy or a myopathy, but these must be rare. Residual effects of polyneuropathy are also seen in patients with the eosinophilia-myalgia syndrome; the latter has been traced to the ingestion of *adulterated* L*-tryptophan*, which had been used in nonprescription drugs for insomnia (page 1490). In several instances that we have seen, this syndrome had caused quadriplegia and simulated GBS. There may be an eosinophilic infiltrate in nerves, but the neuropathy is probably the result of a direct toxic mechanism. The ingestion of adulterated *rapeseed oil* (toxic-oil syndrome) produces the same effects. A sensory neuropathy resulting from excessive *pyridoxine* ingestion, alluded to above, is still seen among individuals who take huge doses of vitamin supplements. *Amitriptyline* is capable of producing paresthesias, but the effect seems to be idiosyncratic and infrequent. *Vacor*, a phenylnitrosurea rodenticide, has been used from time to time as a suicidal agent. It gives rise to a profound sensory and autonomic neuropathy with abdominal pain and hyperglycemia due to acute pancreatitis.

As a rare complication of *gold* therapy, a predominantly motor polyneuropathy has been reported, as mentioned in Chap. 43. In most cases the cumulative dose of gold has exceeded 1 g, but in a few instances the neuropathy has occurred with 0.5 g. Painful distal burning is the initial complaint, and weakness and wasting follow; the onset of weakness, although usually insidious, can be abrupt enough to simulate GBS. There have been trigeminal, facial, and oculomotor palsies. One of the unusual features is a marked rise in CSF protein concentration.

The anesthetic agent *trichloroethylene*, as with *stilbamidine*, has a predilection for cranial nerves, particularly the fifth. The neurotoxicity is apparently due to dichloroacetylene, formed as a decomposition product of trichloroethylene. The neuropathic potential of nitrous oxide has already been mentioned.

Subacute Asymmetrical and Multifocal Polyneuropathies (Mononeuropathy Multiplex)

Several systemic conditions are commonly accompanied by a subacute affection of *multiple individual nerves*, occurring almost simultaneously and giving rise to a distinctive clinical picture. The most notable examples of this syndrome are associated with diabetes, polyarteritis nodosa, cryoglobulinemia and other vasculitides such as Churg-Strauss syndrome, and the uncommon form of idiopathic vasculitis that is confined to the peripheral nervous system. Less frequently, sarcoidosis, forms of HIV-related neuropathy, and Lyme disease present in this fashion. Leprosy, a special case in this group, is discussed further on.

Diabetic Neuropathy About 15 percent of patients with diabetes mellitus have both symptoms and signs of neuropathy, but nearly 50 percent have either neuropathic symptoms or nerve conduction abnormalities. Neuropathy is most common in diabetics more than 50 years of age; it is uncommon in those under 30 years of age and rare in childhood. Dyck and colleagues (1993) studied 380 diabetics—27 percent with type 1 (insulin-dependent) diabetes and 73 percent with type 2 (non-insulin-dependent); symptomatic polyneuropathy was found in 15 percent of the first group and 13 percent of the second. The percentages were far higher when patients were examined electrophysiologically.

Several clinical syndromes have been delineated: (1) acute diabetic ophthalmoplegia that affects the third and less often the sixth nerve; (2) acute mononeuropathy of limbs or trunk including a painful thoracolumbar radiculopathy; (3) a rapidly evolving, painful, asymmetrical, predominantly motor multiple neuropathy affecting the upper lumbar roots and the proximal leg muscles and usually undergoing remission ("diabetic amyotrophy"); (4) a more symmetrical, proximal motor weakness and wasting, often without pain and with variable sensory loss that pursues a subacute or chronic course; (5) a distal, symmetrical, primarily sensory polyneuropathy affecting feet and legs more than hands in a chronic, slowly progressive manner (the commonest of the diabetic neuropathies); and (6) an autonomic neuropathy involving bowel, bladder, and circulatory reflexes; and (7) a painful thoracoabdominal radiculopathy. These forms of neuropathy often coexist or overlap, particularly the autonomic and distal symmetrical types and the subacute proximal neuropathies [items (3) and (4) in the above classification].

The first five types of neuropathy listed above, and possibly the seventh type as well, are thought to be due to infarction of nerves related to a diabetic microvasculopathy; in other words, they are all special types of so-called *mononeuropathy multiplex*. The remaining types are also associated with small blood vessel disease but also with a poorly understood metabolic abnormality.

Acute Diabetic Mononeuropathies *Diabetic ophthalmoplegia* is a not uncommon occurrence, usually in a patient with well-established diabetes. It presents as an isolated, painful third nerve palsy with sparing of pupillary function. In the first autopsied patient reported by Dreyfus et al, there was an ischemic lesion in the center of the retro-orbital portion of the third nerve. Subsequently, a similar case was described by Asbury et al. Less often, the sixth nerve is involved. The disorder is described on page 286. Isolated affection of practically all the major peripheral nerves has been described in diabetes, but the ones most commonly involved are the *femoral*, *sciatic*, and *peroneal nerves* in about that order of frequency. Rarely, a nerve in the upper extremity is affected. As mentioned, the acute mononeuropathies, cranial and peripheral, are presumably due to infarction of the nerve, and it is in the third nerve that this pathologic basis has been most convincingly established. Recovery is the rule but may take many months.

Multiple Mononeuropathies and Radiculopathies A painful unilateral or asymmetrical multiple neuropathy tends to occur in older patients with relatively mild or even unrecognized diabetes. The affection of several single nerves in a random distribution (mononeuritis multiplex) often emerges during periods of transition, when severe hyper- or hypoglycemia arises, when insulin treatment is being initiated, or when there has been rapid weight loss. In the most characteristic lumbar type, pain, which can be severe, begins in the low back or hip and spreads to the thigh and knee on one side. It usually has a deep, aching character with superimposed lancinating jabs, and there is a propensity for the discomfort to be most severe at night. Weakness and atrophy are evident in the pelvic girdle and thigh muscles, although the distal muscles of the leg may also be affected. The patellar reflex is lost on one or both sides. The upper extremities are only rarely affected. Deep and superficial sensation may be intact or mildly impaired, conforming to either a multiple nerve or root distribution or both. Recovery from this type of neuropathy is the rule, although months and even years may elapse before it is complete. There is a tendency for the same syndrome to recur after an interval of months or years in the opposite limb. The EMG shows denervation in the L2-L3 and sometimes adjacent myotomes. This form of neuropathy is often referred to as diabetic amyotrophy, a term that draws attention to one facet of the syndrome but is otherwise uninformative. A vasculitic mechanism has been proposed by PJB Dyck and others but is not uniformly accepted. There is no doubt that an identical painful lumbofemoral neuropathy occurs in nondiabetics; possibly this form is also vasculitic. A retroperitoneal hematoma that has compressed upper lumbar roots, carcinomatous meningitis, and neoplastic and sarcoid infiltration of the lumbar plexus enter into the differential diagnosis, but the features of the diabetic illness are usually so distinctive as to permit a confident diagnosis on clinical grounds alone.

Also observed in diabetics is a proximal symmetrical leg weakness, wasting, and reflex loss of more insidious onset and gradual evolution. The proximal muscles of the lower limbs, particularly the iliopsoas, quadriceps, and hamstrings, are involved in varying degrees. The muscles of the scapulae and upper limbs, usually the deltoid and triceps, are affected less frequently. Pain is not a consistent feature, as it is in the acute asymmetrical type, and sensory changes, if present, are distal, symmetrical, and usually mild in degree.

With this definition of two types of subacute proximal diabetic neuropathy, it must be emphasized that there is a great deal of overlap between them and that distal parts of the affected limb are often involved to a lesser degree. Nor can they be distinguished on pathologic or electrophysiologic grounds. Whether they should be considered as separate entities is questionable.

Attention has also been drawn to a syndrome of severe *thoracoabdominal radiculopathy* characterized by severe pain and dysesthesia. Almost always the diabetes has been of long-standing (Kikta et al). The pain is distributed over one or several adjacent segments of the chest or abdomen; it may be unilateral or less often bilateral and is usually associated with recent weight loss. Superficial sensory loss can be detected over the involved area in most patients. The pathology of this state is not known but is presumed to be an ischemic radiculopathy on the basis of the EMG changes, which characteristically consist of fibrillations of the paraspinal and abdominal wall muscles in one or more adjacent myotomes, corresponding to the painful area. Recovery may be protracted, but the ultimate prognosis for recovery is good. The differential diagnosis includes pre-eruptive herpes zoster and sarcoid infiltration of nerve roots.

Distal Polyneuropathy The *distal, symmetrical, primarily sensory form* is the most common type of diabetic neuropathy. Although it is a chronic process, sometimes unnoticed by the patient, we include it here for the sake of presenting the diabetic neuropathies as a unified topic. When the polyneuropathy becomes symptomatic, the main complaints are persistent and often distressing numbness and tingling, usually confined to the feet and lower legs and worse at night. The ankle jerks are absent, and sometimes the patellar reflexes as well. As a rule the sensory signs are confined to the distal parts of the lower extremities, but in severe cases the hands may be involved and the sensory loss may spread to the anterior aspect of the lower abdomen, giving rise to confusion in diagnosis (Said et al). Trophic changes in the form of deep ulcerations and neuropathic degeneration of the joints (Charcot joints) are occasionally encountered, presumably due to severe sensory denervation and injuries. Muscle weakness is usually mild, but in some patients a distal sensory neuropathy is combined with a proximal weakness and wasting of the types described above. Treatment of the acral pain may be a major problem and is discussed further on.

In another group of patients the clinical picture may be dominated by loss of deep sensation, ataxia, and atony of the bladder, with only slight weakness of the limbs, in which case it resembles tabes dorsalis (hence the term *diabetic pseudotabes*). The similarity is even closer if lancinating pains in the legs, unreactive pupils, and neuropathic arthropathy are present.

Autonomic Neuropathy Symptoms of *autonomic involvement* include pupillary and lacrimal dysfunction, impairment of sweating and vascular reflexes, nocturnal diarrhea, atonicity of the gastrointestinal tract and bladder, sexual impotence, and postural hypotension. The basis of this type of involvement is not well understood. Duchen and associates, who studied the sympathetic ganglia in diabetics with autonomic symptoms, described vacuoles and granular deposits in neurons and little if any neuronal degeneration; there was also a loss of myelinated nerve fibers in the vagus and splanchnic nerves and loss of neurons in the intermediolateral columns of the spinal cord.

In all forms of diabetic neuropathy, the CSF protein may be elevated from 50 to 150 mg/dL and sometimes even higher.

Pathology and Pathophysiology Thomas and Tomlinson have reviewed the neuropathology of diabetic polyneuropathy. Loss of myelinated nerve fibers is the most prominent finding in the distal symmetrical type of polyneuropathy. In addition, segmental demyelination and remyelination of remaining axons are apparent in teased nerve fiber preparations. The latter findings are probably too severe and widespread in some cases to be simply a reflection of axonal degeneration. Occasionally, repeated demyelination and remyelination leads to onion-bulb formations of Schwann cells and fibroblasts, as it does in the relapsing inflammatory neuropathies. Unmyelinated fibers are also reduced in number in some specimens. Similar lesions are found in the posterior roots and posterior columns of the spinal cord and in the rami communicantes and sympathetic ganglia. Under the electron microscope, the basement membranes of intraneural capillaries are seen to be thickened and duplicated.

Many uncertainties persist about the pathogenesis of the diabetic neuropathies. Both the cranial (diabetic ophthalmoplegia) and peripheral mononeuropathies as well as the painful, asymmetrical, predominantly proximal neuropathy of sudden onset are thought to be ischemic in origin, secondary to disease of the vasa nervorum; obliterative vascular lesions were illustrated by Raff and coworkers and multiple small infarcts were found in the nerve trunks. In the other forms of diabetic neuropathy, a metabolic basis, as yet undefined, has long been favored, but the observations of Dyck and of Johnson and their associates suggest that these and all other forms of diabetic neuropathy might have the same vascular basis. These authors described multiple foci of fiber loss throughout the length of the peripheral nerves, beginning high in the proximal segments and becoming more frequent and severe in the distal segments. This pattern of change differs from that observed in diffuse metabolic disease of Schwann cells and in dying-back neuropathy and suggests an ischemic etiology. Fagerberg noted that the fascicular capillaries and epineural arterioles have thickened and hyalinized basement membranes, similar to the microvascular changes seen in the retina and other organs. Occlusion of vessels and frank infarction of nerve was not observed, so that a vascular pathogenesis remains somewhat unsettled. Inflammatory changes in diabetic nerves have not been as impressive in our material as in the above cited and that of Said et al.

The several biochemical findings and their interpretations have been reviewed by Thomas and Tomlinson and by Brown and Greene. The latter authors advanced the idea that persistent hyperglycemia inhibits sodium-dependent myoinositol transport. Low levels of intraneural myoinositol reduce phosphoinositide metabolism and sodium-potassium ATPase activity. Others have emphasized a deficiency of aldose reductase and an elevation of polyols (particularly sorbitol) as being causally important. After reading these articles, one can only conclude that a convincing biochemical pathogenesis has yet to be formulated.

Treatment The only meaningful preventive treatment is the maintenance of the blood glucose concentration in a normal range, since the prevailing view is that there is some relationship between peripheral nerve damage and inadequate regulation of the diabetes. This view is supported by the findings of the National Diabetic Complications Trial, in which 715 patients with type 1 diabetes were followed for 6 to 10 years. There was a clear relation between strict glucose control, by means of an intravenous insulin infusion system, and a reduction in painful neuropathic symptoms, retinopathy, and nephropathy. However, this came at the price of a threefold increase in hypoglycemic reactions (see also Samanta and Burden). Whether similar protective effects apply to type 2 diabetes is not known. Culebras and associates reported therapeutic success with an aldose reductase inhibitor called *albrestatin*. The drug was given intravenously over a period of 5 days, after which 7 of 10 patients declared that their weakness, sensory loss, and pains had diminished; there was also improvement in nerve conduction velocities. Others have made similar but uncontrolled observations (see Thomas and Tomlinson). Some recent interest has centered on the use of gangliosides, which are normal components of neuronal membranes and can be administered exogenously. The authors have had no experience with either of these agents and cannot vouch for them.

In the long term, the distressing paresthesias of the distal extremities are best managed with amitriptyline or one of the newer generation of antidepressants, such as sertraline or fluoxetine, which are better tolerated. Shooting, stabbing pain also responds to some degree to carbamazepine or phenytoin, but in general the results are unimpressive. Neurontin may give somewhat better results, perhaps in part because high doses are well tolerated (Gorson et al). Nerve blocks and epidural injections have been helpful in only a few patients. In the proximal asymmetrical, truncal, or ophthalmoplegic neuropathies, the severe pain usually lasts for only a short period and requires the judicious use of analgesics, as outlined in Chap. 8. *Prognosis* in patients with the distal, symmetrical sensory neuropathy is uncertain, but in the other types improvement and eventual recovery may be expected over a period of months or years.

Ischemic Neuropathy A number of patients with atherosclerotic ischemic disease of the legs will be found to have localized sensory changes or impairment of reflexes. Usually the other effects of ischemia—claudication and pain at rest, absence of distal pulses, and trophic skin changes—are so prominent that the neurologic changes may be overlooked. In experimental studies of peripheral nerve ischemia, lesions of nerve are produced only by combined occlusion of the aorta and many limb vessels because of the profusely ramifying neural vasculature. In our own experience comprising 12 patients with one critically ischemic leg, the neuropathy was characterized by a pronounced distal predominance—sensory loss in the feet (worse than the symptoms might suggest) and mild weakness of the toes, and the ankle reflex was lost or depressed (Weinberg et al). Although paresthesias, numbness, and deep aching pain were characteristic, the patients were more limited by symptoms of their vascular claudication than the neuropathic ones. Restoration of circulation to the limb by surgical or other means, including gene therapy, has resulted in some improvement of the regional neuropathy. The literature on this subject is to be found in the writings of Chalk et al and Eames and Lange listed in the References.

A poorly understood but presumably localized ischemic neuropathy occurs in the region of arteriovenous shunts that have been placed for the purpose of dialysis. Complaints of transient diffuse tingling of the hand are not uncommon soon after placement of the shunt, but only a few patients develop persistent forearm weakness and numbness and burning in the fingers, reflecting variable degrees of ulnar, radial, and median nerve and muscle ischemia. The role of an underlying uremic polyneuropathy in facilitating this neuropathy is unclear.

Bendixen and colleagues have described a progressive, symmetrical polyneuropathy due to systemic cholesterol embolism. An inflammatory and necrotizing arteritis surrounds embolic cholesterol material within small vessels and appears to account for the progression. This neuropathic process is probably more often discovered at autopsy than in the clinic, being eclipsed during life by the cerebral manifestations of cholesterol embolism. The entire illness closely simulates the generalized polyneuropathy of polyarteritis.

Angiopathic (Arteritic) Neuropathies A number of focal and multifocal asymmetrical neuropathies are known to be caused by arteritis of small and medium-sized vessels. Approximately one-third of all cases of mononeuropathy multiplex can be traced to a *systemic vasculitis of the vasa nervorum*. Included in this category are polyarteritis nodosa, the Churg-Strauss syndrome (allergic bronchial asthma and eosinophilia), rheumatoid arthritis, lupus erythematosus, systemic sclerosis, cryoglobulinemia, Wegener granulomatosis, and an idiopathic variety. This subject has been thoroughly reviewed by Chalk et al; Dyck, Benstead et al; Said; and Kissell. A small-vessel arteritis is also the putative mechanism in the multiple mononeuropathies that complicate Lyme disease and AIDS. In Said's series of 200 cases of vasculitis affecting the peripheral nerves, 36 percent were due to polyarteritis nodosa, 21 percent to rheumatoid arthritis, and 4 percent to other connective tissue diseases; in 35 percent there were no signs of vasculitis beyond the peripheral nerves.

Polyarteritis Nodosa with Neuropathy Perhaps 75 percent of cases of polyarteritis nodosa show involvement of the small nutrient arteries of peripheral nerves (autopsy figures), but a symptomatic form of neuropathy develops in only about half this number. Involvement of the peripheral nerves may be the principal clue to the diagnosis of the underlying disease when, up to that time, the main components of the clinical picture—abdominal pain, hematuria, fever, eosinophilia, hypertension, vague limb pains, and possibly asthma—had not fully declared themselves or had been misinterpreted.

The neuropathy associated with polyarteritis nodosa may be diffuse and more or less symmetrical in distribution as a result of the cumulation of many small nerve infarctions, i.e., simulating a polyneuropathy. In these cases, careful clinical and electrophysiologic examinations disclose elements of mononeuritis that have been engrafted on the ostensibly generalized process, for example, an asymmetrical foot or wrist drop, or a disproportionate affection of one nerve in a limb, such as ulnar palsy with relative sparing of function of the adjacent median nerve. More often it takes the form, throughout its course, of a *mononeuropathy multiplex*, i.e., a random infarction of two or more individual nerves. The onset in this latter form is usually abrupt, with symptoms of pain or numbness in the distribution of an affected nerve, followed in hours or days by motor or sensory loss in the distribution of that nerve, and then by involvement, in a saltatory fashion, of other peripheral nerves. Both spinal and cranial nerves may be affected. No two cases are identical. The CSF is usually normal because the roots are not involved. Muscle biopsy, taken near the motor point so as to include nerve twigs, shows perivascular inflammation, necrosis and cellular infiltration of arterial vessel walls, and vascular occlusion, changes that are needed to corroborate the clinical impression when systemic manifestations of the disease are not evident. On the basis of the smaller size of affected vessels and the presence of perinuclear antinuclear cytoplasmic autoantibodies (p-ANCA), Lhote et al have differentiated a "microscopic polyarteritis"—an entity with which we have had little experience. Rapidly progressive glomerulonephritis and lung hemorrhage are the main features, neuropathy occurring less frequently than in typical polyarteritis.

Mononeuropathy multiplex due to polyarteritis calls for treatment with corticosteroids and cyclophosphamide. We have used intravenous methylprednisolone, 1.5 mg/kg, for several days, followed by oral treatment, and cyclophosphamide, 1 g/m^2 once a month for several months, but other equivalent regimens have been suggested. Azathioprine is a reasonable alternative if cyclophosphamide is not tolerated. Treatment must be continued for at least several months. In intractable cases and in those with systemic involvement, treatment with methotrexate may be indicated. Spontaneous remission and therapeutic arrest are known, but many cases have a fatal outcome. The palsies and sensory loss of the mononeuropathies generally persist even when the systemic disease is brought under control.

Churg-Strauss and Hypereosinophilic Syndrome These systemic illnesses involve multiple individual peripheral nerves, much as in polyarteritis, but they are characterized by an excess of circulating and tissue eosinophils and a tendency to involve the lungs and skin, in contrast to the renal and bowel infarctions in polyarteritis nodosa. They segregate into two varieties with a considerable degree of pathologic and clinical overlap: the Churg-Strauss necrotizing vasculitis with asthma and vasculitic skin lesions, and a more benign asthma-eosinophilia syndrome that is less aggressive and has a greater tendency for the eosinophils to infiltrate other tissues. A medication (zafirlukast) that is used in Europe to treat asthma is said to have precipitated several cases of Churg-Strauss disease.

The Churg-Strauss type has many similarities to polyarteritis; indeed, the original paper by Churg and

Strauss in 1951 was meant in part to distinguish the two diseases on the basis of "allergic granulomas" and eosinophilic infiltrates that involved many organs. The diffuse subcutaneous nodules created by these granulomas and vasculitic skin lesions, a marked eosinophilia of peripheral blood, and the occurrence of late-life asthma are the characteristic features of the Churg-Strauss syndrome. Similar lesions within the skin are found from time to time in other diseases such as Wegener granulomatosis, lupus erythematosus, rheumatoid disease, lymphoma, and endocarditis, but the eosinophilic infiltration is less pronounced than that of the Churg-Strauss syndrome. We have seen other types of cutaneous disease, the most impressive being a massive leukocytoclastic vasculitis of the skin (necrotic polymorphonuclear cells surrounding venules)—large hemorrhagic lesions developing simultaneously with an eosinophilia and multiple mononeuropathies. Usually, in the patient with Churg-Strauss syndrome, there is a progression from rhinitis or asthma, which may have been present for years, to eosinophilia and organ infiltration, particularly a pneumonitis. The neuropathy, which then develops in approximately three-quarters of the patients, most often appears in the context of fever and weight loss and takes the form of an acute, painful mononeuritis multiplex. The granular cytoplasmic pattern of antineutrophil cytoplasmic autoantibody (c-ANCA) of the same type that occurs in Wegener granulomatosis is usually found (see below). The substrate for the neuropathy, a vasculitis involving the vasa nervorum, can be detected in sural nerve biopsy, the special feature possibly being a more intense eosinophilic infiltration than is usually seen in polyarteritis nodosa.

The *idiopathic eosinophilic syndrome* comprises a heterogeneous group of disorders, the common features of which are a persistent and extreme degree of eosinophilia and eosinophilic infiltration of many organ systems. Neuropathy occurs in half of the cases, taking the form of a painful sensorimotor process with axonal damage or of a mononeuritis multiplex (see Moore et al). The pathologic appearance is one of infiltration of the nerves by eosinophils rather than a vasculitis. The clinical effects are attributable to the infiltration itself or to a postulated tissue-damaging effect of the eosinophilic cell.

Both the Churg-Strauss and the idiopathic hypereosinophilic syndrome are best treated with high doses of corticosteroids, after which the peripheral eosinophilia as well as tissue damage should abate. Further immunosuppressive agents in the form of azathioprine, chlorambucil, or cyclophosphamide have been used intermittently in fulminant or refractory cases, which includes most of the cases that we have seen.

Wegener Granulomatosis (Necrotizing Granulomatous Vasculitis) This disorder has given rise to two neuropathic syndromes—one a symmetrical or asymmetrical polyneuropathy indistinguishable from the other angiopathic neuropathies described above, the other involving the lower cranial nerves directly as they exit the skull and pass through the retropharyngeal tissues. The finding of c-ANCA is relatively specific for Wegener granulomatosis and Churg-Strauss disease, as mentioned above (Specks et al) and helps to differentiate these diseases from carcinoma, chordoma, sarcoidosis, and zoster. This vasculitis and its effect on the lower cranial nerves is discussed further on page 1462.

Essential Mixed Cryoglobulinemia This process has been associated with a vasculitic mononeuritis multiplex as well as a more generalized polyneuropathy. In many cases, glomerulonephritis, arthralgias, and purpura are conjoined, reflecting the systemic nature of the vasculopathy, but the mononeuritis may occur in isolation. The evolution in our cases has been slower than in the typical vasculitic neuropathies, sometimes weeks or longer elapsing between attacks of mononeuritis. The neurologic disorder has become quiescent for long periods, during which time considerable improvement may occur. There is no evident relationship between the mode of onset or severity of the neuropathy and the concentration of cryoprecipitable proteins in the serum; the latter can be detected by cooling the serum and demonstrating a precipitation of IgG and IgM proteins that redissolve upon warming to 37°C. This requires that the blood sample be carefully transported to the laboratory in a warm water bath. Garcia-Bragado and colleagues have suggested that the neuropathy is stabilized by corticosteroids and cyclophosphamide. In our experience, plasma exchange has also been beneficial, but this measure has not been systematically tested. The relationship of some cases to hepatitis C infection is mentioned below, and other aspects of the condition are discussed under "Neuropathies Associated with Paraproteinemias," further on.

Rheumatoid Arthritis Some 1 to 5 percent of patients with rheumatoid arthritis have involvement of one or more nerves at some time in the course of their disease. Apart from pressure neuropathies due to thickened tendons and destructive joint changes, there is a form of rheumatoid arteritis that results in acute ischemic necrosis and demyelination of single or multiple nerves. The arteritis is of small-vessel fibrinoid type and immune globulins are demonstrable in the walls of the vessel. Most of the affected patients have had severe rheumatic disease for many years and are strongly seropositive. In addition to the neuropathy, such patients often have rheumatoid nodules, skin vasculitis, weight loss, fever, a high titer of rheumatoid factor, and low serum complement.

There are also rare forms of chronic progressive polyneuropathy that complicate rheumatoid arthritis; they are described further on, under the chronic polyneuropathies associated with the connective tissue diseases.

Lupus Erythematosus Approximately 10 percent of patients with lupus will exhibit symptoms and signs of peripheral nerve involvement. Usually the neuropathy appears in the established and more advanced stages of the disease, but rarely it has been the initial presentation. In several of our cases the polyneuropathy has taken the form of a symmetrical, progressive sensorimotor paralysis, beginning in the feet and legs and extending to the arms, evolving over a period of several days or weeks and at times simulating GBS. In a few, weakness and areflexia were more prominent than the sensory loss; the latter involved mainly vibratory and position senses. A more common syndrome in our experience has been a progressive or relapsing disease that cannot be distinguished clinically from chronic inflammatory demyelinating polyneuropathy (discussed further on). Multiple mononeuropathies have also been reported, as has involvement of the autonomic nervous system. An elevation of CSF protein in some cases suggests root involvement. Sural nerve biopsies regularly show vascular changes consisting of endothelial thickening and mononuclear inflammatory infiltration in and around the small vessels. In the nerves, axonal degeneration is the most common change, but a chronic demyelinating pathology has also been described (Rechthand et al). Vascular injury from deposition of immune complexes is the likely mechanism.

Isolated (Nonsystemic) Vasculitic Neuropathy In contrast to the aforementioned disorders, which characteristically involve several tissues and organs in addition to the peripheral nerves, a necrotizing vasculitis may affect the peripheral nerves exclusively. In our hospitals a case of this type appears about yearly, i.e., about as often as the systemic vasculitides as a cause of neuropathy. This disease takes the form of a multiple mononeuropathy and, less often, of a subacute symmetrical or asymmetrical polyneuropathy; ANCA is found in some cases. The neuropathy tends to be indolent and less lethal than the systemic forms of vasculitic neuropathy and generally does not require treatment with cyclophosphamide (Dyck et al, 1987). Steroids in high doses often prevent progression of the disease. The main difficulty in diagnosis arises when the EMG performed early in the course of illness shows conduction block that simulates a demyelinating polyneuropathy.

Other Vasculitic Neuropathies In the past, administration of pooled serum for the treatment of infections often led to brachial neuritis (page 1430) and less often to an immune mononeuritis multiplex, presumably from deposition of antibody-antigen complexes in the walls of the vasa nervorum. A similar "serum sickness" may occur after viral infections that have caused arthritis, rash, and fever. The neuropathy that emerges with hepatitis C infection may also be of this type, perhaps mediated by a frequently associated cryoglobulinemia. Interferon, which has been effective in treating the hepatitis, may also ameliorate the neuropathy, but greater success has been reported with cyclophosphamide. Pooled immunoglobulin for the treatment of diverse neuromuscular diseases has not, to our knowledge, led to a serum-sickness neuropathy, but one of our patients with Churg-Strauss disease developed a fulminating vasculitic skin eruption when treated in this way.

The increasing appearance of vasculitic neuropathy with *HIV infection*, including the type that is independent of CMV infection, has already been mentioned; these cases tend to improve spontaneously or with corticosteroids. It has been stated that the CMV virus should be suspected if the number of CD4 cells in the blood is below 200/mm^3 in a patient with AIDS; in about half of these cases the CSF shows a polymorphonuclear predominance. Also, from time to time a patient with a lymphoproliferative disorder such as Hodgkin disease will develop mononeuritis multiplex that is found by biopsy to be due to vasculitis.

The role of vasculitis in obscure axonal polyneuropathies in elderly patients is controversial. We have not found, as suggested by Chia and colleagues, an unexpected vasculitis in the nerve biopsies of such patients. The majority of our cases with severe neuropathy that is not explained by a known systemic disease (diabetes, cancer, or a paraproteinemia, etc.) or an overt toxic exposure remain unexplained after nerve biopsy.

Sarcoidosis Sarcoidosis is a rare cause of subacute or chronic polyneuropathy or polyradiculopathy of asymmetrical type (Zuniga et al). It may be associated with lesions in muscles (polymyositis) or with signs of central nervous system (CNS) involvement (stalk of the pituitary with diabetes insipidus, cerebellum with ataxia, and a myelopathy).

Involvement of a single nerve with sarcoid most often takes the form of a facial palsy; in other cases, multiple cranial nerves are affected successively (see page 1454). Weakness and reflex and sensory loss in the distribution of one or more spinal nerves or roots may be added. The occurrence of large, irregular zones of sensory loss over the trunk is said to distinguish the neuropathy of sarcoidosis from other forms of mononeuropathy multiplex. This type of sensory loss, particularly when accompanied by pain, should also suggest a diagnosis of diabetic radiculopathy (see above).

Lyme Disease Neuropathy develops in 10 to 15 percent of patients with this disease, and it takes several forms. Cranial nerve involvement is well known; uni- or bilateral facial palsy is by far the most frequent (page 1453), but other cranial nerves can be affected as well. Almost any of the somatic roots may be affected, most often the cervical or lumbar ones. An aseptic meningitis, essentially a meningoradiculitis, and an associated pleocytosis are particularly characteristic (although the same occurs in HIV and CMV neuritis). Some of the CSF cells may have immature features that suggest a lymphomatous meningitis. The radicular pain may simulate that of cervical or lumbar disc disease. The triad of cranial nerve palsies, radiculitis, and aseptic meningitis is highly characteristic of Lyme disease and develops early in its disseminated phase, i.e., from 1 to 3 weeks following the tick bite or the appearance of the typical rash.

As to polyneuropathies, the clinical situation is more complex, since several patterns have been recognized: (1) a syndrome of multiple mononeuropathies (involvement of a single major nerve in the limbs, resulting in an isolated foot or wrist drop, is distinctly rare); (2) a lumbar or brachial plexopathy (also rare); (3) a predominantly sensory polyneuropathy in which paresthesias and loss of superficial sensation in the feet and legs are coupled with loss of ankle jerks; and (4) an axonal polyneuropathy (Halperin and Loggigian). The last form is mainly sensory as well and is sometimes accompanied by a mild encephalopathy. Electrophysiologic testing indicates that the various peripheral nerve syndromes frequently overlap. All of them occur as late complications of Lyme disease, several months or even years after the initial infection (if untreated). The late neuropathic syndromes respond less favorably to treatment than the acute syndrome.

There are virtually no adequate pathologic studies of the peripheral nerves, since the disease is not fatal. No one has demonstrated the infective agent in the nerves, although this has been suggested as the mechanism of the lesions, and the pathophysiology of the peripheral neuropathy remains obscure. With treatment (see below) the neuropathic symptoms gradually recede.

An intensely painful lumbosacral polyradiculitis has long been known in Europe as the Bannwarth syndrome (also Garin-Bujadoux syndrome) and is probably due to a spirochete different from the one that causes Lyme disease in North America. In the Bannwarth syndrome and in occasional cases of Lyme disease, there is a characteristic type of cauda equina involvement, with sciatic, hip, and buttock pain and bladder difficulty. Less frequent is a cervical polyradiculopathy, with shoulder and arm pain. Headache and a brisk pleocytosis accompany the pain and the latter may precede the neuropathy by many days or weeks. The neuropathy may occur in any region of the body or migrate from one part to another.

It should be noted that a similar syndrome of lumbar polyradiculitis has been caused by the herpes and Epstein-Barr viruses and most often by an opportunistic CMV infection in patients with AIDS.

Diagnosis requires serologic testing. Testing by enzyme-linked immunosorbent assay (ELISA) is not altogether satisfactory because it frequently yields false-positive results. Western blot testing is more specific. The knowledge that the patient has lived in or visited an endemic area and more specifically has had a tick bite with the characteristic rash or has a history of nonneurologic manifestations of Lyme disease (cardiac, arthritic) supports the diagnosis. Indeed, one should be cautious in making this diagnosis unless a primary Lyme syndrome is described. The co-occurrence of bifacial palsy in any of these contexts also makes Lyme a likely diagnosis. Treatment of the neuropathic disease is with intravenous antibiotics, preferably ceftriaxone 2 g daily for 1 month.

Sjögren-Sicca Syndrome This is a chronic, slowly progressive autoimmune disease characterized by lymphocytic infiltration of the exocrine glands and resulting in keratoconjunctivitis sicca and xerostomia (dry eyes and mouth). The latter features may be combined with rheumatoid arthritis or with a wide range of other abnormalities, notably lymphoma, vasculitis, renal tubular defects, and most often by several types of polyneuropathy (see review by Kaplan et al). Grant et al collected 54 patients with sicca complex and peripheral neuropathy and found that the neuropathy had been the presenting problem in 87 percent. The sicca symptoms were usually mild and often were reported only upon specific inquiry. A symmetrical sensory polyneuropathy or ganglionopathy was the most common type. Sensorimotor polyneuropathy, polyradiculoneuropathy, autonomic neuropathy, or mononeuropathy (most often of the trigeminal nerve, as described by Kaltrieder and Talal) are less common types. We have observed yet another neuropathic syndrome, taking the form of an asymmetrical sensory loss, mostly of position sense and involving the upper limbs predominantly, in association with tonic pupils and trigeminal anesthesia.

Nerve biopsies in some cases have revealed a necrotizing vasculitis, inflammatory cell infiltrates, and focal nerve fiber destruction. Usually, the CSF protein is normal and there is no cellular reaction.

The sensory polyneuropathy of the Sjögren syndrome—more an inflammatory ganglionitis or sensory neuronopathy (see Griffin et al)—is of particular interest to neurologists, since most cases will first be seen by them. More than 90 percent of the patients are women. The main clinical features are a widespread sensory loss that may include the trunk and a profoundly diminished kinesthetic sense, giving rise to a characteristic sensory limb and gait ataxia. Loss of pain and temperature sensation is variable. Tendon reflexes are abolished. In time, many of these patients develop autonomic abnormalities such as bowel atony, urinary retention, loss of sweating, and pupillary changes. The sensorimotor polyneuropathic syndrome begins with paresthesias of the feet and is usually mild in degree.

The evaluation of all these cases, but particularly those with ganglionitis, should include a Schirmer or Rose Bengal test (page 562) to demonstrate the absence of tearing. If this test is positive, it may be followed by a biopsy of the lip to demonstrate the inflammatory changes in the small salivary glands. Many patients will have serologic abnormalities such as antinuclear antibodies (anti-Ro, also termed SS-A, and anti-La, or SS-B) or increased monoclonal immunoglobulins, particularly of the IgM subclass. The frequency of Sjögren-specific antibodies varies greatly between series; they may be useful as screening tests, but the lip biopsy is a far more sensitive diagnostic procedure. The sedimentation rate is often elevated. As already mentioned, the main differential diagnostic entity is paraneoplastic sensory neuropathy-ganglionitis.

Mellgren and also Leger and their colleagues have stressed the point that a proportion of unexplained polyneuropathies in middle and late life are caused by Sjögren syndrome. The latter authors found typical Sjögren abnormalities in the lip biopsies of 7 of 32 patients with chronic axonal polyneuropathy that could not otherwise be classified. Several other studies have corroborated this finding of inflammatory disruption of the minor salivary glands in obscure neuropathies in women and some men. But this has not been the experience in our clinic, where lip biopsies are routinely performed in patients with sensory neuropathies and rarely show the features of Sjögren disease.

Treatment of the sicca complex and the neuropathic manifestations is symptomatic. Corticosteroids, cyclophosphamide, and chlorambucil have been used when the neuropathy is severe and are indicated when the vasculitis involves renal and pulmonary structures. The recent review of the neurologic manifestations of Sjögren syndrome by Lafitte is recommended.

Idiopathic and Other Sensory Ganglionopathies (Chronic Ataxic Neuropathy) In addition to the pansensory syndrome described above and those that evolve more rapidly as paraneoplastic, postinfectious, or toxic processes (page 1388), there is an idiopathic condition characterized by severe global sensory loss and ataxia. We have encountered several patients with a nondescript distal sensory neuropathy and pronounced ataxia resembling the cases described by Dalakas. The numbness and sensory loss progressed over months and spread to proximal parts of the arms and legs and then to the trunk (either in an escutcheon pattern or as a sensory level). The face and top of the skull were finally involved. Despite severe ataxia and areflexia, muscular power remained normal. Pain was not a problem. Within a year, these patients became completely disabled from the ataxia, unable to walk or even feed themselves. Autonomic failure was another feature in a few of the cases, and one became deaf. Extensive examinations for an *occult cancer, paraproteinemia, Sjögren disease, Refsum disease, autoimmune diseases, and all potential causes of an ataxic neuropathy*, proved to be negative, but it is, of course, possible that some patients had as yet undiscovered tumors.

The motor nerve conduction studies have been normal or slightly affected and the sensory potentials were eventually lost over time (but they may be normal when first tested early in the illness). A puzzling feature in two patients has been an unexpected preservation of many sensory nerve potentials even after a year of illness. In these cases the process is apparently situated in the dorsal roots or the centrally directed sensory axons rather than in the dorsal ganglia. In a few instances there has been a signal change in the posterior columns of the spinal cord. The spinal fluid has generally shown a moderately elevated protein concentration.

Pathologic examination of the sensory ganglia has exposed an inflammatory process identical to that of Sjögren disease in a few cases. Our attempts at treatment using plasma exchanges, IVIG, corticosteroids, and immunosuppressive agents have been unsuccessful.

Migrant Sensory Neuritis (of Wartenberg) The defining feature of this syndrome is a searing and pulling sensation that involves a small cutaneous area of a limb and is evoked by extending or stretching the limb, as occurs when reaching for an object with the extended arm and open hand, kneeling, or pointing the foot. The pain is momentary but leaves in its wake a patch of numbness. Cutaneous sensory nerves must be involved during such a maneuver. Often these are proximal to the most terminal sensory distribution of the nerve, encompassing, for example, a patch on the lateral edge of the hand and the proximal fifth finger or a larger region over the patella (the sites of affection in three of our patients). Recovery of the numbness takes several weeks but may persist if the symptoms are induced repeatedly. Except for patches of cutaneous analgesia, the examination is normal. Selected sensory nerves may show abnormalities in conduction. Matthews and Esiri have listed the many areas that may be affected in a single patient and have described an increase in the endoneurial connective tissue in a biopsied sural nerve. The illness comes in attacks over many years, without symptoms between attacks, sometimes suggesting a diagnosis of multiple sclerosis.

Sensory Perineuritis Under this title, Asbury and colleagues, in 1972, described a patchy, painful, partially remitting affection of distal cutaneous sensory nerves. The pathologic picture was one of inflammatory scarring restricted to the perineurium, with compression of the contained nerve fibers. As with the Wartenberg syndrome (above), the reflexes and motor function are unaffected and digital nerves as well as the medial and lateral branches of the superficial peroneal nerve are the ones most often involved. Matthews and Squier have described a trigeminal and occipital distribution, and one of the patients of Asbury et al also had scalp lesions. A Tinel sign can characteristically be elicited by tapping the skin overlying the involved cutaneous nerves and is indicative of partial nerve damage. The differential diagnosis is from all forms of painful sensory neuropathy. The diagnosis can only be established by biopsy of a very distal cutaneous branch of a sensory nerve. A special group of patients with "burning feet" may have a small-fiber neuropathy that affects intradermal nerve fibers (see further on).

Since the original report by Asbury, the pathologic changes that characterize perineuritis have been described in a number of polyneuropathies, including diabetes and cryoglobulinemia, and in patients with nutritional diseases and malignancy (Sorenson et al). Moreover, the patients displayed a diversity of clinical patterns of neuropathy, mainly mononeuritis multiplex and demyelinating neuropathy. These findings indicate that perineuritis is possibly a nonspecific change. However, a proportion of the idiopathic cases seem to respond to corticosteroids.

Celiac-Sprue Disease Among the multitude of odd neurologic manifestations of this disease (see pages 1228 and 1198) the best known are a cerebellar ataxia and myoclonus. In addition, Hadjivassiliou and colleagues have reported nine patients with a range of neuromuscular disorders in all of whom the neurologic symptoms antedated the diagnosis of the bowel disorder. A nondescript sensorimotor neuropathy was the most frequent complication, but one patient was said to have a mononeuritis multiplex. Antigliadin antibodies and histologic examination of a duodenal biopsy confirmed the diagnosis, and the authors suggested that a search be made for these antibodies in patients with polyneuropathies of obscure origin. It is not clear how many of their cases could be attributed to nutritional deficiency.

Numerous other systemic diseases have reportedly been conjoined with peripheral neuropathy, among them, temporal arteritis. In most of these anecdotal reports it is impossible to interpret the pathogenesis of the nerve disorder.

Syndrome of Polyradiculopathy with or without Meningeal Disease

Patients with disease of multiple spinal nerve roots present with a distinctive constellation of findings, quite different from those of polyneuropathy or multiple mononeuropathies. Muscle weakness due to polyradiculopathy is characteristically asymmetrical and variably distributed in proximal and distal parts of the limbs, reflecting the fact that the involved muscles have a common root innervation (for example, the combination of hamstring and gastrocnemius, or of iliopsoas, quadriceps, and obturators). However, muscles with similar innervation are not necessarily affected to the same degree because of the disproportionate contribution of a given root to each muscle. Sensory loss tends also to be similarly patchy and to involve the proximal segments of limbs as often as the distal ones; as a rule, the sensory findings are less prominent than the weakness. In keeping with the spotty affection of nerve roots, certain tendon reflexes may be spared; a normal ankle jerk combined with an absent knee jerk, for example, is particularly suggestive of a polyradiculopathy (or a lumbar plexopathy). Pain with diseases of the nerve roots is common but not invariable and takes the form of sharp jabs projected into the region innervated by the involved root. As with mononeuritis multiplex, the cumulative effect of multiple root lesions can simulate a polyneuropathy; the tendency for polyradiculopathy to involve proximal muscles is the most helpful distinguishing feature.

An elevated CSF protein and a pleocytosis usually accompany neoplastic or inflammatory meningeal diseases that implicate the nerve roots. Often what appears to be a polyneuropathy on clinical grounds turns out to have an electrophysiologic pattern of root disease at many spinal levels. McGonagle and colleagues estimate that polyradiculopathies account for 5 percent of all cases referred to their laboratory. Careful EMG testing is the most useful ancillary examination and the pattern of muscle denervation can be ascertained by this test. Foremost among the EMG findings is the preservation of sensory nerve potentials in nerves that supply weak and denervated muscles. This demonstrates that the lesion is located proximal to the dorsal root ganglion and spares the peripheral sensory axons. The proximal location of the lesion can be corroborated by finding evidence of denervation in the paraspinal, gluteal, or rhomboid muscles, which are innervated by nerves that arise proximal to their respective plexuses.

Some of the diseases that affect nerve roots solely or predominantly have already been discussed. They can be grouped into three broad categories: diseases of the spinal column that compress roots, infiltrative diseases of the meninges that secondarily involve the roots as they course through the subarachnoid space, and primary neuropathies, usually inflammatory, infectious, or diabetic, that have a predilection for the radicular portion of the nerves.

Among the acute and subacute meningeal radiculopathies, neoplastic infiltration (carcinomatous and lymphomatous) is the most common. Others are Lyme disease, sarcoidosis, herpes genitalis, arachnoiditis and the AIDS-related cauda equina neuritis caused by CMV or independently by EBV. In the past, meningeal syphilis was a common cause. Diseases of the spine, exemplified by lumbar stenosis and cervical spondylosis, commonly impinge on nerve roots, as discussed in Chap. 11. Metastatic carcinoma of the vertebral bodies may compress roots by encroaching on posterolateral recesses of the canal and proximal neural foramina. A chronic lumbosacral radiculopathy associated with a greatly widened lumbar subarachnoid space and dural eventrations surrounding nerve roots may complicate ankylosing spondylitis (see page 221).

Finally, it should be mentioned that one is confronted from time to time by a subacute or chronic polyradiculopathy with an abnormal CSF, in which extensive examination fails to identify any of the diseases enumerated above. This idiopathic form is seen once or twice yearly on our services. Particularly difficult in this respect is a polyradiculopathy that involves the motor roots exclusively, being distinguishable from motor neuron disease by the complete absence, over a long period of time, of widespread denervation or of progressive upper motor neuron signs and differing from anti-GM_1 and related immune motor neuropathies by the absence of conduction block.

SYNDROME OF CHRONIC SENSORIMOTOR POLYNEUROPATHY

In these syndromes, impairment of sensation, weakness, and muscular atrophy progress over a period of many months or years. Within this overall category, two groups are readily distinguished. In the first and *less chronic* of the two groups ("early chronic"), the neuropathy develops over a period of many months or a year or two. Comprising this group are the *acquired* paraneoplastic (which may also appear subacutely), chronic demyelinative, certain metabolic, and the immune-mediated polyneuropathies. Leprous neuritis is the one infectious member of this group and also the one exception to the rule that all chronic neuropathies are more or less symmetrical in distribution. The polyneuropathies that make up the second group are *far more chronic* than the first, evolving over many years ("late chronic"). Constituting this second group are mainly the *heredodegenerative* diseases of the peripheral nervous system.

Acquired ("Early") Forms of Chronic Polyneuropathy

Neuropathies Associated with Paraproteinemias

The occurrence of a chronic sensorimotor polyneuropathy in association with an abnormality of immunoglobulin is being recognized with increasing frequency. The excess protein, also called paraprotein, which gives rise to polyneuropathy, may be an isolated abnormality or a by-product of a plasma cell malignancy, notably multiple myeloma, plasmacytoma, or Waldenstrom macroglobulinemia or one of the special forms of neuropathy associated with acquired amyloidosis. The latter group is discussed further on with the genetic forms of amyloidosis. Several lines of evidence suggest that a pathogenetically active antibody against components of myelin or axon is present in at least some of these cases.

Monoclonal Gammopathy of Undetermined Significance (MGUS, Benign Monoclonal Gammopathy) In recent years, a category of polyneuropathy with isolated monoclonal and polyclonal gammopathies has been added to those of multiple myeloma and solitary plasmacytoma (see reviews of Kyle and Dyck and of Thomas and Willison). This non-neoplastic group is far more common than the malignant one and in our own experience, the monoclonal proteins underlie the largest group of otherwise unexplained neuropathies in older adults. Forssman and colleagues first described a patient with a benign IgM paraproteinemia and a neuropathy, an association that was treated as coincidental until Kahn established a compelling statistical association between them.

These polyneuropathies occur in patients with a monoclonal protein in the blood of less than 3 g/100 mL (usually less than 1.8 g/100 mL), in whom there is no evidence of multiple myeloma or other malignant disease. It should be emphasized that routine serum protein electrophoresis fails to detect the majority of these paraproteins; immunoelectrophoresis (SPEP) or the more sophisticated immunofixation (IEP) testing is required. The bone marrow shows a normal or only mildly increased proportion of plasma cells, which are the ostensible source of the paraprotein, and the plasma cells are not "atypical," as they are in myeloma. Insofar as myeloma becomes manifest in fewer than one-third of patients many years after the gammopathy has been recognized, the condition is now termed monoclonal gammopathy of undetermined significance (MGUS), although the older term, "benign monoclonal gammopathy," is less cumbersome.

Some 6 percent of patients referred to the Mayo Clinic with peripheral neuropathy of unknown cause and as many as 20 percent in our experience and in other series have proved to have a monoclonal paraproteinemia of this type. Despite the fact that IgG is the most frequent paraprotein, the polyneuropathy is associated more often with the IgM class. Combining three large series of patients with neuropathy and monoclonal paraproteinemias (62 patients of Yeung et al, 65 patients of Gosselin et al, and 34 of Simovic et al), there were 96 with IgM, 50 with IgG, and 15 with IgA subclass, or isotype paraproteins. Most have had a *kappa* light chain component. In our experience and that of others, the IgM group has tended to have more sensory findings and a demyelinative type of EMG abnormality compared with the IgG group. However, with the exception of the anti-MAG syndrome (see below), we have not found the degree difference in clinical features and response to treatment that has been reported by others (Simovic et al).

An identical but infrequent condition exists in which only the light chain component of an immunoglobulin is produced by the plasma cells and the paraprotein is found exclusively in the urine (similar to the Bence-Jones protein of myeloma). A proportion of all these patients will develop myeloma or Waldenstrom disease within 10 years, but in the large majority of our patients there has been no transformation to a malignancy.

The neuropathy of monoclonal gammopathy affects mainly males in the sixth and seventh decades of life. The onset is insidious, with numbness and paresthesias of the feet and then of the hands, followed by a symmetrical weakness and wasting of these parts. In some patients sensory signs predominate and the tendon reflexes are preserved or only diminished in the early part of the illness. The neuropathy is usually slowly progressive, rarely remitting and relapsing. The Raynaud phenomenon is observed in some, even in the absence of a cryoprotein. The CSF typically shows an elevation of the protein concentration in the range of 50 to 100 mg/dL, not due to passive diffusion of the paraprotein into the CSF.

The majority of reported cases of monoclonal gammopathy have a demyelinating or mixed axonal-demyelinating pattern by EMG, but we found 16 patients with predominantly axonal features in a series of 36 consecutive cases during a 5-year period. With the exception of less severe sensory loss and reduced but preserved tendon reflexes in some of the axonal cases, the axonal and demyelinating groups could not be distinguished on clinical grounds or by their response to therapy (Gorson et al). Sural nerve biopsies have shown an extensive loss of myelinated fibers of all sizes; unmyelinated fibers are mostly spared; hypertrophic changes are present in about half the cases (Smith et al). The latter authors found the monoclonal IgM antibody bound to the surviving myelin sheaths, and Latov and coworkers have shown that the serum IgM fraction displays antimyelin activity.

Although more than a dozen specific antibodies against myelin have been identified in these neuropathies, the most important ones, present in 50 to 75 percent of patients with IgM-associated neuropathies, are those that react with a myelin-associated glycoprotein (MAG) or with related glycolipid or sulfatide components of myelin, referred to as SGPG and SPLPG. An association has been reported between the latter antibodies and infection with CMV. Deep sensory loss with gait imbalance and a Romberg sign are common findings in the IgM group with anti-MAG activity, but weakness tends to appear late in the illness. Other, mainly IgM antineural antibodies have a more tentative connection to polyneuropathy. Polyclonal IgM antibodies against the GM_1 antigen of myelin are linked with multifocal motor conduction block, described under "Chronic Inflammatory Demyelinating Polyradiculoneuropathy (CIDP)," below. It is reasonable to assume that IgG monoclonal gammopathies are also capable of causing chronic neuropathies, but the evidence is less compelling; it has been suggested that in many reported instances this association is coincidental. Certainly IgG gammopathies are frequent in older individuals; when treated similarly to the IgM group, they seem to respond as well or better.

In most cases of uncomplicated monoclonal gammopathy, plasma exchange provides transient improvement for several weeks to months, somewhat more so in patients with IgG and IgA types of neuropathy than in those with the IgM type (Dyck et al, 1991). The treatment regimen is the same as for GBS, a total volume of approximately 250 mL/kg being exchanged in each of four to six treatments.

In patients found to have serum activity against specific components of myelin (MAG), plasma exchange alone has effected transient improvement in 40 percent but sustained periods of improvement in only 10 percent of our patients. This discouraging outcome is particularly true for slowly progressive cases of severe ataxia with marked distal sensory loss. In some patients, the response to immunosuppression with intravenous cyclophosphamide or fludarabine, or oral chlorambucil, coupled with plasma exchanges has been somewhat better. Improvement with high doses of infused immunoglobulin (IVIG) has not been effective according to some reports, but half of our cases with typical paraproteinemia and 20 percent of those with anti-MAG neuropathy have improved for at least a brief time. In almost all instances the plasma exchanges and immunosuppressive treatment must be repeated at intervals of one to several months as determined by the clinical course. This group of neuropathies does not appear to respond to corticosteroids.

Osteosclerotic Myeloma (POEMS Syndrome) and Multiple Myeloma The neuropathy of *multiple myeloma* has already been mentioned, under "Paraneoplastic Neuropathy." Polyneuropathy complicates 13 to 14 percent of cases of multiple myeloma and has a disproportionately high association with the osteosclerotic form. An abnormal and excessive gamma globulin (with mainly the *kappa* light chain component in multiple myeloma and *lambda* in the osteosclerotic type) is found in the serum of 80 percent of patients with myelomatous neuropathy.

In many patients with osteosclerotic myeloma, the sensorimotor polyneuropathy—which tends to be of moderate severity—is associated with organomegaly, endocrinopathy, elevated *M* protein, and skin changes (mainly hypertrichosis and skin thickening) making up the acronym *POEMS* (also referred to as the Crow-Fukase syndrome in Japan, where the disease is prevalent). The neuropathy in these patients is not fundamentally different from that of patients in whom the systemic features are lacking. Also, in many cases, there is the lymphadenopathy of Castleman disease, as discussed earlier. A characteristic feature of the osteosclerotic related polyneuropathy is a greatly elevated CSF protein. The diagnosis can be suspected from the presence of a paraprotein in the blood, often polyclonal or biclonal rather than monoclonal, and possessing a lambda light chain component. The diagnosis requires the demonstration of the osteosclerotic myeloma by a radiographic survey of the long bones, pelvis, spine, and skull (a bone scan may miss the sclerotic lesions) and a bone marrow examination, which shows a moderate elevation in the proportion of well-differentiated plasma cells. In most of our cases there have been several bone lesions concentrated in the ribs and spine; the skull and long bones may harbor such lesions as well, or the lesions may be single. The neuropathy that complicates a solitary plasmacytoma may improve markedly following irradiation of the bone lesion; multiple lesions are treated with chemotherapy (melphalan and prednisone) and some improvement or stabilization in the neuropathy can be expected. Treatment with plasma exchange yields uncertain results.

Waldenstrom Macroglobulinemia *Macroglobulinemia* was the term applied by Waldenstrom to a systemic condition occurring mainly in elderly persons and characterized by fatigue, weakness, and a bleeding diathesis. Immunoelectrophoretic examination of the blood discloses a marked increase in the IgM plasma fraction. A significant proportion of patients with hyperproteinemia have a hyperviscosity state manifest by a diffuse slowing of retinal and cerebral circulation (*Bing-Neel syndrome*)—giving rise to episodic confusion, coma, and sometimes strokes—in addition to peripheral neuropathy. The latter may evolve subacutely but is more often chronic in nature, and either asymmetrical in a multiple nerve trunk pattern (particularly at the onset of the neuropathy) or in a symmetrical and distal sensorimotor pattern. Our few cases have been of the latter type, very slowly progressive, and limited to the feet and legs, with mild sensory ataxia and loss of knee and ankle jerks. The CSF protein is usually elevated and the globulin fraction increased. In a case recorded by Rowland et al, the polyneuropathy was purely motor and simulated motor neuron disease; other cases of this type, albeit rare, have been brought to our attention.

Cryoglobulinemia As mentioned previously in the section on vasculitic neuropathies, *cryoglobulinemia* is characterized by a serum protein that precipitates on cooling. The cryoglobulins are usually IgG or IgM. Cryoglobulinemia may occur without any apparent associated condition (essential cryoglobulinemia) but as frequently it accompanies a wide variety of disorders such as myeloma, lymphoma, connective tissue disease, chronic infection, and, particularly, hepatitis C. Peripheral neuropathy occurs in a small proportion of both types of cases. Occasionally the neuropathy evolves over a period of a few days and remits rapidly. More often it takes the form of a distal symmetrical sensorimotor loss, which develops insidiously in association with the Raynaud phenomenon and purpuric eruptions of the skin. Initially, the neuropathic symptoms consist only of pain and paresthesias that may be precipitated by exposure to cold. Later, weakness and wasting develop, more in the legs than in the arms and more or less in the distribution of the vascular changes. Less often, there is a mononeuropathy multiplex, with severe denervation in the territory of the involved nerves (Garcia-Bragado et al). In a few of our cases, the two neuropathic syndromes have been combined.

Any of the paraproteinemic states may be associated with amyloid polyneuropathy. This subject is accorded a separate section, below.

The pathology of the neuropathies associated with macroglobulinemia and cryoglobulinemia has been incompletely studied, and the mechanisms by which these disorders cause neuropathy are quite uncertain. One presumes that some component of the paraprotein acts as an antineural antibody or that deposition of the protein is toxic. In our most thoroughly autopsied case, there was widespread distal axonal degeneration of nondescript type without amyloid deposition or inflammatory cells; yet in other reported cases, amyloid has been found. Immune deposits of IgM had impregnated the inner layers of the perineurium in the case reported by Ongerboer de Visser and colleagues. Dalakas and Engel have made similar observations. Possibly the neuropathy of cryoglobulinemia is due to the intravascular deposition of cryoglobulins, causing a vasculitic ischemia, as alluded to earlier (Chad et al).

In the macroglobulinemic neuropathies, the use of prednisone, the alkylating agent chlorambucil, cyclophosphamide, or plasma exchange has at times led to improvement in the systemic and neuropathic symptoms, although recovery has been incomplete.

Primary (Nonfamilial, AL) Amyloid Neuropathy There are sporadic instances, far more common than familial ones, in which a peripheral neuropathy is associated with amyloid deposition in the heart, kidneys, and gastrointestinal tract (called *primary systemic amyloidosis* to distinguish it from the inherited varierties). In most cases, the amyloid is derived from a paraproteinemia, but the proportion of "benign" and malignant sources of the protein varies from one series to another. In the large series of Kyle and Bayrd, 26 percent of patients with primary amyloidosis had a plasma cell dyscrasia. In 90 percent of cases of primary amyloidosis, there is a monoclonal protein (rarely polyclonal) in the blood; macrophage enzymes cleave the larger immunoglobulin molecules to form light chains that make up the actual amyloid deposits in tissue, or the plasma cells produce light chains directly ("light-chain disease"). Lambda light chain predominates in the idiopathic variety and kappa light chain in myeloma. In a few cases the light chain is found only in the urine (Bence Jones protein). In primary amyloidosis there is no evidence of preceding or coexisting disease (except the association with paraproteinemia or multiple myeloma), in distinction to secondary amyloidosis, which is associated with chronic infection or other chronic disease outside the nervous system. As a rule, secondary amyloidosis is not associated with neuropathy. Familial amyloidosis, a third variety, is at times associated with neuropathy (see page 1423).

Primary amyloidosis is mainly a disease of older men, the median age at the time of diagnosis being 65 years. In our clinical material, the majority of the patients with AL have had peripheral neuropathy, but in other series fewer than one-third were affected in this way (Kyle and Dyck). The neuropathic symptoms and signs are similar to those of hereditary amyloid polyneuropathy, but the progress of the disease is considerably more rapid. The initial symptoms are sensory—numbness, paresthesias, and often acral pain—and the signs are characteristic of involvement of small-diameter sensory fibers (loss of pain and thermal sensation). Weakness follows, initially limited to the feet but becoming more extensive as the disease progresses and eventually affecting the hands and arms. Loss of large fiber–mediated sensation may appear. Twenty-five percent of patients have a carpal tunnel syndrome from infiltration of the flexor retinaculum.

Autonomic involvement can be severe and becomes evident early in the course of the illness; several of our patients presented with disturbances of gastrointestinal motility, especially episodic diarrhea, or with orthostatic symptoms and also with impotence and bladder disturbances. The pupils may react slowly, and there may be a reduction in sweating. An infiltrative *amyloid myopathy* occurs as a rare complication of the disease; it presents as an enlargement and induration of many muscles, particularly those of the tongue (macroglossia), pharynx, and larynx. Progression of the illness is relatively rapid, the mean survival being 12 to 24 months. A more indolent neuropathy that evolves over years is not likely to be due to amyloid, though we have seen a few such cases. Death is usually due to the renal, cardiac, or gastrointestinal effects of amyloid deposits, the manifestations of which are already evident in at least half of the patients who present with neuropathy. A nephrotic syndrome is particularly characteristic.

Analysis of the serum and urine, searching for an abnormal paraprotein (found in most of our patients), followed by a microscopic examination of abdominal fat pad, gingival, or rectal biopsy for amyloid, are the most useful screening tests. If a sensory neuropathy or evidence of organ infiltration is evident, biopsy of the sural nerve or the involved viscera has a high diagnostic yield for amyloid. The liver is positive in all cases and the kidney has amyloid infiltration in about 85 percent. In several of our patients with a clinical syndrome typical of amyloid neuropathy, amyloid was not found in the sural nerve; only after sequential biopsy of numerous sites (fat pad, kidney, liver) was the diagnosis established. If the sural nerve is severely depopulated of nerve fibers, the amount of congophilic staining and the characteristic birefringence may be meager and yield a spuriously negative result. It is also critical to assure the accuracy of congophilic staining by comparison with positive and negative control tissue from the same laboratory. The CSF has a normal or moderately elevated protein concentration.

The prognosis is dismal and attempts at immunomodulation, immunosuppression (which may help the renal disease), or removal of amyloid by plasma exchange have been marginally effective. The most recent approach has been with stem cell replacement (harvested from the patient) after bone marrow suppression with high doses of melphalan. Several such patients have survived for several years with marked improvement in the neuropathy. The pain may be treated with transcutaneous fentanyl patches or with oral narcotic medications, and orthostasis responds to the use of leg stockings and mineralocorticoids.

The differential diagnosis of acquired amyloid neuropathy includes the more slowly evolving familial types (see further on), the myelomatous varieties, toxic and nutritional small-fiber neuropathies, and an idiopathic small-fiber sensory neuropathy, which we have encountered more frequently than amyloidosis.

Chronic Inflammatory Demyelinating Polyradiculoneuropathy (CIDP) This form of polyneuropathy was separated from acute inflammatory polyradiculopathy, or GBS, by Austin in 1958 on the basis of a chronic relapsing course, enlargement of nerves, and responsiveness to steroids. Undoubtedly there are clinical similarities between these disorders. Both are widespread polyradiculoneuropathies, usually with cytoalbuminologic dissociation of the CSF; both exhibit nerve conduction abnormalities with the characteristics of a demyelinating neuropathy (reduced conduction velocity and partial conduction block in motor nerves). Pathologically, both show a similar type of inflammatory change. But there are also important differences, the most evident of which are their modes of evolution and prognosis. As a rule, CIDP begins insidiously and evolves slowly, either in a steadily progressive or stepwise manner, attaining its maximum severity after several months or even a year or longer. From the beginning it may be asymmetrical. In only a small proportion of patients (16 percent in the series of McCombe et al, and the same proportion in our own series) does the disease evolve at a tempo that mimics GBS. Thereafter it runs a persistent relapsing or fluctuating course, or it may simply worsen slowly and progressively.

In contrast to acute GBS, many cases of CIDP respond favorably to the administration of prednisone. Antecedent infections can be identified far less regularly in patients with CIDP than in those with GBS. Finally, CIDP may be distinct immunologically, insofar as certain HLA antigens (A1, B8, DRw3, Dw3) reportedly occur with greater frequency in patients with CIDP than in the normal population or in patients with GBS (Adams et al). However, as mentioned above, Hughes has described a group of patients with polyneuritis in whom weakness progressed steadily for 4 to 12 weeks and who responded to corticosteroids, thus blurring the distinction between GBS and CIDP and suggesting that the two are related rather than separate entities.

The EMG findings of demyelination in CIDP essentially define the illness—multifocal conduction block as described in Chap. 45, prolonged distal latencies (distal block), nerve conduction slowing to less than 80 percent of normal in several nerves, loss of late responses, and dispersion of the compound muscle action potentials; one or more of these changes have been present in more than three-quarters of our patients (Gorson et al). In the early stages of the disease these changes must be carefully sought by testing multiple nerves at several sites along the course of each nerve. After several months, these findings are often associated with some degree of axonal change (30 percent of our series), but the fundamental process continues to be one of multiple foci of demyelination. Even more salient findings in such patients are the absence of denervation changes despite weakness and reduced amplitude of the motor action potential, and weakness of a muscle that can be made to contract by stimulating the nerve distally, indicative of a demyelinating conduction block at a proximal site.

Several large series of CIDP have been reported. Dyck and colleagues (1975) studied 53 patients in whom the neuropathy progressed for more than 6 months. The clinical course was monophasic and slowly progressive in about one-third of their patients, stepwise and progressive in another third, and relapsing in the remaining third. The periods of worsening or improvement were measured in weeks or months. Infections and inoculations in the 3 months preceding the onset of CIDP were no more frequent than in the population at large. Weakness of the limbs, particularly of the proximal leg muscles, or numbness, paresthesias, and dysesthesias of the hands and feet were the initial symptoms. In 45 of the 53 patients, the signs were those of a mixed sensorimotor polyneuropathy with weakness of the shoulder, upper arm, and thigh muscles in addition to motor and sensory loss in the distal parts of the limbs. In 5 patients the neuropathy was purely motor, and in 3, purely sensory. Cranial nerve abnormalities were distinctly unusual. Enlarged, firm nerves were found in 6 patients; thus CIDP has to be distinguished from other chronic and recurrent neuropathies, particularly the hereditary ones.

In the series of McCombe et al, comprising 92 patients, two major subgroups were recognized—*relapsing* (corresponding to the relapsing and stepwise progressive groups of Dyck et al) and *nonrelapsing* (corresponding to Dyck's monophasic and gradually progressive groups). In our own series of more than 100 patients, we have been impressed with unusual patterns of clinical presentation in one-third of patients. Numbness and weakness of the hands before the feet are similarly affected, unusual in other polyneuropathies, occurred in about 10 percent of our cases (Gorson et al). A sensory ataxic form, a purely motor form, and mononeuropathies superimposed on a mild generalized polyneuropathy each accounted for approximately 7 percent of the cases. A small proportion, fewer than 10 percent, began as acute GBS but continued to progress or relapsed in the following months.

Other comprehensive accounts have been given by Barohn, Cornblath, Dyck, and Hughes and their associates. All these authors place the demyelinating neuropathies that progress for over 8 to 12 weeks within the CIDP category. Also recognized is the frequency (up to one-quarter of the patients in some series, far less often in our experience) with which systemic conditions such as paraproteinemia, lymphoma, an undifferentiated reactive adenopathy, and lupus accompany the neuropathy. These associations create problems in nosology that can be reconciled by labeling a given case as "CIDP with paraproteinemia" or whatever the underlying disease may be, thus separating it from the idiopathic-inflammatory variety.

Several polyneuropathies that share many of the features of CIDP have been given separate names because of some unique clinical or electrophysiologic attribute. These include *multifocal motor neuropathy* and *multifocal conduction block*. The latter seems to be clearly a type of CIDP; its main feature is a block of sensory and motor conduction across the same site in a limited number of nerves. Multifocal motor neuropathy, on the other hand, shows multiple focal sites of block of motor conduction alone, without any change in sensory conduction. The distinction between these two entities has been obscured by the finding of mild but consistent demyelination in sensory nerve biopsies from patients with multifocal motor neuropathy (Corse et al). Both of these syndromes may begin with a partial mononeuropathy, an uncharacteristic finding in most cases of CIDP. While these conditions are best considered for the moment as types of CIDP, there is a high concordance of multifocal motor neuropathy with a particular antibody, anti-GM_1, against a ganglioside component of peripheral myelin (Pestronk et al). For this reason, some view this illness as belonging to the class of paraproteinemic neuropathies (see above and Simmons et al).

The CSF protein is elevated in 80 percent of patients with CIDP, typically in the range of 75 to 200 mg/dL. In a few instances there is papilledema and a pseudotumor syndrome, corresponding to extremely high levels of CSF protein (usually >/1000 mg/dL). Elevation of the CSF gamma globulin and a mild lymphocytic pleocytosis are said to occur in some 10 percent of patients (more consistently in those who are HIV-seropositive), a considerably higher percentage than in our series.

In biopsy material (sural nerve), a few of the patients are found to have interstitial and perivascular infiltrates of inflammatory cells, although one expects that most would show these changes if sufficient nerves could be sampled. As in GBS, the demyelination appears to be effected by T cells and macrophages within the endoneurium but also in the perineurium. Myelinated fibers are lost to a varying degree, and many of the remaining ones are seen to be undergoing degeneration or show the changes of segmental demyelination or demyelination-remyelination. So-called onion-bulb formations are conspicuous in the recurrent and relapsing cases. The few complete autopsy studies have shown only minimal or patchy inflammation and a considerable degree of axonal damage. The presence of endoneurial and subperineurial edema has been emphasized by Prineas and McLeod and by Pollard.

The status of a predominantly axonal polyneuropathy that simulates CIDP and responds to the same immunomodulating treatments is unclear (Uncini et al; Gorson and Ropper). The present authors have the impression that it is an immune mediated neuropathy in the spectrum of CIDP.

Treatment Several trials have shown benefit from the intravenous infusion of high doses of gamma globulin (2 g/kg in divided infusions over 4 or 5 days), and we can verify this. More than half of our patients have responded to this treatment, albeit for only several weeks to months, after which the infusions must be repeated. However, efforts to spare patients the side effects of indefinite prednisone administration make this mode of therapy a reasonable alternative. Some patients have been treated with repeated infusions for many years without ill effects. IVIG is also effective in the treatment of multifocal motor neuropathy, but sustained improvement usually requires the addition of another immunosuppressant, such as oral cyclophosphamide. Patients who require treatment at such short intervals as to be impractical have sometimes benefited from the addition of small doses of prednisone. The main drawbacks of IVIG are its expense and the several hours required for its infusion; rare instances of nephrotic syndrome, aseptic meningitis (both now infrequent), serum sickness, thrombolic arterial occlusion, and hypotension have been reported, particularly if the infusion is too rapid.

Close to half of these patients also respond well to plasma exchange. In a prospective double-blind trial, Dyck and colleagues found that plasma exchange, administered twice weekly for 3 weeks, had a beneficial effect on both the neurologic disability and nerve conduction. The response to plasma exchange in our patients has been comparable to that obtained with IVIG and with steroids, some patients responding to only one type of treatment. However, the beneficial effects in many patients begin to subside in 10 to 14 days. In some cases these responses last longer, as reported by Dyck and by Hahn et al. For this reason we prefer to try plasma exchange or immune globulin before committing a patient to long-term treatment with prednisone. When the response is clear, three or four brief series of plasma exchange or infusions of immune globulin often suffice, again supplemented by small doses of prednisone when frequent treatments become impractical. When these measures prove unsatisfactory, we have added cyclophosphamide or cyclosporine, but we have been unable to draw any firm conclusions as to their effectiveness.

Corticosteroids were formerly the mainstay of therapy, but most patients become dependent on the medication and the general approach has shifted to utilizing these medications as a third resort, or as an adjunct to one of the above-mentioned treatments. A usual regimen begins with 80 mg of prednisone that is tapered over months to the lowest effective dose. We have not had much success with daily doses of less than 25 mg. A number of patients will not respond to corticosteroids within 1 or 2 months but will do so if treatment is continued. The drug produces a tremor or may exaggerate the one caused by the neuropathy. Should a sustained trial of prednisone therapy prove unsuccessful, a course of azathioprine (for at least 3 months), 3 mg/kg in a single daily dose, has been recommended (Dalakas and Engel), but a controlled trial has failed to show benefit from this combination and we have had little success with it.

Some patients who have failed to benefit from the aforementioned treatments have improved in response to the administration of α-interferon (Gorson et al). We have no explanation for the remarkable improvement and continued good health of a few patients after a severe bacterial infection (Ropper).

It has been stated that patients with discrete relapses have a better prognosis than those with a progressive course. In McCombe's series, 73 percent were said to have made a good recovery, but the long-term outcome in this disease has generally been poor in our experience, involving decades of disability and dependence on treatment. In a small number of patients, fewer than 10 percent, the disease burns out after many years and treatment can be withdrawn.

Uremic Polyneuropathy Polyneuropathy is probably the most common complication of chronic renal failure. Robson estimated that it complicates end-stage renal failure in two-thirds of patients about to begin dialysis therapy. Bolton's figures are much the same; 70 percent of patients being dialyzed regularly had uremic polyneuropathy, and in 30 percent the neuropathy was of moderate or severe degree. As in the original description by Asbury, Victor, and Adams, the neuropathy takes the form of a painless, progressive, symmetrical sensorimotor paralysis of the legs and then of the arms. In some patients, the neuropathy begins with burning dysesthesias of the feet or with sensations of creeping, crawling, and itching of the legs and thighs, which tend to be worse at night and are relieved by movement ("restless legs" syndrome, page 412). Renal failure accompanied by diabetes may give rise to a particularly severe neuropathy.

The combination of muscle weakness and atrophy, areflexia, sensory loss, and the graded distribution of the neurologic deficit in the limbs leaves little doubt about the neuropathic nature of the disorder. Usually the neuropathy evolves slowly over many months, at times in subacute fashion. Rare instances of a more acute sensorimotor polyneuropathy have been reported as well, occurring mainly in diabetics receiving peritoneal dialysis (see page 1388; Asbury et al; Ropper). Also, a uremic polymyositis with hypophosphatemia has been described (Layzer). The neuropathy has been observed with all types of chronic kidney disease. More important to the development of neuropathy than the nature of the renal lesion is the duration and severity of the renal failure and symptomatic uremia (not merely azotemia).

With long-term hemodialysis, the symptoms and signs of polyneuropathy stabilize, but they improve in relatively few patients. In fact, rapid hemodialysis may occasionally worsen the polyneuropathy temporarily. Peritoneal dialysis appears to be more successful than hemodialysis in improving the neuropathy but this has not been studied systematically. Complete recovery, occurring over a period of 6 to 12 months, usually follows successful renal transplantation, for the reason given below.

The pathologic findings are those of a nonspecific axonal degeneration. In rapidly progressive cases, there is a tendency for the large fibers to be affected; this is evident particularly on electrophysiologic testing. The changes are most intense in the distal segments of the nerves, with the expected chromatolysis of their cell bodies.

The cause of uremic polyneuropathy is unknown. The "middle molecule" theory is the most plausible. The end stage of renal failure is associated with the accumulation of toxic substances in the range of 300 to 2000 mol wt. Furthermore, the concentration of these substances, which include methylguanidine and myoinositol, has been shown to correlate with the degree of neurotoxicity (Funck-Brentano et al). These toxins (and the clinical signs of neuropathy) are not greatly reduced by chronic hemodialysis. On the other hand, the transplanted kidney effectively eliminates substances of wide-ranging molecular weights, which would account for the invariable improvement of neuropathy after transplantation.

Alcoholic–Nutritional and Subacute Diabetic Neuropathy In all patients with alcoholic-nutritional polyneuropathy who for some reason remain untreated, the weakness and atrophy of the legs, and to a lesser extent the arms, may reach an extreme degree. Thus this disease, though subacute in its evolution, becomes a frequent cause of chronic polyneuropathy. Certain cases of diabetic neuropathy behave similarly.

Leprous Polyneuritis This is the classic example of an infectious neuritis, being due to the direct invasion of nerves by the acid-fast *Mycobacterium leprae*. The disease is still frequent in India and Central Africa, but there are many lesser endemic foci, including parts of South America and of Florida, Texas, and Louisiana that border on the Gulf of Mexico.

The initial lesion in leprosy is an innocuous-appearing skin macule or papule, which is often hypopigmented and lacking in sensation and is caused by the invasion of cutaneous nerves by *M. leprae*. The disease may progress no further than this stage, which is spoken of as *indeterminate leprosy*, or it may evolve in several ways, depending mainly upon the resistance of the host. The bacilli may be locally invasive, producing a circumscribed epithelioid granuloma that implicates cutaneous and subcutaneous nerves and results in a characteristic patch of superficial sensory loss (*tuberculoid leprosy*). The subcutaneous sensory nerves may be palpably enlarged. If a large nerve in the vicinity of the granuloma is invaded (the ulnar, median, peroneal, posterior auricular, and facial nerves are most frequently affected in this way), a sensorimotor deficit in the distribution of that nerve is added to the patch of cutaneous anesthesia.

Lack of resistance permits the proliferation and hematogenous spread of bacilli and the diffuse infiltration of skin, ciliary bodies, testes, lymph nodes, and nerves (*lepromatous leprosy*). Widespread invasion of the cutaneous nerves produces a symmetrical pattern of pain and temperature loss, involving the pinnae of the ears as well as the dorsal surfaces of hands, forearms, and feet and anterolateral aspects of the legs—a distribution that is apparently determined by the relative coolness of these parts of the skin. Eventually the anesthesia spreads to involve most of the cutaneous surface. Extensive sensory loss is followed by loss of motor function owing to invasion of muscular nerves where they lie closest to the skin (the ulnar nerve is the most vulnerable). There is a loss of sweating in areas of sensory loss, but otherwise the autonomic nervous system is unaffected. In distinction to other polyneuropathies, tendon reflexes are usually preserved in leprosy despite widespread sensory loss. Probably this depends upon sparing of the muscular and larger sensory nerves. Because of widespread anesthesia, injuries may pass unrecognized, with resultant infections, trophic changes, and loss of tissue. Variations in host immunity result in patterns of disease having both tuberculoid and lepromatous characteristics (dimorphous leprosy).

All forms of leprosy require long-term treatment with sulfones (dapsone being the most commonly used), rifampin, and clofazimine. The skin lesions of lepromatous leprosy are responsive to thalidomide, which itself may cause a sensory neuropathy (page 1286; Barnhill and McDougall).

Polyneuropathy with Hypothyroidism Although characteristic disturbances of skeletal muscle are known to complicate hypothyroidism (see Chap. 51), the demonstration of a polyneuropathy has been infrequent. However, a number of elderly myxedematous patients complain of weakness and numbness of the feet, legs, and, to a lesser extent, hands, for which no other explanation can be found. Loss of reflexes, diminution in vibratory, joint-position, and touch-pressure sensations, and weakness in the distal parts of the limbs are the usual findings. The neuropathic manifestations are seldom severe. Nerve conduction velocities are significantly diminished, and the protein content of the CSF is usually increased, to more than 100 mg/dL in some patients; possibly this is a reflection of the increased protein content of the serum. The subjective improvement and complete or near-complete reversibility of neuropathic signs following treatment with thyroid hormones provides convincing evidence of a hypothyroid etiology. In biopsies of nerve, an edematous protein infiltration of the endoneurium and perineurium, a kind of metachromatic mucoid material, has been seen. Dyck and Lambert noted segmental demyelination in teased fiber preparations. In electron-microscopic sections, a slight increase in glycogen, acid mucopolysaccharides, and aggregates of glycogen and cytoplasmic laminar bodies in Schwann cells have been observed by others.

Polyneuropathy of sensorimotor type has also been observed in association with chronic lymphocytic thyroiditis and alopecia (Hart et al).

Chronic Benign Sensory Polyneuropathy of the Elderly The authors have observed numerous cases of a benign, relatively nonprogressive sensory polyneuropathy in elderly patients. Tingling paresthesias of feet and lower legs, sensory loss, and absent ankle reflexes are the usual findings. The hands may be mildly affected but leg weakness and imbalance are absent or trifling. Laboratory studies may be normal or reveal minimally altered sensory conduction, but the evaluation has usually not been extensive, and therefore it is difficult to say if Sjögren syndrome or another underlying disease is responsible.

The most common variant of this form of chronic sensory polyneuropathy is one that affects mainly elderly women, who complain of slowly progressive (over years) *burning and numbness of the feet*, ascending to the ankles or midcalves. There are few findings on examination; often only a mild loss of pinprick and thermal sensation, and ankle reflexes that may or may not be reduced. There is little or no progression over the years.

Electrophysiologic tests are likewise normal or virtually so, a few showing diminished sural nerve potentials and minor changes of motor amplitudes. When these changes cannot be ascribed to diabetes, malnutrition, or medications, a substantial group of patients is left in need of symptomatic relief. Some have been helped by gabapentin or by antidepressants (amitryptiline, desipramine, or sertraline) and capsaicin cream applied nightly to the soles and toes. Surprisingly, a few of the more severe cases have apparently responded to gamma globulin infusions, but these observations require corroboration (Gorson and Ropper, 1995). In a number of such cases with burning feet, the intradermal sensory nerves are said to be depleted in skin biopsy specimens, but the meaning of this finding is not certain (Periquet et al).

Syndrome of Multiple Symmetrical Lipomas with Sensorimotor Polyneuropathy Whereas the usual cutaneous lipomas have no neurologic accompaniments, this clinical curiosity, known as Lannois-Bensaude disease, consists of symmetrical lipomas of the neck and shoulders that are associated with polyneuropathy and sometimes deafness. A mitochondrial disorder is suspected. Details can be found in the review by Neumann.

GENETIC ("LATE") FORMS OF CHRONIC POLYNEUROPATHY

In this category of chronic polyneuropathy, symptoms evolve gradually over a period of many years. The neuropathic disease may be remarkably restricted, as in familial analgesia with foot ulcers, or extensive, as in chronic amyloidosis and familial peroneal muscular atrophy. The time of onset of these very chronic neuropathies is often uncertain, although the heredofamilial types are obviously present from early life. In infants, the condition may be mistaken for muscular dystrophy or infantile muscular atrophy until sensory testing becomes possible. In the developing child, whose musculature naturally increases in power and volume, it may be difficult to decide whether the disease is progressive. Ataxia of the limbs may be pronounced at a stage when sensory loss exceeds paresis. As characteristic as the chronicity is a symmetry of neurologic findings and EMG abnormalities (except one variety that causes a susceptibility to compression neuropathies).

Pes cavus and, in extreme forms, talipes equinus are strong indicators of the early onset of inherited polyneuropathy. In the later stages of these neuropathies, trophic changes of skin and bone in distal parts of the limbs indicate involvement of small (pain) fibers, and the presence of deformed and degenerated joints (Charcot joint) indicates a loss of large proprioceptive fibers. The mutilating effects are the result of repeated injury to analgesic parts and to a lack of autonomic vascular reflexes. The atrophy of muscle and trophic changes in the skin are more marked than in the acute and subacute forms of polyneuropathy; for this reason, the more chronic syndrome must be differentiated from the other forms of severe muscular atrophy, i.e., motor system disease, the distal type of muscular dystrophy, and syringomyelia.

The CSF protein content may remain mildly or moderately elevated over a period of years. Most of the inherited neuropathies are axonal in nature when studied by EMG with the notable exception of the commonest variety, Charcot-Marie-Tooth disease type 1. Another distinctive feature of hereditary neuropathy is the uniformity of the electrophysiologic changes, e.g., the same degree of slowing of nerve conduction velocity in all the nerves of the lower limbs, a feature that distinguishes this group from all acquired neuropathies.

There has been much difficulty in classifying the chronic familial polyneuropathies. The time-honored clinical classification divides them into two broad groups, each with several subgroups: (1) a mixed sensorimotor group, the prototype of which is Charcot-Marie-Tooth disease, and (2) a predominantly sensory type, often with autonomic involvement and trophic lesions. Recent genetic findings have not greatly simplified the matter of classification but have permitted the creation of a nosology that more or less parallels the clinical one. The proposed classifications in Tables 46-1 and 46-2 represent an attempt to conciliate the clinical and genetic data.

Of this large and varied group, only the sensorimotor Charcot-Marie-Tooth type is likely to be seen with any regularity by neurologists and general physicians. Some hereditary neuropathies are associated with certain abnormalities of the CNS, whereas most neuropathies are relatively pure. Logically, we have discussed several of the hereditary polyneuropathies in which a metabolic abnormality has been discovered in Chap. 37. The other inherited neuropathies are considered here.

Inherited Polyneuropathies of Predominantly Sensory Type

Common to the several diseases comprised by this group are insensitivity to pain, lancinating pains, and ulcers of the feet and hands, leading to osteomyelitis, osteolysis, stress fractures, and recurrent episodes of cellulitis. Since similar symptoms and signs occur in syringomyelia, leprosy, and tabes dorsalis, there is considerable uncertainty in older writings on this subject as to whether the reported cases were examples of one of these diseases or of hereditary neuropathy. According to Dyck, it was Leplat in 1846 who first described plantar ulcers (*mal perforant du pied*), followed by Nelaton in 1852. Morvan in 1883 reported his observations of adult patients who had developed suppuration of the pulps of insensitive fingers (whitlows). It is now generally agreed that Morvan's cases were examples of syringomyelia, whereas the family described by Nelaton was probably an example of the recessive form of childhood sensory polyneuropathy, since familial syringomyelia in children is practically unknown. We agree with Dyck that most such cases are examples of sensory polyneuropathy.

Mutilating Hereditary (Dominant) Sensory Polyneuropathy in Adults The characteristic features of this group of polyneuropathies are an autosomal dominant mode of inheritance and onset of symptoms in the second decade or later. Characteristically there is involvement mainly of the feet, with calluses of the soles and, later, episodes of blistering, ulceration, and lymphangitis followed by osteomyelitis and osteolysis, shooting pains, distal sensory loss with greater affection of pain and thermal sensation than of touch and pressure, loss of sweating, diminution or absence of tendon reflexes, and only slight loss of muscle power.

The plantar ulcer overlying the head of a metatarsal bone is the most dreaded complication, since it may develop into an osteomyelitis. Infection of the pulp of the fingers and paronychias are uncommon. Some patients have a mild pes cavus and weakness of the peroneal and pretibial muscles, with foot drop and steppage gait. Lancinating pains may occur in the legs, thighs, and shoulders, and, exceptionally, the pain may last for days or longer and be as disabling as that of tabes dorsalis; however, in the majority of patients there is no pain whatsoever. Neural deafness was present in one of Denny-Brown's patients. In the latter case, which was studied postmortem, there was a loss of small nerve cells in the lumbosacral dorsal root ganglia; the dorsal roots were thin, and the fibers in the posterior columns of the spinal cord and peripheral nerves were diminished in number. Myelinated and unmyelinated fibers were both affected. Both axonal degeneration and segmental demyelination have been demonstrated in teased nerve preparations. Sensory nerve conduction may be absent or is uniformly slow in every nerve tested.

Recessive Mutilating Sensory Polyneuropathy of Childhood Here the pattern of inheritance is autosomal recessive. Onset is in infancy and early childhood and walking is delayed; there is pes cavus deformity and the first movements are ataxic. Ulcerations of the tips of toes and fingers and repeated infections of these parts result in the formation of paronychias and whitlows. The tendon reflexes are absent, but muscular power is well preserved. All sensory modalities are impaired (touch-pressure somewhat more than pain-temperature), mainly in the distal parts of the limbs but also over the trunk. In addition, there are reports of several sibships in which multiple members had a sensory neuropathy manifest by a generalized insensitivity to pain of the type described below. The lesions and electrophysiologic findings are similar to those in the dominantly inherited sensory neuropathy.

In both types of hereditary sensory neuropathy, measures must be taken to prevent stress fractures, acral mutilation, and infection. This is more difficult in the small child who does not understand the problem.

Congenital Insensitivity to Pain In *congenital indifference to pain*, a syndrome in which the patient throughout life is unreactive to the pain of injury, there is no loss of the ability to distinguish pinprick and other noxious stimuli from nonnoxious ones. Furthermore, the nervous system of such individuals seems to be normal. There is, however, another variety characterized by universal analgesia (Swanson and colleagues). This latter type is inherited as an autosomal recessive trait and at least one form involves the gene for a nerve growth factor receptor located on chromosome 1q immediately adjacent to the site of the mutation for Charcot-Marie-Tooth disease type 1B. During childhood, one of the patients of Swanson et al had high fever when the environmental temperature was raised, and the other possibly had orthostatic hypotension. One of the patients died in his 12th year and was found to have an absence of small neurons in the dorsal root ganglia, an absence of Lissauer's tracts, and a decrease in size of the descending spinal tracts of the trigeminal nerves. Sweat glands were present in the skin but were not innervated.

Other Forms of Inherited Sensory Neuropathy Included here are the neuropathy of Friedreich ataxia, which is discussed in Chap. 39; the Riley-Day syndrome, which is discussed further on in this chapter; and the neuropathies in which there are recognized metabolic abnormalities, including familial amyloidosis. Also, we have seen unclassifiable examples of an almost pure sensory or sensorimotor type. Some years ago a young man and woman with universal anesthesia affecting head, neck, trunk, and limbs came to our attention (Adams et al); all forms of sensation were absent. The patients were areflexic but retained nearly full motor power; the movements were ataxic. Autonomic functions were impaired but not abolished. In a sural nerve biopsy, nearly all fibers—large and small, myelinated and unmyelinated—had disappeared. Surprisingly, there were no trophic changes of any kind. Another of our families with ulcers and loss of digits had a symmetrical sensory and motor polyneuropathy of the extremities with areflexia. The inheritance was of autosomal dominant type, with onset in adolescence. Donaghy and others have described a unique variant of the recessively inherited form of sensory neuropathy in which there was an associated neurotrophic keratitis and a selective loss of small myelinated fibers in sural nerve biopsies. We continue to observe variant and unclassifiable cases such as these every year.

Inherited Polyneuropathies of Mixed Sensorimotor-Autonomic Types

Peroneal Muscular Atrophy [Charcot-Marie-Tooth Disease, or CMT Types 1 and 2; Hereditary Motor-Sensory Neuropathy, or HMSN Types I and II (Dyck); and Related Conditions] The hallmarks of this class of polyneuropathies (Table 46-2) are genetic transmission, complete symmetry, slow progression, and axon-myelin fiber loss (Dyck). These are the most common forms of inherited peripheral neuropathy and indeed among the most common of all inherited neurologic diseases. The frequency of the disease cannot be stated with precision because of its clinical heterogeneity, but overall the usually quoted prevalence is 1 in 2500 of the population, the most frequent subtype occurring in 1 in 4000. More than 15 subtypes have been described but only a few occur with any regularity.

Because the disease was described in 1886 almost simultaneously by Tooth in England and by Charcot and Marie in France, all their names were attached to it, even though similar cases had been recorded earlier by Eulenberg (1856), Friedreich (1873), Ormerod (1884), and Osler (1880). Because of secondary changes in the spinal cord and the occasional association of this disease with Friedreich ataxia, early observers considered it to be a hereditary myelopathy and did not class it with the neuropathies, but the evidence that supports this latter nosologic grouping is now unassailable. The two important advances in our understanding of this disease, since the original descriptions, have been the separation of the main subtypes on the basis of their electrophysiologic (EMG) features, and the assignment of the loci of certain genotypes to regions that code for components of peripheral nerve myelin.

Genetic Transmission The pattern of inheritance of Charcot-Marie-Tooth disease is most often autosomal dominant, with almost complete penetrance (the frequency of clinical expression of a genotype); less often it is autosomal recessive and rarely X-linked dominant or X-linked recessive (Table 46-2). Some cases arise as de novo mutations (Hoogendijk et al). Most kinships with autosomal dominant inheritance have been linked to a gene locus on chromosome 17p (the demyelinating type referred to below); however, other kinships are linked to chromosome 1 (the axonal type), and still others are linked to neither, implicating additional and as yet undiscovered loci. Kindreds that are connected to chromosomes 1 or 17 cannot be distinguished from one another on clinical grounds.

Seventy percent of CMT type 1 cases result from duplication of the gene for a peripheral myelin protein (PMP 22) on chromosome 17. Other studies of the PMP 22 and PO (another myelin protein) gene expression in CMT1 and CMT3 cases (Dejerine-Sottas disease) have yielded discordant results because mutations on different loci, including on chromosome 1, lead to different presentations, as noted in Table 46-2. The disease termed *hereditary liability to pressure palsies* also displays an aberration on chromosome 17, but in the form of a deletion rather than a duplication of the gene for PMP 22. This disease is discussed further on, under "Brachial Plexus Neuropathies." Yet an additional X-linked variant derives from a mutation of the gene for connexin, another component of myelin.

Undoubtedly further studies of genes and gene products will continue to advance our understanding of the inherited neuropathies, but for the present, clinicians are still best served by the descriptive clinical classification outlined in Table 46-1—acknowledging, of course, the heterogeneity of this class of disorders.

Clinical and Electrophysiologic Features Dyck and Lambert and Harding and Thomas have subdivided CMT disease into two types: hereditary motor sensory neuropathy (HMSN) I and II (or CMT1 and 2). This subdivision was made on the basis of conduction velocity in the median or ulnar nerve—slow (mean conduction velocity less than 38 m/s) in type 1 and normal or near normal in type 2. Electromyographers therefore refer to these respectively as the demyelinating and axonal types. In both, the compound muscle action potentials and sensory potentials are greatly reduced in amplitude, and in type 2 there are findings of denervation. In type 1 there is severe slowing of nerve conduction, but the type of conduction block that characterizes the acquired demyelinating neuropathies is not found. In distinction to acquired diseases, *the EMG findings, particularly the pronounced slowing of conduction in CMT1, are uniform throughout the peripheral nervous system.*

The classic form of CMT has its onset during late childhood or adolescence, although neurologists are increasingly aware that some cases, particularly type 2,

Table 46-2
Classification of the main inherited neuropathies

Neuropathy	*Inheritance*	*Gene*	*Clinical Features*	*Pathology*	*Nerve Conduction*
CMT 1A[a] (HSMN I)-demyelinating type	Dominant, sporadic; 1 in 5000, half of all inherited neuropathies	Duplication of 17p11.2 (PMP 22 gene), few due to point mutation	Motor-sensory, pes cavus, diminished relfexes, may have enlarged nerves	Demyelinative with onion bulbs	Uniformly slow conduction
1B	Dominant, 1 in 80,000	Point mutation 1q22-23 (PO gene)	Motor-sensory	Demyelinative with onion bulbs	Slow conduction
CMT 2 (axonal type)	Dominant	Chromosome 1 p, 3 q	Motor and sensory neuropathy, later onset than type 1, no nerve enlargement	Axonal loss	Low CMAPs, normal or minimally slowed conduction velocities
CMT X[a]	X-linked dominant, 1 in 20,000 (rarely recessive)	Point mutation or deletion Xq13.1 (connexin)	Motor-sensory, more severe in males, late childhood-early adolescent onset	Demyelinative with axonal degeneration	Mildly slowed velocities
Hereditary neuropathy with liability1 to pressure palsies (HNPP)[a]	Dominant, sporadic, 1 in 10,000 (may be under-recognized)	Deletion and other mutations at 17p11.2 (PMP22 gene)	Multiple focal palsies at common compression sites, plexopathy	"Tomaculous" swellings of nerve (redundant myelin)	Focal conduction block at compression sites, mild generalized slowing
Familial brachial plexopathy (HNA)	Rare	Chromosome 17 q 23, gene error unknown	Recurrent painful brachial plexopathy	Unknown	Multifocal plexus abnormalities
HMSN III (Dejerine-Sottas type)	Variable inheritance and sporadic	PO or PMP22 sites, point mutations (17p11.2)	Severe, predominantly sensory, hypertrophic nerves, childhood nest	Severe demyelination	Very slow conduction

Key: CMT Charcot-Marie-Tooth; HSMN; hereditary motor sensory neuropathy.
[a] Genetic testing available.

may not attract attention until middle life. Difficulty running, frequent weakness and sprains of the ankles, or stumbling and slapping of the feet are noted by the parents of younger children. Older patients have difficulty dating the onset of symptoms. With milder forms, they may not even be aware of having a neuropathic illness. In some cases the striking and widespread changes on EMG only come to light when this test is performed for the diagnosis of an unrelated problem or a parent becomes aware of his neuropathy when a child proves to have the disease. Type 1 cases have a peak appearance during the first decade. Peak onset of type 2 is in the second decade and even later in many cases; an onset in middle adult life is not unknown. Both motor and sensory signs are said to be more severe in the first type (Harding and Thomas).

Essentially, the chronic degeneration of peripheral nerves and roots results in distal muscle atrophy, beginning in the feet and legs and later involving the hands. The extensor hallucis and digitorum longus, the peronei, and the intrinsic muscles of the feet are affected early and produce pes cavus and *pied en griffe* (high arches and hammertoes). Later, all muscles of the legs and sometimes the lower third of the thigh become weak and atrophic. The thin legs have been likened to those of a stork or, if the lower thigh muscles are affected, to an "inverted champagne bottle." Eventually the nerves to the calf muscles degenerate and the ability to plantar flex the feet is lost. After a period of years, atrophy of the hand and forearm muscles develops. The hands later become clawed. The wasting seldom extends above the elbows or above the middle third of the thighs. Paresthesias and cramps are invariably present to some degree and there is always some impairment, usually slight, of deep and superficial sensation in the feet and hands, shading off proximally. Rarely, the sensory loss is severe, and perforating ulcers may appear. The tendon reflexes are absent in the involved limbs. The illness progresses very slowly and seems to stabilize for long periods so that it may evolve over decades.

The walking difficulty, which is the main disability, is due to a combination of sensory ataxia and weakness. Foot drop and instability of the ankles are additional handicaps. The feet and legs may ache after use and cramps may be troublesome, but otherwise pain is exceptional; the feet are often cold, swollen, and blue, secondary to inactivity of the muscles of the feet and legs and their dependent position. There is usually no disturbance of autonomic function. Fixed pupils, optic atrophy, nystagmus and endocrinopathies, epilepsy, and spina bifida, which have been reported occasionally in association with peroneal muscular atrophy, probably represent coincidental congenital disorders. The only distinguishing clinical feature between types 1 and 2, and this is present in only a minority of cases, is enlargement of the nerves in type 1, most easily appreciated by palpation of the greater auricular nerves.

The clinical heterogeneity of CMT disease has been alluded to above. In combination with tremor, it may be difficult to draw a line between this disease and the Roussy-Lévy syndrome, now considered to be a variant of CMT (see further on). Restricted forms are known to affect only the peroneal and pectoral or scapular muscles (scapuloperoneal form of Dawidenkow). The *"familial claw foot with absent tendon jerks"* of Symonds and Shaw is another variant.

Laboratory data, except for the uniform and pronounced slowing of nerve conduction in CMT1 (often in the range of 20 m/s) or near normal velocities with evidence of denervation in type 2, are of little help. The CSF is usually normal. Genetic testing for the most common (type 1A) PMP duplication mutation and for the X-linked and 1B varieties are available, and it should now be possible to identify many more cases, including sporadic ones. It is seldom necessary to resort to nerve biopsy to establish the diagnosis.

Pathologic Findings Degenerative changes in the nerves result in depletion of the population of large sensory and motor fibers, leaving only the condensed endoneurial connective tissue. As far as one can tell, axons and myelin sheaths are both affected, the distal parts of the nerve more than the proximal. In type I, the nerves may be enlarged, with "onion-bulb" formations of Schwann cells and fibroblasts, as in Déjerine-Sottas disease (type III HMSN in the Dyck classification). This change can often be seen in sural nerve biopsies. Anterior horn cells are slightly diminished in number and some are chromatolyzed. Dorsal root ganglion cells suffer a similar fate. The disease involves sensory posterior root fibers with degeneration of the posterior columns of Goll more than of Burdach. The autonomic nervous system remains relatively intact. The muscles contain large fields of atrophic fibers (group atrophy). Some of the larger fibers have a target appearance and may show degenerative changes. This muscle lesion is of the denervative type. Claims of a coincidental myelopathy and degeneration of spinocerebellar and corticospinal tracts probably indicate that the associated disease was really Friedreich ataxia or some other combination of chronic myelopathy and neuropathy.

Treatment No specific treatment is known. Stabilizing the ankles by arthrodeses is indicated if foot drop is severe and the disease has reached the point where it is not progressing. Fitting the legs with light braces and the shoes with springs, to overcome foot drop, can be helpful.

Differential diagnosis involves the distal dystrophies (page 1505), late forms of familial motor system disease, Friedreich ataxia (page 1145), Roussy-Lévy syndrome (see below) and other familial polyneuropathies, and, in adults, CIDP and the paraproteinemic neuropathies, discussed earlier.

Hypertrophic Neuropathy of Infancy (Déjerine-Sottas Disease or HMSN III of Dyck) This type of neuropathy is inherited as an autosomal recessive trait. It begins in childhood or infancy, earlier than the classic form of peroneal muscular atrophy. Walking is delayed in onset and then progressively impaired. Pain and paresthesias in the feet are early symptoms, followed by the development of symmetrical weakness and wasting of the distal portions of the limbs. Talipes equinovarus postures with claw feet and later claw hands are common. All modalities of sensation are impaired in a distal distribution, and the tendon reflexes are absent. Miotic, unreactive pupils, nystagmus, and kyphoscoliosis have been observed in some cases. The trunk and other cranial nerves are spared. The ulnar, median, radial, posterior neck, and peroneal nerves stand out like tendons and are easily followed with the gently roving finger. The enlarged nerves are not tender. Unlike other forms of CMT, the CSF protein is persistently elevated in Déjerine-Sottas disease because the spinal roots are affected. Nerve conduction velocities are markedly reduced, even when there is little or no functional impairment. Patients are usually much more disabled than with peroneal muscular atrophy and are confined to wheelchairs at an early age. Treatment is purely symptomatic.

It is important to emphasize that the occurrence of hypertrophic neuropathy is not confined to this particular inherited disease. If one groups all patients in whom the nerves are diffusely enlarged (incorrectly called "hypertrophic," since it is mainly the epineural and perineural connective tissue that enlarges), several different diseases, both genetic and acquired, are included. The identifying histologic lesion in these cases is the "onion bulb," which consists of a whorl of overlapping, intertwined, attenuated Schwann cell processes that encircle naked or finely myelinated axons. Enlarged nerves have been described in some cases of recurrent demyelinating polyneuritis, familial amyloidosis, Refsum disease (HMSN type IV of Dyck), peroneal muscular atrophy type I, and other diseases. As was first noted by Thomas, any pathologic process that causes recurrent segmental demyelination and subsequent repair and remyelination may have this effect. In some patients with a history of early childhood hereditary polyneuropathy, the nerves are not yet palpably enlarged, but the characteristic Schwann cell abnormalities can be seen in a biopsy of a cutaneous nerve.

Hereditary Areflexic Dystasia (Roussy-Lévy Syndrome) In 1926 Roussy and Lévy reported seven cases of a dominantly inherited malady that had not previously been described. Its close relation to Friedreich ataxia and the amyotrophy of Charcot-Marie-Tooth disease was recognized. For many years thereafter the existence of this entity was disputed and only recently, on the basis of molecular genetic testing, have these relationships been clarified.

The condition in question is a sensory ataxia (dystasia) with pes cavus and areflexia, affecting mainly the lower legs and progressing later to involve the hands. Some degree of sensory loss, mainly of vibratory and position sense, has been described in all cases. Atrophy of the muscles of the legs and postural tremor become prominent eventually. None of the patients has had evidence of cerebellar ataxia. Kyphoscoliosis is described in several. Although the feet may be cold or slightly discolored, no autonomic defects are documented. The nerves are not palpably enlarged. Electrocardiographic abnormalities similar to those of Friedreich ataxia have been noted in one family. The onset in many patients is during infancy, possibly dating from birth, and the course is benign; all descendants of the original Roussy-Lévy family were still able to walk during their seventh decade of life.

On clinical and pathologic grounds, Dyck et al placed the Roussy-Lévy kinships within the category of the demyelinating type of Charcot-Marie-Tooth disease (CMT1). The mode of inheritance of the two syndromes, their benign course, pattern of neurologic signs, slow nerve conduction, and biopsy features (demyelination of nerve fibers with onion bulb formation) are much the same. This view has been reinforced by the recent genetic findings of Planté-Bordeneuve et al. In affected members of the original Roussy-Lévy family, these investigators identified a point mutation in the domain of the myelin protein gene Po, on chromosome 17 p 11.2, the same gene that is implicated in CMT and Déjerine-Sottas disease.

Chronic Polyneuropathy with Hereditary Spastic Paraplegia From time to time we have observed children and young adults with unmistakable progressive spastic paraplegia superimposed on which was a sensorimotor polyneuropathy of extremely chronic evolution. Sural nerve biopsy in two of our cases disclosed a typical "hypertrophic" polyneuropathy. In another case only loss of nerve fibers was found. Cavanaugh and colleagues and Harding and Thomas have reported similar patients. Our patients were severely disabled, being barely able to stand on their atrophic legs. The disease is slowly progressive. The patients described by Cavanaugh and coworkers had mainly sensory deficits and were not disabled.

While few in number, some cases of chronic polyneuropathy are combined with optic atrophy, with or without deafness or retinitis pigmentosa, and Dyck has classed these in separate groups. Jaradeh and Dyck have also described a hereditary motor-sensory polyneuropathy with the later development of a parkinsonian or a choreic-dystonic syndrome that responded to L-dopa. Most cases of this type have had an autosomal recessive inheritance.

Inherited Polyneuropathies with a Recognized Metabolic Disorder

Refsum Disease (Heredopathia Atactica Polyneuritiformis; HMSN IV of Dyck) This rare disorder is inherited as an autosomal recessive trait and has its onset in late childhood, adolescence, or early adult life. Diagnosis is based on a combination of clinical manifestations—retinitis pigmentosa, cerebellar ataxia, and chronic polyneuropathy—coupled with an increase in blood phytanic acid. Cardiomyopathy and neurogenic deafness are present in most patients, and pupillary abnormalities, cataracts, and ichthyotic skin changes (particularly on the shins) are added features in some. Anosmia and night blindness with constriction of the visual fields may precede the neuropathy by many years; usually the latter develops gradually, sometimes rapidly. The polyneuropathy is sensorimotor, distal, and symmetrical in distribution, affecting the legs more than the arms. All forms of sensation are reduced and tendon reflexes are lost. The CSF protein is increased, sometimes markedly.

Although the nerves may not be palpably enlarged, "hypertrophic" changes with onion-bulb formation are invariable pathologic features. The metabolic defect is in the utilization of dietary phytol; a failure of oxidation of phytanic acid—a tetramethylated 16-carbon fatty acid—results in its accumulation. The relation between the increased phytanic acid and the polyneuropathy is uncertain. Clinical diagnosis is confirmed by the finding of increased phytanic acid in the blood; the normal level is less than 0.3 mg/dL, but in patients with this disease it constitutes 5 to 30 percent of the total fatty acids of the serum lipids. Diets low in phytol may be beneficial, but this is difficult to judge, for after an acute attack there is sometimes a natural remission. The effects of plasma exchange have also been difficult to interpret. In some patients there is a very slow and gradual progression of the disease, and in others a more rapid progression with death from cardiac complications. Diagnosis is confirmed by measuring serum and urinary phytanic acid.

Ataxia, Retinitis Pigmentosa, and Peripheral Neuropathy without Increase in Phytanic Acid (NARP) Like Tuck and McLeod, we have observed several cases over a period of years in which the clinical picture was almost identical to that of Refsum disease, but changes in phytanic acid could not be detected. A mild ichthyosis, sensorineural deafness, ataxia of mixed tabetic-cerebellar type, areflexia, and retinitis pigmentosa were the main findings. None of our cases had a positive family history. Sural nerve biopsy showed loss of large fibers. Biochemical abnormalities in the blood or cultured fibroblasts have not been detected. There was a mitochondrial disorder in most of the recently studied cases. This, the so-called NARP syndrome, was described in detail on page 1043. The onset of the disease has been in adolescence with slow progression.

Abetalipoproteinemia (Bassen-Kornzweig Syndrome) This rare autosomal recessive disorder has been described in Chap. 37 (page 1021) with the inherited metabolic disorders of the nervous system. It is mentioned here because the brunt of the neurologic disorder falls upon the peripheral nerves; *acanthocytosis* is an identifying feature. The first neurologic finding is diminution or absence of tendon reflexes, detected as early as the second year of life. Later, when the patient is able to cooperate in sensory testing, a loss of vibratory and position sense is found in the legs. Cerebellar signs (ataxia of gait, trunk, and extremities; titubation of the head; and dysarthria), muscle weakness, ophthalmoparesis, Babinski signs, and loss of pain and temperature sense are other characteristic neurologic abnormalities, in more or less this order of frequency. Mental backwardness occurs in some patients. There are no signs of autonomic disorder. Irregular progression occurs over a few years and many patients are unable to stand and walk by the time they reach adolescence.

Skeletal abnormalities include pes cavus and kyphoscoliosis, which are secondary to the neuropathy. Constriction of the visual fields and ring scotomata are manifestations of the macular degeneration and retinitis pigmentosa. Cardiac enlargement and failure are serious late complications.

Neuropathologic findings consist of demyelination of peripheral nerves and degeneration of nerve cells in the spinal gray matter and cerebellar cortex. Diagnosis is confirmed by the finding of acanthocytes, low serum cholesterol, and β (low-density)-lipoproteins. What is known about the pathogenesis and treatment is discussed in Chap. 37. A deficiency of vitamin E, due to malabsorption, may be an important factor, and large doses of the vitamin should be tried as therapy.

A closely related disease, also with familial hypobetalipoproteinemia, has been described by van Buchem and coworkers. It too is associated with a malabsorption syndrome, an ill-defined weakness, ataxia, dysesthesia of the legs, and Babinski signs. There is no sensory loss.

Tangier Disease This is an exceedingly rare familial disorder, named for the island off the Virginia coast, where the first-described cases resided. It is inherited as an autosomal recessive trait. The genetic abnormality is situated in the gene for the so-called ATP-cassette transporter protein. It is marked by a deficiency of high-density lipoprotein, low cholesterol, diminution of phospholipids, and high triglyceride concentrations in the serum. Perhaps because of these abnormalities, the patients are disposed to early and severe atherosclerosis. The presence of enlarged, yellow-orange (cholesterol-laden) tonsils is said to be a frequent manifestation. About half of the reported cases have had neuropathic symptoms, taking the form of an asymmetrical sensorimotor neuropathy that fluctuates in severity. The polyneuropathy may come in attacks—that is to say, it is recurrent. In the two sisters reported by Engel and coworkers, the onset of symptoms was in childhood and in infancy, respectively. The sensory loss is predominantly for pain and temperature and extends over the entire body; at times it is limited to the face and upper extremities, simulating syringomyelia (pseudosyringomyelia). Tactile and proprioceptive sensory modalities tend to be preserved.

The muscular weakness, if present, affects either the lower or upper extremities or both, particularly the hand muscles, which may undergo atrophy and show denervation potentials by EMG. In one of our patients, only a facial diplegia was present, and the pain and temperature loss was restricted to the head, neck, and arms. Nerve conduction is slowed. Tendon reflexes are often lost or diminished. Transient ptosis and diplopia have been reported.

Fat-laden macrophages are present in the bone marrow and elsewhere. No complete pathologic studies are available. There is no known treatment. Dietary measures may help, particularly in preventing atherosclerosis, but whether they influence the neuropathy is uncertain.

Fabry Disease (Anderson-Fabry Disease) The genetic and metabolic aspects of this sex-linked disorder have already been considered with the inherited metabolic diseases (page 1037). Here we offer some additional remarks about the painful neuropathic component.

The pain, which is usually the initial symptom in childhood and adolescence, often has a burning quality or occurs in brief lancinating jabs, mostly in the fingers and toes, and may be accompanied by paresthesias of the palms and soles. Changes in environmental temperature and exercise may induce pain. These abnormalities are due to the accumulation of glycolipid (ceramide trihexoside) in peripheral nerves, both perineurally and intraneurally, as well as in cells of the spinal ganglia and the anterior and intermediolateral horns of the spinal cord. Ohnishi and Dyck have demonstrated a preferential loss of small myelinated and unmyelinated fibers and small neurons of dorsal root ganglia. Involvement of the latter cells and the associated degenerative changes in the afferent fibers are thought to be the likely cause of the painful sensory phenomena (Kahn).

Later in the illness there is progressive impairment of renal function and cerebral and myocardial infarction. But the most characteristic feature is an eruption of dark red macules and papules, up to 2 mm in diameter, over the trunk and limbs, most closely clustered over the thighs and lower trunk and the around the umbilicus (*angiokeratoma corporis diffusum*).

Phenytoin, carbamazepine, or gabapentin and amitriptyline may be helpful in alleviating the pain and dysesthesias, but there is no specific therapy for the disease.

Polyneuropathy of Acromegaly and Gigantism *Nerve entrapment*, particularly of the median nerve, is a well-known feature of acromegaly. Pickett and colleagues identified a carpal tunnel syndrome in 56 percent of acromegalics. Also recognized as a complication of acromegaly, but not due to multiple nerve entrapments, is a *polyneuropathy* characterized by paresthesias, loss of tendon reflexes in the legs, and atrophy of slight degree in the distal leg muscles. Sometimes there are enlarged nerves. In the case reported by Stewart, the enlargement was the result of hypertrophic changes in the endoneurial and perineurial tissues, similar to those that occur in other so-called hypertrophic neuropathies of inflammatory or heredofamilial origin. In cases of extreme gigantism, a more severe polyneuropathy has been reported, to the point of causing Charcot joints (Daughady). We have also observed a severe motor neuropathy in a patient with Pyle disease, a metaphyseal dysplasia that resembles acromegaly.

Metachromatic Leukodystrophy (See also Chap. 37.) In this disease the congenital absence of the degradative enzyme sulfatase leads to massive accumulation of sulfatide throughout the central and peripheral nervous systems and to a lesser extent in other organs. The abnor-

4. **Cranial neuropathy with corneal lattice dystrophy** This unusual form of amyloid neuropathy was first described in three Finnish families by Meretoja—hence "Finnish type." Subsequently, it was reported from several different parts of the world in families of other than those of Finnish heritage.

The disease usually begins in the third decade, with lattice corneal dystrophy. Vitreous opacities are not observed, and visual acuity is little affected. Peripheral neuropathy may not be evident until the fifth decade, at which time the facial nerves, particularly their upper branches, become affected. The nerves of the limbs are involved even later and to a much lesser extent than in other amyloid neuropathies. At postmortem examination, deposits of amyloid are found in virtually every organ, but mainly in the kidneys and blood vessels and in the perineurium of affected nerves.

Pathologic Findings In familial amyloid polyneuropathy, amyloid deposits are demonstrable in the blood vessels, the interstitial (endoneurial) tissues of the peripheral somatic and autonomic nerves, and in the spinal and autonomic ganglia and roots. There is a loss of nerve fibers, the unmyelinated and small myelinated fibers being more depleted than the large myelinated ones. The anterior horn and sympathetic ganglion cells are swollen and chromatolysed due to involvement of their axons, and the posterior columns of the spinal cord degenerate.

The pathogenesis of the fiber loss in the familial type, as in the acquired type, is not fully understood. On the basis of their findings in a sporadic case of amyloid polyneuropathy with diabetes mellitus, Kernohan and Woltman suggested that amyloid deposits in the walls of the small arteries and arterioles interfere with the circulation in the nerves and that amyloid neuropathy is essentially an ischemic neuropathy. In other cases, however, the vascular changes are relatively slight and the degeneration of the nerve fibers appears to be related to their compression and distortion by the endoneurial deposits of amyloid. Amyloid is also seen in the tongue, gums, heart, gastrointestinal tract, kidneys, and many other organs, where it may possibly act as a tissue toxin.

Neuropathies Associated with AIDS These patients are prone to several types of neuropathy, including a predominantly sensory type that may be painful, a lumbosacral polyradiculopathy, cranial and limb mononeuropathies, CIDP, GBS, and, rarely, a vasculitic mononeuritis multiplex—none of which differs from the idiopathic or conventional varieties of these neuropathies, except that there is often a pleocytosis. Unique to the AIDS patient are the CMV cauda equina neuritis and an acute or subacute painful infiltrative lymphocytic neuropathy—a component of the diffuse infiltrative lymphocytosis (DILS) with CD8 cells (Moulingier et al). Polyneuropathy may also be induced by antiviral agents that are used in the treatment of HIV infection, as discussed in Chap. 33.

Problems in Diagnosis of the Chronic Polyneuropathies

This is the group that has given the present authors the most difficulty. The cause of most of the acute and many of the subacute and relapsing forms can usually be established by the clinical and laboratory methods presently available in large centers. It is the early and late chronic cases that continue to baffle the neurologist and general physician, despite the respectable advances that have been made in the field of genetics.

Diagnosis of Early Chronic Polyneuropathies A *sensorimotor paralysis*, which evolves over several weeks (subacutely) or more slowly, over many months or a year or two, and involves legs more than arms and distal parts more than proximal should, in an adult, always lead to a search for diabetes, occult neoplasia (carcinoma, lymphoma, multiple myeloma, or plasmacytoma), HIV infection, paraproteinemia (including amyloid neuropathy), and CIDP. In exceptional cases, a neoplastic process remains hidden for as long as 2 or 3 years after the onset of neuropathy. In our experience, an environmental toxin, endocrine disorder (except for diabetes), or nutritional cause is seldom identified, despite the frequent attribution of obscure polyneuropathies to such causes. Nonetheless, history of exposure to industrial or hobbyist toxins, sociopathy or psychopathy that would lead to toxin ingestion, or foreign travel should be sought and testing should include heavy metals in obscure cases. Unusual causes of nutritional deficiency, such as celiac-sprue disease and other malabsorption syndromes (Whipple disease, Crohn disease, chronic hepatic disease, intestinal bypass surgery), have usually been obvious enough when present, so that the experienced clinician rarely overlooks them. Vitamin B_{12} deficiency should be sought in any case of large-fiber neuropathy. A difficult type of case is that of an older person with a mild, nonprogressive sensorimotor polyneuropathy in whom there is evidence of mild hypothyroidism, marginally low vitamin B_{12} and folic acid levels in the blood, a somewhat unbalanced diet, perhaps an excessive alcohol intake, and an abnormal glucose tolerance curve. It is easy to imagine but hard to prove that any one of these factors is relevant.

In the *purely or predominantly sensory polyneuropathies*—some painful, some not, some with marked ataxia—an association with occult carcinoma, an IgM paraproteinemia, amyloidosis, or Sjögren syndrome are the primary considerations. Rarely, milder neuropathy may be seen with biliary cirrhosis. When the symptoms are confined to the feet and legs, a sporadic example of hereditary sensory neuropathy must be considered if the condition is of very long standing. Intoxications with pyridoxine or metals account for a few chronic sensory neuropathies. Despite all these considerations, we still regularly encounter patients in whom the cause is not disclosed by any of the available tests. We have watched helplessly as some of these patients become reduced to a bed and wheelchair existence and others suffer from pain until they turn to and become dependent on opiates.

In our experience, the *subacute and chronically evolving demyelinating neuropathies* that are suspected clinically and then confirmed by slowed conduction velocity, conduction block, and relatively normal needle EMG studies generally turn out to be variants of CIDP. Some others are associated with a paraproteinemia. Often the electrophysiologic tests point to a combined axonal and demyelinating process, the latter reflected in prolonged distal latencies, conduction slowing or block, and loss of late responses. Marked weakness and reduced muscle action potential amplitudes in the face of minimal denervation, even if present in only a few nerves, also indicate at least a component of focal demyelination. Most of the mixed axonal-demyelinating cases in which one eventually arrives at a diagnosis will also be related to an immune (paraproteinemic) or inflammatory (CIDP) process; for the moment, it is useful to place these in the demyelinating category since many will respond the same measures as are used in the treatment of purely demyelinating CIDP.

Laboratory tests that are useful in the investigation of this group of neuropathies are listed in Table 46-3.

Table 46-3
Laboratory tests for the investigation of subacute and chronic polyneuropathies—in addition to electromyography[a]

Serum glucose, glucose tolerance test, and glycosylated hemoglobin-A1C (diabetes)
Anti-Hu antibody (paraneoplastic neuropathies)
Immunoelectrophoresis or immunofixation of serum and urine (paraproteinemic and amyloid neuropathies)
Anti-MAG and antisulfatide antibodies (immune sensory neuropathies)
Anti-GM_1 antibody (multifocal motor conduction block)
Vitamin B_{12} and methylmalonic acid levels (B_{12} deficiency or nitrous oxide exposure)
HIV antibody
Lyme antibody
Heavy metal levels in blood and tissue (toxic neuropathies)
BUN
Thyroid hormone
Sedimentation rate, ANA, cryoglobulins, c-ANCA, rheumatoid factor, anti-SSA/SSB Sjögren antibodies, eosinophil count (vasculitides), antigliadin antibodies (sprue)
Serum carotene, vitamin E, pyridoxine levels (nutritional deficiencies and vitamin excess)
Genetic testing for Charcot-Marie-Tooth disease, type 1 and for hereditary liability to pressure palsy and brachial plexopathy (inherited neuropathies)
Spinal fluid protein determination and cell content (CIDP, neoplastic and granulomatous meningitis)

[a] The use of each test is guided by clinical circumstances.

Diagnosis of Late Chronic Polyneuropathies The majority of the more chronic and very gradually progressive polyneuropathies (i.e., evolving over 10 or more years) prove to be heredofamilial or sporadic mutations of the genes that are responsible for the inherited types. The observations of Dyck and coworkers, referred to in the introduction to this chapter, are of interest in this respect. In a series of 205 patients who were referred to the Mayo Clinic with neuropathies of unknown cause, 86 were found to have an inherited form of the disease. With appropriate genealogic data, the diagnosis of the hypertrophic polyneuropathy of Déjerine-Sottas and the peroneal muscular atrophy of Charcot-Marie-Tooth, the two major types, can usually be made on clinical grounds alone. Sporadic cases become more difficult. Dyck and associates found that direct examinations of the patients' kin—using all available clinical data, EMG, nerve conduction studies, CSF examination, and nerve and muscle biopsy—was often successful in revealing a hereditary basis for the neuropathy. We, too, have found that in perplexing cases, routine examination of other family members, searching for mild reflex or foot abnormalities or atrophy of leg muscles, has often clarified the diagnosis. DNA testing for the classic forms of Charcot-Marie-Tooth disease is now available in commercial laboratories and has increased the diagnostic yield.

A few young patients have come to our attention in whom a gradually progressive polyneuropathy that evolved over almost a decade turned out to be an acquired chronic inflammatory demyelinating condition. The absence of a family history of neuropathy or of high arches and heterogeneous slowing of both nerve conduction velocities and reductions in motor amplitudes on the EMG were hints to the nature of the condition.

Finally, it should be stated again that even after the most assiduous clinical and laboratory investigation of patients with chronic neuropathy, at least one-third of these disorders currently remain unexplained.

Problems in Diagnosis of Recurrent and Relapsing Polyneuropathy

Several types of neuropathy are particularly prone to recurrence: chronic inflammatory-demyelinating neuropathy (CIDP), Refsum disease, Tangier disease, and the porphyric type, in which the attacks recur spontaneously or because of the administration of barbiturates or other drugs. Approximately 5 percent of patients with GBS have one or more relapses, in which the clinical and pathologic changes differ in no meaningful way from those of the acute monophasic form of the disease. Some instances of mononeuritis multiplex, especially when associated with cryoglobulinemia, are characterized by remission and relapse, although the remissions are incomplete. A common cause of relapse is the withdrawal of corticosteroids in CIDP patients who are dependent on these drugs; similarly, lapses in the treatment of paraproteinemic neuropathies cause fluctuations in symptoms. Enlargement of nerves may occur with repeated attacks, and it is probable that some patients classed originally as having one form of Déjerine-Sottas disease fall into this category. Also, it is obvious that patients who have recovered from an episode of alcoholic-nutritional or toxic polyneuropathy may develop a recurrence of their disease if they are subjected again to intoxication or nutritional deficiency.

Neuropathic symptoms that fluctuate in relation to environmental factors such as cold (cryoglobulinemia), heat (Fabry and Tangier diseases), or intermittent exposure to heavy metal or other type of poisoning may simulate a relapsing polyneuropathy.

MONONEUROPATHY, MONONEUROPATHY MULTIPLEX, AND PLEXOPATHY

The distinguishing feature of this group of neuropathies is that either one or several individual peripheral nerves are involved by a disease process. The diagnosis rests on the finding of motor, reflex, or sensory changes confined to the territory of a single nerve; of several individual nerves affected in a random manner (*mononeuritis or mononeuropathy multiplex*); or of a plexus of nerves or part of a plexus (*plexopathy*). Certain neuropathies of this type—traceable to polyarteritis nodosa and other vasculitides, leprosy, sarcoid, or diabetes—have already been discussed and are the main causes of diseases in this category. In addition to the signs of mononeuritis multiplex, pain, sometimes local erythema over the infarction, and irregularly elevated CSF protein with pleocytosis are the main features (e.g., Lyme disease; see Chap. 32). A subacute or chronic inflammatory neuropathy and the immune neuropathy caused by antibodies to GM_1 should also be considered.

The reader should refer to Table 48-1 (page 1468), which lists the roots, nerves, and muscles that are involved in particular movements.

Brachial Plexus Neuropathies

Brachial plexus neuropathies, usually unilateral, comprise an interesting group of neurologic disorders. Some may develop without apparent cause and manifest themselves by sensorimotor derangements ascribable to one or more of the cords of the plexus. Others result from trauma in which the arm is hyperabducted or the shoulder violently separated from the neck. Difficult births are an important source of such traction injuries. Rarely, the brachial plexus or other peripheral nerves may be damaged at the time of an electrical injury, either from lightning or from a household or industrial source. There may be impairment of function of the brachial plexus or portions thereof developing many months or years after radiation therapy. Direct compression of parts of the plexus by adjacent skeletal anomalies (cervical rib, fascial bands, narrowed thoracic outlet) or infiltration by breast or apical lung tumors represents another category of brachial plexus injury. A subcutaneous or intramuscular injection of vaccine or foreign serum may be followed by a brachial plexopathy, usually partial.

Brachial plexus neuritis of obscure origin, also called *neuralgic amyotrophy* or *Parsonage-Turner syndrome*, stands as a special clinical entity, often difficult to distinguish from other types of brachial pain. Some of these cases, surprisingly, are familial; others occur in small outbreaks. There are plexus lesions of presumed toxic nature, such as those following heroin injection. Granulomatous diseases such as sarcoid and secondary inflammatory processes related to lymphoma may implicate the plexus.

In summary, most brachial plexus disorders are due to trauma, infiltration by tumor, compression, obscure infections (possibly viral), and the delayed effects of radiotherapy (page 1431).

In assessing the type and degree of plexus injury, electrophysiologic testing is of particular importance. Early after a traumatic injury or other acute disease of the plexus, the only electrophysiologic abnormality may be an absence of late responses (F wave). After 7 to 10 days or longer, as the process of wallerian degeneration proceeds, sensory potentials are lost and the amplitudes of compound muscle action potentials are variably reduced, in proportion to the severity of axonal loss. Fibrillation potentials, indicative of denervation, then begin to appear in the corresponding muscles. Even later, usually after several weeks, signs of reinnervation can be detected. In more chronic cases, all of these features may be evident when the patient is first studied. The pattern of denervated muscles allows a distinction to be made between a plexopathy, radiculopathy, and mononeuritis multiplex based on the known patterns of innervation. If denervation changes are found in the paraspinal muscles, the source of weakness and pain is in the intraspinal roots. This localization is corroborated by finding preserved sensory potentials in nerves that are unaffected by lesions central to the ganglion. MRI may expose infiltrative lesions of the plexus (it is normal in so-called plexitis or neuralgic amyotrophy), but small nodular lesions may escape detection, and one then defers to the clinical data if these suggest an infiltrative or compressive lesion.

For the anatomic plan of the brachial (and lumbosacral) plexus and their relations to blood vessels and bony structures, one of the more detailed monographs on the peripheral nerves should be consulted. In the examination of individual nerves, the illustrated manual of Devinsky and Feldmann and the one published by the Guarantors of Brain are particularly useful and are listed in the references.

For quick orientation, it is enough to remember that the brachial plexus is formed from the anterior and posterior divisions of cervical roots 5, 6, 7, and 8 and the first thoracic nerve roots (see Fig. 46-4). The fifth and sixth cervical roots merge into the upper trunk, the seventh root forms the middle trunk, and the eighth cervical and first thoracic roots form the lower trunk. Each trunk divides into an anterior and posterior division. The posterior divisions of each trunk unite to form the posterior cord of the plexus. The anterior divisions of the upper and middle trunks unite to form the lateral cord. The anterior division of the lower trunk forms the medial cord. Two important nerves emerge from the upper trunk (dorsal scapular nerve to the rhomboid and levator scapulae muscles, and long thoracic nerve to the anterior serratus). The posterior cord gives rise mainly to the radial nerve. The medial cord gives rise to the ulnar nerve, medial cutaneous nerve to the forearm, and medial cutaneous nerve to the upper arm. This cord lies in close relation to the subclavian artery and apex of the lung and is the part of the plexus most susceptible to traction injuries and to compression by tumors that invade the costoclavicular space. The median nerve is formed by the union of parts of the medial and lateral cords.

Lesions of the Whole Plexus The entire arm is paralyzed and hangs uselessly at the side; the sensory loss is complete below a line extending from the shoulder diagonally downward and medially to the middle third of the upper arm. Biceps, triceps, radial periosteal, and finger reflexes are abolished. The usual cause is vehicular trauma.

Upper Brachial Plexus Paralysis This is due to injury to the fifth and sixth cervical nerves and roots, the most common causes of which are forceful separation of the head and shoulder during difficult delivery, pressure on the supraclavicular region during anesthesia, injections of foreign serum or vaccines, and idiopathic brachial plexitis (see below). The muscles affected are the biceps, deltoid, supinator longus, supraspinatus and infraspinatus, and rhomboids. The arm hangs at the side, internally rotated and extended at the elbow. Movements of the hand and forearm are unaffected. The prognosis for spontaneous recovery is generally good, though this may be incomplete; injuries of the upper brachial plexus and spinal roots incurred at birth (Erb-Duchenne palsy) may persist throughout life.

Lower Brachial Plexus Paralysis This is usually the result of traction on the abducted arm in a fall or during an operation on the axilla, infiltration or compression by tumors arising from the apex of the lung (superior sulcus or Pancoast syndrome), or compression by cervical ribs or bands. Injury may occur during birth, particularly with breech deliveries (Déjerine-Klumpke paralysis). There is weakness and wasting of the small muscles of the hand and a characteristic claw-hand deformity. Sensory loss is limited to the ulnar border of the hand and the inner forearm; if the first thoracic motor root is involved, there may be an associated paralysis of the cervical sym-

Figure 46-4

Diagram of the brachial plexus: the components of the plexus have been separated and drawn out of scale. Note that peripheral nerves arise from various components of the plexus: roots [indicated by cervical roots 5, 6, 7, 8, and thoracic root 1]; trunks (upper, middle, lower); divisions (anterior and posterior); and cords (lateral, posterior, and medial). The median nerve arises from the heads of the lateral and medial cords. (From Haymaker and Woodhallby permission.)

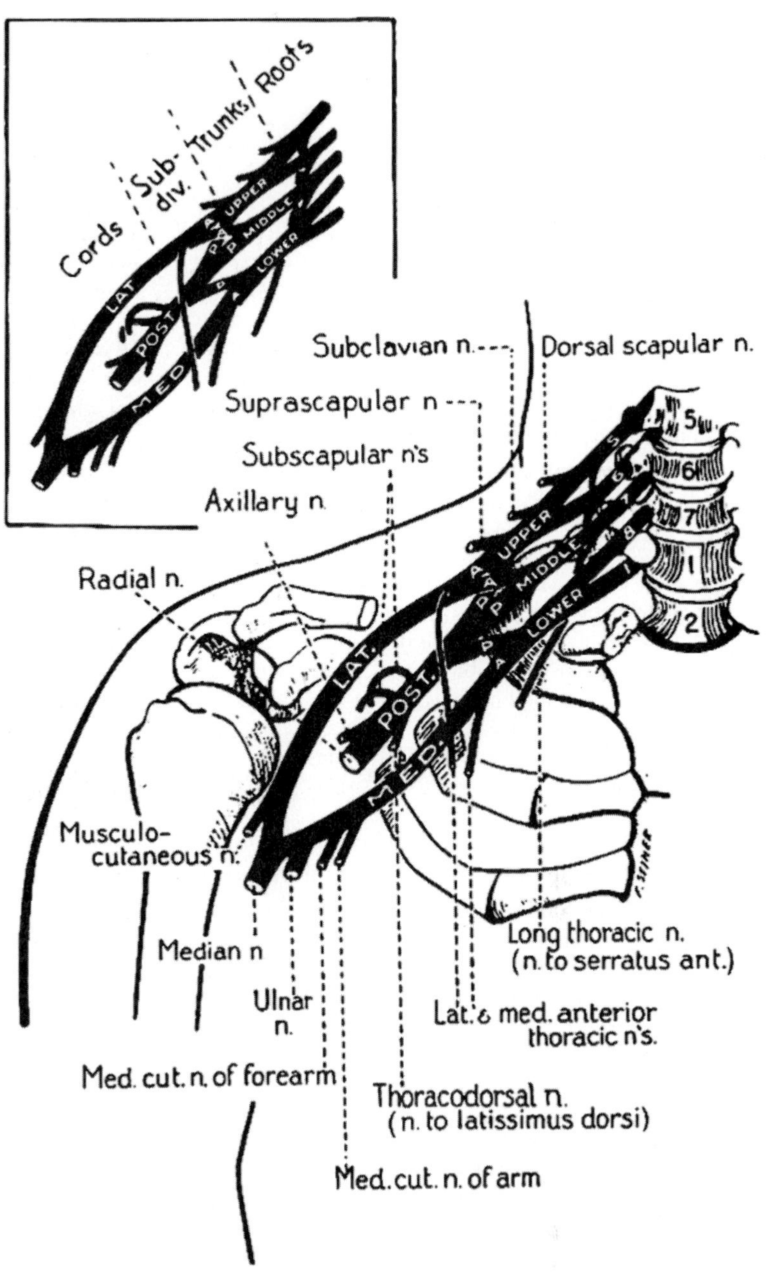

pathetic nerves with a Horner syndrome. Invasion of the lower plexus by tumors is usually painful; postradiation lesions are more likely to cause paresthesias without pain (Lederman and Wilbourn).

Infraclavicular Lesions Involving Cords of the Brachial Plexus (See Fig. 46-4.) A lesion of the *lateral cord* causes weakness of the muscles supplied by the musculocutaneous nerve and the lateral root of the median nerve; it manifests itself mainly as a weakness of flexion and pronation of the forearm. The intrinsic muscles of the hand innervated by the medial root of the median nerve are spared. A lesion of the *medial cord* of the plexus causes weakness of muscles supplied by the medial root of the median nerve and the ulnar nerve. The effect is that of a combined median and ulnar nerve palsy.

A lesion of the *posterior cord* results in weakness of the deltoid muscle, extensors of the elbow, wrist, and fingers, and sensory loss on the outer surface of the upper arm.

One group of infraclavicular injuries, often iatrogenic, results from damage to the subclavian or axillary vessels and the formation of pseudoaneurysms or hematomas. Small puncture wounds—as might occur with catheterization of the subclavian vein, anesthetic block of the brachial plexus, or transaxillary arteriography—are likely to produce this type of injury. Compression of the plexus evolves subacutely, up to 3 weeks at times, although once started, the deterioration may be rapid. Prompt recognition of the condition and early decompression are essential.

Other frequent causes of injury to the cords are dislocation of the head of the humerus, direct axillary trauma (stab wounds), pressure of a cervical rib or band, and supraclavicular compression during anesthesia. All cords of the plexus may be injured, or they may be affected in various combinations.

Costoclavicular (Thoracic Outlet) Syndrome This is discussed in Chap. 11 (page 227).

Brachial Plexus Neuropathy (Neuralgic Amyotrophy, Brachial Neuritis or Plexitis, Parsonage-Turner Syndrome) This illness, of obscure nature, may develop abruptly in an otherwise healthy individual; it may also complicate an infection, an injection of vaccine or antibiotic, childbirth, surgical procedures of any type, or the use of heroin. Magee and DeJong in 1960 and Tsairis and coworkers in 1972 reported large series of cases and amplified a well-known clinical picture that the authors have observed repeatedly. Our patients have nearly all been adults ranging from 20 to 65 years of age. Males are slightly more susceptible (2.4:1). Beginning as an ache in and around the shoulder, at the root of the neck or base of the skull, and suspected at first of being only a "wry neck," the pain rapidly becomes more severe. It is made worse by movements that involve the muscles in the region, and the patient searches for a comfortable position. After a period of 3 to 10 days there is a rapid development of muscular weakness and sensory and reflex impairment. With the development of weakness and soon afterwards of atrophy, the pain tends to subside. In a few cases, the neurologic disorder occurs with little or no antecedent pain. Possibly, in some, the pain is not followed by demonstrable weakness. Unlike restricted radicular lesions, which almost never cause complete paralysis of a muscle, certain muscles involved in brachial neuritis—such as the serratus anterior, deltoid, biceps, or triceps—may be totally or almost totally paralyzed. Rarely are all the muscles of the arm involved (4 of 99 cases of Tsairis et al). Recovery of paralysis and restoration of sensation are usually complete in a matter of 6 to 12 weeks but sometimes not for a year or longer. In 5 to 10 percent of cases, there is residual weakness and wasting of the affected muscles, and a similar number have had a recurrence on the same or the opposite side.

Motor nerve conduction becomes impaired in 7 to 10 days. The lesions are presumably of axonal type, and signs of denervation follow. A small proportion of cases are bilateral, usually sequentially, rather than simultaneously, and recurrences have been reported. Most of the neurologic deficits in our cases have been localized around the shoulder and upper arm; rarely the hand has been affected predominantly. Either the biceps or triceps reflex may be abolished. In a few of our cases there has been an additional median, radial, or posterior interosseous nerve palsy that can be isolated by EMG to a site distal to the plexus (see below).

The term *neuralgic amyotrophy* was applied to this symptom complex by Parsonage and Turner, who wrote extensively on the subject. Their term for the condition is not entirely inappropriate, since the clinical and EMG findings suggest a lesion of the peripheral nerves of the shoulder girdle and upper arm rather than the cords of the plexus. Actually, the exact site of the pathologic changes has not been established. Such patients usually have no fever, leukocytosis, or increased sedimentation rate. Occasionally there is a mild pleocytosis (10 to 50 white blood cells per cubic millimeter) and slightly increased protein in the CSF.

There are probably *highly restricted forms* of the same disorder that affects only one or two nerves of the brachial plexus. The most common of these is an isolated palsy of the serratus anterior (long thoracic nerve). The suprascapular, axillary, posterior interosseus, and phrenic nerves are other common solitary sites of affection. In the case of a unilateral phrenic nerve paralysis, there is mild dyspnea on exertion and one hemidiaphragm is found to be elevated on the chest film. When the process is not progressive and no mediastinal lesion can be detected, the phrenic palsy can be assumed to fall into this idiopathic category.

Duchowny and colleagues have described a patient in whom a typical brachial neuritis occurred as part of a febrile illness that proved to be due to CMV infection, and the same has been observed in patients with AIDS. A few outbreaks have been recorded and prompted the suggestion that the Coxsackie virus is the cause. The therapeutic use of interleukin-2 and interferon has apparently precipitated a few cases. Formerly, when animal antisera were in common use, this entity was rather frequent, but now it is rare. About 3 to 10 days after the administration of horse tetanus antitoxin, for example, there occurred the acute onset of severe pain in the shoulder and upper arm on one side, sometimes on both sides. The pain coincided with or followed, within a day or two, the development of other systemic manifestations of serum sickness. Several days after the onset of pain, as with brachial neuritis of idiopathic type, weakness about the shoulder was noted, usually in the distribution of the upper (lateral) trunk of the brachial plexus. Or there would be only an isolated mononeuropathy (most often of the axillary, suprascapular, musculocutaneous, or long thoracic nerve). Plexitis following vaccines is similar. It has been seen after injection of tetanus toxoid, typhoid-paratyphoid vaccine, and triple vaccine (pertussis, diphtheria, and tetanus).

Plexitis also occurs as an uncommon idiopathic complication of the *postpartum state* (Lederman and Wilbourn). Some of these instances are repetitive or bilateral and some are familial, but otherwise the plexitis has no distinguishing features from the idiopathic type of brachial neuritis.

One must differentiate brachial plexitis from the following conditions: (1) spondylosis or ruptured disc with root involvement, particularly the C5 and C6 roots, in which paralysis is rarely as severe as it is in plexitis; (2) brachialgia from bursitis or "rotator cuff syndrome"; (3) polymyalgia rheumatica; (4) entrapment neuropathies, particularly of the subscapular or dorsal scapular nerve; (5) carcinomatous plexopathy; (6) radiation plexopathy; and, rarely, (7) sarcoid and other granulomatous infiltrations. The special case of plexopathy in patients with a genetic proclivity to pressure palsies is discussed below.

Pathologic data are sparse, but Suarez and coworkers have reported collections of intense mononuclear inflammation in fascicles of the plexus obtained by biopsy. Lymphocytes could be found endoneurially and perivascularly in the epineurium. The disease has not been reproduced in the experimental animal. Therapy is purely symptomatic, but we have often embarked on a course of steroids and, in a few cases, other immunosuppressants when the illness continued to advance over many weeks. This approach has a beneficial effect on pain. Steroids have also been successful in some cases of lumbosacral plexitis and is favored by Suarez and colleagues.

Heredofamilial Plexopathy and Pressure Palsies Rarely, an acute *recurrent brachial neuropathy* occurs in families. The pattern of inheritance is autosomal dominant, and the attacks occur most commonly in the second and third decades of life. The authors have observed this syndrome in three generations of a family, some members having had three to five attacks at ages ranging from 3 to 45 years. Lower cranial nerve involvement and mononeuropathies in other limbs were conjoined in some instances (see Taylor). Again, the clinical course is benign. We have also seen the contemporaneous onset of brachial plexitis in an adult brother and sister who shared the same household but had no family history of a similar problem. A shared susceptibility to viral or environmental agents was suspected.

Madrid and Bradley have examined the sural nerves from two patients with familial recurrent brachial neuropathy. In teased single nerve fibers, they found sausage-like segments of thickened myelin and redundant loops of myelin with secondary constriction of the axon. In addition, nerve fibers showed a considerable degree of segmental demyelination and remyelination. They called this aberration of myelin formation "tomaculous neuropathy" (from *tomaculum*, "sausage"). These changes were not observed in the sural nerve of a sporadic case of recurrent acute brachial plexus neuropathy. The tomaculous change probably reflected a susceptibility to pressure palsies.

The genetic vulnerability to brachial neuropathy is closely related to the *hereditary neuropathy with liability to pressure palsies* reported by Earl and colleagues and by others. In the nerves of such patients, Behse and associates have found sausage-like swellings of the myelin sheaths, like those observed in familial brachial plexus neuropathy. However, the two inherited focal neuropathies—brachial plexus neuropathy and liability to pressure palsies—rarely overlap clinically. Almost invariably, patients with recurrent pressure palsies also show signs of a generalized polyneuropathy, including pes cavus and hammertoes in some cases and slowed or reduced motor nerve conduction. Moreover, within affected kinships, those who are free of pressure palsies may show signs of polyneuropathy. The molecular defect in patients with hereditary pressure palsies and recurrent brachial palsies has been identified as a DNA deletion on chromosome 17 (page 1417). Thus there is a linkage of these disorders with the autosomal dominant type of Charcot-Marie-Tooth disease (CMT1), which is associated with a DNA duplication at the same locus (Verhalle et al).

Brachial Neuropathy following Radiation Therapy
This is usually a complication of irradiation of the axilla

for carcinoma of the breast. Stoll and Andrews studied a group of 117 such patients who were treated with high-voltage, small-field therapy and had received either 6300 or 5775 cGy in divided doses. Of those receiving the larger dose, 73 percent developed weakness and sensory loss in the hand and fingers between 4 and 30 months after treatment, most of them after 12 months. In one autopsied case, the brachial plexus was ensheathed in dense fibrous tissue; distal to this zone, both myelin and axons had disappeared (secondary to wallerian degeneration), presumably as a result of entrapment of nerves in fibrous tissue; possibly a vascular factor was also operative.

Kori and coworkers, who analyzed the brachial plexus lesions in 100 patients with cancer, also found that doses exceeding 6000 cGy were associated with radiation damage. Usually the upper plexus was involved and was associated with a painless lymphedema. In patients who received lower doses, the development of brachial plexopathy usually indicated tumor infiltration; these lesions affected the lower plexus more than the upper; they were often painful and accompanied by a Horner syndrome (see also Lederman and Wilbourn). Rarely, radiation may give rise, many years later, to a malignant tumor of nerve or the surrounding connective tissue. Myokymic discharges and fasciculations are particularly suggestive of radiation damage.

Herpes Zoster Plexitis, Neuritis, and Ganglionitis

(See Chap. 33.)

Brachial Mononeuropathies (See Table 48-1)

Long Thoracic Nerve (of Bell) This nerve is derived from the fifth, sixth, and seventh cervical nerves and supplies the serratus anterior muscle, which fixates the lateral scapula to the chest wall. Paralysis of this muscle results in an inability to raise the arm over the head and winging of the medial border of the scapula when the outstretched arm is pushed forward against resistance. The nerve is injured most commonly by carrying heavy weights on the shoulder or by strapping the shoulder on the operating table. As stated above, the neuropathy sometimes followed immunization. At times it may be the only affected nerve in a brachial plexus neuropathy of either the inherited or idiopathic variety (Phillips).

Suprascapular Nerve This nerve is derived from the fifth (mainly) and sixth cervical nerves and supplies the supraspinatus and infraspinatus muscles. Lesions may be recognized by the presence of atrophy of these muscles and weakness of the first 15 degrees of abduction (supraspinatus) and of external rotation of the arm at the shoulder joint (infraspinatus). The latter is tested by having the patient flex the forearm and then, pinning the elbow to the side, asking him to swing the forearm backward against resistance. This nerve is often involved as part of a brachial plexus neuropathy of either the sporadic or inherited type. It may be affected during infectious illnesses and may be injured in gymnasts or as a result of local pressure, from carrying heavy objects on the shoulder ("meat-packer's neuropathy"). An entrapment syndrome has also been reported; it is characterized by pain and weakness on external rotation of the shoulder joint with atrophy of the infraspinatus muscle (Table 46-1). Decompression of the nerve where it enters the spinoglenoid notch relieves the condition.

Axillary Nerve This nerve arises from the posterior cord of the brachial plexus (mainly from the C5 root, with a smaller contribution from C6) and supplies the teres minor and deltoid muscles. It may be involved in dislocations of the shoulder joint, fractures of the neck of the humerus, serum- and vaccine-induced neuropathies, and brachial neuritis; in other instances, no cause may be apparent. The anatomic diagnosis depends on recognition of paralysis of abduction of the arm (in testing this function, the angle between the side of the chest and the arm must be greater than 15 degrees and less than 90 degrees), wasting of the deltoid muscle, and slight impairment of sensation over the outer aspect of the shoulder.

Musculocutaneous Nerve The origin of this nerve is from the fifth and sixth cervical roots. It is a branch of the lateral cord of the brachial plexus and innervates the biceps brachii, brachialis, and coracobrachialis muscles. Lesions of the nerve result in wasting of these muscles and weakness of flexion of the supinated forearm. Sensation may be impaired along the radial and volar aspects of the forearm (lateral cutaneous nerve). Isolated lesions of this nerve are usually the result of fracture of the humerus.

Radial Nerve This nerve is derived from the sixth to eighth (mainly the seventh) cervical roots and is the distal extension of the posterior cord of the brachial plexus. It innervates the triceps, brachioradialis, and supinator muscles and continues below the elbow as the posterior interosseous nerve, which innervates the extensor muscles of the wrist and fingers, the abductor of the thumb, and the extensors of the fingers at both joints. A complete radial nerve lesion results in paralysis of extension of the elbow, flexion of the elbow with the forearm midway between pronation and supination (due to paralysis of the brachioradialis muscle), supination of the forearm, extension of the wrist and fingers, and extension and abduction of the thumb in the plane of the palm. If the lesion is confined to the posterior interosseous nerve, only the extensors of the wrist and fingers are affected. Sensation is impaired over the posterior aspects of the forearm and over a small area on the radial aspect of the dorsum of the hand.

The radial nerve may be compressed in the axilla ("crutch palsy") but more frequently at a lower point, where the nerve winds around the humerus (Table 46-4); pressure palsies incurred during an alcoholic stupor and fractures of the humerus commonly injure the nerve at the latter site. It is susceptible to lead intoxication and is frequently involved as part of a neuralgic amyotrophy.

Median Nerve This nerve originates from the fifth cervical to the first thoracic roots but mainly from the sixth cervical root and is formed by the union of the medial and lateral cords of the brachial plexus. It innervates the pronators of the forearm, long finger flexors, and abductor and opponens muscles of the thumb and is a sensory nerve to the palmar aspect of the hand. Complete interruption of the median nerve results in inability to pronate the forearm or flex the hand in a radial direction, paralysis of flexion of the index finger and terminal phalanx of the thumb, weakness of flexion of the remaining fingers, weakness of opposition and abduction of the thumb in the plane at a right angle to the palm (abductor and flexor pollicis brevis), and sensory impairment over the radial two-thirds of the palm and dorsum of the distal phalanges of the index and third fingers. The nerve may be injured in the axilla by dislocation of the shoulder and in any part of its course by stab, gunshot, or other types of wounds. Incomplete lesions of the median nerve between the axilla and wrist may result in causalgia (see further on).

Table 46-4
Entrapment neuropathies

Nerve	*Site of entrapment*
Suprascapular	Spinoglenoid notch
Lower trunk or medial cord of branchial plexus	Cervical rib or band at thoracic outlet
Median	
Wrist	Carpal tunnel
Elbow	Between heads of pronator teres (pronator syndrome)
Ulnar	
Wrist	Guyon's canal (ulnar tunnel)
Elbow	Bicipital groove, cubital tunnel
Posterior interosseous nerve	Radial tunnel—at point of entrance into supinator muscle (arcade of Frohse)
Lateral femoral cutaneous (meralgia paresthetica)	Inguinal ligament
Obturator	Obturator canal
Posterior tibial	Tarsal tunnel; medial malleolus–flexor retinaculum
Interdigital plantar (Morton metatarsalgia)	Plantar fascia: heads of third and fourth metatarsals

Carpal Tunnel Syndrome Compression of the nerve at the wrist (*carpal tunnel syndrome*) is the most common disorder affecting the median nerve and the most frequent nerve entrapment syndrome. This is usually due to excessive use of the hands and occupational exposure to repeated trauma. Infiltration of the transverse carpal ligament with amyloid (as occurs in multiple myeloma) or thickening of connective tissue in rheumatoid arthritis, acromegaly, mucopolysaccharidosis, and hypothyroidism are less commonly identified causes. It is not uncommon for the condition to make its appearance during pregnancy. In elderly individuals, the cause of the carpal tunnel syndrome is often not apparent.

Dysesthesias and pain in the fingers, referred to for many years as "acroparesthesiae" and attributed to cervical ribs, came to be recognized as a syndrome of median nerve compression only in the early 1950s. According to Kremer and colleagues, it was McArdle, in 1949, who first suggested that the cause of this syndrome was a compression of the median nerve at the wrist and that the symptoms would be relieved by division of the flexor retinaculum forming the ventral wall of the carpal tunnel. The paresthesias are characteristically worse during the night. As pointed out in Chap. 11, the pain in carpal tunnel syndrome often radiates into the forearm and even into the region of the biceps and rarely to the shoulder. The syndrome is essentially a sensory one; the loss or impairment of superficial sensation affects the thumb, index, and middle fingers (especially the index finger) and may or may not split the ring finger (splitting does not occur with a plexus or root lesion). Weakness and atrophy of the abductor pollicis brevis and other median-innervated muscles occur in only the most advanced cases of compression. Electrophysiologic testing confirms the diagnosis and explains cases in which operation has failed (see also the review by Stevens).

Surgical division of the carpal ligament with decompression of the nerve is curative. Splinting of the wrist, to avoid flexion, almost always relieves the discomfort but denies the patient the full use of the hand. It is a useful temporizing measure, however, as is the injection of hydrocortisone into the carpal tunnel.

Another site of compression of the median nerve is at the elbow, where the nerve passes between the two heads of the pronator teres, or just above that point behind the bicipital aponeurosis. It gives rise to the pronator syndrome, in which forceful pronation of the forearm produces an aching pain (Table 46-4). There is weakness of the abductor pollicis brevis and opponens muscles and numbness of the first three digits and palm.

Ulnar Nerve This nerve is derived from the eighth cervical and first thoracic roots. It innervates the ulnar flexor of the wrist, the ulnar half of the deep finger flexors, the adductors and abductors of the fingers, the adductor of the thumb, the third and fourth lumbricals, and muscles of the hypothenar eminence. Complete ulnar paralysis is manifest by a characteristic claw-hand deformity; wasting of the small hand muscles results in hyperextension of the fingers at the metacarpophalangeal joints and flexion at the interphalangeal joints. The flexion deformity is most pronounced in the fourth and fifth fingers, since the lumbrical muscles of the second and third fingers, supplied by the median nerve, counteract the deformity. Sensory loss occurs over the fifth finger, the ulnar aspect of the fourth finger, and the ulnar border of the palm.

The ulnar nerve is vulnerable to pressure in the axilla from the use of crutches, but it is most commonly injured at the elbow by fracture or dislocation involving the joint. *Delayed ("tardive") ulnar palsy* may occur many years after an injury to the elbow that had resulted in a cubitus valgus deformity of the joint. Because of the deformity, the nerve is stretched in its groove over the ulnar condyle, and its superficial location renders it vulnerable to compression. A shallow ulnar groove, quite apart from abnormalities of the elbow joint, may expose the nerve to compressive injury. Anterior transposition of the ulnar nerve is a simple and effective form of treatment for these types of ulnar palsy. Compression of the nerve may occur just distal to the medial epicondyle, where it runs beneath the aponeurosis of the flexor carpi ulnaris (*cubital tunnel*). Flexion at the elbow causes a narrowing of the tunnel and constriction of the nerve. This type of ulnar palsy is treated by incising the aponeurotic arch between the olecranon and medial epicondyle. Yet another site of ulnar nerve compression is in the ulnar tunnel, at the wrist. Prolonged pressure on the ulnar part of the palm may result in damage to the deep palmar branch of the ulnar nerve, causing weakness of small hand muscles but no sensory loss. This site is most often implicated in patients who hold tools or implements tightly in the hand for long periods (we have seen it in machinists and cake decrators). The lesion is localizable by nerve conduction studies.

A characteristic syndrome of burning pain and associated symptoms (causalgia) may follow incomplete lesions of the ulnar nerve (or other major nerves of the limbs) and is described further on.

Lumbosacral Plexus and Crural Neuropathies

The twelfth thoracic, first to fifth lumbar, and first, second, and third sacral spinal nerve roots compose the lumbosacral plexuses and innervate the muscles of the lower extremities (see Fig. 46-5). The following are the common plexus and crural nerve palsies.

Lumbosacral Plexus Lesions Extending as it does from the upper lumbar area to the lower sacrum and passing near several lower abdominal and pelvic organs, this plexus is subject to a number of special injuries and diseases, most of them secondary. The cause of involvement may be difficult to ascertain because the primary disease is often not within reach of the palpating fingers, either from the abdominal side or through the anus and vagina; even refined radiologic techniques may not reveal it. Diagnosis involves exclusion of spinal root (cauda equina) lesions by EMG, examination of CSF, CT myelography, and MRI. The clinical findings help to focus studies on the appropriate part of the lumbosacral plexus.

The main effects of upper lumbar plexus lesions are weakness of flexion and adduction of the thigh and extension of the leg, with sensory loss over the anterior thigh and leg; these effects must be distinguished from the symptoms and signs of femoral neuropathy (see below). Lower plexus lesions weaken the posterior thigh, leg, and foot muscles and abolish sensation over the first and second sacral segments (sometimes the lower sacral segments also). Lesions of the entire plexus, which occur infrequently, cause a weakness or paralysis of all leg muscles, with atrophy, areflexia, anesthesia from the toes to the perianal region and autonomic loss with warm, dry skin. Usually there is edema of the leg as well.

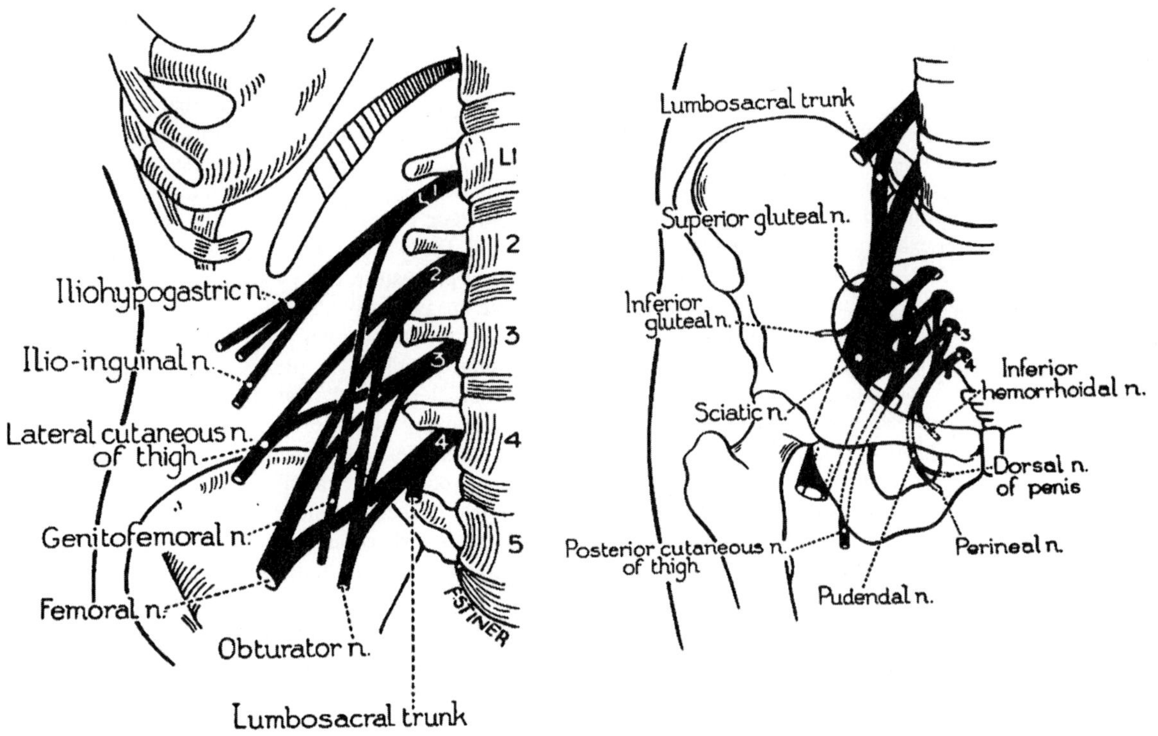

Figure 46-5

Diagram of the lumbar plexus (left) and the sacral plexus (right). The lumbosacral trunk is the liaison between the lumbar and the sacral plexuses. (From Haymaker and Woodhall by permission.)

The types of lesions that involve the lumbosacral plexus are rather different from those affecting the brachial plexus. Trauma is a rarity except with massive pelvic, spinal, and abdominal injuries because the plexus is so well protected. Occasionally a pelvic fracture will damage the sciatic nerve as it issues from the plexus. In contrast, some part of the plexus may be damaged during surgical procedures on abdominal and pelvic organs, often for reasons that may not be entirely clear. For example, hysterectomy has on a number of occasions led to neurologic consultation in our hospitals because of numbness and weakness of the anterior thigh. Either the cords of the upper part of the plexus or the femoral nerve was compressed by retraction against the psoas muscle or, in vaginal hysterectomy (when thighs are flexed, abducted, and externally rotated), the femoral nerve was compressed against the inguinal ligament. A similar type of injury may be associated with childbirth. Lumbar sympathectomy has also been associated with upper plexus lesions, of which the most disabling sequelae are burning pain and hypersensitivity of the anterior thigh. Appendectomy, pelvic explorations, and hernial repair may injure branches of the upper plexus (ilioinguinal, iliohypogastric, and genitofemoral nerves), with severe pain and slight sensory loss in the distribution of one of these nerves. The pain may last for months or a year or more.

The lumbar plexus may be compressed by an aortic atherosclerotic aneurysm. Usually there is pain that radiates to the hip, the anterior thigh, and occasionally the flank. Slight weakness in hip flexion and altered sensation over the anterior thigh are found on examination. Plexus involvement with tumors is commonplace and at times presents special difficulties in diagnosis. Carcinoma of either the cervix or prostate may seed itself along the perineurial lymphatics and cause pain in the groin, thigh, knee, or back without much in the way of sensory, motor, or reflex loss. The pain is more often unilateral than bilateral. The CSF and spinal canal (by MRI) are normal. Testicular, uterine, ovarian, and colonic tumors or retroperitoneal lymphomas, by extending along the paravertebral gutter, implicate various parts of the lumbosacral plexus. Instances of endometriosis that involve the plexus have also been reported. The neurologic symptoms are projected at a distance in the leg and may or may not be confined to the territory of any one nerve. Pelvic and rectal examinations may be negative, and CT scanning and MRI may be necessary to show such lesions. If all these examinations are negative, exploratory laparotomy may have to be undertaken.

In cancer patients, it is sometimes difficult to distinguish the effects of radiation on the lumbosacral plexus from those of metastatic tumor, as is the case in relation to the brachial plexus. Thomas and colleagues found that the earliest symptom in metastatic lumbosacral plexopathy was pain, whereas in radiation plexopathy it was weakness. Plexopathy from metastatic tumor was usually unilateral and detectable by CT scanning; radiation plexopathy was usually bilateral and not evident in CT scans. Fasciculations and myokymia were more likely to be seen in patients with radiation plexopathy, which seemingly occurs more frequently in patients with diabetic neuropathy.

Reference has already been made to femoral nerve injury during parturition, but other *puerperal complications* are also observed. Back pain in the latter part of pregnancy is common, but there are rare instances in which the patient complains of severe pain in the back of one or both thighs during labor and after delivery has numbness and weakness of the leg muscles, with diminished ankle jerks. *Parturitional lumbosacral plexus injuries* occur with a frequency of 1 per 2000 deliveries. This type of plexus injury is usually unilateral and is manifest by pain in the thigh and leg and symptoms and signs of involvement of the superior gluteal and sciatic nerves (Feasby et al). The attribution of these symptoms to pressure of the fetal head on the sacral plexus(es) is conjectural. A limited plexopathy, ocurring after difficult vaginal delivery, mainly impairs sensation in the perineum and sphincteric function (Ismael et al). The perineal muscles may show signs of denervation. Protrusion of an intervertebral disc may also occur during delivery.

A *neuralgic amyotrophy* or *lumbosacral plexitis*, analogous to the brachial variety, is observed from time to time. Bradley and coworkers have recorded such cases. After causing widespread unilateral or bilateral sensory, motor, and reflex changes in a leg, lumbosacral plexitis may leave the patient with dysesthesias as troublesome as those that follow herpes zoster (which may also occur at this level). Some patients have had an exploration of the cauda equina (for ruptured disc), even though loss of sweating and warmth of the feet should have indicated interruption of autonomic fibers by lesions in peripheral nerves. (Lesions that are confined to nerve roots spare autonomic functions.) The sedimentation rate may be elevated. Immunosuppressant drugs were beneficial in 4 of 6 cases (Bradley et al). Sarcoidosis is another cause and may be responsive to corticosteroids. *Diabetic amyotrophy*, due to involvement of the lumbar plexus(es), has a vascular origin (page 1397), and there are probably also nondiabetic vascular lesions that give rise to lumbar and upper leg pain and weakness in proximal muscles. The plexus lesions of polyarteritis nodosa, unilateral or bilateral, may also be manifest as a mononeuropathy multiplex. The incidence of mononeuropathy multiplex in diabetics is augmented by an associated occlusive vascular disease of the lower extremities. Diabetic mononeuropathy multiplex is discussed in an earlier part of this chapter and protruded intervertebral disc syndromes are described in Chap. 11.

Lateral Cutaneous Nerve of the Thigh This is a sensory nerve that originates from the second and third lumbar roots and supplies the anterolateral aspect of the thigh, from the level of the inguinal ligament almost to the knee. The nerve penetrates the psoas muscle, crosses the iliacus, and passes into the thigh by coursing between the attachments of the lateral part of the inguinal ligament to the anterior superior iliac spine. Compression (entrapment) may occur at the point where it passes between the two prongs of attachment of the inguinal ligament.

Compression of the nerve results in uncomfortable paresthesias and sensory impairment in its cutáneous distribution, a common condition known as *meralgia paresthetica* (*meros*, "thigh"). Usually numbness and mild sensitivity of the skin are the only symptoms, but occasionally there is a persistent distressing burning pain. Perception of touch and pinprick are reduced in the territory of the nerve; there is no weakness of the quadriceps or diminution of the knee jerk. The symptoms are characteristically worsened in certain positions and after prolonged standing or walking. Occasionally, for an obese person, sitting is the most uncomfortable position. Obesity, pregnancy, and diabetes mellitus are contributory factors. Most often the neuropathy is unilateral; Ecker and Woltman found only 20 percent of their cases to be bilateral.

Most of our patients with meralgia paresthetica request no treatment once they learn of its benign character. Weight loss and adjustment of restrictive clothing or correction of habitual postures that might compress the nerve are sometimes helpful. A few with the most painful symptoms have demanded a neurectomy or section of the nerve, but it is always wise to perform a lidocaine block first, so that the patient can decide whether the persistent numbness is preferable. In one specimen of nerve obtained at operation, we found a discrete traumatic neuroma. Hydrocortisone injections at the point of entrapment have helped in a few cases.

Obturator Nerve This nerve arises from the third and fourth and to a lesser extent the second lumbar roots. It supplies the adductors of the thigh and contributes to the innervation of the internal and external rotators. The adductors have the added function of flexing the hip. The nerve may be injured by the fetal head or forceps during the course of a difficult labor or compressed by an obturator hernia. Rarely, it is affected in diabetes, polyarteritis nodosa, and osteitis pubis and by retroperitoneal spread of carcinoma of the cervix, uterus, and other tumors (Rogers et al).

Femoral Nerve This nerve is formed from the second, third, and fourth lumbar roots. Within the pelvis it passes along the lateral border of the psoas muscle and enters the thigh beneath Poupart's ligament, lateral to the femoral artery. Branches arising within the pelvis supply the iliacus and psoas muscles. Just below Poupart's ligament the nerve splits into anterior and posterior divisions. The former supplies the pectineus and sartorius muscles and carries sensation from the anteromedial surface of the thigh; the posterior division provides the motor innervation to the quadriceps and the cutaneous innervation to the medial side of the leg from the knee to the internal malleolus.

Following injury to the femoral nerve, there is weakness of extension of the lower leg, wasting of the quadriceps muscle, and failure of fixation of the knee. The knee jerk is abolished. If the nerve is injured proximal to the origin of the branches to the iliacus and psoas muscles, there is weakness of hip flexion. The adductor of the thigh (innervated by the obturator nerve) is spared, distinguishing femoral neuropathy from an L3 radiculopathy.

The commonest cause of femoral neuropathy is diabetes. The nerve may be involved by pelvic tumors. Not uncommon is injury of the nerve during pelvic operations. Usually this is the result of improper placement of retractors, which may compress the nerve directly or indirectly by undue pressure on the psoas muscle. Bleeding into the iliacus muscle or the retroperitoneum, observed in patients receiving anticoagulants and in hemophiliacs, is a relatively common cause of isolated femoral neuropathy (Goodfellow et al). The presenting symptom of iliacus hematoma is pain in the groin spreading to the lumbar region or thigh, in response to which the patient assumes a characteristic posture of flexion and lateral rotation of the hip. A palpable mass in the iliac fossa and the signs of femoral nerve compression (quadriceps weakness and loss of knee jerk) follow in a day or two. Infarction of the nerve may occur in the course of diabetes mellitus and polyarteritis nodosa. Not infrequently acute femoral neuropathy is of indeterminate cause.

Sciatic Nerve This nerve is derived from the fourth and fifth lumbar and first and second sacral roots, for which reason a ruptured disc at these levels may simulate sciatic neuropathy (sciatica). The sciatic nerve supplies motor innervation to the hamstring muscles and all the muscles below the knee through its two divisions, the tibial and peroneal nerves (see below); the sciatic nerve conveys sensory impulses from the posterior aspect of the thigh, the posterior and lateral aspects of the leg, and the entire sole. In complete sciatic paralysis, the knee cannot be flexed and all muscles below the knee are paralyzed. Weakness of gluteal muscles and pain in the buttock and posterior thigh point to nerve involvement in the pelvis. Lesions beyond the sciatic notch spare the gluteal muscles but not the hamstrings. Partial compressive lesions are more common and tend to involve peroneal-innervated muscles more than tibial ones, giving the impression of a peroneal palsy.

As mentioned, rupture of one of the lower lumbar intervertebral discs is perhaps the commonest cause of sciatica although it does not directly involve the sciatic nerve. The associated motor and sensory findings allow localization of the root compression (L4-5 disc compressing L5 root: pain in posterolateral thigh and leg with numbness over the inner foot and weakness of dorsiflexion of the foot and toes; L5-S1 disc compressing S1 root: pain in posterior thigh and leg, numbness of lateral foot, weakness of foot dorsiflexion and loss of ankle jerk).

The sciatic nerve is commonly injured by fractures of the pelvis or femur, fracture/dislocation of the hip, gunshot wounds of the buttock and thigh, and the injection of toxic substances into the lower gluteal region. Total hip arthroplasty is another common cause. Tumors of the pelvis (sarcomas, lipomas) or gluteal region may compress the nerve. Sitting for a long period with legs flexed and abducted (lotus position) under the influence of narcotics or barbiturates or lying flat on a hard surface in a sustained stupor may severely injure one or both sciatic nerves or branches thereof. The nerve may be involved by neurofibromas and infections and by ischemic necrosis in diabetes mellitus and polyarteritis nodosa. Cryptogenic forms also occur and are actually more frequent than those of identifiable cause. Partial lesions of the sciatic nerve occasionally result in causalgia (see further on).

Common Peroneal Nerve Just above the popliteal fossa the sciatic nerve divides into the tibial nerve (*medial*, or *internal*, *popliteal nerve*) and the common peroneal nerve (*lateral*, or *external*, *popliteal nerve*). The latter swings around the head of the fibula to the anterior aspect of the leg, giving off the musculocutaneous branch (to the peroneal muscles) and continuing as the *anterior tibial*, or *deep peroneal*, *nerve*. Branches of the latter supply the dorsiflexors of the foot and toes and carry sensory fibers from the dorsum of the foot and lateral aspect of the lower half of the leg. There was weakness of dorsiflexion of the foot in all of the 116 cases of common peroneal neuropathy reported by Katirji and Wilbourn, and numbness of the dorsum of the foot was present in most cases. Weakness of eversion of the foot is usually demonstrable; inversion, a function of the L-5 root and the tibial nerve, is spared. Pain is variable; it was quite severe in a few of our patients.

Pressure during an operation or sleep or from tight plaster casts, obstetric stirrups, habitual and prolonged crossing of the legs while seated, and tight knee boots are the most frequent causes of injury to the common peroneal nerve. The point of compression of the nerve is where it passes over the head of the fibula. Emaciation increases the incidence of these types of compressive injury. The nerve may also be affected in diabetic neuropathy and injured by fractures of the upper end of the fibula. A Baker cyst, which consists of inflamed synovium extending into the retropopliteal space, and it may be damaged by muscle swelling or small hematomas behind the knee in asthenic athletes.

Tibial Nerve This, the other of the two divisions of the sciatic nerve (it divides in the popliteal fossa), supplies all of the calf muscles—i.e., the plantar flexors and invertors of the foot and toes—after which it continues as the posterior tibial nerve. This nerve passes through the tarsal tunnel, an osseofibrous channel that runs along the medial aspect of the calcaneus and is roofed by the flexor retinaculum. The tunnel also contains the tendons of the tibialis posterior, flexor digitorum longus, and flexor hallucis longus muscles and the vessels to the foot. The posterior tibial nerve terminates under the flexor retinaculum and divides into medial and lateral plantar nerves (supplying the small muscles of the foot).

Complete interruption of the tibial nerve results in a calcaneovalgus deformity of the foot, which can no longer be plantar-flexed and inverted. There is loss of sensation over the plantar aspect of the foot.

The posterior tibial nerve may be compressed in the tarsal tunnel (entrapment syndrome) by thickening of the tendon sheaths or the adjacent connective tissues or by osteoarthritic changes. Tingling pain and burning over the sole of the foot develop after standing or walking for a long time. Usually there is no motor deficit. Relief is obtained by severing the flexor retinaculum.

Entrapment Neuropathies

Reference has been made in several places in the preceding pages to entrapment neuropathies. A nerve passing through a tight canal is trapped and subjected to constant movement or pressure, forces not applicable to nerves elsewhere. The epineurium and perineurium become greatly thickened, strangling the nerve, with the additional possibility of demyelination. Function is gradually impaired, sensory more than motor, and the symptoms fluctuate with activity and rest. The most frequently compressed nerves are the median, ulnar, peroneal, tibial, and plantar in approximately that order. It is well to keep in mind the systemic processes that enhance pressure palsies by infiltration of the nerve or surrounding tissues. The main ones are hypothyroidism, amyloid, pregnancy, and hereditary liability to pressure palsies.

Listed in Table 46-4 are the more common entrapment neuropathies and the locations of compression. Detailed accounts of these disorders are contained in the monographs of Dawson and colleagues and of Asbury and Gilliat, listed in the References.

Causalgia and Reflex Sympathetic Dystrophy

(See also pages 148 and 230.) *Causalgia* was the name applied by Weir Mitchell to a rare (except in time of war) type of peripheral neuralgia consequent upon trauma, with partial interruption of the median or ulnar nerve and perhaps less often, the sciatic or peroneal nerve. It is characterized by persistent, severe pain in the hand or foot, most pronounced in the digits, palm of the hand, or sole. The pain has a burning quality and frequently radiates beyond the territory of the injured nerve. The painful parts are exquisitely sensitive to contactual stimuli, so the patient cannot bear the pressure of clothing or drafts of air; even ambient heat, cold, noise, or emotional stimuli intensify the causalgic symptoms. The affected extremity is kept protected and immobile, often wrapped in a cloth moistened with cool water. Sudomotor, vasomotor, and, later, trophic abnormalities are usual accompaniments of the pain. The skin of the affected part is moist and warm or cool and soon becomes shiny and smooth, at times scaly and discolored.

A number of theories have been proposed to explain the causalgic syndrome. For many years it was attributed to a short-circuiting of impulses, the result of an artificial connection between efferent sympathetic and somatic afferent pain fibers at the point of the nerve injury. The demonstration that the causalgic pain could be abolished by depletion of neurotransmitters at sympathetic adrenergic endings shifted the presumed site of sympathetic-afferent interaction to the nerve terminals and suggested that the abnormal cross-excitation is chemical rather than electrical in nature. An explanation favored in recent years is that an abnormal adrenergic sensitivity develops in injured nociceptors and that circulating or locally secreted sympathetic neurotransmitters trigger the painful afferent activity. Another theory holds that a sustained period of bombardment by sensory pain impulses from one region results in the sensitization of central sensory structures. "True causalgia" of this type can be counted upon to respond favorably, if only temporarily, to procaine block of the appropriate sympathetic ganglia and, over the longer run, to regional sympathectomy. Prolonged cooling and the intravenous injection of guanethidine into the affected limb (with the venous return blocked for several minutes) may alleviate the pain for days or longer. Epidural infusions, particularly of analgesics or ketamine, infusion of bisphosphonates and spinal cord stimulators are other forms of treatment (Kemler). The roles of the central and sympathetic nervous systems in causalgic pain have been critically reviewed by Schott and by Schwartzman and McLellan.

The term *causalgia* is best reserved for the syndrome described above—i.e., persistent burning pain and abnormalities of sympathetic innervation consequent upon trauma to a major nerve in an extremity. Others have applied the term to a wide range of conditions that are characterized by persistent burning pain but have only an inconstant association with sudomotor, vasomotor, and trophic changes and an unpredictable response to sympathetic blockade. These latter states, which have been described under a plethora of titles (Sudeck atrophy of bone, minor causalgia, shoulder-hand syndrome, algoneurodystrophy), may follow nontraumatic lesions of the peripheral nerves or even lesions of the CNS ("mimocausalgia").

Also, we have no explanation for the so-called causalgia-dystonia syndrome (Bhatia et al) in which a fixed dystonic posture is engrafted on a site of causalgic pain. The clinical features of both the causalgic and dystonic elements of the syndrome were somewhat unusual in the cases of these investigators. The degree of injury was often trivial or nonexistent and no signs of a neuropathic lesion were evident. Remarkably, both the causalgia and dystonia spread from their initial sites to widely disparate parts of the limbs and body. The syndrome did not respond to any form of treatment, although some patients recovered spontaneously. Its origin is not explained.

Traumatic Interruption of Nerves

The management of such lesions is best delegated to specialized neurosurgeons, but several aspects involve the neurologist. Surgical advances have allowed the successful apposition of severed nerve ends. The current recommendations are that a sharp and clean division should be repaired by end-to-end suturing of the stumps within 72 h. In cases where the nerve is found on exploration to be bluntly severed with ragged ends, most surgeons recommend tacking the free ends to adjacent connective tissue planes and attempting repair in 2 to 4 weeks. The majority of injuries however, are blunt and retain some continuity of the nerve. If such continuity of the nerve across the traumatized region can be demonstrated by electrophysiologic examination, operation is not necessary. In the absence of improvement in the clinical and electrophysiologic features after several months (up to 6 months for plexus lesions) surgical repair may facilitate limited healing.

REFERENCES

ADAMS RD, SHAHANI BT, YOUNG RR: A severe pansensory familial neuropathy. *Trans Am Neurol Assoc* 98:67, 1973.

ALI Z, CARROLL M, ROBERTSON KP, FOWLER CJ: The extent of small fibre sensory neuropathy in diabetics with plantar foot ulceration. *J Neurol Neurosurg Psychiatry* 52:94, 1989.

AMERICAN ACADEMY OF NEUROLOGY AIDS TASK FORCE: Research criteria for diagnosis of chronic inflammatory demyelinating polyneuropathy (CIDP). *Neurology* 41:617, 1991.

ANDRADE C, CANIJO M, KLEIN D, KAELIN A: The genetic aspect of the familial amyloidotic polyneuropathy: Portuguese type of paraamyloidosis. *Humangenetik* 7:163, 1969.

ARAKI S, MAWATARI S, OHTA M, et al: Polyneurotic amyloidosis in a Japanese family. *Arch Neurol* 18:593, 1968.

ASBURY AK, ALDREDGE H, HERSHBERG R, et al: Oculomotor palsy in diabetes mellitus. A clinicopathologic study. *Brain* 93:555, 1970.

Asbury AK, Arnason BGW, Adams RD: The inflammatory lesion in acute idiopathic polyneuritis. *Medicine* 48:173, 1969.

Asbury AK, Cornblath DR: Assessment of current diagnostic criteria for Guillain-Barré syndrome. *Ann Neurol* 27:521, 1990.

Asbury AK, Fields HL: Pain due to peripheral nerve damage: An hypothesis. *Neurology* 34:1587, 1984.

Asbury AK, Gilliat RW (eds): *Peripheral Nerve Disorders.* London, Butterworth, 1984.

Asbury AK, Picard EH, Baringer JR: Sensory perineuritis. *Arch Neurol* 26:302, 1972.

Asbury A, Thomas PK: *Peripheral Nerve Disorders*, 2nd ed. London, Butterworth & Heinemann, 1995.

Asbury A, Victor M, Adams RD: Uremic polyneuropathy. *Arch Neurol* 8:113, 1963.

Austin JH: Observations on the syndrome of hypertrophic neuritis (the hypertrophic interstitial radiculoneuropathies). *Medicine* 35:187, 1956.

Barnhill RL, McDougall AC: Thalidomide: Use and possible mode of action in reactional lepromatous leprosy and in various other conditions. *J Am Acad Dermatol* 7:317, 1982.

Barohn RJ, Kissel JT, Warmolts JR, Mendell JR: Chronic inflammatory polyradiculoneuropathy: Clinical characteristics, course, and recommendations for diagnostic critieria. *Arch Neurol* 46:878, 1989.

Bendixen BH, Younger DS, Hair LS, et al: Cholesterol emboli neuropathy. *Neurology* 42:428, 1992.

Bhatia KP, Bhatt MH, Marsden CD: The causalgia-dystonia syndrome. *Brain* 116:843,1993.

Bolton CF: Peripheral neuropathies associated with chronic renal failure. *Can J Neurol Sci* 7:89, 1980.

Bouldin TW, Hall CO, Krigman MR: Pathology of disulfiram neuropathy. *Neuropathol Appl Neurobiol* 6:155, 1980.

Bradley WG, Chad D, Verghese JP, et al: Painful lumbosacral plexopathy, with elevated sedimentation rate: A treatable inflammatory syndrome. *Ann Neurol* 15:457, 1984.

Brashear A, Unverzaght FW, Farber MO, et al: Ethylene oxide neurotoxicity: A cluster of 12 nurses with peripheral and central nervous system toxicity. *Neurology* 46:992, 1996.

Brostoff SW, Levit S, Powers JM: Induction of experimental allergic neuritis with a peptide from myelin P_2 basic protein. *Nature* 268:752, 1977.

Brown MJ, Greene DA: Diabetic neuropathy: Pathophysiology and management, in Asbury AK, Gilliat RW (eds): *Peripheral Nerve Disorders.* Boston, Butterworth, 1984, pp 126–153.

Cavanaugh NPC, Eames RA, Galvin RJ, et al: Hereditary sensory neuropathy with spastic paraplegia. *Brain* 102:79, 1979.

Chad D, Periser K, Bradley WG, et al: The pathogenesis of cryoglobulinemic neuropathy. *Neurology* 32:725, 1982.

Chalk CH, Dyck PJ: Ischemic neuropathy, in Dyck PJ, Thomas PK, Griffin JW, et al (eds): *Peripheral Neuropathy*, 3rd ed. Philadelphia, Saunders, 1993, pp 980–989.

Chalk CH, Dyck PJ, Conn DL: Vasculitic neuropathy, in Dyck PJ, Thomas PK, Griffin JW, et al (eds): *Peripheral Neuropathy*, 3rd ed. Philadelphia, Saunders, 1993, pp 1424–1436.

Chia, L, Fernandez A, Lacroix D, et al: Contribution of nerve biopsy findings to the diagnosis of disabling neuropathy in the elderly. A retrospective review of 100 consecutive patients. *Brain* 119:1091, 1996.

Cornblath DR, McArthur JC, Kennedy PGE, et al: Inflammatory demyelinating peripheral neuropathies associated with human T-cell lymphotropic virus type III infection. *Ann Neurol* 21:32, 1987.

Corse AM, Chaudhry V, Crawford TO, et al: Sensory nerve pathology in multifocal motor neuropathy. *Ann Neurol* 39:319, 1996.

Croft PB, Wilkinson M: The incidence of carcinomatous neuromyopathy in patients with various types of carcinoma. *Brain* 88:427, 1965.

Culebras A, Alio J, Herrera J-L, Lopez-Fraile IP: Effect of aldose reductase inhibitor on diabetic peripheral neuropathy. *Arch Neurol* 38:133, 1981.

Dalakas MC: Chronic idiopathic ataxic neuropathy. *Ann Neurol* 19:545, 1986.

Dalakas MC, Engel WK: Chronic relapsing (dysimmune) polyneuropathy: Pathogenesis and treatment. *Ann Neurol* 9:134, 1981.

Dalakas MC, Engel WK: Polyneuropathy with monoclonal gammopathy: Studies of 11 patients. *Ann Neurol* 10:45, 1981.

Dalmau J, Graus F, Rosenbaum MK, Posner JB: Anti-Hu–associated paraneoplastic encephalomyelitis/sensory neuropathy: A clinical study of 71 patients. *Medicine* 71:59, 1992.

Daughady WH: Extreme gigantism: Analysis of growth velocity and occurrence of severe peripheral neuropathy with neuropathic joints. *N Engl J Med* 297:1267, 1977.

Dawidenkow S: Über die neurotische Muskelatrophie Charcot-Marie: Klinisch-genetische Studien. *Z Neurol* 107:259; 108:344, 1927.

Dawson DM, Hallett M, Millender LH: *Entrapment Neuropathies*, 2nd ed. Boston, Little, Brown, 1990.

Delank HW, Koch G, Kohn G, et al: Familiare amyloid Polyneuropathie typus Wohlwill-Corino Andrade. *Aerztl Forsch* 19:401, 1965.

Denny-Brown D: Hereditary sensory radicular neuropathy. *J Neurol Neurosurg Psychiatry* 14:237, 1951.

Devinsky O, Feldmann E: *Examination of the Cranial and Peripheral Nerves.* New York, Churchill Livingstone, 1988.

Donaghy M, Hakin RN, Bamford JM, et al: Hereditary sensory neuropathy with neurotrophic keratitis. *Brain* 110:563, 1987.

Dreyfus PM, Hakim S, Adams RD: Diabetic ophthalmoplegia: Report of a case with post-mortem study and comments on vascular supply of human oculomotor nerve. *AMA Arch Neurol Psychiatry* 77:337, 1957.

Duchen LW, Anjorin A, Watkins PJ, Mackay JD: Pathology of autonomic neuropathy in diabetes mellitus. *Ann Intern Med* 92:301, 1980.

Duchowny M, Caplan L, Siber G: Cytomegalovirus infection of the adult nervous system. *Ann Neurol* 5:458, 1979.

Dyck PJ, Benstead TJ, Conn DL, et al: Nonsystemic vasculitic neuropathy. *Brain* 110:843, 1987.

Dyck PJ, Chance P, Lebo R, Carney JA: Hereditary motor and sensory neuropathies, in Dyck PJ, Thomas PK, Griffin JW, et al (eds): *Peripheral Neuropathy*, 3rd ed. Philadelphia, Saunders, 1993, pp 1094–1136.

DYCK PJ, DAUBE J, O'BRIEN P, et al: Plasma exchange in chronic inflammatory demyelinating polyneuropathy. *N Engl J Med* 314:461, 1986.

DYCK PJ, KARNES JL, O'BRIEN P, et al: The spatial distribution of fiber loss in diabetic polyneuropathy suggests ischemia. *Ann Neurol* 19:440, 1986.

DYCK PJ, KARNES JL, O'BRIEN P, RIZZA R: Fiber loss is primary and multifocal in sural nerves in diabetic polyneuropathy. *Ann Neurol* 19:425, 1986.

DYCK PJ, KRATZ KM, KARNES JL, et al: The prevalence by staged severity of various types of diabetic neuropathy, and nephropathy, in a population based cohort. *Neurology* 43:817, 1993.

DYCK PJ, LAIS AC, OHTA M, et al: Chronic inflammatory polyradiculoneuropathy. *Mayo Clin Proc* 50:621, 1975.

DYCK PJ, LAMBERT EH: Lower motor and primary sensory neuron disease with peroneal muscular atrophy. *Arch Neurol* 18:603, 1968.

DYCK PJ, LAMBERT EH: Polyneuropathy associated with hypothyroidism. *J Neuropathol Exp Neurol* 29:631, 1970.

DYCK PJ, LOW PA, WINDEBANK AJ, et al: Plasma exchange in polyneuropathy associated with monoclonal gammopathy of undetermined significance. *N Engl J Med* 325:1482, 1991.

DYCK PJ, OVIATT KF, LAMBERT EH: Intensive evaluation of referred unclassified neuropathies yields improved diagnosis. *Ann Neurol* 10:222, 1981.

DYCK PJ, PRINEAS J, POLLARD J: Chronic inflammatory demyelinating polyradiculoneuropathy, in Dyck PJ, Thomas PK, Griffin JW, et al (eds): *Peripheral Neuropathy*, 3rd ed. Philadelphia, Saunders, 1993, pp 1498–1517.

DYCK PJB, ENGELSTAD J, NORELL J, DYCK PJ: Microvasculitis in non-diabetic lumbosacral radiculoplexus neuropathy (LSRPN): Similarity to the diabetic variety. (DLSRPN). *J Neuropath Exp Neurol* 59:525, 2000.

EAMES RA, LANGE LS: Clinical and pathologic study of ischaemic neuropathy. *J Neurol Neurosurg* 30:215, 1967.

EARL CJ, FULLERTON PM, WAKEFIELD GS, SCHUTTA HS: Hereditary neuropathy with liability to pressure palsies. *Q J Med* 33:481, 1964.

ECKER AD, WOLTMAN WH: Meralgia paresthetica: A report of one hundred and fifty cases. *JAMA* 110:1650, 1938.

EKBOM KA: Restless legs syndrome. *Neurology* 10:858, 1960.

ENGEL WK, DORMAN JD, LEVY RI, FREDRICKSON DS: Neuropathy in Tangier disease. *Arch Neurol* 17:1, 1967.

ENGLAND AC, DENNY-BROWN D: Severe sensory changes and trophic disorders in peroneal muscular atrophy (Charcot-Marie-Tooth type). *Arch Neurol Psychiatry* 67:1, 1952.

FAGERBERG S-E: Diabetic neuropathy: A clinical and histological study on the significance of vascular affections. *Acta Med Scand* 164(suppl 345):1, 1959.

FALLS HF, JACKSON JH, CAREY JG, et al: Ocular manifestations of hereditary primary systemic amyloidosis. *Arch Ophthalmol* 54:660, 1955.

FARCAS P, AVNUM L, FRISHER S, et al: Efficacy of repeated intravenous immunoglobulin in severe unresponsive Guillain-Barré syndrome. *Lancet* 350:1747, 1997.

FEASBY TE, BURTON SR, HAHN AF: Obstetrical lumbosacral plexus injuries. *Muscle Nerve* 15:937, 1992.

FEASBY TE, GILBERT JJ, BROWN WF, et al: An acute axonal form of Guillain-Barré polyneuropathy. *Brain* 109:1115, 1986.

FISHER CM: An unusual variant of acute idiopathic polyneuritis (syndrome of ophthalmoplegia, ataxia and areflexia). *N Engl J Med* 255:57, 1956.

FISHER CM, ADAMS RD: Diphtheritic polyneuritis: A pathological study. *J Neuropathol Exp Neurol* 15:243, 1956.

FORRESTER C, LASCELLES RG: Association between polyneuritis and multiple sclerosis. *J Neurol Neurosurg Psychiatry* 42:864, 1979.

FORSSMAN O, BJORKMAN G, HOLLENDER A, ENGLUND NE: IgM-producing lymphocytes in peripheral nerve in a patient with benign monoclonal gammopathy. *Scand J Haematol* 11:332, 1973.

FRENCH COOPERATIVE GROUP: Efficiency of plasma exchange in Guillain-Barré syndrome. *Ann Neurol* 22:753, 1987.

FUNCK-BRENTANO JL, CUEILLE GF, MAN NK: A defense of the middle molecule hypothesis. *Kidney Int* 13(suppl 8):S31, 1978.

GARCIA-BRAGADO F, BERNANDEZ JM, NAVARRO C, et al: Peripheral neuropathy in essential mixed cryoglobulinemia. *Arch Neurol* 45:1210, 1988.

GARLAND H: Diabetic amyotrophy *BMJ* 2:1287, 1955.

GOODFELLOW J, FEARN CB, MATTHEWS JM: Iliacus haematoma: A common complication of haemophilia. *J Bone Joint Surg* 49B:748, 1967.

GORSON KC, ALLAM G, ROPPER AH: Chronic inflammatory demyelinating polyneuropathy: clinical features and response to treatment in 67 consecutive patients with and without monoclonal gammopathy. *Neurology* 48:321, 1997.

GORSON KC, ROPPER AH: Axonal neuropathy associated with monoclonal gammopathy of undetermined significance. *J Neurol Neurosur Psychiatry* 63:21 63, 1997.

GORSON KC, ROPPER AH, CLARK BD, et al: Treatment of chronic inflammatory demyelinating polyneuropathy with interferon-alpha 2a. *Neurology* 50:84, 1998.

GORSON KC, ROPPER AH, MUREILLO M, BLAIR R: Prospective evaluation of MRI lumbosacral root enhancement in acute Guillain-Barré syndrome. *Neurology* 47:813, 1996.

GORSON KC, ROPPER AH, WEINBERG DH: Upper limb predominant, multifocal inflammatory demyelinating neuropathy. *Muscle Nerve* 22:758, 1999.

GORSON KC, SCHOTT C, RAND WM, et al: Gabapentin in the treatment of painful diabetic neuropathy: a placebo-controlled, double-blind, crossover trial. *J Neurol Neurosurg Psychiatry* 66:251, 1999.

GOSSELIN S, KYLE RA, DYCK PJ: Neuropathy associated with monoclonal gammopathy of undetermined significance. *Ann Neurol* 30:54, 1991.

GRANT I, HUNDER GG, HOMBURGER HA, DYCK PJ: Peripheral neuropathy associated with sicca complex. *Neurology* 48:855, 1997.

GRIFFIN JW, CORNBLATH DR, ALEXANDER B, et al: Ataxic sensory neuropathy and dorsal root ganglionitis associated with Sjögren's syndrome. *Ann Neurol* 27:304, 1990.

GRIFFIN JW, LI CY, HO TW, et al: Guillain-Barré syndrome in northern China: The spectrum of neuropathological changes in clinically defined cases. *Brain* 118:577, 1995.

GUARANTORS OF BRAIN: *Aids to the Examination of the Peripheral Nervous System*, 2nd ed. London, Baillière-Tindall, 1986.

GUILLAIN-BARRÉ STUDY GROUP: Plasmapheresis and acute Guillain-Barré syndrome. *Neurology* 35:1096, 1985.

HADJIVASSILIOU M, CHATTOPADHYAY AK, DAVIES-JONES GA, et al: Neuromuscular disorder as presenting feature of coeliac disease. *J Neurol Neurosurg Psychiat* 63:770, 1997.

HAFER-MACKO CE, SHEIKH KA, LI CY, et al: Immune attack on the Schwann cell surface in acute inflammatory demyelinating polyneuropathy. *Ann Neurol* 39:625, 1996.

HAHN AF, BOLTON CF, PILLAY N, et al: Plasma exchange therapy in chronic inflammatory demyelinating polyneuropathy. *Brain* 119: 1055, 1996.

HAHN AF, BOLTON CF, ZOCHODNE D, FEASBY TE: Intravenous immunoglobulin treatment in chronic inflammatory demyelinating polyneuropathy. *Brain* 119:1067, 1996.

HARDING AE, THOMAS PK: The clinical features of hereditary motor and sensory neuropathy: Types I and II. *Brain* 103:259, 1980.

HARDING AE, THOMAS PK: Peroneal muscular atrophy with pyramidal features. *J Neurol Neurosurg Psychiatry* 47:168, 1984.

HART ZH, HOFFMAN W, WINBAUM E: Polyneuropathy, alopecia areata, and chronic lymphocytic thyroiditis. *Neurology* 29:106, 1979.

HARTUNG H-P, REINERS K, SCHMIDT B, et al: Serum interleukin-2 concentrations in Guillain-Barré syndrome and chronic idiopathic demyelinating polyneuropathy: Comparison with other neurological diseases of presumed immunopathogenesis. *Ann Neurol* 30:48, 1991.

HARTUNG H-P, STOLL G, TOYKA KV: Immune reactions in the peripheral nervous system, in Dyck PJ, Thomas PK, Griffin JW, et al (eds): *Peripheral Neuropathy*, 3rd ed. Philadelphia, Saunders, 1993, pp 418–444.

HAYMAKER W, KERNOHAN JW: The Landry-Guillain-Barré syndrome: Clinicopathologic report of fifty fatal cases and critique of the literature. *Medicine* 28:59, 1949.

HENSON RA, URICH H: *Cancer and the Nervous System*. Oxford, Blackwell, 1982, pp 368–405.

HONOVAR M, THARAKAN JK, HUGHES RAC, et al: A clinicopathological study of Guillain-Barré syndrome: Nine cases and literature review. *Brain* 114:1245, 1991.

HOOGENDIJK JE, HENSELS GW, GABREEL S, et al: De novo mutation in hereditary motor and sensory neuropathy, type 1. *Lancet* 339:1081, 1992.

HORWICH MS, CHO L, PORRO RS, POSNER JB: Subacute sensory neuropathy: A remote effect of carcinoma. *Ann Neurol* 2:7, 1977.

HUGHES RAC: *Guillain–Barré Syndrome*. London, Springer–Verlag, 1990.

HUGHES RAC: Ineffectiveness of high-dose intravenous methylprednisolone in Guillain-Barré syndrome. *Lancet* 338:1142, 1991.

HUGHES R, SANDERS E, HALL S, et al: Subacute idiopathic demyelinating polyradiculoneuropathy. *Arch Neurol* 49:612, 1992.

IKEDA S-I, HANYU N, HONGO M, et al: Hereditary generalized amyloidosis with polyneuropathy: Clinicopathological study of 65 Japanese patients. *Brain* 110:315, 1987.

ILLA I, GRAUS F, FERRER I, ENRIQUEZ J: Sensory neuropathy as the initial manifestation of primary biliary cirrhosis. *J Neurol Neurosurg Psychiatry* 52:1307, 1989.

ISMAEL SS, AMARENCO G, BAYLE B, KERDRAON J: Postpartum lumbosacral plexopathy limited to autonomic and perineal manifestations: Clinical and electrophysiologic study of 19 patients. *J Neurol Neurosurg Psychiatry* 68:771, 2000.

JANKOVIC J, VAN DER LINDEN C: Dystonia and tremor induced by peripheral trauma: Predisposing factors. *J Neurol Neurosurg Psychiatry* 51:1512, 1988.

JARADEH S, DYCK PJ: Hereditary motor sensory neuropathy with treatable extrapyramidal features. *Arch Neurol* 49:175, 1992.

JOHNSON PC, DOLL SC, CROMEY DW: Pathogenesis of diabetic neuropathy. *Ann Neurol* 19:450, 1986.

KAHN P: Anderson-Fabry disease: A histopathological study of three cases with observations on the mechanism of production of pain. *J Neurol Neurosurg Psychiatry* 36:1053, 1973.

KAHN SN, RICHES PG, KOHN J: Paraproteinemia in neurological disease: Incidence, association and classification of monoclonal immunoglobulins. *J Clin Pathol* 33:617, 1980.

KALTRIEDER HB, TALAL N: The neuropathy of Sjögren's syndrome: Trigeminal nerve involvement. *Ann Intern Med* 70:751, 1961.

KANTARJIAN AD, DEJONG RN: Familial primary amyloidosis with nervous system involvement. *Neurology* 3:399, 1953.

KAPLAN JG, ROSENBERG R, REINITZ E, et al: Invited review: Peripheral neuropathy in Sjögren's syndrome. *Muscle Nerve* 13:573, 1990.

KATIRJI MB, WILBOURN AJ: Common peroneal mononeuropathy: A clinical and electrophysiologic study of 116 lesions. *Neurology* 38:1723, 1988.

KELLY JJ, ADELMAN LS, BERKMAN E, BHAN I: Polyneuropathies associated with IgM monoclonal gammopathies. *Arch Neurol* 45:1355, 1988.

KEMLER MA, BAREUDSE GA, VAN KLEEF M, et al: Spinal cord stimulation in patients with chronic reflex sympathetic dystrophy. *New Engl J Med* 343:618, 2000.

KENNETT RP, HARDING AE: Peripheral neuropathy associated with the sicca syndrome. *J Neurol Neurosurg Psychiatry* 49:90, 1986.

KERNOHAN JW, WOLTMAN HW: Amyloid neuritis. *Arch Neurol Psychiatry* 47:132, 1942.

KIKTA DG, BREUER AC, WILBOURN AJ: Thoracic root pain in diabetes: The spectrum of clinical and electromyographic findings. *Ann Neurol* 11:80, 1982.

KING R: *Atlas of Peripheral Nerve Pathology*, London, Arnold, 1999.

KISSEL JT: Vasculitis of the peripheral nervous system. *Semin Neurol* 14:361, 1994.

KORI SH, FOLEY KM, POSNER JB: Brachial plexus lesions in patients with cancer: 100 cases. *Neurology* 31:45, 1981.

Koski CL, Gratz E, Sutherland J, et al: Clinical correlation with anti-peripheral nerve myelin antibodies in Guillain-Barré syndrome. *Ann Neurol* 19:573, 1986.

Kremer M, Gilliatt RW, Golding JSR, Wilson TG: Acroparaesthesiae in the carpal-tunnel syndrome. *Lancet* 2:590, 1953.

Kyle RA, Bayrd ED: Amyloidosis: Review of 236 cases. *Medicine* 54:271, 1975.

Kyle RA, Dyck PJ: Amyloidosis and neuropathy, in Dyck PJ, Thomas PK, Griffin JW, et al (eds): *Peripheral Neuropathy*, 3rd ed. Philadelphia, Saunders, 1993, pp 1294–1309.

Lafitte C: Manifestations neurologique du syndrome de Gougerot-Sjögren primitif. *Rev Neurol* 154:658, 1998.

Latov N, Gross RB, Kastelman J, et al: Complement-fixing antiperipheral nerve myelin antibodies in patients with inflammatory polyneuritis and with polyneuropathy and paraproteinemias. *Neurology* 31:1530, 1981.

Layzer RB: *Neuromuscular Manifestations of Systemic Disease: Contemporary Neurology Series*. Vol 25. Philadelphia, Davis, 1984.

Lederman RJ, Wilbourn AJ: Brachial plexopathy: Recurrent cancer or radiation? *Neurology* 34:1331, 1984.

Leger JM, Bouche P, Cervera P, Hauw JJ: Primary Sjögren syndrome in chronic polyneuropathy presenting in middle or old age. *J Neurol Neurosurg Psychiatry* 59:1276, 1995.

Lederman RJ, Wilbourn AJ: Postpartum neuralgic amyotrophy. *Neurology* 47:1213, 1996.

Lewis RA, Sumner AJ, Brown MJ, Asbury AK: Multifocal demyelinating neuropathy with persistent conduction block. *Neurology* 32:958, 1982.

Lewis T, Pickering GW: Circulatory changes in the fingers in some diseases of the nervous system with special reference to the digital atrophy of peripheral nerve lesions. *Clin Sci* 2:149, 1936.

Lhermitte F, Fritel D, Cambier J, et al: Polynevrites au cours de traitements par la nitrofurantoine. *Presse Med* 71:767, 1963.

Lhote F, Cohen P, Genereau T, et al: Microscopic polyangiitis: clinical aspects and treatment. *Ann Med Interne* 147:165, 1996.

Loggigian EL, Kaplan RF, Steere AC: Chronic neurologic manifestations of Lyme disease. *N Engl J Med* 323:1438, 1990.

Logina I, Donaghy M: Diphtheritic polyneuropathy: a clinical study and comparison with Guillain-Barré syndrome. *J Neurol Neurosurg Psychiatry* 67:433, 1999.

Low PA, Dyck PJ, Lambert EH: Acute panautonomic neuropathy. *Ann Neurol* 13:412, 1983.

Madrid R, Bradley WG: The pathology of neuropathies with focal thickening of the myelin sheath (tomaculous neuropathy). *J Neurol Sci* 25:415, 1975.

Magee KR, DeJong RN: Paralytic brachial neuritis. *JAMA* 174: 1258, 1960.

Marquez S, Turley JJ, Peters WJ: Neuropathy in burn patients. *Brain* 116:471, 1993.

Matthews WB, Esiri M: The migrant sensory neuritis of Wartenberg. *J Neurol Neurosurg Psychiatry* 46:1, 1983.

Matthews WB, Squier MV: Sensory perineuritis. *J Neurol Neurosurg Psychiatry* 51:473, 1988.

McCombe PA, McLeod JG, Pollard JD, et al: Peripheral sensorimotor and autonomic polyneuropathy associated with systemic lupus erythematosus. *Brain* 110:533, 1987.

McCombe PA, Pollard JD, McLeod JG: Chronic inflammatory demyelinating polyradiculoneuropathy: A clinical and electrophysiological study of 92 cases. *Brain* 111:1617, 1987.

McGonagle TK, Levine SR, Donofrio PD, Albers JW: Spectrum of patients with EMG features of polyradiculopathy without neuropathy. *Muscle Nerve* 13:63, 1990.

McKhann GM, Griffin JW, Cornblath DR, et al: Plasmapheresis and Guillain-Barré syndrome: Analysis of prognostic factors and the effect of plasmapheresis. *Ann Neurol* 23:347, 1988.

Mellgren SI, Conn DL, Stevens JC, Dyck PJ: Peripheral neuropathy in primary Sjögren's syndrome. *Neurology* 39:390, 1989.

Meretoja J: Familial systemic paramyloidosis with lattice dystrophy of the cornea, progressive cranial neuropathy, skin changes and various internal symptoms: A previously unrecognized heritable syndrome. *Ann Clin Res* 1:314, 1969.

Moore PM, Harley JB, Fauci AS: Neurologic dysfunction in the idiopathic hypereosinophilic syndrome. *Ann Intern Med* 102:109, 1985.

Moulingier A, Authier F-J, Baudrimont M, et al: Peripheral neuropathy in human immunodeficiency virus-infected patients with the diffuse infiltrative lymphocytosis syndrome. *Ann Neurol* 41:438, 1997.

Nathan PW: Painful legs and moving toes: Evidence on the site of the lesion. *J Neurol Neurosurg Psychiatry* 41:934, 1978.

Neumann M: Neurological multisystem manifestation in multiple symmetric lipomatosis: A clinical and electrophysiologic study. *Muscle Nerve* 18:693, 1995.

Ohnishi A, Dyck PJ: Loss of small peripheral sensory neurons in Fabry disease. *Arch Neurol* 31:120, 1974.

Ongerboer de Visser BW, Feltkamp-Vroom TM, Feltkamp CA: Sural nerve immune deposits in polyneuropathy as a remote effect of malignancy. *Ann Neurol* 14:261, 1983.

Osterman PO, Fagius J, Safwenberg J, et al: Early relapses after plasma exchange in acute inflammatory polyradiculoneuropathy. *Lancet* 2:1161, 1986.

Pallis CA, Scott JT: Peripheral neuropathy in rheumatoid arthritis. *BMJ* 1:1141, 1965.

Parsonage MJ, Turner JWA: Neuralgic amyotrophy: The shoulder girdle syndrome. *Lancet* 1:973, 1948.

Pascoe MK, Low PA, Windebank AJ, Litchy WJ: Subacute diabetic proximal neuropathy. *Mayo Clin Proc* 72:1123, 1997.

Periquet MI, Novak V, Collins MP, et al: Painful sensory neuropathy: Prospective evaluation using skin biopsy. *Neurology* 52: 1641, 1999.

Pestronk A, Chaudhry V, Feldman EL, et al: Lower motor neuron syndromes defined by patterns of weakness, nerve conduction abnormalities, and high titers of antiglycolipid antibodies. *Ann Neurol* 27:316, 1990.

Phillips LH: Familial long thoracic nerve palsy: A manifestation of brachial plexus neuropathy. *Neurology* 36:1251, 1986.

Pickett JBE, Layzer RB, Levin SR, et al: Neuromuscular complications of acromegaly. *Neurology* 25:638, 1975.

Planté-Bordeneuve V, Guichon-Mantel A, Lacroix C, et al: The Roussy-Lévy family: from the original description to the gene. *Ann Neurol* 46:770, 1999.

Prineas JW, McLeod JG: Chronic relapsing polyneuritis. *J Neurol Sci* 27:427, 1976.

Raff MC, Sangalang V, Asbury AK: Ischemic mononeuropathy multiplex associated with diabetes mellitus. *Arch Neurol* 18:487, 1968.

Rechthand E, Cornblath DR, Stern BJ, Meyerhoff JO: Chronic demyelinating polyneuropathy in systemic lupus erythematosus. *Neurology* 34:1375, 1984.

Refsum S: Heredopathia atactica polyneuritiformis: A familial syndrome not hitherto described. *Acta Psychiatr Scand Suppl* 38:1, 1946.

Robson JS: Uraemic neuropathy, in Robertson RF (ed): *Some Aspects of Neurology*. Edinburgh, Royal College of Physicians, 1968, pp 74–84.

Rogers LR, Borkowski JW, Albers KH, et al: Obturator mononeuropathy caused by pelvic cancer: six cases. *Neurology* 43:1489, 1993.

Ropper AH: The Guillain-Barré syndrome. *N Engl J Med* 326: 1130, 1992.

Ropper AH: Accelerated neuropathy of renal failure. *Arch Neurol* 50:536, 1993.

Ropper AH: Further regional variants of acute immune polyneuropathy. *Arch Neurol* 51:671, 1994.

Ropper AH: Chronic demyelinating polyneuropathy: Improvement after sepsis. *Neurology* 46:848, 1996.

Ropper AH: Unusual clinical variants and signs in Guillain-Barré syndrome. *Arch Neurol* 43:1150, 1986.

Ropper AH, Gorson KC: Neuropathies associated with paraproteinemias. *N Engl J Med* 338:1601, 1998.

Ropper AH, Kehne SM: Guillain-Barré syndrome: Management of respiratory failure. *Neurology* 35:1662, 1985.

Ropper AH, Wijdick EFM, Truax BT: *Guillain-Barré Syndrome*. Philadelphia, Davis, 1991.

Rowland LP, Defendini R, Sheman W, et al: Macroglobulinemia with peripheral neuropathy simulating motor neuron diseases. *Ann Neurol* 11:532, 1982.

Rukavina JG, Block WD, Jackson CE, et al: Primary systemic amyloidosis: A review and an experimental genetic and clinical study of 29 cases with particular emphasis on the familial form. *Medicine* 35:239, 1956.

Said G: Perhexiline neuropathy: A clinicopathologic study. *Ann Neurol* 3:259, 1978.

Said G: Vasculitic neuropathy, in Hartung HP (ed), *Peripheral Neuropathies: Balliére's Clinical Neurology*: Part I, Vol 4. London, Balliére Tindall, 1995, pp 489–503.

Said G, Elgrably F, Lacroix C, et al: Painful proximal diabetic neuropathy: inflammatory nerve lesions and spontaneous favorable outcome. *Ann Neurol* 41:762, 1997.

Said D, Slama G, Selva J: Progressive centripetal degeneration of axons in small fiber type diabetic polyneuropathy: A clinical and pathological study. *Brain* 106:791, 1983.

Samanta A, Burden AC: Painful diabetic neuropathy. *Lancet* 1:348, 1985.

Saraiva MJM, Costa PP, Goodman DS: Genetic expression of a transthyretin mutation in typical and late-onset Portuguese families with familial amyloidotic polyneuropathy. *Neurology* 36:1413, 1986.

Schaumburg HH, Berger AR, Thomas PK: *Disorders of Peripheral Nerves*, 2nd ed. Philadelphia, Davis, 1992.

Schaumburg HH, Kaplan J, Windebank A, et al: Sensory neuropathy from pyridoxine abuse. *N Engl J Med* 309:445, 1983.

Schott GD: Mechanisms of causalgia and related clinical conditions. *Brain* 109:717, 1986.

Schwartzman RJ, McLellan TL: Reflex sympathetic dystrophy: A review. *Arch Neurol* 44:555, 1987.

Shahani BT, Young RR, Adams Rd: Neuropathic tremor: Evidence on the site of the lesion. *Electroencephalogr Clin Neurophysiol* 34:800, 1973.

Simmons Z, Albers JW, Bromberg MB, Feldman EL: Long-term follow-up of patients with chronic demyelinating polyradiculoneuropathy without and with monoclonal gammopathy. *Brain* 118:359, 1995.

Simovic D, Gorson KC, Ropper AH: Comparison of IgM-MGUS and IgG-MGUS polyneuropathy. *Acta Neurol Scand* 97:194, 1998.

Skjeldal OH, Nyberg-Hansen R, Stokke O: Neurological disorders and phytanic acid metabolism. *Acta Neurol Scand* 78:324, 1988.

Smith IS, Kahn SN, Lacey BW, et al: Chronic demyelinating neuropathy associated with benign IgM paraproteinemia. *Brain* 106:169, 1983.

Sorenson EJ, Sima AAF, Blaivas M, et al: Clinical features of perineuritis. *Muscle Nerve* 20:1153, 1997.

Specks U, Wheatley CL, McDonald TJ, et al: Anticytoplasmic autoantibodies in the diagnosis and follow-up of Wegener's granulomatosis. *Mayo Clin Proc* 64:28, 1989.

Spencer PS, Schaumburg HH, Ludolph AC (eds): *Experimental and Clinical Neurotoxicology*. New York, Oxford University Press, 1999.

Spillane JW, Nathan PW, Kelly RE, Marsden CD: Painful legs and moving toes. *Brain* 94:541, 1971.

Staunton H, Dervan P, Kale R, et al: Hereditary amyloid polyneuropathy in northwest Ireland. *Brain* 110:1231, 1987.

Sterman AB, Schaumberg HH, Asbury AK: The acute sensory neuropathy syndrome: A distinct clinical entity. *Ann Neurol* 7:354, 1980.

Stevens JC: The electrodiagnosis of the carpal tunnel syndrome. *Muscle Nerve* 12:99, 1987.

Stewart BM: The hypertrophic neuropathy of acromegaly: A rare neuropathy associated with acromegaly. *Arch Neurol* 14:107, 1966.

Stoll BA, Andrews JT: Radiation induced peripheral neuropathy. *BMJ* 1:834, 1966.

Suarez GA, Giannini C, Bosch EP, et al: Immune brachial plexus neuropathy: Suggestive evidence for inflammatory-immune pathogenesis. *Neurology* 46:559, 1996.

Sun SF, Steib EW: Diabetic thoracoabdominal neuropathy: Clinical and electrodiagnostic features. *Ann Neurol* 9:75, 1981.

SWANSON AG, BUCHAN GC, ALVORD EC JR: Anatomic changes in congenital insensitivity to pain: Absence of small primary sensory neurons in ganglia, roots and Lissauer's tract. *Arch Neurol* 12:12, 1965.

SYMONDS CP, SHAW ME: Familial clawfoot with absent tendon jerks: A "forme-fruste" of the Charcot-Marie-Tooth disease. *Brain* 49:387, 1926.

TAYLOR RA: Heredofamilial mononeuritis multiplex with brachial predilection. *Brain* 83:113, 1960.

THÉVENARD A: L'Acropathie ulcero-mutilante familiale. *Rev Neurol* 74:193, 1942.

THOMAS JE, CASCINO TL, EARLE JD: Differential diagnosis between radiation and tumor plexopathy of the pelvis. *Neurology* 35:1, 1985.

THOMAS PK, TOMLINSON DR: Diabetic and hypoglycemic neuropathy, in Dyck PJ, Thomas PK, Griffin JW, et al (eds): *Peripheral Neuropathy*, 3rd ed. Philadelphia, Saunders, 1993, pp 1219–1250.

THOMAS PK, WILLISON JH: Paraproteinemic neuropathy, in McLeod JG (ed): *Inflammatory Neuropathies: Bailliére's Clinical Neurology*. Vol 3. London, Bailliére-Tindall, 1994, p 129.

TRIGGS WJ, CROS D, GOMINAK SC, et al: Motor nerve inexcitability in Guillain-Barré syndrome. *Brain* 115:1291, 1992.

TSAIRIS P, DYCK PJ, MULDER DW: Natural history of brachial plexus neuropathy: Report on 99 cases. *Arch Neurol* 27:109, 1972.

TUCK RR, MCLEOD JG: Retinitis pigmentosa, ataxia, and peripheral neuropathy. *J Neurol Neurosurg Psychiatry* 46:206, 1983.

UCHUYA M, GRAUS F, VEGA F, et al: Intravenous immunoglobulin treatment in paraneoplastic neurological syndromes with antineuronal antibodies. *J Neurol Neurosurg Psychiatry* 60:388, 1996.

UNCINI A, SABATELLI M, MIGNOGNA T, et al: Chronic progressive steroid responsive axonal polyneuropathy: A CIDP variant or a primary axonal disorder. *Muscle Nerve* 19:365, 1996.

VALLAT JM, DEMASCAREL A, BORDESSOULE D, et al: Non-Hodgkin malignant lymphomas and peripheral neuropathies C13 cases. *Brain* 118:1233, 1995.

VAN ALLEN MW, FROHLICH JA, DAVIS JR: Inherited predisposition to generalized amyloidosis. *Neurology* 19:10, 1969.

VAN BUCHEM FSP, POL G, DE GIER J, et al: Congenital β-lipoprotein deficiency. *Am J Med* 40:794, 1966.

VAN DER MECHÉ FGA, SCHMITZ PIM, AND THE DUTCH GUILLAIN-BARRÉ STUDY GROUP: A randomized trial comparing intravenous immune globulin and plasma exchange in Guillain-Barré syndrome. *N Engl J Med* 326:1123, 1992.

VERHALLE D, LÖFGREN A, NELIS E, et al: Deletion in the CMT1A locus on chromosome 17 p11.2 in hereditary neuropathy with liability to pressure palsies. *Ann Neurol* 35:704, 1994.

VISSER LH, VAN DER MECHÉ FGA, VAN DOORN PA, et al: Guillain-Barré syndrome without sensory loss (acute motor neuropathy). *Brain* 118:841, 1995.

WAKSMAN BH, ADAMS RD: Allergic neuritis: An experimental disease of rabbits induced by the injection of peripheral nervous tissue and adjuvants. *J Exp Med* 102:213, 1955.

WALDENSTROM J: The porphyrias as inborn errors of metabolism. *Am J Med* 22:758, 1957.

WARTENBERG R: *Neuritis, Sensory Neuritis, and Neuralgia*. New York, Oxford University Press, 1958, pp 233–247.

WEINBERG DH, SIMOVIC D, ROPPER AH, ISNER J: Chronic Ischemic monomelic neuropathy. *Neurology* 50:A207, 1998.

WEINSHILBOUM RM, AXELROD J: Reduced plasma dopamine-hydroxylase activity in familial dysautonomia. *N Engl J Med* 285:938, 1971.

WILLIAMS IR, MAYER RF: Subacute proximal diabetic neuropathy. *Neurology* 26:108, 1976.

WINDEBANK AJ, BLEXRUD MO, DYCK PJ, et al: The syndrome of acute sensory neuropathy: Clinical features and electrophysiologic and pathologic changes. *Neurology* 40:584, 1990.

WINDEBANK AJ, BONKOVSKY HL: Porphyric neuropathy, in Dyck PJ, Thomas PK, Griffin JW, et al (eds): *Peripheral Neuropathy*, 3rd ed. Philadelphia, Saunders, 1993, pp 1161–1168.

WULFF CH, HANSEN K, STRANGE P, TROJABORG W: Multiple mononeuritis and radiculitis with erythema, pain, elevated CSF protein, and pleocytosis: Bannwarth's syndrome. *J Neurol Neurosurg Psychiatry* 46:485, 1983.

YEUNG KB, THOMAS PK, KING RHM, et al: The clinical spectrum of peripheral neuropathies associated with benign monoclonal IgM and IgA paraproteinemias. *J Neurol* 238:383, 1991.

YOUNG RR, ASBURY AK, CORBETT JL, ADAMS RD: Pure pandysautonomia with recovery. *Brain* 98:613, 1975.

ZOCHODNE DW, BOLTON CF, WELLS GA: Critical illness polyneuropathy: A complication of sepsis and multiple organ failure. *Brain* 110:819, 1987.

ZUNIGA G, ROPPER AH, FRANK J: Sarcoid peripheral neuropathy. *Neurology* 41:1558, 1991.

Chapter 47

DISEASES OF THE CRANIAL NERVES

The cranial nerves are susceptible to a number of special diseases, some of which never affect the spinal peripheral nerves. For this reason alone they deserve to be considered separately. Certain of them have already been discussed: namely, disorders of olfaction, in Chap. 12; of vision and extraocular muscles, in Chaps. 13 and 14; of cochlear and vestibular function, in Chap. 15; and craniofacial pain in Chap. 10. There remain to be described the disorders of the facial (seventh) nerve and of the lower cranial nerves (IX to XII) as well as certain aspects of disordered trigeminal (fifth) nerve function. These are considered below.

The Fifth, or Trigeminal, Nerve

Anatomic Considerations The fifth nerve (Fig. 47-1) is a mixed sensory and motor nerve. It conducts sensory impulses from the greater part of the face and head; from the mucous membranes of the nose, mouth, and paranasal sinuses; and from the cornea and conjunctiva. It also innervates the dura of the anterior and middle cranial fossae. The cell bodies of the sensory part of the nerve lie in the gasserian, or semilunar, ganglion. This, the largest sensory ganglion in humans, lies in the medial part of the middle cranial fossa at the base of the cranium. The central axons of the ganglion cells form the sensory root. These fibers, on entering the mid pons, divide into short ascending and long descending branches. The former are concerned mainly with tactile and light pressure sense and synapse with second-order neurons in the principal sensory nucleus. Proprioceptive afferents from facial muscles and the masseter terminate in the mesencephalic nucleus. The fibers that mediate pain and temperature sensation do not end in these nuclei but form the long descending branches of the spinal trigeminal tract. The latter pathway, which contains both facilitatory and inhibitory fibers, together with its nucleus, extends from the junction of the pons and medulla to the uppermost segments (C2 or C3) of the spinal cord (facial pain has been relieved after medullary trigeminal tractotomy). From all parts of the principal sensory and spinal nuclei, second-order fibers cross to the opposite side and ascend to the thalamus. They come to lie in the most medial part of the spinothalamic tract and lateral part of the medial lemniscus. These systems of fibers are called the *trigeminothalamic tract*. In addition, the secondary trigeminal neurons project to the facial and hypoglossal nuclei bilaterally, the salivatory nuclei, the cuneate nuclei of the upper cervical segments, and other cranial nerve nuclei. The main sensory and spinal trigeminal nuclei receive fibers from the reticular formation, the thalamus, the nucleus solitarius, and the sensory cortex. The spinal nucleus is a continuation of the spinal tract of Lissauer and substantia gelatinosa; the main sensory nucleus is a continuation of the nucleus of the medial lemniscus.

The peripheral branches of the gasserian ganglion form the three sensory divisions of the nerve. The first (ophthalmic) division passes through the superior orbital fissure; the second (maxillary) division leaves the middle fossa through the foramen rotundum; and the third (mandibular), through the foramen ovale.

The motor portion of the fifth nerve, which supplies the masseter and pterygoid muscles, has its origin in the trigeminal motor nucleus in the midpons; the exiting fibers pass underneath the gasserian ganglion and become incorporated into the mandibular nerve. The masseter and pterygoid muscles are utilized in chewing and are implicated in a number of brainstem reflexes, the best known of which is the jaw jerk. Tapping the chin with the jaw muscles relaxed stimulates proprioceptive afferents that terminate in the mesencephalic nucleus of the midbrain, which sends collaterals to the motor nucleus of the fifth nerve and causes the masseters to contract. This reflex is enhanced in spastic bulbar (pseudobulbar) palsy. Another pontine reflex that utilizes

Figure 47-1

Scheme of the trigeminal nuclei and some of the trigeminal reflex arcs. I, ophthalmic division; II, maxillary division; III, mandibular division. (From Carpenter MB, Sutin J: Human Neuroanatomy, 8th ed. Baltimore, Williams & Wilkins, 1982, by permission.)

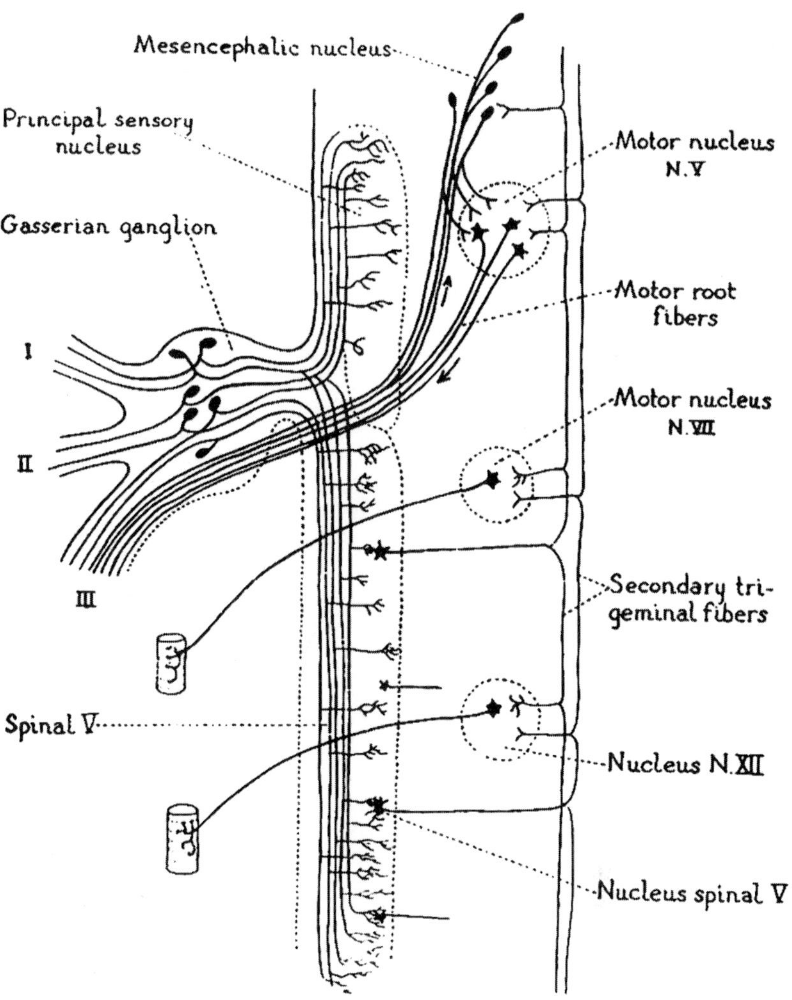

afferent trigeminal sensory nerves is the blink reflex. Tapping of the brow or bridge of the nose evokes bilateral blink through activation of the orbicularis oculi muscles (facial nerve efferents). Touching the eyelids and cornea (corneal reflex) does the same.

Because of their wide anatomic distribution, complete interruption of both the motor and sensory fibers of the trigeminal nerve is rarely observed. On the other hand, partial affection of the trigeminal nerve, particularly of the sensory part, is not uncommon. The various cranial nerve and brainstem syndromes in which the fifth nerve is involved are listed in Tables 47-1 and 47-2 and 31-4.

Diseases Affecting the Fifth Nerve A variety of diseases may affect the peripheral branches of the trigeminal nerves, the gasserian (semilunar) ganglion, and the roots (sensory and motor). These have been ably described by Hughes. The most frequent, and at the same time the most elusive from the standpoint of its pathologic basis, is *trigeminal neuralgia (tic douloureux)*, which is also discussed on page 196. This condition has been known since ancient times, having been described by Arateus in the first century A.D., by John Locke in 1677, by Nicolaus Andre in 1756, and by John Fothergill in 1776 (according to Katusic et al). The overall incidence rate for both sexes combined is 4.3 per 100,000 persons per year, but it is higher for women than for men (in a ratio of 3:2) and is much higher in the elderly. The mean age of onset is 52 to 58 years for the idiopathic form and 30 to 35 years for the symptomatic forms, the latter being caused by trauma or vascular, neoplastic, and demyelinative diseases. The nature of the pain, its unilaterality and tendency to involve the second and third

Table 47-1
Extramedullary cranial nerve syndromes (see also Tables 31-4 and 47-3)

Site	*Cranial nerves involved*	*Eponymic syndrome*	*Usual cause*
Sphenoidal fissure	III, IV, ophthalmic, V, VI	Foix	Invasive tumors of sphenoid bone, aneurysms
Lateral wall of cavernous sinus	III, IV, ophthalmic (occasionally maxillary), V, VI	Tolosa-Hunt Foix	Aneurysms or thrombosis of cavernous sinus; invasive tumors from sinuses and sella turcica; sometimes recurrent, benign granulomatous reactions, responsive to steroids
Retrosphenoidal space	II, III, IV, V, VI	Jacod	Large tumors of middle cranial fossa
Apex of petrous bone	V, VI	Gradenigo	Petrositis, tumors of petrous bone
Internal auditory meatus	VII, VIII		Tumors of petrous bone (dermoids, etc.), acoustic neuroma
Pontocerebellar angle	V, VII, VIII, and sometimes IX		Acoustic neuromas, meningiomas
Jugular foramen	IX, X, XI	Vernet	Tumors and aneurysms
Posterior laterocondylar space	IX, X, XI, XII	Collet-Sicard	Tumors of parotid gland, carotid body; secondary and lymph node tumors, tuberculous adenitis, carotid artery dissection
Posterior retroparotid space	IX, X, XI, XII, and Bernard-Horner syndrome	Villaret MacKenzie	Same as above, and granulomatous lesions (sarcoid, fungi)
Posterior retroparotid space	X and XII, with or without XI	Tapia	Parotid and other tumors of, or injuries to, the high neck

divisions of the trigeminal nerve, an intensity that makes the patient grimace or wince (tic), the presence of an initiating or trigger point, the lack of demonstrable sensory or motor deficit, and its response in more than half of the cases to carbamazepine, phenytoin, and other drugs are characteristic. The diagnosis of the idiopathic form of trigeminal neuralgia and its differentiation from symptomatic forms—as well as from cluster headache, dental neuralgia, temporomandibular pain, and atypical facial pain—is usually not difficult, especially if there is a trigger point and no demonstrable evidence of sensory or motor impairment. The treatment of idiopathic trigeminal neuralgia is considered on page 198.

In rare instances trigeminal neuralgia is preceded or accompanied by hemifacial spasm, a combination that Cushing called *tic convulsif*. This is often indicative of a tumor (cholesteatoma), an aneurysmal dilatation of the basilar artery, or an arteriovenous malformation that compresses both the trigeminal and facial nerves. Trigeminal neuralgia and glossopharyngeal neuralgia (pain in the tonsillar region) may also be combined in these disease states, but these conditions are usually idiopathic.

Of the conditions that damage the branches of the trigeminal nerve, cranial injuries and fractures are the most common. The most superficial branches—the supratrochlear, supraorbital, and infraorbital—are the ones usually involved. The sensory loss is present from the time of the injury, and partial regeneration may be attended by constant pain, often demanding nerve block and sectioning. Stilbamidine and trichloroethylene are known to cause sensory loss, tingling, burning, and itching exclusively in the trigeminal sensory territory.

Of the various inflammatory and infectious diseases that affect the trigeminal nerves or ganglia, *herpes zoster* ranks first (page 799). *Herpes simplex virus* has been isolated from the ganglion in as many as 50 percent of routine autopsies, but in nearly all patients this virus is associated only with lesions of the skin and lips. Middle ear infections and osteomyelitis of the apex of the petrous bone may spread to the ganglion and root, also implicating the sixth cranial nerve (*Gradenigo syndrome*).

Table 47-2
Intramedullary (brainstem) syndromes involving cranial nerves

Eponym[a]	*Site*	*Cranial nerves involved*	*Tracts and nuclei*	*Signs*	*Usual cause*
Weber syndrome	Base of midbrain	III	Corticospinal tract	Oculomotor palsy with crossed hemiplegia	Vascular occlusion, tumor, aneurysm
Claude syndrome	Tegmentum of midbrain	III	Red nucleus and brachium conjunctivum	Oculomotor palsy with contralateral cerebellar ataxia and tremor	Vascular occlusion, tumor, aneurysm
Benedikt syndrome	Tegmentum of midbrain	III	Red nucleus, corticospinal tract, and brachium conjunctivum	Oculomotor palsy with contralateral cerebellar ataxia, tremor, and corticospinal signs	Infarct, hemorrhage, tuberculoma, tumor
Nothnagel syndrome	Tectum of midbrain	Unilateral or bilateral III	Superior cerebellar peduncles	Ocular palsies, paralysis of gaze, and cerebellar ataxia	Tumor
Parinaud syndrome	Dorsal midbrain		Supranuclear mechanism for upward gaze and other structures in periaqueductal gray matter	Paralysis of upward gaze and accommodation; fixed pupils	Pinealoma, hydrocephalus, and other lesions of dorsal midbrain
Millard-Gubler syndrome and Raymond-Foville syndrome	Base of pons	VII and often VI	Corticospinal tract	Facial and abducens palsy and contralateral hemiplegia; sometimes gaze palsy to side of lesion	Infarct, or tumor
Avellis syndrome	Tegmentum of medulla	X	Spinothalamic tract; sometimes descending pupillary fibers, with Bernard-Horner syndrome	Paralysis of soft palate and vocal cord and contralateral hemianesthesia	Infarct, or tumor
Jackson syndrome	Tegmentum of medulla	X, XII	Corticospinal tract	Avellis syndrome plus ipsilateral tongue paralysis	Infarct, or tumor
Wallenberg syndrome	Lateral tegmentum of medulla	Spinal V, IX, X, XI	Lateral spinothalamic tract Descending pupillodilator fibers Spinocerebellar and olivocerebellar tracts	Ipsilateral V, IX, X, XI palsy, Horner syndrome and cerebellar ataxia; contralateral loss of pain and temperature sense	Occlusion of vertebral or posterior-inferior cerebellar artery

[a]See Silverman and associates for references to orginal reports.

The trigeminal root may be compressed or invaded by intracranial meningiomas, acoustic neuromas, trigeminal neuromas (Fig. 47-2), cholesteatomas, and chordomas. Sinus tumors and metastatic disease may also implicate the nerve, causing pain and a gradually progressive sensory loss. The ophthalmic division of the fifth nerve may be involved in the wall of the cavernous sinus in combination with the third, fourth, and sixth nerves by a variety of processes, including thrombosis of the cavernous sinus. Tumors of the sphenoid bone (myeloma, metastatic carcinoma, squamous cell carcinoma, and lymphoepithelioma of the nasopharynx) may involve branches of the trigeminal nerve at their foramina of entry or exit. The mandibular division may be compressed by the roots of an impacted third molar (wisdom) tooth. We have several times observed numbness of the chin and lower lip (infiltration of the mental nerve) as the first indication of metastatic carcinoma of the breast and prostate and from multiple myeloma. Massey and colleagues have described 19 such cases ("numb-chin syndrome"). A perineural spread of tumor from squamous cell skin cancers of the face is discussed further on, under "Multiple Cranial Nerve Palsies."

Figure 47-2

Trigeminal neuroma (schwannoma) that caused only minor sensory changes on the face seen on a gadolinium-enhanced MRI. The dumbbell-shaped tumor is pinched at the foramen ovale.

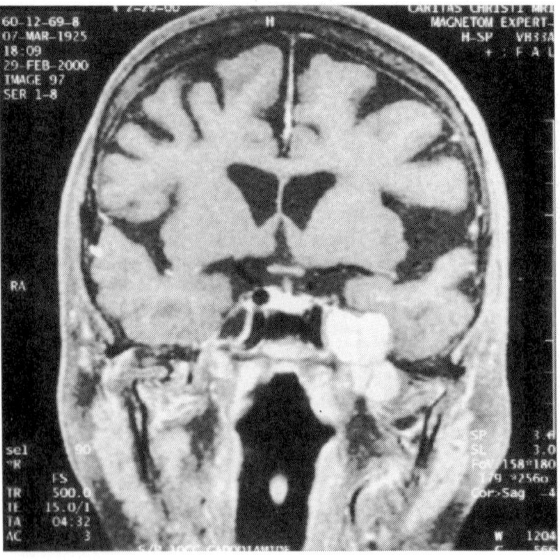

Loss of facial sensation can occur as part of a widespread sensory neuropathy that occurs as a remote effect of cancer or as part of Sjögren disease (pages 727 and 1403). Far more common is the association between *isolated trigeminal neuropathy* and immune-mediated connective tissue disease. Of 22 such cases described by Lecky and colleagues, 9 had either scleroderma or mixed connective tissue disease, and a similar number had either organ- or non-organ-specific serum autoantibodies. The symptoms may involve the other side years later. Hughes has also reported cases of trigeminal neuropathy with scleroderma, lupus erythematosus, and Sjögren disease. We have seen several patients with Sjögren disease in whom the trigeminal neuropathy and the associated antibodies or inflammation of the minor salivary glands were evident well before the characteristic sicca syndrome or other systemic manifestations of the disease. The condition may remain troublesome for years. Pathologic data are limited but point to an inflammatory lesion of the trigeminal ganglion or sensory root.

Every neurologist from time to time encounters idiopathic instances of slowly evolving unilateral or bilateral trigeminal neuropathy in which there is a sensory impairment confined to the territory of the trigeminal nerve, sometimes associated with pain and paresthesias and disturbances of taste. Spillane and Wells stressed the importance of this isolated trigeminal neuropathy (it has been called "Spillane's trigeminal neuritis" in some texts). Four of their 16 patients had an associated paranasal sinusitis, but subsequent reports have failed to substantiate a causal relationship between sinusitis and cranial neuritis. One wonders how many of these individuals had an occult connective tissue disease. A less common form of idiopathic trigeminal sensory neuropathy has a more acute onset and a tendency to resolve completely or partially, in much the same manner as Bell's palsy, with which it is sometimes associated (Blau et al). A recurrent variety of uncertain origin has been reported in the dental literature. We have had experience with patients whose facial numbness was a component of an upper cervical disc syndrome that included numbness on the same side of the body. Cases such as these are reported in the literature.

A pure unilateral trigeminal motor neuropathy is a clinical rarity. Chia has described five patients in whom an aching pain in the cheek and unilateral weakness of mastication were the main features. Electromyography (EMG) showed denervation changes in the ipsilateral masseter and temporalis muscles. The outcome was apparently favorable.

In most cases of trigeminal neuropathy except those due to tumor, the results of gadolinium-enhanced MRI are normal, as is the cerebrospinal fluid. The function of the nerve may be studied by the electrical recording of blink reflexes. A few laboratories have developed an evoked potential test specifically of the trigeminal nerve.

The Seventh, or Facial, Nerve

The seventh cranial nerve is mainly a motor nerve supplying all the muscles concerned with facial expression on one side. The sensory component is small (the nervus intermedius of Wrisberg); it conveys taste sensation from the anterior two-thirds of the tongue and probably cutaneous sensation from the anterior wall of the external auditory canal. The taste fibers at first traverse the lingual nerve (a branch of the mandibular) and then join the chorda tympani, which conveys taste sensation to the nucleus of the tractus solitarius. Secretomotor fibers innervate the lacrimal gland through the greater superficial petrosal nerve and the sublingual and submaxillary glands through the chorda tympani (Fig. 47-3).

Several other anatomic facts are worth remembering. The motor nucleus of the seventh nerve lies ventral and lateral to the abducens nucleus, and the intrapontine

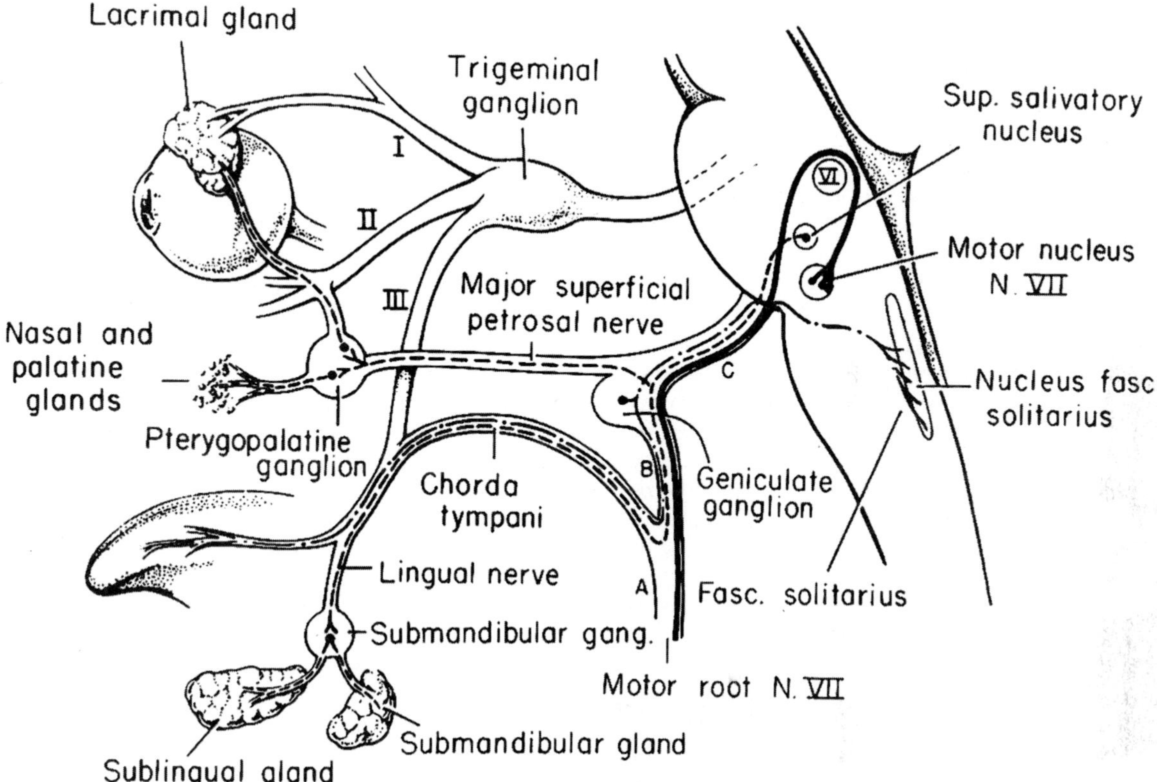

Figure 47-3

Scheme of the seventh cranial (facial) nerve. The motor fibers are represented by the heavy black line. Parasympathetic fibers are represented by regular dashes; special visceral afferent (taste) fibers are represented by long dashes and dots. A, B, and C denote lesions of the facial nerve at the stylomastoid foramen, distal to the geniculate ganglion, and proximal to the geniculate ganglion. Disturbances resulting from lesions at each of these sites are described in the text. (From Carpenter MB, Sutin J: Human Neuroanatomy, 8th ed. Baltimore, Williams & Wilkins, 1982, by permission.)

fibers of the facial nerve hook around and pass ventrolaterally to the abducens nucleus before emerging from the pons, just lateral to the corticospinal tract. The facial nerve enters the internal auditory meatus with the acoustic nerve and then bends sharply forward and downward around the anterior boundary of the vestibule of the inner ear. At this angle (*genu*) lies the sensory ganglion (named *geniculate* because of its proximity to the genu). The nerve continues its course in its own bony channel, the facial canal, within which, just distal to the geniculate ganglion, it provides a branch to the pterygopalatine ganglion, i.e., the greater superficial petrosal nerve; somewhat more distally, it gives off a small branch to the stapedius muscle and is joined by the chorda tympani. It makes its exit from the skull at the stylomastoid foramen, then passes through the parotid gland and subdivides into five branches that supply the facial muscles, the stylomastoid muscle, and the posterior belly of the digastric muscle.

A complete interruption of the facial nerve at the stylomastoid foramen paralyzes all muscles of facial expression. The corner of the mouth droops, the creases and skin folds are effaced, the forehead is unfurrowed, the palpebral fissure is widened, and the eyelids will not close. Upon attempted closure of the lids, both eyes roll upward (Bell's phenomenon), but the one on the paralyzed side remains visible. The lower lid sags also, and the punctum falls away from the conjunctiva, permitting tears to spill over the cheek. Food collects between the teeth and cheek, and saliva may dribble from the corner of the mouth. The patient complains of a heaviness or numbness and sometimes an aching pain in the face, but sensory loss can usually not be demonstrated. Taste, however, is intact because the lesion is beyond the site where the chorda tympani has separated from the main trunk of the facial nerve.

If the lesion is in the facial canal above the junction with the chorda tympani but below the geniculate ganglion, all the above symptoms occur; in addition, taste is lost over the anterior two-thirds of the tongue on the same side. If the nerve to the stapedius muscle is involved, there is hyperacusis (painful sensitivity to loud sounds). With a stethoscope in the patient's ears, a tuning fork at the bell is louder on the side of the paralyzed stapedius muscle. If the geniculate ganglion or the motor root proximal to it is involved, lacrimation and salivation may be reduced. Lesions at this point may also affect the adjacent eighth nerve, causing deafness, tinnitus, or dizziness. Intrapontine lesions that paralyze the face often affect the abducens nucleus and the corticospinal and sensory tracts (Millard-Gubler syndrome; Table 47-2).

If the peripheral facial paralysis has existed for some time and return of motor function has begun but is incomplete, a kind of contracture (in reality a continuous diffuse myokymic contraction) may appear. The palpebral fissure becomes narrowed and the nasolabial fold deepens. Attempts to move one group of facial muscles result in contraction of all of them (associated movements, or synkinesis). Spasms of facial muscles may develop and persist indefinitely, being initiated by every facial movement. However, this condition, called *hemifacial spasm*, occurs most often in adults who have never had a facial palsy and may be related to compression of the nerve by a tortuous blood vessel on the surface of the ventral pons as discussed further on (page 1455).

Anomalous regeneration of the seventh nerve fibers, following a Bell's palsy or other injury, may result in other curious disorders. The most common is the "jaw-winking" phenomenon (also called Wartenberg's or inverse Marcus-Gunn sign), in which jaw movements, especially lateral movements (pterygoid muscle), cause an involuntary closure of the eyelid. If regenerating fibers originally connected with the orbicularis oculi become connected with the orbicularis oris, closure of the lids may cause a retraction of the corner of the mouth; or if visceromotor fibers originally innervating the salivary glands later come to innervate the lacrimal gland, anomalous tearing (crocodile tears) occurs whenever the patient salivates. A similar mechanism explains gustatory sweating of the cheek and upper lip. With the passage of time, the corner of the mouth and even the tip of the nose may become pulled to the affected side.

Bell's Palsy The most common disease of the facial nerve is Bell's palsy (incidence rate of 23 per 100,000 annually, according to Hauser et al). This disorder affects men and women more or less equally and occurs at all ages and all times of the year. There is controversy regarding an increased incidence in women during the third trimester of pregnancy, particularly in the 2 weeks preceding delivery and in the first 2 weeks postpartum; up to a threefold increase has been cited by some authors, but others have failed to find this disproportionate number of cases. Supporting such a proclivity for facial palsy are scattered reports of a recurrence with each pregnancy. Bell's palsy is probably more common in diabetics and possibly in hypertensives than in the normal population.

As one might expect, the opportunity to examine the facial nerve in the course of Bell's palsy occurs very rarely. Only a handful of such cases are on record, all showing varying degrees of degeneration of nerve fibers.

One case was said to show inflammatory changes, but these may have been misinterpreted (see Karnes).

Regarding causation of Bell's palsy, a viral agent has long been suspected (Baringer). Only in the past few years, however, has such a mechanism been established with a reasonable degree of certainty for the majority of cases formerly considered to be idiopathic. Burgess and colleagues identified the genome of herpes simplex virus (HSV) in the geniculate ganglion of an elderly man who died 6 weeks after the onset of Bell's palsy. More recently, Murakami and coworkers, using the polymerase chain reaction (PCR) technique to amplify viral genomic sequences, identified HSV type I in the endoneurial fluid surrounding the seventh nerve in 11 of 14 cases of Bell's palsy; the fluid was obtained during surgical decompression of the nerve in severe cases. The same investigators have produced facial paralysis by inoculating HSV into the ears and tongues of mice; virus antigens were then found in the facial nerve and geniculate ganglion. Varicella zoster virus (VZV) was not found in any of the Bell's palsy patients but was isolated from patients with the Ramsay-Hunt syndrome (page 799 and further on). Control patients with fracture or infections of the temporal bone yielded neither HSV or VZV gene sequences. In the light of these findings, the term *idiopathic facial paralysis*, until now the accepted synonym for Bell's palsy, is not entirely appropriate and should perhaps be changed to *herpes simplex* or *herpetic facial paralysis*.

The onset of Bell's palsy is acute; about one-half of the cases attain maximum paralysis in 48 h and practically all cases within 5 days. Pain behind the ear may precede the paralysis by a day or two and in a few patients is quite intense and persistent. In a small proportion of patients, a hypesthesia in one or more branches of the trigeminal nerve can be demonstrated. The explanation of this finding is not clear. Impairment of taste is present to some degree in almost all patients but rarely persists beyond the second week of paralysis. As indicated above, it means that the lesion has extended to or above the point where the chorda tympani fibers join the facial nerve. Hyperacusis or distortion of sound in the ipsilateral ear indicates paralysis of the stapedius muscle. Unlike the fifth nerve in idiopathic trigeminal neuritis, the facial nerve in Bell's palsy is often seen to display enhancement on the gadolinium-enhanced MRI. Correspondingly, there is a mild increase of lymphocytes and mononuclear cells in the CSF in a few of the cases.

Fully 80 percent of patients recover within a few weeks or in a month or two. Recovery of taste precedes recovery of motor function; if the former occurs in the first week, it is a good prognostic sign. Early recovery of some motor function in the first 5 to 7 days is the most favorable prognostic sign. Electromyography may be of value in distinguishing temporary conduction defects from a pathologic interruption of nerve fibers; if there is evidence of denervation after 10 days, one may expect a long delay in the onset of recovery (3 months, on the average). Recovery then proceeds by regeneration of nerve, a process that may take 2 years or longer and is often incomplete.

Idiopathic Bell's palsy is said to recur in 8 percent of cases (van Amstel and Devriese; Pitts et al), presumably as a result of reactivation of the herpesvirus. The palsy reemerges during an infection or pregnancy or for no apparent reason. The interval between episodes is unpredictable but has been 10 years, on average. Other recurrent forms of facial paralysis occur with Lyme disease and sarcoidosis, and in a familial variety as mentioned below.

Protection of the eye during sleep, massage of the weakened muscles, and a splint to prevent drooping of the lower part of the face are the measures generally employed in the management of such cases. There is no evidence that surgical decompression of the facial nerve is effective, and it may be harmful. The administration of prednisone (40 to 60 mg/day) during the first week to 10 days after onset may be beneficial; it is thought to decrease the possibility of permanent paralysis from swelling of the nerve in the tight facial canal. The recent finding of viral genome surrounding the seventh nerve suggests that antiviral agents may be useful in the management of Bell's palsy. Several small trials suggest that acyclovir, used alone, is no more effective than corticosteroids. The use of both medications together is under study. The treatment of facial palsy due to VZV (Ramsay-Hunt syndrome) with these drugs is discussed below.

Other Causes of Facial Palsy Lyme disease commonly involves the facial nerve, as indicated on pages 768 and 1403. The mechanism is not thought to be a direct spirochetal infection. The diagnosis is likely when there has been a tick bite with erythema marginatum or arthritis. Several of our cases have had almost simultaneous facial palsy and sensory neuropathy. Human immunodeficiency virus (HIV) infection is an infrequent cause of facial palsy. The facial palsy of both Lyme and HIV infections is associated with a pleocytosis; serologic and CSF examination may be useful if there is a suspicion of either process. Rarely, chickenpox in children may be followed in 1 to 2 weeks by facial paralysis. Tuberculous infection of the mastoid and middle ear or of the petrous bone is a cause of facial paralysis in parts of the world where tuberculosis is particularly common. Facial palsy may occur in infectious mononucleosis and was observed occasionally in poliomyelitis. The facial nerve is frequently involved in leprosy. Bilateral involvement of the facial nerve is commented on below.

The *Ramsay Hunt syndrome*, due presumably to herpes zoster of the geniculate ganglion, consists of a facial palsy associated with a vesicular eruption in the external auditory canal, other parts of the cranial integument, and mucous membrane of the oropharynx. Often the eighth cranial nerve is affected as well, causing vertigo and deafness (see pages 189 and 799). Murakami et al have shown that the virus can be detected even before the emergence of typical vesicles by collecting exudate from the skin of the pinna on a Schirmer strip (otherwise used to quantitate tearing) and applying PCR techniques. In this way, in a manner of a few hours, they documented VZV infection in 71 percent of patients with Ramsay-Hunt syndrome without vesicles. Treatment with a combination of corticosteroids and acyclovir has been recommended based on a randomized trial (Whitley et al).

Tumors of the parotid gland or ones that invade the temporal bone (carotid body, cholesteatoma, and dermoid) or granulomatosis at the base of the brain (histiocytosis) may produce a facial palsy; the onset is insidious and the course progressive. Fracture of the temporal bone (usually with damage to the middle or internal ear), otitis media, and middle ear surgery are relatively uncommon causes. Acoustic neuromas, neurofibromas, glomus jugulare tumors, and aneurysmal dilatations of the vertebral or basilar artery may involve the facial nerve. Pontine lesions, most often vascular or neoplastic, may cause facial palsy, usually in conjunction with other neurologic signs. Amyloidosis of the type associated with crystal lattice deposits in the cornea may involve the facial nerves. An autosomal dominant form of facial palsy, multiple truncal café-au-lait spots, and mild developmental delay have been described by Johnson and colleagues. Weakness of only a portion of the facial musculature, associated with numbness in the same region, may be the result of perineural tumor invasion by squamous cell or other skin cancers (see further on, under "Multiple Cranial Nerve Palsies").

Bell's palsy may be bilateral, but rarely is the involvement on the two sides simultaneous. Contemporaneous *bilateral facial paralysis* (facial diplegia) is most often a manifestation of the Guillain-Barré syndrome and may also occur in Lyme disease (page 1472). There are numerous other causes of bilateral facial palsy, all of them infrequent (Keane). It is reported in approximately 7 of every 1000 patients with sarcoidosis (*uveoparotid fever*, or *Heerfordt syndrome*), where the paralysis on each side tends to be separated by weeks or longer. It is a feature of the Möbius syndrome; even less common is the *Melkersson-Rosenthal syndrome*, consisting of the triad of recurrent facial paralysis, facial (particularly labial) edema, and, less constantly, plication of the tongue. The syndrome begins in childhood or adolescence and may be familial. Biopsy of the lip may reveal a granulomatous inflammation. Causes of *recurrent Bell's palsy* have been listed above and are summarized by Pitts and colleagues.

Muscles innervated by the facial nerve may be affected by lesions of the supranuclear pathways, which disinhibit or otherwise derange brainstem reflex activity. In the condition referred to as "apraxia of the eyelids," the patients cannot close the eyelids voluntarily, but they will still close reflexively in response to stimulation of the supraorbital branch of the trigeminal nerve (by a tap on the brow or bridge of the nose or by touching the cornea). As described in Chap. 45, under "Blink Reflexes," these are trigeminofacial reflexes. Actually, the blink reflex is expressed by two electrical responses, one early and mainly ipsilateral (termed R1) and the other late and bilateral (R2). The late response (to a tap on the brow), which is lost in Parkinson disease and is enhanced in pseudobulbar palsy, utilizes large fiber bundles in the supraorbital nerves; the early response (corneal reflex) utilizes the small fiber bundles in the long ciliary nerves. Derangement of one of these reflexes or of the jaw jerk is found in 25 percent of patients with multiple sclerosis. In pseudobulbar palsy, tapping the tendinous insertions into the orbicularis oris elicits a buccal (trigeminofacial) reflex, which may spread to cause closure of the eyes.

All forms of nuclear or peripheral facial palsy must be distinguished from the supranuclear type. In the latter, the frontalis and orbicularis oculi muscles are involved less than those of the lower part of the face or not at all, since the corticopontine innervation of the upper facial muscles is bilateral, and that of the lower facial muscles, mainly contralateral (a finding attributed to Broadbent). In supranuclear lesions there may be a dissociation of emotional and voluntary facial movements (page 56); often, some degree of paralysis of the arm and leg or an aphasia (in dominant hemisphere lesions) is conjoined. A developmental malformation of the perisylvian regions of the cortex may present as facial diplegia and pharyngeal paralysis, essentially a pseudobulbar palsy.

An obscure disorder is the *facial hemiatrophy of Romberg*. It occurs mainly in females and is characterized by a disappearance of fat in the dermal and subcutaneous tissues on one or both sides of the face. It usually begins in adolescence or early adulthood and is slowly progressive. In its advanced form, the affected side of the face is gaunt and the skin thin, wrinkled, and rather dark; the hair may turn white and fall out, and the sebaceous glands become atrophic; the muscles and bones are not involved as a rule. The condition is a form of *lipodystrophy*, but the localization within a dermatome indicates the operation of some neural factor (possibly a growth factor) of unknown nature. A variegated coloration of the iris and a congenital oculosympathetic paralysis are found in some cases. Rarely certain central nervous system abnormalities (mainly focal seizures and ventricular dilatation) referable to the homolateral hemisphere are conjoined (Hosten). The significance of these associations is unclear. Wilson and Hoxie have pointed out the frequent coexistence of facial asymmetry in adults with congenital or early-onset superior oblique palsy and compensatory head tilt or torticollis.

Hemifacial Spasm The facial muscles on one side may be involved in painless irregular clonic contractions of varying degree (*hemifacial spasm*). This condition develops in the fifth and sixth decades, affects women more than men, and is usually without known antecedent cause. It usually proves to be due to a compressive lesion of the facial nerve (most often by a tortuous branch of the basilar artery that lies on the ventral surface of the pons and forms a loop under the proximal nerve, and rarely by a basilar artery aneurysm, or by a acoustic nerve tumor or meningioma). Less often it is a transient or permanent sequela of a Bell's palsy, as stated earlier. The spasm usually begins in the orbicularis oculi muscle and gradually spreads to other muscles on that side of the face, including the platysma. The paroxysm may be induced or aggravated by voluntary and reflexive movements of the face.

There was for a time controversy concerning the pathogenesis of "idiopathic" hemifacial spasm. Jannetta attributes all cases to a compression of the root of the facial nerve by an aberrant looped blood vessel. Microsurgical decompression of the root with the interposition of a pledget between the vessel and the root has relieved the facial spasm in most of his cases. These results were corroborated by Barker and associates in a series of 705 patients, followed postoperatively for an average period of 8 years; 84 percent achieved an excellent result. Similar results were obtained in a prospective series of 83 patients by Illingworth and colleagues (cure of 81 of 83 patients).

The pathophysiology of the spasm is believed to be nerve root compression and segmental demyelination. The demyelinated axon is capable of activating adjacent nerve fibers by ephaptic transmission ("artificial synapse" of Granit et al). Another possible source of the spasm is ectopic excitation arising in injured fibers. Nielsen and Jannetta, who offer the same explanation (and treatment) for trigeminal neuralgia, have shown that ephaptic transmission disappears after the nerve is decompressed.

Surgical decompression of a vascular loop, which involves exploration of the posterior fossa, is not without risk. The facial muscles may be weakened, sometimes permanently. Another complication has been deafness due to injury of the adjacent eighth nerve. Also, there is a modest risk of recurrence of the spasms, usually within 2 years of the operation (Piatt and Wilkins). Operative success depends on tight dural closure to prevent CSF leakage from the posterior fossa.

The authors believe that patients with idiopathic hemifacial spasm should first be treated medically. Alexander and Moses noted that carbamazepine (Tegretol), in a dosage of 600 to 1200 mg/day, controlled the spasm in two-thirds of the patients. Baclofen or gabapentin can be tried if carbamazepine fails. Some patients cannot tolerate these drugs, have only brief remissions, or fail to respond; they may be treated with botulinum toxin injected into the orbicularis oculi and other facial muscles. The hemifacial spasms are relieved for 4 to 5 months and injections can be repeated without danger. Some patients have been injected repeatedly for more than 5 years without apparent adverse effects.

Other Disorders of the Facial Nerve *Facial myokymia* is a fine rippling activity of all the muscles of one side of the face. It develops most often in the course of multiple sclerosis or a brainstem glioma. It has also been seen in the course of diseases of the facial nerve, e.g., in Guillain-Barré syndrome (GBS), in which case it is usually bilateral. We have seen it more often in the recovery stage than in the early phase of GBS. The fibrillary nature of the involuntary movements and their arrhythmicity tend to distinguish them from the coarser intermittent facial spasms and contracture, tics, tardive dyskinesia, and clonus. The EMG pattern is one of spontaneous asynchronous discharge of adjacent motor units, appearing singly or in doublets or triplets at a rate varying from 30 to 70 cycles per second. Demyelination of the intrapontine part of the facial nerve and possibly supranuclear disinhibition of the facial nucleus have been the postulated mechanisms. But the observation of facial myokymia in GBS informs us that the abnormal movement may have its origin in a lesion at any point along the nerve (see pages 1467 and 1568 for further discussion of myokymia).

A clonic or tonic contraction of one side of the face may be the sole manifestation of a cerebral cortical seizure. An involuntary recurrent spasm of both eyelids (*blepharospasm*) may occur with dystonia but is most frequent in elderly persons as an isolated phenomenon, and there may be varying degrees of spasm of the other facial muscles (see page 114). Relaxant and tranquilizing drugs are of little help in this disorder, but injections of botulinum toxin into the orbicularis oculi muscles give temporary or lasting relief. A few of our patients have been helped (paradoxically) by L-dopa; baclofen, clonazepam, and tetrabenazine in increasing doses may be helpful. In the past, failing these measures, the periorbital muscles were destroyed by injections of doxorubicin or surgical myectomy (Hallett and Daroff). With the advent of botulinum treatment, there is no longer a need to resort to extreme surgical measures. In some cases, blepharospasm subsides spontaneously. Rhythmic unilateral myoclonia, akin to palatal myoclonus, may be restricted to facial, lingual, or laryngeal muscles.

Hypersensitivity of the facial nerve occurs in tetany; spasm of the facial muscles is elicited by tapping in front of the ear (Chvostek sign).

The Ninth, or Glossopharyngeal, Nerve

This nerve arises from the lateral surface of the medulla by a series of small roots that lie just rostral to those of the vagus nerve. The glossopharyngeal, vagus, and spinal accessory nerves leave the skull together through the jugular foramen and are then distributed peripherally. The *ninth nerve* is mainly sensory, with cell bodies in the inferior, or petrosal, ganglion (the central processes of which end in the nucleus solitarius) and the small superior ganglion (the central fibers of which enter the spinal trigeminal tract and nucleus). Within the nerve are afferent fibers from baroreceptors in the wall of the carotid sinus and from chemoreceptors in the carotid body. The baroreceptors are involved in the regulation of blood pressure, and chemoreceptors are responsible for the ventilatory responses to hypoxia. The somatic efferent fibers of the ninth nerve are derived from the nucleus ambiguus, and the visceral efferent (secretory) fibers, from the inferior salivatory nucleus. These fibers contribute in a limited way to the motor innervation of the striated musculature of the pharynx (mainly of the stylopharyngeus, which elevates the pharynx), the parotid gland, and the glands in the pharyngeal mucosa (see the discussion of swallowing on page 581).

It is commonly stated that this nerve mediates sensory impulses from the faucial tonsils, posterior wall of the pharynx, and part of the soft palate as well as taste sensation from the posterior third of the tongue. However, an isolated lesion of the ninth cranial nerve is a rarity, and the effects are not fully known. In one personally observed case of bilateral surgical interruption of the ninth nerves, verified at autopsy, there had been no demonstrable loss of taste or other sensory or motor impairment. This suggests that the tenth nerve may be responsible for these functions, at least in some individuals. The role of the ninth nerve in the reflex control of blood pressure and ventilation has been mentioned above.

One may occasionally observe a glossopharyngeal palsy in conjunction with vagus and accessory nerve involvement due to a tumor in the posterior fossa or an aneurysm of the vertebral artery. The nerves are compressed as they pass through the jugular foramen. Hoarseness due to vocal cord paralysis, some difficulty in swallowing, deviation of the soft palate to the sound side, anesthesia of the posterior wall of the pharynx, and weakness of the upper trapezius and sternomastoid muscles make up the clinical picture (see Table 47-1, jugular foramen syndrome). On leaving the skull, the ninth, tenth, and eleventh nerves lie adjacent to the internal carotid artery, where they can be damaged by a dissection of that vessel.

Glossopharyngeal neuralgia, first described by Weisenburg in 1910, is a syndrome that resembles trigeminal neuralgia in many respects except that the unilateral stabbing pain is localized to the root of the tongue and throat. It is far less common than trigeminal neuralgia. Sometimes the pain overlaps the vagal territory beneath the angle of the jaw and external auditory meatus. It may be triggered by coughing, sneezing, swallowing, and pressure on the tragus of the ear (see page 198). Temporary blocking of the pain by anesthetizing the tonsillar fauces and posterior pharynx with 10% lidocaine spray is diagnostic. Rarely, herpes zoster may involve the glossopharyngeal nerve. Fainting as a manifestation of vagoglossopharyngeal neuralgia is described on page 395.

The same drugs that have been found helpful in the treatment of tic douloureux may be used to treat glossopharyngeal neuralgia, but their efficacy has been difficult to judge. Resnick and colleagues have reported the results of microvascular decompression of the ninth nerve in 40 patients; in 32 of these, relief of symptoms was complete and was sustained during an average follow-up of 4 years; 3 patients remained with permanent weakness of structures thought to be innervated by the ninth nerve. A similar high rate of success has been achieved by others. If syncope is associated with the pain, it can be expected to cease with abolition of the attacks of pain. Syncope can also occur when the ninth nerve is involved by tumors of the parapharyngeal space; most of these are squamous cell carcinomas and both the ninth and tenth nerves are implicated. Section of rootlets of the ninth nerve has reportedly reduced or abolished the episodes of fainting.

The Tenth, or Vagus, Nerve

This nerve has an extensive sensory and motor distribution. It has two ganglia: the *jugular*, which contains the cell bodies of the somatic sensory nerves (innervating the skin in the concha of the ear), and the *nodose*, which contains the cell bodies of the afferent fibers from the pharynx, larynx, trachea, esophagus, and the thoracic and abdominal viscera. The central processes of these two ganglia terminate in relation to the nucleus of the spinal trigeminal tract and the tractus solitarius, respectively. The motor fibers of the vagus are derived from two nuclei in the medulla—the nucleus ambiguus and the dorsal motor nucleus. The former supplies somatic motor fibers to the striated muscles of the larynx, pharynx, and palate; the latter supplies visceral motor fibers to the heart and other thoracic and abdominal organs. The distribution of vagal fibers is illustrated in Fig. 47-4, and their participation in swallowing is described on page 581.

Complete interruption of the intracranial portion of one vagus nerve results in a characteristic paralysis. The soft palate droops on the ipsilateral side and does not rise in phonation. The uvula deviates to the normal side on phonation, but this is an inconstant sign. There is loss of the gag reflex on the affected side and of the *curtain movement* of the lateral wall of the pharynx, whereby the faucial pillars move medially as the palate rises in saying "ah." The voice is hoarse, often nasal, and the vocal cord on the affected side lies immobile in a "cadaveric" position, i.e., midway between abduction and adduction. With partial lesions, movements of abduction are affected more than those of adduction (Semon's law). There may also be a loss of sensation at the external auditory meatus and back of the pinna. Usually no change in visceral function can be demonstrated. If the pharyngeal branches of both vagi are affected, as in diphtheria, the voice has a nasal quality, and regurgitation of liquids through the nose occurs during the act of swallowing.

Complete bilateral paralysis is said to be incompatible with life, and this is probably true if the nuclei are completely destroyed in the medulla by poliomyelitis or some other disease. However, in the cervical region, both vagi have been blocked with procaine in the treatment of intractable asthma, without mishap. Moreover, Johnson and Stern report a case of bilateral vocal cord paralysis in association with familial hypertrophic polyneuropathy, and Plott relates the history of three brothers with congenital laryngeal abductor paralysis due to bilateral dysgenesis of the nucleus ambiguus. Bannister and Oppenheimer have called attention to defects of phonation and laryngeal stridor as early features of autonomic failure in multiple system atrophy (page 1137). We have seen several such patients in whom stridor was a prominent feature of the illness and required tracheostomy for survival.

The vagus nerve may be implicated at the meningeal level by tumors and infectious processes and within the medulla by vascular lesions (e.g., the lateral medullary syndrome of Wallenberg or a cavernous angioma), by motor system disease, and occasionally by tumors. Dysphagia is then invariably present. Herpes zoster may attack this nerve, either alone or together with the ninth nerve as part of a jugular foramen syndrome. The vagus is often affected along with the glossopharyngeal nerve by dissection of the carotid artery at the base of the skull. The vagus nerves may be damaged in the course of thyroid surgery and may be involved in cases of advanced alcoholic or diabetic neuropathy. Polymyositis and dermatomyositis, which cause hoarseness and dysphagia by direct involvement of laryngeal and pharyngeal muscles, may simulate disease of the vagus nerves.

A fact of some importance is that the left recurrent laryngeal nerve may be damaged as a result of thoracic disease. There is no dysphagia with lesions at this point in the nerve since the branches to the pharynx (but not to the larynx) have already been given off. An aneurysm of the aortic arch, an enlarged left atrium, mediastinal lymph nodes from bronchial carcinoma, and a mediastinal or superior sulcus lung tumor are much more frequent causes of an isolated vocal cord palsy than are intracranial diseases.

It is estimated that in one-quarter to one-third of all cases of paralysis of the recurrent laryngeal nerve no cause can be established, i.e., they are idiopathic. The highest incidence is in the third decade, and males are more susceptible than females. Of the 21 cases reported by Blau and Kapadia, 5 recovered completely and 5 partially

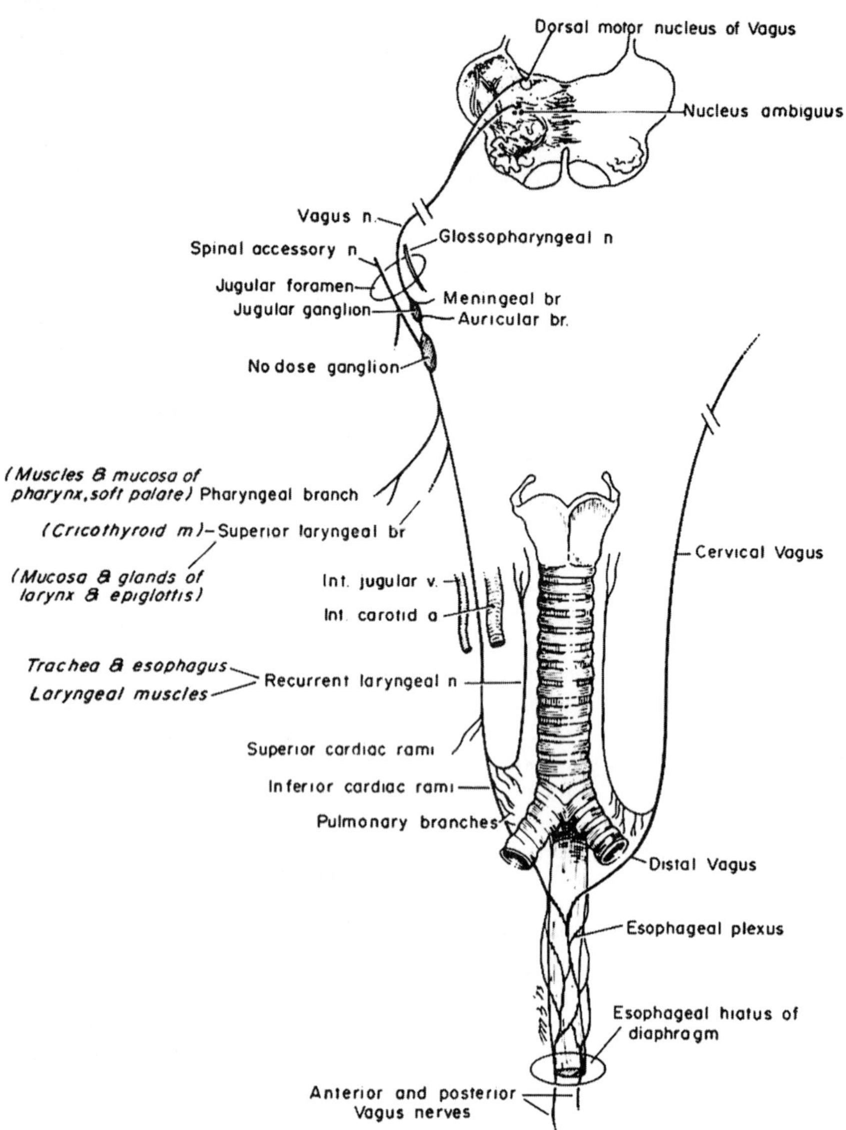

Figure 47-4

Anatomic features of the vagus nerve. Note the relationship to the spinal-accessory and glossopharyngeal nerves at the jugular foramen and the long course of the left recurrent laryngeal nerve, which is longer than the right.

within a few months; no other disease appeared in the 8-year period that followed. Palsies of the superior and recurrent laryngeal nerves, occurring as part of isolated vagal neuropathies, have been described by Berry and Blair. A few were bilateral, and again the majority of the cases were idiopathic and had much the same prognosis as isolated palsies of the recurrent laryngeal nerve.

Laryngeal neuralgia is a rare entity, in which paroxysms of pain are localized over the upper portion of the thyroid cartilage or hyoid bone on one or both sides. It is evoked by coughing, yawning, talking, or sneezing. In the case reported by Brownstone and coworkers it was relieved by carbamazepine.

When confronted with a case of vocal cord palsy, the physician must attempt to determine the site of the lesion. If it is intramedullary, there are usually ipsilateral cerebellar signs, loss of pain and temperature sensation over the ipsilateral face and contralateral arm and leg, and an ipsilateral Bernard-Horner syndrome. If the lesion is extramedullary but intracranial, the glossopharyngeal and spinal accessory nerves are frequently involved (jugular foramen syndrome, Table 47-1). If it is extracranial in the posterior laterocondylar or retroparotid space, there may be a combination of ninth, tenth, eleventh, and twelfth cranial nerve palsies and a Bernard-Horner syndrome. Combinations of these lower cranial nerve palsies, which have a variety of eponymic designations (see Table 47-1), are caused by various types of tumor, both primary and metastatic, or by chronic inflammations or granulomas involving lymph nodes at the base of the skull. If there is no palatal weakness and no pharyngeal or palatal sensory loss, the lesion is below the origin of the pharyngeal branches, which leave the vagus nerve high in the cervical region. The usual site of disease is then the mediastinum.

The 11th, or Accessory, Nerve

This is a purely motor nerve, actually of spinal rather than cranial origin. Its fibers arise from the anterior horn cells of the upper four or five cervical segments and enter the skull through the foramen magnum. Intracranially, the accessory nerve travels for a short distance with the part of the 10th nerve that is derived from the caudalmost cells of the nucleus ambiguus; together, the two roots are referred to as the *vagal-accessory nerve* or *cranial root of the accessory nerve*. The two roots leave the skull through the jugular foramen. The aberrant vagus fibers then rejoin the main trunk of the vagus, and the fibers derived from the cervical segments of the spinal cord form the external ramus and innervate the sternocleidomastoid and trapezius muscles. Only the latter fibers constitute the accessory nerve in the strict sense. In patients with torticollis, however, division of the upper cervical motor roots or the spinal accessory nerve has often failed to ablate completely the contraction of the sternomastoid muscle. This suggests a wider innervation of the muscle, perhaps by fibers of apparent vagal origin that join the accessory nerve for passage through the jugular foramen.

A complete lesion of the accessory nerve results in weakness of the sternocleidomastoid muscle and upper part of the trapezius (the lower part of the trapezius is innervated by the third and fourth cervical roots through the cervical plexus). This can be demonstrated by asking the patient to shrug his shoulders; the affected trapezius will be found to be weaker, and there will often be evident atrophy of its upper part. With the arms at the sides, the shoulder on the affected side droops and the scapula is slightly winged; the latter defect is accentuated with lateral movement of the arm (with serratus anterior weakness, winging of the scapula occurs on forward elevation of the arm). When the patient turns his head forcibly against the examiner's hand, preferably from the deviated to the straight-ahead position, the sternomastoid of the opposite side does not contract firmly beneath the fingers. This muscle can be further tested by having the patient press his head forward against resistance or lift his head from the pillow.

Motor system disease, poliomyelitis, syringomyelia, and spinal cord tumors may involve the cells of origin of the spinal accessory nerve. In its intracranial portion, the nerve is usually affected along with the ninth and tenth cranial nerves by herpes zoster or by lesions of the jugular foramen (glomus tumors, neurofibromas, metastatic carcinoma, jugular vein thrombosis). Tumors at the foramen magnum may also damage the nerve. In the posterior triangle of the neck, the 11th nerve can be damaged during surgical operations and by external compression or injury. Compressive-invasive lesions of this nerve may be visualized by computed tomography (CT) or MRI of the posterior cervical space.

A benign disorder of the 11th nerve, akin to Bell's palsy, has been described by Spillane and by Eisen and Bertrand; it begins with pain that subsides in a few days and is followed by weakness and atrophy in the distribution of the nerve. Also, a recurrent form of spontaneous accessory neuropathy has been described (Chalk and Isaacs). About one-quarter to one-third of 11th nerve lesions are estimated to be of this idiopathic type; most but not all of the patients recover. As in the case of idiopathic brachial plexopathy, ideas about its origin are speculative.

Bilateral sternomastoid and trapezius palsy, which occurs with primary disease of muscles—e.g., polymyositis and muscular dystrophy—may be difficult to distinguish from a bilateral affection of the accessory nerves or the motor nuclei (progressive bulbar palsy).

Hypoglossal Nerve

This is also a pure motor nerve, which supplies the somatic musculature of the tongue. It arises as a series of rootlets that issue from the medulla between the pyramid and inferior olivary complex. The nerve leaves the skull through the hypoglossal foramen and innervates the genioglossus muscle, which acts to protrude the tongue;

the styloglossus, which retracts and elevates its root; and the hypoglossus, which causes the upper surface to become convex. Complete interruption of the nerve results in paralysis of one side of the tongue. The tongue curves slightly to the healthy side as it lies in the mouth, but on protrusion it deviates to the affected side, owing to the unopposed contraction of the healthy genioglossus muscle. By pushing against the tongue in the cheek, one can judge the degree of one-sided weakness. The tongue cannot be moved with natural facility. The denervated side becomes wrinkled and atrophied, and fasciculations and fibrillations can be seen.

Lesions of the hypoglossal nerve roots are rare. Occasionally an intramedullary lesion damages the emerging fibers of the hypoglossal nerve, corticospinal tract, and medial lemniscus. The result is paralysis and atrophy of one side of the tongue, together with spastic paralysis and loss of vibration and position sense in the opposite arm and leg. Poliomyelitis and motor system disease may destroy the hypoglossal nuclei. Lesions of the basal meninges and the occipital bones (platybasia, invagination of the occipital condyles, Paget disease) may involve the nerve in its extramedullary course, and it is sometimes damaged in operations on the neck. A dissecting aneurysm of the carotid artery was shown by Goodman and coworkers to have compressed the hypoglossal nerve, with resultant weakness and atrophy. Lance and Anthony have described the simultaneous occurrence of nuchal-occipital pain and ipsilateral numbness of the tongue, provoked by the sudden, sharp turning of the head ("neck-tongue syndrome"). The phenomenon is attributed to compression, in the atlantoaxial space, of the second cervical root, which carries some of the sensory fibers from the tongue, via the hypoglossal nerve, to the C2 segment of the spinal cord.

The tongue may be red and smooth in vitamin deficiency states. *Glossodynia* (burning pain of the tongue), a condition most frequently seen in the elderly, may or may not be accompanied by redness and dryness but not by weakness. A habit of tongue-thrusting and teeth-clenching is often associated. The facile ascription of these motor abnormalities to a psychogenic mechanism does not accord with the authors' experience (see also Quinn).

Syndrome of Bulbar Palsy

This syndrome is the result of weakness or paralysis of muscles that are supplied by the motor nuclei of the lower brainstem, i.e., the motor nuclei of the fifth, seventh, and ninth to twelfth cranial nerves. (Strictly speaking, the motor nuclei of the fifth and seventh nerves lie outside the "bulb," which is the old name for the medulla oblongata.) Involved are the muscles of the jaw and face; the sternomastoids and upper parts of the trapezii; and the muscles of the tongue, pharynx, and larynx. If weakness develops rapidly, as may happen in Guillain-Barré syndrome, diphtheria, or poliomyelitis, there is no time for muscle atrophy. Myasthenia gravis and polymyositis may on rare occasions produce such a picture. The more chronic diseases—e.g., progressive bulbar palsy (a form of motor system disease) and the childhood form of Fazio-Londe—result in marked wasting and fasciculation of the facial, tongue, sternomastoid, and trapezius muscles. These disorders must be differentiated from pseudobulbar palsy (see page 517).

MULTIPLE CRANIAL NERVE PALSIES

As one can readily understand, several cranial nerves may be affected by a single disease process. One of the clinical problems that arises is whether the lesion lies within or outside the brainstem. Lesions lying on the surface of the brainstem are characterized by involvement of adjacent cranial nerves (often occurring in succession and often painful) and by late and only slight if any involvement of the long sensory and motor pathways and segmental structures lying within the brainstem. The opposite is true of intramedullary, intrapontine, and intramesencephalic lesions. The extramedullary lesion is more likely to cause bone erosion or to be associated with encroachment on cranial nerves (seen radiographically). Lesions within the brainstem that involve cranial nerves often produce a crossed sensory or motor paralysis (cranial nerve signs on one side of the body and tract signs on the opposite side). In this way, a number of distinctive syndromes, to which eponyms have been attached, are produced. These are listed in Table 47-2. The special problems of multiple cranial nerve palsies of the ocular motor nerves are addressed in Chap. 14.

Involvement of multiple cranial nerves outside the brainstem is frequently the result of trauma (sudden onset), localized infections such as herpes zoster (less acute onset), Wegener granulomatosis, sarcoidosis, or other types of granulomatous disease (subacute onset), or compression by tumors and saccular aneurysms (chronic development). The main causes of multiple cranial nerve palsies of extramedullary origin are listed in Table 47-3. *The sequential painless affection of contiguous or noncontiguous nerves over several days or weeks is particularly characteristic of meningeal carcinomatosis*

Table 47-3
Causes of extramedullary multiple cranial nerve palsies

Processes based on the meninges (meningoradiculitis)
- Carcinomatous and lymphomatous meningitis
- Infectious radiculitis (tuberculous, fungal, syphilitic, Lyme, etc.)
- Idiopathic pachymeningitis

Lesions affecting nerves at the skull base
- Metastasis of solid tumor or lymphomatous infiltration
- Local spread from nasopharyngeal tumor, chordoma, sarcoma
- Trauma
- Vascular occlusion or dissection (carotid artery, jugular vein thrombosis)
- Paget disease, basilar invagination, Arnold-Chiari and other bony disorders

Processes within nerves
- Perineural invasion of spindle cell, basal cell, parotid, and squamous cell cancer
- Granulomas and infectious diseases (sarcoid, Wegener granulomatosis, diphtheria, HIV, Lyme disease, idiopathic)
- Herpes zoster and other viral and postinfectious inflammatory lesions (GBS)
- Mixed connective tissue disease

Idiopathic
- Tolosa-Hunt-like syndrome affecting nonorbital nerves
- Melkersson-Rosenthal syndrome

or lymphomatosis. The eighth nerve is commonly incorporated in the neoplastic meningeal infiltrations. Among the solid tumors that cause local compression of nerves, neurofibromas, schwannomas, meningiomas, cholesteatomas, carcinomas, cordomas, and chondromas have all been observed. Nasopharyngeal carcinoma (Schmincke tumor or lymphoepithelioma) may implicate several cranial nerves in succession (mainly the fifth and sixth), as do basilar invagination and adult-onset Chiari malformation. On occasion, several lower cranial nerves are involved on one side by a carotid artery dissection. In France, a successive involvement of all cranial nerves on one side is called the Garcin syndrome or hemibasal syndrome. It has been reported in chondromas and chondrosarcomas of the clivus but presumably may occur with nasopharyngeal carcinomas as well.

Multiple or single cranial nerve palsies of abrupt onset may precede or accompany infectious mononucleosis and sometimes other viral or mycoplasmal diseases. DeSimone and Snyder have assembled a series of 20 such cases associated with mononucleosis; bilateral facial paralysis was the most common presentation, bilateral optic neuritis the next, and in three cases, three or four cranial nerves were involved. The prognosis is excellent. The main causes of bilateral facial palsy have been discussed earlier in the chapter. A purely motor disorder without atrophy always raises the question of myasthenia gravis. Owing to their anatomic relationships, the multiple cranial nerve palsies form a number of distinctive syndromes, listed in Table 47-1 and discussed in Chap. 31, on intracranial neoplasms (see also Table 31-4). MRI of cervical and basal cranial regions has greatly facilitated the diagnosis of tumors involving these nerves.

From time to time one observes an acute form of multiple cranial neuropathy of undetermined cause. Juncos and Beal have reported on 14 patients of this type, along with 6 well-documented cases of the Tolosa-Hunt orbitocavernous sinus syndrome with oculomotor palsies. In the former group, the onset was with facial pain and headache (temporofrontal), followed within days by abducens palsy (12 of 14), oculomotor palsy (6 of 14), trigeminal palsy (5 of 14), facial weakness (4 of 14), and less often by involvement of the eighth, ninth, and tenth cranial nerves (unilaterally in most instances). Increased protein of CSF and pleocytosis occurred in several. The prompt relief of pain upon administration of steroids was similar to that obtained in the Tolosa-Hunt syndrome. The mode of recovery, which usually occurred within a few months, was also much the same in the two groups of patients. Juncos and Beal concluded that the clinical features of the two groups overlapped and that their separation into two syndromes was arbitrary. We have also seen a relapsing form of this illness in young adults, responsive on each occasion to steroids. Numerous tests of the CSF by the polymerase chain reaction revealed no viruses. Conceivably, some of these cases represent a variant form of the Guillain-Barré syndrome, inasmuch as they may be preceded by a nonspecific infection and accompanied by areflexia, evanescent paresthesias or weakness of the extremities, and an elevated CSF protein without pleocytosis. Others probably are examples of the same entity described by Juncos and Beal. As a more chronic affliction, we have observed 10 cases in which cranial nerves were affected sequentially over a period of many years (*polyneuritis cranialis multiplex*). Two were later found to have tuberculosis of cervical lymph nodes (presumably scrofula), and three had sarcoidosis. No cause was determined in the rest. Symonds had a similar experience. It is usually worth obtaining a biopsy of an enlarged cervical lymph node in these circumstances. Corticosteroid treatment seemed to have been helpful.

The special case of painless multiple oculomotor palsies is discussed in Chap. 14. The main causes are Guillain-Barré syndrome, botulism, myasthenia gravis, thyroid ophthalmopathy, and diphtheria. In cases of chronic evolution, oculopharyngeal dystrophy and mitochondrial myopathy (progressive external ophthalmoplegia) must also be considered.

The *cavernous sinus syndrome*, discussed on pages 288 and 911, consists of various combinations of oculomotor palsies and upper trigeminal sensory loss, usually accompanied by signs of increased pressure or inflammation of the venous sinus. Cranial nerves are affected first on one side only, but any of the processes that infiltrate or obstruct the sinus may spread to the other side. The main causes are septic or aseptic thrombosis of the venous sinus due to trauma, hypercoagulable states or adjacent infections in adjacent structures, carotid artery aneurysm, and neoplastic infiltration. Keane has summarized his experience with 151 instances of cavernous sinus syndrome and found trauma and surgical procedures to be the commonest causes, followed by neoplasms (specifically those originating in the nasopharynx), pituitary tumors, metastases, and lymphomas.

A special cause of multiple cranial nerve palsies that has been brought to our attention is an infiltration along the distal nerves in the skin and subcutaneous tissues by squamous cell carcinomas of the face, especially the spindle cell and other atypical varieties. This type of perineural spread first causes unilateral palsies related to the superficial branches of the fifth and seventh cranial nerves in one region of the face and then extends to the base of the skull and to the ventral brainstem. According to Clouston and colleagues, who present five cases in detail, the initial symptoms are usually pain and numbness in the area underlying the skin lesion and facial weakness confined to the same regions of the face; this pattern is a result of the proximity of fifth and seventh nerve branches in the skin and subcutaneous tissues. Various combinations of oculomotor palsies may follow as a result of tumor entry into the orbit via the infraorbital branch of the maxillary nerve. Occasionally there is no pain. We have also observed a similar regional pattern of extracranial involvement of trigeminal and facial nerves with mixed cell tumors of the parotid gland.

The question of *viral infections of cranial nerves* is always raised by these acute palsies of the facial, trigeminal, and auditory nerves, especially when the affection is bilateral, involves several nerves in combination, or is associated with a pleocytosis. Actually, the only proved viral etiology in this group of cases is that of the herpes simplex and herpes zoster infections causing Bell's palsy, as discussed earlier in the chapter. Since perceptive deafness, vertigo, and other cranial nerve palsies have been observed in conjunction with the postinfectious encephalomyelitides of *Mycoplasma*, varicella, measles, rubella, mumps, and scarlet fever and also with GBS, an immune-mediated mechanism must be considered. However, as elaborated in Chaps. 33 and 36, new techniques that identify small components of the genome of these organisms indicate that some cases formerly thought to be postinfectious in nature may be true infections of the nerve. The same may be said of the single and multiple cranial nerve palsies that are sometimes associated with HIV and CMV infections. Nothing is known of the pathology of the cranial nerve lesion nor has a virus been isolated in these latter diseases. Treatment of the parainfectious cases is symptomatic; fortunately the prognosis for recovery is excellent.

In the *Tolosa-Hunt* cases in which the orbital or cavernous sinus has been biopsied, a nonspecific granuloma has been found. *Sarcoid* and *tuberculosis* have been the causes of a few cases, as noted above. In *Wegener granulomatosis*, multiple cranial nerve palsies, usually lower ones, are reported. The administration of cyclophosphamide has led to remission (page 1401).

REFERENCES

ALEXANDER GE, MOSES H: Carbamazepine for hemifacial spasm. *Neurology* 32:286, 1982.

BANNISTER R, OPPENHEIMER DR: Degenerative diseases of the nervous system associated with autonomic failure. *Brain* 95:457, 1972.

BARINGER JH: Herpes simplex virus and Bell palsy. *Ann Intern Med* 124:63, 1996.

BARKER FG, JANNETTA PJ, BISSONETTE DJ, et al: Microvascular decompression for hemifacial spasm. *J Neurosurg* 82:201, 1995.

BERRY H, BLAIR RL: Isolated vagus nerve palsy and vagal mononeuritis. *Arch Otolaryngol* 106:333, 1980.

BLAU JN, HARRIS M, KENNET S: Trigeminal sensory neuropathy. *N Engl J Med* 281:873, 1969.

BLAU JN, KAPADIA R: Idiopathic palsy of the recurrent laryngeal nerve: A transient cranial mononeuropathy. *BMJ* 4:259, 1972.

BRODAL A: *The Cranial Nerves*. Springfield, IL, Charles C Thomas, 1959.

BROWNSTONE PK, BALLENGER JJ, VICK NA: Bilateral superior laryngeal neuralgia. *Arch Neurol* 37:525, 1980.

BURGESS RC, MICHAELS L, BALE JF JR, SMITH RJ: Polymerase chain reaction amplification of herpes simplex viral DNA from the geniculate ganglion of a patient with Bell's palsy. *Ann Otol Rhinol Laryngol* 103:775, 1994.

CHALK C, ISAACS H: Recurrent spontaneous accessory neuropathy. *J Neurol Neurosurg Psychiatry* 53:621, 1990.

CHIA L-G: Pure trigeminal motor neuropathy. *BMJ* 296:609, 1988.

CLOUSTON PD, SHARPE DM, CORBETT AJ, et al: Perineural spread of cutaneous head and neck cancer: Its orbital and central neurologic complications. *Arch Neurol* 47:73, 1990.

DESIMONE PA, SNYDER D: Hypoglossal nerve palsy in infectious mononucleosis. *Neurology* 28:844, 1978.

DEVINSKY O, FELDMANN E: *Examination of the Cranial and Peripheral Nerves*. New York, Churchill Livingstone, 1988.

EISEN A, BERTRAND G: Isolated accessory nerve palsy of spontaneous origin: A clinical and electromyographic study. *Arch Neurol* 27:496, 1972.

GOODMAN JM, ZINK WL, COOPER DF: Hemilingual paralysis caused by spontaneous carotid artery dissection. *Arch Neurol* 40:653, 1983.

GRANIT R, LESKELL L, SKOGLAND CR: Fibre interaction in injured or compressed region of nerve. *Brain* 67:125, 1944.

HALLETT M, DAROFF RB: Blepharospasm: Report of a workshop. *Neurology* 46:1213, 1996.

HAUSER WA, KARNES WE, ANNIS J, KURLAND LT: Incidence and prognosis of Bell's palsy in the population of Rochester, Minnesota. *Mayo Clin Proc* 46:258, 1971.

HOSTEN N: MR of brain involvement in progressive facial hemiatrophy (Romberg disease): Reconsideration of a syndrome. *Am J Neuroradiol* 15:145, 1994.

HUGHES RAC: Diseases of the fifth cranial nerve, in Dyck PJ, Thomas PK, Lambert EH, et al (eds): *Peripheral Neuropathy*, 3rd ed. Philadelphia, Saunders, 1993, pp 801–817.

ILLINGWORTH RD, PORTER DG, JAKUBOWSKI J: Hemifacial spasm: A prospective long-term follow up of 83 patients treated by microvascular decompression. *J Neurol Neurosurg Psychiatry* 60:73, 1996.

JANNETTA PJ: Posterior fossa neurovascular compression syndromes other than neuralgias, in Wilkins RH, Rengachary SS (eds): *Neurosurgery*, 2nd ed. New York, McGraw-Hill, 1996, pp 3227–3233.

JOHNSON JA, STERN LZ: Bilateral vocal cord paralysis in a patient with familial hypertrophic neuropathy. *Arch Neurol* 38:532, 1981.

JOHNSON VP, MCMILLIN JM, ACETO T, BRUINS G: A newly recognized neuroectodermal syndrome of familial alopecia, anosmia, deafness, and hypogonadism. *Am J Med Genet* 15:497, 1983.

JUNCOS JL, BEAL MF: Idiopathic cranial polyneuropathy. *Brain* 110:197, 1987.

KARNES WE: Diseases of the seventh cranial nerve, in Dyck PJ, Thomas PK, Lambert EH, et al (eds): *Peripheral Neuropathy*, 3rd ed. Philadelphia, Saunders, 1993, pp 818–836.

KATUSIC S, BEARD CM, BERGSTRALH E, KURLAND LT: Incidence and clinical features of trigeminal neuralgia, Rochester, Minnesota, 1945–1984. *Ann Neurol* 27:89, 1990.

KEANE JR: Bilateral seventh nerve palsy: Analysis of 43 cases and review of the literature. *Neurology* 44:1198, 1994.

KEANE JR: Cavernous sinus syndrome: Analysis of 151 cases. *Arch Neurol* 53:967, 1996.

LANCE JW, ANTHONY M: Neck-tongue syndrome on sudden turning of the head. *J Neurol Neurosurg Psychiatry* 43:97, 1980.

LECKY BRF, HUGHES RAC, MURRAY NMF: Trigeminal sensory neuropathy. *Brain* 110:1463, 1987.

MASSEY EW, MOORE J, SCHOLD SC JR: Mental neuropathy from systemic cancer. *Neurology* 31:1277, 1981.

MAYO CLINIC DEPARTMENT OF NEUROLOGY: *Clinical Examinations in Neurology*, 7th ed. St Louis, Mosby-Year Book, 1998.

MURAKAMI S, HONDA N, MIZOBUCHI M, et al: Rapid diagnosis of varicella zoster virus in acute facial palsy. *Neurology* 51:1202, 1998.

MURAKAMI S, MIZOBUCHI M, NAKASHIRO Y, et al: Bell palsy and herpes simplex virus: Identification of viral DNA in endoneurial fluid and muscle. *Ann Intern Med* 124:27, 1996.

NIELSEN VK, JANNETTA PJ: Pathophysiology of hemifacial spasm: Effects of facial nerve decompression. *Neurology* 34:891, 1984.

PIATT JH, WILKINS RH: Treatment of tic douloureux and hemifacial spasm by posterior fossa exploration: Therapeutic implications of various neurovascular relationships. *Neurosurgery* 14:462, 1984.

PITTS DB, ADOUR KK, HILSINGER RL: Recurrent Bell's palsy analysis of 140 patients. *Laryngoscope* 98:535, 1988.

PLOTT D: Congenital laryngeal-abductor paralysis due to nucleus ambiguus dysgenesis in three brothers. *N Engl J Med* 271:593, 1964.

QUINN JH: Glossodynia. *J Am Dent Assoc* 70:1418, 1965.

RESNICK DK, JANNETTA PJ, BISSONETTE D, et al: Microvascular decompression for glossopharyngeal neuralgia. *Neurosurgery* 36:64, 1995.

SILVERMAN JE, LIU GT, VOLPE NJ, GALETTA SL: The crossed paralyses. *Arch Neurol* 52:635, 1995.

SPILLANE JD: Isolated unilateral spinal accessory nerve palsy of obscure origin. *BMJ* 2:365, 1949.

SPILLANE JD, WELLS CEC: Isolated trigeminal neuropathy: A report of 16 cases. *Brain* 82:391, 1959.

SWEET WH: The treatment of trigeminal neuralgia (tic douloureux). *N Engl J Med* 315:174, 1986.

SYMONDS C: Recurrent multiple cranial nerve palsies. *J Neurol Neurosurg Psychiatry* 21:95, 1958.

VAN AMSTEL AD, DEVRIESE PP: Clinical experience with recurrences of Bell's palsy. *Arch Otorthinolaryngol* 245:302, 1998.

WHITLEY RJ, WEISS H, GNANN JW, et al: Acyclovir with and without prednisone for the treatment of herpes zoster: A randomized, placebo-controlled trial. *Ann Intern Med* 125:376, 1996.

WILSON ME, HOXIE J: Facial asymmetry in superior oblique muscle palsy. *J Pediatr Ophthalmol Strabismus* 30:315, 1993.

Chapter 48

PRINCIPLES OF CLINICAL MYOLOGY: DIAGNOSIS AND CLASSIFICATION OF MUSCLE DISEASES—GENERAL CONSIDERATIONS

Skeletal, or voluntary, muscle constitutes the principal organ of locomotion as well as a vast metabolic reservoir. Disposed in more than 600 separate muscles, this tissue makes up as much as 40 percent of the weight of adult human beings. An intricacy of structure and function undoubtedly accounts for its diverse susceptibility to disease, for which reason the following anatomic and physiologic facts are provided, as an introduction to the several chapters on muscle disease.

A single muscle is composed of thousands of muscle fibers that extend for variable distances along its longitudinal axis. Each fiber is a relatively large and complex multinucleated cell varying in length from a few millimeters to several centimeters (34 cm in the human sartorius muscle) and in diameter from 10 to 100 μm. Some fibers span the entire length of the muscle; others are joined end to end by connective tissue. Each muscle fiber is enveloped by an inner plasma membrane (the sarcolemma) and an outer basement membrane. The nuclei of each cell, which are oriented parallel to the longitudinal axis of the fiber and may number in the thousands, lie beneath the plasma membrane (sarcolemma)—hence they are termed *subsarcolemmal* or just *sarcolemmal nuclei*.

The cytoplasm (sarcoplasm) of the cell is abundant and contains myofibrils, various organelles such as mitochondria, and ribosomes; each myofibril is enveloped in a membranous net, the sarcoplasmic reticulum (Fig. 45-3). Extensions of the plasma membrane into the fiber form the transverse tubular system (T tubules), which are extracellular channels of communication with the intracellular sarcoplasmic reticulum (SR). The SR and T tubules are anatomically independent but functionally related membrane systems. The junctional gap between the T tubules and SR is occupied by protein formations that are attached to the SR and are referred to as *junctional feet*; the latter have been identified as ryanodine receptors and are responsible for the release of calcium from the SR (Franzini-Armstrong).

The myofibrils are composed of longitudinally oriented interdigitating filaments (myofilaments) of contractile proteins (actin and myosin) and regulatory proteins (tropomyosin, troponin, and nebulin). The series of biochemical events by which these proteins, under the influence of Ca ions, accomplish the contraction and relaxation of muscle is described in Chap. 45. Droplets of stored fat, glycogen, various proteins, many enzymes, and myoglobin, the latter imparting the red color to muscle, are contained within the sarcoplasm or its organelles.

Although the muscle fiber represents an indivisible anatomic and physiologic unit, disease may affect only one part of it, leaving the remainder to become dysfunctional or to atrophy, degenerate, or regenerate, depending on the nature and severity of the disease process.

The individual muscle fibers are enveloped by delicate strands of connective tissue (endomysium), which provide their support and permit unity of action. Capillaries, of which there may be several for each fiber, and nerve fibers lie within the endomysium. Muscle fibers are bound into groups or *fascicles* by similar reticular tissue and sheets of collagen (perimysium), which also bind together groups of fascicles and surround the entire muscle (epimysium). The latter connective tissue tunics are also richly vascularized; different types of muscle have different arrangements of arteries and veins; fat cells (lipocytes) are embedded within the interstices. The muscle fibers are attached at their ends to tendon fibers, which in turn connect with the skeleton. By this means muscle contraction maintains posture and imparts movement.

Other notable characteristics of muscle are its natural mode of contraction—i.e., through innervation—and the necessity of intact innervation for the maintenance of its normal trophic state. Each muscle fiber receives a nerve twig from a motor nerve cell in the anterior horn of the spinal cord or nucleus of a cranial nerve; the nerve twig joins the muscle fiber at the *neuromuscular junction* or *motor end plate*. As was pointed out on page 47, groups of muscle fibers with a common innervation from one anterior horn cell constitute the *motor unit*, which is the basic physiologic unit in all reflex, postural, and voluntary activity.

Acetylcholine (ACh), ACh receptors, and acetylcholinesterase (AChE), which play a special role in neuromuscular transmission, are concentrated at the neuromuscular junction. ACh is synthesized in the motor nerve terminal and stored in vesicles as packets, or "quanta," each containing a relatively fixed number of molecules (about 10,000). Quanta of ACh are released at the nerve ending, diffuse into the narrow synaptic cleft, and combine with specialized receptors on the postsynaptic membrane. Small numbers of quanta of ACh are released spontaneously, producing miniature end-plate potentials (MEPPs) of about 0.5 mV. A nerve impulse depolarizes the presynaptic membrane and causes an ingress of Ca^{2+} into the nerve terminal through voltage-gated calcium channels, thereby triggering the release of many ACh quanta and producing a much larger end-plate potential (EPP). This wave of depolarization is propagated along the sarcolemma and transverse tubules to the interior of the fibers and leads to muscle contraction (see Chap. 45). The process of ACh release is terminated by action of the enzyme AChE, which breaks down ACh at the neuromuscular junction. For the details of the exocytosis of the synaptic vesicles and their reconstitution, the reader is referred to the chapter on transmitter release in the text of Kandel and colleagues, listed in the References.

In addition to motor nerve endings, muscle contains several types of sensory endings, all of them acting as mechanoreceptors: free nerve endings subserve the sensation of deep pressure-pain; Ruffini and pacinian corpuscles are pressure sensors; and the Golgi tendon organs and muscle spindles are tension receptors and participate in the maintenance of muscle tone and in reflex activity (page 48). The Golgi receptors are located mainly at the myotendon junctions; pacinian corpuscles are also localized at the tendon site but are sparse in muscle itself. Muscle spindles, specialized groups of small muscle fibers, regulate muscle contraction and relaxation, as described on page 48. All these receptors are present in highest density in muscles that are involved in fine movements.

All muscles are not equally susceptible to disease, despite the apparent similarity of their structure. In fact, practically no disease affects all muscles in the body, and each disease has as one of its features a characteristic topography within the musculature. The topographic differences between diseases provide incontrovertible evidence of structural or physiologic differences between muscles that are not presently disclosed by the light or electron microscope. The factors responsible for the selective vulnerability of certain muscles are not known. Several hypothetical explanations come to mind. One factor may relate simply to fiber size; consider, for example, the large diameter and length of the fibers of the glutei and paravertebral muscles in comparison with the smallness of the ocular muscle fibers. The number of fibers composing a motor unit may also be of significance; in the ocular muscles, a motor unit contains only 6 to 10 muscle fibers (some even less), but a motor unit of the gastrocnemius contains as many as 1800 fibers. Also, the eye muscles have a much higher metabolic rate and a richer content of mitochondria than the large trunk muscles. Differences in patterns of vascular supply may permit some muscles to withstand the effects of hypoxia or vascular occlusion better than others. Histochemical studies of skeletal muscles have disclosed that within any one muscle, there are subtle metabolic differences between fibers—certain ones (type 1 fibers) being richer in oxidative and poorer in glycolytic enzymes, and others (type 2 fibers) being the opposite. The eye muscles do not contain dystrophin, a membrane-anchoring protein that is deficient in Duchenne and related forms of muscular dystrophy, which may explain the muscles' lack of involvement in these diseases. Doubtless other differences will be discovered.

These anatomic and biochemical properties of muscle suggest some of the ways in which this tissue can be affected by disease. Thus, one may envisage causative agents or genetic defects that affect different components of sarcoplasm: the filamentous proteins; the mitochondrial enzymes; the sarcoplasmic reticulum; the specialized channels for the entry of calcium, sodium, or chloride; the transverse tubules; or the sarcolemma itself. The endomysial connective tissue could be the primary pathway in disease, since it so closely invests the muscle fiber. Endomysial fibroblasts of eye muscles contain an abundance of glycosaminoglycans, which may render them susceptible to thyroid diseases. Finally, the nerve or its cell of origin in the spinal cord is known to bear the brunt of certain pathologic processes, paralyzing all the muscle fibers that it innervates and depriving them of the unique trophic influence that nerve normally has upon muscle.

Normal muscle possesses the capacity, albeit limited, to regenerate, a point often forgotten. Complete destruction of the muscle fiber is not followed by regeneration. Partial destructive processes of the muscle fiber, e.g., inflammatory or metabolic, are usually followed by fairly complete restoration of the muscle cells provided that some part of each fiber has survived and the endomysial sheaths of connective tissue have not been disrupted. Unfortunately, many pathologic processes of muscle are chronic and unrelenting. Under such conditions, any regenerative activity fails to keep pace with the disease and the loss of muscle fibers is permanent. The bulk of the muscle is then replaced by fat and collagenous connective tissue, as typically seen in the muscular dystrophies.

APPROACH TO THE PATIENT WITH MUSCLE DISEASE

The number and diversity of diseases of striated muscle greatly exceeds the number of symptoms and signs by which they express themselves clinically; thus, different diseases share certain common symptoms and even syndromes. To avoid excessive repetition in the description of individual diseases, we shall discuss in one place all their clinical manifestations, a subject that is appropriately called *clinical myology.*

The physician is initially put on the track of a myopathic disease by eliciting complaints of muscle weakness or fatigue, pain, limpness or stiffness, spasm, cramp, twitching, or a muscle mass or change in muscle volume. Of these, the symptom of weakness is by far the most frequent and at the same time the most elusive. As remarked in Chap. 24, when speaking of weakness, the patient often means excessive fatigability. Although fatigability may be a feature of muscle diseases—particularly those affecting the neuromuscular junction, such as myasthenia gravis—it is far more frequently a complaint of patients with chronic systemic disease or with anxiety and depression. To distinguish between fatigability and weakness, one must assess the patient's capacity to perform certain common activities such as walking, running, climbing stairs, and arising from a sitting, kneeling, squatting, or reclining position. Difficulty in performing these tasks signifies weakness rather than fatigue. The same is true of difficulty in working with the arms above shoulder level. Particular complaints may reveal a localized muscle weakness; e.g., drooping of the eyelids, diplopia and strabismus, change in facial expression and voice, and difficulty in chewing, closing the mouth, and swallowing indicate a paresis of the levator palpebrae, extraocular, facial, laryngeal, masseter, and pharyngeal muscles, respectively. Of course, these impairments of muscle function may be due to a neuropathic or central nervous system (CNS) disturbance rather than to a myopathic one, but usually these conditions can be separated by the methods indicated further on in this chapter and in Chaps. 3 and 24.

Evaluation of Muscle Weakness and Paralysis

Reduced strength of muscle contraction—manifest by diminished power of single contractions and resistance to opposition (peak power) and by endurance during the sustained performance of demanded movements (i.e., work)—is the indubitable sign of muscle disease. In such testing, the physician may encounter difficulty in enlisting the patient's cooperation. The tentative, hesitant performance of the asthenic or hypersuggestible individual or the hysteric or malingerer poses difficulties that can be surmounted by the techniques described in Chap. 3. In infants and small children, who cannot follow commands, one assesses muscle power by their resistance to passive manipulation or observing their performance while they are engaged in certain activities. The patient may be reluctant to fully contract the muscles in a painful limb, and indeed pain itself may cause a slight reflex diminution in the power of contraction (algesic paresis). Estimating the strength of isometric contractions that do not require the painful part to be moved is a way around this difficulty. Sometimes the weakness of a group of muscles becomes manifest only after a period of activity; e.g., the feet and legs may "drag" only after the patient has walked a long distance. The physician, upon being told this by the patient, should conduct the examination under circumstances that duplicate the complaint(s).

Weakness of muscle contraction acquires added significance when it is associated with other abnormalities, such as tenderness or atrophy of muscle, change in tendon reflexes, twitching, and spasm. Also, severe weakness of certain muscle groups may result in abnormalities of posture and gait. A waddling gait indicates affection of the medial glutei (or dysplasia of hip joints); excessive lumbar lordosis and protuberance of the abdomen indicate weakness of the iliopsoas and abdominal muscles; kyphoscoliosis points to an asymmetrical weakness of the paravertebral muscles; and flaring of the shoulder blades is a sign of weakness of the lower trapezii, serratus magnus, and rhomboid muscles. Equinovarus deformities of the feet may be the result of fibrous contracture (pseudocontracture) of the calf muscles.

Ascertaining the extent and severity of muscle weakness requires a systematic examination of the main groups of muscles from forehead to feet. The patient is asked to contract each group with as much force as possible, while the examiner opposes the movement and offers a graded resistance in accordance with the degree of residual power (isokinetic contraction). Alternatively, the patient is asked to produce a maximal contraction, and the examiner estimates power by the force needed to "break" or overcome it (isometric contraction or maximum voluntary isometric contraction). If the weakness is unilateral, one has the advantage of being able to compare it with the strength on the normal side. If it is bilateral, the physician must refer to a concept of what constitutes normalcy, based on experience in muscle testing. These methods of manual muscle testing, while adequate in most clinical situations, may not be sufficiently refined for the evaluation of certain muscle diseases.

In order to quantitate the degree of weakness, which indicates the severity of affection, and to compare one examination with another, which is necessary to determine the course of the disease and the effects of therapy, a rating scale should be used. Most widely used is the one proposed by the Medical Research Council (MRC) of Great Britain, which recognizes six grades of muscle strength, as follows: 0, complete paralysis; 1, minimal contraction; 2, active movement with gravity eliminated; 3, weak contraction against gravity; 4, active movement against gravity and resistance; and 5, normal strength. Further gradations may be added, specified as 4+ for barely detectable weakness and 4− for easily detected weakness, 3+ and 3−, and so on. This allows 10 gradations of power. With practice, one can distinguish true weakness from unwillingness to cooperate, feigned or neurasthenic weakness, and inhibition of movement by pain.

Ocular, facial, lingual, pharyngeal, laryngeal, cervical, shoulder, upper arm, lower arm and hand, truncal, pelvic, thigh, and lower leg and foot muscles are examined sequentially. The anatomic significance of each of the actions tested—i.e., what roots, nerves, and muscles are involved—can be determined by referring to Table 48-1. A practiced examiner can survey the strength of these muscle groups in 2 to 3 min. A word of caution: in manually resisting the patient's attempts to contract the large and powerful trunk and girdle muscles, the examiner may fail to detect slight degrees of weakness, particularly in well-muscled individuals. These muscle groups are best tested by having the patient squat and kneel and then assume the erect posture, arise from and step onto a chair without using the hands, walk on his toes and heels, and lift a heavy object (textbook of medicine) over his head. The strength of muscles of the hand can be quantified with a dynamometer; for research purposes, similar but more sophisticated devices exist for other muscle groups (see Fenichel et al).

Qualitative Changes in the Contractile Process

In the *myasthenic states* there is a rapid failure of contraction in the most affected muscles during sustained activity. For instance, after the patient looks at the ceiling for a few minutes, the eyelids progressively droop; after the patient closes his eyes and rests the levator palpebrae muscles, the ptosis lessens or disappears. Similarly, holding the eyes in a far lateral position will induce diplopia and strabismus. These effects, in combination with restoration of power by the administration of neostigmine or edrophonium (Tensilon), are the most valid clinical criteria for the diagnosis of myasthenia gravis (page 1542).

In addition to myasthenic weakness, there are other abnormalities that may be discovered by observing, during one or a series of maximal actions of a group of muscles, the speed and efficiency of contraction and relaxation. In myxedema, for example, a stiffness and slowness of contraction in a muscle such as the quadriceps may be seen on change in posture (*contraction myoedema*); often it is associated with prolonged duration of the tendon reflexes and myoedema, which can be elicited by direct percussion of a muscle. Slowness in relaxation of muscles is another feature of hypothyroidism, accounting for the complaint of uncomfortable tightness of proximal limb muscles. A curious *rippling phenomenon* in muscles called *myokymia*, inherited as an autosomal dominant trait, has been observed in several families (Chap. 55). After a period of relaxation, a stiffening and rippling occurs in the contracting or stretched muscles. The stiffness is reduced by dantrolene but not by tocainamide. Acquired forms of myokymia are due to

Table 48-1
Actions of the principal muscles and their nerve root supply[a]

Action tested	*Roots*	*Nerves*	*Muscles*
CRANIAL			
Closure of eyes, pursing of lips, exposure of teeth	Cranial 7	Facial	Orbicularis oculi Orbicularis oris
Elevation of eyelids, movement of eyes	Cranial 3, 4, 6	Oculomotor, trochlear, abducens	Levator palpebrae, extraocular
Closing and opening of jaw	Cranial 5	Motor trigeminal	Masseters Pterygoids
Protrusion of tongue	Cranial 12	Hypoglossal	Lingual
Phonation and swallowing	Cranial 9, 10	Glossopharyngeal, vagus	Palatal, laryngeal, and pharyngeal
Elevation of shoulders, anteroflexion and turning of head	Cranial 11 and upper cervical	Spinal accessory	Trapezius, sternomastoid
BRACHIAL			
Adduction of extended arm	***C5***, C6	Brachial plexus	Pectoralis major
Fixation of scapula	C5, C6, C7	Brachial plexus	Serratus anterior
Initiation of abduction of arm	***C5***, C6	Brachial plexus	Supraspinatus
External rotation of flexed arm	***C5***, C6	Brachial plexus	Infraspinatus
Abduction and elevation of arm up to 90°	***C5***, C6	Axillary nerve	Deltoid
Flexion of supinated forearm	C5, C6	Musculocutaneous	Biceps, brachialis
Extension of forearm	C6, ***C7***, C8	Radial	Triceps
Extension (radial) of wrist	C6	Radial	Extensor carpi radialis longus
Flexion of semipronated arm	C5, ***C6***	Radial	Brachioradialis
Adduction of flexed arm	C6, ***C7***, C8	Brachial plexus	Latissimus dorsi
Supination of forearm	C6, C7	Posterior interosseous	Supinator
Extension of proximal phalanges	***C7***, C8	Posterior interosseous	Extensor digitorum
Extension of wrist (ulnar side)	***C7***, C8	Posterior interosseous	Extensor carpi ulnaris
Extension of proximal phalanx of index finger	***C7***, C8	Posterior interosseous	Extensor indicis
Abduction of thumb	***C7***, C8	Posterior interosseous	Abductor pollicis longus and brevis
Extension of thumb	***C7***, C8	Posterior interosseous	Extensor pollicis longus and brevis
Pronation of forearm	C6, C7	Median nerve	Pronator teres
Radial flexion of wrist	C6, C7	Median nerve	Flexor carpi radialis
Flexion of middle phalanges	C7, ***C8***, T1	Median nerve	Flexor digitorum superficialis
Flexion of proximal phalanx of thumb	C8, ***T1***	Median nerve	Flexor pollicis brevis
Opposition of thumb against fifth finger	C8, ***T1***	Median nerve	Opponens pollicis
Extension of middle phalanges of index and middle fingers	C8, ***T1***	Median nerve	First, second lumbricals
Flexion of terminal phalanx of thumb	***C8***, T1	Anterior interosseous nerve	Flexor pollicis longus

Table 48-1 (*Continued*)
Actions of the principal muscles and their nerve root supply[a]

Action tested	*Roots*	*Nerves*	*Muscles*
Flexion of terminal phalanx of second and third fingers	C8, T1	Anterior interosseous nerve	Flexor digitorum profundus
Flexion of distal phalanges of ring and little fingers	C7, ***C8***	Ulnar	Flexor digitorum profundus
Adduction and opposition of fifth finger	C8, ***T1***	Ulnar	Hypothenar
Extension of middle phalanges of ring and little fingers	C8, ***T1***	Ulnar	Third, fourth lumbricals
Adduction of thumb against second finger	C8, ***T1***	Ulnar	Adductor pollicis
Flexion of proximal phalanx of thumb	***C8***, T1	Ulnar	Flexor pollicis brevis
Abduction and adduction of fingers	C8, ***T1***	Ulnar	Interossei
CRURAL			
Hip flexion from semiflexed position	***L1***, ***L2***, L3	Femoral	Iliopsoas
Hip flexion from externally rotated position	L2, L3	Femoral	Sartorius
Extension of knee	L2, ***L3***, ***L4***	Femoral	Quadriceps femoris
Adduction of thigh	***L2***, ***L3***, L4	Obturator	Adductor longus, magnus, brevis
Abduction and int. rotation of thigh	***L4***, ***L5***, S1	Superior gluteal	Gluteus medius
Extension of thigh	***L5***, ***S1***, S2	Inferior gluteal	Gluteus maximus
Flexion of knee	L5, ***S1***, S2	Sciatic	Biceps femoris Semitendinosus Semimembranosus
Dorsiflexion of foot (medial)	***L4***, L5	Peroneal (deep)	Anterior tibial
Dorsiflexion of toes (proximal and distal phalanges)	***L5***, S1	Peroneal (deep)	Extensor digitorum longus and brevis
Dorsiflexion of great toe	***L5***, S1	Peroneal (deep)	Extensor hallucis longus
Eversion of foot	L5, S1	Peroneal (superficial)	Peroneus longus and brevis
Plantar flexion of foot	***S1***, S2	Tibial	Gastrocnemius, soleus
Inversion of foot	L4, ***L5***	Tibial	Tibialis posterior
Flexion of toes (distal phalanges)	L5, ***S1***, ***S2***	Tibial	Flexor digitorum longus
Flexion of toes (middle phalanges)	***S1***, ***S2***	Tibial	Flexor digitorum brevis
Flexion of great toe (proximal phalanx)	S1, S2	Tibial	Flexor hallucis brevis
Flexion of great toe (distal phalanx)	L5, ***S1***, ***S2***	Tibial	Flexor hallucis longus
Contraction of anal sphincter	S2, S3, S4	Pudendal	Perineal muscles

[a] Predominant root(s) supplying a particular muscle are indicated in bold italic type.
Source: Modified from Walton by permission.

diverse processes including nerve injury and regeneration (particularly in the face), hypothyroidism, and obscure causes.

A prolonged failure of relaxation with afterdischarge is characteristic of the *myotonic phenomenon*, which typifies certain diseases—congenital myotonia (of Thomsen), myotonic dystrophy (of Steinert), and the paramyotonia of von Eulenberg (Chap. 54). True myotonia, with its prolonged discharges of action potentials, requires strong contraction to elicit, is more evident after a period of relaxation, and tends to disappear with repeated contractions (pages 1363 and 1553). This persistence of contraction is demonstrable also by tapping a muscle (*percussion myotonia*), a phenomenon easily distinguished from the electrically silent local bulge (*myoedema*) induced by tapping the muscle of a myxedematous or cachetic patient and from the brief fascicular contraction that is induced by tapping a normal or partially denervated muscle; the latter is referred to as *idiomuscular contraction*. It should be noted that in patients with hyperactive tendon reflexes, striking the muscle rather than its tendon can elicit a stretch reflex. *Paradoxical myotonia* refers to an increase in the degree of myotonia during a series of contractions (the reverse of what happens in the usual type of myotonia). It occurs in some cases of von Eulenberg paramyotonia.

An increment in power with a series of several voluntary contractions in the absence of myotonia is a feature of the *inverse myasthenic (Lambert-Eaton) syndrome*, which is associated in about 50 percent of cases with small-cell carcinoma of the lung. The same increment occurs in botulism. In both instances there is an electromyographic (EMG) equivalent—a rapid increase in the voltage of a series of action potentials with appropriate stimulation (pages 1359 and 1547).

The effect of cold on muscle contraction may also prove informative; either paresis or myotonia, lasting for a few minutes, may be evoked or enhanced by cold, as in the paramyotonia of von Eulenberg.

Myotonia and myoedema must also be distinguished from the recruitment and spread of involuntary spasm induced by strong and repeated contractions of limb muscles in patients with *mild or localized tetanus* or with the "stiff-man" syndrome, and with dystonia. These are not primary muscle phenomena but are neural in origin, due to an abolition of inhibitory mechanisms.

The repeated contraction of forearm or leg muscles after the application of a tourniquet (exceeding arterial pressure) to the proximal part of a limb will often elicit latent tetany (carpopedal spasms). Its special mode of development in conditions that decrease the concentration of ionized calcium—as well as its duration, its enhancement by hyperventilation, and the association of tingling, prickling paresthesias—separate tetany from ordinary cramp and also from true physiologic contracture.

In practice, the term *contracture* is applied to all states of fixed muscle shortening. Several distinct types can be recognized. In *true contracture* a group of muscles, after a series of strong contractions, may remain shortened for many minutes because of failure of the metabolic mechanism necessary for relaxation; in this shortened state, the EMG remains relatively silent, in contrast to the high-voltage, rapid discharges observed with cramp, tetanus, and tetany. True contracture occurs in McArdle disease (phosphorylase deficiency), in which it is aggravated by arterial occlusion, but it has been seen in phosphofructokinase deficiency and possibly in another disease, as yet undefined, where the tourniquet has no effect and phosphorylase seems to be present. Yet another type of exercise-induced contracture, described originally by Brody, has been attributed by Karpati and coworkers to a deficiency of calcium adenosine triphosphatase in the sarcoplasmic reticulum. These various forms of contracture are described further in Chap. 55. True contracture is to be distinguished from paradoxical myotonia (see above) and from cramp, which in certain conditions (dehydration, tetany, pathologic cramp syndrome, amyotrophic lateral sclerosis) may be initiated by one or a series of strong voluntary muscle contractions.

It is appropriate here to comment on *pseudocontracture (myostatic or fibrous contracture)*. This is the common form of muscle and tendon shortening that follows prolonged fixation and complete inactivity of the normally innervated muscle (as in a broken limb immobilized by a cast or flaccid weakness of a limb that is allowed to remain immobile). Here the shortened state of the muscle, which may persist for days or weeks, has no clearly established anatomic, physiologic, or chemical basis. Far more frequent is a fibrosis of muscle, a state following chronic fiber loss and immobility of muscle. Depending on the predominant position, certain muscles are both weakened and shortened. Flexor fibrous contracture of the arms is a prominent feature of the Emery-Dreifuss form of muscular dystrophy. It also accounts for the rigidity and kyphoscoliosis of the spine which are so frequently a part of myopathic diseases. The latter state is distinguished from *ankylosis* by the springy nature of the resistance, coincident with increased tautness of muscle and tendon during passive motion, and from *Volkmann contracture*, in which there is evident fibrosis of muscle and surrounding tissues due to ischemic injury, usually after a fracture of the elbow.

Arthrogryposis multiplex congenita, described on page 1530, is another form of fibrous contracture, involving multiple muscle groups. This syndrome appears in the newborn, in association with several different types of neuromuscular disease that have two features in common—onset during intrauterine life and a primary alteration of one of the components of the "final common motor pathway." Most often the cause is a loss or failure of development of anterior horn cells, as in Werdnig-Hoffman disease, but occasionally the abnormality is in the nerve roots, peripheral nerves, motor end plates, or muscle. Contractures and fixity of the limbs result from immobility of the developing joints, consequent upon muscle weakness during fetal development. The *rigid spine syndrome* is yet another form of fibrous contracture, due presumably to an unusual axial muscular dystrophy. Rigidity of the spine is a predominant and early feature.

Topography or Patterns of Myopathic Weakness

In almost all the diseases under consideration, some muscles are affected and others spared, each disease displaying its own pattern. Moreover, the topography or distribution of involvement tends to follow the same pattern in all patients with the same disease. Thus, topography or pattern of involvement becomes a central diagnostic attribute of muscular disease.

The following patterns of muscle involvement constitute a core of essential clinical knowledge in this field:

1. *Ocular palsies presenting more or less exclusively as ptosis, diplopia, and strabismus*, sometimes in association with exophthalmos and pupillary change. As a rule, primary diseases of muscle do not involve the pupil, and in most instances their effects are bilateral. In lesions of the third, fourth, or sixth cranial nerves, the neural origin is disclosed by the pattern of ocular muscle palsies, abnormalities of the pupil, or both. When weakness of the orbicularis oculi (muscles of eye closure) is added to weakness of eye opening (ptosis), it nearly always signifies a primary disease of muscle or of neuromuscular transmission.

In the more *subacute and chronic* development of relatively pure affection of eye muscles, myasthenia gravis, progressive external ophthalmoplegia (ocular myopathy), oculopharyngeal muscular dystrophy, and exophthalmic (hyperthyroid) ophthalmopathy are the most frequent causes. In the disorder known as progressive external ophthalmoplegia, only eye muscles may be affected. All the extraocular muscles, including the levators of the eyelids, become paretic over a period of years, but there is usually no diplopia, since the weakness evolves slowly and in a balanced pattern. Only many years later may other muscles be involved. This disorder has been shown in most cases to be a form of mitochondrial myopathy, but there appear to be other types as well. Oculopharyngeal dystrophy involves primarily the levators of the eyelids and, to a somewhat lesser extent, other eye muscles and pharyngeal-upper esophageal striated muscles. It begins in middle or late adult life and later, and—like progressive external ophthalmoplegia—tends later to involve girdle and proximal limb muscles.

There are several other less common chronic myopathies in which external ophthalmoplegia is associated with involvement of other muscles or organs, namely, the congenital ophthalmoplegia of the Goldenhar-Gorlin syndrome (Aleksic et al); the Kearns-Sayre syndrome (retinitis pigmentosa, heart block, short stature, generalized weakness, and ovarian hypoplasia); other congenital myotubular and mitochondrial myopathies; nuclear ophthalmoplegia with bifacial weakness (Möbius syndrome); and the myotonic dystrophy of Steinert. Rarely, eye muscle weakness may occur at a late stage in other dystrophies, such as the facioscapulohumeral type. Trichinosis is an occasional cause.

Acute bilateral ophthalmoplegia raises an entirely different set of diagnostic considerations. It may be an expression of the Fisher syndrome of ophthalmoplegia, areflexia, and ataxia (page 1381) and of other variants of the Guillain-Barré syndrome or of botulism, diphtheria, rarely tick paralysis, and occlusion of the basilar artery or its branches. Trichinosis is a very rare cause.

2. *Bifacial palsy presenting as an inability to smile, expose the teeth, and close the eyes.* Varying degrees of bifacial weakness are observed in myasthenia gravis, usually conjoined with ptosis and ocular palsies. However, weakness of facial muscles may be combined with myasthenic weakness of the masseters and other bulbar muscles without involvement of ocular muscles. The same is true of myotonic dystrophy. More severe or complete facial palsy occurs in facioscapulohumeral dystrophy, sometimes presenting several years before weakness of the shoulder girdle muscles. Bifacial weakness is also a feature of congenital myopathies

(centronuclear, nemaline, carnitine deficiency) and the Möbius syndrome (in combination with abducens palsies).

More *acute and subacute bifacial palsies* are usually attributable to the Guillain-Barré syndrome (always with other signs of neuropathy), sarcoid, Lyme disease, tick paralysis, the Melkersson-Rosenthal syndrome (page 1454), AIDS, or polymyositis (rare), or are part of a cranial polyneuritis of unknown cause (page 1461), all discussed in the preceding chapter. Rarely, Bell's palsy is simultaneously bilateral (it is more often sequential), and these same considerations apply. Advanced scleroderma, Parkinson disease, or a pseudobulbar state can immobilize the face to the point of simulating myopathic or neuropathic paralysis, but always in a context that makes the cause obvious.

3. *Bulbar (oropharyngeal) palsy presenting as dysphonia, dysarthria, and dysphagia with or without weakness of jaw or facial muscles.* Myasthenia gravis is the most frequent cause of this syndrome and must also be considered whenever a patient presents with the solitary finding of a hanging jaw or fatigue of the jaw while eating or talking; usually, however, ptosis and ocular palsies are conjoined. Dysphagia may be an early and prominent sign of polymyositis as well as inclusion body myositis and may appear in patients with myotonic dystrophy, due to upper esophageal atonia.

Combinations of these palsies are also observed as an *acute syndrome* in botulism, in brainstem stroke, and at the outset of the Guillain-Barré syndrome. Diphtheria and bulbar poliomyelitis are now rare diseases that may present in this way. Progressive bulbar palsy (motor neuron disease) may also be the basis of this syndrome (page 1154); the diagnosis is most obvious when the tongue is withered and twitching. Syringobulbia, basilar invagination of the skull, and certain types of Chiari malformation may reproduce some of the findings of bulbar palsy by involving the lower cranial nerves. Rare cases of hereditary progressive aphonia include the X-linked Kennedy syndrome of bulbospinal atrophy (page 1161). Spastic bulbar paralysis, or pseudobulbar palsy, is readily distinguished by the presence of hyperactive facial and gag reflexes, lack of muscle atrophy, and the associated clinical findings (pages 517 and 547). One must also keep in mind restricted extrapyramidal diseases, such as Wilson disease and dystonia, that cause the mouth to be kept open and the face and bulbar musculature to appear immobile. The mechanism of swallowing and the ways in which it is disturbed are discussed on page 581.

4. *Cervical palsy presenting with inability to hold the head erect or to lift the head from the pillow.* The patient may be unable to hold up his head, owing to weakness of the posterior neck muscles, or to lift it from a pillow because of weakness of the sternocleidomastoids and other anterior neck muscles. In advanced forms of this syndrome, the head may hang with chin on chest unless it is held up by the patient's hands.

The "*hanging, or dropped, head syndrome*" with weakness of the posterior neck muscles occurs most often in idiopathic polymyositis and inclusion body myositis and is often combined with mild dysphagia, dysphonia, and weakness of girdle muscles. Myasthenic patients commonly complain of an inability to hold up their heads late in the day; both flexors and extensors of the neck are found to be weak. The same symptom may be a feature of motor neuron disease, but it is rarely the presenting problem. Occasionally this pattern is observed in patients with nemaline rod myopathy or with a poorly defined local myopathic process that has no distinguishing histopathologic or histochemical features. The latter condition is observed not infrequently in elderly persons. There is severe but relatively nonprogressive weakness of the neck extensors and only mild weakness of shoulder girdle and proximal arm muscles. Katz and colleagues suggest the designation "isolated neck extensor myopathy" in preference to "dropped head syndrome."

The major types of progressive muscular dystrophy, when advanced, usually affect the anterior neck muscles disproportionately. Rarely, syringomyelia, spinal accessory neuropathy, some form of meningoradiculitis, and loss of anterior horn cells in conjunction with systemic lymphoma or carcinoma may differentially paralyze the various neck muscles.

5. *Weakness of respiratory and trunk muscles.* Usually the diaphragm and chest and trunk muscles are affected in association with shoulder and proximal limb muscles, but occasionally weakness of the respiratory muscles is the initial or the dominant manifestation of disease. Selective involvement of the intercostal muscles and diaphragm, giving rise to dyspnea and diminished vital capacity, may first bring the patient to the pulmonary clinic. We have observed this to happen in patients with motor system disease, glycogen storage disease (acid maltase deficiency), and polymyositis. Unilateral paralysis of the diaphragm may result from compression of the phrenic nerve in the thorax by tumor or aortic aneurysm; an idiopathic or postinfectious variety may be related to brachial plexitis. The paravertebral

muscles may be severely affected in some types of muscular dystrophy, but usually in association with pelvicrural and shoulder muscle weakness. Nocturnal dyspnea, sleep apnea, and respiratory arrest may occur, particularly in myasthenics and patients with glycogen storage myopathies. And, of course, respiratory failure may threaten life in severe myasthenia gravis and Guillain-Barré syndrome, as it can in poliomyelitis. As a general rule, in the acute neuromuscular paralyses, the cervical and shoulder muscles and the diaphragm, all of which share a common innervation, show a similar degree of weakness. Asking the patient to expand his chest and count aloud a consecutive series of numbers on one breath (less than 20 equates with a vital capacity of less than 1500 mL) can help to detect this pattern of muscle weakness. Paradoxical inward movement of the abdomen with inspiration is another sign of diaphragmatic weakness. Disorders of breathing and ventilation are also discussed on pages 576 to 581.

6. *Bibrachial palsy, sometimes presenting as a dangling-arm syndrome*. Weakness, atrophy, and fasciculations of the hands, arms, and shoulders characterize the common form of motor system disease, namely, amyotrophic lateral sclerosis. Primary diseases of muscle hardly ever weaken these parts disproportionately. Rarely, a diffuse weakness of both arms and the shoulder muscles may occur in the early stages of Guillain-Barré syndrome, paraneoplastic disease, and amyloid neuropathy, in special forms of IgM-related paraproteinemic or inflammatory neuropathy, and in porphyric polyneuropathy, but it soon becomes part of a more generalized paralysis.

7. *Bicrural palsy presenting as lower leg weakness with inability to walk on the heels and toes, or as paralysis of all leg and thigh muscles*. Symmetrical weakness of the lower legs is usually due to polyneuropathy, although peroneal, anterior tibial, and thigh muscles are often weakened in muscular dystrophy. Diabetic polyneuropathy or carcinomatous or lymphomatous radiculopathy may cause asymmetrical weakness of thigh and pelvic muscles, often with pain and little sensory change. Chronic inflammatory demyelinating polyneuropathy (CIDP) may do the same. In total leg and thigh weakness, one first thinks of a spinal cord disease, in which case there is usually impaired sphincteric function of the bladder and bowel as well as loss of sensory function below a certain level on the trunk. Motor system disease may begin in the legs, asymmetrically and distally as a rule, and affect them out of proportion to other parts. Thus the differential diagnosis of leg weakness involves more diseases than are involved in the restricted paralyses of other parts of the body.

8. *Limb-girdle palsies presenting as inability to raise the arms or to arise from a squatting, kneeling, or sitting position*. Polymyositis, inclusion body myositis, dermatomyositis, and the progressive muscular dystrophies most often manifest themselves in this fashion. The Duchenne, Becker, and limb-girdle types of dystrophy tend first to affect the muscles of the pelvic girdle, gluteal region, and thighs, resulting in a lumbar lordosis and protuberant abdomen, a waddling gait, and difficulty in arising from the floor and climbing stairs without the assistance of the arms. Facioscapulohumeral dystrophy affects the muscles of the face and shoulder girdles foremost and is manifest by incomplete eye closure, inability to whistle and to raise the arms above the head, winging of the scapulae, and thinness of the upper arms ("Popeye" effect). In the milder forms of polymyositis, weakness may be limited to the neck muscles or those of the shoulder or pelvic girdles. In a similar vein, early or mild forms of dystrophy may selectively involve only the peroneal and scapular muscles (scapuloperoneal dystrophy). A number of other diseases of muscle may express themselves by a disproportionate weakness of girdle and proximal limb musculature. A metabolic myopathy, such as the adult form of acid maltase deficiency and the familial (hypokalemic) type of periodic paralysis, may affect only the pelvic and thigh muscles. In a number of the congenital polymyopathies (central core, nemaline, myotubular, etc.), a relatively nonprogressive weakness affects girdle muscles more than distal ones. These are discussed in Chap. 52. Proximal muscles are occasionally implicated in progressive spinal muscular atrophy, as in the syndrome first described by Wohlfart and coworkers and by Kugelberg and Welander, which unfortunately adds to confusion in diagnosis.

Similarly, a *pure quadriceps femoris weakness* may be the expression of several diseases. If bilateral, it usually indicates a polymyositis, an early stage of inclusion body myositis (may be unilateral or asymmetrical), or a restricted dystrophy. In thyrotoxic and steroid myopathies, the major effects are on the quadriceps muscles. If unilateral or bilateral with loss of patellar reflex and sensation over the inner leg, this condition is due most often to a femoral neuropathy, as from diabetes, or to an upper lumbosacral plexus lesion. Injuries to the hip and knee cause rapid disuse atrophy of the quadriceps muscles.

9. *Distal bilateral limb palsies presenting usually as foot drop with steppage gait (with or without pes cavus),*

weakness of all lower leg muscles, and later wrist drop and weakness of hands. The principal cause of this neuromuscular syndrome is a familial polyneuropathy, such as the peroneal muscular atrophy of Charcot-Marie-Tooth or the hypertrophic polyneuropathy of Déjerine and Sottas (see Chap. 46). Chronic nonfamilial polyneuropathies, particularly paraproteinemic and inflammatory ones and exceptionally some forms of familial progressive muscular atrophy and distal types of progressive muscular dystrophy (Gowers, Milhorat, Welander, and Miyoshi types) may also present in this way. In myotonic dystrophy, there may be weakness of the leg muscles as well as the forearms, sternomastoids, face, and eyes. Despite these exceptions, the generalization that girdle weakness without sensory changes is indicative of myopathy and that distal weakness is indicative of neuropathy is clinically useful.

10. *Generalized or universal paralysis: limb (but usually not cranial) muscles, involved either in attacks or as part of a persistent, progressive deterioration.* When acute in onset and episodic, this syndrome is usually a manifestation of familial hypokalemic or hyperkalemic periodic paralysis. One variety of the hypokalemic type is associated with hyperthyroidism, another with hyperaldosteronism (Chap. 54). In a setting of a critical illness with multiple organ failure or sepsis, generalized weakness of variable degree may occur from either a neuropathy ("critical illness neuropathy") or a severe and widespread myopathy that is thought to be caused by the use of high doses of corticosteroids, perhaps exaggerated by the concomitant use of neuromuscular blocking agents. Generalized paresis (rather than paralysis) that has an acute onset and lasts many weeks is at times a feature of a severe form of idiopathic or parasitic (trichinosis) polymyositis and rarely of pharmaceutical agents, particularly those used to reduce hypercholesterolemia. Idiopathic polymyositis and rarely inclusion body myositis may involve all limb and trunk muscles but usually spare the facial and ocular muscles, whereas the weakness in trichinosis is mainly in the ocular and lingual muscles. In infants and young children, a chronic and persistent generalized weakness of all muscles except those of the eyes always raises the question of Werdnig-Hoffman spinal muscular atrophy or, if mild in degree and relatively nonprogressive, of congenital myopathy or polyneuropathy. In these diseases of infancy, paucity of movement, hypotonia, and retardation of motor development may be more obvious than weakness. As a rule, universal weakness of muscle does not occur in the muscular dystrophies.

Widespread ascending paralysis (progressing from the arms to the legs), developing over a few days, with involvement of cranial (including ocular) muscles, is usually due to an inflammatory demyelinating or axonal polyneuritis (Guillain-Barré syndrome) and occasionally to porphyric or diphtheric polyneuropathy, tick paralysis, or severe hypophosphatemia. Certain inflammatory neuropathies evolve subacutely, and this may also be true in patients undergoing peritoneal dialysis for end-stage renal failure or with toxic exposure to certain heavy metals. An even more insidious onset and slow (months to years) progression of paralysis, atrophy, and fasciculation of limb and trunk muscles without sensory loss characterize motor system disease. Here the eye muscles are always spared. Mild degrees of generalized weakness are features of nemaline and central core polymyopathy as well as a number of metabolic myopathies, such as thyrotoxic myopathy, glycogen storage diseases, and rickets.

11. *Paralysis of single muscles or a group of muscles.* This is usually neuropathic, less often spinal or myopathic. Muscle disease does not need to be considered except possibly in certain instances of pressure-ischemic necrosis of muscle, as in so-called monoplegic alcoholic myopathy or diabetic muscle infarction and focal inclusion body myositis, which has a predilection for certain sites, namely parts of the quadriceps and the forearm muscles, particularly the long finger flexors (flexor digitorum profundus).

From this exposition of the topographic aspects of weakness, one can appreciate that each neuromuscular disease exhibits a predilection for particular groups of muscles. As a corollary, a given pattern of weakness should always suggest certain possibilities of disease and exclude others.

Of course, just as in the neuropathies, diagnosis also depends on features of the paralysis other than its topography—the age of onset and tempo of progression, the coexistence of medical disorders, and certain laboratory findings (serum concentrations of muscle enzymes, EMG, and biopsy findings) and particularly its genetic determinants also figure prominently in the delineation of muscle diseases.

Muscle Fatigue, Lack of Endurance, and Exercise Intolerance

As stated in an earlier part of this chapter and in Chap. 24, fatigue is an abstruse symptom, always needing analysis and interpretation. When not attended by manifest reduction in muscle power, it is usually nonmuscular in origin. It may, on medical investigation, prove to be a manifestation of infection, metabolic or endocrine disorder, or neoplasia. More often, when expressed as a feeling of weariness and disinclination to undertake or sustain mental and physical activity, it is indicative of neurasthenia, a psychiatric manifestation common to states of chronic anxiety and depression or simply to boredom and lack of purpose. Recently, the elusive syndrome of lifelong exercise intolerance, often accompanied by muscle cramps during exercise, has been traced in a limited number of cases to mutations in the cytochrome b gene of the mitochondrial DNA (Andreu et al), and syndromes have been attributed to a deficiency of myoadenylate—but these are very rare. The subject of fatigue as a physiologic phenomenon and as a clinical feature of many psychiatric and medical diseases, including those that are predominantly myopathic, is considered fully in Chap. 24.

Muscle Tone

All normal muscles display a slight resistance to stretch when fully relaxed. When stretched to their limit and released, they recoil, mainly because of the elasticity of the fibers and their connective tissue sheaths. In addition, the trunk and proximal limb musculature is intermittently or constantly activated in the maintenance of attitudes and postures. To relax—i.e., to completely disengage a muscle from all its natural activities—requires practice and seems increasingly difficult in the elderly, in whom it merges with oppositional, or paratonic, rigidity ("gegenhalten," page 77). A reduced innervation of muscle, atrophy, or loss of contracting fibers are causes of "hypotonia." In infants this state has come to be accepted as a mark of neuromuscular disease; the infant is said to be "floppy."

The assessment of muscle tone is of special importance in infants (the "floppy baby"), mainly because of the difficulty in testing strength at this age. Tone can be assessed by lifting the infant in a prone position; if the child is hypotonic, the head and legs cannot be supported against gravity and therefore dangle. Or, when held under the arms, the hypotonic infant slips through the examiner's hands. André-Thomas introduced the term *passivité* to refer to the amplitude of the flapping movement of the hand or foot when the limb is shaken and *extensibilité* to denote the reduced resistance of a relaxed muscle to slow passive stretch. In our opinion these are but different ways of testing muscle tone. Diminution in tone is observed in infants suffering from Werdnig-Hoffman disease or the congenital myopathies as well as in those with a benign type of hypotonia; diminished tone may also be seen in sickly infants with a variety of systemic diseases. In adults, hypotonia is a feature of many of the myopathies and neuropathies, all of which reduce the number of contracting motor units.

The finding of generalized excessive tone, apart from that observed as a consequence of extrapyramidal rigidity, is rare in infants. A purely myopathic form of hypertonia is difficult to substantiate (the exceptions being tetanus and hypocalcemic tetany). Various types of disease may lead to fibrous contracture and arthrogryposis, as stated earlier. An axial myopathy is the basis of the "rigid spine syndrome." For the most part, the muscle stiffness syndromes are due to continuous overactivity of motor units, the extreme forms being the "stiff-man" and the Isaacs syndromes and several related conditions (Chap. 55).

Changes in Muscle Volume

Diminution or increase in muscle bulk stands as another feature of disease that can be observed in all except the most obese patients. There are, of course, innate differences in muscle development, a greater salience of muscle in the male than in the female, and differences due to use and disuse. In general, the relative size of muscles is a genetic trait; in some families, muscles, like the skeleton, are large and in others, small. Greatly increased size and strength of muscles (hypertrophia musculorum vera) is observed in cultists devoted to bodybuilding (although, as a rule, they are exercising muscles that are large from birth); in congenital myotonia (circus freaks with phenomenal muscular development often have this disease); in instances of a rare pathologic cramp syndrome; in the Bruck-DeLange syndrome of congenital hypertrophy of muscle, athetosis, and mental retardation; and in some patients destined to develop muscular dystrophy. In some of the latter patients, the muscle enlargement is in reality a pseudohypertrophy, in which the increase in size is accompanied by weakness. Here large and small fibers are mixed with fat cells, which have replaced many of the degenerated muscle fibers; other muscles in the same patient are atrophied. Other dystrophies (Becker, Emery-Dreifuss) may also cause pseudohypertrophy. Rarely, we have seen it in amyloidosis, sarcoidosis, eosinophilic myositis, and certain of the congenital myopathies. Hypothyroidism is often accompanied by an increase in volume of certain muscles, simulating hypertrophia musculorum vera and congenital myotonia. Enlargement of muscles in only one limb may be due to an arteriovenous malformation, neurofibroma, or the Klippel-Trénaunay-Weber syndrome. A single muscle, most often the gastrocnemius, may become hypertrophied after partial injury to its nerve root (see Mielke et al); this is seen most often in relation to disc compression or surgical injury of the S1 nerve root.

Denervation is invariably attended by atrophy. Lesions of the peripheral nerve or anterior horn cells, if complete, lead to a loss of bulk of up to 85 percent of the original volume within 3 to 4 months, although some shrinkage of muscle becomes evident before that time. The most severe degrees of atrophy are observed in the chronic polyneuropathies, motor system diseases, and muscular dystrophies. The distribution of the atrophy corresponds to the paresis. Cachexia, malnutrition, male hypogonadism, and lipodystrophy tend to reduce muscle bulk without a proportionate reduction in the power of contraction (*pseudoatrophy*). Of interest is the fact that a number of myopathic diseases result in severe weakness with little or no atrophy; these are polymyositis, myasthenia gravis, periodic paralyses, steroid myopathy, hypothyroidism, and Addison disease.

Twitches, Spasms, and Cramps

Fascicular twitches at rest (fasciculations), if pronounced and combined with muscular weakness and atrophy, usually signify motor neuron disease (amyotrophic lateral sclerosis, progressive muscular atrophy, or progressive bulbar palsy); but they may be seen in other diseases that involve the gray matter of the spinal cord (e.g., syringomyelia or tumor) as well as in lesions of the anterior roots (e.g., protruded intervertebral disc) and in certain peripheral neuropathies. Widespread fasciculations may occur with severe dehydration and electrolyte imbalance after an overdose of neostigmine or with organophosphate poisoning. Slow and persistent fasciculations, spreading in a wave-like pattern along the entire length of a muscle and associated with slight reduction in the speed of contraction and relaxation, are part of the syndrome of continuous muscular activity (page 1568).

Fasciculations that occur with muscular contraction, in contrast to those at rest, indicate a state of heightened irritability of muscle; this may occur for no discernible reason or as a sequela of denervation that leaves muscle with some paralyzed motor units, so that during contraction small and increasingly larger units are not enlisted smoothly. *Benign fasciculations*, a common finding in otherwise normal individuals, can be distinguished by the lack of muscular weakness and atrophy. The recurrent twitches of the eyelid or muscles of the thumb experienced by most normal persons are often referred to as "live flesh" or myokymia but are more closely related to benign fasciculations. *Myokymia* is a less common condition, alluded to earlier, in which repeated twitchings impart a rippling appearance to the muscle. Another form of rippling, as mentioned above, is familial and associated with an unspecified type of myopathy (Chap. 55).

Muscle cramps, despite their common occurrence, are a poorly understood phenomenon. They occur at rest or with movement (action cramps) and are frequently reported in motor system disease, tetany, dehydration after excessive sweating and salt loss, metabolic disorders (uremia and hemodialysis, hypocalcemia, hypothyroidism, and hypomagnesemia), and certain muscle diseases (e.g., rare cases of Becker muscular dystrophy and congenital myopathies). Gospe and colleagues have reported a familial (X-linked recessive) type of myalgia and cramps associated with a deletion of the first third of the dystrophin gene, the one lacking in Duchenne dystrophy; strangely, there was no weakness or evidence of dystrophy. Lifelong, severe cramping of undetermined type has also been seen in a few families. Far more frequent than all these types of cramping is the benign form (*idiopathic cramp syndrome*), in which no other neuromuscular disturbance can be found. Most often cramps in otherwise normal individuals occur at night and affect the muscles of the calf and foot, but they may occur at any time and may involve any muscle group. Some patients state that cramps are more frequent when the legs are cold and daytime activity has been excessive. Cramps of this type are extremely common; they are provoked by the abrupt stretching of muscles, are very painful, and tend to wax and wane before they disappear. The EMG counterpart is a high-frequency discharge. Although of no pathologic significance, the cramps in extreme cases are so persistent and so readily provoked by innocuous movements as to be disabling. Cramps of all types need to be distinguished from *sensations of cramp* without muscle spasm. The latter is a dysesthetic phenomenon.

In contrast to cramp is the physiologic contracture, observed in McArdle disease and carnitine palmitoyl transferase deficiency, in which increasing muscle shortening and pain gradually develop during muscular activity. Unlike cramping, it does not occur at rest, the pain is less intense, and the EMG of the contracted muscle is relatively silent.

Cramps are also to be distinguished from the malignant and progressive form of painful spasm known

alternative consideration. Muscle enzymes in the serum may be relatively normal. Electromyography and biopsy are helpful in diagnosis.

4. *The patient with diffuse myalgia and fatigability*. Features that exclude a polymyositis are (*a*) lack of reduced peak power of contraction and (*b*) normal EMG, serum enzymes, and muscle biopsy. Hypothyroidism, McArdle disease, hyperparathyroidism, steroid myopathy, adrenal insufficiency, hyperinsulinemia, and early rheumatoid arthritis must be ruled out by appropriate studies (see Chap. 51). Most of our patients with diffuse myalgia and fatigability have proved to be neurasthenic or depressed and rarely myopathic.

5. *The patient with a clinical picture of polymyositis* in whom the muscle biopsy discloses a noncaseating granulomatous reaction consistent with sarcoid (see further on, page 1490).

Treatment *Corticosteroids* are the first line of therapy for both PM and DM. Prednisone, 1 mg/kg, is given in three or four divided doses per day. The response to corticosteroids is monitored by careful testing of strength and measurement of CK. In patients who respond, the serum CK decreases before the weakness subsides; with relapse, the serum CK rises before weakness returns. Once recovery has begun and the dosage has been reduced to 20 mg daily, it is appropriate to try an alternate-day schedule with double this amount (i.e., 40 mg). This schedule reduces the side effects of corticosteroids. After cautious reduction of prednisone over a period of 6 months to a year or longer, the patient can usually be maintained on doses of 7.5 to 20 mg daily, with the aim of eventual discontinuation of the drug. Corticosteroids should not be discontinued prematurely, for the relapse that may follow is often more difficult to treat than the original symptoms. In acute and particularly severe cases, treatment may be facilitated by the use initially of high-dose pulse methylprednisolone (1 g infused over 2 h each day for 3 days). This form of treatment should be regarded as a temporary measure until oral prednisone becomes effective.

Some patients who cannot tolerate or are refractory to prednisone may respond favorably to oral *azathioprine* (150 to 300 mg/day), with care being taken to keep the white blood cell (WBC) level above 3000/mm^3, or to *methotrexate* (5 to 10 mg/week in three divided oral doses, increased by 2.5 mg per week, to a total dose of 20 mg weekly). Preferably the methotrexate or azathioprine should be given along with relatively small daily doses (15 to 25 mg) of prednisone. Some clinicians favor, from the beginning, a combination of prednisone in low dosage and one of the immunosuppressant drugs; this approach is generally necessary when systemic vasculitis or interstitial pneumonitis is coupled with DM. The steroid-sparing effects of azathioprine may also be useful in patients requiring long-term immunosuppressant therapy. *Cyclophosphamide*, which is a useful drug in the treatment of Wegener granulomatosis, polyarteritis, and perhaps other vasculitides, is said to be of lesser value in PM, but several of our rheumatologist colleagues recommend it and we have seen good responses in adults. *Cyclosporine* has also been used in recalcitrant cases; it has no advantages over other immunosuppressant drugs but has a number of potentially serious side effects, including nephrotoxicity.

In *patients with DM* who respond poorly to corticosteroids and other immunosuppressants or are severely affected early on, the addition of intravenous immunoglobulin infusions (IVIG) often proves to be effective—although several courses of treatment at monthly intervals may be required to achieve sustained improvement. In several controlled studies of small numbers of DM patients (Dalakas; Mastaglia et al), practically all showed improvement in muscle strength and skin changes and a reduction in CK concentration. PM has also been reported to respond favorably to treatment with IVIG, but further controlled studies are required to corroborate these reports and to establish, in both PM and DM, optimal doses and modes of administration. It is noteworthy that IVIG has rarely been effective in PM or DM when used alone or as initial therapy. Whole-body radiation is said to be helpful in a few drug-resistant cases, but the side effects of this treatment are forbidding.

Prognosis Except for patients with malignancy, the prognosis in adult PM and DM is favorable. Only a small proportion of patients with PM succumb to the disease, and then usually from a pulmonary or cardiac complication. The period of activity of disease varies considerably but is usually around 2 years in both the child and adult groups. As indicated above, the majority improve with corticosteroid therapy, but many are left with varying degrees of weakness of the shoulders and hips. Approximately 20 percent of our patients have recovered completely, and long-term remissions have been achieved in about an equal number. The extent of recovery is roughly proportional to the acuteness and severity of the disease and the duration of symptoms prior to institution of therapy. Patients with acute or subacute PM in whom treatment is begun soon after the onset of symptoms have the best prognosis. In the series of DeVere and Bradley, in which patients were treated early, there was remission in over 50 percent of cases, whereas in the series of Riddoch and Morgan-Hughes, who were treated more than 2 years after onset of the disease, the remission rate was considerably lower.

Even in patients with a coexistent malignancy, muscle weakness may lessen and serum enzyme levels decline in response to corticosteroid therapy, but weakness returns after a few months and may then be resistant to further treatment. As already stated, if the tumor is successfully removed, the muscle symptoms may remit. The mortality after several years ranges around 15 percent, being higher in childhood DM, in PM with connective tissue diseases, and, of course, with malignancy.

INCLUSION BODY MYOSITIS

Inclusion body myositis (IBM) is the third major form of idiopathic inflammatory myopathy (after PM and DM). Its defining features, the intracytoplasmic and intranuclear inclusions, were first described in 1965 by Adams and colleagues, who also drew attention to a number of clinical features now considered characteristic of this myopathy. Since then many cases have been reported, and we are seeing more instances of this disease than of PM and DM combined. Garlepp and Mastaglia concluded that approximately one-third of the cases of inflammatory myopathy, especially in men, are of this type. By 1994, more than 240 sporadic cases and 59 familial ones had been recorded in the medical literature (Mikol and Engel). A set of clinical and pathologic diagnostic criteria for the disease has recently been proposed by Griggs et al.

The disease predominates in males (in a ratio of 3:1) and has its onset in middle or late adult life. Practically all instances occur sporadically, but inherited forms, both autosomal recessive and dominant, have been reported (Cole et al, Neville et al). The muscle weakness in familial IBM begins in early childhood and usually spares the quadriceps. Also, muscles in the familial form, unlike in the sporadic cases, lack inflammatory changes—for which reason the designation *familial inclusion body myopathy* would be more appropriate. Many but not all forms of autosomal recessive inclusion body myopathy are caused by a gene defect at chromosome 9p1-q1 (Argov et al). One must express some skepticism about the validity of linking sporadic and familial cases on the basis of the histopathologic findings. Diabetes, a variety of autoimmune diseases, and a relatively mild polyneuropathy are associated in about 20 percent of the sporadic cases, but an association with malignancy or connective tissue disease has not been established.

Clinical Manifestations The illness is characterized by a steadily progressive, painless muscular weakness and atrophy which may be generalized or affect the limbs selectively and often asymmetrically. Either the proximal or distal muscles may be mainly affected, or the limbs may be involved more or less evenly. In about 20 percent of cases, the disease begins with focal weakness of the quadriceps, finger or wrist flexors, or lower leg muscles on one or both sides and spreads to other muscle groups only after many months or years. Selective weakness of the flexor pollicis longus is particularly characteristic. The tendon reflexes are normal initially but diminish in about half the patients with progression of the disease. Interestingly, the knee jerks may be depressed or lost even without severe quadriceps weakness. Dysphagia is common (Wintzen et al), and some type of cardiovascular abnormality is seen in a few cases.

Laboratory and Muscle Biopsy Features The CK is normal or slightly elevated. The EMG abnormalities are much like those found in PM (see above). In addition, a small proportion of IBM patients display a neuropathic EMG pattern, mainly with fibrillation potentials, particularly in the distal limb muscles.

Diagnosis ultimately depends on the muscle biopsy, which discloses structural abnormalities of muscle fibers and inflammatory changes, identical to but usually of lesser severity than those observed in idiopathic PM. The infiltrating cells are particularly T cells of the CD8 type. However, definitive diagnosis depends upon the finding, by histochemical techniques, of intracytoplasmic vacuoles and eosinophilic inclusions in both the cytoplasm and nuclei of degenerating muscle fibers. The vacuoles contain and are rimmed by basophilic granular material, a point of difference from the vacuoles seen in some cases of PM. The inclusions are congophilic, i.e., they stain positively for β-amyloid protein, the detection of which is enhanced by the use of fluorescence illumination (Askanas et al). Ultrastructural studies show that this protein accumulates at or near foci of abnormal tubulofilamentous structures in both the nuclei and cytoplasm. The nature of these diverse myopathic changes is obscure. The tubulofilamentous inclusions have suggested a viral origin, but a virus has never been isolated and serologic studies have failed to substantiate a viral causation except for one patient in whom adenovirus type 2 was isolated from a biopsy specimen (Mikol and Engel).

Treatment Inclusion body myositis has not responded in any consistent fashion to treatment with corticosteroids or other immunosuppressive drugs or to IVIG. Indeed, the disease should be suspected in recalcitrant cases of apparent polymyositis. Because a few patients improve slightly or cease worsening with steroids, a several-month trial is often recommended (Lotz et al). The level of CK and the degree of leukocyte infiltration of muscle diminish with corticosteroid treatment despite a lack of clinical improvement. On this basis, Barohn and coworkers suggest that the inflammatory response is not a primary cause of muscle destruction. Sayres and colleagues concluded in a review of 32 patients that low-dose methotrexate and corticosteroids may slow the progression of disease, but this regimen has not been widely adopted. In a few cases there has been improvement in response to IVIG, especially in the weakened muscles involved in swallowing. The disease in most patients is relentlessly progressive, however, and no method of treatment has altered the long-term prognosis. Plasma exchange and leukocytopheresis have been tried, with generally discouraging results.

Other Inflammatory Myopathies

Included under this heading are a large number of unrelated myositides—certain rare forms of focal myositis and relatively minor changes in muscle that occur in the course of inflammatory diseases of blood vessels or disseminated or systemic infections or thymoma. Most of them do not warrant consideration in a textbook of neurology but are described in detail in monographs devoted to muscle disease (see Banker).

We have made exceptions of three diseases, eosinophilic myositis and fasciitis, orbital myositis, and sarcoid, which are described below.

Eosinophilic Myositis and Fasciitis This term has been applied to four separable but possibly overlapping clinical entities: (1) eosinophilic fasciitis, (2) eosinophilic monomyositis (sometimes multiplex), (3) eosinophilic polymyositis, and (4) the eosinophilia-myalgia syndrome.

Eosinophilic Fasciitis This condition was originally reported by Shulman in 1974. He described two men with a scleroderma-like appearance of the skin and flexion contractures at the knees and elbows associated with hyperglobulinemia, elevated sedimentation rate, and eosinophilia. Biopsy revealed greatly thickened fascia, extending from the subcutaneous tissue to the muscle and infiltrated with plasma cells, lymphocytes, and eosinophils; the muscle itself appeared normal and the skin lacked the characteristic histologic changes of scleroderma. One of Shulman's patients recovered in response to prednisone.

The many reports that followed have fully substantiated and amplified Shulman's original description. The disease predominates in men, in a ratio of 2:1. Symptoms appear between the ages of 30 and 60 years in most cases and are often precipitated by heavy exercise (Michet et al). Initially there may be low-grade fever and myalgia, followed by the subacute development of diffuse cutaneous thickening and limitation of movement of small and large joints. In some patients, proximal muscle weakness and eosinophilic infiltration of muscle can be demonstrated (Michet et al). Repeated examinations of the blood disclose an eosinophilia in most but not all patients.

In many patients the disease remits spontaneously or responds well to corticosteroids. A small number relapse and do not respond to treatment, and some have developed aplastic anemia and a form of lympho- or myeloproliferative disease.

Eosinophilic Monomyositis Painful swelling of a calf muscle or, less frequently, some other muscle has been the chief characteristic of this disorder. A painful mass forms within the muscle. Biopsy discloses inflammatory necrosis and edema of the interstitial tissues; the infiltrates contain variable numbers of eosinophils. This disorder is typified by one of our cases—a young woman who developed such an inflammatory mass first in one calf and then, 3 months later, in the other. The response to prednisone in this patient was dramatic; the swelling and pain subsided in 2 to 3 weeks, and power of contraction was then found to be normal. When the connective tissue and muscle are both damaged, a chaotic regeneration of fibroblasts and myoblasts may occur, forming a pseudotumor mass that may persist indefinitely.

Eosinophilic Polymyositis Layzer and associates have described a third form of this disorder, which they classified as a true subacute polymyositis. Their patients were adults in whom a predominantly proximal weakness of muscles had evolved over a period of several weeks. The other features of the muscle disorder were also typical of polymyositis except that the inflammatory infiltration was predominantly eosinophilic. Moreover, in each case the muscle disorder was part of a severe and widespread systemic illness typical of the *hypereosinophilic syndrome*. The systemic manifestations included a striking eosinophilia of the blood (20 to 55 percent of the WBCs), cardiac involvement (conduction disturbances and congestive failure), vascular disorder (Raynaud phenomenon, subungual hemorrhages), pulmonary infiltrates, strokes, anemia, neuropathy, and hypergammaglobulinemia. The muscles were swollen and painful. There was a favorable response to corticosteroids in two patients, but in a third the outcome was fatal within 9 months. Layzer and associates related the syndrome to eosinophilic pulmonary disease. They felt that a lack of necrotizing arteritis distinguished it from polyarteritis nodosa and Churg-Strauss disease. No infective agent could be isolated. An allergic mechanism seems a likely cause of the lesions, and in the present authors' view one cannot exclude an angiitis as a cause of all of the lesions.

The last two of these syndromes (mono- and polymyositis) have overlapping features, as shown by Stark's cases, in which a monomyositis was accompanied by several of the systemic features described by Layzer et al.

The Eosinophilia-Myalgia Syndrome Beginning in 1980, a number of sporadic reports documented a lingering systemic illness characterized by severe generalized myalgia and eosinophilia of the peripheral blood following the ingestion of L-tryptophan. In late 1989 and early 1990, there occurred a massive outbreak of eosinophilia-myalgia, as this syndrome came to be called, 1269 cases being reported to the Centers for Disease Control (Medsger). The outbreak was traced to the use of nonprescription L-tryptophan tablets supplied by a single manufacturer and contaminated by a ditryptophan aminal of acetaldehyde (Mayeno et al).

The syndrome was more frequent in women. The onset was relatively acute, with fatigue, low-grade fever, and eosinophilia ($>1000/mm^3$). Muscle pain and tenderness, cramps, weakness, paresthesias of the extremities, and induration of the skin were the main clinical features. A severe axonal neuropathy with slow and incomplete recovery was associated in some cases. Biopsies of the skin fascia, muscle, and peripheral nerve disclosed a microangiopathy and an inflammatory reaction in connective tissue structures—changes like those observed in scleroderma, eosinophilic fasciitis, and the *toxic oil syndrome*. The latter syndrome, caused by the ingestion of contaminated rapeseed oil (in Spain, 1981), gave rise to a constellation of clinical and pathologic changes that were similar if not identical to those caused by L-tryptophan (Ricoy et al; page 1281). The two syndromes are also closely linked chemically. Mayeno and colleagues have identified two trace contaminants in the L-tryptophan consumed by patients with the eosinophilia-myalgia syndrome.

The cutaneous symptoms and eosinophilia of this syndrome responded to treatment with prednisone and other immunosuppressive drugs, but other symptoms did not. The severe axonal neuropathy in our patients improved over several years, but incompletely and leaving patients chairbound.

Acute Orbital Myositis Among the many cases of idiopathic orbital inflammatory disease (pseudotumor of the orbit, page 287), there is a small group in whom the inflammatory process appears to be localized to the extraocular muscles. To this latter group the term *acute orbital myositis* has been applied. The abrupt onset of orbital pain that is made worse by eye motion, redness of the conjunctiva adjacent to the muscle insertions, diplopia caused by restrictions of ocular movements, lid edema, and mild proptosis are the main clinical features. It may spread from one orbit to the other. The erythrocyte sedimentation rate is usually elevated and the patient may feel generally unwell, but only rarely can the ocular disorder be related to a connective tissue disease or any other specific systemic disease. Computed tomography and magnetic resonance imaging have proved to be particularly useful in demonstrating the swollen ocular muscles or muscle and separating orbital myositis from the many other remitting inflammatory orbital and retro-orbital conditions (Dua et al). As a rule, acute orbital myositis resolves spontaneously in a matter of a few weeks or a month or two, although it may recur in the same or the opposite eye. Administration of steroids appears to hasten recovery.

Sarcoid Myopathy, Granulomatous Myositis, and Localized Nodular Myositis Although there are undoubted examples of muscle involvement in patients with sarcoidosis, they seem to us to be less frequent and less certain than would appear from the medical literature. In some cases, sarcoid myopathy becomes evident as a slowly progressive, occasionally fulminant, painless proximal weakness. The CK and angiotensin-converting enzyme levels are elevated. Muscle biopsy discloses the presence of numerous noncaseating granulomas. It is important to note that such lesions may also be found in patients with sarcoidosis who have no weakness. Treatment with moderate doses of corticosteroids (prednisone,

25 to 50 mg daily) is usually effective, but in patients who do not respond, an immunosuppressive agent such as cyclosporine may have to be given in addition.

Much more puzzling to the authors have been cases of myopathy with the clinical features of idiopathic polymyositis and the presence of noncaseating granulomas in the muscle biopsy but with no evidence of sarcoidosis of the nervous system, lungs, bone, skin, or lymph nodes. Such cases call into question the validity of a muscle granuloma as a criterion of sarcoidosis, but the matter cannot be settled until we have better laboratory tests than are now available. These cases are presently being classified as *granulomatous myositis* and, if limited to one or a small group of muscles, *localized nodular myositis* (Cumming et al). We suspect that such lesions have several clinical associations. In one syndrome, described by Namba and colleagues, this type of myositis was combined with myasthenia gravis, myocarditis, and thyroiditis. It has, on a few occasions, been associated with Crohn disease. Electron microscopy in some instances has disclosed muscle fiber invasion by lymphocytes, suggesting a cell-mediated immune reaction. Very rarely, a granulomatous myositis may complicate tuberculosis or syphilis.

REFERENCES

ADAMS RD, KAKULAS BA, SAMAHA FA: A myopathy with cellular inclusions. *Trans Am Neurol Assoc* 90:213, 1965.

ANTONY JH, PROCOPIS PG, OUVRIER RA: Benign acute childhood myositis. *Neurology* 29:1068, 1979.

ARGOV Z, TIRAM E, EISENBERG GI, et al: Various types of hereditary inclusion body myopathies map to chromosome 9p1-q1. *Ann Neurol* 41:548, 1997.

ASKANAS V, ENGEL WK, ALVAREZ RB: Enhanced detection of Congo-red-positive amyloid deposits in muscle fibers of inclusion body myositis and brain of Alzheimer's disease using fluorescence technique. *Neurology* 43:1265, 1993.

BANKER BQ: Dermatomyositis of childhood: Ultrastructural alterations of muscle and intramuscular blood vessels. *J Neuropathol Exp Neurol* 34:46, 1975.

BANKER BQ: Other inflammatory myopathies, in Engel AG, Franzini-Armstrong C (eds): *Myology*, 2nd ed. New York, McGraw-Hill, 1994, pp 1461–1486.

BANKER BQ: Parasitic myositis, in Engel AG, Franzini-Armstrong C (eds): *Myology*, 2nd ed. New York, McGraw-Hill, 1994, pp 1438–1460.

BANKER BQ, VICTOR M: Dermatomyositis (systemic angiopathy) of childhood. *Medicine* 45:261, 1966.

BAROHN RJ, AMATO AA, SAHENK Z, et al: Inclusion body myositis: Explanation for poor response to immunosuppressive therapy. *Neurology* 45:1302, 1995.

COLE AJ, KUZNIESKY R, KARPATI G, et al: Familial myopathy with changes resembling inclusion body myositis and periventricular leukoencephalopathy. *Brain* 111:1025, 1988.

CUMMING WJK, WEISER R, TEOH R, et al: Localized nodular myositis: A clinical and pathological variant of polymyositis. *Q J Med* 46:531, 1977.

DALAKAS MC: Intravenous immune globulin therapy for neurological diseases. *Ann Neurol* 126:721,1997.

DALAKAS MC, ILLA I, PEZESHKPOUR GH, et al: Mitochondrial myopathy caused by long-term zidovudine therapy. *N Engl J Med* 322:1098, 1990.

DEVERE R, BRADLEY WG: Polymyositis, its presentation, morbidity and mortality. *Brain* 98:637, 1975.

DUA HS, SMITH FW, SINGH AK, FORRESTER JV: Diagnosis of orbital myositis by nuclear magnetic resonance imaging. *Br J Ophthalmol* 71:54, 1987.

EMSLIE-SMITH AM, MAYENO AN, NAKANO S, et al: 1,1-Ethylidenebis[tryptophan] induces pathologic alterations in muscle similar to those observed in the eosinophilia-myalgia syndrome. *Neurology* 44:2390, 1994.

ENGEL AG, ARAHATA K: Mononuclear cells in myopathies: Quantitation of functionally distinct subsets, recognition of antigen-specific cell-mediated cytotoxicity in some diseases and implications for the pathogenesis of the different inflammatory myopathies. *Hum Pathol* 17:704, 1986.

ENGEL AG, EMSLIE-SMITH AM: Inflammatory myopathies. *Curr Opin Neurol Neurosurg* 2:695, 1989.

ENGEL AG, HOHLFELD R, BANKER BQ: The polymyositis and dermatomyositis syndromes, in Engel AG, Franzini-Armstrong C (eds): *Myology*, 2nd ed. New York, McGraw-Hill, 1994, pp 1335–1383.

GAMBOA ET, EASTWOOD AB, HAYS AP, et al: Isolation of influenza virus from muscle in myoglobinuric polymyositis. *Neurology* 29:556, 1979.

GARLEPP MJ, MASTAGLIA FL: Inclusion body myositis. *J Neurol Neurosurg Psychiatry* 60:251, 1996.

GHERARDI R, BAUDRIMONT M, LIONNET F, et al: Skeletal muscle toxoplasmosis in patients with acquired immunodeficiency syndrome: A clinical and pathological study. *Ann Neurol* 32:535, 1992.

GRIGGS RC, ASKANAS V, DIMAURO S, et al: Inclusion body myositis and myopathies. *Ann Neurol* 38:705, 1995.

GROSS B, OCHOA J: Trichinosis: A clinical report and histochemistry of muscle. *Muscle Nerve* 2:394, 1979.

HART MN, LINTHICUM DS, WALDSCHMIDT MM, et al: Experimental autoimmune inflammatory myopathy. *J Neuropathol Exp Neurol* 46:511, 1987.

KAKULAS BA, ADAMS RD: *Diseases of Muscle: Pathological Foundations of Clinical Myology*, 4th ed. Philadelphia, Harper & Row, 1985.

KASS EH, ANDRUS SB, ADAMS RD, et al: Toxoplasmosis in the human adult. *Arch Intern Med* 89:759, 1952.

KISSEL JT, MENDELL JR, RAMMOHEN KW: Microvascular deposition of complement membrane attack complex in dermatomyositis. *N Engl J Med* 314:329, 1986.

LAYZER RB, SHEARN MA, SATYA-MURTI S: Eosinophilic polymyositis. *Ann Neurol* 1:65, 1977.

LOTZ BP, ENGEL AG, NISHINO H, et al: Inclusion body myositis: Observations in 40 patients. *Brain* 112:727, 1989.

LUNDBERG A: Myalgia cruris epidemica. *Acta Paediatr Scand* 46:18, 1957.

MASTAGLIA FL, OJEDA VJ: Inflammatory myopathies. *Ann Neurol* 17:278, 317, 1985.

MASTAGLIA FL, PHILLIPS BA, ZILKO PJ: Immunoglobulin therapy in inflammatory myopathies. *J Neurol Neurosurg Psychiatry* 65:107, 1998.

MAYENO AN, BELONGIA EA, LIN F, et al: 3-(phenylamino)alanine, a novel aniline derived amino acid associated with the eosinophilia-myalgia syndrome: A link to the toxic oil syndrome? *Mayo Clin Proc* 67:1134, 1992.

MAYENO AN, LIN F, FOOTE CS, et al: Characterization of "peak E," a novel amino acid associated with eosinophilia-myalgia syndrome. *Science* 250:1707, 1990.

MEDSGER TA JR: Tryptophan-induced eosinophilia-myalgia syndrome. *N Engl J Med* 322:926, 1990.

MICHET CJ JR, DOYLE JA, GINSBURG WW: Eosinophilic fasciitis: Report of 15 cases. *Mayo Clin Proc* 56:27, 1981.

MIKOL J, ENGEL AG: Inclusion body myositis, in Engel AG, Franzini-Armstrong C (eds): *Myology*, 2nd ed. New York, McGraw-Hill, 1994, pp 1384–1398.

NAMBA T, BRUNNER MG, GROG N: Idiopathic giant cell polymyositis: Report of a case and review of the syndrome. *Arch Neurol* 31:27, 1974.

NEVILLE HE, BAUMBACH LL, RINGEL SP, et al: Familial inclusion body myositis: Evidence for autosomal dominant inheritance. *Neurology* 42:897, 1992.

PACHMAN LM: An update on juvenile dermatamyositis. *Curr Opin Rheumatol* 7:437, 1995.

RICOY JR, CABELLO A, RODRIGUEZ J, TELLEZ I: Neuropathological studies on the toxic syndrome related to adulterated rapeseed oil in Spain. *Brain* 106:817, 1983.

RIDDOCH D, MORGAN-HUGHES JA: Prognosis in adult polymyositis. *J Neurol Sci* 26:71, 1973.

SAYRES ME, CHOU SM, CALABRESE LH: Inclusion body myositis: Analysis of 32 cases. *J Rheumatol* 19:1385, 1992.

SHULMAN LE: Diffuse fasciitis with hyperglobulinemia and eosinophilia: A new syndrome? *J Rheumatol* 1(suppl):46, 1974.

SIGURGEIRSSON B, LINDELOF B, EDHAG O, ALLANDER E: Risk of cancer in patients with dermatomyositis or polymyositis. *N Engl J Med* 326:363, 1992.

SIMPSON DM, KATZENSTEIN DA, HUGHES MD, et al: Neuromuscular function in HIV infection: Analysis of a placebo-controlled combination antiretroviral trial. *AIDS* 12:2425, 1998.

STARK RJ: Eosinophilic polymyositis. *Arch Neurol* 36:721, 1979.

THOMAS MR, LANCASTER R: Polymyositis presenting with dyspnea, greatly elevated muscle enzymes but no apparent muscular weakness. *Br J Clin Pract* 44:378, 1990.

TONIN P, LEWIS P, SERVIDEI S, DIMAURO S: Metabolic causes of myoglobinuria. *Ann Neurol* 27:181, 1990.

WALTON JN: The idiopathic inflammatory myopathies and their treatment. *J Neurol Neurosurg Psychiatry* 54:285, 1991.

WALTON JN, ADAMS RD: *Polymyositis*. London, Livingstone, 1958.

WHITAKER JN, ENGEL WK: Vascular deposits of immunoglobulin and complement in idiopathic inflammatory myopathy. *N Engl J Med* 286:333, 1972.

WINTZEN AR, BOTS GTH, DEBAKKER HM, et al: Dysphagia in inclusion body myositis. *J Neurol Neurosurg Psychiatry* 51: 1542, 1988.

Chapter 50

THE MUSCULAR DYSTROPHIES

The muscular dystrophies are progressive hereditary degenerative diseases of skeletal muscles. The innervation of the affected muscles, in contrast to that of the neuropathic and spinal atrophies, is sound. Indeed, final proof that these disorders originate in muscle itself comes from the demonstration of intact spinal motor neurons, muscular nerves, and nerve endings in the presence of severe degenerative changes in the muscle fibers. The symmetrical distribution of muscular weakness and atrophy, intact sensibility, preservation of cutaneous reflexes, and heredofamilial incidence are the characteristic features of this group of diseases and serve to set them apart on clinical grounds alone.

Some clinicians and researchers have applied the term *muscular dystrophy* to other degenerative diseases of muscle, such as those in animals due to vitamin E deficiency and the coxsackieviruses and certain inherited metabolic diseases in humans; we would discourage this practice as one leading to terminologic confusion. The intensity of the degenerative changes and cellular response and the vigor of the regenerative changes distinguish the latter diseases histologically and also imply a fundamental difference in pathogenesis. We therefore reserve the term *dystrophy* for the purely degenerative muscular disease of hereditary type and refer to the others as myopathies or polymyopathies. The more benign and relatively nonprogressive myopathies—such as central core, nemaline, mitochondrial, and centronuclear diseases— present a greater difficulty in classification. Like the dystrophies, they are primarily diseases of muscle and are heredofamilial in nature; but again we prefer to place them in a separate category because of their nonprogressive or slowly progressive course and the distinctive histochemistry and ultrastructure (Chap. 52).

Historical Background The differentiation of dystrophic diseases of muscle from those secondary to neuronal degeneration was an achievement of neurologists of the second half of the nineteenth century. Isolated cases of muscular dystrophy had been described earlier, but no distinction was made between neuropathic and myopathic disease. Thus, Little had described what appears to be Duchenne muscular dystrophy in lectures given at the Royal Orthopedic Hospital in 1843 and 1844. Meryon in 1852 gave the first clear description of progressive weakness and atrophy of muscle in young boys who, at autopsy, had an intact spinal cord and nerves—a fact that led him to postulate an "idiopathic disease of muscles, dependent perhaps on defective nutrition." In 1855, the French neurologist Duchenne described the progressive muscular atrophy of childhood that now bears his name. However, it was not until the second edition of his famous monograph in 1861 that the "hypertrophic paraplegia of infancy" was recognized as a distinct syndrome of unknown pathology, with speculation about the nature of hypertrophy of muscles. By 1868 he was able to write a comprehensive description of 13 cases and recognized that the disease was muscular in origin and restricted to males. Gowers in 1879 gave a masterful account of 21 personally observed cases and called attention to the characteristic way in which such patients arose from the floor (Gowers sign).

Leyden in 1876 and Möbius 1879 reported a nonhypertrophic form of disease that began in the pelvic girdle muscles and could affect both sexes. Erb, in 1891, crystallized the clinical and histologic concept of a group of diseases due to primary degeneration of muscle, which he called *muscular dystrophies*. The first descriptions of facioscapulohumeral dystrophy were published by Landouzy and Déjerine in 1894; of progressive ocular myopathy, by Fuchs in 1890; of myotonic dystrophy, by Steinert and by Batten and Gibb in 1909; of distal dystrophy, by Gowers in 1888, by Milhorat and Wolff in 1943, and by Welander in 1951; and of oculopharyngeal dystrophy, by Victor, Hayes, and Adams in 1962.

In addition to these classic forms of dystrophy, a number of variant syndromes have come to light. Bramwell in 1922 described hereditary quadriceps myopathy; Dreifuss in 1961 and Emery in 1966 placed on record a sex-linked humeroperoneal dystrophy; and Seitz in 1957 distinguished a form of scapuloperoneal dystrophy with cardiomyopathy from the larger group of scapuloperoneal syndromes. References to these and other writings of historical importance can be found in the works of Kakulas and Adams, of Walton et al., and of Engel and Franzini-Armstrong (see References).

In the more recent history of the dystrophies, the most notable event has been the discovery by Kunkel, in 1986, of the dystrophin gene and its protein product. Since then there has been an extraordinary accumulation of molecular-genetic, ultrastructural, and biochemical information about the muscular dystrophies which has greatly broadened our understanding of their mechanisms and causation. It has also clarified a number of uncertainties as to their clinical presentations and has necessitated a revision of traditional forms of classification. Newer classifications (Table 50-1) separate the muscular dystrophies according to the conventional clinical types and their patterns of mendelian inheritance as well as to the presence and locus of the abnormal gene and the defective gene product. Each type of dystrophy is described below, in accordance with this scheme.

Duchenne Muscular Dystrophy (Severe Generalized Muscular Dystrophy of Childhood)

This is the most frequent and best known of the childhood muscular dystrophies. It begins in early childhood and runs a relatively rapid, progressive course. The incidence rate is in the range of 13 to 33 per 100,000 yearly or about one in 3300 live male births in every part of the world. There is a strong familial liability; since the disease is transmitted as an X-linked recessive trait, it occurs predominantly in males. Approximately 30 percent of patients have a negative family history and are said to represent spontaneous mutations. However, careful examination of their mothers will show slight involvement in as many as half of the so-called mutant cases, as pointed out by Roses and coworkers.

Occasionally a severe proximal muscular dystrophy occurs in young girls. This may have several explanations: (1) If the female has only one X chromosome, as occurs in the Turner (XO) syndrome, and if that chromosome carries the defective gene, she would develop the same affection as the male. (2) This could also happen through operation of the so-called Lyon principle, i.e., inactivation of the normal paternal X chromosome in a large proportion of embryonic cells. However, most cases of female childhood dystrophy prove to be of autosomal recessive limb-girdle type.

Clinical Features Duchenne muscular dystrophy is usually recognized in the third year of life and almost always before the sixth year, but nearly half of the patients show evidence of disease before beginning to walk. Many of them are backward in other ways (psychomotor retardation), and the muscle weakness may at first be overlooked. An elevated creatine kinase (CK) may be the first clue. In another group of young children, an indisposition to walk or run when they would be expected to do so brings them to medical attention; or, having achieved these motor milestones, they appear to be less active than usual and are prone to falls. Increasing difficulty in walking, running, and climbing stairs, swayback, and waddling gait become ever more obvious as time passes. The iliopsoas, quadriceps, and gluteal muscles are involved initially; then the pretibial muscles weaken (foot drop and toe walking). Muscles of the pectoral girdle and upper limbs are affected after the pelvicrural ones; the serrati, lower parts of pectorals, latissimus dorsi, biceps, and brachioradialis muscles are affected, more or less in the order mentioned.

Enlargement of the calves and certain other muscles is progressive in the early stages of the disease, but most of the muscles, even the ones that are originally enlarged, eventually decrease in size; only the gastrocnemii, and to a lesser extent the lateral vasti and deltoids, are consistently large, and this peculiarity may attract attention before the weakness becomes evident. The enlarged muscles have a firm, resilient ("rubbery") feel and as a rule are slightly less strong and more hypotonic than healthy ones (pseudohypertrophy). Rarely, all muscles are at first large and strong, even the facial muscles, as in one of Duchenne's cases (a "Farnese Hercules"); this is a true hypertrophy.

Muscles of the pelvic girdle, lumbosacral spine, and shoulders become weak and wasted, accounting for certain clinical peculiarities. Weakness of abdominal and paravertebral muscles accounts for the lordotic posture and protuberant abdomen when standing and the rounded back when sitting. Bilateral weakness of the extensors of the knees and hips interferes with equilibrium and with activities such as climbing stairs or rising from a chair or from a stooped posture. In standing and walking, the patient places his feet wide apart in order to increase his base of support. To rise from a sitting position, he first

Table 50-1
The muscular dystrophies

Disease	*Pattern of inheritance*	*Chromosomal locus*	*Altered gene product*
Duchenne/Becker	Sex-linked recessive	Xp21	Dystrophin
Emery-Dreifuss	Sex-linked recessive	Xq28	Emerin
Myotonic dystrophy (dystrophia myotonica)	Autosomal dominant	19q13.2–19q13.3	Myotonin protein kinase
Proximal myotonic myopathy (PROMM)	Autosomal dominant	3q	—
Congenital muscular dystrophy (CMD)			
Classic merosin-positive CMD	Autosomal recessive	—	—
Classic merosin-negative CMD	Autosomal recessive	6q22–23	Merosin (laminin α-2)
Fukuyama CMD	Autosomal recessive	9q31–33	Fukutin
Walker-Warburg syndrome	Autosomal recessive	—	—
Muscle-eye-brain disease	Autosomal recessive	1p32–34	—
CMD with rigid spine syndrome (CMD-RSS)	Autosomal recessive	1p35–36	—
Facioscapulohumeral	Autosomal dominant	4q35	—
Scapuloperoneal	Autosomal dominant	12	—
Limb-girdle muscular dystrophy (LGMD)			
LGMD 1A	Autosomal dominant	5q22.3–5q31.3	—
LGMD 1B (Bethlem myopathy)	Autosomal dominant	1q11–21	—
LGMD 1C	Autosomal dominant	3p25	Caveolin 3 (CAV 3)
LGMD 2A	Autosomal recessive	15q15.1–21.1	Calcium-activated neutral protease (calpain 3 or CANP3)
LGMD 2B	Autosomal recessive	2p 13 17q11–12 9q31–33	Dysferlin — —
LGMD 2C (SCARMD 1)	Autosomal recessive	13q13 (pericentromeric)	γ-Sarcoglycan, 35 kDa
LGMD 2D (SCARMD 2)	Autosomal recessive	17q12–q21.33	α-Sarcoglycan, 50 kDa (adhalin)
LGMD 2E	Autosomal recessive	4q12	β-Sarcoglycan, 43 kDa (hetarosin)
LGMD 2F	Autosomal recessive	5q33–34	δ-Sarcoglycan
Distal myopathies			
Late adult type 1 (Welander)	Autosomal dominant	14	—
Early adult type 1 (Nonaka)	Autosomal recessive	—	—
Early adult type 2 (Miyoshi)	Autosomal recessive	2p12–14	Dysferlin
Oculopharyngeal	Autosomal dominant	14q11.2–14q13	—
Progressive external ophthalmoplegia	Autosomal dominant	Mitochondrial	—

flexes his trunk at the hips, puts his hands on his knees, and pushes the trunk upward by working the hands up the thighs. In rising from the ground, the child first assumes a four-point position by extending the arms and legs to the fullest possible extent and then works each hand alternately up the corresponding thigh (a sign traditionally attached to Gowers' name). In getting up from a recumbent position, the patient turns his head and trunk and pushes himself sideways to a sitting position. S. A. K. Wilson used an alliterative phrase to describe the characteristic abnormalities of stance and gait—the patient "straddles as he stands and waddles as he walks."

The waddle is due to bilateral weakness of the gluteus medius. Calf pain is a not infrequent complaint. Weakening of the muscles that fix the scapulae to the thorax (serratus anterior, lower trapezius, rhomboids) causes a winging of the scapulae, and the scapular angles can sometimes be seen above the shoulders when one is facing the patient.

Later, weakness and atrophy spread to the muscles of the legs and forearms. The muscles that are selectively affected include the neck flexors, wrist extensors, brachioradialis, costal part of the pectoralis major, latissimus dorsi, biceps, triceps, anterior tibial, and peroneal muscles. The ocular, facial, bulbar, and hand muscles are usually spared, although weakness of the facial and sternomastoid muscles and of the diaphragm occurs in the late stages of the disease. As the trunk muscles atrophy, the bones stand out like those of a skeleton. The space between the lower ribs and iliac crests diminishes with affection of the abdominal muscles.

The limbs are usually loose and slack, but as the disability progresses, fibrous contractures appear as a result of the limbs remaining in one position and the imbalance between agonists and antagonists. Early in the ambulatory phase of the disease, the feet assume an equinovarus position due to shortening of the posterior calf muscles, which act without the normal opposition of the pretibial and peroneal muscles. Later, the hamstring muscles become permanently shortened because of a lack of counteraction of the weaker quadriceps muscles. Similarly, contractures occur in the hip flexors because of the relatively greater weakness of hip extensors and abdominal muscles. This leads to a pelvic tilt and compensatory lordosis to maintain standing equilibrium. The consequences of these contractures account for the habitual posture of the patient with Duchenne dystrophy: lumbar lordosis, hip flexion and abduction, knee flexion, and plantar flexion. As they become severe, these contractures contribute importantly to the eventual loss of ambulation. Scoliosis, due to unequal weakening of the paravertebral muscles, and flexion contractures of the forearms appear, usually after walking is no longer possible.

The tendon reflexes are diminished and then lost as muscle fibers disappear, the ankle reflexes being the last to go. The bones are thin and demineralized, and the appearance of ossification centers is delayed. Smooth muscles are spared, but the heart is usually affected. Various types of arrhythmia may appear. The electrocardiogram (ECG) shows prominent R waves in the right precordial leads and deep Q waves in the left precordial and limb leads, the result of cardiac fiber loss and replacement fibrosis of the basal part of the left ventricular wall (Perloff et al). Death is usually the result of pulmonary infections and respiratory failure and sometimes cardiac decompensation. Mild degrees of mental retardation, which is nonprogressive, are observed in many cases. Death usually occurs during late adolescence, and not more than 20 to 25 percent of patients survive beyond the twenty-fifth year. The last years of life are spent in a wheelchair; finally the patient becomes bedfast.

As mentioned above, Roses and colleagues have studied the female carriers of the disease (i.e., the mothers of affected boys) and report a slight weakness and enlargement of the calves as well as elevated CK values and abnormalities of the electromyogram (EMG) and muscle biopsy—all slight in degree—in over 80 percent. A small number of carriers manifest a moderate degree of myopathy that may mimic limb-girdle dystrophy. The muscle fibers of such patients (referred to as *manifesting* or *symptomatic* carriers) show a unique mosaic immunostaining pattern—some fibers containing dystrophin and others lacking it (Hoffman et al). This diagnostic information is particularly helpful in genetic counseling.

Becker-Type Muscular Dystrophy

This is another well-characterized dystrophy, closely related to the Duchenne type. It had long been noted that mixed with the Duchenne group of cases were certain relatively benign ones. In 1955, Becker and Keiner proposed that the latter be separated as a distinct entity; it is now known as Becker muscular dystrophy. Its incidence is difficult to ascertain, probably 3 to 6 per 100,000 male births. Like the Duchenne form, it is an X-linked disorder, practically limited to males and transmitted by females. It causes weakness and hypertrophy in the same muscles as the Duchenne dystrophy, but the onset is much later (mean age, 12 years; range, 5 to 45 years); the average age at which the patient becomes unable to walk is 25 to 30 years; death usually occurs in the fifth decade, but some patients live to an advanced age. If maternal uncles are affected by the disease and are still walking, the diagnosis is relatively easy. Cardiac involvement is less frequent than in Duchenne dystrophy and mentation is usually normal. Kuhn and associates have added a genealogy in which early myocardial disease and cramping myalgia were prominent features.

The serum CK values are 25 to 200 times normal, which, with the EMG and muscle biopsy findings, helps to exclude a hereditary spinal muscular atrophy. The EMG shows fibrillations, positive waves, low-amplitude and polyphasic motor unit potentials, and sometimes high-frequency discharges. The female carrier may occasionally display the same abnormalities as in Duchenne dystrophy, but to a much milder degree.

Pathology In the early stages of Duchenne dystrophy, the most distinctive features are prominent segmental degeneration and phagocytosis of single fibers or groups of fibers and evidence of regenerative activity (basophilia of sarcoplasm, hyperplasia and nucleolation of sarcolemmal nuclei, and the presence of myotubes and myocytes). The necrosis excites a regenerative or restorative process, which explains the forking of fibers and clustering of small fibers with prominent nuclei. The necrotic sarcoplasm and sarcolemma are removed by mononuclear phagocytic (macrophage) cells. There may also be a few T lymphocytes in the region; the blood vessels are normal. There is a hyalinization of the sarcoplasm of many degenerating and nondegenerating fibers. In longitudinal sections, these are seen as "contraction bands," expressive of the irritability of dystrophic muscle. This phenomenon may be present before there is any significant degree of degeneration and is more extensive in Duchenne than in any of the other dystrophies. Eventually there are histologic changes that are common to all types of advanced muscular dystrophies: loss of muscle fibers, residual fibers of larger and smaller size than normal—all in haphazard arrangement, and increase in lipocytes and fibrosis.

Hypertrophy of muscle is believed to be a result of work-induced enlargement of sound fibers in the face of adjacent fiber injury. But examples of true hypertrophy of entire muscles prior to the first sign of weakness may occur and are difficult to explain. Those large fibers may be present when at most only a few degenerating fibers are present. Pseudohypertrophy is due to lipocytic replacement of degenerated muscle fibers, but in its earlier stages the presence of many enlarged fibers contributes importantly to the enlargement of muscle. Thus a true hypertrophy appears to give way to pseudohypertrophy. The increase in lipocytes, fibrosis, and thickening of the walls of blood vessels are secondary changes. Smallness of residual fibers (possibly atrophy) is a prominent histologic feature. It is uncertain if this represents a gradual failure of cell metabolism and reduction in volume of all sarcoplasmic constituents or a stage in the regeneration of the damaged muscle fiber. The fibers do eventually degenerate and disappear, owing presumably to an exhaustion of regenerative capacity after repeated injuries or more and more extensive necrosis.

In the late stage of the dystrophic process, only a few scattered muscle fibers remain, almost lost in a sea of fat cells. It is of interest that the late or burned-out stage of chronic polymyositis resembles muscular dystrophy in that the fiber population is depleted, the residual fibers are of variable size but otherwise normal, and fat cells and endomysial fibrous tissue are increased; lacking only are the hypertrophied fibers of dystrophy. This resemblance informs us that many of the typical changes of muscular dystrophy are nonspecific, reflecting only the chronicity of the myopathic process. Finally, it should be restated that in all forms of muscular dystrophy the spinal neurons and their axons in the roots and peripheral nerves are essentially normal.

Etiology of Duchenne-Becker Dystrophy As mentioned earlier, the most important development in our understanding of the Duchenne and Becker muscular dystrophies has been the discovery by Kunkel of the abnormal gene on the X chromosome that is shared by these disorders and of the gene product. *Dystrophin* is the name that has been applied to the protein encoded by the affected gene (Hoffman et al). The biochemical assay of this protein and its histochemical demonstration near the sarcolemma have made possible the accurate diagnosis of the Duchenne and Becker phenotypes and have clarified the relationship between these two disorders. Whereas dystrophin is absent in patients with the Duchenne phenotype, it is present but structurally abnormal in the Becker type. Moreover, the phenotype that falls between the classic Duchenne and Becker forms (intermediate or "outlier" types) is characterized by a lower than normal amount of dystrophin. As noted, the Duchenne and Becker dystrophies and their intermediate forms are spoken of as *dystrophinopathies*.

A slightly different form of dystrophin, originating in a different part of the gene, is found in neurons of the cerebrum and brainstem and in astrocytes, Purkinje cells, and Schwann cells at nodes of Ranvier (Harris and Cullen). A deficiency of this dystrophin may in some way explain the mild mental retardation. It will be interesting to learn how such a deficiency might impair brain development and whether it might explain some cases of mental deficiency without muscular dystrophy.

Figure 50-1, taken from Sunada and Campbell, is useful in understanding the pathogenesis of the dystrophinopathies (as well as certain limb-girdle and congenital dystrophies described further on). In normal skeletal and cardiac muscle, dystrophin is localized to the cytoplasmic face of the sarcolemma, where it interacts with F-actin of the cytoskeleton (the filamentous

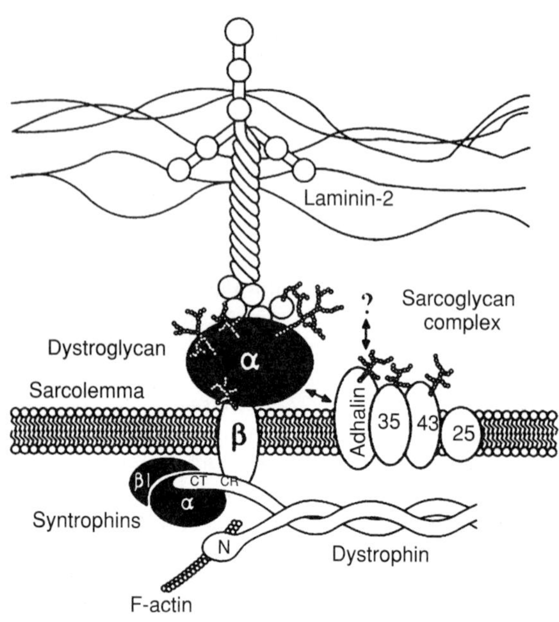

Figure 50-1

The molecular organization of the dystrophin-glycoprotein complex in the sarcolemma. Details in text. CT, carboxy terminal; CR, cystein-rich domain; N, amino terminal. (Reproduced, with permission, from Sunada and Campbell.)

reinforcing structure of the muscle cell). Dystrophin is also tightly bound to a complex of sarcolemmal proteins, known as dystrophin-associated proteins (DAPs) and glycoproteins (DAGs). Of special biologic importance in this complex are the proteins adhalin (defective in a particular limb-girdle dystrophy) and a 156-kDa glycoprotein called α-dystroglycan. The latter actually lies just outside the muscle cell and links the sarcolemmal membrane to the extracellular matrix (the inner portion of the basement membrane) by binding with merosin, a subunit of laminin. Thus, in this scheme, the dystrophin-glycoprotein complex functions as a transsarcolemmal structural link between the subsarcolemmal cytoskeleton and the extracellular matrix.

The loss of dystrophin leads to a loss of DAPs and disruption of the dystroglycan-protein complex. This disruption is thought to render the sarcolemma susceptible to breaks or tears during muscle contraction (Matsumura and Campbell)—a hypothesis consistent with the ultrastructural abnormalities that characterize Duchenne dystrophy, as first demonstrated by Mokri and Engel. The latter authors showed that there were defects of the plasma membrane (sarcolemma) in a large proportion of nonnecrotic hyalinized muscle fibers, allowing ingress of extracellular fluid and calcium. The entrance of calcium is believed to activate proteases and to increase protein degradation. The membrane defects and the associated alterations in the underlying region of the fiber represent an early and basic pathologic change in Duchenne dystrophy and account for the leakage into the serum of CK and other enzymes of muscle.

The identification of dystrophin has made possible a number of highly refined tests for the diagnosis of Duchenne and Becker dystrophies as well as the carrier state. Analysis of the dystrophin gene, in DNA obtained from white blood cells or 50 mg of skeletal muscle, can demonstrate the gene mutations in Duchenne and Becker patients and discriminate between these diseases with great accuracy. Analysis of dystrophin protein by immunostaining and immunoblot methods is the definitive method for discriminating between Duchenne, Becker, the carrier state, and other muscle disorders. Byers and colleagues have developed an enzyme-linked immunosorbent assay (ELISA) to measure the dystrophin levels in muscle biopsy samples. This assay is a rapid and relatively inexpensive tool for establishing the diagnosis of Duchenne-Becker muscular dystrophy and distinguishing it from unrelated disorders.

Other Dystrophinopathies Refined testing for the dystrophin protein has also brought to light several rarer types of *dystrophin abnormalities*. One, described by Gospe and coworkers, takes the form of a familial X-linked *myalgic-cramp-myoglobinuric syndrome*, with a deletion of the first third of the dystrophin gene at the Xp21 locus. The muscle changes are mild and relatively nonprogressive. Another dystrophinopathy takes the form of an *X-linked cardiomyopathy*, characterized by progressive heart failure in young persons without clinical evidence of skeletal muscle weakness; biopsy of skeletal muscle reveals reduced immunoreactivity to dystrophin (Jones and de la Monte). In yet another type, a glycerol-kinase deficiency is associated with varying degrees of adrenal hypoplasia, mental retardation, and myopathy. A number of defects in the glycoproteins that are associated with the dystrophin complex but do not involve dystrophin per se are described further on.

Emery-Dreifuss Muscular Dystrophy

This is another X-linked muscular dystrophy, relatively benign in comparison with the Duchenne type. It was described originally by Emery and Dreifuss and more recently by Hopkins and by Merlini and their colleagues.

The age of onset varies from childhood to late adolescence or adulthood. The weakness affects first the upper arm and pectoral girdle musculature and later the pelvic girdle and the distal muscles in the lower extremities. A consistent and distinguishing feature of the disease is the early appearance of contractures in the flexors of the elbow, extensors of the neck, and posterior calf muscles. Facial muscles are affected occasionally. There is no hypertrophy or pseudohypertrophy, and mentation is intact. A severe cardiomyopathy with variable sinoatrial and atrioventricular conduction defects is a common accompaniment. The course is generally benign, like that of Becker dystrophy, but weakness and contractures are severe in some cases, and sudden death is a frequent occurrence.

The X-linked *scapuloperoneal muscular atrophy with cardiopathy* (Mawatari and Katayama) and the X-linked scapuloperoneal syndrome described by Thomas and coworkers (1972) are probably variants of this disease. The latter disorder, like Emery-Dreifuss dystrophy, has been localized by linkage analysis to chromosome Xq28, and the gene product, called *emerin*, has been identified. The two disorders are probably allelic.

The humeroperoneal myopathy described by Gilchrist and Leshner is phenotypically much the same as the Emery-Dreifuss syndrome, though it is genetically distinct, being inherited as an autosomal dominant trait.

Facioscapulohumeral Muscular Dystrophy (Landouzy-Déjerine, Relatively Mild Restricted Muscular Dystrophy; FSH)

This is a slowly progressive dystrophy involving primarily the musculature of the face and shoulders, often with long periods of nearly complete arrest. The pattern of inheritance is usually autosomal dominant.

Although less common than the Duchenne and myotonic dystrophies, this disease is not rare (an estimated yearly incidence rate of 5:100,000). The age of onset is usually between 6 and 20 years; cases with onset in early adult life are occasionally encountered. As a rule, the first manifestations are difficulty in raising the arms above the head and winging of the scapulae, although in many cases bifacial weakness may have attracted attention, even in early childhood. There is involvement especially of the orbicularis oculi, the zygomaticus, and the orbicularis oris, whereas the masseters as well as the temporalis, extraocular, pharyngeal, and respiratory muscles are spared. Weakness and atrophy of the involved muscles are the major physical findings; pseudohypertrophy occurs only rarely and is slight. There is an inability to close the eyes firmly, to purse the lips, and to whistle; the lips have a peculiar looseness and tendency to protrude. The lower parts of the trapezius muscles and the sternal parts of the pectorals are almost invariably affected. By contrast, the deltoids may seem to be unusually large and strong, an appearance that may be mistaken for pseudohypertrophy. The advancing atrophic process involves the sternomastoid, serratus magnus, rhomboid, erector spinae, latissimus dorsi, and eventually the deltoid muscles. The bones of the shoulders become salient; the scapulae are winged and elevated ("angel-wing" appearance), and the clavicles are prominent. The anterior axillary folds slope down and out as a result of wasting of the pectoral muscles. Usually the biceps waste less than the triceps, and the brachioradialis muscles even less, so that the upper arm may be thinner than the forearm ("Popeye" effect). Pelvic muscles are involved later and to a milder degree, giving rise to a slight lordosis and pelvic instability. The pretibial muscles weaken, and foot drop is added to the waddling gait. Beevor's sign, an upward movement of the umbilicus on flexing the neck due to weakness of the lower abdominal muscles, is reportedly common (Awerbuch et al), but we have not seen it in early cases.

Early in the disease, the muscular weakness may be asymmetrical (winging of only one scapula). Many of the patients with milder degrees of this form of dystrophy are unaware that they have the disease. This was true of nearly half of the very large series of patients described by Tyler and Stephens in the Utah Mormon population. At any one point the disease may become virtually arrested. Nevertheless, 15 to 20 percent of patients eventually become wheelchair-bound (Tawil et al).

An occasional feature of this group of diseases is the congenital absence of a muscle (one pectoral, brachioradialis, or biceps femoris) or part of a muscle in patients who later develop the typical affection. Also, the external ocular muscles are known to become affected occasionally, late in the illness. Cardiac involvement is rare, but in a few of the cases tachycardia, cardiomegaly, and arrhythmias (ventricular and atrial extrasystoles) have occurred. Mental function is normal. Serum CK values are normal or slightly elevated.

At a molecular level, facioscapulohumeral dystrophy is now defined by its consistent association with deletions of variable size on chromosome 4q. No genes have been identified despite extensive sequencing of the deleted region, and it has been postulated that the deletions interfere with the expression of a gene or genes located proximal to the deletions (see Tawil et al).

A probable variant is characterized by an early onset and relatively rapid progression and an association with facial diplegia, sensorineural deafness, and sometimes exudative retinal detachment (Coats disease). Using fluorescein angiography, Fitzsimmons and others found a variety of other retinal abnormalities—comprising telangiectases, occlusion, leakage, and microaneurysms—in 56 of 75 persons with the usual form of facioscapulohumeral dystrophy, suggesting that these retinal abnormalities are an integral part of the disease.

Scapuloperoneal Muscular Dystrophy

Beginning with Brossard in 1886, there have been numerous reports of a distinctive pattern of progressive muscular weakness and wasting that typically involves the muscles of the neck, shoulders, and upper arms and anterior tibial and peroneal groups, causing foot drop. The nature of this disorder has been a matter of controversy, some claiming it to be a progressive muscular dystrophy and others, a muscular atrophy of spinal or neuropathic type. Probably both are correct in that either process can produce the same pattern of weakness. Davidenkow, who wrote extensively on this subject, described a form of familial scapuloperoneal weakness and atrophy associated with areflexia and distal sensory loss (a spinal-neuronopathic form), and others have confirmed these findings (see discussions of Thomas et al and of Munsat and Serratrice). Nevertheless, Thomas and colleagues (1975) established a myopathic form. The onset of symptoms in their six patients was in early or middle adult life, with difficulty in walking due to bilateral foot drop; symptoms referable to scapulohumeral involvement came later. Progression was slow and none of the patients became severely incapacitated. Autosomal dominant inheritance seemed likely.

More recently, Wilhelmsen and associates have defined the genetic defect in a large family with autosomal dominant scapuloperoneal syndrome (14 affected persons in a 44-member pedigree). Onset was in early adult life with difficulty in walking and climbing stairs, due to foot drop, followed by weakness of the proximal arm muscles. In 3 members, the disease was relentlessly progressive, but in the others it was relatively benign. In addition to the nonspecific histologic features of muscular dystrophy, some fibers showed eosinophilic hyaline inclusions and rimmed vacuoles. Linkage analysis has localized the gene to chromosome 12, proving that it is not simply an allelic variant of facioscapulohumeral or other type of muscular dystrophy.

Limb-Girdle Muscular Dystrophies (Scapulohumeral and Pelvifemoral Muscular Dystrophies; Erb-Type Dystrophies; LGMD Types 1 A-B and 2 A-E)

(See Table 50-1.) Clearly there is a large group of patients with muscular dystrophy who do not fit into the Duchenne-Becker, facioscapulohumeral, or scapuloperoneal categories described above. Children of both sexes in this group lack the hypertrophy of calves and other muscles; adults with late-onset forms have either pelvic or shoulder girdle involvement or both, and their facial muscles are spared. Insofar as Wilhelm Erb first called attention to these types of dystrophy, they were classified by Walton and Nattrass as the "limb-girdle dystrophies of Erb." This grouping has been problematic from the time it was proposed, because, like the scapuloperoneal group, it is heterogenous—the only unifying feature being the presence of limb-girdle weakness with sparing of the facial muscles. The inheritance has been variable, but the autosomal recessive forms are the most common. Either the shoulder girdle or pelvic girdle muscles may be first affected (traditionally these forms have been referred to as the Erb juvenile atrophic and Leyden-Möbius types, respectively). The weakness and atrophy may become evident during either during late childhood or early adult life and spread from shoulders to hips or vice versa.

The later the onset of this group of disorders, the more likely that the course will be benign; dominant inheritance and lack of family history are also features favoring slow progression. In the latter group, while the EMG is myopathic, the CK values are only moderately elevated and may even be normal in the most chronic forms. Cardiac involvement is infrequent, and mental function is normal.

As indicated earlier in this chapter, the status of this group of limb-girdle dystrophies as a clinical-genetic entity is being steadily eroded. The delineation of the progressive spinal muscular atrophies and the congenital and metabolic myopathies has considerably narrowed the category of limb-girdle dystrophies as originally described. During the past decade, with the application of molecular genetic techniques, progress in this direction has accelerated greatly. At the time of writing, at least eight forms of autosomal recessive and three forms of autosomal dominant limb-girdle dystrophies have been defined—most with a distinct chromosomal locus and gene and, in seven of them, an identifiable gene product (Bushby). This information is summarized in

Table 50-1 and the better-characterized types are discussed below.

Severe Childhood Autosomal Recessive Muscular Dystrophy (Sarcoglycanopathy; SCARMD; LGMD 2C, D, and E) This is perhaps the best-defined form of limb-girdle dystrophy. Clinically it resembles the severe form of Duchenne dystrophy in practically all respects, including the presence of calf hypertrophy, cardiomyopathy, and marked elevation of CK in the early stages of the illness. The obvious distinction from Duchenne dystrophy is the autosomal recessive pattern of inheritance (affection of both girls and boys in the same sibship). The largest and best-studied group of this severe, recessive pelvic-pectoral dystrophy (99 children in 28 families), has come from Tunisia (Ben Hamida et al). It also occurs commonly in other Arab countries and has been observed repeatedly in Brazil but less in Europe and North America.

The basic defect in SCARMD is in one of three dystrophin-associated glycoproteins (DAGs)—α-, β-, and γ-sarcoglycan (see Fig. 50-1); α-sarcoglycan (50 DAG) is also called adhalin, from the Arabic word *adhal*, meaning muscle. A primary deficiency of adhalin is due to a defective gene mapped to chromosome 17q21 (Roberds et al). A primary defect in β-sarcoglycan (43 DAG or hetarosin) has been mapped to chromosome 4q12, and of γ-sarcoglycan (35 DAG) to the pericentromeric region of chromosome 13q. When SCARMD is due to a primary defect in 43 DAG or 25 DAG, it may in addition show a deficiency of adhalin, but the latter is incomplete and represents a secondary effect, possibly explained by the proximity of the defective genes to the adhalin gene.

From a practical point of view, there is no difficulty in distinguishing SCARMD from a dystrophinopathy. In addition to the difference in inheritance, the former can be readily diagnosed by showing a loss of sarcolemmal immunostaining for adhalin. Clinically it is not possible to distinguish one sarcoglycanopathy from another; this can be accomplished only by appropriate immunostaining.

Autosomal Recessive Muscular Dystrophy Linked to Chromosomes 15q and 2p (LGMD 2A and B) These forms of limb-girdle dystrophy have been described in several large kindreds, in Indiana (among the Amish people), on the island of Réunion in the Indian Ocean, and in Brazil, affecting males and females equally. Both the shoulder and pelvic girdles were affected. The weakness varied considerably in severity but differed from SCARMD in its later age of onset (usually between 8 and 15 years) and loss of ambulation (around 30 years). In one form of the disease, called LGMD 2A, the abnormal gene has been mapped to chromosome 15q and the gene product has been identified as calcium-activated neutral protease, or calpain. This "calpainopathy" accounts for about 40 percent of patients with LGMD. Frequently, and early in the course of disease, there are Achilles tendon contractures and very high serum CK levels (at least 10 times normal)—features that may permit distinction from the sarcoglycanopathies on clinical grounds.

Yet another gene for a recessive limb-girdle dystrophy of slow progression has been identified in a Palestinian and Sicilian family and mapped to chromosome 2p. The gene product appears to be the protein dysferlin, which localizes to the muscle fiber membrane. Noteworthy is the fact that this same protein is also involved in the predominantly distal form of Miyoshi muscular dystrophy, described further on. Early involvement of the gastrocnemius muscle (inability to walk on tiptoe) and extraordinarily high levels of CK, as in calpainopathy, are clues to the latter.

Autosomal Dominant Limb-Girdle Dystrophies Localized to Chromosomes 21q and 5q (LGMD 1B) In 1976, Bethlem and van Wijngaarden described an autosomal dominant, early-onset limb-girdle dystrophy in 28 members of three unrelated Dutch families. Flexion contractures of the elbows, ankles, and interphalangeal joints of the fingers were present from the beginning stages of weakness but neither the weakness nor the contractures were disabling. Unlike Emery-Dreifuss dystrophy, contractures of the neck and spine were not present. Uniformity of clinical expression, slow progression with long periods of arrest, and normal longevity are other important features of the illness. Mohire and coworkers have proposed the designation *Bethlem myopathy*. A similar disease has now been reported from many parts of the world. Linkage analysis has assigned the gene locus of this myopathy to the distal part of chromosome 21q. The Dutch families described by van der Kooi et al were also shown to have an autosomal dominant pattern of inheritance. Clinically the dystrophy was much the same as described by Bethlem, except that more than half of the affected members in van der Kooi's families developed abnormalities of cardiac rhythm in their later years, necessitating pacemaker implantation. In the latter cases the gene abnormality has been localized to chromosome 1q.

Yet another type of autosomal dominant limb-girdle dystrophy of late onset has been found in a large North Carolina family (49 affected members in a pedigree of 218 persons). Mean age at onset was 27 years. Proximal leg weakness, with or without proximal arm weakness, and elevated CK values were the main clinical characteristics. Speer and colleagues have linked the abnormal gene to chromosome 5q.

Progressive External Ophthalmoplegia (Ocular Myopathy of von Graefe-Fuchs; Kearns-Sayre syndrome; PEO)

This is a slowly progressive myopathy primarily involving and often limited to the extraocular muscles. Usually the levators of the eyelids are the first to be affected, causing ptosis, followed by progressive ophthalmoparesis. This disorder usually begins in childhood, sometimes in adolescence, and rarely in adult life (as late as 50 years). Males and females are equally affected; the pattern of inheritance is autosomal dominant in some and recessive or uncertain in others. Once started, the disease progresses relentlessly until the eyes are motionless. Simultaneous involvement of all extraocular muscles permits the eyes to remain in a central position, so that strabismus and diplopia are uncommon (in rare instances one eye is affected before the other). As the patient attempts to raise his eyelids and to see under them, the head is thrown back and the frontalis muscle is contracted, wrinkling the forehead (hutchinsonian facies). The eyelids are abnormally thin because of atrophy of the levator muscles. The orbicularis oculi muscles are frequently involved in addition to the extraocular muscles. Thus, in progressive external ophthalmoplegia, as in myasthenia gravis and myotonic dystrophy, there is a characteristic combination of weakness of eye closure and eye opening, a combination that is nearly always myopathic. Other facial muscles, masseters, sternocleidomastoids, deltoids, or peronei are variably weak and wasted in about 25 percent of cases.

The absence of myotonia, cataracts, and endocrine disturbances distinguishes progressive external ophthalmoplegia from myotonic dystrophy, with which it might be confused because of the ptosis. The more extensive forms of the disease may resemble a mild form of facioscapulohumeral muscular dystrophy, and, indeed, Landouzy and Déjerine described ocular palsy in one of their cases. The characteristic feature of progressive external ophthalmoplegia is that ptosis and ocular paralysis precede involvement of other muscles by many years. The relatively early age of onset and absence of dysphagia set it apart from the oculopharyngeal form of dystrophy, and the lack of retinal degeneration and the normality of growth, mentation, and cerebrospinal fluid (CSF) protein distinguish it from the related mitochondrial disorder, Kearns-Sayre syndrome.

Opinions vary as to whether all cases of progressive external ophthalmoplegia should be assigned a myopathic origin. Dystrophy and partial denervation are difficult to distinguish on the basis of the appearance of the biopsied eye muscle, as pointed out by Ringel and associates. (Denervation of eye muscles does not result in grouped atrophy.) The categorization of progressive external ophthalmoplegia is complicated further by its frequent association with a variety of neurologic abnormalities and atypical pigmentary degeneration of the retina. This has led to the reclassification of many of these cases as mitochondrial diseases. The purely myopathic origin of some cases is proven by intactness of neurons in the brainstem nuclei and normality of the cranial nerves. From the available data, the authors believe it possible to separate at least two distinctive syndromes from this group. One of these is the restricted oculopharyngeal dystrophy of late onset, which is described below. Another rather uniform syndrome comprises childhood ophthalmoplegia, pigmentary degeneration of the retina, varying degrees of heart block, short stature, and elevated CSF protein (Kearns and Sayre). Because of its special histopathologic features, this latter syndrome is discussed with the congenital mitochondrial myopathies (page 1043).

Oculopharyngeal Dystrophy

This disease is inherited as an autosomal dominant trait and is unique in respect to its late onset (usually after the 45th year) and the restricted muscular weakness, manifest mainly as a bilateral ptosis and dysphagia. E. W. Taylor first described the disease in 1915 and assumed that it was due to a nuclear atrophy (oculomotor-vagal complex); Victor and colleagues, in 1962, showed that the descendants of Taylor's cases had a late-life myopathy (myopathic EMG and biopsy). One of the families that we described was subsequently traced through 10 generations to an early French-Canadian immigrant, who was the progenitor of 249 descendants with the disease (Barbeau). Other families showing a dominant (rarely recessive) pattern of inheritance and a number of sporadic cases have been observed in many parts of the world.

Associated with slowly progressive ptosis is difficulty in swallowing and change in voice. Swallowing becomes so difficult that food intake is limited, resulting in cachexia. The latter is ameliorated by cutting the cricopharyngeus muscles and, failing this measure, by a gastrostomy or nasogastric tube. Later in the disease, in some families, the external ocular muscles and shoulder and pelvic muscles become weakened and atrophic to a varying extent. In the few autopsied cases, a loss of fibers of modest proportions was widespread in these and many other muscles. Rimmed vacuoles in the sarcoplasm and, by electron microscopy, intranuclear tubular filaments are characteristic but not specific histologic findings (these features are seen in several other myopathies, particularly in inclusion body myositis). The brainstem nuclei and cranial nerves are normal. As in the other mild and restricted muscular dystrophies, the serum CK and aldolase levels are normal, and the EMG is altered only in the affected muscles. The gene locus has been mapped to chromosome 14q (Brais et al), and DNA testing is now available. The gene product remains to be identified.

Myotonic Dystrophy (Dystrophia Myotonica)

This, the commonest adult form of muscular dystrophy, was described in 1909 by Steinert, who considered it to be a variant of congenital myotonia (Thomsen disease), and, in the same year, by Batten and Gibb, who recognized it as a separate clinical entity. It is distinguished by an autosomal dominant pattern of inheritance with a high level of penetrance, a unique topography of the muscle atrophy, an associated myotonia, and the occurrence of dystrophic changes in nonmuscular tissues (lens of eye, testicle and other endocrine glands, skin, esophagus, heart, and, in some cases, the cerebrum). Certain muscles—namely the levator palpebrae, facial, masseter, sternomastoid, and forearm, hand, and pretibial muscles—are consistently involved in the dystrophic process. In this sense, dystrophia myotonica is a distal type of myopathy. It is possible that Gowers' case of an 18-year-old youth with weakened and wasted anterior tibial and forearm muscles and sternomastoids, in conjunction with paresis of the orbicularis and frontalis muscles, was an example of this disease, differing from the simple distal muscular dystrophy described later by Welander and others (see further on).

Despite the clinical variability of myotonic dystrophy, the defective gene segregates as a single locus at chromosome 19q13.3 in every population that has been studied. At this locus there is a specific molecular defect—an unstable trinucleotide sequence (cytosine, thymine, guanidine, or CTG) that is larger in affected individuals than in normal siblings or unaffected control subjects. Myotonin protein kinase is the product encoded by the myotonic dystrophy gene. The size of this lengthened DNA fragment (the "fat gene") varies among affected siblings and increases in size through successive generations, in parallel with earlier occurrence and increasing severity of the disease (genetic anticipation).

Clinical Features In most instances of myotonic dystrophy, the muscular wasting does not become evident until early adult life, but it may present in childhood, usually with facial weakness and ptosis. Also, a severe, *neonatal (congenital) form* of the disease is now well known and is described further on.

In the common early-adult form of the disease, the small muscles of the hands along with the extensor muscles of the forearms are often the first to become atrophied. In other cases, ptosis of the eyelids and thinness and slackness of the facial muscles may be the earliest signs, preceding other muscular involvement by many years. Atrophy of the masseters leads to narrowing of the lower half of the face, and the mandible is slender and malpositioned so that the teeth do not occlude properly. This—along with the ptosis, frontal baldness, and wrinkled forehead—imparts a distinctive physiognomy that, once seen, can be recognized at a glance. The sternomastoids are almost invariably thin and weak and are associated with an exaggerated forward curvature of the neck ("swan neck"). Atrophy of the anterior tibial muscle groups, leading to foot drop, is an early sign in some families.

Pharyngeal and laryngeal weakness results in a weak, monotonous, nasal voice. The uterine muscle may be weakened, interfering with normal parturition, and the esophagus is often dilated because of loss of muscle fibers in the striated as well as smooth muscle parts. Megacolon occurs in some patients. Diaphragmatic weakness and alveolar hypoventilation, resulting in chronic bronchitis and bronchiectasis, are common features, as are cardiac abnormalities; the latter are most often due to disease of the conducting apparatus, giving rise to bradycardia and a prolonged PR interval. Patients with extreme bradycardia or high degrees of atrioventricular block may die suddenly; for such subjects, insertion of a pacemaker has been recommended (Moorman et al). Mitral valve prolapse and left ventricular dysfunction (cardiomyopathy) are less frequent abnormalities.

The disease progresses slowly, with gradual involvement of the proximal muscles of the limbs and muscles of the trunk. Tendon reflexes are lost or much reduced. Contracture is rarely seen, and the thin, flattened hands are consequently soft and pliable. Most patients are confined to a wheelchair or bed within 15 to 20 years, and death occurs before the normal age from pulmonary infection, heart block, or heart failure.

The phenomenon of *myotonia*, which expresses itself in prolonged idiomuscular contraction following brief percussion or electrical stimulation and in delay of relaxation after strong voluntary contraction, is the third striking attribute of the disease. Not as widespread as in myotonia congenita (Thomsen disease—see page 1553), it is, nonetheless, easily elicited in the hands and tongue in almost all cases and in the proximal limb muscles in half of the cases. Gentle movements do not evoke it (eye blinks, movements of facial expression, and the like are not impeded), whereas strong closure of the lids and clenching of the fist are followed by a long delay in relaxation.

Myotonia may precede weakness by several years. Indeed, Maas and Paterson claimed that many cases diagnosed originally as myotonia congenita eventually prove to be examples of myotonia dystrophica. Of interest is the fact that in congenital or infantile cases of myotonic dystrophy, the myotonic phenomenon is not elicited until later in childhood, after the second or third year of life (see below). Moreover, the patient often becomes accustomed to the myotonia and does not complain about it. The relation of myotonia to the dystrophy is not direct. Certain muscles that show the myotonia best (tongue, flexors of fingers) are seldom weak and atrophic. There may be little or no myotonia in certain families that show the other characteristic features of myotonic dystrophy.

The fourth major characteristic is the association of dystrophic changes in nonmuscular tissues. The most common of these are lenticular opacities, which are found by slit-lamp examination in 90 percent of patients. At first dust-like, they then form small, regular opacities in the posterior and anterior cortex of the lens just beneath the capsule; under the slit lamp they appear blue, blue-green, and yellow and are highly refractile. Microscopically, the crystalline material (probably lipids and cholesterol, which cause the iridescence) lies in vacuoles and lacunae among the lens fibers. In older patients a stellate cataract slowly forms in the posterior cortex of the lens.

Mild to moderate degrees of mental retardation are not infrequent, and the brain weight in several of our patients was 200 g less than in normals of the same age. Late in adult life, some patients become suspicious, argumentative, and forgetful. In some families, a hereditary sensorimotor neuropathy may be added to the muscle disease (Cros et al).

Other nonspecific abnormalities, such as hyperostosis of the frontal bones and calcification of the basal ganglia, both readily discerned by CT scanning, seem to be more common in patients with myotonic dystrophy than in normal persons.

Progressive frontal alopecia, beginning at an early age, is a characteristic feature in both men and women with this disease. Testicular atrophy with androgenic deficiency, reduced libido or impotence, and sterility are frequent manifestations. In some patients gynecomastia and elevated gonadotropin excretion are found. Testicular biopsy may show atrophy and hyalinization of tubular cells and hyperplasia of Leydig cells. Thus all the clinical characteristics of the Klinefelter syndrome may be present. However, the nuclei of skin or bone marrow cells only rarely show the "sex chromatin mass" (Barr body). The majority of patients have the usual sex chromatin constitution. Ovarian deficiency occasionally develops in the female patient but is seldom severe enough to interfere with menstruation or fertility. The prevalence of clinical or chemical diabetes mellitus is only slightly increased in patients with myotonic dystrophy, but an increased insulin response to a glucose load has proved to be a common abnormality. Numerous surveys of other endocrine functions have yielded rather little of significance.

In an extensive clinical experience with this form of dystrophy, we have been impressed with the variability of its clinical expression. In many patients, intelligence has been unimpaired and the myotonia and muscle weakness have been so mild that the patients were unaware of any difficulty. Pryse-Philips and associates emphasized these features in their description of a large Labrador kinship in which 27 of 133 patients had only a partial syndrome and only minor muscle symptoms at the time of examination.

Pathologic Features There are several unusual myopathologic features. Peripherally placed sarcoplasmic masses and circular bundles of myofibrils (ringbinden) are common. Central nucleation may be marked. In many of the muscle spindles there is an excess of intrafusal fibers (particularly in the congenital form, see below). In addition, one observes necrosis of single muscle fibers and many atrophic fibers. Many of the terminal arborizations of the peripheral nerves are unusually elaborate and elongated. The spindle and nerve changes may be secondary to the myotonia or to an associated terminal neuropathy.

Congenital Myotonic Dystrophy Brief reference was made earlier to this distinctive and potentially lethal form of myotonic dystrophy. That it occurs not infrequently is evident from Harper's (1975) study of 70 personally observed patients and 56 others gathered from the medical literature. Profound hypotonia and facial diplegia at birth are the most prominent clinical features; myotonia is notable for its absence. The drooping of the eyelids, the tented upper lip ("carp mouth"), and the open jaw impart a characteristic appearance, which allows immediate recognition of the disease in the newborn infant and in the child. Difficulty in sucking and swallowing, bronchial aspiration (due to palatal weakness), and respiratory distress (due to diaphragmatic and intercostal weakness and pulmonary immaturity) are present in varying degrees of severity; the latter disorders are responsible for a previously unrecognized group of neonatal deaths (24 such deaths among sibs of affected patients in Harper's study). In surviving infants, delayed motor and speech development, swallowing difficulty, mild to moderately severe mental retardation, and talipes or generalized arthrogryposis are common. Once adolescence is attained, the disease follows the same course as the later form. As stated above, clinical myotonia in the congenital form of the disease becomes evident only later in childhood, although EMG study may disclose myotonic discharges in early infancy. The diagnosis may be suspected by the simple test of eliciting myotonia in the mother. Electrocardiographic changes occur in one-third of the patients.

The affected parent in the congenital form of this disease is always the mother, in whom the disease need not be severe; electrophysiologic testing will bring out the myotonia in the mother if it is inevident on percussion of muscle. In cases of adult onset, transmission is maternal or paternal. These data suggest that in addition to inheriting the myotonic dystrophy gene, the congenital cases also receive some maternally transmitted factor, the nature of which is presently unknown. The prenatal diagnosis of myotonic dystrophy is readily accomplished by examination for CTG repeats in the amniotic fluid or in a biopsy of chorionic villi. However, it is not possible to predict whether a fetus with an expansion mutation will have congenital myotonic dystrophy or myotonic dystrophy of other type.

Proximal Myotonic Myopathy (PROMM) Under this title, Ricker and colleagues have described a myopathy characterized by autosomal dominant inheritance, proximal muscle weakness, myotonia, and cataracts. Seventeen families, containing 50 affected members, have been studied by these authors. Onset was between 20 and 40 years, with intermittent myotonic symptoms of the hands and proximal leg muscles, followed by a mild, slowly progressive weakness of the proximal limb muscles without significant atrophy. Cataracts developed in half the patients and cardiac arrhythmias in only two. Ptosis, weakness of facial, jaw, and distal limb muscles, and mental abnormalities were notably absent.

Histologically the appearance was that of a nonspecific myopathy, without ringbinden or subsarcolemmal masses. The gene defect for this disease has been mapped to chromosome 3q. Analysis of leukocyte and muscle DNA discloses no expansion of the CTG component of the myotonic dystrophy gene.

The Distal Muscular Dystrophies (Welander, Miyoshi Types)

Included under this heading is a group of slowly progressive distal myopathies with onset principally in adult life. Weakness and wasting of the muscles of the hands, forearms, and lower legs, especially the extensors, are the main clinical features. Although cases such as these had been reported by Gowers and others, their differentiation from myotonic dystrophy and peroneal muscular atrophy was unclear until relatively recent times.

One type of distal dystrophy, inherited as an *autosomal dominant* trait, was recorded by Milhorat and Wolff in 1943. They studied 12 individuals of one family affected by "a progressive muscular dystrophy of atrophic distal type." The onset was between 26 and 43 years; within 5 to 15 years the patients had become disabled. There was one autopsy, confirming the dystrophic nature of the disease.

Welander's account of a similar disorder, based on the study of 249 patients from 72 Swedish pedigrees, appeared in 1951 (not to be confused with the Kugelberg-Welander juvenile spinal muscular atrophy affecting proximal muscles—see page 1161). In her series, the mode of inheritance was also autosomal dominant. Weakness developed first in the small hand muscles and then spread to the distal leg muscles, causing a steppage gait. Fasciculations, cramps, pain, sensory disturbances, and myotonia were notably absent. Senile cataracts appeared after the age of 70 in three patients and can be discounted as having special significance. No endocrine disorders were detected. Dystrophic changes were demonstrated in three autopsies and 22 biopsy specimens. The central nervous system and peripheral nerves were normal. Progression of the disease was very slow; after 10 years or so some wasting of proximal muscles was seen in a few of the patients. Markesbery and colleagues reported a late-onset distal myopathy in which weakness began in the distal leg muscles and later spread to the hands; there was also cardiomyopathy and heart failure.

A second type of distal dystrophy characterized by an *autosomal recessive* pattern of inheritance is particularly prevalent in Japan (Miyoshi et al, Nonaka et al). Onset of the disease is in early adult life, with weakness and atrophy of the leg muscles, most prominent in the peroneal or the gastrocnemius and soleus muscles. Over many years the weakness extends to the thighs, gluteal muscles, and arm muscles, including the proximal ones. Serum CK concentrations are greatly increased in the early stages of the disease. In this "Miyoshi type" of dystrophy, gene linkage to chromosome 2p12-14 has been established; the mutation leads to an absence of the muscle protein dysferlin, a membrane protein that is not thought to be part of the dystrophin complex (Matsuda et al). Of interest is the fact, mentioned earlier, that one of the limb-girdle dystrophies (2B) has been linked to the same chromosomal locus and also lacks the dysferlin protein (Table 50-1).

An apparently separate form of distal myopathy with autosomal dominant inheritance and onset before 2 years of age has been described by Magee and DeJong and by van der Does de Willebois and coworkers. Whether these infantile-onset cases represent a true muscular dystrophy has not been established beyond doubt.

Congenital Muscular Dystrophy (Fukuyama, Walker-Warburg, Merosin Deficient, Rigid Spine, and Other Types)

Early in the twentieth century there were scattered reports of congenital myopathy, but the status of this condition was difficult to evaluate, mainly because of a lack or incompleteness of pathologic examinations. Some cases may have represented congenital myotonic dystrophy, described above, or one of the congenital myopathies, described in Chap. 52. In 1957 Banker and her associates described two patients (siblings), one dying 1 1/2 h after birth and the other at the age of 10 months of a congenital muscular dystrophy with arthrogryposis. The pathologic changes consisted of muscle fiber degeneration, variation in fiber size, fibrosis, and fat cell replacement. The central and peripheral nervous systems were intact. The severity of the degenerative changes was such that a developmental disorder of muscle could be excluded.

Pearson and Fowler, in 1963, reported a brother and sister with similar clinical and pathologic findings, and Walton et al described yet another patient, aged 4 years. By 1967 Vassella and colleagues were able to collect 27 cases from the medical literature and to add 8 cases of their own. The high incidence of sibling involvement pointed to an autosomal recessive inheritance.

Defined as a muscle dystrophy already present at birth, often with contractures of proximal muscles and trunk, the severity of the weakness and degree of progression have varied widely. Of the eight cases reported by Rotthauwe and others, one had a benign course, but the others all had weakness and hypotonia at birth, and difficulty in sucking and swallowing had interfered with nutrition. Their oldest patients, aged 14 and 23 years, and several others had walked, but at a late age. In the Finnish series of Donner and associates, congenital dystrophy accounted for 9 percent of the 160 cases of neuromuscular disease seen at their hospital over a decade. The weakness and hypotonia were generalized, and three had ECG abnormalities. The CK values were elevated and the EMGs were myopathic.

In the 1960s a series of papers issued from Japan relating the details in over 100 patients with congenital dystrophy (Fukuyama et al). A feature of these cases was the coexistence of severe mental retardation and developmental anomalies of the cerebral cortex. Hyperlucency in the periventricular white matter (by computed tomography) was frequently observed in these patients. In another group of cases, congenital muscular dystrophy was associated with lissencephaly as well as cerebellar and retinal malformations (Walker-Warburg syndrome; see Dobyns et al). In a series of 19 Finnish cases reported by Santavuori and coworkers, congenital muscular dystrophy was associated with retinal degeneration and optic atrophy, hydrocephalus, pachygyria-polymicrogyria, and hypoplastic or absent septum pellucidum and corpus callosum ("muscle-eye-brain disease"). Lebenthal and colleagues described a large Arab pedigree with congenital muscular dystrophy and patent ductus arteriosus. Some patients had contractures at birth; in others contractures developed at a later age. The EMG disclosed a myopathic pattern, and CK levels were moderately elevated.

In recent years the classification and relationships of the congenital muscular dystrophies have been clarified to some extent by a number of molecular genetic studies (see Table 50-1). The most frequent congenital muscular dystrophy in the Caucasian population is the classic (Occidental) type, so called because it is characterized exclusively by muscle involvement. (Occasionally there are abnormal white matter signals on magnetic resonance imaging.) Tomé and others have shown that in approximately half such patients, merosin is completely absent (merosin-negative). Merosin, the predominant isoform of α-laminin in the basement membrane of the muscle fiber, is closely bound to α-dystroglycan, which in turn is bound to the dystrophin cytoskeleton (Fig. 50-1). An absence of merosin interrupts this linkage and leads to muscle degeneration. The diagnosis of merosin deficiency can be made by immunostaining of chorionic villi cells prenatally and skeletal muscle postnatally. Merosin-negative congenital muscular dystrophy has been mapped to chromosome 6q22, clearly distinguishing it from the Fukuyama, or merosin-positive, type on both genetic and clinical grounds (Table 50-1).

An additional member of the group of merosin-positive congenital muscular dystrophies is one termed *rigid spine syndrome*. The term was first proposed by Dubowitz and the clinical syndrome, as outlined by Flanigan et al, consists of (1) infantile hypotonia with early weakness of neck muscles and poor head control; (2) stabilization with only slight decrease of muscle strength but marked loss of muscle bulk; (3) prominent contractures of spinal muscles, resulting in scoliosis and rigidity in flexion and, to a lesser extent, contractures of limb joints; (4) respiratory insufficiency with onset before adolescence; and (5) normality of intellectual and cardiac function. Recently the locus for congenital muscular dystrophy with rigid spine syndrome (CMD-RSS) was mapped to 1p35–36 (Moghadaszdeh et al).

In the Fukuyama type of congenital muscular dystrophy, the abnormal gene has been mapped to 9q31–33, and the altered gene product has been identified (fukutin). The so-called muscle-eye-brain disease (MEB) is genetically distinct; the chromosomal locus is at 1p32–34. The status of the Walker-Warburg syndrome is uncertain. Its relationship to the Fukuyama or the MEB syndrome is not clear, since the genetic defect has not been established.

Problems in Diagnosis

The following are some of the common problems that arise in the diagnosis of muscular dystrophy:

1. *The diagnosis of muscular dystrophy in a child who has just begun to walk or in whom walking is delayed.* Tests of peak power on command cannot be used with reliability in small children. The most helpful points in identifying Duchenne dystrophy are (*a*) unusual difficulty in climbing stairs or arising from a crouch or from a recumbent position on the floor, showing greater weakness at the hips and knees than at the ankles; (*b*) unusually large, firm calves; (*c*) male sex; (*d*) high serum CK, aldolase, and myoglobin; (*e*) myopathic EMG; (*f*) biopsy findings; and (*g*) special methods of testing for dystrophin protein (see previous discussions).

2. *The adult patient with diffuse or proximal muscle weakness of several months' duration, raising the question of polymyositis versus dystrophy.* Even biopsy may be misleading in showing a few inflammatory foci in an otherwise dystrophic picture. The main points that help to distinguish polymyositis from dystrophy have been indicated in Chap. 49. As a rule, polymyositis evolves more rapidly than dystrophy and is associated with high CK and aldolase values (higher than any dystrophy except the Duchenne and distal Miyoshi types), and the EMG shows many fibrillation potentials (rare in adult forms of muscular dystrophy). With these points in mind, there may still be uncertainty, in which instance a trial of prednisone is indicated for a period of 6 months. Unmistakable improvement favors polymyositis; questionable improvement (physician's and patient's judgment not in accord) leaves the diagnosis unsettled.

3. *An adult with a slowly evolving proximal weakness.* In addition to facioscapular and limb-girdle dystrophies, several of the congenital polymyopathies discussed in Chap. 52 may begin to cause symptoms or to worsen in adult years. These include central core and nemaline myopathy. Examples of mild forms of acid maltase or debrancher enzyme deficiency with glycogenosis, progressive late-stage hypokalemic polymyopathy, mitochondrial myopathy, and carnitine polymyopathy have been reported in the adult. Muscle biopsy and histochemical staining of the muscle usually provide the correct diagnosis.

4. *The occurrence of subacute or chronic symmetrical proximal weakness in an adolescent or adult that raises the question of spinal muscular atrophy* (Kugelberg-Welander type—see page 1161) as well as of polymyositis and muscular dystrophy. Electromyography and muscle biopsy usually settle the matter. Some of the same problems arise in an adult with distal dystrophy.

5. *Weakness of a shoulder or one leg of some weeks' standing, with increasing atrophy.* Here one must differentiate between a mononeuritis or radiculitis, the beginning of motor system disease (progressive spinal muscular atrophy), and rarely the early stage of a muscular dystrophy. The first two may develop silently, in mild form, and attract notice only when wasting begins

(denervation atrophy takes 3 to 4 months to reach its peak). Points in favor of these acquired diseases are (*a*) confinement of the disease to muscles originally affected and sparing of other muscles and (*b*) an EMG showing denervation effects. Biopsy is seldom performed under such circumstances, for, by temporizing, the problem eventually settles itself. Invariably muscle dystrophy becomes bilateral and symmetrical; mononeuritis stabilizes and recovers; and spinal muscular atrophy declares itself by the presence of fasciculations and relatively rapid progression of weakness.

6. *The distinction, in the child or adolescent, between dystrophy and one of the congenital myopathies is considered in relation to the latter disorders (Chap. 52).*

Treatment There is no specific treatment for any of the muscular dystrophies; the physician is forced to stand by helplessly and witness the unrelenting progression of weakness and wasting. The various vitamins (including vitamin E), amino acids, testosterone, and drugs such as penicillamine, recommended in the past, have all proved to be ineffective. The administration of prednisone appears to retard the tempo of progression of Duchenne dystrophy for a period of up to 3 years (Fenichel et al). The optimal dose is 0.75 mg/kg given daily, but it must often be reduced because of intolerable side effects (weight gain, cushingoid appearance, behavioral and gastrointestinal disorders).

Quinine has a mild curare-like action at the motor end plate and thus relieves myotonia. Although symptomatic relief of the myotonia is usually achieved, the drug has no effect on progression of the muscle atrophy or other degenerative aspects of myotonic dystrophy. The usual dose is 0.3 to 0.6 g orally, repeated as needed about every 6 h. Mild toxic symptoms such as tinnitus may develop before enough quinine has been given to relieve the myotonia. Some patients find the side effects more distressing than the myotonia and prefer not to take quinine except on occasions when the myotonia is troublesome in a particular activity. Also, procainamide (0.5 to 1.0 g four times daily) and phenytoin are sometimes useful in alleviating myotonia, but the former is dangerous, even in patients with a pacemaker. Quinine and procainamide slow conduction through the AV node, whereas phenytoin does not have this effect. Testosterone has been found to increase muscle mass and creatine excretion in patients with myotonic dystrophy but was of no value in preserving strength or lessening myotonia (Griggs et al).

Respiratory failure occurs in virtually all patients affected with Duchenne dystrophy after they become wheelchair-bound as well as in some of the other dystrophic diseases. It may be so insidious as to become evident only as sleep apnea, as a retention of carbon dioxide that causes morning headache, or as a progressive weight loss that reflects the excessive work of breathing. If there are frequent episodes of oxygen desaturation, some improvement in daytime strength and alertness can be attained by assisting ventilation at night. This may be accomplished in early stages by a negative-pressure cuirass-type of device that expands the chest wall periodically or, more conveniently, by nasal positive pressure (so-called NIPPV or BIPAP) and later by positive-pressure ventilation through a fenestrated tracheostomy that allows nighttime ventilation but leaves the patient free to speak and breathe through normal mechanisms during the day. However, in patients free of respiratory failure, with vital capacities between 20 and 50 percent of predicted values, a randomized trial of nasal mechanical ventilation failed to demonstrate improvement or prolonged survival (Raphael et al). In sum, the clinical impression remains that more severely affected patients can be managed at home for prolonged periods with respiratory assistance. Needless to say, the common complications of muscular dystrophy—notably pulmonary infections and cardiac decompensation—must be treated symptomatically. Surgical management of cataracts is indicated when they become mature.

In recent years there has been a flurry of interest in the injection of human myoblasts with a full complement of dystrophin into the muscles of Duchenne patients. The difficulties of injecting every dystrophic muscle are obvious, and no convincing evidence of the efficacy of such injections even into individual muscles has been forthcoming.

Until such time as gene therapy becomes practical for muscular dystrophy, physicians must rely on physical methods of rehabilitation. Vignos, who reviewed the studies that evaluated muscle-strengthening exercises, has offered evidence that maximal resistance exercises, if begun early, can strengthen muscles in Duchenne, limb-girdle, and facioscapulohumeral dystrophies. None of the muscles were weaker at the end of a year than at the beginning. Cardiorespiratory function after endurance exercise was not significantly improved. Contractures were reduced by passive stretching of the muscles 20 to 30 times a day and by splinting at night. If contractures have already formed, fasciotomy and tendon lengthening are indicated in patients who are still ambulatory. Maintenance of ambulation and upright posture will delay scoliosis. Preventive measures were more successful than restorative ones.

From such observations it is concluded that two factors are of importance in the management of patients with muscular dystrophy: avoiding prolonged bed rest and encouraging the patient to maintain as full and normal a life as possible. These help to prevent the rapid worsening associated with inactivity and to conserve a healthy attitude of mind. Obesity should be avoided; this requires careful attention to diet. Swimming is a useful exercise. Massage and electrical stimulation are probably worthless. The education of children with muscular dystrophy should continue, with the aim of preparing them for a sedentary occupation.

REFERENCES

ANGELINI C, FANIN M, PEGORARO E, et al: Clinical-molecular correlation in 104 mild X-linked muscular dystrophy patients: Characterization of sub-clinical phenotypes. *Neuromuscul Disord* 4:349, 1994.

ARAHATA K, ISHIURA S, ISHIGURO T, et al: Immunostaining of skeletal and cardiac muscle surface membrane with antibody against Duchenne muscular dystrophy peptide. *Nature* 333:861, 1988.

ASLANIDIS C, JANSEN G, AMEMIYA C, et al: Cloning of the essential myotonic dystrophy region and mapping of the putative defect. *Nature* 355:548, 1992.

AWERBUCH GI, NIGRO MA, WISHNOW R: Beevor's sign and facioscapulohumeral dystrophy. *Arch Neurol* 47:1208, 1990.

BANKER BQ: The congenital muscular dystrophies, in Engel AG, Franzini-Armstrong C (eds): *Myology*, 2nd ed. New York, McGraw-Hill, 1994, pp 1275–1289.

BANKER BQ, VICTOR M, ADAMS RD: Arthrogryposis multiplex due to congenital muscular dystrophy. *Brain* 80:319, 1957.

BARBEAU A: The syndrome of hereditary late onset ptosis and dysphagia in French Canada, in Kuhn EE (ed): *Progressive Muskeldystrophies, Myotonie, Myasthenie*. New York, Springer-Verlag, 1966.

BATTEN FE, GIBB HP: Myotonia atrophica. *Brain* 32:187, 1909.

BECKER PE, KEINER F: Eine neue X-chromosomale muskeldystrophie. *Arch Psychiatr Z Neurol* 193:427, 1955.

BEN HAMIDA M, FARDEAU M, ATTIA N: Severe childhood muscular dystrophy affecting both sexes and frequent in Tunisia. *Muscle Nerve* 6:469, 1983.

BETHLEM J, VAN WIJNGAARDEN GK: Benign myopathy with autosomal dominant inheritance: A report on three pedigrees. *Brain* 99:91, 1976.

BRAIS B, XIE Y-G, SANSON M, et al: The oculopharyngeal muscular dystrophy locus maps to the region of the cardiac a and b myosin heavy chain gene on chromosome 14q11.2-q 13. *Hum Mol Genet* 4:429, 1995.

BUSHBY KMD: Making sense of the limb girdle muscular dystrophies. *Brain* 122:1403, 1999.

BUXTON J, SHELBOURNE P, DAVIES J, et al: Detection of an unstable fragment of DNA specific to individuals with myotonic dystrophy. *Nature* 355:547, 1992.

BYERS TJ, NEUMANN PE, BEGGS AH, KUNKEL LM: ELISA quantitation of dystrophin for the diagnosis of Duchenne and Becker muscular dystrophies. *Neurology* 42:570, 1992.

CAMPBELL KP: Three muscular dystrophies: Loss of cytoskeleton-extra cellular matrix linkage. *Cell* 80:675, 1995.

CHAKRABARTI A, PEARSE JMS: Scapuloperoneal syndrome with cardiomyopathy: Report of a family with autosomal dominant inheritance and unusual features. *J Neurol Neurosurg Psychiatry* 44:1146, 1981.

CROS D, HARNDEN P, POUGET J, et al: Peripheral neuropathy in myotonic dystrophy: A nerve biopsy study. *Ann Neurol* 23:470, 1988.

DAVIDENKOW S: Scapuloperoneal amyotrophy. *Arch Neurol Psychiatry* 41:694, 1939.

DOBYNS WB, PAGON R, ARMSTRONG D, et al: Diagnostic criteria for Walker-Warburg syndrome. *Am J Med Genet* 32:195, 1989.

DONNER M, RAPOLA J, SOMMER H: Congenital muscular dystrophy: A clinicopathological and follow-up study of 13 patients. *Neuropediatrie* 6:239, 1975.

DUBOWITZ V: Rigid spine syndrome: A muscle syndrome in search of a name. *Proc R Soc Med* 66:219, 1973.

EMERY AEH, DREIFUSS FE: Unusual type of benign X-linked muscular dystrophy. *J Neurol Neurosurg Psychiatry* 29:338, 1966.

ENGEL AG, FRANZINI-ARMSTRONG C (eds): *Myology*, 2nd ed. New York, McGraw-Hill, 1994.

ENGEL AG, YAMAMOTO M, FISCHBECK KH: Dystrophinopathies, in Engel AG, Franzini-Armstrong C (eds): *Myology*, 2nd ed. New York, McGraw-Hill, 1994, pp 1133–1187.

FENICHEL GM, FLORENCE JM, PESTRONK A, et al: Long-term benefit from prednisone therapy in Duchenne muscular dystrophy. *Neurology* 41:1874, 1991.

FITZSIMMONS RB, GURWIN EB, BIRD AC: Retinal vascular abnormalities in facioscapulohumeral muscular dystrophy. *Brain* 110:631, 1987.

FLANIGAN KM, KERR L, BROMBERG MB, et al: Congenital muscular dystrophy with rigid spine syndrome: A clinical, pathological, and genetic study. *Ann Neurol* 47:152, 2000.

FUKUYAMA Y, OSAWA M, SAITO K (eds): *Congenital Muscular Dystrophies*. Amsterdam, Elsevier, 1997.

GILCHRIST JM, LESHNER RT: Autosomal dominant humeroperoneal myopathy. *Arch Neurol* 43:734, 1986.

GOSPE SM JR, LAZARO RP, LAVA NS, et al: Familial X-linked myalgia and cramps: A nonprogressive myopathy associated with a deletion in the dystrophin gene. *Neurology* 39:1277, 1989.

GOWERS WR: *Pseudohypertrophic Muscular Paralysis*. London, Churchill Livingstone, 1879.

GRIGGS RC, MENDELL JR, MILLER RG: *Evaluation and Treatment of Myopathies*. Philadelphia, Davis, 1995.

GRIGGS RS, PANDYA S, FLORENCE JM, et al: Randomized controlled trial of testosterone in myotonic dystrophy. *Neurology* 39:219, 1989.

HARLEY HG, BROOK JD, RUNDLE SA, et al: Expansion of an unstable DNA region and phenotypic variation in myotonic dystrophy. *Nature* 355:545, 1992.

HARPER PS: Congenital myotonic dystrophy in Britain. *Arch Dis Child* 50:505, 514, 1975.

HARPER PS: *Myotonic Dystrophy*. Philadelphia, Saunders, 1979.

HARRIS JB, CULLEN MJ: Ultrastructural localization and possible role of dystrophin, in Kakulas BA, Howell JM, Rosas AD (eds): *Duchenne Muscular Dystrophy*. New York, Raven Press, 1992.

HOFFMAN EP, ARAHATA K, MINETTI C, et al: Dystrophinopathy in isolated cases of myopathy in females. *Neurology* 42:967, 1992.

HOFFMAN EP, BROWN RH JR, KUNKEL LM: Dystrophin: The protein product of the Duchenne muscular dystrophy locus. *Cell* 51:919, 1987.

HOFFMAN EP, FISCHBECK KH, BROWN RH, et al: Characterization of dystrophin in muscle-biopsy specimens from patients with Duchenne's or Becker's muscular dystrophy. *N Engl J Med* 318:1363, 1988.

HOPKINS LC, JACKSON JA, ELIAS LJ: Emery-Dreifuss humeroperoneal muscular dystrophy: An X-linked myopathy with unusual contractures and bradycardia. *Ann Neurol* 10:230, 1981.

JONES HR, DE LA MONTE SM: Case Records of the Massachusetts General Hospital; Case 22-1998. *N Engl J Med* 339:182, 1998.

KAKULAS BA, ADAMS RD: *Diseases of Muscle: Pathological Foundations of Clinical Myology*, 4th ed. Philadelphia, Harper & Row, 1985.

KEARNS TP, SAYRE GP: Retinitis pigmentosa, external ophthalmoplegia and complete heart block. *Arch Ophthalmol* 60:280, 1958.

KUGELBERG E, WELANDER L: Heredofamilial juvenile muscular atrophy simulating muscular dystrophy. *Arch Neurol Psychiatry* 75:500, 1956.

KUHN E, FIEHN W, SCHRODER JM, et al: Early myocardial disease and cramping myalgia in Becker type muscular dystrophy: A kindred. *Neurology* 29:1144, 1979.

KUNKEL LM: Analysis of deletions in DNA from patients with Becker and Duchenne muscular dystrophy. *Nature* 322:73, 1986.

LEBENTHAL E, SCHOCHET SR, ADAM A, et al: Arthrogryposis multiplex congenita: 23 cases in an Arab kindred. *Pediatrics* 16:891, 1970.

MAAS O, PATERSON AS: Myotonia congenita, dystrophia myotonica, and paramyotonia. *Brain* 73:318, 1950.

MAGEE KR, DEJONG RN: Hereditary distal myopathy with onset in infancy. *Arch Neurol* 13:387, 1965.

MARKESBERY WR, GRIGGS RC, LEACH RP, LAPHAM LW: Late onset hereditary distal myopathy. *Neurology* 23:127, 1974.

MATSUDA C, AKOI M, HAYASHI YK, et al: Dysferlin is a surface membrane-associated protein that is absent in Miyoshi myopathy. *Neurology* 53:1119, 1999.

MATSUMURA K, CAMPBELL KP: Dystrophin glycoprotein complex: Its role in the molecular pathogenesis of muscular dystrophies. *Muscle Nerve* 17:2, 1994.

MAWATARI S, KATAYAMA K: Scapuloperoneal muscular atrophy with cardiopathy. *Arch Neurol* 28:55, 1973.

MERLINI L, GRANATA C, DOMINICI P, BONFIGLIOLI S: Emery-Dreifuss muscular dystrophy: Report of five cases in a family and review of the literature. *Muscle Nerve* 9:481, 1986.

MILHORAT AT, WOLFF HG: Studies in diseases of muscle: XIII. Progressive muscular dystrophy of atrophic distal type; report on a family; report of autopsy. *Arch Neurol Psychiatry* 49:655, 1943.

MIYOSHI K, KAWAI H, IWASA M, et al: Autosomal recessive distal muscular dystrophy as a new type of progressive muscular dystrophy. *Brain* 109:31, 1986.

MOGHADASZDEH B, DESGUERRE I, TOPALOGLU H, et al: Identification of a new locus for a peculiar form of congenital muscular dystrophy with early rigidity of the spine, on chromosome 1p35-36. *Am J Hum Genet* 62:1439, 1998.

MOHIRE MD, TANDAN R, FRIES TJ, et al: Early-onset benign autosomal dominant limb-girdle myopathy with contractures (Bethlem myopathy). *Neurology* 38:573, 1988.

MOKRI B, ENGEL AG: Duchenne dystrophy: Electron microscopic findings pointing to a basic or early abnormality in the plasma membrane of the muscle fiber. *Neurology* 25:1111, 1975.

MOORMAN JR, COLEMAN RE, PACKER DL, et al: Cardiac involvement in myotonic muscular dystrophy. *Medicine* 64:371, 1985.

MUNSAT TL, SERRATRICE G: Facioscapulohumeral and scapuloperoneal syndromes, in Vinken PJ, Bruyn GW, Klawans H (eds): *Handbook of Clinical Neurology*, vol 18 (new series). Amsterdam, Elsevier Science, 1992, pp 161–176.

NEVIN S: Two cases of muscular degeneration occurring in late adult life with a review of the recorded cases of late progressive muscular dystrophy (late progressive myopathy). *J Med* 5:51, 1936.

NONAKA I, SUNOHARA N, SATOYOSHI E, et al: Autosomal recessive distal muscular dystrophy: A comparative study with distal myopathy with rimmed vacuole formation. *Ann Neurol* 17:52, 1985.

PEARSON CM, FOWLER WG: Hereditary nonprogressive muscular dystrophy inducing arthrogryposis syndrome. *Brain* 86:75, 1963.

PERLOFF JK, ROBERTS WC, DELEON AC, et al: The distinctive electrocardiogram of Duchenne's muscular dystrophy. *Am J Med* 42:179, 1967.

PRYSE-PHILIPS W, JOHNSON GJ, LARSEN B: Incomplete manifestations of myotonic dystrophy in a large kinship in Labrador. *Ann Neurol* 11:582, 1982.

RAPHAEL JC, CHEVRET S, CHASTANG C, et al: Randomised trial of preventive nasal ventilation in Duchenne muscular dystrophy. French Multicentre Cooperative Group on Home Mechanical Ventilation Assistance in Duchenne de Boulogne Muscular Dystrophy. *Lancet* 343:1600, 1994.

RICKER K, KOCH MC, LEHMANN-HORN F, et al: Proximal myotonic myopathy: A new dominant disorder with myotonia, muscle weakness, and cataracts. *Neurology* 44:1448, 1994.

RICKER K, KOCH MC, LEHMANN-HORN F, et al: Proximal myotonic myopathy. *Arch Neurol* 52:25, 1995.

Ringel SP, Wilson WB, Barden MT: Extraocular muscle biopsy in chronic progressive ophthalmoplegia. *Ann Neurol* 6:326, 1979.

Roberds SL, Leturcq F, Allamand V, et al: Missense mutation in the adhalin gene linked to autosomal recessive muscular dystrophy. *Cell* 78:625, 1994.

Roses MS, Nicholson MT, Kircher CS, Roses AD: Evaluation and detection of Duchenne's and Becker's muscular dystrophy carriers by manual muscle testing. *Neurology* 27:20, 1977.

Rotthauwe HW, Mortier W, Beyer H: Neuer Typ einer recessiv X-chromosomal verebten Muskeldystrophie: Scapulo-humero-distale Muskeldystrophie mit fruhzeitigen Kontrakturen und Herzrhythmusstorungen. *Humangenetik* 16:181, 1972.

Santavuori P, Somer H, Sainio A, et al: Muscle-eye-brain disease (MEB). *Brain Dev* 11:147, 1989.

Seitz D: Zur nosologischen Stellung des sogenannten scapulo-peronealen Syndroms. *Dtsch Z Nervenheilkd* 175:547, 1957.

Speer MC, Yamaoka LH, Gilchrist JH, et al: Confirmation of genetic heterogeneity in limb-girdle muscular dystrophy: Linkage of an autosomal dominant form to chromosome 5q. *Am J Hum Genet* 50:1211, 1992.

Steinert TH: Über das klinische und anatomische Bild des Muskelschwunds der Myotoniker. *Dtsch Z Nervenheilkd* 37:58, 1909.

Sunada Y, Campbell KP: Dystrophin-glycoprotein complex: Molecular organization and critical roles in skeletal muscle. *Curr Opin Neurol* 8:379, 1995.

Swash M, Heathfield KWG: Quadriceps myopathy: A variant of the limb-girdle dystrophy syndrome. *J Neurol Neurosurg Psychiatry* 46:355, 1983.

Tawil R, Figlewicz DA, Griggs RC, et al: Facioscapulohumeral dystrophy: A distinct regional myopathy with a novel molecular pathogenesis. *Ann Neurol* 43:279, 1998.

Thomas PK, Calne B, Elliott CF: X-linked scapuloperoneal syndrome. *J Neurol* 35:298, 1972.

Thomas PK, Schott GD, Morgan-Hughes JA: Adult onset scapuloperoneal myopathy. *J Neurol Neurosurg Psychiatry* 38:1008, 1975.

Tomé FMS, Evangelista T, LeClerc A, et al: Congenital muscular dystrophy with merosin deficiency. *CR Acad Sci* 317: 351, 1994.

Tyler FH, Stephens FE: Studies in disorders of muscle: II. Clinical manifestations and inheritance of facioscapulohumeral dystrophy in large family. *Ann Intern Med* 32:640, 1950.

van der Does de Willebois AEM, Bethlem J, Meyer AEFH, Simons AJR: Distal myopathy with onset in early infancy. *Neurology* 18:383, 1968.

van der Kooi AJ, Ledderhof TM, De Voogt WG, et al: A newly recognized autosomal dominant limb girdle muscular dystrophy with cardiac involvement. *Ann Neurol* 39:363, 1996.

van der Kooi AJ, van Meegan M, Ledderhof TM, et al: Genetic localization of a newly recognized autosomal dominant limb-girdle muscular dystrophy with cardiac involvement (LGMD 1B) to chromosome 1q11-21. *Am J Hum Genet* 60:891, 1997.

Vassella F, Mumenthaler M, Rossi E, et al: Congenital muscular dystrophy. *Dtsch Z Nervenheilkd* 190:349, 1967.

Victor M, Hayes R, Adams RD: Oculopharyngeal muscular dystrophy: A familial disease of late life characterized by dysphagia and progressive ptosis of the eyelids. *N Engl J Med* 267:1267, 1962.

Vignos PJ: Physical models of rehabilitation in neuromuscular disease. *Muscle Nerve* 6:323, 1983.

Walton JN, Karpati G, Hilton-Jones D (eds): *Disorders of Voluntary Muscle*, 6th ed. Edinburgh, Churchill Livingstone, 1994.

Walton JN, Nattrass FS: On the classification, natural history and treatment of myopathies. *Brain* 77:169, 1954.

Welander L: Myopathia distalis tarda hereditaria. *Acta Med Scand* 141 (suppl 265):1, 1951.

Wilhelmsen KC, Blake DM, Lynch T, et al: Chromosome 12-linked autosomal dominant scapuloperoneal muscular dystrophy. *Ann Neurol* 39:507, 1996.

Wohlfart G, Fex J, Eliasson S: Hereditary proximal spinal muscle atrophy simulating progressive muscular dystrophy. *Acta Psychiatr Neurol* 30:395, 1955.

Chapter 51

THE METABOLIC AND TOXIC MYOPATHIES

Three classes of metabolic disease of muscle are recognized—one in which a muscle disorder is traceable to a primary, or hereditary, metabolic abnormality; another in which the myopathy is secondary to a disorder of endocrine function, i.e., to disease of the thyroid, parathyroid, pituitary, or adrenal gland; and a third group, due to a large variety of myotoxic drugs and other chemical agents. The latter two groups are relatively common and more likely to come initially to the attention of the internist rather than the neurologist.

The primary hereditary metabolic myopathies are of special interest because they reveal certain aspects of the complex chemistry of muscle fibers. Indeed, each year brings to light some new genetically determined enzymopathy of muscle. And a number of diseases, formerly classified as dystrophic or degenerative, are consistently being added to the enlarging list of metabolic myopathies. There are now so many of them that only the most representative forms can be presented in a textbook of neurology. Complete accounts of this subject can be found in the section on metabolic disorders in Engel and Franzini-Armstrong (eds.), *Myology*, and in the chapter by DiMauro and colleagues in the *Handbook of Clinical Neurology* (see References).

PRIMARY METABOLIC DISORDERS OF MUSCLE

The chemical energy for muscle contraction is provided by the hydrolysis of adenosine triphosphate (ATP) to adenosine diphosphate (ADP); ATP is restored by phosphocreatine and ADP acting in combination. These reactions are particularly important during brief, high-intensity exercise. During periods of prolonged muscle activity, rephosphorylation requires the availability of carbohydrates, fatty acids, and ketones, which are catabolized in mitochondria. Glycogen is the main sarcoplasmic source of carbohydrate, but blood glucose (from the catabolism of liver glycogen) also moves freely in and out of muscle cells as needed during sustained exercise. The fatty acids in the blood, derived mainly from adipose tissue and intracellular lipid stores, constitute the other major source of energy. Carbohydrate is metabolized during aerobic and anaerobic phases of metabolism, the fatty acids only aerobically.

Resting muscle derives approximately 70 percent of its energy from the oxidation of long-chain fatty acids. As stated above, during a short period of intense exercise, the muscle utilizes carbohydrate derived from glycogen stores; myophosphorylase is the enzyme that initiates the metabolism of glycogen. With longer aerobic exercise, blood flow to muscle and the availability of glucose and fatty acids is increased. At first, glucose is the main source of energy; later, with exhaustion of the glycogen stores, energy is provided by oxidation of fatty acids.

Thus, muscle failure at a certain phase of exercise is predictive of the type of energy failure. A rising blood concentration of β-hydroxybutyrate reflects the increasing oxidation of fatty acids, and an increase in blood lactate reflects the anaerobic metabolism of glucose. The cytochrome oxidative mechanisms are essential in both aerobic and anaerobic muscle metabolism; these mechanisms are considered in Chap. 37, in relation to the mitochondrial diseases, and are referred to here only briefly.

It follows from these observations that the efficiency and endurance of muscle depend on a constant supply of glycogen, glucose, and fatty acids and the enzymes committed to their metabolism. Biochemical derangements in their metabolism give rise to a large number of muscle disorders, the most important of which are elaborated in the following pages.

Glycogen Storage Myopathies

An abnormal accumulation of glycogen in the liver and kidneys was described by von Gierke in 1929; shortly thereafter, Pompe (1932) reported a similar disorder involving cardiac and skeletal muscle. Major contributions to our understanding of glycogen metabolism were made by McArdle, by Cori and Cori, and by Hers, who discovered the deficiency of acid maltase in Pompe disease and enunciated the concept of inborn lysosomal diseases (see Chap. 37). Since then, many nonlysosomal enzyme deficiencies have been identified and have become the basis of the classification presented in Table 51-1. These enzymatic deficiencies alter the metabolism of many cells but most strikingly those of the liver, heart, and skeletal muscle. In about half of the affected individuals, a chronically progressive or intermittent myopathic syndrome is the major manifestation of the disease. With the exception of the rare phosphoglycerate kinase deficiency (X-linked recessive inheritance), *all the glycogenoses are inherited as autosomal recessive traits*. The most impressive and common of these glycogen storage diseases from the standpoint of the clinical neurologist are α-1,4-glucosidase (acid mal-tase) and myophosphorylase deficiencies.

Acid Maltase Deficiency (Glycogenosis Type II)

The gene encoding acid maltase has been mapped to the distal portion of the long arm of chromosome 17 (17q23). A deficiency of this enzyme takes three clinical forms, of which the first (Pompe disease) is the most malignant. The latter develops in infancy, between 2 and 6 months; dyspnea and cyanosis call attention to enlargement of the heart, and the liver may be enlarged as well. The skeletal muscles are found to be weak and hypotonic, though their bulk may be increased. The tongue may be enlarged, giving the infant a cretinoid appearance. Hepatomegaly, while often present, is not pronounced. Exceptionally, the heart is relatively normal in size, and the central nervous system and muscles bear the brunt of the disorder. The clinical picture then resembles infantile muscular atrophy (Werdnig-Hoffmann disease) and, to add to difficulty in differential diagnosis, occasionally there are fasciculations. The disease is rapidly progressive and ends fatally in a few months. The electromyogram (EMG) is myopathic, but there are fibrillation potentials, heightened insertional activity, and pseudomyotonia as well. Large amounts of glycogen accumulate in muscle, heart, liver, and neurons of the spinal cord and brain. All tissues lack alpha glucosidase (acid maltase).

In the second (childhood) form, onset is during the second year, with delay in walking and slowly progressive weakness of shoulder, pelvic girdle, and trunk muscles. The toe walking, waddling gait, enlargement of calf muscles, and lumbar lordosis resemble those of Duchenne dystrophy. Cardiomyopathy is exceptional. Hepatomegaly is less frequent than in the infantile form, and mental retardation was present in only 2 of 18 cases reported by DiMauro et al. Death occurs between 3 and 24 years of age, usually from ventilatory insufficiency.

In the third, or adult, form there is a more benign truncal and proximal limb myopathy. The weakness is slowly progressive over years, and death is usually the result of paralysis of respiratory muscles. At times the only severe weakness is of the diaphragm, as in the case reported by Sivak and colleagues. The liver and heart are not enlarged. Creatine kinase (CK) values are increased, as they are in all forms of the disease. The EMG discloses a number of abnormalities—brief motor unit potentials, fibrillation potentials, positive waves, bizarre high-frequency discharges, and occasional myotonic discharges (without clinical evidence of myotonia). The disease must be differentiated from other chronic adult polymyopathies, such as polymyositis and the endocrine myopathies, and from motor neuron disease.

The diagnosis is readily confirmed by muscle biopsy. The sarcoplasm is vacuolated and most vacuoles contain periodic acid–Schiff (PAS)-positive diastase-digestible material; they stain intensely for acid phosphatase. The glycogen particles lie in aggregates; electron microscopy shows some of them to occupy lysosomal vesicles (i.e., this is a lysosomal storage disease) and others to lie free. The myofibrils are disrupted, and some muscle fibers degenerate. The glycogen accumulation is more pronounced in type 1 fibers. As indicated above, in the more severe infantile form of acid maltase deficiency, heart muscle and the large neurons of the spinal cord and brainstem may also accumulate glycogen and degenerate. The difference in severity between infant and adult forms may relate to the completeness of enzyme deficiency, but possibly other factors are at work. More than one of the three types may occur in the same family.

The adult with threat of respiratory failure should be observed frequently with measurements of vital capacity and blood gases. Umpleby and coworkers have reported that a low-carbohydrate, high-protein diet may be beneficial. A few of our patients died unexpectedly during sleep. Respiratory support (rocking bed, nasal positive pressure, and cuirass as discussed on page 1508) may prolong life.

Table 51-1
The glycogenoses affecting skeletal muscle[a]

Glycogenosis type (proper name)	*Defective enzyme*	*Chromosomal locus*	*Onset of disease[b]*	*Hypotonia*	*Exercise intolerance (myalgia, cramps, stiffness, ± myoglobinuria)*	*Early fatigue and second wind*	*Myopathy ± atrophy*	*Severe respiratory muscle weakness*
II (Pompe)	Acid maltase	17q23	I	+			+	+
II	Acid maltase	17q23	C				+	+
II	Acid maltase	17q23	A				+	+
III (Cori-Forbes)	Debrancher	1p21	C-A	+			+	
IV (Andersen)	Branching		I-C	+			+	
V (McArdle)	Myophosphorylase	11q13	C, Ad, A		+	+	+	
VII (Tarui)	Phosphofructokinase	1q cent–q32	C-A		+	+	+	
VIII	Phosphorylase B kinase	16q12–q13; 7p12	I, C, Ad, A	+	+		+	
IX	Phosphoglycerate-kinase	Xq13	I, C-A		+		+	
X	Phosphoglycerate-mutase	7	A		+			
XI	Lactic dehydrogenase	11	Ad-A		+	+		

[a]All types: elevated CK; myopathic EMG, with increased irritability and myotonia.

[b]I, infancy; C, childhood; Ad, adolescence; A, adult.

Additional features (not charted above): feeding difficulties, II Pompe; retarded growth, III; neurologic abnormalities, II Pompe, IX; seizures, VIII, IX; hypoglycemic seizures, III; jaundice, VII, IX; cirrhosis, IV; generalized scaling erythema, XI; firm consistency of muscle, II Pompe; elevated serum aspartate aminotransferase and lactic dehydrogenase, II; elevated serum bilirubin, VII, IX; failure of LDH to rise proportionally to elevation of CK, XI; fasting hypoglycemia, III; hemolytic anemia and reticulocytosis, VII, IX; hemoglobinuria, IX; excessive rise in serum pyruvates during ischemic exercise test, XI.

Contractures	*Organomegaly*	*Myoglobinuria*	*Positive ischemic exercise test*	*Enzyme-deficient cells for assay*	*Membrane-lined vacuoles with glycogen*	*Increased glycogen in subsarcolemma and intermyofibrillar areas*	*Intra- and extra-vacuolar acid phosphatase*	*Amylopectin deposits*	*Histochemistry*
	+			Muscle, WBC, chorionic villus, amniotic fluid	+	+	+		
				Muscle	+	+	+		
				Muscle	+	+	+		
+	±	+		Muscle, WBC, fibroblasts		+			
+	+			Muscle, WBC fibroblasts, amniotic fluid		+	+	+	
+		+	+	Muscle, WBC		+			Absence of myophosphorylase
+		+	+	Muscle, RBC		+		+	Absence of phosphofructokinase
	+	+	+	Muscle		+			
	+	+	+	Muscle, RBC		±			
		+	+	Muscle		+			
		+	+	Muscle		+			

Myophosphorylase Deficiency (Type V Glycogenosis; McArdle Disease); Phosphofructokinase Deficiency (Type VII Glycogenosis; Tarui Disease) These disorders are considered together, since they are clinically identical and both express themselves by the development of muscle cramps (actually true contractures, page 1470) in response to exercise—a feature that distinguishes them from other glycogenoses. In both these diseases an otherwise normal child, adolescent, or adult begins to complain of weakness and stiffness and sometimes pain on using the limbs. Muscle contraction and relaxation are normal when the patient is in repose, but strenuous exercise, either isometric (lifting heavy weights) or dynamic (climbing stairs or walking uphill), causes the muscles to shorten (contracture), since they are unable to relax. After vigorous exercise, episodes of myoglobinuria are common, complicated by renal failure in some instances. With mild sustained activity, the patient experiences progressive fatigue and weakness, which diminish following a brief pause. The patient can then resume his activities at the original pace ("second-wind" phenomenon). During the second-wind phase, the patient copes with his symptoms by increasing cardiac output and substituting free fatty acids and blood-borne glucose for muscle glycogen (Braakhekke et al).

The primary abnormality in *McArdle* disease is a deficiency of myophosphorylase, which prevents the conversion of glycogen to glucose-6-phosphate. Phosphofructokinase deficiency (*Tarui disease*) interferes with the conversion of glucose-6-phosphate to glucose-1-phosphate; the defect in the latter condition is also present in red blood cells (Layzer et al). The gene for myophosphorylase has been localized to the long arm of chromosome 11 (11q13), and analysis of DNA from the patient's leukocytes can be used for diagnosis. The muscle (M) subunit of the phosphofructokinase protein localizes to a gene defect on chromosome 1. This defect predominates in Ashkenazi Jewish men.

Clinical variants of these disorders are known. Some patients, with no previous symptoms of cramps or myoglobinuria, develop progressive weakness of limb muscles in the sixth or seventh decade. One of these older patients had come to our attention because of chronically elevated levels of CK and mild muscle cramping after climbing stairs. In others, rapidly progressive weakness became evident in infancy, with early death from respiratory failure. These unusual forms are not directly related to severity of the enzyme deficiencies.

The contracted muscles in these disorders, unlike muscles in other involuntary spasms, no longer use energy, and they are more or less electrically silent (i.e., no electrical activity is recorded from maximally contracted muscle during cramps induced by ischemic exercise); moreover, they do not produce lactic acid. This shortened state is spoken of as *pharmacologic contracture*. Ischemia contributes to this condition by denying glucose to the muscle, which cannot function adequately on fatty acids and nonglucose substrates. These features are the basis of the *forearm ischemic exercise test*, which is useful if performed carefully in the diagnosis of both McArdle and Tarui disease. An indwelling catheter is placed in the antecubital vein and a basal blood sample is obtained. Above the elbow, a sphygmomanometer cuff is inflated to exceed arterial pressure. After 1 min of vigorous hand exercise (30 closures against an ergometer), blood samples are obtained at 1 and 3 min. Normal individuals show a three- to five-fold increase in blood lactate. In patients with either McArdle or Tarui disease, the lactate fails to rise. This procedure has reportedly caused a localized rhabdomyolysis (Meinck et al), for which reason Griggs and associates recommend that the test be carried out *without* a blood pressure cuff. Problems with consistency in conducting the test and processing blood samples for lactate limit its validity unless the test is performed by experienced personnel. Definitive diagnosis depends upon histochemical stains of biopsied muscle, which reveal an absence of phosphorylase activity (in McArdle disease) or of phosphofructokinase activity (in Tarui disease).

The only known treatment is a planned reduction and intermittency in physical activity. Fructose and creatine taken orally are said to be helpful in some cases. Improvement has also been reported after the administration of glucagon (Kono et al) and after a high-protein diet (Slonim and Goans), but these effects are not consistent.

Other Forms of Glycogenosis (See Table 51-1.) Of the remaining types of glycogen storage disease, type III (*debranching enzyme deficiency; Cori-Forbes disease*) affects muscle, but not consistently. The childhood form is characterized mainly by a benign hepatopathy, but sometimes there is also diminished muscle strength and tone. An adult form beginning in the third and fourth decades presents with proximal and distal myopathy. The course is slowly progressive and may be associated with wasting of the leg and hand muscles. In the series reported by DiMauro and colleagues, several of the patients who developed weakness during adult life complained of rapid fatigue and aching of muscles, occurring with exertion and beginning at an early age. Serum CK values were elevated, and the EMG showed a myopathic picture as well as increased insertional activity, pseudomyotonic discharges, and fibrillation potentials. Rarely in the adult form, glycogen also accumulates in the peripheral nerves, giving rise to mild symptoms of polyneuropathy. The enzymatic defect is one of amylo-1,6-glucosidase deficiency.

Disturbance of skeletal muscle is much less prominent in type IV glycogenosis (*branching enzyme deficiency*, or *Andersen disease*). This is a rapidly progressive disease of infancy and early childhood, characterized by cirrhosis and chronic hepatic failure, usually with death in the second or third year. Hepatomegaly due to accumulation of an abnormal polysaccharide is a universal finding. Muscle weakness and atrophy, hypotonia, and contractures occur less regularly and are usually overshadowed by the liver disease. The diagnostic hallmark of this myopathy is the presence of basophilic, intensely PAS-positive polysaccharide granules in skin and muscle.

The remaining nonlysosomal glycogenoses (types VIII through XI) need only be mentioned briefly. They are all rare and clinically heterogenous, and a myopathy—characterized by intolerance to exercise, cramps, myoglobinuria, elevated CK, and sometimes renal failure—has been observed in only a small proportion of them. Phosphoglycerate kinase deficiency (type IX glycogenosis) differs in that it is inherited as a sex-linked recessive trait. The defective gene has been localized to chromosome Xq13. Hemolytic anemia—becoming evident soon after birth—mental retardation, seizures, and tremor are other features that set this glycogenosis apart from the others. The myopathic features of the lysosomal and nonlysosomal glycogenoses are listed in Table 51-1. Detailed accounts of these glycogenoses can be found in the monographs of Griggs and associates and of Engel and Franzini-Armstrong (chapters by DiMauro and Tsujino and by Engel and Hirschhorn); see References.

Disorders of Lipid Metabolism Affecting Muscle

Although it has long been known that lipids are an important source of energy in muscle metabolism (along with glucose), it was only in 1970 that W. K. Engel and others reported the storage of lipid in muscle fibers, attributable to a defect in the oxidation of long-chain fatty acids. The subjects of their report were twin sisters who had experienced intermittent cramping of muscles associated with myoglobinuria after vigorous exercise. In 1973, A. G. Engel and Angelini described a young woman with progressive myopathy, lipid storage predominantly in type 1 muscle fibers, and a deficiency of muscle carnitine, a cofactor required for the oxidation of fatty acids. Since that time, highly sophisticated biochemical techniques have greatly enhanced the study of fatty acid metabolism and the identification of many of the primary defects.

Biochemistry of Fatty Acid Metabolism Carnitine (beta-hydroxy-gamma-*N*-trimethylamino-butyrate), derived from lysine and methionine, plays a central role in the metabolism of fatty acids. About 75 percent of carnitine comes from dietary sources (red meat and dairy products); the remainder is synthesized in the liver and kidneys. Practically all of the body carnitine is stored in muscle, where it has two main functions: (1) transporting long-chain fatty acyl-CoAs from the cytosol compartment of the muscle fiber into the mitochondria, where they undergo β-oxidation, and (2) preventing the intramitochondrial accumulation of acyl-CoAs, thus protecting the cell from the membrane-destabilizing effects of these substances.

In order to be oxidized, the long-chain fatty acids undergo a series of biochemical transformations. First they are activated to corresponding acyl-CoA esters by acyl-CoA synthetase, located on the outer mitochondrial membrane. Since the inner mitochondrial membrane is impermeable to acyl-CoA esters, they are transferred into the mitochondria as acylcarnitine esters. This is accomplished by carnitine palmitoyl transferase I (CPT I), also located on the outer mitochondrial membrane. A second carnitine palmitoyl transferase (CPT II), bound to the inner face of the inner mitochondrial membrane, reconverts the acyl-carnitines to fatty acyl-CoAs, which undergo β-oxidation within the mitochondrial matrix. The steps in the transport of long-chain fatty acids into the mitochondrial matrix (the carnitine cycle) are described in detail in the reviews of DiMauro et al, of DiDonato, and of Roe and Coates, listed in the References. Isoforms of carnitine palmityltransferase are critically involved in this process at the inner and outer membranes of the mitochondria.

Clinical Features of Disordered Fatty Acid Metabolism Despite the many biochemical abnormalities that have been defined in the fatty acid metabolic pathways, there are essentially three clinical patterns by which these defects are expressed:

1. One constellation of symptoms referred to as the *encephalopathic* syndrome has its onset in infancy or early childhood. Its very first manifestation may be sudden death (sudden infant death syndrome, or SIDS), or there may be vomiting, lethargy and coma, hepatomegaly, cardiomegaly, muscular weakness, and hypoketotic hypoglycemia, with hyperammonemia, i.e., a Reye-like syndrome. Undoubtedly, instances of this syndrome have not been recognized as abnormalities of fatty acid metabolism but have been designated incorrectly as the Reye syndrome or as SIDS. They are discussed in Chap. 37.

2. A second (*myopathic*) syndrome appears in late infancy, childhood, or adult life and takes the form of a progressive myopathy, with or without cardiomyopathy. The myopathy may follow upon episodes of hypoketotic hypoglycemia or may develop de novo.

3. The third syndrome is one that usually begins in the second decade of life. It is induced by a sustained period of physical activity or fasting and is characterized by repeated episodes of *rhabdomyolysis* with or without myoglobinuria.

Summarized below are the disorders of fatty acid metabolism that affect skeletal muscle:

Primary Systemic Carnitine Deficiency To date, this is the only form of carnitine deficiency that can be considered primary. Its main clinical features are progressive lipid storage myopathy and cardiomyopathy, sometimes associated with the signs of hypoketotic hypoglycemia. There is no dicarboxylic aciduria, in distinction to the secondary β-oxidation defects, in all of which dicarboxylic aciduria is present. The cardiomyopathy, which is fatal if untreated, responds dramatically to oral administration of L-carnitine, 2 to 6 g/day. This disorder is inherited as an autosomal recessive trait. In these families there is frequently a history of sudden unexplained death in siblings, so that early identification of affected children is essential.

Carnitine Palmityltransferase (CPT) Deficiency This disease is also inherited as an autosomal recessive trait. The gene encoding CPT has been mapped to chromosome 1q12. There are three types of CPT deficiency, referred to as types I, IIA, and IIB. Type I is the most common. It affects males predominantly, beginning in the second decade of life. Attacks of myalgia, cramps, and muscle weakness, "tightness," and stiffness are precipitated by sustained (though not necessarily intense) exercise and less often by a prolonged period of fasting. Fever, anesthesia, drugs, emotional stress, and cold are rare precipitating events. The attacks vary greatly in frequency. They are usually accompanied by myoglobinuria, and renal failure occurs in about one-fourth of cases (DiMauro et al). The attacks are not aborted by rest and, once initiated, there is no second-wind phenomenon. There are no warning signs of an impending attack. Any muscle group may be affected. Persistence of weakness after an attack is uncommon. Serum CK rises to high levels not only during attacks of myoglobinuria but also after vigorous exercise without myoglobinuria. A mild form is more likely to occur in females.

In type I deficiency, necrosis of muscle fibers, particularly type I fibers, occurs during attacks, followed by regeneration. Between attacks, muscle is normal. In type IIA, lipid bodies accumulate in the liver, and in type IIB, excess lipid is detected in heart, liver, kidneys, and skeletal muscle.

During attacks, CPT is either undetectable or greatly reduced in muscle. Dicarboxylic aciduria is absent. Assays are available for the measurement of CPT I and II in circulating lymphocytes and cultured fibroblasts.

There is no specific therapy except that directed at the myoglobinuria and its renal complications. A high-carbohydrate, low-fat diet, ingestion of frequent meals, and additional carbohydrate before and during exercise appear to reduce the number of attacks. Patients need to be instructed about the risks of prolonged exercise and skipped meals.

Secondary Systemic Carnitine Deficiency This is occasionally the result of severe dietary deprivation or impaired hepatic and renal function. Such instances have been observed in patients with alcoholic-nutritional diseases and kwashiorkor, in premature infants receiving parenteral nutrition, in patients with chronic renal failure undergoing dialysis, and rarely as a complication of valproate therapy. However, most cases of systemic carnitine deficiency are due to defects of β-oxidation, described below.

Other Rare Lipid Myopathies

Defects of β-Oxidation Rarely do these defects affect muscle alone or predominantly. Practically always, other features of disordered fatty acid metabolism—liver disease, hypoketotic hypoglycemia, Reye-like syndrome, SIDS, and so on—are present in some combination. All of the β-oxidative defects are characterized by dicarboxylic aciduria. The abnormal organic acid(s) in each case are determined by analysis of blood and urine; identification of the specific enzyme deficiency requires tissue analysis (liver and muscle homogenates, cultured fibroblasts). At the time of this writing, no less than eight specific defects of β-oxidation affecting muscle have been described; they are tabulated below.

Carnitine Acylcarnitine Translocase Deficiency This condition causes muscular weakness, cardiomyopathy, hypoketotic hypoglycemia, and hyperammonemia, which develop in early infancy, with death in the first month of life.

Long-Chain Acyl-CoA Dehydrogenase Deficiency (LCAD) The presentation is in infancy, with recurrent episodes of fasting hypoglycemic coma, muscle weakness, and myoglobinuria, and sometimes sudden death. Survivors may develop a progressive myopathy. Administration of carnitine improves the cardiac disorder and prevents metabolic attacks.

Medium-Chain Acyl-CoA Dehydrogenase Deficiency (MCAD) This is a cause of SIDS and a Reye-like syndrome. About half of survivors develop a lipid-storage myopathy in childhood or adult life. The abnormal gene has been mapped to chromosome 1p31. Oral L-carnitine may be of therapeutic value.

Short-Chain Acyl-CoA Dehydrogenase Deficiency (SCAD) This myopathy in a limb-girdle distribution may appear initially in older children and adults, or it may follow episodic metabolic disorders in infancy.

Long-Chain Hydroxyacyl-CoA Dehydrogenase Deficiency (HAD) This is a disease of infancy marked by episodes of Reye-like syndrome, hypoketotic hypoglycemia, lipid storage myopathy, cardiomyopathy, and sometimes sudden death.

Short-Chain Hydroxyacyl-CoA Dehydrogenase Deficiency (SCHAD) This presents as an episodic disorder like the one described above (HAD), but having its onset in adolescence. Recurrent attacks may be associated with myoglobinuria.

Multiple Acyl-CoA Dehydrogenase Deficiency (MADD); Glutaric Aciduria Type II (GA II) Some cases are caused by a deficiency of electron transfer flavoprotein (ETF) and others by a deficiency of electron transfer flavoprotein-coenzyme Q oxidoreductase (ETF-QO).

In the severest form of MADD, infants are born prematurely and many die within the first week of life; added to the common metabolic abnormalities are multiple congenital defects and a characteristic "sweaty feet" odor. In less severe cases, the congenital anomalies are absent. In the least severe form, the onset may be in late infancy (with episodic metabolic disturbances) or in childhood or adult life (with a lipid storage myopathy and a deficiency of serum and muscle carnitine). The prenatal diagnosis of GA II is suggested by the finding of large amounts of glutaric acid in the amniotic fluid. In the milder forms of the disease, oral riboflavin (100 to 300 mg/day) may be helpful.

Muscle Coenzyme Q10 Deficiency This condition presents as a slowly progressive lipid storage myopathy from early childhood. The basic defect is in coenzyme Q10 in the respiratory chain of muscle mitochondria. The feeding of coenzyme 10 has improved the myopathy.

Multisystem Triglyceride Storage Disease (Chanarin Disease) This abnormality of lipid metabolism is distinct from the β-oxidation defects. A progressive myopathy is combined with ichthyosis and neurologic manifestations, such as developmental delay, ataxia, neurosensory hearing loss, and microcephaly. The lipid material is stored in muscle as triglyceride droplets that are nonlysosomal and non-membrane-bound.

Mitochondrial Myopathies The genetic aspects of mitochondrial diseases and the diverse and overlapping clinical syndromes that constitute this category—including the myopathic ones—are discussed in Chap. 37.

THE ENDOCRINE MYOPATHIES

Thyroid Myopathies

Several myopathic diseases are related to alterations in thyroid function: (1) chronic thyrotoxic myopathy, (2) exophthalmic ophthalmoplegia (infiltrative ophthalmopathy), (3) myasthenia gravis associated with diffuse toxic goiter or with hypothyroidism, (4) periodic paralysis associated with toxic goiter, and (5) muscle hypertrophy and slow muscle contraction and relaxation associated with myxedema and cretinism. Although they are not common, we have encountered several examples of these diseases in a single year in a large general hospital.

Chronic Thyrotoxic Myopathy This disorder, first noted by Graves and Basedow in the early nineteenth century, is characterized by progressive weakness and wasting of the skeletal musculature, occurring in conjunction with overt or covert (masked) hyperthyroidism. The thyroid disease is usually chronic and the goiter is of the nodular rather than the diffuse type. Exophthalmos and other classic signs of hyperthyroidism are often present but need not be. This complication of hyperthyroidism is most frequent in middle age, and men are more susceptible than women. Some degree of myopathy has been found in more than 50 percent of thyrotoxic patients. The onset is insidious and the weakness progresses over weeks and months. The muscular disorder is most often mild to moderate in degree, but it may be so severe as to suggest progressive spinal muscular atrophy (motor system disease). Muscles of the pelvic girdle and thighs are weakened more than others (Basedow paraplegia), though all are affected to some extent, even the bulbar muscles and rarely the ocular ones. However, the shoulder and hand muscles show the most conspicuous atrophy. Tremor and twitching during contraction may occur, but we have not seen fasciculations. The tendon reflexes are of average briskness, possibly more lively than normal. Both the contraction and relaxation phases of the tendon reflexes are shortened, but usually this cannot be detected by the clinician. Serum concentrations of muscle enzymes are not increased and may be reduced. Usually the EMG is normal, without fibrillation potentials, though occasionally the action potentials are abnormally brief or polyphasic. Biopsies of muscle, except for slight atrophy of both type 1 and 2 fibers and an occasional degenerating fiber, have been normal. Administration of neostigmine has no effect. Muscle power and bulk are gradually restored when thyroid activity is reduced to normal levels.

Exophthalmic Ophthalmoplegia (Graves Ophthalmopathy) These terms refer to the concurrence of weakness of the external ocular muscles and exophthalmos in patients with Graves disease (pupillary and ciliary muscles are always spared). The exophthalmos varies in degree, sometimes being absent at an early stage of the disease, and is not in itself responsible for the muscle weakness. Often there is orbital pain. Both the exophthalmos and the weakness of the extraocular muscles may precede the signs of hyperthyroidism or may follow effective treatment of the disorder. The extraocular muscle palsies (and exophthalmos) may occasionally be unilateral, especially at the onset of the illness. Any of the external eye muscles may be affected, usually one more than others, accounting for strabismus and diplopia; the inferior and medial recti are the most frequently affected, but upward movements are usually limited as well. The typical but not invariable sign of lid retraction imparts a staring appearance. Subtle exophthalmos can be appreciated by standing above and behind the seated patient and observing the relative positions of the lids and the eyelashes. Conjunctival edema and vascular engorgement over the insertions of the medial and lateral rectus muscles can be appreciated by inspecting the globe in its extreme lateral positions. In advanced cases, the enlarged muscle insertions themselves can be appreciated. These swollen muscles are visible on orbital ultrasound, CT, and MRI.

Examination of the eye muscles in biopsy and autopsy material has shown prominent fibroblastic tissue, many degenerated fibers, and infiltrations of lymphocytes, mononuclear leukocytes, and lipocytes; hence the term *infiltrative ophthalmopathy*. These histopathologic findings are suggestive of a specific autoimmune disease—a hypothesis supported by the finding of serum antibodies that react with extracts of eye muscles (Kodama et al). Possibly the antibodies target glycosaminoglycans of the orbital fibroblasts. β-Adrenergic sensitivity of muscle fibers caused by excessive thyroid hormone has been also postulated. Other factors may be involved, such as the small size of oculomotor motor units, the absence of dystrophin, and the rich mitochondrial content of these specialized muscles. The condition often runs a self-limited course, as does the exophthalmos, and therapy is difficult to evaluate. Certainly the maintenance of a euthyroid state is desirable (Dresner and Kennerdell).

If the exophthalmos is slight, topical applications of adrenergic blocking agents (guanethidine eye drops, 5%) and ophthalmic ointment to prevent corneal drying are adequate. Severe exophthalmos, marked by periorbital and conjunctival edema, and the extraocular muscle weakness may be partially controlled by high doses of corticosteroids (about 80 mg prednisone per day). Because of the hazards of protracted corticosteroid therapy, it should be reserved for patients who would otherwise require surgical intervention. In a number of such cases it has been possible for the patient treated with corticosteroids to weather the crisis and avoid the damaging effects of extreme exophthalmos and risks of surgery. Exophthalmos of a degree that threatens to injure the cornea or cause blindness requires tarsorrhaphy or decompression by removal of the roof of the bony orbit.

Thyrotoxic Periodic Paralysis This disorder resembles familial periodic paralysis (page 1562) and consists of attacks of mild to severe weakness of the muscles of the trunk and limbs; usually the cranial muscles are spared. The weakness develops over a period of a few minutes or hours and lasts for part of a day or longer. In some series of patients with periodic paralysis, as many as half have had hyperthyroidism and many of them have been Asian males. Unlike the typical hypokalemic form, thyrotoxic periodic paralysis is not a familial disorder, and its onset is usually in early adult life. Nevertheless, in most of the thyrotoxic cases, the serum potassium levels have been low during the attacks of weakness, and the administration of 100 to 200 mg of potassium chloride has terminated the attacks. Propranolol in doses of 160 mg daily in divided doses is helpful in preventing the attacks. Effective treatment of the hyperthyroidism abolishes the periodic attacks of weakness in more than 90 percent of cases. Other aspects of periodic paralysis are discussed in Chap. 54.

Myasthenia Gravis with Hyperthyroidism Myasthenia is discussed fully in Chap. 53. Here only a few remarks are made on its special relationship to thyrotoxicosis. Myasthenia gravis, in its typical autoimmune, anticholinesterase-responsive form, may accompany hyper- or, rarely, hypothyroidism, which are also considered to be autoimmune diseases. Approximately 5 percent of myasthenic patients have hyperthyroidism, and the frequency of myasthenia gravis in hyperthyroid patients is 20 to 30 times that in the general population. Either condition may appear first, or they may coincide. The weakness and atrophy of chronic thyrotoxic myopathy may be added to the myasthenia without appearing to affect the requirement for or response to neostigmine. By contrast, hypothyroidism, even of mild degree, seems to aggravate the myasthenia gravis, greatly increasing the need for pyridostigmine and at times inducing a myasthenic crisis. Also, in the latter case, thyroxine is beneficial and, with respect to myasthenia, restores the patient to the status that existed before the onset of thyroid insufficiency. The myasthenia should be regarded as an autoimmune disease independent of the thyroid disease, and each must be treated separately.

Hypothyroid Myopathy Abnormalities of skeletal muscle—consisting of diffuse myalgia and increased volume, stiffness, and slowness of contraction and relaxation—are common manifestations of hypothyroidism, whether in the form of myxedema or cretinism. These changes probably account for the large tongue and dysarthria that one observes in myxedema. The presence of action myospasm and myokymia (both of which are rare) and of percussion myoedema and slowness of both the contraction and relaxation phases of tendon reflexes assists the examiner in making a bedside diagnosis. Cretinism in association with these muscle abnormalities is known as the *Kocher-Debré-Semelaigne syndrome*, and myxedema in childhood or adult life with muscle hypertrophy as the *Hoffmann syndrome*; the latter simulates hypertrophia musculorum vera and myotonia congenita. In neither cretinism nor myxedema, however, is there evidence of true myotonia, either by clinical test or by EMG, although muscle action potentials are myopathic and often show bizarre high-frequency discharges. Serum transaminase values are normal, but CK levels are usually elevated, often markedly so. Serum globulin may also be increased. Muscle biopsies have disclosed only the presence of large fibers or an increase in the proportion of small fibers (either type 1 or 2) and slight distention of the sarcoplasmic reticulum and subsarcolemmal glycogen (probably all due to disuse atrophy).

The administration of thyroxine corrects the muscle disturbance.

Pathogenesis of the Thyroid Myopathies How thyroid hormone affects the muscle fiber is still a matter of conjecture. Clinical data indicate that thyroxine influences the contractile process in some manner but does not interfere with the transmission of impulses in the peripheral nerve, across the myoneural junction, or along the sarcolemma. In hyperthyroidism this functional disorder enhances the speed of the contractile process and reduces its duration, the net effect being fatigability, weakness, and loss of endurance of muscle action. In hypothyroidism, muscle contraction is slowed, as is relaxation, and its duration is prolonged.

The speed of the contractile process is thought to be related to the quantity of myosin adenosinetriphosphatase (ATPase), which is increased in hyperthyroid muscle and decreased in hypothyroid muscle. The speed of relaxation depends on the rate of release and reaccumulation of calcium in the endoplasmic reticulum. This is slowed in hypothyroidism and increased in hyperthyroidism (Ianuzzo et al). The myopathic effects of hypothyroidism need always to be distinguished from those of a neuropathy, which may rarely complicate hypothyroidism (page 1414).

Corticosteroid Polymyopathies

The widespread use of adrenal corticosteroids has created a class of muscle diseases similar to the one that occurs in the Cushing syndrome (Müller and Kugelberg). A deficiency of corticosteroids, as occurs in Addison disease, also causes generalized weakness, but without an identifiable muscle disease.

Corticosteroid Myopathy The prolonged use of corticosteroids causes the proximal limb and girdle musculature to become weak, to the point where the patient has difficulty in elevating the arms and arising from a sitting, squatting, or kneeling position; walking, particularly up stairs, may also be hampered. The EMG is either normal or mildly myopathic, with small and abundant action potentials but no fibrillations. Biopsies disclose only a slight variation in fiber size, with atrophic fibers, mainly of type 2b, but little or no fiber necrosis and no inflammatory cells. Electron microscopically, there are aggregates of mitochondria, accumulations of glycogen and lipid, and slight myofibrillar loss (disuse atrophy). The serum CK and aldolase are usually normal. These changes are the same as those that characterize Cushing disease and may suggest that diagnosis (page 715).

There is only a poor correlation between the total dose of corticosteroid and the severity of muscle weakness.

Nevertheless, in patients who develop this type of myopathy, the corticosteroid dosage has usually been high and sustained over a period of months or years. All corticosteroids may produce the disorder, although fluorinated ones are said to be more culpable than others. Discontinuation or reduction of corticosteroid administration leads to gradual improvement and recovery. The mechanism by which corticosteroids cause muscle weakness is not known. In corticosteroid-treated animals, there is a measurable decrease in amino acid uptake and protein synthesis.

Acute Steroid Myopathy (Critical Illness Myopathy; Acute Quadriplegic Myopathy) In addition to the well-known proximal myopathy induced by the long-term use of steroids, an acute and severe myopathy has been recognized. It is seen most often in critical care units, typically among patients with severe intractable asthma but also among others with numerous systemic diseases who are being treated with high doses of corticosteroids—and rarely in those with sepsis and shock alone. The use of neuromuscular blocking agents plays an important complementary role in the genesis of this myopathy, being a factor in over 80 percent of reported cases, but it is uncertain whether they alone can produce a similar process (see reviews by Gorson and Ropper, by Lacomis et al, and by Barohn et al).

The severe muscle weakness becomes evident when the systemic illness subsides, and it greatly slows weaning from the ventilator. The tendon reflexes are normal or diminished and there may be confounding features of a polyneuropathy, which can also be induced by critical illness and sepsis (page 1388). Most of our patients have recovered over a period of many weeks after the offending agent has been withdrawn, but a few have remained weak for as long as a year. Patients who acquire this problem have generally been exposed to high doses of corticosteroids, albeit for brief periods in some cases. Exceptional instances have been reported in which the myopathy was induced by doses as low as 60 mg prednisone administered for 5 days, but we have not encountered cases such as these. Likewise, the amount of simultaneous exposure to neuromuscular blocking agents, when they have been implicated, has varied, the total dose falling in the range of 500 to 4000 mg of pancuronium or its equivalent.

Serum CK is usually elevated, at least early in the process. The EMG discloses the characteristic features of a myopathy; often there are fibrillations as well, attributable to separation of the motor end-plate region from intact segments of muscle fibers. Polyneuropathy and residual neuromuscular blockade can be excluded by appropriate electrophysiologic studies. Muscle biopsy shows varying degrees of necrosis and vacuolation affecting mainly type 2 fibers. There is a striking loss of thick (myosin) filaments that is thought by some to be highly characteristic of the process. The most severe degrees of muscle necrosis have been accompanied by massively elevated CK levels and by myoglobinuria and renal failure.

Several experimental observations explain the apparent additive effect on muscle of steroids and neuromuscular blocking agents. Animals exposed to high doses of steroids after muscle denervation display a selective loss of myosin, which is characteristic of this disease. The depletion of myosin is reversed by reinnervation but not by withdrawal of the corticosteroids. Furthermore, denervation of muscle has been found to induce an increase in glucocorticoid receptors in the muscle. Dubois and Almon have postulated that exposure to neuromuscular blocking agents creates a functional denervation, rendering the muscle fiber vulnerable to the damaging effects of steroids. It is curious that this myopathy has not been seen with high-dose corticosteroid administration for neurologic diseases such as multiple sclerosis, but the observation of Panegyres and colleagues of a myasthenic patient who developed a severe, myosin-depleted myopathy following high doses of methylprednisolone supports a dual action of denervation (at the postsynaptic membrane) and glucocorticoids.

Adrenocortical Insufficiency

Generalized weakness and fatigability are characteristic of adrenocortical insufficiency, whether it be *primary* in type, i.e., due to *Addison disease* (infectious, neoplastic, or autoimmune destruction of the adrenal glands or adrenal hemorrhage) or secondary to a pituitary deficiency of adrenocorticotropic hormone (ACTH). The weakness and fatigability are related to the water and electrolyte disturbances and hypotension. Rarely, a permanent contracture of hamstring muscles develops, preventing upright stance. Biopsy has not disclosed any abnormalities of muscle, and postmortem examination of the muscle in one such case showed no changes. The EMG is normal, and the tendon reflexes are retained. Addisonian weakness (and hyperkalemic paralysis) respond to glucocorticoid and mineralocorticoid replacement.

Primary Aldosteronism Production of an excess of aldosterone by adrenal adenomas has been the subject of many articles, one of the earliest and most notable being that of Conn. Muscular weakness has been observed in three-quarters of the reported cases, and in nearly half of them there was either hypokalemic periodic paralysis or tetany. Chronic potassium deficiency may express itself either by periodic weakness or by a chronic myopathic weakness. An associated alkalosis causes the tetany.

Diseases of Parathyroid Glands and Vitamin D Deficiency

A small proportion of patients with parathyroid adenomas complain of weakness and fatigability. Vicale described the first example of this disorder and remarked on the muscular atrophy and weakness and the pain on passive or active movement. The tendon reflexes were retained. A few scattered muscle fibers had undergone degeneration. Claims for a denervative process are disputed. We have not been impressed with either a myopathy or neuropathy in this disease.

In *hypoparathyroidism*, muscle cramping is prominent but there are no other neuromuscular manifestations. In both hypoparathyroidism and pseudohypoparathyroidism—the latter with characteristic skeletal abnormalities and, in some instances, mental backwardness—the most important muscle abnormality is *tetany*. This is due to low ionized serum calcium, which depolarizes axons more than muscle fibers (see page 1465).

In *osteomalacia*, due to vitamin D deficiency and disorders of renal tubular absorption, muscle weakness and pain have been common complaints, similar to those in patients with primary hyperparathyroidism and uremia (see Layzer for further comment).

More striking than any of the foregoing disturbances, in our view, has been a chronic proximal myopathy in conjunction with hypophosphatemia and solitary bone cysts. In two of our patients, removal of the cyst restored serum phosphorus levels and cured the muscle weakness. Hypophosphatemic myopathic weakness has also been noted in a number of our patients in a critical care unit. The onset can be so abrupt when precipitated by hyperalimentation solutions as to simulate the Guillain-Barré syndrome. The oral administration of phosphates to raise the serum phosphorus has been beneficial in the nonneoplastic cases. Some of the latter are accompanied by pain and stiffness. Presumably the phosphorus depletion in these disorders had limited the phosphorylation reactions and the synthesis of ATP.

Diseases of the Pituitary Gland

Proximal muscle weakness and atrophy have been recorded as late developments in many acromegalic patients. Formerly thought to be due to neuropathy, these symptoms have been convincingly shown by Mastaglia and colleagues to be the result of a chronic polymyopathy. The serum CK is slightly elevated in some cases, and myopathic potentials are observed in the EMG. Biopsy specimens have shown atrophy and reduced numbers of type 2 fibers and necrosis of only a few fibers. Treatment of the pituitary adenoma and correction of the hormonal changes restores strength. A mild peripheral neuropathy of sensorimotor type has also been reported in a few acromegalic patients but is less frequent than the carpal tunnel syndrome.

MYOPATHIES DUE TO DRUGS AND TOXINS

A vast number of drugs and other chemical agents have been identified as myotoxic. Curry and colleagues, in 1989, found reports (in the English literature alone) of about a hundred drugs that had caused rhabdomyolysis and myoglobinuria. The list continues to grow, and additional myotoxic agents can be expected to appear as new drugs are introduced. It is not practical to describe the myotoxins individually; they are categorized and their main features are listed in Table 51-2.

Toxic agents produce myopathic changes in several ways. They may act directly on muscle cells, either diffusely or locally, as occurs with intramuscular injections, or the muscle damage can be secondary to a diverse number of factors—electrolyte disturbances (hypokalemia), renal failure, excessive energy requirements of muscle (as occur with drug-induced seizures and malignant hyperthermia), or inadequate delivery of oxygen and nutrients (drug-induced coma with compressive-ischemic injury of muscle).

Several clinical features mark a myopathy as toxic in nature: lack of pre-existing muscular symptoms; delay in onset of symptoms after exposure to a putative toxin; lack of any other cause for the myopathy; and often complete or partial resolution of symptoms after withdrawal of the toxic agent. Pathologically, this group of disorders is characterized by nonspecific myopathic changes, which in severe degrees take the form of myonecrosis (rhabdomyolysis) and myoglobinuria; the latter is the

Table 51-2
Features of toxin-induced myopathies

Myopathic syndrome	*Agent*	*Risk factors*
Necrotizing myopathy (rhabdomyolysis)	1. Alcohol abuse	1. Cyclosporine/gemfibrozil
	2. Clofibrate, gemfibrozil	2. Renal failure
	3. Epsilon-aminocaproic acid	3. Therapy duration >4 weeks
	4. Lovastatin, pravastatin, simvastatin	
	5. Hypervitaminosis E	5. Uncontrolled self-medication
	6. Organophosphates	6. Accidental insecticide exposure
	7. Snake venoms	
	8. High-dose corticosteroids in critical illness	
	9. Mushroom poisoning (*Amanita phalloides*)	
	10. Cocaine	
Myoglobinuria	Wide variety of agents (see text)	
Steroid myopathy	1. Acute	High IV steroid doses, ventilated patients on pancuronium
	2. Chronic	2. Daily prednisone >10 mg
Hypokalemic myopathy	1. Diuretics	Fasting, exercise
	2. Laxatives	
	3. Licorice, carbenoxolone	
	4. Amphotericin B, toluene	
	5. Alcohol abuse	
Amphiphillic cationic drug myopathy (lysosomal storage, "lipidosis")	1. Chloroquine, hydroxychloroquine, quinacrine, plasmocid	1. Daily chloroquine dose > 500 mg
	2. Amiodarone	
	3. Perhexiline	
Impaired protein synthesis	Ipecac syrup, emetine	Eating disorders, >600 mg in 10 days
Antimicrotubular myopathy	1. Colchicine	1. Chronic renal failure
	2. Vincristine	
Inflammatory myopathy	1. D-penicillamine	
	2. Procainamide	
	3. Cimetidine? Ciguatera toxin?	
Fasciitis, perimyositis, microangiopathy	1. Toxic oil syndrome	1. Rapeseed oil, Spain, 1981
	2. Eosinophilia-myalgia syndrome	2. Tryptophan products, 1989
Mitochondrial myopathy	1. Zidovudine	
	2. Germanium	
Various	1. Cyclosporine	
	2. Labetalol	
	3. Anthracycline antibiotics	
	4. Rifampin, amiodarone	
Myopathy due to IM injections	1. Acute: IM injection of various drugs—e.g., cephalothin, lidocaine, diazepam	
	2. Chronic: Repeated IM injections—e.g., pethidine, pentazocine, intravenous drug abuse, antibiotics (in children)	Genetic factor ?

Clinical features	*Pathology*	*Laboratory findings*[a]
Acute/subacute painful proximal myopathy; tendon reflexes usually preserved	Necrosis, regeneration	CK ↑ ↑, myoglobinuria +/−
5. Painless	5. Paracrystalline inclusion bodies	
7. Severe, acute intoxication		
	9. Loss of myosin	
Severe muscle pain, swelling flaccid, quadriparesis, areflexia possible, acute renal failure	Severe necrosis, regeneration	CK ↑ ↑ ↑, myoglobinuria +++
Severe proximal and distal weakness	Type 1 and 2 fibers; vacuolar changes, regeneration,	CK ↑ ↑, myoglobinuria +
2. Proximal atrophy, weakness	2. Type 2 fiber atrophy	Blood lymphocytosis
Weakness may be periodic, reflexes may be depressed or absent, rarely severe myoglobinuria	Necrosis, regeneration, vacuolization	CK ↑ ↑, myoglobinuria +/−, hypokalemia
Proximal muscle pain and weakness, sensorimotor neuropathy, cardiomyopathy	1. Chloroquine: vacuole formation, optically dense structures	CK ↑
Myalgia, proximal weakness, cardiomyopathy	Focal mitochondrial loss, vacuoles	CK ↑
Proximal weakness, peripheral neuropathy; CK may be normal	Vacuolar myopathy (rimmed vacuoles)	CK ↑
Proximal muscle pain, weakness, skin changes possible	Inflammation, necrosis, regeneration,	CK ↑, myoglobinuria +/−
Myalgia, skin changes, peripheral neuropathy, other systems also affected	Vasculitis, connective tissue infiltration	Eosinophilia
Proximal myalgia and weakness	1. Ragged red fibers, necrosis, regeneration	CK normal or ↑
3. Humans: only cardiomyopathy		
Local pain, swelling, sometimes abscess formation	Focal necrosis	CK ↑
Induration and contracture of injected muscles	Marked fibrosis and myopathic changes	Normal

[a]CK (serum creatinine kinase): ↑ (mild), ↑ ↑ (moderate), ↑ ↑ ↑ (marked) elevations; myoglobinuria: +/− (may be present).
Source: Adapted from Victor and Sieb by permission.

most frequent and serious myotoxic syndrome and is discussed below, along with its more important causes.

Necrotizing Polymyopathy (Rhabdomyolysis) with Myoglobinuria In any disease that results in rapid destruction of striated muscle fibers (rhabdomyolysis), myoglobin and other muscle proteins may enter the bloodstream and appear in the urine. The latter is "cola"-colored (burgundy red or brown), much like the urine in hemoglobinuria. In hemoglobinuria, however, the serum is initially pink, because hemoglobin (but not myoglobin) is bound to haptoglobin, and this complex is not excreted in the urine as readily as myoglobin (also, the hemoglobin molecule is three times as large as the myoglobin molecule). The hemoglobin-haptoglobin complex is removed from the blood plasma over a period of hours, and if hemolysis continues, the haptoglobin may be depleted, so that hemoglobinuria is present without grossly evident hemoglobinemia. Differentiation of the two pigments in urine is difficult; both are guaiac-positive and may be detected by a "dipstick." Only very small differences are seen on spectroscopic examination. The most sensitive means of detecting myoglobin is by radioimmunoassay.

Many of the causes of myonecrosis and myoglobinuria have already been mentioned. Myoglobinuria may be detected in cases of acute inflammatory myopathy, in several types of glycogenosis (Table 51-1), in carnitine palmityltransferase deficiency, and as a result of poisoning or therapeutic use of a vast array of drugs (including the combination of steroids and pancuronium, discussed above), toxins, and venoms (see Table 51-2). Myoglobinuria is an important feature of many other conditions: crush injury; extensive infarction of muscle; excessive use or repeated injury of muscles (as occurs in status epilepticus, generalized tetanus, malignant neuroleptic syndrome, agitated delirium, prolonged marching, conga drumming, or simply excessive exercise—although the latter always suggests an underlying metabolic disease of muscle); electrical and lightning injuries; etc. Two noteworthy conditions that are characterized by myonecrosis and myoglobinuria are acute alcoholic intoxication and malignant hyperthermia. The former is described below and the latter in Chap. 54, with the membrane channel disorders.

Regardless of the cause of the rhabdomyolysis, the affected muscles become painful and tender within a few hours. Power of contraction is diminished. Sometimes the skin and subcutaneous tissues overlying the affected muscles (nearly always of the limbs and sometimes of the trunk) are swollen and congested. There may be a low-grade fever. Apart from the discoloration of the urine, albumin excretion rises, and there is a leukocytosis. If myoglobinuria is mild, recovery occurs within a few days and there is only a residual albuminuria. When myoglobinuria is severe, renal damage may ensue and lead to anuria. The mechanism of the renal damage is not clear; probably it is not simply a mechanical obstruction of tubules by precipitated myoglobin. It is more likely to occur with massive rhabdomyolysis and very high CK levels in the serum. Alkalinization of the urine by ingestion or infusion of sodium bicarbonate is said to protect the kidneys by preventing myoglobin casts, but in severe cases it is of doubtful value, and the sodium may actually be harmful if anuria has already developed. Therapy is the same as for the anuria that follows shock (see *Harrison's Principles of Internal Medicine*).

Alcoholic Myopathy Several forms of muscle weakness have been ascribed to alcoholism. In one type, a painless and predominantly proximal weakness develops over a period of several days or weeks in the course of a prolonged drinking bout and is associated with severe degrees of *hypokalemia* (serum levels <2 meq/L). The urinary excretion of potassium is not significantly increased; depletion is probably the result of vomiting and diarrhea, which usually precede the onset of muscular weakness. In addition, serum levels of liver and muscle enzymes are markedly elevated. Biopsies from severely weakened muscles show single-fiber necrosis and vacuolation. Treatment consists of the administration of potassium chloride intravenously (about 120 meq daily for several days), after which oral administration suffices. Strength returns gradually in 7 to 14 days, and enzyme levels return to normal concomitantly.

Another type of myopathic syndrome, occurring acutely at the height of a prolonged drinking bout, is manifest by severe pain, tenderness, and edema of the muscles of the limbs and trunk, accompanied in severe cases by renal damage and hyperpotassemia (Hed et al). The muscle affection is generalized in some patients and remarkably focal in others. A swollen, painful, tender limb or part of a limb may give the appearance of a deep phlebothrombosis or lymphatic obstruction. Myonecrosis is reflected by high serum levels of CK and aldolase and the appearance of myoglobin in the urine, leading in some cases to fatal myoglobinuric nephrosis. In a general hospital, alcoholism is the commonest cause of rhabdomyolysis and myoglobinuria. Some patients recover within a few weeks, but others require several months, and relapse during another drinking spree occurs frequently. Restoration of motor power is attendant upon regeneration but may be complicated by polyneuropathy and other syndromes of neuromuscular disability associated with alcoholism. Haller and Drachman have produced rhabdomyolysis (with elevated CK and myoglobinuria) in rats by subjecting the animals to a brief fast following a 2- to 4-week exposure to alcohol, suggesting that a similar mechanism may be operative in alcoholic individuals.

Perkoff and his associates described what is presumably another form of acute muscular disorder in alcoholics, characterized by severe muscular cramps and diffuse weakness, occurring in the course of a sustained drinking bout. They noted a number of biochemical abnormalities in these patients as well as in asymptomatic alcoholics who had been drinking heavily for a sustained period before admission to the hospital—elevated serum levels of CK, myoglobinuria, and a diminished rise in blood lactic acid in response to ischemic exercise, as occurs in McArdle disease. In distinction to the latter, however, myophosphorylase levels were not consistently reduced in the alcoholic patients. How these biochemical abnormalities are related to muscle cramps and weakness is a matter of speculation.

From time to time one observes in alcoholics the subacute or chronic evolution of painless weakness and atrophy of the proximal muscles of the limbs, especially of the legs, with only minimal signs of neuropathy in the distal segments of the legs and feet. Cases such as these have been referred to as *chronic alcoholic myopathy*, implying a direct toxic effect of alcohol on muscle, but the data are insufficient to warrant such an assumption. Some of these cases have shown necrosis of individual muscle fibers and other signs of polymyositis; most cases seen by the authors have proved to be neuropathic in nature. This has been the experience of others as well (Faris and Reyes; Rossouw et al). Treatment follows along the lines indicated for nutritional-alcoholic neuropathy (page 1214), and complete recovery can be expected if the patient abstains from alcohol and maintains a regimen of good nutrition.

REFERENCES

Barohn RJ, Jackson CE, Rogers SJ, et al: Prolonged paralysis due to non-depolarizing neuromuscular blocking agents and corticosteroids. *Muscle Nerve* 17:647, 1994.

Braakhekke JP, De Bruin MI, Stegeman DF, et al: The second wind phenomenon in McArdle's disease. *Brain* 109:1087, 1986.

Conn JW: Aldosteronism in man: Some clinical and climatological aspects. *JAMA* 183:871, 1963.

Cori GT, Cori CF: Glucose-6-phosphatase of the liver in glycogen storage disease. *J Biol Chem* 199:661, 1952.

Curry SC, Chang D, Connor D: Drug and toxin-induced rhabdomyolysis. *Ann Emerg Med* 18:1068, 1989.

DiDonato S: Disorders of lipid metabolism affecting skeletal muscle: Carnitine deficiency syndromes, defects in the catabolic pathway, and Chanarin disease, in Engel AG, Franzini-Armstrong C (eds): *Myology*, 2nd ed. New York, McGraw-Hill, 1994, pp 1587–1609.

DiMauro S, Melis-DiMauro P: Muscle carnitine palmitoyltransferase deficiency and myoglobinuria. *Science* 182:929, 1973.

DiMauro S, Tonin P, Servidei S: Metabolic myopathies, in Vinken PJ, Bruyn GW (eds): *Handbook of Clinical Neurology*. Vol 18. Amsterdam, North Holland, 1992, pp 479–526.

Dresner SC, Kennerdell JS: Dysthyroid orbitopathy. *Neurology* 35:1628, 1985.

Dubois DC, Almon RR: A possible role for glucocorticoids in denervation atrophy. *Muscle Nerve* 4:370, 1981.

Engel AG, Angelini C: Carnitine deficiency of human skeletal muscle with associated lipid storage myopathy: A new syndrome. *Science* 179:899, 1973.

Engel AG, Franzini-Armstrong C (eds): *Myology*, 2nd ed. New York, McGraw-Hill, 1994, pp 1533–1768.

Engel WK, Vick NK, Glueck J, Levy RI: A skeletal muscle disorder associated with intermittent symptoms and a possible defect in lipid metabolism. *N Engl J Med* 282:697, 1970.

Faris AA, Reyes MG: Reappraisal of alcoholic myopathy: Clinical and biopsy study on chronic alcoholics without muscle weakness or wasting. *J Neurol Neurosurg Psychiatry* 34:86, 1971.

Gorson KC, Ropper AH: Generalized paralysis in the intensive care unit: Emphasis on the complications of neuromuscular blocking agents and corticosteroids. *J Int Care Med* 11:219, 1996.

Griggs RC, Mendell JR, Miller RG: *Evaluation and Treatment of Myopathies*. Philadelphia, Davis, 1995.

Haller RG, Drachman DB: Alcoholic rhabdomyolysis: An experimental model in the rat. *Science* 208:412, 1980.

Hed R, Lundmark C, Fahlgren H, Orell S: Acute muscular syndrome in chronic alcoholism. *Acta Med Scand* 171:585, 1962.

Hers HG: Alpha-glucosidase deficiency in generalized glycogen storage disease (Pompe's disease). *Biochem J* 86:11, 1963.

Ianuzzo D, Patel P, Chen V, et al: Thyroidal trophic influence on skeletal muscle myosin. *Nature* 270:74, 1977.

Illingworth B, Cori GT: Structure of glycogens and amylopectins: III. Normal and abnormal human glycogen. *J Biol Chem* 199:653, 1952.

Illingworth B, Larner J, Cori GT: Structure of glucogens and amylopectins: I. Enzymatic determination of chain length. *J Biol Chem* 199:631, 1952.

Kodama K, Sikorska H, Bandy-Dafoe P, et al: Demonstration of circulating autoantibody against a soluble eye-muscle antigen in Graves' ophthalmopathy. *Lancet* 2:1353, 1982.

Kono N, Mineo I, Simsumi S, et al: Metabolic basis of improved exercise tolerance: Muscle phosphorylase deficiency after glucagon administration. *Neurology* 34:1417, 1984.

LACOMIS D, GIULIANI MJ, VAN COTT A, KRAMER DJ: Acute myopathy of intensive care: Clinical, electromyographic, and pathological aspects. *Ann Neurol* 40:645, 1996.

LARNER J, ILLINGWORTH B, CORI GT, CORI CF: Structure of glycogens and amylopectins: II. Analysis by stepwise enzymatic degradation. *J Biol Chem* 199:641, 1952.

LAYZER RB: *Neuromuscular Manifestations of Systemic Disease.* Philadelphia, Davis, 1985.

LAYZER RB, ROWLAND LP, RANNEY HM: Muscle phosphofructokinase deficiency. *Arch Neurol* 17:512, 1967.

MASTAGLIA FL, BARWICH DD, HALL R: Myopathy in acromegaly. *Lancet* 2:907, 1970.

MCARDLE B: Myopathy due to a defect in muscle glycogen breakdown. *Clin Sci* 10:13, 1951.

MEINCK HM, GOEBEL HH, RUMPF KW, et al: The forearm ischaemic work test—Hazardous to McArdle patients? *J Neurol Neurosurg Psychiatry* 45:1144, 1982.

MÜLLER R, KUGELBERG E: Myopathy in Cushing's syndrome. *J Neurol Neurosurg Psychiatry* 22:314, 1959.

PANEGYRES PK, SQUIER M, MILLS KR, NEWSOM-DAVIS J: Acute myopathy associated with large parenteral dose of corticosteroid in myasthenia gravis. *J Neurol Neurosurg Psychiatry* 56:702, 1993.

PERKOFF GT, HARDY P, VELEZ-GARCIA E: Reversible acute muscular syndrome in chronic alcoholism. *N Engl J Med* 274:1277, 1966.

ROE CR, COATES PM: Mitochondrial fatty acid oxidation disorders, in Scriver CR, Beaudet AL, Sly WS, Valle D (eds): *The Metabolic and Molecular Bases of Inherited Disease*, 7th ed. New York, McGraw-Hill, 1995, pp 1501–1533.

ROSSOUW JE, KEETON RJ, HEWLETT RH: Chronic proximal muscular weakness in alcoholics. *S Afr Med J* 50:2095, 1976.

SIVAK ED, SALANGA VD, WILBOURN AJ, et al: Adult onset acid maltase deficiency presenting as diaphragmatic paralysis. *Ann Neurol* 9:613, 1981.

SLONIM AE, GOANS PH: Myopathy in McArdle's syndrome: Improvement with a high protein diet. *N Engl J Med* 312:355, 1985.

SLONIM AE, WEISBERG MD, BENKE P: Reversal of debrancher deficiency myopathy by the use of high protein nutrition. *Ann Neurol* 11:420, 1982.

SPECTOR RH, CARLISLE JA: Minimal thyroid ophthalmopathy. *Neurology* 37:1803, 1987.

UMPLEBY AM, WILES CM, TREND PS, et al: Protein turnover in acid maltase deficiency before and after treatment with a high protein diet. *J Neurol Neurosurg Psychiatry* 50:587, 1987.

VICALE CT: The diagnostic features of a muscular syndrome resulting from hyperparathyroidism, osteomalacia owing to renal tubular acidosis, and perhaps to related disorders of calcium metabolism. *Trans Am Neurol Assoc* 74:143, 1949.

VICTOR M, SIEB JP: Myopathies due to drugs, toxins, and nutritional deficiency, in Engel AG, Franzini-Armstrong C (eds): *Myology*, 2nd ed. New York, McGraw-Hill, 1994, pp 1697–1725.

Chapter 52

THE CONGENITAL NEUROMUSCULAR DISORDERS

Included under this title are two sizable groups of muscle diseases—one is a group of congenital deformities that involve muscle, and the other is a unique class of hereditary muscle diseases known as the congenital myopathies. Insofar as all of the disorders comprising these categories develop in utero, i.e., are congenital, it may be helpful, by way of introduction, to summarize briefly the main facts about the development and aging of muscle. Such diseases are of particular importance in pediatric neurology, for most of them attract notice at an early age.

The Development and Aging of Muscle

The commonly accepted view of the embryogenesis of muscle is that muscle fibers form originally by fusion of myoblasts soon after the latter differentiate from somatic mesodermal cells. Muscle connective tissue derives from somatopleural mesoderm. The myoblasts, which are postmitotic, are spindle-shaped mononuclear cells that fuse to form muscle fibers. After fusion, a series of transcriptive cellular events leads to myofibril formation. The newly formed fibers are thin, centrally nucleated tubes (appropriately called *myotubes*) in which myofilaments begin to be produced from polyribosomes. As myofilaments become organized into myofibrils, the nuclei of the muscle fiber are displaced peripherally to a subsarcolemmal position. Once the nuclei assume a peripheral position, the myofiber is formed. The detailed mechanisms whereby myoblasts seek one another, the manner in which each of a series of fused nuclei contribute to the myotube, the formation of actin and myosin fibrils, and the differentiation of a small residue of satellite cells on the surface of the fibers are reviewed by Franzini-Armstrong and Fischman.

The mechanisms that determine the number and arrangement of fibers in each muscle are not as well understood. Presumably the myoblasts themselves possess the genetic information that controls the program of development, but within any given species there are wide familial and individual variations, which account for obvious differences in the size of muscles and their power of contraction.

The number of fibers assigned to each muscle is probably attained by birth, and growth of muscle thereafter depends mainly on the enlargement of fibers. Although the nervous system and musculature develop independently, muscle fibers continue to grow after birth only when they are active and under the influence of nerve. Measurements of muscle fiber diameters from birth to old age show the growth curve ascending rapidly in the early postnatal years and less rapidly in adolescence, reaching a peak during the third decade. After puberty, growth of muscle is less in females than in males, and such differences are greater in the arm, shoulder, thigh, and pelvic muscles than in those of the leg; growth in ocular muscles is about equal in the two sexes. At all ages, disuse of muscle decreases fiber size by as much as 30 percent (at the expense of myofibrils), and overuse increases the size by about the same amount (work hypertrophy). Normally, type 1 (oxidative enzyme–rich) fibers are slightly smaller than type 2 (phosphorylative enzyme–rich) fibers; the proportions of the two fiber types vary in different muscles in accordance with their natural functions.

During late adult life and the senium, the number of muscle fibers diminishes and variation in fiber size increases. The variations are of two types: *group atrophy*, in which clusters of 20 to 30 fibers are all reduced in diameter to about the same extent, and *random single-fiber atrophy*. Also, there is enlargement of other fibers. The exercising of young animal muscle causes a hypertrophy of high-oxidative type 1 fibers and an increase in the proportion of low-oxidative type 2 fibers; aging muscle lacks this capacity—exercise produces only an increase in the proportion of type 2 fibers (Silbermann et al). No such data are available in humans, but clinical observation informs us that with aging, the capacity of muscle to respond to intense, sustained exercise is diminished. Also, muscle cells, like other cells of postmitotic type, are subject to aging changes (lipofuscin accumulation, autophagic vacuolization, enzyme loss) and to death. Group atrophy, present in 90 percent of gastrocnemii in individuals more than 60 years of age, represents denervation effect from loss of lumbar motor neurons and peripheral nerve fibers.

Derangements of the Life Cycle of Muscle Fibers

These have not been fully ascertained, but one can envision the following possibilities: (1) failure of myoblasts to differentiate in a given region, manifest by a congenital absence of muscle; (2) congenital hypoplasia, local or universal; (3) congenital hyperplasia, local or universal; (4) faulty intrinsic development, leading to certain disfigurations of fibers (improper arrangement of nuclei, myofilaments, and other organelles, particularly mitochondria; this conceivably could reduce viability, i.e., cause abiotrophy); and (5) denervation effect of aging, as noted above.

Denervation from spinal or nerve disease at every age has roughly the same effect—namely, atrophy of muscle fibers (first in random distribution, then in groups) and later degeneration. Segmental necrosis at all ages excites a regenerative response from sarcolemmal and satellite cells in the intact parts of the fibers. Presumably, if this occurs repeatedly, the regenerative potential wanes, with ultimate death of the fiber—leading to permanent depopulation of fibers and muscle weakness.

CONGENITAL DEFORMITIES INVOLVING MUSCLE

Congenital Fibrous Contractures of Muscle and Joint Deformities

Arthrogryposis Multiplex Congenita *Multiple congenital contractures, multiple congenital articular rigidities*, and *amyoplasia congenita* are some of the names that have been applied to congenital deformity and rigidity of many joints. This disorder, now generally referred to as *arthrogryposis* (literally, curved joints), has been estimated to occur once in 3000 births. The joint deformities result from a lack of movement during fetal development and can therefore be produced by any disorder that immobilizes the developing embryo—whether it be of anterior horn cells, peripheral nerves, the motor end plate (as in an infant born to a myasthenic mother), or muscle. Often there are associated developmental defects of the nervous system and somatic structures—low-set ears, wide and flat nose, micrognathia, and high-arched palate; less often, there is a short neck, congenital heart disease, hypoplasia of the lungs, and cryptorchidism.

Of the many conditions that underlie arthrogryposis, *developmental abnormalities of the anterior horn cells* (mainly Werdnig-Hoffman disease, as discussed in Chap. 39) are by far the most common. A failure in development of anterior horn cells results in an uneven smallness and paresis of limb muscles. The unopposed contraction of relatively normally innervated muscles sets the fixed deformities. In the less common myopathic form, the nervous system is intact and the disease is that of a polymyopathy or congenital muscular dystrophy. It is of interest that in the myopathic variety, the limbs are fixed in a position of flexion at the hips and knees and adduction of the legs, in contrast to the variable postures of the myelopathic (anterior horn cell) form. Also, the latter type is more frequently conjoined with multiple anomalies than the myopathic type. In addition to these two well-recognized types, occasional cases of arthrogryposis are attributable to a neonatal neuropathy, neonatal myasthenia gravis, and the Prader-Willi syndrome (intrauterine hypotonia).

An infant with arthrogryposis should be evaluated with an electromyogram (EMG), interpreted by an experienced electromyographer for the presence of denervation or myopathic potentials, and particularly with a biopsy of muscle to detect group atrophy or one of the characteristic congenital polymyopathies described further on in this chapter. These tests may be difficult to interpret in the premature and term infant; in many circumstances, there is value in delaying them until several weeks of post-term development. If the initial evaluation is unrevealing, an imaging study of the brain, to detect malformations that may portend malformations, and high-resolution banding of chromosome structure (to detect Prader-Willi syndrome) may prove useful.

Fibrous Contractures This term refers to a fixation of limb posture due to a developmental lack or destruction of muscles, with shortening and fibrosis of supporting tissue and ligaments. A surprising number of deformities in infants and children are traceable to the shortening and fibrosis of muscles. The most common are congenital clubfoot (talipes), congenital torticollis, congenital elevation of the scapula (Sprengel deformity), and congenital dislocation of the hips. In all these conditions the postural distortion is produced and maintained either by a weakened, fibrotic muscle or by a normal one that is contracted and shortened because of the absence of a countervailing antagonist. Trauma to a muscle during intrauterine life or at birth leads to fibrosis and to fibrous contracture in some cases.

Congenital Clubfoot Here the deformity may be one of plantar flexion of the foot and ankle (talipes equinus), inversion (talipes varus or clubfoot), eversion (talipes valgus or splayfoot), or dorsiflexion of foot and ankle (talipes calcaneus). About 75 percent of all cases are equinovarus. Usually both feet are affected. Multiple incidence in one family may occur. Several explanations of cause and pathogenesis have been offered: fetal malposition, an embryonic abnormality of tarsal and metatarsal bones, a primary defect in nerves or anterior horn cells of the spinal cord, or a congenital dystrophy of muscle. No one theory explains all cases; available pathologic data exclude a single cause and pathogenesis. In some instances clubfoot is the only recognizable congenital abnormality, but more often it occurs as a manifestation of generalized arthrogryposis (see below) and is an indicator of a more widespread involvement of the central nervous system. (See Kakulas and Adams and also Banker for pertinent literature on the subject.)

Congenital Torticollis (Wryneck) This disorder begins during the first months of life and, unlike the dystonic torticollis of adults, is due to shortening of the sternomastoid muscle, which is firm and taut. The head is inclined to one side and the occiput slightly rotated to the side of the affected muscle. This disorder is nonfamilial and is usually ascribed to injury of the sternomastoid at birth. Whether the injury is a purely mechanical one to the muscle itself or is due to ischemia stemming from arterial or venous occlusion is not entirely clear. It gives rise to a sternomastoid tumor (actually a pseudotumor) that appears, on exploration, as a pale, spindle-shaped swelling of the muscle belly. The histologic findings are similar to those of Volkmann contracture, i.e., replacement of the muscle fibers by relatively acellular connective tissue, so that an ischemic mechanism appears most likely.

Congenital Absence of Muscles

It is well known that some individuals are born without certain muscles. This pertains not only to certain inconstant and functionally unimportant muscles, such as the palmaris longus, but also to more constant and important ones as well. The muscles found to be absent most frequently are the pectoralis, trapezius, serratus anterior, and quadriceps femoris, but many others are found to be missing in isolated cases.

Congenital absence of muscle is usually associated with congenital anomalies of neighboring nonmuscular tissues. For example, congenital absence of the pectoral muscle is often accompanied by aplasia or hypoplasia of the mammary gland as well as syndactyly and microdactyly. Agenesis of the pectoral muscle may also be associated with scoliosis, webbed fingers, and underdevelopment of the ipsilateral arm and hand (Poland syndrome). Another unusual syndrome consists of congenital absence of portions of the abdominal muscles ("prune belly") in association with arthrogryposis and a defect of ureters, bladder, and genital organs.

Restricted Nuclear Amyotrophies

In another group of restricted palsies, the essential abnormality appears to lie in the nervous system (nuclear amyotrophies). One of the most frequent is congenital ptosis, due to an innervatory defect of the levator palpebrae muscles. Complete paralysis of all muscles supplied by the oculomotor nerve, due apparently to hypoplasia of the third nerve nuclei, may be observed in several members of a family and occasionally in only one member. A congenital Horner syndrome is well known and may be familial; it is associated with depigmentation of the iris (heterochromia iridis). Bilateral abducens palsy is often associated with bifacial palsy in the newborn and is known as the *Möbius syndrome*; this usually nonfamilial anomaly, the cause of which is thought to be a nuclear hypoplasia or aplasia, is discussed with the developmental disorders (page 1079). In these familial nuclear amyotrophies the muscles develop independently of the nervous system but have no prospect of attaining their natural growth and function—and indeed of surviving—because of failure of innervation. It is a kind of congenital denervation hypotrophy. Of course, a primary muscle defect may also give rise to bifacial weakness, as in facioscapulohumeral muscular dystrophy.

RELATIVELY NONPROGRESSIVE CONGENITAL POLYMYOPATHIES

Beginning in 1956, with the account by Shy and Magee of a patient whose muscle fibers showed a peculiar central densification of sarcoplasm ("cores"), a new class of hereditary diseases of muscle has been delineated. The more common and better-defined members of this group are the central core, nemaline (rod-body), and centronuclear myopathies and myopathy with tubular aggregates. As the names imply, in each of these diseases there is a distinctive morphologic abnormality that expresses itself early in life by a lack of muscle bulk, hypotonia, weakness of the limbs, and often mild dysmorphic features of other parts of the body. A variety of other morphologic types have been described, but they are relatively uncommon and some are of dubious specificity; these latter types are mentioned only briefly. A detailed account can be found in the chapter by Fardeau and Tomé in *Myology*. Further study has revealed that the diseases of this group are not confined to infancy and early childhood and some of them, especially those present at birth, are not as benign as their early descriptions implied.

Each of the entities mentioned above has been observed at a later age, even in middle adult life; if the disease is mild, there is often no way of deciding whether it had been present since birth. *Lack of progression or extremely slow progression characterizes most of the congenital myopathies*, in contrast to the more rapid pace of many muscular dystrophies, Werdnig-Hoffmann disease, and other forms of hereditary motor system disease of childhood and adolescence. Exceptionally, an example of more rapid progression of a congenital myopathy has been reported, and, prior to the use of histochemical and electron microscopic techniques, such patients were usually considered to have a benign muscular dystrophy. Familial occurrence has also been established, so the clinical line of separation between this group of diseases and some of the more slowly progressive muscular dystrophies remains ambiguous. There is no specific treatment for any of the congenital myopathies.

As mentioned earlier, the lesions in the congenital myopathies are revealed most clearly by the systematic application of histochemical stains to frozen sections and by phase and electron microscopy. Some of the abnormalities are also disclosed by the conventional stains used in light microscopy, but as a group their identification has been the product of newer histologic techniques.

A word of caution about the specificity of some of the morphologic changes and the classifications of the congenital myopathies based upon them. It is treacherous to assume that a change in a single organelle or a subtle change in the sarcoplasm of a muscle fiber can be relied upon to characterize a pathologic process. Indeed, as more careful studies were made of this class of disease, the specificity of the lesions came to be questioned. Central cores are sometimes found in the same muscle as nemaline bodies, and so on, and each of the denotative lesions has been reported in association with other conditions. Nevertheless, the prominence of the morphologic change in any individual case, along with certain characteristic clinical features, permits an accurate diagnosis to be made.

Central Core Myopathy In the original family described by Shy and Magee, 5 members (4 males) in three successive generations were affected, suggesting an autosomal dominant pattern of inheritance. The youngest was 2 years old; the oldest, 65 years. In each, there was weakness and hypotonia ("floppy infant") and a general delay in motor development, particularly in walking, which was not achieved until the age of 4 to 5 years; always the patient had had difficulty in arising from a chair, climbing stairs, and running. The weakness was greater in proximal than in distal muscles, though the latter did not escape, and shoulder-girdle muscles were affected less than those of the pelvic girdle. Facial, bulbar, and ocular muscles were spared. The tendon reflexes were hypoactive and symmetrical. Muscle atrophy was not a prominent feature, though poor muscular development was present in one patient and has since been reported in others. There were no fasciculations, cramps, or myotonia, but cramps following exercise have been described in other families. The electrocardiograms were normal.

The disease is rare, but as additional cases were discovered, milder forms of the disease came to be recognized, and in some of them the symptoms first appeared in adult life. Originally some of these patients were thought to have limb-girdle dystrophy because of the disproportionate involvement of proximal muscles. In other families, such as the one reported by Patterson and colleagues, the disease was first recognized in middle adult life, with the rapid evolution of a proximal myopathy. These represent the two extremes of the clinical state. Dislocation of the hips, pes cavus or pes planus, and kyphoscoliosis have been found in a few children. In the majority of cases the progress of the disease is extremely slow, with slight worsening over many years.

The EMG reveals only brief, small-amplitude motor unit potentials with a normal interference pattern. Serum concentration of CK is normal or only slightly elevated, as it is in all the congenital myopathies.

Every patient with central core disease is a potential candidate for the development of malignant hyperthermia and should wear a bracelet or be otherwise identified to indicate his vulnerability to this anesthetic-induced complication. The gene for central core disease has been mapped to chromosome 19q13.1, where it is tightly linked to the ryanodine receptor gene—a mutation of which is also implicated in the causation of malignant hyperthermia (see Chap. 54).

Pathologically, the majority of the fibers appear normal in size or enlarged, and no focal destruction or loss of fibers can be found. The unique feature of the disease is the presence in the central portion of each muscle fiber of a dense, amorphous condensation of myofibrils or myofibrillar material. This altered zone characteristically lacks mitochondria and other organelles and gives a positive periodic acid–Schiff (PAS) reaction and a dark blue color with the Gomori trichrome stain, contrasting with the normal blue-green color of the peripheral fibrils. Within the core, there is a lack of phosphorylase and oxidative enzymes. Most of the cores are in type 1 fibers, which predominate. These cores run the length of the muscle fiber, thus differing from the multiple cores or minicores that are seen in oculopharyngeal and other forms of muscular dystrophy.

Nemaline Myopathy This disorder also expresses itself by hypotonia and impaired motility in infancy and early childhood, but—unlike the case in central core disease—the muscles of the trunk and limbs (proximal greater than distal) as well as the facial, lingual, and pharyngeal muscles are strikingly thin and hypoplastic. Several forms have been observed. One is congenital, with generalized weakness in the neonatal period, making breathing and feeding difficult. The limbs are flaccid and areflexic. Pneumonia and death occur within weeks to months. In forms that permit survival, the weakness is less severe, involving mainly the proximal muscles. Tendon reflexes are diminished or absent. The young child with this disease usually suffers from inanition and frequent respiratory infections, which may shorten life. Strength slowly improves with growth, the latter process evidently overcoming the advance of the disease. A slender appearance, narrow face, open mouth, narrow, arched palate, and kyphoscoliosis are regular but not invariable accompaniments of nemaline myopathy. Pes cavus or clubfoot may be added. Some of the milder cases reach adulthood, at which time a cardiomyopathy may threaten life. A. G. Engel as well as W. K. Engel and Reznick have observed individuals who first showed signs of the disease in middle age; the weakness was mainly in proximal muscles, and the dysmorphic and skeletal abnormalities of the childhood form were lacking. The EMG is "myopathic," and serum enzymes are normal or only slightly elevated.

Nemaline myopathy appears to be genetically heterogeneous. The pattern of inheritance is most often autosomal dominant, with variable penetrance. In a few families an autosomal recessive or an X-linked pattern of inheritance has been suggested. The localization of the gene (in the autosomal dominant type) to chromosome 1q21–23 should clarify the uncertainties about inheritance and perhaps explain the relationships between the different forms of the disease. More recently, the alpha-tropomyosin gene (TPM3) has been reassigned to the same locus.

A Gomori trichrome–stained section of frozen muscle discloses the characteristic lesion, which can be seen under the light microscope. Myriads of bacillus-like rods, singly and in small packets, are seen beneath the plasma membrane of the muscle fiber. They are composed of material that resembles that of Z bands under the electron microscope, and often actin filaments are attached, just as they are to Z bands. The type 1 fibers, which usually predominate, are smaller than normal, as in central core disease. The size of the motor neurons is said to be reduced. The cause of the disease is unknown, but probably the weakness is related to a smallness and reduction in the number of muscle fibers and possibly to focal interruption of their cross striations, particularly the Z bands.

Centronuclear or Myotubular Myopathy In this familial disease, hypotonia and weakness become manifest soon after birth or in infancy or early childhood. Rarely, in the mildest form, the diagnosis does not become evident until adult years. All the striated skeletal muscles are involved to some degree. Ptosis and ocular palsies are combined with weakness of facial, masticatory, lingual, pharyngeal, laryngeal, and cervical muscles in most of the infants with this disease, but not in the adults. In the limbs, distal weakness keeps pace with proximal weakness. The limbs remain thin and areflexic throughout life. Motor development is necessarily retarded, though some improvement with maturation can occur; later, however, motor functions that had been acquired may be lost as the disease slowly advances. Several patients have shown signs of cerebral abnormality, with seizures and an abnormal electroencephalogram (EEG), but this may not be part of the disease. Needle EMG examination shows the usual myopathic pattern, as well as positive sharp waves and fibrillation potentials in some cases. Abundant spontaneous activity should suggest the diagnosis of centronuclear myopathy (Griggs et al). Heckmatt and colleagues have classified this disorder into three types, based on severity, mode of presentation, and genetic pattern: (1) a severe neonatal X-linked recessive type; (2) a less severe early-infantile, late-infantile, or childhood autosomal recessive type; and (3) a still milder late childhood–adult autosomal dominant type. The gene for the X-linked form has been localized to chromosome Xq28, making possible the identification of carriers.

The outstanding pathologic features of the disease are the smallness of muscles and their constituent fibers and central nucleation. In one group of centronuclear myopathies, there is hypotrophy of type 1 fibers (Bethlem et al, Karpati et al). Surrounding most of the centrally placed nuclei is a clear zone, in which there is a lack of organization of contractile elements. Because of central nucleation, the disease has incorrectly been referred to as *myotubular myopathy*, implying an arrest in development of muscle at the myotubular stage. Actually, the nature of the pathologic process is obscure. The small, centrally nucleated fibers do not really resemble typical myotubes. Also, there is evidence, from electron microscopic studies, of changes in the central parts of the fibers (lack of enzymatic activity in the clear zones surrounding the nuclei), leading in all probability to fiber loss. Such changes argue against a purely developmental abnormality.

Myopathy with Tubular Aggregates The accumulation of tubular aggregates in the subsarcolemmal or more interior regions of muscle fibers was first observed in patients with hypokalemic periodic paralysis and myotonia congenita and later with a number of diverse conditions, such as chronic drug intoxication, hypoxia, and congenital myasthenic syndromes. However, tubular aggregates are also the defining feature of several purely myopathic syndromes: (1) a slowly progressive muscular weakness, in a limb-girdle distribution, with onset in childhood or early adult life; inheritance is either autosomal dominant or recessive in type. (2) A childhood onset of proximal weakness, easy fatigability, and myasthenic features; heredity is autosomal recessive. This syndrome may respond to pyridostigmine. (3) Muscle pain, cramps, and stiffness induced by exercise; the cases to date have been sporadic.

The histologic changes are readily overlooked in paraffin sections. Cryostat sections show masses of material that is basophilic with hematoxylin and eosin and bright red with Gomori trichrome and shows an intense reaction with NADH dehydrogenase. By electron microscopy, the bundles of tubular aggregates are sharply demarcated from myofibrils.

Other Congenital Myopathies The foregoing congenital myopathies—central core, nemaline, centronuclear, and tubular aggregate types—are well-defined clinical-pathologic entities. In addition, other far less common types have been described, each named according to a distinctive dysmorphic alteration of organelles in muscle fibers in histochemical and electron microscopic preparations. In none of these additional types has the pattern of inheritance or the gene locus been identified. Some of these myopathies—*multicore (minicore), fingerprint body, sarcotubular*—have been reported in only a few cases, quite insufficient to allow their categorization as disease entities. Two other types—*congenital fiber type disproportion* and *congenital fiber type predominance*—originally designated as congenital myopathies, have proved to be nonspecific histochemical alterations observed in many infants and children with congenital developmental abnormalities, delays in motor development, and other conditions. Other alleged congenital myopathies include so-called *reducing body, trilaminar, and cap disease, zebra body and familial myopathy with lysis in type 1 fibers*, among others. They most likely represent nonspecific reactions in muscle or fixation artifacts; as yet there is no evidence that any one of them represents a clinical pathologic entity.

Myofibrillar Myopathy During the past few decades the field of chronic noninflammatory myopathies has been muddied by a plethora of reports describing a variety of curious inclusions in muscle fibers, under a bewildering array of terms: *myopathy with inclusion bodies, atypical myopathy with myofibrillar aggregates; autosomal dominant myopathy with myofibrillar inclusions; cardioskeletal myopathy with intrasacroplasmic dense granulofilamentous material; cytoplasmic body myopathy; spheroid body myopathy; myopathy with characteristic sarcoplasmic bodies and skeleton (desmin) filaments; myopathy with Mallory-body-like inclusions; and familial cardiomyopathy with subsarcolemmal vermiform deposits*. Implied by these reports was the notion that each of these structural abnormalities represented a new and distinctive myopathy.

More recently, in a careful light microscopic evaluation of both published reports and their own cases, Nakano and Engel and their colleagues convincingly demonstrated that the many reported structural changes were the consequence of a single pathologic process—a focal dissolution of myofibrils, followed by an accumulation of the products of the degradative process. These authors proposed the term *myofibrillar myopathy* to encompass the entire spectrum of pathologic changes.

The diagnosis of myofibrillar myopathy (by biopsy) is usually made in adult life. Men and women are equally affected. Slowly progressive weakness of the muscles of limbs and trunk is the main clinical feature. Both proximal and distal muscles are affected, more in the legs than in the arms. Hyporeflexia is usual. Cardiac involvement, usually abnormalities of conduction, is present in about one-half the patients. The pattern of inheritance is most often autosomal dominant, but autosomal recessive and X-linked inheritance is well known.

Genetically there is considerable heterogeneity. At the time of writing, no fewer than five chromosomal loci for myofibrillar myopathy have been documented, and more are likely to exist (Engel). Predictably, therefore, a more sharply defined disease or diseases will emerge with further study of the category of myofibrillar myopathy.

THE SPINAL MUSCULAR ATROPHIES OF INFANCY AND CHILDHOOD

Obviously this important group of diseases, appearing as they do in the same periods of life as the congenital polymyopathies described above and certain of the congenital muscular dystrophies, must figure in the differential diagnosis of early-onset muscle weakness. Indeed, they represent the main problems faced by the clinical myologist. Their hereditary nature, their progressivity to fatal issue or delayed motor attainments, and their tendency in certain instances to produce disabling contractures are shared with the primary muscle diseases. Fortunately the proper application of current laboratory techniques sets them apart in most instances. In deference to their neuronal origin, the authors have decided to place them with the other degenerative diseases (see pages 1158–1162).

REFERENCES

Banker BQ: Congenital deformities, in Engel AG, Franzini-Armstrong C (eds): *Myology*, 2nd ed. New York, McGraw-Hill, 1994, pp 1905–1937.

Banker BQ, Victor M, Adams RD: Arthrogryposis multiplex due to congenital muscular dystrophy. *Brain* 80:319, 1957.

Bethlem J, Arts WF, Dingemans KP: Common origin of rods, cores, miniature cores, and focal loss of cross striations. *Arch Neurol* 35:555, 1978.

DeReuck J, Adams RD: The metrics of muscle, in Kakulas BA (ed): *Basic Research in Myology*. International Congress Series. Excerpta Medica Foundation, 1973, pp 1–11.

Engel AG: Myofibrillar myopathy. *Ann Neurol* 46:681, 1999.

Engel AG, Angelini C, Gomez MR: Fingerprint body myopathy. *Mayo Clin Proc* 47:377, 1972.

Engel WK, Reznick JS: Late onset rod-myopathy: A newly recognized, acquired, and progressive disease. *Neurology* 16: 308, 1966.

Fardeau M, Tomé FMS: Congenital myopathies, in Engel AG, Franzini-Armstrong C (eds): *Myology*, 2nd ed. New York, McGraw-Hill, 1994, pp 1487–1532.

Franzini-Armstrong C, Fischman DA: Morphogenesis of skeletal muscle fibers, in Engel AG, Franzini-Armstrong C (eds): *Myology*, 2nd ed. New York, McGraw-Hill, 1994, pp 74–96.

Griggs RC, Mendell JR, Miller RG: *Evaluation and Treatment of Myopathies*. Philadelphia, Davis, 1995.

Heckmatt JZ, Sewry CA, Hodes D, Dubowitz V: Congenital centronuclear (myotubular) myopathy. *Brain* 108:941, 1985.

Henderson JL: The congenital facial diplegia syndrome: Clinical features, pathology and aetiology. *Brain* 62:381, 1939.

Jerusalem F, Engel AG, Gomez MR: Sarcotubular myopathy. *Neurology* 23:897, 1973.

Kakulas BA, Adams RD: *Diseases of Muscle: The Pathological Foundations of Clinical Myology*, 4th ed. Philadelphia, Harper & Row, 1985.

Karpati G, Carpenter S, Nelson RF: Type 1 muscle fiber atrophy and central nuclei. *J Neurol Sci* 10:489, 1970.

Lichtenstein BW: Congenital absence of the abdominal musculature: Associated changes in the genitourinary tract and the spinal cord. *Am J Dis Child* 58:339, 1939.

Nakano S, Engel AG, Waclawik AJ, et al: Myofibrillar myopathy with abnormal foci of desmin positivity: I. Light and electron microscopy analysis of 10 cases. *J Neuropathol Exp Neurol* 44:549, 1996.

Patterson VH, Hill TRG, Fletcher PJH, Heron JR: Central core disease: Clinical and pathological progression within a family. *Brain* 102:581, 1979.

Robertson WC, Kawamura Y, Dyck PJ: Morphometric study of motoneurons in congenital nemaline myopathy and Werdnig-Hoffmann disease. *Neurology* 28:1057, 1978.

Shy GM, Gonatos NK, Perez M: Two childhood myopathies with abnormal mitochondria. *Brain* 89:133, 1966.

Shy GM, Magee KR: A new congenital non-progressive myopathy. *Brain* 79:610, 1956.

Silbermann M, Finkelbrand S, Weiss A, et al: Morphometric analysis of aging skeletal muscle following endurance training. *Muscle Nerve* 6:136, 1983.

Tomlinson BF, Walton JN, Rebeiz JJ: The effects of aging and cachexia upon skeletal muscle: A histopathologic study. *J Neurol Sci* 8:201, 1969.

Chapter 53

MYASTHENIA GRAVIS AND RELATED DISORDERS OF THE NEUROMUSCULAR JUNCTION

Included under this title is a group of diseases affecting the neuromuscular junction, the most important of which is myasthenia gravis. As a group, these disorders exhibit several striking features, the essential one being a fluctuating weakness and fatigability of muscle. There is usually some degree of weakness at all times, but it is made worse by activity. The weakness and fatigability reflect physiologic abnormalities of the neuromuscular junction that are demonstrated by clinical signs and special electrophysiologic testing.

MYASTHENIA GRAVIS

The main feature of myasthenia gravis, usually referred to simply as myasthenia, is a fluctuating weakness of certain voluntary muscles, particularly those innervated by motor nuclei of the brainstem, i.e., ocular, masticatory, facial, deglutitional, and lingual. Manifest weakening during continued activity, quick restoration of power with rest, and dramatic improvement in strength following the administration of anticholinesterase drugs such as neostigmine are the other notable clinical features.

Historical Note Several students of medical history affirm that Willis, in 1672, gave an account of a disease that could be none other than myasthenia gravis. Others give credit to Wilks (1877) for the first description and for having noted that the medulla was free of disease, in distinction to other types of bulbar paralysis. The first reasonably complete accounts were those of Erb (1878), who characterized the disease as a bulbar palsy without an anatomic lesion, and of Goldflam (1893); for many years thereafter, the disorder was referred to as the *Erb-Goldflam syndrome*. Jolly (1895) was the first to use the name *myasthenia gravis*, to which he added the term *pseudoparalytica* to indicate the lack of structural changes at autopsy. Also it was Jolly who originally demonstrated that myasthenic weakness could be reproduced by repeated faradic stimulation of the relevant motor nerve and that the "fatigued" muscle would still respond to galvanic stimulation. Interestingly, he suggested the use of physostigmine as a form of treatment, but there the matter rested until Reman, in 1932, and Walker, in 1934, demonstrated the therapeutic value of the drug.

Campbell and Bramwell (1900) and Oppenheim (1901) each analyzed over 60 cases and crystallized the clinical concept of the disease. The relationship between myasthenia gravis and tumors of the thymus gland was first noted by Laquer and Weigert in 1901, and in 1949 Castleman and Norris gave the first detailed description of the pathologic changes in the gland.

In 1905 Buzzard published a careful clinicopathologic analysis of the disease, commenting on both the thymic abnormalities and the infiltrations of lymphocytes (called lymphorrhages) in muscle. He postulated that an "autotoxic agent" caused the muscle weakness, the lymphorrhages, and the thymic lesions. He also commented on the close relation of myasthenia gravis to Graves disease and Addison disease, which are also now considered to have an autoimmune basis. In 1960, Simpson and, independently, Nastuk and coworkers theorized that an autoimmune mechanism must be operative in myasthenia gravis. Finally, in 1973 and subsequently, the autoimmune nature of myasthenia gravis was established through a series of investigations by Patrick and Lindstrom, Fambrough, Lennon, and Engel and their colleagues (see further on, under "Etiology and Pathogenesis").

These and other references to the early historical features of the disease are to be found in the reviews by

Viets and by Kakulas and Adams; Engel's monograph (1999) is an excellent modern reference.

Clinical Manifestations

Myasthenia gravis, as the name implies, is a muscular weakness with a (formerly) grave prognosis. Repeated or persistent activity of a muscle group exhausts its contractile power, leading to a progressive paresis, and rest restores strength, at least partially. These are the identifying attributes of the disease; their demonstration, assuming that the patient cooperates fully, is sometimes enough to establish the diagnosis.

The onset is usually insidious, but there are instances of fairly rapid development, sometimes initiated by an emotional upset or infection (usually respiratory). In most patients, however, a precipitating event cannot be identified. Symptoms may first appear during pregnancy or, more commonly, in the puerperium or in response to drugs used during anesthesia. Thymic abnormalities of several types are closely connected with the disease, as elaborated further on, and weakness may begin months or years after removal of a thymoma. Once the disease has begun, a slow progression follows. Usually the muscles of the eyes—and somewhat less often of the face, jaws, throat, and neck—are the first to be affected, but in rare cases the initial complaint may be referable to the limbs. However, as the disease advances, it often spreads to other muscles.

The special vulnerability of certain muscles is another characteristic of myasthenia gravis, accounting for its common modes of clinical presentation. Weakness of the levator palpebrae or extraocular muscles is the initial manifestation of the disease in about half the cases, and these muscles are involved eventually in more than 90 percent. Ocular palsies and ptosis (weakness of eyelid opening) are usually accompanied by weakness of eye closure, a combination observed regularly only in this disease and in muscular dystrophy. Certain ocular signs are characteristic of myasthenia. Usually the diplopia that is demonstrated by red-glass testing (pages 282 to 286) does not correspond to a particular innervation but is the result instead of weakness that randomly involves several muscles in both eyes. Sustained upgaze will usually induce or exaggerate ptosis. Cogan has described a twitching of the upper eyelid that appears a moment after the patient moves his eyes from a downward to the primary position. Or, after sustained upward gaze, one or more twitches may be observed with closure of the eyelids or during horizontal movements of the eyes. Repeated ocular versions induced by tracking a target or by an optokinetic stimulus will cause progressive paresis of the muscles utilized for these movements. Unilateral painless ptosis without ophthalmoplegia or pupillary abnormality in an adult will most often prove to be due to myasthenia. Attempts to overcome the ptosis may impart a staring expression of the opposite eye. Bright sunlight is said to aggravate the ocular signs and cold, to improve them.

Muscles of facial expression, mastication, swallowing, and speech are frequently affected (80 percent), and in 5 to 10 percent they are the first or only muscles to be involved. Even less frequent is the initial or early involvement of the flexors and extensors of the neck, muscles of the shoulder girdle, and flexors of the hips. Of the trunk muscles, the erector spinae are the most frequently affected. In the most advanced cases, all muscles are weakened, including the diaphragmatic, abdominal, and intercostal muscles and even the external sphincters of the bladder and bowel. The incidence of involvement of any group of muscles closely parallels the likelihood of their having been initially affected by the disease. Clinically, myasthenia gravis may be conceived as a fluctuating oculofaciobulbar palsy. In patients with weakness of the trunk and limbs, the clinical rule holds firm that the proximal muscles are far more vulnerable than distal ones, as they are in almost all other forms of myopathy.

To reiterate the topographic attributes of the illness, drooping of the eyelids and intermittent diplopia are the most common complaints. In fact, the presence of *normal pupillary responses to light and accommodation in the face of weakness of the extraocular muscles, levators, and orbicularis oculi is virtually diagnostic of myasthenia*, especially if strength is restored after a period of rest. Facial mobility and expression are altered. The natural smile becomes transformed into a snarl. The jaw may sag, so that it must be propped up by the patient's hand. Chewing tough food may be difficult, and the patient may have to terminate a meal because of inability to masticate and swallow. It may be more difficult to eat after talking, and the voice fades and becomes nasal after sustained conversation. Women may complain of inability to fix their hair because of fatigue of the shoulders, or of difficulty in applying lipstick because they are unable to purse and roll their lips. Weakness of the neck muscles causes fatigue in holding up the head. Another characteristic feature of myasthenic weakness is its tendency to increase as the day wears on or with repeated use of an affected muscle group, but patients seldom volunteer this information. A few are worse on awakening, especially if they have not received medication during the night. A temporary increase in weakness has reportedly followed vaccination, menstruation, and exposure to extremes of temperature. A peculiarity of myasthenic muscle contraction is a sudden lapse of sustained posture or interruption of movement resulting in a kind of irregular tremor, similar to that of normal muscle nearing the point of exhaustion. A dynamometer demonstrates the rapidly waning power of contraction of a series of hand grips, and repetitive stimulation of a motor nerve at slow rates while recording muscle action potentials reflects the same decremental disorder in a more quantitative fashion (see Fig. 45-5*A* and further on).

Weakened muscles in myasthenia gravis undergo atrophy to only a minimal degree or not at all. Tendon reflexes are seldom altered. Even repeated tapping of a tendon does not usually tax muscles to the point where contraction fails. Smooth and cardiac muscles are not involved.

Other neural functions are preserved. The weakened muscles, especially those of the eyes and back of the neck, may ache, but pain is seldom an important complaint. Paresthesias of the face, hands, and thighs are reported very infrequently and are not accompanied by demonstrable sensory loss. Anosmia and ageusia have been mentioned as rare findings, but whether they are coincidental has not been decided. The tongue may display one central and two lateral longitudinal furrows (trident tongue), as pointed out originally by Buzzard.

Certain *statistical features* of the disease are of clinical significance. Its prevalence is variously estimated to be from 43 to 84 per million of the population and the annual incidence rate, approximately one per 300,000. The disease may begin at any age, but onset in the first decade is relatively rare (only 10 percent of cases occur under the age of 10 years). The peak age of onset is between 20 and 30 years in women and between 50 and 60 years in men. Under the age of 40, females are affected two to three times as often as males, whereas in later life, the incidence in males is higher (3:2). Of patients with thymomas, the majority are older (50 to 60 years), and males predominate.

The *course of the illness* is extremely variable. Rapid spread from one muscle group to another occurs in some, but in others the disease remains unchanged for months before progressing. Remissions may take place without explanation, but these happen in less than half the cases and seldom last longer than a month or two. If the disease remits for a year or longer and then recurs, it tends to be progressive. Remission is more likely to occur in the early years of the disease than later. Relapse may be occasioned by the same events that preceded the onset of the illness. In Simpson's opinion, and this coincides with our observations, the danger of death from myasthenia gravis is greatest in the first year after onset of the disease. A second period of danger in progressive cases is from 4 to 7 years after onset. After this time the disease tends to stabilize and the risk of severe relapse diminishes. Fatalities then relate mainly to respiratory complications (infection, aspiration). The mortality rate in the first years of illness, formerly in excess of 30 percent, is now less than 5 percent, and with appropriate therapy, most patients are able to lead productive lives. The course is altered by thymectomy (see further on).

To facilitate clinical staging of therapy and prognosis, the following classification, introduced by Osserman, has been widely adopted (the relative incidence of each type is indicated):

I. Ocular myasthenia (15 to 20 percent)
II. *A.* Mild generalized myasthenia with slow progression; no crises; drug-responsive (30 percent)
   B. Moderately severe generalized myasthenia; severe skeletal and bulbar involvement but no crises; drug response less than satisfactory (25 percent)
III. Acute fulminating myasthenia; rapid progression of severe symptoms with respiratory crises and poor drug response; high incidence of thymoma; high mortality (15 percent)
IV. Late severe myasthenia; symptoms same as III, but resulting from steady progression over 2 years from class I to class II (10 percent)

Other authors (Compston et al) have classified the disease according to age of onset, presence or absence of thymoma, antibody level against acetylcholine receptors (AChR), and association with HLA haplotypes: (1) myasthenia gravis with thymoma—no sex or HLA association, high AChR antibody titer; (2) onset before age 40, no thymoma—female preponderance and an increased association with HLA A1, B8, and DRW3 antigens; (3) onset after age 40, no thymoma—male preponderance, increased association with HLA A3, B7, and DRW2 antigens, low AChR antibody titer. The latter group includes a proportion of older men with purely ocular symptoms (Osserman type I).

The *prognosis and response to treatment* vary with the pattern of muscle involvement and severity, though it remains difficult to predict the outcome in an individual case. According to Bever and coworkers, an increasing duration of purely ocular myasthenia is associated with a decreasing risk of late generalization of weakness. These authors found, in a retrospective study of 108 such patients, that only 15 percent of the observed generalizations occurred after 2 years of ocular manifestations alone. They also found that a higher age at onset was associated with a higher incidence of fatal respiratory crises; in general, patients with a younger age of onset ran a more benign course. Grob and colleagues, who observed the course of 1036 patients for a mean duration of 12 years, found that the clinical manifestations remained confined to the extraocular muscles and orbiculares oculi in 16 percent. Their data indicated further that if localized ocular myasthenia had been present for only a month, there was a 60 percent likelihood that the disease would become generalized. If the ocular myasthenia remained localized for a year, there was only a 16 percent likelihood that it would eventually become generalized. These authors found that in two-thirds of 750 patients with generalized myasthenia gravis, the disease attained its maximum severity within a year of onset, and in 83 percent of patients, within 3 years. By contrast, in our experience, 17 of 37 ocular cases became generalized within a period of 6 years (Weinberg et al). As a rule, the progression of symptoms was more rapid in male than in female patients.

It is not widely recognized that isolated muscle groups may occasionally remain *permanently weak* even when the ocular and generalized weakness has resolved. The muscles most often affected in this way are the anterior tibials, triceps, and portions of the face.

The long-term outlook for *myasthenic children* is generally good, and their life expectancy is only slightly reduced. Rodriguez and colleagues followed a group of 149 children for an average of 17 years; 85 of them had thymectomies. Approximately 30 percent of the non-thymectomized and 40 percent of the thymectomized patients underwent remission and were free of symptoms. The remission usually occurred in the first 3 years. Those with bulbar symptoms and no ocular or generalized weakness had the most favorable outcome.

Thymic and Other Associated Disorders *Thymic tumors* occur in 10 to 15 percent of patients with myasthenia gravis, and lymphofollicular hyperplasia of the thymic medulla in 65 percent. Thymomas with malignant characteristics may spread locally in the mediastinum and to regional lymph nodes, but rarely metastasize. (N.B.: thymic tumors can be missed in plain films and should be sought by CT scanning of the chest.) The significance of thymic disorders are discussed below and in relation to thymectomy on page 1545.

A biologic trait of interest is the coexistence of myasthenia gravis and other autoimmune diseases. *Thyrotoxicosis* (5 percent of myasthenic patients—page 1520), lupus erythematosus, rheumatoid arthritis, Sjögren syndrome, mixed connective tissue disease, anticardiolipin antibody, and polymyositis are all associated with myasthenia more often than can be explained by chance. Aplastic anemia of autoimmune type has also been reported, particularly with thymoma. In the series of patients reported by Kerzin-Storrar and associates, 30 percent had a maternal relative with one of these or other disorders of autoimmune nature, suggesting that myasthenia gravis patients inherit a susceptibility to autoimmune disease.

There have been numerous case reports of the concurrence of myasthenia and multiple sclerosis, again suggesting a common autoimmune basis, but the statistical association is not certain. A large proportion of young women with myasthenia have moderately elevated titers of antinuclear antibody without the clinical manifestations of lupus. *Antibody against striated muscle* has been found in almost half the patients with onset of myasthenia after age 40 (without thymoma) and in 84 percent of myasthenics with thymoma (Compston et al).

Familial occurrence is known but rare. Many of these cases prove to have a genetically determined myasthenic syndrome and not the acquired autoimmune form of myasthenia gravis (see further on).

Pathologic Features Reference has already been made to the involvement of the *thymus gland* in myasthenia gravis. True neoplasms of the gland are found in about 10 to 15 percent of patients, and fully 65 percent of the remaining patients show a striking degree of hyperplasia of lymphoid follicles, with active germinal centers confined to the medulla of the thymus. The proportion with hyperplasia is even higher in younger patients. The cells in the centers of the follicles are histiocytes; they are surrounded by helper T lymphocytes, B lymphocytes, and plasma cells; IgG is elaborated in the germinal follicles. The changes in the thymus gland resemble the reaction in the thyroid in Hashimoto thyroiditis. Since the latter has been reproduced in animals by injecting extracts of thyroid with Freund adjuvants, it is probable that the so-called thymitis of myasthenia gravis is of similar autoimmune nature. Immunosuppression with steroids causes involution of the thymus.

Aside from lymphoid hyperplasia, two forms of thymic tumors have been described: one is composed of reticular (histiocytic) cells like those in the center of the follicles, and the other is predominantly lymphocytic and specified as lymphosarcomatous. Some of the tumors are composed of spindle-shaped cells. Overlapping types are common in our material. Thymic tumors may be unattended by myasthenia, though myasthenia eventually developed in all of our cases, sometimes 15 to 20 years after the tumor was first recognized and removed surgically. According to Brill et al, the severity of myasthenic symptoms is no different in patients with thymoma from that in patients without a tumor.

As regards the *nervous system*, all current studies, including 40 autopsies at our hospitals, confirm Erb's original contention that myasthenia gravis is a disease without a central nervous system lesion. The brain and spinal cord are normal unless damaged by hypoxia and hypotension from cardiorespiratory failure. The *muscle fibers* are generally intact, although in fatal cases with extensive paralysis, isolated fibers of esophageal, diaphragmatic, and eye muscles may undergo segmental necrosis with variable regeneration (Russell). Scattered aggregates of lymphocytes (lymphorrhages) are also observed, as originally noted by Buzzard, but none of these changes in muscle explain the widespread and severe weakness. The lymphorrhages, which are found more frequently in the tumor cases, are not confined to the vicinity of the motor end plates.

Of central importance are the ultrastructural alterations of the *motor end plate*. These changes, elegantly demonstrated by A. G. Engel and associates, consist of a reduction in the area of the nerve terminal, a simplification of the postsynaptic region (sparse, shallow, abnormally wide or absent secondary synaptic clefts), and a widening of the primary synaptic cleft (Fig. 53-1). The number and size of the presynaptic vesicles and their quanta of ACh are within the normal range. The observation of regenerating axons near the junction, the many simplified junctions, and the absence of nerve terminals supplying some postsynaptic regions suggested to Engel and coworkers that there was an active process of degeneration and repair of the neuromuscular junction in myasthenia gravis.

Etiology and Pathogenesis The establishment of an *immunologic mechanism*, operative at the neuromuscular junction, has been the most significant development in our understanding of myasthenia gravis. Almost accidentally, it was discovered by Patrick and Lindstrom that repeated immunization of rabbits with ACh receptor protein obtained from the electric eel caused a muscular weakness, which Lennon and colleagues recognized as being similar to that of myasthenia gravis. Soon thereafter Fambrough and coworkers demonstrated the basic defect in myasthenia gravis—a marked reduction in the number of ACh receptors on the postsynaptic membrane of the neuromuscular junction. These observations were followed by the creation of an experimental model of the disease and the demonstration that experimentally induced myasthenia had clinical, pharmacologic, and electrophysiologic properties identical with those of human myasthenia gravis—i.e., decreased miniature end-plate potentials (MEPPs), decremental response on neuromuscular stimulation at 3 Hz, and correlation of weakness with the number of labeled antibodies attached to the receptor sites (Engel et al). It was also shown that humoral antibodies to receptor protein could transfer the myasthenic weakness to normal animals and that the weakness as well as the physiologic abnormalities could be reversed by the administration of anticholinesterase drugs. Thus, the accumulated evidence satisfied the criteria for the diagnosis of an autoantibody-mediated disorder (Drachman).

The present view of the disease is that the myasthenic weakness and fatigue are due to the failure of effective neuromuscular transmission. Normally, binding of ACh to the ACh receptor produces a localized electrical end-plate potential of sufficient amplitude to generate a muscle action potential and trigger contraction of the muscle fiber. At myasthenic junctions, because of the greatly reduced number of receptors and the competitive activity of anti-AChR antibodies (see below), the end-plate potentials are of insufficient amplitude to generate action potentials in some fibers (page 1347). Blocked transmission at many end plates results in a reduction in the contractile power of the whole muscle. This deficiency is reflected first in the ocular and cranial muscles, the most continuously active muscles, whose motor units have the fewest ACh receptors. Fatigue is understandable as the result of the normal decline in the amount of ACh released with each successive impulse.

Antibodies to ACh receptor protein have been found to be present in approximately 85 percent of patients with generalized myasthenia and in 60 percent of those with ocular myasthenia (Newsom-Davis). Antibodies are also present in infants with neonatal myasthenia gravis and in animal species known to have a naturally occurring myasthenia. The presence of receptor antibodies has proved to be a sensitive and reliable test of the disease, as discussed further on, under "Measurement of Receptor Antibodies in Blood."

How the antibodies act at the receptor surface of the end plate has also been investigated, but the matter is not entirely settled. Neuromuscular transmission can be impaired in several ways: (1) The antibodies may block the binding of ACh to the ACh receptors. (2) Serum IgG from myasthenic patients has been shown to induce a two- to threefold increase in the degradation rate of ACh receptors. This may be the result of the capacity of antibodies to cross-link the receptors, which are gathered

Figure 53-1

A. *End plate from a patient with myasthenia gravis. The terminal axon contains abundant presynaptic vesicles, but the postsynaptic folds are wide and there are few secondary folds. The loose junctional sarcoplasm is filled with microtubules and ribosomes. The synaptic cleft (asterisk) is widened. (From Santa et al by permission.)* B. *Normal end plate for comparison. (Courtesy of Dr. A. G. Engel.)*

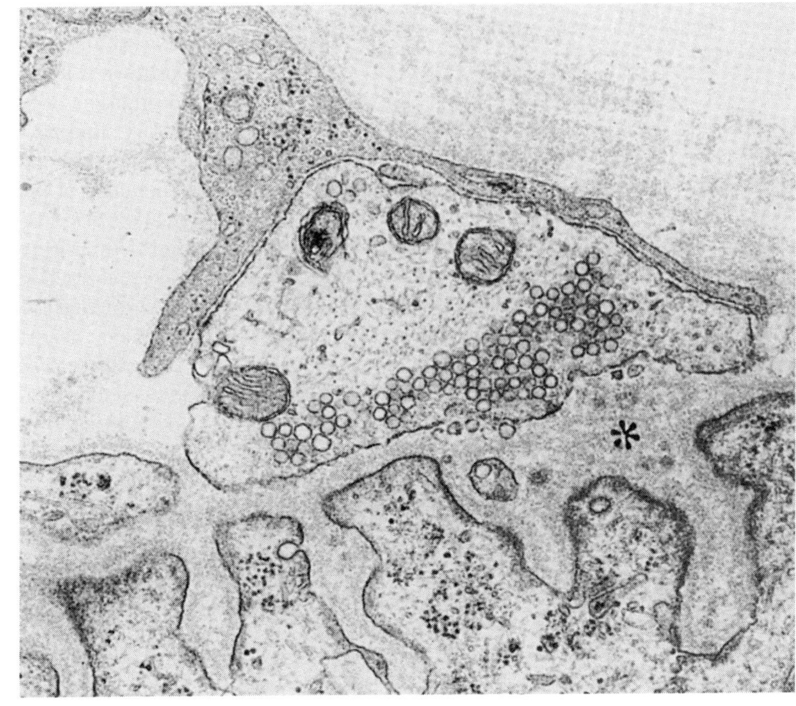

A

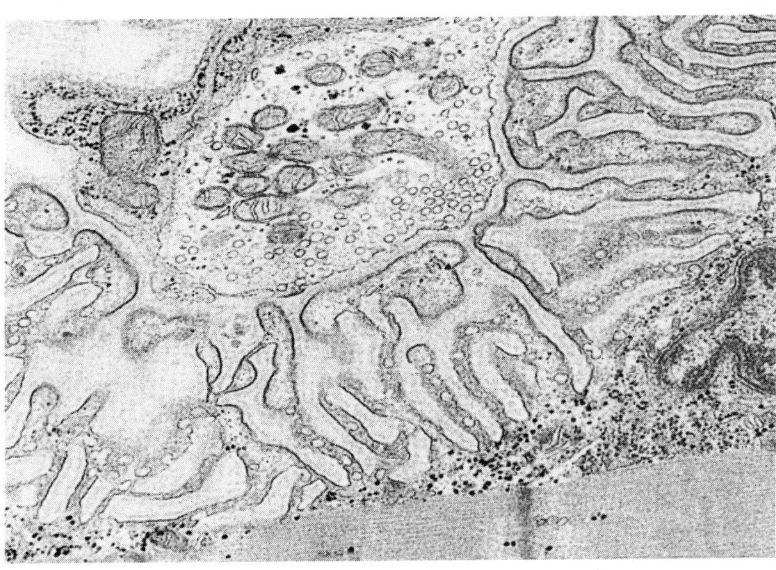

B

into clusters in the muscle membrane, internalized by a process of endocytosis, and degraded. (3) Antibodies may cause a complement-mediated destruction of the postsynaptic folds (Engel and Arahata). The latter two mechanisms would be expected to reduce the number of ACh receptors at the synapse.

Although the evidence that an autoimmune mechanism is responsible for the functional disorder of muscle in myasthenia gravis appears to be incontrovertible, the source of the autoimmune response has not been established. Because most patients with myasthenia gravis have thymic abnormalities and a salutary response to thymectomy, it is logical to implicate this gland in the pathogenesis of the disease. Both T and B cells from the myasthenic thymus are particularly responsive to the ACh receptor, more so than analogous cells from peripheral blood. Moreover, the thymus contains "myoid cells" (resembling striated muscle) that bear surface ACh receptors. That thymic myoid cells are the foci of immunologic stimulation in myasthenia gravis is unlikely for several reasons, the most obvious being that such cells are even more abundant in the normal than in the myasthenic thymus (Schluep et al). Another suggestion, unconfirmed, is that a virus with a tropism for thymic cells that have ACh receptors might injure such cells and induce antibody formation. It might at the same time have a potential for oncogenesis, accounting for the 10 percent or more of myasthenic patients with thymic tumors. Scadding and associates have suggested a somewhat different mode of thymic involvement; they have shown that thymic lymphocytes from patients with myasthenia gravis can synthesize anti-ACh receptor antibody, both in culture and spontaneously.

Diagnosis In patients who present with a changeable diplopia and the typical myasthenic facies—unequally drooping eyelids, relatively immobile mouth turned down at the corners, a smile that looks more like a snarl, a hanging jaw supported by the hand—the diagnosis can hardly be overlooked. However, only a minority of patients present in this stage of the disease, and seldom is there a clear recognition, even by the patient, that the muscles tire during activity. Ptosis, diplopia, difficulty in speaking or swallowing, or weakness of the limbs are at first mild and inconstant. However, the finding that sustained activity of small cranial muscles results in weakness (e.g., increasing droop of eyelids while looking at the ceiling or diplopia when fixating in lateral or vertical gaze or reading for 2 to 3 min) and that contraction improves after a brief rest is virtually diagnostic, even in the early stages of the disease. Any other affected group of muscles may be critically tested in similar fashion. The characteristic ocular signs have already been described. If the diagnosis remains in doubt, the measurement of specific antibody (anti-AChR), electromyography, and certain pharmacologic tests (see below) are necessary.

Electrophysiologic Testing The rapid reduction in the amplitude of compound muscle action potentials evoked during repetitive stimulation of a peripheral nerve at a rate of 3 per second (*decrementing response*, as shown in Fig. 45-5*A*) and reversal of this response by neostigmine or edrophonium has been a reliable confirmatory finding in the majority of cases; it can be obtained from the facial, hand, or proximal limb muscles, which may or may not be clinically weak. During a progressive phase of the disease or during steroid therapy, a slight initial incrementing response may be obtained, not to be confused with the marked incrementing response after voluntary contraction that characterizes the Lambert-Eaton syndrome (see further on).

Single-fiber electromyography (EMG) represents an even more sensitive method of detecting the defect in neuromuscular transmission by demonstrating increased variability of the interpotential interval ("jitter"—see page 1366) or blocking of successive discharges from single muscle fibers belonging to the same motor unit. This test requires a great deal of cooperation from the patient in sustaining contraction of a muscle at just the right amplitude in order to isolate single muscle fibers from the same unit. With patience on the part of the electromyographer, it is also possible to detect such pairs by electrically stimulating a nerve. Also characteristic of the myasthenic syndrome is the postactivation potentiation of single evoked action potentials, followed by exhaustion. Since the eye muscles exert a pull on the globe, which is reflected in intraocular tension, the increase of the latter in response to edrophonium can also be measured, although this test is rarely performed. Nerve conduction velocities and distal latencies are usually normal.

Equally valuable at this point are the edrophonium (Tensilon) and neostigmine tests, which are performed in the following manner.

Edrophonium (Tensilon) and Neostigmine Tests After the strength of certain cranial muscles (usually the levator palpebrae or an extraocular muscle) or limb muscles (by dynamometry) or vital capacity has been measured, 10 mg (1 mL) of edrophonium is injected intravenously. Initially 1 mg (0.1 mL) is given; if this dose is tolerated and no definite improvement in strength occurs after 45 s, another 3 to 6 mg is injected. If there is no response after another 45 s, the remaining amount is given over approximately 1 min. Most patients who respond do so after 5 mg has been administered. The clinical effect persists for no more than 4 to 5 min. The mild muscarinic effects of edrophonium (nausea, vomiting, bowel activation, sweating, salivation) can be blocked by pretreatment with atropine 0.8 mg subcutaneously. A positive test consists of visible (objective) improvement in muscle contractility, complete fusion of diplopia, or total resolution of fatigable ptosis. The report of subjective improvement alone is not dependable, and one must also be distrustful of equivocal test results, which may occur with ocular palsies due to tumors, thyroid disease, Guillain-Barré syndrome, progressive supranuclear palsy, or carotid aneurysms (pseudo-ocular myasthenia). In some patients who later prove to have myasthenia gravis, the edrophonium test (and EMG and AChR antibody measurements) may be entirely normal during the first episode or even after several episodes of ocular myasthenia. Only later, for inexplicable reasons, do these tests become positive. Finally, it should be noted that the drug carries a rare risk of ventricular fibrillation and cardiac arrest, so that testing is preferably carried out in a hospital setting, where emergency respiratory support is available.

The use of the edrophonium test in the diagnosis of so-called cholinergic crisis is discussed further on.

Neostigmine is sometimes preferable to edrophonium because the longer duration of its effect allows more deliberate and repeated testing. Neostigmine methylsulfate is injected intramuscularly in a dose of 1.5 mg. Atropine sulfate (0.8 mg) should be given several minutes in advance to counteract muscarinic effects. Neostigmine may be given intravenously in a dose of 0.5 mg but again should always be preceded by atropine sulfate to obviate the annoying muscarinic side effects and the danger of cardiac arrhythmias. Objective and subjective improvement occurs in 10 to 15 min, reaches its peak at 20 min, and lasts 2 or 3 h, allowing for careful testing of neurologic improvement. A negative test does not exclude myasthenia gravis but is a strong point against the diagnosis (see below). A trial of oral prostigmine, 15 mg every 4 h during the day, is sometimes recommended in doubtful cases, but we have been misled more often than helped by it.

Measurement of Receptor Antibodies in Blood As stated earlier, this is in general a sensitive and highly specific test. The radioimmunoassay method has been the most accurate and widely used. Serum antibody against ACh receptor can be found in 80 to 90 percent of patients with generalized myasthenia gravis and about 60 percent of those whose symptoms are restricted to the ocular muscles (Vincent and Newsom-Davis). Adult myasthenics whose serum is persistently negative for AChR antibodies do not differ clinically or electromyographically from patients with serum antibodies. In general, persistently negative AChR antibody tests are more frequently found in ocular myasthenia than in patients with generalized weakness. Patients with thymoma and severe generalized myasthenia are practically always seropositive. Interestingly, the antibody titers remain elevated during clinical remissions. The reason for persistent seronegativity in some patients is not well understood. Some instances are due to antibody production against unusual epitopes on or near the acetylcholine receptor; their detection requires a special panel of tests.

Each of the commonly used diagnostic tests proves to be about equally reliable. Kelly and coworkers obtained positive results with single-muscle-fiber recording in 79 percent, with the antireceptor antibody test in 71 percent, and with the edrophonium test in 81 percent. Combined, they confirmed the diagnosis in 95 percent of clinically suspected cases.

In keeping with the observation by some myasthenic patients that their weakness improves in the cold, a test has been devised in which an ice pack is placed over the ptotic eyelid. Sethi and colleagues found that the ptosis was diminished in 8 of 10 patients, but we have been unsuccessful in demonstrating this effect with consistency.

Other diagnostic tests performed routinely in all patients thought to have myasthenia gravis include CT of the chest (for thymus enlargment or thymoma), tests of thyroid function, and, in selected patients, magnetic resonance imaging of the cranium and orbits (to rule out compressive and inflammatory lesions of the cranial nerves and ocular muscles).

Special Diagnostic Problems We have sometimes been puzzled by the following clinical problems:

1. *The concurrence of myasthenia gravis and thyrotoxicosis.* As indicated on page 1520, thyrotoxicosis may produce its own type of myopathy. There is no certain evidence that thyrotoxicosis aggravates myasthenia gravis; some have even observed a seesaw relationship which we have not confirmed. Hypothyroidism, however, does worsen myasthenia gravis. The ophthalmoplegia of thyrotoxicosis can usually be distinguished by the presence of an associated exophthalmos (early in the disease, exophthalmos may be absent) and the lack of response to neostigmine. Lupus erythematosus and polymyositis are distinguished by lack of involvement of extraocular muscles. Finding the signs of these diseases in combination with those of myasthenia usually indicates the concurrence of two independent autoimmune diseases.

2. *The neurasthenic patient who complains of weakness when actually referring to fatigability*. There is no ptosis, strabismus, or dysphagia, though a neurotic individual may complain of diplopia (usually of momentary duration, when drowsy) and also of tightness in the throat (globus hystericus). A number of such patients claim improvement with neostigmine, but objective weakness and reversal thereof is always uncertain. Conversely, myasthenia may be mistaken for hysteria or other emotional illness, mainly because the physician is unfamiliar with myasthenia (or with hysteria) and has been overly impressed with the precipitation of the illness by an emotional crisis.

3. *Progressive external ophthalmoplegia and other restricted myopathies, including the congenital myasthenic states*. These may be mistaken for myasthenia gravis. It should be emphasized that the extraocular muscles and levator palpebrae may be permanently damaged by myasthenia and cease to respond to neostigmine. Another possibility is that restricted ocular myasthenia may not respond to anticholinesterase drugs from the beginning and the diagnosis of myasthenia is erroneously excluded. One must then turn to other muscles for clinical and electromyographic confirmation of the diagnosis.

4. *Illnesses with dysarthria and dysphagia, but without ptosis or obvious strabismus*. These may be mistaken for multiple sclerosis, polymyositis, inclusion body myositis, stroke, motor neuron disease, or some other neurologic disease.

5. *The initial manifestations of botulism*—blurred vision, diplopia, ptosis, strabismus, and ophthalmoparesis—may be mistaken for myasthenia gravis of acute onset. In botulism, however, the pupils are usually large and unreactive, and the eye signs are followed in rapid succession by involvement of bulbar, trunk, and limb muscles.

6. *The oculopharyngeal-brachial and Fisher variants of the Guillain-Barré syndrome* (GBS), in their early stages, have many of the features of myasthenia gravis, including ptosis that may be partially responsive to anticholinesterase drugs. The loss of tendon reflexes or the rapid development of ataxia in GBS and detailed electrophysiologic testing distinguishes the two conditions.

7. *Intoxication with organophosphate insecticides*, because of their capacity to induce a cholinergic crisis, may be confused with a myasthenic crisis (see further on).

Treatment The treatment of this disease involves the careful use of two groups of drugs—anticholinesterases and immunosuppressants—thymectomy, and, in special circumstances, plasma exchange and intravenous immune globulin.

Anticholinesterase Drugs The two drugs that have given the best results in ameliorating myasthenic weakness are neostigmine (Prostigmin) and pyridostigmine (Mestinon), the latter being preferred by most clinicians and patients. The usual dose of pyridostigmine is 30 to 90 mg q6h (typically a 60-mg pill is tried first); the oral dose of neostigmine ranges from 7.5 to 45 mg given every 2 to 6 h. Delayed-action forms of both drugs are available but should be given at bedtime only to patients who complain of weakness during the night or early morning hours. The dosage of these drugs and their frequency of administration vary considerably from patient to patient, but we agree with Drachman that the maximal useful dosage of pyridostigmine rarely exceeds 120 mg q3h.

For mild cases without thymic tumor and for purely ocular myasthenia, the use of anticholinesterase drugs may be adequate and the only form of therapy necessary for some period of time. Although these drugs seldom relieve symptoms completely (the response of ocular symptoms is incomplete), most such patients are able to remain functional. Small doses of corticosteroids are often necessary for complete relief of diplopia (see further on).

If the response to anticholinesterase drugs is poor and progressively larger doses are not relieving symptoms, there is always the danger of a so-called *cholinergic crisis*. This consists of a relatively rapid increase in muscular weakness, usually coupled with the muscarinic effects of the anticholinesterase drug (nausea, vomiting, pallor, sweating, salivation, colic, diarrhea, miosis, bradycardia). An impending cholinergic effect is betrayed by constriction of pupils (they should not be allowed to contract to less than 2 mm). If the blood pressure falls, 0.6 mg atropine sulfate should be given slowly by the intravenous route. Edrophonium may be used to determine whether weakness is due to an excess of anticholinesterase medications or whether little change signifies a cholinergic excess. This test has been misleading and undoubtedly has contributed to an overestimation of the frequency and importance of the cholinergic crisis. In our own experience with more than 60 cases of severe myasthenia in an intensive care unit, we have been persuaded of the occurrence of a cholinergic crisis only rarely. Infection or the natural course of the disease (myasthenic crisis as discussed below) has been a far more common cause of severe weakness and respiratory failure.

Thymectomy Thymectomy, first introduced by Blalock, is advisable as an elective procedure in practically all patients with uncomplicated myasthenia gravis between puberty and approximately 55 years of age who, after a period of treatment with anticholinesterase drugs, are responding poorly and require increasing doses of medication. The remission rate after thymectomy in nontumor patients is approximately 35 percent provided that the procedure is done in the first year or two after onset of the disease, and another 50 percent will improve to some extent (Buckingham et al). The remission rate is progressively lower if operation is postponed beyond this time. The response to thymectomy is usually not evident for several months and is maximal by 3 years. In favorably responding cases, levels of circulating receptor antibody are reduced or disappear entirely. If possible, thymectomy should be postponed until puberty because of the importance of the gland in the development of the immune system, but juvenile myasthenia is also quite responsive.

A suprasternal approach has been developed and results in less postoperative pain and morbidity; however, the transsternal approach is preferable because it assures a more complete removal of thymic tissue. In patients with myasthenia restricted to the ocular muscles for a year or longer, the prognosis is so good that thymectomy is unnecessary. The operation is best performed in a hospital where there is close collaboration between the thoracic surgeon and the neurologist. If the patient is very weak preoperatively, a course of plasma exchange or immune globulin should precede the surgical procedure. After operation, respiratory assistance must be available. Neostigmine may be given every 3 to 6 h. Usually the dose requirement is about 75 percent of that taken before surgery. As improvement occurs, the dosage of neostigmine can be reduced.

The benefit of thymectomy in children has already been described under "Clinical Manifestations." Thymectomy is also a safe and effective treatment in nontumorous patients with late-onset myasthenia. In 12 such patients, Olanow and associates reported complete remission in 9 and clinical improvement in the remainder. Evidence of benefit in older patients is less convincing than in the younger group, in part because the thymus is atrophic, but some of our patients over age 60 have benefited.

Removal of the thymus gland is also indicated in practically all patients in whom *thymoma* is detected by CT scanning of the chest. The tumor can be locally invasive but rarely metastasizes. The operative approach is through the anterior thorax, with adequate exposure to remove all the tumor tissue. If the tumor cannot be removed completely, the remaining tissue should be treated with focused radiation. Local spread and lymph node invasion has been treated with combinations of chemotherapy including cisplatin. Park and colleagues have concluded from a large retrospective study that chemotherapy offers some benefit in terms of survival, but this remains a controversial area.

Corticosteroids For the myasthenic patient with moderate to severe generalized weakness in whom a remission has not been induced by thymectomy or who is responding inadequately to anticholinesterase drugs, the long-term administration of corticosteroids is the most consistently effective form of treatment (Pascuzzi et al). One must contend with the side effects of long-term corticosteroid therapy, and we hesitate to undertake such a program in children or patients with severe diabetes or other diseases that are likely to be aggravated by this form of immunosuppression. Corticosteroids alone or in combination with azathioprine (see below) are often adequate to control ocular myasthenia.

The usual form of corticosteroid therapy is prednisone (or corresponding doses of prednisolone), beginning with 15 to 20 mg/day and increasing the dose gradually until a satisfactory clinical response or a daily dose of 50 to 60 mg is reached. With higher doses or more rapid elevations of the doses, worsening in the first week is common, and hospitalization and careful observation for respiratory difficulty is advisable. Improvement occurs in the following few weeks. Once the maximal effect from prednisone has been attained, the dosage can be reduced slowly over months to the lowest point at which it is still effective. The usual practice is then to institute an alternate-day schedule, which diminishes the side effects. Our patients have done better with a modest difference in dose from one day to the next, rather than omitting an alternate-day dose entirely. Potassium supplements and antacids should be prescribed liberally, as with any chronic corticosteroid regime. At the outset of steroid therapy, anticholinesterase drugs are given simultaneously; as the patient improves, the dosage may be adjusted downward.

Azathioprine (Imuran) and Cyclosporine Azathioprine is a useful drug as an adjunct to steroids and in patients who cannot tolerate or fail to respond to prednisone. It has been possible to manage the disease effectively with azathioprine alone. Treatment begins with 50 mg (1 tablet) daily for a few days; if this is well tolerated, the dosage is raised to 2 to 3 mg/kg per day

(150 to 250 mg daily). The number of positive responses is much the same as with prednisone. However, improvement occurs much more slowly with azathioprine, and a significant response may not be evident for many months to a year (Witte et al). The Myasthenia Gravis Clinical Study Group has found that the most severe forms of the disease, often resistant to prednisone or azathioprine alone, benefit from the combination of the two medications. Liver function and the white blood cell count should be monitored regularly.

The clinical effects of the immunosuppressive agent cyclosporine are much like those of azathioprine but become evident more rapidly, in a matter of a month or two (Tindall et al). It is given in two divided doses daily, to a total of about 6 mg/kg. The use of this drug is restricted by its serious side effects (hypertension, nephrotoxicity) and its high cost.

Plasma Exchange and Intravenous Immune Globulin For the patient with severe myasthenia that is refractory to treatment with anticholinesterase drugs, thymectomy, and prednisone, one must resort to other measures. Striking temporary remissions (2 to 8 weeks) may be obtained by the use of *plasma exchange*. This form of treatment may be lifesaving during a myasthenic crisis, as noted below. It is also useful before and after thymectomy and at the start of immunosuppressive drug therapy. The number and volume of exchanges required in these circumstances is somewhat arbitrary, but they tend to be less than those required for Guillain-Barré syndrome; several exchanges of 2 to 3.5 L each (totaling approximately 125 mL/kg), performed over a week, usually suffice. The removed plasma is replaced with albumin and saline. It has been estimated that a 2-L exchange will remove 80 percent of circulating antibodies and that this will be reflected in reduced ACh antibody levels in 3 to 5 days. However, there is only a rough correlation between a reduction in the titer of circulating antibody and the degree of clinical improvement. In a crisis requiring plasma exchanges and mechanical ventilation, it has been our practice to discontinue or curtail the use of anticholinesterase drugs and resume them as the patient is being weaned from the ventilator. Also, it appears that sensitivity to these drugs may be enhanced in the hours after an exchange, so that their dosages must be adjusted accordingly. Plasma exchange also reduces the weakness that is often induced by the institution of high-dose corticosteroids.

A few patients respond so well to plasma exchange and find the side effects of steroids so intolerable that they choose to be maintained with two to three exchanges every few months. Immunoadsorption, a technique that removes antibodies and immune complexes by running blood over a tryptophan column, is less cumbersome than conventional plasma exchange, but experience with this procedure is as yet limited.

Intravenous immune globulin is also a useful measure in the short-term control of acutely worsening myasthenia. The usual dose is 2 g/kg given in divided doses over 3 to 5 days. However, neither plasma exchange nor immune globulin has been subjected to systematic study or comparison, and it should be re-emphasized that while these measures are invaluable in deteriorated patients or those in crisis, they offer only short-term benefit and are not used regularly in the treatment of most patients.

Myasthenic Crisis A rapid deterioration of the myasthenia itself, termed *myasthenic crisis*, can bring the patient to the brink of respiratory failure and quadriparesis in a matter of hours. A respiratory infection or excessive use of sedative drugs or drugs with a potential for blocking neuromuscular transmission may precede the myasthenic crisis. We have encountered numerous cases in which oropharyngeal weakness has led to aspiration pneumonia and precipitated a rapid deterioration of power in the limbs and diaphragm. Just as frequently, a precipitating event is not evident. Rarely, a respiratory arrest is the first manifestation of crisis. Such events may occur at any time after the diagnosis of myasthenia, but about half of them are evident within 18 months. In experience with 53 patients in myasthenic crisis seen over a period of 12 years at the Columbia-Presbyterian Medical Center, infection, usually pneumonia, was the most frequent precipitating event, but no cause could be determined in almost one-third of the patients (Thomas et al).

Incipient respiratory failure is marked usually by a reduction of vital capacity, often accompanied by restlessness, anxiety, diaphoresis, or tremor. Once the diaphragm fails, movements of the chest wall and abdomen become paradoxical (the abdomen moves inward during inspiration) or there may be shallow excursions of the chest, alternating with paradoxical movements. In an emergency, after clearing of the airway, such a patient can be supported briefly by a tight-fitting face mask and manual bag breathing.

Management of the crisis entails timely and careful intubation followed by mechanical ventilation in a critical care unit that is prepared to attend to the medical and neurologic needs of such a patient. One must cope with both the oropharyngeal weakness that endangers the airway and the diaphragmatic weakness. Anticholinergic drugs are best withdrawn at this point. The use of plasma exchange appears to hasten improvement and weaning from the ventilator. Intravenous gamma globulin may be a useful alternative but has not been studied extensively. Some of our colleagues have used high-dose corticosteroid infusions, but this measure has not been particularly successful in our hands and, in the short run, carries the risk of inducing widespread worsening of the weakness (Panegyres et al). Patients may respond to plasma exchange or immunoglobulin infusions in 1 or 2 days, but more often a week or more is required for recovery. It is generally best to wait 2 or 3 weeks before committing such a patient to tracheostomy.

When weaning from the ventilator is anticipated, anticholinesterase agents are reintroduced slowly, and treatment with corticosteroids can be instituted if necessary. *Oral doses of 60 mg pyridostigmine or 15 mg neostigmine are roughly equivalent to 0.5 to 1 mg neostigmine intravenously and 1.5 to 2 mg intramuscularly.* The management of the critically ill myasthenic patient has been reviewed by Fink.

Most patients with myasthenic crisis will take several weeks to recover, and a few of our patients have remained ventilator-dependent for months. Again, in the experience from Columbia-Presbyterian, half of the patients could be safely extubated within 2 weeks and three-quarters by a month (Thomas et al). There were 7 deaths among 53 patients, reflecting the gravity of this syndrome; this mortality accords with our experience. Atelectasis, severe anemia, congestive heart failure, and clostridial diarrhea (associated with antibiotic use) portend a prolonged period of intubation. From time to time one encounters a patient in whom respiration and ambulation do not improve for months after a myasthenic crisis. In our experience these have been middle-aged or older patients, usually women, in whom an element of hyperthyroidism or hypothyroidism may have been added. They became wasted as the proximal limb and axial muscles, including the diaphragm, failed to recover their power, even though the ocular and oropharyngeal muscles had improved. The role of corticosteroids in producing a concomitant proximal myopathy is a frequent problem that can be solved by careful EMG examination.

Management of Anesthesia and Pregnancy in the Myasthenic Patient These special problems should be mentioned here. Surgical procedures of any type are often sufficiently stressful to produce decompensation of the disease. If the patient is unable to take medications orally, anticholinesterase agents may be given intramuscularly (one-thirtieth of the oral dose of pyridostigmine and one-tenth the oral dose of neostigmine). If corticosteroids were being used, they should be continued and the dose generally kept unchanged; large "stress" doses are generally not necessary. Neuromuscular blocking agents of the noncompetitive type may have a very prolonged effect and should be avoided as part of the anesthetic regimen if possible. If they are necessary for some reason, a period of mechanical ventilation should be anticipated. In contrast, the dose of succinylcholine (which is not recommended) required to produce muscle relaxation may be larger than usual. Any drug whose use is contemplated in the anesthetic and postsurgical management of the myasthenic patient should be checked against the list of drugs that might exaggerate myasthenic weakness (see below).

Pregnancy is usually uncomplicated in myasthenic women. However, the use of intravenous cholinesterase inhibitors is contraindicated because of the possibility of inducing uterine contractions, and cytotoxic drugs are generally not used because of the potential for causing fetal abnormalities. Also, magnesium is not recommended for the treatment of eclampsia because of its neuromuscular blocking effects. Delivery usually proceeds normally, and breast-feeding is not thought to be a problem with regard to the transmission of AChR antibodies. The issues of neonatal myasthenia and reduced intrauterine movements are considered below.

Other Disorders of Neuromuscular Transmission

Considered here are several disorders of neuromuscular transmission characterized clinically by muscular weakness and fatigability but differing in causation and mechanism from acquired autoimmune myasthenia gravis. The Lambert-Eaton myasthenic syndrome, neonatal myasthenia, the congenital myasthenic syndromes, and the myasthenic syndromes induced by drugs and toxins are the main representatives of this group of disorders. Two important members of this group—botulism and organophosphate poisoning—are described elsewhere (pages 1274 and 1281, respectively).

The Myasthenic-Myopathic Syndrome of Lambert-Eaton This special form of myasthenia, observed most often with oat-cell carcinoma of the lung, was first described by Lambert, Eaton, and Rooke in 1956 and by

Eaton and Lambert in 1957. Unlike the case in myasthenia gravis, the muscles of the trunk, shoulder girdle, pelvic girdle, and lower extremities are the ones that most frequently become weak and fatigable; the EMG findings and poor response to anticholinesterase drugs also serve to differentiate it from myasthenia gravis. Often the first symptoms are difficulty in arising from a chair, climbing stairs, and walking; the shoulder muscles are affected later. While ptosis, diplopia, dysarthria, and dysphagia may occur, presentation with these symptoms is distinctly unusual. Increasing weakness after exertion stamps the condition as myasthenic, but as originally pointed out, *there may be a temporary increase in muscle power during the first few contractions*. The tendon reflexes are often diminished, but abolition of the reflexes should raise the question of an associated carcinomatous polyneuropathy. Fasciculations are not seen. Other complaints are paresthesias, aching pain (suggesting arthritis), and a number of autonomic disturbances, such as dryness of the mouth, constipation, difficult micturition, and impotence. There may be other neurologic manifestations of neoplasia (polyneuropathy, polymyositis or dermatomyositis, multifocal leukoencephalopathy, cerebellar degeneration, as discussed on pages 721–728).

The onset is usually subacute and the course variably progressive. The myasthenia may precede discovery of the tumor by months or years. About 60 percent of patients have an associated small-cell lung cancer, but the syndrome has also occurred with carcinoma of the breast, prostate, stomach, and rectum and with lymphomas. Males are affected more often than females (5:1). In about one-third of patients, no tumor is found; most of these cases are associated with other autoimmune diseases. The condition may occur in children, usually without relation to tumor. In the tumor cases, death usually occurs in a few months or years from the effect of the tumor itself.

As mentioned above, the response to neostigmine and pyridostigmine is poor and unpredictable. On the other hand, *d*-tubocurarine, suxamethonium chloride, gallamine, and other muscle relaxants have a deleterious effect; when given during anesthesia, they may increase the weakness dramatically and even lead to fatality.

Electrodiagnostic studies have shown no abnormality in the peripheral nerves. A single stimulus of nerve may yield a low-amplitude muscle action potential (in contrast to myasthenia gravis, in which it is normal or nearly so), whereas at fast rates of stimulation (50 per second) as shown in Fig. 45-5*B* and with strong voluntary contraction (for 15 s or longer), there is a marked increase in the amplitude of action potentials (incrementing response). Single-fiber recordings show an increase in "jitter," as in myasthenia gravis (page 1366).

In patients with the Lambert-Eaton syndrome, there is an increased incidence of HLA-B8 and -DR3 haplotypes, as may occur in other autoimmune diseases. Elmquist and Lambert, from a series of studies of excised muscle, deduced that there is a defect in the release of ACh quanta from the presynaptic nerve terminals, akin to that in paralysis due to botulinum toxin, magnesium excess, and neomycin (see further on). When injected into mice, serum IgG from patients with this syndrome transfers the physiologic abnormality (reduction in nerve-evoked quantal release of ACh). The presynaptic vesicles themselves appear to be normal in electron micrographs. In contrast to myasthenia gravis, the extent of the receptor surface in the myasthenic syndrome is actually increased (A. G. Engel), and no receptor antibody is present. The fundamental physiologic defect in Lambert-Eaton myasthenic syndrome has been attributed to a loss of voltage-sensitive calcium channels on the presynaptic motor nerve terminal; the calcium channels are cross-linked and aggregated by the patients's IgG autoantibodies, with an ultimate reduction in the number of functioning channels (Fukunaga et al). Muscle biopsy is normal or shows only the same slight, nonspecific changes as in myasthenia gravis.

Recognition of the Lambert-Eaton syndrome should lead to a search for occult tumor, especially of the lung. If found, it should of course be treated; this alone may result in improvement in the neurologic syndrome. If none is found, the search should be repeated at regular intervals, since the tumors tend to be small and may be inapparent until autopsy.

Treatment Guanidine hydrochloride (20 to 30 mg/kg/day in divided doses) has proved to be more effective in increasing strength than neostigmine or pyridostigmine. Subsequently, guanidine was largely replaced by 3,4-diaminopyridine, 20 mg orally five times daily, in conjunction with pyridostigmine (Lundh et al). Streib and Rothner were able to achieve long-term improvement with prednisone. Dau and Denys obtained the best results in nontumor cases with repeated courses of plasmapheresis in combination with prednisone and azathioprine. Intravenous immune globulin has also been effective in a few cases. Because of the unpredictable side effects of diaminopyridine (seizures, confusional state, paresthesias), some clinicians prefer alternate-day administration of prednisone and azathioprine—prednisone 25 to 60 mg/day, and azathioprine 2.3 to 2.9 mg/kg body weight daily—supplemented by intravenous immune globulin. The response to treatment tends to be slow, over a period of months to a year. Some patients recover fully; in others, restoration of power is incomplete.

Diagnosis A syndrome of symmetrical weakness and fatigability of proximal muscles—coupled with dry mouth, sphincter disturbances, aching muscles, and diminished reflexes—should be diagnostic. The only illnesses with which it might be confused are polymyositis and hysterical paralysis, where the patient may do better with encouragement on successive voluntary contractions, and arthritis, where pain hampers the first movements more than successive ones. Then the electrodiagnostic tests are of value.

Neonatal Myasthenia Gravis An estimated 12 to 20 percent of babies born to myasthenic mothers show signs of myasthenia (hypotonia, weak cry and suck). This is a transitory phenomenon with a mean duration of 18 days, and recovery is usually complete within 2 months of birth (rarely longer), without later relapse. Uncommonly, the myasthenic mother experiences reduced intrauterine movements, suggesting a dangerous degree of myasthenia in the fetus. A few of these children will be born with arthrogryposis, the result of a sustained period of intrauterine immobility, and this complication tends to recur in subsequent births. It has long been assumed that this neonatal myasthenia is due to the passive transplacental transfer of anti-AChR antibodies. This explanation seems unlikely, insofar as maternal AChR antibodies are transferred from mother to fetus in all AChR antibody–positive pregnancies. Moreover, the severity of the neonatal myasthenia gravis does not correlate with the severity or duration of the mother's illness or with the serum level of the maternal AChR antibody. In fact, neonatal myasthenia may occur when the mother is in remission.

The use of plasma exchange and anticholinesterase drugs may be useful in hastening recovery from neonatal myasthenia.

Congenital Myasthenic Syndromes Sporadically in the medical literature, there have appeared reports of a benign congenital myopathy in which myasthenic features could be recognized in the neonatal period or soon thereafter. The affected infants had been born to nonmyasthenic mothers and were described under headings such as "Myasthenia Gravis in the Newborn" and "Familial Infantile Myasthenia" (Greer and Schotland; Robertson et al).

In the 1970s and 1980s, when the autoimmune basis of myasthenia gravis was established and its morphologic and physiologic features were defined, the differences between this disease and the familial infantile forms became evident. Since then, at least six distinct and rare congenital myasthenic syndromes have been delineated on the basis of their electrophysiologic and ultrastructural features, and a number of others have been partially characterized. Each of these new forms of congenital myasthenia is featured by a unique synaptic or pre- or postsynaptic defect, involving the resynthesis or packaging of ACh or a paucity of synaptic vesicles (presynaptic defect); a deficiency of end-plate ACh esterase (synaptic defect); or a kinetic abnormality of the ACh receptor channels, with or without AChR deficiency (postsynaptic defects). In three-fourths of the cases the defect is postsynaptic, in 13 percent it is synaptic, and in 8 percent it is presynaptic. Mainly this has been the accomplishment of A. G. Engel, who has systematically defined and classified these disorders in a series of extensive investigations of more than 100 cases of congenital myasthenia. A detailed and current account of this work can be found in Engel's chapter on the subject in his monograph *Myasthenia Gravis and Myasthenic Disorders*. The following clinical features are more or less applicable to all of the congenital myasthenic syndromes.

In the neonate, the most important clue to the disease is an increase in ptosis and in bulbar and respiratory weakness with crying. Later in infancy these symptoms, as well as fluctuating ocular palsies and abnormal fatigability, are brought out by other types of sustained activity. Motor milestones may be delayed. In some cases, the myasthenic weakness and fatigability become evident only in the second and third decades of life. The intravenous edrophonium test is inconsistently positive in a few forms of congenital myasthenia but is usually negative. There is usually a decremental EMG response at low-frequency stimulation (2 Hz). *A positive ACh receptor antibody test excludes the diagnosis of a congenital myasthenic syndrome*. Some forms of the syndromes respond to treatment with anticholinesterase drugs; others do not. All congenital myasthenic syndromes are inherited as an autosomal recessive trait.

Myasthenic Weakness due to Antibiotics and Other Drugs and to Natural Environmental Toxins Many drugs may cause a myasthenic syndrome or a worsening of myasthenia gravis by their action on pre- or postsynaptic structures. This is most likely to happen in patients who are already receiving some other drug or drugs for a variety of illnesses and have hepatic or renal disease. The myasthenic state in these conditions is acute and lasts hours or days, with full recovery provided that the patient does not succumb to respiratory failure. The ocular, facial, and bulbar muscles are involved as well as other muscles. The treatment in all instances is to provide respiratory support, discontinue the offending drug, and attempt to reverse the block at the end plate by infusions of calcium gluconate, potassium supplements, and the administration of anticholinesterases along the lines suggested by Argov and Mastaglia.

There are more than 30 drugs in current clinical use (other than anesthetic agents) that may interfere with neuromuscular transmission in otherwise normal individuals. Of these, the most important are the aminoglycoside antibiotics. Myasthenic weakness has been reported with 18 different antibiotics but particularly with neomycin, kanamycin (less so with gentamicin), colistin, streptomycin, polymyxin B, and certain tetracyclines (McQuillen et al; Pittinger et al). It has been shown that these drugs impair transmitter release by interfering with calcium-ion fluxes at nerve terminals. They are especially dangerous when given to myasthenic patients, but they may be used if necessary in a patient who is already receiving ventilatory support. Also, several of the immunosuppressant drugs—such as adrenocorticotropic hormone (ACTH), prednisone, and possibly azathioprine—worsen myasthenia temporarily by depolarizing nerve terminals or impairing release of ACh.

Other drugs—such as anticholinesterase agents, particularly insecticides and nerve gases—cause paralysis by binding to cholinesterase and blocking the hydrolysis of ACh. The end plate remains depolarized and is refractory to neural stimuli. As mentioned, the most notable of these drugs or toxins are botulinum toxin, which binds to cholinergic motor endings, blocking quantal release of ACh; black widow spider venom, which causes a massive release of ACh, resulting in muscular contraction and then paralysis from a lack of ACh; *d*-tubocurarine, which binds to ACh receptors; suxamethonium and decamethonium, which also bind to ACh receptors; organophosphates, which bind irreversibly to ACh esterases; and malathion and parathion, which inhibit ACh esterase. The actions of all these agents except for the organophosphate "nerve gases" are transitory.

The administration of *d*-penicillamine has also caused a type of myasthenia. The weakness is typical in that rest increases strength—as do neostigmine and edrophonium—and the electrophysiologic findings are also the same. In such cases, Vincent and others found anti-ACh receptor antibodies in the serum; hence, one must assume that this is a form of induced autoimmune myasthenia gravis. In these respects it differs from the weakness caused by aminoglycosides (see review of Swift). Rarely, typical autoimmune myasthenia gravis develops as part of a chronic graft-versus-host disease in long-term (2- to 3-year) survivors of allogeneic marrow transplants.

A large group of naturally occurring environmental neurotoxins are known to act at the neuromuscular junction and to induce muscle paralysis with a distribution like that of myasthenia gravis. Venoms of snakes, spiders, and ticks are common and well-known animal poisons, as are ciguatera and related toxins (from fish that have ingested certain dinoflagellates), curare (from plants), and *Clostridium botulinum*—all of which are discussed in other parts of this book (see Chap. 43). Poisoning by these natural neurotoxins constitutes an important public health hazard in many parts of the world but particularly in the tropics. This class of disorders of neuromuscular transmission has been reviewed by Senanayake and Roman.

REFERENCES

Argov Z, Mastaglia FL: Disorders of neuromuscular transmission caused by drugs. *N Engl J Med* 301:409, 1979.

Bever CT Jr, Aquino AV, Penn AS, et al: Prognosis of ocular myasthenia. *Ann Neurol* 14:516, 1983.

Brill V, Kojic J, Dhanani A: The long-term clinical outcome of myasthenia gravis in patients with thymoma. *Neurology* 51:1198, 1998.

Buckingham JM, Howard FM Jr, Bernatz PE, et al: The value of thymectomy in myasthenia gravis: A computer-assisted matched study. *Ann Surg* 184:453, 1976.

Buzzard EF: The clinical history and postmortem examination of 5 cases of myasthenia gravis. *Brain* 28:438, 1905.

Cogan DG: Myasthenia gravis: A review of the disease and a description of lid twitch as a characteristic sign. *Arch Ophthalmol* 74:217, 1965.

Cohen MS, Younger D: Aspects of the natural history of myasthenia gravis: Crisis and death. *Ann NY Acad Sci* 377:670, 1981.

Compston DAS, Vincent A, Newsom-Davis A, Batchelor JR: Clinical, pathological, HLA antigen, and immunological evidence for disease heterogeneity in myasthenia gravis. *Brain* 103:579, 1980.

Dau PC, Denys EH: Plasmapheresis and immunosuppressive therapy in the Eaton-Lambert syndrome. *Ann Neurol* 11:570, 1982.

Drachman DB: How to recognize an antibody-mediated autoimmune disease: Criteria, in Waksman BH (ed):

Immunologic Mechanisms in Neurologic and Psychiatric Disease. *Res Publ Assoc Res Nerv Ment Dis* 68:183, 1990.

Drachman DB: Myasthenia gravis. *N Engl J Med* 330:1797, 1994.

Drachman DB: Myasthenic antibodies cross-link acetylcholine receptors to accelerate degradation. *N Engl J Med* 298:136, 186, 1978.

Eaton LM, Lambert EH: Electromyography and electric stimulation of nerves and diseases of motor unit: Observations on myasthenic syndrome associated with malignant tumors. *JAMA* 163:1117, 1957.

Elmquist D, Lambert EH: Detailed analysis of neuromuscular transmission in a patient with the myasthenic syndrome, sometimes associated with bronchial carcinoma. *Mayo Clin Proc* 43:689, 1968.

Engel AG: Congenital myasthenic syndromes, in Engel AG (ed): *Myasthenia Gravis and Myasthenic Disorders*. New York, Oxford University Press, 1999, pp 251–297.

Engel AG (ed): *Myasthenia Gravis and Myasthenic Disorders*. New York, Oxford University Press, 1999.

Engel AG, Lambert EH, Howard FM: Immune complexes (IgG and C3) at motor end-plate in myasthenia gravis. *Mayo Clin Proc* 52:267, 1977.

Engel AG, Lambert EH, Santa T: Study of long-term anticholinesterase therapy. *Neurology* 23:1273, 1973.

Engel AG, Tsujihata M, Lambert EH, et al: Experimental autoimmune myasthenia gravis: A sequential and quantitative study of the neuromuscular junction ultrastructure and electrophysiologic correlations. *J Neuropathol Exp Neurol* 35:569, 1976.

Engel AG, Tsujihata M, Lindstrom JM, Lennon VA: The motor end plate in myasthenia gravis and in experimental autoimmune myasthenia gravis. *Ann N Y Acad Sci* 274:60, 1976.

Engel AL, Arahata K: The membrane attack complex of complement at the endplate in myasthenia gravis. *Ann N Y Acad Sci* 505:326, 1987.

Fambrough DM, Drachman DB, Satyamurti S: Neuromuscular junction in myasthenia gravis: Decreased acetylcholine receptors. *Science* 182:293, 1973.

Fink ME: Treatment of the critically ill patient with myasthenia gravis, in Ropper AH (ed): *Neurological and Neurosurgical Intensive Care*, 3rd ed. New York, Raven, 1993, pp 351–362.

Fukunaga H, Engel AG, Osane M, et al: Paucity and disorganization of presynaptic membrane active zones in the Lambert-Eaton myasthenic syndrome. *Muscle Nerve* 5:686, 1982.

Greer M, Schotland M: Myasthenia gravis in the newborn. *Pediatrics* 26:101, 1960.

Grob D, Brunner NG, Namba T: The natural course of myasthenia gravis and effect of therapeutic measures. *Ann N Y Acad Sci* 377:652, 1981.

Kakulas BA, Adams RD: *Diseases of Muscle: Pathological Foundations of Clinical Myology*, 4th ed. Philadelphia, Harper & Row, 1985.

Kelly JJ, Daube JR, Lennon VA: The laboratory diagnosis of mild myasthenia gravis. *Ann Neurol* 12:238, 1982.

Kerzin-Storrar L, Metcalfe RA, Dyer PA: Genetic factors in myasthenia gravis: A family study. *Neurology* 38:38, 1988.

Lambert EH, Eaton LM, Rooke ED: Defect of neuromuscular transmission associated with malignant neoplasm. *Am J Physiol* 187:612, 1956.

Lambert EH, Lindstrom JM, Lennon VA: End-plate potentials in experimental autoimmune myasthenia gravis in rats. *Ann N Y Acad Med* 274:300, 1976.

Lennon VA: Immunologic mechanisms in myasthenia gravis—A model of a receptor disease, in Franklin E (ed): *Clinical Immunology Update—Reviews for Physicians*. New York, Elsevier/North-Holland, 1979, pp 259–289.

Lennon VA, Lindstrom JM, Seybold ME: Experimental autoimmune myasthenia gravis in rats and guinea pigs. *J Exp Med* 141:1365, 1975.

Lindstrom JM, Lambert EH: Content of acetylcholine receptor and antibodies bound to receptor in myasthenia gravis, experimental autoimmune myasthenia gravis, and Eaton-Lambert syndrome. *Neurology* 28:130, 1978.

Lundh H, Nilsson O, Rosen I: Treatment of Lambert-Eaton syndrome: 3,4-Diaminopyridine and pyridostigmine. *Neurology* 34:1324, 1984.

Mayer RF, Williams IR: Incrementing responses in myasthenia gravis. *Arch Neurol* 31:24, 1974.

McQuillen MP, Cantor HE, O'Rourke JR: Myasthenic syndrome associated with antibiotics. *Arch Neurol* 18:402, 1968.

Meyers KR, Gilden DH, Rinaldi CF, Hansen JL: Periodic muscle weakness, normokalemia, and tubular aggregates. *Neurology* 22:269, 1972.

Mossman S, Vincent A, Newsom-Davis J: Myasthenia gravis without acetylcholine receptor antibody: A distinct disease entity. *Lancet* 1:116, 1986.

Myasthenia Gravis Clinical Study Group: A randomized clinical trial comparing prednisone and azathioprine in myasthenia gravis: Results of the second interim analysis. *J Neurol Neurosurg Psychiatry* 56:1157, 1993.

Nastuk WL, Plescia OJ, Osserman KE: Changes in serum complement activity in patients with myasthenia gravis. *Proc Soc Exp Biol Med* 105:177, 1960.

Newsom-Davis J: Diseases of the neuromuscular junction, in Asbury AK, McKhann GM, McDonald WI (eds): *Diseases of the Nervous System*, 2nd ed. Philadelphia, Saunders, 1992, pp 197–212.

Olanow CW, Lane RJM, Roses AD: Thymectomy in late-onset myasthenia gravis. *Arch Neurol* 39:82, 1982.

Osserman KE: *Myasthenia Gravis*. New York, Grune & Stratton, 1958.

Panegyres PM, Squier M, Mills KR, Newsom-Davis J: Acute myopathy associated with large parenteral dose of corticosteroid in myasthenia gravis. *J Neurol Neurosurg Psychiatry* 56:72, 1993.

Park HS, Shin DM, Lee JS, et al: Thymoma. A retrospective study of 87 cases. *Cancer* 73:2491, 1994.

Pascuzzi RM, Coslett HB, Johns TR: Long-term corticosteroid treatment of myasthenia gravis: Report of 116 cases. *Ann Neurol* 15:291, 1984.

Patrick J, Lindstrom JP: Autoimmune response to acetylcholine receptor. *Science* 180:871, 1973.

PATRICK J, LINDSTROM JP, CULP B, MCMILLAN J: Studies on purified eel acetylcholine receptor and antiacetylcholine receptor antibody. *Proc Natl Acad Sci USA* 70:3334, 1973.

PEREZ MC, BUOT WL, MERCADO-DONGUILAN C: Stable remissions in myasthenia gravis. *Neurology* 31:32, 1981.

PITTINGER CB, ERYASE Y, ADAMSON R: Antibiotic induced paralysis. *Anesth Analg* 49:487, 1970.

REMAN L: Zur Pathogenese und Therapie der Myasthenia gravis pseudoparalytica. *Dtsch Z Nervenheilkd* 128:66, 1932.

REUTHER P, FULPIUS BW, MERTENS HB, HERTEL G: Anti-acetylcholine receptor antibody under long-term azathioprine treatment in myasthenia gravis, in Dau PC (ed): *Plasmapheresis and the Immunobiology of Myasthenia Gravis*. Boston, Houghton Mifflin, 1979, pp 329–348.

ROBERTSON WC, CHUN RWM, KORNGUTA SE: Familial infantile myasthenia. *Arch Neurol* 37: 117, 1980.

RODRIGUEZ M, GOMEZ MR, HOWARD FM: Myasthenia gravis in children: Long-term followup. *Ann Neurol* 13:504, 1983.

RUSSELL DS: Histological changes in myasthenia gravis. *J Pathol Bacteriol* 65:279, 1953.

SANTA T, ENGEL AG, LAMBERT EH: Histometric study of neuromuscular junction ultrastructure: I. Myasthenia gravis. *Neurology* 22:71, 1972.

SCADDING GK, VINCENT A, NEWSOM-DAVIS J, HENRY K: Acetylcholine receptor antibody synthesis by thymic lymphocytes: Correlation with thymic histology. *Neurology* 31:935, 1981.

SCHLUEP M, WILLCOX N, VINCENT A, et al: Acetylcholine receptors in human thymic cells in situ: An immunohistological study. *Ann Neurol* 22:212, 1987.

SENANAYAKE N, ROMAN GC: Disorders of neuromuscular transmission due to natural environmental toxins. *J Neurol Sci* 107:1, 1992.

SETHI KD, RIVNER MH, SWIFT TR: Ice pack test for myasthenia gravis. *Neurology* 37:1383, 1987.

SIMPSON JA: Myasthenia gravis: A new hypothesis. *Scot Med J* 5:419, 1960.

STREIB EW, ROTHNER D: Eaton-Lambert myasthenic syndrome: Long-term treatment of 3 patients with prednisone. *Ann Neurol* 10:448, 1981.

SWIFT TR: Disorders of neuromuscular transmission other than myasthenia gravis. *Muscle Nerve* 4:334, 1981.

THOMAS CE, MAYER SA, GUNGOR Y, et al: Myasthenic crisis: Clinical features, mortality, complications, and risk factors for prolonged intubation. *Neurology* 48:1253, 1997.

TINDALL RSA, PHILLIPS JT, ROLLINS JA, et al: A clinical therapeutic trial of cyclosporine in myasthenia gravis. *Ann NY Acad Sci* 681:539, 1993.

VIETS HR: A historical review of myasthenia gravis from 1672 to 1900. *JAMA* 153:1273, 1953.

VINCENT A, NEWSOM-DAVIS J: Acetylcholine receptor antibody as a diagnostic test for myasthenia gravis: Results in 153 validated cases and 2967 diagnostic assays. *J Neurol Neurosurg Psychiatry* 48:1246, 1985.

VINCENT A, NEWSOM-DAVIS J, MARTIN V: Antiacetylcholine receptor antibodies in *d*-penicillamine associated myasthenia gravis. *Lancet* 1:1254, 1978.

VINCENT A, WRAY D (eds): *Neuromuscular Transmission. Basic and Applied Aspects*. New York, Manchester Press, 1990.

WALKER MB: Treatment of myasthenia gravis with physostigmine. *Lancet* 1:1200, 1934.

WEINBERG DH, RIZZO JF, HAYES MT, et al: Ocular myasthenia gravis: Predictive value of single-fiber electromyography. *Muscle Nerve* 22:1222, 1999.

WITTE AS, CORNBLATH DR, PARRY GJ, et al: Azathioprine in the treatment of myasthenia gravis. *Ann Neurol* 15:602, 1984.

YAMAMOTO T, VINCENT A, CIULLA TA, et al: Seronegative myasthenia gravis: A plasma factor inhibiting agonist-induced acetylcholine receptor function copurifies with IgM. *Ann Neurol* 30:550, 1991.

Chapter 54

THE HEREDITARY MYOTONIAS AND PERIODIC PARALYSES (THE CHANNELOPATHIES)

Grouping the hereditary myotonias with the periodic paralyses is a relatively new development in the classification of muscle diseases. In the medical literature, until quite recently, the myotonias stood alone or were thought to be related in some undefined way to the muscular dystrophies. In a similar vein, the periodic paralyses (better called *episodic paralyses*) have usually been considered with other types of metabolic myopathy. Recent molecular genetic studies, notably those of Rüdel, Lehmann- Horn, and Ricker and their associates, have identified the fundamental defects in the myotonias and episodic paralyses and clarified their relationships, and several new forms of nondystrophic myotonia have been defined. It is now known that all these diseases are caused by mutations in genes that code for chloride, sodium, or calcium channels in muscle fiber membranes, and all are now referred to as *ion channel diseases,* or, colloquially, as "channelopathies." The main features of the ion channel diseases are summarized in Table 54-1. Individual members of the group are described below.

CHLORIDE CHANNEL DISEASES

Myotonia Congenita (Thomsen Disease)

This is an uncommon disease of skeletal muscle that begins in early life and is characterized by myotonia, muscular hypertrophy, a nonprogressive course, and dominant inheritance. It is set apart from myotonic dystrophy, which has a different genetic basis and is characterized by a progressive degeneration of muscle fibers (see page 1503).

History This disorder was first brought to the attention of the medical profession in 1876 by Julius Thomsen, a Danish physician who himself suffered from the disease, as did 20 other members of his family over four generations. His designation of *ataxia muscularis* was not apt, but his description left no doubt as to the nature of the condition, which featured "tonic cramps in voluntary muscles associated with an inherited psychical indisposition." The association of the latter condition was not borne out by subsequent studies and is now thought to be fortuitous. Strumpell in 1881 assigned the name *myotonia congenita* to the disease, and Westphal in 1883 referred to it as *Thomsen's disease*. Erb provided the first description of its pathology and called attention to two additional unique features, muscular hyperexcitability and hypertrophy. In 1923, Nissen, Thomsen's great-nephew, extended the original genealogy to 35 cases in seven generations. In 1948, Thomasen updated the subject in a monograph that is still a useful clinical reference.

Clinical Features Tonic spasm of muscle after forceful voluntary contraction stands as the cardinal feature of the disease and is most pronounced after a period of inactivity. Repeated contractions "wear it out," so to speak, and later movements in a series become more swift and effective. Rarely the converse is observed—where only the later movements of a series induce myotonia (*myotonia paradoxica*); but usually this is a feature of cold-induced paramyotonia congenita (see further on). Unlike cramp, the spasm is painless, but after prolonged activity, nocturnal myalgia—a pinching-aching sensation in the overactive muscles—may develop and prove distressing. Close observation reveals a softness of the muscles during rest, and the initial contraction appears not to be significantly slowed unless there is pre-existent myotonia.

The congenital nature of the dominant form of the disease may be evident even in the crib, where the

Table 54-1
Inherited myotonia and periodic paralyses (the channelopathies)

Channelopathy	*Chloride*	*Chloride*	*Chloride*	*Sodium*	*Sodium*
Disease	**Myotonia congenita (Thomsen)**	**Generalized myotonia (Becker)**	**Myotonia levior (DeJong)**	**Hyperkalemic periodic paralysis**	**Normokalemic periodic paralysis**
Inheritance	Dominant	Recessive	Dominant	Dominant	Dominant
Gene locus	7q32	7q32	7q32	17q	17q
Gene	CLCN1	CLCN1	CLCN1	SCN4A	SCN4A
Channel protein	CLC1	CLC1	CLC1	α subunit	α subunit
Myotonia (electrical)	++	++	+	+/−	+/−
Myotonia (clinical)	++	+++	+	+/−	+/−
Paramyotonia (clinical)	—	—	—	+/−	+/−
Episodic paralysis	—	—	—	+++	+++
Onset	Congenital to late childhood	Late childhood or earlier	Adolescence	First decade	First decade
Precipitating factors					
Appears during exercise	—	—	—	—	—
Increases with exercise	—	—	—	—	—
Appears after exercise	++	++	+	++	++
Fasting	—	—	—	+	—
Carbohydrate load	—	—	—	—	—
Potassium load	—	—	—	++	+/−
Cold	—	—	—	++	+
Emotional stress	+	+	—	++	+
Pregnancy	+	+	—	++	—
Anesthetics (halothane, succinylcholine)	—	—	—	—	—
"Warmup" phenomenon	++	++	+	+	+
Transient weakness following myotonia	+	++	—	—	—
Persistent weakness following myotonia	—	—	—	—	—
Exercise-induced myalgia	—	—	—	—	—
Involvement of cranial muscles	+	+	—	—	+/−
Lid lag and blepharospasm	+	+	—	—	—
Muscle hypertrophy	+	++	—	—	+
Permanent myopathy	—	+	—	+	+
Serum CK during attack	Normal to borderline	Increased 2 to 3 times	Normal	Increased	Increased
Serum K during attack	Normal	Normal	Normal	Increased	Normal
Serum K between attacks	Normal	Normal	Normal	Normal	Normal
Significant myopathology (vacuolar myopathy)	—	—	—	++	++
Treatment	Mexiletine if required	Mexiletine if required	No treatment necessary	During attack, glucose; for prevention, high-CHO, low-K diet	Large doses of Na

Table 54-1 *(Continued)*
Inherited myotonia and periodic paralyses (the channelopathies)

Sodium	*Sodium*	*Sodium*	*Sodium*	*Calcium*	*Calcium*
Paramyotonia congenita	**Myotonia fluctuans**	**Myotonia permanens**	**Acetazolamide-responsive myotonia**	**Hypokalemic periodic paralysis**	**Malignant hyperthermia**
Dominant	Dominant	Dominant	Dominant	Dominant	Dominant
17q	17q	17q	17q	1q31–32	1q13.1
SCN4A	SCN4A	SCN4A	SCN4A	DHP receptor	RYR1
α subunit	α subunit	α subunit	α subunit	Dihydropyridine α subunit	Ryanodine receptor
++	++	+++	++	—	—
—	+	+++	++	—	—
+++	+	+++	+	—	—
+/−	—	—	—	+++	—
Paramyotonia at birth	Adolescence	Early childhood	First decade	Early childhood to third decade	All ages
+++	—	+++	+	—	+
+++	—	++	+	—	+
—	+	+	+	+	—
—	—	—	+	—	—
—	—	—	—	+	—
+/−	++	++	++	—	—
+++	+/−	+/−	+/−	+	—
+	+	+	—	+	—
++	+/−	—	—	+	—
++	++	++	—	—	++++
—	++	—	+	+	—
++	—	+	—	—	—
++	—	+	—	—	—
+	+	—	++	—	—
+++	++	++	+	+	++
+	—	++	—	—	—
—	—	+++	—	—	—
—	—	++	—	+	—
Increased 5 to 10 times	Increased 2 to 4 times	Increased	Increased	Normal to slightly increased	Markedly increased
Normal	Normal	Normal	Normal	Decreased	Normal
Normal	Normal	Normal	Normal	Normal	Normal
—	—	++	—	++	Rhabdomyolysis cores
Mexiletine if needed	Mexiletine if needed	Procainamide, mexiletine	Acetazolamide, carbohydrates	KCl during and acetazolamide between attacks	Intravenous dantrolene

infant's eyes are noted to open slowly after it has been crying or sneezing, and its legs are conspicuously stiff as the child tries to take its first steps. In other cases, the myotonia becomes evident only later in the first or second decade. The muscles are generously proportioned and may become hypertrophied, but seldom to the degree observed in the recessive form of the disease, described further on. Despite their muscular appearance, these patients are inept in athletic pursuits.

When severe, the myotonia tends to affect all skeletal muscles but is especially prominent in the lower limbs. Attempts to walk and run are sometimes impeded to the extent that the patient stumbles and falls. Other limb and trunk muscles are also thrown into spasm, as are those of the face and upper limbs. Occasionally a sudden noise or fright may cause generalized stiffness and falling. Small, gentle movements such as blinking or elicitation of a tendon reflex do not initiate myotonia, whereas strong closure of the eyelids, as in a sneeze, sets up a spasm that may prevent complete opening of the eyes for many seconds. Spasms of extraocular muscles occur in some instances, leading to strabismus. If the patient has not spoken for a time, there is sometimes a striking dysarthria. Arising at night, the patient cannot walk without first moving his legs for a few minutes. After a period of rest, the patient may have difficulty in arising from a chair or climbing stairs. Loosening of one set of muscles after a succession of contractions does not prevent the appearance of myotonia in another set, nor in the same ones if used in another pattern of movement. Contrary to conventional teaching, exposure to cold does not worsen myotonia that is due to this mutation of chloride channels. Smooth and cardiac muscles are never affected. Intelligence is normal. Lacking also are the narrow face, frontal balding, cataracts, and endocrine changes of myotonic dystrophy (page 1503). Myotonia that is evident in infancy is far more likely to represent myotonia congenita than myotonic dystrophy, in which myotonia rarely has its onset in the first few years of life.

Myotonia can be induced in most cases by tapping a muscle belly with a percussion hammer (percussion myotonia). Unlike the lump or ridge produced in hypothyroid or cachectic muscle (myoedema), the myotonic contraction involves an entire fasciculus or an entire muscle and, unlike the phenomenon of idiomuscular irritability, it persists for several seconds. If tapped, the tongue shows a similar reaction. An electrical stimulus delivered to the motor point in a muscle also induces a prolonged contraction (Erb's myotonic reaction).

Biopsy reveals no abnormality other than enlargement of muscle fibers, and this change occurs only in hypertrophied muscles. As often happens in fibers of increased volume, central nucleation is somewhat more frequent than in normal muscle. The large fibers contain increased numbers of normally structured myofibrils. In well-fixed biopsy material examined under the electron microscope, Schroeder and Adams were unable to discern any significant morphologic changes. There are no changes in the peripheral or central nervous system.

Pathogenesis In view of the absence of morphologic changes and the prominence of the myotonic phenomenon in individual muscle fibers, one must assume the existence of a physiologic change in the sarcolemma or some other part of the conducting apparatus of the muscle fibers. It persists after the administration of curare. Electromyography (EMG) shows that the tension in contracting muscle fibers is slow to diminish, due to persistence of very fine electrical potentials (Fig. 45-8). Some of the latter are the same size as fibrillation potentials, but others are larger (normal motor unit potentials). The small potentials indicate independent, incoordinate activity of single fibers. Their activity continues after the volley of nerve impulses that initiated the contraction has ceased. Denny-Brown and Foley, stimulating single muscle fibers directly, obtained this myotonic afterdischarge only by a volley of stimuli, never by a single stimulus, and the series of myotonic fibrillation potentials progressively diminished in size—these physiologic findings matching the clinical ones. Percussion elicits myotonia because it, too, provides a brief but relatively intense repetitive excitation. Thus myotonia can be distinguished electrophysiologically from contracture of other types (e.g., that produced by perfusion of muscle with *Veratrum* alkaloids). In addition, Denny-Brown and Nevin noted that strong myotonia in one group of muscles may evoke reflex afterspasm in antagonist and synergist muscles—a reaction that depends on the operation of spinal mechanisms. This impairs efficiency and power of movement.

The biophysical basis of myotonia is now reasonably well understood. Intrinsic proteins, embedded in the lipid bilayer of the muscle membrane, function as gates or filters for the passage of particular ions—sodium (Na^+), calcium (Ca^{2+}), chloride (Cl^-)—each of which flows through its separate channel. Bryant, on the basis of in vitro studies of myotonic goat muscle, attributed the myotonic excitability (repetitive firing and afterdischarge) to a reduced chloride conductance in the transverse tubular system. Subsequent studies of human myotonic muscle, by Lipicky and Bryant, demonstrated a similarly low chloride conductance. Abnormal sodium channel reopenings are also implicated in the membrane hyperexcitability of the myotonic muscle fibers. As indicated earlier, the genes encoding these muscle ion channels and the gene protein products have now been identified (see Table 54-1).

Myotonia Levior This is the name applied by DeJong to a dominantly inherited form of myotonia congenita in which the symptoms are of milder expression and later onset than those of Thomsen disease. In two patients of a myotonia levior family, Lehmann-Horn and coworkers have identified a mutation of the chloride ion channel (CLCN1)—that is, the same genetic defect that characterizes Thomsen disease. Thus it appears that myotonia levior is simply a mild form of Thomsen disease.

Diagnosis In patients who complain of spasms, cramping, and stiffness, myotonia must be distinguished from several of the disorders described in Chap. 55—myokymia, persistent muscle activity and the cramp-fasciculation syndromes, periodic hyperkalemic paralysis, the Schwartz-Jampel syndrome, the pathologic cramp syndrome, the "stiff-man" syndrome—as well as the contracture of phosphorylase or phosphofructose kinase deficiency. In none of these disorders is there percussion myotonia or the typical EMG abnormality. The only exception is the Schwartz-Jampel syndrome of hereditary stiffness combined with short stature and muscle hypertrophy. This is probably a form of myotonia and should be set apart from myokymia and the syndrome of continuous muscle activity (page 1568).

Diagnostic uncertainty may arise in those patients who later prove to have myotonic dystrophy when only myotonia is noted in early life. The myotonia in these latter cases is usually mild, and in several families that we have followed, some degree of weakness and a typical facies could be perceived even in early childhood. Also, in paramyotonia congenita (see further on), there is myotonia of early onset, but again it tends to be mild, involving mainly the orbicularis oculi, levator palpebrae, and tongue; the diagnosis is seldom in doubt because of the cold-induced episodes of paralysis.

Also to be differentiated is the myotonia induced by certain drugs—occasionally by beta-blocking agents or diuretics (especially during pregnancy) and more regularly by depolarizing, relaxing, and anesthetic agents and drugs used in the treatment of hypercholesterolemia. Their effects are usually short-lived.

In patients with very large muscles, one must consider not only myotonia congenita but also familial hyperdevelopment, hypothyroid polymyopathy, hypertrophic polymyopathy (hypertrophia musculorum vera), and the Bruck-DeLange syndrome (congenital hypertrophy of muscles, mental retardation, and extrapyramidal movement disorder). The demonstration of myotonia by percussion and EMG study usually resolves the problem, although it should be noted that in exceptional cases of Thomsen disease, the persistence of contraction may be difficult to demonstrate. In hypothyroidism, the EMG may show bizarre high-frequency (pseudomyotonic) discharges (page 1364). However, true myotonia does not occur, myoedema is prominent, and—along with other signs of thyroid deficiency—there is slowing of contraction and relaxation of tendon reflexes not seen in myotonia congenita.

Treatment Quinidine sulfate, 0.3 to 0.6 g, procainamide, 250 to 500 mg qid, and mexiletine, 100 to 300 mg tid, are clearly beneficial in myotonia congenita. Phenytoin, 100 mg tid, has also been useful in some cases. The cardiac antiarrhythmic drug tocainide (1200 mg daily) has also proved to be beneficial, but it sometimes causes agranulocytosis and is no longer recommended.

Generalized Myotonia (Becker Disease)

This is a second form of myotonia congenita, inherited as an autosomal recessive trait. Like the dominant form, it is caused by an allelic mutation of the gene encoding the chloride ion channel of the muscle fiber membrane. The clinical features of the dominant and recessive types are similar except that myotonia in the recessive type does not become manifest until 10 to 14 years of age or even later and tends to be more severe than the myotonia of the dominant type. The myotonia appears first in the lower limbs and spreads to the trunk, arms, and face. Hypertrophy is invariably present. There may be an associated mild distal weakness and atrophy; this was found in the forearms in 28 percent of Becker's 148 patients and in the sternomastoids in 19 percent. Dorsiflexion of the feet was limited and fibrous contractures were common. Weakness may also be present in the proximal leg and arm muscles. The most troublesome aspect of the disease is the transient weakness that follows initial muscle contraction after a period of inactivity. Progression of the disease continues to about 30 years of age, and according to Sun and Streib, the course of the illness thereafter remains unchanged. The creatine kinase (CK) may be elevated. Testicular atrophy, cardiac abnormality, frontal baldness, and cataracts—the features that characterize myotonic dystrophy—are conspicuously absent.

SODIUM CHANNEL DISEASES

Included in this category are the following hereditary muscle disorders: hyperkalemic periodic paralysis, normokalemic periodic paralysis, paramyotonia congenita, myotonia fluctuans, myotonia permanens, and acetazolamide-responsive myotonia. All of them have been mapped to chromosome 17q23 and are due to mutations in the gene encoding the alpha subunit of the sodium channel in skeletal muscle (SCN4A). The first three are the better-known members of the group: the three latter disorders have been defined only in recent years and are included on the basis of shared clinical abnormalities and molecular defects.

Primary Hyperkalemic Periodic Paralysis

This type of periodic paralysis was first described and distinguished from the more common (hypokalemic) form by Tyler and colleagues, in 1951. Five years later, Gamstorp described two additional families with this disorder and named it *adynamia episodica hereditaria*. As further examples were reported, it was noted that in many of them there were minor degrees of myotonia, which brought the condition into relation with paramyotonia congenita (see further on).

There are three distinct variants of hyperkalemic periodic paralysis: (1) without myotonia, (2) with myotonia, and (3) with paramyotonia. The three clinical variants, which are elaborated below, are found to breed true. Presumably in all three, rises in extracellular potassium (K) fail to inactivate the aberrant sodium (Na) channel.

Clinical Manifestations The pattern of inheritance is autosomal dominant. Onset is usually in infancy and childhood. Characteristically, the attacks of weakness occur before breakfast and later in the day, when the patient is resting in a chair about 20 to 30 min after exercise. The paresis begins in the legs, thighs, and lower back and spreads to the hands, forearms, and shoulders. Only in the severest attacks are the neck and cranial muscles involved. Respiratory muscles are usually spared. As the muscles become inexcitable, tendon reflexes are diminished or lost. Attacks usually last 15 to 60 min, and recovery can be hastened by mild exercise. After an attack, mild weakness may persist for a day or two. In severe cases, the attacks may occur every day; during late adolescence and the adult years, when the patient becomes more sedentary, the attacks may diminish and cease. In certain muscle groups, if myotonia coexists, it is difficult to separate the effects of paresis from those of myotonia. Indeed, when an attack of paresis is prevented by continuous movement, firm, painful lumps may form in the calf muscles. Some patients with repeated attacks may be left with a permanent weakness and wasting of the proximal limb muscles.

During the attack of weakness, serum K rises, usually up to 5 to 6 mmol/L. This is associated with an increased amplitude of T waves in the electrocardiogram (ECG), and there is a fall in the serum Na level (due to entry of Na into muscle). With increased urinary excretion of K, the serum K falls and the attack terminates. Between attacks, serum K is normal. The attacks of paralysis are alike in the three clinical variants of the disease. Usually the presence of myotonia can only be detected electromyographically. In the paramyotonic form, the attacks are associated with paradoxical myotonia—that is, myotonia induced by exercise and also by cold.

The *provocative test*, undertaken when the patient is functioning normally, consists of the oral administration of 2 g of KCl in a sugar-free liquid repeated every 2 h for four doses if that many are necessary to provoke an attack. The test is given in the fasting state, ideally just after exercise. The weakness typically has a latency of 1 to 2 h after the administration of K. The patient must be carefully monitored by ECG and frequent serum K estimations. The test should never be undertaken in the presence of an attack of weakness or reduced renal function or in diabetics requiring insulin.

The *treatment* of this syndrome is the same as that for paramyotonia congenita, described further on.

Normokalemic Periodic Paralysis This is a rare form of episodic paralysis that resembles the hyperkalemic form in practically all respects except for the fact that serum potassium does not increase, even during the most severe attacks. However, some patients with normokalemic periodic paralysis are sensitive to potassium loading (Poskanzer and Kerr); other kindreds are not (Meyers et al). The disorder is also transmitted as an autosomal dominant trait, and the basic defect has proved to stem from the same mutation as that of hyperkalemic periodic paralysis.

Paramyotonia Congenita (Von Eulenberg)

In this disease, attacks of periodic paralysis are associated with myotonia, which may be paradoxical in type—that is, it develops during exercise and worsens as the exercise continues. Characteristically, a widespread myotonia, often coupled with weakness, is induced by exposure to cold. In some patients the myotonia can be elicited even in a warm environment. The weakness may be diffuse, as in hyperkalemic periodic paralysis, or limited to the part of the body that is cooled. Once started, the weakness persists for several hours, even after the body is rewarmed. Percussion myotonia can be evoked in the tongue and thenar eminence. Immersion of the arm and hand in ice water elicits both myotonia and weakness after a period of about 30 min. According to Haass and colleagues, myotonia that is constantly present in a warm environment diminishes with repeated contraction, whereas myotonia induced by cold increases with repeated contraction (paradoxical myotonia).

Like hyperkalemic periodic paralysis, paramyotonia congenita is transmitted as an autosomal dominant trait, and both diseases have been linked to the same gene (SCN4A), which encodes the alpha subunit of the muscle membrane sodium channel; the two diseases are caused by allelic mutations.

Laboratory Findings In both hyperkalemic periodic paralysis and paramyotonia congenita, the serum K is usually above the normal range, but paralysis has been observed at levels of 5 meq/L or even lower. Each patient appears to have a critical level of serum K, which, if exceeded, will be associated with weakness. The administration of KCl, raising serum K to above 7 meq/L but to a level that has no effect on normal individuals, invariably induces an attack in the patient. The EMG shows myotonic discharge in all muscles, even at normal temperatures. The CK may be elevated.

In vitro studies of muscle from patients with cold-induced stiffness and weakness have shown that as temperature is reduced, the muscle membrane is progressively depolarized, to the point where the fibers are inexcitable (Lehmann-Horn et al). A sodium channel blocker (tetrodotoxin) prevents the cold-induced depolarization. In patients with paramyotonia—but not in those with hyperkalemic periodic paralysis—Subramony and colleagues have observed a diminution of the compound muscle action potential in response to the cooling of muscle, settling the argument as to whether the two syndromes (hyperkalemic paralysis and paramyotonia) are the same or different.

Some patients with paramyotonia, like those with other forms of periodic paralysis, may in later life slowly develop a mild myopathy that causes persistent weakness.

There are either no histologic changes or at most only a few vacuoles in some of the muscle fibers. By electron microscopy, aggregates of tubules are seen in the muscle fibers in this as well as in normokalemic periodic paralysis. Fiber necrosis occurs in long-standing cases with fixed weakness.

Treatment Many attacks of primary hyperkalemic paralysis and of paramyotonia congenita are too brief and mild to require treatment. If attacks are severe, intravenous calcium gluconate (1 to 2 g) often restores power. If, after a few minutes, this treatment is unsuccessful, intravenous glucose or glucose and insulin and hydrochlorothiazide should be tried.

The continuous use of diuretics such as hydrochlorothiazide (about 0.5 g daily), keeping the serum K below 5 meq/L, prevents attacks. When the myotonia is more troublesome than the weakness, procainamide or the lidocaine derivative tocainide, in doses of 400 to 1200 mg daily, is useful; as mentioned, the latter carries the risk of agranulocytosis. Acetazolamide has proved effective in treating myotonia but aggravates cold-induced weakness. Mexiletine 200 mg tid is perhaps the best alternative, since it prevents both cold- and exercise-induced myotonia.

Other Sodium Channel Disorders Several other forms of hereditary periodic paralysis have been linked to mutations of the gene encoding the alpha subunit of the skeletal muscle sodium channel. One of these, first described by Ricker and colleagues, has been designated *myotonia fluctuans*, because the muscle stiffness fluctuated in severity from day to day in affected family members. In other respects the clinical features resembled those of myotonia congenita, including provocation of attacks of myotonia by exercise. The muscle stiffness was only slightly sensitive to cold but was markedly aggravated by ingestion of potassium and, interestingly, never progressed to muscular weakness or paralysis.

Myotonia permanens is the name given to another sodium channel disorder, characterized by the presence of severe, persistent myotonia and marked hypertrophy of muscles, particularly of the neck and shoulders. The EMG discloses continuous muscle activity. This disease was discovered in the course of genotyping a patient who earlier had been reported by Spaans and associates as an example of "myogenic" Schwartz-Jampel syndrome.

Trudell and colleagues, in 1987, studied 14 patients from a large kindred with autosomal dominant myotonia, the main feature of which was periodic worsening of myotonia accompanied by muscle pain and stiffness, most severe in the face and hands. The symptoms were enhanced by cold (suggesting paramyotonia), and severe stiffness and palpable rigidity followed within 15 min of K ingestion. Neither of these measures provoked muscle weakness. Muscle biopsy disclosed a normal ratio of types 1, 2A, and 2B fibers, further distinguishing this disorder from typical myotonia congenita, where 2B fibers may be reduced in number. All patients in this family who were treated with the carbonic anhydrase inhibitor acetazolamide (Diamox) had a dramatic resolution of symptoms within 24 h—hence the name *acetazolamide-responsive myotonia.* This disorder has now been linked to a specific molecular alteration of the sodium channel gene (Ptáček et al).

Rosenfeld et al have described yet another form of *painful congenital myotonia* attributable to a novel mutation in the sodium channel α-subunit gene (SCN4A). Affected members of this family experienced debilitating pain, particularly severe in the intercostal muscles. Also, the pain was resistant to treatment with acetazolamide and other antimyotonic drugs (mexiletine and tocainamide) and could not be provoked by ingestion of potassium-rich foods—differing in these ways from the patients described by Trudell and (Ptáček and their associates.

Finally, in regard to the channelopathies, it should be mentioned that the marine toxins (ciguatoxin, tetrodotoxin, saxitoxin, etc.), as discussed in Chap. 43, produce their effects on the peripheral and central nerves by blocking sodium channels but have little obvious effect on muscle function.

CALCIUM CHANNEL DISEASE

Hypokalemic Periodic Paralysis

This is the best-known form of periodic paralysis. The history of the disease is difficult to trace, but the first unmistakable account was probably that of Hartwig in 1874, followed by the accounts of Westphal (1885) and Oppenheim (1891). Goldflam (in 1895) first called attention to the remarkable vacuolization of the muscle fibers. In 1937, Aitken and associates described the occurrence of low serum potassium during attacks of paralysis and reversal of the paralysis by the administration of potassium, thus setting the stage for subsequent differentiation of the normo- and hyperkalemic forms of periodic paralysis. For English-speaking readers, Talbott's monograph serves as the best historical review of the subject and includes all cases that had been reported prior to 1941; the recent reviews by Layzer and by Lehmann-Horn and Engel and their associates bring the subject up to date.

The usual pattern of inheritance is autosomal dominant with reduced penetrance in women (male-to-female ratio of 3 or 4 to 1). Fontaine and Ptáček and their coworkers have localized the disease to chromosome 1q31–q32, a region containing the gene that encodes the α-1 subunit of the calcium channel of skeletal muscle. This subunit, which is part of the dihydropyridine receptor complex, is located in the transverse tubular system. This region is believed to act both as a voltage sensor that controls calcium release from the sarcoplasmic reticulum, thus mediating muscle excitation-contraction coupling, and as a calcium-conducting pore. How the reduced calcium channel function relates to hypokalemia-induced attacks of muscle weakness is not known.

Clinical Manifestations The disease may have its onset at any time from early childhood to the third decade of life. In Talbott's review of 152 cases, there were 40 in which symptoms began before the 10th year of life and 92 before the 16th year. The typical attack comes on during the second half of the night or the early morning hours, after a day of unusually strenuous exercise; a meal rich in carbohydrates favors its development. Excessive hunger or thirst, dry mouth, palpitation, sweating, diarrhea, nervousness, and a sense of weariness or fatigue are mentioned as prodromata but do not necessarily precede an attack. Usually the patient awakens to discover a mild or severe weakness of the limbs. However, diurnal attacks also occur, especially after a nap following a large meal. The attack evolves over minutes to several hours; at its peak, it may render the patient so helpless as to be unable to call for assistance. Once established, the weakness lasts a few hours if mild or several days if severe.

The distribution of the paralysis varies. Limbs are affected earlier and often more severely than trunk muscles, and proximal muscles are possibly more susceptible than distal ones. The legs are often weakened before the arms, but exceptionally the order is reversed. The muscles most likely to escape are those of the eyes, face, tongue, pharynx, larynx, diaphragm, and sphincters, but on occasion even these may be involved. When the attack is at its peak, tendon reflexes are reduced or abolished and cutaneous reflexes may also disappear. Sensation is preserved. As the attack subsides, strength generally returns first to the muscles that were last to be affected. Headache, exhaustion, diuresis, and occasionally diarrhea may follow the attack. Myotonia is not seen; indeed, EMG evidence of myotonia excludes the diagnosis of hypokalemic periodic paralysis.

Attacks of paralysis tend to occur every few weeks and to lessen in frequency with advancing age. Rarely, death may occur from respiratory paralysis or derangements of the conducting system of the heart. Mainly, such cases were reported in the era before modern intensive care.

Atypical forms include weakness of one limb or certain groups of muscles, bibrachial palsy (inability to lift one's arms or to comb one's hair), and transient weakness during accustomed activities. Earlier descriptions of daily brief attacks, some associated with exposure to cold or coupled with muscular hypertrophy or exophthalmic goiter, preceded recognition of the other types of periodic paralysis and cannot be evaluated. Some of our patients had a talipes deformity from early life. A number of patients developed a slowly progressive proximal myopathy, with vacuolated and degenerated fibers and myopathic action potentials, during middle adult life, in some instances long after attacks of periodic paralysis had ceased.

Andersen and coworkers first drew attention to a distinct form of periodic paralysis characterized by the triad of periodic potassium-sensitive weakness, ventricular dysrhythmias, and dysmorphic features (short stature, scaphocephaly, hypertelorism, broad nose, low-set ears, short index fingers, and small mandible). More recently Sansone et al have described 11 additional patients with Andersen's syndrome from five kindreds. These authors have pointed out that attacks of paralysis could be associated with hypo-, normo-, or hyperkalemia and that a prolonged QT interval is an integral feature (and sometimes the only sign in an individual from a typical kindred). Noteworthy is the fact that an association between this form of periodic paralysis and mutations in either the sodium or calcium channel genes responsible for typical hyperkalemic and hypokalemic periodic paralysis has not been established. Stevens has described a family, traced through five generations, with hypokalemic periodic paralysis as well as myotonia, peroneal muscle atrophy, impaired sensation, and ataxia. One cannot determine whether these are chance associations of two hereditary diseases.

Laboratory Findings The attacks are accompanied by reduction in serum K levels, as low as 1.8 meq/L, but usually at levels that would not be associated with paresis in normal subjects. Some episodes occur with near normal levels of K, and weakness persists for a time after the serum level has been restored. The fall in serum K is associated with little or no increase in urinary K excretion. Presumably, large volumes of the K enter the muscle fibers during an attack. The serum K levels return to normal during recovery. Although the shifts in K are of undoubted importance in the pathogenesis of muscle weakness, the marked sensitivity to small reductions of serum K suggests that other factors are also operative and that the fall in K may be a secondary phenomenon.

The muscular paralysis is associated with a decrease in and eventual loss of muscle action potentials, and there is failure of all attempts to excite them by supramaximal stimulation of peripheral nerve and strong voluntary effort. Decline in strength precedes loss of motor unit potentials and the failure of propagation of action potentials over the surface of the fiber. The polarization potentials of muscle fibers measured by intracellular recordings are normal despite the failure of impulse propagation by the sarcolemma. One would expect the muscle fiber to be hyperpolarized as K moves into it, but, if anything, it is actually hypopolarized. Rüdel and associates attribute the latter change to an increased Na conductance. The ECG changes also begin at levels of K that are slightly below normal (about 3 meq/L); they consist of prolonged PR, QRS, and QT intervals and flattening of T waves.

Diagnosis at a time when the patient is normal may be facilitated by provocative tests. With the patient carefully monitored, including ECG, the oral administration of 50 to 100 g of glucose or loading with 2 g of NaCl every hour for seven doses, followed by vigorous exercise, brings on an attack, which then can be terminated by 2 to 4 g of oral KCl.

Pathologic Changes The nervous system is entirely normal. The muscle fibers are uniformly somewhat large, but the most striking change, particularly in the late degenerative phases of the disease, is vacuolization of the sarcoplasm. The myofibrils are separated by round or oval vacuoles containing clear fluid, presumably water, and a few PAS-positive granules. There are pathologic changes in myofibrils and mitochondria as well, and focal increases in muscle glycogen. Isolated muscle fibers may undergo segmental degeneration. Electron microscopic studies have shown that the vacuoles arise as a result of proliferation and degeneration of membranous organelles within the sarcoplasmic reticulum and transverse tubules (A. G. Engel).

Treatment The daily administration of 5 to 10 g of KCl orally in an unsweetened aqueous solution prevents attacks in many patients, and apparently this program can be maintained indefinitely. When this fails, a low-carbohydrate, low-salt, high-K diet combined with a slow-release K preparation may be effective. A low-sodium diet (160 meq/day), avoidance of large meals and exposure to cold, acetazolamide 250 mg three times daily, and chlorothiazide 500 mg daily may also be helpful in preventing attacks.

For an acute attack, 0.25 meq KCl/kg should be given orally or, if this is not tolerated, some other K salt. This dose may be insufficient, and if there is no improvement in 1 or 2 h, KCl may have to be given intravenously—0.05 to 0.1 meq/kg IV initially in a bolus at a safe rate, followed by 20 to 40 meq KCl in 5% mannitol, avoiding glucose or NaCl as the carrier solution. For the late progressive polymyopathy that follows many severe attacks of periodic paralysis, Dalakas and Engel report successful restoration of strength by the administration of the carbonic anhydrase inhibitor dichlorphenamide. Regular exercise (not too strenuous) to keep the patient fit is desirable. To prevent an attack, the drugs of choice are said to be imipramine or acetazolamide.

Secondary Kalemic Periodic Paralyses

In addition to the hereditary kalemic paralyses described above, transitory episodes of weakness are known to be associated with a number of acquired derangements of potassium metabolism (mainly hypokalemia), such as thyrotoxicosis, aldosteronism, 17α-hydroxylase deficiency (Yazaki et al), barium poisoning (Lewi and Bar-Khayim), glycyrrhizic acid ingestion (a substance in licorice that has mineralocorticoid activity), and abuse of thyroid hormone (Layzer). Other forms of secondary hypokalemic weakness have been observed in patients suffering from chronic renal and adrenal insufficiency or disorders due to a loss of potassium, as occurs with excessive use of diuretics or laxatives (the commonest cause in practice). Renal failure with hyperkalemia can also induce paralysis.

Thyrotoxicosis with Periodic Paralysis This, a form of secondary hypokalemic periodic paralysis, occurs mainly in young adult males (despite the higher incidence of thyrotoxicosis in women), with a predilection for those of Japanese and Chinese extraction. In Japan, Okinaka and associates found that 8.9 percent of males with thyrotoxicosis had periodic paralysis but only 0.4 percent of females; for the Chinese, the corresponding figures were 13.0 and 0.17 percent (McFadzean and Yeung). The paralytic disorder is unrelated to the severity of the hyperthyroidism. In patients with the familial forms of periodic paralysis, the induction of hyperthyroidism is said not to increase the frequency or intensity of attacks. Therefore it seems likely that thyrotoxicosis has unmasked another type of hereditary periodic paralysis, although a familial occurrence in the thyrotoxic cases is exceptional. Clinically, the attacks of paralysis are much the same as those of familial hypokalemic type except for a greater liability to cardiac irregularity. As in the familial form, the paralyzed muscles are inexcitable, due possibly to overactivity of the Na-K pump, according to Layzer. Potassium chloride restores power in paralytic attacks, and treatment of the hyperthyroidism prevents their recurrence (see page 1520).

Hypokalemic Weakness in Primary Aldosteronism Hypokalemic weakness due to hypersecretion of the major adrenal mineralocorticoid aldosterone was first described by Conn and associates in 1955. In *primary aldosteronism*, the cause of the hypersecretion is in the adrenal gland itself—usually an adrenal cortical adenoma, less often adrenal cortical hyperplasia. The disorder is not common (occurring in about 1 percent of unselected hypertensive patients), but its recognition is essential, since it can be treated effectively. Persistent aldosteronism is frequently associated with hypernatremia, polyuria, and alkalosis, which predispose the patient to attacks of tetany as well as to hypokalemic weakness. Conn and associates (1964), in an analysis of 145 patients with primary aldosteronism, found that persistent muscular weakness was a major complaint in 73 percent; intermittent attacks of paralysis occurred in 21 percent and tetany in 21 percent. These manifestations were much more frequent in women than in men, in contrast to the preponderance of men among patients with hypokalemic periodic paralysis of familial type. Rarely, as already noted, primary aldosteronism is produced by the chronic ingestion of licorice; this is due to its content of glycyrrhizic acid, a potent mineralocorticoid (Conn et al 1968).

The muscle fibers of patients with primary aldosteronism show necrosis and vacuolation. Ultrastructurally, the necrotic areas are characterized by a dissolution of myofilaments with degenerative vacuoles; nonnecrotic fibers contain membrane-bound vacuoles and show dilatation of the sarcoplasmic reticulum and abnormalities of the transverse tubular system, suggesting that a vulnerability of the latter structures may be responsible for the muscle fiber necrosis (Atsumi et al).

Malignant Hyperthermia

This refers to a syndrome that is observed during general anesthesia, characterized, if not treated properly, by rapidly rising body temperature, muscular rigidity and a high mortality. Since the original report by Denborough and Lovell in 1960, as larger experience was gained with this entity, it proved to be a metabolic polymyopathy inherited as a dominant trait, rendering the individual vulnerable to any potent volatile anesthetic agent, particularly halothane and to the muscle relaxant succinylcholine. Malignant hyperthermia occurs approximately once in the course of 50,000 instances of general anesthesia.

The clinical picture is dramatic. As halothane or a similar inhalational anesthesia is induced or suxamethonium is given for muscular relaxation, the jaw muscles unexpectedly become tense rather than relaxed, and soon the rigidity extends to all of the muscles. Thereafter the body temperature rises to 42 or 43°F—with coincidental tachypnea and tachycardia. Arterial CO_2 may exceed 100 mmHg, and blood pH may fall to 7.00 or below. There may be gross myoglobinuria, and serum CK often reaches extraordinarily high levels. Circulatory collapse and death may ensue (in approximately 10 percent of cases), or the patient may survive, with gradual recovery. In some cases there is the same sequence of events (increased temperature and acidosis) without muscular spasm. With the patient's early death, the muscle may appear normal by light microscopy. After the patient's survival for several days, samples of muscle reveal scattered segmental necrosis and phagocytosis of sarcoplasm without inflammation. Regenerative activity is in progress. Multicores are frequently found in the muscle of patients who have had such episodes.

The pathogenesis of this reaction has been the subject of a number of investigations. During the rigor phase, oxygen consumption in muscle increases 3-fold and serum lactate, 15- to 20-fold. Muscle from affected individuals is abnormally sensitive to caffeine, which induces contracture in vitro. It has been postulated that halothane acts in a manner similar to caffeine—that is, to release calcium from the sarcoplasmic reticulum and prevent its reaccumulation, thus interfering with relaxation of the muscle. There is a breed of pigs, inbred for muscular development, in which muscle spasm (true contracture) and hyperthermia follow the administration of anesthetic agents. The latter increase O_2 consumption by 50 to 60 percent and deplete the adenosine triphosphate of muscle fibers. These swine have an inherited defect in the ryanodine receptor, a protein component of the calcium channel of the sarcoplasm that is sensitive to both caffeine and ryanodine. One of several similar defects is found in only 10 percent of human cases. It has been proposed that other yet unidentified allelic mutations of this receptor or another that controls the structure of the calcium channel account for the remainder. The cause of the fever is not known; it is probably due to the muscle spasm, but an effect of the anesthetic on heat-regulating centers cannot be excluded.

Clues as to which patients are at risk for this condition come from several sources. Other members of the family may have collapsed or died during anesthesia. Some of the susceptible individuals exhibit certain myopathic and musculoskeletal abnormalities (Isaacs and Barlow). As to the latter, short stature, ptosis, strabismus, highly arched palate, dislocated patellae, and kyphoscoliosis have been noted in some families (King-Denborough syndrome). Duchenne-Becker muscular dystrophy may also be associated. Central core (multicore) myopathy (page 1533) is frequently complicated by malignant hyperthermia. This is understandable insofar as both disorders have been linked to the gene encoding the ryanodine receptor; the two diseases are allelic (Quane et al).

Treatment consists of discontinuation of anesthesia at the first hint of masseter spasm or rise of temperature. The intravenous administration of dantrolene, which inhibits the release of calcium from the sarcoplasmic reticulum, may be lifesaving. An infusion of 1 mg/kg is given initially and increased slowly until symptoms subside, the total dosage not to exceed 10 mg/kg. Other measures should include body cooling, intravenous hydration, sodium bicarbonate infusions to correct acidosis, and mechanical hyperventilation to decrease respiratory acidosis. Halothane and other volatile anesthesic agents and succinylcholine should thereafter be avoided in such individuals, and any surgical procedures, if necessary, should be done under nitrous oxide, fentanyl, thiopental (or other barbiturate), or local anesthesia. Intravenous dantrolene, 2.5 mg/kg given slowly 1 h prior to anesthesia, prevents the syndrome.

Malignant Neuroleptic Syndrome

This state, in which hyperthermia occurs as an idiosyncratic reaction to neuroleptic drugs, is also accompanied by widespread myonecrosis. It is discussed in Chap. 43.

REFERENCES

Andersen ED, Krasilnikoff PA, Overvad H: Intermittent muscular weakness, extrasystoles, and multiple developmental anomalies. *Acta Paediatr Scand* 60:559, 1971.

Atsumi T, Ishikawa S, Miyatake T, Yoshida M: Myopathy and primary aldosteronism: Electron microscopic study. *Neurology* 29:1348, 1979.

Becker PE: Genetic approaches to the nosology of muscle disease: Myotonias and similar diseases: Pt 7. Muscle, in Bergsma D (ed): *The Clinical Delineation of Birth Defects*. Baltimore, Williams & Wilkins, 1971.

Bryant SH: Cable properties of external intercostal muscle fibers from myotonic and nonmyotonic goats. *J Physiol* 204:539, 1969.

Cannon SC, Brown RH Jr, Corey DP: A sodium channel defect in hyperkalemic periodic paralysis: Potassium-induced failure of inactivation. *Neuron* 6:619, 1991.

Conn JW, Knopf RF, Nesbit RM: Clinical characteristics of primary aldosteronism from an analysis of 145 cases. *Am J Surg* 107:159, 1964.

Conn JW, Rovner DR, Cohen EL: Licorice-induced pseudoaldosteronsim: Hypertension, hypokalemia, aldosteronopenia and suppressed plasma renin activity. *JAMA* 205:492, 1968.

Dalakas MC, Engel WK: Treatment of "permanent" muscle weakness in familial hypokalemic periodic paralysis. *Muscle Nerve* 6:182, 1983.

DeJong JGY: Myotonia levior, in Kuhn E (ed): *Progressive Muskeldystrophie-Myotonie-Myasthenie*. Heidelberg, Springer, 1966, pp 255–259.

Denborough MA, Lovell RRH: Anaesthetic deaths in a family. *Lancet* 2:45, 1960.

Denny-Brown D, Foley JM: Evidence of a chemical mediator in myotonia. *Trans Assoc Am Physicians* 62:187, 1949.

Denny-Brown D, Nevin S: The phenomenon of myotonia. *Brain* 64:1, 1941.

Engel AG: Evolution and content of vacuoles in primary hypokalemic periodic paralysis. *Mayo Clin Proc* 45:774, 1970.

Fontaine B, Vale Santos JM, Jurkat-Rott JK, et al: Mapping of hypokalemic periodic paralysis (hypo PP) to chromosome 1q31-q32 by a genome-wide search in three European families. *Nature Genet* 6:267, 1994.

Frank JP, Harati Y, Butler JJ, et al: Central core disease and malignant hyperthermia syndrome. *Ann Neurol* 7:11, 1980.

Gamstorp I: Adynamia periodica hereditaria. *Acta Paediatr Scand* (Suppl 108) 45:1–126, 1956.

Haass A, Ricker K, Rüdel R, et al: Clinical study of paramyotonia congenita with and without myotonia in a warm environment. *Muscle Nerve* 4:388, 1981.

Isaacs H, Barlow MB: Malignant hyperpyrexia. *J Neurol Neurosurg Psychiatry* 36:228, 1973.

Layzer RB: *Neuromuscular Manifestations of Systemic Disease*. Philadelphia, Davis, 1985.

Lehmann-Horn F, Engel AG, Ricker K, Rüdel R: The periodic paralyses and paramyotonia congenita, in Engel AG, Franzini-Armstrong C (eds): *Myology*, 2nd ed. New York, McGraw-Hill, 1994, pp 1303–1334.

Lehmann-Horn F, Mailänder V, Heine R, George AL: Myotonia levior is a chloride channel disorder. *Hum Mol Genet* 4:1397, 1995.

Lehmann-Horn F, Rüdel R, Ricker K: Membrane defects in paramyotonia congenita (Eulenberg). *Muscle Nerve* 10:633, 1987.

Lewi Z, Bar-Khayim Y: Food poisoning from barium carbonate. *Lancet* 2:342, 1964.

Lipicky RJ, Bryant SH: Ion content, potassium flux, and cable properties of myotonic, human, external intercostal muscle. *Trans Am Neurol Assoc* 96:34, 1971.

Lipicky RJ, Bryant SH: Sodium, potassium, and chloride fluxes in intercostal muscle from normal goats and goats with hereditary myotonia. *J Gen Physiol* 50:89, 1966.

McFadzean AJS, Yeung R: Periodic paralysis complicating thyrotoxicosis in Chinese. *BMJ* 1:451, 1967.

Meyers KR, Gilden DH, Rinaldi CF, Hansen JL: Periodic muscle weakness, normokalemia, and tubular aggregates. *Neurology* 22:269, 1972.

Nissen K: Beiträge zur Kenntnis der Thomsen'schen Krankheit (Myotonia congenita), mit besonderer Berücksichtigung des hereditären Momentes und seinen Beziehungen zu den Mendelschen Vererbungsregeln. *Z Klin Med* 97:58, 1923.

Okinaka S, Shizume K, Iinos S, et al: The association of periodic paralysis and hyperthyroidism in Japan. *J Clin Endocrinol Metab* 17:1454, 1957.

Poskanzer DC, Kerr DNS: A third type of periodic paralysis with normokalemia and favorable response to NaC1. *Am J Med* 31:328, 1961.

Ptáček LJ, Tawil R, Griggs RC, et al: Dihydropyridine receptor mutations cause hypokalemic periodic paralysis. *Cell* 77:963, 1994.

Ptáček LJ, Tawil R, Griggs RC, et al: Sodium channel mutations in acetazolamide-responsive myotonia congenita, paramyotonia congenita, and hyperkalemic periodic paralysis. *Neurology* 44:1500, 1994.

Quane KA, Healy JMS, Keating KE, et al: Mutations in the ryanodine receptor gene in central core disease and malignant hyperthermia. *Nature Genet* 5:51, 1993.

Ricker K, Moxley RT, Heine R, Lehmann-Horn F: Myotonia fluctuans: A third type of muscle sodium channel disease. *Arch Neurol* 51:1095, 1994.

Rosenfeld J, Sloan-Brown K, George AL: A novel muscle sodium channel mutation causes painful congenital myotonia. *Ann Neurol* 42:811, 1997.

Rüdel R, Lehmann-Horn F, Ricker K, et al: Hypokalemic periodic paralysis: In vitro investigation of muscle fiber membrane parameters. *Muscle Nerve* 7:110, 1984.

Sansone V, Griggs RC, Meola G, et al: Andersen's syndrome: A distinct periodic paralysis. *Ann Neurol* 42:305, 1997.

Schroeder JM, Adams RD: The ultrastructural morphology of the muscle fiber in myotonic dystrophy. *Acta Neuropathol* 10:218, 1968.

Spaans F, Theunissen P, Reekers AD, et al: Schwartz-Jampel syndrome: 1. Clinical, electromyographic, and histologic studies. *Muscle Nerve* 13:516, 1990.

STEVENS JR: Familial periodic paralysis, myotonia, progressive amyotrophy, and pes cavus in members of a single family. *Arch Neurol Psychiatry* 72:726, 1954.

STREIB EW: Paramyotonia congenita: Successful treatment with tocainide: Clinical and electrophysiologic findings in seven patients. *Muscle Nerve* 10:155, 1987.

STREIB EW: Successful treatment with tocainide of recessive generalized congenital myotonia. *Ann Neurol* 19:501, 1986.

SUBRAMONY SH, WEE AS, MISHRA SK: Lack of cold sensitivity in hyperkalemic periodic paralysis. *Muscle Nerve* 9:700, 1986.

SUN SF, STREIB EW: Autosomal recessive generalized myotonia. *Muscle Nerve* 6:143, 1983.

TALBOTT JH: Periodic paralysis: A clinical syndrome. *Medicine* 20:85, 1941.

THOMASEN E: *Myotonia, Thomsen's Disease, Paramyotonia, Dystrophia Myotonica*. Aarhus, Denmark, Universitetsforlaget i Aarhus, 1948.

THOMSEN J: Tonische Krämpfe in willkürlich beweglichen Muskeln in Folge von ererbter psychischer disposition (Ataxia muscularis?). *Arch Psychiatr Nervenkr* 6:706, 1876.

TRUDELL RG, KAISER KK, GRIGGS RC: Acetazolamide-responsive myotonia congenita. *Neurology* 37:488, 1987.

TYLER FH, STEPHENS FE, GUNN FD, PERKOFF GT: Studies on disorders of muscle: VII. Clinical manifestations and inheritance of a type of periodic paralysis without hypopotassemia. *J Clin Invest* 30:492, 1951.

YAZAKI K, KURIBAYASHI T, YAMAMURA Y, et al: Hypokalemic myopathy associated with a 17 α-hydroxylase deficiency: A case report. *Neurology* 32:94, 1982.

Chapter 55

DISORDERS OF MUSCLE CHARACTERIZED BY CRAMP, SPASM, PAIN, AND LOCALIZED MASSES

Quite apart from spasticity and rigidity, which are due to a disinhibition of spinal motor mechanisms, there are forms of muscular stiffness and spasm that can be traced to abnormalities of the lower motor neuron and its spinal inhibitory mechanisms or to the sarcolemma of the muscle fiber and its intrinsic conducting apparatus. Thus, muscles may go into spasm because of an unstable depolarization of motor axons, which sends volleys of impulses across neuromuscular junctions—as occurs in myokymia, hypocalcemic tetany, and pseudohypoparathyroidism. In other states, discussed in the preceding chapter, the innervation of muscle may be normal but contraction persists despite attempts at relaxation (myotonia). Or, after one or a series of contractions, the muscle may be slow in decontracting, as occurs in paradoxical myotonia and hypothyroidism; in the contracture of McArdle phosphorylase deficiency and phosphofructokinase deficiency, muscle, once contracted, may lack the energy to relax.

Each of these conditions evokes the complaint of cramp or spasm, which is variably painful and interferes with free and effective voluntary activity. Each condition has its own identifying clinical and electromyographic (EMG) characteristics, and most of them respond favorably to therapy. A premium is therefore attached to the clinical differentiation of these phenomena.

Muscle Cramp

This subject has already been introduced in Chap. 48, where it was pointed out that everyone at some time or other has experienced muscle cramps. Usually they occur during the night, after a day of unusually strenuous activity; less often they occur during the day, either during a period of relaxation or occasionally after a strong voluntary contraction or postural adjustment. A random restless or stretching movement will induce a hard contraction of a single muscle (most frequently of the foot or leg) that cannot be voluntarily relaxed. The muscle is visibly and palpably taut and painful, and the condition is readily distinguished from an illusory cramp, in which the sensation of cramp is experienced with little or no contraction of muscle. The latter phenomenon may occur in normal persons as well as in those with certain peripheral nerve diseases. Massage and vigorous stretch of the cramped muscle will cause the spasm to yield, though for a time the muscle remains excitable and subject to recurrent cramps. Visible fasciculations may precede and follow the cramp, indicating an excessive excitability of the terminal branches of motor neurons supplying the muscle. Sometimes the cramp is so strong that the muscle appears to have been injured; it remains sore to touch and painful upon use for a day or longer. Cramps of precordial chest muscles or diaphragm may arouse fear of heart or lung disease. In the EMG, the cramp is marked by bursts of high-frequency, high-voltage action potentials and the precramp phase by runs of activity in motor units. Why cramps should be painful is not known; probably the demands of the overactive muscle exceed metabolic supply, causing a relative ischemia and accumulation of metabolites. Overwork of muscle with or without impairment of circulation is also painful. Between cramps, the muscles are normal clinically and electromyographically.

Cramps are known to increase in frequency under certain conditions and with certain diseases. They are frequent during pregnancy for reasons not fully understood. Dehydration and sweating predispose to cramping and are a constant threat to athletes, who try to prevent them by ingesting electrolyte solutions. Exertional cramps are frequent in motor system disease and hypothyroidism and less so in chronic polyneuropathies. Patients undergoing hemodialysis are subject to cramps, which can be suppressed by intravenous hypertonic saline or hypertonic glucose. Rapid rehydration after dehydration is another provocative factor. Focal cramping occurs after partial nerve or root injury and with diseases involving anterior horn cells.

The mechanism of muscle cramping is obscure. In a number of cases with exercise-induced stiffness and muscle pain, sometimes progressing to cramp, below-normal levels of myoadenylate deaminase have been found. The significance of this observation is uncertain. This enzyme, which is present in high concentration in muscle, is thought to function primarily during aerobic exercise and facilitate the regeneration of adenosine triphosphate from adenosine diphosphate through the action of adenylate kinase. Others assert that low levels of this enzyme are not specific, occurring in such unrelated disorders as hypokalemic periodic paralysis and spinal muscular atrophy (see Layzer for details).

Quinine sulfate, 300 mg at bedtime and repeated in 4 h if necessary, or 300 mg tid for diurnal cramping is an effective medication; diphenhydramine hydrochloride (Benadryl) 50 mg or procainamide 0.5 to 1.0 g can be substituted if quinine is not tolerated. Phenytoin, carbamazepine, propoxyphene, and sometimes clonazepam are even more useful in alleviating repeated daytime cramping.

Tetany, Pseudotetany, and Related Cramp Syndromes

As pointed out on page 1352, a reduction in ionizable calcium and magnesium is associated with involuntary cramplike spasms; in their mildest form they appear as distal carpopedal spasms, but they may involve any of the muscles except the extraocular ones. Stimulation of a muscle through its nerve at certain frequencies (15 to 20 times per second) characteristically reproduces the spasms, and hyperventilation and ischemia increase the tendency. Indeed, the Trousseau sign—carpal spasms with occlusion of the blood supply to the arm—takes advantage of the latter phenomenon. That hypocalcemic tetany is attributable to an unstable depolarization of the axonal membrane of the nerve fiber is shown by (1) the sensitivity of nerve to percussion (tapping over the facial nerve near its foramen of exit induces a facial twitch, or Chvostek sign), (2) the appearance of fast-frequency doublets and triplets of motor unit potentials in the EMG, (3) evocation of spasm by application of a tourniquet to proximal parts of a limb (causing ischemia of segments of nerve beneath the tourniquet), and (4) the regular association of tingling, prickling paresthesias from excitation of sensory nerve fibers. Hypocalcemia also causes a lesser change in the muscle fibers themselves; hence nerve block does not completely eradicate tetany.

A condition resembling tetany but without measurable hypocalcemia is the aforementioned benign cramp syndrome (*pseudotetany*). In the most severe forms, all skeletal muscles are intermittently locked in spasm, and almost any strong postural or voluntary movement leads to cramp. When this phenomenon is repeated again and again, the overly active muscles begin to hypertrophy. In about half of the authors' cases, stimulation of nerve at 15 or more per second produced cramp discharges, as in tetany. Biopsies have disclosed no abnormalities of the muscle fibers except for a few ringbinden (circumferential bands of myofibrils encircling a normal core of longitudinally oriented myofibrils). Calcium and diazepam are of no therapeutic value, but some patients respond to phenytoin, quinine, procainamide, or chlorpromazine.

Satoyoshi has described a group of such patients who, in addition to the widespread severe cramping of muscle, also showed universal alopecia, amenorrhea, intestinal malabsorption, and sometimes epiphyseal destruction and retarded growth; the serum calcium in these patients was normal, and the EMG showed only high-frequency discharges. A familial (autosomal dominant) form of the benign cramp syndrome has been reported by Jusic and coworkers; the cramps affected the distal limb muscles, began in childhood and adolescence, and persisted throughout life. Another such family with cramps beginning somewhat later in life and affecting the anterior neck, arm, and abdominal muscles as well as those of the thigh and calf has been described by Ricker and Moxley. Also, as mentioned in Chap. 50, a familial myalgic-cramp syndrome has been associated with deletion of part of the dystrophin gene (but with little or no dystrophic weakness). A tendency to cramp and pain has also been noted in a number of the congenital myopathies and in some families with Duchenne and Becker dystrophies.

States of Persistent Fasciculation, Myokymia, Continuous Muscle Activity, Neuromyotonia, "Stiff-Man" Syndrome, and Schwartz-Jampel Syndrome

This is a confusing group of clinical states, all characterized by some degree of regional continuous muscular activity, that in some cases cannot be fully differentiated from one another.

Benign Fasciculations As is well known, a few random fasciculations in the muscles of the calf or elsewhere are to be seen in most normal individuals.

They are of no significance but can be a source of worry to physicians and nurses who have heard or read that fasciculations are an early sign of amyotrophic lateral sclerosis. A simple clinical rule is that fasciculations in relaxed muscle are never indicative of motor system disease unless there is an associated weakness, atrophy, or reflex change.

Frequently a normal individual experiences intermittent twitching of a muscle (or even part of a muscle), such as one of the muscles of the thenar eminence, eyelids, calves, or orbicularis oculi. It may continue for days. Lay persons refer to it as "live flesh." Also, penicillin may destabilize the polarization of distal motor endings and cause twitching. Electromyographically, these benign fasciculations tend to be more constant in location and more frequent and rhythmic than the ominous fasciculations of amyotrophic lateral sclerosis, but such distinctions are not entirely reliable. Quantification of the motor unit size may be helpful in these circumstances by demonstrating normally modeled units in the benign form and abnormally large units due to reinnervation in the case of motor neuron disease (see page 1364).

Occasionally, *benign fasciculations* are widespread and may last for months or even years. In several of our patients they have recurred in bouts separated by months and lasting several weeks. No reflex changes, sensory loss, nerve conduction, EMG abnormality (other than fasciculations), or increase in serum muscle enzymes are found. Low energy and fatigability in some of these patients may suggest an endogenous depressive illness, yet the fasciculations are indeed prominent. Commonly there is a sense that the muscles affected by the twitching are weak, and several of our patients have complained of migratory zones of paresthesias. Pain, of aching or burning type, increases during activity and ceases during rest. Fatigue and a sense of weakness are frequent complaints. We suspect that this fasciculatory state reflects a disease of the terminal motor nerves, for a few of our patients have shown slowing of distal latencies, and Cöers and associates have found degeneration and regeneration of motor nerve terminals. Carbamazepine, and to a lesser extent phenytoin, has been helpful in reducing the fasciculations and weak sensations in affected muscles. In the cases reported by Hudson and colleagues, and this conforms to our experience, the condition, even after years, did not progress to spinal muscular atrophy or amyotrophic lateral sclerosis. Eventual recovery can be expected.

There are, in addition to the aforementioned benign states, three major syndromes of abnormal muscle activity: (1) *Myokymia*, a state of successive contractions of motor units, imparting an almost continuous undulation or rippling of the overlying body surface. This phenomenon may fluctuate in severity and may be localized or widespread; in the latter case, it is associated with slight weakness. (2) *A state of persistent muscle spasm* that is arrested by spinal anesthesia and procaine nerve block. The latter has been called "stiff-man" syndrome. (3) A rare inherited syndrome of continuous muscle activity associated with skeletal abnormalities, the *Schwartz-Jampel* syndrome.

Myokymia This state of abnormal muscle activity, as defined above, may be generalized or limited to one part of the body, such as the muscles of the shoulders or of the lower extremities. It is observed most often with regeneration of peripheral nerve following injury, as in the facial palsy of Guillain-Barré syndrome. In the EMG, myokymic discharges consist of groups of 2 to 10 potentials, firing at 5 to 60 Hz and recurring regularly at 0.2- to 10-s intervals. They arise in the most peripheral parts of the axon of chronically damaged nerves. In some patients, cramping is associated and, indeed, muscles about to cramp may twitch or show spontaneous rippling contractions; the cramping may be associated with sweating. Thus, myokymia, fasciculation, and cramping are closely related but not identical conditions.

Ricker and Burns and their associates have described a rare familial disorder (autosomal dominant) in which muscles display an unusual sensitivity to stretch, manifest by rippling waves of muscle contraction; percussion of muscles yields a pronounced and painful local mounding. The EMG discloses neither myotonic discharges nor the action potentials of cramp, indicating that the basic abnormality is in the muscle membrane.

Continuous Muscle Activity (Isaacs Syndrome) The relation of myokymia to the state called *continuous muscle fiber activity* is ambiguous. Sporadically, in the neurologic literature, there have been described patients whose muscles at some point begin to "work" continuously (see Isaacs). Terms such as *neuromyotonia* and *widespread myokymia with delayed muscle relaxation* are additional names that have been applied to what is essentially the same condition. At the moment, there is little reason to distinguish one from another except in gradations of severity. In each case the excessive and spontaneous activity can be attributed to hyperexcitability of terminal parts of motor nerve fiber, possibly as a result of a partial loss of motor innervation and compensatory collateral sprouting of surviving axons (Cöers et al, Valli et al). Twitching, spasms, and rippling of muscles (myokymia) are evident, the latter being the main clinical sign. In advanced cases there is generalized muscle stiffness and a sense of weakness. Complaints of muscle aching are usual, but severe myalgia is uncommon. The tendon reflexes may be reduced or abolished. Any muscle group may be affected. The stiffness and slowness of movement make walking laborious ("armadillo syndrome"); in extreme cases, all voluntary movement is blocked. The muscle activity persists throughout sleep.

General and spinal anesthesia do not always suppress the muscular activity, but curare does; nerve block usually has no effect or may reduce the activity, as in the case of Lütschg and colleagues. The EMG findings are much the same as those described above.

This syndrome arises in childhood or adult life, in association either with a polyneuropathy or with an inherited type of episodic ataxia that is variably responsive to acetazolamide or remits spontaneously. An inherited form of continuous muscle activity has been traced to a gene mutation on chromosome 12 and is attributed to a peripheral nerve K channel abnormality (Gutmann and Gutmann). In addition to the association with polyneuropathy, continuous muscular activity has also been described with lung cancer and thymoma, with or without myasthenia, in which cases an immune mechanism has been inferred (see reviews by Thompson and by Newsom-Davis and Mills). An association of continuous muscle fiber activity with psychosis or a severe sleep disorder was first described by Morvan under the name *chorée fibrillaire* (see Serratrice and Azalay). Most cases appear to be idiopathic, however.

Treatment with phenytoin or carbamazepine often abolishes the continuous muscular activity and causes a return of reflexes. Many of the idiopathic cases, as already noted, will improve spontaneously after several years, but plasma exchange may be tried if the symptoms are intractable.

"Stiff-Man" Syndrome This is a condition of persistent spasms, particularly of the lower limbs, forcing the patient eventually to lie helplessly in bed with the feet in equinus position and the legs extended. It was originally described by Moersch and Woltman in 1956 as "stiff-man" syndrome. Since then, many examples have been reported all over the world and the term "stiff-person" syndrome has been used to indicate its occurrence is women. The onset is insidious, usually in middle life, and men and women are affected equally. No genetic predisposition is known. At first the stiffness and spasms are intermittent; then, gradually, they become more or less continuously active in the proximal limb and axial trunk muscles and increasingly painful. The spasms impart a robotic appearance to walking and an exaggerated lumbar lordosis. Attempts to move an affected part passively yield an almost rock-like immobility, perceptibly different from spasticity, paratonia, or extrapyramidal rigidity. Muscles of respiration and swallowing and those of the face may be involved in the more advanced cases, but trismus, a common feature of tetanus, does not occur. We have seen brief periods of cyanosis and respiratory arrest during episodes of intense spasm, and one of our patients died during such an episode. Eye muscles are rarely affected. Any noise or other sensory stimulus or attempted passive or voluntary movement precipitates severely painful spasms of all the involved musculature. The tendon reflexes are normal if they can be tested. A similar stiffness of one limb (*"stiff-limb" syndrome*) has been differentiated from the generalized variety by Barker and colleagues, but it seems to us to be part of the same illness, especially since most of the localized cases have antibodies to glutamic acid decarboxylase, as described below. This limited form of spasm is similar to localized tetanus.

A central origin of the muscle spasms is suggested by their disappearance during sleep, during general anesthesia, and with proximal nerve block. The electrophysiologic features differ from those of myokymia and continuous muscle fiber activity syndrome in that the EMG in stiff-man syndrome consists entirely of normal motor units, with no evidence of distal motor nerve disturbance.

Of interest is the finding that more than half of the cases of stiff-man syndrome have circulating autoantibodies that are reactive with glutamic acid decarboxylase (GAD), the synthesizing enzyme for GABA (Solimena et al). These findings suggest an imbalance between the spinal inhibitory (GABAergic) input and the excitatory input to alpha motor neurons. This interpretation is supported by the fact that the spasms worsen under the influence of drugs that (1) enhance aminergic activity, facilitating long-latency spinal reflexes, and (2) inhibit catecholaminergic or GABAergic transmitters. An autoimmune mechanism is further suggested by the high incidence of insulin-dependent diabetes with detectable antibodies to islet cells; some patients have thyroiditis, pernicious anemia, or immune-mediated vitiligo.

In the stiff-man syndrome, diazepam in doses of 50 to 250 mg/day, increased gradually, is most effective; clonazepam or baclofen are sometimes effective as well.

In keeping with the presumed autoimmune mechanism, plasma exchange, high-dose corticosteroids, or intravenous gamma globulin are helpful in some patients, albeit for only several weeks or months. Two of our patients have required infusions of gamma globulin for several years at intervals of 6 to 12 weeks and became disabled if the dose of diazepam was reduced below 200 mg/day.

Clinically, the stiff-man syndrome must be distinguished from tetanus (page 1271 and further on), the Isaacs syndrome (see above), and the rare syndrome of subacute myoclonic spinal neuronitis, described on page 1315. In both the stiff-man syndrome and myoclonic spinal neuronitis, the intense spasms and stiffness of muscles are due to disinhibition of interneurons (possibly via GABAergic Renshaw cells) in the gray matter of the spinal cord. These syndromes of continuous muscle activity, except perhaps the stiff-man syndrome, are, as a rule, usually distinguishable clinically and electromyographically from extrapyramidal and corticospinal abnormalities such as dystonia, dyskinesia, rigidity, and spasticity.

Congenital Neonatal Rigidity A "stiff-infant" syndrome, observed by Dudley and colleagues in four families of mixed heritage, should probably be included in this general category. The condition came to medical attention because of respiratory distress due to a generalized muscular rigidity beginning at about 2 months of age. The rigidity spread slowly from cervical muscles to those of the trunk and limbs, and, as it persisted, slight hypertrophy developed. The use of respiratory aid and a feeding gastrostomy enabled the infants to survive. The rigidity slowly diminished in the second year of life. The clinical course was unlike that of tetanus. In fatal cases there were zones of fiber loss, with fibrosis in skeletal and cardiac muscles, and a greater than normal variation in fiber size. Altered Z lines were observed electronmicroscopically in some fibers.

Schwartz-Jampel Syndrome Blepharospasm, dwarfism, pinched face with low-set ears, blepharophimosis, high-arched palate, receding chin, diffuse metaphyseal and epiphyseal bone dysplasia with flattened vertebrae, and a generalized muscular disorder of stiffness and continuous muscle fiber activity were crystallized as a syndrome by Schwartz and Jampel in 1962. It has also been reported under the name of *myotonic chondrodystrophy*. Intelligence is usually preserved. There may be percussion myotonia. The stiff muscles disturb gait. Muscle stiffness is the result of frequent, almost continuous muscle activity with a combination of normal motor units as well as high-frequency discharges and afterdischarges similar to those seen in Isaacs syndrome. Some of the discharges probably arise from muscle fibers themselves, since the activity is not obliterated by curare. Agents such as procainamide, which block sodium channels in muscle, inhibit the discharges, just as they do in some other myotonic disorders. However, Spaans and associates, who have reviewed the clinical, EMG, and histologic features of 30 cases of this syndrome, report a diminished chloride conductance by the sarcolemma, which can be suppressed by procainamide or even better by mexiletine.

The disorder is usually inherited as an autosomal recessive trait. Electronmicroscopic studies of muscle have yielded inconsistent findings: dilated T system, Z-band streaming, and dilatation of mitochondria; in addition, in the patient reported by Fariello and colleagues, muscle biopsy disclosed signs of denervation (group atrophy). In the latter case, treatment with procainamide, phenytoin, diazepam, and barbiturates was ineffective.

The condition described by Aberfeld and coworkers, of two siblings in whom myotonia was combined with dwarfism, diffuse bone disease, and unusual ocular and facial abnormalities and thought by them to represent a unique disorder, is probably a variant of the Schwartz-Jampel syndrome.

Muscle Contracture, Pseudomyotonia, Tetanus, and Related States

Physiologic Contracture due to Phosphorylase Deficiency (McArdle) and Phosphofructokinase Deficiency (Tarui) These are examples of an entirely different type of painful shortening and hardness of muscle. In both these diseases, an otherwise normal child, adolescent, or adult begins to complain of weakness and stiffness and sometimes pain on using the limbs. Muscle contraction and relaxation are normal when the patient is in repose, but strenuous activity, especially under conditions of ischemia, causes the muscles to shorten gradually, due to a failure of relaxation. The contracted muscles in these disorders—unlike muscles in cramp, continuous muscular activity syndromes, or myotonia and other involuntary spasms—no longer use energy. During contracture, the muscles are more or less electrically silent in the EMG. This condition is spoken of as *pharmacologic* or *physiologic contracture*. McArdle and Tarui disease are discussed more fully beginning on page 1515.

Pseudomyotonia This phenomenon is observed in *hypothyroidism*, where the muscle fibers contract and relax slowly. This response is readily demonstrated in eliciting tendon reflexes, particularly the Achilles reflex. The muscles are large and subject to myoedema; when used, they may show waves of slow contraction. The basis of this disorder appears to be a slowness in the reaccumulation of calcium ions in the endoplasmic reticulum and in the disengagement of thin actin and thick myosin filaments. The EMG may show afterpotentials following voluntary contraction, but they do not resemble the typical waning discharges ("myotonic runs") of true myotonia.

A closely related syndrome, wherein painless contracture is induced by exercise, has been described by Lambert and Goldstein, and by Brody. Whereas muscle contraction is normal, the relaxation phase becomes increasingly slow during exercise. Lambert and coworkers referred to it as an unusual type of myotonia, and Brody, as a decrease of relaxing factor. The slow relaxation of muscles has also been attributed to a decreased uptake of calcium by the sarcoplasmic reticulum.

Tetanus This disorder is characterized by persistent spasms of skeletal muscles, owing to the effect of the tetanus toxin on spinal neurons (Renshaw and other cells), the natural function of which is to inhibit the motor neurons. As the condition develops, activities that normally excite the neurons (i.e., voluntary contraction and startle from visual and auditory stimulation) all evoke involuntary spasms. Sleep tends to quiet them, and they are suppressed by spinal anesthesia and curare. The EMG shows the expected interference pattern of action potentials. Once the muscle is involved in persistent contraction, it is said that the shortened state is not abolished by procaine block or severance of nerve (in animals), but this so-called *myostatic contracture* has not been demonstrated in humans.

The effect on the inhibitory neurons is analogous to that of strychnine (see page 1271 for a full description of tetanus and its treatment). There is also an action of the tetanus toxin at the neuromuscular junction, which has been more difficult to evaluate in the face of its powerful central action. Having injected this toxin locally in animals, Price and associates have demonstrated its localization at motor end plates. It binds with ganglioside in the axon membrane and is transported by retrograde flow to the spinal cord, where it induces local tetanus effects. Neurons that innervate slow-twitch type 1 muscle fibers are more sensitive than those supplying fast-twitch type 2 fibers. Presynaptic vesicles increase, acetylcholine (ACh) is blocked, and terminal axon injury may paralyze muscle fibers. Fibrillation potentials and axonal sprouting follow. The similarities to stiff-man syndrome have already been mentioned.

Black Widow Spider Bite The toxin produced by this spider, within a few minutes of the bite, leads to cramps and spasms and then a painful rigidity of abdominal, trunk, and leg muscles. The spasms are followed by weakness. There is also vasoconstriction, hypertension, and autonomic hyperactivity. If death does not occur in the first 24 to 48 h, recovery is complete.

The spider venom has a presynaptic localization and rapidly releases quanta of ACh. The vesicles are depleted. There is some evidence that the venom prevents endocytosis of the vesicles by inserting itself into the presynaptic membranes, causing a disturbance of ionic conductance channels (Swift).

Treatment, which is more or less empiric, consists of calcium gluconate infusions. Intravenous magnesium sulfate also helps to reduce the release of ACh and control the convulsions that sometimes occur. There is a reconstituted antiserum that is available in regions where such envenomation is frequent.

Malignant Hyperthermia This condition is also characterized by an acute onset of generalized muscular rigidity accompanied by a rapid rise in body temperature, metabolic acidosis, and myoglobinuria. It is invariably induced by anesthetic agents and other drugs and is fully discussed on page 1563.

Myalgic States

Many of the muscle diseases described in the preceding pages are associated with aching and discomfort. These are particularly prominent in conditions that are accompanied by cramp and biochemical contracture (phosphorylase and phosphofructokinase deficiency). Ischemia of muscle—that is, intermittent claudication—is also painful, as is dystonia in some cases. Muscle weakness that imposes persistent abnormal postures on the limbs may cause stretch injury of muscles and tendons. This is observed in a number of the congenital myopathies and dystrophies. In all these conditions, clinical study will usually disclose the source or sources of the pain.

Diffuse muscle pain, which merges with malaise, is a frequent expression of a large variety of systemic infections—e.g., influenza, brucellosis, dengue, Colorado tick fever, glanders, measles, malaria, relapsing fever, rheumatic fever ("growing pains"), salmonellosis, toxoplasmosis, trichinosis, tularemia, and Weil disease. When the pain is intense, especially if it is localized to one side of the lower chest and abdomen, the most likely diagnostic possibility is epidemic myalgia (also designated as *pleurodynia*, "devil's grip," and *Bornholm disease*, due to coxsackievirus infection, page 787). Poliomyelitis may be accompanied by intense pain at the onset of neurologic involvement, and later the paralyzed muscles may ache. This is true also of the Guillain-Barré syndrome, in which the pain may precede weakness by several days. Little is known about the pathologic basis of the muscular pain in these diseases; it is not due to muscle inflammation. Muscle pain is a frequent but not a necessary accompaniment of polymyositis and dermatomyositis.

Polymyalgia Rheumatica The major consideration in elderly and middle-aged patients with pain in proximal muscles of the limbs is polymyalgia rheumatica. This subject is mentioned briefly in other sections of this book in relation to back and extremity pain (page 230) and to temporal arteritis, to which it is closely connected (page 193). The muscular soreness may be diffuse or asymmetrical, particularly in the proximal arms and shoulders. Every movement is reported as stiff and painful. The periarticular tissues and their muscular attachments are affected primarily and may be tender, but this is difficult to interpret, since it may be found in otherwise normal individuals. The sedimentation rate is greatly elevated in the majority of patients, and a 48-h trial of prednisone, by alleviating muscle pain, confirms the diagnosis. In the context of muscle pain, systemic symptoms such as weight loss, headache, and fatigue are particularly suggestive of polymyalgia rheumatica.

Fibromyalgia This would appear, by definition, to represent an inflammation of the fibrous tissues of the muscles, fascia, aponeuroses, and possibly nerves as well. Unfortunately, the pathologic basis of this state remains obscure. Only some clinical facts are at hand. During the first movements after a period of inactivity, a muscle or group of muscles may become painful and tender, particularly after exposure to cold, dampness, or minor trauma, but often for no reason that can be discerned. One looks in vain for signs of tendinous or arthritic disease. The neck and shoulders are the most common sites. Sometimes firm, tender areas, up to several centimeters in diameter, can be palpated within the muscles ("fibrositic nodules"), and active contraction or passive stretching of the involved muscles increases the pain—points said to be of diagnostic value, but still disputed. Symptoms such as mental and physical fatigue, insomnia, giddiness, and headache are frequently associated and raise the suspicion of an anxiety state or depression. Often the condition clears up in a few weeks; local heat and massage and local injections of anesthetics or steroids are found to give comfort while symptoms are present.

The chronic form of fibromyalgia presents far greater problems, usually disabling the patient and causing a change in accustomed habits and employment. It has become one of the prime diagnoses made by rheumatologists and physiatrists, but the patient may first come to the attention of a neurologist. Muscle pain is the primary symptom, with fatigue and the other aforementioned complaints added as an afterthought by the patient, or the muscular symptoms are elicited in exploring a case of chronic fatigue syndrome (pages 231 and 528). There is a great preponderance of women among these patients, and in the majority the illness is not predated by any particular factor, although a few have a viral prodrome or recently preceding trauma.

Most definitions of the syndrome have been circular or somewhat arbitrary. Those now in general use are similar to the one proposed by a committee of the American College of Rheumatology. The basis for diagnosis is the presence of widespread pain including focal areas of pain (trigger points) that can be produced by 4 kg of digital pressure in 11 of 18 typical locations over muscles, tendons, or bone—these are concentrated around the shoulders and paraspinal regions—and there is no requirement for the presence of the several common systemic complaints that accompany the illness in most patients (fatigue, difficulty concentrating, sleeping difficulty, or anxiety). Often there is said to be a knot or fibrous band at the site of tenderness, but this is difficult to objectify.

There is controversy regarding the nature of these pressure points and the validity of methods used to elicit them, since mechanical dolorimetry often suggests that these patients have a reduced tolerance to pain at all sites. But there is also uncertainty regarding the relationship of the symptoms to underlying depression. In the past, similar pains were associated with cases of irritable bowel or irritable bladder syndromes, dysmenorrhea, chronic headache, and cold intolerance. Depending upon how broad a definition one allows for the widespread pain and painful trigger points, most or all patients in our experience manifest many of the same complaints as those with the chronic fatigue syndrome, which is discussed in Chap. 24. Authorities on the subject, however, have claimed that in the majority of patients, formal assessment by modern criteria fails to confirm the presence of depression and that, when depression does coexist with the muscular complaints, the two are discordant temporally and in severity. While we acknowledge that antidepressants often give disappointing results and that in our practice there have been several young women with fibromyalgia who appeared to be well adjusted and lacked depression, these are the exceptions. The literature eschews the use of corticosteroids for treatment of the pain, but we have had occasion to see two patients whose symptoms were relieved when these medications were used for other purposes. It can be said in conclusion that fibromyalgia remains a problematic illness, defined by a pattern of pain that justifies its name. Despite attempts to objectify the physical symptoms, psychiatric factors should not be overlooked. This condition is a "favorite" illness with physiotherapists, who claim that their physical measures are helpful, as they may be. Rarely, a similar syndrome is the forerunner of what proves, after some days, with the onset of neurologic signs, to be a radiculitis, brachial neuritis, or outbreak of herpes zoster (see Goldenberg).

Other Myalgic States An impressive polymyalgia is one that follows excessive exercise. Often the patient observes that aching pain occurs not at the time of activity but some hours or even a day or two later, resembling the discomfort following the excessive use of unconditioned muscles. The muscles are sore and there is an intolerance of exercise and physical exertion. This is a natural phenomenon and is self-limiting. When such a state persists indefinitely and a program of conditioning exercises does not alleviate the pain, it represents a special category of disease. In a few instances an increased sedimentation rate or other laboratory aids may clarify the diagnosis, and muscle biopsy may reveal a nonspecific interstitial nodular myositis or the giant-cell arteritis associated with polymyalgia rheumatica. However, this cluster of symptoms most often occurs without explanation, and one can only suspect an obscure infection or a subtle aberration of muscle metabolism, presently impossible to demonstrate. Reference was made earlier to the finding of a *myoadenylate deaminase deficiency* in some of these cases. Sometimes a rapid rise of CK after strenuous exercise will provide a clue. There is also a group of patients who have idiopathic leg pain during rest after activity. Some families afflicted in this way are forced to live a sedentary existence. The condition does not respond to analgesics. In two cases, a deficiency of Ca-ATPase was found and reportedly alleviated by a calcium channel blocker such as verapamil, 120 mg qid (Walton; Taylor et al). It must be distinguished from Fabry disease (page 1422), from the syndromes of painful legs and moving toes, and from the restless leg syndrome of Ekbom (page 412).

The problem of a muscular pain-fasciculation syndrome was discussed earlier. In thin, asthenic adults who exhibit rather vague polymyalgia without other abnormalities, with or without cramps and fasciculations, the authors have found it difficult to exclude hysteria or other neurosis and depression. Before concluding that the condition has a psychiatric basis, it is important in every such individual to search for evidence of a rheumatic disease, brucellosis, or the myopathy that may accompany hypothyroidism, hyperparathyroidism and renal tubular acidosis, hypophosphatemia, hypoglycemia, and the intrinsic phosphorylase or phosphofructokinase defect. Patients with these latter diseases often complain of soreness, stiffness, and lameness after strenuous muscular effort. According to Mills and Edwards, *the most valuable screening tests are the sedimentation rate and serum CK concentration.* Other patients probably have an obscure metabolic myopathy, presently undiagnosable. In every reported series, such as that of Serratrice and coworkers, about half of the cases with diffuse myalgia are undiagnosable. This coincides with our own experience.

LOCALIZED MUSCLE MASSES

Masses may be found in one or many muscles in a variety of clinical settings, and the clinical findings in each one have a different significance.

Muscle rupture is usually caused by a violent strain attended by an audible snap and then a bulge, which appears when the muscle contracts. A weakening in contractile power and mild discomfort are usually noted by the patient. The biceps and soleus muscles are most often affected. Treatment is immediate surgical repair; if that is delayed, little can be done for the condition.

Hemorrhage into muscle may occur as a consequence of trauma, as a complication of the use of anticoagulants, in hematologic diseases, or after a minor trauma in a patient with Zenker degeneration of muscle who is convalescing from typhoid fever or some other infection. Runners may acquire painful localized hematomas in leg muscles.

Tumors include *desmoid tumor* (a benign massive growth of fibrous tissue observed most often in parturient women and after surgery), *rhabdomyosarcoma* (a highly malignant tumor with strong liability to local recurrence and metastasis), *liposarcoma*, and *angioma*. Large neurofibromas or neurofibrosarcomas beneath large muscles such as the hamstring may be difficult to differentiate by physical examination or magnetic resonance imaging (MRI) from masses within the muscle. *Pseudotumorous* growths, sometimes massive, may follow injury of a muscle. Interlacing regenerating muscle fibers and fibroblasts compose the mass. Excision of the entire muscle had been undertaken in several cases in the belief that the growth was a rhabdomyosarcoma, whereas it is actually a benign reaction to trauma (Kakulas and Adams).

Thrombosis of arteries or, more often, of *veins* causes congestion and infarction of muscle. A special type of *muscle infarction* occurs in patients with complicated and poorly controlled diabetes mellitus (Banker and Chester). Usually the infarction involves the anterior thigh, occasionally other muscles of the lower limb. The major symptoms are the sudden onset of pain and swelling of the thigh, with or without the formation of a tender, palpable mass. Recurrent infarction of the same or opposite thigh is characteristic. The stereotypical clinical picture obviates the need for diagnostic muscle biopsy. The extensive infarction of muscle is due to the occlusion of many medium-sized muscular arteries and arterioles, most likely the result of embolization of atheromatous material from eroded plaques in the aorta or iliac arteries. Recognition of this complication and immobilization of the limb are of prime practical importance, since muscle biopsy and early ambulation may cause serious hemorrhage into the infarcted tissue.

The *pretibial syndrome*, also well recognized, follows direct trauma or excessive activity (marching, exercising of unconditioned muscles). There is swelling of the extensor hallucis longus, extensor digitorum longus, and anterior tibial muscles. Being tightly enclosed by the bones and pretibial fascia, the swelling leads to ischemic necrosis and myoglobinuria. Permanent weakness of this group of muscles can be prevented by incising the pretibial fascia.

Myositis Ossificans This condition involves the deposition of bone within the substance of a muscle. Two types are recognized. One is a localized form that appears in a single muscle or group of muscles after trauma, and the other is a progressive, widespread ossifying process, entirely unrelated to trauma, in many muscles of the body.

Localized (Traumatic) Myositis Ossificans After a muscle tear, a single blow to the muscle, or repeated minor trauma, a painful area develops in the muscle. It is gradually replaced by a mass of cartilaginous consistency, and within 4 to 7 weeks' time a solid mass of bone can be felt and seen in radiographs. As would be expected, this most frequently happens in vigorous adult men; the inner thigh muscles (in those who ride horses) and to a lesser extent the pectoralis major and biceps brachii are the most common sites of the abnormality. The mass tends to subside after several months if the patient desists from the activity that produced the trauma.

Generalized Myositis Ossificans This disease, first described by Munchmeyer in 1869, has since been referred to by his name or as *myositis ossificans progressiva*. It is rare, although Lutwak, in 1964, was able to collect 264 cases from the literature. The cause is unknown, but the disease is probably inherited as an autosomal dominant trait. It consists of widespread bone formation along the fascial planes of muscles and has its onset in infancy and childhood in 90 percent of cases. Biopsies of early indurated swellings have revealed extensive proliferation of interstitial connective tissue in which little inflammatory cell reaction is found. Within a few weeks, the connective tissue becomes less cellular and retracts, compressing the adjacent muscle fibers. Osteoid and cartilage formation occur at a later stage, developing in the connective tissue and enclosing relatively intact muscle fibers.

Nearly 75 percent of all reported cases have been associated with congenital anomalies, the most frequent of which is a failure of development of the great toes or thumbs and less often other digits. Less frequently, there is hypogenitalism, deafness, and an absence of upper incisors. The first symptom is often a firm swelling and tenderness in a paravertebral or cervical muscle. There is, in addition, a mild discomfort during muscle contraction, and the overlying skin may be reddened and slightly swollen. Trauma may be recalled as the initiating factor, but as the months pass, other muscles not injured in any recognizable way become similarly involved. At first, radiographs reveal no important changes, but within 6 to 12 months, calcium deposits are observed, and one can feel stony-hard masses within the muscles. As the disease advances, limitation of movement and deformities become increasingly evident. Calcified bridges between adjacent muscles and across joints lead to rigidity of the spine, jaw, and limbs, scoliosis, and limited expansion of the thorax. Ultimately, the patient is virtually "changed to stone."

The principal problem in *diagnosis* is to differentiate generalized myositis ossificans from calcinosis universalis. The latter usually occurs in relation to scleroderma or polymyositis and is characterized by calcium deposits in the skin, subcutaneous tissues, and connective tissue sheaths around the muscles; in myositis ossificans, there is actual bone formation within the muscles. The pathologic data are often too meager to justify this sharp distinction. The prolonged ingestion of large doses of vitamin D may also result in the deposition of masses of calcium salts around muscles, joints, and subcutaneous tissue. Calcific deposits, perhaps true ossification, may occur in the soft tissues around the hips and knees of paraplegics and rarely following a hemiplegia ("paralytic myositis ossificans").

The disease may undergo spontaneous remissions and may stabilize for many years, during which the patient is capable of adequate function. In other cases, progression leads to marked debilitation and respiratory embarrassment, the final illness often being a terminal pneumonia or other infection.

The administration of a diphosphonate [ethane-1-hydroxy-1,1-diphosphate (EHDP), 10 to 20 mg/kg orally], a compound that inhibits the deposition of calcium phosphate, has been said to cause regression of new swellings and to prevent calcification (Russell et al). Some of the calcium deposits in calcinosis universalis have receded in response to prednisone, and because of the unclear relationship of this disease to generalized myositis ossificans, it is probably advisable to try this form of therapy as well. Excision of bony deposits may be undertaken if it is certain that they are the cause of particular disabilities.

REFERENCES

Aberfeld DC, Hinterbuchner LP, Schneider M: Myotonia, dwarfism, diffuse bone disease, and unusual ocular and facial abnormalities (a new syndrome). *Brain* 88:313, 1965.

Banker BQ: Other inflammatory myopathies, in Engel AG, Franzini-Armstrong C (eds): *Myology*, 2nd ed. New York, McGraw-Hill, 1994, pp 1461–1486.

Banker BQ, Chester CS: Infarction of thigh muscle in the diabetic patient. *Neurology* 23:667, 1973.

Barker RA, Reeves T, Thom M, et al: Review of 23 patients affected by the stiff man syndrome: Clinical subdivision into stiff trunk (man) syndrome, stiff limb syndrome, and progressive encephalomyelitis with rigidity. *J Neurol Neurosurg Psychiatry* 65:633, 1998.

Brody IA: Muscle contracture induced by exercise: A syndrome attributable to decreased relaxing factor. *N Engl J Med* 281:187, 1969.

Burns RJ, Bretag AH, Blumbergs PC, Harbord MG: Benign familial disease with muscle mounding and rippling. *J Neurol Neurosurg Psychiatry* 57:344, 1994.

Cöers C, Telerman-Toppet N, Durda J: Neurogenic benign fasciculations, pseudomyotonia, and pseudotetany. *Arch Neurol* 38:282, 1981.

Conner JM, Evans DA: Genetic aspects of fibrodysplasia ossificans progressiva. *J Med Genet* 19:35, 1982.

Denny-Brown D, Foley JM: Evidence of a chemical mediator in myotonia. *Trans Assoc Am Physicians* 62:187, 1949.

Denny-Brown D, Nevin S: The phenomenon of myotonia. *Brain* 64:1, 1941.

Dudley MA, Dudley AW, Bernstein LH, et al: Progressive neonatal rigidity: Biochemical aspects of a new familial myopathy. *J Neuropathol Exp Neurol* 38:311, 1979.

Fariello R, Meloff K, Murphy EG, et al: A case of Schwartz-Jampel syndrome with unusual muscle biopsy findings. *Ann Neurol* 3:93, 1978.

Goldenberg DL: Fibromyalgia syndrome and its overlap with chronic fatigue syndrome, in Dawson DM, Sabin TD (eds): *Chronic Fatigue Syndrome*. Boston, Little, Brown, 1993, pp 75–90.

Gutmann L, Gutmann L: Axonal channelopathies: An evolving concept in the pathogenesis of peripheral nerve disorders. *Neurology* 47:18, 1996.

Hudson AJ, Brown WF, Gilbert JJ: The muscular pain-fasciculation syndrome. *Neurology* 28:1105, 1978.

Isaacs H: Continuous muscle fibre activity in an Indian male with additional evidence of terminal motor fibre abnormality. *J Neurol Neurosurg Psychiatry* 30:126, 1967.

Jusic A, Dogan S, Stojanovic V: Hereditary persistent distal cramps. *J Neurol Neurosurg Psychiatry* 35:379, 1972.

Kakulas BA, Adams RD: *Diseases of Muscle: Pathological Foundations of Clinical Myology*, 4th ed. Philadelphia, Harper & Row, 1985.

Lambert EH, Goldstein NP: An unusual form of "myotonia." *Physiologist* 1:51, 1957.

Lance JW, Burke D, Pollard J: Hyperexcitability of motor and sensory neurons in neuromyotonia. *Ann Neurol* 5:523, 1979.

Layzer RB: Muscle pain, cramps, and fatigue, in Engel AG, Franzini-Armstrong C (eds): *Myology*, 2nd ed. New York, McGraw-Hill, 1994, pp 1754–1768.

Lütschg J, Jerusalem F, Ludin HP, et al: The syndrome of "continuous muscle fiber activity." *Arch Neurol* 35:198, 1978.

Lutwak L: Myositis ossificans progressiva: Mineral, metabolic and radioactive calcium studies of the effects of hormones. *Am J Med* 37:269, 1964.

Mills KR, Edwards RHT: Investigative strategies for muscle pain. *J Neurol Sci* 58:73, 1983.

Moersch FP, Woltman HW: Progressive fluctuating muscular rigidity ("stiff-man syndrome"): Report of a case and some observations in 13 other cases. *Mayo Clin Proc* 31:421, 1956.

Newsom-Davis J, Mills KR: Immunological associations of acquired neuromyotonia (Isaacs' syndrome). *Brain* 116:453, 1993.

Price DL, Griffin JW, Peck K: Tetanus toxin: Evidence for binding at presynaptic nerve endings. *Brain Res* 121:379, 1977.

RICKER K, MOXLEY RT: Autosomal dominant cramping disease. *Arch Neurol* 47:810, 1990.

RICKER K, MOXLEY RT, ROHKAMM R: Rippling muscle disease. *Arch Neurol* 46:405, 1989.

RUSSELL RGG, SMITH R, BISHOP MC, et al: Treatment of myositis ossificans progressiva with a diphosphonate. *Lancet* 1:10, 1972.

SATOYOSHI E: A syndrome of progressive muscle spasm, alopecia and diarrhea. *Neurology* 28:458, 1978.

SCHWARTZ O, JAMPEL R: Congenital blepharophimosis associated with a unique generalized myopathy. *Arch Ophthalmol* 68:52, 1962.

SERRATRICE G, AZULAY JP: Que reste-t-il de la chorée fibrillaire de Morvan? *Rev Neurol* 150:257, 1994.

SERRATRICE G, GASTAUT JL, SCHIANO A, et al: A propos de 210 cas de myalgies diffuses. *Semin Hop Paris* 56:1241, 1980.

SOLIMENA M, FOLLI F, APARISI R, et al: Autoantibodies to GABA-ergic neurons and pancreatic beta cells in stiff-man syndrome. *N Engl J Med* 322:1555, 1990.

SPAANS F, THEUNISSEN P, REEKERS AD, et al: Schwartz-Jampel syndrome: 1. Clinical, electromyographic, and histologic studies. *Muscle Nerve* 13:516, 1990.

SWIFT TR: Disorders of neuromuscular transmission other than myasthenia gravis. *Muscle Nerve* 4:334, 1981.

TAYLOR DJ, BROSNAN MJ, ARNOLD DL, et al: Ca-ATPase deficiency in a patient with an exertional muscle pain syndrome. *J Neurol Neurosurg Psychiatry* 51:1425, 1988.

THOMPSON PD: Stiff muscles. *J Neurol Neurosurg Psychiatry* 56:121, 1993.

VALLI G, BARBIERI S, STEFANO C, et al: Syndromes of abnormal muscular activity: Overlap between continuous muscle fiber activity and the stiff-man syndrome. *J Neurol Neurosurg Psychiatry* 46:241, 1983.

WALTON J: Diffuse exercise-induced pain of undetermined cause relieved by verapamil. *Lancet* 1:993, 1981.

WETTSTEIN A: The origin of fasciculations in motor neuron disease. *Ann Neurol* 5:295, 1979.

Part 6

PSYCHIATRIC DISORDERS

To understand mental disorders, one must know something of how the brain functions, know something of human psychology, and at the same time be sensitive and responsive to other human beings and have a sincere desire to help them. The first two of these objectives require special study; the latter are more innate qualities, found in all good physicians. Indeed, the attributes that exalt our profession are sympathy for the sick and the willingness to put the patient's welfare ahead of our own—attributes that meet their greatest challenge in dealing with the mentally ill.

Mental disorders pose a number of special problems not met in other fields of medicine. In the first place, there are such wide variations in personality, character, and behavior that the point where normal ends and abnormal begins is often difficult to ascertain. Second, the methods of studying mental illness are quite subjective, depending mainly on the physician's perceptions of the inner secrets and purposes of the patient and on the patient's powers of description and narration in revealing his symptoms; these latter capacities vary with intelligence, personality, education, and cerebral function. Finally, and most vexing to the neurologist, the clinical entities to be presented in the following chapters are for the most part unverifiable; neither by laboratory test nor by postmortem examination can one reliably corroborate their existence.

In attempting to study mental disorder, one must be aware of another, more abstruse and essentially theoretical problem. Here, physicians find that there are two different and seemingly antithetical approaches to disordered nervous function—one proceeding along strictly medical or neurologic lines, the other psychologic. They must learn to utilize two types of data, one drawn from observations of the patient's behavior, the other from the patient's introspections. It must be emphasized that the terms *neurologic* and *psychologic* in this context do not necessarily refer to the activities of neurologists and psychiatrists. They are merely convenient terms for two distinct modes of approach to mental disorders; both may be and frequently are used by the neurologist and the psychiatrist, as will be made clear.

The neurologic approach begins with the premise that all clinical manifestations of a nervous disorder are expressions of a pathologic process (disease) within the nervous system. This process may be obvious (such as a tumor or cerebral infarct), or it may be impossible to detect with the light or even the electron microscope (such as the encephalopathy of delirium tremens). In all instances the pathologic process is traceable to some genetic, chemical, or physical factor acting on the brain, and the visible lesion represents only an advanced and often irreversible stage of a dynamic morbid process. The particular clinical effect, qua symptom or sign—whether it be paralysis, sensory loss, visual or auditory impairment, ataxia, aphasia, tremor, confusion, coma, convulsion, or hallucination—depends on the nature of the lesion and its locus within the nervous system. The clinical manifestations, therefore, are interpretable in terms of neuroanatomy, neuropathology, neurophysiology, and neuropsychology.

The symptoms and signs of the disease, i.e., the expressions of the pathologically altered nervous system, take two forms, either of loss of function, or negative effects (as might occur with a hemiplegia), or of overactivity, i.e., positive effects, due to disinhibition of intact parts of the brain or to seizure activity. In many cerebral disorders, however, such distinctions between negative and positive effects cannot be made with certainty; in relation to processes such as perceiving, thinking, remembering, symbolization, etc., we lack the knowledge that would enable us to reduce them to this basic formulation. Here, the advancing field of neuropsychology with its special methodologies, in combination with functional magnetic resonance imaging (MRI), promises to be of particular value.

This brings us face to face with other problems that are posed by more complex diseases of the brain. In a syndrome such as dementia or partial aphasia, for example, the deficit symptoms may be much the same from patient to patient, whereas the unbalanced behavior may differ, even with the same disease in the same parts of the cerebrum. Only with some knowledge of the patient's natural endowment, education, premorbid personality, stability of emotional control, etc., can such differences be understood.

In cerebral diseases causing complex disorders of perception, speech, and thinking, there is usually both an impairment of introspective ability (lack of insight) and a change in behavior. This dual loss provides the most certain proof that activities of the mind and behavior depend on the same physiologic processes in the brain. It leads inevitably to a psychophysical monism, the position on the mind-body problem most acceptable to neurologists. Admittedly, this theoretical concept has not had universal acceptance. Western philosophers, from Plato in ancient times through Descartes and, more recently, Sherrington and Eccles, have generally been dualists, holding that body and mind are independent systems, each susceptible to its own disorders. One of the ideas most difficult to appreciate, though it follows clearly from the neurologic concept of disordered nervous function, is that there is no essential difference between diseases called physical or organic and others called functional or mental. Every disorder of function must have a structural basis. The difficulty in psychiatric disease is that the physical basis is subcellular and not observable by traditional histopathologic methods.

The methodology of the *neurologic approach* or *medical model*, which was for a long time espoused by our colleague and teacher Mandel Cohen and is now endorsed by many others, was described in Chap. 1. It utilizes the standard procedures of history taking and physical examination, supplemented by biochemical, physiologic, and psychologic tests. Pathologic examination provides the final confirmation of diagnosis. The goals of this neurologic methodology and of neuropathology (defined broadly as the scientific study of diseases of the nervous system) are to determine whether or not a disease exists in the patient and, if so, to determine its prognosis and the possibilities of prevention and therapy. A complete concept of a disease must incorporate all its essential elements—genetic, biochemical, physiologic, and psychologic as well as pathologic. This concept of "disorders of mind arising in brain" is subscribed to by most modern psychiatrists (Andreasen).

A second mode of approach to disordered mental function and behavior, which one may term the *psychologic approach*, has as its main premise that the disordered function is understandable solely in terms of a reaction to previous or present life experiences. Certain abnormalities of behavior, emotional immaturity, and inability to adjust to the challenges and opportunities of everyday life are thought to stem from an inadequate development of personality, distressing experiences in early life, or both. Some of these experiences are remembered (i.e., "conscious"); others are said to be suppressed or forgotten (i.e., "subconscious or unconscious," according to psychoanalytic theory) and recalled with difficulty or by repeated questioning or through the free-association method of psychoanalysis. In either case, the principal approach is to construct a kind of psychologic autobiography of the individual, with particular emphasis on early life experiences, and to search it for the roots of the present psychologic difficulty. Psychiatrists of this persuasion have formulated a number of psychologic mechanisms whereby symptoms are produced, and they speak of them in a language rather unfamiliar to most physicians—e.g., conflict, repression, conversion, projection, displacement of affect, conditioning, and arrest or fixation of libido. Some of the more narrowly trained psychoanalysts cast all mental disorder in psychologic terms and believe that anatomic, biochemical, and pathologic considerations have no place in such a formulation. The purpose of this approach is not only to determine causality—namely, psychogenesis—but also to understand the patient's current behavior in the light of past experiences and to use this understanding to effect change. By frank discussion, the physician endeavors to demonstrate the relationship of the patient's symptoms to abnormal behavior patterns and reactions, and, by a kind of re-education, i.e., psychotherapy, to assist in bringing about an understanding of the problems and improved ways of coping with them.

A HOLISTIC AND ECLECTIC POSITION

It seems to the present authors that both the neurologic and the psychologic concepts and approaches have their place in medicine. But the two methods operate at different levels and are of principal use in different types of nervous aberrations.

In the diagnosis of a disease of the nervous system, one begins always with a careful recording of the symptoms and signs and their temporal aspects, obtained through a detailed history and physical and ancillary examinations. The interpretation of such data by the use of anatomic and physiologic data leads to diagnosis. Here the psychologic method is of little value and the neurologic method stands as the only valid system of analysis. It permits one to approach the problem of nervous system disease as one does any other medical problem.

It must be acknowledged, however, that special difficulties attend the diagnosis of psychiatric diseases. These illnesses are expressed mainly by symptoms—complaints about distressing thoughts or feelings, or behavior that is disturbing to others. Seldom are there objectifiable signs. Often patients are not consistent in what they say, and their behavior may change with time. Symptoms are always more liable to varied interpretation than are signs. Nevertheless the physician must rely on the methodology of medicine, with due allowance for these added difficulties.

In theorizing about disease and investigating its causes, this broad neurologic or medical approach is essential, for it accepts data from all the medical sciences and is able to incorporate all the biologic as well as psychologic facts. It is supported by the realization that every known psychiatric symptom is reproduced by known cerebral diseases, and every major neurologic disease of the cerebrum may be attended by symptoms of psychiatric disease. Here, too, the psychologic method has limited application, and although yielding useful data concerning the patient's background and the evolution of particular symptoms and their form and content, it will not provide a complete explanation of disease.

By contrast, in the diagnosis and management of certain disorders of personality, character, and social maladjustments, which constitute such a large and important part of medicine and psychiatry, the psychologic approach achieves great credence. Worry over loss of a job or the illness of a child, the death of a loved one, or domestic difficulty, with all their potential physiologic disturbances, are acceptable to every thoughtful physician as derangements consequent upon the social situation. Indeed, only when such worries and stresses are beyond the patient's control or the connection between the social problem and its physical effects is not perceived do they become medical problems. These are suitably looked upon as reactions to life's difficulties and dealt with entirely at a psychologic level. Furthermore, in the management of all diseases, knowledge of the patient's intelligence, education, personality, and general reactions to life experiences is quite indispensable. This is a province of medicine where the psychologic approach is of inestimable value, and the physician who knows the patient and how to deal with him as a troubled individual functions with great effectiveness.

This brings us to one of the crucial problems in neurology and psychiatry—that of defining a disease of the nervous system and distinguishing it from a social or psychologic maladjustment. Failure to do this has resulted in much confusion as to the legitimate spheres of medical activity and has been an obstacle to research. The present authors define a disease of the nervous system as any condition in which there is a visible lesion or in which there is reasonable evidence of its existence on the basis of stereotypy of clinical expression and of genetic and collateral laboratory data. Goodwin and Guze offer a slightly different definition of psychiatric disease—as any cluster of symptoms and signs that occur with such consistency as to permit the prediction of their outcome. An abnormal psychologic reaction is defined as a disorder of psychic function and behavior caused by a maladjustment in social relations or a disordered response to life's difficulties not based directly on a known disease process or lesion.

Simple as this division might seem, it is not easily applied to every abnormal neuropsychiatric state. How does one interpret disturbances of impulse control, hyperactivity, timidity, seclusiveness, suspiciousness, inability to learn at the accustomed pace, failure to read or master arithmetic at the usual age, criminality, and inadequacy in adjustment to school, work, marriage, and society? Some of these disturbances, as pointed out in Chap. 28, are surely due to specific retardations in development; others may be due to innate personality (genetically based) traits, lack of proper training and education, unstable home environment, etc. Obviously, with such complex phenomena, it may at times be impossible to separate cause and effect. An individual whose nervous system is affected by disease and who is unable to learn or to form stable social relationships may create an abnormal environment. Or a serious environmental stress may decompensate a patient with underlying nervous system disease.

Also, certain mental abnormalities have an uncertain status vis-à-vis this division and are currently subject to double interpretations, depending on one's premises. A persistent anxiety state without obvious cause in a previously healthy adult would be viewed by some psychiatrists as a reaction of fear to some unconscious threat. Others would consider it a genetic disease closely allied to endogenous depression, in which some biochemical disturbance, as mysterious as was hyperthyroidism a century ago, has developed de novo. Since the nature of the condition is unsettled, it is treated by physicians using both psychologic methods and drugs. Anyone who proposes to investigate it, we would argue, should do so with a completely open mind and be prepared to review critically any reasonable hypothesis as to its cause.

As to the major psychiatric disorders—depression, mania, paranoia, and schizophrenia—they are regarded by most psychiatrists and neurologists as genetically determined diseases of the nervous system, the mechanism, anatomy, and biochemistry of which are still obscure. Environmental stress at times seems important in their evocation and exacerbation but is obviously not an essential or sufficient factor. Only a few psychiatrists still insist that such states represent deviant ways of living or abnormal psychologic reactions. It seems reasonable to assume that the more comprehensive methodology of the neurologic and medical sciences will eventually lead to their solution. Similarly, certain socially delicate issues such as gender identity and homosexuality will probably prove to have explanations in both psychologic and anatomic terms.

When the clinical specialties of psychiatry and neurology are viewed in terms of these theories about disease and psychosocial reactions, it is obvious that they have overlapping interests. Diseases such as schizophrenia and manic-depressive psychosis, while of interest to neurologists, will remain indubitably in the province of psychiatrists. The latter have the training in psychotherapeutic methods and expertise in neuropharmacology that are needed in the care of such patients. Also, the psychiatrist must stand as the spokesman for the medical position on the countless ills related to social and behavioral maladjustments in modern life. The vast array of well-defined cerebrospinal diseases is the prerogative of the neurologist, but he, too, must be sensitive to their psychologic aspects.

Psychosomatic Medicine It is difficult to appreciate the evolution of psychiatry, particularly in America, without mentioning psychosomatic medicine. Beginning in the 1930s there was great interest in a large category of disease referred to for decades as psychosomatic. Included here were peptic ulcer, mucous and ulcerative colitis, hay fever, bronchial asthma, urticaria, angioneurotic edema, essential hypertension, hyperthyroidism, rheumatoid arthritis, amenorrhea, and migraine—diseases in which a stressful life situation or emotional upset appeared to be associated with their development, exacerbation, or prolongation. More than 70 years have passed since these ideas were first proclaimed, and an enormous literature followed, with the establishment of pathetically few unassailable facts. It became clear that the so-called psychosomatic diseases are not neuroses in that they have different symptoms, and in most instances there is a known and easily demonstrable pathologic basis. Even peptic ulcer, an old psychosomatic favorite, is now traced to a bacterial infection. No complete proof of psychic causation of any of the psychosomatic diseases has been found. Treatment has been concerned mainly with the relief of symptoms and has been directed for the most part by nonpsychiatric specialists. There is no evidence that the therapeutic results obtained by psychiatrists are better than those of a competent internist.

This extended application of the concept of psychosomatic disorders is still extant. The psychiatric literature is permeated with references to personality types that predispose to disease. Our criticism is that it tends to overemphasize the psychologic aspects out of all proportion to the somatic. One must concede that anxiety and related states raise the blood pressure and probably are associated with other physiologic changes, but the majority of assertions regarding personality types and psychologic states in relation to physical diseases remain unproven. The current societal preoccupation with "stress" as a cause or trigger for all manner of medical and neurologic disease, including disordered function of the immune system, is an extension of this still tenuous concept. As pointed out by Wolff in his scholarly exposition of the "mind-body" relationship, the fallacy of "psychogenic" or "psychosomatic" concepts is that they imply a mind acting in opposition to the body. Nevertheless, interest in the psychosomatic diseases has focused attention on the importance of psychosocial factors in the diseased patient and not merely on the disease in isolation. This has had a salutary influence in medicine. First suggested by Claude Bernard and ably espoused and elaborated by Walter Cannon and Adolph Meyer is the view that the patient must always be regarded as a complex psychobiologic unit functioning in relation to the immediate physical and social environment. Disease represents a faulty or inadequate adaptation of the organism to the environment. Interestingly, the terms *psychosomatic* and *psychophysiologic* are not listed in the fourth edition of the American Psychiatric Association's official diagnostic manual, the *Diagnostic and Statistical Manual of Mental Disorders* (DSM-IV). A few of the disorders originally called psychosomatic now appear under the categories of "somatoform disorders" or "psychological factors affecting physical conditions"; these are discussed in subsequent chapters.

The reader seeking further information as to the status of psychosomatic or psychophysiologic disorders is referred to the review by Rogers and Reich.

PLAN OF PSYCHIATRY SECTION

In the chapters that follow there will be a consideration of the neuroses, the affective disorders, the sociopathies, the schizophrenias, and the paranoid states. The magnitude of these disorders and their clinical and social importance can hardly be overestimated. Some 20 to 30 percent of all individuals will at some period of their lives experience psychiatric symptoms and seek medical help for them. The headings that guide our exposition of neuropsychiatric illnesses might be questioned, but the justification for their selection is that each can be diagnosed by a competent physician and each diagnosis, once made, has been validated by follow-up studies. All physicians should know something about these categories of psychiatric disease. Neurologists in particular need to be familiar with them, if only for the purposes of differentiating them from other neurologic diseases and initiating intelligent management.

Emphasis throughout these chapters will be on the biologic characteristics and the diagnosis of each state. This approach is in keeping with a significant change in American psychiatry, namely, the development of rigorous criteria for the diagnosis of psychiatric disorders.

The stimulus for this development can be largely traced to the studies of the Washington University group, in St. Louis (Feighner, Robins, Guze, and their colleagues; see also the monographs of Goodwin and Guze and of Rakoff et al). Many of the diagnostic formulations proposed by these workers were adopted, in 1980, by DSM-III (and later its revised form, DSM-III-R, and DSM-IV). The prevention of suicide, the choice of appropriate therapy, communication with the patient's family and physician, predictions about the course of the illness (prognosis)—all begin with accurate diagnosis. In addition to their practical clinical value, strict diagnostic criteria are important in psychiatric research.

Mainly, in the chapters that follow, we adhere to conventional psychiatric terms, since they are the ones most widely used in psychiatry and are familiar to most physicians. The DSM has introduced a plethora of new terms, and these will be alluded to where they may possibly be preferable to the older and better-known ones.

In adhering to the bias of neurologic medicine, we do not wish to depreciate the importance of psychologic medicine or of psychiatry. Our position on this matter has been fully stated in the preceding pages and needs no further elaboration. Theoretic aspects of personality and psychopathology and symptom formation will be given little space because of our ignorance of such psychologic mechanisms. Although many of these psychiatric conditions are regarded as diseases of the nervous system, because of their ubiquity and chronicity they should be treated by psychiatrists. The reader will find them well presented in the references at the end of each chapter.

REFERENCES

American Psychiatric Association: *Diagnostic and Statistical Manual of Mental Disorders*, 4th ed (DSM-IV). Washington, DC, APA, 1994.

Andreasen N: Linking mind and brain in the study of mental illness: A project for a scientific psychopathology. *Science* 275:1586, 1997.

Feighner JP, Robins E, Guze SB, et al: Diagnostic criteria for use in psychiatric research. *Arch Gen Psychiatry* 26:57, 1972.

Goodwin DW, Guze SB: *Psychiatric Diagnosis*, 5th ed. New York, Oxford University Press, 1996.

Guze SB: *Why Psychiatry Is a Branch of Medicine*. New York, Oxford University Press, 1992.

McHugh PR: Psychiatric misadventures. *American Scholar* 61:4, 1992.

Rakoff V, Stancer HC, Kedward HB (eds): *Psychiatric Diagnosis*. New York, Brunner-Mazel, 1977.

Rogers MP, Reich P: Psychosomatic medicine and consultation-liaison psychiatry, in Nicholi AM (ed): *The New Harvard Guide to Psychiatry*, 2nd ed. Cambridge, MA, Harvard University Press, 1988, pp 387–417.

Wolff HG: The mind-body relationship, in Bryson L (ed): *An outline of Man's Knowledge of the Modern World*. New York, McGraw-Hill, 1960.

Chapter 56

THE NEUROSES AND PERSONALITY DISORDERS

From time immemorial, in every society, it has been realized that there are many mentally troubled individuals who are neither insane nor feebleminded. They differ from normal persons in being plagued by feelings of inferiority and self-doubt, suspicion about the motives of others, low energy, inexplicable fatigue, shyness, irritability, moodiness, sense of guilt, and unreasonable worries and fears; or they behave in ways that are upsetting to those around them and to society at large. Yet none of these conditions precludes their partaking in many of the everyday affairs of life, such as attending school, working, marrying, and rearing a family. As these conditions were more carefully documented, the ones that caused an individual much personal distress came to be called *psychoneuroses* and, later, *neuroses*, and those that created societal difficulties were called *psychopathies* and, more recently, *sociopathies*.

The question of the purity and homogeneity of these mental states has excited a lively polemic in the psychiatric literature. The neuroses as a group appeared to be so diverse as to require subdivision (in the fourth edition of the *Diagnostic and Statistical Manual of Mental Disorders*, or DSM-IV) into no less than seven different types, as elaborated further on. And the psychopathies, in older classifications, came to include conditions as disparate as extreme asociality, criminality, sexual perversions, and drug and alcohol addictions.

Originally, Freud referred to the neuroses as psychoneuroses, and the subject became enmeshed in psychoanalytic theory. The assumption was that an undercurrent of anxiety arising in unconscious conflict was the explanation of all the different types of neurosis as well as the psychopathies. Later, psychiatrists uncommitted to psychoanalytic theory attributed them to social forces leading to maladaptive behavior in childhood. These notions were not acceptable to biologically oriented psychiatrists, with the result that the term *psychoneurosis* was expunged from later editions of the DSM and even the term *neurosis* was replaced by terms such as *anxiety disorders*, *phobic states*, and *obsessive-compulsive disorder*. These terms are presently being applied to any mental disorder with the following characteristics: (1) symptoms that are distressing to the affected individual and regarded by him as unacceptable or alien; (2) reality testing (the patient's evaluation of the relationship between himself and the outside world) that remains intact; (3) symptomatic behavior that does not seriously violate social norms, although personal functioning may be considerably impaired; (4) a disturbance that is enduring—not a transitory reaction to stress; and (5) absence of a discernible organic cause.

The foregoing definition of the anxiety and allied disorders, or neuroses, has the virtue of being descriptive without committing one to any hypothesis of causation. It retains the historical connotation of neurosis and provides a terminologic link between psychiatrists throughout the world.

The genesis of the neuroses, a matter that has occupied psychiatrists for many years, remains elusive. It is generally conceded that such disorders do not arise de novo in otherwise normal individuals. Their antecedents are thought to be abnormalities in personality development, possibly molded by stressful events in the life of the individual and influenced by genetic factors (Noyes et al). Yet there are undoubtedly traits of this nature that arise in several individuals from the same family. Thus an informative discussion of such disorders requires a brief digression into the origins of normal personality development and departures therefrom.

Personality Disorders

The concept of *personality* and its development were introduced in Chap. 28. There it was pointed out that the term embraces the totality of a person's physical and mental attributes, his observable behavior and reportable subjective experience—the sum of which distinguishes one individual from all others. Thus it includes elements of the individual's character, intelligence, instinctual drives, temperament, sentiments, behavior, motor control, and memories—in short, all forces from within the organism, as well as the reactions to prevailing influences of the environment that govern behavior. The term *character* is almost synonymous with personality but is less useful because of its moralistic connotation.

The roots of personality are multiple. Certain personality traits—such as boldness and timidity, novelty seeking and excitability, level of energy and activity, fearfulness and fearlessness, social adaptability and rigidity or stubbornness, etc.—are already evident in the first months of life. Monozygotic twins are alike (but not absolutely identical) in these respects, even when reared apart. Gesell and his colleagues, in their studies of infants (see Chap. 28), observed individual differences that are clearly innate; each of these characteristics is genetically determined, like intelligence. Probably a multiplicity of genes set the general pattern of each person's innate characteristics. In addition, these patterns are subject to incessant modification through familial, educational, social, and other environmental influences. The personalities that result are as individualistic as fingerprints. One example of a genetic predisposition to a human personality trait has been found in the expression of thrill seeking, exploration, and excitability. According to Cloninger et al (1996), pleomorphism of the dopamine receptor gene on chromosome 11 accounts in small measure for the genetic variability of this personality type; a long allele at this locus expresses higher degrees of risk taking and short alleles are associated with personalities that are more rigid, deliberate, and orderly. Findings such as these suggest that similar polymorphisms contribute to other traits such as anxiety, obsessiveness, etc., but only in part. The notion, expressed by authors such as Kandel, that genetics will explain a large part of mental function and mental illness sounds reasonable enough, but the data that are necessary to established this prediction are far from complete.

Pertinent to the subject matter of this chapter is the assumption that in approximately 15 percent of the general population, certain personality traits are so pronounced as to be distressing to the individual and disturbing to others, even though the patient is not manifestly sociopathic or psychotic. Some of these traits first become sources of difficulty during childhood, in relation to eating, behavior during play, school attendance, etc. They may be aggravated by parental abuse, adoption, divorce, and other persistently distressing circumstances. Perhaps, during maturation, the development of certain portions of the personality has lagged or become dissociated from the personality synthesis, or these aspects are repressed to the point of having a diminished or distorted influence on behavior. How this happens and why the deviations take such a variety of forms is not known. Psychodynamic explanations abound, but—being based only on anecdotal evidence—are difficult or impossible to validate. They tend to emphasize psychologic conflict and to de-emphasize genetic and biologic factors. The extent to which these deviations reflect past experience or a genetically predetermined pattern is unsettled.

Another unsolved problem is whether each of the personality types listed in Table 56-1 (taken from the list of personality disorders accepted by the American Psychiatric Association) is predictive or determinative of a particular type of neurosis or psychosis. In this regard, two broad groups of personality disorders can be recognized. In one group—comprising the paranoid, schizoid, cyclothymic, and obsessive-compulsive personality types—there is a probable relationship to a major type of psychiatric illness. Thus, among patients who develop paranoid schizophrenia, a considerable number will have had the attributes described under "paranoid personality type." Similarly, among patients who develop schizophrenia of another type, the history will frequently disclose a pre-existent schizoid personality. In fact, it may be difficult to judge where the personality disorder left off and the schizophrenic illness began. It seems clear from several family studies that the cyclothymic personality is related to manic-depressive disease. Obsessive-compulsive personality is related not only to obsessive-compulsive neurosis, as one might expect, but also to depressive disease. A relationship exists between sociopathy and the development of alcoholism and of criminality.

In other personality disorders, such relationships are far less evident. Care must be taken to distinguish between "hysterical personality" (called "histrionic personality" in DSM-IV) and the disease *hysteria*, or "somatiform disorder." Some patients with the disease hysteria have a histrionic personality, but this is far from a tight relationship. Similarly, the features of hysterical personality can be observed in individuals who never exhibit "conversion" symptoms (see further on)—and the latter may occur in patients who do not have a hysterical personality. Also, the evidence that asthenic, inadequate, and passive-aggressive or passive-dependent

Table 56-1
Personality disorders

Type[a]	*Characteristics*	*Type*[a]	*Characteristics*
Paranoid (16)	Chronic wariness, suspiciousness, litigiousness; hypersensitivity, jealousy, envy; lack of insight or humor; tendency to blame others; sense of self-importance and entitlement	Asthenic (1)	Chronic weakness, easy fatigability, sense of vulnerability, oversensitive to physically and emotionally taxing situations, little ambition or aggression; low energy level; anhedonia
Cyclothymic (3)	Recurring periods of depression (low energy, pessimism, hopelessness, despair) and elation (high energy, ambition, enthusiasm, optimism) not readily explained by circumstances	Passive-aggressive (78)	Obstructive behavior, stubborness, intentional errors or omissions; intolerance of authority with struggles over control often creating difficulties in medical settings; externalization of conflicts and blaming others for untoward events
Schizoid (30)	Isolation, seclusiveness, secretiveness; discomfort in relationships; often eccentric and lacking in energy; few friends; detachment; inability to express ideas and feelings, especially anger	Inadequate (17)	Chronic inability to meet ordinary life demands in the absence of mental retardation; severe dependency on others; tendency to become institutionalized or to become dependent on institutions
Explosive (4)	Outbursts of rage and aggression not in keeping with usual personality, often in response to minor provocation; sense of loss of control followed by regret	Antisocial (32)	Unsocialized or antisocial behavior in conflict with society; selfishness, callousness, impulsiveness, lack of loyalty, and little guilt; low frustration tolerance; tendency to blame others; long history of interpersonal and social difficulties and arrests
Obsessive-compulsive (anankastic) (21)	Chronic worries about standards; excessive concern about self-image; tension in relationships, leading to isolation; inability to relax and excessive inhibitions; overly meticulous, conscientious, and perfectionist; predisposition to depression and obsessive-compulsive neurosis	Passive-dependent (30)	Lack of self-confidence, indecisiveness, tendency to cling to and seek support from others
		Immature (12)	Ineffectual responses to social, psychologic, and physical demands; lack of stamina; poor adaptation to ordinary situations; a "loser"
Hysterical (103)	Immaturity, histrionic behavior, excitability, emotional instability, sexualization of relationships, low frustration tolerance, and shallow interpersonal ties; dependency	Unspecified (14)	

[a]Figures in parentheses represent the number of diagnoses of each personality disorder out of a total of 361 patients with the diagnosis of personality disorder at the Psychiatric Service of the University of Iowa (Winokur and Crowe).

personalities are associated with a major psychiatric illness is rather weak. In this sense, these are "eccentric" personality traits, which in themselves may be lifelong sources of personal distress and difficulties in functioning but which do not, as a rule, lead to the development of any specific psychiatric illness.

It need hardly be stressed that many of the terms listed in Table 56-1 and specifying the several well-recognized personality types are used indiscriminately by lay persons as well as by physicians to judge the personalities and character of others. The defining features of the personality disorders, as listed in the table, fall short of meeting the diagnostic criteria for the neuroses. Yet, an understanding of these personal peculiarities and their less obtrusive traits may be of great help to the physician. This knowledge makes it possible to appreciate their role as sources of perennial complaint, self-concern, and family discord and to explain a patient's reactions, which may have interfered with diagnostic and therapeutic procedures during a medical illness.

Personality disorders are pervasive, enduring, and little influenced by the physician, although often the contacts between physician and patient over many years and repeated reassurance and explanations of how best to cope with difficulties may in themselves serve as a stabilizing force; and, of course, one should never underestimate the power of maturation to ameliorate the turmoil of adolescence and to settle the mind. The use of medications to influence some aspect of personality should be avoided unless there is evidence that the peculiarity of personality has elaborated into a full-blown neurosis.

In the following pages, prototypes of the clinically recognized neuroses and sociopathies are described, along with current hypotheses of their pathogenesis.

THE NEUROSES

Though considered to be the most frequent of mental illnesses, the neuroses are among the least understood. They were established as clinical entities in the late nineteenth century, but there are still major unresolved issues with respect to their nature, classification, and etiology. Descriptively the neurotic disorders include the following syndromes: (1) anxiety neurosis; (2) phobic neurosis, which includes phobia of illness, social phobia, agoraphobia, etc.; (3) obsessive-compulsive neurosis; (4) hysteria; and (5) hypochondriasis. Former classifications included additional types called neurasthenia (dysthymia or depressive neurosis), which is better considered with the depressive illnesses, and "depersonalization neurosis" (dissociative disorders), which is probably a form of hysterical neurosis. Although each of these syndromes is clinically identifiable and separable when occurring in pure form, experience shows that most patients experience symptoms of more than one type and therefore are said to have "mixed neuroses." In the most recent classification, i.e., in DSM-IV, all of the neuroses have been replaced by three broad categories of disorders: (1) the *anxiety disorders* (which include panic states, with and without agoraphobia, and the phobic and obsessive-compulsive neuroses); (2) the *somatiform disorders* (comprising hysterical neurosis, or conversion disorder, and hypochondriasis); and (3) the *dissociative disorders*.

It is evident from these and several other attempts at classification that a single definition—one that would satisfactorily explain the attributes of all the neuroses—is still to come. Syndromes as different as hypochondriasis and panic reaction do not lend themselves to a unitary explanation. If there is a central feature of the neuroses, it is thought to be anxiety, which runs as a kind of leitmotif through all of them. Even in hysterical neurosis and sociopathy, in which patients seem indifferent to their disabilities, there is often a strong undercurrent of anxiety. Psychodynamic theories that attempt to provide a unified explanation of these diverse neurotic states have been reviewed by Nemiah.

Incidence

In an epidemiologic survey sponsored by the National Institute of Mental Health, it was estimated that approximately one-third of the population of the United States, at some point during their lives, have some type of mental disorder. In this survey, mental disorders related to chronic alcoholism were the most common, followed by anxiety, mood, obsessive-compulsive, phobic, conversion, and so-called posttraumatic stress disorders. A different view of the relative frequency of mental disorders is provided by an analysis of 1045 consecutive psychiatric consultations at the New England Center Hospital (now New England Medical Center) during the years 1955 and 1956. In this institution, a tertiary referral hospital, the dominant psychiatric syndrome in about 20 percent of patients was an anxiety state. In addition, symptoms of anxiety were present in some cases of depression, hysteria, and schizophrenia. In contrast, frank hysteria was diagnosed in only 6 percent of cases, and all the other neuroses—together with schizophrenia, alcoholic psychoses, sociopathic states, and the dementias—made up only 10 percent. As indicated on page 1608, depression in one form or another was the most common psychiatric illness (50 percent); psychiatric disease either was absent or could not be diagnosed in the remaining 14 percent of this series.

Other epidemiologic studies have also disclosed a strikingly high incidence of anxiety disorders in the general population (see review of Winokur and Coryell). Lifetime prevalence figures for anxiety disorder indicate that at least 11 percent of the population is so affected—i.e., some 25 million persons in the United States. Such information as is available suggests that the incidence of the neuroses is much the same in an urban population (midtown New York) and a rural one (Stirling County, Nova Scotia), indicating that socioeconomic, racial, and cultural factors are of relatively little importance. Further, in times of calamity, such as the bombing of London, the incidence of neurotic symptoms was said not to have increased. Thus one tends to dismiss as an oversimplification the notion that neuroses are merely by-products of life in civilized society or reactions to environmental stress (see also Chap. 24).

Except for hysteria, which, with the qualifications to be indicated, is mainly a disease of women, neuroses of all types occur in both sexes. The onset is in late childhood, adolescence, and early adult life. Admittedly, neurotic symptoms may be recognized for the first time after this age, but a good clinical rule is to suspect any mental illness that appears for the first time after the age of 40 years to be either a depression or a dementia due to degenerative or other organic disease of the brain.

ANXIETY NEUROSIS AND PANIC ATTACKS

The term *anxiety neurosis* was introduced by Freud in the latter part of the nineteenth century to describe a syndrome consisting of general irritability, anxious expectation, anxiety attacks, somatic equivalents of anxiety, and nightmares. In anxiety neurosis, this symptom complex constitutes the entire illness. However, as indicated earlier, this syndrome may also be a part of several other psychiatric diseases—manic-depressive psychosis, schizophrenia, hysteria, and phobic neurosis. Its closest link is with depression, which it resembles in another respect—namely, *there is a strong hereditary factor in both*, as pointed out by Mandel Cohen and colleagues in 1940. The term used in DSM-IV is *anxiety disorder*, of which phobias, obsessive-compulsive disorder, panic attacks, and so-called posttraumatic stress disorder are the important subdivisions. We still prefer the term *anxiety neurosis*.

Clinical Presentation

Anxiety neurosis is a chronic disease, punctuated by recurrent attacks of acute anxiety or panic. The acute attacks are the hallmark of the disease, and many psychiatrists are reluctant to make a diagnosis of anxiety neurosis in their absence. Because of the clinical peculiarities of panic attacks and particularly their episodic nature, they are of special interest to neurologists and general physicians. Fully developed, panic attacks are almost as dramatic as convulsive seizures. They begin with distressing feelings of dread and foreboding. The patient is assailed by a sense of strangeness, as though his body had changed or the surroundings were unreal (depersonalization; derealization). He is frightened, most often by the prospect of imminent death (*angor animi*) or of losing his mind or self-control. There may be a feeling of smothering. "I am dying," "This is the end," "Oh, my God, I'm going," or "I can't breathe" are the characteristic expressions of alarm and panic. The heart races, breathing comes in rapid gasps, pupils are dilated, and the patient sweats and trembles. The palpitation and breathing difficulties are so prominent that a cardiologist is often called. The symptoms abate spontaneously after 15 to 30 min, leaving the patient shaken, tense, perplexed, and often embarrassed. There is no element of confusion, and after the episode, there is full memory of the event.

Most anxiety attacks are of lesser severity than the one described above. The patient complains of faintness, palpitations, or a feeling of postural instability, referred to as dizziness. Breathlessness, vague chest or upper abdominal discomfort, a feeling as if the heart were beating too hard, and asthenia are other common symptoms. The feelings may be of sufficient intensity to cause the patient to fall to his knees or to seek to lie down, although the symptoms do not subside with assumption of a supine position. Certain attacks may vaguely simulate epilepsy insofar as the patient is so apprehensive that he cannot think clearly. In all such cases there is a constant uneasiness that the spells may occur in public; hence the patient may be fearful of leaving his home, lest help not be available should an attack occur (agoraphobia).

Except in minor details, all the attacks are alike in any one individual. Between attacks, some patients feel relatively well, but many complain of the symptoms of anxiety in lesser but persistent fashion. Cohen and White listed the following symptoms in order of frequency: palpitation, 97 percent; easy fatigue, 93 percent; breathlessness, 90 percent; nervousness, 88 percent; chest pain, 85 percent; sighing, 79 percent; dizziness, 78 percent; apprehensiveness, 61 percent; headache, 58 percent; paresthesias, 58 percent; weakness, 56 percent; insomnia, 53 percent; unhappiness, 50 percent.

Hyperventilation is a special though not invariable feature of the anxiety attack. Hyperventilation itself, by reducing the P_{CO_2}, will cause giddiness, paresthesias of the fingers, tongue, and lips, and at times frank tetany. Patients may become frightened and cry during a period of forced overbreathing. Contrary to the popular belief, in only a minority of patients does a 3-min period of commanded deep breathing reproduce the symptoms of an anxiety attack.

Anxiety attacks may occur at infrequent intervals or several times a day. They may occur in situations where there are no easily recognizable sources of fear, as when the patient is sitting quietly at home or is asleep. In other instances, a trying or upsetting experience induces an attack, which is nonetheless excessive for the condition that provoked it. In some patients, attacks are provoked by confinement to a closed space (claustrophobia)—an elevator, for example—or by crowded surroundings, as in church or in a restaurant or theater. An anxiety state not infrequently follows an accident and may, according to Modlin, be a source of disability. Symptoms of anxiety and depression may be prominent features of the postconcussive syndrome (page 945).

Anxiety neurosis may begin with an acute panic attack, but more frequently the onset is insidious—feelings of tenseness, vague apprehension, fatigue, weakness, and giddiness having been present for weeks or months before the first panic attack. From the history alone, two patterns of chronic anxiety neurosis are discernible. In one, there is a nearly lifelong history of poor exercise tolerance, little stamina, inability to do heavy physical work or participate in vigorous sports, tenseness, nervousness, and intolerance of crowds. In the other, the patient is vigorous and symptom-free before the anxiety state begins. The latter type usually has its origin in a late-life "anxious depression." Most patients with chronic symptoms first consult a physician with complaints referable to the cardiorespiratory system, but in a significant number the initial symptoms are gastrointestinal (dyspepsia, loss of appetite, or "irritable colon"). The former symptoms often come to light during military service and have been designated, since the American Civil War, as *neurocirculatory asthenia*, "irritable heart," or "soldier's heart."

The physical examination between acute attacks yields relatively little of diagnostic value. The common findings, disclosed by the study of Cohen and associates, were slight tachycardia, sighing respirations, yawning, flushed face and neck, tremor of the outstretched hands, and brisk tendon jerks. The patient tends to be restless and abrupt in movement, expressive of an inner uneasiness. During a panic attack, there may be manifest agitation and a tendency to leave the current venue, and blood pressure is almost invariably elevated.

The onset of both acute and chronic anxiety neurosis is rare before 18 or after 35 to 40 years of age (average age of onset, 25 years). The condition is twice as frequent in women as in men, and there is a high familial incidence. In one study (Wheeler et al) there was a prevalence of 49 percent among the grown children of patients with anxiety neurosis, compared with a prevalence of about 5 percent in the general population. Slater and Shields found that there was a concordance rate of 40 percent in identical twins, compared with 4 percent in dizygotic twins. Among the relatives of index cases, the mothers suffered from anxiety neurosis more often than the fathers; in the latter, alcoholism was more frequent than in the population at large (Modlin). The pattern of inheritance has not been established, but it most closely approximates that of autosomal dominance with incomplete penetrance.

The course of anxiety neurosis is variable. The symptoms fluctuate in severity without apparent relation to environmental stress. A 20-year follow-up study by Wheeler and associates showed that symptoms of anxiety neurosis were still present in 88 percent but were moderately or severely disabling in only 15 percent. Most of the patients were able to work and to enjoy a reasonably normal family and social life. Their only liability to further psychiatric illness was to recurrent anxiety neurosis or anxious depression; so-called psychosomatic illnesses and other psychiatric illnesses did not occur more frequently than in the general population. The life span of patients with anxiety neurosis is not shortened. Those with pure, uncomplicated anxiety neurosis rarely commit suicide.

Etiology and Pathogenesis

Anxiety neurosis has been attributed to a genetic abnormality, to constitutional weakness of the nervous system, to social and psychologic factors, some of which have already been discussed, and, more recently, to certain physiologic and biochemical derangements; but none of these factors provides a completely satisfactory explanation of the primary disorder. The symptoms of an anxiety attack resemble those of fear in many ways, though nearly always the former symptoms are longer in duration and less distinct. The most important difference, however, is that the cause of fear is known to the patient, whereas that of anxiety is not.

On the physiologic and biochemical side, it has been observed that anger provokes an excessive secretion of norepinephrine, whereas fear is accompanied by increased secretion of epinephrine. Actually fear activates the whole autonomic nervous system, and the increase in epinephrine is more than counterbalanced by a parasympathetic discharge. Attention has been focused on the locus ceruleus and upper brainstem nuclei as the possible anatomic substratum of anxiety (Judd et al). Others have implicated serotoninergic centers. Evidently the responsiveness of the autonomic nervous system remains heightened with chronic anxiety, and a number of stimuli (cold, pain, muscular effort) may produce abnormal responses in pulse, respiration, oxygen consumption, and work performance. Another interesting abnormality (first noted by Cohen et al) is that the blood lactic acid levels in response to exercise are higher than normal. The presence of these derangements does not necessarily mean that they are causal; they could be secondary to the poor physical condition and apprehension associated with the syndrome. Nevertheless, several investigators have found that infusions of lactic acid can trigger panic attacks in persons with anxiety neurosis (Liebowitz et al). Subsequently, a number of other theories of causation have been proposed based on the reported provocation of panic attacks by several different substances—carbon dioxide, yohimbine, gamma aminobutyric acid (GABA), and isoproterenol.

Studies correlating cerebral function and blood flow indicate that when panic is induced by an intravenous injection of sodium lactate, there is an immediate increase in blood flow to the cortex of both temporal lobes. In states of fear, the tips of the temporal lobes and also the amygdaloid nuclei become activated. In the relaxed period between panic attacks, the right limbic system and the parahippocampal gyrus are abnormally active.

Of potential importance is the recent finding of a connection between anxiety traits and polymorphisms of the serotonin transporter gene on chromosome 17 (Lesch et al). These authors estimated that this particular allelic difference contributes perhaps 10 percent to the overall neurotic tendency and implied that numerous other genes may participate in a similar way. Others have not found this particular association or have found it only in patients with generalized anxiety but not those with panic attacks. Therefore the precise relationship of this and other genetic abnormalities to anxiety neurosis cannot be stated at this moment.

Differential Diagnosis

Shorn of the psychologic components of apprehension and fear, the anxiety attack consists essentially of an excessive autonomic discharge. Some of the autonomic symptoms are duplicated by chromaffin tumors, hyperthyroidism, and the menopause. The prominence of chest pain and respiratory distress during an acute anxiety attack may be mistaken for myocardial ischemia, in which case the patient is often subjected to a series of studies of cardiac function. Another form of the illness—in which dizziness, instability of gait, and fear of losing consciousness are the most prominent features—may be mistaken for a neuro-otologic problem. On the other hand, headache is a relatively minor part of the acute symptom complex, and the diagnosis should be suspect if headache is a prominent feature. (Chronic headache may be part of chronic anxiety state or anxious depression.) Other medical diseases that simulate certain elements of an anxiety state are pulmonary embolism, cardiac arrhythmias, hypoglycemia, hypoparathyroidism, alcohol and nicotine withdrawal, and complex partial seizures. Strict adherence to the diagnostic criteria of these disease states readily permits their differentiation from acute anxiety, but diagnosis may be difficult if the symptoms of anxiety persist for hours or days on end.

Of greater importance is the relationship of anxiety neurosis to other psychiatric illnesses, particularly to depression. Symptoms of depression are frequently added to those of anxiety neurosis, and the majority of patients with depression have symptoms of anxiety. Indeed, some psychiatrists believe that anxiety neurosis is only an allelic variant of depression. As has been mentioned, an anxiety state appearing for the first time after the fortieth year usually proves to be a depression. The uncovering of paranoid symptoms in a patient with an anxiety state should always raise the question of depression, as should the presence of symptoms such as overwhelming fatigue, self-depreciation, and feelings of hopelessness. A relatively small number of patients with a condition diagnosed as anxiety neurosis or alcoholism by competent psychiatrists have committed suicide.

Schizophrenia may begin with prominent anxiety symptoms. Here the diagnosis rests on finding the characteristic thought disorder of schizophrenia, which may emerge only after several interviews. Hysteria may include anxiety symptoms, though they are seldom prominent, as do also phobic and obsessive-compulsive neuroses, but each has other distinguishing attributes.

Treatment

Certain medications, particularly anxiolytics and antidepressants, are often highly effective in suppressing panic attacks and creating a sense of well-being. Among these, the benzodiazepine alprazolam (2 to 6 mg/day) is currently favored, but lorazepam is almost as effective and is considered slightly less likely to cause dependence. In mild cases, the benzodiazepines may be used intermittently rather than several times daily, but they tend to be less useful once a panic attack has become established. The panic attacks tend to recur when the medications are discontinued, even after prolonged (6 to 12 months) administration. Tricyclic antidepressants and the newer drugs that raise serotonin concentrations in the nervous system (selective serotonin reuptake inhibitors, or SSRIs) are also quite effective in the treatment of panic attacks and agoraphobia. These drugs become necessary for symptoms of anxiety that persist for more than several weeks. They are given in doses similar to those used to treat depression (see Chap. 57). Buspirone, a specific serotonin 5-HT_2 agonist, has been promoted as particularly effective in the treatment of anxiety and as a surrogate for benzodiazepines, but its effects have seemed to us to be slight. During the initial weeks of administration of antidepressants, an anxiolytic is usually required until the antidepressant becomes effective. Propranolol, 10 to 20 mg tid, blocks many of the autonomic accompaniments of anxiety, but its effects on the other symptoms are uncertain. In general, it is preferable not to prescribe drugs for prolonged low-grade anxiety.

Behavioral therapy (progressive exposure of the patient to panic-provoking situations) is said to be beneficial, particularly if agoraphobia is a major symptom. Relaxation activities, including biofeedback and meditation, help many patients, although persistence is required in performing these at least once daily and they do not seem to help once a panic attack has begun.

So-called cognitive-behavioral psychotherapy, which is discussed in relation to the treatment of depression (page 1620), also appears to be useful in the treatment of panic disorder (Andreasen and Black). A cardiac consultation and some simple tests (electrocardiogram, chest films) may be needed to reinforce the benign nature of the cardiac and respiratory symptoms and to alleviate the patient's fear of heart disease. These and other current concepts of the treatment of anxiety are discussed by Peroutka and by Goodwin and Guze. Anxiety symptoms arising in relation to a particular threatening event carry a better prognosis.

PHOBIC NEUROSIS

In this state, patients (women more than men) are overwhelmed by an intense and irrational fear of some animal, object, social situation, or disease. Though acknowledging that there are no rational grounds for a particular fear (hence it is not a delusion) and that such provocative stimuli are innocuous, the patient is nonetheless powerless to suppress it. This disorder was known to Hippocrates, who drew a distinction between normal and morbid fears. Westphal in 1871 was the first to give morbid fears the status of a disease.

Mild phobias of darkness, solitude, snakes, thunder and lightning, and high places are commonplace in childhood; some persist into adult life and may be culturally acceptable. Unlike an anxiety attack, such a phobia always focuses on an object or situation. The patient is chronically fearful of a particular animal or situation and may be extremely anxious or panic-stricken and incapacitated when placed in a situation that evokes the phobia. These situations are avoided at all costs. For example, it may be impossible for the patient to leave the house or neighborhood unaccompanied, mingle in a crowd, walk across a bridge, or travel by air. This fear of being in places or situations from which escape might be difficult or extremely embarrassing is spoken of as *agoraphobia* and results in a homebound state. Agoraphobia, however, may be a feature of other psychiatric disorders, the commonest being anxiety with panic attacks. The patient may be unable to eat certain foods, eat in public, have sexual intercourse, urinate in the presence of others, etc. Phobias are essentially *obsessive fears* and should probably be included in this category of neurosis. The most common phobia is probably claustrophobia (the fear of being confined in a close space, such as an elevator or a magnetic resonance scanner). Other phobias, as remarked earlier, are those of open (agoraphobia), closed, or high places, dogs, cats, dirt, sprays and other contaminants, air travel, the acquired immunodeficiency syndrome (AIDS), cancer, insanity, and death. Feelings of helplessness, pessimism, and despondency, the hallmarks of a depressive illness, may result. Often there are obsessive-compulsive tendencies as well, and some patients are hypochondriacal. The present authors have observed a number of patients whose phobic (or obsessive-compulsive) neurosis decompensated as an endogenous depression developed. Recovery from the depression returned them to their earlier and milder phobic state. All of these features suggest a linkage between these neuroses and depression.

OBSESSIVE-COMPULSIVE NEUROSIS

Like the pure phobic states, a neurosis dominated by obsessions and compulsions is relatively rare, occurring in less than 5 percent of patients seeking help in a psychiatric outpatient clinic. Minor compulsions (not stepping on cracks in the sidewalk, etc.), like minor phobias, are common in children, cause little or no distress, and tend to disappear in later life. A few, such as rechecking a locked door or a gas stove, may persist throughout life. Also, certain habits and rigid, obsessional ways of thinking, stubbornness, extreme punctuality, and excessive attention to detail are frequent and persistent but excite little attention medically unless they interfere with some diagnostic procedure or the treatment of some disease.

Obsessive-compulsive neurosis, or *disorder*, as it is now designated in DSM-IV, begins, as do the other neuroses, in adolescence or early adult years, although treatment may not be sought until middle age is reached. The two sexes are equally affected. The onset is usually gradual and cannot be accurately dated, but in some cases it is precipitated by a particular event in the patient's life, such as the death of a relative. The family history often discloses a high incidence of obsessional personality in other members. In most instances, the obsessive-compulsive neurosis is engrafted onto a personality in which rigidity, inflexibility, and lack of adaptability are prominent. These traits are manifest in the individual's punctuality and in his dependability and reliability in the affairs of everyday life. There is always a prevailing undercurrent of insecurity.

Obsessions may be defined as imperative and distressing thoughts and impulses that persist in the patient's mind despite a desire to resist and to be rid of them. Obsessions take various forms. The most common are *intellectual obsessions*, in which phrases, rhymes, ideas, or vivid images (these are often absurd, blasphemous, obscene, and sometimes frightening) constantly intrude into consciousness; *impulsive obsessions*, in which the mind is dominated by an impulse to kill oneself, to stab one's children, or to perform some other objectionable act; and *inhibiting obsessions*, in which every act must be ruminated upon and analyzed before it is carried out—a state aptly called *doubting mania*. Every effort at distraction fails to rid the patient of the obsessive thought. It engulfs the mind, rendering him miserable and inefficient. Probably the most disturbing obsessions are the impulsive ones, in which patients constantly struggle with the fear that they will put some terrible thought into action. Even as they tell of the obsession, they reveal their underlying anxiety and seek reassurance that they will not yield to it. Fortunately, such patients rarely obey their pathologic impulses.

Compulsions are acts that result from obsessions. These are single acts or a series of acts (rituals) that the patient must carry out in order to put his mind at ease. Examples are repeated checking of the gas jets or the locks on doors, adjusting articles of clothing, repeated hand washing, using a clean handkerchief to wipe objects that have been touched by others, tasting foods in specific ways, touching objects in a particular sequence, etc.

Certain motor disturbances—namely, habit spasms or tics—are, in a sense, *motor compulsions*. They consist of repetitious movements of the shoulders, arms, hands, and certain of the facial muscles (see Chap. 6). One feature that separates quasi-voluntary tics from involuntary movements of extrapyramidal type is the patient's feeling that the tics must be carried out to relieve tension. Unlike compulsions, however, tics are not usually based on obsessive thoughts—except perhaps the Gilles de la Tourette syndrome, in which multiple tics are combined with compulsive utterances, often offensive ones (see below).

In all these obsessions and compulsions and in the phobias, patients recognize the irrationality of their ideas and behavior yet are powerless to control them, much as they desire to do so. It is this insight into the obsessional experience and the struggle against it that distinguish obsessions from delusions.

The majority of patients with obsessive-compulsive neurosis are tense, irritable, and apprehensive. They suffer a curious feeling of insufficiency or incompetency in being unable to expel their troublesome thoughts. The most distraught emotional state, as mentioned above, is related to the fear that an idea may eventuate in reality. These patients may complain of typical anxiety attacks; after the condition has persisted for a time, they may become depressed. Fatigue, anorexia, and general lack of interest, which are often present, are probably related to the secondary effects of anxiety and depression.

Mechanisms of Phobic and Obsessive Neuroses

For many years, a number of psychoanalytic conceptualizations of obsessional neurosis as the product of intrapsychic conflicts held sway. Only relatively recently has a neurobiologic model been advanced. Patients with this condition are found to have enlarged ventricular-cerebral ratios (Behar et al) and a reduction in the volume of the caudate nuclei, although these observations require corroboration. Weilburg and associates have described a left-sided lesion (on magnetic resonance imaging) in the head of the caudate nucleus and putamen in a patient with obsessive-compulsive disorder, and positron emission tomography studies have demonstrated increased metabolic activity in both caudate nuclei. Many similar studies implicated the caudate nuclei, but the anatomic observations are by no means uniform. The orbitofrontal cortex and amygdala were reported to be shrunken in some cases. In a study of 13 patients who developed elements of obsessiveness and compulsive disorder after incurring focal brain lesions, Berthier et al found lesions in diverse loci, including the cingulate, frontal, and temporal cortices as well as the basal ganglia. Two of the most accurately localized lesions in their series were a hamartoma of the right parahippocampal gyrus and an infarction in the posterior putamen. The presence of brain injuries and seizure disorders in other patients made a precise localization problematic.

Some insight into acquired obsessive-compulsive disorder may also be gleaned from its occurrence in a poststreptococcal tic disorder termed PANDAS (pediatric autoimmune psychiatric disorders associated with streptococcal infections, page 118). This disorder is presumably related to Sydenham chorea, in which tics and similar movement disorders as well as behavioral abnormalities also occur. Imaging studies have implicated the basal ganglia in the latter situations. Functional imaging studies in patients with PANDAS have yielded variable findings, but generally there has been increased activity in the caudate nucleus and orbitofrontal cortex in association with compulsive thoughts.

The *Gilles de la Tourette syndrome* of multiple tics, including vocal ones, beginning in childhood or adolescence and lasting more than a year, is also closely related to obsessive-compulsive disorder. The two conditions often coexist; more than half of Tourette patients have obsessive-compulsive disorder, and both are believed to be inherited as an autosomal dominant trait, with 50 to 70 percent penetrance. There is also a questionable relationship of the Tourette syndrome to the attention deficit–hyperactivity syndrome of children, conduct disorder, stuttering, and phobic states (Kurlan). Dopamine antagonists are the drugs of choice in management of the Tourette syndrome. These observations have given rise to a number of etiologic hypotheses revolving around serotoninergic and dopaminergic neurotransmitter systems (Black; Baxter; Behar et al). In the present authors' opinion, the pathophysiology of Tourette syndrome, both the persistent and transitory or intermittent types, and their relationship to obsessive-compulsive disorder have yet to be established (see page 117 for more extensive comments on the Tourette syndrome).

The neurochemical alterations in obsessive-compulsive disorder have also been studied actively. Most of the conclusions have been based on the responses to medications, notably to the serotonin reuptake inhibitors, e.g., clomipramine. These agents are found to be of therapeutic benefit, as have stereotactic neurosurgical lesions in the cingulate gyri.

Diagnosis

Since the prevailing emotional state in patients with phobias and obsessions is one of anxiety and depression, it is necessary to distinguish between phobic and obsessional neuroses, anxiety neurosis, and depressive illnesses. In phobic and obsessional neuroses, the depression tends to be inconstant and closely related to a sense of weariness and helplessness in overcoming the irrational fears and obsessive thinking. As the latter improve, the depression lightens. In uncomplicated anxiety states, baseless and indefinable fears are common but never so persistent or disabling as in phobic and obsessional neurosis; also, the indecisiveness and compulsive tendencies are lacking. Schizophrenia must be considered when an adolescent or young adult begins to harbor peculiar ideas or becomes hypochondriacal, but then a careful mental examination reveals the other characteristic disturbances of the underlying disease (Chap. 58).

Treatment

This is best left to the psychiatrist. At least there should be a trial of therapy using behavioral modification techniques. In the case of phobic neurosis, the aim of such treatment is to reduce the patient's fear to the extent that exposure to the phobic situation can be tolerated. A popular form of therapy is *systematic desensitization* (Wolpe), which consists of graded exposure of the patient to the object or situation that arouses fear. Psychotherapy, if undertaken, need not be intensive, consisting instead of repeated explanation, reassurance, and guidance in dealing with symptoms.

Currently, certain medications, such as the tricyclic antidepressants or the SSRI fluoxetine, are considered to be the most effective form of therapy—abolishing or greatly reducing obsessions and compulsions in more than half the patients.

Cases of obsessional neurosis that are cyclic in nature, with exacerbations and remissions and with no apparent relationship to environmental factors, have the best prognosis. Some psychiatrists treat this cyclic form like cyclic depression, with antidepressant drugs and electroconvulsive therapy (ECT). It is not certain that these measures accomplish more than can be attributed to the spontaneous changes in the disease. More often the course of obsessional neurosis is steady and severely disabling, and in these patients the outlook for recovery has been poor (Berg; Pollitt). As with phobic neurosis, several reports have indicated that the compulsive rituals can often be abolished by the techniques of behavior therapy—based on the graduated exposure of the patient to the fear-inducing stimulus. Much in vogue is so-called cognitive-behavioral psychotherapy, alluded to earlier and discussed in the next chapter (page 1620). This too is best left to the experienced psychiatrist (see also chapter by March).

Cingulotomy has produced symptomatic improvement in both phobic and obsessional neuroses. This measure, if it is to be used at all, should be considered only as a last resort in exceptionally severe cases, in which the patient has failed to respond to all other methods of treatment and is totally disabled.

HYSTERIA (BRIQUET DISEASE; SOMATIZATION DISORDER)

Although hysteria has been known since ancient times, many writers credit the first description of the syndrome (on somewhat uncertain grounds) to the French physician Briquet in 1859. Later, Charcot elaborated certain manifestations of the disease and interested Freud and Janet in it. Charcot believed that the symptoms could be produced and relieved by hypnosis (mesmerism). Janet postulated a *dissociative state* of mind to account for certain features such as trance and fugue states. Freud and his students conceived of hysterical symptoms as a product of "ego defense mechanisms," in which psychic energy, generated by unconscious psychic conflicts, is converted into physical symptoms. This latter concept was widely accepted, to the point where the term *conversion* became incorporated into the nomenclature of the neuroses and the terms *conversion symptoms* and *conversion reaction* came to be equated with the disease hysteria. In the present authors' opinion, the term *conversion*, if it is used at all, should refer only to certain *unexplained symptoms*, such as amnesia, paralysis, blindness, aphonia, etc., that mimic neurologic disease. We see no merit in the dichotomy, based on unsubstantiated psychodynamic theory, of a conversion type as separate from a dissociative type, as claimed by the DSM classification. Nemiah, who is in other respects partial to the psychoanalytic interpretation, agrees. In our view, the term *hysteria* is best reserved for a *disease* that is practically confined to women and is characterized further by a distinctive age of onset, natural history, and many somatic symptoms and signs, which typically include "conversion symptoms," dissociative reactions, and states of "multiple personality."

The term *hysteria* has a number of other connotations, most of them pejorative. Lay people refer to individuals with tantrums or loss of self-control in the face of an emotional crisis as "hysterical." Some psychiatrists dub any dramatic, histrionic, manipulative, or "seductive" behavior as hysterical (referring to the *hysterical personality*). Others equate hysteria with hypersuggestibility and susceptibility to hypnosis. These are traditional ideas based on the incorrect belief that these qualities are the defining attributes of the disease. As indicated earlier, some patients with hysteria also have the hysterical personality (i.e., they are histrionic, emotionally labile, egocentric, "seductive," and dependent), but many such individuals never develop conversion symptoms.

In clinical neurology one encounters two types of hysteria: (1) a chronic illness marked by multiple and often dramatically presented symptoms and somatic abnormalities, for which no cause is evident (mainly in girls and women), and (2) an illness predominantly of men but also of women who develop physical symptoms or remain inexplicably disabled for the purpose of obtaining compensation, influencing litigation, avoiding military duty or imprisonment, etc. This latter state is called *compensation neurosis*, *compensation hysteria*, or *hysteria with sociopathy*.

Classic Hysteria

This neurosis, which accounts for 1 to 2 percent of admissions to a neurologic service, usually has its onset in the teens or early twenties. However, a few cases may begin before puberty. Once established, the diagnosis remains unchanged over many years but the symptoms recur intermittently, though with lessening frequency, throughout the adult years, even to an advanced age. No doubt there are cases of lesser severity in which symptoms occur only a few times or perhaps only once, just as there are mild forms of other diseases. The patient may be seen for the first time during middle life or later, and the earlier history may not at first be forthcoming. Careful probing, however, will almost invariably reveal that the earliest manifestations of the illness had appeared before the age of 25 years.

Other important data are also brought to light by eliciting a careful past history. During late childhood and adolescence, the normal activities of the patient, including education, have often been interrupted by periods of ill-defined illness. Rheumatic fever or some obscure disease may have been suspected. Later in life, problems in work adjustment and marriage are frequent. There is a notably high incidence of marital incompatibility, separation, and divorce. The patient's life history is punctuated by symptoms that do not conform to recognizable patterns of medical and surgical disease. For these, many forms of therapy, including surgical operations, will have been performed. Rarely has adult life been reached without at least one abdominal operation, which was usually done because of vague abdominal pain, persistent nausea and vomiting, or some gynecologic complaint. Often the indications for the surgical procedures are unclear; moreover, the same symptoms or others often recurred to complicate the convalescence. The biographies of these patients are also replete with disorders that center about menstrual, sexual, and procreative functions. Menstrual periods may be painfully prostrating, irregular, or excessive. Sexual intercourse may be painful or unpleasant. Pregnancies may be difficult; the usual vomiting of the first trimester may persist all through the gestational period, with weight loss and prostration; labor may be unusually difficult and prolonged, and all manner of unpredictable complications are said to have occurred during and after parturition.

Hysteria is, then, a polysymptomatic disorder, involving almost every organ system. The most frequent symptoms, all statistically significant, that were elicited during a study of 50 unmistakable cases of female hysteria as compared with a control group of 50 healthy women included the following: headache, blurred vision, lump in the throat, loss of voice, dyspnea, palpitation, anxiety attacks, anorexia, nausea and vomiting, abdominal pain, food allergies, severe menstrual pain, urinary retention, sexual indifference, painful intercourse, paresthesias, dizzy spells, nervousness, and easy crying (Purtell et al).

The examination of the female hysteric demonstrates a number of characteristic findings, mostly in the sphere of mental status. There is a lack of precision in relating the details of the illness. Questions regarding the chief complaint usually elicit a vague reply or the narration of a series of incidents or problems, many of which prove to have little or no relevance to the question. Memory defects (amnesic gaps) are usually demonstrated while the history is being taken; the patient appears to have forgotten important segments of the history, some of which she had clearly described in the past and are part of the medical record. However, unlike the situation in a psychotic illness, the patient's ideas about most aspects of her life are rational and coherent, and there is no evidence of hallucinations, delusions, disturbance in logical thinking, or loss of appreciation of the reality of the situation. The manner of the patient is often amiable and even ingratiating. Incongruity of affect is notable; the description of symptoms may be dramatic and exaggerated and not in accord with the facts as elicited from other members of the family. Or a rather casual demeanor is manifest, the patient insisting that everything in her life is quite normal and controlled, when, in fact, her medical record is checkered with instances of dramatic behavior and unexplained illness. This calm attitude toward a turbulent illness and seemingly disabling physical signs is so common that it has been singled out as an important characteristic of hysteria, *la belle indifference*. Other patients, however, are obviously tense and anxious, and report frank anxiety attacks; or the patient may be effusive in her enthusiasms, fickle and flighty, always putting on an act, and demanding constant attention. Her emotional reactions are superficial and she creates scenes that are disturbing to others but are quickly forgotten. If physical signs are present, attempts by the physician to disprove their somatic nature usually meet with anxiety and protest. Claims of early-life sexual abuse are common and often prove to be figments of the imagination. Antisocial behavior occurs in a minority of patients.

There are no pathognomonic physical findings. Although many writers have commented on the rather youthful, girlish appearance and coquettish ("seductive") manner of the patients, these by no means characterize all of them. The so-called stigmata of hysteria—i.e., corneal anesthesia; absence of gag reflex; spots of pain and tenderness over the scalp, sternum, breasts, lower ribs, and ovaries—are often suggested by the examiner and are too inconsistent to be of much help in the diagnosis. The variation and pleomorphism of the physical signs are limited only by the patient's ability to produce them by voluntary effort. Accordingly, symptoms and signs that are beyond volitional control cannot be accepted as manifestations of hysteria. Often the patient's physical signs are an imitation of those of another member of the family or are evoked by a stressful event in the patient's personal life. However, this may not be disclosed at the time of the first examination. The present authors place great weight on the importance of *hypersuggestibility*, in keeping with older studies that emphasized these patients' unusual susceptibility to suggestion and hypnosis. Interesting in this regard were the observations of Charcot's students, who noted that on their wards the patients' symptoms disappeared in his absence.

When diagnosis is based on the totality of the clinical picture and not on the "discrepancy method," it can be quite accurate. In a follow-up study of a cohort of 56 patients with so-called conversion disorder (exclusive of pseudoseizures), only two developed a neurologic lesion (cerebral infarct; multiple sclerosis) that in retrospect was related to the initial episode (Couprie et al). Our experience has been similar.

Special Hysterical Syndromes

A few hysterical syndromes occur with great regularity, and every physician may expect to encounter them. They constitute some of the most puzzling diagnostic problems in medicine.

Hysterical Pain This may involve any part of the body; generalized or localized headache, "atypical facial pain," vague abdominal pain, and chronic back pain with camptocormia are the most frequent and troublesome. In many of these patients the response to analgesic drugs has been unusual, and some of them are addicted. The hysterical patient may respond to a placebo as though it were a potent drug, but it should be pointed out that this is a notoriously unreliable means of distinguishing hysterical pain from that of other diseases. A greater error is to mistake the pain of osteomyelitis, metastatic carcinoma, or brain tumor—before other symptoms have developed—for a manifestation of hysteria. There are several helpful diagnostic features of hysterical pain: the patient's inability to give a clear, concise description of the type of pain; the location of the pain, which does not conform to the pattern of pain in the familiar medical syndromes; the dramatic elaborations of its intensity (speaking in inflated metaphors—"like a giant knife stabbing") and effects; its persistence, either continuous or intermittent, for long periods of time; the absence of other diseases that could account for pain; the assumption of bizarre attitudes and postures; and, most important, the coexistence of other clinical features or previous attacks of hysterical nature.

Hysterical Vomiting This is often combined with pain and tenderness in the lower abdomen and results in unnecessary appendectomies and removal of pelvic organs in adolescent girls and young women. The vomiting often occurs after a meal, leaving the patient hungry and ready to eat again; it may be induced by unpleasant circumstances. Some of these patients can vomit at will, regurgitating food from the stomach like a ruminant animal. Vomiting may persist for weeks with no cause being found. Weight loss may occur, but seldom to the degree anticipated. As remarked above, the usual first-trimester vomiting of pregnancy may continue throughout the entire 9 months, and occasionally pregnancy will be interrupted because of it. Anorexia may be a prominent symptom and must be differentiated from anorexia nervosa, another disease of young women (page 1064).

Hysterical Seizures, Trances, and Fugues These conditions seem to be less frequent than in the days of Charcot, when *la grande attaque d'hysterie* was often exhibited before medical audiences. Nevertheless, such attacks do occur and must be distinguished from cerebral cortical seizures and catalepsy. To witness an attack is of great assistance in diagnosis. The lack of an aura, initiating cry, hurtful fall, and incontinence; the presence of peculiar movements such as grimacing, squirming, thrashing and flailing of the limbs, side-to-side motions of the head, and striking at or resisting those who offer assistance; the retention of consciousness during a motor seizure that involves both sides of the body; the long duration of the seizure, its abrupt termination by strong sensory stimulation, lack of postictal confusion, and failure to produce a rise in creatine kinase and prolactin—are all typical of the hysterical attack. Sometimes hyperventilation will initiate an attack and is therefore a useful diagnostic maneuver. Both epilepsy, particularly of frontal-lobe type, and hysteria may occur in the same patient, a combination that invariably causes difficulty in diagnosis.

Hysterical trances or fugues, in which the patient wanders about for hours or days and carries out complex acts, may simulate temporal lobe epilepsy or any of the conditions that lead to confusional psychosis or stupor. Here the most reliable point of differentiation comes from observation of the patient, who, if hysterical, is likely to indicate a degree of alertness and promptness of response not seen in temporal lobe seizures or confusional states. Following the episode, an interview with the patient—under the influence of hypnosis, strong suggestion, or midazolam or amobarbital—will often bring to light memories of what happened during the episode. This helps to exclude the possibility of an epileptic fugue.

Hysterical Paralyses, Gait, and Tremors Hysterical palsies may involve an arm, a leg, one side of the body, or both legs. If the affected limb can be moved at all, muscle action is weak and tremulous. Movements are characteristically slow, tentative, and poorly sustained; often it can be demonstrated that the strength of voluntary movement is proportional to the resistance offered by the examiner, thus imparting a "give-way" character. One can feel agonist and antagonist muscles contracting simultaneously, and when the resistance is suddenly withdrawn, there is no follow-through or rebound, as is normally the case. Other indicators have been devised to demonstrate inconsistency with normal physiologic principles and a conscious lack of cooperation. These discrepancies are elicited by testing an agonist, antagonist, or fixator movement while the patient is focused on making an effort with another group of muscles (e.g., the Hoover sign, see page 65). The muscular tone in the affected limbs is usually normal, but rigidity may sometimes be found. A seeming lack of effort and full compliance with the examiner's requests during the testing of muscle strength, while common in hysterical patients, is not confined to them; one encounters such findings not infrequently during the examination of suggestible but nonhysterical patients who harbor a neurologic disease. Walking may be impossible, there may be a veritable astasia-abasia, or the gait may be bizarre (page 130). Weakness and poor balance are combined elements in both the quadriparetic and hemiparetic forms. In Keane's series of 60 cases of hysterical gait, the hemiparetic and monocrural forms were twice as frequent as the quadriparetic. The gait disorder is difficult to describe because of its variability. Sudden falls without voluntary protective movements and inconsistencies of balance are helpful features. The discrepancy between the inability to walk and to move the legs is, of course, not unique to hysteria; it also occurs in so-called frontal lobe apraxia and in ataxia from midline cerebellar lesions. Maintenance of the limb(s) in a rigid posture for a long time may result in a bed-bound, crippled state with flexion pseudocontractures of the limbs. The tendon reflexes are usually normal, but with hysterical rigidity and contractures, the abdominal and plantar reflexes may be suppressed.

Anesthesia or hypesthesia is almost always inadvertently suggested by the physician's examination. Seldom is sensory loss a spontaneous complaint, although "numbness" and paresthesias are not uncommon. The sensory loss may involve one or more limbs below a sharp line (stocking and glove distribution), or may involve precisely one-half of the body, or vibratory sense may be lost over precisely one-half of the skull. Touch, pain, taste, smell, vision, and hearing may all be affected on that side, which is an anatomic impossibility from a single lesion.

The features of hysterical tremor have been described on page 105. To be emphasized are the cessation of tremor with distracting tasks—e.g., complex finger movement patterns on the side opposite the tremor (such as touching the fourth, second, and fifth fingers in sequence rapidly), refixation of the eyes on a target, and walking on the outside of the heels, and the ability of the examiner to "chase" the tremor to proximal or distal parts of the limb by holding and immobilizing other parts.

Hysterical Blindness This dramatic event may affect one eye or both and may be coupled with hemiparesis or appear in isolation. The symptoms usually develop suddenly, often after an altercation or other emotionally charged event. The patient stares straight ahead blandly when undisturbed but may squint or move the head as if straining to see when asked to view an object. Some such individuals can reduce reflexive blinking in response to a visual threat, but the psychic nature of the problem may be recognized by a nurse who observes the patient reaching for a cup or the phone. The preservation of vision is confirmed by the presence of normal pupillary reflexes and optokinetic nystagmus, although one occasionally encounters a patient who has learned to suppress the latter response as well. The presence of visual evoked responses confirms the intactness of retino-occipital connections. The patient expresses little concern about her condition, which is usually short-lived. Cortical blindness and variants of the Balint syndrome (pages 489 and 491) from bioccipital infarcts are the main diagnostic considerations.

Convergence spasm, occurring as an isolated phenomenon, is practically always of hysterical nature (page 288). Another related phenomenon involves the *self-administration of mydriatic eyedrops* by health care personnel. The patient arrives on the emergency ward complaining of reduced vision (expected) or with headache and claiming to have an intracranial mass. This behavior is perhaps more sociopathic (malingering) than hysterical.

Hysterical Amnesia Patients brought to a hospital in a state of amnesia, not knowing their own identity, are usually hysterical females or sociopathic males involved in a crime. Usually, after a few hours or days, with encouragement, they divulge their life history. Epileptic patients or victims of a concussion, transient global amnesia, or acute confusional psychosis do not come to a hospital asking for help in establishing their identity. Moreover, the complete loss of memory for all previous life experiences by patients who are otherwise able to comport themselves normally is not observed in any other condition.

In the *Ganser syndrome* (amnesia, disturbance of consciousness, and hallucinations), patients pretend to have lost their memory or to have become insane. They act in an absurd manner, in the way they believe that an insane or demented person should act, and give a senseless or only approximate answer to every question asked of them.

Unexplained Hyperpyrexia Among patients who turn up on every medical service with unexplained fever, there are always a few hysterics. One cannot help but be impressed with the number of student nurses, nurses, and nurses' aides among this group of patients. Most of them will be found to have no fever if the nurse or doctor checks the temperature. Others have oral temperatures of 37 to 38°C (99 to 100°F), which must be regarded as normal for some individuals. Finally, there are a few cases of hyperpyrexia that appear to be of psychogenic origin; in these the possibility of some obscure hypothalamic disorder cannot be excluded. Diagnosis is assisted by a longitudinal history and the elicitation of the other symptoms and signs of hysteria.

Dermatitis Factitia (Hysterical Dermatoneurosis) This condition is seen more often in the sociopath than in the hysterical patient. The skin eruptions induced by the patient are characterized by erythema, ulcerations, gangrene, and variable degrees of dermatitis. Usually a caustic or irritant chemical or a sharp instrument such as a nail file has been used. The lesions are most commonly observed on parts of the body accessible to the right hand, i.e., right side of the face, neck, anterior trunk, anterior surface of left arm. They are multiple, sharply outlined, appear at variable intervals of time, and do not conform to any of the standard dermatologic diseases. They resist all treatment until the skin is protected from the persistent manipulations of the patient, and then they heal promptly.

Hysteria in Men (Compensation Neurosis in Men and Women)

As stated above, hysterical symptoms do occur in men, most often in those trying to avoid legal difficulties or military service or attempting to obtain disability payments, veterans' and other pensions, or, most often, compensation following injury. Sociopaths may also present with this type of illness. Unless such a factor can be identified, the diagnosis of hysteria in the male should be made with great caution. In compensation neurosis, as in the classic form of hysteria, multiple symptoms are often noted; many of the symptoms are the same as those listed under female hysteria. Or the patient may be monosymptomatic (e.g., "seizures"), and the symptoms, particularly chronic pain, may be confined to the neck, head, arm, or low back. The description of symptoms tends to be lengthy and circumstantial, and the patient fails to give details that are necessary for diagnosis. A tangible gain from the illness may be discovered by simple questioning. This is usually in the form of monetary compensation, which, surprisingly, is sometimes less than the patient could earn if he returned to work. Many such patients are actively engaged in litigation when first seen. Another interesting feature is the frequency with which the patient expresses extreme dissatisfaction with the medical care given him; he is often hostile toward the physicians and nurses. Many of these patients have already been subjected to an excessive number of hospitalizations, and rather dramatic mishaps have allegedly occurred in carrying out diagnostic and therapeutic procedures. The majority of these patients have been suspected and many have been accused of malingering, a closely related disorder that is discussed further on, with the sociopathies (page 1602).

Women who suffer injury at work or are involved in auto accidents may exhibit the same symptoms and signs of compensation neurosis as men.

Etiology and Pathogenesis Psychoanalytic theory, which holds that both conversion and dissociative symptoms are based on particular psychodynamic mechanisms, is impossible to affirm or refute. Sociologic and educational factors are probably important, for it is generally agreed that hysterical women as a group are less intelligent and less educated than nonhysterical women. A genetic causation must also be considered. Family studies have disclosed that about 20 percent of first-degree relatives of female hysterics have the same illness, an incidence 10 times that in the general population. This supports the idea that hysteria is a disease and not merely a surfacing of a basic personality disorder (see Goodwin and Guze).

Whether conversion symptoms are consciously produced by the patient or arise unconsciously, without the patient's awareness, is a question that has been debated endlessly, without resolution. Babinski attributed the symptoms to hypersuggestibility. In fact, he defined hysteria as an illness whose symptoms could be induced (and removed) by suggestion. There is strong evidence to support this idea, since most patients can be readily hypnotized and their symptoms temporarily eliminated by this procedure, or by an interview and examination under the influence of midazolam or amytal.

As pointed out by Carothers and by Guze and colleagues, hysteria and sociopathy are closely related. Hysteria is a disease of women and sociopathy mainly of men; as restated by Cloninger and colleagues, they may constitute expressions of a single underlying variable. This relationship is supported by family studies. First-degree male relatives of hysterical women have an increased incidence of sociopathy and alcoholism; among first-degree female relatives of convicted male felons, there is an increased prevalence of hysteria. Moreover, careful histories of sociopathic girls reveal that many of them develop the full syndrome of hysteria. Women felons often present a mixed picture of hysteria and sociopathy, according to Cloninger and Guze.

Diagnosis The method of diagnosis subject to the least error is the one employed in medicine generally, i.e., obtaining an informative history (from the patient as well as from sources other than the patient) and performing physical and mental status examinations. The characteristic age of onset; the longitudinal history of recurrent multiple complaints, as outlined above; the attitude of the patient and the manner of presenting her symptoms; the incongruity of affect and clinical state; the discrepancy between the neurologic deficit and the signs on examination; the impossibility of explaining the patient's signs on an anatomic or physiologic basis; and the absence of symptoms and signs of other medical and surgical disease will permit an accurate diagnosis in the majority of cases.

There is a significant overlap of hysteria and other medical and neurologic diseases. There are on record seven studies (between 1962 and 1985) in which patients with an initial diagnosis of hysteria by general physicians were followed for many years; 13 to 34 percent of them turned out eventually to have an "organic condition" which, in retrospect, explained the initial symptoms (see Couprie et al). This means that the original clinical diagnosis of hysteria is often erroneous. When the diagnostic criteria in these cases are closely analyzed, it appears that diagnosis was often made solely by the "discrepancy method"—i.e., the patient's symptoms or signs were not deemed to be credible manifestations of disease, based on the clinical experience of the examiner. (Of course, this assumes that the examiner has a wide experience; for the novice, many syndromes are unknown or incomprehensible.) The third and even less reliable method of diagnosis is dependent on purely psychologic criteria. In decreasing order of reliability, in the opinion of Lazare and of Gatfield and Guze, are the presence of (1) sociopathy or schizophrenia (present in 33 to 50 percent); (2) a model for the conversion symptom from some previous illness in the patient or in another important person in the patient's life ("modeling," in the language of Raskin et al); (3) emotional stress before onset of hysterical symptoms; (4) disturbed sexuality; (5) an assumed symbolism of the symptom, expressive of repressed wishes; (6) secondary gain; and (7) hysterical personality. In our case material, these psychologic factors have been inconsistent and often misleading.

So-called projective tests (the Rorschach and Thematic Apperception Tests), which for a time were popular with dynamic psychiatrists, are not helpful in diagnosis and are now used very little. The presence of extreme suggestibility and the tendency to dramatize symptoms (as measured by one part of the Minnesota Multiphasic Personality Inventory) is helpful in diagnosis but not pathognomonic of the disease; these traits appear under certain conditions in individuals who never develop hysteria.

Treatment of Hysteria

This may be considered from two aspects: the correction of the long-standing basic personality defect and relieving the recently acquired physical symptoms. Little or nothing can be done about the former. Psychoanalysts have attempted to modify it by long-term re-education, but their results are unavailable, and there are no control studies for the few reports of therapeutic success. One has the impression that in most cases the underlying illness is so pervasive and deeply rooted that nothing can be accomplished except to grant that the patient is inadequate in certain respects and requires medical support. Many psychiatrists, for this reason, are inclined to regard the female hysteric with a lifelong history of ill health as having a severe personality disorder—i.e., sociopathy. In other, less severe cases and especially in those in whom hysterical symptoms have appeared under the pressure of a major crisis, explanatory and supportive psychotherapy appears to be helpful, and the patients have been able thereafter to resume their places in society.

The acute symptoms can usually be controlled by persuasion. Here the best tactic is to treat the patient as though she has had an illness and is now in the process of recovering. The earlier this is done after the development of symptoms, the more likely they are to be relieved. In chronically bedridden patients, strong pressure to get out of bed and resume function must be applied. Compensation and litigation neuroses are quite difficult to treat, and settlement of the patient's claim ("the green poultice") is usually necessary before the symptoms subside.

The following principles should govern the treatment of classic female hysteria:

1. Hysteria must be treated as a tangible, definite illness. In our view, the patient should not be told, "There's nothing wrong with you," "It's all in your mind," or "It's your nerves." This at once alienates the patient, and she almost invariably terminates her relations with the physician. The patient should not be dismissed as a malingerer or a faker of illness.

2. Simple, understandable language should be employed in interviews with these patients; abstruse psychologic terms should be avoided. It is unnecessary to employ the term *hysteria* in discussions with these patients or their families, since it has a derogatory connotation that the physician should not imply.

3. The care of the patient should be entrusted to one physician.

4. All indicated examinations and laboratory procedures for the investigation of the chief complaints should be conducted before actual treatment is begun. Once treatment is started, one should avoid, if possible, checking or repeating physical or laboratory examinations.

5. Persuasion and suggestion, both direct and indirect, should be employed. Illustratively, the patient should be repeatedly encouraged, told that she is improving, and urged to resume work or household duties and to continue participation in routine activities. Medication should be withheld.

6. A regimen of physical therapy should be instituted, utilizing an experienced therapist and setting simple goals for success.

7. There should be several interviews in which the patient is permitted to direct the discussion. She should be assured of the privacy of the interview, of the impersonal, "morally neutral" position of the physician, and of the advantages of "thinking things out more thoroughly." Any questions that the patient asks should be answered truthfully, in accordance with the physician's knowledge, in simple, direct terms.

8. Every illness in such patients should be evaluated objectively, so as not to overlook any medical or surgical disease, which may strike a hysterical patient just as it does any other person. Surgical procedures should be used only if strict criteria of surgery-requiring disease are satisfied.

How successful this program will be over a long period of time is not known. The eradication of some recently acquired hysterical symptom is relatively easy. The real test of therapy, however, is whether it enables the patient to adjust satisfactorily to family and society and to perform daily activities effectively, and whether it prevents addiction, unnecessary medical treatments, and operations. Estimates of the recurrence rate of hysterical symptoms vary widely, from 12 to 80 percent. In the series of Gatfield and Guze and of Merskey, the recurrence of somatic symptoms of similar or of other types was as high as in sociopathies. We have seen patients with monosymptomatic hysteria (paraparesis, bizarre gait, crippling dystonia) that persisted for years on end.

Hypochondriasis

Hypochondriasis (hypochondriacal neurosis) is the morbid preoccupation with bodily functions or physical signs and sensations, leading to the fear or belief of having serious disease. Hallmarks of this condition are the failure of repeated examinations to disclose any physical basis for the patient's symptoms and the failure of reassurance to affect either the patient's symptoms or his conviction of being sick.

It is estimated that 85 percent of hypochondriasis is secondary to other mental disorders, chiefly depression, but also schizophrenia and the neuroses. In about 15 percent of cases, however, there appears to be no associated illness (*primary hypochondriasis*). Most patients in this latter category are habitues of medical outpatient clinics, who are passed from specialist to specialist, perplexing and angering doctors along the way, because their symptoms defy both satisfactory diagnosis and cure. Often referred to by house officers as "crocks," these patients seldom benefit from conventional therapy.

Of a different order are the hypochondriacal reactions that one encounters in otherwise normal individuals during periods of stress. Medical students, for example, traditionally develop symptoms of a variety of diseases during their first exposure to clinical medicine. However, when an adolescent or young adult develops hypochondriacal symptoms that are not related to such forms of situational stress, one should suspect a more serious underlying disorder, such as depression or schizophrenia.

The first step in the management of hypochondriasis is to determine whether it is part of another psychiatric syndrome. As a rule, this question can best be answered by a psychiatrist, and it is advisable to have each case evaluated from this point of view. If depressive symptoms are an important part of the clinical picture, the patient should be given a trial of antidepressant medication. Particularly troublesome are young adults who present with a fixed somatic delusion such as a belief that the tongue is swollen, the jaw is not properly aligned, or the penis is ulcerated when in fact no such abnormalities are present. The malignant aspect of such an illness is the persistence of the symptom and disability that extends for years, all tests having been negative. Probably these patients should be treated like schizophrenics, which many of them probably are.

The treatment of primary hypochondriasis is difficult if not impossible unless the physician keeps in mind the personality of the patient and the therapeutic goals. For a variety of reasons, these patients need to retain their symptoms, so that the usual concept of "curing" is inapplicable. The presence of symptoms provides the context for a relationship with a physician. It is the continuation of this relationship, which is often the only dependable human contact in the patient's life, that motivates some hypochondriacs. Thus it is understandable why this type of hypochondriac is seldom moved to improve by reassurances that vigor and health will be restored. Such patients are best managed by physicians who realize that these are patients who do not necessarily want or expect a cure, who are content with small gains and the avoidance of unnecessary surgery, and who have an interest in the way symptoms persist rather than in any improvement.

THE SOCIOPATHIES AND SEXUAL PERVERSIONS

Antisocial Personality (Sociopathy)

Of all the abnormal personality types listed in Table 56-1, the antisocial is the best defined and the one most likely to cause trouble in the family and community. Formerly sociopathy was referred to as psychopathic personality, constitutional psychopathy, and chronic psychopathic inferiority and was defined (in DSM-III) as a state in which the individual "is always in trouble, profiting not from experience or punishment, unable to empathize with family or friends or to maintain loyalties to any person, group or code. He is likely to be shallow, callous, and hedonistic, showing marked emotional immaturity with lack of sense of responsibility, lack of judgment, and an ability to rationalize his behavior so that it appears warranted, reasonable and justified." Also included under this heading were certain instances of sexual deviation and of addiction.

Since Prichard, in 1835, first described this condition under the term *imoral* insanity, there have been many attempts to give it a more precise definition and to avoid using it as a psychiatric wastebasket. At the turn of the century, Koch introduced the term *psychopathic inferiority*, implying that it was a constitutionally determined deviation in personality. Later the term *psychopathic personality* came into common use. Some authors used this last term indiscriminately to embrace all forms of deviant personality. Subsequently the term came to be used in a more restricted sense to define a subgroup of antisocial or aggressive psychopaths (*antisocial personality disorder,* DSM-IV). Aubrey Lewis has given a lucid account of the history of the concept of sociopathy.

By far the best modern study of sociopathy is that of L. N. Robins, based on a 30-year follow-up study of 524 cases from a child guidance clinic and 100 controls. Other investigations of note are those of Cleckley, of McCord and McCord, and of Guze and coworkers, who studied psychiatric illness in large numbers of felons and their first-degree relatives. The descriptions that follow and the quotation above are taken largely from these writings and those of Reid.

Clinical State This condition, unlike many psychiatric disorders, is manifest by the age of 12 to 15 years and frequently earlier. It consists essentially of deviant behavior in which individuals seem driven to make trouble in everything they do. Every code imposed by family, school, religion, and society is broken. Seemingly the sociopath acts on impulse, but after committing the unsocial act, he shows no remorse. The most frequent antisocial activities are theft, incorrigibility, truancy, running away overnight, associating with undesirable characters, staying out late, indiscriminate sexual relations, repeated fighting, recklessness and impulsivity, lying without cause, vandalism, abuse of drugs and alcohol, and, later, inability to work steadily or keep a job. Of children or adolescents who exhibited 10 or more of these antisocial symptoms, 43 percent were classed as sociopaths in adulthood. If only 8 or 9 of these traits were present, 29 percent were so classed; if 6 or 7, 25 percent; and 3 to 5, only 15 percent. Conversely, not a single adult sociopath was observed who did not manifest antisocial symptoms in earlier life. Interestingly, a number of other problems of childhood and adolescence—such as enuresis, dirty appearance, sleepwalking, irritability, nail biting, oversensitivity, poor eating habits, nervousness, being withdrawn or seclusive, unhappiness, tics, and fears—were not predictive of adult sociopathy. None of Robins's patients was mentally defective. However, there is an increased incidence of sociopathic traits among the large population of sociocultural retardates (discussed in Chap. 28).

As noted above, more than half the deviant children in Robins's study (even those with 10 or more antisocial manifestations) had lost most of their sociopathic traits by adulthood. This does not mean that they remained psychiatrically normal, however. Of those who did not become adult sociopaths, the large majority developed other adult psychiatric illnesses, particularly addiction to alcohol. Only in the group of children with less than three antisocial symptoms did a reasonable number (one-third) remain well in adult life. Because sociopathic behavior in children may terminate spontaneously or evolve into other disorders, it is advised (in DSM-IV) that the diagnosis of antisocial personality disorder be reserved for adults; the same behavior pattern in children is designated as *conduct disorder*.

Robins's criteria for making the diagnosis sociopathy in the adult were persistent disturbances in so-called life areas, as exemplified by at least five of the following: poor work record, marital difficulties, inability to function as a responsible parent, financial irresponsibility and dependency, illegal occupations, multiple arrests, abuse of alcohol, sexual promiscuity, vagrancy, leading a "wild life," social isolation, disciplinary problems in the armed forces, lack of guilt, more than nine somatic complaints or a complaint of medical disability, use of aliases, pathologic lying, recklessness, aggressiveness and belligerency, and suicide attempts. These findings in the adult were the same, whether the patients were drawn from the community at large, from a mental hospital, or from a group of prisoners (or parolees or probationers). Only 12 percent of Robins's adult sociopaths were in prison at the time of their follow-up examination. In each of the groups of adult sociopaths, the manifestations of antisocial behavior in childhood were much the same.

Also of interest are Robins's findings that sociopaths show an unusually high incidence of "conversion" symptoms as well as depressive symptoms and anxiety, and that the neurotic symptoms are in proportion to the sociopathic ones—i.e., the larger the number of antisocial manifestations, the larger the number of neurotic symptoms or the greater the disability from them. The latter symptoms and many other somatic complaints frequently bring the sociopath to the attention of the physician.

The manifestations of sociopathic behavior in children and adults were five to ten times more frequent in males than in females. Among the latter there was a high incidence of hysterical manifestations—further evidence that female hysteria may be the counterpart of male sociopathy. In Robins's series, a search for evidence of encephalitis, often postulated as the basis of sociopathy, was not revealing, nor was there any proof of other brain damage.

It has been shown that electroencephalographic (EEG) abnormalities, taking the form of mild to moderate bilateral slowing, are more frequent in criminals and sociopaths than in the normal population. Furthermore, the biologic parents of sociopaths also show a higher frequency of such EEG abnormalities than the general population. These and other findings suggest that there may be a genetic predisposition to antisocial personality. In a Danish study (Christiansen), "inappropriate nonpsychotic impulse-ridden behavior" was found to be five times more frequent in first-degree biologic relatives than in the general population. Criminality was two times more frequent in monozygotic twins than in dizygotic ones. This study also found a relationship between hysteria and sociopathy. More direct evidence of a genetic factor has been provided by Cadoret's studies of adoptees who were separated at birth from antisocial biologic parents; later observations disclosed a higher incidence of antisocial behavior in the adoptees than in controls. Cadoret's study also suggested that childhood hyperactivity and classic female hysteria were phenotypic manifestations of the antisocial personality genotype. The presence of a chromosomal abnormality, e.g., XYY, which has been found in a small number of sex deviants, has not been studied in a controlled manner in sociopaths.

Surveys of the families of sociopaths have also disclosed a high incidence of broken homes, alcoholism, and poverty. Two factors that seem most closely related to the development of sociopathy are a lack of parental discipline and having an antisocial or alcoholic father. However, as Robins's study has shown, if any of these factors are causal, they must be mediated through the occurrence of deviant behavior in childhood. In the absence of the latter, broken homes, slum neighborhoods, etc., do not lead to adult sociopathy.

Cadoret and his colleagues have presented convincing evidence for gene-environment interaction in the development of adolescent antisocial behavior. They analyzed data from three large adoption studies and found a significant increase in antisocial behaviors when both a genetic factor and an adverse environmental factor were present; the increase with both factors acting together was much greater than the predicted increase from either factor acting alone.

Prognosis This is of interest for several reasons. One is the relation between deviant behavior in childhood and adolescence and the development of sociopathy and other psychiatric illnesses in adult life, which has already been discussed. In addition, it should be noted that improvement of gross antisocial behavior in adult sociopaths is possible, occurring in somewhat more than one-third of such individuals. Improvement occurs most frequently between the ages of 30 and 40 years (median age, 35). This bears out the Gluecks' contention that repetitive criminality diminishes with age. Improvement of sociopathic behavior does not necessarily mean that these individuals have become well adjusted but rather that they have married and are maintaining a home and working. Probably maturation, marriage, assumption of family responsibilities, and fear of imprisonment are the main stabilizing forces; at least these are the ones proffered by sociopaths to explain their improvement.

There is no information as to the best methods of *treatment*. Most psychiatrists have been discouraged by the results of psychotherapy, but whether behavioral therapy, psychoanalysis, or drugs have more to offer cannot be determined from available data. Medical efforts should be directed to evaluating the patient's neurologic status, assessing his intelligence, and explaining the nature of the disorder to parents and social agencies. This task is best performed by a psychiatrist, acting as a spokesman for the medical profession.

Malingering

This problem arises frequently in connection with both hysteria and sociopathy, and the physician should know how to deal with it. It is not a medical diagnosis except under the rare circumstances in which a patient is caught in the act of producing a sign of disease or confesses to having done so. The term *malingering* refers to the *conscious and deliberate feigning of illness or disability in order to attain a desired goal.* It does not occur as an isolated phenomenon, and its occurrence must be interpreted as a sign of a serious personality disturbance, often one that prevents effective work or military service, though noteworthy exceptions to this statement can be found.

Certainly there is a close similarity between hysteria and malingering, but the nature of the relationship is nebulous, and there may be great difficulty in establishing a clinical differentiation. As Jones and Llewellyn have observed:

> *Nothing . . . resembles malingering more than hysteria; nothing, hysteria more than malingering. In both alike we are confronted with the same discrepancy between fact and statement, objective sign and subjective symptom—the outward aspect of health seemingly giving the lie to all the alleged functional disabilities. We may examine the hysterical person and the malingerer, using the same tests, and get precisely the same results in one case as the other.*

Most authors cite the following as the main points of difference between the two conditions:

1. The conscious or unconscious quality of the motivation, which always seems more unconscious in the hysteric and more conscious in the malingerer.

2. The influence of persuasion, which is usually effective in hysteria and not in the malingerer.

3. The attitude of the patient. The hysteric appears more genuinely ill and invites examination; the malingerer seems less ill and evades examination. The tendency of the sociopath to malinger has already been mentioned. Most of the more obvious cases of malingering seen by the present authors have been in sociopaths, for which reason discussions of the two conditions have been juxtaposed.

In the malingerer one observes pain, hyperesthesia, anesthesia, limping gait, tremor, contracture, paralysis, amaurosis, deafness, stuttering, mutism, amnesia, epileptiform seizures and fugues, unexplained gastrointestinal bleeding, and unexplained skin lesions—in short, the same array of symptoms and signs, singly or in combination, as in the patients with compensation hysteria. A particular form of sociopathy or malingering, which consists essentially of deceiving the medical profession, has been described under the title of *Munchausen's syndrome*—named, not altogether aptly, after a seventeenth-century German soldier, Baron von Munchhausen, who invented incredible tales of adventure and daring. Ireland and colleagues, who analyzed 59 well-documented cases (45 men, 14 women), list the following characteristic features, which will be recognized at once by all neurologists with extensive hospital experience: feigned severe illness of a dramatic and emergency nature; factitious evidence of disease, surreptitiously produced by interference with diagnostic procedures or by self-mutilation; a history of many hospitalizations (sometimes more than a hundred); extensive travel or visits to innumerable physicians; evidence of laparotomy scars and cranial burr holes; pathologic lying; aggressive, unruly, evasive behavior; and, finally, departure from the hospital against medical advice.

Unlike the usual forms of compensation hysteria, an ulterior motive is not readily discernible. The psychopathology of this syndrome is quite obscure. It has been regarded as a form of sociopathy, malingering, and compensation hysteria, but the distinctions between them are too ambiguous to be of clinical value. Probably the medical profession has placed too great a reliance on degree of conscious awareness of deception. In such unstable and immature individuals, the terms *conscious*, *unconscious*, and *deception* are too vague and subjective to serve as useful guides in practical work.

Intermittent Explosive Disorder

Designated by this title is an uncommon disorder, the characteristic feature of which is the occurrence of repetitive, unpredictable outbursts of violent, aggressive behavior out of all proportion to the provoking situation. This condition needs to be set apart from the uncontrollable outbursts of violent behavior that sometimes are associated with mental retardation, schizophrenia, drug addiction, or alcoholism, or those that follow serious head injuries or other brain diseases.

Some persons with intermittent explosive disorder have, from early childhood, reacted to frustration with a loss of self-control, striking out in blind rage at anyone who crossed them (*episodic dyscontrol syndrome*); as adults, they may inflict serious injury or kill. Lesser degrees are recognized as expressions of "hot temper." Sometimes such behavior appears to be a continuation of the temper tantrums of earlier childhood.

The causes of aggressive violence are poorly understood. There appears to be a heritable tendency (Cadoret et al); males predominate and a sex-linked form, extending over several generations, has been described. In some patients, a seizure disorder can be identified, particularly temporal lobe epilepsy, which is not excluded by a normal EEG. Arresting examples, occurring in patients with temporal lobe tumors and encephalitis, raise the possibility that all cases have a pathologic basis. Adrenergic hyperactivity has been suggested and supported to some extent by these patients' response to propranolol (see Chap. 25 on the limbic system).

These cases aside, the authors believe that most instances of explosive disorder represent a variant of the sociopathy described above. In DSM-IV, intense outbursts of anger and physical violence are important features of a diagnostic category called *borderline personality disorder*, the other manifestations of which include "a pervasive pattern of instability of mood, interpersonal relationships, and self-image." Elliott, and Jenkins and Maruta report a beneficial effect of propranolol. Others find lithium, carbamazepine, and phenytoin to be helpful in controlling and preventing attacks.

Psychosexual Disorders

Although sexual perversions are usually included in the section on neurosis or sociopathy in most textbooks of psychiatry, it is a mistake to assume that every sexually perverse individual is neurotic or psychopathic, a position emphasized by Kinsey and colleagues in their two texts. Some psychiatrists would define any sexual activity that does not lead to reproduction as perverse, but this would place even masturbation and sexual intercourse with contraceptives in this category. Yet all would agree that unusual sexual practices that become ends in themselves are deviant in western society.

Much has been written in the psychoanalytic literature about the physiologic development of the sexual instinct from childhood to adult life, and arrests of development are one way of looking at some of the sexual aberrations listed below.

Included under the heading of psychosexual disorders are a variety of psychologically determined sexual deviations, the most common of which are (1) *transsexualism* (the wish to be rid of one's own genitalia and live as a member of the other sex) and (2) *paraphilias* or what were formerly referred to as *sexual deviations*. Included in this latter category are *fetishism* (the use of nonliving objects to achieve sexual excitement), *frotteurism* (intense sexual urges involving touching and rubbing against a nonconsenting person), *pedophilia* (sexual activity with a prepubescent child), *transvestism* (habitual dressing in the clothes of the opposite sex), *zoophilia*, *exhibitionism*, *voyeurism*, *sexual masochism*, and *sadism*. These represent special problems rarely encountered by the neurologist and are not included here for that reason. The reader seeking information on these subjects and on sexual dysfunctions is referred to the chapters by Levine and by Green and Blanchard in the *Comprehensive Textbook of Psychiatry* and to the discussion of sexual disorders in DSM-IV.

Alcohol and Drug Addiction

These conditions are unquestionably associated with sociopathy, as indicated above, but they also represent special problems of immense proportions and are therefore discussed in Chaps. 42 and 43.

ANOREXIA NERVOSA AND BULIMIA

Anorexia nervosa is a behavioral disorder of previously healthy girls and young women, mainly from the upper and middle social classes, who become extremely emaciated as a result of voluntary starvation. It is rare in Asians and African-Americans and rarely occurs in males. Herzog reminds us that it was Richard Morton who first described the condition in 1649, under the title of "nervous phthisis," a "nervous consumption" resulting from "sadness and anxious cares"—a title that embodied enigmatic roots in psychologic derangements. Bulimia (literally ox-hunger), to which it is closely related, was not isolated as an eating disorder until the latter part of the nineteenth century.

As a rule, anorexia nervosa begins shortly after puberty—sometimes later, but seldom after 30 years of age. Some of the patients have been overweight in childhood, especially in the prepubertal period. Dieting is much talked about and may have been encouraged, especially by mothers who want their daughters to become more attractive. Sometimes there appears to be a precipitating event, such as leaving home, a disruption of family life, or other stress. Whatever the provocation, it leads to an obsessive refusal to eat. What is more important, the abnormal eating habits persist even when the patient has become painfully thin, and when counseled to eat normally, she will use every artifice to starve herself. Food is hidden instead of being eaten, vomiting may be provoked after a meal, or the bowel may be emptied by laxatives. No amount of persuasion will induce the patient to take adequate amounts of food. The patient shows no concern about her obvious emaciation and remains active. If left alone, these patients waste away, and about 5 percent have succumbed to some intercurrent infection or other complication, placing it among the most lethal of psychiatric conditions.

On physical examination, one is struck with the degree of emaciation; it exceeds that of most of the wasting diseases. Often 30 percent or more of the body weight will have been lost by the time the patient's family insists on medical consultation. A fine lanugo covers the face, body, and limbs. The skin is thin and dry, without its normal elasticity, and the nails are brittle. Pubic hair and breast tissue (except for loss of fat) are normal, and in this respect anorexia nervosa is unlike hypopituitary cachexia (Simmonds disease). The extremities are often cold and blue. There are no neurologic signs of nutritional deficiency. The patient is alert and cheerfully indifferent to her condition. Any suggestion that she is unattractively thin or seriously depleted is rejected.

Amenorrhea is practically always present and may precede the extreme weight loss. Luteinizing hormone (LH) concentrations are reduced to pubertal or prepubertal levels. Clomiphene citrate fails to stimulate a rise in LH, as it does normally. Administration of gonadotropic releasing factor raises the LH and FSH levels, suggesting a hypothalamic disorder. The basal metabolic rate is low; T3 and T4 are low, while levels of physiologically inactive 3,3,5-triiodothyronine (reverse T3) are normal or increased. Plasma thyrotropin (TSH) and growth hormone levels are normal. Serum cortisol levels are usually normal; excretion of 17-hydroxysteroids is slightly reduced. In sum, there is evidence of hypothalamic-pituitary dysfunction; probably this is not primary but is secondary to starvation. These abnormalities are summarized in the review by Becker and colleagues. However, Scheithauer and colleagues found no definite changes in the pituitary gland in 12 fatal cases. CT scanning shows slight to moderate enlargement of the lateral and third ventricles, which return to normal size as the anorexia subsides.

The etiology of anorexia nervosa is unknown, although there is no dearth of hypotheses. Holland and coworkers reported a strikingly high concordance in monozygotic twins as compared with dizygotic twins, indicating that constitutional factors are important. Earlier signs of hysterical tendencies, obsessional personality traits, and depression are mentioned as being frequent in some reported series but not in others. Certain polymorphisms in the serotonin transporter gene, of types different from those that have been tentatively attached to anxiety and to obsessive traits, have also been reported. The meaning of these genetic findings is difficult to interpret. A functional imaging study has shown activation of the left insula, amygdala, and cingulate when high-calorie drinks were imbibed by anorectic women (Ellison et al), but this may conceivably have reflected anxiety that the authors termed "calorie fear" rather than a specific biologic feature of the disease.

Reports concerning the percentage of first-degree relatives with manic-depressive disease are also contradictory. An increased prevalence of neurosis or alcoholism has been noted in other members of the family. However, all psychiatrists seem agreed that the patient does not have symptoms that conform to any of the major neuroses or psychoses. Certainly loss of appetite, lack of self-esteem and interest in personal appearance, and self-destructive behavior—common features of anorexia nervosa—are also symptoms of depressive illness, yet most of the patients do not look or admit to being dejected. Moreover, endogenous depression affects both sexes. The pathologic fear of becoming fat and the obsession with weight might be interpreted as a phobic or obsessional neurosis. A characteristic personality disorder has not been defined, however.

The fact that anorexia nervosa is practically confined to females must figure in any acceptable explanation of the syndrome. Among psychiatric disorders, only hysteria has this sexual predilection. Yet most psychiatrists do not believe anorexia nervosa to be a manifestation of hysteria. The racial-social relationships of the syndrome are noteworthy. Undoubtedly important is the fact that anorexia nervosa has its onset in relation to the menarche, at a time when the female exhibits rather large fluctuations in appetite and weight. This suggests an imbalance between the satiety center, believed to lie in the ventromedial hypothalamus, and the feeding center, in the lateral hypothalamus (McHugh). The intestinal hormone cholecystokinin may be implicated; it is released when food enters the intestine and may function as a feedback mechanism, acting on the satiety center and inhibiting food intake. Obesity before or around puberty is more pronounced in girls than in boys. It is as though the appetite-satiety mechanism of the female hypothalamus were unstable.

The most effective treatment consists of winning the patient's confidence, supportive psychotherapy, assignment of one individual to sit with the patient as each meal is eaten, and a gradual increase of a balanced diet (Anderson). Extreme cases may require hospitalization. If the patient refuses to eat, tube feeding is the only alternative, and she must understand that it is simply a question of eating voluntarily or being tube-fed. As weight is gained over several weeks, the patient usually becomes more normal in her attitude and will continue to recover on this regimen at home. The menses will not return until considerable weight has been gained (about 10 percent above the weight at the time of the menarche). Our colleagues report an increased success with such a regime when imipramine or fluoxetine is added. Others have found these drugs to be ineffective except in patients with prominent symptoms of depression.

Becker and her colleagues have recently reviewed the problem of eating disorders. They emphasize the potentially devastating effect on health of the many medical complications to which severely anorectic patients are prone and the need to evaluate and treat these complications at the same time that nutritional therapy is undertaken. In particular, an electrocardiogram is essential in order to exclude a prolonged QT interval—the presence of which contraindicates the use of tricyclic antidepressants and increases the risk of ventricular tachycardia.

On average, 50 percent of patients recover completely or almost completely (Steinhausen and Seidel). In the remainder, the outcome is quite unfavorable. They either relapse after an initial period of improvement or remain chronically anorectic. Many patients are said to lapse into a chronic neurotic state characterized by a persistent preoccupation with food, weight, and dieting. It is not generally appreciated that chronic anorexia nervosa significantly shortens life; after a mean follow-up period of 12 years, 11 percent of a group of 84 patients had died (Deter and Herzog), and 15 percent after 20 years (Ratnasuriya et al). Suicide is a major contributor to this high mortality rate (Sullivan).

The few adolescent boys that we have seen with this syndrome have recovered on antidepressant medication. A few cases, due to tumors within the hypothalamus, have been mentioned in Chap 27.

The association of *anorexia* with disease involving the appetite centers has not been established, though the cases of Lewin and colleagues and of White and Hain are suggestive. Martin and Reichlin, in citing these rare cases, attribute the anorexia and cachexia to lesions of the lateral hypothalamus. A rare disorder of infants has been described under the title of diencephalic syndrome. Progressive and ultimately fatal emaciation (failure to thrive), despite normal food intake, in an otherwise alert and cheerful infant is the main clinical feature. The lesion has usually proved to be a low-grade astrocytoma of the anterior hypothalamus or optic nerve (Burr et al). See Chap. 27 for further discussion and references.

Bulimia This is a related eating disorder characterized by massive binge eating followed by the induction of vomiting and excessive use of laxatives. Insofar as the central psychologic disturbance is the pursuit of thinness at all costs, it is generally conceived as a variant of anorexia nervosa. Indeed, binge eating is a frequent manifestation of anorexia nervosa, although it also occurs as the only, or predominant, eating disorder. However, a close relationship with the menarche as well as emaciation and endocrinologic disturbances are not as evident in bulimic patients as in those with anorexia nervosa. Pope and colleagues have reported considerable success in 19 of 20 bulimic patients treated with imipramine and followed for 2 years; the newer antidepressants appear to be equally effective. In general, the therapeutic benefit of these drugs is considerably greater in cases of bulimia than in anorexia nervosa.

REFERENCES

American Psychiatric Association: *Diagnostic and Statistical Manual of Mental Disorders* (DSM-IV). Washington DC, APA, 1994.

Anderson AE: *Practical Comprehensive Treatment of Anorexia Nervosa and Bulimia*. Baltimore, Johns Hopkins University Press, 1985.

Andreasen NC, Black DW: *Introductory Textbook of Psychiatry*, 2nd ed. Washington DC, American Psychiatric Press, 1995.

Baxter LR: Neuroimaging in obsessive-compulsive disorder: Seeking the mediating neuroanatomy, in Jenike MA, Baer L, Minichiello WE (eds): *Obsessive-Compulsive Disorders: Theory and Management*, 2nd ed. Chicago, Mosby-Year Book, 1990, pp 167–188.

Becker AE, Grinspoon SK, Klibanski A, Herzog DB: Eating disorders. *N Engl J Med* 340:1092, 1999.

Behar D, Rapoport JL, Berg CJ, et al: Computerized tomography and neuropsychological test measures in adolescents with obsessive-compulsive disorder. *Am J Psychiatry* 141:363, 1984.

Berg I: School phobia in children of agoraphobic women. *Br J Psychiatry* 128:86, 1976.

Berthier ML, Kulisevsky J, Gironell A, et al: Obsessive-compulsive disorder associated with brain lesions: Clinical phenomenology, cognitive function and anatomic correlates. *Neurology* 47:353, 1996.

Black JL: Obsessive compulsive disorder: A clinical update. *Mayo Clin Proc* 67:266, 1992.

Briquet P: *Traite clinique et therapeutique a l'hysterie*. Paris, Ballière, 1859.

Burr IM, Slonim AE, Danish RK: Diencephalic syndrome revisited. *J Pediatr* 88:429, 1976.

Cadoret RJ: Psychopathology in adopted-away offspring of biologic parents with antisocial behavior. *Arch Gen Psychiatry* 35:176, 1978.

Cadoret RJ, Cain C, Crowe RR: Evidence for gene-environment interaction in the development of adolescent antisocial behavior. *Behav Genet* 13:301, 1983.

Cadoret RJ, Leve LD, Devor E: Genetics of aggressive and violent behavior. *Psychiatr Clin North Am* 20:301, 1997.

Cannon WB: *Bodily Changes in Pain, Hunger, Fear and Rage*, 2nd ed. New York, Appleton, 1920.

Carothers JC: Hysteria, psychopathy and the magic word. *Mankind Q* 16:93, 1975.

Christiansen KO: Crime in a Danish twin population. *Acta Genet Med Gemellol* 19:323, 1970.

Cleckley H: *The Mask of Sanity*. St. Louis, Mosby, 1955.

Cloninger CR, Adolfsson R, Svrakic NM: Mapping genes for human personality. *Nature Genet* 12:3, 1996.

Cloninger CR, Guze SB: Psychiatric illness and female criminality: The role of sociopathy and hysteria in the antisocial woman. *Am J Psychiatry* 127:303, 1970.

Cloninger CR, Reich T, Guze SB: The multifactorial model of disease transmission: III. Familial relationship between sociopathy and hysteria (Briquet's syndrome). *Br J Psychiatry* 127:23, 1975.

Cohen ME, White PD: Life situations, emotions, and neurocirculatory asthenia (anxiety neurosis, neurasthenia, effort syndrome). *Proc Assoc Res Nerv Ment Dis* 29:832, 1950.

Cohen ME, White PD, Johnson RE: Neurocirculatory asthenia, anxiety neurosis or the effort syndrome. *Arch Intern Med* 81:260, 1948.

Couprie W, Wijdicks EFM, Rooijmans HGM, van Gijn J: Outcome in conversion disorder: A follow up study. *J Neurol Neurosurg Psychiatry* 58:750, 1995.

Deter H-C, Herzog W: Anorexia nervosa in a long-term perspective: Results of the Heidelberg-Mannheim study. *Psychosom Med* 56:20, 1994.

Easton JD, Sherman DG: Somatic anxiety attacks and propranolol. *Arch Neurol* 33:689, 1976.

Elliott FA: Propranolol for the control of belligerent behavior following acute brain damage. *Ann Neurol* 1:489, 1977.

Ellison Z, Foong J, Howard R, et al: Functional anatomy of calorie fear in anorexia nervosa. *Lancet* 352:1192, 1998.

Gatfield PD, Guze SB: Prognosis and differential diagnosis of conversion reactions: A follow-up study. *Dis Nerv Syst* 23:623, 1962.

Glueck S, Glueck E: *Criminal Careers in Retrospect*. New York, Commonwealth Fund, 1943.

Goodwin DW, Guze SB: *Psychiatric Diagnosis*, 5th ed. New York, Oxford University Press, 1996.

Green R, Blanchard R: Gender identity disorders, in Sadock BJ, Sadock VA (eds): *Kaplan and Sadock's Comprehensive Textbook of Psychiatry*, 7th ed. Philadelphia, Lippincott Williams & Wilkins, 2000, pp 1646–1662.

Guze S: The role of follow-up studies: The contribution to diagnostic classification as applied to hysteria. *Semin Psychiatry* 2:392, 1970.

Guze SB, Goodwin DW, Crane JB: Criminal recidivism and psychiatric illness. *Am J Psychiatry* 127:832, 1970.

Herzog DB: Eating disorders, in Nicholi AM (ed): *The New Harvard Guide to Psychiatry*, 2nd ed. Cambridge, MA, Harvard University Press, 1988, pp 434–445.

Holland AJ, Sicotte N, Treasure J: Anorexia nervosa: evidence for a genetic basis. *J Psychosom Res* 32:561, 1988.

Ireland P, Sapira JD, Templeton B: Munchausen's syndrome. *Am J Med* 43:579, 1967.

Jenkins SC, Maruta T: Therapeutic use of propranolol for intermittent explosive disorders. *Mayo Clin Proc* 62:204, 1987.

Jones AB, Llewellyn LJ: *Malingering*. Philadelphia, Lippincott, 1918.

Judd FK, Brurrows GD, Norman TR: The biological basis of anxiety: An overview. *J Affective Disord* 9:271, 1985.

Kandel ER: A new intellectual framework for psychiatry. *Am J Psychiatry* 155:457, 1998.

Keane JR: Hysterical gait disorders: 60 cases. *Neurology* 39:586, 1989.

Kinsey AC, Pomeroy WB, Martin CE, Gebhard PH: *Sexual Behavior of the Human Female*. Philadelphia, Saunders, 1948.

Kinsey AC, Pomeroy WB, Martin CE, Gebhard PH: *Sexual Behavior of the Human Male*. Philadelphia, Saunders, 1948.

Kurlan R: Tourette's syndrome: Current concepts. *Neurology* 39:1625, 1989.

Lazare A: Current concepts in psychiatry: Conversion symptoms. *N Engl J Med* 305:745, 1981.

Lesch K-P, Bengel D, Heils A, et al: Association of anxiety-related traits with polymorphism in the serotonin transporter gene regulatory region. *Science* 274:1527, 1996.

Levine SB: Paraphilias, in Sadock BJ, Sadock VA (eds): *Kaplan and Sadock's Comprehensive Textbook of Psychiatry*, 7th ed. Philadelphia, Lippincott Williams & Wilkins, 2000, pp 1631–1646.

Lewis A: Psychopathic personality: A most elusive category. *Psychol Med* 4:133, 1974.

Liebowitz MR, Fryer AJ, Goerman JM, et al: Lactate provocation of panic attacks. *Arch Gen Psychiatry* 41:764, 1984.

March JS: Cognitive-behavioral psychotherapy, in Sadock BJ, Sadock VA (eds): *Kaplan and Sadock's Comprehensive Textbook of Psychiatry*, 7th ed. Philadelphia, Lippincott Williams & Wilkins, 2000, pp 2806–2813.

McCord W, McCord J: *The Psychopath*. Princeton, NJ, Van Nostrand, 1964.

McHugh PR: Food intake and its disorders, in Asbury AK, McKhann GM, McDonald WI (eds): *Diseases of the Nervous System*, 2nd ed. Philadelphia, Saunders, 1992, pp 529–536.

Merskey H: *The Analysis of Hysteria*. London, Ballière Tindall, 1979.

Meyer JK: Paraphilias, in Kaplan HI, Sadock BJ (eds): *Comprehensive Textbook of Psychiatry*, 6th ed. Baltimore, Williams & Wilkins, 1995, pp 1334–1347.

Michaels R, Marzuk PM: Progress in psychiatry. *N Engl J Med* 329:552, 1993.

Modlin HC: Postaccident anxiety syndrome: Psychosocial aspects. *Am J Psychiatry* 123:1008, 1967.

Nemiah JC: The psychodynamic basis of psychopathology: Psychoneurotic disorders, in Nicholi AM Jr (ed): *The New Harvard Guide to Psychiatry*. Cambridge, MA, Harvard University Press, 1988, pp 208–258.

Noyes R, Clarkson C, Crowe R, et al: A family study of generalized anxiety disorder. *Am J Psychiatry* 144:1019, 1987.

Pauls DL, Leckman JF: The inheritance of Gilles de la Tourette's syndrome and associated behaviors: Evidence for autosomal dominant transmission. *N Engl J Med* 315:993, 1986.

Peroutka SJ: The selection of anxiolytics in clinical neurology, in Plum F (ed): *Advances in Contemporary Neurology*. Philadelphia, Davis, 1988, pp 135–152.

Pollitt J: Natural history of obsessional states. *BMJ* 1:194, 1957.

Pope HG, Hudson JI, Jones JM, et al: Bulimia treated with imipramine: A placebo-controlled double-blind study. *Am J Psychiatry* 140:554, 1983.

Purtell JJ, Robins E, Cohen ME: Observations on clinical aspects of hysteria. *JAMA* 146:902, 1951.

Raskin M, Talbott JA, Meyerson AT: Diagnosis of conversion reactions: Predictive value of psychiatric criteria. *JAMA* 197:530, 1966.

Ratnasuriya RH, Eisler I, Szmukler GJ, Russell GFM: Anorexia nervosa: Outcome and prognostic factors after 20 years. *Br J Psychiatry* 158:495, 1991.

Reid W (ed): *The Psychopath: A Comprehensive Study of Antisocial Disorders and Behaviors*. New York, Brunner-Mazel, 1978.

Robins E, Purtell JJ, Cohen ME: Hysteria in men. *N Engl J Med* 246:677, 1952.

Robins LN: *Deviant Children Grown Up: A Sociological and Psychiatric Study of Sociopathic Personality*. Huntington, NY, Krieger, 1974.

Scheithauer BW, Kovacs KT, Jariwala LK, et al: Anorexia nervosa: An immunohistochemical study of the pituitary gland. *Mayo Clin Proc* 63:23, 1988.

Slater B, Shields J: Genetical aspects of anxiety, in Lader MH (ed): *Studies of Anxiety*. London, Royal Medico-Psychological Association, 1969, pp 62–71.

Slater E: A heuristic theory of neurosis. *J Neurol Neurosurg Psychiatry* 7:48, 1944.

Steinhausen HC, Seidel R: The Berlin follow-up study of eating disorders in adolescence, Part 2: Intermediate-term catamnesis after 4 years. *Nervenarzt* 65:26, 1994.

Sullivan PE: Mortality in anorexia nervosa. *Am J Psychiatry* 152:1073, 1995.

von Korff M, Eaton W, Keyl P: The epidemiology of panic attacks and panic disorder. *Am J Epidemiol* 122:970, 1985.

Weilburg JB, Mesulam M-M, Weintraub S, et al: Focal striatal abnormalities in a patient with obsessive-compulsive disorder. *Arch Neurol* 46:233, 1989.

Wheeler EO, White PD, Reed EW, Cohen ME: Neurocirculatory asthenia (anxiety neurosis, effort syndrome, neurasthenia): A twenty year follow-up study of one hundred and seventy-three patients. *JAMA* 142:878, 1950.

White LF, Hain RF: Anorexia in association with a destructive lesion of the hypothalamus. *Arch Pathol* 68:275, 1959.

Winokur G, Coryell W: Anxiety disorders: The magnitude of the problem, in Coryell W, Winokur G (eds): *The Clinical Management of Anxiety Disorders*. New York, Oxford University Press, 1991, pp 3–9.

Winokur G, Crowe RR: Personality disorders, in Freedman AM, Kaplan HI, Sadock BJ (eds): *Comprehensive Textbook of Psychiatry*, 2nd ed. Baltimore, Williams & Wilkins, 1976, pp 1279–1297.

Wolpe J: *Psychotherapy by Reciprocal Inhibition*. Stanford, CA, Stanford University Press. 1958.

Chapter 57

REACTIVE DEPRESSION, ENDOGENOUS DEPRESSION, AND MANIC-DEPRESSIVE DISEASE

There are four major categories of psychosis: (1) the confusional-delirious states, (2) the psychoses associated with focal or multifocal cerebral lesions, (3) the affective disorders (manic-depressive and depressive psychoses), and (4) the schizophrenias. The first two categories are discussed in Chaps. 20 and 22. The latter two groups make up the subject matter of this and the following chapter.

Depression is the cause of more grief and misery than any other single disease to which humankind is subject. This view, expressed by Kline almost forty years ago, is still shared by everyone in the field of mental health. Although depression has been known for over 2000 years (melancholia is described in the writings of Hippocrates), there is still uncertainty as to its medical status. Is depression a disease state (kraepelinian concept) or a type of psychologic reaction (meyerian concept)? In other words, is it basically a biologic derangement or a response to psychosocial stress with which a person cannot cope? These two disparate concepts are not irreconcilable. An eclectic position is that both are correct—i.e., that there are two basic forms of depression: exogenous and endogenous. *Exogenous (or reactive) depressions* have an overt external cause, such as the loss of a loved one, loss of one's fortune or position, or a disabling or life-threatening illness. In this framework, *grief* would exemplify a reactive or exogenous depression. In contrast, the *endogenous depressions* have no apparent external cause; they seem to occur in susceptible individuals as a response to some unknown biologic alteration. In respect to endogenous depression and manic-depressive psychosis, the genetic and neurochemical data (cited further on) support the kraepelinian view of a disease state. Nonetheless, a lay concept persists, perpetuated perhaps by some process-oriented psychiatrists, that events in one's life, either distant or current, underlie both types of depressive illness. An unfortunate consequence of this view is the assumption that an inability to deal with these stresses represents a personal failure of sorts and may inhibit the acceptance of psychiatric help.

A few additional remarks are necessary to explain the grouping of entities to be considered in this chapter. *A depressed or dysphoric mood* is the symptom that relates all of them, but it is the setting in which the depression occurs as well as differences in certain clinical attributes that underline the distinction of a number of separable clinical states. Taken together, they are the most frequent of all psychiatric illnesses. In a tertiary general referral hospital, as indicated on page 1587, they accounted for an estimated 50 percent of psychiatric consultations and 12 percent of all admissions. Grief reactions are ubiquitous, but only exceptionally do they require psychiatric referral.

Depressive states are so often associated with obscure physical symptoms that they are more likely to come to the attention of general physicians and internists than are other psychiatric entities. Moreover, they are frequently misdiagnosed, the symptoms being mistakenly attributed to anemia, low blood pressure, hypothyroidism, migraine, tension headaches, a chronic pain syndrome, chronic infection, emotional problems, worry, and stress. Neurologists in particular are likely to encounter depressed patients who complain of fatigue and weakness, chronic headache, and difficulty in thinking or remembering. An important reason why all physicians should be knowledgeable about depressive illnesses is the danger of suicide, which may be attempted and successfully accomplished before the depression is recognized. Timely diagnosis may prevent such a tragedy—one that is all the more regrettable since most depressive illnesses can be successfully treated.

Nosology and Classification

As remarked in Chap. 24, the term *depression* embraces more than a feeling of sadness and unhappiness. It stands for *a complex of disturbed feelings* (called *mood*, or *affective, disorder*)—which includes despair, hopelessness, a sense of worthlessness, and thoughts of self-harm—associated with decreased energy and libido, loss of interest in life's events, impaired concentration, various abnormalities of behavior, and prominent physical complaints—the most important of which are insomnia, either anorexia or overeating, headache, and various types of regional pain. At one extreme are depressive symptoms of psychotic proportions (including paranoid or somatic delusions), which create chaos in the lives of the patient and those close to him. At the other extreme are the common feelings of unhappiness, anhedonia (loss of pleasurable responses), discouragement, and resentment that occur in almost everyone as a reaction to the disappointments of everyday life, such as loss of employment, a failure to gain recognition, or unsuccessful sexual or social adjustment, all of which are closely linked in their duration to the persistence of the precipitant factors.

Some *mood*, or *affective, disorders* take the form of a relatively pure, uncomplicated depressive illness; others are mixed with symptoms of anxiety and agitation. Because of an apparent tendency to appear for the first time in middle and late adult life, the latter syndrome was referred to in the past as *involutional melancholia*. This term takes license with the concept of involution, for such an illness may occur at any time in adult life, with no relationship to the climacteric (Winokur and Cadoret).

Some depressions are clearly reactions to real and imaginary life situations. If a depression arises in proximate relation to the loss of a family member, the condition is called *grief*; if in relation to a life-threatening or disabling medical or neurologic disorder, it is referred to as *induced* or *reactive depression*. As indicated in the preceding chapter, depression may complicate phobic and obsessive-compulsive states and even hysteria; in a sense the depression in these circumstances is also secondary or reactive. Then there are depressions that present as *hypochondriasis*; although the latter psychiatric syndrome may rarely occur as a protracted and obstinate neurosis, the coexistence of an underlying depression must always be considered in assessing a hypochondriacal patient.

An abnormally elevated mood, or *mania*, is about one-third as frequent as depression. It also may develop as a relatively pure, recurrent clinical state, or it may alternate or be intertwined with depression, in which case it has classically been referred to as *manic-depressive disease* (*bipolar disorder* in the classification of the *Diagnostic and Statistical Manual of Mental Disorders*, or DSM-IV). Prolonged milder forms of moodiness and depression, lasting for years, have been classified as *dysthymia*. *Hypomania* and *cyclothymic disorder* are the names given to milder forms of mania and bipolar disorder, respectively. The DSM-IV classification also acknowledges the existence of mixed *schizoaffective states* with attributes of depression and schizophrenia. These fall into the category of either dysthymic personality disorders, episodic hypomania, or reactive depression, in our view. Distinguishing these various types of depressive illness is of therapeutic as well as theoretical importance insofar as a particular type of depressive illness may respond better to one form of treatment than to another.

As already indicated, when depression masquerades as a chronic pain or fatigue state or some other medical condition, it has been called "masked depression" or "depressive equivalent." In the following pages the masked depression as a diagnostic problem is emphasized. Finally, the neurologist should always bear in mind the possibility of an incipient dementia presenting as a depression, although the reverse, a masked depression causing difficulty with thinking and memory (pseudodementia) is more common.

To summarize, from a general medical standpoint there are four main depressive illnesses with which the physician should be acquainted:

1. Grief reaction
2. Reactive or secondary depression in relation to a medical or neurologic disease
3. Endogenous or primary depression (with or without agitation and anxiety) and manic-depressive disease
4. Depression in relation to a fixed personality trait or neurosis

The foregoing classification of depression and mania does not strictly follow the DSM-IV classification but is nonetheless in harmony with it. Also, the nosology in this chapter is in keeping with the classification proposed by Winokur.

Grief Reactions

Discussion of the depressive illnesses may suitably begin with the most common form, the grief reaction. Analysis of the typical grief reaction discloses the following characteristics (according to Lindemann): (1) an intense subjective sensation of mental pain accompanied by a feeling of exhaustion, (2) preoccupation with the image of the deceased, (3) a sense of guilt concerning the relationship to the deceased, (4) sometimes an inexplicable and unwarranted hostility toward friends and relatives, and (5) a loss of or change in the usual pattern of conduct. Bereaved persons have difficulty in initiating or organizing their daily affairs and tend to perform them in an automatic and uninterested fashion ("going through the motions" is a common description).

The authors cannot vouch for the validity of each of these characteristics, especially the third and fourth, but accept them as reasonable. There is no doubt, however, that a sense of exhaustion and disorganization of daily activities are to some extent invariable accompaniments. As a rule, the grief reaction lasts for a period of 4 to 12 weeks, by which time it begins to abate, with a gradual resumption of normal activities, which come to occupy the mind more and more of the time and to expel thoughts of the deceased. Grieving is to be regarded as a natural reaction to personal tragedy; its absence in circumstances where it should be called forth is believed by psychiatrists to be abnormal. However, the overt expressions of grief are highly individual, depending on personality as well as cultural and other factors.

Distortions of the normal reaction to personal loss are not infrequent; they are referred to as *pathologic grief.* The most frequent distortion is *prolongation of the reaction*—i.e., there is no sign of resolution by the end of a 3-month period. Mothers who have lost a child tend to suffer for an unduly long period of time, and the elderly who have lost a spouse may never recover completely. Patients with a history of previous depressive episodes may also remain in mourning longer than usual. In general, when a bereaved person has shown no improvement within 3 to 4 months of the loss, one should suspect a pathologic grief reaction that calls for psychiatric consultation. Unlike the normal grief reaction, prolonged grief is not an unusual setting for suicide.

In other variations of the grief reaction, the bereaved person may show little or no immediate reaction to the loss (the "stiff-upper-lip" attitude, much admired in Anglo-Saxon culture), or the bereaved may even become hyperactive and undertake a series of ill-advised social and economic ventures. Occasionally patients will acquire the same symptoms as the deceased and may be convinced that they have the same disease. This may be the origin of some of the hypochondriacal ideas that accompany depressive reactions. The identification of this variant of grieving requires only that the examiner, after excluding the presence of disease in the patient for want of clinical evidence, inquire about the illness that took the life of the deceased.

Management of the usual grief reaction consists of maintaining a sympathetic attitude and helping the bereaved person to acknowledge the loss and to face the changes required as a result of it. Stoicism should not be encouraged or reinforced. To express sadness through tears, anguish, and even hostility is helpful for many individuals. The practice of treating grief-stricken patients with antidepressants is seldom effective, for it attempts to suppress what is a natural and necessary human reaction. Early on, undue restlessness, anxiety, and insomnia can be relieved by anxiolytic and sedative medication. Diazepam, lorazepam, or—if there is a great deal of associated anxiety—alprazolam are suitable for daytime sedation and can be used at bedtime for sleep. These drugs have a wide margin of safety, which decreases the danger of their use as a means of committing suicide. The possibility of suicide must be entertained in managing all depressed patients, including mourners, and care must be taken not to supply them with large amounts of sedative medication.

Antidepressants can be utilized if the grief reaction is unusually prolonged or disabling, although they can generally be avoided. In treating patients of this latter type, the help of a psychiatrist should be enlisted to determine whether the plan of treatment is sound; often these patients require specialized psychiatric help.

Other Reactive Depressions

Patients reacting to a medical or neurologic illness seldom express feelings of sadness or despair without mentioning physical concomitants, such as easy fatigability, anxiety, tension headaches, dizziness, loss of appetite, reduced interest in life and love, trouble in falling asleep, or premature awakening. It follows that whenever these symptoms become manifest in the course of medical disease, they should arouse suspicion of a depressive reaction (see Table 57-1).

Chronic pain is a particularly frequent somatic manifestation of depression. The pain may be based on an attendant disease but is prolonged, disabling, sometimes vague in nature, and recalcitrant to straightforward medical and surgical approaches. In other words, depressed mood exacerbates and prolongs pain of any type. All patients with chronic pain syndromes should be evaluated psychiatrically, as pointed out in Chap. 8.

Table 57-1
Depression secondary to neurologic, medical, and surgical diseases and drugs

1. *Neurologic diseases*
   a. Neuronal degenerations—Alzheimer, Huntington, and Parkinson disease
   b. Focal CNS disease—strokes, brain tumors and trauma, multiple sclerosis
2. *Metabolic and endocrine diseases*
   a. Corticosteroids, excess or deficiency
   b. Hypothyroidism, rarely thyrotoxicosis
   c. Cushing syndrome
   d. Addison disease
   e. Hyperparathyroidism
   f. Pernicious anemia (vitamin B_{12} deficiency)
   g. Chronic renal failure/dialysis
   h. B-vitamin deficiencies
3. *Myocardial infarction, open heart surgery, and other operations*
4. *Infectious diseases*
   a. Brucellosis
   b. Viral hepatitis, influenza, pneumonia
   c. Infectious mononucleosis
5. *Cancer, particularly pancreatic*
6. *Parturition*
7. *Medications*
   a. Analgesics and anti-inflammatory agents (other than steroids)—indomethacin, phenacetin, and phenylbutazone
   b. Amphetamines (when withdrawn)
   c. Antibiotics, particularly cycloserine, ethionamide, griseofulvin, isoniazid, nalidixic acid, and sulfonamide
   d. Antihypertensive drugs—clonidine, methyldopa, propranolol, reserpine
   e. Cardiac drugs—digitalis, procainamide
   f. Corticosteroids and ACTH
   g. Disulfiram
   h. L-Dopa
   i. Methysergide
   j. Oral contraceptives
8. *Alcoholism*

In a number of major medical illnesses, depressive symptoms occur with such frequency as to become almost part of the disease. They constitute important diagnostic and therapeutic problems. Contrariwise, in certain chronic, occult diseases, symptoms such as lassitude and fatigue may resemble and be mistaken for a depressive reaction. Hypothyroidism, infectious mononucleosis, infectious hepatitis, carcinoma of the head of the pancreas, metastatic carcinoma of the liver, malnutrition, polymyalgia rheumatica, and frontal lobe tumors, especially meningiomas, may simulate depression for several weeks or months before the diagnosis becomes evident. Sedative drugs, beta-adrenergic blocking agents, beta-interferon, and the phenothiazines may evoke a depressive reaction; corticosteroids can induce a peculiar psychiatric state in which confusion, insomnia, and either an elevation of mood or depression are combined. A depressed mood may also emerge during the tapering-off period of steroid medication.

Of particular significance is the depression that occurs on learning of a medical or neurologic disease. Often such an emotional reaction, which the physician may tend to ignore, is the dominant manifestation of a disease that threatens the life pattern and independence of the patient. Recognition by the patient that he has suffered a stroke or that he has cancer, multiple sclerosis, or Parkinson disease is almost always followed by some degree of reactive depression, often with an element of anxiety.

A prime example is the depression that follows myocardial infarction (Wishnie et al). Usually it begins toward the end of the patient's stay in the acute-care ward. In the beginning, it may attract little attention, being obscured by bed rest and sedative medication. Once the patient is home, fatigability that approaches exhaustion is the main complaint and interferes with accustomed activities; it may be described as weakness and falsely attributed to a failing heart. Symptoms of irritability, anxiety, and despondency are next in order of frequency, followed by insomnia and feelings of aimlessness and boredom. Although most of these patients ultimately recover without medical assistance (the disorder, in this sense, is self-limited), the depression exacts a high toll in terms of mental suffering.

An analogous depressive reaction occurs in patients with stroke. It appears that patients with left anterior cerebral lesions, involving predominantly the lateral frontal cortex or basal ganglia (as judged by CT scanning) and examined within several weeks of the stroke, have a greater frequency and severity of depression than patients with lesions in any other location (Starkstein et al; Robinson). According to these authors, lesions of the right hemisphere do not show this correlation with depression but do show a higher association with pathologic cheerfulness or mania. House et al, in a British community-based study of stroke survivors, failed to confirm these findings, perhaps because the infarcts were small in size (more than half the patients had never been admitted to hospital) and many patients were examined for the first time only at 6 and 12 months after their strokes. Levine and Finkelstein have reported the occurrence of psychotic depression with hallucinations and delusions in patients with right temporoparietal infarcts. Our own experience suggests a not surprising relationship between the degree of motor and language disability and the severity of poststroke depression but a less predictable relationship to the location of the lesion. Also not surprisingly, strokes in the anterior (carotid) circulation give rise to more emotional changes than those in the posterior circulation. The possible predisposing effects of minor previous episodes, family history of depressive illness, medications, etc., have not been studied systematically.

Parkinson disease is complicated by a depressive reaction in approximately one-quarter of the cases. In this disorder, weakness and fatigability, the principal psychologic manifestations, are added to the bradykinesia, and the resulting therapeutic problem becomes formidable. Another hazard in Parkinson disease is the tendency for L-dopa itself to provoke a depression in a limited number of patients, sometimes with suicidal tendencies, paranoid ideation, and psychotic episodes. The treatment of depression with monoamine oxidase (MAO) inhibitors is contraindicated in patients receiving L-dopa. Huntington chorea is often associated with depression, even before the movement disorder and dementia become conspicuous; in one series, 10 of 101 patients with Huntington disease either committed suicide or attempted it. Also, Alzheimer disease is often accompanied by depressive symptoms, in which instance it is difficult or impossible to evaluate the relative contributions of the mood disorder and the dementia.

ENDOGENOUS DEPRESSION AND MANIC-DEPRESSIVE DISEASE

Definitions and Epidemiology

Manic-depressive disease is a disorder of mood consisting of prolonged episodes of depression, mania, or both. A traditional view of this disease was that of a periodic or cyclic condition in which one major mood swing was followed by an equal but opposite excursion. This is seldom the case, however. Episodes of depression are twice as frequent as manic ones, and the most common form of the illness is characterized by episodic depression alone. Recurrence of episodes of pure mania without interspersed episodes of depression is well known but relatively uncommon. As a consequence, manic-depressive psychosis has been divided into two subtypes: a *unipolar group*, in which only an endogenous depressive illness occurs, and a *bipolar group*, in which mania occurs with or without depression.

In addition, there are *mixed affective states*, in which symptoms of both depression and mania occur within a single episode of the illness. *Dysthymia* (formerly referred to as *depressive neurosis* or *neurotic depression*) is the name given to an extremely chronic and intermittent but relatively mild depressive illness. *Cyclothymic disorder* is the term applied to another mild affective syndrome in which there are swings in mood between hypomania and depression, the latter being of insufficient severity to meet the criteria for a major depressive episode. *Seasonal affective disorder* refers to a depression that recurs at a similar time each year, most often the winter; it is in most ways similar to the usual depressive illness except that it may respond to therapy with natural light. A rapid-cycling form of manic-depressive disease has been recognized in which four or more circumscribed episodes occur in a year. Like other variants of the disease, it tends to have an aberrant response to medication. Still other patients present with atypical features; instead of anorexia, weight loss, and insomnia, for example, they sleep and eat excessively. These patients are also difficult to treat. In adolescents, the latter symptoms are difficult to differentiate from the Kleine-Levin syndrome (page 598).

Manic-depressive psychosis was given its name by Kraepelin in 1896, and it was with him that our current clinical concept of this disorder originated. He viewed the manic and depressive attacks as opposite poles of the same underlying process and pointed out that, unlike dementia praecox (his name for schizophrenia), manic-depressive psychosis entails no intellectual deterioration with recurrent episodes.

The prevalence of manic-depressive disease cannot be stated with precision, mainly because of differing criteria for diagnosis. The apparent increase of the disease in the past 50 years probably reflects a growing awareness of the condition, among both physicians and the laity. Studies of large groups of patients from isolated areas of Iceland and the Danish islands of Bornholm and Samsø indicate that 5 percent of men and 9 percent of women will develop symptoms of depression, mania, or both at some time during their lives (Goodwin and Guze). The estimate for an American urban community (New Haven, Connecticut) is higher; the lifetime expectancy for an attack of major depression is 8 to 12 percent in men and twice this number in women (Weissman and Myers).

Manic-depressive disease occurs most frequently in middle and later adult years, with a peak age of onset between 55 and 65 for both sexes. However, a significant proportion of patients experience the first attack in childhood, adolescence, or early adult life. Depression is also a significant problem in the elderly; Blazer and Williams, who studied 997 persons over the age of 65 in North Carolina, found symptoms of a major depressive illness in 3.7 percent. The disease is two or three times more frequent among women. There is no known explanation for this difference, but some have speculated that just as many men are depressed, only they deny it or turn to alcohol. It was reported in the 1930s to be more common in individuals of Jewish and Irish ethnicity and among those in upper socioeconomic strata, but subsequent studies have not confirmed these findings. The bipolar variety occurs in about 10 percent of patients with affective disorder. Patients in the bipolar group have an earlier age of onset, more frequent and shorter cycles of illness, and a greater prevalence of affective disorder among their relatives than do patients with unipolar disease (Winokur).

Clinical Presentation

The fully developed endogenous depression may evolve within a few days, or, more often, it emerges more gradually, on a background of vague prodromal symptoms that had been present for months. A detailed description of the symptoms and signs of depression is given in Chap. 24. Here it need only be repeated that the patient expresses feelings of sadness, unhappiness, discouragement, hopelessness, and despondency, with loss of self-esteem. Reduced energy and activity, typically expressed as mental and physical exhaustion, is universally present, to the point of catatonia in the most severe cases. There is heightened irritability as well as a lack of interest in all activities that formerly were pleasurable. The patient tends to move slowly, sighing is frequent, and speech is reduced. The mental life of such an individual may narrow to a single-minded concern about his physical or mental decline or both. In dialogue, the patient's rejoinders become so stereotyped that the listener can soon predict exactly what is going to be said. There is a poverty of ideation as well as a notable absence of insight. Consciousness is clear, and though there is usually no evidence of a schizophrenic type of thought disorder, delusional ideas and less often hallucinations may be prominent in some patients, justifying the term *depressive psychosis*. The delusions are generally congruent with the patient's mood and are not as fixed or bizarre as those of schizophrenia or paranoia. In our experience, delusions are more common in older patients and tend to appear only after weeks or months of more typical symptoms of depression. In younger patients, delusions may take the form of beliefs or fears such as a concern about cancer or AIDS. Hallucinations, when they occur, are usually vocal and accusatory; their presence should always raise the possibility of an associated structural disease, drug intoxication, or alcoholic auditory hallucinosis.

Frequently, agitation and irascibility, rather than physical inactivity and mental slowness, are the principal behavioral abnormalities. The source of the agitation is an underlying anxiety state. Pacing the floor and wringing the hands, particularly in the early morning hours, are characteristic. Such patients tend to be overtalkative and vexed in their manner of expression, irritable, short-tempered, impatient, and intolerant of minor problems—changes noted mainly by family members. Attempts at reassurance may meet with initial success, only to be dispelled in the next rush of doubts. These patients remain impervious to reason and logic in respect to their symptoms, even though they are reasonable and logical to a variable degree in other areas of their lives. At its worst the illness takes the form of a depressive stupor; the patient becomes mute, indifferent to nutritional needs, and neglectful even of bowel and bladder functions (anergic depression). The condition at this time resembles catatonia. Such patients must be fed and their other needs attended to until therapy [usually electroconvulsive therapy (ECT)] brings about improvement.

The most important concern in patients with late-life depression is the risk of suicide. Since many of these individuals have reputations for being sound, dependable, and stable and deny being depressed, one's inclination is to doubt the possibility of self-destruction. *Such patients (and younger ones in whom suicidal ideation is suspected) should be questioned forthrightly on this subject*: Do they feel that life is not worthwhile? Have there been thoughts of suicide? Do they think themselves capable of committing suicide? Have they made such plans or made suicide attempts before? Do they own a firearm? Are they fearful of dying? Are they concerned about leaving their family without support? Do they have a religious view on suicide and share a religious proscription against it? Is there a family history of suicide? These questions relate to features that have been shown to put depressed individuals at risk of suicide. If, from their answers, they are judged to carry a risk of suicide, they should be directed to a psychiatrist.

The *manic state* is, in most ways, the mirror opposite of the depressed state, being characterized by a flight of ideas, motor and speech hyperactivity, and an increased appetite and sex urge. After a minimum of sleep, the patient awakes with enthusiasm and expectation. The manic individual appears to possess great drive and confidence yet lacks the ability to carry out his plans. Headstrong, impulsive, socially intrusive behavior is characteristic. The patient's judgment may be so impaired that he may make reckless investments, spend fortunes in gambling, and embark on extravagant shopping sprees. Setbacks do not perturb the patient, but rather act as goads to new activities. Euphoria and expansiveness sometimes bubble over into delusions of power and grandeur, which, in turn, may make the patient offensively aggressive. Up to a point, the patient's mirth and good spirits may be contagious, and others may join in the laughter; however, if the patient is thwarted, the warmth and good humor can suddenly change to anger. Irritability rather than elation may become the prevailing mood. The threshold for paranoid thinking is low, which makes the patient sensitive and suspicious. Personal neglect may reach the point of dishevelment and poor hygiene. In its most advanced form, a condition described as "delirious mania," the patient becomes totally incoherent and altogether disorganized in behavior. At this stage visual and auditory hallucinations and paranoid delusions may be rampant; furthermore, as the term *delirium* implies, the patient may be disoriented, with a clouded sensorium. Fortunately, this extreme is rarely encountered. As mentioned earlier, one observes patients with repeated attacks of mania without depression at any time, but this is rare.

Hypomania represents a milder degree of the disorder, but this term is also used loosely to depict behavior in a normally functioning individual who is unusually energetic and active. In this latter sense hypomania is a personality trait found in many talented and productive persons and need not arouse concern unless it is excessive and out of character for the individual. This is best determined by questioning the family.

First attacks of either depression or mania last an average of 6 months if untreated, although the range of duration of attacks varies greatly. With modern therapy, this can be reduced by more than half in most patients. Although most attacks of manic-depressive disease subside in a matter of months, a significant number, unipolar patients more than bipolar ones, remain chronically ill for long periods of time. According to Winokur and colleagues, 14 percent of their bipolar patients had not recovered after 2 years and 5 percent after 5 years. Comparative figures for primary unipolar patients were 19 and 12 percent, respectively. More than one-half of all depressed patients have one or more recurrences. Variables that are predictive of an unfavorable outcome are high degrees of neuroticism, long duration of illness before treatment, strongly positive family history, and presence of depression-provoking circumstances (Hirschfeld et al).

Diagnosis

According to DSM-IV, the essential diagnostic criteria of endogenous depression ("major depressive syndrome") consist of a dysphoric mood or loss of interest or pleasure in all usual activities (including sexual activity) in combination with at least four of the following seven symptoms: (1) disturbance of appetite and change in weight; (2) sleep disorder; (3) psychomotor retardation or agitation; (4) decreased energy and fatigue; (5) self-reproach, feelings of worthlessness or guilt; (6) indecisiveness, complaints of memory loss and difficulty in concentrating; and (7) thoughts of death or suicide or actual suicide attempts. Each of the four diagnostic symptoms should have been present for at least 2 weeks.

Adherence to the aforementioned criteria undoubtedly facilitates diagnosis, but not infrequently a single one of these symptoms so dominates the clinical picture as to suggest the diagnosis of another disease state and obscure the presence of an underlying depression. As mentioned earlier, depressed patients who are referred to the neurologist tend to complain inordinately of physical and cognitive symptoms and to minimize or deny the purely affective ones.

Complaints of fatigue, weakness, malaise, or widespread aches and pains, for example, suggest a variety of medical diseases, such as Addison disease, hypothyroidism, chronic infection, polymyositis, early rheumatoid arthritis, etc. Often the fatigue state is misinterpreted as muscular weakness, and this directs a medical search for neuromuscular or other neurologic disease. Similarly, complaints of persistent headache may suggest the presence of intracranial disease. Complaints of poor memory, inability to concentrate, and other cognitive impairments raise the question of a dementia—until it is found, by careful examination, that mental competence belies the patient's appraisal of his own presumed defects.

Hypochondriacal preoccupation with bowel and digestive functions accounts for repeated visits to the medical clinic. In one study, 21 of 120 such hypochondriacal patients were subsequently diagnosed as being depressed. Persistent insomnia may be the major complaint of the depressed patient. Early awakening is typical, and the morning hours are then the worst period of the day. Other patients have difficulty falling asleep, especially if there is an associated anxiety state. A complaint in the male of loss of libido and impotence is another monosymptomatic presentation; only with probing inquiry about other disturbances common to depression will the diagnosis become evident.

A number of psychologic testing scales are used to detect and score the severity of depression. Although they are utilized mainly for clinical studies and less for diagnostic purposes, several of them can be quite helpful in particular circumstances, since they are sensitive to one or another aspect of depression. They do not supplant the clinical examination in determining if an individual is depressed but may be helpful in differentiating depression from dementia and in detecting depression in cases where physical complaints are more prominent than psychic ones. The ones most familiar to neurologists are the Hamilton scale and the Beck scale, but others are used for research purposes.

In our experience, the following are some of the common and troublesome clinical situations in which it may prove difficult to recognize an underlying depression:

1. *Patients with chronic pain.* The association of chronic pain and depression has long been known. Patients who show this association are far from a homogeneous group. The special case of chronic headache, confronted often by neurologists, is mentioned below. In some patients with chronic pain, the symptoms and signs of depression are quite apparent. If the pain has been present for less than a year and had its onset at the same time as other depressive symptoms, response to antidepressant treatment is likely to be favorable.

Far more difficult to understand and to manage are patients with persistent pain as the only complaint; the head, face, and lower back are the most common loci. If an exhaustive search for the source of the pain proves unsuccessful, the conclusion is reached that the pain is "psychogenic." This attribution of pain to some obscure psychologic mechanism is hardly helpful, for usually no amount of exploration will reveal its source. Nevertheless, in a small proportion of such patients, pain will be alleviated by antidepressant drugs, suggestive, at least in these cases, of a linkage of the pain and depression.

In this group of patients, the problem is frequently made even more difficult by repeated surgical operations as well as dependency on analgesic drugs, which in themselves deplete energy and have other adverse effects. Such patients are to be found among those disabled after multiple operations for prolapsed intervertebral disc or arthritic hips or those with atypical facial pain. Where pain is the initial event (postherpetic neuralgia, for example), followed by chronicity of pain, abuse of drugs, chronic fatigue, and depressive symptoms, we tend to view the latter symptoms as reactive and direct our therapeutic efforts to the relief of both the pain and depression.

Intractable headaches may be the most prominent manifestation of depression. *Weeks or months of unremitting daily tension-type headaches in the context of a normal examination are highly suggestive of depression at any age.*

2. *Depression and alcoholism.* These are commonly associated, and it is important to determine which is primary and which is secondary. A depressive syndrome developing for the first time on a background of alcoholism (*secondary depression*) is a very common clinical occurrence. In a large series of alcoholics studied by Cadoret and Winokur, a secondary depression occurred in 30 of 61 females and in 41 of 112 males; moreover, once the alcoholism was established, depression became evident much earlier in the women than in the men. The opposite occurrence (i.e., the development of alcoholism on the background of a primary depression) is less common. Again, women are disproportionately affected. Moreover, women with primary depression and subsequent alcoholism have a higher incidence of affective disorder in first-degree relatives (Schuckit et al). As mentioned earlier, these differences may be spurious; Winokur's family studies suggest that the same genetic predisposition leads to depression in females and alcoholism and sociopathy in men.

3. *Depression in childhood and adolescence.* We have frequently observed depressive states in children, and they have often been misdiagnosed by both pediatricians and psychiatrists. The common manifestations have been chronic headache, refusal to go to school, withdrawal from social activities, anorexia, vomiting and weight loss, and scholastic failure. Nearly all of our cases of so-called male anorexia nervosa have proven to be due to depressive states. Puberty is a time of onset in many cases, but we have seen the disease in late childhood, and it is extremely frequent in high school and college students. It is a tragic mistake not to appreciate this fact and to be treating the patient for some presumed non-affective nervous symptoms, only to have the patient commit suicide. This has happened to more than a dozen of the children of our colleagues.

4. *Anxiety neurosis, hypochondriasis, and pseudodementia.* There are several other clinical circumstances in which an underlying depressive illness may not be immediately apparent but must always be suspected. One of these is the relatively acute development of anxiety or hypochondriacal symptoms in a young person. These symptoms are discussed in detail in the preceding chapter. The complaint of severe chronic fatigue without medical explanation should raise the same suspicion (Chap. 24). And always to be kept in mind in an elderly person with seemingly early signs of dementia is that this may, on closer examination, turn out to be a severe depressive illness (pseudodementia, page 453).

5. Depressive states with prominent affective and hallucinatory-delusional symptoms and disordered thinking—the so called schizothymic or schizoaffective syndrome. As will be pointed out in the next chapter, most such states will eventually be identified as instances of manic-depressive disease. However, they do bring into question the validity of our current classification of major psychoses.

Etiology

The following are the main theories, not mutually exclusive, that have been proposed to explain the origin of depression.

Genetic Factors The capacity to experience sadness and depression is common to all people. Although there is no question that depression can be provoked by misfortune and stressful life events, some individuals are more liable to depression than others who are subjected to similar psychosocial forces. In general, there seems to be a familial diathesis for most depressive illness, but especially for unipolar and bipolar affective disorder. Adopted children whose biologic parents had affective disorder were at greater risk of developing this disease than adoptees whose biologic parents were not affected (Mendlewicz and Rainer; Cadoret). The frequency of these illnesses is increased in the relatives of affected patients (prevalence rate of 14 to 25 percent in first-degree relatives). Furthermore, the type of illness tends to breed true, at least in the bipolar form, which is more common among relatives of bipolar patients than among relatives of unipolar patients. Similarly, the morbidity risk among first-degree relatives is increased (15 percent, in comparison to 1 to 2 percent risk in the general population). If all twin studies are taken together, 72 percent of monozygotic twins are concordant for bipolar disease, compared with 14 percent of same-sex dizygotic twins; comparative figures for unipolar disease are 40 percent and 11 percent, respectively (see Goodwin and Guze). All of these findings are indicative of a genetic factor. Although the exact pattern of inheritance has not been defined, the authors, from their personal experience, believe that a dominant mode of heredity with incomplete penetrance is likely. The gene(s) for manic-depressive disease remain to be discovered, and current theory holds that several of them are likely to be involved. One of the first indications that specific genes may alter the susceptibility to depression has been presented by Ogilvie and colleagues. They found that allelic variations in the serotonin transporter gene (the main target of the selective serotonin antidepressants) were associated with a greatly increased (sevenfold) risk of major depression. Not all studies agree on these points. Other hypotheses postulate susceptibility loci on chromosomes 18, 21, and X. As already stated, a single gene locus seems highly unlikely (see Sanders et al). However, findings such as these tie the genetic hypotheses to the biochemical ones, which are described next.

Biochemical Theories The biogenic monoamines (norepinephrine, serotonin, and dopamine) are the key elements in these theories. Following the observations that the tricyclic antidepressants and the MAO inhibitors exert their effect by increasing norepinephrine and serotonin at central adrenergic receptor sites in the limbic system and hypothalamus and that depression-provoking drugs (such as reserpine) deplete biogenic amines at these sites, the theory followed that naturally occurring depressions might be associated with a deficiency of these latter substances. Furthermore it was observed that depressed patients and their first-degree relatives, as well as healthy individuals, develop a greatly depressed mood after dietary depletion of the monoamine precursor tryptophan. Also noteworthy is the finding that concentrations of 3-methoxy-4-hydroxyphenylglycol (MHPG), a metabolite of norepinephrine, are subnormal in the cerebrospinal fluid (CSF) of patients with endogenous depression and elevated in manic states. Some neurochemical imaging studies, still preliminary, corroborate these findings. This view is supported by the finding that 5-hydroxyindoleacetic acid (5-HIAA), a deaminated metabolite of serotonin, is reduced in the CSF of depressed patients (Carroll et al). However, the aforementioned CSF findings have not been consistent; in some patients with depressive illnesses, the CSF concentrations of bioamine metabolites are entirely normal. Most of the neurochemical theories of depression have

PIRODSKY DM, COHN JS: *Clinical Primer of Psychopharmacology: A Practical Guide*, 2nd ed. New York, McGraw-Hill, 1992.

ROBINS E: *The Final Months: A Study of the Lives of 134 Persons Who Committed Suicide*. Oxford, Oxford University Press, 1981.

ROBINSON RG: Mood disorders secondary to stroke. *Semin Clin Neuropsychiatry* 2:244, 1997.

SADOCK BJ, SADOCK VA (eds): *Kaplan and Sadock's Comprehensive Textbook of Psychiatry*, 7th ed. Philadelphia, Lippincott Williams & Wilkins, 2000.

SANDERS AR, DETERA-WADLEIGH SD, GERSHON ES: Molecular genetics of mood disorders, in Charney DS, Nestler EJ, Bunney BS (eds): *Neurobiology of Mental Illness*. New York, Oxford University Press, 1999, pp 299–316.

SCHLESSER MA, WINOKUR G, SHERMAN BM: Hypothalamic-pituitary-adrenal axis activity in depressive illness. *Arch Gen Psychiatry* 37:737, 1980.

SCHUCKIT M, PITTS FN, REICH T, et al: Alcoholism: I. Two types of alcoholism in women. *Arch Gen Psychiatry* 20:301, 1969.

STARKSTEIN SE, FEDOROFF P, BERTHIER ML, ROBINSON RG: Manic-depressive and pure manic states after brain lesions. *Biol Psychiatry* 29:149, 1991.

STARKSTEIN SE, ROBINSON RG, PRICE TR: Comparison of cortical and subcortical lesions in the production of poststroke mood disorders. *Brain* 110:1045, 1987.

THOMSON KC, HENDRIE HC: Environmental stress in primary depressive illness. *Arch Gen Psychiatry* 26:130, 1972.

WEISSMAN NM, MYERS JK: Affective disorders in a U.S. urban community. *Arch Gen Psychiatry* 35:1304, 1978.

WILLNER P: Dopamine and depression: A review of recent evidence. *Brain Res Rev* 6:211, 225, 237, 1983.

WINOKUR G: *Mania and Depression: A Classification of Syndrome and Disease*. Baltimore, Johns Hopkins University Press, 1991.

WINOKUR G, CADORET RJ: The irrelevance of the menopause to depressive disease, in Sachar EJ (ed): *Topics in Psychoendocrinology*. New York, Grune & Stratton, 1975, pp 59–66.

WINOKUR G, CORYELL W, KELLER M, et al: A prospective follow-up of patients with bipolar and primary unipolar affective disorder. *Arch Gen Psychiatry* 50:457, 1993.

WISHNIE HA, HACKETT TP, CASSEM NH: Psychological hazards of convalescence following myocardial infarction. *JAMA* 215:1292, 1971.

Chapter 58

THE SCHIZOPHRENIAS AND PARANOID STATES

SCHIZOPHRENIA

Schizophrenia is among the most serious of all unsolved diseases. This was the opinion expressed almost 50 years ago in *Medical Research: A Mid-century Survey*, sponsored by the American Foundation. Because of a worldwide lifetime prevalence of about 0.85 percent and particularly because of its onset early in life, its chronicity, and the associated social, vocational, and personal disabilities, the same conclusion is probably justified today (Carpenter and Buchanan).

Definitions Neurologists and psychiatrists currently accept the idea that schizophrenia comprises a group of closely related disorders characterized by a particular type of disordered thinking, affect, and behavior. The syndromes by which these disorders manifest themselves differ from those of delirium, confusional states, dementia, and depression in ways that will become clear in the following exposition. Unfortunately, diagnosis depends on the recognition of characteristic psychologic disturbances largely unsupported by physical findings and laboratory data. This inevitably results in a certain diagnostic imprecision. In other words, any group of patients classified as schizophrenic will to some extent be "contaminated" by patients with diseases that only resemble schizophrenia, whereas variant or incomplete cases of schizophrenia may not have been included. Moreover, there is not full agreement as to whether all the conditions called schizophrenic are the expression of a single disease process. In America, for example, *paranoid schizophrenia* is usually considered to be a subtype of the common syndrome, whereas in Europe it is thought to be a separate disease.

Historical Background Present views of the disease we now call schizophrenia originated with Emil Kraepelin, a Munich psychiatrist, who first clearly separated it from manic-depressive psychosis. He called it *dementia praecox* (adopting the term introduced earlier by Morel) to refer to a deterioration of mental function, at an early age, from a previous level of normalcy. At first, Kraepelin believed that "catatonia" and "hebephrenia," which had previously been described by Kahlbaum and by Hecker, respectively, as well as the paranoid form of schizophrenia, were separate diseases, but later, by 1898, he had concluded that these were all subtypes of a single disease. Onset in adolescence and early adult life and the chronic course, often ending in marked deterioration of the personality, were emphasized as the defining attributes of all forms of the disease.

Early in the twentieth century, the Swiss psychiatrist Eugen Bleuler substituted the term *schizophrenia* for *dementia praecox*. This was an improvement insofar as the term *dementia* was already being used to specify the clinical effects of another category of disease, but unfortunately the new name implied a "split personality" or "split mind," a feature thought by Morton Prince to be typical of a neurosis. Nonetheless *schizophrenia* became and still is the accepted name for the disease. By the "splitting" of psychic functions, Bleuler meant the lack of correspondence between ideation and emotional display—the inappropriateness of the patient's affect in relation to his thoughts and behavior. (By contrast, in manic-depressive disease, the patient's mood and affect accurately express his morbid thoughts.) He also introduced the terms *autism* ("thinking divorced from reality") and *ambivalence* to describe particular aspects of schizophrenia, and called attention to a fourth syndrome, that of *simple schizophrenia*.

Bleuler believed that all the schizophrenic syndromes were composed of primary or basic symptoms, easily remembered as the "four A's" (loose *a*ssociations, flat *a*ffect, *a*mbivalence, and *a*utism), and of secondary or "partial phenomena" such as delusions, hallucinations, negativism, stupor, etc. However interesting this formulation proved to be, the psychologic abnormalities are so difficult to define precisely that this arbitrary division has been of only mnemonic value.

Other early theories were those of Adolf Meyer and Sigmund Freud. Meyer, who introduced the "psychobiologic approach" to psychiatry, sought the origins of schizophrenia, as well as other psychiatric syndromes, in the personal and medical history of patients and their habitual reactions to life events. Freud viewed schizophrenia as a manifestation of a "weak ego" and an inability to use the ego defenses to handle anxiety and instinctual forces—the result of a fixation of libido at an early ("narcissistic") stage of psychosexual development. Berze in 1914 singled out the "insufficiency and lowering of all psychic activity" as being the fundamental defect in schizophrenia and attributed it to organic damage of unknown nature. None of these theories has been corroborated, and none ever gained wide acceptance.

In 1937, Langfeldt advanced the important concept that schizophrenia consists principally of two different types of psychosis—namely, (1) a type that corresponds to the disease considered briefly above, i.e., Kraepelin's dementia praecox and Bleuler's schizophrenia (characterized essentially by early onset of anhedonia and asociality and by a poor prognosis), and (2) a type that occurs acutely, on a background of a stable premorbid personality, often with clouding of consciousness, prominent delusions and hallucinations, and demonstrable precipitating factors. For the second type, which could be a manifestation of several diseases, Langfeldt proposed the term *schizophreniform psychosis*. Cases of the latter type tend to have a favorable prognosis. Subsequent studies validated this distinction, as indicated further on.

A more contemporary biologic approach to the phenomenology of schizophrenia has involved the isolation of the many persistent mental and behavioral features and subjecting them to factor analysis. This has disclosed three clusterings of symptoms: (1) so-called negative symptoms of *diminished psychomotor activity* (poverty of speech and spontaneous movement, flatness of affect); (2) a *"disorganization" syndrome*, or thought disorder (fragmentation of ideas, loosening of associations, tangentiality, and inappropriate emotional expression); and (3) *reality distortion*, comprising hallucinations and delusions or so-called positive symptoms (Liddle; Liddle and Barnes). A separation of behavior into "positive" and "negative" symptoms was at one time thought to be useful in distinguishing among the types of schizophrenia and perhaps to reflect dysfunction of different neurochemical systems, but this view is an oversimplification (see review by Andreasen). Although there may still be disagreement as to whether each of these groups of symptoms is primary or secondary, positive or negative, they do lend themselves to objective study and correlation with other biologic parameters. And these syndromes correspond more or less with the more conventional clinical views of schizophrenia, described below.

Epidemiology Schizophrenia has been found in every racial and social group so far studied. The reported incidence rates vary considerably because not all psychiatrists have used the same diagnostic criteria. On average, 35 new cases per 100,000 population appear annually (Jablensky). As indicated above, studies of prevalence suggest that, at any given time, 0.85 percent of the world population is suffering from schizophrenia, and expectancy rates are estimated to be as high as 1000 per 100,000 (i.e., one chance in 100 that a person will manifest the condition during his or her lifetime).

Schizophrenic patients occupy about half the beds in mental hospitals—more hospital beds than are allocated to any other single disease. They constitute 20 to 30 percent of all new admissions to psychiatric hospitals (100,000 to 200,000 new cases per year in the United States); at any one time, about 300,000 such patients are in hospitals and 1.5 million are living outside. The age of admission to hospital is between 20 and 40, with a peak at 28 to 34 years. The economic burden created by this disease is enormous—in 1990, the direct and indirect costs in the United States were estimated to be $33 billion (Rupp and Keith).

The incidence of schizophrenia has remained more or less the same over the past several decades. Males and females are affected with equal frequency. For unknown reasons, the incidence is higher in social classes showing high mobility and disorganization. It has been suggested that deteriorating function caused by the disease results in a "downward drift" to the lowest socioeconomic stratum, where one finds poverty, crowding, limited education, and associated handicaps; but the same data have been used to support the idea that schizophrenia can be caused by such social factors. The fertility of schizophrenics, formerly lowered by institutionalization, is now approaching that of the general population, which will probably result in an increase in their number.

The Clinical Syndrome of Schizophrenia

Included in the early definitions of the disease, both of Kraepelin and of Bleuler, were a characteristic premorbid personality, an insidious onset of the more flagrant symptoms in adolescence or early adult life, and a chronic but fluctuating course with a tendency to progressive deterioration. Both regarded hallucinations and delusions as secondary or accessory symptoms that could be absent, as in their "dementia praecox simplex" or "simple schizophrenia." They emphasized the absence of primary disturbances of perception, orientation, memory, and other cognitive functions, which played such a large role in other cerebral diseases. Embodied in both their definitions was the concept of disease (rather than a psychopathologic reaction) characterized by a poor prognosis and a unique constellation of symptoms different from those of delirium, confusion, depression, mania, dementia, and other brain diseases.

Attempts to apply these diagnostic criteria met with difficulty, especially when hallucinations and delusions were absent. In order to overcome this difficulty, Schneider proposed that the distinction between primary and accessory manifestations be abandoned. He attached importance and reliability to the occurrence of auditory hallucinations, perceptual delusions (misinterpretation of what the patient hears and feels), and disturbances of thinking, often reflected in the experience that one's thoughts and actions are being broadcast and are not one's own but influenced by some outside agency (experiences of alienation and influence). This constellation of symptoms, which was precise and easy to recognize, came to be known as *Schneider's first-rank symptoms of active schizophrenia.*

Strict adherence to Schneider's diagnostic criteria, when applied to a group of patients admitted to the hospital with a diagnosis of schizophrenia, served to distinguish two groups of patients—those with and those without first-rank symptoms (Taylor). The former responded more poorly to treatment and required a more prolonged period in hospital and higher doses of neuroleptic drugs than the latter. The two groups correspond closely to the two categories of schizophrenic disorders recognized by Robins and Guze on the basis of prognosis. The Schneider-positive, poor-prognosis schizophrenia (also referred to as *nuclear* or *process schizophrenia*) corresponds closely to kraepelinian schizophrenia; many of the Schneider-negative patients with good prognosis are probably suffering from some other nonschizophrenic illness or the so-called schizophreniform illness of Langfeldt or manic-depressive disease ("hypomanic psychosis") (see Chap. 57).

From the neurologic point of view, the central abnormality in schizophrenia appears to be a special disorder in the perception of one's self in relation to the external world. It is unlike the condition that prevails in delirium and other confusional states, dementia, and depression. Some patients with chronic schizophrenia, before the onset of a flagrant psychosis or when in remission, show none of the schneiderian first-rank symptoms and—during brief testing of mental status—might even pass for normal. But on long-term observation they are vague and preoccupied with their own thoughts. They seem unable to think in the abstract, to fully understand figurative statements such as proverbs, or to separate relevant from irrelevant data. There is a circumstantiality and tangentiality about their remarks. They fail to communicate their ideas clearly. Their thinking no longer respects the logical limits of time and space. Parts are confused with the whole or are clustered together or condensed in an illogical way. Opposites may be considered as identical, and conceptual relationships are distorted. In an analysis of a problem or a situation, there is a tendency to be overinclusive rather than underinclusive (as happens in dementia). In conversation and in writing, the trend of an argument or thought sequence is often interrupted abruptly, with a resulting disorder of verbal communication. Such disorders of thinking are reflected in the patient's behavior; there is a general deterioration in functioning, social withdrawal and at times bizarre actions, idleness, self-absorption, and aimlessness. Lack of initiative, drive, and interest, blunting of affect, and anhedonia are subtle features that may pass unnoticed.

In more severely affected schizophrenics, thinking is even more disintegrated. They appear to be totally preoccupied with their inner psychic life (autism) and may do no more than utter a series of meaningless phrases or neologisms, or their speech may be reduced to a "word salad." They are unable to attend to any task or to concentrate, and their performance is interrupted by sudden "blocking" or by insertion of some extraneous idea or inexplicable act, somewhat like that observed in a severely confused or delirious patient. At times these patients are talkative and exhibit odd behavior; at other times they are quiet and idle; in the extreme, the patients are mute or assume and maintain imposed postures or remain immobile (catalepsy). With remission, they may remember much of what has happened or they may have only fragmentary memories of events that occurred during the exacerbation of their illness.

Highly characteristic of schizophrenia is the patient's expression of remarkably unusual experiences and ideas. The patient may express the thought that his body is somehow separated from his mind, that he does feel like himself, that his body belongs to someone else, or that he is unsure of his own identity or even sex. These experiences have been called *depersonalization*. *Thought insertion*, wherein it seems to the patient that an idea has been implanted into his mind, or *thought withdrawal*, wherein an idea has been extracted from his mind by an outside agency, are other parts of this state. Closely related, and characteristic of schizophrenia, are the ideas of being under the control of some external agency or being made to speak or act in ways that are dictated by others, often through the medium of radar, telepathy, and so on (*passivity feelings*). Frequently, there are *ideas of reference*—that the remarks or actions of others are subtly or overtly directed to the patient. Finally, the patient may feel that the world about him is changed or unnatural, or his perception of time may be altered, not in a brief episode like the *jamais vu* of a temporal lobe seizure, but continuously. This is the phenomenon of *derealization*.

Auditory hallucinations are frequent; they consist of voices that comment on the patient's character and activities and are usually accusatory, threatening, or claiming control of the patient's actions. The voices may or may not be recognized; they may belong to one person or two or more persons who converse with the patient or with one another. Seldom can the voices be localized to a point outside the patient. Instead, they seem to come from within the patient, in which case they cannot be distinguished from his own feelings and thoughts. Certain somatic hallucinations and delusions may predominate. Visual, olfactory, and other types of hallucinations also occur but are much less frequent. The patient believes in the reality of these hallucinations and often weaves them into a delusional system.

Of recent interest has been the belated affirmation of the importance of negative symptoms in schizophrenia. Liddle and Barnes, looking objectively at all aspects of schizophrenic thought and behavior, divided them into four groups: (1) flat affect, diminution in expressive gestures, latency of response, physical asynergia, reduced spontaneous movements, apathy, restricted recreational activities, inability to feel intimate or close, and motor retardation. These negative symptoms correlated with reduced blood flow in the frontal lobes and a bad prognosis. (2) Disorganization of thought, incoherence, inappropriate affect, illogicality, bizarre behavior, aggression, agitation, and tangentiality. These abnormalities are nonfrontal. (3) Hallucinations and delusions that the patient's mind is being read and that his thoughts are being extracted from his mind or being controlled or broadcasted. (4) Suspicion, hostility, and delusions of reference. These authors also found an overlap of symptoms from one syndrome to another, i.e., the four syndromes can coexist in various combinations. However valid such subdivisions prove to be, they are of importance in offering a more neurologic approach to schizophrenia and in directing attention to the functional anatomy and physiology of particular neuronal systems in the brain (see further on; also Friston et al).

The behavior of the individual experiencing these ideas and feelings is correspondingly altered. Early in the course of the illness, normal activities may be slowed or interrupted. No longer does the patient function properly in school or at work. Associates and relatives are likely to find the patient's complaints and ideas disturbing. The patient may be idle for long periods—preoccupied with inner ruminations—and may withdraw socially. A panic or frenzy of excitement may lead to an emergency ward visit (a high degree of anxiety occurring for the first time in a young person should always raise the suspicion of a developing schizophrenia); or the patient may become mute and immobile, i.e., *catatonic*. However, attacks of catatonia are infrequent, and lack of will, drive, assertiveness, etc., is more characteristic of the disease.

Much has been made of the change in affect. Usually the affect is said to be "flat," i.e., the patient's manner is bland or apathetic; he may casually express ideas that would be disturbing to a normal person, even smiling or laughing over a morbid idea. To the authors, this has not been an impressive feature of the illness. Often one observes agitation and an appropriate display of emotion in response to a threatening hallucination or delusion, although later there appears increasing indifference and preoccupation, as though the patient had become inured to the abnormal thoughts and feelings.

Other behavioral and delusional features are discussed in relation to the special types of schizophrenia.

Subtypes of Schizophrenia

Psychiatrists have traditionally distinguished a number of subtypes of schizophrenia, although the usefulness of these distinctions has been questioned in recent years. Indeed, the various types may overlap or change during the course of the illness. And there are cases that do not conform entirely to the conventional subtypes or display characteristics of more than one type (referred to as *undifferentiated* or mixed types). Despite these caveats, the subtyping of schizophrenia still has descriptive value and carries the imprimatur of DSM-IV, for which reasons the traditional categories are briefly reviewed here.

Simple Schizophrenia In this least florid form, the patient exhibits thought disorder, bland affect, social withdrawal, and reduction in speech and movement, all of which impair work performance; however, hallucinations and delusions are absent. Poverty of psychomotor activity is the dominant feature. At this stage the diagnosis is often uncertain. A disorder of thinking may be difficult to elicit, but from time to time a peculiar idea emerges in conversation or is discovered in letters. Objective study of thinking, by means of formal psychologic tests (Solovay et al), has shown it in most instances to be "disorganized, confused, and ideationally fluid with many peculiar words and phrases." This is a refinement of Bleuler's characterization of "loosening of associations." Terms such as *schizoid*, *schizotypal*, *latent*, or *borderline schizophrenia* have been applied to this form of the illness. This seems to be an extension of the childhood schizoid personality traits into adolescence. Eventually, an outbreak of flagrant hallucinations and delusions occurs—an acute schizophrenic episode that brings the patient to the attention of a physician. The patient usually needs to be hospitalized and be given medication because of a suicidal or, rarely, homicidal attempt or some other unexpected behavioral abnormality. As a rule, a remission follows within a few weeks or months, during which the patient is again able to function, but at a level below that which is expected on the basis of his natural abilities and intelligence, and he continues to be lacking in normal drive, initiative, and enterprise, much as he was before the outbreak. These patients attract notice because they behave in an odd manner, tending to remain by themselves ("loners"), making no effort to adjust to a social group at school or to find work, "have dates," or establish a family unit. If the parents do not provide support and protection, such persons drift from one menial job to another, always shy, withdrawn, and relatively indifferent to their surroundings. Some individuals of this type roam the streets and live in appalling conditions on the fringes of society.

Catatonic Schizophrenia This, the most readily differentiated type of schizophrenia, is now quite rare. Characterized by an extreme diminution in psychomotor activity, it was originally described by Kahlbaum and considered to be a mental disturbance sui generis until Kraepelin recognized that it was another form of schizophrenia. In about 60 percent of cases, the onset is relatively acute. In the remainder, after a long prodrome of slackening interest, apathy, and dreamy preoccupation, a state of dull stupor supervenes, with mutism, inactivity, refusal of food, and a tendency to maintain one position "like a mummy" (*catalepsy*). The facial expression is vacant, the lips are pursed; the patient lies supine without motion or sits for hours with hands on knees and head bowed (catalepsy). If a limb is lifted by the examiner, it will sometimes be held in that position for hours (*flexibilitas cerea*). Urine and feces are retained or there is incontinence. The patient must be tube-fed (or will eat mechanically) and has to be dressed and undressed. Pinprick or pinch induces no reaction. Extreme negativism, every command being resisted, characterizes some cases. Echolalia and echopraxia are observed occasionally. Yet these patients may be fully aware of what is said to them or happening around them and will reproduce much of this information during a spontaneous remission or one induced by intravenous sodium amytal. Even if untreated, the patient, after weeks or months in this state, begins to talk and act more normally, and there is then rapid recovery. In certain phases of catatonia there may be a period of excitement and impulsivity, during which the patient may be suicidal or homicidal.

As mentioned, and for reasons that are unclear, this form of schizophrenia is now seen infrequently, and there is increasing recognition of the fact that many of its features are often manifestations of a depressive illness rather than of schizophrenia.

Disorganized, or Hebephrenic, Schizophrenia This was believed by Kraepelin to be a particularly malignant form. It tends to occur at an earlier age than the other varieties, hence the prefix *hebe* ("youth"). The thought disorder is pronounced—there is a striking incoherence of ideas and a grossly inappropriate affect; the frequent occurrence of hallucinations and delusions leaves little doubt that the patient is psychotic. The visual and auditory illusions and hallucinations are usually more in the nature of symbolic interpretations than abnormal perceptions. Kraepelin remarked on the changeable, fantastic, and bizarre character of the delusions. Motor symptoms, in the form of grimacing, stereotyped mannerisms, and other oddities of behavior, are prominent. In hebephrenic patients, since early life, there is likely to have been a history of tantrums and of being overly pious, shy, fearful, solitary, conscientious, and idealistic—traits that may have marked these individuals as odd. This latter state corresponds to what was referred to earlier on as a *schizoid personality* but could just as well represent the early phase of the disease itself (see Chap. 56).

Paranoid Schizophrenia This is one of the most frequent types. The mean age of onset is 42 years, later than that of the preceding types (Winokur). The central feature is the preoccupation with one or more delusions, accompanied by auditory hallucinations and related to a single theme. More often than not, the delusional-hallucinatory content is persecutory, but it may also be religious, depressive, grandiose, or bizarrely hypochondriacal in nature. Delusional jealousy may be added. Many such patients settle into a chronic hallucinatory psychosis with disorders of thinking, featured by mistrust and suspiciousness. They appear cold, aloof, and indifferent.

Many psychiatrists, impressed with the lack of schizoid traits in the premorbid period and in the family history, have insisted that paranoid schizophrenia is a separate disease. The studies of Rosenthal and colleagues tend to bear them out. Also, the clinical and family studies of Winokur indicate that simple, catatonic, and hebephrenic schizophrenias are probably different illnesses from paranoid schizophrenia.

There are, of course, other psychiatric illnesses in which paranoid delusions appear, notably manic-depressive psychosis, dementia, and delirium. Alcoholic auditory hallucinosis stands as a separate illness (page 1240). There is, in addition, a special form of *delusional disorder (paranoia)* in which the individual is consumed by a single persecutory, grandiose, or amorous delusional system without any other disorder of thinking. An exotic form is known as *folie à deux*, in which two closely related persons share a delusional system. These several types of paranoia are discussed further on in this chapter.

Acute Schizophreniform Psychosis A special problem arises in the diagnosis of a rapidly evolving psychotic syndrome with florid hallucinations and delusions that clear in several weeks or less, with or without treatment. This so-called *acute schizophrenia* most often turns out to be the initial attack of mania or intoxication with a psychotropic-hallucinogenic drug, for which reason it is not accorded a separate subtype of schizophrenia. The resolution of the diagnostic dilemma often depends on the patient's premorbid status and the course of events that follows the acute episode. This topic is discussed further on under "Diagnosis," below.

Suicide in Schizophrenia That schizophrenia of all types carries a significant risk of suicide is not generally appreciated. In a 30- to 40-year follow-up study of schizophrenic and manic-depressive patients, Winokur and Tsuang found that in each group the proportion of patients who had committed suicide was the same (about 10 percent). Suicide occurs most often among young schizophrenics living apart from their families who are frightened and overwhelmed by their symptoms and the difficulties of independent existence. Sometimes suicide is a response to terrifying and commanding vocal hallucinations. The schizophrenic may also be homicidal, usually acting upon a delusion that he or she has been wronged by the victim. Incidents of this type are unpredictable, but the presence of escalating paranoia should be a warning.

Remissions and Exacerbations Some schizophrenic patients are subject to periodic exacerbations of their illness, sometimes at regular intervals, as though their illness were determined by a metabolic disorder. Functional remissions are more frequent and lasting when medication is given and long institutionalization is avoided. A small proportion of patients (about 10 percent, according to Kety and Matthysse), after an acute schizophrenic episode, have a long-lasting and fairly complete remission before lapsing into a chronic form of the illness. Unfortunately, these latter patients, at the time of their acute psychosis, cannot be distinguished from those who will have a permanent remission.

Modern therapeutic programs have reduced the number of patients in mental hospitals by 1 to 2 percent per year. However, readmission rates have also risen (revolving-door phenomenon), and the total number of very young and very old patients in hospitals has even increased slightly. The life expectancy of schizophrenics is somewhat reduced, possibly because of the malnutrition, neglect, and exposure to infections that occur in some public institutions and from living on the streets or in marginal circumstances.

Neurologic and Neuropsychologic Abnormalities in Schizophrenia

The early findings of Kraepelin and of Bleuler, that many schizophrenic patients will, on detailed examination, show some neurologic abnormalities, have been amply substantiated by Stevens, Kennard, Hertzig and Birch, Tucker and colleagues, and Woods. They have all found a much higher frequency of "soft neurologic signs" in schizophrenics than in a normal population. The soft signs to which they refer include impersistence in assigned tasks, astereognosis and graphesthesia, sensory extinction, hyperreflexia and hyporeflexia, slight tendency to grasping, mild impairment of coordination and disturbances of balance, abnormal (choreiform) movements, abnormalities of motor activity, adventitial and overflow movements, anisocoria, esotropia, and faults in visual auditory integration. Some of these signs were objectified by the Goldstein-Scherer object-sorting test and the Halstead-Reitan tactual performance test. Signs of this type were noted in 50 percent of patients and correlated with the degree of cognitive disorder. Also evident in about one-half of schizophrenics are defects in ocular tracking movements (Levin et al). These take the form mainly of slowed smooth pursuits and intrusions of saccades during pursuit; some relatives of schizophrenics show these eye signs when carefully tested. "Hard signs" (such as unilateral motor or sensory defects) are not seen. Electroencephalographic (EEG) abnormalities have been noted in about one-third of all patients but are generally minor. The meaning of these slight EEG abnormalities is conjectural. They are more frequent in the group of schizophrenic patients who have a positive family history and are found to have enlarged ventricles (Murray et al).

Sophisticated psychometric testing has disclosed abnormalities not so much in intelligence and memory (which are only slightly reduced in 20 to 30 percent of cases) as in other psychologic functions. Alertness is not impaired, but the ability to maintain attention, as measured by continuous performance tasks, is reduced (Seidman). Except where muteness is a feature, no measurable alteration of language function or calculation has been reported. In tests of verbal and visual pattern learning, problem solving, and memorizing, Cutting found a surprising degree of impairment in both acute and chronic schizophrenic patients (and in patients with retarded depression) not attributable to electroconvulsive therapy, seizures, drugs, or other diseases. In the acute schizophrenic patient, verbal memory was more affected than visual pattern memory, in agreement with the findings of Flor-Henry that left-hemispheric functions are more reduced than right-sided ones; in the chronic schizophrenic, there was evidence of bihemispheral impairment.

Theories of Causation and Mechanism

Although there is no universal agreement as to the cause of the disease, an increasing weight of evidence favors a genetic basis. There is also emerging evidence that a genetic proclivity may be manifest by alterations in certain neurochemical pathways of the brain. Other biologic, brain developmental, and psychosocial factors are also considered important. The evidence for each is presented below. A more detailed analysis of potential causes than can be given here may be found in the reviews of Waddington, of Carpenter and Buchanan, of Harrison, and, most recently, of Pearlson.

Genetic Factors The early studies of Kallmann showed that the frequency of schizophrenia in 5000 siblings of schizophrenic patients was 11 percent, in contrast to 1 percent (or slightly less) in the general population. In 90 sets of fraternal twins of whom one had schizophrenia, the incidence of disease in the other twin was also 11 percent, the same as in nontwin siblings; however, in 62 sets of monozygotic twins, the incidence in the second twin was 68 percent. In other words, the closer the relatedness of a family member to a schizophrenic, the greater the risk of schizophrenia for that individual. Thus, the risk that the child of a schizophrenic parent will develop schizophrenia is the same as that for the sibling of a schizophrenic patient (i.e., 11 percent); if one sibling and one parent have schizophrenia, the risk is 17 percent; if both parents are schizophrenic, the chances are 46 percent that the child will have the disease. Subsequent family and twin studies have repeatedly confirmed these findings (see Goodwin and Guze for a more complete tabulation). It is noteworthy that the penetrance of this inherited trait appears to be less than for manic-depressive disease.

Although the importance of genetic factors in the etiology of schizophrenia is undeniable, a mendelian pattern of inheritance has not been determined. Nor have any chromosomal loci or gene abnormalities been unequivocally incriminated by molecular genetic or linkage analysis (Kendler). Several sites, particularly on chromosomes 6 and 13, seem to confer some susceptibility to developing the disease but are in themselves inadequate to explain its occurrence. One of these, an allelic variation in the gene that codes for serotonin receptors, is appealing because it ties genetic with neurochemical changes, as discussed further on.

There has been much discussion in the medical literature concerning the relative importance of genetic and environmental factors in the causation of the disease. The lack of complete concordance between monozygotic twins and the fact that approximately 80 percent of patients diagnosed as schizophrenic have no other family members with the disease indicate that factors other than genetic ones must play a role. In the study of Rosenthal et al, a group of children of schizophrenics were removed at an early age from their natural parents and placed in adoptive homes; these children were compared with a group of adopted children whose natural parents had no known psychiatric disease. Follow-up observations disclosed that the incidence of schizophrenia in the first group of children was about twice that in the second. In two similar studies, both Karlsson and Heston showed that children who were separated early in life and reared apart from schizophrenic parents had the same disposition to schizophrenia (11 percent) as children of schizophrenics raised in the homes of their biologic parents. Fischer approached the problem differently. Monozygotic twins, only one of whom was schizophrenic, were identified and their children were studied; the incidence of schizophrenia in the children of the nonschizophrenic member of the twin pair was the same as that in the children of the schizophrenic member.

Developmental Abnormalities The neuropsychiatric literature contains numerous bits of evidence that schizophrenia is a developmental disorder consequent upon brain injury during the intrauterine or neonatal period. Reportedly there is an increased incidence of complications during the gestational period and birth of schizophrenics. Others have proposed that damage to the temporal lobes from intrauterine or perinatal injury or a genetic factor that predicates both the injury and mental disorder is involved. In the northern latitudes, more schizophrenics are born in the winter months and to women who were exposed to influenza during midpregnancy—inviting speculation that a viral infection may have damaged the fetal brain. Mortenson and colleagues found that being born in an urban region, particularly in February or March, carried with it a higher risk for developing the disease than having an affected parent or sibling. They suggested that these inexplicable demographic features accounted for more cases than did inheritance. Jones and colleagues reported on a cohort of 5362 infants who were followed prospectively since their birth in 1946. As a group, the 30 individuals who later developed schizophrenia were delayed in the attainment of motor milestones and speech and exhibited greater social withdrawal and schoolroom anxiety as well as lower scholastic achievement. Thus it appears that schizophrenic patients are not normal in early childhood, but whether their abnormalities are already early manifestations of schizophrenia or risk factors for the disease has not been determined.

Notably lacking in all these reports are neuropathologic data. However, in recent years a number of reports, using special cell-labeling studies, have found cytoarchitectonic abnormalities in the brains of schizophrenics. For example, Akbarian and colleagues, following previous similar findings, have described a maldistribution of interstitial neurons in the frontal lobe white matter. These cells have their origin in the embryologic subplate that guides neuronal migration, and the inference is that the abnormally migrating cells have formed aberrant neuronal connections. Benes and colleagues observed that the number of small neurons was reduced in at least one layer (usually layer II) of the anterior cingulate cortex. These are GABA-releasing (inhibitory) neurons. She also noted that the arrays of macrocolumns of cortical neurons were smaller in the occipital lobes (vertical axons increased in number), but without gliosis. These observations suggest a developmental rather than an acquired lesion, and the absence of gliosis supports but does not prove the hypothesis that the developmental disorder occurs prenatally. Other aspects pertaining to developmental changes and neuronal density are discussed further on.

Neurotransmitter and Metabolic Abnormalities When certain hallucinogens, such as mescaline and lysergic acid diethylamide (LSD), were first observed to induce hallucinations and abnormalities of thinking, it was hoped that these drugs might provide experimental models of schizophrenia. This hope was never realized, but there are instances, difficult to interpret, in which these drugs induced a prolonged relapse in a schizophrenic patient. Similarly, when methionine, a potent source of methyl groups, was observed to exacerbate the symptoms of some schizophrenic patients, it was thought that a primary metabolic fault had been discovered; increased serum concentrations of dimethoxyphenylethylamine and *N*-methylated indoleamines lent support to this idea. Again, none of these observations has been unequivocally corroborated.

The leading *biochemical hypothesis* has been based on the response of psychotic symptoms to phenothiazine medications, which allegedly implicate the dopaminergic system of the temporal lobe (see review of Carlsson). The evidence for this hypothesis is circumstantial but is supported by observations that antipsychotic drugs reduce the electrical activity of mesolimbic dopaminergic neurons in experimental models. Further, there have been several demonstrations of increased concentrations of dopamine or its metabolite, homovanillic acid, in schizophrenic brains obtained at autopsy. The finding that dopamine receptors are organized in two systems, one mesolimbic and the other mesocortical, led to an expanded but purely speculative hypothesis that an excess of dopaminergic activity in the mesolimbic system gives rise to the positive symptoms of schizophrenia—i.e., psychosis—whereas a diminished activity in the mesocortical system accounts for the negative symptoms. The involvement of the mesolimbic system, which plays a role in attention, has prompted further speculation that the thought disorder of schizophrenia is attributable to a breakdown of the normal "filtering" of stimuli reaching cognition. Yet another theory, seeking to explain the late-adolescent onset of schizophrenia, supposes that intrauterine damage to temporal lobe dopaminergic pathways is somehow unmasked by the developmental changes that occur during this period of life.

Since the antipsychotic drugs display an affinity for dopamine receptors, it has been widely concluded that these drugs produce their therapeutic effects (and side effects) by receptor blockade. Other hypotheses have proposed a reduction in dopaminergic transmission, implicating neurotransmitters such as norepinephrine, acetylcholine, serotonin (see below), and gamma-aminobutyric acid (GABA), which interact or maintain a balance with dopamine. The many hypotheses concerning the role of dopamine receptors and other neurotransmitters in the pathophysiology of schizophrenia, none of them entirely convincing, have been reviewed by Sedvall and Farde.

Second only to the dopaminergic hypotheses of schizophrenia are the serotoninergic hypotheses. As with the dopaminergic model, attention was drawn to mechanisms relating to serotonin when a new class of antipsychotics (clozapine, risperidone), which have effects on the latter system, were found to ameliorate the psychosis. Several groups have reported alterations in serotonin receptors in the brains of schizophrenics (see below). A further connection is based on the finding by Williams and colleagues of an allelic variation in the gene on chromosome 13 encoding for a serotonin receptor (5-HT_{2A}) that confers a susceptibility to schizophrenia. A similar finding has been reported in a Japanese population. The variation in this gene is not sufficient to cause schizophrenia, if for no other reason than that many patients who are homozygous for the suspect allele do not have the disease and the allelic variations do not alter its protein product. Perhaps a nearby region relating to the receptor may be at fault through linkage disequilibrium (see commentary by Harrison and Geddes).

Also, there have been many attempts to isolate some metabolite or toxic substance from the blood of schizophrenic patients that could reproduce the clinical state when injected into nonschizophrenic subjects. Such positive results as were claimed have not been verified. From time to time an aminoaciduria, a folate or vitamin B_{12} deficiency, or some other condition has been discovered in a psychotic patient who is said to have schizophrenia, but isolated findings of this sort in patients in whom the diagnosis can be questioned have little meaning. Usually such symptomatic psychoses are of brief duration, which is the reason why, in the American Psychiatric Association's *Diagnostic and Statistical Manual of Mental Disorders* (DSM-IV), one of the diagnostic criteria of schizophrenia is that the symptoms must have been continuous for at least 6 months.

A great variety of physiologic and endocrine differences between schizophrenic and normal subjects have been claimed. None has proved to be significant. Since psychoses may complicate corticosteroid administration and certain endocrine disorders (Cushing syndrome, thyrotoxicosis), there have been many attempts to uncover such abnormalities in the schizophrenic patient. All have failed.

Psychosocial Factors The notion that psychosocial factors play an important role in the genesis of schizophrenia was a recurrent theme in older psychiatric writings but is now given little credence. Prominent in these early writings was Freud's view, already mentioned, that the schizophrenic process represents a fixation at an early autoerotic stage of sexual development. There is no way of affirming or refuting this proposition. The same can be said for the many suggestions that disturbed intrafamily relationships were responsible for engendering schizophrenic traits or possibly provoking psychosis in persons who are genetically vulnerable. Behind all these suggestions was the notion that disturbed interpersonal relations in the family in some way interfered with the normal maturation of personality. Adolf Meyer believed that schizophrenia was a reaction to a series of traumatic life situations—a maladaptive response to some organic, psychologic, or sociologic factor. Others have stressed the importance of disturbed interpersonal relationships. However, with all these hypotheses, proof is totally lacking that such environmental factors are unique to the development of schizophrenia. Furthermore, the extent to which these aberrations of family relationships are primary or secondary cannot be ascertained.

The often cited observations of Harlow on the deleterious effects of maternal and peer deprivation in primates suggested the notion that similar deprivations in humans were responsible for the development of schizophrenia. However, such severe degrees of familial deprivation have rarely been documented in humans; when they were, as in some orphans, the effects were only transitory.

Neuropathologic and Neurophysiologic Findings

Kraepelin conceived of schizophrenia (*dementia praecox*, in his terminology) as a disease process that was organic and progressive. For the following hundred years this insightful clinical judgment stimulated neuropathologists in a search for its histologic basis. Alzheimer and his pupils, who had access to Kraepelin's pathologic material, made a study of 55 cases, including 18 of the uncomplicated and 6 of the acute type. They noted hypertrophy ("ameboid" change) of the astrocytes, to which importance was attached because this change was not found in cases of manic-depressive psychosis. Further, in the cerebra of deteriorated schizophrenics, an outfall of neurons in the second and third laminae of the frontal cortex was described, along with nuclear swelling, shrinkage of cell bodies, and deposits of lipofuscin. Similar findings were subsequently described by others.

Dunlap, in 1928, in a critical analysis, repudiated all earlier interpretations of these alterations. He pointed out that many changes, such as the dark "sclerotic" nerve cells, were artifacts and that lipofuscin was a nonspecific age change. He asserted also that the neuronal loss described by Alzheimer was based on impression and could not be corroborated by quantitative methods. Similarly, the claim of Oscar Vogt of neuronal loss in the cortex was rejected by his contemporaries, Spielmeyer and Scholz, who were unable to find any consistent cellular abnormality in schizophrenia. Spielmeyer, in a critical study of the problem in 1930, concluded that such changes as had been described up to that time could not be clearly distinguished from the normal, and that the more marked changes in some cases were likely due to coincidental causes (age, complicating disease, etc.). Corsellis, on the basis of yet another review of the neuropathologic data in 1976, found no reasons to deviate from Spielmeyer's view. The uncertain meaning of the neuropathologic findings was responsible for the enigmatic categorization of schizophrenia as a "functional" disorder, i.e., a disorder with no structural basis.

The advent of computed tomography and subsequently of magnetic resonance imaging of the brain provided a new stimulus to the anatomic study of schizophrenia. Johnstone et al were the first to describe ventricular enlargement and sulcal widening in 18 patients and correlate these findings with dulling of intellect and affect. In a study of 58 chronic schizophrenics under the age of 50 years, Weinberger and colleagues found enlargement of the lateral ventricles in 40 percent. In 9 of 11 CT studies, the third ventricle was found to be enlarged, and in 14 of 17 studies, the sulci were widened. In 15 pairs of monozygotic twins, one of whom had schizophrenia, the anterior hippocampi were found to be smaller and the lateral and third ventricles larger in the affected twin (Suddath et al). Shenton and colleagues have demonstrated a reduction in the volume of gray matter in the posterior part of the left superior temporal gyrus, which includes Heschl's gyri and the planum temporale. The degree of volumetric reduction correlated with the severity of the thought disorder. The reduction in volume of the superior temporal gyrus has also been associated with the occurrence of auditory hallucinations (Barta et al). Other MRI studies have shown a volumetric change in the gray matter of the left hippocampus, parahippocampal gyrus, and amygdala (in right-handed patients). Equally compelling is the finding that young individuals having two or more relatives with the disease, and therefore being at risk for developing schizophrenia, have certain volumetric brain changes detected by imaging studies (Lawrie et al). In unaffected relatives, the left hippocampal-amygdaloid region was smaller than in normals and slightly larger than in affected relatives.

In summarizing the many cerebral changes observed in schizophrenics, Harrison concluded that some are quite consistent. These include mild enlargement of the lateral and third ventricles; decreased cortical volume, perhaps disproportionate in the temporal lobe; and—microscopically—diminution in size of cortical and hippocampal neurons; a diminished number of neurons in the dorsal thalamus; and a notable absence of gliosis. There has been a general sense that the number of neurons in the gray matter is normal, but the pyramidal cells are smaller and more densely packed, resulting in a thinning of laminae II and III. The cytoarchitectonic changes have been the most difficult to interpret and to confirm. Capricious methods such as the rapid Golgi stain indicate that density of dendritic spines is decreased in the frontal and temporal cortex of chronic schizophrenics. The observations of Benes et al, pointing to cytoarchitectonic developmental disorders in fetal life, have already been mentioned under "Developmental Abnormalities."

There are also a number of neurochemical changes in the striatum and cortex, mainly in dopamine content and dopamine receptor density, but all are probably attributable to treatment with dopamine blocking drugs. The exception may be a decrease in 5-HT_{2A} receptors in the cortex, which is found even in untreated patients.

Detailed neuropsychologic testing has disclosed deficits in attention and abnormalities of the P300 waves (cortical "event-related" potentials). These deficits correlate with reduced cognitive activation activity in functional MRI. It is unclear, however, if these changes represent primary defects or are secondary to an inherent lack of motivation.

From these neuroradiologic findings, Murray and coworkers have asked whether there are at least two types of this disease—one with ventricular enlargement and a negative family history and the other (approximately two-thirds of the whole group) with normal ventricles and a positive family history. In the first group of sporadic, "acquired" schizophrenia, environmental factors, such as birth injury and EEG abnormalities (see below), were thought to be more frequent.

A special problem in all morphologic studies relates to the accuracy of the clinical diagnosis and whether the study was made on the brains of patients in the early or late (deteriorated) stage of the disease. As pointed out by Davison and Bagley, many of the psychologic and behavioral characteristics of schizophrenia occur in Wilson disease, Huntington chorea, temporal lobe epilepsy, chronic alcoholism, and other metabolic encephalopathies, such as the neuronal storage diseases. Hence one may be observing a clinical syndrome of multiple etiologies, some with an identifiable morphologic substratum. Theoretically, true schizophrenia may be affecting the same regions of the brain but presently without a consistent demonstrable cytopathology.

Despite the uncertainties that still surround this subject, there can be no doubt, from the anatomic data outlined above, that schizophrenia is a neurologic disease and has lost its status as a purely "functional psychosis."

Finally, attention should be drawn to the regional alterations of cerebral blood flow in chronic stable schizophrenic patients, as revealed by positron emission tomography (PET) and functional MRI. Weinberger and colleagues and Liddle and Barnes have reported a decrease in blood flow in the prefrontal areas during cognitive performances. Friston and associates found consistent abnormalities in the left parahippocampal region in all forms of chronic schizophrenia. Studies of regional glucose metabolism and postmortem norepinephrine measurements have yielded equivocal data, although most patients show a reduction in glucose metabolism in the thalamus and frontal cortex. Several lines of investigation point more to the medial part of the left temporal lobe and related limbic and frontal systems as being the focus of a developmental abnormality (see Tsuang et al and Friston et al for pertinent references). According to Sabri et al, the inconsistent findings on functional imaging may be accounted for by correlations between certain blood flow patterns and specific symptoms. For example, the formal thought disorder corresponded to increased flow in the frontal and temporal regions, while delusions and hallucinations were associated with reduced flow in the cingulate, left frontal, and temporal areas. Silbersweig et al have performed PET studies in schizophrenics while they were experiencing auditory hallucinations. They found an increased blood flow mainly in both thalami, left hippocampus and the right striatum, but also in the parahippocampal, orbitofrontal, and cingulate areas. One drug-naive patient with visual and auditory hallucinations showed activation.

Diagnosis

From a neurologic standpoint, the main distinction to be made is between an acute schizophrenia-like psychosis (schizophreniform reaction; "good-prognosis" schizophrenia) and the chronic disease schizophrenia (nuclear or "process" schizophrenia). The *acute schizophreniform illness* takes the form of a delusional-hallucinatory syndrome in which there is little if any disturbance of consciousness. Although such a syndrome is characteristic of schizophrenia, it may occur in the manic phase of manic-depressive disease, encephalitis, temporal lobe epilepsy, chronic amphetamine intoxication, withdrawal from alcohol after a sustained period of intoxication, phencyclidine (PCP), lysergic acid diethylamide (LSD), and other drug intoxications; it is rarely seen in certain endocrine and metabolic disorders, in which consciousness is not impaired. Whenever this syndrome is recognized, therefore, these several causes need to be differentiated. At our hospitals, less than one out of five of the acute schizophreniform psychoses has proved to be due to the disease schizophrenia. This distinction is made by the premorbid history and the course of the illness. If the patient had been reclusive, withdrawn and socially maladept and does not seem to recover fully from the acute psychosis, then the diagnosis of schizophrenia is appropriate. Lacking these features, and in particular with a full remission, one assumes the occurrence of hypomania or of a toxic-metabolic psychosis, which can usually be detected by laboratory screening for drugs and endocrine diseases. Only 10 percent of patients with classic schizophrenia will have such an acute episode.

It is the present authors' opinion that the status of acute schizophrenia and of the so-called schizothymic and schizoaffective states brings to light a crucial nosologic problem. Namely, is the traditional separation of depressive disease, manic-depressive disease, and schizophrenia biologically sound? The suggestion is that they are linked in some way by these transitional forms. Neurologists should keep an open mind about these and other theoretical problems that lack a firm genetic and neuropathologic basis.

The presence of a chronic delusional-hallucinatory syndrome always raises the possibility of schizophrenia, but it must be remembered that in either chronic schizophrenia or the remittent form of the disease, delusions and hallucinations may be either absent or too subtle to be detected during a brief examination. Other data are required for diagnosis. Feighner and colleagues, who first drew up a set of diagnostic criteria for research in the major psychiatric syndromes (which were subsequently incorporated in successive editions of the DSM), stated that the diagnosis of schizophrenia is tenable only in the presence of (1) a chronic illness of at least 6 months' duration and a failure (after an acute episode) to return to the premorbid level of psychosocial adjustment, (2) delusions or hallucinations without significant perplexity or disorientation (i.e., without clouding of consciousness), (3) verbal productions that are so illogical and confusing as to make communication difficult (if the patient is mute, diagnosis should be deferred), and (4) at least three of the following manifestations: (a) among adults, the lack of a partner or spouse; (b) poor premorbid social adjustment or work history; (c) family history of schizophrenia; or (d) onset of illness prior to age of 40 years. Important negatives include the absence of a family history of manic-depressive disease, absence of an earlier illness with depressive or manic symptoms, and absence of alcoholism, drug abuse, or other organic disease within a year of onset of the psychosis.

While the Feighner criteria are so strict as to exclude certain patients with a schizophrenic illness, those who are included will be found to constitute a fairly homogeneous group. Morrison and colleagues, who used these criteria, noted that after a 10-year period there was practically no change in diagnosis; they had reliably separated schizophrenia, schizophreniform psychosis (in which only the acute delusional-hallucinatory syndrome was present), and manic-depressive psychosis.

In addition to the acute schizophreniform psychosis described above, the authors have encountered the greatest difficulties in the diagnosis of schizophrenia in the following clinical situations:

1. A patient with a normal family and premorbid history *with an acute illness* having many of the typical features of schizophrenia but *associated with confusion, forgetfulness,* and/or *clouding of consciousness*. Mood change may be prominent. Thus the illness combines the features of an affective disorder, schizophrenia, and a confusional state. This syndrome is characteristic of corticosteroid psychosis (drug-induced or Cushing disease), thyrotoxic psychosis, puerperal psychosis, phencyclidine intoxication, and so-called combat fatigue of wartime. Usually recovery is complete, and schizophrenia is excluded by the fact that the patient remains well.

2. *Adolescents and young adults whose social relationships are disorganized* and who are unusually sensitive, resentful, rebellious, fearful, discouraged, in trouble with school authorities and the law, using drugs, etc. The latter may have caused seizures, hallucinations, and withdrawal symptoms or may have resulted in addiction. Such patients are usually classified as having a borderline personality or "character disorder" that appears to go back several years; if they are incorrigible, unable to profit by experience, amoral, and in trouble with social agencies, they are called *sociopaths*. This type of personality disorder and social maladjustment usually turns out not to be schizophrenia. The most dependable means of determining this fact at the time the patient is first seen is the strict application of the Feighner criteria for the diagnosis of schizophrenia.

3. There is the opposite type of diagnostic problem, arising in *an individual who has been only marginally competent because of personality problems and many vague neurotic and hypochondriacal symptoms*, often requiring prolonged psychotherapy. Many such individuals will indeed be found to have simple schizophrenia (called "pseudoneurotic" at one time). Here also errors in diagnosis usually result from a failure to assess mental status carefully and to ascertain the life profile of the disorder.

4. *A chronic delusional-hallucinatory state in a chronic alcoholic patient*. Usually the history will disclose that the illness began when alcohol was withdrawn, after a period of sustained drinking, and at first took the form of an acute auditory hallucinosis, characterized by threatening, exteriorized auditory hallucinations to which the patient's emotional reaction was appropriate. Only later do a few of these patients drift into a quiet hallucinatory, mildly paranoid state, with rather bland affect. Evidence of the prepsychotic schizoid personality cannot be detected, and there is usually no family history of schizophrenia. Cases of this type that we have studied had their onset between 45 and 50 years of age, i.e., much later than the age of onset of schizophrenia. For these reasons, this alcoholic, schizophrenia-like illness

should be differentiated from the paranoid type of schizophrenia.

5. *A patient who is confused or stuporous and seemingly negativistic, refusing or unable to speak, to execute commands, or to be activated in any way.* If signs of focal cerebral or brainstem disease are absent, one is tempted to make a diagnosis of catatonic schizophrenia, not appreciating that catatonia as a phenomenon may be indistinguishable from akinetic mutism (page 370) and may also appear with widespread disease of the associational cortices and with severe depression, certain confusional states, and hysteria. The error can be avoided if one makes diagnoses on the basis of positive findings, not on the absence of data. The authors have seen cases of hypoxic and other metabolic encephalopathies, Schilder disease, certain storage diseases, and Creutzfeldt-Jakob disease mistaken for schizophrenia because of failure to adhere to this principle.

6. *A patient with temporal lobe epilepsy* who, apart from intermittent psychomotor seizures, has long periods (weeks or months) of hallucinations, delusions, bizarre behavior, and disorganization of thinking. Such a mental disturbance often reflects the presence of a persistent state of temporal lobe seizures (temporal lobe status), which in some cases have been demonstrated by depth electrodes to originate in the amygdaloid or other medial temporal areas. Other types of psychopathology, such as sexual deviations, may also be associated with temporal lobe epilepsy. The nature of the disturbances of emotionality and mentation in such patients is discussed in Chaps. 16 and 25.

7. *Schizophrenics with prominent depressive symptoms who have made repeated suicide attempts* pose an exceptionally difficult problem in diagnosis. They were referred to in the past as *schizothymic*, and to this day it is not certain whether they have schizophrenia, a relatively mild chronic depressive illness (dysthymia), depressive disease, or both schizophrenia and depression ("schizoaffective"). When in remission, patients with affective disorders are usually normal, whereas those with schizophrenia and many with schizoaffective states are not.

8. *One should always be hesitant to make the diagnosis of schizophrenia during childhood*, although such a diagnosis has been entertained in children who have a variety of developmental and adjustment problems and who at some time become psychotic, i.e., they become excited, depressed, or hallucinatory and express bizarre ideas. There is no evidence that such children go on to have schizophrenia later in life. And although what are thought to be "schizoid" traits may be recognized in childhood, a frank psychosis is hardly ever recorded at this age. Of particular importance in such children is to exclude the presence of metabolic errors, mental retardation, or an early onset depressive illness. Similarly, childhood autism and particularly its milder forms (Asperger syndrome, page 1098) should not be confused with schizophrenia. The fact that the incidence of schizophrenia is not increased in the families of autistic children supports the idea that the two are separate diseases.

Treatment

The aims of treatment are to suppress psychotic symptoms, ameliorate the disorder of thinking and the apathetic state, prevent relapse, and optimize social adjustment. It is often possible, once the diagnosis of schizophrenia is established and the optimal regimen of medication decided upon, for a general physician to share the responsibility for following the patient with a psychiatric social worker or nurse. The physician soon becomes accustomed to the particular pattern of the patient's behavior and can help support the patient and his family during difficult periods. Relapse with psychotic decompensation demands drug therapy, and if there is a hazard of injury or suicide or difficulty in management at home, hospitalization becomes necessary. Many general hospitals and specialized psychiatric institutions have facilities for the management of such cases; state hospitals and other institutions are able to provide long-term treatment. The aim of hospitalization is to protect the patient, relieve the family of the need for constant vigilance and supervision, and assure the administration of drugs until the exacerbation spends itself. Later, instead of mere custodial care, the patient needs a supervised program of planned activities, vocational and milieu therapy, etc., in a "halfway house," which involves the patient as a contributing member during the more chronic phases of the disease. If medication is successful in preventing progressive decompensation, the patient can often return to the family and community. It is helpful to have a competent social worker maintain frequent contact with the patient and his family.

The modern era of treatment of schizophrenia began in 1952, with the demonstration of the antipsychotic properties of the dopaminergic blocking agent chlorpromazine. Treatment consists essentially of the administration of this drug or one of several similar antipsychotic medications.

The various classes of antipsychotic drugs, their mode of action, and neurologic ("neuroleptic") side effects have been discussed in Chap. 43 (pages 1263 to 1265).

In recent years several "atypical" antipsychotic agents that have complex effects on dopamine and serotonin systems (clozapine, risperidone, quetiapine, etc., as noted below) have been added to the standard dopaminergic antagonists such as the phenothiazines and butyrophenones. They all serve to calm the patient, blunt his emotional responses, reduce hallucinosis and aggressive and impulsive behavior, leaving cognitive functions relatively intact. The main side effects, pertaining mostly to the phenothiazine group, are summarized in Table 58-1 and on page 1264. The antipsychotic action of these drugs is more impressive in the short and intermediate term, although some data suggest that they are also of value in preventing relapses. Negative symptoms (apathy and withdrawal) respond less well than positive ones, and it is generally acknowledged that 10 to 20 percent of patients respond little or not at all to medication.

The optimal daily dose for treatment of an acute psychotic episode is in the range of 10 to 20 mg daily of haloperidol or the equivalent amount (400 to 800 mg) of a phenothiazine such as chlorpromazine. The administration of much higher doses is popular with some psychiatrists but entails serious risks, and the advantages of this practice have not been demonstrated in controlled trials (see Kane and Marder). The same dose or lower doses are used to maintain remission. Attempts are then made to individualize and eventually to lower the dosage until the patient's behavior suggests that a relapse is imminent. Long-acting piperazine phenothiazines, given subcutaneously every week or two, are used in patients who are unable to take oral medication or refuse to do so.

Table 58-1
Neurologic side effects of the neuroleptic-antipsychotic drugs

Reaction	*Clinical features*	*Period of maximum risk*	*Proposed mechanism*	*Treatment*
Acute dystonias	Spasm of muscles of tongue, face, neck, back	1–5 days	Dopamine excess? Acetylcholine excess?	Antiparkinson agents are diagnostic and curative (IM or IV, then PO)
Parkinson syndrome	Bradykinesia, rigidity, masked facies, shuffling gait, variable tremor	5–30 days (may persist)	Dopamine blockade	Antiparkinson agents (PO); dopamine agonists risky?
"Rabbit" syndrome	Perioral tremor, flexed posture; usually reversible	Months or years	Unknown	Antiparkinson agents: reduce dose of neuroleptic
Akathisia	Motor restlessness with anxiety or agitation	1–60 days (commonly persists)	Adrenergic excess?	Reduce dose or change drug; low doses of propranolol[a]; antiparkinson agents or benzodiazepines may help
Neuroleptic malignant syndrome	Catatonia, stupor, fever, unstable pulse and blood pressure, myoglobinemia, elevated CPK[b]; can be fatal	Weeks	Unknown	Stop neuroleptic; antiparkinson agents usually fail; bromocriptine and dantrolene often help; expert supportive care crucial, ICU best
Tardive dyskinesia	Oral-facial dyskinesia, choreoathetosis, often slowly reversible, rarely progressive	6–24 months (worse on withdrawal)	Dopamine excess?	Prevention best; treatment unsatisfactory; slow, spontaneous remission

Abbreviations: IM, intramuscularly; IV, intravenously; PO, per os (orally); ICU, intensive care unit.

[a]There may be an increased risk of hypotension on interaction between high doses of propranolol and some antipsychotic agents; clonidine may also be effective at doses of 0.2–0.8 mg/day but carries a high risk of hypotension, and tolerance (loss of efficacy) may develop.

[b]CPK, creatine-phosphokinase in serum, released from hypertonic muscle.

Source: Adapted from Baldessarini and Cole, by permission.

Clozapine, *olanzapine, risperidone*, and *quetiapine* are more recently introduced drugs with incompletely defined pharmacologic properties but with narrower affinities for certain receptors. They have been shown to produce clinical improvement in about half of patients who have proved to be unresponsive to other antipsychotic medications. The drugs bind to and inhibit serotonin receptors (Meltzer and Nash) but have a lower affinity for striatal dopamine receptors, thus providing a major advantage—the absence of immediate or tardive extrapyramidal side effects. This has led some psychiatrists to use one of these drugs, rather than a phenothiazine, as a first choice. About 1 percent of patients treated with clozapine develop leukopenia, which may prove fatal; there appears to be less risk with olanzapine, but leukopenia and agranulocytosis have been reported in rare instances. Orthostatic hypotension, tachycardia, fever, and hypersalivation may be troublesome in the first days and weeks of therapy. *Risperidone*, another of the newer antischizophrenic drugs, is a potent serotonin and dopamine receptor antagonist. Low doses of this drug reportedly attenuate the negative symptoms of schizophrenia (apathy, emotional withdrawal, lack of social interaction), and the incidence of extrapyramidal side effects is low provided that the dosage is kept below 6 mg daily. Dosages of these antipsychotic drugs are indicated in Table 58-2.

Antidepressants and lithium have been used in schizophrenic patients with prominent affective symptoms. Electroconvulsive therapy (ECT) is now seldom used except in patients who are catatonic or severely agitated or who have prominent affective symptoms, or, in exceptional instances, where there has been no response to medication.

Many of the extrapyramidal side effects of haloperidol and the phenothiazines can be prevented or at least minimized by the simultaneous parenteral administration of antihistaminic drugs—e.g., diphenhydramine (Benadryl), 25 mg tid—and the anticholinergic drugs used in the treatment of Parkinson disease—e.g., benztropine mesylate (Cogentin), 0.2 mg tid. However, the latter drugs must be given cautiously, for they may interfere with the action of the antipsychotic drugs and, if given in large doses, may themselves induce a toxic confusional state. If it becomes necessary to treat the extrapyramidal side effects, it is usually possible to eliminate the anticholinergic drugs after 2 to 3 months without a return of symptoms. In chronically medicated patients, 20 to 40 percent of whom develop tardive dyskinesias, an increased dose of the antipsychotic drug may suppress the dyskinesia, but only temporarily. The most dreaded complication of pharmacotherapy is the neuroleptic malignant syndrome. The nature and management of this syndrome and other tardive dyskinesias have been discussed on page 1265.

Supportive psychotherapy (repeated explanation, reassurance, encouragement) is of course necessary, as in any prolonged illness, and the family needs the same type of help. The physician should be understanding and sympathetic but also firm and professional. The general purpose of psychotherapy is to help the patient get a grasp on reality and to strengthen his self-esteem and psychologic defenses. Psychoanalytic therapy has little to offer as a primary mode of treatment.

Outcome With modern drug therapy and supportive psychiatric management, fully 60 percent of schizophrenic patients will recover sufficiently to return to their homes and become socially adjusted to a varying degree (about half of this group can engage in some occupation). About 30 percent remain helpless and severely handicapped and 10 percent remain hospitalized.

Table 58-2
Newer antipsychotic drugs with limited extrapyramidal side effects

Medication	*Brand name*	*Initial dose*	*Target or maximal dose*	*Potential side effects*[a]
Olanzapine	Zyprexa	5 mg	10 mg	Orthostatic hypotension, transaminase elevation, hyperprolactinemia
Quetiapine	Seroquel	25 mg bid	300 mg	Orthostatic hypotension, cataracts, transaminase elevation
Clozapine	Clozaril	12.5 mg bid	300 mg	Agranulocytosis, transient fever, anticholinergic activity, hyperglycemia
Risperidone	Risperidol	1 mg bid	3 mg bid	Orthostatic hypotension

[a]All have the potential to cause tardive dyskinesias and neuroleptic malignant syndrome (Table 58-1), but these complications are thought to be less frequent than with phenothiazines and haloperidol.

DELUSIONAL DISORDER (PARANOIA)

The term *paranoid* (*para* = beside, *nous* = mind) literally means a mind beside itself (Day and Manschreck). It designates patients who show "fixed suspicions, persecutory delusions, dominant ideas or grandiose trends logically elaborated and with due regard for reality once the false interpretation or premise has been accepted. Further characteristics are formally correct conduct, adequate emotional reactions, and coherence of the train of thought" (Rosanoff).

In other words, in pure paranoia (*delusional disorder* in DSM-IV), there is supposed to be no mental defect other than the delusional system—no dementia, hallucinations, or emotional disturbance. In past years, a large group of the mentally ill were classified as paranoid. But with advancing knowledge of mental illness, fewer and fewer have been left in this category.

The trouble that psychiatrists have taken to couch this definition in negatives implies that paranoia is frequently a feature of other forms of mental illness, notably schizophrenia, manic-depressive disease, Alzheimer disease, Lewy-body disease, toxic or alcoholic psychosis, general paresis, etc. This fact about paranoia was known from the beginning, when Heinroth originally described it in 1818 and classified it as a limited disorder of the intellect. Krafft-Ebing, in his monograph on the subject, took pains to distinguish two syndromes: (1) "original paranoia," developing about the time of puberty and attributable to heredity (surely paranoid schizophrenia by present-day criteria), and (2) acquired paranoia, developing in later life, particularly in the involutional period (the condition under discussion). Kraepelin, in agreement with the ideas of Kahlbaum, distinguished between paranoia and dementia praecox but remarked that approximately 40 percent of patients who developed paranoia early in life went on to become schizophrenic. The others represented true paranoia or a closely related condition which he called paraphrenia, a term no longer used. In DSM-IV, this disorder is classified as "delusional (paranoid) disorder" and defined as a *persistent* delusion that is not part of any other mental disorder. Furthermore, the delusions are nonbizarre, i.e., they involve situations that could occur in real life, such as being followed, poisoned, infected, loved at a distance, or deceived by a spouse, or having a disease.

Figures on the frequency of true paranoia are probably not reliable because they are of necessity based on hospital records. Doubtless there are many individuals with mild forms of the disorder who have never crossed the threshold of a mental hospital. They are relatively harmless and in their communities are judged to be mildly "cracked," or monomaniacs. Males and females are about equally affected. Among psychiatric hospital patients, true isolated paranoia is rare (0.1 percent of admissions, according to Winokur).

Clinical Manifestations

It would be inappropriate in a neurology text to give an account of all the many ways in which paranoiacs behave. A simple paradigm will suffice—that of a middle-aged man of uneasy, brooding, asocial, eccentric nature who gradually develops a dominating idea or belief of his own importance, of having in his possession special powers that make him the envy of others, who become bent on persecuting him. As the delusion grows, he becomes more preoccupied, less efficient, and increasingly suspicious of others, with a tendency to interpret every one of their words, gestures, or actions as having some reference to himself. Only when his behavior becomes noticeably bizarre or when he does something to annoy others does his condition come to medical attention. On examining such a person, one is impressed with his capacity for careful reasoning, which betrays good intelligence. Whatever the type of delusional theme—erotomanic (a delusion that another person, usually of higher status, is in love with the patient), grandiose, jealous, persecutory, or somatic, the last being the most common—the patient's arguments are logical and buttressed cogently by evidence. The patients express their false beliefs with certainty and conviction and are totally unaccepting of all arguments that impugn their rationality. Also, the views of such patients about matters other than their delusions can be quite sensible.

As was said, the illness usually does not lead to hospitalization, and if admitted to hospital, the patient does not stay long. The querulous paranoiacs are the most annoying. They usually remain in the community, flooding the mails with copies of documents accusing people falsely, incessantly writing to newspapers, and expressing their worthless opinions about anything and everything. As the years pass, the patient changes little, though a few such patients may later break down and begin to hallucinate and finally end in a deteriorated state much like that of schizophrenia. This trend supports Bleuler's opinion that the illness is often a variant of schizophrenia.

Regarding causation, there have been several interesting but unverifiable ideas. The Freudian school attributed paranoia to repressed homosexuality and fixation at the narcissistic level. Meyer invoked a long-standing personality disorder, the *paranoid constitution*. He used the term to refer to persons with a lifelong tendency to hold biased views, to be overly concerned about what others think of them, and to attribute deliberate intentions to indifferent actions. This behavior seems but an exaggeration of a mild suspiciousness that is part of the personality makeup of many individuals. Manschreck has presented a detailed discussion of the proposed psychologic mechanisms of paranoia.

The authors' experience with pure paranoia in a general hospital has been rather limited. One sees deluded patients, to be sure, but usually their abnormal ideas have centered on personal persecution, health and bodily functions, infidelity of a spouse, theft of possessions, and the like. The claim that poisoning by carbon monoxide has left the person with ill-defined defects in concentration and other mental functions or the belief that there exists an unobservable parasitic skin infestation have been common delusions in our experience. One of our patients, functioning normally in every other way, carried the unshakable idea that people were sneaking into her house at night and when she was away and rearranging the furniture. Physicians under our care have woven delusional ideas around tenuous scientific theories; these ideas have applied to personal life events as well as physical and psychologic symptoms, and in some cases have resulted in peculiar regimens of self-medication. Rarely, a patient comes to the hospital for some other medical reason and it is found that he or she has been living quietly in the community, preoccupied with a bizarre delusional system yet appearing neither depressed nor schizophrenic. Certainly one often sees delusions in depressed patients who decompensate as their depression worsens.

Sharply separated from the more or less pure delusional disorders are the ones that occur as part of a confusional state or delirium. Delusions occurring in the latter setting are characteristically bizarre, changeable, poorly systematized, and, with rare exceptions, transitory; they are usually associated with many other aberrations of mental function. The same can be said for delusions that occur in the course of a dementing disease. Persons without known mental illness may experience a brief delusional episode, notably after an extensive surgical procedure or the administration of sedative drugs. Such events are common, of course, in elderly persons with an incipient or well-compensated dementia ("beclouded dementia," page 440). Rarely, one of the degenerative dementing diseases of middle and late life (Alzheimer, Huntington, and especially Lewy-body) presents with a delusional disorder. Certain drugs have a tendency to produce paranoia in otherwise nonpsychotic individuals; phencyclidine, amphetamine, and cocaine are the main offenders seen in patients arriving in emergency departments, and ketamine-like or anticholinergic drugs are often responsible in hospitalized patients. These "organic delusions" have been discussed by Cummings.

Management

The methods and objectives of psychotherapy are discussed fully by Manschreck (see References). We have no way of deciding whether psychotherapy has influenced this state. In a general hospital, where most of our paranoid patients have been depressed or manic, we have several times been gratified by the effects of antidepressant medication. In the treatment of patients with pathologic jealousy, Mooney has found phenothiazine drugs to be useful.

From what has been said, the clinical analysis of patients with delusions requires a careful study of mood and intelligence to rule out manic-depressive psychosis and dementia. If either of these two states exists, the treatment proceeds along the lines discussed in Chaps. 57 and 21. A matter of practical importance is for the physician to evaluate carefully the nature of the delusional ideas and try to judge whether the patient is homicidal or suicidal. Occasionally, physicians and others have been killed or maimed by paranoiacs who thought they were being mistreated.

PUERPERAL (POSTPARTUM) PSYCHOSES

Parturition, associated as it is with many biologic disturbances such as the effects of pain, drugs, eclampsia, hemorrhage, infection, and an abrupt hormonal adjustment, is frequently associated with a disturbance of mood. Obstetricians have repeatedly observed that the woman may feel extraordinarily well immediately postpartum, only to lapse in the following days into a weepy, depressed state in which she may be distressed by lack of feeling for her newborn infant. Usually this lasts for only a few days ("postpartum blues"), being quelled by the return home, responsibility for the infant, nursing, etc. In some patients the depressive symptoms persist for months (see below).

The period after childbirth is also one in which there is a strong disposition to psychosis. Opinion varies as to whether there is a special *puerperal psychosis*. Most psychiatrists believe that the psychotic break that may occur at this time is either a confusional-delirious state or a schizophreniform or depressive psychosis, and that these illnesses do not differ from those occurring at other times in life.

Additionally there occurs a psychosis that cannot be categorized in this way. Usually it has its onset between 48 and 72 h after a delivery that may have been complicated by excessive bleeding or infection. The patient alternates between periods of noisy hyperactivity and of mutism and inactivity. She is disoriented and incapable of thinking clearly. The baby is rejected as not belonging to her (instances of infanticide are not unknown). Although the illness has some features of delirium, it may merge with a schizophrenic or depressive type of psychosis that persists for months. Our experience is like that of Boyd, who found in a series of cases that about 40 percent were predominantly affective, 20 percent schizophreniform, and the remainder self-limited confusional psychoses of the type described above.

Also, in some patients, a typical depressive illness has followed each of several pregnancies, disabling the patient for weeks to months at a time. Some women with manic-depressive disease have had their early depressive attacks only after delivery. Also, as consultants to the Boston Lying-In Hospital, we had observed a number of patients with an acute postpartum schizophrenic episode. These patients were without family history or prepsychotic schizoid personality and seemed to have a better prognosis than one usually expects in schizophrenia, i.e., they had "good prognosis" schizophrenia. These are only impressions, however.

In the diagnosis of postpartum psychosis, one must also keep in mind the possibility of eclampsia, the consequences of pituitary infarction, cerebral vein thrombosis or transitory stroke of arterial type, ergot-induced psychosis, and hypotensive-hypoxic cerebral injury.

THE ENDOCRINE PSYCHOSES

One of the most provocative observations in contemporary psychiatry is that apparently normal individuals may become psychotic when they develop hyper- or hypothyroidism or the Cushing syndrome (or less often, adrenal insufficiency), or when they receive therapeutic doses of corticosteroids. If these conditions were no more than examples of drug-induced psychosis, they would be interesting enough. The fact is, however, that they differ considerably from the usual toxic deliria or confusional states. The syndrome, somewhat reminiscent of puerperal psychosis and some cases of "combat fatigue" seen in wartime, comprises features that are suggestive of manic-depressive psychosis or schizophrenia on the one hand and of confusional psychosis on the other. These endocrine psychoses have far-reaching medical significance, for they provide artificial models of psychoses created by the manipulation of metabolic and by exogenous factors.

Corticosteroid and Adrenocorticotropic Hormone Psychosis First described in arthritic patients being treated with cortisone, these syndromes are now occurring far less frequently than when this hormone was introduced into medical practice. Presumably, ACTH and cortisone are now more purified, and there are more reliable data as to safe dosage. The psychosis usually develops over a period of a few days after the patient has received the hormone for a week or more. The features are extremely variable. Depression and insomnia are the most frequent symptoms, but some patients become elated, agitated, excited, and talkative, as though under pressure to speak, while others are mute; or the prevailing emotional response may be one of anxiety and panic. Thinking may be illogical, tangential, and incoherent. Hallucinations and sensory misinterpretations may appear. Clouding of the sensorium and disorientation, the hallmarks of deliria and the confusional psychoses, have not been prominent in the ACTH and corticosteroid psychoses. However, the state of awareness is not altogether normal, and at times the patient is frankly bewildered. In the motor sphere there may be incessant activity or immobility, resistiveness, and even negativism verging on catatonia. If administration of the hormone is discontinued as soon as symptoms appear, the psychosis subsides gradually over several days to weeks, with complete recovery.

In patients with Cushing disease, mental changes are frequent. There is a combination of affective disorder and impairment of cognitive function, easily elicited during mental status testing. The lateral and third ventricles are enlarged. Among athletes taking anabolic steroids, some develop affective and psychotic symptoms—reduced sleep, irritability, paranoid delusions, auditory hallucinations, and euphoria or depression. Mental changes in *Addison disease* are frequent but varied. Irritability, confusion, disorientation, and convulsions, with or without symptoms of hypoglycemia, are the main features. The mechanisms are not well understood.

The mechanism of acute steroid psychosis is also obscure. From the few available studies it has been learned that the occurrence of the psychosis is not related to the premorbid personality. Although the dosage of ACTH or corticosteroid has usually been high, there has been no close correlation between the dosage and the occurrence, severity, and duration of the psychosis. Nor does the mental disturbance appear to be related to the rapidity and intensity of the therapeutic response to ACTH and cortisone. The notion that dexamethasone is less often associated with psychosis than other corticosteroids is unproven. Lithium is often effective in controlling the symptoms, allowing continuation of the corticosteroid therapy. The dose is the same as for manic states (page 1619; see also Falk et al).

Thyroid Psychosis A great deal has been said about the pervasive effects of abnormal thyroid function on all organs, including the neuromuscular apparatus and central nervous system. These effects are discussed in Chap. 40, under acquired metabolic diseases of the nervous system (pages 1199 to 1202).

The hyperthyroid patient often shows minor changes in emotions and mentation. Restlessness, irritability, apprehension, emotional lability, and at times even agitation and a generalized chorea may occur. Either of two trends may be observed in the relatively rare thyrotoxic patient who develops a psychosis. There may be a manic state, with its characteristic increase in psychomotor activity, overtalkativeness, and flight of ideas, or there may be depression, with its somber mood, weeping, and anxiety. Visual and auditory hallucinations may be present in both groups. The clinical picture is seldom clear. Usually the psychiatrist finds something more than simple mania or agitated depression, i.e., some clouding of the sensorium with perplexity and confusion, suggestive of delirium. The condition is said to be related to the premorbid personality, some personality types being more vulnerable, but this point is disputed; it is not directly related to the severity of the thyrotoxicosis. Careful studies of cerebral blood flow and metabolism during and after the psychosis have not been done. Treatment of the hyperthyroidism does not result in prompt arrest of the psychic disorder; recovery usually takes place over a period of months. One must distinguish this illness from other types of recurrent psychosis that happen to be coincidental with or precipitated by hyperthyroidism.

With *myxedema* there is a characteristic slowness and thickness of speech, drowsiness, hypothermia, mental dullness, listlessness and apathy, irritability, and sometimes suspiciousness. The patient may sleep most of the time, having to be awakened for meals. A disturbance of memory and the lack of genuine symptoms of depression, such as feelings of hopelessness and loss of self-esteem, help to distinguish the mental disorder of myxedema from that of a depressive illness. Nevertheless, unless one thinks of myxedema in all cases of psychomotor retardation, the diagnosis will be missed. Reduced cerebral blood flow and metabolism have been found in myxedema; with specific therapy, these functions are restored to normal.

An entirely different type of mental disturbance, characterized by intermittent delirium and stupor, associated with myoclonus and probably autoimmune in nature, may occur in patients with Hashimoto thyroiditis (page 1200).

REFERENCES

Akbarian S, Kim JJ, Potkin SG, et al: Maldistribution of interstitial neurons in prefrontal white matter of the brains of schizophrenic patients. *Arch Gen Psychiatry* 53:425, 1996.

American Foundation: *Medical Research: A Mid-century Survey*. Boston, Little, Brown, 1956.

American Psychiatric Association: *Diagnostic and Statistical Manual of Mental Disorders* (DSM-IV). Washington, DC, APA, 1994.

Andreasen NC: Symptoms, signs, and diagnosis of schizophrenia. *Lancet* 346:477, 1996.

Baldessarini RJ, Cole JO: Chemotherapy, in Nicholi AM Jr (ed): *The New Harvard Guide to Psychiatry*, 2nd ed. Cambridge, MA, Harvard University Press, 1988, pp 481–533.

Barta PE, Pearlson GD, Powers RE, et al: Auditory hallucinosis and smaller superior temporal gyral volume in schizophrenia. *Am J Psychiatry* 146:1456, 1990.

Benes FM, Davidson J, Bird ED: Quantitative cytoarchitectural studies of the cerebral cortex of schizophrenics. *Arch Gen Psychiatry* 43:31, 1986.

Bleuler E: *Dementia Praecox or the Group of Schizophrenias*. Zinkin J (trans). New York, International Universities Press, 1950.

Boyd DA: Mental disturbances with childbearing. *Am J Obstet Gynecol* 43:148, 1942.

Brown R, Colter N, Corsellis JAN, et al: Postmortem evidence of structural brain changes in schizophrenia: Differences in brain weight, temporal horn area, and parahippocampal gyrus compared with affective disorder. *Arch Gen Psychiatry* 43:36, 1986.

Carlsson A: The current status of the dopamine hypothesis of schizophrenia. *Neuropsychopharmacology* 1:179, 1988.

Carpenter WT, Buchanan RW: Schizophrenia. *N Engl J Med* 330:681, 1994.

Corsellis JAN: Psychoses of obscure pathology, in Blackwood W, Corsellis JAN (eds): *Greenfield's Neuropathology*. London, Edward Arnold, 1976, pp 903–915.

CUMMINGS JL: Organic delusions. *Br J Psychiatry* 46:184, 1985.

CUTTING J: Memory in functional psychoses. *J Neurol Neurosurg Psychiatry* 42:1031, 1979.

DAVISON K, BAGLEY CR: Schizophrenia-like psychoses associated with organic disorders of the nervous system: Review of literature, in Herrington RN (ed): *Br J Psychiatry, Spec Publ No 4, Curr Probl Neuropsychiatry* 1969, pp 113–184.

DAY M, MANSCHRECK TC: Delusional (paranoid) disorders, in Nicholi AM Jr (ed): *The New Harvard Guide to Psychiatry*, 2nd ed. Cambridge, MA, Harvard University Press, 1988, pp 296–308.

DUNLAP CR: The pathology of the brain in schizophrenia. *Res Publ Assoc Res Nerv Ment Dis* 5:371, 1928.

FALK WE, MANKE MW, POSKANZER DC: Lithium prophylaxis of corticotropin-induced psychosis. *JAMA* 241:1011, 1979.

FEIGHNER JP, ROBINS E, GUZE SB, et al: Diagnostic criteria for use in psychiatric research. *Arch Gen Psychiatry* 26:57, 1972.

FISCHER M: Psychoses in the offspring of schizophrenic twins and their normal co-twins. *Br J Psychiatry* 118:43, 1971.

FLOR-HENRY P: Lateralized temporo-limbic dysfunction and psychopathology. *Ann N Y Acad Sci* 280:777, 1976.

FRISTON KJ, LIDDLE PF, FRITH CD, et al: The left medial temporal region and schizophrenia: A PET study. *Brain* 115:367, 1992.

GOODWIN DW, GUZE SB: *Psychiatric Diagnosis*, 5th ed. New York, Oxford University Press, 1996.

HARLOW H: *Learning to Love*. New York, Jason Aronson, 1974.

HARRISON PJ: The neuropathology of schizophrenia. A critical review of the data and their interpretation. *Brain* 122:593, 1999.

HARRISON PJ, GEDDES JR: Schizophrenia and the 5-HT_{2A} receptor gene. *Lancet* 347:1274, 1996.

HEATH RB: Psychosis and epilepsy: Similarities and differences in the anatomico-physiologic substrate, in Koella WP, Trumble MR (eds): *Advances in Biologic Psychiatry*. Vol 8. New York, Karger, 1982, pp 166–216.

HERTZIG MA, BIRCH HC: Neurological organization in psychiatrically disturbed patients. *Arch Gen Psychiatry* 19:528, 1968.

HESTON L: Psychiatric disorders in foster home-reared children of schizophrenic mothers. *Br J Psychiatry* 112:819, 1966.

JABLENSKY A: Epidemiology of schizophrenia: A European perspective. *Schizophr Bull* 12:52, 1986.

JOHNSTONE EC, CROW TJ, FRITH CD, et al: The dementia of dementia praecox. *Acta Psychiatr Scand* 57:305, 1978.

JONES P, RODGERS B, MURRAY R, MARMOT M: Child developmental risk factors for adult schizophrenia in the British 1946 birth cohort. *Lancet* 344:1398, 1994.

KALLMANN FJ: The genetic theory of schizophrenia: An analysis of 691 twin index families. *Am J Psychiatry* 103:309, 1946.

KANE JM, MARDER SR: Psychopharmacologic treatment of schizophrenia. *Schizophr Bull* 19:287, 1993.

KARLSSON JL: *The Biologic Basis of Schizophrenia*. Springfield, IL, Charles C Thomas, 1966.

KARNOSH LJ, HOPE JM: Puerperal psychosis and their sequelae. *Am J Psychiatry* 94:537, 1937.

KENDLER KS: Molecular genetics of schizophrenia, in Charney DS, Nestler EJ, Bunney BS (eds): *Neurobiology of Mental Illness*. New York, Oxford University Press, 1999, pp 203–213.

KENNARD M: Value of equivocal signs in neurological diagnosis. *Neurology* 10:753, 1960.

KETY SS, MATTHYSSE S: Genetic and biochemical aspects of schizophrenia, in Nicholi AM Jr (ed): *The New Harvard Guide to Psychiatry*. Cambridge, MA, Harvard University Press, 1988, pp 139–151.

KRAEPELIN E: Robertson GM (ed): *Dementia Praecox and Paraphrenia*. Barclay RM (trans). Edinburgh, Livingstone, 1919.

LANGFELDT G: The prognosis in schizophrenia and the factors influencing the course of the disease. *Acta Psychiatr Neurol Scand* Suppl 13, 1937.

LANGFELDT G: The prognosis in schizophrenia. *Acta Psychiatr Neurol Scand* Suppl 110, 1956.

LAWRIE SM, WHALLEY H, KESTELMAN JN, et al: Magnetic resonance imaging of brain in people at high risk of developing schizophrenia. *Lancet* 353:30, 1999.

LEVIN S, JONES A, STARK L, et al: Identification of abnormal patterns in eye movements of schizophrenic patients. *Arch Gen Psychiatry* 39:1125, 1982.

LIDDLE PF: The symptoms of chronic schizophrenia: A re-examination of the positive-negative dichotomy. *Br J Psychiatry* 151:145, 1987.

LIDDLE PF, BARNES TRE: Syndromes of chronic schizophrenia. *Br J Psychiatry* 157: 558, 1990.

MANSCHRECK TC: Delusional disorder and shared psychotic disorder, in Sadock BJ, Sadock VA (eds): *Kaplan and Sadock's Comprehensive Textbook of Psychiatry*, 7th ed. Philadelphia, Lippincott Williams & Wilkins, 2000, pp 1243–1264.

MELTZER HY, NASH JF: Effects of antipsychotic drugs on serotonin receptors. *Pharmacol Rev* 43:587, 1991.

MEYER A: Fundamental conceptions of dementia praecox, in *Collected Papers of Adolph Meyer*. Vol 2. Baltimore, Johns Hopkins University Press, 1950.

MOONEY H: Pathologic jealousy and psychochemotherapy. *Br J Psychiatry* 111:1023, 1975.

MORRISON J, WINOKUR G, CROWE R, CLANCY J: The Iowa 500: The first follow-up. *Arch Gen Psychiatry* 29:677, 1973.

MORTENSON PB, PEDERSEN CB, WESTERGAARD T, et al: Effects of family history and place and season of birth on the risk of schizophrenia. *N Engl J Med* 340:603, 1999.

MUELLER PS: Neuroleptic malignant syndrome. *Psychosomatics* 26:654, 1985.

MURRAY RM, LEWIS SW, REVELEY AM: Towards an etiologic classification of schizophrenia. *Lancet* 1:1023, 1985.

PEARLSON GD: Neurobiology of Schizophrenia. *Ann Neurol* 48:556, 2000.

POPE H, LIPINSKI J: Differential diagnosis of schizophrenic and manic-depressive illness. *Arch Gen Psychiatry* 35:811, 1978.

ROBINS E, GUZE SB: Establishment of diagnostic validity in psychiatric illness: Its application to schizophrenia. *Am J Psychiatry* 126:983, 1970.

ROSANOFF AJ: *Manual of Psychiatry*. New York, Wiley, 1920.

ROSENTHAL D, WENDER PH, KETY SS, et al: Parent-child relationships and psychopathologic disorder in the child. *Arch Gen Psychiatry* 32:466, 1975.

Rosenthal D, Wender PH, Kety SS, et al: The adopted-away offspring of schizophrenics. *Am J Psychiatry* 128:307, 1971.

Rupp A, Keith SJ: The costs of schizophrenia: Assessing the burden. *Psychiatr Clin North Am* 16:413, 1993.

Sabri O, Ekworth R, Schreckenberger M, et al: Correlation of positive symptoms exclusively to hyperperfusion or hypoperfusion of cerebral cortex in never-treated schizophrenics. *Lancet* 349:1735, 1997.

Schneider K: *Clinical Psychopathology*. Hamilton MW (trans). New York, Grune & Stratton, 1959.

Sedvall G, Farde L: Chemical brain anatomy in schizophrenia. *Lancet* 346:743, 1995.

Seidman LJ: Schizophrenia and brain dysfunction: An integration of recent neurodiagnostic findings. *Psychol Bull* 94:195, 1983.

Shenton ME, Kikinis R, Jolesz FA, et al: Abnormalities of the left temporal lobe and thought disorder in schizophrenia. *N Engl J Med* 327: 604, 1992.

Silbersweig DA, Stern E, Frith C, et al: A functional neuroanatomy of hallucinations in schizophrenia. *Nature* 378:176, 1995.

Solovay MR, Shenton ME, Holzman PS: Comparative studies of thought disorders: I. Mania and schizophrenia. *Arch Gen Psychiatry* 44:13, 1987.

Spielmeyer W: The problem of the anatomy of schizophrenia. *J Nerv Ment Dis* 72:241, 1930.

Stevens JR: An anatomy of schizophrenia? *Arch Gen Psychiatry* 29:177, 1973.

Suddath RL, Christison GW, Torrey EF, et al: Anatomical abnormalities in the brains of monozygotic twins discordant for schizophrenia. *N Engl J Med* 322:789, 1990.

Taylor MA: Schneiderian first-rank symptoms and clinical prognostic features in schizophrenia. *Arch Gen Psychiatry* 26:64, 1972.

Tsuang MT, Faraone SV, Day M: Schizophrenic disorders, in Nicholi AM Jr (ed): *The New Harvard Guide to Psychiatry*, 2nd ed. Cambridge, MA, Harvard University Press, 1988, pp 259–295.

Tucker CJ, Campion EW, Silberfarb PM: Sensorimotor functions and cognitive disturbance in psychiatric patients. *Am J Psychiatry* 132:17, 1975.

Waddington JL: Schizophrenia: Developmental neuroscience and pathobiology. *Lancet* 341:531, 1993.

Weinberger DR, Berman KF, Zec RF: Physiologic dysfunction of the dorsolateral prefrontal cortex in schizophrenia: Regional cerebral blood flow evidence. *Arch Gen Psychiatry* 43:114, 1986.

Weinberger DR, Torry EF, Neophytides AN, Wyatt RJ: Lateral cerebral ventricular enlargement in chronic schizophrenia. *Arch Gen Psychiatry* 36:735, 1979.

Williams J, Spurlock G, McGuffin P, et al: Association between schizophrenia and T102C polymorphism of the 5-hydroxytryptamine type 2a-receptor gene. *Lancet* 347:1294, 1996.

Winokur G: Delusional disorder (paranoia). *Compr Psychiatry* 18:511, 1977.

Winokur G, Tsuang M: The Iowa 500: Suicide in mania, depression and schizophrenia. *Am J Psychiatry* 132:650, 1975.

Woods BT: Neurologic soft signs in psychiatric disorders, in Joseph AB, Young RR (eds): *Movement Disorders in Neurology and Neuropsychiatry*. Cambridge, MA, Blackwell, 1992, pp 438–448.

INDEX

Note: Page numbers in italics indicate figures; those followed by t indicate tables.

ISBN 0-07-067497-3
90000
9 780070 674974
US Edition

ISBN 0-07-116333-6

IE Edition